The American Psychiatric Publishing Textbook of Psychiatry

FIFTH EDITION

EDITORIAL BOARD

INTERNATIONAL EDITORIAL ADVISORY BOARD

The American Psychiatric Publishing Textbook of Psychiatry

FIFTH EDITION

Edited by

Robert E. Hales, M.D., M.B.A.
Stuart C. Yudofsky, M.D.
Glen O. Gabbard, M.D.

With Foreword by
Alan F. Schatzberg, M.D.

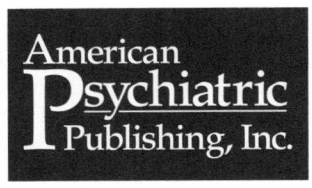

American Psychiatric Publishing, Inc.

Washington, DC
London, England

Diagnostic criteria included in this book are reprinted, with permission, from the *Diagnostic and Statistical Manual of Mental Disorders*, 4th Edition, Text Revision. Copyright 2000, American Psychiatric Association.

Copyright © 2008 American Psychiatric Publishing, Inc.
ALL RIGHTS RESERVED

Manufactured in the United States of America on acid-free paper
12 11 10 09 08   5 4 3 2 1
Fifth Edition

Typeset in Adobe's AvantGarde and Palatino.

American Psychiatric Publishing, Inc.
1000 Wilson Boulevard
Arlington, VA 22209-3901
www.appi.org

Library of Congress Cataloging-in-Publication Data
The American Psychiatric Publishing textbook of psychiatry / edited by Robert E. Hales, Stuart C. Yudofsky, Glen O. Gabbard; with foreword by Alan F. Schatzberg. — 5th ed.
    p. ; cm.
    Rev. ed. of: The American Psychiatric Publishing textbook of clinical psychiatry / edited by Robert E. Hales, Stuart C. Yudofsky. 4th ed. c2003.
    Includes bibliographical references and index.
    ISBN 978-1-58562-257-3 (hardcover : alk. paper)
    1. Psychiatry.   I. Hales, Robert E. II. Yudofsky, Stuart C. III. Gabbard, Glen O. IV. American Psychiatric Publishing. V. American Psychiatric Publishing textbook of clinical psychiatry. VI. Title: Textbook of psychiatry.
    [DNLM: 1. Mental Disorders.   2. Psychiatry.   WM 140 A5126 2008]
    RC454.A419 2008
    616.89—dc22
                                                                                              2007038178

British Library Cataloguing in Publication Data
A CIP record is available from the British Library.

To our teachers, our patients, and our students
and
to the family members of those among us
with mental illnesses—

We are continuously enlightened
by your inquiries and insights
and inspired by your devotion and courage.

CONTENTS

PART I

INTERVIEWING AND TESTING

PART II

BASIC SCIENCE AND DEVELOPMENT

PART III

PSYCHIATRIC DISORDERS

PART IV

PSYCHIATRIC TREATMENTS

PART V

SPECIAL PATIENT POPULATIONS

PART VI

IMPORTANT CLINICAL ISSUES

CONTRIBUTORS

Berry Anderson, B.S.N., R.N.
Clinical Research Manager, Central Study Coordinator for National Institute of Mental Health Optimization of Transcranial Magnetic Stimulation for the Treatment of Depression (OPT-TMS Depression) Study, Brain Stimulation Laboratory, Institute of Psychiatry, Medical University of South Carolina, Charleston, South Carolina

Linda B. Andrews, M.D.
Associate Dean for Graduate Medical Education, Director of Residency Education, Psychiatry, Baylor College of Medicine, Houston, Texas

Richard Balon, M.D.
Professor of Psychiatry, Associate Residency Training Director, Department of Psychiatry and Behavioral Neurosciences, Wayne State University School of Medicine, Detroit, Michigan

L. Jarrett Barnhill, M.D.
Professor of Psychiatry and Director of the Developmental Neuropharmacology Clinic, Department of Psychiatry, Division of Child and Adolescent Psychiatry, University of North Carolina, Chapel Hill, North Carolina

Aaron T. Beck, M.D.
Professor of Psychiatry, University of Pennsylvania School of Medicine, Philadelphia, Pennsylvania

Judith V. Becker, Ph.D.
Professor of Psychology and Psychiatry, Department of Psychology, The University of Arizona, Tucson, Arizona

Heather A. Berlin, D.Phil., M.P.H.
Postdoctoral Fellow, Department of Psychiatry, Mount Sinai School of Medicine, New York, New York

Jed E. Black, M.D.
Associate Professor, Sleep Medicine Division, Stanford University; Medical Director, Stanford Sleep Medicine Clinic, Stanford, California

Dan G. Blazer, M.D., Ph.D.
J.P. Gibbons Professor of Psychiatry and Behavioral Sciences, Duke University School of Medicine, Durham, North Carolina

Jeffrey J. Borckardt, Ph.D.
Assistant Professor, Departments of Psychiatry and Anesthesiology, Medical University of South Carolina, Charleston, South Carolina

James A. Bourgeois, O.D., M.D., F.A.P.M.
Alan Stoudemire Professor of Psychosomatic Medicine, Department of Psychiatry and Behavioral Sciences, University of California, Davis Medical Center, Sacramento, California

Vivien K. Burt, M.D., Ph.D.
Professor of Psychiatry, Geffen School of Medicine, University of California, Los Angeles; Director, Women's Life Center Semel Institute for Neuroscience and Human Behavior, Los Angeles, California

Daniel J. Buysse, M.D.
Professor of Psychiatry, University of Pittsburgh School of Medicine; Director, Neuroscience Clinical and Translational Research Center, Department of Psychiatry, Western Psychiatric Institute and Clinic, Pittsburgh, Pennsylvania

Cameron S. Carter, M.D.
Professor of Psychiatry and Psychology; and Director, Imaging Research Center, University of California, Davis, School of Medicine, Sacramento, California

Prabhakara V. Choudary, Ph.D., F.R.S.C.
Professor of Psychiatry and Behavioral Sciences, Center for Neuroscience, University of California, Davis, California

John F. Clarkin, Ph.D.
Professor of Clinical Psychology in Psychiatry, Weill Medical College of Cornell University, The New York Presbyterian Hospital, White Plains, New York

Paul D. Cox, M.D.
Associate Clinical Professor, Department of Psychiatry and Behavioral Sciences, University of California–Davis School of Medicine, Sacramento, California

Stephen J. Cozza, M.D.
Associate Professor, Department of Psychiatry, and Associate Director, Center for the Study of Traumatic Stress, F. Edward Hébert School of Medicine, Uniformed Services University of the Health Sciences, Bethesda, Maryland

Glen C. Crawford, M.D.
Director of Medical Services and Clinical Support Services, Staff Child and Adolescent Forensic Psychiatrist, U.S. Naval Hospital, Naples, Italy; Assistant Professor of Psychiatry, F. Edward Hébert School of Medicine, Uniformed Services University of the Health Sciences, Bethesda, Maryland

Mantosh J. Dewan, M.D.
Professor and Chair, Department of Psychiatry and Behavioral Sciences, SUNY Upstate Medical University, Syracuse, New York

Jack Drescher, M.D.
Training and Supervising Analyst, William Alanson White Institute; Adjunct Clinical Assistant Professor, New York University Postdoctoral Program in Psychotherapy and Psychoanalysis; and Clinical Assistant Professor of Psychiatry, New York Medical College, Vahalla, New York

Mina K. Dulcan, M.D.
Margaret C. Osterman Professor of Child Psychiatry and Psychiatrist-in-Chief, Children's Memorial Hospital; Head of Adolescent Psychiatry, Northwestern Memorial Hospital; and Head of Child and Adolescent Psychiatry and Professor of Psychiatry and Behavioral Sciences and Pediatrics, Feinberg School of Medicine, Northwestern University, Chicago, Illinois, Head, Child and Adolescent Psychiatry, Northwestern University, Feinberg School of Medicine, Children's Memorial Hospital

Laura B. Dunn, M.D.
Assistant Professor of Psychiatry, Division of Geriatric Psychiatry, Department of Psychiatry (116A-1), University of California, San Diego, California

Marc D. Feldman, M.D.
Clinical Professor of Psychiatry, Department of Psychiatry and Behavioral Medicine, The University of Alabama, Tuscaloosa, Alabama

Milton J. Foust Jr., M.D.
Assistant Professor of Psychiatry, Medical University of South Carolina, Charleston, South Carolina

Glen O. Gabbard, M.D.
Brown Foundation Chair of Psychoanalysis and Professor of Psychiatry, Baylor College of Medicine, Houston, Texas

Albert C. Gaw, M.D.
Medical Director of Quality Management, Community Behavioral Health Services, Department of Public Health, City and County of San Francisco; Clinical Professor, Department of Psychiatry, University of California San Francisco, California

Ralph J. Gemelli, M.D.
Clinical Associate Professor of Psychiatry, George Washington University School of Medicine, Washington, DC; Clinical Associate Professor of Psychiatry, Uniformed Services University of the Health Sciences, F. Edward Hébert School of Medicine, Bethesda, Maryland

Mark S. George, M.D.
Distinguished Professor of Psychiatry, Radiology, and Neurosciences; Director, Medical University of South Carolina (MUSC) Center for Advanced Imaging Research; Director, Brain Stimulation Laboratory; MUSC Director, South Carolina Brain Imaging Center of Excellence; Chairman, National Institute of Mental Health Optimization of Transcranial Magnetic Stimulation for the Treatment of Depression (OPT-TMS Depression) Study

Ira D. Glick, M.D.
Professor, Department of Psychiatry and Behavioral Sciences, Stanford University School of Medicine, Stanford, California

Roger P. Greenberg, Ph.D.
Professor and Head, Psychology Division, Department of Psychiatry and Behavioral Sciences, SUNY Upstate Medical University

John G. Gunderson, M.D.
Professor of Psychiatry, Harvard Medical School, Boston; and Director, Psychosocial and Personality Research, McLean Hospital, Belmont, Massachusetts

Robert E. Hales, M.D., M.B.A.
Joe P. Tupin Endowed Chair, and Professor and Chair, Department of Psychiatry and Behavioral Sciences, University of California-Davis School of Medicine, Sacramento, California

Katherine A. Halmi, M.D.
Professor of Psychiatry, Director Eating Disorder Program, New York Presbyterian Hospital—Westchester Division, White Plains, New York

Eric Hollander, M.D.
Esther and Joseph Klingenstein Professor, Chair of Psychiatry; Director, Seaver and NY Autism Center of Excellence; Director of Clinical Psychopharmacology; Director, Compulsive, Impulsive, and Anxiety Disorders Program; Mount Sinai School of Medicine, New York, New York

Jinger G. Hoop, M.D.
Assistant Professor, Department of Psychiatry and Behavioral Medicine, Medical College of Wisconsin, Milwaukee, Wisconsin

Diane B. Howieson, Ph.D.
Associate Professor of Neurology, Oregon Health and Science University, Portland, Oregon

Robin A. Hurley, M.D., F.A.N.P.A.
Associate Chief of Staff, Mental Health, W.G. "Bill" Hefner VAMC, Salisbury, North Carolina; Co-Director, Education, VISN 6 Mental Illness Research, Education and Clinical Center, and Associate Professor, Departments of Psychiatry and Radiology, Wake Forest University School of Medicine; Clinical Associate Professor, Baylor College of Medicine, Salisbury, North Carolina

Bradley R. Johnson, M.D.
Assistant Professor of Psychiatry, University of Medicine College of Medicine, Tucson, Arizona; and Chief of Psychiatry, Arizona Community Protection and Treatment Center, Arizona State Hospital, Phoenix, Arizona

Billy E. Jones, M.D., M.S.
President, B Jones Consulting Service, New York, New York; Vice President and Chief Medical Director, Care Management Technologies Division, Comprehensive NeuroScience, Inc., Morrisville, North Carolina; Clinical Professor of Psychiatry and Behavioral Sciences, New York Medical College, Vahalla, New York

John A. Joska, M.D., M.Med.(Psych.), F.C.Psych.(S.A.)
Senior Specialist and Lecturer, Department of Psychiatry and Mental Health, University of Cape Town, South Africa

Paul H. Kartheiser, M.D.
Attending Child and Adolescent Psychiatrist, Dorothea Dix Hospital, Raleigh, North Carolina; Assistant Professor of Psychiatry, Division of Child and Adolescent Psychiatry, Department of Psychiatry, University of North Carolina, Chapel Hill, North Carolina

H. Florence Kim, M.D.
Assistant Professor, Medical Director, Neuropsychiatry Programs, Department of Psychiatry and Behavioral Sciences, Baylor College of Medicine, Houston, Texas

Kimberly G. Klipstein, M.D.
Director, Behavioral Medicine and Consultation Psychiatry, Department of Psychiatry, and Assistant Professor of Psychiatry, Mount Sinai School of Medicine, New York, New York

James A. Knowles, M.D., Ph.D.
Professor of Psychiatry, Zilkha Neurogenetic Institute, Keck School of Medicine, University of Southern California, Los Angeles, California

James L. Levenson, M.D.
Professor of Psychiatry, Medicine, and Surgery, Virginia Commonwealth University School of Medicine, Richmond, Virginia

Susan G. Lazar, M.D.
Adjunct Professor, Department of Psychiatry, George Washington University School of Medicine, Washington, D.C.; Adjunct Professor, Department of Psychiatry, Uniformed Services University of the Health Sciences, F. Edward Hébert School of Medicine, Bethesda, Maryland; Training and Supervising Analyst, Washington Psychoanalytic Institute, Washington, D.C.

Martin H. Leamon, M.D.
Associate Professor of Clinical Psychiatry, Department of Psychiatry and Behavioral Sciences, University of California, Davis; Medical Director, Sacramento County Mental Health Treatment Center, Sacramento, California

Raphael J. Leo, M.D.
Associate Professor, Department of Psychiatry, State University of New York at Buffalo, School of Medicine and Biomedical Sciences; and Director, Consultation-Liaison Services, Erie County Medical Center, Buffalo, New York

José R. Maldonado, M.D., F.A.P.M., F.A.C.F.E.
Associate Professor of Psychiatry and Behavioral Sciences; Chief, Medical and Forensic Psychiatry Section; Director, Medical Psychotherapy Clinic, Department of Psychiatry and Behavioral Sciences, Stanford University School of Medicine; Medical Director, Consultation/Liaison Service, Stanford University Medical Center, Stanford, California

Lauren B. Marangell, M.D.
Brown Foundation Chair, Psychopharmacology of Mood Disorders; Associate Professor of Psychiatry; and Director, Mood Disorders Research, Menninger Department of Psychiatry, Baylor College of Medicine; Associate Director of Research, South Central MIRECC, Department of Veterans Affairs, Houston, Texas

John C. Markowitz, M.D.
Research Psychiatrist, New York State Psychiatric Institute; and Clinical Professor of Psychiatry, Weill Medical College of Cornell University, New York, New York

James M. Martinez, M.D.
Clinical Research Physician, Eli Lilly and Company, Indianapolis, Indiana; Assistant Professor of Psychiatry, and Associate Director, Mood Disorders Center, Menninger Department of Psychiatry, Baylor College of Medicine, South Central MIRECC, Department of Veterans Affairs, Houston, Texas

Melissa Martinez, M.D.
Assistant Professor of Psychiatry, Menninger Department of Psychiatry, Baylor College of Medicine, Houston, Texas

A. Kimberley McAllister, Ph.D.
Associate Professor of Neuroscience, Center for Neuroscience, University of California–Davis, Davis, California

Joel McClough, Ph.D.
Director, 9–11 Bereavement/Families Forward Program, Institute for Trauma and Stress, New York University School of Medicine

Benjamin H. McCommon, M.D.
Assistant Clinical Professor of Psychiatry, Columbia University, and Attending Psychiatrist, New York Presbyterian Hospital, New York, New York

Barbara E. McDermott, Ph.D.
Associate Professor of Clinical Psychiatry, University of California, Davis School of Medicine, Department of Psychiatry and Behavioral Sciences, Division of Psychiatry and the Law, Sacramento; Research Director, Clinical Demonstration/Research Unit, Napa State Hospital, Napa, California

Ilan Melnick, M.D.
Assistant Professor Department of Psychiatry, Miller School of Medicine, University of Miami, Miami, Florida

Michael J. Minzenberg, M.D.
Assistant Professor, Imaging Research Center, University of California, Davis, School of Medicine, Sacramento, California

Hugh Myrick, M.D.
Associate Professor of Psychiatry, Medical University of South Carolina, Ralph H. Johnson VAMC, Charleston, South Carolina

Ziad H. Nahas, M.D., M.S.C.R.
Associate Professor; Director, Mood Disorders Program; Medical Director, Brain Stimulation Laboratory, Medical University of South Carolina, Charleston, South Carolina

Jeffrey H. Newcorn, M.D.
Associate Professor of Psychiatry and Pediatrics and Director, Division of Child and Adolescent Psychiatry, Mount Sinai Medical Center, New York, New York

Stephen C. Noctor, Ph.D.
Research Scientist, Institute for Regenerative Medicine, Department of Neurology, University of California–San Francisco, San Francisco, California

Brooke S. Parish, M.D.
Assistant Professor of Psychiatry, Department of Psychiatry, University of New Mexico, Albuquerque, New Mexico

Cameron D. Quanbeck, M.D.
Assistant Clinical Professor of Psychiatry, University of California Davis Medical Center, Sacramento, California

Stephen Rayport, M.D., Ph.D.
Associate Professor of Clinical Neuroscience, Department of Psychiatry, Columbia University College of Physicians and Surgeons; Research Psychiatrist, Department of Molecular Therapeutics, New York State Psychiatric Institute, New York, New York

Phillip J. Resnick, M.D.
Professor of Psychiatry and Director, Division of Forensic Psychiatry, Case Western Reserve University School of Medicine, Cleveland, Ohio

Michelle Riba, M.D., M.S.
Clinical Professor and Associate Chair for Integrated Medicine and Psychiatry Services, Department of Psychiatry, University of Michigan Medical School, Ann Arbor, Michigan; Zonal Representative (Area 2, USA), World Psychiatric Association, and Past President, American Psychiatric Association

Eva C. Ritvo, M.D.
Associate Professor, Department of Psychiatry, Miller School of Medicine University of Miami, Miami Beach, Florida

Laura Weiss Roberts, M.D., M.A.
Professor and Chairman, Charles E. Kubly Professor of Psychiatry and Behavioral Medicine, Department of Psychiatry and Behavioral Medicine, Medical College of Wisconsin

Alan F. Schatzberg, M.D.
Kenneth T. Norris Jr. Professor and Chairman, Department of Psychiatry and Behavioral Sciences, Stanford University School of Medicine, Stanford, California

Paul E. Schulz, M.D.
Associate Professor, Department of Neurology, Baylor College of Medicine, Houston, Texas

Charles L. Scott, M.D.
Associate Professor of Clinical Psychiatry and Chief of Psychiatry and the Law, University of California, Davis School of Medicine, Department of Psychiatry and Behavioral Sciences, Division of Psychiatry and the Law, Sacramento, California

Jeffrey S. Seaman, M.S., M.D.
Residency Training Director, Associate Professor of Psychiatry, Department of Psychiatry and Behavioral Sciences, University of Oklahoma Health Sciences Center, Oklahoma City, Oklahoma

Mark E. Servis, M.D.
Roy T. Brophy Professor and Vice Chair for Education, Department of Psychiatry and Behavioral Sciences, University of California Davis, School of Medicine, Sacramento, California

Daniel W. Shuman, J.D.
Professor of Law, Southern Methodist University, Dedman School of Law, Dallas, Texas

Daphne Simeon, M.D.
Associate Professor, Co-Director, Compulsive Impulsive Disorders Program; Director, Depersonalization and Dissociation Program, Mount Sinai School of Medicine, New York, New York

Robert I. Simon, M.D.
Clinical Professor of Psychiatry; Director, Program in Psychiatry and Law, Georgetown University School of Medicine, Washington, D.C.; Chair, Department of Psychiatry, Suburban Hospital, Bethesda, Maryland

Andrew E. Skodol, M.D.
President, Institute for Mental Health Research, Phoenix, Arizona

David Spiegel, M.D.
Willson Professor and Associate Chair of Psychiatry and Behavioral Sciences, Department of Psychiatry and Behavioral Sciences, Stanford University School of Medicine; Medical Director, Center for Integrative Medicine, Stanford University Medical Center, Stanford, California

Patrick J. Strollo Jr., M.D.
Associate Professor of Medicine, University of Pittsburgh School of Medicine; Medical Director, Sleep Medicine Center, University of Pittsburgh Medical Center, Pittsburgh, Pennsylvania

Stephen M. Sonnenberg, M.D
Clinical Professor, Department of Psychiatry, Baylor College of Medicine, Houston, Texas; Adjunct Professor, Department of Psychiatry, Uniformed Services University of the Health Sciences, F. Edward Hébert School of Medicine, Bethesda, Maryland; Training and Supervising Analyst, Houston–Galveston Psychoanalytic Institute, Austin, Texas

Brett N. Steenbarger, Ph.D.
Clinical Associate Professor, Department of Psychiatry and Behavioral Sciences, SUNY Upstate Medical University, Syracuse, New York

Dan J. Stein, M.D., Ph.D.
Professor and Chair, Department of Psychiatry, University of Cape Town, South Africa; Visiting Professor, Department of Psychiatry, Mount Sinai School of Medicine, New York, New York

Kira Stein, M.D.
Clinical Instructor, David Geffen School of Medicine, University of California Los Angeles, California

Jill D. Stinson, Ph.D.
Psychology Resident, Fulton State Hospital, Fulton, Missouri

James J. Strain, M.D.
Professor of Psychiatry, Mount Sinai School of Medicine, New York, New York

Katherine H. Taber, Ph.D., F.A.N.P.A.
Assistant Co-Director for Education, VISN 6 Mental Illness Research, Education and Clinical Center; Research Health Scientist, W.G. "Bill" Hefner VAMC, Salisbury, North Carolina; Research Professor, Division of Biomedical Sciences, Edward Via Virginia College of Osteopathic Medicine, Blacksburg, Virginia; Adjunct Associate Professor, Department of Physical Medicine and Rehabilitation; Baylor College of Medicine, Houston, Texas

Michael E. Thase, M.D.
Professor of Psychiatry, University of Pittsburgh Medical Center, Pittsburgh, Pennsylvania

Amy M. Ursano, M.D.
Assistant Professor of Psychiatry, Department of Psychiatry, Division of Child and Adolescent Psychiatry, University of North Carolina, Chapel Hill, North Carolina

Robert J. Ursano, M.D.
Professor and Chairman, Department of Psychiatry, Uniformed Services University of the Health Sciences, F. Edward Hébert School of Medicine, Bethesda, Maryland; teaching faculty, Washington Psychoanalytic Institute, Washington, D.C.

W. Martin Usrey, Ph.D.
Associate Professor of Neurology, Center for Neuroscience, University of California–Davis, Davis, California

Sophia Vinogradov, M.D.
Professor in Residence, University of California–San Francisco School of Medicine, San Francisco, California

Elizabeth A. Wilde, Ph.D.
Assistant Professor, Department of Physical Medicine and Rehabilitation, Baylor College of Medicine, Houston, Texas

John W. Winkelman, M.D., Ph.D.
Assistant Professor of Psychiatry, Harvard Medical School, Boston, Massachusetts; Medical Director, Sleep Health Center, Brigham and Women's Hospital, Brighton, Massachusetts

Arnold Winston, M.D.
Professor of Psychiatry, Albert Einstein College of Medicine, Department of Psychiatry and Behavioral Sciences, Bronx, New York; Chairman, Department of Psychiatry and Behavioral Sciences, Beth Israel Medical Center, New York, New York

Jesse H. Wright, M.D., Ph.D.
Professor and Chief of Adult Clinical Psychiatry, University of Louisville, School of Medicine, Norton Psychiatric Center, Louisville, Kentucky

Tara M. Wright, M.D.
Assistant Professor of Psychiatry, Medical University of South Carolina, Ralph H. Johnson VAMC, Charleston, South Carolina

Irvin D. Yalom, M.D.
Professor of Psychiatry and Behavioral Sciences, Emeritus, Stanford University School of Medicine, Palo Alto, California

Jong H. Yoon, M.D.
Assistant Professor, Imaging Research Center, University of California, Davis, School of Medicine, Sacramento, California

Stuart C. Yudofsky, M.D.
D.C. and Irene Ellwood Professor and Chairman, Menninger Department of Psychiatry and Behavioral Sciences, Baylor College of Medicine; Chairman, Department of Psychiatry, The Methodist Hospital, Houston, Texas

Sean H. Yutzy, M.D.
Associate Professor of Psychiatry, Department of Psychiatry, University of New Mexico, Albuquerque, New Mexico

Phyllis G. Zee, M.D., Ph.D.
Professor of Neurology, Northwestern University, Chicago, Illinois

Disclosure of Interests

The contributors have declared all forms of support received within the 12 months prior to manuscript submittal that may represent a competing interest in relation to their work published in this volume, as follows:

L. Jarrett Barnhill, M.D.   *Consultant:* Abbott, GlaxoSmithKline; *Speakers' Bureau:* Ortho-McNeil.

Aaron T. Beck, M.D.   The author may receive a portion of profits from sale of software "Good Days Ahead" for computer-assisted CBT discussed in this text. The publisher of the software is Mindstreet, LLC, Louisville, KY.

Jed E. Black, M.D.   *Consultant/Grant Support:* Takeda, Boehringer-Ingelheim, Jazz Pharmaceuticals, GlaxoSmithKline, Cephalon.

Jeffrey J. Borckardt, Ph.D.   *Grant Support:* National Institute of Neurological Disorders and Stroke, Cyberonics, Neurosciences Institute.

Vivien K. Burt, M.D., Ph.D.   *Speakers' Bureau:* Eli Lilly, GlaxoSmithKline, Forest Pharmaceuticals, Wyeth Ayerst; *Advisory Board:* Eli Lilly; *Consultant:* Eli Lilly, Forest Pharmaceuticals, Wyeth Ayerst.

Daniel J. Buysse, M.D.   *Consultant/Speakers' Bureau:* Actelion, Cephalon, Eli Lilly, GlaxoSmithKline, Merck, Neurocrine, Neurogen, Pfizer, Respironics, sanofi-aventis, Sepracor, Servier, Stress Eraser, Takeda.

Mina K. Dulcan, M.D.   *Consultant/Advisory Board:* Eli Lilly.

Mark S. George, M.D.   *Grant Support/Speakers' Bureau:* GlaxoSmithKline, Parke-Davis; *Consultant:* Aventis, Jazz Pharmaceuticals, Argolyn Pharmaceuticals, Abbott; *Formal Research Collaborations:* Dantec (Medtronic); *Clinical Research Grant/Consultant:* Neutonus (now Neuronetics); *Grant Support/Speakers' Bureau/Advisory Board:* Cyberonics; *Advisory Board:* NeuroPace; *Grant Support/Advisory Board:* Cephos.

Robert E. Hales, M.D., M.B.A.   Chair of industry-sponsored symposium sponsored by Bristol-Myers Squibb at the APA Annual Meeting.

Eric Hollander, M.D.   *Grant Support:* Pfizer, Ortho-McNeil, Abbott.

Bradley R. Johnson, M.D.   *Speakers' Bureau:* AstraZeneca, Forest Pharmaceuticals.

Billy E. Jones, M.D., M.S.   Employed by Comprehensive Neuroscience, Inc.

James L. Levenson, M.D.   *Advisory Board:* Eli Lilly.

Lauren B. Marangell, M.D.   *Grant Support:* Bristol-Myers Squibb, Eli Lilly, Cyberonics, Neuronetics, National Institute of Mental Health, Stanley Foundation; *Consultant/Honoraria:* Eli Lilly, GlaxoSmithKline, Cyberonics, Pfizer, Medtronic, Forest, Aspect Medical Systems, Novartis.

John C. Markowitz, M.D.   *Royalties:* American Psychiatric Press, Perseus/Basic Books, Franco Angeli, Editions Médecine & Hygiène Société, Oxford University Press; *Consultant:* Ono Pharmaceuticals; *Salary:* Forest Laboratories.

James M. Martinez, M.D.   *Research Support:* Aspect Medical Systems, AstraZeneca, Bristol-Myers Squibb, Cyberonics, Eli Lilly, Forest Pharmaceuticals, Neuronetics, sanofi-aventis, National Institute of Mental Health, Stanley Foundation; *Speakers' Bureau:* AstraZeneca, Bristol-Myers Squibb, Cyberonics, Eli Lilly, Forest Pharmaceuticals, GlaxoSmithKline, Janssen, Pfizer, Wyeth Ayerst; *Consultant:* Cyberonics.

Melissa Martinez, M.D.   *Research Support:* Cyberonics, Eli Lilly, sanofi-aventis, Aspect Medical Systems, Bristol-Myers Squibb, Neuronetics.

Michael J. Minzenberg, M.D.   *Research Support:* Elan, Cephalon.

Ziad H. Nahas, M.D., M.S.C.R.   *Grant Support:* National Institute of Mental Health, Neuronetics, Cyberonics, Medtronic, Eli Lilly, Neurospace; *Consultant:* Neuronetics, Cyberonics, Avanir Pharmaceutical, Aventis Pharmaceutical, Neuropace; *Speakers' Bureau:* Cyberonics.

Jeffrey H. Newcorn, M.D.   *Advisory Board/Consultant:* Abbott, McNeil, Eli Lilly, Shire, Novartis, Cortex, Pfizer, Lupin; *Research Support:* McNeil, Eli Lilly, Shire, Novartis; *Speakers' Bureau:* Novartis, Shire

Brooke S. Parish, M.D.   *Financial Interest/Stock Ownership:* 100 shares, Merck.

Jeffrey S. Seaman, M.S., M.D.   *Clinical Trials:* Bristol-Myers Squibb, Cephalon.

Paul E. Schulz, M.D.   *Speakers' Bureau:* Pfizer, Forest Pharmaceuticals.

Dan J. Stein, M.D., Ph.D.   *Grant Support/Consultant Honoraria:* AstraZeneca, Eli Lilly, GlaxoSmithKline, Lundbeck, Orion, Pfizer, Pharmacia, Rocher, Servier, Solvay, Sumitomo, Wyeth.

Patrick J. Strollo Jr., M.D.   *Grant Support:* ResMed, Respironics.

Michael E. Thase, M.D.   *Advisory/Consultant:* AstraZeneca, Bristol-Myers Squibb, Cephalon, Cyberonics, Eli Lilly, GlaxoSmithKline, Janssen, MedAvante, Neuronetics, Novartis, Organon, Sepracor, Shire US, Supernus, Wyeth; *Speakers' Bureau:* AstraZeneca, Bristol-Myers Squibb, Cyberonics, Eli Lilly, GlaxoSmithKline, Organon, Sanofi Aventis, Wyeth; *Expert Testimony:* Jones Day (Wyeth litigation), Phillips Lytle (GlaxoSmithKline litigation); *Equity Holdings:* MedAvante, Inc.

Robert J. Ursano, M.D.   *Consultant:* Abbott, GlaxoSmithKline; *Speakers' Bureau:* McNeil.

John W. Winkelman, M.D., Ph.D.   *Advisory Board/Speakers' Bureau:* Boehringer-Ingelheim, Cephalon, GlaxoSmithKline, Pfizer, sanofi-aventis, Sepracor, Schwarz-Pharma, Takeda.

Jesse H. Wright, M.D., Ph.D.   The author may receive a portion of profits from sale of software "Good Days Ahead" for computer-assisted CBT discussed in this text. The publisher of the software is Mindstreet, LLC, Louisville, KY.

Stuart C. Yudofsky, M.D.   Co-chairman for educational symposium at American Psychiatric Association annual meeting sponsored by Bristol-Myers Squibb.

Phyllis G. Zee, M.D.   *Consultant/Advisory Board:* Boehringer-Ingelheim, GlaxoSmithKline, Jazz, sanofi-aventis, Takeda.

The following contributors stated that they had no competing interests during the year preceding manuscript submission: Berry Anderson, B.S.N., R.N.; Linda B. Andrews, M.D.; Richard Balon, M.D.; Judith V. Becker, Ph.D.; Heather A. Berlin, D.Phil., M.P.H.; Dan G. Blazer, M.D., Ph.D.; James A. Bourgeois, O.D., M.D., F.A.P.M.; Cameron S. Carter, M.D.; Prabhakara V. Choudary, Ph.D., F.R.S.C.; John F. Clarkin, Ph.D.; Paul D. Cox, M.D.; Stephen J. Cozza, M.D.; Glen C. Crawford, M.D.; Mantosh J. Dewan, M.D.; Jack Drescher, M.D.; Laura B. Dunn, M.D.; Marc D. Feldman, M.D.; Milton J. Foust Jr., M.D.; Glen O. Gabbard, M.D.; Albert C. Gaw, M.D.; Ralph J. Gemelli, M.D.; Ira D. Glick, M.D.; Roger P. Greenberg, Ph.D.; John G. Gunderson, M.D.; Katherine A. Halmi, M.D.; Jinger G. Hoop, M.D.; Diane B. Howieson, Ph.D.; Robin A. Hurley, M.D., F.A.N.P.A.; John A. Joska, M.D., M.Med.(Psych.), F.C.Psych.(S.A.); Paul H. Kartheiser, M.D.; H. Florence Kim, M.D.; Kimberly G. Klipstein, M.D.; James A. Knowles, M.D., Ph.D.; Susan G. Lazar, M.D.; Martin H. Leamon, M.D.; Raphael J. Leo, M.D.; José R. Maldonado, M.D., F.A.P.M., F.A.C.F.E.; A. Kimberley McAllister, Ph.D.; Joel McClough, Ph.D.; Benjamin H. McCommon, M.D.; Barbara E. McDermott, Ph.D.; Ilan Melnick, M.D.; Hugh Myrick, M.D.; Stephen C. Noctor, Ph.D.; Cameron D. Quanbeck, M.D.; Stephen Rayport, M.D., Ph.D.; Phillip J. Resnick, M.D.; Michelle Riba, M.D., M.S.; Eva C. Ritvo, M.D.; Laura Weiss Roberts, M.D., M.A.; Alan F. Schatzberg, M.D.; Charles L. Scott, M.D.; Mark E. Servis, M.D.; Daniel W. Shuman, J.D.; Daphne Simeon, M.D.; Robert I. Simon, M.D.; Andrew E. Skodol, M.D.; Stephen M. Sonnenberg, M.D.; David Spiegel, M.D.; Brett N. Steenbarger, Ph.D.; Kira Stein, M.D.; Jill D. Stinson, Ph.D.; James J. Strain, M.D.; Katherine H. Taber, Ph.D., F.A.N.P.A.; Amy M. Ursano, M.D.; W. Martin Usrey, Ph.D.; Sophia Vinogradov, M.D.; Elizabeth A. Wilde, Ph.D.; Arnold Winston, M.D.; Tara M. Wright, M.D.; Irvin D. Yalom, M.D.; Jong H. Yoon, M.D., Ph.D.; Sean H. Yutzy, M.D.

FOREWORD

Alan F. Schatzberg, M.D.

Any living entity must adapt and change in order to survive and prevail. This axiom applies as uniformly to medical specialties and to medical textbooks as it does to plants and animals. Paralleling the field of psychiatry over the past 20 years, *The American Psychiatric Publishing Textbook of Psychiatry* (the Textbook) continues to change, adapt, survive, and thrive into its Fifth Edition. Given the "two-decade milestone" of the Textbook, I felt that my understanding of the new Edition would be enhanced through an appreciation of what has been changed and what has been preserved from the previous four editions. The Editors of the First Edition of the Textbook included John Talbott, M.D., in addition to Drs. Hales and Yudofsky, who have remained with the Textbook through this edition.

In the Preface to the First Edition, the Editors explicitly proclaimed their goal as "...to assemble a textbook that presents, as comprehensively as is possible in a single volume, the clinically relevant topics in psychiatry.... We have thus endeavored to present a psychiatric text that may be used in a fashion similar to that of several other standard textbooks in other fields such as internal medicine, general surgery, pediatrics, endocrinology, and pharmacology: a text that is not only useful as a standard educational reference for psychiatrists and psychiatry residents, but that is also purchased and used extensively by medical students, residents, and more advanced professionals from other disciplines and specialties" (Talbott, Hales, and Yudofsky 1988, p. xvii). The Editors set for themselves an extraordinary challenge. As early as 1980, the most widely used psychiatric textbook of that era, *The Comprehensive Textbook of Psychiatry*, Third Edition (Kaplan, Freedman, and Sadock 1980), comprised three large volumes and 3,365 pages! Notwithstanding the exponential increase in the database and scope of the field of psychiatry over the past two decades, the Editors of *The American Psychiatric Publishing Textbook of Psychiatry* have stuck to their guns throughout the entirety of the five editions by maintaining a one-volume format with a remarkable consistency in the number of pages for each edition (i.e., 1,280 pages in Edition I; 1,610 pages in Edition II; 1,702 pages in Edition III; 1,648 pages in Edition IV; and 1,672 pages in Edition V).

With the aforementioned as prelude, I considered the following three questions in assessing the achievements of this edition of the Textbook: First, how well have the Editors accomplished the twin goals articulated in the Preface to the First Edition: maintaining a single-volume format while including the profusion of recently discovered, relevant information so essential for the practicing clinician? Second, has important information been omitted in order to accommodate the single-volume format? And third, are the unprecedented research advances in psychiatry since publication of the previous edition of the Textbook 5 years ago integrated into the chapters? At the top of my long list of such advances are 1) neuropsychiatric diagnostics and imaging, 2) basic behavioral sciences, and 3) evidence-based brief psychotherapies.

Neuropsychiatric Diagnostics and Imaging

Let us first consider the related topics of neuropsychiatric diagnostics and neuroimaging in the Fifth Edition of the Textbook (Hales, Yudofsky, and Gabbard 2008, pp. 19–72). Chapter 2, "Laboratory Testing and

Imaging Studies in Psychiatry," by Drs. Kim, Schulz, Wilde, and Yudofsky, is entirely revised and extensively expanded from the previous edition. Written by two neuropsychiatrists, a neurologist, and a neuropsychologist, this chapter conveys a salutary reminder that psychiatric disorders are, first and foremost, brain illnesses. The authors make the important point that because a vast range of neurological and medical illnesses can give rise to psychiatric symptomatologies, a careful and comprehensive neuropsychiatric history and physical examination with judicious clinical laboratory testing constitute the primary and most important steps in the psychiatric evaluation. They further emphasize that a meticulous history and physical examination often can obviate expensive and invasive laboratory testing and diagnostic imaging. Also, because psychiatric symptoms tend not to be specific to a particular etiology, the practitioner must be particularly vigilant in identifying biological disorders that are reversible with treatment. A strength of this chapter is the review of those screening laboratory tests that have been demonstrated to be cost effective (e.g., serum glucose and blood urea nitrogen concentrations, creatinine clearance, urinalysis). Additionally, thyroid screening of female mood disorder patients older than age 50 years is justified because of the high prevalence of hypothyroidism in this group. The practicing clinician will find Table 2–2, a summary of laboratory screening tests useful in the neuropsychiatric workup, particularly valuable, with reference ranges that are difficult to locate in single sources (e.g., luteinizing hormone and follicle-stimulating hormone ranges for men and women). The authors go on to address a series of specific clinical presentations, providing guidelines for recommended diagnostic testing for patients with fluctuating mental status of acute onset, for patients in cognitive decline, for patients who abuse mind-altering substances, for patients with new-onset psychosis, for patients with new-onset depressive or manic symptoms, for patients with new-onset anxiety symptoms, and for patients with a range of other neuropsychiatric presentations. Similarly, the thorough review of medication monitoring and maintenance and the unusually clear presentation of pharmacogenetics and pharmacogenomics are remarkably comprehensive and up to date. I also commend to the reader's close review Table 2–12, in which investigational biological markers are presented and critiqued, as this table affords a unique and realistic glimpse into the future of psychiatric practice. The remainder of Chapter 2 is an equally lucid and thoughtful presentation of electrophysiological and neuroimaging studies in psychiatry. In an era in which considerable confusion prevails in regard to clinical rationales for specific diagnostic tests, the authors are careful to present full and current data on indications for and limitations of each specific test. For example, the authors note that 20% of patients with epilepsy will have normal electroencephalograms, while 2% of patients without epilepsy will have spike and wave formations. Particularly useful are the explanations of the comparative indications for magnetic resonance imaging (MRI) versus computed tomography (CT), and specifically Table 2–16, which compares SPECT, PET, and fMRI from the perspectives of resolution, scan time, and cost. New technologies such as diffusion tensor imaging (DTI) are also introduced to the reader.

Chapter 5, "Neuroanatomy For The Psychiatrist," by Drs. Katherine H. Taber and Robin A. Hurley, is an excellent complement to Chapter 2. I fully agree with the assertion made by the authors at the beginning of this extraordinary chapter: "As structural and functional neuroimaging and genetics become more entwined in modern medicine, it has become more evident that practicing psychiatrists need to understand basic neuroanatomy and its relationship to psychiatric disease" (Ibid., p. 157). Thereafter, in the most systematic and original fashion, Drs. Taber and Hurley deploy a vivid series of brain imaging graphics to elucidate regional brain structures and to link these regions and systems to brain function and dysfunction. Table 5–1 extensively reviews functional anatomy pertinent to psychiatry and summarizes the functional impairments that commonly occur when the respective regions suffer injury. The authors make the important observation that the brain is the organ of our field. I commend this chapter as the best available resource to the resident studying for certification boards or to the practitioner who desires a practical review that links brain structures, systems, and functions.

In summary, I conclude that Chapters 2 and 5 have exceeded my expectations and requirements for a comprehensive and up-to-date presentation of diagnostics and neuroimaging.

Basic Behavioral Sciences

Although the four previous editions of *The American Psychiatric Publishing Textbook of Psychiatry* each contained a section titled "Theoretical Foundations," the Fifth Edition is the first to have an individual section devoted to basic science and brain development. This enhancement is doubtlessly in justifiable recognition in the unprecedented explosion in behavioral neurosciences since the turn of this century.

Chapter 4, "Cellular and Molecular Biology of the Neuron," by Drs. A. Kimberley McAllister, W. Martin Usrey, Stephen C. Noctor, and Stephen Rayport, begins with the following premise: "Neuropsychiatric disorders are due to disordered functioning of neurons and, in particular, their synapses" (Ibid, p. 123). The authors argue that many neuropsychiatric disorders arise from aberrations in neurodevelopmental mechanisms, particularly in the initial assembly of the brain during infancy, and that these dysfunctions are most likely to be intrinsically or genetically based. They further posit that with maturation of the individual, life experience becomes the dominant force in shaping neuronal connections and regulation and, therefore, that neuropsychiatric dysfunction is usually experience-based. By contrast, geriatric neuropsychiatric disorders derive from neurodegenerative processes that "may unravel neural circuits by aberrantly engaging neurodevelopmental mechanisms" (Ibid., p. 123). McAllister and colleagues also maintain that the rapid rate of recent discoveries in the field has begun to yield insight into "how therapeutic interventions to correct aberrant neuronal growth and differentiation during development and maturation, or later to normalize neuronal signaling, may translate into revolutionary treatments for neuropsychiatric disorders" (Ibid., p. 114). Consistent with the chapter's title, they devote the largest proportion of their text to an explication of the cellular and molecular functioning of the neuron. With almost poetic economy of expression, the authors sum up neuronal functioning as follows: "Individual neurons in the brain receive signals from thousands of neurons and, in turn, send information to thousands of others.... CNS neurons may be seen as part of dynamic cellular ensembles that shape their participation from one network to another as information is used in varied tasks. The sophistication of these networks depends on both the properties of the neurons themselves and the patterns and strength of their connections" (Ibid., p. 124). Addressing such broad topics as the cellular composition of the brain, neuronal shape, neuronal excitability, rapid postsynaptic responses, organization of postsynaptic receptors at synapses, and synaptic modulation in learning and memory, the authors bring to life the cellular and molecular functioning of the CNS neuron.

A second major consideration of Chapter 4 is the development of neurons, which is a "hot" current topic and has promise for opening new avenues for both understanding and treating psychiatric illnesses. The authors of this chapter are renowned scientists, each of whom has made original and seminal contributions to the chapter's subject, and this is especially evident in the sections covering the birth and migration of neurons, the identification of neuronal progenitor cells (Dr. Noctor), the migration and organization of brain neurons, synapse formation, neuronal maturation and survival, experience-dependent synaptic refinement, and neurotrophic and neurotoxic actions of neurotransmitters. From my perspective, Chapter 4 is a *tour de force* of presentation, organization, and relevance. I particularly appreciated the creative and compelling graphical depictions of synaptic transmission, including neurotransmitter transporters.

Psychiatric genetics is a second key area of exponential growth in the 5 years since publication of the Fourth Edition of the *Textbook of Psychiatry*. I reasoned that coverage of this subject would be another major test of the Editors' success in maintaining the scientific currency of the Fifth Edition while keeping the length down to a single volume. In Chapter 6, "Genetics," the authors note that the goal of psychiatric genetics is to identify susceptibility genes and elucidate the neural mechanisms by which genetic variation influences the risk of mental illness in an individual. The authors' expressed objectives for their chapter are 1) to present the fundamental principles of classical and molecular human genetics, 2) to summarize the results of selected studies aimed at deciphering genetic contributions to the most common and disabling psychiatric illnesses, and 3) to speculate about the future of psychiatric genetics research, with particular emphasis on new psychiatric drug development based on genetic etiological findings rather than disease phenotypes or symptoms. Highlights of this chapter include up-to-date and comprehensive reviews of the evidence supporting the genetic transmission of prevalent psychiatric disorders and the hereditary risks for the development of these conditions, particularly evidence from twin and adoption studies. This chapter is unusually strong in its presentation of genetic linkage analysis and association studies, realms that students and practitioners of psychiatry must understand (but often do not). I particularly appreciated the highly topical presentation of candidate genes for schizophrenia (there are at least 18) and Table 6–3, which summarizes this complex subject so well. In my opinion, no area of psychiatric genetics is more productive and exiting than that of mood disorders. As outlined in Table 6–5, there are currently 12 candidate genes for bipolar disorder and at least 5 candidate genes for major depressive disorder. Chapter author Prabhakara V. Choudary, Ph.D., is a leading scientist in this realm, with pioneering research on two candidate genes for major depressive disorder. Indeed, one of the most important scientific discoveries of the past 5 years was reported in Caspi and co-workers' paper on the serotonin transporter gene, *SLC6A4* (Caspi, Sugden, and Moffitt et.al. 2003). Caspi and associates devised an experiment to answer, in part, the fundamental question of why certain people are more vulnerable to developing depression as the result of life stress. Specifically, they investigated a functional polymorphism in the promoter region of the *SLC6A4* serotonin transporter gene, which is responsible for the reuptake of serotonin at brain synapses. The polymorphism entails a short ("s") allele of the transporter that is less efficient at than the long ("l") allele. Analyzing a cohort of 1,037 subjects from Great Britain for the association of life stress and major depression, Caspi and colleagues found that the short ("s") polymorphism in the promoter region of the serotonin transporter gene increased the influence of stressful life events on the development of depression. Thus, they isolated and demonstrated a genetic–environmental interaction in which the influence of stress on the development of depression is affected by a subject's genetic makeup. I was pleased to note that this notable research finding was discussed not only in the chapter on genetics but also in the chapter on cellular and molecular biology of the neuron *and* the chapter on mood disorders—evidence of an excellent integration of basic neuroscience and clinical psychiatry in the Fifth Edition of the Textbook.

Evidence-Based Brief Psychotherapies

The third area of area of accelerated expansion of psychiatric knowledge over the past 5 years has been in evidence-based psychotherapies, and I was curious to see how the Editors responded, in the Fifth Edition of their Textbook, to this growth. Drs. Hales and Yudofsky have been the sole Editors of the Textbook over its previous two editions, and their subspecialty interest is neuropsychiatry. As it turns out, Hales and Yudofsky made significant changes in the Fifth Edition in recognition of the advances and expansion of knowledge in psychotherapies. Glen Gabbard, M.D., noted psychoanalyst and highly regarded researcher, theoretician, and author on psychodynamic psychiatry, was invited to be the third Editor for the Fifth Edition of the Textbook. Dr. Gabbard was given the responsibility to develop a revised and expanded consideration of psychotherapies. New to the Fifth Edition are individual chapters on supportive psychotherapy and combining psychotherapy and pharmacotherapy, in addition to chapters on brief psychotherapies, psychodynamic psychotherapy, interpersonal psychotherapy, cognitive

therapy, couples and family therapy, and group therapy. The authors of these chapters represent a veritable "Who's Who" of experts in the respective therapies, and they have done an outstanding job of crafting chapters that allow readers to incorporate the knowledge and skills imparted by the text into their practices.

Comprising 46 pages, Chapter 31, "Cognitive Therapy," by Drs. Jesse H. Wright, Michael E. Thase, and Aaron T. Beck is as thorough and well-wrought a chapter on this important subject as I have read anywhere. One of the best parts of this chapter is the section documenting the effectiveness of cognitive therapy (CT). The authors point out that more than 350 randomized controlled trials of CT have been conducted and that CT has been demonstrated to compare favorably with other treatments for depression (including psychopharmacology); for anxiety disorders; for the symptoms of certain eating disorders, including bulimia nervosa and binge-eating disorder; and even for psychotic symptoms.

Chapter 33, "Combining Psychotherapy and Pharmacotherapy," by Drs. Michelle Riba and Richard Balon also reviews the available published literature documenting that combining these treatments improves outcomes for patients with major depression, bipolar disorder, bulimia nervosa, and nicotine dependence. This chapter also does an excellent job of distinguishing between integrated and split treatments and of providing practical and helpful guidelines on such topics as questions to ask a patient in the initial telephone call for an appointment, key ingredients of the first session of combined treatment, and special issues involving medications.

I found the cluster of chapters on psychotherapy not to be repetitive, but rather integrated and complementary, and this reflects well on both the chapter authors' and Dr. Gabbard's editing. The net result is that Fifth Edition's presentation of psychotherapies essentially represents "a book within a book" and a product that manages to exhibit both economy of scale and completeness.

Conclusion

In summary, I believe that the Fifth Edition of *The American Psychiatric Publishing Textbook of Psychiatry* is an altogether worthy reflection of the robust and remarkable progress of the field of psychiatry over the past several decades. The Editors have worked hard on updating, bridging, and integrating such classical topics as psychoanalytical psychotherapy with recent discoveries in cell biology, molecular biology, and genetics. In addition, the Editors have preserved in the

Fifth Edition the organizational concepts that were delineated in the First Edition, including the single-volume format. The net result is that the Textbook has not only survived to its Fifth Edition but has flourished. I found myself enjoying the chapter presentations of the Fifth Edition, which so keenly reflect the state of the art in psychiatric diagnosis and treatment in 2008, while also looking ahead with eager anticipation to the achievements and transformations that inevitably will follow in the years to come—substantive and thrilling advances that are certain to be embraced and skillfully presented in future editions of the Textbook. I trust that you, the reader, will enjoy this book as much as I have, and I congratulate Drs. Hales, Yudofsky, and Gabbard, and all of the other editors and contributors, for a job well done.

References

Caspi A, Sugden K, Moffitt TE, et al: Influence of life stress on depression: moderation by a polymorphism in the 5-HTT gene. Science 301:386–389, 2003

Kaplan HI, Freedman AM, Sadock BJ (eds): Comprehensive Textbook of Psychiatry, 3rd Edition. Baltimore, MD, Williams & Wilkins, 1980

Hales RE, Yudofsky SC, Gabbard GO (eds): The American Psychiatric Publishing Textbook of Psychiatry, 5th Edition. Washington, DC, American Psychiatric Publishing, 2008

Talbott JA, Hales RE, Yudofsky SC (eds): The American Psychiatric Press Textbook of Psychiatry. Washington, DC, American Psychiatric Press, 1988

PREFACE

The Fifth Edition of *The American Psychiatric Publishing Textbook of Psychiatry* has undergone the most comprehensive and significant change in its 20-year history. Although it remains a one-volume, clinically oriented textbook of psychiatry that has been crafted for use primarily by practicing psychiatrists and advanced psychiatry residents who may be studying for their board examinations, the Textbook also remains a standard educational reference for physicians in other specialties, such as family practice, internal medicine, and neurology. This year we added our good friend and distinguished colleague, Glen O. Gabbard, M.D., as a co-editor. Dr. Gabbard is a prolific author of professional and trade books and has written and edited two major textbooks that have greatly influenced the field of psychiatry: *Psychodynamic Psychiatry in Clinical Practice* and *Gabbard's Treatments of Psychiatric Disorders*, both now in their fourth editions. Dr. Gabbard will also be publishing a new, comprehensive textbook in 2008 on psychotherapies. His addition as an editor has provided a useful clinical and scientific balance to Dr. Yudofsky's expertise in neuropsychiatry and Dr. Hales' interests in clinical psychiatry.

We are grateful to Alan Schatzberg, M.D., senior editor of *The American Psychiatric Publishing Textbook of Psychopharmacology*, for writing such a scholarly and inspirational Foreword for this edition. His research experience in the field of psychopharmacology is truly exceptional.

With the burgeoning psychiatric knowledge gained during the last 20 years, the size of the Textbook has grown from 1,344 pages and 38 chapters in 1988 to 1,672 pages and 44 chapters in this edition. A total of 8 new chapters were added for the Fifth Edition. Following Glen Gabbard's recommendations, we added chapters on supportive psychotherapy, combining psychotherapy and pharmacotherapy, and treatment of gay, lesbian, bisexual, and transgender patients. New chapters were added in the field of neuroscience: cellular and molecular biology (which is also included in the Fifth Edition of *The American Psychiatric Publishing Textbook of Neuropsychiatry and Behavioral Neurosciences*) and neuroanatomy for the psychiatrist. We also added a new chapter on human sexuality and changed the orientation of the violence chapter to assessment of dangerousness. Because of the development of new nonpharmacological somatic treatments in psychiatry, a chapter was added to address this topic.

This edition includes 66 new contributors, with the total number of contributors increasing from 88 to 104. Fifteen of the chapters have completely new authors. In summary, 23 of the 44 chapters either address new topics or have new authors, making the Fifth Edition the most completely revised edition yet.

We have maintained close contact with many of the professionals who purchased the previous editions of the Textbook and have benefited from their comments and suggestions. Work on the Fifth Edition began in earnest in late 2005. This edition represents the culmination of a nearly 3-year effort to provide the most useful and up-to-date clinical information in the field. In addition to new authors and chapters, all previous chapters have been extensively updated to include the latest references and research findings. Included with this edition is access to an electronic version of the book, along with a PowerPoint presentation of all tables, figures, and key clinical points for every chapter. An important feature of *The American Psychiatric Publishing Textbook of Psychiatry* since its inception has been the combination of senior and junior authors for selected chapters. For instance, Chapter 10, "Schizophrenia and Other Psychotic Disorders," is authored by two bright and energetic assistant professors, Michael Minzenberg, M.D., and Jong Yoon, M.D., and a senior professor, Cameron Carter, M.D. Similarly, Chapter 12, "Anxiety Disorders," features Professor and Chair Eric Hollander, M.D., together with Associate Professor Daphne Simeon, M.D. We have found that the addition of more junior authors has infused the chapters with new research insights and fresh perspectives on the subject matter. The senior authors have been able to temper these new ideas with their considerable wisdom and vast research and clinical experience. We believe that these collaborations enrich the appeal of the chapters to readers at all levels of educational and clinical experience. We also believe that these collaborations have enriched the diversity and quality of material presented in the Textbook.

All chapters were reviewed by a member of our editorial board and by the editors. The editorial board represents a wide range of clinical and research interests and includes senior psychiatrists, an early-career psychiatrist, and a senior psychiatry resident. We wanted our textbook to be relevant to our more junior colleagues and feel that Drs. Florence Kim (an assistant professor) and Julie Young (a third-year psychiatry resident) have helped us a great deal to achieve this goal.

For this edition we also included an international editorial advisory board. This group of distinguished psychiatrists represents some of the preeminent academicians and researchers from around the world. Their main task will be to review carefully the Fifth Edition and to recommend chapters and portions of chapters for inclusion in an essentials version of the book to be published in 2010. It is hoped that the essentials version will gain wide acceptance by our colleagues in other countries.

An enhancement to this edition is a companion Web site at www.PsychiatryOnline.com/Psychiatry that offers online access to the full text of the Textbook and a downloadable PowerPoint presentation containing all tables, figures, and key clinical points for every chapter. Also available is an interactive study guide—available both in print and at the companion Web site—including more than 300 questions and annotated answers corresponding to textbook chapters. The online version offers 20 AMA PRA Category 1 Credits™ and has been approved by the American Board of Psychiatry and Neurology as part of a comprehensive lifelong learning program, which is mandated by the American Board of Medical Specialties as a necessary component of maintenance of certification.

We hope that you will enjoy reading the Fifth Edition of the *Textbook of Psychiatry* as much as we enjoyed crafting and editing the volume. Please contact one of us if you have suggestions on how the Sixth Edition could be made even better.

Robert E. Hales, M.D., M.B.A.
Sacramento, California

Stuart C. Yudofsky, M.D.
Houston, Texas

Glen O. Gabbard, M.D.
Houston, Texas

About the Cover Image

The cover image is a watercolor representation of a microscopic section of the human hippocampus, whose principal function is the acquisition of new factual knowledge. Since that is the purpose of this textbook as well, the editors felt that this was a fitting image for the Fifth Edition.

The artist, Peter Shahrokh, Ph.D., M.B.A., has graduate degrees in English literature and business and currently works in the University of California, Davis Office of Architects and Engineers commissioning new buildings for the campus.

ACKNOWLEDGMENTS

We wish to thank many people for their invaluable assistance with the Fifth Edition of *The American Psychiatric Publishing Textbook of Psychiatry.* First, we are grateful to the outstanding authors who produced exceptional chapters and who labored to respond with good humor to our many editorial suggestions and critiques of their chapters. Also, our distinguished editorial board worked closely with us in designing a clinically focused and scientifically substantiated volume.

The outstanding staff at APPI has been highly encouraging and effective with all aspects of this project. Ron McMillen, CEO, and John McDuffie, Editorial Director, have been perennially insightful and invaluable to the concept, organization, and content of all editions of the Textbook. Greg Kuny, Managing Editor assisted us with key structural elements of the book and coordinated the entire production process. The Project Editor, Rebecca Richters, had the daunting challenge of overseeing the line-by-line editing of all of the manuscripts and asking for additional information or clarification from our authors. Special thanks go to Ann Eng, Senior Editor, who designed and coordinated the layout of the book, and to Judy Castagna, Manufacturing Manager, for ensuring that the published book was a high-quality product. The original cover artwork was painted by a talented Northern California artist, Dr. Peter Shahrokh. Thanks also go to Kathy Stein, the highly competent Director of Financial and Business Operations, and the always pleasant and helpful Bessie Jones, Acquisitions Coordinator, who aided us with numerous administrative and technical requirements for the publication of this edition. Finally, Bob Pursell, Director of Sales and Marketing, has organized an outstanding program for publicizing our Textbook to the field through various promotional efforts.

The organizational headquarters for this edition of the Textbook of Psychiatry was located at the University of California, Davis School of Medicine in Sacramento. Carrie Stafford handled all the correspondence and the majority of the calls to our authors and editorial board members. Her dedication and commitment to the publication of this edition are greatly appreciated. Susan Mortensen assisted me greatly in completing the final editing and review of the page proofs and in assembling the international advisory board. Susan also prepared the Study Guide question and answers, and Dr. James Bourgeois and Narri Shahrokh were outstanding co-authors who helped one of us (REH) write and edit the Study Guide. I would also like to thank Cristina and Alain Camu for allowing me to work at their wonderful home in Porto Ercole (Grosseto), Italy, where I reviewed the page proofs and wrote the initial drafts of the study guide questions.

Finally, and of most importance, we acknowledge the many people with psychiatric disorders, their families, and those who have dedicated their lives to caring for them through clinical service, research, and education. These brave and exemplary people have provided us with the inspiration, motivation, and knowledge for the crafting of this textbook.

Robert E. Hales, M.D., M.B.A.
Sacramento, California

Stuart C. Yudofsky, M.D.
Houston, Texas

Glen O. Gabbard, M.D.
Houston, Texas

INTERVIEWING AND TESTING

THE PSYCHIATRIC INTERVIEW AND MENTAL STATUS EXAMINATION

Linda B. Andrews, M.D.

Requisite Physician Preparation

An effective psychiatric interview allows the clinician both to connect with a patient and to gather pertinent data. Although medical technology has advanced tremendously in recent years and has increased the amount of laboratory and neuroimaging information available to assist psychiatrists in making more accurate diagnoses and developing more specific treatment plans for patients, these tests cannot supplant the importance of gathering critical data via the traditional psychiatric interview. The psychiatric interview is the single most important method of arriving at an understanding of a patient who exhibits the signs and symptoms of a psychiatric illness (Scheiber 2003). Patients usually communicate the most important aspects of their illnesses to their physicians during the doctor–patient interview. The psychiatrist listens and then responds to the patient in an effort to understand the patient's problems in the context of the patient's culture and environment (MacKinnon and Yudofsky 1991; MacKinnon et al. 2006). The psychiatric interview is similar to the general medical interview in that both include the patient's chief complaint, history of

present illness, past history, social and family history, and review of systems. However, the psychiatric interview differs from the traditional medical interview because the psychiatric interview also includes a more thorough examination of the patient's developmental history, including the patient's feelings about important life events and exploration of the patient's significant interpersonal relationships, patterns of adaptation, and character traits (MacKinnon et al. 2006; Scheiber 2003). The psychiatric interview includes a formal examination of the patient's mental status as well.

Connecting with a patient and gathering pertinent data via the psychiatric interview requires considerable preparation and practice. Psychiatric interviewing is a skill founded on extensive knowledge of normal and abnormal human behavior (MacKinnon et al. 2006). It is optimal for a training psychiatrist to observe others interviewing many patients and to be observed and critiqued while interviewing many patients before practicing independently. In medical education, such observation and supervision should occur often during both medical school and psychiatric residency training. Optimally, similar observation opportunities should continue throughout one's professional practice of psychiatry.

Conduct of the Psychiatric Interview

Goals and Purpose

The psychiatrist should consider a number of important issues in preparation for conducting a psychiatric interview with an adult patient. The psychiatrist must establish the goals and purpose for the psychiatric interview. What exactly does the psychiatric interviewer hope to accomplish during the psychiatric interview? The psychiatrist should be prepared to communicate clearly his or her interview goals to the patient. The psychiatrist should also be prepared to ascertain the patient's goals and expectations for the interview. Just as the psychiatrist has prepared for the interview, the patient, most likely, has also prepared. If the psychiatric interviewer and the patient wish to complete a successful interview, it is very helpful, and probably necessary, for the psychiatric interviewer and the patient to agree on the purpose of the interview. Relevant questions to establish the goals and purpose of the interview include the following:

- Is this interview being conducted for diagnostic or therapeutic purposes?
- Will the psychiatrist see this patient for this interview alone with the expressed goal to establish a psychiatric diagnosis, or does this interview represent the first of many appointments with this patient within a newly developed therapeutic or treatment relationship?
- What does the psychiatric interviewer know about the patient and the patient's expectations for this interview?
- What does the patient know about the psychiatrist or the psychiatrist's goals for this encounter?
- What does the patient expect to happen during and after this interview?

Guidelines for the Interview

The interviewer must understand many other parameters before beginning the actual interview:

- Under what circumstances is the psychiatric interview occurring?
- Who requested and who made arrangements for the psychiatric interview to take place?
- Will the results of the psychiatric interview be confidential?
- Is the patient participating voluntarily in the interview?

- How much time does the psychiatrist have to conduct the psychiatric interview?
- Does the psychiatric evaluation consist of one or more than one actual meetings with the patient?
- Where will the psychiatric interview occur?
- Does the psychiatrist or patient expect other persons to be interviewed as part of the psychiatric evaluation?
- Is the patient expected to pay for the psychiatric interview? If so, how will the fee be determined and how will the billing be handled?

Different answers to each of these questions will significantly influence how the psychiatrist conducts the psychiatric interview, what results the psychiatrist obtains from the psychiatric interview, and what the psychiatrist does with the obtained results.

Pre-Interview Contact

The psychiatrist must decide whether he or she should have telephone or E-mail contact with the patient before, during, and after the formal psychiatric evaluation. In the current age of electronic communication, patients may expect to communicate with their physicians via E-mail. As with most guidelines for conducting the psychiatric interview and mental status examination, no absolute rule exists about communications with patients outside of the actual psychiatric interview. Patients should be clearly instructed about how they should handle medical or psychiatric emergencies that might occur before or after the formal evaluation or between appointments if the psychiatrist and patient plan to meet more than once. Most commonly, this involves the psychiatrist either giving the patient an after-hours contact number or instructing the patient to go to a particular hospital emergency department in the case of a true medical or psychiatric emergency. For patient questions other than emergencies, each psychiatrist must decide for him- or herself how to manage phone calls and E-mails.

Process of the Psychiatric Interview

Once all of the questions have been answered, the psychiatrist is ready to begin the actual psychiatric interview and mental status examination. The first—and perhaps most important—task is to establish rapport with the patient being interviewed (Table 1–1). Establishing an effective working relationship will be necessary to accomplish all of the other tasks discussed throughout this chapter. Creating such a working relationship requires that the psychiatrist and the patient collaborate together in the service of learning about the patient and gathering information. Without this effective doctor–patient connection, the psychiatrist will most likely be unsuccessful in obtaining the requisite information to develop a thorough and accurate differential diagnosis and to design and implement an effective treatment plan. Developing this working alliance with the patient is generally accomplished by communicating respect and empathy to the patient. Communicating respect includes an appropriate introduction of one's self to the patient and respectfully asking the patient how he or she wishes to be addressed during the interview. Respectful and empathic communication involves making appropriate eye contact, observing nonverbal cues, and limiting interruptions.

Empathic communications show the patient that the psychiatrist is trying to listen and observe from the patient's perspective. The psychiatrist is attempting to understand the patient's experience from the patient's point of reference. This often requires that the psychiatrist acknowledge when his or her own thoughts, feelings, perceptions, or experiences differ from the patient's. The psychiatrist, then, should deliberately choose to focus on the patient's experiences and needs rather than on his or her own experiences or needs.

Early in the interview, the psychiatric interviewer should ask questions that create opportunities for expanding his or her emotional connection with the patient. For example, an empathic response by the psychiatric interviewer to a patient who shares that his 70-year-old grandmother has just died from complications of heart disease might be "Were you and your grandmother close?" Examples of less empathic responses by the psychiatric interviewer might be "My grandmother is about to celebrate her 90th birthday next month" or "Does anyone else in your family have heart disease?" The more empathic response focuses on the patient's emotional experience of his grandmother's death. The first less empathic response focuses on the interviewer more than the patient. The second less empathic response focuses away from the patient's emotional experience and more toward data gathering. If the psychiatrist has very limited time within which to complete the interview, and/or if this exchange were to occur toward the end of the interview time, the third response might be acceptable and even necessary.

Based on an empathic connection with the patient, the psychiatrist should be able to adjust his or her interview style to match the needs of a particular patient

TABLE 1–1.	Tasks for the therapist conducting a psychiatric interview

1. Establish goals.
2. Establish rapport.
3. Develop a collaborative doctor–patient relationship.
4. Communicate empathically.
5. Maintain appropriate boundaries.
6. Communicate in a language that the patient understands, and avoid psychiatric jargon.
7. Monitor the emotional intensity of the interview and adjust as necessary.
8. Gather pertinent psychiatric history data.
9. Perform a mental status examination.
10. Assess patient reliability.
11. Assess patient safety.
12. Develop a plan for possible emergencies.
13. Review previous records and other available data.
14. Interview others as appropriate.
15. Document accurately.
16. Manage time.

at any particular point in the interview. This empathic connection should also allow the psychiatrist to follow a patient's cues or leads as appropriate. Doing so demonstrates to the patient that the psychiatric interviewer is listening and responding to the patient in real time. Empathic attunement also allows the psychiatrist to focus on more emotionally relevant topics. Open-ended questions generally assist in this effort and allow a patient to give more detailed and emotionally meaningful responses to such questions.

Empathic communication may also allow the psychiatric interviewer to recognize when a patient is becoming overwhelmed with the emotional load of the interview and to reduce the intensity of the interview by using more focused, close-ended questions. This type of question more often generates a brief, even "yes" or "no" response from the patient. Such questions generally focus on gathering factual data from the patient rather than on understanding emotional meaning for the patient. Close-ended questions are also useful when interviewing patients with disturbances of thought content or production, perceptual disturbances, or cognitive deficits. Empathic attunement also allows the psychiatrist to recognize when an interview should be stopped before completion because a patient has become acutely agitated, dangerous, or medically compromised. Gathering data should never supersede keeping a patient safe during an interview.

Empathic and respectful communication should allow the patient to understand the psychiatrist's questions or comments. The psychiatrist should adjust his or her use of words to match the patient's intellectual abilities, perceived educational level, and language and cultural needs. The psychiatrist should avoid the use of medical jargon. The psychiatrist should enlist the assistance of a translator when necessary. The psychiatrist should ask additional questions to help clarify the meaning of a patient's words or nonverbal gestures that seem to be unclear to the psychiatric interviewer. The psychiatrist can demonstrate that he or she is actively listening to the patient by verifying that he or she has heard the patient correctly. For example, following a patient's response to a question about his noncompliance with his medication, the psychiatrist might say "So, you had wanted to fill the prescription and take the medication as prescribed, but you did not do so because you could not afford the prescription. Is that correct?" This type of clarification and verification allows the psychiatrist to demonstrate that he or she is listening carefully to the patient, which will hopefully enhance the patient's trust in the psychiatrist and build the collaborative nature of the doctor–patient relationship. It also allows the patient to correct any errors in the psychiatrist's understanding of the patient, which should lead to improved overall patient care. In this example, the psychiatric interviewer might be able to use this clarification to discuss further the difficult subject of the patient's financial limitations.

As the psychiatrist gathers information throughout the interview, he or she should remain cognizant of assessing the patient's reliability. Information obtained during the psychiatric interview is only as valid as the information's source. The psychiatrist should generally begin every interview assuming that the patient being interviewed will tell the truth to the best of his or her ability and will, therefore, be a reliable interviewee. However, as the interview progresses—and especially if, when interviewing others in the course of completing the assessment, the psychiatrist obtains information that conflicts with the patient's reported story—the psychiatrist ultimately will need to decide whether the patient is a reliable source of information. Confirming information given by the patient with information that can be verified by medical records or other valid sources should help the psychiatrist determine the patient's overall reliability.

Although the interviewer cannot ever anticipate or control every possible exchange that might take place with a new patient, the psychiatric interviewer should begin each relationship with a new patient by having some personally and professionally established guidelines about self-disclosure. For most first interviews, the psychiatrist will remain focused on gathering information about the patient and would rarely intend to be self-disclosing at this juncture in the physician–patient relationship. If the relationship with the patient were to develop into a therapeutic relationship, then the psychiatrist would need to judge whether, and when, self-disclosure might be beneficial in deepening the collaborative therapeutic relationship with the patient.

Similarly, if, during a psychiatric interview, a patient becomes agitated or threatening toward the psychiatrist, the psychiatrist must rather abruptly adjust his or her interview focus to manage this acute situation. Flexible interviewing strategies, such as rearranging the chairs in the examination room, opening the door, letting a patient stand during the interview, or inviting a professionally trained colleague or comforting family member to join the interview, may allow the patient to continue the interview and provide additional safety for both the patient and the interviewer.

Documentation is an important and necessary responsibility for the physician caring for patients. When conducting a psychiatric interview, the psychiatrist should determine ahead of time if and how records of the interview will be kept. If the interview is being conducted for trainee examination purposes only, the records will most likely be destroyed upon completion of the interview. If the interview occurs within a training setting, the psychiatric trainee may be required to take extensive notes or to audiotape or videotape the psychiatric interview. Patients must give informed consent to be audiotaped or videotaped. In a clinical setting, the psychiatrist should explain to the patient that he or she will take notes that will become part of the patient's medical record, but that the content of these notes are covered by the Health Insurance Portability and Accountability Act of 1996 and will be privacy protected to the fullest extent allowed by law.

During the psychiatric interview itself, the psychiatrist should take notes to ensure that an accurate recording of the dialogue is kept but should not take such voluminous notes so as to interfere with establishing and maintaining rapport or remaining empathically connected to the patient. For most clinicians, the skill of effectively taking notes during a patient interview develops over time with much practice. Each clinician must find his or her own comfortable balance between accurately recording data and remaining empathically attuned to the patient. Clinicians must also determine whether the notes taken during the psychiatric interview itself will become the official chart notes, or if they will serve as process notes used for supervision purposes, after which the interviewer will create an abbreviated summary note that will become an actual part of the patient's medical record. In most settings, the patient will have the right to view his or her medical record.

Ideally, the psychiatrist will review all of the available patient data prior to conducting the psychiatric interview of the patient. If this is not possible, the psychiatrist should at least review these records before developing a final diagnosis and treatment plan. This review would include reading any available medical records or psychiatric records as well as the results of all laboratory tests, neuropsychological testing, or neuroimaging scans that have been performed.

A thorough psychiatric interview could also include interviewing other individuals who have firsthand knowledge of the patient. This could include, but is not limited to, family members, teachers, colleagues, other physicians, or other health care providers. Whenever possible, the psychiatric interviewer should inform and obtain consent from the patient to interview these other individuals. It is best not to keep secrets from the patient, either about who else is being interviewed or about information provided by these other individuals when they are interviewed.

Throughout the interview, the psychiatrist must remain cognizant of time constraints. The psychiatric interviewer should have decided before beginning the interview whether he or she plans to make diagnostic and treatment recommendations during the first interview or if these issues will be presented to and discussed with the patient at a subsequent visit. If the psychiatric interviewer plans to discuss diagnosis and treatment during the first appointment, then the interviewer should manage the interview to leave adequate time toward the end for patient questions and to discuss significant diagnostic and treatment issues. If the psychiatrist has decided to have this discussion at the next appointment, then he or she should leave a few minutes at the end of this first appointment to allow the patient to ask questions and to schedule the next appointment together.

Content of the Psychiatric Interview

Once the introductions, instructions, and consents have been completed, the psychiatrist may focus on obtaining information from the patient (Table 1–2). If time allows, the interviewer should cover all key elements of the psychiatric history and mental status examination. For the psychiatric history, these key elements include the chief complaint or primary reason for the evaluation, history of the present illness, past psychiatric history, family psychiatric history, past medical history, family medical history, social history, developmental history, and a review of systems. For the mental status examination, these key elements include general appearance, orientation, speech, motor, affect, mood, thought production, thought content, perceptions, suicidal/homicidal ideation, memory/cognition, insight, and judgment.

Chief Complaint and History of Present Illness

It is usually best to begin the interview with a relatively open-ended, unstructured question to elicit the patient's chief complaint or primary concern. Examples of this type of question include the following: "How are you doing today?" "What brings you to the clinic today?" or "Are you having any troubles today?" These types of questions allow the patient to direct the conversation initially and to decide what is discussed first between the patient and the doctor. If possible, the psychiatrist will allow the patient adequate time to present his or her chief complaint, or primary concern, in a relatively uninterrupted manner.

Using information learned initially from the patient, the psychiatric interviewer should slowly direct the questions to obtain more details about the chief complaint and allow the chief complaint to be expanded to include a more thorough discussion of the history of present illness. The interviewer assumes, and this is usually the case, that the chief complaint and the history of the present illness will be linked in some important way. It is extremely important to spend adequate time and effort to flesh out considerable details about the history of the present illness. Otherwise, upon completing the interview, the psychiatrist's understanding of the patient will be simply a list of facts and data points without the important personal connecting thread to develop and create this pa-

TABLE 1–2.   Outline of the psychiatric interview
1. Chief complaint
2. History of present illness
3. Past psychiatric history
4. Past medical history
5. Social history
6. Developmental history
7. Family psychiatric and medical history
8. Review of systems

tient's story at this point in time. Questions about the history of present illness should include a review of current psychiatric symptoms: their onset, frequency, intensity, duration, precipitating factors, relieving or aggravating factors, and associated symptoms.

Past Psychiatric History

Expanding the history of present illness to inquire whether such symptoms have ever occurred before will lead to questions about the patient's past psychiatric history. This discussion should include past symptom frequency, intensity, and duration; precipitating, relieving, or aggravating factors; and associated symptoms. The review of the patient's past psychiatric history should include questions about past treatment with medications, therapy, or electroconvulsive therapy; previous hospitalizations; previous treatment for alcohol or substance abuse or dependence; and previous suicidal or homicidal ideation or attempts. With respect to previous medications, the psychiatrist should ask the patient to list all previously taken medications, including their dosages, side effects, length of treatment, compliance with treatment, and, if relevant, reason(s) for stopping treatment. With respect to psychotherapy, the psychiatrist should ask the patient to describe all previous experiences in psychotherapy, including therapy type, format, frequency, duration, and adherence. With respect to treatment for substance abuse, the psychiatrist should ask the patient to describe his or her substance use history, including quantity; frequency; route of administration; pattern of use; functional, interpersonal, or legal consequences of use; tolerance or withdrawal phenomena; and experience in any previous addiction treatment programs, including type and duration of the program and the patient's compliance with or completion of any such addiction treatment program (Vergare et al. 2006). The psychiatric interviewer should try to understand the patient's opinion about the efficacy of all previous treatments. The psy-

chiatrist should avoid recommending a treatment deemed by the patient to have been previously unsuccessful. The psychiatrist should pay particular attention to treatments that have been successful in the past, because the patient is more likely to respond to such treatments again in the future. Family members' positive responses to a particular treatment may also predict a good response for the patient being evaluated.

Family Psychiatric History

The interviewer should gather detailed information about the patient's family psychiatric history, including the presence or absence of psychiatric illnesses in parents, grandparents, siblings, aunts, uncles, cousins, and children. A patient should be made aware that his or her risk for developing certain psychiatric illnesses, including schizophrenia, bipolar disorder, major depressive disorder, obsessive-compulsive disorder, and panic disorder, increases if his or her family members have or have had these illnesses. The psychiatric interviewer may need to use less medical jargon when inquiring about the patient's family psychiatric history, because family stories and lore about family members' previous experiences with mental illness vary widely. For example, after asking "Is there a history of schizophrenia in your family?" the interviewer might follow up with a question such as "Has anyone in your family ever had a nervous breakdown or been placed in a mental hospital or institution?" The patient may or may not be aware of the formal diagnostic terms for psychiatric illnesses.

Medical History

The interviewer must inquire about the patient's past and current medical problems. Specifically, the psychiatrist needs to know what medications the patient takes regularly and if the patient is allergic to any medications or other things. Inquiry about medications should also include over-the-counter medications, herbal or energy supplements, vitamins, and complementary or alternative medical treatments (Vergare et al. 2006). The patient should be asked about any history of side effects to medications taken. Even if the patient denies any medical problems, it is important for the psychiatrist to ask specific questions about several medical illnesses, such as diabetes mellitus, seizure disorder, hypo- or hyperthyroidism, and cardiac disease, because a patient having any of these illnesses may alter the psychiatrist's diagnostic impressions or treatment plans. For example, if a patient with hypothyroidism presents with decreased energy and hypersomnia, the psychiatrist should inquire if the patient is taking thyroid medication and has had a recent thyroid hormone panel checked before assuming these symptoms could only be related to a primary depressive disorder. Also, if the psychiatrist interviewing the patient believed the patient had schizophrenia and intended to prescribe an atypical antipsychotic agent, the psychiatrist would need to ask if the patient had a history of diabetes, cardiac disease, or obesity, because several of the atypical antipsychotic medications can elevate the patient's blood sugar, exacerbate an existing cardiac condition, or cause weight gain. The psychiatrist should also inquire about a family history of medical problems.

Social History

Gathering information about the patient's social history is an extremely important part of the psychiatric interview because stability or instability in the patient's surroundings may dramatically affect the status of the patient's psychiatric illness. The psychiatric interviewer should inquire about the patient's living situation:

- Does the patient have a stable place of residence that is safe and affordable?
- Has anything about the patient's living situation changed recently?
- Are any changes expected in the near future?
- Does the patient have a reliable source of income?
- Is the patient working?
- Does the patient rely on some sort of subsidy, such as Medicare, Medicaid, or Social Security disability, for financial resources?
- Does the patient have an adequate support system, including family, friends, neighbors, and so on?
- Is the patient's support system reliable and available in times of need?
- Is the patient married, single, divorced, separated?
- Does the patient have children?
- Does the patient have family nearby and available to help?
- What is the nature of the patient's relationship with his or her family—that is, is the family supportive and helpful or intrusive and difficult?

Understanding the family system and dynamics is particularly important. If prescribed treatment plans require the patient to change behaviors, the psychiatrist must understand how such behavior changes might affect other family members. Even if a patient wishes to change his or her problematic behaviors, the family's willingness to support such change will be critical. The family's resistance to such change may severely undermine the patient's efforts for change.

The psychiatrist should ask about the patient's level of education. Skilled psychiatrists can often estimate a patient's educational level without asking specific questions, based on the patient's use of vocabulary and general fund of knowledge. However, it is wise to ask specific questions about the patient's level of education, to ensure that the interviewer does not misinterpret a patient's answers as indicative of neuropsychiatric deficits when they really represent a lower level of education. Similarly, the interviewer should gather some information about the patient's ethnic and cultural beliefs, because symptoms considered to be problematic and indicative of serious psychiatric illness in Western cultures are often believed to be normal behaviors in other cultures. The psychiatrist should ask the patient if he or she has strong connections to or receives support from a particular faith or spiritual group. Does the patient have any religious or other beliefs about psychiatry and psychiatric medications that might influence the efficacy of prescribed treatments?

The interviewer should ask the patient if he or she has any habits that could negatively affect the efficacy of any psychiatric treatments prescribed, such as tobacco use, alcohol use, or sexual promiscuity. When inquiring about these types of habits, the interviewer must ask specific questions to elicit meaningful answers. Patients do not generally easily or openly discuss behaviors about which they have some concern, embarrassment, or shame. For example, if the interviewer has reason to believe that the patient uses alcohol excessively, instead of asking "Do you drink much?" the interviewer should ask a series of specific questions that do not allow the patient to generalize his or her answers or to avoid answering the questions directly. The examiner should consider asking some of the following questions:

- Do you drink alcohol daily?
- How many drinks do you drink each night?
- Have you ever thought you should cut back on your drinking?
- Have you ever felt annoyed by people criticizing your drinking?
- Have you ever felt guilty about your drinking?
- Have you ever had to drink first thing in the morning to relieve a hangover?
- Have you ever blacked out from alcohol use?
- Have you ever had a legal problem, such as a DWI, from drinking too much?

A similarly detailed series of questions should be asked if the examiner suspects other drug use or abuse. Tobacco use can alter the metabolism of several psychiatric medications, so the examiner should ask every patient about smoking. The interviewer should also ask the patient about any current or pending legal problems. The interviewer should also ask whether the patient is now serving or has ever served in the U.S. military. If yes, the interviewer should ask the patient to describe his or her experiences in the military. Patients who serve or did serve in the military may be eligible for specialized medical and psychological services through the federal government. Questions about domestic violence should be covered at some time during the interview, and for many psychiatrists, doing so concurrent with discussions about the patient's social history seems most appropriate. As is the case with other sensitive topics, the psychiatric interviewer will likely need to ask very specific questions regarding domestic violence or other abusive relationships, because many patients will be reticent to discuss this with the interviewer, especially during their first meeting. The psychiatric interviewer should consider asking some of the following questions:

- Is your home a safe place to live?
- Has anyone in your family ever hit you?
- Have you ever gone to an emergency department because you were injured during a fight with your spouse/partner?
- Has anyone in your family forced you to have sexual contact with them against your wishes?

Developmental History

Gathering information about the patient's developmental history is another critical aspect of the psychiatric interview. Understanding a patient's development will greatly improve the likelihood that the psychiatrist will be able accurately to contextualize the patient's current psychiatric symptoms. A truly thorough developmental history will include questioning along a number of developmental continua, including motor, language, physical, sexual, emotional, and moral. The psychiatrist should ask about any unusual perinatal events and whether the patient achieved most developmental milestones, such as talking, walking, reading, and so on, in a normal fashion. Sometimes, a patient will not remember this information, but family members, especially parents or siblings, can be particularly helpful in obtaining a thorough and accurate developmental history. Psychiatrists often focus most on the patient's emotional development, because problems in this arena most dramatically influence the patient's subsequent psychiatric symptomatology. In this regard, most psychiatric interviewers ask the patient some of the following questions:

- Who lived in the home with you in early childhood?
- Are both of your parents still living?
- Did your family unit seem safe and stable to you?

Also, the psychiatrist will try to ascertain the quality of the patient's attachments to parental figures, the patient's experiences of various separations in childhood, and the quality of the patient's peer relationships, considering issues of attachment, trust, and intimacy to be of critical importance. Many adult manifestations of personality health or disorder relate significantly to the presence or absence of and the quality of these early childhood relationships. The psychiatric interviewer should ask if the patient experienced any verbal, emotional, physical, or sexual abuse as a child or teenager.

Because development extends beyond the childhood years, the psychiatric interviewer should assess the patient's ongoing development through adolescence and early, middle, and late adulthood, as appropriate, including an assessment of patterns of response to normal life transitions and major life events as well as the quality of ongoing interpersonal relationships. Some important areas to consider include how the patient handled the following events: moving away from home for the first time, going to college, getting married, having children, losing a job, losing a parent, and so on. Most psychiatrists include questions about sexual orientation in the social history portion of the interview as well.

Review of Systems

The psychiatric interviewer should complete this portion of the evaluation by reviewing any general medical systems or psychiatric illness categories that have not previously been discussed. The psychiatric interviewer should ask every patient about his or her sleep and appetite patterns, weight regulation, and sexual functioning (MacKinnon et al. 2006). The psychiatric interviewer should also ask every patient at least one or two questions about thought, mood, anxiety, substance use, and cognitive disorders, if these have not already been covered elsewhere.

The Mental Status Examination

The psychiatric interviewer completes the mental status examination by combining a series of observations with a series of formal questions (Table 1–3). The purpose of the mental status examination is to provide as clear a picture as possible of the patient's actual mental state at the time of the psychiatric interview or evaluation. It is truly a "state" rather than "trait" examination, meaning that it describes the patient's mental function at a given moment in time and does not necessarily represent a historical perspective of the patient's mental illness. It is, therefore, quite common, and probably expected, that the patient's mental status examination will differ from interview to interview. For this reason, the psychiatrist can use changes in a patient's mental status examination across multiple appointments to help clarify diagnostic questions and/or to update treatment decisions. Careful documentation and appropriate use of standard terminology of the mental status examination may allow these diagnostic and therapeutic decisions to be made even when different practitioners see the patient over time.

General Appearance

The psychiatric interviewer should observe the patient's general appearance throughout the interview. The interviewer's report should include some comment on the patient's posture, grooming, clothing, and body habitus. When reporting this portion of the mental status examination, the interviewer may simply state that the patient's general appearance is within normal limits or may include specific mention of any particular abnormality. If the psychiatrist has been treating a patient over time, he or she should mention any changes in the patient's general appearance, particularly as these may correlate with changes in the patient's overall mental health.

Orientation

When a psychiatrist interviews a patient for the first time, he or she should complete some formal assessment of orientation, asking the patient his or her full name, the full date (number, month, and year), and the place where the interview is occurring (city, state, building, floor, clinic name). In subsequent appointments with the same patient, the interviewer may decide to only ask these very specific orientation questions again if the patient's attention or focus seems to have changed from previous meetings.

TABLE 1–3.   Outline of the mental status examination

1. General appearance
2. Orientation
3. Speech
4. Motor activity
5. Affect and mood
6. Thought production
7. Thought content
8. Perceptual disturbances
9. Suicidal and homicidal ideation
10. Attention, concentration, and memory
11. Abstract thinking
12. Insight/judgment

Speech

The psychiatrist should include commentary about the patient's speech as part of the formal mental status examination. For example, the psychiatrist should describe the patient's rate, volume, articulation, coherence, and spontaneity of speech as observed throughout the psychiatric interview. Because several psychiatric illnesses can affect a patient's speech, particularly the rate of speech, slowing it down or speeding it up, monitoring a patient's speech remains important throughout a course of treatment.

Motor Activity

The mental status examination should include specific mention of the patient's motor behavior. This should include comment on the patient's gait and station, gestures, abnormal movements, tics, and overall general body movements as witnessed throughout the entire interview. Some psychiatric illnesses, such as bipolar disorder, manic phase, may produce a tendency toward exaggerated movements, whereas others, such as schizophrenia or major depressive disorder, may produce a tendency toward sluggish or diminished body movements. Monitoring changes in motor activity over time may help the clinician track the patient's illness progression over time, including compliance with and response to psychiatric medications.

Affect

The psychiatrist should observe and then comment on the patient's affect. *Affect* describes the patient's expressed emotional state that the psychiatrist observes throughout the interview. Words such as sad, sullen, bubbly, or agitated could be used. The interviewer should note if the patient's affect changes throughout the interview. If so, the interviewer should include comment about whether the changes are congruent to the interview content and appropriate for the interview setting. The interviewer should also note whether the affect changes occur gradually or abruptly. The lack of affective responsivity may occur in several psychiatric illnesses, such as depressive or thought disorders. Affective lability and instability may occur in other psychiatric illnesses, such as during a manic phase of bipolar disorder or alcohol intoxication. A patient's affect might also be inappropriate, such as when it does not match with the expressed content of the current conversation, for example, when a patient laughs while recounting a friend's death. The psychiatric interviewer should note whether the patient's affect and affect changes are appropriate.

Mood

Reporting the patient's mood is the only element of the mental status examination that actually is historical and not observed. The interviewer should ask the patient to report his or her mood for the past few days and weeks. The psychiatric interviewer can only know this by asking the patient. Information about *mood* cannot be obtained simply by observation during the psychiatric interview. Whenever possible, the psychiatric interviewer should use words directly reported by the patient, such as "The patient states that her mood has been gloomy over the past few weeks." It is helpful for the psychiatrist to compare the patient's reported mood with the psychiatrist's observation of the patient's affect during the psychiatric interview. Because a patient's affect is normally more fluid and more likely to fluctuate in response to surrounding circumstances, the patient's reported mood and manifest affect may or may not be congruent at all times. However, if the patient's mood and affect never seem to be congruent, the psychiatrist might comment on this observation to gather the patient's perspective. Patients who use denial as the defense mechanism to avoid dealing with their problems or who have poor insight into their problems may not realize that their pleasant, even cheerful, outward affective expression does not match with their reported depressed mood.

Thought Production

Thought process or *production* describes how the patient's thoughts are expressed during the psychiatric interview. The psychiatric interviewer should com-ment on the patient's thought production rate and flow, including comments about whether the patient's thinking is logical, goal-directed, circumstantial, tangential, or shows loosening of associations or flight of ideas (i.e., ideas are not connected one to the next). A patient's flow of thought can usually be described somewhere on the continuum between goal-directed and disconnected. Disorganizing psychiatric illnesses, such as thought disorders and bipolar disorder, manic type, most commonly cause loosely connected or disorganized thought production. Stimulant intoxication or manic episodes can also cause excessively rapid thought production.

Thought Content

A description of the patient's thought content should include mention of important themes and the presence or absence of delusional or obsessional thinking and suicidal or homicidal thoughts. *Delusional thinking* includes fixed false beliefs that are persecutory, erotomanic, grandiose, somatic, or jealous in content. Patients with delusions believe that their fixed false beliefs are reality. Thought disorders, such as schizophrenia or schizoaffective disorder, are the most likely causes of bizarre delusions over a long period of time. Alcohol or drug intoxication may cause acute changes in thought content, including paranoid ideation or even delusional thinking. *Obsessions* are defined as recurrent, persistent thoughts that intrude involuntarily into a person's thinking. Obsessions appear to be senseless and are not based in reality. They most commonly occur in obsessive-compulsive disorder but may also occur in eating disorders or other impulse control disorders. Patients with obsessions recognize that their intrusive thoughts are not normal. A patient's awareness that these thoughts are senseless, as opposed to believing them to be reality, distinguishes obsessions from delusions.

Perceptual Disturbances

The psychiatric interviewer must inquire about the patient's perceptual abilities. Asking questions about perceptual disturbances can be particularly challenging for the novice interviewer, because the questions may seem strange and even intrusive to the psychiatric interviewer him- or herself. The interviewer must ask if the patient sees, hears, smells, or feels anything that is not based on an actual sensory stimulus. Of course, the interviewer probably should word the question more clearly to a patient, such as "Do you ever see things that other people don't see?" or "Do you ever hear voices talking to you and then realize that no one is actually in the room with you?" Perceptual disturbances such as hearing, seeing, smelling, or feeling things in the absence of an actual sensory stimulus are called *hallucinations*. Hallucinations most typically occur as part of a psychotic illness, such as schizophrenia, or during intoxication or withdrawal from alcohol or illicit drugs. During a psychiatric interview, the interviewer may be able to observe a patient who is responding to internal stimuli because the patient is answering a question even though a question has not been asked or is turning to talk to someone in a different part of the room when another person is not actually present. A patient may or may not acknowledge or admit to having such perceptual disturbances. Often the patient is so frightened by the auditory or visual hallucinations that he or she denies hearing voices or seeing things even when the psychiatric interviewer is convinced that the patient has such perceptual disturbances. Patients often will only admit to these hallucinations after establishing some sort of therapeutic relationship with the doctor, after several appointments together.

Suicidal and Homicidal Ideation

A competent psychiatric interview should always include an assessment of suicidality and homicidality. The suicide assessment is particularly critical for patients with a personal or family history of suicide attempts or a family history of completed suicide and should include exploring for the presence or absence of current suicidal ideation, intent, and plan. The homicide assessment is particularly critical for patients with a prior history of violence or trouble with the law. If, during a psychiatric interview, the psychiatrist learns that a patient is actively suicidal or homicidal, the psychiatrist must redirect his or her interviewing efforts to manage this acute situation. Such management might be to organize admission to a psychiatric hospital for an acutely suicidal patient or to call the police to get assistance with an acutely agitated or homicidal patient. The interviewer should be knowledgeable about state laws regarding the duty to warn, should a patient threaten to harm another person.

Attention, Concentration, and Memory

As part of the mental status examination, the psychiatric interviewer should assess the patient's attention, concentration, and memory. Theoretically, this could be done without asking any specific questions but based solely on the patient's participation in the entire psychiatric interview. This is most possible for a patient whose memory is completely intact or for a more experienced clinician. However, most clinicians will ask at least a few testing questions before concluding that the patient's attention, concentration, and memory are within normal limits. Some tests include the following:

- "Please spell the word 'world' forward for me. Now spell the word 'world' backwards."
- "Start with the number 100, subtract 7, and continue to count backward by 7s until I tell you to stop."
- "Who is the current president of the United States? Who was president before him? Who were the previous four presidents of the United States before him?"

The psychiatric interviewer must carefully choose the questions to assess attention, concentration, and memory to ensure that the questions match the patient's educational level and cultural background. Patients with lower educational levels and with non-Western cultural backgrounds may be at particular risk to perform poorly on these questions. For patients who appear to have cognitive deficits, it is recommended that the psychiatric interview include a formal Mini-Mental State Examination (MMSE), which includes a specific set of questions whose answers are scored and compared with a 30-point maximum score. Patients with cognitive disorders as well as cognitive impairment secondary to other psychiatric disorders usually have lower MMSE scores (Folstein et al. 1975). Several psychiatric disorders, in addition to actual cognitive disorders, can cause attention, concentration, memory, and other cognitive changes. Such deficits caused by psychiatric disorders, such as attention-deficit disorder or major depressive disorder, may improve with appropriate treatment. Therefore, for patients who have lower MMSE scores, the psychiatrist should repeat the MMSE at each subsequent appointment and track the patient's performance over time to monitor for cognitive changes. Upon receiving appropriate consent, the psychiatric interviewer might choose to expand his or her understanding about the patient's apparent cognitive problems by speaking with family members who live with or near the patient.

Abstract Thinking

Some psychiatric conditions, including serious thought disorders, traumatic brain injury, and chronic alcohol or substance abuse, can impair patients' ability to perform abstract thinking. Therefore, as part of the mental status examination, most psychiatrists perform some assessment of abstraction abilities. Most often, the psychiatric interviewer will ask the patient to interpret a proverb by saying something similar to the following, "Please tell me what this saying might mean, as if you were trying to explain its meaning to a small child. 'Don't cry over spilled milk' or 'People who live in glass houses shouldn't throw stones.'" Patients with less than an eighth-grade education or patients who have not yet fully acculturated into the Western culture may struggle with this type of question, regardless of any superimposed psychiatric illness. Therefore, a psychiatrist must be guarded in interpreting the meaning of a patient's concrete responses to this type of question. The psychiatrist should incorporate data from the entire interview when determining whether a patient's thinking is more concrete than would otherwise be expected for the patient's level of education or acculturation.

Insight/Judgment

Toward the end of the psychiatric interview and mental status examination, the interviewer should consider the degree to which the patient understands and appreciates the impact of his or her psychiatric illness on the rest of the patient's life. Psychiatrists refer to this capacity to understand one's illness as *insight*. Patients with greater insight into their illnesses generally demonstrate greater compliance with treatment recommendations. Patients with poorer insight into their illnesses tend to comply less well with treatment recommendations. Compliance can also serve as a measure of judgment. Psychiatrists assume that patients with better judgment will be more compliant with treatment recommendations.

Some interviewers ask questions to assess judgment more formally. In the past, these questions would tend to be about hypothetical situations, such as "What would you do if you found a stamped, addressed envelope on the sidewalk?" or "What would you do if you were in a movie theater and smelled smoke?" However, asking questions that are pertinent and more probable in their likelihood of occurrence is probably a more helpful approach and will likely provide a better assessment of the patient's judgment. Suggested questions include "What would you do if you ran out of your medications 1 week before your next scheduled doctor's appointment?" or "What would you do if you developed severe diarrhea 2 days after starting a new medication for your depression?" These questions allow the physician to test the patient's judgment and also introduce an effective way to discuss such important treatment issues as compliance and medication side effects.

Diagnostic Formulation and Treatment Planning

The steps involved in consolidating a diagnostic formulation and developing a treatment plan are listed in Table 1–4.

In beginning to consolidate an understanding of the patient, the psychiatrist may decide to complete various rating scales to help document the presence or absence of symptoms or to quantify the severity of specific illnesses identified. A wide variety of such rating scales exists and should be chosen carefully and specifically for each patient (MacKinnon et al. 2006).

TABLE 1–4.	Steps in developing a diagnostic formulation and treatment plan
1.	Complete rating scales, if indicated.
2.	Review laboratory, neuroimaging, and neuropsychological testing results.
3.	Incorporate significant physical examination findings.
4.	Assimilate psychiatric history data into a biopsychosocial formulation.
5.	Develop a working diagnosis.
6.	Determine the optimal treatment setting.
7.	Recommend biopsychosocial treatment goals and plan.
8.	Ensure that the patient understands the treatment goals and plan.
9.	Verify that the patient can afford the treatment recommendations.
10.	Document if the patient refuses treatment.
11.	Make follow-up arrangements.

The biopsychosocial formulation allows the interviewer to assimilate the primary biological, psychological, and social factors into a brief but integrated understanding of the patient. The primary function of the biopsychosocial formulation is to provide a succinct conceptualization of the patient and thereby guide a treatment plan. The biopsychosocial formulation is a hypothesis or set of hypotheses that attempt to explain the patient's symptoms. If the psychiatric interviewer sees the patient over time, the biopsychosocial formulation should be revised regularly as new data appear (Kassaw and Gabbard 2002; Perry et al. 1987). The biopsychosocial formulation is generally relatively short but includes the key biological, psychological, and social elements from the psychiatric history and mental status examination that are most pertinent to understanding this patient at this point in time. Particularly for the psychological portion of the formulation, the psychiatrist should not try to make the formulation all-inclusive but should focus on one or two key themes at the core of the patient's problems, identify key developmental experiences and relevant stressors, and use the here-and-now transference and countertransference data from the interview to link the patient's past and present problems (Kassaw and Gabbard 2002).

An example of an abbreviated biopsychosocial formulation follows.

> A 45-year-old white, strong, athletic man, who is the president of a prominent company, presents 4 weeks after his first myocardial infarction, reporting decreased sleep, energy, and concentration; increased irritability; and angry outbursts at his wife and son. He has a family history of mood disorders and alcohol abuse. He has not yet been able to return to work because of ongoing medical complications following the myocardial infarction. The patient seems to be unaware of his feelings of fear and helplessness to change his situation. He has begun drinking daily, despite being told by his cardiologist that he should not drink at all. The patient is likely developing symptoms of depression and increased alcohol use because he has lost two of his most reliable sources of self-esteem—his work and his physical strength. He feels impotent and unable to cope via his previously successful strategy of dealing with stress simply by working more.

Using the biopsychosocial formulation as a guide, the psychiatrist should next develop a working diagnosis using the five-axis classification system delineated in DSM-IV-TR (Table 1–5; American Psychiatric Association 2000).

The psychiatrist does not necessarily need to explain to the patient, in great detail, the entire five-axis diagnostic assessment. However, the psychiatrist does need to explain to the patient, in language that the patient can understand, a summary of the psychiatrist's diagnostic impression along with some discussion of the patient's prognosis given this (or these) psychiatric diagnosis(es).

In developing a treatment plan, the psychiatrist should include relevant biological, psychological, and social treatment recommendations. The first treatment decision involves determining the appropriate setting in which treatment should occur. Specifically, can the patient and his or her illness be managed in the outpa-

TABLE 1–5.	DSM-IV-TR multiaxial assessment and differential diagnosis
Axis I	All primary psychiatric disorders of thought, mood, anxiety, cognition, and substance abuse and other conditions that might be a focus of clinical attention
Axis II	Personality disorders and disorders first diagnosed in childhood, including mental retardation
Axis III	Concurrent general medical conditions
Axis IV	Psychosocial and environmental problems
Axis V	Global assessment of functioning based on a standard scoring system from 1 to 100, with 1 being severe impairment of function and 100 being no impairment of function

Source. Adapted from American Psychiatric Association 2000, pp. 27–33.

tient setting? If not, the psychiatric interviewer must make the necessary arrangements to hospitalize the patient. Once the setting has been determined, the psychiatrist can proceed in creating a biopsychosocial treatment plan.

The biological portion of the treatment plan may include performing or arranging for a physical examination to be performed. Next, the psychiatrist should determine any laboratory tests as well as any neuroimaging studies that should be completed. The biological portion of the biopsychosocial treatment plan should also include the list of any psychiatric medications that the patient is currently taking with explicit instructions about whether those medications will be continued and, if so, how they should be taken. It should include instructions for any medication blood levels or other laboratory tests that the patient will need to obtain following the first appointment. The biological portion of the treatment plan should also include a discussion about any medical illness management issues that need to be addressed, such as referral to an internist to improve hypertension or diabetes mellitus control or referral to a dietitian for weight loss management.

The psychological portion of the treatment plan should include recommendations for indicated neuropsychological testing as well as a discussion of all possible psychotherapeutic interventions. Neuropsychological testing may reveal important information about the patient's cognitive abilities and personality. The psychiatric interviewer should explain, in language that the patient can understand, if a particular psychotherapy is being recommended, why it is being recommended, and how the patient is expected to participate in that psychotherapy. Psychotherapy treatment options should include individual psychotherapy, group psychotherapy, couples therapy, or family therapy as indicated by the patient's particular treatment needs. Individual psychotherapy recommendations could include long- or short-term psychodynamic psychotherapy; brief focused therapies, such as cognitive-behavioral therapy, interpersonal psychotherapy, or dialectical behavior therapy; and long- or short-term supportive psychotherapy. The psychotherapeutic treatment plan must be specifically tailored to each patient. The treatment recommendations may include more than one form of psychotherapy. The key to successful psychotherapy depends on carefully selecting patients suited to the particular psychotherapy chosen. Two principal assessments must be made when recommending psychotherapy: 1) Are the patient's clinical symptoms likely to respond to the particular therapy being recommended, and 2) If considering psychodynamic therapy, does the patient have the psychological characteristics suitable for the psychodynamic approach (Gabbard 2004)?

The patient's ability to afford the recommended psychotherapy, both from a financial and a time perspective, must be considered when developing a final treatment plan. If the patient's financial resources are limited, the psychiatrist should familiarize him- or herself with any lower-fee psychotherapy services available within the area.

The social portion of the treatment plan may include recommendations to improve the patient's living, work, financial, or support network situations, as relevant to the particular patient. For example, involving a social worker to assist the patient in obtaining job retraining or in applying for Social Security disability may be important. The social treatment plan might include a day treatment program or a social skills development program to expand the patient's opportunities for regular social interactions. The psychiatrist might decide that helping a patient reconnect with his or her church community for support is important. The psychiatrist should give the patient referral contact information for local mental health support group chapters, such as the local chapter of the National Alliance for the Mentally Ill. The social treatment plan might also include recommendations for the patient to quit smoking or to attend Alcoholics Anonymous groups.

Each portion of the treatment plan must be carefully tailored to meet an individual patient's needs.

Implementation of each treatment recommendation should be plausible and feasible. The patient's potential resistance for any element of the treatment plan should be addressed as directly as possible, to minimize opportunities for the patient to sabotage the treatment plan. The psychiatrist should ensure that the patient fully understands each aspect of the treatment plan. The patient should be given ample opportunity to ask questions and to consider alternative options, if acceptable treatment substitutes exist.

The psychiatrist should document if the patient refuses any portion of the treatment plan. The psychiatrist should attempt to understand why a patient refuses to comply with a particular treatment recommendation and, depending on the reason, should decide whether that treatment element can be discarded or is critical to the patient's overall treatment response and illness recovery. If the psychiatrist believes that the patient's treatment refusal will cause serious harm to the patient or others or that the patient's psychiatric illness will deteriorate significantly without treatment, the psychiatrist might need to pursue mandated treatment, including possibly pursuing appointing another person to serve as the patient's guardian to force treatment adherence.

Finally, the psychiatrist and patient should discuss and agree on a follow-up plan. The follow-up plan should include a discussion about any assignments for the patient before the next visit, such as gathering old records or having laboratory tests completed, and any assignments for the psychiatrist before the next visit, such as speaking to a physician who previously cared for the patient or reviewing pending laboratory results. Whenever possible, the date and time of the next appointment should be determined before the patient leaves the psychiatrist's office. Last, as discussed previously, the psychiatrist should give the patient specific contact information for his or her office and instructions about how to handle any urgent or emergent situations regarding the patient's mental health that might arise before the next appointment.

Conclusion

The psychiatric interview, including the mental status examination, continues to be one of the most important tools for patient assessment, even with recent advances in medical technology. As is the case with all critical medical skills, psychiatrists must maintain their expertise through continued education and regular practice.

Key Points

- Establish rapport and communicate respect. Introduce yourself, use patient's name, make eye contact, and limit interruptions.

- Use empathic connection to guide and adjust interview to match the particular patient and situation. Follow the patient's leads or cues whenever possible and use open-ended questions to increase depth of understanding and information gathered (fewer topics covered, greater depth). Use focused questions to increase breadth of understanding and information gathered (more topics covered, less depth). Increase focus of questions for patients with disturbances of thought content or production, perceptual disturbances, or cognitive deficits. Abbreviate the interview for acutely agitated, dangerous, or medically compromised patients. Use words that the patient can understand—avoid medical jargon; assess the patient's education, language, and cultural needs; and use a translator when necessary. Clarify and verify that the patient understands you and that you understand the patient.

- Assess the patient's safety, including assessment of suicide risk in every patient. Assess dangerousness early and often during an interview with a potentially dangerous patient.

- Take notes to record necessary data, but do not let note taking interfere with your ability to establish and maintain rapport with the patient. Review available medical records and test results before completing your assessment and developing your treatment plan. Interview other relevant persons in the patient's life.

- Cover all key elements of the psychiatric history and mental status examination. Psychiatric history includes chief complaint, history of present illness, past psychiatric history, past medical history, social history, developmental history, family psychiatric and medical history, and review of systems. For the mental status examination, observe or assess the following aspects of behavior and thought: general appearance; orientation; speech; motor activity; affect and mood; thought production; thought content; perceptual disturbances; suicidal or homicidal ideation; attention, concentration, and memory; abstract thinking; and insight/judgment.

- Formulate the data gathered during psychiatric interview and develop a biopsychosocial formulation and a thorough differential diagnosis, including information for all five DSM-IV-TR axes. Develop a treatment plan that includes appropriate biological, psychological, and social interventions and considers the patient's overall prognosis. Ensure that the patient understands the treatment goals and plan, and verify that the patient can afford the treatment recommendations. Document if the patient refuses treatment. Establish follow-up plans (e.g., next appointment, tests to complete).

Suggested Readings

MacKinnon RA, Yudofsky SC: Principles of the Psychiatric Evaluation, 2nd Edition. Philadelphia, PA, JB Lippincott, 1991

MacKinnon RA, Michels R, Buckley PJ: The Psychiatric Interview in Clinical Practice, 2nd Edition. Washington, DC, American Psychiatric Publishing, 2006

References

American Psychiatric Association: Diagnostic and Statistical Manual of Mental Disorders, 4th Edition, Text Revision. Washington, DC, American Psychiatric Association, 2000

Folstein MF, Folstein SE, McHugh PR: "Mini-Mental State": a practical method for grading the cognitive state of patients for the clinician. J Psychiatr Res 12:189–198, 1975

Gabbard GO: Long-Term Psychodynamic Psychotherapy. Washington, DC, American Psychiatric Publishing, 2004

Kassaw K, Gabbard GO: Creating a psychodynamic formulation from a clinical evaluation. Am J Psychiatry 159:721–726, 2002

MacKinnon RA, Yudofsky SC: Principles of the Psychiatric Evaluation, 2nd Edition. Philadelphia, PA, JB Lippincott, 1991

MacKinnon RA, Michels R, Buckley PJ: The Psychiatric Interview in Clinical Practice, 2nd Edition. Washington, DC, American Psychiatric Publishing, 2006

Perry S, Cooper AM, Michels R: The psychodynamic formulation: its purpose, structure and clinical application. Am J Psychiatry 144:543–551, 1987

Scheiber SC: The psychiatric interview, psychiatric history, and mental status examination, in The American Psychiatric Publishing Textbook of Clinical Psychiatry, 4th Edition. Edited by Hales RE, Yudofsky SC. Washington, DC, American Psychiatric Publishing, 2003, pp 155–188

Vergare MJ, Binder RL, Cook IA, et al: Practice guideline for the psychiatric evaluation of adults, 2nd Edition. Am J Psychiatry 163:1–36, 2006

2

LABORATORY TESTING AND IMAGING STUDIES IN PSYCHIATRY

H. Florence Kim, M.D.
Paul E. Schulz, M.D.
Elisabeth A. Wilde, Ph.D.
Stuart C. Yudofsky, M.D.

Laboratory and diagnostic testing traditionally have not held a central role in the diagnosis and treatment of patients with psychiatric disorders. This contrasts with the other specialties of modern medicine, which have come to rely heavily on laboratory and imaging modalities to provide the necessary information to diagnose and treat patients with disorders such as cancer, heart disease, and pulmonary problems.

Psychiatric diagnoses, on the other hand, continue to be made primarily on clinical grounds, with laboratory and diagnostic testing being relegated to informing clinicians about medical causes of psychiatric symptoms that might be excluded from the differential of diagnoses or used to monitor psychotropic drug levels during treatment. Yet clinical laboratory and diagnostic imaging is on the threshold of a new era.

New methods such as pharmacogenetic and pharmacogenomic testing are becoming widespread and more widely available for clinical use. Research into structural and functional neuroimaging abnormalities in psychiatric disorders are providing valuable information about the possible pathophysiology underlying these disease states and hold promise for eventual use as routine diagnostic modalities. Research into the use of combined laboratory and imaging modalities is leading us to our eventual goal of early identification, treatment, and ultimately prevention of psychiatric illnesses. In this chapter, we present what is currently available for clinical diagnostic testing and imaging of psychiatric patients and what the future holds for these modalities as the arsenal of diagnostic modalities grows ever larger for the clinical psychiatrist.

Approach to Screening Laboratory and Diagnostic Testing of Psychiatric Patients

Laboratory assessment is essential to the workup of the psychiatric patient because any number of neurological and medical illnesses can give rise to psychiatric symptomatology. A careful neuropsychiatric history and physical examination and judicious clinical laboratory testing are still the first and very important steps in the workup. They can focus or even obviate neuroimaging or electrophysiological testing, which can be expensive, invasive, and physically and emotionally uncomfortable to the patient.

Moreover, psychiatric symptoms that on the surface may appear to be similar may, in fact, have dissimilar etiologies. For example, hallucinations can occur in the context of schizophrenia as well as in Alzheimer's disease, Parkinson's disease, frontotemporal dementia, delirium from other chronic medical illnesses, and alcohol withdrawal. Table 2–1 lists some of the many medical and neurological illnesses that may present with prominent neuropsychiatric symptoms. Clinical laboratory assessment and diagnostic testing can help determine which of these many causes is responsible for a patient's hallucinations. Importantly, a number of these etiologies may have potentially curative remediations, and hence accurate diagnosis is critical.

TABLE 2–1.   Selected medical conditions with psychiatric manifestations

Neurological

    Cerebrovascular disease

    Multiple sclerosis

    Multiple systems atrophy

    Parkinson's disease

    Progressive supranuclear palsy

    Alzheimer's disease

    Frontotemporal dementias

    Dementia associated with Lewy bodies

    Seizure disorder

    Huntington's disease

    Traumatic brain injury

    Anoxic brain injury

    Migraine headache

    Sleep disorders (narcolepsy, sleep apnea)

    Normal pressure hydrocephalus

Neoplastic

    Central nervous system tumors, primary and metastatic

    Pancreatic carcinoma

    Paraneoplastic syndromes

    Endocrine tumors

    Pheochromocytoma

Infectious

    HIV

    Neurosyphilis

TABLE 2–1.   Selected medical conditions with psychiatric manifestations *(continued)*

Infectious *(continued)*

    Creutzfeldt-Jakob disease

    Systemic viral and bacterial infections

    Viral and bacterial meningitis and encephalitis

    Tuberculosis

    Infectious mononucleosis

    Pediatric autoimmune neuropsychiatric disorder associated with streptococcal infections (PANDAS)

Nutritional

    Vitamin deficiencies

    B_{12}: pernicious anemia

    Folate: megaloblastic anemia

    Nicotinic acid deficiency: pellagra

    Thiamine deficiency: Wernicke-Korsakoff syndrome

    Trace mineral deficiency (zinc, magnesium)

Autoimmune

    Systemic lupus erythematosus

    Sarcoidosis

    Sjogren syndrome

    Behcet's syndrome

Endocrine/metabolic

    Wilson's disease

    Fluid and electrolyte disturbances (syndrome of inappropriate antidiuretic hormone secretion [SIADH], central pontine myelinolysis)

    Porphyrias

    Uremias

    Hypercapnia

    Hepatic encephalopathy

    Hyper-/hypocalcemia

    Hyper-/hypoglycemia

    Thyroid and parathyroid disease

    Diabetes mellitus

    Pheochromocytoma

    Pregnancy

    Gonadotropic hormonal disturbances

    Panhypopituitarism

Drugs and toxins

    Environmental toxins: organophosphates, heavy metals, carbon monoxide

    Drug or alcohol intoxication/withdrawal

    Adverse effects of prescription and over-the-counter medications

Source.   Adapted from Ringholz 2001; Sadock and Sadock 2007; Wallach 2000.

A complete psychiatric assessment, including a medical and psychiatric history, physical examination, and mental status examination, must be conducted before the initiation of any clinical and diagnostic testing. Such initial assessments will guide the clinician in his or her choices for relevant, cost-effective laboratory testing. Laboratory costs accounted for 10%–12% of total health care costs in 1990, and unnecessary tests should be avoided if they are unlikely to alter the patient's treatment and outcome (Sheline and Kehr 1990).

Screening Laboratory Testing

At present, there are no consensus guidelines for the initial laboratory screening of psychiatric patients without known medical illnesses. Clinicians are generally guided by the history, physical examination, and mental status examination and by their own clinical judgment to decide what tests are appropriate to obtain.

Some studies of patient populations with general medical illnesses have shown that the history and review of systems obtained from the patient are superior to the physical examination in the diagnosis and management of patients and that screening laboratory testing can be the least helpful modality (Barnes et al. 1983; Hampton et al. 1975). Furthermore, other studies indicate that there is little relationship between physical complaints and the presence of physical disease (Honig et al. 1991; Koran et al. 1989).

Which screening laboratory tests, then, are most helpful for the psychiatric patient? Several studies have been conducted to investigate the utility of screening laboratory testing in the psychiatric patient, although most of these have been conducted in a retrospective manner, drawing from varied patient populations (Barnes et al. 1983; Catalano et al. 2001; Dolan and Mushlin 1985; Hall et al. 1980; Korn et al. 2000; Mookhoek and Sterrenburg-vdNieuwegiessen 1998; Sheline and Kehr 1990; White and Barraclough 1989; Willett and King 1977). Based on these varied studies, it appears that patients with psychiatric complaints alone, without other medical problems or complaints, will benefit from a few screening tests such as serum glucose concentration, blood urea nitrogen (BUN) concentration, creatinine clearance, and urinalysis (Anfinson and Kathol 1992). More extensive screening panels appear to be unnecessary. Screening of female psychiatric patients older than 50 years of age, especially those with mood symptoms, may be justified due to a high prevalence of hypothyroidism in the patients. Thyroid screening of men and younger women, among whom the prevalence of thyroid dysfunction is estimated to be 0.1%, should be limited to patients with two or more clinical signs of hypothyroidism (Anfinson and Stoudemire 2000).

More extensive laboratory screening may be required for several categories of patients: elderly individuals, institutionalized persons, persons of low socioeconomic status, individuals with a high degree of self-neglect, persons with alcohol or drug dependence, and those with cognitive impairment or fluctuating mental status (Anfinson and Kathol 1992; Hall et al. 1978; Koran et al. 1989; Sox et al. 1989). These patients may be less able to give a coherent or complete clinical history, or to have higher burden of complex medical illnesses, and thus require more "detective" work in the form of laboratory workup.

In these situations, screening laboratory tests will vary according to the patient's clinical presentation, the clinical situation (outpatient clinic vs. emergency department vs. inpatient setting) and concomitant medical illnesses. Laboratory screening becomes anything but routine for the patients in these categories, and it must be tailored to the patient's specific presenting complaints and physical findings. Table 2–2 presents a list of screening laboratory tests that clinicians often use during the initial evaluation of the patient with psychiatric complaints.

Screening Chest Radiographs

In several studies, investigators have retrospectively reviewed the utility of the screening chest radiograph in the evaluation of psychiatric patients. Data from several studies suggest that there is little evidence that a routine chest radiograph will yield beneficial information for a patient without respiratory or neurological symptoms (Brown and Gaar 1995; Gomez-Gil et al. 2002; Harms and Hermans 1994; Hughes and Barraclough 1980; Liston et al. 1979; Mookhoek and Sterrenburg-vdNieuwegiessen 1998). These data, in addition to the absence of current screening guidelines for chest radiographs in the general population, indicate that the *routine* screening chest radiograph is not indicated for a person being evaluated for the presence of a psychiatric disorder. However, chest radiographs are clearly indicated for specific clinical situations. For example, for an elderly patient with sudden onset of fever, shortness of breath, chest pain, or delirium, a chest radiograph should be ordered on an emergency basis.

Screening Electrocardiograms

Several studies have shown that the routine performance of screening electrocardiograms on young, medically healthy psychiatric patients who do not

TABLE 2–2. Useful screening labs in the workup of the neuropsychiatric patient

Type	Test	Reference range	Indication	Comments
Hematological studies	Coomb's test, direct and indirect	Positive/negative	Hemolytic anemias secondary to psychiatric medications	Evaluation of drug-induced hemolytic anemias, such as those secondary to chlorpromazine, phenytoin, levodopa, and methyldopa
	Ferritin (serum)	20–323 ng/mL 16–283 ng/mL	Cognitive/neuropsychiatric workup	Decreased: iron-deficiency anemia; most-sensitive test Elevated: anemias other than iron-deficiency
	Folate Plasma Red cell	3.1–12.4 ng/mL 186–645 ng/mL	Alcohol abuse	Utilized in vitamin B_{12} deficiencies associated with psychosis, paranoia, fatigue, agitation, dementia, delirium
	Hemoglobin	Male: 13.8–17.2 g/dL Female: 12.1–15.1 g/dL	Cognitive/neuropsychiatric workup	Decreased: alcohol abuse, cirrhosis, liver disease
	Hematocrit	Male: 40.7%–50.3% Female: 44.3%–63.1%	Cognitive/neuropsychiatric workup	
	Iron (serum)	45–160 µg/dL 30–160 µg/dL	Cognitive/neuropsychiatric workup	Decreased: iron-deficiency anemia, other normochromic anemias
	Iron-binding capacity	220–420 µg/dL	Cognitive/neuropsychiatric workup	Decreased: hemochromatosis, liver cirrhosis, thalassemia Elevated: iron-deficiency anemia, acute and chronic blood loss, acute liver damage
	Mean corpuscular volume	$87 \pm 5 \text{ m}^3$	Alcohol abuse	Elevated: alcoholism and vitamin B_{12} and folate deficiency
	Partial thromboplastin time	21–32 secs	Treatment with antipsychotics, heparin	Monitor anticoagulant therapy; Elevated: in presence of lupus anticoagulant and anticardiolipin antibodies

TABLE 2–2.   Useful screening labs in the workup of the neuropsychiatric patient *(continued)*

Type	Test	Reference range	Indication	Comments
Hematological studies *(continued)*	Platelets	$1.8\text{–}6.6 \times 10^3/\mu L$ $140\text{–}144 \times 10^3/\mu L$	Use of psychotropic medications	Decreased by certain psychotropic medications (carbamazepine, clozapine, phenothiazines)
	Porphobilinogen deaminase (erythrocyte uroporphyrinogen-1-synthetase)	2.1–4.3 mU/g Hgb	Porphyrias	Decreased: Porphyria synthesizing enzyme in red blood cells (RBCs) in patients with acute intermittent porphyria
	Prothrombin time	8.2–10.3 secs	Cognitive/medical workup	Elevated: significant liver damage (cirrhosis)
	Reticulocyte count	0.5%–1.5%	Cognitive/medical workup	Decreased: megaloblastic or iron-deficiency anemia and anemia of chronic disease, alcoholism Indicator of effective RBC production
	White blood cell (WBC) count	$3.8\text{–}9.8 \times 10^3/\mu L$	Use of psychiatric medications	Leukopenia and agranulocytosis associated with certain psychotropic medications, such as phenothiazines, carbamazepine, clozapine Leukocytosis associated with lithium and neuroleptic syndrome
Serum chemistries/ vitamins	Acid phosphatase	0–0.7 IU/L	Cognitive/medical workup	Elevated: prostate cancer, benign prostatic hypertrophy, excessive platelet destruction, bone disease
	Alanine aminotransferase (ALT)/serum glutamate pyruvate transaminase (SGPT)	7–53 IU/L	Neuropsychiatric workup	Elevated: hepatitis, cirrhosis, liver metastasis Decreased: B_6/pyridoxine deficiency
	Albumin	3.6–5.0 g/dL	Cognitive/medical workup	Elevated: dehydration

TABLE 2–2. Useful screening labs in the workup of the neuropsychiatric patient *(continued)*

Type	Test	Reference range	Indication	Comments
Serum chemistries/ vitamins *(continued)*	Alkaline phosphatase	38–126 IU/L	Cognitive/neuropsychiatric workup Use of psychiatric medications	Elevated: Paget's disease, hyperparathyroidism, hepatic disease, liver metastases, heart failure, phenothiazine use Decreased: pernicious anemia (vitamin B_{12} deficiency)
	Ammonia	11–35 µmol/L	Cognitive/neuropsychiatric workup	Elevated: hepatic encephalopathy, liver failure, Reye's syndrome; increases with gastrointestinal hemorrhage and severe congestive heart failure
	Amylase	25–115 IU/L	Eating disorders	May be elevated in bulimia nervosa
	Aspartate aminotransferase (AST)/serum glutamic oxaloacetic transaminase (SGOT)	11–47 IU/L	Cognitive/neuropsychiatric workup	Elevated: heart failure, hepatic disease, pancreatitis, eclampsia, cerebral damage, alcoholism Decreased: pyridoxine (vitamin B_6) deficiency and terminal stages of liver disease
	Bicarbonate	21–29 mEq/L	Panic disorder Eating disorder	Decreased: hyperventilation syndrome, panic disorder, anabolic steroid abuse May be elevated in patients with bulimia nervosa, in laxative abuse, psychogenic vomiting
	Bilirubin	0.3–1.1 mg/dL	Cognitive/neuropsychiatric workup	Elevated: hepatic disease
	Blood urea nitrogen	7–35 mg/dL	Delirium	Elevated: renal disease, dehydration

TABLE 2–2. Useful screening labs in the workup of the neuropsychiatric patient *(continued)*

Type	Test	Reference range	Indication	Comments
Serum chemistries/ vitamins *(continued)*	Calcium	8.6–10.3 mg/dL	Cognitive/neuropsychiatric workup Mood disorders Psychosis Eating disorders	Elevated: hyperparathyroidism, bone metastases Elevation associated with delirium, depression, psychosis Decreased: hypoparathyroidism, renal failure Decrease associated with depression, irritability, delirium, chronic laxative abuse
	Chloride	97–110 mmol/L	Eating disorder Panic disorder	Decreased: patients with bulimia, psychogenic vomiting Mild elevation in hyperventilation syndrome, panic disorder
	CO_2 content (plasma)	22–32 mmol/L	Cognitive/neuropsychiatric workup Delirium	
	Creatinine phosphokinase (CPK)	≤150 U/L	Delirium	Elevated: neuroleptic malignant syndrome, intramuscular injection rhabdomyolysis (secondary to substance abuse), patients in restraint, patients experiencing dystonic reactions; asymptomatic elevations with use of antipsychotic drugs
	Creatinine	0.8–1.8 g/day	Cognitive/neuropsychiatric workup	Elevated: renal disease (see blood urea nitrogen)
	Gamma-glutamyl transpeptidase (serum)	11–50 IU/L 7–32 IU/L	Alcohol abuse	Elevated: alcohol abuse, cirrhosis, liver disease

TABLE 2–2.   Useful screening labs in the workup of the neuropsychiatric patient (continued)

Type	Test	Reference range	Indication	Comments
Serum chemistries/ vitamins (continued)	Glucose	65–109 mg/dL	Panic attacks Anxiety Delirium Depression	Very high fasting blood sugar associated with delirium Very low fasting blood sugar associated with delirium, agitation, panic attacks, anxiety, depression
	Lactate dehydrogenase	100–250 IU/L	Cognitive/neuropsychiatric workup	Elevated: myocardial infarction, pulmonary infarction, hepatic disease, renal infarction, seizures, cerebral damage, megaloblastic (pernicious) anemia Factitious elevations secondary to rough handling of blood specimen tube
	Magnesium (serum)	65–109 mg/dL	Alcohol abuse Cognitive/neuropsychiatric workup	Decreased: alcoholism; low levels associated with agitation, delirium, seizures
	Phosphorus (serum)	2.5–4.5 mg/dL	Cognitive/neuropsychiatric workup	Increased: acute porphyria
	Potassium	3.3–4.9 mmol/L	Cognitive/neuropsychiatric workup Eating disorders	Increased: hyperkalemic acidosis Increase associated with anxiety in cardiac arrhythmia Decreased: cirrhosis, metabolic alkalosis, laxative abuse, diuretic abuse Decrease common in bulimic patients and in psychogenic vomiting, anabolic steroid abuse
	Protein (total)	6.5–8.5 g/dL	Cognitive/neuropsychiatric workup	Increased: multiple myeloma, myxedema, lupus

TABLE 2–2.   Useful screening labs in the workup of the neuropsychiatric patient *(continued)*

Type	Test	Reference range	Indication	Comments
Serum chemistries / vitamins *(continued)*	Sodium	135–145 mmol/L	Cognitive/neuropsychiatric workup	Decreased: water intoxication; SIADH; use of carbamazepine; myxedema, congestive heart failure, diarrhea, polydipsia, renal failure Increased: diabetes insipidus; anabolic steroids
	Vitamin A (serum)	360–1,200 mg/L	Depression Delirium	Hypervitaminosis A is associated with a variety of mental status changes, headache
	Vitamin B$_{12}$ (serum)	200–1,100 pg/mL	Cognitive/neuropsychiatric workup Dementia Mood disorder	Part of workup of megaloblastic anemia and dementia B$_{12}$ deficiency associated with psychosis, paranoia, fatigue, agitation, dementia, delirium Often associated with chronic alcohol abuse
	Zinc (serum)	75–120 µg/dL	Cognitive/neuropsychiatric workup	
Endocrine studies	Adrenocorticotropic hormone	<60 pg/mL	Cognitive/neuropsychiatric workup	Changes with steroid abuse; may be elevated in seizures, psychosis, Cushing's disease, and in response to stress
	Beta human chorionic gonadotropin	Negative	Pregnancy test	Prior to initiation of teratogenic psychotropic medications
	Cortisol	6–30 mg/dL	Cognitive/neuropsychiatric workup Mood disorders	Excess levels may indicate Cushing's disease; associated with anxiety, depression, and a variety of other conditions
	Catecholamines, urinary and plasma Homovanillic acid, vanillylmandelic acid	<540 µg/day	Panic attacks Anxiety	Elevated: pheochromocytoma

TABLE 2–2. Useful screening labs in the workup of the neuropsychiatric patient *(continued)*

Type	Test	Reference range	Indication	Comments
Endocrine studies *(continued)*	Estrogens (total)	Male: 29–127 pg/mL Female: 35–650 pg/mL (varies over menstrual cycle)	Mood disorder	Decreased: menopausal depression and premenstrual syndrome; variable changes in anxiety
	Follicle-stimulating hormone	Male: 1.1–13.5 mIU/mL Female: 0.4–22.6 mIU/mL (varies over menstrual cycle)	Depression	High normal in anorexia nervosa, higher values in postmenopausal women; low levels in patients with panhypopituitarism
	Growth hormone	Male: <1 ng/mL Female: <10 ng/mL	Depression Anxiety Schizophrenia	Blunted response to insulin-induced hypoglycemia in depressed patients; increased response to dopamine agonist challenge in schizophrenic patients; elevated in some anorexic patients
	Luteinizing hormone	Male: 1.4–7.7 mIU/mL Female: 1.6–62.0 mIU/mL (varies over menstrual cycle)	Depression	Decreased: patients with panhypopituitarism Decrease associated with depression
	Parathyroid hormone	12–72 pg/mL	Anxiety Cognitive/neuropsychiatric workup	Low level causes hypocalcemia and anxiety Dysregulation associated with wide variety of organic mental disorders
	Prolactin	Male: 1.6–18.8 ng/mL Female: 1.4–24.2 ng/mL	Use of antipsychotic medications Cocaine use Pseudoseizures	Antipsychotics, by decreasing dopamine, increase prolactin synthesis and release, especially in women Elevated: cocaine withdrawal Lack of prolactin elevation after seizure suggestive of pseudoseizure

TABLE 2–2. Useful screening labs in the workup of the neuropsychiatric patient *(continued)*

Type	Test	Reference range	Indication	Comments
Endocrine studies *(continued)*	Testosterone (serum)	Male: 270–1,070 ng/dL Female: 6–86 ng/dL	Impotence Inhibited sexual desire	Elevated: anabolic steroid abuse May be decreased in impotence and inhibited sexual desire Used in follow-up of sex offenders treated with medroxyprogesterone Decreased: medroxyprogesterone treatment
	Thyroid function tests Thyroid-stimulating hormone Thyroxine (T$_4$) Triiodothyronine (T$_3$) Thyroxine-binding globulin capacity T$_3$ resin uptake	2–11 µU/mL 4–11 µg/dL 75–220 ng/dL 12–28 µg/dL 25%–35%	Cognitive/neuropsychiatric workup Depression	Detection of hypo- or hyperthyroidism Abnormalities can be associated with depression, anxiety, psychosis, dementia, delirium, lithium treatment
Autoimmune studies	Antinuclear antibody	Negative at 1:10 dilution	Cognitive/neuropsychiatric workup	Most sensitive test for systemic lupus erythematosus (SLE; detects up to 95% of cases); specificity is low in rheumatic diseases in general (50%) Elevated: SLE and drug-induced lupus (e.g., secondary to phenothiazines, anticonvulsants); SLE can be associated with delirium, psychosis, mood disorders
	AntiDNA antibody	None detected	Cognitive/neuropsychiatric workup	Positive in 40%–80% of SLE patients High titers characteristic of SLE; low titers in other rheumatic diseases
	Erythrocyte sedimentation rate	<20 mm/hour	Cognitive/neuropsychiatric workup	Elevated: nonspecific indicator of infectious, inflammatory, autoimmune, or malignant disease; sometimes recommended in the evaluation of anorexia nervosa

TABLE 2–2.   Useful screening labs in the workup of the neuropsychiatric patient *(continued)*

Type	Test	Reference range	Indication	Comments
Autoimmune studies *(continued)*	Lupus anticoagulant	Negative	Use of phenothiazines	An antiphospholipid antibody, which has been described in some patients using phenothiazines, especially chlorpromazine; often associated with elevated partial thromboplastin time; associated with anticardiolipin antibodies
	Rheumatoid factor	0.0–20.0 IU/mL	Neuropsychiatric workup	Use in evaluation of stroke in young person or vasculitis
Cerebrospinal fluid (CSF) studies	Acid-fast bacilli stain	None detected	Neuropsychiatric workup	Useful for diagnosis of tuberculous meningitis
	Cell count (CSF)	0–2 WBCs 0–5 RBCs	Neuropsychiatric workup	Lymphocytes present in tuberculous meningitis Polymorphonuclear leukocytes (PMNs) present in bacterial meningitis
	Culture and sensitivities		Neuropsychiatric workup	For evaluation of bacterial meningitis/encephalitis
	Glucose (CSF)	65–109 mg/dL	Neuropsychiatric workup	Decreased: bacterial, tuberculous and fungal meningitis
	Immunoglobulin (Ig) G	<4 mg/dL	Neuropsychiatric workup	Elevated in 70% of multiple sclerosis (MS) patients
	Myelin basic protein	0.07–4.10 ng/mL	Neuropsychiatric workup	Elevated in 70%–90% of MS patients during an acute exacerbation; also elevated in other demyelinating diseases

TABLE 2–2.   Useful screening labs in the workup of the neuropsychiatric patient *(continued)*

Type	Test	Reference range	Indication	Comments
Cerebrospinal fluid (CSF) studies *(continued)*	Protein electrophoresis (CSF and serum) Prealbumin Albumin Alpha-1 globulin Alpha-2 globulin Beta globulin Gamma globulin	2%–7% 56%–76%	Neuropsychiatric workup	Oligoclonal bands positive in 85%–95% of patients with definite MS; most sensitive marker of MS Use in evaluation of inflammatory and hypercoagulable states
	Opening pressure	<7 mm Hg (100 mm water)	Neuropsychiatric workup	Elevated: in pseudotumor cerebri, meningitis, subarachnoid hemorrhage or other head trauma
	Protein (CSF)	6.5–8.5 g/dL	Neuropsychiatric workup	Elevated: bacterial, tuberculous, and fungal meningitis Must obtain serum protein levels as reference
Serological studies	Cytomegalovirus (CMV) (serum and CSF)	Positive/negative	Altered mental status/ Neuropsychiatric workup	CMV can produce anxiety, confusion, mood disorders CMV IgG and IgM
	Epstein-Barr virus (EBV) (serum and CSF)	Positive/negative	Cognitive/neuropsychiatric workup Anxiety Mood disorders	Part of herpes virus group EBV is causative agent for infectious mononucleosis, which can present with depression, fatigue, and personality change EBV may be associated with chronic mononucleosis-like syndrome associated with chronic depression and fatigue
	Hepatitis A viral antigen (serum)	Positive/negative	Mood disorders Cognitive/neuropsychiatric workup	Less severe, better prognosis than hepatitis B; may present with anorexia, depression
	Hepatitis B surface antigen Hepatitis B core antigen	Positive/negative	Mood disorders Cognitive/neuropsychiatric workup	Active hepatitis B infection indicates greater degree of infectivity and of progression to chronic liver disease

TABLE 2–2. Useful screening labs in the workup of the neuropsychiatric patient *(continued)*

Type	Test	Reference range	Indication	Comments
Serological studies *(continued)*	Hepatitis C core antibody	Positive/negative	Mood disorders Cognitive/neuropsychiatric workup	High rates of depression related to interferon treatment
	HIV-1 p24 antigen (serum)	Positive/negative	Altered mental status/neuropsychiatric workup	Positive ELISA confirmed via Western blot or immunofluorescence assay
	Lyme titer (serum)		Altered mental status	Evaluation of meningitis due to Lyme disease (*Borrelia burgdorferi*) Elevated: IgM and IgG antibodies Suspected cause of meningitis with elevated lymphocytes, elevated protein and IgG oligoclonal bands in CSF
	Syphilis test (rapid plasma reagin test, venereal disease research laboratory slide test) (serum and CSF)	Nonreactive	Neuropsychiatric workup	Positive in syphilis
Urine tests	Myoglobin	0–1 mg/L	Phenothiazine use Substance abuse Use of restraints	Elevated: neuroleptic malignant syndrome; phencyclidine, cocaine, or lysergic acid diethylamide intoxication; and in patients in restraints
	Urinalysis Specific gravity pH Protein Glucose Occult blood Ketones Bilirubin Nitrite Urobilinogen Microscopic	 1.005–1.030 5.0–8.5 Negative Negative Negative Negative Negative Negative 0.1–1.0 ≤2 WBC/high power field (hpf), ≤2 RBC/hpf	Cognitive/neuropsychiatric workup Pretreatment workup of lithium Drug screening	Provides clues to cause of various cognitive disorders (assessing general appearance, pH, specific gravity, bilirubin, glucose, blood, ketones, protein, etc.); specific gravity may be affected by lithium

TABLE 2–2.   Useful screening labs in the workup of the neuropsychiatric patient *(continued)*

Type	Test	Reference range	Indication	Comments
Urine tests *(continued)*	Urine porphyrins Uroporphyrin Coproporphyrin Porphobilinogen	0–4 μmol/mol Cr 0–22 μmol/mol Cr 0–8.8 μmol/L	Altered mental status	Elevated: acute intermittent porphyria, especially during acute attack
	Urine catecholamines, metanephrines, vanillylmandelic acid	0.0–7.0	Altered mental status, anxiety	Elevated: pheochromocytoma; metanephrines most reliable screening test for pheochromocytoma
Toxicology	Alcohol		Altered mental status Anxiety	Elevated blood alcohol level varies by state law (>0.08%–0.15%) Tolerance likely if blood alcohol level >0.10% but intoxication symptoms absent Elevated gamma-glutamyltransferase and liver function tests Detectable for up to 12 hours in urine
	Amphetamines	Positive/negative	Altered mental status	Detectable for up to 48 hours in urine
	Barbiturates	Positive/negative	Altered mental status	
	Benzodiazepines	Positive/negative	Altered mental status Suicide attempts	Detectable for up to 3 days in urine
	Caffeine	Positive/negative	Anxiety/panic disorder	Evaluation of patients with suspected caffeinism
	Cannabis	Positive/negative	Altered mental status	Detectable up to 4 weeks chronic users
	Cocaine	Positive/negative	Altered mental status	Elevated levels of benzoylecgonine (metabolite) present Detectable up to 48 hours in urine
	Inhalants		Altered mental status	

TABLE 2–2.   Useful screening labs in the workup of the neuropsychiatric patient *(continued)*

Type	Test	Reference range	Indication	Comments
Toxicology *(continued)*	Nicotine	Positive/negative	Anxiety Nicotine addiction	Evaluation of anxiety in smokers Elevated levels of cotinine (metabolite) can be detected in blood, saliva, or urine
	Opiates/narcotics	Positive/negative	Altered mental status	Elevated SGOT and CPK
	Phencyclidine	Positive/negative	Altered mental status	Detectable up to 8 days in urine
	Salicylates		Organic hallucinosis Suicide attempts	Toxic levels may be seen in suicide attempts; high levels may cause organic hallucinosis
Other diagnostic tests/procedures	CO$_2$ inhalation, sodium bicarbonate infusion		Anxiety/panic disorder	Provocative test Panic attacks induced in subgroup of patients
	Doppler ultrasound		Impotence Cognitive/neuropsychiatric workup	Carotid occlusion, transient ischemic attack, reduced penile blood flow in impotence
	Echocardiogram		Panic disorder	10%–40% of patients with panic disorder have mitral valve prolapse
	Electroencephalogram		Cognitive/neuropsychiatric workup	Evaluation of seizures, brain death, lesions Shortened REM latency in depression High-voltage activity in excitement, functional nonorganic cases (e.g., dissociative states), alpha activity present in the background, which responds to auditory and visual stimuli Biphasic or triphasic slow bursts seen in dementia of Creutzfeldt-Jakob disease

TABLE 2–2.   Useful screening labs in the workup of the neuropsychiatric patient *(continued)*

Type	Test	Reference range	Indication	Comments
Other diagnostic tests/procedures *(continued)*	Holter monitor		Panic disorder	Evaluation of panic-disordered patients with palpitations and other cardiac symptoms
	Nocturnal penile tumescence		Impotence	Quantification of penile circumference changes, penile rigidity, frequency of penile tumescence Evaluation of erectile function during sleep Erections associated with REM sleep Helpful in differentiation between organic and functional causes of impotence

Note.   Reference values given in conventional units; may vary between laboratories.
ELISA=enzyme-linked immunosorbent assay; REM=rapid eye movement; SGOT=serum glutamic-oxaloacetic transaminase; SIADH=syndrome of inappropriate antidiuretic hormone secretion.

Source.   Adapted from Alpay and Park 2000; Anfinson and Stoudemire 2000; Fadem and Simring 1998; Methodist Health Care System 2001; Sadock and Sadock 2007; Wallach 2000.

have cardiovascular symptoms is unnecessary (Hollister 1995). However, studies differ regarding the importance of electrocardiography in the elderly, with some finding an increased prevalence of electrocardiographic abnormalities in people over age 50. Furthermore, the conclusions of these studies differ with regard to the clinical importance or outcome that these abnormalities might have for the patient's health (Hall et al. 1980; Harms and Hermans 1994; Hollister 1995; Mookhoek and Sterrenburg-vdNieuwegiessen 1998). However, all agree that, regardless of age, an electrocardiogram is indicated when the history, review of systems, or findings from the physical examination suggest cardiovascular disease, or if a patient is initiating treatment with a psychotropic drug, such as a tricyclic antidepressant (TCA) or an antipsychotic, that is known to alter cardiac function or increase cardiac conduction times.

Screening Electroencephalograms

The electroencephalogram (EEG) can be very useful when a patient has altered mental status, such as delirium or encephalopathy. It can be useful for distinguishing between possible diagnoses. For example, it can diagnose complex partial status epilepticus. It can also be useful for diagnosing metabolic encephalopathy, which is generally due to a systemic illness that is having an effect on the nervous system, such as a urinary tract infection, endocrine disorder, toxin(s), or metabolic derangement(s). The EEG is also useful for distinguishing some specific etiologies of encephalopathy. For example, it might show the di- and triphasic waves characteristic of renal failure, hepatic failure, or anoxia. In the patient who is frankly comatose, the EEG can be very valuable for identifying the level of nervous system impairment. For example, it can show an alpha coma pattern or a theta coma pattern characteristic of brain stem lesions producing coma or may show a delta coma pattern characteristic of bihemispheric disease. In the patient who appears to be obtunded, the EEG can be useful for demonstrating whether a patient is catatonic, and hence has a normal awake-looking EEG, versus encephalopathic, where there might be diffuse slowing or triphasic waves (metabolic encephalopathy).

Although the acute computed tomography (CT) scan has generally superseded the EEG for diagnosing strokes, strokes may not be demonstrable in the first 24 hours after they occur. In that setting, an EEG may be useful for diagnosing a focal deficit before it is visible on a CT scan. Thus, it might be useful, for example, to distinguish a functional right hemiparesis and aphasia due to a stroke that is not yet visible on a head CT. When these symptoms are due to a large middle cerebral artery stroke, there will be focal slowing on the EEG. The EEG will be normal, in contrast, in a functional hemiparesis and aphasia.

Screening Structural Neuroimaging Examinations

A screening head CT scan is very easy to perform, takes only a few minutes, produces little discomfort, and has a fairly high resolution and sensitivity. It can thus be easily performed in any psychiatric patient admitted with clinical features that do not appear to be classic for the disorder diagnosed. For example, if a patient has late-onset depression or mood disorder, then a head CT scan can be useful for screening for vascular disease, demyelinating disease, subdural hematoma, subarachnoid hemorrhage, and so on.

Magnetic resonance imaging (MRI) of the brain has the advantage over the head CT of being more sensitive. It is much more likely to detect vascular disease and demyelinating disease. It is also useful for detecting mild neurodegenerative changes that might point to degenerative dementias. However, MRI does take longer (about 45 minutes) than CT scans, and it is at least twice as expensive. In most places, MRI is also not available at night and hence is not useful for rapid screening.

Overall Role of Screening Laboratory and Diagnostic Testing

The consensus of studies evaluating the role and value of laboratory testing is that patients who have psychiatric signs and symptoms but who do not exhibit other physical complaints or symptoms will benefit from a small screening battery that includes serum glucose concentration, BUN concentration, creatinine clearance, and urinalysis. Female patients over age 50 will also benefit from a screening thyroid-stimulating hormone (TSH) test regardless of the presence or absence of mood symptoms. Broader screening panels are generally unnecessary and costly. However, for psychiatric patients who have concomitant physical complaints or findings on physical examination, more extensive laboratory workup may become necessary. Likewise, more extensive laboratory workup is warranted for patients who are of higher risk, such as elderly or institutionalized patients or those with low socioeconomic status, self-neglect, alcohol or drug dependence, or cognitive impairment. Imaging may also be helpful when atypical features are present, such as an older age at onset of psychiatric illness, or when cognitive impairment is present.

Laboratory Approach to Specific Clinical Situations in Psychiatry

In this section, we discuss the specific clinical situations that may arise with the psychiatric patient that would warrant more extensive laboratory and diagnostic workup. These situations include, but are not limited to, new-onset psychosis, new-onset mood symptoms, anxiety symptoms, altered mental status, cognitive decline, and substance abuse.

New-Onset Psychosis

A careful evaluation is important for a patient with a first episode of psychosis in order to rule out the many possible medical and neurological causes of psychosis. Routine screening tests often include serum chemistries including sodium, potassium, chloride, carbon dioxide, BUN, and creatinine; liver function tests such as total protein, total and direct bilirubin, serum aspartate transaminase/serum glutamic-oxaloacetic transaminase (AST/SGOT), and alanine aminotransferase/serum glutamate pyruvate transaminase (AAT/SGPT); complete blood count (CBC) with platelets and differential; TSH; a rapid plasma reagin for syphilis; HIV serology; serum alcohol level; urinalysis; and urine toxicology screen for drugs of abuse. Other tests to consider during the initial workup include structural neuroimaging (head CT or brain MRI) and electroencephalography. If appropriate, the clinician should also consider ordering a urine pregnancy test and baseline electrocardiogram, especially if he or she is planning to initiate or change antipsychotic medication. If these initial tests do not immediately yield an etiology, the clinician may also consider a lumbar puncture to analyze cerebrospinal fluid (CSF) for the presence of red and white blood cells, protein, and glucose; opening pressure; and bacterial culture, cryptococcal antigen, and viral serologies. Antinuclear antibodies, rheumatoid factor, erythrocyte sedimentation rate, urine porphyrins, blood cultures, and assays for heavy metals (manganese and mercury) and bromides are other tests to

consider. There are many causes of psychosis that need to be considered, including central nervous system (CNS) or systemic infections, temporal lobe epilepsy, substance intoxication and withdrawal, metabolic or endocrine disorders, CNS tumors, and heavy metal poisoning. Table 2–3 summarizes some of the recommended tests in the diagnostic approach to a patient with new-onset psychosis.

Mood Disturbance: Depressive or Manic Symptoms

A thorough laboratory screening is also recommended for the evaluation of adult patients with new-onset mood symptoms such as depression or mania. Tests might include TSH, serum chemistries, CBC, urinalysis, and urine toxicology screen for drugs of abuse. If appropriate, the clinician should also consider ordering a urine pregnancy test and electrocardiogram, especially if he or she is considering starting a mood-stabilizing medication. Measuring levels of therapeutic drugs can be helpful to confirm the presence of a drug if noncompliance is suspected or if therapeutic effect is not obtained, to determine whether toxicity may be contributing to the patient's clinical presentation, or to determine whether drug interactions have altered the desired therapeutic levels (Wallach 1992). Serum trough levels of mood stabilizers such as lithium, valproate, or carbamazepine and TCAs can be obtained to monitor therapeutic response in accordance with therapeutic levels. (See sections on "Medication Monitoring and Maintenance" and "Pharmacogenetics and Pharmacogenomics" for additional information.)

Neuroimaging and electroencephalography are often helpful as well in understanding the etiology of a patient's mood symptoms. Multiple neurological and medical disorders have mood manifestations that may often be the presenting complaint. For example, stroke, seizure disorders, Parkinson's disease, Huntington's disease, frontotemporal dementia, and thyroid and other endocrine abnormalities may all present with depression, mania/hypomania, or psychosis as the primary complaint, with only subtle physical and cognitive manifestations that may be missed by cursory clinical examination. Further workup with laboratory tests, structural and sometimes functional imaging, and electroencephalography can uncover medical or neurological etiologies, thus providing the patient with effective treatment or prophylaxis against further episodes. The diagnostic approach to a patient with new-onset depressive or manic symptoms is summarized in Table 2–4.

TABLE 2–3.   Recommended diagnostic workup for a patient with new-onset psychosis

Routine screening

Complete blood count with differential and platelets

Serum chemistries, including liver and renal function tests

Thyroid-stimulating hormone

Rapid plasma reagin

HIV serology

Erythrocyte sedimentation rate

Serum alcohol level

Urine toxicology screen

Head computed tomography or brain magnetic resonance imaging scan

Electroencephalogram

Urine pregnancy test

Baseline electrocardiogram

Therapeutic drug levels

Consider per clinical suspicion

Antinuclear antibody

Rheumatoid factor

Blood cultures

Serum B_{12} and folate levels

Metal assays: serum and urine copper, serum ceruloplasmin; lead; mercury; manganese

Cerebrospinal fluid analysis: red blood cell count; white blood cell count; protein; glucose; opening pressure; bacterial cultures; cryptococcal antigen; viral serologies

Urine porphyrins

TABLE 2–4.   Recommended diagnostic workup for a patient with new-onset depressive or manic symptoms

Routine screening

Complete blood count with differential and platelets

Serum chemistries, including liver and renal function tests

Thyroid-stimulating hormone

Rapid plasma reagin

HIV serology

Urinalysis

Urine toxicology screen

Serum alcohol level (if suspected)

Urine pregnancy test

Electrocardiogram

Therapeutic drug levels (if patient is already on psychiatric medications)

Consider per clinical suspicion

Structural neuroimaging (brain magnetic resonance imaging)

Electroencephalogram

TABLE 2–5.   Recommended diagnostic workup for a patient with new-onset anxiety symptoms

Routine screening

Serum chemistries, including liver and renal function tests

Serum glucose

Thyroid-stimulating hormone

Referral for cardiac evaluation: electrocardiogram, Holter monitoring, stress test and/or echocardiogram

Consider per clinical suspicion

Referral for respiratory evaluation: chest radiograph; pulmonary function tests

Electroencephalogram

Urine porphyrins and vanillylmandelic acid levels

Urine metanephrines

Blood gas

Anxiety

The initial workup for anxiety symptoms should include serum chemistries, serum glucose, and TSH and other endocrine measures (Table 2–5). Many different medical diseases can also manifest with anxiety, including angina and myocardial infarction, mitral valve prolapse, substance intoxication and withdrawal, and metabolic and endocrine disorders such as thyroid abnormalities, pheochromocytoma, and hypoglycemia. Neurological disorders, such as many forms of dementia, can also present with anxiety. A cardiac workup is important because cardiac symptoms may masquerade as panic attacks and are often misdiagnosed as such, especially in female patients. Therefore, electrocardiography, Holter monitoring, stress test, and/or echocardiography may be necessary. Respiratory function should also be evaluated with a chest radiograph or pulmonary function tests to rule out chronic obstructive pulmonary disease as a contributory factor. Other tests to consider if one has clinical suspicion include electroencephalography, urine porphyrins, and urine vanillylmandelic acid.

Altered Mental Status

Patients with a fluctuating mental status of acute onset most likely will have one or more underlying medical or neurological causes for their impaired consciousness. This often constitutes a medical emergency, and comprehensive laboratory and diagnostic testing are indicated on an emergency basis, as summarized in Table 2–6. In addition to a complete physical examination and as much history as can be obtained from the patient and ancillary sources, the clinician should order serum chemistries, CBC, erythrocyte sedimentation rate, HIV serology, urinalysis and urine toxicology, electrocardiogram, and chest radiograph. A CT scan, blood cultures, lumbar puncture with CSF analysis, and EEG can be helpful as well, if clinically indicated. Many medical and neurological disorders can cause impairment in mental status, including seizures, CNS and systemic infection, kidney or liver failure, cardiac arrhythmias, stroke, myocardial infarction, and substance intoxication and withdrawal.

As noted previously, the EEG can be very helpful in the workup of patients with encephalopathy. It can diagnose seizures. It can also suggest that an encephalopathy is due to a nonneurological etiology. For example, it can show a metabolic etiology (metabolic encephalopathy), which often suggests that systemic issues are at the root of encephalopathy. Such etiologies include electrolyte disturbances, infections, and toxins.

The head CT scan can also be helpful in the workup of the patient with altered mental status. It can detect subdural hematomas or subarachnoid hemorrhage, and a CT with contrast can suggest infections such as meningitis or an abscess. Strokes do not typically present as altered mental status. However, a right middle cerebral artery stroke or a thalamic stroke can occasionally present with altered mental status, and the head CT scan can be very useful for detecting these etiologies.

Cognitive Decline

Dementias

Laboratory testing is a major component of the comprehensive evaluation of cognitive decline. The current American Academy of Neurology (2007) practice recommendations for evaluation of reversible causes of dementia include testing for vitamin B_{12} deficiency and hypothyroidism. These laboratory tests are recommended in addition to structural imaging (noncontrast head CT or MRI studies) and evaluation of depression to rule out so-called pseudodementia, or dementia-like symptoms that stem from depression. Syphilis serology screening is necessary only in pa-

TABLE 2–6.	Recommended diagnostic workup for a patient with altered mental status

Routine screening

Serum chemistries, including liver and renal function tests
Complete blood count
Erythrocyte sedimentation rate
HIV serology
Antinuclear antibody
Rheumatoid factor
B_{12}
Folate
Rapid plasma reagin
Urinalysis
Urine toxicology
Serum alcohol level
Therapeutic drug levels
Electrocardiogram
Chest radiograph
Head computed tomography scan
Electroencephalogram

Consider per clinical suspicion

Cerebrospinal fluid analysis: red blood cell count; white blood cell count; protein; glucose; opening pressure; bacterial cultures; cryptococcal antigen; viral serologies
Urine porphyrins
Serum ammonia level
Brain magnetic resonance imaging
Arterial blood gases
Blood cultures

tients with dementia who are at risk for neurosyphilis. Neuropsychological testing is also recommended. It can be very useful for differentiating between dementia and pseudodementia, for distinguishing among the many types of dementia, and for determining whether a patient is responding to treatment.

Other imaging modalities—such as linear and volumetric imaging, single photon emission computed tomography (SPECT), and positron emission tomography (PET)—are not recommended routinely at this time because there are insufficient data on the validity of these tests to diagnose illnesses that lead to cognitive disorders and dementia. However, PET and SPECT are approved to distinguish between Alzheimer's dementia and frontotemporal dementia.

Likewise, there are no serum or CSF biomarkers or genetic tests currently recommended for routine use in the diagnosis of dementia, although the clinical utility of several tests is being investigated. These are discussed in the section titled "Investigational Biological and Genetic Markers" later in the chapter. One exception is the immunoassay for CSF 14–3–3 protein, which is useful for the confirmation of Creutzfeldt-Jakob disease in a patient with rapidly progressive dementia and pathognomonic neurological symptoms (i.e., myoclonic jerks). False-positive results can occur with some other neurological conditions such as viral encephalitis, stroke, and paraneoplastic neurological disorders. Table 2–7 lists the laboratory and diagnostic tests that would be included in the workup of a patient with cognitive impairment.

TABLE 2–7.   Recommended diagnostic workup for a patient with cognitive decline

Routine screening

Complete blood count with differential and platelets

Serum chemistries including liver and renal function tests

Erythrocyte sedimentation rate

Antinuclear antibody

Rheumatoid factor

B_{12} and folate levels

Thyroid-stimulating hormone

Structural neuroimaging studies (head computed tomography or brain magnetic resonance imaging scan)

Consider per clinical suspicion

Rapid plasma reagin

HIV serology

C-reactive protein

Cerebrospinal fluid (CSF) analysis: red blood cell count; white blood cell count; protein; glucose; opening pressure; bacterial cultures; cryptococcal antigen; viral serologies; CSF 14–3–3 protein immunoassay (if Creutzfeldt-Jakob disease is suspected); CSF tau and Abeta 42 levels for frontotemporal dementia vs. Alzheimer's disease

Urine porphyrins

Functional neuroimaging studies (single photon emission computed tomography or positron emission tomography)

Electroencephalogram

Apolipoprotein E genotyping

Neuropsychological testing

Fasting lipids, triglycerides, and blood sugar when a vascular etiology is suspected

---

Mild Cognitive Impairment

There are no current clinical recommendations for the laboratory assessment of patients who have mild cognitive impairment. By definition, such patients do not yet meet criteria for dementia. However, patients with mild cognitive impairment are at very high risk for developing dementia or Alzheimer's disease (Petersen et al. 2005). However, the utility of a diagnostic workup, aside from cognitive screening, is as yet unknown. Patients who have symptoms of mild cognitive impairment will likely benefit from a thyroid screen. Other laboratory tests typically ordered for the evaluation of dementia may be of use should signs and symptoms be elicited from the history, review of systems, or physical examination. For example, it may be useful to measure folate and vitamin B_{12} levels in a patient with mild cognitive impairment who has a long history of alcohol abuse or who is discovered to have peripheral neuropathy on the neurological examination. Because one-third of patients with mild cognitive impairment progress to Alzheimer's disease over 3 years (Petersen et al. 2005), many clinicians feel it prudent to order the same tests they would to rule out reversible causes of dementia. However, as of yet, there are no studies that have proven the clinical utility of this strategy.

Substance Abuse

In a study of 345 consecutive patients who presented to the emergency department of an urban teaching hospital with primary psychiatric complaints, 141 of these patients (41%) had positive urine toxicology screens for substances of abuse, and 90 (26%) had positive ethanol screens (Olshaker et al. 1997). Clearly, laboratory testing is essential to the evaluation, monitoring, and subsequent treatment of patients who abuse alcohol, prescribed addictive medications, or illicit drugs.

Laboratory detection of drugs of abuse, as well as test results indicative of end-organ damage related to the abuse, can provide valuable hard evidence for the treating clinician, which can be used to inform and monitor his or her patient's progress. These data are also frequently useful in confronting the denial of substance abuse by the patient or his or her family. Laboratory testing can be conducted with blood and urine specimens or with saliva and hair samples. Urine specimens are typically preferred, because the detectable length of time that a particular drug of abuse and its metabolites are present is longer in urine than in blood. However, some substances, such as alcohol or barbiturates, are best detected in blood specimens.

The length of time that a drug of abuse is detectable in the urine varies based on the amount and duration of

TABLE 2–8. **Substances of abuse**

Agent	Toxic level	Urine detection time
Alcohol	300 mg/dL at any time or >100 g ingested	7–12 hours
Amphetamines		48 hours
Barbiturates	>6 μg/mL	24 hours (short-acting) 3 weeks (long-acting)
Benzodiazepines	Varies with medication Lorazepam: >25–100 mg Diazepam: >250 mg	3 days
Cannabis	50–200 μg/kg	4–6 weeks
Cocaine	>1.2 g	6–8 hours 2–4 days (metabolites)
Opiates	Varies with medication Heroin: >100–250 mg Codeine: >500–1,000 mg Morphine: >50–100 μg/kg	2–3 days
Phencyclidine	>10–20 mg	1–2 weeks

Source. Adapted from Wallach 2000.

substance consumed, kidney and liver function, and the specific drug itself. Laboratory methodologies vary. If the screening tests yield a positive result, follow-up with more specific tests, including quantitative analyses, can be ordered for confirmation. Table 2–8 reviews common drugs of abuse, length of detection time, and common psychiatric manifestations of each.

Medication Monitoring and Maintenance

Measuring levels of therapeutic drugs to evaluate for toxicity and effective levels can be extremely helpful in the workup and treatment of the psychiatric patient. Therapeutic drug monitoring should be used to confirm the presence and level of the drug if noncompliance is suspected, if the desired therapeutic effect is not obtained, or if signs or symptoms of toxicity occur; to determine whether toxicity may be contributing to the patient's clinical presentation; or to determine whether drug interactions have altered desired levels of therapeutic drugs (Wallach 1992). Serum trough levels of mood stabilizers (such as lithium, valproate, or carbamazepine) and TCAs can be obtained to monitor therapeutic response in accordance with therapeutic levels for acute exacerbation and maintenance treatment of bipolar disorder.

Mood Stabilizers

Blood tests are important for screening for end-organ damage before the initiation of treatment with these mood stabilizers. Follow-up testing during maintenance treatment is recommended at regular intervals, although the utility of these routine screens in detecting asymptomatic end-organ damage—such as an increase in liver function with valproate or renal impairment with lithium—is unclear. No clear consensus exists as to the appropriate interval for routine monitoring during the use of mood stabilizers. Most experts recommend screening every 3–6 months; however, some experts recommend that clinical monitoring of signs of toxicity may be more effective than periodic screening. That may especially be the case for drugs like valproate for which the routine monitoring of liver function tests may have little predictive value in terms of hepatotoxicity (Marangell et al. 2002; Pellock and Willmore 1991; Willmore et al. 1991). Although there is a lack of consensus regarding the recommended screening tests, a potential set of guidelines, which most authors appear to support, is listed in Table 2–9. The table shows the psychotropic medications for which therapeutic drug monitoring may be useful as well as therapeutic and toxic drug levels and ancillary tests that are recommended to monitor for the prevention of end-organ damage.

TABLE 2–9. Medication monitoring

Medication type	Medication	Therapeutic range	Toxic level	Recommended screening
Mood stabilizer	Lithium	0.8–1.2 mEq/L	>1.5 mEq/L	Initiation: sodium, potassium, calcium, phosphate, BUN, creatinine, TSH, T$_4$, CBC, urinalysis, beta-HCG if appropriate; ECG in patient older than 50 years or with preexisting cardiac disease Maintenance: TSH, BUN/creatinine recommended every 6 months; ECGs as needed in patient older than 40 years or with preexisting cardiac disease
	Valproate	50–150 µg/mL	>150 µg/mL	Initiation: CBC with platelets, LFTs; beta-HCG if appropriate Maintenance: LFTs, CBC recommended every 6 months
	Carbamazepine	8–12 µg/mL	>12 µg/mL	Initiation: CBC with platelets, LFTs, BUN/creatinine Maintenance: CBC with platelets, LFTs, BUN/creatinine
Tricyclic antidepressant (TCA)	Imipramine + desipramine	125–250 ng/mL	>500 ng/mL or >1 g ingested	Desipramine is metabolite of imipramine Initiation: ECG in patient older than 40 years or with preexisting cardiac disease for all TCAs
	Doxepin + metabolite desmethyldoxepin	100–275 ng/mL	>500 ng/mL	Initiation: ECG in patient older than 40 years or with preexisting cardiac disease for all TCAs
	Amitriptyline + nortriptyline	75–225 ng/mL	>500 ng/mL	Initiation: ECG in patient older than 40 years or with preexisting cardiac disease for all TCAs
	Nortriptyline only	50–150 ng/mL	>50 ng/mL	Initiation: ECG in patient older than 40 years or with preexisting cardiac disease for all TCAs
Antipsychotics	Olanzapine, quetiapine, risperidone, ziprasidone			Fasting serum glucose Triglycerides

Note. BUN=blood urea nitrogen; CBC=complete blood count; ECG=electrocardiogram; HCG=human chorionic gonadotropin; LFT=liver function test; T$_4$=thyroxine; TSH=thyroid-stimulating hormone.

Source. Adapted from Wallach 2000; Hyman SE, Arana GW, Rosenbaum JF. Handbook of Psychiatric Drug Therapy, 3rd Edition. Boston, MA, Little, Brown and Co., 1991. Used with permission.

Tricyclic Antidepressants

Drug levels of TCAs may also be obtained, although it is unclear whether blood levels of antidepressants correlate with therapeutic response. Four TCAs—imipramine, desipramine, amitriptyline, and nortriptyline—have been well studied, and generalizations can be made about the relationship of drug levels to therapeutic response. For imipramine, optimal response rates occur as blood levels reach 200–250 ng/mL, and levels greater than 250 ng/mL often produce more side effects but no change in antidepressant response (American Psychiatric Association Task Force on the Use of Laboratory Tests in Psychiatry 1985). Nortriptyline, in contrast, appears to have a specific therapeutic window between 50 and 150 ng/mL, and poor clinical response occurs both above and below that window. Desipramine also appears to have a linear relationship between drug concentration and clinical outcome, with plasma concentrations greater than 125 ng/mL being significantly more effective. Amitriptyline has been fairly well studied; however, some studies have found a linear relationship similar to that of imipramine, others have found a curvilinear relationship, and others have found no relationship between blood levels and clinical outcomes (American Psychiatric Association Task Force on the Use of Laboratory Tests in Psychiatry 1985). For the other TCAs that have been less well studied, drug levels can still be useful to confirm the presence of the drug or to confirm extremely high serum levels (Hyman and Arana 1991).

Neuroleptics

The monitoring of blood levels for neuroleptics is not routinely used in clinical practice. Different methods for monitoring neuroleptic drugs have been developed, but a reliable therapeutic range has not been established because there does not appear to be a consistent relationship between blood levels of neuroleptics and clinical response (Curry 1985). However, there are several clinical situations in which it may be useful to obtain blood levels of neuroleptics.

Blood level monitoring may be useful to confirm the presence of the neuroleptic when adherence is a concern. It may be used to ascertain the presence of drug interactions in a patient who has relapsed or experienced an exacerbation of symptoms after a period of stabilization and who has been taking drugs that may interact with neuroleptics, such as carbamazepine or fluoxetine. It may also be helpful to obtain drug levels in patients who develop excessive side effects to moderate dosages of neuroleptics (Bernardo et al. 1993).

Diagnostic and laboratory monitoring are important components of care for patients receiving neuroleptic medications. In patients who are over the age of 50, or who have preexisting cardiac disease, a screening electrocardiogram should be ordered before institution of antipsychotic medications, such as thioridazine or ziprasidone, that may cause prolongation of the QT_c interval (a marker for potentially life-threatening cardiac arrhythmias such as torsades de pointes). Follow-up electrocardiograms should be ordered for any patient receiving treatment with antipsychotic medications in whom symptoms indicative of cardiac compromise appear. It is also recommended that screening laboratory studies be performed at regular intervals (every 6 months) to test for glucose and metabolic dysregulation (hyperlipidemias, diabetes, hypothyroidism), which are often associated with atypical antipsychotic medications.

Pharmacogenetics and Pharmacogenomics

Recent progress in drug metabolism research has resulted in newly available tests that may have significant clinical utility for psychopharmacology. Human drug metabolism is highly variable, making it difficult to predict therapeutic dosage levels and ranges, and can lead to unanticipated adverse outcomes, toxicity, and therapeutic failure. Clearly, adverse drug reactions are a serious problem, as estimated by a meta-analysis of serious adverse drug reactions (Lazarou et al. 1998). It was estimated that in 1994, more than 2 million hospitalized patients had serious adverse drug reactions, with more than 100,000 resulting in death in the United States alone.

Most psychiatric drugs are metabolized by microsomal enzymes called the cytochrome P450 (CYP) enzyme system. The CYP enzymes are a superfamily of more than 20 related enzymes, although only six metabolize more than 90% of all medications (Streetman 2000). These six enzymes that are important to human drug metabolism are CYP1A2, CYP2C9, CYP2C19, CYP2D6, CYP2E1, and CYP3A. Enzymes are identified by numbers and letters that identify the family and subfamily grouping. For example, CYP2D6 is in family 2 and subfamily 2D and is structurally related to CYP2C19 in the same family, but it is not similar to CYP3A, which is in a different family (Streetman 2000).

The majority of CYP enzyme metabolism occurs in the liver, although metabolism can occur elsewhere in the body, such as the small intestine (CYP3A4), the brain (CYP2D6), and the lung (CYP1A1). The CYP enzyme system, in addition to metabolizing drugs, also metabolizes exogenous substances, such as environmental toxins and dietary nutrients, and endogenous substances, such as steroids and prostaglandins. Through drug metabolism, a medication is made more hydrophilic or water soluble in order to be excreted by the kidneys. Table 2–10 lists many of the psychiatric drugs that are metabolized by selected CYP enzymes (substrates) as well as those that may decrease enzyme activity (inhibitors). CYP drug metabolism is highly variable due to several factors, including genetic polymorphisms, effects of concomitant medications (inhibition or induction of enzymes), physiological or disease status, and environmental or exogenous factors such as toxins and diet (Ingelman-Sundberg et al. 1999).

Pharmacogenetics is the study of genetic variation as it relates to drug response and metabolism. Research in pharmacogenetics to date has focused largely on genes that encode receptors targeted by drugs such as the serotonin and dopamine receptor subtypes or those that encode CYP enzymes. Research on the latter has been significantly more helpful to our understanding of the genetic basis of variability in medication response than the former.

The pharmacokinetic effects of the CYP enzyme system, specifically CYP2D6 and CYP2C19 polymorphisms, on psychiatric medications have been studied extensively. The allele sequence that produces normally functioning enzyme is coded by the wild-type gene (given the suffix "*1"). Thereafter, differing genetic sequence polymorphisms are numbered sequentially (i.e.,*2, *3). Thus, multiple copies of a functional CYP enzyme gene can occur, resulting in enzyme overactivity. Conversely, polymorphisms may be inactivating, resulting in decreased CYP enzyme activity or even a complete loss of activity.

Four general phenotypes have been used to describe the outcomes of these CYP genetic polymorphisms (Table 2–11): ultrarapid metabolizers, extensive metabolizers, intermediate metabolizers, and poor metabolizers. Extensive metabolizers have the normal two copies of fully active CYP enzyme alleles for a particular microsomal enzyme. Poor metabolizers do not have the active enzyme gene allele, resulting in increased concentrations of medications due to reduced metabolism, and may have more adverse effects at usual, recommended dosages. In contrast, ultrarapid metabolizers will have multiple copies of the functional enzyme allele, resulting in increased rate of drug metabolism, and may not reach therapeutic concentrations at the recommended dosage.

TABLE 2–10. Psychiatric drug metabolism by specific P450 enzymes

Enzyme	CYP2D6	CYP2C19

Substrates (drugs metabolized by specific enzyme)	Antidepressants
	  Amitriptyline
	  Desipramine
	  Duloxetine
	  Imipramine
	  Fluoxetine
	  Fluvoxamine
	  Nortriptyline
	  Paroxetine
	  Sertraline
	  Trazodone
	  Venlafaxine
	Antipsychotics
	  Aripiprazole
	  Clozapine
	  Haloperidol
	  Fluphenazine
	  Perphenazine
	  Olanzapine
	  Risperidone
	  Thioridazine
	Other drugs
	  Donepezil
	  Methadone
		Antidepressants
		  Citalopram
		  Escitalopram
		  Amitriptyline
		  Clomipramine
		  Imipramine
		Other drugs
		  Diazepam

Inhibitors	Antidepressants
	  Amitriptyline
	  Bupropion
	  Desipramine
	  Fluoxetine
	  Paroxetine
	  Sertraline
	Antipsychotics
	  Thioridazine
	  Clomipramine
	  Clozapine
		Amitriptyline
		Citalopram
		Clomipramine
		Fluvoxamine
		Fluoxetine

Source.   Data adapted from Kirchheiner et al. 2001; Streetman 2000.

There is significant ethnic variability in allele frequencies, with 4%–10% of Caucasians completely lacking the CYP2D6 enzyme compared with only 1%–3% of African Americans and Chinese. Similarly, discrepancy in allele frequencies occur for the CYP2C19 enzyme, with up to 20% of Asians lacking the active enzyme gene allele compared with only 2%–5% of Caucasians (de Leon et al. 2006).

Genotyping tests for CYP enzyme DNA sequence variants are now available. They utilize DNA microarray assays to detect single nucleotide polymorphisms

TABLE 2-11. Drug metabolizer phenotype classification

Type	Number of active enzyme gene alleles	Expected response to substrate drug
Poor metabolizer	None	Reduced metabolism of drug may result in increased concentrations and more adverse effects
Intermediate metabolizer	One active and one inactive allele, or two gene alleles with reduced activity	Lesser degree of adverse effects related to reduced metabolism
Extensive metabolizer (normal)	2	Expected response to standard medication dosage
Ultrarapid metabolizer	>2	Rapid clearance of medications, so may not reach therapeutic concentrations at recommended dosages

Source. Adapted from Ingelman-Sundberg et al. 1999; Mrazek 2006.

(SNPs) or DNA sequence variations in the genes encoding CYP enzymes. These tests are not yet in routine clinical practice because of prohibitive costs and lack of insurance reimbursement. As studies become available that provide evidence of health care cost savings, CYP genotyping has the potential to revolutionize psychiatric approaches to medication management. These tests in their current form are most helpful when phenotype closely mirrors genotype. Genotyping only needs to be performed once in a patient's life. If performed prior to initiation of medications, it could prevent adverse drug reactions.

In the future, perhaps specific dosing adjustment recommendations can be compiled for a patient based on his or her drug metabolism genotype profile. The sensitivity for predicting poor metabolizers in Caucasian populations is 99% for the CYP2D6 enzyme genotyping test and 98%–100% for the CYP2C19 test (Brosen et al. 1995; Sachse et al. 1997; Sagar et al. 1998). Data on the effects of genotyping on treatment outcomes and health care costs are not yet available, but the potential benefits of genotyping are numerous. For example, genotyping may eventually obviate the need for costly and lengthy drug trials, potentially allowing the physician to choose the best medication for the patient at treatment outset. Furthermore, for medications with narrow therapeutic windows, genotyping may reduce the frequency of toxicity and other adverse events.

Limited data exist regarding antidepressant effectiveness based on CYP genotype. Even fewer data are available for antipsychotic efficacy and CYP genotype. Preliminary antidepressant dosage recommendations are being developed based on CYP drug metabolism phenotype. A recent report by Kirchheiner et al. (2001) presented preliminary practical dosage recommendations for several antidepressant medications according to metabolizer status. Recommended dosages for poor metabolizers were 20%–70%, dosages for intermediate metabolizers were 80%–90%, and dosages for ultrarapid metabolizers were 100%–130% of those recommended for extensive metabolizers of CYP2D6 or CYP2C19. Several other antidepressants are metabolized by CYP3A4, including mirtazapine, nefazodone, sertraline, and trazodone. However, poor and ultrarapid metabolizers of CYP3A4 have not been identified due to the relative lack of variability in the 3A4 gene; thus, dosing recommendations have not been developed for CYP3A4.

In general, dosages of TCAs are reduced by 50% for poor metabolizers of CYP2D6 or CYP2C19 substrates, with less dramatic dosage reductions for selective serotonin reuptake inhibitors (de Leon 2006; Kirchheiner et al. 2001). A very small proportion of poor metabolizers are lacking both CYP2D6 and CYP2C19 functional alleles. These patients are likely to have adverse reactions to most available antidepressant medications. Thus, the use of antidepressant medications such as bupropion and mirtazapine, which are not dependent on these metabolic pathways, would be prudent in these patients (de Leon et al. 2006).

Similar guidelines for practical dosage recommendations for antipsychotic medications have yet to be defined, largely because data on their clinical efficacy based on CYP genotyping are extremely limited. A conservative estimate is to lower the dosage of typical antipsychotics and risperidone by one-half in CYP2D6 poor metabolizers (de Leon 2006).

Interpretation of clinical drug response in the context of CYP genotyping is still fraught with complications because the effects of medical comorbidities, environment, and medication interactions must be addressed. Concomitant medications can be powerful inducers or inhibitors of CYP metabolism and must also be taken into account when predicting drug response. Despite these complications, these advances in pharmacogenetics bring us one step closer to the "individualized" or "personalized" approach to medicine, with the potential to reduce possible adverse events, costly trials of ineffective medication treatments, and hasten recovery times.

Cerebrospinal Fluid Studies

Laboratory examination of CSF can be helpful in the diagnosis of some neuropsychiatric disorders. CSF studies are often employed in the secondary evaluation of a psychiatric patient when a neurological and possibly reversible cause is suspected, including infections, such as encephalitis or meningitis, which may be caused by bacteria; acid-fast bacilli (e.g., tuberculosis); spirochetes (e.g., syphilis, Lyme disease); viruses (e.g., herpes simplex, cytomegalovirus, Epstein-Barr virus, West Nile virus); prions (e.g., Creutzfeldt-Jakob disease); or fungi (e.g., *Cryptococcus*). CSF analysis can also reveal subarachnoid hemorrhage, which can present with altered mental status, headache, coma, and/or focal findings.

Spinal fluid analysis can also be useful for investigating inflammatory etiologies for neuropsychiatric complaints. These include autoimmune demyelinating disorders (e.g., multiple sclerosis or acute demyelinating encephalomyelitis) and autoimmune neuronal disorders (systemic lupus erythematosus). CSF analysis can also reveal disorders of CSF production that produce elevated (e.g., pseudotumor cerebri) or low pressure. Finally, CSF analysis can be very useful for identifying neoplastic processes within the nervous system, including direct tumor invasion (e.g., lymphoma), carcinomatous meningitis (e.g., prostate cancer), or a paraneoplastic syndrome.

The utility of spinal fluid analysis is being investigated for the diagnosis or differentiation between various neurodegenerative dementias. CSF tau and A beta 1–42 levels can sometimes distinguish between Alzheimer's disease and frontotemporal dementia. Spinal fluid analysis is not sensitive or specific enough to be a diagnostic test, but it can be a useful adjuvant. Other spinal fluid markers are the subject of intense investigation, with the goal of identifying one capable of diagnosing neurological and psychiatric disorders.

Typical tests ordered for evaluation of CSF are listed in Table 2–2. CSF is obtained through lumbar puncture and should always be accompanied by a blood sample drawn simultaneously and sent for protein, glucose, and serum protein electrophoresis. Except under emergency conditions, lumbar puncture should not be performed until a head CT scan has been obtained to rule out increased intracranial pressure or a mass lesion in a position that could produce herniation after a lumbar puncture. A lumbar puncture can be obtained fluoroscopically if it cannot be readily obtained due to the large size of the patient or lumbar spinal abnormalities.

Investigational Biological and Genetic Markers

There is considerable interest in isolating biological markers for psychiatric illnesses for the purposes of improving the accuracy of diagnosis, predicting treatment response, identifying patients at risk, and ultimately preventing the development of these disorders. Great strides have been made in discovering the genetic markers and pathophysiology underlying many primary neurological disorders, such as the dementias (Alzheimer's type and frontotemporal) and movement disorders (Huntington's disease, Parkinson's disease, and spinocerebellar ataxias). Sadly, no genetic or biological marker has yet been identified for any of the primary psychiatric disorders, although many studies are currently being undertaken. Table 2–12 lists some of the biomarkers being researched at this time.

Neuroendocrine Testing

Much research has been conducted on the relationship of endocrine abnormalities to primary psychiatric disorders. This has been engendered by the observation that both endogenous endocrine disorders, such as Cushing's syndrome or hypo- and hyperthyroidism, as well as the administration of exogenous hormones, such as glucocorticoid steroids, can produce mood and psychotic episodes identical to those of endogenous primary mood and psychotic disorders. In general, neuroendocrine evaluation measures 1) basal hormone levels; 2) circadian secretion patterns; and 3) secretion response to a hormonal challenge or provocation. The challenge or provocation tests have received the most attention. For this method, a hypothalamic releasing factor, such as thyrotropin-releasing hormone (TRH), corticotropin-releasing hormone (CRH), gonadotro-

TABLE 2–12. Selected investigational biological and genetic markers

Type	Biomarker	Disease	Comments
Genetic markers	Chromosome 4p16.3	Huntington's disease	Trinucleotide (CAG) repeat
	Chromosome 4q21–22	Parkinson's disease	Some familial cases linked to mutation of the alpha-synuclein gene
	Chromosome 13	Wilson's disease	Copper transport gene
	Chromosome 21	Alzheimer's disease	Amyloid precursor protein mutations
	Chromosomes 1, 12	Alzheimer's disease	Presenilin 1 and 2
	Chromosome 17q21–23	Frontotemporal dementias	Familial cases with mutations in the *tau* gene
	Chromosome 18p, 18q, 21q, 12q, 4p	Bipolar disorder	Genetic linkages in families with bipolar disorder
Biochemical markers	CSF B-amyloid$_{1-42}$	Alzheimer's disease	May be reduced in the CSF of patients with Alzheimer's disease compared with elderly control subjects
	CSF tau	Alzheimer's disease	May be elevated in the CSF of patients with Alzheimer's disease compared with control subjects
	CSF AD7C-NTP	Alzheimer's disease	
	CSF 14–3–3 protein	Creutzfeldt-Jakob disease	Elevated in CSF of patients with Creutzfeldt-Jakob disease, recent stroke, herpes encephalitis
Catecholamines and metabolites	Dopamine, plasma homovanillic acid	Schizophrenia, depression	Decreases with antipsychotic treatment
	Norepinephrine, MHPG (3-methoxy-4-hydroxyphenylglycol)	Major depression, bipolar disorder	Low CSF levels associated with increased risk of suicidal behavior. Urine levels may predict antidepressant response
Indoleamines and metabolites	Serotonin, 5-hydroxyindoleacetic acid (5-HIAA)	Depression, suicide, violence	Low CSF levels associated with suicidal behavior, aggression, impulsivity, depression, seizures, alcoholism High CSF levels associated with anxiety

TABLE 2–12. Selected investigational biological and genetic markers (*continued*)

Type	Biomarker	Disease	Comments
Amino acids	Tryptophan, tyrosine, glycine, glutamate	Mood disorders	Low serum levels in depression Dietary neurotransmitter precursors being studied as treatment for depression
Enzymes	Monoamine oxidase, dopamine-beta-hydroxylase, catechol-O-methyltransferase, adenyl cyclase, guanyl cyclase, nitric oxide synthase, tyrosine hydroxylase	Mood and anxiety disorders, psychotic disorders	Numerous targets of antidepressant and mood stabilizer therapy
Psychoimmunological markers	Cytokine levels, immunoglobulin levels	Mood disorders	Proinflammatory cytokines are hypothesized to induce depression by their influence on the HPA system
Neuroendocrine markers	Dexamethasone suppression test (DST)	Major depression	Limited clinical utility Posttreatment DST cortisol nonsuppression predictive of poor outcome and higher relapse risk
	Thyrotropin-releasing hormone stimulation test	Major depression	Helpful in thyroid disorder diagnosis, but limited psychiatric utility Blunted response in up to 30% of depressed patients

Note. CSF=cerebrospinal fluid; HPA=hypothalamic-pituitary-adrenal.

pin-releasing hormone (GnRH), or growth hormone–releasing hormone (GH-RH), is administered to stimulate the release of corresponding downstream pituitary hormone (TRH → TSH, CRH → adrenocorticotropic hormone, GnRH → follicle-stimulating hormone and luteinizing hormone, and GH-RH → growth hormone).

Several psychiatric disorders have been associated with abnormal secretion in response to these hormonal challenges. The best known of these challenge tests is the dexamethasone suppression test, in which secretion of serum cortisol is measured at several time points for 24 hours after a "challenge" of dexamethasone administration. An abnormal response is a failure to suppress serum cortisol levels below 5 μg/dL. Initially, this test was believed to be useful in the diagnosis of melancholic depression (Carroll 1984). However, it has limited sensitivity, because it is positive in only 40%–50% of depressed patients (Wallach 2000). Furthermore, there are multiple factors that can interfere with the test results, including drugs that can cause nonsuppression, such as barbiturates, carbamazepine, and chronic alcohol use, as well as those that can enhance suppression, such as high-dosage benzodiazepines, corticosteroids, and dextroamphetamine. Medical conditions such as pregnancy, systemic infections, endocrine and liver disease, and other severe medical illnesses may result in a false-positive test (Wallach 2000).

Unfortunately, neither the dexamethasone suppression test nor any other neuroendocrine testing method has clinical applications at this time. Given that neuroendocrine systems are highly complex feedback loops, affected by numerous endogenous and environmental factors, perhaps these tests will attain clinical utility in the future as we better understand the workings and relationships of these psychoneuroendocrine systems.

Electrophysiological Testing

Standard Electroencephalogram

The standard EEG is a noninvasive recording of electrical activity of the brain. Electrodes placed on the scalp record extracellular current flow of neurons. The EEG is used in the evaluation of the psychiatric patient to exclude the contribution of a general medical condition, such as epilepsy or delirium, to a patient's clinical presentation. In general, an abnormal EEG will consist of one or more of the following: 1) paroxysmal activity indicative of transient, episodic neuronal discharges as seen in epilepsy; 2) nonparoxysmal slowing of

activity, as seen in delirium; 3) asymmetric activity as observed with mass lesions or infarction; or 4) sleep abnormalities consistent with sleep apnea, rapid eye movement sleep behavior disorder, or narcolepsy.

No clear guidelines exist for the use of electroencephalographic evaluation in routine screening of the psychiatric patient. An EEG would be prudent to obtain in a patient with new-onset psychosis, episodic behavioral disturbance, or altered mental status. In a patient with altered mental status, the EEG can be diagnostically useful because it can differentiate between a diffuse encephalopathy, nonmotoric status epilepticus, or focal lesion (Boutros and Struve 2004). A normal EEG does not exclude seizure disorder from the differential diagnosis, because 20% of patients with epilepsy will have normal EEGs, and 2% of patients without epilepsy will have spike and wave formations (Engel 1992). The diagnosis of epilepsy is a clinical one, based on observation of the patient or the report of someone who has observed the patient having a seizure. Although the EEG can support the diagnosis, it cannot exclude it. Several techniques can be implemented in order to increase the diagnostic yield of the EEG, including sleep deprivation, serial EEGs, 24-hour electroencephalographic monitoring, or adjustments in electrode placement, including nasopharyngeal, sphenoidal, and anterior temporal electrodes. Despite the fact that electroencephalography is widely available, noninvasive, inexpensive, and useful for diagnosing neurological disorders, it has fairly limited utility in the differentiation of psychiatric disorders.

Polysomnography

Polysomnography entails the recording of multiple physiological variables during sleep to determine the presence of sleep disorders. It is a useful technique to implement in the psychiatric patient if a sleep disorder is suspected to be responsible for or exacerbating psychiatric symptoms. Hypnagogic hallucinations, which occur at the interface between sleep and wakefulness, can often be mistaken for symptoms of a primary psychotic disorder. Furthermore, there is considerable overlap in symptoms of depression and sleep disorders, such as insomnia, daytime fatigue, or excessive daytime sleepiness. A typical polysomnogram will consist of an EEG, electrocardiogram, electro-oculogram, and electromyogram and measurement of respiratory airflow and oxygenation, blood pressure, and body temperature. Again, no definitive guidelines exist as to the usefulness of polysomnography in the clinical workup of the psychiatric patient. Although psychiatric disorders often go hand in hand with disturbed sleep, sleep studies are not ordered for the routine evaluation of the psychiatric patient. Instead, a polysomnogram is ordered when there is clinical suspicion of parasomnia or hypersomnia (narcolepsy), a breathing disorder such as sleep apnea, or limb movements during sleep.

Evoked Potentials

Auditory, visual, somatosensory, or cognitive stimuli can be used to evoke electrical potentials that can be recorded. Repetitive stimuli result in small-magnitude electrical changes that are mathematically manipulated or "averaged," resulting in the evoked potential. Evoked potential testing provides clinically useful information about processing of sensory stimuli, which is helpful in discerning medical versus psychogenic causes of some symptoms. For example, visual evoked potentials can be useful to differentiate psychogenic blindness from true blindness, and auditory evoked potentials can be used to differentiate psychogenic deafness from catatonia in a mute, unresponsive patient.

Initial evoked potentials are followed by other evoked potential components such as midlatency evoked responses and even later event-related potentials. The latter have been the focus of much research, because they are elicited by a psychological event. For example, the P300 event-related potential, a positive peak that occurs 250–500 msec poststimulus, has been found to be abnormal in amplitude and latency in multiple psychiatric disorders.

Quantitative EEG

Quantitative EEG uses 1–2 minutes of a resting EEG that is analyzed using fast Fourier transform to quantify the power at each frequency of the EEG averaged across the entire sample (Hughes and John 1999). For each of the four frequency bands (delta [1.5–3.5 Hz], theta [3.5–7.5 Hz], alpha [7.5–12.5 Hz], and beta [12.5–20 Hz]), results obtained include absolute power (total microV2), relative power (percentage of total power for each band), coherence (synchronization between bands), and symmetry between bands. Thus, quantification allows comparison of these variables between patient groups. Despite numerous studies of quantitative EEG in dementias, cerebrovascular disease, schizophrenia, mood and anxiety disorders, learning disorders, and substance abuse disorders, there are few data available to support its use in the clinical evaluation of psychiatric patients. However, this analytical tool holds great promise for the future.

Neuroimaging Studies in Psychiatry

Brain imaging research in psychiatry has exploded in the past two decades, spurred on by increasingly sophisticated neuroimaging modalities. Although neuroimaging does not yet play a diagnostic role for any of the primary psychiatric disorders, it is still an integral part of the clinical workup for psychiatric patients to rule out underlying medical causes of psychiatric symptoms. In this section, we discuss current clinical and research neuroimaging modalities as they relate to psychiatric disorders.

Current neuroimaging methods provide both structural and functional data about the brain. Structural imaging techniques such as CT and MRI provide a fixed image of the brain's anatomy and spatial distribution. Newer functional neuroimaging techniques such as PET and SPECT provide information about brain metabolism, blood flow, the presynaptic uptake of transmitter precursors, neurotransmitter transporter activity, and postsynaptic receptor activity. Functional scans should always be interpreted in the context of the underlying structural images. With these techniques, one can find a grossly normal brain, structurally speaking, with abnormal function. Alternately, one can have abnormal brain structures that can lead to reduced or increased metabolic function (e.g., a brain tumor).

Structural Neuroimaging Modalities

Computed Tomography

CT scanning enlists a focused beam of X-rays that passes through the brain at many angles. The many images evoked are then joined together to provide a cross-sectional view of the brain. The X-rays are attenuated as they pass through tissue, which absorbs their energy. The degree of energy absorbed varies, based on the radiodensity of the tissue. This differential X-ray attenuation is transformed into a two-dimensional grayscale map of the brain by computers, with bone appearing most radiopaque, or white, and air the least radiopaque, or black. Brain tissue, CSF, and water have varying degrees of radiopacity (Figure 2–1).

CT has many advantages. It is widely available, less expensive than MRI, has a quick scanning time, and is relatively more comfortable and convenient than other structural imaging modalities. Thus, CT is quick and efficient and is used to rule out life-threat-

Tissue		Relative attenuation values (in Hounsfield units)	Appearance on CT
Metal		1,000	White
Bone/calcium		100–1,000	
Blood			
	Acute	80–85	
	Subacute	25–50	
	Chronic	0–25	
Gray matter		35–40	
White matter		25–30	
Water		0	
Fat		–100	
Air		–1,000	Black

FIGURE 2–1.   Computed tomography (CT) tissue attenuation values and appearance.

Source.   Adapted from J Levine lecture "Structural Neuroimaging in Psychiatry," given as part of the Neuroimaging in Psychiatry lecture series, Department of Psychiatry, Baylor College of Medicine, March 2006.

ening conditions such as skull fracture, hemorrhage, or brain tumor.

CT also has limitations. A brain CT scan involves some radiation exposure. Deep brain structures, including those of the posterior fossa such as brain stem and cerebellum, are poorly visualized with CT because of the surrounding bony structures. Furthermore, discrimination between gray and white matter in the brain is limited due to their similar radiodensities.

Magnetic Resonance Imaging

MRI relies upon nuclear magnetic resonance. Hydrogen nuclei in the body have paramagnetic properties, and their spins align when placed in a static magnetic field. The magnetic field is pulsed, causing the hydrogen protons to align. When the magnetic pulses are terminated, the protons relax toward their original positions and release energy at a detectable radiofrequency. The collective magnetic behavior of the realigning hydrogen atoms within the magnetic field constitutes T1, or longitudinal relaxation, and T2, or transverse relaxation. The bulk of the MRI signaling comes from hydrogen atoms in water. MRI can distinguish between hydrogen nuclei in free water and those in blood, fat, or muscle based on differential relaxation rates in different tissues. These resonant frequencies are nonionizing and not harmful. The quality of the images produced is determined by the strength of the static magnet. Most clinical MRI scanners use a superconducting magnet of 1.5 tesla strength, although MRI

scanners for research use often use 3.0 tesla or more.

In clinical practice, T2-weighted images can be very useful for visualizing lesions because they show edema as an increase in signal intensity. T1-weighted images are useful for demonstrating structural anatomy. Gradient echo images can reveal past hemorrhages. Fluid attenuated inversion recovery images are useful for removing fluids like CSF, but retaining fluid changes as observed with the gliosis of past infarcts. One can thus observe, for example, the extent of past small-vessel ischemic changes. Table 2–13 lists the characteristic appearance of tissue signals on T1- and T2-weighted MRI images. Figure 2–2 illustrates axial MRI images of a patient with bipolar disorder compared with an age-matched control patient.

Comparison of CT and MRI

MRI has many advantages over CT. First and foremost, it has superior visualization of brain tissue, providing enhanced gray/white matter discrimination versus CT and allowing quantitative or volumetric measurement of brain regions. Deep brain structures such as the cerebellum and brain stem are better visualized with MRI. Furthermore, axial, coronal, and sagittal images may be acquired. MRI image acquisition is complex, and depending on parameters, can produce T1-, T2-, or proton density–weighted images, spin-echo, and inversion-recovery images. Table 2–14 provides a summary comparison of CT and MRI imaging modalities. Figure 2–3 is a comparison of images available with CT versus MRI.

TABLE 2–13.   Tissue signal on T1 versus T2 weighting

	T1	T2
Paramagnetic substances (contrast, melanin)	High/bright	Low/dark
Fat	High	Low
Protein	High	Low
Water/cerebrospinal fluid	Low	High
Calcium/bone	Low	Low
Gray matter	Low–intermediate	Intermediate–high
White matter	Intermediate–high	Low–intermediate

Source.   Adapted from J Levine lecture "Structural Neuroimaging in Psychiatry," given as part of the Neuroimaging in Psychiatry lecture series, Department of Psychiatry, Baylor College of Medicine, March 2006.

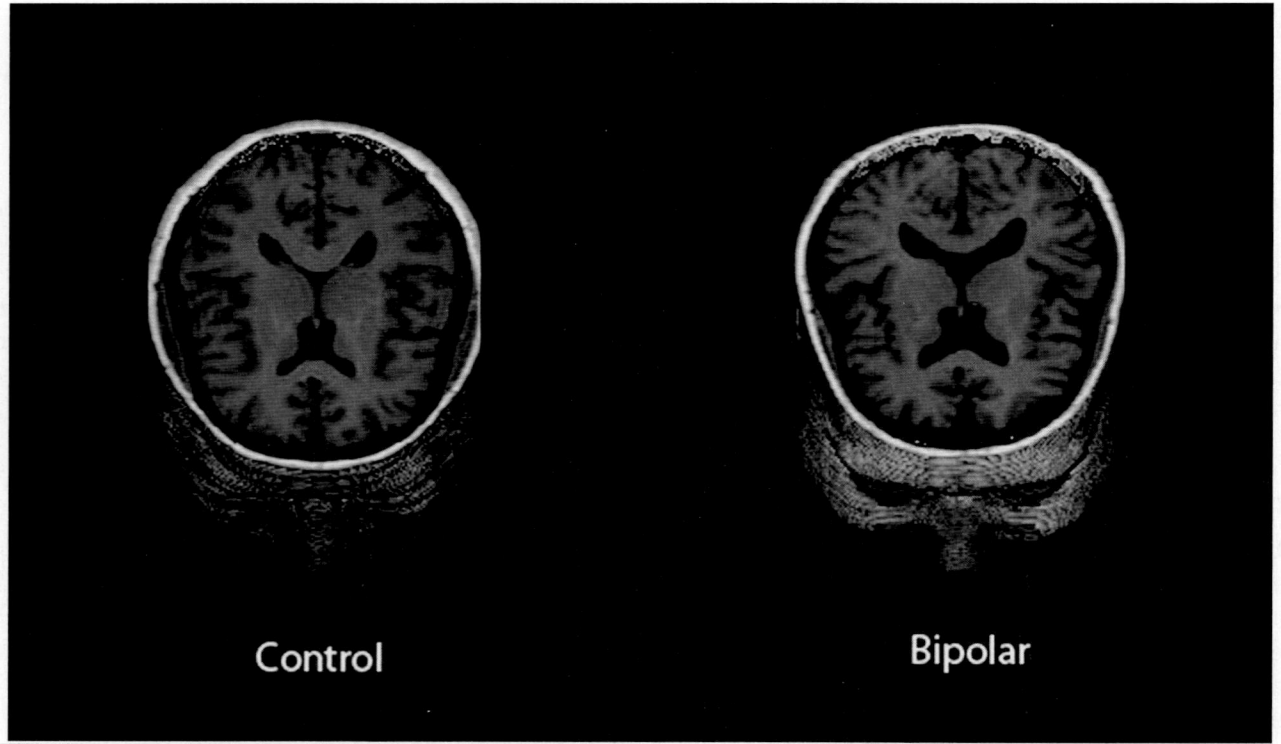

FIGURE 2–2.   MRI comparison axial cuts, bipolar disorder patient versus matched control.

MRI (T1-weighted) images of a 58-year-old healthy control patient *(left)* as compared with a patient of comparable age with bipolar disorder *(right)* but without any significant medical or substance abuse history. Although not diagnostic, common findings in neuroimaging research studies with bipolar disorder patients include diffuse gray matter loss, enlargement of the ventricles, and mild prefrontal volume loss.

Source.   Images courtesy of Elisabeth A. Wilde, PhD, Department of Physical Medicine and Rehabilitation, Baylor College of Medicine, Houston, Texas.

TABLE 2–14.   Comparison of computed tomography (CT) and magnetic resonance imaging (MRI)

	CT	MRI
Mechanism	X-ray attenuation	Proton magnetic resonance
Imaging planes	Axial (transverse) only	Axial, coronal, sagittal
Image acquisition time	Short (5–10 minutes)	Longer (45 minutes)
Slice thickness	2–5 mm	1–3 mm
Spatial resolution	1–2 mm	<1 mm
Cost	$300–$500	$800–$1,000
Advantages	Widely available Rapid acquisition Useful in evaluating for acute, life-threatening conditions such as hemorrhage or trauma	No radiation exposure Gray–white contrast excellent Excellent visualization of posterior fossa
Disadvantages	Radiation exposure Limited visualization of posterior fossa	Unable to use if metal or pacemakers present Slow acquisition

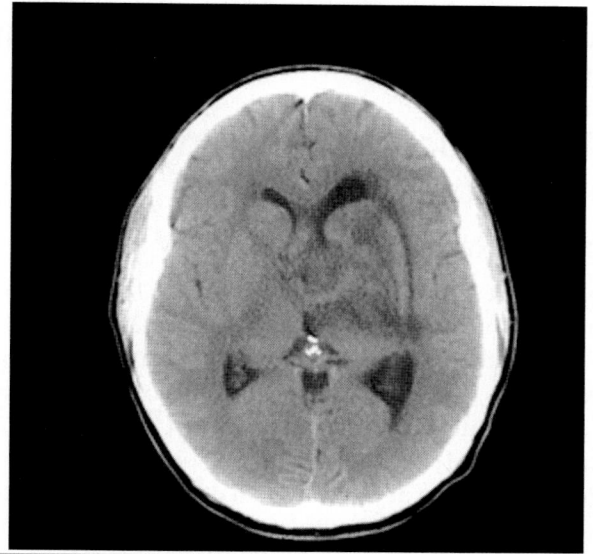 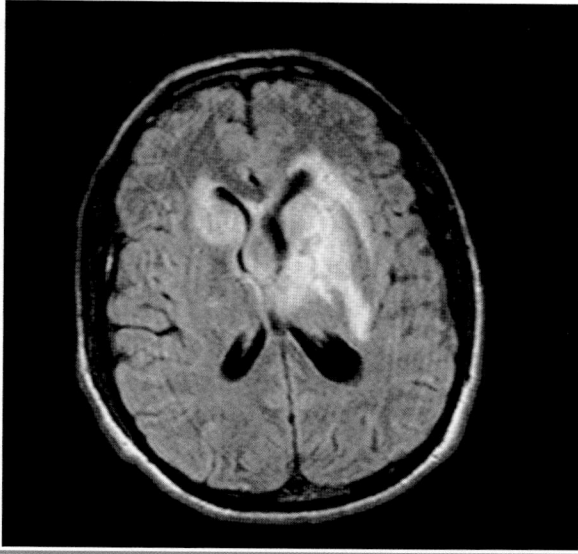

FIGURE 2–3.   **Side-by-side comparison of structural imaging modalities: CT and MRI.**
The sensitivity of head CT versus MRI of the brain in the same patient is demonstrated here in a patient who presented with memory loss. Head CT scan at *left* shows a large area of decreased density consistent with edema. It is difficult to ascertain whether there is an underlying mass or what its shape might be. The image on the *right* is from a brain MRI (T2 image) and also demonstrates an area of increased intensity of about the same shape as the CT abnormality. The patient was found to be HIV positive, and a subsequent brain biopsy demonstrated that the mass was a B-cell lymphoma.
Source.   Images courtesy of Paul E. Schulz, MD, Department of Neurology, Baylor College of Medicine, Houston, Texas.

Clinical Use of CT and MRI in Psychiatry

For the primary psychiatric disorders, the clinical use of structural neuroimaging such as CT and MRI is largely limited to the identification of medical causes of psychiatric symptomatology. Structural imaging is ordered to evaluate for evidence of tangible abnormalities such as stroke, brain tumor, trauma, or developmental abnormalities that might underlie psychiatric symptoms. The clinical utility of structural imaging modalities has been evaluated in several retrospective studies (Agzarian et al. 2006; Hollister and Shah 1996; McClellan et al. 1988; Moles et al. 1998). There appears to be little justification for routine screening of psychiatric patients (Agzarian et al. 2006; McClellan et al. 1988). In one retrospective study by McClellan et al. (1988), all psychiatric inpatients during a 3-year period were screened with CT scans. In this period, 261 patients with both primary psychotic disorders and mood disorders and without focal neurological signs were screened. Of these, 88% of the CT scans were normal, 10% (27) showed only cortical atrophy, and 1.5% (4) had anomalies unrelated to the psychiatric condition. Given these results, the authors concluded there was no justification for routine screening by CT of psychiatric patients without focal neurological signs.

Similarly, in a more recent study, 397 consecutive psychiatric patients without focal neurological signs were screened with CT scans over a 2-year period, and 95% (377) of these scans were normal. Although 5 of the 20 abnormal scans showed cortical atrophy, all of the abnormal findings were considered to be unrelated to the patient's psychiatric condition and symptoms. The authors concluded that routine screening with CT scan is unlikely to be helpful for the evaluation of psychiatric patients without neurological signs on clinical examination (Agzarian et al. 2006; Moles et al. 1998). Moles et al. (1998) retrospectively attempted to identify which clinical features of psychiatric patients might be predictive of abnormal CT findings that would influence treatment recommendations. The authors found that an abnormal cognitive examination (Folstein Mini-Mental State Examination was used in this study), an abnormal neurological examination, and age were the most sensitive predictors of abnormal CT findings that would influence treatment.

The clinical utility of MRI in the evaluation of adult psychiatric patients has been addressed in a few studies (Erhart et al. 2005; Hollister and Shah 1996). In a retrospective chart review of psychiatric patients referred for brain MRI evaluation (excluding those referred for evaluation of dementia) over a 6-year period, 15% (38

of 253) had MRI findings that modified treatment recommendations. For 6 patients (2%), MRI identified a new medical condition requiring treatment. Thus, the authors concluded that MRI evaluation can be valuable in patients with suspected underlying medical problems causing psychiatric manifestations (Erhart et al. 2005). In a study of CT and MRI scans ordered in a psychiatric hospital over a 2-year period, 17% (12 of 68) of scans were abnormal. The authors concluded that brain imaging scans are indicated for psychiatric patients with cognitive impairment (to evaluate for dementia), a first psychotic break, personality change in a patient older than 50 years, or new or unexplained focal neurological signs (Hollister and Shah 1996).

Although evidence is limited, structural neuroimaging appears to be indicated for the following clinical situations for psychiatric patients: new or unexplained focal neurological signs, cognitive changes or impairment, new-onset psychosis, or prior to the initiation of electroconvulsive therapy. For psychiatric patients older than 50 years, any change in mental status, mood, personality, or behavior may warrant an MRI (Rauch and Renshaw 1995). A CT is valuable when evaluating for suspected hemorrhage or skull fracture or when MRI is contraindicated (e.g., metal implants) (Table 2–15).

Other Structural Imaging Techniques

Magnetic Resonance Spectroscopy

Magnetic resonance spectroscopy (MRS) is based on the same nuclear magnetic resonance principles as MRI, but rather than relying on the resonance of hydrogen protons, MRS detects other signals of interest, including protium (^{1}H), phosphorus 31 (^{31}P), lithium 7 (^{7}Li), fluorine-19 (^{19}F), and carbon-13 (^{13}C). MRS provides information about neuronal damage by measuring several markers of cellular integrity and function, including N-acetyl aspartate, creatinine, choline, and myoinositol. Each of these compounds produces a characteristic spectral peak, thus allowing quantification and distribution of the compound within regions of the brain. MRS has been applied extensively to research of numerous psychiatric disorders and is even used to assess pharmacokinetics and pharmacodynamics of psychotropic medications. Its clinical use, however, is currently somewhat limited for primary psychiatric disorders. However, it is quite useful in the neurological arena for brain tumor typing and grading, differentiating brain tumor from infection or inflammation, stroke management, and seizure disorders.

TABLE 2–15. Indications for computed tomography (CT), prior to or instead of magnetic resonance imaging (MRI)

Noncontrast CT

Evaluation of new-onset or acute neurological abnormality

Acute stroke

Subarachnoid hemorrhage

Trauma

Mass with edema, hydrocephalus, mass effect

Evaluation of ventricular size

Sinus disease

CT with or without contrast

Bone pathology (with or without contrast)

Source. Adapted from J Levine lecture "Structural Neuroimaging in Psychiatry," given as part of the Neuroimaging in Psychiatry lecture series, Department of Psychiatry, Baylor College of Medicine, March 2006.

Diffusion Tensor Imaging

Diffusion tensor imaging (DTI) is based on structural MRI and is a tool to map white matter fiber tracts of the brain. DTI measures the diffusion of water in brain tissues, allowing one to quantify a tissue's orientation and structure. This is especially useful in mapping white matter and neural fiber tracts of the brain. In DTI, diffusion-weighted pulse sequences that are sensitive to the random motion of water are used to quantify how water diffuses along axes. A matrix of water diffusion speed, the diffusion tensor, is calculated for every voxel in an image. The speed of water diffusion is generally constant in all directions. However, in white matter, water diffusion is faster parallel to axons rather than perpendicular to axons, ostensibly because myelin sheaths and white matter tracts constrain and direct water diffusion (Taber et al. 2002). Alterations in diffusion are used to identify damage to the structural integrity of white matter tracts as seen in traumatic brain injury, stroke, or multiple sclerosis. This information can also be used to map white matter tracts that have been compromised by pathology or developmental anomaly.

DTI is a fairly new imaging technique. It is the subject of intense psychiatric and neurological research, including dementias and cognitive disorders, schizophrenia, mood disorders, substance use disorders, and brain injury. It should prove promising in the future, but at this time its clinical utility is limited. Figures 2–4 and 2–5 illustrate the white matter tracts that can be visualized with DTI in various disorders.

Functional Neuroimaging Modalities

Single Photon Emission Computed Tomography

SPECT provides images of cerebral blood flow and brain activity. For this particular scan, a radioactive tracer attached to a drug, generally Technetium-99m-HMPAO (hexamethylpropylene amine oxime) or technetium-99m-ECD (ethyl cysteinate dimer), is administered intravenously. HMPAO and ECD are lipophilic drugs and are able to diffuse across the blood-brain barrier and into neurons. Once inside the cell, they are converted into hydrophilic compounds and are unable to diffuse out of the cell. Physical decay of the radionuclide attached to HMPAO or ECD leads to high-energy photon emissions that are measured by a SPECT detector. A computer creates visual images from this information, using various algorithms and filtering techniques to correct background noise and motion. Tracer uptake and cerebral blood flow are high in the gray matter, where neuronal bodies and synapses reside, and are low in the white matter, which is composed of metabolically less active axons. Thus, the cortex and subcortical structures will appear bright, or "hot," on SPECT, whereas white matter will appear "cold" and dark. The ventricles will appear even darker.

Positron Emission Tomography

PET assesses glucose metabolism within the brain. In this technique, radioactive tracer administered intravenously enters neurons and decays, thereby emitting positrons that collide with electrons within the tissue. Each collision produces two high-energy photons, which travel in paths at a 180° angle from each other. The PET image is constructed from the simultaneous emission of these pairs of photons. For example, PET utilizing the radiotracer ^{18}F-2-fluorodeoxyglucose provides direct information about cerebral glucose metabolism by calculating average glucose metabolic rate per volume. PET can also be applied to study of regional blood flow, neuroreceptor imaging, and neurotransmitter kinetics.

Comparison of SPECT and PET

SPECT is more widely available than other functional imaging modalities, less expensive, and technically easier than PET imaging. Because PET tracers have much shorter half-lives than those of SPECT tracers, they require an on-site cyclotron and radiopharmaceutical laboratory for compounding immediately prior to

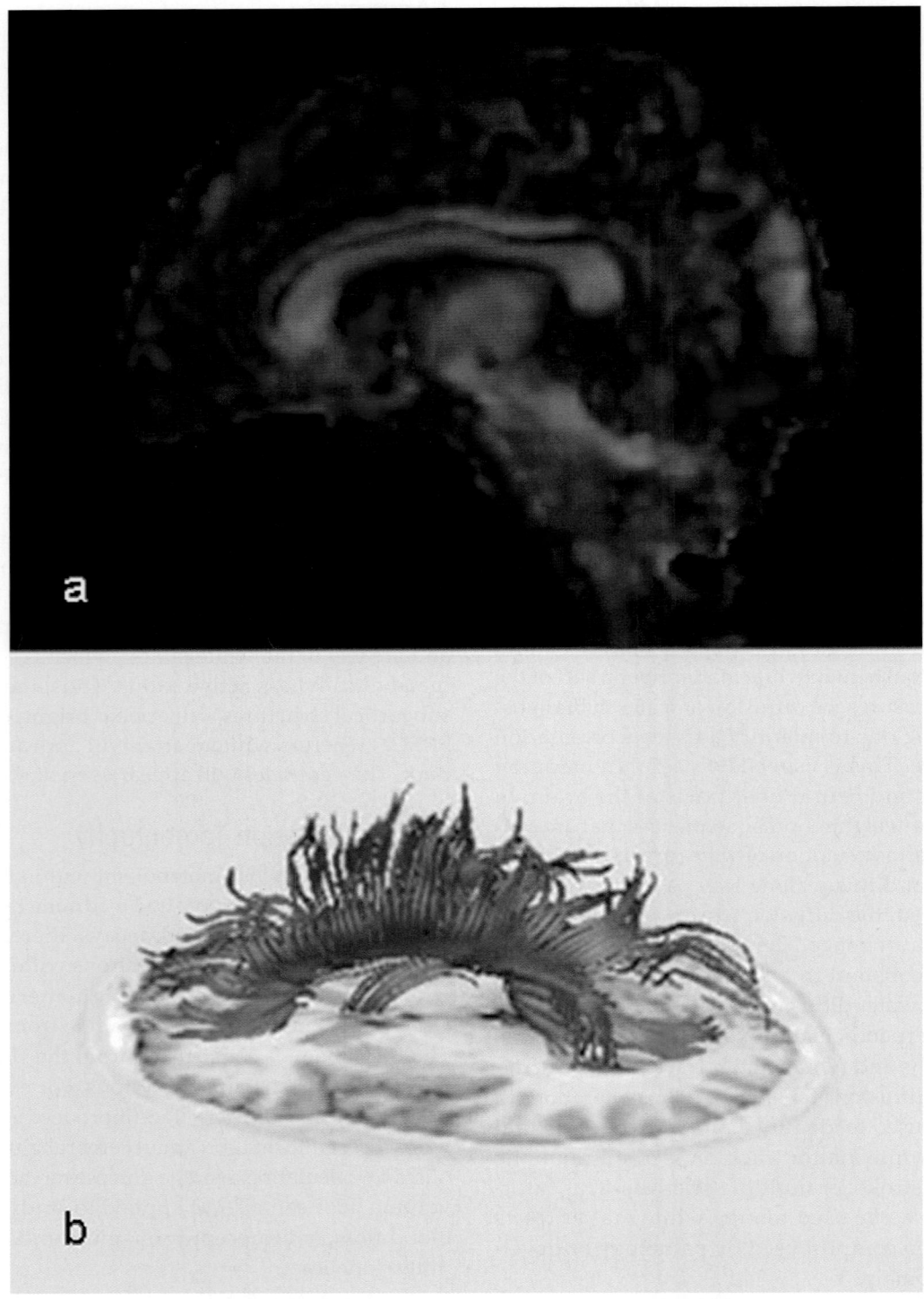

FIGURE 2–4.   Diffusion tensor imaging (DTI).

A, Fractional anisotropy color map derived from DTI in the sagittal plane. *Red* indicates white matter fibers coursing in a right-left direction, *blue* indicates fibers running in a superior-inferior direction, and *green* reflects fibers oriented in an anterior-posterior direction. **B,** Fiber tracking using DTI of the total corpus callosum overlaid on a T1-weighted inversion recovery image from the same brain.

Source.   Images courtesy of Elisabeth A. Wilde, PhD, Department of Physical Medicine and Rehabilitation, Baylor College of Medicine, Houston, Texas.

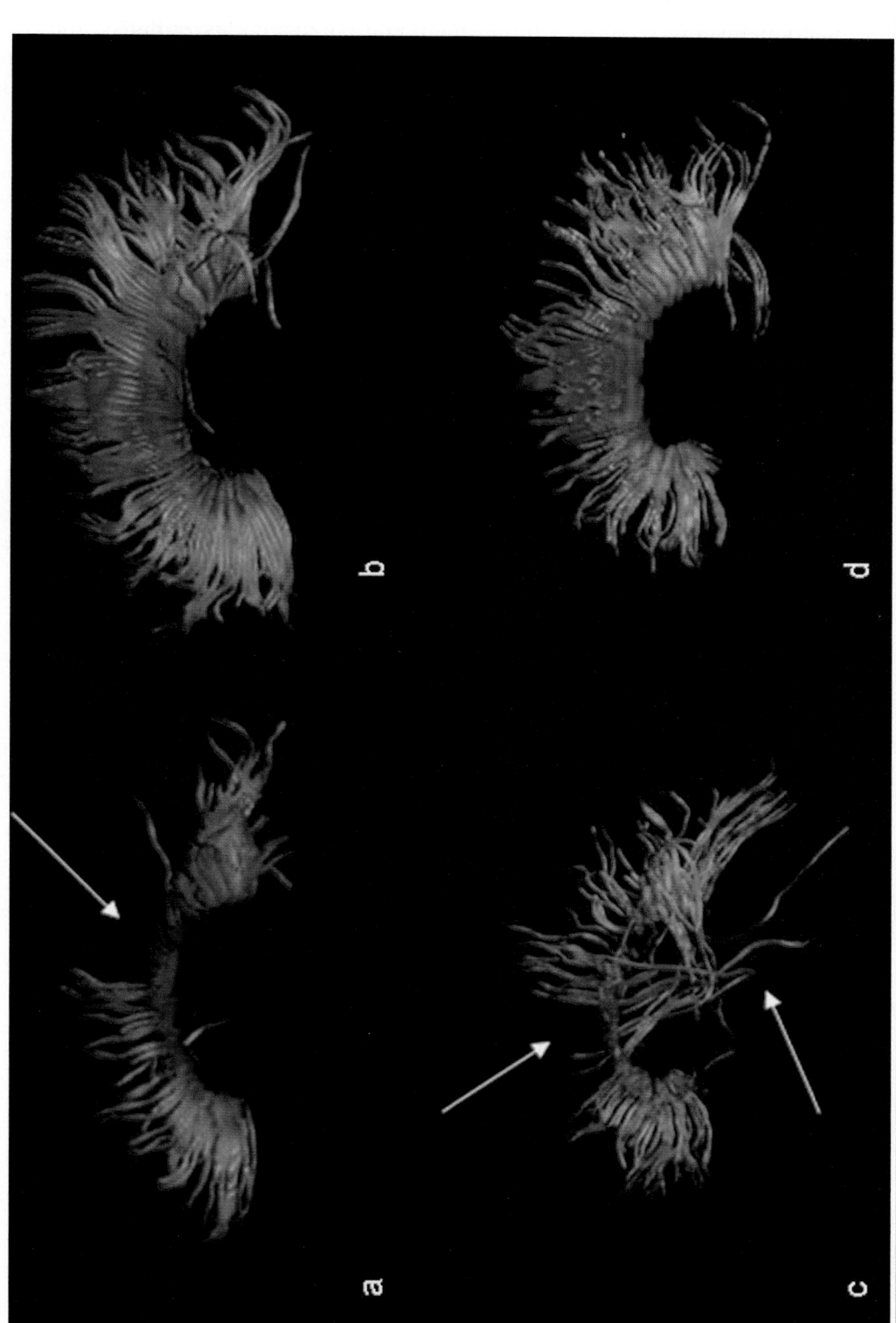

FIGURE 2–5.   Diffusion tensor imaging (DTI) in traumatic brain injury and bipolar disorder.

Fiber tracking of the corpus callosum in **A,** a 16-year-old male patient who sustained severe traumatic brain injury and **B,** an uninjured young man of the same age. The *arrow* indicates the absence of fibers emanating from the posterior body of the corpus callosum. Note also the reduced length and number of fibers emanating from other aspects of the corpus callosum body, likely resulting from injury to the white matter in this area. The mean fractional anisotropy of the fibers in this system was significantly reduced. In addition to quantitative measures of anisotropy, DTI can be used to examine aberrant fiber patterns such as that demonstrated in a 55-year-old female bipolar patient (**C**) as compared with the expected pattern demonstrated in a woman of comparable age without history of illness (**D**). Interestingly, the patient had no significant abnormalities evident on conventional magnetic resonance imaging.

Source.   Images courtesy of Elisabeth A. Wilde, PhD, Department of Physical Medicine and Rehabilitation, Baylor College of Medicine, Houston, Texas.

each study. In comparison, SPECT tracers are stable for 4–6 hours after preparation. Thus, although temporal and spatial resolution is generally superior with PET, it is used less often for clinical reasons due to practical considerations of tracer acquisition, insurance reimbursement, and cost. Both imaging modalities provide only limited visualization of anatomic structures; thus, they often require structural MRI to be superimposed on the functional scan. Table 2–16 provides a comparison of SPECT, PET, and functional MRI modalities.

Clinical Use of PET and SPECT in Psychiatry

Increasingly, structural and functional imaging are used together in the evaluation of neuropsychiatric and neurological disorders. For the primary psychiat-ric disorders, functional imaging techniques hold promise for the future but currently have limited clinical utility. However, for broader neuropsychiatric problems such as evaluation of suspected cognitive impairment and the dementias, epilepsy, and traumatic brain injury, functional neuroimaging is playing an increasingly useful role. Functional imaging techniques such as SPECT and PET are now being used in several clinical situations, including the evaluation of dementia, presurgical evaluation of medically refractory seizures, vascular disease to localize compromised vascular reserve, and brain injury. The exact clinical utility of SPECT and PET for some of these circumstances remains debatable. Figure 2–6 provides a comparison of structural versus functional neuroimaging modalities, and Figure 2–7 compares SPECT and PET images.

TABLE 2–16. Comparison of SPECT, PET, and fMRI

	SPECT	PET	fMRI
Measures	Cerebral perfusion	Cerebral glucose metabolism	Oxygen saturation of blood
Typical radiotracer half-life	^{99m}Tc $T_{1/2}$ = 6 hrs	^{18}F $T_{1/2}$ = 110 min ^{15}O $T_{1/2}$ = 2 min ^{13}N $T_{1/2}$ = 10 min ^{11}C $T_{1/2}$ = 20 min	N/A
Temporal resolution	Fair	Good	Great
Spatial resolution	6–9 mm	4–5 mm	3 mm
Scan time	30 min	8 min	30–60 min
Cost	$1,500	$4,000	$800–$1,000
Advantages	Less expensive Technically easier method Relative stability of radiotracer	More precise and direct quantification of brain function Shorter radiation exposure time Markers for some receptors or enzymes of interest may be available	No ionizing radiation exposure Ability to scan subject multiple times Superior temporal and spatial resolution
Disadvantages	Limited structural anatomic visualization Radiation exposure	Limited structural anatomic visualization Prohibitive cost Short half-life of radiotracer Radiation exposure Problematic for diabetes patients due to glucose load from tracer (fluorodeoxyglucose-PET)	Limited clinical utility

Note.   fMRI=functional magnetic resonance imaging; PET=positron emission tomography; SPECT=single photon emission computed tomography.

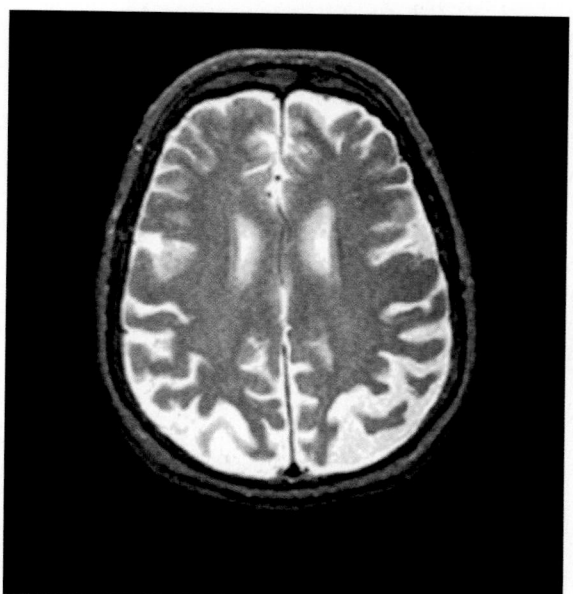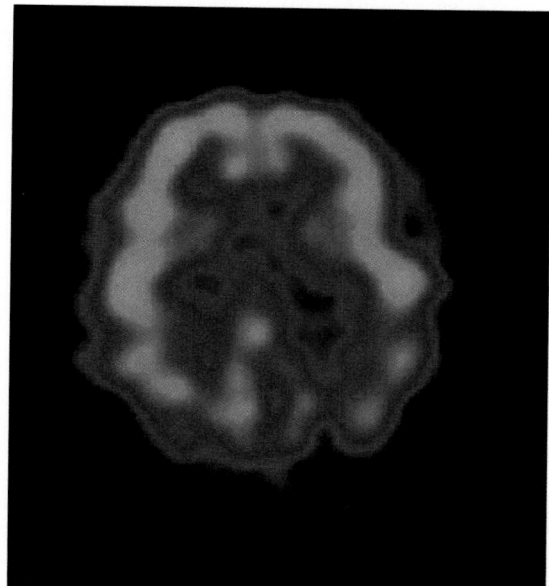

FIGURE 2–6.   Side-by-side comparison of structural and functional neuroimaging: magnetic resonance imaging (MRI) and positron emission tomography (PET).

Axial image of brain MRI (fluid attenuated inversion recovery images [FLAIR] sequence) and corresponding PET scan of a patient with Alzheimer's disease. The MRI image on the *left* shows prominent atrophic change in the posterior regions of the brain, consistent with striking reduction of metabolic activity in the posterior parietal lobes on PET imaging.

Source.   Image courtesy of Ziad Nahas, MD, MSCR, Department of Psychiatry, Medical College of South Carolina, Charleston, South Carolina.

Cognitive Decline and Dementia

SPECT and PET can be helpful in the workup of a patient who is experiencing cognitive decline but shows normal or nonspecific brain structural changes on MRI. Functional imaging can be particularly helpful for providing clues regarding anatomic areas of involvement and thus clues as to the type of early or mild dementia that is present. In this case, the PET or SPECT can reveal areas of reduced brain metabolic activity in areas that the MRI suggests are structurally normal.

PET and SPECT can be particularly useful to the clinician for differentiating between disorders such as Alzheimer's disease and frontotemporal dementia. Alzheimer's disease is often associated with bilateral, symmetric, posterior temporal, and parietal lobe perfusion defects, whereas frontotemporal dementia is generally associated with reduced perfusion of the frontal and/or lateral temporal lobes bilaterally. In contrast, patients with multi-infarct dementia may show patchy perfusion defects corresponding to the site of strokes, whereas patients with depression, which may take the form of a pseudodementia, may show normal brain perfusion or only mildly reduced prefrontal perfusion.

Epilepsy

SPECT and PET can be used to identify seizure foci in the interictal period or to localize deep subcortical foci that may not be apparent on EEG. They are also useful techniques for the presurgical localization of seizure foci in patients with medically refractory seizures. SPECT is often used rather than PET in this clinical situation because the relative stability of radioactive tracers (usable up to 4–6 hours after preparation) is helpful for imaging of seizure activity. SPECT is used in the context of partial or focal seizures in order to identify a localized brain region that can be removed surgically to eradicate the seizures. Seizures can be localized both during the ictal and interictal phases.

Seizures are associated with intense increases in glucose metabolism and regional cerebral blood flow. Thus, the seizure foci appear bright or hypermetabolic on SPECT scan during the seizure (ictal scan) and are dark or hypometabolic between seizures (interictal phase = interictal scan). Ictal scans are the most sensitive but most difficult method of localizing seizures. Radioactive tracer is injected within the first minute of seizure onset and accumulates in the brain. The SPECT images are acquired after cessation of seizure activity and subsequent recovery of the patient, usually an hour later.

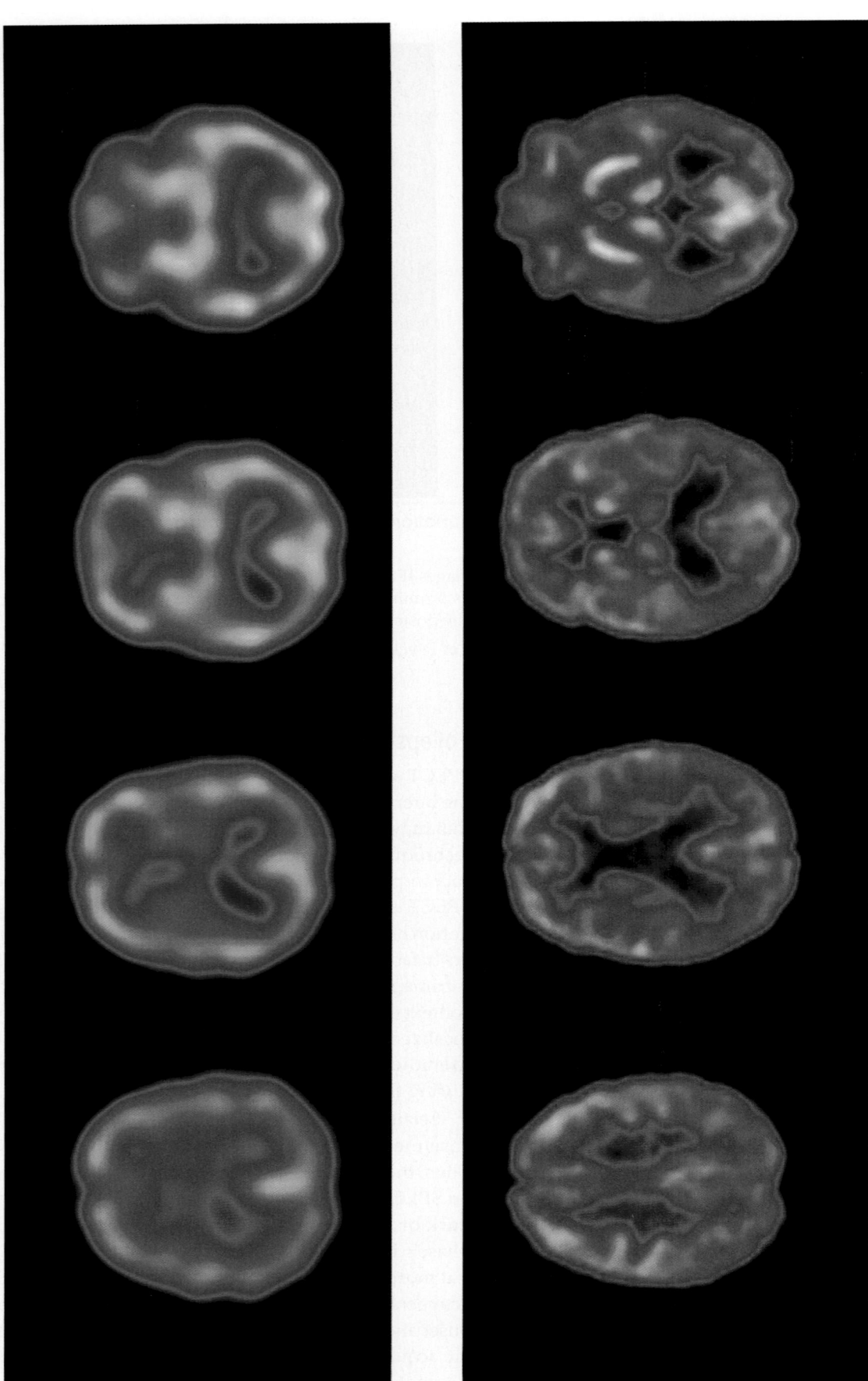

FIGURE 2–7. Side-by-side comparison of single photon emission computed tomography (SPECT) versus positron emission tomography (PET).

SPECT (*top row*) and PET images from two patients with clinically similar degrees of mild cognitive impairment. The PET scan demonstrates parietal changes, suggesting that this patient is at greater risk of developing Alzheimer's disease. The PET scan also demonstrates much better resolution than the SPECT scan.

Source. Images courtesy of Paul E. Schulz, MD, Department of Neurology, Baylor College of Medicine, Houston, Texas.

An easier but less sensitive method of localizing seizures with SPECT or PET is scanning between seizures in order to look for hypometabolic areas. These hypometabolic areas are believed to be a result of neuronal damage that occurs as a result of the seizure. Ictal and interictal scans are now often used together to localize a focus that is hypermetabolic on ictal scan but hypometabolic on interictal scan (Henry and van Heertum 2003).

Stroke

SPECT is an extremely sensitive test for stroke: it is able to visualize perfusion defects and define the size of the stroke. However, CT is still used in the acute setting because it is quick and easy to obtain. In addition, CT is superior to SPECT in differentiating between hemorrhagic and nonhemorrhagic stroke, which is essential to know prior to starting thrombolytic medications. SPECT holds great promise for the evaluation and treatment of stroke, and its role will likely expand dramatically in the future.

Traumatic Brain Injury

Studies have found SPECT to be more sensitive than CT or MRI in the diagnosis of traumatic brain injury. Structural neuroimaging modalities can detect serious head injuries but often do not detect mild traumatic brain injuries. Patients with mild traumatic brain injuries often complain of persistent neuropsychiatric symptoms despite having normal CT or MRI scans. Because of its increased sensitivity, SPECT may show regional cerebral blood flow hypoperfusion despite normal CT or MRI scans (Audenaert et al. 2003; Bonne et al. 2003). However, the prognosis of patients with an abnormal SPECT is unclear. It may be further complicated by difficulties in recognizing which specific SPECT abnormalities are attributable to brain injury as opposed to motion artifact, normal variation, and processing errors. Thus, the clinical utility of the SPECT scan in mild traumatic brain injury is not clear and requires further investigation. Figures 2–8, 2–9, and 2–10 illustrate the uses of SPECT and PET in brain-injured patients.

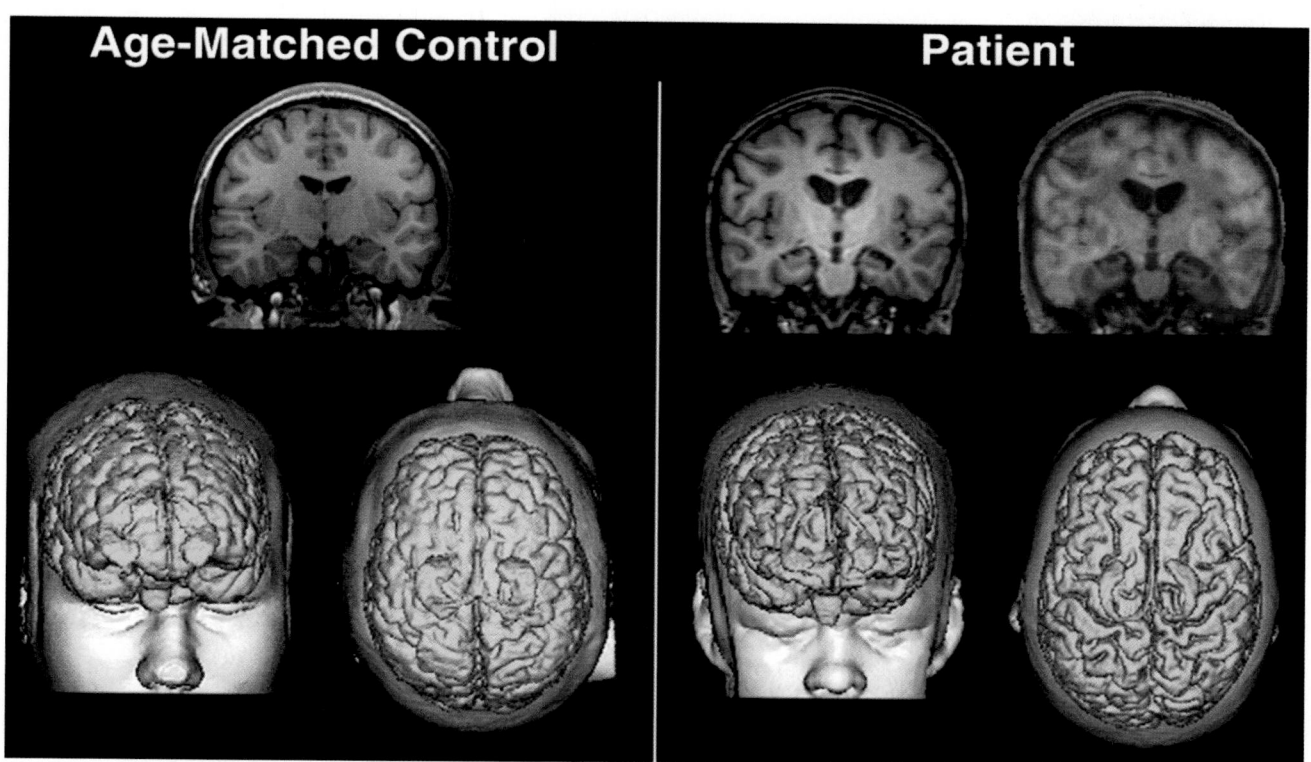

FIGURE 2–8. Structural magnetic resonance imaging (MRI) and positron emission tomography (PET) imaging of a healthy control subject and a patient with traumatic brain injury.

Coronal slices *(MRI)* and three-dimensional reconstruction of the cortical surface *(pink)* and hippocampi *(yellow)* of a typically developing adolescent male *(left)* and an adolescent male with traumatic brain injury *(right)*. Note the significant cortical and hippocampal atrophy in the patient as compared with the age-matched control. The *top right* image portrays PET findings overlaid on the MRI. PET reveals significant bilateral metabolic defects in the patient's mesial temporal areas as indicated by the absence of "warm" colors. *Red* represents areas of the greatest metabolic activity, followed by *orange, yellow, green, blue,* and *violet*.
Source. Images courtesy of Erin Bigler, PhD, University of Utah, Salt Lake City, Utah.

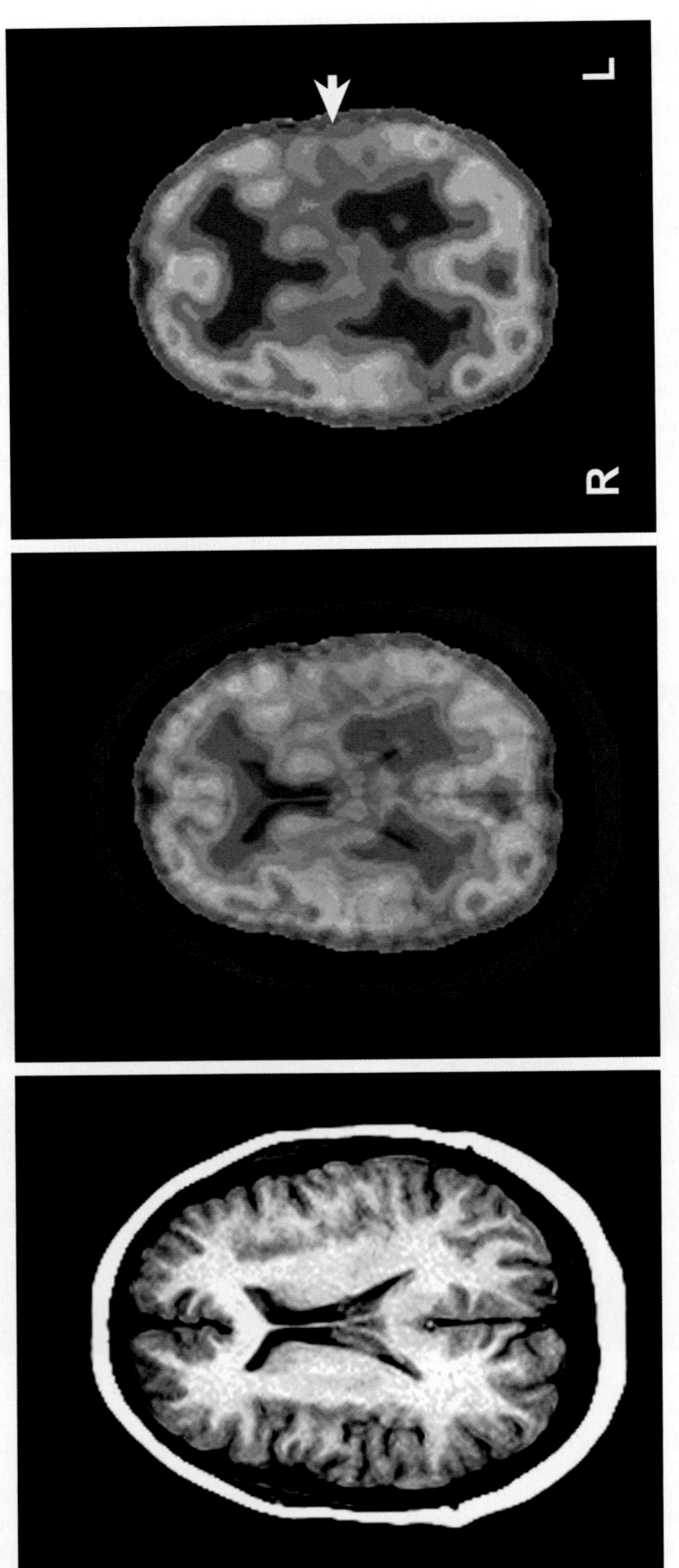

FIGURE 2–9. Structural magnetic resonance imaging (MRI) and positron emission tomography (PET) imaging of a patient with hypoxic brain injury.

Despite the absence of significant findings on structural imaging, PET reveals areas of significant hypometabolism in the left temporal area as indicated by the *arrow*. *Red* represents areas of the greatest metabolic activity, followed by *orange, yellow, green, blue,* and *violet.* The *center image* is a fusion of the MRI and PET images.

Source. Images courtesy of Erin Bigler, PhD, University of Utah, Salt Lake City, Utah.

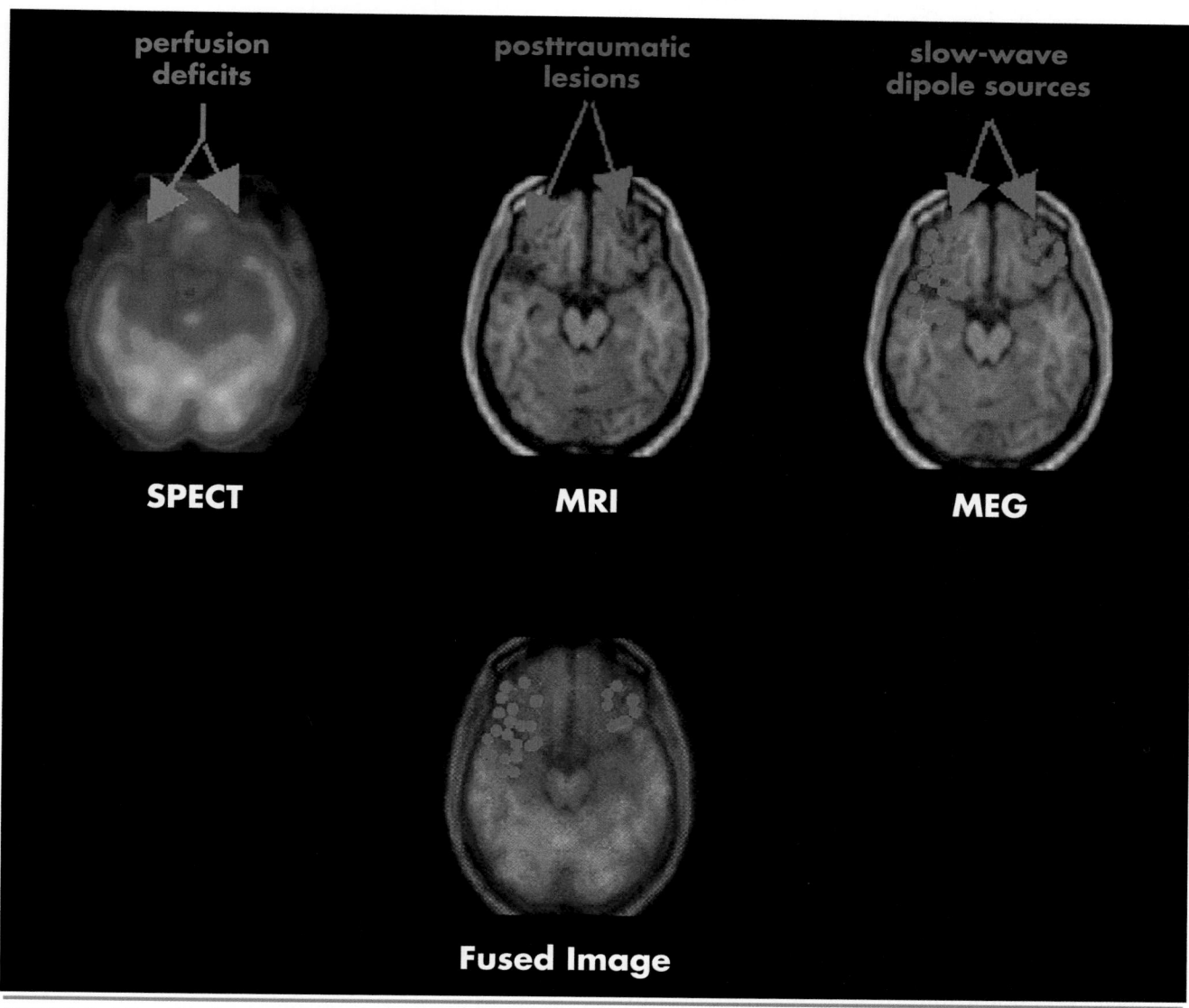

FIGURE 2–10.   Single photon emission computed tomography (SPECT), structural magnetic resonance imaging (MRI), and magnetoencephalography (MEG) imaging of a patient with traumatic brain injury.

Findings from multiple neuroimaging modalities in a patient with traumatic brain injury reveal structural and functional deficits in the inferior frontal and temporal regions, common sites of focal injury in head trauma. Functional imaging reveals even more extensive defects in perfusion *(SPECT, left)* and dipole abnormality *(MEG, right)* than the areas of focal injury evident on structural *MRI (center)*. The fused image *(bottom)* displays the results of the SPECT and MEG overlaid on the MRI.

Source.   Images courtesy of Erin Bigler, PhD, University of Utah, Salt Lake City, Utah.

Neuroreceptor Imaging

Recently, there has been a great deal of research regarding the use of radiolabeled neuroreceptor ligands in SPECT and PET imaging to study the distribution and density of neuroreceptors in the brain of patients with psychiatric disorders. Many experimental neurochemical targets have been investigated with SPECT and PET radioligands, including dopamine transporters, postsynaptic dopamine receptors (D_1 and D_2), several serotonin receptors (5-HT$_{1A}$ and 5-HT$_{2A}$) and

transporters (SERT), γ-aminobutyric acid-A receptors, acetylcholine receptors, and histamine receptors.

Functional Magnetic Resonance Imaging

Functional MRI (fMRI) measures the level of oxygenation in brain tissue to map the neuroanatomical activation that occurs with various challenges. Several fMRI techniques have been developed, but the most widely used one is the blood oxygenation level–dependent

(BOLD) technique. BOLD fMRI is based on the magnetic susceptibility of blood, whose hemoglobin fluctuates between a paramagnetic, deoxygenated state in resting state blood and an isomagnetic, oxygenated state. Deoxyhemoglobin acts as an endogenous contrast agent. Increased neuronal activity in response to a sensorimotor, cognitive, or behavioral challenge results in an increase in regional cerebral blood flow and subsequent decrease in regional deoxyhemoglobin concentration. Oxygen saturation changes in blood due to cognitive challenge or sensory stimuli result in a corresponding change in T2-weighted magnetic resonance signal intensity, thus allowing neuronal activation to be mapped neuroanatomically through the BOLD signal. fMRI images are obtained when the subject is at rest and when the subject is engaged in a sensorimotor or cognitive task and then compared to determine changes in regional cerebral blood flow. Structural MRI can be obtained simultaneously, and these images can be interleaved with the fMRI images to more precisely pinpoint neuroanatomical locations of regional activation.

fMRI has many advantages compared with other functional imaging techniques in that it provides superior spatial and temporal resolution, is minimally invasive, and does not involve exposure to harmful ionizing radiation. It is being used extensively in research to understand the neurocircuitry involved in psychotic disorders, mood and anxiety disorders, substance use disorders, and cognitive and developmental disorders. Furthermore, the effects of psychotropic medications are being studied via fMRI, with the hope of understanding the regional brain effects of acute and chronic treatment with these medications. Despite the insights into structure–function relations that fMRI has revealed, it is not yet used as a diagnostic or treatment modality. This probably has to do with difficulties standardizing stimuli and determining stimuli that differentiate between different disorders. Figures 2–11, 2–12, and 2–13 illustrate research uses of fMRI.

Magnetoencephalography

Magnetoencephalography (MEG) measures extracranial magnetic signals generated by the positive ionic flow of cortical pyramidal cells in the brain. These extracranial neuromagnetic fields are about 10^{-8} to 10^{-9} of the earth's magnetic field (Reite et al. 1999). In order to be identified, they require expensive superconducting technology as well as magnetic shielding to screen out competing magnetic fields from the earth, sun, and environment. Magnetoencephalography is noninvasive, does not entail exposure to ionizing radiation, and has excellent spatial and temporal resolution. It is currently being studied in several psychiatric disorders and has been used to localize epileptiform activity by co-registration with structural MRI data. It has also been used in conjunction with evoked potentials to presurgically map auditory and somatosensory cortical areas to be avoided during neurosurgical procedures (Hund et al. 1997). Magnetoencephalography is also being used to study possible cortical reorganization, cerebral lateralization, and auditory sensory memory abnormalities in patients with psychotic disorders.

Neuroimaging of Psychiatric Disorders

Structural and functional neuroimaging of psychiatric disorders has exploded in recent decades, given the many new and powerful imaging techniques that are now available. Yet these marked advances have led to few conclusive findings about the pathophysiology and workings of the mysterious human brain. A comprehensive discussion of the research findings to date in the neuroimaging of the major psychiatric disorders is beyond the scope of this chapter. However, Table 2–17 summarizes the structural and functional neuroimaging findings in selected psychiatric disorders that may be of interest to the psychiatric clinician.

Conclusion

Laboratory assessment and imaging studies are particularly important to the evaluation of the psychiatric patient. Their influence and scope, although of limited clinical use in the past, have the potential to increase tremendously, as promising new modalities become more widely available and demonstrate ever-increasing clinical possibilities.

Judicious choice of laboratory testing, guided by a complete psychiatric assessment—including a thorough medical and psychiatric history, review of systems, and physical examination—may often uncover an unsuspected medical or neurological etiology underlying primarily psychiatric symptomatology. Likewise, structural and functional neuroimaging are powerful tools that can provide evidence of tangible abnormalities that might underlie psychiatric symptoms. One hopes that through advances in neuroimaging and laboratory testing, promising genetic and biological markers will be discovered and will attain a level of clinical utility so that a new and important dimension may be added to the uses of laboratory testing: the identification, biological treatment, and ultimately prevention of psychiatric illnesses.

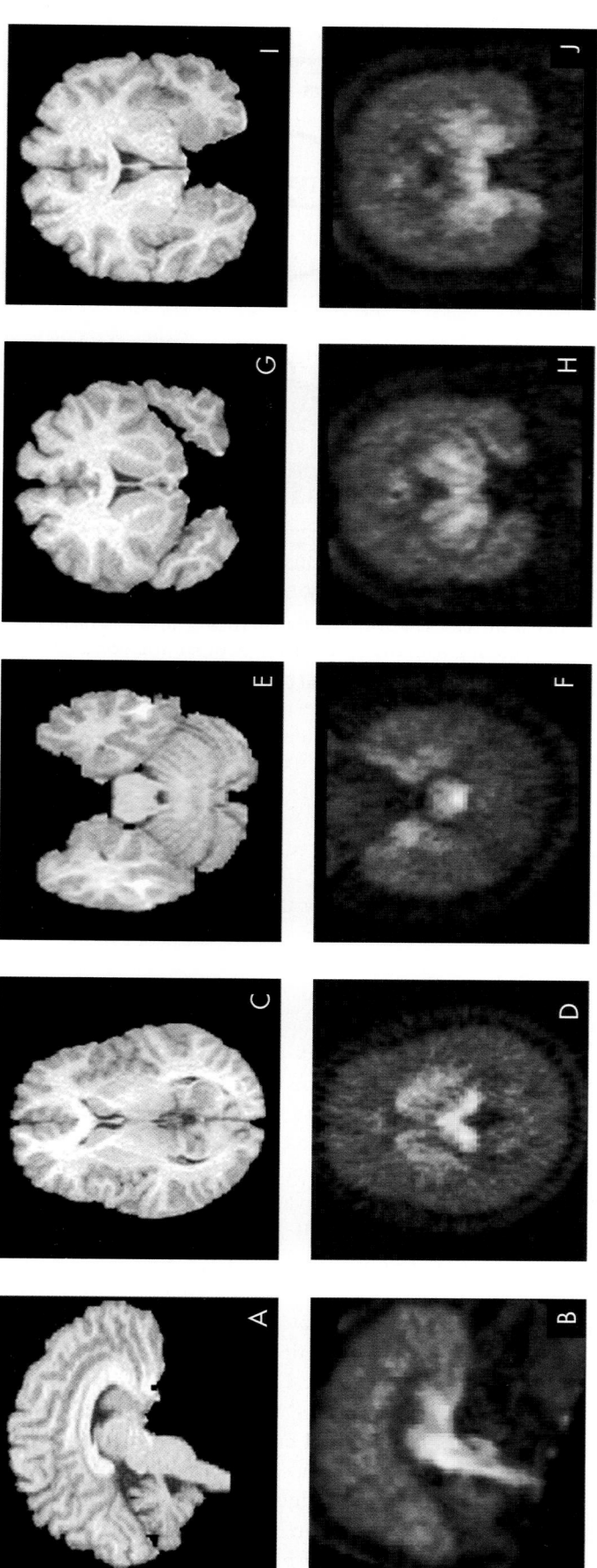

FIGURE 2–11. Neuroreceptor imaging.

Magnetic resonance imaging (*top*) and co-registered positron emission tomography images (*bottom*) acquired from 40 to 100 minutes following injection of 14.9 mCi $[^{11}C]$DASB in a 40-year-old healthy male volunteer. **A, B:** Sagittal plane close to the midline, showing accumulation of activity in the midbrain, thalamus, and caudate. This picture also illustrates the low level of activity in the cerebellum. Activity concentration is also seen in the cortical gray matter (cingulate cortex). **C, D:** Transaxial plane, illustrating activity concentration in thalamus and striatum. **E, F:** Transaxial plane at the level of the midbrain. The very high activity concentration is seen at the level of the dorsal raphe. The amygdala is also seen on this plane. **G, H:** Coronal plane at the level of the anterior striatum, illustrating the ventrodorsal gradient of SERT in the striatum. This view also shows activity concentration in cingulate and temporal cortices. **I, J:** Coronal plane at the level of the postcommissural striatum, illustrating activity concentrations in the caudate and putamen, in the thalamus, and in the amygdala.

Source.   Images courtesy of Gordon Frankle, MD, Department of Psychiatry, University of Pittsburgh, Pittsburgh, Pennsylvania.

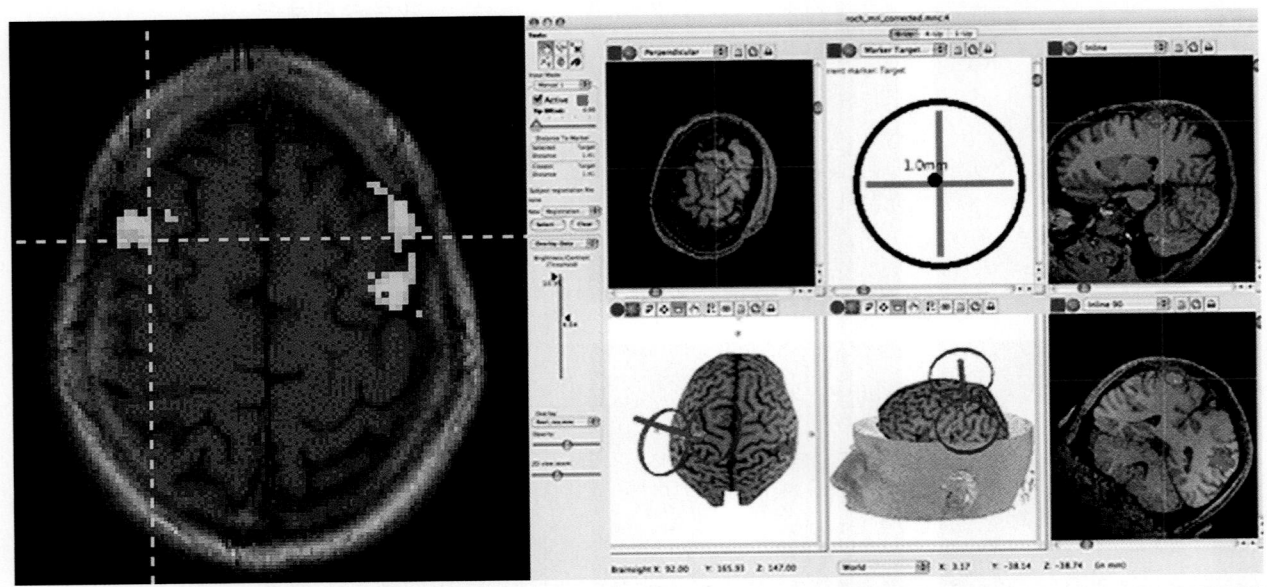

FIGURE 2–12. Functional magnetic resonance imaging of working memory.

Increased regional blood flow evident in prefrontal cortex while a subject is performing the Sternberg Task *(left image)*. Corresponding images in Brainsight™ Frameless used for stereotactic targeting with transcranial magnetic stimulation *(right images)*.

Source. Images courtesy of Ziad Nahas, MD, MSCR, Department of Psychiatry, Medical College of South Carolina, Charleston, South Carolina.

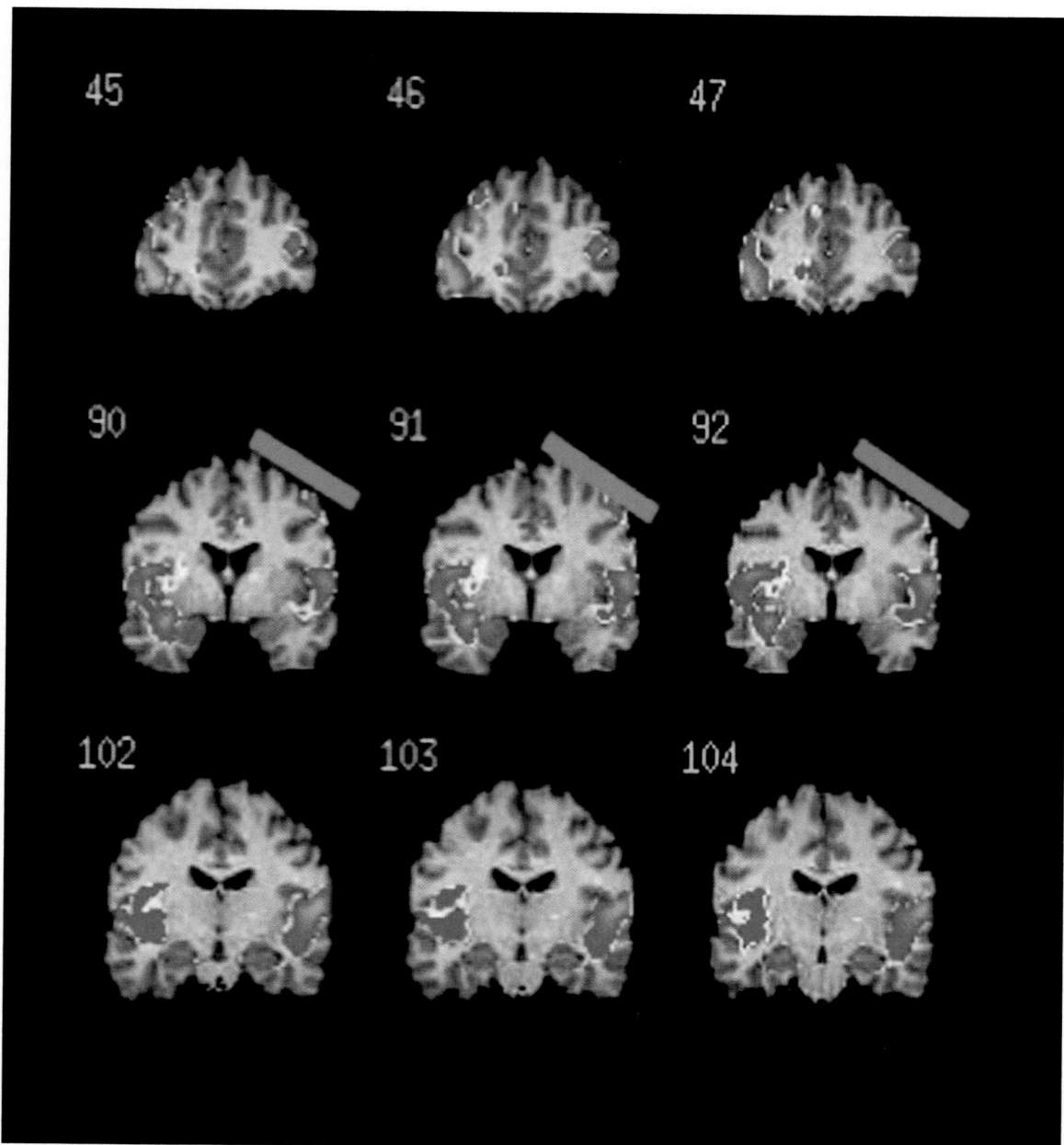

FIGURE 2–13. Functional magnetic resonance (fMRI) and transcranial magnetic stimulation (TMS) as a neuroscience tool.

fMRI interleaved with TMS over left prefrontal cortex in healthy volunteers illustrating both local and transsynaptic functional connectivity of cortical-subcortical networks.

Source. Images courtesy of Ziad Nahas, MD, MSCR, Department of Psychiatry, Medical College of South Carolina, Charleston, South Carolina.

TABLE 2–17. Summary of neuroimaging findings in selected psychiatric disorders

Disorder/imaging modality	Findings
Schizophrenia and primary psychotic disorders	
Structural imaging studies	Ventricular enlargement; abnormalities in medial temporal lobe structures and superior temporal gyrus (Shenton et al. 2001). Majority of studies report frontal lobe abnormalities (prefrontal gray matter and orbitofrontal regions) (Shenton et al. 2001). Subcortical abnormalities involving cavum septum pellucidum, basal ganglia, corpus callosum, and thalamus (Shenton et al. 2001). Ventricular enlargement and decreased gray matter volumes in first-episode schizophrenic patients (Lim et al. 1996).
Functional imaging studies	Positron emission tomography shows relative hypometabolism in the prefrontal cortex (Buchsbaum et al. 1982; Tamminga et al. 1992). Metabolic abnormalities of limbic areas (temporal lobe, anterior cingulum) (Nordahl et al. 2001; Tamminga et al. 1992).
Magnetic resonance spectroscopy	Decreased NAA levels in frontal, temporal, and thalamic regions (Bertolino et al. 1998; Deicken et al. 1998; Nasrallah et al. 1994; Yurgelun-Todd et al. 1996). Antipsychotic medications associated with selective increase in *N*-acetyl aspartate in dorsolateral prefrontal cortex (Bertolino et al. 2001).
Mood disorders	
Structural imaging studies	Abnormal signal hyperintensities in frontal cortex and basal ganglia (Videbech 1997). Ventricular enlargement and increased sulcal prominence in patients with bipolar disorder and unipolar depression (Elkis et al. 1995).
Functional imaging studies	Depression: hypometabolism in limbic and dorsolateral prefrontal cortical regions, but hypermetabolism of ventrolateral frontal cortex (Brody et al. 2001; Ketter et al. 1996).
Magnetic resonance spectroscopy	Major depression: increased choline levels in basal ganglia and anterior cingulate (Renshaw et al. 2001; Soares et al. 1999).
Anxiety disorders/obsessive-compulsive disorder (OCD)	
Structural imaging studies	OCD: unclear findings; no volume differences in striatal or ventricular regions (Aylward et al. 1996)
Functional imaging studies	Hypermetabolism in the orbitofrontal cortex and anterior cingulum (Nordahl et al. 1989; Swedo et al. 1989). Successful treatment of OCD associated with decreased metabolism in orbitofrontal cortex, anterior cingulum, and caudate nucleus (Baxter et al. 1992; Benkelfat et al. 1990; Swedo et al. 1992).

Key Points

- Laboratory testing of the psychiatric patient in the past has been utilized mainly to uncover medical or neurological causes of psychiatric symptoms.

- The consensus of studies evaluating the role and value of laboratory testing is that patients who have psychiatric signs and symptoms but who do not exhibit other physical complaints or symptoms will benefit from a small screening battery that includes serum glucose concentration, BUN concentration, creatinine clearance, and urinalysis. Female patients older than 50 years will also benefit from a screening TSH test regardless of the presence or absence of mood symptoms.

- More extensive laboratory screening may be necessary for psychiatric patients who do have concomitant physical complaints or findings on physical examination or for patients who are of higher risk, such as elderly or institutionalized patients or those with low socioeconomic status, self-neglect, alcohol or drug dependence, or cognitive impairment.

- Newer laboratory testing methods such as pharmacogenetic testing and testing for investigational genetic and biological markers have the potential to transform and dramatically increase the importance of laboratory testing in the workup of the psychiatric patient.

- Imaging may also be helpful when atypical features are present, such as an older age at onset of psychiatric illness, or when cognitive impairment is present.

- Neuroimaging does not yet play a diagnostic role for any of the primary psychiatric disorders, but it is still an integral part of the clinical workup for psychiatric patients to rule out underlying medical causes of psychiatric symptoms.

- Current neuroimaging methods provide both structural and functional data about the brain. Structural imaging techniques such as CT and MRI provide a fixed image of the brain's anatomy and spatial distribution. Newer functional neuroimaging techniques such as PET and SPECT provide information about brain metabolism, blood flow, the presynaptic uptake of transmitter precursors, neurotransmitter transporter activity, and postsynaptic receptor activity.

- Functional scans should always be interpreted in the context of the underlying structural images.

Suggested Readings

Baumann P, Hiemke C, Ulrich S, et al: The AGNP-TDM Expert Group consensus guidelines: therapeutic drug monitoring in psychiatry. Pharmacopsychiatry 37:243–265, 2004

Cabeza R, Nyberg L: Imaging cognition II: an empirical review of 275 PET and fMRI studies. J Cogn Neurosci 12:1–47, 2000

de Leon J, Armstrong SC, Cozza KL: Clinical guidelines for psychiatrists for the use of pharmacogenetic testing for CYP450 2D6 and CYP450 2C19. Psychosomatics 47:75–85, 2006

Yudofsky SC, Kim HF (eds): Neuropsychiatric Assessment (Review of Psychiatry Series; Oldham JM and Riba MB, series eds). Washington, DC, American Psychiatric Publishing, 2004

References

Agzarian MJ, Chryssidis S, Davies RP, et al: Use of routine computed tomography brain scanning of psychiatry patients. Australas Radiol 50:27–28, 2006

Alpay M, Park L: Laboratory tests and diagnostic procedures, in Psychiatry: Update and Board Preparation. Edited by Stern TA, Herman JB. New York, McGraw-Hill, 2000, pp 251–266

American Academy of Neurology: American Academy of Neurology practice guidelines for dementia. Continuum 13(2):Appendix A, 2007

American Psychiatric Association Task Force on the Use of Laboratory Tests in Psychiatry: Tricyclic antidepressants: blood level measurements and clinical outcome. An APA Task Force report. Am J Psychiatry 142:155–162, 1985

Anfinson TJ, Kathol RG: Screening laboratory evaluation in psychiatric patients: a review. Gen Hosp Psychiatry 14:248–257, 1992

Anfinson TJ, Stoudemire A: Laboratory and neuroendocrine assessment in medical-psychiatric patients, in Psychiatric Care of the Medical Patient, 2nd Edition. Edited by Stoudemire S, Fogel BS, Greenberg D. New York, Oxford University Press, 2000, pp 119–145

Audenaert K, Jansen HM, Otte A, et al: Imaging of mild traumatic brain injury using 57Co and 99mTc HMPAO SPECT as compared to other diagnostic procedures. Med Sci Monit 9:MT112–117, 2003

Aylward EH, Harris GL, Hoehn-Saric R, et al: Normal caudate nucleus in obsessive-compulsive disorder assessed by quantitative neuroimaging. Arch Gen Psychiatry 53:577–584, 1996

Barnes RF, Mason JC, Greer C, et al: Medical illness in chronic psychiatric outpatients. Gen Hosp Psychiatry 5:191–195, 1983

Baxter LR Jr, Schwartz JM, Bergman KS, et al: Caudate glucose metabolic rate changes with both drug and behavior therapy for obsessive-compulsive disorder. Arch Gen Psychiatry 49:681–689, 1992

Benkelfat C, Nordahl TE, Semple WE, et al: Local cerebral glucose metabolic rates in obsessive-compulsive disorder patients treated with clomipramine. Arch Gen Psychiatry 47:840–848, 1990

Bernardo M, Palao DJ, Arauxo A, et al: Monitoring plasma level of haloperidol in schizophrenia. Hosp Community Psychiatry 44:115, 118, 1993

Bertolino A, Callicott JH, Elman I, et al: Regionally specific neuronal pathology in untreated patients with schizophrenia: a proton magnetic resonance spectroscopic imaging study. Biol Psychiatry 43:641–648, 1998

Bertolino A, Callicott JH, Mattay VS, et al: The effect of treatment with antipsychotic drugs on brain N-acetylaspartate measures in patients with schizophrenia. Biol Psychiatry 49:39–46, 2001

Bonne O, Gilboa A, Louzoun Y, et al: Cerebral blood flow in chronic symptomatic mild traumatic brain injury. Psychiatry Res 124:141–152, 2003

Boutros N, Struve F: Electrophysiological testing, in Neuropsychiatric Assessment. Edited by Yudofsky SC, Kim HF (Review of Psychiatry Series; Oldham JM and Riba MB, series eds). Washington, DC, American Psychiatric Publishing, 2004, pp 69–104

Brody AL, Barsom MW, Bota RG, et al: Prefrontal-subcortical and limbic circuit mediation of major depressive disorder. Semin Clin Neuropsychiatry 6:102–112, 2001

Brosen K, de Morais SM, Meyer UA, et al: A multifamily study on the relationship between CYP2C19 genotype and s-mephenytoin oxidation phenotype. Pharmacogenetics 5:312–317, 1995

Brown D, Gaar SJ: Alaska services for children and youth with dual sensory impairments final performance report, October 1, 1992 to September 30, 1995. Washington, DC, U.S. Department of Education, Office of Educational Research and Improvement, Educational Resources Information Center, 1995

Buchsbaum MS, Ingvar DH, Kessler R, et al: Cerebral glucography with positron tomography: use in normal subjects and in patients with schizophrenia. Arch Gen Psychiatry 39:251–259, 1982

Carroll BJ: Problems with diagnostic criteria for depression. J Clin Psychiatry 45:14–18, 1984

Catalano G, Catalano MC, O'Dell KJ, et al: The utility of laboratory screening in medically ill patients with psychiatric symptoms. Ann Clin Psychiatry 13:135–140, 2001

Curry S: The strategy and value of neuroleptic drug monitoring. J Clin Psychopharmacol 5:263–271, 1985

de Leon J: Psychopharmacological treatment based on individual drug metabolism: CYP2D6 poor metabolizers. CNS Spectr 11:8–12, 2006

de Leon J, Armstrong S, Cozza KL: Clinical guidelines for psychiatrists for the use of pharmacogenetic testing for CYP450 2D6 and CYP450 2C19. Psychosomatics 47:75–85, 2006

Deicken RF, Zhou L, Schuff N, et al: Hippocampal neuronal dysfunction in schizophrenia as measured by proton magnetic resonance spectroscopy. Biol Psychiatry 43:483–488, 1998

Dolan JG, Mushlin AI: Routine laboratory testing for medical disorders in psychiatric inpatients. Arch Intern Med 145:2085–2088, 1985

Elkis H, Friedman L, Wise A, et al: Meta-analyses of studies of ventricular enlargement and cortical sulcal prominence in mood disorders: comparisons with controls or patients with schizophrenia. Arch Gen Psychiatry 52:735–746, 1995

Engel J Jr: The epilepsies, in Cecil Textbook of Medicine, 19th Edition, Vol 2. Edited by Wyngaarden JB, Smith LH, Bennett JC. Philadelphia, PA, WB Saunders, 1992, pp 2202–2213

Erhart SM, Young AS, Marder SR, et al: Clinical utility of magnetic resonance imaging radiographs for suspected organic syndromes in adult psychiatry. J Clin Psychiatry 66:968–973, 2005

Fadem B, Simring S: High Yield Psychiatry. Baltimore, MD, Williams & Wilkins, 1998

Gomez-Gil E, Trilla A, Corbella B, et al: Lack of clinical relevance of routine chest radiography in acute psychiatric admissions. Gen Hosp Psychiatry 24:110–113, 2002

Hall RC, Popkin MK, Devaul RA, et al: Physical illness presenting as psychiatric disease. Arch Gen Psychiatry 35:1315–1320, 1978

Hall RC, Gardner ER, Stickney SK, et al: Physical illness manifesting as psychiatric disease, II: analysis of a state hospital inpatient population. Arch Gen Psychiatry 37:989–995, 1980

Hampton JR, Harrison MJ, Mitchell JR, et al: Relative contributions of history-taking, physical examination, and laboratory investigation to diagnosis and management of medical outpatients. Br Med J 2:486–489, 1975

Harms H, Hermans P: Admission laboratory testing in elderly psychiatric patients without organic mental syndromes: should it be routine? Int J Geriatr Psychiatry 9:133–140, 1994

Henry TR, van Heertum RL: Positron emission tomography and single photon emission computed tomography in epilepsy care. Semin Nucl Med 33:88–104, 2003

Hollister LE: Electrocardiographic screening in psychiatric patients. J Clin Psychiatry 56:26–29, 1995

Hollister LE, Shah NN: Structural brain scanning in psychiatric patients: a further look. J Clin Psychiatry 57:241–244, 1996

Honig A, Tan ES, Weenink A, et al: Utility of a symptom checklist for detecting physical disease in chronic psychiatric patients. Hosp Community Psychiatry 42:531–533, 1991

Hughes J, Barraclough BM: Value of routine chest radiography of psychiatric patients. Br Med J 281:1461–1462, 1980

Hughes JR, John ER: Conventional and quantitative electroencephalography in psychiatry. J Neuropsychiatry Clin Neurosci 11:190–208, 1999

Hund M, Rezai AR, Kronberg E, et al: Magnetoencephalographic mapping: basic of a new functional risk profile in the selection of patients with cortical brain lesions. Neurosurgery 40:936–942, discussion 942–943, 1997

Hyman SE, Arana GW: Handbook of Psychiatric Drug Therapy. Boston, MA, Little, Brown, 1991

Ingelman-Sundberg M, Oscarson M, McLellan RA: Polymorphic human cytochrome P450 enzymes: an opportunity for individualized drug treatment. Trends Pharmacol Sci 20:342–349, 1999

Ketter TA, George MS, Kimbrell TA, et al: Functional brain imaging, limbic function, and affective disorders. The Neuroscientist 2:55–65, 1996

Kirchheiner J, Brosen K, Dahl ML, et al: CYP2D6 and CYP2C19 genotype-based dose recommendations for antidepressants: a first step towards subpopulation-specific dosages. Acta Psychiatr Scand 104:173–192, 2001

Koran LM, Sox HC Jr, Marton KI, et al: Medical evaluation of psychiatric patients, I: results in a state mental health system. Arch Gen Psychiatry 46:733–740, 1989

Korn CS, Currier GW, Henderson SO: "Medical clearance" of psychiatric patients without medical complaints in the emergency department. J Emerg Med 18:173–176, 2000

Lazarou J, Pomeranz BH, Corey PN: Incidence of adverse drug reactions in hospitalized patients: a meta-analysis of prospective studies. JAMA 279:1200–1205, 1998

Lim KO, Tew W, Kushner M, et al: Cortical gray matter volume deficit in patients with first-episode schizophrenia. Am J Psychiatry 153:1548–1553, 1996

Liston EH, Gerner RH, Robertson AG, et al: Routine thoracic radiography for psychiatric inpatients. Hosp Community Psychiatry 30:474–476, 1979

Marangell LB, Martinez JM, Silver JM, et al: Concise Guide to Psychopharmacology. Washington, DC, American Psychiatric Publishing, 2002

McClellan RL, Eisenberg RL, Giyanani VL, et al: Routine CT screening of psychiatry inpatients. Radiology 169:99–100, 1988

Methodist Health Care System: Laboratory Medicine Handbook, 4th Edition. Hudson, OH, Lexi-Comp, 2001

Moles JK, Franchina JJ, Sforza PP: Increasing the clinical yield of computerized tomography for psychiatric patients. Gen Hosp Psychiatry 20:282–291, 1998

Mookhoek EJ, Sterrenburg-vdNieuwegiessen IM: Screening for somatic disease in elderly psychiatric patients. Gen Hosp Psychiatry 20:102–107, 1998

Mrazek DA: The context of genetic testing in clinical psychiatric practice. CNS Spectr 11:3–4, 2006

Nasrallah HA, Skinner TE, Schmalbrock P, et al: Proton magnetic resonance spectroscopy (1H MRS) of the hippocampal formation in schizophrenia: a pilot study. Br J Psychiatry 165:481–485, 1994

Nordahl TE, Benkelfat C, Semple WE, et al: Cerebral glucose metabolic rates in obsessive compulsive disorder. Neuropsychopharmacology 2:23–28, 1989

Nordahl TE, Carter CS, Salo RE, et al: Anterior cingulate metabolism correlates with Stroop errors in paranoid schizophrenia patients. Neuropsychopharmacology 25:139–148, 2001

Olshaker JS, Browne B, Jerrard DA, et al: Medical clearance and screening of psychiatric patients in the emergency department. Acad Emerg Med 4:124–128, 1997

Pellock JM, Willmore LJ: A rational guide to routine blood monitoring in patients receiving antiepileptic drugs. Neurology 41:961–964, 1991

Petersen RC, Thomas RG, Grundman M, et al: Vitamin E and donepezil for the treatment of mild cognitive impairment. N Engl J Med 352:2379–2388, 2005

Rauch SL, Renshaw PF: Clinical neuroimaging in psychiatry. Harv Rev Psychiatry 2:297–312, 1995

Reite M, Teale P, Rojas DC: Magnetoencephalography: applications in psychiatry. Biol Psychiatry 45:1553–1563, 1999

Renshaw PF, Parow AM, Hirashima F, et al: Multinuclear magnetic resonance spectroscopy studies of brain purines in major depression. Am J Psychiatry 158:2048–2055, 2001

Ringholz GR: Differential Diagnosis. Lecture presented at Current Neurology conference, Houston, Texas, November 2001

Sachse C, Brockmoller J, Bauer S, et al: Cytochrome P450 2D6 variants in a Caucasian population: allele frequencies and phenotypic consequences. Am J Hum Genet 60:284–295, 1997

Sadock BJ, Sadock VA: Laboratory tests in psychiatry, in Kaplan and Sadock's Synopsis of Psychiatry, 10th Edition. Baltimore, MD, Lippincott Williams & Wilkins, 2007, pp 255–267

Sagar M, Seensalu R, Tybring G, et al: CYP2C19 genotype and phenotype determined with omeprazole in patients with acid-related disorders with and without Helicobacter pylori infection. Scand J Gastroenterol 33:1034–1038, 1998

Sheline Y, Kehr C: Cost and utility of routine admission laboratory testing for psychiatric inpatients. Gen Hosp Psychiatry 12:329–334, 1990

Shenton ME, Dickey CC, Frumin M, et al: A review of MRI findings in schizophrenia. Schizophr Res 49:1–52, 2001

Soares JC, Boada F, Spencer S, et al: NAA and choline measures in the anterior cingulate of bipolar disorder patients (abstract). Biol Psychiatry 45 (8 suppl):119S, 1999

Sox HC Jr, Koran LM, Sox CH, et al: A medical algorithm for detecting physical disease in psychiatric patients. Hosp Community Psychiatry 40:1270–1276, 1989

Streetman DS: Metabolic basis of drug interactions in the intensive care unit. Crit Care Nurs Q 22:1–13, 2000

Swedo SE, Pietrini P, Leonard HL, et al: Cerebral glucose metabolism in childhood-onset obsessive-compulsive disorder: revisualization during pharmacotherapy. Arch Gen Psychiatry 49:690–694, 1992

Swedo SE, Schapiro MB, Grady CL, et al: Cerebral glucose metabolism in childhood-onset obsessive-compulsive disorder. Arch Gen Psychiatry 46:518–523, 1989

Taber KH, Pierpaoli C, Rose SE, et al: The future for diffusion tensor imaging in neuropsychiatry. J Neuropsychiatry Clin Neurosci 14:1–5, 2002

Tamminga CA, Thaker GK, Buchanan R, et al: Limbic system abnormalities identified in schizophrenia using positron emission tomography with fluorodeoxyglucose and neocortical alterations with deficit syndrome. Arch Gen Psychiatry 49:522–530, 1992

Videbech P: MRI findings in patients with affective disorder: a meta-analysis. Acta Psychiatr Scand 96:157–168, 1997

Wallach J: Interpretation of Diagnostic Tests. Boston, MA, Little, Brown, 1992

Wallach J: Interpretation of Diagnostic Tests, 7th Edition. Philadelphia, PA, Lippincott Williams & Wilkins, 2000

White AJ, Barraclough B: Benefits and problems of routine laboratory investigations in adult psychiatric admissions. Br J Psychiatry 155:65–72, 1989

Willett AB, King T: Implementation of laboratory screening procedures on a short-term psychiatric inpatient unit. Dis Nerv Syst 38:867–870, 1977

Willmore LJ, Triggs WJ, Pellock JM: Valproate toxicity: risk-screening strategies. J Child Neurol 6:3–6, 1991

Yurgelun-Todd DA, Renshaw PF, Gruber SA, et al: Proton magnetic resonance spectroscopy of the temporal lobes in schizophrenics and normal controls. Schizophr Res 19:55–59, 1996

3

THE ROLE OF PSYCHIATRIC MEASURES IN ASSESSMENT AND TREATMENT

John F. Clarkin, Ph.D.
Diane B. Howieson, Ph.D.
Joel McClough, Ph.D.

The current methodology and content of psychiatric diagnosis, the growing specificity of treatment planning in regard to both medication and psychosocial interventions, and the nature of the health care delivery system all influence the context that determines the use of psychological tests and rating scales to inform assessment and treatment planning. Two major forces have influenced treatment planning in the recent past: 1) the use of a diagnostic system, since 1980, that has been strong on reliability and relatively uneven on validity and 2) the impact of changes in the priorities and structure of the health care delivery system that place emphasis on cost saving and delivery of services deemed "medically necessary." Psychological assessment has evolved under these influences, resulting in a diversification of assessment approaches and foci.

In this chapter we discuss the objectives, forms, and utility of psychological assessment and provide an outline for considering the main areas of assessment. We review the most valid and established tests within this structure and present a clinical decision tree that relates both to the referral of patients for testing and to the selection of appropriate tests. Also, we review recent developments in the use of psychological testing in systems of care and "evidence-based" mental health treatment.

We wish to thank the authors who assisted on previous versions of this chapter: S.W. Hurt, S. Mattis, and E. Fertuck.

Definition and Development of Psychological Assessment Instruments

Three types of instruments are currently used in the assessment of patient functioning: psychological tests, rating scales, and semistructured interviews (Table 3–1). Psychological tests are standardized methods of sampling behaviors in a reliable and valid way. The test stimuli, the method of presenting these stimuli, and the method of scoring the responses are carefully standardized to ensure reliability. The actual test stimuli can be constructed in numerous ways. For example, test items on the Wechsler Adult Intelligence Scale—Third Edition (WAIS-III; Wechsler 1997a), a widely used intelligence test, include factual questions (e.g., "What does ponder mean?"), and each answer is scored 2 (i.e., to contemplate), 1 (i.e., to wonder), or 0 (i.e., to fret). The restandardized Minnesota Multiphasic Personality Inventory–2 (MMPI-2; Butcher et al. 1989), a highly developed and widely used symptom and personality test, consists of questions about presence or absence of specific feelings, thoughts, and experiences (e.g., "I usually feel that life is worthwhile," an item on Scale 2) in a true/false format. Test stimuli on the Rorschach (Rorschach 1949), a projective test of personality styles and characteristics, are amorphous inkblots (Figure 3–1). The patient is asked to tell the examiner what the blots look like or what they remind the patient of. The response is recorded verbatim and scored with a standardized system.

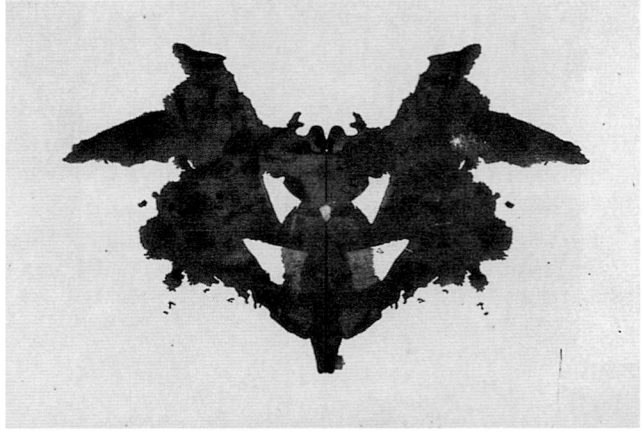

FIGURE 3–1. Rorschach, Card I.

Source. Reprinted with permission from Rorschach H: *Rorschach Test.* Psychodiagnostics Plates. Copyright Verlag Hans Huber, Hoegrefe AG, Bern, Switzerland, 1921, 1948, 1994.

TABLE 3–1. Three types of psychological assessment instruments

Type	Example
Psychological tests	Wechsler Adult Intelligence Scale–Third Edition Minnesota Multiphasic Personality Inventory–2
Rating scales	Brief Psychiatric Rating Scale
Semistructured interviews	Structured Clinical Interview for DSM-IV Axis I Disorders International Personality Disorder Examination

Behavior rating scales are standardized devices that allow various informants or observers (e.g., therapist, nurse on a clinical inpatient unit, relatives, trained observers) to rate the behavior of the patient in specified areas. To aid the observer in a reliable rating of the behavior, anchor points are provided in one of several ways. For example, on the Brief Psychiatric Rating Scale (BPRS; Overall and Gorham 1962), somatic concern, defined as the "degree of concern over present bodily health," is rated by the interviewer on a seven-point scale from "not present" to "extremely severe." Commonly used rating scales, to be discussed later in this chapter, include the BPRS, the Hamilton Rating Scale for Depression (HRSD; Hamilton 1960, 1967), and the Katz Adjustment Scales (Katz and Lyerly 1963).

Semistructured interviews are standardized by controlling the questions, including specifying what kind of probes can be used, and standardizing the scoring of the patient's response, often by using rating scales as described earlier. Although developed for research, these interviews have clinical usefulness in the reliable assessment of diagnostic criteria. As an example of a semistructured interview item, the following is a question from the Structured Clinical Interview for DSM-IV Axis I Disorders (SCID-I; First et al. 1995): "In the last month, has there been a period of time when you were feeling depressed or down most of the day nearly every day?" The subject's response is rated on a scale of 1 (absent or false), 2 (subthreshold), or 3 (threshold, or true). Useful semistructured interviews include the Schedule for Affective Disorders and Schizophrenia (SADS; Endicott and Spitzer 1979), the SCID-I, and the International Personality Disorder Examination (IPDE; Loranger 1999).

The science of assessment depends on the development of instruments that meet certain standards. Chief among these standards are those for reliability and various types of validity. Standardization of administration and scoring to minimize the influence of factors unrelated to the area of assessment is essential for establishing reliability. The degree to which a test meets acceptable standards for reliability is evaluated by readministering the test at later times to determine if individual scores remain stable; developing alternative forms of the test that, when compared, provide roughly equivalent scores for an individual; and demonstrating that any subgroup of items from the test yields a score comparable with an equivalent number of items in any other subgroup of items. These procedures for establishing reliability are generally referred to as test–retest reliability, alternate form reliability, and split-half reliability, respectively (Table 3–2).

Demonstration of adequate test reliability is only the first step in test development. It establishes that the test items are sufficiently closely related to one another to provide relatively stable measurements. However, a test's reliability does not guarantee its validity. Establishing a test's validity requires demonstration that the test measures what it is intended to measure. Three major types of validity can be assessed: content validity, criterion-related validity, and construct validity. *Content validity* can be achieved only if the content of the test can be said to adequately sample the area of interest. For example, an intelligence test must contain items that tap several areas of intellectual functioning, such as knowledge of words, arithmetic ability, abstracting ability, knowledge of social conventions, and so forth, in order to meet acceptable standards for content validity. *Criterion-related validity* refers to the test's relationship to independent criteria of an individual's ability in a particular area (i.e., concurrent validity) or to the ability of the test to make predictions about future behavior (i.e., predictive validity). For example, a test of the severity of depressive symptoms would achieve concurrent validity if scores on the test were closely related to a trained observer's rating of the severity of the depression, and it would achieve predictive validity if scores on the test were found to be related to the likelihood that a given individual would respond to a specific treatment for reducing depressive symptoms. *Construct validity* can be achieved only by demonstrating that the test specifically measures a theoretical construct of interest and that scores on the test are unrelated to similar areas.

If a clinician needs to determine whether a test will be valid with a patient from another culture, there are specific psychometric procedures the instrument should have undergone. These include translation of

Type	Description
TABLE 3–2.	**Types of reliability and validity**
	Reliability
Test–retest	Test yields comparable scores at two proximate points in time
Alternate form	Two forms of the same test yield comparable scores
Split-half	Subgroups of items yield scores comparable with those of other subgroups of items
	Validity
Content	Items adequately sample the content area
Criterion related	Test score correlates with other measurements of the same area of activity
Construct	Test measures a theoretical construct and is unrelated to similar but different constructs

the test from English to the patient's native language, subsequent norming and validation of the translated test, and demonstration of the new test's relevance to the target cultural group (Geisinger 1994).

Despite the importance of cultural factors in the assessment process, few tests have been adequately developed to address the test biases that could influence important clinical decisions such as diagnosis, severity of psychopathology, and intelligence/achievement levels. However, the MMPI-2 is an instrument that has been restandardized and normed on adolescents, ethnic minority groups, non-English cultures, and the elderly (Butcher 1998). It is recommended for personality assessment in diverse cultures. Also, intelligence can be assessed in a culturally and linguistically fair manner by using nonverbal tests of intelligence or by utilizing an interpreter during the testing process.

For further information on the general principles of assessment, tests, and test construction, one may consult Anastasi (1982) and Cronbach and Meehl (1955). Also, the Mental Measurements Yearbooks, edited by Buros (1971, 1978), provide excellent reviews of existing instruments. One can also consult Newman and Ciarlo (1994) for criteria that can be used to select instruments for various tasks. A useful compendium to this chapter and extensive review of psychiatric measures is the Second Edition of the *Handbook of Psychiatric Measures* (Rush et al. 2008).

Goals of Assessment

The role of assessment has always been closely linked to the need to conceptualize and implement successful intervention strategies for the remediation of psychological disorders. As a consequence, the goals of assessment should constantly be revised as new treatment methods are developed. Common assessment goals are listed in Table 3–3.

Diagnostic assessment remains the primary reason for clinical psychiatric referral. DSM-IV (American Psychiatric Association 1994) and its text update, DSM-IV-TR (American Psychiatric Association 2000) provide a focus for diagnostic issues and simultaneously capitalize on and fuel a growing interest in the issues of accurate diagnosis. Much of the research stimulated by the development and implementation of DSM-III (American Psychiatric Association 1980) and its successors focused on the sensitivity and specificity of the diagnostic criteria with the aim of identifying groups of symptoms that are optimally responsive to the growing armamentarium of psychiatric and psychological interventions. This kind of research represented a shift from the idiographic approach, typical of earlier psychiatric research, to a more nomothetic approach. Under the latter approach, the goals of assessment are to relate the individual features of test performance to patterns of performance typical of certain diagnostic groups rather than to highlight the unique aspects of any one individual's performance (Hurt et al. 1991).

This shift in emphasis suggests that assessment is much more likely to be tailored to specific aspects of the referral and to the salient dimensions of information that constitute the differential. For example, depressed mood is featured as a criterion for a number of DSM-IV-TR disorders, including major depression, atypical depression, bipolar disorder, dysthymia, adjustment disorder with depressed mood, schizoaffective disorder, and borderline personality disorder. Because each of these different disorders is optimally responsive to a different treatment, and because attempts to ameliorate the depressed mood itself may require different intervention strategies for some of these disorders, the goal of differential diagnosis takes on added value. The clinical psychologist, therefore, must carefully choose the instruments for the assessment in light of the need for distinguishing among these disorders.

Differential treatment planning, then, is at the heart of the assessment process and provides the rationale for the diagnostic effort. In the absence of treatment

TABLE 3–3. Specific objectives of assessment
1. Screening for psychiatric disturbance
2. Clarification of diagnostic uncertainty following clinical interview
3. Specification of the severity of symptoms and other difficulties
4. Assessment of patient strengths
5. Informing differential treatment assignment
6. Role-inducing the patient into a therapeutic stance
7. Monitoring the impact of treatment over time
8. Assessment of barriers to learning for educational planning
9. Assessment of quality and cost-effectiveness of systems of care

specificity, there is little justification for an intensive focus on diagnosis. Although the science of differential therapeutics is in its infancy, the proliferation of medication and treatment approaches and modalities has spawned a growing literature on the assessment of various characteristics and dimensions that are thought to be essential to the understanding of and rational treatment planning for the various disorders. Often, there is a close relationship between Axis I diagnosis and medication treatment targets (e.g., major depression). The relationship between diagnosis and psychotherapy is likewise closely related with certain Axis I disorders such as anxiety and depression. However, there are many nondiagnostic patient issues that affect the psychotherapeutic selection and process. A recent extensive review of this area suggested that there are six major patient variables that are central to psychotherapy treatment planning: functional impairment, subjective distress, social support, problem complexity and chronicity, reactance, and coping styles (Beutler et al. 2000).

A ready example of this kind of development can be found in the literature on depression. Drawing on the infrahuman learning literature, A.T. Beck and Young (1985) argued that cognitions such as hopelessness, helplessness, and worthlessness are essential for understanding depression. This cognitive theory of depression has been sufficiently well elaborated to lead to the development of rating scales that are sensitive to these cognitions and to the design of an appropriate treatment approach.

Clinical Decision Tree

Psychiatrists should be clear about the precise areas for assessment before referring a patient for testing. Likewise, clinical psychologists should pursue testing with efficiency and utilize instruments that will answer the referral questions with precision, reliability, and validity. Both psychiatrists and psychologists should make use of a clinical decision tree that informs their differential therapeutic procedures.

At the present state of knowledge, we suggest that before referring a patient for assessment, the psychiatrist should complete a semistructured interview (or methodical clinical interview) that elicits information about which DSM-IV-TR criteria (on both Axis I and Axis II) the patient meets. Armed with this diagnostic information, the clinical psychologist can pursue questions about the patient along any one or mix of the axes that we describe in this chapter—symptoms, personality traits, cognitive functioning, psychodynamics, and environment and social adjustment—by selecting and administering tests, interviews, and rating scales with the overall goal of informed differential therapeutics. Which of the five axes the psychologist pursues will depend on which DSM-IV-TR criteria the patient meets and the nature of the pathology that requires further explication.

Psychological assessment currently takes many forms. Depending on the objective of the assessment, the clinician can decide on the types of tests, the number of tests, and the level of expertise required to complete the assessment. The most common forms of assessment include screening, diagnostic/treatment planning assessment, and neurocognitive/neuropsychological assessment.

Psychological screening is typically done with self-report instruments during the initial evaluation and periodically during and after the treatment process to assess the severity, complexity, and type of distress in a quick, cost-effective manner. The scoring and interpretation of these instruments are straightforward and can be done with reliability and validity by most clinicians. The Symptom Checklist–90—Revised (SCL-90-R; Derogatis 1977, 1983), discussed later in this chapter, is commonly used and recommended for initial and periodic screening in psychiatric settings. If a screening and standard psychiatric interview do not adequately clarify the referral question, referral to a psychologist for more elaborate assessment may be recommended.

The indications for assessment vary with the setting in which the assessment is conducted and the typical patient encountered in that setting. In clinical psychiat-ric settings, assessment is most often requested to aid in reducing uncertainty regarding diagnosis and in evaluating the severity of specific symptoms or symptom complexes (e.g., depression, suicide intent, thought disorder). Such an assessment plays an important role in providing information on patients that can be usefully generalized by facilitating comparisons between patients or by tracking the severity of symptoms under the impact of treatment. This assessment may form the basis for recommended treatments, help in establishing goals for the general treatment plan, or assist in determining treatment progress and the need for further intervention.

Historically, inpatient settings have focused on the question of differential diagnosis. In day hospital settings, referrals often emphasize the need for assessment of specific cognitive, vocational, and social assets that can be adaptively employed in helping the patient return to full participation in community life.

In general outpatient settings, psychological assessment can uniquely address a variety of clinical issues. Common referral questions include the following:

- *"Does this patient exhibit a thought disorder indicative of a diagnosis of psychosis?"* The answer to this question will clarify whether and what type of medication may be required and the form of psychosocial intervention that is optimal (e.g., an exploratory or supportive psychotherapy).

- *"What is the cognitive ability (e.g., intelligence) of this patient?"* This common referral question will inform clinicians as to whether the patient may require special education and/or whether the patient has the intellectual capacity to benefit from psychosocial interventions, which usually require at least average intelligence.

- *"What type of personality characteristics does this patient have, and how might these affect the patient's ability to utilize treatment—in particular, psychotherapy?"* Factors such as the presence of a personality disorder, a treatment-resistant personality profile, a tendency toward deception, and level of psychological sophistication can all predict treatment dropout, adherence, and success rates. Behavior therapists working in a phobia clinic may be particularly interested in the interaction between fear and situation so as to successfully plan a program of desensitization. A psychoanalyst may refer a patient for psychological assessment early in treatment to determine the patient's capacity for long-term psychodynamic psychotherapy and to assess the status of various transference paradigms that would help him or her to tailor the patient's treatment.

Neurocognitive and neuropsychological assessments are increasingly valuable forms of assessment that measure impairments in how patients process information and examine how these impairments might be affected by brain–behavior relationships. In neurology clinics, referral for assessment is frequently made to more specifically identify the nature and degree of impairment, particularly in children and elderly persons. Because the symptoms overlap, a common question for referral is, "Does this geriatric patient have dementia or depression?" Different answers to this question will lead to quite different treatment approaches. Another common referral question is, "Is this patient's cognitive profile indicative of possible brain damage, such as from a stroke?" Finally, neuropsychological assessment can be used to answer the question, "Does this patient have a learning disability that affects his or her ability to perform academically?" Because of the training in administration, scoring, and interpretation required with neuropsychological batteries, this type of assessment demands the expertise of a clinical psychologist or clinical neuropsychologist and the administration of several tests (a battery) in a reliable and standardized manner. Furthermore, the scoring, interpretation, and synthesis of the information require supervised training. Therefore, these assessments, unlike screening assessments, require the expertise of a clinical psychologist.

Cultural Factors in Psychological Assessment

The results from the psychological tests described previously must be carefully considered in the context of the patient's culture, subculture, gender, age, and linguistic competence. The Multicultural Assessment Procedure (Ridley et al. 1998) is a flexible and pragmatic clinical procedure that allows clinicians to meaningfully incorporate cultural data into the assessment process. The principles of the procedure can be applied to all clinical data, whether from a standard interview or from psychological testing. The four phases of the procedure are reviewed in Table 3–4.

Major Areas of Assessment

To further the overall goal of clinical assessment (i.e., differential treatment planning), one must consider the most important content areas of assessment. The assessment procedures chosen should depend on the

---

TABLE 3–4. The Multicultural Assessment Procedure

1. *Identify cultural data during the initial interview.* Cultural variables include level of acculturation, economic issues, history of oppression, language, experience of racism and prejudice, sociopolitical issues (e.g., citizenship status, level of political activity), methods of child rearing, religious and spiritual practices, family composition, and cultural values (e.g., attitudes toward time, property, family, work, gender, sexuality, leisure).

2. *Interpret the cultural data.* Arrive at a working hypothesis regarding the impact of cultural variables on the patient's clinical presentation. The working hypothesis requires careful consideration of the relative contributions of the patient's current stressors, clinical presentation, experience with racism, psychiatric history, and reality testing.

3. *Incorporate the cultural data.* Measure the working hypothesis against additional data and criteria, such as medical evaluation, psychological tests, and DSM-IV-TR diagnostic criteria.

4. *Arrive at a sound assessment decision.* Once the working hypothesis has been tested with additional data, devise an assessment and treatment plan that meaningfully and fairly incorporates the cultural data.

---

nature of the patient's difficulties revealed or suspected during routine psychiatric examination. They should be carried out in the context of the major dimensions of human functioning relevant to diagnosis and treatment planning. The areas or dimensions of human functioning that seem most central for diagnosis and treatment planning include 1) symptoms and related Axis I disorders, 2) cognitive functioning, 3) personality traits and disorders, 4) psychodynamics, and 5) environmental demands and social adjustment. In the subsections that follow we review the best available instruments in each of these five areas.

Assessment of Axis I Constellations and Related Symptoms

As psychiatric nomenclature has undergone revision, assessment tools have been developed that rely on interviews and self-reports (Table 3–5), providing data that are immediately relevant to diagnosis.

TABLE 3–5. Instruments for the assessment of DSM-IV Axis I disorders and related symptom patterns

Instrument	General classification	Description	Scoring features
DSM-IV Axis I disorders			
Structured Clinical Interview for DSM-IV Axis I Disorders (SCID-I); Patient Edition (SCID-I/P); Non-Patient Edition (SCID-I/NP); Clinician Version (SCID-CV)	Semistructured interview	Three-point rating scales of symptoms	Oriented to diagnosis using DSM-IV
Related symptom patterns			
Minnesota Multiphasic Personality Inventory—2	Self-report	567-item checklist, true/false format	*T* scores for 13 criterion scales
Symptom Checklist–90—Revised	Self-report	90-item checklist, 5-point intensity scales	*T* scores for 9 symptom clusters
Brief Symptom Inventory	Self-report	53-item checklist, 5-point intensity scales	*T* scores for 9 symptom clusters
Brief Psychiatric Rating Scale	Clinical interview	16 items, 7-point severity scales	5 factor scores and total scores
Personality Assessment Inventory	Self-report	344 items, true/false format	4 validity scales, 10 clinical scales covering symptoms and severe personality disorders
Millon Clinical Multiaxial Inventory—III	Self-report	175 items, true/false format	3 validity scales, 22 clinical scales covering Axis I and II areas

The SADS represents this tradition. Developed in the 1970s at the New York State Psychiatric Institute, the SADS was designed as a semistructured interview instrument to gather information pertinent to the classification of psychiatric disorders. Its primary purpose was to provide information that was sufficient to classify patients into relatively homogeneous subgroups for the purposes of research (Endicott and Spitzer 1979). These classifications were explicated through use of the Research Diagnostic Criteria (Feighner et al. 1972), which specified explicit symptomatic criteria for 23 psychiatric disorders. These criteria served as the forerunner to DSM-III and have, in the main, been incorporated into that version of psychiatric nomenclature. Using the same semistructured interview format and item rating procedures, Spitzer et al. (1992) developed the SCID-I (First et al. 1995), which directly orients the diagnostic process to the Axis I and Axis II categories of the DSM system. The SCID-I is designed specifically for use in research settings and is available

in three editions that differ based on the type of subjects being interviewed. The SCID-I/P (Patient Edition) is simply the SCID-I designed for subjects who have been identified as psychiatric patients; the SCID-I/NP is the Non-Patient Edition and is intended for research subjects who identify themselves as nonpsychiatric patients, often seen in general medical, primary care, or community settings. The third research version is the SCID-I/P With Psychotic Screen, designed for psychiatric patients who most likely do not require a comprehensive assessment of psychotic disorders. The SCID-Clinician Version (SCID-CV; First et al. 1997b) covers only the diagnoses most frequently encountered in clinical practice and excludes most of the specifiers and subtypes found in the research versions. In addition, the Mood and Substance Abuse modules in the clinician version are greatly simplified.

With their explicit focus on psychiatric classification, the SADS and the SCID have acquired all of the problems inherent in adopting the present psychiatric nomenclature as the reference point for assessment. Chief among these problems is the insufficient validation of the diagnostic categories themselves. However, as tools for investigating the range, severity, frequency, and duration of symptomatic disturbance and for training in the formal interview assessment of psychopathology, these instruments are an important part of the assessment armamentarium.

Omnibus Measures of Symptoms

A number of instruments have been developed for the assessment of a wide variety of symptoms (see Table 3–5). These measures depend on either self-report or interview methods for data collection.

Minnesota Multiphasic Personality Inventory

The MMPI (Hathaway and McKinley 1967) and its successor, the MMPI-2 (Hathaway and McKinley 1989), are probably the most widely used assessment instruments in existence. There are several reasons for the MMPI's extensive use, including its efficiency (the patient spends 1–2 hours taking the test, which can then be computer scored), the extensive data accumulated with the test, its normative base, the use of validity scales that indicate the patient's test-taking attitude, and its impressive cross-cultural validation. Although labeled as a personality test, the MMPI was constructed to assess what are now categorized as Axis I conditions and, to a lesser extent, a few dimensions of personality not represented on Axis II.

The MMPI was developed in the 1940s by J. Charnley McKinley, a psychiatrist, and Starke R. Hathaway, a psychologist. Items were generated from lists of psychiatric symptoms and complaints found in the current textbooks of psychiatry and previously constructed personality inventories. Beginning with a large pool of such items, McKinley and Hathaway used the method of contrasting criterion groups to construct several psychopathological scales. For example, a Hypochondriasis scale measuring the degree of concern with bodily health was developed on the basis of items frequently endorsed by patients with hypochondriasis uncomplicated by psychosis or other psychiatric disorders. The patients' responses to the MMPI items were contrasted with those of friends or relatives who visited the University Hospitals in Minneapolis, Minnesota. Using this method of criterion-keyed scoring, McKinley and Hathaway constructed nine clinical scales: Hypochondriasis (Scale 1), Depression (Scale 2), Hysteria (Scale 3), Psychopathic Deviance (Scale 4), Masculinity–Femininity (Scale 5), Paranoia (Scale 6),

Psychasthenia (Scale 7), Schizophrenia (Scale 8), and Mania (Scale 9) (Table 3–6). Items were worded so that persons with an elementary school education could take the test, and norms were established for determining the degree of disturbance typical of psychopathological groups. For example, an item on Scale 2 (i.e., Depression) reads as follows: "I find it hard to keep my mind on a task or job (True)."

TABLE 3–6.   Scales of the Minnesota Multiphasic Personality Inventory—2

Scale	Characteristics of high scorers
Validity scales	
Lie	Dishonest, deceptive, and/or defended
Infrequency	Exhibit randomness of responses or psychotic psychopathology
Correction/ defensiveness	Defensive through presenting themselves as healthier than they are
Clinical scales	
Hypochondriasis	Somatizers, possible medical problems
Depression	Dysphoric, possibly suicidal
Hysteria	Highly reactive to stress, anxious, and sad at times
Psychopathic deviance	Antisocial, dishonest, possible drug abusers
Masculinity– femininity	Exhibit lack of stereotypical masculine interests, aesthetic and artistic
Paranoia	Exhibit disturbed thinking, ideas of persecution, possibly psychotic
Psychasthenia	Exhibit psychological turmoil and discomfort, extreme anxiety
Schizophrenia	Confused, disorganized, possible hallucinations
Hypomania	Manic, emotionally labile, unrealistic self-appraisal
Social introversion	Very insecure and uncomfortable in social situations, timid

In addition to the clinical scales, validity scales were developed to assess the test-taking attitudes of the patient. McKinley et al. (1948) focused on the assessment of defensiveness or of minimizing symptoms and problems (faking good) and maximizing or exaggerating problems (faking bad). Validity scales were constructed to evaluate these dimensions, which are helpful in interpreting the severity of symptomatic complaints on the clinical scales.

The MMPI has been revised and restandardized as the MMPI-2. Revisions include the deletion of objectionable items and the rewording of other items to reflect more modern language usage, as well as the addition of several new items focusing on suicide, drug and alcohol abuse, Type A behavior, interpersonal relations, and treatment compliance. Restandardization of the norms was based on a randomly solicited national sample of 1,138 males and 1,462 females.

Clinical interpretation of the MMPI-2 is not, however, simply a matter of noting a scale that is high relative to these norms and assigning that diagnosis to the patient (e.g., a patient with a high Schizophrenia [Scale 8] score would not necessarily receive a schizophrenia diagnosis). Instead, relying on an extensive clinical database, typical symptomatic and personality dysfunctions are described on the basis of two- and three-point codes (Greene 1991). For example, individuals with a 2–4–8 three-point code (scores above 70 on Scales 2, 4, and 8) are described as typically distrustful of people, keeping others at a distance, afraid of emotional involvement, using projection and rationalization as defenses, argumentative and sensitive to anything that can be construed as a demand, and unpredictable and changeable in behavior and attitudes (Marks and Seeman 1963). Research has indicated that many patients with this code exhibit symptoms that fulfill criteria for borderline personality disorder (Hurt et al. 1985).

Personality Assessment Inventory

The Personality Assessment Inventory (PAI; Morey 1991) focuses on clinical syndromes that have been staples of psychopathological nosology and have retained their importance in contemporary diagnostic practice. Items were written with careful attention to their content validity, which was designed to reflect the phenomenology of the clinical construct across a broad range of severity. An initial pool of 2,200 items was generated from the research literature, classic texts, DSM, and other diagnostic manuals and from the clinical experience of practitioners who participated in the project. This pool of items was finally reduced to 344 items covering 4 validity scales, 11 clini-

cal syndromes, 5 treatment planning areas, and the 2 major dimensions of the interpersonal complex. All items are rated with a four-point Likert-type response format. For example, on the borderline scale is the following item: "I'm too impulsive for my own good." Final clinical validation was carried out on the data from 235 subjects from 10 clinical sites and 2 community and 2 college student samples.

The Millon Clinical Multiaxial Inventory

The Millon Clinical Multiaxial Inventory–III (MCMI-III; Millon et al. 1997)) is a 175-item true/false self-report instrument that yields scores on 11 clinical personality patterns closely related to Millon's theory of personality and psychopathology, the personality disorder diagnoses of DSM-IV Axis II, and nine clinical syndromes. Probably the major difficulty with this instrument is psychometric in nature, because there is much item overlap in the scales resulting in difficulties in interpretation. In the MCMI-II (Millon 1987), a revision of the original scale, two new personality disorder scales were introduced and two of the original personality scales were modified. For the third version of the instrument, 95 new items were added, but it is unclear how they differ from items previously included. It has been suggested that the MCMI-III should be best used primarily as a measure of Millon's theoretical conceptualization of personality and secondarily as a means of identifying personality disorder diagnoses according to DSM-IV criteria (Kaye and Shea 2000).

Symptom Checklist–90—Revised

The SCL-90-R (Derogatis 1994) is a relatively recent revision of a much-used self-report instrument designed to provide information about a broad range of complaints typical of individuals with psychological symptomatic distress. Briefer than the MMPI-2 and the PAI, the SCL-90-R contains only 90 items and can be administered in 30 minutes and scored by computer. These items are combined into nine symptom scales: 1) somatization, 2) obsessive-compulsive behavior, 3) interpersonal sensitivity, 4) depression, 5) anxiety, 6) hostility, 7) phobic anxiety, 8) paranoid ideation, and 9) psychoticism. In addition, three global indices are compiled: 1) general severity, 2) positive symptom distress index, and 3) total positive symptoms. The criterion group method was not used in the development of this test; rather, the content validity and internal consistency of the items guided the construction of the scales.

A companion instrument, the Hopkins Psychiatric Rating Scale (Derogatis et al. 1974), can be used to rate material obtained through direct interview of the patient on each of the nine symptom dimensions of the SCL-90-R. No structured interview procedure is associated with the Hopkins scale, so formal training in the interview assessment of psychopathology is essential to the accuracy of the assessment. Eight additional dimensions are covered in the interview.

The Brief Symptom Inventory (BSI; Derogatis 1993) is a 53-item self-report form of the SCL-90-R that assesses the same nine symptom dimensions and three global indices but is composed of a subset of items selected from the SCL-90-R with the heaviest loadings on the nine primary symptoms dimensions so that the same symptom constructs could be reliably and validly measured. The psychometric properties of the BSI are comparable with the SCL-90-R, and it has the advantage of increased ease of administration, taking only 8–10 minutes to complete. The scale is appropriate for a broad range of individuals and offers an excellent brief assessment of the patient's clinical status.

Brief Psychiatric Rating Scale

Another widely used rating scale for a range of psychiatric symptoms is the BPRS (Overall and Gorham 1962), which was developed mainly for the assessment of symptoms with an inpatient population. Areas rated include somatic concern, anxiety, emotional withdrawal, conceptual disorganization, guilt, tension, mannerisms and posturing, grandiosity, depressive mood, hostility, suspiciousness, hallucinatory behavior, motor retardation, uncooperativeness, unusual thought content, blunted affect, excitement, and disorientation.

The MMPI-2, PAI, SCL-90-R, BSI, Hopkins Psychiatric Rating Scale, and BPRS represent efforts to develop procedures for the general assessment of psychopathology that meet standards of test construction. These procedures provide coverage of symptomatically distressing areas that are independent of psychiatric classifications. However, through the extensive use of these procedures in psychiatric settings, a large body of literature has developed that relates the findings of these tests to diagnostic categories favored in such settings.

Specific Areas of Symptomatology

In addition to the omnibus measures of symptomatology, there are a number of instruments that assess one area of symptomatology in depth (Table 3–7). The major constellations of symptoms that may require assessment are 1) substance abuse, including abuse of food, alcohol, and drugs; 2) affects such as anxiety, elation, and depression; 3) thought disorder; and 4) suicidal intentions and behaviors.

Substance Abuse

Psychological distress and dysfunction arising from the abuse of a wide variety of substances is perhaps the chief reason for seeking psychological or psychiatric treatment. The treatment of alcoholism, drug abuse, and eating disorders, combined with the income lost, probably consumes more health dollars than does any other group of disorders. Thus, the identification of these disorders deserves careful attention. The threat to the validity of self-report screening instruments to detect substance abuse is such that these instruments should be buttressed by the assessment of biological markers (e.g., urine and blood) and reports from other informants. However, it is helpful to review the instruments that have been used for this purpose (see Table 3–7). The prominent instruments in this area are the MacAndrew Alcoholism Scale (MacAndrew 1965), the Addiction Potential Scale from the MMPI-2 (Weed et al. 1992), and Scales B (Alcohol Dependence) and T (Drug Dependence) from the MCMI-III.

The assessment of substance abuse potential is reflected in omnibus symptom rating scales such as the MMPI-2, which contains an item key, the MacAndrew Alcoholism Scale, for identifying patients who have histories of alcohol abuse or who have the potential to develop problems with alcohol (Hoffmann et al. 1974). A more thorough instrument, the Alcohol Use Inventory (Horn et al. 1986), is a self-administered test standardized on over 1,200 admissions to an alcoholism treatment program. It contains 24 scales that measure alcohol-related problems and considers the subjects' responses in four separate domains: benefits from drinking, style of drinking, consequences of drinking, and concerns associated with drinking.

The Addiction Severity Index (McLellan et al. 1980) is a 142-item multidimensional, semistructured interview designed to be used as a guide for initial assessment and treatment planning for patients presenting with substance abuse disorders in both inpatient and outpatient settings. Information is gathered on seven problem areas frequently affected by substance abuse: medical status, employment and support, drug use, alcohol use, legal status, family or social status, and psychiatric status. Items include both objective indicators and subjective assessment of problem severity. Its major strengths include its coverage of a wide range of abused substances, its focus on multiple problem areas, and its extensive normative data.

TABLE 3–7. Instruments for the assessment of specific symptom areas

Instrument	General classification	Description	Scoring features
Substance abuse			
Alcohol Use Inventory	Self-report	228 items rated on 2- to 6-point scales	17 primary scales in four areas and 7 second-order factor scales
Addiction Severity Index	Semistructured interview	142 items rated on 5-point subjective assessment scale and 10-point severity scale	7 functional areas of problems with substances
University of Rhode Island Change Assessment	Self-report or interview	32 items, 5-point scale	4 scores corresponding to 4 stages of change
Eating Disorders Inventory—2	Self-report	91 forced-choice items rated on a 6-point frequency scale	8 subscales and 3 provisional scales for issues and features pertinent to eating disorders
Affects			
State–Trait Anxiety Inventory	Self-report	Two 20-item scales, 4-point frequency ratings	Total scores for state and trait anxiety
S-R Inventory of Anxiousness	Self-report	14-item responses on 5-point severity scales to 11 situations	Focus on intensity and quality of situations arousing anxiety
Fear Questionnaire	Self-report	17 items reflecting specific phobias rated on 9-point avoidance scales	Total scores for agoraphobia, social phobia, and blood and injury phobias
Beck Anxiety Scale	Self-report	21 items, 4-point scale	Total score
Panic Disorder Severity Scale	Clinical interview	7 items, 5-point scale	Total score
Beck Depression Inventory	Self-report	20 items, 4-point intensity scales	Total score
Hamilton Rating Scale for Depression	Clinical interview	17–24 items, 3- to 5-point severity scales	Total score
Geriatric Depression Scale	Self-report	30 items, yes/no, 10 negatively keyed, 20 positively keyed	Total number of depressive responses endorsed
Manic-State Rating Scale	Observer rating	26 items, each scored for frequency and intensity	Total score
State–Trait Anger Inventory	Self-report		Total scores for state and trait anger

TABLE 3–7. Instruments for the assessment of specific symptom areas *(continued)*

Instrument	General classification	Description	Scoring features
Affects *(continued)*			
Anger, Irritability, and Assault Questionnaire	Self-report	42 questions, 5 time frames, 210 items	5 subscales, 3 overarching scales
Suicidal behavior			
Suicide Intent Scale	Self-report	15 items, 3-point categorical scales	Total score
Index of Potential Suicide	Self-report or semistructured interview	50 items, 5-point severity scales	Total score and 6 subscores
Reasons for Living Inventory	Self-report	6 factors	Total score
Thought disorder			
Thought Disorder Index	Content rating	22 categories at 4 levels of severity	Total score
Positive and Negative Syndrome Scale	Semistructured interview	30 items, 7-point scale	3 scale scores, option for composite score and conversion to *T* scores
Scale for Assessment of Positive Symptoms	Observer rating	30 items, 6-point scale	4 global domain scores, summary score, and composite score

The University of Rhode Island Change Assessment (McConnaughy et al. 1983) is a measure developed to assess a patient's readiness to change to address issues related to the use of drugs, alcohol, and nicotine. The instrument is based on Prochaska et al.'s (1992) Readiness to Change Stage model. According to the model, behavioral change is related to a sequential series of stages associated with various motivational states and decisions. The subscales define four stages of change: Precontemplation, Contemplation, Action, and Maintenance. Treatment recommendations can therefore be based on the patient's stage of change readiness.

Garner (1992) developed a multidimensional self-report measure to assess attitudes, behaviors, and traits associated with anorexia nervosa and bulimia nervosa. This inventory, the Eating Disorders Inventory–2, consists of 91 items rated on 6-point frequency scales that form 11 subscales. The items were chosen to reflect important clinical aspects of anorexia and were retained if they successfully discriminated between anorexic, normal-weight, and obese males and females. Internal reliability, construct validity, and treatment response data have been reported, and the inventory can be a useful screening instrument for identifying inpatients with potentially serious eating disorders. Normative data are available for individuals with anorexia, bulimia, junior high boys and girls, high school boys and girls, and college-age men and women.

Affects

The content, range, and management of emotional expression constitute a symptomatic area of focus for the evaluation of psychopathology and are important in the differential diagnosis of a wide variety of psychiatric disorders. The main affects of interest are anxiety, depression, aggression, and elation.

As one factor in the larger context of the total personality, anxiety can be assessed with the 16–Personality Factor Inventory (Cattell et al. 1970), the Eysenck Personality Inventory (Eysenck and Eysenck 1969), and the Taylor Manifest Anxiety Scale (Taylor-Spence and Spence 1966), a scale derived from the MMPI.

Other instruments assess only anxiety or other forms of fearfulness and thus may be more clinically useful as dimensional measures of the severity of anxiety or in the identification of specific situational anxiety that will become the focus of intervention. The Anxiety Status Inventory is a rating scale for anxiety developed for clinical use adhering to an interview guide, and the Self-Rating Anxiety Scale is a compan-

ion self-report instrument, both developed by Zung (1971). Both scales assess a wide range of anxiety-related behaviors: fear, panic, physical symptoms of fear, nightmares, and cognitive effects. These scales are recommended for the serial measurement of the effects of therapy on anxiety states. Hamilton (1959) devised an anxiety rating scale that is parallel to the HRSD but is less frequently used.

The Beck Anxiety Scale (A.T. Beck et al. 1988) is a 21-item self-report questionnaire with a focus on somatic anxiety symptoms, such as heart pounding, nervousness, inability to relax, and dizziness or light-headedness. Items are rated on a 4-point scale ranging from 0 (not at all) to 3 (severely: I could barely stand it). This measure takes approximately 5 minutes to complete and was designed specifically to discriminate between anxiety and depression. Although the measure does not discriminate well among anxiety disorders, it has been found to be sensitive to change as a result of treatment (G.K. Brown et al. 1997). Because of its ease of administration, it is well suited for use as a measure of health care delivery systems in the treatment of anxiety.

The State-Trait Anxiety Inventory (Spielberger et al. 1970) is a self-report instrument in which patients are asked to report on anxiety in general (i.e., trait) and at particular points in time (i.e., state). The Endler S-R Inventory of Anxiousness (Endler et al. 1962) is a self-report measure of the interaction between the patient's anxiety and environmental situations such as interpersonal, physically dangerous, and ambiguous situations. This instrument has been widely used as a therapy outcome measure and is recommended as an instrument that may be helpful in tailoring treatment to the specific circumstances of the patient's anxiety.

The Liebowitz Social Anxiety Scale (Liebowitz 1987) is a clinician-administered semistructured interview that assesses social phobias. The instrument covers a wide range of fears and avoidance across social and performance situations. It has potential clinical usefulness in the development of a fear hierarchy and the assessment of treatment progress for patients with social phobias. A similar instrument is the Brief Social Phobia Scale (Davidson et al. 1991), an 11-item semistructured interview constructed to assess severity and treatment response of social phobias.

The measurement of the severity of obsessive-compulsive symptoms is often accomplished with the widely used Yale-Brown Obsessive Compulsive Scale (Y-BOCS; Goodman et al. 1989). There are two subscales in this clinician-administered semistructured interview, an Obsessions subscale and a Compulsions subscale. The instrument has been demonstrated to reliably discriminate between subjects with and without obsessive-compulsive disorder and to be sensitive to change.

A simple and brief instrument designed to assess the overall severity of DSM-IV panic disorder is the Panic Disorder Severity Scale (Shear et al. 1997). Using a scripted interview, the scale provides ratings of DSM-IV panic symptoms and consists of seven items: panic frequency, distress during panic, panic-focused anticipatory anxiety, phobic avoidance of situations, phobic avoidance of physical sensations, impairment in work functioning, and impairment in social functioning. It is modeled on the Y-BOCS and is sensitive to change with treatment. A useful self-report instrument for quantifying the presence and severity of posttraumatic stress disorder (PTSD) symptoms is the Posttraumatic Stress Diagnostic Scale devised by Foa (1995). This instrument can be used for screening and can be supplemented with an associated clinician-administered structured interview, the Clinician-Administered PTSD Scale (Blake et al. 1990), when the accuracy of patient self-report data is in doubt.

The Beck Depression Inventory (BDI; A.T. Beck et al. 1996) is probably the most widely used self-report inventory of depression. The original scale was administered in an interviewer-assisted manner, but a later version is completely self-administered. The 21 items of the inventory were selected to represent symptoms commonly associated with a depressive disorder. The rating of each item relies on the endorsement of one or more of four statements listed in order of symptom severity. Item categories include mood, pessimism, crying spells, guilt, self-hate and accusations, irritability, social withdrawal, work inhibition, sleep and appetite disturbance, and loss of libido. The content of the BDI emphasizes pessimism, a sense of failure, and self-punitive wishes. This emphasis is consistent with Beck's cognitive view of depression and its causes. This self-report instrument is frequently used in conjunction with the HRSD, which allows a clinician to rate the severity of depressive symptoms during an interview with the patient. In contrast to the BDI, the HRSD is more systematic in assessing neurovegetative signs. Although only rough interview guidelines for using the HRSD are available, interrater reliability is generally good.

The Geriatric Depression Scale (Yesavage and Brink 1983) is a commonly used instrument to screen for depressive illness in geriatric patients. The scale was developed to address the unique challenges inherent in the identification of depression in elderly patients. The scale is formatted to be easy to read and re-

spond to; does not contain somatic items that are often shared with nondepressed elderly people and those with medical problems (e.g., decreased energy, decreased libido, and sleep difficulties); and focuses on symptoms with maximum discriminatory power with geriatric populations, such as poor self-image, poor motivation, past versus future orientation, cognitive problems, and agitation. Studies suggest that the scale has excellent reliability and validity and demonstrates good sensitivity and specificity for depression.

The Manic-State Rating Scale (Beigel et al. 1971) is a 26-item observer-rated scale that is useful for patients with bipolar depression. Eleven items reflecting elation–grandiosity and paranoid–destructive features of manic patients have produced the most consistent results and have been applied successfully in the prediction of inpatient lengths of stay (Young et al. 1978). The scale has demonstrated adequate reliability and concurrent validity, and it can detect clinical change (Janowsky et al. 1978). Secunda et al. (1985) used similar items from several instruments employed in the National Institute of Mental Health Clinical Research Branch Collaborative Program on the Psychobiology of Depression to develop indices for responsiveness to lithium treatment in manic patients. A newer rating scale, the Internal State Scale (Bauer et al. 1991), is a self-report instrument that allows individuals to rate the present state of 17 items reflecting bipolar symptomatology.

Aggressive behavior, including aggressive imagery and hostile affect, is an important area in treatment planning both for the individual patient and for the general concepts that the inventory assesses. The Buss-Durkee Hostility Inventory (Buss and Durkee 1957) is a 75-item self-report questionnaire that measures different aspects of hostility and aggression. There are eight subscales: assault, indirect hostility, irritability, negativism, resentment, suspicion, verbal hostility, and guilt. Some norms exist for clinical populations. Megargee et al. (1967) developed an overcontrolled hostility scale using MMPI items. A review of studies involving this scale (Greene 1991) suggests that it can be used to screen for patients who display excessive control of their hostile impulses and are socially alienated. Spielberger (1991) developed a State–Trait Anger Expression Inventory that takes about 15 minutes to complete. This 44-item scale divides behavior into state anger (i.e., current feelings) and trait anger (i.e., disposition toward angry reactions), and the latter area has subscales for angry temperament and angry reaction (sample items include "How I feel right now: I feel irritated" or "How I generally feel: I fly off the handle").

The Overt Aggression Scale–Modified (OAS-M; Coccaro et al. 1991) is a semistructured clinician interview that assesses aggression, irritability, and suicidality in the past week. The OAS-M is intended for outpatients, and it is adapted from the original Overt Aggression Scale, which was developed for inpatients (Yudofsky et al. 1986). Given its focus on actual behaviors and the time span of the previous week, the instrument would be most useful in assessing patient change in these areas.

The Anger, Irritability, and Assault Questionnaire (Coccaro et al. 1991) is a 42-question self-report questionnaire designed to assess several aspects of impulsive aggression putatively related to serotonergic function. The instrument focuses primarily on the inability to control aggression and is composed of five subscales: Irritability, Labile Anger, Direct Assault, Verbal Assault, and Indirect Assault. Each question is rated on five time frames—past week, past month, adulthood, adolescence, and childhood—resulting in 210 items. The Irritability, Assault, and Labile Anger subscales are adapted from the Buss-Durkee Hostility Inventory and the Affective Lability Scales (Harvey et al. 1989). Available psychometric data suggest fairly strong short-term test–retest reliability as well as adequate construct validity with related measures.

Thought Disorder

One approach to the reliable assessment of cognition is the use of semistructured interviews such as the SADS and the SCID. The presence or absence of disorders of thinking such as thought derailment or frank hallucinations or delusions is determined during the course of an extensive interview. There are obvious problems with this approach. Many individuals may not wish to reveal frank delusional experiences, or they may be unaware of the presence of more subtle varieties of disordered thinking. Although other commonly used measures of disordered thinking such as the Positive and Negative Syndrome Scale (Kay et al. 1987) and the Scale for the Assessment of Positive Symptoms (Andreasen 1984) supplement the information obtained from the clinical interview with collateral information from caretakers, review of clinical records, and direct behavioral observation prior to rating the presence or absence of a symptom, problems in the accuracy of judgments remain. To avoid these pitfalls, an alternative approach is to obtain a sample of the thought process. The test most widely used in examinations for thought disorders has been the Rorschach inkblot test, which was developed by the Swiss psychiatrist Hermann Rorschach. In this test, a relatively ambiguous stimulus (a colored or achromatic "inkblot") is used, and, without additional instruction, individuals are asked to state what the blot looks like to them. Responses are scored for location (i.e., the area of the card that elicits a response), determinants (i.e., form, movement, color, and shading), form quality (i.e., the degree to which percepts are congruent with the area chosen), and content (e.g., human, animal, object). Exner (1974, 1978) developed a scoring system for the Rorschach test that attempts to integrate the best aspects of prior systems.

Holzman and his colleagues have published extensively on the relationship of various forms of thought disorder and its severity to psychiatric diagnosis and treatment (Solovay et al. 1986). Although the scoring scheme can be applied to any record of verbal production, its most frequent application has been in the context of verbal records from the administration of such tests as the WAIS-III and the Rorschach. In its present version, the Thought Disorder Index (Solovay et al. 1986) considers 22 forms of thought disturbance ranging across four levels of severity as the basis for a total score. The total score has been found to distinguish psychotic from nonpsychotic patients, and more severe forms of thought disorder have been most frequently associated with schizophrenic disorders. One report indicates a strong relationship between the degree of hypertrophy of the left posterior superior temporal gyrus, noticeable with magnetic resonance imaging, and the severity of thought disorder in schizophrenia patients (Shenton et al. 1992).

In addition to the work of Holzman and his colleagues, Harrow and associates have developed another battery, consisting of three tests, to quantify thought disorder. This work has considered patients with clinical diagnoses of schizophrenia, affective disorder, and schizoaffective disorder. In a series of studies, these investigators addressed the persistence of thought disorders in treated groups who had been followed for a period of 2–4 years (Harrow and Quinlan 1985; Marengo and Harrow 1985).

Suicidal Behavior

The suicide potential of patients has obvious treatment and management implications for the clinician. Suicidal threats, suicidal planning and/or preparation, suicidal ideation, and recent parasuicidal behavior are all direct indicators of current risk and should be assessed thoroughly and specifically in the clinical interview (Simon 2006). In addition, self-report instruments that focus specific and detailed attention on known predictors of suicidal behavior are sometimes clinically useful. Thus it is recommended that the assessment of suicidal behavior be embedded in an assessment package that involves interview and use of instruments (Bongar 1991).

With that caveat in mind, suicidal assessment instruments that are frequently used include the Beck Hopelessness Scale and the Beck Suicide Intent Scale. In addition, it should be noted that the Koss–Butcher critical item set revised on the MMPI is a list of 22 items that are related specifically to depressed suicidal ideation. These critical items should not be seen as scales but rather as markers of particular item content that might be significant in assessing the individual patient (Butcher 1989).

The Suicide Intent Scale (A.T. Beck et al. 1974), the Index of Potential Suicide (Zung 1974), and the Suicide Probability Scale (Cull and Gill 1986) are three widely used instruments. A complementary approach has been taken, culminating in the development of the Reasons for Living Inventory (Linehan et al. 1983). Of practical interest is that the Fear-of-Suicide subscale in the inventory differentiates between those who have only considered suicide and those who have made previous suicide attempts. Individuals scoring high on reasons for living and on subscales measuring survival and coping skills, responsibility to family, and child-related concerns were less likely to attempt suicide.

Assessment of Cognitive Functioning

Neuropsychological assessment is a branch of psychological assessment with the aim of understanding the relationship between the brain and behavior. Because neuropsychological assessments in the 1950s and 1960s preceded neuroimaging of the brain by computed tomography scan or magnetic resonance imaging, the initial role of neuropsychological assessments was to help diagnose whether someone had "brain damage" and the locus of the lesion. With the current range of powerful tools for showing structural and physiological changes in the brain, the role of neuropsychological assessments has progressed to that of evaluating the cognitive and psychosocial consequences of damage to the brain that often is well localized. These assessments continue to be used to establish diagnoses in some cases. Additionally, they may be used to identify a patient's cognitive strengths and weaknesses or ability to work, to formulate a treatment or intervention, or to determine competency.

The core feature of most neuropsychological assessments is the examination of cognitive functioning; however, emotional and social functioning are important aspects of the examination as well. Many of the commonly used instruments for assessing cognition, such as the various versions of the Wechsler Intelligence Scales, were designed to predict someone's academic or occupational potential but have proved useful for examining cognitive strengths and weaknesses associated with brain disorders. Other tests have been developed specifically for the examination of brain–behavior relationships. Like other psychological tests, these instruments must be reliable and valid. Ideally, a neuropsychological test would assess one circumscribed cognitive domain or one area of brain function for ease of interpretation. In fact, cognition is too complex for this goal to be fully achieved. Most neuropsychological tests described as measuring a particular cognitive function actually measure interrelated cognitive functions. Drawing a conclusion about the reason for poor performance on a test requires knowing where the breakdown occurred and may require using multiple tests with overlapping cognitive requirements to look for common failures. For example, if a patient cannot perform written arithmetic calculations, it is important to know whether the failure is an inability to know how to calculate or one of a number of other interpretations: an inability to read the arithmetic symbols associated with the problems, an inability to align numbers spatially on the page, or a general level of confusion. The interpretation of the pattern of performance on a range of cognitive tests and knowledge of the cognitive profile of neurological diseases or brain injuries require skill by a psychologist trained in this specialty area.

Assessment of an individual's performance on cognitive tests involves interpreting the pattern of performance. In the case of someone with a marked cognitive deficit, the question of whether the patient can perform a task might be answered with a "yes" or "no." In other cases, the loss may be less obvious, and the question may be the degree of cognitive deficit; thus making this determination requires assumptions. One assumption involves estimating the expected performance on tests for the patient in question. This estimation is derived from all pertinent information about the person's premorbid intellectual ability, including education, school grades, occupation, and highest level of functioning. Reading vocabulary, such as measured by the National Adult Reading Test, now in its second edition (H. Nelson and Willison 1991), or its American version (Grober and Sliwinski 1991), frequently is used to estimate premorbid intellectual ability because reading vocabulary correlates well with verbal intelligence and is unaffected by many types of brain damage except those causing language problems or substantial dementia. Unless the patient has had a previous examination, the patient's performance is measured against a standard, usually a normative group composed of intact people of the same age and demographic background. Using this comparison, a person's performance can be classified as within expectation or below expectation. For example, a patient with a high school education and average grades who has worked in a semiskilled job might be assumed to be of average premorbid intellectual ability, whereas a college graduate with excellent grades who becomes a high-level administrator might be assumed to be of at least high average intellectual ability.

Another assumption is that people tend to perform at a similar level across a range of cognitive tests. Thus, a drop in performance on one or more tests raises the question of an acquired deficit. This process is referred to as "deficit measurement" (Lezak et al. 2004). Of course, people have varying strengths and weaknesses, and a person may not have performed at the same level on all cognitive tests premorbidly. Performance below expectation can be presumed to be an acquired deficit if the deficit would be expected based on the patient's disease or condition or if the impairment represents a large discrepancy with other test performances. No exact standard is well established for defining a discrepancy as large. Some clinicians use 1.5 standard deviations below the expected score, some use 2 standard deviations, and some use clinical judgment.

Representative neuropsychological tests are described here (Table 3–8). For a more complete discussion of neuropsychological tests, see Lezak et al. (2004). Normative data on many neuropsychological tests may be found in Mitrushina et al. (2005) and Strauss et al. (2006).

Attention

Attentional abilities are critical cognitive functions, because without proper attention many other cognitive abilities fail. Attention takes many forms. Simple attention is the act of focusing on a stimulus. More complex forms of attention require sustaining attention over an extended time, dividing attention over more than one stimulus, and maintaining attention under conditions of interference. Attention-deficit disorder is a disorder with childhood onset in which impaired attention is the cardinal feature. Many psychiatric disorders have impaired attention as a disabling symptom, as do many neurological disorders. Inattention to the contralateral side of personal space can occur with le-

sions in many different brain regions but are most common and persistent with right-hemisphere lesions (Heilman et al. 2003). Other forms of attentional disorders are common after traumatic brain injury, stroke, neurodegenerative disorders, and even normal aging (Leclercq and Zimmermann 2002). Information processing speed is a related function and is impaired in many brain disorders.

Instruments used to measure attention vary according to the aspect of attention under investigation. One of the most frequently used tests is *digit span,* in which the person is asked to repeat numbers in increasing series lengths, thereby measuring capacity of holding information in mind. Tests of *contralateral neglect* often require patients to respond to every occurrence of a stimulus while stimuli are presented in both sides of personal space. *Cancellation tests* may be used in which the patient is to cross out every occurrence of a stimulus, such as a letter, in rows of varying stimuli. Patients with unilateral neglect may omit more target items on one side of the page, whereas patients with a general attentional disorder may omit items sporadically throughout the test. Complexity can be added by asking patients to cancel every occurrence of two items, such as two letters, which requires divided attention.

Visual Search and Attention Test

The Visual Search and Attention Test (Trenerry et al. 1990) is a cancellation test with rows of characters of which some are the target character to be cancelled. On the most difficult test trial, a variety of symbols are printed in different-colored inks, and the target is defined by both the symbol and color, thus requiring attention to both dimensions. In addition to total score, the test is scored separately for left- and right-side performance to assess for unilateral neglect.

Vigilance tests are designed to measure sustained attention, and the best examples are computerized tests in which the patient is asked to push a button every time a target stimulus appears on the screen (L.H. Beck et al. 1956). Subjects also can be asked to make a response every time a letter, or combination of letters, is presented in an audiotape (Cicerone 1997).

Continuous Performance Test

The computerized Continuous Performance Test (Conners 2000), now in its second edition, requires that the subject press a key whenever any letter except the letter "X" appears on the screen. During the 13 minutes of the test, stimuli are presented at random intervals so that response times cannot be anticipated. Scores are provided for a number of measures, includ-

TABLE 3–8.   Representative instruments for examining various cognitive domains

Cognitive domain	Instrument	Description
Attention	Continuous Performance Test	Computerized sustained-attention test
	Visual Search and Attention	Cancellation test requiring divided attention
	Auditory Consonant Trigrams	Working memory for letters following interference
Memory	Rey Auditory Verbal Learning Test	Word-list learning test
	California Verbal Learning Test II	Word-list learning with a semantic encoding feature
	Complex Figure Test	Visuospatial memory for a complex design
	Brief Visual Attention Test—Revised	Visuospatial memory for a series of simple designs
Language	Boston Diagnostic Aphasia Examination	Comprehensive receptive and expressive language test
	Boston Naming Test	Naming familiar items
Visual perception	Judgment of Line Orientation	Matching orientation of straight lines
	Hooper Visual Organization Test	Visual synthesis of parts to whole
Constructional abilities	Wechsler Adult Intelligence Scale Block Design	Reconstructing designs with blocks
	Complex Figure Test	Copying a complex geometric design
Reasoning	The Category Test	Conceptual and spatial reasoning
	Wisconsin Card Sorting Test	Concept formation and cognitive flexibility
	Raven's Progressive Matrices	Pattern matching using analogy problems
Executive functions	Tower of London	Planning using a problem-solving test
	Letter Fluency	Initiation and maintenance of strategies for generating items
	Trail Making Test	Set-switching using a visuographic sequence test
	Stroop Test	Response inhibition

ing reaction times and errors of omission and commission. Errors of omission are interpreted as attentional problems, whereas errors of commission may represent impulsivity or disinhibition.

Working memory is the ability to hold information in mind while performing a mental operation (Baddeley 1986). It requires both maintenance of attention and temporary memory storage. Deficits in working memory occur particularly with lesions of the prefrontal cortex (Koechlin et al. 1999). Many cognitive tasks require adequate working memory. Repeating digits backward or mentally solving arithmetic problems requires holding numbers in mind while manipulating them. The WAIS-III Letter-Number Sequence Test involves mentally rearranging numbers and letters after hearing them read aloud. The Auditory Consonant Trigram test (Stuss et al. 1989) asks subjects to repeat three consonants after a period of interfering verbal activity ranging up to 36 seconds, which is intended to prevent rehearsal.

Memory

Memory, like attention, is central to all cognitive functions. It is not surprising that patients or the people close to them may attribute a variety of cognitive and behavioral problems to failing memory, so a careful interview is important for establishing the type of memory problem (Howieson and Lezak 2002). For example, many elders will report a memory problem when referring to difficulty coming up with the name of a familiar person or a word, which is a retrieval problem that can be distinct from an inability to form or retrieve new memories and may have different diagnostic implications.

For memories to occur, information must have been registered, stored, and retrieved. Encoding of memories according to associations at the time of learning improves their ability to be retrieved. Remote memory disorders are rare. By contrast, the ability to learn and retrieve new information frequently is impaired in people with damage to the brain. New learning and retention are mediated by the medial temporal lobe, particularly the hippocampal formation and adjacent cortices, and diencephalon (Squire 1994). Any disorder that affects these brain regions can produce impairment in forming new memories. Verbal memory deficits are more pronounced with left-hemisphere damage, whereas nonverbal, such as visuospatial, memory deficits are more pronounced with right-hemisphere damage, although these differences may not always be evident (Loring et al. 2000).

Memory tests designed to assess new learning and retention often involve lists of words, stories, or designs. Patients who have a pronounced impairment in immediate memory may have failed to register or encode the material, whereas those whose poor performance shows up mainly on delayed recall tests may have problems with retention or retrieval. Poor encoding can lead to less effective retrieval. Memory tests that include both free recall and recognition memory often can identify the patient whose problems are mainly retrieval and not retention—that is, their recognition memory is intact but their free recall is impaired. Careful selection of memory tests may help identify the underlying problem.

California Verbal Learning Test

The California Verbal Learning Test II (Delis et al. 2000) is a word-list learning test designed to assess the use of encoding strategies. Each of the 16 words belongs to one of four categories, and the category items are presented in random order. Patients who recognize the associations and use them to cluster the words according to meaning have a strategic advantage for later recall. Recall of the words is tested under both uncued and cued conditions and both free recall and recognition.

Visuospatial memory is frequently assessed by having the subject copy designs and recall them later, such as the Visual Reproduction test of the various versions of the Wechsler Memory Scale (Wechsler 1997b) or the Complex Figure Test, described later. However, when copy of the material is piecemeal or fragmented, poor recall performance may be due to poor processing rather than to poor memory. In these cases, a test that uses simpler designs, such as the Benton Visual Retention Test (Sivan 1992), or one that requires recognition rather than drawing may be selected.

Language

Verbal skills may be impaired when any of the brain regions involved in language processing is injured. In most people these regions are concentrated in the temporal, parietal, and frontal lobes of the left hemisphere. Although a number of aphasic syndromes have been well described, patients often do not fit neatly into one of these classic syndromes. The Boston Diagnostic Aphasia Examination (Goodglass et al. 2000) is a comprehensive examination of discrete verbal skills. Other language tests may focus on just one language function. The Token Test assesses language comprehension using multi-step commands (De Renzi and Faglioni 1978). The quality of verbal expression can be assessed by a variety of tests in which the patients express ideas, such as the Comprehension and Vocabulary tests in the WAIS-III. Among the most common language problems in nonaphasic patients is the ability to retrieve words for naming. Anyone who examines elders knows that word-finding difficulty is a frequent complaint associated with normal aging. In a more pronounced form it is a common problem associated with Alzheimer's disease and other diseases of the temporal lobes. The Boston Naming Test (Goodglass et al. 2000) is a confrontational naming test that presents for naming line drawings of familiar objects. Rapidity of word retrieval may be assessed with a variety of verbal fluency tests, including those designed to assess the ability to generate words that begin with a particular letter or are members of the same semantic category, such as animals. Because fluency tests require the generation of strategies and maintenance of effort, they often are described as executive tests.

Perception

A wide range of reliable visual perceptual tests have been developed, although fewer are designed to study auditory, tactile, and olfactory perception. Spatial perception in the most basic form can be examined with the Judgment of Line Orientation Test (Benton et al. 1994), which assesses the perception of angular relationships using matching of straight lines presented at the same angles. The perception of formed objects often is examined with matching tasks in which the patient indicates which of a series of forms matches a target form. The forms may be geometric figures or faces (Benton et al. 1994). Speed in matching forms is examined with the Symbol Search test in the WAIS-III. The more complex task of synthesizing parts into a whole is measured with the Hooper Visual Organization Test (Hooper 1983), in which disarranged fragments of drawings of an object are presented for recognition.

Constructional Abilities

Like any complex activity, constructional tasks require several skills. In the case of visual constructional tasks commonly used in neuropsychological evaluations, these skills include visual processing, planning, and organization in the execution of a drawing or a construction. Many of these tests have a prominent spatial component. Patients with right-hemisphere lesions often produce fragmented constructions with serious distortions. Lesions in other brain regions may affect other features of the production (Pillon 1981). For instance, patients with frontal lesions may use a disorganized approach and repeat elements. Understanding the qualitative feature of the performance is important for understanding the nature of the deficit.

Complex Figure Test

A good example of a constructional task that provides insight into the type of breakdown in constructional ability is the Complex Figure Test, sometimes called the Rey-Osterreith Complex Figure (Rey 1941) and translated in Corwin and Bylsma (1993). A complex geometric design is presented for copy. The copy can be approached many different ways, and the relative lack of structure of the task is one of its best features. The approach to copying the test gives information about visuospatial processing, planning, organization, and other qualitative features. A recall is commonly obtained, so that the test provides a host of information.

Another commonly used constructional task is Block Design from the WAIS-III. The task is to reconstruct with blocks two-color designs as presented in a booklet. Patients with visuospatial deficits find this test very challenging, whereas those whose major problems are with organization and planning may perform this test better than the Complex Figure because is it more structured—that is, there are fewer options for approaching the task.

Reasoning

The ability to form conclusions, draw inferences, or make judgments depends on logical thought. The more severe the brain dysfunction, the more likely reasoning is affected. A visual reasoning test from the WAIS-III is Picture Completion. The object is to identify the missing feature in pictures of familiar objects or scenes. Patients who name features not intended to be in the picture have failed to make correct inferences. As an example, one item is a picture of a leaf with a detail missing and some patients say that "the tree" is missing. Many neuropsychological tests of reasoning also assess concept formation and cognitive flexibility, such as the Category Test (Reitan and Wolfson 1993). To succeed at this test, the subject must identify the target feature in a set of designs that produces correct responses based on feedback for each response. The correct principle varies during the set of six problem sets. A related test of concept formation and cognitive flexibility is the Wisconsin Card Sorting Test (Grant and Berg 1948). Subjects match cards according to feedback about the correctness of their sorts. A key feature is that after 10 correct sorts, the correct sorting principle changes without warning, and subjects must change their sorting strategy accordingly. Because of the lack of warning about the change, this test places a strong emphasis on cognitive flexibility.

Delis-Kaplan Executive Function System Sorting Test

Another concept formation test that uses semantic as well as perceptual features as sorting principles is the Delis-Kaplan Executive Function System Sorting Test (Delis et al. 2001). Six cards, each with a word and several distinct perceptual features, are presented to the subject, and the task is to sort the cards into two piles so that the cards in each pile have a common characteristic. The object is to sort the cards as many ways as possible. The main measures are the number of correct sorts and the quality of the description of the sorts.

Executive Functions

Higher-order cognitive processes such as goal setting, planning, organization, adaptive responding, and self-monitoring fall under the umbrella of *executive functions*. Often executive functions are assumed to be mediated by the frontal lobes, but many executive tests are sensitive to damage in other parts of the brain (Lezak et al. 2004). Patients with psychiatric disorders often have executive impairment. The major obstacle to examining executive functions is that the examination process is so structured that goal setting and other behaviors that normally require self-direction are fixed by the examiner. Motivation and initiation are among the most difficult to assess in a structured examination, and the patient's facility in these areas may best be obtained from history (Lezak et al. 2004). Nevertheless, tests have been developed to measure potential for specific executive domains. *Fluency tests* are used to indicate initiation and maintenance of behavior. They ask subjects to produce as many items of a designated type as they can think of, which requires initiation and maintenance of strategies for successful performance. In addition to the verbal fluency tests described earlier, *design fluency* tests look at the ability to generate unique designs according to the requirements of the tests. The Ruff Figural Fluency Test (Ruff et al. 1987) presents a series of squares with five dots in each and asks the subject to make patterns by connecting any two or more dots. The object is to make as many unique designs as possible within the time limit. Some cognitive tests are self-administered, such as written arithmetic problems, and the effort exerted by the patient may reflect the ability to maintain behavior. As mentioned earlier, the Complex Figure Test is a good measure of planning and organization, at least for visuospatial material. Traditionally, planning has been examined with mazes, but various tower instruments have come into favor. These are similar to the familiar Tower of Hanoi puzzle.

The Tower of London

The Tower of London (Culbertson and Zillmer 2001) problems consist of moving beads on rods to predetermined positions by moving only one at a time and using as few moves as possible. The best performance is obtained by thinking through the necessary moves before beginning the task so as to eliminate unnecessary moves. Keeping the series of moves in mind requires good working memory.

Brief Batteries

A number of brief batteries are available for use in screening or to address specific conditions. One widely used instrument, the Repeatable Battery for

Assessment of Neuropsychological Status (Randolph et al. 1998), usually takes about 30 minutes to administer. Tests in the battery are identical or similar to commonly used neuropsychological tests and consist of measures of attention, speed of processing, recent memory, confrontational naming, semantic fluency, and visuospatial processing. Normative data for individual tests are available from Lezak et al. (2004), and age- and education-corrected normative information has been published for community-dwelling older adults (Beatty et al. 2003; Duff et al. 2003).

Assessment of Personality Traits and Disorders

In developing a treatment plan for a specific patient, the psychiatrist must assess personality traits for various reasons. Personality traits or disorders may 1) be the focus of intervention, 2) exacerbate or be related to the incidence of certain symptoms (e.g., depression), or 3) either help or hinder the development of a therapeutic relationship with the patient.

Dimensional Assessment of Personality

The dimensional assessment of personality using psychological tests has been characterized by a nomothetic approach in which specific personality dimensions (e.g., introversion) are assessed. The dimensions chosen for assessment are typically derived from a personality theory, and individuals are expected to show quantitative differences on these various dimensions. The number of items relevant to a particular dimension that are endorsed is thought to reflect important aspects of that individual's personality style. Within the field of personality measurement, much attention has been paid to the generalizability of such measures. Efforts to investigate the relationship between self-report measures of interpersonal behavior and actual behavior in interpersonal situations continue to contribute to the refinement of this important area of psychological assessment.

Several widely used and psychometrically sound instruments are available for the assessment of personality (Table 3–9). Such tests include the 16–Personality Factor Inventory, the Eysenck Personality Inventory, the Multidimensional Personality Questionnaire (MPQ; Tellegen 1982), and the California Personality Inventory (Gough 1956). These instruments were de-

TABLE 3–9. Instruments for the assessment of personality traits and disorders

Instrument	General classification	Description	Scoring features
Neuroticism, Extroversion, and Openness Personality Inventory—Revised	Self-report	240 items, 5-point scale	5 domain scales and 30 facet scales
16–Personality Factor Inventory	Self-report	3 equivalent forms of 106–187 items each	Scaled scores for 16 personality traits
Eysenck Personality Inventory	Self-report	57 yes/no items, parallel forms	Scores on extraversion and neuroticism
Schedule for Nonadaptive and Adaptive Personality	Self-report	12 primary traits and 3 temperament dimensions	
Dimensional Assessment of Personality Pathology—Basic Questionnaire	Self-report	18 scales	Scores on 18 scales
California Personality Inventory	Self-report	468 items	Scores on 18 scales and 4 special scales
Millon Clinical Multiaxial Inventory—III	Self-report	175 items, true/false format	Base rate scores on 22 clinical scales
Multidimensional Personality Questionnaire	Self-report	300 items	11 subscales and 3 higher-order scales
Structural Interview for the DSM-IV Personality Disorders	Semistructured interview	3-point rating scales	Yields DSM-IV Axis II diagnoses
International Personality Disorder Examination	Semistructured interview	Semistructured interview for patient and self-report by family member on the patient	Dimensional and categorical scales on DSM-IV Axis II personality disorders
Structured Clinical Interview for DSM-IV Axis II Personality Disorders	Semistructured interview	3-point rating scales	Categorical scales on DSM-IV Axis II personality disorders
Diagnostic Interview for DSM-IV Personality Disorders	Semistructured interview	3-point rating scales	Categorical scales on DSM-IV Axis II personality disorders
Personality Disorder Interview—IV	Semistructured interview	3-point rating scales	Dimensional and categorical scales on DSM-IV Axis II personality disorders
Structural Analysis of Social Behavior	Self-report	36–72 statements of interpersonal behavior rated true/false	Internalized attitudes regarding self and significant others

TABLE 3–9. Instruments for the assessment of personality traits and disorders *(continued)*

Instrument	General classification	Description	Scoring features
Wisconsin Personality Disorders Inventory—IV	Self-report	214 items, 10-point scale	Dimensional and categorical scales on DSM-IV Axis II personality disorders based on Structural Analysis of Social Behavior perspective
Shedler-Westen Assessment Procedure	Q-sort methodology	200 descriptive statements, 7-point scale, sorted according to fixed distribution	Yields categorical and dimensional DSM-IV diagnoses based on prototypes

signed for the validation of personality constructs rather than for the assessment of psychopathology, although they have been employed in clinical settings with limited success. However, these instruments, and their designers, have not been oriented toward psychopathology, and there is no explicit theory of personality disorder that underlies the interpretation of results from these tests.

The Neuroticism, Extroversion, and Openness Personality Inventory (NEO-PI), a carefully constructed instrument measuring five central facets of personality, has gained recognition (Wiggins and Pincus 1992), and its clinical use will probably increase. The revised version, the NEO-PI-R (Costa and McCrae 1992), provides a measure of five facets of personality: neuroticism, extraversion, openness, agreeableness, and conscientiousness. Each of the facets also includes six subscales. For example, the six facets of neuroticism include anxiety, anger/hostility, depression, self-consciousness, impulsiveness, and vulnerability. The revised version completes the earlier instrument by providing facet scales for agreeableness and conscientiousness.

The MPQ is a 300-item, factor-analytically developed self-report instrument designed to assess 11 primary personality dimensions as well as 3 higher-order traits, namely Positive Affectivity, Negative Affectivity, and Constraint. *Positive Affectivity* is believed to include a group of personality traits that reflect temperamental and behavioral traits conducive to joy, excitement, vigor, and states of general positive engagement. Alternatively, *Negative Affectivity* is primarily associated with negative affect states, such as anger, hostility, and anxiety. The higher-order factor *Constraint* refers to temperamental and behavioral traits related to response inhibition or self-restraint. The MPQ was rigorously developed and tested and has demonstrated gen-

erally excellent psychometric properties, including internal consistency and test–retest reliability. The MPQ is also associated with a robust amount of data suggesting that the major components of the instrument are subject to genetic influences (Markon et al. 2002; Tellegen et al. 1988).

In this era of searching for efficient care, some consideration should be given to the use of screening instruments that can be administered rapidly to assess for the potential for personality disorders, disorders that retard and complicate the treatment of Axis I disorders. Four screening instruments deserve consideration: the IPDE Screen (Lenzenweger et al. 1997), the Iowa Personality Disorder Screen (Pfohl and Langbehn 1994), the self-directedness subscale from the Temperament and Character Inventory (Cloninger et al. 1993; Svrakic et al. 1993), and a screen for personality disorders developed from the Inventory of Interpersonal Problems (Pilkonis et al. 1996).

Interpersonal Aspects of Personality

One particular school of personality research that has concerned itself with pathological expressions of personality factors has focused explicitly on interpersonal behavior. Adherents of this view of psychopathology emphasize the centrality of the problems that people experience with others, for it is in this area that all symptoms are activated, reinforced, and (for some persons) caused. The assessment of interpersonal behavior can be central to understanding the patient's social world, with its pleasures and disappointments as well as its barriers to success in love and work, and can be used as a forecast of the kind of relationship the patient will form with the clinician.

This interpersonal tradition dates back to psychologist Timothy Leary's circumplex model (Leary 1957). Underlying the expression of all interpersonal styles are the two major orthogonal axes of power and affiliation. Each interpersonal style is seen as involving varying degrees of the expression of power and affiliation leading to 16 modes of interaction. These 16 modes are organized along the circumference of a circle defining eight broad categories that are used in interpersonal diagnosis: ambitious–dominant, gregarious–extroverted, warm–agreeable, unassuming–ingenuous, lazy–submissive, aloof–introverted, cold–quarrelsome, and arrogant–calculating. This system is more than merely descriptive. Theoretically, one is able to predict not only the kind of interpersonal style that the patient expresses but also the kind of behavior that this style tends to elicit from others. Behavior on one side of the circle tends to elicit from others behaviors on the opposite side of the circle. For example, a patient who is ambitious–dominant tends to elicit lazy–submissive behavior from others. In terms of differential therapeutic treatment planning, this model suggests not only that the patient will behave in a certain fashion but also that this behavior will elicit therapist behavior found on the opposite side of the circle. It has been suggested that interpersonal diagnosis can thus highlight transference and possible countertransference reactions in therapies that are interpersonal in orientation. Furthermore, the theory indicates what kinds of counterbehavior the therapist should engage in to dislodge the patient from his or her predominant mode of interaction.

There are several instruments that have been developed from this basic interpersonal theory. In a series of investigations, Lorr and McNair (1965) generated the most recent version of the Interpersonal Behavior Inventory. This inventory has been judged to be psychometrically sound and a useful clinical device for the assessment of patient characteristics and therapy outcome (Wiggins and Pincus 1992). The instrument is a clinical rating by professionals but in principle could be employed in a self-report format. The Interpersonal Style Inventory (Lorr and Youniss 1973) is a self-report instrument for persons ages 14 years and older. A large number (300) of true/false statements are employed to assess interpersonal involvement, socialization, self-control, stability, and autonomy. Techniques of rational scale construction, including validity factor analyses, were employed. Norms were established based on 1,500 college and high school students.

Also in the same tradition, Benjamin (1988) developed an instrument for the assessment of interpersonal behavior, the Structural Analysis of Social Behavior, and a computer-based scoring system, marketed under the trade name INTREX, which is self-administered. The Structural Analysis of Social Behavior can also be used by clinicians to record their impressions about the patient. A related coding scheme has been developed for use by trained observers to record the patient's actual interactions with others, such as family members, during the course of treatment.

Assessment of Personality Disorders

A relatively new approach to the assessment of personality disorders is to construct instruments, either self-report or semistructured interviews, that evaluate the presence or absence of specific personality traits described in Axis II of DSM-IV-TR. DSM-IV-TR neither defines nor develops from any particular theory of personality. Instead, it identifies clusters (in most cases, those with little empirical validation) of personality traits that are considered sufficiently maladaptive to warrant the personality disorder designation. *Personality traits* are described as enduring patterns of perceiving, relating to, and thinking about the environment and oneself that are exhibited or manifested in a wide range of important social and interpersonal contexts. When these traits are inflexible and maladaptive and cause either significant impairment in social or occupational functioning or subjective distress, they are defined as a personality disorder in DSM-IV-TR. The most promising instruments of this type include the Personality Diagnostic Questionnaire–4 (PDQ-4; Hyler 1994; Hyler et al. 1988); the MCMI-III (Millon et al. 1997); the Structured Clinical Interview for DSM-IV Axis II Personality Disorders (SCID-II; First et al. 1997a); the IPDE (Loranger 1999); and the Structural Interview for the DSM-IV Personality Disorders (SIDP-IV; Pfohl et al. 1997).

The PDQ-4 is an 85-item true/false self-report inventory of Axis II diagnostic criteria, and the test yields scores on each of the 10 personality disorder categories of DSM-IV. Several improvements of the original PDQ have been implemented, including the addition of two validity scales designed to identify those who are "faking good" and those who may be lying, not taking the questions seriously, or responding in a random fashion. The items of the PDQ-4 have also been rearranged in an effort to reduce the instrument's transparency. The instrument has a high false-positive rate, meaning that many patients who meet the PDQ-4 criteria do not actually have a personality disorder. In addition, patients typically report a number of traits and will often meet criteria for several diagnostic categories; therefore the PDQ-4 may be more useful as a screening measure.

The MCMI-III is another useful self-report instrument that covers personality disorders; see previous discussion under "Omnibus Measures of Symptoms."

There are several new self-report questionnaires that assess personality and personality pathology that have been carefully constructed with attention to psychometric properties. These include the Schedule for Nonadaptive and Adaptive Personality (Clark 1993), the Dimensional Assessment of Personality Pathology–Basic Questionnaire (Schroeder et al. 1994), and the Wisconsin Personality Disorders Inventory–IV (Klein et al. 1993). The latter is unique in that it is a self-report measure designed to provide a dimensional and categorical assessment of the DSM-IV personality disorders from the interpersonal perspective of Benjamin's Structural Analysis of Social Behavior. Available psychometric studies suggest good initial reliability and validity, although correlations with other measures of personality disorder are moderate.

There are five semistructured interviews that have been designed to assess, via the patient's report and the clinical judgment of the interviewer, the presence of Axis II disorders: the IPDE, the SIDP-IV, the SCID-II, the Diagnostic Interview for DSM-IV Personality Disorders (Zanarini et al. 1987), and the Personality Disorder Interview–IV (Widiger et al. 1995).

The IPDE is a semistructured interview that yields both dimensional and categorical scores for DSM-IV Axis II criteria based on 99 sets of questions. An important feature of this semistructured interview, which takes approximately 1–2 hours to administer, is that the criteria are assessed in related clusters such as self-concept, affect expression, reality testing, impulse control, interpersonal relations, and work. The interview goes beyond a simple listing of the criteria and in many cases provides multiple questions designed to help the interviewer gain a broad appreciation of the criterion under assessment. A parallel version of the interview has been constructed for use with informants, in recognition of the fact that information from patients themselves, especially around personality issues, may be distorted. Initial reliability data are impressive, and validity studies are under way. The instrument is likely to be widely used. In fact, it has been translated into several languages, is available in an ICD-10 version, and was used in an international study approved by the World Health Organization and the former Alcohol, Drug Abuse, and Mental Health Administration (Loranger et al. 1991).

The SIDP-IV is a semistructured interview designed to assess DSM-IV Axis II disorders both categorically and dimensionally. The 101 sets of questions are thematically organized into 10 topic areas: Interests and Activities, Work Style, Close Relationships, Social Relationships, Emotions, Observational Criteria, Self-Perception, Perception of Others, Stress and Anger, and Social Conformity. A 107-question modular version organized by personality disorder is also available. A rating form provides a three-point rating scale for each criterion. Ratings are based on the clinical assessment of the interview data. The authors of the interview recommend that it be used in conjunction with a general psychiatric interview in which major (i.e., Axis I) psychiatric disorders have been diagnosed, so that lifelong personality traits can be distinguished from episodic psychiatric disorders. The authors also recommend gathering information from an informant who knows the patient well. Although the measure can be scored dimensionally, the authors do not explicitly endorse that procedure.

The SCID-II is concerned with the assessment of Axis II personality disorders. The interview format is determined by the DSM-IV disorders and provides no guide for elaborating the assessment of the criteria. One reported advantage of the SCID-II for some clinicians is its slightly shorter administration time compared with other semistructured Axis II interviews.

The Diagnostic Interview for DSM-IV Personality Disorders is a 108-question interview developed to categorically assess DSM-IV personality disorders. The questions are organized according to personality disorder and appear in both yes/no and open-ended formats. Information on administration and scoring, as well as the psychometric properties of the instrument, is limited.

The Personality Disorder Interview–IV is similar to the SIDP-IV in that it is available in a thematic and a modular version. The thematic version is organized into nine topical areas including Attitudes Toward Self, Attitudes Toward Others, Security of Comfort with Others, Friendships and Relationships, Conflicts and Disagreements, Work and Leisure, Social Norms, Mood, and Appearance and Perception. Few psychometric studies exist, and the measure's real strength appears to be its comprehensive and detailed manual.

There are several problems with this relatively new approach of assessing personality disorders guided solely by DSM-IV and DSM-IV-TR. First, Axis II is neither an empirically nor a theoretically derived compilation of personality traits that lead to, cause, or constitute psychopathology. Rather, it is a somewhat arbitrary collection of traits that are thought to be important markers of pathology. Thus, any instrument guided solely by DSM-IV will leave serious questions of internal consistency, content validity, and construct validity largely unanswered. Most probably, attempts to assess these important test characteristics within the context of DSM-IV are likely to be carried out with these instruments.

The Shedler-Westen Assessment Procedure (SWAP-200; Westen and Shedler 1999a, 1999b) is an innovative and creative alternative approach to the assessment and classification of Axis II pathology. The SWAP-200 is an assessment tool that uses the Q-sort method. In brief, a *Q-sort* is a set of statements (based on the DSM, clinical observation, the literature, and so on) describing various aspects of personality that are printed on individual index cards. A clinician who knows the patient very well arranges the cards into categories based on the degree to which the statement describes the patient. The cards are sorted from those that are inapplicable to those that are extremely descriptive. Obviously, this approach depends on the judgment of the clinician rather than the patient's self-report. The SWAP-200 consists of 200 personality descriptive statements that clinicians sort into eight categories with values of 0–7. Clinicians must assign a specific number of statements to each category, resulting in a fixed distribution. Completion of the SWAP-200 takes approximately 45 minutes. Psychometric studies support the validity of the instrument for assessing personality disorders, and it appears to be one alternative approach that may offer a solution to the inherent problems of diagnosis based on DSM-IV.

Assessment of Psychodynamics

The assessment of factors relevant to psychodynamic and psychoanalytic theory and treatment approaches has a long history in the clinical psychological literature. The development of the "standard battery," including the WAIS-III, the Rorschach, and the Thematic Apperception Test (Table 3–10), has its origins in the efforts of clinical psychologists to provide an assessment of such psychodynamic factors as drives, unconscious wishes, conflicts, and defenses. For those clinicians committed to the psychodynamic model, assessments

that focus exclusively on overt behaviors will be less than totally satisfactory.

The importance of providing information about personality dynamics and structure that are outside the conscious awareness of the examinee has been the single most significant rationale for the continued use of projective tests. In part, therefore, the value of such assessments varies directly with the degree to which maladaptive and symptomatic behaviors are presumed to be beyond the conscious control of the examinee. A second rationale for the continued use of these tests is that the unstructured nature of the tests provides a singular opportunity to assess the degree to which organization of behavior is dependent on a high degree of structure in the examination procedure itself. The assessment of both of these factors is of clear relevance to a treatment method that attempts to explore and alter unconscious determinants of behavior and for which success depends on introducing as little structure into the treatment as is realistically possible.

The most widely used assessment procedure for the examination of patients over a range of ego functions and dynamic factors is the Rorschach inkblot test, described earlier. Scoring systems have been developed by many authors, and Exner (1974, 1978) created a scoring system that attempts to integrate the best aspects of earlier systems. From these scores, inferences are drawn concerning the patient's self-image, identity, defensive structure, reality testing, affective control, amount and degree of fantasy life, degree of thought organization, and potential for impulsive acting out.

The Thematic Apperception Test is another widely used projective process for assessing the patient's self-concept in relation to others. Originally developed by Murray (1943), the test consists of a set of 30 pictures depicting one or more individuals. The patient is asked to make up a story based on each picture. The stories generated are then scored for the individual's needs as reflected in the feelings and impulses attributed to the major character in each story and the interactions with the environment leading to a resolution. As currently used, the stories are most often examined for the patient's self–other concepts as revealed in the interaction and outcome of the story line.

In an effort to systematically assess concepts related to psychodynamic theory in a manner amenable to the objective self-report of patients, two instruments have been developed: the Inventory of Personality Organization (IPO; Clarkin et al. 2001) and the Defense Style Questionnaire (Bond and Wesley 1996). Kernberg (1996) theorized that personality "organi-

TABLE 3–10. Instruments for the assessment of psychodynamics and patient enabling factors

Instrument	General classification	Description	Scoring features
Rorschach	Unstructured or projective test	10 ambiguous inkblots, responses scored on multiple criteria	Accuracy of form, location, use of color, shading, etc., provide summary scores
Thematic Apperception Test	Unstructured or projective test	30 ambiguous scenes	Affects, outcomes, and other qualities
Inventory of Personality Organization	Self-report	83 items, 5-point scale	3 primary scales and 2 supplementary scales
Defense Style Questionnaire	Self-report	88 items, 9-point scale	4 scales
Minnesota Multiphasic Personality Inventory—2	Self-report	566-item checklist, true/false format	T scores for 13 criterion scales
Symptom Checklist–90—Revised	Self-report	90-item checklist, 5-point intensity scales	T scores for 9 symptom clusters
Millon Clinical Multiaxial Inventory—III	Self-report	175 items, true/false format	Base rate scores for 22 clinical scales

zation" falls into three broad classes, specifically the neurotic, borderline, and psychotic levels of organization. Specific personality disorders delineated within the DSM-IV nomenclature (e.g., borderline, narcissistic, histrionic, antisocial, paranoid, schizoid, schizotypal, and dependent) as well as others from the psychoanalytic tradition (e.g., hypochondriasis, sadomasochistic, and malignant narcissism), arise from within the borderline level of personality organization. This level of organization is characterized by marked identity diffusion, predominance of primitive psychological defenses, and broadly intact reality testing.

Identity diffusion refers to a psychological structure that is characterized by a poorly integrated internalized concept of self and a poorly integrated internalized concept of significant others. *Primitive psychological defenses* are those defensive propensities that distort the individual's interpersonal interactions and interfere with functioning. These defensive operations primarily include the mechanisms of splitting and projective identification. Other dominant primitive mechanisms that complement or reinforce splitting and projective identification include denial, devaluation, and omnipotent control. These rigid and inflexible defenses suggest more severe psychopathology and are distinguished from healthier variants of defensive operations characteristic of neurotic personality organization, such as repression, reaction formation, and suppression. *Reality testing*, in this model,

"refers to the capacity to differentiate self from nonself, intrapsychic from external stimuli, and to maintain empathy with ordinary social criteria of reality" (Kernberg 1996, p. 120). Previous efforts to implement this model within an interview format (Kernberg 1981) were extended by Kernberg and his colleagues with the development of the IPO.

The IPO is an 83-item self-report measure consisting of three primary clinical scales and two secondary scales. The three primary clinical scales (57 items) are relevant to the central dimensions of Kernberg's personality organization model (i.e., identity diffusion, primitive psychological defenses, and reality testing). The two secondary scales (29 items) operationalize the supplementary diagnostic components of Kernberg's model (i.e., aggression and moral values). All IPO items have a five-point Likert-type format (1=never true to 5=always true). The Primitive Defenses subscale contains 16 items, the Identity Diffusion subscale contains 21 items, the Reality Testing subscale contains 20 items, the Moral Values subscale contains 11 items, and the Aggression subscale contains 18 items. As reported by Lenzenweger et al. (2001), initial psychometric characteristics of the three primary clinical scales in a large nonclinical sample of young adults suggest that the three primary dimensions display adequate internal consistency as well as short-term test–retest reliability. In addition, initial criterion validation, derived from a nonclinical sample, is quite supportive of the

IPO (Lenzenweger et al. 2001). An unpublished study by McClough et al. of the basic psychometric properties of the five subscales of the IPO, as well as its construct validity, in a clinical sample of patients diagnosed with borderline personality disorder also supports the adequate reliability and validity of the measure (McClough JF, Clarkin JF, Lenzenweger MF, et al: "The Inventory of Personality Organization (IPO): Psychometric Properties and Criterion Relations With Affect, Constraint, Aggression, and Psychopathology in a Clinical Sample of Borderline Personality Disorder Patients," unpublished, 2005).

The Defense Style Questionnaire is designed to dimensionally assess conscious derivatives of defense mechanisms. The underlying assumption of the scale is that people are sufficiently aware of their characteristic style(s) of dealing with stress and conflict that they can provide an accurate report of their defensive functioning. The 88-item questionnaire provides scores on four defensive functioning styles: Maladaptive Action, Image-Distorting, Self-Sacrificing, and Adaptive. Each of the styles consists of several defense mechanisms. For instance, the Maladaptive Action style consists of projection, regression, projective identification, inhibition, acting out, somatization, withdrawal, fantasy, help rejecting, undoing, consumption, and complaining, whereas the Adaptive style consists of humor, sublimation, suppression, and affiliation. Initial psychometric data are greatly limited, but the reliability of the measure appears to be good, and these defensive styles have been shown to be related to treatment response.

Assessment of Environmental Demands and Social Adjustment

The interaction between the patient and the pressures of the environment is now acknowledged in the standard diagnostic system (DSM-IV-TR) by a rating on Axis IV. Probably the most substantiated area with empirical data indicating the impact of the patient–environment interaction is the investigation of expressed emotion and its influence on the course of schizophrenia. This work suggests that certain elements in the home environment of a patient with schizophrenia can adversely affect the course of the illness. Expressed emotion can be assessed by the Camberwell Family Interview (G.W. Brown and Rutter 1966), a 1-hour semistructured interview of a relative of the patient. The scoring scheme for this instrument is not readily accessible and is therefore not usable in standard clinical situations.

In measuring both stress and the patient's ability to cope with stress, one can assess the stimuli, the individual's response to the stimuli, or the interaction of the person with stressful stimuli (Table 3–11). The Jenkins Activity Survey (Jenkins et al. 1967) is the prototype of an interaction-based measure of stress, focusing on the cognitive and perceptual characteristics of the individual that mediate responses to stress. This instrument has been shown to have predictive validity in studies of reaction to coronary heart disease. The Derogatis Stress Profile (Derogatis 1982) is helpful in evaluating stimuli from work and home and can be used to assess health as well as characteristic attitudes and coping mechanisms. The Recent Life Changes Questionnaire (Holmes and Rahe 1967) is a standardized measure designed to assess major life circumstances and their impact on mental and physical health. It is the most widely used measure that assesses the relationship between psychological symptoms and the environmental context in which they often exist. Similar stress and life events measures include the Daily Hassles Scale (Lazarus and Folkman 1989), the Life Experiences Survey (Sarason et al. 1978), and the Perceived Stress Scale (Cohen et al. 1983). These three measures emphasize the critical role the patient's subjective interpretation of life events plays in relation to adjustment.

TABLE 3–11. **Instruments for the assessment of environmental stressors**

Instrument	General classification	Description	Scoring features
Social Adjustment Scale— Self Report	Self-report	42 questions, rated on 5-point scale of severity	Mean score for 7 areas and an overall score
Dyadic Adjustment Scale	Self-report	31 items, 4 dimensions	Total score
Marital Satisfaction Inventory	Self-report	280 items	T scores on 11 scales

We use the term *social adjustment* to indicate the skill of the individual in handling interpersonal situations, whether at home, in school, or in the work setting. The term has been used more narrowly to indicate the community and social adjustment of diagnosed psychiatric patients, who often have severe illnesses such as schizophrenia and major affective disorder (Weissman and Sholomskas 1982). Notable assessment instruments in this area include the Katz Adjustment Scale—Relative's Form (Katz and Lyerly 1963), the Social Adjustment Scale–Self-Report (Weissman and Bothwell 1976), and the Dyadic Adjustment Scale (Spanier 1976).

The Katz Adjustment Scale–Relative's Form is a relative's self-report inventory of the patient's symptomatic behavior and social adjustment in the community. The scale has sections on symptoms and social behavior, performance of socially expected tasks, relative's expectation for the performance of these tasks, the patient's leisure-time activities, and the relative's satisfaction with the performance of these free-time activities.

The Social Adjustment Scale–Self-Report contains 42 questions covering instrumental and affective qualities in role performance, social and leisure activities, relationships with extended family, marital role, parental role, family unit, and economic independence. Norms are available for nonpatient community samples, acutely ill and recovered depressed outpatients, schizophrenic patients, and drug-addicted patients. The Social Support Questionnaire (Sarason et al. 1983) is an efficient method for assessing social satisfaction. This instrument provides information about available resources of support and the patient's level of satisfaction with this support system.

Several widely used rating scales of overall psychosocial functioning (i.e., symptoms, social and occupational functioning) that rate patients on a hypothetical continuum from psychological sickness to mental health are the Global Assessment Scale (GAS; Endicott et al. 1976), the Global Assessment of Functioning Scale (GAF), and the Social and Occupational Functioning Assessment Scale (SOFAS; Goldman et al. 1992). The GAS is a revision of Luborsky's (1962) Health Sickness Rating Scale. It is a 100-point single item rating scale divided into 10 equal intervals, 1–10, 11–20, and so on, up to 91–100. The scale is designed to be completed by the clinician after compiling clinical information from all available sources (e.g., patient and informant interview, review of records). To make a rating, the clinician chooses the lowest interval that describes the patient's level of functioning during the previous week and then selects a specific scale point within that interval. The final scale score is comprised of a single number. The GAF is a revision of the GAS and comprises Axis V on the multiaxial system of DSM-IV. The SOFAS is also a derivative of the GAS, but with an exclusive focus on the patient's level of social and occupational functioning. All three rating scales are extremely easy to use, appropriate for use in numerous contexts, and shown to be reliable. The scales can be used for treatment planning, tracking changes over time, the assessment of treatment effects, the validation of other measures, the prediction of outcome, and the evaluation of quality of life. The advantage of the SOFAS is that ratings are not directly influenced by psychological symptoms to the same extent as the GAS and GAF.

Related to overall psychosocial functioning is the concept of quality of life. The construct of *quality of life* is relatively new to the psychological literature, and disagreements exist regarding its definition. Nevertheless, there is a consensus that quality of life is multidimensional in nature and includes the psychological, social functioning, and physical domains (and their combinations). Quality-of-life measures such as the Quality of Life Interview (Lehman 1988), the Quality of Life Scale (Heinrichs et al. 1984), and the Wisconsin Quality of Life Index (Becker et al. 1993) are disease specific and intended for patients who are severely or persistently mentally ill. Generic measures appropriate for use with any patient group include the Quality of Life Enjoyment and Satisfaction Questionnaire (Endicott et al. 1993), the Quality of Life Index (Ferrans and Powers 1985), and the Quality of Life Inventory (Frisch 1994). The Psychosocial Adjustment to Illness Scale (Derogatis 1986) and the Spitzer Quality of Life Index (Spitzer et al. 1981) are health-related measures and assume that the patient is dealing with a medical condition. The measures are more or less equivalent, and the choice of instrument should be based on the research question or clinical issue being considered. Regardless, these scales are useful for assessing change over time and as measures of therapeutic outcome.

The whole area of the quality of marital adjustment is relevant to treatment planning for married individuals with psychiatric disorders such as phobias and mood disorders (Clarkin et al. 1992), as well as those couples who present with marital difficulties. Two useful self-report instruments in this area are the Dyadic Adjustment Scale and the Marital Satisfaction Inventory (Snyder et al. 1981).

Assessment of Therapeutic Enabling Factors

Accurate diagnosis is not sufficient for determining optimal specific treatments. Although the patient's diagnosis helps to narrow the focus, optimal treatment planning depends on nondiagnostic factors such as characteristics of the patient that will affect the acceptance, use, and absorption of the treatment that is recommended. Psychological tests can be useful in assessing these dimensions. From a review of the comparative psychotherapy outcome research data (Beutler 1983; Beutler and Clarkin 1990; Gaw and Beutler 1995), one can isolate five areas of assessment: 1) problem severity, 2) motivational distress, 3) problem complexity, 4) resistance potential or reactance level, and 5) coping style.

Problem severity is defined as a continuum of functioning ranging from little impairment to incapacitation. Instruments reviewed in this chapter assessing symptoms and general functioning are appropriate tools for measuring problem severity. *Motivational distress* is the degree of subjective disturbance experienced by the patient in reference to his or her problems. Motivational distress is important because it motivates help-seeking activity such as psychotherapy in order to reduce discomfort. The BSI is an efficient method of assessing aspects of patient self-defined problem severity. The global severity index from the BSI can be used as an estimate of subjective or motivational distress. It is suggested that when the global severity index value exceeds a T score of 63, a treatment that is designed to reduce subjective distress is indicated (Derogatis 1993). If distress levels are low, the clinician must consider whether to confront the patient with the contradiction of low distress in the face of impairment. The MMPI-2 can also be used to assess motivational distress. For example, Scale 7 (Psychasthenia) is an index of psychological turmoil and discomfort (Graham 1990). Scores above 70 on the F scale may suggest good motivation for treatment. Individuals whose high scores on the F scale are matched with elevations on the L and K scales tend to resist and react to authority and, inferentially, to therapists.

Problem complexity relates to the pervasiveness and endurance of the problem. A complex problem is pervasive and enduring—that is, it is chronic and transsituational rather than situation specific. The BSI offers information on the degree to which the problem spreads across symptom domains, which is one aspect of complexity. The MMPI-2 two-point code types (Graham 1990) and the Axis II indicators from the MCMI-II may also shed light on the spread and chronicity of problems.

Reactance is a construct from social psychology that indicates the degree to which an individual is resistant or oppositional to interpersonal demands such as the recommendations or advice of a mental health professional. One of the most promising instruments for assessing reactance is the Therapeutic Reactance Scale (Dowd et al. 1991). This is a 28-item self-report instrument for which there have been two normative studies.

Coping style refers to the manner in which an individual manages or deals with anxiety that arises from interpersonal or intrapersonal conflict. The MMPI-2 is useful in defining the patient's coping styles along an internalizing–externalizing dimension. Externalizing patterns are indicated by the Hysteria, Psychopathic Deviance, Paranoia, and Mania scales. Internalizing coping styles are indicated by the Hypochondriasis, Depression, Psychasthenia, and Social Introversion scales.

Psychological Assessment in the Contemporary Health Care Climate

There is the potential for psychological assessment to become integral to the mental health care system because of its methodological rigor and psychometric sophistication. Rapidly escalating health care costs have forced businesses, legislators, and consumers to identify cost containment as a top priority (Moreland et al. 1994). For better or worse, third-party payers are demanding that services become time limited, problem focused, and "medically necessary." Traditional psychological assessment, by these standards, has been seen as a superfluous and unnecessary cost and has therefore been forced to significantly change its focus.

Psychological assessment has survived in this era and will continue to do so insofar as it contributes to cost-containment mechanisms, quality improvement, and consumer satisfaction in health care settings (Moreland et al. 1994). Consequently, certain areas of priority have begun to be addressed in systematic and rigorous ways, the hallmark of sound psychological assessment: 1) treatment planning, 2) ongoing assessment of the impact of treatment and assessment of outcome, 3) quality assurance within and across institutions, and 4) screening for psychiatric disturbance.

In the arena of *treatment planning*, psychological assessment can systematically inform clinicians and reviewers about the most cost-effective treatment. Such assessment involves questions such as "What level of care is most appropriate for this patient at this time—inpatient, partial hospital, intensive outpatient, or outpatient?"

Once treatment has begun, routine, standardized psychological assessment can *track the progress and impact of treatment* among individuals and groups. Many efficient, easy-to-administer omnibus measures have been developed that can quickly (via computerized databases) assess changes in patients' symptoms, behaviors, quality of life, and functional levels during the treatment process. With these data, informed decisions can be made about whether the current treatment is effective or whether another treatment should be considered. Consider, for example, a depressed patient with a BDI score of 24 and few Reasons for Living at the outset of treatment. If these measures were readministered by the clinician at monthly intervals, that clinician would obtain reliable and valid indicators of the impact of treatment. Possession of such indicators would enable the clinician to communicate convincingly with reviewers about the current treatment's effectiveness and the continued need for treatment.

In regard to the ongoing impact of treatment, outcome assessment addresses the immediate and long-term stability of improvements in patients and groups. At the end of treatment and after, psychological assessment can be utilized to address questions such as "How permanent are the patient's improvements in symptoms of depression?" and "With improvements in mood, has the patient's ability to work and have relationships improved (functional level)?" Insofar as recidivism, relapse, and short-term treatment effects constitute a major financial drain, any health care system serious about containing costs must grapple with long-term outcomes in terms of patients' functional levels after treatment has ended, even if the treatments appear to adequately improve symptoms and behavior in the short term.

At present, *quality assurance* appears to be primarily defined by the satisfaction of the health care consumer; however, it can be argued that this aspect is not, by itself, an adequate measure of quality. Notwithstanding, psychological assessment has the ability to systematically track patient satisfaction for accrediting agencies that require such information (e.g., the Joint Committee on Health Care Accreditation). Ideally, these data can be observed in concert with other outcome data, such as symptoms, behaviors, and quality of life. Several instruments exist to measure consumer's satisfaction with health care as well as their perceptions of the quality of care. These measures include the Patient Satisfaction Questionnaire (Marshall et al. 1993), the Patient Judgment System (Nelson et al. 1989), the Client Satisfaction Questionnaire–8 (Larsen et al. 1979), and the Service Satisfaction Scale–30 (Greenfield and Attkisson 1989).

Within the past several years, mental health tracking systems have been developed to collect data that are useful for clinicians (treatment planning), administrators (efficiency of clinicians in delivering care), and third-party payers, employers, and accrediting agencies (patient satisfaction and outcome assessment). By gathering systematic and sequential data, these systems provide information for utilization review regarding the need for additional treatment. Such data can also be used to assess clinicians' performance in relation to cost and to identify clinicians who are effective or ineffective in conducting interventions with different types of individuals. Mental health tracking systems focus on patient processes and outcomes of interest to employers as well. These include alleviation of symptom distress, reduction of health care expenses, and reduction of absenteeism.

In summary, the role of the psychological assessment system in determining the cost-effectiveness of treatments for mental and physical health will likely become more prominent in the new century's health care as the demand for rigorous and systematic documentation of treatment effects remains a priority. Given this scenario, one can predict that psychological assessment will continue to evolve to address individual, group, and institutional variables; will become more rapid and focused; will rely heavily on computerized administration, scoring, and database management; and will address not only symptoms and behavior in the short term but also functional level and quality of life in the long term. In addition, psychological and biological assessments will continue to become more integrated (e.g., neuropsychological assessment). Finally, considering these trends, psychiatrists will need to become better educated and trained regarding the principles and uses of rigorous, empirically sound psychological assessment.

Key Points

- Three types of instruments are used in the assessment of patient functioning: psychological tests, rating scales, and semistructured interviews.

- Tests should meet the standards of both reliability and validity.

- Establishing a test's reliability requires demonstration that the test items are sufficiently closely related to one another to provide relatively stable measurements. Three major types of reliability can be assessed: test–retest reliability, alternate form reliability, and split-half reliability.

- Establishing a test's validity requires demonstration that the test measures what it is intended to measure. Three major types of validity can be assessed: content validity, criterion-related validity, and construct validity.

- Assessment has the following objectives: 1) screening for psychiatric disturbance, 2) clarification of diagnostic uncertainty following clinical interview, 3) specification of the severity of symptoms and other difficulties, 4) assessment of patient strengths, 5) informing differential treatment assignment, 6) role-inducing the patient into a therapeutic stance, 7) monitoring the impact of treatment over time, 8) assessment of barriers to learning for educational planning, and 9) assessment of quality and cost-effectiveness of systems of care.

- Cultural factors may influence subjects' response to assessment instruments.

- Major content areas of assessment include symptoms, cognitive functioning, personality disorders and traits, psychodynamics, and environmental demands and social adjustment.

- Therapeutic enabling factors are aspects of the patient that affect the acceptance, use, and absorption of the treatment.

- The major therapeutic enabling factors are problem severity, motivational distress, problem complexity, reactance, and coping style.

Suggested Readings

Beutler LE, Groth-Marnat G (eds): Integrative assessment of adult personality. 2nd Edition. New York, Guilford, 2003

Harrow M, Quinlan D (eds): Disordered Thinking and Schizophrenic Psychopathology. New York, Gardner, 1985

Hersen M (ed): Psychological Assessment in Clinical Practice. New York, Brunner-Routledge, 2004

Maruish ME (ed): The Use of Psychological Testing for Treatment Planning and Outcomes Assessment, Vol 3, 3rd Edition. Mahwah, NJ, Lawrence Erlbaum, 2004

Rush AJ, First MB, Blacker D (eds): Handbook of Psychiatric Measures, 2nd Edition. Arlington, VA, American Psychiatric Publishing, 2008

References

American Psychiatric Association: Diagnostic and Statistical Manual of Mental Disorders, 3rd Edition. Washington, DC, American Psychiatric Association, 1980

American Psychiatric Association: Diagnostic and Statistical Manual of Mental Disorders, 4th Edition. Washington, DC, American Psychiatric Association, 1994

American Psychiatric Association: Diagnostic and Statistical Manual of Mental Disorders, 4th Edition, Text Revision. Washington, DC, American Psychiatric Association, 2000

Anastasi A: Psychological Testing, 5th Edition. New York, Macmillan, 1982

Andreasen NC: Scale for the Assessment of Positive Symptoms (SAPS). Iowa City, University of Iowa, 1984

Baddeley A: Working Memory. Oxford, United Kingdom, Clarendon Press, 1986

Bauer MS, Crits-Christoph P, Ball WA, et al: Independent assessment of manic and depressive symptoms by self-rating: scale characteristics and implications for the study of mania. Arch Gen Psychiatry 48:807–812, 1991

Beatty WW, Mold JW, Gontkovsky ST: RBANS performance: influences of sex and education. J Clin Exp Neuropsychol 25:1065–1069, 2003

Beck AT, Young JE: Depression, in Clinical Handbook of Psychological Disorders. Edited by Barlow DH. New York, Guilford, 1985, pp 202–244

Beck AT, Schuyler D, Herman I: Development of suicidal intent scales, in The Prediction of Suicide. Edited by Beck AT, Resnick HLP, Lettieri DJ. Bowie, MD, Charles Press, 1974, pp 2045–2056

Beck AT, Epstein N, Brown G, et al: An inventory for measuring clinical anxiety: psychometric properties. J Consult Clin Psychol 56:893–897, 1988

Beck AT, Steer RA, Brown GK: Beck Depression Inventory Manual, 2nd Edition. San Antonio, TX, Psychological Corporation, 1996

Beck LH, Bransome ED Jr, Mirsky AF, et al: A continuous performance test of brain damage. J Consult Psychol 20:343–350, 1956

Becker M, Diamond R, Sainfort F: A new patient focused index for measuring quality of life in persons with severe and persistent mental illness. Qual Life Res 2:239–251, 1993

Beigel A, Murphy DL, Bunney WE Jr: The Manic-State Rating Scale: scale construction, reliability, and validity. Arch Gen Psychiatry 25:256–262, 1971

Benjamin LS: SASB Short Form User's Manual. Salt Lake City, University of Utah, 1988

Benton A, Sivan A, Hamsher K: Contributions to Neuropsychological Assessment: A Clinical Manual, 2nd Edition. New York, Oxford University Press, 1994

Beutler LE: Eclectic Psychotherapy: A Systematic Approach. New York, Pergamon, 1983

Beutler LE, Clarkin JF: Systematic Treatment Selection: Toward Targeted Therapeutic Interventions. New York, Brunner/Mazel, 1990

Beutler LE, Clarkin JF, Bongar B: Guidelines for the Systematic Treatment of the Depressed Patient. New York, Oxford University Press, 2000

Blake DD, Weathers FW, Nagy LN, et al: A clinician ratings scale for assessing current and lifetime PTSD: the CAPS-1. Behavior Therapist 18:187–188, 1990

Bond M, Wesley S: Manual for Defense Style Questionnaire. Montreal, Quebec, Canada, McGill University, 1996

Bongar B: The Suicidal Patient: Clinical and Legal Standards of Care. Washington, DC, American Psychological Association, 1991

Brown GK, Beck AT, Newman CF, et al: A comparison of focused and standard cognitive therapy for panic disorder. J Anxiety Disord 11:329–345, 1997

Brown GW, Rutter M: The measurement of family activities and relationships: a methodological study. Hum Relat 19:241–263, 1966

Buros OK (ed): The Seventh Mental Measurements Yearbook. Highland Park, NJ, Gryphon, 1971

Buros OK (ed): The Eighth Mental Measurements Yearbook. Highland Park, NJ, Gryphon, 1978

Buss AH, Durkee A: An inventory for assessing different kinds of hostility. J Consult Psychol 21:343–349, 1957

Butcher JN: The Minnesota Report: Adult Clinical System MMPI-2. Minneapolis, University of Minnesota Press, 1989

Butcher JN: Objective study of abnormal personality in cross-cultural settings: the Minnesota Multiphasic Personality Inventory (MMPI-2). J Cross Cult Psychol 29:189–211, 1998

Butcher JN, Dahlstrom WG, Graham JR, et al: Manual for the Restandardized Minnesota Multiphasic Personality Inventory (MMPI-2): An Administrative and Interpretive Guide. Minneapolis, University of Minnesota Press, 1989

Cattell RB, Eber HW, Tatsuoka MM: Handbook for the Sixteen Personality Factor Inventory. Champaign, IL, Institute for Personality and Ability Testing, 1970

Cicerone K: Clinical sensitivity of four measures of attention to mild traumatic brain injury. Clin Neuropsychol 11:266–272, 1997

Clark LA: Manual for the Schedule for Nonadaptive and Adaptive Personality (SNAP). Minneapolis, University of Minnesota Press, 1993

Clarkin JF, Haas GL, Glick ID: Family and marital therapy, in Handbook of Affective Disorders, 2nd Edition. Edited by Paykel ES. London, England, Churchill Livingstone, 1992, pp 487–500

Clarkin JF, Foelsch PA, Kernberg OF: The Inventory of Personality Organization. White Plains, NY, Weill Medical College of Cornell University, 2001

Cloninger CR, Svrakic DM, Przybeck TR: A psychobiological model of temperament and character. Arch Gen Psychiatry 50:975–990, 1993

Coccaro EF, Harvey PD, Kupsaw-Lawrence E, et al: Development of neuropharmacologically based behavioral assessments of impulsive aggressive behavior. J Neuropsychiatry Clin Neurosci 3:S44–S51, 1991

Cohen S, Kamarck T, Mermelstein R: A global measure of perceived stress. J Health Soc Behav 24:385–396, 1983

Conners C: Continuous Performance Test II. Toronto, Ontario, Canada, Multi-Health Systems, 2000

Corwin J, Bylsma F: Translations of excerpts from Andre Rey's Psychological Examination of Traumatic Encephalopathy and P.A. Osterreith's The Complex Figure Copy Test. Clin Neuropsychol 7:3–21, 1993

Costa LD, McCrae RR: NEO PI-R: Professional Manual. Odessa, FL, Psychological Assessment Resources, 1992

Cronbach L, Meehl P: Construct validity in psychological tests. Psychol Bull 42:281–301, 1955

Culbertson W, Zillmer E: Tower of London: Drexel University (TOL$_{DX}$). North Tonawanda, NY, Multi-Health Systems, 2001

Cull JG, Gill WS: Suicide Probability Scale (SPS) Manual. Los Angeles, CA, Western Psychological Services, 1986

Davidson JRT, Potts NLS, Richichi EA, et al: The Brief Social Phobia Scale. J Clin Psychiatry 52:48–51, 1991

De Renzi E, Faglioni P: Normative data and screening power of a shortened version of the Token Test. Cortex 14:41–49, 1978

Delis D, Kaplan E, Kramer JH, et al: California Verbal Learning Test—2nd Edition (CVLT-II) Manual. Edited by Corporation TP. San Antonio, TX, Harcourt Brace, 2000

Delis D, Kaplan E, Kramer J: Delis-Kaplan Executive Function System. San Antonio, TX, Psychological Corporation, 2001

Derogatis LR: The SCL-90-R. Baltimore, MD, Clinical Psychometric Research, 1977

Derogatis LR: Self-report measures of stress, in Handbook of Stress. Edited by Goldberger L, Breznitz S. New York, Free Press, 1982, pp 270–294

Derogatis LR: SCL-90-R: Administration, Scoring, and Procedures Manual II. Baltimore, MD, Clinical Psychometric Research, 1983

Derogatis LR: The Psychological Adjustment to Illness Scale (PAIS). J Psychosom Res 30:77–91, 1986

Derogatis LR: Brief Symptom Inventory (BSI): Administration, Scoring, and Procedures Manual, 3rd Edition. Minneapolis, MN, National Computer Systems, 1993

Derogatis LR: SCL-90-R, Brief Symptom Inventory, and matching clinical rating scales, in Psychological Testing, Treatment Planning, and Outcome Assessment. Edited by Maruish M. New York, Lawrence Erlbaum, 1994

Derogatis LR, Lipman RS, Rickels K, et al: The Hopkins Symptom Checklist (HSCL): a measure of primary symptom dimensions, in Psychological Measurements in Psychopharmacology, Vol 7: Modern Problems of Pharmacopsychiatry. Edited by Pichot P. Basel, Switzerland, S Karger, 1974, pp 79–110

Dowd ET, Milne CR, Wise SL: The Therapeutic Reactance Scale: a measure of psychological reactance. J Consult Clin Psychol 69:541–545, 1991

Duff K, Patton D, Schoenberg MR, et al: Age- and education-corrected independent normative data for the RBANS in a community dwelling elderly sample. Clin Neuropsychol 17:351–366, 2003

Endicott J, Spitzer RL: Use of the Research Diagnostic Criteria and the Schedule for Affective Disorders and Schizophrenia to study affective disorders. Am J Psychiatry 136:52–56, 1979

Endicott J, Spitzer RL, Fleiss JL, et al: The Global Assessment Scale: a procedure for measuring overall severity of psychiatric disturbance. Arch Gen Psychiatry 33:766–771, 1976

Endicott J, Nee J, Harrison W, et al: Quality of Life Enjoyment and Satisfaction Questionnaire: a new scale. Psychopharmacol Bull 29:321–326, 1993

Endler NS, Hunt J McV, Rosenstein AJ: An S-R inventory of anxiousness (monogr no 536). Psychological Monographs: General and Applied 76:1–31, 1962

Exner JE Jr: The Rorschach: A Comprehensive System, Vol 1. New York, Wiley, 1974

Exner JE Jr: The Rorschach: A Comprehensive System, Vol 2. New York, Wiley, 1978

Eysenck HJ, Eysenck SB: The Structure and Measurement of Personality. San Diego, CA, RR Knapp, 1969

Feighner JP, Robins E, Guze SB, et al: Diagnostic criteria for use in psychiatric research. Arch Gen Psychiatry 26:57–63, 1972

Ferrans CE, Powers MJ: Quality of Life Index: development and psychometric properties. Adv Nurs Sci 8:15–24, 1985

First MB, Spitzer RL, Gibbon M, et al: Structured Clinical Interview for DSM-IV Axis I Disorders—Patient Edition (SCID-I/P). New York, Biometrics Research Department, New York State Psychiatric Institute, 1995

First MB, Gibbon M, Spitzer RL, et al: User's Guide for the Structured Clinical Interview for DSM-IV Axis II Personality Disorders (SCID-II). Washington, DC, American Psychiatric Press, 1997a

First MB, Spitzer RL, Gibbon M, et al: Structured Clinical Interview for DSM-IV Axis I Disorders—Clinician Version (SCID-CV). Washington, DC, American Psychiatric Press, 1997b

Foa EB: Posttraumatic Stress Diagnostic Scale: Manual. Minneapolis, MN, National Computer Systems, 1995

Frisch MB: Manual and Treatment Guide for the Quality of Life Inventory. Minneapolis, MN, National Computer Systems, 1994

Garner DM: Eating Disorder Inventory 2: Professional Manual. Odessa, FL, Psychological Assessment Resources, 1992

Gaw KF, Beutler LE: Integrating treatment recommendations, in Integrative Assessment of Adult Personality. Edited by Beutler LE, Berren MR. New York, Guilford, 1995, pp 280–319

Geisinger KF: Cross-cultural normative assessment: translation adaptation issues influencing the normative interpretation of assessment instruments. Psychol Assess 6:312–314, 1994

Goldman HH, Skodol AE, Lave TR: Revising Axis V for DSM-IV: a review of measures of social functioning. Am J Psychiatry 149:1148–1156, 1992

Goodglass H, Kaplan E, Barresi B: Boston Diagnostic Aphasia Examination, 3rd Edition. Philadelphia, PA, Lippincott Williams & Wilkins, 2000

Goodman WK, Price LH, Rasmussen SA, et al: The Yale-Brown Obsessive Compulsive Scale, I: development, use, and reliability. Arch Gen Psychiatry 46:1006–1011, 1989

Gough HG: California Psychological Inventory. Palo Alto, CA, Consulting Psychologists Press, 1956

Graham JR: MMPI-2: Assessing Personality and Psychopathology. New York, Oxford University Press, 1990

Grant D, Berg E: A behavioral analysis of the degree of reinforcement and ease of shifting to new responses in a Weigl-type card sorting problem. J Exp Psychol 38:404–411, 1948

Greene RL: The MMPI-2/MMPI: An Interpretive Manual. Needham Heights, MA, Allyn & Bacon, 1991

Greenfield TK, Attkisson CC: Steps toward a multifactorial satisfaction scale for primary care and mental health services. Eval Program Plann 12:271–278, 1989

Grober E, Sliwinski M: Development and validation of a model for estimating premorbid verbal intelligence in the elderly. J Clin Exp Neuropsychol 13:933–949, 1991

Hamilton M: The assessment of anxiety states by rating. Br J Med Psychol 32:50–55, 1959

Hamilton M: A rating scale for depression. J Neurol Neurosurg Psychiatry 23:51–56, 1960

Hamilton M: Development of a rating scale for primary depressive illness. Br J Soc Clin Psychol 6:278–296, 1967

Harrow M, Quinlan D (eds): Disordered Thinking and Schizophrenic Psychopathology. New York, Gardner, 1985

Harvey PD, Greenberg BR, Serper MR: The Affective Lability Scales: development, reliability, and validity. J Clin Psychol 45:786–793, 1989

Hathaway SR, McKinley JC: Minnesota Multiphasic Personality Inventory Manual, Revised Edition. New York, Psychological Corporation, 1967

Hathaway SR, McKinley JC: Minnesota Multiphasic Personality Inventory—2. Minneapolis, University of Minnesota Press, 1989

Heilman K, Watson R, Valenstein E: Neglect and related disorders, in Clinical Neuropsychology. Edited by Heilman K, Valenstein E. New York, Oxford University Press, 2003, pp 296–346

Heinrichs DW, Hanlon TE, Carpenter WT: The Quality of Life Scale: an instrument for rating the schizophrenic deficit syndrome. Schizophr Bull 10:388–397, 1984

Hoffmann H, Loper RG, Kammeier ML: Identifying future alcoholics with MMPI alcoholism scales. Q J Stud Alcohol 35:490–498, 1974

Holmes TH, Rahe RH: The social readjustment rating scale. J Psychosom Res 11:213–218, 1967

Hooper H: Hooper Visual Organization Test Manual. Los Angeles, CA, Western Psychological Services, 1983

Horn JL, Wanberg KW, Foster FM: Alcohol Use Inventory. Minneapolis, MN, National Computer Systems, 1986

Howieson D, Lezak M: Separating memory from other cognitive disorders, in The Handbook of Memory Disorders. Edited by Baddeley A, Kopelman M, Wilson B. West Sussex, England, Wiley, 2002, pp 637–654

Hurt SW, Clarkin JF, Frances A, et al: Discriminate validity of the MMPI for borderline personality disorder. J Pers Assess 49:56–61, 1985

Hurt SW, Reznikoff M, Clarkin JF: Psychological Assessment, Psychiatric Diagnosis, and Treatment Planning. New York, Brunner/Mazel, 1991

Hyler SE: Personality Diagnostic Questionnaire—4. New York, New York State Psychiatric Institute, 1994

Hyler SE, Rieder RO, Williams JBW, et al: The Personality Diagnostic Questionnaire: development and preliminary results. J Personal Disord 2:229–237, 1988

Janowsky D, Judd L, Huey L, et al: Naloxone effects on manic symptoms and growth-hormone levels (letter). Lancet 2:320, 1978

Jenkins CD, Rosenman RH, Friedman J: Development of an objective psychological test for the determination of the coronary-prone behavior pattern in employed men. J Chronic Dis 20:371–379, 1967

Katz MM, Lyerly SB: Methods for measuring adjustment and social behavior in the community, I: rationale, description, discriminative validity and scale development. Psychol Rep Monogr 13:503–535, 1963

Kay SR, Fiszbein A, Opler LA: Positive and Negative Syndrome (PANSS) for schizophrenia. Schizophr Bull 13:261–276, 1987

Kaye AL, Shea MT: Personality disorders, personality traits, and defense mechanisms measures, in Handbook of Psychiatric Measures. Washington, DC, American Psychiatric Association, 2000, pp 734–736

Kernberg OF: Structural interviewing. Psychiatr Clin North Am 4:169–195, 1981

Kernberg OF: A psychoanalytic theory of personality disorders, in Major Theories of Personality Disorder. Edited by Clarkin JF, Lenzenweger MF. New York, Guilford, 1996, pp 106–140

Klein MH, Benjamin LS, Rosenfeld R, et al: The Wisconsin Personality Disorders Interview: development, reliability, and validity. J Personal Disord 7:285–303, 1993

Koechlin E, Basso G, Pietrini P, et al: The role of the anterior prefrontal cortex in human cognition. Nature 399:148–151, 1999

Larsen DL, Attkisson CC, Hargreaves WA, et al: Assessment of client/patient satisfaction: development of a general scale. Eval Program Plann 2:197–207, 1979

Lazarus RS, Folkman S: Manual: Hassles and Uplifts Scale, Research Edition. Palo Alto, CA, Mind Garden, 1989

Leary T: Interpersonal Diagnosis of Personality. New York, Ronald Press, 1957

Leclercq M, Zimmermann P: Applied Neuropsychology of Attention: Theory, Diagnosis and Rehabilitation. New York, Psychology Press, 2002

Lehman AF: Quality of Life Interview for the chronically mentally ill. Eval Program Plann 11:51–62, 1988

Lenzenweger MF, Loranger AW, Korfine L, et al: Detecting personality disorders in a nonclinical population: application of a two-stage procedure for case detection. Arch Gen Psychiatry 54:345–351, 1997

Lenzenweger MF, Clarkin JF, Kernberg OF, et al: The Inventory of personality organization: psychometric properties, factorial composition, and criterion relations with affect, aggressive dyscontrol, psychosis proneness, and self-domains in a nonclinical sample. Psychol Assess 13:577–591, 2001

Lezak M, Howieson D, Loring D: Neuropsychological Assessment, 4th Edition. New York, Oxford University Press, 2004

Liebowitz MR: Social phobia. Mod Probl Pharmacopsychiatry 22:141–173, 1987

Linehan MM, Goodstein JL, Nielson SL, et al: Reasons for staying alive when you are thinking of killing yourself: the Reasons for Living Inventory. J Consult Clin Psychol 51:276–286, 1983

Loranger AW: International Personality Disorder Examination (IPDE) Manual. Odessa, FL, Psychological Assessment Resources, 1999

Loranger AW, Hirschfeld RMA, Sartorius N, et al: The WHO/ADAMHA international pilot study of personality disorders: background and purpose. J Personal Disord 5:296–306, 1991

Loring DW, Hermann BP, Lee GP, et al: The Memory Assessment Scales and lateralized temporal lobe epilepsy. J Clin Psychol 56:563–570, 2000

Lorr M, McNair DM: Expansion of the interpersonal behavior circle. J Pers Soc Psychol 2:823–830, 1965

Lorr M, Youniss RP: An inventory of interpersonal style. J Pers Assess 37:165–173, 1973

Luborsky L: Clinicians' judgments of mental health. Arch Gen Psychiatry 7:407–417, 1962

MacAndrew C: The differentiation of male alcohol outpatients from nonalcoholic psychiatric patients by means of the MMPI. Q J Stud Alcohol 26:238–246, 1965

Marengo J, Harrow M: Thought disorder: a function of schizophrenia, mania, or psychosis? J Nerv Ment Dis 173:35–41, 1985

Markon KE, Krueger RF, Bouchard TJ, et al: Normal and abnormal personality traits: evidence for genetic and environmental relationships in the Minnesota Study of Twins Reared Apart. J Pers 70:661–693, 2002

Marks IM, Seeman W: The Actuarial Description of Abnormal Personality. Baltimore, MD, Williams & Wilkins, 1963

Marshall GN, Hays RD, Sherbourne CD, et al: The structure of patient satisfaction with outpatient medical care. Psychol Assess 5:477–483, 1993

McConnaughy EA, Prochaska JO, Velicer WF: Stages of change in psychotherapy: measurement and sample profiles. Theory, Research, and Practice 20:368–375, 1983

McKinley JC, Hathaway SR, Meehl PE: The MMPI-VI: K scale. J Consult Psychol 12:20–31, 1948

McLellan AT, Luborsky L, Woody GE, et al: An improved diagnostic evaluation instrument for substance abuse patients: the Addiction Severity Index. J Nerv Ment Dis 168:26–33, 1980

Megargee EI, Cook PE, Mendelsohn GA: Development and validation of an MMPI scale of assaultiveness in overcontrolled individuals. J Abnorm Psychol 72:519–528, 1967

Millon T: Millon Clinical Multiaxial Inventory—II: Manual for the MCMI-II. Minneapolis, MN, National Computer Systems, 1987

Millon T, Davis R, Millon C: MCMI-III Manual, 2nd Edition. Minneapolis, MN, National Computer Systems, 1997

Mitrushina M, Boone K, Razani J, et al: Handbook of Normative Data for Neuropsychological Assessment, 2nd Edition. New York, Oxford University Press, 2005

Morey LC: Personality Assessment Inventory. Odessa, FL, Psychological Assessment Resources, 1991

Moreland KL, Fowler RD, Honaker LM: Future directions in the use of psychological assessment for treatment planning and outcome assessment: predictions and recommendations, in The Use of Psychological Testing for Treatment Planning and Outcome Assessment. Edited by Maruish ME. Hillsdale, NJ, Lawrence Erlbaum, 1994, pp 581–602

Murray HA: Thematic Apperception Test Manual. Cambridge, MA, Harvard University Press, 1943

Nelson EC, Hays RD, Larson C, et al: The Patient Judgment System: reliability and validity. Qual Rev Bull 15:185–191, 1989

Nelson H, Willison J: The National Adult Reading Test: Test Manual, 2nd Edition. Windsor, United Kingdom, NFER Nelson, 1991

Newman FL, Ciarlo JA: Criteria for selecting psychological tests/instruments, in Use of Psychological Testing for Treatment Planning and Outcome Assessment. Edited by Maruish M. Malvern, PA, LEA Publishers, 1994, pp 98–110

Overall JE, Gorham DR: The Brief Psychiatric Rating Scale. Psychol Rep 10:799–812, 1962

Pfohl B, Langbehn D: Iowa Personality Disorder Screen (Version 1.2). Iowa City, University of Iowa, Department of Psychiatry, 1994

Pfohl B, Blum N, Zimmerman M: Structured Interview for DSM-IV Personality (SIDP-IV). Washington, DC, American Psychiatric Press, 1997

Pilkonis PA, Kim Y, Proitetti JM, et al: A screen scale for personality disorders developed from the Inventory of Interpersonal Problems. J Personal Disord 10:355–369, 1996

Pillon B: [Visuo-constructive problems and methods of compensation: results for 85 patients with brain lesions.] Neuropsychologia 19:375–383, 1981

Prochaska JO, DiClemente CC, Norcross JC: In search of how people change: applications to addictive behaviors. Am Psychol 47:1102–1114, 1992

Randolph C, Tierney MC, Mohr E, et al: The Repeatable Battery for the Assessment of Neuropsychological Status (RBANS): preliminary clinical validity. J Clin Exp Neuropsychol 20:310–319, 1998

Reitan R, Wolfson D: The Halstead-Reitan Neuropsychological Test Battery: Theory and Clinical Applications, 2nd Edition. Tucson, AZ, Neuropsychology Press, 1993

Rey A: L'examen psychologique dans les cas d'encephalopathie traumatique. Archives de Psychologie 28:286–340, 1941

Ridley CR, Li LC, Hill CL: Multicultural assessment: reexamination, reconceptualization and practical application. Couns Psychol 26:827–910, 1998

Rorschach H: Psychodiagnostics. New York, Grune & Stratton, 1949

Ruff R, Light R, Evans R: The Ruff Figural Fluency Test: a normative study with adults. Dev Neuropsychol 3:37–52, 1987

Rush AJ, First MB, Blacker D (eds): Handbook of Psychiatric Measures, 2nd Edition. Arlington, VA, American Psychiatric Publishing, 2008

Sarason IG, Johnson JH, Seigel JM: Assessing the impact of life changes: development of the Life Experiences Survey. J Consult Clin Psychol 46:932–946, 1978

Sarason IG, Levine HM, Basham RB, et al: Assessing social support: the Social Support Questionnaire. J Pers Soc Psychol 44:127–139, 1983

Schroeder ML, Wormworth JA, Livesley WJ: Dimensions of personality disorder and the five-factor model of personality, in Personality Disorders and the Five-Factor Model of Personality. Edited by Costa PT, Widiger TA. Washington, DC, American Psychological Association, 1994, pp 117–127

Secunda S, Katz M, Swann A, et al: Mania: diagnosis, state measurement, and prediction of treatment response. J Affect Disord 8:113–121, 1985

Shear MK, Brown TA, Barlow DH, et al: Multicenter collaborative Panic Disorder Severity Scale. Am J Psychiatry 154:1571–1575, 1997

Shenton ME, Kikinis R, Frenc AJ, et al: Abnormalities of the left temporal lobe and thought disorder in schizophrenia: a quantitative magnetic resonance imaging study. N Engl J Med 327:604–612, 1992

Simon RI: Suicide risk: assessing the unpredictable, in American Psychiatric Publishing Textbook of Suicide Assessment and Management. Edited by Simon RI, Hales RE. Washington, DC, American Psychiatric Publishing, 2006, pp 1–32

Sivan A: Benton Visual Retention Test, 5th Edition. San Antonio, TX, Psychological Corporation, 1992

Snyder DK, Wills RM, Keiser TW: Empirical validation of the Marital Satisfaction Inventory: an actuarial approach. J Consult Clin Psychol 49:262–268, 1981

Solovay MR, Shenton ME, Gasperetti C, et al: Scoring manual for the Thought Disorder Index. Schizophr Bull 12:483–496, 1986

Spanier GB: Measuring dyadic adjustment: new scales for assessing the quality of marriage and similar dyads. J Marriage Fam 38:15–28, 1976

Spielberger CD: State-Trait Anger Expression Inventory, Revised Research Edition. Odessa, FL, Psychological Assessment Resources, 1991

Spielberger CD, Gorsuch RR, Luchene RE: State-Trait Anxiety Inventory. Palo Alto, CA, Consulting Psychologists Press, 1970

Spitzer WO, Dobson AJ, Hall J, et al: Measuring the quality of life of cancer patients: a concise QL-Index for use by physicians. J Chronic Dis 34:585–597, 1981

Spitzer RL, Williams J, Gibbon M, et al: Structured Clinical Interview for DSM-III-R (SCID): User's Guide. Washington, DC, American Psychiatric Press, 1992

Squire LR: Declarative and nondeclarative memory: multiple brain systems supporting learning and memory, in Memory Systems 1994. Edited by Schacter DL, Tulving E. Cambridge, MA, MIT Press, 1994, pp 203–231

Strauss E, Spreen O, Sherman L: A Compendium of Neuropsychological Tests, 3rd Edition. New York, Oxford University Press, 2006

Stuss D, Stethem L, Hugenholtz H, et al: Traumatic brain injury: a comparison of three clinical tests and analysis of recovery. Clin Neuropsychol 3:145–156, 1989

Svrakic DM, Whitehead C, Przybeck TR, et al: Differential diagnosis of personality disorders by the seven-factor model of temperament and character. Arch Gen Psychiatry 50:991–999, 1993

Taylor-Spence JA, Spence KW: The motivational components of manifest anxiety: drive and drive stimuli, in Anxiety and Behavior. Edited by Spielberger CD. New York, Academic Press, 1966, pp 291–326

Tellegen A: Brief Manual for the Multidimensional Personality Questionnaire. Minneapolis, University of Minnesota, 1982

Tellegen A, Lykken DT, Bouchard TJ, et al: Personality similarity in twins reared apart and together. J Pers Soc Psychol 54:1031–1039, 1988

Trenerry M, Corsson B, DeBoe J, et al: Visual Search and Attention Test. Lutz, FL, Psychological Assessment Resources, 1990

Wechsler D: Wechsler Adult Intelligence Scale—III Administrative and Scoring Manual. San Antonio, TX, Psychological Corporation, 1997a

Wechsler D: Wechsler Memory Scale—Third Edition Manual. San Antonio, TX, The Psychological Corporation, 1997b

Weed NC, Butcher JN, McKenna T, et al: New measures for assessing alcohol and drug abuse with the MMPI-2: the APS and AAS. J Pers Assess 58:389–404, 1992

Weissman MM, Bothwell S: Assessment of social adjustment by patient self-report. Arch Gen Psychiatry 33:1111–1115, 1976

Weissman MM, Sholomskas D: The assessment of social adjustment by the clinician, the patient, and the family, in The Behavior of Psychiatric Patients: Quantitative Techniques for Evaluation. Edited by Burdock EI, Sudilovsky A, Gershon S. New York, Marcel Dekker, 1982, pp 177–209

Westen D, Shedler J: Revising and assessing Axis II, part I: developing a clinically and empirically valid assessment method. Am J Psychiatry 156:258–272, 1999a

Westen D, Shedler J: Revising and assessing Axis II, part II: toward an empirically based and clinically useful classification of personality disorders. Am J Psychiatry 156:273–285, 1999b

Widiger TA, Mangine S, Corbitt EM, et al: Personality Disorder Interview-IV: A Semi-Structured Interview for the Assessment of Personality Disorders. Odessa, FL, Psychological Assessment Resources, 1995

Wiggins JS, Pincus AL: Personality: structure and assessment. Annu Rev Psychol 43:473–504, 1992

Yesavage JA, Brink TL: Development and validation of a geriatric depression screening scale: a preliminary report. J Psychiatr Res 17:37–49, 1983

Young RC, Biggs JT, Ziegler VE, et al: A rating scale for mania: reliability, validity and sensitivity. Br J Psychiatry 133:429–435, 1978

Yudofsky SC, Silver JM, Jackson W, et al: The Overt Aggression Scale for the objective rating of verbal and physical aggression. Am J Psychiatry 143:35–39, 1986

Zanarini MC, Frankenburg FR, Chauncey DL, et al: The Diagnostic Interview for Personality Disorders: interrater and test-retest reliability. Compr Psychiatry 28:467–480, 1987

Zung WWK: A rating instrument for anxiety disorders. Psychosomatics 12:371–379, 1971

Zung WWK: Index of Potential Suicide (IPS): a rating scale for suicide prevention, in The Prediction of Suicide. Edited by Beck AT, Resnick HLP, Lettieri DJ. Bowie, MD, Charles Press, 1974, pp 221–249

BASIC SCIENCE AND DEVELOPMENT

4

CELLULAR AND MOLECULAR BIOLOGY OF THE NEURON

A. Kimberley McAllister, Ph.D.
W. Martin Usrey, Ph.D.
Stephen C. Noctor, Ph.D.
Stephen Rayport, M.D., Ph.D.

Neuropsychiatric disorders are due to disordered functioning of neurons and, in particular, their synapses (Charney et al. 2004; Graham et al. 2002; Waxman 2005). Many neuropsychiatric disorders arise from aberrations in neurodevelopmental mechanisms. In the initial stages of brain development, cell–cell interactions are the dominant force in the assembly of the brain (Wichterle et al. 2002). As circuits form, individual neurons and connections are pruned on an activity-dependent basis, driven by intrinsic activity and competition for trophic factors. Neurogenesis does not stop with maturation but in fact continues in some brain regions and appears to be required for mood regulation (Santarelli et al. 2003; Warner-Schmidt and Duman 2006). With further maturation, experience becomes the dominant force in shaping neuronal connections and regulating their efficacy. In the mature brain, these neurodevelopmental mechanisms are harnessed in muted form and mediate most plastic processes (Black 1995; Kandel and O'Dell 1992). Neuropsychiatric disorders arising from problems in early brain development are more likely to be

intrinsically or genetically based, whereas those arising during later stages are more likely to be experience-based (Toga and Thompson 2005). In senescence, neurodegenerative processes may unravel neural circuits by aberrantly engaging neurodevelopmental mechanisms (Luo and O'Leary 2005).

Experience is so pivotal in fine-tuning neural connectivity that aberrant experience—particularly during critical periods in development—may give rise to or exacerbate neuropsychiatric disorders. For example, monocular occlusion or strabismus in young animals results in permanent pathological connectivity of the visual system (Hubel et al. 1977). In humans, failure to achieve conjugate gaze in childhood results in permanent visual loss. In mice, early blockade of the serotonin transporter with fluoxetine engenders an anxious phenotype when the mice grow up (Ansorge et al. 2004). In humans, early life stress engenders greater vulnerability to depression in adult life (Caspi et al. 2003). Similar but subtler changes occur in adulthood during learning. From work on the simple nervous systems of organisms such as the marine snail

Aplysia (Kandel 2001b), it is known that changes in synaptic connections encode memories. Here, too, abnormal experiences may permanently alter patterns of neuronal connectivity. In the human brain, imaging studies have begun to reveal changes in regional brain activity that occur after learning and that are suggestive of changes in the strength of neuronal connections (Maguire et al. 2000; Pantev et al. 1998; Sadato et al. 1996). Some functional neuropsychiatric disorders have now been shown to have a direct impact on brain structure; for example, posttraumatic stress disorder has been associated with alterations in hippocampal size (Kitayama et al. 2005).

In this chapter, we focus first on the cellular function of neurons and then on how they develop. The accelerating pace of recent advances begins now to offer a glimmer of how therapeutic interventions to correct aberrant neuronal growth and differentiation during development and maturation, or later to normalize neuronal signaling, may translate into revolutionary treatments for neuropsychiatric disorders.

Cellular Function of Neurons

Individual neurons in the brain receive signals from thousands of neurons and, in turn, send information to thousands of others. Whereas activity in peripheral sensory neurons may represent particular bits of information, activity of networks of neurons in the central nervous system (CNS) represents integrated sensory and associational information. CNS neurons may be seen as part of dynamic cellular ensembles that shift their participation from one network to another as information is used in varied tasks. The sophistication of these networks depends on both the properties of the neurons themselves and the patterns and strength of their connections.

Cellular Composition of the Brain

Brain cells comprise two principal types: *neurons* and *glia.* Neurons are the substrate for most information processing, whereas glia are classically believed to play a supporting role. Neurons are highly differentiated cells that show considerable heterogeneity in shape and size; in fact, there are more types of neurons than types of cells in any other part of the body. Some are among the largest cells in the body, as in the case of the upper motor neurons that project to the lumbar

spinal cord and have axons that are a meter or more in length; others are among the smallest cells in the body, as in the case of the granule cells of the cerebellum. Neurons are quite numerous, and they interconnect via synapses that are still more numerous. The human brain contains 10^{12}–10^{13} neurons. Each neuron forms an average of 10^3 connections, which is a minimal estimate, so the brain has on the order of 10^{15}–10^{16} synapses. In childhood and continuing throughout the life span to a more limited extent, the numbers of neurons and synapses show dramatic changes. During early development, neurogenesis can occur at a rate of up to 250,000 neurons per minute. In childhood, there is considerable refinement in neural circuits, associated with programmed cell death, or apoptosis, and a reduction in the number of synapses. In adulthood, neurogenesis continues, but in a very limited way. In later life, neurodegenerative disorders produce losses in the number of neuron and synapses.

Glial cells can be divided into three classes: 1) astrocytes, 2) oligodendrocytes, and 3) microglia. *Astrocytes* have three traditional functions: they provide the scaffolding of the brain, form the blood–brain barrier, and guide neuronal migration during development. Evidence is accumulating, however, that astroglial cells are more dynamic than previously suspected and are capable of cell–cell signaling over long distances (Dani et al. 1992; Fellin and Carmignoto 2004; Murphy et al. 1993). Moreover, they can influence neuronal activity, enhance neuronal connectivity, and play critical roles in regulating neuronal excitability during normal processes as well as in disease states (Araque et al. 1999; Mennerick and Zorumski 1994; Nedergaard 1994; Pfrieger and Barres 1997). And they are neural progenitor cells (Noctor et al. 2002). *Oligodendrocytes* produce the myelin sheath that speeds conduction of the action potential along axons. In patients with multiple sclerosis, which results from an immune attack on the principal protein of the myelin sheath, myelin basic protein, there is a failure in action potential conduction (Graham and Lantos 2002). *Microglia* are the macrophages of the brain: quiescent until activated by brain injury.

Neuronal Shape

Neurons share a common organization dictated by their function, which is to receive, process, and transmit information. The great Spanish neuroanatomist Santiago Ramón y Cajal called this *dynamic polarization* (Ramón y Cajal 1894). Although neurons show a wide diversity of sizes and shapes, they generally have four well-defined regions (Figure 4–1): 1) dendrites, 2) cell body, 3) axon, and 4) synaptic specializations. Each re-

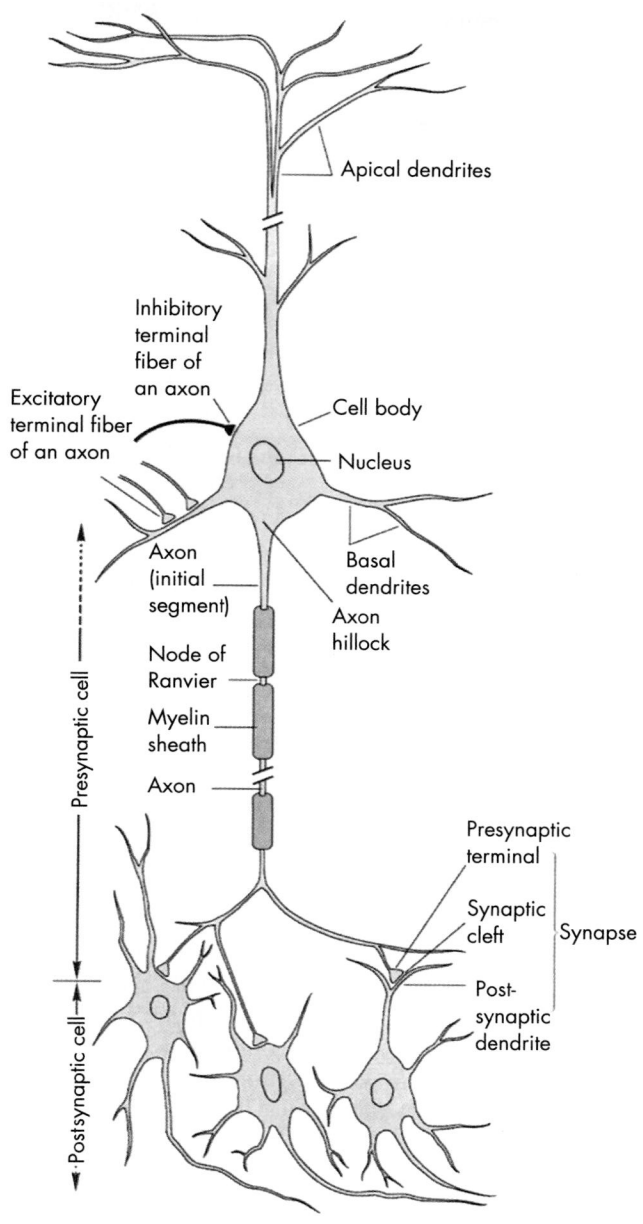

FIGURE 4–1. Functional organization of the neuron.

Neurons have distinct cellular regions subserving the input, integration, conduction, and output of information: the dendrites, cell body, axon, and synaptic specializations, respectively. Excitatory and inhibitory neurotransmitters released by other neurons induce depolarizing or hyperpolarizing current flow in dendrites. These currents converge in the cell body, and if the resulting polarization is sufficient to bring the initial segment of the axon to threshold, an action potential is initiated. The action potential travels down the axon, speeded by myelination, to reach the synaptic terminals. Axon terminals form synapses with other neurons or effector cells, renewing the cycle of information flow in postsynaptic cells. As in all cells, the cell body (or perikaryon) is also the repository of the neuron's genetic information (in the nucleus) and the principal site of macromolecular synthesis.

Source.   Reprinted from Kandel ER: "Nerve Cells and Behavior," in *Principles of Neural Science, 4th Edition.* Edited by Kandel ER, Schwartz JH, Jessell TM. New York, McGraw-Hill, 2000, pp. 19–35. Copyright 2000, The McGraw-Hill Companies, Inc. Used with permission.

gion has distinct functions. *Dendrites* receive signals from other neurons, process and modify this information, and then convey these signals to the cell body. As in all cells, the *cell body* contains the genetic information resident in the nucleus that codes for the fabrication of the necessary elements of cellular function, as well as sites for their manufacture, processing, and transport. The *axon* makes highly specific connections and conveys information over long distances to its terminals. Finally, *synaptic specializations* comprise the active zone and synaptic terminal on the presynaptic axon and the postsynaptic density on the postsynaptic dendrite.

A neuron's shape is determined by the cytoskeleton. The cytoskeleton is composed primarily of three filamentous components: 1) microtubules, 2) neurofilaments, and 3) actin (Pigino et al. 2006). *Microtubules* are composed of tubulin subunits and form a scaffold that determines the shape of the neuron. These tubules form bundles that extend throughout the major processes of the neuron and are stabilized by microtubule-associated proteins, called MAPs. *Neurofilaments* are the most abundant cytoskeletal components of the axon and are much more stable than microtubules. These neurofilaments are constituents of neurofibrillary tangles, characteristic of Alzheimer's disease. Finally, *actin* filaments form a dense network concentrated just under the cell membrane. Together with a large number of actin-binding proteins, this network facilitates cell motility and formation of synaptic specializations and allows for plasticity of axonal and dendritic structures (Dillon and Goda 2005). In addition to its important structural role, the cytoskeleton is essential for intracellular trafficking of proteins and organelles and facilitates the selective transport of axonal and dendritic proteins (Burack et al. 2000; Kamal and Goldstein 2002). Thus, cytoskeletal defects are likely to cause devastating neuronal damage—impairing axonal and dendritic transport and cell signaling, and eventually causing cell death (Hirokawa and Takemura 2003). Many neurodegenerative disorders are associated with defects in the trafficking of molecules or synaptic function (Cummings 2003).

Neuronal Excitability

Neurons are capable of transmitting information because they are electrically and chemically excitable. This excitability is conferred by a number of classes of ion channels that are selectively permeable to specific ions and that are regulated by voltage (voltage-gated channels), neurotransmitter binding (ligand-gated channels), or by pressure or stretch (mechanically gated channels) (reviewed in Hille 2001). In general, neuronal ion channels conduct ions across the plasma membrane at extremely rapid rates—100 million ions may pass through a single channel in a second. This large flow of current causes rapid changes in membrane potential and is the basis for the action potential, the substrate for information transfer *within* neurons, and for fast synaptic responses, the substrate for information transfer *between* neurons. Ligand-gated channels are often targets for psychiatric drugs, anesthetics, and neurotoxins. As expected, diseases caused by defects in ion channels are diverse and devastating. For example, in myasthenia gravis the immune system mounts an attack on nicotinic acetylcholine receptors; in hyperkalemic periodic paralysis, muscle stiffness and weakness following exercise result from a point mutation in voltage-gated Na^+ channels; and in episodic ataxia, the generalized ataxia triggered by periods of stress results from a point mutation in a delayed-rectifier voltage-gated K^+ channel (reviewed in Koester and Siegelbaum 2000).

Neurotransmitters released by one neuron at synapses activate receptors (ligand-gated channels) on dendrites of other neurons and induce ion flux across the membrane. The resulting electrical signals spread passively over some distance, often reaching the cell body in this way. In addition to passive conductances, localized regenerative mechanisms similar to those that give rise to the action potential (discussed later in this section) amplify dendritic input signals, boosting them so that they can reach the cell body (Eilers and Konnerth 1997; Magee and Carruth 1999; Yuste and Tank 1996). In the cell body, these synaptic inputs combine and, if sufficient, depolarize the initial segment of the axon, or axon hillock, which is the part of the axon closest to the cell body that has the lowest threshold for activation. When a threshold level of depolarization is reached, the action potential is initiated. The action potential, or spike, is an electrical wave that propagates down the axon. In the axon terminals, this wave triggers an influx of calcium (Ca^{2+}), which leads to exocytosis of neurotransmitters from synaptic vesicles at specialized sites called *active zones*. The released neurotransmitter reaches and activates closely apposed receptors in the postsynaptic density on the postsynaptic cell's dendrites. Ultimately, this information flow reaches effector cells, principally motor fibers that mediate movement and thus generate behavior. Action potentials also back-propagate into dendrites (Johnston et al. 2003), which contributes to the crucial postsynaptic depolarization necessary for long-term potentiation (LTP).

The ability of neurons to generate an action potential derives from the presence of strong ionic gradients across the membrane; sodium (Na^+) and chloride (Cl^-) are highly concentrated outside the membrane, while potassium (K^+) is highly concentrated inside. These gradients are generated by the continuous action of membrane pumps energized by the hydrolysis of adenosine triphosphate (ATP). Also in the membrane are voltage-gated ion channels that regulate the flow of Na^+, K^+, and Ca^{2+} ions across the membrane. At rest, K^+ and Cl^- channels are open so that K^+ and Cl^- gradients determine the membrane potential, causing the cell to be negative inside by about –50 mV to –75 mV. However, if the membrane is depolarized past the threshold potential for generating an action potential, voltage-gated Na^+ channels open rapidly. Because inflow of Na^+ depolarizes the membrane, this confers a regenerative property—once a threshold potential is reached, increased Na^+ influx leads to further depolarization, which opens more Na^+ channels, further enhancing Na^+ influx, and so on. Thus, once threshold is reached, the membrane potential switches to +50 mV very rapidly. The membrane potential stays depolarized for only about a millisecond, because Na^+ channels then show a time-dependent inactivation (Figure 4–2). Simultaneously, voltage-dependent K^+ channels, which are also activated by depolarization but more slowly, increase their permeability. Because K^+ flows along its concentration gradient out of the cell, this, together with reduction in Na^+ current, leads to the repolarization of the membrane. Thus, the membrane potential peaks at a depolarized level determined by the Na^+ gradient and then rapidly returns to the resting potential, determined by the K^+ gradient. Once the membrane is repolarized, Na^+ inactivation wears off (the time this takes accounts for the refractory period of the neuron, a brief period when the threshold for firing an action potential is elevated), and the cell can fire again.

The regenerative property of the action potential not only serves to amplify threshold potentials (its principal function in dendrites) but also confers long-distance signaling capabilities in the axon (Figure 4–3). When the membrane potential peaks under the control of the increase in Na^+ permeability, adjacent regions of the axon become sufficiently depolarized so that they, in turn, are brought to threshold and generate an action potential. As successive axonal segments are depolarized, the action potential conducts at great speed down the axon. This is further enhanced by myelination, which increases the rate of conduction severalfold by restricting the current flow required for action potential generation to the gaps between myelin segments, the nodes of Ranvier (see Figures 4–1 and 4–3). Because

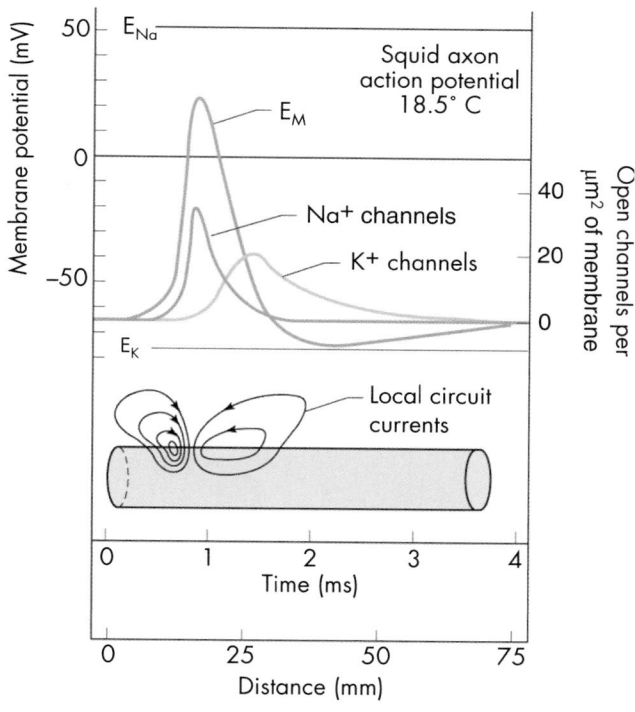

FIGURE 4–2. Opening of ion channels gives rise to the action potential.

The upper traces show the two principal currents shaping the action potential, sodium (Na^+) and potassium (K^+) currents. Once a neuron reaches threshold for firing an action potential, voltage-activated Na^+ channels open, giving rise to a rapid inward Na^+ current and to the rapid rising phase of the action potential (green trace; membrane potential, E_M). Once the membrane is depolarized, Na^+ channels rapidly inactivate, reducing the Na^+ current (purple trace) and thereby contributing to the falling phase of the action potential. Then, outward K^+ current (yellow trace) activates, driving the falling phase of the action potential. K^+ channels are slow to open but stay open for much longer than Na^+ channels, pulling the E_M back to the resting level. E_{Na} and E_K represent the reversal potentials for Na^+ and K^+, respectively, to which the opening of channels drives the membrane potential (E_M). The lower schematic shows the local circuit currents that underlie the propagation of the action potential. The intense loop on the left spreads the depolarization to the right into unexcited membrane, which then renews the cycle, depolarizing the next segment and thereby propagating the action potential. *Source.* Reprinted from Hille B, Catterall WA: "Electrical Excitability and Ion Channels," in *Basic Neurochemistry: Molecular, Cellular and Medical Aspects*, 7th Edition. Edited by Siegel GJ, Albers RW, Brady S, Price DL. Burlington, MA, Elsevier Academic, 2006, pp. 95–109. Copyright 2006. Used with permission from Elsevier.

of its all-or-none characteristics and ability to conduct over long distances, the action potential provides a high-quality digital signaling mechanism in neurons.

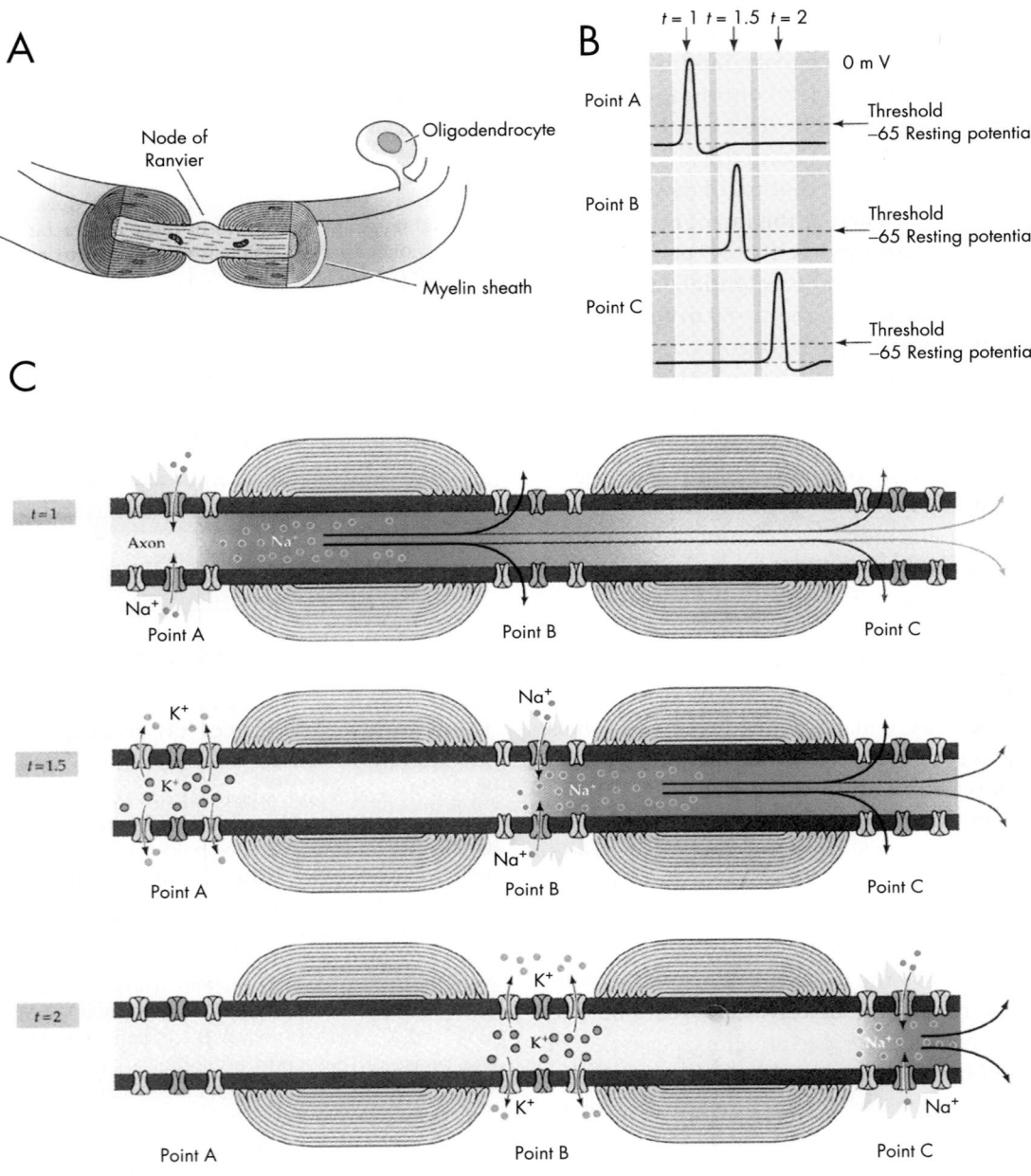

FIGURE 4–3.   Action potential conduction in myelinated axon.

Panel A.   Schematic of a myelinated axon. Oligodendrocytes produce the insulating myelin sheath that surrounds the axon in segments. Myelination restricts current flow to the gaps between myelin segments, the nodes of Ranvier, where sodium (Na^+) channels are concentrated. The result is a dramatic enhancement of the conduction velocity of the action potential. *Panel B.*   Because Na^+ channels are activated by membrane depolarization and also cause depolarization, they have regenerative properties. This underlies the "all-or-nothing" properties of the action potential and also explains its rapid spread down the axon. The action potential is an electrical wave; as each node of Ranvier is depolarized, it in turn depolarizes the subsequent node. *Panel C.*   The Na^+ current underlying the action potential is shown in three successive images at 0.5-millisecond intervals and corresponds to the current traces in Panel B. As the action potential (*red shading*) travels to the right, Na^+ channels go from closed to open to inactivated to closed. In this way, an action potential initiated at the initial segment of the axon conducts reliably to the axon terminals. Because Na^+ channels temporarily inactivate after depolarization, there is a brief refractory period following the action potential that blocks backward spread of the action potential and thus ensures reliable forward conduction.

Source.   Reprinted from Purves D, Augustine GJ, Fitzpatrick D, et al. (eds): *Neuroscience,* 3rd Edition. Sunderland, MA, Sinauer Associates, 2004, p. 64. Used with permission.

Although the information that a neuron integrates comes from synaptic input, how the neuron processes that information depends on its intrinsic properties (Llinás 1988; London and Häusser 2005). Many CNS neurons have the ability to generate their own patterns of activity in the absence of synaptic input, firing either at a regular rate (pacemaker firing) or in clusters of spikes (burst firing) (McCormick and Bal 1997). This endogenous activity is driven by specialized ion channels with their own voltage and time dependence that periodically bring the initial segment of the axon to threshold. These channels can be modulated by the membrane potential of the cell or by second-messenger systems. Depending on the activation of these specialized channels, neurons may profoundly change how they respond to a given synaptic input. For example, a thalamic neuron fires as a pacemaker when stimulated from slightly depolarized levels, whereas it fires in bursts of action potentials when stimulated from hyperpolarized levels (Llinás and Jahnsen 1982; Sherman 2001) (Figure 4–4). Changes in second-messenger levels may also profoundly affect the activity or response properties of neurons, lending still a greater repertoire to the functioning of individual neurons. Thus, synaptic inputs may not only evoke a response in a postsynaptic neuron but also shape intrinsic firing patterns, cause a cell to shift from one mode of activity to another, or modulate responses to other synaptic inputs.

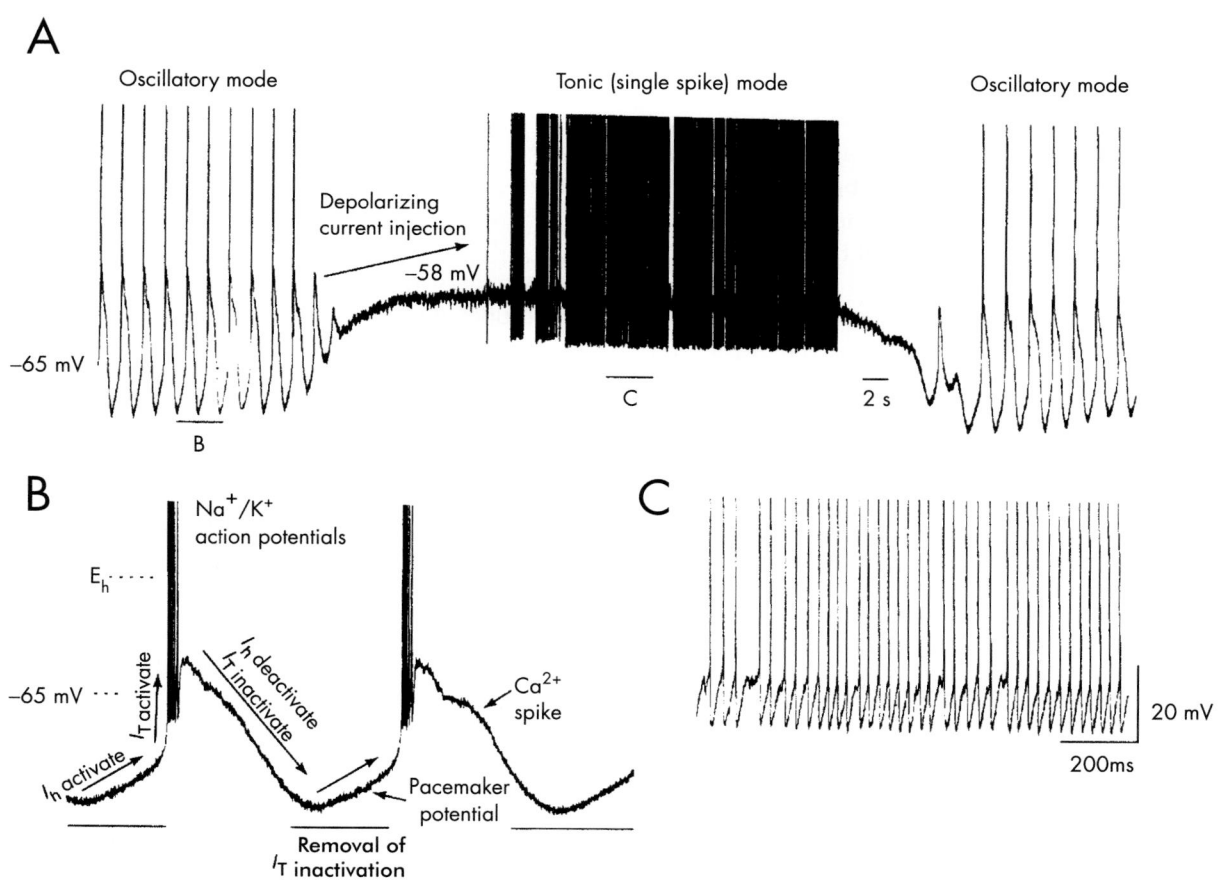

FIGURE 4–4. Intrinsic properties determine neuronal responses.

Many CNS neurons respond differently to the same inputs, depending on their level of depolarization. *Panel A.* Thalamic neurons spontaneously generate bursts of action potentials, resulting from interactions between an inward pacemaker current and a calcium (Ca^{2+}) current. Depolarization of these neurons changes their firing to a tonic mode. *Panel B.* Action potential bursts at higher time resolution from trace in Panel A. *Panel C.* Higher time resolution of currents in the tonic mode from Panel A. I_h and I_T = the currents through a hyperpolarization-activated channel and a T-type calcium channel, respectively.
Source. Reprinted from McCormick DA: "Membrane Potential and Action Potential," in *Fundamental Neuroscience,* 2nd Edition. Edited by Squire LR, Roberts JL, Spitzer NC, et al. San Diego, CA, Academic Press, 2003, pp. 139–161. Copyright Elsevier 2004. Used with permission.

Signaling Between Neurons

Neurons communicate with one another at specialized sites of close membrane apposition called *synapses.* The prototypic axodendritic synapse connects a presynaptic axon terminal with a postsynaptic dendrite. This arrangement is typical for projection neurons that convey information from one region of the brain to another. In contrast, local circuit interneurons interact with neighboring neurons. While interneurons may make axodendritic and axosomatic connections, they can also form several other kinds of synaptic contacts that greatly increase their functional sophistication (Figure 4–5). In some cases, dendrites may synapse with dendrites (*dendrodendritic* connections) or cell bodies with cell bodies (*somasomatic* connections), forming local neural circuits that convey information without action potential firing. Axons may synapse onto the axon terminals of other axons (*axoaxonic* connections) and modulate transmitter release by presynaptic inhibition or facilitation. Some neurons may function both as interneurons and as projection neurons, the most prominent example being the medium spiny γ-aminobutyric acid (GABA) neurons of the striatum, which comprise about 95% of the neurons in the region (Smith and Bolam 1990).

A minority of local connections are mediated by electrical synapses that do not require chemical neurotransmitters at all. Electrical synapses are formed by multisubunit channels, called *gap junctions,* that link the cytoplasm of adjacent cells (Bennett et al. 1991; Sohl et al. 2005), allowing both small molecules and ions carrying electrical signals to flow directly from one cell to another. Electrical synapses couple dendrites or cell bodies of adjoining cells of the same kind, typically dendrite to dendrite or soma to soma. During embryonic development, the ability to pass small molecules, including second messengers, between cells is important for the generation of morphogenic gradients (Dealy et al. 1994). During early brain development, such gradients regulate cell proliferation and establish patterns of connectivity (Kandler and Katz 1995). In the mature brain, electrical synapses act to synchronize the electrical activity of groups of neurons and mediate high-frequency transmission of signals (Bennett 1977; Brivanlou et al. 1998; Tamas et al. 2000). Glial cells are also connected by gap junctions, which link these cells into large syncytia, providing avenues for intercellular propagation of chemical signals mediated by small molecules and ions, such as Ca^{2+}. The importance of gap junctions for glial cell function is underscored by the fact that the X-linked form of Charcot-Marie-Tooth disease results from a single mutation

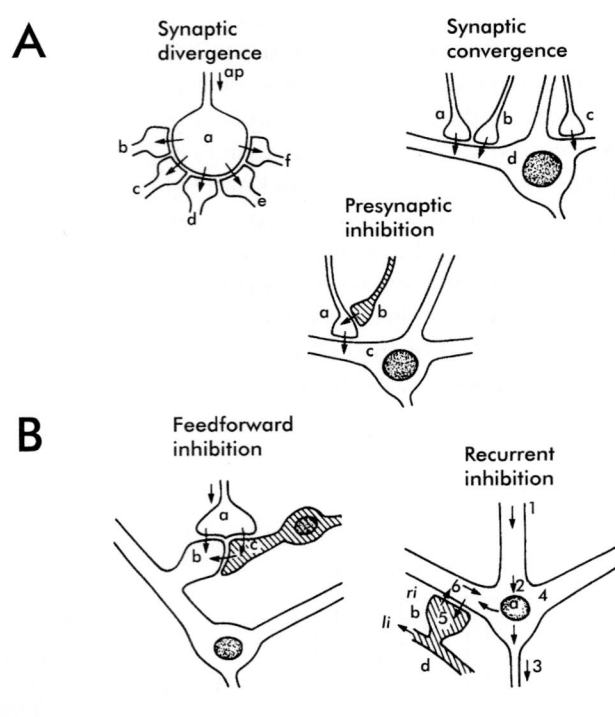

FIGURE 4–5. Modes of interneuronal communication.

Panel A. Different connection patterns dictate how information flows between neurons. In synaptic divergence, one neuron (a) may disseminate information to several postsynaptic cells (b–f) simultaneously (information flow is shown by *arrows*). Alternatively, in the case of synaptic convergence, a single neuron (d) may receive input from an array of presynaptic neurons (a–c). In presynaptic inhibition, one neuron (b) can modulate information flowing between two other neurons (from a to c) by influencing neurotransmitter release from the presynaptic neuron's terminals; this can be inhibitory (as shown) or facilitatory. *Panel B.* Neurons may modulate their own actions. In feedforward inhibition, the presynaptic cell (a) may directly activate a postsynaptic cell (b) and at the same time modulate its effects via activation of an inhibitory cell (c), which in turn inhibits the cell (b). In recurrent inhibition, a presynaptic cell (a) activates an inhibitory cell (b) that synapses back onto the presynaptic cell (a), limiting the duration of its activity. ap = action potential; *li* = lateral inhibition; *ri* = recurrent inhibition.
Source. Adapted from Shepherd GM, Koch C: "Introduction to Synaptic Circuits," in *The Synaptic Organization of the Brain,* 3rd Edition. Edited by Shepherd GM. New York, Oxford University Press, 1990, pp. 3–31.

in a connexin gene required for formation of gap junctions between Schwann cells (reviewed in Schenone and Mancardi 1999).

Most CNS synaptic connections are mediated by chemical neurotransmitters. Although chemical synapses are slower than electrical ones, they allow for signal amplification, may be inhibitory as well as excitatory, are susceptible to a wide range of modulation, and can modulate the activities of other cells through the release of transmitters activating second-messenger cascades. There are primarily two classes of neurotransmitters in the nervous system: 1) small molecule transmitters and 2) neuropeptides. In general, *small molecule transmitters* mediate fast synaptic transmission; are stored in small, clear synaptic vesicles; and include glutamate, GABA, glycine, acetylcholine, serotonin, dopamine, norepinephrine, epinephrine, and histamine. The cellular and molecular mechanisms of release of these synaptic vesicles are described in the remainder of this section. In contrast, the *neuropeptides* are a very large family of neurotransmitters that modulate synaptic transmission, are stored in large dense-core vesicles, and include somatostatin, the hypothalamic-releasing hormones, endorphins, enkephalins, and the opioids. Interestingly, small molecule transmitters and neuropeptides are often released from the same neuron and can act together on the same target (Hökfelt 1991).

Small neurotransmitter molecules are stored in small, clear, membrane-bound granules called *synaptic vesicles* (Figure 4–6). Each synaptic vesicle contains several thousand neurotransmitter molecules. When an action potential invades the presynaptic region, the depolarization activates voltage-dependent Ca^{2+} channels and triggers transmitter release (Figure 4–7). The subsequent Ca^{2+} influx raises the local Ca^{2+} concentration near the active zone, promoting synaptic vesicle fusion and neurotransmitter release via *exocytosis*. Neurotransmitter then diffuses a short distance across the synaptic cleft and binds to postsynaptic receptors. The dynamics and modulation of synaptic transmission are fundamental to alterations in synaptic connections that underlie both normal and pathological learning and memory. Recently, the molecular machinery (Figure 4–8) involved in synaptic transmission has been increasingly clarified (Sudhof 2004). Interestingly, several potent neurotoxins act directly on this machinery. Current theory is that synaptic transmission comprises a large number of consecutive steps that occur both pre- and postsynaptically. Within the general events described in Figure 4–7, synaptic vesicles undergo a six-step cycle:

1. Vesicles dock at active zones before exocytotic release.
2. Priming occurs, whereby vesicles become ready to respond to increases in intracellular Ca^{2+}. (The potent neurotoxins botulinum and tetanus toxin block

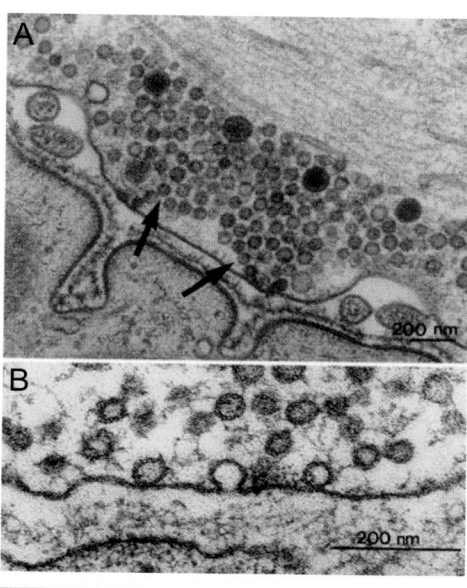

FIGURE 4–6. Synaptic ultrastructure.

Neuromuscular junctions from frog sartorius muscle were flash-frozen milliseconds after high potassium treatment to increase synaptic transmission. ***Panel A.*** Synaptic vesicles are clustered at two active zones (*arrows*), which are sites where vesicles fuse with the plasma membrane to release their neurotransmitter. ***Panel B.*** At higher magnification and after stimulation, omega profiles of vesicles in the process of releasing their neurotransmitter are visible.

Source. Reprinted from Schwarz TL: "Release of Neurotransmitters," in *Fundamental Neuroscience,* 2nd Edition. Edited by Squire LR, Roberts JL, Spitzer NC, et al. San Diego, CA, Academic Press, 2003, pp. 197–224; original source Heuser JE: "Synaptic Vesicle Endocytosis Revealed in Quick-Frozen Frog Neuromuscular Junctions Treated With 4-Aminopyridine and Given a Single Electrical Shock." *Society for Neuroscience Symposia* 2:215–239, 1977. Copyright 1977. Used with permission.

synaptic transmission by proteolysis of key molecules involved in priming.)
3. Triggered by an influx in Ca^{2+}, fusion/exocytosis then occurs in less than a millisecond, releasing the neurotransmitter into the synaptic cleft.
4. Endocytosis recovers the synaptic vesicle membrane.
5. Synaptic vesicles are refilled with neurotransmitter, driven by an acidic intravesicular gradient.
6. The filled synaptic vesicles are transported back to the active zone to complete the cycle.

Neurotransmitter activity is typically limited in duration by several mechanisms that rapidly remove released neurotransmitter from the synapse. First, simple diffusion out of the synaptic cleft limits the duration of action of all neurotransmitters. Second,

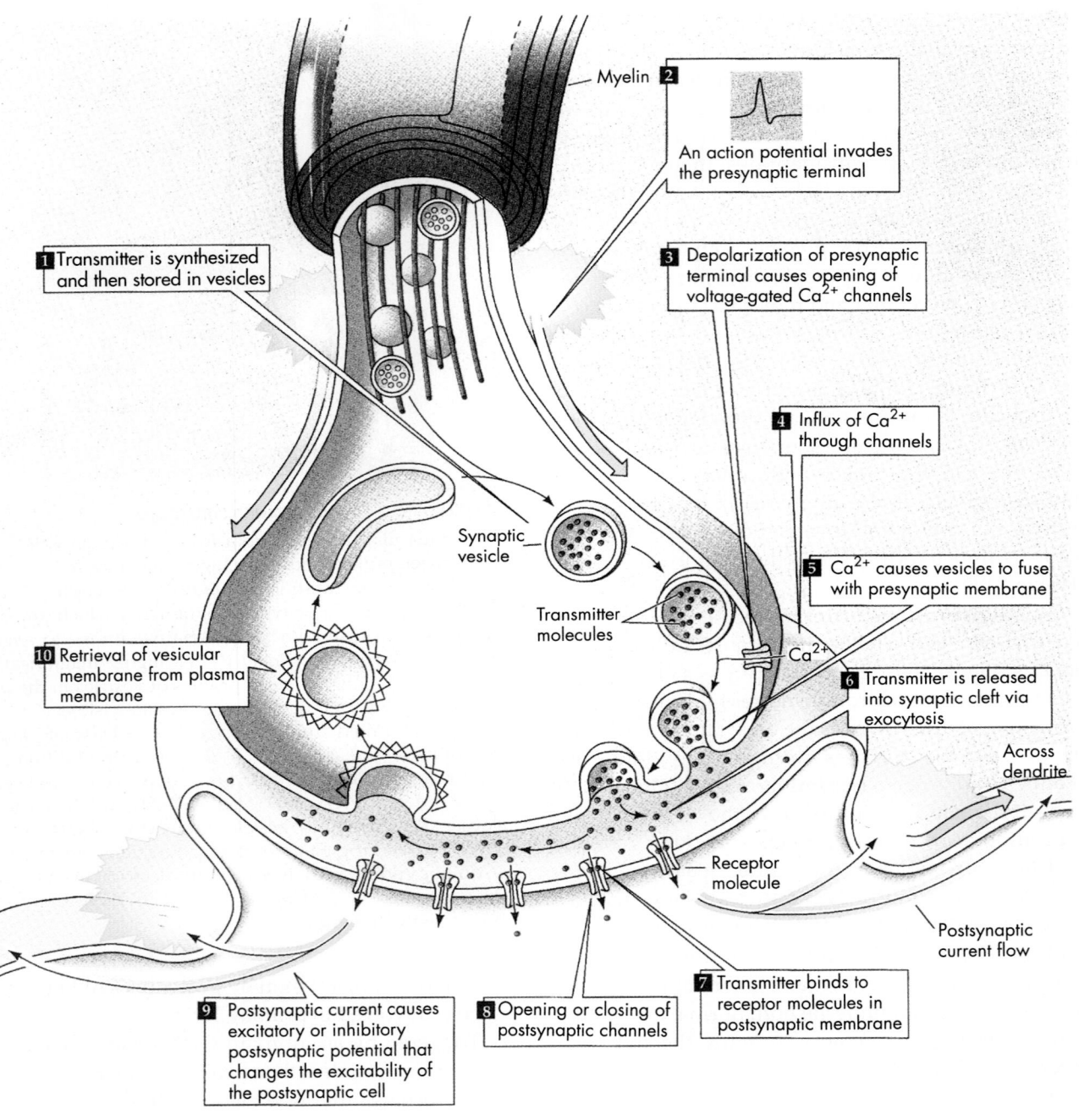

FIGURE 4–7. Steps in synaptic transmission at a chemical synapse.

Essential steps in the process of synaptic transmission are numbered. Ca^{2+} = calcium.

Source. Reprinted from Purves D, Augustine GJ, Fitzpatrick D, et al. (eds): *Neuroscience,* 3rd Edition. Sunderland, MA, Sinauer Associates, 2004, p. 97. Used with permission.

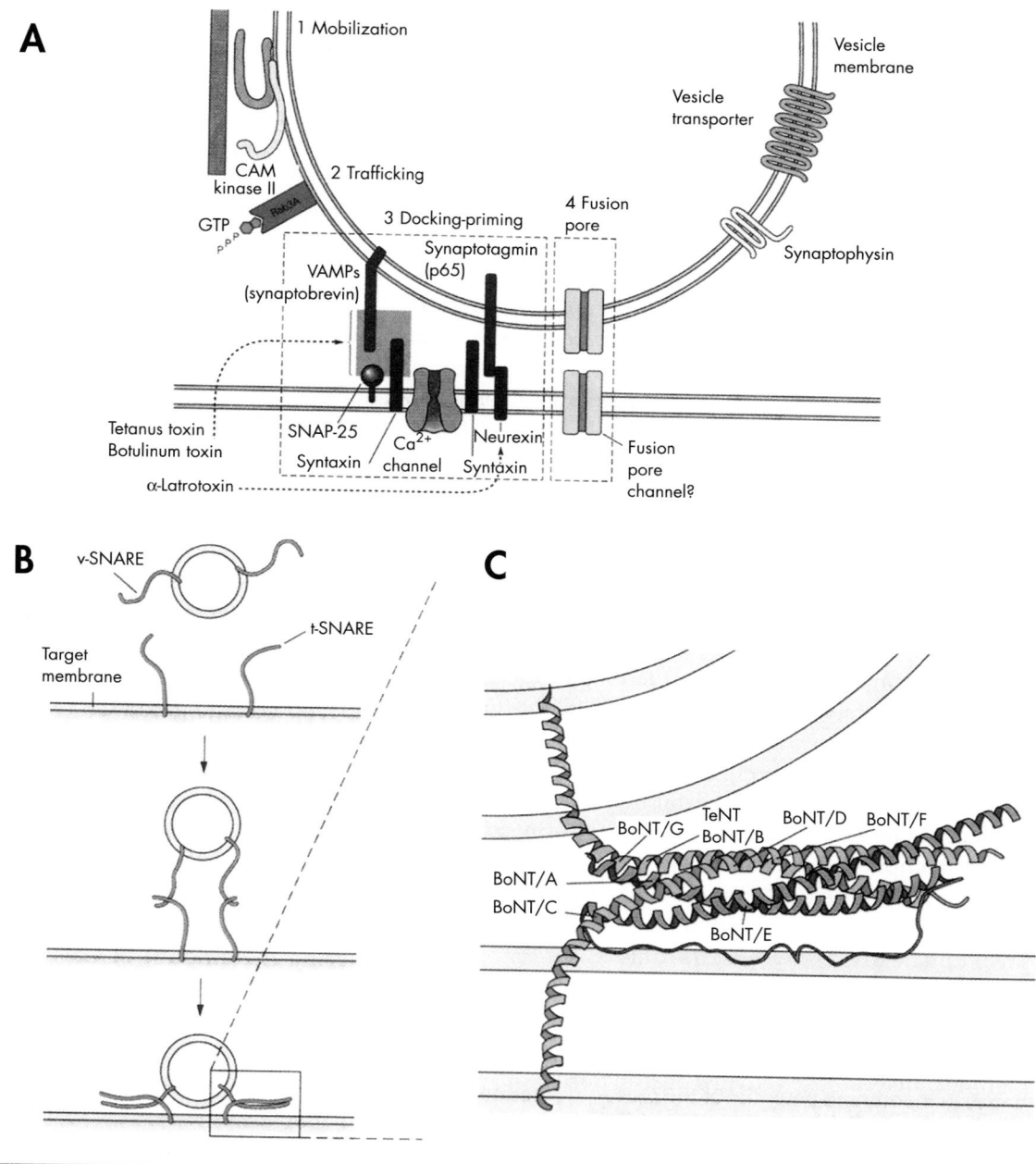

FIGURE 4–8.   Molecular events in synaptic vesicle docking and fusion.

A coordinated set of proteins is involved in the positioning of vesicles at the presynaptic membrane and in controlling release by membrane fusion. *Panel A.*   Many of the recently cloned synaptic vesicle proteins are integral to this process. Some of these proteins interact with the cytoskeleton to position the vesicles at the terminal, while other proteins are integral to the fusion process. In addition, several of these synaptic vesicle proteins are targets for neurotoxins that function by influencing neurotransmitter release. *Panel B.*   The current theory for how synaptic vesicles fuse with the membrane and release neurotransmitter is called the SNARE hypothesis. Both the synaptic vesicles and the plasma membrane express specific proteins that mediate docking and fusion: v-SNAREs (synaptic vesicles) and t-SNAREs (plasma membrane). Vesicles are brought close to the membrane through interactions between VAMP (synaptobrevin), syntaxin, and SNAP-25. *N*-ethylmaleimide-sensitive fusion protein (NSF) then binds to the complex to facilitate fusion. Calcium (Ca^{2+}) influx is required to stimulate fusion, but the precise binding partner for calcium and the exact events leading to fusion remain obscure. *Panel C.*   The crystal structure of the fusion complex, as shown here, is consistent with the SNARE hypothesis. BoNT = botulinum toxin; TeNT = tetanus toxin. *Source.*   Adapted from Kandel ER, Siegelbaum SA: "Transmitter Release," in *Principles of Neural Science,* 4th Edition. Edited by Kandel ER, Schwartz JH, Jessell TM. New York, McGraw-Hill, 2000, pp. 253–279. Copyright 2000, The McGraw-Hill Companies, Inc. Used with permission.

neurotransmitters may be enzymatically degraded; for example, acetylcholine is hydrolyzed by acetylcholinesterase bound to the postsynaptic membrane adjacent to the receptors. Finally, although the monoamine and amino acid neurotransmitters are also metabolized, they are principally removed from the synaptic cleft by rapid reuptake mechanisms, whereby they are repackaged in synaptic vesicles or metabolized (Masson et al. 1999).

The monoamine neurotransmitter transporters (Figure 4–9), which mediate this rapid reuptake process, are the sites of action of a number of drugs and neurotoxins (Gainetdinov and Caron 2003). Prominent among these are the tricyclic antidepressants, selective serotonin reuptake inhibitors (SSRIs), the psychostimulants, and the neurotoxin 1-methyl-4-phenyl-1,2,3,4-tetrahydropyridine (MPTP). The tricyclics block serotonin and norepinephrine reuptake, and the SSRIs, as their name suggests, block serotonin reuptake. Other newer antidepressants block feedback inhibition of release, thereby increasing synaptic serotonin levels. Cocaine prevents dopamine and serotonin reuptake, whereas amphetamine both slows reuptake of dopamine and serotonin and induces dopamine release (Ramamoorthy and Blakely 1999; Sulzer et al. 2005). Molecular studies have also suggested that cocaine binding and dopamine reuptake occur at separate sites on the transporter, suggesting the possibility that cocaine action could be successfully blocked without impeding normal reuptake (Lin et al. 2000). Mice lacking the dopamine transporter (DAT) show a profound persistence of synaptic dopamine so that they appear as if they are permanently on psychostimulants (Giros et al. 1996); psychostimulants have no effect on these animals, confirming that the dopamine transporter is critical to the action of these drugs. MPTP is taken up by the dopamine transporter selectively; once in dopamine neurons, it increases oxidative stress, leading to the demise of the neurons and behaviorally to parkinsonism (Pifl et al. 1996).

Rapid Postsynaptic Responses

The action of a neurotransmitter depends on the properties of the postsynaptic receptors to which it binds. Postsynaptic receptors activated by neurotransmitter fall into two classes: 1) ionotropic and 2) metabotropic (discussed in the following section). Ionotropic receptors are directly linked to an ion channel; these receptors undergo a conformational change upon neurotransmitter binding that opens the channel. This results in either depolarization, giving rise to an excitatory postsynaptic potential, or hyperpolarization, giving rise to an inhibitory postsynaptic potential. The

neuromuscular junction is the prototypic excitatory synapse; simultaneous binding of two acetylcholine molecules opens a channel in the receptor that is permeable to both Na^+ and K^+ (Karlin and Akabas 1995). This results in a strong depolarization of the postsynaptic membrane mediated by Na^+ influx (and moderated by K^+ efflux), leading to an action potential in the motor fiber that evokes contraction. Ligand-gated channels are found at synapses such as the neuromuscular junction, where rapid and reliable activation of the postsynaptic cell is required. At the neuromuscular junction, the postsynaptic response is sufficiently strong so that there is a one-to-one translation of motor neuron spikes into muscle fiber spikes, thus ensuring reliable muscle contraction.

Unlike the neuromuscular junction, CNS neurons function in dynamic networks (Vogels et al. 2005) so that generally no individual cell has so strong a synaptic connection with another cell that it alone brings it to threshold. Rather, groups of neurons—active in concert—converge on a postsynaptic neuron to generate multiple postsynaptic potentials. These potentials may summate within regions of the postsynaptic neuron (*spatial summation*) if they occur sufficiently close together in time to cause the postsynaptic neuron to fire. As a rule, fast ligand-gated channels mediate the flow of information representing patterns of sensory input and associations between sensory modalities, underlying central representations that ultimately give rise to motor outputs. In the CNS, glutamate receptors mediate most fast excitatory transmission; GABA and glycine are the most common inhibitory neurotransmitters.

Glutamate Receptors

Excitatory postsynaptic potentials are mediated by two classes of ionotropic glutamate receptors: *N*-methyl-D-aspartate (NMDA) receptors and non-NMDA, or α-amino-3-hydroxy-5-methylisoxazole-4-propionic acid (AMPA), receptors (Hassel and Dingledine 2006). Ionotropic glutamate receptors are multimeric proteins, usually composed of four subunits. NMDA receptors are formed from combinations of NR1 and NR2 subunits; the NR1 subunit is universally expressed in neurons, whereas the NR2, which comes in several subtypes, is heterogeneously expressed both during development and among different neurons, giving rise to different response properties (Schoepfer et al. 1994). NMDA receptors depolarize cells by opening channels that principally allow Ca^{2+} to enter the cell. The most striking property of NMDA receptors is that the ion channel is usually blocked by Mg^{2+} at membrane potentials more negative than about 40 mV (MacDermott et al. 1986; Nowak et al. 1984). As a re-

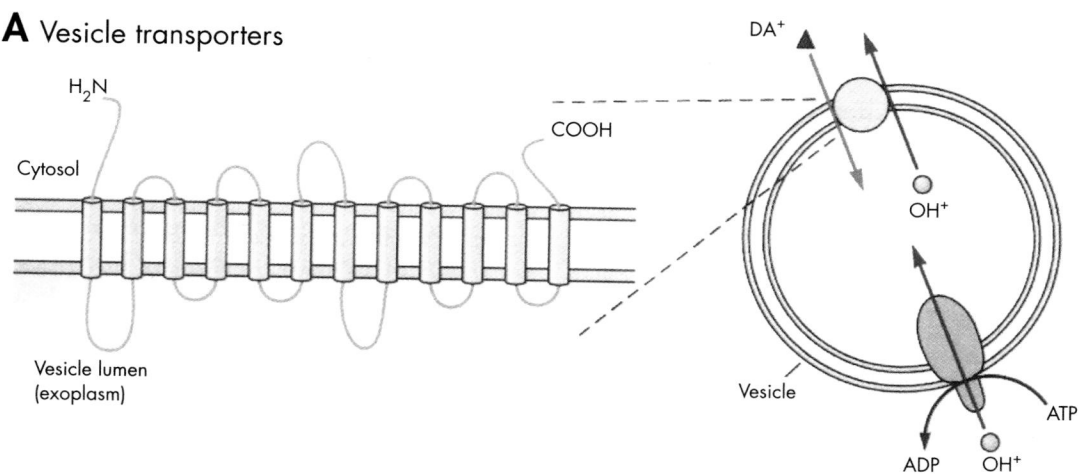

A Vesicle transporters

B Glutamate uptake

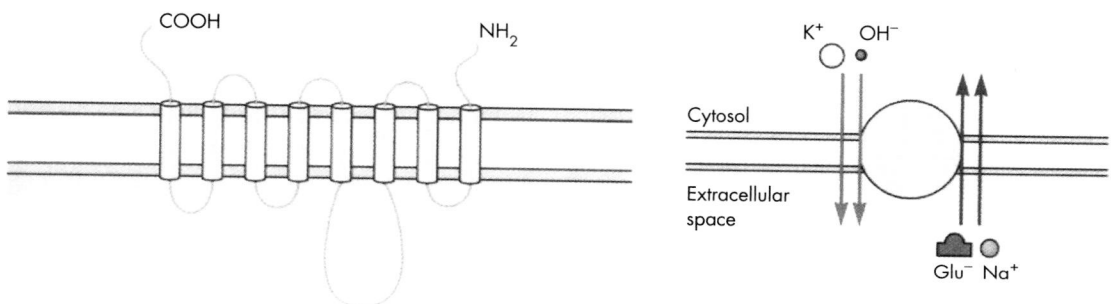

C Uptake of other transmitters

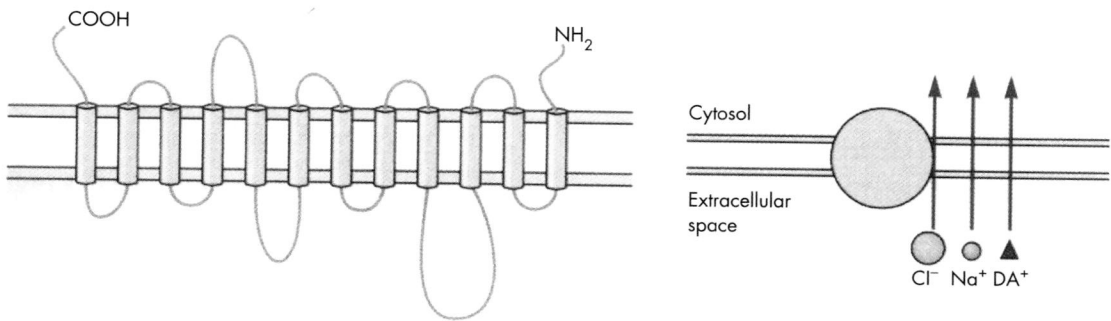

FIGURE 4–9. Neurotransmitter transporters.

Synaptic transmission in the CNS is terminated for the most part by reuptake of neurotransmitter by specific transporters with shared molecular motifs. These transporters carry neurotransmitters across membranes against concentration gradients, and thus require metabolic energy. Most often, this energy is provided by cotransport of an ion down its concentration gradient. *Panel A.* One family of transporters in synaptic vesicles serves to load neurotransmitter or transmitter precursors into synaptic vesicles. *Panel B.* A second family of transporters in the plasma membrane with eight transmembrane domains handles amino acid neurotransmitters, such as glutamate and γ-aminobutyric acid. *Panel C.* A third family of transporters in the plasma membrane with 12 transmembrane domains handles the monoamines dopamine, norepinephrine, and serotonin.
Source. Reprinted from Schwartz JH: "Neurotransmitters," in *Principles of Neural Science,* 4th Edition. Edited by Kandel ER, Schwartz JH, Jessell TM. New York, McGraw-Hill, 2000, pp. 280–297. Copyright 2000, The McGraw-Hill Companies, Inc. Used with permission.

sult, at the resting potential of most neurons, the NMDA receptor channel is occluded. For current to flow through NMDA channels, glutamate must bind to the receptor and the membrane must be depolarized simultaneously to displace the Mg^{2+}. This dual requirement underlies the unique role of NMDA receptors in processes as varied as synaptogenesis, learning and memory, and even cell death. NMDA receptors are also likely to be critical for proper mental functioning. NMDA receptor hypofunction has been implicated as a pathogenic mechanism in schizophrenia (Coyle 2006), and transgenic mice with reduced NMDA receptor expression display aberrations in behavior similar to those seen in patients with schizophrenia (Gainetdinov et al. 2001).

The non-NMDA glutamate receptors are further divided into AMPA receptors and kainate receptors on the basis of their affinities for these glutamate analogs. AMPA receptors are formed from combinations of subunits GluR1 to GluR4, and kainate receptors are formed from combinations of GluR5 to GluR7 plus KA1 and KA2. The complexity in the types of possible glutamate receptors is further increased by the existence of flip and flop conformations of GluR1 to GluR4 subunits and posttranslational editing of glutamate receptor mRNA. Non-NMDA receptors generally gate channels that allow Na^+ but not Ca^{2+} to cross the membrane. The GluR2 subunit of the AMPA receptor channel is responsible for blocking Ca^{2+} passage. Neurons that express such Ca^{2+}-permeable AMPA receptors may be particularly vulnerable to excitotoxic cell death in disease states such as amyotrophic lateral sclerosis (Van Den Bosch et al. 2006). Ca^{2+}-permeable AMPA receptors mediate non–NMDA-dependent long-term potentiation, which has been implicated in anxiety states (Mahanty and Sah 1998).

GABA Receptors

Inhibitory postsynaptic potentials in the brain are mediated primarily by GABA receptors (Olsen and Betz 2006). Several classes of GABA receptors have been identified. $GABA_A$ receptors are ionotropic receptors that form Cl^--selective channels and mediate fast synaptic inhibition in the brain. $GABA_B$ receptors are metabotropic receptors that tend to be slower acting and play a modulatory role; they are often found on presynaptic terminals, where they inhibit transmitter release. $GABA_A$ receptors are members of the nicotinic acetylcholine receptor superfamily. The $GABA_A$ receptor-channel complex is composed of a mixture of five subunits from α, β, γ, and ρ families. This gives rise to receptors with varying properties, depending on the specific receptor subunit composition. Because most of the subunit families have multiple subtypes, some of which can undergo RNA splicing, there is the potential for an extraordinary diversity of $GABA_A$ receptor function. During early development, intracellular chloride levels are high, so $GABA_A$ receptors in fact mediate excitation (H. Lee et al. 2005). Recent studies indicate that at some synapses, in particular those projecting onto the initial segments of cortical pyramidal neurons, GABA may continue to be depolarizing in adulthood (Szabadics et al. 2006).

The mRNA sequences for individual or multiple receptor subunits can be injected into oocytes or cultured mammalian cells, and the properties of the subsequently expressed receptor subunit combinations elucidated. This approach has shown how the properties of a particular $GABA_A$ receptor depend on the subunit composition as well as on interactions among the subunits. Site-directed mutagenesis has been applied to localize binding sites of specific ligands on receptor subunits. Benzodiazepines bind to a recognition site formed by the α and γ subunits. The α_1 subunits mediate the sedating effects of benzodiazepines and are targeted selectively by the newer-generation soporifics such as zolpidem, while the α_2 subunits mediate the anxiolytic effects. The clinical actions of benzodiazepines, along with two other classes of CNS-depressant drugs, barbiturates and anesthetic steroids, as well as ethanol seem to be related to their ability to bind to $GABA_A$ receptors and to enhance $GABA_A$ receptor currents (Yamakura et al. 2001). Individual $GABA_A$ channels do not open continuously in the presence of GABA but rather flicker open and closed, often in bursts. Benzodiazepines increase GABA current by increasing the frequency of channel openings without altering open time or conductance. Barbiturates prolong the channel open time without altering opening frequency or conductance. Steroids such as androsterone and pregnenolone increase the open time and the frequency of bursts. Despite the different mechanisms of action, each drug enhances GABAergic transmission, accounting for their shared properties as anticonvulsants. In fact, they may directly counteract a GABA deficit due to a reduction in GABA transporter numbers in epileptogenic cortex that may be etiological in epilepsy (During et al. 1995).

Metabotropic Receptors

Longer-term modulatory effects are generally mediated by metabotropic receptors (Greengard 2001). These nonchannel-linked receptors regulate cell function via activation of G proteins that couple to second-messenger cascades. Although other non-channel-linked receptors may also be catalytic, in the CNS only G protein–linked receptors are found. In fact, the majority of neurotransmitters and neuromodulators exert their effects through binding to G protein receptors. G protein–linked receptors are so named because they couple to intracellular guanosine triphosphate (GTP)-binding regulatory proteins. G proteins are formed from a complex of three membrane-bound proteins (Gαβγ); when the receptor is activated, the α subunit (Gα) binds GTP and dissociates from a complex of the β and γ subunits (Gβγ). Both Gα and Gβγ may go on to trigger subsequent events. Activated G proteins have a life span of seconds to minutes; Gα auto-inactivates by hydrolyzing its bound GTP, after which it reaggregates with Gβγ, returning to the resting state. Continued transmitter binding to the receptor may reinitiate the cycle.

G proteins are the first link in signaling cascades that either directly activate protein kinases—enzymes that phosphorylate cellular proteins (Walaas and Greengard 1991)—or raise intracellular Ca^{2+} and indirectly activate kinases (Figure 4–10) (Ghosh and Greenberg 1995). Proteins undergo conformational changes when they are phosphorylated that may lead to either their activation or inactivation. Proteins affected may include membrane channels, cytoskeletal elements, and transcriptional regulators of gene expression. In this way, modulatory actions mediated by second messengers control most cellular processes. The potential for amplification, combined with divergence and convergence of signals, provides the requisite mechanisms for enduring changes in neuronal function, especially for mechanisms essential for learning and memory and for development. The three major second-messenger cascades involving G proteins and their interaction with Ca^{2+} are schematized in Figure 4–10.

As these G protein–coupled receptors are the targets of many therapeutic and abused drugs, understanding their regulation is of paramount clinical importance. Major advances have been made in defining the mechanisms mediating downregulation of G protein–coupled receptors (Tsao and von Zastrow 2000). Receptor downregulation is generally induced by prolonged activation of receptors, leading to receptor internalization. For example, prolonged activation of dopamine type 1 (D_1) receptors in striatal neurons by agonist injection in vivo causes rapid internalization of dopamine receptors (Dumartin et al. 1998). This receptor internalization is mediated by highly specific dynamin-dependent and dynamin-independent mechanisms (Vickery and von Zastrow 1999). Determining the mechanisms of G protein receptor downregulation may identify targets for

development of new classes of drugs useful for the therapeutic manipulation of G protein receptor signaling. For instance, mutant mice lacking β-arrestin 2 show no tolerance to opioids (Bohn et al. 1999).

The slower actions of metabotropic receptors are responsible for altering neuronal excitability and the strength of synaptic connections, often reinforcing neural pathways involved in learning (Bailey and Kandel 2004). Activation of these receptors generally does not change the membrane potential at all. Rather, receptor binding activates second-messenger cascades that can dramatically alter the response properties of other receptors. Most profoundly, second messengers may translocate to the nucleus, where they may control gene expression, exerting longer-term changes in cell function via the activation of genes in a temporal sequence (Girault and Greengard 2004). Many long-term adaptations, such as those induced by psychotropic agents, appear to be mediated by adaptations in metabotropic receptor signaling. For instance, the antidepressant effects of SSRIs are due not to the immediate surge in serotonin associated with the blockade of the serotonin reuptake transporter (SERT) but rather to longer-term adaptations in signaling mediated by serotonin 5-HT_{1A} and 5-HT_{2A} receptors (Blier and Abbott 2001). Dopaminergic actions in cortex, implicated in the modulation of working memory (Goldman-Rakic et al. 2000), result in long-term adaptations in cortical signaling (Seamans and Yang 2004).

Gases as Transcellular Modulators

Surprisingly, nitric oxide (NO), a gas, has been shown to mediate interneuronal signaling, functioning as a second messenger with neurotransmitter properties (Brenman and Bredt 1997; Schulman 1997). NO is extremely short-lived and is rapidly synthesized on demand from arginine by the enzyme nitric oxide synthase (NOS). NOS is activated by increases in intracellular Ca^{2+} concentration. Unlike conventional intracellular messengers that are localized to the postsynaptic cell, where they have their effects, NO diffuses across membranes to adjacent presynaptic or postsynaptic cells and activates guanylyl cyclase, raising levels of cyclic guanosine 3′,5′-monophosphate (cGMP) and in turn triggering the production of other intracellular messengers. NO, as well as carbon monoxide (CO) and arachidonic acid, other transcellular modulators, may coordinate pre- and postsynaptic changes in synaptic plasticity (Meffert et al. 1996; O'Dell et al. 1994). Excitotoxicity due to excessive activation of the NMDA class of glutamate receptors appears to be mediated in part by NO (Dawson et al. 1994).

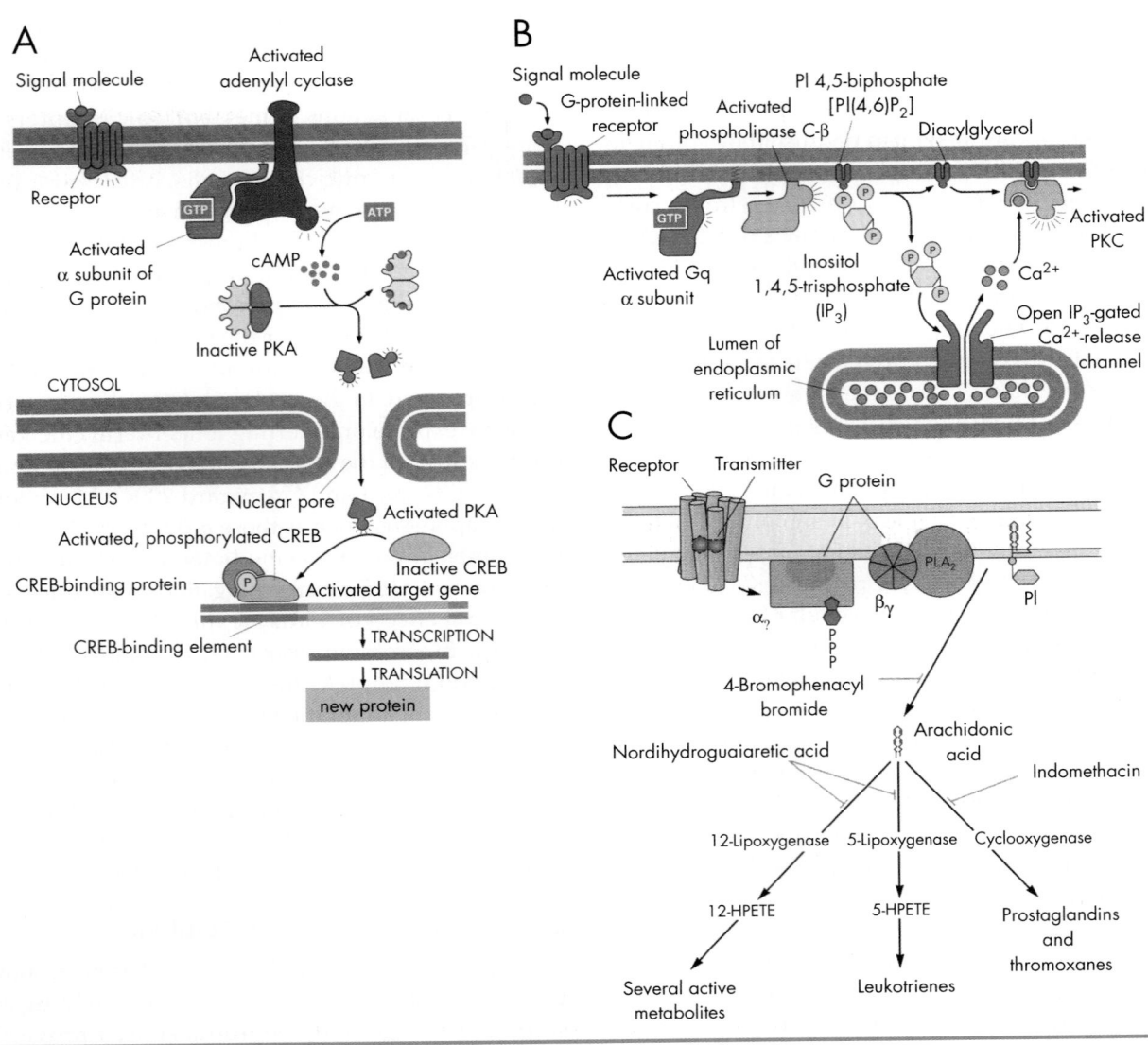

FIGURE 4–10.   Major intracellular signaling pathways in neurons.

Ligand binding to receptors activates three major signaling pathways via G proteins. *Panel A.*   In the cyclic adenosine mono-phosphate (cAMP) system, a G protein link couples ligand binding to activation of adenylyl cyclase. This in turn generates cAMP, which binds to the regulatory units (R) of cAMP-dependent protein kinase, releasing the catalytic subunits (activated protein kinase A). After being phosphorylated (activated, phosphorylated CREB), CREB binds to cAMP response elements (CREB-binding element) to regulate gene expression. *Panel B.*   In the inositol phospholipid system, G proteins activate phospholipase C, which hydrolyzes membrane phospholipids to produce two second messengers, diacylglycerol and inositol 1,4,5-triphosphate (IP$_3$). IP$_3$ triggers the release of calcium (Ca^{2+}) from the endoplasmic reticulum. Ca^{2+}, in turn, triggers the translocation of protein kinase C (PKC) to the cell membrane, where it is activated by diacylglycerol. Because it becomes membrane bound with activation, PKC may be especially important in the modulation of membrane channels. Ca^{2+} released from intracellular stores may act similarly to Ca^{2+} that enters from outside the cell (not shown), allowing temporal coincidence through activation of voltage-dependent Ca^{2+} channels. *Panel C.*   In the arachidonic acid system, G proteins may couple to phospholipase A$_2$ (PLA$_2$), forming arachidonic acid by hydrolysis of membrane phospholipids. Arachidonic acid is either a second messenger in its own right or a precursor of the lipoxygenase pathway giving rise to a family of membrane-permeant second messengers. The cyclooxygenase pathway is principally important outside the brain in prostaglandin production. HPETE = hydroperoxyeicosatetraenoic acid; PI = phosphatidylinositol.

Source.   Panels A and B reprinted from Alberts B, Johnson A, Lewis J, Raff M, Roberts K, Walter P: *Molecular Biology of the Cell.* New York, Garland Science, 2002. Copyright Garland Science/Taylor & Francis LLC, 2002. Used with permission. Panel C reprinted from Siegelbaum SA, Schwartz JH, Kandel ER: "Modulation of Synaptic Transmission: Second Messengers," in *Principles of Neural Science,* 4th Edition. Edited by Kandel ER, Schwartz JH, Jessell TM. New York, McGraw-Hill, 2000, pp. 229–252. Copyright 2000 The McGraw-Hill Companies, Inc. Used with permission.

Organization of Postsynaptic Receptors at Synapses

Most neurotransmitter receptors are clustered at postsynaptic sites closely apposed to the presynaptic terminal. Several laboratories have made remarkable progress in identifying the molecular components of the postsynaptic scaffold that holds synaptic receptors in place (Figure 4–11) (Lee and Sheng 2000; O'Brien et al. 1998). One of the most abundant proteins in the postsynaptic density is PSD-95 (a postsynaptic density protein of 95 kd). PSD-95 is a cytoplasmic protein that contains three domains important for protein binding, called *PDZ domains* (named after the initials of the first three proteins found to share a common sequence of 80–90 amino acids important for their stabilization at the postsynaptic membrane). These domains of PSD-95 bind to the NMDA receptor, to the Shaker K^+ channel, and to cell adhesion proteins called *neuroligins.* In contrast, AMPA receptors bind a distinct PDZ domain protein called GRIP, and metabotropic glutamate receptors interact with HOMER. These PDZ proteins are believed to cluster neurotransmitter receptors and other important components of the synapse at the postsynaptic density and to mediate rapid insertion or removal of receptors from the synapse, as may occur during synaptic plasticity (Kennedy and Ehlers 2006).

Synaptic Modulation in Learning and Memory

Learning and memory require both short- and long-term changes at synapses. In addition to rapid signals, neurotransmitters activate second-messenger systems that profoundly increase the range of responses a neuron shows to synaptic input. Second messengers activate kinases that both amplify and prolong signals by phosphorylating other proteins. Phosphorylated proteins remain active—often for a much longer period than agonist remains bound to receptor—until they are dephosphorylated by protein phosphatases. Because second messengers trigger numerous cellular functions, activation of a single receptor may trigger a coordinated cellular response involving several systems. This may include activity-dependent modulation of genomic transcription, leading to enduring changes in cellular function.

Sensitization in *Aplysia*

Investigations using the marine mollusk *Aplysia californica* have been fundamental to current understanding of the cellular mechanisms of learning and mem-

ory (Hawkins et al. 2006; Kandel 2001a). Because its nervous system is composed of relatively few neurons that are identifiable from animal to animal, changes in *Aplysia* behavior can be traced to alterations in individual synaptic connections. *Aplysia* exhibits a simple defensive behavior, the gill-withdrawal reflex, that shows several elementary forms of learning. Mild stimulation to the siphon skin overlying the gill leads to its reflex withdrawal. If a shock is delivered to the tail, the reflex shows sensitization; subsequent siphon stimulation elicits a more brisk reflex. If siphon stimulation is paired with tail shock, the animal shows associative learning manifested in an increased reflex response to the mild siphon stimulation. In effect, *Aplysia* learns that mild siphon stimulation predicts tail shock.

Sensitizing stimuli to the tail activate serotonergic facilitator neurons that synapse on sensory neuron terminals. The serotonin released produces presynaptic facilitation by activating adenylyl cyclase via a G protein link; cyclic adenosine monophosphate (cAMP) binds to the regulatory subunits of cAMP-dependent protein kinase A (PKA), releasing the catalytic subunits, which phosphorylate a class of voltage-dependent K^+ channels (S-K^+ channels) and inactivate them. Because less K^+ current is evoked, the membrane remains depolarized a bit longer with a given action potential, there is more Ca^{2+} influx, and thus more transmitter release. Associative learning appears to be due to facilitator neuron activation closely following sensory neuron activation. The spike-triggered Ca^{2+} influx in the sensory neuron terminal and serotonin-activated second-messenger systems, when activated together, produce enhanced protein kinase C (PKC) activity. This is termed *activity-dependent enhancement of presynaptic facilitation,* and it provides the coincidence detection inherent in associative learning (Figure 4–12A, *Short term*). In all of these short-term forms of learning, the mechanisms involve covalent modification of existing proteins, principally by phosphorylation.

In contrast, long-term memory requires changes in gene transcription. The same mechanisms that mediate short-term sensitization initiate long-term memory formation. In long-term as in short-term sensitization, the memory is encoded by a strengthening of sensorimotor synapses. There is increased transmitter release, and S-K^+ channels are closed, leading to increased Ca^{2+} influx. Synaptic vesicles are trafficked to release sites, accounting for about a third of the increment in synaptic strength, with the balance mediated by growth of new varicosities (Kim et al. 2003). With such structural changes, there is an absolute requirement for gene tran-

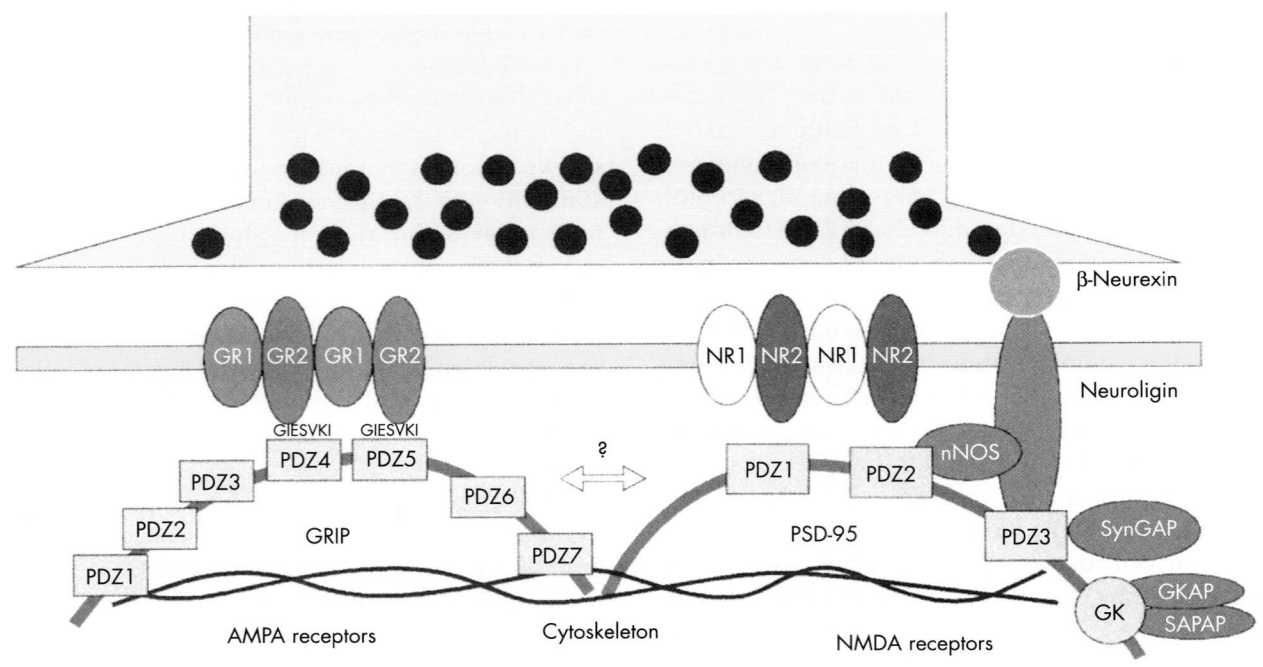

FIGURE 4–11. Selected molecular components of a typical CNS glutamatergic synapse.

α-Amino-3-hydroxy-5-methylisoxazole-4-propionic acid (AMPA) receptor subunits are tethered to GRIP through PDZ domain interactions, and the *N*-methyl-D-aspartate (NMDA) receptor subunits are bound to PSD-95. Both GRIP and PSD-95 also interact with the cytoskeleton, providing a protein scaffold for glutamate receptors in the postsynaptic density. This scaffold may regulate the dynamic, activity-dependent insertion or removal of glutamate receptors from CNS synapses. GIES-VKI = the amino acids critical for binding GR2 to PDZ4 and PDZ5; nNOS = neuronal nitric oxide synthase.
Source.   Reprinted from O'Brien RJ, Lau LF, Huganir RL: "Molecular Mechanisms of Glutamate Receptor Clustering at Excitatory Synapses." *Current Opinion in Neurobiology* 8:364–369, 1998. Copyright 1998. Used with permission from Elsevier.

scription and the synthesis of new proteins. cAMP affects gene transcription by binding to the cAMP response element–binding protein (CREB), which then binds to regulatory cAMP response element sites to activate gene transcription (Figure 4–12A, *Long term*). CREB in turn induces ubiquitin transcription, which leads to the cleavage of the regulatory subunit of cAMP-dependent protein kinase and an enduring up-regulation of the kinase. Ultimately, the changes triggered by repeated sensory input, activation of facilitatory interneurons, serotonin application, or cAMP injection lead to enduring structural changes involving the growth of new processes and increased numbers and size of synapses. These morphological changes are mediated in part by cell adhesion molecules, akin to ones that play crucial roles in the assembly of the nervous system. Changes in gene expression lead to protein synthesis at the cellular but not synaptic level, raising the question as to how specific connections are strengthened selectively. Once sensitization has been initiated by repeated serotonin application, subsequent

serotonin stimulation at the level of single synapses appears to mark the synapses for growth (Figure 4–12B). Additionally, neurons appear to be capable of limited local protein synthesis at synapses, providing further means for synapse-specific plasticity (Brittis et al. 2002). Thus, short-term changes in synaptic strength translate into enduring structural changes through interactions among second-messenger systems orchestrating gene transcription.

Long-Term Potentiation

Since the pioneering observations more than 50 years ago on patient H.M., who following bilateral hippocampal resection was no longer able to encode memories, studies of memory have focused on the circuitry of the hippocampus (Lynch 2004). This focus was further strengthened, more than 30 years ago, by the discovery that brief high-frequency stimulation of hippocampal pathways leads to LTP of the synaptic connections (Bliss and Lomo 1973). In intact animals, LTP may last for days to weeks, and thus has come to be seen as the

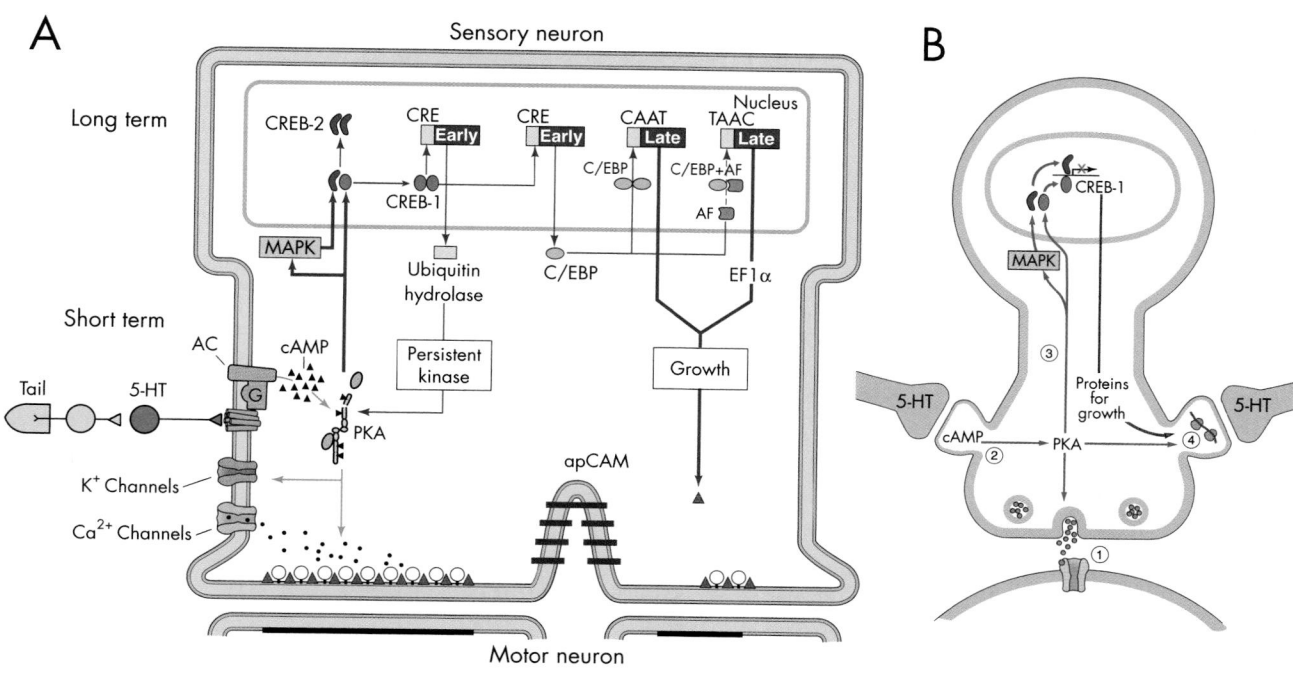

FIGURE 4–12. Molecular mechanisms of short-term and long-term memory storage.

Panel A. Schematic shows a single synaptic connection between a sensory and motor neuron in the neural circuit mediating defensive gill-withdrawal reflex in the marine snail *Aplysia californica.* Serotonin (5-HT) triggers an increase in synaptic strength, which underlies the animal's heightened reflex withdrawal response when stressed. In short-term sensitization (lasting on the order of an hour), one electric shock to the tail activates 5-HT interneurons (*blue*), activating serotonin receptors (also in *blue*) that activate protein kinase A (PKA), which phosphorylates existing proteins, leading to a short-term enhancement of synaptic transmission. With repeated stress, persistent elevation of cyclic adenosine monophosphate (cAMP) levels engages nuclear regulatory pathways. PKA, in turn, activates another kinase (MAPK), and together they phosphorylate cAMP response element–binding protein 2 (CREB-2), releasing active CREB-1. CREB-1 then activates directly and indirectly a series of genes in temporal sequence, locking in the activation of PKA via ubiquitin hydrolase and encoding proteins necessary for synaptic growth. One example is *Aplysia* cell-adhesion molecule (apCAM), a molecule important in synaptic development, which plays a similar role in the further growth of synaptic connections with learning. ***Panel B.*** The signaling mechanisms involved in sensitization are summarized in broader strokes in this schematic: 1) sensory neurons activate motor neurons via exocytic release of the excitatory transmitter glutamate; 2) stress stimuli activate protein kinase, which both enhances transmitter release locally and 3) translocates to the nucleus to orchestrate long-term changes. The proteins for growth are utilized at synapses marked by 5-HT stimulation, leading to long-term strengthening of stressed synapses.
Source. Reprinted from Kandel ER: "The Molecular Biology of Memory Storage: A Dialogue Between Genes and Synapses." *Science* 294:1030–1038, 2001, with permission from AAAS and the Nobel Foundation. Copyright Nobel Foundation 2000.

crucial synaptic process underlying memory formation. In the hippocampus, each of the three major synaptic circuits shows LTP, with distinct but shared mechanisms. At the most studied synapse, the Schaffer collateral synapse made by the projections of CA3 onto CA1 pyramidal neurons (Figure 4–13), LTP is initiated by Ca^{2+} influx into the postsynaptic neuron via NMDA receptors. Although glutamate released by CA3 neurons acts on NMDA and AMPA receptors, only high-frequency firing activates sufficient numbers of AMPA receptors to depolarize the postsynaptic membrane, relieve the voltage-dependent Mg^{2+} block of the NMDA receptor, and allow Ca^{2+} influx, initiating LTP (Blitzer

et al. 2005). Because NMDA receptor activation requires both binding of neurotransmitter and postsynaptic depolarization, the NMDA receptor provides the molecular coincidence detector originally postulated by Donald Hebb (1949), who predicted that alterations in synaptic strength would involve coordinated pre- and postsynaptic activity.

The influx of Ca^{2+} into the postsynaptic CA3 neuron activates Ca^{2+}/calmodulin-dependent protein kinase II (CaMKII), which mediates the phosphorylation of AMPA receptors, increasing their sensitivity (Lisman et al. 2002). CaMKII is capable of autophosphorylation and locks itself in an active catalytic state. This provides

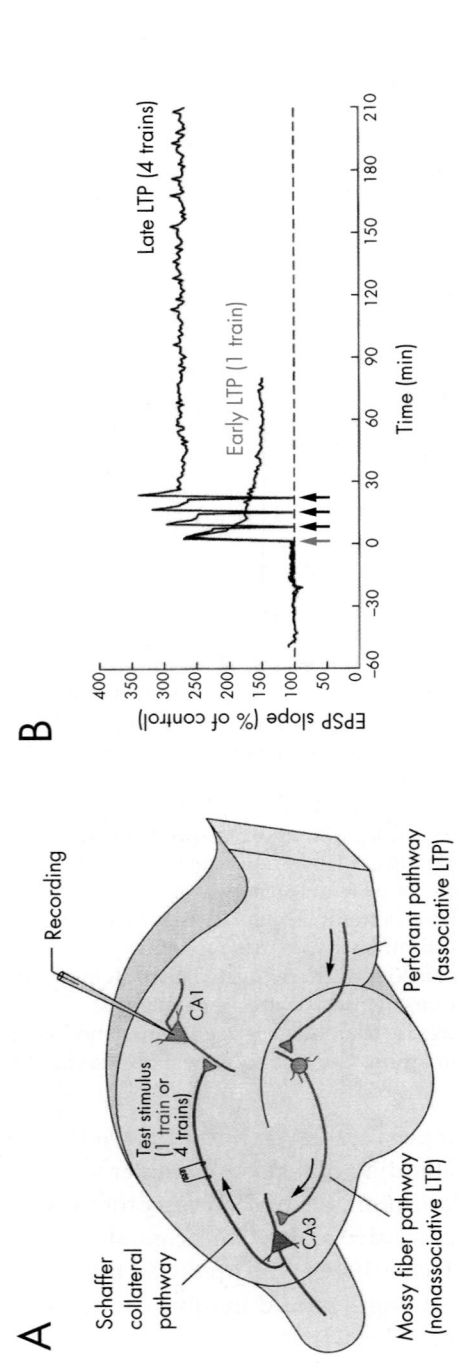

FIGURE 4–13.   Long-term potentiation (LTP) in the hippocampus.

Panel A.   A brain slice preparation from the rodent hippocampus is shown with the postsynaptic recording electrode in a CA1 pyramidal cell and a presynaptic stimulating electrode (coil) on the Schaffer collateral pathway axon of a CA3 pyramidal cell. *Panel B.*   Stimulating the Schaffer collateral pathway at low frequency (once a minute) causes the CA3 axon terminals to release glutamate, which evokes a stable excitatory response (measured as the rising slope of the excitatory postsynaptic potential, EPSP; the control response is normalized to 100%). A single tetanus (*blue arrow*, 100 stimuli in 1 second) evokes early LTP, which is weak and lasts on the order of an hour. In contrast, with four tetani (*blue and black arrows*), the postsynaptic response is dramatically increased. Late LTP lasts for over 24 hours, as would be required for a synaptic mechanism encoding long-term memory.

Source.   Adapted from Kandel ER: "Cellular Mechanisms of Learning and the Biological Basis of Individuality," in *Principles of Neural Science*, 4th Edition. Edited by Kandel ER, Schwartz JH, Jessell TM. New York, McGraw-Hill, 2000, pp. 1247–1279. Copyright 2000, The McGraw-Hill Companies, Inc. Used with permission.

a molecular basis for early LTP. Ca^{2+} also activates calcineurin (PP2b), a phosphatase, which modulates PP1, which in turn can dephosphorylate CaMKII and block LTP. Calcineurin's action is modulated by cAMP, which acting through PKA blocks PP1 activity (Blitzer et al. 1998). This pathway, which is activated by catecholamines and Ca^{2+}, serves a gating function. Dopamine acting via D$_1$ receptors is required for late LTP (Huang and Kandel 1995). Switching off calcineurin in adult mice enhances LTP in the hippocampus and spatial learning (Malleret et al. 2001), arguing further for the significance of LTP for memory. Interestingly, however, mice with genetic deletion of calcineurin in the forebrain show working memory deficits reminiscent of those seen in schizophrenia (Miyakawa et al. 2003).

LTP is composed of at least two phases: early and late LTP. Early LTP lasts for the first 3 hours after induction and does not require protein synthesis. In contrast, late LTP lasts for several hours and requires both gene transcription and protein translation. As is true for long-term synaptic enhancement in *Aplysia,* late LTP involves activation of CamKII, production of cAMP, and activation of gene transcription through a CREB-dependent process. LTP can also stimulate the growth of new synaptic connections. Such changes are likely to underlie the more permanent synaptic alterations necessary for learning and memory (Bailey and Kandel 2004). In early LTP, synaptic strengthening occurs postsynaptically via increased sensitivity of existing AMPA receptors. As memory is encoded in late LTP, AMPA receptors are inserted in functionally silent synapses, and altogether new postsynaptic structures develop (Lisman et al. 2002) (Figure 4–14). In particular, *silent* synapses—synapses that contain only NMDA receptors before induction of LTP—may be activated by activity-dependent insertion of new AMPA receptors. Increases in AMPA receptor function at previously silent synapses after LTP-inducing stimuli have been visualized directly by following the trafficking of AMPA receptors tagged with green fluorescent protein (GFP) (Shi et al. 1999). Relatively subtle changes in AMPA receptor trafficking are crucial, as has been shown in the amygdala for fear conditioning (Rumpel et al. 2005).

Whereas the *induction* of LTP is postsynaptic and depends on Ca^{2+} and the activation of CaMKII, the *expression* of LTP involves coordinated pre- and postsynaptic changes. Such an LTP-dependent increase in synaptic transmission has been visualized using antibody uptake (Malgaroli et al. 1995) and demonstrated in recordings from single synapses that have shown that the expression of LTP is associated with an increase in the numbers of synaptic vesicles released (Bolshakov

et al. 1997). The question then arises: How do postsynaptic events triggered by NMDA receptor activation lead to changes in presynaptic neurotransmitter release? A retrograde second messenger that could diffuse across the synapse and act on the presynaptic terminal seems to be required. Several experiments indicate that NO or CO can convey such a retrograde signal, diffusing from postsynaptic to nearby presynaptic sites, and activate guanylyl cyclase to induce an elevation in cGMP in the presynaptic terminal (Wang et al. 2005). Neurotrophins may also act as retrograde signals in LTP (McAllister et al. 1999).

How is the strengthening of synapses by LTP kept in check? Hippocampal synapses also show long-term depression (LTD), which involves a similar array of mechanisms activated by low-frequency synaptic activation (Anwyl 2006). LTD may be mediated by a decrease in neurotransmitter release and/or a decrease in postsynaptic responsiveness due to lowered numbers or sensitivity of glutamate receptors. Thus, through a dynamic balance between LTP and LTD, memories of irrelevant information may be eliminated and lasting memories fine-tuned. The regulation of synaptic strength appears to be controlled in the hippocampus by the predominant theta rhythm. Stimulation at the theta frequency produces LTP, whereas stimulation that is slower or specifically associated with the troughs of the rhythm produces LTD (Huerta and Lisman 1996). Possibly, alterations in brain rhythms, implicated in several neuropsychiatric disorders (Behrendt and Young 2004; Spencer et al. 2004), act in part via modulation of synaptic plasticity.

Development of Neurons
Birth and Migration

The human nervous system is the most complex organ system in vertebrates and contains a greater variety of cell types than is found in any other organ. Remarkably, the diversity of cell types that regulate every aspect of our lives is accomplished during a brief span of development encompassing just 3–4 months in humans. It is therefore not surprising that this critical period of gestation is sensitive to interference through environmental factors and pathogens, as well as genetic mutations. For example, extrinsic factors such as alcohol exposure have been shown to decrease neuronal production and, in severe cases, to produce microcephaly and mental retardation (M.W. Miller 1989). In addition, mutations in the doublecortin gene have been shown to dramatically interfere with neocortical

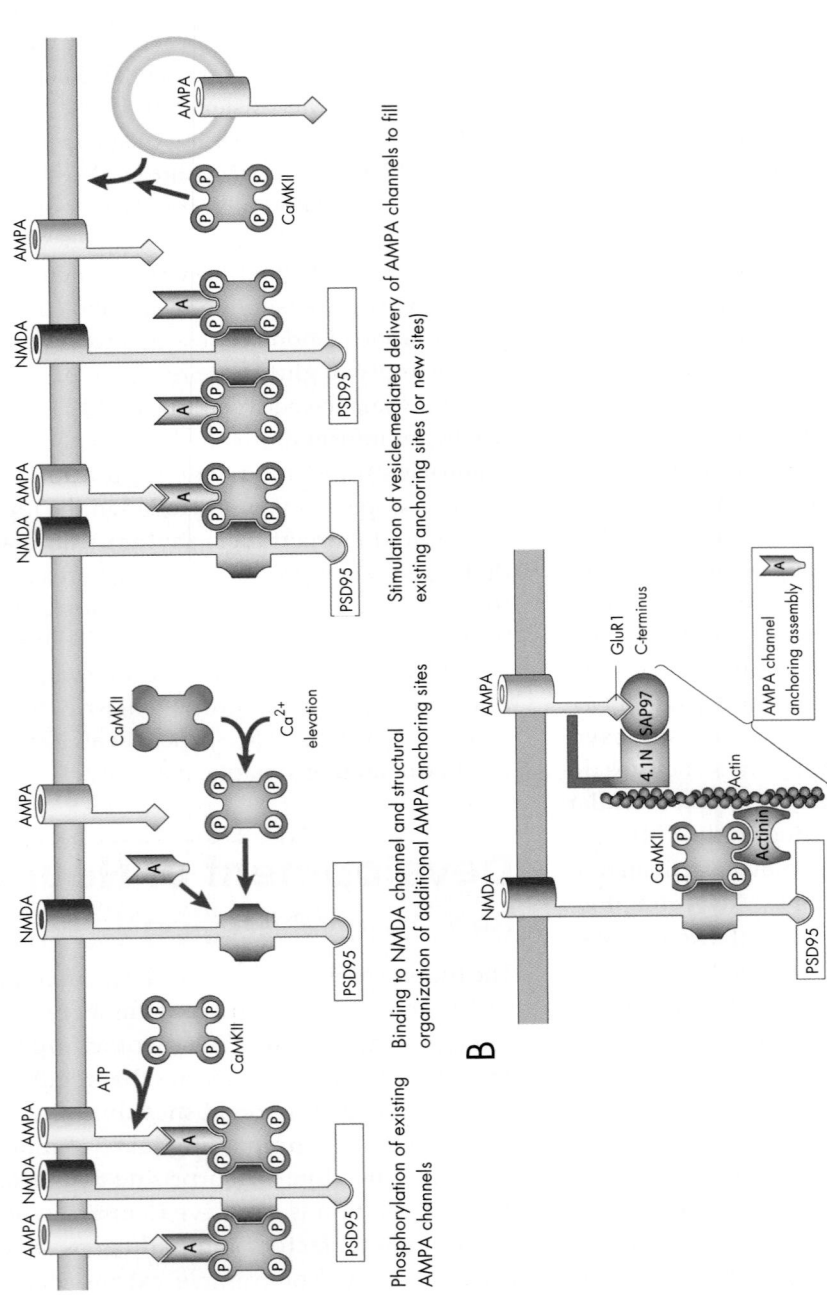

FIGURE 4–14. Molecular basis for long-term potentiation in the postsynaptic membrane of a CA1 pyramidal neuron.

Panel A. With sufficient stimulation (or coincident postsynaptic depolarization), *N*-methyl-D-aspartate (NMDA)–type glutamate receptors are activated and Ca^{2+} fluxes into the cell. Ca^{2+} activates calcium/calmodulin-dependent protein kinase II (CaMKII), which increases the responsiveness of α-amino-3-hydroxy-5-methylisoxazole-4-propionic acid (AMPA)–type glutamate receptors. CaMKII can phosphorylate itself, locking it in the active mode. With continued activity, CaMKII organizes the further insertion of AMPA receptors into the postsynaptic membrane. *Panel B.* AMPA receptor recruitment to the postsynaptic membrane is mediated by the contractile protein actin. Actin is a ubiquitous contractile protein, the same protein involved peripherally in muscle contraction. CaMKII thus plays a pivotal role at all steps in the enhancement of synaptic transmission with long-term potentiation.

Source. Reprinted from Lisman J, Schulman H, Cline H: "The Molecular Basis of CaMKII Function in Synaptic and Behavioural Memory." *Nature Reviews Neuroscience* 3:175–190, 2002. Copyright 2002. Used with permission from Macmillan Publishers Ltd.

development, resulting in epilepsy and in severe cortical malformations such as lissencephaly (des Portes et al. 1998; Gleeson et al. 1998).

The principal cell types in the brain, neurons and glia, are generated in two proliferative zones that line the ventricular system during development, after which they migrate into the overlying cortical mantle. Each proliferative zone is comprised of a different class of progenitor cells. The ventricular zone (VZ), which is adjacent to the ventricular lumen during CNS development, consists primarily of pseudostratified columnar epithelial cells (Boulder Committee 1970). These cells were first characterized in the late nineteenth century and have gone by various names but are now called *radial glial cells* (Rakic 1971). Radial glia are bipolar cells with a soma located in the VZ, a long, thin ascending process that often contacts the pial surface of the developing brain (Misson et al. 1988a), and a short descending process that contacts the ventricular lumen. The nucleus of radial glial cells undergoes a characteristic to-and-fro motion within the VZ, termed *interkinetic nuclear migration.* During progression through the cell cycle, the nucleus is positioned at the top of the VZ during S-phase and at the surface of the ventricular lumen during M-phase, where division is completed (Sauer 1935). A second proliferative zone, the subventricular zone (SVZ), appears just above the VZ at the onset of neurogenesis in many CNS regions (Boulder Committee 1970). SVZ progenitor cells are generated by VZ precursor cells but have distinguishing features. SVZ cells are multipolar, they do not maintain contact with the pial and ventricular surfaces as do radial glial cells, they do not undergo interkinetic nuclear migration as they proceed through the cell cycle, and they divide away from the ventricular lumen (Takahashi et al. 1995).

Identification of Neuronal Progenitor Cells

Early studies of nervous system development described mitotic cells adjacent to the ventricle that were assumed to be neuronal progenitor cells (Ramón y Cajal 1911). Nevertheless, the exact identity of the neural progenitor cells remained elusive until recent advances in molecular biology provided new tools with which to study nervous system development. Replication-incompetent retroviruses carrying reporter genes (Sanes et al. 1986) and the delivery of plasmid DNA to progenitor cells through electroporation to modify gene expression (Saito and Nakatsuji 2001) are now common tools in many laboratories. These techniques can deliver genes and fluorescent reporter proteins, such as GFP. Fluorescent reporter proteins have proven invalu-

able for detailed characterization of targeted cells in living tissue. Thus, it has become possible to study the expression of mRNA and protein, as well as the physiological properties of the labeled cells. Furthermore, it is now possible to study the behaviors of labeled precursor cells through time-lapse imaging in cultured tissue.

Retroviral lineage studies performed in the 1980s and 1990s reported clones containing either neuronal or glial cells, but rarely both (Luskin et al. 1988; Walsh and Cepko 1990). Although radial glial cells divide during neurogenesis (Misson et al. 1988b), they were thought to serve primarily as migratory guides for immature neurons (Rakic 1971). Thus, it was commonly thought that distinct classes of progenitor cells generate neuronal and glial cells. However, new studies have shown that neuronal and glial cell lineages are not as divergent as previously thought. Indeed, it has now been shown that in addition to guiding neuronal migration, radial glial cells also serve as neuronal progenitor cells in several regions of the developing mammalian brain, including the ventral telencephalon (Anthony et al. 2004; Halliday and Cepko 1992), the dorsal telencephalon (Malatesta et al. 2000; Miyata et al. 2001; Noctor et al. 2001), and the spinal cord (Anthony et al. 2004), as well as in other species (Alvarez-Buylla et al. 1990). In addition to generating neurons, radial glia also generate the SVZ progenitor cells that subsequently divide in the SVZ to generate two neurons (Noctor et al. 2004). The SVZ was previously thought to be the site of gliogenesis, but recent evidence shows that SVZ progenitor cells provide a major contribution to neurogenesis (Haubensak et al. 2004; Kriegstein and Noctor 2004; Letinic et al. 2002; Miyata et al. 2004; Tarabykin et al. 2001), particularly during the genesis of the upper neocortical layers as originally proposed by Smart (1973).

Radial glial cells are present along the entire axis of the developing CNS (Ramón y Cajal 1911), raising the possibility that they might be universal neural progenitor cells. However, evidence suggests that while cerebellar Purkinje neurons are generated by radial glial cells in the VZ (Miale and Sidman 1961), cerebellar granule cells are generated by a distinct class of neural progenitor cells that reside in the external granular layer (EGL) of the developing cerebellum (Kamei et al. 1998; Miale and Sidman 1961). Nevertheless, EGL progenitors in the cerebellum may be homologous to SVZ progenitors in the neocortex. Thus, the lineage relationship between EGL precursors and radial glial cells in the developing cerebellum should be worked out in future research.

When neurogenesis is complete, radial glial cells migrate away from the proliferative zones into the cortical mantle and transform into mature astrocytes in several brain regions (Schmechel and Rakic 1979). Individual radial glial cells have been shown to generate neurons before transforming into astrocytes (Noctor et al. 2004). Astrocytes remain capable of division in the postnatal brain and, interestingly, have been shown to generate neurons in specific regions of the adult brain such as the hippocampus (Doetsch et al. 1999; Seri et al. 2001). It not yet known if adult neurogenic astrocytes are descended from embryonic radial glial cells, but it is likely that a specific astroglial lineage may serve as neuronal progenitor cells throughout life. Identification and characterization of these important progenitor cells have fundamentally altered our understanding of developmental processes in the brain. More importantly, this research has identified a potential source of cells for replacement strategies in the treatment of neurodegenerative disorders.

Regulation of Proliferation

A number of factors, including neurotransmitter substances, growth factors, and even hormones, are present in proliferative regions of the brain and are known to regulate cell division in the developing and adult brain. For example, it has been shown that the classical neurotransmitters GABA and glutamate differentially regulate proliferation in the ventricular and subventricular zones during neocortical development (Haydar et al. 2000; LoTurco et al. 1995). Proliferative VZ radial glial cells are coupled to one another through connexin gap junction channels (LoTurco and Kriegstein 1991). New evidence indicates that waves of Ca^{2+} activity in radial glial cells are transmitted through connexin channels (gap junctions) and may be instrumental in regulating the proliferation of radial glial cells and thereby neurogenesis (Weissman et al. 2004). Finally, proteins such as β-catenin, a structural component of the adherens junctions that form between progenitor cells in the VZ, have been shown to promote proliferation versus differentiation of progenitor cells during cortical development (Chenn and Walsh 2002). These varied factors thus work in conjunction to regulate the proliferative behavior of progenitor cells during specific stages of brain development.

Determination of Cell Fate

The determination of cell fate occurs at regional, local, and cellular levels. The expression of different transcription factors along the rostrocaudal axis of the developing nervous system reveals one mechanism by which cortical cells acquire specific identities (Schuurmans and Guillemot 2002). Although all radial glial cells share characteristic morphological features, they nonetheless constitute a heterogeneous population based on protein expression patterns (Kriegstein and Gotz 2003). This may explain how different regions of the developing telencephalon generate different classes of cortical cells. For example, excitatory pyramidal cells and astrocytes are generated by Pax6-expressing cells in the dorsal telencephalon, while inhibitory interneurons are generated by Dlx-1/2–expressing cells in the ganglionic eminences of the embryonic ventral telencephalon (Anderson et al. 1997). The expression of transcription factors such as Dlx-1/2 is likely an early step in the commitment of telencephalic cells to a specific fate. The expression of these factors may even correlate with the phenotype of specific neuronal subtypes. Indeed, new evidence indicates that subregions of the ganglionic eminences express different transcription factors and give rise to interneuron subtypes (Nery et al. 2002). Local environmental factors also play a role in determining the fate of neurons in the developing cortex. Transplantation studies demonstrate that the laminar fate of cortical neurons can be altered when transplantation of cortical precursor cells occurs during specific phases of the cell cycle (McConnell and Kaznowski 1991). Furthermore, expression of transcription factors is crucial for the normal differentiation of cortical neurons. For example, the absence of the transcription factor Foxg1 during cortical neurogenesis induces deep-layer cortical neurons to adopt the phenotype of Cajal-Retzius neurons that are normally found in the superficial layer 1 of the neocortex (Hanashima et al. 2004).

The generation of sufficient numbers of the diverse cell types in the nervous system is accomplished through two basic types of progenitor cell divisions: symmetrical and asymmetrical (Gotz and Huttner 2005). Symmetrical divisions generate two daughter cells that are similar, whereas asymmetrical divisions generate two daughter cells that differ from one another. Recent evidence indicates that these types of divisions might occur in different proliferative zones—asymmetrical divisions occur more frequently at the surface of the ventricular lumen, while symmetrical divisions occur more frequently in the SVZ (Noctor et al. 2004).

Radial glial cells divide asymmetrically at the ventricular lumen to generate either a single neuron or an SVZ progenitor that will subsequently generate two neurons. Therefore, each radial glial cell division can generate either one neuron directly or two neurons indirectly (Figure 4–15). Determination of daughter cell fate after radial glial divisions, for either neuronal or

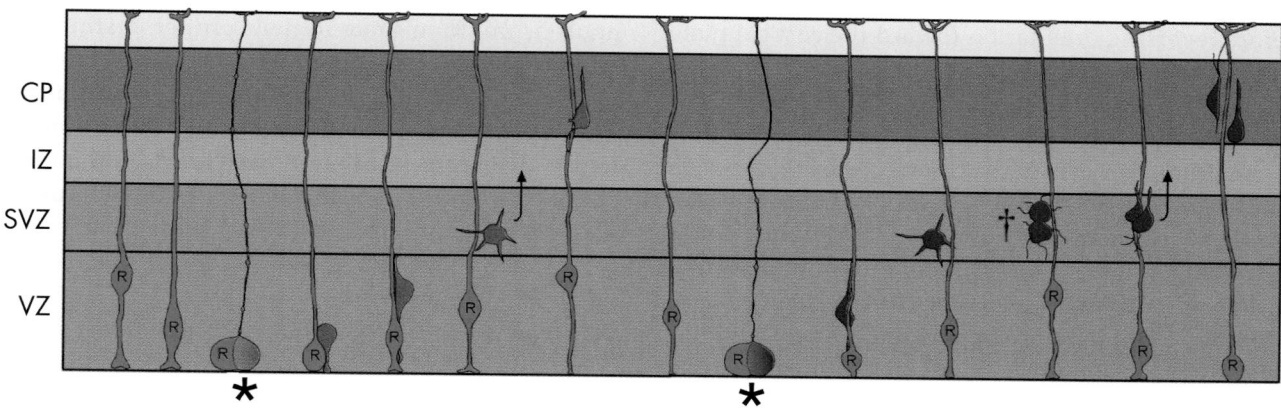

FIGURE 4–15. Key events in the generation of cortical neurons during embryogenesis.

Radial glial cells (R, shown in *green*) undergo interkinetic nuclear migration and divide asymmetrically at the ventricular surface (*) to self-renew and to generate neurons either directly (*red cell*) or indirectly through the generation of an intermediate progenitor cell (*blue*). Intermediate progenitor cells subsequently undergo terminal symmetrical division in the subventricular zone (SVZ, †) to generate two neurons. CP = cortical plate; IZ = intermediate zone; SVZ = subventricular zone; VZ = ventricular zone.

Source. Reprinted from McAllister AK, Usrey WM, Noctor SC, Rayport S: "Cellular and Molecular Biology of the Neuron," in *The American Psychiatric Publishing Textbook of Neuropsychiatry and Clinical Neurosciences,* 5th Edition. Washington, DC, American Psychiatric Publishing, 2008, pp. 3–43.

SVZ progenitors, thus affects the total number of neurons generated at a given time. A shift toward neuronal fate would decrease the total numbers of neurons being generated, whereas a shift toward SVZ progenitor fate for the radial glial daughter cells would double the neuronal output at a given time. Regulation of daughter cell fate during neurogenesis may thus affect the neuronal density for a given neocortical layer or structure. Invertebrate studies have revealed a number of important fate-determining molecules that are differentially segregated to nascent daughter cells during progenitor cell divisions. Some of these molecules, such as Notch and Numb, are also expressed in mammalian proliferative zones, and research into their role in determining daughter cell fate continues (Pearson and Doe 2004).

Migration

Neurons in the adult brain are organized into complex, intricately interconnected groups of nuclei and laminae. One of the remarkable aspects of brain development is that neurons are not born in their final locations. Instead, neurons are generated in proliferative zones surrounding the ventricular lumen and then must migrate substantial distances, up to 7,000 μm or longer, to reach their destination. Despite the complexity of the task, this feat is achieved with such regularity and precision that there is little variation in the archi-

tectonic pattern of brain structures from one person to the next, and even between species. In the developing neocortex, cortical neurons are generated in an inside-out sequence such that the deepest layers of the cerebral cortex form first, and subsequent waves of migrating neurons traverse the established layers as they migrate into the cortical mantle. Thus, as development proceeds, neurons must migrate progressively longer distances and through increasing numbers of cortical cells. Migration relies on cell–cell adhesion ligand molecules that signal between the radial glial fibers and migrating neurons (Hatten 1990). Neuronal migration is also regulated by a number of extracellular signaling molecules, such as neurotransmitter substances acting through the NMDA receptor (Komuro and Rakic 1993) and reelin protein acting through its constituent receptor molecules (Tissir and Goffinet 2003).

Recent experiments employing time-lapse imaging of fluorescently labeled cells in cultured brain tissue have revealed that the patterns of neuronal migration in the neocortex are more complex than originally thought. Neurons undergo several distinct stages of migration that can be identified based on the morphology and position of the neurons. After being generated, the cortical neurons leave the ventricular surface and rapidly ascend to the SVZ, where they acquire a multipolar morphology and remain stationary for one day or longer. After sojourning in the SVZ (Bayer and

Altman 1991), many cortical neurons make a retrograde movement back toward the ventricular lumen before reversing orientation toward the cortical plate and commencing radial migration (Noctor et al. 2004) (Figure 4–16). Similar ventricle-directed movements have been reported for GABAergic interneurons during their migration into the dorsal cortex (Nadarajah and Parnavelas 2002). The similarity in the ventricle-directed movements of these distinct cell types indicates that excitatory and inhibitory neurons are capable of responding to similar cues during their cortical migrations, and it hints at a potential source of important migration-guidance molecules located near the ventricular lumen of the developing brain.

Different forms of migration have been identified in other regions of the developing brain, such as the tangential migration of interneurons from the ganglionic eminences of the ventral telencephalon into the dorsal telencephalon. Interneurons do not appear to migrate along radial glial fibers during their journey from the ventral into the dorsal telencephalon. But it has yet to be determined whether they rely on cellular guides, such as developing axonal pathways in the intermediate zone of the developing cortex, or rather are guided solely along gradients of chemoattractive and repulsive factors (Marin and Rubenstein 2003). The picture is further complicated because interneurons migrate along several different complex pathways en route to their destination in the dorsal cortex (Kriegstein and Noctor 2004). The significance of these divergent pathways has yet to be determined, but it is possible that specific interneuron subtypes respond to different migration cues and thus adopt different routes of migration. Yet another form of migration, termed *chain migration*, has been identified for olfactory bulb interneurons as they migrate from their birthplace in the cortical SVZ along the rostral migratory stream into the olfactory bulb (Lois et al. 1996).

Despite differences in the identified forms of migration, each appears to rely on a shared set of intracellular molecules that are involved in the extension of leading processes and the transportation of cellular structures such as the nucleus (Feng and Walsh 2001). Neuronal migration is thus a complex interplay between the migrating cell and its environment that relies on intracellular machinery as well as extrinsic signaling factors. Given the complexity of this task, it is not surprising that a number of nervous system malformations have been identified that result from defects in neuronal migration (Feng and Walsh 2001). These range from severe brain malformations such as lissencephaly to periventricular nodular heterotopia to more moderate cases involving small ectopic clusters of neurons. In each case, varying proportions of neurons fail to migrate to their proper destinations. Afflicted individuals present with mental retardation in severe cases. Mild malformations are often associated with epilepsy. The lifelong impact of these neurological disorders on affected individuals and families cannot be overstated and necessitates our further search for the root causes of these conditions.

Synapse Formation

When an axonal growth cone reaches a target cell, a complex series of interactions commences, ultimately resulting in the formation of a synapse. Although there is still much to be learned about the formation of synapses in the CNS, the basic process of synaptogenesis at the neuromuscular junction (NMJ; the synapse between a motor neuron and a muscle cell) has been well described (Figure 4–17). Both the motor neuron and the muscle cell have the necessary molecular machinery prefabricated before synapse formation (Sanes and Lichtman 1999). The motor neuron growth cone functions like a protosynapse, showing activity-dependent neurotransmitter release. Noninnervated postsynaptic cells have transmitter receptors distributed over much of their surface, and within minutes of initial contact, a rudimentary form of synaptic transmission begins. Over subsequent days, connections become stronger and stabilize as the growth cone matures into a presynaptic terminal, gathering the cellular elements necessary for focused release of neurotransmitter at active zones. In parallel, the postsynaptic cell concentrates receptors at the site of contact, removing them from other regions, and over the course of days it develops postsynaptic specializations.

Although there are many differences between the NMJ and CNS synapses, the general principles of synapse formation appear to be conserved. As at the NMJ, presynaptic and postsynaptic proteins are present in axons and dendrites, respectively, of CNS neurons prior to synapse formation. Presynaptic proteins are transported in at least two separate multiprotein-containing transport vesicles that are mobile before synapse formation—one carries a subset of active zone proteins and another carries synaptic vesicles and additional active zone proteins (Ziv and Garner 2004). Postsynaptic proteins are also trafficked in transport vesicles prior to synapse formation; NMDA receptor transport vesicles also contain SAP102, a scaffolding protein found at young synapses (Washbourne et al. 2004b). These mobile transport vesicles accumulate rapidly at new sites of contact between presynaptic

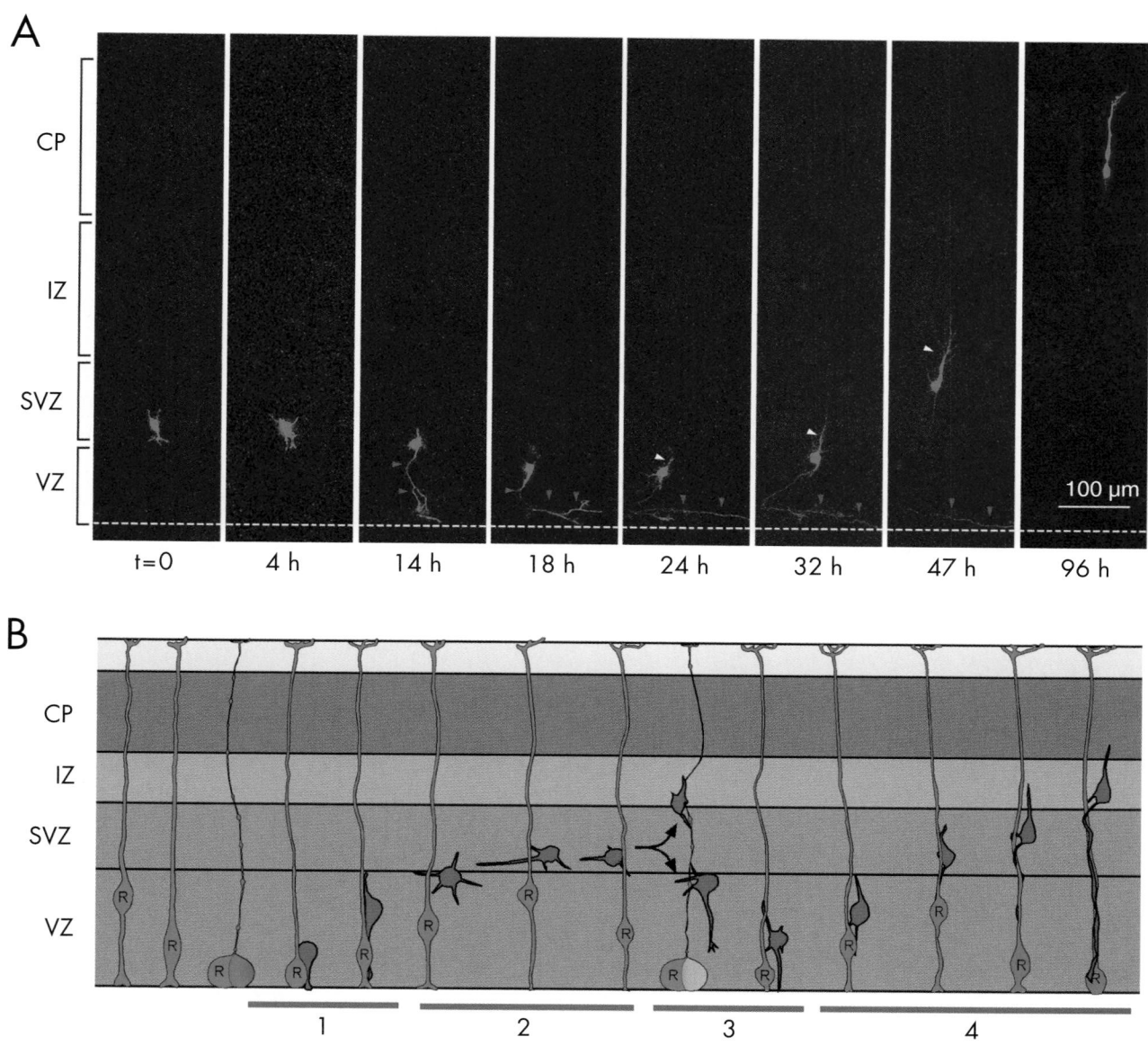

FIGURE 4–16. Migration phases of neocortical neurons during development.

During development, neocortical neurons exhibit four distinct phases in migration. *Panel A.* A time-lapse sequence of a retrovirally labeled neuron expressing the reporter protein green fluorescent protein (GFP) undergoing migration from the proliferative zone to the cortical plate in a cultured brain slice. The sequence begins when the neuron is in the second phase, which consists of migratory arrest for 24 hours or more (shown here at the end of phase two, t = 0 hours), followed by a third phase of retrograde migration toward the ventricle (t = 14–18 hours) and a final phase of polarity reversal and migration toward the cortical plate (CP) (t = 24–96 hours). Before initiating the final phase of radial migration, the neuron develops a leading process oriented toward the CP (*white arrowhead*). After 96 hours in culture, the migrating neuron had reached its destination at the top of the cortical plate. These neurons often leave a trailing axon in the ventricular zone (VZ, *red arrowheads*). *Panel B.* Schematic depicting a neuron (shown in *dark green*) undergoing the four phases of migration: 1) After being generated by its mother radial glial cell (R, shown in *light green*), the neuron commences initial radial migration, 2) migratory arrest in the SVZ, 3) retrograde migration, and 4) secondary radial migration. IZ = intermediate zone; SVZ = subventricular zone.

Source. Reprinted from McAllister AK, Usrey WM, Noctor SC, Rayport S: "Cellular and Molecular Biology of the Neuron," in *The American Psychiatric Publishing Textbook of Neuropsychiatry and Clinical Neurosciences,* 5th Edition. Washington, DC, American Psychiatric Publishing, 2008, pp. 3–43.

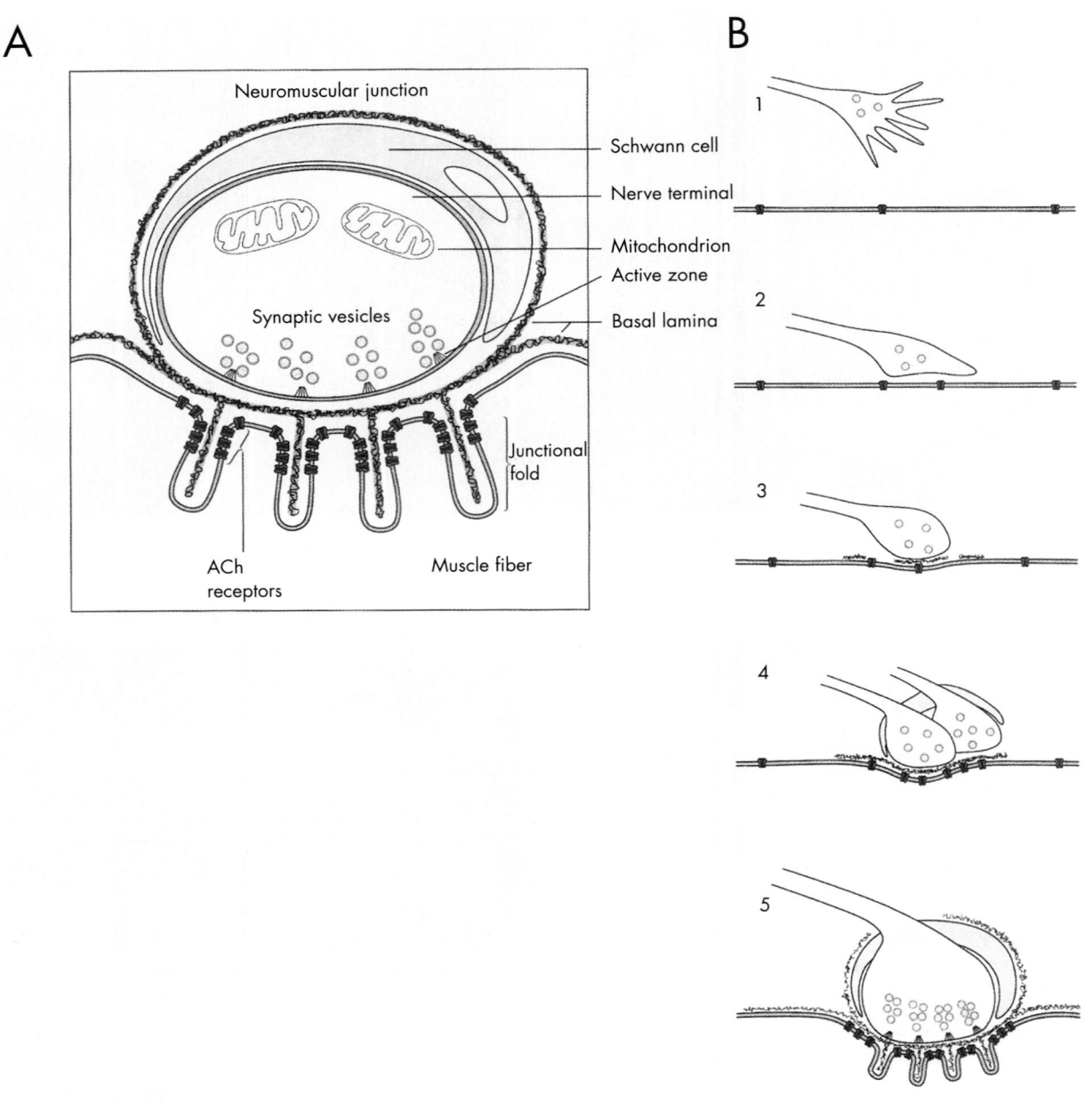

FIGURE 4–17.   Synapse formation of the neuromuscular junction (NMJ).

Panel A.   Schematic view of the molecular components of a typical NMJ. At a mature NMJ, the presynaptic terminal is separated from the postsynaptic muscle cell by the synaptic cleft. Synaptic vesicles filled with acetylcholine (ACh) are clustered at active zones, where they can fuse with the plasma membrane upon depolarization to release their transmitter into the synaptic cleft. Acetylcholine receptors are found postsynaptically, and glial cells called Schwann cells surround the synaptic terminal.
Panel B.   Stages in the formation of the NMJ: 1) An isolated growth cone from a motor neuron is guided to the muscle by axon guidance cues. 2) The first contact is an unspecialized physical contact. 3) However, synaptic vesicles rapidly cluster in the axon terminal, acetylcholine receptors start to cluster under the forming synapse, and a basal lamina is deposited in the synaptic cleft. 4) As development proceeds, multiple motor neurons innervate each muscle. 5) Over time, however, all but one of the axons are eliminated through an activity-dependent process, and the remaining terminal matures.
Source.   Reprinted from Sanes JR, Jessell TM: "The Formation and Regeneration of Synapses," in *Principles of Neural Science,* 4th Edition. Edited by Kandel ER, Schwartz JH, Jessell TM. New York, McGraw-Hill, 2000, pp. 1087–1114. Copyright 2000, The McGraw-Hill Companies, Inc. Used with permission.

and postsynaptic CNS neurons. Axodendritic contact is followed within minutes by the rapid and simultaneous recruitment of synaptic vesicles and NMDA receptors to new synapses (Washbourne et al. 2002). This early recruitment of NMDA receptors, but not AMPA receptors, to new synapses has been described in multiple systems; the resulting synapses are electrically "silent" until AMPA receptors are inserted (Isaac 2003). In the hours following contact, scaffolding proteins are also recruited to nascent synapses by as-yet-unknown mechanisms (Kim and Sheng 2004).

In order for synapses to form so quickly, specific contacts between axons and dendrites must initiate intracellular signals that lead to rapid recruitment of pre- and postsynaptic proteins. In the past few years, our understanding of the molecular signals that cause the initial recruitment of synaptic proteins to new sites of axodendritic contact has increased dramatically (Scheiffele 2003; Waites et al. 2005). In general, there are three major classes of signals that regulate synapse formation: adhesion molecules, diffusible molecules, and molecules secreted from glial cells. The first class of these synaptogenic molecules are the cell adhesion molecules, which include integrins, neural cell adhesion molecules (NCAMs), nectins, cadherins, neurexin-neuroligin, synaptic cell adhesion molecules (SynCAMs), and the ephrins (Washbourne et al. 2004a). Although models are rapidly evolving with ongoing research, to date the most current model is that initial cadherin-based adhesion stabilizes transient, dynamic axodendritic contacts long enough to allow other classes of synaptogenic molecules to interact and activate intracellular cascades that recruit synaptic proteins. After rapid cadherin-based adhesion, trans-synaptic molecules such as neuroligin and SynCAM then lead to simultaneous bidirectional signaling in the axon and dendrite; this kind of signaling could be critical for the rapid and simultaneous recruitment of synaptic transport vesicles and NMDA receptor transport packets to new axodendritic contacts. Recent studies have begun to provide strong evidence that a lack, or abnormal expression, of trans-synaptic adhesion molecules may cause neurodevelopmental disorders. For example, intense interest has recently been focused on the possibility that mutations in one or more of the genes that encode neuroligins—a synaptogenic molecule that mediates both presynaptic and postsynaptic differentiation—cause autism (Chih et al. 2004).

The second class of synaptogenic molecules is diffusible molecules—brain-derived neurotrophic factor (BDNF) and members of the Wnt and TGFβ families (Salinas 2005). Less is known about how and when, after initial contact, these molecules influence the recruitment of synaptic proteins to new contacts. Finally, the role of glial cells in regulating synapse formation has been an area of recent intense research (Allen and Barres 2005). Glial cells potently influence synapse formation and function through the secretion of thrombospondins, cholesterol, and tumor necrosis factor–alpha (TNFα). In sum, although this field is making remarkably rapid progress in identifying synaptogenic molecules, there is not yet a clear understanding of how these many molecules interact to initiate synapse formation. Moreover, little is known about the molecular mechanisms of synapse stabilization or elimination in the CNS—processes that are critical for learning and memory and that are likely to give rise to cellular deficits in neurodegenerative disorders.

Neuronal Maturation and Survival

Maturation of the postsynaptic cell requires de novo protein synthesis, as do learning-dependent, long-term changes in the adult CNS. Immediate-early response genes (IEGs) (Morgan and Curran 1989, 1995) are among the first genes activated by postsynaptic depolarization, stimulated by elevations in Ca^{2+}, cAMP, cGMP, inositol 1,4,5-triphosphate (IP_3), or diacylglycerol (DAG) (see Figure 4–10). The prototype of this family of proto-oncogenes is *c-fos*. Transcription of IEGs leads to the synthesis of proteins that modulate or induce transcription of other genes that induce structural changes in the cell. For instance, nerve growth factor (NGF) synthesis may be controlled by *c-fos* transcription; lesions of the sciatic nerve lead to a rapid increase in levels of fos, which binds to the transcription initiation site for NGF and causes NGF production (Hengerer et al. 1990). Long-term sensitization in *Aplysia* (Barzilai et al. 1989), hippocampal LTP (Cole et al. 1989; Wisden et al. 1990), and structural plasticity of dendrites and dendritic spines are also associated with the specific activation of other IEGs such as Arc and CREB (Lyford et al. 1995; Steward and Worley 2002). Current models for synaptic plasticity propose that local activation of IEGs by correlated activity at individual synapses may lead to local protein synthesis specifically at those strengthened synapses. This local protein synthesis has been proposed to play a role in synaptic plasticity and memory consolidation (Steward and Worley 2002).

Interactions between presynaptic and postsynaptic neurons can act to enhance and modulate their differentiation. For example, secretion of trophic factors by postsynaptic cells can determine whether innervating presynaptic neurons survive or undergo apoptosis. More subtle regulation of presynaptic cell differentiation occurs as well. In the developing sympathetic nervous system, young neurons are exclusively noradrenergic before synapse formation. Depending on the target tissue, they may be induced to become cholinergic, retaining only traces of the noradrenergic phenotype (Landis 1990). This target-dependent effect is mediated by the release of a soluble cholinergic-differentiation factor by the postsynaptic cells. Once synaptic contact is established, cholinergic activation of the postsynaptic cell by presynaptic spikes suppresses the release of cholinergic differentiation factor. Thus, synapse formation may trigger far-reaching changes, both pre- and postsynaptically, extending to the choice of neurotransmitter by a presynaptic neuron.

In many areas of the vertebrate nervous system, neurons are initially produced in excess. To survive, neurons must receive an adequate supply of one or more trophic factors produced by their target neurons. Competition for limited supplies of these factors ensures that surviving neurons will be correctly connected and that the number of neurons will be matched to the size of the target. In general, cells deprived of neurotrophic factors undergo apoptosis, a genetically programmed form of cell death characterized by cytoplasmic shrinkage, chromatin condensation, and degradation of DNA into oligonucleosomal fragments (Edwards et al. 1991). Unlike necrosis, this process does not stimulate an inflammatory response. Apoptosis is an active process that requires RNA and protein synthesis (Oppenheim et al. 1991; Scott and Davies 1990). Data are accumulating to support the remarkable hypothesis that apoptosis is the default program for most cells and that widespread cell suicide is prevented only by the continual presence of survival signals that suppress the intrinsic cell death program (Raff et al. 1993). The best-studied neuronal example is the dependence of sympathetic and sensory neurons on NGF, which is produced by the target tissue. Although approximately half of the sympathetic neurons normally undergo apoptosis, exogenously applied NGF prevents most of the cells from dying; in contrast, neutralizing antibodies to NGF produce widespread sympathetic cell death (Raff et al. 1993).

Several families of growth factors and their receptors have been identified, including the neurotrophins that bind to members of the Trk family of receptor tyrosine kinases (Figure 4–18). These include NGF, BDNF, and neurotrophins 3, 4/5, and 6. Another family includes ciliary neurotrophic factor, growth-promoting activity, and leukemia inhibitory factor. Addi-

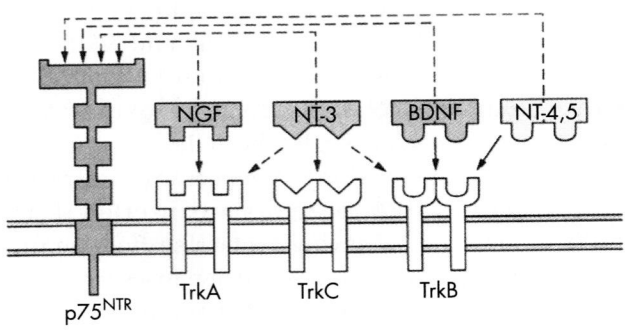

FIGURE 4–18.   Neurotrophins and their receptors.

Neurotrophins exert their effects through binding to two types of receptors: the low-affinity nerve growth factor receptor (also called p75) and the high-affinity tyrosine kinase receptors (the Trk receptors). Nerve growth factor (NGF) binds primarily to TrkA, and brain-derived neurotrophic factor (BDNF) and neurotrophin 4/5 (NT-4,5) bind primarily to TrkB. The specificity of neurotrophin 3 (NT-3) is less precise; although it mostly binds to TrkC, it can also bind to TrkA and TrkB under some cellular contexts. In addition, all of the neurotrophins bind to p75.

Source.   Adapted from Jessell TM, Sanes JR: "The Generation and Survival of Nerve Cells," in *Principles of Neural Science*, 4th Edition. Edited by Kandel ER, Schwartz JH, Jessell TM. New York, McGraw-Hill, 2000, pp. 1041–1062. Copyright 2000, The McGraw-Hill Companies, Inc. Used with permission.

tional neurotrophic factors include basic fibroblast growth factor and glia cell line–derived neurotrophic factor. Transgenic mice with targeted null mutations in neurotrophic genes or their receptors have been produced and have abnormalities in selected populations of neurons (Davies 1994). Neuronal survival factors are not exclusively target-derived. Sources also include innervating neurons, glial cells, and circulating hormones. The ability of trophic factors to promote neuronal survival has been attributed to the phosphatidylinositide 3'-OH kinase/c-Akt kinase cascade acting through at least two components of the intracellular cell death pathway, Bad and caspase-9, and the transcription factor NF-κB (Datta et al. 1999). In addition to their clear roles as survival factors, neurotrophins can also promote cell death through the activation of the p75 receptor, which competes with the Trk receptors for binding to the neurotrophins. Thus, a neuron's decision to live or die is determined by a balance between neurotrophin binding to Trk and p75 receptors (Miller and Kaplan 2001).

The cellular mechanisms of apoptosis appear to involve a complex interplay of several signaling cascades (Putcha and Johnson 2004; Sastry and Rao 2000).

In the worm *Caenorhabditis elegans, ced-3* and *ced-4* are required for apoptosis (Ellis et al. 1991). The gene product of *ced-3* is a cysteine protease and has a mammalian homologue called interleukin-1b converting enzyme (ICE). A large number of cysteine proteases have recently been discovered in many species that play diverse roles in cell death; these proteins are classified as members of the large caspase (for cysteine-requiring aspartate protease) family of proteins. Some of the caspases are considered the final effector proteins in the cell death cascade. In contrast to the cell death genes *ced-3* and *ced-4, ced-9* acts to prevent apoptosis in normally surviving *C. elegans* cells. A mutation in *ced-9* leads to widespread apoptosis and death of the embryo (Hengartner et al. 1992). The *ced-9* gene found in worms is homologous to the human oncogene *Bcl-2,* which is overexpressed in human B cell lymphomas (Tsujimoto et al. 1984). The human gene can block cell death in several in vivo and in vitro systems and has been transferred to *C. elegans,* where, remarkably, it can substitute for *ced-9* and prevent apoptosis of *C. elegans* cells. These studies have led to the current "central dogma" of apoptosis: a protein called Egl-1 is induced in cells destined to undergo apoptosis; Egl-1 interacts with Ced-9, displacing the adapter Ced-4, which then activates Ced-3 and causes cell death (Putcha and Johnson 2004). In recent years, results suggest that there may be several apoptotic pathways that depend on cell type and the inducing agent; however, most of these pathways appear to converge at the ICE/caspase step. Although some of the more specific steps in the cell death pathway remain unclear, the basic molecular mechanisms of apoptosis show a remarkable conservation across evolution.

The molecular events that underlie apoptosis in neuronal and nonneuronal cells are likely to include an array of initiators, mediators, and inhibitors, but several common features are emerging. There is evidence that reactive oxygen species can trigger apoptosis in neurons (Greenlund et al. 1995), and *Bcl-2* may prevent apoptosis by suppressing free-radical production (Hockenbery et al. 1990; Kane et al. 1993). This hypothesis has led to attempts to use antioxidants and inhibitors of free-radical production as therapeutic agents in several neurodegenerative diseases, trauma, and stroke. For example, superoxide dismutase (a free-radical scavenger) protects neurons from ischemic injury. Transgenic mice that overexpress superoxide dismutase have smaller infarcts after arterial occlusion (Kinouchi et al. 1991). Mutations in the Cu/Zn superoxide dismutase gene are associated with certain forms of familial amyotrophic lateral sclerosis, sug-

gesting that oxygen radicals may be responsible for motor neuron degeneration in patients with this disease (Rosen et al. 1993).

Experience-Dependent Synaptic Refinement

Normal sensory experience is essential to the maturation of neural connections in both the peripheral and central nervous systems. Sensory experience shapes the development of many diverse brain regions during a specific time window during development called the *critical period.* The process of synaptic refinement assumes clinical significance as it continues to be important throughout the life span, providing mechanisms for activity-dependent modification of neuronal structure and connectivity that may be the basis for learning, memory, and forgetting. The integral role of sensory activity in brain development and the ability of experience to alter perception have been most extensively documented in the visual system. In the visual system, overlapping visual input from the two eyes must be combined in an orderly way to maximize acuity and stereopsis (Figure 4–19). In animals with binocular vision, such as humans, cats, and monkeys, visual stimuli from a specific region of visual space activate neurons in the contralateral visual cortex. Neurons in the left hemi-retinas of right and left eyes both convey signals to the left cortex, and similarly, neurons in the right hemi-retinas convey signals to the right cortex (Figure 4–19A). Thus, visual information emanating from the same external source is temporally separated into right eye– and left eye–specific pathways and then reunited in the same cortical hemisphere.

How is this visual information recombined? The eye-specific segregation of inputs from each retina is maintained in the visual thalamus, or lateral geniculate nucleus (LGN), and in the projection layers of the visual cortex, but then eventually converges in other layers of the primary visual cortex (V1). In geniculate-recipient layers of V1 in the adult, inputs from the two eyes project to separate columns of cells. The ocular dominance columns (OD columns) thus formed are arranged adjacent to each other in alternate stripes dominated by one eye or the other (Figure 4–19) (Hubel and Wiesel 1977). The pattern of stripes formed on the surface of the cortex resembles those of a zebra (Figure 4–19B, D). Output neurons in the OD columns project to other cortical layers, where the visual information derived from inputs to both eyes is recombined and stereopsis clues are extracted. How separate signals from each eye are handled in parallel, recombined,

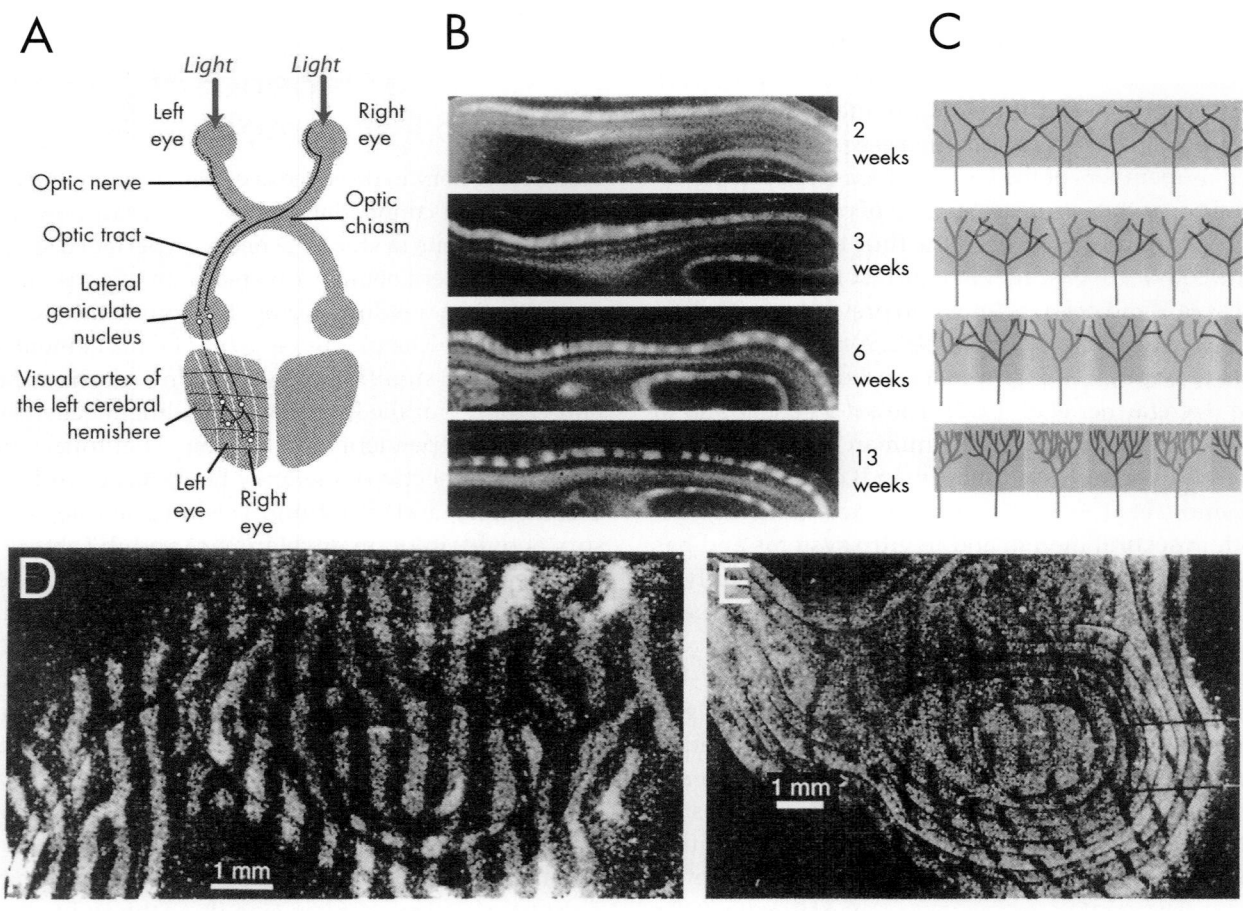

FIGURE 4–19.   Ocular dominance columns in visual cortex.

Panel A.   In the human visual pathway, optic fibers from each eye split at the optic chiasm, half going to each side of the brain. In this schematic drawing, fibers conveying visual information from the left sides of each retina are shown projecting to the left lateral geniculate nucleus (LGN). LGN neurons (in different layers) in turn project to ipsilateral visual cortex (principally to layer 4c). In the geniculate-recipient layers of the mature visual cortex, inputs from the eyes segregate into ocular dominance (OD) columns. *Panel B.*   Radioactive proline injections into one eye of a 2-week-old kitten uniformly label layer 4 in coronal sections of visual cortex, indicating that afferents from that eye are evenly distributed in cortex at this age. However, over the next few weeks, similar injections show a segregation of geniculate afferents into OD columns. *Panel C.*   Schematic diagram of the formation of OD columns within layer 4 of cortex during normal development. *Panel D.*   One eye of a normal monkey was injected with a radioactive tracer that was transported transsynaptically along the visual pathways. Cortical areas receiving inputs from the injected eye are labeled white, revealing an alternating pattern of evenly spaced stripes (section cut tangentially through layer 4c). *Panel E.*   Monocular deprivation alters the development of OD columns. Here the tracer was injected into the nondeprived eye, revealing broader stripes and thus an expansion of the area innervated by the nondeprived eye. Thus, normal experience is a prerequisite to the correct wiring of the cortex.

Source.   Panel A reprinted from Kandel ER, Jessell T: "Early Experience and the Fine Tuning of Synaptic Connections," in *Principles of Neural Science.* Edited by Kandel ER, Schwartz JHS, Jessell TM. Stamford, CT, Appleton & Lange, 1991, pp. 945–958. Copyright 1991, The McGraw-Hill Companies, Inc. Used with permission.
Panel B adapted from LeVay S, Stryker MP, Shatz CJ: "Ocular Dominance Columns and Their Development in Layer IV of the Cat's Visual Cortex: A Quantitative Study." *Journal of Comparative Neurology* 179:223–244, 1978. Used with permission.
Panel C reprinted from Purves D, Augustine GJ, Fitzpatrick D, et al. (eds): *Neuroscience.* Sunderland, MA, Sinauer Associates, 1997, p. 427. Used with permission.
Panels D and E reprinted from Hubel DH, Wiesel TN, LeVay S: "Plasticity of Ocular Dominance Columns in Monkey Striate Cortex." *Philosophical Transactions of the Royal Society of London—Series B: Biological Sciences* 278:377–409, 1977. Used with permission.

and separated again is representative of a more general pattern in the processing of visual information (Livingstone and Hubel 1988).

Although there are some conflicting reports (Crowley and Katz 2002), most evidence suggests that during development, OD columns arise through activity-dependent processes (Hubel and Wiesel 1977). Initially, geniculate axons carrying information from both eyes overlap. However, as development proceeds, these axons slowly begin to segregate into OD columns (Figure 4–19B, C). During this period, the pattern of distinct stripes, evenly divided between the two eyes, depends on normal visual activity. If vision in one eye is impaired or there is strabismus, input from the normal or dominant eye comes to control most of the visual cortex, and the other eye becomes functionally blind (Figure 4–19E). In the cortex, the OD columns of the normal or dominant eye expand at the expense of those of the impaired eye. The columnar segregation of inputs carrying information from each eye is activity dependent (Constantine-Paton et al. 1990; Shatz and Stryker 1988). It depends on discordant inputs from the two retinas; segregation fails if all visual input to the cortex is blocked (with tetrodotoxin) or artificially synchronized in both eyes (by simultaneous electrical stimulation) (Shatz 1990).

Different patterns of electrical activity from each eye, as occur normally, mediate OD segregation. But segregation also requires the activity of postsynaptic cortical cells; infusion of the inhibitory drug muscimol (a $GABA_A$ agonist) causes a reversal of ocular dominance so that, paradoxically, the weak rather than the strong eye gains the larger cortical influence (Reiter and Stryker 1988). Thus, appropriate segregation of cortical inputs requires the coordination of both normal presynaptic activity and postsynaptic responses. Similar activity dependence is also found in retinal axons impinging on LGN cells (Goodman and Shatz 1993). Indeed, activity-dependent segregation of sensory inputs into functional columns appears to be an inherent property of topographical projections in sensory systems. In frogs, which have neither binocular vision nor OD columns, when an extra eye is transplanted into a tadpole, the optic fibers from the third eye compete with the other eye innervating that side of the brain, producing OD columns (Constantine-Paton and Law 1978).

The cellular and molecular mechanisms underlying activity-dependent synaptic refinement are just beginning to be elucidated. Many of these mechanisms are remarkably similar to the cellular mechanisms that underlie learning and memory in the adult brain. In the visual system, geniculate afferents are believed to undergo segregation into OD columns based on a Hebbian learning rule (Hebb 1949), whereby neurons that fire together are selectively strengthened. This rule predicts that neurons that fire synchronously will strengthen their synapses, whereas asynchronous firing will weaken synapses. LTP and LTD are attractive candidates for mediating the process of OD column formation (Bear and Rittenhouse 1999). In addition to activity, other factors may also act to selectively strengthen coincidentally active synapses. One of the most attractive candidates for such a role is the neurotrophin family of growth factors. The neurotrophins are produced in limiting amounts by cortical neurons, their expression is increased by activity, and they can increase synaptic strength as well as alter dendritic and axonal arborizations of cortical neurons (Huberman and McAllister 2002). Consistent with this hypothesis, either infusion of excess neurotrophins or blockade of the neurotrophins prevents the formation of OD columns (Cabelli et al. 1995, 1997). Thus, the neurotrophins are in a prime position to mediate experience-dependent synaptic refinement during development. Finally, in recent years, a critical role for inhibitory neurons in mediating activity-dependent changes in circuitry has been revealed. Experience-dependent plasticity is deficient in transgenic mice that have decreased GABAergic transmission (Hensch and Fagiolini 2005), and the end of the critical period for activity-dependent plasticity correlates strongly with the development of inhibitory synaptic transmission in multiple systems (Berardi et al. 2003).

Neurotrophic and Neurotoxic Actions of Neurotransmitters

Neurotransmitters themselves may have trophic or toxic roles in the shaping of neurons and their interconnections (Lipton and Kater 1989). Excitatory neurotransmitters such as glutamate trigger Ca^{2+} influx that controls the progress of growth cones. Local intracellular levels of Ca^{2+} act within a narrow window. When levels are low, growth cones are quiescent; when levels rise, growth cones begin to move. Above a certain level, however, further elevations of Ca^{2+} arrest growth and cause retraction or destruction of neuronal processes (al-Mohanna et al. 1992). This can be countered by inhibitory neurotransmitters as well as by provision of neurotrophic factors (Kater et al. 1989; Mattson and Kater 1989).

Higher levels of glutamate produce excitotoxicity, perhaps reflecting the pathological functioning of these developmental signaling systems (Kater et al. 1989). Alternatively, excitotoxicity may have a normal function in regulating cell numbers and connectivity. Excitotoxicity appears to be mediated acutely by the entry of Na^+ through AMPA channels. This leads to neuronal swelling (resulting in brain edema). Sustained Ca^{2+} entry through NMDA receptor channels causes a delayed mode of excitotoxicity that kills neurons, probably by activation of intracellular proteases and/or generation of free radicals, including NO (Arundine and Tymianski 2003; Choi 1994; Dawson et al. 1994). In addition to mediating Na^+ influx and swelling, AMPA receptors may be coupled to the IP_3/DAG pathway, leading also to increases in intracellular Ca^{2+} and C kinase activation.

Excitotoxicity figures prominently in neuronal loss in strokes, status epilepticus, hypoglycemia, and head trauma (Choi and Rothman 1990). These brain insults are linked in that all lead to neuronal depolarization, which results in excessive electrical activity, evoking excessive increases in glutamate release. In each case, elevated levels of extracellular glutamate are present in experimental models, and their cytopathology can be mimicked by intracerebral injections of excitatory amino acids. The same neurons spared in these disease states are also less affected in the experimental models, probably because they have fewer excitatory amino acid receptors. Injured neurons show increased intracellular levels of Ca^{2+}, and excitatory amino acid antagonists, particularly those blocking NMDA receptors or channels, prevent or dramatically reduce neuronal loss in these conditions.

Similarities between other neuropsychiatric disorders and idiopathic neurodegenerative disorders suggest a pervasive role for excitotoxic mechanisms (Arundine and Tymianski 2003). Intriguingly, a growing body of findings implicates excitotoxic mechanisms in the pathology of Huntington's disease. The neuropathology of Huntington's disease is mimicked by the injection of excitatory amino acids, and the same classes of striatal neurons are spared in both cases (Wexler et al. 1991).

Perspectives

Brain development is not determined merely by cell-autonomous genetic programs but is instead highly interactive, depending on complex hierarchies of signaling factors operating that progressively restrict cell fate. Once cells have achieved a specific phenotype and have arrived at an appropriate location, competition for survival factors provides another opportunity for environmental influence over developmental out-

come. The cellular development of the brain is therefore not strictly lineage dependent but rather involves a remarkable degree of interactive signaling. In many brain areas, pruning of exuberant synaptic contacts on an activity-dependent basis is yet another example of a mechanism by which experience can refine structural aspects of brain development. One consequence of these developmental mechanisms is that no two outcomes will be exactly the same, even in a case of twins with identical genetic makeup. Another consequence is the potential for pathological disruption of normal development by physical, chemical, or infectious agents in the fetal or neonatal period.

It is becoming increasingly clear that the adult brain retains a significant degree of plasticity throughout life and that changes in cortical organization can be induced by behaviorally important, temporally coincident sensory inputs (Buonomano and Merzenich 1998). Behavioral training of adult owl monkeys in discrimination of the temporal features of a tactile stimulus can alter the spatial and temporal response properties of cortical neurons. When adult owl monkeys are rewarded for responding to a 30-Hz tactile stimulation of one finger, there is a progressive increase in the area of somatosensory cortex over which neurons respond to the 30-Hz stimulation.

The kinds of changes that take place in the organization of somatosensory cortex also occur in primary auditory cortex. Owl monkeys trained for several weeks to discriminate small differences in the frequency of sequentially presented tones demonstrate progressive improvement in performance with training. At the end of the training period, the amount of cortex responding to behaviorally relevant frequencies is increased. In control studies with equivalent stimulation procedures in which stimuli are unattended, no significant representational changes are recorded. Thus, attended, rewarded behaviors can induce changes in the organization of primary sensory cortex that are correlated with an improvement in perceptual acuity. These experiments begin to suggest ways in which life experiences, including psychotherapy (Etkin et al. 2005), can potentially modify cortical function and alter perception or behavior.

These plastic changes appear to share a common molecular language, first expressed during development involving activity-dependent mechanisms. Neural activity is essential to activity-dependent synaptic refinement, LTP, LTD, and excitotoxicity (Bailey et al. 2000; Brown et al. 1990; Choi and Rothman 1990; Constantine-Paton et al. 1990; Lipton and Kater 1989). The key player is the NMDA receptor, which requires both agonist binding and depolarization for activation. This appears to be the essential requirement for pairing specificity, a mode of synaptic plasticity initially postulated by Hebb (1949), whereby simultaneous activation of presynaptic and postsynaptic elements strengthens connections. In contrast, correlation of presynaptic activity with postsynaptic inhibition may selectively weaken connections (Reiter and Stryker 1988). The Ca^{2+} influx mediated by the NMDA receptor may trigger changes in the strength of synapses, in time leading to more permanent structural changes in synapse number. At higher levels, Ca^{2+} may arrest the growth of neurites, cause their retraction, or selectively lesion the susceptible cell.

Many neuropsychiatric disorders no doubt play out in this context. To consider a few examples, most of which have been mentioned already, striatal degeneration in Huntington's disease appears to be due to the overproduction of huntingtin, a synaptic vesicle–associated protein (DiFiglia et al. 1995) that among a multiplicity of actions may trigger NMDA receptor–mediated excitotoxicity (Rego and de Almeida 2005). In Parkinson's disease, a selective loss of dopaminergic neurons in the substantia nigra may be the delayed result of a viral process, lesioning by dopaminergic neurotoxins exemplified by MPTP, or a deficiency in BDNF or glia cell line–derived neurotrophic factor, both of which may be essential for the survival of dopaminergic neurons (Cardoso et al. 2005). In Alzheimer's disease, the loss of cholinergic neurons may result from a deficiency or perhaps aberrant handling of NGF once it is taken up by neurons in the basal forebrain (Pereira et al. 2005). Clearly, elucidation of the cellular and molecular events that occur during normal brain development, maturation, and aging, as well as those that underlie neuropsychiatric disorders, will greatly enhance approaches to their treatment and prevention (Cummings 2003).

Perhaps the most exciting and revolutionary possible intervention to treat neuropsychiatric diseases is the potential use of stem cells to repair the damaged brain (Lee et al. 2000). Despite tremendous efforts by the neuroscience community during the last century, there are currently no feasible therapies for repairing the damaged adult human brain. Clearly, treatment of many neuropsychiatric diseases would be greatly enhanced if new neurons could be added to a particular damaged brain region and stimulated to differentiate into the appropriate neuronal type and to form appropriate connections. There are currently two approaches to achieving this goal. First, pluripotent stem cells are being used, with increasing success, to repopulate damaged brain regions. For example, adult rats with symptoms similar to Parkinson's disease can regain function after implantation of dopaminergic neurons created in vitro from fetal rat neuronal precursors (Studer et al. 1998). Second, newly discovered intrinsic repair mechanisms in the adult brain are being studied for their therapeutic potential. Neurogenesis has been discovered in several regions of the adult brain, including the dentate gyrus of the hippocampal formation (Fuchs and Gould 2000). These neurons migrate within the brain regions, differentiate, and form functional connections. Moreover, experience, learning, and physical exercise enhance neuronal proliferation in the adult (Fuchs and Gould 2000; Kempermann et al. 2004). The discovery of neurogenesis in the adult brain suggests that the adult brain may have intrinsic mechanisms for repair that could be manipulated to treat neurodegenerative disorders (Kozorovitskiy and Gould 2003; Lie et al. 2004).

As the mechanisms of neuropsychiatric disorders are resolved at the cellular and molecular levels and the tremendous potential of stem cell research is harnessed, it is likely that revolutionary treatments for many neuropsychiatric diseases will be forthcoming.

Key Points

- Neuropsychiatric disorders result from disordered functioning of neurons and in particular their synapses.

- Neurons receive synaptic input from thousands of other neurons and in turn transmit information to thousands of other neurons.

- Learning and memory involve both short- and long-term synaptic changes, characteristically induced by high-frequency activation.

- Neurotransmitter receptors couple to second messenger systems that profoundly increase the range of responses a neuron shows to synaptic input, extending to changes in gene transcription.

- During development, neurons and glia are generated in proliferative zones lining the ventricular system and then migrate into the overlying cortical mantle.

- The determination of cell fate occurs at regional, local, and cellular levels.

- Neurotransmitters themselves may have trophic or toxic roles in the shaping of neurons and their interconnections.

- Neurons are initially produced in excess; their survival depends on trophic factors produced by their targets.

- Normal sensory experience is essential to the maturation of neural connections.

- Behaviorally relevant, temporally coincident sensory input induces changes in cortical synaptic connectivity.

- In both development and learning, the NMDA receptor is the coincidence detector, requiring both neurotransmitter binding and depolarization for activation.

- NMDA receptors mediate the influx of Ca^{2+} and trigger changes in synaptic strength and numbers.

- Ca^{2+} regulates the growth or retraction of neurites and programmed cell death.

- Adult neurogenesis may provide intrinsic mechanisms that could be harnessed for the treatment of neurodegenerative disorders.

Suggested Readings

Charney DS, Nestler EJ, Bunney BS (eds): Neurobiology of Mental Illness, 2nd Edition. New York, Oxford University Press, 2004

Cummings JL: Toward a molecular neuropsychiatry of neurodegenerative diseases. Ann Neurol 54:147–154, 2003

Graham DI, Lantos PL (eds): Greenfield's Neuropathology, 7th Edition. London, Arnold, 2002

Kandel ER, Schwartz JH, Jessel TM (eds): Principles of Neural Science, 5th Edition. In press, 2007

Purves D, Augustine GJ, Fitzpatrick D, et al. (eds): Neuroscience, 3rd Edition. Sunderland, MA, Sinauer Associates, 2004

Siegel GJ, Albers RW, Brady S, et al. (eds): Basic Neurochemistry: Molecular, Cellular and Medical Aspects, 7th Edition. New York, Elsevier, 2006

Waxman SG: From Neuroscience to Neurology: Neuroscience, Molecular Medicine, and the Therapeutic Transformation of Neurology. Boston, MA, Elsevier Academic Press, 2005

References

Allen NJ, Barres BA: Signaling between glia and neurons: focus on synaptic plasticity. Curr Opin Neurobiol 15:542–548, 2005

al-Mohanna FA, Cave J, Bolsover SR: A narrow window of intracellular calcium concentration is optimal for neurite outgrowth in rat sensory neurones. Brain Res Dev Brain Res 70:287–290, 1992

Alvarez-Buylla A, Kirn JR, Nottebohm F: Birth of projection neurons in adult avian brain may be related to perceptual or motor learning. Science 249:1444–1446, 1990

Anderson SA, Eisenstat DD, Shi L, et al: Interneuron migration from basal forebrain to neocortex: dependence on Dlx genes. Science 278:474–476, 1997

Ansorge MS, Zhou M, Lira A, et al: Early life blockade of the 5-HT transporter alters emotional behavior in adult mice. Science 306:879–881, 2004

Anthony TE, Klein C, Fishell G, et al: Radial glia serve as neuronal progenitors in all regions of the central nervous system. Neuron 41:881–890, 2004

Anwyl R: Induction and expression mechanisms of postsynaptic NMDA receptor-independent homosynaptic long-term depression. Prog Neurobiol 78:17–37, 2006

Araque A, Parpura V, Sanzgiri RP, et al: Tripartite synapses: glia, the unacknowledged partner. Trends Neurosci 22:208–215, 1999

Arundine M, Tymianski M: Molecular mechanisms of calcium-dependent neurodegeneration in excitotoxicity. Cell Calcium 34:325–337, 2003

Bailey C, Kandel E: Synaptic growth and the persistence of long-term memory: a molecular perspective, in The Cognitive Neurosciences, 3rd Edition. Edited by Gazzaniga MS. Cambridge, MA, MIT Press, 2004, pp 647–663

Bailey CH, Giustetto M, Huang YY, et al: Is heterosynaptic modulation essential for stabilizing Hebbian plasticity and memory? Nat Rev Neurosci 1:11–20, 2000

Barzilai A, Kennedy TE, Sweatt JD, et al: 5-HT modulates protein synthesis and the expression of specific proteins during long-term facilitation in *Aplysia* sensory neurons. Neuron 2:1577–1586, 1989

Bayer SA, Altman J: Neocortical Development. New York, Raven, 1991

Bear MF, Rittenhouse CD: Molecular basis for induction of ocular dominance plasticity. J Neurobiol 41:83–91, 1999

Behrendt RP, Young C: Hallucinations in schizophrenia, sensory impairment, and brain disease: a unifying model. Behav Brain Sci 27:771–830, 2004

Bennett MVL: Electrical transmission: a functional analysis and comparison to chemical transmission, in Handbook of Physiology, Vol I: The Nervous System. Bethesda, MD, American Physiological Society, 1977, pp 357–416

Bennett MVL, Barrio LC, Bargiello TA, et al: Gap junctions: new tools, new answers, new questions. Neuron 6:305–320, 1991

Berardi N, Pizzorusso T, Ratto GM, et al: Molecular basis of plasticity in the visual cortex. Trends Neurosci 26:369–378, 2003

Black IB: Trophic interactions and brain plasticity, in The Cognitive Neurosciences. Edited by Gazzaniga MS. Cambridge, MA, MIT Press, 1995, pp 9–17

Blier P, Abbott FV: Putative mechanisms of action of antidepressant drugs in affective and anxiety disorders and pain. J Psychiatry Neurosci 26:37–43, 2001

Bliss TV, Lomo T: Long-lasting potentiation of synaptic transmission in the dentate area of the anaesthetized rabbit following stimulation of the perforant path. J Physiol 232:331–356, 1973

Blitzer RD, Connor JH, Brown GP, et al: Gating of CaMKII by cAMP-regulated protein phosphatase activity during LTP. Science 280:1940–1942, 1998

Blitzer RD, Iyengar R, Landau EM: Postsynaptic signaling networks: cellular cogwheels underlying long-term plasticity. Biol Psychiatry 57:113–119, 2005

Bohn LM, Lefkowitz RJ, Gainetdinov RR, et al: Enhanced morphine analgesia in mice lacking beta-arrestin 2. Science 286:2495–2498, 1999

Bolshakov VY, Golan H, Kandel ER, et al: Recruitment of new sites of synaptic transmission during the cAMP-dependent late phase of LTP at CA3-CA1 synapses in the hippocampus. Neuron 19:635–651, 1997

Boulder Committee: Embryonic vertebrate central nervous system: revised terminology. Anatomical Record 166:257–261, 1970

Brenman JE, Bredt DS: Synaptic signaling by nitric oxide. Curr Opin Neurobiol 7:374–378, 1997

Brittis PA, Lu Q, Flanagan JG: Axonal protein synthesis provides a mechanism for localized regulation at an intermediate target. Cell 110:223–235, 2002

Brivanlou IH, Warland DK, Meister M: Mechanisms of concerted firing among retinal ganglion cells. Neuron 20:527–539, 1998

Brown TH, Kairiss EW, Keenan CL: Hebbian synapses: biophysical mechanisms and algorithms. Annu Rev Neurosci 13:475–511, 1990

Buonomano DV, Merzenich MM: Cortical plasticity: from synapses to maps. Annu Rev Neurosci 21:149–186, 1998

Burack MA, Silverman MA, Banker G: The role of selective transport in neuronal protein sorting. Neuron 26:465–472, 2000

Cabelli RJ, Hohn A, Shatz CJ: Inhibition of ocular dominance column formation by infusion of NT-4/5 or BDNF. Science 267:1662–1666, 1995

Cabelli RJ, Shelton DL, Segal RA, et al: Blockade of endogenous ligands of trkB inhibits formation of ocular dominance columns. Neuron 19:63–76, 1997

Cardoso SM, Moreira PI, Agostinho P, et al: Neurodegenerative pathways in Parkinson's disease: therapeutic strategies. Curr Drug Targets CNS Neurol Disord 4:405–419, 2005

Caspi A, Sugden K, Moffitt TE, et al: Influence of life stress on depression: moderation by a polymorphism in the 5-HTT gene. Science 301:386–389, 2003

Charney DS, Nestler EJ, Bunney BS (eds): Neurobiology of Mental Illness, 2nd Edition. New York, Oxford University Press, 2004

Chenn A, Walsh CA: Regulation of cerebral cortical size by control of cell cycle exit in neural precursors. Science 297:365–369, 2002

Chih B, Afridi SK, Clark L, et al: Disorder-associated mutations lead to functional inactivation of neuroligins. Hum Mol Genet 13:1471–1477, 2004

Choi DW: Calcium and excitotoxic neuronal injury. Ann N Y Acad Sci 747:162–171, 1994

Choi DW, Rothman SM: The role of glutamate neurotoxicity in hypoxic-ischemic neuronal death. Annu Rev Neurosci 13:171–182, 1990

Cole AJ, Saffen DW, Baraban JM, et al: Rapid increase of an immediate early gene messenger RNA in hippocampal neurons by synaptic NMDA receptor activation. Nature 340:474–476, 1989

Constantine-Paton M, Law MI: Eye-specific termination bands in tecta of three-eyed frogs. Science 202:639–641, 1978

Constantine-Paton M, Cline HT, Debski E: Patterned activity, synaptic convergence, and the NMDA receptor in developing visual pathways. Annu Rev Neurosci 13:129–154, 1990

Coyle JT: The neurochemistry of schizophrenia, in Basic Neurochemistry: Molecular, Cellular and Medical Aspects, 7th Edition. Edited by Siegel GJ, Albers RW, Brady S, et al. Burlington, MA, Elsevier Academic, 2006, pp 875–885

Crowley JC, Katz LC: Ocular dominance development revisited. Curr Opin Neurobiol 12:104–109, 2002

Cummings JL: Toward a molecular neuropsychiatry of neurodegenerative diseases. Ann Neurol 54:147–154, 2003

Dani JW, Chernjavsky A, Smith SJ: Neuronal activity triggers calcium waves in hippocampal astrocyte networks. Neuron 8:429–440, 1992

Datta SR, Brunet A, Greenberg ME: Cellular survival: a play in three Akts. Genes Dev 13:2905–2927, 1999

Davies AM: The role of neurotrophins in the developing nervous system. J Neurobiol 25:1334–1348, 1994

Dawson TM, Zhang J, Dawson VL, et al: Nitric oxide: cellular regulation and neuronal injury. Prog Brain Res 103:365–369, 1994

Dealy CN, Beyer EC, Kosher RA: Expression patterns of mRNAs for the gap junction proteins connexin43 and connexin42 suggest their involvement in chick limb morphogenesis and specification of the arterial vasculature. Dev Dyn 199:156–167, 1994

des Portes V, Pinard JM, Billuart P, et al: A novel CNS gene required for neuronal migration and involved in X-linked subcortical laminar heterotopia and lissencephaly syndrome. Cell 92:51–61, 1998

DiFiglia M, Sapp E, Chase K, et al: Huntingtin is a cytoplasmic protein associated with vesicles in human and rat brain neurons. Neuron 14:1075–1081, 1995

Dillon C, Goda Y: The actin cytoskeleton: integrating form and function at the synapse. Annu Rev Neurosci 28:25–55, 2005

Doetsch F, Caille I, Lim DA, et al: Subventricular zone astrocytes are neural stem cells in the adult mammalian brain. Cell 97:703–716, 1999

Dumartin B, Caille I, Gonon F, et al: Internalization of D1 dopamine receptor in striatal neurons in vivo as evidence of activation by dopamine agonists. J Neurosci 18:1650–1661, 1998

During MJ, Ryder KM, Spencer DD: Hippocampal GABA transporter function in temporal-lobe epilepsy. Nature 376:174–177, 1995

Edwards SN, Buckmaster AE, Tolkovsky AM: The death programme in cultured sympathetic neurones can be suppressed at the posttranslational level by nerve growth factor, cyclic AMP, and depolarization. J Neurochem 57:2140–2143, 1991

Eilers J, Konnerth A: Dendritic signal integration. Curr Opin Neurobiol 7:385–390, 1997

Ellis RE, Yuan JY, Horvitz HR: Mechanisms and functions of cell death. Annu Rev Cell Biol 7:663–698, 1991

Etkin A, Pittenger C, Polan HJ, et al: Toward a neurobiology of psychotherapy: basic science and clinical applications. J Neuropsychiatry Clin Neurosci 17:145–158, 2005

Fellin T, Carmignoto G: Neurone-to-astrocyte signalling in the brain represents a distinct multifunctional unit. J Physiol 559:3–15, 2004

Feng Y, Walsh CA: Protein-protein interactions, cytoskeletal regulation and neuronal migration. Nat Rev Neurosci 2:408–416, 2001

Fuchs E, Gould E: Mini-review: in vivo neurogenesis in the adult brain: regulation and functional implications. Eur J Neurosci 12:2211–2214, 2000

Gainetdinov RR, Caron MG: Monoamine transporters: from genes to behavior. Annu Rev Pharmacol Toxicol 43:261–284, 2003

Gainetdinov RR, Mohn AR, Caron MG: Genetic animal models: focus on schizophrenia. Trends Neurosci 24:527–533, 2001

Ghosh A, Greenberg ME: Calcium signaling in neurons: molecular mechanisms and cellular consequences. Science 268:239–247, 1995

Girault JA, Greengard P: Principles of signal transduction, in Neurobiology of Mental Illness, 2nd Edition. Edited by Charney DS, Nestler EJ, Bunney BS. New York, Oxford University Press, 2004, pp 41–65

Giros B, Jaber M, Jones SR, et al: Hyperlocomotion and indifference to cocaine and amphetamine in mice lacking the dopamine transporter. Nature 379:606–612, 1996

Gleeson JG, Allen KM, Fox JW, et al: Doublecortin, a brain-specific gene mutated in human X-linked lissencephaly and double cortex syndrome, encodes a putative signaling protein. Cell 92:63–72, 1998

Goldman-Rakic PS, Muly EC 3rd, Williams GV: D(1) receptors in prefrontal cells and circuits. Brain Res Brain Res Rev 31:295–301, 2000

Goodman CS, Shatz CJ: Developmental mechanisms that generate precise patterns of neuronal connectivity. Cell 72 (suppl):77–98, 1993

Gotz M, Huttner WB: The cell biology of neurogenesis. Nat Rev Mol Cell Biol 6:777–788, 2005

Graham D, Lantos P: Greenfield's Neuropathology, 7th Edition. London, Arnold, 2002

Greengard P: The neurobiology of slow synaptic transmission. Science 294:1024–1030, 2001

Greenlund LJ, Deckwerth TL, Johnson E Jr: Superoxide dismutase delays neuronal apoptosis: a role for reactive oxygen species in programmed neuronal death. Neuron 14:303–315, 1995

Halliday AL, Cepko CL: Generation and migration of cells in the developing striatum. Neuron 9:15–26, 1992

Hanashima C, Li SC, Shen L, et al: Foxg1 suppresses early cortical cell fate. Science 303:56–59, 2004

Hassel B, Dingledine R: Glutamate, in Basic Neurochemistry: Molecular, Cellular and Medical Aspects, 7th Edition. Edited by Siegel GJ, Albers RW, Brady S, et al. Burlington, MA, Elsevier Academic, 2006, pp 267–290

Hatten ME: Riding the glial monorail: a common mechanism for glial-guided neuronal migration in different regions of the developing mammalian brain. Trends Neurosci 13:179–184, 1990

Haubensak W, Attardo A, Denk W, et al: Neurons arise in the basal neuroepithelium of the early mammalian telencephalon: a major site of neurogenesis. Proc Natl Acad Sci U S A 101:3196–3201, 2004

Hawkins RD, Kandel ER, Bailey CH: Molecular mechanisms of memory storage in Aplysia. Biol Bull 210:174–191, 2006

Haydar TF, Wang F, Schwartz ML, et al: Differential modulation of proliferation in the neocortical ventricular and subventricular zones. J Neurosci 20:5764–5774, 2000

Hebb DO: The Organization of Behavior: A Neuropsychological Theory. New York, Wiley, 1949

Hengartner MO, Ellis RE, Horvitz HR: *Caenorhabditis elegans* gene ced-9 protects cells from programmed cell death. Nature 356:494–499, 1992

Hengerer B, Lindholm D, Heumann R, et al: Lesion-induced increase in nerve growth factor mRNA is mediated by c-fos. Proc Natl Acad Sci U S A 87:3899–3903, 1990

Hensch TK, Fagiolini M: Excitatory-inhibitory balance and critical period plasticity in developing visual cortex. Prog Brain Res 147:115–124, 2005

Hille B: Ion Channels of Excitable Membranes, 3rd Edition. Sunderland, MA, Sinauer Associates, 2001

Hille B, Catterall WA: Electrical excitability and ion channels, in Basic Neurochemistry: Molecular, Cellular and Medical Aspects, 7th Edition. Edited by Siegel GJ, Albers RW, Brady S, et al. Burlington, MA, Elsevier Academic, 2006, pp 95–109

Hirokawa N, Takemura R: Biochemical and molecular characterization of diseases linked to motor proteins. Trends Biochem Sci 28:558–565, 2003

Hockenbery D, Nunez G, Milliman C, et al: Bcl-2 is an inner mitochondrial membrane protein that blocks programmed cell death. Nature 348:334–336, 1990

Hökfelt T: Neuropeptides in perspective: the last ten years. Neuron 7:867–879, 1991

Huang YY, Kandel ER: D1/D5 receptor agonists induce a protein synthesis-dependent late potentiation in the CA1 region of the hippocampus. Proc Natl Acad Sci U S A 92:2446–2450, 1995

Hubel DH, Wiesel TN: Ferrier lecture: functional architecture of macaque monkey visual cortex. Proc R Soc Lond B Biol Sci 198:1–59, 1977

Hubel DH, Wiesel TN, LeVay S: Plasticity of ocular dominance columns in monkey striate cortex. Philos Trans R Soc Lond B Biol Sci 278:377–409, 1977

Huberman AD, McAllister AK: Neurotrophins and visual cortical plasticity. Prog Brain Res 138:39–51, 2002

Huerta PT, Lisman JE: Low-frequency stimulation at the troughs of theta-oscillation induces long-term depression of previously potentiated CA1 synapses. J Neurophysiol 75:877–884, 1996

Isaac JT: Postsynaptic silent synapses: evidence and mechanisms. Neuropharmacology 45:450–460, 2003

Jessell TM, Sanes JR: The generation and survival of nerve cells, in Principles of Neural Science, 4th Edition. Edited by Kandel ER, Schwartz JH, Jessell TM. New York, McGraw-Hill, 2000, pp 1041–1062

Johnston D, Christie BR, Frick A, et al: Active dendrites, potassium channels and synaptic plasticity. Philos Trans R Soc Lond B Biol Sci 358:667–674, 2003

Kamal A, Goldstein LS: Principles of cargo attachment to cytoplasmic motor proteins. Curr Opin Cell Biol 14:63–68, 2002

Kamei Y, Inagaki N, Nishizawa M, et al: Visualization of mitotic radial glial lineage cells in the developing rat brain by Cdc2 kinase-phosphorylated vimentin. Glia 23:191–199, 1998

Kandel ER: Cellular mechanisms of learning and the biological basis of individuality, in Principles of Neural Science, 4th Edition. Edited by Kandel ER, Schwartz JH, Jessell TM. New York, McGraw-Hill, 2000a, pp 1247–1279

Kandel ER: Nerve cells and behavior, in Principles of Neural Science, 4th Edition. Edited by Kandel ER, Schwartz JH, Jessell TM. New York, McGraw-Hill, 2000b, pp 19–35

Kandel ER: The molecular biology of memory storage: a dialog between genes and synapses. Biosci Rep 21:565–611, 2001a

Kandel ER: The molecular biology of memory storage: a dialogue between genes and synapses. Science 294:1030–1038, 2001b

Kandel ER, Jessell T: Early experience and the fine tuning of synaptic connections, in Principles of Neural Science. Edited by Kandel ER, Schwartz JHS, Jessell TM. Stamford, CT, Appleton & Lange, 1991, pp 945–958

Kandel ER, O'Dell TJ: Are adult learning mechanisms also used for development? Science 258:243–245, 1992

Kandel ER, Siegelbaum SA: Transmitter release, in Principles of Neural Science, 4th Edition. Edited by Kandel ER, Schwartz JH, Jessell TM. New York, McGraw-Hill, 2000, pp 253–279

Kandler K, Katz LC: Neuronal coupling and uncoupling in the developing nervous system. Curr Opin Neurobiol 5:98–105, 1995

Kane DJ, Sarafian TA, Anton R, et al: Bcl-2 inhibition of neural death: decreased generation of reactive oxygen species. Science 262:1274–1277, 1993

Karlin A, Akabas MH: Toward a structural basis for the function of nicotinic acetylcholine receptors and their cousins. Neuron 15:1231–1244, 1995

Kater SB, Mattson MP, Guthrie PB: Calcium-induced neuronal degeneration: a normal growth cone regulating signal gone awry (?). Ann N Y Acad Sci 568:252–261, 1989

Kempermann G, Wiskott L, Gage FH: Functional significance of adult neurogenesis. Curr Opin Neurobiol 14:186–191, 2004

Kennedy MJ, Ehlers MD: Organelles and trafficking machinery for postsynaptic plasticity. Annu Rev Neurosci 29:325–362, 2006

Kim E, Sheng M: PDZ domain proteins of synapses. Nat Rev Neurosci 5:771–781, 2004

Kim JH, Udo H, Li HL, et al: Presynaptic activation of silent synapses and growth of new synapses contribute to intermediate and long-term facilitation in *Aplysia*. Neuron 40:151–165, 2003

Kinouchi H, Epstein CJ, Mizui T, et al: Attenuation of focal cerebral ischemic injury in transgenic mice overexpressing CuZn superoxide dismutase. Proc Natl Acad Sci U S A 88:11158–11162, 1991

Kitayama N, Vaccarino V, Kutner M, et al: Magnetic resonance imaging (MRI) measurement of hippocampal volume in posttraumatic stress disorder: a meta-analysis. J Affect Disord 88:79–86, 2005

Koester J, Siegelbaum S: Propagated signaling: the action potential, in Principles of Neural Science, 4th Edition. Edited by Kandel ER, Schwartz JH, Jessell TM. New York, McGraw-Hill, 2000, pp 167–169

Komuro H, Rakic P: Modulation of neuronal migration by NMDA receptors. Science 260:95–97, 1993

Kozorovitskiy Y, Gould E: Adult neurogenesis: a mechanism for brain repair? J Clin Exp Neuropsychol 25:721–732, 2003

Kriegstein AR, Gotz M: Radial glia diversity: a matter of cell fate. Glia 43:37–43, 2003

Kriegstein AR, Noctor SC: Patterns of neuronal migration in the embryonic cortex. Trends Neurosci 27:392–399, 2004

Landis SC: Target regulation of neurotransmitter phenotype. Trends Neurosci 13:344–350, 1990

Lee H, Chen CX, Liu YJ, et al: KCC2 expression in immature rat cortical neurons is sufficient to switch the polarity of GABA responses. Eur J Neurosci 21:2593–2599, 2005

Lee SH, Sheng M: Development of neuron-neuron synapses. Curr Opin Neurobiol 10:125–131, 2000

Lee SH, Lumelsky N, Studer L, et al: Efficient generation of midbrain and hindbrain neurons from mouse embryonic stem cells. Nat Biotechnol 18:675–679, 2000

Letinic K, Zoncu R, Rakic P: Origin of GABAergic neurons in the human neocortex. Nature 417:645–649, 2002

LeVay S, Stryker MP, Shatz CJ: Ocular dominance columns and their development in layer IV of the cat's visual cortex: a quantitative study. J Comp Neurol 179:223–244, 1978

Lie DC, Song H, Colamarino SA, et al: Neurogenesis in the adult brain: new strategies for central nervous system diseases. Annu Rev Pharmacol Toxicol 44:399–421, 2004

Lin Z, Wang W, Uhl GR: Dopamine transporter tryptophan mutants highlight candidate dopamine- and cocaine-selective domains. Mol Pharmacol 58:1581–1592, 2000

Lipton SA, Kater SB: Neurotransmitter regulation of neuronal outgrowth, plasticity and survival. Trends Neurosci 12:265–270, 1989

Lisman J, Schulman H, Cline H: The molecular basis of CaMKII function in synaptic and behavioural memory. Nat Rev Neurosci 3:175–190, 2002

Livingstone M, Hubel D: Segregation of form, color, movement, and depth: anatomy, physiology, and perception. Science 240:740–749, 1988

Llinás R: The intrinsic electrophysiological properties of mammalian neurons: insights into central nervous system function. Science 242:1654–1664, 1988

Llinás R, Jahnsen H: Electrophysiology of mammalian thalamic neurones in vitro. Nature 297:406–408, 1982

Lois C, Garcia-Verdugo JM, Alvarez-Buylla A: Chain migration of neuronal precursors. Science 271:978–981, 1996

London M, Häusser M: Dendritic computation. Annu Rev Neurosci 28:503–532, 2005

LoTurco JJ, Kriegstein AR: Clusters of coupled neuroblasts in embryonic neocortex. Science 252:563–566, 1991

LoTurco JJ, Owens DF, Heath MJ, et al: GABA and glutamate depolarize cortical progenitor cells and inhibit DNA synthesis. Neuron 15:1287–1298, 1995

Luo L, O'Leary DD: Axon retraction and degeneration in development and disease. Annu Rev Neurosci 28:127–156, 2005

Luskin MB, Pearlman AL, Sanes JR: Cell lineage in the cerebral cortex of the mouse studied in vivo and in vitro with a recombinant retrovirus. Neuron 1:635–647, 1988

Lyford GL, Yamagata K, Kaufmann WE, et al: Arc, a growth factor and activity-regulated gene, encodes a novel cytoskeleton-associated protein that is enriched in neuronal dendrites. Neuron 14:433–445, 1995

Lynch MA: Long-term potentiation and memory. Physiol Rev 84:87–136, 2004

MacDermott AB, Mayer ML, Westbrook GL, et al: NMDA-receptor activation increases cytoplasmic calcium concentration in cultured spinal cord neurones. Nature 321:519–522, 1986

Magee JC, Carruth M: Dendritic voltage-gated ion channels regulate the action potential firing mode of hippocampal CA1 pyramidal neurons. J Neurophysiol 82:1895–1901, 1999

Maguire EA, Gadian DG, Johnsrude IS, et al: Navigation-related structural change in the hippocampi of taxi drivers. Proc Natl Acad Sci U S A 97:4398–4403, 2000

Mahanty NK, Sah P: Calcium-permeable AMPA receptors mediate long-term potentiation in interneurons in the amygdala. Nature 394:683–687, 1998

Malatesta P, Hartfuss E, Gotz M: Isolation of radial glial cells by fluorescent-activated cell sorting reveals a neuronal lineage. Development 127:5253–5263, 2000

Malgaroli A, Ting AE, Wendland B, et al: Presynaptic component of long-term potentiation visualized at individual hippocampal synapses. Science 268:1624–1628, 1995

Malleret G, Haditsch U, Genoux D, et al: Inducible and reversible enhancement of learning, memory, and long-term potentiation by genetic inhibition of calcineurin. Cell 104:675–686, 2001

Marin O, Rubenstein JL: Cell migration in the forebrain. Annu Rev Neurosci 26:441–483, 2003

Masson J, Sagn C, Hamon M, et al: Neurotransmitter transporters in the central nervous system. Pharmacol Rev 51:439–464, 1999

Mattson MP, Kater SB: Excitatory and inhibitory neurotransmitters in the generation and degeneration of hippocampal neuroarchitecture. Brain Res 478:337–348, 1989

McAllister AK, Katz LC, Lo DC: Neurotrophins and synaptic plasticity. Annu Rev Neurosci 22:295–318, 1999

McConnell SK, Kaznowski CE: Cell cycle dependence of laminar determination in developing neocortex. Science 254:282–285, 1991

McCormick DA, Bal T: Sleep and arousal: thalamocortical mechanisms. Annu Rev Neurosci 20:185–215, 1997

Meffert MK, Calakos NC, Scheller RH, et al: Nitric oxide modulates synaptic vesicle docking/fusion reactions. Neuron 16:1229–1236, 1996

Mennerick S, Zorumski CF: Glial contributions to excitatory neurotransmission in cultured hippocampal cells. Nature 368:59–62, 1994

Miale IL, Sidman RL: An autoradiographic analysis of histogenesis in the mouse cerebellum. Exp Neurol 4:277–296, 1961

Miller FD, Kaplan DR: Neurotrophin signalling pathways regulating neuronal apoptosis. Cell Mol Life Sci 58:1045–1053, 2001

Miller MW: Effects of prenatal exposure to ethanol on neocortical development, II: cell proliferation in the ventricular and subventricular zones of the rat. J Comp Neurol 287:326–338, 1989

Misson JP, Edwards MA, Yamamoto M, et al: Identification of radial glial cells within the developing murine central nervous system: studies based upon a new immunohistochemical marker. Brain Res Dev Brain Res 44:95–108, 1988a

Misson JP, Edwards MA, Yamamoto M, et al: Mitotic cycling of radial glial cells of the fetal murine cerebral wall: a combined autoradiographic and immunohistochemical study. Brain Res 466:183–190, 1988b

Miyakawa T, Leiter LM, Gerber DJ, et al: Conditional calcineurin knockout mice exhibit multiple abnormal behaviors related to schizophrenia. Proc Natl Acad Sci U S A 100:8987–8992, 2003

Miyata T, Kawaguchi A, Okano H, et al: Asymmetric inheritance of radial glial fibers by cortical neurons. Neuron 31:727–741, 2001

Miyata T, Kawaguchi A, Saito K, et al: Asymmetric production of surface-dividing and non-surface-dividing cortical progenitor cells. Development 131:3133–3145, 2004

Morgan JI, Curran T: Stimulus-transcription coupling in neurons: role of cellular immediate-early genes. Trends Neurosci 12:459–462, 1989

Morgan JI, Curran T: Immediate-early genes: ten years on. Trends Neurosci 18:66–67, 1995

Murphy TH, Blatter LA, Wier WG, et al: Rapid communication between neurons and astrocytes in primary cortical cultures. J Neurosci 13:2672–2679, 1993

Nadarajah B, Parnavelas JG: Modes of neuronal migration in the developing cerebral cortex. Nat Rev Neurosci 3:423–432, 2002

Nedergaard M: Direct signaling from astrocytes to neurons in cultures of mammalian brain cells. Science 263:1768–1771, 1994

Nery S, Fishell G, Corbin JG: The caudal ganglionic eminence is a source of distinct cortical and subcortical cell populations. Nat Neurosci 5:1279–1287, 2002

Noctor SC, Flint AC, Weissman TA, et al: Neurons derived from radial glial cells establish radial units in neocortex. Nature 409:714–720, 2001

Noctor SC, Flint AC, Weissman TA, et al: Dividing precursor cells of the embryonic cortical ventricular zone have morphological and molecular characteristics of radial glia. J Neurosci 22:3161–3173, 2002

Noctor SC, Martinez-Cerdeno V, Ivic L, et al: Cortical neurons arise in symmetric and asymmetric division zones and migrate through specific phases. Nat Neurosci 7:136–144, 2004

Nowak L, Bregestovski P, Ascher P, et al: Magnesium gates glutamate-activated channels in mouse central neurones. Nature 307:462–465, 1984

O'Brien RJ, Lau LF, Huganir RL: Molecular mechanisms of glutamate receptor clustering at excitatory synapses. Curr Opin Neurobiol 8:364–369, 1998

O'Dell TJ, Huang PL, Dawson TM, et al: Endothelial NOS and the blockade of LTP by NOS inhibitors in mice lacking neuronal NOS. Science 265:542–546, 1994

Olsen R, Betz H: GABA and glycine, in Basic Neurochemistry: Molecular, Cellular and Medical Aspects, 7th Edition. Edited by Siegel GJ, Albers RW, Brady S, et al. Burlington, MA, Elsevier Academic, 2006, pp 291–301

Oppenheim A, Altuvia S, Kornitzer D, et al: Translation control of gene expression. J Basic Clin Physiol Pharmacol 2:223–231, 1991

Pantev C, Oostenveld R, Engelien A, et al: Increased auditory cortical representation in musicians. Nature 392:811–814, 1998

Pearson BJ, Doe CQ: Specification of temporal identity in the developing nervous system. Annu Rev Cell Dev Biol 20:619–647, 2004

Pereira C, Agostinho P, Moreira PI, et al: Alzheimer's disease-associated neurotoxic mechanisms and neuroprotective strategies. Curr Drug Targets CNS Neurol Disord 4:383–403, 2005

Pfrieger FW, Barres BA: Synaptic efficacy enhanced by glial cells in vitro. Science 277:1684–1687, 1997

Pifl C, Giros B, Caron MG: The dopamine transporter: the cloned target site of parkinsonism-inducing toxins and of drugs of abuse. Adv Neurol 69:235–238, 1996

Pigino G, Kirkpatrick L, Brady S: The cytoskeleton of neurons and glia, in Basic Neurochemistry: Molecular, Cellular and Medical Aspects, 7th Edition. Edited by Siegel GJ, Albers RW, Brady S, et al. Burlington, MA, Elsevier Academic, 2006, pp 123–137

Purves D, Augustine GJ, Fitzpatrick D, et al: Neuroscience. Sunderland, MA, Sinauer Associates, 1997

Purves D, Augustine GJ, Fitzpatrick D, et al: Neuroscience. Sunderland, MA, Sinauer Associates, 2004

Putcha GV, Johnson EM Jr: Men are but worms: neuronal cell death in *C elegans* and vertebrates. Cell Death Differ 11:38–48, 2004

Raff MC, Barres BA, Burne JF, et al: Programmed cell death and the control of cell survival: lessons from the nervous system. Science 262:695–700, 1993

Rakic P: Guidance of neurons migrating to the fetal monkey neocortex. Brain Res 33:471–476, 1971

Ramamoorthy S, Blakely RD: Phosphorylation and sequestration of serotonin transporters differentially modulated by psychostimulants. Science 285:763–766, 1999

Ramón y Cajal S: Les nouvelles idées sur la structure du système nerveux chez l'homme et chez les vertébrés. Paris, France, C. Reinwald, 1894

Ramón y Cajal S: Histologie du système nerveux de l'homme et des vertébrés. Paris, France, Maloine, 1911

Rego AC, de Almeida LP: Molecular targets and therapeutic strategies in Huntington's disease. Curr Drug Targets CNS Neurol Disord 4:361–381, 2005

Reiter HO, Stryker MP: Neural plasticity without postsynaptic action potentials: less-active inputs become dominant when kitten visual cortical cells are pharmacologically inhibited. Proc Natl Acad Sci U S A 85:3623–3627, 1988

Rosen DR, Siddique T, Patterson D, et al: Mutations in Cu/Zn superoxide dismutase gene are associated with familial amyotrophic lateral sclerosis. Nature 362:59–62, 1993

Rumpel S, LeDoux J, Zador A, et al: Postsynaptic receptor trafficking underlying a form of associative learning. Science 308:83–88, 2005

Sadato N, Pascual-Leone A, Grafman J, et al: Activation of the primary visual cortex by Braille reading in blind subjects. Nature 380:526–528, 1996

Saito T, Nakatsuji N: Efficient gene transfer into the embryonic mouse brain using in vivo electroporation. Dev Biol 240:237–246, 2001

Salinas PC: Signaling at the vertebrate synapse: new roles for embryonic morphogens? J Neurobiol 64:435–445, 2005

Sanes JR, Jessell TM: The formation and regeneration of synapses, in Principles of Neural Science, 4th Edition. Edited by Kandel ER, Schwartz JH, Jessell TM. New York, McGraw-Hill, 2000, pp 1087–1114

Sanes JR, Lichtman JW: Development of the vertebrate neuromuscular junction. Annu Rev Neurosci 22:389–442, 1999

Sanes JR, Rubenstein JL, Nicolas JF: Use of a recombinant retrovirus to study post-implantation cell lineage in mouse embryos. Embo J 5:3133–3142, 1986

Santarelli L, Saxe M, Gross C, et al: Requirement of hippocampal neurogenesis for the behavioral effects of antidepressants. Science 301:805–809, 2003

Sastry PS, Rao KS: Apoptosis and the nervous system. J Neurochem 74:1–20, 2000

Sauer FC: Mitosis in the neural tube. J Comp Neurol 62:377–405, 1935

Scheiffele P: Cell-cell signaling during synapse formation in the CNS. Annu Rev Neurosci 26:488–508, 2003

Schenone A, Mancardi GL: Molecular basis of inherited neuropathies. Curr Opin Neurol 12:603–616, 1999

Schmechel DE, Rakic P: A Golgi study of radial glial cells in developing monkey telencephalon: morphogenesis and transformation into astrocytes. Anat Embryol (Berl) 156:115–152, 1979

Schoepfer R, Monyer H, Sommer B, et al: Molecular biology of glutamate receptors. Prog Neurobiol 42:353–357, 1994

Schulman H: Nitric oxide: a spatial second messenger. Mol Psychiatry 2:296–299, 1997

Schuurmans C, Guillemot F: Molecular mechanisms underlying cell fate specification in the developing telencephalon. Curr Opin Neurobiol 12:26–34, 2002

Schwartz JH: Neurotransmitters, in Principles of Neural Science, 4th Edition. Edited by Kandel ER, Schwartz JH, Jessell TM. New York, McGraw-Hill, 2000, pp 280–297

Scott SA, Davies AM: Inhibition of protein synthesis prevents cell death in sensory and parasympathetic neurons deprived of neurotrophic factor in vitro. J Neurobiol 21:630–638, 1990

Seamans JK, Yang CR: The principal features and mechanisms of dopamine modulation in the prefrontal cortex. Prog Neurobiol 74:1–58, 2004

Seri B, García-Verdugo JM, McEwen BS, et al: Astrocytes give rise to new neurons in the adult mammalian hippocampus. J Neurosci 21:7153–7160, 2001

Shatz CJ: Impulse activity and the patterning of connections during CNS development. Neuron 5:745–756, 1990

Shatz CJ, Stryker MP: Prenatal tetrodotoxin infusion blocks segregation of retinogeniculate afferents. Science 242:87–89, 1988

Shepherd GM, Koch C: Introduction to synaptic circuits, in The Synaptic Organization of the Brain. Edited by Shepherd GM. New York, Oxford, 1990, pp 3–31

Sherman SM: Tonic and burst firing: dual modes of thalamocortical relay. Trends Neurosci 24:122–126, 2001

Shi SH, Hayashi Y, Petralia RS, et al: Rapid spine delivery and redistribution of AMPA receptors after synaptic NMDA receptor activation. Science 284:1811–1816, 1999

Smart IH: Proliferative characteristics of the ependymal layer during the early development of the mouse neocortex: a pilot study based on recording the number, location and plane of cleavage of mitotic figures. J Anat 116:67–91, 1973

Smith AD, Bolam JP: The neural network of the basal ganglia as revealed by the study of synaptic connections of identified neurones. Trends Neurosci 13:259–265, 1990

Sohl G, Maxeiner S, Willecke K: Expression and functions of neuronal gap junctions. Nat Rev Neurosci 6:191–200, 2005

Spencer KM, Nestor PG, Perlmutter R, et al: Neural synchrony indexes disordered perception and cognition in schizophrenia. Proc Natl Acad Sci U S A 101:17288–17293, 2004

Squire LR, Roberts JL, Spitzer NC, et al (eds): Fundamental Neuroscience, 2nd Edition. San Diego, CA, Academic Press, 2003

Steward O, Worley P: Local synthesis of proteins at synaptic sites on dendrites: role in synaptic plasticity and memory consolidation? Neurobiol Learn Mem 78:508–527, 2002

Studer L, Tabar V, McKay RDG: transplantation of expanded mesencephalic precursors leads to recovery in parkinsonian rats. Nat Neurosci 1:290–205, 1998

Sudhof TC: The synaptic vesicle cycle. Annu Rev Neurosci 27:509–547, 2004

Sulzer D, Sonders MS, Poulsen NW, et al: Mechanisms of neurotransmitter release by amphetamines: a review. Prog Neurobiol 75:406–433, 2005

Szabadics J, Varga C, Molnar G, et al: Excitatory effect of GABAergic axo-axonic cells in cortical microcircuits. Science 311:233–235, 2006

Takahashi T, Nowakowski RS, Caviness VS Jr: Early ontogeny of the secondary proliferative population of the embryonic murine cerebral wall. J Neurosci 15:6058–6068, 1995

Tamas G, Buhl EH, Lorincz A, et al: Proximally targeted GABAergic synapses and gap junctions synchronize cortical interneurons. Nat Neurosci 3:366–371, 2000

Tarabykin V, Stoykova A, Usman N, et al: Cortical upper layer neurons derive from the subventricular zone as indicated by Svet1 gene expression. Development 128:1983–1993, 2001

Tissir F, Goffinet AM: Reelin and brain development. Nat Rev Neurosci 4:496–505, 2003

Toga AW, Thompson PM: Genetics of brain structure and intelligence. Annu Rev Neurosci 28:1–23, 2005

Tsao P, von Zastrow M: Downregulation of G protein-coupled receptors. Curr Opin Neurobiol 10:365–369, 2000

Tsujimoto Y, Yunis J, Onorato-Showe L, et al: Molecular cloning of the chromosomal breakpoint of B-cell lymphomas and leukemias with the t(11;14) chromosome translocation. Science 224:1403–1406, 1984

Van Den Bosch L, Van Damme P, Bogaert E, et al: The role of excitotoxity in the pathogenesis of amyotrophic lateral sclerosis. Biochim Biophys Acta 1762:1068–1082, 2006

Vickery RG, von Zastrow M: Distinct dynamin-dependent and -independent mechanisms target structurally homologous dopamine receptors to different endocytic membranes. J Cell Biol 144:31–43, 1999

Vogels TP, Rajan K, Abbott LF: Neural network dynamics. Annu Rev Neurosci 28:357–376, 2005

Waites CL, Craig AM, Garner CC: Mechanisms of vertebrate synaptogenesis. Annu Rev Neurosci 28:251–274, 2005

Walaas SI, Greengard P: Protein phosphorylation and neuronal function. Pharmacol Rev 43:299–349, 1991

Walsh C, Cepko CL: Cell lineage and cell migration in the developing cerebral cortex. Experientia 46:940–947, 1990

Wang HG, Lu FM, Jin I, et al: Presynaptic and postsynaptic roles of NO, cGK, and RhoA in long-lasting potentiation and aggregation of synaptic proteins. Neuron 45:389–403, 2005

Warner-Schmidt JL, Duman RS: Hippocampal neurogenesis: opposing effects of stress and antidepressant treatment. Hippocampus 16:239–249, 2006

Washbourne P, Bennett JE, McAllister AK: Rapid recruitment of NMDA receptor transport packets to nascent synapses. Nat Neurosci 5:751–759, 2002

Washbourne P, Dityatev A, Scheiffele P, et al: Cell adhesion molecules in synapse formation. J Neurosci 24:9244–9249, 2004a

Washbourne P, Liu XB, Jones EG, et al: Cycling of NMDA receptors during trafficking in neurons before synapse formation. J Neurosci 24:8253–8264, 2004b

Waxman SG: From Neuroscience to Neurology: Neuroscience, Molecular Medicine, and the Therapeutic Transformation of Neurology. Boston, MA, Elsevier Academic Press, 2005

Weissman TA, Riquelme PA, Ivic L, et al: Calcium waves propagate through radial glial cells and modulate proliferation in the developing neocortex. Neuron 43:647–661, 2004

Wexler NS, Rose EA, Housman DE: Molecular approaches to hereditary diseases of the nervous system: Huntington's disease as a paradigm. Annu Rev Neurosci 14:503–529, 1991

Wichterle H, Lieberam I, Porter JA, et al: Directed differentiation of embryonic stem cells into motor neurons. Cell 110:385–397, 2002

Wisden W, Errington ML, Williams S, et al: Differential expression of immediate early genes in the hippocampus and spinal cord. Neuron 4:603–614, 1990

Yamakura T, Bertaccini E, Trudell JR, et al: Anesthetics and ion channels: molecular models and sites of action. Annu Rev Pharmacol Toxicol 41:23–51, 2001

Yuste R, Tank DW: Dendritic integration in mammalian neurons, a century after Cajal. Neuron 16:701–716, 1996

Ziv NE, Garner CC: Cellular and molecular mechanisms of presynaptic assembly. Nat Rev Neurosci 5:385–399, 2004

5

NEUROANATOMY FOR THE PSYCHIATRIST

Katherine H. Taber, Ph.D., F.A.N.P.A.
Robin A. Hurley, M.D., F.A.N.P.A.

As science and technology have improved with time, so has their application to psychiatry and mental illness. Conditions once believed to be the result of environmental influences are now understood for their biological basis and heritability. As structural and functional neuroimaging and genetics become more entwined in modern medicine, it has become more and more evident that practicing psychiatrists need to understand basic neuroanatomy and its relationship to psychiatric disease. The purpose of this chapter is to serve as a visual refresher. Medical informatics research has found that appropriate use of images and color-coding of information promote assimilation of large amounts of dense, detailed scientific knowledge. Thus, we have integrated colored visual graphics as a means to review neuroanatomical detail. The primary learning venue is thus the figures, with limited text to clarify some details. For more detailed anatomical maps and circuit drawings, the interested reader may refer to the reference list at the end of the chapter.

A basic understanding of the cortical and subcortical anatomy involved in executive function, memory, and emotion is essential to understanding the latest in the biological basis of psychiatric illness and to proper appreciation of neuroimaging findings in patients. In addition, a familiarity with the symptoms of emo-tional, memory, and cognitive dysfunction associated with anatomical lesions can help the psychiatrist know when to ask for imaging in a patient, when to call for a neurological or neuropsychiatric consultation, and when to suspect medical conditions that may account for the psychiatric symptoms (e.g., traumatic brain injury, stroke, multiple sclerosis, poison/toxin exposure). These anatomical images and the accompanying brief descriptive material not only can familiarize the clinician with normal imaging anatomy pertinent to a psychiatrist but also can serve as a base for more in-depth reference/study. Although important for many functions, the cranial nerves, motor pathways, and peripheral sensory tracts are not central to general psychiatric conditions and therefore are not discussed.

Emotion, cognition, and memory are currently believed to occur through circuits or networks that are interconnected throughout the brain. Lesions at any point in a circuit can potentially give rise to identical symptoms (Burruss et al. 2000; Dalgleish 2004; Taber et al. 2004; Tekin and Cummings 2002).

Although this chapter focuses on the larger brain structures, any lesion along the small tracts between regions can also produce similar deficits. Major neuropsychiatric symptoms associated with damage to various subcortical structures are summarized. These summaries were derived from a more comprehensive review, which can be consulted for more detail (Naumescu et al. 1999).

Shown next are planes of sections of the brain (Figure 5–1), anatomic orientations (Figure 5–2), and the major divisions of the brain (Figure 5–3).

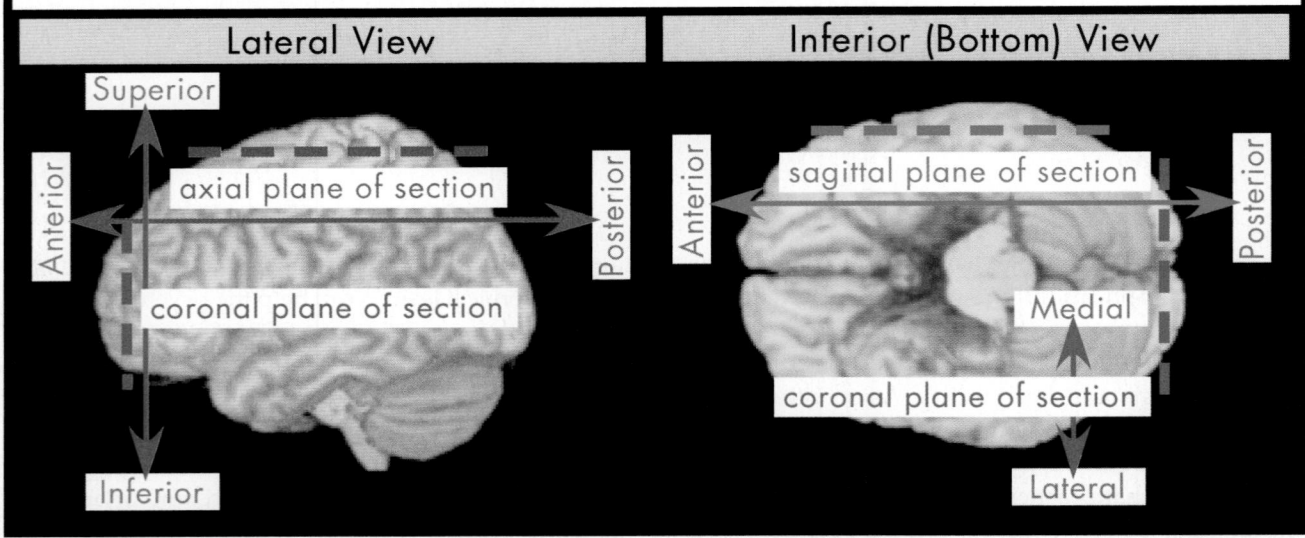

Planes of Section

In medical practice, the most common way to view the brain is the two-dimensional sections provided by magnetic resonance imaging (MRI) and computed tomography (CT). While it is possible to image the brain in virtually any orientation, the axial plane of section is used most often, as it allows the entire brain to be captured in the fewest number of sections. Anatomists prefer the coronal plane of section because many structures, particularly small ones, are more easily recognized. Note that both the axial and sagittal planes of section go from the front (anterior) to the back (posterior) of the brain. Axial goes from one side to the other (medial to lateral). Sagittal goes from top (superior) to bottom (inferior).

FIGURE 5–1. Planes of section.

Source. Used with permission from Mid-Atlantic Mental Illness Research, Education, and Clinical Center.

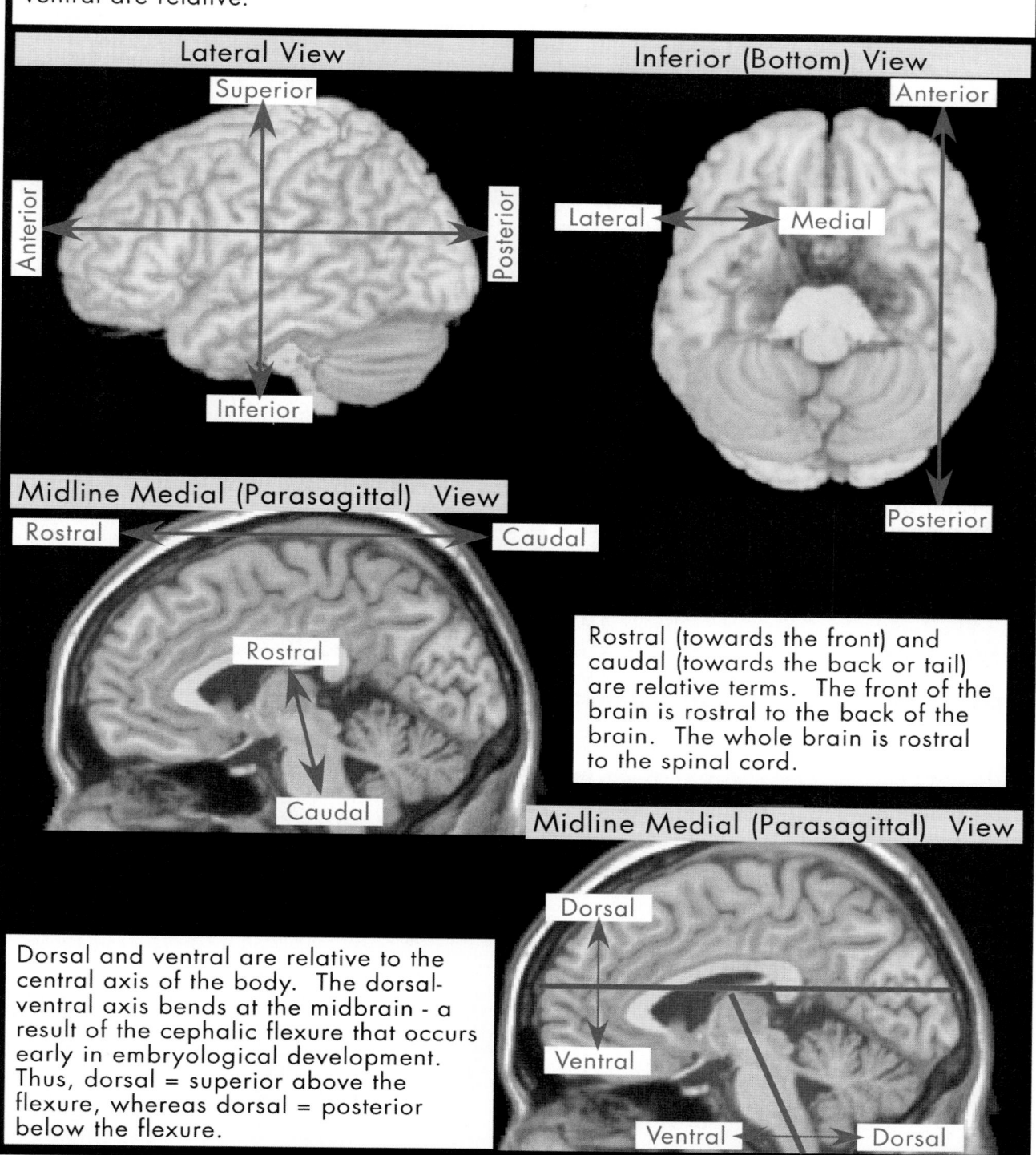

Anatomic Orientations and Directions

Several sets of terms are used to describe directions in the brain. Some of them are invariant, whereas others are named relative to a particular axis. Superior - inferior, anterior - posterior, and medial - lateral do not change. Rostral - caudal and dorsal - ventral are relative.

Lateral View

Superior
Anterior
Posterior
Inferior

Inferior (Bottom) View

Anterior
Lateral
Medial
Posterior

Midline Medial (Parasagittal) View

Rostral
Caudal
Rostral
Caudal

Rostral (towards the front) and caudal (towards the back or tail) are relative terms. The front of the brain is rostral to the back of the brain. The whole brain is rostral to the spinal cord.

Midline Medial (Parasagittal) View

Dorsal
Ventral
Ventral
Dorsal

Dorsal and ventral are relative to the central axis of the body. The dorsal-ventral axis bends at the midbrain - a result of the cephalic flexure that occurs early in embryological development. Thus, dorsal = superior above the flexure, whereas dorsal = posterior below the flexure.

FIGURE 5–2. Anatomic orientations and directions.

Source. Used with permission from Mid-Atlantic Mental Illness Research, Education, and Clinical Center.

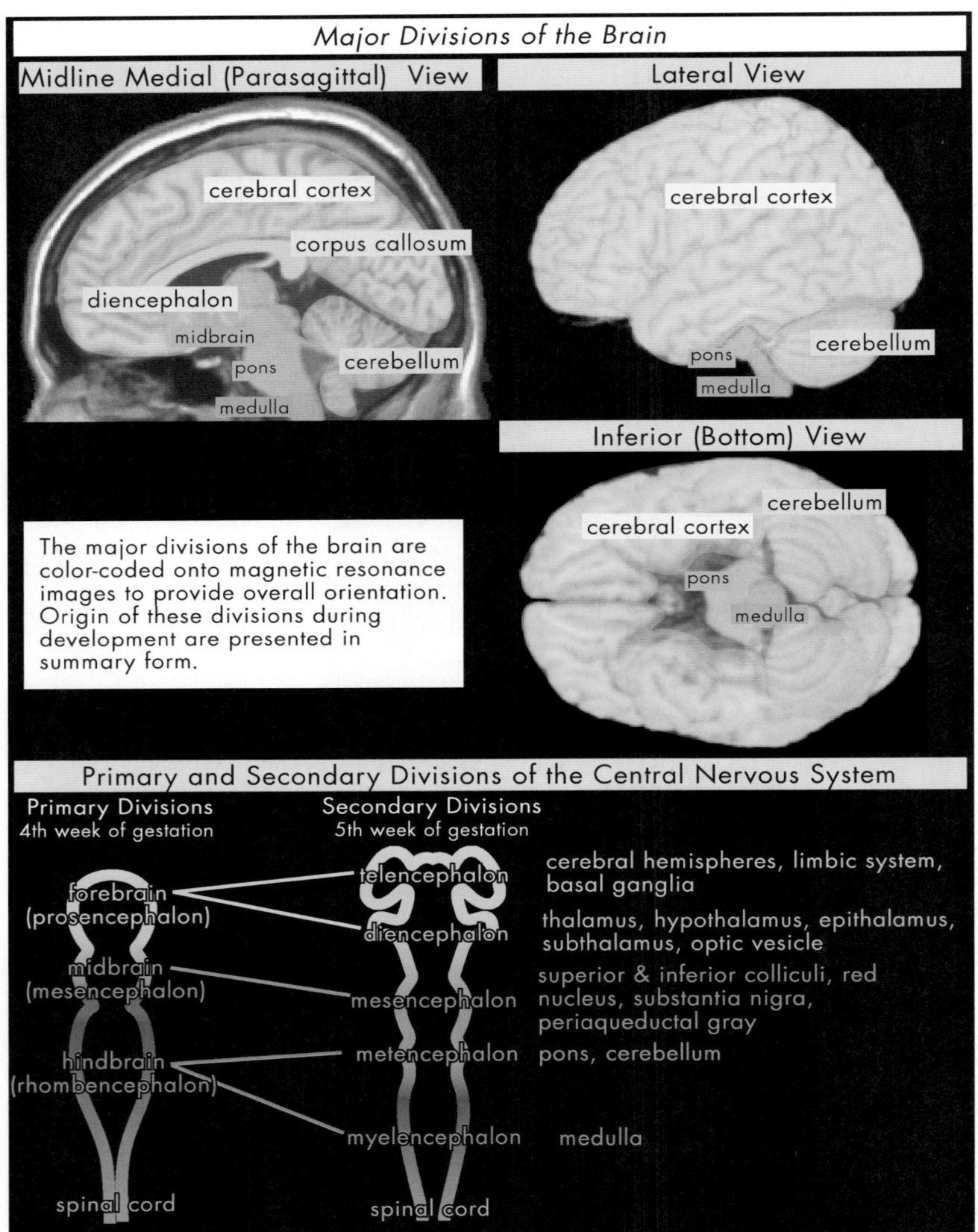

FIGURE 5–3. Major divisions of the brain.

Source. Used with permission from Mid-Atlantic Mental Illness Research, Education, and Clinical Center.

Cerebral Cortex

The largest division of the human brain is the cerebral cortex, containing billions of neurons and close to one trillion glial cells. Anatomists divide the cerebral cortex into either four or five lobes. All recognize the frontal, temporal, parietal, and occipital lobes. Some consider the limbic lobe to be a fifth lobe; others consider it to be contained within the temporal and frontal lobes and diencephalon. The neocortex (telencephalon) is the newest of brain structures in the evolutionary hierarchy and serves as the "modulator" for the more primitive functions housed in the lower structures of the brain. In keeping with traditional anatomic discussions, each lobe of the cerebral cortex has many defined functions; those most critical to emotion, cognition, and memory will be elucidated here. However, it is vital to remember that no area of cortex functions in isolation; all areas work in series with areas in other lobes, subcortical structures, and in a larger system of circuits. Each cortical circuit has both excitatory and inhibitory influences. In most individuals (including approximately two-thirds of left-handed persons), verbal information is processed in the left hemisphere; nonverbal and visuospatial information are processed primarily in the right hemisphere (Mesulam 2000; Pincus and Tucker 2002). Not all individual functions of each cortical area are covered in this brief review. This work is intended to give the reader a very basic framework upon which to build further neuroanatomical study and for use as a quick-reference guide to the more commonly observed functions.

Frontal Lobe

The frontal lobes are the largest of the major cortical lobes. They contain five key areas for neuropsychiatric function (e.g., executive function, personality, intellect, working memory, speech) and motor functions. The frontal operculum contains Broca's area on the left (responsible for fluency of speech). The right frontal operculum adds emotion to speech—gesturing, prosody, and inflection. Lesions to Broca's area result in a nonfluent aphasia, characterized by difficulty in producing fluent speech, defective naming, and impaired repetition. Patients usually are aware of the deficits, and comprehension of spoken speech is intact. Right frontal operculum lesions result in an "expressive aphasia" with loss of emotion in the speech. Comprehension remains intact.

The superior mesial region contains the anterior cingulate and the medial portion of the supplementary motor area. These areas subserve initiation and synchronization of speech and complex movements. Lesions to this region can result in akinetic mutism, with restricted efforts to communicate, an expressionless face, and limited body/arm movements. With unilateral lesions, this decrease in motivated movements can be temporary, eventually subsiding. The cingulate is extensively involved in the circuit of Papez and the limbic system, both of which are discussed later in this chapter.

The orbital and inferior mesial regions are integrally involved in social conduct, insight, judgment, and mood. The orbital cortex functions to allow restraint of emotional reactions to environmental situations. Injury to this region can cause severe disruption of social conduct, including defects in planning, judgment, and decision making. Lesions of this region can produce an inability to feel autonomic response to traumatic or anxious situations. A classic case study is that of Phineas Gage (Damasio et al. 1994).

The dorsolateral prefrontal region is highly critical for focused attention, concentration, working memory, management of retrograde memory recall, and mood. In particular, the left hemisphere is more attuned to verbal memory management and the right to nonverbal and visuospatial tasks. Lesions can be associated with intellectual deficits, loss of memory for frequency of time and events, inability to maintain focus or attention, and inability to shift focus (e.g., schizophrenia).

The supplemental motor cortex, frontal eye fields, and primary motor cortex are all contained in the frontal lobes. They are important for visually guided movements and targeting, initiation of desired movements, and movement of muscle groups. For further details, the interested reader is referred to Mesulam (2000) and Tranel (2002).

Temporal Lobe

The temporal lobes are essential to many emotion and memory circuits. They are integrally involved in hearing, naming of objects, formation and management of memory, and visual recognition. Some temporal lobe functions show significant hemispheric lateralization. The left lateral inferior region is important for visual recognition, with lesions leading to prosopagnosia (an agnosia for faces). The right lateral inferior region is involved in visuospatial recognition, with lesions resulting in loss of recognition of objects in time and space. The left lateral anterior region is important for naming of objects. Injury to this region can cause an agnosia for objects (as compared with faces or people). The right lateral anterior region also participates in naming of objects, as well as management of retrograde episodic memory. Lesions lead not only to deficits in naming of objects but also to loss of personal past events in time and detail. The dorsolateral cortex is the primary auditory cortex. Central deafness occurs with bilateral lesions. The temporoparietal junction is discussed in the following section (see "Parietal Lobe," below). The mesial temporal region contains the hippocampal complex and the amygdala, which are reviewed later in this chapter (see "Limbic System" section). The insula contains the olfactory cortex. A loss of smell can occur with bilateral lesions. Olfactory hallucinations commonly occur with mesial temporal lobe seizures, presumably due to the close proximity of the seizure focus.

Parietal Lobe

The parietal lobes are crucial to sensation, speech, understanding, and other intellectual functions. As study of the brain progresses, the integral ties between the parietal and frontal lobes are becoming more apparent. They are critical for maintaining focused attention and directing focus and attention in time and space. The left temporoparietal junction contains Wernicke's area. This area is critical for comprehension of speech, production of sensical speech, and for verbal repetition. Lesions lead to a Wernicke's aphasia (fluent paraphasic speech) with frequent errors in word choice, impaired repetition, and defective aural comprehension. The right hemispheric equivalent is important for recognition and processing of music and voice. Deficits include amusia (nonrecognition of music and voice). Bilateral lesions lead to auditory agnosia with an inability to recognize/identify any type of sounds. The left inferior parietal lobule supports speech conduction, verbal repetition, sensical speech production, object naming, reading aloud, spelling, and writing to dictation. Lesions can produce a conduction aphasia with impaired repetition, fluent paraphasic speech, defective object naming, impaired oral reading, inability to spell or write to dictation, tactile object agnosia, and acalculia. The right inferior parietal lobule is essential for audiovisual awareness and deficit recognition. Neglect syndromes can occur with lesions in these areas. These include an unawareness of audio and visual modalities, neglect of intra- and extrapersonal space, anosognosia, denial of a paretic limb or loss of tactile modalities. Body schema disturbances and anosognosia can occur with bilateral lesions. The superior parietal lobule contains the sensory association cortex bilaterally. This cortex is vital for sensory integration and recognition in the contralateral side of the body. Loss of sensory integration and recognition can occur with lesions. The primary sensory cortex, essential for receiving body sensations, also lies within this lobule. It is directly posterior to the central sulcus. Deficits can produce numbness of the contralateral side of the body.

Occipital Lobe

The occipital lobes are essential for vision. The primary visual cortex receives the optic radiations. It is critical for vision, color perception, whole-object integration/imaging, and reading. Interhemispheric connections between the right and left support visual information integration. Lesions can produce visual-field cuts (i.e., blindness), disintegration of whole-object imaging, and color blindness. The adjacent visual association cortex is important for visual orientation, peripheral gaze direction, visual guidance, and visual scanning within the environment. The areas above the calcarine sulcus/fissure are called the dorsal component. Lesions of these areas can lead to Balint's syndrome, characterized by visual disorientation, ocular apraxia, and optic ataxia. There can also be defective motion perception and decreased depth perception (partial or mild for unilateral lesions). The areas below the calcarine sulcus/fissure are called the ventral component. Left-sided lesions can produce left hemiachromatopsia, apperceptive visual agnosia, and defective facial imagery. Right-sided lesions can result in right hemiachromatopsia, "pure" alexia, and impaired mental imagery. Bilateral lesions can cause full-field achromatopsia, visual object agnosia, impaired mental imagery, and prosopagnosia.

Basal Forebrain

The basal forebrain lies posterior to the frontal lobes, and includes the inferior surface between the orbital portion of frontal cortex and the hypothalamus. The portion below the anterior commissure has been called the substantia innominata. Important structures include the nucleus basalis (of Meynert), the septal nuclei, the diagonal band of Broca, and the nucleus accumbens. The diagonal band of Broca connects the septal nuclei to the hippocampal complex. The septal nuclei are large producers of acetylcholine. These structures are intimately involved in memory formation, storage and retrieval. Severe memory deficits can be seen with lesions, including anterograde memory loss, inability to integrate learned information, and a tendency to confabulate answers. Alzheimer's disease and anterior communicating artery aneurysm rupture/repair are both associated with basal forebrain loss/injury.

Shown next are the lobes (Figure 5–4), major gyri and sulci (Figure 5–5), and functions of the cerebral cortex (Figure 5–6), followed by a general mapping of Brodmann areas (Figure 5–7) and a simplified variability map for Brodmann area 17 (primary visual cortex) (Figure 5–8).

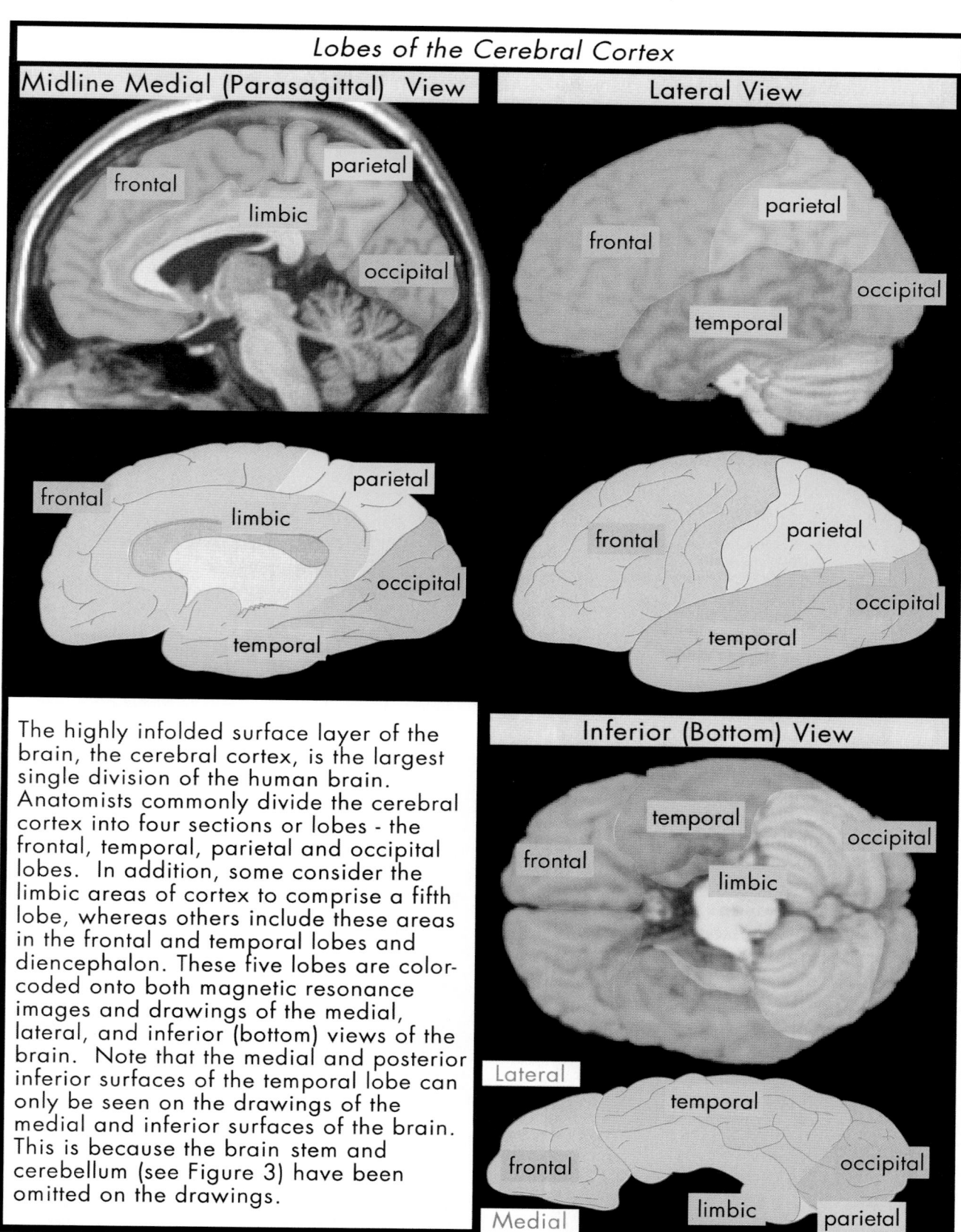

Lobes of the Cerebral Cortex

Midline Medial (Parasagittal) View

frontal · parietal · limbic · occipital

frontal · parietal · limbic · occipital · temporal

Lateral View

frontal · parietal · occipital · temporal

frontal · parietal · occipital · temporal

The highly infolded surface layer of the brain, the cerebral cortex, is the largest single division of the human brain. Anatomists commonly divide the cerebral cortex into four sections or lobes - the frontal, temporal, parietal and occipital lobes. In addition, some consider the limbic areas of cortex to comprise a fifth lobe, whereas others include these areas in the frontal and temporal lobes and diencephalon. These five lobes are color-coded onto both magnetic resonance images and drawings of the medial, lateral, and inferior (bottom) views of the brain. Note that the medial and posterior inferior surfaces of the temporal lobe can only be seen on the drawings of the medial and inferior surfaces of the brain. This is because the brain stem and cerebellum (see Figure 3) have been omitted on the drawings.

Inferior (Bottom) View

temporal · occipital · frontal · limbic

Lateral

temporal · frontal · occipital · limbic · parietal

Medial

FIGURE 5–4. Lobes of the cerebral cortex.

Source. Used with permission from Mid-Atlantic Mental Illness Research, Education, and Clinical Center.

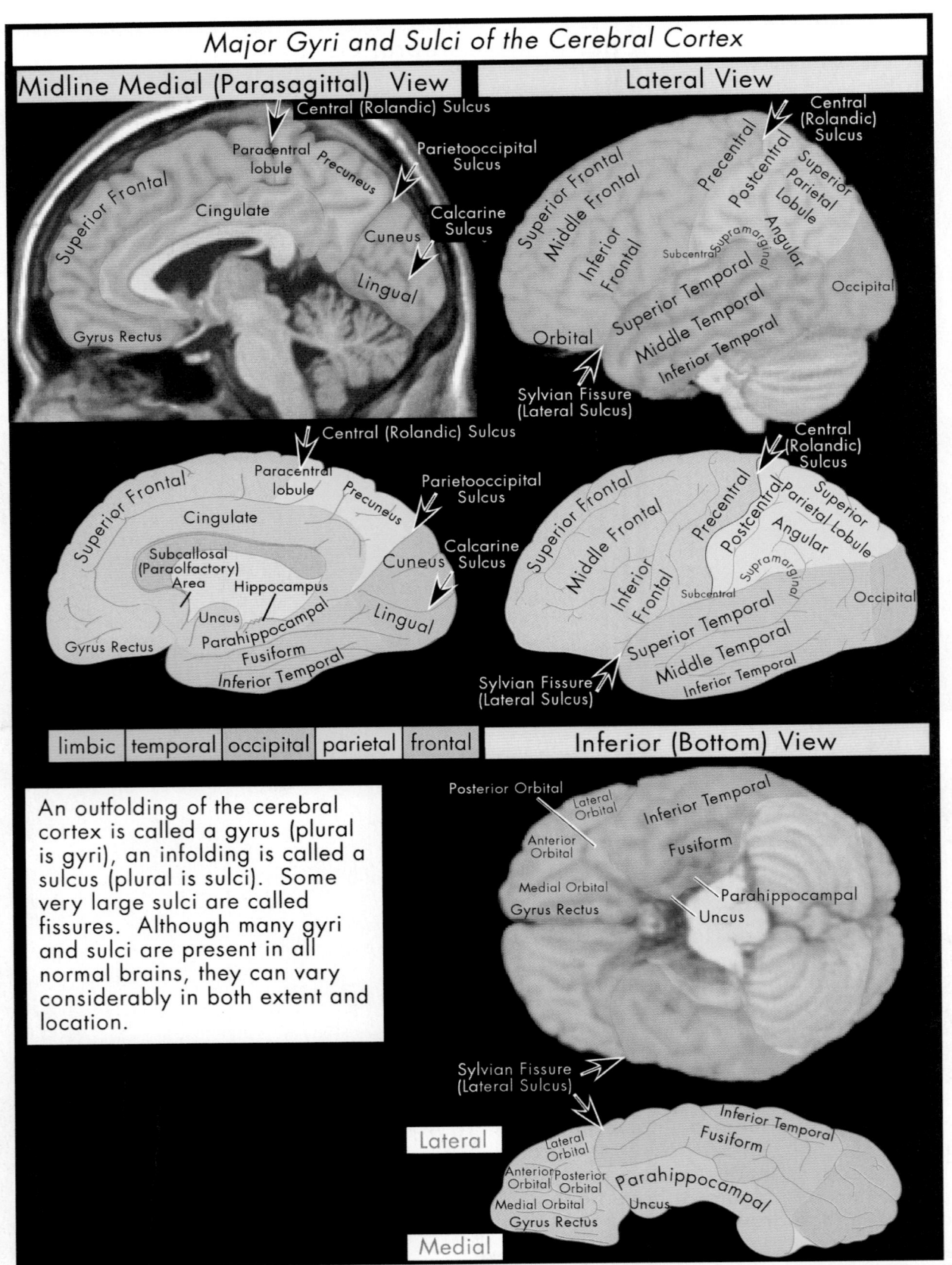

FIGURE 5–5. Major gyri and sulci of the cerebral cortex.

Source. Used with permission from Mid-Atlantic Mental Illness Research, Education, and Clinical Center.

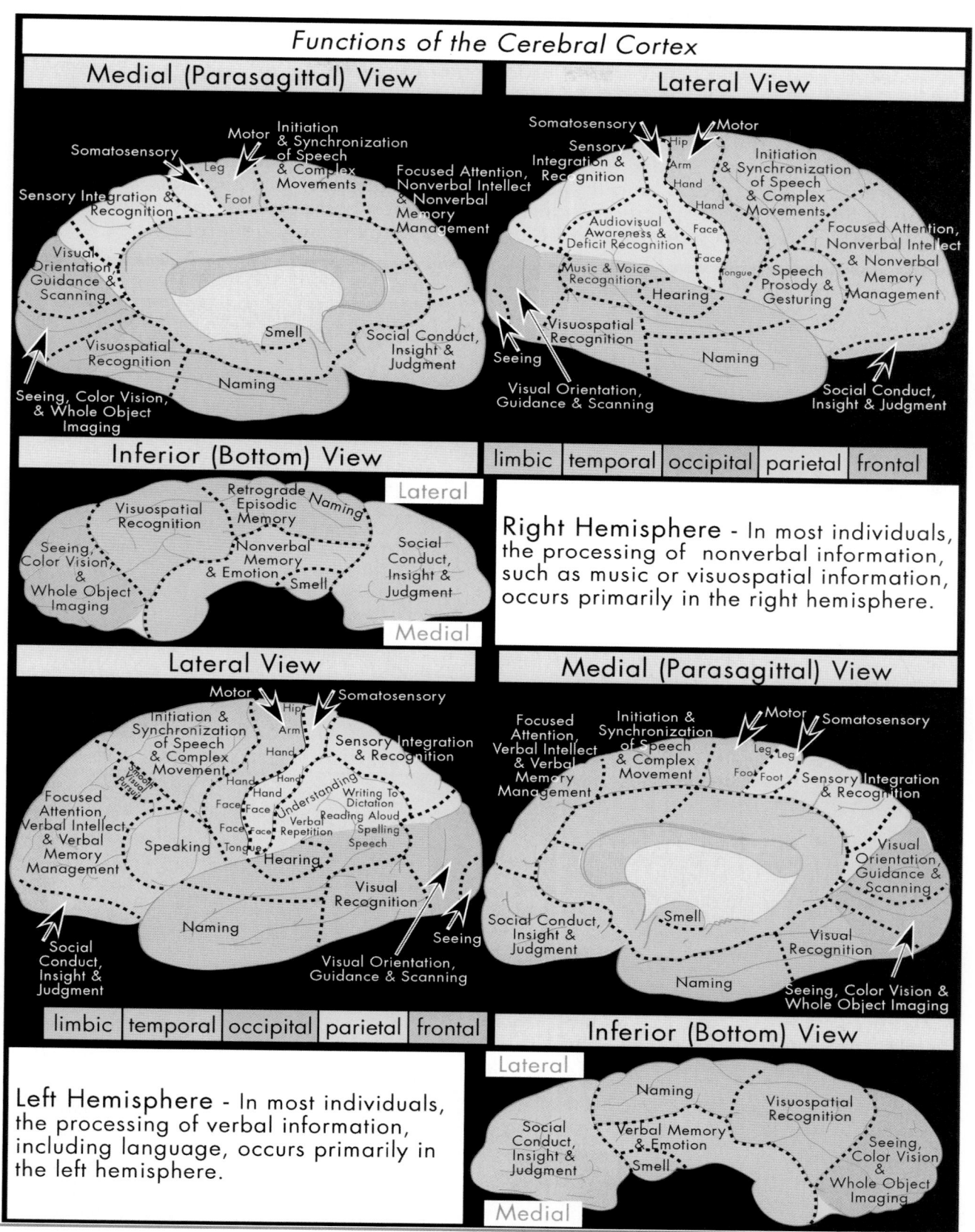

FIGURE 5–6. Functions of the cerebral cortex.

Source. Used with permission from Mid-Atlantic Mental Illness Research, Education, and Clinical Center.

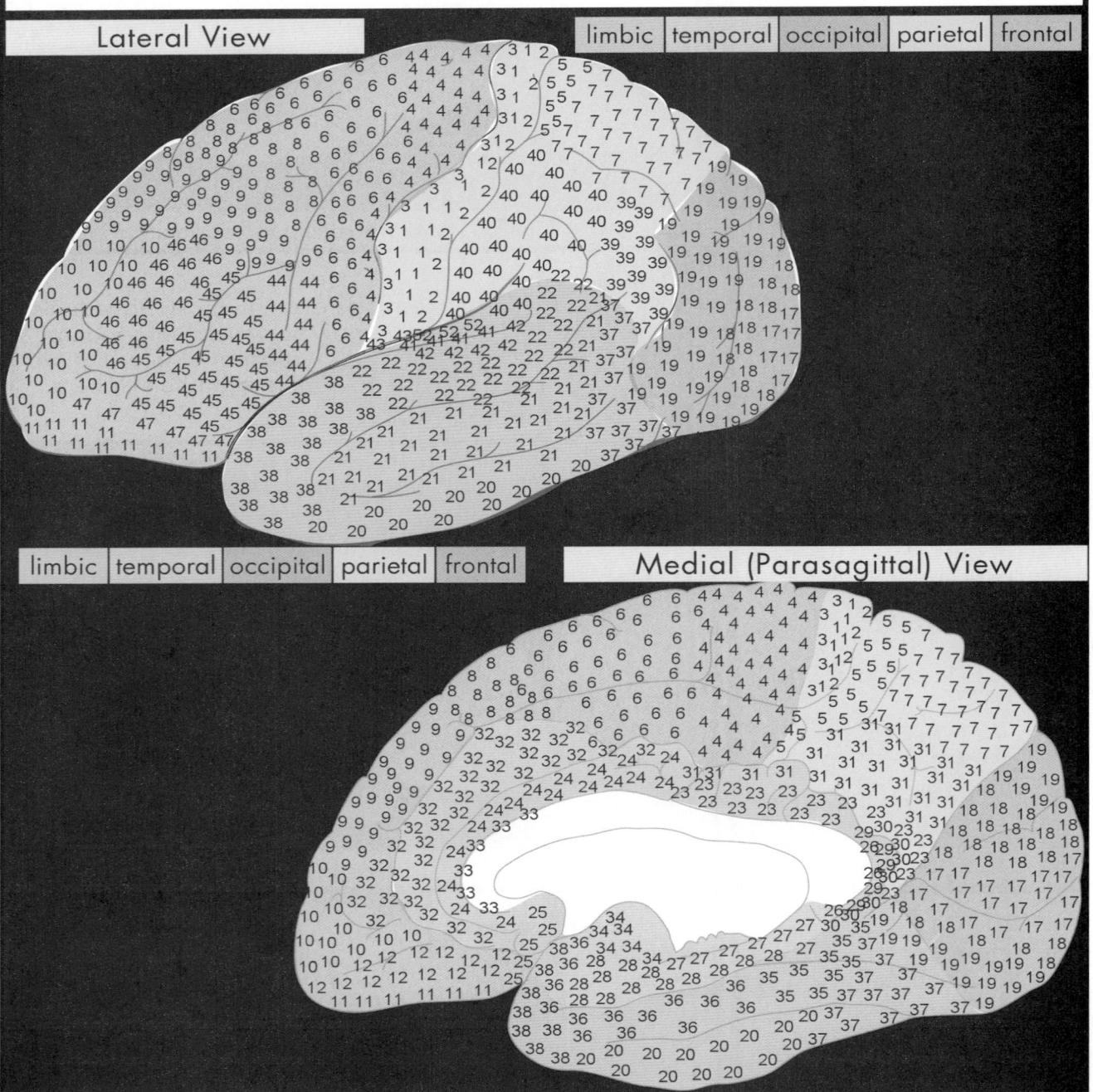

Brodmann Areas

In the early part of the 20th century, Brodmann defined cortical areas based upon features such as the size, shape, and distribution of neurons (cytoarchitecture). An approximation of these areas is provided in the illustrations below. Versions of this system are still widely used (Zeki 2005). While useful, it is important to always keep in mind that Brodmann's work was based upon analysis of a single brain. Brains vary greatly in size, shape, and infolding patterns. Research has shown a wide range in the extent of a specific Brodmann area when compared across individuals (Figure 8). Thus, such maps should be used only as extremely general guides.

FIGURE 5–7. Brodmann areas.

Source. Used with permission from Mid-Atlantic Mental Illness Research, Education, and Clinical Center.

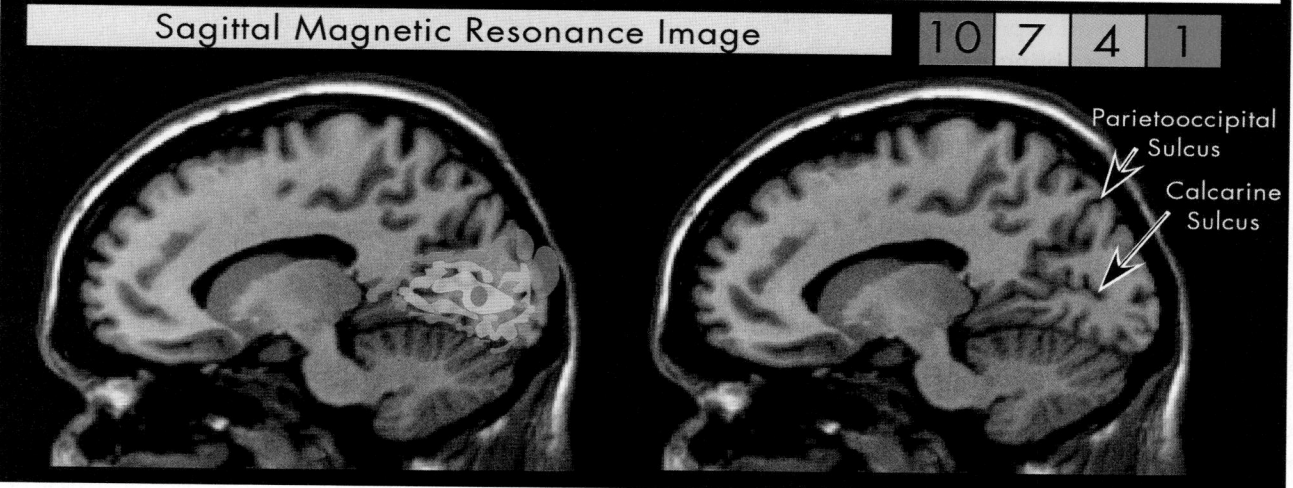

Variability in Brodmann Areas

Multiple studies have compared the extent of particular Brodmann areas across individuals (Amunts et al. 2000; Amunts et al. 2004; Uylings et al. 2005). There is considerable variability, even in areas dedicated to essential sensory functions such as primary visual cortex (Brodmann area 17). Individuality is even greater in areas subserving more complex functions. Variability (or probability) maps have been created by transforming each studied brain into a common anatomic space, so that the areas can be superimposed. This illustration is a simplification of published variability maps for Brodmann area 17 (primary visual cortex), which borders the calcarine sulcus in the occipital lobe. The colors indicate the number of individual brains (out of 10 brains) that overlapped.

Sagittal Magnetic Resonance Image 10 7 4 1

Parietooccipital Sulcus

Calcarine Sulcus

FIGURE 5–8. Variability in Brodmann areas.

Source. Used with permission from Mid-Atlantic Mental Illness Research, Education, and Clinical Center.

Subcortical Areas

Basal Ganglia

The basal ganglia are a group of small interconnected subcortical nuclei made up of the caudate nucleus, putamen, globus pallidus, claustrum, subthalamus, and substantia nigra. The caudate nucleus and putamen are often called the *corpus striatum,* and the globus pallidus and putamen are called the *lentiform nucleus.* Together, the structures of the basal ganglia are familiar to psychiatrists from disorders such as Huntington's chorea and Parkinson's disease or as the targets of many poison/toxin exposures. These nuclei serve a key role as a site for bringing emotion, executive function, motivation, and motor activity together. There are many input and output circuits that traverse these areas, including the three frontal lobe circuits of dorsolateral, orbitofrontal, and anterior cingulate gyrus (Burruss et al. 2000; Tekin and Cummings 2002; Tisch et al. 2004). Lesions within these structures result in syndromes of hypokinetic or hyperkinetic movements as well as cognitive and emotional dysfunction. The basal ganglia contain significant acetylcholine, dopamine, γ-aminobutyric acid (GABA), and neuropeptide projections. The dopaminergic projections have been pharmacological targets for schizophrenia and Parkinson's disease.

Caudate Nucleus

The caudate nuclei are C-shaped structures, each having a head, body, and tail. They arch to follow the walls of the lateral ventricles and terminate in the amygdaloid nuclei bilaterally. The caudate nucleus and putamen together are thought of as the input nuclei, receiving projections from the cerebral cortex, thalamus, and substantia nigra pars compacta. The major outputs for the caudate nucleus and putamen are the globus pallidus and substantia nigra pars reticulata. Neuropsychiatric symptoms of injury to the caudate nucleus are numerous and can be divided into behavioral, emotional, memory, language, and other symptoms. More commonly reported deficits include disinhibition, disorganization, executive dysfunction, apathy, depression, memory loss, atypical aphasia,

psychosis, personality changes, and predisposition for delirium.

Putamen

The putamen is the most lateral of the basal ganglia structures. It is separated from the caudate nucleus by the anterior limb of the internal capsule. The putamen and the caudate nucleus are considered input nuclei. (See "Caudate Nucleus" section above for afferent and efferent projections.) Neuropsychiatric symptoms of lesions to the putamen include primarily language and behavioral deficits (e.g., atypical aphasia, obsessive-compulsive traits, executive dysfunction). However, hemineglect, depression, and memory loss have been reported.

Globus Pallidus

The globus pallidus lies medial to the putamen and has two divisions (internal and external). The globus pallidus is functionally considered an output nucleus. Primary output is to the subthalamus and thalamus via GABAergic pathways. The neuropsychiatric symptoms most often associated with lesions to the globus pallidus are emotional. The most commonly reported symptoms are anxiety, depression, apathy, psychosis, and central pain. Less often reported symptoms include amnesia and cognitive deficits.

Substantia Nigra

The substantia nigra nuclei of the midbrain are dark because they contain melanin. They are divided into the pars compacta and pars reticulata. The former sends dopaminergic projections to the caudate nucleus and putamen. The latter receives input from the striatum and sends efferents to the thalamus, subthalamus, and reticular formation. Reported neuropsychiatric symptoms of lesions to the substantia nigra include primarily behavioral and emotional deficits (e.g., apraxia, ataxia, aggression, and depression), with less frequent reports of memory and cognitive deficits.

Shown next are illustrations of the major subcortical structures (Figure 5–9) and the basal forebrain (Figure 5–10). An axial atlas (Figures 5–11 through 5–16), color-coded to the major subcortical structures depicted in Figure 5–9, is then presented.

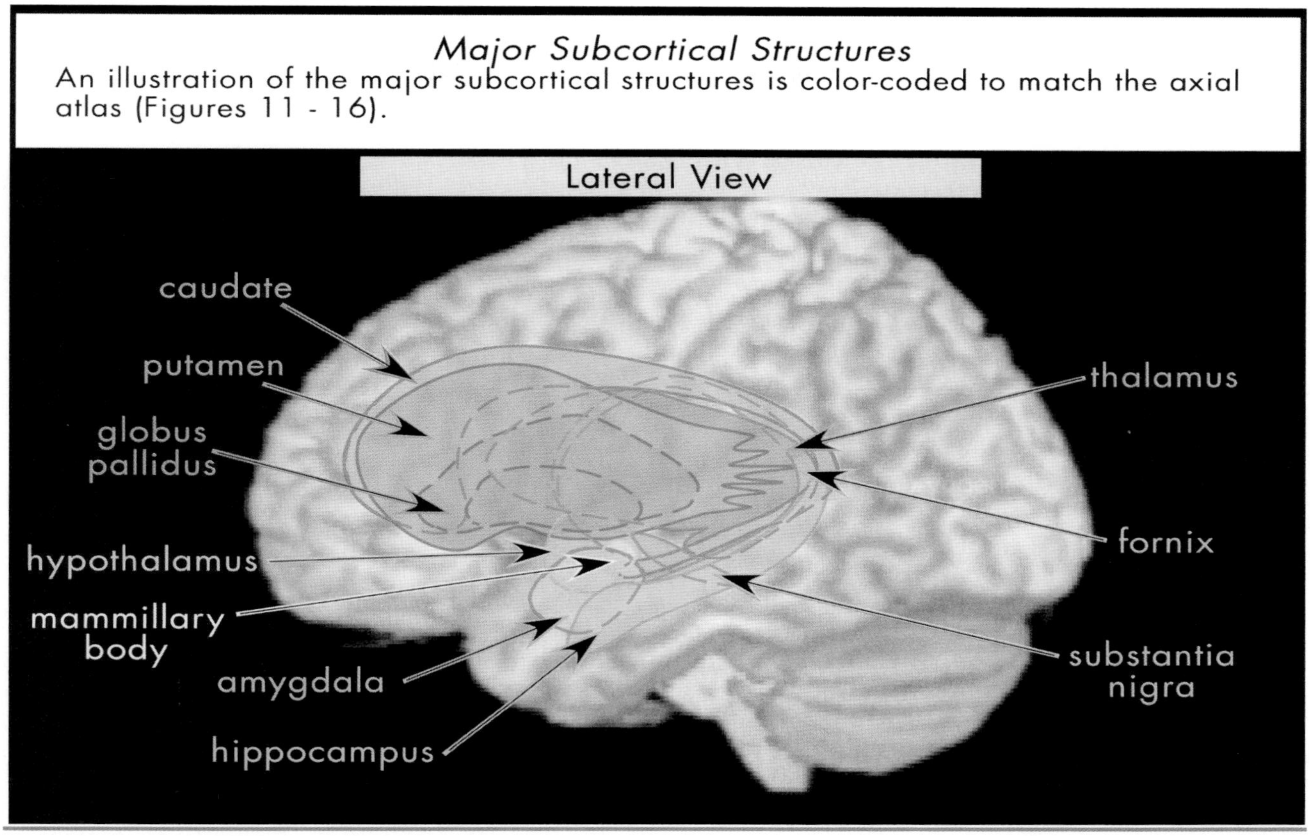

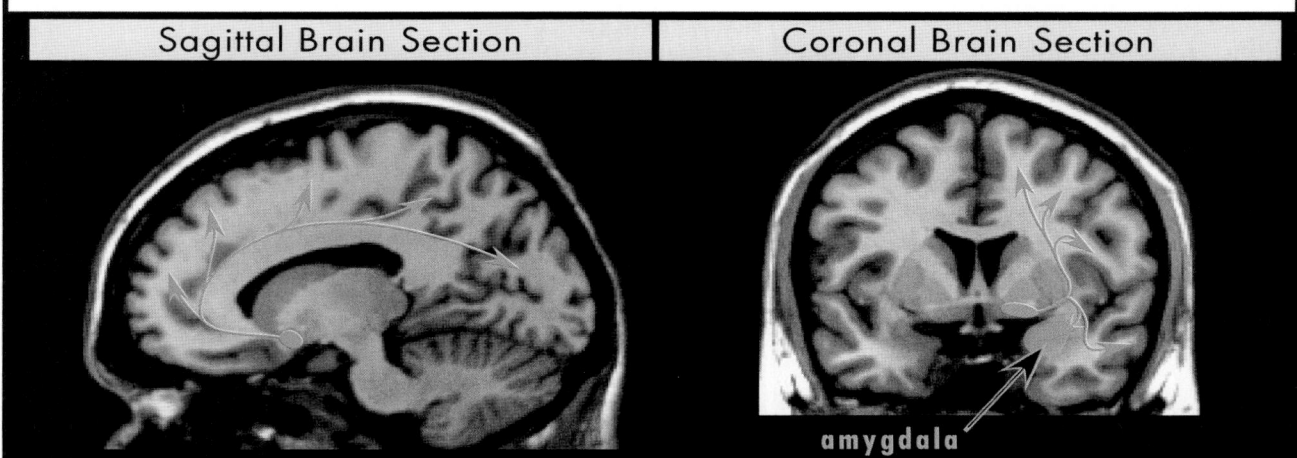

Major Subcortical Structures
An illustration of the major subcortical structures is color-coded to match the axial atlas (Figures 11 - 16).

Lateral View

caudate

putamen

globus pallidus

hypothalamus

mammillary body

amygdala

hippocampus

thalamus

fornix

substantia nigra

FIGURE 5–9. Major subcortical structures.

Source. Used with permission from Mid-Atlantic Mental Illness Research, Education, and Clinical Center.

Basal Forebrain
The basal forebrain area (basal nucleus of Meynert, nucleus of the diagonal band, septal nuclei) contains many cholinergic neurons. The general location of this important region and its projections to cortical and subcortical areas are indicated on sagittal and coronal magnetic resonance images.

Sagittal Brain Section

Coronal Brain Section

amygdala

FIGURE 5–10. Basal forebrain.

Source. Used with permission from Mid-Atlantic Mental Illness Research, Education, and Clinical Center.

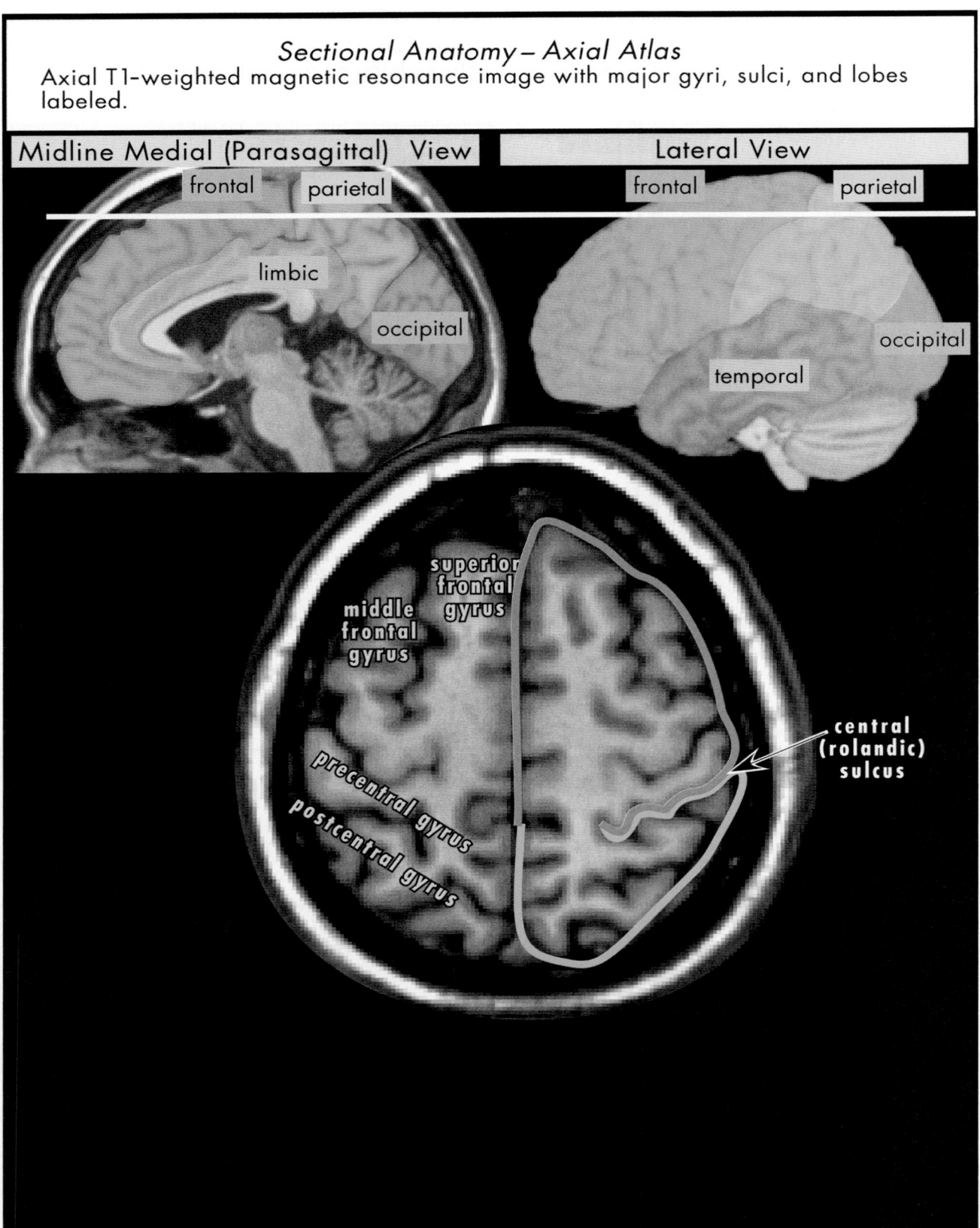

FIGURE 5–11.   Sectional anatomy—axial atlas: dorsal frontal and parietal cortices.

Source.   Used with permission from Mid-Atlantic Mental Illness Research, Education, and Clinical Center.

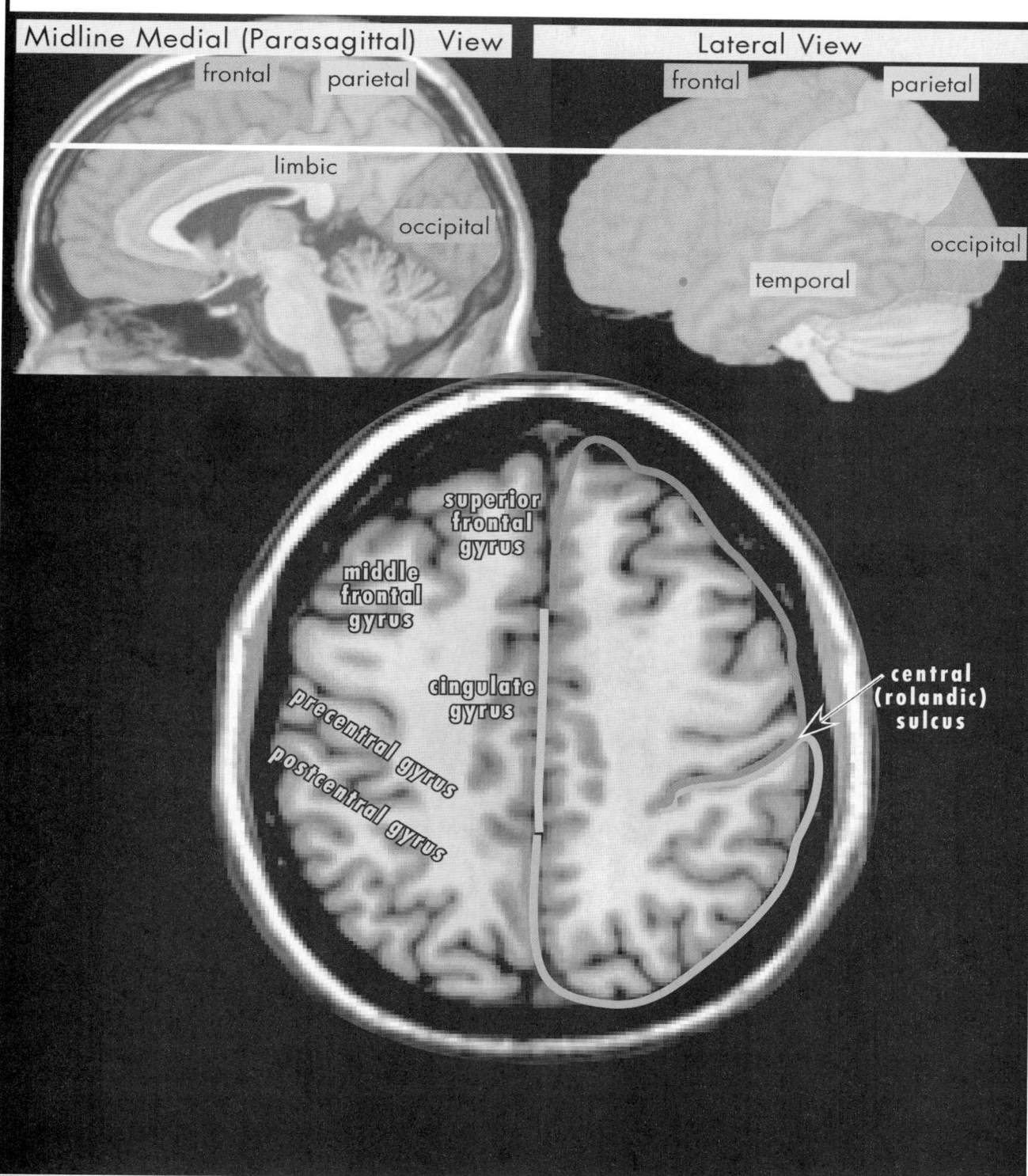

FIGURE 5–12. Sectional anatomy—axial atlas: cingulate cortex.

Source. Used with permission from Mid-Atlantic Mental Illness Research, Education, and Clinical Center.

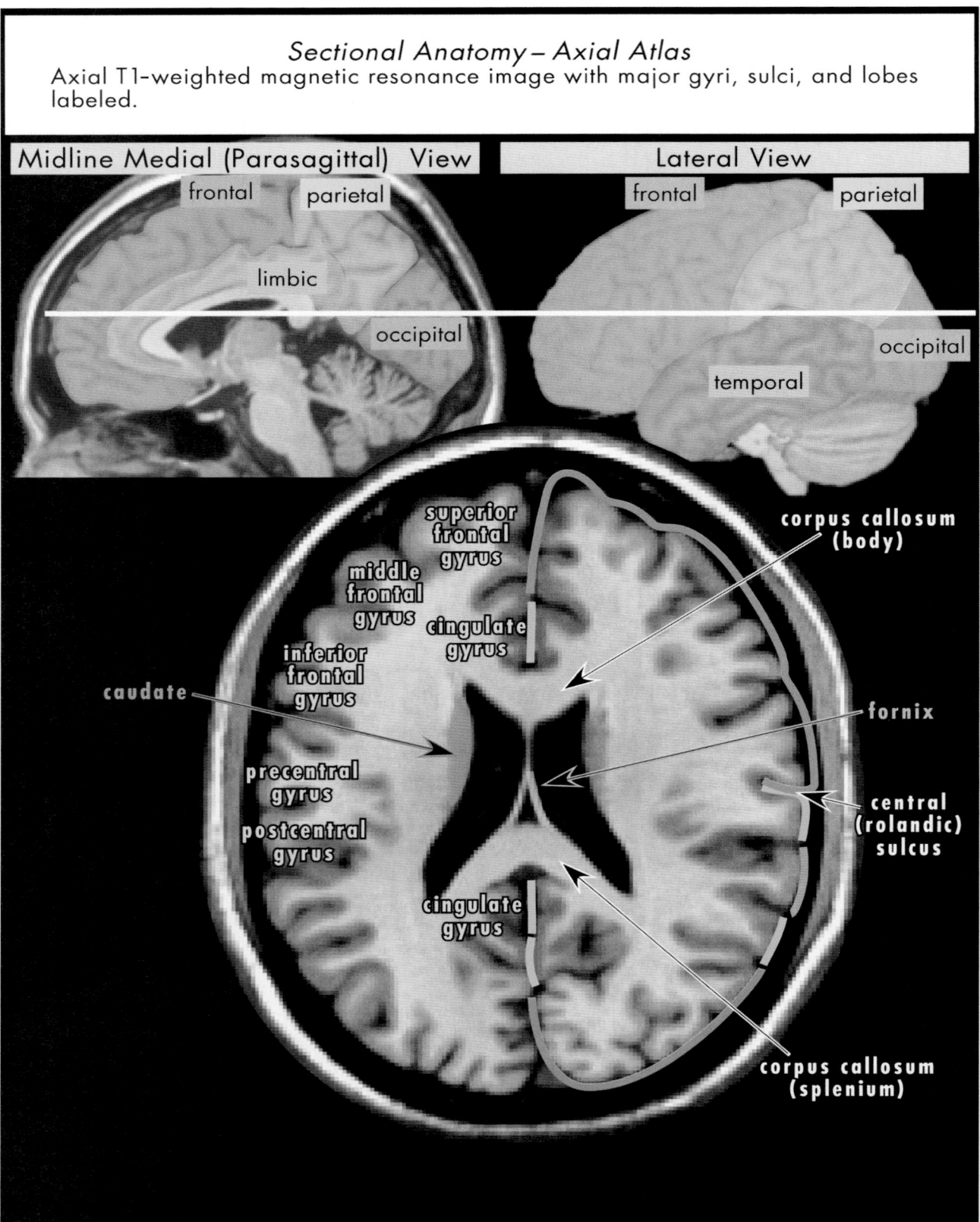

FIGURE 5–13. Sectional anatomy—axial atlas: dorsal occipital and parietal cortices, caudate.

Source. Used with permission from Mid-Atlantic Mental Illness Research, Education, and Clinical Center.

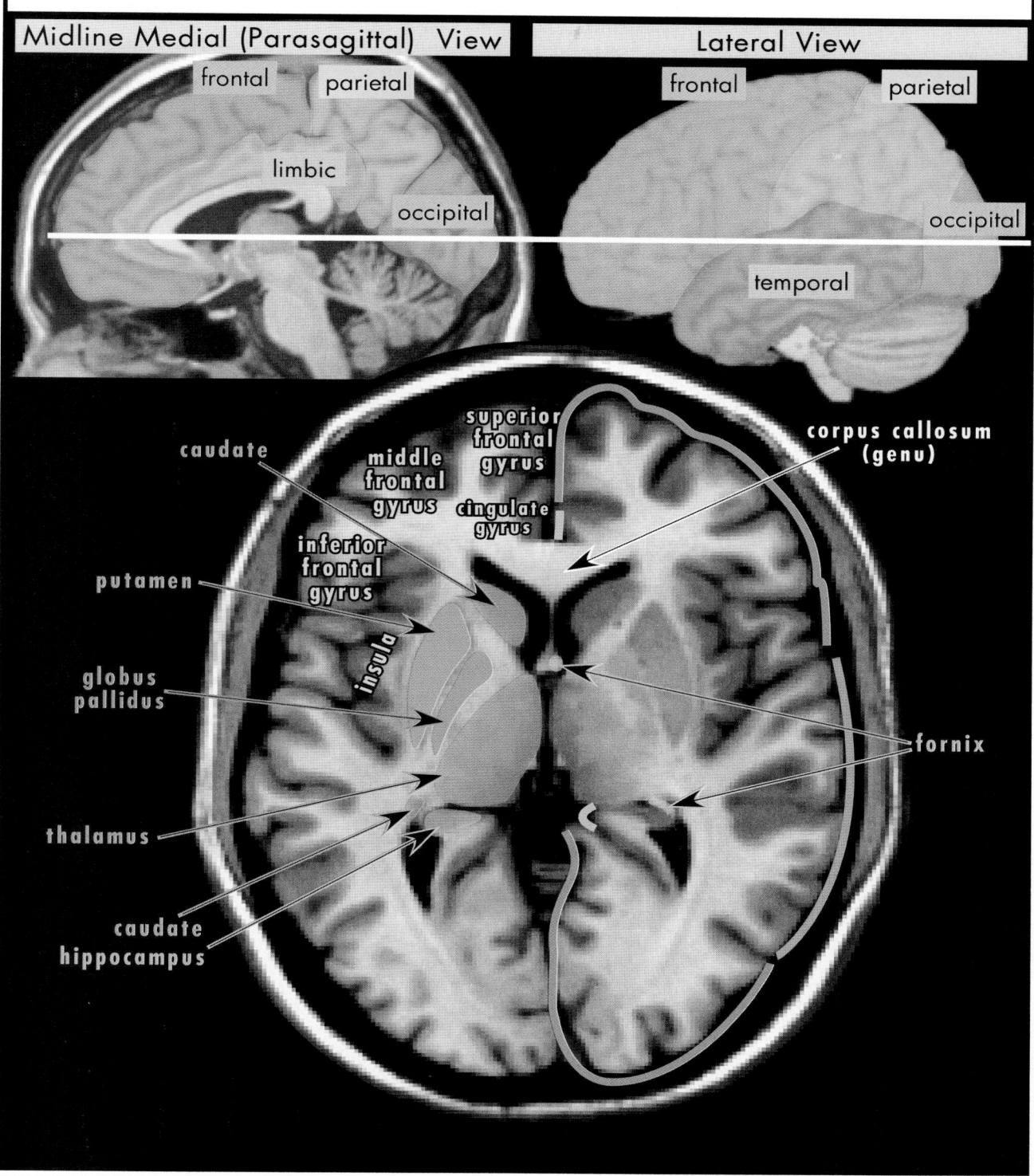

FIGURE 5–14. Sectional anatomy—axial atlas: insular cortex, basal ganglia, thalamus.

Source. Used with permission from Mid-Atlantic Mental Illness Research, Education, and Clinical Center.

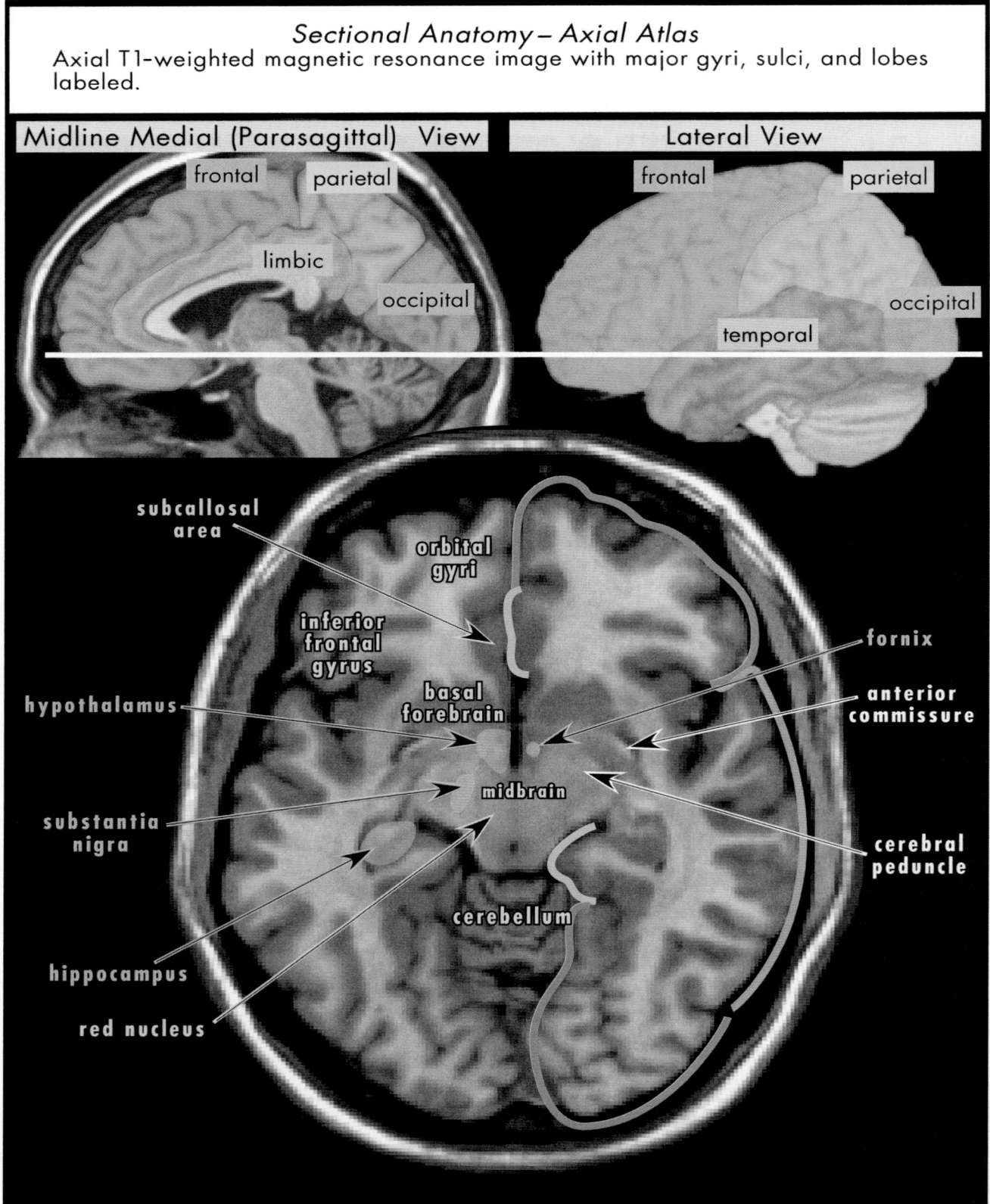

FIGURE 5–15. **Sectional anatomy—axial atlas: orbital cortex, basal forebrain, hippocampus, midbrain.**
Source.   Used with permission from Mid-Atlantic Mental Illness Research, Education, and Clinical Center.

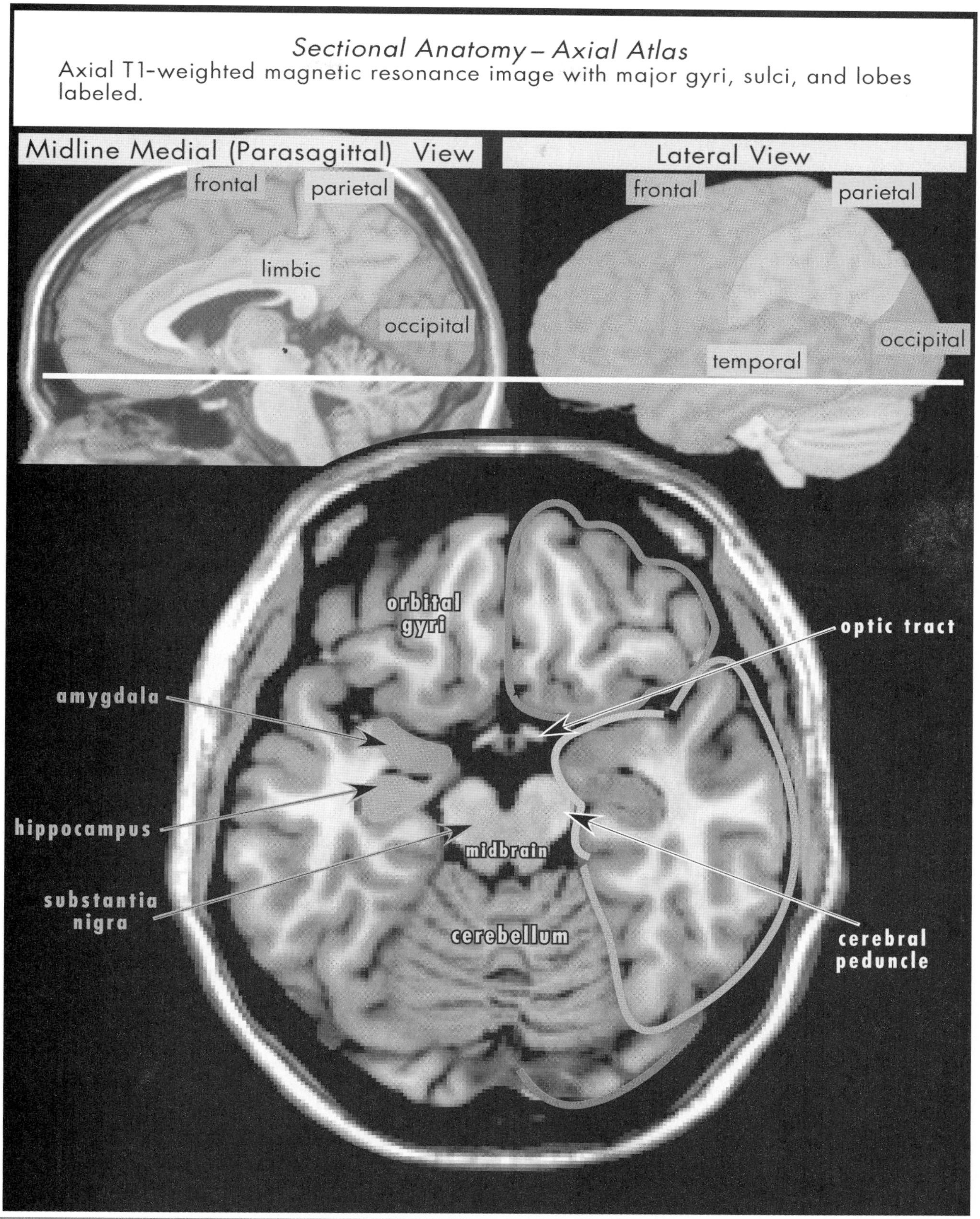

Sectional Anatomy – Axial Atlas
Axial T1-weighted magnetic resonance image with major gyri, sulci, and lobes labeled.

FIGURE 5–16.   **Sectional anatomy—axial atlas: orbital cortex, hippocampus, amygdala, midbrain.**
Source.   Used with permission from Mid-Atlantic Mental Illness Research, Education, and Clinical Center.

Limbic System

The term *limbic system* is most often used to describe the areas of brain involved in the production of emotion, memory, or aggression (Dalgleish 2004; Heimer and Van Hoesen 2006; Morgane and Mokler 2006). Originally suggested by Broca (*"le grand lobe limbique"*), the name is purely descriptive of the anatomic location of these structures (*limbus* means "border," and these structures border the neocortex). Papez suggested that these areas were important for memory and emotion, rather than just smell, as had been previously believed. MacLean applied the name "limbic system" to the circuit of Papez, reasoning that these structures are placed to integrate signals from the external and internal worlds. Commonly, these structures are divided into an outer and an inner lobe. Other areas closely associated with these, and often considered part of the limbic system, include the mammillary bodies and parts of the thalamus. Some authors also include other areas, such as the orbitofrontal cortex and hypothalamus.

Shown next are illustrations of the limbic lobes (Figure 5–17) and the circuit of Papez (Figure 5–18), color-coded to match the summary of subcortical structures (see Figure 5–9) and the sectional axial atlas (see Figures 5–11 through 5–16).

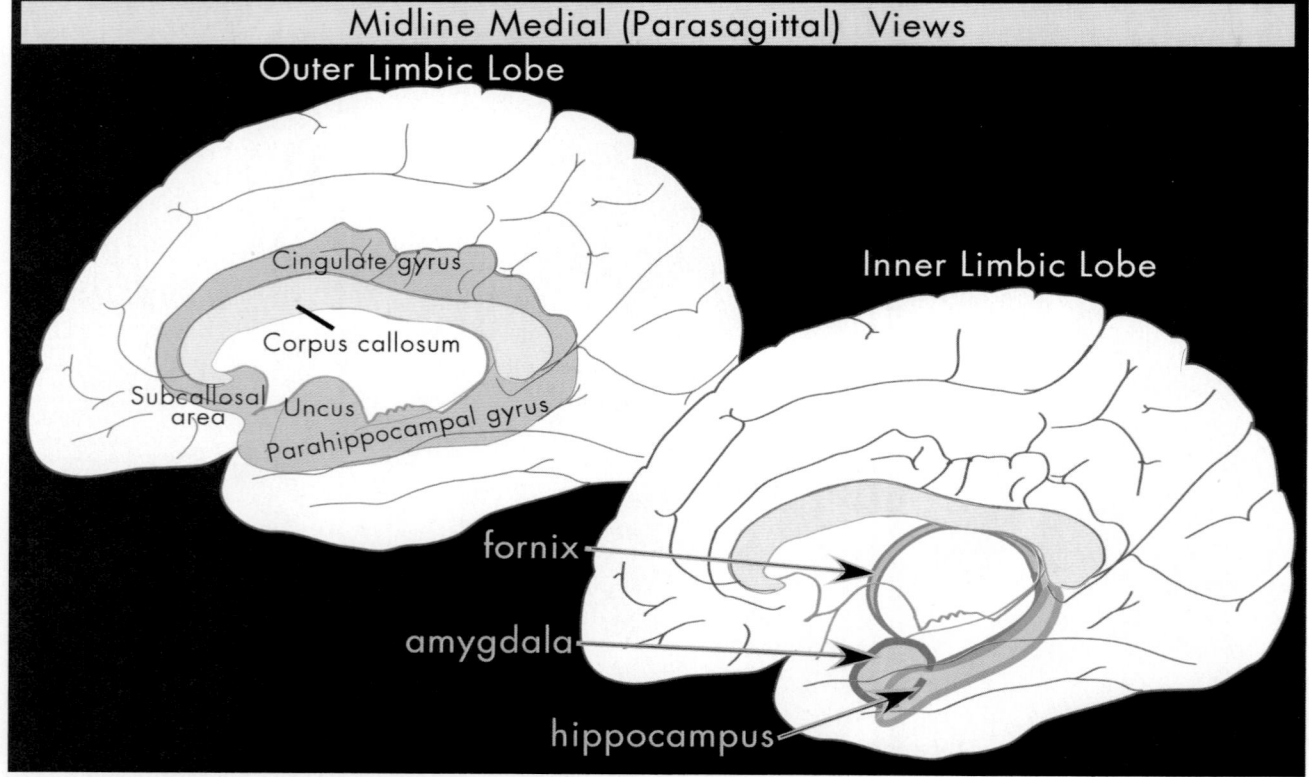

The Limbic Lobes

The location and names of the structures that make up the outer (surface of brain) and inner (deep structures) limbic lobes are illustrated on schematic diagrams of the medial surface of the right cerebral hemisphere. Structures are color-coded to match the summary of subcortical structures (Figure 9) and the sectional axial atlas (Figures 11 – 16).

Midline Medial (Parasagittal) Views

Outer Limbic Lobe

Cingulate gyrus

Corpus callosum

Subcallosal area   Uncus

Parahippocampal gyrus

Inner Limbic Lobe

fornix

amygdala

hippocampus

FIGURE 5–17.   Limbic lobes.

Source.   Used with permission from Mid-Atlantic Mental Illness Research, Education, and Clinical Center.

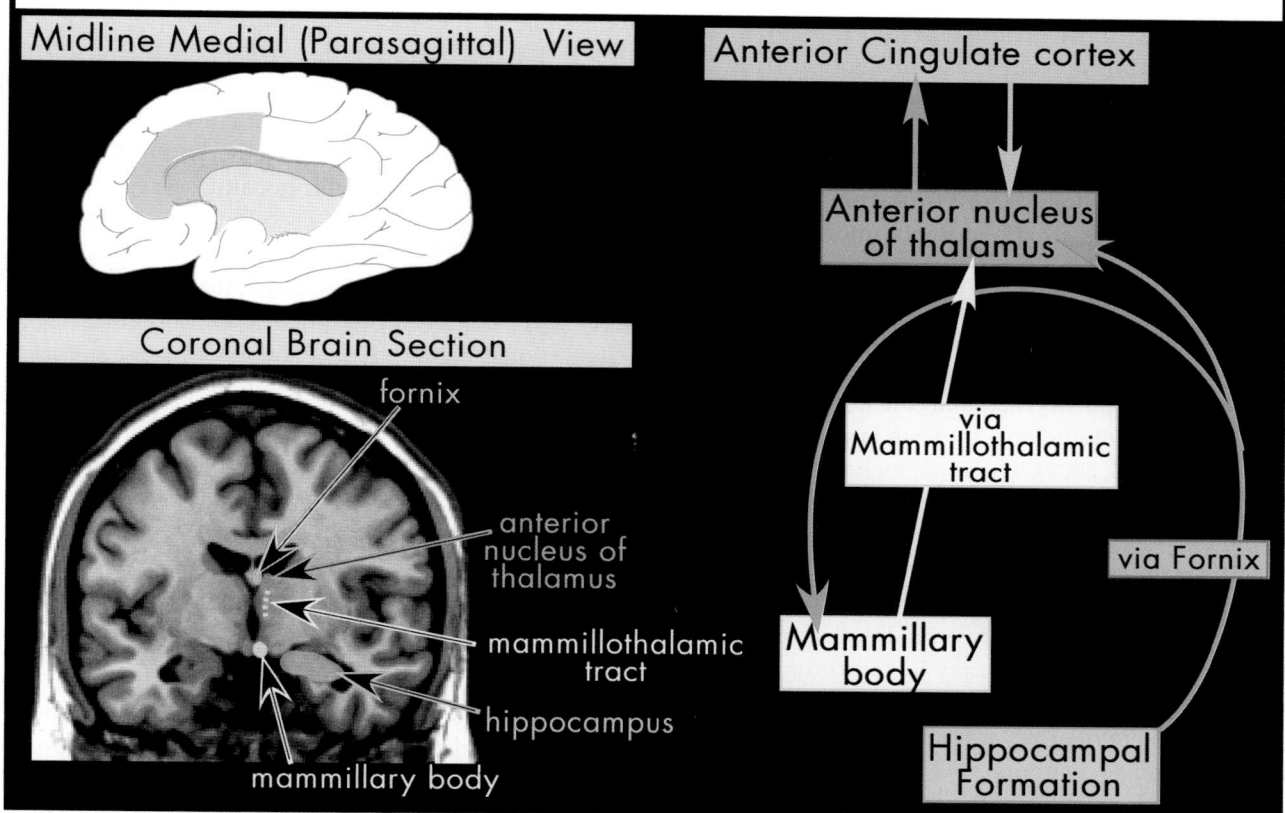

FIGURE 5–18. Circuit of Papez.

Source. Used with permission from Mid-Atlantic Mental Illness Research, Education, and Clinical Center.

Hippocampal Formation and Parahippocampal Cortex

The hippocampal formation and parahippocampal cortex (or gyrus) are collectively considered to be the "memory structures." They function, in essence, to form and direct the storage of memories. The parahippocampus extends from the cingulate cortex to the amygdala. The main body of the hippocampal formation extends from the crus of the fornix to the amygdala, located in the medial temporal lobe. Neuropsychiatric symptoms of lesions to the hippocampal formation are primarily memory deficits. These include anterograde and retrograde amnesia, inability to form new memories, and temporally graded amnesia.

The fornix is the major fiber tract of the hippocampal formation. It is made up of both afferent and efferent hippocampal fibers. Neuropsychiatric symptoms of lesions to the fornix are memory deficits, and they overlap symptoms that follow damage to the hippocampal formation, including impaired recent memory, syndrome of transitory amnesia, and long-term anterograde amnesia.

Amygdala

The amygdala lies at the juncture of the tail of the caudate nucleus and the anteriormost ends of the parahippocampus and hippocampus. It sends projections to the basal forebrain and striatum, hypothalamus, thalamus, midbrain, and brain stem. Neuropsychiatric symptoms of lesions to the amygdala are primarily behavioral and emotional and include passivity or aggression; hypersexuality; hyperorality; hyperphagia; decreased fear, anxiety, or startle; and decreased link between emotion and memory.

Mammillary Bodies

The mammillary bodies are two small round nuclei that lie in the posterior portion of the diencephalon. They receive afferents from the hippocampus and send efferents to the brain stem and thalamus. The mammillothalamic tract is the projection from the mammillary bodies to the anterior nucleus of the thalamus. Neuropsychiatric symptoms with lesions of the mammillary body or its tract are primarily memory deficits and psychosis. Confabulation and anterograde memory loss are the most common.

Thalamus

The thalamus is medial to the caudate nucleus and putamen and lateral to the third ventricle. The superior and medial portions contain the anterior nucleus, the medial dorsal nucleus, and the lateral dorsal nucleus (Taber et al. 2004). These nuclei have intimate interconnections with the limbic system. Injury to the medial portion of the left thalamus is associated with deficits in language, verbal intellect, and verbal memory. Injury to the right thalamus is associated with deficits in visuospatial and nonverbal intellect and visual memory. Medial thalamus may be important for temporal aspects of memory. Bilateral damage is associated with severe memory impairment ("thalamic amnesia") as well as dementia. The memory deficits may result from destruction of the tracts connecting these thalamic nuclei with limbic structures. Injury to the anterior and medial thalamus can also result in disturbances of autonomic functions, mood, and the sleep–wake cycle.

Hypothalamus

The hypothalamus lies ventral to the thalamus around the third ventricle. It has projections to and from the orbitofrontal cortex, the limbic circuits, the thalamus, the reticular formation, and the autonomic and endocrine systems. Thus, it is a key structure in bridging internal homeostasis and the outside environment. Behavioral, emotional, and memory symptoms as well as other deficits are associated with lesions to the hypothalamus. Examples of commonly reported symptoms are aggression, violence, anorexia, depression, impaired short-term memory, dementia, gelastic (laughing) seizures, and altered sleep–wake cycle.

Pons

The pons lies in the posterior fossa between the midbrain and the medulla oblongata. It contains nuclei and tracts that are necessary for arousal (reticular formation) and affective stability. The raphe nuclei (found at the midline along the entire brain stem) send serotonergic projections to structures throughout the brain, including the thalamus, hippocampus, basal ganglia, and frontal cortex. The locus coeruleus is also found in the pons. It sends noradrenergic projections to the limbic system, hypothalamus, thalamus, cerebellum, and cerebral cortex. Neuropsychiatric symptoms from pontine lesions include behavioral, emotional, language, memory, and other deficits. Commonly reported deficits include disinhibition, disturbed sleep–wake cycles, anxiety, depression, emotional lability, cognitive deficits, central pain, personality changes, and psychosis.

Cerebellum

The cerebellum lies ventral to the temporal and occipital lobes and the pons, surrounding the fourth ventricle. In addition to its extensive connections with the motor system, the cerebellum projects (via the thalamus) to cingulate, dorsomedial prefrontal, and dorsolateral prefrontal cortices (Middleton and Strick 2000; Schmahmann and Pandya 1997a, 1997b; Taber et al. 2005).

Recent work indicates that cerebellar lesions, particularly to the posterior cerebellum and vermis, can result in a range of cognitive and emotional deficits including executive dysfunction, visuospatial deficits, personality changes, and linguistic abnormalities (Konarski et al. 2005; Rapoport et al. 2000; Schmahmann 2004; Taber et al. 2005; Turner and Schiavetto 2004).

Shown next are illustrations of the surface anatomy and circuits (Figure 5–19) and sectional anatomy (Figure 5–20) of the prefrontal cortex, followed by a summary of functional anatomy pertinent to psychiatry (Table 5–1).

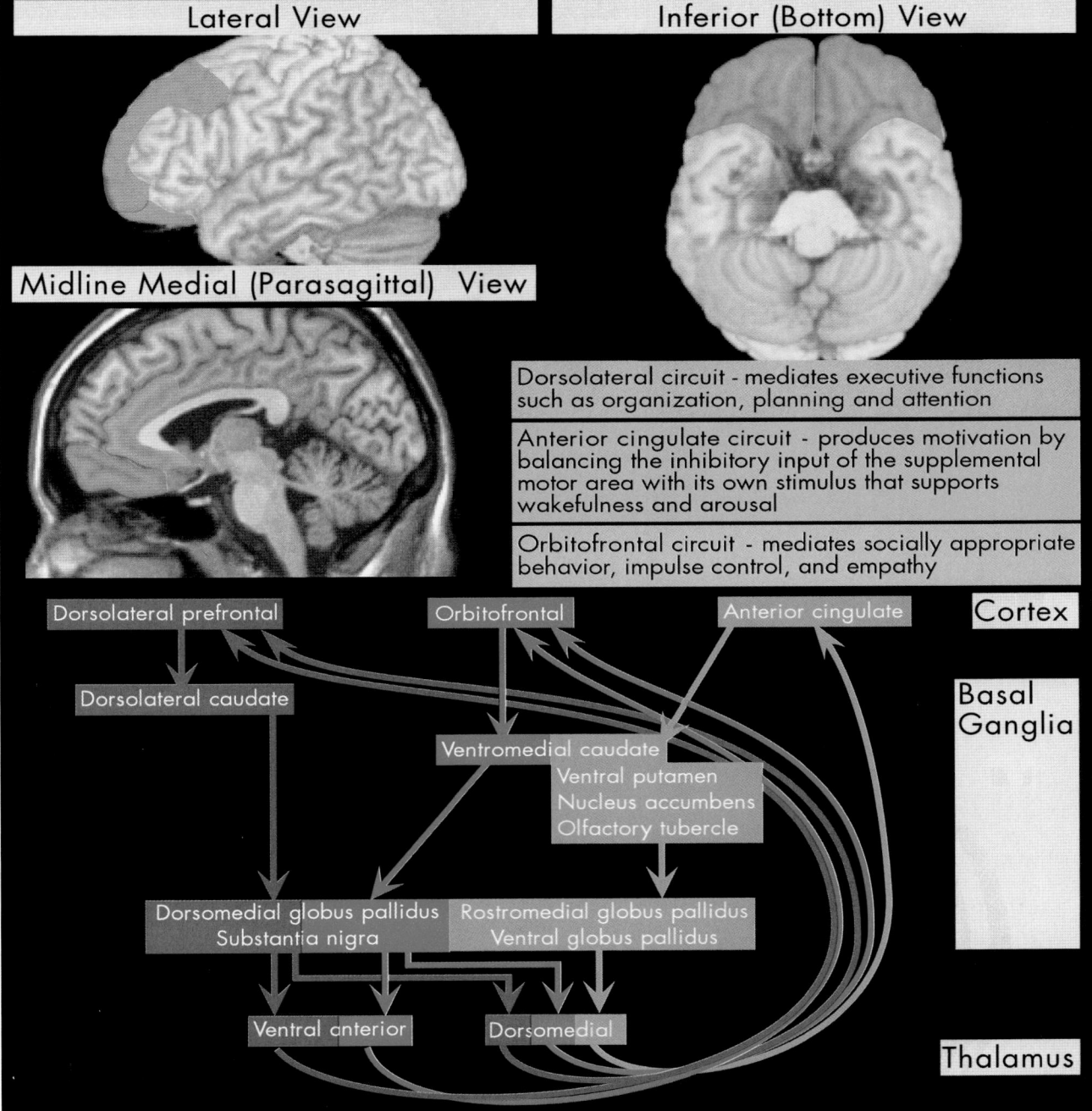

Prefrontal Cortex—Surface Anatomy and Circuits

In psychiatry, the prefrontal cortex is generally divided into three principal areas. Each area has reciprocal connections with subcortical structures that form cortico-subcortical circuits. These circuits are formed by chains of neurons with cell bodies in gray matter structures (both cortical and subcortical) connected by the axons that form the white matter. Recently, the evidence supporting a similar reciprocal circuit to the cerebellum has strengthened, although its functions are still controversial.

Lateral View

Inferior (Bottom) View

Midline Medial (Parasagittal) View

Dorsolateral circuit - mediates executive functions such as organization, planning and attention

Anterior cingulate circuit - produces motivation by balancing the inhibitory input of the supplemental motor area with its own stimulus that supports wakefulness and arousal

Orbitofrontal circuit - mediates socially appropriate behavior, impulse control, and empathy

Dorsolateral prefrontal   Orbitofrontal   Anterior cingulate   Cortex

Dorsolateral caudate

Basal Ganglia

Ventromedial caudate
Ventral putamen
Nucleus accumbens
Olfactory tubercle

Dorsomedial globus pallidus   Rostromedial globus pallidus
Substantia nigra   Ventral globus pallidus

Ventral anterior   Dorsomedial   Thalamus

FIGURE 5–19.   **Prefrontal cortex—surface anatomy and circuits.**

Source.   Used with permission from Mid-Atlantic Mental Illness Research, Education, and Clinical Center.

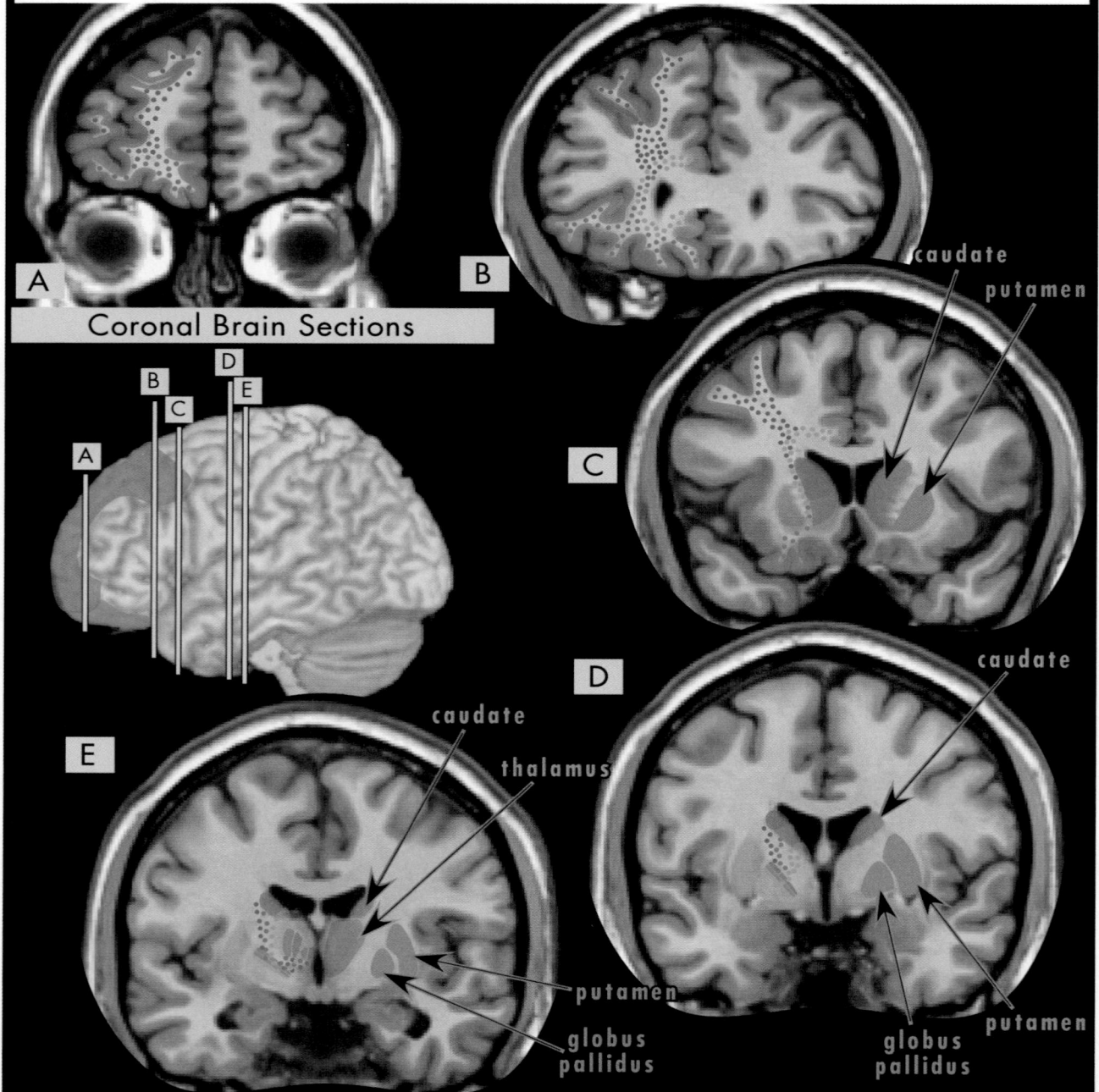

FIGURE 5–20.   Prefrontal cortex—sectional anatomy.

Source.   Used with permission from Mid-Atlantic Mental Illness Research, Education, and Clinical Center.

TABLE 5–1.   Summary of functional anatomy pertinent to psychiatry

Brain region or structure	Functions of interest	Common consequences of injury
Cortical areas		
Frontal lobe—executive functions, personality, intellect, speech, motor functions, memory		
Frontal operculum		
Left (Broca's area)	Adds fluency to speech	Broca's aphasia (nonfluent speech)—difficulty with naming, awareness of deficit, deficit in repetition, comprehension is intact
Right	Adds emotion to speech—gesturing, speech prosody	Expressive aphasia—loss of emotion in speech, comprehension is intact
Superior mesial region	Initiation and synchronization of speech and complex movements	Akinetic mutism—no efforts to communicate, empty face, limited body/arm movements (may resolve if injury is to one side)
Orbital and inferior mesial region	Social conduct, insight, judgment—allows one to withhold emotional responses to situation	Severe disruption of social conduct, including defects in planning, judgment, and decision making; impaired ability to add feelings to actions; inability to feel autonomic response to traumatic or anxious situations (similar to psychopathic traits)
Dorsolateral prefrontal region		
Left	Focused attention, verbal intellect, verbal memory management	Intellectual deficits, loss of memory for frequency of time and events, inability to maintain focus or attention, inability to shift focus (e.g., schizophrenia)
Right	Focused attention, nonverbal intellect, nonverbal memory management	
Motor cortex	Allows physical movement of muscle groups	Paralysis of contralateral side
Temporal lobe—hearing, naming of objects, memory, emotion, visual recognition		
Lateral inferior region		
Left	Visual recognition	Prosopagnosia—agnosia for faces (varying degrees depending on lesion size)
Right	Visuospatial recognition	Loss of recognition of objects in time and space

TABLE 5–1. Summary of functional anatomy pertinent to psychiatry *(continued)*

Brain region or structure	Functions of interest	Common consequences of injury
Temporal lobe—hearing, naming of objects, memory, emotion, visual recognition *(continued)*		
Lateral anterior region		
Left	Naming of objects	Naming deficits, especially for natural objects (vs. manmade)
Right	Naming of objects, retrograde episodic memory	Naming deficits, memory loss for past events in time
Dorsolateral area (small)	Hearing	Deafness if bilateral
Mesial temporal region		
Hippocampal complex (hippocampus, parahippocampal gyrus)		Anterograde declarative memory loss, procedural memory spared
Left	Formation and storage of verbal declarative (autobiographical) memory	Amnesia for verbal material (e.g., spoken words, written material)
Right	Formation and storage of nonverbal declarative (autobiographical) memory	Amnesia for nonverbal material (e.g., complex auditory or visual patterns)
Amygdala	Adds emotion to memory, important for recognition of emotion	Loss of emotional attachment to memories, emotional dyscontrol (e.g., Klüver-Bucy syndrome)
Occipital lobe—vision, visual association (support) areas		
Primary visual cortex	Vision, color perception, whole object imaging, reading—connects right to left visual information	Visual field cuts
Visual association cortex	Visual orientation, peripheral gaze direction, visual guidance, visual scanning	
Dorsal component (primary visual cortex and visual association cortex above calcarine sulcus)		Balint's syndrome—visual disorientation, ocular apraxia, optic ataxia, defective motion perception, no depth perception (partial or mild for unilateral lesions)

TABLE 5–1. Summary of functional anatomy pertinent to psychiatry *(continued)*

Brain region or structure	Functions of interest	Common consequences of injury
Occipital lobe—vision, visual association (support) areas *(continued)*		
Ventral component (primary visual cortex and visual association cortex below calcarine sulcus)		
Left		Left hemiachromatopsia, apperceptive visual agnosia, defective facial imagery, "pure" alexia
Right		Right hemiachromatopsia, "pure" alexia, impaired mental imagery
Bilateral		Full field achromatopsia, visual object agnosia, impaired mental imagery, prosopagnosia
Parietal lobe—sensation, speech, understanding, academics		
Temporoparietal junction		
Left (Wernicke's area)	Sensical speech production, verbal repetition, aural comprehension	Wernicke's aphasia (fluent paraphasic speech)—frequent errors in word choice, impaired repetition, defective aural comprehension
Right	Recognition and processing of music and voice	Amusia—nonrecognition of music and voice
Bilateral		Auditory agnosia—inability to recognize any sounds
Inferior parietal lobule		
Left	Speech conduction, verbal repetition, sensical speech production, object naming, reading aloud, spelling, writing to dictation, ability to calculate	Conduction aphasia—impaired repetition, fluent paraphasic speech, defective object naming, impaired oral reading, inability to spell or write to dictation, tactile object agnosia, acalculia
Right	Audiovisual awareness, deficit recognition	Neglect—unawareness of audio and visual modalities, neglect of intra- and extrapersonal space Anosognosia—denial of acquired motor, sensory, or cognitive deficit (e.g., denial of paretic limb)
Bilateral		Body schema disturbances, anosognosia
Optic tracts	Vision	Visual field loss

TABLE 5–1.   Summary of functional anatomy pertinent to psychiatry *(continued)*

Brain region or structure	Functions of interest	Common consequences of injury
Parietal lobe—sensation, speech, understanding, academics *(continued)*		
Superior parietal lobule		
Sensory association cortex	Sensory integration and recognition for contralateral side of body	Loss of sensory integration and recognition
Sensory cortex	Somatosensory for contralateral side of body	Numbness of contralateral side
Other cortical structures		
Insula (located beneath the frontal operculum)	Smell	Loss of smell if lesion is bilateral
Basal forebrain (common site of pathology in Alzheimer's disease; anterior communicating artery aneurysm rupture or repair may injure this area)	Memory formation, storage and retrieval (large acetylcholine supply)	Severe memory deficits—deficits particularly in anterograde memory, cannot integrate learned information, confabulation
Subcortical areas		
Basal ganglia—movement, emotion		
Caudate	Voluntary motor movements, planning and programming of movement, suppression of involuntary movement, anterograde memory, contribution to mood	Hemiparesis if lesioned close to the internal capsule; gross abnormal involuntary movement, subcortical dementia, depression, loss of planning and programming of movement
Left	Fluent, articulate speech production, comprehension, repetition of speech	Fluent paraphasic, dysarthric speech with poor comprehension and impaired repetition
Globus pallidus	Functions as a unit with the caudate	Lesions produce similar picture as the caudate, more vulnerable to poisons/toxins
Putamen	Functions as a unit with the caudate and globus pallidus	Lesions produce similar picture as the caudate or globus pallidus, more vulnerable to poisons/toxins
Substantia nigra	Modulates involuntary movement, muscle tone, and posture	Fine abnormal involuntary movement, decreased muscle tone, loss of postural control
Subthalamic nucleus		

TABLE 5–1. Summary of functional anatomy pertinent to psychiatry *(continued)*

Brain region or structure	Functions of interest	Common consequences of injury
Thalamus—"relay station" for the entire basal ganglia and cerebral cortex		
Limbic nuclei		
Medial dorsal Anterior Lateral dorsal	Memory, emotion Problem-solving skills	Severe anterograde amnesia, especially for declarative memory (memory for facts, time, and events), confabulation, disturbance of problem solving
Motor nuclei		
Ventroanterior Ventrolateral	Motor stabilization	Paralysis or difficulty executing movement
Sensory nuclei		
Ventroposteromedial Ventroposterolateral	Somatosensory	Loss of sensory functions—may include loss of balance or ability to walk secondary to inability to "feel the feet"
Medial geniculate	Receives the cochlear nerve, origin of the auditory radiations to the temporal lobe: hearing	Deafness if lesions are bilateral
Lateral geniculate	Receives the optic tract, origin of the optic radiation to the occipital cortex: vision	Blindness in the contralateral field of vision
Pulvinar	Connections to lateral and medial geniculate—interconnections of the visual and auditory systems with the parietal cortex	Disconnection of visual and auditory information
Hypothalamus	Temperature control, sleep, water metabolism, hormone secretion, blood pressure control, satiety, maintenance of balance, circadian rhythms Modulates physiological reaction to emotional stimuli	Hyper-/hypothermia, insomnia, polydipsia, hormone hyper-/hyposecretion, hyper-/hypotension, hunger, hyper-/hyporeaction to emotional stimuli (e.g., excessive startle response)

TABLE 5–1. Summary of functional anatomy pertinent to psychiatry *(continued)*

Brain region or structure	Functions of interest	Common consequences of injury
Pineal body/gland	Contains no nerve tracts—secretes hormones directly into the bloodstream, inhibits endocrine gland production (pituitary islets of Langerhans, parathyroids, adrenals, gonads), circadian rhythm function—most active in the dark Also releases melatonin, serotonin, norepinephrine	Hormonal dysfunction in the endocrine system (pituitary, pancreas, adrenal glands, parathyroids, or gonads)
Reticular activating system (RAS)—consciousness	Nuclei and tracts for this system are in medulla, pons, and midbrain. It receives stimuli from the hypothalamus, basal ganglia, vestibular system, and sensory input from the body. It projects to thalamus and cerebral cortex. The RAS controls the degree of consciousness and alertness (e.g., sleep, stupor).	
Midbrain—consciousness, fiber tracts, cranial nerves		
Tectum—superior and inferior colliculi		
Tegmentum—cerebral peduncles (basis pedunculi)		
Red nucleus		
Cranial nerve 3 and nucleus		
Cranial nerve 4 and nucleus		
Pons—mood, motor and sensory tracts, wakefulness		
Locus coeruleus	Number 1 producer of norepinephrine in the brain—sleep, wakefulness, control of mood	Hyper-/hyposomnia, emotional lability (including pathological crying)
Raphe nucleus	Contains the tracts that directly connect to the thalamus, basal ganglia, and hypothalamus—motor and mood control, production of serotonin	Motor lesions; behavioral changes, including emotional dyscontrol
Central pons	Contains the reticular core—alertness	Stupor
Cranial nerves 4, 5, and 6 and nuclei	Eye muscles, motor and facial nerves	Deficits depend on which cranial nerve is lesioned

TABLE 5–1. Summary of functional anatomy pertinent to psychiatry *(continued)*

Brain region or structure	Functions of interest	Common consequences of injury
Cerebellum—equilibrium, muscle tone		
Flocculonodular lobe Central nodulus Paired flocculus	Truncal equilibrium	Instability, incoordination of head and trunk
Anterior lobe (includes vermis)	Gross head and body movement, muscle tone	Movement decomposition, ataxia, gait alternation, nystagmus, dysarthria, slurred speech
Posterior lobe (includes vermis)	Voluntary muscle coordination	Cognitive and emotional deficits in addition to motor dysfunctions listed for anterior lobe
Brain stem (medulla oblongata)—ascending and descending fiber tracts, respiratory centers		
Cranial nerves 8–12 and nuclei, as well as respiratory and cardiac centers		With increased pressure of lesion, herniation, coma, and death

Source. From Nolte 2002; Tranel 2002.

Conclusion

In summary, this chapter presents the practicing psychiatrist with an overview of the basic structures of the brain and common orientation guides to assist in reading anatomical literature/neuroimaging reports. A color-coded atlas is provided for visual learning. The chapter also includes a basic summary of functional anatomy as it relates to the cortex and the larger subcortical areas most pertinent to emotional, behavioral, and memory/cognitive performance. These neurobehavioral functions happen by way of circuits that start and end in the cortical areas, with pathways that traverse the brain. The circuits, although quite extensive, are believed to have both direct and indirect loops, pathways, and supporting elements. Often, lesions in multiple positions along a circuit can give the same clinical presentation, thus making the relationship between brain and behavior all the more confusing. It is critical for the practicing psychiatrist to have a basic awareness of the major anatomical structures that have known associations to emotion, memory, cognition, and behavior. Those structures include the cortical lobes, limbic system, basal ganglia, thalamus, hypothalamus, pons, and cerebellum. A fundamental understanding of this anatomy will assist the practicing clinician in the diagnostic assessment of patients with potential or known illnesses/lesions causing psychiatric symptoms.

Key Points

- The dorsolateral prefrontal region is important for cognition, executive function, and focused attention.

- The orbital prefrontal region is important for social conduct, insight, judgment, and mood.

- The mesial region of the temporal lobe contains the hippocampus, the parahippocampus, and the amygdala.

- The hippocampal complex is the key to memory formation and storage functions.

- The parietal lobe is important for sensation, speech production/conduction, and deficit recognition.

- The basal ganglia are critical for suppression/modulation of involuntary movements and contribute to memory, cognition, behavior, and mood.

- The thalamus is the key "relay station" for memory, emotion, cognition, behavior, motor, and sensory functions.

- The hypothalamus modulates physiological response to emotional stimuli, temperature control, sleep, water metabolism, hormone secretion, satiety, and circadian rhythms.

- The pons contains the locus coeruleus (norepinephrine production) and portions of the reticular formation (alertness).

- The cerebellum is important for equilibrium and fine motor coordination and is associated with cognition.

Suggested Readings

Hurley RA, Taber KH: Windows to the Brain: Insights From Neuroimaging. Arlington, VA, American Psychiatric Publishing, 2008

Nolte J: The Human Brain. St. Louis, MO, Mosby, 2002

Snell RS: Clinical Neuroanatomy for Medical Students, 6th Edition. Philadelphia, PA, Lippincott Williams & Wilkins, 2005

Tekin S, Cummings JL: Frontal-subcortical neuronal circuits and clinical neuropsychiatry: an update. J Psychosom Res 53:647–654, 2002

Harel BT, Tranel D: Functional neuroanatomy: neuropsychological correlates of cortical and subcortical damage, in The American Psychiatric Publishing Textbook of Neuropsychiatry and Behavioral Neurosciences, 5th Edition. Edited by Yudofsky SC, Hales RE. Arlington, VA, American Psychiatric Publishing, 2008, pp 45–91

References

Amunts K, Malikovic A, Mohlberg H, et al: Brodmann's areas 17 and 18 brought into stereotaxic space—Where and how variable? Neuroimage 11:66–84, 2000

Amunts K, Weiss PH, Mohlberg H, et al: Analysis of neural mechanisms underlying verbal fluency in cytoarchitectonically defined stereotaxic space—the roles of Brodmann areas 44 and 45. Neuroimage 22:42–56, 2004

Burruss JW, Hurley RA, Taber KH, et al: Functional neuroanatomy of the frontal lobe circuits. Radiology 214:227–230, 2000

Dalgleish T: The emotional brain. Nat Med 5:582, 2004

Damasio H, Grabowski T, Frank R, et al: The return of Phineas Gage: clues about the brain from the skull of a famous patient. Science 264:1102–1105, 1994

Heimer L, Van Hoesen GW: The limbic lobe and its output channels: implications for emotional functions and adaptive behavior. Neurosci Biobehav Rev 30:126–147, 2006

Konarski JZ, McIntyre RS, Grupp LA, et al: Is the cerebellum relevant in the circuitry of neuropsychiatric disorders? J Psychiatry Neurosci 30:178–186, 2005

Mesulam M: Principles of Behavioral and Cognitive Neurology. New York, Oxford University Press, 2000

Middleton FA, Strick PL: Basal ganglia and cerebellar loops: motor and cognitive circuits. Brain Res Rev 31:236–250, 2000

Morgane PJ, Mokler DJ: The limbic brain: continuing resolution. Neurosci Biobehav Rev 30:119–125, 2006

Naumescu I, Hurley RA, Hayman LA, et al: Neuropsychiatric symptoms associated with subcortical brain injuries. Int J Neuroradiol 5:51–59, 1999

Nolte J: The Human Brain. St. Louis, MO, Mosby, 2002

Pincus JH, Tucker GJ: Behavioral Neurology. New York, Oxford University Press, 2002

Rapoport M, van Reekum R, Mayberg H: The role of the cerebellum in cognition and behavior: a selective review. J Neuropsychiatry Clin Neurosci 12:193–198, 2000

Schmahmann JD: Disorders of the cerebellum: ataxia, dysmetria of thought, and the cerebellar cognitive affective syndrome. J Neuropsychiatry Clin Neurosci 16:367–378, 2004

Schmahmann JD, Pandya DN: Anatomic organization of the basilar pontine projections from prefrontal cortices in rhesus monkey. J Neurosci 17:438–58, 1997a

Schmahmann JD, Pandya DN: The cerebrocerebellar system. Int Rev Neurobiol 41:31–60, 1997b

Taber KH, Wen C, Khan A, et al: The limbic thalamus. J Neuropsychiatry Clin Neurosci 16:127–132, 2004

Taber KH, Strick PL, Hurley RA: Rabies and the cerebellum: new methods for tracing circuits in the brain. J Neuropsychiatry Clin Neurosci 17:133–139, 2005

Tekin S, Cummings JL: Frontal-subcortical neuronal circuits and clinical neuropsychiatry: an update. J Psychosom Res 53:647–654, 2002

Tisch S, Silberstein P, Limousin-Dowsey P, et al: The basal ganglia: anatomy, physiology, and pharmacology. Psychiatr Clin North Am 27:757–799, 2004

Tranel D: Functional neuroanatomy: neuropsychological correlates of cortical and subcortical damage, in The American Psychiatric Publishing Textbook of Neuropsychiatry, 4th Edition. Edited by Yudofsky SC, Hales RE. Washington, DC, American Psychiatric Publishing, 2002, pp 71–113

Turner R, Schiavetto A: The cerebellum in schizophrenia: a case of intermittent ataxia and psychosis. Clinical, cognitive, and neuroanatomical correlates. J Neuropsychiatry Clin Neurosci 16:400–408, 2004

Uylings HB, Rajkowska G, Sanz-Arigita E, et al: Consequences of large interindividual variability for human brain atlases: converging macroscopical imaging and microscopical neuroanatomy. Anat Embryol (Berl) 210:423–431, 2005

Zeki S: Introduction: cerebral cartography 1905-2005. Philos Trans R Soc Lond B Biol Sci 360:651–652, 2005

6

GENETICS

Prabhakara V. Choudary, Ph.D., F.R.S.C.
James A. Knowles, M.D., Ph.D.

Most important discoveries are usually not solved in one "Eureka" moment, as movie scripts
sometimes suggest,…but require scientists to make not one, but a number of original discoveries and to persist in pursuing them until a discovery is complete.

Daniel E. Koshland Jr.

The goal of psychiatric genetics is to identify susceptibility genes and elucidate the neural mechanisms by
which genetic variation influences the risk of a mental
illness in an individual. As impressive advances have
marked this field over the past decade, even more significant breakthroughs are anticipated over the coming years. In this chapter, we recite the fundamental
principles of classical and molecular human genetics;
summarize the results of select studies aimed at deciphering genetic contributions to schizophrenia, mood
disorders, and related psychiatric diseases; and conclude with thoughts on how a combination of traditional and modern approaches may shape the future of
psychiatric genetics research and facilitate new drug
development with genetic etiological findings rather
than disease phenotype/symptoms as the basis.

Searches for susceptibility genes until now have relied primarily on two approaches: 1) linkage mapping,
which tracks the segregation of chromosomal regions
marked by random genetic variants in families with
complex diseases, where families can range from simple sib pairs to large extended pedigrees; and 2) association studies, which search populations for differences in the frequency of common genetic variants
between ethnically matched case and control subjects
to find variants that are strongly associated with the
disease phenotype (Baron 2002; Owen 2005). Association studies survey single nucleotide polymorphisms

PVC and JAK gratefully acknowledge the support of the National Institute of Mental Health (NIMH) (RO1-MH60912, RO1-
MH50214), the National Institute on Drug Abuse (RO1-DA12190, DA12853), the National Institute on Aging (RO1-
AG15473), and the National Alliance for Research on Schizophrenia and Depression; and of the Pritzker Neuropsychiatric
Disorders Research Fund L.L.C. and the NIMH (Silvio O. Conte Center for Mood Disorders Research #2P50-MH060398-07),
respectively. The authors have no competing financial interests.

(SNPs) and copy number variants (CNVs). Commonly known as "chromosomal abnormalities" or "insertions" (or duplications) and "deletions," CNVs involve extra or missing pieces of genomic DNA (Cohen 2007; Lupski et al. 1991). In a major break with the past, however, the association studies now increasingly tend to explore genetic variation using genomewide human SNP arrays, which feature probes for about a million each of SNPs and CNVs on a single array. The genomewide strategies, with their unparalleled power and high-throughput capacity, are beginning to redefine how regulation of gene expression is examined and polymorphisms are genotyped, especially in terms of speed and throughput.

Linkage studies have implicated several genomic regions, a few of which have been replicated in independent samples, although none has been confirmed. The replicated regions include chromosomes 1q, 2q, 6q, 8p, 10p, 13q, and 22q in schizophrenia; and 1q, 2, 4q, 6, 8, 13q, 16p, 18p, 18q, and 22q in manic-depressive (bipolar) illness. Because replication is the bedrock of credibility of a genotype–phenotype association and consequent reliable risk predictability, only the findings with independent replication are discussed here. Also indicated are loci and candidate genes with independent validation by microarray, in situ hybridization (ISH), and/or animal models. Admittedly, while some candidate genes might eventually turn out to be true causal genes, preliminary reports awaiting replication or lacking clear-cut evidence are beyond the scope of this chapter. Similarly, mandated size restrictions have limited the citations to the most recent and/or pioneering references, with rare exceptions.

However, a comprehensive listing of genetic association findings of psychiatric disorders and other diseases, including studies that were not replicated or were refuted, can be found in recent reviews listed under each disorder, and more readily in the public databases—the Online Mendelian Inheritance in Man (OMIM; http://www.ncbi.nlm.nih.gov/omim)—accessible from and linked to the National Center for Biotechnology Information (NCBI) *Entrez* cross-database (http://www.ncbi.nlm.nih.gov/gquery/gquery.fcgi), and the Genetic Association Database (http://geneticassociationdb.nih.gov).

Underlying the optimism for impending breakthroughs in psychiatric genetics are the remarkable advances revolutionizing the field of human molecular genetics, starting with the positional cloning of the genes for Mendelian (monogenic) disorders. A total of 10,432 gene loci are now established, and 11,782 genes (with sequences known) causing 2,164 clinical diseases (phenotype description, with molecular basis known) identified (http://www.ncbi.nlm.nih.gov/omim/mimstats.html), although some genes can be related to more than one disease. The transmission patterns of almost all of the 2,164 human genetic diseases can be predicted from knowing how genetic information is transmitted to offspring during meiosis (Mendel's laws). The identification of the genes that cause three relatively common diseases—cystic fibrosis (an autosomal recessive disease); neurofibromatosis type I (an autosomal dominant disease); and Duchenne muscular dystrophy (an X-linked disease)—illustrates the power of genetics in determining the cause of human disease. In each of these Mendelian disorders, molecular biological techniques facilitated 1) determining chromosomal location of the disease genes, 2) isolating the genes in both complementary DNA and genomic DNA forms, 3) identifying the disease-causing mutations, and 4) in vitro production of abnormal protein products of the disease genes for further study. Unlike Mendelian disorders, however, psychiatric disorders lack clear-cut inheritance patterns and are therefore classified as "complex" genetic disorders. In addition, psychiatric disorders lack etiological homogeneity, well-defined (or stable) phenotypes, validating diagnostic tests, or reproducible associations of chromosomal rearrangement syndromes, making disease gene discovery more difficult.

A unique resource that is proving immensely useful in this regard is the sequence of the human reference genome, aptly dubbed the "Book of Life," or rather a wiki, where individual chromosomes constitute the "chapters." The Human Genome Project (http://ornl.gov/sci/techresources/Human_Genome/project/about.shtml) was launched formally in 1990, focusing initially on sequencing the human genome. Working drafts (covering 94%–96%) of the sequence of the haploid genome have been published simultaneously by a public research team (Lander et al. 2001) and a private team (Venter et al. 2001). The latest sequence and related information can be accessed through each of the public genome browsers listed at the end of the chapter (see Online Resources). The sequences of the genomes of 1,717 model organisms, such as the yeast, roundworm, fruit fly, pufferfish, mouse, and monkey—which currently are either complete, in draft assembly mode, or in progress (see http://www.ncbi.nlm.nih.gov/genomes/static/gpstat.html)—will provide comparative information that is vital to understanding the complex functioning of the human genome.

The unprecedented insights gleaned into the molecular secrets of life with the help of human genome sequence promise to reshape medical practice. An important discovery that resulted from the human genome sequence analysis with direct relevance to psychiatric genetics is that the mutation rate in males is twice as high as that in females. Of note in this regard is the reported strong monotonic increase in risk for sporadic (nonfamilial) schizophrenia resulting from de novo mutations occurring with advancing paternal age (Malaspina et al. 2002).

By current estimates, the human genome comprises only 20,000 to 25,000 genes, a number markedly lower than the previous estimate of 100,000 to 250,000. A roundworm or a fruit fly has about one-half of this number of genes, and the yeast has about one-sixth. Arguably, an intricate and complex organization and expression of the genome, coupled with functional diversity, appear to set humans apart from the rest of the living beings. Remarkably, most of the evolutionarily new genes code for the functions of the brain, immune system, and tissue-specific developmental regulation. Of the approximately 3 billion base pairs (bp) in the human genome, only 1% account for coding sequences (exons) of genes, while 24% account for intervening sequences (introns), and 75% for intergenic sequences.

These studies further found that chromosomes differ from each other once every 1,000 base pairs on average and estimated that humans consequently would diverge from each other genomically by about 0.1%.

However, the 4 million differences recently discovered between the maternal and paternal chromosome sets of an individual (Levy et al. 2007) peg the combined (diploid) genomic variation between humans at 0.5%. Most of the genetic variation[1] occurs in the form of SNPs. To identify the variants, their genomic locations, and their distribution patterns among people within populations and among populations from different geographical parts of the world, the 3-year International HapMap project was initiated in 2002 and completed in 2005 (International HapMap Consortium 2005, 2007). The HapMap, however, does not establish disease associations of genetic variants but rather assembles information useful in linking genetic variants to the risk for specific illnesses. As of March 2007, the NCBI db-SNP (Build 127), the repository of all SNPs, contained a total of 11,811,594 RefSNP clusters, of which 5,689,286 have been validated (http://www.ncbi.nlm.nih.gov/SNP/snp_summary.cgi). These include the SNP collection containing all processed data from phases I and II of the HapMap project (release #22, August 2007, NCBI B36 assembly, dbSNP b127) as well as genotypes from the Affymetrix 500k genotyping array.

The new resources are steadily improving our ability to identify, isolate, and characterize the genes responsible for some of the complex disorders. A notable success in this regard is in the field of cancer genetics, where genes for different classes and forms of cancer have been identified and utilized in the screening of families with multiple individuals who developed

---

[1] Structural variations of the genome are at the root of natural phenotypic traits, disease vulnerability, and genetic disorders. Variations can occur in the form of SNPs, variable number of tandem repeats (VNTRs; e.g., mini- or macrosatellites), transposable elements (Alu sequences), or chromosomal rearrangements (Freeman et al. 2007). The Human Genome Project has provided us with the primary structure (sequence) of a reference genome, and the HapMap and genomewide association (GWA) studies flag SNPs, but other possible variations remain unknown. However, crucial to its apt application in molecular medicine and eventually in "personalized" medicine is a comprehensive understanding of the genome, including its higher-order structural features and all possible variations, functions, and interactions with the environment and individual lifestyles. A post–genomic era undertaking, the Copy Number Variation Project (Freeman et al. 2007) aims at establishing a comprehensive atlas and characterizing CNVs, which can heavily influence physiology; and the Human Genome Structural Variation Working Group (2007) identifies the remainder of the normal structural variations (e.g., duplications, deletions, inversions, insertions) and integrates them into the human genome sequence. A complementary community project, ENCODE (ENCyclopedia Of DNA Elements), is tasked with the goal of cataloging all functional elements in the human genome. The functional elements comprise genomic sequences that encode proteins as well as those that do not, and the regulatory elements (ENCODE Project Consortium 2007). Determining and comparing every functional element (DNA sequence) across various mammalian species (29 targeted so far), including humans, will permit comprehension of how cells decipher the instructions inscribed in the genome and how evolution has shaped various species (Check 2007). A recent collaborative model taking shape is a public–private partnership, GAIN (Genetic Association Information Network). It addresses the nuts and bolts of GWA studies by setting robust standards for selecting studies, subjects, methods, quality control, and data analysis, and organizing data banking and sharing (GAIN Collaborative Research Group 2007).

breast cancer, leading to delineation of the complex mode of inheritance of the disease. However, when only those families with a young age at onset were examined, an autosomal dominant mode of inheritance was observed. This finding led to the linkage of the breast cancer 1 gene (*BRCA1*) to chromosome 17, subsequent cloning of the gene, and detection of more than 130 disease-causing mutations in the gene (Couch and Weber 1996). Since then, a second breast cancer gene, *BRCA2*, has been localized to chromosome 13 and cloned. These epoch-making discoveries led to the development of a widely used genetic test for breast cancer risk based on the mutations in *BRCA1* and *BRCA2* genes. However, the diagnostic test has recently been found to miss about 12% of breast cancer patients with a family history of severe breast or ovarian cancer because the test is designed to detect coding sequence mutations but not changes in the rest of the sequence and deletions and duplications (Walsh et al. 2006). Even before the recognition of the limitations of the two-gene test (due to its narrow specificity), van de Vijver et al. (2002) devised a gene-expression signature based on a 70-gene panel, which proved to be more powerful than conventional systems, which were based on clinical and histological criteria in predicting the disease outcome in young patients with breast cancer. In parallel, Ramaswamy et al. (2003) developed molecular signatures for identifying metastasis in primary solid tumors and distinct molecular phenotypes in acute megakaryoblastic leukemia, as demonstrated by Bourquin et al. (2006).

There have also been several large-scale genome-wide scans for linkage in other complex disorders, such as diabetes (for a review, see McCarthy 2003), multiple sclerosis (Rubio et al. 2000), and asthma (Hakonarson and Halapi 2002). Unlike the case in psychiatric disorders, a biological test (e.g., pathology, blood glucose) is available for validating association findings for each of these diseases. The work in type 2 diabetes mellitus has led to the identification of calpain-10 as a putative disease gene, one of the first for a polygenic form of a disorder. However, a recent study of 59 families from northern Sweden consisting of 129 cases of type 2 diabetes and 19 subjects with impaired glucose tolerance validated 2q37 linkage with a lod score of 3.19, but found no evidence of the association of the previously reported SNP in Calponin-10 gene in a case–control cohort from the same population (Einarsdottir et al. 2006). Genetic linkage studies in psychiatry are expectedly more difficult due to the diagnostic uncertainties involved.

Psychiatric Genetics: Aims and Methods

Studies of genetic contribution to psychiatric disorders, constituting the core of psychiatric genetics, have also led researchers in several related directions, including the search for environmental etiological factors, the refinement of psychiatric nosology, the investigation of normal and abnormal psychological and behavioral traits, and the development of effective methods for the prevention and treatment of psychiatric disorders.

Aims

Genetic investigation in psychiatry has the following goals:

1. To establish and specify the genetic component of the etiology of psychiatric syndromes and thus determine a) to what extent a psychiatric disorder is genetically caused, b) the DNA variation underlying each genetic contribution, c) the biopsychosocial abnormalities associated with the gene or genes involved, and d) the processes by which genetic abnormalities lead to symptoms.
2. To establish and specify the nongenetic component of the etiology of psychiatric syndromes and thus identify environmental factors that, acting independently of or interacting with vulnerable genotypes, produce or increase the likelihood of a disorder.
3. To validate the boundaries of diagnostic entities and subtypes within entities by determining a) the similarities in genetic variations between disorders, or between subtypes of a disorder, to establish groupings of genetically related disorders (e.g., a schizophrenia spectrum) or to split disorders established on clinical phenomenology (e.g., different subtypes of schizoaffective disorder); and b) the characteristics (e.g., severity, subject's age at onset) of a disorder that increase its heritability, thereby helping to identify diagnostic boundaries that more closely correspond to biological boundaries.
4. To specify the genetic contribution to traits and psychological symptoms, independent of their role as components of defined psychiatric syndromes.
5. To develop methods of preventing or treating psychiatric disorders based on knowledge of genetic and environmental factors in their etiology. These methods include genetic counseling, alteration of the necessary/permissive environment for persons at risk, and gene therapy.

Methods

Research methods have evolved for each of the aims of genetic investigation. Over the past two decades, the methodologies have been especially productive in determining to what extent a psychiatric disorder is genetically caused (Table 6–1). New techniques hold the promise of determining the location, nature, and product of the genetic contribution to many disorders. Genetic investigation of a psychiatric disorder attempts to answer numerous interrelated questions such as the following:

- Is the illness familial?
- Is this familiality caused by genetic factors?
- What are the various clinical expressions of the abnormal gene(s)?
- What are the earliest manifestations of the predisposition to illness?
- What environmental variables increase or decrease the chances of predisposed individuals developing the disorder?
- What is the mode of transmission?
- Where is (are) the abnormal gene(s)?
- What is the biological, physiological, and psychological outcome of the genetic abnormality?

Different techniques, each with its own advantages and disadvantages as described below, are utilized in attempts at answering these questions.

Is the Illness Familial?—Family Risk Studies and Epidemiological Studies

Family risk studies are designed to determine the extent to which an illness runs in families because genetic diseases show increased rates of illness among relatives, although not all familial traits are genetic (e.g., language skill). Research by the pioneers of psychiatric genetics in the early part of the twentieth century found higher rates of schizophrenia and bipolar illness among family members of affected individuals than in the general population. As diagnostic criteria have been developed and validated, such studies have continued for the psychoses as well as for other diagnostic entities—for example, schizophrenia (Kendler et al. 1985), affective disorders (Andreasen et al. 1987), panic disorder (Noyes et al. 1986), and simple phobias (Fyer et al. 1990).

The methodology of conducting such studies has sufficiently developed to meet higher research standards. In the studies conducted in the early part of the twentieth century, nonrepresentative hospitalized cases were sampled, and data on family members were collected indirectly. Diagnoses were made on the basis of global clinical impressions by investigators who were not blind to the diagnoses of other family members. The results were then compared with control subjects diagnosed by other investigators. The current state-of-the-art family risk study does the following:

1. Samples patients (termed *probands* or *index cases*) in an unbiased way to obtain a sample that is representative of all patients with the disorder.
2. Either interviews family members directly or obtains detailed descriptions of a family member's illness through records and multiple informants.
3. Arrives at diagnoses while blind to the disease status of the index case.
4. Uses operationalized diagnostic criteria (such as those in DSM-IV-TR [American Psychiatric Association 2000]).
5. Demonstrates reliability in both the information gathering and the diagnostic processes.
6. Compares the data on familial psychopathology, using appropriate statistical analyses, with the rate of psychopathology in the family members of a matched control group investigated simultaneously with the same methodology.

Investigations that use these techniques have not only supported the original studies demonstrating the familial nature of many psychiatric illnesses but also yielded much more precise estimates of the prevalence of various forms of psychopathology among relatives. From these studies have emerged the concepts of a spectrum of illnesses related to schizophrenia, the affective disorder spectrum, and associations between clinically distinct disorders such as anorexia nervosa and affective disorders.

Calculation of the extent of psychiatric disorders among the relatives of probands begins with determining the rates through the process of family interviews. Since some family members will not have passed through the age at risk for the disorder, it would be an underestimate of the eventual rate of psychopathology among relatives to assume that these individuals will remain well. Therefore, the data usually are reported in terms of *lifetime morbid risk*, which is an estimate of the eventual rate of illness among relatives, were they to be followed through the age at risk. Various methods are used to calculate lifetime morbid risk, all based on knowledge of the cumulative incidence of cases for a certain disorder through the life span. A simple method, the *Weinberg abridged method*, determines morbid risk by dividing the number of ill relatives by a new denominator (called a *bezugsziffern*). This denominator is deter-

TABLE 6–1. Evidence in support of genetic transmission of various psychiatric disorders

Illness	Genetic transmission supported by			
	Family risk studies	Twin studies	Adoption studies	Molecular studies
Schizophrenia	+	+	+	+
Bipolar disorder	+	+	+	+
Major depression	+	+	(+)	+
Panic disorder and agoraphobia	+	+		+
Generalized anxiety disorder	+	+		
Simple phobia	+	+		
Social phobia	+	+		
Obsessive-compulsive disorder	(+)	+		+
Posttraumatic stress disorder		+		
Anorexia nervosa	+	+		+
Briquet's syndrome/somatization disorder and sociopathy	+	(+)	+	
Alcoholism	+	(+)	+	+
Personality disorders				
Antisocial	+			
Schizotypal	+	+		+
Borderline		+		
Avoidant	+			
Dependent	+			
Alzheimer's disease	+	(+)		+

Note. Evidence discussed, with references, in text. +=most or all findings support genetic transmission; (+)=some findings support genetic transmission, but others do not.

mined by counting all relatives, then subtracting out the relatives below the age at risk, and subtracting out one-half of the number of relatives within the age at risk (Gottesman and Shields 1982). A more precise method used in modern studies is that of *survival analysis,* which is used to plot the time of onset of the disorder among relatives and, through this, to estimate the proportion of relatives who eventually will be affected (Kalbfeish and Prentice 1980). If the cumulative incidence of a disorder is not known, as is currently the case, for example, with most personality disorders, lifetime morbid risk calculations cannot legitimately be made.

When the lifetime morbid risks for first-degree relatives of ill and control probands are determined, a *rel-ative risk* for first-degree relatives of ill probands can be calculated. As seen in Table 6–2, which is based on selected methodologically sound studies, this relative risk varies from approximately 3 to 25 for the psychiatric disorders studied, indicating significant familial aggregation for all of them. From these data, it appears that bipolar disorder, schizophrenia, panic disorder, and alcoholism are familial disorders.

As was noted earlier, however, such rates of illness may be influenced by environmental conditions shared by family members. Thus, the extent to which a disorder is familial cannot be immediately taken as an indication of the extent to which it is genetically determined. Family studies are quite useful for ruling out a

TABLE 6–2. Relative risks for psychiatric disorders

Disorder	Relative risk	Reference
Bipolar disorder	24.5	Weissman et al. 1984
Schizophrenia	18.5	Kendler et al. 1985
Bulimia nervosa	9.6	Kassett et al. 1989
Panic disorder	9.6	Crowe et al. 1983
Alcoholism	7.4	Merikangas 1989
Generalized anxiety disorder	5.6	Noyes et al. 1987
Anorexia nervosa	4.6	Strober et al. 1985
Simple phobia	3.3	Fyer et al. 1990
Social phobia	3.2	Fyer et al. 1993
Somatization disorder	3.1	Cloninger et al. 1986
Major depression	3.0	Weissman et al. 1984
Agoraphobia	2.8	Crowe et al. 1983

Note. Other studies may have relative risk ratios that differ considerably from those in these studies, especially if different diagnostic criteria were used. However, the methodological soundness of studies referenced here prompted our selection of them for discussion in the text and in this comparison.

genetic basis of a disorder but can only provide support, not proof, of the existence of heritable factors. There may also be *assortative mating,* a tendency for those with a psychiatric disorder to mate preferentially, usually with those who have similar psychopathology, or in other nonrandom ways, thus increasing the likelihood that their children will inherit a genetic predisposition to the disorder beyond what would be the case if only one parent was affected. Unless recognized, this could lead to a familial pattern that overestimates the genetic effect.

Large-scale epidemiological studies, such as the National Institute of Mental Health (NIMH) Epidemiologic Catchment Area (ECA) study (Robins et al. 1984) and the National Comorbidity Survey (NCS) (R.C. Kessler et al. 1994), can contribute to the value and interpretation of the familial data. With the use of structured interview schedules and standardized diagnostic criteria, estimates of the population prevalence of disorders can be determined and compared with the data obtained from the family studies. Some studies blend the techniques of epidemiology and family risk, studying geographical, ethnic, or cultural isolates (Egeland et al. 1987).

In isolated populations, we expect greater genetic homogeneity for the psychiatric disorder present because all or most cases of the disorder may stem from a common progenitor who is the single source of the pathogenic gene(s). In addition, higher environmental homogeneity is likely, and because the variation of a trait explained by genetic factors is actually the sum of the environmental and genetic factors, decreasing the environmental variance increases the genetic variance. There may also be a higher prevalence of certain disorders in such populations. These elevated rates may be caused by an increased frequency of the abnormal genotype or a higher rate of expression of the gene (i.e., increased penetrance). Isolated kindreds showing a high incidence of the disorder provide the best samples for the segregation and linkage analytic techniques described later, which can identify and localize a potent genetic contributory factor.

Do Genetic Factors Contribute to the Illness?— Twin and Adoption Studies

Once a psychiatric disorder is found to be familial, twin and adoption studies are utilized to determine relative contributions of genetics and environment to the etiology of the disorder.

Twin studies. Twin studies examine the concordance, or the coincidence, of a disorder in monozygotic, genetically identical (MZ) twins and in dizygotic, fraternal (DZ) twins, the latter sharing on average one-half of their genes, as do siblings. One strategy involves comparing concordance in MZ pairs and same-sex DZ pairs. If the rearing environment has predisposed an index case to illness, then the co-twin, whether MZ or DZ, also should be at risk, and the rates for both MZ and DZ twins should be equally elevated (compared with the population rate). If, on the other hand, pathogenic genes have predisposed the index twin to illness, then an MZ co-twin would be at a higher risk than a DZ co-twin. The concordance rate for MZ twins would be higher than that for DZ twins, and the latter should show similar concordance rate as siblings.[2]

One assumption of this strategy is that MZ and DZ twins have the same degree of similarity of familial environment—in other words, that MZ twins do not share environmental similarity any more than DZ twins do in ways that would increase the MZ concordance for psychiatric disorders. It is obvious that in some ways MZ twins are treated more similarly (e.g., being dressed alike). It is also clear that in many families MZ twins receive very similar emotional and attitudinal input from their parents. However, reflecting the complexity of the issue, evidence indicates that temperamental characteristics of MZ twins (which may be genetic in origin) generate this similarity in rearing. The available empirical evidence does support the assumption of an equal environment in both female and male twin pairs.

Because it is difficult to determine the degree to which shared environment could account for the increased MZ concordance rates of twins raised in the same home, studies of twins raised apart in uncorrelated (i.e., randomly assigned) environments would be useful. Ideally, the concordance rates of MZ and DZ pairs raised apart could be compared, but even having only such a sample of MZ twins would allow for comparison of their concordance rates with those of MZ twins raised in the same home. However, systematic samples of such twins are difficult to obtain, and case reports of concordance are more likely to be noted and published than are those of discordant pairs.

A third way to use the concordance rates for twins to address the question of genetic versus environmental factors is to examine the extent to which MZ twins are discordant for a disorder. Given that MZ twins are

genetically identical, any degree of discordance implies that there are nongenetic etiological factors that can either produce or unmask the disorder. For example, these findings could result from "phenocopies," cases that appear to have the disorder in question but have an environmentally determined, pathogenically distinct illness that mimics the genetically determined disease. Another possibility is that environmental conditions might be necessary to add to or to interact with genetic factors to produce the illness, leading to MZ twins being both predisposed genetically for the disorder, but discordant on the basis of having experienced different environments. Huntington's disease has a nearly 100% MZ concordance rate, whereas common psychiatric disorders such as schizophrenia and bipolar disorder have rates that approximate 50% and 65%, respectively.

These twin strategies produce quantitative data that are tempting to translate into estimates of the extent to which a disorder is genetically caused. The *heritability* of a psychiatric disorder is defined as the portion of a trait's variation in the population that is accounted for by genetic factors. Two types of heritability have been defined: *broad-sense heritability*—the portion accounted for by all genetic influences; and *narrow-sense heritability*—the portion accounted for by additive genetic variance only. Broad-sense heritability is calculated by doubling the difference in rates of concordance observed in the MZ and DZ twin pairs for a disease or trait. For instance, if the concordance rates found in a twin study of schizophrenia were 47.5% and 17.5% for MZ and DZ twin pairs, respectively, then the estimated broad-sense heritability would be 60% [$2 \times (47.5 - 17.5)$]. Broad-sense heritability includes the influence of gene dominance and epistasis (interactions between genes), whereas narrow-sense heritability estimates the amount of genetic influence that is likely to be passed on to offspring.

Questions regarding the interpretation of MZ twin concordance rates may be resolved by another twin strategy, the study of the offspring of discordant MZ twins. If the ill twin has a purely environmentally caused disorder, then the offspring of the well co-twin should not be at elevated risk (unless he or she is exposed to the pathogenic environmental insults that his

---

[2] There are two methods of calculating concordance: pairwise and probandwise. In the pair method, every pair is counted only once; in the proband method, pairs are counted twice if each twin was an ill proband sampled for the study independently, and this usually results in somewhat higher concordances. Many geneticists regard the latter method as preferable because the rates can be compared with population rates (Gottesman and Shields 1982). In this chapter, probandwise rates are given unless otherwise noted.

or her aunt or uncle, but not his or her parent, experienced). On the other hand, if the ill and well twins share a genetic predisposition to the illness, but one had not experienced certain precipitating or contributing environmental insults, then the well co-twin will be a carrier of liability for the illness, and his or her offspring will be at elevated risk. This strategy was pioneered by Fischer (1971) and extended by Gottesman and Bertelsen (1989), who found that the offspring of nonschizophrenic MZ co-twins and the offspring of their ill co-twins had an equal morbid risk for the illness, suggesting that much of the discordance between the twins could be attributed to differential exposure to environmental factors.

Adoption studies.   Adoption studies are based on the knowledge that adoption separates the two major influences parents have on their children, namely, genes and rearing. It offers researchers a naturalistic "experiment" that has the potential to answer the questions of whether a disorder is familial because of genetic transmission or because of the shared environment. Four types of adoption studies have been used:

1. *Adoptee study method:* the study of adopted-away children of a parent with a disorder.
2. *Cross-fostering strategy:* the study of children born of nondisordered parents adopted into a family with a disordered parent.
3. *Adoptees' family method:* the study of the adoptive and the biological relatives of disordered adoptees.
4. *MZ twins reared apart:* the study of MZ twins reared apart, as discussed previously (see "Twin Studies").

Such research is much easier to conceptualize than execute. State-of-the-art investigations using these strategies must use systematic sampling, adoptee control subjects, careful attention to make diagnoses blind to the diagnosis of the index case, and operationalized diagnostic criteria. Pioneering studies were conducted by Rosenthal, Kety, Wender, and Schulsinger, with later collaboration by Kendler in an investigation of schizophrenia in a Danish sample (Kety 1988; Kety et al. 1994; Parnas et al. 1982; Rosenthal et al. 1968, 1970; Schulsinger et al. 1979; Wender et al. 1974, 1986). Adoption studies have been carried out for mood disorders, alcoholism, drug abuse, sociopathy, attention-deficit/hyperactivity disorder, and other psychiatric conditions as well as for IQ and personality variables.

Although adoption permits ideal separation of genetic factors from environmental influences, it suffers from certain methodological drawbacks. Because few children are adopted away immediately after birth, usually some familial environmental influences of undetermined significance can exist, which are difficult to measure. Also, "environment" does not necessarily begin at birth; and the uterine environment of an affected mother may have a significant role in the transmission of the illness, which may be examined by comparing the risk to the children of affected mothers with the risk to the children of affected fathers; or in the adoptee's family method the risk to paternal half-siblings may be compared with maternal half-siblings.

Another major difficulty stems from the unusual nature of adoption itself. The types of parents or the circumstances that lead parents to give up their children may alter the representative nature of the sample. Thus, the investigator comparing the adopted-away children of ill parents with the adopted-away children of "normal" control subjects must accept the fact that the control parents might themselves be ill in some way and that the rates of psychiatric illness in both groups of adoptees might be unusually high. Similarly, the investigator studying the biological and adoptive parents of adoptees with disorders cannot legitimately use differences in the rates of illness between these two groups to prove a genetic hypothesis, given that adoptive parents are often psychiatrically screened by adoption agencies. Thus, the biological relatives of the disordered adoptees and the biological relatives of the control adoptees must be compared, again encountering the problem of high rates of psychopathology among the control relatives.

These methodological difficulties, unless they are overcome by removing ill probands from the control group, tend to lead to a rejection or minimization of the genetic hypothesis (a *type II error*). Thus, it is somewhat surprising that so many adoption studies have yielded results strongly supportive of genetic factors in the etiology of psychiatric disorders, while it is not surprising that the diagnostic evaluations from these studies have been strongly contested because of the high rates of illness diagnosed among the control subjects.

What Are the Various Clinical Expressions of the Abnormal Gene(s)?—Spectrum Studies

In most of the family studies conducted on the major psychiatric disorders, investigators have found an increase not only in the disorder in question but also in other types of psychopathology. At times, this increase has been in milder or related syndromes of the major disorder, such as dysthymia in the relatives of patients with major depression or unipolar depression in the relatives of patients with bipolar disorder. In other illnesses, more distant syndromes have appeared—an increase in mood disorders in the relatives of patients with eating disorders and in sociopathy in the relatives of patients with somatization disorder.

As evidence has accumulated suggesting that genetic factors account for the increased familial incidence of major psychiatric disorders, a hypothesis has been put forth that the other syndromes found to be increased among relatives are also the result of the same genetic predisposition. This concept has been expressed as the "spectrum" of disorders related to, for example, schizophrenia or bipolar disorder. As discussed below, the former is said to include schizotypal personality, paranoid personality, schizoaffective disorder (by DSM-III-R [American Psychiatric Association 1987] criteria), and atypical psychosis; the latter, bipolar II disorder, recurrent major depressive disorder, cyclothymia, dysthymia, schizoaffective disorder (Research Diagnostic Criteria [RDC; Spitzer et al. 1978] bipolar type), and possibly others.

The diagnostic trend in American psychiatry, first prominently represented in DSM-III (American Psychiatric Association 1980) and continued in the subsequent editions, has been to narrow the boundaries of Axis I disorders and to develop alternative categories (e.g., atypical psychosis, psychosis not otherwise specified) for less severe or mixed-symptom cases. It was hoped that these restrictions would produce more symptomatically and etiologically homogeneous categories, an especially appropriate development for the study of treatment effects and biological markers, for which a sample of "pure" cases could be recruited.

For many types of genetic studies, however, determining, for all family members, who in the family is ill and who is well is often of utmost importance. Studies attempting to determine the mode of transmission (i.e., segregation analysis) and linkage studies are most obviously affected by misclassification. Because problems are posed by both overinclusion and overexclusion, the issue of which phenotypic syndromes are manifestations of the genotype is essential. In practice, the spectrum of disorders found in the current or prior studies to be increased in the family members of index cases, as compared with similarly diagnosed control families, is often entered into one or more data analyses as alternative manifestations of the genotype. The spectrum concept has thus been developed and used in genetic research studies.

Such application of spectrum findings has problems too. Even if the assumption of genetic relatedness between the disorders is correct, some of the individual cases may be genetically connected, but not others; consider, for example, the various causes of major de-

pression among relatives of a patient with bipolar disorder. Also, there may not be a direct genetic link between the disorders, even if there is a familial association. The syndromes in the spectrum may be a result of environmental influences associated with index families (e.g., the effect of early parental depression or suicide on children); or, even if genetically caused, they may be the product of assortative mating (consider, for example, the case of sociopathic individuals mating with schizophrenic or depressed patients, leading to increased sociopathy in the offspring).

The problems of using spectrum diagnoses become even more acute when this genetic causation is assumed to apply in a clinical situation. For heterogeneous illnesses, the etiological factors most often at work in index families may not be those represented in the population at large. Thus, whereas a schizophrenic patient's first-degree relative with a schizotypal personality disorder may very likely share the genetic predisposition to schizophrenia, the schizotypal individual without such a family history may be much less likely to have the same genetic makeup. The determination of the extent to which a spectrum illness is associated with the "index" disorder must include identification of that spectrum illness in family studies of other index disorders and in family studies that take the spectrum diagnosis as the index disorder. An example of this process has occurred with schizotypal personality disorder, first described as occurring in the families of schizophrenic patients and thus classified as part of the schizophrenic spectrum. In addition, an equal increase of schizotypal personality disorder in the families of mood disorder patients has been shown. Family studies of schizotypal disorder itself have shown increased rates of both schizotypal personality disorder and schizophrenia in relatives of schizotypal personality disorder probands.

What Are the Early Manifestations of and Environmental Risk Factors for the Illness?— High-Risk Studies

High-risk research, or the study of children at risk, is a strategy that begins with a factor of known or putative importance for the development of psychopathology and examines, through controlled studies, the influence of that factor on exposed infants or children. Such a design has been used to delineate the effects of maternal alcohol consumption during pregnancy on low birth weight. It has also been used to identify the early development of psychopathology among the offspring of parents with psychiatric disorders. This strategy entails selection of parent probands with an accurately diagnosed disorder, evaluation of psychopathology in the co-parents, and usually a longitudinal evaluation of the children with a battery of psychological and biological measures, as well as a record of environmental conditions during development. These studies can investigate 1) presymptomatic differences between the high-risk group and the control group and whether such abnormalities predict later psychopathology, 2) early manifestations of psychopathology in subjects who later develop the same disorder that their parents experienced, 3) the childhood psychopathological syndromes that may be genetically related to the adult psychiatric disorders of either or both parents, and 4) environmental variables that are associated with the development of illness in the genetically predisposed group.

Investigating presumably predisposed individuals in the well state for hidden psychological or physiological differences that could play a role in their development of the illness (e.g., psychological or physiological differences in the response of sons of alcoholic parents to alcohol) avoids one of the major pitfalls of studying already ill individuals—namely, that abnormalities found in ill subjects may be a sequelae of the illness or of its treatment rather than aspects of an intrinsic vulnerability. Investigations of the first manifestations of an illness (such as attentional deficits in the children of schizophrenic parents) may be helpful in establishing the nature of a genetically determined "core deficit" in evolving illnesses such as schizophrenia. Examining the rates of specific childhood disorders in the at-risk group (e.g., the rates of separation anxiety in the children of parents with panic disorder) can establish links between childhood and adult syndromes in the same way that family and adoption studies can identify a spectrum of adult disorders with a possibly shared genetic causation.

In high-risk studies, the environment can be controlled (Nagler 1985), but it is usually studied by evaluating the influence of spontaneously occurring environmental events in a genetically predisposed population. These events could be those with a predisposing potential, such as parental loss, or those that might protect a vulnerable individual, such as experiences of competence and success. This application of high-risk studies parallels the study of discordant MZ twins for environmental variables that account for their discordance.

Major problems in the execution and interpretation of high-risk studies include the influence of co-parent psychopathology that may not be randomized be-

cause of assortative mating, the large sample of children that must be studied in low-prevalence disorders such as schizophrenia to achieve meaningful statistical results, the difficulty of identifying pathogenic environmental stressors when these are nonspecific and cumulative, and the difficulty of elucidating the influence of any environmental variable when it is not known as to who among the offspring are truly genetically predisposed. In the future, when DNA variations have been found that are clearly thought to increase the risk of developing a psychiatric disorder, a new generation of high-risk studies will explore the early manifestations of the variation and the influence of environmental factors in the offspring and relatives of probands.

What Is the Mode of Transmission?— Segregation Analysis

When family, twin, and adoption studies show a role for genetic factors in the pathogenesis of a disorder, then *segregation analysis* can be attempted to determine the mode of transmission of those genetic factors. It is done by studying the pattern of inheritance of the disorder in a collection of families and comparing it to known patterns of inheritance. Mutations at any single gene are inherited in a dominant or recessive manner and may be autosomal or sex-linked. If the disorder is transmitted in families in one of these patterns, a single-gene mutation could be its cause.

For example, approximately 50% of the offspring of parents affected with one of the dominant monogenic disorders (e.g., Huntington's disease or acute intermittent porphyria) are themselves affected. Affected offspring always have an affected parent (unless the offspring's condition represents a new mutation, which is rare). If a group of families with a particular disorder all have this pattern of transmission, then the disorder is caused by a single dominant gene. For the recessive disorders (e.g., phenylketonuria or cystic fibrosis), each affected individual will have unaffected parents who must nonetheless be carriers, and approximately 25% of the offspring of two carrier parents will be affected. Often, the incidence of consanguineous marriages (inbreeding) is increased in these families. In the sex-linked recessive disorders (e.g., hemophilia), all of the daughters of an affected father are unaffected carriers, and 50% of their sons in turn will be affected. Furthermore, no father-to-son transmission occurs.

Segregation analysis was originally developed as a test for recessive inheritance: segregation ratios in sibships were observed and compared with the ratio of 25% affected to 75% unaffected, predicted by Mendel's first law. Subsequently, this modest approach has been expanded into a sophisticated mathematical analysis. Qualitative notions such as dominant and recessive inheritance have given way to quantitative estimates of gene frequency, gene transmission probability, and genotype penetrance. Moreover, the laws of Mendelian inheritance have been replaced by models for single-gene transmission that incorporate intermediate types of gene effect. When these estimates and models are varied, they predict different phenotypic resemblances between different classes of relatives (MZ twins, DZ twins, full sibs, half sibs, and parents and offspring). These predictions are then statistically compared with the observed concordance between relatives, allowing the investigator to determine "best-fit" models. If there is an extremely close fit between the predictions and the observations, then the model's mode of inheritance and quantitative estimates are supported. If even the best-fit model for a certain mode of transmission shows little resemblance to the observed concordances, then it can be ruled out as a possible mode of transmission. However, it is important to note that segregation analysis relies on pooled data from many nuclear families and assumes genetic homogeneity across these families. This assumption is not always warranted (disorders may be phenotypically identical but etiologically distinct) and may lead to spurious results, such as the false rejection of monogenic transmission.

Unfortunately, segregation analyses of common psychiatric disorders do not confirm one of the simple Mendelian or sex-linked patterns described above. For this reason, the psychiatric disorders belong to the group of "complex" (i.e., non-Mendelian) genetic disorders. Other complex genetic disorders include hypertension and diabetes. Complex patterns can arise from multiple genetic phenomena. The first of these is *genetic heterogeneity*. If a disorder can be caused by an abnormal gene at two (or more) genetic loci, and one of these causes the disorder in a recessive pattern and the other in a dominant pattern, then a segregation analysis of all those with the disorder will support neither model. Genetic heterogeneity is suspected because it has been shown in so many other medical disorders for which the genetic causes have been determined. Complex patterns may also occur because of environmental influences. There may be individuals who have the disorder but do not have any genetic predisposition. These individuals are said to have a *phenocopy* of the genetic form of the disorder. Likewise, individuals who carry the disease gene may not have the disorder because of *reduced penetrance* of the gene. The psychiatric disorders are thought to show many of the above phenomena, complicating segregation analysis. All of the major psychiatric disorders can be mimicked by medical illnesses; thus, other phenocopies, indistinguishable clinically, are suspected.

Another cause of complex inheritance patterns is termed *polygenic* or *multifactorial inheritance*. A polygenic disease results when multiple genes, none of which has a very strong effect by itself, interact with one another (polygenic inheritance) or when multiple genes, some of which might have a major effect, interact with various environmental factors (multifactorial inheritance) to cause the disorder (Kidd 1981). Because polygenic and multifactorial models have many variables, they produce a wide variety of possible values for familial concordances and thus can often fit quite closely with the observed data. In other words, monogenic disorders can be characterized by specific segregation ratios (i.e., rates of disorder in relatives), whereas polygenic disorders cannot. However, newer methods of segregation analysis that use Monte Carlo Markov Chain methods may provide insights into how many genes contribute to polygenic traits or disease.

A few predictions stemming from polygenic models differ from those of monogenic models. In polygenic disorders, the proband is at risk of being affected with increasing severity of illness, whereas relatives face a greater risk of being affected in higher numbers. In addition, the risk of illness drops off precipitously as one moves from MZ twins to first- and second-degree relatives, and affected relatives are often found on both maternal and paternal sides (Gottesman and Shields 1982). Also, monogenic disorders tend to have low population prevalence. This suggests that common diseases (i.e., those occurring in more than 1% of the population) are likely to be polygenic, as are many traits that have been genetically studied (e.g., intelligence, height, skin color) (Lamason et al. 2005).

In summary, segregation analysis has shown that most psychiatric disorders do not show a simple monogenic pattern of any variety. This finding leads to increased consideration of (but not proof for) polygenic inheritance and of confounding factors such as heterogeneity, reduced penetrance, and phenocopies. The technique may be of greater value if more discrete disorders are discovered, or if it is used to study the genetics of specific symptoms or physiological phenomena.

Where Is the Abnormal Gene?—Genetic Linkage Analysis and Association Studies

Two general approaches permit the discovery of genetic factors responsible for the pathogenesis of a disease: 1) genome scans followed by subsequent positional cloning and 2) candidate gene association studies. In the first approach, the broad chromosomal location of an abnormal gene is identified, perhaps containing hundreds of genes, without reference to the abnormal protein for which it codes, by the use of a genome scan and genetic linkage analysis (described in the next paragraph). Examples of linkage findings in schizophrenia can be found in recent reviews by Shastry (2002), Sklar (2002), McDonald and Murphy (2003), Kendler (2003), and Shih et al. (2004). Additional genetic analysis can then lead to a smaller region and eventually to the DNA variations that underlie the disease. Researchers using the positional cloning approach have elucidated the pathogenesis of hundreds of genes for the Mendelian genetic disorders, including cystic fibrosis, neurofibromatosis type I, Duchenne muscular dystrophy, and the early-onset forms of familial Alzheimer's disease.

Genetic linkage analysis is a technique based on exceptions to Mendel's second law (Suarez and Cox 1985). This empirical observation, also known as the law of independent assortment, states that alleles (specific gene configurations) at different genetic loci are inherited independently of one another. This clearly applies to loci lying on different chromosomes. This law also often applies to loci lying on the same chromosome because of the exchange of genetic material between homologous chromosomes that occurs during the meiotic phase of gametogenesis in a process known as crossing over. To understand this phenomenon (Figure 6–1), consider the possible gametes (i.e., reproductive cells) that may result from the mating of two parents, one of which is heterozygous at two loci, A and B, on a given paired chromosome (a_1b_1/a_2b_2), and the other which is homozygous at both loci (a_2b_2/a_2b_2). In the absence of crossing over, the gametes that are produced include only a_1b_1 and a_2b_2. If crossing over occurs between loci A and B, two new gametes, known as *recombinants,* are produced by the mother (a_1b_2 and a_2b_1), and alleles at loci A and B may appear

to be assorting independently in this family, even though they are on the same chromosome.[3] Consequently, within a given pedigree, the parental gametes (in the example above, a_1b_1 and a_2b_2) will be disproportionately represented if loci A and B are located near each other, and alleles at these loci will appear to violate Mendel's second law. Loci A and B may then be said to be "linked" (Figure 6–1). By extension, if linkage can be established between a hypothetical disease locus and a marker locus with known chromosomal location, then the approximate location of the disease locus can be inferred, and ultimately the disease gene can be isolated.

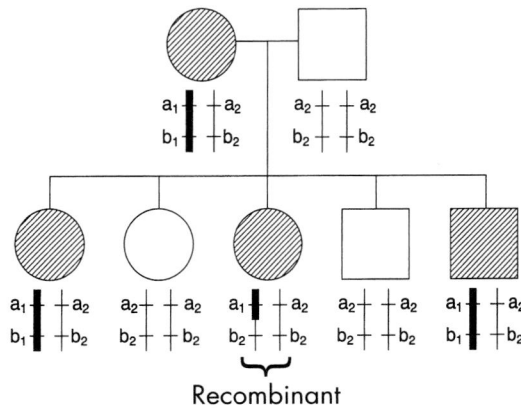

Recombinant

FIGURE 6–1. Genetic linkage and recombination.

Depicted is a hypothetical family (*circles:* females; *squares:* males) transmitting an autosomal dominant disease. The disease locus A (containing either the defective allele a_1 or its normal counterpart a_2) lies close to a marker locus B (containing marker alleles b_1 and b_2). The mother is affected with the disease (*shaded symbol*) and is heterozygous at both the disease and the marker loci. The father is unaffected (*open symbol*) and is homozygous at both loci. Because the disease and marker loci are genetically linked (i.e., they lie near each other), crossing over rarely occurs between them. Most children who inherit the disease allele a_1 also receive the b_1 marker allele from their mother. Occasionally, a recombination event (i.e., "crossing over") occurs in the mother, and she transfers a chromosome bearing the b_2 marker allele along with the disease allele (as occurred in the daughter labeled "recombinant"). The frequency of such recombinants increases as the distance between the disease and marker locus increases.

---

[3]However, crossing over rarely occurs between loci lying near one another. The frequency with which recombination results is roughly proportional to the distance between the affected loci. For example, a recombination frequency of 1% per meiosis corresponds to a functional distance of 1 centimorgan and a physical distance of approximately 1 million DNA base pairs.

Several approaches are available for determining linkage between disease and marker loci. One approach, known as the likelihood method (Morton 1955), may be used to 1) examine co-segregation of the disease and marker phenotypes within a pedigree; 2) determine the probability (likelihood [L]) of achieving the observed distribution of phenotypes, given estimates for the proportion of recombinant gametes among gametes (i.e., the recombination fraction), θ, ranging from 0.0 to 0.5 (the latter representing no linkage); and 3) calculate the odds ratio (defined as the ratio $L[\theta]\backslash L[\theta = 0.5]$)—that is, the relative likelihood of the evidence for linkage versus the evidence for no linkage. By convention, the odds ratio is expressed as its base 10 logarithm (known as the *lod score*), so that linkage data from several families can be pooled and their respective contributions added to obtain a combined probability of linkage. For monogenic diseases that have Mendelian patterns of inheritance, when the lod score at the best estimate of θ (best being defined as that estimate that yields the highest lod score) is greater than +3, linkage is confirmed; when it is less than –2, linkage is rejected. The lod scores required to confirm or reject linkage for the psychiatric disorders need to be of greater magnitude because of the complex pattern of inheritance. Corrections for the testing of multiple-disease models are also required.

If some but not all families have linkage to a particular marker, a statistical test can be performed to determine whether there is evidence for genetic heterogeneity within a disorder. This appears to be the case with Charcot-Marie-Tooth disease (peroneal muscular atrophy). Once linkage is established, knowledge of the genotype can then permit presumptive presymptomatic identification of affected persons in individual pedigrees at risk for the disease, given appropriate information about family members.

Although the likelihood method is a statistically powerful approach for detecting linkage, it relies on several assumptions that may not be warranted. These assumptions include random mating, no association between particular disease and marker alleles within the population, and genetic homogeneity of the illness across pedigrees. Also included is specification of genetic parameters (i.e., mode of inheritance, gene frequencies, and genotype penetrances) for both the disease loci and the marker loci. To circumvent these hurdles, several nonparametric methods for finding

genetic loci have been developed. In general, these methods trade the need to specify a genetic model for the ability to detect linkage under a known model with the likelihood method. The first of these, the affected sib-pair method (Suarez et al. 1978), posits that siblings who are both affected with a genetic disorder should be identical in the region of the genome that causes the disorder. In the other areas of the genome, the siblings should, on average, share one-half of their genetic material. Multiple sib pairs are tested, and the number of pairs who are identical for a given marker provides a statistical measure of support for linkage. This method makes no assumptions about the mode of inheritance. By sampling only sib pairs in which both members are clearly affected, it avoids considering either ambiguous cases or well individuals. (For disorders with reduced penetrance, the latter may be genetically vulnerable but are thought to represent instances of recombination.)

The sib-pair method, despite its advantages, also suffers from certain limitations. Although it can use information from sibships, it is forced to disregard other information present in extended pedigrees and does not provide an estimate of genetic distance to the disease. It is also nearly equivalent to a parametric analysis assuming complete penetrance and a recessive mode of inheritance. Although it is most powerful in detecting linkage in rare recessive disorders, this technique may only be powerful enough to detect linkage in major psychiatric disorders if the illness is linked to a marker locus for most families.

In the likelihood and affected sib-pair methods, linkage refers to a correlation between two loci, and not to their associated alleles within families. Candidate-gene genetic association studies look for correlations between certain alleles at a locus and the population of individuals with disease. Although certain allele pairings of linked loci are likely to be disproportionately represented within any given kindred, as recombination occurs, this eventually will result in an even distribution of disease-marker allele combinations within the population at large. When the disease gene and marker loci are relatively far apart, such distribution will occur over the course of a few generations. On the other hand, if marker loci are close to a mutation that has spread through the population, this equilibrium may not have occurred.[4] Thus, an association between a disease and a particular allele within

---

[4] It has been estimated that approximately 69 generations, or 2,000 years, are necessary for the frequency of an allele combination to go to half of its equilibrium value for two loci that are separated by 1 centimorgan.

the population (linkage disequilibrium) suggests that the location of the disease gene and the marker locus is within a small genetic region. The advantage of this method over linkage analysis is that it may be sensitive to genes with small phenotypic effects. The drawbacks of this method are that the ability to detect a genetic association declines rapidly as genetic distance increases and that this method, like linkage analysis, is affected by genetic heterogeneity. The choice of the genetic control group is also critical. If individuals with the illness are from genetic backgrounds that differ from those of the control subjects with whom they are compared, the observed differences in allele frequencies may be due to racial differences rather than to differences in disease status (*population stratification*). Newer statistical approaches have been developed to address this potential artifact.

Historically, various marker loci have been used for genetic linkage mapping. The first markers were blood antigens from both erythrocytes (ABO, Rh, and MNS) and leukocytes (human leukocyte antigen [HLA]) that could be measured serologically; serum proteins and isozymes that could be measured electrophoretically; and common anomalies such as color blindness. The major shortcomings of these marker loci were their paucity (only about 30 are known) and their irregular distribution throughout the genome. In the early 1980s, the first markers using DNA polymorphisms, the restriction fragment length polymorphisms (RFLPs), came into vogue. The RFLP markers detect variations in DNA sequence that create or abolish recognition sites for enzymes that cut DNA sequences at specific locations (i.e., restriction endonucleases). Because a restriction endonuclease site is either present or absent in a given chromosome (i.e., there are only two possible alleles), the RFLP markers limit the frequency of heterozygotes to 50%. The variation in DNA sequence that underlies most RFLPs is an SNP, as discussed below.

Driven by the minimal information available from having only two alleles and the laborious effort required for generating RFLP data, a second generation of polymorphic DNA markers (i.e., microsatellites or simple sequence repeats) was developed and mapped to various chromosomes. These markers use the naturally occurring variations in the length of dinucleotide (also tri-, tetra-, pentanucleotide) repeat elements present in the genomic DNA. For example, an individual might have the DNA sequence >GATT(CA)$_{12}$GCTA< on one of his homologous chromosome pairs and >GATT(CA)$_{16}$GCTA< on the other. After these DNA fragments have been selectively amplified 100,000-fold and labeled with radioactive nucleotides using the polymerase chain reaction (PCR), they can be separated by length (32 bp vs. 40 bp) and detected by autoradiography. The inheritance pattern of these fragments can then be followed up in families who have the disease of interest (Figure 6–2). The microsatellite markers have multiple alleles (e.g., [CA]$_{12}$ to [CA]$_{30}$) and therefore ensure that pedigree members are quite likely to be heterozygous for the marker loci. As illustrated in Figure 6–1, individuals who are heterozygous at a marker locus are essential for linkage studies. At the current microsatellite loci, 65%–85% of the individuals will be heterozygous. These markers are also densely and uniformly distributed in the human genome (approximately every 6 kilobases), and genotypes for the pedigree members can be determined in a day or two using PCR. High-density maps of each chromosome have been created using more than 8,000 of these markers (Broman et al. 1998).

The third-generation polymorphic markers are the SNPs. In these single base-pair variations, one chromosome might have a "G," while another has an "A" in its place, irrespective of the rest of the DNA sequence which may be exactly identical. Individual SNPs can thus be regarded as independent location-specific markers along the genome. Furthermore, as was noted earlier, SNPs occurring in the cutting sites of restriction endonucleases cause RFLPs. In humans, any two unrelated genomes are estimated to differ by 1 bp in every 290 to 1,000 bp. Given the 3.08 billion bp estimated size of the human genome, approximately 3 million sequence positions can be nonidentical between any two unrelated individuals, and 90% of the variations would be SNPs. Although microsatellite markers have more alleles and thus can be more informative in linkage analyses, the bi-allelic nature of SNP markers makes automated computer scoring of alleles much more reliable. Further, since SNP markers are much more common, it is possible to overcome the lack of information from any single SNP by typing multiple SNPs in a given gene; that way the higher laboratory throughput of SNP genotypes provides more information than microsatellite markers. In addition, some of the SNPs will embody actual DNA variations that influence phenotypic traits and will thus boost the power to detect them. Last, high-density SNP maps will enable genomewide association (GWA) studies in which several thousand SNP markers are genotyped in a collection of pedigrees (Risch and Merikangas 1996).

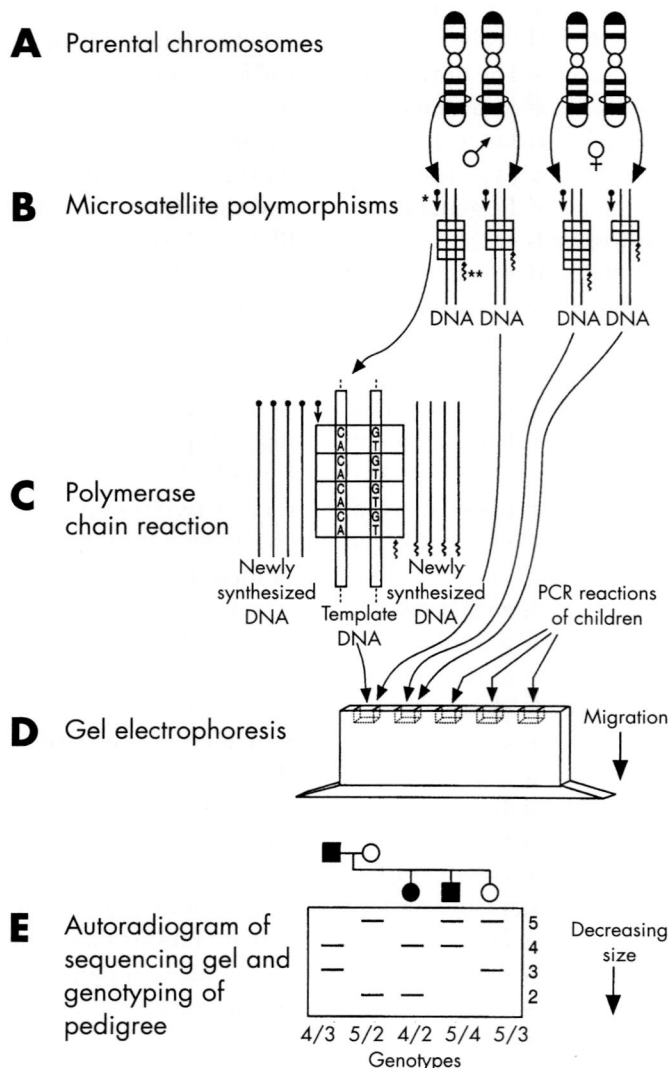

FIGURE 6–2. Schematic representation of a microsatellite marker.

Note. **Panel A.** Autosomal homologous chromosome pairs from parents in a pedigree to be genotyped. **Panel B.** The DNA sequence on the long arm of the chromosome is examined in greater detail, revealing the variable repeating DNA sequence termed a *microsatellite marker.* For a dinucleotide repeat, each box represents two nucleotides (e.g., CA). Differing numbers of repeats of this dinucleotide are frequently found in different individuals. The example shows a father with four and three repeats and a mother with five and two repeats. (This is a simplification; most commonly there are 15–20 repeats.) **Panel C.** Using DNA primers (* and **), one of which is radiolabeled, and a heat-stable DNA polymerase, repetitive cycles of DNA denaturation and replication exponentially amplify (105-fold) the DNA sequence bound by the primers. This process is termed the *polymerase chain reaction* (PCR) and is shown for only one of the two chromosomes of the father. Because the length of the fragment amplified is bounded by the primers, which are attached to nonrepeating sequences outside the microsatellite region, the length of the product of this reaction from each chromosome will be determined by the number of repeats. **Panel D.** The amplified DNA fragments are separated on the basis of size by gel electrophoresis. **Panel E.** The presence of the bands is determined by autoradiography. Individuals have two bands that correspond to the lengths of the amplified fragments. Each band is a marker for this region of the long arm of its own chromosome. The inheritance of these fragments can then be followed through all members of a pedigree whose DNA is available for the PCR reaction. Genotypes for each of the members of the hypothetical pedigree are shown under the autoradiogram. If an autosomal dominant disease is depicted by solid symbols, allele 4 would be linked to the disorder in this pedigree. This linkage, if statistically significant, indicates that the microsatellite marker is located close to the disease gene.

Problems of Diagnosis and Classification in Genetic Investigations

Most genetic studies are severely hampered by any ambiguity in knowing who has and who does not have the illness under examination. For example, accurate diagnosis of every family member is essential for all forms of segregation analysis and for almost all molecular genetic studies. Changes in the diagnoses of pedigree members can have profound effects on the evidence for linkage, as would be apparent in the studies of bipolar disorder.

Various versions of diagnostic criteria have been developed for psychiatric disorders. However, these criteria often exclude ambiguous cases rather than clarify their status. Moreover, even when the diagnostic criteria are reliable as for many psychiatric disorders, the robustness of diagnostic categories as specific entities remains to be proven. Lastly, the finding that the schizophrenic population is pharmacologically heterogeneous (Ban 2004) adds to diagnostic uncertainties. Thus, a lack of clear-cut diagnosis continues to confound genetic investigations.

The high prevalence of psychiatric disorders and the existence of many known medical disorders that can produce major psychiatric syndromes (e.g., various "symptomatic schizophrenias") are reasons to believe that most psychiatric diagnostic categories are clinical syndromes, identifying patients with a variety of etiological abnormalities. A diagnosis of Huntington's disease or Duchenne muscular dystrophy is known to specify a group with a specific etiology and pathogenesis, whereas a diagnosis of schizophrenia or major depressive disorder is not. If the diagnostic entities that psychiatry has established are not etiologically homogeneous, then searching for the modes of transmission or genetic linkages of these disorders may be likened to the genetic study of pneumonia, renal failure, or dropsy. Thus, even the most reliable criteria available for psychiatric disorders, validated to the best of our current ability, may fail to identify certain individuals with the disease (especially those with milder or deviant forms) and also may fail by falsely identifying some individuals with a "similar disease" (if there are multiple diseases that lead to a common clinical picture) as affected.

Most psychiatric disorders are complex in origin, with multiple interacting genetic and environmental contributors and stochastic effects (i.e., polygenic or multifactorial inheritance). In these cases, for linkage studies to succeed, the diagnostic schema must identify a group in which most patients share some specific abnormal genetic component, and this may not be the case with the current nomenclature. Psychiatric nosology has of course aimed at identifying illnesses with the specificity needed by genetic analysis, and it has explored the validity of various diagnostic systems by using broad versus narrow definitions, exclusion criteria, definitions of "functional impairment" and "secondary cases," and correction factors for diagnostic instability. The relative failure of this attempt may be inevitable for a nosology based on clinical phenomenology, for which greater knowledge of the biological pathogenesis of psychiatric disorders may be necessary. To capitalize on the new advances in genetic methodology, psychiatry may need to discover, in addition to the symptoms of the illness, subtypes of current diagnostic categories that have one or more specific measurable biochemical or physiological traits, known as "intermediate phenotypes" or "endophenotypes" (Berrettini 2005; Braff and Light 2005; Flint and Munafo 2007; Gottesman and Gould 2003; Hasler et al. 2004). The examples include precipitation of panic attacks with lactate infusion, and association of schizophrenia with deviant eye tracking. This development may be fostered by the emerging advances in neuroradiography, neurophysiology, neurochemistry, and the specification of cognitive deficits.

However, certain aspects of psychiatric disorders that make accurate diagnosis problematic will likely persist; these include late age at onset, intermittent expression of symptoms, progressive variation of symptoms over time (e.g., major depressive disorder becoming bipolar disorder), and the influence of environmental factors on the emergence (i.e., penetrance) of these disorders or in producing phenocopies. Also, as discussed earlier in the subsection "What Are the Various Clinical Expressions of the Abnormal Gene(s)?—Spectrum Studies," all major conditions have mild or intermediate forms (e.g., schizotypal personality disorder, schizoaffective disorder); and such cases may at times represent *formes frustes* that are genetically associated with the major disorder. There are benefits to counting these cases as affected in genetic studies, but even more etiological heterogeneity is likely in these milder and intermediate syndromes than in the major ones; and considering such cases as affected can result in misleading results regarding specific genetic determinations (such as mode of transmission or linkage).

Genetics of Psychiatric Disorders

Schizophrenia

Family Studies

Beginning with the pioneering work of Rudin (1916), Kallmann (1946/1994), and others in the Berlin school, more than 5,000 affected individuals and relatives have been examined for the risk of schizophrenia (Riley and Kendler 2006). These studies, more than 25 to date, have consistently reported elevated morbid risks for schizophrenia in the first-degree relatives of schizophrenic probands (parents, mean = 5.6%; sibs, 10.1%; children, 12.8%) compared with those in the general population (0.9%), suggesting that schizophrenia is familial (Gottesman and Shields 1982). Subsequent studies, meeting modern criteria for the collection of family data, have corroborated the earlier findings. The observed lower risk to parents, at odds with Mendelian inheritance—all first-degree relatives sharing 50% of their genes should show equal risk— may be reflecting reproductive fitness effects.

It would appear that schizophrenia, regardless of whether broadly or narrowly defined, is familial. Furthermore, schizoaffective disorder (as defined in DSM-III-R), paranoid personality disorder, atypical psychosis, and schizotypal personality disorder also aggregate in the relatives of schizophrenic probands, indicating possible boundaries of the phenotypic spectrum (Kendler et al. 1985). Additional studies have extended this boundary to other clinical conditions (qualitative phenotypes) and clinical and subclinical signs (quantitative phenotypes). It appears that even bipolar disorder may be elevated in the relatives of schizophrenic probands, at least in some families (Pope and Yurgelun-Todd 1990)—possibly those with schizophrenia "spectrum conditions" (Baron and Gruen 1991)—or when the mood disorder is associated with psychotic symptoms (Decina et al. 1991).

Elevated quantitative phenotypes that are clinically apparent in the relatives of schizophrenic probands include 1) positive symptoms measured by the Thought Disorder Index (Shenton et al. 1989); 2) negative symptoms measured by the Scale for the Assessment of Negative Symptoms (Tsuang et al. 1991); 3) neuropsychological signs such as deficits in abstraction (as measured by the Wisconsin Card Sorting Test) and in short-term verbal memory (Franke et al. 1992); and 4) neurological soft signs (Kinney et al. 1991).

Subclinical phenotypes that are elevated in the relatives of schizophrenic probands include 1) disturbances in thinking, social relatedness, volition, and affective expressivity as measured by a psychometric index derived from the Minnesota Multiphasic Personality Inventory (MMPI) (Moldin et al. 1990a); 2) eye movement dysfunction on smooth pursuit (Trillenberg et al. 2004) and visual fixation tasks (Amador et al. 1995); 3) impairments in suppression of the 50 msec preattentional component (P50) of the auditory evoked potential in a conditioning testing paradigm (Clementz et al. 1998); and 4) attentional disturbances as measured by the Continuous Performance Test (CPT) (Keefe et al. 1997), the Forced-Choice Span of Apprehension Task (SPAN), and the Digit Symbol Substitution Test (DSST) (Laurent et al. 2000).

Family studies have also provided clues to the genetic boundaries of other psychotic and related disorders. Thus, risk for both schizophrenia and bipolar disorder may be elevated in the relatives of probands with schizoaffective disorder (Coryell and Zimmerman 1988), psychotic affective illness may be elevated in the relatives of patients with schizophreniform disorder (Pulver et al. 1991), and schizophrenia may be elevated in the relatives of patients with schizotypal personality disorder (Battaglia et al. 1995). Three large independent family studies conducted a meta-analysis of relative risk and found the odds ratios of 16, 5, and 4 for developing schizophrenia, schizotypal personality disorder, and other nonaffective psychoses, respectively, in first-degree relatives of probands with schizophrenia (Kendler and Gardner 1997).

Family studies may help in elucidating etiologically homogeneous subgroupings in schizophrenia. For example, specific environmental exposures, structural brain abnormalities, and/or age at onset may predict more or less "familial" forms of the disorder: probands who had obstetrical complications may be at a lower familial risk than those who did not (Bersani et al. 1995). Similarly, siblings of probands with a negative family history may have greater ventricular enlargement (Silverman et al. 1998). One exception to this supposition may be males with a very early onset, who may be at elevated familial risk (Pulver et al. 1990). Similarly, females with an especially early onset (before age 22 years) may be at an elevated familial risk (Sham et al. 1994). Age at onset has not been universally associated with familial risk of illness in all studies. Prognostic features may predict other types of familial risk: for example, probands with good social, occupational, and residential outcome may have elevated family risks for unipolar illness.

On the other hand, family studies may help to eliminate nongenetic subgroupings. For example, in one study, paranoid versus nonparanoid subtypes of schizophrenia, neither bred true nor could be distinguished by differential rates of schizophrenia or mood disorder in the relatives of probands. Likewise, there may be no individual symptoms in probands that result in differential risk for schizophrenia in relatives (Kendler et al. 1994).

Finally, family studies performed on special populations may shed light on (epigenetic) etiological factors contributing to disease expression. The recent observation of a 4- to 15-fold increase in the morbid risk for schizophrenia among siblings of (British-born) second-generation African Caribbean schizophrenic probands compared with the siblings of their white counterparts suggests the interaction of a particularly vulnerable genetic background with risk-conferring environmental factors, in a phenomenon known as phenotype amplification (Weiss 1993). Cantor-Graae and Selten (2005), in a meta-analysis, have synthesized findings of studies appearing in MEDLINE between 1977 and 2003 implicating personal or family history of migration as a risk factor and suggested a potential role for psychosocial adversity in the etiology of schizophrenia.

Thus, family studies have contributed a great deal to defining the (clinical and subclinical) schizophrenia spectrum, clarifying the nosological relationship of other psychotic disorders to schizophrenia, and addressing the issues of etiological heterogeneity and etiology. They have provided confirmation that schizophrenia is familial. It bears emphasizing, however, that even well-designed family studies cannot distinguish between genetic and environmental influences on familial aggregation of a complex disorder such as schizophrenia. Therefore, other strategies, including twin and adoption studies, are needed. Shih et al. (2004) have recently reviewed the evidence from family, twin, and adoption studies for genetic contribution to adult psychiatric disorders, including schizophrenia.

Twin Studies

If the contribution of genetic factors is crucial to the pathogenesis of schizophrenia, it is imperative that MZ and DZ co-twins of probands with schizophrenia differ in their risk for the disorder. In fact, this has been consistently observed since the initial twin studies conducted by Luxenberger almost 60 years ago. Up until 1986, 817 MZ twin pairs and 1,016 same-sex DZ twin pairs were studied, with weighted mean probandwise concordances of 59.2% and 15.2%, respectively, and therefore a broad-sense heritability of 88% (Kendler 1986). Nonetheless, estimates of proband-

wise concordance have varied, possibly reflecting differences in diagnostic criteria, case sampling, and zygosity assessment across studies. For example, broader diagnoses and more severe illness in probands—fewer positive symptoms, more negative symptoms, poorer premorbid social competence (Onstad et al. 1991)—both yield higher concordance rates. More recently, five large meta-analysis studies using explicit operational diagnostic criteria found DSM-III-R schizophrenia concordances of 50% for MZ and 4% for DZ pairs and found the best fit to a model with a narrow-sense heritability of 88% (83% using ICD-10 diagnoses) (Cardno and Gottesman 2000).

In addition to establishing the importance of genetic factors, estimates of concordance may also shed light on the boundaries of schizophrenia; by identifying which operational definition of schizophrenia maximizes the difference between MZ and DZ concordance rates, investigators may determine a genetically validated definition of the disorder. In a reanalysis of the Maudsley twin study reported by Gottesman and Shields (1972), the maximum difference in rates occurred when DSM-III schizophrenia, affective disorder with mood-incongruent delusions, atypical psychosis, and schizotypal personality disorder were considered affected (Farmer et al. 1987). However, it is likely that not all of the genetic factors of these disorders are shared; analysis of a Finnish twin sample testing a multiple threshold model in which schizophrenia has the highest liability and affective and other psychoses have a lower liability found no support for the model (Cannon et al. 1998).

To summarize, the risk of schizophrenia in MZ co-twins of affected probands is at least three times that in DZ co-twins and about 40–60 times that in the general population. Just as noteworthy, however, is that only about half of MZ twin pairs are concordant for schizophrenia despite genetic identity. Monochorionic MZ twins are more likely to be concordant than are dichorionic MZ twins, perhaps because the former share not only identical genes but also a similar in utero environment (J. O. Davis and Phelps 1995). Although many nonschizophrenic MZ co-twins of affected probands show a variety of psychiatric disorders, including "neurotic" and character disorders and "schizoid" conditions, many (up to 43% in one series [Fischer 1971]) appear to harbor no psychiatric disorder. Moreover, the offspring of nonschizophrenic MZ co-twins may be at as high a risk for schizophrenia as are the offspring of their affected siblings, implying that these co-twins carry the schizophrenic genotype despite their "normal" appearance. These findings argue against phenocopies as the sole explanation for MZ twin discordance in schizophrenia. An additional argument against phenocopies is that discordant and concordant MZ twin pairs do not differ with respect to family risk, nor do they differ in birth order, birth weight, or condition at birth (Onstad et al. 1992). These findings also suggest a range of phenotypes compatible with the schizophrenic genotype and suggest an additive (or interactive) relation between genes and epigenetic (environmental) factors in the pathogenesis of the disorder.

Discordant MZ twins also provide a clue to the timing of these epigenetic factors and their effect on brain development. Differences between discordant MZ twins in dermatoglyphic patterns established in utero have suggested that a second-trimester environmental stressor combines with genetic risk in a "two-hit" model of disease pathogenesis (Rosa et al. 2000). Other studies of discordant MZ twin pairs have shown differences in left hemisphere hypodensity on computed tomography (CT) scan (Reveley et al. 1987); smaller anterior pes hippocampi on magnetic resonance imaging (MRI) (Suddath et al. 1990); and diminished activation of the dorsolateral prefrontal cortex while performing the Wisconsin Card Sorting Test, as measured by regional cerebral flood flow (Weinberger et al. 1992), smooth pursuit eye tracking (Litman et al. 1997), and electroencephalogram patterns (Stassen et al. 1999). Altered expression of genes regulating neurodevelopment (*TRAF4, Neurod1,* histone deacetylase 3), encoding a circadian pacemaker (*PER1*), and several others involved in regulating chromatin function and signaling mechanisms not only supports association of schizophrenia with abnormalities in oligodendroglia but also suggests a role for epigenetic mechanisms and altered circadian rhythms in schizophrenia (Aston et al. 2004).

Adoption Studies

All four types of adoption study have been applied to schizophrenia: adoptee study method, cross-fostering, adoptee's family method, and the study of MZ twins reared apart (see discussion of adoption studies earlier in this chapter). Despite varying methodology, these studies have consistently suggested a role for genetic influences in schizophrenia.

The adoptee study method was initially used by Heston (1966), who found a significantly greater risk for schizophrenia among the offspring of schizophrenic mothers separated at birth than among the adopted-away offspring of control mothers. This finding has been replicated in a Danish sample studied by Wender et al. (1974), which has withstood blind reanalysis with DSM-III criteria, and in a Finnish sample studied by Tienari et al. (2000), which has incorporated modern techniques such as direct blind interview of adoptees and detailed examination of adoptive families, the latter permitting an analysis of genotype–environmental interactions.

The sole cross-fostering study to date found equivalent rates of severe psychiatric illness among adoptees from biological parents without psychiatric illness, regardless of whether or not their adoptive parents had schizophrenia; both adoptee groups had significantly lower rates of illness than those in a group of adoptees from biological parents with schizophrenia and related disorders (Wender et al. 1974). In addition to providing evidence for the etiological importance of genetic factors in schizophrenia, this cross-fostering study argues against a causal role for rearing factors associated with parent psychosis, except perhaps in the presence of a susceptible genotype.

The adoptee's family method has been used in a series of studies conducted by Kety and colleagues in Denmark. They found that schizophrenia and related disorders were more common in the biological relatives of 34 schizophrenic adoptees (13 of 150 vs. 3 of 156, $P < 0.01$), whereas the rates for these disorders, being low in both, did not differentiate the adoptive relatives of either adoptee group. The Danish adoption study has withstood reanalysis with DSM-III criteria and has since been replicated with a second cohort of 41 index and control adoptees (Kety 1988). The biological relatives of schizophrenic adoptees have shown higher rates not only of schizophrenia but also of DSM-III-diagnosed schizotypal and paranoid personality disorders, again expanding the boundaries of the schizophrenic syndrome (Kendler and Gruenberg 1984). Overall, the biological relatives of schizophrenic adoptees have shown a 10-fold increase in the risk for schizophrenia and spectrum disorders over the biological relatives of control subjects (Kety et al. 1994). Finally, two studies of MZ twins reared apart have shown high pairwise concordance for schizophrenia, providing further evidence for a genetic component in the etiology of this disorder (Gottesman and Shields 1982).

High-Risk Studies

High-risk studies have examined both early characteristics that distinguish the offspring of schizophrenic parents from control subjects, and premorbid features that predict which of those offspring will go on to develop schizophrenia. By the age of 1 year, high-risk infants were more likely than control infants to show "anxious" attachment behavior and sensorimotor deficits. By two, they were seen to be more passive and less attentive in play. Later, they show progressively less social competence. These findings have been taken as evidence of an inherited neurointegrative defect in schizophrenia (Fish et al. 1992). Alternatively, the findings might reflect developmental delays caused by obstetrical complications (such as low birth weight), which frequently befall schizophrenic mothers. In fact, psychopathology at age 6 years (especially among males) has been associated with low socioeconomic status, low Apgar score, and neonatal neurological abnormality (McNeil and Kaij 1987).

Older high-risk children have shown defective emotional rapport and disturbed cognition in unblinded clinical interviews, diminished attention on measures such as the CPT and the digit cancellation task, and greater impairment on the aforementioned psychometric index derived from the MMPI. These abnormalities support the Bleulerian notion of a primary affective, associational, and attentional disturbance in schizophrenia. Moreover, because these abnormalities characterize high-risk individuals who go on to develop either schizophrenia or schizotypal personality disorder, they support the genetic relatedness of these disorders. Because the abnormalities described herein affect only about 10%–25% of high-risk offspring (Watt et al. 1984), they appear to be somewhat removed from a core monogenic defect (if present) in schizophrenia. On the other hand, smooth pursuit eye movement dysfunction has been reported to characterize approximately 50% of the teenage children of schizophrenic parents and thus may more closely reflect the schizophrenic diathesis (Mather 1985).

Premorbid psychosocial predictors of schizophrenia (vs. schizotypal personality disorder) among adopted-away high-risk children have included communication deviance within the adoptive family (Tienari et al. 1994). Such observations do not clarify, however, whether this intrafamilial deviance is causative of, or reactive to, greater psychopathology among juvenile adoptees destined to develop more severe psychopathology in adulthood. Premorbid physiological predictors of adult schizophrenia among high-risk children have included obstetrical complications; soft neurological signs such as impaired balance, left-right confusion, and motor overflow in childhood; and autonomic hypoarousal in adolescence (Cannon et al. 1990). Moreover, adult correlates of schizophrenia (vs. schizotypal personality disorder) among high-risk offspring have included ventricular enlargement (especially of the third ventricle) on CT scan (Cannon

et al. 1994). It is tempting to speculate that these clinical and radiological findings reflect a common perinatal neurological insult that contributes to disease expression. This speculation is supported not only by prospective studies of high-risk individuals but also by retrospective studies of schizophrenic patients (Hultman et al. 1997) and by studies of discordant MZ twins. In these studies, poorer outcome has been associated with the triad of obstetrical complications, neurological dysfunction, and ventricular enlargement (the latter perhaps reflecting primarily enlargement *ex vacuo* of the temporal horn of the lateral ventricle in association with smaller anterior pes hippocampi). Nonetheless, many of these findings await replication and should be viewed with caution.

Mode of Inheritance

Several models for the genetic transmission of schizophrenia have been proposed, including monogenic/single major locus; oligogenic; and polygenic/multifactorial models. For example, Bššk (1953) was able to account for observed frequencies of schizophrenia in a geographical isolate in northern Sweden by proposing a dominant gene (with a frequency of 0.07) with homozygous penetrance of 100% and limited heterozygous penetrance (20%). Similarly, Karlsson (1988) suggested that a dominant gene with reduced penetrance (25%) could account for most cases of schizophrenia in Iceland. The reproductive disadvantage of schizophrenia (Larson and Nyman 1973), however, would seem to select strongly against a dominant gene.

A recessive monogenic model (with reduced penetrance) predicts that the incidence of schizophrenia among the offspring of two schizophrenic parents would be comparable to the probandwise concordance for MZ twins, and, in fact, this is what has been observed (Kringlen 1978). Similarly, a recessive model could allow for the maintenance of the abnormal gene in the population, despite reduced reproductive fitness of those individuals with the illness (Erlenmeyer-Kimling and Paradowski 1966). Normal rates of consanguinity in most families with schizophrenia, however, argue against recessive transmission of the disorder (Rosenthal 1970; but see Chaleby and Tuma 1987 regarding special populations).

Sex-linked models have been proposed by DeLisi and Crow (1989), who suggested that a schizophrenia susceptibility gene might reside on the X chromosome on the basis of sex differences in the clinical presentation of the illness, with a later onset and more benign course in women perhaps attributable to demonstration of random inactivation of X chromosomes carrying mutant alleles. Alternatively, these authors argued X chromosome inheritance on the basis of cytogenetic anomalies (including X chromosome aneuploidies—XXY, XXX—as well as a fragile site at Xq27) associated with schizophrenia-like psychoses. They attributed the observation that schizophrenia appears to be transmitted on the X chromosome in some families, and, given cases of male-to-male transmission, on an autosome in others, to be compatible with a susceptibility gene for the disorder residing in the "pseudoautosomal" region of the sex chromosomes (i.e., a region of sequence homology between X and Y chromosomes wherein recombination may occur during male meiosis [Burgoyne 1982]). "Pseudoautosomal" transmission would predict an increased frequency of same-sex sibling pairs affected with schizophrenia when illness is inherited through the paternal lineage, and, in fact, this has been observed (Crow et al. 1989).

Monogenic models, however, have difficulty accounting for the sharp drop in risk for schizophrenia as we move from MZ twins to first- and second-degree relatives. Oligogenic models involving the epistatic interaction of two or three gene loci may better account for these data (Risch 1990). Likewise, monogenic models are hard-pressed to account for the observed increased risk of schizophrenia in relatives, given either increased severity in the proband or a greater number of other affected relatives (Gottesman and Shields 1982). These observations, on the other hand, are compatible with a polygenic/multifactorial model. Furthermore, O'Rourke et al. (1982) argued against a single-locus, two-allele model by citing its inability to account for the observed distribution in the rates of schizophrenia among four classes of relatives of schizophrenia probands (parents, siblings, and MZ and DZ co-twins) in 21 studies meeting criteria of adequacy. Finally, several segregation analyses have similarly rejected monogenic models or, at least, have been unable to reject polygenic models (Vogler et al. 1990). Finally, multiple genomewide searches for schizophrenia have been performed with linkage analysis, yet the relationship between observed genetic risk and a specific variant, protein alteration, or biological process remains to be demonstrated (Riley and Kendler 2006).

These results are compatible, however, with a so-called mixed model involving a major locus in the setting of a multifactorial background (Tsuang et al. 1991). Moreover, they do not preclude the possibility that major loci underlie certain aspects of the schizophrenia phenotype. Thus, admixture analysis, a strategy complementary to segregation analysis that examines the population distribution of a quantitative

phenotype for multimodality (each mode presumably reflecting the mean phenotypic consequence of a particular genotype), has provided preliminary evidence for a major gene underlying the aforementioned psychometric index derived from the MMPI (Moldin et al. 1990b) and smooth pursuit eye movement dysfunction (Clementz et al. 1992).

Linkage, Association, and Gene Expression Analyses

Over the past decade, several genetic loci and candidate genes have been implicated in the pathogenesis of schizophrenia, and some have been partially replicated (for review, see Riley and Kendler 2006; Sklar 2002). While none of these regions has yet yielded a confirmed gene for schizophrenia, evidence is strong for several of them (Table 6–3). Of overall importance, however, is the overlap of several of these loci/candidate genes with those reported for bipolar disorder (see section "Mood [Affective] Disorders" below).

Mood (Affective) Disorders

The major mood disorders—bipolar disorder (also known as manic depressive illness) and major depression (also called unipolar depressive disorder)—have been found to be highly familial in several European and American studies, since the conceptualization of bipolar illness 35 years ago. First-degree relatives of bipolar probands have an elevated morbid risk for both bipolar and major depressive illnesses, whereas relatives of major depression probands have an elevated risk for major depression but not bipolar disorder (Weissman et al. 1984). In these studies, there have been inconsistent findings of increased rates of alcoholism and sociopathy among relatives. Schizoaffective disorder, especially schizoaffective disorder with manic symptoms, has also frequently been found to be associated with a high rate of bipolar disorder among relatives.

In addition to finding these high rates of familial incidence of mood disorders, some studies have also noted that the risk for family members and the morbid risk in the population have increased for those born in later decades versus earlier decades of the twentieth century (Gershon et al. 1987; Klerman et al. 1985). This has been termed an *age-period-cohort effect*, and it has been found to be present in many countries (Weissman et al. 1992). The cause of this ominous trend remains undetermined.

The results of a very large NIMH collaborative study (2,226 interviewed relatives) that used the RDC,

TABLE 6–3. Candidate genes for schizophrenia

Candidate gene symbol	Name	Chromosome band	Biological function	Evidence*	References
SELENBP1	Selenium-binding protein 1	1q21–q22	Rapid cell outgrowth	G B P	Glatt et al. 2005; Prabakaran et al. 2007
RGS4	Regulator of G protein signaling	1q23.3	G protein signaling	L G	Brzustowicz et al. 2000; Gurling et al. 2001; Mirnics et al. 2001b
DISC1	Disrupted in schizophrenia 1	1q42.1	Cognition/cortical development	L A	Clapcote et al. 2007; Ekelund et al. 2004; Hennah et al. 2005; Hodgkinson et al. 2004; Kamiya et al. 2005; Lipska et al. 2006; Millar et al. 2005; Morris et al. 2003; Sawa and Snyder 2005; Sawamura et al. 2005
MAL	Myelin and lymphocyte protein	2cen–q13	Myelin biogenesis/function	G	Hakak et al. 2001; Tkachev et al. 2003
MDH1	Malate dehydrogenase	2q13.3	Metabolic regulation	G F	Burlina and Visentin 1965; Hakak et al. 2001; Middleton et al. 2002; Vawter et al. 2004
GAD1	Glutamate dehydrogenase 1	2q31.1	Cognition	A G	Addington et al. 2004; Akbarian et al. 1995; Goldman-Rakic 1994; Guidotti et al. 2005; Hashimoto et al. 2003; C. M. Lewis et al. 2003; Volk et al. 2000; Weinberger et al. 1986
DTNBP1	Dysbindin	6p22.3	Lysosomal biogenesis	L A G	Straub et al. 2002; Talbot et al. 2004
NRG1	Neuregulin	8p21–p12	Neural plasticity/ NRG1–ErbB signaling	L A G	Brzustowicz et al. 1999; Law et al. 2006; Pulver et al. 1995; Stefansson et al. 2002
PPP3CC	Protein phosphatase 3	8p21.3	Calcium signaling	A M	Gerber et al. 2003
HSPA12A	Heat shock 70kDa protein 12A	10q26.12	Neuron development/maturation	A G	D. A. Lewis et al. 2004; Pongrac et al. 2004
HTR2A	Serotonin receptor 2A	13q14.1–q32	Synaptic transmission	L	Blouin et al. 1998; Brzustowicz et al. 1999; Chumakov et al. 2002; Lin et al. 1995; Lohmueller et al. 2003

TABLE 6–3. Candidate genes for schizophrenia *(continued)*

Candidate gene symbol	Name	Chromosome band	Biological function	Evidence*	References
AKT1	RAC-alpha serine/threonine-protein kinase	14q32.32	Neuronal survival	L	Norton et al. 2006
MAG	Myelin-associated glycoprotein	19q13.1	Myelination	G	Aston et al. 2004; Hakak et al. 2001; Tkachev et al. 2003
COMT	Catecholamine methyltransferase	22q11.21	Cognition	A G	Egan et al. 2001; Funke et al. 2005; Shifman et al. 2002; Straub and Weinberger 2006
PRODH	Proline dehydrogenase	22q11.21	Apoptosis	A F M	Bender et al. 2005; Gogos et al. 1999
PLP1	Proteolipid protein 1	Xq21.3–q22	Myelination	G	Hakak et al. 2001; Hof et al. 2003; Tkachev et al. 2003
APOL	Apolipoprotein gene cluster	22q13.1–q12.3	Lipid/fatty acid metabolism	G	Mimmack et al. 2002

*Evidence key: A=association study; B=blood lymphocytes; F=functional activity; G=gene expression; L=linkage analysis; M=animal model.
Additional sources.

URLs: OMIM (http://www.ncbi.nlm.nih.gov/entrez/query.fcgi?db=OMIM); GAD (geneticassociationdb.nih.gov).
Review articles: Harrison and Weinberger 2005; D. A. Lewis and Gonzalez-Burgos 2006; D. A. Lewis et al. 2005; Mirnics and Pevsner 2004; Mirnics et al. 2000, 2001a, 2006; Norton et al. 2006; O'Donovan et al. 2003; Owen 2005; Owen et al. 2004; Riley and Kendler 2006; Ross et al. 2006; Straub and Weinberger 2006.

as reported by Andreasen et al. (1987) for interviewed relatives, are summarized in Table 6–4. These data confirm the above findings. This study also found that first-degree relatives of schizoaffective probands with depressive features had a somewhat elevated rate (2.5%) of schizophrenia and a zero prevalence of bipolar I disorder. These findings, being quite different from those for schizoaffective disorder of bipolar type, provided evidence that certain types of schizoaffective disorder may not be related to bipolar disorder. In this study, the authors decided to report rates of illness rather than morbid risk figures because the age and sex distributions across relative groups were similar, and the presence of the age-period-cohort effect could prevent accurate morbid risk calculations.

Many other family studies have also attempted to use variations in the rate of affected relatives to validate subtypes of major depression. This is an effort, in part, to find a phenotype(s) that could be a discrete illness and correspond to Mendelian inheritance pattern or show linkage to genetic markers. This search has investigated various definitions of endogenous depression, pharmacological response, severity of illness, suicidality, presence of psychotic features, rapid cycling, associated illnesses (e.g., alcoholism, anxiety disorder), decreased rapid eye movement (REM) latency, early age at onset, and recurrent episodes. Except for the last three, most of these factors have not been consistently shown to increase familial risk. In two studies, reduced REM latency was also associated with higher familial rates (Giles et al. 1988; Mendlewicz et al. 1989). In addition, in more than six studies on depressed and/or bipolar probands, early age at onset (before age 20 years) has been shown to be associated with an increased rate of illness by two- to three-fold among adult relatives (vs. relatives of other depressed probands). The increase is even greater for early-onset cases among relatives (Kupfer et al. 1989). The corresponding increase in a study of prepubertal depression was 14-fold (Weissman et al. 1988). Last, two family studies (Bland et al. 1986; Rice et al. 1987a) reported increased familial risk for probands with recurrent major depressive disorder. Age at onset and recurrence appear to act independently to increase risk. When probands had recurrent disease and an age at onset below the sample median (about 50), their relatives had more than five times higher risk of major depressive disorder than did relatives of later-onset, single-episode probands (Bland et al. 1986).

Similar efforts to distinguish subtypes of major depression, but beginning with differences in familial background rather than proband characteristics, were made by Winokur et al. (1975). In this work, patients with major depression who have a first-degree relative with bipolar disorder are considered bipolar disorder-related, whereas others with major depression are divided into familial pure depressive disorder (i.e., first-degree relative with affective illness), depressive spectrum disease (i.e., first-degree relative with alcoholism or antisocial personality), and sporadic depressive disease (i.e., no family history of depression, antisocial personality, or alcoholism). Additional studies that used this typology have found a more favorable short-term (i.e., 6-month) outcome with pure depressive disorder, and those subjects with depressive spectrum disease were found to have less severe depression (but more alcoholism and social maladjustment) on long-term (i.e., 11-year) follow-up.

Twin studies have supported the importance of genetic factors in the transmission of the major mood disorders. Summed data from early twin studies that did not distinguish between bipolar disorder and major depression give a 65% pairwise concordance rate for MZ twin pairs and a 14% rate for DZ pairs (Nurnberger and Gershon 1982). The MZ rate for bipolar disorder was higher than that for major depression, but the study sample sizes were much smaller. One of the studies that found highest heritability of bipolar disorder, using strict criteria, observed a pairwise concordance rate of 58% for MZ pairs compared with 17% for DZ pairs, in a total of 110 pairs (broad-sense heritability of 82%) (Bertelsen et al. 1977). A meta-analysis of five twin studies of major depression, with a starting sample of more than 21,000 individuals, estimated that the additive genetic contribution to developing the disorder was 37%, and the rest of the variance was explained by individual-specific environmental effects, whereas none was attributable to shared familial environmental effects (Sullivan et al. 2000). Two twin studies of major depression suggested that heritability of major depression is higher in females than in males (Bierut et al. 1998; Kendler et al. 2001), particularly when using a broad disease definition, but this was not observed in the above meta-analysis.

The few adoption studies of major mood disorders are confounded by differences in sampling and therefore have produced somewhat conflicting data. The lone study of adopted-away offspring found that the children of mothers with bipolar disorder or major depression had a higher rate of major mood disorder than did the adopted-away children of mothers with other psychiatric conditions (Cadoret 1978). Mendlewicz and Rainer (1977) found a significantly increased risk for affective illness in the biological par-

TABLE 6–4.   National Institute of Mental Health Collaborative Study of Affective Disorders: rates of illness in interviewed first-degree relatives

Diagnoses in relatives (%)	Diagnosis of proband					
	Bipolar I	Bipolar II	Unipolar	Schizoaffective —depressive	Schizoaffective— bipolar	Schizophrenia
Bipolar I	3.9	4.2	22.8	0.2	0.5	1.0
Bipolar II	1.1	8.2	26.2	0	0.4	0.4
Unipolar	0.6	2.9	8.4	20.3	0.2	0.3
Schizoaffective— depressed	0	3.7	21.0	0	0	2.5
Schizoaffective— bipolar	3.6	5.8	25.4	0	0.7	0.7

Source.   Data from Andreasen et al. 1987.

ents of bipolar adoptee probands, compared with their adoptive parents or with the biological parents of control subjects. Wender et al. (1986) studied a group of adoptees with mixed mood disorder diagnoses (bipolar, unipolar, neurotic depression, "affect reaction") and found an increase in suicide and some mood disorders among their biological, but not their adoptive, relatives when each was compared with his or her corresponding control subject. In contrast, von Knorring et al. (1983), in a similar design, found no differences between the biological parent groups and noted an excess of psychiatric illness in the adoptive parents of the index cases, who were primarily adoptees with nonbipolar depression.

Many psychiatric disorders have been associated with bipolar disorder and/or major depression in family and twin studies; thus, an "affective disorder spectrum" is thought to include dysthymia, cyclothymia, schizoaffective disorder (RDC), alcoholism, and eating disorders. Newer studies convincingly add attention-deficit/hyperactivity disorder, nicotine addiction, and even migraine to this list. In addition, certain personality traits (e.g., rigidity) appear to be increased among relatives (Maier et al. 1992). However, preferential mating between those persons with mood disorders plus the frequency of secondary depressions complicating almost all severe illnesses makes it difficult to determine whether these associations actually reflect joint etiological determinants.

High-risk studies of children of parents with major mood disorders have quite consistently found high rates of social and psychiatric impairment. Controlled studies of specific diagnoses have noted an increased prevalence of major depression, conduct disorder, at-

tention-deficit/hyperactivity disorder, anxiety disorder, substance abuse, and school problems, as well as poorer social functioning among these children. These high-risk offspring displayed an earlier age at onset of depression (mean age=12–13 years) than depressed control subjects whose parents were not depressed (mean age at onset=16–17 years).

The mode of transmission of the mood disorders currently is an area of intense research activity. One hypothesis that has been repeatedly tested without conclusive results is that major depression and bipolar disorder are mild and severe forms, respectively, of the same disorder, either by being on the same continuum of vulnerability to illness (polygenic or multifactorial model) or by being phenotypic variants of the same (abnormal) genotype at a single major locus. The prevalence data from family studies usually have been consistent with multiple-threshold polygenic models, but some data sets have been equally consistent with multiple-threshold single major locus models.

Pedigree and segregation analyses, which are more powerful techniques, have tended to reject single autosomal locus transmission, but the best-fitting genetic model in the largest segregation analysis of bipolar disorder was to a dominant, Mendelian major locus (Spence et al. 1995). In contrast, a segregation analysis of the Amish pedigrees could rule out autosomal dominant transmission under some circumstances (Pauls et al. 1995). Another segregation analysis failed to correspond well to either multifactorial-polygenic or single major locus models, leading the authors to conclude that bipolar disorder, although highly familial, has a "complex" mode of transmission (Rice et al. 1987b). Likewise, for major depression, segregation analyses have not resolved the mode of inheritance. Two older studies found evidence of a single major locus effect with non-Mendelian transmission probabilities (Price et al. 1987), whereas a newer study of early-onset recurrent depression (before age 25 years) found evidence for non-Mendelian inheritance of a recessive single major locus effect with a narrow diagnosis (recurrent major depressive disorder) and evidence for a Mendelian co-dominant major locus with residual parental and spousal effects with a broader diagnostic definition (Marazita et al. 1997).

Capitalizing on the availability of a large sample that is informative for genetic linkage analysis in the NIMH Genetics Initiative for Bipolar Disorder, Dick et al. (2003) conducted a genomewide linkage analysis on 1,152 individuals from 250 families segregating for bipolar disorder and related illnesses. They found significant linkage to two regions: 17q, at the marker *D17S928*; and 6q, near the marker *D6S1021*. Suggestive evidence of linkage was observed in three regions: 2p, 3q, and 8q.

Recently, in an attempt to simultaneously analyze bipolar illness, psychosis, suicidal behavior, and panic disorder, Cheng et al. (2006) conducted a genomewide scan on a large bipolar pedigree of 1,060 individuals from 154 multiplex families in the NIMH Genetics Initiative. Standard diagnostic models identified chromosomes 10q25, 10p12, 16q24, 16p13, and 16p12 with strongest linkage signals; while phenotypic subtypes—suicidal behavior, panic disorder, and psychosis—identified 6q25, 7q21, and 16p12, respectively. Some regions suggestive of linkage were also found by two phenotypic subtypes—psychosis (1p13; 1p21; 2p25; 4p16; 5p15; 6p25; 10p11; 13q32; and 19p13) and suicidal behavior (4p16; 10q25). Of these, chromosomes 1p, 1q, 6q, 8p, 13q, and 16p have been linked to bipolar disorder. The phenotypic subtype–based approach used by Cheng et al. (2006) is consistent with the convergent genomics paradigm that etymological dissection of a complex disease phenotype into component endophenotypes can reduce heterogeneity and simplify etiological analysis of polygenic diseases, including psychiatric disorders.

Overall, although the history of linkage studies on bipolar disorder is relatively short and is fraught with weak or inconsistent findings, genome scans, as described below, have identified several regions of interest on different chromosomes. Currently, the regions with the best support for containing a disease gene for bipolar disorder include 1q25–q32, 4q, 6q, 13q31–q32, 18p11, 18q21–q23, 21q22, and 22q11–q13 (reviewed in Hayden and Nurnberger 2006). Interestingly, several

of these loci overlap with those observed in schizophrenia, fueling a continuing nosological debate (K.L. Davis and Haroutunian 2003).

Genetic Association Studies of Depression

There have also been numerous genetic association studies of bipolar disorder and major depression. Meta-analyses of some of these have been reviewed recently by Craddock and Forty (2006) and Hayden and Nurnberger (2006), and gene–environment interaction by Lesch (2004); these are summarized in Table 6–5. However, one recent GWA study merits discussion here for its diligent experimental design and skillful execution.

In a landmark feasibility study of 14,000 cases of seven common diseases and 3,000 shared controls, the Wellcome Trust Case Consortium (WTCCC 2007) identified 24 genetic risk factors. The study, hailed by *Nature* as the "biggest pot of (genetics) gold yet," is the most dramatic demonstration to date of the power of the GWA approach.

Bipolar disorder was one of the seven diseases addressed in this study. The others were coronary artery disease, Crohn's disease, hypertension, rheumatoid arthritis, type 1 diabetes, and type 2 diabetes. The bipolar study, like the others, included 2,000 cases and 3,000 matched controls. The results showed the strongest signal with rs420259 at chromosome 16p12, in a recessive genetic model. However, despite its significance (P value of 6.3×10^{-8}) in genotype testing, the association was not supported by the expanded reference-group analysis, signifying the need for independent replication. Nonetheless, the authors noted several pathologically relevant genes localized to this locus: *COG7, GGA2, EARS2, UBFD1, NDUFAB1, PALB2, DCTN5, PLK1,* and *ERN2*. Fascinatingly, none of these genes had been reported previously, but some shared the same physiological pathways with previous candidate genes and some were related to completely novel pathways.

Of the nine candidate genes located at 16p12, two are involved in Golgi-related functions. *Cog7* codes for Golgi-localized protein complex, which is essential for Golgi apparatus structure and its function in intracellular transport and glycosylation; and *GGA2* encodes a member of the Golgi-localized, gamma-adaptin ear-containing, ARF-binding (GGA) family of ubiquitous coat proteins. It regulates movement of cargo molecules and assembly of clathrin-coated vesicles. Again, proteins encoded by two genes are associated with mitochondrial function. *NDUFAB1* encodes NADH-ubiquinone oxidoreductase 1 α/β subcomplex 1, the first enzyme complex in the electron transport chain of mitochondria; and *EARS2* codes for putative mitochondrial glutamyl-tRNA synthetase. *DCTN5* encodes dynactin 5 (p25), which is involved in slow axonal transport (Dillman et al. 1996), and known to interact with *DISC1*, a candidate gene with replicated association in both bipolar disorder and schizophrenia. *PALB2*, a breast cancer susceptibility gene with checkpoint functions, plays a role in the Fanconi anemia–DNA repair pathway and breast cancer predisposition (Rahman et al 2007). *ERN2*, coding for endoplasmic reticulum to nucleus signaling 2, is an endoplasmic reticulum (ER) stress-response gene. *PLK1* codes for polo-like kinase 1 (*Drosophila* homolog), a regulator of mitotic spindle function. *UBFD1* encodes ubiquitin-binding protein homolog, a member of the ubiquitin family domain containing 1.

Found significant in the expanded reference group analysis is *KCNC2*, encoding Shaw-related K(+) channel. Noting its strong association with channelopathies, the authors suggested its possible involvement in episodic disturbances of mood and behavior. In a surprise agreement with published reports, some of the SNPs implicated GABA neurotransmission (rs7680321; *GABRB1*; C/T allele), glutamate neurotransmission (rs1485171; *GRM7*; G/T allele), and synaptic function (rs11089599; *SYN3*; G/T allele), all of which have been previously implicated in bipolar disorder, schizophrenia, and (albeit in a different direction for some) major depression. Remarkably, all three SNPs are located in introns.

Other Approaches

Over the past decade, several nontraditional approaches have been taking the center stage in attempts to identify genetic factors for schizophrenia and elucidate the pathophysiological role of molecular variations. Specifically, one approach that has become highly popular and promising since its debut in 1995 is the microarray technology (Lockhart et al. 1996; Schena et al. 1995). By simultaneous assay of the global expression pattern of several thousand genes (transcripts) using microarrays, the hidden networks of molecular interactions and biological processes can be uncovered and interpreted in an appropriate biological context. By far the most successful example of the application of this nascent technology is demonstrated in cancer research (Lossos et al. 2004; van de Vijver et al. 2002), and there is considerable enthusiasm for reaching similar goals in psychiatric diseases and human behavior (for reviews, see Mirnics et al. 2006; Watson et al. 2000). Microarray assays of postmortem brains have implicated a number of candidate genes and neurobio-

logical pathways in the etiology of major psychiatric disorders. Despite considerable divergence among the overall findings reported by the studies, which can only be resolved by larger sample sizes and several more studies, a trend is definitely emerging to build consensus on a few of the candidate genes, which are summarized in Table 6–5; and functional implications of these findings may be found in Chapter 4, "Cellular and Molecular Biology of the Neuron." Validation of candidate genes by independent methods (e.g., genetic linkage/association studies) will further reinforce microarray findings and vice versa (Kennedy et al. 2003; Mirnics and Pevsner 2004).

With a putative gene identified and validated, understanding how it can influence the risk for the psychiatric disorder depends on defining the variation(s) in cognate DNA sequence. According to the convergent functional genomics model (Niculescu et al. 2000), multiple lines of converging evidence would bring a candidate gene into greater focus for further characterizations, including exploration of biological significance. A strategy of proven value in this regard has been to use genetic engineering techniques and 1) create a mouse lacking the gene (knockout) or 2) deliberately introduce specific variations into the mouse genome (site-directed mutagenesis), and then study the effect of genetic manipulation on the behavior of the mouse. Notwithstanding the limitation that human behavior in its full complexity is hard to reproduce in a mouse model, the fact that knockout mice have been produced for several neuropsychiatric candidate genes identified to date attests to the practical value of animal models in psychiatric genetics research (Clapcote et al. 2007; Low and Hardy 2007; Role and Talmage 2007; http://www.jax.org). Another emerging trend is the use of short interfering RNA (siRNA) to silence gene transcripts in vivo to study loss of function of a candidate gene in animals. Yet another approach is to study individuals carrying genotypic variation at a candidate disease locus and attempt to correlate the genetic change with behaviors, traits, and/or endophenotypes.

Comprehensive reviews of experimental designs and data analysis procedures and discussions of merits and limitations of the application of microarrays to postmortem human brain studies of psychiatric diseases can be found in recent articles (Bunney et al. 2003; Jackson et al. 2005; Mirnics and Pevsner 2004; Mirnics et al. 2006).

Anxiety Disorders

Anxiety disorders are a group of conditions marked by intense, often unrealistic, and extreme states of fear

TABLE 6–5.   Candidate genes for mood (affective) disorders

Candidate gene symbol	Name	Chromosome band	Biological function	Evidence*	References
Bipolar disorder					
DISC1	Disrupted in schizophrenia 1	1q42.1	Cognition/cortical development	L A B G	Berrettini 2000; Blackwood et al. 2001; Curtis et al. 2003; Detera-Wadleigh et al. 1999; Macgregor et al. 2004; Maeda et al. 2006; McInnis et al. 2003; Palo et al. 2007
MAL	Myelin and lymphocyte protein	2cen–q13	Myelin biogenesis/function	G	Iwamoto et al. 2004; Ogden et al. 2004; Tkachev et al. 2003
SST	Somatostatin	3q28	GABA signaling	G	Konradi et al. 2004; Nakatani et al. 2006; Sun et al. 2006
FAT	FAT tumor suppressor homolog 1	4q34–q35	Adhesion/signaling	L A D	Adams et al. 1998; Badenhop et al. 2003; Blair et al. 2006
HEY2	Hairy/enhancer-of-split related YRPW motif 2	6q22	Neurogenesis/transcription	A	Dick et al. 2003; Middleton et al. 2004; Schulze et al. 2004
BDNF	Brain-derived neurotrophic factor	11p13–p12	CNS development	A F	Geller et al. 2004; Lohoff et al. 2005; Neves-Pereira et al. 2002; Rybakowski et al. 2006; Sklar et al. 2002
DAOA (G72)/G30	D-amino acid oxidase activator	13q34–q31	NMDA receptor pathway	L A	Badner and Gershon 2002; Chen et al. 2004; Hattori et al. 2003; Potash et al. 2003; Schumacher et al. 2004
MAG	Myelin-associated glycoprotein	19q13.1	Myelination	G	Iwamoto et al. 2004; Ogden et al. 2004; Tkachev et al. 2003
TRPM2	Transient receptor potential cation channel M2	21q22.3	Calcium homeostasis	L A S	McQuillin et al. 2006
COMT	Catecholamine methyltransferase	22q11.2	Cognition	A	Badner and Gershon 2002; Lachman et al. 1996; Rotondo et al. 2002

TABLE 6–5. Candidate genes for mood (affective) disorders *(continued)*

Candidate gene symbol	Name	Chromosome band	Biological function	Evidence*	References
Bipolar disorder *(continued)*					
ADRBK2 (GRK3)	G-protein coupled receptor kinase 3	22q11.13; 22q12.1	GPR signaling	L A M	Barrett et al. 2003; Kelsoe et al. 2001; Niculescu et al. 2000; Potash et al. 2003
APOL	Apolipoprotein gene cluster	22q13	Lipid/fatty acid metabolism	G Q	Middleton et al. 2005
Major depressive disorder					
CREB1	cAMP-responsive element binding protein 1	2q34	cAMP signaling	A	Zubenko et al. 2002, 2003
FGF2	Fibroblast growth factor 2	4q26–q27	Neuroprotection	G I Q D	Choudary et al. 2005; S. J. Evans et al. 2004
SLC1A2	Glial high-affinity glutamate transporter 2	11p13–p12	Glutamate removal	G	Choudary et al. 2005
SLC6A4	Serotonin transporter	17q11.1–q12	Neurotransmission	A	Caspi et al. 2003; Hoefgen et al. 2005; Ogilvie et al. 1996; Taylor et al. 2005; Willeit et al. 2003
MAG	Myelin-associated glycoprotein	19q13.1	Myelination	G	Aston et al. 2005

*Evidence key: A=association study; B=blood lymphocytes; D=drug studies; F=functional activity; G=gene expression; I=in situ hybridization; L=linkage analysis; M=animal model; Q=quantitative polymerase chain reaction (qPCR); S=sequencing.

Additional sources.

URLs: OMIM (http://www.ncbi.nlm.nih.gov/entrez/query.fcgi?db=OMIM); GAD (geneticassociationdb.nih.gov).

Review articles: Farmer et al. 2007; Hayden and Nurnberger 2006; Kato 2007; Craddock and Forty 2006; Levinson 2006.

and phobia that interfere with an individual's activities and normal functioning. The NIMH epidemiological study of anxiety disorders found 1-year prevalence rates of 12.6%, thus ranking anxiety as the most common category of illness (Regier et al. 1993). Diagnostic terms and concepts of anxiety disorders have changed considerably over the past decade and a half, diminishing the relevance of older studies in this area. However, whenever studied, "anxiety neurosis" was found to be highly familial, with up to two-thirds of families showing cases in first-degree relatives. Studies that used DSM-III-R diagnostic categories have reported increased familial rates for panic disorder and agoraphobia, generalized anxiety disorder, simple and social phobias, and obsessive-compulsive disorder (OCD). The considerable number of chromosomal regions implicated in panic disorder, phobias, and anxiety disorders attest to the existence of a significant genetic basis for these disorders (see Villafuerte and Burmeister 2003).

Panic Disorder

Several family studies have detected a higher rate of panic disorder in the relatives of affected probands than in the relatives of control subjects. The relative risk to first-degree relatives of panic disorder probands ranged between 2.6- and 20-fold, with a median value of 7.8-fold. This has been seen consistently in all studies, including several overseas studies. For example, Middeldorp et al. (2005), in a study of 2,287 Australian and 1,185 Dutch twins and sibs, found an upper heritability estimate of 40% and 50% for generalized anxiety disorder and social phobia, respectively, and 46% for same-sex sibs only, indicating different familial factors for men and women. Several twin studies of panic disorder have been done. The earliest were performed by Torgersen (1983, 1990) and Skre et al. (1993), who found broad-sense heritability estimates between 30% and 62%. The higher estimates of heritability are likely to be overestimates because of the absence of observed DZ pairs concordant for panic disorder in the early studies. The best-fitting bivariate model predicted that approximately half of this additive genetic effect was shared in common between panic and generalized anxiety disorder (Scherrer et al. 2000). Genome scans of panic disorder and/or agoraphobia identified a recessive locus on 7p15 (Knowles et al. 1998) and a dominant locus on 13q when the affected phenotype for the analysis was panic disorder, mitral valve prolapse, serious headache, thyroid problems, or kidney or bladder problems (Hamilton et al. 2003; Weissman et al. 2000).

Major anxiety disorders, including phobias and panic disorder, are complex traits sharing at least one susceptibility locus (e.g., 4q31–q34 at marker *D4S413* [Kaabi et al. 2006]). This region, also harboring the neuropeptide Y receptor gene, *NPY1R* (4q31–q32), has been linked to anxiolytic-like effects in rats (Sorensen et al. 2004). Another candidate is chromosome 9q31 at marker *D9S271*, which has been linked not just to panic disorder but to anxiety in general in 62 Icelandic families genotyped with 976 microsatellite markers and validated in a subset of 25 extended families (Thorgeirsson et al. 2003). Multivariate structural equation modeling in 9,270 adult subjects from the Virginia Adult Twin Study of Psychiatric and Substance Use Disorders population indicate that *GAD1* variants may contribute to individual differences in neuroticism and influence susceptibility across a range of anxiety disorders as well as major depression (Hettema et al. 2006). Individuals with panic disorder are more sensitive to the anxiogenic effects of multiple substances, including cholecystokinin (CCK), lactate, and inhaled carbon dioxide (Caldirola et al. 1997). Family studies of carbon dioxide sensitivity have shown larger increases of anxiety symptoms in the first-degree relatives of panic disorder patients as compared with healthy control subjects (van Beek and Griez 2000), and segregation analysis suggested a single major locus for the transmission of carbon dioxide sensitivity (Cavallini et al. 1999).

The possibility of a genetic relation between adult and childhood anxiety disorders has been prompted by the high rates of separation anxiety and school phobia reported by adults with panic disorder. Offspring of parents with panic disorder appear more likely to have separation anxiety disorder, panic disorder, or agoraphobia, regardless of whether their parents suffer from depression. Offspring of parents with major depression, on the other hand, were more likely to have social phobia, separation anxiety disorder, major depression, or disruptive behavior disorders, irrespective of whether or not their parents have panic disorder. A genetic relation is also likely between panic disorder and mood disorders, particularly bipolar disorder, because the incidence of panic disorder in families with bipolar disorder is more tightly linked to chromosome 18 (MacKinnon et al. 1998).

Obsessive-Compulsive Disorder

OCD is a severe psychiatric illness characterized by intrusive and senseless thoughts and impulses (obsessions) and by repetitive behaviors (compulsions) (Willour et al. 2004). It is estimated to affect nearly 5 million people in the United States (Karno et al. 1988). Evidence for a strong genetic component and environmental susceptibility factors in OCD comes from twin studies, family genetics studies, and segregation analyses (for review, see Alsobrook et al. 2002). The results of family studies of OCD are largely inconsistent (Mataix-Cols 2006), except that early-onset OCD, like early-onset mood disorder, seems highly familial. Substantial comorbidity of Gilles de la Tourette's syndrome is seen with OCD, and family studies together suggest a shared genetic diathesis (Barr and Sandor 1998; Leckman and Chittenden 1990).

Twin studies of OCD also indicate involvement of genetic factors. Carey and Gottesman (1981) found significant MZ–DZ differences (87% vs. 47%, respectively), giving a heritability estimate of 80%, which is similar to the results found earlier in a Japanese OCD investigation and in other studies. Several segregation analyses of OCD suggest that a single, possibly dominant, major locus may best account for the familial aggregation. Recently, Hu et al. (2006) confirmed linkage of *SLC6A4* promoter gain-of-function genotypes to OCD by demonstrating that the *HTTLPR L(A)L(A)* genotype exerts a moderate (1.8-fold) effect on the risk for OCD. The short variant of the serotonin transporter gene (*SLC6A4*; 17q11.1–q12) polymorphism, designated *5-HTTLPR,* reduces the transcriptional efficiency of the *SLC6A4* gene promoter, culminating in decreased serotonin transporter expression and serotonin uptake in lymphoblasts (Lesch et al. 1996). Transporter-facilitated uptake of serotonin is the site of action of widely used uptake-inhibiting antidepressant and antianxiety drugs, commonly known as the selective serotonin reuptake inhibitors (SSRIs). The lone known environmental factor with a potential to interact with genetic vulnerability to OCD is poststreptococcal autoimmunity (pediatric autoimmune neuropsychiatric disorders associated with streptococcal infections) (Leonard and Swedo 2001).

Other Anxiety Disorders (Generalized Anxiety Disorder, Phobias, Posttraumatic Stress Disorder)

Family studies of generalized anxiety disorder, simple phobias, and social phobia, but not posttraumatic stress disorder (PTSD), have found familial aggregation. Noyes et al. (1987) noted that increased rates of generalized anxiety disorder were specific and that they were not found among the relatives of patients with panic disorder. Fyer et al. (1990) reported a rate of 31% for simple phobia in first-degree relatives compared with 11% in control subjects (relative risk=3.3).

For social phobia, two studies (Fyer et al. 1993; Reich et al. 1988) found a threefold increase in this disorder in the relatives of probands, the latter reporting rates of 16% vs. 5% in the control group. When subtypes of social phobia were studied, an approximately 10-fold increase in the rate of generalized social phobia (and avoidant personality disorder), but not discrete and nongeneralized social phobia, was observed in the first-degree relatives of patients with social phobia of each respective subtype as compared with the relatives of control subjects (Stein et al. 1998). There is extensive comorbidity of these disorders in probands (Goldenberg et al. 1996), but the disorders "breed true" when the families of probands without comorbidity are studied (Fyer et al. 1995). Finally, no increase in PTSD was found in the families of PTSD probands analyzed for depression using family history, but it has been reported to increase the risk to develop PTSD after rape (Davidson et al. 1998).

Twin studies showed a 28%–40% heritability rate for agoraphobia, social phobia, and animal phobia (Nelson et al. 2000), with males showing marginally lower rates, and 15%–20% for generalized anxiety in both males and females, with no evidence of sex-specific genetic factors (Hettema et al. 2001). Overall, however, molecular genetic studies of these disorders are few and inconclusive. A quantitative gene expression profiling of various brain regions in six inbred mouse strains with anxiety-like behavioral phenotypes led Hovatta et al. (2005) to the identification of 17 candidate genes. In lentivirus-mediated gene transfer experiments to validate candidate genes, they detected increased anxiety-like behavior in the mouse brain in response to local overexpression of glyoxalase-1 and glutathione reductase-1, and decreased anxiety-like behavior consequent to local inhibition of glyoxalase-1 expression via RNA interference, leading to the conclusion that both of these genes may be involved in oxidative stress metabolism, linking this pathway to anxiety-related behavior.

Drug Dependence

Numerous studies (reviewed in Merikangas et al. 1989) show that alcoholism is highly familial and that the risk to first-degree relatives is increased approximately sevenfold. This work has been extended to other drugs of abuse, with most having an eightfold increased risk to first-degree relatives. A study of the siblings of the probands in the Collaborative Study on the Genetics of Alcoholism (COGA) found similar results (Bierut et al. 1998). Both studies found evidence of specific transmission of risk for each drug of abuse, in addition to general factors that predispose to all drugs.

Several adoption studies also provide evidence that genetic factors, as well as environmental ones, are involved in the etiology of alcoholism. Goodwin (1979) found elevated rates of alcoholism among both the adopted-away daughters of alcoholic persons and control adoptees, whereas Cadoret et al. (1985) found higher rates in the daughters of index cases compared with control subjects. Data from a large Swedish sample also support a genetic predisposition to alcoholism in women and men (Cloninger et al. 1981), as well as the possible importance of certain environmental factors, such as lower occupational status of the adoptive father. In the COGA study, the risk of alcoholism in siblings of alcoholic females was observed to be slightly higher than for siblings of alcoholic males, suggesting a higher genetic predisposition in the females (Reich et al. 1998). In several studies, alcoholism in the adoptive environment was not found to increase the risk among adoptees.

Twin studies support the hypothesis that substance abuse disorders are highly heritable and that genetic factors predispose to abuse in general and to specific substances. In addition, it appeared that genetic factors influencing alcoholism do not completely overlap between the two sexes (Prescott 2002). This is consistent with the animal work on alcoholism (see later discussion in this section). Furthermore, the sex-specific genetic factors appear to overlap with those that predispose individuals to developing major depression (Prescott et al. 2000). Substantial overlap between the genetic factors for alcoholism and nicotine use (heritability of 50%–70% in many studies) has been observed in twin studies (True et al. 1999). Last, overlap has been observed between genetic factors for major depression and nicotine use in females (Kendler et al. 1993), suggesting that a set of genes may act in a sex-specific manner in predisposing to major depression, nicotine dependence, and alcoholism. Further, notwithstanding their relatively low magnitudes, the consistent changes observed in the expression of candidate genes in the frontal cortex across alcoholic individuals may be indicative of an important alcohol response.

There are a multitude of molecular studies of substance abuse disorders. These studies have been reviewed recently (Lachman 2006; Nestler and Malenka 2004; Oroszi and Goldman 2004; Rhodes and Crabbe 2005). The genes well studied for their influence on the development of a substance abuse disorder encode alcohol dehydrogenase (*ADH2*), which metabolizes ethanol to acetaldehyde, and aldehyde dehydrogenase

(*ALDH2*), which converts acetaldehyde to acetate (Radel and Goldman 2001). Acetaldehyde is toxic, and genetic variations that increase its synthesis or decrease its breakdown cause a reaction of facial flushing, headache, palpitations, hypotension, tachycardia, nausea, and vomiting. Such variants have been observed in the Asian population and appear to be protective against developing alcoholism (Thomasson et al. 1991). Chai et al. (2005) examined *ADH2*, *ADH3*, and *ALDH2* polymorphisms in a sample of Korean men, 72 with alcoholism and 38 without alcoholism. Forty-eight of the alcoholic men had Cloninger type 1 alcoholism, and 24 had Cloninger type 2. The frequency of *ADH2*1* and *ADH3*2* alleles was significantly higher in type 2 alcoholism than in type 1 alcoholism or in control subjects. The frequency of the *ALDH2*1* allele was significantly higher in alcohol-dependent men than in controls, suggesting that the genetic characteristics of alcohol metabolism in type 1 alcoholism may be intermediary between nonalcoholism and type 2 alcoholism.

Most of the candidate gene work on substance abuse has confirmed the role of the genes in the dopamine pathway. However, despite the key role of dopamine in reward behavior and addiction, the findings are controversial, and studies have reached very different conclusion (Koob and Nestler 1997; Rhodes and Crabbe 2005). The *DRD1*, *DRD3*, *DRD4*, *DRD5*, *DAT1*, and *MAOA* genes have also been studied for genetic association, but largely with negative results (for a review, see Rhodes and Crabbe 2005).

Herman et al. (2003) showed association between the *SLC6A4* short form of the promoter polymorphism and alcohol consumption in a college population. Munafo et al. (2005) replicated the finding of the short allele's association with increased alcohol consumption in 755 unrelated individuals (ages 33–73 years), who were recruited as part of a study of genetic associations with smoking cessation. There was suggestive evidence of a genotype–sex interaction. Post hoc analysis indicated that just the presence of the short allele, regardless of copy number, is sufficient to increase alcohol consumption in men, while heterozygosity conferred higher consumption rates on women. Feinn et al. (2005), in a meta-analysis of data collected from 17 published studies including 3,489 alcoholics and 2,325 controls, also found significant association of the frequency of the short allele of *SLC6A4* with alcohol dependence; a comorbid psychiatric condition, an early onset, or a more severe alcoholism subtype further increased the association. Radel et al. (2005) genotyped alcohol-dependent and unaffected individuals in a

Southwestern Native American sample ($n = 433$) and a Finnish sample ($n = 511$) for 6 SNPs in the *GABA-A* receptor gene cluster on chromosome 5q34. Sib-pair linkage, case–control association analyses, and linkage disequilibrium mapping with haplotypes demonstrated sib-pair linkage of *GABA-A* receptor genes to alcohol dependence in both samples. Three polymorphisms of *GABRA6*, including a pro[385]ser substitution, were implicated in haplotype localization.

Multiple candidate genes for nicotine use have been investigated, but there are no replicated positive findings even from methodologically sound studies (for a review, see Al Koudsi and Tyndale 2005). Alcohol and nicotine dependence have been the subject of many genome scans (Uhl 2004). A genome scan of 105 families from the COGA study found evidence for linkage of chromosomes 1, 2, and 7 (highest lod score = 3.49) and for a protective locus on chromosome 4, which contains the *ADH* gene cluster (Reich et al. 1998). A subsequent analysis suggested that the locus on chromosome 1 predisposes to both alcoholism and major depression (Nurnberger et al. 2001), which is what was predicted by the family and twin study discussed earlier. Lappalainen et al. (2004) fine-mapped the region and found the strongest TDT evidence for marker *D1S406* and three additional markers all within less than 350 kb, suggesting that one or more alcoholism susceptibility genes reside on chromosome 1 in a region approximately delimited by markers *D1S1170* and *D1S2779*.

A second genome scan of 172 sibling pairs from a Southwestern American Indian tribe found evidence for loci on both copies of chromosome 4, which contains the *GABAB1* gene, and chromosome 11, which contains the genes for *TH* and *DRD4* (Long et al. 1998). One genome scan has been published for nicotine dependence; this study of 130 families from New Zealand and an additional 91 families from Virginia found the strongest evidence for linkage on chromosome 2 (Straub et al. 1999) and detected weaker signals on chromosomes 4, 10, 16, 17, and 18.

A molecular genetic approach that has worked particularly well in understanding the biology of substance abuse is the use of animal models. Berrettini et al. (1994) were able to map three loci in mice for oral morphine preference by breeding mice from progenitor strains that differed in their morphine preference. The effect of one of these loci, on mouse chromosome 10, has been replicated in another sample, and the linked region contains a candidate gene, encoding the mu opiate receptor. Two sex-specific loci for alcohol preference in mice have also been mapped (Melo et al.

1996). Interestingly, the locus for alcohol preference in female mice demonstrates genomic imprinting (is only active when passed from one parental line—in this case from the mother). Neither locus for alcohol preference overlaps with the three loci for morphine preference, suggesting the genetic basis for each addictive disorder is distinct.

Recently, however, valuable insights were also gleaned in substance abuse research, especially alcoholism, by gene expression profiling using microarrays. Molecular determinants of an alcoholism trait (characterized by craving, dependence, and tolerance) are inherently difficult to study in humans. By contrast, rodent models, particularly isogenic strains of mice with a high or low degree of preference for voluntary consumption of alcohol, offer a unique opportunity to decipher molecular complexities underlying the genetic predisposition to alcohol consumption. Consequently, a majority of the microarray studies analyzed well-established rodent models of alcoholism, whereas far fewer studies investigated human postmortem brains. However, the animal and human studies together are yielding data that are gradually converging on the neurobiological pathways associated with alcoholism and/or substance abuse/addiction or comorbidity with depression.

Mulligan et al. (2006), in a 107 microarray-based meta-analysis of a behavioral phenotype, found several functional groups, including mitogen-activated protein kinase signaling and transcription regulation pathways, to be significantly overrepresented among the 3,800 nonoverlapping candidate genes. Four of the candidate genes, *Pknox2*, *Scn4b*, *9030425E11Rik*, and *1110032A03Rik*, were correlated with alcohol preference in a BXD recombinant inbred population (Phillips et al. 1994), and five had putative transcriptional activity: *Carm1*, *Pknox2*, *Tcf12*, *Zfp29*, and *Limd1*.

In another approach, candidate behavior genes were identified by associating regional expression with behavioral phenotypes of anxiety, drug-naive and ethanol-induced distance traveled across a grid floor, and seizure susceptibility (Letwin et al. 2006). Here, multiple genes within the glutamatergic signaling pathway (i.e., *N*-methyl-D-aspartate/glutamate receptor subunit 2C, calmodulin, solute carrier family 1 member 2, and glutamine synthetase) showed a phenotype-dependent and region-specific pattern. In addition, glutamatergic signaling genes, including those found here, in various combinations, have been implicated in seizures (Eid et al. 2004), ethanol-induced locomotion (Roberto et al. 2004), and major depressive disorder (Choudary et al. 2005).

Extending their previous findings, Liu et al. (2006) identified novel genes involved in cell adhesion, apoptosis, and neural diseases that were altered by long-term alcohol abuse. Eighteen of the 20 cell adhesion candidate genes were downregulated. Cell adhesion molecules play critical roles in the development of the central nervous system, synapse formation, and immune responses. Ethanol has previously been shown to change neural cell–cell adhesion in vitro (Charness et al. 1994). Most of the published results also show concordant downregulation of the myelination (4 genes) and calpain/calpastatin systems. In the Liu et al. (2006) study, 10 out of 11 myelination-related genes were downregulated, and the 11th gene was upregulated. Genes encoding the major component of the myelin sheath, proteolipid protein 1, and several encoding minor components (UDP glycosyltransferase 8, CNP, CD9 antigen, and claudin 11) were also downregulated, affirming that myelin structure is compromised by chronic alcohol abuse. Relatively small expression changes in the frontal cortex of alcoholic human brain seem quite consistent across individuals and likely represent important alcohol-responsive genes.

The rapidly growing number of microarray studies; application of global unbiased data analysis strategies; proteomic analyses; and integration of animal models, behavioral phenotypes, and QTLs together signal a new era in alcoholism research and are setting a model for psychiatric genetics research in general. As a result, the optimism is rational and justified that gene signatures based on improved understanding of the molecular basis will soon become available for early diagnosis of alcoholism. Numerous studies addressing the molecular basis of substance abuse disorders have been reviewed recently (Lachman 2006; Nestler and Malenka 2004; Oroszi and Goldman 2004; Rhodes and Crabbe 2005). Interestingly, several genes have been proposed as risk factors for both alcoholism and Alzheimer's disease—for example, transferrin (van Rensburg et al. 2004), calpain3, presenilin 1, and a glial specific gene (*PAWR*) (Guo et al. 1998).

Suicide and Impulsive Behavior

Many family studies have found familial clustering of suicides and suicide attempts (Brent and Mann 2005). This has been observed in studies of completers that used either friends (Shafii et al. 1985), individuals from the community (Brent et al. 1996), or nonsuicidal diagnostically matched control subjects (Tsuang 1983). Although it is difficult to control for the psychiatric co-

morbidity that also runs in the families of the victims, Brent et al. (1996) found a fourfold increased risk of suicide attempts and completions in the relatives of suicide probands as compared with the relatives of control subjects from the community. In the Amish, 73% of suicides occur in 16% of the pedigrees, even though some of the nonsuicide pedigrees are just as severely affected with bipolar disorder (Egeland and Sussex 1985). This pattern of increased risk to relatives of suicide probands as compared with relatives of control subjects—even beyond the risk conferred by an Axis I disorder—is also seen for relatives of suicide attempters.

Several lines of evidence suggest that a portion of this familial clustering is due to genetic factors (Savitz et al. 2006). One study of 176 twin pairs found 11% (7 of 62) of MZ and 1% (2 of 114) of DZ twin pairs to be concordant for suicide (Roy et al. 1991). Another study found concordance rates of attempted suicide among co-twins of suicide victims to be 38% (10 of 26) for MZ and 0% (0 of 9) for DZ twin pairs (Roy et al. 1995). The largest twin study of suicidal behavior interviewed 2,718 twin pairs and found the best estimate of heritability of reporting any suicidal ideation, persistent thoughts, and suicide plans or attempts to be about 44% and that of reporting serious attempts to be 55% (Statham et al. 1998). Adoption studies provide additional support for the hypothesis that genetic factors contribute to suicide (Wender et al. 1986).

Many studies suggest that altered serotonin metabolism may underlie both the trait of impulsivity and suicidal behavior. However, investigation of several genes in the serotonergic system (e.g., *TPH, 5-HT1B*, and *5-HT2A*) showed no clear genetic association with suicide. Some studies showed stronger results in patients with violent attempts, suggesting that the genetic association could be with a predisposition to violence rather than with suicide.

Perhaps the clearest link between a genetic mutation and human behavior with a psychiatric illness comes from the study of Brunner's syndrome in a large Dutch family (Brunner et al. 1993b). This X-linked syndrome is characterized by borderline mental retardation along with aggressive and violent impulsive behavior in affected males. Some of these behaviors include arson, exhibitionism, and attempted rape and suicide. A linkage study of the X chromosome found a lod score of 3.69 at the *MAOA* locus, and 24-hour urinalysis of three affected males showed abnormal monoamine metabolism (Brunner et al. 1993b). Subsequent analysis of *MAOA* revealed that affected males in the family have a cytosine to thymidine mutation at position 936, changing a glutamine codon to a termination codon, and cell culture assays showed the lack of MAOA enzymatic activity in the affected males (Brunner et al. 1993a). Further proof of the effect of this gene on behavior came from the aggressive behavior observed in a transgenic mouse strain in which the *MAOA* gene was deleted (Cases et al. 1995).

Merali et al. (2004), on the basis of quantitative PCR data, suggested a possibility that the CRH and GABA(A) receptor subunit changes, or the disturbed coordination between these GABA(A) receptor subunits, may contribute to depression and/or suicidality or may be a secondary effect of the illness/distress associated with it. The latter possibility was corroborated by the finding of Choudary et al. (2005) that frontal cortical levels of *GABA(A)α1* and *GABA(A)β3* transcripts in suicide completers are elevated with concomitant upregulation of several glutamate and GABA(A) receptor subunits in postmortem brains of individuals with major depressive disorder.

Consistent decreases in the expression of the spermine/spermidine N(1)-acetyltransferase gene (*SAT1*; Xp22.1) were found in the frontal cortex of suicide completers with or without major depression as a comorbid condition, and RT-PCR, immunohistochemistry, and Western blot analyses validated the finding in independent samples of adjacent areas (Sequeira et al. 2006). The variant of polyamine-responsive element regulatory region in *SAT1* (*SAT*342A/C) has a significant effect on brain expression levels of *SAT1*, the rate-limiting enzyme in the catabolism of polyamines. The *SAT*342C allele showed a higher frequency among suicide cases in an independent sample of 181 male suicide completers and 80 male control subjects, suggesting that this allele may partially increase predisposition to suicide.

Neuropsychiatric Disorders

The neuropsychiatric disorders—Gilles de la Tourette's syndrome, Huntington's disease, Lesch-Nyhan syndrome, Parkinson's disease—and Alzheimer's disease are not considered here. Up-to-date reviews can be found in several recent articles (Bertram and Tanzi 2004; Finkbeiner et al. 2006; Kamboh 2004) and in the companion book, *The American Psychiatric Publishing Textbook of Neuropsychiatry and Clinical Neurosciences*, 5th Edition (Yudofsky and Hales 2008).

Epigenetics

Parallels between neuropsychiatric disorders and other medical conditions suggest potential epigenetic regula-

tion of gene expression (e.g., gene–environment interactions) without altering the primary structure of genomic DNA. For example, schizophrenia bears many similarities to type 1 diabetes mellitus. Both disorders are associated with a modest increase in risk to first-degree relatives (λ_s of 15), an intermediate concordance among MZ twins (approximately 50%), and a combined effect of several major susceptibility loci. Perhaps the most important of these loci for type 1 diabetes mellitus is the class II major histocompatibility complex (MHC) locus (Davies et al. 1994), governing, among other things, the host response to viral infection. Not surprisingly, infection by a common agent, *Coxsackievirus*, and molecular mimicry between viral and host antigens have been implicated in the pathogenesis of type 1 diabetes mellitus (Solimena and De Camilli 1995). Likewise, several studies have suggested a role for both class II MHC locus (Nimgaonkar et al. 1995) and viral infection (Kaufmann and Ziegler 1987) in schizophrenia, implicating a common mechanism (Wright et al. 1995). The availability of suitable cohorts of subjects with schizophrenia, such as those originally identified through the landmark Child Health and Development Study (1959–1966; van den Berg et al. 1988), who have been followed up since early in gestation, and from whom both subject DNA and maternal prenatal serum samples have been obtained, should permit validation of class II MHC variation and specific intrauterine viral exposure. More recent studies have pursued epigenetic models of animals for schizophrenia vulnerability in relation to 1) the role of MHC class I molecules implicated in synaptic plasticity and developmental regulation of neurons (Oliveira et al. 2004); and 2) pharmacological correction of methionine-induced schizophrenia-like epigenetic molecular and behavioral neuropathologies in mice (Tremolizzo et al. 2005).

Besides, we now know that the total gene count in different organisms is not considerably different. The question then is: What makes each organism unique and each cell type different, and how is the information that is embedded in the genome decoded? The key seems to lie in the "cellular state" of a cell, which to a large extent can be deduced from its methylation/chromatin state. Accordingly, intense attempts are under way to define the functions of histone methylation and chromatin organization in the genome across diverse mammalian cell types. Pursuing this goal, Barski et al. (2007) created high-resolution profiles of histone methylations in the human genome, and Mikkelsen et al. (2007) independently constructed genomewide maps of chromatin state in both undifferentiated and differentiated cells. Both groups used a similar experimental approach—that is, sequencing ChIP (chromatin-immunoprecipitated) DNA using the ultra-throughput Illumina/Solexa method. The results shed new light on the topography of the regulatory elements (e.g., enhancers, insulators, repressors) and suggest that promoters could assume any of three functional forms—active, repressed, or poised for alternative developmental fates, depending on the biological context.

Nosology

As genetic variations underlying neuropsychiatric disorders are revealed, our notions of the boundaries between these disorders may need to be revised. With only linkage results in hand, we already have indications that disorders such as bipolar disorder and schizophrenia, once thought to be distinct, in fact overlap (Craddock et al. 2006). Thus, some groups studying bipolar disorder have found linkage in the same region of chromosome 6 implicated in schizophrenia; conversely, other groups studying schizophrenia have found evidence for linkage in the same region of chromosome 18 implicated in bipolar disorder. In addition, many of the replicated findings for both disorders identify the same chromosomal regions. Likewise, linkage analyses of panic disorder have found positive lod scores in some of the same chromosomal regions, corroborating pathway analyses that suggest an overlap between mood and anxiety disorders.

The possibility of a continuum between bipolar disorder and schizophrenia has been debated since the time of Kraepelin. Perhaps these disorders do lie on a continuum or share some, but not all, of a set of epistatic loci. Regardless of how, the lines between diagnostic categories will certainly need to be redrawn as the molecular basis for each disorder becomes clearer (see www.dsm5.org).

Genetic Counseling

With increasing awareness among patients, families, psychiatrists, and the general public about the hereditary aspects of psychiatric illness, interest in genetic counseling is steadily growing. The aims of those seeking genetic counseling for psychiatric disorder are manifold, and these as well as the data and techniques involved must be understood by physicians before attempting such an endeavor or referring patients for it. It is often not the patient who seeks genetic counseling; or, if such is the case, it quite likely happens at the insistence of others. Family members

and prospective spouses frequently ask for genetic information 1) to learn about the risk for themselves or their offspring, 2) to obtain advice on decisions of marriage or pregnancy, 3) to gain an understanding of a devastating illness in a family member, or 4) to reduce their sense of guilt or to ascribe guilt to others. Patients themselves, when they do seek this type of help, usually do so in the context of an ongoing therapeutic relationship. They may be seeking to understand the cause of their illness, to discover the implications it has for their descendants (present and future), or to determine whether it is "curable." A wealth of information is available on this subject at www.ornl.gov/sci/techresources/Human_Genome/medicine/genecounseling.shtml.

The components, or stages, of counseling as described by Tsuang (1978) are as follows:

- Diagnosis
- Family history
- Estimation of the risk of recurrence
- Evaluation of the aims, intelligence, and emotions of the counselee
- Helping the counselee to understand the risk of recurrence in the context of the burden of the disorder
- Formation of a plan of action
- Follow-up

Accurate diagnosis is essential, and careful review of the patient's history as well as diagnostic interviews with relatives may reveal diagnostic issues that have genetic implications (e.g., depressive disorder with early onset, or "symptomatic schizophrenia" from temporal lobe epilepsy).

With the diagnosis established, there are various methods of estimating the risk of recurrence. Risk rates for siblings, offspring, and other classes of relatives, such as those presented in this chapter, are available. These, however, are averages that are known not to apply under certain circumstances. For example, the risk for schizophrenia is increased in families by severity of the proband's illness, the presence of schizophrenic relatives besides the proband, and psychiatric illness in the proband's mate (Gottesman and Shields 1982). More sophisticated analyses can take into account information such as the number of ill relatives, subclinical or "spectrum" illnesses, and the age at risk for onset of illness, but such computerized programs need to assume an underlying mode of transmission. With the mode of transmission remaining unknown for most psychiatric disorders, such assumptions can affect risk estimates considerably (up to 10-fold). Thus, establishing accurate risk estimates in family members for most psychiatric disorders is also not possible currently, and therefore caution is warranted in counseling in the face of uncertainty.

When knowledge is lacking on the mode of transmission and the ability to identify family members at risk for the psychiatric disorders, it could (at times) be reconstructed from the other surviving family members. In the case of a disease with full penetrance, known dominant inheritance, and a closely linked marker, accurate assignments of the probability of an individual being affected can be made using a computerized linkage program, with the caveat that the program assumes no heterogeneity (Ott 1974).

The genetic counselor, especially one who is psychiatrically trained, has a unique opportunity to provide a great deal of important aid beyond estimating the risks of recurrence. This includes evaluating and helping the counselee, especially by reducing the amount of misinformation, confusion, guilt, and fear regarding the illness. The counselor also may be able to offer a plan with the potential for reducing or preventing the transmission of the illness but should recognize that counseling, although often successful in its educational goals, is unlikely to affect reproductive decisions (S. Kessler 1989). In doing this work, the counselor combines the skills of a geneticist, internist, psychiatrist, psychotherapist, marital counselor, and family therapist.

Psychopharmacogenetics

Psychopharmacogenetics refers to the study of genetic differences in the behavioral response to pharmacological agents. Behavioral differences may result from both pharmacokinetic variability (i.e., genetic differences in the absorption and degradation of drugs) and pharmacodynamic variability (i.e., genetic differences in tissue sensitivity to drugs). These differences can be used to predict both efficacy and potential adverse effects of various pharmacological agents (Bondy 2005). Most psychopharmacogenetic studies have focused on antidepressants and neuroleptics. Plasma levels of one of the tricyclics, nortriptyline, appear to be under genetic control, given that MZ twins have higher relative concentrations of the drug than DZ twins following administration of identical oral doses (Alexanderson et al. 1969). Variation in *CYP2D6* and *CYP2C19* alters the metabolism of many tricylic antidepressants (and some SSRIs), and dosage reductions have been suggested for individuals who carry alleles that make them poor metabolizers of these agents (Rasmussen et

al. 2006); these genotypes can be determined using microarrays (Murphy et al. 2001).

Plasma levels of the monoamine oxidase inhibitor phenelzine are also under genetic control: a polymorphism in the hepatic enzyme *N*-acetyltransferase that is responsible for degradation of the drug has been identified and appears to be inherited in a Mendelian fashion. Individuals with the less active isozyme ("slow acetylators") appear to be more prone to side effects from phenelzine (D. A. Evans et al. 1965) and, in at least one study, have shown greater therapeutic response to moderate doses of the drug. Also, the tendency to respond to a specific class of antidepressants seems familial (Franchini et al. 1998).

Although this might reflect the aforementioned pharmacokinetic differences in the rates of metabolism of these drugs, it is equally plausible that there are genetically distinct biological types of depression associated with different drug responses. Also, several studies suggest that variations in *5-HTTLPR* may predict response to SSRIs. In one study, 102 individuals with psychotic depression were treated with fluvoxamine with or without pindolol and were genotyped for the *5-HTTLPR* polymorphism. Individuals homozygous for the short form of the polymorphism (s/s) did not respond as quickly or as well as those with genotypes of l/s and l/l when treated with fluvoxamine alone (Smeraldi et al. 1998). All three genotypic groups responded similarly in the fluvoxamine plus pindolol treatment group. These findings have been replicated in an elderly patient population suffering from major depression treated with fluvoxamine (Zanardi et al. 2001), paroxetine (Pollock et al. 2000), or sertraline (Durham et al. 2004).

The genetic factors associated with the response and the side effects to the atypical neuroleptic clozapine have been investigated extensively. Ten studies examined the effect of variation in the 5-HT$_{2A}$ gene (*HTR2A*) on clozapine response with mixed results, as were studies of the other serotonin receptor genes and *DRD3* and *DRD4* (Lane et al. 2005). Genetic factors also appear to be important in the likelihood of developing an agranulocytotic reaction to clozapine. Lieberman et al. (1990) found increased frequencies of the HLA antigens B38, DR4, and DQw3 in Ashkenazi Jews who developed agranulocytosis. Further work has supported the association of *HLA-B38* and clozapine-induced agranulocytosis (Meged et al. 1999). Finally, genetic variations in *DRD3* and *HTR2C* have been associated with akathisia and tardive dyskinesia (Eichhammer et al. 2000; Segman et al. 2000).

Prevention and Treatment

As the molecular mechanisms underlying neuropsychiatric disorders become clearer, points of potential clinical intervention will also become apparent. They may be divided into those involving primary, secondary, and tertiary prevention, referring to interventions that prevent disease, prevent its evolution, or prevent its complications, respectively. Among primary preventive interventions are genetic counseling and gene therapy. Preconceptional decision making will need to change, as genetic counseling takes stock of complex disorders for which risks are relative, susceptibilities are multiple, and outcomes are uncertain. Prospects for gene therapy of disorders that afflict the postmitotic brain, once thought impossible, now appear feasible. Highly selective neurotropic, defective viral vectors (e.g., adenoviruses, lentiviruses, herpesviruses) have emerged as likely agents for wild-type gene transfer into the nervous system (Kaplitt and Makimura 1997). The possibility that gene transfer into the central nervous system might be effective has gained support from the observation that certain "stem-like" neural cells retain their pleuripotentiality until late in development (Snyder et al. 1997). Among secondary preventive interventions are targeted environmental manipulations in at-risk subjects, that is, reductions in exposure to relevant epigenetic factors, be they viruses, nutritional deficiencies, or early losses, in individuals with particular genetic susceptibilities. Ironically, in this regard, the very complexities that vex the study of complex disorders bode well for their treatment. Finally, the long delay between in utero exposure and adult onset for many neuropsychiatric disorders provides a large window for tertiary preventive interventions. For example, pharmacological studies of animal models of schizophrenia, such as those involving perinatal damage to the anterior hippocampus, suggest that early intervention with anticonvulsants may forestall the development of limbic dopaminergic supersensitivity (and presumably "positive" symptoms), whereas epidemiological studies of patients with schizophrenia suggest that early intervention, after the development of "positive" symptoms, with neuroleptic or electroconvulsive therapy may forestall the development of "negative" symptoms.

Conclusion

Progress in human genetics in general, and psychiatric genetics in particular, is occurring at an ever-increasing pace. No doubt only some of the future developments we have predicted will be borne out, and other, unimagined developments will occur. We need to consider only the disparity between the depiction of the late twentieth century evident in early science fiction films and our current reality to know that prognostication is a clumsy art, at best. Robust GWA findings, genome sequence information (of humans and several model organisms), powerful informatics tools to process massive data efficiently, target-specific gene/siRNA/nanoparticle delivery systems, and novel pathways as drug targets are converging and raising our hopes of at last unravelling the genetic underpinnings of complex diseases in the near future. Underlying this exuberance is the growing new culture of cooperation among national and international researchers and between academia and industry to forge partnerships and pool samples, analytical tools, and data. The new trend of cooperative research, in turn, is enabling us to see the big picture of biology and address the unsolved old, knotty scientific problems with new vigor. GWA breakthroughs that have been achieved within the past 20 months using such collaborative models include the identification of risk loci of coronary heart disease, Crohn's disease, breast cancer, prostate cancer, glaucoma, age-related macular degeneration, adult-onset diabetes, and obesity. Judging by this unprecedented record of achievements, and aided by the combined power of GWA, gene expression profiling, and various "-omics" studies, the prospect of identifying the genetic bases of neuropsychiatric diseases no longer seems endlessly elusive as in the decades past. Adding to our excitement is the little-explored frontier of RNA biology, which is just beginning to yield glimpses of its hidden repertoire (e.g., riboswitches, RNA chaperones, short interfering RNA [siRNA], microRNA [miRNA], Piwi-interacting RNA [piRNA], RNA interference [RNAi], and RNA trans-splicing), which were never before dreamt of. We believe that these epoch-making developments together promise a golden era of psychiatric genetics to all, in Albert Szent-Györgyi's words, "who see what everyone else has seen and think what no one else has thought before."

Key Points

- Multiple genes, each with a small effect, contribute to a psychiatric disease.

- Environmental influences, interacting with genetic factors, have a definite role in psychiatric illnesses.

- None of the psychiatric diseases has a confirmed disease gene as yet, but there are promising candidate genes for each disorder.

- *DISC1, NRG1, OLIG2, COMT, G72, APOL* cluster, and *SELENBP1* are strong candidate genes for schizophrenia.

- *SLC6A4, BDNF,* and *NMDAR* are promising candidate genes for bipolar illness.

- The fibroblast growth factor (FGF) system and GABA glutamate system appear to be involved in genetic etiology of major depressive disorder.

- Dysregulation of synaptic function, myelination, and oligodendrocyte function seem to be common to several psychiatric disorders.

- At the genetic level, bipolar disorder increasingly seems to share more common features with schizophrenia than with major depressive disorder.

- The HapMap project provides a bridge between linkage mapping and single nucleotide polymorphisms (SNPs).

- Combining data on linkage, SNP association, regulation of gene expression, and protein and RNA functions can be a powerful strategy for discovering psychiatric disease genes.

- It remains to be seen whether blood/peripheral blood leukocytes (PBLs) can serve as an alternative tissue that can be noninvasively accessed for routine diagnosis of psychiatric illnesses.

- Epigenetics likely has a greater role in the etiology of psychiatric illnesses than is now apparent.

- It pays to play by the rules of ethics.

Suggested Readings

Akil H: Stressed and depressed. Nat Med 11:116–118, 2005

Bunney WE, Bunney BG, Vawter MP, et al: Microarray technology: a review of new strategies to discover candidate vulnerability genes in psychiatric disorders. Am J Psychiatry 160:657–666, 2003

Burton PR, Tobin MD, Hopper JL: Key concepts in genetic epidemiology. Lancet 366:941–951, 2005

Cordell HJ, Clayton DG: Genetic association studies. Lancet 366:1121–1131, 2005

Couzin J, Kaiser J: Genome-wide association. Closing the net on common disease genes. Science 316:820–822, 2007

Dawn Teare M, Barrett JH: Genetic linkage studies. Lancet 366:1036–1044, 2005

Holden C: Future brightening for depression treatments. Science 302:810–813, 2003

Hopper JL, Bishop DT, Easton DF: Population-based family studies in genetic epidemiology. Lancet 366:1397–1406, 2005

Insel TR: Shining light on depression. Science 317:757–758, 2007

Kennedy JL, Farrer LA, Andreasen NC, et al: The genetics of adult-onset neuropsychiatric disease: complexities and conundra? Science 302:823–826, 2003

Palmer LJ, Cardon LR: Shaking the tree: mapping complex disease genes with linkage disequilibrium. Lancet 366:1223–1234, 2005

Online Resources

Cold Spring Harbor Laboratory. Available at: http://www.cshl.org. Accessed September 10, 2007.

Ensembl Genome Browser. A joint project between the European Molecular Biology Laboratory–European Bioinformatics Institute (EMBL-EBI) and the Sanger Institute to develop a software system that produces and maintains automatic annotation on selected eukaryotic genomes. Available at: http://www.ensembl.org/index.html. Accessed December 20, 2006.

Entrez cross-database search page. A retrieval system designed for searching several linked databases using keywords. Available at: http://www.ncbi.nlm.nih.gov/gquery/gquery.fcgi. Accessed December 20, 2006.

Ethics in biomedical research. Available at http://www.hhmi.org/bioethics. Accessed September 10, 2007.

Mental Health Research Association. Available at http://www.narsad.org. Accessed September 10, 2007.

Wellcome Trust Case Control Consortium. Available at: http://www.wtccc.org.uk. Accessed September 10, 2007.

Genetic Association Database. An archive of human genetic association studies of complex diseases and disorders. Available at: http://geneticassociationdb.nih.gov. Accessed December 20, 2006.

UCSC Genome Browser at the University of California Santa Cruz. Reference sequence and working draft assemblies for a large collection of genomes, and a portal to the National Human Genome Research Institute's ENCODE (ENCyclopedia Of DNA Elements) project. Available at: http://www.genome.ucsc.edu. Accessed December 20, 2006.

Human Genome Collection. An archive of all articles published in *Nature* on human genome sequence. Available at: http://www.nature.com/nature/supplements/collections/humangenome/index.html. Accessed December 20, 2006.

Human Genome Project. The sequences of the 3 billion chemical base pairs that make up human DNA and genes. Available at: http://ornl.gov/sci/techresources/Human_Genome/project/about.shtml. Accessed December 20, 2006.

International HapMap Organization. A catalog of genetic similarities and differences in human beings. Available at: www.hapmap.org. Accessed December 20, 2006.

NIH Knockout Mouse Project (KOMP). A comprehensive and public resource comprised of mice containing a null mutation in every gene in the mouse genome. Available at: http://www.nih.gov/science/models/mouse/knockout/index.html. Accessed December 20, 2006.

Online Mendelian Inheritance in Man (OMIM). A catalog of human genes and genetic disorders by McKusick VA et al. Available at: http://www.ncbi.nlm.nih.gov/entrez/query.fcgi?db=OMIM. Accessed December 20, 2006.

Talking Glossary. A glossary of genetic terms. Available at: http://genome.gov/10002096. Accessed December 20, 2006.

References

Adams LJ, Mitchell PB, Fielder SL, et al: A susceptibility locus for bipolar affective disorder on chromosome 4q35. Am J Hum Genet 62:1084–1091, 1998

Addington AM, Gornick M, Sporn AL, et al: Polymorphisms in the 13q33.2 gene G72/G30 are associated with childhood-onset schizophrenia and psychosis not otherwise specified. Biol Psychiatry 55:976–980, 2004

Akbarian S, Kim JJ, Potkin SG, et al: Gene expression for glutamic acid decarboxylase is reduced without loss of neurons in prefrontal cortex of schizophrenics. Arch Gen Psychiatry 52:258–266, 1995

Al Koudsi N, Tyndale RF: Genetic influences on smoking: a brief review. Ther Drug Monit 27:704–709, 2005

Alexanderson B, Evans DA, Sjoqvist F: Steady-state plasma levels of nortriptyline in twins: influence of genetic factors and drug therapy. BMJ 4:764–768, 1969

Alsobrook JP 2nd, Zohar AH, Leboyer M, et al: Association between the COMT locus and obsessive-compulsive disorder in females but not males. Am J Med Genet 114:116–120, 2002

Amador XF, Malaspina D, Sackeim HA, et al: Visual fixation and smooth pursuit eye movement abnormalities in patients with schizophrenia and their relatives. J Neuropsychiatry Clin Neurosci 7:197–206, 1995

American Psychiatric Association: Diagnostic and Statistical Manual of Mental Disorders, 3rd Edition. Washington, DC, American Psychiatric Association, 1980

American Psychiatric Association: Diagnostic and Statistical Manual of Mental Disorders, 3rd Edition, Revised. Washington, DC, American Psychiatric Association, 1987

American Psychiatric Association: Diagnostic and Statistical Manual of Mental Disorders, 4th Edition, Text Revision. Washington, DC, American Psychiatric Association, 2000

Andreasen NC, Rice J, Endicott J, et al: Familial rates of affective disorder. A report from the National Institute of Mental Health Collaborative Study. Arch Gen Psychiatry 44:461–469, 1987

Aston C, Jiang L, Sokolov BP: Microarray analysis of postmortem temporal cortex from patients with schizophrenia. J Neurosci Res 77:858–866, 2004

Aston C, Jiang L, Sokolov BP: Transcriptional profiling reveals evidence for signaling and oligodendroglial abnormalities in the temporal cortex from patients with major depressive disorder. Mol Psychiatry 10:309–322, 2005

Badenhop RF, Moses MJ, Scimone A, et al: Genetic refinement and physical mapping of a 2.3 Mb probable disease region associated with a bipolar affective disorder susceptibility locus on chromosome 4q35. Am J Med Genet B Neuropsychiatr Genet 117:23–32, 2003

Badner JA, Gershon ES: Meta-analysis of whole-genome linkage scans of bipolar disorder and schizophrenia. Mol Psychiatry 7:405–411, 2002

Ban TA: Neuropsychopharmacology and the genetics of schizophrenia: a history of the diagnosis of schizophrenia. Prog Neuropsychopharmacol Biol Psychiatry 28:753–762, 2004

Baron M, Gruen RS: Schizophrenia and affective disorder: are they genetically linked? Br J Psychiatry 159:267–270, 1991

Baron M: Manic-depression genes and the new millennium: poised for discovery. Mol Psychiatry 7:342–358, 2002

Barr CL, Sandor P: Current status of genetic studies of Gilles de la Tourette syndrome. Can J Psychiatry 43:351–357, 1998

Barrett TB, Hauger RL, Kennedy JL, et al: Evidence that a single nucleotide polymorphism in the promoter of the G protein receptor kinase 3 gene is associated with bipolar disorder. Mol Psychiatry 8:546–557, 2003

Barski A, Cuddapah S, Cui K, et al: High-resolution profiling of histone methylations in the human genome. Cell 129:823–837, 2007

Battaglia M, Bernardeschi L, Franchini L, et al: A family study of schizotypal disorder. Schizophr Bull 21:33–45, 1995

Bender HU, Almashanu S, Steel G, et al: Functional consequences of PRODH missense mutations. Am J Hum Genet 76:409–420, 2005

Berrettini WH: Susceptibility loci for bipolar disorder: overlap with inherited vulnerability to schizophrenia. Biol Psychiatry 47:245–251, 2000

Berrettini WH: Genetic bases for endophenotypes in psychiatric disorders. Dialogues Clin Neurosci 7:95–101, 2005

Berrettini WH, Ferraro TN, Alexander RC, et al: Quantitative trait loci mapping of three loci controlling morphine preference using inbred mouse strains. Nat Genet 7:54–58, 1994

Bersani G, Taddei I, Venturi P, et al: [Familial occurrence and obstetric complications in siblings discordant for schizophrenia]. Minerva Psichiatr 36:127–132, 1995

Bertelsen A, Harvald B, Hauge M: A Danish twin study of manic-depressive disorders. Br J Psychiatry 130:330–351, 1977

Bertram L, Tanzi RE: Alzheimer's disease: one disorder, too many genes? Hum Mol Genet 13 (Spec No 1):R135–R141, 2004

Bierut LJ, Dinwiddie SH, Begleiter H, et al: Familial transmission of substance dependence: alcohol, marijuana, cocaine, and habitual smoking: a report from the Collaborative Study on the Genetics of Alcoholism. Arch Gen Psychiatry 55:982–988, 1998

Blackwood DH, Fordyce A, Walker MT, et al: Schizophrenia and affective disorders-cosegregation with a translocation at chromosome 1q42 that directly disrupts brain-expressed genes: clinical and P300 findings in a family. Am J Hum Genet 69:428–433, 2001

Blair IP, Chetcuti AF, Badenhop RF, et al: Positional cloning, association analysis and expression studies provide convergent evidence that the cadherin gene FAT contains a bipolar disorder susceptibility allele. Mol Psychiatry 11:372–383, 2006

Bland RC, Newman SC, Orn H: Recurrent and nonrecurrent depression. A family study. Arch Gen Psychiatry 43:1085–1089, 1986

Blouin JL, Dombroski BA, Nath SK, et al: Schizophrenia susceptibility loci on chromosomes 13q32 and 8p21. Nat Genet 20:70–73, 1998

Bondy B: Pharmacogenomics in depression and antidepressants. Dialogues Clin Neurosci 7:223–230, 2005

Bourquin JP, Subramanian A, Langebrake C, et al: Identification of distinct molecular phenotypes in acute megakaryoblastic leukemia by gene expression profiling. Proc Natl Acad Sci U S A 103:3339–3344, 2006

Braff DL, Light GA: The use of neurophysiological endophenotypes to understand the genetic basis of schizophrenia. Dialogues Clin Neurosci 7:125–135, 2005

Brent DA, Mann JJ: Family genetic studies, suicide, and suicidal behavior. Am J Med Genet C Semin Med Genet 133:13–24, 2005

Brent DA, Bridge J, Johnson BA, et al: Suicidal behavior runs in families. A controlled family study of adolescent suicide victims. Arch Gen Psychiatry 53:1145–1152, 1996

Broman KW, Murray JC, Sheffield VC, et al: Comprehensive human genetic maps: individual and sex-specific variation in recombination. Am J Hum Genet 63:861–869, 1998

Brunner HG, Nelen M, Breakefield XO, et al: Abnormal behavior associated with a point mutation in the structural gene for monoamine oxidase A. Science 262:578–580, 1993a

Brunner HG, Nelen MR, van Zandvoort P, et al: X-linked borderline mental retardation with prominent behavioral disturbance: phenotype, genetic localization, and evidence for disturbed monoamine metabolism. Am J Hum Genet 52:1032–1039, 1993b

Brzustowicz LM, Honer WG, Chow EW, et al: Linkage of familial schizophrenia to chromosome 13q32. Am J Hum Genet 65:1096–1103, 1999

Brzustowicz LM, Hodgkinson KA, Chow EW, et al: Location of a major susceptibility locus for familial schizophrenia on chromosome 1q21–q22. Science 288:678–682, 2000

Bššk JA: A genetic neuropsychiatric investigation of a North Swedish population. Acta Genetica Medica Statistica 4:1–100, 1953

Bunney WE, Bunney BG, Vawter MP, et al: Microarray technology: a review of new strategies to discover candidate vulnerability genes in psychiatric disorders. Am J Psychiatry 160:657–666, 2003

Burgoyne PS: Genetic homology and crossing over in the X and Y chromosomes of mammals. Hum Genet 61:85–90, 1982

Burlina A, Visentin B: [Research on enzyme pathology in schizophrenic states, 1: malate dehydrogenase of the blood]. Riv Anat Patol Oncol 27:380–386, 1965

Cadoret RJ: Evidence for genetic inheritance of primary affective disorder in adoptees. Am J Psychiatry 135:463–466, 1978

Cadoret RJ, O'Gorman TW, Troughton E, et al: Alcoholism and antisocial personality. Interrelationships, genetic and environmental factors. Arch Gen Psychiatry 42:161–167, 1985

Caldirola D, Perna G, Arancio C, et al: The 35% CO_2 challenge test in patients with social phobia. Psychiatry Res 71:41–48, 1997

Cannon TD, Mednick SA, Parnas J: Antecedents of predominantly negative- and predominantly positive-symptom schizophrenia in a high-risk population. Arch Gen Psychiatry 47:622–632, 1990

Cannon TD, Mednick SA, Parnas J, et al: Developmental brain abnormalities in the offspring of schizophrenic mothers, II: structural brain characteristics of schizophrenia and schizotypal personality disorder. Arch Gen Psychiatry 51:955–962, 1994

Cannon TD, Kaprio J, Lonnqvist J, et al: The genetic epidemiology of schizophrenia in a Finnish twin cohort. A population-based modeling study. Arch Gen Psychiatry 55:67–74, 1998

Cantor-Graae E, Selten JP: Schizophrenia and migration: a meta-analysis and review. Am J Psychiatry 162:12–24, 2005

Cardno AG, Gottesman II: Twin studies of schizophrenia: from bow-and-arrow concordances to star wars Mx and functional genomics. Am J Med Genet 97:12–17, 2000

Carey G, Gottesman II: Twin and family studies of anxiety, phobic, and obsessive disorders, in Anxiety: New Research and Changing Concepts. Edited by Klein DF, Rabkin J. New York, Raven, 1981, pp 117–136

Cases O, Seif I, Grimsby J, et al: Aggressive behavior and altered amounts of brain serotonin and norepinephrine in mice lacking MAOA. Science 268:1763–1766, 1995

Caspi A, Sugden K, Moffitt TE, et al: Influence of life stress on depression: moderation by a polymorphism in the 5-HTT gene. Science 301:386–389, 2003

Cavallini MC, Perna G, Caldirola D, et al: A segregation study of panic disorder in families of panic patients responsive to the 35% CO_2 challenge. Biol Psychiatry 46:815–820, 1999

Chai YG, Oh DY, Chung EK, et al: Alcohol and aldehyde dehydrogenase polymorphisms in men with type I and type II alcoholism. Am J Psychiatry 162:1003–1005, 2005

Chaleby K, Tuma TA: Cousin marriages and schizophrenia in Saudi Arabia. Br J Psychiatry 150:547–549, 1987

Charness ME, Safran RM, Perides G: Ethanol inhibits neural cell-cell adhesion. J Biol Chem 269:9304–9309, 1994

Check E: Genome project turns up evolutionary surprises. Nature 447:760–761, 2007

Chen YS, Akula N, Detera-Wadleigh SD, et al: Findings in an independent sample support an association between bipolar affective disorder and the G72/G30 locus on chromosome 13q33. Mol Psychiatry 9:87–92, 2004

Cheng R, Juo SH, Loth JE, et al: Genome-wide linkage scan in a large bipolar disorder sample from the National Institute of Mental Health genetics initiative suggests putative loci for bipolar disorder, psychosis, suicide, and panic disorder. Mol Psychiatry 11:252–260, 2006

Choudary PV, Molnar M, Evans SJ, et al: Altered cortical glutamatergic and GABAergic signal transmission with glial involvement in depression. Proc Natl Acad Sci U S A 102:15653–15658, 2005

Chumakov I, Blumenfeld M, Guerassimenko O, et al: Genetic and physiological data implicating the new human gene G72 and the gene for D-amino acid oxidase in schizophrenia. Proc Natl Acad Sci U S A 99:13675–13680, 2002

Clapcote SJ, Lipina TV, Millar JK, et al: Behavioral phenotypes of Disc1 missense mutations in mice. Neuron 54:387–402, 2007

Clementz BA, Grove WM, Iacono WG, et al: Smooth-pursuit eye movement dysfunction and liability for schizophrenia: implications for genetic modeling. J Abnorm Psychol 101:117–129, 1992

Clementz BA, Geyer MA, Braff DL: Poor P50 suppression among schizophrenia patients and their first-degree biological relatives. Am J Psychiatry 155:1691–1694, 1998

Cloninger CR, Bohman M, Sigvardsson S: Inheritance of alcohol abuse. Cross-fostering analysis of adopted men. Arch Gen Psychiatry 38:861–868, 1981

Cloninger CR, Martin RL, Guze SB, et al: A prospective follow-up and family study of somatization in men and women. Am J Psychiatry 143:873–878, 1986

Cohen J: Genomics. DNA duplications and deletions help determine health. Science 317:1315–1317, 2007

Coryell W, Zimmerman M: The heritability of schizophrenia and schizoaffective disorder. A family study. Arch Gen Psychiatry 45:323–327, 1988

Couch FJ, Weber BL: Mutations and polymorphisms in the familial early onset breast cancer (BRCA1) gene. Breast Cancer Information Core. Hum Mutat 8:8–18, 1996

Craddock N, Forty L: Genetics of affective (mood) disorders. Eur J Hum Genet 14:660–668, 2006

Craddock N, O'Donovan MC, Owen MJ: Genes for schizophrenia and bipolar disorder? Implications for psychiatric nosology. Schizophr Bull 32:9–16, 2006

Crow TJ, DeLisi LE, Johnstone EC: Concordance by sex in sibling pairs with schizophrenia is paternally inherited. Evidence for a pseudoautosomal locus. Br J Psychiatry 155:92–97, 1989

Crowe RR, Noyes R, Pauls DL, et al: A family study of panic disorder. Arch Gen Psychiatry 40:1065–1069, 1983

Curtis D, Kalsi G, Brynjolfsson J, et al: Genome scan of pedigrees multiply affected with bipolar disorder provides further support for the presence of a susceptibility locus on chromosome 12q23–q24, and suggests the presence of additional loci on 1p and 1q. Psychiatr Genet 13:77–84, 2003

Davidson JR, Tupler LA, Wilson WH, et al: A family study of chronic post-traumatic stress disorder following rape trauma. J Psychiatr Res 32:301–309, 1998

Davies AJ, Bone AJ, Wilkin TJ, et al: Serum biopterin—a novel marker for immune activation during pre-diabetes in the BB rat. Diabetologia 37:466–470, 1994

Davis KL, Haroutunian V: Global expression-profiling studies and oligodendrocyte dysfunction in schizophrenia and bipolar disorder. Lancet 362:758, 2003

Davis JO, Phelps JA: Twins with schizophrenia: genes or germs? Schizophr Bull 21:13–18, 1995

Decina P, Mukherjee S, Lucas L, et al: Patterns of illness in parent-child pairs both hospitalized for either schizophrenia or a major mood disorder. Psychiatry Res 39:81–87, 1991

DeLisi LE, Crow TJ: Evidence for a sex chromosome locus for schizophrenia. Schizophr Bull 15:431–440, 1989

Detera-Wadleigh SD, Badner JA, Berrettini WH, et al: A high-density genome scan detects evidence for a bipolar-disorder susceptibility locus on 13q32 and other potential loci on 1q32 and 18p11.2. Proc Natl Acad Sci USA 96:5604-5609, 1999

Dick DM, Foroud T, Flury L, et al: Genomewide linkage analyses of bipolar disorder: a new sample of 250 pedigrees from the National Institute of Mental Health Genetics Initiative. Am J Hum Genet 73:107–114, 2003

Dillman JF III, Dabney LP, Karki S, et al: Functional analysis of dynactin and cytoplasmic dynein in slow axonal transport. J Neurosci 16:6742-6752, 1996

Durham LK, Webb SM, Milos PM, et al: The serotonin transporter polymorphism, 5HTTLPR, is associated with a faster response time to sertraline in an elderly population with major depressive disorder. Psychopharmacology (Berl) 174:525–529, 2004

Egeland JA, Sussex JN: Suicide and family loading for affective disorders. JAMA 254:915–918, 1985

Egeland JA, Gerhard DS, Pauls DL, et al: Bipolar affective disorders linked to DNA markers on chromosome 11. Nature 325:783–787, 1987

Eichhammer P, Albus M, Borrmann-Hassenbach M, et al: Association of dopamine D3-receptor gene variants with neuroleptic induced akathisia in schizophrenic patients: a generalization of Steen's study on DRD3 and tardive dyskinesia. Am J Med Genet 96:187–191, 2000

Eid T, Thomas MJ, Spencer DD, et al: Loss of glutamine synthetase in the human epileptogenic hippocampus: possible mechanism for raised extracellular glutamate in mesial temporal lobe epilepsy. Lancet 363:28–37, 2004

Einarsdottir E, Mayans S, Ruikka K, et al: Linkage but not association of calpain-10 to type 2 diabetes replicated in northern Sweden. Diabetes 55:1879–1883, 2006

Egan MF, Goldberg TE, Kolachana BS, et al: Effect of COMT Val108/158 Met genotype on frontal lobe function and risk for schizophrenia. Proc Natl Acad Sci U S A 98:6917–6922, 2001

Ekelund J, Hennah W, Hiekkalinna T, et al: Replication of 1q42 linkage in Finnish schizophrenia pedigrees. Mol Psychiatry 9:1037–1041, 2004

ENCODE Project Consortium: Identification and analysis of functional elements in 1% of the human genome by the ENCODE pilot project. Nature 447:799–816, 2007

Erlenmeyer-Kimling LE, Paradowski W: Selection and schizophrenia. Am Nat 100:651–665, 1966

Evans DA, Davison K, Pratt RT: The influence of acetylator phenotype on the effects of treating depression with phenelzine. Clin Pharmacol Ther 6:430–435, 1965

Evans SJ, Choudary PV, Neal CR, et al: Dysregulation of the fibroblast growth factor system in major depression. Proc Natl Acad Sci U S A 101:15506–15511, 2004

Farmer AE, McGuffin P, Gottesman II: Twin concordance for DSM-III schizophrenia. Scrutinizing the validity of the definition. Arch Gen Psychiatry 44:634–641, 1987

Farmer A, Elkin A, McGuffin P: The genetics of bipolar affective disorder. Curr Opin Psychiatry 20:8–12, 2007

Feinn R, Nellissery M, Kranzler HR: Meta-analysis of the association of a functional serotonin transporter promoter polymorphism with alcohol dependence. Am J Med Genet B Neuropsychiatr Genet 133:79–84, 2005

Finkbeiner S, Cuervo AM, Morimoto RI, et al: Disease-modifying pathways in neurodegeneration. J Neurosci 26:10349–10357, 2006

Fischer M: Psychoses in the offspring of schizophrenic monozygotic twins and their normal co-twins. Br J Psychiatry 118:43–52, 1971

Fish B, Marcus J, Hans SL, et al: Infants at risk for schizophrenia: sequelae of a genetic neurointegrative defect. A review and replication analysis of pandysmaturation in the Jerusalem Infant Development Study. Arch Gen Psychiatry 49:221–235, 1992

Flint J, Munafo MR: The endophenotype concept in psychiatric genetics. Psychol Med 37:163–180, 2007

Franchini L, Serretti A, Gasperini M, et al: Familial concordance of fluvoxamine response as a tool for differentiating mood disorder pedigrees. J Psychiatr Res 32:255–259, 1998

Franke P, Maier W, Hain C, et al: Wisconsin Card Sorting Test: an indicator of vulnerability to schizophrenia? Schizophr Res 6:243–249, 1992

Freeman JL, Perry GH, Feuk L, et al: Copy number variation: new insights in genome diversity. Genome Res 16:949–961, 2007

Funke B, Malhotra AK, Finn CT, et al: COMT genetic variation confers risk for psychotic and affective disorders: a case control study. Behav Brain Funct 1:19, 2005

Fyer AJ, Mannuzza S, Gallops MS, et al: Familial transmission of simple phobias and fears. A preliminary report. Arch Gen Psychiatry 47:252–256, 1990

Fyer AJ, Mannuzza S, Chapman TF, et al: A direct interview family study of social phobia. Arch Gen Psychiatry 50:286–293, 1993

Fyer AJ, Mannuzza S, Chapman TF, et al: Specificity in familial aggregation of phobic disorders. Arch Gen Psychiatry 52:564–573, 1995

GAIN Collaborative Research Group: New models of collaboration in genome-wide association studies: the Genetic Association Information Network. Nat Genet 39:1045–1051, 2007

Geller B, Badner JA, Tillman R, et al: Linkage disequilibrium of the brain-derived neurotrophic factor Val66Met polymorphism in children with a prepubertal and early adolescent bipolar disorder phenotype. Am J Psychiatry 161:1698–1700, 2004

Gerber DJ, Hall D, Miyakawa T, et al: Evidence for association of schizophrenia with genetic variation in the 8p21.3 gene, PPP3CC, encoding the calcineurin gamma subunit. Proc Natl Acad Sci U S A 100:8993–8998, 2003

Gershon ES, Hamovit JH, Guroff JJ, et al: Birth-cohort changes in manic and depressive disorders in relatives of bipolar and schizoaffective patients. Arch Gen Psychiatry 44:314–319, 1987

Giles DE, Biggs MM, Rush AJ, et al: Risk factors in families of unipolar depression, I: psychiatric illness and reduced REM latency. J Affect Disord 14:51–59, 1988

Glatt SJ, Everall IP, Kremen WS, et al: Comparative gene expression analysis of blood and brain provides concurrent validation of SELENBP1 upregulation in schizophrenia. Proc Natl Acad Sci U S A 102:15533–15538, 2005

Gogos JA, Santha M, Takacs Z, et al: The gene encoding proline dehydrogenase modulates sensorimotor gating in mice. Nat Genet 21:434–439, 1999

Goldenberg IM, White K, Yonkers K, et al: The infrequency of "pure culture" diagnoses among the anxiety disorders. J Clin Psychiatry 57:528–533, 1996

Goldman-Rakic PS: Working memory dysfunction in schizophrenia. J Neuropsychiatry Clin Neurosci 6:348–357, 1994

Goodwin DW: Alcoholism and heredity. A review and hypothesis. Arch Gen Psychiatry 36:57–61, 1979

Gottesman II, Bertelsen A: Confirming unexpressed genotypes for schizophrenia. Risks in the offspring of Fischer's Danish identical and fraternal discordant twins. Arch Gen Psychiatry 46:867–872, 1989

Gottesman II, Gould TD: The endophenotype concept in psychiatry: etymology and strategic intentions. Am J Psychiatry 160:636–645, 2003

Gottesman II, Shields J: Schizophrenia and Genetics: A Twin Vantage Point. New York, Academic Press, 1972

Gottesman II, Shields J: Schizophrenia: The Epigenetic Puzzle. Cambridge, England, Cambridge University Press, 1982

Guidotti A, Auta J, Davis JM, et al: GABAergic dysfunction in schizophrenia: new treatment strategies on the horizon. Psychopharmacology (Berl) 180:191–205, 2005

Guo H, Jin YX, Ishikawa M, et al: Regulation of beta-chemokine mRNA expression in adult rat astrocytes by lipopolysaccharide, proinflammatory and immunoregulatory cytokines. Scand J Immunol 48:502–508, 1998

Gurling HM, Kalsi G, Brynjolfsson J, et al: Genomewide genetic linkage analysis confirms the presence of susceptibility loci for schizophrenia, on chromosomes 1q32.2, 5q33.2, and 8p21–22 and provides support for linkage to schizophrenia, on chromosomes 11q23.3–24 and 20q12.1–11.23. Am J Hum Genet 68:661–673, 2001

Hakak Y, Walker JR, Li C, et al: Genome-wide expression analysis reveals dysregulation of myelination-related genes in chronic schizophrenia. Proc Natl Acad Sci U S A 98:4746–4751, 2001

Hakonarson H, Halapi E: Genetic analyses in asthma: current concepts and future directions. Am J Pharmacogenomics 2:155–166, 2002

Hamilton SP, Fyer AJ, Durner M, et al: Further genetic evidence for a panic disorder syndrome mapping to chromosome 13q. Proc Natl Acad Sci U S A 100:2550–2555, 2003

Harrison PJ, Weinberger DR: Schizophrenia genes, gene expression, and neuropathology: on the matter of their convergence. Mol Psychiatry 10:40–68, 2005

Hashimoto T, Volk DW, Eggan SM, et al: Gene expression deficits in a subclass of GABA neurons in the prefrontal cortex of subjects with schizophrenia. J Neurosci 23:6315–6326, 2003

Hasler G, Drevets WC, Manji HK, et al: Discovering endophenotypes for major depression. Neuropsychopharmacology 29:1765–1781, 2004

Hattori E, Liu C, Badner JA, et al: Polymorphisms at the G72/G30 gene locus, on 13q33, are associated with bipolar disorder in two independent pedigree series. Am J Hum Genet 72:1131–1140, 2003

Hayden EP, Nurnberger JI Jr: Molecular genetics of bipolar disorder. Genes Brain Behav 5:85–95, 2006

Hennah W, Tuulio-Henriksson A, Paunio T, et al: A haplotype within the DISC1 gene is associated with visual memory functions in families with a high density of schizophrenia. Mol Psychiatry 10:1097–1103, 2005

Herman AI, Philbeck JW, Vasilopoulos NL, et al: Serotonin transporter promoter polymorphism and differences in alcohol consumption behaviour in a college student population. Alcohol Alcohol 38:446–449, 2003

Heston LL: Psychiatric disorders in foster home reared children of schizophrenic mothers. Br J Psychiatry 112:819–825, 1966

Hettema JM, Prescott CA, Kendler KS: A population-based twin study of generalized anxiety disorder in men and women. J Nerv Ment Dis 189:413–420, 2001

Hettema JM, An SS, Neale MC, et al: Association between glutamic acid decarboxylase genes and anxiety disorders, major depression, and neuroticism. Mol Psychiatry 11:752–762, 2006

Hodgkinson CA, Goldman D, Jaeger J, et al: Disrupted in schizophrenia 1 (DISC1): association with schizophrenia, schizoaffective disorder, and bipolar disorder. Am J Hum Genet 75:862–872, 2004

Hoefgen B, Schulze TG, Ohlraun S, et al: The power of sample size and homogenous sampling: association between the 5-HTTLPR serotonin transporter polymorphism and major depressive disorder. Biol Psychiatry 57:247–251, 2005

Hof PR, Haroutunian V, Friedrich VL Jr, et al: Loss and altered spatial distribution of oligodendrocytes in the superior frontal gyrus in schizophrenia. Biol Psychiatry 53:1075–1085, 2003

Hovatta I, Tennant RS, Helton R, et al: Glyoxalase 1 and glutathione reductase 1 regulate anxiety in mice. Nature 438:662–666, 2005

Hu XZ, Lipsky RH, Zhu G, et al: Serotonin transporter promoter gain-of-function genotypes are linked to obsessive-compulsive disorder. Am J Hum Genet 78:815–826, 2006

Hultman CM, Ohman A, Cnattingius S, et al: Prenatal and neonatal risk factors for schizophrenia. Br J Psychiatry 170:128–133, 1997

Human Genome Structural Variation Working Group: Completing the map of human genetic variation. Nature 447:161–165, 2007

International HapMap Consortium: A haplotype map of the human genome. Nature 437:1299–1320, 2005

International HapMap Consortium: A second generation human haplotype map of over 3.1 million SNPs. Nature 449:851–861, 2007

Iwamoto K, Kakiuchi C, Bundo M, et al: Molecular characterization of bipolar disorder by comparing gene expression profiles of postmortem brains of major mental disorders. Mol Psychiatry 9:406–416, 2004

Jackson ES, Wayland MT, Fitzgerald W, et al: A microarray data analysis framework for postmortem tissues. Methods 37:247–260, 2005

Kaabi B, Gelernter J, Woods SW, et al: Genome scan for loci predisposing to anxiety disorders using a novel multivariate approach: strong evidence for a chromosome 4 risk locus. Am J Hum Genet 78:543–553, 2006

Kalbfeish JD, Prentice RL: The Statistical Analysis of Failure Time Data. New York, Wiley, 1980

Kallmann FJ: The genetic theory of schizophrenia. An analysis of 691 schizophrenic twin index families. 1946. Am J Psychiatry 151:188–198, 1994

Kamboh MI: Molecular genetics of late-onset Alzheimer's disease. Ann Hum Genet 68:381–404, 2004

Kamiya A, Kubo K, Tomoda T, et al: A schizophrenia-associated mutation of DISC1 perturbs cerebral cortex development. Nat Cell Biol 7:1167–1178, 2005

Kaplitt MG, Makimura H: Defective viral vectors as agents for gene transfer in the nervous system. J Neurosci Methods 71:125–132, 1997

Karlsson JL: Partly dominant transmission of schizophrenia in Iceland. Br J Psychiatry 152:324–329, 1988

Karno M, Golding JM, Sorenson SB, et al: The epidemiology of obsessive-compulsive disorder in five US communities. Arch Gen Psychiatry 45:1094–1099, 1988

Kassett JA, Gershon ES, Maxwell ME, et al: Psychiatric disorders in the first-degree relatives of probands with bulimia nervosa. Am J Psychiatry 146:1468–1471, 1989

Kato T: Molecular genetics of bipolar disorder and depression. Psychiatry Clin Neurosci 61:3–19, 2007

Kaufmann CA, Ziegler RJ: The viral hypothesis of schizophrenia, in Receptors and Ligands in Psychiatry. Edited by Sen AK, Lee T. Cambridge, England, Cambridge University Press, 1987, pp 187–208

Keefe RS, Silverman JM, Mohs RC, et al: Eye tracking, attention, and schizotypal symptoms in nonpsychotic relatives of patients with schizophrenia. Arch Gen Psychiatry 54:169–176, 1997

Kelsoe JR, Spence MA, Loetscher E, et al: A genome survey indicates a possible susceptibility locus for bipolar disorder on chromosome 22. Proc Natl Acad Sci U S A 98:585–590, 2001

Kendler KS: Genetics of schizophrenia, in American Psychiatric Association Annual Review, Vol 5. Edited by Frances AJ, Hales RE. Washington, DC, American Psychiatric Press, 1986, pp 25–41

Kendler KS: The genetics of schizophrenia: chromosomal deletions, attentional disturbances, and spectrum boundaries. Am J Psychiatry 160:1549–1553, 2003

Kendler KS, Gardner CO: The risk for psychiatric disorders in relatives of schizophrenic and control probands: a comparison of three independent studies. Psychol Med 27:411–419, 1997

Kendler KS, Gruenberg AM: An independent analysis of the Danish Adoption Study of Schizophrenia, VI: the relationship between psychiatric disorders as defined by DSM-III in the relatives and adoptees. Arch Gen Psychiatry 41:555–564, 1984

Kendler KS, Gruenberg AM, Tsuang MT: Psychiatric illness in first-degree relatives of schizophrenic and surgical control patients. A family study using DSM-III criteria. Arch Gen Psychiatry 42:770–779, 1985

Kendler KS, Neale MC, MacLean CJ, et al: Smoking and major depression. A causal analysis. Arch Gen Psychiatry 50:36–43, 1993

Kendler KS, Neale MC, Heath AC, et al: A twin-family study of alcoholism in women. Am J Psychiatry 151:707–715, 1994

Kendler KS, Gardner CO, Neale MC, et al: Genetic risk factors for major depression in men and women: similar or different heritabilities and same or partly distinct genes? Psychol Med 31:605–616, 2001

Kennedy JL, Farrer LA, Andreasen NC, et al: The genetics of adult-onset neuropsychiatric disease: complexities and conundra? Science 302:822–826, 2003

Kessler RC, McGonagle KA, Zhao S, et al: Lifetime and 12-month prevalence of DSM-III-R psychiatric disorders in the United States. Results from the National Comorbidity Survey. Arch Gen Psychiatry 51:8–19, 1994

Kessler S: Psychological aspects of genetic counseling, VI: a critical review of the literature dealing with education and reproduction. Am J Med Genet 34:340–353, 1989

Kety SS: Schizophrenic illness in the families of schizophrenic adoptees: findings from the Danish national sample. Schizophr Bull 14:217–222, 1988

Kety SS, Wender PH, Jacobsen B, et al: Mental illness in the biological and adoptive relatives of schizophrenic adoptees. Replication of the Copenhagen Study in the rest of Denmark. Arch Gen Psychiatry 51:442–455, 1994

Kidd KK: Genetic models for psychiatric disorders, in Genetic Research Strategies for Psychobiology and Psychiatry. Edited by Gershon ES, Matthysse S, Breakefield XO, et al. Pacific Grove, CA, Boxwood Press, 1981, pp 369–382

Kinney DK, Yurgelun-Todd DA, Woods BT: Hard neurologic signs and psychopathology in relatives of schizophrenic patients. Psychiatry Res 39:45–53, 1991

Klerman GL, Lavori PW, Rice J, et al: Birth-cohort trends in rates of major depressive disorder among relatives of patients with affective disorder. Arch Gen Psychiatry 42:689–693, 1985

Knowles JA, Fyer AJ, Vieland VJ, et al: Results of a genome-wide genetic screen for panic disorder. Am J Med Genet 81:139–147, 1998

Konradi C, Eaton M, MacDonald ML, et al: Molecular evidence for mitochondrial dysfunction in bipolar disorder. Arch Gen Psychiatry 61:300–308, 2004

Koob GF, Nestler EJ: The neurobiology of drug addiction. J Neuropsychiatry Clin Neurosci 9:482–497, 1997

Kringlen E: [The status of schizophrenia research]. Tidsskr Nor Laegeforen 98:65–69, 1978

Kupfer DJ, Frank E, Carpenter LL, et al: Family history in recurrent depression. J Affect Disord 17:113–119, 1989

Lachman HM: An overview of the genetics of substance use disorders. Curr Psychiatry Rep 8:133–143, 2006

Lachman HM, Morrow B, Shprintzen R, et al: Association of codon 108/158 catechol-O-methyltransferase gene polymorphism with the psychiatric manifestations of velo-cardio-facial syndrome. Am J Med Genet 67:468–472, 1996

Lamason RL, Mohideen MA, Mest JR, et al: SLC24A5, a putative cation exchanger, affects pigmentation in zebrafish and humans. Science 310:1782–1786, 2005

Lander ES, Linton LM, Birren B, et al: Initial sequencing and analysis of the human genome. Nature 409:860–921, 2001

Lane HY, Hsu SK, Liu YC, et al: Dopamine D3 receptor Ser9Gly polymorphism and risperidone response. J Clin Psychopharmacol 25:6–11, 2005

Lappalainen J, Kranzler HR, Petrakis I, et al: Confirmation and fine mapping of the chromosome 1 alcohol dependence risk locus. Mol Psychiatry 9:312–319, 2004

Larson CA, Nyman GE: Differential fertility in schizophrenia. Acta Psychiatr Scand 49:272–280, 1973

Laurent A, Biloa-Tang M, Bougerol T, et al: Executive/attentional performance and measures of schizotypy in patients with schizophrenia and in their nonpsychotic first-degree relatives. Schizophr Res 46:269–283, 2000

Law AJ, Lipska BK, Weickert CS, et al: Neuregulin 1 transcripts are differentially expressed in schizophrenia and regulated by 5' SNPs associated with the disease. Proc Natl Acad Sci U S A 103:6747–6752, 2006

Leckman JF, Chittenden EH: Gilles de La Tourette's syndrome and some forms of obsessive-compulsive disorder may share a common genetic diathesis. Encephale 16 Spec No:321–323, 1990

Leonard HL, Swedo SE: Paediatric autoimmune neuropsychiatric disorders associated with streptococcal infection (PANDAS). Int J Neuropsychopharmacol 4:191–198, 2001

Lesch KP: Gene-environment interaction and the genetics of depression. J Psychiatry Neurosci 29:174–184, 2004

Lesch KP, Bengel D, Heils A, et al: Association of anxiety-related traits with a polymorphism in the serotonin transporter gene regulatory region. Science 274:1527–1531, 1996

Letwin NE, Kafkafi N, Benjamini Y, et al: Combined application of behavior genetics and microarray analysis to identify regional expression themes and gene-behavior associations. J Neurosci 26:5277–5287, 2006

Levinson DF: Meta-analysis in psychiatric genetics. Curr Psychiatry Rep 7:143–151, 2005

Levinson DF: The genetics of depression: a review. Biol Psychiatry 60:84–92, 2006

Levy S, Sutton G, Ng PC, et al: The diploid genome sequence of an individual human. PLoS Biol 5(10):e254 [Epub ahead of print], 2007

Lewis CM, Levinson DF, Wise LH, et al: Genome scan meta-analysis of schizophrenia and bipolar disorder, part II: schizophrenia. Am J Hum Genet 73:34–48, 2003

Lewis DA, Gonzalez-Burgos G: Pathophysiologically based treatment interventions in schizophrenia. Nat Med 12:1016–1022, 2006

Lewis DA, Volk DW, Hashimoto T: Selective alterations in prefrontal cortical GABA neurotransmission in schizophrenia: a novel target for the treatment of working memory dysfunction. Psychopharmacology (Berl) 174:143–150, 2004

Lewis DA, Hashimoto T, Volk DW: Cortical inhibitory neurons and schizophrenia. Nat Rev Neurosci 6:312–324, 2005

Lieberman JA, Yunis J, Egea E, et al: HLA-B38, DR4, DQw3 and clozapine-induced agranulocytosis in Jewish patients with schizophrenia. Arch Gen Psychiatry 47:945–948, 1990

Lin MW, Curtis D, Williams N, et al: Suggestive evidence for linkage of schizophrenia to markers on chromosome 13q14.1–q32. Psychiatr Genet 5:117–126, 1995

Lipska BK, Peters T, Hyde TM, et al: Expression of DISC1 binding partners is reduced in schizophrenia and associated with DISC1 SNPs. Hum Mol Genet 15:1245–1258, 2006

Litman RE, Torrey EF, Hommer DW, et al: A quantitative analysis of smooth pursuit eye tracking in monozygotic twins discordant for schizophrenia. Arch Gen Psychiatry 54:417–426, 1997

Liu J, Lewohl JM, Harris RA, et al: Patterns of gene expression in the frontal cortex discriminate alcoholic from nonalcoholic individuals. Neuropsychopharmacology 31:1574–1582, 2006

Lockhart DJ, Dong H, Byrne MC, et al: Expression monitoring by hybridization to high-density oligonucleotide arrays. Nat Biotechnol 14:1675–1680, 1996

Lohmueller KE, Pearce CL, Pike M, et al: Meta-analysis of genetic association studies supports a contribution of common variants to susceptibility to common disease. Nat Genet 33:177–182, 2003

Lohoff FW, Sander T, Ferraro TN, et al: Confirmation of association between the Val66Met polymorphism in the brain-derived neurotrophic factor (BDNF) gene and bipolar I disorder. Am J Med Genet B Neuropsychiatr Genet 139:51–53, 2005

Long JC, Knowler WC, Hanson RL, et al: Evidence for genetic linkage to alcohol dependence on chromosomes 4 and 11 from an autosome-wide scan in an American Indian population. Am J Med Genet 81:216–221, 1998

Lossos IS, Czerwinski DK, Alizadeh AA, et al: Prediction of survival in diffuse large-B-cell lymphoma based on the expression of six genes. N Engl J Med 350:1828–1837, 2004

Low NC, Hardy J: What is a schizophrenic mouse? Neuron 54:348–349, 2007

Lupski JR, de Oca-Luna RM, Slaugenhaupt S, et al: DNA duplication associated with Charcot-Marie-Tooth disease type 1A. Cell 66:219–232, 1991

Macgregor S, Visscher PM, Knott SA, et al: A genome scan and follow-up study identify a bipolar disorder susceptibility locus onchromosome1q42. Mol Psychiatry 9:1083–1090, 2004

MacKinnon DF, Xu J, McMahon FJ, et al: Bipolar disorder and panic disorder in families: an analysis of chromosome 18 data. Am J Psychiatry 155:829–831, 1998

Maeda K, Nwulia E, Chang J: Differential expression of disrupted-in-schizophrenia (DISC1) in bipolar disorder. Biol Psychiatry 60:929–935, 2006

Maier W, Lichtermann D, Minges J, et al: Personality traits in subjects at risk for unipolar major depression: a family study perspective. J Affect Disord 24:153–163, 1992

Malaspina D, Corcoran C, Fahim C, et al: Paternal age and sporadic schizophrenia: evidence for de novo mutations. Am J Med Genet 114:299–303, 2002

Marazita ML, Neiswanger K, Cooper M, et al: Genetic segregation analysis of early onset recurrent unipolar depression. Am J Hum Genet 61:1370–1378, 1997

Mataix-Cols D: Deconstructing obsessive-compulsive disorder: a multidimensional perspective. Curr Opin Psychiatry 19:84–89, 2006

Mather JA: Eye movements of teenage children of schizophrenics: a possible inherited marker of susceptibility to the disease. J Psychiatr Res 19:523–532, 1985

McCarthy MI: Growing evidence for diabetes susceptibility genes from genome scan data. Curr Diab Rep 3:159–167, 2003

McDonald C, Murphy KC: The new genetics of schizophrenia. Psychiatr Clin North Am 26:41–63, 2003

McInnis MG, Lan TH, Willour VL, et al: Genome-wide scan of bipolar disorder in 65 pedigrees: supportive evidence for linkage at 8q24, 18q22, 4q32, 2p12, and 13q12. Mol Psychiatry 8:288–298, 2003

McNeil TF, Kaij L: Swedish high-risk study: sample characteristics at age 6. Schizophr Bull 13:373–381, 1987

McQuillin A, Bass NJ, Kalsi G, et al: Fine mapping of a susceptibility locus for bipolar and genetically related unipolar affective disorders, to a region containing the C21ORF29 and TRPM2 genes on chromosome 21q22.3. Mol Psychiatry 11:134–142, 2006

Meged S, Stein D, Sitrota P, et al: Human leukocyte antigen typing, response to neuroleptics, and clozapine-induced agranulocytosis in Jewish Israeli schizophrenic patients. Int Clin Psychopharmacol 14:305–312, 1999

Melo JA, Shendure J, Pociask K, et al: Identification of sex-specific quantitative trait loci controlling alcohol preference in C57BL/6 mice. Nat Genet 13:147–153, 1996

Mendlewicz J, Rainer JD: Adoption study supporting genetic transmission in manic—depressive illness. Nature 268:327–329, 1977

Mendlewicz J, Sevy S, de Maertelaer V: REM sleep latency and morbidity risk of affective disorders in depressive illness. Neuropsychobiology 22:14–17, 1989

Merali Z, Du L, Hrdina P, et al: Dysregulation in the suicide brain: mRNA expression of corticotropin-releasing hormone receptors and GABA(A) receptor subunits in frontal cortical brain region. J Neurosci 24:1478–1485, 2004

Merikangas KR: Genetics of alcoholism: a review of human studies, in Genetics of Neuropsychiatric Diseases. Edited by Wetterberg I. London, England, Macmillan, 1989, pp 269–280

Merikangas KR, Spence MA, Kupfer DJ: Linkage studies of bipolar disorder: methodologic and analytic issues. Report of MacArthur Foundation Workshop on Linkage and Clinical Features in Affective Disorders. Arch Gen Psychiatry 46:1137–1141, 1989

Middeldorp CM, Birley AJ, Cath DC, et al: Familial clustering of major depression and anxiety disorders in Australian and Dutch twins and siblings. Twin Res Hum Genet 8:609–615, 2005

Middleton FA, Mirnics K, Pierri JN, et al: Gene expression profiling reveals alterations of specific metabolic pathways in schizophrenia. J Neurosci 22:2718–2729, 2002

Middleton FA, Pato MT, Gentile KL, et al: Genomewide linkage analysis of bipolar disorder by use of a high-density single-nucleotide-polymorphism (SNP) genotyping assay: a comparison with microsatellite marker assays and finding of significant linkage to chromosome 6q22. Am J Hum Genet 74:886–897, 2004

Middleton FA, Pato CN, Gentile KL, et al: Gene expression analysis of peripheral blood leukocytes from discordant sib-pairs with schizophrenia and bipolar disorder reveals points of convergence between genetic and functional genomic approaches. Am J Med Genet B Neuropsychiatr Genet 136:12–25, 2005

Mikkelsen TS, Ku M, Jaffe DB, et al: Genome-wide maps of chromatin state in pluripotent and lineage-committed cells. Nature 448:553–560, 2007

Millar JK, Pickard BS, Mackie S, et al: DISC1 and PDE4B are interacting genetic factors in schizophrenia that regulate cAMP signaling. Science 310:1187–1191, 2005

Mimmack ML, Ryan M, Baba H, et al: Gene expression analysis in schizophrenia: reproducible up-regulation of several members of the apolipoprotein L family located in a high-susceptibility locus for schizophrenia on chromosome 22. Proc Natl Acad Sci U S A 99:4680–4685, 2002

Mirnics K, Pevsner J: Progress in the use of microarray technology to study the neurobiology of disease. Nat Neurosci 7:434–439, 2004

Mirnics K, Middleton FA, Marquez A, et al: Molecular characterization of schizophrenia viewed by microarray analysis of gene expression in prefrontal cortex. Neuron 28:53–67, 2000

Mirnics K, Middleton FA, Lewis DA, et al: Analysis of complex brain disorders with gene expression microarrays: schizophrenia as a disease of the synapse. Trends Neurosci 24:479–486, 2001a

Mirnics K, Middleton FA, Stanwood GD, et al: Disease-specific changes in regulator of G-protein signaling 4 (RGS4) expression in schizophrenia. Mol Psychiatry 6:293–301, 2001b

Mirnics K, Levitt P, Lewis DA: Critical appraisal of DNA microarrays in psychiatric genomics. Biol Psychiatry 60:163–176, 2006

Moldin SO, Gottesman II, Erlenmeyer-Kimling L, et al: Psychometric deviance in offspring at risk for schizophrenia, I: initial delineation of a distinct subgroup. Psychiatry Res 32:297–310, 1990a

Moldin SO, Rice JP, Gottesman II, et al: Psychometric deviance in offspring at risk for schizophrenia, II: resolving heterogeneity through admixture analysis. Psychiatry Res 32:311–322, 1990b

Morris JA, Kandpal G, Ma L, et al: DISC1 (Disrupted-In-Schizophrenia 1) is a centrosome-associated protein that interacts with MAP1A, MIPT3, ATF4/5 and NUDEL: regulation and loss of interaction with mutation. Hum Mol Genet 12:1591–1608, 2003

Morton NE: Sequential tests for the detection of linkage. Am J Hum Genet 7:277–318, 1955

Mulligan MK, Ponomarev I, Hitzemann RJ, et al: Toward understanding the genetics of alcohol drinking through transcriptome meta-analysis. Proc Natl Acad Sci U S A 103:6368–6373, 2006

Munafo MR, Lingford-Hughes AR, Johnstone EC, et al: Association between the serotonin transporter gene and alcohol consumption in social drinkers. Am J Med Genet B Neuropsychiatr Genet 135:10–14, 2005

Murphy GM Jr, Pollock BG, Kirshner MA, et al: CYP2D6 genotyping with oligonucleotide microarrays and nortriptyline concentrations in geriatric depression. Neuropsychopharmacology 25:737–743, 2001

Nagler S: Overall design and methodology of the Israeli high-risk study. Schizophr Bull 11:31–37, 1985

Nakatani N, Hattori E, Ohnishi T, et al: Genome-wide expression analysis detects eight genes with robust alterations specific to bipolar I disorder: relevance to neuronal network perturbation. Hum Mol Genet 15:1949–1962, 2006

Nelson EC, Grant JD, Bucholz KK, et al: Social phobia in a population-based female adolescent twin sample: comorbidity and associated suicide-related symptoms. Psychol Med 30:797–804, 2000

Nestler EJ, Malenka RC: The addicted brain. Sci Am 290:78–85, 2004

Neves-Pereira M, Mundo E, Muglia P, et al: The brain-derived neurotrophic factor gene confers susceptibility to bipolar disorder: evidence from a family based association study. Am J Hum Genet 71:651–655, 2002

Niculescu AB 3rd, Segal DS, Kuczenski R, et al: Identifying a series of candidate genes for mania and psychosis: a convergent functional genomics approach. Physiol Genomics 4:83–91, 2000

Nimgaonkar VL, Rudert WA, Zhang XR, et al: Further evidence for an association between schizophrenia and the HLA DQB1 gene locus. Schizophr Res 18:43–49, 1995

Norton N, Williams HJ, Owen MJ: An update on the genetics of schizophrenia. Curr Opin Psychiatry 19:158–164, 2006

Noyes R Jr, Crowe RR, Harris EL, et al: Relationship between panic disorder and agoraphobia. A family study. Arch Gen Psychiatry 43:227–232, 1986

Noyes R Jr, Clarkson C, Crowe RR, et al: A family study of generalized anxiety disorder. Am J Psychiatry 144:1019–1024, 1987

Nurnberger JI Jr, Gershon ES: Genetics, in Handbook of Affective Disorders. Edited by Paykel ES. New York, Guilford, 1982, pp 126–145

Nurnberger JI Jr, Foroud T, Flury L, et al: Evidence for a locus on chromosome 1 that influences vulnerability to alcoholism and affective disorder. Am J Psychiatry 158:718–724, 2001

O'Donovan MC, Williams NM, Owen MJ: Recent advances in the genetics of schizophrenia. Hum Mol Genet 12:R125–R133, 2003

Ogden CA, Rich ME, Schork NJ, et al: Candidate genes, pathways and mechanisms for bipolar (manic-depressive) and related disorders: an expanded convergent functional genomics approach. Mol Psychiatry 9:1007–1029, 2004

Ogilvie AD, Battersby S, Bubb VJ, et al: Polymorphism in serotonin transporter gene associated with susceptibility to major depression. Lancet 347:731–733, 1996

Oliveira AL, Thams S, Lidman O, et al: A role for MHC class I molecules in synaptic plasticity and regeneration of neurons after axotomy. Proc Natl Acad Sci U S A 101:17843–17848, 2004

Onstad S, Skre I, Torgersen S, et al: Subtypes of schizophrenia—evidence from a twin-family study. Acta Psychiatr Scand 84:203–206, 1991

Onstad S, Skre I, Torgersen S, et al: Birthweight and obstetric complications in schizophrenic twins. Acta Psychiatr Scand 85:70–73, 1992

Oroszi G, Goldman D: Alcoholism: genes and mechanisms. Pharmacogenomics 5:1037–1048, 2004

O'Rourke DH, Gottesman II, Suarez BK, et al: Refutation of the general single-locus model for the etiology of schizophrenia. Am J Hum Genet 34:630–649, 1982

Ott J: Estimation of the recombination fraction in human pedigrees: efficient computation of the likelihood for human linkage studies. Am J Hum Genet 26:588–597, 1974

Owen MJ: Genomic approaches to schizophrenia. Clin Ther 27 (suppl A):S2–S7, 2005

Owen MJ, Williams NM, O'Donovan MC: The molecular genetics of schizophrenia: new findings promise new insights. Mol Psychiatry 9:14–27, 2004

Palo OM, Antila M, Silander K, et al: Association of distinct allelic haplotypes of DISC1 with psychotic and bipolar spectrum disorders and with underlying cognitive impairments. Hum Mol Genet [Epub ahead of print], 2007

Parnas J, Schulsinger F, Schulsinger H, et al: Behavioral precursors of schizophrenia spectrum: a prospective study. Arch Gen Psychiatry 39:658–664, 1982

Pauls DL, Bailey JN, Carter AS, et al: Complex segregation analyses of old order Amish families ascertained through bipolar I individuals. Am J Med Genet 60:290–297, 1995

Phillips TJ, Crabbe JC, Metten P, et al: Localization of genes affecting alcohol drinking in mice. Alcohol Clin Exp Res 18:931–941, 1994

Pollock BG, Ferrell RE, Mulsant BH, et al: Allelic variation in the serotonin transporter promoter affects onset of paroxetine treatment response in late-life depression. Neuropsychopharmacology 23:587–590, 2000

Pongrac JL, Middleton FA, Peng L, et al: Heat shock protein 12A shows reduced expression in the prefrontal cortex of subjects with schizophrenia. Biol Psychiatry 56:943–950, 2004

Pope HG Jr, Yurgelun-Todd D: Schizophrenic individuals with bipolar first-degree relatives: analysis of two pedigrees. J Clin Psychiatry 51:97–101, 1990

Potash JB, Zandi PP, Willour VL, et al: Suggestive linkage to chromosomal regions 13q31 and 22q12 in families with psychotic bipolar disorder. Am J Psychiatry 160:680–686, 2003

Prabakaran S, Wengenroth M, Lockstone HE, et al: 2-D DIGE analysis of liver and red blood cells provides further evidence for oxidative stress in schizophrenia. J Proteome Res 6:141–149, 2007

Prescott CA: Sex differences in the genetic risk for alcoholism. Alcohol Res Health 26:264–273, 2002

Prescott CA, Aggen SH, Kendler KS: Sex-specific genetic influences on the comorbidity of alcoholism and major depression in a population-based sample of US twins. Arch Gen Psychiatry 57:803–811, 2000

Price RA, Kidd KK, Weissman MM: Early onset (under age 30 years) and panic disorder as markers for etiologic homogeneity in major depression. Arch Gen Psychiatry 44:434–440, 1987

Pulver AE, Brown CH, Wolyniec P, et al: Schizophrenia: age at onset, gender and familial risk. Acta Psychiatr Scand 82:344–351, 1990

Pulver AE, Brown CH, Wolyniec PS, et al: Psychiatric morbidity in the relatives of patients with DSM-III schizophreniform disorder: comparisons with the relatives of schizophrenic and bipolar disorder patients. J Psychiatr Res 25:19–29, 1991

Pulver AE, Lasseter VK, Kasch L, et al: Schizophrenia: a genome scan targets chromosomes 3p and 8p as potential sites of susceptibility genes. Am J Med Genet 60:252–260, 1995

Radel M, Goldman D: Pharmacogenetics of alcohol response and alcoholism: the interplay of genes and environmental factors in thresholds for alcoholism. Drug Metab Dispos 29:489–494, 2001

Radel M, Vallejo RL, Iwata N, et al: Haplotype-based localization of an alcohol dependence gene to the 5q34 {gamma}-aminobutyric acid type A gene cluster. Arch Gen Psychiatry 62:47–55, 2005

Rahman N, Seal S, Thompson D et al: PALB2, which encodes a BRCA2-interacting protein, is a breast cancer susceptibility gene. Nature Genet 39:165–167, 2007

Ramaswamy S, Ross KN, Lander ES, et al: A molecular signature of metastasis in primary solid tumors. Nat Genet 33:49–54, 2003

Rasmussen JO, Christensen M, Svendsen JM, et al: CYP2D6 gene test in psychiatric patients and healthy volunteers. Scand J Clin Lab Invest 66:129–136, 2006

Regier DA, Narrow WE, Rae DS, et al: The de facto US mental and addictive disorders service system. Epidemiologic Catchment Area prospective 1-year prevalence rates of disorders and services. Arch Gen Psychiatry 50:85–94, 1993

Reich T, Cloninger CR, Van Eerdewegh P, et al: Secular trends in the familial transmission of alcoholism. Alcohol Clin Exp Res 12:458–464, 1988

Reich T, Edenberg HJ, Goate A, et al: Genome-wide search for genes affecting the risk for alcohol dependence. Am J Med Genet 81:207–215, 1998

Reveley MA, Reveley AM, Baldy R: Left cerebral hemisphere hypodensity in discordant schizophrenic twins. A controlled study. Arch Gen Psychiatry 44:625–632, 1987

Rhodes JS, Crabbe JC: Gene expression induced by drugs of abuse. Curr Opin Pharmacol 5:26–33, 2005

Rice J, Endicott J, Knesevich MA, et al: The estimation of diagnostic sensitivity using stability data: an application to major depressive disorder. J Psychiatr Res 21:337–345, 1987a

Rice J, Reich T, Andreasen NC, et al: The familial transmission of bipolar illness. Arch Gen Psychiatry 44:441–447, 1987b

Riley B, Kendler KS: Molecular genetic studies of schizophrenia. Eur J Hum Genet 14:669–680, 2006

Risch N: Linkage strategies for genetically complex traits, I: multilocus models. Am J Hum Genet 46:222–228, 1990

Risch N, Merikangas K: The future of genetic studies of complex human diseases. Science 273:1516–1517, 1996

Roberto M, Schweitzer P, Madamba SG, et al: Acute and chronic ethanol alter glutamatergic transmission in rat central amygdala: an in vitro and in vivo analysis. J Neurosci 24:1594–1603, 2004

Robins LN, Helzer JE, Weissman MM, et al: Lifetime prevalence of specific psychiatric disorders in three sites. Arch Gen Psychiatry 41:949–958, 1984

Role LW, Talmage DA: New order for thought disorders. Nature 448:263–265, 2007

Rosa A, Fananas L, Bracha HS, et al: Congenital dermatoglyphic malformations and psychosis: a twin study. Am J Psychiatry 157:1511–1513, 2000

Rosenthal D: Genetic Theory and Abnormal Behavior. New York, McGraw-Hill, 1970

Rosenthal D, Wender PH, Kety SS, et al: Schizophrenics' offspring reared in adoptive homes. J Psychiatr Res 6:377–391, 1968

Ross CA, Margolis RL, Reading SA, et al: Neurobiology of schizophrenia. Neuron 52:139–153, 2006

Rotondo A, Mazzanti C, Dell'Osso L, et al: Catechol O-methyltransferase, serotonin transporter, and tryptophan hydroxylase gene polymorphisms in bipolar disorder patients with and without comorbid panic disorder. Am J Psychiatry 159:23–29, 2002

Roy A, Segal NL, Centerwall BS, et al: Suicide in twins. Arch Gen Psychiatry 48:29–32, 1991

Roy A, Segal NL, Sarchiapone M: Attempted suicide among living co-twins of twin suicide victims. Am J Psychiatry 152:1075–1076, 1995

Rubio JP, Speed TP, Bahlo M, et al: The current state of multiple sclerosis genetic research. Ann Acad Med Singapore 29:322–330, 2000

Rudin E: Zur Vererbung und Neuenstehung der Dementia Praecox. Berlin, Germany, Springer-Verlag, 1916

Rybakowski JK, Borkowska A, Skibinska M, et al: Illness-specific association of val66met BDNF polymorphism with performance on Wisconsin Card Sorting Test in bipolar mood disorder. Mol Psychiatry 11:122–124, 2006

Savitz JB, Cupido CL, Ramesar RS: Trends in suicidology: personality as an endophenotype for molecular genetic investigations. PLoS Med 3:e107, 2006

Sawa A, Snyder SH: Genetics. Two genes link two distinct psychoses. Science 310:1128–1129, 2005

Sawamura N, Sawamura-Yamamoto T, Ozeki Y, et al: A form of DISC1 enriched in nucleus: altered subcellular distribution in orbitofrontal cortex in psychosis and substance/alcohol abuse. Proc Natl Acad Sci U S A 102:1187–1192, 2005

Schena M, Shalon D, Davis RW, et al: Quantitative monitoring of gene expression patterns with a complementary DNA microarray. Science 270:467–470, 1995

Scherrer JF, True WR, Xian H, et al: Evidence for genetic influences common and specific to symptoms of generalized anxiety and panic. J Affect Disord 57:25–35, 2000

Schulze TG, Buervenich S, Badner JA, et al: Loci on chromosomes 6q and 6p interact to increase susceptibility to bipolar affective disorder in the national institute of mental health genetics initiative pedigrees. Biol Psychiatry 56:18–23, 2004

Schulsinger F, Kety SS, Rosenthal D, et al: A family study of suicide, in Origin, Prevention and Treatment of Affective Disorders. Edited by Schou M, Stromgren E. New York, Academic Press, 1979, pp 277–287

Schumacher J, Jamra RA, Freudenberg J, et al: Examination of G72 and D-amino-acid oxidase as genetic risk factors for schizophrenia and bipolar affective disorder. Mol Psychiatry 9:203–207, 2004

Segman RH, Heresco-Levy U, Finkel B, et al: Association between the serotonin 2C receptor gene and tardive dyskinesia in chronic schizophrenia: additive contribution of 5-HT2Cser and DRD3gly alleles to susceptibility. Psychopharmacology (Berl) 152:408–413, 2000

Sequeira A, Gwadry FG, Ffrench-Mullen JM, et al: Implication of SSAT by gene expression and genetic variation in suicide and major depression. Arch Gen Psychiatry 63:35–48, 2006

Shafii M, Carrigan S, Whittinghill JR, et al: Psychological autopsy of completed suicide in children and adolescents. Am J Psychiatry 142:1061–1064, 1985

Sham PC, Jones P, Russell A, et al: Age at onset, sex, and familial psychiatric morbidity in schizophrenia. Camberwell Collaborative Psychosis Study. Br J Psychiatry 165:466–473, 1994

Shastry BS: Schizophrenia: a genetic perspective (review). Int J Mol Med 9:207–212, 2002

Shenton ME, Solovay MR, Holzman PS, et al: Thought disorder in the relatives of psychotic patients. Arch Gen Psychiatry 46:897–901, 1989

Shifman S, Bronstein M, Sternfeld M, et al: A highly significant association between a COMT haplotype and schizophrenia. Am J Hum Genet 71:1296–1302, 2002

Shih RA, Belmonte PL, Zandi PP: A review of the evidence from family, twin and adoption studies for a genetic contribution to adult psychiatric disorders. Int Rev Psychiatry 16:260–283, 2004

Silverman JM, Smith CJ, Guo SL, et al: Lateral ventricular enlargement in schizophrenic probands and their siblings with schizophrenia-related disorders. Biol Psychiatry 43:97–106, 1998

Sklar P: Linkage analysis in psychiatric disorders: the emerging picture. Annu Rev Genomics Hum Genet 3:371–413, 2002

Sklar P, Gabriel SB, McInnis MG, et al: Family based association study of 76 candidate genes in bipolar disorder: BDNF is a potential risk locus. Brain-derived neurotrophic factor. Mol Psychiatry 7:579–593, 2002

Skre I, Onstad S, Torgersen S, et al: A twin study of DSM-III-R anxiety disorders. Acta Psychiatr Scand 88:85–92, 1993

Smeraldi E, Zanardi R, Benedetti F, et al: Polymorphism within the promoter of the serotonin transporter gene and antidepressant efficacy of fluvoxamine. Mol Psychiatry 3:508–511, 1998

Snyder EY, Park KI, Flax JD, et al: Potential of neural "stem-like" cells for gene therapy and repair of the degenerating central nervous system. Adv Neurol 72:121–132, 1997

Solimena M, De Camilli P: Coxsackieviruses and diabetes. Nat Med 1:25–26, 1995

Sorensen G, Lindberg C, Wortwein G, et al: Differential roles for neuropeptide Y Y1 and Y5 receptors in anxiety and sedation. J Neurosci Res 77:723–729, 2004

Spence MA, Flodman PL, Sadovnick AD, et al: Bipolar disorder: evidence for a major locus. Am J Med Genet 60:370–376, 1995

Spitzer RL, Endicott J, Robins E: Research diagnostic criteria: rationale and reliability. Arch Gen Psychiatry 35:773–782, 1978

Stassen HH, Coppola R, Gottesman II, et al: EEG differences in monozygotic twins discordant and concordant for schizophrenia. Psychophysiology 36:109–117, 1999

Statham DJ, Heath AC, Madden PA, et al: Suicidal behaviour: an epidemiological and genetic study. Psychol Med 28:839–855, 1998

Stefansson H, Sigurdsson E, Steinthorsdottir V, et al: Neuregulin 1 and susceptibility to schizophrenia. Am J Hum Genet 71:877–892, 2002

Stein MB, Chartier MJ, Hazen AL, et al: A direct-interview family study of generalized social phobia. Am J Psychiatry 155:90–97, 1998

Straub RE, Weinberger DR: Schizophrenia genes—famine to feast. Biol Psychiatry 60:81–83, 2006

Straub RE, Sullivan PF, Ma Y, et al: Susceptibility genes for nicotine dependence: a genome scan and follow-up in an independent sample suggest that regions on chromosomes 2, 4, 10, 16, 17 and 18 merit further study. Mol Psychiatry 4:129–144, 1999

Straub RE, MacLean CJ, Ma Y, et al: Genome-wide scans of three independent sets of 90 Irish multiplex schizophrenia families and follow-up of selected regions in all families provides evidence for multiple susceptibility genes. Mol Psychiatry 7:542–559, 2002

Strober M, Morell W, Burroughs J, et al: A controlled family study of anorexia nervosa. J Psychiatr Res 19:239–246, 1985

Suarez BK, Cox NJ: Linkage analysis for psychiatric disorders, I: basic concepts. Psychiatr Dev 3:219–243, 1985

Suarez BK, Rice J, Reich T: The generalized sib pair IBD distribution: its use in the detection of linkage. Ann Hum Genet 42:87–94, 1978

Suddath RL, Christison GW, Torrey EF, et al: Anatomical abnormalities in the brains of monozygotic twins discordant for schizophrenia. N Engl J Med 322:789–794, 1990

Sullivan PF, Neale MC, Kendler KS: Genetic epidemiology of major depression: review and meta-analysis. Am J Psychiatry 157:1552–1562, 2000

Sun X, Wang JF, Tseng M, et al: Downregulation in components of the mitochondrial electron transport chain in the postmortem frontal cortex of subjects with bipolar disorder. J Psychiatry Neurosci 31:189–196, 2006

Talbot K, Eidem WL, Tinsley CL, et al: Dysbindin-1 is reduced in intrinsic, glutamatergic terminals of the hippocampal formation in schizophrenia. J Clin Invest 113:1353–1363, 2004

Taylor WD, Steffens DC, Payne ME, et al: Influence of serotonin transporter promoter region polymorphisms on hippocampal volumes in late-life depression. Arch Gen Psychiatry 62:537–544, 2005

Thomasson HR, Edenberg HJ, Crabb DW, et al: Alcohol and aldehyde dehydrogenase genotypes and alcoholism in Chinese men. Am J Hum Genet 48:677–681, 1991

Thorgeirsson TE, Oskarsson H, Desnica N, et al: Anxiety with panic disorder linked to chromosome 9q in Iceland. Am J Hum Genet 72:1221–1230, 2003

Tienari P, Wynne LC, Moring J, et al: The Finnish adoptive family study of schizophrenia. Implications for family research. Br J Psychiatry Suppl (23):20–26, 1994

Tienari P, Wynne LC, Moring J, et al: Finnish adoptive family study: sample selection and adoptee DSM-III-R diagnoses. Acta Psychiatr Scand 101:433–443, 2000

Tkachev D, Mimmack ML, Ryan MM, et al: Oligodendrocyte dysfunction in schizophrenia and bipolar disorder. Lancet 362:798–805, 2003

Torgersen S: Genetic factors in anxiety disorders. Arch Gen Psychiatry 40:1085–1089, 1983

Torgersen S: Comorbidity of major depression and anxiety disorders in twin pairs. Am J Psychiatry 147:1199–1202, 1990

Tremolizzo L, Doueiri MS, Dong E, et al: Valproate corrects the schizophrenia-like epigenetic behavioral modifications induced by methionine in mice. Biol Psychiatry 57:500–509, 2005

Trillenberg P, Lencer R, Heide W: Eye movements and psychiatric disease. Curr Opin Neurol 17:43–47, 2004

True WR, Xian H, Scherrer JF, et al: Common genetic vulnerability for nicotine and alcohol dependence in men. Arch Gen Psychiatry 56:655–661, 1999

Tsuang MT: Genetic counseling for psychiatric patients and their families. Am J Psychiatry 135:1465–1475, 1978

Tsuang MT: Risk of suicide in the relatives of schizophrenics, manics, depressives, and controls. J Clin Psychiatry 44:396–397, 398–400, 1983

Tsuang MT, Gilbertson MW, Faraone SV: The genetics of schizophrenia. Current knowledge and future directions. Schizophr Res 4:157–171, 1991

Uhl GR: Molecular genetics of substance abuse vulnerability: remarkable recent convergence of genome scan results. Ann N Y Acad Sci 1025:1–13, 2004

van Beek N, Griez E: Reactivity to a 35% CO_2 challenge in healthy first-degree relatives of patients with panic disorder. Biol Psychiatry 47:830–835, 2000 van den Berg BJ, Christianson RE, Oechsli FW: The California Child Health and Development Studies of the School of Public Health, University of California at Berkeley. Paediatr Perinatal Epidemiol 2:265–282, 1988

van de Vijver MJ, He YD, van't Veer LJ, et al: A gene-expression signature as a predictor of survival in breast cancer. N Engl J Med 347:1999–2009, 2002

van Rensburg SJ, Berman P, Potocnik F, et al: 5- and 6-glycosylation of transferrin in patients with Alzheimer's disease. Metab Brain Dis 19:89–96, 2004

Vawter MP, Ferran E, Galke B, et al: Microarray screening of lymphocyte gene expression differences in a multiplex schizophrenia pedigree. Schizophr Res 67:41–52, 2004

Venter JC, Adams MD, Myers EW, et al: The sequence of the human genome. Science 291:1304–1351, 2001

Villafuerte S, Burmeister M: Untangling genetic networks of panic, phobia, fear and anxiety. Genome Biol 4:224, 2003

Vogler GP, Gottesman II, McGue MK, et al: Mixed-model segregation analysis of schizophrenia in the Lindelius Swedish pedigrees. Behav Genet 20:461–472, 1990

Volk DW, Austin MC, Pierri JN, et al: Decreased glutamic acid decarboxylase67 messenger RNA expression in a subset of prefrontal cortical gamma-aminobutyric acid neurons in subjects with schizophrenia. Arch Gen Psychiatry 57:237–245, 2000

von Knorring AL, Cloninger CR, Bohman M, et al: An adoption study of depressive disorders and substance abuse. Arch Gen Psychiatry 40:943–950, 1983

Walsh T, Casadei S, Coats KH, et al: Spectrum of mutations in BRCA1, BRCA2, CHEK2, and TP53 in families at high risk of breast cancer. JAMA 295:1379–1388, 2006

Watson SJ, Meng F, Thompson RC, et al: The "chip" as a specific genetic tool. Biol Psychiatry 48:1147–1156, 2000

Watt NF, Anthony EJ, Wynne LC, et al (eds): Children at Risk for Schizophrenia: A Longitudinal Perspective. Cambridge, England, Cambridge University Press, 1984

Weinberger DR, Berman KF, Zec RF: Physiologic dysfunction of dorsolateral prefrontal cortex in schizophrenia, I: regional cerebral blood flow evidence. Arch Gen Psychiatry 43:114–124, 1986

Weinberger DR, Berman KF, Suddath R, et al: Evidence of dysfunction of a prefrontal-limbic network in schizophrenia: a magnetic resonance imaging and regional cerebral blood flow study of discordant monozygotic twins. Am J Psychiatry 149:890–897, 1992

Weiss KM: Genetic Variation and Human Disease. Cambridge, England, Cambridge University Press, 1993

Weissman MM, Wickramaratne P, Merikangas KR, et al: Onset of major depression in early adulthood. Increased familial loading and specificity. Arch Gen Psychiatry 41:1136–1143, 1984

Weissman MM, Warner V, Wickramaratne P, et al: Early onset major depression in parents and their children. J Affect Disord 15:269–277, 1988

Weissman MM, the Cross-National Collaborative Group: The changing rate of major depression: cross-national comparisons. JAMA 268:3098–3105, 1992

Weissman MM, Fyer AJ, Haghighi F, et al: Potential panic disorder syndrome: clinical and genetic linkage evidence. Am J Med Genet 96:24–35, 2000

Wellcome Trust Case Control Consortium: Genome-wide association study of 14,000 cases of seven common diseases and 3,000 shared controls. Nature 447:661–678, 2007

Wender PH, Rosenthal D, Kety SS, et al: Crossfostering. A research strategy for clarifying the role of genetic and experiential factors in the etiology of schizophrenia. Arch Gen Psychiatry 30:121–128, 1974

Wender PH, Kety SS, Rosenthal D, et al: Psychiatric disorders in the biological and adoptive families of adopted individuals with affective disorders. Arch Gen Psychiatry 43:923–929, 1986

Willeit M, Praschak-Rieder N, Neumeister A, et al: A polymorphism (5-HTTLPR) in the serotonin transporter promoter gene is associated with DSM-IV depression subtypes in seasonal affective disorder. Mol Psychiatry 8:942–946, 2003

Willour VL, Yao Shugart Y, Samuels J, et al: Replication study supports evidence for linkage to 9p24 in obsessive-compulsive disorder. Am J Hum Genet 75:508–513, 2004

Winokur G, Cadoret R, Baker M, et al: Depression spectrum disease versus pure depressive disease: some further data. Br J Psychiatry 127:75–77, 1975

Wright P, Takei N, Rifkin L, et al: Maternal influenza, obstetric complications, and schizophrenia. Am J Psychiatry 152:1714–1720, 1995

Yudofsky SC, Hales RE: The American Psychiatric Publishing Textbook of Neuropsychiatry and Clinical Neurosciences, 5th Edition. Washington, DC, American Psychiatric Publishing, 2008

Zanardi R, Serretti A, Rossini D, et al: Factors affecting fluvoxamine antidepressant activity: influence of pindolol and 5-HTTLPR in delusional and nondelusional depression. Biol Psychiatry 50:323–330, 2001

Zubenko GS, Hughes HB 3rd, Maher BS, et al: Genetic linkage of region containing the CREB1 gene to depressive disorders in women from families with recurrent, early onset, major depression. Am J Med Genet 114:980–987, 2002

Zubenko GS, Maher B, Hughes HB 3rd, et al: Genome-wide linkage survey for genetic loci that influence the development of depressive disorders in families with recurrent, early onset, major depression. Am J Med Genet B Neuropsychiatr Genet 123:1–18, 2003

7

NORMAL CHILD AND ADOLESCENT DEVELOPMENT

Ralph J. Gemelli, M.D.

Toward an Integrated Theoretical Model of Mental Development

Theories of normal development were, and still are, obviously constructed by the minds of developmental researchers, who are influenced by their own individual life experiences. These experiences always produce inevitable biases about which aspects of development are of high importance and which are of lesser or no importance in the normal development of the child.

The multiplicity of psychoanalytically oriented and other theories of human development becomes quite apparent when one attempts to teach a course on normal development to psychiatric residents or psychology graduate students. Teachers who are aware of this multiplicity of theories are faced with a collection of partial theories, which they typically present to the student. Piaget's (1954a) theory of cognitive development, Erikson's (1959) psychosocial task theory, and Freud's (S. Freud 1923/1963) psychosexual theory are examples of theories that focus on certain aspects of mental development without addressing the many other maturational events that occur during the developmental process. Students implicitly or explicitly are tasked with attempting to integrate these theories into a coherent picture of the developmental process that can be used in the evaluation and treatment of psychiatric patients.

In this chapter I present a possible theoretical model and organizational outline that bring together many of the particular theories on normal mental development and assemble them into a reasonable integrated "quilt." This model, which is more fully elaborated in my textbook *Normal Child and Adolescent Development* (Gemelli 1996), can be used to organize and understand how children's minds undergo normal maturation and developmental change. In adapting the biopsychosocial theoretical model to an object relations–structural view of the mind, I present each aspect of normal development not as a unique characteristic that appears at a specific age, but rather as a capacity that emerges during a certain period and then continues to evolve from one developmental phase to the next. Presenting child development in this way illustrates how the developmental process is continuous, in that each phase of development builds upon the previous phase and leads to the next. Table 7–1 lists the mastery areas for each developmental phase.

Biopsychosocial Stimuli

Each of the capacities, abilities, characteristics, or emotions listed in Table 7–1 emerges from transactions among biological, social, and psychological stimuli, which are defined as follows:

- *Biological stimuli* are the sensory stimuli that emanate from the infant's physical nature, both in health and in disease. For example, some biological stimuli emanate from inside the infant's body such as the physiological stimuli that produce the sensation of thirst.

- *Social stimuli* are all the sensory stimuli that emanate from sources external to the infant's body, brain, and mind. These would be stimuli emanating from people, things, and events that produce changes in one or more of the infant's sensory modalities.
- *Psychological stimuli* are mental sensory stimuli emanating from
    1. the infant's mental *nature,* which is composed of the infant's innate needs, a collection of emotions, temperamental characteristics, innate processing capacities, and the contributions emanating from the process of maturation.
    2. the infant's life experiences, emerging during the process of receiving *nurturance* from the infant's social environment, which generate the *experiential mental structures* we name as thoughts, perceptions, conceptions, and memories.

Object Relationships and Experiential Mental Structural Representations

In this adaptation of the traditional biopsychosocial scientific model to an *object relations–structural model* of how the mind matures and develops, the human infant is viewed as developing within one or more *object* (which unfortunately stands for people) *relationships.* The child's mind generates mental structural representations of these object relationships that become the child's unique representations of his or her living experiences.

These mental structural representations, together with the ongoing influences of the social environment, forever affect the child's current and future object relationships, in that new representations trigger transformations of one or more existing representations. The developmental process is not a series of additions but rather an ongoing transformation of mental representations. Accordingly, the developing child's representational world forever influences both how he or she perceives the current social world and also the kind of thoughts, feelings, and memories that are generated in response to these perceptions. Thus, for example, a 4-year-old girl's internalization of her conception of her parents being married will transform her preexisting mental representations of her mother and her father. These transformed representations of her parents will now influence how she emotionally and cognitively reacts to each parent and to both parents as a married couple.

Innate and experiential representational structures

TABLE 7–1. Components of each developmental phase

- Maturation and Development of Innate Needs
- Maturation and Development of Physical Capabilities
- Maturation and Development of Cognitive Abilities
- Maturation and Development of Temperamental Characteristics
- Maturation and Development of Emotions
- Maturation and Development of Verbal Language Abilities
- Maturation and Development of the Preexisting Representational World
- Development of the Self and Object Relationships
- Development of the Superego
- Development of Adaptational Capabilities

(or *mental structures* for short) imbue the human mind with continuity: being able to store representations of the past, the child brings to each new living experience a capacity to predict, transfer, and expect that the present will be based in part on the past. In addition, the human mind is able to be open to entirely unexpected new experiences, termed *developmental discontinuities* (R. Tyson 1986). A *discontinuity* is a specific time in the child's life cycle in which unexpected physical and/or cognitive abilities emerge or unexpected social events occur (e.g., the child's life is changed by entering a new school or by meeting a new playmate), none of which appear to be the result of prior competencies or social interactions. These discontinuities create disequilibrium in a child's inner mental world, which in turn triggers transformations of existing mental structures, ultimately resulting in changes in the child's thinking, feeling, remembering, and behaving. The tasks of constructing, reconstructing, and transforming mental representations take place through the process of cognition.

Cognition and Memory

Innate mental processing structures enable infants to begin to carry out the process of cognition. *Cognition* is any mental process that generates new or experiential information (as opposed to information that is innate). A *mental process* is defined as a simple or complicated mental action or series of mental actions that are not directly observed but are inferred to be present in order to explain the products of their actions (e.g., dreaming would be the action and the dream the product [Pulver 1988]). All mental processes occur outside of conscious awareness. The *innate processing structures* present in infants are processes that generate the infant's initial perceptions, conceptions, and memories and those that store and retrieve memories.

A *conception* is defined as a mental structure that is formed when a perception becomes understood to some degree, or is given meaning, by the developing child (Gemelli 1996). Conceptions are ideas, wishes, fantasies, beliefs, and so on. The complexity of an infant's conceptions is a function of that infant's cognitive capabilities, which at birth are only beginning to undergo maturational growth.

Another experiential informational structure is a *memory,* defined as the mind's storage unit for information gained through living experiences. Through memories, infants progressively store a personal history of their living experiences. This personal history then becomes available to them through the process of remembering. The human mind encodes incoming stimuli into perceptions, and possibly conceptions, and temporarily stores this encoded information in short-term working memory. Eventually this coded memory may be stored as a long-term memory structure. Long-term memories are later retrievable through the process of remembering. In terms of how the human mind stores and retrieves information, there are two types of long-term memory structures: implicit ones and explicit ones (Clyman 1991; Schacter 1992; Squire 1986, 1992; Terr 1994).

Implicit memory (Solms and Turnbull 2002) is defined as

> the way in which the brain encodes an experience and then influences later behavior without requiring conscious awareness, recognition, recall, or an inner experience of a [consciously] "retrieved memory." Thus, the skill of riding a bicycle can be demonstrated even if the youngster has no [conscious] recall of when s/he learned to ride. This is implicit memory without explicit recall. (Siegel 1993, p. 6)

The second type of memory is *explicit memory,* which is the way in which the brain encodes an experience and then influences later behavior with conscious awareness of the inner experience of a retrieved memory (Siegel 1993). This conscious retrieval or remembering of facts or events can usually be stated in words. Consequently, explicit memories are storage units for information that is received after a child becomes verbal (i.e., at about age 2–2½ years).

Developmental Change

Developmental change can be defined as a mental process in which the child's mind constructs new mental representations and retains them as long-term memories. These changes can be triggered by *maturation* (i.e., the process in which new cognitive abilities and emotions emerge through chronological, genetically controlled growth and differentiation of various parts of the brain), by events in the child's *social environment,* or by both.

Nurturance in the human context is defined as caretaking activities provided to the child by one or more people in his or her environment that ensure the child's 1) physical survival and 2) development as a socialized member of his or her society. One characteristic of the human infant is that, for any degree of physical and *mental maturation* to emerge, a life-sustaining amount of physical *nurturance* (e.g., nutrition, thermal regulation, physical activity, protection against bodily injury) must be provided by the infant's caretakers.

Developmental change begins as the developing child's mind processes the transactions among biological, social, and psychological stimuli and then generates one or more of the following as initial inputs: perceptions, conceptions (i.e., wishes, fantasies, or beliefs), feelings, or memories. Next, the child's mind processes, integrates, and transforms these internal responses to generate a new mental representation. This new representation becomes a *potential* piece of developmental change—for only if the child stores the new representation as a long-term memory does developmental change occur. Subsequently when recalling this memory, the child will invariably begin to practice and consolidate this new knowledge by engaging in new learning experiences.

Therefore, the process of mental development is one of sequential developmental changes and associated new learning experiences—a process in which infants gradually acquire knowledge about their minds and bodies, their caretakers, and others (Harrison and Tronick 2007).

Mental Organizing Principles

We view the mind as an organized biological system because, in its normal development and functioning, it possesses the qualities of regulation and order rather than those of unregulation and chaos. One organizing principle of the human mind is termed the *representational principle.* This principle states that each infant will mentally process sensory inputs and generate *individualized* perceptual, wishful, and emotional *repre-*

*sentations—not exact replicas—*of these sensory inputs. These unique representations become the substance of the developing infant's implicit memories and the older child's implicit and explicit memories.

Infants are innately endowed with a group of emotions. The stimulation of each of these emotions is tied to the stimulus seeking–stimulus avoiding principle (or *stimulus principle* for short), which is another of the operating principles by which the human mind is organized. In essence, this principle states that infants will automatically seek quantities and qualities of stimulation that are within their *optimal stimulation range.* This stimulation range is unique for each infant. Each infant's upper and lower thresholds of stimulation are defined by that infant's individual innate endowment and individual stimulus barriers (S. Freud 1900/1963).

As the developing infant's cognitive capacities mature, the results of three new organizing principles generate new developmental changes: the transference-assimilation principle, the accommodation-transformation principle, and the hierarchical restructuring principle.

Assimilation is the mental process in which a child "takes in" a current perception or conception into a preexisting representation. In trying to assimilate this perception or conception, the child attempts to achieve a sense of knowing or a sense of familiarity regarding the new perception or conception. If a child is not able to assimilate a new perception or conception, a state of uncertainty occurs. The child may abandon the activity if he or she is not motivated to continue for a variety of reasons. However, if what the child perceives or conceives is within the child's zone of proximal development (see subsection with that title below), the process of accommodation may be activated. *Accommodation* occurs when the child perceives the new perception or conception as being novel, and, in integrating this perception or conception, either reconstructs or transforms an existing representation or constructs an entirely new one. Successful accommodation leads to new developmental changes, because new representational mental structures are constructed.

The transference-assimilation principle states that infants, in formulating a perception or conception from current biological, social, or psychological stimuli, will unconsciously or automatically activate their database—stored within their long-term memories—of representations of people and things to generate predictive expectancies and transfer these expectancies onto the new perception or conception (Panksepp 2004). This transference was defined by Lichtenberg and Kindler (1994) as "an expectancy of a human response or a situation involving humans and inanimate objects that may require very little cueing in actuality to seem confirmed" (p. 406). Thus, for example, an infant is propelled to automatically or unconsciously transfer one or more aspects of a previously stored representation of a person onto a new person who is currently being perceived. This transference becomes the first inner referent for how the infant views the new person, a view initially colored by the wishes, feelings (including fears), conceptual beliefs, or fantasies that are contained within the representation that the infant has constructed of someone in his or her past. Following the transference of expectations, the infant then attempts to assimilate the new perception or conception into a prior representation.

When the new perception or conception cannot be assimilated into a prior representation, the accommodation-transformation principle is activated and accommodation to the new perception or conception occurs, resulting in either the reconstruction or transformation of an existing representation or the construction of an entirely new one.

The third principle that comes into play, often triggered by a new maturational cognitive advance, is the hierarchical restructuring principle. This principle states that as a child's cognitive abilities continue to mature and his or her mind continues to reconstruct prior representations to reflect a more advanced level of cognitive integration and comprehension, the child's mind will reorganize its representations into a hierarchy that reflects the child's unique preferences. Pine (1989) described this process as a slow and progressive reorganization of a child's inner (or representational) world in which the child prioritizes his or her innate needs (e.g., an attachment relationship with his or her parents and siblings may be ranked ahead of the child's assertively seeking new relationships outside his or her family), emotions (e.g., the expression of anger may be ranked ahead of the expression of loving feelings), personal interests (e.g., school may be ranked ahead of sports), and parental developmental taskings (e.g., parental taskings of the child to do well in school may be ranked ahead of parental taskings to be considerate to friends).

Zone of Proximal Development

Although an infant may receive enough parental encouragement to convert developmental changes into new learning experiences, the parents may or may not expose the infant to the type of social environment that will enable him or her to activate this developmental change in practice and consolidate this knowledge through the process of learning. For example, a 6-month-old boy might manifest the following maturational changes: he can sit up without his parent's support and at the same time grasp an object offered to him. These maturational changes generate new transactions between the infant and his parents, and he eventually acquires a new developmental change: he constructs a representation of the pleasurable experiences generated by his sitting and grasping behaviors. During infancy, in order for infants to be motivated to engage in potential new learning experiences, the parents must provide objects that the infant is physically able to grasp or situations that the infant can understand. In other words, they must provide objects and interactional experiences that are within the infant's *zone of proximal development* (Vygotsky 1978). Vygotsky emphasized that an infant is stimulated to apply already achieved developmental changes to new learning experiences when the parents provide objects and

experiences that are just proximal to (or slightly ahead of) the infant's cognitive and physical capabilities. As Kagan (1984) noted, infants learn within a range or zone that has as its borders the completely learned and the completely bizarre (or too novel).

Developmental Tasks

Developmental tasks have been defined (Erikson 1959) for each phase of the life cycle from infancy through adulthood (Table 7–2). These tasks determine what knowledge and behaviors the infant will be more or less expected to acquire and master in order to become a productive member of society, and how each child must adapt his or her innate and maturationally emerging needs, emotions, temperamental characteristics, and cognitive capabilities to society's rules and guidelines concerning their proper verbal and behavioral expression.

TABLE 7–2. Developmental phases and key tasks

Developmental phase	Key task	Associated normogenic belief
Infancy (birth–18 months)	Basic Trust	"I trust my parents and others."
Toddlerhood (18 months–3 years)	Autonomy	"I like to explore, but sometimes I get afraid when I can't see my mom or dad."
Early childhood (3–6 years)	Curiosity	"I am very curious, and my parents like that."
Late childhood (6–12 years)	Industry	"I like to show my friends what I can do."
Adolescence (12–19 years)	Identity	"I know who I am, and I'm not exactly like my parents."

Infancy Phase of Mental Development (Birth to Age 18 Months)

Major Developmental Tasks of Infancy

During the infancy phase, which I define as extending from birth through age 18 months, the major developmental tasks are as follows (Miller 1991):

1. Infants develop the awareness that they are separate from and are valued and loved by their parents.
2. Infants develop the awareness that their parents can be trusted to feed, shelter, protect, and stimulate them in more emotionally pleasurable than emotionally displeasurable ways.

3. Infants develop the awareness that they are engaged in relationships with their parents in which both act and react to each other.

Functions of the Social Environment

During the first years of life, infants learn that there exists a social world of people, animals, and inanimate objects that emit stimuli that vary in their frequency, intensity, and complexity. As infants begin to differentiate these "social stimuli," they slowly learn that the social environment performs many functions; these functions are in the service of society's goals of nurturing, protecting, educating, and making them socialized members of society. Throughout all phases of the life cycle, five functions support parents as they engage to provide a dynamically changing, developmentally enhancing, transactional goodness of fit with their children.

Providing Truthful Information About the Infant's Body and Surrounding World

One major developmental task of infancy for infants is to become aware that they can trust their parents (Erikson 1959). Parents instill such a sense of trust in their infants by becoming consistently reliable conveyors of truthful information about the world the infant has entered (Magnusson and Allen 1983). An infant eventually learns that when she experiences a specific type of internal stimulation (which later she will learn is named hunger), her mother provides her with substances that cause this internal stimulation to be pleasurably abated.

Providing Stimulus Modulation and Protection

Infants are innately endowed with the ability to gratify their innate needs, one of which is to assertively seek social stimuli. Infants are not innately endowed, however, with the knowledge that their self-initiated activities can also expose them to emotionally displeasurable and even life-threatening situations.

Infants are preprogrammed to sense and comprehend their parents' behavioral and emotional signals. Within days after birth, they display the ability to "read" their parents' looks of apprehension, an ability that Emde and Buchsbaum (1989) called *social referencing* but that I label *emotional referencing*.

Parents must also provide the social function of modulating the quality of the stimulation to which their infant is exposed so that they can keep the overall stimulation within the infant's optimal range. For example, they must protect their infant from the following:

1. Receiving too much stimulation
2. Receiving insufficient stimulation
3. Receiving overly repetitive and potentially monotonous stimulation
4. Receiving stimulation in a sensory modality that the infant will process into perceptions that are overstimulating (e.g., some infants are overly sensitive to loud auditory stimuli)

Providing Encouragement, Support, and Admiration

Infants will turn to their parents for behavioral and emotional feedback when they are in the midst of or have recently completed a behavior stimulated by one of their innate needs (e.g., sucking on the mother's breast nipple), new maturational advances (e.g., initiating crawling), or new developmental achievements (e.g., eating with a spoon). Parents must respond to these infant behaviors with encouragement and admiration. These parental responses become the crucial ingredients of infants' steady construction of internal perceptions of themselves as admirable and valuable. When these perceptions are stored as long-term memories, they become the forerunners of infants' future positive self-esteem.

Providing Truthful Information About Achieving Gratification of Innate Needs

Although infants are preprogrammed to gratify their own innate needs, they do not know what knowledge they must acquire and what behaviors they must master in order to become a productive member of society, nor do they know how they must adapt the expression of their innate needs and maturationally emerging capabilities to society's rules and guidelines. These behaviors are taught to infants and children by their parents (e.g., how to use the eating utensils preferred by their society, how to use speech to properly express anger).

Providing Adaptive Solutions to Emotionally Displeasurable Life Events

Parens (1987) described two types of displeasurable experiences for the developing infant:

1. Benignly displeasurable experiences are those in which the intensity of an infant's displeasurable feelings is not so severe as to prevent the infant from habituating, assimilating, or accommodating to the stimuli and ultimately adapting his or her needs to the situation at hand.
2. Excessively displeasurable experiences are traumatic experiences—that is, those that cause an excessive and sustained degree of displeasurable feelings and that cannot be terminated or withdrawn from by an infant, child, or adult (e.g., a severe physical injury).

Parents try to protect their children from traumatic experiences. However, children gradually discover that benignly emotionally displeasurable experiences are a part of life, and that their parents are not omnipotent in being able to spare them from these experiences.

The Organizational Mental Structures of the Id, Ego, Superego, and Self

S. Freud (1923/1963) conceptualized the mind as developing into three major structures: the id, ego, and superego. Although the self was also described by Freud, its more complete definition is attributed to post-Freudian developmentalists such as Kohut (1971), Kernberg (1982), and Havens (1986). The id, ego, superego, and self are conceptualized as complex organizational mental structures, each of which carries out a set of mental functions. (A *mental function* is defined as the mind's application of one or more mental structures, mental processes, or both for the purpose of attaining one of the mind's goals.) The theoretical constructs of the id, ego, superego, and self are more complex than the mental representational structures labeled as perceptions, conceptions, emotions, and memories.

Id

The id, as the "container" of the infant's innate needs, has the goal of generating psychological stimuli (i.e., defined as sensory stimuli emanating from within the infant's mind). For example, the innate need to eat generates the sensation of hunger.

Ego

The ego is the collection of the individual infant's emotions, temperamental characteristics, and cognitive, verbal, and physical capabilities. The ego receives biopsychosocial stimuli and engages these stimuli in a transactional and transformational process with the mind's prior representations and conceptions and then generates mental and behavioral "products" or information (i.e., perceptions, conceptions, emotions, verbal language, surface behaviors, and memories) for the self.

To summarize, the ego performs a variety of *ego functions* (Table 7–3) (Greenspan 1989; Hartman 1939; Kernberg 1987; Rapaport 1959). The ego operates silently and hence unconsciously. Infants and children will never directly experience their egos; they will experience them only indirectly through observing the products of their egos—namely, their own mental and behavioral abilities and surface and verbal behaviors.

Superego

The third complex organizational structure is the *superego* (S. Freud 1923/1963). The superego—or its synonym, the conscience—is another "container" of specific mental functions. The superego's functions, however, are organized under the goal of providing the developing child with an inner source of familial and societal rules and standards, as well as an inner source of self-esteem. Unlike the id and ego, which are viewed as existing from birth, the superego does not begin to fully function as an effective internal author-

TABLE 7–3. Ego functions
• Reception of biopsychosocial stimuli
• Integration and transformation of biopsychosocial sensory stimuli with existing mental representations
• Generation of emotions
• Formation of perceptions and conceptions
• Production of verbal language
• Formation, storage, and recall of memories
• Utilization of defense mechanisms
• Generation of transference reactions
• Activation of all surface behaviors

ity over the id and ego until about age 5 years. Even then, it must undergo many more years of development before it functions most effectively.

Self

Viewed as present from birth, the fourth complex organizational structure is the *self*. The self is defined as the supraordinate organizational structure of the mind; according to this view, it exerts overriding control of the id, ego, and superego. The self not only occupies the conscious mental domain but also occupies, or has ongoing access to, the preconscious and unconscious mental domains. As such, the self, not the ego, becomes the *source of agency* of the child's developing mind. The self therefore makes both conscious and unconscious decisions about whether to act, to deploy a defense mechanism, to repress a thought or feeling, or to relinquish an operative defense mechanism to allow a repressed long-term memory to enter consciousness.

Maturation and Development of Innate Needs: The Oral Phase

Innate Physiological Needs

Infants' innate need to gratify their physiological requirements (i.e., hunger, thirst, elimination, tactile stimulation, equilibrium, thermal control, and sleep) and their ability to generate feelings and activate distress signals in response to the stimulation and gratification or failure of gratification of these needs indicate that infants "greet" their parents with active, preprogrammed behavioral abilities that are then developed through the unique relationship with their parents that we label the attachment relationship.

Satisfying innate needs.   From birth to age 18 months, infants seek oral sensual stimulation and gratification (Brenner 1965). The sensual pleasure achieved through oral stimulation motivates infants to use their mouths to acquire new knowledge about biological stimuli (e.g., the oral mucosa and tongue) and social stimuli (e.g., the mother's breast nipple). S. Freud (1923/1963) called this period of development the *oral phase* and labeled infants' sensual pleasure as *oral eroticism*. He viewed infants as possessing a sexual drive that propelled them to seek sensual pleasure and, following maturation of the sexual drive, sexual pleasure.

In interactions between each of their innate needs (i.e., as aspects of their nature) and their parents' and others' responses to them (i.e., the nurturing element), infants eventually construct mental representations of each innate need, how their parents responded to that need, and what emotions both the parents and the infant experienced in expressing and meeting those needs. This is a good example of how infants' socialization experiences trigger developmental changes—namely, infants' construction of new mental representations of significant enough emotional valence to be retained as long-term memories.

Signaling when innate needs are not met.   Crying—an innate behavior that triggers socializing transactions between an infant and its parents or caretakers—has been proposed by several developmentalists (Ainsworth et al. 1978; Bowlby 1969; Lamb 1981) to be an innate capability that generates an innate or preprogrammed response in other humans (both children and adults), especially the infant's parents, who are biologically ready to enter into an emotional state of mind in reference to their infant that is very similar to the innate and emotional reactions to the initial stage of falling in love (Mayes 2006). When adult caretakers respond appropriately and consistently to infants' crying signals, infants learn to perceive their caretakers as predictable and reliable soothers of their distress.

In addition to signaling hunger, temperature-related discomfort, and the need for stimulating interactions with the parents, crying is also used as an active means by which infants attempt to shut out their reception of 1) sensory stimuli that have reached their unique upper or lower stimulation thresholds or 2) sensory stimuli being received through a specific sensory modality (e.g., auditory stimuli) that generate a level of stimulation that is above their upper stimulation threshold. Consequently, crying helps infants adapt to their social world in that it gives them a means of controlling their level of stimulation and thus helps them to self-regulate their emotions.

Need to Assertively Explore the Social Environment

Infants' need to act assertively.   Infants are equipped with an innate assertiveness, or "assertiveness system" (Stechler and Halton 1987), which internally motivates them to explore the social environment in a manner that is directed, focused, and not easily prohibited or deflected from its goal.

Parents' interpretation of their infant's assertiveness.   For an infant to experience the joy of causing things to happen in his or her environment, the parents must want the infant to learn about his or her assertive abilities. While allowing the infant a certain amount of flexibility in initiating his or her assertiveness, parents must also behave as consistently reliable sources of stimulus modulation and protection to prevent the infant's assertiveness from leading to displeasurable feelings or physical pain. Winnicott (1965) described this function of parents as providing a *holding environment*.

Human Motivation: The Central Role of Emotions

The pleasurable emotions (joy, excitement, pleasurable anxiety) that infants begin to experience in activating certain transactions with their parents and being allowed by their parents to assert themselves are the major motivators in infants' continued assertiveness in seeking new stimuli. Being assertively active and reactive within a transactional relationship with each parent whom an infant is learning to trust is one of the major developmental tasks of infancy. In slowly achieving this task, infants begin to categorize their representations of experiences in which they were assertive into those that generated pleasurable feelings and those that generated displeasurable feelings. These representations are then stored as long-term implicit memories and become future motivators of other actions (Schacter 1992; Terr 1994). Emotions, therefore, now occupy the place of prominence in answering the centuries-old question of what motivates the infant to act or not act. The answer is that the human infant, and the developing child and future adult, is motivated to engage in those activities that generate emotional pleasure and to avoid those that produce emotional displeasure.

Maturation and Development of Physical Capabilities

Since the 1940s, the virtual explosion of researchers' interest in systematically observing infant behavior (Dowling and Rothstein 1989; Lichtenberg and Kindler 1994; Stern 1985) has provided a large body of evidence demonstrating that infants are equipped with a sophisticated, genetically endowed perceptual apparatus that selectively orients them to attend to other human beings (Schaffer 1984).

Reflexive Abilities

Infants' preprogrammed or innate reflexes are automatic, involuntary responses that appear to orient them toward reacting to, as well as stimulating transactions with, their parents. Two tactile reflexes are especially important in early infant–parent transactions: 1) the sucking reflex, stimulated by stroking the infant's lips, which causes the infant to produce a sucking movement of the lips and mouth; and 2) the rooting reflex, produced by stroking the infant's cheek or lips, which causes the infant to turn its head toward the stimulus and initiate a snapping movement with the mouth.

Perceptual Abilities

An infant's innate perceptual apparatus is highly developed at birth. In this section, I address four specific innate perceptual abilities—visual, auditory, olfactory, and intermodal perceptual matching behaviors—in which infants display selective biases.

Visual. Shortly after birth, infants show a preference for disks with facial patterns painted on them over disks with nonfacial patterns (Fantz 1963; Kagan 1984). Also by this age, infants are more attracted to a moving rather than a stationary face (Girton 1979). Schaffer (1984) noted that faces easily attract the infant's attention because the infant is perceptually preprogrammed to respond selectively to the human face.

Auditory. Fantz (1961) and Hutt et al. (1968) showed that within the first days of life, infants preferentially respond to sounds that demonstrate auditory patterns similar to human speech over other types of sounds. Mills and Melhuish (1974) demonstrated that 3-week-old infants choose to suck on a nipple when the sucking is associated with their mother's voice.

Olfactory. Infants' innate abilities to form olfactory perceptions also show an early preferential bias for, and a discrimination of, human tastes.

Intermodal perceptual matching. It has been proposed that infants, from the first month of life, possess the ability to perform intermodal perceptual matching, defined as "the capacity to know or comprehend that two identical objects are similar even when they are perceived through different sensory modalities, such as touch and vision" (Dowling 1981, p. 293). In possessing this ability, infants are able to match, for example, a voice (which is heard) with a mouth (which is seen).

Maturation and Development of Cognitive Capabilities

Cognitive processes within the unconscious mental domain mostly follow *primary process* rules of thinking, characterized by the absence of logic, the existence of contradictions, the absence of time, and the inability to recognize negatives. Primary process thinking is irrational and magical. Conversely, cognitive processes within the preconscious and conscious domains primarily follow *secondary process* rules of thinking, characterized by laws of logic, identification of causal factors, and the permanence of elapsed time.

Piaget viewed infants as being innately active seekers of knowledge—as innately motivated learners, using their innate reflexes and innate abilities to form perceptions to act on their social world. In the process, they acquire knowledge. Piaget postulated that children become more intelligent as their cognitive maturational competencies evolve with increasing age.

According to Piaget, there are four major phases of cognitive maturation and development, each of which is qualitatively and quantitatively different from the preceding phase (Table 7–4). The age spans listed for the phases are only approximations of when most children can be expected to show the specific cognitive developmental achievements characteristic of that particular phase. This phasic theory has been labeled *epigenetic,* since Piaget fostered a theory of genetic epistemology, which is the "study of the manner in which a subject comes to attain objective knowledge of the world" (Case 1992, p. 164). (*Genetic* here refers to the progressive unfolding of new cognitive dynamic mental structures in accordance with a set plan, and *epistemology* refers to the study of the limits of children's acquisition of knowledge at each phase in the life cycle.) In essence, Piaget's cognitive genetic epistemological theory was an epigenetic one, as were Freud's and Erikson's theories.

TABLE 7–4.	Piaget's phases of cognitive maturation and development

- Sensorimotor phase (birth to age 2 years)
- Preoperational phase (ages 2–7 years)
- Concrete operational phase (ages 7–12 years)
- Formal operational phase (age 12 years and onward)

Acquiring Knowledge in the Sensorimotor Phase

According to Piaget, infants' innately endowed reflexes—defined as biological stimuli in the biopsychosocial model—become activated at birth and mediate the acquisition of their earliest knowledge of the world. Piaget put forth the following postulates for understanding how infants use their innate reflexes to acquire knowledge about their body and the environment:

1. *Infants' innately endowed reflexive apparatuses are not only exquisitely reactive to any available sensory stimulation, but also active in seeking out more and more complex stimuli with which to interact.* Thus, infants possess an intrinsic motivation to acquire knowledge. According to Piaget's theory, "action, not perceptual abstraction, is the primary source of information about the world" (Bidell and Fischer 1992, p. 105).
2. *Newborns' and growing infants' perceptions trigger innate reflexive surface behaviors.* For example, any object that touches the lips of a 1-day-old infant will stimulate the infant's innate sucking reflex, and sustained sucking will occur.
3. *Once an inborn reflex has been activated, an infant's maturing mind seeks to repeat the reflex.* Different stimuli initiate innate reflexes, as infants continually use these reflexes to acquire new knowledge and become "intelligent." For example, at birth, when an infant is hungry, any object that touches the infant's mouth will activate its sucking reflex (provided that it does not overly stimulate or harm the infant). By age 3 days, however, only a nipple on a bottle with palatable fluid within it or a breast nipple that produces milk will continue to be sucked on for any length of time. The infant has already begun to learn to differentiate stimuli that touch its mouth.
4. *Infants continue to acquire knowledge and learn by acting on and reacting to their environment; in this way, motor actions become the initial basic triggers for acquiring new knowledge.* Through repeated sucking actions, the infant learns that a nipple that is sucked on produces fluid that, when swallowed, relieves a displeasurable feeling (hunger) and produces a pleasurable feeling (satiation). In actively seeking to repeat the sucking reflex, the infant learns that sucking on certain types of nipples gives satisfaction. The repetition of these behaviors makes up a set of experiences that eventually become an internal mental representation called a *nipple schema.* This schema then becomes a new unit of knowledge for the infant (Table 7–5).
5. *Infants are motivated to initiate action when existing schemata cannot be used to integrate and comprehend new perceptions.* This process of acquiring new knowledge by changing a preexisting schema into a new schema involves the following mental processes:
   a. *Habituation*—According to the *habituation principle,* when infants become selectively focused on a stimulus that appears novel in some way, their response to that stimulus will decrease over time as the stimulus is repeated without producing noxious effects. The infant eventually reacts to the stimulus with a sense of boredom. Habitation is not discussed by Piaget but needs to be included here, because habituation is even more basic than Piaget's processes of assimilation and accommodation.
   b. *Assimilation*—In effect, assimilation helps the infant achieve a sense of pleasure in knowing and mastering an external experience by making it equal to an existing inner experience.
   c. *Accommodation*—An infant's or child's accommodations are always limited by the cognitive phase he or she has reached developmentally.
   d. *Circular reaction*—In this mental process, which can sometimes be observed behaviorally, an infant continues trying to assimilate a new object into an old schema, and then eventually accommodates the new perception into a new schema.

TABLE 7–5.	Schema or mental representations

- The mind forms representations of what is perceived.
- The day's representations are stored in short-term memory.
- The mind "erases" representations that have little emotional content and stores representations that have high emotional content.
- The stored representations become long-term memories.

Discrepant Events

The processes of assimilation and accommodation are optimized when new experiences are initially perceived as both similar and dissimilar to preexisting schemata. These types of new experiences are called *discrepant events,* defined as "events that are a partial transformation of existing schemata" (Kagan 1984, p. 37). Discrepant events attract and sustain a child's attention and concentration more than do nondiscrepant events and produce a pleasurable emotional response in infants and children.

Maturation and Development of Temperamental Characteristics

Temperament can be defined as the style in which infants express the following temperamental characteristics (Goldsmith et al. 1987):

1. *Activity,* in stimulating the environment
2. *Reactivity,* in responding to environmental stimulation
3. *Emotionality,* in terms of the thresholds of stimulation that generate each emotion, the behavioral style in which each emotion is expressed, the intensity of each emotion, and the time it takes to return levels of stimulation to the infant's optimal stimulation range and thereby achieve emotional self-regulation
4. *Sociability,* in terms of initiating social responses from others and responding to social communications

An infant's emotional style is how the infant expresses a particular emotion and recovers from it. For example, one 2-month-old infant might become angry more quickly and take much longer to calm herself than another infant of the same age. Also, the style in which infants express one emotion may not necessarily be the same style in which they express other emotions.

Researchers have found evidence indicating that infants' temperamental characteristics (Table 7–6) (Mitchell 1993) also undergo maturation. Both innate and maturationally emerging temperamental characteristics operate as psychological stimuli that interact with the social environment and ultimately lead infants to construct representations of each of their temperamental traits. For example, a 6-year-old boy told a playmate, "When I get angry, I need more time than my older brother does to calm down."

In the earliest formal research on temperament, Thomas and Chess (1977) launched a longitudinal study of a group of 133 infants born into white, middle-class, mostly professional families in New York City. From 1966 to 1980, Korn and Gannon (1984) studied another cohort of 98 infants born into Puerto Rican working-class families. In both studies, temperament was defined as the style of an infant's reactions to his or her environment, but did not include the infant's emotions generated in specific stimulating situations or how the infant's styles of emotional and behavioral response to stimulation might vary as his or her specific emotions varied. Campos et al. (1983), in reviewing these studies, noted that although these researchers believed that infants with a low threshold for crying would also have a low threshold for other emotions (e.g., anger), some infants might have a lower threshold for crying but a high threshold for anger. As noted in Table 7–6, Thomas and Chess focused on 10 categories of temperament. From these were derived three topological characterizations of infants: easy, difficult, and slow to adapt (Chess and Thomas 1989; Thomas and Chess 1977). The infants' temperamental reaction patterns were evaluated primarily through parent and teacher report, not by direct observations of the infants.

Chess and Thomas (1989) found that these topological characterizations sometimes, but not always, predicted and correlated highly with the traits shown in young adulthood. However, in the majority of cases the 3-year-old child viewed as being difficult tended to exhibit those same traits as a young adult.

In summary, temperamental characteristics, as innately present and maturationally emerging aspects of infants' mental nature, develop in the context of the socializing parental environment. By age 18 months, when infants develop an objective awareness of their own temperamental characteristics, they begin to become consciously aware that their parents support some of their temperamental traits but not others.

Maturation and Development of Emotions

Role of Emotions

Infants at birth are capable of generating several distinct emotions in response to sensory stimuli. Their primary emotions are joy, fear, anger, sadness, disgust, and surprise. These emotions are characterized both by their early appearance and by their attendant prototypic and universal facial expressions (M. Lewis and Brooks-Gunn 1979).

Emde (1983) noted that, throughout this process, infants are preprogrammed to monitor their experi-

TABLE 7–6.   Phenomenological categories of infant temperament: action and reaction patterns

Activity level	Quantity, quality, and proportion of active to inactive periods
Rhythmicity	Regulation of irregularity of biological functions (e.g., hunger, sleep, wakefulness, excretion)
Approach–withdrawal	Assertiveness in approaching unfamiliar or unexpected situations versus inhibition and withdrawal
Adaptability	Time duration of achieving adaptation to a stimulating experience
Threshold	Minimum strength of stimulus needed to evoke a response
Intensity of emotional response	Behavior intensity of emotions as observed in various situations
Quality of emotional states	Presence of pleasurable emotions (e.g., joy, excitement) versus displeasurable emotions (e.g., fear, anger)
Distractibility	Degree to which extraneous stimuli alter behaviors
Ability to complete a task	Attention span and persistence at a task
Attention span–persistence	Ability to focus attention on a novel stimulus and persist at attempts to achieve mastery despite distracting stimuli

Source.   Studies of Thomas and Chess (1977) and Chess and Thomas (1989).

ences according to what is *emotionally pleasurable* and *emotionally displeasurable.* Within the biopsychosocial model, the infant is innately motivated to seek to repeat emotionally pleasurable experiences—especially those that generate competency pleasure—and to avoid those experiences that generate displeasurable emotions.

Eventually, infants build a memory bank of *conceptual mental representations* of their different emotions, how they expressed them, and how their parents responded to them. In this way, their inner world of emotional representations is constructed, leading to developmental change and later learning experiences. As Stern (1985) expressed it, "For each separate emotion, the infant comes to recognize and expect a characteristic constellation of things happening" (p. 89).

Parents' Interpretations of Infants' Emotions

Infants' emotions are open to interpretation by their parents and are strongly influenced by the parents' aspirations, beliefs, and projections of their own feelings, given that pre-self-aware infants do not possess an objective sense of being separate selves in a world of parents and others. As Shapiro and Hertzig (1988) expressed it, "the very young [infant's] emotional expression tells us little of his or her emotional experience. Nevertheless, parents and others respond to the infant's emotional expressions as if they were a reflection of subjective experience" (p. 108).

Infants' Ability to Perceive Others' Emotions

Emde (1983) noted that pre-self-aware infants are able to perceive emotional information emanating from their parents and to use this information for emotional referencing. This ability to engage in emotional referencing propels infants to spontaneously seek and actively scan their parents' faces for emotional information as they assertively seek a novel stimulus, demonstrating infants' ever-present need to use their parents' emotions to help them regulate their own levels of stimulation so that they remain within their optimal stimulation range.

Development of the Self and Object Relationships

Developing Self-Value While Engaging in Transactional Relationships With Others

Perhaps the most important social function parents must fulfill is that of instilling within their infants self-esteem. This self-esteem is developed in a nurturant arena in which infants are given the physical space and an interesting and novel environment in which to perform and produce (Greenspan 1996). While the parents are fulfilling this and other social functions, they are operating as *selfobjects.*

Kohut and Wolf (1978) defined *selfobject* as an object that is experienced as part of oneself and that one expects to control in the same manner that one controls one's own body and mind. Pre-self-aware infants perceive their parents as being both separate objects and a part of their own self-absorbed experience—that is, as selfobjects.

Normally developing infants and children are thought to need their parents to function as both *idealizing* and *mirroring selfobjects* (Kohut 1971, 1977; Kohut and Wolf 1978). Eventually, children learn to perform these mirroring and idealizing social functions for themselves. However, when parents fail to provide these functions in early life, children can grow up with serious deficits in their ability to provide these functions for themselves.

As idealizing selfobjects, parents fulfill the infants' need to idealize and otherwise view the parents as all-powerful and perfect. As mirroring selfobjects, parents fulfill the infant's need to be given and to receive acceptance and admiration for his or her performances, something that pre-self-aware infants cannot provide for themselves because they are unable to recognize their own competencies. Infants then incorporate this parental acceptance and admiration into their gradually developing self-representation. If infants do not receive this acceptance and admiration (e.g., if they are not given tasks that are within their innate and maturing abilities to perform, for which they can then be admired), they will not begin to establish a sense of self-value and will fail to develop self-esteem.

No matter what the infant's appearance, proud parents exclaim, "Isn't my baby just wonderful!" Before infants have any conscious ability to understand any concept of value, they subjectively experience a sense of esteem when they gaze into their parents' eyes and, regardless of how they are functioning at the moment, see a gleam of satisfaction, admiration, and joy. This non-performance-related idealizing and positive mirroring from the parents becomes the crucial social stimulus involved in infants' development of self-esteem.

The second source of infants' sense of value is performance-related idealizing and positive mirroring responses from their parents. Parents give these responses when they observe their infant's expression of competency pleasure and when parents spontaneously respond to their infant's pleasing behaviors prior to their infant's evidencing any competency pleasure. When infants are able to master a novel stimulus or to effect an interesting change in their environments in an assertive manner, they are likely to display a smile, designated a *mastery smile*. This innately developing smile tends to be generated whenever infants experience an emotion of competency pleasure and

does not require an audience. However, parents usually are quite happy to see a mastery smile on their infant's face and are very willing to respond with a performance-confirming, positive mirroring smile of their own, coupled with an idealizing facial expression and a "You're great!" verbal response. Each mastery smile and complementary parental mirroring smile, with or without idealizing behaviors, fuels the infant's development of a sense of value and associated self-esteem. In forming memories of these mirroring smiles and idealizing responses, the infant begins to look for and transferentially to expect a positive mirroring smile in the parents and/or an idealizing response after the infant displays a mastery smile. Parents' provision of performance-related positive mirroring must involve their use of empathy in assessing when to positively mirror their infant's competency pleasure and when to emotionally signal that the infant is beginning to engage in a potentially displeasurable or dangerous situation.

Developing a Sense of Separateness

In addition to parents' wish to instill a sense of value in their infants, they also want to instill a sense of separateness. Awareness of both qualities develops concurrently while infants are engaged in transactional relationships with each of their parents. These transactions include the following.

Transactions related to infants' innate needs. Infants discover their true selves when they begin to construct representations of their innate needs, emotions, temperamental characteristics, and cognitive abilities as belonging to themselves and come to believe (through experiences with their parents) that they will be respected and gratified.

Low-stimulation, everyday caretaking activities with parents. Another set of experiences that lead to infants' development of a sense of separateness while engaged in relationships with their parents are those that take place when infants are relatively quiet and unstimulated. Pine (1985) identified a range of these everyday experiences: touching, rocking, seeing, smiling, and sucking.

Bodily contact. Infants experience a sense of separateness when they are engaged in transactional relationships with their parents that involve the infants' body wholeness. *Body wholeness* is a term used to describe each individual's "sense of being a nonfragmented, physical whole with boundaries and locus of integrated action" (Stern 1985, p. 71). These boundaries are conveyed by each individual's skin and sensoriperceptive organs.

Parental responses to infants' gender.   As infants develop their self-representations, giving rise to an objective self (at about age 18 months), they will construct an early gender representation. This early gender identity is the mental conceptual representation of how infants define themselves as being a member of the category male or female. As they grow older, infants will learn what it means to be male or female within their family and eventually will define for themselves gender role behaviors in discovering what it means to be masculine or feminine.

The Attachment Relationship

An *attachment relationship* is the specific relationship that forms between infants and their parents in a particular context (Bowlby 1988). The *attachment context* is one in which infants are completely dependent on the specific behaviors of their parents for survival. In this mutually activating and stimulating relationship, socializing transactions occur between infants and their parents (Oppenheim and Goldsmith 2007).

The goals of the attachment relationship are 1) to ensure the infant's maturational survival and 2) to ensure the infant's development as a socialized member of the society in which he or she is being nurtured. The first goal can be attained without attainment of the second—that is, survival can occur without socialization—but the result is often a child who can survive only in an isolated environment. Thus, the socialization process is necessary for each child to attain full psychological development (i.e., to become a person with a capacity to be self-aware and subsequently to understand one's self in an ever-expanding integrated autobiography of one's life story). This self-awareness capacity has been defined by Fonagy (1999) as the *mentalizing function,* which is the capacity to understand one's mind and the mind of others as being complex, with different emotions, beliefs, conflicts, and the like.

The Triadic Attachment Relationship

The older *dyadic model* of attachment has been gradually replaced by a newer *triadic model* that addresses the attachment relationship as taking place among the mother, the father, and the infant (Herzog 1982; Lamb 1981).

During the first 6 months of an infant's life, the father's attachment is both similar to and different from that of the mother. A father provides more physical, spontaneous interactions as well as more novel and complex behavioral interactions (Parke and Tinsley 1981). Greenberg and Morris (1974), however, found that fathers develop unique bonds to their infant within the first 3 days of the infant's life. They labeled this strong, emotionally positive bonding experienced by fathers as *engrossment.* An engrossed father experiences feelings of elation, preoccupation, absorption, and interest in his infant. Greenberg and Morris noted that engrossed fathers also reported a strong desire to look at, touch, and stimulate their infants.

Recent findings concerning shared father–mother attachment to the infant can be summarized as follows:

1. Infants can form multiple attachments; the strength of the attachment to each parent is a function of the quantity and quality of transactions with that parent.
2. A lower quantity of high-quality care provided by a parent is more important for attachment to the mother or father than a higher quantity of poor-quality care.
3. Fathers can fulfill traditional mother-only attachment roles. Data now exist that demonstrate a stronger attachment between the infant and the father when the mother spends less time with her infant.
4. In two-career families, when the husband has supported his wife's pursuit of a career, daughters often grow up believing that the female role presents an opportunity to develop both career and motherly ambitions.

Maternal bonding.   Maternal bonding is defined as "the establishment of a long-lasting, affectionate attachment of a mother toward her infant as the result of the mother's skin-to-skin contact with her newborn during a hormonally sensitive period lasting for a few hours after birth" (Campos et al. 1983, p. 820).

Maternal attunement.   Maternal attunement (Emde 1983; Stern 1985) is similar to father engrossment in that its etiology is thought to be a genetically induced, preprogrammed capacity in the mother that is released through the nurturing experience. *Attunement* is defined as the ability in the mother to "tune in" to her infant in a form of behavior that is more similar to matching than to imitation (Stern 1985).

Beebe and Sloate (1982) identified various attunement transactions. One example is *mutual gaze.* At birth, infants show visual preference for patterns and are capable of following a bright light with their eyes. By age 7 days, eye-to-eye contact between infant and mother is observed, with the development of selective visual gaze for the mother's face.

A good early maternal attunement is also indicated by *maternal play stimulation*—a regular rhythm in the mother's vocal, facial, and kinesthetic interactions with her infant. The attuned mother is empathically aware of her infant's specific attention–inattention and activity–inactivity rhythmic cycles.

Phases in the Attachment Relationship

Following engrossment and maternal bonding and attunement is the longitudinal unfolding of the attachment relationship (Ainsworth 1964; Ainsworth et al. 1978). This can be roughly divided into the following three phases.

Phase 1: Emergent social responsiveness (birth–2 months).

Much of the actual surface behaviors that transpire between infants and parents in this phase have to do with infants' achieving homeostasis. (*Homeostasis* was defined by Greenspan [1979] as an infant's capacity to regulate states; form basic cycles and rhythms of sleep, wakefulness, and alertness; organize internal and external experience [e.g., habituate to stimuli, organize patterns]; and integrate a number of modalities into more complex patterns [e.g., developing self-soothing behaviors].) Thus, it appears that infants, even in their first 2 months of life, are transactional social beings—that is, they are equipped to react to and produce reactions in their socializing environment.

Phase 2: Discriminating social responsiveness (ages 2–6 months): the social smile.

At age 2 or 3 months, infants develop the ability to raise their heads, which allows them to further control and direct their visual gazing. Stern (1985) observed that "by controlling their own direction of gaze, [infants] self-regulate the level and amount of social stimulation to which they are subject" (p. 21).

A major maturational advance signifying the development of infants' perceptual discrimination associated with a growing internal mental representation of their parents is the appearance of the *selective social smile*. This smile is given preferentially to the parents or to other significant caretakers, including siblings, with whom the infant has been involved since birth. The selective smile can emerge anywhere between ages 4 weeks and 12 weeks, and it also indicates that the infant is capable of recognition memory. A stranger's face will now be recognized as different from that of the infant's mother or father, and the infant reacts with wariness and will not smile as readily at the stranger. The selective social smile is considered an important sign of a healthy attachment relationship between an infant and his or her primary caretakers.

Phase 3: Active seeking of proximity to primary caretakers (age 6 months and onward): psychological birth.

Near age 5–6 months, there appears to be a maturational advance in infants' innate need to assertively explore their social environment for novel stimuli. At this stage, they become preoccupied with inanimate things. In Mahler's (1975) theory, at about age 6 months, the infant's *psychological birth* occurs. Mahler noted that 6-month-old infants appear more alert and are more goal-directed in their assertive pursuits than before. These new behaviors, which for Mahler ushered in the separation–individuation process, appeared to Mahler as indicating the infant's psychological birth, a sort of infant "hatching." Mahler divided the separation–individuation process into three subphases: 1) differentiation, 2) early practicing and practicing proper, and 3) rapprochement.

The first subphase—*differentiation*—is so labeled because it signifies infants' beginning development of a sense of separateness from the mother. Infants also begin to differentiate where their body ends and their mother's begins, manifested in their pulling at their mother's hair, ears, or nose and putting food into their mother's mouth (Mahler 1975).

Another behavior that emerges at ages 5–6 months is wariness of strangers. Traditionally this has been designated as *stranger anxiety* or *stranger distress* (Emde et al. 1979). At this age, infants experience a displeasurable emotional state, manifested by their reaching out and seeking proximity to the mother or father, whenever a strange face appears in front of them.

A month or so after the emergence of stranger anxiety, at about age 8 months, infants manifest a new anxiety—*separation anxiety*—or, as it is called by Kagan (1979), *separation distress*. At this stage, infants show fretfulness, reach out toward or seek proximity to a parent, and cry when a parent leaves them.

In infants involved in a developmentally enhancing fit with their parents, the emergence of moderate levels of stranger anxiety and separation anxiety is an indication that they have become *selectively attached*. These anxieties motivate them to be assertive in taking the initiative to maintain physical proximity to the parents. By age 10 months, most infants have formed selective attachments to a small number (usually three or four) of specific people (e.g., mother, father, siblings, babysitters, other relatives, family friends), with the strongest attachment usually to the mother (Shapiro and Hertzig 1988).

Bowlby (1988) phenomenologically described three principal patterns of attachment:

1. The pattern of attachment consistent with healthy development is *secure attachment,* in which children are confident that their parents (or parent figures) will be available, responsive, and helpful should they encounter adverse or frightening situations. With this assurance, children feel (assertively) bold in their explorations of the world and also competent in dealing with it.
2. In a second pattern, *anxious resistant attachment,* the child is uncertain whether his or her parents will be available or responsive or helpful when called upon. Because of this uncertainty, the child is always prone to separation anxiety, tends to be clinging, and is anxious about exploring the world.
3. In a third pattern, *anxious avoidant attachment,* the child has no confidence that when he or she seeks care, he or she will be responded to, but, on the contrary, expects to be rebuffed. Such children attempt to live their lives without the love and support of others. The most extreme cases result from rejection and ill-treatment or prolonged institutionalization. Clinical evidence suggests that if it persists, this pattern can lead to a variety of personality problems, ranging from compulsive self-sufficiency to persistent delinquency.

Maturation and Development of Adaptational Capabilities

In their assertive exploration of their environments, infants use some of the same behaviors used when responding to stimuli perceived as threatening. Parents must learn to differentiate between their infants' *aggressive assertiveness* and *reactive aggressive responses* to perceived threatening stimuli.

When confronted with threatening or distress-inducing stimuli (Lichtenberg 1989), infants' innate need to signal their distress is triggered. This in turn propels them to activate preprogrammed behaviors (e.g., crying, taste aversion, gaze aversion, auditory aversion, touch aversion), thereby generating both *fight responses* (i.e., aggressive and antagonistic behaviors to ward off the source of perceived danger) and *flight responses* (i.e., withdrawing and avoiding behaviors). The fight responses generate the displeasurable feelings of crying distress, anger, and disgust, and the flight responses generate the displeasurable feelings of crying distress, fear, and, later, shame and a subdued demeanor (Lichtenberg 1989).

Toddlerhood Phase of Mental Development (Ages 18 Months–3 Years)

Major Developmental Tasks of Toddlerhood

During each phase of the life cycle, the developing child constructs and develops subcomponents of his or her overall identity. These continually developing subcomponents are the building blocks of the toddler's continuously growing overall identity.

By the end of toddlerhood, children will have constructed the following:

1. An autonomous identity, in that they believe that they are separate individuals who can be autonomous, despite their wish at times to be dependent on their parents or significant others.
2. A gender identity, in that they believe that they are either boys or girls.

Functions of the Social Environment

In nurturing their toddler to develop autonomous and gender identities, parents must be attuned to and fulfill the following functions:

- Protect the toddler in his or her *assertive explorations* from experiencing too many episodes of distressful over- or understimulation.
- Teach the toddler how to gratify his or her *needs and wishes* within the family and social environment while keeping within the limits and rules set by the parents' society.
- Provide empathically attuned encouragement, support, and admiration for the toddler's growing *autonomy* while at the same time teaching the toddler that his or her autonomy has limits and restrictions.

Maturation and Development of Innate Needs: The Anal Phase

S. Freud (1923/1963) hypothesized a progression in body parts or *zones* through which infants and children seek sensual, and ultimately sexual, pleasure. In the *oral phase* of infancy, sensual pleasure was experienced through the lips and oral mucosa. In the toddlerhood phase—Freud's *anal and urethral phase*—the toddler's anal and urethral mucosa become the erogenous zones.

Maturation and Development of Physical Capabilities

Between 18 months and 3 years, toddlers walk fairly well, experiment with running, and learn more each day about how their hands can manipulate new objects and parts of their own bodies. Toddlers derive particular competency pleasure from discovering actions that they can make recur. In this sense, they are developing the concept of "I" as an active agent who can bring about changes in the environment. Toddlers' activity, as motivated by their innate need to be assertive, has been noted to be the most important trigger for the development of a sense of self (McDevitt 1987), in that through activity, toddlers slowly become aware of themselves as agents who make things happen (Pine 1985).

For example, a 10-month-girl took her first steps when she stood up, using a toy with wheels designed to aid in walking as support. Her mother witnessed this first walking event and responded with an enthusiastic smile. This event will lead the girl to construct a conceptual belief (or *belief* for short) about her new walking behavior. When something awakes her recall of this belief, triggering a *self-state* in which she is concentrating on walking, the girl will expect to feel competency pleasure and also expect that her parents will smile enthusiastically when she exhibits new walking behaviors. This use of a developmental change—the previously constructed conceptual belief about walking—to practice new walking-related behaviors is defined as the process of *learning.*

Maturation and Development of Cognitive Capabilities

Emergence of Objective Self-Awareness

At age 18 months, due to maturation of cognitive capacities, toddlers rather suddenly become able to be objective and to observe themselves as separate people in a world of others. At this point, the child's *objective self* is born (i.e., a self-representation is constructed), and with it appears a beginning understanding of the concepts *I, you,* and *we.* This objective self-awareness is in contrast to the infant's (before 18 months) subjective, or entirely self-absorbed, self-awareness (Stechler 1982).

Lewis and Brooks-Gunn (1979) described the toddler's progressive awareness of being a separate self in a world of others as a parallel process involving the toddler's concurrent acquisition of knowledge of self and others. Thus, toddlers construct, and become aware of having, object (e.g., parent) representations.

Toddlers' emerging *objective self-awareness* can be observed in their behaviors. Kagan (1981, 1989) described the following behaviors that emerge between ages 17 and 24 months:

1. *An appreciation of right and wrong, good and bad, valued and not valued.* Through their growing capacity to discriminate between good and bad behaviors and their ability to realize that parents attribute value to events, inanimate objects, and people, toddlers begin to recognize that they are individuals and that people are valued on the basis of what they do (Rochlin 1965).

2. *The recognition, through inferential thinking, that results have causes.* As toddlers begin to understand that events have causes (Greenspan 1979), they become motivated to understand the causes for the events they observe.

3. *The use of early forerunners of empathy to motivate and guide behaviors.* By age 2 years, toddlers are able to infer the emotional state of another person in their efforts to understand the effects of their own behavior on others (Brothers 1989). This is a precursor to true empathy. At this earlier stage, toddlers engage in the unconscious process of *projective identification,* through which they infer that someone else experiences the same feelings they themselves would experience in the same situation; thus, they project their own feelings onto others and then identify with the projected feelings.

   Parents, through constant verbalization of their thoughts and feelings about what they believe is occurring in their toddler's minds, play a crucial role in the process by which toddlers develop self-awareness. In this process, *toddlers first discover their minds by finding their individual minds in their parents' minds.*

4. *The beginning construction of standards.* After about age 18 months, toddlers increasingly recognize the existence of standards that dictate whether a behavior is good or bad.

5. *The use of verbal language to identify actions.* By age 2 years, toddlers are beginning to discover that they have a mind that senses, perceives, feels, thinks, and remembers (Leslie 1987). They also become aware of being able to speak and to use words to identify and differentiate their own characteristics and actions from the characteristics and actions of others.

6. *The ability to visually recognize one's separateness as a person.* Lewis and Brooks-Gunn (1979) documented how, at about age 18 months, toddlers will look in a mirror after their face has been altered by a spot of rouge on the nose and be able to touch the spot, an ability they did not possess earlier. Because they recognize that something in the reflection is not "just right," it is thought that they are able to recognize that the reflection in the mirror is not exactly their own. By age 3 years, however, those same children will immediately know that their face has been altered and that the altering hides in some way their true facial image. Most children at this age will touch the spot, laugh, and immediately assume that someone wants them to pretend to be a clown, hide their identity, or some such activity.

Continued Development of Conceptual Thinking

The major cognitive advances emerging during this phase of childhood are discussed in the following subsections.

Ability to symbolize.   The ability to form symbols emerges with toddlers' maturation of conceptual thinking (Klein 1930/1975; Werner and Kaplan 1963). One characteristic of toddlers' symbolizing is that they cannot distinguish between the symbol and what it symbolizes. For example, a toddler attributes a symbolic meaning to a dog puppet, imbuing it with the quality of being alive (this is called *animism*).

Ability to understand concepts expressed in verbal language.   By age 2 years, toddlers' ability to form symbolic conceptions and learn words enables them to begin to store explicit memories—information encoded in verbal form; in visual, auditory, tactile, and olfactory perceptions and conceptions; or in a combination of these forms.

Ability to form fantasies.   Fantasies are constructed from the same ingredients as beliefs: current sensations, perceptions, thoughts, emotions, and wishes, as well as the memories of any or all of these, including earlier fantasies and beliefs that are associated with the current experience. A fantasy conceptualizes what and how a person wishes his or her world could be and incorporates the way that person would change things and people so that his or her wishes would come true.

Ability to form beliefs.   A *belief* is a conception that establishes the relationship between two or more inanimate objects, aspects of nature's laws, or people. A be-

lief's truthfulness can be judged on a spectrum from being highly truthful to being completely false (Meissner 1992). The belief allows the toddler to make declarative statements about his or her social and inanimate worlds. Thus, a belief of a 3-year-old child might be, "The earth moves," or "The sun makes the earth warm."

Ability to form categories.   A *category* can be defined as "the symbolic representation of the qualities shared by a set of events" (Kagan 1989, p. 230). Toddlers automatically construct categories as another function of their maturing cognitive abilities. Although parents can, and often do, directly teach their toddlers to place people and things into categories, most of toddlers' categories arise through their automatic categorical constructions.

Development of self-reflection.   Toddlers develop the ability to revise old conceptions through a process called *self-reflection.* By age 2½ years, toddlers can use their new ability for self-reflection to think about prior beliefs and fantasies about themselves, their parents, and objects and transform them. In addition, through self-reflection, toddlers slowly begin to prioritize their wishes, beliefs, and fantasies.

Use of primary process and secondary process thinking.   The further development and differentiation of toddlers' *primary process* (magical, absence of logical connections) thinking from their *secondary process* (reality based, logical) thinking is enhanced by the development of their ability to 1) use self-reflective, intuitive, and logical thinking; 2) use verbal language; and 3) create and use symbols.

Primary process symbolic representations allow toddlers and children up to about age 6 or 7 years to use magical thinking to deal with displeasurable life events. A toddler's use of a teddy bear is an example of the child's creation of a transitional object (Winnicott 1953/1971, 1959/1989). A *transitional object* is so called because it allows toddlers to make the transition from the infancy phase—in which they developed *basic trust* and a *sense of separateness and value* without mistrust—to the toddler phase—during which they must begin to exercise their separateness and value through acting *autonomously* without excessive doubt and separation anxiety (Erikson 1959). The transitional object is not just a substitute for the mother or father but also a magical creation by the toddler. It is a symbolic representation of the parent and is imbued with magical powers to soothe, protect, and empower the toddler to continue to explore the world. Transitional objects are most often created by toddlers between ages 15 months and 2 years. These objects may persist in the child's life up to ages 4–5 years.

Deferred imitation. During the period from 18 months to 3 years, toddlers begin to demonstrate what Piaget (1954b/1981) called *deferred imitation*. In deferred imitation, instead of needing to imitate an observed behavior immediately, toddlers may spontaneously attempt to imitate and repeat the behavior at a later time, often hours and sometimes days later.

Inability to understand conservation. Children are unable to understand the concepts of conservation of mass and number until about age 3 years. For example, a 2-year-old boy who is shown two same-sized circular apple pies, one cut into four pieces and the other cut into eight pieces, and is asked which pie he wants will choose the eight-piece pie, "because there is more pie."

Psychic equivalence mode of viewing external reality. The inability to understand conservation of both mass and number points to a more general cognitive inability in toddlers: the inability to perceive two physical dimensions of an object and to understand that both dimensions are properties of the same object. This inability to take in two simultaneously perceived dimensions was called in the old literature egocentrism or an egocentric view of the world. *Egocentrism* is the belief that one's own point of view or perception of an object or event is the only point of view that can exist for that object or event. The more modern view is that if a toddler "sees it, it is real." There is a *psychic equivalency* between what is thought or felt and external reality. This psychic equivalence mode of thinking prevents a toddler from comprehending how, if he or she sees a house as "big," the toddler's mother can see it as "small."

Play. In toddlerhood, the quality and meaning of toddlers' play changes greatly (Waelder 1930/1976a, 1932/1976b). Play may be thought of as the primary means by which toddlers and children up to age 6 years teach themselves. The function of play for toddlers is threefold:

1. *To act out, in playful fantasy, a pleasurable life experience using toys, other adults, and children as symbols for the real experience, acquiring new knowledge in the process.*
2. *To practice delaying the behavioral or verbal expression of wishes and feelings that are causing developmental conflicts with parents.* Toddlers use play to deal with situations of developmental conflict. A *developmental conflict* is a disparity between a toddler's current wish and the wishes of his or her parents connected to the socialization of the toddler (Brenner 1979). In these situations, toddlers experience a benignly dis-

pleasurable level of anxiety caused by their fear of losing their parents' positive mirroring and attributions of value and love if they were to suddenly express in behavior or speech their restricted wishes.

3. *To unconsciously attempt to reconstruct a pathogenic belief, especially one resulting from a traumatic experience.* Toddlers who have experienced a traumatic event construct a conception of that event that becomes a pathogenic belief. This belief is usually repressed and relegated to the dynamic unconscious to keep the child from remembering the highly displeasurable emotions (i.e., the feelings of intense separation anxiety and rage and the sense of helplessness) associated with the trauma (Ross 2007).

The *repetition principle* states that the human mind is unconsciously motivated to attempt to recreate an event in the present that is similar to a past traumatic event that has led to construction and retention of one or more posttraumatic pathogenic beliefs. In toddler posttraumatic play, the toddler enacts a role in which he or she feels in control of emotions and achieves *competency pleasure* (i.e., wherein the toddler is a victor) as opposed to feeling the rage, panic, and sense of incompetence and helplessness associated with being the victim of trauma. The repetition principle is enacted when toddlers are exposed to an experience that in some way reminds them of a repressed traumatic memory. Completely unconscious of this remembering, toddlers remain unaware of how their unconscious traumatic memory is being worked on through their play re-creation; they are aware only of being motivated to create what they believe is a new scene (Terr 1994).

Maturation and Development of Temperamental Characteristics

Infants and toddlers undergo changes in temperament as a result of maturation of temperamental characteristics (Baldwin and Baldwin 1978). One such maturational change involves modifications in the child's optimal stimulation range and the point at which the child signals distress when he or she is over- or understimulated. This maturation enables toddlers to habituate to more stimulating experiences with their parents, siblings, and others.

Maturation and Development of Emotions

When a toddler achieves self-awareness and begins to recognize himself or herself as 1) a separate agent of assertive behaviors who expresses innate needs and interests in the environment, 2) a constructor of memories, 3) a possessor of an intact and whole body, and 4) a possessor of emotions in response to sensations and perceptions (Izard 1971, 1972), the toddler begins to construct emotional conceptions about his or her emotionally tinged experiences within the environment.

Self-aware toddlers' ability to cognitively appraise their interactions with others enables them to generate a new set of emotions: the emotions of shame and shyness, followed later by the emotions of guilt, contempt, and hatred (Demos 1981; Emde 1984; Harris et al. 1986; Henry 1973; Hoffman 1983; Zajonic 1980). These five emotions are called *social emotions*. To generate these emotions, the child must first be able to cognitively appraise what behaviors are expected of him or her (Emde et al. 1991).

Maturation and Development of Verbal Language Abilities

Development of Verbal Language

Two components of toddlers' earliest language are *syntax* (the structure and rules of language) and *semantics* (the meaning of language). Comprehension of the verbal message precedes the expression of the words and the understanding of the rules of verbal language. Thus, toddlers will know what they mean to say before they know how to say it. Evidenced by the fact that, by age 4 or 5 years, children have a 2,000-word vocabulary, it would seem that children ages 2–5 years have a "word hunger."

Speech as Facilitator of an Autonomous Identity

The ability to use speech as a language to communicate one's wishes, feelings, and conceptions of oneself and others facilitates toddlers' development of their self-representation, specifically by facilitating their development of an autonomous identity. This is accomplished by the effect of speech development on the following aspects of toddlers' developing autonomous identity.

An enhancer of self-esteem.   A parent's image of his or her toddler is mirrored in how that parent speaks to the toddler. Parents' words communicate their esteem for their child. In time, toddlers learn that their words are valued and responded to by their parents with love and support.

A means of exhibiting self-assertion and autonomy.   Speech emerges at the same time that toddlers are furthering their locomotive skills, developing their ability to defer imitation and to symbolize, and discovering that they are separate people in a world of others. Also in the midst of these advances, toddlers are becoming more autonomous, and they revel in being able to assert their autonomy through use of the word "no."

A means of expressing self and object (other) interdependence.   In acquiring speech, toddlers discover that they can share so much more of what they perceive externally and internally. As Stern (1985) expressed it,

> With each word, children solidify their mental commonality with the parent and later with other members of the language culture…. Language, then, provides a new way of being related to others by sharing personal knowledge with them, coming together in the domain of verbal relatedness. (pp. 172–173)

A vehicle to achieve self-inhibition and to demonstrate mechanisms of defense.   Shortly after speech acquisition begins to accelerate (i.e., around age 2½ years), toddlers are observed to generate inner speech (i.e., speech not spoken before an audience) (Berk 1994). Toddlers typically repeat aloud the shoulds and should nots they have been taught by their parents, learned about from siblings and playmates, and arrived at through their own empathic and inferential thinking.

Speech also enables toddlers to put defense mechanisms into operation. For example, verbalized denial can be useful as an adaptive mechanism (operating as a defense mechanism) in dealing with others. Many of the defense mechanisms toddlers use are the ones they see and hear their parents use.

Maturation and Development of the Preexisting Representational World

Once mental development begins at age 18 months, the developing mind, in storing a record of toddlers' experienced past, makes its own contributions to its continued development. As toddlers begin to construct, store, and retrieve explicit memories, these become differentiated into two types: semantic memories and episodic memories (Nelson 1990). *Semantic memories* store information about abstract concepts or events in time (Siegel 1993). An example of an abstract concept would be a 3-year-old girl's retention of the fact that wooden blocks can be used to build towers; an example of an event in time would be a 4-year-old boy's retention of the fact that on Halloween, children dress in costumes. *Episodic memories* involve the retention of information about a child's life experiences. These memories refer to something that happened at a specific time and in a specific place (Nelson 1993a, 1993b).

When toddlers reach age 2½ years, the parents begin to influence what episodic memories their toddlers will retain as part of their *autobiographical memories* (i.e., long-term explicit memories that become the memorial part of toddlers' ever-growing self-representation). Parents influence the development and recall of these memories when they engage in *memory talk,* through which they help the toddler organize his or her memory fragments of particular events into narratives the child can understand (Nelson 1993a, 1993b). In composing these narratives, parents help reinforce their toddlers' retrieval mechanisms and impart a sense of meaning and importance to the individual memories. By engaging in memory talk, parents communicate to their toddler that they have the child's life in their minds.

As noted earlier, toddlers view external reality primarily through two modes: the *psychic equivalence* mode (i.e., what the toddler thinks about reality *is* reality) and the *pretend* or *pretense* mode. The pretense mode has elements of magical thinking and fantasy formation. Consequently, toddlers' autobiographical memories are a mixture of psychic equivalence and pretense modes (Fonagy et al. 2002; Tessler 1986, 1991). As toddlers age, their parents help them (as I describe in the next phase of childhood) to integrate these two modes of viewing external reality and in the process restructure memories formed in the earlier ways of perceiving internal reality.

Development of the Self and Object Relationships

Development of Autonomous and Gender Identities

Identity is developed through all phases of the life cycle. In a Lego metaphor, children add new interlocking blocks at each phase in the life cycle that become new parts of their overall identity. This exercise involves more than interconnecting the new blocks with the preexisting blocks; it is a mental process of transforming preexisting blocks as one result of adding new blocks or mental representations. What is old is transformed by what is new. Thus, children continue to develop their emerging composite identity with the ultimate goal of establishing an emancipated identity by the end of adolescence.

Formation of a Gender Identity

Somewhere between the ages of 18 months and 2 years, after toddlers have attained self-awareness, they construct a gender identity (Emde 1983; Lewis and Brooks-Gunn 1979). According to Meyer (1982), *gender identity* can be defined as

> a psychological construct [or conceptual belief] which refers to a basic sense of maleness or femaleness or a conviction that one is male or female. (p. 382)

In becoming aware of being a separate person who possesses a particular gender, toddlers, by age 2 years, are engaged in a process of *gender categorization,* forming early categories of what it means to be a boy or a girl (Meyer 1980). Toddlers are propelled to identify with their same-gender parent; boys wonder about being a man just like their father, and girls wonder about being a woman just like their mother (Erikson 1963). This process of identifying with the same-gender parent helps toddlers begin to consolidate an early gender identity. Kagan (1984) described the process of identification as one in which toddlers, in possessing a conscious awareness of being a separate self, begin (at times consciously and at other times unconsciously) to infer that if they share some qualities with a parent, then they must automatically share other qualities with that parent as well.

Mastery Over Bodily Functions: Toilet Training

As mentioned earlier, Freud called the period coinciding with toddlerhood the anal and urethral stage (S. Freud 1923/1963). With this designation, he emphasized the pleasure toddlers experience in holding and letting go of urine and feces, but underemphasized toddlers' need to have mastery of their bodies. Toilet-trained toddlers possess within their self-representation a new awareness of their self-competency, self-agency, and self-responsibility.

Advances and Regressions in Achievement of Autonomy

For every advance in a toddler's capabilities, parents can describe an episode in which their toddler gave up that advance and returned to an earlier behavior. This return is called *regression.* The overall human developmental process is one in which advances, regressions, progressions, and plateaus in various biological, psychological, and social competencies take place.

The Rapprochement Subphase of Separation–Individuation

As toddlers experience the joy of being autonomous explorers and experimenters, they struggle with the gradual realization that their growing autonomy from their parents does not protect them from experiencing stranger and separation anxiety. In addition, parents do not always positively mirror and admire their toddler's explorations and new experiments.

All of these new discoveries cause toddlers to experience somewhat of a "breakup" of their initial loving attachment with their parents. They begin to have episodes of being quite angry at their parents. This period, which occurs approximately between ages 18 and 24 months, was labeled the *rapprochement subphase* by Mahler (1975) in her separation–individuation developmental theory. The use of the term *rapprochement* (or its synonym, *reconciliation*) points to the need for toddlers to get through this relative "breakup" with their parents.

In addition, because toddlers want to view their parents as all-powerful protectors, they are slowly constructing an *ideal object representation* of each parent. This representation is an internal view of the parents the way toddlers wish their parents could be. In conjunction with constructing ideal object representations—which exist concurrently with toddlers' more general object representations of loving, admiring, and supportive parents—toddlers also construct an *ideal self-representation* that exists concurrently in their representational world with their more general self-representation. Toddlers' ideal self-representation is an internal view of themselves the way they wish they could be.

The difficulty for toddlers occurs in situations in which they feel angry toward their parents but at the same time love them and idealize them. The rapprochement crisis becomes difficult because toddlers must face their own ambivalent feelings toward their parents, a fact of human experience that is not easy for toddlers to tolerate and understand. When the rapprochement crisis occurs, toddlers, in perceiving reality in the psychic equivalence mode, still tend to think that each person can experience only the emotion he or she is showing and/or verbalizing at the moment. Thus, when the mother is angry, toddlers literally think, "What you see is what you get"; they do not understand that the mother's loving feelings have not gone away. This is because toddlers segregate their loving object representations from their angry object representations of each parent, by means of the maturationally emerging process of *splitting*. In splitting, children retain two diametrically opposed images of a parent: one as all good and imbued with pleasurable emotions, and the other as all bad and imbued with displeasurable emotions. When one emotion is dominant, the other is nonexistent in their current view of their parents. The angry mother becomes a great threat, because the loving mother is "gone." Likewise, when toddlers feel angry toward their mothers, they reject them and avoid them, because toddlers believe that their anger is completely justified.

If, by about age 3 years, toddlers have had more loving than angry transactions with each parent, they will mentally integrate their good and bad representations of each parent and construct an *emotionally constant positive object representation* of each (Fraiberg 1969; hereafter referred to as *positive object constancy*). In achieving this integration, they will possess an object representation of their mother and father as loving, admiring, and supportive even when that parent is angry with or absent from them. The toddler's emotionally constant maternal and paternal object representations are no longer ambivalent (Solnit and Neubauer 1986), meaning that the toddler no longer questions whether the parents truly love and value him or her. Although toddlers continue to experience ambivalent feelings toward their parents, they now have a basic conviction that their parents ultimately love them.

Integration occurs also in reference to the toddler's identity: 3-year-old children integrate their feelings of self-love and self-hatred into a predominantly self-loving representation. They now begin to view themselves as valued and loved even though they may have angry and hateful feelings toward their parents. This *emotionally constant positive self-representation* (hereafter referred to as *positive self-constancy*) gives birth to the cohesive self (Kohut and Wolf 1978); that is, toddlers achieve an objective self-awareness in which they believe that their admiring and valuing parents (in their functioning as selfobjects) will continue to provide these mirroring representations even though the parents may at times disappoint and anger them (Tolpin 1971, 1978).

The establishment of positive self-constancy and positive object constancy brings the rapprochement crisis to a successful resolution. In normal developmental situations, positive self-constancy and positive object constancy become protective factors preventing toddlers from resurrecting their ideal self-representations and ideal object (parent) representations to their old place of prominence.

Development of the Superego

Through play, toddlers practice how to be social and construct beliefs about which behaviors are good versus which are bad. These beliefs can be called *standards* (Kagan 1984). If toddlers did not possess some innate need to be valued and loved, their adoption of their parents' and society's standards would be based entirely on the rewards and punishments they received from their parents in reference to each of their innate needs. Kagan (1984) has suggested that toddlers possess an innate need to choose the good over the bad. In learning what is good and right, toddlers want to choose good behaviors as goals in themselves, not only so they can have their survival needs met but also because they appear to have an innate sense of morality.

Development of Adaptational Capabilities

Development of New Defense Mechanisms

Defense mechanisms, by definition, are activated by the unconscious mental domain. Having access to both the conscious and unconscious domains, the toddler's unconscious self scans all of the child's mental activity and activates a defense mechanism when a mental event threatens to enter the child's consciousness that will generate highly displeasurable emotions, especially intense disintegration anxiety and/or separation anxiety.

TABLE 7–7. **Characteristics of defense mechanisms**

Defense mechanisms...

- Are innate.

- Evolve chronologically as an aspect of maturation in the psychological domain.

- Evolve outside of voluntary control and awareness.

- Produce external behaviors or certain ways of talking.

- Are recognized by their systematic distortion of those events that are known to have occurred, are occurring, or are expected to occur.

- Restore emotional self-regulation, allowing an unpleasurable emotional state to no longer be consciously experienced.

- Are the psychological counterparts of immune mechanisms (e.g., just as people differ in their immune response to inoculation with live bacilli, so they also differ in their defensive responses to unpleasurable emotional states).

Characteristics and functions of defense mechanisms. Functioning as mental safety valves, defense mechanisms (Table 7–7) enable the toddler to regain a momentary state of emotional self-regulation and a sense of control when an intensely unpleasurable emotion threatens to break into consciousness. However, these mechanisms will always distort the toddler's perception of reality to some degree and are useful to toddlers only when their deployment is fairly transient in duration. In all definitions of defense mechanisms, it is acknowledged that use of these mechanisms should be transient, because they are mental processes that suspend the toddler's necessary and healthy engagement in resolving external and internal developmental conflicts.

Types of defense mechanisms. The defense mechanisms that emerge during toddlerhood are as follows:

- *Repression*—The unconscious automatic barring from consciousness wishes, feelings, and memories that are associated with a highly displeasurable emotional state. When repression is fully effective, the repressed mental event is relegated to a toddler's unconscious but may be revived in the future by a sensation or perception that relates to the repressed mental content.
- *Projective identification*—An unconsciousness automatic process that is a primitive forerunner of the future capacity for empathy. In this process, a toddler unconsciously projects onto a parent or another person an intolerable mental possession (e.g., a wish, a feeling, a pathogenic belief) and then, in inferring that the other person wishes, feels, or believes in accordance with the projected content, attempts to manipulate that person to show the projected wish, feeling, or belief (Kernberg 1976; Meissner 1980). (For an extensive discussion of projective identification, see Sharff 1992.)
- *Projection*—The unconscious and automatic barring from one's consciousness a wish, feeling, or belief while consciously being convinced that the wish, feeling, or belief is possessed by a parent or another.
- *Introjection*—The unconscious taking in of another's wish or feeling while consciously believing it is one's own (i.e., the opposite of projection).
- *Turning against the self*—Unconsciously and automatically barring from one's consciousness a wish, feeling, belief, or fantasy and then turning that mental content against oneself.
- *Identification*—According to P. Tyson and Tyson (1991, p. 329), *identification* is

changing the shape of one's self-representation to become more like the perception of an admired person or of some aspect of an admired person.

When used as a defense mechanism, identification allows toddlers to unconsciously affiliate themselves with parental behaviors that are causing them to experience repeated episodes of intensely displeasurable emotions, often at a traumatic level. When toddlers cannot use fight-or-flight behaviors, or when their posttraumatic play fails to relieve their misery, toddlers can achieve some sense of mastery of these traumatic experiences by identifying with the aggressor (A. Freud 1936/1966).

Effect of Parents' Use of Defense Mechanisms on Their Toddlers' Use of Defense Mechanisms

An important aspect of the maturation and development of defense mechanisms in toddlers is how often and what types of defense mechanisms are used by parents in their interactions with their children. Psychologically aware, healthy parents intrinsically allow their child to develop and use defense mechanisms as a way of coping with life's demands and the inevitable external and internal conflicts with parents and others. However, they eventually coax their child to relinquish defense mechanisms in the context of the protected and trusting relationship created by the ongoing transactional goodness-of-fit attachment.

Early Childhood Phase of Mental Development (Ages 3–6 Years)

By age 3 years, when children's representational worlds have begun to be "occupied" by representational composite images of both parents, memories of life experiences, and beliefs concerning emotions and rules of behavior, their minds will refer to and will be influenced by this inner world in processing more complex transactions involving biopsychosocial stimuli. An *information-processing model* (Berg 1992; Kail and Bisanz 1992) can be useful in conceptualizing how mental developmental change—as a final output of children's mental processing of biopsychosocial transactions—occurs. Mental processing of biopsychosocial stimuli is thought to involve six steps:

1. Reception of biopsychosocial stimuli
2. Generation of initial emotional responses and cognitive and emotional processing of transactions among biopsychosocial stimuli that evoke children's representational perceptions, conceptions (i.e., wishes, fantasies, and beliefs), emotions, and memories
3. Processing of mental contents into internal motivators that trigger generation of one or more of the following *initial output responses* (where *output* is either a mental output or a surface behavioral output):
   a. Initiate an action or surface behavior (e.g., a 3-year-old boy walks toward his mother or decides to play with a novel game)
   b. Initiate speaking (e.g., a 3-year-old girl tells her mother, "I don't want to go to the store")
   c. Delay acting or speaking while consciously and privately contemplating one's thoughts and emotions as internal "mental actions" (e.g., a boy remembers a game similar to the one he is looking at and then recalls how much fun he had playing this game with his father)
   d. Delay acting or speaking while unconsciously activating a mental mechanism of defense, which usually involves behaving or talking in a certain way (e.g., a 3-year-old girl unconsciously projects her angry feelings onto her older brother and then complains to her mother that her older brother is angry at her)
   e. Delay acting or speaking while unconsciously activating the defense mechanism of somatization (e.g., a child with asthma experiences distressful overstimulation and begins to experience an asthmatic episode)
4. Activation of the capacity for self-in-relation-to-other observation, which enables children to observe the effectiveness of their initial output response (i.e., one of outputs a–e above) in achieving their goals in their current interactions with others
5. Activation of the capacity for self-reflection, which enables children to reflect upon this feedback information to determine whether they are achieving their goals at the moment, and if not, whether they should generate a different response
6. Construction of a new representation involving their final output responses and the responses or lack of responses from others in their social environment

Once children have generated a final output response, they move on to the sixth processing step, construction of a new representation or transformation and reconstruction of a preexisting representation. If stored as a long-term memory, this final representation will become a new mental developmental change.

Major Developmental Tasks of Early Childhood

If their first 3 years of life have gone reasonably well, children will continue to develop the following representations, which are part of their positive self-constancy and object constancy:

1. An *autonomous* and *valued identity*
2. A *gender identity* as male or female

Children's autonomous identity and gender identity are developed in the context of their belief that their parents can be trusted to continue to support, admire, protect, and love them. In addition, by age 3 years, young children begin to have experiences that enable them to construct the following additions to their self-representations, resulting in new pieces of their overall identity:

1. A *sexual identity*—A collection of beliefs, fantasies, and emotions that defines children's awareness of being able to seek sensual–sexual gratification from other individuals and that prohibits such gratification based on the rules of the family and society.
2. A *peer identity*—A collection of beliefs, fantasies, and emotions that defines children's awareness of being able to interact, cooperatively play, and negotiate conflicts with other children as a member of a peer group.
3. A *superego* or *conscience*—Children's dawning awareness that they can control their behaviors by choosing between right and wrong behaviors relatively independently of the presence of their parents.

Functions of the Social Environment

Fostering Children's Healthy Narcissism in Conjunction With Their Developing Reciprocal Relationships With Others

In a mutually satisfying goodness-of-fit process, parents help their children to gradually learn that there are times that they can achieve a certain degree of gratification of their needs in a manner that is emotionally pleasurable and there are other times that the gratification of their needs must be delayed because such gratification places them in conflict with the wishes of their parents or others. Parents provide appropriate instruction to assist their children in initiating delays

in their actions so that they can think about various behavioral solutions to these conflicts.

Development of a True Self

When a goodness of fit exists between children and their parents, children are said to be developing a true self-representation of their true self (Kohut 1971; Winnicott 1959/1989). A true self means that children are basically true to their innate needs. They do not have to avoid perceiving and learning about their own needs. A child's true self emerges in the context of maturing and developing within a family and social environment in which the child has learned how to gratify—or to delay the immediate gratification of—his or her needs in ways that, in most situations, please both the child and the parents.

Sensitively aware parents assist in their children's struggle to develop a true self vis-à-vis their periodically resurrected wishes to be perfect or to idealize their parents as being perfect in the following two ways:

1. *Remaining aware of their child's aspirations, both conscious and unconscious, to be perfect.* Any parental aspirations to be perfect or to raise a child who will worship the parent as being perfect must, if present, be relinquished. If not, children will begin to identify with their parents' idealizing view of them, especially when parents do not accept their children's performances, and will have great difficulty in relinquishing their periodic wish to have perfect parents.
2. *Allowing their child both to periodically view him- or herself as perfect and to periodically view the parents as perfect.* Parents intuitively know that their children will sometimes need to view themselves as perfect (e.g., in the context of having been confronted with a new limitation or a disappointment) and their parents as perfect. Rather than immediately confronting grandiose or idealizing fantasies, psychologically aware parents will allow them to persist temporarily but will refrain from supporting those false views. Instead, they will help their child express his or her real feelings of anger or disappointment, thereby supporting the child's true self.

The development and ascendancy to a position of prominence of a true self (over an ideal self), therefore, protects young children from wanting to abandon the reality of their current relationships—conflicts and all—with their parents and others. Such abandonment would lead them to seek narcissistic gratification in attempting to live the fantasy of being perfect and not needing their parents to guide and protect them, or to resurrect the fantasy of having a perfect parent figure whom they can worship and who will take care of them and protect them from experiencing any developmental anxieties.

Healthy and Unhealthy Narcissism

Narcissism is generally defined as self-love (P. Tyson and Tyson 1984). *Healthy narcissism* is synonymous with toddlers' first objective awareness of being valued and loved by their parents. It leads to healthy self-esteem but also to children's development of esteem and love for their parents. Thus, in normal development, children's healthy narcissistic investment in themselves goes hand in hand with their loving investment in their parents. Stated another way, narcissistic self-love and object love develop concurrently.

According to Kohut (1971), the central mechanisms "I am perfect" and "You are perfect, and I am a part of you" are the two basic narcissistic configurations used to preserve a part of the original experience of narcissistic perfection (i.e., the early toddler's sense of experiencing no limitations in assertively exploring the world). Later, in the rapprochement phase, toddlers must face the developmental crisis of confronting limitations. They resolve this crisis by taking the "road" of emotional self-constancy and object constancy while still keeping within their minds a potential "detour," which is their "I am perfect" representation—their ideal self-representation—and their "You are perfect, and I am a part of you" representation—their ideal object representation. They use this "detour" to lead them to a periodic refuge from particularly tough days when they must face a limitation or a disappointment.

However, young children involved in a poorness of fit may develop a false self by staying permanently on the "I am perfect" or "You are perfect, and I am a part of you" road as they journey through childhood, adolescence, and adult life. Or, in the case of severe and sustained emotional and/or physical abuse, one or both parents may "inject" into the child's mind an "alien self." In response, the child will invariably generate a belief in his or her own omnipotence and will then continually attempt to control others, taking pleasure in their irritation, anger, or sadness in resisting or succumbing to his or her controlling and demeaning behaviors.

Children who enjoy a goodness-of-fit relationship with their parents have parents who do not seek to maintain an illusion of perfection in themselves or their children. Rather, both parents and children find acceptable ways to reasonably gratify each of their innate needs in an emotionally pleasurable fashion. In this context, the term *reasonable* indicates that parents and children arrive at compromises between what they want and what they realize is possible, while maintaining an attachment relationship with each other.

Maturation and Development of Innate Needs: The Early Genital Phase

At about age 3 years, children begin to focus much more on their genital regions. Whereas toddlers were interested in looking at and exploring their bodies and genital apparatus (which served the purpose of their constructing a gender identity), young children seek sensual pleasure by manipulating their penile or clitoral area. Children discover masturbation in the natural process of exploring their genital regions.

S. Freud (1923/1963) documented a progressive maturation of what he called children's *sexual drive.* This progression began with seeking sensual pleasure through oral mucosal stimulation (the *oral phase*), to seeking sensual pleasure through anal and urethral stimulation (the *anal phase*), to seeking sensual and truly sexual pleasure through stimulation of the sexual organs (the *phallic phase*). (Freud named this latter phase after the male genitalia because he believed that the penis—the phallus—dominated the thinking of both boys and girls. Later researchers [Galenson 1993; Kestenberg 1968; Parens et al. 1976; Roiphe and Galenson 1981; P. Tyson 2005] have shown, however, that girls demonstrate just as much interest in their own genitals as boys do in theirs. Both boys and girls are interested in the genitals of each other.)

Maturation and Development of Physical Capabilities

From age 3 to age 5 years there is a significant increase in children's body weight, size, and motor coordination—that is, walking and running abilities, hand–eye coordination, and leg–eye coordination (Ames and Ilg 1976a, 1976b, 1976c, 1979). Children age 3 years also begin to reveal whatever athletic abilities they possess as they show maturation of large- and small-muscle mass. Three-year-olds undergo a "strength spurt" over the next 2 years, and by 5 years of age they are much stronger as a result of large-muscle development.

Maturation and Development of Cognitive Capabilities

Ways Self-Reflective/Mentalizing Parents Help Their Children Develop Reality-Based Thinking

Up until about age 3 years, children's capacity to evaluate reality—what is going on around them (social variables), what is going on in their bodies (biological variables), and what is going on in their minds (psychological variables)—has been primarily influenced by their attachment figures. The capacity of parents to be self-reflective enables them, to varying degrees, to internally or mentally reflect upon the biopsychosocial stimuli that their children are processing. Greenspan (1998) wrote,

> No human being…is equally reflective across the entire range of experience. No one possesses the ability to step back and examine with uniform subtlety and flexibility feelings of love, loss, aggression, fear, anger, dependency, intimacy, and the rest. (p. 166)

Because adults differ in how much they are aware—and how effective they are in being aware—of the emotions, thoughts, and memories going through their minds, parents can be separated into two groups:

1. Psychologically aware parents who have developed a capacity for *mentalization* and have to some degree the ability to use empathy, intuition, and fantasy to reflect upon the biopsychosocial stimuli in their own minds and the minds of their children. These parents are fully aware that their minds mediate what they think, feel, and do behaviorally and are similarly aware that their children have separate minds that mediate what they think, feel, remember, and do behaviorally.
2. Parents who have not developed a capacity for mentalization and are quite deficient in being aware of what is going on in their own minds and in the minds of their children and others. In lacking this awareness, these parents are significantly hampered in differentiating their concepts (beliefs and fantasies) about the external world (their "psychic reality") from their assessments of and understandings about external reality.

By age 4–4½ years, children have established a "theory of mind"—meaning that they now realize that someone else can have a view of a person, object, or event that differs from their own. They can understand how another child looking at a dollhouse from a phys-ical vantage point different from their own can see a different view of the dollhouse.

By age 4½ years, children will continue to use symbolic objects in play to construct a *compensatory fantasy*, a fantasy that helps them to avoid becoming consciously aware of a developmental anxiety they are feeling. However, in now mentalizing, they are more readily able to think concurrently about what they are pretending in their minds (an aspect of their psychic reality) and what they are perceiving in the external world, including their body (their external reality). With this awareness of the relationship between internal (psychic reality) and external reality there now will be a pretense present in their play that was not present when they were younger. Consequently, they now use play to *pretend about* another reality, whereas before about age 4½ to 5 years, their play automatically *became* an alternative reality.

Maturing of the Mind's Executive Functions

In recent years, developmentalists have identified many of the cognitive functions that mature during the first 4 years of life and continue to be used by children. These functions, named *executive ego functions*, are used by the child's self, which I discussed earlier as the mind's superordinate or executive organizational structure. The self functions unconsciously and exerts an overriding organizing and regulating control over the id, ego, and superego. These executive functions, as outlined by Brown (2006), mediate how the mind organizes tasks (Table 7–8).

In most 4- to 5-year-old children, executive functions are called into action throughout the day. When one or more of these self-management components do not operate properly (e.g., the child appears unable to apply him- or herself with a sustained effort to assigned tasks), the child may be diagnosed as having a learning disability, an attention-deficit disorder, or a conduct disorder.

Maturation and Development of Temperamental Characteristics

Longitudinal studies of infant and child temperament (Chess and Thomas 1986; Kagan 1989) have demonstrated that some children will show continuity or temporal stability in certain temperamental characteristics they exhibited in infancy into their sixth year of life, whereas other children will show discontinuity or temporal instability between their infant temperamental characteristics and the temperamental characteristics they manifest by age 6 years.

TABLE 7–8.   Executive ego functions
• **Activation**—organizing, prioritizing, and getting to work
• **Focus**—tuning in, sustaining focus, and shifting attention when appropriate
• **Effort**—regulating alertness, sustaining effort, and adjusting processing speed
• **Emotions**—managing frustration and modulating emotion
• **Memory**—holding on to and working with information; retrieving memories
• **Action**—monitoring and regulating one's actions

Source.   Brown 2006.

Temperamental characteristics, like any other innate and maturing capacity in children, will mature and develop in the context of the transactional relationship between children and their parents.

Maturation and Development of Emotions

Construction of Rules for Emotional Display

In early childhood, children's emotions undergo significant maturation and development. As I described earlier, these maturational and developmental changes can be conceptualized within the framework of how emotions continue to be children's main organizers for 1) energy mobilization, 2) self-regulation, 3) social adaptation, and 4) enhancing developmental change (Emde 1999).

Emotions as Energy Mobilizers

As young children use both their unconscious implicit memories and their unconsciously repressed dynamic explicit memories as energy mobilizers in deciding to act or not act, they begin to learn more about what specific behavioral strategies they can use to express or withhold their emotions. In early childhood, children begin to construct *emotional display rules* (Maletesta and Haviland 1982) or *emotional control structures* (Clyman 1991)—the rules and procedures that govern 1) whether it is permissible to verbally express different emotions and 2) how each emotion is allowed to be expressed.

Traumatic Emotional Memories as Unconscious Energy Mobilizers

Explicit emotional autobiographical memories of a traumatic experience will be relegated to a child's unconscious. The resulting *unconscious dynamic memory* (where *dynamic* refers to the mind's use of defense mechanisms, notably repression, to push the explicit emotional autobiographical memory out of the conscious domain and into the unconscious one) does not lose its explicit content but instead becomes incorporated into the primary process thinking mode of the unconscious (Person 1995; Terr 1994). These types of memories exert a silent influence on children's perceptions of their current experiences and lead them to unconsciously enact certain behaviors in an attempt to re-create aspects of and repeat the original trauma in a new, mastery-achieving way. In this case, the intensely displeasurable unconscious emotions associated with the repressed memory act as an unconscious energy mobilizer. In effect, the unconscious mind causes a child to repeat certain behaviors associated with the trauma as a way of remembering it in action instead of in thought.

Emotions as Self-Regulators

In early childhood, children also use their emotions as organizers for developing their capacity for self-regulation. In this respect, they are assisted by a maturational advance occurring at about age 3 or 4 years, when they become able to consciously experience not only a wider range of emotions but also different *shades* of emotions (Lane and Schwartz 1987). Being happy is no longer one state; children can now perceive within themselves and in others that there are *degrees* of happiness (Emde 1999; Pally 1998). Children also become more capable of perceiving shades of emotions in their parents, which allows them to better assess what to do to keep interactions with their parents within a mutually pleasurable range (e.g., they can tell the difference between a low level of anger and a high level of anger when a parent says "Enough!") and what to do to return an interaction to a pleasurable range when it has become displeasurable. Children now begin to become more proficient at using their own emotions as *internal signals of distress* and using the displeasurable emotions of their parents as their possible *external signals of distress*.

One feeling in particular that becomes important for children to regulate is anxiety. Children between 4 and 5 years gradually become more proficient not only in recognizing when they feel anxious but also in discriminating what they are anxious about.

Emotions as Facilitators of Social Adaptation

In the period from ages 3 to 5 years, children use their emotions as they continue to improve their social adaptation. In so doing, they attempt to achieve an internal adaptation to their innate needs and an external adaptation to the developmental taskings and rules of their parents and society. Young children usually achieve self-regulation and social adaptation concurrently. More often than not, their internal adaptation is not achieved at the expense of their external adaptation. For example, children do not adapt to their innate need to be assertive while completely disregarding their external adaptation to their parents' rules about limits on their assertive will.

Maturation and Development of Verbal Language Abilities

Starting around age 3 years, children begin to use thought, speech, and behaviors to achieve a belief in their own ability to anticipate and predict what will happen in the future. Also, they begin to remember their past—known as *reproductive memory*—and to ask questions of themselves and their parents about why things happened. In this process, children begin to engage in *reconstructive memory* (Perry 1992; Piaget and Inhelder 1973), in which they generate a fantasy based on a recalled memory and reconstruct the memory to enhance its pleasurable emotionality in some way or to change its displeasurable emotionality into a pleasurable one. Many of these memories and their reconstructions are expressed in children's stories (Beal and Flavell 1984; Hudson 1990, 1993).

Maturation and Development of the Preexisting Representational World

Between the ages of 4 and 5 years, children's mentalizing or self-reflective functions continue to develop. By age 4½ years, children have begun to engage in what will be a lifelong conscious and unconscious mental activity—the ordering of their own motivations from highest to lowest priority in terms of importance. Motives are hierarchically organized primarily on the basis of wished-for emotional states and feared emotional states (Westen 1997). Wished-for emotional states are connected in the child's mind with conscious and unconscious representations of people, places, and things to pursue, and feared emotional states are connected internally with representations of people, places, and things to avoid.

Development of the Self and Object Relationships

By age 3 years, children have begun to construct the sequence of subidentities that make up their overall identity. Thus, by the time they enter the early childhood phase, they will have constructed enough of a beginning autonomous identity to enable them to explore away from their parents while tolerating their separation anxiety. Also, the attainment of a growing positive self-constancy enables young children to begin to value and love themselves as their parents value and love them.

Development of a Sexual Identity: Emergence of the Early Genital Phase

In addition to continuing to learn what it means to be a boy or a girl in their society through continuing to develop their gender identity, 3-year-old children begin to construct a *sexual identity.* A sexual identity is the view of oneself that has to do with all of the emotions, fantasies, beliefs, and behaviors that are involved in the innate need to seek pleasurable sensual–sexual gratification. Stoller (1976, 1985) defined *core gender identity,* established by age 3 years, as children's "unquestioned, unthinking conviction—a piece of identity—that they are male or female" (Stoller 1985, p. 55).

Exhibitionism of genitals.   In the initial unfoldings of the early genital phase, children are quite intensely exhibitionistic. In admiring their own clothed and nude body in the mirror, they are intensely joyous in receiving mirroring smiles of admiration from both parents. For example, a 4-year-old boy entered his parents' bedroom one morning and proudly showed his erect penis, stating, "See, Dad, mine goes up just like yours!"

The basic difference between the exhibitionism of boys and that of girls in the early genital phase is that boys have a ready organ on which to focus. The penis is outside, visible, and manipulatable; boys can make it "grow" by making it erect. Although girls do not have such an externally visible organ on which to focus, their genital region is as easily accessible and manipulated. Girls 3–4 years old ask their parents to name their genital parts. However, often girls' genitals are left nameless. Vulva, labia, clitoris, vagina, cervix, and uterus are terms rarely heard by children of either sex. This is a problem for little girls because, as Balsam (quoted in Long 2005) noted, "naming offers the possibility of developing a clearer mental image, while silence creates mystery and fosters anxiety about bodily functions" (Long 2005, p. 1171).

Girls eventually learn that their vagina is an organ that is primarily a cavity and that their reproductive organs are internal, in contrast to boys' external penis and scrotum with its testicles.

Girls between ages 3 and 4 years gradually become aware that they have a clitoris, primarily through learning how to manipulate their genital region, but initially do not have a clear sense of its shape and stimulation properties.

Curiosity about genitals.   Parents begin to teach their children about the limits on their sexual curiosity; in the process, they teach them about a developmental task associated with constructing a sexual identity: the necessity of learning about body privacy.

Erikson (1963) labeled the psychosocial task in early childhood as the need for children to attain a belief that they can express their *initiative* and *curiosity* without experiencing an overriding feeling of *guilt*. Erikson was referring to the danger of guilt feelings that may be evoked if children's interests and actions associated with the early genital phase are not supported and protected by their parents.

Body damage anxiety.   Body damage anxiety is another of the developmental anxieties that S. Freud (1923/1963) defined as inevitable. It results from children fearing the possibility of a new developmental calamity in which their body is damaged, particularly their genitals or genital area. Freud, in emphasizing the penis as the predominant body part that both boys and girls highly value, named this fear *castration anxiety.* However, developmental researchers (Mayer 1995) now believe that the term *body damage anxiety* better reflects a more generic anxiety in the boy and the girl.

Choice of sexual object.   Between ages 3 and 4 years, children begin to make a sexual object choice. This occurs as they begin to expand on their earlier masturbatory fantasies, which contained their early attractions to either the same gender or the opposite gender for sexual gratification. If the former, they begin to make a homosexual object choice; if the latter, they begin to make a heterosexual object choice.

Children with a heterosexual object choice are sexually aroused by the opposite-gender parent, while children with a homosexual object choice experience sexual excitation in being physically close to the same-gender parent.

Emergence of the triangular phase.   Young children's sexual object choice becomes the main organizer for their developing sexual identity, as well as a basic aspect of 4- to 5-year-old children's progression into the *triangular phase* (Mayer 1995; P. Tyson 1982). This was called the *oedipal phase* in the past. However, Person (2005) and others have suggested that the term should be *triangular,* because *oedipal* refers to the legendary Oedipus myth, which concerns only boys, not girls.

The triangular phase is the phase during which the heterosexual child fantasizes about replacing his or her same-gender parent and engaging in an exclusive, sexually tinged relationship with his or her opposite-gender parent. It comprises a mixture of behaviors based on what children have learned—and carry within their object representations of their parents and others—about what constitutes being a man and a woman. It is also based on what *inferences* children make about what it means to be a husband or wife, father or mother.

Triangular behavior in the heterosexual boy culminates in his wish to "marry Mom" or at least have an exclusive relationship with her that excludes Dad. The heterosexual little girl who is beginning to include herself in the category of "women who seek men for sensual–sexual pleasure" now views her mother as a rival for her father's affections. She fantasizes about marrying her father, of having a baby with him, and of sending her mother away. However, it is unclear in her mind just how she and her father will physically produce a baby. The heterosexual girl's burgeoning sexual identity in being attractive to men develops, for the most part, in what she perceives in the eyes of her father and other important men in her life (e.g., her uncles, male teachers). The same dynamic occurs in boys: their sexual identity "develops" in the eyes of their mothers.

Relative relinquishment of triangular wishes.   Triangular wishes in heterosexual children decrease when children begin to put aside (but do not completely give up) their wishes to have what the same-gender parent has and do what the same-gender parent does (Table 7–9). Because boys love their mothers and fathers, they are helped in relinquishing the wish to replace the father, and they are encouraged in identifying with and wanting to grow up to be like their father, when the father is respected and loved by the mother and the mother is respected and loved by the father. Similar dynamics need to exist for girls; they are helped in identifying with and growing up to be like their mother when their father respects and loves their mother and their mother respects and loves their father. This decreased intensity of children's triangular wishes does not resolve those wishes forever, however. This is only their first and relative relinquishment; triangular wishes involving the child and the

TABLE 7–9.	First resolution of triangular wishes (age 6–7 years)

- Child relinquishes wishes to occupy the same-gender parent's space

- Child reaffirms his or her identification with the same-gender parent

- Separation–body damage anxieties greatly diminish

parents return when children enter puberty, at about age 12 or 13 years.

A healthy resolution of the triangular phase in heterosexual children will enhance the identification process with the same-gender parent and other same-gender individuals in their lives. Children's gender identity becomes more consolidated as they become comfortable in demonstrating their correct gender-role behaviors.

Many adults cannot remember any aspects of their own triangular phase—or of their lives before ages 5–6 years, for that matter. One reason is that, for many adults, the triangular phase was *not* associated with high emotional content, either displeasurable or pleasurable. As a result, many of the triangular experiences were not major events in their life.

Development of a Peer Identity

It is during early childhood (ages 3–6 years) that the need for peer interaction becomes a crucial ingredient in fostering children's confidence in performing outside of their individual families and in taking the initiative in solving problems, resolving interpersonal conflicts (thereby maintaining the capacity for emotional regulation [P. Tyson 2005]), and gradually learning about the concept of sharing.

Development of the Superego

As noted earlier, the *superego* is a metaphorical, theoretical mental construct that comprises specific mental functions that share the common quality of providing an inner source of children's, society's, and families' standards, ethical rules, and moral values, as well as children's internalized mental representations of the responses of parents and others when the children have and have not obeyed these standards and rules. So if a 4-year-old girl's object representation of her mother's response to her following and not following the rules in her superego is imbued with hostility, her early superego will retaliate for her transgressions with much hostility and be only minimally admiring, if admiring at

all, when she does obey the rules within her superego.

By ages 2–3 years, the normally disciplined child's motivation to obey to avoid punishment has minimal carryover (Damon 1988). At about age 3 years, conventional morality begins (Kohlberg 1981). If the establishment of positive self-constancy and object constancy has led to children's construction of primarily loving object representations of their parents, children will be motivated to obey their parents' rules to keep receiving the love they have learned to expect. However, every child regresses and breaks rules if the parent is away or is unavailable to the child. As the superego begins to come into being, children experience guilt when 1) they know what is a right and what is a wrong behavior, 2) they believe they have a choice between the two behaviors, and 3) they have made the bad choice. Children do not like guilt; it makes them feel they are bad and potentially unloved. In their first experiences of feeling guilty, they will try to blame someone else for their own wrong statement or behavior.

Children also begin to experience *superego anxiety*—that is, the anxiety they feel when they think about doing or saying something that is forbidden by their conscience. This superego anxiety is another internal distress signal that warns the child that guilt will ensue if a forbidden action or verbalization being considered by the child occurs.

A healthy superego must be nurtured by parents, teachers, and peers. The principal sign of a functioning healthy or normal superego in a child is manifestation of *self-responsibility* (in the child's following, most of the time, the rules of his or her family, school, etc.) and *self-love* (in the child's feeling proud and lovable when he or she has followed the rules and standards of his or her superego).

Development of Adaptational Capabilities

Repression is defined as an automatic unconscious mental process, viewed as an activity of children's ego under the direction of the self, that bars from their conscious awareness 1) wishes and feelings that, if gratified, would produce either parental (external) disapproval or superego (internal) disapproval (once the superego becomes an internal structure), and 2) memories of experiences that are associated with an intensely displeasurable emotional state.

Repression begins to emerge at around age 18 months but does not become a predominant defense mechanism until children reach about age 3 years. At that age, a child's superego begins to function more as an internal structure, and the child must begin to deal with the rules or standards that the superego brings to bear. When the superego generates guilt in response to a forbidden wish, feeling, verbalization, action, or recalled memory that is so excessive that it generates a level of displeasure that exceeds a child's stimulation threshold, then the forbidden wish, feeling, verbalization, action, or recalled memory and associated guilt will be repressed. Both the emotion of guilt and the aspect of the superego that is stimulating that guilt will remain unconscious (Blum 1985).

Repression helps children adapt and continues to be used throughout life. However, it can be used too much—that is, it can be used to repress those childhood wishes (e.g., triangular-phase wishes) that should normally be partially relinquished during development or to repress wishes and feelings associated with traumatic events that need to be worked through and eventually mastered.

Late Childhood Phase of Mental Development (Ages 6–12 Years)

Major Developmental Tasks of Late Childhood

The major developmental tasks of late childhood are as follows:

1. To continue to add to and reconstruct a *peer identity,* particularly in being able to begin to relate cooperatively and competitively to peers in the formal grade-school setting
2. To construct a beginning *social identity* (the beginning belief that one is a member of various categories within one's society as a whole)

Traditionally, age 7 years was thought of as the age at which children were capable of true reasoning and learning true social responsibility, because children ages 6–7 years were found to be able to use secondary process, logical, and reasonable thinking more consistently than they used primary process magical thinking.

By ages 5½–7 years, children have developed the following components of their overall identity:

1. *Autonomous identity*—They are able to see themselves as being separate while maintaining a positive self-constancy and object constancy.
2. *Gender identity*—They are able to view themselves as a boy or a girl and have already constructed

many beliefs, fantasies, and categories relating to what it means to be a boy or a girl. They continue to identify with both parents and others in learning more about their gender identity.
3. *Sexual identity*—They have made a sexual object choice and are sexually attracted to same-gender or opposite-gender individuals. Heterosexual children have "put aside" their heterosexual early triangular wishes toward sexually stimulating objects. At the same time, both heterosexual and homosexual children look toward their parents and others in authority for more information about the social rules pertaining to sexual stimulation and gratification, and they are permitted some measure of sexual gratification through masturbation.
4. *Peer identity*—During toddlerhood, most children have had some contact with other children (e.g., siblings, others). At around age 3 years, many children begin some kind of out-of-the-home school activity, usually involving 2–3 hours per day. In this activity, children begin to think about and compare themselves with peers. As they create a new mental category, "children," and a related category, "my friends," a peer identity begins to be constructed.

Erikson (1963, 1968) proposed that from ages 6 to 11 years, children's developmental task is to develop a belief in their ability to be *industrious* and perform in front of peers instead of a belief of being *inferior* in front of peers and others. Erikson described a developmental conflict arising in children between wanting to be industrious and avoiding being industrious because of a belief that being industrious generates internal problems (e.g., excessive separation, body damage, and/or superego anxiety) or external problems (e.g., various forms of criticism and/or abandonment by parents, siblings, or peers).

Further Development of a Peer Identity

The development of children's peer identity further develops their 1) *autonomous identity,* in being able to assertively perform and produce in front of their peers and expecting and receiving a certain degree of admiration and affirmation from them; 2) *gender identity,* in being able to act like others of their gender and be accepted by their peers; and 3) *sexual identity,* in being able to continue to learn about the social rules between peers in terms of sexual stimulation and sexual gratification.

Development of a Social Identity

As 5½- to 6½-year-old children start to recognize that they are members of various categories within their society as a whole (e.g., citizen, American, New Yorker, student at Our Lady of Victory School), they begin to construct new categories. In addition, children construct other representations that define many of the procedures and skills that are required to function in their society outside of the family home.

By age 5½ years, children are motivated to relate to their family group, play group, or class group, and they learn that they must follow rules and that they will be judged by the other members of the group. Group rules, standards, ethics, and principles become ingredients to be added to the child's developing superego. Once children (at ages 6–7 years) begin to use their superego anxiety signals as the "voice" of their parents when their parents are not around, they are truly becoming autonomously social.

Functions of the Social Environment

The dominant triggering social variable in the biopsychosocial model of mental development from 6–11 years of age is the social requirement (in most countries, it is a law) for all children to attend school. In essence, going to school is the "job" of late childhood (Table 7–10).

Beginning around age 2½ years, children hear of the day when they will go to "regular" or "big boys' and girls'" school, something that initially occurs between ages 2½ and 3½ years when children go to a 2- to 3-hour daily nursery class. This is followed between ages 3½ and 4½ years by children attending a half-day or full day of prekindergarten class, and at age 5½–6½ years by children attending kindergarten. Finally, children begin formal grade school between ages 6 and 7 years. However, even before children walk into their first day of first grade, they will have constructed conceptual beliefs and fantasies about what grade school will be like and what it will mean to them, and they will be primed to generate positive transferences toward their teacher and classmates. In many ways, school is a "classroom" for the further development of peer and social identities.

Maturation and Development of Innate Needs

Need for Fulfillment of Physiological Needs Related to Bodily Regulation and Physical Survival

One requirement for attending first grade is that children be able to take over the proper fulfillment of their

---

TABLE 7–10. **Preparations for beginning first grade (age 5½–6½ years)**

- From infancy: "I trust my teachers."

- From toddlerhood: "I feel good about being autonomous from my parents."

- From early childhood: "I like being curious and assertively inquisitive."

- Now: "I can be industrious and present my work to others, and I'll do well and be liked."

---

physiological needs (e.g., dress warmly if it is winter, regulate their level of stimulation while playing in the schoolyard, take care of their need for food in eating lunch and snacks at the designated times, ensure that they get enough sleep so that they will not be drowsy in class).

Need to Assertively Explore the Social Environment

At about age 6 or 7 years, normally developing children appear to undergo what Shapiro and Hertzig (1988) called a *biodevelopmental shift.* This refers to children's maturation of physical, cognitive, language, emotional, and defense mechanisms that appear to fuel children's activation of the innate need to exhibit their autonomous identity in the social world.

Need for Human Attachment in Emotionally Pleasurable Interactions

Children ages 5½–6½ years have developed positive self-constancy and positive object constancy, providing them with an inner representational world, or world of mind, that is a source of comfort during physical separations from the family. These self- and object-constant representations also lead them to generate *positive transference reactions* to new peers and teachers at school.

In normally developing children (as in normally developing adolescents and adults), development of attachment and development of autonomy are mutually enhancing processes: a child's true self develops in the context of his or her maintaining attachment relationships with others who have developed (e.g., parents, teachers) or are developing (e.g., peers) their true selves. When both attachment and autonomy needs are gratified concurrently, children develop more normally than when one of these two develops at the expense of the other. Quite often, children who maintain attachments to their parents at the expense of their autonomous development have parents who are overprotective and biased against their children's autonomous growth.

Need for Emotionally Pleasurable Sensory–Sexual Stimulation and Gratification

Freud labeled the period between ages 6 and 11 years as the period of *latency*—specifically, sexual latency (S. Freud 1905/1963). He believed that this was a period of relative "quietness" of sexual instinctual wishes in children, in which the children's oedipal (now renamed the *early triangular*) wishes are beginning to be mastered and recede in prominence until puberty (ages 11–13 years), when some triangular wishes return and must be relinquished once again.

Children continue to develop a sexual identity by learning more about how *not* to express their sexual ideas and fantasies. Children ages 5½–8 years receive emphatic admonitions from parents and teachers—who, as concerned adults, desire to protect children from pedophiles (adults who seek children for sexual stimulation and pleasure)—cautioning them that children should never go anywhere with strangers and should never allow anyone—even a known teacher, parent, or coach—to touch them (other than a normal hug), ask them to undress, or ask them to show any part of their bodies. Concurrently, their parents are emphasizing privacy at home, by respecting each other's rooms, not witnessing nudity, not allowing or inviting the child to come into the bathroom while the parent is urinating or defecating, and establishing similar prohibitions. In school, teachers are making sure that boy–girl pairs are not hiding together, going to the bathroom together, and so forth. All of these messages from the adults in their society make 5½- to 11-year-olds avoid excessive masturbation, because such *excessive sexual stimulation* makes it more difficult for them to obey these warnings and prohibitions about sexual exposure and stimulation. Also, sexual stimulation greatly interferes with the process of learning.

Need to Signal Distress When Experiencing Emotionally Displeasurable Over- or Understimulation and to Initiate Other Fight-or-Flight Behavioral and Mental Responses

In late childhood, children become more able to organize how they activate distress signals and how they can tolerate more of a delay before activating a fight-or-flight response. New defense mechanisms maturationally emerge between ages 5½ and 11 years, namely isolation of emotion, sublimation, reaction formation, and displacement. Fantasy formation also becomes a standard mechanism of defense. In addition, 5½- to 11-

year-old children's ability to use both conscious thinking and unconscious defense mechanisms to delay action and ponder responses makes their representational world of stored knowledge more available to them than ever before.

Maturation and Development of Physical Capabilities

Brain frontal lobe maturation mediates neuronal systems that contribute to children's self-regulatory and self-soothing capabilities. At birth, an infant's total brain volume is only 10% of what it will be at age 20 years, while by age 7 years, brain volume has reached 90% of the volume it will be at age 20 years (Schechter and Combrinck-Graham 1991; Shapiro and Perry 1976). Frontal lobe maturation is associated with an increased ability to recall and to use executive control structures (e.g., steps for accomplishing a task) and emotional display rules (e.g., rules about verbalization of sad feelings) to accomplish tasks and to use speech in the service of self-regulation and self-soothing.

Another aspect of this biodevelopmental shift at age 7 years is the completion of major nerve tract myelination (Brodal 1969), allowing children to become more adept at controlling large-muscle groups. Children ages 6–10 years have better balance and have become better runners, jumpers, bicycle riders, and tumblers than they were at age 5 years (Schechter and Combrinck-Graham 1991).

Myelination of nerve tracts also enhances 7-year-old children's fine-motor abilities as well as visual–auditory and visual–motor coordination. Maturation of temporospatial capabilities enables 5½- to 7-year-old children to discriminate right from left and days from months or years and to begin to understand that past, present, and future are different points along a temporal continuum. These advances assist children in further developing their positive self-constancy.

Maturation and Development of Cognitive Capabilities

Emergence of More Complex Mental Operations

Piaget labeled the period between ages 6 and 11 years the *concrete operational phase* of cognitive development, referring to children's ability to carry out complex thinking processes about concrete events but not about abstract phenomena. Whenever children are able to figure out the solutions to various problems presented to them in their minds, they are developing their self-confidence in their thinking abilities. They may verbalize this pride to their parents (e.g., a 7-year-old boy says, "Dad, I used to have to write down all my numbers. Now I can add them in my mind!"). The cognitive capabilities that mature and develop between 6 and 11 years of age are as follows:

1. *Ability to understand others' perspectives.* As noted earlier, children's ability to take on another person's perspective undergoes a remarkable advance beginning at around age 4½ years, when children first integrate the pretense and psychic equivalence modes of dealing with reality. At that point, children discover that other people can have views or intentions that differ from their own.

2. *Ability to develop more complex categories.* Children also have a new ability to classify objects according to their logical or reasonable similarities or differences. Eight- to 10-year-olds become immersed in classifying and collecting all sorts of objects (Shapiro and Hertzig 2003). Boys collect baseball cards, DVDs of adventure movies, basketball T-shirts, and so forth. Girls collect hair fasteners, slogan T-shirts, princess costumes, and the like.

3. *Ability to reason logically and to understand relational rules.* Children from the first grade (age 5½–6½ years) to the sixth grade (age 11 years) are increasingly becoming logical thinkers. They seek to understand the relationships between things; for example, they now know that bigger and taller are linked through the common relation of height.

4. *Increased ability to use secondary process thinking.* As 6- to 7-year-old children's cognitive abilities enable them to think more and act less, they begin to use more secondary process thinking in reacting to novel perceptions. They compare new perceptions with preexisting representations and analyze them completely within their minds.

5. *Ability to understand concept of reversibility.* In late childhood, children's cognitive ability to understand reversible (mental) operations (i.e., that for every action or mental operation, there is another that cancels it) emerges. For example, they can now understand equations such as $8 \times 6 = 48$ and $48 \div 8 = 6$. Children also begin to use the concept of reversibility to understand new phenomena. For example, when they do something wrong, they can "undo" the wrong by doing something good.

6. *Ability to compare past and present.* Children in the concrete operational stage (ages 6–11 years) reevaluate and achieve new understandings of their memories (i.e., their previously acquired knowledge). In a process of ongoing reconstruction of prior representations, they acquire new knowledge through the internal process of comparing present and past knowledge, or as Piaget (1967) put it, a "reshaping through thought of previous material."

7. *Ability to understand conservation of mass and number.* Children ages 6–7 years now understand the concept of conservation of both quantity (mass) and number. Applying the principle of conservation of mass gives children a new understanding of how each person remains a whole person, unique and separate, despite changes in his or her appearance or emotional state. The concept of conservation of number states that an object's properties or attributes remain the same despite transformations in the object's appearance.

Differentiation of Primary and Secondary Process Thinking: Development of Masking and Latent Symbols

In late childhood, children's primary process or pretend thinking remains evident in the way they use symbolic thinking (a 7-year-old observes, "That tree is like a statue"), remember night dreams and daytime fantasies (an 8-year-old girl confides, "I had this great dream last night"), write and verbalize scripts or stories (a 10-year-old boy says, "Here is a story I wrote about parents"), and develop new interest in activities such as drawing, painting, and building models.

In late childhood, there is a gradual masking of primary process magical thinking within children's symbolic representations, whether through speech, play, fantasies, written stories, drawings, paintings, or models. Before age 5½ years, children could not distinguish between their symbols and what they symbolized. They now are becoming much more aware of how their symbols may reveal wishes and feelings that they 1) do not wish to acknowledge to themselves and/or 2) do not wish to reveal to their parents or others.

Consequently, although 6- to 7-year-old children continue to symbolize aspects of themselves, others, and events, their symbols are less transparent than before. They not only hide from themselves something that they would rather put out of their conscious mind, but also prevent others from figuring out what they are avoiding. These *masking symbols* (Sarnoff 1987) are adaptive in that they allow children a means of concealing certain facts of their life that they would be anxious about revealing directly to themselves or others in either speech or behavior.

The anxiety is associated with their expectation that the truthful verbalization of a wish, feeling, or memory will be met with some degree of disapproval. This expectation of disapproval is one of the motivations for 6- to 7-year-old children's interest in forming secrets.

What is true about latent and manifest fantasies also holds for children's *pathogenic beliefs.* Pathogenic beliefs are not wishful but rather "compelling, grim, and maladaptive" (Weiss 1993). Pathogenic beliefs inhibit the development of children's overall identity—specifically, their development of a true self-representation. A pathogenic belief is constructed from experiences in which a child's wishes and feelings have led to highly displeasurable levels of developmental anxiety, rage, and the like. Children's inferences—that is, their personal explanations for why the emotionally painful experience happened to them—become the substance of their pathogenic beliefs. For example, the pathogenic belief that a 9-year-old boy might construct in response to periodically being physically hit by his father might be something like, "My father hits me a lot because he hates me; he hates me because he says I was born bad. And he's right. Now I'm always bad!"

Maturation and Development of Temperamental Characteristics

As noted earlier, temperament is now accepted as part of infants' innately endowed characteristics (Thomas and Chess 1977). Behavioral inhibition to the unfamiliar, for example, is a characteristic that shows temporal stability from infancy through age 7 years (Kagan 1989). However, Kagan found that some infants' inhibition to the unfamiliar could be gradually modified by their attachment relationship with their parents (Kagan 1989).

Despite Kagan's research, the continuity versus discontinuity of temperamental characteristics is an area of ongoing controversy. Rutter (1986) found little stability in temperamental characteristics in longitudinal studies of temperament from infancy to ages 9–11 years. He cited evidence suggesting that a child's attachment relationship may 1) maintain stability of temperament, 2) accentuate certain temperamental traits, or 3) change a child's temperament from infancy to late childhood. Chess and Thomas (1989) have suggested that alterations in children's temperaments may be attributable not only to the parenting received but also to maturational changes in the children's temperament in the context of the parenting environment.

Maturation and Development of Emotions

Between 6 and 11 years of age, children increasingly become aware of "blends" of feelings and of how new emotions can block out old remembered ones (Lane and Schwartz 1987). Children also become more consciously aware of their ambivalent feelings toward their parents and others. Finally, they begin to use their intuition and empathy more fully in appreciating the emotional states of others based on their own similar wishes and experiences. This increased capacity for empathy results in part from their new cognitive ability to recognize that others can have perspectives different from their own.

Because older children have the capacity to reflect on much more of their complicated emotional representational worlds than ever before, their rules for displaying those emotions must become more sophisticated. Children must also begin to transfer their emotional display rules from their family setting into the classroom, onto the ball field, into the synagogue or church, and so on.

Beginning at ages 6–7 years and continuing throughout late childhood, children are also becoming more aware of their anxious emotions or developmental anxiety. They learn to use developmental anxiety as an internal signal that warns them to become vigilant about an external threat (e.g., a physically dangerous person) or an internal threat (e.g., their own building rage toward a little sister who has just destroyed their new video game but whom they are forbidden to physically strike).

Maturation and Development of Verbal Language Abilities

Children now begin to think more before they speak and in the process develop their ability to delay the gratification of a feeling and to experience the feeling and think about why they are feeling this way. This form of regulating one's feelings has been called *mentalized affectivity* by Fonagy (1999).

If children are to believe in the value of their speech in solving internal and external conflicts, it is crucial for their parents to continually request verbal communication from them.

Maturation and Development of the Preexisting Representational World

By the time children reach the first grade (age 6 or 7 years), their representational world has become a crucial source of information that they use to strike a balance between their internal adaptation to their innate needs, wants, and wishes and their external adaptation to the demands, guidelines, and developmental taskings of their parents, peers, teachers, and others. In this process, children will call upon their preexisting representational world (psychological stimuli) of beliefs, fantasies, emotional control procedures, and other mental contents in an attempt to achieve the following:

1. Use their memories to generate transference predictions about their daily experiences with people.
2. Discover which of their transference predictions about people seem to be true, thus reinforcing their prior experiences with people.
3. Discover which of their transference predictions do not seem to be true, thus challenging their prior experiences with people.

In normally developing children, transference reactions involve a transfer of positive or negative feelings, thoughts, wishes, and conceptions from a person or experience in the past onto a person or experience in the present. In particular, children will transfer what they believe to be true—whether that truth is emotionally pleasurable or displeasurable—onto their current encounters in an attempt to assimilate the new experiences and to achieve an immediate sense of intellectual mastery. Negative transference reactions are motivated by children's attempts to avoid experiences in the present that remind them of past experiences that were highly displeasurable, or even traumatic.

From 8 years onward, children increasingly think about their past, and many of their memories from the first 8 years of life undergo reconstructive revision, or *representational reorganization* (Karmiloff-Smith 1979). As a result, older children will restructure and transform prior memories, reprioritizing them and adjusting the relative importance assigned to certain memories as being crucial in shaping their life—which experiences were most valuable in the past, and which experiences they will seek to repeat in the future.

It is difficult to know how much of what children report as happening to them represents actual memories constructed in the past and how much represents a more recent reconstruction and transformation of past memories (M. L. Lewis 1995; Terr 1994). In fact, children's reconstruction of their past is just that: a composite memory consisting of an original memory (i.e., the initially constructed memory of an experience) plus one or more reconstructions of that original memory (Perry 1992). Thus, at any point in time, what children remember about their past is what they currently believe about what happened in the past.

Development of the Self and Object Relationships

Children's attainment of an autonomous and valued identity enables them to approach grade school with a sense of taking pleasure in being curious and taking the initiative in approaching the learning process (Erikson 1963). Between ages 5½ and 11 years, children begin to show "in miniature" an early picture of the personality they will have as an adult. Longitudinal data reveal that the highest correlation of childhood behavior predicting future adult behavior exists for this age period, especially for children between the ages of 8 and 11 years (Roff and Wirt 1984).

Colarusso (1992) has noted that children's acceptance or rejection by their peers is an important indication of whether children are developing normally. In my view, this is true only if children are exposed to peers who share many of the same developmental taskings, standards, moral values, and behaviors for adapting to conflicts. Beginning around age 6–7 years, children discover that both physical games (e.g., sports) and nonphysical games (e.g., board games) can be competitive. They also learn that games have rules. Once they understand the concept of games, children begin constructing their own games and setting rules that help them gratify a wish through the game that would be more difficult to gratify more directly.

Throughout late childhood (ages 5½ to 11 years), children often undergo periods of being quite discouraged about their limitations. The child now perceives that he or she does not always get an A on every test, or that he or she is not the best in gymnastics class. In response to the realization that he or she will never attain perfection, the child may give up, saying, "School stinks!" or "I don't care anymore about going to soccer" (Thompson 1996). Once again, psychologically attuned parents—and teachers and coaches—must tolerate children's discouragement while being firm in not allowing them to avoid activities that might bring them face to face with their limitations and imperfections. As children reach 10 or 11 years of age, compensatory fantasies and their abject discouragement about not being perfect begin to give way to the development of more realistically attainable ambitions and ideals. Kohut and Wolf (1978) suggested that a child's transformed ideal self-image eventually becomes, as a new representation within his or her overall self-representation, that child's more realistic *ambitions*, whereas a child's ideal parent images become the child's more realistic but still somewhat idealistic *goals*. For 10- to 11-year-old children to begin to transmute their periodic perfectionistic images of both themselves and their parents, they must believe that their parents value them despite their limitations and imperfections. When they believe this, children can use their parents' realistic view of them to begin to transform their perfect self-image and perfect parental images into more realistically attainable ambitions and ideals.

Continued Development of Gender and Sexual Identities

Development of Gender Identity

One motivating force that propels 6- to 7-year-old children to identify with their same-gender parent is their need to feel more competent as a boy or girl and to feel a sense of power. Between ages 6 and 11 years, children learn that there are three types of mechanisms through which power or prestige may be gained in society: first, there is *intrinsic power,* which comes from being loved and valued unconditionally by their parents; second, there is *attributed power,* which is based on their performance in mastering stimuli presented to them during their first 6 years of life; and third, there is *formal or bestowed power,* which is power given by some social organization (Horner 1989).

During the first few years of grade school, children construct the new category of "people with power" and then further refine this general category into different types of power. Police officers, ministers, priests, presidents, and so on all have different types of power and manifest that power in different ways. Children feel that they have power in their particular gender through identification with those whom they perceive as being powerful.

By ages 9–10 years, boys still want to be with boys and girls with girls. This segregation helps older children "put aside" in their minds the issue of sexual object choice and instead do more work on consolidating gender-appropriate identifications and constructing more categories of what it means to be their gender.

Development of Sexual Identity

Sexual identity development in late childhood comes under the sway of society's message that no direct sexual activity between children is permitted. Indirect activity does take place, however. The school classroom and playground become the places where children covertly and overtly develop their sexual identities concurrently with their peer and social identities.

Despite the edict heard from first through eighth grade—"Boys with the boys and girls with the girls"—heterosexual children have a secret and emotional interest in the opposite gender. Sexual undercurrents begin in the first grade and extend through the sixth grade (about ages 11–12 years). Girls ages 5½–9 years may speak of having a "boyfriend" in their class, but they are easily embarrassed when someone reminds them of this stated admission. The same occurs in boys, but boys tend to be much less open about their interest in a "girlfriend." Boys may fantasize about what kissing a girl might be like, but they will fight with any friend who teases them about wanting to kiss a girl.

Development of the Superego

By ages 6–7 years, as children partially relinquish their early triangular wishes toward the same-gender parent, they both acknowledge their parents' authority and power over them and identify with parental authority (Loewald 1979). In doing the latter, they are literally infusing their superego with authority, something they may not have bargained for! They then begin to learn how to listen to the voice of their superego as the authority of their parents, lest they feel the unpleasurable feeling of guilt. If they have repressed their early triangular wishes only out of fear of parental retaliation, their superego will become an unwelcome internalized parent against which they will begin to rebel. Normally developing 6- to 7-year-old children, however, will experience their superego as an ally—residing within their heart or brain (labeled by Stillwell et al. [1991] as a *brain or heart conscience*)—that begins to perform two basic functions: 1) to regulate and control their behavior relatively independently of external restraints, and 2) to become a source of self-esteem that is relatively independent of external feedback.

Obviously, this goal is greatly assisted if parents and authority figures point out children's transgressions firmly but also kindly and empathically, without overly embarrassing or demeaning them. Such authority figures 1) verbalize their criticism without assassinating children's self-esteem, 2) give punishments that are reasonable, and 3) treat children with respect, even though they do not always obey the rules they should have learned.

Most children's peer groups are selected by both children and their parents on the basis of their matching the children's standards and values. By ages 7–8 years, a moral code of fairness with a sense of group justice is becoming internalized within children's conscience. Latency-age children are motivated to internalize their peer group's rules and standards of fairness because of their need for peer group approval

(Coie 1990) and their fear of peer group rejection (Asher and Coie 1990; Putallaz and Dunn 1990).

Sullivan (1953) emphasized the importance of the *close chum* or close friend, during the period between ages 8 and 10 years, in helping children further modify their conscience. Through this relationship, children have a chance to share their worries about not living up to some of the high demands concerning behavior that have been internalized within their conscience. The first real close relationship with a friend becomes the child's first real experience with making the problems, worries, and anxieties of a peer their own. In this sense, such relationships are felt by Sullivan (1953) to be a precursor to children's eventual ability to enter into mature intimate heterosexual loving relationships in young adult life. In an adult intimate relationship, mutual concern, acceptance of each other's imperfections, and willingness to be vulnerable and dependent are all necessary for genuine love and trust to develop.

Development of Adaptational Capabilities: Evolution of New Defense Mechanisms

The predominant defense mechanisms used by children in late childhood are fantasy formation, isolation of emotion, sublimation, reaction formation, displacement, and suppression.

Fantasy formation is used more than ever before as an adaptive defense by children in this age period. Instead of verbally or behaviorally expressing an anxiety-provoking wish or feeling that is associated with a developmental anxiety, children construct an unconscious latent fantasy that expresses the wish or feeling in a way that brings gratification. This latent fantasy stays repressed while a disguised manifest fantasy is experienced in consciousness.

Isolation of emotion is an automatic barring from consciousness of an emotion that, if expressed, would produce an intolerable level of developmental anxiety. When this defense is used, there is only the conscious awareness of the thoughts being experienced at the moment, but without the associated feelings connected with those thoughts.

Sublimation is an automatic unconscious process in which gratification of a wish is achieved by changing the object or aim of the wish. The object or aim is altered from one that may have been socially objectionable to one that is socially acceptable.

Reaction formation is an automatic unconscious process that bars from consciousness an unacceptable wish or feeling and produces in consciousness the op-

posite wish or feeling. It is a predominant defense mechanism for children ages 3–11 years. As with all defenses, it is adaptive when used for a short period of time.

Displacement is an automatic unconscious mental mechanism that displaces the expression of a wish or feeling from the original person or object that is causing high levels of developmental anxiety to another, less anxiety-provoking person or object. For example, a boy may displace his anger at his father onto his friend and become angry at him for a trivial reason.

Suppression is the conscious and willful attempt to put mental contents out of one's conscious awareness. It is the only specific mechanism of defense that is defined as consciously volitional. Vaillant (1977) noted that with suppression, the child says, "I will think about it tomorrow," and the next day he or she remembers to think about it. Thus, when children use suppression, they are deliberately and temporarily postponing—but not deciding to permanently avoid—thinking or talking about conflictual thoughts, wishes, and feelings. Parents can support either an adaptive or a maladaptive use of suppression. They can remind their children that something that was suppressed was not supposed to be suppressed forever.

Adolescence Phase of Mental Development (Ages 12–19 Years)

Adolescence as a developmental period, and adolescents as members of society, have both been the subject of considerable interest, speculation, and, regrettably, bad press. In most societies, it is during adolescence that young individuals truly begin to assert their own views and preferences as separate from those of their parents and teachers; accordingly, it is during adolescence that they begin to make their presence known as future adults who will eventually take a place within society.

The biopsychosocial stimuli of adolescence can be understood as follows. The biological changes that take place at the onset of adolescence—which is called *puberty*—are quite striking and, in many families, become more of a triggering stimulus than the biological changes associated with prior developmental phases. Adolescents also enter puberty with a much more complex representational world. This world is a source of psychological stimuli with which adolescents can engender quite elaborate internal responses—beliefs, fantasies, feelings, and memories—to their own biological pubertal changes. A society's developmental taskings for its adolescents will profoundly influence the further development of adolescents' sexual identity and the consolidation of the various aspects of their overall identity (i.e., their autonomous, gender, sexual, peer, and social identities) into an emancipated identity. All in all, each adolescent will emerge from this phase at about age 18 or 19 years with an emancipated identity that is defined by the way in which he or she has cognitively processed the transactions between these biological, psychological, and social stimuli.

Major Developmental Tasks of Adolescence

The major developmental tasks of adolescence are as follows:

1. Construction of an emancipated identity
2. Construction of realistic ambitions and reasonable ideals
3. Further development of a sexual identity
4. Further development of a social identity

Maturation and Development of Physical Capabilities

Puberty is defined as the life-cycle phase in which the external bodily changes, defined as *secondary sexual characteristics,* make their appearance. These characteristics are induced by sex hormones (estrogen or androgen) (Frank and Cohen 1979; Sugar 1993). Secondary sexual characteristics differ from primary sexual characteristics in that the latter encompass changes that create the capacity for procreation (Bloch 1995). The entrance into adolescence, in most cultures, is signified by the external physical changes that occur at the onset of puberty, rather than the new internal physical and physiological changes that make procreation possible.

Secondary sexual characteristics in boys include an increase in the size of the genitals; the appearance of pubic, axillary, and facial hair; the deepening of the voice; and bone and muscle growth. In girls, secondary sexual characteristics include breast growth, pelvic and hip changes, the appearance of pubic and axillary hair, and the onset of menses (Tanner 1970).

The "surgent" maturation at puberty of 11- to 13-year-old boys' innate need for sensual–sexual pleasurable gratification causes them to experience genital body sensations that physically are quite compelling. Boys awaken most mornings and notice that they have

an erection. Likewise, 11- to 13-year-old girls have their first episode of menstruation. They wake up many mornings with obvious genital sensations that coincide with the fact that their breasts are developing and their pubic hair is beginning to show. They may avoid processing these new body perceptions or even fail to notice some of the subtle bodily changes that accompany these sexual sensations.

The rate at which boys' and girls' primary and secondary sexual characteristics mature differs (Khatchadourian 1977). At age 13 years, overall physical and secondary sexual development in girls is often 1½–2 years ahead of that in boys.

The age at onset of menstruation in girls has been decreasing throughout time. Around 1880, the age at onset was 15 or 16 years; in 1925, 13 or 14 years; and in 1985, 12 years of age (Kestenbaum 1979). Pregnancy becomes possible in girls by age 14 or 15 years; mature sperm are in evidence in boys by age 15 or 16 years (Khatchadourian 1977). Thus, procreation is possible by about midadolescence (Tanner 1978).

Indeed, pubertal bodily changes compel adolescents to look at their bodies. This increased body awareness becomes an important biological triggering stimulus that causes adolescents to have many internal responses (psychological stimuli) and to encounter many external responses (social stimuli) to their changing body appearance. Adolescents' mental processing of these biopsychosocial transactions will lead to new developmental changes in their body image. The developmental changes that take place in adolescents' body image become a crucial aspect of what they believe about themselves as valued, as well as sexually attractive, individuals.

Maturation and Development of Cognitive Capabilities

What Piaget termed the *formal cognitive phase,* during which formal thinking emerges, begins at about age 11 or 12 years, and it is not fully completed until about age 16 years. Some adolescents and adults, however, may never fully achieve the formal phase of cognitive maturation and development (Blackburn and Papalia 1992).

Emergence of Hypothetical Thinking

Pubertal cognitive advances associated with formal thinking operations include the following:

1. The ability to be able to reason regarding a hypothesis based on verbal propositions. At age 12 years,

adolescents can begin to understand the idea or concept inherent in a hypothesis without having to see physical proof in order to achieve this understanding. They can, therefore, understand either–or and if–then statements.

2. The ability to combine propositions and isolate variables to test a hypothesis. This new increase in cognitive ability to analytically solve problems leads adolescents to construct executive control structures that are much more complex than before. This type of thinking is the deductive reasoning of the scientist.

3. The ability to use thoughts and increasingly believe in the power of thoughts in planning for the future (Overton et al. 1992). Whereas latency-age children tend to be preoccupied with the present, adolescents in the formal operational phase become concerned with hypothetical, remote, and future concerns. Young adolescents begin to develop the ability to integrate past, present, and future when thinking about an issue or a problem.

4. The ability to classify objects and people based on propositional or hypothetical reasoning. Prior to age 12 years, children use their cognitive abilities to construct and reconstruct numerous categories that they have stored as memories within their representational worlds. By age 12 or 13 years, adolescents are capable of thinking about the similarities between categories based not only on concrete evidence they can see but also on mental propositions they can form.

5. The ability to be increasingly creative in thinking and more sophisticated in the use of symbolic thinking. Adolescents begin to become aware that they formulate ideas that are uniquely their own (Noy 1979). Their ability to arrive at creative ideas to aid them in reevaluating previous behavioral patterns helps adolescents to "resolve internal conflicts by utilizing new ways of understanding and coping" (Schneider 1992, p. 414).

6. The ability to form personal opinions and to construct individual standards and moral values, along with an increase in the capability to separate what is theoretically possible from what is realistically possible. P. Tyson and Tyson (1991) remarked on adolescents' development of a *cognitive egocentrism*. In so doing, they were addressing adolescents' resurrection of the wish for an ideal self (e.g., to be a grandiosely wise person) whose creative ideas (e.g., about government, the meaning of life, poverty) should be listened to as important contributions to the world scene.

Construction of the Concept of an Unconscious Mental Domain

Adolescents' eventual discovery that they possess an unconscious mental domain is a slowly evolving process that begins during adolescence and is achieved in most adolescents by age 16 or 17 years. Once achieved, the recognition that not every action, belief, or opinion can be readily explained through conscious mental activity assists adolescents in modifying their demand that their actions, beliefs, and opinions be easily supported by the facts as they consciously know them.

Maturation and Development of Emotions: Development of Emotional Self-Awareness

Emotions continue to serve adolescents in energy mobilization, self-regulation, and social adaptation.

Emotions as Energy Mobilizers

Adolescents experience a new emotion in adolescence—cognitive dissonance—as they reexamine and reflect on their beliefs and standards. For example, an adolescent girl will scan her beliefs and standards for logical consistency, and if she detects inconsistency, she automatically tries to rearrange or alter them to attain coherence among her beliefs and between her beliefs and behaviors. Failure to do so results in a special feeling state we might call *cognitive dissonance*, which is not identical to *guilt* (which follows recognition that one's voluntary actions deviate from a standard) (Kagan 1984).

As an emotion, this cognitive dissonance might be named *cognitive confusion* or even *cognitively generated ambivalent feelings*. Adolescents experience ambivalent feelings: one feeling is the competency pleasure in discovering the cognitive dissonance, and another is frustration and even anger that such dissonance exists. Cognitive dissonance acts as an energy mobilizer in motivating adolescents to reflect on the logical inconsistency between a belief or standard they possess and information being obtained through new experiences.

The advances in their formal thinking operations enable adolescents to become aware of much more *complex emotions* within themselves and others. Fischer et al. (1990) noted that adolescents have entered a "new developmental tier," characterized by cognitive advances in abstract thinking. The expression and appreciation of affect begin to take on a more complex meaning. Beyond the basic emotions of anger, sadness, fear, joy, and love, for example, adolescents can appreciate more complex, adult-like "scripts" for emotions, such as jealousy and resentment, as well as the concept of deeply hidden or repressed emotions (Fischer et al. 1990).

Emotions as a Means of Self-Regulation

By the time they reach age 12 years, adolescents have already been using their emotions as internal signals to assist them in guiding their actions in order to remain within their optimal stimulation range. The new awareness of emotional blends upsets adolescents' ability to use their emotions as signals of distress. For some time during adolescence, therefore, adolescents find that their own emotional signals are difficult to decipher.

Emotions as an Aid in Achieving Social Adaptation

More than ever before in their lives, adolescents are able to use the emotional communications of others to guide their actions. This is attributed to their growing ability to manifest true empathy in relation to other persons. They can use empathy and intuitive thinking to view an interpersonal situation involving themselves by seeing themselves through the eyes of another (Lane and Schwartz 1987).

Maturation and Development of Verbal Language Abilities

In the psychologically aware family, the parents begin to allow their young adolescents a new "language space" in which they permit them to verbalize their thoughts and emotions within the family without always encouraging them to think before they speak. It is as if parents are encouraging their young teens to move back to the speech dominance of early childhood and away from the thought dominance of late childhood.

When a family does not want to hear an adolescent's emotions, it is often because the family does not want the adolescent to think about and question certain family relationships. The adolescents may be discovering a family myth (Viorst 1986)—that is, a specific belief overtly endorsed and covertly reinforced by family members even in the face of direct contradictory evidence—for example, "Mother is a terrific mom" (even though her three children and her husband do everything around the house while she sits in a chair depressed, chain-smoking, and lamenting her fate).

Development of the Self-Representation and of Object Representations

Constructing an Emancipated Identity While Maintaining Transactional Relationships With Important Others

The attainment of an *emancipated identity* is the major developmental task of adolescence; as such, it is not fully achieved until the completion of adolescence, at age 18 or 19 years. Although Erikson did not use the term *emancipated,* his definition of identity in adolescence is the same as that delineated in Table 7–11.

In this definition of an emancipated identity, the first component is the main organizer of adolescents' achieving a sense of true emancipation. Achieving a belief in being truly separate and autonomous speaks to the issue of which mental structure is responsible for activating and organizing the adolescent's self-autonomy.

Young teens embark on this process of establishing an emancipated identity when they begin to question many of the beliefs, standards, and values that they had previously internalized as long-term memory structures within their representational world. This reevaluation or reassessment of prior knowledge is necessary if they are to become adults who truly believe that they possess their own beliefs, goals, ambitions, standards, and values, versus adults who are always trying to agree with (i.e., be a "clone") or rebel against (i.e., be a "rebel") either their real parents or the internalized representation of their parents.

Blos (1985) viewed adolescents as eventually achieving an emancipated identity through engaging in the "second individuation process of adolescence." The first individuation process began in toddlerhood, where there was more of a need to establish "a relative independence from external objects, while the second, the adolescent step of individuation, aims at the independence from internalized, infantile objects" (Blos 1985, p. 145). These internalized infantile objects (here Blos's use of *infantile* refers to prepubertal) are the positive object-constant parental representations that normally developing pubertal adolescents bring to their adolescent state of development. These preadolescent parental and other important object representations enabled the infant, toddler, preschooler, and grade-school child to explore autonomously and with industry away from his or her parents. Now, in adolescence, these object representations must be *transformed* and *restructured,* not relinquished or replaced. The process

---

TABLE 7–11. **Components of an emancipated identity**

1. Being separate and autonomous from one's parents and significant figures—especially the parents—while maintaining supportive transactional relationships with the parents and important others.

2. Believing in one's self-value while possessing individual points of view, ideals, and values different from those of respected parents, teachers, coaches, and similar significant figures.

3. Possessing sex-role behaviors congruent with one's sexual object choice in demonstrating heterosexuality or homosexuality.

4. Possessing social behaviors and beliefs that enable one to be comfortable in adopting a social role. (This social role gives older adolescents a continued sense of trust in entering society and committing to a particular lifestyle—for example, as a college student, an employee, or a provider of community service.)

5. Attaining an appreciation of the progressive continuity in life between one's past, one's present, and one's fantasies and ambitions for the future.

---

by which this occurs in great part involves transferring object relations conflicts into structural conflicts, which I describe below.

Object Relations Conflicts and Structural Conflicts

Dorpat (1976) observed the difference between internal object relations conflicts and structural conflicts. Adults who possess internal object relations conflicts are those with an identity that is either forever attempting to please its parental (and other persons of importance) object representations or forever rebelling against pleasing these object representations.

Young adolescents, in the process of reevaluating and reassessing their representational world and their current relationships with their parents and siblings, inevitably experience internal object relations conflicts. These conflicts must be externalized by bringing them into the open—that is, by adolescents engaging in conversations with their parents and other important people in their lives.

Generational Conflicts

The transformation of internal object relations conflicts into structural conflicts is, in essence, the psycho-

logical work of adolescence (Dahl 1995). Internal object relations conflicts also contribute to the emergence of generational conflicts—that is, conflicts between adolescents' prior and current internalized views of their parents (contained within their object representations of the parents) and their current needs, beliefs, or wishes.

Generational conflicts inevitably are expressed through a certain degree of normal rebellion. Rebellion in adolescents has been romanticized by some adults and overemphasized by some psychiatrists and psychologists who see only a selected population of emotionally disturbed adolescents (Offer and Schonert-Reichl 1992). Generational conflicts are a normal part of the adolescent's developmental process.

Adoption of a False Identity

Erikson delineated the overall psychosocial conflict that is inevitable during adolescence as one of establishing an *emancipated identity* versus succumbing to role, self, or *identity confusion*. Significant identity confusion leads adolescents to adopt a false identity that has been attained through some combination of internal rebellion—against unloving and critically harsh parental representations contained within their superegos—and external rebellion—against unloving and critically harsh voices currently emanating from others (e.g., parents, siblings, teachers).

A false identity is established in abnormally developing adolescents when they are unable to integrate the diverse social, peer, gender, and sexual roles that they assume at one time or another throughout their adolescence. This can occur in adolescents who have never attained positive self-constancy and object constancy (normally first attained at about age 3 years) and hence are very mistrustful, because they believe that people will abandon or hurt them in some way.

These adolescents often manifest an external rebellion: they search for a new person, group, cult, or organization through which they can discard their previously internalized negative self-constancy and object constancy and its associated overly critical standards, values, and so on. The new person or group provides these adolescents with an identity that helps them repress their sense of role confusion and even identity diffusion (Erikson 1968). These adolescents resurrect the generational gap as an impasse and a life preoccupation; they also resurrect—as a permanent solution for their conflicts—their childhood-derived ideal self-representations and ideal parent representations.

Parents' Role in Facilitating Formation of Emancipated Identity

Parents must empathize with the adolescent's need to confront parental values, standards, and beliefs in order to support their adolescent's verbalization and resolution of conflict.   When parents are able to express their own views, they encourage their teenager to do the same. When there is disagreement, parents need to model for their teenager an important socially adaptive behavior: constructive arguing and conflict resolution. Collins and Laursen (1992) made the following points:

1. Conflicts tend to emerge in interpersonal relationships that are closer rather than more distant or superficial.
2. The interdependencies between adolescents and their parents—developed before the onset of adolescence—inevitably lead to generational conflict.
3. Verbalization of conflicts can be developmentally enhancing or developmentally inhibiting in relation to adolescents' construction and development of an emancipated identity. Verbalization of conflicts is more developmentally enhancing when parents gradually use less of their authoritative power to resolve conflicts with the adolescent and instead begin to solve conflicts by working out compromises, instituting "time-outs" to allow each to reformulate his or her opinion, and engaging in negotiations.

Parents need to be consistent in expressing their values and standards.   Parents must be relatively consistent in expressing their values, attitudes, ideals, and points of view to provide their adolescent with a frame of reference to test out his or her own views, ideals, and beliefs by entering into verbal conflict with his or her parents. Parents must appreciate that their teenager will often fluctuate between wanting to agree and wanting to disagree with them.

Parents need to encourage their adolescent's continued involvement with a peer group and not be overly competitive with that peer group.   Parents who appreciate the crucial role of the peer group in facilitating the adolescent's development of an emancipated identity do not set up a competition between themselves and the peer group's attitudes, values, and so on. The majority of normally developing adolescents do not join peer groups whose values, attitudes, and rules of behavior differ greatly from those of their parents.

Further Development of Sexual and Social Identities

The first and perhaps most significant catalyst that sets into operation the process of establishing an emancipated self is puberty. This is the first step in adolescents' construction of a sexual identity. Having attained a solid gender identity (i.e., a basic sense of maleness or femaleness and associated identifications with gender-role behaviors) and sexual identity (in which they make their sexual object choice), adolescents begin to discover and consider embarking upon new behaviors as they enter the world of sexual activity.

Young adolescents experience a new variant of the developmental anxiety discussed earlier as *disintegration anxiety* (i.e., anxiety associated with not receiving positive mirroring and admiration for one's characteristics or performances). Throughout development, the body has been an important source of positive or negative self-esteem, and this is no less true in adolescence. Young adolescents feel anxious that their bodily changes will not be accepted by their parents, teachers, and peers. This form of disintegration anxiety can be thought of as *body reflection anxiety* about not being viewed as a potentially sexually attractive individual.

Pubertal Changes

Important rite-of-passage events for 12- to 13-year-old boys are buying their first underarm deodorant and their first athletic supporter.

Both pubertal boys and girls experience some anxiety about having to take a shower in public locker rooms (e.g., at school, at a health club). Girls worry about their breast size (that they are either too big or too small) and the presence or absence of axillary and pubic hair (Bloch 1995). Boys worry about their axillary, chest, and pubic hair growth. All boys are aware of penis size (Sugar 1993) and may avoid taking a locker next to a boy in the class who is taller than they are because they believe that the taller boy will have a bigger penis.

Girls ages 11 or 12 years approach buying their first brassiere as a rite of passage into adolescence. When doing so, they experience some anxiety about not being developed enough or being too developed. Again, their anxiety is primarily what they see reflected in the eyes of others in reference to their new sexual bodily appearance. Pubertal girls will want to go to the store with their mothers, who are more psychologically attuned to this experience, and will avoid going with their fathers.

Both pubertal boys and girls become preoccupied

with how to dress their sexually maturing bodies. They now embark on the important personal task of shopping for and selecting their own clothes (Rizzuto 1992). In working on eventual self-emancipation, young teens assert their separation from their parents by shopping with peers and in the process communicate to their parents that their adolescent body no longer belongs to the parents (Rizzuto 1992).

As a triggering biological stimulus, menarche propels adolescent girls to begin to more seriously contemplate a feminine sexual identity (Ritvo 1976). P. Tyson and Tyson (1991) emphasized the importance of menarche as a potent conceptual organizer of the pubertal girl's image of her female body.

Around the time of the expected onset of menarche, the sensitively aware mother initiates an interest in discussing her daughter's use of tampons and the body events associated with having a period. The mother will attempt to find out what her daughter knows about menarche and what fantasies and possible worries she is currently having about beginning her periods. In these discussions, the mother communicates to her daughter that she wants her daughter to understand and respect her body (Kestenberg 1968). This strengthens the daughter's gender identity, consolidating her identification with females. And as Dahl (1995) further observed, "Through the experience of her mother's bodily care, the girl's relationship to her own body is established" (pp. 201–202).

Reemergence of the Early Triangular Phase

In partially resolving their triangular wishes at around age 5–6 years, heterosexual children relinquished their wish to have an exclusive sensual–sexual relationship with the opposite-gender parent and began to identify with the same-gender parent. During early adolescence, the reawakening of adolescents' sexual drives restimulates the previous early triangular wishes.

In addition, however, a negative triangular conflict exists for heterosexual adolescents with their same-gender parent (Blos 1985). Girls' *negative triangular wishes* are their wishes to be dependent on and taken care of by their mother. These wishes evolve from girls' infant and childhood attachment relationship with their mother. In essence, throughout development, much of a mother's role as an empathically attuned, admiring object for her daughter (or an admiring selfobject) is subsumed in this concept of the negative triangular conflict. The *negative triangular conflict* for the heterosexual girl is one in which she experiences love for and a wish to be dependently cared for in a passive surrender to her mother, but, at the

same time, fears that these passive–dependent feelings indicate that she may be drifting from her previous heterosexual object choice to a homosexual object choice. The negative triangular conflict becomes stimulated in early adolescence because of the concurrent stimulation and return of the *positive triangular conflict.*

At around age 12 years, the physical and sexual changes that boys experience propel them to a new realization that they are becoming men. This brings their attention to the developmental task of putting more energy into developing their sexual identity. More often than not in contemporary American society, the heterosexual boy in his early teens learns that the male who is assertive in seeking and winning the girl is demonstrating a healthy heterosexual sexual identity (a derivative of his positive oedipal complex), and the boy who wants his father or another man to take care of him or find him a girlfriend is demonstrating a diminished or even "wimpy" heterosexual sexual identity. But the heterosexual teenage boy's negative triangular conflict is between his love and passive surrender to his father's potent caring and his fear that such passive dependency will cause him to lose his potency or even to become homosexual. Teenage heterosexual and homosexual boys fight hard to establish their assertive potency, whereas they fear passivity and impotency. As one grandmother told her grandson when he asked her advice about what to do when he liked a girl in his high school class, "Men are hunters" (M. Avallone, personal communication, August 1960).

Young adolescents' positive triangular wishes cause them to experience various anxieties: *body damage anxiety* at the hands of the same-gender parent, *superego anxiety* (for contemplating a wish to dispose of the symbol of family authority), and a certain degree of *disintegration anxiety* in reference to possibly losing the same-gender parent as a mirroring source of admiration (i.e., as an admiring selfobject).

So what do pubertal adolescents do? Katan (1951) noted that they must engage in a mental process of *object removal.* This process entails more than adolescents' simple displacement of their sexual desires toward the same-gender parent onto new sexual objects outside the family. It is an adaptive defense mechanism that involves the unconscious transfer of a highly displeasurable wish or feeling from one person or situation onto another person or situation that is associated with less emotional displeasure.) The normal pubertal adolescent's object removal is not reversible. For example, a boy will remove his mother from his "list" of possible sexual love objects and begin to look for an appropriate nonincestuous love object. If he does not engage in incestuous object removal, he is left with two other developmentally inhibiting options: 1) he can fight his positive triangular wishes by regressing to pre-pubertal behaviors, avoiding any contact with girls his age and instead socializing with prepubertal boys, or 2) he can resist experiencing sexual sensations by fighting his body (e.g., he may automatically overeat and become grossly overweight, or he may attempt to become extremely thin in an unconscious attempt to avoid developing any degree of sexual attractiveness in body appearance). Parents do not have to look too hard to notice their pubertal boy's desire to distance himself from physically close encounters with his mother.

Heterosexual pubertal boys' need to avoid close physical contact with their mother is motivated by the societal rule prohibiting incest. It may also be motivated by boys' healthy prepubertal attachment relationship to their mother, which, as I described earlier, has been hypothesized by Erickson (1993) to serve as a protective factor against the threat or risk of incest.

The normally developing pubertal boy will tend to avoid his mother and to spend more time with his father and other men. As his relationship with his father becomes stronger, he begins to relinquish his positive triangular wishes for the second time in his life, and as he becomes more aware of his emotional closeness with his father, he begins to deal with the issue of asserting his heterosexuality and his position in the category of "heterosexual men." When the pubertal boy is physically close to his father and other men and male peers, he may become a bit anxious: too much physical and emotional closeness makes him worry that he may be drifting toward homosexuality. His negative triangular wishes toward his father will, throughout his adolescence, cause him some measure of anxiety.

As girls between ages 12 and 15 years turn away from their fathers, there is a general reaction against their regressing to a more emotionally close and dependent relationship with their mothers. The young adolescent girl becomes anxious about wanting and needing her mother to help her develop her sexual identity. This anxiety is related to the girl's worry that she will become too dependent on her mother, thereby losing her "hard-won activity" (Dahl 1995) and burgeoning self-emancipation. As a result, girls in early adolescence undergo a period in which they turn away from involvement with their mothers, often developing a close relationship with a particular same-age peer.

In early adolescence (ages 12–15 years), as heterosexual teenagers are attempting to establish a heterosexual identity and to construct a set of standards for sexual behavior, they are assisted in this process by be-ing able to masturbate. Masturbation (Laufer and Laufer 1984) becomes a means of discharging sexual tension. However, when adolescents discover in their masturbatory fantasies a wish (i.e., an incestuous wish) that they sense is wrong or forbidden—either externally by society or internally by the superego—they can gradually begin to relinquish the wish. Positive triangular wishes are never truly destroyed (Loewald 1979), but only wane significantly; they must be repeatedly addressed throughout life.

As dating begins, teenagers want their parents, particularly the opposite-gender parent, to acknowledge them as a sexually attractive person, since the adolescents' internalization of a belief in having a competent and attractive heterosexual identity continues to develop under the admiring gaze of the opposite-gender parent.

Initiation of Sexual Activity

The issue of when loss of virginity should "normally" take place is a problematic one. Virginity lasting up until age 25–30 years or older may indicate not abnormal heterosexual or homosexual development but rather a conscious moral or value choice in a person who has achieved self-emancipation. Adolescents need to be helped in limiting their exposure to too much sexual stimulation, because each adolescent has his or her own "clock" concerning sexual activity.

For adolescents who so choose, the first experience with sexual activity can be quite self-centered. They are initially focused on their own sexual performance rather than on caring and concern for their partner's feelings. They seek admiring feedback about how they have performed. And some adolescents may masturbate to completely avoid heterosexual or homosexual activity because of their concern about loss of virginity, pregnancy, or HIV or other sexually transmitted diseases.

Development of the Superego
Construction of Realistic Ambitions and Reasonable Ideals

Normally developing adolescents begin to attain self-emancipation when they begin to accept their wish to take authority for directing their life from their parents. Adolescents' wish to compete with their parents for authority of their own lives and win the battle of becoming an emancipated self generates guilt (Loewald 1979); the guilt comes from their viewing their wish to sever the relationship of parent and child as a wrongful behavior or sin that demands atonement.

This guilt is alleviated when older adolescents (ages 16–19 years) reconstruct their superegos to become truly their own ethical standards and beliefs.

Before the emancipated self emerges, changes must occur in adolescents' conscience, as well as concurrent changes in their long-standing periodic resurrection of childhood wishes to be perfect and to have perfect parents.

Throughout adolescence, the conscience grows more and more internalized, gradually becoming better able to achieve its main two functions:

1. To regulate and control behavior relatively independently of external restraints
2. To become a source of self-esteem that is relatively independent of others' evaluations of one's worth and value

Throughout adolescence, teenagers evaluate the moral rules and values defined by peers, teachers, and other adults. Some of these rules and values are internalized and become further building blocks of the developing conscience (Sugar 1992).

Psychologically attuned parents recognize when their teenager is struggling with the wish to find rules about life by which he or she can live, and they encourage these conflictual conversations and help their young adolescent realize when he or she has set unattainable standards of behavior for him- or herself.

A "Confused Conscience"

The process of idealizing and de-idealizing parents goes on for much of middle to late adolescence. The process becomes most prominent in 16- to 19-year-old adolescents when their positive triangular wishes begin to wane and their relationship and identification with the same-gender parent becomes stronger. A process of de-idealization of both parents now begins in which adolescents ultimately give up any residual wishes to have perfect and all-powerful parents to protect them from life's challenges.

Once again, the peer group rescues teenagers from feeling too disappointed and anxious about becoming emancipated, and they can eventually relinquish their view of their parents as all-protecting and all-admiring. In so doing, teenagers feel, for a while, a sense of loss in losing their parents as a source of admiration and positive self-esteem (Table 7–12). A period of transience ensues during which adolescents turn inward and look toward the peer group and occasionally other adults to assist them in controlling their behavior; for example, peer group rules and attitudes about dating

TABLE 7–12. Adolescence phase: the function of superego as an internal regulator of behavior

- As the teenager grows older (ages 16–18 years), emancipation is looming—and the peer group increasingly assumes a role in facilitating emancipation from the parents.

- Parental rules previously internalized within the teen's superego become less of an influence in maintaining rules and values.

- In the teen's reconsidering of parental rules and values, "old" ones are less compelling.

- While conscience is weakened, the teen alternates between seeking isolation and turning to his or her peer group for help with self-control, which leaves the teen vulnerable to the dictates of a "group superego."

become very important. A narcissistic stage occurs wherein adolescents alternate between overly admiring themselves and being overly critical of their own imperfections and their lack of some of the abilities and attributes they admire in other adolescents.

Eventually, in late adolescence, teenagers begin to relinquish their wish to be perfect or have their parents be perfect. Their ideal images of the same-gender parent had stimulated their negative oedipal wishes toward this parent. In eventually relinquishing this wish as being realistically unattainable, adolescents will construct realistic (i.e., de-idealized) ambitions and reasonable ideals for themselves.

Attainment of an Integrated Conscience

The older teen's more highly developed superego now enables him or her to experience true structural conflicts. The superego becomes a more realistic and friendlier internal guide for behavioral choice and an internal source of admiration when older adolescents attain more realistic ambitions. Stillwell et al. (1991) labeled this more developed superego in late adolescence as the *integrated conscience*, in which good dominates evil.

Development of Adaptational Capabilities: Emergence of More Socially Mature Mechanisms of Defense

Parents must work at 1) creating a communication space within their homes and 2) being models of how to socially communicate. The first requirement involves figuring out ways to help teenagers keep a certain amount of communication going between themselves and their parents, which entails not allowing too much time to go by during which teenagers are silent around the family. The second requirement involves the parents' modeling how teenagers should verbalize their feelings and conflicts and what constitutes socially acceptable defense mechanisms.

Specific defense mechanisms have been shown to be associated with healthy adult functioning (Vaillant 1971, 1974), particularly in adults who have a good capacity to adapt to different social, educational, and professional situations. These mechanisms include the following:

- *Intellectualization*—Intellectualization is an automatic process in which thoughts about a topic causing emotional displeasure remain within adolescents' consciousness while the emotionally displeasurable feelings are relegated to their unconscious mental domain. Intellectualization is a derivative of the defense mechanism of *isolation of emotion*. It is useful to think of intellectualization as a prominent adolescent defense mechanism, because adolescents are quite adept at using their new formal-thinking capacities to suppress or repress displeasurable feelings.
- *Humor*—Humor is used as a defense mechanism throughout adolescence, especially in late adolescence. In humor, the forbidden wish is expressed but not acted upon. Humor that affects others unpleasantly, such as satire and practical jokes, can often be thought of as displacement or passive aggression.
- *Anticipation*—Anticipation is the automatic delay of action accompanied by the conscious experiencing of thoughts and feelings associated with a future event or an encounter with a person.

Transitioning From Adolescence to Young Adulthood: Criteria for Adulthood

The word *adolescence* literally means "becoming an adult." Hence, the end of adolescence is usually defined by what society associates with adult behavior and adult psychological maturity. This is quite difficult to clearly define. As Blos (1979) noted, "Behavior alone never renders a reliable assessment of an individual's developmental status, nor does it reveal the working of his motivational system" (p. 85).

Whether an older adolescent 18–19 years of age pursues more education after high school or does not, it seems that adolescence has been prolonged based on criteria used to determine the entrance into young adulthood. These "rites of passage" criteria are quite difficult to describe, because the basic issues of importance for middle to late adolescence are, for the most part, very similar to those for young adulthood.

The following criteria can be used to define the end of adolescence and the beginning of adult functioning. These criteria represent the developmental tasks that must be mastered at around age 18 or 19 years. In each of these tasks, mastery of the task is relative—that is, in order for development into adulthood to be smooth and nonconflictual, there must be *more* rather than *less* mastery of the task. All four tasks below lead to new possessions within the older adolescent's self-representation. This self-representation defines the emancipated self.

Establishment of Autonomy From Parents (Self-Autonomy)

Toward the end of adolescence, the individual begins to assert control over his or her own life, believing in his or her ability to function apart from parents or other adults. However, this emancipated or fully autonomous identity is not that of a person who is an island unto him- or herself. Self-autonomy occurs in the context of being comfortable with needing to be in emotionally intimate relationships with others (Miller 1991).

By late adolescence, parents have for the most part been de-idealized and have come to be viewed more as advisers, guides, and friends. Parents are no longer automatically viewed as having all the answers, nor are they viewed as being completely "out of it." Superego anxiety is less intense, because the superego is less perfectionistic.

Establishment of Realistic Goals (Realistic Self-Image)

Through a progressive relinquishment of wishes for perfection, signified by the ability to set reasonable goals and to tolerate the realization that every goal will not be achieved, the adolescent begins to manifest more self-responsibility, in that imperfections, setbacks, or faults do not generate blaming of others.

Establishment of a Stable Sexual Identity

This goal is often delayed due to the older adolescent's decision to avoid sexual activity in order to pursue higher education or vocational goals. In 18- to 19-year-olds who have become sexually active, this criterion addresses their growing capacity to make a mutually caring choice of a heterosexual or a homosexual partner and to treat that partner's body with kindness and respect rather than as a vehicle for demonstrating their sexual potency.

Establishment of a Sense of Continuity Between Past Life Experiences and Current Motivations and Beliefs

Individuals in late adolescence can gain a new understanding of the relative influence of past experiences on current wishes, motivational goals, and beliefs. This understanding often entails seeking out the life histories of other family members to help one understand present problems.

Conclusion

Developmental psychiatry defines as its area of study the biological, psychological, and social variables inherent in the genesis of both normal and abnormal behavior and mental activity.

Developmental psychopathology, by contrast, attempts to acquire a body of data that will help in predicting which children, as a result of possessing specific conscious and unconscious pathogenic beliefs,

fantasies, emotions, and long-term memories, will develop abnormally in the future.

My hope is that the object relations–structural modification of the biopsychosocial model used in this chapter's presentation of normal development will assist students and professionals in mental health fields of study both in evaluating, diagnosing, understanding, and treating psychopathology present in their adult patients.

A knowledge of normal development can assist the mental health professional in considering that certain behaviors in his or her adult patient may represent a conscious or unconscious attempt to gratify wishes that were appropriate in childhood but that may not be appropriate in a well-functioning adult. In identifying these childhood developmental wishes and including them in formulating a treatment plan, the therapist can help the adult patient to realize and eventually accept that adults can only have two overall goals or "positions" in life—either 1) to stay "stuck" in repeating behaviors that do not lead to the gratification of adult needs, or 2) to move ahead and (often with a therapist's help) engage in the process of developmental change, thereby transforming pathogenic beliefs and attitudes into new normogenic ones. No adult can go back to childhood and receive from his or her parents and others what was not received from them as a child. Unfortunately, however, many adults continue to try.

Key Points

The following terms and concepts are key to an understanding of normal child and adolescent development:

- **Accommodation–transformation principle**—The principle that becomes activated when stimuli create perceptions or conceptions that cannot be assimilated into prior representations. When this occurs, the infant will either change a preexisting representation to include the new perception or conception or add a new representation to his or her mental world.

- **Attachment relationship**—The specific relationship that develops between infants and their parents.

- **Belief**—A type of conception that, as a representational mental structure, establishes the relationship between two or more inanimate objects, aspects of nature's laws, or people (e.g., the child and his or her mother).

- **Child protective factor**—A characteristic within the child, the parents, the child–parent relationship, and/ or the society in which the child is living that helps the child and the parents achieve developmental adaptations and maintain their goodness-of-fit transactions.

- **Developmental continuity**—The term used to address the fact that a great part, but not all, of psychological development is dependent on what took place in the past.

- **Developmental discontinuity**—An event in a person's life that is unexpected and not predictable from what has occurred in the person's past.

- **Developmentally enhancing adaptation**—An adaptation by the child that enhances the child's sense of competency, pleasure in mastering a task, and feelings of joyful pride.

- **Disintegration anxiety**—The internally generated fear that if anyone knew how imperfect or impotent the child believes himself or herself to be, others would totally reject him or her.

- **Experiential mental structures**—The emotions (e.g., shame, guilt), thoughts (perceptions and conceptions), and memories (short- and long-term) that are the result of the mind's processing of transactions between biopsychosocial stimuli.

- **Hierarchical restructuring principle**—The principle that states that as a child's cognitive abilities continue to mature and his or her mind continues to reconstruct prior representations to reflect a more advanced level of cognitive integration and comprehension, the child's mind will reorganize its representations into a hierarchy that reflects the child's unique preferences.

- **Inner mental world or representational world**—The inner world we refer to as an individual's mind, which is in contrast to the outer world of people and things.

- **Mentalizing function**—The capacity to use self-reflection to become aware of possessing a mind and to gradually understand one's own mind and the minds of others as being complex, with different emotions, beliefs, and conflicts.

- **Normal developmental external conflict**—An aspect of normal development that occurs when there is a disparity between the child's current need, wish, and/or impulse and the desires of the parents or others with whom the child is relating.

- **Normal developmental internal conflict**—An aspect of normal development that occurs when there is a disparity between what the child desires to do, fantasizes about, or believes and an inner voice that prohibits or warns the child that a developmental calamity will occur if the child acts upon his or her impulse, desire, and/or fantasy.

- **Normogenic belief**—A belief, developed by the child, that enhances the child's psychological development. Such a belief enables the child to generate positive expectancies about new life events and people.

- **Pathogenic belief**—A belief, developed by the child, that interferes with the child's psychological development. Such a belief functions as an internal inhibiting factor in that it causes the child to generate negative expectancies about new life events and people.

Suggested Readings

Cozolino L: The Neuroscience of Psychotherapy: Building and Rebuilding the Human Brain. New York, WW Norton, 2002

Fonagy P, György G, Jurist EL, et al (eds): Affect Regulation, Mentalization, and the Development of the Self. New York, Other Press, 2002

Gazzaniga MS: The Ethical Brain. New York, Dana Press, 2005

Gemelli R: Normal Child and Adolescent Development. Washington, DC, American Psychiatric Press, 1996

Kandel ER: In Search of Memory: The Emergence of a New Science of the Mind. New York, WW Norton, 2006

Person ES, Cooper AM, Gabbard GO (eds): The American Psychiatric Publishing Textbook of Psychoanalysis. Washington, DC, American Psychiatric Publishing, 2005

Rich HL: In the Moment: Celebrating the Everyday. New York, HarperCollins, 2002

Solms M, Turnbull O: The Brain and the Inner World: An Introduction to the Neuroscience of Subjective Experience. New York, Other Press, 2002

References

Ainsworth MD: Patterns of attachment behavior shown by the infant in interaction with his mother. Merrill-Palmer Quarterly 10:51–58, 1964

Ainsworth MD, Belehar M, Waters E, et al: Patterns of Attachment: A Psychological Study of the Strange Situation. Hillsdale, NJ, Lawrence Erlbaum, 1978

Ames LB, Ilg FL: Your Three-Year-Old. New York, Dell Publishing, 1976a

Ames LB, Ilg FL: Your Four-Year-Old. New York, Dell Publishing, 1976b

Ames LB, Ilg FL: Your Five-Year-Old. New York, Dell Publishing, 1976c

Ames LB, Ilg FL: Your Six-Year-Old. New York, Dell Publishing, 1979

Asher SR, Coie JD: Peer Rejection in Childhood. New York, Cambridge University Press, 1990

Baldwin JD, Baldwin JI: Open peer commentary: the stage question in cognitive-developmental theory. The Behavioral and Brain Sciences 2:182–183, 1978

Beal CR, Flavell JH: Development of the ability to distinguish communicative intention and literal message meaning. Child Dev 55:920–928, 1984

Beebe B, Sloate P: Assessment and treatment difficulties in mother-infant attunement in the first three years of life: a case history. Psychoanalytic Inquiry 1:601–624, 1982

Berg C: Perspectives for viewing intellectual development throughout the life course, in Intellectual Development. Edited by Sternberg J, Berg C. New York, Cambridge University Press, 1992, pp 1–16

Berk LE: Why children talk to themselves. Sci Am 271:5, 1994

Bidell TR, Fischer KW: Beyond the stage debate: action, structure, and variability in Piagetian theory and research, in Intellectual Development. Edited by Sternberg R, Berg C. New York, Cambridge University Press, 1992, pp 100–141

Blackburn JA, Papalia DE: The study of adult cognition from the Piagetian perspective, in Intellectual Development. Edited by Sternberg R, Berg C. New York, Cambridge University Press, 1992, pp 141–160

Bloch HS: Adolescent Development, Psychopathology, and Treatment. New York, International Universities Press, 1995

Blos P: The Adolescent Passage: Developmental Issues. New York, International Universities Press, 1979

Blos P: Son and Father, Before and After the Oedipus Complex. New York, Free Press, 1985

Blum HP: Superego formation, adolescent transformation, and the adult neurosis. J Am Psychoanal Assoc 33:887–909, 1985

Bowlby J: Attachment and Loss, Vol 1: Attachment. New York, Basic Books, 1969

Bowlby J: Developmental psychiatry comes of age. Am J Psychiatry 145:1–10, 1988

Brenner C: An Elementary Textbook of Psychoanalysis. New York, International Universities Press, 1965

Brenner C: The components of psychic conflict and its consequences in mental life. Psychoanal Q 48:547–567, 1979

Brodal A: Neurological Anatomy. London, Oxford University Press, 1969

Brothers L: A biological perspective on empathy. Am J Psychiatry 146:10–19, 1989

Brown TE: Inside the ADD mind. Additude Attention Deficit 6:34–38, 2006

Campos J, Barrett KC, Lamb ME, et al: Socio-emotional development, in Handbook of Child Psychology, 4th Ed, Vol 2: Infant Development. Edited by Haith M, Campos J. New York, Wiley, 1983, pp 785–915

Case R: Neo-Piagetian theories of child development, in Intellectual Development. Edited by Sternberg RJ, Berg CA. New York, Cambridge University Press, 1992, pp 161–197

Chess S, Thomas A: Temperament in Clinical Practice. New York, Guilford, 1986

Chess S, Thomas A: Temperament and its functional significance, in The Course of Life, Vol 2: Early Childhood. Edited by Greenspan SI, Pollock GH. Madison, CT, International Universities Press, 1989, pp 163–227

Clyman R: The procedural organization of emotions: a contribution from cognitive science to the psychoanalytic theory of therapeutic action. J Am Psychoanal Assoc 39:349–383, 1991

Coie JD: Toward a theory of peer rejection, in Peer Rejection in Childhood. Edited by Asher SR, Coie JD. New York, Cambridge University Press, 1990, pp 365–403

Colarusso CA: Child and Adult Development. New York, Plenum, 1992

Collins W, Laursen B: Conflicts and relationships during adolescence, in Conflict in Child and Adolescent Development. Edited by Shantz CU, Hartup WW. New York, Cambridge University Press, 1992, pp 216–242

Dahl EK: Daughters and mothers. Psychoanal Study Child 50:187–204, 1995

Damon W: The Moral Child. New York, Free Press, 1988

Demos EV: Affect in early infancy: physiology or psychology? Psychoanalytic Inquiry 1:533–574, 1981

Dorpat T: Structural conflict and object relations conflict. J Am Psychoanal Assoc 24:855–873, 1976

Dowling S: Abstract report from the literature on neonatology. Psychoanal Q 50:290–296, 1981

Dowling S, Rothstein A (eds): The Significance of Infant Observational Research for Clinical Work With Children, Adolescents and Adults. Madison, CT, International Universities Press, 1989

Emde RN: The prerepresentational self and its affective core. Psychoanal Study Child 38:165–192, 1983

Emde RN: The affective self: continuities and transformations from infancy, in Frontiers of Infant Psychiatry, Vol 2. Edited by Call JD, Galenson E, Tyson RL. New York, Basic Books, 1984, pp 38–54

Emde RN: Moving ahead: integrating influences of affective processes for development and for psychoanalysis. Int J Psychoanal 80(Pt 2):317–339, 1999

Emde RN, Buchsbaum HK: A psychoanalytic theory of affect, III: emotional development and signaling in infancy, in The Course of Life, Vol 1: Infancy. Edited by Greenspan SI, Pollock GH. Madison, CT, International Universities Press, 1989, pp 193–227

Emde RN, Gaensbauer TJ, Harmon RJ: Emotional Expression in Infancy. New York, International Universities Press, 1979

Emde RN, Biringen Z, Clyman RB, et al: The moral self of infancy: affective core and procedural knowledge. Developmental Review 11:251–290, 1991

Erickson MT: Rethinking Oedipus: an evolutionary perspective of incest avoidance. Am J Psychiatry 150:411–415, 1993

Erikson E: Identity and the Life Cycle. New York, Norton, 1959

Erikson E: Childhood and Society, Revised Edition. New York, Norton, 1963

Erikson E: Identity, Youth and Crisis. New York, Norton, 1968

Fantz RL: The origin of form perception. Scientific American 204:62–72, 1961

Fantz R: Pattern vision in newborn infants. Science 140:296–297, 1963

Fischer KW, Carnochan P, Shaver PR: How emotions develop and how they organize development. Cognition and Emotion 4:81–121, 1990

Fonagy P: The Process of Change and the Change of Processes: What Can Change in a "Good" Analysis. Keynote Address to the Spring Meeting of Division 39 of the American Psychological Association, New York, 16 April 1999. Available at: http://www.dspp.com/papers/fonagy.htm. Accessed September 2007.

Fonagy P, György G, Jurist EL, et al (eds): Affect Regulation, Mentalization, and the Development of the Self. New York, Other Press, 2002

Fraiberg S: Object constancy and mental representation. Psychoanal Study Child 24:9–47, 1969

Frank RA, Cohen DJ: Psychosocial concomitants of biological maturation in preadolescence. Am J Psychiatry 136:1516–1524, 1979

Freud A: The Ego and the Mechanisms of Defense, Vol 2 (1936), in The Writings of Anna Freud. New York, International Universities Press, 1966

Freud S: The interpretation of dreams (1900), in The Standard Edition of the Complete Psychological Works of Sigmund Freud, Vols 4 and 5. Translated and edited by Strachey J. London, Hogarth Press, 1963, pp 1–610

Freud S: Three essays on the theory of sexuality (1905), in The Standard Edition of the Complete Psychological Works of Sigmund Freud, Vol 7. Translated and edited by Strachey J. London, Hogarth Press, 1963, pp 135–243

Freud S: The ego and the id (1923), in The Standard Edition of the Complete Psychological Works of Sigmund Freud, Vol 19. Translated and edited by Strachey J. London, Hogarth Press, 1963, pp 12–66

Galenson E: Sexuality in infancy and preschool-aged children, in Child and Adolescent Psychiatric Clinics of North America, Vol 2. Edited by Yates A. Philadelphia, PA, WB Saunders, 1993

Gemelli R: Normal Child and Adolescent Development. Washington, DC, American Psychiatric Publishing, 1996

Girton M: Infants' attention to intrastimulus motion. J Exp Child Psychol 28:416–423, 1979

Goldsmith H, Buss A, Plomin R, et al: Roundtable: what is temperament? four approaches. Child Dev 58:505–529, 1987

Greenberg M, Morris N: Engrossment: the newborn's impact upon the father. Am J Orthopsychiatry 44:520–531, 1974

Greenspan SI: Intelligence and Adaptation: An Integration of Psychoanalytic and Piagetian Developmental Psychology. New York, International Universities Press, 1979

Greenspan SI: The development of the ego: biological and environmental specificity in the psychopathological developmental process and the selection and construction of ego defenses. J Am Psychoanal Assoc 37:605–639, 1989

Greenspan SI: A developmental approach to intelligence. AACAP News 27(5), 1996

Greenspan SI: The Growth of the Mind: And the Endangered Origins of Intelligence. New York, Basic Books, 1998

Harris PL, Donnelly K, Guz GR, et al: Children's understanding of mixed and masked emotions, in Transitional Mechanisms in Child Development. Edited by de Ribaupierre E. Cambridge, UK, Cambridge University Press, 1986, pp 125–141

Harrison AM, Tronick EZ: Understanding therapeutic change. J Am Psychoanal Assoc 55:853–875, 2007

Hartman H: Ego Psychology and the Problem of Adaptation. New York, International Universities Press, 1939

Havens L: A theoretical basis for the concepts of self and authentic self. J Am Psychoanal Assoc 34:363–378, 1986

Henry J: On Shame, Vulnerability and Other Forms of Self-Destruction. New York, Vantage Books, 1973

Herzog JM: On father hunger: the father's role in the modulation of aggressive drive and fantasy, in Father and Child. Edited by Cath SW, Gurwitt AR, Ross JM. Boston, MA, Little, Brown, 1982, pp 163–174

Hoffman M: Affective and cognitive processes in moral internalization, in Social Cognition and Social Development. Edited by Higgens ET, Ruble DN, Hartnup WW. Cambridge, UK, Cambridge University Press, 1983, pp 236–274

Horner AJ: The Wish for Power and the Fear of Having It. Northvale, NJ, Jason Aronson, 1989

Hudson JA: The emergence of autobiographic memory in mother-child conversations, in Knowing and Remembering in Young Children. Edited by Fivush R, Hudson JA. New York, Cambridge University Press, 1990, pp 166–196

Hudson JA: Understanding events: the development of script knowledge, in The Development of Social Cognition. Edited by Bennett M. New York, Guilford, 1993, pp 142–167

Hutt SJ, Hutt C, Lenard H, et al: Auditory responsivity in the human neonate. Nature 218:888–890, 1968

Izard CE: The Face of Emotion. New York, Appleton-Century-Crofts, 1971

Izard CE: Patterns of Emotions. New York, Academic Press, 1972

Kagan J: The form of early development. Arch Gen Psychiatry 36:1047–1054, 1979

Kagan J: The Second Year: The Emergence of Self-Awareness. Cambridge, MA, Harvard University Press, 1981

Kagan J: The Nature of the Child. New York, Basic Books, 1984

Kagan J: Unstable Ideas: Temperament, Cognition and Self. Cambridge, MA, Harvard University Press, 1989

Kail R, Bisanz J: The information-processing perspective on cognitive development in childhood and adolescence, in Intellectual Development. Edited by Sternberg J, Berg C. New York, Cambridge University Press, 1992, pp 229–261

Karmiloff-Smith A: Problem solving procedures in the construction and representation of closed railway circuits. Archives de Psychologie 67:37–59, 1979

Katan A: The role of displacement in agoraphobia. Int J Psychoanal 32:41–50, 1951

Kernberg OF: Object Relations Theory and Clinical Psychoanalysis. New York, Jason Aronson, 1976

Kernberg OF: Self, ego, affects and drives. J Am Psychoanal Assoc 30:893–917, 1982

Kernberg OF: An ego psychology-object relations theory approach to the transference. Psychoanal Q 51:197–221, 1987

Kestenbaum CJ: Current sexual attitudes, societal pressure, and the middle-class adolescent girl, in Adolescent Psychiatry, Vol 7. Edited by Feinstein SC, Giovacchini PL. Chicago, IL, University of Chicago Press, 1979, pp 147–157

Kestenberg JS: Outside and inside, male and female. J Am Psychoanal Assoc 16:457–520, 1968

Khatchadourian H: The Biology of Adolescence. San Francisco, CA, Freeman, 1977

Klein M: The importance of symbol-formation in the development of the ego (1930), in The Writings of Melanie Klein, Vol 1. London, Hogarth Press, 1975, pp 219–232

Kohlberg LA: The Philosophy of Moral Development, Moral Stages, and the Ideal of Justice: Essays on Moral Development, Vol 1. San Francisco, CA, Harper & Row, 1981

Kohut H: The Analysis of the Self: A Systematic Approach to the Psychoanalytic Treatment of Narcissistic Personality Disorders. New York, International Universities Press, 1971

Kohut H: Restoration of the Self. New Haven, CT, International Universities Press, 1977

Kohut H, Wolf E: The disorders of the self and their treatment: an outline. Int J Psychoanal 59:413–425, 1978

Korn S, Gannon S: Temperament, cultural variation and behavior disorder in preschool children. Child Psychiatry Hum Dev 13:203–212, 1984

Lamb ME (ed): The Role of the Father in Child Development, 2nd Edition. New York, Wiley, 1981

Lane RD, Schwartz GE: Levels of emotional awareness: a cognitive-developmental theory and its application to psychopathology. Am J Psychiatry 144:133–143, 1987

Laufer M, Laufer ME: Adolescence and Developmental Breakdown. New Haven, CT, Yale University Press, 1984

Leslie AM: Pretense and representation: the origins of "theory of mind." Psychol Rev 94:412–426, 1987

Lewis M, Brooks-Gunn J: Social Cognition and the Acquisition of Self. New York, Plenum, 1979

Lewis ML: Memory and psychoanalysis: a new look at infantile amnesia and transference. J Am Acad Child Adolesc Psychiatry 34:405–417, 1995

Lichtenberg JD: Psychoanalysis and Motivation. Hillsdale, NJ, Analytic Press, 1989

Lichtenberg JD, Kindler AR: A motivational systems approach. J Am Psychoanal Assoc 42:405–421, 1994

Loewald HW: The waning of the Oedipus complex. J Am Psychoanal Assoc 27:751–775, 1979

Long KD: Panel report: The changing language of female development. Journal of the American Psychoanalytic Association 53(4):1161–1174, Fall 2005. Available at: http://apsa.org/Portals/1/docs/JAPA/534/McDermott%20Long-PAN-P-1161-1174.pdf. Accessed October 2007.

Magnusson D, Allen V: Human Development: An Interactional Approach. New York, Academic Press, 1983

Mahler MS: On human symbiosis and the vicissitudes of individualization. J Am Psychoanal Assoc 23:740–763, 1975

Maletesta C, Haviland J: Learning display rules: the socialization of emotion expression in infancy. Child Development 53:991–1003, 1982

Mayer LM: Towards female gender identity. J Am Psychoanal Assoc 43:17–39, 1995

Mayes LC: Arousal regulation, emotional flexibility, medial amygdala function, and the impact of early experience: comments on the paper of Lewis et al. Ann N Y Acad Sci 1094:178–192, 2006

McDevitt JB: The emergence of hostile aggression and its defensive and adaptive modifications during the separation-individualization process. J Am Psychoanal Assoc 31 (suppl):273–300, 1987

Meissner W: A note in projective identification. J Am Psychoanal Assoc 28:43–68, 1980

Meissner WW: The pathology of belief systems. Psychoanalysis and Contemporary Thought 15:99–129, 1992

Meyer JK: Body ego, selfness, and gender sense: the development of gender identity. Psychiatr Clin North Am 3:21–36, 1980

Meyer JK: The theory of gender identity disorders. J Am Psychoanal Assoc 30:381–419, 1982

Miller JB: Woman's Growth in Connection: Writings From the Stone Center. New York, Guilford, 1991

Mills M, Melhuish E: Recognition of mother's voice in early infancy. Nature 252:123–124, 1974

Mitchell SA: Aggression and the endangered self. Psychoanal Q 62:351–352, 1993

Nelson K: Event knowledge and the development of language functions, in Research in Child Language Disorders. Edited by Miller J. New York, Little, Brown, 1990, pp 125–141

Nelson K: Narrative and memory in early childhood. Paper presented at annual meeting of the American Academy of Child and Adolescent Psychiatry, San Antonio, TX, October 1993a

Nelson K: The psychological and social origins of autobiographical memory. Psychological Science 4:7–14, 1993b

Noy P: Form creation in art: an ego-psychological approach to creativity. Psychoanal Q 48:229–256, 1979

Offer D, Schonert-Reichl K: Debunking the myths of adolescence: findings from recent research. J Am Acad Child Adolesc Psychiatry 31:1003–1014, 1992

Oppenheim D, Goldsmith DF (eds): Attachment Theory in Clinical Work With Children. New York, Guilford, 2007

Overton WF, Steidl JH, Rosenstein D, et al: Formal operations as regulatory context in adolescence, in Adolescent Psychiatry, Vol 18. Edited by Feinstein SC. Chicago, IL, University of Chicago Press, 1992, pp 502–513

Pally R: Emotional processing: the mind–body connection. Int J Psychoanal 79(Pt 2):349–362, 1998

Panksepp J (ed): Textbook of Biological Psychiatry. Hoboken, NJ, John Wiley & Sons, 2004

Parens H: Aggression in Our Children. New York, Jason Aronson, 1987

Parens H, Pollack L, Stern J, et al: On the girl's entry into the oedipus complex. J Am Psychoanal Assoc 24:79–107, 1976

Parke R, Tinsley B: The father's role in infancy: determinants of involvement in caregiving and play, in The Role of the Father in Child Development. Edited by Lamb M. New York, Wiley, 1981, pp 45–76

Perry NW: How children remember and why they forget. The Advisor 5:1–16, 1992

Person ES: By Force of Fantasy. New York, Basic Books, 1995

Person ES: A new look at core gender and gender role identity in women. Journal of the American Psychoanalytic Association 53(4):1045–1058, Fall 2005. Available at: http://apsa.org/Portals/1/docs/JAPA/534/Person%20Intro-P.%201045-1058.pdf. Accessed October 2007.

Piaget J: The Psychology of Intelligence. London, Routledge & Kegan Paul, 1950

Piaget J: The Construction of Reality in the Child. New York, Basic Books, 1954a

Piaget J: Intelligence and Affectivity: Their Relationship During Child Development, Revised (1954b). Palo Alto, CA, Annual Reviews, 1981

Piaget J: Biologie et Connaissance [Biology and Knowledge]. Paris, Gallimard, 1967

Piaget J, Inhelder B: Memory and Intelligence. New York, Basic Books, 1973

Pine F: Developmental Theory and Clinical Process. New Haven, CT, Yale University Press, 1985

Pulver S: Psychic structure, function, process, and content: toward a definition. J Am Psychoanal Assoc 36 (suppl):165–188, 1988

Putallaz M, Dunn SE: The importance of peer relations, in Handbook of Developmental Psychopathology. Edited by Lewis M, Miller SM. New York, Plenum, 1990, pp 227–236

Rapaport D: Introduction: a historical survey of psychoanalytic ego psychology. Psychol Issues 1:5–17, 1959

Ritvo S: Adolescent to woman. J Am Psychoanal Assoc 24:127–138, 1976

Rizzuto A: The adolescent's sartorial dilemmas, in Adolescent Psychiatry, Vol 18. Edited by Feinstein SC. Chicago, IL, University of Chicago Press, 1992, pp 440–448

Rochlin G: The dread of abandonment. Psychoanal Study Child 16:451–470, 1965

Roff JD, Wirt RD: Childhood social adjustment, adolescent status, and young adult mental health. Am J Orthopsychiatry 54:595–602, 1984

Roiphe H, Galenson E: Infantile Origins of Sexual Identity. New Haven, CT, International Universities Press, 1981

Ross JM: Trauma and abuse in the case of Little Hans. J Am Psychoanal Assoc 55:779–799, 2007

Rutter M: Meyerian psychobiology, personality development and the role of life experiences. Am J Psychiatry 143:1077–1087, 1986

Sarnoff C: Psychotherapeutic Strategies in Late Latency Through Early Adolescence. Northvale, NJ, Jason Aronson, 1987

Schacter DL: Understanding implicit memory: a cognitive neuroscience approach. Am Psychol 47:559–569, 1992

Schaffer H: The Child's Entry Into a Social World. New York, Academic Press, 1984

Schechter M, Combrinck-Graham L: The normal development of the seven-to-ten-year-old, in The Course of Life, Vol 3. Edited by Greenspan S, Pollack G. New Haven, CT, International Universities Press, 1991

Schneider S: Impingement of cultural factors on identity formation in adolescence, in Adolescent Psychiatry, Vol 18. Edited by Feinstein SC. Chicago, IL, University of Chicago Press, 1992, pp 407–418

Shapiro T, Hertzig ME: Normal growth and development, in American Psychiatric Press Textbook of Psychiatry. Edited by Talbott JA, Hales RE, Yudofsky SC. Washington, DC, American Psychiatric Press, 1988, pp 91–122

Shapiro T, Hertzig ME: Normal child and adolescent development, in The American Psychiatric Publishing Textbook of Psychiatry, 4th Edition. Edited by Hales RE, Yudofsky SC. Washington, DC, American Psychiatric Publishing, 2003, pp 67–105

Shapiro T, Perry R: Latency revisited. Psychoanal Study Child 31:79–105, 1976

Sharff J: Projective and Introjective Identification and the Use of the Therapist's Self. Northvale, NJ, Jason Aronson, 1992

Siegel DJ: Childhood memory. Paper presented at the annual meeting of the American Academy of Child and Adolescent Psychiatry, San Antonio, TX, October 1993

Solms M, Turnbull O: The Brain and the Inner World: An Introduction to the Neuroscience of Subjective Experience. New York, Other Press, 2002

Solnit AJ, Neubauer PB: Object constancy and early triadic relationships. J Am Acad Child Adolesc Psychiatry 25:23–29, 1986

Squire LR: Mechanisms of memory. Science 232:1612–1619, 1986

Squire LR: Declarative and non-declarative memory: multiple brain systems supporting learning and memory. Journal of Cognitive Neuroscience 43:232–243, 1992

Stechler G: The dawn of awareness. Psychoanalytical Inquiry 1:503–543, 1982

Stechler G, Halton A: The emergence of assertion and aggression during infancy: a psychoanalytic systems approach. J Am Psychoanal Assoc 35:821–838, 1987

Stern D: The Interpersonal World of the Infant. New York, Basic Books, 1985

Stillwell BM, Galvin M, Kopta SM: Conceptualization of conscience in normal children and adolescents, ages 5 to 17. J Am Acad Child Adolesc Psychiatry 30:16–21, 1991

Stoller RJ: Primary femininity. J Am Psychoanal Assoc 24 (suppl):59–78, 1976

Stoller RJ: Presentations of Gender. New Haven, CT, Yale University Press, 1985

Sugar M: Late adolescent development and treatment, in Adolescent Psychiatry, Vol 18. Edited by Feinstein SC. Chicago, IL, University of Chicago Press, 1992, pp 131–155

Sugar M: Adolescent sexuality. Child Adolesc Psychiatr Clin N Am 2:407–415, 1993

Sullivan HS: The Interpersonal Theory of Psychiatry. New York, W W Norton, 1953

Tanner JM: Physical growth, in Carmichael's Manual of Child Psychology, Vol 1, 3rd Edition. Edited by Mussen PH. New York, Wiley, 1970, pp 77–155

Tanner JM: Foetus Into Man. Cambridge, MA, Harvard University Press, 1978

Terr L: Unchained Memories: True Stories of Traumatic Memories, Lost and Found. New York, Basic Books, 1994

Tessler M: Mother-child talk in a museum: the socialization of a memory. Unpublished manuscript, City University of New York Graduate Center, New York, 1986

Tessler M: Making memories together: the influence of mother-child joint encoding on the development of autobiographical memory style. Unpublished doctoral dissertation, City University of New York Graduate Center, New York, 1991

Thomas A, Chess S: Temperament and Development. New York, Brunner/Mazel, 1977

Thompson MG: How to support our middle schoolers, grades 4 through 9. Paper presented at the Langley School Parent Education Lecture Series, McLean, VA, March 1996

Tolpin M: On the beginnings of a cohesive self: an application of the concept of transmuting internalization to the study of the transitional object and signal anxiety. Psychoanal Study Child 26:316–352, 1971

Tolpin M: Self-objects and oedipal objects. Psychoanal Study Child 33:167–184, 1978

Tyson P: A developmental line of gender identity, gender role and choice of love object. J Am Psychoanal Assoc 30:59–84, 1982

Tyson P: Affects, agency, and self-regulation: complexity theory in the treatment of children with anxiety and disruptive behavior disorders. J Am Psychoanal Assoc 53:159–187, 2005

Tyson P, Tyson RL: Narcissism and superego development. J Am Psychoanal Assoc 32:75–98, 1984

Tyson P, Tyson R: Psychoanalytic Theories of Development. New Haven, CT, Yale University Press, 1991

Tyson RL: The roots of psychopathology and our theories of development. J Am Acad Child Adolesc Psychiatry 25:12–22, 1986

Vaillant GE: Theoretical hierarchy of adaptive ego mechanisms. Arch Gen Psychiatry 24:107–118, 1971

Vaillant GE: The natural history of male psychological health, II: some antecedents of healthy adult adjustment. Arch Gen Psychiatry 31:15–22, 1974

Vaillant GE: Adaptation to Life. Boston, MA, Little, Brown, 1977

Viorst J: Necessary Losses. New York, Simon & Schuster, 1986

Vygotsky LS: Mind in Society: The Development of Higher Psychological Processes. Cambridge, MA, Harvard University Press, 1978

Waelder R: The principle of multiple function: observations on overdetermination (1930), in Psychoanalysis: Observation, Theory, Application. Edited by Guttman SA. New York, International Universities Press, 1976a, pp 68–83

Waelder R: The psychoanalytic theory of play (1932), in Psychoanalysis: Observation, Theory, Application. Edited by Guttman SA. New York, International Universities Press, 1976b, pp 84–100

Weiss J: How Psychotherapy Works: Process and Technique. New York, Guilford, 1993

Werner H, Kaplan B: Symbol Formation: An Orgasmic-Developmental Approach to Language and the Expression of Thought. New York, Wiley, 1963

Westen D: Towards a clinically and empirically sound theory of motivation. Int J Psychoanal 78(Pt 3):521–548, 1997

Winnicott DW: Transitional objects and transitional phenomena (1953), in Playing and Reality. New York, Basic Books, 1971, pp 1–25

Winnicott DW: The fate of the transitional object (1959), in Psychoanalytic Explorations. Edited by Winnicott C, Shepherd R, Davis M. Cambridge, MA, Harvard University Press, 1989, pp 53–58

Winnicott DW: The Maturational Process and the Facilitating Environment. New York, International Universities Press, 1965

Zajonic R: Feeling and thinking: preferences need no inferences. Am Psychol 35:151–175, 1980

PSYCHIATRIC DISORDERS

8

DELIRIUM, DEMENTIA, AND AMNESTIC AND OTHER COGNITIVE DISORDERS

James A. Bourgeois, O.D., M.D., F.A.P.M.
Jeffrey S. Seaman, M.S., M.D.
Mark E. Servis, M.D.

Delirium, dementia, and amnestic and other cognitive disorders are classified as cognitive disorders in DSM-IV-TR (American Psychiatric Association 2000). As a group, they represent psychiatric disturbances formerly described as exclusively due to "organic" as opposed to "functional" etiological factors. As research into the etiology and treatment of other psychiatric disorders has progressed, the artificial distinction between *organic* (an anachronistic term in current clinical practice) and *functional* psychiatric illness has blurred substantially. Nonetheless, these cognitive disorders generally have clear structural and functional disturbances in brain function as their primary causes. Psychological factors are still very relevant in the patient's experience of symptoms and his or her behavioral and emotional response to illness. Delirium, dementia, and the other cognitive disorders make clear the need for psychiatric evaluation based on the biopsychosocial model of psychiatric illness.

In the management of cognitive disorders, there is a high likelihood of the psychiatrist's involvement with other specialty physicians in the often-complex medical and surgical presentations of these patients. Thorough evaluation of psychiatric, neurological, general medical/surgical, and psychosocial variables is essential to render appropriate care. One cognitive disorder may predispose a patient to other cognitive disorders. For example, it is common to discover that a patient with delirium also has a preexisting dementia. Although delirium, dementia, and amnestic and other cognitive disorders are discussed in this chapter as separate pathological entities, the alert physician must be mindful of the possible comorbidity of more than one cognitive disorder in a given patient.

Recent research and clinical developments have enabled advances in pathophysiology, prevention efforts, and treatments for cognitive disorders. Interventions are now available to significantly reduce the suffering caused by and at times improve the clinical outcomes of these disorders. Skill in management of these disorders is expected of all psychiatrists and is the *sine qua non* of those practicing psychosomatic medicine.

Delirium

Two millennia ago, physicians understood delirium. They knew it occurred in hypo- and hyperactive forms (*lethargus* and *phrenitis*), attributed both forms to brain disease, and recommended both physiological and psychological treatments (Lipowski 1991). In modern times, varying terms have been used for delirium, such as *acute confusional disorder, metabolic encephalopathy*, and *intensive care unit (ICU) psychosis*. The term chosen was often more dependent on the specialty of the physician than it was on the clinical picture itself. Lipowski (1983) led the effort to remedy this by reintroducing the term *delirium* in DSM-III (American Psychiatric Association 1980), departing from the less specific *organic mental disorder* used in DSM-II (American Psychiatric Association 1968). The use of explicit diagnostic criteria in DSM-III and subsequent versions has sought to standardize delirium as a clinical entity. The first practice guideline for delirium (American Psychiatric Association 1999) further enhanced consensus.

Current and future progress is viable due to the robust foundation prepared by thought leaders in delirium, namely Engel, Lipowski, Trzepacz, and Inouye, among others. Novel hypotheses and discoveries from a growing array of delirium researchers are seeking to blend in with the established framework yet simultaneously challenge it where necessity dictates. Fittingly, there has been a global surge in studies since the previous edition of this text, yielding exciting possibilities and hopefully new realities in our struggle to mitigate delirium.

Definition

Delirium is an acute brain disorder manifested by a syndromal array of neuropsychiatric symptoms. Engel and Romano (1959) portrayed delirium as a "syndrome of cerebral insufficiency," analogous to heart failure or renal insufficiency. They were the first to assert delirium not only complicated the treatment of concurrent systemic illnesses but also carried "the serious possibility of permanent irreversible brain damage" in its own right. In other words, Engel and Romano proposed delirium is *brain failure*—a "new" conceptualization fundamental to an updated understanding of delirium.

The DSM-IV-TR model describes delirium as an acute, *reversible* neuropsychiatric syndrome *caused* by general medical conditions and/or exogenous substances. A recent survey (Ely et al. 2004b) confirmed many clinicians believe delirium to be transient and lacking in long-term consequences on the brain. This belief system is in direct conflict, however, with current scientific evidence on several fronts. For one, delirium has been shown to markedly and *independently* affect patient outcomes such as length of stay, subsequent institutionalization, and death, among others (i.e., Edelstein et al. 2004; Marcantonio et al. 2005; Thomason et al. 2005). Equally striking are studies (McCusker et al. 2001; Rockwood et al. 1999; Serrano-Duenas and Bleda 2005) demonstrating new and permanent cognitive deficits *postrecovery* that may be linked to hypothesized pathological processes occurring within the delirious brain (Gaudreau and Gagnon 2005; Munford and Tracey 2002; Pratico et al. 2005).

Clinical Features

Delirium is not always a "fortunate complication" of being hospitalized and seriously ill. The 50% of patients who recall their delirious episode rate the experience as highly distressing (Breitbart et al. 2002a). The families and staff caring for the delirious patient rate their experiences as quite miserable as well (Morita et al. 2004).

DSM-IV-TR Diagnosis of Delirium

The DSM-IV-TR diagnostic criteria for delirium require a disturbance in *consciousness/attention* and a change in *cognition* that develop *acutely* and *tend* to fluctuate (Table 8–1). Lipowski (1983, 1987) characterized delirium as a disorder of attention, wakefulness, cognition, and motor behavior. The disruption of attention is often considered the core symptom. Patients struggle to sustain attentional focus, are easily distracted, and often vary in their level of alertness. Sleep and wake cycles are disrupted as well, with patients frequently having grossly fragmented sleep and loss of normal circadian rhythm. The impairment in cognition can be across a wide spectrum—from subtle to overt and from focal to global. Deficits can occur in perception, memory, language, processing speed, and executive functioning. The reported frequencies of these clinical features are shown in Table 8–2.

Delirium Subtypes

Consistent with the ancient descriptions of phrenitis and lethargus, hyperactive and hypoactive subtypes of delirium have been reported. Liptzin and Levkoff (1992) first characterized delirious patients with restlessness, hypervigilance, rapid speech, irritability, and combativeness as *hyperactive*, whereas those showing slowed speech and kinetics, apathy, and reduced alert-

TABLE 8–1.	DSM-IV-TR diagnostic criteria for delirium due to ... *[indicate the general medical condition]*

A. Disturbance of consciousness (i.e., reduced clarity of awareness of the environment) with reduced ability to focus, sustain, or shift attention.

B. A change in cognition (such as memory deficit, disorientation, language disturbance) or the development of a perceptual disturbance that is not better accounted for by a preexisting, established, or evolving dementia.

C. The disturbance develops over a short period of time (usually hours to days) and tends to fluctuate during the course of the day.

D. There is evidence from the history, physical examination, or laboratory findings that the disturbance is caused by the direct physiological consequences of a general medical condition.

Coding note: If delirium is superimposed on a preexisting vascular dementia, indicate the delirium by coding 290.41 vascular dementia, with delirium.

Coding note: Include the name of the general medical condition on Axis I, e.g., 293.0 delirium due to hepatic encephalopathy; also code the general medical condition on Axis III (see DSM-IV-TR Appendix G for codes).

TABLE 8–2.   Range of reported frequencies of clinical features of delirium

Clinical features	Range (%)
Poor attention/vigilance	100
Memory impairment	64–100
Clouding of consciousness	45–100
Disorientation	43–100
Acute onset	93
Disorganized thinking/thought disorder	59–95
Diffuse cognitive impairment	77
Language disorder	41–93
Sleep disturbance	25–96
Delusions	18–68
Mood lability	43–63
Psychomotor changes	38–55
Perceptual changes/hallucinations	17–55

Source.   Modified with permission from Meagher DJ, Trzepacz PT: "Delirium Phenomenology Illuminates Pathophysiology, Management, and Course." *Journal of Geriatric Psychiatry and Neurology* 11:150–156, 1998. Includes data from Voyer et al. 2006.

ness were designated *hypoactive*. The mixed type vacillated or included elements of the two other subtypes. Hypoactive patients tend to be older (McCusker et al. 2001; Peterson et al. 2006), to have more severe cognitive disturbances (Koponen et al. 1989c), to be less likely to be diagnosed (Inouye et al. 2001), and to have a poorer prognosis (Andrew et al. 2005; Liptzin and Levkoff 1992). The likelihood of developing a particular subtype seems to be influenced by several variables, including age, location, and comorbidities. For instance, more than 80% of delirious patients with end-stage disease admitted to palliative care units in Scotland had the hypoactive type (Spiller and Keen 2006). There does seem to be an overall trend, however, with the mixed type as most prevalent, followed by the hypo- and then hyperactive variants (Peterson et al. 2006; Rooij et al. 2005).

Etiopathogenesis

One key to sustained progress in understanding delirium is a *refutation* of the misleading model wherein de-

lirium is believed to be *caused* by the comorbid systemic disease. We suggest instead that comorbid disease states, environmental stressors, and certain medications may *precipitate* delirium in vulnerable patients. The vast number and disparate nature of the identified precipitants (Elie et al. 1998) innately argue against most of them having *direct* causality for delirium. Furthermore, it is recognized clinically that delirium often persists *well after* the precipitants have been successfully addressed and removed. This occurs most typically in patients clinically estimated to have less cerebral reserve.

We have postulated that precipitants can initiate a cascade of neurochemical and metabolic events in the brain. More robust patients can resist this cascade and not become delirious or, if they do become delirious, recover rapidly and without sequelae. Variations on this theme may exist where selected precipitants have partial causal links, such as medications with hefty anticholinergic or prodopaminergic activity.

Notably, the question remains of how and where to fit delirium tremens and sedative withdrawal states into the larger delirium paradigm. There are behavioral similarities manifested between these clinical states and "regular" delirium, yet neurochemistry, electroencephalographic patterns, and treatments are more disparate than similar. We defer this discussion to other venues.

Neuronal Integrity

Engel and Romano's recommendation in 1959 to examine the functional integrity of the neuron and brain energy metabolism during delirium is still valid. Few studies have sought to further clarify the etiopathogenesis of delirium since Engel and Romano's work in the mid-1940s, perhaps in part due to the practice of deferring to "underlying medical causes." Nonetheless, several hypotheses seeking to elucidate the causative cascade for delirium have been advanced in recent years and are presented in brief.

Role of Oxygen

The clinical importance of oxygen in the pathogenesis of delirium has been demonstrated in several studies. Among *healthy young* adults, concentration and short-term learning are degraded when the partial pressure of oxygen (PaO_2) drops to 45–60 mm Hg, and frank delirium reliably occurs at a PaO_2 of 35–45 mm Hg (Gibson et al. 1981). Delirium would likely have developed at a higher PaO_2 had this study been in a less robust population. In one retrospective analysis of ICU patients, three measures of oxygenation (hemoglobin, hematocrit, pulse oximetry) and two of metabolic stress (sepsis, pneumonia) were worse in patients prior to developing delirium despite no difference in illness severity between groups (Seaman et al. 2006). Not all studies have found these differences, however, and a large, carefully designed prospective study (Agnoletti et al. 2005) is under way to clarify this question.

The importance of oxidative metabolism in delirium is also evident in patients with sepsis. Delirious patients with sepsis have lower hemoglobin, lower cerebral blood flow (CBF), lower metabolic rate for O_2, and lower cerebral O_2 delivery compared with *matched* nondelirious septic patients (Maekawa et al. 1991).

Cardiovascular and Respiratory Reserves

A broad decline in cardiovascular and respiratory reserves occurs with age. By age 85 years, vital capacity is reduced by 30%–40% and the arterial–alveolar gradient widens; by age 90 years, basal PaO_2 drops to 70 mm Hg, the ventilatory response to acute hypoxia is blunted, and maximum heart rate and cardiac output are decreased (Pack and Millman 1988). Oxygen delivery to the brain in times of increased metabolic stress can also be limited by the reduced capacity for compensatory changes in carotid and vertebral vessel dynamics due to vasculopathy. In support of this, Rudolph et al. (2005) found that elevated atherosclerotic scores for the internal carotids and ascending aorta significantly increased postoperative delirium risk. The frail elderly patient, in part by these reasons, can be viewed as being exquisitely vulnerable to sliding into "brain insufficiency" (Tune 1991)—much like patients with "brittle" congestive heart failure.

Oxygen Demand and Anemia

Brown (2000) noted the hospitalized patient's homeostasis is threatened by the increased O_2 demand from acute illness and fever (Fink 1997). Anemia is also commonly encountered among hospitalized patients, which can further limit O_2 delivery to the brain. Of interest, the clinical threshold to transfuse is often based on providing a baseline minimum for the brain and kidneys. Although the "baseline minimum" hematocrit may be enough to keep the brain alive and to avoid watershed strokes, it may *not be enough* to support normal function, particularly for the patient with limited cerebral reserve. As shown later, keeping the brain alive but not at an adequate functional level (i.e., delirium) may have dire consequences.

Anoxia

A proposed causal link between metabolic derangements and the development of delirium has been presented in Brown (2000) and Bourgeois et al. (2003) and is summarized in Figure 8–1.

Additional Selective Mechanisms

In one hypoxic encephalopathy model, dopamine release was shown to increase 500-fold, whereas γ-aminobutyric acid (GABA) release was increased only fivefold (Globus et al. 1988a). This massive increase in dopamine results from a breakdown in adenosine triphosphate–dependent transporters (decreased reuptake) during anoxic depolarization (Pulsinelli and Duffy 1983) as well as decreases in metabolism through the reduced activity of the O_2-dependent catechol-*O*-methyltransferase (Gibson et al. 1981). Another potential mechanism underlying the increase in dopamine is reduced activity of dopamine-β-hydroxylase. This enzyme is also O_2 dependent; thus, in hypoxic conditions, less dopamine is converted to norepinephrine (Gibson et al. 1981).

Perhaps as an evolutionary programmed act of self-preservation, a global shift of CBF and cerebral metabolic rate from cortical to subcortical areas occurs

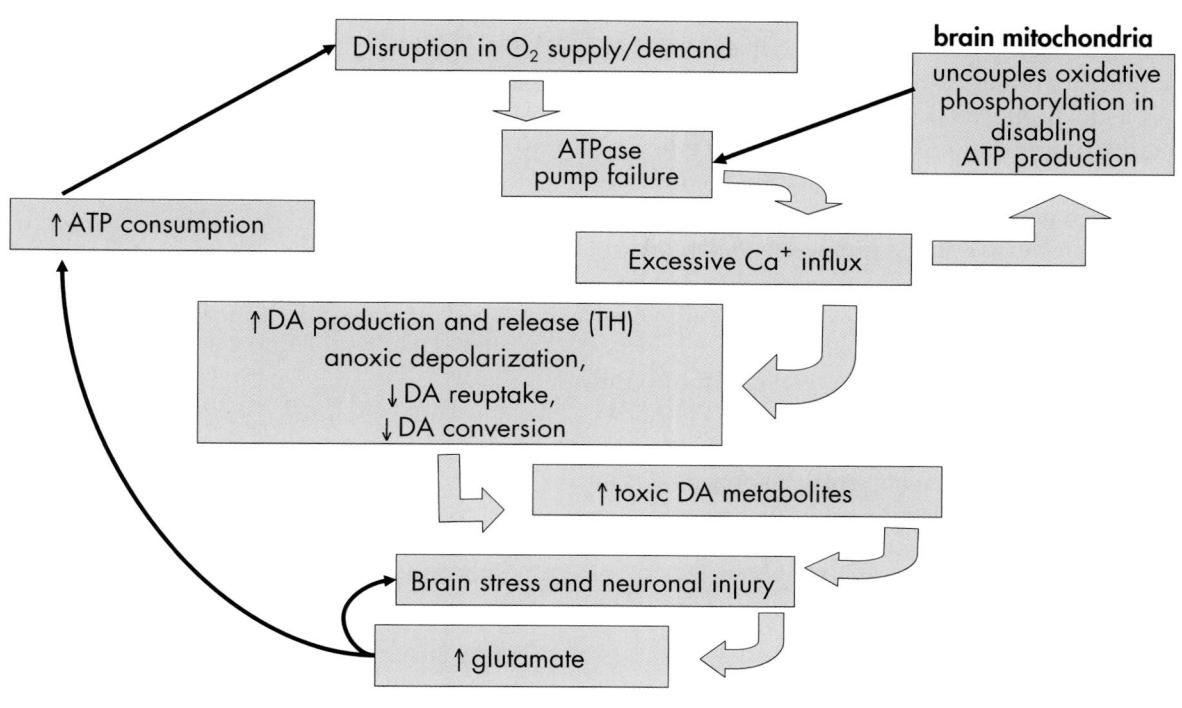

FIGURE 8–1. Hypothesized delirium cascade: dopamine–oxygen link.

ATP=adenosine triphosphate; Ca^+=calcium; DA=dopamine; O_2=oxygen; TH=tyrosine hydroxylase.

in hepatic encephalopathy patients (Lockwood et al. 1991). Regional differences in CBF in subclinical hepatic encephalopathy patients have also been reported (Trzepacz 1994), with the largest reduction in the right dorsolateral prefrontal cortex.

Neurotransmitter Roles

Regarding specific changes in neurotransmitters in delirium, the two most accepted are a reduction in acetylcholine activity and an excess of dopamine activity (Trzepacz 2000). Acetylcholine has long been known to be decreased in delirium (Itil and Fink 1966) as well as in hypoxia (Gibson and Blass 1976). Arousal, the sleep–wake cycle, attention, learning, and memory are heavily dependent on acetylcholine via its nicotinic and muscarinic receptors (Picciotto and Zoli 2002; Trzepacz 2000). Both human (Itil and Fink 1966) and animal (Trzepacz et al. 1992) models of delirium have utilized anticholinergic medications to induce delirium with the resultant hyperactivity, psychosis (humans), cognitive impairment, and electroencephalographic slowing. It is important to note GABAergic interactions with acetylcholine appear critical in serving cognitive and attentional processes (Picciotto and Zoli 2002).

Dopamine is considered to have important roles in attention, mood, motor activity, perception, and executive functioning. Dopamine may be particularly valuable in facilitating cortical circuit activity during times of change, stress, or disequilibrium (Grace 2002). Excess dopamine activity can lead to delirium, as seen with drugs such as L-dopa or cocaine. Dopamine agonists have also been shown to cause electroencephalographic slowing despite motoric hyperactivity (Ongini et al. 1985). Moreover, interplay between dopamine and acetylcholine exists, as evidenced experimentally by the finding that D_2 antagonists enhance acetylcholine release (Ikarashi et al. 1997) and clinically by the utility of antipsychotics in reversing anticholinergic-precipitated delirium (Itil and Fink 1966). Additional potent regulators of dopamine function (i.e., tonic/phasic balance) include complex relationships among $GABA_A$ and $GABA_B$, glutamate, adenosine A_{2A} receptors, nitric oxide (NO), and D_2 autoreceptors (Grace 2002; Williams 2002).

Glutamate excess is notably also seen in hypoxia (Benveniste et al. 1984). The glutamate transporter fails in periods of energy deprivation, with a resultant loss of reuptake compounded by massive glutamate efflux. The excess glutamate then induces neuronal injury and necrosis in conjunction with calcium over-load, reactive oxygen species, and the mitochondrial permeability transition cascade (Coyle et al. 2002). Dopamine excess may also be necessary for glutamate to exert its toxic effect (Globus et al. 1988b).

Gaudreau and Gagnon (2005) proposed a neural circuit, as shown in Figure 8–2, whereby the interactions between neurons utilizing dopamine, acetylcholine, glutamate, and GABA regulate the thalamocortical glutaminergic tract. Sensory overload, confusion, psychosis, and altered arousal levels can result when this tract is in a state of dysregulation.

Future efforts may include investigation into the role of corticotropin-releasing factor (CRF) and its non–hypothalamic-pituitary-adrenal axis receptor, CRF-2. CRF likely has diverse stress-response roles in the brain, potentially including a stimulatory effect on arousal and vigilance via its activation of the locus coeruleus (DeSouza and Grigoriadis 2002).

Melatonin

New evidence has emerged suggesting that melatonin dysregulation may have a contributory role in delirium. Shigeta et al. (2001) found that delirious patients had abnormal plasma melatonin, whereas nondelirious patients did not show these abnormalities. Balan et al. (2003) reported lower levels of the melatonin metabolite 6-sulfatoxymelatonin (6-SMT) in hyperactive delirious patients, but higher levels in hypoactive patients.

Factors associated with decreased formation of melatonin include disruption of the day/light cycle, first postoperative day, corticosteroids, and benzodiazepines. Conversely, sepsis, food restriction, and opioids increase melatonin formation (Bourne and Mills 2006). Elderly individuals are known to have lower nocturnal melatonin levels, which may be yet another factor underlying their vulnerability to delirium. Finally, melatonin and 6-SMT have direct antioxidant activity, stimulate other antioxidants, and suppress NO formation (Bourne and Mills 2006). These properties could have relevance for recovery potential in delirium.

Neuroanatomic Loci

There is no single neuroanatomic locus for delirium, although reports have focused on prefrontal and right-sided brain lesions (summarized in Trzepacz 2000). Overall, delirium may have associations with specific brain regions (i.e., bifrontal and right prefrontal cortex, right anterior thalamus, right posterior parietal cortex, basal ganglia, and lingual gyrus), yet lesions anywhere can precipitate delirium.

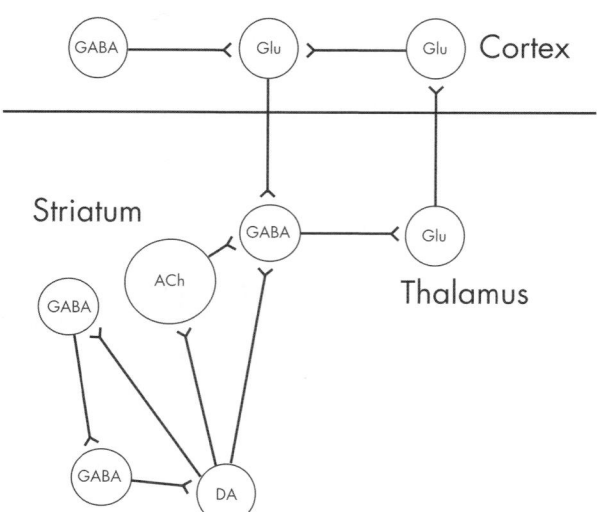

FIGURE 8–2.   Gaudreau and Gagnon delirium circuit hypothesis.

ACh = acetylcholine; DA = dopamine; GABA = γ-aminobutyric acid; Glu = glutamate.

Source.   Reprinted from Gaudreau JD, Gagnon P: "Psychogenic Drugs and Delirium Pathogenesis: The Central Role of the Thalamus." *Medical Hypotheses* 64:471–475, 2005. Copyright 2005, Elsevier, Inc. Used with permission.

Epidemiology

Inpatient Studies

Delirium is epidemic among hospitalized patients, especially in the elderly. Inouye (2006) estimated that delirium annually complicates the hospitalizations of 2.5 million elderly Americans, is present for about 17 million inpatient days, and will cost Medicare alone $7 billion in 2006, *excluding* the substantial postdischarge morbidity costs. Delirium was also shown to *directly* increase hospital costs by 40% (Milbrandt et al. 2004). In a 2005 paper, Pandharipande et al. calculated that delirium may directly increase ICU costs by up to $20 billion per year.

Inpatient studies have reported a delirium prevalence of 12%–40% among geriatric patients (Francis and Kapoor 1992; Inouye and Charpentier 1996; Inouye et al. 1998; O'Keeffe and Lavan 1997), 10%–15% across patients of all ages (Cameron et al. 1987), and 37% among postoperative patients (Dyer et al. 1995). Delirium has been found to be even more common in elderly patients with hip fractures (Gustafson et al. 1988; Marcantonio et al. 2000), hospitalized AIDS patients (F. Fernandez et al. 1989), terminally ill cancer patients (Gagnon et al. 2000; Massie et al. 1983), ICU patients (Pisani et al. 2003), and patients undergoing stem cell transplantation (Fann et al. 2000).

Diagnostic and Liaison Challenges

Most delirium cases are either never diagnosed (Elie et al. 2000; Levin 1951; Rockwood et al. 1994) or misdiagnosed (Armstrong et al. 1997). This is particularly worrisome because poor recognition of delirium is associated with increased hospital mortality (Andrew et al. 2005). Diagnosis can also be difficult because some delirious patients remain "fluent" despite marked cognitive impairment (C.A. Ross et al. 1991). Delirium can also fluctuate. A patient may be in a "lucid interval" for the physician's visit and yet be frankly delirious at other times. Furthermore, primary physicians may feel reluctant to consult a psychiatrist because delirium is often viewed as a syndrome caused by the patient's systemic illness(es). Hence it is the more troublesome behavioral cases that are more likely to generate consultation requests or receive delirium-specific treatment (Engel and Romano 1959; Meagher et al. 1996).

Clinical Evaluation

History

A thorough history provides the majority of the diagnostic information (Table 8–3). Several factors can obscure the clinical picture, however, and thus a meticulous approach is indispensable. The referral problem is frequently characterized as psychosis, depression, noncompliance, or unruly behavior. A savvy consultation psychiatrist can serve to promptly identify and recharacterize the clinical question. Furthermore, the consultant may also be called later in the course of a delirium and thus need to retrospectively search for history and hospital course data.

Central to the history gathering is establishing what the patient's premorbid baseline was, whether a recent change occurred, and when. Not only is this information key in distinguishing delirium from dementia, but it may also serve to identify precipitants. Prime sources of information are those who have known the patient for some time, such as family and treatment team members. Review of the patient's current medical or surgical illness is also essential. Assessment of the treatment environment with a focus on variables that could confuse, disorient, and disrupt circadian cycles is standard. These variables may include visual or hearing aids; light, dark, and noise cycles; communi-

TABLE 8–3. Evaluation of delirium
Standard
Vital signs
Complete history
Medication review: recent past and current
Neurological examination
Bedside testing: months of the year backward (5), verbal Trails B (10), clock drawing, A-test for vigilance
As clinically warranted
Laboratory work: complete blood count, electrolytes, blood urea nitrogen, creatinine, glucose, calcium, pulse oximetry or arterial blood gas, urinalysis, drug screen, liver function test with serum albumin, cultures, HIV screening, cerebrospinal fluid examination
Tests: chest X-ray, electrocardiogram, brain imaging, electroencephalogram

cation efforts and assistive devices; familiar versus unfamiliar caretakers, objects, and routines; and depersonalization factors.

Medication Review

Every delirium evaluation warrants a medication review inclusive of current and recently discontinued drugs, whether prescription, over-the-counter, herbal, or illicit. Medications with anticholinergic properties should be avoided as possible. The potential for drug–drug interactions should be reviewed (i.e., look it up). Adverse interactions include both pharmacodynamic (e.g., toxic synergies) and pharmacokinetic (e.g., cytochrome P450 system induction/inhibition, competition for serum protein binding, decreased clearance in renal or hepatic disease) effects. It is necessary to further consider the unique metabolism or medication sensitivity in special populations—such as the young, the old, and the malnourished as well as those with renal or liver compromise or those with AIDS. Elder patients with delirium have reduced plasma esterases (phase 1 metabolic enzymes). This esterase reduction, in turn, was reported to show a strong inverse relationship with hospital mortality for delirious patients (White et al. 2005). This group also demonstrated that delirious patients have lower plasma albumin and increased C-reactive protein. The C-reactive protein is relevant because inflammatory cytokines suppress P450 enzyme synthesis (Abdel-Razzak et al. 1993).

Interview and Observation

The interview itself should focus on establishing a global image of the patient's cognitive functioning. It is helpful to observe the patient for decreased attention capacity, psychosis, short-term memory deficits, disorientation, executive dysfunction, and changes in mood or kinetics. Bedside examinations (e.g., the A test for vigilance) and tests sensitive to frontal lobe dysfunction (Royall et al. 1998) are quick and easy to administer. These tests have not been validated as delirium screens but can function to rapidly illuminate key cognitive domains. Not surprisingly, one group (Adamis et al. 2005a) found that the clock drawing test was unable to predict delirium when scored with a scheme that correlated with Folstein et al.'s (1975) Mini-Mental State Exam (MMSE) rather than with executive functioning (i.e., the CLOX 1; Royall et al. 1998).

In regard to the MMSE, one study (C.A. Ross et al. 1991) reported the mean MMSE score to be 14.3 for delirious patients, versus 29.6 for control subjects. The first elements of the MMSE in their relatively young cohort to show deficits were the reverse calculation, orientation, and recall items. A single MMSE is not sensitive (33%) for identifying delirium, however, and is incapable of discriminating delirium from dementia (Trzepacz et al. 1986). Serial MMSEs, on the other hand, can help identify improvement or worsening of delirium (O'Keeffe et al. 2005; Tune and Folstein 1986) and assist in delirium screening when baseline MMSEs are clearly known (Fayers et al. 2005).

Rating Scales

Diagnostic and rating tools are critical for objectifying and unifying diagnostic and research efforts in delirium. The most-cited and -validated instruments are the Delirium Rating Scale (DRS) and the Delirium Rating Scale—Revised–98 (DRS-R-98; Trzepacz et al. 1988a, 2001), the Confusion Assessment Method (CAM; Inouye et al. 1990), and the Memorial Delirium Assessment Scale (MDAS; Breitbart et al. 1997).

The DRS-R-98 is a 16-item, 46-point clinician-rated scale. It can serve to diagnose, rate severity, and track delirium changes over time. The best cutoff score is 15 for the severity subscale and 18 for the total score (sensitivity and specificity in the mid-90 percentiles). It has excellent internal validity and has the capacity to discriminate delirium from dementia. This scale is an upgraded version of the original DRS, which lacked expanded functionality for doing repeat measurements or for discriminating motoric subtypes (hypo- or hyperactive).

The CAM is designed for detection of delirium by nonpsychiatrists. It is an algorithm-based tool that operationalizes DSM diagnostic criteria. Sensitivity and specificity are both above 90%, and kappa with the DRS is excellent, at 0.92 (Adamis et al. 2005b). Interrater reliability between trained lay interviewers (Monette et al. 2001), nurses (Pun et al. 2005), and experts is high. The 5-minute CAM-ICU (Ely et al. 2001) can be used for ventilated patients and was found to have a sensitivity of 73% and specificity of 100% compared with the CAM in one validation study (McNicoll et al. 2005). Inouye et al. (2005) also aptly demonstrated the viability of a short chart-based tool for delirium with a sensitivity of 74% and specificity of 83% compared with the CAM.

Breitbart's MDAS is a 10-item, 30-point clinician scale best suited for rating severity. A cutoff score of 13 offers a sensitivity of 71% and a specificity of 94%. The MDAS correlates very well with the DRS and clinician's severity ratings, and the scale is well suited for serial administration. It is often used as a severity scale along with the diagnostic CAM or DRS.

Neurological Examination

Unexplained or new focal neurological signs beyond cognitive disturbances are atypical in delirium and warrant discussion with a neurologist. Neuroimaging should be considered for patients with head injuries, focal findings, cancer, stroke risk, AIDS, and atypical presentations (e.g., young, healthy, lack of identifiable precipitants). Nonspecific abnormalities visible on neuroimaging such as periventricular white matter disease, varying degrees of generalized atrophy, and ventricular enlargement are common among the delirious elderly (Koponen et al. 1989a) and are often described as "chronic, age-related changes." Such white matter disease and cortical atrophy could foreseeably be investigated as markers of reduced cerebral reserve. In line with this, the degree of generalized cortical atrophy has been more closely linked to delirium risk than has the presence of focal cortical lesions alone (Tsai and Tsuang 1979). The question remains as to whether the association between depression and elevated delirium risk in the elderly (Leung et al. 2005) represents a cerebral reserve deficit that is reversible (major depression) or resilient (vascular depression; Krishnan et al. 1997).

Laboratory Tests

Laboratory tests are important but are not the foundation of a delirium evaluation. Tests are thus warranted on an individually tailored basis. Not only is such a practice fiscally responsible, but it also avoids the error of pursuing clinically irrelevant and/or false-positive results. Evaluations may include a complete blood count, electrolytes, blood urea nitrogen, creatinine, glucose, calcium, pulse oximetry or arterial blood gas, and urinalysis (see Table 8–3). Other tests commonly obtained are urine drug screens, liver function tests with serum albumin, cultures, chest X-ray, and electrocardiogram. Cerebrospinal fluid examination should also be considered for cases in which meningitis or encephalitis is suspected as well as for atypical cases of delirium.

Electroencephalography

Utilizing electroencephalography, Romano and Engel (1944) first demonstrated delirious patients had progressive disorganization of rhythms and generalized slowing (Figure 8–3). Delirious patients specifically have slowing of the peak and average frequencies in addition to increased theta and delta but decreased alpha rhythms (Koponen et al. 1989b). This same pattern of electroencephalographic slowing has been elicited in an animal model of delirium (Trzepacz et al. 1992) by decreasing acetylcholine or increasing dopamine activity (Keane and Neal 1981). The pattern is also seen in humans with hypoxic encephalopathy (Engel et al. 1945). The electroencephalographic changes interestingly correlate with cognitive dysfunction and memory and attention deficits but not with psychomotor subtype (Koponen et al. 1989b; Trzepacz 1994). It is also important to realize that there are instances when the electroencephalogram (EEG) may be read as "normal" in a delirious patient but is actually *abnormal* for the individual when compared with the baseline EEG—particularly for those patients whose usual electroencephalographic frequencies reside in the fast range (Engel and Romano 1959).

In contrast to the electroencephalographic changes observed in delirium, patients with sedative/alcohol withdrawal delirium are known to have a pattern characterized by low-voltage fast activity (Kenard et al. 1945).

The EEG is useful in the uncommon situation where one is trying to distinguish delirium from other psychiatric states, for example, catatonia, depression, conversion disorder, and malingering. EEG changes normalize before cognitive dysfunction clears (Trzepacz et al. 1992), whereas cognitive testing remains sensitive throughout the course of the delirium (Trzepacz et al. 1988b). Nondelirious elderly patients can additionally exhibit electroencephalographic slowing, particularly if they have dementia (Obrist 1979).

Differential Diagnosis

Delirium needs to be distinguished most frequently from dementia (Table 8–4). Dementia has an insidious rather than an acute onset, features chronic memory and executive disturbances, and—unless it is Lewy body dementia (LBD) or there is a superimposed delirium—tends to not fluctuate. A nondelirious dementia patient typically has intact attention and alertness. Dementia is also characterized by impoverished speech and thinking, as opposed to the confused or disorganized pattern seen in delirium. "Beclouded dementia" describes delirium that develops in a patient who already has dementia. Beclouded dementia should be approached like any other case of delirium (Trzepacz et al. 1998), albeit with the understanding such patients are highly sensitive to precipitants and medications.

Other possibilities to consider in the differential diagnosis include drug intoxication and withdrawal, schizophrenia, catatonia, and Bell's mania (Table 8–5). A thorough history, physical examination, and toxicology screen should identify most intoxication cases. Stimulants, hallucinogens, and dissociative drugs are commonly abused agents capable of mimicking or precipitating delirium. It is worth noting that agents such as mescaline and lysergic acid diethylamide do not cause diffuse electroencephalographic slowing like that seen in delirium (Engel and Romano 1959). The *first episode* of a psychotic disorder can also be difficult to differentiate from delirium, particularly if the mental status change developed acutely without a prolonged prodrome. Attentional difficulties, disorganization, and diffuse cognitive dysfunction can occur in both illnesses. A trial of antipsychotics and observation may suffice if no localizing neurological abnormalities or identifiable deliriogenic precipitants are present in an otherwise healthy young person. If the cause was delirium, it typically clears rapidly in this population. On the other hand, it is likely the first episode of a primary psychotic disorder if the negative signs of schizophrenia persist with residual delusions or hallucinations, but attention and cognitive function improve. Catatonia can be difficult to differentiate at times, particularly if there are no motor findings (Seaman 2005). Serial examinations, a trial of intravenous lorazepam, and an EEG are often most helpful. Another rare possibility to consider is brief psychotic disorder, a poorly understood condition associated with various stressors (e.g., sleep deprivation). Finally, Bell's mania is a syndrome presenting as an extreme manic episode with the cognitive and attentional disturbances of delirium. History gathering is essential in

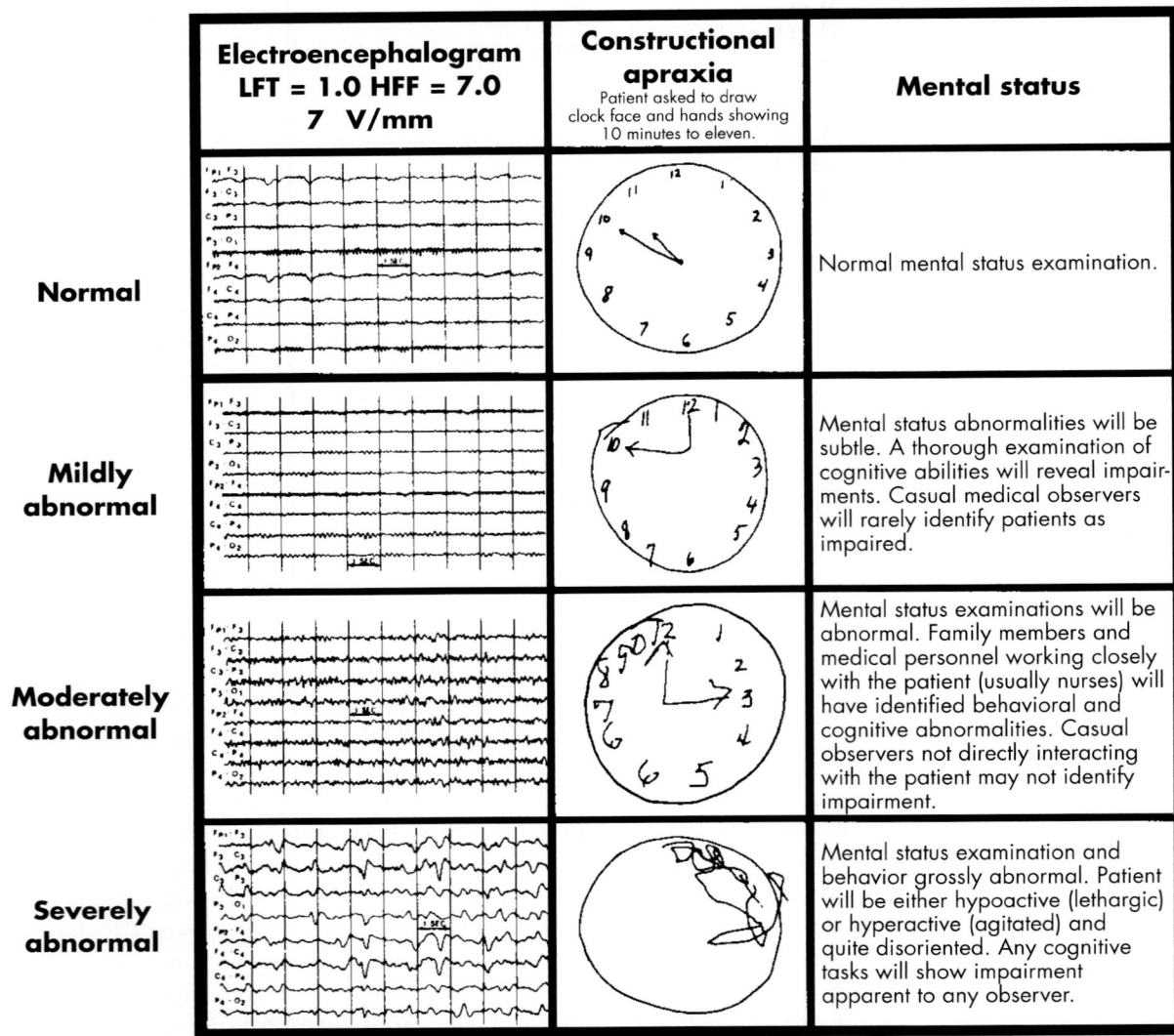

FIGURE 8–3. Comparison of electroencephalogram, constructional apraxia, and mental status in delirium.

TABLE 8–4. Delirium versus dementia

Feature	Delirium	Dementia
Onset	Acute	Insidious
Cognitive dysfunction	Acute/acutely worse	Chronic
Attention	Disrupted	Intact (except Lewy body dementia and end-stage disease)
Fluctuation	Common	No (except Lewy body dementia)
Speech	Disorganized/confused	Impoverished

diagnosing this illness, which is best treated with both antipsychotics and mood-stabilizing agents or electroconvulsive therapy (ECT) (Fink 1999).

Risk Factors: Precipitants and Baseline Vulnerability

Inconsistency abounds in the published and clinical language as to what constitutes a cause versus a risk factor of delirium. This arbitrariness is reflected in the current DSM and in the 1999 American Psychiatric Association treatment guidelines. The phrases "cause," "risk factor," "associated conditions," and "underlying etiology" have been and often still are used interchangeably and without scientific or literary discipline. Critically, the cerebral etiopathology of delirium

TABLE 8–5.   **Delirium differential beyond dementia**

Diagnosis	Similarities	Differences
Depression	Withdrawn, hypoactive	Intact attention, insidious, EEG
Catatonia	Hypo- or hyperactive, odd behavior, limited or no speech	Motor findings, resolves with lorazepam/ECT, EEG
Bell's mania	Hyperactive, confused	Responsive to ECT, other manic symptoms and history, EEG
First-break schizophrenia	Disorganized, poor attention, diffuse cognitive dysfunction	Young age, no precipitants, persistent psychotic symptoms after confusion cleared, EEG
Drug/alcohol intoxication or withdrawal	Hypo- or hyperactive, hallucinations, poor attention	Positive drug screen or history, EEG

Note.   ECT = electroconvulsive therapy; EEG = electroencephalogram.

has yet to be sufficiently elucidated, and thus we cannot identify a cause. The term *precipitant*, however, can be justifiably used to subsume risk factors that are generally transient or acute (e.g., a urinary tract infection). Similarly, *baseline vulnerability* is a term coined by Inouye to describe the risk factors that are, by definition, chronic and innate to the patient (e.g., cerebral atrophy). Echoing O'Keeffe (1999), we advocate there are numerous and widely varying precipitants that can activate delirium in susceptible (high baseline vulnerability) patients.

Inouye and Charpentier (1996) eloquently supported this concept in their landmark 1996 study (Figure 8–4). They separated out baseline risks present at admission (e.g., prior cognitive impairment) from precipitants affecting the patient after admission (e.g., new-onset respiratory insufficiency). Robust patients with less baseline vulnerability ("more cerebral reserve") were more resilient to new precipitants after admission. The reverse was true as well. The more baseline vulnerability patients had, the higher the likelihood they would develop delirium if their frail homeostasis ("less cerebral reserve") was stressed with additional precipitants. Hence, the brain–delirium relationship was demonstrated to behave much like other organ failure systems.

One of the most common precipitants of delirium is medication. Numerous medications across many classes have been noted to precipitate delirium (Brown and Stoudemire 1998). The commonly used benzodiazepine lorazepam has been shown to independently increase delirium development in ICU patients (Pandharipande et al. 2006; Figure 8–5). Importantly, the capacity of a medication to exert anticholinergic activity has been shown to correlate with its propensity to trigger delirium (L. Han et al. 2001). A 1992 study found that 14 of the 25 drugs most commonly prescribed for elderly patients (i.e., furosemide, digoxin, Dyazide, Lanoxin, dipyridamole, theophylline, warfarin, prednisone, nifedipine, isosorbide dinitrate, codeine, cimetidine, captopril, and ranitidine) had detectable anticholinergic effects (Tune et al. 1992). It is important to note although that a single medication may have a low serum level of anticholinergic activity (SAA) by itself, the combined effect of several such medications (Tune et al. 1992) may precipitate delirium in a susceptible individual. One group (Mussi et al. 1999) suggested that a total SAA greater than 20 pmol/mL atropine equivalents confers a risk for delirium. Mulsant et al. (2003), however, reported that a much lower SAA of greater than or equal to 2.8 pmol/mL in community-dwelling elderly increased their likelihood of cognitive impairment (MMSE score less than 24) by 13 times. Last, some general anesthetic agents such as isoflurane and ketamine are potent inhibitors of nicotinic acetylcholine receptors and thus may be pertinent for examining postoperative delirium risk (Fodale and Santamaria 2003).

Prospective studies have identified many other precipitants and baseline risks for delirium (Table 8–6). Two of the most frequently reported are preexisting cognitive decline and advanced age. In a cohort of patients with an average age of 86 years, Voyer et al. (2006) illustrated a dose–response relationship between the degree of prior cognitive impairment and subsequent likelihood of developing delirium.

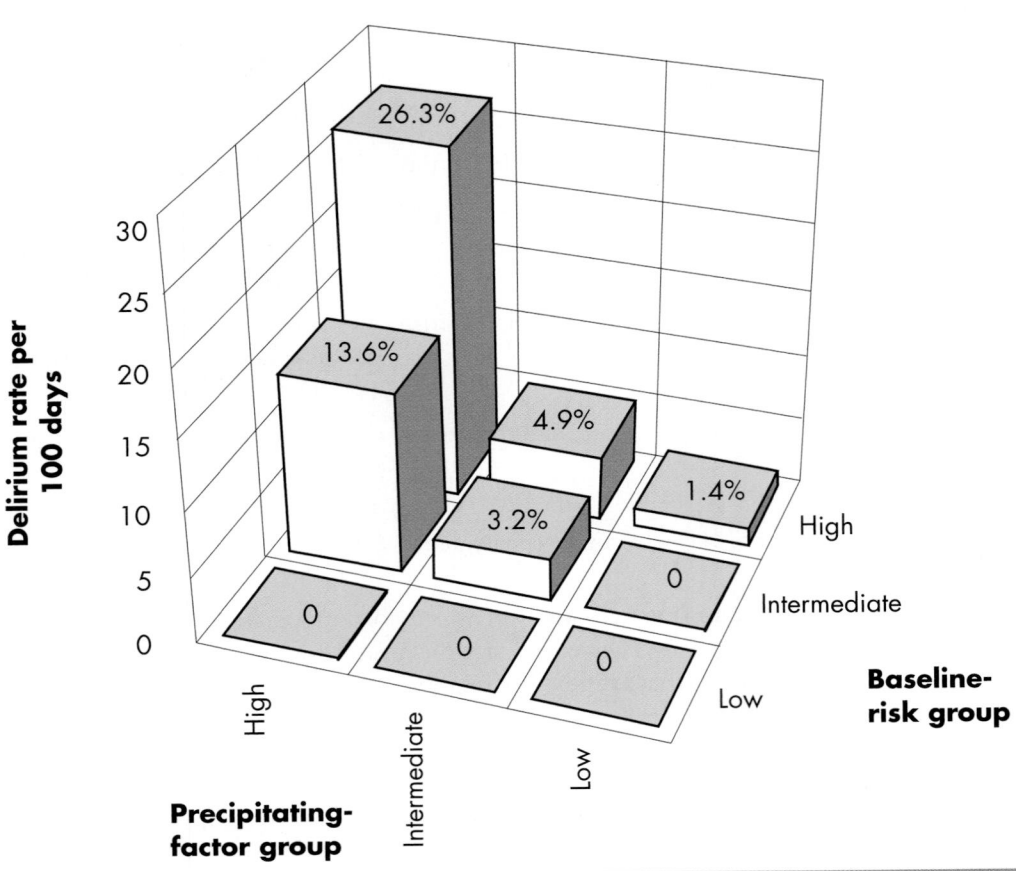

FIGURE 8–4.   Interrelationship of baseline and precipitating factors in delirium.

Source.   Adapted from Inouye SK, Charpentier PA: "Precipitating Factors for Delirium in Hospitalized Elderly Persons: Predictive Model and Interrelationship With Baseline Vulnerability." *Journal of the American Medical Association* 275:852–857, 1996. Copyright 1996, American Medical Association. Used with permission.

Prognosis

Mortality

Lipowski (1983) described delirium as a "grave prognostic sign," and a wealth of published data support this view. Many dozens of studies have reported elevated death rates for delirious inpatients, and a few studies of delirious patients discharged to postacute facilities (i.e., Bellelli and Trabucchi 2006) are now available. When the most robust studies were combined in a meta-analysis (Cole and Primeau 1993), patients with delirium were reported to have an average 1-month mortality of 14.2% (vs. 4.8% in control subjects) and a 6-month mortality of 22.2% (vs. 10.6% in control subjects).

Seven studies have been published that used multivariate and logistic regression analyses to demonstrate that delirium *independently* increased mortality risk in their groups. Caraceni et al. (2000) showed that delirium predicted a shorter survival time in cancer pa-

tients receiving palliative care. A second study (Kelly et al. 2001) found a direct mortality effect for patients whose delirium failed to improve and/or was rated as severe. A group from Taiwan (Lin et al. 2004) found a hazard ratio of 2.6 and an odds ratio of 13 for delirium's impact on ICU patient mortality. Ely et al. (2004a; Figure 8–6) uncovered a 6-month mortality hazard ratio of 3.2 for ICU patients who had been delirious while on the ventilator. Leslie et al. (2005b) strengthened this claim further by reporting that death rates increased in step with delirium severity during the index hospitalization 1 year after hospitalization. A large study from Finland tracked a combined elderly sample (most subjects older than 85 years) from nursing homes and geriatric hospital wards for 2 years. In this group, delirium was an independent predictor of death at 1 and 2 years (Pitkala et al. 2005). Marcantonio et al. (2005) prospectively tracked 504 patients in skilled-nursing facilities. They discovered that 25% of those who were delirious at admission had died by 6 months compared

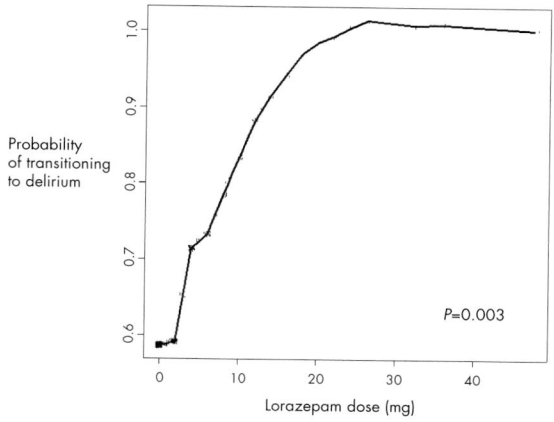

Lorazepam and the Probability of Transitioning to Delirium

Probability of transitioning to delirium

$P=0.003$

Lorazepam dose (mg)

FIGURE 8–5.   Lorazepam and the probability of transitioning to delirium.

Source.   Reprinted from Pandharipande P, Shintani A, Peterson J, et al: "Lorazepam Is an Independent Risk Factor for Transitioning to Delirium in Intensive Care Unit Patients." *Anesthesiology* 104:21–26, 2006. Copyright 2006, Lippincott Williams & Wilkins. Used with permission.

with 5.7% of those without delirium at admission. In contrast, other studies have not found delirium to independently affect mortality in their samples (Dolan et al. 2000; Francis and Kapoor 1992; Levkoff et al. 1992; O'Keeffe and Lavan 1997).

Delirium unfortunately accounts for 10%–23% of palliative terminal sedation, compounding the strain on patients, family, and caregivers (Fainsinger et al. 2000). The Steering Committee for the European Association for Palliative Care recently recommended the inclusion of delirium in making a prognosis for advanced cancer patients (Maltoni et al. 2005). This group included delirium within the top group of clinical prognostic indicators along with dyspnea, performance status, and anorexia-cachexia syndrome. To summarize, it appears delirium likely exerts an independent mortality risk for select populations and serves as a "medical alarm" for many others.

Morbidity

Delirium also often portends poor clinical outcomes. The length of hospital stay is longer (Ely et al. 2004a; Thomason et al. 2005), the readmission rate higher (Marcantonio et al. 2005), and the loss of independent living more common (Adamis et al. 2006; Bourdel-Marchasson et al. 2004; Francis and Kapoor 1992; Pitkala et al. 2005) among patients who had been delirious. These differences persist even after control for variables such as illness severity, preexisting chronic

cognitive impairment, and activities of daily living status. Delirium also independently predicted increased nursing home placements and decreased ability to perform activities of daily living (Inouye et al. 1998; Marcantonio et al. 2000; O'Keeffe and Lavan 1997). Overall, a meta-analysis (Cole and Primeau 1993) found that patients with delirium had a mean length of hospital stay of 20.7 days (vs. 8.9 days for control subjects) and a reduced rate of independent living 6 months after admission of 56.8% (vs. 91.7% in control subjects). The longer length of stay has in turn been shown to increase health care costs for delirious patients (Franco et al. 2001).

Patients who experience delirium during hospitalization also have less functional improvement 2 years after orthopedic surgery, experience a higher rate of major postoperative and hospital-acquired complications, and do less well in rehabilitation compared with patients without delirium (Dolan et al. 2000; Gustafson et al. 1988; Marcantonio et al. 2000; O'Keeffe and Lavan 1997; Rogers et al. 1989). Importantly, Edlund et al. (2001) found that patients who only develop delirium postoperatively have better survival rates and functional recoveries than those who were already delirious prior to femoral neck fixation surgery. Clearly, delirium is not just a marker of poor prognosis but is actually a *vital determinant of hospital outcomes* (Inouye et al. 1998).

These published findings, as well as clinical experience, have led this author (JSS) to doubt the doctrine that delirium is a transient and reversible syndrome. A search for additional understanding on how and why delirium has a profound impact on hospital outcomes and long-term morbidity identified few reports and studies of relevance.

Permanent Cognitive Dysfunction

Clinical studies.   A few authors have suggested that long-term morbidity could be due to cerebral damage from the disease of delirium (Engel and Romano 1959; O'Keeffe and Lavan 1997). Others have speculated that delirium may unmask a subtle, previously unidentified dementia, which would account for most of the functional and progressive decline observed (Francis and Kapoor 1992; Koponen et al. 1989c). Alternatively, Inouye (1998) stated that "the long-term deleterious effects are most likely related to the duration, severity, and underlying cause(s) of the delirium as well as the vulnerability of the host" (p. 757). In the same paragraph, she also noted that future studies are needed to establish "whether delirium itself leads to permanent neurologic damage" (p. 757). Numerous studies have sought to answer these questions, although many of

TABLE 8–6.   Risk factors for delirium

Baseline type (less modifiable)	Precipitant type (more modifiable)
Dementia	Blood urea nitrogen/creatinine >18
Preexisting cognitive impairment	Abnormal Na$^+$, K$^+$, or blood glucose levels
Age	Anticholinergics
Cerebral atrophy	Hypoxia
Illness severity	Windowless intensive care unit
Vision or hearing impairment	Malnutrition
Impaired functional status	Hyper- or hypothermia
Orthopedic, thoracic, or aortic aneurysm surgery	Infection
	Uremia
Fracture	Preoperative depression
Lower education level	Perioperative and intraoperative hypotension
Smoking history	Anemia
Previous delirium	Disseminated intravascular coagulation
Previous stroke	More than three new medications begun
Diabetes mellitus	Benzodiazepines >2 mg lorazepam equivalents
Vascular depression?	Corticosteroids >15 mg dexamethasone equivalents
	Opioids >90 mg morphine equivalents
	Many chemotherapy and immunosuppressive agents
	Many medications with strong anticholinergic activity
	Several Parkinson's disease medications
	Numerous isolated reports of varying medications

Source.   Benoit et al. 2005; Brown and Stoudemire 1998; Centeno et al. 2004; Culp et al. 2004; Edlund et al. 2001; Foy et al. 1995; Francis et al. 1990; Gaudreau et al. 2005; Gustafson et al. 1988; Henon et al. 1999; Inouye and Charpentier 1996; Inouye et al. 1993; Leung et al. 2005; Lundstrom et al. 2003; Marcantonio et al. 1994; Minden et al. 2005; Pompei et al. 1994; Rockwood 1989; Rogers et al. 1989; Schor et al. 1992; Williams-Russo et al. 1992; L.M. Wilson 1972.

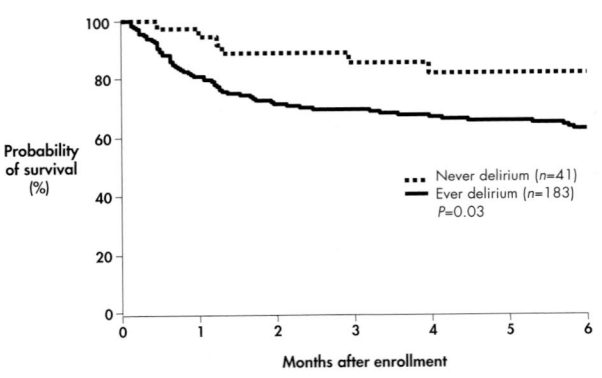

FIGURE 8–6.   Delirium and mortality in intensive care unit patients.

Source.   Ely et al. 2004a.

these efforts have been limited by design problems.

Several groups have reported MMSE score decreases or increased dementia rates for older patients tracked for 1 year (Katz et al. 2001; Koponen et al. 1989b), 2 years (Dolan et al. 2000; Francis and Kapoor 1992; Rahkonen et al. 2000; Wacker et al. 2006), 3 years (Rahkonen et al. 2001), and 5 years (Lundstrom et al. 2003) after an index hospitalization with delirium versus comparison groups. The studies in this set, however, each had several design limitations, such as insufficient measures of cognitive functioning, large dropout rates, insufficient serial examination for delirium, retrospective design, no use of objective rating scales, nonblinded raters, unsubstantiated baseline cognitive status, and unsatisfactory comparison groups. The consistent trend from their reports nonetheless is in favor of cognitive decline.

There are a few studies with more rigorous methodology. Serrano-Duenas and Bleda (2005) tracked patients with Parkinson's disease for 5 years. Only patients without initial depression or dementia were included. For the patients who experienced an incident delirium while hospitalized, their cognitive function declined more rapidly than that of the control subjects over the 5-year span, as did their Kaplan-Meier survival curve. Rockwood et al. (1999) designed a study to examine this question in a prospective fashion, used recognized rating scales, and sufficiently established a predelirium cognitive baseline. They followed 203 consecutively admitted patients 65 and older across a period of 3 years. Nondemented patients with delirium developed dementia at a rate of 18% per year versus 6% for those who did not have delirium at the index admission. Another well-designed project (McCusker et al. 2001) found that delirium exerted an independent effect in lowering cognitive function 1 year after hospitalization, even after controlling for many covariables. In sum, clinical experience in conjunction with these findings suggests that delirium can resolve completely, resolve gradually, or illuminate or *induce* a permanent cognitive disorder.

Hypothesized mechanisms. If delirium can lead to permanent cognitive decline in some patients, it would be worthy to elucidate how this occurs so that interventions can be suitably designed. In hypoxic conditions and during times of excessive dopamine turnover, the metabolism of dopamine shifts to more toxic oxidative pathways, generating cytotoxic quinones (Graham 1978) or reactive aldehyde intermediates such as DOPAL (3-,4-dihydroxyphenylethanol), but this does not occur with other catecholamines. Consistent with this, preexisting lesions of the substantia nigra have been found to protect projection areas during hypoxia (Globus et al. 1986). For these toxic agents to injure neurons, they first must overwhelm the cell's protective mechanisms—for example, superoxide dismutase, catalase, glutathione peroxidase, and reduced glutathione (Graham 1984). It would be valuable to examine whether these and other protective systems are reduced in patients at high risk for delirium and, as Brown (2000) posited, whether these toxic metabolites are related to the permanent cognitive sequelae of delirium.

K. Wilson et al. (2005) reported that delirious elderly inpatients with lower insulin growth factor (IGF)-1 levels at admission developed delirium more often than did control subjects. IGF-1 is important because it inhibits toxic cytokines. The newly coined "cholinergic anti-inflammatory pathway" (Czura et al. 2003; Pavlov et al. 2003) looks intriguing for a role in regulating tissue damage beyond inflammatory diseases, such as for sepsis and organ failure; this could include brain failure (delirium). Essentially the vagus nerve releases acetylcholine, which binds specific nicotinic-acetylcholine receptors on macrophages, which in turn inhibit the release of toxic cytokines, including tumor necrosis factor, interleukin-1, interleukin-6, and interleukin-18. Patients with low acetylcholine or vagal activity could thus potentially be at risk for an excessive cytokine response. As this area of exploration advances, it would be worthy to track delirium, vagal

tone/acetylcholine activity, cytokine levels, and long-term cognitive changes. Pandharipande et al. (2005) intriguingly asked if delirium could also impart its mortality effects in part through this brain–immune system interaction.

The reactive species NO promotes cell injury when activated by tumor necrosis factor or ischemia. One striking study (Harmon et al. 2005) found evidence of greater NO_x levels (stable end products of NO: NO_3 and NO_2) pre-, intra-, and postoperatively in patients who later developed *new and persistent cognitive deficits* up to 3 months after coronary artery bypass graft. NO is also known to facilitate dopamine neurotransmission (Grace 2002).

Duration

Average delirium episodes of 3–13 days are typically reported, although 20 days was the mean in a sample of patients with "beclouded" dementia (Koponen et al. 1989c). Persistence beyond 30 days has been described to occur in as many as 13%–50% of delirious elderly (Marcantonio et al. 2000). Patients with hypoactive delirium have been shown to have longer episodes than those with the mixed or hyperactive subtypes (Kelly et al. 2001). Studies have also noted some delirium symptoms persist at time of discharge in as many as 60%–96% of elderly patients who experienced delirium during their stay (Kelly et al. 2001). One investigation (Kiely et al. 2004) found that half of the 15% patients in skilled-nursing facilities with delirium at the time of admission remained delirious 1 month into their stay. Independent predictors of the delirium persistence included age older than 85 years, preexisting cognitive impairment, and severe delirium (MDAS score >5).

Treatment and Prevention

The precipitant–vulnerability brain-failure model presented earlier can serve to guide modern delirium management. Once the delirium diagnosis is made, the first task of the psychiatrist is to *not* recommend that the primary team "search for an underlying cause of delirium" and to recommend antipsychotics if the patient is agitated. Our first task in delirium treatment is to be a *diligent observer* and an *active learner*. Active data collection enables the physician to more selectively seek to address modifiable precipitants and to choose when and which pharmacological agents would best serve the patient.

Modifiable precipitants may be an undetected urinary tract infection, pneumonia, organ failure, sepsis, select medications, or a host of other variables (see Table 8–6). Anticholinergics, benzodiazepines, cortico-steroids, powerful dopamine agonists, and some opioids are best limited when feasible (Morita et al. 2005), although uncertainty remains in this arena (Gaudreau et al. 2005). The fundamental goal of treating delirium is not to control agitation or hallucinations alone, *it is to prevent and reverse the delirium and thus mitigate associated morbidity and mortality risks.*

Nonpharmacological Interventions

Several comprehensive, primarily nonpharmacological intervention protocols have been published. Regrettably, only a few of these reports are methodologically robust. One large, well-designed study was Inouye et al.'s (1999) Elder Life Program. This prevention program selected 426 nondelirious patients at risk for delirium and sought to address baseline cognitive impairment, sleep, mobility, vision, hearing, and dehydration (Table 8–7). The authors reported a decline in delirium incidence in the intervention group compared with a usual-care group (10% vs. 15%). The cost of the program was $327 per patient; it saved an average of $6,341 for each patient who did not develop delirium. One year after discharge, the intervention group demonstrated a 15% reduction in costs and lengths of stay at nursing homes compared with the control group (Leslie et al. 2005a).

A cleverly designed and blinded study from Sweden (Lundstrom et al. 2005) consisted of delirium education for the medical staff on the intervention ward, with emphasis on recognition, prevention, unspecified treatments, and individualized care. Significant separation between the intervention group and the usual-care group was found for presence of delirium at day 7 (30.2% vs. 59.7%), mean length of stay (9.4 days vs. 13.4 days), *and mortality rate* (3% vs. 15%).

An early prevention study (Gustafson et al. 1991) using the less specific Organic Brain Syndrome Scale described a reduction in delirium incidence, duration, severity, and hospital length of stay for postoperative patients. This protocol consisted chiefly of oxygen therapy and prevention of perioperative hypotension. Cole et al. (2002), on the other hand, found their comprehensive nonpharmacological intervention program to be *ineffective* in reducing delirium incidence. In general, environmental and nursing measures are most valuable in delirium management when they target modifiable precipitants and promote delirium recognition and education.

Pharmacotherapy

Although tailored environmental manipulations and supportive care are crucial, medications offer further advantages. First, interventions directed at delirium precipitants should be instituted. Unless the delirium clears very rapidly or is mild, the concurrent use of delirium-specific treatments is recommended. Elevated dopamine levels are known to occur in delirium; thus, the judicious use of dopamine-receptor antagonists is rational. Although further study is needed, patients with the nonagitated, hypoactive subtype of delirium may be among the *most important to treat* with delirium-specific medication (Platt et al. 1994), considering their poor prognosis.

Haloperidol has been the most studied treatment for delirium. The American Psychiatric Association (1999) practice guideline supported haloperidol as a first-line agent for delirium because of its minimal anticholinergic effects, minimal orthostasis, limited sedation, and flexibility in dosing and administration with oral, intramuscular, and intravenous routes. Both oral and intravenous forms have been used for more than 40 years and have an extensive track record of safety and efficacy in even the most severely ill medical and surgical patients (Cassem and Sos 1978). Haloperidol has also been proven clearly superior to benzodiazepines given alone in delirium (Breitbart et al. 1996).

The recommended dosage of haloperidol (American Psychiatric Association 1999) is 1–2 mg every 2–4 hours as needed, with further titration until desired effects are seen. Once stabilized, patients are often transitioned to a twice-daily or a daily bedtime oral dose, which is then continued or slowly tapered until the delirium has resolved. Patients with AIDS are sensitive to developing extrapyramidal symptoms (Breitbart et al. 1988); thus, low dosages of haloperidol or atypical antipsychotics with lower risk are recommended.

In severe delirium refractory to boluses, continuous haloperidol infusions of 3–25 mg/hour have been used safely (Riker et al. 1994), although the practice guideline suggested a ceiling of 5–10 mg/hour. Electrocardiographic monitoring is recommended with continuous infusion because of concerns about torsades de pointes, although no specific dosage threshold has been designated (American Psychiatric Association 1999; Sharma et al. 1998). Awareness and management of risk factors for QTc prolongation (hypokalemia, hypomagnesemia, bradycardia, congenital long-QT syndrome, preexisting cardiac disease, and drug–drug interactions) are advised (Gury et al. 2000). Prolonged QTc intervals beyond 450 msec or 25% above baseline should prompt a cardiology consultation, a dosage reduction, or discontinuation of the antipsychotic agent (American Psychiatric Association 1999).

TABLE 8–7.   **Risk factors for delirium and intervention protocols**

Targeted risk factor and eligible patients	Standardized intervention protocols
Cognitive impairment[a]	
All patients, protocol once daily; patients with baseline MMSE score of <20 and orientation score of <8, protocol three times daily	Orientation protocol: board with names of care-team members and day's schedule; communication to reorient to surroundings Therapeutic activities protocol: cognitively stimulating activities three times daily (e.g., discussion of current events, structured reminiscence, word games)
Sleep deprivation	
All patients; need for protocol assessed once daily	Nonpharmacological sleep protocol: at bedtime, warm drink (milk or herbal tea), relaxation tapes or music, and back massage Sleep-enhancement protocol: unitwide noise-reduction strategies (e.g., silent pill crushers, vibrating beepers, and quiet hallways) and schedule adjustments to allow sleep (e.g., rescheduling of medications and procedures)
Immobility	
All patients; ambulation whenever possible, and range-of-motion exercises when patient is chronically nonambulatory, bed- or wheelchair-bound, or immobilized (e.g., because of an extremity fracture or deep venous thrombosis) or has been prescribed bed rest	Early mobilization protocol: ambulation or active range-of-motion exercises three times daily; minimal use of immobilizing equipment (e.g., bladder catheters, physical restraints)
Visual impairment	
Patients with <20/70 visual acuity on binocular near-vision testing	Vision protocol: visual aids (e.g., glasses or magnifying lenses) and adaptive equipment (e.g., large illuminated telephone keypads, large-print books, fluorescent tape on call bell), with daily reinforcement of their use
Hearing impairment	
Patients with <7 of 12 whispers on Whisper Test	Hearing protocol: portable amplifying devices, earwax disempaction, and special communication techniques, with daily reinforcement of these adaptations
Dehydration	
Patients with ratio of blood urea nitrogen to creatinine of >17, screened for protocol by geriatric nurse–specialist	Dehydration protocol: early recognition of dehydration and volume repletion (e.g., encouragement of oral intake fluids)

[a]Orientation score consists of first 10 items on the Mini-Mental State Exam (MMSE).
Source.   Adapted with permission from Inouye SK, Bogardus ST Jr, Charpentier PA, et al.: "A Multicomponent Intervention to Prevent Delirium in Hospitalized Older Patients." *New England Journal of Medicine* 340:669–676, 1999. Copyright 1999, Massachusetts Medical Society. All rights reserved.

Other, more rarely utilized agents for delirium include propofol (Mirenda and Broyles 1995), other typical antipsychotics, intravenous ondansetron (a 5-HT$_3$ antagonist; Bayindir et al. 2000), and valproic acid (Bourgeois et al. 2005; Ichikawa et al. 2005).

At least 19 English-language reports are available regarding atypical antipsychotics for delirium (Table 8–8). Only one of those 19 reports, however, was a randomized, double-blind trial (risperidone), and it was powered as a pilot only. Specialists in psychosomatic medicine have been successfully using these agents in clinical practice for the past decade despite scanty literature support and other pressures. The advantages are the lowered risk of extrapyramidal symptoms or electrocardiographic abnormalities (Titier et al. 2004), mood-modulating effects, and possibly enhanced efficacy in select patients. These agents also may exert their effectiveness via blockade at 5-HT$_{2A}$, D$_4$, and α_1 receptors and agonism at 5-HT$_{1A}$ (H.Y. Meltzer 2002). Interestingly, olanzapine, risperidone, and ziprasidone may also enhance net cholinergic activity in the prefrontal cortex (Ichikawa et al. 2002; Parada et al. 1997) via several serotonin–acetylcholine receptor interactions (Kennedy et al. 2001).

Amisulpride, which is not available in the United States, has also been reported to be as effective as quetiapine in an open trial (Lee et al. 2005), with an average of 6 days to stabilization. Overall, there remains a dearth of sound clinical trials to examine whether there is efficacy, let alone a tiered efficacy, for the treatment of delirium with antipsychotics.

Controversy abounds regarding the use of antipsychotics in elderly patients with dementia (Carson et al. 2006; Liperoti et al. 2005), and this was recently fueled by the U.S. Food and Drug Administration (FDA; 2005) warnings regarding increased stroke and mortality risks for this population (Schneider et al. 2005, 2006). This concern has spread by proximity to patients with delirium. Interestingly, a risk stratification has not been found between different antipsychotic medications, inclusive of haloperidol (Herrmann et al. 2004b; Schneider et al. 2005). The pressure *not to treat* and *to limit the treatment* of delirious elderly persons with this class of medications has existed for several years; however, consensus does not seem to have been reached on this issue. The relative risk in treating versus not treating elder delirious patients with antipsychotics has not been sufficiently examined. Based on the stroke and mortality risks ether by the FDA, it may only require small effect sizes (i.e., reduction of morbidity and mortality) to seemingly favor delirium treatment.

Cholinergic Modulation

Shifting gears, Tune's SAA has been used to demonstrate that numerous commonly used medications have anticholinergic effects (Tune et al. 1992). Delirious patients have been shown in several studies to have higher SAA levels than control subjects (Tune and Egeli 1999). An interesting new and unreplicated discovery is of unidentified endogenous anticholinergic substances in hospitalized elderly (Flacker and Wei 2001). Furthermore, there appears to be a substantial interplay between acetylcholine systems in the brain and anesthetic agents (Pratico et al. 2005).

Armed with this knowledge, there has been a resurgent interest in utilizing procholinergic agents in delirium, specifically acetylcholinesterase/butyrylcholinesterase inhibitors. Interest for this treatment option was initially sluggish due to limitations with physostigmine use (American Psychiatric Association 1999) and scattered case reports of acetylcholinesterase inhibitors precipitating delirium (Trzepacz et al. 1996). More recently, there have been several case reports and small case series noting improvements in beclouded dementia (Wengel et al. 1998), opioid-precipitated delirium (Slatkin and Rhiner 2004; Slatkin et al. 2001), postsurgical delirium (Gleason 2003; Liptzin et al. 2005), and antipsychotic-resistant delirium (Dautzenberg et al. 2004a; Wengel et al. 1999). In a progressive study, 5 mg of donepezil daily was not effective in preventing delirium versus placebo in a relatively healthy, low-risk population (Liptzin et al. 2005). These agents may, nonetheless, have a prophylactic role in reducing delirium risk in vulnerable populations (Dautzenberg et al. 2004b; Moretti et al. 2004) or in cases of treatment-resistant delirium.

Duration of treatment is practitioner dependent, with no data-driven guidelines. It has been this author's (JSS) practice to recommend a 50% reduced dosage for 1 week after symptoms improve for those patients with prolonged and slowly recovering courses of delirium or for those estimated to have low cerebral reserve. Patients who fully recover quickly do not seem to require continued antidelirium medications, assuming the precipitants were able to be assuaged.

Prevention

An absolute duty in the management of delirium is prevention (Lipowski 1983). Several studies have identified and tracked risk factors with which to develop predictive instruments, also called risk-stratification models (Freter et al. 2005; Inouye and Charpentier 1996; Marcantonio et al. 1994). Four risk factors—vision impairment, severe illness, preexisting cogni-

TABLE 8–8.   Reports of atypical antipsychotics in the treatment of delirium

	Quetiapine[a]	Risperidone[b]	Aripiprazole[c]	Olanzapine[d]
Number of reports	7	7	1	5
Number of RPCDBs	0	1	0	0
Total subjects	75	163	14	139
Average daily dosage*	118 mg	1.7 mg	9 mg	6 mg
Average dosage range	45–211 mg	0.5–4.0 mg	5–15 mg	2.5–20.0 mg
Average days to response**	6.5 days	3.8 days	6 days	4.8 days

Note.   RPCDB = randomized, double-blind study with a control group.
[a]Reports for quetiapine: K.Y. Kim et al. 2003; Lee et al. 2005; Pae et al. 2004; Sasaki et al. 2003; Schwartz and Masand 2000; Torres et al. 2001.
[b]Reports for risperidone: C.S. Han and Kim 2004; Horikawa et al. 2003; J.Y. Kim et al. 2005; Liu et al. 2004; Mittal et al. 2004; Parellada et al. 2004; Toda et al. 2005.
[c]Report for aripiprazole: Straker 2005.
[d]Reports for olanzapine: Breitbart et al. 2002b; Gupta et al. 2004; K.S. Kim et al. 2001; Sipahimalani and Masand 1997; Skrobik et al. 2004.
*Weighted by sample size.
**Weighted by *N*, best estimates for some reports, response equal to or below scale cutoff.

Source.   Reprinted from Seaman J: "Diagnosis and Treatment of Delirium in 2006." *Psychiatric Times* 23(6):1–2, 2006. Copyright 2006, CMP Media LLC. Used with permission.

tive impairment, and dehydration—were used in one predictive model (Inouye et al. 1993). Nine percent of the low-risk patients (i.e., those with none of the four factors) later developed delirium compared with 23% of those with one or two factors and 83% of those with three or four factors.

Ideally, patients could be quickly screened for delirium at intake (Monette et al. 2001) and scored with a predictive model. Patients would be eligible for prophylactic interventions if judged to be at high risk for developing delirium. Such screening practices would be much like what is currently done to reduce the risks of other illnesses (e.g., subcutaneous heparin for pulmonary-embolus prophylaxis). Candidates for preventive interventions could include both pharmacological and nonpharmacological measures.

There are now two published trials using haloperidol as a prophylaxis against delirium, although both have methodological limitations. The first study (Kaneko et al. 1999) reported that 10% of their intravenous haloperidol group (5 mg/day) developed delirium over 4 postoperative days, compared with 32% of the control group. These investigators did not use an objective rating scale, nor did they report who rated the patients. The second study (Kalisvaart et al. 2005) did not find a difference in delirium incidence with the use of oral haloperidol prophylaxis (0.5 mg tid) versus placebo, but they did find reduced severity and du-

ration of delirium as well as a shorter hospital stay among those in the treatment group. Data confounders were the low dosage and comprehensive geriatric consultations for both study groups, which likely diluted treatment effects. Of interest, several reports have noted that haloperidol has favorable immune-modulating effects (Moots et al. 1999; Song et al. 2000), which may drive the lower mortality of ventilated patients treated with haloperidol (Milbrandt et al. 2005).

Additional hypothesized mechanisms are emerging and may become targets of future biological therapies for delirium. One group (J.R. Maldonado et al. 2003) used dexmedetomidine in a postoperative sedation protocol. They reported a stunning 5% 3-day incidence of delirium in the group receiving the α_2 agonist versus a 51% incidence for those who received standard sedation protocols. A full-scale study is under way at the time of this manuscript preparation. A second group also found dexmedetomidine to be effective in preventing postoperative agitation or delirium in a rare study in children by a margin of 61%–26% (Shukry et al. 2005). The mechanisms underlying the potential effectiveness of this α_2 agonist remain elusive but may be associated with sleep regulation pathways. Additional hypotheses point to the reduced intraoperative anesthetic requirements with dexmedetomidine use and its role in modulating autonomic reactivity to surgery (Shukry et al. 2005).

Finally, as interventions for cerebral ischemia advance, it would seem reasonable to explore their use in delirium as well. Exogenous phosphocreatine delays adenosine triphosphate depletion during hypoxia and doubles the latency of anoxic depolarization, which is intimately linked to brain damage in hypoxia. In one animal model of Huntington's disease, phosphocreatine exerted neuroprotective effects, presumably against N-methyl-D-aspartate (NDMA)–related neuronal degeneration (Ferrante et al. 2000). Efforts to decrease brain metabolic requirements, as well as adenosine-receptor agonists (P1:A$_1$), NMDA receptor antagonists, calcium antagonists, and free-radical scavengers may also be worthy of examination. On the other hand, agonism of some metabotropic (mGluR) receptors for glutamate (Group 2 and 3) may have a protective role in excitotoxicity (Coyle et al. 2002).

Delirium: Summary

The era of contentment with our understanding of delirium has thankfully expired. Aggressive examination of this pervasive and destructive disorder is under way as we question delirium's etiopathogenesis and neurotoxicity, which in turn will inform data-driven prevention and treatment strategies. Continued cultivation of an objectively defined paradigm for delirium may lead us to the day when we can routinely prevent delirium and offer better protection for our patients against spiraling functional and cognitive decline.

Dementia

The dementias are a heterogeneous group of psychiatric disorders characterized by loss of previous levels of cognitive, executive, and memory (anterograde and/or retrograde) function in a state of full alertness. The loss of socioeconomic productivity and burdens to family caregivers are profound. With the increasing age of the population, the prevalence of dementia is expected to double by 2030 (Doraiswamy et al. 1998). Dementia directly increases health care expenditures and complicates the management of comorbid medical conditions. Patients with dementia have increased rates of institutionalization and mortality. The average duration from diagnosis to death is 3–10 years (Doraiswamy et al. 1998).

The biopsychosocial management of dementia is an integral part of primary care medicine, neurology, and psychiatry practice. Dementia uniquely challenges the psychiatrist's diagnostic, psychopharmacological, and psychotherapeutic skills. Because of the progressive nature of most dementias, the likelihood of physician involvement in medicolegal matters such as institutionalization and determination of decreased cognitive capacity for decision making is high. Although the typical course of most dementias is progressive cognitive and functional decline until death, physicians are now urged to view the dementias as treatable illnesses. Contemporary advances in psychopharmacology equip the physician with a greater range of medications to maximize function, delay disease progression, and minimize disruption to patients and caregivers. Early identification of cases is now imperative, given that prompt evaluation and diagnosis facilitate early use of cognition-enhancing and neuroprotective therapies and supportive care to the patient and family. Thorough evaluation and management of comorbid systemic and neuropsychiatric illness are essential to foster the best clinical outcomes.

Clinical Features of the Dementias

DSM-IV-TR Classification of Dementias

According to DSM-IV-TR, core features of the dementias include multiple cognitive deficits (anterograde and/or retrograde memory impairment and aphasia, apraxia, agnosia, or disturbance in executive functioning) that cause impairment in role functioning and represent a significant decline (American Psychiatric Association 2000). Dementia subtypes specified in DSM-IV-TR are shown in Table 8–9. Although the dementias share core features, specific dementia syndromes differ in terms of the sequence of presentation of these and additional associated clinical features.

Cortical Versus Subcortical Dementias

A distinction is made between dementias with primarily cortical and those with primarily subcortical pathology (Table 8–10). Whereas all dementias exhibit the same core clinical features, cortical and subcortical dementias often differ in their specific clinical presentation. Cortical dementia is characterized by prominent memory impairment (recall *and* recognition), language deficits, apraxia, agnosia, and visuospatial deficits (Doody et al. 1998; Paulsen et al. 1995). Subcortical dementia features greater impairment in recall memory, decreased verbal fluency without anomia, bradyphrenia (slowed thinking), depressed mood, affective lability, apathy, and decreased attention/concentration (Doody et al. 1998; Paulsen et al. 1995). Cortical dementias generally lack prominent motor signs, whereas subcortical dementias typically feature such signs (Geldmacher and Whitehouse 1997). The corti-

TABLE 8–9.	Diagnostic features of the dementias

Features common to all dementias:

Multiple cognitive deficits that do not occur exclusively during the course of delirium, including memory impairment and aphasia, apraxia, agnosia, or disturbed executive functioning that represent a decline from previous level of functioning and impair role functioning

Dementia of the Alzheimer's type, additional features:

Gradual onset and continuing cognitive decline, deficits are not due to other central nervous system, systemic, or substance-induced conditions and not better attributed to another Axis I disorder

Vascular dementia, additional features:

Focal neurological signs and symptoms or laboratory/radiological evidence indicative of cerebrovascular disease etiologically related to deficits

Dementia due to other general medical conditions, additional features:

Clinical evidence that cognitive disturbance is direct physiological consequence of one of the following: HIV, head trauma, Parkinson's disease, Huntington's disease, Pick's disease, Creutzfeldt-Jakob disease, or another general medical condition (includes Lewy body dementia)

Substance-induced persisting dementia, additional features:

Deficits persist beyond usual duration of substance intoxication or withdrawal with clinical evidence that deficits are etiologically related to the persisting effects of substance use

Dementia due to multiple etiologies, additional feature:

Clinical evidence that the disturbance has more than one etiology

Dementia not otherwise specified, additional feature:

Dementia that does not meet criteria for one of the specified types above

Source. Adapted from American Psychiatric Association 2000.

TABLE 8–10.	Cortical and subcortical dementia types

Cortical dementias

Dementia of the Alzheimer's type (DAT)
Frontotemporal dementia, including dementia due to Pick's disease
Dementia due to Creutzfeldt–Jakob disease
Dementia due to chronic subdural hematoma

Subcortical dementias

Dementia due to HIV
Dementia due to Parkinson's disease
Dementia due to Huntington's disease
Dementia due to multiple sclerosis

Dementias with cortical and subcortical features

Vascular dementia (formerly multi-infarct dementia)*
Vascular dementia (poststroke dementia)*
Mixed dementia (DAT + vascular dementia)
Lewy body variant of Alzheimer's disease*
Lewy body dementia*
Dementia due to fragile X–associated tremor/ataxia syndrome
Dementia due to normal-pressure hydrocephalus

*Relative amount of cortical and subcortical features is dependent on location of neuropathology.

pairment in addition to the aforementioned "subcortical" symptoms (Cummings and Benson 1988). This is illustrated in some vascular dementia (VaD) syndromes (Roman 2002). The likely functional and anatomic connection between subcortical pathology and frontal lobe deficiency syndromes involves interruption of frontal–subcortical circuits that subsume executive function (the dorsolateral prefrontal–subcortical circuit), behavioral disinhibition (the orbital frontal–subcortical circuit), and apathy/depression (the medial-frontal [cingulate]–subcortical circuit) (Roman 2002).

Cortical Dementias

Dementia of the Alzheimer's type (DAT), the most common dementia, is estimated to affect nearly 2 million white Americans (Hy and Keller 2000). There is an important conceptual and semantic distinction between the DSM-IV-TR diagnoses of DAT and Alzheimer's disease (AD) (Rabins et al. 1997). DAT is a clinical diagnosis, based on the findings of insidious onset and gradual, steady progression of cognitive deficits. Because symptoms and signs consistent with DAT may be present with other types of neuropathology, a clinical diagnosis of AD should be made only after medical evaluation fails to reveal other causes for the dementia symptoms (Rabins et al. 1997). Even so, the clinical

cal–subcortical dichotomy is not absolute, however, because aphasia, apraxia, and agnosia (in isolation) have a low sensitivity in distinguishing cortical from subcortical dementia, and several dementia types may express both cortical and subcortical features at some point in the course of illness (Kramer and Duffy 1996). In addition, the term *fronto-subcortical dementia* is used to describe dementia syndromes with frontal lobe im-

diagnosis of AD can be *definitively* validated only by microscopic examination of neural tissue, typically at autopsy, for characteristic neuropathology (Rabins et al. 1997). A *clinical* diagnosis of AD (after ruling out other dementia causes) is pathologically validated in 70%–90% of cases (Rabins et al. 1997). The reader should keep these distinctions in mind, because many literature references use the terms *Alzheimer's disease* or *Alzheimer's dementia* interchangeably and somewhat presumptively to describe cases that have not yet gone to autopsy. For simplicity, in this chapter the abbreviation DAT is used to refer to the clinical illness that is not yet validated by autopsy, and AD is used for literature addressing neuropathologically validated illness. Established and proposed risk factors for DAT are shown in Table 8–11 (Blennow et al. 2006; Moceri et al. 2000).

Amnesia and other cognitive symptoms may be present early in the disease, although poor insight regarding memory loss is common. Decreased visual attention may be a key factor in cognitive impairment (Rizzo et al. 2000). The patient may become spatially disoriented and wander aimlessly. Apraxias for self-care behaviors may be evident. Deficits in memory, concentration, attention, and executive functions eventually render the patient unable to maintain employment or safely operate a motor vehicle.

The noncognitive symptoms in dementia are also referred to as the behavioral and psychological symptoms of dementia (Lawlor 2004). These include psychiatric symptoms and behavioral manifestations that cross the boundaries of DSM-IV-TR categories of psychiatric disorders. Over the course of a case of dementia, the symptoms tend to fluctuate as the patient's cognitive status changes. Mood symptoms that occur before cognitive deficits may represent a prodromal state (Berger et al. 1999). Depressive disorders have been reported in up to 86% of patients with DAT, with a median estimate of 19% (Aalten et al. 2003; Zubenko et al. 2003). Depression is more common in mild DAT, whereas psychosis is more common in moderate to severe DAT (Rabins et al. 1997; Rao and Lyketsos 1998). Apathy is common and may occur in the absence of full-syndrome depression; apathy, agitation, dysphoria, and aberrant motor behavior all increase with illness progression and increasing cognitive impairment (Aalten et al. 2003; Lyketsos et al. 2002). The construct of "minor depression" (a mood disorder subsyndromal for major depression) with comorbid dementia has been associated with significant psychological and functional impairment (Starkstein et al. 2005). Disinhibited social and sexual behavior, assaultiveness, and inappropriate laughter or tearfulness are common.

TABLE 8–11. Established and proposed risk factors for dementia of the Alzheimer's type

Increased age
Female gender
Head trauma
Small head size
Family history
Low childhood intelligence
Limited education
Childhood rural residence
Large sibships
Smoking
Never having married
Depression
Diabetes mellitus
Increased total cholesterol
Vascular disease
Hypertension
Increased platelet membrane fluidity
Apolipoprotein E (APOE) ε4 allele on chromosome 19
Abnormalities on chromosomes 1, 6, 12, 14, and 21
Trisomy 21

Evening agitation ("sundowning") may be a notably disruptive symptom and has been linked to disturbed circadian rhythms and a phase delay of body temperature in DAT (Volicer et al. 2001). Other motor symptoms include motor slowing, extrapyramidal symptoms, gait disturbances, dysarthria, myoclonus, and seizures (Goldman et al. 1999; Rabins et al. 1997). Parkinsonian symptoms are associated with a more rapid progression of the disease (R.S. Wilson et al. 2000).

Psychosis is common in DAT; the early appearance of psychosis correlates with more rapid cognitive decline (Ropacki and Jeste 2005; Wilkosz et al. 2006). Visual hallucinations are the most common perceptual disturbance (Class et al. 1997). The prevalence of delusions in DAT is as high as 73%; delusions of persecution, theft, reference, and jealousy are common (Rao and Lyketsos 1998; Ropacki and Jeste 2005). Wilkosz et al. (2006) have proposed a model of psychosis in DAT with two distinct subtypes: one with persecutory delusions and the other characterized by misidentification delusions and hallucinations. Depression, behavioral disturbances, and psychosis are often recurrent.

The neuropathology of AD includes β-amyloid deposits, neuritic plaques, and neurofibrillary tangles (NFTs; Figure 8–7) (Felician and Sandson 1999; Jellinger 1996). Amyloid precursor protein (APP, coded on chromosome 21) is cleaved by proteases (β and γ secretases), producing insoluble β-amyloid (Haass and De Strooper 1999; Jellinger 1996). APP processing may be partially controlled by cholinergic mechanisms (Small 1998b). Inhibition of β and γ secretases and presenilin proteins 1 and 2 (proteins coded for on chromosomes 1 and 14, respectively, which appear to modulate secretase activity) may decrease cleavage of APP, thereby decreasing production of insoluble β-amyloid (Haass and De Strooper 1999).

β-Amyloid activates macrophages and microglia, producing inflammation that accelerates neuronal damage, although β-amyloid has itself been reported to be toxic to cultured neurons (Breitner 1996; Smits et al. 2000). Oxidative stress appears to increase the rate of neuronal death; this process may be blocked by vitamin E (Felician and Sandson 1999). Increased CSF prostaglandin E2 has been found in AD, supporting the possibility that prostaglandin production may play a significant role in the pathogenesis of illness; this process might be blocked by the use of nonsteroidal anti-inflammatory drugs (Montine et al. 1999). Amyloid deposition in cerebral vessels is also seen (Cummings et al. 1998).

Diffuse plaques are β-amyloid depositions without surrounding neuronal degeneration (Felician and Sandson 1999). *Neuritic plaques* (a core of β-amyloid surrounded by dystrophic neurites) are surrounded by immune-activated microglia and reactive astrocytes (Felician and Sandson 1999; Smits et al. 2000). Neuritic plaque density is increased in several regions of the cortex, hippocampus, entorhinal cortex, amygdala, and cerebral vessels in AD and continues to increase with disease progression (Felician and Sandson 1999; Haroutunian et al. 1998).

NFTs, intraneuronal bundles of phosphorylated tau proteins, are an early pathological change in the hippocampus, amygdala, and entorhinal cortex (Felician and Sandson 1999). Dementia severity is proportional to the density of NFTs (Felician and Sandson 1999; Jellinger 1996). With accumulated neuron damage, presynaptic terminal density is decreased (Cummings et al. 1998). The pathophysiological events in AD are represented schematically in Figure 8–8 (Felician and Sandson 1999).

The apolipoprotein E (APOE) ε4 allele on chromosome 19 affects the rate of β-amyloid production and the clinical manifestations of AD in a dose-dependent fashion; homozygotes have a higher risk, earlier onset, and faster rate of decline than do heterozygotes and noncarriers (Blennow et al. 2006; Caselli et al. 1999; Craft et al. 1998). Adults without dementia who carried the APOE ε4 allele were found to exhibit decreased verbal memory performance and minor hippocampal damage (Bottino and Almeida 1997; Small

et al. 1999). The APOE ε2 allele may confer protection against AD, whereas the APOE ε3 allele appears to not change AD risk (Rebeck and Hyman 1999).

The hippocampus is an early locus of pathology in AD. There is a correlation between hippocampal neuron and volume loss and an increase in hippocampal NFTs (Bobinski et al. 1996). This suggests that hippocampal atrophy in AD is due to primary neurofibrillary pathology, because hippocampal volume decreases were not correlated with an increased density of amyloid plaques. Volumetric measurements of the hippocampus on magnetic resonance imaging (MRI) predict memory loss in both normal aging and AD (Jack et al. 2000; Petersen et al. 2000).

Central cholinergic hypofunction follows neuronal loss in the nucleus basalis of Meynert, medial septum, and diagonal band of Broca (collectively part of the cholinergic basal forebrain), clinically correlating with decreased attention and memory (Whitehouse 1986). Decreased central acetylcholinesterase activity has been found on positron emission tomography (PET) scanning in AD (Kuhl et al. 1999). With progression of AD, a deficiency in central cholinergic function leads to a relative hyperdopaminergic condition correlating with the emergence of psychotic symptoms (Rao and Lyketsos 1998). The connections between the hippocampus and adjacent temporal lobe structures and those between the basal forebrain and the rest of the cortex suffer disproportionate degeneration in AD (Geula 1998).

Other neurotransmitter systems affected in AD include serotonin (neuronal loss and NFTs in the dorsal raphe and central septal nucleus) and norepinephrine (neuronal loss in the locus coeruleus with compensatory increased noradrenergic metabolism and/or hypersensitive noradrenergic autoreceptors) (Herrmann et al. 2004a). In one study, AD patients demonstrated lower $5-HT_{2A}$ receptor binding in the anterior cingulate, prefrontal cortex, and sensorimotor cortex on PET scanning, consistent with serotonergic neuronal degeneration (C.C. Meltzer et al. 1999). Noradrenergic dysregulation in DAT may be implicated in many of the behavioral sequelae, including depression, aggression/agitation, and psychosis (Herrmann et al. 2004a).

Later stages of AD affect various areas of the cortex, forming the anatomic substrates for clinical deficits in construction, language, and problem solving (Paulsen et al. 1995). Delacourte et al. (1999) demonstrated a temporal and spatial sequence of neurofibrillary degeneration in AD as follows: initial changes in the transentorhinal cortex; then the entorhinal cortex, hippocampus, anterior inferior and medium temporal

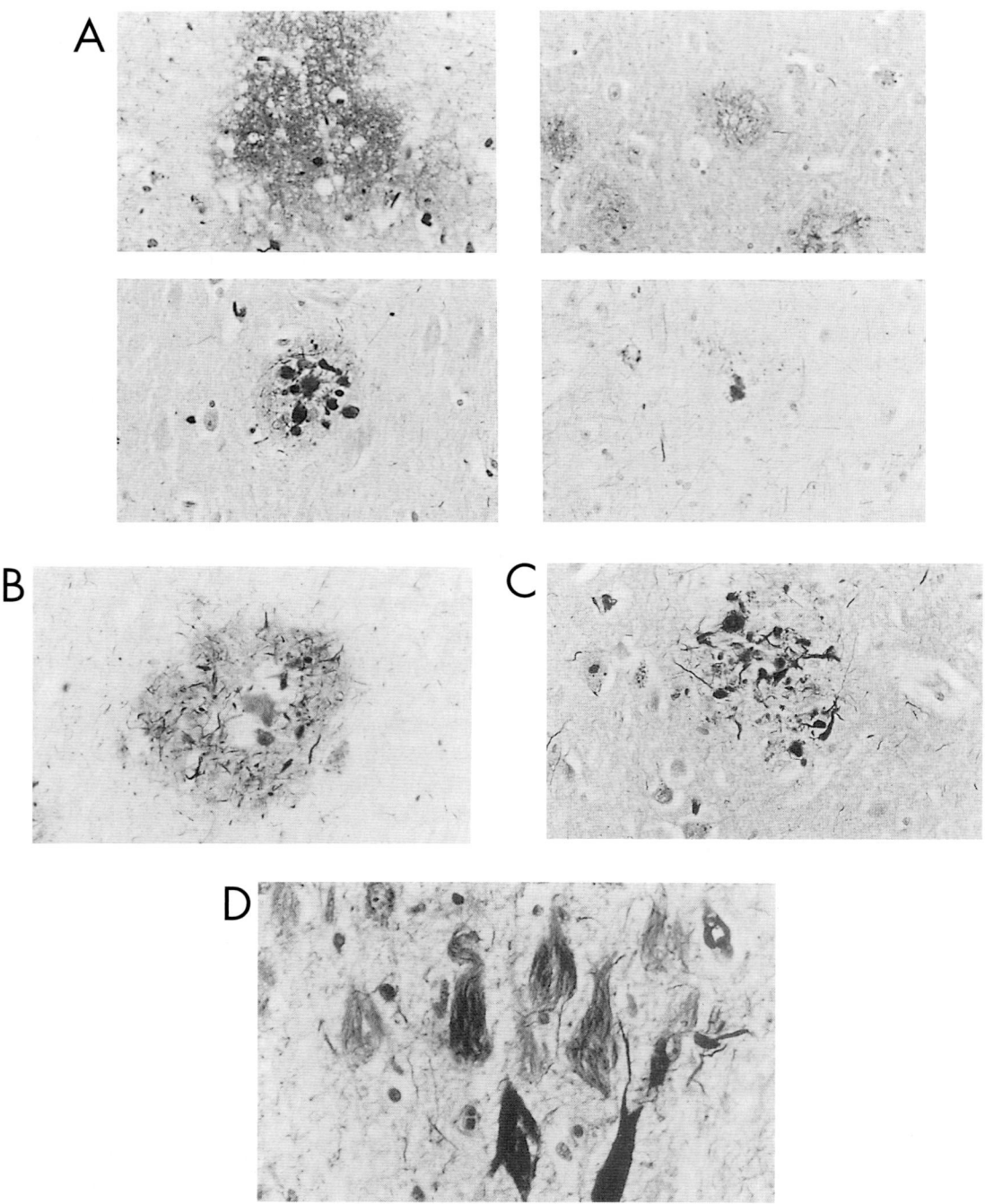

FIGURE 8–7.   Histopathology images: β-amyloid plaques, neuritic plaques, and neurofibrillary tangles in Alzheimer's disease.

A, Four recognized stages of neuritic plaque development revealed by the Bielschowsky silver technique. *Top left:* Diffuse plaque composed mostly of β-amyloid (Aβ) peptide without increased density of neurites. *Top right:* Primitive plaque consisting of Aβ peptide accumulation and increased numbers of nonenlarged neurites. *Bottom left:* Mature plaque with a densely stained central Aβ amyloid core surrounded by greatly enlarged dystrophic neurites. *Bottom right:* Burned-out (end-stage) plaque consisting of an isolated mass of Aβ amyloid. **B,** The classic mature neuritic plaque, about 100 μm in diameter, containing a pale staining amyloid core at its center that is surrounded by a halo of dystrophic (enlarged) neurites. Bielschowsky silver technique. **C,** A mature neuritic plaque with enlarged dystrophic neurites but no amyloid core. **D,** High magnification view of neurofibrillary tangles, which appear coarse and stain darkly by the Bielschowsky silver technique.

Source.   Reprinted from Davis RL, Robertson DM (eds): *Textbook of Neuropathology,* 3rd Edition, Baltimore, MD, Williams & Wilkins, 1997. Copyright 1997, Williams & Wilkins. Used with permission.

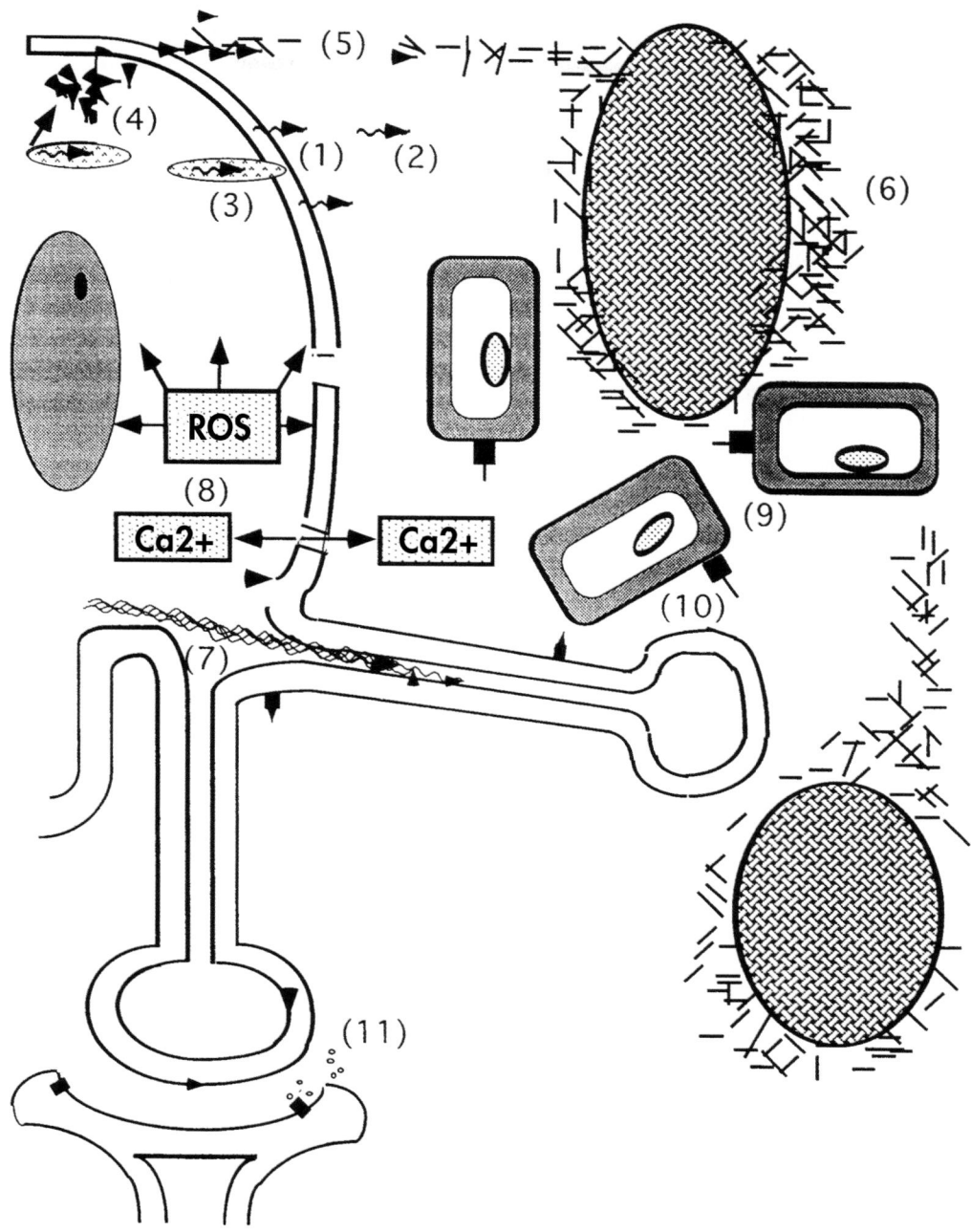

FIGURE 8–8.   Schematic view of the main pathological events in Alzheimer's disease.

Amyloid precursor protein (APP) *(1)* is released into the media after cleavage by α-secretase to form the soluble α APP *(2)*. Conversely, APP may be internalized *(3)* and cleaved by β- and γ-secretases to form β-amyloid (Aβ) fragments *(4)*. The protein Aβ aggregates *(5)* in fibrillar nonsoluble material to compose the core of the neuritic plaque *(6)*. Neurofibrillary tangles form *(7)*. The neurotoxicity of tau and amyloid results in oxidative stress, with increased intracellular reactive oxygen species (ROS), and disruption of structures involved in ion homeostasis such as ion-motive adenosine triphosphatases *(8)*. Inflammatory responses with reactive glial cells *(9)* lead to production of cytokines and complement. Possibly playing key roles are membrane receptors such as class A scavenger receptor or receptor for advanced glycation end products *(10)*. Global decrease occurs in neurotransmitters, including acetylcholine *(11)*. *Potential pharmacological targets:* β-amyloid protein metabolism *(1– 5)* and aggregation *(6)*; tau protein metabolism *(7)*; oxidative stress, acting via calcium channels *(8)*; inflammatory response *(9, 10)*; neurotransmitter modulation *(11)*; and neuroprotection.

Source.   Reprinted with permission from Felician O, Sandson TA: "The Neurobiology and Pharmacotherapy of Alzheimer's Disease." *Journal of Neuropsychiatry and Clinical Neuroscience* 11:19–31, 1999. Copyright 1999, American Psychiatric Press, Inc.

cortex, polymodal association areas, unimodal areas, and primary motor or sensory areas; and, finally, all remaining neocortical areas. Volumes of the hippocampus, parahippocampal gyrus, fusiform gyrus, medial inferior and superior temporal gyrus, and cortex have been shown to be smaller in patients with AD than in control subjects (Bottino and Almeida 1997).

Reduced activation of the bilateral mid-inferotemporal and posterior inferotemporal regions on functional MRI has been reported in normal subjects at high genetic risk for AD (Smith et al. 1999). In the parietal cortex, patients with AD were found to have decreased glucose metabolism both at rest and after stimulation, whereas the relatively more preserved areas of the visual and auditory cortex showed decreased glucose metabolism only under stimulation (Pietrini et al. 1999). Reduced temporoparietal cortex blood volume has also been reported (Harris et al. 1996). Functional impairment of the parietal-occipital cortex has been demonstrated in a study examining visuospatial perception in AD (Tetewsky and Duffy 1999). Abnormal occipital cortex function has been reported in AD on the basis of reduced regional cortical blood flow observed during PET scanning (Mentis et al. 1996).

Higher educational attainment may lead to cognitive reserve that operates to forestall the clinical onset of memory decline in incipient AD (Stern et al. 1999). This "cognitive reserve" concept was supported in a study using PET scanning (Alexander et al. 1997). For equal levels of dementia severity, patients with higher levels of premorbid intellectual function showed greater decreases in cerebral metabolism in the prefrontal, premotor, and left superior parietal association areas.

Frontotemporal dementia (FTD), including dementia due to Pick's disease, features an earlier age at onset than DAT, executive dysfunction, attentional deficits, loss of insight, aphasia, and personality changes (typically increased extroversion) with relatively spared memory and visuospatial functions (Boeve 2006; Kertesz and Munoz 2002; Mendez et al. 2006). Patients may exhibit "childlike" exuberance, "catastrophic" reactions to trivial events, decreased social awareness, disinhibition, distractibility, aphasia, perseveration, carbohydrate cravings, and frontal lobe release signs and may have a poorer response to cholinesterase inhibitors than do patients with AD (Duara et al. 1999; Kertesz and Munoz 2002). Consensus criteria for the diagnosis of FTD have been developed that include the following core diagnostic features: insidious onset and gradual progression, early decline in social interpersonal conduct, early impairment in regu-

lation of personal conduct, early emotional blunting, and early loss of insight (Neary et al. 1998). FTD patients' deficits on full neuropsychological assessment include tests of complex executive function, such as the Wisconsin Card Sorting Test and the Stroop test (Kertesz and Munoz 2002). Neuropathological findings in FTD are restricted to the frontal and anterior temporal lobes and include characteristic Pick inclusion bodies, NFTs, and ballooned cells, all containing tau protein (Jellinger 1996; Kertesz and Munoz 2002).

Dementia due to Creutzfeldt-Jakob disease (CJD), also called "spongiform encephalopathy," is a prion-mediated infection. It manifests as a rapidly progressive cortical dementia accompanied by myoclonus and may first appear with psychosis (Dunn et al. 1999; Zerr et al. 2000). In patients with CJD, the EEG shows a characteristic pattern of repetitive sharp waves or slow spikes followed by synchronous triphasic sharp waves (Dunn et al. 1999; Zerr et al. 2000). In classic CJD, the cortex is diffusely affected, with a general loss of cortical substance and a spongy atrophic appearance (Dunn et al. 1999).

Dementia due to chronic subdural hematoma may present with focal neurological signs, personality changes, various cognitive impairments (including decreased memory, language disturbances, difficulty with abstraction, problems with calculation, and poor social judgment), lethargy, and/or agitation (G. W. Ross and Bowen 2002). The syndrome may have a relatively sudden onset and may show fluctuation in clinical status; a history of trauma may be absent in one-third of affected patients (G. W. Ross and Bowen 2002).

Subcortical Dementias

Dementia due to HIV initially manifests as decreases in psychomotor and information processing speed, verbal memory, learning efficiency, and fine motor function with later cortical symptoms of decreased executive function, aphasia, apraxia, and agnosia (Maldonado et al. 2000). In advanced stages, ataxia, spasticity, increased muscle tone, and incontinence may develop (Maldonado et al. 2000). Dementia has been reported in up to 30% of HIV-positive patients, may present early in the course of illness, increases suicide risk, and may compromise compliance with antiviral regimens (Cohen and Jacobson 2000; Maldonado et al. 2000). More recent estimates of the incidence of dementia due to HIV are somewhat lower, possibly due to the neuroprotective effects of early, aggressive antiviral treatment (d'Arminio Monforte et al. 2000; Goodkin et al. 2001). Dementia due to HIV results from neurotoxicity mediated by HIV-infected macrophages (which serve as the site for viral replication) (McDaniel et al. 2000; Smits et al. 2000).

Dementia due to Parkinson's disease (PD) is seen in as many as 60% of patients with PD and features bradyphrenia, apathy, poor retrieval memory, decreased verbal fluency, and attention deficits (Levy and Cummings 2000; Marsh 2000). Although dementia due to PD is classified as a primarily subcortical dementia, cortical symptoms of executive dysfunction, visuospatial impairment, agnosia, anomia, aphasia, and apraxia may be seen in patients with PD dementia who develop cortical Lewy bodies (Hurtig et al. 2000; Levy and Cummings 2000). Increased age, greater severity of neurological symptoms, and the APOE ε2 allele have been associated with an increased risk of dementia in patients with PD (Harhangi et al. 2000; Hughes et al. 2000). Cognition may improve with treatment for the common comorbid mood disorders (Levy and Cummings 2000). Psychosis can be induced by antiparkinsonian treatment of the motor symptoms of PD. Dementia due to PD features deposition of α-synuclein or tau protein in the substantia nigra and commonly involves Lewy bodies in the substantia nigra, cortex, and subcortex, with resulting deficits in dopaminergic, noradrenergic, cholinergic, and serotonergic neurotransmission (Levy and Cummings 2000; Marsh 2000).

Dementia due to Huntington's disease features abulia and impairments in retrieval memory, cognitive speed, concentration, verbal learning, and cognitive flexibility (Boeve 2006; Ranen 2000). With progression, more global impairment in memory, visuospatial function, and executive function may follow (Ranen 2000). Comorbid mood disturbance, anxiety (including obsessive-compulsive symptoms), and psychotic symptoms are common (Boeve 2006; Tost et al. 2004). These patients have a high risk for personality change, irritability, aggressive behavior, and suicide (Ranen 2000; Rosenblatt and Leroi 2000). The dementia results from cell loss in primary sensory and association areas, entorhinal cortex, caudate nucleus, and putamen (Jellinger 1996; Ranen 2000).

Dementia due to multiple sclerosis is seen in as many as 65% of multiple sclerosis patients (Schwid et al. 2000). Clinical features include deficits in memory, attention, information processing speed, learning, and executive functions; language and verbal intelligence are relatively spared (Schwid et al. 2000). Cognitive impairment may present early in the course of multiple sclerosis, and progression is roughly proportional to the number of central nervous system (CNS) demyelinating lesions (Schwid et al. 2000).

Dementias With Cortical and Subcortical Features

VaD broadly includes dementias resulting from vascular pathology that have as a final common pathway the loss of functional cortex. Because VaD exists on a continuum extending from the essentially subcortical pathology formerly described as "multi-infarct dementia" to the primarily cortical pathology in "poststroke dementia" (i.e., dementia following a single stroke), it is problematic to attempt to fit all VaDs (thus inclusively defined) into the "cortical versus subcortical" dichotomy. This already problematic distinction between multi- and single-infarct dementias is further obscured by the inclusion of dementia following a single stroke within the classification of VaD in much of the clinical literature (Kaye 1998). In other literature, the term *vascular dementia* generally refers to dementia following multiple infarcts. Even DSM-IV-TR is somewhat equivocal on this issue; the heading of "Vascular Dementia (Formerly Multi-Infarct Dementia)" would implicitly exclude dementia following a single stroke, yet the detailed diagnostic criteria for VaD in DSM-IV-TR would include it. A reasonable (albeit cumbersome) solution would be for clinicians to describe all dementias due to vascular pathology as "vascular dementia," with further specification as "multi-infarct" or "poststroke" as appropriate to the clinical situation, remaining mindful of the semantic imprecision in the clinical literature.

Additionally, the boundary between AD and the broad category of VaD is itself quite permeable. The term "mixed dementia" is used to describe cases with co-existing DAT and VaD (Langa et al. 2004). It has been estimated that approximately 25% of DAT cases also feature concurrent vascular pathology and could be reasonably classified as mixed dementia (Langa et al. 2004). Cerebral infarcts in established AD are associated with greater overall severity of dementia and poorer neuropsychological testing performance (Heyman et al. 1999). The distinction between AD and VaD is further complicated by the findings of Zhu et al. (2000) that mild dementia and cognitive impairment are themselves associated with an increased risk of stroke in subjects older than age 75 years.

Multi-infarct VaD is characterized by abrupt onset, decreased executive functioning, gait disturbance, affective lability, and parkinsonian symptoms (Choi et al. 2000; Patterson et al. 1999). Risk factors include increased age, hypertension, diabetes mellitus, atherosclerotic heart disease, hypertriglyceridemia, and hyperlipidemia (Curb et al. 1999; G.W. Ross et al. 1999). Because the cognitive deficits follow a series of discrete lesions, progression is "stepwise," with relative

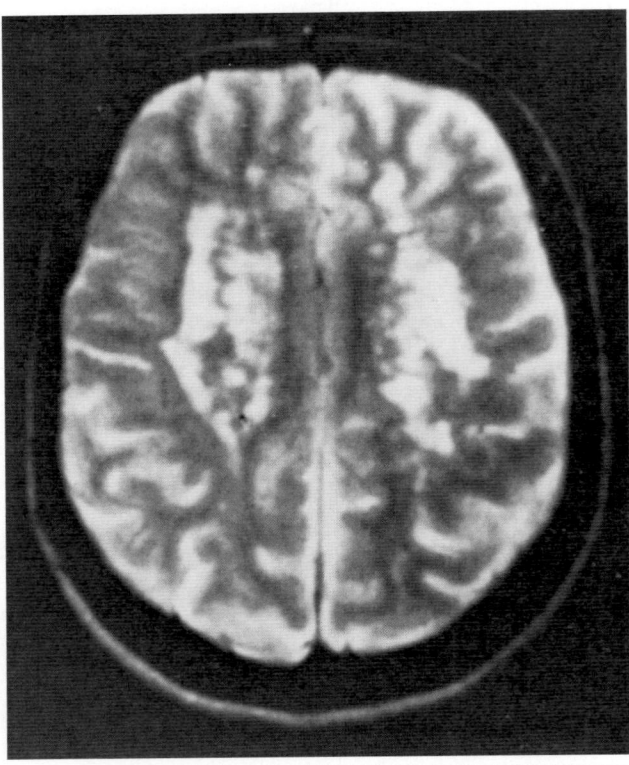

FIGURE 8–9.   T2 magnetic resonance image of vascular dementia, multi-infarct type, in a patient with diabetes mellitus and hypertension.

The bilateral, symmetrical pattern of white matter lesions is characteristic of small vessel arterial disease. Enlarged sulci are consistent with associated perenchymal loss.

Source.   Reprinted with permission from Yock DH: *Imaging of CNS Disease: A CT and MRI Teaching File.* St. Louis, MO, Mosby–Year Book, Inc., 1991.

stability of cognitive status between vascular insults as opposed to the gradual progression of deficits seen in AD. The progression of multi-infarct VaD may be affected by risk factor modification and antiplatelet therapy (Rabins et al. 1997). Lesions are generally located in the subcortical nuclei, frontal lobe white matter, thalamus, and internal capsule and are associated with a characteristic appearance on MRI of periventricular hyperintensities on the T2 images (Figure 8–9; Choi et al. 2000). However, periventricular hyperintensities are also seen in normal aging and in other types of dementia and thus, in isolation, represent a nonspecific finding (Smith et al. 2000). Diffusion-weighted MRI has been shown to be a more sensitive method of evaluating small-vessel ischemic disease in VaD (Choi et al. 2000). The syndrome of cerebral autosomal dominant arteriopathy with subcortical infarcts and leukoencephalopathy is a syndrome of small-vessel vascular disease due to mutation in the *NOTCH3* gene and

has been described as an archetype of pure subcortical VaD (Peters et al. 2005).

Poststroke VaD—dementia occurring as the acute or subacute consequence of a single stroke—may be difficult to clearly distinguish from multi-infarct VaD that follows a series of vascular events. Poststroke dementia is associated with apraxia, neglect, hemianopsia, facial paralysis, and extremity weakness (de Koning et al. 1998). Poststroke VaD was found to independently increase the risk of stroke recurrence (Moroney et al. 1997). Poststroke dementia was found in 24% of a series of 300 stroke patients (de Koning et al. 1998). Left-hemisphere lesions were associated with a decreased incidence of poststroke dementia, whereas hemorrhagic stroke carried an increased risk of subsequent dementia. Another study found poststroke dementia in 26% of a series of 453 patients (Desmond et al. 2000). Major dominant-hemisphere stroke, left-hemisphere location, internal carotid artery distribution, diabetes mellitus, prior cerebrovascular accident (CVA), older age, less education, and nonwhite race were found to be risk factors for poststroke dementia (Desmond et al. 2000). Major depression is common with poststroke dementia, with anterior left-hemisphere stroke posing the highest risk (Robinson 1998). The risk for poststroke dementia associated with major depression is highest in the first year (Robinson 1998). Deficits in orientation, language, visuoconstruction, and executive functions are common but may improve with treatment of the poststroke depression (Robinson 1998).

Lewy body variant (LBV) of AD and LBD have a significant degree of phenomenological overlap and may be difficult to differentiate clinically (Leverenz and McKeith 2002). The more general term *dementia with Lewy bodies* is often used to denote the continuum of LBV, LBD, and dementia due to PD (Boeve 2006; Gomez-Isla et al. 1999). There also is considerable overlap between dementia due to PD and LBD. One recent study showed a higher rate of family history of dementia in LBD compared with PD with dementia (Papapetropoulos et al. 2006).

Clinically, LBV and LBD share the common features of fluctuation of mental status, well-formed visual hallucinations, delusions, depression, apathy, anxiety, and extrapyramidal symptoms (Heyman et al. 1999; Lopez et al. 2000a). Visual hallucinations occur early in the course of illness, even with mild levels of cognitive impairment (Ballard et al. 2001; Leverenz and McKeith 2002). In comparison with AD, LBV exhibits greater deficits in attention, verbal fluency, and visuospatial functioning and increased parkinsonian symptoms

(Lopez et al. 2000a; McKeith et al. 2000). LBV has also been associated with more rapid cognitive decline, earlier institutionalization, and shorter survival time (Lopez et al. 2000a; Serby et al. 2003). The clinical distinction between LBV and AD may be more apparent in the moderate/severe stages of dementia (Lopez et al. 2000b). LBD also features impaired executive functioning, disinhibited social behavior, syncope, and increased sensitivity to antipsychotic agents (manifested by drowsiness, further cognitive decline, and neuroleptic malignant syndrome) (Aarsland et al. 2005; McKeith et al. 2000). Progression is usually more rapid in LBD than in AD, although psychotic symptoms in LBV and LBD may be improved by treatment with cholinesterase inhibitors, whereas psychotic symptoms may paradoxically worsen with antipsychotic agents (Ballard et al. 2001; Leverenz and McKeith 2002; Levy and Cummings 2000). LBV and LBD are also associated with neuroleptic sensitivity, characterized by sedation, immobility, rigidity, postural instability, falls, and decreased cognitive status (Basksys 2004).

A similar degree of overlap is seen in the neuropathology of LBV and LBD. Pathologically, LBV is characterized by the presence of Lewy bodies (intraneuronal eosinophilic inclusion bodies) in subcortical and cortical structures in addition to AD neuropathology (Figure 8–10) (Gomez-Isla et al. 1999). LBV has a lower density of NFTs in the neocortex than does AD (Heyman et al. 1999). LBD also features subcortical and cortical Lewy bodies, with a relative absence of NFTs and other AD neuropathology (Litvan and McKee 1999). Occipital lobe metabolic rates in LBD have been found to be lower than those in AD, a finding that correlates with the prominence of visual hallucinations in LBD (Ishii et al. 1998). Both LBV and LBD are characterized by a marked loss of choline acetyltransferase activity, independent of AD pathology, and show more choline acetyltransferase activity loss than does pure AD (Tiraboschi et al. 2000).

Dementia due to fragile X–associated tremor/ ataxia syndrome (FXTAS) is a newly described syndrome that features frontal lobe and subcortical dementia symptoms in concert with motor anomalies in the grandfathers of children with the fragile X syndrome (Jacquemont et al. 2003). Patients experience amnesia, executive function deficits, and psychomotor slowing. Notable neurological symptoms include rigidity, tremor, and ataxia. Patients exhibit a progressive neurological and cognitive decline. Due to the prominent motor symptoms, this syndrome bears some resemblance to PD with dementia. Neuroimag-

ing has revealed generalized cortical and cerebellar atrophy and increased signal intensity on the middle cerebellar peduncles (Brunberg et al. 2002). The laboratory test for FXTAS dementia is an alteration on the *FMR1* gene at Xq 27.3 on Southern Blot and polymerase chain reaction.

Dementia due to normal-pressure hydrocephalus is associated with amnesia, decreased psychomotor movement, gait apraxia (often described as a "magnetic" gait, where patients are unable to lift their feet to initiate walking), and incontinence (G. W. Ross and Bowen 2002). Neuroimaging reveals ventricular dilatation that is disproportionate to the sulcal widening. Cognitive and motor symptoms may improve following a tap of cerebrospinal fluid or shunting procedures.

Epidemiology

The risk of dementia increases exponentially with age, from 1% for those younger than 65 years to 25%–50% for those older than 85 years (Jorm and Jolley 1998). The annual risk of dementia is 0.5% between ages 60 and 69 years, 1% between 70 and 74 years, 2% between 75 and 79 years, 3% between 80 and 84 years, and 8% thereafter (Rabins et al. 1997). The prevalence of dementia was found to be 3.9% for patients older than 60 years in a general hospital population (Lyketsos et al. 2000a). The risk for patients between ages 60 and 64 years was 2.6%; this risk increased to 8.9% for those older than 85 years. Reported estimates of the relative frequency of the different dementia types in study populations of dementia patients include 50%–90% DAT, 8%–20% VaD, and 7%–26% LBD, with other subtypes less common (Lyketsos et al. 2000b; Roman 2002). Poststroke VaD has been estimated in up to 41% of patients following stroke (Roman 2002). Reversible dementias are estimated to account for 1%–10% of dementias; examples of potentially reversible dementias are shown in Table 8–12 (Gliatto and Caroff 2001; Tager and Fallon 2001).

Comorbidity and Differential Diagnosis

The patient with cognitive impairment may have psychiatric illnesses other than or in addition to dementia. Clinical history and examination need to be focused to consider these other diagnostic possibilities. The psychiatric differential diagnosis of dementia is shown in Table 8–13.

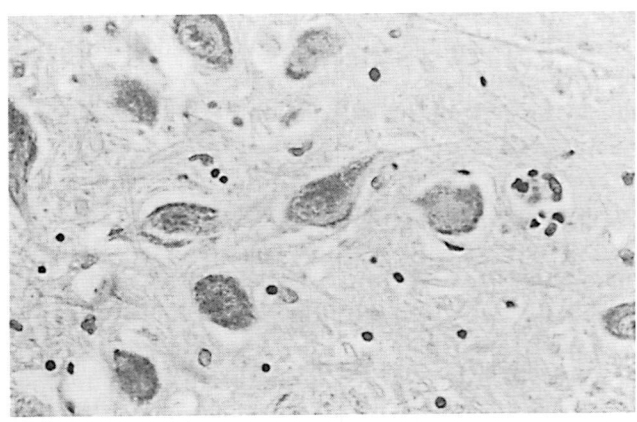 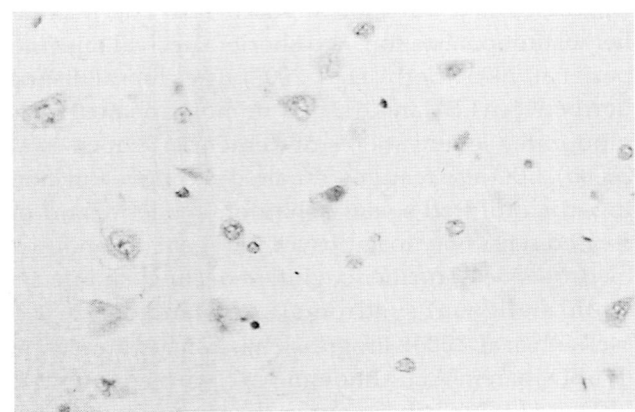

FIGURE 8–10.   **Histopathology images: Lewy body variant of Alzheimer's disease.**

In this patient with dementia, the number of plaques and tangles in the neocortex was borderline for the diagnosis of Alzheimer's disease. *Left,* The substantia nigra showed a moderate degree of nerve cell loss and small numbers of Lewy bodies. *Right,* Ubiquitin immunohistochemistry revealed multiple Lewy bodies in nerve cells of the cingulate gyrus.

Source.   Reprinted from Davis RL, Robertson DM (eds): *Textbook of Neuropathology,* 3rd Edition. Baltimore, MD, Williams & Wilkins, 1997. Copyright 1997, Williams & Wilkins. Used with permission.

TABLE 8–12.   **Potentially reversible etiologies of dementia**

Structural central nervous system factors

Vascular dementia
Head trauma
Subdural hematoma
Normal-pressure hydrocephalus
Multiple sclerosis

Psychiatric illnesses

Major depression
Substance dependence

Systemic/metabolic factors

Hypothyroidism
Hypercalcemia
Hypoglycemia
Thiamine, niacin, B_{12} deficiency
Renal failure
Hepatic failure
Medications

Infectious diseases

HIV
Central nervous system infection

TABLE 8–13.   **Psychiatric differential diagnosis of dementia**

Mild cognitive impairment
Delirium
Mood disorders
Amnestic disorders
Substance use disorders
Psychotic disorders
Mental retardation

impairment on formal testing and the patients' ability to function in their environments are significantly less than in patients with full-syndrome dementia (Portet et al. 2006). This may represent a transitional condition for many patients who will eventually develop dementia (G.W. Ross and Bowen 2002). The rate of conversion from MCI to DAT is estimated at 10%–15% per year (Blennow et al. 2006). Whether this condition warrants antidementia treatment at this stage is controversial. Magnetic resonance spectroscopy (MRS) has been reported to be helpful in predicting which cases of MCI are likely to progress to DAT (Modrego et al. 2005).

Mild Cognitive Impairment

Mild cognitive impairment (MCI) is a milder cognitive disorder that has varied definitions in the literature (G.W. Ross and Bowen 2002). Patients have memory complaints, and formal testing reveals objective evidence of cognitive impairment, but both the degree of

Delirium

Dementia increases the risk for delirium from numerous systemic conditions (e.g., urinary tract infections, pneumonia, dermatological infections, dehydration, constipation) after surgery and as a side effect of medications, particularly anticholinergic medication (Rabins et al. 1997). Delirium in the elderly patient with dementia may present with decreased psychomotor activity (Daniel 2000). Episodes of delirium may be more prolonged in dementia. Given that aberrant motor behaviors, such as repetitive pacing, are uncommon in early dementia, their presence in a patient with mild dementia is suggestive of a superimposed delirium (Mega et al. 1996). Digit span and memory registration, although preserved until late in the course of dementia, may be initially impaired in delirium (Small 1998a). Hallucinations are more common in delirium than in dementia. Electroencephalography may be helpful in differentiating delirium from dementia, because an abnormal EEG is more suggestive of delirium. Onset of symptoms following a systemic medical illness, a recent change in medication, or some other perturbation is strongly suggestive of delirium.

Mood Disorders

Depressed patients may appear to have cognitive impairment, a phenomenon described as "pseudodementia." Such patients will often have a history of mood disorders (Raskind 1998). Although pharmacological treatment of the mood disorder can improve cognitive function, the improvement may be incomplete and/or temporary (Butters et al. 2000; Raskind 1998). Depressed dementia patients may communicate their mood state indirectly, with agitation and insomnia, rather than through specific mood complaints (Small 1998a). Depressed dementia patients may underreport the severity of their depressive symptoms relative to the observations of caregivers. Depressive disorders coexisting with dementia can increase the use of inpatient psychiatric resources beyond that for either condition alone (Kales et al. 1999). Patients with depression plus dementia have a high rate of depression in first-degree relatives, independent of any family risk for dementia (Strauss and Ogrocki 1996).

Amnestic Disorders

Amnestic disorders can be profoundly impairing, but the diagnosis of dementia requires impairment in other spheres of mental activity beyond loss of memory function. Conditions characterized by "pure" amnesia (e.g., carbon monoxide poisoning, Wernicke's encephalopathy, transient global amnesia) should be considered.

Substance Abuse/Dependence

Substance use disorders can lead to dementia, especially after a long history of alcohol dependence. Active management of substance abuse and dependence

should be accomplished in the context of other psychiatric interventions for substance-dependent dementia patients.

Psychotic Disorders and Mental Retardation

Schizophrenia will very rarely be first diagnosed in an elderly patient and will feature prominent psychotic symptoms at the onset of illness, not after several years of cognitive losses. Mental retardation, although increasing the risk for dementia (e.g., trisomy 21), represents a stable state of decreased cognitive function.

Clinical Evaluation

History

A clinical history should first be obtained from the patient directly, initially without the presence of other family members. History taking should address recent cognitive function; examples include function at work, at home, while driving, and while performing other high-risk activities (Patterson et al. 1999). A complaint of memory loss may be predictive of a later diagnosis of DAT, even without demonstrable memory deficits on initial clinical examination (Geerlings et al. 1999). A personal and family history of psychiatric illness should be obtained, specifically to include dementia and neurological illness with high risk for dementia. Because the patient is most reliable in the early stages of illness, the physician should then separately interview family members and synthesize the separate histories obtained to derive the most balanced view of the patient's functioning.

The medical history should address all chronic systemic illnesses, with particular attention to conditions that increase risk for DAT, VaD, and other dementia types. Specific examples of such systemic illnesses include hypertension, diabetes mellitus, hyperlipidemia, PD, multiple sclerosis, and prior CVA (Geldmacher and Whitehouse 1997). Recent systemic illnesses that may put the patient at risk for delirium also need to be explored. The medication history should address both psychotropic and nonpsychotropic medications taken before the onset of the cognitive and behavioral symptoms (Doraiswamy et al. 1998). The use of nonprescription medications (especially antihistamines and sedatives) and herbal preparations also needs to be explored.

The social history should address the patient's living circumstances, presence of supportive family members and/or of other significant persons living nearby, financial and insurance resources, participation in social activities, and personal relationships.

Collateral history obtained from family members should focus on concerns about the patient's cognitive function and overt behavior. Problematic symptoms such as paranoia, agitation, physical violence, and inattentive and dangerous operation of dangerous machinery need to be addressed, as well as access to weapons and any threats made to self or others. Any complaint of neglect or abuse, or any physical examination findings suggestive of inappropriate care, should be reported promptly to the agency responsible for performing on-site evaluation of neglect or abuse of adults. Aggressive and/or delusional patients may be at greatest risk of such maltreatment (Cummings and Masterman 1998). Dementia patients are also at increased risk for syncope and loss of consciousness, which can result in head trauma, hip fracture, or other injuries. Any report of falls in dementia patients requires a full evaluation for injuries.

Mental Status Examination

Formal assessment of cognitive function must be added to routine evaluation of mood and affect, level of consciousness, psychomotor activity, speech production, thought content, and thought processes. It is recommended that the clinician use a cognitive assessment instrument such as the MMSE. A score of 24 or less on the MMSE, when correlated with clinical findings, is highly suggestive of dementia, but education and other patient-specific variables must be taken into close account (Patterson et al. 1999). A cutoff score of 22 is advised in the elderly nursing home population; the MMSE may overestimate dementia in patients with less education, age older than 85, or a history of depression (Dufouil et al. 2000). Conversely, patients with high levels of education and other evidence of premorbid high intellectual function may score in the "unimpaired" range on the MMSE despite decreased functional status. Serial administrations of the MMSE can quantify the progress or stability of dementia; a typical decline in MMSE scores in DAT is 2–4 points per year in untreated patients (Folstein et al. 1975; Rabins et al. 1997). Adjunctive tests of cognitive function include clock drawing, category generation (e.g., having the patient name as many animals as possible in 1 minute; 16 is a cutoff score), and the "go, no-go" test (the patient is instructed to tap once if the examiner taps once, and to not tap if the examiner taps twice). The Neuropsychiatric Inventory is a 12-item behavioral rating scale to assess noncognitive symptoms of dementia (Aalten et al. 2003). A series of structured questions administered to the patient's caretaker are used to assess the following behavioral domains:

delusions, hallucinations, agitation/aggression, dysphoria/depression, anxiety, apathy, irritability, euphoria, disinhibition, aberrant motor behavior, nighttime behavioral disturbance, and appetite/eating abnormalities (Aalten et al. 2003). For each item, severity is rated from 1 to 3 and frequency is rated from 1 to 4; these are summed for a total score. Depression rating scales (e.g., the Hamilton Rating Scale for Depression [Hamilton 1960], the Geriatric Depression Scale [Yesavage et al. 1983]) are recommended to assist in distinguishing dementia from depression and in monitoring response to antidepressants (Katz 1998). Suicide risk increases in the elderly population, and clinical assessment of other suicide risk factors (e.g., substance abuse, isolation, past suicidal behavior, access to weapons) needs to be integrated into the physician's clinical examination.

Physical Examination

Assessment of vision and hearing should not be overlooked (Doraiswamy et al. 1998). Relative sensory deprivation due to uncorrected vision and/or hearing deficits can cause spuriously poor performance on formal cognitive testing. Loss of visual acuity and severe cognitive impairment in patients with DAT can increase visual hallucinations (Chapman et al. 1999). Neurological examination should include assessment of gait, frontal lobe release signs, movement disorders, sensory function, and focal neurological deficits (Doraiswamy et al. 1998). Physical examination should address blood pressure, orthostatic hypotension, cardiovascular disease, cerebrovascular disease, signs of metabolic illnesses, marginal hygiene, poor nutritional status, weight loss, and dehydration. Treatment of vascular risk factors has been shown to decrease the risk of dementia, including DAT and VaD (Alagiakrishnan et al. 2006; Peila et al. 2006).

Laboratory Tests

Laboratory tests may be modified on a case-by-case basis. Tests to consider are shown in Table 8–14 (Patterson et al. 1999; Rabins et al. 1997). Serum drug levels of medications associated with altered mental status (e.g., tricyclics, anticonvulsants, digitalis, antiarrhythmics) should be obtained if clinically indicated. A 12-lead electrocardiogram should be considered, especially if there is a history of cardiac and/or vascular disease.

When CJD is suspected, cerebrospinal fluid samples should be obtained for testing for the neuronal proteins 14–3–3 and γ-enolase (Zerr et al. 2000). CJD is characterized by a classic electroencephalographic ap-

TABLE 8–14. **Laboratory tests for dementia workup**

Electrolytes, blood urea nitrogen, creatinine, calcium

Liver-associated enzymes

Glucose

Complete blood count

Thyroid profile with thyroid-stimulating hormone assay

Erythrocyte sedimentation rate, antinuclear antibody panel

Prothrombin time/partial thromboblastin time

B_{12} and folate

Syphilis serology

Urinalysis and urine toxicology

Pulse oximetry

Medication levels (e.g., tricyclic antidepressants, anticonvulsants, digitalis, antiarrhythmics)

HIV

pearance of repetitive sharp waves or slow spikes followed by synchronous triphasic sharp waves, although the six different phenotypes of this illness may present with different combinations of EEG findings (Zerr et al. 2000). Lumbar puncture should also be considered if there is a clinical suspicion of normal-pressure hydrocephalus, metastatic carcinoma, or unusually early onset and/or rapid progression of deficits (Small 1998a). Other laboratory tests to consider in specific cases include serum ammonia, heavy metals, and cortisol; carotid Doppler studies; chest X-ray; and mammography (Patterson et al. 1999; Rabins et al. 1997).

Neuroimaging

Neuroimaging is increasingly routine in the evaluation of dementia. Computed tomography (CT) is generally more readily available and of lower cost than MRI, although MRI's superior resolution has led to its greater use in dementia evaluation (G. W. Ross and Bowen 2002). A diagnosis of VaD requires confirmatory neuroimaging (Roman 2002). Contrast-enhanced CT and gadolinium-enhanced MRI are recommended less highly. In cases of suspected DAT, hippocampal atrophy may serve as a sensitive early marker for cognitive decline (Figure 8–11) (Jack et al. 2000; Petersen et al. 2000). When more quantitative techniques for assessing hippocampal size and appearance become more widely available, they are likely to increase specificity.

Cortical atrophy and ventriculomegaly do not by themselves confirm dementia and, in isolation, are not specific findings (Doraiswamy et al. 1998; Small 1998a). Progressive cerebral atrophy and ventriculomegaly are more likely in DAT than in VaD and have been reported to correlate with declines in performance on the MMSE (Patterson et al. 1999). If initial neuroimaging reveals hippocampal and/or cortical atrophy that correlates with the clinical presentation and gradual course of DAT, then serial neuroimaging to follow progress is not routinely necessary. Periventricular hyperintensities on MRI may be seen in DAT as well as in VaD; their significance in DAT is unclear, because they may not correlate independently with cognitive changes (Doody et al. 1998; Smith et al. 2000). Decreased white matter volume has been associated with DAT (Smith et al. 2000). If initial imaging shows white matter lesions typical of VaD that correlate with clinical findings, a follow-up CT or MRI could be considered if the patient later presents with an abrupt decrease in mental status suggestive of delirium and/or a new CVA. Diffusion-weighted MRI, which has been shown to be more sensitive than CT in imaging the ischemic small-vessel disease in VaD, may be used to monitor progression of these patients (Choi et al. 2000). Functional neuroimaging (e.g., single photon emission computed tomography, PET scanning, and in vivo proton MRS), although not currently widely available, holds promise in the evaluation of the cortical pathology of dementia, particularly when combined with genetic assessment of patients at risk for clinical dementia (Weiss et al. 2003; Figures 8–12 and 8–13). Functional neuroimaging techniques may reveal a specific pattern of parietal and temporal deficits in DAT that could lead the physician to consider earlier treatment with antidementia pharmacotherapy (Small and Leiter 1998).

Multidisciplinary Referrals

Neuropsychological consultation may be helpful in early dementia cases when cognitive deficits are subtle on clinical examination and may identify MCI cases at risk for later dementia (Griffith et al. 2006). Recall, delayed recall, verbal fluency, and visuomotor ability deficits are predictive of dementia (Bottino and Almeida 1997). Neuropsychological assessment may be especially useful in patients in whom the capacity for autonomy (e.g., driving, medical informed consent) appears equivocal on interview alone. Executive dysfunction (especially when confirmed by neuropsychological assessment) may correlate significantly with loss of capacity for decision making (Marson et al. 1999).

Social work intervention may be of substantial benefit. Family therapy can assist the patient and family to adjust to the reduced social expectations and impairments of the patient. Social workers may facilitate

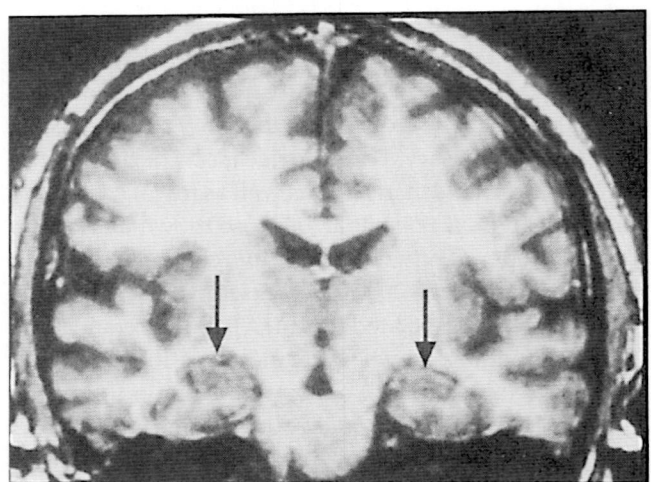 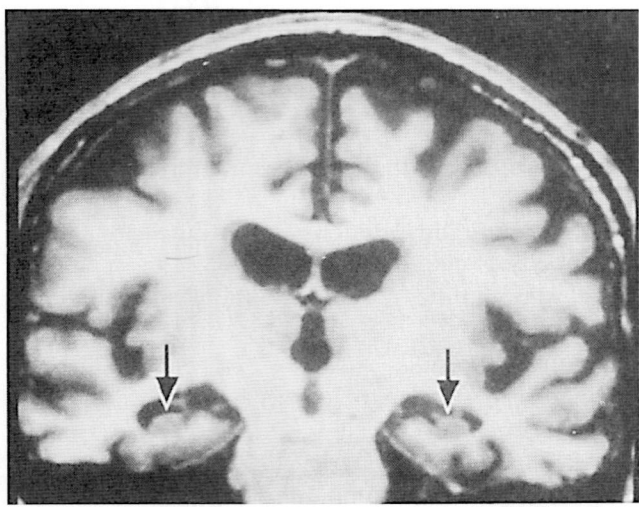

FIGURE 8–11. Magnetic resonance image of hippocampal volume *(arrows)* in a healthy control subject *(left)* and a patient with Alzheimer's disease and hippocampal atrophy *(right)*.

Source. Reprinted with permission from Foster NL, Minoshima S, Kuhl DE: "Brain Imaging in Alzheimer Disease," in *Alzheimer Disease*, 2nd Edition. Edited by Terry RD, Katzman R, Bick KL, et al. Philadelphia, PA, Lippincott Williams & Wilkins, 1999, p. 69, Figures 2A and 2B. Copyright 1999, Lippincott Williams & Wilkins.

patient and family access to supportive social services to assist the patient in staying with his or her family, to secure institutional placement, and to explore funding sources for institutional care.

Psychiatric nurses may be invaluable in the area of home visitation and outreach. A system of care in which the psychiatric nurse calls on the patient at home may be established for patients with dementia. The psychiatric nurse assesses mental status, helps with the management of psychotropic medications, and evaluates the residence for safe living circumstances, which may help to avoid unneeded hospitalization and to forestall nursing home placement.

Occupational, recreational, and physical therapy may be very helpful with in vivo assessment of the patient's ability to function safely and independently in various physical and social environments, as part of a comprehensive patient safety evaluation (Grossberg and Lake 1998). Occupational therapists may assist in assessment of the patient's ability to drive safely.

Management

Clinical Management

Attention to comorbid systemic and neuropsychiatric illnesses is the first priority in clinical management of the dementia patient. Close collaboration with the patient's other physician(s) is essential for managing medical illnesses that increase the risk for cognitive deficits. Examples include the neurologist in the case of a patient with PD or multiple sclerosis and the internist in the case of a patient with VaD or HIV. Management of pain may decrease agitated behavior in patients with dementia. Psychopharmacological approaches to anxiety, psychotic, and mood disorders are discussed in detail later (see "Pharmacotherapy"). Substance abuse interventions consisting of medical detoxification, participation in Alcoholics Anonymous or other 12-Step recovery programs, judicious use of agonist therapies, and close attention to comorbid substance-induced mood and anxiety disorders are necessary in the dementia patient with comorbid substance abuse or dependence.

Early frank discussion of diagnosis, prognosis, and management, with clinical follow-ups scheduled at least every 3 months, are advised. Every visit should include an evaluation of whether the patient can still safely live at home. More frequent visits should be scheduled to monitor response and side effects when psychotropic medications are prescribed. Supportive psychotherapy may assist the patient in dealing with grief and loss. Admission to a psychiatry inpatient unit skilled in dealing with dementia patients may be needed for severely regressed, suicidal, violent, or psychotic patients, especially if complex psychopharmacological regimens and/or ECT is considered (Rabins et al. 1997).

Psychoeducation can be very valuable, especially

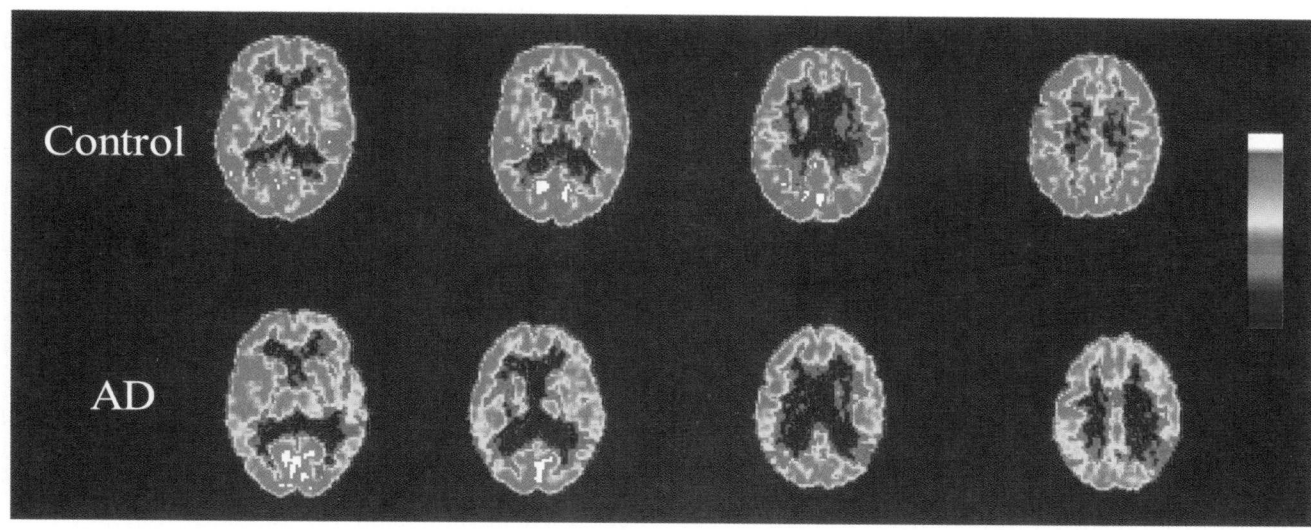

FIGURE 8–12.   Fluorodeoxyglucose positron emission tomography study of a healthy older control subject and a patient with Alzheimer's disease (AD).

The patient demonstrates bilateral temporal and parietal hypometabolism with some involvement of the posterior cingulate gyrus and relative preservation of primary cortex and basal ganglia. Metabolic activity is greatest in the visual cortex.
Source.   Reprinted with permission from Valk PE, Bailey DL, Townsend DW, et al.: *Positron Emission Tomography: Basic Science and Clinical Practice.* London, Springer-Verlag, 2003, pp. 343, 344.

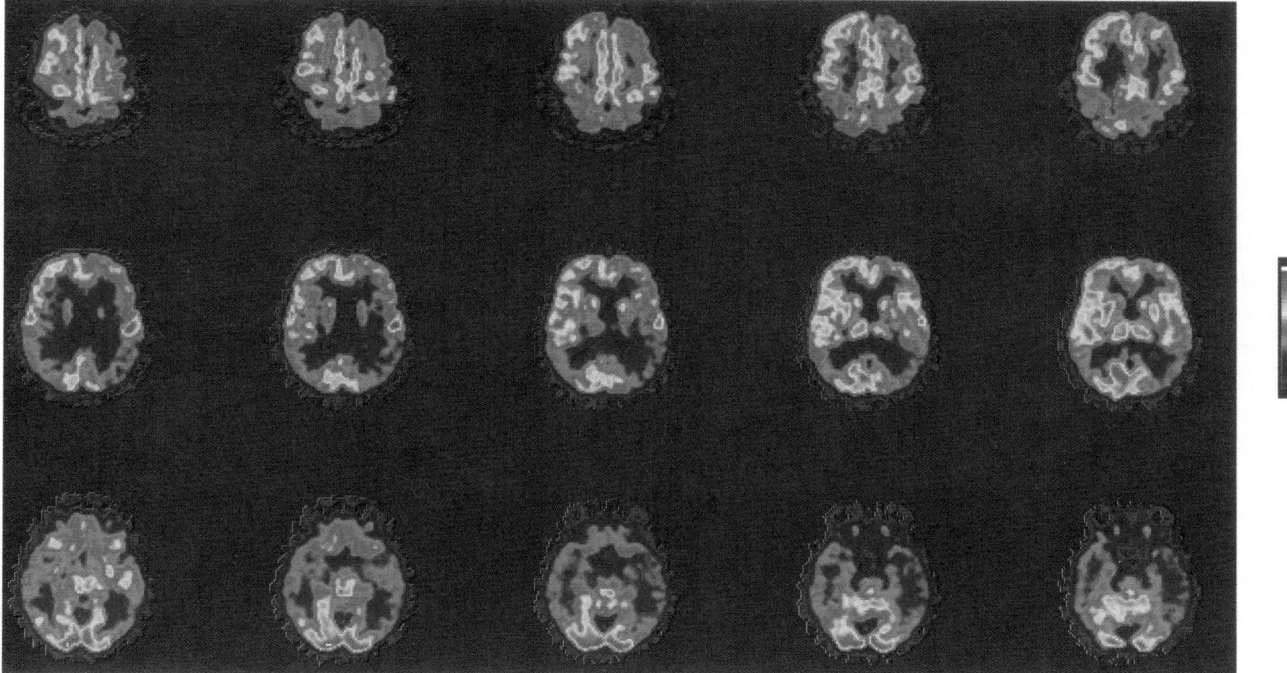

FIGURE 8–13.   Fluorodeoxyglucose positron emission tomography study of a patient with late-stage Alzheimer's disease.

This patient shows widespread hypometabolism that is still most pronounced in temporal and parietal cortex and maximal in the left hemisphere *(right side of the image).* There is relative preservation of metabolism in visual cortex and sensorimotor cortex bilaterally.
Source.   Reprinted with permission from Valk PE, Bailey DL, Townsend DW, et al.: *Positron Emission Tomography: Basic Science and Clinical Practice.* London, Springer-Verlag, 2003, pp. 343, 344.

for family caregivers (Grossberg and Lake 1998). *The 36-Hour Day: A Family Guide to Caring for Persons With Alzheimer's Disease, Related Dementing Illnesses, and Memory Loss in Later Life* (Mace and Rabins 1981) is often helpful to both patients and families. Support and advocacy groups are available through the Alzheimer's Association (1-800-621-0379; www.alz.org) (Rabins et al. 1997). The Alzheimer's Association can facilitate patient enrollment in the Safe Return Program, a nationwide program that assists in the identification and return of dementia patients who wander. The patient should always carry and/or wear identification (e.g., a MedicAlert bracelet) and can be registered with the local police department. Physicians should inform caregivers of the increased risk of depression in primary caregivers of dementia patients and facilitate respite opportunities for caregivers (Grossberg and Lake 1998).

A recent major review of the psychological approaches to the neuropsychiatric disturbances in dementia demonstrated that behavior management strategies, caregiver and residential staff education, and (possibly) cognitive stimulation techniques had an adequate evidence base supporting their prolonged effectiveness (Livingston et al. 2005). Environmental and behavioral management may include provision of adequate lighting, music, access to pets, and appropriate levels of psychological stimulation. Because of the decreased psychological flexibility of the dementia patient, the home should be organized to allow for simplicity of routines, with prominent display of calendars, schedules, and the photographs and names of people close to the patient. Events that trigger problematic behaviors should be identified and minimized (Parnetti 2000). For safety, childproofing devices may be considered. Vehicle keys, power tools, and sharp household objects should be secured. Weapons should be removed from the home or at least be secured in a locked cabinet.

Legal issues should be addressed early in the course of the illness, while the patient can still direct his or her wishes. These matters include the completion of medicolegal documents such as living wills, durable powers of attorney, and advance directives (Grossberg and Lake 1998). The physician may be asked to comment on the patient's capacity to make legally binding decisions. Neuropsychological testing may be of help. The capacity for medical decision making needs to be considered as well. The physician is advised to thoroughly evaluate the patient's clinical status at the time a medical decision is needed to ensure that the patient understands the implications of his or

her medical choices. The capacity to vote is generally preserved in mild DAT, whereas patients with moderate disease may require specific assessment of this capacity (Applebaum et al. 2005).

Driving or the operation of other dangerous machinery is often a point of great contention. Many patients will maintain the motor skills for driving despite showing substantial cognitive deficits on the clinical interview and on formal mental status testing (Rabins 1998). Even in mild dementia, the statistical risk of motor vehicle accidents is increased (Dubinsky et al. 2000). Physicians are advised to acquaint themselves with the disclosure laws regarding notification of dementia diagnoses to state motor vehicle departments. A road competency test may be advisable. A useful clinical guideline to consider is that driving is not advised whenever a dementia diagnosis leads the clinician to institute pharmacotherapy for dementia and/ or when the MMSE score is less than 24. Other contraindications could be the presence of paranoia, agitation, or assaultive behavior.

Institutional placement is often a painful decision. To many patients, the loss of the home environment, even when clearly necessary to preserve safety, is a devastating experience that usually leads to further confusion, behavioral regression, and increased risk of depression. The lack of or loss of a primary caregiver may predict earlier institutionalization (Patterson et al. 1999). The physician should make every reasonable effort to maintain the patient in his or her home environment. An important intervention is respite care for caregivers. Various respite models to consider include in-home caregivers (e.g., the visiting nurse model) and adult day care centers/senior centers (in which the patient attends a supervised therapeutic environment for the business day and returns home at night).

However, the patient may ultimately regress to a point at which life without 24-hour supervision is not safe. Specific examples of behaviors that cannot safely be managed at home include exhibiting assaultive or threatening behavior, leaving dangerous appliances on inappropriately, continuing to drive despite prohibitions, and being unable to maintain feeding, drinking, dressing, and toileting functions. When placement is necessary, an institution that specializes in the care of dementia patients is advised. A secured unit may be required to prevent wandering. Treatment models emphasizing behavioral modification can decrease agitated behavior and minimize the need for pharmacological therapy and physical restraint (Teri et al. 2000). Physicians and family members should clarify with nursing home facilities what degree of medical morbidity can be managed in these institutions, because medical illnesses may lead to more frequent changes in care setting, promoting further behavioral regression with each change of venue.

Pharmacotherapy

Anticholinesterase agents act through inhibition of acetylcholinesterase, increasing the net amount of synaptic acetylcholine available for neurotransmission (Table 8–15). Anticholinesterase agents are advised early in the course of DAT and may reduce the rate of cognitive decline (Blennow et al. 2006). Once initiated and well tolerated at the highest recommended dosages, anticholinesterase agents should be continued indefinitely, with regular monitoring of cognitive, emotional, and functional behavioral status. Although their effects may be relatively modest, more often involving a slowing of decline than a reversal of cognitive losses, they represent a major breakthrough in psychopharmacology (Bonner and Peskind 2002; Trinh et al. 2003). There is some early evidence that anticholinesterase agents may have a neuroprotective function on the hippocampus in DAT (Hashimoto et al. 2005; Krishnan et al. 2003).

Anticholinesterase agents should also be considered (along with antipsychotics) in managing dementia-related psychotic symptoms (Rao and Lyketsos 1998). These agents can also be safely combined with antidepressants, which may lead to greater symptomatic improvement, given that catecholamine abnormalities may be related to some of the symptoms of dementia (Tune and Sunderland 1998). Cholinergic side effects seen with anticholinesterase agents include nausea, abdominal discomfort, vomiting, loose stools, muscle cramps, muscle weakness, increased sweating, and bradycardia. Acetylcholinesterase inhibitors should be discontinued before surgery in which succinylcholine may be used because of the risk of prolonged paralysis.

Anticholinesterase agents may also be used for other dementing illnesses (e.g., dementia due to PD, LBV, LBD, and CJD; VaD; and mixed VaD and DAT); they may be particularly helpful with the psychotic symptoms of LBV and LBD (Roman et al. 2005; Simard and van Reekum 2004). One hypothesis that may explain the benefit of anticholinesterase agents for other dementias is the "cholinergic-vascular hypothesis," where it has been postulated that the main effect of anticholinesterase agents is on increased CBF (Claassen and Jansen 2006). Combination regimens consisting of an anticholinesterase agent and other agents more directly protective against neuronal degenera-

tion (e.g., memantine, antioxidants, anti-inflammatory agents, hormones) with psychotropic medications (to address specific neuropsychiatric symptoms) are emerging as treatment for DAT. Tacrine, donepezil, rivastigmine, and galantamine are FDA approved for DAT, although tacrine has been associated with hepatotoxicity and is now rarely used clinically.

Donepezil is started at 5 mg/day, which may be increased to 10 mg/day in 1–6 weeks. It has been shown to slow the rate of decline or to improve cognitive performance in mild, moderate, or severe DAT (Winblad et al. 2006). Donepezil has been found to maintain improvements in cognition when continued for up to 98 weeks (Rogers and Friedhoff 1998). In addition, emotional and behavioral symptoms of dementia may improve (Weiner et al. 2000).

Rivastigmine is a cholinesterase inhibitor with effects on both acetylcholinesterase and butyrylcholinesterase (Stahl 2000). Because of its effects on butyrylcholinesterase, it is theoretically of additional benefit in advanced DAT, when glial proliferation leads to greater CNS concentrations of butyrylcholinesterase (Stahl 2000). Rivastigmine is started at 1.5 mg twice daily for 2 weeks; the dosage may be gradually raised every 2 weeks to a maximum recommended dosage of 6 mg twice daily (Kumar et al. 2000; Spencer and Noble 1998).

Galantamine is a cholinesterase inhibitor that also allosterically modulates nicotine cholinergic receptors, theoretically further enhancing acetylcholine release (Raskind et al. 2000; Stahl 2000). This agent may enhance the release of other CNS neurotransmitters important in dementia (Stahl 2000), thereby leading to further improvements in emotional and behavioral symptoms. Galantamine is initially started at 4 mg twice a day, with dosage increases to 8 mg twice daily and 12 mg twice daily after 4-week intervals. In several clinical trials lasting up to 12 months, galantamine has been associated with improved cognitive, behavioral, and global function as well as reduced caregiver distress (Cummings et al. 2004; Rockwood et al. 2006).

Memantine is an NMDA antagonist that blocks glutamate-medicated excitotoxicity (Winblad and Poritis 1999). Physiological receptor activation is not affected, but pathological excitotoxicity is inhibited (Reisberg et al. 2003). Dosages start at 5 mg/day and are increased to 10 mg bid for moderate to severe DAT to reduce clinical behavioral disturbances and to reduce caregiver distress, and it may delay institutionalization (Reisberg et al. 2003; Wimo et al. 2003). Side effects reported include dizziness, headache, constipation, falls, and confusion (Hartman and Mobius 2003; Tariot

TABLE 8–15. Dementia pharmacotherapy

Medication class	Target symptom(s)	Starting dosage	High dosage
Cholinesterase inhibitors	Decreased cognition, delusions, hallucinations		
Tacrine		10 mg qds	40 mg qds
Donepezil		5 mg/day	10 mg/day
Rivastigmine		1.5 mg bid	6 mg bid
Galantamine		4 mg bid	12 mg bid
NMDA antagonist	Decreased cognition		
Memantine		5 mg/day	10 mg bid
Antioxidants			
α-Tocopherol		1,000 IU bid	
Selegiline		5 mg/day	10 mg/day
Antidepressants	Depression, irritability, anxiety		
Fluoxetine		10 mg/day	40 mg/day
Paroxetine		10 mg/day	40 mg/day
Sertraline		25 mg/day	200 mg/day
Citalopram		10 mg/day	40 mg/day
Escitalopram		5 mg/day	20 mg/day
Venlafaxine (extended release)		37.5 mg/day	350 mg/day
Mirtazapine		7.5 mg/day hs	45 mg/day hs
Duloxetine		20 mg bid	30 mg bid
Trazodone		25 mg/day hs	400 mg/day hs
Bupropion		37.5 mg bid	200 mg bid
Anxiolytic	Anxiety, irritability		
Buspirone		5 mg tid	20 mg tid
Anticonvulsants	Irritability, agitation		
Carbamazepine		100 mg/day	[a]
Valproate		125 mg/day	[b]
Oxcarbazepine		150 mg bid	600 mg bid
Antipsychotics	Delusions, hallucinations, disorganized thoughts, agitation		
Risperidone		0.25 mg/day hs	3 mg/day hs
Olanzapine		2.5 mg/day hs	10 mg/day hs
Quetiapine		25 mg/day hs	150 mg bid
Ziprasidone		20 mg/day hs	40 mg bid
Aripiprazole		5 mg/day	15 mg/day
Clozapine		25 mg bid	100 mg bid

TABLE 8–15. **Dementia pharmacotherapy** *(continued)*

Medication class	Target symptom(s)	Starting dosage	High dosage
Additional medications (consider as adjunctive therapy on case-by-case basis)			
β-Blockers			
Psychostimulants			
Nonsteroidal anti-inflammatory drugs			
Antiplatelet agents			
Antihypertensives			
Calcium channel blockers			
Statins			
Warfarin			
Neuroprotective agents			
Hormones			
Highly active antiretroviral therapy (HAART)			

[a]Upper limit of dosage to give serum drug level of 8–12 ng/mL.
[b]Upper limit of dosage to give serum drug level of 50–60 ng/mL.

et al. 2004a). Memantine is usually used in concert with a cholinesterase inhibitor; this combination is generally well tolerated (Hartman and Mobius 2003). Memantine has also been shown to benefit cognitive function in VaD (Mobius and Stoffler 2003).

Antioxidants can be considered for their neuroprotective effects. Selegiline (a selective monoamine oxidase B inhibitor), 5–10 mg/day, is used in mild to moderate DAT for its antioxidant properties and its effect of increasing CNS catecholamine levels (Sano et al. 1997). Selegiline may have a positive effect on both cognition and behavior (Lawlor et al. 1997). A tyramine-restricted diet is not required at dosages up to 10 mg/day. Selegiline must be used cautiously because of its risk of drug–drug interactions and orthostatic hypotension. Its use is contraindicated with selective serotonin reuptake inhibitors (SSRIs), tricyclic antidepressants, and meperidine.

α-Tocopherol, 1,000 IU bid, may slow the progression of moderate DAT, because its antioxidant properties may protect against neuronal damage caused by amyloid deposition (Felician and Sandson 1999). Although generally well tolerated, it has been associated with decreased coagulation function in patients with vitamin K deficiency (Rabins et al. 1997). Either selegiline or α-tocopherol may delay a poor outcome in dementia (e.g., death, institutionalization, inability to perform activities of daily living; Sano et al. 1997). One study showed a reduced risk of DAT in patients with high dietary intake of the two antioxidants vitamins C

and E, although there are insufficient data for the effects of vitamin C for dementia in isolation (Engelhart et al. 2002).

Antidepressants should be used for comorbid depressive disorders, depressive and anxiety symptoms that do not qualify for a full depressive or anxiety disorder diagnosis, sleep disturbances, and agitation. Because of their generally benign side-effect profile and their effectiveness, SSRIs are the preferred class of antidepressants in dementia patients and should be started at lower dosages than in healthy adults. Initial dosages can be doubled after 2–4 weeks if necessary, and a trial should continue for at least 12 weeks once the usual adult dosage has been reached (Class et al. 1997). Paroxetine has more clinically significant anticholinergic activity than the other SSRIs and should be used with caution. SSRIs may also have utility in managing sexual disinhibition in dementia (Stewart and Shin 1997).

Other antidepressants to consider include bupropion, trazodone, mirtazapine, duloxetine, and venlafaxine extended release. Blood pressure must be monitored in patients using venlafaxine because of the risk of hypertension. Tricyclics should be used with caution in dementia because of the cognitive toxicity that may result from anticholinergic side effects. "Pseudodementia" due to depression should be managed with antidepressants and follow-up cognitive assessment.

Psychostimulants as adjunctive therapy with antidepressants may be considered for refractory mood symptoms and/or apathy; methylphenidate 2.5–5 mg/day is a recommended starting dosage (Rabins et al. 1997). An alternative agent is modafinil, with dosages starting at 100 mg to a maximum to 400 mg in the morning. ECT should be considered for cases of treatment-refractory depression; however, because of the risk for post-ECT delirium and amnesia, ECT treatments should be given no more frequently than twice per week, with unilateral electrode placement (Rabins et al. 1997).

Anxiolytics may be used for anxiety or agitation. Because of the high risk of further memory impairment, sedation, and falls, physicians should avoid the use of benzodiazepines in dementia patients (Rabins et al. 1997). The clinician might consider buspirone, 5 mg tid, and increase dosage gradually to an upper limit of 20 mg tid (Alexopoulos et al. 1998).

Anticonvulsants may be indicated for agitated and aggressive behavior or for emotional lability (Class et al. 1997). A recommended starting dosage of carbamazepine for the elderly patient with dementia is 100 mg/day, which can be titrated to achieve a serum drug level of 8–12 ng/mL (Rabins et al. 1997). Side effects include ataxia, sedation, confusion, and (rarely) bone marrow suppression (Rabins et al. 1997).

Divalproex sodium can be started at 125 mg/day and titrated upward to yield a serum drug level of 50–60 ng/mL (Rabins et al. 1997). Divalproex sodium is associated with gastrointestinal distress, ataxia, and (less frequently) hyperammonemia, hepatotoxicity, or bone marrow suppression (Rabins et al. 1997). Monitoring of complete blood count and of liver-associated enzymes is recommended with the use of carbamazepine and valproate (Rabins et al. 1997). Oxcarbazepine may be a safer alternative to carbamazepine; initial dosages of 150 mg bid may be gradually increased to a maximum of 600 mg as needed.

β-Blockers may have a role in the management of aggression and agitation in dementia, especially those cases that are refractory to other psychopharmacological management (Herrmann et al. 2004a). Both propranolol (dosage range, 30–520 mg/day) and pindolol (dosage range, 40–60 mg/day) have been reported to control aggression and agitation (Herrmann et al. 2004a). Caution must be exercised due to the risks of bradycardia/syncope and exacerbation of comorbid chronic obstructive pulmonary disease, diabetes mellitus, and peripheral vascular disease in these patients (Herrmann et al. 2004a).

Antipsychotics are indicated for paranoid thinking, hallucinations, delirium, and agitation. Initial dosages in elderly patients with dementia should be less than those used in younger patients because of the risks of sedation and further cognitive decline. Although conventional antipsychotic agents are often used as first-line treatment for agitation, they are associated with frequent adverse side effects in patients with dementia (Alexopoulos et al. 1998; Daniel 2000).

The atypical antipsychotic agents risperidone, olanzapine, quetiapine, ziprasidone, and aripiprazole are recommended in dementia with agitation and psychosis because of their clinical efficacy and (when compared with conventional antipsychotics) greater tolerability and lower risk of extrapyramidal symptoms and neuroleptic malignant syndrome; clozapine is not generally recommended as a first-line antipsychotic in dementia due to the risk of agranulocytosis and its propensity to increase the risk of delirium and seizures (Carson et al. 2006; Mintzer et al. 2006; Sink et al. 2005). Reduced starting and maximum dosages (e.g., risperidone dosage range of 0.25–3 mg/day at bedtime) are recommended to minimize side effects (Daniel 2000). Nighttime dosing is preferred, because sleep is facilitated and the risk of daytime sedation is minimized. Risperidone dosages ranging from 0.75 to 1.75 mg/day were associated with only a 2.6% risk of tardive dyskinesia at 1-year follow-up (Jeste et al. 2000). In patients with feeding tubes or other limitations affecting their use of solid medications, risperidone liquid can be considered. For rapid oral absorption, oral disintegrating risperidone or olanzapine and oral liquid risperidone are useful. Olanzapine and ziprasidone are available in intramuscular preparations. Suggested dosages for olanzapine are 2.5–10.0 mg/day at bedtime; quetiapine dosages can range from 25 mg/day at bedtime to 150 mg bid, ziprasidone may be dosed between 20 mg at night to 40 mg bid, aripiprazole from 5 to 15 mg/day, and clozapine from 25 to 100 mg bid (Daniel 2000).

Generally, olanzapine and quetiapine are more sedating than the other atypical antipsychotics. Olanzapine has been associated with gait disturbance in dementia patients (Lawlor 2004; Tariot et al. 2004b). Quetiapine may minimize risk of motor side effects in psychosis with PD and LBD, as well as in other dementias, and be safer than clozapine (Baskys 2004; Keys and De Wald 2005b). Clozapine may be used in cases of PD and LBD (due to its relatively lower likelihood of exacerbating movement disorders) and in cases where psychosis is refractory to other agents (Keys and De Wald 2005b; Leverenz and McKeith 2002).

The atypical antipsychotics have been associated with weight gain, increased serum glucose, emergence of diabetes mellitus, and hyperlipidemia. This risk is particular high for olanzapine and clozapine (Keys and De Wald 2005b). Use of these medications of dementia should be accompanied by monitoring for these conditions (Keys and De Wald 2005a).

Recent concern has been raised over the increased risk of both CVA and death in dementia patients who are treated with atypical antipsychotics; there does not seem to be a differential risk among the agents of this class (Schneider et al. 2005; Sink et al. 2005). This increased risk of adverse cerebrovascular events with atypical antipsychotics has not been seen in all studies (Herrmann et al. 2004b; Liperoti et al. 2005). Risk for these complications may be greater in the immediate post-CVA period (Keys and De Wald 2005b). Speculation of causality of this finding has included the atypical antipsychotics' effect on arrhythmia potential (Titier et al. 2004), serotonin blood vessels, thrombus formation, and orthostasis (Keys and De Wald 2005a). This concern has led to a 2005 Health Advisory Warning from the FDA (Sink et al. 2005). As a result, physicians should consider avoiding indefinite treatment with atypical antipsychotics for dementia-related psychosis and agitation and discontinue these medications promptly if clinical improvement is not seen (Sink et al. 2005). The risk of death from haloperidol was similar to that from the atypical antipsychotics; thus, renewed use of the typical antipsychotics may not be a viable alternative to mitigate this risk (Sink et al. 2005).

Follow-up monitoring should include examination for medication-induced movement disorders with the Abnormal Involuntary Movement Scale. If problems with compliance lead the physician to consider depot antipsychotics, reduced dosages (e.g., fluphenazine decanoate, 1.25–3.75 mg IM monthly) can be considered. In the United States, the use of antipsychotic medication in nursing home patients with dementia is regulated by the Omnibus Budget Reconciliation Act of 1987, which requires clear documentation of clinical indications and consideration of alternative interventions (Rabins et al. 1997). Dosage decreases or trial discontinuations of antipsychotics should be considered as the illness progresses. Atypical antipsychotics may still be indicated even in severe dementia; in one study, risperidone 1 mg/day led to improvement in objective behavioral measures (particularly decreased aggression) without further decrements in cognitive function or self-care (Katz et al. 1999).

Antiplatelet therapy and/or ergot mesylates (e.g., hydergine 3 mg/day initially to a maximum of 9 mg/day) may be considered for cases of VaD and may stabilize or improve cognitive function (Meyer et al. 1995). Hydergine may be associated with nausea and

other gastrointestinal symptoms; its use is contraindicated in patients with psychotic symptoms (Rabins et al. 1997). Other systemic interventions may be indicated in VaD, such as the statins, warfarin (in cases with atrial fibrillation), antihypertensives, calcium channel blockers, neuroprotective agents, and vascular surgery for hemodynamically significant carotid stenosis.

Hormones may have an adjunctive role in dementia, although this is controversial. A large meta-analysis of the effects of postmenopausal hormone replacement on cognition concluded that hormone replacement therapy produced improvement in verbal memory, vigilance, reasoning, and motor speed in women with menopausal symptoms (LeBlanc et al. 2001). Estrogen replacement and raloxifene, an estrogen receptor modulator, have been associated with decreased dementia risk but have not been shown to be effective for cognitive functioning in cases of established DAT (LeBlanc et al. 2001; Yaffe et al. 2005).

However, the Women's Health Initiative Memory Study demonstrated that estrogen plus progesterone increased the risk of probable dementia in women older than 65 years and did not prevent MCI in this group (Shumaker et al. 2003); a small risk of clinically meaningful cognitive decline was associated with the combination (Rapp et al. 2003). This major study's results cast doubt on the current role for hormonal therapy or dementia in women. Medroxyprogesterone may be used to manage disinhibited sexual acting-out behavior in male patients with AD (Rabins et al. 1997).

Future exploration in pharmacotherapy will likely target DAT but would be expected to have applicability to other dementia types as well. Areas of active interest include neurotrophic factors (e.g., nerve growth factor), modification of amyloid metabolism (likely targeting the activities of APP), and reduction of oxidative stress and inflammation (Aisen and Davis 1997).

Highly active antiretroviral therapy for underlying HIV infection is an essential part of the management of HIV dementia and can reverse cognitive losses (Cohen and Jacobson 2000; McDaniel et al. 2000). The cognitive effects of this therapy may be further enhanced in combination with ibuprofen (Gendelman et al. 1998). Psychostimulants may be helpful in HIV-associated fatigue and decreased concentration and memory (Maldonado et al. 2000; McDaniel et al. 2000).

Dementia: Summary

The dementias are a heterogeneous group of clinical syndromes, unified by their common findings of deterioration in cognitive and executive functions. Physicians need to be alert to the need for a thorough history, targeted evaluation, and psychopharmacological and psychosocial management in patients with these clinical syndromes. Modern clinical interventions, including anticholinesterase agents in concert with other psychopharmacological agents, should be aggressively used early in the disease process to maintain the patient's cognitive functional status. Advances in basic science research point to possible new directions in the pathophysiology and psychopharmacological management of this major public health problem.

Amnestic and Other Cognitive Disorders

Amnestic Disorders

Amnestic disorders are characterized by a loss of memory due to the direct physiological effects of a general medical condition or due to the persisting effects of a substance. The amnestic disorders share a common symptom presentation of memory impairment but are differentiated by etiology. Amnestic disorders are secondary syndromes caused by systemic medical illness, primary cerebral disease or trauma, substance use disorders, or adverse medication effects. The impairment must be sufficient to compromise social and occupational functioning, and it should represent a significant decline from the previous level of functioning.

Epidemiology

Limited data are available on the prevalence and incidence of amnestic disorders (Harper et al. 1995). Memory impairment due to head trauma is probably the most common etiology, with more than 500,000 patients hospitalized annually in the United States for head injury. Alcohol abuse and associated thiamine deficiency are historically common etiologies, but some studies suggest that the incidence of alcohol-induced amnestic disorders is decreasing, whereas that of amnestic disorders due to head trauma is increasing (Kopelman 1995).

Etiology

The DSM-IV-TR diagnostic classification for amnestic disorders is based on etiology. Amnestic disorders can be diagnosed as resulting from a general medical condition (Table 8–16), as due to the effects of a substance (Table 8–17), or as "not otherwise specified." The most common etiologies are listed in Table 8–18 and usually involve bilateral damage to areas of the brain involved

---

TABLE 8–16. DSM-IV-TR diagnostic criteria for amnestic disorder due to ... *[indicate the general medical condition]*

A. The development of memory impairment as manifested by impairment in the ability to learn new information or the inability to recall previously learned information.

B. The memory disturbance causes significant impairment in social or occupational functioning and represents a significant decline from a previous level of functioning.

C. The memory disturbance does not occur exclusively during the course of a delirium or a dementia.

D. There is evidence from the history, physical examination, or laboratory findings that the disturbance is the direct physiological consequence of a general medical condition (including physical trauma).

Specify if:

Transient: if memory impairment lasts for 1 month or less

Chronic: if memory impairment lasts for more than 1 month

Coding note: Include the name of the general medical condition on Axis I, e.g., 294.0 amnestic disorder due to head trauma; also code the general medical condition on Axis III (see DSM-IV-TR Appendix G for codes).

---

in memory. These areas include the dorsomedial and midline thalamic nuclei, the hippocampus, the amygdala, the fornix, and the mammillary bodies. Unilateral damage may sometimes be sufficient to produce memory impairment, particularly in the case of left-sided temporal lobe and thalamic structures (Benson 1978). Several iatrogenic causes, such as medication effects, ECT, and the ICU setting, lack clearly identified neuroanatomic damage (Jones et al. 2000).

Clinical Features

Patients with amnestic disorders either are impaired in their ability to learn and recall new information (anterograde amnesia) or are unable to recall previously learned material (retrograde amnesia). The deficits in short-term or recent memory seen in anterograde amnesia can be assessed by asking the patient to recall three objects after a 5-minute distraction. Whereas anterograde amnesia is nearly always present, retro-

TABLE 8–17. DSM-IV-TR diagnostic criteria for substance-induced persisting amnestic disorder

A. The development of memory impairment as manifested by impairment in the ability to learn new information or the inability to recall previously learned information.

B. The memory disturbance causes significant impairment in social or occupational functioning and represents a significant decline from a previous level of functioning.

C. The memory disturbance does not occur exclusively during the course of a delirium or a dementia and persists beyond the usual duration of substance intoxication or withdrawal.

D. There is evidence from the history, physical examination, or laboratory findings that the memory disturbance is etiologically related to the persisting effects of substance use (e.g., a drug of abuse, a medication).

Code [specific substance]–induced persisting amnestic disorder: (291.1 alcohol; 292.83 sedative, hypnotic, or anxiolytic; 292.83 other [or unknown] substance)

TABLE 8–18. Causes of amnestic disorders

Head trauma

Wernicke-Korsakoff syndrome

Alcohol-induced blackouts

Benzodiazepines

Barbiturates

Intrathecal methotrexate

Methylenedioxymethamphetamine (MDMA; "Ecstasy")

Seizures

Herpes simplex encephalopathy

Klüver-Bucy syndrome

Electroconvulsive therapy

Carbon monoxide poisoning

Heavy metal poisoning

Hypoxia

Hypoglycemia

Cerebrovascular disorders

Cerebral neoplasms

grade amnesia is more variable and depends on the location and severity of brain damage. Both immediate recall (as tested by digit span) and remote memory for distant past events are usually preserved. Memory for the physical traumatic event that caused the deficit is often lost. Orientation may be impaired, because it is dependent on the ability to store information regarding time, date, location, and circumstance. The patient may therefore present as confused and disoriented but without the fluctuation in level of consciousness associated with delirium. Orientation to self is nearly always preserved in amnestic disorders.

Most patients with amnestic disorders lack insight into their deficits and may vehemently deny the presence of memory impairment despite clear evidence to the contrary. This lack of insight may lead to anger, accusations, and occasionally agitation. More commonly, patients present with apathy, lack of initiative, and diminished affective expression suggestive of altered personality function.

Confabulation is often associated with amnestic disorders. Confabulation is characterized by responses to questions that not only are inaccurate but also are often so bizarre and unrealistic as to appear psychotic. Historically, confabulation was considered to represent

an attempt by these patients to "cover up" their deficits in memory, but this explanation is probably overly simplistic. The presence and degree of confabulation are usually correlated not with the severity of memory deficits but rather with the loss of self-corrective and monitoring functions, as seen in bifrontal lobe disease (Mercer et al. 1977). Confabulation in amnestic disorders is usually seen during the early stages of the illness and tends to disappear over time.

The onset of amnesia may be sudden or gradual, depending on etiology. Head trauma, vascular events, and specific neurotoxic exposures such as carbon monoxide poisoning are associated with acute mental status changes. Prolonged substance use, sustained nutritional deficiency, and chronic neurotoxic exposures may produce a more gradual and sustained decline in memory function, eventually leading to a clinically diagnosable impairment.

Selected Amnestic Disorders

Head injury. Severe neurological and psychiatric symptoms can result from head injury, even in the absence of radiological evidence of structural damage. Amnesia after head injury typically includes both anterograde (or ongoing) amnesia and retrograde amnesia for a period ranging from a few minutes to several years before the injury. As anterograde amnesia fades and the patient regains the ability to learn and recall new information, retrograde amnesia "shrinks," usually remaining only for the very short period (seconds to minutes) before the injury. A prolonged retrograde amnesia is an indication of ongoing anterograde amnesia, whereas a short period of retrograde amnesia is associated with recovery (Benson and McDaniel 1991). Severe injuries may result in permanent deficits, although some recovery of memory function can be seen up to 24 months after head trauma.

Korsakoff's syndrome.   Korsakoff's syndrome is an amnestic disorder caused by thiamine deficiency usually associated with excessive, prolonged ingestion of alcohol. It can occur in other malnourished conditions, such as marasmus, gastric carcinoma, and HIV (Kopelman 1995). Korsakoff's syndrome is associated with an acute phase of illness—known as Wernicke's encephalopathy—that presents with ophthalmoplegia, peripheral neuropathy, ataxia, nystagmus, and delirium. Although these acute neurological symptoms respond to aggressive thiamine repletion, a residual, persistent amnestic syndrome usually remains. The associated neuroanatomical abnormalities in Korsakoff's syndrome include bilateral sclerosis of the mammillary bodies (Benson 1978) and punctate lesions of the gray nuclei in the periventricular regions of the third and fourth ventricles and the sylvian aqueduct (Victor et al. 1989). Some investigators have questioned whether there are distinctive pathophysiological differences between Wernicke-Korsakoff syndrome and the cognitive impairment and dementia due to chronic alcohol neurotoxicity (Blansjaar and Van Dijk 1992). Given the high prevalence of missed diagnoses of Wernicke-Korsakoff syndrome and the insidious, progressive course of the illness, in which each episode gives rise to cumulative damage, all alcohol-dependent patients should be treated with thiamine.

Transient global amnesia.   Transient global amnesia (TGA) is a form of amnestic disorder characterized by an abrupt episode of profound anterograde amnesia and a variable inability to recall events that occur during the episode. These episodes typically last for only a few minutes or hours, ending with a rapid, spontaneous restoration of intact cognitive function. Mean duration of the amnestic period is 4.2 hours; periods greater than 12 hours are exceptional. The patient's level of consciousness and orientation to self are unaffected during the episode (Shuping et al. 1980). Patients are often bewildered and confused during the episodes and may ask repeated questions about their

circumstances. No data are available to suggest that TGA is associated with focal neurological features or with any comorbid psychiatric illness. TGA is more common in men and usually occurs after age 50. In women episodes are often associated with anxiety and an emotional precipitating event. In younger patients, a history of headaches may constitute an important risk factor (Quinette et al. 2006). The etiology is unclear, but most experts believe that it is associated with cerebrovascular disease and episodic vascular insufficiency of the mesial temporal lobe. Other etiologies of TGA, including brain tumors, cardiac arrhythmias, migraine, thyroid disorders, general anesthesia, sexual intercourse, polycythemia vera, epilepsy, and myxomatous mitral valvular disease, have also been reported (Hodges and Warlow 1990a; Pai and Yang 1999). The most common angiographic findings are in the vertebrobasilar system, specifically occlusion or stenosis of the posterior cerebral artery. TGA generally has a good prognosis, with only 8% of patients experiencing a second episode (Hodges and Warlow 1990b).

Benzodiazepine persisting amnestic disorder. Several medications have been associated with amnestic syndromes, with benzodiazepines receiving the most attention. Benzodiazepines can cause anterograde amnesia and may interfere with memory consolidation and retrieval. Risk factors include high dosage, intravenous administration, and use of high-potency, short-half-life agents such as triazolam (Scharf et al. 1987). These effects may be enhanced by the concurrent use of alcohol (Linnoila 1990). The resulting memory impairment is not associated with the degree of sedation or psychomotor impairment (Roache and Griffiths 1985). Amnestic sleep-related eating disorders can be seen, with transient amnesia for nocturnal eating (Morgenthaler and Silber 2002).

Differential Diagnosis

Memory deficits seen in amnestic syndromes are frequently a feature of delirium and dementia. In delirium, the memory disturbance is accompanied by a disturbed level of consciousness and usually fluctuates with time. More pervasive signs of cerebral dysfunction, such as difficulty focusing or sustaining attention, are present. In dementia, memory impairment is accompanied by additional cognitive impairments such as aphasia, apraxia, agnosia, and disturbances in executive functioning.

In dissociative or psychogenic forms of amnesia, the memory loss usually does not involve deficits in learning and recalling new information. Patients typically present with a circumscribed inability to recall previously learned and personal information, often regarding the patient's own identity or a traumatic or stressful event. These deficits persist even as the patient continues to function normally in the present. Interestingly, changes in limbic function are observed on PET in patients with psychogenic amnesia (Yasuno et al. 2000). Patients with malingering or factitious disorders can present with amnestic symptoms that also fit the profile for dissociative amnesia. Systematic memory testing of these patients will often yield inconsistent results.

Treatment

As in delirium and dementia, the primary goal of treatment in amnestic disorders is to identify and treat the underlying cause or pathological process. There are no definitively effective treatments for amnestic disorder that are specifically aimed at reversing apparent memory deficits. Fortunately, these deficits are often temporary—as in transient amnestic syndromes—or are partially or completely reversible—as in head trauma, thiamine deficiency, or anoxia. Acute management should include continuous reorientation of the patient by means of verbal redirection, clocks, calendars, and familiar stimuli. Individual supportive psychotherapy for the patient, and family counseling to assist and educate caregivers, is also helpful. Chronic reversible amnestic syndromes may be managed with cognitive rehabilitation and therapeutic milieus intended to promote recovery from brain injury. More severe and permanent deficits may require supervised living environments to ensure appropriate care.

Mild Cognitive Impairment

MCI is a clinical syndrome defined as cognitive decline that is greater than expected for a patient's age and education level but that does not interfere with normal functioning. A classification has been proposed that differentiates between amnestic or single memory MCI, multiple-domain MCI, and single nonmemory MCI (Petersen 2004). Prevalence in population-based epidemiological studies ranges from 3% to 19% in adults older than 65 years (Gauthier et al. 2006; G.W. Ross and Bowen 2002). Some patients with MCI remain stable or return to normal over time, but more than half progress to dementia within 5 years. The amnestic subtype in particular has a high probability of progressing to DAT (Ganguli et al. 2004) and could constitute a prodromal stage of this disorder, although the multiple-domain subtype has higher sensitivity for both DAT and VaD (Rasquin et al. 2005). The rate of progression to DAT may be predicted by the severity

of memory impairment at baseline, the severity of hippocampal atrophy, and the presence of an ε4 allele of the *APOE* gene (Geda et al. 2006). Comorbid depression with MCI more than doubles the risk of developing DAT, and patients with a poor response to antidepressants appear to be at an even greater risk (Modrego and Ferrandez 2004).

Neuropathological features of MCI mimic the early changes associated with DAT, with NFTs in the ventromedial temporal lobe being the probable substrate for memory decline (Petersen et al. 2006). The diagnosis of MCI involves assessment of multiple cognitive domains, with particular attention to episodic and semantic memory. A self-administered screening battery, the Computer-Administered Neuropsychological Screen for Mild Cognitive Impairment, may be a reliable, valid screening tool in determining whether more intensive testing for MCI is warranted (Tornatore et al. 2005). Although there are no pharmacological treatments at present that are capable of delaying the long-term progression of MCI to dementia, there is some evidence for short-term symptomatic benefits with acetylcholinesterase inhibitors (Saykin et al. 2004). Secondary prevention by controlling risk factors such as systolic hypertension, atrial fibrillation, and low folate levels may help prevent conversion to VaD (Ravaglia et al. 2006).

Postconcussion Syndrome

Postconcussion syndrome (PCS) is defined as a condition arising from traumatic brain injury that produces deficits in three areas of CNS function: somatic, psychological, and cognitive. The most common somatic symptom is headache, but fatigue, dizziness, blurred vision, and photophobia can also occur. Psychological symptoms include anxiety, depression, apathy, and emotional lability. Cognitive symptoms include decreased concentration, decreased verbal fluency, and impairments in working memory. The American Psychiatric Association's current criteria for postconcussional disorder (PCD), a similar diagnosis in Appendix B of DSM-IV-TR, require that there be an "acquired impairment in cognitive functioning, accompanied by specific neurobehavioral symptoms, that occurs as a consequence of closed head injury of sufficient severity to produce a significant cerebral concussion" (American Psychiatric Association 2000, p. 760). The most important differential diagnosis is usually malingering, and several psychiatric and neurological tests are available to assist the clinician. The Halstead-Reitan battery is reported to be 93.8% reliable in detecting patients who are intentionally trying to fake cognitive symptoms of head trauma (Mittenberg et al. 1996). Additional psychological testing that can be helpful includes the Minnesota Multiphasic Personality Inventory–2, the Dissimulation Scale, the Ego Strength Scale, and the Fake Bad Scale (Hall et al. 2005).

Neuropathological features of PCS probably relate to the primary pathological injury seen in brain trauma with axonal sheering and tensile strain damage to neurons due to rotational acceleration forces. Clinically significant concussions usually produce no detectable findings on neuroimaging because of the diffuse nature of the damage. The release of inhibitory neurotransmitters such as GABA can produce a cascade of further postinjury neuronal damage, with excessive calcium influx into damaged neurons, release of cytokines, oxidative free-radical damage, damage to cell wall receptors, and inflammation (Rao and Lyketsos 2002). Most symptoms of PCS resolve within 1 month, with only 7%–15% of patients having persistent symptoms after 1 year (McHugh et al. 2006). Risk factors for persistent PCS symptoms include female gender, age greater than 40 years, history of alcohol abuse, prior head injury, and significant comorbid medical or psychiatric illness (Ryan and Warden 2003). Treatment of PCS should be conservative, with education about PCS symptoms and positive prognoses associated with good outcomes (Corrigan et al. 2003). Patients with persistent somatic headache symptoms benefit from standard headache therapy ranging from nonsteroidal anti-inflammatory drugs to prophylactic migraine medications such as fluoxetine and verapamil (Hall et al. 2005). Supportive psychotherapy and short-term use of antidepressants may be helpful for persistent psychological symptoms of anxiety or depression. Physicians must be careful in prescribing psychoactive medications that may have deleterious CNS side effects that delay neuronal recovery or worsen memory impairment, as with haloperidol or benzodiazepines. Psychostimulants, dopamine agonists, and cholinesterase inhibitors have been used to treat the cognitive deficits of PCS, but they only result in mild and transient benefit for most patients (Hall et al. 2005).

Conclusion

The cognitive disorders represent a heterogeneous group of clinical syndromes that can generate incalculable agony from the threatened and often realized loss of a highly prized portion of our personhood: the capacity to think and remember. Psychiatrists need to be mindful of the broad differential diagnosis of patients presenting with cognitive impairment. It is advised that care of these patients be firmly grounded in the biopsychosocialspiritual model, thorough history taking; directed mental status examinations; rational use of laboratory tests, electroencephalography, and neuroimaging; and comprehensive interventions. A commitment to remain current in the rapidly evolving knowledge base for the cognitive disorders is necessary to competently employ psychopharmacological and behavioral interventions. Tremendous and exciting research advances continue to build momentum and will yield improved options for the diagnosis, treatment, and prevention of cognitive impairment.

Key Points

DELIRIUM

- Delirium is an acute brain disorder manifested by a syndromal array of neuropsychiatric symptoms.
- Delirium is epidemic among hospitalized patients, especially in the elderly.
- Numerous and widely varying precipitants can activate delirium in vulnerable patients.
- Delirium likely exerts an independent mortality risk for select populations and serves as a "medical alarm" for many others.
- Delirium can resolve completely, resolve gradually, or lead to a permanent cognitive disorder.
- The fundamental goal of treating delirium is to prevent and reverse delirium and thus mitigate associated morbidity and mortality risks.

DEMENTIA

- Dementia is characterized by amnesia and one or more other impairment(s) in cognition.

- Cortical dementias feature notable aphasia, apraxia, agnosia, and visuospatial deficits plus amnesia that is not helped by cueing, whereas subcortical dementias feature apathy, affective lability, depressed mood, bradyphrenia, and decreased attention/concentration plus amnesia that is helped by cueing.

- Compared with DAT, FTD is characterized by executive dysfunction, disinhibition, attentional deficits, and personality changes with relatively preserved memory and visuospatial function.

- LBD and LBV are characterized by fluctuations in mental status, well-formed visual hallucinations, delusions, depression, apathy, anxiety, extrapyramidal symptoms, and neuroleptic sensitivity.

- MCI patients have memory symptoms validated by clinical examination and/or testing that is significantly less impairing than full-spectrum dementia; whether this condition warrants medication treatment for cognitive symptoms is controversial.

- Neuroimaging is a routine expectation in the workup of dementia.

- A common clinical combination of medications for DAT is an anticholinesterase agent with memantine.

AMNESTIC AND OTHER COGNITIVE DISORDERS

- Amnestic disorders are characterized by an inability to learn and recall new information (anterograde amnesia) or an inability to recall previously learned information (retrograde amnesia).

- Common causes of amnestic disorder include head injury, transient global amnesia, and benzodiazepines.

- MCI is defined as cognitive decline greater than expected for a patient's age and education level but without the deficits in normal functioning associated with dementia.

- MCI is a risk state for dementia, with more than half of patients with the amnestic subtype of MCI progressing to dementia within 5 years.

- PCS is a constellation of somatic, psychological, and cognitive symptoms resulting from head trauma that usually resolve within 1 month, although persistent symptoms may continue for 1 year in 7%–15% of patients.

Suggested Readings

American Psychiatric Association: Practice guideline for the treatment of patients with Alzheimer's disease and other dementias of late life. Am J Psychiatry 154 (suppl): 1–39, 1997

American Psychiatric Association: Practice guideline for the treatment of patients with delirium. Am J Psychiatry 156 (suppl):1–20, 1999

Barber R, Ballard C, McKeith IG, et al: MRI volumetric study of dementia with Lewy bodies: a comparison with AD and vascular dementia. Neurology 54:1304–1309, 2000

Blesa R, Davidson M, Kurz A, et al: Galantamine provides sustained benefits in patients with "advanced moderate" Alzheimer's disease for at least 12 months. Dement Geriatr Cogn Disord 15:78–87, 2003

Bookheimer SY, Strojwas MH, Cohen MS, et al: Patterns of brain activation in people at risk for Alzheimer's disease. N Engl J Med 343:450–456, 2000

Brodaty H, Ames D, Snowdon J, et al: A randomized placebo-controlled trial of risperidone for the treatment of aggression, agitation, and psychosis of dementia. J Clin Psychiatry 64:134–143, 2003

Fontaine CS, Hynan LS, Koch K, et al: A double-blind comparison on olanzapine versus risperidone in the acute treatment of dementia-related behavioral disturbances in extended care facilities. J Clin Psychiatry 64:726–730, 2003

Grigoletto F, Zappala G, Anderson DW, et al: Norms for the Mini-Mental State Examination in a healthy population. Neurology 53:315–320, 1999

Folstein MF (ed): The Neurobiology of Primary Dementia. Washington, DC, American Psychiatric Publishing, 2005

ICU Delirium and Cognitive Impairment Study Group (www.icudelirium.org)

Kashima H, Kato M, Yoshimasu H, et al: Current trends in cognitive rehabilitation for memory disorders. Keio J Med 48:79–86, 1999

Levenson JL (ed): American Psychiatric Publishing Textbook of Psychosomatic Medicine. Washington, DC, American Psychiatric Publishing, 2005

Levy ML, Cummings JL, Fairbanks LA, et al: Longitudinal assessment of symptoms of depression, agitation, and psychosis in 181 patients with Alzheimer's disease. Am J Psychiatry 153:1438–1443, 1996

Nadler JD, Relkin NR, Cohen MS, et al: Mental status testing in the elderly nursing home population. J Geriatr Psychiatry Neurol 8:177–183, 1995

Olichney JM, Galasko D, Salmon DO, et al: Cognitive decline is faster in Lewy body variant than in Alzheimer's disease. Neurology 51:351–357, 1998

Paulsen JS, Salmon DP, Monsch AU, et al: Discrimination of cortical from subcortical dementias on the basis of memory and problem-solving tests. J Clin Psychol 51:48–58, 1995

Paulsen JS, Salmon DP, Thal LJ, et al: Incidence of and risk factors for hallucinations and delusions in patients with probable AD. Neurology 54:1965–1971, 2000

Perry RJ, Hodges JR: Differentiating frontal and temporal variant frontotemporal dementia from Alzheimer's disease. Neurology 54:2277–2284, 2000

Pollock BG, Mulsant BH, Rosen J, et al: Comparison of citalopram, perphenazine, and placebo for the acute treatment of psychosis and behavioral disturbances in hospitalized, demented patients. Am J Psychiatry 159:460–465, 2002

Porter RJ, Lunn BS, Walker LLM, et al: Cognitive deficit induced by acute tryptophan depletion in patients with Alzheimer's disease. Am J Psychiatry 157:638–640, 2000

Rabinowitz J, Katz IR, De Deyn PP, et al: Behavioral and psychological symptoms in patients with dementia as a target for pharmacotherapy with risperidone. J Clin Psychiatry 65:1329–1334, 2004

Rainer MK, Masching AJ, Ertl MG, et al: Effect of risperidone on behavioral and psychological symptoms and cognitive function in dementia. J Clin Psychiatry 62:894–900, 2001

Starkstein SE, Petracca G, Chemerinski E, et al: Syndromic validity of apathy in Alzheimer's disease. Am J Psychiatry 158:872–877, 2001

Tariot PN, Erb R, Podgorski CA, et al: Efficacy and tolerability of carbamazepine for agitation and aggression in dementia. Am J Psychiatry 155:54–61, 1998

Tariot PN, Solomon PR, Morris JC, et al: A 5-month, randomized, placebo-controlled trial of galantamine in AD. Neurology 54:2269–2276, 2000

Terao T, Shimomura T, Izumi Y, et al: Two cases of quetiapine augmentation for donepezil-refractory visual hallucinations in dementia with Lewy bodies. J Clin Psychiatry 64:1520–1521, 2003

Terry RD, Katzman R, Bick KL, et al (eds): Alzheimer Disease, 2nd Edition. Philadelphia, PA, Lippincott Williams & Wilkins, 1999

Tschanz JT, Welsh-Bohmer KA, Skoog I, et al: Dementia diagnosis from clinical and neuropsychological data compared: the Cache County study. Neurology 54:1290–1296, 2000

Yudofsky SC, Hales RE (eds): American Psychiatric Publishing Textbook of Neuropsychiatry and Clinical Neurosciences, 4th Edition. Washington, DC, American Psychiatric Publishing, 2002

References

Aalten P, de Vugt ME, Lousberg R, et al: Behavioral problems in dementia: a factor analysis of the Neuropsychiatric Inventory. Dement Geriatr Cogn Disord 15:99–105, 2003

Aarsland D, Perry R, Larsen JP, et al: Neuroleptic sensitivity in Parkinson's disease and parkinsonian dementias. J Clin Psychiatry 66:633–637, 2005

Abdel-Razzak Z, Loyer P, Fautrel A, et al: Cytokines downregulate expression of major cytochrome P-450 enzymes in adult human hepatocytes in primary culture. Mol Pharmacol 44:707–715, 1993

Adamis D, Morrison C, Treloar A, et al: The performance of the clock drawing test in elderly medical inpatients: does it have utility in the identification of delirium? J Geriatr Psychiatry Neurol 18:129–133, 2005a

Adamis D, Treloar A, MacDonald AJ, et al: Concurrent validity of two instruments (the CAM and the DRS) in the detection of delirium among older medical inpatients. Age Ageing 34:72–75, 2005b

Adamis D, Treloar A, Martin FC, et al: Recovery and outcome of delirium in elderly medical inpatients. Arch Gerontol Geriatr 43:289–298, 2006

Agnoletti V, Ansaloni L, Catena F, et al: Postoperative delirium after elective and emergency surgery: analysis and checking of risk factors. A study protocol. BMC Surg 5:12, 2005

Aisen PS, Davis KL: The search for disease-modifying treatment for Alzheimer's disease. Neurology 48 (5 suppl 6):S35–S41, 1997

Alagiakrishnan K, McCracken P, Feldman H: Treating vascular risk factors and maintaining vascular health: is this the way towards successful cognitive ageing and preventing cognitive decline? Postgrad Med J 82:101–105, 2006

Alexander GE, Furey ML, Grady CL, et al: Association of premorbid intellectual function with cerebral metabolism in Alzheimer's disease: implications for the cognitive reserve hypothesis. Am J Psychiatry 154:165–172, 1997

Alexopoulos GS, Silver JM, Kahn DA, et al: Treatment of Agitation in Older Patients With Dementia: A Postgraduate Medicine Special Report. Minneapolis, MN, McGraw-Hill, 1998, pp 1–88

American Psychiatric Association: Diagnostic and Statistical Manual of Mental Disorders, 2nd Edition. Washington, DC, American Psychiatric Association, 1968

American Psychiatric Association: Diagnostic and Statistical Manual of Mental Disorders, 3rd Edition. Washington, DC, American Psychiatric Association, 1980

American Psychiatric Association: Diagnostic and Statistical Manual of Mental Disorders, 4th Edition. Washington, DC, American Psychiatric Association, 1994

American Psychiatric Association: Practice guideline for the treatment of patients with delirium. Am J Psychiatry 156 (suppl):1–20, 1999

American Psychiatric Association: Diagnostic and Statistical Manual of Mental Disorders, 4th Edition, Text Revision. Washington, DC, American Psychiatric Association, 2000

Andrew MK, Freter SH, Rockwood K: Incomplete functional recovery after delirium in elderly people: a prospective cohort study. BMC Geriatr 5:1471–1423, 2005

Applebaum PS, Bonnie RJ, Karlawish JH: The capacity to vote of persons with Alzheimer's disease. Am J Psychiatry 162:2094–2100, 2005

Armstrong SC, Cozza KL, Watanabe KS: The misdiagnosis of delirium. Psychosomatics 38:433–439, 1997

Balan S, Leibovitz A, Zila SO, et al: The relation between the clinical subtypes of delirium and the urinary level of 6-SMT. J Neuropsychiatry Clin Neurosci 15:363–366, 2003

Ballard CG, O'Brien JT, Swann AG, et al: The natural history of psychosis and depression in dementia with Lewy bodies and Alzheimer's disease: persistence and new cases over 1 year of follow-up. J Clin Psychiatry 62:46–49, 2001

Baskys A: Lewy body dementia: the litmus test for neuroleptic sensitivity and extrapyramidal symptoms. J Clin Psychiatry 65 (suppl):16–22, 2004

Bayindir O, Akpinar B, Can E, et al: The use of the 5-HT3-receptor antagonist ondansetron for the treatment of postcardiotomy delirium. J Cardiothorac Vasc Anesth 14:288–292, 2000

Bellelli G, Trabucchi M: Outcomes of older people admitted to postacute facilities with delirium. J Am Geriatr Soc 54:380–381, 2006

Benoit AG, Campbell BI, Tanner JR, et al: Risk factors and prevalence of perioperative cognitive dysfunction in abdominal aneurysm patients. J Vasc Surg 42:884–890, 2005

Benson DF: Amnesia. South Med J 71:1221–1227, 1231, 1978

Benson DF, McDaniel KD: Memory disorders, in Neurology in Clinical Practice, Vol 2. Edited by Bradley WG, Daroff RB, Fenichel GM, et al. Boston, MA, Butterworth-Heinemann, 1991, pp 1389–1406

Benveniste H, Drejer J, Schousboe A, et al: Elevation of the extracellular concentrations of glutamate and aspartate in rat hippocampus during transient cerebral ischemia monitored by intracerebral microdialysis. J Neurochem 43:1369–1374, 1984

Berger A-K, Fratiglioni L, Frosell Y, et al: The occurrence of depressive symptoms in the preclinical phase of AD: a population-based study. Neurology 53:1998–2002, 1999

Blansjaar BA, Van Dijk JG: Korsakoff minus Wernicke syndrome. Alcohol Alcohol 27:435–437, 1992

Blennow K, de Leon MJ, Zetterberg H: Alzheimer's disease. Lancet 368:387–403, 2006

Bobinski M, Wegel J, Wisniewski HM, et al: Neurofibrillary pathology: correlation with hippocampal formation atrophy in Alzheimer disease. Neurobiol Aging 17:909–919, 1996

Boeve BF: A review of the non-Alzheimer dementias. J Clin Psychiatry 67:1983–2001, 2006

Bonner LT, Peskind ER: Pharmacological treatments of dementia. Med Clin North Am 86:657–674, 2002

Bottino CM, Almeida OP: Can neuroimaging techniques identify individuals at risk of developing Alzheimer's disease? Int Psychogeriatr 9:389–403, 1997

Bourdel-Marchasson I, Vincent S, Germain C, et al: Delirium symptoms and low dietary intake in older patients are independent predictors of institutionalization: a 1-year prospective population-based study. J Gerontol A Biol Sci Med Sci 59A:350–354, 2004

Bourgeois JA, Seaman JS, Servis ME: Delirium, dementia, and amnestic disorders, in The American Psychiatric Publishing Textbook of Clinical Psychiatry, 4th Edition. Edited by Hales RE, Yudofsky SC. Washington, DC, American Psychiatric Publishing, 2003, pp 259–308

Bourgeois JA, Koike AK, Simmons JE, et al: Adjunctive valproic acid for delirium and/or agitation on a consultation-liaison service: a report of six cases. J Neuropsychiatry Clin Neurosci 17:232–238, 2005

Bourne RS, Mills GH: Melatonin: possible implications for the postoperative and critically ill patient. Intensive Care Med 32:371–379, 2006

Breitbart W, Marotta R, Call P: AIDS and neuroleptic malignant syndrome. Lancet 2:1488–1489, 1988

Breitbart W, Marotta R, Platt MM, et al: A double-blind trial of haloperidol, chlorpromazine, and lorazepam in the treatment of delirium in hospitalized AIDS patients. Am J Psychiatry 153:231–237, 1996

Breitbart W, Rosenfeld B, Roth A, et al: The Memorial Delirium Assessment Scale. J Pain Symptom Manage 13:128–137, 1997

Breitbart W, Gibson C, Tremblay A: The delirium experience: delirium recall and delirium-related distress in hospitalized patients with cancer, their spouses/caregivers, and their nurses. Psychosomatics 43:183–194, 2002a

Breitbart W, Tremblay A, Gibson C: An open trial of olanzapine for the treatment of delirium in hospitalized cancer patients. Psychosomatics 43:175–182, 2002b

Breitner JC: The role of anti-inflammatory drugs in the prevention and treatment of Alzheimer's disease. Annu Rev Med 47:401–411, 1996

Brown TM: Basic mechanisms in the pathogenesis of delirium, in The Psychiatric Care of the Medical Patient, 2nd Edition. Edited by Stoudemire A, Fogel BS, Greenberg DB. New York, Oxford University Press, 2000, pp 571–580

Brown TM, Stoudemire A: Psychiatric Side Effects of Prescription and Over-the-Counter Medications. Washington, DC, American Psychiatric Press, 1998

Brunberg JA, Jacquemont S, Hagerman RJ, et al: Fragile X permutation carriers: characteristic MR imaging findings of adult male patients with progressive cerebellar and cognitive dysfunction. Am J Neuroradiol 23:1757–1766, 2002

Butters MA, Becker JT, Nebes RD, et al: Changes in cognitive functioning following treatment of late-life depression. Am J Psychiatry 157:1949–1954, 2000

Cameron DJ, Thomas RI, Mulvihill M, et al: Delirium: a test of the Diagnostic and Statistical Manual III criteria on medical inpatients. J Am Geriatr Soc 35:1007–1010, 1987

Caraceni A, Nanni O, Maltoni M, et al: Impact of delirium on the short term prognosis of advanced cancer patients. Italian Multicenter Study Group on Palliative Care. Cancer 89:1145–1149, 2000

Carson S, McDonagh MS, Peterson K: A systematic review of the efficacy and safety of atypical antipsychotics in patients with psychological and behavioral symptoms of dementia. J Am Geriatr Soc 54:354–361, 2006

Caselli RJ, Graff-Radford NR, Reiman EM, et al: Preclinical memory decline in cognitively normal apolipoprotein E-epsilon4 homozygotes. Neurology 53:201–207, 1999

Cassem NH, Sos J: Intravenous use of haloperidol for acute delirium in intensive care settings. Paper presented at 131st Annual Meeting of the American Psychiatric Association, Washington, DC, May 1978

Centeno C, Sanz A, Bruera E: Delirium in advanced cancer patients. Palliat Med 18:184–194, 2004

Chapman FM, Dickinson J, McKeith I, et al: Association among visual hallucinations, visual acuity, and specific eye pathologies in Alzheimer's disease: treatment implications. Am J Psychiatry 156:1983–1985, 1999

Choi SH, Na DL, Chung CS, et al: Diffusion-weighted MRI in vascular dementia. Neurology 54:83–89, 2000

Claassen JAHR, Jansen RWMM: Cholinergically mediated augmentation of cerebral perfusion in Alzheimer's disease and related cognitive disorders: the cholinergic-vascular hypothesis. J Gerontol A Biol Sci Med Sci 61A:267–271, 2006

Class CA, Schneider L, Farlow MR: Optimal management of behavioural disorders associated with dementia. Drugs Aging 10:95–106, 1997

Cohen MAA, Jacobson JM: Maximizing life's potential in AIDS: a psychopharmacological update. Gen Hosp Psychiatry 22:375–388, 2000

Cole MG, Primeau FJ: Prognosis of delirium in elderly hospital patients. Can Med Assoc J 149:41–46, 1993

Cole MG, McCusker J, Bellavance F, et al: Systematic detection and multidisciplinary care of delirium in older medical inpatients: a randomized trial. Can Med Assoc J 167:753–759, 2002

Corrigan JD, Wolfe M, Mysiw WF, et al: Early identification of mild traumatic brain injury in female victims of domestic violence. Am J Obstet Gynecol 188:71–76, 2003

Coyle JT, Leski ML, Morrison JH: The diverse roles of L-glutamic acid in brain signal transduction, in Neuropsychopharmacology: The Fifth Generation of Progress. Edited by Davis KL, Charney D, Coyle JT, et al. Philadelphia, PA, Lippincott Williams & Wilkins, 2002, pp 71–90

Craft S, Teri L, Edland SD, et al: Accelerated decline in apolipoprotein E-epsilon 4 homozygotes with Alzheimer's disease. Neurology 51:149–153, 1998

Culp KR, Wakefield B, Dyck et al: Bioelectric impedance analysis and other hydration parameters as risk factors for delirium in rural nursing home patients. J Gerontol A Biol Sci Med Sci 59:813–817, 2004

Cummings JL, Benson DF: Psychological dysfunction accompanying subcortical dementias. Ann Rev Med 39:53–61, 1988

Cummings JL, Masterman DL: Assessment of treatment-associated changes in behavior and cholinergic therapy of neuropsychiatric symptoms in Alzheimer's disease. J Clin Psychiatry 59 (suppl 13):23–30, 1998

Cummings JL, Vinters HV, Cole GM, et al: Alzheimer's disease: etiologies, pathophysiology, cognitive reserve, and treatment opportunities. Neurology 51 (1 suppl 1): S2–S17; discussion S65–S67, 1998

Cummings JL, Schneider L, Tariot PN: Reduction of behavioral disturbances and caregiver distress by galantamine in patients with Alzheimer's disease. Am J Psychiatry 161:532–538, 2004

Curb JD, Rodriguez BL, Abbott RD, et al: Longitudinal association of vascular and Alzheimer's dementias, diabetes, and glucose tolerance. Neurology 52:971–975, 1999

Czura CJ, Friedman SG, Tracey KJ: Neural inhibition of inflammation: the cholinergic anti-inflammatory pathway. J Endotoxin Res 9:409–413, 2003

Daniel DG: Antipsychotic treatment of psychosis and agitation in the elderly. J Clin Psychiatry 61 (suppl 14):49–52, 2000

d'Arminio Monforte A, Duca PG, Vago L, et al: Decreasing incidence of CNS AIDS-defining events associated with antiretroviral therapy. Neurology 54:1856–1859, 2000

Dautzenberg PLJ, Mulder LJ, OldeRikkert MGM, et al: Adding rivastigmine to antipsychotics in the treatment of a chronic delirium. Age Ageing 33:516–517, 2004a

Dautzenberg PLJ, Mulder LJ, OldeRikkert MGM, et al: Delirium in elderly hospitalized patients: protective effects of chronic rivastigmine usage. Int J Geriatr Psychiatry 19:641–644, 2004b

Davis RL, Robertson DM (eds): Textbook of Neuropathology, 3rd Edition. Baltimore, MD, Williams & Wilkins, 1997

de Koning I, van Kooten F, Dippel DW, et al: The CAMCOG: a useful screening instrument for dementia in stroke patients. Stroke 29:2080–2086, 1998

Delacourte A, David JP, Sergeant N, et al: The biochemical pathway of neurofibrillary degeneration in aging and Alzheimer's disease. Neurology 52:1158–1165, 1999

Desmond DW, Moroney JT, Paik MC, et al: Frequency and clinical determinants of dementia after ischemic stroke. Neurology 54:1124–1131, 2000

DeSouza EB, Grigoriadis DE: Corticotropin-releasing factor: physiology, pharmacology, and role in central nervous system disorders, in Neuropsychopharmacology: The Fifth Generation of Progress. Edited by Davis KL, Charney D, Coyle JT, et al. Philadelphia, PA, Lippincott Williams & Wilkins, 2002, pp 91–107

Dolan MM, Hawkes WG, Zimmerman SI, et al: Delirium on hospital admission in aged hip fracture patients: prediction of mortality and 2-year functional outcomes. J Gerontol 55:M527–M534, 2000

Doody RS, Massman PJ, Mawad M, et al: Cognitive consequences of subcortical magnetic resonance imaging changes in Alzheimer's disease: comparison to small-vessel ischemic vascular dementia. Neuropsychiatry, Neuropsychology, and Behavioral Neurology 11:191–199, 1998

Doraiswamy PM, Steffens DC, Pitchumoni S, et al: Early recognition of Alzheimer's disease: What is consensual? What is controversial? What is practical? J Clin Psychiatry 59 (suppl):6–18, 1998

Duara R, Barker W, Luis CA: Frontotemporal dementia and Alzheimer's disease: differential diagnosis. Dement Geriatr Cogn Disord 10 (suppl):37–42, 1999

Dubinsky RM, Stein AC, Lyons K: Practice parameter: risk of driving and Alzheimer's disease (an evidence-based review). Neurology 54:2205–2211, 2000

Dufouil C, Clayton D, Brayne C, et al: Population norms for the MMSE in the very old: estimates based on longitudinal data. Mini-Mental State Examination. Neurology 55:1609–1613, 2000

Dunn NR, Alfonso CA, Young RA, et al: Creutzfeldt-Jakob disease appearing as paranoid psychosis. Am J Psychiatry 156:2016–2017, 1999

Dyer CB, Ashton CM, Teasdale TA: Postoperative delirium: a review of 80 primary data-collection studies. Arch Intern Med 155:461–465, 1995

Edelstein DM, Aharonoff GB, Karp A, et al: Effect of postoperative delirium on outcome after hip fracture. Clin Orthop Relat Res 1:195–200, 2004

Edlund A, Lundstrom M, Brannsrom B, et al: Delirium before and after operation for femoral neck fracture. J Am Geriatr Soc 49:1335–1340, 2001

Elie M, Cole MG, Primeau FJ, et al: Delirium risk factors in elderly hospitalized patients. J Gen Intern Med 13:204–212, 1998

Elie M, Rousseau F, Cole M, et al: Prevalence and detection of delirium in elderly emergency room department patients. Can Med Assoc J 163:977–981, 2000

Ely EW, Inouye SK, Bernard GR, et al: Delirium in mechanically ventilated patients: validity and reliability of the confusion assessment method for the intensive care unit (CAM-ICU). JAMA 286:2703–2710, 2001

Ely EW, Shintani A, Truman B, et al: Delirium as a predictor of mortality in mechanically ventilated patients in the intensive care unit. JAMA 291:1753–1762, 2004a

Ely EW, Stephens RK, Jackson JC, et al: Current opinions regarding the importance, diagnosis, and management of delirium in the intensive care unit: a survey of 912 healthcare professionals. Crit Care Med 32:106–112, 2004b

Engel GL, Romano J: Delirium: a syndrome of cerebral insufficiency. J Chronic Dis 9:260–277, 1959

Engel GL, Webb JP, Ferris EB: Quantitative electroencephalographic studies of anoxia in humans: comparisons with acute alcohol intoxication and hypoglycemia. J Clin Invest 24:691–697, 1945

Engelhart MJ, Geerlings MI, Ruitenberg A, et al: Dietary intake of antioxidants and risk of Alzheimer disease. JAMA 287:3223–3229, 2002

Fainsinger RL, Waller A, Bercovici M, et al: A multicentre international study of sedation for uncontrolled symptoms in terminally ill patients. Palliat Med 14:257–265, 2000

Fann JR, Roth-Roemer S, Burington B, et al: Delirium in patients undergoing hematopoietic stem cell transplantation: epidemiology, risk factors, and outcomes. Symposium presented at the annual meeting of the Academy of Psychosomatic Medicine, Palm Springs, CA, November 2000

Fayers PM, Hjermstad MJ, Ranhoff AH, et al: Which Mini-Mental State Exam items can be used to screen for delirium and cognitive impairment? J Pain Symptom Manage 30:41–50, 2005

Felician O, Sandson TA: The neurobiology and pharmacotherapy of Alzheimer's disease. J Neuropsychiatry Clin Neurosci 11:19–31, 1999

Fernandez F, Levy JK, Mansell PW: Management of delirium in terminally ill AIDS patients. Int J Psychiatry Med 19:165–172, 1989

Ferrante RJ, Andreason OA, Jenkins BG, et al: Neuroprotective effects of creatine in a transgenic mouse model of Huntington's disease. J Neurosci 20:4389–4397, 2000

Fink M: Cytopathic hypoxia in sepsis. Acta Anaesthesiol Scand 110 (suppl):87–95, 1997

Fink M: Delirious mania. Bipolar Disord 1:54–60, 1999

Flacker JM, Wei JY: Endogenous anticholinergic substances may exist during acute illness in elderly medical patients. J Gerontol 56:M353–M355, 2001

Fodale V, Santamaria LB: Drugs of anesthesia, central nicotinic receptors and postoperative cognitive dysfunction. Acta Anaesthesiol Scand 47:1180–1182, 2003

Folstein MF, Folstein SE, McHugh PR: "Mini-Mental State": a practical method for grading the cognitive state of patients for the clinician. J Psychiatr Res 12:189–198, 1975

Foster NL, Minoshima S, Kuhl DE: Brain imaging in Alzheimer disease, in Alzheimer Disease, 2nd Edition. Edited by Terry RD, Katzman R, Bick KL, et al. Philadelphia, PA, Lippincott Williams & Wilkins, 1999

Foy A, O'Connell D, Henry D, et al: Benzodiazepine use as a cause of cognitive impairment in elderly hospital inpatients. J Gerontol 50A:M99–M106, 1995

Francis J, Kapoor WN: Prognosis after hospital discharge of older medical patients with delirium. J Am Geriatr Soc 40:601–606, 1992

Francis J, Martin D, Kapoor WN: A prospective study of delirium in hospitalized elderly. JAMA 263:1097–1101, 1990

Franco K, Litaker D, Locala J, et al: The cost of delirium in the surgical patient. Psychosomatics 42:68–73, 2001

Freter SH, Dunbar MJ, MacLeod H, et al: Predicting postoperative delirium in elective orthopaedic patients: the Delirium Elderly At-Risk (DEAR) instrument. Age Ageing 34:169–171, 2005

Gagnon P, Allard P, Masse B, et al: Delirium in terminal cancer: a prospective study using daily screening, early diagnosis, and continuous monitoring. J Pain Symptom Manage 19:412–426, 2000

Ganguli M, Dodge HH, Shen C, et al: Mild cognitive impairment, amnestic type: an epidemiologic study. Neurology 63:115–121, 2004

Gaudreau JD, Gagnon P: Psychogenic drugs and delirium pathogenesis: the central role of the thalamus. Med Hypotheses 64:471–475, 2005

Gaudreau JD, Gagnon P, Harel F, et al: Fast, systematic, and continuous delirium assessment in hospitalized patients: the nursing delirium screening scale. J Pain Symptom Manage 29:368–375, 2005

Gauthier S, Reisberg B, Zaudig M, et al: Mild cognitive impairment. Lancet 367:1262–1270, 2006

Geda YE, Knopman DS, Mrazek DA, et al: Depression, apolipoprotein E genotype, and the incidence of mild cognitive impairment: a prospective cohort study. Arch Neurol 63:435–440, 2006

Geerlings MI, Jonker C, Bouter LM, et al: Association between memory complaints and incident Alzheimer's disease in elderly people with normal baseline cognition. Am J Psychiatry 156:531–537, 1999

Geldmacher DS, Whitehouse PJ Jr: Differential diagnosis of Alzheimer's disease. Neurology 48 (5 suppl 6):S2–S9, 1997

Gendelman HE, Zheng J, Coulter CL, et al: Suppression of inflammatory neurotoxins by highly active antiretroviral therapy in human immunodeficiency virus–associated dementia. J Infect Dis 178:1000–1007, 1998

Geula C: Abnormalities of neural circuitry in Alzheimer's disease: hippocampus and cortical cholinergic innervation. Neurology 51 (1 suppl 1):S18–S29; discussion S65–S67, 1998

Gibson GE, Blass JP: Impaired synthesis of acetylcholine in brain accompanying mild hypoxia and hypoglycemia. J Neurochem 27:37–42, 1976

Gibson GE, Pulsinelli W, Blass JP, et al: Brain dysfunction in mild to moderate hypoxia. Am J Med 70:1247–1254, 1981

Gleason OC: Donepezil for postoperative delirium. Psychosomatics 44:437–438, 2003

Gliatto MF, Caroff SN: Neurosyphilis: a history and clinical review. Psychiatr Ann 31:153–161, 2001

Globus MY, Ginsberg M, Dietrich WD, et al: Substantia nigra lesion protects against ischemic damage in the striatum. Neurosci Lett 68:169–174, 1986

Globus MY, Busto R, Dietrich WD, et al: Effect of ischemia on the in vivo release of striatal dopamine, glutamate, and gamma-aminobutyric acid studied by intracerebral microdialysis. J Neurochem 51:1455–1464, 1988a

Globus MY, Busto R, Martinez E, et al: Intra-ischemic extracellular release of dopamine and glutamate is associated with striatal vulnerability to ischemia. Neurosci Lett 91:36–40, 1988b

Goldman WP, Baty JD, Buckles VD, et al: Motor dysfunction in mildly demented AD individuals without extrapyramidal signs. Neurology 53:956–962, 1999

Gomez-Isla T, Growdon WB, McNamara M, et al: Clinicopathological correlates in temporal cortex in dementia with Lewy bodies. Neurology 53:2003–2009, 1999

Goodkin K, Baldewicz TT, Wilkie FL, et al: Cognitive-motor impairment and disorder in HIV-1 infection. Psychiatr Ann 31:37–44, 2001

Graham DG: Oxidative pathways for catecholamines in the genesis of neuromelanin and cytotoxic quinones. Mol Pharmacol 14:633–643, 1978

Graham DG: Catecholamine toxicity: a proposal for the molecular pathogenesis of manganese neurotoxicity and Parkinson's disease. Neurotoxicology 5:83–96, 1984

Grace AA: Dopamine, in Neuropsychopharmacology: The Fifth Generation of Progress. Edited by Davis KL, Charney D, Coyle JT, et al. Philadelphia, PA, Lippincott Williams & Wilkins, 2002, pp 119–132

Griffith HR, Netson KL, Harrell LE, et al: Amnestic mild cognitive impairment: diagnostic outcomes and clinical prediction over a two-year tie period. J Int Neuropsychol Soc 12:166–175, 2006

Grossberg GT, Lake JT: The role of the psychiatrist in Alzheimer's disease. J Clin Psychiatry 59 (suppl 9):3–6, 1998

Gupta N, Sharma P, Prabhakar S: Olanzapine for delirium in parkinsonism: therapeutic benefits in lieu of adverse consequences. Neurol India 52:274–275, 2004

Gury C, Canceil O, Iaria P: Antipsychotic drugs and cardiovascular safety: current studies of prolonged QT interval and risk of ventricular arrhythmia (abstract). Encephale 26:62–72, 2000

Gustafson K, Berggren D, Brannstrom B, et al: Acute confusional states in elderly patients treated for femoral neck fractures. J Am Geriatr Soc 36:525–530, 1988

Gustafson K, Brannstrom B, Berggren D, et al: A geriatric-anaesthesiologic program to reduce acute confusional states in elderly patients treated for femoral neck fractures. J Am Geriatr Soc 39:655–662, 1991

Haass C, De Strooper B: The presenilis in Alzheimer's disease: proteolysis holds the key. Science 286:916–919, 1999

Hall R, Hall R, Chapman M: Definition, diagnosis, and forensic implications of postconcussional syndrome. Psychosomatics 46:195–202, 2005

Hamilton M: A rating scale for depression. J Neurol Neurosurg Psychiatry 23:51–56, 1960

Han CS, Kim YK: A double-blind trial of risperidone and haloperidol for the treatment of delirium. Psychosomatics 45:297–301, 2004

Han L, McCusker J, Cole, M, et al: Use of medications with anticholinergic effect predicts clinical severity of delirium symptoms in older medical inpatients. Arch Intern Med 161:1099–1105, 2001

Harhangi BS, de Rijk MC, van Duijn CM, et al: APOE and the risk of PD with or without dementia in a population-based study. Neurology 54:1272–1276, 2000

Harmon D, Eustace N, Ghori K, et al: Plasma concentrations of nitric oxide products and cognitive dysfunction following coronary artery bypass surgery. Eur J Anesthesiol 22:269–276, 2005

Haroutunian V, Perl DP, Purohit DP, et al: Regional distribution of neuritic plaques in the nondemented elderly and subjects with very mild Alzheimer disease. Arch Neurol 55:1185–1191, 1998

Harper C, Fornes P, Duyckaerts C, et al: An international perspective on the prevalence of the Wernicke-Korsakoff syndrome. Metab Brain Dis 10:17–24, 1995

Harris GJ, Lewis RF, Satlin A, et al: Dynamic susceptibility contrast MRI of regional cerebral blood volume in Alzheimer's disease. Am J Psychiatry 153:721–724, 1996

Hartman S, Mobius HJ: Tolerability of memantine in combination with cholinesterase inhibitors in dementia therapy. Int Clin Psychopharmacol 18:81–85, 2003

Hashimoto M, Kazui H, Matsumoto K, et al: Does donepezil treatment slow the progression of hippocampal atrophy in patients with Alzheimer's disease? Am J Psychiatry 162:676–682, 2005

Henon H, Lebert F, Durieu I, et al: Confusional state in stroke: relation to preexisting dementia, patient characteristics, and outcome. Stroke 30:773–779, 1999

Herrmann N, Lanctot KL, Khan LR: The role of norepinephrine in the behavioral and psychological symptoms of dementia. J Neuropsychiatry Clin Neurosci 16:261–276, 2004a

Herrmann N, Mamdani M, Lanctot: Atypical antipsychotics and risk of cerebrovascular accidents. Am J Psychiatry 161:1113–1115, 2004b

Heyman A, Fillenbaum GG, Gearing M, et al: Comparison of Lewy body variant of Alzheimer's disease with pure Alzheimer's disease. Neurology 52:1839–1844, 1999

Hodges JR, Warlow CP: Syndromes of transient global amnesia: towards a classification. A study of 153 cases. J Neurol Neurosurg Psychiatry 53:834–843, 1990a

Hodges JR, Warlow CP: The aetiology of transient global amnesia. A case-control study of 114 cases with prospective follow-up. Brain 113 (pt 3):639–657, 1990b

Horikawa N, Yamazaki T, Miyamoto K, et al: Treatment for delirium with risperidone: results of a prospective open trial with 10 patients. Gen Hosp Psychiatry 25:289–292, 2003

Hughes TA, Ross HF, Musa S, et al: A 10-year study of the incidence of and factors predicting dementia in Parkinson's disease. Neurology 54:1596–1602, 2000

Hurtig HI, Trojanowski JQ, Galvin J, et al: Alpha-synuclein cortical Lewy bodies correlate with dementia in Parkinson's disease. Neurology 54:1916–1921, 2000

Hy LX, Keller DM: Prevalence of AD among whites: a summary by levels of severity. Neurology 55:198–204, 2000

Ichikawa J, Dai J, O'Laughlin IA, et al: Atypical, but not typical, antipsychotic drugs increase cortical acetylcholine release without an effect in the nucleus accumbens or striatum. Neuropsychopharmacology 26:325–339, 2002

Ichikawa J, Chung YC, Dai J, et al: Valproic acid potentiates both typical and atypical antipsychotic-induced prefrontal cortical dopamine release. Brain Res 1052:56–62, 2005

Ikarashi Y, Takahashi A, Ishimaur H, et al: Regulation of dopamine D1 and D2 receptors on striatal acetylcholine release in rats. Brain Res Bull 43:107–115, 1997

Inouye SK: Delirium in hospitalized older patients. Acute Hospital Care 14:745–764, 1998

Inouye SK: Current concepts: delirium in older persons. N Engl J Med 354:1157–1165, 2006

Inouye SK, Charpentier PA: Precipitating factors for delirium in hospitalized elderly persons: predictive model and interrelationship with baseline vulnerability. JAMA 275:852–857, 1996

Inouye SK, VanDyck CH, Alessi CA, et al: Clarifying confusion: the confusion assessment method: a new method for detection of delirium. Ann Intern Med 113:941–948, 1990

Inouye SK, Viscoli CM, Horwitz RI, et al: A predictive model for delirium in hospitalized elderly medical patients based on admission characteristics. Ann Intern Med 119:474–481, 1993

Inouye SK, Rushing JT, Foreman MD, et al: Does delirium contribute to poor hospital outcomes? A three-site epidemiologic study. J Gen Intern Med 13:234–242, 1998

Inouye SK, Bogardus ST, Charpentier PA, et al: A multicomponent intervention to prevent delirium in hospitalized older patients. N Engl J Med 340:669–676, 1999

Inouye SK, Foreman MD, Mikon LC, et al: Nurses' recognition of delirium and its symptoms: comparison of nurse and researcher ratings. Arch Intern Med 161:2467–2473, 2001

Inouye SK, Leo-Summers L, Zhang Y, et al: A chart-based method for identification of delirium: validation compared with interviewer ratings using the confusion assessment method. J Am Geriatr Soc 53:312–318, 2005

Ishii K, Imamura T, Sasaki M, et al: Regional cerebral glucose metabolism in dementia with Lewy bodies and Alzheimer's disease. Neurology 51:125–130, 1998

Itil T, Fink M: Anticholinergic drug-induced delirium: experimental modification, quantitative EEG and behavioral correlations. J Nerv Ment Dis 6:492–507, 1966

Jack CR, Petersen RC, Xu YC, et al: Prediction of AD with MRI-based hippocampal volume in mild cognitive impairment. Neurology 54:1397–1403, 2000

Jacquemont S, Hagerman RJ, Leehy, M, et al: Fragile X permutation tremor/ataxia syndrome: molecular, clinical, and neuroimaging correlates. Am J Hum Genet 72:869–878, 2003

Jellinger KA: Structural basis of dementia in neurodegenerative disorders. J Neural Transm 47 (suppl):1–29, 1996

Jeste DV, Okamoto A, Napolitano J, et al: Low incidence of persistent tardive dyskinesia in elderly patients with dementia treated with risperidone. Am J Psychiatry 157:1150–1155, 2000

Jones C, Griffiths R, Humphris G: Disturbed memory and amnesia related to intensive care. Memory 8:79–94, 2000

Jorm AF, Jolley D: The incidence of dementia: a meta-analysis. Neurology 51:728–733, 1998

Kales HC, Blow FC, Copeland LA, et al: Health care utilization by older patients with coexisting dementia and depression. Am J Psychiatry 156:550–556, 1999

Kalisvaart KJ, DeJonghe JFM, Bogaards MJ, et al: Haloperidol prophylaxis for elderly hip-surgery patients at risk for delirium: a randomized placebo-controlled study. J Am Geriatr Soc 53:1658–1666, 2005

Kaneko T, Cai J, Ishikura T, et al: Prophylactic consecutive administration of haloperidol can reduce the occurrence of postoperative delirium in gastrointestinal surgery. Yonago Acta Med 42:179–184, 1999

Katz IR: Diagnosis and treatment of depression in patients with Alzheimer's disease and other dementias. J Clin Psychiatry 59 (suppl 9):38–44, 1998

Katz IR, Jeste DV, Mintzer JE, et al: Comparison of risperidone and placebo for psychosis and behavioral disturbances associated with dementia: a randomized, double-blind trial. Risperidone Study Group. J Clin Psychiatry 60:107–115, 1999

Katz IR, Curyto KJ, TenHave T, et al: Validating the diagnosis of delirium and evaluating its association with deterioration over a one-year period. Am J Geriatr Psychiatry 9:148–159, 2001

Kaye JA: Diagnostic challenges in dementia. Neurology 51 (1 suppl 1):S45–S52; discussion S65–S67, 1998

Keane PE, Neal H: The effect of injections of dopaminergic agonists into the caudate nucleus on the electrocortigram of the rat. J Neurosci Res 6:237–241, 1981

Kelly KG, Zisselman M, Cutillo-Schmitter T, et al: Severity and course of delirium in medically hospitalized nursing facility residents. Am J Geriatr Psychiatry 9:72–77, 2001

Kenard MA, Bueding E, Wortis WB: Some biochemical and electroencephalographic changes in delirium tremens. Q J Stud Alcohol 6:4–14, 1945

Kennedy JS, Zager A, Bymaster F, et al: The central cholinergic system profile of olanzapine compared with placebo in Alzheimer's disease. Int J Geriatr Psychiatry 16:S24–S32, 2001

Kertesz A, Munoz DG: Frontotemporal dementia. Med Clin North Am 86:501–518, 2002

Keys MA, DeWald C: Clinical perspective on choice of atypical antipsychotics in elderly patients with dementia, part I. Annals of Long-Term Care: Clinical Care and Aging 13(2):26–32, 2005a

Keys MA, DeWald C: Clinical perspective on choice of atypical antipsychotics in elderly patients with dementia, part II. Annals of Long-Term Care: Clinical Care and Aging 13(3):30–38, 2005b

Kiely DK, Bergmann MA, Jones RN, et al: Characteristics associated with delirium persistence among newly admitted post-acute facility patients. J Gerontol A Biol Sci Med Sci 59A:344–349, 2004

Kim JY, Jung IK, Han C, et al: Antipsychotics and dopamine transporter gene polymorphisms in delirium patients. Psychiatry Clin Neurosci 59:183–188, 2005

Kim KS, Pae CU, Chae JH, et al: An open pilot trial of olanzapine for delirium in the Korean population. Psychiatry Clin Neurosci 55:515–519, 2001

Kim KY, Bader GM, Kotlyar V, et al: Treatment of delirium in older adults with quetiapine. J Geriatr Psychiatry Neurol 16:29–31, 2003

Kopelman MD: The Korsakoff syndrome. Br J Psychiatry 166:154–173, 1995

Koponen H, Hurri L, Stenback U, et al: Computed tomography findings in delirium. J Nerv Ment Dis 177:226–231, 1989a

Koponen H, Partanen J, Paakkonen A, et al: EEG spectral analysis in delirium. J Neurol Neurosurg Psychiatry 52:980–985, 1989b

Koponen H, Stenback U, Mattila E, et al: Delirium among elderly persons admitted to a psychiatric hospital: clinical course during the acute stage and one-year follow-up. Acta Psychiatr Scand 79:579–585, 1989c

Kramer JH, Duffy JM: Aphasia, apraxia, and agnosia in the diagnosis of dementia. Dementia 7:23–26, 1996

Krishnan KR, Hays JC, Blazer DG: MRI-defined vascular depression. Am J Psychiatry 154:497–501, 1997

Krishnan KRR, Charles HC, Doraiswamy PM, et al: Randomized, placebo-controlled trial of the effects of donepezil on neural markers and hippocampal volumes in Alzheimer's disease. Am J Psychiatry 160:2003–2011, 2003

Kuhl DE, Koeppe RA, Minoshima S, et al: In vivo mapping of cerebral acetylcholinesterase activity in aging and Alzheimer's disease. Neurology 52:691–699, 1999

Kumar V, Anand R, Messina J, et al: An efficacy and safety analysis of Exelon in Alzheimer's disease patients with concurrent vascular risk factors. Eur J Neurol 7:159–169, 2000

Langa KM, Foster NL, Larson EB: Mixed dementia: emerging concepts and therapeutic implications. JAMA 292:2901–2908, 2004

Lawlor BA: Behavioral and psychological symptoms in dementia: the role of atypical antipsychotics. J Clin Psychiatry 65 (suppl):5–10, 2004

Lawlor BA, Aisen PS, Green C, et al: Selegiline in the treatment of behavioural disturbance in Alzheimer's disease. Int J Geriatr Psychiatry 12:319–322, 1997

LeBlanc ES, Janowsky J, Chan BKS, et al: Hormone replacement therapy and cognition: systematic review and meta-analysis. JAMA 285:1489–1499, 2001

Lee KU, Won WY, Lee HK, et al: Amisulpride versus quetiapine for the treatment of delirium: a randomized, open prospective study. Int Clin Psychopharmacol 20:311–314, 2005

Leslie DL, Zhang Y, Bogardus ST, et al: Consequences of preventing delirium in hospitalized older adults on nursing home costs. J Am Geriatr Soc 53:405–409, 2005a

Leslie DL, Zhang Y, Holford TR, et al: Premature death associated with delirium at 1-year follow-up. Arch Intern Med 165:1657–1662, 2005b

Leung JM, Sands LP, Mullen EA, et al: Are preoperative depressive symptoms associated with postoperative delirium in geriatric surgical patients? J Gerontol A Biol Sci Med Sci 60A:1563–1568, 2005

Levin M: Delirium: a gap in psychiatric teaching. Am J Psychiatry 107:689–694, 1951

Levkoff SE, Evans DA, Liptzin B, et al: Delirium: the occurrence of and persistence of symptoms among elderly hospitalized patients. Arch Intern Med 152:334–340, 1992

Leverenz JB, McKeith: Dementia with Lewy bodies. Med Clin North Am 86:519–535, 2002

Levy ML, Cummings JL: Parkinson's disease, in Psychiatric Management in Neurological Disease. Edited by Lauterbach EC. Washington, DC, American Psychiatric Press, 2000, pp 41–70

Lin SM, Liu CY, Wang CH, et al: The impact of delirium on the survival of mechanically ventilated patients. Crit Care Med 32:2254–2259, 2004

Linnoila MI: Benzodiazepines and alcohol. J Psychiatr Res 24 (suppl):121–127, 1990

Liperoti R, Gambassi G, Lapane KL, et al: Cerebrovascular events among elderly nursing home patients treated with conventional or atypical antipsychotics. J Clin Psychiatry 66:1090–1096, 2005

Lipowski ZJ: Transient cognitive disorders (delirium, acute confusional states) in the elderly. Am J Psychiatry 140:1426–1436, 1983

Lipowski ZJ: Delirium (acute confusional states). JAMA 258:1789–1792, 1987

Lipowski ZJ: Delirium: how its concept has developed. Int Psychogeriatr 3:115–120, 1991

Liptzin B, Levkoff SE: An empirical study of delirium subtypes. Br J Psychiatry 161:843–845, 1992

Liptzin B, Laki A, Garb JL, et al: Donepezil in the prevention and treatment of postsurgical delirium. Am J Geriatr Psychiatry 13:1100–1106, 2005

Litvan I, McKee A: Clinicopathological case report. Dementia with Lewy bodies (DLB). J Neuropsychiatry Clin Neurosci 11:107–112, 1999

Liu CY, Juang YY, Liang HY, et al: Efficacy of risperidone in treating the hyperactive symptoms of delirium. Int Clin Psychopharmacol 19:165–168, 2004

Livingston G, Johnston K, Katona C, et al: Systemic review of psychological approaches to the management of neuropsychiatric symptoms of dementia. Am J Psychiatry 162:1996–2021, 2005

Lockwood AH, Yap EW, Rhoades HM, et al: Altered cerebral blood flow and glucose metabolism in patients with liver disease and minimal encephalopathy. J Cereb Blood Flow Metab 11:331–336, 1991

Lopez OL, Wisniewski S, Hamilton RL, et al: Predictors of progression in patients with AD and Lewy bodies. Neurology 54:1774–1779, 2000a

Lopez OL, Hamilton RL, Becker JT, et al: Severity of cognitive impairment and the clinical diagnosis of AD with Lewy bodies. Neurology 54:1780–1787, 2000b

Lundstrom M, Edlund A, Bucht G et al: Dementia after delirium in patients with femoral neck fractures. J Am Geriatr Soc 51:1002–1006, 2003

Lundstrom M, Edlund A, Karlsson S, et al: A multifactorial intervention program reduces the duration of delirium, length of hospitalization, and mortality in delirious patients. J Am Geriatr Soc 53:622–628, 2005

Lyketsos CG, Sheppard JM, Rabins PV: Dementia in elderly persons in a general hospital. Am J Psychiatry 157:704–707, 2000a

Lyketsos CG, Steinberg M, Schantz JT, et al: Mental and behavioral disturbances in dementia: findings from the Cache County Study on Memory in Aging. Am J Psychiatry 157:708–714, 2000b

Lyketsos CG, Lopez O, Jones B, et al: Prevalence of neuropsychiatric symptoms in dementia and mild cognitive impairment: results from the Cardiovascular Health Study. JAMA 288:1475–1483, 2002

Mace NL, Rabins PV: The 36-Hour Day: A Family Guide to Caring for Persons with Alzheimer's Disease, Related Dementing Illnesses, and Memory Loss in Later Life. Baltimore, MD, Johns Hopkins University Press, 1981

Maekawa T, Fujii Y, Sadamitsu D, et al: Cerebral circulation and metabolism in patients with septic encephalopathy. Am J Emerg Med 9:139–143, 1991

Maldonado JL, Fernandez F, Levy JK: Acquired immunodeficiency syndrome, in Psychiatric Management in Neurological Disease. Edited by Lauterbach EC. Washington, DC, American Psychiatric Press, 2000, pp 271–295

Maldonado JR, VanDerStarre PJ, Wysong A: Postoperative sedation and the incidence of ICU delirium in cardiac surgery patients. ASA Annual Meeting Abstracts. Anesthesiology 99:A465, 2003

Maltoni M, Caraceni A, Brunelli C, et al: Prognostic factors in advanced cancer patients: evidence-based clinical recommendations—a study by the steering committee of the European Association for Palliative Care. J Clin Oncol 23:6240–6248, 2005

Marcantonio ER, Goldman L, Mangione CM, et al: A clinical predictive rule for delirium after elective noncardiac surgery. JAMA 271:134–139, 1994

Marcantonio ER, Flacker JM, Michaels M, et al: Delirium is independently associated with poor functional recovery after hip fracture. J Am Geriatr Soc 48:618–624, 2000

Marcantonio ER, Kiely DK, Simon SE, et al: Outcomes of older people admitted to postacute facilities with delirium. JAGS, 53:963–969, 2005

Marsh L: Neuropsychiatric aspects of Parkinson's disease. Psychosomatics 41:15–23, 2000

Marson DC, Annis SM, McInturff B, et al: Error behaviors associated with loss of competency in Alzheimer's disease. Neurology 53:1983–1992, 1999

Massie MJ, Holland J, Glass E: Delirium in terminally ill cancer patients. Am J Psychiatry 140:1048–1050, 1983

McCusker J, Cole M, Dendukuri N, et al: Delirium in older medical inpatients and subsequent cognitive and functional status: a prospective study. Can Med Assoc J 165:575–583, 2001

McDaniel JS, Chung JY, Brown L, et al: Practice guideline for the treatment of patients with HIV/AIDS. Work Group on HIV/AIDS. American Psychiatric Association. Am J Psychiatry 157 (suppl):1–62, 2000

McHugh T, Laforce R, Gallagher P, et al: Natural history of the long-term cognitive, affective and physical sequelae of mild traumatic brain injury. Brain Cogn 60:209–211, 2006

McKeith IG, Ballard CG, Perry RH, et al: Prospective validation on consensus criteria for the diagnosis of dementia with Lewy bodies. Neurology 54:1050–1058, 2000

McNicoll L, Pisani MA, Ely EW, et al: Detection of delirium in the intensive care unit: comparison of confusion assessment method for the intensive care unit with confusion assessment method ratings. J Am Geriatr Soc 53:495–500, 2005

Meagher DJ, O'Hanlon D, O'Mahony E, et al: A study of environmental strategies in the study of delirium. Br J Psychiatry 168:512–515, 1996

Mega MS, Cummings JL, Fiorello T, et al: The spectrum of behavioral changes in Alzheimer's disease. Neurology 46:130–135, 1996

Meltzer HY: Mechanism of action of atypical antipsychotic drugs, in Neuropsychopharmacology: The Fifth Generation of Progress. Edited by Davis KL, Charney D, Coyle JT, et al. Philadelphia, PA, Lippincott Williams & Wilkins, 2002, pp 819–831

Meltzer CC, Price JC, Mathis CA, et al: PET imaging of serotonin type 2A receptors in late-life neuropsychiatric disorders. Am J Psychiatry 156:1871–1878, 1999

Mendez MF, Chen AK, Shapiro JS, et al: Acquired extroversion with bitemporal variant of frontotemporal dementia. J Neuropsychiatry Clin Neurosci 18:100–107, 2006

Mentis MJ, Horwitz B, Grady CL, et al: Visual cortical dysfunction in Alzheimer's disease evaluated with a temporally graded "stress test" during PET. Am J Psychiatry 153:32–40, 1996

Mercer B, Wepner W, Gardner H, et al: A study of confabulation. Arch Neurol 34:429–433, 1977

Meyer JS, Muramatsu K, Mortel KF, et al: Prospective CT confirms differences between vascular and Alzheimer's dementia. Stroke 26:735–742, 1995

Milbrandt E, Deppen S, Harrison P, et al: Costs associated with delirium in mechanically ventilated patients. Crit Care Med 32:955–962, 2004

Milbrandt EB, Kersten A, Kong L, et al: Haloperidol use is associated with lower hospital mortality in mechanically ventilated patients. Crit Care Med 33:226–229, 2005

Minden SL, Carbone LA, Barsky A, et al: Predictors and outcomes of delirium. Gen Hosp Psychiatry 27:209–214, 2005

Mintzer J, Greenspan A, Caers I, et al: Risperidone in the treatment of Alzheimer disease: results from a prospective clinical trial. Am J Geriatr Psychiatry 14:280–291, 2006

Mirenda J, Broyles G: Propofol as used for sedation in the ICU. Chest 108:539–548, 1995

Mittal D, Jimerson NA, Neely EP, et al: Risperidone in the treatment of delirium: results from a prospective open-label trial. J Clin Psychiatry 65:662–667, 2004

Mittenberg W, Rotholc A, Russell E, et al: Identification of malingered head injury on the Halstead-Reitan battery. Arch Clin Neuropsychol 11:271–281, 1996

Mobius HJ, Stoffler A: Memantine in vascular dementia. Int Psychogeriatr 15 (suppl):207–213, 2003

Moceri VM, Kukull WA, Emanuel I, et al: Early life risk factors and the development of Alzheimer's disease. Neurology 54:415–420, 2000

Modrego PJ, Ferrandez J: Depression in patients with mild cognitive impairment increases the risk of developing dementia of Alzheimer type: a prospective cohort study. Arch Neurol 61:1290–1293, 2004

Modrego PJ, Fayed N, Pina MA: Conversion from mild cognitive impairment to probable Alzheimer's disease predicted by brain magnetic resonance spectroscopy. Am J Psychiatry 162:667–675, 2005

Monette J, Galbaud du Fort G, Fung SH, et al: Evaluation of the Confusion Assessment Method (CAM) as a screening tool for delirium in the emergency room. Gen Hosp Psychiatry 23:20–25, 2001

Montine TJ, Sidell KR, Crews BC, et al: Elevated CSF prostaglandin E2 levels in patients with probable AD. Neurology 53:1495–1498, 1999

Moots RJ, AlSaffar Z, Hutchinson D, et al: Old drug, new tricks: haloperidol inhibits secretion of proinflammatory cytokines. Ann Rheum Dis 58:585–587, 1999

Moretti R, Torre P, Antonello RM, et al: Cholinesterase inhibition as a possible therapy for delirium in vascular dementia: a controlled, open 24-month study of 246 patients. Am J Alzheimers Dis Other Demen 19:333–339, 2004

Morgenthaler TI, Silber MH: Amnestic sleep-related eating disorder associated with zolpidem. Sleep Med 3:323–327, 2002

Morita T, Hirai K, Sakaguchi Y, et al: Family perceived distress from delirium-related symptoms of terminally ill cancer patients. Psychosomatics 45:107–113, 2004

Morita T, Takigawa C, Onishi H, et al: Opioid rotation from morphine to fentanyl in delirious cancer patients: an open-label trial. J Pain Symptom Manage 30:96–103, 2005

Moroney JT, Bagiella E, Tatemichi TK, et al: Dementia after stroke increases the risk of long-term stroke recurrence. Neurology 48:1317–1325, 1997

Mulsant BH, Pollack BG, Kirshner M, et al: Serum anticholinergic activity in a community-based sample of older adults. Arch Gen Psychiatry 60:198–203, 2003

Munford RS, Tracey KJ: Is severe sepsis a neuroendocrine disease? Mol Med 8:437–442, 2002

Mussi C, Ferrari R, Ascari S, et al: Importance of serum anticholinergic activity in the assessment of elderly patients with delirium. J Geriatr Psychiatry Neurol 12:82–86, 1999

Neary D, Snowden JS, Gustafson L, et al: Frontotemporal lobar degeneration: a consensus on clinical diagnostic criteria. Neurology 51:1546–1554, 1998

Obrist WD: Electroencephalographic changes in normal aging and dementia, in Brain Function in Old Age. Edited by Hoffmeister F, Mhuller C. New York, Springer-Verlag, 1979, pp 102–111

O'Keeffe ST: Delirium in the elderly. Age Ageing 28:5–8, 1999

O'Keeffe ST, Lavan J: The prognostic significance of delirium in older hospital patients. J Am Geriatr Soc 45:174–178, 1997

O'Keeffe ST, Mulkerrin EC, Nayeem K, et al: Use of serial Mini-Mental Status Examinations to diagnose and monitor delirium in elderly hospital patients. J Am Geriatr Soc 53:867–870, 2005

Ongini E, Caporali MG, Massotti M: Stimulation of dopamine D1 receptors by SKF 38393 induces EEG desynchronization and behavioral arousal. Life Sci 37:2327–2333, 1985

Pack AI, Millman RP: The lungs in later life, in Pulmonary Diseases and Disorders, 2nd Edition. Edited by Fishman AP. New York, McGraw-Hill, 1988, pp 80–90

Pae CU, Lee SJ, Lee CU, et al: A pilot trial of quetiapine for the treatment of patients with delirium. Hum Psychopharmacol 19:125–127, 2004

Pai M, Yang S: Transient global amnesia: a retrospective study of 25 patients. Chin Med J 62:140–144, 1999

Pandharipande P, Jackson J, Ely EW: Delirium: acute cognitive dysfunction in the critically ill. Curr Opin Crit Care 11:360–368, 2005

Pandharipande P, Shintani A, Peterson J, et al: Lorazepam is an independent risk factor for transitioning to delirium in intensive care unit patients. Anesthesiology 104:21–26, 2006

Papapetropoulos S, Lieberman A, Gonzalez, J, et al: Family history of dementia: dementia with Lewy bodies and dementia in Parkinson's disease. J Neuropsychiatry Clin Neurosci 18:113–116, 2006

Parada MA, Hernandez L, Puig de Parada M, et al: Selective action of acute systemic clozapine on acetylcholine release in the rat prefrontal cortex by reference to the nucleus accumbens and striatum. J Pharmacol Exp Ther 281:582–588, 1997

Parellada E, Baeza I, de Pablo J, et al: Risperidone in the treatment of patients with delirium. J Clin Psychiatry 65:348–353, 2004

Parnetti L: Therapeutic options in dementia. J Neurol 247:163–168, 2000

Patterson CJS, Gauthier S, Bergman H, et al: The recognition, assessment, and management of dementing disorders: conclusions form the Canadian Consensus Conference on Dementia. Can Med Assoc J 160 (suppl):S1–S14, 1999

Paulsen JS, Butters N, Sadek JR, et al: Distinct cognitive profiles of cortical and subcortical dementia in advanced illness. Neurology 45:951–956, 1995

Pavlov VA, Wang H, Czura CJ, et al: The cholinergic anti-inflammatory pathway: a missing link in neuroimmunomodulation. Mol Med 9:125–134, 2003

Peila R, White LR, Masaki K, et al: Reducing the risk of dementia: efficacy of long-term treatment of hypertension. Stroke 37:1165–1170, 2006

Peters N, Opherk C, Danek A, et al: The pattern of cognitive performance in CADASIL: a monogenic condition leading to subcortical ischemic vascular dementia. Am J Psychiatry 162:2078–2085, 2005

Petersen RC: Mild cognitive impairment as a diagnostic entity. J Intern Med 256:183–194, 2004

Petersen RC, Jack CR, Xu Y-C, et al: Memory and MRI-based hippocampal volumes in aging and AD. Neurology 54:581–587, 2000

Petersen RC, Parisi JE, Dickson DW, et al: Neuropathological features of amnestic mild cognitive impairment. Arch Neurol 63:665–672, 2006

Peterson JF, Pun BT, Dittus RS, et al: Delirium and its motoric subtypes: a study of 624 critically ill patients. J Am Geriatr Soc 54:479–484, 2006

Picciotto MR, Zoli M: Nicotinic receptors in aging and dementia. J Neurobiol 53:641–655, 2002

Pietrini P, Furey ML, Alexander GE, et al: Association between brain functional failure and dementia severity in Alzheimer's disease: resting versus stimulation PET study. Am J Psychiatry 156:470–473, 1999

Pisani MA, McNicoll L, Inouye SK: Cognitive impairment in the intensive care unit. Clin Chest Med 24:727–737, 2003

Pitkala KH, Laurila JV, Strandberg TE, et al: Prognostic significance of delirium in frail elderly people. Dement Geriatr Cogn Disord 19:158–163, 2005

Platt MM, Breitbart W, Smith M, et al: Efficacy of neuroleptics for hypoactive delirium. J Neuropsychiatry 6:66, 1994

Pompei P, Foreman M, Rudberg MA, et al: Delirium in hospitalized older persons: outcomes and predictors. J Am Geriatr Soc 42:809–815, 1994

Portet F, Ousset PJ, Visser PJ et al.: Mild cognitive impairment in medical practice: critical review of the concept and new diagnostic procedure. Report of the MCI Working Group of the European Consortium on Alzheimer's Disease (EADC). J Neurol Neurosurg Psychiatry 77:714–718, 2006

Pratico C, Quattrone D, Lucanto T, et al: Drugs of anesthesia acting on central cholinergic system may cause postoperative cognitive dysfunction and delirium. Med Hypotheses 65:972–982, 2005

Pulsinelli WA, Duffy TE: Regional energy balance in rat brain after transient forebrain ischemia. J Neurochem 40:1500–1503, 1983

Pun BT, Gordon SM, Peterson JF, et al: Large-scale implementation of sedation and delirium monitoring in the intensive care unit: a report from two medical centers. Crit Care Med 33:1199–1205, 2005

Quinette P, Guillery-Girard B, Dayan J, et al: What does transient global amnesia really mean? Review of the literature and thorough study of 142 cases. Brain 129:1640–1658, 2006

Rabins PV: Alzheimer's disease management. J Clin Psychiatry 59 (suppl 13):36–38, 1998

Rabins PV, Blacker D, Bland A, et al: Practice guideline for the treatment of patients with Alzheimer's disease and other dementias of late life. American Psychiatric Association. Am J Psychiatry 154 (suppl):1–39, 1997

Rahkonen T, Luukkainen-Markkula R, Paanila S, et al: Delirium episode as a sign of undetected dementia among community dwelling elderly subjects: a 2 year follow up study. J Neurol Neurosurg Psychiatry 69:519–521, 2000

Rahkonen T, Eloniemi-Sulkava U, Halonen P, et al: Delirium in the nondemented oldest old in the general population: risk factors and prognosis. Int J Geriatr Psychiatry 16:415–421, 2001

Ranen NG: Huntington's disease, in Psychiatric Management in Neurological Disease. Edited by Lauterbach EC. Washington, DC, American Psychiatric Press, 2000, pp 71–92

Rao V, Lyketsos CG: Delusions in Alzheimer's disease: a review. J Neuropsychiatry Clin Neurosci 10:373–382, 1998

Rao V, Lyketsos CG: Psychiatric aspects of traumatic brain injury. Psychiatr Clin North Am 25:43–69, 2002

Rapp SR, Espeland MA, Shumaker SA, et al: Effect of estrogen plus progestin on global cognitive function in postmenopausal women. The Women's Health Initiative Memory Study: a randomized controlled trial. JAMA 289:2663–2672, 2003

Raskind MA: The clinical interface of depression and dementia. J Clin Psychiatry 59 (suppl):9–12, 1998

Raskind MA, Peskind ER, Wessel T, et al: Galantamine in AD: a 6-month randomized, placebo controlled trial with a 6-month extension. The Galantamine USA-1 Study Group. Neurology 54:2261–2268, 2000

Rasquin SM, Lodder J, Visser PJ, et al: Predictive accuracy of MCI subtypes for Alzheimer's disease and vascular dementia in subjects with mild cognitive impairment: a 2-year follow-up study. Dement Geriatr Cogn Disord 19:113–119, 2005

Ravaglia G, Forti P, Maioli F, et al: Conversion of mild cognitive impairment to dementia: predictive role of mild cognitive impairment subtypes and vascular risk factors. Dement Geriatr Cogn Disord 21:51–58, 2006

Rebeck GW, Hyman BT: Apolipoprotein and Alzheimer's disease, in Alzheimer's Disease, 2nd Edition. Edited by Terry RD, Katzman R, Bick KL, et al. Philadelphia, PA, Lippincott Williams & Wilkins, 1999, pp 339–346

Reisberg B, Doody R, Stoffler A, et al: Memantine in moderate-to-severe Alzheimer's disease. N Engl J Med 348:1333–1341, 2003

Riker RR, Fraser GL, Cox PM: Continuous infusion of haloperidol controls agitation in critically ill patients. Crit Care Med 22:433–440, 1994

Rizzo M, Anderson SW, Dawson J, et al: Visual attention impairments in Alzheimer's disease. Neurology 54:1954–1959, 2000

Roache JD, Griffiths RR: Comparison of triazolam and pentobarbital: performance impairment, subjective effects, and abuse liability. J Pharmacol Exp Ther 234:120–133, 1985

Robinson RG: The Clinical Neuropsychiatry of Stroke: Cognitive, Behavioral, and Emotional Disorders Following Vascular Brain Injury. New York, Cambridge University Press, 1998

Rockwood K: Acute confusion in elderly medical patients. J Am Geriatr Soc 37:150–154, 1989

Rockwood K, Cosway S, Stolee P, et al: Increasing the recognition of delirium in elderly patients. J Am Geriatr Soc 42:252–256, 1994

Rockwood K, Cosway S, Carver, D, et al: The risk of dementia and death after delirium. Age Ageing 28:551–556, 1999

Rockwood K, Fay S, Song X, et al: Attainment of treatment goals by people with Alzheimer's disease receiving galantamine: a randomized controlled trial. Can Med Assoc J 174:1099–1105, 2006

Rogers SL, Friedhoff LT: Long-term efficacy and safety of donepezil in the treatment of Alzheimer's disease: an interim analysis of the results of a US multicentre open label extension study. Eur Neuropsychopharmacol 8:67–75, 1998

Rogers MP, Liang MH, Daltroy LH, et al: Delirium after elective orthopedic surgery: risk factors and natural history. Int J Psychiatry Med 19:109–121, 1989

Roman GC: Vascular dementia revisited: diagnosis, pathogenesis, treatment, and prevention. Med Clin North Am 86:3477–3499, 2002

Roman GC, Wilkinson DG, Doody RS, et al: Donepezil in vascular dementia: combined analysis of two large-scale clinical trials. Dement Geriatr Cogn Disord 20:338–344, 2005

Romano J, Engel GL: Delirium, part 1: electroencephalographic data. Arch Neurol Psychiatry 51:356–377, 1944

Rooij SE, Schuurmans MJ, VanderMast RC, et al: Clinical subtypes of delirium and their relevance for daily clinical practice: a systematic review. Int J Geriatr Psychiatry 20:609–615, 2005

Ropacki SA, Jeste DV: Epidemiology of risk factors for psychosis of Alzheimer's disease: a review of 55 studies published from 1990 to 2003. Am J Psychiatry 162:2022–2030, 2005

Rosenblatt A, Leroi I: Neuropsychiatry of Huntington's disease and other basal ganglia disorders. Psychosomatics 41:24–30, 2000

Ross CA, Peyser CE, Shapiro I, et al: Delirium: phenomenological and etiologic subtypes. Int Psychogeriatr 3:135–147, 1991

Ross GW, Bowen JD: The diagnosis and differential diagnosis of dementia. Med Clin North Am 86:455–476, 2002

Ross GW, Petrovitch H, White LR, et al: Characterization of risk factors for vascular dementia: the Honolulu–Asia Aging Study. Neurology 53:337–343, 1999

Royall DR, Cordes JA, Polk M: CLOX: an executive clock drawing task. J Neurol Neurosurg Psychiatry 64:588–594, 1998

Rudolph JL, Babikian VL, Birjiniuk V, et al: Atherosclerosis is associated with delirium after coronary artery bypass graft surgery. J Am Geriatr Soc 53:462–466, 2005

Ryan LM, Warden DL: Post concussion syndrome. Int Rev Psychiatry 15:310–316, 2003

Sano M, Ernesto C, Thomas RG, et al: A controlled trial of selegiline, alpha-tocopherol, or both as treatment for Alzheimer's disease. The Alzheimer's Disease Cooperative Study. N Engl J Med 336:1216–1222, 1997

Sasaki Y, Matsuyama T, Inoue S, et al: A prospective, open-label, flexible-dose study of quetiapine in the treatment of delirium. J Clin Psychiatry 64:1316–1321, 2003

Saykin AJ, Wishart HA, Rabin LA, et al: Cholinergic enhancement of frontal lobe activity in mild cognitive impairment. Brain 127:1574–1583, 2004

Scharf MB, Saskin P, Fletcher K: Benzodiazepine-induced amnesia: clinical laboratory findings. J Clin Psychiatry Monogr 5:14–17, 1987

Schneider LS, Dagerman KS, Insel P: Risk of death with atypical antipsychotic drug treatment for dementia: meta-analysis of randomized placebo-controlled trials. JAMA 294:1934–1943, 2005

Schneider LS, Dagerman KS, Insel P: Efficacy and adverse effects of atypical antipsychotics for dementia: meta-analysis of randomized, placebo-controlled trials. Am J Geriatr Psychiatry 14:191–210, 2006

Schor JD, Levkoff SE, Lipsitz LA, et al: Risk factors for delirium in hospitalized elderly. JAMA 267:827–831, 1992

Schwartz TL, Masand PS: Treatment of delirium with quetiapine. Prim Care Companion J Clin Psychiatry 2:10–12, 2000

Schwid SR, Weinstein A, Wishart HA, et al: Multiple sclerosis, in Psychiatric Management in Neurological Disease. Edited by Lauterbach EC. Washington, DC, American Psychiatric Press, 2000, pp 249–270

Seaman J: Seeing catatonia (letter). J Neuropsychiatry Clin Neurosci 17:558–559, 2005

Seaman J, Schillerstrom J, Carroll D, et al: Impaired oxidative metabolism precipitates delirium: a study of 101 ICU patients. Psychosomatics 47:56–61, 2006

Serby M, Brickman AM, Haroutunian V: Cognitive burden and excess Lewy-body pathology in the Lewy-body variant of Alzheimer's disease. Am J Geriatr Psychiatry 11:371–374, 2003

Serrano-Duenas M, Bleda MJ: Delirium in Parkinson's patients: a five year follow-up study. Parkinsonism Relat Disord 11:387–392, 2005

Sharma ND, Rosman HS, Padhi D, et al: Torsades de pointes associated with intravenous haloperidol in critically ill patients. Am J Cardiol 81:238–240, 1998

Shigeta H, Yasui A, Nimura Y, et al: Postoperative delirium and melatonin levels in elderly patients. Am J Surg 182:449–454, 2001

Shukry M, Clyde MC, Kalarickal PL, et al: Does dexmedetomidine prevent emergence delirium in children after sevoflurance-based general anesthesia? Pediatr Anesth 15:1098–1104, 2005

Shumaker SA, Legault C, Rapp SR, et al: Estrogen plus progestin and the incidence of dementia and mild cognitive impairment in postmenopausal women. The Women's Health Initiative Memory Study: a randomized clinical trial. JAMA 289:2651–2662, 2003

Shuping JR, Rollinson RD, Toole JF: Transient global amnesia. Ann Neurol 7:281–285, 1980

Simard M, van Reekum R: The acetylcholinesterase inhibitors for treatment of cognitive and behavioral symptoms in dementia with Lewy bodies. J Neuropsychiatry Clin Neurosci 16:409–425, 2004

Sink KM, Holden KF, Yaffe K: Pharmacological treatment of neuropsychiatric symptoms on dementia: a review of the evidence. JAMA 293:596–608, 2005

Sipahimalani A, Masand PS: Use of risperidone in delirium: case reports. Ann Clin Psychiatry 9:105–107, 1997

Skrobik YK, Bergeron N, Dumont M, et al: Olanzapine vs haloperidol: treating delirium in a critical care setting. Intensive Care Med 30:444–449, 2004

Slatkin N, Rhiner M: Treatment of opioid-induced delirium with acetylcholinesterase inhibitors: a case report. J Pain Symptom Manage 27:268–273, 2004

Slatkin N, Rhiner M, Bolton TM: Donepezil in the treatment of opioid-induced sedation: report of six cases. J Pain Symptom Manage 21:425–438, 2001

Small GW: Differential diagnosis and early detection of dementia. Am J Geriatr Psychiatry 6 (2 suppl 1):S26–S33, 1998a

Small GW: The pathogenesis of Alzheimer's disease. J Clin Psychiatry 59 (suppl 9):7–14, 1998b

Small GW, Leiter F: Neuroimaging for diagnosis of dementia. J Clin Psychiatry 59 (suppl 11):4–7, 1998

Small GW, Chen ST, Komo S, et al: Memory self-appraisal in middle-aged and older adults with the apolipoprotein E-4 allele. Am J Psychiatry 156:1035–1038, 1999

Smith CD, Andersen AH, Kryscio RJ, et al: Altered brain activation in cognitively intact individuals at high risk for Alzheimer's disease. Neurology 53:1391–1396, 1999

Smith CD, Snowdon DA, Wang H, et al: White matter volumes and periventricular white matter hyperintensities in aging and dementia. Neurology 54:838–842, 2000

Smits HA, Boven LA, Pereira CF, et al: Role of macrophage activation in the pathogenesis of Alzheimer's disease and human immunodeficiency virus type 1-associated dementia. Eur J Clin Invest 30:526–535, 2000

Song C, Lin A, Kenis G, et al: Immunosuppressive effects of clozapine and haloperidol: enhanced production of the interleukin-1 receptor antagonist. Schizophr Res 42:157–164, 2000

Spencer CM, Noble S: Rivastigmine. A review of its use in Alzheimer's disease. Drugs Aging 13:391–411, 1998

Spiller JA, Keen JC: Hypoactive delirium: assessing the extent of the problem for inpatient specialist palliative care. Palliat Med 20:17–23, 2006

Stahl SM: The new cholinesterase inhibitors for Alzheimer's disease, Part 1: their similarities are different. J Clin Psychiatry 61:710–711, 2000

Starkstein SE, Jorge R, Mizrahi R, et al: The construct of minor and major depression in Alzheimer's disease. Am J Psychiatry 162:2086–2093, 2005

Stern Y, Albert S, Tang MX, et al: Rate of memory decline in AD is related to education and occupation: cognitive reserve? Neurology 53:1942–1947, 1999

Stewart JT, Shin KJ: Paroxetine treatment of sexual disinhibition in dementia. Am J Psychiatry 154:1474, 1997

Straker D: Aripiprazole for the treatment of delirium. Webb Fellow Presentation, 52nd Annual Meeting of the Academy of Psychosomatic Medicine, Santa Ana Pueblo, NM, November 2005

Strauss ME, Ogrocki PK: Confirmation of an association between family history of affective disorder and the depressive syndrome in Alzheimer's disease. Am J Psychiatry 153:1340–1342, 1996

Tager FA, Fallon BA: Psychiatric and cognitive features of Lyme disease. Psychiatr Ann 31:173–181, 2001

Tariot PN, Farlow MR, Grossberg GT: Memantine treatment in patients with moderate to severe Alzheimer's disease already receiving donepezil. JAMA 291:317–324, 2004a

Tariot PN, Profenno LA, Ismail MS: Efficacy of atypical antipsychotics in elderly patients with dementia. J Clin Psychiatry 65 (suppl):11–15, 2004b

Teri L, Logsdon RG, Peskind E, et al: Treatment of agitation in AD: a randomized, placebo-controlled clinical trial. Neurology 55:1271–1278, 2000 (erratum in Neurology 56:426, 2001)

Tetewsky SJ, Duffy CJ: Visual loss and getting lost in Alzheimer's disease. Neurology 52:958–965, 1999

Thomason JW, Shintani A, Peterson JF, et al: Intensive care unit delirium is an independent predictor of longer hospital stays: a prospective analysis of 261 nonventilated patients. Crit Care 9:R375–R381, 2005

Tiraboschi P, Hansen LA, Alford M, et al: Cholinergic dysfunction in diseases with Lewy bodies. Neurology 54:407–411, 2000

Titier K, Canal M, Deridet E, et al: Determination of myocardium to plasma concentration ratios of five antipsychotic drugs: comparison with their ability to induce arrhythmia and sudden death in clinical practice. Toxicol Appl Pharmacol 199:52–60, 2004

Toda H, Kusumi I, Sasaki Y, et al: Relationship between plasma concentration levels of risperidone and clinical effects in the treatment of delirium. Int Clin Psychopharmacol 20:331–333, 2005

Tornatore JB, Hill E, Laboff JA, et al: Self-administered screening for mild cognitive impairment: initial validation of a computerized test battery. J Neuropsychiatry Clin Neurosci 17:98–105, 2005

Torres R, Mittal D, Kennedy R: Use of quetiapine in delirium: case reports. Psychosomatics 42:347–349, 2001

Tost H, Wendt CS, Schmitt A, et al: Huntington's disease: phenomenological diversity of a neuropsychiatric condition that challenges traditional concepts in neurology and psychiatry. Am J Psychiatry 161:28–34, 2004

Trinh N-H, Hoblyn J, Mohanty S, et al: Efficacy of cholinesterase inhibitors in the treatment of neuropsychiatric symptoms and functional impairment in Alzheimer disease: a meta-analysis. JAMA 289:210–216, 2003

Trzepacz PT: The neuropathogenesis of delirium: a need to focus our research. Psychosomatics 35:374–391, 1994

Trzepacz PT: Is there a final common neural pathway in delirium? Focus on acetylcholine and dopamine. Semin Clin Neuropsychiatry 5:132–148, 2000

Trzepacz PT, Maue FR, Coffman G, et al: Neuropsychiatric assessment of liver transplantation candidates: delirium and other psychiatric disorders. Int J Psychiatry Med 7:101–111, 1986

Trzepacz PT, Baker RW, Greenhouse J: A symptom rating scale for delirium. Psychiatry Res 23:89–97, 1988a

Trzepacz PT, Brenner RP, Coffman G, et al: Delirium in liver transplantation candidates: discriminant analysis of multiple test variables. Biol Psychiatry 24:3–14, 1988b

Trzepacz PT, Leavitt M, Congioli K: An animal model for delirium. Psychosomatics 33:404–414, 1992

Trzepacz PT, Ho V, Mallavarapu H: Cholinergic delirium and neurotoxicity associated with tacrine for Alzheimer's dementia. Psychosomatics 37:299–301, 1996

Trzepacz PT, Mulsant BH, Amanda Dew M, et al: Is delirium different when it occurs in dementia? A study using the delirium rating scale. J Neuropsychiatry Clin Neurosci 10:199–204, 1998

Trzepacz PT, Mittal D, Torres R, et al: Validation of the Delirium Rating Scale–Revised–98: comparison with the delirium rating scale and cognitive test for delirium. J Neuropsychiatry Clin Neurosci 13:229–242, 2001

Tsai L, Tsuang MT: The Mini-Mental State Test and computerized tomography. Am J Psychiatry 136:436–439, 1979

Tune LE: Postoperative delirium. Int Psychogeriatr 3:325–332, 1991

Tune LE, Egeli S: Acetylcholine and delirium. Dement Geriatr Cogn Disord 10:342–344, 1999

Tune LE, Folstein MF: Postoperative delirium. Adv Psychosom Med 15:51–68, 1986

Tune LE, Sunderland T: New cholinergic therapies: treatment tools for the psychiatrist. J Clin Psychiatry 59 (suppl 13):31–35, 1998

Tune LE, Carr S, Hoag E, et al: Anticholinergic effects of drugs commonly prescribed for the elderly: potential means for assessing risk of delirium. Am J Psychiatry 149:1393–1394, 1992

U.S. Food and Drug Administration: FDA public health advisory: deaths with antipsychotics in elderly patients with behavioral disturbances. Rockville, MD, U.S. Food and Drug Administration, April 11, 2005. Available at: http://www.fda.gov/cder/drug/advisory/antipsychotics.htm

Valk PE, Bailey DL, Townsend DW, et al: Positron Emission Tomography: Basic Science and Clinical Practice. London, England, Springer-Verlag, 2003

Victor M, Adams RD, Collins GH: The Wernicke-Korsakoff Syndrome and Related Neurologic Disorders Due to Alcoholism and Malnutrition, 2nd Edition. Philadelphia, PA, FA Davis, 1989

Volicer L, Harper DG, Manning BC, et al: Sundowning and circadian rhythms in Alzheimer's disease. Am J Psychiatry 158:704–711, 2001

Voyer P, Cole MG, McCusker J, et al: Prevalence and symptoms of delirium superimposed on dementia. Clin Nurs Res 15:46–66, 2006

Wacker P, Nunes PV, Cabrita H, et al: Postoperative delirium is associated with poor cognitive outcome and dementia. Dement Geriatr Cogn Disord 21:221–227, 2006

Weiner MF, Martin-Cook K, Foster BM, et al: Effects of donepezil on emotional/behavioral symptoms in Alzheimer's disease patients. J Clin Psychiatry 61:487–492, 2000

Weiss U, Bacher R, Vonbank H, et al: Cognitive impairment: assessment with brain magnetic resonance imaging and proton mass spectroscopy. J Clin Psychiatry 64:235–242, 2003

Wengel SP, Roccaforte WH, et al: Donepezil improves symptoms of delirium in dementia: implications for future research. J Geriatr Psychiatry Neurol 11:159–161, 1998

Wengel SP, Burke WJ, Roccaforte WH: Donepezil for postoperative delirium associated with Alzheimer's disease. J Am Geriatr Soc 47:379–380, 1999

White S, Calver BL, Newsway V, et al: Enzymes of drug metabolism during delirium. Age Ageing 34:603–608, 2005

Whitehouse PJ: The concept of subcortical and cortical dementia: another look. Ann Neurol 19:1–6, 1986

Wilkosz PA, Miyahara S, Lopez OL, et al: Prediction of psychosis onset in Alzheimer disease: the role of cognitive impairment, depressive symptoms, and further evidence of psychosis subtypes. Am J Geriatr Psychiatry 14:352–360, 2006

Williams M: Purinergic neurotransmission, in Neuropsychopharmacology: The Fifth Generation of Progress. Edited by Davis KL, Charney D, Coyle JT, et al. Philadelphia, PA, Lippincott Williams & Wilkins, 2002, pp 191–206

Williams-Russo P, Urquhart BL, Sharrock NE, et al: Postoperative delirium: predictors and prognosis in elderly orthopedic patients. J Am Geriatr Soc 40:759–767, 1992

Wilson K, Broadhurst C, Diver M, et al: Plasma insulin growth factor-1 and incident delirium in older people. Int J Ger Psychiatry 20:154–159, 2005

Wilson LM: Intensive care delirium: the effect of outside deprivation in a windowless unit. Arch Intern Med 130:225–226, 1972

Wilson RS, Bennett DA, Gilley DW, et al: Progression of parkinsonian signs in Alzheimer's disease. Neurology 54:1284–1289, 2000

Wimo A, Winblad B, Stoffler A, et al: Resource utilization and cost analysis of memantine in patients with moderate to severe Alzheimer's disease. Pharmacoeconomics 21:327–340, 2003

Winblad B, Poritis N: Memantine in severe dementia: results of the 9M-BEST Study (Benefit and Efficacy in Severely Demented Patients during Treatment with Memantine). Int J Geriatr Psychiatry 14:135–146, 1999

Winblad B, Kilander L, Eriksson S, et al: Donepezil in patients with severe Alzheimer's disease: double-blind, parallel group, placebo-controlled study. Lancet 367:1057–1063, 2006

Yaffe K, Krueger K, Cummings SR, et al: Effect of raloxifene on prevention of dementia and cognitive impairment in older women: the Multiple Outcomes of Raloxifene Evaluation (MORE) randomized trial. Am J Psychiatry 162:683–690, 2005

Yasuno F, Nishikawa T, Nakagawa Y, et al: Functional anatomical study of psychogenic amnesia. Psychiatry Res 99:43–57, 2000

Yesavage JA, Brink TL, Rose TL, et al: Development and validation of a geriatric depression screening scale: a preliminary report. J Psychiatr Res 17:37–49, 1983

Yock DH: Imaging of CNS Disease: A CT and MRI Teaching File. St. Louis, MO, Mosby Year Book, 1991

Zerr I, Schultz-Schaeffer WJ, Giese A, et al: Current clinical diagnosis in Creutzfeldt-Jakob disease: identification of uncommon variants. Ann Neurol 48:323–329, 2000

Zhu L, Fratiglioni L, Guo Z, et al: Incidence of stroke in relation to cognitive function and dementia in the Kungsholmen Project. Neurology 54:2103–2107, 2000

Zubenko GS, Zubenko WN, McPherson S: A collaborative study of the emergency and clinical features of the major depressive syndrome of Alzheimer's disease. Am J Psychiatry 160:857–866, 2003

9

SUBSTANCE-RELATED DISORDERS

Martin H. Leamon, M.D.
Tara M. Wright, M.D.
Hugh Myrick, M.D.

Psychoactive substance use has been part of people's lives for millennia (Austin 1978). About half of the world population uses at least one psychoactive substance, and although most do so without difficulties, for others problems arise that are related to the substance use (United Nations Office on Drugs and Crime 2005). Worldwide, drug and alcohol use disorders (excluding tobacco) are the sixth leading cause of disease burden in adults, whereas tobacco use and exposure to tobacco smoke are the leading preventable causes of death (World Health Organization 2003). Nationally (again excluding tobacco), 63% of American adults report that alcohol or drug addiction in themselves, family, or close friends has had an impact on their lives (Peter D. Hart Research Associates 2004). This chapter presents an overview of substance-related disorders, primarily focusing on those substances that are abused for their psychoactive effects, with additional material contained in the "Suggested Readings" listed at the end of the chapter.

Classification Systems

DSM-IV-TR defines a *substance* as "a drug of abuse, a medication, or a toxin" (American Psychiatric Association 2000) and classifies disorders attributable to substance use according to the schema in Table 9–1.

TABLE 9–1.	DSM-IV-TR classification of substance-related disorders
Substance-related disorders	
Substance use disorders	
Dependence	
Abuse	
Substance-induced disorders	
Intoxication	
Withdrawal	
Others (see Table 9–6)	

Eleven classes of substances that include the commonly recognized abusable drugs are described, and then other medications or toxins that could cause disorders are grouped into the class of other or unknown. The specific substance-related disorders are the substance-induced disorders of *intoxication* and *withdrawal* (Tables 9–2 and 9–3) and the substance use disorders of *abuse* and *dependence* (Tables 9–4 and 9–5).

Other substance-induced disorders are classified with their phenomenologically similar disorders, for example, substance-induced mood disorder is included in the DSM-IV-TR mood disorders section. Not all types of disorders are recognized for all classes of substances (Table 9–6).

TABLE 9–2.   DSM-IV-TR diagnostic criteria for substance intoxication

A. The development of a reversible substance-specific syndrome due to recent ingestion of (or exposure to) a substance.   **Note:**   Different substances may produce similar or identical syndromes.

B. Clinically significant maladaptive behavioral or psychological changes that are due to the effect of the substance on the central nervous system (e.g., belligerence, mood lability, cognitive impairment, impaired judgment, impaired social or occupational functioning) and develop during or shortly after use of the substance.

C. The symptoms are not due to a general medical condition and are not better accounted for by another mental disorder.

TABLE 9–3.   DSM-IV-TR diagnostic criteria for substance withdrawal

A. The development of a substance-specific syndrome due to the cessation of (or reduction in) substance use that has been heavy and prolonged.

B. The substance-specific syndrome causes clinically significant distress or impairment in social, occupational, or other important areas of functioning.

C. The symptoms are not due to a general medical condition and are not better accounted for by another mental disorder.

TABLE 9–4.   DSM-IV-TR diagnostic criteria for substance abuse

A. A maladaptive pattern of substance use leading to clinically significant impairment or distress, as manifested by one (or more) of the following, occurring within a 12-month period:

   (1) recurrent substance use resulting in a failure to fulfill major role obligations at work, school, or home (e.g., repeated absences or poor work performance related to substance use; substance-related absences, suspensions, or expulsions from school; neglect of children or household)

   (2) recurrent substance use in situations in which it is physically hazardous (e.g., driving an automobile or operating a machine when impaired by substance use)

   (3) recurrent substance-related legal problems (e.g., arrests for substance-related disorderly conduct)

   (4) continued substance use despite having persistent or recurrent social or interpersonal problems caused or exacerbated by the effects of the substance (e.g., arguments with spouse about consequences of intoxication, physical fights)

B. The symptoms have never met the criteria for substance dependence for this class of substance.

TABLE 9–5.   DSM-IV-TR diagnostic criteria for substance dependence

A maladaptive pattern of substance use, leading to clinically significant impairment or distress, as manifested by three (or more) of the following, occurring at any time in the same 12-month period:

(1) tolerance, as defined by either of the following:
   (a) a need for markedly increased amounts of the substance to achieve intoxication or desired effect
   (b) markedly diminished effect with continued use of the same amount of the substance

(2) withdrawal, as manifested by either of the following:
   (a) the characteristic withdrawal syndrome for the substance (refer to criteria A and B of the criteria sets for withdrawal from the specific substances)
   (b) the same (or a closely related) substance is taken to relieve or avoid withdrawal symptoms

(3) the substance is often taken in larger amounts or over a longer period than was intended

(4) there is a persistent desire or unsuccessful efforts to cut down or control substance use

(5) a great deal of time is spent in activities necessary to obtain the substance (e.g., visiting multiple doctors or driving long distances), use the substance (e.g., chain-smoking), or recover from its effects

(6) important social, occupational, or recreational activities are given up or reduced because of substance use

(7) the substance use is continued despite knowledge of having a persistent or recurrent physical or psychological problem that is likely to have been caused or exacerbated by the substance (e.g., current cocaine use despite recognition of cocaine-induced depression, or continued drinking despite recognition that an ulcer was made worse by alcohol consumption)

TABLE 9–6.   DSM-IV-TR diagnoses associated with class of substances

	Dependence	Abuse	Intoxication	Withdrawal	Intoxication delirium	Withdrawal delirium	Dementia	Amnestic disorder	Psychotic disorders	Mood disorders	Anxiety disorders	Sexual dysfunctions	Sleep disorders
Alcohol	X	X	X	X	X	X	X	X	X	X	X	X	X
Amphetamines	X	X	X	X	X				X	X	X	X	X
Caffeine			X								X		X
Cannabis	X	X	X		X				X		X		
Cocaine	X	X	X	X	X				X	X	X	X	X
Hallucinogens	X	X	X		X				X*	X	X		
Inhalants	X	X	X		X		X		X	X	X		
Nicotine	X			X									
Opioids	X	X	X	X	X				X	X		X	X
Phencyclidine	X	X	X		X				X	X	X		
Sedatives, hypnotics, or anxiolytics	X	X	X	X	X	X	X	X	X	X	X	X	X
Polysubstance	X												
Other	X	X	X	X	X	X	X	X	X	X	X	X	X

Note.   X indicates that the disorder is recognized in DSM-IV-TR.
*Includes hallucinogen persisting perception disorder (flashbacks).
Source.   Adapted from American Psychiatric Association 2000, p. 193.

The World Health Organization's (2006) *International Statistical Classification of Diseases and Related Health Problems*, 10th Revision (ICD-10) is similar to DSM-IV-TR in its recognition of intoxication, withdrawal, and dependence syndromes. Instead of the disorder of substance abuse, however, ICD-10 includes the disorder of harmful use, which has somewhat broader diagnostic criteria (Table 9–7).

Another classification system, used only for alcohol, is that of high-risk and low-risk drinking (Table 9–8) (National Institute on Alcohol Abuse and Alcoholism 2005). Unlike the DSM-IV-TR system, which focuses on the behavioral consequences of dysfunctional use, the high-/low-risk system focuses exclusively on volumetric and frequency criteria, based on the association of these parameters with risks of general medical sequelae to alcohol use (Rehm et al. 2003).

A word on terminology is in order. The words *dependence, abuse, addiction,* and others are often used with different meanings when discussing psychoactive substance use, potentially leading to confusion and misunderstanding (O'Brien et al. 2006). For the purposes of this chapter, the uncapitalized terms *dependence* and *addiction* are used interchangeably, and the uncapitalized term *abuse* is used to refer to substance use that leads to problems at any level. In DSM-IV-TR, the diagnoses are capitalized, thus leading to the commonly encountered but somewhat paradoxical situation in which Substance Dependence and Substance Abuse are both forms of substance abuse. It is also important to keep in mind the potential differences between lay, pharmacological, and psychiatric meanings of the term *intoxication*—the psychiatric disorder requires the impact of the substance effect to be "clinically significant" and "maladaptive." Last, many clinicians and patients consider treatment for substance dependence to be a process that involves a reorientation of all areas of a patient's life—a process termed *recovery*. At times, this chapter uses the terms *recovery* and *treatment* synonymously.

Neurobiology

A number of different neuronal circuits and neurotransmitters have been implicated in the process of addiction. Recent theories suggest that the process of becoming addicted to a substance includes a usurpation of the brain circuits involved in the pursuit and acquisition of normal "survival-relevant natural goals… [or] 'rewards,'" such as food or mating opportunities (Hyman 2005, p. 1414). The firing of dopamine-releas-

TABLE 9–7. ICD-10 classification of substance use disorders

Mental and behavioral disorders due to psychoactive substance use (F10–F19)

Acute intoxication

Harmful use
"A pattern of psychoactive substance use that is causing damage to health. The damage may be physical (e.g., hepatitis from self-administration of injected psychoactive substances) or mental (e.g., episodes of depressive disorder secondary to heavy consumption of alcohol)" (World Health Organization 2006).

Dependence syndrome

Withdrawal state

Others (e.g., withdrawal state with delirium, psychotic disorder, amnesic syndrome)

TABLE 9–8. Maximum alcohol consumption for low-risk drinking

For healthy men up to age 65 years
No more than 4 drinks in a day *and*
No more than 14 drinks in a week

For healthy women up to age 65 years
No more than 3 drinks in a day *and*
No more than 7 drinks in a week

For healthy adults older than 65 years
No more than 1 drink in a day *and*
No more than 7 drinks in a week

Recommend lower limits or abstinence as medically indicated; for example, for patients who
Take medications that interact with alcohol
Have a health condition exacerbated by alcohol
Are pregnant (advise abstinence)

Source. Adapted from National Institute on Alcohol Abuse and Alcoholism 2005. Public domain.

ing neurons, with cell bodies in the ventral tegmental area and axon terminals in the nucleus accumbens, serves to mark the importance or salience of a reward as well as signaling that a rewarding event is about to occur. Many, if not all, addictive substances produce a measure of firing that is much greater than that produced by more mundane survival-relevant ones. Further processing of the stimulus by prefrontal cortical areas leads to associative learning that attributes an unduly high level of significance to the substance effect and substance use–related cues (Kalivas and Volkow 2005). In addition to dopamine, the neurotransmitters glutamate, γ-aminobutyric acid (GABA), and opioid neuropeptides are important in this circuitry (Figure 9–1).

The eventual circuitry changes resulting from the intracellular accumulation of gene transcription products and other neuronal modifications result in the substance use changing from intentional to compulsive and out of control (Nestler 2005). Interestingly, the circuitry involved with relapse (i.e., the reinstitution of substance use following a period of cessation of use in an addicted person) overlaps but is not identical to that involved in the initial addiction, and there seem to be different pathways involved if the relapse is triggered by stress, exposure to substance-related cues, or direct substance use (Weiss 2005).

There is ample epidemiological and experimental evidence that susceptibility to addiction is influenced by genetics and that the genetic contribution is determined by multiple genes and is modulated by environmental influences (Kreek et al. 2005; Nader and Czoty 2005; Velleman et al. 2005). The questions of which genes are involved for which substances and what environmental factors increase or decrease susceptibility are matters of active research. One of the environmental factors does seem to be the type of drug used. The 2004 National Survey on Drug Use and Health revealed large differences between substances in the percentage of past-year users meeting criteria for abuse or dependence (Table 9–9) (Substance Abuse and Mental Health Services Administration 2005).

Looking at lifetime risk, the National Comorbidity Survey (NCS) conducted in the early 1990s found that around one-third of people who had ever smoked a cigarette developed nicotine dependence; 15% of those who had ever drunk alcohol developed alcohol dependence; and 15% of those who had ever tried other drugs developed drug dependence (Anthony et al. 1994).

Approach to the Patient

A patient with a substance use disorder may present in a number of different ways, and in a general psychiatric practice he or she may present with complaints of mood problems, anxiety, sleep difficulties, or symptoms of another Axis I or Axis II psychiatric disorder. For this reason, all patients should be routinely and consistently screened for substance use disorders. A number of instruments exist, and different ones may be used depending on the specific clinical setting

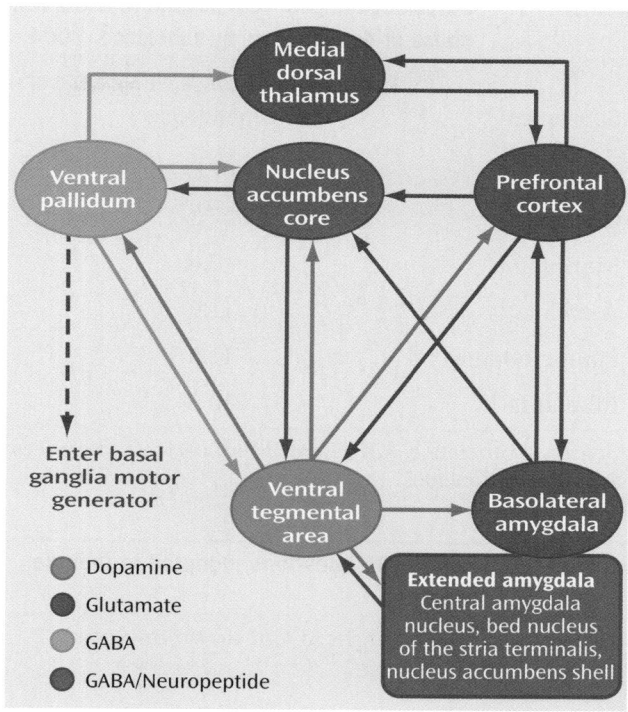

FIGURE 9–1. Neural circuitry implicated in the process of addiction.

GABA = γ-aminobutyric acid.

Source. Reprinted from Kalivas PW, Volkow ND: "The Neural Basis of Addiction: A Pathology of Motivation and Choice." *American Journal of Psychiatry* 162:1403–1413, 2005. Used with permission.

(Dyson et al. 1998; McPherson and Hersch 2000; Workgroup on Substance Use Disorders 2006). One such instrument is the CAGE-D (Table 9–10); the patient's answers to the questions can serve as a springboard into further discussion of substance use (Dyson et al. 1998). One should inquire about all classes of substances (e.g., alcohol, opioids, sedative/hypnotics, stimulants, cannabis, nicotine), including prescription medications as well as legal and illegal substances, because a patient may not regard abuse of some substances to be as significant as that of others.

There is a large societal stigma against people with substance use disorders, and patients may be quite averse to acknowledging substance-related problems. Additionally, patients may be hesitant to disclose illegal activities. Questions must be asked with nonjudgmental empathy and caring professional interest. Confrontational challenging is not always useful and may disrupt therapeutic rapport (Miller et al. 1993). The basic areas of inquiry are listed in Table 9–11. Obtaining information from collateral sources with the patient's consent and repeated assessments and history taking

TABLE 9–9. Percentage of past-year substance users with abuse or dependence, by substance: 2004

Substance	Percentage of users with abuse or dependence
Heroin	67.8
Cocaine	27.8
Marijuana	17.6
Alcohol	11.9
Hallucinogens	11.6
Inhalants	10.3

Source. Substance Abuse and Mental Health Services Administration 2005.

TABLE 9–10. The CAGE questions, adapted to include drugs

Have you felt you ought to **C**ut down on your drinking or drug use?

Have people **A**nnoyed you by criticizing your drinking or drug use?

Have you felt bad or **G**uilty about your drinking or drug use?

Have you ever had a drink or used drugs first thing in the morning to steady your nerves or to get rid of a hangover (**E**ye-opener)?

Note. The regular CAGE questions simply omit the "or drug use/or used drugs" phrases. In general, two or more "yes" answers indicate the need for further evaluation. In the psychiatric setting, the questions may also be used as a springboard to further discussion of the role substance use plays in the patient's life, regardless of initial patient response.

Source. Reprinted from Brown RL, Rounds LA: "Conjoint Screening Questionnaires for Alcohol and Drug Abuse." Wisconsin Medical Journal 94:135–140, 1995. Used with permission.

TABLE 9–11. Basic components of substance use disorder evaluation

1. Chronology of substance use: onset, fluctuations over time, development of tolerance, episodes of withdrawal, periods of abstinence, resumption of use, most recent use

2. History of formal substance abuse treatment, attendance at self-help meetings or groups

3. Perceptions of substance-related difficulties, problems, or complications

4. Full psychiatric and general medical histories, including medication history

5. Legal history, including substance-related legal problems

6. Family and social histories, including psychiatric or substance-related disorders in family members, diagnosed/treated or not

7. General psychiatric examination, including screening for other psychiatric disorders, and a mental status examination

8. General physical examination

9. Laboratory studies, as indicated by substances used

Source. Adapted from Workgroup on Substance Use Disorders 2006. Used with permission.

Treatment: General Principles

Intoxication and Withdrawal

Severe intoxications can be life threatening and may require emergent general medical care. Detailed discussion of such care is beyond the scope of this chapter, and the interested reader is referred to specialized emergency medicine texts. When necessary, treatment of withdrawal is generally accomplished by one or a combination of two general methods (Center for Substance Abuse Treatment 2006). In the first, a cross-tolerant, less harmful, and usually longer-acting medication is substituted for the drug of abuse (e.g., methadone for heroin, nicotine for tobacco smoke, diazepam for alcohol). The dosage is adjusted until withdrawal symptoms are minimized, and then the medication is gradually tapered off. In the second method, non-cross-tolerant medications are used to reduce withdrawal-associated symptoms (e.g., clonidine for opioid withdrawal, bupropion for nicotine withdrawal).

over time may be necessary to gain a sufficiently detailed picture of the patient's use to make accurate treatment recommendations.

The approach to assessment for intoxication and withdrawal varies according to substance. In general, however, a high degree of clinical vigilance should be maintained when treating patients in inpatient general medical or psychiatric settings. Sometimes the first indication of a substance use disorder occurs several days into a hospital stay, with the emergence of agitation, confusion, or delirium due to an unanticipated withdrawal syndrome.

However, it should be noted that treatment of substance withdrawal alone does little to improve outcomes for patients with substance use disorders. The time during the treatment of withdrawal should also be used to enhance motivation and initiate treatment for abuse or dependence.

Substance Use Disorders

The type of treatment employed for substance abuse ideally depends on the patient's acceptance of or motivation for treatment, the severity of the patient's substance-related problems, and other, yet-to-be-identified factors. Unfortunately, in many locations, the type of treatment is determined solely by availability and financial constraints (Substance Abuse and Mental Health Services Administration 2005).

The Stages of Change model is useful for conceptualizing a patient's motivation to address substance use problems. The model, derived from research on tobacco cessation, divides the recovery process into sequential stages, with stage-specific goals to achieve before progression (Table 9–12) (Prochaska and DiClemente 1992). The practitioner matches interventions to the patient's stage to enhance commitment to change and to increase the probability of successful change in substance use. Accordingly, a patient with severe addiction who is in the Contemplation stage is less likely to respond to strong recommendations to enter inten-

sive treatment (which may provoke refusal and rejection of further attempts to help) and is more likely to develop motivation for treatment if initially engaged in specific discussion about the advantages and disadvantages of recovery as contrasted with continued substance use and an addicted lifestyle.

At times, however, patients with substance-related criminal charges may be legally coerced into treatment. In most such situations, the treatment is to some extent voluntary or at least selected as an option by the entrant (Klag et al. 2005). Although the research base is diverse and incomplete, it does not appear that patients mandated into treatment by the legal system have particularly worse outcomes, and they may have better outcomes than similar groups of nonmandated patients (Kelly et al. 2005; Klag et al. 2005).

A patient sufficiently motivated is ideally enrolled in a treatment program of an intensity commensurate with his or her level of problems. The Patient Placement Criteria algorithm developed by the American Society of Addiction Medicine assigns a patient within five levels of care (with sublevels) based on six dimensions (Table 9–13) (Mee-Lee et al. 2001). Patients matched to treatment placements based on this algorithm have been shown to have better outcomes than mismatched patients, and although further research continues, it already has been widely implemented (Magura et al. 2003).

TABLE 9–12. Stages of change

Stage	Patient presentation	Stage task	Change strategy
Precontemplation	No intention of changing In "denial" or resistant	Increase doubt and awareness of problem	Nonjudgmental, respectful assessments Consciousness-raising, provide information Low intensity of interaction
Contemplation	Aware of problem Ambivalent about change	Tip the decisional balance	Acknowledge the ambivalence Weigh pros and cons of change vs. risks and benefits of problem Reinforce advantages of change Responsibility for change lies with the patient
Preparation	Intends to change Confusion about best way to do so	Determine best course of action	Offer menu of choices, co-create plan De-mystify change process Inspire realistic hope
Action	Actual behavior change "Treatment"	Implement collaborative, realistic plan	Monitor progress Reinforce incremental success Problem-solve
Maintenance	Behavior changed	Develop new lifestyle Avoid relapse	Watch for overblown expectations Be alert for "seemingly irrelevant decisions" Support realistic hopes

Source. Prochaska and DiClemente 1992.

TABLE 9-13. **American Society of Addiction Medicine Patient Placement Criteria levels and dimensions**

Patient assessment dimensions

1. Intoxication/withdrawal potential
2. Biomedical conditions and complications
3. Emotional, behavioral, or cognitive conditions and complications
4. Readiness to change
5. Relapse, continued use, or continued problem potential
6. Recovery environment

Levels of care*

Level 0.5	Early intervention
Level I	Outpatient treatment
Level II	Intensive outpatient/partial hospitalization
Level III	Residential/inpatient treatment
Level IV	Medically managed intensive inpatient treatment

*Within each general level of care are a number of more refined sublevels.

Source.   Mee-Lee et al. 2001.

For some individuals, recovery from substance use disorders occurs without formal treatment. Given the limited number of studies in this area, as well as methodological issues within and between studies, it is difficult to make conclusive generalizations about spontaneous or natural recovery at this time, other than to acknowledge that it can happen (Ellingstad et al. 2006; Moos and Moos 2006; Sobell et al. 2000).

Psychotherapies

Psychosocial, psychotherapeutic, or behavioral interventions are the mainstays for recovery from substance use disorders. Even methadone or buprenorphine maintenance therapy for opioid dependence includes psychosocial intervention as an essential part of the treatment, in addition to the regular administration of the opioid agonist or partial agonist (Workgroup on Substance Use Disorders 2006).

The most prevalent and widely used psychosocial interventions are the mutual self-help groups based on the 12 Steps of Alcoholics Anonymous (AA) (Tables 9–14 and 9–15) (Peter D. Hart Research Associates 2001; Substance Abuse and Mental Health Services Administration 2005). In studies of alcohol dependence, more

TABLE 9-14. **The Twelve Steps**

1. We admitted we were powerless over alcohol*— that our lives had become unmanageable.
2. Came to believe that a Power greater than ourselves could restore us to sanity.
3. Made a decision to turn our will and our lives over to the care of God as we understood Him.
4. Made a searching and fearless moral inventory of ourselves.
5. Admitted to God, to ourselves, and to another human being the exact nature of our wrongs.
6. Were entirely ready to have God remove all these defects of character.
7. Humbly asked Him to remove our shortcomings.
8. Made a list of all persons we had harmed and became willing to make amends to them all.
9. Made direct amends to such people wherever possible, except when to do so would injure them or others.
10. Continued to take personal inventory, and when we were wrong, promptly admitted it.
11. Sought through prayer and meditation to improve our conscious contact with God, as we understood Him, praying only for knowledge of His will for us and the power to carry that out.
12. Having had a spiritual awakening as the result of these steps, we tried to carry this message to alcoholics* and to practice these principles in all our affairs.

*Other 12-Step groups replace these words with their appropriate counterparts; for example, Narcotics Anonymous uses "our addiction" and "addicts."

Source.   The Twelve Steps are reprinted with permission of Alcoholics Anonymous World Services, Inc. (AAWS). Permission to reprint the Twelve Steps does not mean that AAWS has reviewed or approved the contents of this publication, or that AAWS necessarily agrees with the views expressed herein. AA is a program of recovery from alcoholism *only*—use of the Twelve Steps in connection with programs and activities which are patterned after AA, but which address other problems, or in any other non-AA context, does not imply otherwise.

frequent AA attendance has been associated with better outcomes. For individuals who find the 12 Steps' emphasis on spirituality unacceptable, lay alternatives do exist, but there is much less research supporting their effectiveness.

A number of professional psychosocial interven-

TABLE 9–15. **Twelve-Step group Web sites**

Alcoholics Anonymous	www.aa.org
Narcotics Anonymous	www.na.org
Cocaine Anonymous	www.ca.org
Marijuana Anonymous	www.marijuana-anonymous.org
Crystal Meth Anonymous (methamphetamine)	www.crystalmeth.org
Dual Recovery Anonymous (co-occurring substance abuse and other psychiatric disorders)	www.draonline.org

Note. Sites were accessed July 9, 2006.

tions and psychotherapies have been shown in large studies to be effective for substance use disorder treatment (Table 9–16). Some of these are suited for the office setting; others are more applicable to a clinic or treatment program setting. Although effectiveness in general has been shown, much work remains to be done in being able to determine exactly which type of psychotherapy is best for which individual patient.

Outcomes

The notion of outcome in the treatment of substance dependence can be approached from a number of different perspectives, and the field has moved beyond the limited, restrictive, and sometimes inappropriate use of abstinence as the sole outcome measure for all purposes (McLellan et al. 2005). In general, the optimal goal for the individual patient with substance dependence is abstinence from all non–medically supervised substance use. Treatment, however, may need to focus sequentially on intermediate objectives, such as moving into the Preparation stage (see Table 9–12), decreased psychiatric hospitalizations, and more drug-free urine tests. Population-based public health outcomes may focus on cost savings, decreased incarcerations, and increased productivity from employment. Outcomes evaluating the efficiency or efficacy of a specific intervention (e.g., psychotherapy, medication) are usually partial or intermediate treatment objectives.

Economically, it is no longer debatable that treatment is effective. A large number of studies, using different methods and conducted at different times, have shown that $1 spent on treatment or intervention saves between $4 and $7 in direct, indirect, or combined costs. Clinical outcomes are nicely summarized by McLellan et al. (2000):

Thus, 1-year postdischarge follow-up studies [of substance abuse treatment show that] 40% to 60% of discharged patients are continuously abstinent, although an additional 15% to 30% have not resumed dependent use during this period. Problems of low socioeconomic status, comorbid psychiatric conditions, and lack of family and social supports are among the most important predictors of poor adherence during addiction treatment and of relapse following treatment. (p. 1693)

Alcohol

Epidemiology

Based on combined data from the 2002–2004 National Surveys on Drug Use and Health, it is estimated that 7.6% (18.2 million) of persons age 12 years or older met the criteria for alcohol dependence or abuse in the past year. Data from the national Epidemiologic Catchment Area (ECA) study of the late 1980s indicate that lifetime prevalence of alcohol dependence is as high as 14.7% (Regier et al. 1990). Estimates of financial impact from loss of productivity due to alcohol-related illness, premature deaths, and alcohol-related crimes are greater than $134 million per year (U.S. Department of Health and Human Services 2000).

Intoxication

The degree of clinical impairment from alcohol intoxication is dependent on the individual's tolerance, the amount and type of alcoholic beverage ingested, and the amount absorbed. Table 9–17 lists blood alcohol levels and typical corresponding clinical features of intoxication in an individual who has not developed any tolerance. A blood alcohol level of 0.4 g/dL is associated with a 50% mortality risk in nonalcoholic persons. In determining how quickly a person's blood alcohol level will decrease, a rule of thumb is that the body metabolizes approximately one drink (approximately 0.015 g/dL) per hour.

Withdrawal

Alcohol withdrawal typically begins 6–8 hours after the last drink, peaks 24–28 hours after the last drink, and generally resolves within 7 days (Myrick and Anton 2004). The spectrum of alcohol withdrawal symptoms is wide, and the more common presentations are outlined in Table 9–18. Only about 5% of individuals with alcohol dependence will develop more than mild to moderate withdrawal symptoms.

Alcohol hallucinosis occurs in 3%–10% of patients with severe alcohol withdrawal. It can present as au-

TABLE 9–16. Empirically based psychosocial interventions

Type	Summary	Example
Motivational enhancement therapy	Directive client-centered approach that focuses on uncovering and resolving ambivalence about changing substance use in a manner that increases the patient's internal motivation for and commitment to change; avoids confronting resistance.	Miller WR, Zweben A, DiClemente CC, et al.: *Motivational Enhancement Therapy Manual.* Rockville, MD, U.S. Department of Health and Human Services, 1994
Cognitive-behavioral therapy	Focuses on relapse prevention and the reversing of maladaptive thoughts and beliefs that support substance use.	Kadden R, Carroll KM, Donovan D, et al.: *Cognitive-Behavioral Coping Skills Therapy Manual.* Rockville, MD, U.S. Department of Health and Human Services, 1994 Carroll KM: *A Cognitive-Behavioral Approach: Treating Cocaine Addiction.* Rockville, MD, U.S. Department of Health and Human Services, 1998
12-Step facilitation therapy	Reinforces the Alcoholics/Narcotics Anonymous approach to abstinence. Outside participation in 12-Step groups essential. May include couples sessions.	Nowinski J, Baker S, Carroll KM: *Twelve Step Facilitation Therapy Manual.* Rockville, MD, U.S. Department of Health and Human Services, 1995
Network therapy	Cognitive-behavioral approach combined with sessions with support network (family, friends, etc.). May be combined with disulfiram.	Galanter M: *Network Therapy for Alcohol and Drug Abuse.* New York, Guilford, 1999
Matrix model	A combination of cognitive-behavioral therapy groups, family education groups, social support groups, individual counseling, regular drug testing, and optional 12-Step attendance.	Rawson RA, Marinelli-Casey P, Anglin MD, et al.: "A Multi-Site Comparison of Psychosocial Approaches for the Treatment of Methamphetamine Dependence." *Addiction* 99:708–717, 2004
Contingency management	Reinforces the achievement of interim goals (e.g., drug-free urine tests) with intermittent tangible rewards of increasing value.	Budney AJ, Higgins ST: *A Community Reinforcement Plus Vouchers Approach: Treating Cocaine Addiction.* Rockville, MD, U.S. Department of Health and Human Services, 1998 Petry NM, Peirce JM, Stitzer ML, et al.: "Effect of Prize-Based Incentives on Outcomes in Stimulant Abusers in Outpatient Psychosocial Treatment Programs: A National Drug Abuse Treatment Clinical Trials Network Study." *Arch Gen Psychiatry* 62:1148–1156, 2005
Brief advice or intervention	5- to 15-minute motivational/educational office-based intervention; may include one or more in-person or telephone follow-up contacts.	National Institute on Alcohol Abuse and Alcoholism: *Helping Patients Who Drink Too Much: A Clinician's Guide.* Rockville, MD, U.S. Department of Health and Human Services, 2005 Fiore MC, Bailey WC, Cohen SJ, et al.: *Treating Tobacco Use and Dependence: Quick Reference Guide for Clinicians.* Rockville, MD, U.S. Department of Health and Human Services, 2000

TABLE 9–16. Empirically based psychosocial interventions *(continued)*

Type	Summary	Example
Group and individual drug counseling	Strong emphasis on abstinence, preventing relapses, problem-solving, and involvement in 12-Step groups.	Boren JJ, Onken LS, Carroll KM (eds): *Approaches to Drug Abuse Counseling.* Rockville, MD, U.S. Department of Health and Human Services, 2000
Integrated treatment	A service delivery model for patients with chronic mental illness and substance abuse in which the same provider team delivers both mental health and substance abuse treatment.	Bellack AS, Bennett ME, Gearon JS, et al.: "A Randomized Clinical Trial of a New Behavioral Treatment for Drug Abuse in People With Severe and Persistent Mental Illness." *Arch Gen Psychiatry* 63:426–432, 2006 Mueser KT, Noorksy DL, Drake RE, et al.: *Integrated Treatment for Dual Disorders: A Guide to Effective Practice.* New York, Guilford, 2003
Couples and family therapies	A number of different models.	Reviewed in Carroll KM, Onken LS: "Behavioral Therapies for Drug Abuse." *Am J Psychiatry* 162:1452–1460, 2005

Note. This listing is intended to be more representative than comprehensive. For general reviews, see Carroll and Onken 2005 or Woody 2003.

TABLE 9–17. Blood alcohol level and corresponding symptoms of intoxication in the nontolerant patient

Blood alcohol level (mg/dL)	Clinical presentation
30	Attention difficulties (mild), euphoria
50	Coordination problems, driving is legally impaired
100	Ataxia, drunk driving
200	Confusion, decreased consciousness
>400	Anesthesia, possible coma, possible death

Source. Adapted from Mack et al. 2003.

TABLE 9–18. DSM-IV-TR diagnostic criteria for alcohol withdrawal

A. Cessation of (or reduction in) alcohol use that has been heavy and prolonged.

B. Two (or more) of the following, developing within several hours to a few days after criterion A:
 (1) autonomic hyperactivity (e.g., sweating or pulse rate greater than 100)
 (2) increased hand tremor
 (3) insomnia
 (4) nausea or vomiting
 (5) transient visual, tactile, or auditory hallucinations or illusions
 (6) psychomotor agitation
 (7) anxiety
 (8) grand mal seizures

C. The symptoms in criterion B cause clinically significant distress or impairment in social, occupational, or other important areas of functioning.

D. The symptoms are not due to a general medical condition and are not better accounted for by another mental disorder.

Specify if: With perceptual disturbances

ditory, visual, or tactile hallucinations in the presence of a clear sensorium. Delirium tremens (DT), or alcohol withdrawal delirium, is characterized by agitation and tremulousness, autonomic instability, fevers, auditory and visual hallucinations, and disorientation. DT usually develops 2–4 days from the person's last drink, and the average duration is less than 1 week. DT has been estimated to occur in 5% of patients admitted for alcohol withdrawal (Mayo-Smith et al. 2004). It must be considered a medical emergency, because the mortality rate can be as high at 20% without prompt and adequate treatment of the severe withdrawal.

Seizures, another complication of alcohol withdrawal, are estimated to occur in 5%–15% of patients.

They usually occur in the first 24 hours from last drink, but they can occur any time in the first 5 days. Alcohol withdrawal seizures are usually grand mal in type. Those with a past history of alcohol withdrawal seizures are at increased risk for seizures in subsequent episodes of alcohol withdrawal.

Diagnosis

There are several questionnaires available for the detection of drinking-related problems. A positive response to any of the questions on the CAGE (see Table 9–10) should lead the clinician to investigate problem drinking with the patient further. The Alcohol Use Disorders Identification Test is another 10-item questionnaire used for the screening of alcohol use disorders (Figure 9–2).

Laboratory data and biological markers can be clues to an alcohol use disorder in a patient. Table 9–19 illustrates possible laboratory abnormalities in the setting of alcohol abuse or dependence. γ-Glutamyltransferase (GGT) has typically been recognized as a liver enzyme whose elevation may be more indicative of alcohol use. The sensitivity of GGT in detecting alcohol abuse is 40%–60%, with a specificity of about 80%. A newer test for heavy alcohol consumption is the relative percentage in serum of the carbohydrate-deficient form of an iron transport protein, carbohydrate-deficient transferrin (%CDT). %CDT is a more sensitive and specific indicator of heavy drinking. The diagnostic specificity of %CDT for recent heavy drinking is approximately 70.0% in patients with non-alcohol-induced liver cirrhosis, 88.2% in hepatitis patients, and 93.5% in patients with a nonspecific elevation of GGT (Hock et al. 2005).

Treatment

Acute Withdrawal

The general management strategies in alcohol detoxification include adjunctive treatment of comorbid medical problems, rehydration, and correction of electrolyte abnormalities (including hypomagnesemia, hypophosphatemia, and hypokalemia). Because nutritional deficiencies are common in individuals with chronic alcoholism, oral multivitamin preparations containing folic acid are routinely administered to early abstinent individuals. The replacement of thiamine, particularly before giving glucose, is especially important to prevent Wernicke's encephalopathy, precipitated by depletion of thiamine reserves.

Benzodiazepines have historically been considered

TABLE 9–19. Laboratory abnormalities associated with harmful levels of drinking

Measurable blood alcohol level
Legal limit for driving is <0.08 mg/mL
Levels >0.3 mg/mL with minimal intoxication may indicate tolerance
Elevated mean corpuscular volume >94 fL
Elevated liver transaminases
γ-Glutamyltransferase >65 IU/L
Less specific
Aspartate aminotransferase >38 IU/L
Alanine aminotransferase >45 IU/L
Elevated relative percent in serum of carbohydrate-deficient transferrin >2.5%
Decreased platelets <140 K/mm^3

the gold standard for the treatment of alcohol withdrawal. They can be administered either via fixed dosage and taper or on an as-needed basis. The Clinical Institute Withdrawal Assessment Scale for Alcohol—Revised is a short test rating the severity of alcohol withdrawal as observed by a health care professional (Figure 9–3). This 10-item assessment tool can be used to quantify the severity of alcohol withdrawal syndrome and to monitor and medicate patients going through withdrawal. Scores of 8 points or fewer correspond to mild withdrawal, scores of 9–15 points correspond to moderate withdrawal, and scores of more than 15 points correspond to severe withdrawal symptoms and an increased risk of DT and seizures. Anticonvulsants can also be used in alcohol detoxification. Valproate and carbamazepine are the best studied, and gabapentin is now also being investigated.

Relapse Prevention

Once an individual has been successfully detoxified from alcohol, maintenance of the abstinence is the next goal. The maintenance of abstinence can be a very difficult goal to achieve; it has been estimated that approximately 50% of alcoholic individuals relapse within 3 months of completion of treatment. Psychosocial support remains the cornerstone in achieving this goal, and recent advances in pharmacotherapy have been a valuable addition. Research has shown that three forms of individual behavioral treatment (cognitive-behavioral therapy, motivational enhance-

Circle the number that comes closest to the patient's answer.

1. How often do you have a drink containing alcohol?	

(0) Never   (1) Monthly or less   (2) Two to four times a month   (3) Two to three times a week   (4) Four or more times a week

2. How many drinks containing alcohol do you have on a typical day when you are drinking?
Code the number of standard drinks[1]

(0) 1 or 2   (1) 3 or 4   (2) 5 or 6   (3) 7 or 8   (4) 10 or more

3. How often do you have six or more drinks on one occasion?

(0) Never   (1) Less than monthly   (2) Monthly   (3) Weekly   (4) Daily or almost daily

4. How often during the last year have you found that you were not able to stop drinking once you had started?

(0) Never   (1) Less than monthly   (2) Monthly   (3) Weekly   (4) Daily or almost daily

5. How often during the last year have you failed to do what was normally expected from you because of drinking?

(0) Never   (1) Less than monthly   (2) Monthly   (3) Weekly   (4) Daily or almost daily

6. How often during the last year have you needed a first drink in the morning to get yourself going after a heavy drinking session?

(0) Never   (1) Less than monthly   (2) Monthly   (3) Weekly   (4) Daily or almost daily

7. How often during the last year have you had a feeling of guilt or remorse after drinking?

(0) Never   (1) Less than monthly   (2) Monthly   (3) Weekly   (4) Daily or almost daily

8. How often during the last year have you been unable to remember what happened the night before because you had been drinking?

(0) Never   (1) Less than monthly   (2) Monthly   (3) Weekly   (4) Daily or almost daily

9. Have you or someone else been injured as a result of your drinking?

(0) No   (2) Yes, but not in the last year   (4) Yes, during the last year

10. Has a relative or friend or doctor or other health worker been concerned about your drinking or suggested you cut down?

(0) No   (2) Yes, but not in the last year   (4) Yes, during the last year

Total Score[2]: _____

---

[1]In determining the response categories it has been assumed that one "drink" contains 10 g alcohol. In countries where the alcohol content of a standard drink differs by more than 25% from 10 g, the response category should be modified accordingly.

[2]The AUDIT is not a diagnostic instrument. A total score of 8–15 indicates moderate problems that may respond to brief intervention. Scores of 16–19 may suggest alcohol abuse or dependence. Scores above 19 suggest alcohol dependence.

FIGURE 9–2. Alcohol Use Disorders Identification Test (AUDIT).

Source. Reprinted from Babor TF, Higgins-Biddle JC, Saunders J, et al.: *AUDIT, the Alcohol Use Disorders Identification Test,* 2nd Edition. Geneva, Switzerland, World Health Organization, 2001. Available at: http://whqlibdoc.who.int/hq/2001/WHO_MSD_MSB_01.6a.pdf Accessed July 30, 2006. May be reproduced without permission for noncommercial purposes.

PAROXYSMAL SWEATS—Observation	PULSE—Measurement	
NOTE: These items yield one score. After assessing Sweats and Pulse Rate, use the highter of the two individual scores for the score.		
0 No sweat visible	**0**	<80
1 Barely perceptible sweating, palms moist	**1**	81–100
2	**2**	101–110
3	**3**	111–120
4 Beads of sweat obvious on forehead	**4**	121–130
5	**5**	131–140
6	**6**	141–150
7 Equivalent to acute panic states as seen in severe delirium or acute schizophrenic reactions	**7**	>151

TREMOR—arms extended and fingers spread apart. Observation	AUDITORY DISTURBANCES—Ask "Are you more aware of sounds around you? Are they harsh? Do they frighten you?"
0 No tremor	**0** Not present
1 Not visible, but can be felt fingertip to fingertip	**1** Very mild sensitivity
2	**2** Mild harshness or ability to frighten
3	**3** Moderate harshness or ability to frighten
4 Moderate, with patient's arms extended	**4** Moderately severe hallucinations
5	**5** Severe hallucinations
6	**6** Extremely severe hallucinations
7 Severe, even with arms not extended	**7** Continuous hallucinations

NAUSEA AND VOMITING—Ask "Do you feel sick to your stomach? Have you vomited?" Observation	VISUAL DISTURBANCES—Ask "Does the light appear to be too bright? Is its color different? Does it hurt your eyes? Are you seeing anything that is disturbing to you? Are you seeing things that you know are not there?" Observation
0 No nausea	**0** Not present
1 Mild nausea with no vomiting	**1** Very mild sensitivity
2	**2** Mild sensitivity
3	**3** Moderate sensitivity
4 Intermittent nausea with dry heaves	**4** Moderately severe hallucinations
5	**5** Severe hallucinations
6	**6** Extremely severe hallucinations
7 Constant nausea, frequent dry heaves and vomiting	**7** Continuous hallucinations

FIGURE 9–3.   Clinical Institute Withdrawal Assessment for Alcohol—Revised (CIWA-Ar).

ANXIETY—Ask "Do you feel nervous?" Observation	HEADACHE, FULLNESS IN HEAD—Ask "Does your head feel different? Does it feel like there is a band around your head?" Do not rate for dizziness or light-headedness. Otherwise, rate severity.
0 No anxiety	**0** Not present
1 Mildly anxious	**1** Very mild
2	**2** Mild
3	**3** Moderate
4 Moderately anxious, or guarded so anxiety is inferred	**4** Moderately severe
5	**5** Severe
6	**6** Very severe
7 Equivalent to acute panic states as seen in severe delirium or acute schizophrenic reactions	**7** Extremely severe

AGITATION—Observation	TACTILE DISTURBANCES—Ask "Have you any itching, pins and needles, any burning, or numbness or do you feel bugs crawling under your skin?"
0 Normal activity	**0** None
1 Somewhat more than normal activity	**1** Very mild itching, pins and needles, burning or numbness
2	**2** Mild itching, pins and needles, burning or numbness
3	**3** Moderate itching, pins and needles, burning or numbness
4 Moderately fidgety and restless	**4** Moderately severe hallucinations
5	**5** Severe hallucinations
6	**6** Extremely severe hallucinations
7 Paces back and forth during most of the interview, or constantly thrashes about	**7** Continuous hallucinations

ORIENTATION AND CLOUDING OF SENSORIUM—Ask "What day is this? Where are you? Who am I?"	MEDICATION GUIDELINES
0 Oriented and can do serial additions	1. Contact physician for CIWA ≥10. Benzodiazepine (or other medication) administration may be indicated.
1 Cannot do serial additions or is uncertain about date	2. Call physician on duty at any time for additional medication or if patient does not improve with treatment.
2 Disoriented for date by no more than 2 calendar days	
3 Disoriented for date by more than 2 calendar days	3. Be cautious when giving benzodiazepine if blood alcohol level >0.15%, because increased or additive CNS depression may occur.
4 Disoriented for place and/or person	

FIGURE 9–3.   Clinical Institute Withdrawal Assessment for Alcohol—Revised (CIWA-Ar). *(continued)*

Note.   CNS = central nervous system.

Source.   Adapted from Sullivan et al. 1989.

ment, and 12-Step facilitation [see Table 9–14]) contribute to sustained abstinence and reduced drinking.

As of July 2007, there were only four medications with U.S. Food and Drug Administration (FDA) approval for use in the maintenance treatment of alcohol dependence: disulfiram, naltrexone, a long-acting intramuscular formulation of naltrexone, and acamprosate. Table 9–20 offers a comparison of these medications.

Disulfiram serves as an alcohol deterrent drug by interrupting the metabolism of alcohol. It inhibits aldehyde dehydrogenase and blocks the breakdown of acetaldehyde to acetate. When a person taking disulfiram consumes alcohol, the level of acetaldehyde increases, causing nausea, vomiting, and changes in blood pressure. The patient's fear of this disulfiram–alcohol reaction is meant to serve as a reinforcement for abstinence (Schuckit and Tapert 2004).

The mechanism of action of naltrexone is not fully understood. It is a competitive antagonist at the opioid receptor and is hypothesized to indirectly block alcohol-induced dopamine release. It is thought to decrease the rewarding effects of alcohol and thereby reduce the craving to drink and loss of control (Sinclair 2001). Naltrexone is effective in increasing the percent of days abstinent, prolonging time to first heavy drinking day, and reducing amount of alcohol consumed per drinking episode (Anton et al. 2006). The long-acting intramuscular formulation of naltrexone is the newest to receive FDA approval for the treatment of alcohol dependence. It offers the benefit of once-monthly injections rather than daily dosing of an oral medication.

The mechanism of action of acamprosate remains unclear. Chronic alcohol use leads to alterations in the balance of neuronal excitation and inhibition in the circuitry discussed earlier in the "Neurobiology" section of this chapter. Acamprosate is thought to interact with glutamate and GABA neurotransmitter systems to help restore this balance. Acamprosate is believed to assist in the maintenance of abstinence and to decrease negative symptoms associated with the acute post-withdrawal period in recently detoxified alcohol-dependent individuals (Wilde and Wagstaff 1997).

TABLE 9–20. Comparison of U.S. Food and Drug Administration–approved medications for the treatment of alcohol dependence

	Disulfiram	Acamprosate	Naltrexone	Extended-release naltrexone injection
Mechanism of action	Alcohol deterrent Inhibits alcohol dehydrogenase	Reduces craving Restores balance between excitatory glutamate and inhibitory γ-aminobutyric acid neurotransmitter systems	Reduces craving Opioid receptor antagonist	Reduces craving Opioid receptor antagonist
Interactions with alcohol	Causes adverse reaction, including flushing, nausea, and vomiting	None	None	None
Major advantages	Physical reaction is a strong disincentive to drinking while taking medication	Generally well tolerated, few drug interactions, is not processed through liver	Generally well tolerated, recent large multisite study supports efficacy	Once-a-month injection can greatly enhance compliance
Major disadvantages	Cannot use in the setting of liver failure Patient must avoid *all* products containing alcohol	Dosing is two tablets three times daily	Cannot use in the setting of liver failure Cannot use concurrently with opioid analgesics	Cannot use in the setting of liver failure Cannot use concurrently with opioid analgesics

For the individual patient, the relative effectiveness of these medications compared with each other or in combination is not fully elucidated. One large randomized, controlled trial of recently abstinent alcoholic individuals (the COMBINE [Combining Medications and Behavioral Interventions] trial) evaluated the efficacy of naltrexone, acamprosate, or both in comparison with placebo. The results of this trial favored the efficacy of naltrexone monotherapy over placebo, acamprosate monotherapy, or combined naltrexone–acamprosate (Anton et al. 2006). According to current guidelines, these medications should be used not as monotherapy but rather as augmentation of psychosocial treatment.

Medical Complications

Heavy alcohol consumption results in serious health sequelae over time, with many cases ultimately resulting in death. Heavy alcohol consumption is known to elevate blood pressure and increase the risk of myocardial infarction. There is an increased risk of cancer, particularly esophageal, head, neck, liver, stomach, colon, and lung. Long-term alcoholism results in damage to the liver, with the end point being cirrhosis and death. Esophageal varices resulting from the long-term abuse of alcohol can also be life threatening because they can rupture, leading to rapid, profuse bleeding.

Wernicke-Korsakoff syndrome occurs as a result of thiamine deficiency in alcoholism. The syndrome can be precipitated by the administration of glucose to asymptomatic individuals with thiamine deficiency. It is therefore of utmost importance to ensure that alcohol-dependent individuals receive supplemental thiamine before administration of glucose in an acute setting. Early symptoms of Wernicke-Korsakoff's include decreased concentration, apathy, mild agitation, and depressed mood. Confusion, amnesia, and confabulation are late signs of severe and prolonged thiamine deficit.

Fetal alcohol syndrome results from a mother consuming alcohol during her pregnancy; no amount of alcohol can be considered safe during pregnancy. In this syndrome, mental retardation is common (44% of children with fetal alcohol syndrome have an IQ of 79 or below). Other congenital defects include wide-set eyes, short palpebral fissure, short and broad-bridged nose, hypoplastic philtrum, thinned upper lip, and flattened midface. Maternal alcohol use with breastfeeding has been shown to impair a child's motor, but not mental, development.

Cannabis

Epidemiology

Cannabis, whether as leaves/flowers (marijuana) or resin (hashish), is the most commonly used illicit drug worldwide (United Nations Office on Drugs and Crime 2005). Overall, use in the United States decreased from the 1970s to the 1990s and then increased into the 2000s, although not to the levels of the 1970s. In 2004, 6.1% of subjects in the National Household Survey on Drug Use and Health reported past-month use of marijuana, with about 35% of those using other illicit drugs as well (Substance Abuse and Mental Health Services Administration 2005). Between 1994 and 2004, the percent of patients admitted to substance abuse treatment in the United States who identified cannabis as their primary substance of abuse increased from 9% to 16% (Substance Abuse and Mental Health Services Administration, Office of Applied Studies 2006). In 2004, that percentage was secondary only to alcohol and opioids; the average age of treatment admissions was about 10 years younger than for alcohol, opiates, or stimulants (mid- to late 20s versus mid- to late 30s).

The issue of cannabis, or more specifically, marijuana, as a "gateway drug" (i.e., a drug whose abuse leads to abuse of other more harmful drugs) has been a topic of debate for decades. In many but not all populations, alcohol and tobacco use precede marijuana use, which in turn precedes opioid or cocaine use. A relationship has consistently been shown between early, regular cannabis use and subsequent abuse of other drugs. Hall and Lynskey (2005) condense the probable explanations of this relationship into three broad hypotheses: 1) cannabis abusers have easier access to and more opportunity to acquire other drugs; 2) certain individuals are predisposed through genetic and environmental influences to abuse both cannabis and other drugs; and 3) the pharmacological effects of cannabis increase the risk of other drug abuse. There is limited evidence to support all three hypotheses and not enough to refute any of them. There is very little evidence to use to evaluate the public health inference that reducing marijuana abuse would significantly reduce the abuse of other drugs.

Intoxication and Withdrawal

Intoxication (Table 9–21) has been associated with increased risk of automobile accidents. No specific treatment is generally indicated. A cannabis withdrawal syndrome has recently been described (Table 9–22). It

TABLE 9–21. Symptoms of cannabis intoxication

Lower doses
  Relaxation
  Euphoria
  Altered time and sensory perception
  Increased appetite

Higher doses
  Hypervigilance or paranoia
  Anxiety or panic
  Derealization or depersonalization
  Hallucinations (auditory or visual)

TABLE 9–22. Cannabis withdrawal symptoms

Most frequently seen
  Cannabis craving
  Anxiety, restlessness, and/or irritability
  Insomnia
  Changes in appetite
  Boredom
  Improved memory

Less frequently seen
  Tremor
  Diaphoresis (sweating)
  Tachycardia
  Gastrointestinal disturbances, including nausea,
    vomiting, and diarrhea
  Change in libido
  Depression

Source. Center for Substance Abuse Treatment 2006 and Copersino et al. 2006.

begins 2–3 days after cessation of use and is generally mild, but the duration has been variable in studies, from 12 to 115 days. No specific treatment is generally needed.

Diagnosis and Treatment

Patients often use cannabis in addition to other substances, and careful history taking may be required to determine a diagnosis of abuse or dependence. The comparatively milder symptoms of cannabis intoxication and withdrawal can lead patients to thinking its use is not "serious" or that abstinence is not necessary.

Despite the widespread use of the drug, there is surprisingly little research on the treatment of cannabis dependence (Budney et al. 2006). What studies there are support the use of brief intervention for problematic use/abuse and cognitive-behavioral, motivational enhancement, and contingency management

approaches for the treatment of dependence. No medications have been shown to be consistently useful for the treatment of cannabis dependence, although investigation continues (Huestis et al. 2007).

Medical Complications

Chronic marijuana use has long been associated with increased risk of paranoia, but there is growing evidence (and debate) about associations between early onset of marijuana use and psychosis or schizophrenia (Moore et al. 2007). Additionally, as would be expected in a product that is burned and smoked, there is an increased risk of certain cancers and pulmonary complications.

Women considering becoming pregnant or who are already so should be strongly advised not to use cannabis. Fetal growth decreases, and subsequent cognitive and behavioral impairments and psychiatric symptoms in the child appear to be epidemiologically related to cannabis abuse during pregnancy (Workgroup on Substance Use Disorders 2006).

Stimulants

Epidemiology

The category of stimulants includes cocaine, amphetamine, and amphetamine-like substances. According to the National Survey on Drug Use and Health there were an estimated 1 million new cocaine users in 2004, and about 1% of the U.S. population ages 12 years or older had used cocaine within the past 30 days (Substance Abuse and Mental Health Services Administration 2005). Amphetamine-type substances come in several different forms. Powdered methamphetamine hydrochloride ("speed," "meth," or "crank") can be snorted, injected, or dissolved in beverages. Pills can be prescription medications such as dexamphetamine or clandestinely manufactured tablets of powdered methamphetamine. Freebase methamphetamine (sometimes called "ice") can be vaporized in a pipe or on aluminum foil and insufflated (smoked), producing as rapid a high as with injection but without having to use needles (Maxwell 2005). The United Nations Office on Drugs and Crime estimated that 30 million people worldwide are using amphetamine-type stimulants, primarily methamphetamine, compared with an estimated 15 million people who use opioids and 13 million who use cocaine (United Nations Office on Drugs and Crime 2004). The geographical spread of methamphetamine use is being seen in both rural and urban settings. Alarmingly, although the total number of past-year and past-month methamphetamine users did not change significantly between 2002 and 2004, the number of past-month methamphetamine users *who met criteria for abuse or dependence* increased from 27.5% in 2002 to 59.3% in 2004 (Substance Abuse and Mental Health Services Administration 2005).

Intoxication

Cocaine and amphetamine intoxication have similar symptoms (Table 9–23). The differences in clinical presentation are due to the respective half-lives of the drugs, which are approximately 40–60 minutes for cocaine and 6–12 hours for methamphetamine. Although bingeing is a common pattern of use for both drugs, the difference in half-lives allows some methamphetamine abusers to maintain low levels of intoxication for longer periods of time. Chronic administration of either drug can induce a paranoid psychotic state. There is some evidence that methamphetamine-induced psychosis can be long lasting and may recur in the absence of further drug use. Individuals may be at risk of acting violently in response to frightening delusions common in induced paranoia. Amphetamine use can also result in delirium manifested by disorientation, confusion, fear, and anxiety.

Withdrawal

As with intoxication, the symptoms of cocaine and amphetamine withdrawal are similar, distinguished primarily by time course (Table 9–24). Methamphetamine withdrawal may be more protracted and less abrupt than cocaine withdrawal. Not uncommonly, clinically significant depressive symptoms can accompany the withdrawal. During the late withdrawal phase, a person may experience brief periods of intense, cue-induced drug craving. These periods of intense cravings are high-risk times for relapse.

Treatment

Psychosocial and behavioral approaches are the mainstays of treatment in stimulant-dependent individuals. There are currently no medications with FDA approval for the treatment of cocaine- or amphetamine-dependent individuals. Several lines of pharmacotherapy have been investigated, including antidepressant agents (e.g., selective serotonin reuptake inhibitors [SSRIs], tricyclics), dopaminergic agents (e.g., pergolide, antipsychotics), and anticonvulsant agents (e.g., carbamazepine). Although initial open-label data have suggested effectiveness, none of these agents has

TABLE 9–23. DSM-IV-TR diagnostic criteria for cocaine or amphetamine intoxication

A. Recent use of cocaine, amphetamine, or a related substance (e.g., methylphenidate).

B. Clinically significant maladaptive behavioral or psychological changes (e.g., euphoria or affective blunting; changes in sociability; hypervigilance; interpersonal sensitivity; anxiety, tension, or anger; stereotyped behaviors; impaired judgment; or impaired social or occupational functioning) that developed during, or shortly after, use of cocaine, amphetamine, or a related substance.

C. Two (or more) of the following, developing during, or shortly after, cocaine, amphetamine, or a related substance use:
  (1) tachycardia or bradycardia
  (2) pupillary dilation
  (3) elevated or lowered blood pressure
  (4) perspiration or chills
  (5) nausea or vomiting
  (6) evidence of weight loss
  (7) psychomotor agitation or retardation
  (8) muscular weakness, respiratory depression, chest pain, or cardiac arrhythmias
  (9) confusion, seizures, dyskinesias, dystonias, or coma

D. The symptoms are not due to a general medical condition and are not better accounted for by another mental disorder.

Specify if: With perceptual disturbances

consistently shown efficacy in decreasing stimulant use in double-blind trials. The National Institute on Drug Abuse has set medication development for the treatment of cocaine abuse as a priority research area.

A more recent line of investigation includes the development of active or passive immunization to produce antibodies that may either block the entrance of cocaine into the brain or speed the catabolism of cocaine so less cocaine is able the reach its site of action. Another line of investigation includes the use of sustained-release stimulants (with less abuse potential), such as methylphenidate, as maintenance strategies, much like the use of methadone in opioid dependence (Shearer et al. 2003). Currently, trials are under way to investigate the efficacy of modafinil, a drug approved for the treatment of narcolepsy, and *N*-acetylcysteine, a mucolytic agent and antidote for acetaminophen toxicity, in the treatment of cocaine dependence. In addition, recent work shows promise for disulfiram, an

TABLE 9–24. DSM-IV-TR diagnostic criteria for cocaine or amphetamine withdrawal

A. Cessation of (or reduction in) cocaine or amphetamine (or a related substance) use that has been heavy and prolonged.

B. Dysphoric mood and two (or more) of the following physiological changes, developing within a few hours to several days after criterion A:

    (1) fatigue

    (2) vivid, unpleasant dreams

    (3) insomnia or hypersomnia

    (4) increased appetite

    (5) psychomotor agitation or retardation

C. The symptoms in criterion B cause clinically significant distress or impairment in social, occupational, or other important areas of functioning.

D. The symptoms are not due to a general medical condition and are not better accounted for by another mental disorder.

alcohol deterrent drug, in reducing cocaine use.

Behavior therapies, including cognitive-behavioral therapy (CBT) and supportive-expressive psychotherapy, have been shown to help retain people in treatment and can lead to abstinence. Positive contingency management procedures have also been shown to help an individual achieve initial abstinence. More recently, the Matrix model has received attention as an effective treatment for stimulant disorders. The Matrix model is a 16-week manualized outpatient treatment that combines cognitive-behavioral therapy materials and techniques, educational materials for patient and family on the effects of stimulants, 12-Step program participation, and positive reinforcement for behavior change and treatment compliance.

Medical Complications

Cocaine-related myocardial ischemia and infarction are the most serious complications of cocaine abuse. Cocaine produces a powerful sympathetic effect via inhibition of presynaptic uptake of norepinephrine and dopamine. Chest pain is the most common symptom in cocaine users presenting to the emergency department, and therefore, individuals presenting with chest pain should be asked about cocaine use. Seven percent to 25% of patients presenting to emergency departments with nontraumatic chest pain will screen positive for cocaine in their urine, and approximately

6% of these individuals will have enzymatic evidence of myocardial infarction. It has been estimated that cocaine use acutely increases the risk of acute myocardial infarction by a factor of 24 in otherwise healthy individuals (Mittleman et al. 1999). This increased risk appears to be unrelated to amount of cocaine used, route, or frequency of use. About 50% of those with cocaine-related myocardial infarction will have no evidence of atherosclerotic coronary artery disease. Cocaine ingestion results in coronary vasoconstriction, increased myocardial oxygen demand, and increased thrombus formation, which contribute to myocardial infarction (Wadland and Ferenchick 2004). Left ventricular hypertrophy and reduced left ventricular systolic dysfunction are also associated with cocaine use.

Acute coronary syndrome and cardiac arrhythmias are common in individuals presenting to emergency departments after the use of methamphetamine (Turnipseed et al. 2003). Methamphetamine use is also a risk factor for stroke, likely because its use can lead to elevations in blood pressure, vasculitis, and vasoconstriction. Numerous case reports in the literature link methamphetamine use with massive intracerebral hemorrhage, even in younger people (Wadland and Ferenchick 2004). There are also reports of inhalation of methamphetamine linked with noncardiogenic pulmonary edema and severe pulmonary hypertension.

Of particular concern has been increased methamphetamine use among men of all sexual orientations with an accompanying increased risk of HIV infection. Methamphetamine, and "ice" in particular, is associated with increases in sex drive, decreases in sexual inhibition, and increases in risky behaviors (e.g., reusing and sharing syringes, unprotected sex, and multiple sex partners).

Opioids

Epidemiology

The 2004 National Survey on Drug Use and Health estimated that 118,000 persons had used heroin for the first time within the past 12 months (Substance Abuse and Mental Health Services Administration 2005). It also estimated that 2.8 million persons used an illicit drug for the first time within the past 12 months, the majority of whom used a prescription opioid pain medication. In the 2004 Monitoring the Future survey of eighth, tenth, and twelfth graders, 9.3% of the seniors reported using hydrocodone without a prescription in the past year, and 5% reported using oxycodone.

Intoxication

The pleasurable sensation derived from the ingestion of an opioid drug is referred to as a "rush." The onset, duration, and intensity of the rush are dependent on the particular drug that is used, how much is used, and the route of administration (oral ingestion, inhalation, intravenous injection). The characteristic symptoms of intoxication are listed in Table 9–25. Nausea, vomiting, and severe itching can also occur. After the initial rush, sedation can last for the next several hours.

Overdose involving opioid drugs is a life-threatening situation. Fatal respiratory depression can occur due to direct suppression of respiratory centers in the midbrain and medulla. Obtaining a urine drug screen can be crucial to identify not only the presence of an opioid but also that of other unsuspected drugs. Benzodiazepines are frequently abused with opioids, and when detected, the benzodiazepine component of the overdose can be reversed with flumazenil. Treatment of an opioid overdose includes general supportive management in addition to the use of naloxone, a pure opioid antagonist that can reverse the central nervous system effects of opioid intoxication and overdose. Table 9–26 reviews the steps necessary in the management of an opioid overdose (Zimmerman 2003).

Withdrawal

Table 9–27 outlines the most common signs and symptoms of opioid withdrawal. The timing of the withdrawal is dependent on the type of opioid used. With cessation of chronic heroin use, withdrawal symptoms begin about 8–12 hours after the last dose, peak between 36 and 72 hours, and subside over about 5 days. With methadone, which has a much longer half-life than heroin, the peak of the withdrawal syndrome is usually between days 4 and 6, with acute symptoms persisting for 14–21 days. With any opioid, after acute withdrawal symptoms have subsided, a protracted abstinence syndrome, including disturbances of mood and sleep, can persist for 6–8 months.

Treatment

Management of acute opioid withdrawal involves a combination of general supportive measures in conjunction with pharmacotherapy. There are several options (Table 9–28). The first option is to convert the patient to an equivalent dose of a longer-acting opioid and gradually taper the dose to minimize withdrawal. Methadone and buprenorphine are frequently used in this manner. In the inpatient setting, the taper is generally completed in 5–7 days, but it may need to be sig-

---

TABLE 9–25. DSM-IV-TR diagnostic criteria for opioid intoxication

A. Recent use of an opioid.

B. Clinically significant maladaptive behavioral or psychological changes (e.g., initial euphoria followed by apathy, dysphoria, psychomotor agitation or retardation, impaired judgment, or impaired social or occupational functioning) that developed during, or shortly after, opioid use.

C. Pupillary constriction (or pupillary dilation due to anoxia from severe overdose) and one (or more) of the following signs, developing during, or shortly after, opioid use:

   (1) drowsiness or coma
   (2) slurred speech
   (3) impairment in attention or memory

D. The symptoms are not due to a general medical condition and are not better accounted for by another mental disorder.

Specify if: With perceptual disturbances

TABLE 9–26. Management of acute opioid overdose

1. Establish and maintain airway. Intubation and mechanical ventilation may be necessary.

2. Naloxone 0.4–0.8 mg may be administered intravenously, intramuscularly, by sublingual injection, or via endotracheal tube to reverse toxic effects.

   (a) Onset of action with intravenous administration is approximately 2 minutes.

   (b) If initial doses of naloxone restore adequate respiration and further therapy is needed, repeat boluses, or a continuous infusion of naloxone can be used.

   (c) The infusion dose is typically one-half to two-thirds of the initial amount of naloxone that reversed the respiratory depression, administered on an hourly basis.

   (d) If the patient has been intubated, a naloxone infusion is not necessary.

3. Monitor for development of pulmonary edema

---

nificantly extended in the outpatient setting to decrease the likelihood of dropout and relapse.

Another option includes the use of a clonidine (an α_2-adrenergic agonist) taper for amelioration of tremor, diaphoresis, and agitation. If an expedited treatment of the withdrawal is desired, then an opioid antagonist, such as naltrexone, can be administered in conjunction

TABLE 9–27.   Signs and symptoms of opioid withdrawal

Early to moderate	Moderate to advanced
Anorexia	Abdominal cramps
Anxiety	Broken sleep
Craving	Hot or cold flashes
Dysphoria	Increased blood pressure
Fatigue	Increased pulse
Headache	Low-grade fever
Irritability	Muscle and bone pain
Lacrimation	Muscle spasm ("kicking the
Mydriasis (mild)	habit")
Perspiration	Mydriasis (with fixed,
Piloerection	dilated pupils at the peak)
(gooseflesh;	Nausea and vomiting
"cold turkey")	
Restlessness	
Rhinorrhea	
Yawning	

Source.   Adapted from Collins and Kleber 2004.

with clonidine. Expedited withdrawal may be advantageous when a patient is withdrawing from a longer-acting agent such as methadone and would otherwise be facing a longer withdrawal treatment. The symptoms of expedited withdrawal may be more severe initially, so frequent patient monitoring and proactive use of adjunctive medications are essential.

With all protocols, adjuvant medications may be used. Nonsteroidal anti-inflammatory drugs may be used for myalgias. Benzodiazepines or other hypnotics may be used for short-term management of insomnia. Cyclobenzaprine (a muscle relaxant) can be used to treat muscle cramps. Dicyclomine (an anticholinergic used to reduce the contraction of muscles in the intestine) is used to treat the gastrointestinal symptoms that occur in acute withdrawal.

Another, less-recommended option is the use of ultrarapid opioid detoxification. This method uses general anesthesia with propofol or conscious sedation with midazolam along with naltrexone (or naloxone or nalmafene), ondansetron (an antiemetic), octreotide (an antidiarrheal), clonidine, and other benzodiazepines. Complications can include flash pulmonary edema, prolonged withdrawal, drug toxicity, rupture of varices, and aspiration pneumonia. A number of deaths have been reported. Ultrarapid detoxification has not been shown to have better substance abuse outcomes than other less risky protocols (Collins and Kleber 2004).

Maintenance treatment with agonist therapy provides relief from opioid withdrawal symptoms and thereby allows psychosocial stabilization. Methadone

TABLE 9–28.   Opioid detoxification medication protocols

Methadone substitution and taper

- *Day 1:* Start with a dose of 10–20 mg. If withdrawal symptoms persist 1 hour after dosing, an additional 5–10 mg of methadone can be given. The initial dose should not exceed 30 mg, and the total 24-hour dose should not exceed 40 mg in the first few days unless is there is clear documentation of the patient using opioids in excess of 40-mg methadone equivalents per day.

- *Days 2–4:* Maintain a stable dose for 2–3 days.

- *Days 5–Completion:* Slowly taper dose by 10%–15% per day.

Buprenorphine substitution and taper

- *Day 1:* Administer buprenorphine 4 mg sublingually after the emergence of mild to moderate withdrawal symptoms. If withdrawal symptoms persist after 1 hour, another 4-mg dose may be given.

- *Days 2–4:* On subsequent days, 8–12 mg may be sufficient to relieve withdrawal symptoms, although higher dosages may be required.

- *Days 5–Completion:* A slow taper has been shown be superior to rapid tapers in some studies, although the rate of taper is not clearly defined.

Clonidine taper

- *Day 1:* 0.1–0.2 mg orally every 4–6 hours up to 1 mg.

- *Days 2–4:* 0.2–0.4 mg orally every 4–6 hours up to 1.2 mg.

- *Days 5–Completion:* Reduce total daily dose by 0.2 mg daily, given in two to three divided doses (the nighttime dose should be reduced last).

- Adjunctive therapy, including nonsteroidal anti-inflammatory drugs for myalgias, benzodiazepines for insomnia, antiemetics, antimotility drugs for intestinal cramping, and muscle relaxants may be necessary.

Note.   For clonidine–naltrexone protocols, consult one of the "Suggested Readings" texts listed at the end of the chapter.

has long been considered the gold standard treatment for maintenance treatment. In late 2002 the FDA also approved buprenorphine for both detoxification and maintenance treatment of opioid dependence. Potential advantages of buprenorphine over methadone include a longer half-life, which decreases the frequency of clinic visits, and a high safety profile with less risk of respiratory depression in overdose. Training programs are available for physicians to become certified to prescribe buprenorphine in office-based settings, not just in the traditional methadone maintenance treatment program. Buprenorphine and methadone have both been shown to be effective maintenance treatments, although some patients report individual preferences for one or the other medication (Mattick et al. 2004).

Medical Complications

One cohort study in South London estimated a standardized morality ratio of 17 for both male and female heroin users (Hickman et al. 2003). In addition to the risk of overdose, medical comorbidities may be consequential. The risk of transmission of HIV, particularly in intravenous opioid users, is a major concern, and an estimated 85% of patients receiving methadone maintenance for opioid dependence in the United States are infected with the hepatitis C virus. Opioid users also can experience decreased immune function, hyperalgesia, and bacterial infections (particularly with intravenous drug use), including abscesses and cellulitis of the skin. Endocarditis with intravenous drug use is another serious concern: more than 50% of these cases will be right-sided, most often involving the tricuspid valve. Sequelae of right-sided endocarditis will often involve the lungs as well.

During pregnancy, opioid withdrawal, even when treated, can increase the risk of miscarriage and premature birth. In addition, there is a very high rate of relapse after detoxification, and risk of cycling between intoxication and withdrawal can be even more dangerous to the fetus. Methadone maintenance has generally been accepted as the standard approach to the pregnant woman (Jarvis and Schnoll 1994). Buprenorphine maintenance is also increasingly being used in pregnant opioid-dependent women. Coordinated care between the substance abuse treatment provider and the obstetrical team is of utmost importance.

Nicotine

Epidemiology

Approximately 42.4% of U.S. adults have ever smoked cigarettes, with half of those (20.9%) being current smokers (Centers for Disease Control and Prevention 2005). The prevalence is higher among men and the poor and decreases with increasing educational levels. Fewer than 9% of adults report past-month cigar and/or smokeless tobacco use. Although tobacco use has been declining in the United States, it is increasing worldwide.

Intoxication and Abuse

Although one can certainly feel ill from too much acute tobacco use (e.g., nausea, dizziness, tachycardia), because there are rarely prolonged maladaptive or clinically significant social sequelae, nicotine intoxication is not a recognized substance-induced disorder. Similarly, neither is nicotine abuse a recognized substance use disorder.

Diagnosis

Although the diagnosis of nicotine dependence is made according to DSM-IV-TR criteria, other rating scales may be useful in treating the disorder. The number of cigarettes smoked per day correlates negatively with ease in quitting and, in many studies, with response to formal treatment. The Fagerström Test for Nicotine Dependence (Figure 9–4) similarly predicts difficulty in quitting.

Treatment and Withdrawal

Given that tobacco use is legal, and its acute use causes minimal behavioral disruption, treatment of nicotine dependence focuses on managing withdrawal and cravings (Table 9–29) and developing other behaviors that promote abstinence and prevent relapse.

Although the long-term (e.g., 12-month) quit rates for a single attempt are less than 10%, the lifetime long-term quit rate is approximately 50%. Accordingly, one of the tasks for the treatment provider is to help the patient deal with relapse and maintain a sense of hope and self-efficacy.

Evidence-based clinical practice guidelines for nicotine dependence are readily available (e.g., Fiore et al. 2000), as are self-help Web sites and phone lines (Table 9–30). Treatment principles are listed in Tables 9–31 and 9–32. The issue of concurrent treatment of nicotine and other substance use disorders continues to be debated (Ziedonis et al. 2006). In two recent review articles, one group recommended concurrent and the other sequential treatments (Kalman et al. 2005; Metz et al. 2005).

Medical Complications

One pharmacological complication especially relevant to psychiatric practice is the induction of hepatic enzymes and drug metabolism by the nonnicotine com-

TABLE 9–29.   DSM-IV-TR diagnostic criteria for nicotine withdrawal

A. Daily use of nicotine for at least several weeks.

B. Abrupt cessation of nicotine use, or reduction in the amount of nicotine used, followed within 24 hours by four (or more) of the following signs:

    (1) dysphoric or depressed mood
    (2) insomnia
    (3) irritability, frustration, or anger
    (4) anxiety
    (5) difficulty concentrating
    (6) restlessness
    (7) decreased heart rate
    (8) increased appetite or weight gain

C. The symptoms in criterion B cause clinically significant distress or impairment in social, occupational, or other important areas of functioning.

D. The symptoms are not due to a general medical condition and are not better accounted for by another mental disorder.

TABLE 9–30.   Smoking cessation information Web sites

- Smokefree.gov (www.smokefree.gov): Tobacco Control Research Branch of the National Cancer Institute, National Institutes of Health. A handheld computer intervention tool software program is available through this site.

- ACS Guide to Quitting Smoking (http://www.cancer.org/docroot/PED/content/PED_10_13X_Guide_for_Quitting_Smoking.asp): American Cancer Society

- TIPS: CDC's Tobacco Information and Prevention Source (http://www.cdc.gov/tobacco): Office on Smoking and Health of National Center for Chronic Disease Prevention and Health Promotion, Centers for Disease Control and Prevention

- Treatobacco.net (http://www.treatobacco.net): Society for Research on Nicotine and Tobacco, World Bank, Cochrane Group, and others

- "Clinical Practice Guideline: Treating Tobacco Use and Dependence" (http://www.ncbi.nlm.nih.gov/books/bv.fcgi?rid=hstat2.chapter.7644): Agency for Healthcare Research and Quality, U.S. Department of Health and Human Services

Note.   Sites accessed July 7, 2006.

TABLE 9–31.   Principles of treatment for nicotine dependence

1. Every patient who uses tobacco should be offered treatment:
    - Patients *willing* to try to quit—evidence-based cessation treatment
    - Patients *unwilling* to try—brief intervention to increase motivation to quit

2. The intensity of counseling is directly related to its effectiveness.
    - Treatments involving person-to-person contact (e.g., individual, group, telephone) are consistently effective, with effectiveness increasing with treatment intensity (e.g., minutes of contact).

3. All patients attempting tobacco cessation should receive
    - Practical counseling (problem solving/skills training).
    - Social support as part of treatment (intratreatment social support).
    - Help in securing social support outside of treatment (extratreatment social support).

4. All patients attempting tobacco cessation should receive adjunctive pharmacotherapy unless contraindicated.
    - First-line pharmacotherapies include bupropion and nicotine gum, inhaler, nasal spray, and patch.
    - Second-line pharmacotherapies include clonidine and nortriptyline.

5. Tobacco dependence treatments are both clinically effective and cost-effective relative to other medical and disease prevention interventions.

Source.   Adapted from U.S. Department of Health and Human Services Public Health Service 2000. Public domain.

---

ponents (probably polycyclic aromatic hydrocarbons) of tobacco smoke. Nicotine-dependent patients hospitalized on nonsmoking units who are stabilized on medications such as haloperidol, valproate, clozapine, oxazepam, and others will experience decreased blood levels of the medications once discharged if they resume smoking.

The cardiovascular, pulmonary, carcinogenic, and other medical complications of nicotine use are well described in the general medical literature and thus are not discussed here.

Questions	Score
1. How soon after you wake up do you smoke your first cigarette? • After 60 minutes　　(0 points) • 31–60 minutes　　(1 point) • 6–30 minutes　　(2 points) • Within 5 minutes　　(3 points)	
2. Do you find it difficult to refrain from smoking in places where it is forbidden? • No　　(0 points) • Yes　　(1 point)	
3. Which cigarette would you hate most to give up? • The first in the morning　　(1 point) • Any other　　(0 points)	
4. How many cigarettes per day do you smoke? • 10 or fewer　　(0 points) • 11–20　　(1 point) • 21–30　　(2 points) • 31 or more　　(3 points)	
5. Do you smoke more frequently during the first hours after awakening than during the rest of the day? • No　　(0 points) • Yes　　(1 point)	
6. Do you smoke if you are so ill that you are in bed most of the day? • No　　(0 points) • Yes　　(1 point)	
Add the scores for questions 1–6 for total score:	

Total score: 1–3 = mild dependence; 4–6 = moderate; >6 = high

FIGURE 9–4. Fagerström Test for Nicotine Dependence.

Source. Adapted from Heatherton et al. 1991.

TABLE 9–32. First-line pharmacotherapies approved for use for smoking cessation by the U.S. Food and Drug Administration*

Agent	Precautions/ contraindications	Side effects	Dosage	Duration	Availability
Bupropion SR	History of seizure History of eating disorders	Insomnia Dry mouth	150 mg every morning for 3 days, then 150 mg twice daily. (Begin treatment 1–2 weeks before quitting.)	7–12 weeks, maintenance up to 6 months	Zyban (prescription only)
Nicotine gum		Mouth soreness Dyspepsia	1–24 cigarettes/day: 2-mg gum (up to 24 pieces/day) 25+ cigarettes/day: 4-mg gum (up to 24 pieces/day)	Up to 12 weeks	Nicorette, different flavors (OTC only)
Nicotine inhaler		Local irritation of mouth and throat	6–16 cartridges/day	Up to 6 months	Nicotrol Inhaler (prescription only)
Nicotine nasal spray		Nasal irritation	8–40 doses/day	3–6 months	Nicotrol NS (prescription only)
Nicotine patch		Local skin reaction Insomnia	21 mg/24 hours 14 mg/24 hours 7 mg/24 hours 15 mg/16 hours	4 weeks then 2 weeks then 2 weeks 8 weeks	Nicoderm CQ, (OTC only) Generic patches (prescription and OTC) Nicotrol (OTC only)
Varenecline		Nausea Sleep disturbance Constipation	Taper up to 1 mg twice a day by day 8. (Begin treatment 1 week pre-quitting.)	12–24 weeks	Chantix (prescription only)

Note. The information contained within this table is not comprehensive. Please see package inserts for the individual medications for additional information. OTC=over the counter.

*Other agents such as rimonabant (cannabinoid-1 receptor antagonist) and selegiline (irreversible monoamine oxidase B inhibitor) are under investigation.

Source. Adapted from Agency for Healthcare Research and Quality 2001.

Sedative-Hypnotics

Epidemiology

Just over 12% of individuals older than 12 years report lifetime abuse of sedative-hypnotic medications (Substance Abuse and Mental Health Services Administration 2005). Benzodiazepines, as well as other sedative-hypnotics, are commonly used in the setting of polysubstance abuse. They may enhance the "high" of other substances or may be used to help a person "come down" from the effects of stimulant drugs. They also can be used alone, particularly when taken in high doses. Barbiturates are more likely to be abused alone.

Intoxication

Signs and symptoms of intoxication are similar to those of alcohol intoxication and can include slurred speech, ataxia, and incoordination. At more severe levels of intoxication, stupor and coma may develop.

With the older nonbenzodiazepine agents, tolerance may develop to a drug's therapeutic effects but not to its toxicity, and a barbiturate overdose can be fatal. An overdose on benzodiazepines alone virtually never leads to death. When they are ingested along with alcohol, major tranquilizers, or opioids, however, the polysubstance overdose can be fatal.

Withdrawal

Abrupt discontinuation of sedative-hypnotics in individuals who are physically dependent on them can lead to significant withdrawal symptoms, the most serious being death. The withdrawal symptoms that occur with benzodiazepines, barbiturates, and nonbarbiturate/nonbenzodiazepine agents are similar to each other as well as to the withdrawal symptoms of alcohol. Table 9–33 identifies the most common signs and symptoms seen in sedative-hypnotic withdrawal. The time course and intensity of withdrawal symptoms depend on the particular drug on which the individual is dependent. With short-acting sedative-hypnotics and benzodiazepines, symptoms can begin between 12 and 24 hours after the last dose and reach peak intensity between 24 and 72 hours. With long-acting drugs, withdrawal symptoms may not peak until the fifth to eighth day.

For patients who were initially prescribed benzodiazepines for the treatment of psychiatric symptoms, those target symptoms may reemerge during withdrawal. Symptom reemergence is not uncommon, occurring in 60%–80% of benzodiazepine-dependent patients initially treated for anxiety and insomnia disorders. Symptom rebound is a brief, intensified return of the target symptoms and is the most common consequence of prolonged benzodiazepine use. Rebound symptoms usually resolve within a few weeks after discontinuation of the benzodiazepine. Protracted withdrawal can occur in a small proportion of patients, usually in the setting of long-term benzodiazepine use. Signs and symptoms of withdrawal can occur for weeks to months and consist of slowly abating symptoms of withdrawal as noted in Table 9–33.

Treatment

Management of severe benzodiazepine overdose includes careful monitoring of the patient's airway and ventilatory support when necessary. Repeated doses of activated charcoal may be particularly helpful in barbiturate or other nonbenzodiazepine ingestions. Flumazenil, a competitive antagonist at the benzodiazepine receptor, may be useful, but if it is not used carefully, the

---

TABLE 9–33. DSM-IV-TR diagnostic criteria for sedative-hypnotic withdrawal

A. Cessation of (or reduction in) sedative, hypnotic, or anxiolytic use that has been heavy and prolonged.

B. Two (or more) of the following, developing within several hours to a few days after criterion A:
   (1) autonomic hyperactivity (e.g., sweating or pulse rate greater than 100)
   (2) increased hand tremor
   (3) insomnia
   (4) nausea or vomiting
   (5) transient visual, tactile, or auditory hallucinations or illusions
   (6) psychomotor agitation
   (7) anxiety
   (8) grand mal seizures

C. The symptoms in criterion B cause clinically significant distress or impairment in social, occupational, or other important areas of functioning.

D. The symptoms are not due to a general medical condition and are not better accounted for by another mental disorder.

Specify if: With perceptual disturbances

---

abruptly induced severe withdrawal can induce seizures in patients dependent on benzodiazepines.

There are four general strategies that can be used for the management of sedative-hypnotic withdrawal, including benzodiazepines. The first option gradually reduces the dosage of the sedative-hypnotic on which the patient is dependent. The second option substitutes a long-acting benzodiazepine (such as chlordiazepoxide) for the agent to which the person is dependent and then tapers the substituted agent. The third option substitutes a long-acting barbiturate (usually phenobarbital) and then tapers that. A fourth option is to use valproate or carbamazepine.

The phenobarbital substitution option has the broadest use for sedative-hypnotic withdrawal and can be used for barbiturate, benzodiazepine, or combined alcohol/sedative-hypnotic withdrawals. Phenobarbital is long-acting, has little variations in blood levels between doses, and has both a low abuse potential and a high therapeutic index. The signs of toxicity (e.g., sustained nystagmus, slurred speech, or ataxia) are reliable and easily observable. The patient's average daily sedative-hypnotic dosage is calculated (Table 9–34) and then divided into three doses spread out over the day. If the patient is using more than one sedative-hypnotic, the total dosage equivalents of phenobarbital for all the substances combined are calculated. Before each dose of phenobarbital, the patient is checked for signs of toxicity, and if any are present, the dose is withheld. If minimal or no signs or symptoms of withdrawal occur, the phenobarbital dosage is decreased by 30 mg each day. If objective signs of withdrawal develop, the daily dosage of phenobarbital is increased by 50%, and the patient is restabilized before continuing the withdrawal.

TABLE 9–34.   Sedative-hypnotics and their phenobarbital withdrawal equivalents

Generic name	Trade name	Common therapeutic uses	Therapeutic dosage range (mg/day)	Dose equal to 30 mg phenobarbital for withdrawal, mg[a]
Benzodiazepines				
Alprazolam	Xanax	Sedative, antipanic	0.75–6	1
Chlordiazepoxide	Librium	Sedative	15–100	25
Clonazepam	Klonopin	Anticonvulsant	0.5–4	2
Clorazepate	Tranxene	Sedative	15–60	7.5
Diazepam	Valium	Sedative	4–40	10
Estazolam	ProSom	Hypnotic	1–2	1
Flunitrazepam[b]	Rohypnol[b]	Hypnotic	0.5–1	0.5
Flurazepam	Dalmane	Hypnotic	15–30	15
Halazepam	Paxipam	Sedative	60–160	40
Lorazepam	Ativan	Sedative	1–6	2
Midazolam	Versed	Intravenous sedation	2.5–7	2.5
Nitrazepam[b]	Mogadon[b]	Hypnotic	5–10	5
Oxazepam	Serax	Sedative	10–120	10
Temazepam	Restoril	Hypnotic	15–30	15
Triazolam	Halcion	Hypnotic	0.125–0.50	0.25
Barbiturates				
Butabarbital	Butisol	Sedative	45–120	100
Butalbital	Fiorinal, Sedapap	Sedative/analgesic[c]	100–300	100
Pentobarbital	Nembutal	Hypnotic	50–100	100
Secobarbital	Seconal	Hypnotic	50–100	100
Other sedative-hypnotics				
Zaleplon	Sonata	Hypnotic	5–20	5
Zolpidem	Ambien	Hypnotic	5–10	5

[a]Phenobarbital withdrawal conversion equivalence is not the same as therapeutic dose equivalency. Withdrawal equivalence is the amount of the drug that 30 mg of phenobarbital will substitute for and prevent serious high-dose withdrawal signs and symptoms.
[b]Although not marketed in the United States, these benzodiazepines are commonly used in many countries.
[c]Butalbital is usually available in combination with opioid and nonopioid analgesics.
Source.   Adapted from Smith and Wesson 2004.

Hallucinogens

Epidemiology

The family of hallucinogens includes drugs that induce a distortion of reality in the user, including alterations of sensory perceptions of sight and sounds as well as changes in emotions. Lysergic acid diethylamide (LSD) is the prototypical hallucinogen. It is an odorless and tasteless synthetic chemical, usually ingested as a solution or dissolved on paper or sugar cubes. Typical hallucinogenic doses are 25–75 micrograms. Analogous lysergic acid derivatives can be extracted from morning glory seeds and ergot, a rye fungus. In 2005, annual use among twelfth graders was 1.8%. Among tenth graders, annual use was 1.5% (National Institute on Drug Abuse 2005a).

Intoxication

LSD interferes with serotonin neurotransporters. It typically induces euphoria in addition to delusions and visual hallucinations; however, the psychological effects it induces can be unpredictable. The experience can be significantly influenced by the user's pre-intoxication mind-set and also by the setting in which the drug is used. "Bad trips" can be marked by feelings of intense fear with avoidant responses. Physical effects include increased body temperature, heart rate, and blood pressure; sleeplessness; and loss of appetite.

Withdrawal

Although hallucinogen withdrawal is not a recognized disorder, withdrawal symptoms of minimal clinical significance (including fatigue, irritability, and anhedonia) are reported by approximately 10% of hallucinogen users.

Treatment

The treatment of acute intoxication with hallucinogens is largely supportive. Providing reassurance, support, and a calm, quiet environment are the mainstays of treatment. For patients with extreme feelings of panic or fear, the use of a benzodiazepine may be warranted.

Medical Complications

A potential complication of hallucinogen use is hallucinogen persisting perception disorder, or "flashbacks." The etiological mechanism underlying flashbacks is not clearly understood, but they have reportedly been precipitated by SSRIs. Flashbacks are spontaneous experiences of the same effects that occurred while a person was intoxicated with a hallucinogen in the past. LSD users may also manifest relatively long-lasting psychoses, such as schizophrenia or severe depression, although such severe reactions are not common.

Phencyclidine and Ketamine

Epidemiology

Phencyclidine (PCP), commonly referred to as "angel dust," inhibits catecholamine reuptake in neurons, leading to adrenergic potentiation (Greydanus and Patel 2003). It was initially developed in the 1950s to be used as an anesthetic, but it was never approved for human use due to its significant adverse effects, including intensely negative psychological ones. It can be used as a liquid, tablet, or powder and can also be sprinkled on a cigarette. Results from the Monitoring the Future survey reveal that in 2005, 2.4% of high school seniors reported a lifetime use of PCP; annual use was reported by 1.3% of seniors, and 30-day use was reported by 0.7% (National Institute on Drug Abuse 2005a).

Ketamine is a derivative of PCP that was first developed in 1965. It is less potent, shorter acting, and is used as a dissociative anesthetic in humans as well as animals. Ketamine is commonly referred to on the street as "Special K," "Vitamin K," "Kit Kat," and "cat Valium." It is available on the street primarily through diversion from legal sources, such as hospitals or veterinary clinics.

Intoxication

Both PCP and ketamine cause anesthesia and behavioral effects, at least in part by selectively reducing the excitatory actions of glutamate on central nervous system neurons mediated by the N-methyl-D-aspartate (NMDA) receptor complex. Acute PCP intoxication can manifest as behavior changes including impulsiveness, unpredictability, psychomotor agitation, impaired judgment, and assaultiveness. Physical findings include hypertension, tachycardia, diminished pain sensation, ataxia, dysarthria, muscle rigidity, and seizures. PCP is the only drug that causes a vertical nystagmus, although it can also cause horizontal or rotatory nystagmus. The spectrum of behavioral effects of ketamine intoxication appears to be similar to that of PCP, although less is published on the treatment of ketamine intoxication.

Withdrawal

Although there is not a specifically defined PCP withdrawal syndrome, about 25% of heavy PCP users report withdrawal symptoms including depression, anxiety, irritability, hypersomnolence, diaphoresis, and tremor.

Treatment

The management of acute intoxication with PCP includes providing a calm environment with minimal stimuli. Objects that can be used to harm oneself or others should be removed from the patient's access. Diazepam or haloperidol may be useful for the management of PCP-induced agitation. Physical restraints should be avoided due to the risk of increasing the likelihood of rhabdomyolysis, which may occur on its own during PCP intoxication.

Medical Complications

With PCP intoxication, death can occur secondary to severe hypertension or hypotension, hypothermia, seizures, or psychotic delirium.

Club Drugs

Epidemiology

"Club drugs" have been categorized as those drugs that are frequently used in all-night parties, "rave" dance clubs, and bars. Drugs that are used in these settings include those that have long been abused, such as marijuana and cocaine, as well as drugs whose abuse is a relatively more recent development. Methylenedioxymethamphetamine (MDMA), γ-hydroxybutyrate (GHB), methamphetamine, flunitrazepam (Rohypnol), and ketamine are among these. In 2000, the National Institute on Drug Abuse launched a broad-based public initiative to inform and educate teens, young adults, parents, and communities about the dangers of club drugs. MDMA, frequently called "Ecstasy" but also referred to as "X," "XTC," "Adam," "Clarity," and "Lover's Speed," is probably the most popular club drug used today.

GHB, also know as "G," Liquid X," "Easy Lay," and "Grievous Bodily Harm," was first synthesized in the 1960s and was used by bodybuilders during the 1980s and 1990s. It was marketed in health food stores as a natural way to promote sleep, slow aging, and build muscle. It is relatively easy to synthesize with ingredients obtained through Internet sites and hardware stores. As its strong addiction potential became evident, it was declared a Schedule I controlled substance by Congress in 2000. GHB is, however, available as a Schedule III prescription medication, Xyrem, through a tightly controlled program for the treatment of narcoleptic cataplexy.

Intoxication

GHB is usually prepared in a liquid formulation that is colorless and odorless. It has a slightly bitter taste that is easy to disguise in drinks. Ingestion results in a "dreamy" stupor and amnesia. Because of these features, GHB has been used to incapacitate victims for sexual assault. Some users describe an alcohol-like buzz known as a "G-ber daze." Higher doses can result in unconsciousness, coma, and death.

MDMA is most commonly taken in tablet form, and its effects are similar to both an amphetamine and a hallucinogen. Users of MDMA report enhanced sensation, increased energy, and a strong sense of relatedness to others. Use also results in elevations of heart rate and blood pressure as well as dilated pupils. Symptoms that a patient reports after MDMA ingestion may also be due to other drugs, because street samples of MDMA have been found to contain caffeine, theophylline, methamphetamine, and other drugs in addition to or instead of actual MDMA.

Withdrawal

Individuals withdrawing from GHB report insomnia, anxiety, tremor, and intense craving. Acute symptoms usually resolve in 3–12 days. Withdrawal from MDMA can result in feelings of fatigue, dysphoria, and depression; loss of appetite; and trouble concentrating.

Treatment and Medical Complications

The management of acute intoxication with GHB is largely supportive, with close monitoring. There are numerous reports in the literature of overdose with GHB leading to coma, respiratory depression, and death. MDMA use has also resulted in death. Dysregulation of body temperature caused by MDMA ingestion, in addition to the high environmental temperatures at raves and increased muscular exertion from prolonged periods of dancing, has resulted in severe rhabdomyolysis. Dehydration is a very serious concern because the drug appears to depress the sense of thirst, and it is used in settings where one may be dancing for hours on end in a crowded, hot club. In addition, deaths involving MDMA use have also been related to cardiac arrhythmias, hypertensive crises, and acute renal failure. Treatment of acute intoxication involves rapid rehydration and core cooling. Lorazepam may be used for agitation, panic, and seizures. It is known that MDMA is a selective serotonergic neurotoxin. Long-term use of MDMA can result in problems with memory and mood.

Inhalants

Epidemiology

Inhalants are often among the first drugs that young children and adolescents experiment with. In 2005, 17.1% of eighth graders, 13.1% of tenth graders, and 11.4% of twelfth graders reported abusing inhalants at least once (National Institute on Drug Abuse 2005a). Frequently termed "whippets," "poppers," or "snappers," inhalants are a diverse group of substances that can be easily purchased over the counter in most stores. The National Institute on Drug Abuse has specified four categories: volatile solvents, nitrites, gases, and aerosols. Examples of common substances include sniffing glue, inhaling paints or sprays, and breathing contents of aerosol spray cans. The route of administration is often to soak a rag in the chemical and then either hold the rag near the face to inhale fumes or put it in a bag and inhale from the bag. Another common route of administration is to pour or spray the inhalant into a bag or balloon directly and then inhale the fumes.

Intoxication and Withdrawal

Most inhalants produce a rapid high that users report as similar to alcohol intoxication. When the amount inhaled is large enough, nearly all solvents and gases produce anesthesia, a loss of sensation, and even unconsciousness. There is no clearly documented withdrawal syndrome from inhalant use.

Treatment and Medical Complications

Consequences of inhalant use can include skin damage (burns and dermatitis). Cardiovascular complications can include arrhythmias, myocardial ischemia from hypoxia, myocardial fibrosis, and ventricular fibrillation. Pulmonary effects from inhalation range from coughing and wheezing to dyspnea, emphysema, and pneumonia. Long-term use of inhalants has also re-

sulted in reports of liver toxicity, metabolic acidosis or alkalosis, acute renal failure, and bone marrow suppression leading to anemia and leukemia. Treatment is supportive and addresses the acute medical complications resulting from inhalant use. Death can result from anoxia, aspiration, asphyxia, cardiac arrhythmias, respiratory depression, and sudden trauma (Ridenour 2005). It has been noted that many AIDS patients with Kaposi's sarcoma had used volatile nitrites before the development of the sarcoma, but whether there is any causal relationship remains unclear. Neurotoxicity and neuropsychiatric complications are the most common reported consequences of inhalant use. Neurological damage can be manifested through ataxia, peripheral and sensorimotor neuropathy, speech problems, and tremor. Psychiatric symptoms resulting from inhalant use include apathy, delirium, dementia, depression, inattention, insomnia, memory loss, and psychosis (Anderson and Loomis 2003).

Anabolic–Androgenic Steroids

Epidemiology

The family of anabolic–androgenic steroids (AASs) includes testosterone and its synthetic derivatives. AASs have long been recognized as substances of abuse in athletes and bodybuilders because the drugs can enhance endurance and performance. They are also abused among male adolescents and young adults to gain muscle mass and lose fat. In 2005, results from the Monitoring the Future study revealed that 2.6% of high school seniors had reported using steroids at least once (National Institute on Drug Abuse 2005b).

AASs can be injected, taken orally, or used transdermally. Use is typically in cycles of administering the drug(s) for weeks or months followed by a scheduled break in use in an attempt to get maximal benefit and to minimize adverse effects. In addition, users will often "stack" by combining several different types of steroids to maximize their effectiveness (National Institute on Drug Abuse 2005b).

Intoxication

Many users report feeling good about themselves while on AASs and may endorse a sense of euphoria. AASs can produce hypomania or mania. It is well known that extreme mood swings, irritability, aggression, and violent behavior can also result from AAS abuse. Paranoid jealousy, extreme irritability, delusions, and impaired judgment stemming from feelings of invincibility have also been reported (Pope and Katz 1988).

Withdrawal

Withdrawal from AASs can result in a constellation of symptoms including low mood, fatigue, restlessness, anorexia, insomnia, decreased libido, and craving for steroids (Brower 2000). These symptoms usually resolve in several weeks, although some persons may develop more persistent symptoms of depression that may respond to treatment with SSRIs. The hypothalamic-pituitary-gonadal axis can be depressed for several months after the cessation of AAS use, contributing to sterility in some and depression in others (Pope and Brower 2004).

Treatment

Despite the medical and psychiatric complications imposed by AAS use, users rarely seek treatment. AAS users may view their use as part of healthy activity when combined with a strenuous exercise regimen and otherwise healthy lifestyle. In addition, users of AASs can be different from other substance abusers in that the desired reward of AASs is not intoxication or a psychoactive effect but a future reward of a more muscular body or athletic success. Motivational issues are different, as are issues regarding relapse to use.

Medical Complications

Major complications resulting from AASs include liver tumors and cancer, jaundice, fluid retention, hypertension, increases in low-density lipoproteins, and decreases in high-density lipoproteins. Kidney tumors, severe acne, and tremulousness are also potential sequelae. Complications in men include testicular atrophy, reduced sperm count, infertility, hair loss, gynecomastia, and increased risk for prostate cancer. In women, hirsutism may occur, including development of facial hair and male-pattern hair loss, menstrual irregularity and/or amenorrhea, clitoral enlargement, and deepening of the voice. AAS use in adolescents may cause premature skeletal maturation (resulting in shorter stature if they use AASs prior to the adolescent growth spurt) and accelerated pubertal changes (National Institute on Drug Abuse 2005b).

Another important consideration is the progression from AAS use to other substances of abuse. There seems to be a particularly prevalent progression in AAS users to opioid dependence. Common reasons cited for initiation of opioid use in AAS users include

counteracting the insomnia and irritability that can occur with AAS use (Arvary and Pope 2000).

Polysubstance Use

Polysubstance use is common; 56% of patients admitted to publicly funded treatment programs in 2002 reported abuse of more than one substance, and more than 70% smoked cigarettes (Office of Applied Studies 2005). If undetected, polysubstance use can complicate the treatment of intoxication and withdrawal. For example, a patient with an opioid overdose remains obtunded despite the administration of naloxone because of concurrent high-dose benzodiazepine use, or a patient in alcohol withdrawal seems to require higher doses of diazepam than expected and the syndrome seems to continue for 2 weeks due to concurrent, undetected benzodiazepine withdrawal.

The disorder of true polysubstance dependence (Table 9–35), however, may be less common and may be associated with poorer outcome and greater impairment than dependence on a single substance (Medina et al. 2006; Schuckit et al. 2001). All substances must be addressed during treatment for the dependence, and the patient may have different levels of motivation for recovery from different substances. (For the issue of treatment for tobacco and other substances, see the section on "Nicotine.")

TABLE 9–35. **DSM-IV-TR diagnostic criteria for polysubstance dependence**

Over the same 12-month period, three or more substances (other than nicotine or caffeine) are repeatedly used.

The diagnostic criteria for substance dependence are not met for any single substance but are met when the substances are considered together.

Note. When multiple substances are used and the criteria for substance dependence are met by each of the substances individually, then each substance dependence diagnosis is listed separately.

Co-Occurring Substance Use Disorders and Other Psychiatric Disorders

Substance use disorders and other psychiatric disorders commonly co-occur, and the relationship is complex and bidirectional. The National Institute of Mental Health's ECA study and the NCS are two large, epidemiological surveys that have evaluated the prevalence of comorbid psychiatric and substance use disorders in community samples. In the ECA study, 45% of individuals with alcohol use disorders and 72% of individuals with a drug use disorder had at least one co-occurring psychiatric disorder (Regier et al. 1990). Likewise, in the NCS, 78% of alcohol-dependent men and 86% of alcohol-dependent women met lifetime criteria for another psychiatric disorder, including drug dependence (Kessler et al. 1994). The co-occurrence of psychiatric and substance use disorders is clinically important because comorbidity has a negative impact on the course, treatment outcome, and prognosis of both syndromes.

Diagnostic Considerations

Accurate diagnosis and differentiation between substance-induced states and primary psychiatric diagnoses is one of the more difficult tasks in assessing patients with co-occurring psychiatric symptoms and substance use disorders. The complex relationships between psychiatric and substance-induced symptoms can often lead to diagnostic uncertainty for several reasons. Some individuals with psychiatric disorders may abuse substances attempting to ameliorate psychiatric symptoms. Chronic and excessive use of some substances may precipitate, trigger, or unmask other latent psychiatric illness. Symptoms of intoxication, withdrawal, or other substance-induced disorders can mimic other psychiatric disorders. Some substances, such as methamphetamine, PCP, LSD, and others, can cause psychiatric symptoms that persist long after the substance has been measurably eliminated from the body. Individuals in acute distress may present with combined symptoms, some attributable to substance abuse and some attributable to another psychiatric disorder.

Clinicians often differentiate transient, substance-induced symptoms from other psychiatric illness through observation during a period of abstinence. The duration of abstinence necessary for accurate diagnosis is based on both the diagnosis being assessed and the substance used. For example, long-half-life drugs (e.g., some benzodiazepines, methadone) may require several weeks of abstinence for withdrawal symptoms to subside so that an accurate diagnosis may be made. Conversely, for shorter-acting substances (e.g., alcohol, cocaine, short-half-life benzodiazepines), both the acute intoxication and withdrawal duration are likely to be shorter, and it may be possible to make valid diag-

noses with shorter periods of abstinence. Sustained psychiatric symptoms during lengthy periods of abstinence, a family history of the particular psychiatric disorder, and the onset of psychiatric symptoms before the onset of substance abuse and dependence all suggest a primary psychiatric illness. Often, considerable patience, persistence, acceptance of ambiguity, and treatment experience with a patient are required to be able to accurately diagnose and treat co-occurring disorders.

Screening patients presenting at either substance abuse or psychiatric treatment settings for both substance use disorders and other psychiatric disorders is essential. Prompt diagnosis and treatment can reduce morbidity, increase treatment efficiency, and improve treatment outcomes. Brief screening tools for substance use disorders that have been found useful in psychiatric settings include the Alcohol Use Disorders Identification Test (see Figure 9–2), the Michigan Alcoholism Screening Test (Selzer 1971), and the Drug Abuse Screening Test (Skinner 1982). The Symptom Checklist (SCL-90) has been found to have moderate specificity and high sensitivity in screening for anxiety and mood disorders in substance use patients (Kennedy et al. 2001). The Psychiatric Research Interview for Substance Use and Mental Disorders (Hasin et al. 1996) can also be used to facilitate determination of the chronological relationships between psychiatric symptoms and substance abuse.

Treatment Considerations

Psychosocial Treatments

Although the treatments for psychiatric and substance abuse disorders have historically largely consisted of separate clinical services, the integration of services results in better treatment for individuals with co-occurring disorders (see Table 9–16). Programs often include a mix of group and individual therapies. CBTs are among the most efficacious treatments for anxiety and depressive disorders as well as for the treatment of substance use disorders. Behavioral therapies such as relaxation and breathing techniques, biofeedback, and meditation are often used in substance abuse treatment facilities and can also be effective in decreasing psychiatric symptoms. Individuals with co-occurring substance abuse and other psychiatric disorders can also benefit from participation in 12-Step groups such as Dual Recovery Anonymous (see Table 9–15).

Pharmacological Treatments

The ideal approach to the pharmacological treatment of these co-occurring conditions would be to use an agent that has no abuse potential, is safe and well tolerated, and is efficacious in both disorders. The benzodiazepines, SSRIs, tricyclic antidepressants (TCAs), monoamine oxidase inhibitors (MAOIs), antipsychotics, and anticonvulsant agents have all been found to be efficacious in treatment studies of specific psychiatric disorders. Unfortunately, there are sparse data in the co-occurring population. Data support the use of SSRI agents in the treatment of co-occurring alcohol dependence and major depression. Higher dosages of SSRIs and TCAs may be required if alcohol use has induced hepatic microsomal enzyme activity. The use of SSRIs in the treatment of particular subtypes of patients with alcohol dependence shows promise, but much work remains to be done. Mirtazapine may be of interest in a population with comorbid alcoholism and depression due to its antagonism of serotonin 5-HT$_3$ receptors, a property that it shares with ondansetron. Although lithium is accepted as the gold standard agent in the treatment of bipolar disorder, anticonvulsant agents have shown some promise in the treatment of co-occurring bipolar and substance use disorders (Myrick et al. 2004). Research investigating the use of psychiatric medications in combination with alcoholism treatment medications such as naltrexone and acamprosate would be of interest.

Active substance abuse or relapse should not be considered an automatic contraindication for the continuance of medications for other psychiatric disorders. Similarly, medication may be indicated for the treatment of substance-induced disorder with prolonged symptoms, such as alcohol-induced depressive disorder or methamphetamine-induced psychotic disorder.

Gender Considerations

In 2001, it was estimated that approximately one-third of the individuals with either alcohol abuse or dependence in the United States were women, as were more than one-third of the illicit drug users (Substance Abuse and Mental Health Services Administration 2002). Alarmingly, in 2003 and 2004, almost 5% of pregnant women were past-month users of illicit drugs (Substance Abuse and Mental Health Services Administration 2005). Gender-related research suggests that women may be more susceptible than men to interpersonal difficulties, trauma, and medical consequences stemming from substance abuse or dependence.

There are differences in the incidence, development, and consequences of alcohol dependence in women compared with men. Women drink alone more often, binge less, have more regular drinking patterns, and drink smaller quantities compared with men. For women in relationships, drinking patterns are more likely to match those of their significant others. Women have been shown to have higher blood alcohol levels than men when ingesting the same amount of alcohol. Lower levels of alcohol dehydrogenase in the gastric mucosa and liver of women compared with men may contribute to this, as may the lower adjusted total body water content and smaller volume of distribution. Some researchers have also suggested that hormonal fluctuations during the menstrual cycle may possibly contribute to the rate of alcohol metabolism, although the data are not clear.

Women are more likely than men to have been introduced to heroin or methamphetamine by a significant other. In addition, women with substance use disorders are more likely to be living with an addicted partner, with obvious treatment implications.

The faster onset of substance-related disorders and medical consequences from substance abuse in women compared with men has been termed the *telescoping effect* (Frezza et al. 1990). Females reach criteria for alcohol dependence from onset of drinking more quickly than males and progress to liver disease with lower levels of drinking over a shorter period of time compared with men. In addition, those women who develop cirrhosis from alcohol dependence have a higher rate of mortality than their male counterparts. A women's risk of breast cancer is also increased by moderate to heavy alcohol consumption.

Reproductive dysfunction is another possible consequence of excessive alcohol use. Alcohol abuse in women can lead to amenorrhea, anovulation, luteal phase dysfunction, and hyperprolactinemia, which in turn can cause menstrual abnormalities and impaired fertility. Alcohol may also increase the risk of spontaneous abortion. Fetal alcohol syndrome, resulting from alcohol use during pregnancy, is well established in medical literature. Illicit drug use during pregnancy often results in lower birth weights and premature delivery.

There is a great degree of co-occurrence of other psychiatric and substance use disorders in women. Compared with men, women with affective and anxiety disorders are more likely to present with a substance use disorder, and women with substance use disorders are more likely to experience depression and anxiety (Chander and McCaul 2003). There may be an etiological role of some anxiety disorders in the initiation of substance abuse in women. Posttraumatic stress disorder secondary to childhood or adult sexual and/or physical abuse is particularly prevalent in women with substance use disorders.

The risk of HIV transmission is of particular concern, because the number of AIDS cases in women has tripled since the mid-1980s. Intravenous drug use as well as heterosexual sex with HIV-infected partners are the major modes of transmission in women. In the past, the prevalence of HIV was highest in men who have sex with men or who use intravenous drugs. The rate of cases acquired through heterosexual sex is now almost equal to that of cases acquired through intravenous drug abuse (Karon et al. 2001).

Women make up approximately 25% of patients in traditional treatment centers for alcohol dependence in the United States. Women with alcohol use disorders are more likely to present for treatment of other problems, such as marital or relationship difficulties, physical illness, or emotional problems. They are more likely to seek treatment in psychiatric or primary care settings than in traditional substance disorder treatment programs. When identifying a woman with a substance use disorder and referring her for treatment, it is important to recognize gender-specific barriers that may impede her ability and willingness to enter and complete treatment. Such barriers include lack of gender and cultural appropriateness in program content, fear of legal consequences (particularly loss of child custody), lack of child care and transportation, inadequate or no health insurance coverage, caretaker roles for dependent family members, and societal intolerance and stigmatization of substance-dependent women (Chasnoff 1991). Some evidence suggests that gender-specific services can improve treatment retention, substance use outcomes, and possibly psychosocial functioning in women when compared with traditional mixed-gender programs, but further research is warranted.

Considerations in Adolescents

The Monitoring the Future survey collects data each year on the attitudes and drug use habits of approximately 50,000 nationally representative students in grades 8, 10, and 12 (Johnston et al. 2006). Alcohol is the most common substance of abuse among adolescents, and marijuana is the most common illicit substance of abuse. In 2005, 47% of twelfth graders reported past-30-day drinking, and 29.2% reported binge drinking (five or more drinks in a row) within 2 weeks of the survey. Fifty percent of American secondary school students have tried an illicit drug by the time of graduation. Results of this survey have shown an approximately 19% decline from 2001 to 2005 in any illicit drug use in the past month by all students combined. Of particular note, cigarette smoking is at its lowest rate in the history of the survey. In 2005, declines were observed in lifetime cigarette use among twelfth and eighth graders and in daily use among twelfth graders. Disapproval of smoking one or more packs of cigarettes a day increased among twelfth graders. Declines in the use of alcohol, methamphetamine, amphetamine, marijuana, and steroids were also seen. In addition to a decline in the lifetime use of MDMA, LSD, and GHB, the perception of the availability of LSD, MDMA, hallucinogens other than LSD, amphetamines, and tranquilizers decreased among twelfth graders.

Recent findings have indicated that a main area of concern is the continued high rates of nonmedical use of prescription pain killers in each grade. In 2005, nonmedical use of hydrocodone and oxycodone within the past year was reported by 9.5% and 5.5% of twelfth-grade students, respectively. Long-term trends show an increase in the abuse of oxycodone from 2002 to 2005 among twelfth graders. Another area of concern is the increase in the use of sedative-hypnotics among twelfth graders since 2001. Between 2002 and 2005, lifetime and past-year use of inhalants increased among eighth graders. This trend is of particular concern because inhalants are abused more often by younger students than by older students.

When evaluating an adolescent with possible substance use disorders, educational status, family functioning, peer relationships, legal status, and use of free time should be assessed, in addition to direct questions about the use of alcohol or drugs and possible psychiatric disorders. Patterns of use, negative consequences, and context and control of use may all be unique in adolescents in comparison with adults. Investigating areas of academic performance, school attendance, and disciplinary problems can be particularly important, because it helps the practitioner ascertain the adolescent's risk of a substance use disorder. Inquiring about a history of physical or sexual abuse is imperative because those adolescents with a history of abuse are at increased risk for a substance use disorder. CRAFFT (Table 9–36) is a useful mnemonic-based questionnaire to screen for possible substance disorders in adolescents (Knight et al. 2002). An answer of "yes" to two or more questions is indicative of harmful substance use.

As in adults, there is a high level of co-occurrence of substance use and other psychiatric disorders in adolescents. Adolescents with anxiety or depression have a higher risk for later substance use. Substance abuse, particularly when comorbid with depression, contributes to an increased rate of adolescent suicide.

TABLE 9–36. CRAFFT questionnaire to identify problem drinking in adolescents

C	Have you ever ridden in **C**ar driven by someone (including yourself) who was "high" or had been using alcohol or drugs?
R	Do you ever use alcohol or drugs to **R**elax, feel better about yourself, or fit in?
A	Do you ever use alcohol/drugs while you are by yourself, **A**lone?
F	Do your family or **F**riends ever tell you that you should cut down on your drinking or drug use?
F	Do you ever **F**orget things you did while using alcohol or drugs?
T	Have you gotten into **T**rouble while you were using alcohol or drugs?

Note.   Two or more "yes" responses indicate harmful substance use and the need for further evaluation.

Source.   Reprinted from Knight JR, Sherritt L, Shrier LA, et al: "Validity of the CRAFFT Substance Abuse Screening Test Among Adolescent Clinic Patients." *Archives of Pediatrics and Adolescent Medicine* 156:607–614, 2002. Used with permission.

The prevalence of substance abuse in those with conduct disorder is estimated to be as high as 80%, with the onset of conduct disorder usually preceding the development of a substance use disorder (Crowley et al. 2001). Attention-deficit/hyperactivity disorder (ADHD) in and of itself does not appear to increase the risk of substance use disorders in adolescents, but rather, substance use appears to be mediated by conduct disorder and bipolar disorder (Biederman et al. 1997). In a recent meta-analysis, although a diagnosis of ADHD did not predict substance abuse, unmedicated and undertreated ADHD did (Wilens et al. 2003).

Psychosocial treatments for substance use disorders in adolescents are similar to those used in adults, except they should be adapted for this specific population. Treatments include CBT, behavioral therapies, brief interventions, psychodynamic interpersonal therapies, family therapies, self-support groups, and 12-Step approaches. CBT assists adolescents in developing greater control, identifying environmental and internal triggers to substance use, and developing strategies for dealing with stressors, triggers, and relapses. Behavioral therapies in adolescents can include operant conditioning methods (with positive and negative reinforcement) as well as behavioral contingency contracts and parent management training. Goals of family therapy include decreasing parental denial, decreasing resistance, and helping the family to initiate and maintain treatment efforts. Participation of the family is crucial in the treatment of an adolescent with a substance use disorder. 12-Step approaches can provide group support from recovering peers and provide reminders of the negative consequences of substance use as well as reminders of the benefits of abstinence. It is important to help a family identify a 12-Step group that is geared specifically toward adolescents. As in adults, the aim of pharmacotherapy in adolescents with sub-stance use disorders includes detoxification, interfering with the physiological and subjective effects of the substance, and treatment of co-occurring psychiatric disorders. A recent small, open-label trial of naltrexone in adolescents found that it was well tolerated and reduced craving and drinking in adolescents who were dependent on alcohol (Deas et al. 2005).

Considerations in Older Adults

Older adults (loosely defined as those 65 years or older) with substance abuse problems face particular challenges compared with younger adults (Oslin 2005). Changes in body composition and metabolism can lead to reversed tolerance, and social and occupational roles change with retirement. Both changes can result in physicians not recognizing or minimizing other symptoms of abuse or dependence. Most of the studies of substance use disorders in older adults have been conducted with alcohol-dependent subjects. Much less is known about use of illicit drugs in this population.

Although the usual treatment modalities (e.g., brief intervention, motivational enhancement, CBT) are indicated in older adults diagnosed with substance use disorders, treatment with age-appropriate components probably results in better outcomes (Blow 2003). Age-specific concerns to be addressed include the presence of multiple medical problems with multiple medications and multiple prescribing physicians; greater access to and greater problems with prescription medications; developmental loss of independence, function, and social supports; and impaired mobility due to either social isolation or general medical conditions, resulting in difficulty accessing clinic or office-based treatment.

Cultural/Ethnic Considerations

Although there have been many definitions of *culture* and *ethnicity*, this section refers to *culture* as "a set of meanings, norms, beliefs and values shared by a group of people" (Ton and Lim 2006, p. 6) and *ethnicity* as "an individual's sense of belonging to a group of people who have a common set of beliefs and customs (culture) and who share a common history and origin" (Ton and Lim 2006, p. 7). An individual's ethnic and cultural identification influences access to specific substances, socially acceptable patterns of substance use, and how someone who abuses substances is viewed in terms of deviancy, marginalization, or acceptance. Ethnic and cultural identification also influences an individual's view of substance abuse as a disorder or illness and of how substance abuse should be dealt with or treated. As a dramatic example, the experience of opioid dependence is likely quite different for a 33-year-old Thai male opium abuser in Bangkok who seeks help from a Buddhist temple program than for a 55-year-old white female hydrocodone abuser in New York contemplating buprenorphine maintenance through her primary care physician's office.

Diagnosing substance abuse or dependence requires the psychiatrist to be knowledgeable or acquire knowledge about a patient's culture, because culture may define the particulars of "major role obligations" and "social or interpersonal problems" (see Table 9–4) or of "important social, occupational, or recreational activities" (see Table 9–5) (American Psychiatric Association 2000).

Often addiction results in the abuser being marginalized or withdrawing from his or her original culture, and as part of treatment, the psychiatrist must know or gain knowledge of what mechanisms exist within the patient's culture that allow reintegration into endogenous support systems and roles. Additionally, a substance abuse treatment program must have ways of negotiating its institutionalized beliefs (e.g., about individuality, diagnoses and disorders, use of medications) with those of the patient to prevent the treatment from becoming more a debate about beliefs than a facilitated collaborative process of recovery (Edwards 1983).

Key Points

- Worldwide drug and alcohol use disorders, excluding tobacco, are the sixth leading cause of disease burden in adults, whereas tobacco use and exposure to tobacco smoke are the leading preventable causes of death.

- Looking at lifetime risk, the NCS, conducted in the early 1990s, found that around one-third of the subjects who had smoked cigarettes at least once developed nicotine dependence, 15% of subjects who had ever drank alcohol developed alcohol dependence, and about 15% of subjects who had ever tried other drugs developed drug dependence.

- Physicians should inquire about all classes of substances (e.g., alcohol, opioids, sedative-hypnotics, stimulants, cannabis, nicotine), including prescription medications, as well as legal and illegal substances, because a patient may not regard abuse of some substances to be as significant as that of others.

- Although psychosocial and behavioral approaches are the cornerstones of treatment for substance dependence, medications are increasingly used to augment the treatment of alcohol, opioid, and nicotine dependence. Developing medications for the treatment of stimulant dependence is a federal research priority.

- There are currently four medications with FDA approval for the maintenance treatment of alcohol dependence: disulfiram, naltrexone, a long-acting intramuscular formulation of naltrexone, and acamprosate.

- The use of buprenorphine for detoxification or maintenance treatment in opioid dependence is increasingly common, in part because buprenorphine can be prescribed in a physician's office with up to 1 month's prescription at a time.

- Although it may take several tries, the overall success rate in helping patients quit smoking is relatively good. The long-term (e.g., 12 months) quit rates for a single attempt are less than 10%, whereas the lifetime long-term quit rate is approximately 50%.

- Polysubstance abuse is common; 56% of patients admitted to publicly funded treatment programs in 2002 reported abuse of more than one substance, and more than 70% smoked cigarettes. If undetected, polysubstance abuse can complicate the treatment of substance intoxication, withdrawal, abuse, or dependence.

- Substance use disorders and other psychiatric disorders commonly co-occur, and the relationship is complex and bidirectional.

- The recent increase in the rates of nonmedical use of prescription pain killers (specifically opioids) in adolescents is notable and concerning.

Suggested Readings

American Journal of Psychiatry, Vol 162, Issue 8, 2005, contains 8 review articles on different aspects of substance use disorders.

Galanter M, Kleber HD (eds): The American Psychiatric Publishing Textbook of Substance Abuse Treatment, 3rd Edition. Washington, DC, American Psychiatric Publishing, 2004

Graham AW, Schultz TK, Mayo-Smith MF, et al (eds): Principles of Addiction Medicine, 3rd Edition. Chevy Chase, MD, American Society of Addiction Medicine, 2003

Kleber HD, Weiss RD, Anton RF Jr, et al: Practice Guidelines for the Treatment of Patients With Substance Use Disorders, 2nd Edition. Washington, DC, American Psychiatric Publishing, 2006

Lowinson JH, Ruiz P, Millman RB, et al (eds): Substance Abuse: A Comprehensive Textbook, 4th Edition. Philadelphia, PA, Lippincott Williams & Wilkins, 2005

Nature Neuroscience, Vol 8, Issue 11, 2005, contains 10 review articles and commentaries. The issue is available online at: http://www.nature.com/neuro/focus/addiction/index.html. Accessed July 2006.

References

Agency for Healthcare Research and Quality: Suggestions for the Clinical Use of Pharmacotherapies for Smoking Cessation. Rockville, MD, U.S. Public Health Service, 2001. Available at: http://www.ahrq.gov/clinic/tobacco/clinicaluse.htm. Accessed July 7, 2006.

American Psychiatric Association: Diagnostic and Statistical Manual of Mental Disorders, 4th Edition, Text Revision. Washington, DC, American Psychiatric Association, 2000

Anderson CE, Loomis GA: Recognition and prevention of inhalant abuse. Am Fam Physician 68:869–874, 2003

Anthony JC, Warner LA, Kessler RC: Comparative epidemiology of dependence on tobacco, alcohol, controlled substances, and inhalants: basic findings from the National Comorbidity Survey. Exp Clin Psychopharmacol 3:244–268, 1994

Anton RF, O'Malley SS, Ciraulo DA, et al: Combined pharmacotherapies and behavioral interventions for alcohol dependence: the COMBINE study: a randomized controlled trial. JAMA 295:2003–2017, 2006

Arvary D, Pope HG Jr: Anabolic-androgenic steroids as a gateway to opioid dependence. N Engl J Med 342:1532, 2000

Austin G: Perspectives on the History of Psychoactive Substance Use (DHEW Publ No [ADM] 79-810). Bethesda, MD, National Institute on Drug Abuse, 1978

Biederman J, Wilens T, Mick E, et al: Is ADHD a risk factor for psychoactive substance use disorders? Findings from a four-year prospective follow-up study. J Am Acad Child Adolesc Psychiatry 36:21–29, 1997

Blow FC: Special issues in treatment: older adults, in Principles of Addiction Medicine, 3rd Edition. Edited by Graham AW, Schultz TK, Mayo-Smith MF, et al. Chevy Chase, MD, American Society of Addiction Medicine, 2003, pp 581–607

Brower KJ: Assessment and treatment of anabolic steroid abuse, dependence, and withdrawal, in Anabolic Steroids in Sport and Exercise. Edited by Yesalis CE. Champaign, IL, Human Kinetics, 2000, pp 305–332

Brown RL, Rounds LA: Conjoint screening questionnaires for alcohol and drug abuse. Wis Med J 94:135–140, 1995

Budney AJ, Moore BA, Rocha HL, et al: Clinical trial of abstinence-based vouchers and cognitive-behavioral therapy for cannabis dependence. J Consult Clin Psychol 74:307–316, 2006

Carroll KM, Onken LS: Behavioral therapies for drug abuse. Am J Psychiatry 162:1452–1460, 2005

Center for Substance Abuse Treatment: Detoxification and Substance Abuse Treatment: Treatment Improvement Protocol (TIP) Series 45. DHHS Publ No (SMA) 06-4131. Rockville, MD, Substance Abuse and Mental Health Services Administration, 2006

Centers for Disease Control and Prevention: Cigarette Smoking Among Adults—United States, 2004. MMWR Morb Mortal Wkly Rep 54:1121–1124, 2005

Chander G, McCaul ME: Co-occurring psychiatric disorders in women with addictions. Obstet Gynecol Clin North Am 30:469–481, 2003

Chasnoff IJ: Drugs, alcohol, pregnancy, and the neonate: pay now or pay later. JAMA 266:1567–1568, 1991

Collins ED, Kleber HD: Opioids: detoxification, in American Psychiatric Publishing Textbook of Substance Abuse Treatment, 3rd Edition. Edited by Galanter M, Kleber HD. Washington, DC, American Psychiatric Publishing, 2004, pp 265–289

Copersino M, Boyd SJ, Tashkin D, et al: Cannabis withdrawal among non-treatment-seeking adult cannabis users. Am J Addict 15:8–14, 2006

Crowley TJ, Mikulich SK, Ehlers KM, et al: Validity of structured clinical evaluations in adolescents with conduct and substance problems. J Am Acad Child Adolesc Psychiatry 40:265–273, 2001

Deas D, May MP, Randall C, et al: Naltrexone treatment of adolescent alcoholics: an open-label pilot study. J Child Adolesc Psychopharmacol 15:723–728, 2005

Dyson V, Appleby L, Altman E, et al: Efficiency and validity of commonly used substance abuse screening instruments in public psychiatric patients. J Addict Dis 17:57–76, 1998

Edwards G: Countries differ in their treatment of drug problems, in Drug Use and Misuse: Cultural Perspectives. Edited by Edwards G, Arif A, Jaffe JH. New York, St. Martin's Press, 1983, pp 176–184

Ellingstad TP, Sobell LC, Sobell MB, et al: Self-change: a pathway to cannabis abuse resolution. Addict Behav 31:519–530, 2006

Fiore MC, Bailey WC, Cohen SJ, et al: Treating Tobacco Use and Dependence. Quick Reference Guide for Clinicians. Rockville, MD, Department of Health and Human Services, U.S. Public Health Service, 2000

Frezza M, di Padova C, Pozzato G, et al: High blood alcohol levels in women: the role of decreased gastric alcohol dehydrogenase activity and first-pass metabolism. N Engl J Med 322:95–99, 1990

Greydanus DE, Patel DR: Substance abuse in adolescents: a complex conundrum for the clinician. Pediatr Clin North Am 50:1179–1223, 2003

Hall W, Lynskey M: Is cannabis a gateway drug? Testing hypotheses about the relationship between cannabis use and the use of other illicit drugs. Drug Alcohol Rev 24:39, 2005

Hasin DS, Trautman KD, Miele GM, et al: Psychiatric Research Interview for Substance and Mental Disorders (PRISM): reliability for substance abusers. Am J Psychiatry 153:1195–1201, 1996

Heatherton TF, Kozlowski LT, Frecker RC, et al: The Fagerström Test for Nicotine Dependence: a revision of the Fagerström Tolerance Questionnaire. Br J Addict 86:1119–1127, 1991

Hickman M, Carnwath Z, Madden P, et al: Drug-related mortality and fatal overdose risk: pilot cohort study of heroin users recruited from specialist drug treatment sites in London. J Urban Health 80:274–287, 2003

Hock B, Schwarz M, Domke I, et al: Validity of carbohydrate-deficient transferrin (%CDT), gamma-glutamyltransferase (gamma-GT) and mean corpuscular erythrocyte volume (MCV) as biomarkers for chronic alcohol abuse: a study in patients with alcohol dependence and liver disorders of non-alcoholic and alcoholic origin. Addiction 100:1477–1486, 2005

Huestis M, Boyd S, Heishman S, et al: Single and multiple doses of rimonabant antagonize acute effects of smoked cannabis in male cannabis users. Psychopharmacology, epub July 10, 2007. Available at: http://dx.doi.org/10.1007/s00213-007-0861-5. Accessed September 6, 2007.

Hyman SE: Addiction: a disease of learning and memory. Am J Psychiatry 162:1414–1422, 2005

Jarvis MA, Schnoll SH: Methadone treatment during pregnancy. J Psychoactive Drugs 26:155–61, 1994

Johnston JD, O'Malley PM, Bachman JG, et al: Monitoring the Future: National Results on Adolescent Drug Use. Overview of Key Findings, 2005. Bethesda, MD, National Institute on Drug Abuse, 2006

Kalivas PW, Volkow ND: The neural basis of addiction: a pathology of motivation and choice. Am J Psychiatry 162:1403–1413, 2005

Kalman D, Morissette SB, George T: Co-morbidity of smoking in patients with psychiatric and substance use disorders. Am J Addict 14:106, 2005

Karon JM, Fleming PL, Steketee RW, et al: HIV in the United States at the turn of the century: an epidemic in transition. Am J Public Health 91:1060–1068, 2001

Kelly JF, Finney JW, Moos R: Substance use disorder patients who are mandated to treatment: characteristics, treatment process, and 1- and 5-year outcomes. J Subst Abuse Treat 28:213–223, 2005

Kennedy BL, Morris RL, Pedley LL, et al: The ability of the Symptom Checklist SCL-90 to differentiate various anxiety and depressive disorders. Psychiatr Q 72:277–288, 2001

Kessler RC, McGonagle KA, Zhao S, et al: Lifetime and 12-month prevalence of DSM-III-R psychiatric disorders in the United States: results from the National Comorbidity Survey. Arch Gen Psychiatry 51:8–19, 1994

Klag S, O'Callaghan F, Creed P: The use of legal coercion in the treatment of substance abusers: an overview and critical analysis of thirty years of research. Subst Use Misuse 40:1777–1795, 2005

Knight JR, Sherritt L, Shrier LA, et al: Validity of the CRAFFT substance abuse screening test among adolescent clinic patients. Arch Pediatr Adolesc Med 156:607–614, 2002

Kreek MJ, Nielsen DA, Butelman ER, et al: Genetic influences on impulsivity, risk taking, stress responsivity and vulnerability to drug abuse and addiction. Nat Neurosci 8:1450–1457, 2005

Mack A, Franklin JE Jr, Frances RJL: Substance use disorders, in American Psychiatric Publishing Textbook of Clinical Psychiatry, 4th Edition. Edited by Hales RE, Yudofsky SC. Washington, DC, American Psychiatric Publishing, 2003, pp 309–378

Magura S, Staines G, Kosanke N, et al: Predictive validity of the ASAM Patient Placement Criteria for naturalistically matched vs. mismatched alcoholism patients. Am J Addict 12:386–397, 2003

Mattick RP, Kimber J, Breen C, et al: Buprenorphine maintenance versus placebo or methadone maintenance for opioid dependence. Cochrane Database Syst Rev (3): CD002207, 2004

Maxwell JC: Emerging research on methamphetamine. Curr Opin Psychiatry 18:235–242, 2005

Mayo-Smith MF, Beecher LH, Fischer TL, et al: Management of alcohol withdrawal delirium: an evidence-based practice guideline. Arch Intern Med 164:1405–1412, 2004

McLellan AT, Lewis DC, O'Brien CP, et al: Drug dependence, a chronic medical illness: implications for treatment, insurance, and outcomes evaluation. JAMA 284:1689–1695, 2000

McLellan AT, McKay JR, Forman R, et al: Reconsidering the evaluation of addiction treatment: from retrospective follow-up to concurrent recovery monitoring. Addiction 100:447–458, 2005

McPherson TL, Hersch RK: Brief substance use screening instruments for primary care settings: a review. J Subst Abuse Treat 18:193–202, 2000

Medina KL, Shear PK, Schafer J: Memory functioning in polysubstance dependent women. Drug Alcohol Depend 84:248–255, 2006

Mee-Lee D, Shulman G, Fishman M, et al (eds): ASAM Patient Placement Criteria for the Treatment of Substance-Related Disorders, 2nd Edition, Revised. Chevy Chase, MD, American Society of Addiction Medicine, 2001

Metz K, Kroger C, Buhringer G: [Smoking cessation during treatment of alcohol dependence in drug and alcohol rehabilitation centers—a review]. Deutsch Gesundheitsw 67:461–467, 2005

Miller WR, Benefield RG, Tonigan JS: Enhancing motivation for change in problem drinking: a controlled comparison of two therapist styles. J Consult Clin Psychol 61:455–461, 1993

Mittleman MA, Mintzer D, Maclure M, et al: Triggering of myocardial infarction by cocaine. Circulation 99:2737–2741, 1999

Moore THM, Zammit S, Lingford-Hughes A, et al: Cannabis use and risk of psychotic or affective mental health outcomes: a systematic review. Lancet 370:319–328, 2007

Moos RH, Moos BS: Rates and predictors of relapse after natural and treated remission from alcohol use disorders. Addiction 101:212–222, 2006

Myrick H, Anton R: Recent advances in the pharmacotherapy of alcoholism. Curr Psychiatry Rep 6:332–338, 2004

Myrick H, Cluver J, Swavely S, et al: Diagnosis and treatment of co-occurring affective disorders and substance use disorders. Psychiatr Clin North Am 27:649–659, 2004

Nader MA, Czoty PW: PET imaging of dopamine D2 receptors in monkey models of cocaine abuse: genetic predisposition versus environmental modulation. Am J Psychiatry 162:1473–1482, 2005

National Institute on Alcohol Abuse and Alcoholism: Helping Patients Who Drink Too Much: A Clinician's Guide. Rockville, MD, U.S. Department of Health and Human Services, 2005

National Institute on Drug Abuse: NIDA InfoFacts: High School and Youth Trends. Bethesda, MD, National Institute on Drug Abuse, 2005a. Available at: http://www.drugabuse.gov/infofacts/HSYouthtrends.html. Accessed May 26, 2006.

National Institute on Drug Abuse: NIDA InfoFacts: Steroids (Anabolic-Androgenic). Bethesda, MD, National Institute on Drug Abuse, 2005b. Available at: http://www.drugabuse.gov/Infofacts/Steroids.html. Accessed May 27, 2006.

Nestler EJ: Is there a common molecular pathway for addiction? Nat Neurosci 8:1445–1449, 2005

O'Brien CP, Volkow N, Li TK: What's in a word? Addiction versus dependence in DSM-V. Am J Psychiatry 163:764–765, 2006

Office of Applied Studies: The DASIS Report: Polydrug Admissions: 2002. Rockville, MD, Office of Applied Studies, Substance Abuse and Mental Health Services Administration, 2005. Available at: http://www.drugabusestatistics.samhsa.gov/2k5/polydrugTX/polydrugTX.pdf. Accessed June 15, 2006.

Oslin DW: Evidence-based treatment of geriatric substance abuse. Psychiatr Clin North Am 28:897–911, 2005

Peter D. Hart Research Associates: The Face of Recovery. Washington, DC, Peter D. Hart Research Associates, 2001. Available at: http://www.facesandvoicesofrecovery.org/pdf/hart_research.pdf. Accessed May 22, 2006.

Peter D. Hart Research Associates: Faces and Voices of Recovery Public Survey, Washington, DC, Peter D. Hart Research Associates, 2004. Available at: http://www.facesandvoicesofrecovery.org/pdf/2004_hart_survey_analysis.pdf. Accessed May 22, 2006.

Pope HG Jr, Brower KJ: Anabolic-androgenic steroids, in The American Psychiatric Publishing Textbook of Substance Abuse Treatment, 3rd Edition. Edited by Galanter M, Kleber HD. Washington, DC, American Psychiatric Publishing, 2004, pp 257–264

Pope HG Jr, Katz DL: Affective and psychotic symptoms associated with anabolic steroid use. Am J Psychiatry 145:487–490, 1988

Prochaska JO, DiClemente CC: Stages of change in the modification of problem behaviors. Prog Behav Modif 28:183–218, 1992

Regier DA, Farmer ME, Rae DS, et al: Comorbidity of mental disorders with alcohol and other drug abuse: results from the Epidemiologic Catchment Area (ECA) Study. JAMA 264:2511–2518, 1990

Rehm J, Room R, Graham K, et al: The relationship of average volume of alcohol consumption and patterns of drinking to burden of disease: an overview. Addiction 98:1209–1228, 2003

Ridenour TA: Inhalants: not to be taken lightly anymore. Curr Opin Psychiatry 18:243–247, 2005

Schuckit MA, Danko GP, Raimo EB, et al: A preliminary evaluation of the potential usefulness of the diagnoses of polysubstance dependence. J Stud Alcohol 62:54–61, 2001

Schuckit MA, Tapert S: Alcohol, in The American Psychiatric Publishing Textbook of Substance Abuse Treatment, 3rd Edition. Edited by Galanter M, Kleber HD. Washington, DC, American Psychiatric Publishing, 2004, pp 151–166

Selzer ML: The Michigan Alcoholism Screening Test (MAST): the quest for a new diagnostic instrument. Am J Psychiatry 127:1653–1658, 1971

Shearer J, Wodak A, van Beek I, et al: Pilot randomized double blind placebo-controlled study of dexamphetamine for cocaine dependence. Addiction 98:1137–1141, 2003

Sinclair JD: Evidence about the use of naltrexone and for different ways of using it in the treatment of alcoholism. Alcohol 36:2–10, 2001

Skinner HA: The drug abuse screening test. Addict Behav 7:363–371, 1982

Smith DE, Wesson DR: Benzodiazepines and other sedative-hypnotics, in The American Psychiatric Publishing Textbook of Substance Abuse Treatment, 3rd Edition. Edited by Galanter M, Kleber HK. Washington, DC, American Psychiatric Publishing, 2004, pp 243–244

Sobell LC, Ellingstad TP, Sobell MB: Natural recovery from alcohol and drug problems: methodological review of the research with suggestions for future directions. Addiction 95:749–764, 2000

Substance Abuse and Mental Health Services Administration: Results from the 2001 National Household Survey on Drug Abuse, Vol 1: Summary of National Findings. Rockville, MD, Office of Applied Studies, 2002

Substance Abuse and Mental Health Services Administration: Findings from the 2004 National Survey on Drug Use and Health. Rockville, MD, Substance Abuse and Mental Health Services Administration, 2005. Available at: http://www.drugabusestatistics.samhsa.gov/nsduh/2k4nsduh/2k4Results/2k4Results.htm#toc. Accessed July 7, 2006.

Substance Abuse and Mental Health Services Administration, Office of Applied Studies: Treatment Episode Data Set (TEDS) Highlights—2004: National Admissions to Substance Abuse Treatment Services, DASIS Series: S-31, DHHS Publ No (SMA) 06-4140, Rockville, MD, Substance Abuse and Mental Health Services Administration, 2006. Available at: http://wwwdasis.samhsa.gov/teds04/tedshigh2k4.pdf. Accessed July 31, 2006.

Sullivan J, Sykora K, Schneiderman J, et al: Assessment of alcohol withdrawal: the Revised Clinical Institute Withdrawal Assessment for Alcohol scale (CIWA-Ar). Br J Addict 84:1353–1357, 1989

Ton H, Lim RF: The assessment of culturally diverse individuals, in Clinical Manual of Cultural Psychiatry. Edited by Lim RF. Washington, DC, American Psychiatric Publishing, 2006, pp 3–31

Turnipseed SD, Richards JR, Kirk JD, et al: Frequency of acute coronary syndrome in patients presenting to the emergency department with chest pain after methamphetamine use. J Emerg Med 24:369–373, 2003

United Nations Office on Drugs and Crime: World Drug Report, Vol 1: Analysis. Vienna, Austria, United Nations, 2004

United Nations Office on Drugs and Crime: World Drug Report 2005. Vienna, Austria, United Nations, 2005

U.S. Department of Health and Human Services: Tenth Special Report to Congress on Alcohol and Health. Bethesda, MD, U.S. Department of Health and Human Services, 2000

U.S. Department of Health and Human Services Public Health Service: Agency for Health Care Policy and Research Supported Clinical Practice Guidelines: Treating Tobacco Use and Dependence (Revised 2000). Rockville, MD, U.S. Department of Health and Human Services, Public Health Service, 2000. Available at: http://www.ncbi.nlm.nih.gov/books/bv.fcgi?rid=hstat2.chapter.7644. Accessed July 1, 2006.

Velleman R, Templeton L, Copello A: The role of the family in preventing and intervening with substance use and misuse: a comprehensive review of family interventions, with a focus on young people. Drug Alcohol Rev 24:93, 2005

Wadland WC, Ferenchick GS: Medical comorbidity in addictive disorders. Psychiatr Clin North Am 27:675–687, 2004

Weiss F: Neurobiology of craving, conditioned reward and relapse. Curr Opin Pharmacol 5:9–19, 2005

Wilde MI, Wagstaff AJ: Acamprosate: a review of its pharmacology and clinical potential in the management of alcohol dependence after detoxification. Drugs 53:1038–1053, 1997

Wilens TE, Faraone SV, Biederman J, et al: Does stimulant therapy of attention-deficit/hyperactivity disorder beget later substance abuse? A meta-analytic review of the literature. Pediatrics 111:179–185, 2003

Woody GE: Research findings on psychotherapy of addictive disorders. Am J Addict 12 (suppl):S19–S26, 2003

Workgroup on Substance Use Disorders: Practice Guideline for the Treatment of Patients With Substance Use Disorders, 2nd Edition. Washington, DC, American Psychiatric Publishing, 2006

World Health Organization: World Health Report 2003. Geneva, Switzerland, World Health Organization, 2003

World Health Organization: International Statistical Classification of Diseases and Related Health Problems, 10th Revision, Version for 2006. Geneva, Switzerland, World Health Organization, 2006. Available at: http://www.who.int/classifications/apps/icd/icd10online. Accessed May 18, 2006.

Ziedonis DM, Guydish J, Williams J, et al: Barriers and solutions to addressing tobacco dependence in addiction treatment programs. Alcohol Res Health 29:228–235, 2006

Zimmerman JL: Poisonings and overdoses in the intensive care unit: general and specific management issues. Crit Care Med 31:2794–2801, 2003

10

SCHIZOPHRENIA

Michael J. Minzenberg, M.D.
Jong H. Yoon, M.D.
Cameron S. Carter, M.D.

Schizophrenia is a serious and lifelong mental disorder that affects 1% of the population worldwide. It is characterized by a range of striking disturbances in mental functioning that are conceptualized as signs and symptoms that can be grouped into discrete categories. These include symptoms of disruption in the experience of reality, such as hallucinations and delusions, which are grouped as positive symptoms. In addition, many patients with schizophrenia show signs of impoverishment in thinking, emotional experience, and social engagement, which are grouped as negative symptoms. A wide range of other signs and symptoms are also observed in this illness, including disorganized thoughts and behaviors, negative mood states, and behavioral impulsivity.

Schizophrenia may be the most devastating mental illness that humans can experience (Mueser and McGurk 2004). Its onset is typically during adolescence or early adulthood, a period when individuals are just beginning to achieve a firm sense of self, to establish enduring relationships, and to make productive contributions to society. Unlike those with illnesses such as Alzheimer's disease, cancer, and heart disease, patients with schizophrenia usually are unable to point to decades of health predating the onset of illness. These aspects of human experience are just a few that are profoundly affected by this illness because

schizophrenia has pervasive consequences for well-being, health (including physical health), and ability to function in society. A large majority of patients with the illness are unable to maintain independent living or gainful employment for any significant period in their lives after the onset of the illness. Once a chronic course is established, patients generally have relapsing periods of overt psychotic symptoms, characterized by disruptions in the capacity to perceive the environment properly, maintain coherent thinking processes, or derive meaning in a manner that can properly guide thoughts, plans, and behaviors. During quiescent periods of the illness, patients continue to have cognitive and social disturbances that sharply limit their capacity for true recovery and reintegration into the community. Schizophrenia also has profound effects on the families who are forced to deal with the illness. The inexplicable, withdrawn, and sometimes antagonistic behavior of these patients creates great stress in most families, who struggle to comprehend the patient and to resolve the patient's needs with those of the rest of the family.

Although clinical providers surely do not experience the same degree of challenge in response to patients with schizophrenia as families do, they too struggle with attempts to provide relief from very serious symptoms while facilitating incremental progress toward reintegration into the community. Overall, the public health effects of schizophrenia are staggering. Although the prevalence of the illness is approximately 1% in the United States (and consistent throughout the world), patients with schizophrenia occupy 25% of all inpatient hospital beds (Terkelsen and Menikoff 1995) and represent 50% of all inpatient admissions (Geller 1992). The overall cost of schizophrenia in the U.S. in 2002 was estimated to be $62.7 billion (Wu et al. 2005). Schizophrenia is one of the top 10 causes of disability-adjusted life years (Murray and Lopez 1996), representing 2.3% of the total burden of disease in developed countries (the fourth leading cause among persons ages 15–44 years) and 0.8% in developing countries (U.S. Institute of Medicine 2001). In the United States (and probably to a lesser extent elsewhere in the world), patients with schizophrenia are also disproportionately found among the chronically homeless, those who undergo the "revolving door" of repeated brief hospitalizations with premature discharge and insufficient postdischarge care, and those languishing in jails and prisons, suggesting a pervasive failure in contemporary society to adequately meet the needs of these patients.

In addition, schizophrenia has historically been the leading subject of study among mental illnesses and typically the focus of investigation for the leading physicians and scientists of each era. It may rightly be considered the Moby Dick of psychiatry, as the disease entity that is the most enigmatic and yet the most disproportionately disruptive to both the individual and society, certainly throughout the West in the past few hundred years. In recent years, many significant advances have been made in characterizing the disorder and its underpinnings in genetic, neurobiological, and environmental factors. This has led to incremental but steady progress in the development of treatment advances, as well as understanding the nature of factors that modify the course of this illness, all in an attempt to lessen the effect of the illness on both the afflicted and the larger society.

Historical Overview

John Haslam (1764–1844), and independently Philippe Pinel (1745–1826), both in early-nineteenth-century Europe, wrote the earliest descriptions of individuals afflicted with the illness that we now clearly recognize as schizophrenia according to the contemporary nosology. However, evidence indicates that a schizophrenia-like illness has been present across both cultures and broad historical periods (Adityanjee et al. 1999; Jeste et al. 1985; Palha and Esteves 1997; Turner 1992). These authors argued that the societies of ancient Egypt, India, China, Mesopotamia, and Greece (at least by the first century A.D.) recognized the illness we now identify as schizophrenia.

Galen (130–200) in the second century A.D. held that mental disorders in general originated from the brain, a prescient notion that has reemerged in the contemporary "remedicalization" of mental illness. By the Middle Ages, asylums for the seriously mentally ill were established in both Europe and the Arab world. The eighteenth century was notable for the emergence of an emphasis on "humane and moral" treatment of the mentally ill. This clinical philosophy was an attempt to remediate the largely neglectful and punitive treatment conditions that existed in mental hospitals throughout Europe at the time. William Tuke (1732–1822) in England and Philippe Pinel in France led this movement by attempting to treat patients in the least restrictive and most socially supportive environment possible, and they used a scientific perspective to support their arguments. These principles also have resurfaced in the modern era—societies have given increased consideration to the individual patient's autonomy and dignity, and psychiatry has worked to establish a firm scientific basis for the understanding and treatment of mental illness.

Later in the eighteenth century, Bénédict Augustin Morel (1809–1873) first used the term *dementia praecox* to describe schizophrenia as a premature dementia, emphasizing the early onset and progressive clinical decline. This appears to be the first biological model of mental illness that explicitly considered hereditary factors (Palha and Esteves 1997). Subsequently, the study of schizophrenia shifted to Germany. Wilhelm Griesinger (1817–1868) achieved an integration of psychiatric illness with other medical illness and explicitly proposed that these were disorders of the brain and suggested that diffuse cerebral pathology may form a unitary basis for a range of psychotic disorders. Karl Ludwig Kahlbaum (1828–1899), who is considered by some as the father of descriptive psychopathology, studied the course of illness in these patients, appropriating methods used to study medical illness. He also categorized the symptoms and derived subtypes of schizophrenia, such as catatonia and hebetic paraphrenia, later termed *hebephrenia* by his colleague Ewald Hecker (1843–1909).

These German psychiatrists were followed in time by three individuals who have had an enduring influence on the description and understanding of schizophrenia throughout the modern era. Emil Kraepelin (1856–1926) has undoubtedly exerted the single greatest influence, evident in part by the "neo-Kraepelinian" orientation of the diagnostic criteria for schizophrenia found in recent editions of DSM (Compton and Guze 1995). He aimed to classify schizophrenia on the basis of a physical etiology and in general to establish the basis for mental illness in the natural sciences. Kraepelin used experimental methods to this end, a result of his training with the experimental psychologist Wilhelm Maximilian Wundt (1832–1920). His ultimate goal was to establish a nosology that would provide direction for prognosis, treatment, and prevention of mental illness. He initially appropriated the term *dementia praecox* from Morel's and Kahlbaum's descriptions of symptom complexes and catatonia. However, Kraepelin placed increasing emphasis on considerations of etiology, clinical course, and outcome. He noted that the age at onset, family history, premorbid personality, and a deteriorating clinical course were useful in the distinction of dementia praecox from manic-depressive illness. This was regarded at the time, and remains, one of the fundamental clinical distinctions in psychiatric nosology (Angst 2002). He emphasized hereditary factors, obstetrical complications, and physical abnormalities, which remain in consideration today as evidence for genetic and neurodevelopmental factors in the illness. Kraepelin observed that clinical features of dementia praecox found in several Asian ethnic groups were similar to those found in Europeans, suggesting a cause for the illness that transcended local environmental conditions.

Kraepelin's understanding of mental illness evolved over the course of his work, which can be seen across the nine editions of his textbook. He first used the term *dementia praecox* in the fourth edition (Kraepelin 1893), and in an 1898 lecture, he indicated that clinical improvement in these patients should be considered temporary because residual symptoms were ubiquitous and relapse inevitable. Interestingly, by the eighth edition of the textbook, he had come to acknowledge that some patients experienced a relatively later onset of illness and/or a significant measure of recovery (Adityanjee et al. 1999). Among groups of symptoms, he emphasized what are now considered negative symptoms as the fundamental disturbance in schizophrenia (Andreasen 1997), presaging the renewed attention to negative symptoms and cognitive dysfunction as the strongest determinants of functional impairment, treatment resistance, and prognosis.

Eugen Bleuler (1857–1939), a Swiss psychiatrist, also has exerted great influence on modern notions of schizophrenia. He introduced the term *schizophrenia*.

He criticized the notion of dementia praecox, noting the late onset and stable course of illness seen in some patients. Nevertheless, he agreed with Kraepelin regarding the cerebral basis for the disease. Bleuler was influenced not only by Wundt but also by the emerging theories of Sigmund Freud (1856–1939) and Carl Jung (1875–1961), emphasizing the psychological aspects of the illness. He considered schizophrenia to be a heterogeneous group of disorders and noted the "weakness of the associative psychic acts" of these patients, defining the primary features of schizophrenia as the "four As": 1) looseness of associations, 2) affective flattening, 3) autism, and 4) ambivalence. This description is essentially an emphasis on cognition, apparent in the link between the term *schizophrenia* (or "split mind") and the formal thought disorder manifest in disturbed associations. Importantly, Bleuler also recognized disturbances in emotion and motivation that were largely neglected by earlier theorists. Although these were considered core clinical features, which constituted diagnostic criteria for the illness, he did not consider them to be pathognomonic. In contrast, he considered symptoms such as hallucinations, delusions, and catatonia to be "accessory" symptoms or psychological reactions to the existence of the primary symptoms.

Bleuler's dichotomy of symptoms parallels the distinction between positive and negative symptoms, which were later appropriated from John Hughlings Jackson's (1835–1911) approach to epilepsy and persisted until the recent addition of disorganized symptoms to the current, empirically derived three-category scheme. Equally important, Bleuler's emphases on illness heterogeneity and the fundamental nature of cognitive dysfunction continue to exert wide influence on how schizophrenia is studied and understood. Bleuler's diagnostic scheme was broader than that of Kraepelin, including types referred to as "latent" and "pseudoneurotic" schizophrenia, as well as the brief schizophreniform psychosis. This wider diagnostic net was endorsed in early editions of DSM, but more recent editions have returned to the narrower Kraepelinian notion of schizophrenia as an illness with early onset and deteriorating course.

The other European figure whose work helped to shape modern notions of schizophrenia is Kurt Schneider (1887–1967). He is best known for outlining a set of "first-rank" symptoms that included many of the most extreme disruptions of reality, such as thought insertion and withdrawal, thought broadcasting, hallucinated voices in argument with each other, and other more severe delusional and passivity experiences reported by patients with schizophrenia. This represented one of the first attempts at establishing a discrete criteria set for the diagnosis. Schneider is credited with a pragmatic approach to diagnosis, facilitating greater precision and reliability, emphasizing symptoms that were easier to define and evaluate in comparison to those of Bleuler. This also had the effect of narrowing the diagnosis of schizophrenia because the first-rank symptoms were clearly pathological, in comparison to some of Bleuler's symptoms, which appeared to be more continuously distributed in the general population. Nevertheless, Schneider also was greatly interested in the subjective experience of the schizophrenic patient. The first-rank symptoms were of interest to Schneider because he thought that the loss of the boundaries of the self, and of psychological autonomy, was fundamental to the illness (Andreasen 1997). These symptoms were incorporated into a range of structured diagnostic interviews that were developed through DSM-III (American Psychiatric Association 1980), including the Feighner criteria (Feighner et al. 1972) and Research Diagnostic Criteria (RDC; Endicott et al. 1978) sets (see section "Diagnosis" later in this chapter).

Clinical Features

As is the case for other complex illnesses with an undefined pathophysiology, no single clinical feature is pathognomonic for schizophrenia. Over the years, the field of schizophrenia phenomenology has emphasized one set of symptoms over others as reflecting core features of schizophrenia. However, no clear consensus has emerged regarding what constitutes this core. Instead, schizophrenia is operationally defined by a large set of signs and symptoms cutting across diverse domains of behavior and mental processes. The variability of clinical features over time for any particular patient with schizophrenia further adds to this complexity. Although active debate continues on the relative merits and validity of the various symptom classification systems that have been proposed, in this chapter we mostly rely on a scheme that segregates clinical findings into positive, negative, and disorganized symptoms (Table 10–1). This system is simple and has received empirical validation in factor analytic studies (Bilder et al. 1985; Liddle 1987). The term *positive symptom* refers to the *presence* of abnormal mental processes, whereas *negative symptom* refers to the *absence* of normal mental function. The *disorganized* category refers to the linguistic and behavioral abnormalities. In addition to the three symptom clusters, we have included two additional groups of symptoms— the cognitive deficits and soft neurological signs—in recognition of the importance of these clinical features of the illness.

TABLE 10–1. Major symptoms in schizophrenia

Positive	Hallucinations	Perception of a real sensory experience in the absence of an external source Most commonly auditory but can occur in all sensory modalities Common attributes of auditory hallucinations: External source Commentary on patient's actions or thoughts Running dialogue between two or more voices
	Delusions	Fixed false beliefs Common types: Paranoid Grandiose Somatic Ideas of reference
Negative	Affect	Diminished expression of emotions (e.g., blunted affect) Apathy or amotivation
	Social	Withdrawal Lack of interest in social contacts
	Cognitive	Alogia/poverty of speech
Disorganized	Speech	Formal thought disorder (e.g., tangentiality)
	Behavior	Purposeless movements or sequence of actions

Positive Symptoms

Three positive symptoms of schizophrenia are generally recognized: hallucinations, delusions, and disorganized speech or behavior (often referred to as *thought disorder*). The fact that the presence of certain types of hallucinations and delusions satisfies criterion A of the DSM-IV-TR (American Psychiatric Association 2000) criteria for schizophrenia (Table 10–2) reflects the relative importance placed on these two symptoms.

Hallucinations

Although hallucinations are encountered in a diverse range of conditions, they have traditionally been viewed as one of the core clinical features of schizophrenia. *Hallucinations* are defined as the perception of a real sensory process in the absence of an external source (e.g., hearing a voice when no one is talking). The perceptual qualities of hallucinations are variable. In some cases, hallucinations are perceived to be indistinguishable from real sensory experiences, whereas in other cases, they are described as only approximating real sensory experiences. It is important to keep in mind that this discussion about the perceptual aspects of hallucinations is distinct from the question of insight. With sufficient insight, a patient may realize that a hallucinatory experience is in fact not real, even if the hallucination fully replicates the sensory qualities of a true sensory experience.

Hallucinations are most frequently reported in the auditory domain. Auditory hallucinations are manifest as voices or other common sounds in the environment such as dogs barking or objects clanging. The presence of a hallucination in other sensory domains is generally more characteristic of other conditions, such as delirium in the case of visual hallucinations and seizures in the case of olfactory hallucinations. However, note that hallucinations can occur in all sensory modalities in schizophrenia, including visual, olfactory, gustatory, and tactile (Goodwin et al. 1971). Some features of auditory hallucinations, either in content or in perceptual quality, may be relatively specific to schizophrenia. For example, DSM-IV-TR specifies that an auditory hallucination, if it is of a single voice making a running commentary of the patient's thoughts or actions or two or more voices conversing with each other, is sufficient to meet criterion A (see Table 10–2). Others have proposed that auditory hallucinations that are perceived as coming from an external source, as opposed to an internal source, may be more specific to schizophrenia. However, these propositions have not been validated (Goodwin et al. 1971).

Delusions

The second core positive symptom is *delusions,* which are defined as fixed false beliefs. A belief is fixed when the individual cannot be dissuaded from believing in its veracity with contradictory evidence or arguments pointing out its implausibility. Another important feature of delusional thinking is the illogical manner in which a conviction is inferred. Delusions also may be vague or poorly formed, such as having a foreboding sense that others have ill intentions or plotting, or may be highly crystallized, such as the specific examples given later in this subsection. The content of delusions also can be quite variable and may involve almost any subject. However, in general, delusions can be grouped into the following common types on the basis of their content: paranoid or persecutory, grandiose, religious, and somatic.

Paranoid or persecutory delusions are perhaps the single most common variety. They involve the conviction that individuals, institutions, or forces are intending the patient harm. The degree of harm can be quite variable—from simply being monitored to being ostracized or singled out for poor treatment to believing that death or torture is imminent. Common examples of paranoid delusions include the conviction that the boss is intentionally targeting the patient for poor treatment, that a family member is trying to poison and kill the patient, and that the Federal Bureau of Investigation has placed the patient under surveillance with concealed listening devices and cameras.

Grandiose delusions refer to self-aggrandizing beliefs (e.g., that the patient has special powers or abilities), often but not necessarily of a bizarre or an unrealistic nature. Common examples of grandiose delusions include the belief that the patient holds a secret that is vital to national security and that the patient's special talents have led others to be jealous. Religious delusions involve religious themes or concepts such as being the son of God.

Somatic delusions refer to false beliefs about the patient's own body parts or internal organs. These delusions commonly involve the belief that a particular body part or organ is dysfunctional or causing the patient harm. Somatic delusions also can include idiosyncratic beliefs about a body part's function. These false beliefs usually involve more than just subjective perceptions (e.g., certainty that one's nose is unattractive), such as specific convictions about the body part that is part of a more elaborate delusional system. Somatic delusions sometimes can tragically lead patients to commit grotesque self-injurious acts on the involved body part.

TABLE 10-2. DSM-IV-TR diagnostic criteria for schizophrenia

A. *Characteristic symptoms:* Two (or more) of the following, each present for a significant portion of time during a 1-month period (or less if successfully treated):

    (1) delusions

    (2) hallucinations

    (3) disorganized speech (e.g., frequent derailment or incoherence)

    (4) grossly disorganized or catatonic behavior

    (5) negative symptoms, i.e., affective flattening, alogia, or avolition

    Note: Only one criterion A symptom is required if delusions are bizarre or hallucinations consist of a voice keeping up a running commentary on the person's behavior or thoughts, or two or more voices conversing with each other.

B. *Social/occupational dysfunction:* For a significant portion of the time since the onset of the disturbance, one or more major areas of functioning such as work, interpersonal relations, or self-care are markedly below the level achieved prior to the onset (or when the onset is in childhood or adolescence, failure to achieve expected level of interpersonal, academic, or occupational achievement).

C. *Duration:* Continuous signs of the disturbance persist for at least 6 months. This 6-month period must include at least 1 month of symptoms (or less if successfully treated) that meet criterion A (i.e., active-phase symptoms) and may include periods of prodromal or residual symptoms. During these prodromal or residual periods, the signs of the disturbance may be manifested by only negative symptoms or two or more symptoms listed in criterion A present in an attenuated form (e.g., odd beliefs, unusual perceptual experiences).

D. *Schizoaffective and mood disorder exclusion:* Schizoaffective disorder and mood disorder with psychotic features have been ruled out because either (1) no major depressive, manic, or mixed episodes have occurred concurrently with the active-phase symptoms; or (2) if mood episodes have occurred during active-phase symptoms, their total duration has been brief relative to the duration of the active and residual periods.

E. *Substance/general medical condition exclusion:* The disturbance is not due to the direct physiological effects of a substance (e.g., a drug of abuse, a medication) or a general medical condition.

F. *Relationship to a pervasive developmental disorder:* If there is a history of autistic disorder or another pervasive developmental disorder, the additional diagnosis of schizophrenia is made only if prominent delusions or hallucinations are also present for at least 1 month (or less if successfully treated).

Classification of longitudinal course (can be applied only after at least 1 year has elapsed since the initial onset of active-phase symptoms):

    Episodic with interepisode residual symptoms (episodes are defined by the reemergence of prominent psychotic symptoms); *also specify if:* **With prominent negative symptoms**

    Episodic with no interepisode residual symptoms

    Continuous (prominent psychotic symptoms are present throughout the period of observation); *also specify if:* **With prominent negative symptoms**

    Single episode in partial remission; *also specify if:* **With prominent negative symptoms**

    Single episode in full remission

    Other or unspecified pattern

Note that the content of delusions often involves more than one type (e.g., belief of being the second coming of the messiah and consequently being persecuted by others). Therapists also may see a broad range in the bizarreness or plausibility of the scenario or content that forms the basis of these beliefs. A common example of a nonbizarre delusion is the conviction that an individual known to the patient is targeting the patient for harm or mistreatment, in the absence of objective evidence supporting this belief, and which may persist even when the patient is confronted with the patent illogicality of his or her inferences. An example of a bizarre delusion may be the belief that a microcomputer chip has been implanted by the police to monitor the patient's thoughts. The DSM-IV-TR criteria (see Table 10–2) specify that a delusion is sufficient to meet criterion A if it is bizarre.

A special class of delusions, ideas of reference, deserves special attention because of its high prevalence and historical importance. Patients with ideas of reference misperceive communications from other persons or entities to be referring to them. Classic examples of this class of delusions include the belief that statements on television or passages in newspaper articles are actually coded messages directed at the patient. More subtle examples include believing that a person on a cellular telephone is talking about the patient. Ideas of reference are an important class of symptoms because they were part of what Schneider referred to as "first-rank symptoms." Other examples of first-rank symptoms include delusions of thought insertion, thought broadcasting, thought withdrawal, and external control of affect and motor acts. As noted earlier, the first-rank symptoms were at one time thought to be specific to schizophrenia. However, subsequent research has not supported this hypothesis.

The cultural context of these expressions is extremely important to the determination of whether they qualify as delusional. Even seemingly bizarre beliefs to an outsider should not be considered a delusion if that belief is commonly shared among the wider community. An example is the widespread acceptance in certain evangelical Christian communities in the possibility of being overtaken by the Holy Spirit and "speaking in tongues" or the belief in ghosts that is common in many cultures.

Negative Symptoms

The negative symptoms of schizophrenia refer to clinical features putatively resulting from the absence of normal mental functions. These include deficits in affective, social, and cognitive realms. Although the positive symptoms have traditionally garnered more attention in the clinical assessment and treatment of schizophrenia, negative symptoms have been long recognized as a core feature of this disorder. Through the work of modern leaders such as William Carpenter, Nancy Andreasen, and Timothy Crow, the field of psychiatry has been steadily rediscovering the importance of negative symptoms in recent years. Once an

acute psychotic state is stabilized with treatment, the negative symptoms may be a stronger indicator of long-term disability. A further indication of their importance is the current absence of clearly effective treatments for these symptoms.

Case 1

Mr. A, a 25-year-old man, has had schizophrenia for 5 years. After leaving the military, he returned to his hometown but was never able to establish a stable life. He was unable to hold down a job and made little effort to maintain relationships with his friends or family. He became homeless and was living in a park when a family acquaintance recognized him and reunited him with his parents. The parents allowed Mr. A to live in their home, but his lack of motivation and absence of structured activity have become points of contention. His parents report that on a typical day, Mr. A does little. He sits around the house, at times watching television, or steps out to smoke a cigarette. He does take short walks in the neighborhood, but he prefers to spend his time by himself. He has difficulty keeping his room clean and orderly. Mr. A requires frequent admonishment from his parents to shower.

During a typical session, Mr. A sits almost motionless, making little eye contact with the doctor. He appears indifferent to the interview and is difficult to engage in a conversation. His grooming is substandard, with noticeable body odor, dirty fingernails, and slightly tattered clothing. His affect is blunted, and he shows no noticeable reactions. His speech is monotonal, and output is notable for poverty of thought (e.g., responds to questions with mostly "yes" or "no" and does not provide any elaborations). He denies experiencing any and all symptoms of psychosis, even though the parents have noted Mr. A talking to himself and responding to internal stimuli.

Affective Deficits

One of the most apparent clinical manifestations of negative symptoms in patients with schizophrenia is the disturbance of normal affective processes. *Blunting of affect* is a term describing the decrease in the amount and range of affective expressivity. This term usually refers to facial expressions in which the normal expressions associated with emotional states are diminished or absent. Other related descriptors are flat and constricted affect, which are defined, respectively, as a total absence of, and a moderate decrease in, affective expressivity. It was once thought that these deficits reflected a fundamental abnormality in the experiencing of emotions, particularly positive emotions or anhedonia. However, recent research has raised significant questions about the validity of this claim. These studies have reported that patients may experience equivalent levels of pleasure. In contrast, some research points to the possibility that patients with a predominance of paranoid delusions may have heightened sensitivity to negative or threatening situations.

Another common affective deficit is apathy, or apparent indifference of the patient to the consequences of his or her own or others' actions and decisions. This can manifest as lack of motivation to initiate or maintain activity. For example, patients with apathy spend an inordinate amount of time at home alone, unable to initiate and engage in a planned activity. Another common manifestation of this deficit may be evident in the patient's lack of interest in events around him or her, such as the clinical interview.

Social Deficits

Deficits in the domain of social functioning are increasingly recognized as important aspects of schizophrenia. Social withdrawal describes the common situation in which the patient has little interest in participating in social events and interacting with people. Patients often describe not needing to spend much time with other people and preferring to be by themselves. They appear to have decreased social drive in that they do not derive pleasure from social interactions that most people experience.

Cognitive Deficits

A more thorough discussion on the many cognitive deficits is presented in the "Cognitive Impairment" section later in this chapter, but here we briefly describe the cognitive features that are often grouped under negative symptoms. Alogia or poverty of speech describes the significant decrease in the amount of unprompted speech given by a patient. Patients with poverty of speech give very short and unelaborated responses to questions. The interviewer often finds himself or herself having to guide the patient with numerous explicit questions to obtain responses with sufficient detail.

Disorganization

The third symptom cluster is disorganization in language or other behavior. The phrase *formal thought disorder* has been defined in a variety of ways, but here we use a more restricted definition of this term, as in the disorganization of the form or flow of thoughts as evident in language output. Various terms can be used in the psychiatric mental status examination to describe formal thought disorder, including (in the order of increasing severity) circumstantiality, derailment, tangentiality, and word salad.

These terms attempt to capture the disruption of the normal processes governing the logical, syntactic, or semantic ordering or association of words and ideas. *Circumstantiality* refers to the preservation of a logical link between each consecutive sentence concomitant with a progressive drifting of ideas away from the original topic. *Derailment* describes a process in which a patient's response is initially topical and logical but then becomes not obviously related. *Tangentiality* refers to the immediate loss of connection between the patient's response and the initial question. Finally, *word salad* describes the highly remarkable phenomenon characterized by a complete absence of a logical link between adjacent words in an utterance. Other common manifestations of formal thought disorder are distractibility (being easily distracted from a conversation by nonrelevant sounds or events), echolalia (repeating verbatim words or statements directed at the patient), clang associations (stringing together words based on phonetic similarities; e.g., fair, share, tear, hair), perseverations (repeating words or phrases), blocking (unable to complete sentences because of apparent internal preoccupation, distraction, or inability to generate words), and neologisms (creation of new words).

Disorganization also can refer to nonlinguistic behaviors such as disordered sequence of or bizarre actions lacking apparent purpose. For example, a patient may approach another person as if to engage in a conversation, but then, without apparent reason or provocation, the patient pulls his sweater over his own head.

Cognitive Impairment

An important recent development has been the rediscovery of the importance of the cognitive deficits in schizophrenia. The earlier schizophrenia phenomenologists such as Kraepelin and Bleuler emphasized cognitive impairments as a key clinical aspect of this illness. In the "Introduction to Etiology and Pathophysiology" section later in this chapter, we focus on the relevance of cognitive deficits to our understanding of the underlying neural dysfunction of schizophrenia. Here, we discuss the clinically relevant aspects of these cognitive deficits.

As a group, patients with schizophrenia show a range of impaired higher cognitive functions, including problems with attention, long-term memory, working memory, abstraction and planning, and language comprehension and production. These cognitive deficits present significant barriers to maintaining occupational and everyday function. Research has shown that cognitive deficits may be the best predictor of functionality over and above other symptom clusters (M.F. Green 1996).

One of the most clinically apparent cognitive deficits is in the domain of attention. In addition to the internal preoccupation and preoccupation associated with hallucinatory and delusional experiences, an individual with schizophrenia experiences difficulty maintaining focused attention on relevant tasks or events. Attentional problems also may manifest in patients as an inability to shift their focus of attention in an appropriate manner, expressed clinically as perseveration.

Working memory, the ability to store and manage information temporarily to rapidly guide thoughts and behavior, has been proposed as a fundamental cognitive deficit in schizophrenia. These theories suggest that many of the clinical features of schizophrenia are manifestations of working memory deficits. For example, thought disorder can be conceived as the inability to maintain a linguistic goal in mind. Problems with multitasking, distractibility, and planning also may involve working memory problems.

Long-term declarative memory deficits have been noted to be an important source of disability in schizophrenia. Although memory problems may not be progressive or as profound as in Alzheimer's dementia, they are nonetheless readily apparent. Common and clinically relevant manifestations of this impairment include forgotten appointments or medication directions, which may directly affect the treatment and stability of the patient.

Soft Neurological Signs

Interestingly, before the age of pharmacological treatments, early schizophrenia researchers noted a heightened prevalence of neurological abnormalities, particularly movement disturbances, in individuals who later developed schizophrenia. Kraepelin described the high prevalence of dyskinesias in the early 1900s. A review of more than 600 case records dating from Victorian England identified the presence of movement disorder in about one-third of the patients with schizophrenia (Turner 1989). In modern research, substantial and growing evidence now indicates a higher prevalence of subtle neurological deficits—most notably, the so-called soft neurological signs (e.g., motor dyscoordination)—in schizophrenia patients (Bombin et al. 2005) (Table 10–3). In one of the most interesting studies to be conducted in this area, close analysis of childhood home videos of patients who later developed schizophrenia found that these "preschizophrenic" subjects had higher rates of motor distur-

bances than did control subjects (Walker et al. 1994). Studies have documented that schizophrenic patients show more neurological soft signs (broadly defined) than do healthy control subjects and that this heightened prevalence cannot be accounted for by medication effects or demographic variables. Positive correlations with clinical indices such as negative—but not positive—symptoms and cognitive deficits have been reported.

Subtypes of Schizophrenia

Over the years, there has been increasing recognition that schizophrenia may constitute a heterogeneous collection of different conditions. This presents a significant challenge not only to our research efforts that seek to uncover the etiology of schizophrenia but also to our efforts to provide targeted and specific treatments. To remedy this situation, several schizophrenia subtype classification schemes have been proposed over the years. All of these are based on the assumptions that 1) clinically evident symptoms reflect underlying brain dysfunction and 2) grouping patients according to shared clinical characteristics will provide more homogeneous groups in terms of identifying underlying pathophysiology and predicting the course of treatment.

Some of the more prominent classification systems share an emphasis on grouping symptoms according to the presence of positive and negative symptoms. One such scheme was exemplified by Crow's proposal, which categorized symptoms into a type I or type II syndrome, approximately equivalent to the positive and negative symptoms, respectively (Crow 1985). Kirkpatrick et al. (2001) proposed a similar binary system, but the emphasis in their system was on identifying patients with what they referred to as the *deficit syndrome*. They proposed that the deficit syndrome represents a distinct and separate disease within the schizophrenia syndrome. The diagnosis was based on the presence of prominent, primary, and enduring negative symptoms. They referred to the remaining patients as non–deficit syndrome patients. Kirkpatrick and colleagues found that the deficit and nondeficit patients could be distinguished on the basis of clinical symptomatology, neurobiological markers of illness, and epidemiological risk factors. For example, they have shown that in comparison with nondeficit patients, deficit patients have worse premorbid functioning, worse course of illness, greater anhedonia, less depression and suicidal ideation, greater likelihood of relatives having schizophrenia, separate

TABLE 10–3.   Soft neurological signs most frequently assessed in schizophrenic patients

Cluster of denomination	Putative neuroanatomic localization	Individual signs assessed
Integrative sensory function	Parietal lobe	Bilateral extinction Audiovisual integration Graphesthesia Right–left confusion Extinction
Motor coordination	Frontal lobe; cerebellum	Intention tremor Balance Gait Hopping Finger–thumb opposition Dysdiadochokinesia Finger-to-nose test
Sequencing of complex motor acts	Prefrontal lobe	Fist-edge-palm test Fist-ring test Oseretsky test Go/no-go test Rhythm tapping (foot or hand)
Primitive reflexes	Frontal lobe	Glabellar tap Jaw jerk Palmomental Corneomandibular Pout/snout Sucking/oral Grasp Forced groping

Source.   Reprinted from Bombin I, Arango C, Buchanan RW: "Significance and Meaning of Neurological Signs in Schizophrenia: Two Decades Later." *Schizophrenia Bulletin* 31:962–977, 2005 (Table 1 [p. 963]). Copyright 2005, Oxford University Press. Used with permission.

season-of-birth effects, and greater impairment in higher-order cognition.

The DSM-IV-TR system is the most frequently used subtype classification system in clinical practice. Empirical research has shown substantial instability over time in diagnostic subtypes, and significant overlap between subtype symptoms, indicating that the validity of this scheme remains to be determined. Nevertheless, it is still worthwhile to familiarize oneself with them, given the advantages of shared terminology conferred by the use of terms with near-universal recognition in psychiatry. DSM-IV-TR recognizes five subtypes of schizophrenia: paranoid, disorganized, catatonic, undifferentiated, and residual (Table 10–4).

Paranoid Schizophrenia

The hallmark of paranoid schizophrenia is the relative prominence of paranoid delusions and auditory hallucinations compared with the other symptoms of schizophrenia. Most important is that the presence of disorganized behavior or speech, catatonia, or flat or inappropriate affect precludes this diagnosis. This subtype has received perhaps the most validation in research, which has suggested that these patients have better premorbid functioning, an older age at onset, higher social and occupational functioning after illness onset, and fewer cognitive and affective deficits.

Case 2

Mr. B, a 32-year-old single man, self-presented to the psychiatric clinic with the chief complaint of concerns that coworkers and others were talking about him and possibly intending to harm him. Since graduating from high school, he has had difficulty maintaining long-term employment because of recurring persecutory fears about his coworkers. On a few occasions, his beliefs resulted in verbal confrontations at work and Mr. B's dismissal from his job.

He presented to the clinic at the urging of his family members. On presentation, he was well groomed and did not show any odd or bizarre behavior. Throughout the interview, Mr. B was irritable and guarded. He had no signs of cognitive impairment, with linear thought process and good abstraction. Mr. B admitted that, on occasion, he had been hearing a voice commenting on his ongoing problems with his coworkers, but he did not want to disclose details about this. When directly questioned about his paranoia, Mr. B firmly held to the veracity of his beliefs that he had been singled out for poor treatment by others.

Toward the end of the interview, we discussed treatment options, including a trial of neuroleptics. Mr. B expressed significant reservations about taking medications and insinuated that the doctor was trying to control his mind. By the end of the session, Mr. B did not consent to medication, but he did agree to a follow-up session. However, he did not show up for this or other sessions.

Disorganized Schizophrenia

As the name implies, the disorganized subtype emphasizes the presence of clinical features related to disorganization. According to DSM-IV-TR, all of the following must be prominent to diagnose this subtype: disorganized speech, disorganized behavior, and flat or inappropriate affect. Additionally, diagnostic criteria for catatonic schizophrenia should not be met. This subtype is thought to represent a more severe form of schizophrenia, with earlier onset, low levels of social and occupational functioning, and poor long-term prognosis. The presence of delusions or hallucinations does not exclude the diagnosis of this subtype, but these symptoms play a less prominent role in psychopathology. The older term *hebephrenic schizophrenia* is synonymous with the disorganized subtype.

Case 3

Mr. C, a 53-year-old homeless man, was well known to the emergency department of a community hospital because he was frequently brought there by the police for a psychiatric evaluation. This time, he was brought to the emergency department after he frightened pedestrians and shopkeepers with his agitated behavior and had a verbal confrontation with the police. The consulting psychiatrist was unable to get a coherent history or chief complaint from Mr. C because of the patient's prominent thought disorder, which is characterized by severe tangentiality and neologism. Throughout the interview, Mr. C incessantly made odd, nonsensical gestures with his hands and arms. Periodically, Mr. C would break from the interview to walk away and stare into space or talk with an imaginary person. Mr. C appeared internally preoccupied.

TABLE 10–4. DSM-IV-TR subtypes of schizophrenia

Paranoid	Prominent hallucinations and delusions Absence of prominent disorganization, flat or inappropriate affect, or catatonia

Disorganized	All of the following:
	    disorganized speech
	    disorganized behavior
	    flat or inappropriate affect
	Diagnostic criteria for catatonic schizophrenia should not be met

Catatonic	Catatonia is the most prominent clinical feature
	At least two of the following:
	    immobility (cataplexy or stupor)
	    motor hyperactivity without purpose or external influence
	    extreme negativism or mutism
	    peculiar voluntary movement or postures
	    stereotyped movements or prominent mannerisms or grimacing
	    echophenomena (echolalia or echopraxia)

Undifferentiated	Criterion A for schizophrenia Diagnostic criteria for the paranoid, disorganized, or catatonic subtypes are not met
Residual	Persistence of negative symptoms or two or more criterion A symptoms in attenuated form Absence of prominent delusions, hallucinations, disorganized speech, and grossly disorganized or catatonic behavior

Catatonic Schizophrenia

Catatonia is a poorly understood clinical syndrome. The term *catatonia* refers to extreme motor states of either stupor or overexcitement that can occur independently of schizophrenia. In catatonic stupor, the patient maintains one body position for a very long time without talking or reacting to others. In this state, some patients may have waxy flexibility, in which a limb or body part is maintained in a posture that is passively positioned by another individual. In catatonic excitement, the patient engages in a series of apparently aimless and exaggerated rapid movements, which also may include acts of minimally directed violent behavior. Note that many clinicians have recognized a significant decrease in the prevalence of catatonic states in recent years such that it is now relatively rare to find classic cases of catatonia. The reason for this decline is unclear. The diagnosis of catatonic schizophrenia is made when catatonia is the most prominent clinical feature and requires the presence of at least two of the following: immobility (cataplexy or stupor); motor hyperactivity without purpose or external influence; extreme negativism or mutism; peculiar voluntary movement or postures, stereotyped movements, or prominent mannerisms or grimacing; and echophenomena (echolalia or echopraxia).

Undifferentiated Schizophrenia

Undifferentiated schizophrenia encompasses cases in which no one cluster of symptoms constituting the paranoid, disorganized, or catatonic subtypes predominates the clinical picture. Consequently, the diagnosis of undifferentiated schizophrenia is made when criterion A for schizophrenia is met (see Table 10–2), and the diagnostic criteria for the paranoid, disorganized, or catatonic subtypes are not met. This is the most frequently encountered subtype in clinical practice.

Residual Schizophrenia

The residual subtype is thought to represent a relatively attenuated state of schizophrenia in which the positive symptoms are relatively quiescent or less symptomatic. Like undifferentiated schizophrenia, this is a subtype diagnosis made by exclusion. The diagnosis is made when negative symptoms persist or two or more symptoms listed in DSM-IV-TR criterion A for schizophrenia (see Table 10–2) are present in an attenuated form, and prominent delusions, hallucinations, disorganized speech, and grossly disorganized or catatonic behavior are absent. Many patients achieve this relatively remitted clinical subtype after sustained effective treatment.

Diagnosis

The contemporary nosology of schizophrenia has been strongly influenced by Kraepelin but reflects emphases of Bleuler and Schneider as well. The origin of this period can be traced to the 1970s with the establishment of two sets of formal criteria for the diagnosis of schizophrenia. The so-called Feighner criteria (Feighner et al. 1972) developed in St. Louis, Missouri, included both cross-sectional and longitudinal criteria, designed primarily to identify individuals with a relatively poor prognosis, reflecting a strong Kraepelinian influence. These investigators limited the maximal age at onset to 40 years and the minimal duration of symptoms to 6 months. This eliminated acute psychosis as a subtype of schizophrenia; affective and substance-related cases also were excluded in this diagnostic scheme. A second diagnostic scheme was developed in New York and referred to as RDC (Endicott et al. 1978). The RDC also excluded persons with major affective disorders and borderline syndromes. The major difference was that the RDC required only 2 weeks' duration for symptoms to meet the criteria for schizophrenia, thus retaining more acute forms of psychotic illness.

These two sets of criteria were very influential in the development of DSM-III and DSM-III-R (American Psychiatric Association 1987), in which both cross-sectional and longitudinal criteria were included. This considerably narrowed the range of pathologies found to meet the diagnosis of schizophrenia, and, in particular, the subtypes referred to as acute, simple, and latent were no longer found in the diagnostic scheme. This constituted a full embrace of Kraepelin's notion of schizophrenia as an illness with a chronic course and clinical deterioration. Another important aspect of the DSM-III changes was the removal of implications about etiology, not only for schizophrenia but also for all diagnoses contained in the manual. Subsequently, all DSM editions have maintained this neutrality with regard to etiology, with an emphasis on descriptive psychopathology instead. This has generally been viewed as advantageous to empirical research by removing presumptions about the source of, or causal factors operating on, the observed phenomenology (or "phenotype," in genetic parlance).

In DSM-IV-TR, the diagnostic manual currently in use in the United States, the emphasis on both cross-sectional and longitudinal criteria continues (see Table 10–2), with a 6-month minimum duration. However, clinical courses that are episodic in manner, including single-episode cases that are followed by full remission, are now recognized. The age criterion has been eliminated. The positive symptom criteria reflect the influence of Schneider's first-rank symptoms as exemplars. The negative and disorganized symptom criteria reflect a renewed prominence given to features originally emphasized by Bleuler. The DSM-IV-TR criteria identify an individual as having schizophrenia if he or she experiences characteristic positive, negative, and/or disorganized symptoms for a significant portion of time during at least 1 month, unless the symptoms are successfully treated; these criterion A symptoms are referred to as *active-phase symptoms*. The patient must have impairment in psychosocial function (work, interpersonal relationships, or self-care). Continuous signs of disturbance must be evident for at least 6 months; this must include at least 1 month of active-phase symptoms but may include periods of prodromal or residual symptoms, which appear as attenuated criterion A symptoms. Major mood disorders (e.g., major depression, bipolar disorder type I), schizoaffective disorder, and substance-related or medical etiologies of the symptoms are to be excluded, and if a pervasive developmental disorder (e.g., autism) is also found, the schizophrenia diagnosis is made only if prominent delusions or hallucinations are also present for at least 1 month. The longitudinal course is classified as episodic, continuous, or single episode, with remission, residual symptoms, and prominent negative symptoms further specified. In addition, subtypes are specified as outlined in the "Subtypes of Schizophrenia" section earlier in this chapter.

It is important to recognize that the development of operationalized diagnostic criteria for the diagnosis of schizophrenia (or any other psychiatric illness, for that matter) has led to a crucial enhancement in the reliability of diagnosis among individual clinicians and across both local and global sites where these patients can be found. Research into the illness has been furthered by the widespread use of a single straightforward and reasonably objective criteria set. However, these criteria sets (those in DSM in particular) were originally designed as a "provisional consensus agreement" among a select group of experts in the field. They were not intended to represent exhaustive sets of clinical features that fully described the illness or accounted for important individual variation that has consequences for treatment or prognosis. Clinicians therefore should not limit their knowledge of what constitutes the illness, much less how to understand the individual patient, to a brief set of diagnostic criteria (Andreasen 1997). In addition, recent diagnostic criteria sets (e.g., DSM-IV-TR) have not attained significant validity by identification of biological substrates of either individual criteria or the set as a whole. This suggests that although most clinicians are likely to agree on whether an individual patient is indeed experiencing a particular illness, advances in elucidating the etiology of the illness (and future treatment targets) must await more refined characterization of the expression of the illness in measures of clinical, behavioral, cognitive, or biological functions (Andreasen 2000). This forms the basis for the recent focus on endophenotypes.

Differential Diagnosis

The diagnosis of schizophrenia continues to rest solely on the history of illness and a thorough mental status examination (Table 10–5). No reliable laboratory tests have yet been established for this illness, but this remains an attainable goal in light of the consistent alterations shown by schizophrenic patients on biochemical, cognitive, and neuroanatomic measures. Along with the history taking and mental status examination, a full physical examination usually should be performed, particularly for new-onset cases, because medical causes of psychotic illness are varied. This list includes intracranial processes such as infections and neoplastic, epileptic, and hypoxic or ischemic disorders; metabolic disorders; and endocrine disorders. The dementias, such as Alzheimer's disease, frontotemporal dementia, Parkinson's disease, Pick's disease, and Huntington's disease, are often associated with psychotic features. Illicit substance use is also quite common in the community and can frequently lead to psychotic symptoms, not only with acute intoxication but also in an intermittent or even a persistent manner with chronic use, particularly with stimulant drugs. Many commonly prescribed medications can also cause psychosis, particularly those with direct effects on the brain, such as steroids, anticholinergics, and medications prescribed for Parkinson's disease. Those cases that present with atypical clinical features, such as late age at onset, clouding of the sensorium (i.e., confusional states), or findings on history or physical examination suggestive of concurrent medical problems should prompt the clinician to pursue alternative causes of illness. Routine laboratory tests that may aid the clinician in ruling out these etiologies include a complete blood count, renal and metabolic panels, liver enzymes, thyroid function, urinalysis, and serological tests for syphilis and HIV. Brain imaging such as magnetic resonance imaging (MRI) or computed tomography (CT) and electroencephalography may be indicated in atypical cases or when the history suggests the need to rule out intracranial pathology unrelated to psychiatric illness.

TABLE 10–5. Differential diagnosis of schizophrenia

Other disorders	Common clinical features	Distinctions from schizophrenia
Axis I diagnoses		
Schizoaffective disorder	Criterion A for schizophrenia, plus at least one lifetime major mood episode (unipolar and bipolar types)	On average, higher function but higher suicide risk; history of major mood episode not found in schizophrenia
Mood disorders with psychosis	Multiple symptoms of mood changes, vegetative symptoms, mood-congruent ideation, and other cognitive changes, with acute or subacute onset and often in response to psychosocial stressors	Mood symptoms are more enduring; more complete interepisodic recovery; psychosis only with severe mood episodes; fuller response to psychotherapy
Delusional disorder	Prominent delusions, with other cognitions and behavior organized around delusion but no other significant psychosis	Psychosis confined to one or more delusions, usually nonbizarre; function largely intact; minimal decline in function or change in symptoms over time; more refractory to treatment
Schizophreniform disorder	Duration of criterion A met for more than 1 month but less than 6 months	Shorter duration than schizophrenia; many ultimately receive schizophrenia diagnosis
Brief psychotic disorder	Psychosis with abrupt onset and duration less than 1 month; often in response to acute stressor	No prodrome; cognition generally intact; better prognosis
Drug-related psychosis	Significant history of drug use, with abuse and often dependence criteria met; associated cyclic impulsivity and interpersonal, occupational, and legal history	Psychosis typically during active periods of drug use, particularly psychostimulants; more complete recovery with sustained abstinence; characteristic medical comorbidity with chronic abuse
Axis II (personality) disorders		
Cluster A: schizotypal, paranoid, schizoid personality disorders	Subpsychotic (positive and/or negative) symptoms with mild to moderate cognitive and social impairment	Less functional decline than schizophrenia; cognition more intact, and rare impulsivity or need for hospitalization
Cluster B: borderline personality disorder	Instability in mood, impulse control, and interpersonal relationships	Less functional decline than schizophrenia; symptoms more sensitive to interpersonal factors; more unstable over time; psychosis only with significant stress
Axis III (medical) disorders		
Dementias (cortical and subcortical)	Slow onset in middle to late adulthood, with progressive cognitive decline; some with prominent motor symptoms	Later onset; cognitive deficits more prominent compared with other symptoms; psychosis primarily in late stages

TABLE 10–5. **Differential diagnosis of schizophrenia** *(continued)*

Other disorders	Common clinical features	Distinctions from schizophrenia
Axis III (medical) disorders *(continued)*		
Acute confusional states (delirium; varied etiologies)	Abrupt onset with risk factors for neurological illness; clouded sensorium; transient psychosis can be in various sensory modes	Premorbid function intact; acute onset; psychotic symptoms less formed; full recovery possible with medical treatment
Iatrogenic psychosis (e.g., steroids, antibiotics, anticholinergics, antiparkinsonian medications)	Acute onset; transient psychosis can be in various sensory modes	Stable premorbid function; acute onset; psychotic symptoms less formed; associated somatic effects of medications; full recovery possible with medical treatment

Although care should be taken to rule out medical causes of psychosis confidently, the major task in differential diagnosis will require distinction of schizophrenia from a range of other psychiatric disorders that also may involve psychotic symptoms. These include schizoaffective disorder; major mood disorders that can present with psychotic features, such as major depression and acute mania among bipolar affective disorder type I patients; delusional disorder; and personality disorders, particularly those in the A or B clusters. To rule out the major mood disorders or schizoaffective disorder, the active phase of psychosis should occur in the absence of an acute mood disorder episode, or alternatively, the mood episodes should be relatively brief in relation to the total duration of the psychotic episode. Most mood disorder patients also maintain or recover significant levels of psychosocial function in between episodes of illness because they do not experience continuous psychotic symptoms or persistently severe mood disturbance. Delusional disorder is distinguished by the lack of other psychotic symptoms, and the content of delusions tend not to be the bizarre thoughts or beliefs often observed in schizophrenia, such as beliefs that monitoring devices are implanted in the patient's body or that the patient is communicating with other species. These individuals also tend to maintain a higher level of function because they largely experience only the circumscribed delusions that meet the criteria for the disorder. Schizophreniform disorder and brief psychotic disorder are also characterized by overt psychotic symptoms. In some cases, a clinician may encounter the patient relatively early in the active psychotic phase of illness, and as a result, one of these diagnoses (both with a briefer duration criterion than that for schizophrenia) is most appropriate to assign initially. However, if psychotic symptoms persist beyond 6 months, then the diagnosis of schizophrenia is most appropriate. It remains to be determined what percentage of individuals with schizophreniform disorder represent patients early in the course of schizophrenia (see section "Related Psychotic Disorders" later in this chapter for discussion of schizoaffective disorder, delusional disorder, schizophreniform disorder, and brief psychotic disorder).

Cluster A ("odd") personality disorders (schizoid, schizotypal, and paranoid) are often referred to as *schizophrenia spectrum disorders* and may be characterized by subthreshold or attenuated psychotic symptoms related to those of schizophrenia. Patients with these personality disorders may show symptoms of social withdrawal, anhedonia, and flat affect quite similar to, but more mild than, the negative symptoms of schizophrenia. However, overt psychotic symptoms are rare (and transient) in these individuals, and their level of function is typically higher, with gainful employment and independent living being the norm. Borderline personality disorder may present with acute, overt psychotic symptoms; however, in this personality disorder, in contrast to schizophrenia, interpersonal stressors are common precipitants of acute psychosis, emotional dysregulation (with lability, multiple negative mood states, and overt antagonism) is nearly ubiquitous, and behavioral impulsivity is present, often including dangerous or hazardous acts such as self-injury and aggressive behavior. Other disorders such as depersonalization disorder, panic disorder, and obsessive-compulsive disorder may present with feelings of unreality or bizarre behavior; however, in each of these disorders, reality testing and social function are preserved, and overt delusions or hallucinations are rare. Finally, factitious disorder and malingering can be found in many clinical settings; the degree to which the clinical picture diverges from well-established profiles found in schizophrenia, along with the identification of secondary gains (e.g., material reward or avoidance of incarceration) attainable as a result of a psychiatric diagnosis or treatment, may call attention to the possibility of these last diagnoses.

Clinical Course

Premorbid Functioning

Any description of the clinical course of schizophrenia should address periods of development occurring well before the onset of overt psychotic symptoms, especially given the neurodevelopmental perspective on this illness (Figure 10–1). Good evidence indicates that in groups of individuals who will later develop schizophrenia, some signs are present long before onset of psychosis, as early as childhood. These signs tend to be subtle and do not warrant a diagnosis of any particular psychiatric disorder.

Nevertheless, retrospective review of clinical and school records and even home film recordings of children who later develop schizophrenia show multiple deficits (Walker et al. 2004). For instance, these children perform lower than their siblings and classmates who do not develop schizophrenia on tests of intelligence and achievement and have poorer grades in school (Jones et al. 1994). This deficit worsens in adolescence as test scores decline further between ages 13 and 16 years. In addition, children who go on to develop schizophrenia have disturbances in social behavior. They are less socially responsive, express less positively valenced emotion, and have poorer social adjustment than do children who maintain health into adulthood. Some of these deficits may be apparent as early as the first year of life. These children also have observable motor deficits, with an increased rate of delayed or abnormal motor development, which includes the attainment of walking. The motor dysfunction of childhood persists throughout the preillness period and into the clinical phase of overt illness. These children typically do not have a diagnosable mental disorder during childhood, even though childhood-onset schizophrenia does exist (Remschmidt 2002).

Prodrome to Schizophrenia

During adolescence, however, those who later develop schizophrenia often begin to undergo changes that are discernible to others, with the onset of significant behavioral and other overt psychiatric symptoms. These include symptoms of depression, social with-drawal, irritability, and antagonistic thoughts and behavior. In this period, these adolescents often come to the attention of school and community clinicians for conduct problems and academic decline. These symptoms are highly nonspecific because they are also characteristic of early symptoms of mood, anxiety, substance use, and personality disorders, all of which can have their onset during this same period. Nevertheless, these symptoms may be retrospectively identified as heralding the onset of the so-called prodrome of schizophrenia, a period of variable duration (usually lasting from several months to a few years) that precedes the onset of schizophrenia in most cases (Phillips et al. 2005). Several clinical signs that can be observed during this period have a high positive predictive value for the later onset of schizophrenia. These largely include subtle attenuated psychotic symptoms that differ from overt psychotic symptoms in frequency or severity. These symptoms may include suspiciousness or perceptual distortions that do not qualify as overtly psychotic. Reality testing is often intact at this stage because many individuals will doubt the veracity of these experiences. Many of these individuals, in adolescence or early adulthood, will at this clinical stage qualify for the diagnosis of schizotypal personality disorder. This schizophrenia spectrum disorder is characterized by symptoms that can be considered either attenuated positive-like or negative-like symptoms, found as a persistent and pervasive pattern in the clinical context of social and interpersonal deficits, and often with clinically significant levels of subjective distress.

Research into the phenomenology and course of individuals in the schizophrenia prodrome is an area of rapidly intensifying interest, given the importance of early and reliable identification of those who will develop schizophrenia. One issue in this work is how to make a positive identification of experiences as pathological within this range of experience because it has been found that "psychotic-like" experiences can be commonly found in the general population at rates that are much higher than the rate of overt psychotic symptoms (Peters et al. 1999). This suggests that for some individuals, these symptoms must resolve without leading to overt psychotic symptoms. A second issue in this research is how to draw the boundary most appropriately between these symptoms and those of full-blown psychosis. Informal criteria for identifying an experience as psychotic usually include the deviant nature of the experience, with a frank break in reality in the perceptual or cognitive/ideational realm; the veracity of this experience is rigidly held, with little

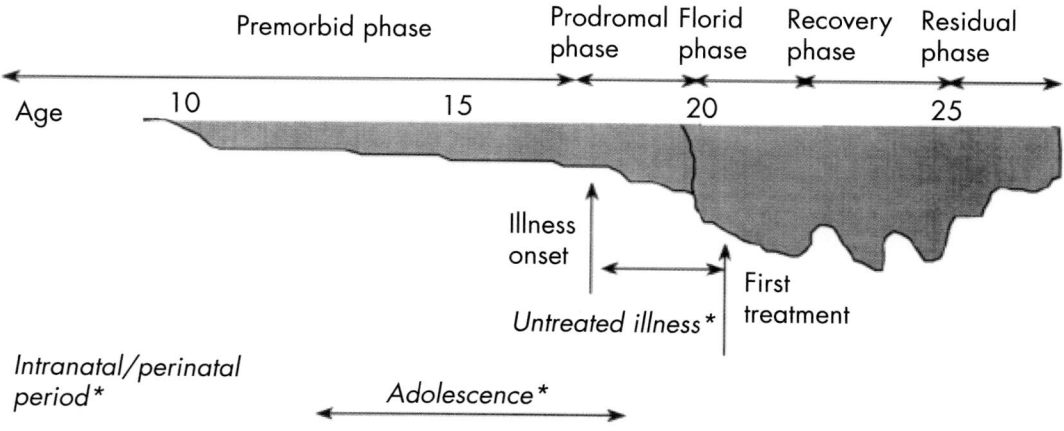

FIGURE 10–1. Natural course of schizophrenia.

Note. Asterisks indicate critical periods for early detection or intervention.

Source. Keshavan MS, Hogarty GE: "Brain Maturational Processes and Delayed Onset in Schizophrenia." *Development and Psychopathology* 11:525–543, 1999 (Figure 1 [p. 526]). Copyright 1999. Reprinted with the permission of Cambridge University Press.

consideration of alternative explanations for the experience. Psychotic symptoms that are clinically significant usually also have some observable effect on other thinking or behavior, such as avoidance of individuals or places that are targets for delusional thinking or behavioral attempts to respond to hallucinations. Despite these discrete criteria, many experiences that patients endorse are on the cusp of psychosis, and it is often difficult to determine whether they should qualify as overtly psychotic. This distinction is important because antipsychotic medication has well-demonstrated efficacy against overt psychotic symptoms, and the use of these medications for psychotic symptoms is usually justified and advantageous. However, the use of these medications to treat symptoms that are below the threshold of psychosis has to date been poorly studied.

This issue takes on greater importance when one considers that early intervention may have potentially profound differences for the course of illness in schizophrenia and even possibly for whether those individuals at risk for schizophrenia convert to the disorder. Several groups around the world are currently evaluating sets of clinical criteria for their value in predicting the conversion to overt psychotic disorders (Phillips et al. 2005) and in some cases have reported prospective rates of conversion as high as 40% in 1 year.

Early Period of Psychotic Illness in Schizophrenia

The crossing of the boundary from the prodrome to schizophrenia proper is an event witnessed with great dismay by patients, families, and care providers alike. It remains an event with obscure causes for most patients, because the precipitants of overt psychosis have not been well established (Broome et al. 2005). In some cases, substance abuse may be a precipitant. Among persons at risk for schizophrenia, cannabis and amphetamines appear to be the most frequently abused substances around the time of onset of psychosis. However, in most cases, the cause of psychosis onset remains unknown. Both genetic and environmental origins have been considered (see section "Introduction to Etiology and Pathophysiology" later in this chapter).

The onset of psychosis can be insidious or abrupt, and those who experience a rapid onset tend to have a more favorable prognosis. This active phase of initial psychotic symptoms is often referred to informally as the *first break*—that is, the break with reality that is a core feature of psychosis. Patients during this phase will experience florid symptoms of hallucinations, delusions, and occasionally disorganized thought and behavior and agitation. At this point, the distress experienced by the patient, family, or both often increases dramatically, prompting entry into treatment. Less often, the patient comes to the attention of the mental health system for involuntary evaluation, as the result of public disturbances or behaviors that are dangerous to the self or others. As treatment for first-episode psychosis proceeds, overt psychotic symptoms commonly abate in the days to few months thereafter. Ample evidence indicates that those patients who experience significant treatment delays have a worse prognosis even when illness severity at presentation is taken into account. This suggests that early intervention is an important treatment goal in schizophrenia.

Longitudinal studies of first-episode psychosis leading to a schizophrenia diagnosis find considerable heterogeneity at follow-up. One review found that approximately one-third of these patients (across 13 prospective studies) experienced a benign course, in contrast to the two-thirds who relapsed, failed to recover, or were rehospitalized, in the first 2 years after a first hospitalization for psychosis (Ram et al. 1992). More recent, longer-term prospective follow-up studies have found considerable heterogeneity in clinical (Bromet and Fennig 1999) and functional status among these patients; significant numbers achieve adequate social and occupational function and quality of life in the several years after onset of psychosis, whereas others experience a decline in these measures (Malla and Payne 2005). For patients who do receive adequate treatment, a *residual phase* follows, during which the range and severity of symptoms can be quite similar to those seen in the prodrome. Psychotic symptoms may persist during this period, although with less intensity and less attendant distress. Over time, most patients will experience a series of acute exacerbations of symptoms occurring episodically as they go into and out of active-phase psychosis. These episodes are often precipitated by environmental stressors, substance abuse, or treatment discontinuation. The degree of remission between these episodes may vary, and there is a tendency in the early phase (the first 5–10 years after onset) of the overt illness for patients to progressively fail to attain the level of function observed prior to each episode (Lieberman et al. 2001). This describes the "clinical deterioration" associated with Kraepelin's construct of schizophrenia and particularly describes the course of patients identified in recent editions of DSM. The chronology, number of acute episodes, and rate of decline during this period do vary considerably among patients. Following this period, however, patients appear to attain a measure of stability in the severity of symptoms, rate of relapse, treatment responsivity, and general level of function.

In addition, a more severe early-onset form of schizophrenia (before age 12 years) has been described. It is quite rare and appears continuous in both clinical and biological features with the more common adult-onset form (Nicolson and Rapoport 1999). Follow-up studies of childhood-onset schizophrenia suggest the following prognostic factors. In general, in comparison to the adult-onset form, childhood-onset schizophrenia has a worse prognosis. Nevertheless, those who experience a more acute onset, a rapid response to acute treatment, and relatively more positive than negative, cognitive, or depressive symptoms have a more favorable prognosis. Premorbid function tends to be more impaired than among adult-onset patients, but those who were observed to be more social and intelligent or have a more "well-integrated" premorbid personality had a better prognosis than did those childhood-onset patients with more impairment on these measures. In addition, a more benign course is observed among those childhood-onset patients who lack a family history of schizophrenia or who have greater family support (Remschmidt 2002).

Long-Term Outcome

Numerous studies have been conducted in an attempt to characterize the long-term outcome of patients with schizophrenia. Hegarty et al. (1994) reviewed 320 studies that included a total of 51,800 patients with schizophrenia, conducted between 1895 and 1992. In these studies, patients were followed for approximately 6 years on average, and 40% were considered to have improved, as indicated by recovery, remission, or clinically stable with minimal symptoms. In those studies in which patients' symptoms were diagnosed with a more narrow criteria set, rates of improvement were lower: 27% on average, probably reflecting the more "Kraepelinian" deteriorating course associated with narrower definitions of the illness. In addition, the rate of improvement was greater for those patients identified after the middle of the twentieth century than for those followed up earlier, likely reflecting treatment advances in this period. Studies reported more recently have indicated lower rates of improvement, possibly reflecting again-narrowed criteria for the diagnosis and possibly more stringent criteria for clinical improvement as well.

Several studies have now been reported in which patients with schizophrenia were identified with contemporary diagnostic criteria and follow-up was obtained over at least 10 years (Jobe and Harrow 2005). Most of these studies have been retrospective chart reviews, typically of patients who were identified initially during hospitalization and then followed up after discharge. The Iowa 500 study followed up 500 psychiatric patients admitted to the Iowa State Psychiatric Hospital between 1934 and 1944 and used the Feighner criteria to identify schizophrenic patients, of whom 200 were followed up an average of 35 years from the index hospitalization (Tsuang and Winokur 1975). These patients were followed up in an era prior to modern antipsychotic medication or modern psychosocial treatment; therefore, this study provided significant documentation of the untreated course of schizophrenia. In this study, the schizophrenic patients were observed to have poorer outcome on all measures, relative to other psychiatric patients and nonpsychiatric surgical patients: 54% had incapacitating symptoms, 67% had never married, 18% were living in institutions, and more than 10% had committed suicide (Tsuang and Winokur 1975). The Chestnut Lodge study followed up 532 patients discharged from this private hospital between 1950 and 1975, for an average of 15 years. Patients were diagnosed by less restrictive DSM-III criteria, yet the findings were broadly similar to those of the Iowa 500. The 163 schizophrenic patients as a group had the following outcomes: 6% recovered, 8% good, 22% moderate, 23% marginal, and 41% continuously incapacitated (McGlashan 1984). A study conducted at the New York State Psychiatric Institute included 552 patients who underwent treatment with psychoanalytically oriented psychotherapy, of whom 99 met DSM-III criteria for schizophrenia. With follow-up between 10 and 23 years, the schizophrenic patients showed poorer outcome compared with other psychiatric patients, had an average DSM Global Assessment of Functioning score of 39, and had a completed suicide rate of 10% (Stone 1986).

Although these studies largely emphasized the relatively poor prognosis of most patients with schizophrenia, other follow-up studies identified subgroups with better outcomes. These studies include Vaillant's study in Boston, Massachusetts, in which the patients identified as completely remitted from an earlier study were then followed up prospectively for 4–16 years. He found that 61% of these patients remained in remission. A study in Edmonton, Alberta, Canada, found that 58% of 92 patients with DSM-II (American Psychiatric Association 1968) schizophrenia experienced full recovery, despite 45% of the full sample having discontinued their psychiatric medication in the 10 months after the index hospitalization. When this same sample was narrowed through the use of stricter Feighner diagnostic criteria, the percentage of patients considered fully recovered was halved (Bland et al. 1978).

Only two long-term follow-up studies were fully prospective in design. The Chicago Follow-Up Study included 73 schizophrenic patients followed up to 20 years. This study found that schizophrenic patients generally fluctuated between moderate and severe disability, but more than 40% showed periods of recovery that often lasted for several years (Harrow and Jobe 2005). Some of these patients were able to function without the benefit of continuous antipsychotic treatment and had tended to have better premorbid function. In addition, a large percentage of the full sample of schizophrenic patients (65%) also had experienced at least one depressive syndrome at 20-year follow-up; the completed suicide rate was 10% at 10 years and higher than 12% at 20 years. The other long-term prospective study of schizophrenic patients, conducted by Carpenter and Strauss (1991), followed up 55 DSM-III-identified schizophrenic patients for 11 years and found no change in their relatively poorer outcome status at 5 and 10 years.

Several long-term follow-up studies have been conducted outside of North America. These studies have typically used *International Classification of Diseases* criteria rather than DSM criteria to identify patients. Some of these studies have found women to have a relatively more benign course of illness compared with men (Angermeyer et al. 1989). One of these studies that is particularly important is the World Health Organization (WHO) study, referred to as the International Pilot Study of Schizophrenia. A total of 1,633 subjects from 14 incidence cohorts and 4 prevalence cohorts in 9 different nations were studied. The most dramatic finding was that outcome in schizophrenia was poorer in fully industrialized countries than in developing countries. Repeated psychotic episodes, for instance, were more common in the developed countries despite the greater availability of modern treatment. The range and severity of symptoms at initial enrollment were not significantly different between sites. This finding has been subject to a great deal of discussion. Some have suggested that a culture of tolerance and benevolence toward those with unusual thoughts and behaviors is more prevalent in developing countries, with a salutary effect of normalizing or "buffering" the patient's psychopathology and maintaining integration in the local community. However, this does not appear to account fully for the differences between these groups of nations (McGrath et al. 2004). Others have suggested that economies that are not fully market-oriented place fewer psychological and practical demands on schizophrenic patients, with less illness exacerbation and less downward social drift as a result. On the whole, in the WHO study, the strongest predictors of poor outcome were social isolation, duration of index episode, history of psychiatric treatment, unmarried status, and history of childhood behavior problems. These factors all may reflect a more severe form of illness at outset.

Etiology and Pathophysiology

The past five decades have borne witness to an impressive period of discovery in the neurobiological basis of schizophrenia. Modern psychiatric research has produced an abundance of evidence supporting the notion that schizophrenia is a disorder primarily related to brain dysfunction. Consequently, the term *functional* brain disorder, which was once commonly used to distinguish schizophrenia and other psychiatric conditions from structurally evident brain disorders found in neurological conditions, has become antiquated. The convergence of disparate modern investigative techniques onto this question has identified tantalizing clues to the neurobiological basis of this condition. However, despite these advances, the full understanding of the causes and the biological pathways leading to schizophrenia remains one of the most enduring challenges facing modern medicine. This state of uncertainty is reflected by the presence of competing theories on the etiology of schizophrenia. The aim of this section is to review and synthesize these major theories and the evidence supporting them.

Before proceeding, a discussion of some of the organizing principles guiding modern schizophrenia research will be helpful in orienting the reader to the research. Two concepts describe the generally accepted framework reflecting the current understanding of the etiology and pathophysiology of schizophrenia. The first is the view that schizophrenia is a neurodevelopmental disorder—that disturbances in the normal growth and maturation of neurons and neural pathways give rise to schizophrenia. The other overarching framework is the diathesis stress model of schizophrenia. This model posits a dynamic interplay between heritable (diathesis) and environmental (stress) factors in determining whether any individual develops this illness. This model is consistent with available data showing that the risk of developing schizophrenia is strongly influenced by genetics, but the eventual development of this illness is also strongly modulated by environmental factors (D. A. Lewis and Levitt 2002; Lieberman et al. 2001).

Genetics

That schizophrenia has a strong genetic component is a readily accepted notion (see Chapter 6 in this volume, "Genetics," by Choudary and Knowles). The degree of risk is proportional to the degree of shared genes (Gottesman 1991). A review of twin studies showed concordance rates between 25% and 50% (Gottesman 1991). Adoption studies showed an elevated risk for schizophrenia among the offspring of mothers with schizophrenia (Kety et al. 1971).

The exact manner in which schizophrenia is heritable and the identity of the specific genes that may give rise to schizophrenia, however, remain topics of significant debate and uncertainty. It is very evident that schizophrenia does not follow simple Mendelian principles of inheritance (McGue and Gottesman 1989). This conclusion follows from the logic that inheritance patterns of diseases following simple Mendelian genetics are relatively easy to detect, and no such pedigree has ever been described for schizophrenia. A complex genetic model of transmission is much more likely to be the case for schizophrenia. Complex diseases involve several genes, each with a modest effect on heritability, acting in concert, in either a linear or a synergistic manner, to confer an overall disease risk (Risch 1990). Additional complexity may arise from partial penetrance of these genes, interactions between genes, and epigenetic neurodevelopmental or environmental factors.

The potential complexity of genetic and nongenetic factors in schizophrenia is illustrated by twin adoption studies. Several have been published, and on the whole, they have been remarkably consistent in reporting approximately 50% concordance rate for monozygotic twins. This result accentuates the importance of both the genetic and the nongenetic factors in conferring disease risk. Even if two individuals share identical genetic makeup, there is only approximately a 50% chance that both will develop schizophrenia. Consequently, nongenetic causes must account for this lack of full concordance. A more recent study has found that this elevated risk may be mediated in part by a stressful environment (Tienari et al. 1994). Similar models of gene–environment interaction leading to disease expression have received empirical validation in other psychiatric disorders (Moffitt et al. 2005). In the following sections, some of the more commonly cited nongenetic factors thought to explain this concordance rate are reviewed.

In the past 10 years, with the development of novel study designs and high throughput methods, we have witnessed a tremendous proliferation in the number of putative schizophrenia risk genes (Figure 10–2). An interesting aspect of this list is that many of these genes are related to neurodevelopmental processes involved in the establishment of neural networks (e.g., neuronal migration and synapse formation or the regulation of synaptic transmission). One such gene that has received a lot of attention is dysbindin *DTNBP1* (Straub et al. 2002). This gene product binds to components of the dystrophin complex, thought to be important in mediating neural synapse structure and function. Another putative schizophrenia gene is neuregulin (*NRG1*) (Stefansson et al. 2002). It is located on 8p21–22 and may have a diverse range of roles in neural transmission, axonal development, and synaptogenesis (Corfas et al. 2004). An important fact to keep in mind is that replications of findings from linkage studies have been relatively rare. However, this may be re-solved by considering that several risk genes are involved, each with only modest effect. A recent meta-analysis of these linkage studies did show some support for the involvement of several regions (Badner and Gershon 2002; C.M. Lewis et al. 2003). Follow-up association studies in many of these regions have been promising, and they have identified several candidate schizophrenia risk genes (Owen et al. 2005).

Environmental Factors

It is very evident from reviewing the genetic literature that nonheritable or environmental factors likely play a significant role in the risk for developing schizophrenia. In this section, we survey studies that have identified several environmental factors that may increase risk for schizophrenia.

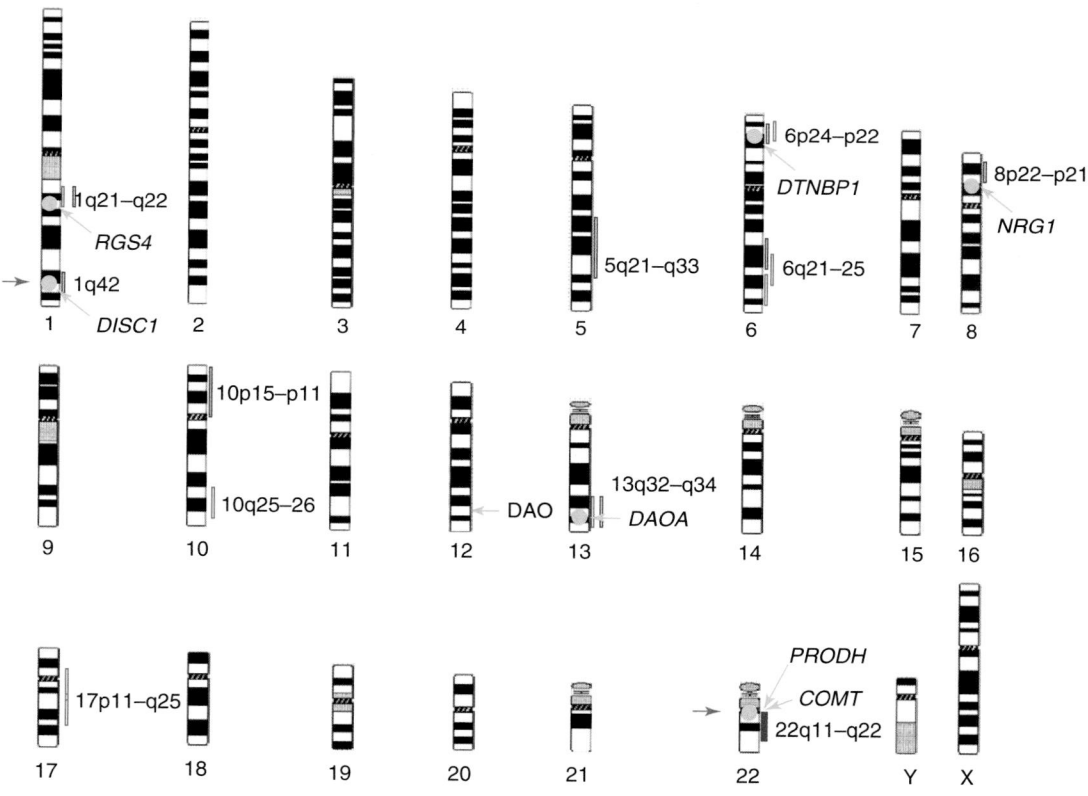

FIGURE 10–2. Candidate schizophrenia genes.

Linkages that reached genomewide significance on their own (*red*) or those that have received strong support from more than one sample (*blue*) are shown. The red arrows refer to the location of chromosomal abnormalities associated with schizophrenia. The *yellow arrows and circles* show the locations of the genes discussed in the source article (Owen et al. 2005).

Source.   Reprinted from Owen MJ, Craddock N, O'Donovan MC: "Schizophrenia: Genes at Last?" *Trends in Genetics* 21:518–525, 2005 (Figure 1 [p. 520]). Copyright 2005, Elsevier Limited. Used with permission.

The idea that fetal neural development represents an especially vulnerable period for the genesis of schizophrenia is supported by observations of higher incidence of obstetric and perinatal complications in patients with schizophrenia in several studies. A recent meta-analytic review categorized these events as 1) complications of pregnancy, 2) abnormal fetal growth and development, and 3) complications of delivery (Cannon et al. 2002). The meta-analysis indicated that each of these categories was significantly associated with increased risk but that the effect sizes were generally modest. Another line of studies has found an association between maternal nutritional status and schizophrenia in the offspring. The Dutch Famine study examined the prevalence of schizophrenia among a cohort of births that occurred during the winter of 1944–1945, a period of severe malnutrition for most citizens in a region of the Netherlands (Susser et al. 1996). The study showed a twofold increased risk for schizophrenia associated with extreme prenatal malnutrition.

Most epidemiological studies investigating environmental risk factors for schizophrenia are limited by the retrospective manner in which data are collected. For example, in the case of maternal exposure to influenza, this information is usually obtained from participants' recollection of influenza infection during pregnancy or the association of a known influenza outbreak in a particular community with the period of pregnancy. The Prenatal Determinants of Schizophrenia Study addressed this limitation by relying on prospectively gathered data, which included maternal serum obtained during prenatal visits and demographic information on the participants (Susser et al. 2000). From the cohort of approximately 12,000 pregnant women, potential cases of schizophrenia were identified from medical and pharmacy records. Of these potential cases, face-to-face diagnostic evaluations by research psychiatrists resulted in the identification of 71 subjects with schizophrenia. This study concluded that influenza infection in the first trimester is associated with a sevenfold increased risk for schizophrenia and related disorders (Brown et al. 2004). Other possible pathogens that were identified in the Prenatal Determinants of Schizophrenia Study include toxoplasmosis and lead.

Another line of research has pointed to the importance of the physical environment and fetal exposures during gestation. Seasonal variation in the prevalence of births leading to schizophrenia has been identified, with an excess of births in winter and spring months (G. Davies et al. 2003). Various theories attempting to account for this finding have been proposed—environmental factors that predisposed to schizophrenia development such as ambient temperature, exposure to infectious agents, and nutritional deficiencies; increased resistance to infections; and other insults conferred by schizophrenia, leading to increased survival in winter months.

Although the worldwide prevalence is thought to be equivalent across nations (Jablensky 2000; Sartorius et al. 1977), numerous findings and theories have suggested a direct relation between specific social and cultural factors and the development or severity of schizophrenia. Some of these factors include immigration status, urbanicity, and socioeconomic status. However, the results of studies examining these factors have been either inconsistent or complicated by confounds that make it very difficult to ascertain whether these factors are causes or effects of illness (e.g., downward drift in socioeconomic status caused by mental illness).

Neurochemical Factors

The serendipitous discovery of the first neuroleptic ushered in the modern era of psychiatry. The effect of this discovery was seen not only in the improved treatment for schizophrenia but also in the research realm. The finding that a pharmacological agent could ameliorate some of the symptoms of schizophrenia motivated researchers to attempt to identify the neurochemical pathways affected by these medications in hopes of determining the underlying pathophysiology of the illness. This line of research has led to the development of influential theories, such as altered function of neurotransmitters, that attempt to account for schizophrenia. Although most researchers now acknowledge that the etiology of schizophrenia cannot be understood solely in terms of neurotransmitter dysfunction, it is clear that dysregulation of neurotransmission is an important aspect in the expression of this disorder.

Dopamine

Chlorpromazine was originally synthesized in the 1950s as an antihistamine for use as a preanesthetic agent. After the French surgeon Henri Laborit noted a particularly calming effect on patients, he recommended chlorpromazine to his psychiatric colleagues for use with agitated patients. They quickly found it beneficial in patients with schizophrenia. They also noted parkinsonian side effects with higher doses. They coined the term *neuroleptic*, literally translated from the French as "seizing the neuron," to reflect their intuition that the mechanism of action somehow involved neural modulation.

The serendipitous discovery of the usefulness of chlorpromazine in schizophrenia led ultimately to the development of the dopamine hypothesis, one of the most influential theories on the etiology of schizophrenia. It posits that the symptoms of this illness are the by-products of dysfunction of dopamine neurotransmission. The main lines of evidence supporting this role for dopamine came from work in the 1960s and 1970s. Carlsson and Lindqvist (1963) determined that the administration of phenothiazines in animals blocks the behavioral effects of dopamine agonists (such as amphetamine) and results in increased turnover of dopamine. Conversely, the administration of amphetamine, which was known to increase synaptic levels of dopamine, resulted in behavioral abnormalities and symptoms reminiscent of schizophrenia. Later work further specified that the most important dopa-

mine receptor may be the D_2 subtype in that clinical potency is best correlated with binding to this receptor subtype (Creese et al. 1976).

Neuroimaging has made significant contributions to our evolving understanding of the neurochemical basis for schizophrenia. Imaging modalities such as positron emission tomography (PET) and single photon emission computed tomography (SPECT) are allowing researchers to assess the functional status of neurotransmitter systems (Figure 10–3). One line of PET studies has led to a more refined hypothesis of dopamine dysregulation. These studies found that the dopaminergic tone associated with schizophrenia may be more complex than previously thought. This newer hypothesis proposes a hyperdopaminergic state in the striatal D_2 system (Abi-Dargham et al. 2000) that gives rise to positive symptoms and a hypodopaminergic state in the prefrontal D_1 system associated with higher-order cognitive deficits (Abi-Dargham et al. 2002).

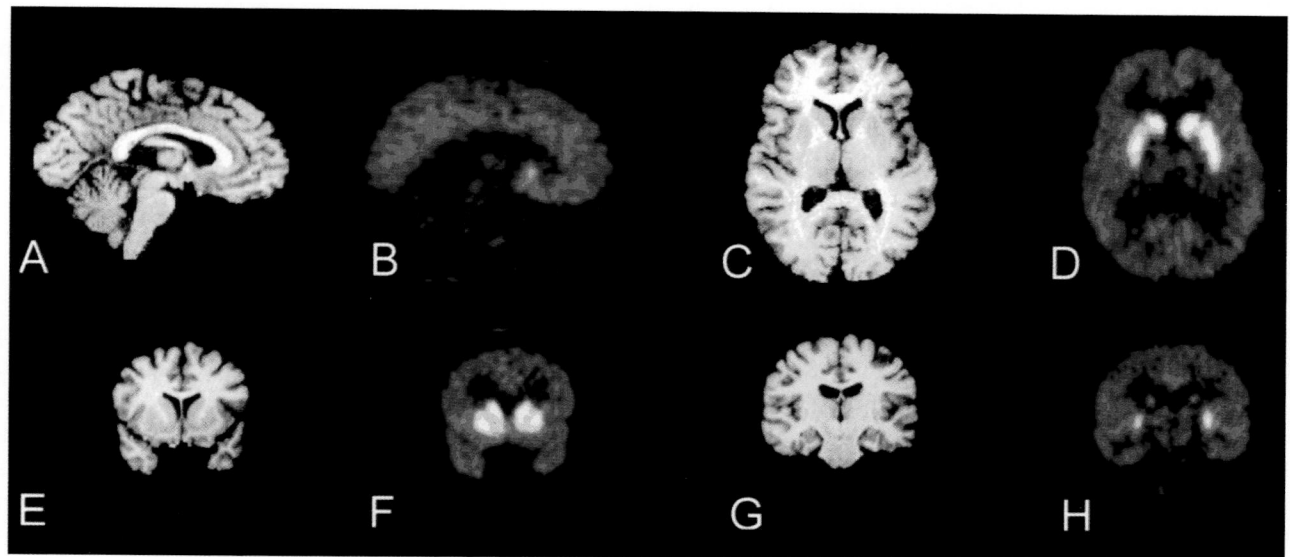

FIGURE 10–3.   Positron emission tomography (PET) images of cognition.

The PET image represents the activity recorded from 30 to 60 minutes after injection of 13.3 mCi in a 37-year-old healthy female volunteer. **A, B,** Sagittal view, illustrating the contrast between cortical and cerebellar activities. **C, D,** Transaxial view, at the level of the head of caudate, putamen, and thalamus. **E, F,** Coronal view, at the level of the anterior striatum, illustrating the lower level of activity in the ventral striatum compared with the caudate and putamen. **G, H,** Coronal view, at the level of the hippocampus, illustrating low levels of activity in thalamus, hippocampus, and parahippocampal gyrus. Putamen and caudate activities are still visualized. NNC 112 = (+)-5-(7-benzofuranyl)-8-chloro-7-hydroxy-3-methyl-2,3,4,5-tetrahydro-1H-3-benzazepine.

Source.   Reprinted from Abi-Dargham A, Mawlawi O, Lombardo I, et al.: "Prefrontal Dopamine D_1 Receptors and Working Memory in Schizophrenia." *Journal of Neuroscience* 22:3708–3719, 2002 (Figure 3 [p. 3713]). Copyright 2002, Society for Neuroscience. Used with permission.

As important as the dopamine hypothesis has been to schizophrenia research, modern psychiatry has appreciated the limitations of this theory. The challenge to the dopamine hypothesis comes from primarily two lines of evidence. First, the dopamine hypothesis does not account for negative symptoms, which are now acknowledged to be essential components of this illness. Dopamine-blocking agents have not been shown to be effective in treating negative symptoms, nor have dopaminergic agents been shown to induce negative symptoms. The second challenge to the dopamine hypothesis comes from the efficacy of the so-called atypical antipsychotics, medications that are thought to act through multiple neurotransmitter systems in addition to dopamine.

Other Monoamines

The observations that the prototypical atypical neuroleptic—clozapine—is often effective in patients who have symptoms refractory to the traditional D_2 receptor-blocking agents and has high affinity for diverse monoaminergic receptors, including serotonergic, histaminergic, muscarinic, and α-adrenergic receptors, in addition to the D_2 receptor, have led to the hypothesis that other neurotransmitter systems may be involved in the pathophysiology of schizophrenia. One of the most important of these other neurotransmitters is serotonin. Serotonin has been implicated by the clinical efficacy of the many atypical agents with high affinity for its receptors. There are 14 known serotonin receptor subtypes, but some of the most important for schizophrenia include the $5-HT_{2C}$, $5-HT_{2A}$, and $5-HT_{1A}$ subtypes.

The acetylcholine system was implicated in the pathophysiology of schizophrenia initially on the basis of the observation that patients with schizophrenia have high rates of use of tobacco products. This led to the hypothesis that the nicotine in tobacco provides some amelioration of symptoms through its action on the acetylcholine system. This hypothesis has received some support by work examining the effects of nicotine on early sensory deficits that were well documented in schizophrenia; nicotine normalized measures of deficient auditory gating in schizophrenia (L.E. Adler et al. 1992).

Glutamate and N-Methyl-D-Aspartate

Glutamate is the most prevalent excitatory neurotransmitter in the brain. Consequently, the function of glutamate is fundamentally different from that of dopamine and the other monoaminergic neurotransmitters, which are primarily modulators of excitatory or inhibitory neurotransmission. The involvement of the glutamate system in the pathophysiology of schizophrenia is inferred primarily from the observation that people intoxicated with agents acting on the glutamate receptor, such as phencyclidine (PCP) and ketamine, often have a behavioral syndrome mimicking schizophrenia. Interestingly, this syndrome can include both positive and negative symptoms of schizophrenia (Javitt and Zukin 1991). PCP and ketamine bind to the N-methyl-D-aspartate (NMDA) class of glutamate receptors, and consequently the main focus of glutamate research has been on this receptor. The NMDA receptor regulation is highly complex with numerous sites of allosteric modulation. One of the most important in terms of psychopathology appears to be the glycine site. Several clinical trials have examined partial (D-cycloserine) and full (glycine, D-serine, and D-alanine) agonists of this site. The pharmacodynamics of cycloserine with the NMDA receptor are complex, with cycloserine acting as an agonist at low and an antagonist at high concentrations. Interestingly, one of the main current uses of cycloserine is in the treatment of tuberculosis, where it is given at high doses, and a relatively common side effect in this setting is psychosis. The results of clinical studies investigating the effects of glycine agonists have been mixed, with some studies showing benefit for both positive and negative symptoms. However, because of the limited number of studies, confirming the importance of the glutamate/NDMA system in schizophrenia will require further investigation.

Gamma-Aminobutyric Acid

The potential role for γ-aminobutyric acid (GABA) in the pathophysiology of schizophrenia follows two separate but related lines of research involving inhibitory interneurons. In the first line of research, the psychotomimetic effects of NMDA antagonists, such as PCP, are thought to be mediated through their action on GABA release. NMDA receptors are found on GABAergic inhibitory interneurons. Activation of these NMDA receptors results in increased GABA release, which then causes suppression of glutamate release from glutamatergic cells. The binding of an antagonist on the NMDA receptor on the inhibitory neurons ultimately results in a hyperglutamatergic state, which is presumed to cause symptoms of psychosis.

In the second line of research, alterations in the neural circuitry of the prefrontal cortex, involving GABA, are thought to give rise to the higher-order cognitive deficits in schizophrenia. Theories on GABA dysfunction in schizophrenia center on the parvalbumin-containing group of inhibitory interneurons.

Studies showing a reduction in the number of parvalbumin cells and underexpression of glutamic acid decarboxylase, a key enzyme in GABA synthesis (Akbarian et al. 1995; Volk et al. 2000), point to a functional deficit in GABA in the prefrontal cortex. Parvalbumin cells can be further subdivided on the basis of differences in histological and putative functional properties. Chandelier cell axons target the axonal initial segment of pyramidal cells in the neocortex and show a limited coverage area of its axons. The wide arbor cells target the soma and proximal portions of the dendrites, and, as the name implies, their axons cover a broad area. With the privileged position of its axonal cartridges, the chandelier cells are thought to potently regulate the timing of output of pyramidal cells within a column, whereas wide arbor cells are thought to inhibit pyramidal cells in neighboring columns (D. A. Lewis 2000). Additionally, chandelier cells can terminate on several hundreds of pyramidal cells, setting the stage for the synchronization of many cells (Figure 10–4) (Cobb et al. 1995; Howard et al. 2005). Taken together, the chandelier and wide arbor cells are thought to coordinate the fine control of the synchrony and spatial extent of pyramidal cell activity in the prefrontal cortex. The disruption of these functions in schizophrenia would be expected to lead to the loss of temporal and spatial organization in neuronal activity necessary for higher-order cognitive processes.

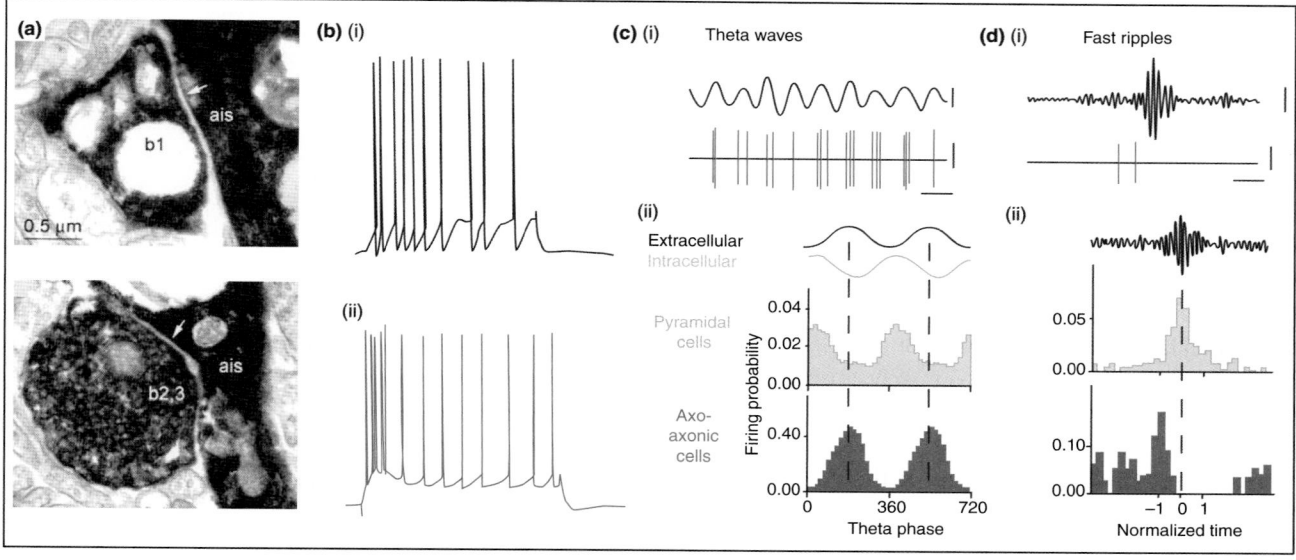

FIGURE 10–4. Chandelier cell ultrastructure and physiology.

(a) Electron micrographs of two of the multiple boutons (labeled *b1* and *b2,3*) from an electrophysiologically recorded, biocytin-filled axo-axonic cell (AAC) synapsing on the biocytin-filled axonal initial segment (AIS) of a postsynaptic pyramidal cell. Arrows indicate synaptic contacts. Note the morphological differences between the boutons. **(b)** Firing pattern of two AACs from rat hippocampus in response to a 500-ms depolarizing pulse. Note that (i) shows a nonadapting pattern, whereas (ii) shows a strongly adapting pattern, documenting that AAC physiology is heterogeneous, even within one species and brain area. **(c,d)** Theta waves (c) and fast ripples (d) in the stratum pyramidale. Extracellularly recorded theta waves and fast ripples are shown in the upper parts of (c,i) and (d,i), respectively, above the simultaneous juxtacellular spike rasters of single AACs in each case. (c,ii) Stratum pyramidale extracellular *(black)* and pyramidal cell intracellular *(blue)* theta rhythms, corresponding to histograms of spike firing probability in pyramidal cells *(blue)* and AACs *(red)*, averaged over several cells. Note that AAC firing is antiphase to pyramidal cell intracellular theta waves and firing but only slightly phase-delayed from extracellular theta waves. (d,ii) Extracellular fast ripples and concomitant spike firing probability in pyramidal cells *(blue)* and AACs *(red)*, averaged over several cells. Note that AACs increase firing probability just before the fast ripple and depress firing after the fast ripple. Scale bars in (c,i): unit, 0.5 mV; theta, 0.2 mV; time, 300 ms. Scale bars in (d,i): unit, 0.5 mV; fast ripple, 0.1 mV; time, 50 ms.

Source.   Reprinted from Howard A, Tamas G, Soltesz I: "Lighting the Chandelier: New Vistas for Axo-Axonic Cells." *Trends in Neurosciences* 28:310–316, 2005 (Figure 3 [p. 313]). Copyright 2005, Elsevier Limited. Used with permission.

Anatomical and Histological Studies

The study of structural abnormalities in the brains of individuals with schizophrenia was once considered a "graveyard" for neuropathologists. The emergence of modern neuroimaging and molecular techniques has led to a renewed interest in this field. Neuroimaging studies have shown consistent evidence of whole-brain volume deficits, and modern neuropathology studies have uncovered provocative clues pointing to alterations in the microscopic neuroanatomy in schizophrenia (Table 10–6).

The advent of modern neuroimaging techniques has allowed detailed analysis of brain structures and has significantly shaped our understanding of the neural basis of schizophrenia. Previously, brain volumes could be measured in a reliable manner only with postmortem samples. The relative ease of use has resulted in a proliferation of in vivo neuroimaging volumetric studies. CT studies documenting significant enlargement of cerebral ventricles and decrease in overall brain volume in subjects with schizophrenia (relative to healthy control subjects) have provided the first compelling neuroimaging results indicating that schizophrenia is a brain-based disorder (Johnstone et al. 1976). These results remain the most reliable and consistent volumetric findings in schizophrenia, with a median reduction in ventricular volume estimated to be 40% (Lawrie and Abukmeil 1998). However, despite the large difference between patients and control subjects, substantial overlap is seen between groups, and this measure cannot be used to differentiate reliably between patients and control subjects. In other words, we do not yet have a good biological diagnostic marker for schizophrenia. More recent MRI volumetric studies have confirmed the results of these earlier CT studies. They also have identified several specific regions of decreased volume, including the prefrontal and medial temporal structures and lateral temporal cortex and thalamus (Harrison 1999). The magnitude of volume difference between subjects with schizophrenia and healthy control subjects is generally modest in these regions, and these results have not been as consistent as the ventricular and whole brain findings. A recent meta-analysis of MRI studies involving first-episode subjects showed highly significant reductions in total brain volume and increased ventricular volume (Steen et al. 2006), suggesting that these findings are not just the result of disease chronicity or medication exposure.

Neuroimaging studies have strongly confirmed

TABLE 10–6. Certainty and doubt in schizophrenia neuropathology

	Strength of evidence
Macroscopic findings	
Enlarged lateral and third ventricles	++++
Decreased cortical volume	++++
The above changes present in first-episode patients	+++
Disproportionate volume loss from temporal lobe (including hippocampus)	+++
Decreased thalamic volume	++
Cortical volume loss affects gray rather than white matter	++
Enlarged basal ganglia secondary to antipsychotic medication	+++
Histological findings	
Absence of gliosis as an intrinsic feature	+++
Smaller cortical and hippocampal neurons	+++
Fewer neurons in dorsal thalamus	+++
Reduced synaptic and dendritic markers in hippocampus	++
Maldistribution of white matter neurons	+
Entorhinal cortex dysplasia	+/–
Cortical or hippocampal neuron loss	+/–
Disarray of hippocampal neurons	+/–
Miscellaneous findings	
Alzheimer's disease is not more common in schizophrenia	++++
Pathology interacts with cerebral asymmetries	++

Note. +/–=weak; +=moderate; ++=good; +++=strong; ++++=shown by meta-analysis.

Source. Reprinted from Harrison PJ: "The Neuropathology of Schizophrenia: A Critical Review of the Data and Their Interpretation." *Brain* 122 (Pt 4):593–624, 1999 (Table 8 [p. 611]). Copyright 1999, Oxford University Press. Used with permission.

that brain abnormalities are indeed associated with schizophrenia. Consequently, interest has been renewed in identifying microscopic neural abnormalities, with modern neuropathology studies identifying alterations not previously appreciated in the brains of individuals with schizophrenia. A review of the literature showed consistent findings, including reduction in cortical neuronal size, reduction in axonal and dendritic arborization, and reduction in the number of thalamic neurons. The latter study has shown highly significant loss in the number of neurons in the mediodorsal nucleus of the thalamus, particularly in the subnucleus that projects to the dorsolateral prefrontal cortex (Popken et al. 2000).

The recent development of diffusion tensor imaging, a magnetic resonance–based technique, is allowing researchers to measure white fiber integrity in the brain. Diffusion tensor imaging has been quickly adopted by schizophrenia researchers to examine white fiber pathology (Kanaan et al. 2005), thereby testing the hypothesis that schizophrenia is a result of diminished connectivity between brain regions. A growing number of studies are finding loss of white fiber integrity in many areas, such as in tracts connecting the prefrontal and temporal cortices (for a review, see Kubicki et al. 2007). However, as expected with such a new technique applied to a complex illness, a large body of studies has not yet replicated these early results. Consequently, the field will have to await future studies in which this promising technology is used before we can assess the importance of this line of research.

Cognitive and Information Processing Deficits

Cognitive deficits have been recognized as an important feature of schizophrenia since the beginning of efforts to systematically study this condition. About 100 years ago, Emil Kraepelin referred to schizophrenia as *dementia praecox*, or premature dementia, to describe the prominent cognitive deficits that he thought formed the core of this condition. As noted earlier, the word *schizophrenia*, originally coined by Eugen Bleuler, is best translated from German as the "splitting of the mind," a term intended to capture the loss of integration of mental processes. The interest in cognition waned in the intervening years as other aspects of the illness became the focal point of research interest. However, in the last 20 years, there has been renewed interest in studying cognitive dysfunction in schizophrenia as a way to understand its pathophysiology. The logic is that cognitive abnormalities represent core deficits of schizophrenia and that the study of core deficits may provide a better index of underlying neural dysfunction.

Evidence that cognition is a core feature of schizophrenia comes from many fronts. First, studies have

documented a fairly strong correlation between cognitive deficits and functional status. This is in distinction to psychotic symptoms, which generally do not correlate well with functional status. Second, cognitive deficits are very common among individuals with schizophrenia. Third, cognitive deficits appear to be an essential aspect of this condition because they predate the onset of psychotic symptoms, and they are present in unaffected first-degree relatives and identical twins. The study of cognition has an additional practical benefit: many paradigms are amenable to experimental controls and manipulation.

An abundance of research now indicates prominent deficits in higher-order cognition in schizophrenia. Disturbances in cognitive control (the coordination of thought and actions), attention, language, and memory have been documented by several researchers who used diverse paradigms. Some investigators have attempted to develop comprehensive cognitive models of schizophrenia that could explain many of the behavioral deficits and symptoms of schizophrenia. Goldman-Rakic (1994) proposed that working memory, the maintenance of information "on-line" to guide behavior, is the fundamental disturbance in schizophrenia. She further proposed that the cognitive deficits and symptoms such as disorganization in speech and actions are manifestations of working memory deficits. Cohen et al. (1999) proposed the context-processing deficit model for schizophrenia. They defined *context* as the conjunction of items, rules, and goals required to guide behavior or decisions. A real-life example of context processing is the ability of a tourist from America, while visiting England, to avoid being hit by a car while crossing a street. He does so by realizing that one needs to look right first and then left before crossing a street in England. In this example, the conjunction of seeing the crossing signal and knowing the rules of the road in England constitutes the context in which actions (looking right and then left) are determined. According to the context-processing model, many of the diverse cognitive deficits seen in schizophrenia can be reduced to this inability to hold diverse representations in mind. Andreasen et al. (1998) proposed the cognitive dysmetria model of schizophrenia, in which the primary deficit is in the inability of patients to coordinate mental activity rapidly and efficiently in a task-appropriate manner.

The first generation of cognitive neuroscience studies focused primarily on traditional areas of research in cognition—namely, higher-order cognitive processes. More recently, the boundaries of inquiry have broadened to include virtually all domains of mental processes impaired in schizophrenia. Consequently, the term *information-processing deficits* may be a more general and appropriate term to describe the diverse studies currently undertaken by schizophrenia researchers. These studies are identifying information-processing deficits in early sensory, affective, and social domains in schizophrenia.

Early Sensory-Processing Deficits

Dysfunction in higher-order cognitive processes has now been firmly established; however, another line of research is investigating the hypothesis that deficits in early sensory processing are a fundamental aspect of schizophrenia. Some have proposed that these early sensory deficits may contribute to higher-order cognitive deficits and have significant effects on the functional status of the affected individuals (Brenner et al. 2002; Javitt et al. 1997; Saccuzzo and Braff 1981). The visual and auditory systems have been the most well studied.

In the visual domain, studies examining the earliest processes in visual perception have detected deficits in schizophrenia. For example, visual masking is a procedure in which the perception of a briefly presented object (target) is reduced by the presentation of another object (mask) shortly before or after. Numerous studies have reported that patients have visual masking deficits, meaning that they have more difficulty, compared with healthy subjects, accurately perceiving the target when a mask is presented (M. Green and Walker 1986). The visual masking deficit has been shown to correlate with negative symptoms (M. Green and Walker 1986) and formal thought disorder (Perry and Braff 1994). Another line of research has found neural correlates of deficits in early visual processing. Several groups that have used evoked response potentials (ERPs) have detected abnormalities in the P1 component of visual evoked responses in schizophrenia.

In the auditory domain, early sensory deficits have been found with auditory ERPs. Patients have abnormalities in the so-called P50 suppression. In healthy subjects, two sounds presented in rapid succession will produce a reduction in the amplitude of the P50 component of the auditory ERP elicited by the second sound (L. E. Adler et al. 1982). This can be viewed as a type of habituation in which the repetition of a sensory event results in a dampening of the neural response. It has been shown that patients do not show this P50 suppression with the second auditory stimulus. This has been interpreted as the inability of patients to gate sensory information properly.

Patients also have been shown to have deficits in mismatch negativity (Shelley et al. 1991). In healthy subjects, the presentation of an "oddball" tone, a deviant tone within a train of brief repetitions of a standard tone, elicits an auditory ERP that is different from the response elicited by the standard tone. Like the P50 suppression, it is thought that mismatch negativity is preattentive in that the mismatch negativity can be elicited regardless of whether the subject is attending to the stimulus.

Affect Processing

With the recognition of the importance of negative symptoms in schizophrenia, increasing attention is being paid to the study of affect and related processes in schizophrenia. In the last 10 years, we have witnessed an exponential increase in the number of studies focusing on this aspect of the illness. These affect studies can be further categorized as those focusing on emotional expression, recognition of emotional signals, and the subjective experiencing of emotions.

Deficits in the emotional expressivity of patients (e.g., blunted or flat affect) are perhaps the single most visibly apparent symptom of schizophrenia. Other than the distressed expressions associated with psychosis, a marked decrease in the emotional expressivity and responsivity of the face occurs in schizophrenia (Berenbaum and Oltmanns 1992). Contrary to the belief that diminished expression of emotion reflects diminished experience of emotion, patients, in general, appear not to have a subjective experiential deficit (Berenbaum and Oltmanns 1992; Earnst and Kring 1999). This is true even in patients with the deficit syndrome or a predominance of blunted affect.

In addition to deficits in the ability to express emotions, individuals with schizophrenia experience difficulty recognizing affect in others. Several studies have found that when presented with a series of pictures of faces depicting the basic emotions, patients have difficulty naming the expressed emotion (Kohler et al. 2000; Schneider et al. 2006). Some researchers have hypothesized that this deficit is one of the basic social communication problems that patients face in everyday life.

An important factor yet to be clarified in this line of work is the specificity of the affect recognition deficit above and beyond a generalized cognitive deficit because some studies have shown the absence (Kohler et al. 2000; Salem et al. 1996), whereas others have shown the presence, of a differential deficit (Schneider et al. 2006).

Social Cognition

As is the case with affect, the interest in examining deficits in social functioning in schizophrenia has greatly expanded. A strong argument can be made that the social deficits of schizophrenia constitute a core feature of this illness because abnormalities in social functions often occur during the prodromal phase (Davidson et al. 1999), at the time of initial diagnosis, and throughout the course of illness (Addington and Addington 2000). Studies on social cognition have identified two general areas of abnormality in schizophrenia: theory of mind and social perceptions (Pinkham et al. 2003). *Theory of mind* refers to the capacity to 1) understand that the mental state (beliefs, intentions, and perspectives) of others is separate and distinct from one's own and 2) make inferences about another's intentions. Theory of mind skills are higher-order cognitive processes requiring the integration of sensory inputs from multiple channels with contextual information. Studies have shown that patients with schizophrenia lack theory of mind skills (Corcoran et al. 1995; Frith and Corcoran 1996). *Social perception,* the ability to recognize information governing appropriate social behavior, also consistently has been shown to be abnormal in schizophrenia. The facial affect recognition deficits previously discussed are an important example of a social perception dysfunction. It is thought that deficits in affect recognition are the cause of patients' inability to decode the emotional state of others. Interestingly, deficits in social cue perception have been shown to be more acute for abstract compared with nonabstract information (Corrigan and Nelson 1998).

Functional Neuroimaging

The discovery that the activity of specific brain regions could be imaged in awake and behaving subjects has been one of the most important developments in the history of psychiatric and schizophrenia research. Especially since the availability of functional MRI (fMRI), functional neuroimaging has been widely adopted by researchers and is now a mainstream method in our search for the neurobiological basis of schizophrenia. Functional neuroimaging allows researchers to identify diseased brain regions and abnormal cognitive processes in schizophrenia by assessing the neural functional correlates of a given cognitive task. The identification of dysfunctional regions provides information that can inform and constrain hypotheses in studies that are using other research methods. For example, the discovery of abnormal engagement of the dorsolateral prefrontal cortex has been very important in guiding postmortem and genetic studies seeking the cellular and molecular basis of higher-order cognitive deficits in schizophrenia.

Functional Imaging Studies of Higher-Order Cognitive Deficits

Although modern functional neuroimaging studies are beginning to uncover the neural correlates of most clusters of clinical features of schizophrenia, including those associated with deficits in early sensory, affective, and social processes mentioned earlier, most functional neuroimaging studies have historically focused on higher-order cognitive deficits. These studies point to abnormalities in several multimodal associative brain regions. These include deficits in the anterior cingulate cortex, superior temporal gyrus, and medial temporal cortex. Since the implementation of the earliest functional neuroimaging studies in schizophrenia in the 1970s (Ingvar and Franzen 1974), there has been special interest in the dorsolateral prefrontal cortex. The dorsolateral prefrontal cortex is thought to be a key region subserving higher-order cognitive processing, and consequently the dorsolateral prefrontal cortex is hypothesized to be one of the most important sites of pathology in schizophrenia. Ingvar and Franzen (1974), and later Weinberger et al. (1986) and Berman et al. (1986), found that the dorsolateral prefrontal cortex is hypoactive in schizophrenia. These results provide the basis for the "hypofrontality" hypothesis of schizophrenia. In the past 20 years, numerous neuroimaging studies have generally supported the notion of a dysfunctional dorsolateral prefrontal cortex in schizophrenia across different imaging modalities and cognitive paradigms (Callicott et al. 2000; Manoach et al. 2000; Perlstein et al. 2001).

Neural Basis of Symptoms

Although functional neuroimaging, particularly fMRI, is a relatively young investigative tool, it has already made significant contributions to our understanding of the neural basis of the clinical features of schizophrenia. Two such clinical features are cognitive disorganization and auditory hallucinations.

Broadly following the theories set forth by Goldman-Rakic and others, which postulate that 1) the ability to maintain information "on line" forms the basis for many higher-order cognitive processes and behaviors and 2) the dorsolateral prefrontal cortex is the key brain region supporting the maintenance of information on line, a series of functional imaging studies has determined that the degree of activation of the dorsolateral prefrontal cortex in schizophrenia is highly correlated with clinical measures of cognitive and behavioral disorganization (Figure 10–5).

Another series of studies is elucidating the neural basis of auditory hallucinations and thereby providing a neurobiological rationale for an effective treatment for this symptom. Auditory hallucinations appear to be the result of abnormal activation of the neural system serving auditory sensory processing. In one study involving patients with schizophrenia with auditory hallucinations, the onset and offset of the hallucinations correlated with the engagement and disengagement of the primary auditory cortex (Figure 10–6) (Dierks et al. 1999).

Functional neuroimaging studies, such as the one cited earlier, have provided support for a novel treatment strategy targeting auditory hallucinations refractory to medications. fMRI studies have shown overactivation in the temporal-parietal cortex during auditory hallucinations. Consequently, it would be logical to hypothesize that treatment of auditory hallucinations could be effected through the deactivation of this region. Hoffman et al. (2005) have proposed to do this with repetitive transcranial magnetic stimulation (rTMS). rTMS is a procedure in which brief repetitive pulses of a magnetic field are applied to a localized region of the cortex. rTMS is believed to reduce excitability in the applied region. A large clinical study reported that rTMS of the left temporal-parietal region is a safe and effective method to reduce the severity of auditory hallucinations in medication-resistant subjects with schizophrenia (Hoffman et al. 2005).

Intervention and Management

Antipsychotic Medications

Brief History of Antipsychotic Development

Pharmacological agents have been the mainstay of treatment of schizophrenia since the mid-twentieth century, even though other medical approaches were in use prior to this time. Indeed, the modern history of approaches to treatment of schizophrenia exemplifies the process of scientific discovery in clinical medicine and the evolution of how this illness has been conceptualized (see Chapter 26 in this volume, "Psychopharmacology," by Martinez et al.). Early in the twentieth century, various pharmacological interventions for schizophrenia, including cocaine, manganese, castor

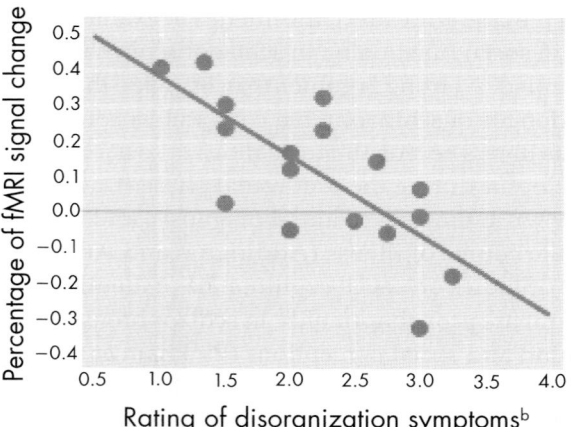

FIGURE 10–5. Relation between disorganization symptoms and change in signal intensity in right dorsolateral prefrontal cortex as a function of working memory load for 17 patients with schizophrenia.[a]

Note. fMRI=functional magnetic resonance imaging.
[a]Working memory was assessed with a sequential-letter task. In the 0-back condition, the target was any letter that matched a prespecified letter. In the 1-back condition, the target was any letter that was identical to the one immediately preceding it. In the 2-back condition, the target was any letter that was identical to the one two trials back. The signal change shown here is the percentage change of the 2-back from the 0-back condition.
[b]Includes conceptual disorganization, mannerisms and posturing, difficulty abstracting, and poor attention from the Positive and Negative Syndrome Scale (Kay et al. 1987).

Source. Reprinted from Perlstein WM, Carter CS, Noll DC, et al.: "Relation of Prefrontal Cortex Dysfunction to Working Memory and Symptoms in Schizophrenia." *American Journal of Psychiatry* 158:1105–1113, 2001 (Figure 2 [p. 1110]). Copyright 2001, American Psychiatric Publishing, Inc. Used with permission.

oil, and sulfur oil, were attempted and reported in the literature. More widely known are the attempts to remediate symptoms of schizophrenia through either sleep induction or insulin-induced coma, the latter of which (introduced by Sakel in 1937) dominated the treatment options for psychiatrists until the 1950s (Ban 2004).

As described earlier, the development of novel adjunct medication for anesthesia yielded the compound chlorpromazine, which was synthesized in 1950 and subsequently observed to induce conscious sedation in agitated patients. It was quickly adopted for use in agitated patients with schizophrenia and found by inpatient clinicians to decrease the need for physical restraint. This phenothiazine compound was the first

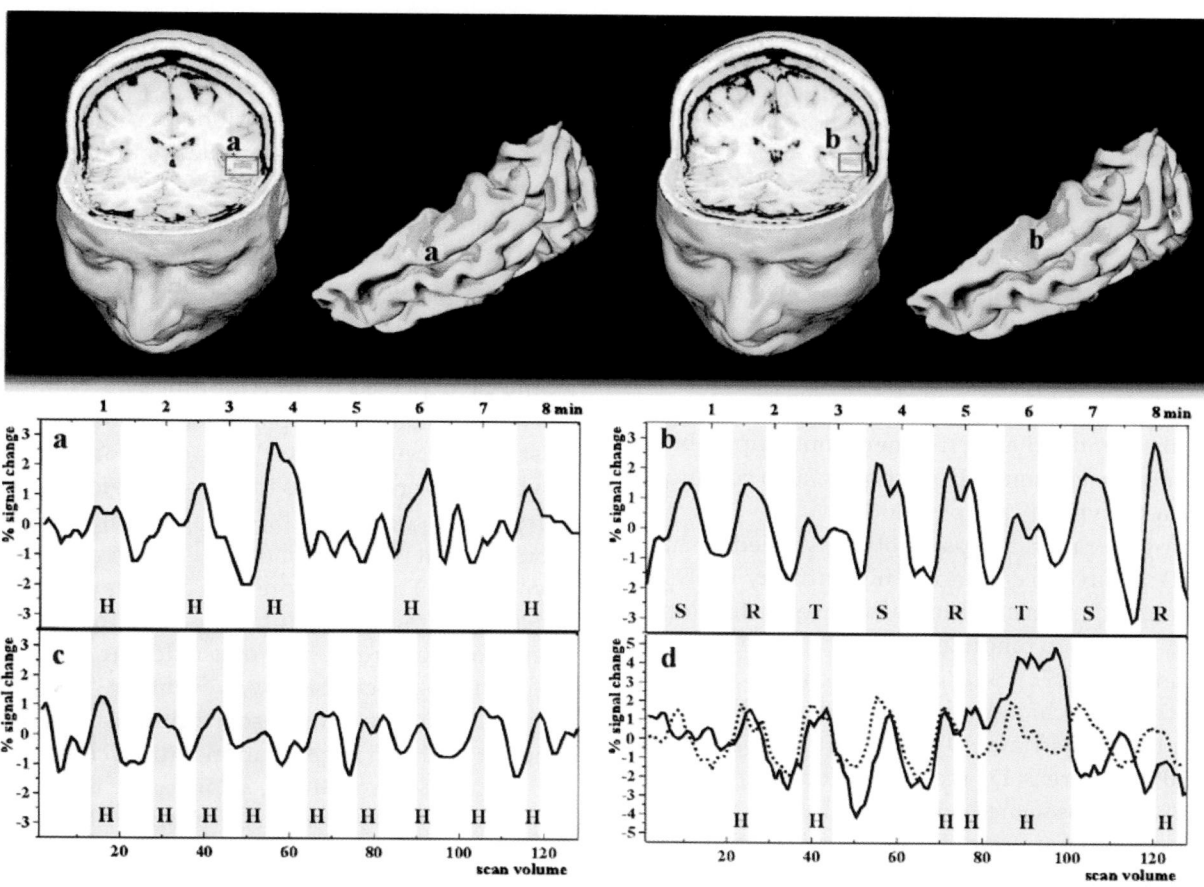

FIGURE 10–6. Activation of Heschl's gyrus during auditory hallucinations and in response to acoustical stimulation.

(Top) Three-dimensional representations of the activation of Heschl's gyrus in patient 1, showing transversal and coronal sections *(left)* and a reconstruction of the gray/white matter boundary of the left temporal lobe *(right)* during hallucinations (a) and acoustical stimulation (b), respectively. (Bottom) Time courses of the blood-oxygen-level-dependent (BOLD) signal for patients 1 (first session) (a and b), 2 (c), and 3 (d), filtered with a high pass of 0.004 Hz and a low pass of 0.05 Hz, from Heschl's gyrus *(solid line)*. The shaded areas indicate experimental conditions (H=hallucinations; S=spoken text; R=reversed speech; T=pulsed tone at 2,000 Hz). For patient 3 (d), the time course of the BOLD signal in Heschl's gyrus *(solid line)* is shown together with the time course of another area in auditory cortex (x=−57, y=−4, z=3) that only responds to acoustic stimulation *(dotted line)* (for acoustical stimulation, the same protocol was used as in [b]).

Source. Reprinted from Dierks T, Linden DE, Jandl M, et al.: "Activation of Heschl's Gyrus During Auditory Hallucinations." *Neuron* 22:615–621, 1999 (Figure 2 [p. 617]). Copyright 1999, Elsevier Limited. Used with permission.

medication for schizophrenia to be tested in placebo-controlled studies, with the landmark report of its superiority in the treatment of schizophrenia emerging several years later. In addition, reserpine (isolated from the rauwolfia plant) was introduced in 1954, but its propensity to induce or worsen depressive symptoms was noted, leading to the examination of its monoaminergic actions and the subsequent articulation of the biogenic amine hypothesis of depression, which paralleled the dopaminergic hypothesis of

schizophrenia. Haloperidol was synthesized in 1958 and introduced the following year; it remains one of the most widely prescribed antipsychotic medications.

Subsequent studies conducted in the 1960s and thereafter further specified the target symptoms responsive to these medications, rates of clinical response, and functional outcome of patients offered these treatments. Basic science investigations established the neurochemical basis for the clinical efficacy of these medications. Initially, Carlsson and Lindqvist

(1963) found that administration of these compounds to rodents led to increased levels of dopamine metabolites and antagonized the behavioral effects of dopamine agonists such as amphetamine and apomorphine. This led Creese et al. (1976) to show that the clinical efficacy of existing antipsychotic medications was directly related to their potency in blocking dopamine receptors, thus refining the dopamine hypothesis of schizophrenia.

Mechanism of Action

To date, more than 30 medications from 11 different chemical classes have been introduced worldwide for the treatment of schizophrenia (Ban 2004). These are generally identified as first-generation antipsychotics or second-generation antipsychotics, also commonly known as "atypical" antipsychotics.

First-generation antipsychotics (typified by haloperidol) all have in common a high affinity for D_2 receptors, and the clinical efficacy of these medications is strongly related to binding affinity for these receptors (Seeman et al. 1976). Studies in which PET was used found that clinical antipsychotic effects occurred at doses at which striatal D_2 receptor occupancy was 65%–70%, whereas D_2 receptor occupancy greater than 80% was associated with a significantly increased incidence of extrapyramidal side effects (EPS) (Remington and Kapur 1999). These studies also have found that at therapeutic doses, first-generation antipsychotics block D_2-like receptors to an equal degree in limbic cortical areas and the striatum, which is also consistent with the relatively narrow range of antipsychotic efficacy in the absence of EPS (Xiberas et al. 2001). The precise cellular feature of altered dopaminergic activity that provides the basis for clinical efficacy remains an active area of investigation. A leading hypothesis suggests that acute administration of these medications is associated with antagonism of D_2 autoreceptors on dopaminergic nerve terminals, leading to a depolarization inactivation of ion channels at those terminals and a resulting incapacity of propagating action potentials to further depolarize the terminal, thus chronically blocking dopamine release into the synapse (Grace et al. 1997).

In contrast, the six second-generation antipsychotics that are currently available in the United States are more heterogeneous in their profile of dopamine receptor antagonism. Risperidone, for example, has D_2 antagonism that is within the range of that for first-generation antipsychotics and, consequently, at therapeutic doses is associated with rates of EPS intermediate between first-generation antipsychotics and other second-generation antipsychotics. Other second-generation antipsychotics, such as clozapine and quetiapine, show minimal D_2 receptor binding at therapeutic doses (Miyamoto et al. 2005). These medications (including the other available second-generation antipsychotics olanzapine, ziprasidone, and aripiprazole) show very heterogeneous profiles of binding at other dopamine receptors.

A leading current hypothesis (the "fast-off" hypothesis) suggests that the relative lack of EPS stemming from the use of these medications may be a result of the relatively faster rate of dissociation of these agents from D_2 receptors. This faster dissociation rate would be expected to more optimally accommodate normal physiological dopamine transmission. In contrast, a competing hypothesis of what constitutes "atypicality" emphasizes the serotonergic receptor activity (5-HT$_{2A}$ and 5-HT$_{2C}$ antagonism and 5-HT$_{1A}$ agonism) that is found among second-generation antipsychotics. These actions are associated with enhanced dopamine and glutamate in prefrontal relative to subcortical areas, and in particular, the ratio of 5-HT$_{2A}$ to D_2 blockade may prevent EPS and remediate negative symptoms of schizophrenia in a manner superior to the first-generation antipsychotics (Meltzer et al. 2003). In addition, aripiprazole is unique as a D_2 partial agonist, which may stabilize elevated rates of dopamine transmission while avoiding a degree of dopamine blockade necessary for EPS.

It also should be emphasized here that all antipsychotics (first- and second-generation antipsychotics) have high-affinity binding at a range of other monoamine receptors in the brain, which may be partly responsible for their efficacy but is well established as the basis for many of their side effects. This includes antagonism at muscarinic, histaminergic, and α-adrenergic receptors, with predictable autonomic effects. In addition, the monoaminergic transporter–blocking effects and 5-HT$_{1A}$ receptor partial agonism or antagonism shown by some second-generation antipsychotics suggest that these medications may exert antidepressant and anxiolytic effects as well (Table 10–7).

Clinical Comparison of Second-Generation Antipsychotics With First-Generation Antipsychotics

Second-generation antipsychotics appear to have efficacy in treatment of positive symptoms that is comparable to that of first-generation antipsychotics (Miyamoto et al. 2005). However, they are consistently superior to first-generation antipsychotics (and placebo) in the treatment of negative symptoms, which,

TABLE 10–7. Relative neurotransmitter receptor affinities for antipsychotics at therapeutic doses

Receptor	Clozapine	Risperidone	Olanzapine	Quetiapine	Ziprasidone	Sertindole	Sulpiride	Amisulpride	Zotepine	Aripiprazole	Haloperidol
D_1	+	+	++	−	+	++	−	−	+	−	+
D_2	+	+++	++	+	+++	+++	++++	++++	++	++++	++++
D_3	+	++	+	−	++	++	++	++	++	++	+++
D_4	++	−	++	−	++	+	−	−	+	+	+++
$5\text{-}HT_{1A}$	−		−	−	+++				++	++	−
$5\text{-}HT_{1D}$	−	+	−	−	+++					+	−
$5\text{-}HT_{2A}$	+++	++++	+++	++	++++	++++	−	−	+++	+++	+
$5\text{-}HT_{2C}$	++	++	++	−	++++	++	−	−	++	+	−
$5\text{-}HT_6$	++	−	++	−	+				++	+	−
$5\text{-}HT_7$	++	+++	−	−	++				++	++	−
α_1	+++	+++	++	+++	++	++	−	−	++	+	+++
α_2	+	++	+	−	−	+	−	−	++	+	−
H_1	+++	−	+++	++	−	+	−	−	++	+	−
M_1	++++	−	+++	++	−	−	−	−	+		−
DA transporter	++		++								−
NA transporter	+		++		++				++	−	
5-HT transporter					++					−	

Note. +/−=weak; +=moderate; ++=good; +++=strong; ++++=shown by meta-analysis.

Source. Adapted from Miyamoto et al. 2005.

as indicated earlier, are important determinants of functional impairment among patients with schizophrenia. In addition, results from the recent Clinical Antipsychotic Trials of Intervention Effectiveness (CATIE) suggested that olanzapine in particular may be more effective than perphenazine (an intermediate-potency first-generation antipsychotic), as well as the other second-generation antipsychotics risperidone, quetiapine, and ziprasidone, in the maintenance of successful treatment of chronic schizophrenia, including the reduction of symptoms and rates of hospital readmission (Lieberman et al. 2005). However, the magnitude of the various reported medication group differences in clinical effects was generally modest, and some of this improvement may in fact be related to

the lower rates of EPS, which are often confounded with negative symptoms in clinical measurement. Some evidence indicates that second-generation antipsychotics (clozapine in particular) show greater efficacy in patients with treatment-refractory schizophrenia (McEvoy et al. 2006; Miyamoto et al. 2005). It is important to note that these last studies were generally conducted in patients who had shown an insufficient prior clinical response to first-generation antipsychotics rather than to other second-generation antipsychotics, and it remains unclear whether similar rates of response to first-generation antipsychotics would be seen after nonresponse to second-generation antipsychotics.

Second-generation antipsychotics also have been

proposed to exert greater effects on the remediation of cognitive deficits in schizophrenia, and this constitutes a fundamental feature of atypicality. However, the empirical literature has been quite inconsistent on this question. Although each of the second-generation antipsychotics has been found to be superior to placebo and first-generation antipsychotics (usually haloperidol) on various tests of attention, memory, executive functions, motor speed, and other cognitive functions, studies finding no differences have been common and have been generally difficult to compare because of methodological differences (Harvey and Keefe 2001). The second-generation antipsychotics may have a lower liability for cognitive performance (compared with first-generation antipsychotics) rather than a greater efficacy. Furthermore, there has been a general lack of hypothesis development to lead investigators from the profile of neurochemical effects to the hypothesized cognitive efficacy of these medications. This is an important area of research because novel medications for schizophrenia are likely to be developed specifically to target cognitive dysfunction. Neurotransmitter systems under consideration as future therapeutic targets for both symptomatic and cognitive remediation currently include glutamate, GABA, acetylcholine, cannabinoid and peptide systems, and brain neurotrophic factors (Miyamoto et al. 2005).

In contrast, the differences between second- and first-generation antipsychotics in side-effect profiles have significant clinical implications. At present, the empirical literature strongly indicates that second-generation antipsychotics are superior to first-generation antipsychotics in the lower incidence of EPS resulting from their use. It appears likely that the incidence of tardive dyskinesia—a persistent, disfiguring, and treatment-refractory movement disturbance that emerges with chronic antipsychotic treatment and that represents an important cause of nonadherence—will be lower with second-generation antipsychotics. Other side effects of first-generation antipsychotic treatment that are lessened or nonexistent with second-generation antipsychotics include hyperprolactinemia and ocular effects in the lens and retina. In contrast, the second-generation antipsychotics as a group have been increasingly associated with significant weight gain, hyperlipidemia, insulin resistance and diabetes mellitus onset, prolonged QTc interval, and other cardiovascular complications (Newcomer 2004). These are important consequences of second-generation antipsychotic treatment and for some patients may lead to serious long-term health risks, as well as antipsychotic nonadherence and subsequent

risk of relapse. Nevertheless, treatment with second-generation antipsychotics appears to be associated with a greater sense of well-being among patients, and this appears to be a major factor in the improved rates of compliance for these medications as a group, compared with first-generation antipsychotics (Naber et al. 2004). It remains to be adequately tested whether these two groups of medications have differential benefits for employment, productivity, or other measures of psychosocial function among patients with schizophrenia (Percudani et al. 2004).

In summary, several recent literature reviews have concluded that the overall clinical advantage of second-generation antipsychotics is either modest in magnitude or inadequately tested and that pharmaceutical industry influence on the study design, initiation, and reporting of clinical trials may have an inordinate effect on the state of the empirical literature (Miyamoto et al. 2005; Tandon and Fleischhacker 2005). This may be the case as well for determinations of comparative efficacy within the second-generation antipsychotic class (Heres et al. 2006). These investigators generally emphasize that both first- and second-generation antipsychotics are superior to placebo in the treatment of most features of schizophrenia, that the selection of medications for individual patients continues to be guided largely by side-effect profiles, and that the full antipsychotic pharmacopoeia should remain in consideration in the approach to an individual patient with schizophrenia.

Treatment of Acute Psychosis

The acute psychotic phase of schizophrenia is characterized by readily detectable positive psychotic symptoms such as hallucinations, frank delusions, and disorganized thought and behavior. It is frequently accompanied by mood symptoms and behavioral activation such as agitation, which may appear as extreme states of anxiety, as well as hostility and aggressive and impulsive behavior. This phase of illness is encountered typically in the medical or psychiatric emergency department but is occasionally seen in outpatient clinic settings. Regardless of the profile of symptoms or clinical setting, the initial response should be a rapid and reliable determination of the acute risk that the patient poses to him- or herself or others, which may be influenced by virtually all of the presenting symptoms (as well as history, etiological factors, and so on). Immediate hospitalization may be indicated both to ensure physical safety and to facilitate the initiation of medications. In addition, the clinician should assess the possibility of other etiologies for psychosis, such as substance-induced and mood-related psychosis, because these disorders are common causes of acute psychosis, particularly when the diagnosis of schizophrenia has not been previously established.

Regardless of the etiology, pharmacological approaches to acute psychosis are well established in the rapid management of psychotic and behavioral symptoms. The mainstay of treatment involves the use of first-generation antipsychotics, often at higher doses than those needed for maintenance treatment of schizophrenia. Repeated doses of first-generation antipsychotics are often necessary in the short term in inpatient settings; however, the literature indicates that either rapid loading or sustained high-dose antipsychotic treatment regimens do not confer added benefit and increase the risk of adverse side effects. Adjunctive medications such as benzodiazepines are frequently used both for their sedating effects and to permit the use of relatively lower doses of antipsychotics. Prophylaxis of EPS with the use of anticholinergic medications is also often indicated, particularly because the incidence of EPS is higher in younger patients (i.e., those most likely to present with a first episode of acute psychosis), and EPS is a common cause of early nonadherence to antipsychotics.

An increasingly used alternative to the first-generation antipsychotics in acute psychosis is the second-generation antipsychotics, particularly those for which therapeutic blood levels can be quickly attained (e.g., olanzapine, risperidone) or those for which parenteral formulations are available (olanzapine, ziprasidone). Current evidence indicates that these medications are probably as effective in acute psychosis as the first-generation antipsychotics and are much better tolerated, suggesting that the second-generation antipsychotics may replace the first-generation antipsychotics for this indication in the future.

Treatment of First-Episode Psychosis

An individual with a first-episode psychosis presenting as an agitated acute psychosis frequently settles into lower doses of either first-generation antipsychotics or second-generation antipsychotics as the inpatient hospital course proceeds (often by increasing the time interval between doses throughout the day), often with adjunct benzodiazepines discontinued prior to discharge. In this setting, or in a first presentation to an outpatient clinic, the relative merits of first-genera-

tion antipsychotics versus second-generation antipsychotics must be considered (as discussed earlier). An increasingly common approach in the outpatient setting is to initiate low to moderate doses of second-generation antipsychotics, primarily in light of the improved patient satisfaction and compliance that may be largely a function of reduced rates of EPS. It should be recalled that this approach largely trades the higher long-term risk of tardive dyskinesia for lower but significant metabolic and cardiovascular risks.

The clinical response rates to both first- and second-generation antipsychotics are high in a first psychotic episode, up to 75% in some well-designed studies (Robinson et al. 2005). To date, the few studies comparing second-generation antipsychotics with first-generation antipsychotics have not found differential response rates, and the comparative efficacy among individual second-generation antipsychotics for first-episode psychosis remains to be studied (Robinson et al. 2005). A large percentage of first-episode patients respond within the first week of treatment, with response rates reaching a plateau in the subsequent 3 months.

In general, the early diagnosis and intervention in schizophrenia have been increasingly advocated. The duration of untreated psychosis has been hypothesized as an important factor in determining the long-term morbidity of schizophrenia because those who experience greater treatment delays tend to have a much worse long-term prognosis (Wyatt and Henter 1998). Others have suggested that individuals with a prolonged duration of untreated psychosis may be experiencing an inherently more severe form of psychopathology and that the treatment delay may reflect rather than cause the relatively worse prognosis (McGlashan 1999). Early treatment before the need for hospitalization has the added benefit of preventing the traumatic effect that admission to an acute inpatient psychiatric unit can have for both patients and their families. Hence the consensus is that the earliest possible intervention is most likely to lead to the most rapid and complete recovery. Many patients with a first psychotic episode who are given a diagnosis of schizophrenia experience excellent resolution of positive symptoms when compared with chronically ill patients experiencing a relapse.

Maintenance Treatment in Schizophrenia

With the resolution of an acute psychotic episode, patients with schizophrenia are transitioned to maintenance treatment to optimize prevention of relapse to acute psychosis and to improve psychosocial function and general recovery. Proper maintenance treatment also often requires considerable clinical attention to the numerous comorbid psychiatric and medical conditions that are prevalent in schizophrenia and an important cause of poor outcomes, including premature death (Escamilla 2001; A.I. Green et al. 2003). Continuous treatment with effective antipsychotic medications is a cornerstone of intervention in this phase, given the need to minimize relapse risk. With successive relapses following antipsychotic discontinuation, the time required to achieve remission on resumption of treatment lengthens, and ultimately a treatment-refractory state may supervene (Lieberman 1993).

Once the diagnosis of schizophrenia is certain, antipsychotic medication should be continued indefinitely, in a manner analogous to the lifelong pharmacological treatment indicated for disorders such as diabetes mellitus and hypertension. In addition to minimizing relapse, sustained treatment with antipsychotics may modify the long-term course of this illness, although this hypothesis remains to be fully tested (Tandon 1998). Alternative strategies such as full antipsychotic withdrawal in schizophrenic patients are associated with significantly increased rates of relapse, as high as 98% at 2 years in one study (Gitlin et al. 2001). In another study, the rate of relapse among schizophrenic patients who self-discontinued their antipsychotic medications was increased fivefold over the rates in those who continued treatment (Robinson et al. 1999). In addition, intermittent dosing is probably less efficacious in preventing relapse in comparison to continuous dosing (Robinson et al. 2005). Baldessarini et al. (1988) found in a review of the older empirical literature that antipsychotic dosages between 50 and 150 mg of chlorpromazine equivalents per day are adequate for most outpatients with chronic schizophrenia.

Problems with treatment adherence are often a significant factor in this phase of treatment with schizophrenic patients. Often, many factors such as intolerable side effects to medication, cognitive dysfunction, social withdrawal, interpersonal conflict, comorbid substance abuse, financial hardship, and other barriers to treatment access sharply limit the capacity of some patients to continue adequate treatment (Fenton et al. 1997). Comprehensive psychosocial support may be necessary for those patients who experience great difficulty adhering to treatment regimens (Zygmunt et al. 2002). In addition, a pharmacological strategy that may be favorable for many of these patients is the tran-

sition to depot forms of antipsychotics. These forms offer comparable symptom relief (largely avoiding first-pass hepatic metabolism, for instance) while EPS, sedation, and other side effects are well controlled, possibly because of slower rates of absorption compared with oral forms of antipsychotics. Treatment adherence is improved as a result of both increased tolerability and less frequent dosing and may lead to lower relapse rates (Davis et al. 1993). At present, among first-generation antipsychotics, haloperidol and fluphenazine are available in decanoate forms for intramuscular administration (typically given at 4-week and 2-week intervals, respectively); risperidone has recently become available as the first second-generation antipsychotic in depot form. Depot antipsychotics are widely and effectively used in Europe and elsewhere and are quite cost-effective; this strategy remains dramatically underused in the maintenance treatment of schizophrenia in the United States.

Treatment-Refractory Schizophrenia

The overall rates of clinical response of schizophrenic patients to antipsychotic medications are within the range observed for outpatients with mood disorders undergoing antidepressant medication treatment. Nonetheless, a significant percentage of schizophrenic patients (up to 40%, depending on how they are identified) can be considered to be poorly responsive to standard antipsychotic medications (Kane et al. 1988). Treatment-refractory states emphasize poor response of positive symptoms to antipsychotic medications, which may increase over time in these patients. In contrast, refractory negative symptoms and cognitive impairment are usually present at the first episode (Meltzer and Pringuey 1998). As indicated earlier, there is increasing awareness of the general need for improved treatment of negative symptoms and cognitive dysfunction.

Evidence is still very minimal to indicate which clinical features observed in an individual patient at the outset of treatment should guide the choice of an individual antipsychotic agent. A typical approach to the patient with no antipsychotic treatment history is for the clinician to initiate one medication on the basis of an optimized side-effect profile, with an attempt to reach an adequate trial (typically defined in treatment guidelines as 4–6 weeks with adequate adherence to 400–600 mg of chlorpromazine equivalents per day) before switching, which may be done in favor of a second medication that is either within or across antipsychotic groups (first- or second-generation antipsychotic). After two such trials with an incomplete clinical response, the rate of response to a standard third antipsychotic trial is quite low, and alternative strategies should be considered.

The available evidence favors clozapine as the most effective antipsychotic for treatment-refractory schizophrenia, although treatment-resistant schizophrenia may respond to other second-generation antipsychotics as well (possibly at lower response rates relative to clozapine) (Conley and Kelly 2001). In addition, most clinicians and experts in this area would agree that previous treatment trials should have included at least one second-generation antipsychotic before clozapine is considered, primarily because of the added burden of frequent clinical monitoring necessary for the early detection of agranulocytosis that occurs in approximately 1% of those taking clozapine. Unfortunately, as many as 40%–70% of patients with treatment-refractory schizophrenia also experience an inadequate response to clozapine. These schizophrenia patients, who have been referred to as "ultrarefractory," have been increasingly studied in clinical trials of antipsychotic augmentation strategies. The public health effect of managing these patients is enormous; one estimate suggests that as a group they may account for up to 97% of the cost of schizophrenia (L.M. Davies and Drummond 1994). At present, among U.S. Food and Drug Administration–approved medications that are widely available in the United States, promising initial results have been obtained for the clinical response of these patients to the addition of lamotrigine and lithium (for schizoaffective patients) (Kontaxakis et al. 2005).

The neurobiological basis for treatment resistance in schizophrenia is an area of increasing scientific interest, given the public health effect of this phenomenon. Patients with treatment-refractory schizophrenia have been found to have relatively greater cortical atrophy on MRI (Stern et al. 1993) and a higher likelihood of altered cortical cell migration (Kirkpatrick et al. 1999), compared with those with treatment-responsive schizophrenia. A more recent focus on the molecular basis for treatment resistance suggests that the activity at the blood–brain barrier may play a key role, as it appears to do in other medically refractory brain diseases. In particular, P-glycoprotein (Pgp) is an important drug efflux transporter that binds most antipsychotic medications, in addition to a range of medications implicated in treatment-refractory cases of various cancers and infections. Competitive inhibitors of Pgp can reverse multidrug resistance in tumor cells

and bacteria, and furthermore, clozapine is not transported by Pgp to any clinically relevant degree, which may provide one explanation for its superiority in treatment-refractory cases. These findings suggest that future attempts to overcome treatment resistance may benefit from adjunctive treatments that enhance brain levels of antipsychotics (Loscher and Potschka 2005).

Other Adjunctive Biological Treatments for Schizophrenia

As implied earlier, a range of other medications are used together with antipsychotics in the various phases of treatment of schizophrenia. Anticholinergic medications are a mainstay of treatment, serving as effective prophylaxis for EPS found in response to not only first-generation antipsychotics but occasionally second-generation antipsychotics (especially risperidone). Some second-generation antipsychotics such as clozapine and olanzapine have significant intrinsic anticholinergic activity, which may be partly responsible for their lower rates of EPS and obviates the need for a second anticholinergic agent. Benzodiazepines are also well used in the treatment of acute psychosis and effective in treating akathisia associated with antipsychotics. They are often used in maintenance treatment of psychotic symptoms and in the treatment of anxiety and insomnia commonly found in these patients. It remains unclear if benzodiazepines allow for the effective use of relatively lower doses of antipsychotics generally across large samples of schizophrenic patients; however, this may be the case for individual patients (Wolkowitz and Pickar 1991). Other adjunctive treatments that target co-occurring symptoms in schizophrenic patients include anticonvulsants (Hosak and Libiger 2002), β-blockers and lithium for aggressive and impulsive behaviors, and antidepressants for both depressive and anxiety disorders that are commonly found in schizophrenia (Escamilla 2001). These important symptoms confer a significant portion of the morbidity and public health effect of schizophrenia, including significant rates of suicide, and adequate treatment of these symptoms is essential to achieve clinical stability and recovery in these patients. Clinicians should remain mindful that the rate of drug–drug interactions increases and adherence decreases with increasing complexity of medication regimens, as for the treatment of medical and psychiatric illness in general.

Electroconvulsive therapy (ECT) is another treatment modality that may continue to have a role in the rapid treatment of acute and subacute states that are refractory to pharmacological intervention, particularly catatonia (Tharyan and Adams 2005). ECT treatment has been refined considerably over the years and now is quite safely administered, with minimal short-term adverse events and no evidence for long-term morbidity associated with its use (Rasmussen et al. 2002). Short-term cognitive dysfunction is common with its use; however, greater cognitive dysfunction is often associated with the illness states for which ECT is indicated (primarily acute treatment-refractory schizophrenia and mood disorders). Nevertheless, access to ECT is limited in many treatment settings, and ECT has no apparent advantage over pharmacological treatment in the maintenance phase of schizophrenia. Another biologically based treatment modality currently being evaluated for patients with schizophrenia is rTMS, which has shown preliminary efficacy in reducing the severity of auditory hallucinations (Hoffman et al. 2000).

Psychosocial Treatments for Schizophrenia

Overview: The Importance of Integrated Treatment for Schizophrenia

Psychosocial treatment is an essential element of the treatment needs of all patients with schizophrenia. In general, all of the interventions described in this subsection are compatible not only with one another but also with pharmacological treatment (Lauriello et al. 2003). Because schizophrenia is a complex disorder that affects virtually every psychological and functional domain, a comprehensive treatment approach to schizophrenia must necessarily address a broad spectrum of problems. Lehman (1999) proposed a framework for evaluating outcomes in schizophrenia, which was based on the findings of a National Institute of Mental Health expert panel. Four domains were identified: clinical, rehabilitative, humanitarian, and public welfare. The clinical domain includes psychopathology and treatment issues. The rehabilitative domain includes social and vocational function. The humanitarian domain includes quality of life, subjective well-being, and other patient-centered measures, and the public welfare domain includes optimizing and resolving the rights of the patients with the welfare of the community at large. It is increasingly recognized that integration of care is associated with maximal benefit for patients with schizophrenia, particularly those who are the sickest and are the highest users of services (Lenroot et al. 2003). A cornerstone of

this perspective is the establishment and maintenance of the alliance not only with the patient but also with families and other care and service providers. This is also of increasing importance given the progressive shifting of the locus of care for the most severely chronically disabled schizophrenic patients—from the large state hospitals of an earlier era to the community in the present.

Case Management and Assertive Community Treatment

Case management is fundamentally a method of coordinating services for the patient in the community. In this model, an individual case manager (typically, a licensed social worker) serves a role somewhat analogous to that of a primary care physician, assessing and prioritizing the needs of the patient, developing an integrated care plan, arranging for provision of this care, and serving as the patient's primary point of contact in the mental health system. Case managers interact with both social service agencies and clinicians to achieve and maintain access to entitlements, social services, and clinical care. Case management aims to maintain the patient in the system of care, to permit the most efficacious treatment in the least restrictive setting, and to optimize outcome, particularly quality of life and social function.

One particularly successful form of case management is referred to in the United States as Assertive Community Treatment (ACT). Candidates for this care are typically identified in community mental health settings as those with the highest service needs (e.g., the most frequent users of emergency or inpatient services) and referred to a multidisciplinary team, often composed of the case manager (licensed social worker or psychologist), psychiatric nurse, psychiatrist, and other psychiatric support staff. These teams have a fixed caseload and a high staff-to-patient ratio, delivering care when and where the patient requires it, including at the patient's residence, clinics and hospitals, and social service agencies, 24 hours a day. ACT approaches have much the same goals as case management in general, with a more aggressive strategy targeted at a select population of the highest users of services. These approaches have been increasingly studied and in most studies appear to reduce the time spent in the hospital (Bustillo et al. 2001) and improve the stability of housing maintenance (Issakidis et al. 1999). This type of intensive case management may particularly benefit the highest users of mental health services (Issakidis et al. 1999).

Cognitive-Behavioral Therapy

Some of the earliest documented experience with cognitive-behavioral therapy (CBT) addressed cases of schizophrenia. CBT was used to treat schizophrenia in the United Kingdom during a period (1970s–1980s) when clinicians in the United States used it primarily for treatment of depression, and CBT remains more popular in the United Kingdom for the treatment of schizophrenia (Turkington et al. 2006). It has been argued that CBT has been prematurely dismissed in the United States in an overgeneralized backlash against psychoanalytic psychotherapy as a treatment for schizophrenia (Turkington et al. 2006). Several features of CBT techniques are highly modified for use with schizophrenic patients. For instance, a relatively greater emphasis is placed on development of the therapeutic alliance as it arises from the patient's perspective. This may include a neutral stance with respect to the patient's delusional content to promote discovery and understanding. The clinician also works to identify and develop alternative explanations of symptoms that are acceptable to both patient and therapist. Another technique involves the use of "peripheral questioning," in which the therapist facilitates the patient to elaborate the belief system, and a related approach of "inference chaining," in which the personalized meaning and string of logic underlying a delusional structure are identified. These strategies are used together with a graded reality testing, with the goal of introducing doubt and possible alternative hypotheses. Cognitive-behavioral therapists attempt to normalize the patient's experience when it is appropriate and in general reduce the effect of positive symptoms. CBT is probably not advisable when the patient is too paranoid, withdrawn, or cognitively impaired to engage in treatment. However, it does not require that the patient accept the diagnosis of schizophrenia in order to be beneficial because it is more focused on symptoms than on the diagnosis per se. It is also very compatible with biological approaches to the understanding and treatment of schizophrenia (Turkington et al. 2006).

CBT is generally very amenable to empirical research. Thus, numerous randomized, controlled studies have shown that CBT is associated with greater improvement in symptom severity relative to both supportive therapy and treatment as usual (Dickerson and Lehman 2006; Turkington et al. 2006). In addition, patients with a first-episode psychosis do appear to benefit from CBT with reduced inpatient days, better treatment adherence, and reduced symptoms, relative to control treatments (Penn et al. 2005).

Cognitive Remediation and Rehabilitation

Cognitive remediation and rehabilitation emphasize the cognitive deficits that are readily evident in schizophrenia and are associated with functional impairment. Techniques include training exercises that have been successfully used in diverse clinical populations such as focal brain-injured and learning-disabled individuals. Computer-based or "pencil-and-paper" tasks guide patients through successive levels of skill in performing cognitive tasks of attention, memory, cognitive flexibility, problem solving, and other functions that are impaired in these patients. Treatment courses typically extend from 1 to 6 months with multiple sessions each week. The evidence to date suggests that certain cognitive functions (such as problem solving) may improve with this type of treatment, and modest effects on social function have been observed in some studies (Bellack et al. 1999).

Social Skills–Based Therapies

Social skills have been defined by Bellack and Mueser (1993) as "specific response capabilities necessary for effective social performance." Deficits in these functions are well established in schizophrenia. Social skills training aims to improve social function in patients by training the behavioral repertoire called on in social settings. One form of training, the basic model, decomposes complex social sequences into simpler components, with subsequent corrective training in which role-playing is used, and the settings should be as naturalistic as possible. In contrast, the social problem-solving model emphasizes improvements in cognitive functions that are thought to underlie social dysfunction. Deficits in receptive and expressive communicatory functions are addressed in the context of treatment adherence, basic social interactions, recreation, and general self-care. The basic model appears to exert benefit for outcome measures that are similar to domains of training; however, it has not been shown to exert a significant effect on improved social adjustment in the community (Dilk and Bond 1996). The social problem-solving model is associated with improvements in measures of social adjustment that may last at least a few years (Liberman et al. 1998).

Vocational Rehabilitation

The rate of continuous employment in a competitive setting (outside of a rehabilitation or "sheltered" work setting) among patients with schizophrenia is probably much lower than 20% in most communities (Lehman 1995). This therefore represents an important goal for improved functional status in schizophrenia. Sheltered work settings provide an environment for patients in which the work and social demands are manageable and the interpersonal environment is accepting of limitations caused by the patient's illness. A contemporary example is the Compensated Work Therapy offered in Department of Veterans Affairs outpatient settings. Other vocational services include more formal job training programs. Individualized placement, with some accommodation of patient preferences; minimization of preemployment screening or pretraining; and sustained periods of support are important to the patient's success. The long-term goal for many patients will be attaining employment in competitive settings in the community. This does appear to be a more frequent outcome after these types of vocational rehabilitation compared with more traditional vocational rehabilitation (Bustillo et al. 2001).

Family Therapy

Interventions that involve working with the families of those with schizophrenia emphasize the importance of the family as the primary environment in which the disease is expressed and modified in a reciprocal manner and that the family is the first line of support for most patients. Intact, adequately functioning family environments offer an important buffer for the symptoms of schizophrenia and are associated with a relatively better prognosis for the patient. Reducing family distress and fostering a collaborative approach to treatment involving the patient, family, and treatment team are important goals for patients at all stages of illness. Earlier studies and models of interaction in families of patients with schizophrenia had been focused on the construct of expressed emotion, in which high rates of expressions critical of the patient were associated with elevated relapse rates. Approaches to these families often include psychoeducation and psychological support, which aid family members in anticipation of the patient's illness expression, and response strategies that help both patient and relatives optimally cope with the patient's illness.

The various forms of family therapy are probably equally efficacious (Penn and Mueser 1996) for all patients with schizophrenia and their families. An earlier review of 14 studies found that family therapy reduced relapse rates considerably (Carpenter 1996), although curiously, the more recent studies did not report benefits for relapse prevention, which may be a result of the relatively low base relapse rates in the comparison treatment groups, who received intensive treatments in some studies (Bustillo et al. 2001). Impor-

tantly, some of the benefit of family therapy may be derived from enhanced adherence to other concurrent treatments. This treatment approach appears cost-effective, may be useful in ethnic and cultural minority families, and in some cases has been structured in treatment manuals, suggesting a potential for wider application in the community (Bustillo et al. 2001).

Individual Psychotherapy

Following the landmark studies by May et al. (1981) and Gunderson et al. (1984), in which no benefit of individual psychoanalytically oriented psychotherapy was found for patients with schizophrenia, this treatment approach has been largely abandoned in the treatment of schizophrenia. At present, individual psychotherapy is generally considered to elevate the risk for psychotic decompensation, probably because of the unstructured and anxiety-provoking nature of this treatment. In contrast, supportive therapy approaches appear to be superior to treatment as usual in studies in which the primary focus is on relative efficacy of CBT. Supportive therapy is a diverse set of approaches to the patient, yet all have in common the goal of providing reassurance, guidance, and an interpersonal environment that is stable, predictable, and tolerant of the patient's expression, symptoms, and problems in living. It is generally less systematic and less symptom-focused than CBT. One particular approach has been termed *personal therapy,* which was developed by Hogarty et al. (1995). It uses techniques that are individualized for the patient, with progressive focus on stress reduction first, followed by cognitive reframing, and later vocational rehabilitation, as the emphasis follows the patient's stage of recovery. Sessions are conducted weekly, with each session typically lasting 30–45 minutes. Empirical evaluation found personal therapy to exert relatively greater benefit for social adjustment compared with other forms of individual or family therapy (Hogarty et al. 1997).

Related Psychotic Disorders

Schizoaffective Disorder

The construct of schizoaffective disorder addresses individuals who have prominent features of both schizophrenia and major mood disorders. The term appears to have originated with Kasanin, who referred to acute schizoaffective psychosis to describe patients with the acute onset of perceptual distortions and "emotional turmoil" that were typically precipitated by a "difficult environmental situation." At that time, these patients were considered to have a subtype of dementia praecox, yet with good premorbid adjustment, rapid recovery, and subsequent achievement of good social and occupational function. This particular definition of schizoaffective disorder appears to resemble the clinical profile of persons who are currently assigned a diagnosis of either acute mania in bipolar affective disorder type I or borderline personality disorder rather than a profile in which DSM-IV-TR criterion A is met for schizophrenia.

The diagnosis of schizoaffective disorder has remained somewhat ambiguous, although it has nevertheless gained in recognition and is increasingly assigned to individuals in clinical settings. The current DSM-IV-TR diagnostic criteria for schizoaffective disorder require an uninterrupted period of illness during which criterion A for schizophrenia is met, along with criteria for depressive, manic, or mixed mood episode. This criterion is the major distinction from schizophrenia per se. During this same period, either delusions or hallucinations must be present for at least 2 weeks in the absence of prominent mood symptoms. This criterion is the major distinction from psychotic mood episodes. Both the reliability and the construct validity of this diagnosis have yet to be adequately established. Several hypothetical ways to conceive of these patients currently exist: 1) as having two coexisting disorders (schizophrenia and a mood disorder), 2) as having primarily schizophrenia with incidental mood symptoms, 3) as having primarily a mood disorder with some features of schizophrenia, or 4) as representing a distinct third group that has only phenomenological similarity to the two major diagnostic origins. Alternatively, patients with schizoaffective disorder may be a heterogeneous group in which some are more accurately deemed to have schizophrenia, whereas others have a mood disorder.

The epidemiological aspects of schizoaffective disorder largely remain to be determined. The base prevalence may be less than 1% in the community, although the disorder is found at much higher rates in clinical settings. The relatives of patients with schizoaffective disorder have an elevated risk for both schizophrenia and mood disorders. Conversely, children with family histories of either schizophrenia or bipolar disorders develop schizoaffective disorder at an elevated rate (Berrettini 2000; Gershon et al. 1988). Individuals with schizoaffective disorder have an elevated rate of winter and spring births compared with the community, like those with schizophrenia and bipolar disorder (Torrey

et al. 1997). A significant percentage of these patients show a deteriorating clinical course with persistent psychosis, although many others show a clinical course more similar to that of bipolar disorder patients (Benabarre et al. 2001). The relative chronology of psychotic and mood symptoms can show varying patterns, being concurrent in some patients and alternating in others; the relative occurrence of these symptom groups can shift over time in individual patients as well.

Overall, the prognosis for schizoaffective patients is intermediate between that for patients with schizophrenia and that for patients with mood disorders. Predictors of poor prognosis in schizoaffective disorder include many of those also established for schizophrenia, including a family history of schizophrenia, poor premorbid function, insidious onset, early age at onset, lack of a clear precipitating factor, predominance of psychotic symptoms, and poor recovery between episodes. With regard to empirical studies of treatment, study samples composed solely of schizoaffective patients are rare; however, many studies of pharmacological treatment in schizophrenia include significant numbers of schizoaffective patients (C.M. Adler and Strakowski 2003). The results from these studies, and the general standards of clinical care in the community, suggest that the treatment for schizoaffective disorder is largely consistent with that for schizophrenia and mood disorders—atypical antipsychotics, mood stabilizers, and antidepressants are used to target the same symptomatology when it is found in schizoaffective disorder (C.M. Adler and Strakowski 2003). Little evidence favors one combination regimen over another in this illness. Patients with treatment-refractory schizoaffective disorder should be approached in a manner similar to that for patients with treatment-refractory schizophrenia or mood disorders.

Delusional Disorder

Delusional disorder is characterized by the presence of one or more nonbizarre delusions in the relative absence of other symptoms of psychosis, and criterion A for schizophrenia has not been met. This is the central DSM-IV-TR diagnostic criterion and the only one that requires the presence of a particular symptom or sign. The delusions tend to be systematized, with associated affect that is consistent with the delusional belief. However, cognitive function and personality features tend to remain intact (although the delusional belief itself may have circumscribed effects on interpersonal function). This diagnosis requires adequate exclusion of other more common psychotic disorders, such as schizophrenia, mood disorders, and dementia, and other medical etiologies. Thus, the DSM-IV-TR criteria require that any associated auditory hallucinations, or affective symptoms, are not prominent, and behavior is not odd or bizarre.

The proper determination of whether a belief is fully delusional is often challenging because it requires a categorical decision about the fixity of the belief, the implausibility or bizarreness of the belief, and the effects of the belief on other thoughts or behavior. The predominant theme of the delusional ideation is used to identify subtypes, such as persecutory, jealous, erotomanic, somatic, grandiose, mixed, and unspecified. The lifetime risk is approximately 0.05%–0.10%, as defined by DSM-IV-TR, with onset in middle to late adulthood. The diagnostic stability of delusional disorder may be relatively low because many patients will develop other psychotic symptoms leading to the diagnosis of schizophrenia. However, the pattern of clinical features and familial aggregation suggest that delusional disorder should not be classified as a subtype of schizophrenia or other psychotic disorders (Cardno and McGuffin 2006).

The pathophysiology of delusional disorder remains obscure, although some preliminary evidence indicates that polymorphisms in genes coding for dopamine receptors (*DRD3* and *DRD4*) are associated with the disorder (Cardno and McGuffin 2006). Most delusional disorder patients experience the delusional belief as "ego-syntonic," which means that the delusional thought is experienced as consistent with the patients' expectations, sense of self, and sense of reality in general. This sharply limits the capacity for insight into the nature of the belief, and as a result, patients generally do not have any incentive to enter mental health treatment because the subjective distress they feel is attributed to a rigid sense of the "state of affairs" in their environment rather than a psychological state in need of remediation. In addition, patients generally do not come to the attention of the mental health system because aggressive behavior or decline in self-care (which would prompt intervention from law enforcement, emergency medical, or social services) is not typical. However, a small percentage of these patients may be at significant risk for aggressive behavior, particularly those with persecutory delusions, which may prompt them to "defend" or retaliate against the perceived source of malevolence. Violent behavior also may result from the relentless pursuit observed in some jealous or erotomanic subtypes of delusional patients. This violence risk is observed among patients with paranoid schizophrenia as well;

however, the relatively preserved cognitive function of the patient with delusional disorder may allow him or her greater capacity to plan and carry out a premeditated act of serious violence. Comorbid substance use can heighten this risk of violence by 10-fold (Smith and Buckley 2006). Involuntary hospitalization is required when the confluence of risk factors indicates that the delusional disorder patient is at significant acute risk for violence. Unfortunately, these patients often become increasingly entrenched in their delusional conviction under stress, and with the act of hospitalization often perceived as antagonistic to their needs, they often refuse treatment while in the hospital and after discharge. However, with a careful approach to the psychological state of this patient, an alliance can be achieved occasionally, often centered around the patient's subjective distress in response to the delusional belief. In response, many patients will agree to a trial of antipsychotic medication, which often relieves the distress as it effectively treats the psychotic symptoms.

The empirical evidence for antipsychotic use in delusional disorder remains scant, and treatment of delusions in this disorder largely proceeds on the basis of established efficacy against delusions in schizophrenia (Smith and Buckley 2006). A tradition to favor pimozide over other first-generation antipsychotics in these cases has arisen out of somewhat obscure origins; no good evidence supports its superiority over other first- or second-generation antipsychotics (Smith and Buckley 2006). The use of psychosocial interventions in delusional disorder has not been studied; most clinicians consider the delusional belief to be essentially unyielding to psychotherapy, but it remains to be seen if psychotherapeutic strategies such as CBT may in fact disrupt the effects of the belief on dangerous behavior or poor decision making.

Schizophreniform Disorder and Brief Psychotic Disorder

The term *schizophreniform psychosis* was initially used by Langfeldt in the 1930s to distinguish patients with schizophrenia who had a relatively better prognosis. Subsequently, the diagnostic category has received relatively little attention in empirical study. In DSM-IV-TR, the criteria for schizophreniform disorder are largely coincident with those for schizophrenia, except that the duration of symptoms in criterion A is shorter—in this case, longer than 1 month but less than 6 months. An earlier comprehensive review of outcome studies found this diagnosis to be heterogeneous and highly unstable (Strakowski 1994). A more recent large study of first-admission patients with a schizophreniform disorder diagnosis found that they were more likely to achieve full remission, and only 19% retained this diagnosis, at 24-month follow-up, with 13% later receiving a mood disorder diagnosis. In contrast, 92% of the subsample who had initially received a schizophrenia diagnosis retained that diagnosis at follow-up (Naz et al. 2003). It appears likely that at the time of diagnosis with this disorder, patients in general are early in the course of overt illness, experiencing psychotic symptoms but without the duration criterion met for schizophrenia. The relatively better prognosis for these patients as a group, compared with patients identified as having schizophrenia at first encounter, may reflect the percentage who go on to identified mood disorders and also that, as a group, these patients have not endured repeated or sustained psychotic episodes and steady functional decline, as would a percentage of any group with a clearly established diagnosis of schizophrenia.

Brief psychotic disorder, on the other hand, is distinguished from schizophrenia as a DSM-IV-TR diagnostic category by the abrupt onset of overt psychotic symptoms (the same set of positive psychotic symptoms as in criterion A for schizophrenia), but the symptoms last for less than 1 month. Individuals whose symptoms meet the criteria for this disorder do not have a history of functional decline or signs that may be retrospectively attributed to a prodrome. In addition, the psychotic symptoms associated with the diagnosis tend to be precipitated more commonly by acute stressors, be associated with acute mood changes, and generally respond well to treatment. These patients as a group also have minimal negative symptoms and a significantly better long-term prognosis than do patients with schizophrenia (on average). As with schizophreniform disorder, this diagnostic entity appears to be highly heterogeneous and reflects both the non-pathognomonic nature of psychotic symptoms and the fact that this diagnosis is established quite early in the course of illness, before certainty can be reached about a specific and enduring diagnosis with resulting implications for treatment and prognosis.

Conclusion

Our understanding of schizophrenia has evolved significantly in the era of modern medicine. This includes significant refinement in how it is identified and a deepened understanding of the natural course of illness, the relation of schizophrenia to boundary conditions, the disturbances in brain structure and function that underlie cognitive and functional deficits, and crucially the genetic and environmental factors that modify the appearance and clinical course of this illness. This progress has accelerated in recent years. The pathophysiology underlying this illness has yet to be definitively elucidated, but advances in neuroscience, genetics, and cognitive science are all being brought to bear on one of the most devastating illnesses to strike at human experience. The grail in this effort will be to attain a measure of effective primary or secondary prevention. For those who have the illness and those who care for them, advances in both psychopharmacological and psychological treatment approaches offer renewed hope that the effects of the illness can be mitigated and that patients may be increasingly able to retain a sense of well-being and a functional role in society. At the level of the individual, the family, and society, the effect of this illness remains enormous, and any breakthrough in prevention and treatment also stands to alleviate a global burden of one of humankind's most significant diseases.

Key Points

- Among medical illnesses, schizophrenia is one of the most serious for the afflicted individual, the family of the patient, and society at large.

- Schizophrenia, like psychiatric illness in general, occurs as a function of both a genetic predisposition and environmental factors.

- Schizophrenia is characterized by cognitive, perceptual, behavioral, and social disturbances and has profound consequences for the individual's capacity for autonomy and function in the community.

- Schizophrenia is currently conceived of as a neurodevelopmental disorder, with disturbances in development across a range of epochs, from early gestation through late adolescence.

- The pathophysiology of schizophrenia involves several anatomical regions and neurotransmitter and other functional systems in the brain.

- The various symptoms and problems in living that schizophrenic patients experience can be treated with the full range of treatment modalities currently available in psychiatry, including pharmacological and psychosocial approaches.

- Although many patients with schizophrenia endure relapsing and remitting periods of illness, with a significant decline in function over the early period of illness, many can retain a measure of well-being, symptom control, and autonomy in the community.

- Research into the causes, clinical course, and treatment of schizophrenia has shown considerable progress in recent times and shows promise for significant advances in the future treatment of this disorder.

Suggested Readings

Andreasen NC: Schizophrenia: the fundamental questions. Brain Res Brain Res Rev 31:106–112, 2000
Compton WM, Guze SB: The neo-Kraepelinian revolution in psychiatric diagnosis. Eur Arch Psychiatry Clin Neurosci 245:196–201, 1995
Lewis DA, Levitt P: Schizophrenia as a disorder of neurodevelopment. Annu Rev Neurosci 25:409–432, 2002
Miyamoto S, Duncan GE, Marx CE, et al: Treatments for schizophrenia: a critical review of pharmacology and mechanisms of action of antipsychotic drugs. Mol Psychiatry 10:79–104, 2005
Mueser KT, McGurk SR: Schizophrenia. Lancet 363:2063–2072, 2004

Online Resources

Schizophrenia.com: http://www.schizophrenia.com (general site, appropriate for families and lay public)
Schizophrenia Research Forum: http://www.schizophreniaforum.org (research-oriented site)

References

Abi-Dargham A, Rodenhiser J, Printz D, et al: Increased baseline occupancy of D2 receptors by dopamine in schizophrenia. Proc Natl Acad Sci U S A 97:8104–8109, 2000
Abi-Dargham A, Mawlawi O, Lombardo I, et al: Prefrontal dopamine D1 receptors and working memory in schizophrenia. J Neurosci 22:3708–3719, 2002
Addington J, Addington D: Neurocognitive and social functioning in schizophrenia: a 2.5 year follow-up study. Schizophr Res 44:47–56, 2000
Adityanjee, Aderibigbe YA, Theodoridis D, et al: Dementia praecox to schizophrenia: the first 100 years. Psychiatry Clin Neurosci 53:437–448, 1999
Adler CM, Strakowski SM: Boundaries of schizophrenia. Psychiatr Clin North Am 26:1–23, 2003
Adler LE, Pachtman E, Franks RD, et al: Neurophysiological evidence for a defect in neuronal mechanisms involved in sensory gating in schizophrenia. Biol Psychiatry 17:639–654, 1982
Adler LE, Hoffer LJ, Griffith J, et al: Normalization by nicotine of deficient auditory sensory gating in the relatives of schizophrenics. Biol Psychiatry 32:607–616, 1992
Akbarian S, Kim JJ, Potkin SG, et al: Gene expression for glutamic acid decarboxylase is reduced without loss of neurons in prefrontal cortex of schizophrenics. Arch Gen Psychiatry 52:258–266, 1995

American Psychiatric Association: Diagnostic and Statistical Manual of Mental Disorders, 2nd Edition. Washington, DC, American Psychiatric Association, 1968

American Psychiatric Association: Diagnostic and Statistical Manual of Mental Disorders, 3rd Edition. Washington, DC, American Psychiatric Association, 1980

American Psychiatric Association: Diagnostic and Statistical Manual of Mental Disorders, 3rd Edition, Revised. Washington, DC, American Psychiatric Association, 1987

American Psychiatric Association: Diagnostic and Statistical Manual of Mental Disorders, 4th Edition, Text Revision. Washington, DC, American Psychiatric Association, 2000

Andreasen NC: The evolving concept of schizophrenia: from Kraepelin to the present and future. Schizophr Res 28:105–109, 1997

Andreasen NC: Schizophrenia: the fundamental questions. Brain Res Brain Res Rev 31:106–112, 2000

Andreasen NC, Paradiso S, O'Leary DS: "Cognitive dysmetria" as an integrative theory of schizophrenia: a dysfunction in cortical-subcortical-cerebellar circuitry? Schizophr Bull 24:203–218, 1998

Angermeyer MC, Goldstein JM, Kuehn L: Gender differences in schizophrenia: rehospitalization and community survival. Psychol Med 19:365–382, 1989

Angst J: Historical aspects of the dichotomy between manic-depressive disorders and schizophrenia. Schizophr Res 57:5–13, 2002

Badner JA, Gershon ES: Meta-analysis of whole-genome linkage scans of bipolar disorder and schizophrenia. Mol Psychiatry 7:405–411, 2002

Baldessarini RJ, Cohen BM, Teicher MH: Significance of neuroleptic dose and plasma level in the pharmacological treatment of psychoses. Arch Gen Psychiatry 45:79–91, 1988

Ban TA: Neuropsychopharmacology and the genetics of schizophrenia: a history of the diagnosis of schizophrenia. Prog Neuropsychopharmacol Biol Psychiatry 28:753–762, 2004

Bellack AS, Mueser KT: Psychosocial treatment for schizophrenia. Schizophr Bull 19:317–336, 1993

Bellack AS, Gold JM, Buchanan RW: Cognitive rehabilitation for schizophrenia: problems, prospects, and strategies. Schizophr Bull 25:257–274, 1999

Benabarre A, Vieta E, Colom F, et al: Bipolar disorder, schizoaffective disorder and schizophrenia: epidemiologic, clinical and prognostic differences. Eur Psychiatry 16:167–172, 2001

Berenbaum H, Oltmanns TF: Emotional experience and expression in schizophrenia and depression. J Abnorm Psychol 101:37–44, 1992

Berman KF, Zec RF, Weinberger DR: Physiologic dysfunction of dorsolateral prefrontal cortex in schizophrenia, II: role of neuroleptic treatment, attention, and mental effort. Arch Gen Psychiatry 43:126–135, 1986

Berrettini WH: Are schizophrenic and bipolar disorders related? A review of family and molecular studies. Biol Psychiatry 48:531–538, 2000

Bilder RM, Mukherjee S, Rieder RO, et al: Symptomatic and neuropsychological components of defect states. Schizophr Bull 11:409–419, 1985

Bland RC, Parker JH, Orn H: Prognosis in schizophrenia: prognostic predictors and outcome. Arch Gen Psychiatry 35:72–77, 1978

Bombin I, Arango C, Buchanan RW: Significance and meaning of neurological signs in schizophrenia: two decades later. Schizophr Bull 31:962–977, 2005

Brenner CA, Lysaker PH, Wilt MA, et al: Visual processing and neuropsychological function in schizophrenia and schizoaffective disorder. Psychiatry Res 111:125–136, 2002

Bromet EJ, Fennig S: Epidemiology and natural history of schizophrenia. Biol Psychiatry 46:871–881, 1999

Broome MR, Woolley JB, Tabraham P, et al: What causes the onset of psychosis? Schizophr Res 79:23–34, 2005

Brown AS, Begg MD, Gravenstein S, et al: Serologic evidence of prenatal influenza in the etiology of schizophrenia. Arch Gen Psychiatry 61:774–780, 2004

Bustillo J, Lauriello J, Horan W, et al: The psychosocial treatment of schizophrenia: an update. Am J Psychiatry 158:163–175, 2001

Callicott JH, Bertolino A, Mattay VS, et al: Physiological dysfunction of the dorsolateral prefrontal cortex in schizophrenia revisited. Cereb Cortex 10:1078–1092, 2000

Cannon M, Jones PB, Murray RM: Obstetric complications and schizophrenia: historical and meta-analytic review. Am J Psychiatry 159:1080–1092, 2002

Cardno AG, McGuffin P: Genetics and delusional disorder. Behav Sci Law 24:257–276, 2006

Carlsson A, Lindqvist M: Effect of chlorpromazine or haloperidol on formation of 3methoxytyramine and normetanephrine in mouse brain. Acta Pharmacol Toxicol (Copenh) 20:140–144, 1963

Carpenter WT Jr: Maintenance therapy of persons with schizophrenia. J Clin Psychiatry 57 (suppl 9):10–18, 1996

Carpenter WT Jr, Strauss JS: The prediction of outcome in schizophrenia, IV: eleven-year follow-up of the Washington IPSS cohort. J Nerv Ment Dis 179:517–525, 1991

Cobb SR, Buhl EH, Halasy K, et al: Synchronization of neuronal activity in hippocampus by individual GABAergic interneurons. Nature 378:75–78, 1995

Cohen JD, Barch DM, Carter C, et al: Context-processing deficits in schizophrenia: converging evidence from three theoretically motivated cognitive tasks. J Abnorm Psychol 108:120–133, 1999

Compton WM, Guze SB: The neo-Kraepelinian revolution in psychiatric diagnosis. Eur Arch Psychiatry Clin Neurosci 245:196–201, 1995

Conley RR, Kelly DL: Management of treatment resistance in schizophrenia. Biol Psychiatry 50:898–911, 2001

Corcoran R, Mercer G, Frith CD: Schizophrenia, symptomatology and social inference: investigating "theory of mind" in people with schizophrenia. Schizophr Res 17:5–13, 1995

Corfas G, Roy K, Buxbaum JD: Neuregulin 1-erbB signaling and the molecular/cellular basis of schizophrenia. Nat Neurosci 7:575–580, 2004

Corrigan PW, Nelson DR: Factors that affect social cue recognition in schizophrenia. Psychiatry Res 78:189–196, 1998

Creese I, Burt DR, Snyder SH: Dopamine receptor binding predicts clinical and pharmacological potencies of antischizophrenic drugs. Science 192:481–483, 1976

Crow TJ: The two-syndrome concept: origins and current status. Schizophr Bull 11:471–486, 1985

Davidson M, Reichenberg A, Rabinowitz J, et al: Behavioral and intellectual markers for schizophrenia in apparently healthy male adolescents. Am J Psychiatry 156:1328–1335, 1999

Davies G, Welham J, Chant D, et al: A systematic review and meta-analysis of Northern Hemisphere season of birth studies in schizophrenia. Schizophr Bull 29:587–593, 2003

Davies LM, Drummond MF: Economics and schizophrenia: the real cost. Br J Psychiatry Suppl (25):18–21, 1994

Davis JM, Kane JM, Marder SR, et al: Dose response of prophylactic antipsychotics. J Clin Psychiatry 54 (suppl): 24–30, 1993

Dickerson FB, Lehman AF: Evidence-based psychotherapy for schizophrenia. J Nerv Ment Dis 194:3–9, 2006

Dierks T, Linden DE, Jandl M, et al: Activation of Heschl's gyrus during auditory hallucinations. Neuron 22:615–621, 1999

Dilk MN, Bond GR: Meta-analytic evaluation of skills training research for individuals with severe mental illness. J Consult Clin Psychol 64:1337–1346, 1996

Earnst KS, Kring AM: Emotional responding in deficit and non-deficit schizophrenia. Psychiatry Res 88:191–207, 1999

Endicott J, Forman JB, Spitzer RL: Research approaches to diagnostic classification in schizophrenia. Birth Defects Orig Artic Ser 14:41–57, 1978

Escamilla MA: Diagnosis and treatment of mood disorders that co-occur with schizophrenia. Psychiatr Serv 52:911–919, 2001

Feighner JP, Robins E, Guze SB, et al: Diagnostic criteria for use in psychiatric research. Arch Gen Psychiatry 26:57–63, 1972

Fenton WS, Blyler CR, Heinssen RK: Determinants of medication compliance in schizophrenia: empirical and clinical findings. Schizophr Bull 23:637–651, 1997

Frith CD, Corcoran R: Exploring "theory of mind" in people with schizophrenia. Psychol Med 26:521–530, 1996

Geller JL: A report on the "worst" state hospital recidivists in the US. Hosp Community Psychiatry 43:904–908, 1992

Gershon ES, DeLisi LE, Hamovit J, et al: A controlled family study of chronic psychoses: schizophrenia and schizoaffective disorder. Arch Gen Psychiatry 45:328–336, 1988

Gitlin M, Nuechterlein K, Subotnik KL, et al: Clinical outcome following neuroleptic discontinuation in patients with remitted recent-onset schizophrenia. Am J Psychiatry 158:1835–1842, 2001

Goldman-Rakic PS: Working memory dysfunction in schizophrenia. J Neuropsychiatry Clin Neurosci 6:348–357, 1994

Goodwin DW, Alderson P, Rosenthal R: Clinical significance of hallucinations in psychiatric disorders: a study of 116 hallucinatory patients. Arch Gen Psychiatry 24:76–80, 1971

Gottesman II: Schizophrenia Genesis: The Origins of Madness. New York, WH Freeman, 1991

Grace AA, Bunney BS, Moore H, et al: Dopamine-cell depolarization block as a model for the therapeutic actions of antipsychotic drugs. Trends Neurosci 20:31–37, 1997

Green AI, Canuso CM, Brenner MJ, et al: Detection and management of comorbidity in patients with schizophrenia. Psychiatr Clin North Am 26:115–139, 2003

Green M, Walker E: Symptom correlates of vulnerability to backward masking in schizophrenia. Am J Psychiatry 143:181–186, 1986

Green MF: What are the functional consequences of neurocognitive deficits in schizophrenia? Am J Psychiatry 153:321–330, 1996

Gunderson JG, Frank AF, Katz HM, et al: Effects of psychotherapy in schizophrenia, II: comparative outcome of two forms of treatment. Schizophr Bull 10:564–598, 1984

Harrison PJ: The neuropathology of schizophrenia: a critical review of the data and their interpretation. Brain 122 (pt 4):593–624, 1999

Harrow M, Jobe TH: Longitudinal studies of outcome and recovery in schizophrenia and early intervention: can they make a difference? Can J Psychiatry 50:879–880, 2005

Harvey PD, Keefe RS: Studies of cognitive change in patients with schizophrenia following novel antipsychotic treatment. Am J Psychiatry 158:176–184, 2001

Hegarty JD, Baldessarini RJ, Tohen M, et al: One hundred years of schizophrenia: a meta-analysis of the outcome literature. Am J Psychiatry 151:1409–1416, 1994

Heres S, Davis J, Maino K, et al: Why olanzapine beats risperidone, risperidone beats quetiapine, and quetiapine beats olanzapine: an exploratory analysis of head-to-head comparison studies of second-generation antipsychotics. Am J Psychiatry 163:185–194, 2006

Hoffman RE, Boutros NN, Hu S, et al: Transcranial magnetic stimulation and auditory hallucinations in schizophrenia. Lancet 355:1073–1075, 2000

Hoffman RE, Gueorguieva R, Hawkins KA, et al: Temporoparietal transcranial magnetic stimulation for auditory hallucinations: safety, efficacy and moderators in a fifty patient sample. Biol Psychiatry 58:97–104, 2005

Hogarty GE, Kornblith SJ, Greenwald D, et al: Personal therapy: a disorder-relevant psychotherapy for schizophrenia. Schizophr Bull 21:379–393, 1995

Hogarty GE, Greenwald D, Ulrich RF, et al: Three-year trials of personal therapy among schizophrenic patients living with or independent of family, II: effects on adjustment of patients. Am J Psychiatry 154:1514–1524, 1997

Hosak L, Libiger J: Antiepileptic drugs in schizophrenia: a review. Eur Psychiatry 17:371–378, 2002

Howard A, Tamas G, Soltesz I: Lighting the chandelier: new vistas for axo-axonic cells. Trends Neurosci 28:310–316, 2005

Ingvar DH, Franzen G: Abnormalities of cerebral blood flow distribution in patients with chronic schizophrenia. Acta Psychiatr Scand 50:425–462, 1974

Issakidis C, Sanderson K, Teesson M, et al: Intensive case management in Australia: a randomized controlled trial. Acta Psychiatr Scand 99:360–367, 1999

Jablensky A: Epidemiology of schizophrenia: the global burden of disease and disability. Eur Arch Psychiatry Clin Neurosci 250:274–285, 2000

Javitt DC, Zukin SR: Recent advances in the phencyclidine model of schizophrenia. Am J Psychiatry 148:1301–1308, 1991

Javitt DC, Strous RD, Grochowski S, et al: Impaired precision, but normal retention, of auditory sensory ("echoic") memory information in schizophrenia. J Abnorm Psychol 106:315–324, 1997

Jeste DV, del Carmen R, Lohr JB, et al: Did schizophrenia exist before the eighteenth century? Compr Psychiatry 26:493–503, 1985

Jobe TH, Harrow M: Long-term outcome of patients with schizophrenia: a review. Can J Psychiatry 50:892–900, 2005

Johnstone EC, Crow TJ, Frith CD, et al: Cerebral ventricular size and cognitive impairment in chronic schizophrenia. Lancet 2:924–926, 1976

Jones P, Rodgers B, Murray R, et al: Child development risk factors for adult schizophrenia in the British 1946 birth cohort. Lancet 344:1398–1402, 1994

Kanaan RA, Kim JS, Kaufmann WE, et al: Diffusion tensor imaging in schizophrenia. Biol Psychiatry 58:921–929, 2005

Kane JM, Honigfeld G, Singer J, et al: Clozapine in treatment-resistant schizophrenics. Psychopharmacol Bull 24:62–67, 1988

Kay SR, Fiszbein A, Opler LA: The Positive and Negative Syndrome Scale (PANSS) for schizophrenia. Schizophr Bull 13:261–276, 1987

Kety SS, Rosenthal D, Wender PH, et al: Mental illness in the biological and adoptive families of adopted schizophrenics. Am J Psychiatry 128:302–306, 1971

Kirkpatrick B, Conley RC, Kakoyannis A, et al: Interstitial cells of the white matter in the inferior parietal cortex in schizophrenia: an unbiased cell-counting study. Synapse 34:95–102, 1999

Kirkpatrick B, Buchanan RW, Ross DE, et al: A separate disease within the syndrome of schizophrenia. Arch Gen Psychiatry 58:165–171, 2001

Kohler CG, Bilker W, Hagendoorn M, et al: Emotion recognition deficit in schizophrenia: association with symptomatology and cognition. Biol Psychiatry 48:127–136, 2000

Kontaxakis VP, Ferentinos PP, Havaki-Kontaxakis BJ, et al: Randomized controlled augmentation trials in clozapine-resistant schizophrenic patients: a critical review. Eur Psychiatry 20:409–415, 2005

Kraepelin E: Psychiatrie: Ein kurzes Lehrbuch für Studirende und Aerzte, 4th Edition. Leipzig, Germany, Abel (Meiner), 1893

Kubicki M, McCarley R, Westin CF, et al: A review of diffusion tensor imaging studies in schizophrenia. J Psychiatr Res 41(1–2):15–30, 2007

Lauriello J, Lenroot R, Bustillo JR: Maximizing the synergy between pharmacotherapy and psychosocial therapies for schizophrenia. Psychiatr Clin North Am 26:191–211, 2003

Lawrie SM, Abukmeil SS: Brain abnormality in schizophrenia: a systematic and quantitative review of volumetric magnetic resonance imaging studies. Br J Psychiatry 172:110–120, 1998

Lehman AF: Vocational rehabilitation in schizophrenia. Schizophr Bull 21:645–656, 1995

Lehman AF: Developing an outcomes-oriented approach for the treatment of schizophrenia. J Clin Psychiatry 60 (suppl 19):30–35; discussion 36–37, 1999

Lenroot R, Bustillo JR, Lauriello J, et al: Integrated treatment of schizophrenia. Psychiatr Serv 54:1499–1507, 2003

Lewis CM, Levinson DF, Wise LH, et al: Genome scan meta-analysis of schizophrenia and bipolar disorder, part II: schizophrenia. Am J Hum Genet 73:34–48, 2003

Lewis DA: GABAergic local circuit neurons and prefrontal cortical dysfunction in schizophrenia. Brain Res Brain Res Rev 31:270–276, 2000

Lewis DA, Levitt P: Schizophrenia as a disorder of neurodevelopment. Annu Rev Neurosci 25:409–432, 2002

Liberman RP, Wallace CJ, Blackwell G, et al: Skills training versus psychosocial occupational therapy for persons with persistent schizophrenia. Am J Psychiatry 155:1087–1091, 1998

Liddle PF: The symptoms of chronic schizophrenia: a re-examination of the positive-negative dichotomy. Br J Psychiatry 151:145–151, 1987

Lieberman JA: Prediction of outcome in first-episode schizophrenia. J Clin Psychiatry 54 (suppl):13–17, 1993

Lieberman JA, Perkins D, Belger A, et al: The early stages of schizophrenia: speculations on pathogenesis, pathophysiology, and therapeutic approaches. Biol Psychiatry 50:884–897, 2001

Lieberman JA, Stroup TS, McEvoy JP, et al: Effectiveness of antipsychotic drugs in patients with chronic schizophrenia. N Engl J Med 353:1209–1223, 2005

Loscher W, Potschka H: Drug resistance in brain diseases and the role of drug efflux transporters. Nat Rev Neurosci 6:591–602, 2005

Malla A, Payne J: First-episode psychosis: psychopathology, quality of life, and functional outcome. Schizophr Bull 31:650–671, 2005

Manoach DS, Gollub RL, Benson ES, et al: Schizophrenic subjects show aberrant fMRI activation of dorsolateral prefrontal cortex and basal ganglia during working memory performance. Biol Psychiatry 48:99–109, 2000

May PR, Tuma AH, Dixon WJ, et al: Schizophrenia: a follow-up study of the results of five forms of treatment. Arch Gen Psychiatry 38:776–784, 1981

McEvoy JP, Lieberman JA, Stroup TS, et al: Effectiveness of clozapine versus olanzapine, quetiapine, and risperidone in patients with chronic schizophrenia who did not respond to prior atypical antipsychotic treatment. Am J Psychiatry 163:600–610, 2006

McGlashan TH: The Chestnut Lodge follow-up study, II: long-term outcome of schizophrenia and the affective disorders. Arch Gen Psychiatry 41:586–601, 1984

McGlashan TH: Duration of untreated psychosis in first-episode schizophrenia: marker or determinant of course? Biol Psychiatry 46:899–907, 1999

McGrath J, Saha S, Welham J, et al: A systematic review of the incidence of schizophrenia: the distribution of rates and the influence of sex, urbanicity, migrant status and methodology. BMC Med 2:13, 2004

McGue M, Gottesman II: A single dominant gene still cannot account for the transmission of schizophrenia. Arch Gen Psychiatry 46:478–480, 1989

Meltzer HY, Pringuey D: Treatment-resistant schizophrenia: the importance of early detection and treatment. Introduction. J Clin Psychopharmacol 18 (2 suppl 1):1S, 1998

Meltzer HY, Li Z, Kaneda Y, et al: Serotonin receptors: their key role in drugs to treat schizophrenia. Prog Neuropsychopharmacol Biol Psychiatry 27:1159–1172, 2003

Miyamoto S, Duncan GE, Marx CE, et al: Treatments for schizophrenia: a critical review of pharmacology and mechanisms of action of antipsychotic drugs. Mol Psychiatry 10:79–104, 2005

Moffitt TE, Caspi A, Rutter M: Strategy for investigating interactions between measured genes and measured environments. Arch Gen Psychiatry 62:473–481, 2005

Mueser KT, McGurk SR: Schizophrenia. Lancet 363:2063–2072, 2004

Murray CJ, Lopez AD: Evidence-based health policy—lessons from the Global Burden of Disease Study. Science 274:740–743, 1996

Naber D, Lambert M, Karow A: [Subjective well-being under antipsychotic treatment and its meaning for compliance and course of disease] [German]. Psychiatr Prax 31 (suppl 2):S230–232, 2004

Naz B, Bromet EJ, Mojtabai R: Distinguishing between first-admission schizophreniform disorder and schizophrenia. Schizophr Res 62:51–58, 2003

Newcomer JW: Metabolic risk during antipsychotic treatment. Clin Ther 26:1936–1946, 2004

Nicolson R, Rapoport JL: Childhood-onset schizophrenia: rare but worth studying. Biol Psychiatry 46:1418–1428, 1999

Owen MJ, Craddock N, O'Donovan MC: Schizophrenia: genes at last? Trends Genet 21:518–525, 2005

Palha AP, Esteves MF: The origin of dementia praecox. Schizophr Res 28:99–103, 1997

Penn DL, Mueser KT: Research update on the psychosocial treatment of schizophrenia. Am J Psychiatry 153:607–617, 1996

Penn DL, Waldheter EJ, Perkins DO, et al: Psychosocial treatment for first-episode psychosis: a research update. Am J Psychiatry 162:2220–2232, 2005

Percudani M, Barbui C, Tansella M: Effect of second-generation antipsychotics on employment and productivity in individuals with schizophrenia: an economic perspective. Pharmacoeconomics 22:701–718, 2004

Perlstein WM, Carter CS, Noll DC, et al: Relation of prefrontal cortex dysfunction to working memory and symptoms in schizophrenia. Am J Psychiatry 158:1105–1113, 2001

Perry W, Braff DL: Information-processing deficits and thought disorder in schizophrenia. Am J Psychiatry 151:363–367, 1994

Peters E, Day S, McKenna J, et al: Delusional ideation in religious and psychotic populations. Br J Clin Psychol 38 (pt 1):83–96, 1999

Phillips LJ, McGorry PD, Yung AR, et al: Prepsychotic phase of schizophrenia and related disorders: recent progress and future opportunities. Br J Psychiatry Suppl 48:S33–44, 2005

Pinkham AE, Penn DL, Perkins DO, et al: Implications for the neural basis of social cognition for the study of schizophrenia. Am J Psychiatry 160:815–824, 2003

Popken GJ, Bunney WE Jr, Potkin SG, et al: Subnucleus-specific loss of neurons in medial thalamus of schizophrenics. Proc Natl Acad Sci U S A 97:9276–9280, 2000

Ram R, Bromet EJ, Eaton WW, et al: The natural course of schizophrenia: a review of first-admission studies. Schizophr Bull 18:185–207, 1992

Rasmussen KG, Sampson SM, Rummans TA: Electroconvulsive therapy and newer modalities for the treatment of medication-refractory mental illness. Mayo Clin Proc 77:552–556, 2002

Remington G, Kapur S: D2 and 5-HT2 receptor effects of antipsychotics: bridging basic and clinical findings using PET. J Clin Psychiatry 60 (suppl 10):15–19, 1999

Remschmidt H: Early onset schizophrenia as a progressive-deteriorating developmental disorder: evidence from child psychiatry. J Neural Transm 109:101–117, 2002

Risch N: Genetic linkage and complex diseases, with special reference to psychiatric disorders. Genet Epidemiol 7:3–16; discussion 17–45, 1990

Robinson D, Woerner MG, Alvir JM, et al: Predictors of relapse following response from a first episode of schizophrenia or schizoaffective disorder. Arch Gen Psychiatry 56:241–247, 1999

Robinson DG, Woerner MG, Delman HM, et al: Pharmacological treatments for first-episode schizophrenia. Schizophr Bull 31:705–722, 2005

Saccuzzo DP, Braff DL: Early information processing deficit in schizophrenia: new findings using schizophrenic subgroups and manic control subjects. Arch Gen Psychiatry 38:175–179, 1981

Sakel M: A new treatment of schizophrenia. Am J Psychiatry 93:829–841, 1937

Salem JE, Kring AM, Kerr SL: More evidence for generalized poor performance in facial emotion perception in schizophrenia. J Abnorm Psychol 105:480–483, 1996

Sartorius N, Jablensky A, Shapiro R: Two-year follow-up of the patients included in the WHO International Pilot Study of Schizophrenia. Psychol Med 7:529–541, 1977

Schneider F, Gur RC, Koch K, et al: Impairment in the specificity of emotion processing in schizophrenia. Am J Psychiatry 163:442–447, 2006

Seeman P, Lee T, Chau-Wong M, et al: Antipsychotic drug doses and neuroleptic/dopamine receptors. Nature 261:717–719, 1976

Shelley AM, Ward PB, Catts SV, et al: Mismatch negativity: an index of a preattentive processing deficit in schizophrenia. Biol Psychiatry 30:1059–1062, 1991

Smith DA, Buckley PF: Pharmacotherapy of delusional disorders in the context of offending and the potential for compulsory treatment. Behav Sci Law 24:351–367, 2006

Steen RG, Mull C, McClure R, et al: Brain volume in first-episode schizophrenia: systematic review and meta-analysis of magnetic resonance imaging studies. Br J Psychiatry 188:510–518, 2006

Stefansson H, Sigurdsson E, Steinthorsdottir V, et al: Neuregulin 1 and susceptibility to schizophrenia. Am J Hum Genet 71:877–892, 2002

Stern RG, Kahn RS, Davidson M: Predictors of response to neuroleptic treatment in schizophrenia. Psychiatr Clin North Am 16:313–338, 1993

Stone MH: Exploratory psychotherapy in schizophrenia-spectrum patients: a reevaluation in the light of long-term follow-up of schizophrenic and borderline patients. Bull Menninger Clin 50:287–306, 1986

Strakowski SM: Diagnostic validity of schizophreniform disorder. Am J Psychiatry 151:815–824, 1994

Straub RE, Jiang Y, MacLean CJ, et al: Genetic variation in the 6p22.3 gene DTNBP1, the human ortholog of the mouse dysbindin gene, is associated with schizophrenia. Am J Hum Genet 71:337–348, 2002

Susser E, Neugebauer R, Hoek HW, et al: Schizophrenia after prenatal famine: further evidence. Arch Gen Psychiatry 53:25–31, 1996

Susser ES, Schaefer CA, Brown AS, et al: The design of the Prenatal Determinants of Schizophrenia Study. Schizophr Bull 26:257–273, 2000

Tandon R: In conclusion: does antipsychotic treatment modify the long-term course of schizophrenic illness? J Psychiatr Res 32:251–253, 1998

Tandon R, Fleischhacker WW: Comparative efficacy of antipsychotics in the treatment of schizophrenia: a critical assessment. Schizophr Res 79:145–155, 2005

Terkelsen KG, Menikoff A: Measuring the costs of schizophrenia: implications for the post-institutional era in the US. Pharmacoeconomics 8:199–222, 1995

Tharyan P, Adams CE: Electroconvulsive therapy for schizophrenia. Cochrane Database Syst Rev (2):CD000076, 2005

Tienari P, Wynne LC, Moring J, et al: The Finnish adoptive family study of schizophrenia: implications for family research. Br J Psychiatry Suppl (23):20–26, 1994

Torrey EF, Miller J, Rawlings R, et al: Seasonality of births in schizophrenia and bipolar disorder: a review of the literature. Schizophr Res 28:1–38, 1997

Tsuang MT, Winokur G: The Iowa 500: field work in a 35-year follow-up of depression, mania, and schizophrenia. Can Psychiatr Assoc J 20:359–365, 1975

Turkington D, Kingdon D, Weiden PJ: Cognitive behavior therapy for schizophrenia. Am J Psychiatry 163:365–373, 2006

Turner TH: Schizophrenia and mental handicap: an historical review, with implications for further research. Psychol Med 19:301–314, 1989

Turner TH: Schizophrenia as a permanent problem: some aspects of historical evidence in the recency (new disease) hypothesis. Hist Psychiatry 3:413–429, 1992

Volk DW, Austin MC, Pierri JN, et al: Decreased glutamic acid decarboxylase67 messenger RNA expression in a subset of prefrontal cortical gamma-aminobutyric acid neurons in subjects with schizophrenia. Arch Gen Psychiatry 57:237–245, 2000

U.S. Institute of Medicine: Neurological, Psychiatric, and Developmental Disorders: Meeting the Challenges in the Developing World. Washington, DC, National Academy of Sciences, 2001

Walker EF, Savoie T, Davis D: Neuromotor precursors of schizophrenia. Schizophr Bull 20:441–451, 1994

Walker E, Kestler L, Bollini A, et al: Schizophrenia: etiology and course. Annu Rev Psychol 55:401–430, 2004

Weinberger DR, Berman KF, Zec RF: Physiologic dysfunction of dorsolateral prefrontal cortex in schizophrenia, I: regional cerebral blood flow evidence. Arch Gen Psychiatry 43:114–124, 1986

Wolkowitz OM, Pickar D: Benzodiazepines in the treatment of schizophrenia: a review and reappraisal. Am J Psychiatry 148:714–726, 1991

Wu EQ, Birnbaum HG, Shi L, et al: The economic burden of schizophrenia in the United States in 2002. J Clin Psychiatry 66:1122–1129, 2005

Wyatt RJ, Henter ID: The effects of early and sustained intervention on the long-term morbidity of schizophrenia. J Psychiatr Res 32:169–177, 1998

Xiberas X, Martinot JL, Mallet L, et al: Extrastriatal and striatal D(2) dopamine receptor blockade with haloperidol or new antipsychotic drugs in patients with schizophrenia. Br J Psychiatry 179:503–508, 2001

Zygmunt A, Olfson M, Boyer CA, et al: Interventions to improve medication adherence in schizophrenia. Am J Psychiatry 159:1653–1664, 2002

11

MOOD DISORDERS

John A. Joska, M.D., M.Med.(Psych.), F.C.Psych.(S.A.)
Dan J. Stein, M.D., Ph.D.

Mood critically affects perception and appraisal of the self and the environment. Changes in mood occur as part of everyday experience, in response to multiple factors. In a proportion of people, mood states can become distressing, and psychopathology ensues. In this chapter, we describe the clinical features of mood disorders, summarize knowledge of their pathogenesis, and outline current approaches to management.

Phenomenology of Mood Disorders

The diagnosis and classification of mood disorders have long been central concerns of psychiatry. Mood problems present in multiple ways, with variation across age, gender, culture, and medical setting. We summarize the current approaches to the phenomenology of mood disorders.

Classification of Mood Disorders

The two major classification systems—DSM-IV-TR (American Psychiatric Association 2000a) and ICD-10 (World Health Organization 1992)—emphasize the importance of having reliable and valid diagnostic criteria for each of the major mood disorders. These classifications also reflect accumulated knowledge about

distinctions between different mood disorders (e.g., unipolar vs. bipolar) and subtypes (e.g., typical vs. atypical).

DSM-IV-TR and ICD-10

The DSM-IV-TR diagnosis of major depressive episode requires the presence of 5 out of a possible 9 symptoms. Further subtypes of major depression are possible, on the basis of the quality of depression, nature of vegetative symptoms, and presence of certain associated features such as the duration of mood symptoms and whether they occur in relation to certain events (e.g., childbirth or seasonal change).

ICD-10 requires the presence of 4 from a list of 10 symptoms for a diagnosis of major depression. Subtle but important differences between DSM-IV-TR and ICD-10 exist: ICD-10 includes "a loss of confidence and self-esteem." In addition, ICD-10 includes somatic symptoms as a defining symptom cluster, whereas DSM-IV-TR does not.

Boundaries

Debate is ongoing about the boundaries between mood and other disorders. Current approaches allow for the diagnosis of comorbid mood and anxiety disorders, yielding data on comorbidity of major depression and anxiety disorders and of bipolar disorder and anxiety disorders (M.P. Freeman et al. 2002). An alternative approach conceptualizes depressive and anxiety symptoms as part of the same construct; mixed anxiety-depressive disorder currently appears only in the research appendix of DSM-IV-TR but is highly prevalent in clinical samples.

Mood and psychotic disorders, too, can be difficult to distinguish. Many patients with severe mood disorders have psychotic symptoms, and many patients with primary psychotic disorders develop mood symptoms or disorders. A categorical approach requires that patients with both disorders are, for example, classified as *schizoaffective*. An alternative approach suggests that these conditions lie on a unitary spectrum of psychopathology, with some patients evolving over time into one category or another.

Again, conceptual difficulties arise with respect to patients who present with both Axis I and Axis II disorders. DSM places mood disorders on Axis I and personality disorders on Axis II. However, the presence of depression—affective instability is a feature of some personality disorders—and the treatment of an Axis I mood disorder may result in changes in personality disorder traits (Akiskal 1996). An alternative approach, therefore, would be to amalgamate both mood disorders and affectively based personality disorders (e.g., borderline) on a single axis.

Subtypes and Forms of Mood Disorders

Assessment of mood disorders requires both a cross-sectional and a longitudinal review. Figure 11–1 summarizes mood disorders according to episode features and specifiers.

Clinical Features of Depression
Mental State Examination

Certain features of depression may be present on the mental state examination. These include a downcast appearance, poor eye contact, and diminished or increased psychomotor activity. Speech may be slow and monotonous, with delays in the production of speech (so-called speech latency or speech pause time). The patient with depression may describe a low mood or may represent it by using particular cultural idioms. Affective expression in depression varies from bland and restricted to anxious, dysphoric, and agitated. Thought may be altered in depression—ranging from slowed flow to poverty of ideation. In psychotic depression, the patient may have loosening of associations, delusions of nihilism ("I am worthless"; "I will be dying shortly"), perceptual disturbances (defamatory and command-type auditory hallucinations are

commonest), and visual hallucinations. Cognitive impairment can occur, with disturbed memory, attention, and executive functions.

Depressed Mood and Anhedonia

Together with low mood, a loss of pleasure—anhedonia—is the other essential feature of a DSM-IV-TR diagnosis of depression. Factor analytic studies have established that low mood and anhedonia are consistently present in individuals with depression and, as such, are critical to its diagnosis (Nelson and Charney 1981). In addition to the presence of depression, factors such as the duration, severity, and intensity of the depression must be considered. Qualitative differences in mood are seen in depressive disorders: an inability to experience a lifting of mood in the presence of typically rewarding events is a key feature of melancholia (lack of "mood reactivity"). This subtype of depression includes the problems of early-morning awakening and diurnal variation in mood (see Figure 11–1).

Cognitive, Neurovegetative, and Behavioral Symptoms

Cognitive impairment in depression includes the errors in information processing and distortions described by a cognitive-behavioral model. These include negative thoughts about the self, the world, and the future. These negative thoughts may begin with vague negative thoughts about the self and the future but ultimately lead to the emergence and expression of suicidal thoughts. Neuropsychological disturbances in depression include poor performance on tests of memory, concentration, and executive functions. In the elderly, this may lead to inappropriate diagnosis of cognitive disorders such as dementia (a condition known as "pseudodementia").

Disturbances of sleep, appetite, and sexual behavior are sometimes referred to as "neurovegetative." Patients describe different sleep patterns in depression, but the presence of terminal insomnia, or early-morning awakening, may be a particularly severe symptom. Appetite is often diminished and, if persistent, will be followed by a significant loss of weight. Sexual interest and activity are also reduced. A small proportion of individuals sleep and eat excessively (hypersomnia and hyperphagia); these symptoms are part of the syndrome of atypical depression (see Figure 11–1).

Duration, Intensity, and Specifiers

Assessment of the depressive episode includes evaluation of the duration of the current episode, the inten-

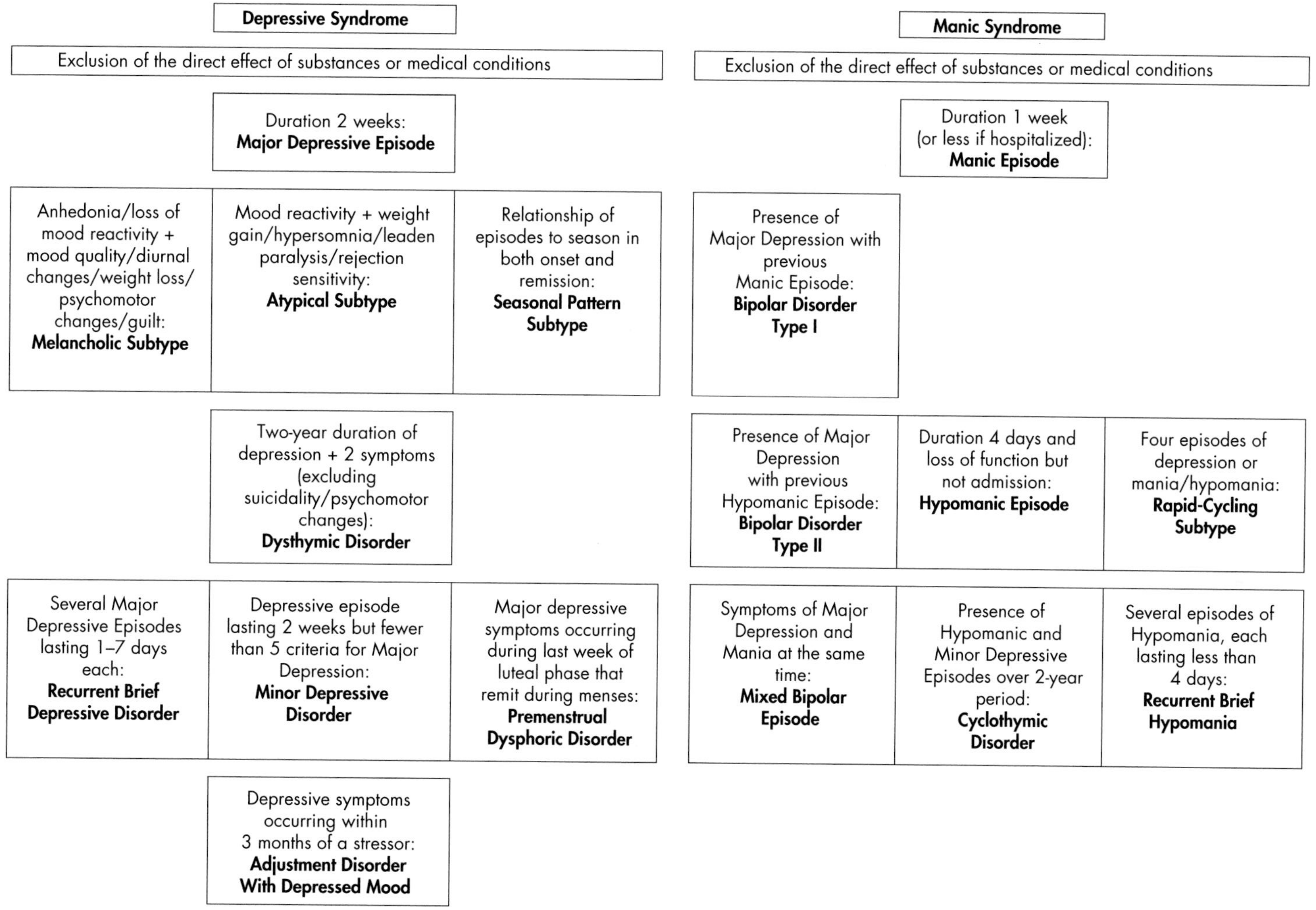

FIGURE 11–1.   Summary of mood disorders, specifiers, and relationships.

sity of the episode, and any episode specifiers. The diagnosis of major depression requires depressive symptoms to be present for most days over a 2-week period. When symptoms have been present for a shorter period, a diagnosis of depressive disorder not otherwise specified or recurrent brief depression may be considered. When depression lasts 2 years or more, the diagnosis of dysthymic disorder is possible.

Although the characterization of an episode as mild, moderate, or severe may seem overly broad, it potentially helps inform management by suggesting which episode may require intensive, combined, or in-patient treatments. In addition, more severe depressive episodes have a tendency to recur more frequently and may require a longer duration of treatment (Kessler et al. 1994).

DSM-IV-TR includes several episode specifiers. Some, which have been mentioned earlier, include subtype specifiers, such as depression with melancholia, atypical features, or catatonic features. Other specifiers indicate when depression occurs: postpartum onset (occurring within 4 weeks of childbirth) or seasonal onset (occurring during a particular season, usually winter). The presence of psychotic symptoms should also be specified.

Major Depressive Disorder

Diagnostic Criteria

The DSM-IV-TR diagnostic criteria for major depressive episode are listed in Table 11–1.

TABLE 11–1. DSM-IV-TR diagnostic criteria for major depressive episode

A. Five (or more) of the following symptoms have been present during the same 2-week period and represent a change from previous functioning; at least one of the symptoms is either (1) depressed mood or (2) loss of interest or pleasure.

Note: Do not include symptoms that are clearly due to a general medical condition, or mood-incongruent delusions or hallucinations.

(1) depressed mood most of the day, nearly every day, as indicated by either subjective report (e.g., feels sad or empty) or observation made by others (e.g., appears tearful). **Note:** In children and adolescents, can be irritable mood.

(2) markedly diminished interest or pleasure in all, or almost all, activities most of the day, nearly every day (as indicated by either subjective account or observation made by others)

(3) significant weight loss when not dieting or weight gain (e.g., a change of more than 5% of body weight in a month), or decrease or increase in appetite nearly every day. **Note:** In children, consider failure to make expected weight gains.

(4) insomnia or hypersomnia nearly every day

(5) psychomotor agitation or retardation nearly every day (observable by others, not merely subjective feelings of restlessness or being slowed down)

(6) fatigue or loss of energy nearly every day

(7) feelings of worthlessness or excessive or inappropriate guilt (which may be delusional) nearly every day (not merely self-reproach or guilt about being sick)

(8) diminished ability to think or concentrate, or indecisiveness, nearly every day (either by subjective account or as observed by others)

(9) recurrent thoughts of death (not just fear of dying), recurrent suicidal ideation without a specific plan, or a suicide attempt or a specific plan for committing suicide

B. The symptoms do not meet criteria for a mixed episode.

C. The symptoms cause clinically significant distress or impairment in social, occupational, or other important areas of functioning.

D. The symptoms are not due to the direct physiological effects of a substance (e.g., a drug of abuse, a medication) or a general medical condition (e.g., hypothyroidism).

E. The symptoms are not better accounted for by bereavement; i.e., after the loss of a loved one, the symptoms persist for longer than 2 months or are characterized by marked functional impairment, morbid preoccupation with worthlessness, suicidal ideation, psychotic symptoms, or psychomotor retardation.

Single-Episode Versus Recurrent Major Depression

Recurrence only follows a previously remitted episode and should not be diagnosed in the presence of residual symptoms of an inadequately treated episode. DSM-IV-TR allows for the addition of interepisode specifiers: with or without full interepisode recovery. This distinction usually depends on the degree of symptom remission assessed by the clinician. The use of rating scales such as the Hamilton Rating Scale for Depression may be useful (Hamilton 1960). Symptom scores of less than 75% of baseline, for example, are considered remitted.

Other Depressive Disorders

Dysthymia

Dysthymic disorder is a common depressive condition, with a lifetime prevalence of up to 6% of the population (J. D. Moore and Bona 2001). It is characterized by milder depressive symptoms than in major depression that persist for at least 2 years, with a symptom-free period of only 2 months in each year (Table 11–2). A major depressive episode may occur after onset of dysthymia (so-called double depression) (J. D. Moore and Bona 2001).

Psychotic Depression

The presence of psychotic symptoms in depression is an indication of severity and a tendency to recurrence (Coryell 1996). Inpatient treatment is usually required because of associated risk. Nihilistic or somatic delusions, together with auditory hallucinations, constitute the commonest psychotic symptoms in major depression. Significant impairment, distress, and sometimes suicide accompany this syndrome. The differential diagnosis includes schizophrenia and schizoaffective disorder.

Seasonal Affective Disorder

Seasonal affective disorder (SAD) is a recent entry to the diagnostic system (Rosenthal et al. 1984). It is now classified as a mood disorder specifier—with seasonal pattern. In major depressive disorder, a seasonal pattern may occur in up to one-third of cases (Table 11–3). Research into the pathophysiology of SAD has focused on the effect of light. Possible derangements include melatonin dysregulation, disrupted circadian rhythm, neurotransmitter dysfunction, and visual sensitivity (Lewy et al. 1988). In addition to the usual treatments for depression, light therapy has been shown to be effective.

Recurrent Brief Depressive Disorder and Minor Depressive Disorder

Recurrent brief depressive disorder and minor depressive disorder are listed in the DSM-IV-TR research appendix. Individuals with recurrent brief depression have an increased risk for suicide compared with the general population. This condition follows a different course from that of major depression (Pezawas et al. 2005). It may well represent a unique subtype of depression for this reason.

Premenstrual Dysphoric Disorder

Premenstrual mood symptoms are common, and about 3%–9% of women meet criteria for premenstrual dysphoric disorder (PMDD) (Halbreich et al. 2003). PMDD is characterized by the onset of severe symptoms, with at least one mood symptom, in the late luteal phase of the menstrual cycle, with remission during the early follicular phase (Table 11–4). The association between depression and derangements of the hypothalamic-pituitary-gonadal (HPG) axis has been established, but the precise nature of the link is unclear. Treatment of PMDD with gonadal hormones has limited effectiveness, whereas intermittent treatment with selective serotonin reuptake inhibitors (SSRIs) is the current pharmacotherapy of choice (Dimmock et al. 2000).

Adjustment Disorder and Bereavement

Even though adjustment disorder and bereavement are covered elsewhere in this book, they deserve a brief mention here. The association between depression and loss is common. However, not all depressive episodes that follow a stressor develop into major depressive episodes. When a stressor has resulted in impaired function or distress, together with depressed mood, then the diagnosis of adjustment disorder with depressed mood is most appropriate.

Similarly, the normal human response to bereavement should not be diagnosed as depression. DSM-IV-TR allows for a 2-month bereavement period, but it does ask clinicians to exercise their judgment when assigning diagnoses. It is regarded as "normal" for bereaved individuals to experience the presence of their loved one in the time after bereavement. This may take the form of hallucinations or vivid dreams. Sleep disturbance, excessive crying, psychomotor changes, and thoughts of death also may occur. The clinician should be guided by the reactions of close family members, cultural norms, and the course of the bereavement. A clinically significant depression may follow in about 15% of people who are bereaved (Clayton 1990).

TABLE 11–2. DSM-IV-TR diagnostic criteria for dysthymic disorder

A. Depressed mood for most of the day, for more days than not, as indicated by either subjective account or observation by others, for at least 2 years. **Note:** In children and adolescents, mood can be irritable and duration must be at least 1 year.

B. Presence, while depressed, of two (or more) of the following:
   (1) poor appetite or overeating
   (2) insomnia or hypersomnia
   (3) low energy or fatigue
   (4) low self-esteem
   (5) poor concentration or difficulty making decisions
   (6) feelings of hopelessness

C. During the 2-year period (1 year for children or adolescents) of the disturbance, the person has never been without the symptoms in criteria A and B for more than 2 months at a time.

D. No major depressive episode (see Table 11–1) has been present during the first 2 years of the disturbance (1 year for children and adolescents); i.e., the disturbance is not better accounted for by chronic major depressive disorder, or major depressive disorder, in partial remission. **Note:** There may have been a previous major depressive episode provided there was a full remission (no significant signs or symptoms for 2 months) before development of the dysthymic disorder. In addition, after the initial 2 years (1 year in children or adolescents) of dysthymic disorder, there may be superimposed episodes of major depressive disorder, in which case both diagnoses may be given when the criteria are met for a major depressive episode.

E. There has never been a manic episode (see Table 11–7), a mixed episode (see DSM-IV-TR p. 365), or a hypomanic episode (see DSM-IV-TR p. 368), and criteria have never been met for cyclothymic disorder.

F. The disturbance does not occur exclusively during the course of a chronic psychotic disorder, such as schizophrenia or delusional disorder.

G. The symptoms are not due to the direct physiological effects of a substance (e.g., a drug of abuse, a medication) or a general medical condition (e.g., hypothyroidism).

H. The symptoms cause clinically significant distress or impairment in social, occupational, or other important areas of functioning.

   Specify if:
      Early onset: if onset is before age 21 years
      Late onset: if onset is age 21 years or older

   Specify (for most recent 2 years of dysthymic disorder):
      With atypical features (see DSM-IV-TR p. 420)

TABLE 11–3. DSM-IV-TR criteria for seasonal pattern specifier

Specify if: **With seasonal pattern** (can be applied to the pattern of major depressive episodes in bipolar I disorder, bipolar II disorder, or major depressive disorder, recurrent)

A. There has been a regular temporal relationship between the onset of major depressive episodes in bipolar I or bipolar II disorder or major depressive disorder, recurrent, and a particular time of the year (e.g., regular appearance of the major depressive episode in the fall or winter). **Note:** Do not include cases in which there is an obvious effect of seasonal-related psychosocial stressors (e.g., regularly being unemployed every winter).

B. Full remissions (or a change from depression to mania or hypomania) also occur at a characteristic time of the year (e.g., depression disappears in the spring).

C. In the last 2 years, two major depressive episodes have occurred that demonstrate the temporal seasonal relationships defined in criteria A and B, and no nonseasonal major depressive episodes have occurred during that same period.

D. Seasonal major depressive episodes (as described above) substantially outnumber the nonseasonal major depressive episodes that may have occurred over the individual's lifetime.

TABLE 11–4. **DSM-IV-TR research criteria for premenstrual dysphoric disorder**

A. In most menstrual cycles during the past year, five (or more) of the following symptoms were present for most of the time during the last week of the luteal phase, began to remit within a few days after the onset of the follicular phase, and were absent in the week postmenses, with at least one of the symptoms being either (1), (2), (3), or (4):

(1) markedly depressed mood, feelings of hopelessness, or self-deprecating thoughts

(2) marked anxiety, tension, feelings of being "keyed up" or "on edge"

(3) marked affective lability (e.g., feeling suddenly sad or tearful or increased sensitivity to rejection)

(4) persistent and marked anger or irritability or increased interpersonal conflicts

(5) decreased interest in usual activities (e.g., work, school, friends, hobbies)

(6) subjective sense of difficulty in concentrating

(7) lethargy, easy fatigability, or marked lack of energy

(8) marked change in appetite, overeating, or specific food cravings

(9) hypersomnia or insomnia

(10) a subjective sense of being overwhelmed or out of control

(11) other physical symptoms, such as breast tenderness or swelling, headaches, joint or muscle pain, a sensation of "bloating," weight gain

Note: In menstruating females, the luteal phase corresponds to the period between ovulation and the onset of menses, and the follicular phase begins with menses. In nonmenstruating females (e.g., those who have had a hysterectomy), the timing of luteal and follicular phases may require measurement of circulating reproductive hormones.

B. The disturbance markedly interferes with work or school or with usual social activities and relationships with others (e.g., avoidance of social activities, decreased productivity and efficiency at work or school).

C. The disturbance is not merely an exacerbation of the symptoms of another disorder, such as major depressive disorder, panic disorder, dysthymic disorder, or a personality disorder (although it may be superimposed on any of these disorders).

D. Criteria A, B, and C must be confirmed by prospective daily ratings during at least two consecutive symptomatic cycles. (The diagnosis may be made provisionally prior to this confirmation.)

Differential Diagnosis of Depressive Disorders

Medical Disorders

Many medical conditions may be associated with depression (Peveler et al. 2002). Some of these are listed in Table 11–5. The mechanism of association may be a result of the condition itself (such as hypothyroidism), a reaction to having a medical condition, a result of the medical treatment of the condition, or a combination of these factors. In some instances, the medical disorder creates the appearance of depression with or without actually causing it. Examples include Parkinson's disease and cerebrovascular disease.

Depression Secondary to Substance Use

The most widespread substance of abuse, alcohol, is a common and independent cause of depressive illness. Patients whose alcohol abuse leads to depression will commonly experience a remission of depressive symptoms after cessation of alcohol use without antidepressant treatment. Other causes of depression secondary to substance and medication use are listed in Table 11–6. The association between substance use and mood disorders has been established in several population surveys—in the Epidemiologic Catchment Area (ECA) study, the use of alcohol increased the likelihood of having major depression twofold and the likelihood of having bipolar disorder nearly fivefold (Regier et al. 1990).

In addition to the possibility that substance abuse leads to depression, depression may lead to substance use (i.e., "self-medication") (Khantzian 1985), or the two disorders may share a common diathesis (e.g., genetic loading). A careful clinical assessment must include a detailed substance use and mood disorder history, with a view to delineating whether mood symptoms occurred in the absence of a period of intoxication or withdrawal. The presence of severe or

TABLE 11–5. Some medical conditions that may cause depression

Neurological disorders
  Epilepsies
  Parkinson's disease
  Multiple sclerosis
  Alzheimer's disease
  Cerebrovascular disease
Infectious disorders
  Neurosyphilis
  HIV/AIDS
Cardiac disorders
  Ischemic heart disease
  Cardiac failure
  Cardiomyopathies
Endocrine and metabolic disorders
  Hypothyroidism
  Diabetes mellitus
  Vitamin deficiencies
  Parathyroid disorders
Inflammatory disorders
  Collagen-vascular diseases
  Irritable bowel syndrome
  Chronic liver disorders
Neoplastic disorders
  Central nervous system tumors
  Paraneoplastic syndromes

TABLE 11–6. Some substances and medications that may cause depression

Central nervous system depressants
  Alcohol
  Barbiturates
  Benzodiazepines
  Clonidine
Central nervous system medications
  Amantadine
  Bromocriptine
  Levodopa
  Phenothiazines
  Phenytoin
Psychostimulants
  Amphetamines
Systemic medications
  Corticosteroids
  Digoxin
  Diltiazem
  Enalapril
  Ethionamide
  Isotretinoin
  Mefloquine
  Methyldopa
  Metoclopramide
  Quinolones
  Reserpine
  Statins
  Thiazides
  Vincristine

chronic symptoms, as well as comorbidity, also may help the clinician determine the primary disorder.

Depression and Other Psychiatric Disorders

A broad range of psychiatric disorders should be considered in the differential diagnosis of major depression. These include the prodrome of schizophrenia, schizoid personality disorder, pervasive developmental disorders, intellectual disability and dementia, and anxiety disorders.

Clinical Features of Mania

Mental State Examination

The presentation of mania is varied. Central to mania, hypomania, or mixed episodes is the presence of either elevated, irritable, or expansive mood. Mania may manifest in obvious ways (e.g., catatonic stupor; violent and aggressive behavior) or in more subtle ways

(e.g., dressing in brighter clothing; agitated psychomotor function). Speech may be pressured. Expansive mood may be elicited when the person describes his or her social interactions; a sense of being connected to the world is often expressed. Affect is often euphoric but may be labile or hostile. Problems with thought include excessive flow of ideas ("flight of ideas"); grandiose, religious, or persecutory delusions; and sometimes bizarre delusions. Perceptual disturbances range from auditory hallucinations (such as hearing the voice of God) to visions of religious and grandiose significance. These mood-congruent symptoms are most common, but incongruent psychosis has been described. Cognitive disturbances include distractibility, poor attention, and executive dysfunction (Table 11–7).

TABLE 11–7. **DSM-IV-TR diagnostic criteria for manic episode**

A. A distinct period of abnormally and persistently elevated, expansive, or irritable mood, lasting at least 1 week (or any duration if hospitalization is necessary).

B. During the period of mood disturbance, three (or more) of the following symptoms have persisted (four if the mood is only irritable) and have been present to a significant degree:

   (1) inflated self-esteem or grandiosity

   (2) decreased need for sleep (e.g., feels rested after only 3 hours of sleep)

   (3) more talkative than usual or pressure to keep talking

   (4) flight of ideas or subjective experience that thoughts are racing

   (5) distractibility (i.e., attention too easily drawn to unimportant or irrelevant external stimuli)

   (6) increase in goal-directed activity (either socially, at work or school, or sexually) or psychomotor agitation

   (7) excessive involvement in pleasurable activities that have a high potential for painful consequences (e.g., engaging in unrestrained buying sprees, sexual indiscretions, or foolish business investments)

C. The symptoms do not meet criteria for a mixed episode (see DSM-IV-TR p. 365).

D. The mood disturbance is sufficiently severe to cause marked impairment in occupational functioning or in usual social activities or relationships with others, or to necessitate hospitalization to prevent harm to self or others, or there are psychotic features.

E. The symptoms are not due to the direct physiological effects of a substance (e.g., a drug of abuse, a medication, or other treatment) or a general medical condition (e.g., hyperthyroidism).

Note: Manic-like episodes that are clearly caused by somatic antidepressant treatment (e.g., medication, electroconvulsive therapy, light therapy) should not count toward a diagnosis of bipolar I disorder.

Mood Disturbance in Mania

Establishing the presence of a disturbed mood in mania is critical to distinguishing mania from other psychiatric conditions. However, this is not always easy, especially when dysphoria is present. Dysphoria is distinct from depression in that it describes a subjective sense of negative, labile, or irritable mood in the absence of persistently low mood and anhedonia. The clinician will need to establish what the premorbid mood state was, how mood changed over time, and whether any associated symptoms were present. For example, patients who engage in excessive goal-directed behavior may be more likely to have mania. Questions around the nature of social relationships, work productivity, and plans for the future may be useful to establish changes in goal-directed behavior. Collateral informants may offer insight into whether mood has been irritable, with interactions characterized by friction and disagreement out of keeping with usual relating. DSM-IV-TR specifies that mood disturbance may be present for only a short time—1 week, or a shorter duration if the person requires hospitalization.

Cognitive, Neurovegetative, and Behavioral Symptoms

Cognitive disturbance in mania includes the nature and content of thinking. When more complex testing methods are used, neuropsychological deficits are also often found. The problem of distractibility is listed as a diagnostic criterion in DSM-IV-TR. This phenomenon may be the result of excessive thought flow or a primary disturbance of information processing and attention. Impairments in memory, executive function, judgment, and visuospatial integration are also frequently encountered (Osuji and Cullum 2005).

Neurovegetative symptoms are usual in mania. Sleep disturbance is characterized by a decreased need for sleep. Libido and appetite are both often increased. Two types of behavior problems in mania may occur: increase in goal-directed behavior and behavior with potential for harm. In some cases, goal-directed behavior leads to increased productivity, increased self-esteem, and even an increase in earnings. This can hinder the patient's insight into the behavior as being abnormal. Harmful behaviors may include excessive spending, gambling, sexual promiscuity, traveling, drug use, or other risk-taking behavior.

Duration, Intensity, and Specifiers

Determining the duration of elevated mood episodes is key to establishing diagnosis. Short-lived episodes may reflect cyclothymic disturbance or rapid cycling, whereas longer episodes may result from treatment resistance or ongoing substance abuse. A life chart may be useful in depicting the nature and extent of mood episodes. Other specifiers include whether the episode was single or recurrent, whether it was postpartum in onset, and whether it was associated with psychosis.

Bipolar I Disorder

Diagnostic Criteria

The diagnostic criteria for bipolar I disorder are listed in Table 11–8. The presence of any past or present manic episode is sufficient to meet criteria. The diagnosis of bipolar disorder should be considered in any patient who presents with depressive symptoms. Certain features may suggest bipolarity: earlier age at onset of symptoms, family history of bipolarity, and presence of atypical depressive symptoms (Perlis et al. 2006).

Single Versus Recurrent Manic Episodes

The recurrence of mania requires a careful reevaluation of contributory factors, such as substance use, poor medication adherence, psychosocial stressors, and medical problems. In addition, a diagnosis of rapid-cycling bipolar disorder should be considered; this requires the presence of at least four discrete mood episodes in a 12-month period. Two further subtypes of rapid cycling have since been added to the nomenclature: ultrarapid cycling (cycles lasting days to weeks) and ultradian cycling (abrupt mood changes in a 24-hour period) (Kramlinger and Post 1996).

Other Bipolar Disorders

Bipolar II Disorder

A diagnosis of bipolar II disorder requires the presence of hypomanic and major depressive episodes (Table 11–9). It is most usual for patients to present with severe depression. Bipolar II disorder should be considered in patients who have atypical features, who abuse substances as a form of self-medication, or who have chaotic relationships. A life chart may be helpful.

Cyclothymia

Cyclothymia is characterized by a 2-year history of changing mood, with both depressive and hypomanic symptoms (Table 11–10). It occurs in about 0.5% of the general population (Weissman and Myers 1978). Patients with cyclothymic disorder do not readily present to mental health services. They may be brought as a result of a suicide attempt, substance abuse, or a relationship issue. Some will later develop manic episodes (6%), and a quarter will go on to develop major depression (Akiskal et al. 1979). There may be a continuum between cyclothymia and intrinsic difficulties in affective regulation and borderline personality disorder, but patients with cyclothymia may respond particularly well to pharmacotherapy.

TABLE 11–8. DSM-IV-TR diagnostic criteria for bipolar I disorder, single manic episode

A. Presence of only one manic episode (see Table 11–7) and no past major depressive episodes.

   Note: Recurrence is defined as either a change in polarity from depression or an interval of at least 2 months without manic symptoms.

B. The manic episode is not better accounted for by schizoaffective disorder and is not superimposed on schizophrenia, schizophreniform disorder, delusional disorder, or psychotic disorder not otherwise specified.

Specify if:

   Mixed: if symptoms meet criteria for a mixed episode (see DSM-IV-TR p. 365)

If the full criteria are currently met for a manic, mixed, or major depressive episode, *specify* its current clinical status and/or features:

   Mild, moderate, severe without psychotic features/severe with psychotic features (see DSM-IV-TR p. 414)

   With catatonic features (see DSM-IV-TR p. 417)

   With postpartum onset (see DSM-IV-TR p. 422)

If the full criteria are not currently met for a manic, mixed, or major depressive episode, *specify* the current clinical status of the bipolar I disorder or features of the most recent episode:

   In partial remission, in full remission (see DSM-IV-TR p. 414)

   With catatonic features (see DSM-IV-TR p. 417)

   With postpartum onset (see DSM-IV-TR p. 422)

TABLE 11–9. **DSM-IV-TR diagnostic criteria for bipolar II disorder**

A. Presence (or history) of one or more major depressive episodes (see Table 11–1).

B. Presence (or history) of at least one hypomanic episode (see DSM-IV-TR p. 368).

C. There has never been a manic episode (see Table 11–7) or a mixed episode (see DSM-IV-TR p. 365).

D. The mood symptoms in criteria A and B are not better accounted for by schizoaffective disorder and are not superimposed on schizophrenia, schizophreniform disorder, delusional disorder, or psychotic disorder not otherwise specified.

E. The symptoms cause clinically significant distress or impairment in social, occupational, or other important areas of functioning.

Specify current or most recent episode:

Hypomanic: if currently (or most recently) in a hypomanic episode (see DSM-IV-TR p. 368)

Depressed: if currently (or most recently) in a major depressive episode (see Table 11–1)

If the full criteria are currently met for a major depressive episode, *specify* its current clinical status and/or features:

Mild, moderate, severe without psychotic features/severe with psychotic features (see DSM-IV-TR p. 412)   **Note:** Fifth-digit codes specified on p. 413 cannot be used here because the code for bipolar II disorder already uses the fifth digit.

Chronic (see DSM-IV-TR p. 417)

With catatonic features (see DSM-IV-TR p. 417)

With melancholic features (see DSM-IV-TR p. 419)

With atypical features (see DSM-IV-TR p. 420)

With postpartum onset (see DSM-IV-TR p. 422)

If the full criteria are not currently met for a hypomanic or major depressive episode, *specify* the clinical status of the bipolar II disorder and/or features of the most recent major depressive episode (only if it is the most recent type of mood episode):

In partial remission, in full remission (see DSM-IV-TR p. 412)   **Note:** Fifth-digit codes specified on p. 413 cannot be used here because the code for bipolar II disorder already uses the fifth digit.

Chronic (see DSM-IV-TR p. 417)

With catatonic features (see DSM-IV-TR p. 417)

With melancholic features (see DSM-IV-TR p. 419)

With atypical features (see DSM-IV-TR p. 420)

With postpartum onset (see DSM-IV-TR p. 422)

Specify:

Longitudinal course specifiers (with and without interepisode recovery) (see DSM-IV-TR p. 424)

With seasonal pattern (applies only to the pattern of major depressive episodes) (see Table 11–3)

With rapid cycling (see DSM-IV-TR p. 427)

Bipolar Spectrum Disorder

There is increasing recognition that many individuals with recurrent depressive episodes also may have subthreshold elevated mood states (Angst and Cassano 2005). The construct of bipolar spectrum disorders emphasizes that symptoms of bipolar disorder occur in a diverse range of conditions more frequently than by chance—such as may occur in some personality disorders, eating disorders, or substance use disorders.

Differential Diagnosis of Bipolar Disorders

Both general medical disorders and other psychiatric disorders should be considered in the differential diagnosis of a manic episode.

Medical Disorders

The emergence of mania or hypomania in the presence of a medical disorder may result from the disorder it-

TABLE 11–10.   DSM-IV-TR diagnostic criteria for cyclothymic disorder

A. For at least 2 years, the presence of numerous periods with hypomanic symptoms (see DSM-IV-TR p. 368) and numerous periods with depressive symptoms that do not meet criteria for a major depressive episode.   **Note:** In children and adolescents, the duration must be at least 1 year.

B. During the above 2-year period (1 year in children and adolescents), the person has not been without the symptoms in criterion A for more than 2 months at a time.

C. No major depressive episode (see Table 11–1), manic episode (see Table 11–7), or mixed episode (see DSM-IV-TR p. 365) has been present during the first 2 years of the disturbance.

   Note: After the initial 2 years (1 year in children and adolescents) of cyclothymic disorder, there may be superimposed manic or mixed episodes (in which case both bipolar I disorder and cyclothymic disorder may be diagnosed) or major depressive episodes (in which case both bipolar II disorder and cyclothymic disorder may be diagnosed).

D. The symptoms in criterion A are not better accounted for by schizoaffective disorder and are not superimposed on schizophrenia, schizophreniform disorder, delusional disorder, or psychotic disorder not otherwise specified.

E. The symptoms are not due to the direct physiological effects of a substance (e.g., a drug of abuse, a medication) or a general medical condition (e.g., hyperthyroidism).

F. The symptoms cause clinically significant distress or impairment in social, occupational, or other important areas of functioning.

self or the associated treatment (Table 11–11). The emergence of a manic episode in an individual older than 35 years should raise the level of suspicion for an underlying medical cause (Larson and Richelson 1988).

Mania Secondary to Substance Use

The use of substances early in the course of bipolar disorder is common (Table 11–12). Furthermore, the use of substances may predict an earlier onset of bipolar disorder and a worse course (Brady and Sonne 1995).

Mania and Other Psychiatric Disorders

When dysphoria or hostility is prominent, diagnoses such as schizophrenia and other psychotic disorders, substance intoxication, antisocial or borderline personality disorder, impulse-control disorders, and intellectual disability should be considered in the differential diagnosis of manic episode. The nature of psychotic symptoms, if present, must be clarified, and a thorough substance misuse history should be taken.

Comorbidity of Mood Disorders

Anxiety Disorders

The co-occurrence of mood disorders with anxiety is extremely common. Nearly 50% of individuals with depression will develop a lifetime anxiety disorder (de Graaf et al. 2003), and anxiety disorders are also commonly comorbid with bipolar disorders (M.P. Freeman et al. 2002).

TABLE 11–11. Some conditions that may cause mania

Neurological disorders
  Epilepsies
  Traumatic brain injury
  Multiple sclerosis
  Cerebrovascular disease
Infectious disorders
  Neurosyphilis
  HIV/AIDS
Neoplastic disorders
  Central nervous system tumors
  Paraneoplastic syndromes
  Traumatic brain injury
Endocrine disorders
  Hypo- and hyperthyroidism
  Diabetes mellitus
  Hypercortisolemia
  Vitamin deficiencies
Inflammatory disorders
  Collagen-vascular diseases

TABLE 11–12. **Some substances and medications that may cause mania**

Central nervous system depressants
  Alcohol

Psychostimulants
  Amphetamines
  Cocaine
  Methylphenidate
  Pseudoephedrine

Central nervous system medications
  Amantadine
  Antidepressants
  Baclofen
  Bromocriptine

Systemic medications
  Anabolic steroids
  Chloroquine
  Corticosteroids
  Dapsone
  Isoniazid
  Metoclopramide
  Theophylline

Anxiety disorders usually precede depressive disorders in onset. Several explanations for this sequence are possible, and more work is needed for a definitive conclusion. In other cases, depression and anxiety symptoms appear to be part of the same syndrome, and DSM-IV-TR includes a disorder of mixed anxiety-depressive disorder in its research appendix.

The association between mania and anxiety also may be heterogeneous in nature. Dysphoria and hostility differ in appearance from anxiety disorders, but there may be underlying psychobiological mechanisms that predispose to their comorbidity. When an anxious individual has used substances to self-medicate the condition, a manic state may be induced.

Schizophrenia

The presence of mood disorders in the context of schizophrenia is important. The coexistence of depression significantly increases the risk of suicide, with rates of up to 10%. When a major mood disturbance has been present throughout the psychosis, then a mood disorder with psychotic features must be diagnosed. If the patient has had a short (2-week) period of psychosis in the absence of mood symptoms within

this disturbance, then DSM-IV-TR schizoaffective disorder should be diagnosed. Other clinical symptoms that may assist in differentiating mood disorders with psychotic features from schizophrenia include bizarreness of delusions and severe thought disorder in schizophrenia and mood congruency of delusions and hallucinations in mood disorders.

Personality Disorders

Personality disorders are commonly associated with mood disorders. Indeed, Cluster B personality disorders, particularly borderline personality disorder, may be characterized by a core disturbance in affect, with both decreased and elevated mood at times. In Cluster A and C personalities, depression may be more common than mania. In the former, more reclusive and eccentric living may provoke depression, whereas in the latter, an anxious and avoidant view of life may be the trigger.

Pediatric Mood Disorders

Depressive Disorders

Depression has a prevalence of up to 14% in adolescents (Birmaher et al. 1996). The clinical presentation may differ between children and adults, and children do not seek help easily, contributing to a previous underestimate of prevalence. Depressed children may show irritability rather than depressed mood. Younger children may have more appetite changes and delusional thinking (Kovacs 1996). Associated features include low self-esteem, negative cognitions, and behavioral difficulties.

It is essential to screen for comorbid conditions, such as learning disability, attention-deficit/hyperactivity disorder (ADHD), disruptive behavior disorders, and anxiety disorders (Emslie et al. 1997). Children with chronic medical problems, including diabetes, asthma, and epilepsy, also have a high rate of depression (Grey et al. 2002).

Bipolar Disorder

The prevalence of bipolar disorder in children and adolescents is about 1% (Keller and Baker 1991). Although manic symptoms have been commonly reported in children, some maintain that bipolar disorder is difficult to diagnose in those younger than 10 years. Bipolar disorder in children is characterized by irritability, cyclical mood changes, and associated ADHD (Biederman et al. 2000). In addition, the clinical course may follow a more chronic, undulating pattern, with fewer discrete mood episodes. Adolescents are more likely to present with typical features of bipolar disorder (Carlson et al. 2003). Differential diagnosis includes ADHD—the presence of elevated mood, grandiosity, flight of ideas, and a decreased need for sleep are features unique to bipolar disorder.

Mood Disorders in Old Age

Age and Illness Presentation

The prevalence of depression rises with age. Rates approaching 25% in the elderly have been cited (Parmelee et al. 1989). First episodes also may occur in late life, as the result of life events, medical conditions, or treatment of these conditions or as a precursor to dementia. General medical conditions must be considered when a mood disorder first occurs in late life. Certain medical conditions, such as Parkinson's disease, other degenerative brain conditions, and endocrine problems, may present with features indistinguishable from depression. Antihypertensives, corticosteroids, and chemotherapies may lead to depression.

Depressive Disorders

With the high prevalence of depression in the elderly, early recognition and treatment are crucial. The clinician should have a high index of suspicion for a depressive disorder if an individual shows a change in cognitive function, neurovegetative symptoms, or suspicious ideation. Loss of cognitive function and general impairment can lead to serious psychosocial problems or "depressive pseudodementia." Terms such as *cognitive impairment secondary to depression* or *depression without sadness* may better describe this entity (Gallo and Rabins 1999). Figures for completed suicide in elderly patients with depression approach 15%. Elderly patients who are unsupported, who are living with a terminal illness, or who live alone are especially at risk.

Cultural Aspects of Depression

The core features of depression exist across cultures and ethnic groups, but the rates of reporting of these symptoms may differ (Kleinman and Good 1985). Idioms of distress may influence the expression of a variety of associated anxiety, psychosomatic, and dissociative symptoms.

Cross-Cultural Equivalence

The development of a diagnostic system that makes use of a set of criteria based on one ethnic group's experiences may not always hold equivalence across a range of cultures. Rating scales have been developed for use in different cultural settings as an adjunct to routine clinical assessment.

Cultural Epidemiology of Depression

Several well-conducted studies have found differing rates of depression across countries and cultures. The World Health Organization Cross-National Study of Mental Disorders in Primary Care found a point prevalence of depressive disorder of 29.5% in Santiago, Chile; 15.9% in Groningen, the Netherlands; and 4.0% in Shanghai, China (Sartorius et al. 1995). Weissman et al. (1996) found a lifetime prevalence of depression of 16.4% in Paris, France; 11.6% in Christchurch, New Zealand; and 4.3% in Puerto Rico. These figures may, however, reflect differences that are a consequence of the methodologies used. For example, rating scales used in these surveys may not have detected local idioms of distress.

Cultural Idioms of Distress

The expression of distress across cultures and regions may reflect important differences in the way that the particular group views mental health, the concept of the body and the self, and the expression of emotion. Unique idioms of distress are recognized in DSM-IV-TR and include feelings of loneliness and the sensation of a "hot or peppery feeling in the head."

Epidemiology

Epidemiology of Mood Disorders

Mood disorders, and depression in particular, are among the most prevalent and disabling of all medical conditions. Although significant advances have been made in epidemiological studies, methodological issues affect our interpretation of the data. Diagnostic instruments differ a great deal in their reliability, validity, and comprehensiveness. Even when studies are carefully done, some data, such as lifetime prevalence, are affected by factors such as recall bias.

Current and Lifetime Prevalence Rates

Selected studies assessing the current and lifetime prevalence of depression and bipolar disorder in the general population are tabulated (Table 11–13). The 1-year prevalence rates of major depression in these studies range from 2.7% in the ECA study to 10.3% in the National Comorbidity Survey (NCS). The lifetime prevalence rates for the same disorder range from 7.8% to 17.1%.

TABLE 11–13. Studies of current and lifetime prevalence of mood disorders

Study	Author	Time frame	Site	N	Instrument	Age (years)	Total	Major depression	Bipolar disorder
ECA	Weissman et al. 1991	1 year Lifetime	United States	18,572	DIS	>18	3.7 7.8	2.7	0.7 (bipolar I)
NCS	Kessler et al. 1994	1 year Lifetime	United States	8,098	CIDI	15–54	11.3 19.3	10.3 17.1	
NEMESIS	Bijl et al. 1998	1 year Lifetime	Netherlands	7,076	CIDI	18–64	7.6 19	5.8 15.4	1.1 1.8
ODIN study	Ayuso-Mateos et al. 2001	Point	Europe	8,764	SCAN	18–64		6.6	
ANMHS	Andrews et al. 2001	1 year	Australia	10,641	CIDI	>18		6.3	
NCS-R	Kessler et al. 2003	1 year Lifetime	United States	9,090	CIDI	>18		6.6 16.2	
WHO WMHCS	Demyttenaere et al. 2004	1 year	Nigeria Japan	4,985 1,663	WMH-CIDI WMH-CIDI	>18 >18	0.8 3.1		

Note. ECA=Epidemiologic Catchment Area study; DIS=Diagnostic Interview Schedule; NCS=National Comorbidity Survey; CIDI=Composite International Diagnostic Interview; NEMESIS=Netherlands Mental Health Survey and Incidence Study; ODIN study=European Outcome of Depression International Network study; SCAN=Schedule for Clinical Assessment in Neuropsychiatry; ANMHS=Australian National Mental Health Survey; NCS-R=National Comorbidity Survey Replication; WHO WMHSC=World Health Organization World Mental Health Survey Consortium; WMH-CIDI=World Mental Health CIDI.

Fewer data are available for bipolar disorder. The ECA study found a prevalence of bipolar disorder type I of 0.7%. Bijl et al. (1998) reported a 1-year prevalence of 1.1% and a lifetime prevalence of 1.8%. When validation studies used the Structured Clinical Interview for DSM-IV, adjusted rates of 0.9% were found (R.D. Goodwin et al. 2006). Higher rates may be seen depending on the diagnostic category used.

Sociodemographic Correlates

The mean age at onset of major depression has been found to be in the late 20s: 27.4 years in the ECA study and 29.9 years reported by de Graaf et al. (2003) in the Netherlands Mental Health Survey and Incidence Study (NEMESIS). In the replication of the National Comorbidity Survey (NCS-R), the median age at onset for mood disorders was 30 years (Kessler et al. 2003). People with bipolar disorder tend to develop symptoms in a bimodal distribution from ages 18 to 44 years (Kessler and Walters 1998).

Depression is twice as common in women (Kessler and Walters 1998). This finding emerges only after adolescence; before this period, rates are similar. Reasons for this gender difference may include hormonal differences, social factors, or an unequal exposure to abuse and stressful life events (Klose and Jacobi 2004). In contrast, the rates of bipolar disorder among men and women appear to be similar (Kessler et al. 1994).

Depression is more common in the unmarried compared with the married person. Kessler et al. (2003) reported that never having been married was associated with a lower rate of depression than having been divorced or widowed. These findings are similar for bipolar disorder. Higher rates of depression in ethnic minorities have been reported, but this effect has been attributed to higher rates of other factors (such as poverty and lack of resources) in these groups. Low socioeconomic status consistently has been shown to be associated with an increased rate of depression (Kessler et al. 1994). Surveys of bipolar disorder in the general population have found a similar result. However, in clinical samples, bipolar disorder appears to be associated with a higher socioeconomic status. The causal factors responsible for these associations remain to be delineated.

Risk Factors for Mood Disorders

Early childhood trauma and adverse life events are associated with an increased risk for developing depression, particularly severe types. Other types of trauma, such as loss of a parent, also have been associated with the development of depression. Some evidence indicates that other types of trauma, such as neglect, predispose to anxiety and other disorders rather than depression (Brown and Eales 1993). In adulthood, the presence of a negative life event has been shown consistently to be a risk factor for major depression. The categories of loss and humiliation appear to predict the onset of depression (Kendler et al. 2003), whereas entrapment and danger may precede anxiety problems.

The risk of developing major depression is significantly higher in relatives of patients with depression. Furthermore, a family history of major depression appears to confer a risk of developing severe, recurrent, and possibly early-onset major depression. Rates of depression among people in the community who have experienced a negative life event are significantly higher in those with a family history (Kendler 1998). Independent of family history, the most consistent sociodemographic risk factor for the development of depression is female gender (R.D. Goodwin et al. 2006).

Interactions between genes and the environment are becoming increasingly delineated. Variants in the gene coding for the serotonin transporter (5-HTT) and adverse life events, for example, appear to interact to predict higher rates of depression and anxiety disorders (Caspi et al. 2003). Similarly, the effect of personality on the development of depression has been examined in several studies, with high levels of neuroticism predicting a likelihood of developing depression (Kendler 1998). Data are too weak to categorically link stress as a direct risk factor for the development of bipolar disorder (R.D. Goodwin et al. 2006).

Global Burden of Mood Disorders

Two landmark studies placed depression into context by comparing it with the burden of other disorders: the Global Burden of Disease (GBD) study (Murray and Lopez 1996) and the Medical Outcomes Study (Wells et al. 1989). The GBD study used the entity of disability-adjusted life-years (DALYs)—a measure of the number of years over which the condition produces disability. The GBD study found that depression results in twice as much disability in middle life as any other condition and that bipolar disorder was the sixth leading cause of disability in this age group (Murray and Lopez 1996). The Medical Outcomes Study made use of the 36-item Short-Form Health Survey in more than 11,000 respondents. It found that depression was as disabling as any other medical condition. In addition, dysthymia was a significant factor in producing disability (Leader and Klein 1996). This added support to the idea that subclinical symptomatology and undetected cases represent a serious worldwide health concern.

Economics of Mood Disorders

The economic cost of mood disorders can be measured in three ways (Greenberg et al. 1996):

1. *The cost of treatment*—In the United States, the cost has been estimated at about $12 billion per annum.
2. *The cost of any increase in mortality attributable to the problem*—Again, in the United States, the cost of mortality may reach $8 billion per annum.
3. *The cost of morbidity, especially loss of earnings and productivity*—This is the largest cost and may amount to about $33 billion per annum in the United States.

Similar figures have been reported for the costs of bipolar disorder. Note that these costs almost certainly underestimate the true costs. As previously mentioned, a range of mood disorders may be regarded as subsyndromal or may not readily present to services. These include dysthymia, cyclothymia, and brief recurrent mood disorders.

Several explanations are available for the costs of depression. First, it has increasingly been recognized that depression may develop early in life; has a peak onset in the late 20s, close to the time of highest productivity; tends to be a chronic and relapsing condition; and is fast becoming one of the most common medical conditions, with an apparent increase in prevalence. The effect of depression in the workplace includes not only the direct loss of working days but also the diminished work performance while at work (W. F. Stewart et al. 2003).

Second, delivery of care to patients with depression and mood disorders is inadequate. The effect of treatment of mood disorders usually results in significant cost savings through reduced use of general medical services (P. S. Wang and Kessler 2006). These costs, however, may be evident only when the costs of treatment are offset against the savings generated by improving work-related productivity (Kessler et al. 2003). Despite these benefits, numerous obstacles to recovery persist. These include patients' delays in seeking help, delays in physicians correctly diagnosing mood disorders, and incorrect use of treatment strategies (P. S. Wang et al. 2003).

To reduce the disease burden of mood disorders, strategies to improve delivery at the primary care level, where most contacts occur, are needed. Psychiatrist-physician collaboration and adherence surveillance may optimize treatment (Katon et al. 1999). The use of a stepped care model, with more intensive interventions being offered to patients with difficult-to-treat depression, should be considered.

Course of Mood Disorders

Course of Major Depression

Current evidence has shown that depression usually begins by age 30 and, in some cases, in adolescence (Oldehinkel et al. 1999). The presence of other conditions, such as anxiety and other depressive disorders, may result in an earlier age at onset (Bittner et al. 2004). Major depression tends to recur—figures range from 72.3% in the NCS (Kessler et al. 1994) to 40%–50% in the NEMESIS (Spijker et al. 2002). Factors that may affect the course of depression include family history, presence of comorbid anxiety, and the age at onset.

Course of Bipolar Disorder

Data have consistently shown that bipolar disorder usually manifests in the early 20s—the mean age at onset in the ECA study and NCS was 21 years (Kessler et al. 1994; Weissman et al. 1991). In retrospective studies, both manic and depressive episodes have been reported to occur between ages 14 and 15 years, suggesting an earlier age at onset than originally thought. These differences may be a result of cohort effects or methodological differences. Following the development of a first hypomanic or manic episode, bipolar disorder tends to be recurrent (Coryell and Winokur 1992).

Pathogenesis of Mood Disorders

Depression is likely to have multiple contributing factors, and here we discuss a range.

Evolutionary Aspects of Mood Disorders

An evolutionary model focuses on the evolutionary origins of behavior and provides different hypotheses about the nature of disordered mood. It is hypothesized that depression has specific adaptive advantages. Depression may allow for time to consider loss, how it may be regained or prevented in the future, and how to develop a strategy for moving forward without the resource (Nesse 2006). The depressed state may provoke a supportive response in others (Bowlby 1973). Price (1967) added that a loss of status may evoke low mood, resulting in diminished exposure to further attack and possibly an increased chance of support. A last theory about the utility of low mood concerns the value of expending resources in an environment with a low potential for yield; environments with readily available reward would engender expansive efforts, whereas those that are less rewarding (or punitive) would encourage a diminished or depressed response (Nesse 1999).

Genetics and Inherited Factors

No single gene has been identified as a major cause of depression or bipolar disorder. Rather, genetic vulnerabilities may be the result of small, additive, and interactive effects of many genes.

Family Studies

Studies have shown that first-degree relatives of patients who have recurrent unipolar depression have an increased risk two to four times that of control subjects for having depression (Gershon et al. 1982; Sullivan and Kendler 2001). Factors that confer a greater degree of heritability (i.e., that yield an increased risk of depression in relatives) are age at onset before 30 years, recurrence, presence of psychotic symptoms, and presence of certain comorbidities (such as panic disorder).

In families of bipolar patients, a spectrum of bipolar and unipolar disorders is found (Baron et al. 1983). These include bipolar I and II disorder, schizoaffective disorder, and recurrent major depression. There does not appear to be a risk of schizophrenia in relatives of bipolar probands. However, first-degree relatives of schizophrenic patients are at increased risk for schizoaffective disorder and recurrent major depression (Gershon 1988).

Twin Studies

Twin studies of recurrent major depression indicate that heritability is approximately 37%—that is, in individuals who share all or almost all of their genetic material, genes account for about 37% of the risk of developing major depression. The effect of the individual environment and the interaction between genes and the said environment probably account for a large portion of the remaining risk. In bipolar disorder, concordances range from 65.1% in monozygotic twins to 14.0% in dizygotic twins. Estimates of heritability of bipolar disorder in monozygotic twins are about 80% (McGuffin et al. 2003).

Adoption Studies

The risk of developing bipolar or unipolar disorder was found to be about 31% in adopted relatives of bipolar patients (Mendlewicz and Rainer 1977). This is similar to the risk of 26% seen in first-degree relatives of affected individuals who have not been adopted.

Molecular Linkage Studies

Molecular linkage genetic studies examine the tendency of two genes to be inherited together in families more frequently than by chance. No major loci have been found, but about 10 minor or susceptibility loci have been identified. In meta-analyses, three areas appear to contribute to the development of bipolar disorder: 13q32, 22q11–13, and the percentriomeric region of 18 (Badner and Gershon 2002; Segurado et al. 2003). Linkage studies of recurrent major depression are less consistent.

Linkage Disequilibrium Studies

Several candidate genes have now been studied. Much focus has been on the 5-HTT, which has several functional variants. Although not all data are consistent, evidence indicates that people with one or more copies of the short allele of the 5-HTT promoter polymorphism are more likely to develop depression or suicidality if they experience stressful life events.

Neurochemistry

Early theories of mood disorders have centered on the monoamine neurotransmitters. As the field has advanced, a range of other neurotransmitters and neurotrophic factors have been explored.

Serotonin System

Serotonin (5-hydroxytryptamine [5-HT]) is synthesized from the essential amino acid tryptophan. Serotonin is metabolized by monoamine oxidase (MAO) to 5-hydroxyindoleacetic acid (5-HIAA). Synaptic serotonin is transported back into the neuron by a reuptake pump. Descending serotonergic projections innervate the spinal cord to modulate pain, whereas ascending fibers project to the limbic system and thalamus. To date, 14 subtypes of serotonin receptors have been cloned (Kroeze et al. 2002). The $5-HT_2$, $5-HT_4$, $5-HT_6$, and $5-HT_{2C}$ receptors appear to be particularly significant in mood disorders. Most of these receptors are found presynaptically, but some are located postsynaptically. Serotonin has an important modulatory effect on dopamine (DA), mainly in the mesolimbic region (Di Matteo et al. 2001). Functions of the serotonin system in the brain include regulating neurovegetative functions, such as sleep, pain sensitivity, sexual function, and appetite (Maes and Meltzer 1995). In addition, serotonin appears to play a neurotrophic role by maintaining structural and synaptic integrity (Duman 2004).

Genetics. Functional variants in the 5-HTT promoter region have been isolated. The so-called short allele of one of the key variants may predispose to depression when environmental stressors are experienced (Caspi et al. 2003).

Biochemistry. Decreased 5-HIAA in the cerebrospinal fluid (CSF) is associated with aggression, impulsivity, and violent suicide (Asberg et al. 1976).

Challenge tests. The release of serotonin facilitates the release of prolactin and corticotrophin. A blunted release of prolactin in response to intravenous tryptophan or clomipramine has been shown to occur in depression (Delgado et al. 1992). Compounds that deplete serotonin or tryptophan are likely to produce depression. The most obvious effects are seen in patients with depression who are serotonin reuptake inhibitor responders, in whom the return of core depressive symptoms is seen.

Postmortem findings. 5-HTT density has been found to be low in frontal cortex, hippocampus, and occipital cortex. Other postmortem findings include reductions in the 5-HT$_{1A}$ receptors in the dorsal and median raphe (Arango et al. 2001).

Norepinephrine System

Norepinephrine (NE) or noradrenaline is synthesized from tyrosine via phenylalanine and DA in neuronal vesicles. NE is released into the synapse in a calcium-dependent process. Removal of released NE is by reuptake pumps for either NE or DA (into dopaminergic neurons) (Torres et al. 2003). NE then may be either reused in vesicles or metabolized by monoamine oxidase into 3-methoxy-4-hydroxymandelic acid. NE neurons originate from several brain-stem nuclei, including the locus coeruleus (Grant and Redmond 1981), and project to fore- and midbrain, cerebellum, and lumbar spinal cord. The effects of NE are modulated in the postsynaptic neuron by metabotropic G-protein-linked receptors. These include β_1- and β_2-adrenergic receptors (stimulatory) and α_1-, α_{2A}-, α_{2B}-, and α_{2C}-adrenergic types (Bylund 1988). The NE system is responsible for modulating behavior and attention, together with the prefrontal cortex. Firing of the locus coeruleus is stimulated by certain stressful situations. Together with the amygdala, NE neurons impart an emotional component to memory (Cahill et al. 2001). This may improve recall of emotionally charged material, but it also may provoke inappropriate memory cueing.

Biochemistry. Investigation of CSF, plasma, and urine for NE and its metabolites in depression has not identified specific correlates of depression. Studies of peripheral platelet and lymphocyte adrenergic receptors have yielded conflicting results. However, the cyclic adenosine monophosphate (cAMP) response to stimulation by a β-stimulant is blunted in depression (Ressler and Nemeroff 1999).

Challenge tests. The use of NE challenge tests in depression has again failed to show specific dysfunction. The daily use of α-methoxy-p-tyrosine (AMPT) in depressed patients who are taking an adrenergic antidepressant is likely to produce a return of depressive symptoms (Delgado et al. 1993).

Dopamine System

DA is synthesized in DA neurons from tyrosine, via two enzymatic steps. Synaptic DA is taken up by both NE and DA reuptake pumps (Torres et al. 2003). DA neurons project mainly from the ventral mesencephalon or from the pituitary gland. Important tracts include the nigrostriatal, mesolimbic, and mesocortical pathways. DA receptors are grouped into the stimulatory D$_1$-like (including D$_1$ and D$_5$) and the inhibitory D$_2$-like (D$_2$, D$_3$, and D$_4$). All are metabotropic and G-protein-coupled. The D$_2$-like receptors are found mainly in limbic brain, whereas D$_1$-like receptors are widespread and especially rich in the striatum. The DA projections are involved in modulating higher centers: nigrostriatal fibers affect motor function, mesolimbic fibers (together with the nucleus accumbens) affect reward and motivation, and mesocortical fibers affect memory and attention (Chen and Zhuang 2003).

Biochemistry. DA plays a role in reward processing and may be dysregulated in depression (Hasler et al. 2004) and mania. The role of DA in mania has been suggested by the manic illness following DA agonist use (e.g., amphetamine compounds). Similarly, DA releasers may be useful in depression, and DA antagonists are effective in treating mania.

Neuropeptides in Mood Disorders

Many neuropeptides are cotransmitters; they are located and released together with a neurotransmitter. Neuropeptide release from large vesicles is usually slower than neurotransmitter release (Baraban and Tallent 2004). Reduced levels of somatostatin and neuropeptide Y have been found in the CSF of depressed patients (Heilig and Widerlov 1995). The role of endogenous opioids in mood disorders is unclear.

Neuroplasticity and Neurotrophic Factors

Stress may have an adverse effect on the brain, particularly the limbic system. Reduction in hippocampal volumes and other structures in depression suggests that maladaptive neuroplastic changes occur during depressive episodes (Campbell et al. 2004). The finding that major depressive mood episodes tend to recur and that subsequent episodes may not follow stress suggests an initial neurotoxicity or impairment of neuroplasticity (Kendler et al. 2000). The expression of brain-derived neurotrophic factor (BDNF), for example, is affected by long-term changes in monoamines (Duman 2004).

Psychoneuroendocrinology

The role of hormones in human emotion and behavior has been suggested by several lines of thought: first, the brain is the major target of most human hormones; second, hormones are released by the brain and are involved in many neural circuits; third, endocrine disorders commonly have neuropsychiatric effects; and last, some exogenous hormones have clear psychotropic effects (e.g., estrogen and thyroid hormone) (Halbreich 1997).

Hypothalamic-Pituitary-Adrenal Axis

Hypothalamic-pituitary-adrenal (HPA) axis stimulation modulates metabolism, reproduction, inflammation, immunity, and hippocampal neurogenesis (Plotsky et al. 1998). A state of reversible depression is induced in more than half of the people with hypercortisolemic conditions, with nearly 10% developing suicidality or psychosis. Conversely, patients with major depression have elevated plasma, CSF, and urine cortisol levels, as well as elevated corticotropin-releasing hormone (CRH). In addition, the dexamethasone suppression test (DST) (failure to suppress cortisol release) is blunted in depression. The test is 90% sensitive to detecting depression but only 30%–50% specific (Copolov et al. 1989). The additional component of CRH stimulation has improved sensitivity and may predict relapse if the DST or CRH test fails to normalize. More recent attention has been directed toward CRH. In depression, CRH is hypersecreted, and early studies have suggested the efficacy of a CRH antagonist (Arborelius et al. 1999).

Mechanisms for this HPA dysregulation are unclear. Corticosteroid receptors, glucocorticoid–neurotransmitter interactions, or the pattern of HPA axis hormone release may be abnormal in depression.

Thyroid Physiology in Depression

Hyperthyroid states are documented to produce emotional lability, irritability, insomnia, anxiety, weight loss, and agitation (Demet et al. 2002). Hypothyroidism typically induces fatigue, memory impairment, irritability, and loss of libido (Chueire et al. 2003). Despite anecdotal evidence to the contrary, studies of hypothyroidism in the general population have not reported an increased rate of depression (Engum et al. 2002). In established depression, approximately one quarter of individuals have thyroid dysfunction—most commonly, an increase in free thyroxine (T_4) (Rubin 1989). Hypofunction of the hypothalamic-pituitary-thyroid (HPT) axis has been linked to poor antidepressant response and earlier recurrence (Joffe and Marriott 2000). HPT axis abnormalities also have been reported in rapid-cycling bipolar disorder, although most first-line mood stabilizers decrease thyroid hormone levels (Baumgartner et al. 1995). The addition of thyroid hormone to tricyclic antidepressants (TCAs) may induce remission in some individuals with depression (Joffe 1997) and stabilize some patients with refractory bipolar disorder (Whybrow et al. 1992).

Hypothalamic-Pituitary-Gonadal Axis

The use of testosterone is controversial—in hypogonadal men, use appears to be associated with improvement in mood (C. Wang et al. 2004), whereas the effects of replacement in older men seem to be associated with only improvement in sexual function (Gray et al. 2005). Exogenous testosterone does not appear to have direct antidepressant properties (Seidman 2006). In studies of men with established depression, conflicting data have been reported (Seidman 2006).

In menopausal women, population-based studies have not shown an increase in major depression, despite anecdotal reports (Avis et al. 1997). In menopausal women who have established depression, the HPG axis appears to be abnormal—in the early phases, axis activity is increased (high luteinizing hormone and follicle-stimulating hormone), and in the subsequent phases, activity is decreased (O'Toole and Rubin 1995).

Two neuroendocrine theories have been proposed to explain the higher prevalence of depression in women: 1) estrogen release sensitizes neurotransmitter systems (Steiner et al. 2003), and 2) the cyclical release causes ongoing changes in neurotransmitter systems that make women more vulnerable to depression (Rubinow et al. 2002). In premenopausal women with major depression, the HPG axis appears to be normal (Amsterdam et al. 1995). Premenstrual dysphoric disorder occurs during the luteal phase and remits during menses. However, no clear luteal-phase-specific physiological changes have been confirmed (Rubinow et al. 2002). Postpartum depression affects 10% of women and is more likely in those with a prior episode (Rubinow et al. 2002). HPG axis function appears to be normal in this state, whereas the HPA axis may be abnormal. Menopausal women often report irritability, crying, mood lability, fatigue, loss of libido, loss of motivation, and anxiety (Steiner et al. 2003). These symptoms may be a result of changes in and withdrawal from estrogens.

Anatomical Pathology

A range of structural and histological pathologies occurs in both depression and bipolar disorder.

Neuronal and Glial Pathology

A reduced number and size of neurons in frontolimbic cortex have been reported (Rajkowska et al. 2001). These regions include dorsolateral prefrontal cortex, orbitofrontal cortex, heteromodal association cortex, and cingulate gyrus. Histopathological findings suggest that neuronal atrophy is the main problem, with an abnormality of development or degeneration rather than loss or apoptosis (Rajkowska 2006). Cell reduction is thought to be related to a decrease or change in dendritic anatomy or altered synaptic contacts, but this has not been systematically studied (Rajkowska 2006).

Postmortem studies of hippocampi have shown that neuronal density is increased, cell size is reduced, and dendritic and glial cell processes are diminished (Rosoklija et al. 2000). These histopathological findings may account for the in vivo findings. Changes of subcortical structures are inconsistent (Rajkowska 2006).

Glial cell changes occur in mood disorders. Many of the brain regions listed earlier are affected by changes in glial cell shape, size, and density. Glial cells have been shown to be increased in size in the prefrontal cortex and limbic region (Rajkowska et al. 2001), with increased density but decreased numbers. In addition, as in the case of neurons, glial dendrites and synapses appear to be diminished in size and number (Rajkowska 2006). Glia bear almost all the same receptors as neurons do, suggesting a role in neuromodulation and neurotransmission beyond that which was originally thought (Cotter et al. 2002).

Clinical studies have shown volumetric loss in cortical, limbic, and subcortical structures, possibly representing atrophy (Soares and Mann 1997). Hippocampal volumes have consistently been shown to be reduced in depression. Patients with unmedicated bipolar disorder appear to have lower N-acetylaspartate (NAA) levels in their hippocampi (representing decreased neuronal viability), whereas treatment with lithium increases NAA levels (G.J. Moore et al. 2000).

Molecular and Cellular Neurobiology

Neuroplasticity and Cellular Resilience

Neuroplasticity (the brain's ability to adapt to stress through changing intra- and interneuronal anatomy) and cellular resilience (the degree to which neurons are able to adapt) are essential components of the development of mood disorders. The secretion of cortisol appears to have an important role in neuroplasticity—the limbic region appears to be reduced in conditions of hypercortisolemia and is reversed by using an antiglucocorticoid (Singh et al. 2006). The limbic region is rich in glucocorticoid receptors. Stress also appears to increase limbic glutamate levels (McEwen 1999). Although N-methyl-D-aspartate (NMDA) receptor antagonists seem to attenuate this process, it is likely that other glutamate receptor subtypes (particularly ionotropic) facilitate neurotoxicity when stress is ongoing or excessive (Singh et al. 2006).

These effects also impair cellular resilience. The decrease of BDNF expression during stress is one way in which this mechanism operates, although BDNF is not directly affected by hypercortisolemia (Lauterborn et al. 1998). Another result of stress is the impairment of neurogenesis (E. Gould and Tanapat 1999). This process occurs in subventricular and subgranular limbic tissue. Some evidence indicates that antidepressant and lithium use may promote neurogenesis (Santarelli et al. 2003). Lithium inhibits several intraneuronal enzymes, including some magnesium-dependent phosphatases and glycogen synthase kinase-3 (Singh et al. 2006).

Neuroimmunity and Mood Disorders

The immune system and cytokines may play a role in mediating mood disorders. Increased cytokine levels in plasma have been linked to depression and depressive behavior (Maes et al. 1993), particularly interleukins 1 and 6. Conversely, patients receiving various cytokines have many depressive symptoms, including depression, anhedonia, and loss of appetite (Singh et al. 2006).

Brain Imaging

A range of structural and functional imaging modalities are now available for investigation of mood disorders. A history of neural localization studies from the first half of the twentieth century laid the foundation for the growing field of neuroimaging—most notably, the work of Moniz (1937), who used neurosurgical ablation to treat melancholia. Current imaging aims to identify pathological substrates that form discrete sites of emotion, as well as the functional pathways that link them (Mayberg 2003).

Structural Imaging

Lesions identified in the brains of individuals with neurological conditions, such as stroke, tumors, or Alzheimer's disease, have shown that certain regions are more likely to play a role in the etiology of depression (Starkstein and Robinson 1993). For example, lesions of the dorsolateral frontal lobe are more likely to cause depressive symptoms than are lesions of the ventral frontal lobe. Similarly, neurodegeneration of the substantia nigra, as seen in Parkinson's disease, is associated with a high risk of developing depression. Because depression may develop as a result of lesions occurring at two discrete sites, the condition may be both heterogeneous and arising from several functionally linked areas. Although there has been some debate, several studies have reported that lesions of the right frontal lobe are more likely to induce mania, whereas lesions of the left frontal lobe are more likely to induce depression (Robinson et al. 1984; Starkstein et al. 1990).

In primary mood disorders, clinicians are unlikely to find pathognomonic major structural abnormalities (Sheline 2003). Gray matter changes have been reported in orbitofrontal cortex with quantitative magnetic resonance imaging (MRI), mainly in the elderly depressed (Ballmaier et al. 2004); loss of volume of the hippocampus also has been found, with the degree of atrophy correlating with disease chronicity and time off treatment (Sheline et al. 2004). Periventricular white matter changes in the elderly, together with ventricular enlargement, also have been documented (Hickie et al. 1997).

Functional Imaging

Functional imaging approaches have added information on putative functional pathways and circuits, especially when similar disease arises from structurally different lesions (Mayberg 2006). The consistent findings are impaired regional blood flow and metabolism of the frontal lobes and cingulate gyrus (Videbech 2000). Some studies have reported an inverse relation between depression severity and prefrontal activity (Ketter et al. 1996).

Both positron emission tomography (PET) and single photon emission computed tomography (SPECT) have used neurochemical markers to identify decreased densities of the 5-HTT in the brain stem (Malison et al. 1998). Several other studies have produced inconsistent findings with respect to other serotonin receptors, as well as the dopamine system. Treatment studies also have been conducted, whereby functional imaging of subjects is performed prior to treatment and then after treatment. In general, these have reported a normalization of pretreatment changes (Mayberg 2006). Most notably, the reduced metabolism seen in the frontal lobes has consistently been found. This occurs when both pharmacotherapies and certain psychotherapies are used in treatment. Studies that have used ligands have been able to show frontal 5-HT_{2A} receptor downregulation following treatment (Mann et al. 2000). When medications are compared with psychotherapy directly, different areas of change have been shown. Decreases in lateral frontal and increases in limbic metabolism have been reported with cognitive-behavioral therapy (CBT), whereas the opposite picture may be seen when medications are used (Mayberg 2006).

Cognitive Processing Models of Depression

Cognitive Deficits in Depression

A range of cognitive changes have been described in studies of depression. These include the speed of cognitive processing, impaired attention, and the bias toward negative stimuli (Williams 1997). Memory problems are also seen in depressed individuals. Delayed recall is impaired more than recognition. Immediate recall seems to be relatively spared. Mood-congruent memory—the phenomenon whereby depressed individuals more readily recall memories when they are matched to negative emotional valence—is also affected. People with depression recall more negative memories (Matt et al. 1992).

Other types of cognitive problems are dysfunctional thoughts and beliefs (Beck 1967). Underlying these, the information-organizing system, or schema, is found. Schemas are ways in which attention, memory, and information are organized. Negative schemas may emerge in response to a stressor.

Kindling and sensitization are important depressive phenomena. In kindling, people with prior depressive episodes are thought to be more likely to carry depressive thoughts and therefore activate subsequent episodes more readily (Post 1992). This theory is supported by evidence that people with recurrent depression develop subsequent episodes despite the absence of a stressor (Kendler et al. 2000).

Cognitive Features of Depression

A common feature of studies of cognition in depression is the bias toward negative information, emotions, and memories. This selective attention may operate at schema level. In this way, negative thoughts and beliefs that prevail during depressive episodes are reinforced by underlying structures that have already been defined by previous negative experiences. The depressed individual will dwell on negative material, such as negative automatic thoughts, but will ascribe meaning that fits with a dysfunctional schema (Beck 1967). More specifically, the person will ruminate on negative thoughts and the potential personal negative consequences: a depressed and self-referent bias. This mode of thinking usually is not disrupted by positive or other external stimuli and leads to a closed loop (Teasdale and Barnard 1993). The ability to shift focus from this negative loop may be a key strategy in treatment. The process whereby the depressed patient accesses negative information from the environment and the inner world could be seen as a selective filter. One strategy in cognitive therapy is to highlight this problem and challenge its use. The individual is then taught to focus on neutral or even positive information.

The other aspect of cognition that needs to be addressed is the slow and effortful thought processing of the depressed individual (Hartlage et al. 1993). Homework tasks that involve mastering small problems and stepwise approaches may go some way to improve this deficit.

Other Psychological Theories of Depression

Several central psychoanalytic and psychodynamic theories of depression and mood disorders have been described.

Sigmund Freud

In depression, Freud said that the superego is dominant as a result of guilt about anger toward loved ones (Freud 1923/1961). He spoke about the defenses of repression, reaction formation, and denial. Conflicts that were experienced early in life were hidden within the unconscious only to emerge later as depression.

Melanie Klein

Klein described an object relations theory whereby an individual moved from a paranoid position toward a depressed position. She maintained that an individual lived with the idea that he or she had destroyed a loved one and that this produced depression in later life (Klein 1940/1975). She was also the first person to speak of the manic defense—that mania might in fact represent a defense against a deeper depressive process.

John Bowlby

Attachment was central to Bowlby's work. The problem of anxious attachment or loss of an attachment was said to evoke depression when loss was experienced in later life (Bowlby 1969, 1980).

A psychoanalytic model of depression may include the following elements: early trauma or loss, leading to unresolved conflicts or anxieties; a lack of integration of these unconscious factors into the conscious life; a pattern of disruptive relationships due to unresolved conflicts or infantile fantasies; and a need to explore these issues through the experience of transference and interpretation in psychotherapy.

Somatic Interventions for Mood Disorders

Antidepressants

Antidepressants are classified according to their activity at monoamine receptors (Table 11–14).

Tricyclics, Tetracyclics, and Monoamine Oxidase Inhibitors

The efficacy of tricyclics, including the tetracyclics, in depression was discovered serendipitously in the 1950s. The TCAs act by reuptake inhibition at both NE and serotonin transporters. This combined effect is probably mediated by active metabolites of the TCAs, as much as by primary drug. However, other receptors are also antagonized by the TCAs: adrenergic, histaminergic, muscarinic, and dopaminergic receptors. These produce many of the undesirable side effects. The anticholinergic side effects (dry mouth and constipation), together with hypotension, somnolence, and cardiac arrhythmias, make these less widely used.

TABLE 11–14. Currently available antidepressants: activity, indications, adverse effects, and dosing

Antidepressant	Examples	Primary activity	Indications	Adverse effects	Dosing
Tricyclic antidepressants (TCAs)	Amitriptyline, desipramine, imipramine	SRI, NRI, Ach-M, Hist, α_1	Major depression, enuresis	Dry mouth, constipation, urinary retention, blurred vision, hypotension, cardiac toxicity, sedation	Commence 25 mg, increase to 100–200 mg/day
Selective serotonin reuptake inhibitors (SSRIs)	Fluoxetine, paroxetine, sertraline	SRI	Major depression, anxiety disorders, impulse-control disorders, bulimia nervosa	Agitation, insomnia, headache, nausea and vomiting, sexual dysfunction, hyponatremia	Usually 20 mg/day (fluoxetine); may increase to 60 mg/day
Monoamine oxidase inhibitors (MAOIs)	Tranylcypromine, moclobemide	MAOI	Major depression, social phobia	Hypertensive crises for older agents, insomnia, nausea, agitation, confusion	Moclobemide: 150–600 mg twice daily after food
Serotonin-norepinephrine reuptake inhibitors (SNRIs)	Venlafaxine, duloxetine	NRI, SRI	Major depression, generalized anxiety disorder	Hypertension (venlafaxine), nausea, insomnia, dry mouth, sedation, sweating, agitation, headache, sexual dysfunction	Venlafaxine: commence at 75 mg/day; increase to 225 mg/day as needed
Norepinephrine and dopamine reuptake inhibitors (NDRIs)	Bupropion	NRI, DRI	Major depression, smoking cessation	Agitation, insomnia, headache, nausea and vomiting, seizures (0.4%)	150 mg twice daily
Serotonin antagonism and reuptake inhibition (SARI)	Nefazodone	SRI, 5-HT$_2$, α_1, NRI	Major depression	Sedation, hepatotoxicity, dizziness, hypotension, paresthesias; priapism (trazodone)	100–300 mg twice daily

TABLE 11–14. Currently available antidepressants: activity, indications, adverse effects, and dosing *(continued)*

Antidepressant	Examples	Primary activity	Indications	Adverse effects	Dosing
Norepinephrine and serotonin specific antidepressant (NASSA)	Mirtazapine	α_2, 5-HT$_3$, 5-HT$_{2A}$, 5-HT$_{2C}$, Hist	Major depression	Weight gain, sedation, dizziness, headache; sexual dysfunction is rare	15–45 mg/day at night
Norepinephrine reuptake inhibition (NRI)	Reboxetine, atomoxetine	NRI	?Major depression, attention-deficit/hyperactivity disorder	Insomnia, sweating, dizziness, dry mouth, constipation, urinary hesitancy, tachycardia	Reboxetine: 4–6 mg twice daily

Note. SRI=serotonin reuptake inhibition; NRI=norepinephrine reuptake inhibition; Ach-M=muscarinic anticholinergic; Hist=histamine blockade; α_1=alpha-1 adrenergic blockade; MAOI=monoamine oxidase inhibition; DRI=dopamine reuptake inhibition; 5-HT$_2$=serotonin type 2 receptor antagonism; α_2=alpha-2 adrenergic blockade; 5-HT$_3$=serotonin type 3 receptor antagonism; 5-HT$_{2A}$=serotonin type 2A receptor antagonism; 5-HT$_{2C}$=serotonin type 2C receptor antagonism.

Other side effects include confusion, urinary retention, and blurred vision in the elderly; and increased appetite and weight gain.

TCAs originally were thought to be more effective in major depression with melancholic features (Paykel 1972). Depression with atypical features may not respond best to TCAs (J.W. Stewart et al. 2002). Care needs to be taken if TCAs are to be used in the elderly, and TCAs are generally not used in children and adolescents in view of lack of efficacy.

Some drug interactions of the TCAs need to be taken into account. Generally, these result from induced or impaired metabolism by the liver microsomal cytochrome P450 system. Care should be taken when any other drug with potential anticholinergic, antiadrenergic, or monoamine inhibition is given. The TCAs generally should be administered in a slow, upward dosage titration. The measurement of plasma levels may be indicated in suspected overdose or poor adherence and to establish a minimum effective dose.

The monoamine oxidase inhibitors (MAOIs) act by the inhibition of the presynaptic enzyme MAO. This produces an increase in synaptic concentrations of all monoamines. The two isoforms are MAO-A and MAO-B. The MAOIs are classified according to the degree of reversibility of binding to MAO and by their binding to the respective isoforms. Tranylcypromine and phenelzine are irreversible inhibitors of both isoforms; selegiline is more selective for MAO-B; moclobemide is a reversible inhibitor of MAO-A (not available in the United States). The inhibition of MAO-A leads to an increase in NE, which may precipitate a hypertensive crisis. For this reason, a diet free of the precursor tyramine is mandatory in patients taking these drugs. Problems in the use of MAOIs have curtailed their use, but a transdermal preparation of selegiline may offer a novel approach to depression, particularly depression with atypical features. Transdermal selegiline has the advantage over older MAOIs in that it does not irreversibly inhibit gut or liver MAO-A, while binding to both forms of MAO in the brain. This preparation may therefore be better tolerated and provide the therapeutic effects of the MAOIs sought by clinicians (Thase 2006). Other adverse effects of the MAOIs include anticholinergic effects, dizziness, nausea, forgetfulness, and myoclonic jerks. Weight gain, muscle cramps, sexual dysfunction, and hypoglycemia are late effects. The MAOIs may interact with a range of medications. Prescribers should be particularly aware of any other medications that may increase adrenergic tone or increase serotonin or dopamine concentrations to dangerous levels. The MAOIs are useful in bipolar depression or atypical depression, but they are not commonly used in view of dietary restrictions and adverse events.

Selective Serotonin Reuptake Inhibitors

The SSRIs are a group of drugs with similar but not identical effects. They are safer in overdose than are TCAs. Activities and dosing are shown in Table 11–15. In general, antidepressant response rates across studies vary from 60% to 75%, with no drug being more effective than another. Some studies have shown that SSRIs are less effective in melancholic depression (P.J. Perry 1996), whereas they are more effective for atypical depression. Neither finding can be conclusively accepted.

Serotonin–Norepinephrine Reuptake Inhibitors

Venlafaxine is an inhibitor of serotonin and NE transporters. It is prescribed in the dosage range of 75–225 mg/day. The extended-release preparation may be administered once daily (Gutierrez et al. 2003). Some elevation of blood pressure may be seen at higher doses, and this should be monitored in patients with a history of hypertension. Duloxetine is a more newly introduced serotonin-norepinephrine reuptake inhibitor that is given in dosages ranging from 20 to 80 mg/day.

Other Antidepressants

Bupropion is an inhibitor of both NE and dopamine reuptake. It also may facilitate presynaptic release of these monoamines. It may spare depressed individuals from the sexual side effects commonly seen with serotonergic agents. It is regarded as having a lower tendency to induce rapid cycling or to induce mania compared with other antidepressants (Stoll et al. 1994). Bupropion is also approved for the treatment of smoking cessation. Adverse effects include anxiety, agitation, dizziness, and nausea. The risk of seizures may be significantly increased, and it should be used with caution in individuals with any predisposing factors for seizures. Dosages should not exceed 400 mg/day.

Mirtazapine is a novel tetracyclic that antagonizes the NE α_2 receptor, as well as the 5-HT$_{2A}$ receptor (noradrenergic and serotonin specific antidepressant) (de Boer et al. 1996). In addition, it blocks 5-HT$_2$ and 5-HT$_3$ receptors, which contribute to anxiolysis. Antihistaminic effects include weight gain and sedation. Patients are given dosages between 15 and 45 mg/day.

Before prescribing an antidepressant, clinicians should be aware of several potentially harmful effects. The antidepressant discontinuation syndrome follows the abrupt cessation of any serotonergic agent—most commonly, SSRIs with a short half-life and venlafaxine.

TABLE 11–15. Selective serotonin reuptake inhibitors (SSRIs): activity, prescribing notes, and dosing

SSRI	Activity	Indications	Notes	Dosing
Fluoxetine	SRI, weak NRI and 5-HT$_{2C}$	Major depression, anxiety disorders, impulse-control disorders, bulimia nervosa	Long half-life (2 weeks), requires long washout before switching; highly protein bound	Usual dose 20 mg/day; increase gradually to 80 mg/day. Start 10 mg in young and old.
Paroxetine	SRI, weak ACh, Hist, and NRI	Major depression, panic disorder, generalized anxiety disorder, OCD	Produces sedation and anticholinergic effects; short half-life, discontinuation a problem	Start 20 mg/day; may increase to 60 mg/day
Sertraline	SRI, weak NRI and DRI	Major depression, PTSD		Start 50 mg/day; may increase to 200 mg/day
Fluvoxamine	NRI, SRI	OCD, depression		Start 50 mg/day; may increase to 200 mg/day
Citalopram	SRI, NRI (weak)	Major depression, panic disorder, and agoraphobia	Low inhibition of cytochrome P450 system; useful when drug interactions may be a problem	Start 20 mg/day; may increase to 60 mg/day
Escitalopram	SRI, NRI (weak)	Major depression, panic disorder, and agoraphobia	Low inhibition of cytochrome P450 system; useful when drug interactions may be a problem	Start 10 mg/day; may increase to 30 mg/day

Note.   SRI=serotonin reuptake inhibition; NRI=norepinephrine reuptake inhibition; 5-HT$_2$=serotonin type 2 receptor antagonism; Ach= anticholinergic; Hist=histamine blockade; OCD=obsessive-compulsive disorder; DRI=dopamine reuptake inhibition; PTSD=posttraumatic stress disorder.

Within a few days, a syndrome of anxiety, tearfulness, dizziness, electric shock–like sensations, irritability, myoclonus, nausea, and tremor may ensue. Clinicians should be mindful of this adverse effect and exercise caution when reducing or stopping such an agent. If this syndrome occurs, clinicians often use substitution and subsequent withdrawal of an agent with a longer half-life.

Sexual dysfunction is another relatively common effect of serotonergic agents. Problems include decreased libido, erectile dysfunction, and delayed ejaculation in men and delayed or absent orgasm in women. The distinction between depression-induced and drug-induced dysfunction can be difficult. If this problem persists, the clinician may be forced to switch to another agent with less potential to cause sexual dysfunction, such as mirtazapine or bupropion.

Mood Stabilizers

In some ways, the term *mood stabilizer* is a misnomer because these drugs have wider uses than for mood disorders. Also, many other drugs (e.g., atypical antipsychotics) have mood-stabilizing properties. However, lithium and the older anticonvulsants remain the archetypal mood stabilizers.

Lithium

In acute mania, lithium remains effective across a range of domains of the illness (Hirschfeld et al. 2002). Treatment response usually can be seen within 5–14 days. Some evidence suggests that lithium is most effective when used in classic or euphoric mania or when the patient has had few lifetime episodes (Bowden 1995). In addition, efficacy appears to be accelerated when dose titration is rapid (Keck et al. 2001). Plasma monitoring is essential in lithium treatment. A range of 0.6–1.2 mEq/L is regarded as therapeutic. Levels greater than that may raise the risk of toxicity, with nausea, vomiting, confusion, myoclonus, seizures, hyperreflexia, and coma. Lower levels may increase the risk of relapse. Other adverse effects of lithium treatment include tremor, cognitive dulling, nausea, weight gain, and sedation.

In the maintenance phase of bipolar illness, lithium has been shown to reduce the risk of relapse (Burgess et al. 2001). More recent studies have confirmed lithium's effectiveness in this regard but also have shown that most patients require more than one drug to achieve stability (Grof 2003). In one study, the combination of lithium and valproate resulted in a significantly lower rate of relapse, compared with monotherapy (Solomon et al. 1997).

Lithium also has been shown to reduce the risk of suicide independently of its mood-stabilizing properties (Baldessarini et al. 2003). In acute bipolar depression, lithium is superior to placebo, although response is usually partial (Zornberg and Pope 1993). This finding often provokes the concomitant use of antidepressants. As for acute mania, plasma levels of lithium need to be greater than 0.8 mEq/L. In unipolar depression, lithium has proven useful in treatment-refractory cases. Rates of improvement of 56%–96% have been reported (M. P. Freeman et al. 2004).

Valproate and Carbamazepine

In the late 1980s, valproate (sodium valproate or divalproex) was found to be superior to placebo in the treatment of acute mania (Bowden et al. 1994). Although studies have failed to show differences in efficacy among agents, the presence of depressive symptoms, impulsivity, hyperactivity, and multiple prior episodes may be associated with a better treatment response for valproate than for lithium (T. W. Freeman et al. 1992; Swann et al. 2002). The usual dose of valproate is 20 mg/kg but this can be increased to 30 mg/kg. Adverse effects include sedation, tremor, nausea and vomiting, hair loss, and weight gain. Rare problems include hepatotoxicity and pancreatitis.

Carbamazepine has been shown in recent studies to be effective in acute mania (Weisler et al. 2004). Adverse effects of carbamazepine include diplopia, blurred vision, ataxia, sedation, and nausea. Rarer problems such as blood dyscrasias, hepatic failure, pancreatitis, and exfoliative dermatitis have been reported. Some data suggest that carbamazepine is effective in maintenance treatment (Dardennes et al. 1995). Small studies have shown some effects of carbamazepine in acute bipolar and unipolar depression, but these were in treatment-refractory cases (Kramlinger and Post 1989). Oxcarbazepine is a similar agent with a lower incidence of side effects, but data on its efficacy are limited.

Other Anticonvulsants

Several newer anticonvulsants have been studied in bipolar illness, including gabapentin, lamotrigine, and topiramate. To date, no trials have conclusively shown that any of these agents is effective in acute mania (Keck and McElroy 2006). In maintenance treatment, lamotrigine has been shown to reduce the incidence of depressive episodes but not manic ones (Bowden et al. 2003). Lamotrigine also has proven effective in acute bipolar depression (Calabrese et al. 1999). Adverse effects of lamotrigine include headache, nausea, and xerostomia. The risk of serious (but rare) rash is reduced with careful dose titration.

Antipsychotic Medications

The antipsychotics as a group have played a significant role in the treatment of mood disorders. They have been used as adjunctive agents, as well as primary agents—in the case of the second-generation antipsychotics. The reader is referred to the chapters on psychotic disorders (see Chapter 10 in this volume, "Schizophrenia," by Minzenberg et al.) and medications in psychiatry (see Chapter 26 in this volume, "Psychopharmacology," by Martinez et al.) for detailed descriptions of the pharmacokinetics and pharmacodynamics of these drugs.

Use in Mood Disorders

In the United States, several antipsychotic agents are registered for use in acute mania: olanzapine, risperidone, quetiapine, ziprasidone, aripiprazole, and chlorpromazine. In addition, olanzapine and aripiprazole are approved for the maintenance treatment of bipolar disorder, and olanzapine is approved for acute bipolar depression. Almost all the antipsychotics are useful in acute mania. Although all first-generation agents are antimanic, chlorpromazine is most studied in this respect (Keck et al. 1998). Likewise, the second-generation agents have been subjected to several controlled trials, and all were found to be effective in acute mania (Strakowski 2003). In addition to being effective primary agents, the second-generation agents seem to increase the rate and degree of antimanic effect when used in combination with a mood stabilizer (Strakowski 2003).

In the maintenance phase, only the medications listed in the previous paragraph are approved in the United States. The first-generation antipsychotics, although widely used in this setting, have not proven effective (Keck et al. 2000). The problem of depression in the long-term course of bipolar disorder has prompted the use of second-generation agents in this phase. To date, olanzapine, aripiprazole, and quetiapine have been studied and have been found to be effective in preventing relapse in bipolar disorder (Marcus et al. 2003; Tohen et al. 2003). When acute bipolar depression is encountered, the first-generation agents have very little effect (Ahlfors et al. 1981). Some effect in acute bipolar depression is seen when second-generation agents are used (Keck et al. 2000), and they may have a role as adjunctive agents. Nevertheless, the mood stabilizers remain the treatments of choice in the

depressive phase of the illness. In unipolar depression, the first-generation agents have been used chiefly when psychotic symptoms are present. However, effective augmentation of antidepressants in nonpsychotic depression recently has been shown with some of the second-generation agents.

An emerging role for second-generation agents has been found in treatment-resistant depression (Shelton et al. 2001). Risperidone is effective in combination with SSRIs in treatment-resistant unipolar depression. Olanzapine in combination with fluoxetine is safe and effective in patients with bipolar depression and those with fluoxetine-resistant depression. Ziprasidone and aripiprazole augmentation of SSRIs has been reported to be effective in treatment-resistant depression in open-label studies.

Adverse Effects

The reader is referred to the chapters on psychotic disorders (see Chapter 10 in this volume, "Schizophrenia," by Minzenberg et al.) and medications in psychiatry (see Chapter 26 in this volume, "Psychopharmacology," by Martinez et al.) for a detailed description of adverse effects of antipsychotics. The long-term problem of tardive dyskinesia (encountered with treatment with first-generation agents) and the metabolic syndrome (seen with certain second-generation agents) should prompt careful consideration of the need for long-term therapy with these agents.

Electroconvulsive Therapy and Transcranial Magnetic Stimulation

Electroconvulsive Therapy

Electroconvulsive therapy (ECT) remains an important part of treatment. ECT evolved out of the field of seizure induction in the 1940s. In the 1950s, it was already recognized as more effective in severe mood disorders and catatonia than in psychosis. The introduction and use of anesthesia in the late 1950s led to safer methods. With the advent of pharmacology, ECT was reserved for more severe cases. More recently, the limitations of drugs have been established, and ECT has again found a place. Research into ECT increased, and a safe method was introduced into practice (Potter et al. 1991).

Mechanism of action. The exact mechanism of action of ECT is unknown. The placement of the electrode(s) and the intensity of the stimulus are crucial components of the mechanism of effect. Clinical and preclinical studies have found some consistent neurotransmitter changes: downregulation of β-adrenergic receptors—a similar effect to antidepressant treatment (Kellar et al. 1981); an increased density of 5-HT$_{2A}$ receptors (Kellar et al. 1981); and an increase in dopaminergic tone (Mann 1998). This latter effect may explain the improvement in motor symptoms of parkinsonism seen after ECT but stands in contrast to ECT's antipsychotic effect. Another postulate of the action of ECT is the stimulation or modulation of the HPA axis. In particular, work has focused on prolactin, with some authors stating that the magnitude of seizure is reflected in the postseizure prolactin level (Lisanby et al. 2000). The interaction of excitatory and inhibitory brain systems is another means of understanding ECT. This idea posits that areas of seizure initiation are functionally inhibited. The seizure therefore induces a change in the excitation-inhibition balance and forms the basis of recovery. This theory has been supported by electroencephalographic changes during effective ECT, which show prefrontal slowing (an increase in delta wave activity) (Sackeim et al. 1996), and some functional imaging studies, which have found reductions in cerebral blood flow after ECT (Saito et al. 1995). These inhibitory changes—particularly in the prefrontal cortex—appear to be linked to efficacy of ECT.

Indications. ECT should be considered if a rapid response is necessary, medication has been ineffective, or the patient has had a history of good response to ECT. It is a highly effective treatment in this setting (Sackeim and Rush 1995). Some evidence suggests that patients with major depression with psychotic features are more likely to respond to ECT (Nobler et al. 1997). ECT also may be used in treatment resistance, or in catatonia, especially when neuroleptic malignant syndrome is encountered (Davis et al. 1991) and benzodiazepines are ineffective. Other neurological indications for ECT include Parkinson's disease and intractable epilepsy.

The presence of intracranial pathology or any contraindication to anesthesia should prompt the clinician to seek alternative treatments. ECT is not contraindicated in elderly persons and may be especially effective and safe in this population.

Adverse effects. Cognitive side effects after ECT are common, although most are transient. A brief period of postictal disorientation is usual. Anterograde amnesia usually resolves in 2–4 weeks (Sackeim 1994). Retrograde amnesia, however, may persist. It is temporarily graded, being most dense for the time preced-

ing the ECT. In rare cases, it may be more extensive and result in memory gaps dating back years (Squire and Slater 1983). The effect of amnesia may be reduced by right unilateral electrode placement, lower dose stimulation, and wider spacing of treatments. A shortening of pulse width also may confer an advantage (Nobler and Sackeim 2006).

Treatment considerations. Patients receiving ECT usually are taking concomitant medications. The use of anticonvulsants and benzodiazepines may impede the treatment—these should be temporarily stopped or reduced. The use of lithium has been associated with prolonged delirium, and it also should be stopped or reduced before treatment. Most antidepressants, other than MAOIs, are safe during a course of ECT. ECT is usually given two to three times per week for between 6 and 12 treatments. Response is typically seen from the sixth treatment; an adequate trial requires at least 10 treatments. Most patients proceed to medication treatment, but some will be either intolerant or nonresponsive to drug treatments (Monroe 1991).

Transcranial Magnetic Stimulation

Repetitive transcranial magnetic stimulation (rTMS) refers to the rapid pulse frequency application of a magnetic field to the head. This results in neuronal depolarization in a "subconvulsive" manner. Some stimulations can, however, produce seizures in vulnerable individuals (Pascual-Leone et al. 1993). The mechanisms of action are not well understood at present. rTMS appears to have antidepressant effects, although results have not always been consistent, and some uncertainties remain about optimal administration (Burt et al. 2002). (See Chapter 27 in this volume, "Nonpharmacological Somatic Treatments," by George et al., for a more detailed discussion of rTMS.)

Novel and Other Somatic Treatments

With the growing body of research into the dysfunction of hormonal and peptide systems in mood disorders, and the established use of hormonal treatments (such as thyroid hormone), novel hormonal and peptide strategies have increasingly been researched.

Hypothalamic-Pituitary-Adrenal Axis Treatments

A range of antiglucocorticoids have been studied in depression, including ketoconazole, metyrapone, and mifepristone. Although few large controlled trials have been done, proof-of-principle studies have been successful.

Thyroid System Treatments

Used as an augmentation, triiodothyronine (T$_3$) produces an antidepressant response in 25%–50% of nonresponders (Aronson et al. 1996). Furthermore, the addition of T$_3$ accelerates the treatment response. This effect seems to be most prominent in women. Thyroid hormone administered at two to three times the normal replacement dose also appears effective in rapid-cycling bipolar disorder (Bauer et al. 2002). Long-term complications may ensue, so clinicians should always exercise caution when this approach is considered.

Testosterone and Gonadal Hormones

The use of testosterone in depression has met with mixed results. Some studies have shown improvement in depressive symptoms in hypogonadal men (Ehrenreich et al. 1999), but not all data are consistent. The effects on prostate enlargement must be considered. In women, estrogen is known to have mood-elevating properties, but this effect has not been shown in controlled studies in depression. In postmenopausal women, estrogen may improve mood symptoms, but its use is limited by adverse effects on uterine and breast tissue.

Vagus Nerve Stimulation

Vagus nerve stimulation (VNS) involves stimulation of the vagus nerve in the neck. The vagus nerve carries both efferent and a large proportion of afferent fibers. The afferent portion is the target of VNS. In this technique, a generator is implanted into the left chest, and a lead is connected to the left cervical vagus nerve. The afferent vagal fibers project to several brain areas implicated in neuropsychiatric disease, including the limbic system. Postulated mechanisms of action include changes in monoamine neurotransmitters, an antidepressant effect secondary to anticonvulsant effect, and longer-term changes in brain anatomy. VNS was initially used in epilepsy but was noted to have antidepressant effects in these patients (George et al. 2000). Although data on VNS are still at an early stage, VNS is now registered for use in the United States. (See Chapter 27 in this volume, "Nonpharmacological Somatic Treatments," by George et al., for a more detailed discussion of VNS.)

Deep Brain Stimulation

In deep brain stimulation (DBS), an electrode is passed into brain tissue and connected to a generator in the chest. Like VNS, DBS was initially used in neurology settings, such as Parkinson's disease. In this patient population, mood changes were observed when brainstem structures were stimulated (Kumar et al. 1998). As better evidence emerges, DBS may play a greater role in the treatment of depression. (See Chapter 27 in this volume, "Nonpharmacological Somatic Treatments," by George et al., for a more detailed discussion of DBS.)

Psychotherapy for Mood Disorders

Cognitive-Behavioral Therapy

The Cognitive Model

In a cognitive model, the depressed individual has negative thoughts about the self, the world, and the future (Beck 1976). These are influenced by genetic factors, early experiences, and the presence of other psychiatric conditions (Clarke et al. 1999). The trigger or activating event is filtered by the individual's orienting scheme. This interacts with a deeper set of structures to produce negative automatic thoughts, reinforcing behaviors, and biological depressive symptoms. The deeper cognitive structures refer to maladaptive beliefs or schemas that the individual has developed over time. Automatic thoughts interact with affect, in that they may either result from affective arousal or produce an affective state. These thoughts emerge into awareness without being checked and are assumed to be true (Thase and Beck 1993). The way in which negative automatic thoughts are structured can be defined in terms of different types of cognitive distortion (Beck and Emery 1985). Examples include all-or-nothing thinking (e.g., "Either I am a success at this job or I am a total failure"); magnification (e.g., "This job is too big for me to do because I am incompetent); and jumping to conclusions (e.g., "If I cannot do this job, I will get fired"). Certain negative thoughts have an associated strong emotion, which amplifies the somatic and behavioral responses. These responses may indicate established neurocircuitry that is prone to reactivate if triggered. The reader is referred to the chapter on CBT (see Chapter 31 in this volume, "Cognitive Therapy," by Wright et al.) for a more detailed discussion on the theory and background of this approach.

CBT Strategies and Techniques

CBT is essentially a brief, structured, and collaborative therapeutic intervention. A therapy may last from 12 to 20 sessions. Each session is structured to include a period of symptom review, intervention performance, and homework setting. Collaboration requires that the patient appreciate the need to give and receive feedback and that the patient–therapist team tackles assignments in a scientific and interactive manner. As the therapy develops, the patient takes on a greater role and ultimately will manage assignments independently. Psychoeducation is a crucial early component and usually makes use of a personally informed explanation of the condition and the therapy. Compliance with homework is associated with a greater treatment response (Burnes and Spangler 2000). Assignments should be described and performed during sessions and then recorded into a book, which is used as a manual. During assessment and early therapy, a record is made of negative automatic thoughts. The therapist may use some during initial feedback but must soon begin to help the patient recognize them. The goal is to identify these thoughts and then begin to challenge their assumed truth in order to modify them. In a patient's workbook, stressors or situations should be recorded. These should include the patient's associated feelings and negative thoughts. As the patient learns to challenge the thoughts, recorded entries may include weighting of the degree to which he or she believed the thought before and after modification. The Socratic technique offers an approach to challenge negative thoughts by means of reasoned inquiry (Beck et al. 1979). The therapist may go on to assist the patient in constructing a case for and a case against these thoughts. An opportunity to provide a reasonable alternative to the negative thought may then follow. For some, the use of imagery or role-playing may better elicit negative automatic thoughts and allow the therapist to analyze and challenge them.

As the therapy progresses, a pattern of thinking may emerge that belies a series of underlying themes. In the same way, these formative beliefs can be challenged. In some instances, they may be related to early experiences. The linking of a current belief system to a past experience may allow a patient to understand the source of negative feelings and thoughts. The introduction of behavioral techniques is particularly important when behavioral inactivation is present (Rehm 1977). Strategies aimed at improving a sense of competence through mastery by offering a series of graded exercises may be included. Similarly, depressed patients have reduced hedonic capacity, and the guided introduction of pleasurable activities may break a negative behavioral cycle. These behavioral tasks should be included in the patient's workbook and feedback about tasks sought at each session.

CBT usually does not require continuation. When symptoms are relieved well in advance of termination, relapse rates are lower than 10% (Thase et al. 1992). In some cases, a continuation phase may be indicated. This phase of therapy aims to eliminate symptoms and reduce risk of relapse (Jarrett and Kraft 1997). A gradual reduction in frequency of sessions is combined with an increase in control by the patient.

In a recent review of meta-analyses, CBT has been shown to produce consistently large effect sizes in the treatment of unipolar depression (Butler et al. 2006). In adults, this effect exceeds that of the antidepressants.

Cognitive-Behavioral Analysis

The cognitive-behavioral analysis system of psychotherapy was developed to treat chronic depression and dysthymia (McCullough 2000). In this therapy, the focus is on the patient's maladaptive style of social problem solving. A link is made between the patient's actions and their consequences. These dysfunctional thoughts and behaviors are purported to arise from early experiences and therefore are automatic and not readily open to challenge. By focusing on behaviors that produce positive outcomes, the therapist can reinforce more adaptive strategies. Four key strategies are used to achieve this goal: 1) situational analysis is used to identify the problematic behavior and then to modify it; 2) in a negative outcome situation, the patient may be offered options; 3) the positive thoughts and feelings that occur with a positive outcome are highlighted; and 4) the interpersonal discrimination exercise teaches the patient to examine expectations in relationships, including the therapeutic relationship, as a means to understand how negative feelings and attitudes may arise in relationships. A significant other list may aid the patient in understanding how important people have influenced his or her thoughts and actions, both positively and negatively (McCullough 2000).

Interpersonal Psychotherapy

Interpersonal therapy (IPT) began as a research tool to investigate depression in the 1970s. What followed was the development of a psychotherapy based on interpersonal theory, which proved to be highly effective in depressive disorders (Klerman et al. 1984; Weissman et al. 2000).

IPT Theory

IPT has its roots in the attachment theory of Bowlby. Building on this approach, the interpersonal theorists noted that social events may be protective and also destructive, if negative in nature. Klerman et al. (1984) described interpersonal events in the social world as complicated bereavement, role disputes (relationship difficulties), role transitions (a loss of any kind), and interpersonal deficits (when social isolation is encountered). These events, when identified by the therapist, form the content of IPT. They need not be causative, merely proximal to the condition. IPT differs from CBT in that it does not make use of homework assignments and differs from psychodynamic therapy in that the therapeutic relationship is not a focus of therapy. IPT has a wide range of indications within mood disorders, all of which have a strong evidence base. IPT has been shown to reduce depressive symptoms in several different settings of major depression, including acute and recurrent major depression (Frank et al. 1990), depression in adolescents and elderly persons (Mufson et al. 1999), depression associated with HIV (Markowitz et al. 1998), depression in primary care (Schulberg et al. 1996), and dysthymia (Markowitz 2003).

IPT Technique

IPT is a brief structured, collaborative therapy that usually lasts between 12 and 20 sessions. It is conventionally separated into early, middle, and termination phases. Central to the early phase are psychiatric assessment and formulation, which take changes in the interpersonal world into account. A clear diagnosis is made, followed by feedback and psychoeducation. The focus is always on depression being a medical condition that is not the patient's fault. The analysis of the patient's interpersonal world is discussed, taking into account recent changes, patient expectations, and relationships that are proximal to the current depressive episode. In the middle phase, the therapist uses the selected interpersonal focus area (see "IPT Theory" earlier in this section) and applies strategies to address it. These may include examining the patient's expectations of the relationship, exploring options in relationships, and role-playing to practice tactics. Each session brings current relationship experiences to the fore. During termination, the patient's competencies are reinforced, and an approach to identifying future depressive triggers is explored. IPT continues to be explored as an effective therapy for various psychiatric conditions.

Psychodynamic Psychotherapy

The basic tenets underlying psychoanalytic and psychodynamic theory are discussed elsewhere in this textbook. Psychodynamic therapy may be effective in mild depression (Gallagher-Thompson and Steffen 1994). Psychodynamic therapy may be necessary when personality factors are implicated in depressive psychopathology—such as when an Axis I condition is comorbid with a personality problem or when depressive personality is diagnosed separately from dysthymia (Gabbard 2000). When other personality disorders occur, such as borderline personality disorder, psychodynamic therapy may offer augmentation to other treatment strategies (American Psychiatric Association 2001).

Principles of Psychodynamic Therapy

Crucial to the consideration of whether to initiate psychodynamic therapy—either brief or long term—are the patient factors that improve chances of the therapy's success. These include a motivation to understand, a tolerance for frustration, significant suffering, and ability to hold a job. As with IPT, brief psychodynamic therapy seeks to define a focus for the therapy. This may involve a loss, a role confusion or change, or relationship stress. Longer-term psychodynamic therapy allows for the therapist to develop a psychodynamic formulation based on a detailed early and current account of events. Within the context of the therapeutic relationship, conflicts and anxieties (in the form of transference and resistance) emerge and offer the therapist an opportunity to analyze the issue. Much of the interaction must be carefully monitored by the therapist, so as to appreciate how he or she may be contributing to the dynamic relationship. Central to psychodynamic therapy is the therapeutic frame, which requires that the therapist retain relative anonymity, that sessions are set in time and place, and that extrasessional contact is dealt with in sessions.

Psychodynamic and Psychoanalytic Approach to Depression

In psychodynamic therapy for the treatment of depression, the therapist must listen carefully to experiences and themes that may have developed into depression. These may include ideas that the patient has internalized anger, has an overdeveloped superego or sense of responsibility, or feels helpless and dependent. Out of these thoughts and feelings, a range of defense mechanisms may have evolved. These include repression, denial, projection, and reaction formation. During the patient's account, patterns of relating may emerge. A core relationship theme may become prominent (Luborsky 1984). This conflict usually will repeat itself within the therapeutic relationship. This affords the therapist the opportunity to understand the patient's contribution to the conflict and a means by which to point out maladaptive defenses. The transference must be understood and brought into the therapy. The termination of psychodynamic therapy inevitably evokes earlier feelings of loss, and the therapist must deal with the unconscious sense of responsibility and anger.

Psychotherapy for Bipolar Disorder

Psychotherapy for bipolar disorder has lagged behind pharmacotherapy, partly because of the pronounced effects that medication alone has on many aspects of the condition. In the past, psychotherapies focused mainly on the depressive episodes and psychological consequences of bipolar disorder. The manic patient's absence of insight and lack of motivation to understand (see "Principles of Psychodynamic Therapy" earlier in this chapter) precluded benefit from psychodynamic therapy. Out of the literature and practice of psychotherapy for schizophrenia arose several therapies recently shown to be of benefit to patients with bipolar disorder.

Psychoeducation

A brief, focused psychoeducational therapy aimed at remitted patients with bipolar disorder is effective in reducing relapse rates (A. Perry et al. 1999). A psychoeducational program should include education about the illness and medication, training in recognition of the signs of early relapse, information about the value of seeking help, and promotion of regular sleep–wake cycles.

Cognitive-Behavioral Therapy

CBT for bipolar disorder has made use of mood diaries, examination of negative thoughts about the illness, and addressing of barriers to treatment adherence. When this type of CBT was added to routine care, the CBT group had fewer bipolar episodes, reduced episode duration, and reduced hospitalizations (Lam et al. 2003). CBT appears to have a greater advantage for depressive episodes than for manic episodes (Scott et al. 2001).

Family Therapy

Family therapy for bipolar disorder has been developed as a family-focused therapy. This therapy, offered as 21 sessions over 9 months, makes use of psychoeducation, communication skills, and problem-solving skills (Miklowitz and Hooley 1998).

Interpersonal and Social Rhythm Therapy

The utility of IPT has been studied in bipolar disorder, and some data support its efficacy. In particular, IPT and social rhythm therapy have been integrated. The combined therapy makes use of the following principles: identifying and managing affective symptoms, linking mood and life events, maintaining regular daily rhythms, linking interpersonal factors to rhythm dysregulation, and mourning the lost healthy self (Frank et al. 2000).

Integrative Management of Mood Disorders

Interest in an integrated approach to the treatment of mood disorders is increasing. An integrated approach includes the use of medication, psychotherapies, and combined approaches. Numerous trials have investigated the treatment of depression, but far fewer studies have focused on the optimal combining or sequencing of different modalities. Practice guidelines and treatment algorithms attempt to synthesize the existing evidence with clinical consensus (Jobson 1997).

Major Depressive Disorder

Treatment Guidelines in Major Depression

Practice guidelines for the treatment of major depression include those published by the American Psychiatric Association (2000b). The Texas Medication Algorithm Project (Crismon et al. 1999), the Sequenced Treatment Alternatives to Relieve Depression study (STAR*D; Fava et al. 2003), and the National Institute of Clinical Excellence (http://www.nice.org.uk/page.aspx?o=mental) have all provided algorithms for the treatment of depression. The Texas Medication Algorithm Project strategies for the treatment of nonpsychotic major depression are shown in Figure 11–2 (Trivedi et al. 2004).

Because no consistent evidence distinguishes between initial monotherapies at this time, a selection strategy might rather use other guides, such as a previously effective agent for that person or a first-degree relative or an agent with effectiveness for a comorbid condition. The goal of treatment is to achieve remission (absence of symptoms) rather than merely response (reduction of at least 50% of symptoms).

The duration of a first treatment trial is often debated. A response should be seen by 10 weeks. When response is partial, an augmentation or a combination

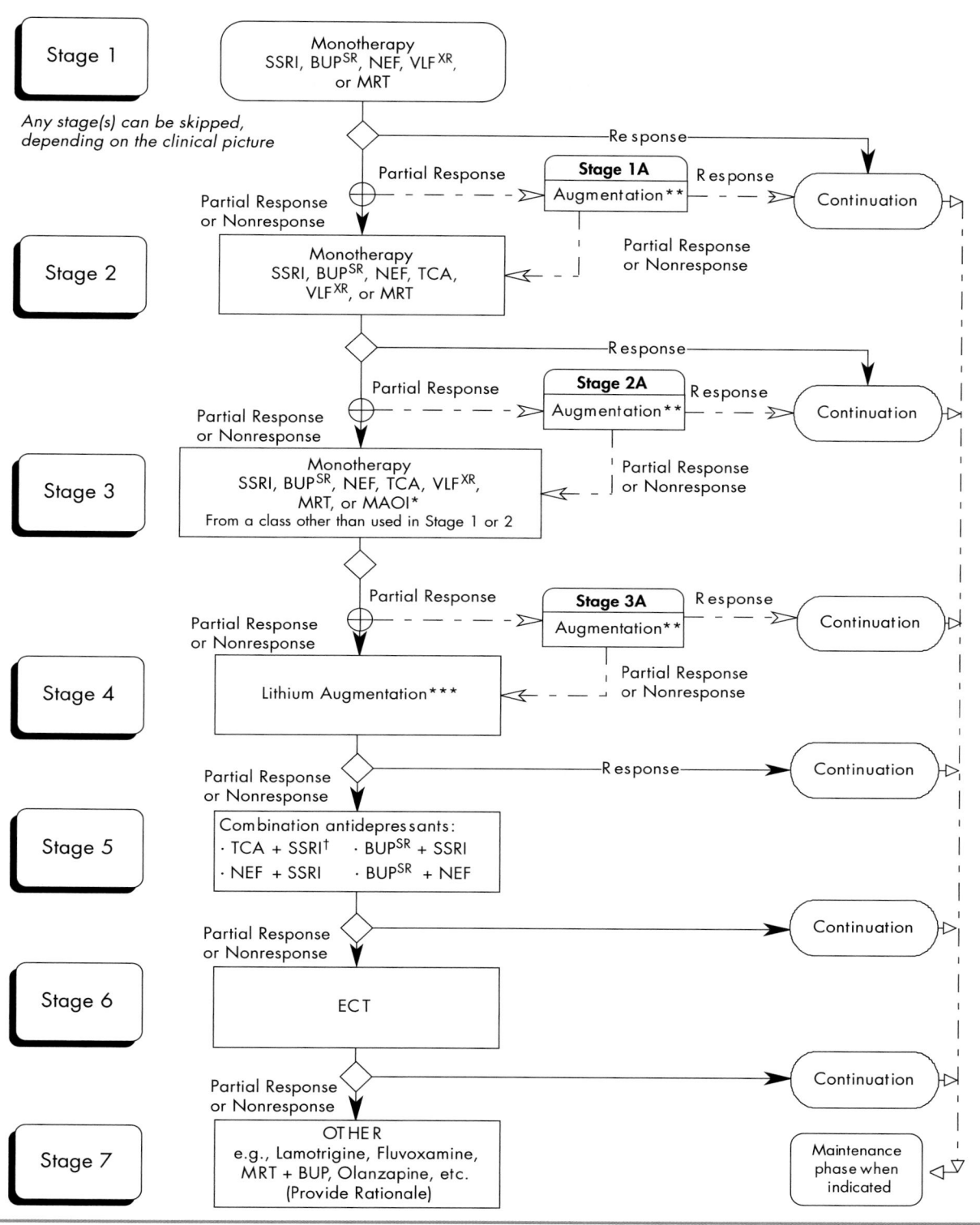

FIGURE 11–2.   Strategies for the treatment of major depression (nonpsychotic).

Note.   SSRI = selective serotonin reuptake inhibitor (fluoxetine, sertraline, paroxetine, citalopram); BUP^{SR} = bupropion sustained release; NEF = nefazodone; VLF^{XR} = venlafaxine extended release; MRT = mirtazapine; TCA = tricyclic antidepressant; MAOI = monoamine oxidase inhibitor; ECT = electroconvulsive therapy.
*Consider TCA/VLF if not tried. **Lithium, thyroid, buspirone. ***Skip if lithium augmentation has already failed.
†Most studied combination.

Source.   Trivedi et al. 2004. Algorithms are revised as new data become available; consult the Texas Implementation of Medication Algorithms (TIMA) Web site (http://www.dshs.state.tx.us/mhprograms/TIMA.shtm) for the most recent versions.

strategy may be used. Fair evidence for lithium, thyroid hormone, and buspirone exists in this regard, and some of the atypical antipsychotics are showing promise as augmenting agents in major depression (Ostroff and Nelson 1999; Shelton et al. 2001). Augmentation should result in response from 4 weeks. If response is adequate, then the strategy should be continued for 4–9 months.

Combined Medication and Psychotherapeutic Approaches

There is empirical evidence for the effectiveness of CBT, IPT, and a cognitive-behavioral analysis system of psychotherapy in the treatment of depression (see "Cognitive-Behavioral Analysis" subsection earlier in this chapter). The combination of medication and psychotherapy is indicated in chronic depressive conditions (Keller et al. 2000). Psychotherapy, particularly a cognitive-behavioral analysis system of psychotherapy, may be considered at stage 1 of the treatment algorithm shown in Figure 11–2 if an individual with chronic depression presents for treatment (Schatzberg et al. 2005). Evidence indicates that individuals with chronic depression and a history of parental loss or abuse in childhood may respond well to psychotherapy (Nemeroff 2003).

Medication Combination and Augmentation

To date, the most evidence on medication combination exists for a combination of TCA and SSRI, but other combinations are used. The evidence is good for the addition of lithium and thyroid hormone and fair for the use of tryptophan (Fava et al. 1994; Joffe and Singer 1990; S. Smith 1998). Other strategies include using ECT (see stage 6 of the depression treatment algorithm in Figure 11–2) and high-dose venlafaxine (D. Smith et al. 2002).

Bipolar Disorder

An integrative approach demands that the clinician appreciate the longitudinal course of the illness, its tendency to recur, and the prominence of depressive episodes. It is useful to understand the management of bipolar disorder from acute-episode and maintenance-phase perspectives.

Treatment Guidelines in Bipolar Disorder

Currently available guidelines include the practice guideline for the treatment of patients with bipolar disorder published by the American Psychiatric Association (2002), the guidelines published by the British Association for Psychopharmacology (G.M. Goodwin et al. 2003), and the Texas Medication Algorithm Project treatment algorithm for patients with bipolar disorder (Suppes et al. 2001). The Texas Medication Algorithm Project treatment strategies for hypomania/mania in bipolar disorder are presented in Figure 11–3. In addition, the prescriber must take into account whether the patient's symptoms have previously responded to an agent, whether rapid cycling is present (use an anticonvulsant), and whether psychotic symptoms are present. The recommended duration of a trial of monotherapy is unclear. A response should be noted by 7–14 days, but remission may take considerably longer. Guidelines for the maintenance phase of the illness are less clear. Common practice and consensus suggest that most clinicians will continue the mood stabilizer that the patient's symptoms responded to in the acute phase and will discontinue any antipsychotics that were used (Bowden et al. 2000).

In acute bipolar depression, the use of antidepressants alone generally should be avoided because of the risk of inducing rapid cycling. Fair evidence indicates that the prescriber should select one of three treatment strategies: lithium, lamotrigine, or a fluoxetine–olanzapine combination. If the episode is severe, combinations of mood stabilizers, ECT, or an antidepressant–mood stabilizer combination may be used. In all cases, thyroid abnormalities and comorbid substance abuse should be ruled out. In the maintenance phase of bipolar depression, there is good evidence for the effectiveness of lamotrigine when depressive episodes are recurrent (Bowden et al. 2003) and for lithium when both manic and depressive episodes recur (Prien et al. 1984). Long-term antidepressant use is associated with a higher risk of recurrence of mania.

Treatment of Bipolar Disorder in Women of Childbearing Age

The clinician must pay special attention to a broad range of needs in women of childbearing age. It is best for women to plan pregnancies to allow for the possible withdrawal of mood stabilizers. In all instances, the clinician must make treatment decisions on the basis of benefits and risks to the fetus. All mood stabilizers are potentially teratogenic, and some may be harmful during lactation (American Psychiatric Association 2002). If drug therapy is considered essential, several strategies may be used to reduce risk to the fetus: using monotherapy at the lowest effective dose, using concomitant folate therapy, and avoiding medication during the first trimester of pregnancy (Iqbal et al. 2001).

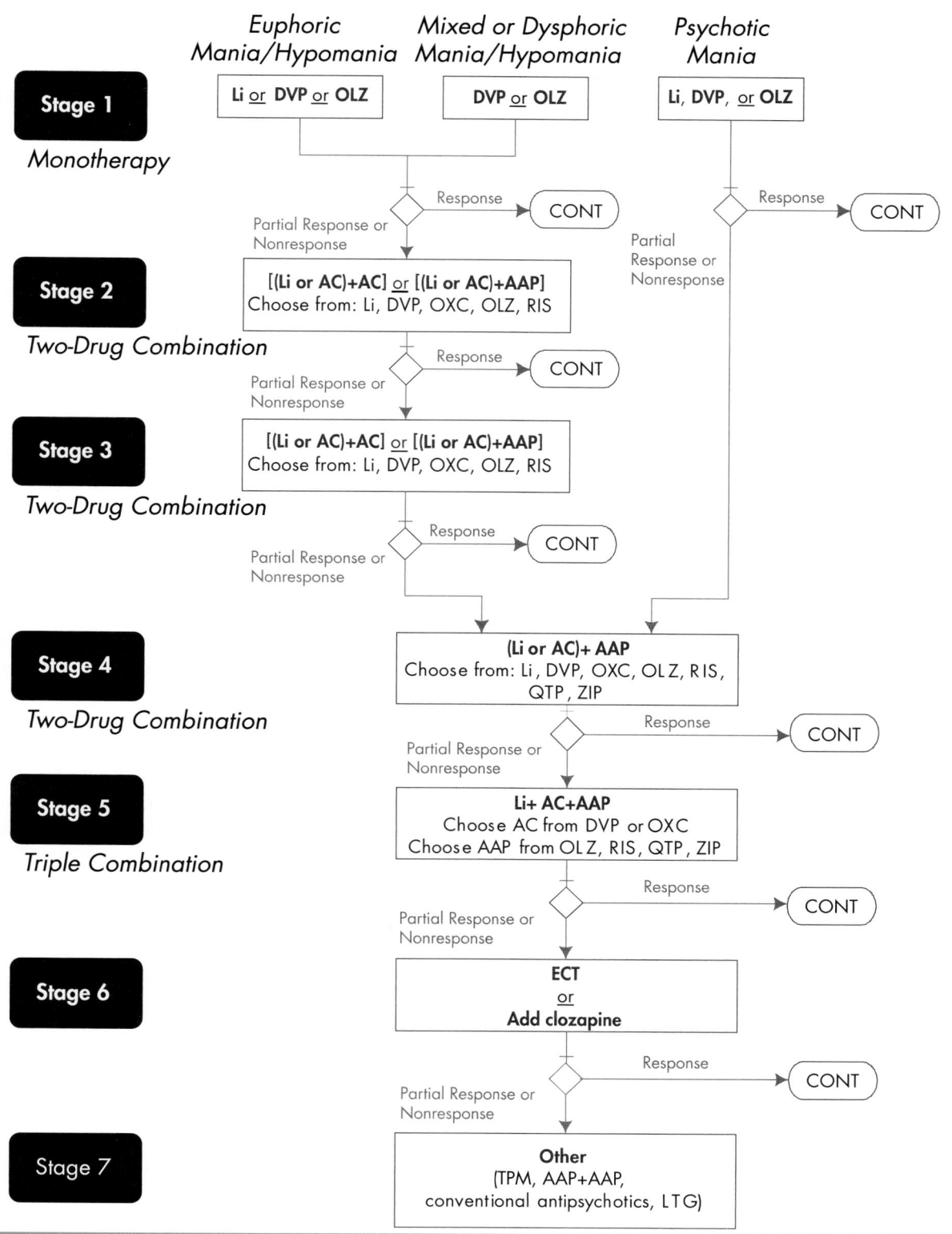

FIGURE 11–3. Strategies for the treatment of bipolar disorder (hypomanic/manic episode).

Note. AC = anticonvulsant; AAP = atypical antipsychotic; CONT = continuation treatment; DVP = divalproex; ECT = electroconvulsive therapy; Li = lithium; OLZ = olanzapine; OXC = oxcarbazepine; QTP = quetiapine; RIS = risperidone; TPM = topiramate; VPA = valproate; ZIP = ziprasidone.

Source. Suppes et al. 2001. Algorithms are revised as new data become available; consult the Texas Implementation of Medication Algorithms (TIMA) Web site (http://www.dshs.state.tx.us/mhprograms/TIMA.shtm) for the most recent versions.

Other Issues in Treatment of Mood Disorders

Treatment in Children and Adolescents

In selecting a treatment for a child with depression, the clinician must consider alternative treatments, including psychotherapies. Much controversy has surrounded the use of antidepressant medication in children and adolescents, with some negative trials of TCAs. To date, several trials have confirmed the effectiveness of SSRIs in childhood depression (Keller et al. 2001; Wagner et al. 2003). The first choice of monotherapy should be an SSRI. Controversy around the risk of suicide has emerged—the U.S. Food and Drug Administration found an increased risk of suicidality (defined as suicidal behavior or ideation) in children taking antidepressants compared with placebo, but no suicides were completed. Indeed, others have reported a decrease in the rates of suicide over the past decade, possibly because of the increased use of antidepressants (M.S. Gould et al. 2003). SSRIs remain an important treatment choice, but careful prescribing and monitoring are recommended.

Treatment in the Elderly

In elderly patients with mood disorders, it is accepted practice to prescribe antidepressants initially at lower dosages and to titrate upward more slowly. Some investigators have argued that this strategy may not improve tolerability but rather may delay response (Roose et al. 1981). Treatment response is often slow, and a period of at least 2–3 months is necessary to ascertain whether treatment response has occurred (Young and Meyers 1992). Among the TCAs, some evidence suggests that nortriptyline may be better tolerated because it has less hypotensive effect (Roose et al.

1981). Some evidence (although limited) indicates that the SSRIs are effective in the elderly. The use of ECT also may need to be considered, and several studies have reported its effectiveness and safety.

Psychosocial treatment in the elderly is equally important. Clinicians may need to carefully consider hospital admission. The risk of displacing the individual may need to be weighed against the need for nursing care. Clearly targeted treatments such as music therapy, occupational therapy, and behavioral modification may need to be considered.

Conclusion

Mood disorders are among the most prevalent of all neuropsychiatric disorders, occurring in up to 20% of people in their lifetime. They are also among the most disabling of all medical conditions, and major depressive disorder in particular, is predicted to become the second leading cause of medical disability by 2020. Understanding of the causes of depressive and bipolar disorders has grown, but remains elusive. At this stage, the contribution of several gene loci, together with the impact of life stress and the ensuing gene–environment interaction, could be seen to underpin most cases of depression. The differentiation of depressive syndromes is critical to understanding the course and clinical management of the condition: Individuals with a major depressive episode in the context of bipolar mood disorder will have a different course and treatment to those with a major depressive episode occurring in the course of unipolar depression. The integration of evidence-based psychotherapies into similarly proven somatic treatments may afford sufferers the best opportunity for recovery.

Key Points

- Depression is a symptom of a syndrome that may have many causes.

- Bipolar disorders can be difficult to diagnose because of the inability to detect past and future episodes.

- The clinical features of depression across cultures may vary, including expressions such as loneliness and somatic complaints.

- Major depression is common, with a lifetime prevalence of about 10%. It also causes about twice as much disability as any other medical condition.

- Major depression is a chronic and recurring illness, with relapses occurring in at least half of patients.

- The causes of depression are multifactorial and usually include genetic and environmental contributions.

- Treatment of major depression consists of selecting an appropriate antidepressant and giving consideration to an effective psychotherapy.

- Bipolar disorders should be treated with mood stabilizers first, with the addition of other agents if response is unsatisfactory.

Suggested Readings

Butler A, Chapman J, Forman E, et al: The empirical status of cognitive-behavioral therapy: a review of meta-analyses. Clin Psychol Rev 26:17–31, 2006

Caspi A, Sugden K, Moffitt T, et al: Influence of life stress on depression: moderation by a polymorphism in the 5-HTT gene. Science 301:386–389, 2003

Fava M, Rush AJ, Trivedi M, et al, for the STAR*D Investigators Group: Background and rationale for the Sequenced Treatment Alternatives to Relieve Depression (STAR*D) study. Psychiatr Clin N Am 26:457–494, 2003

Kessler RC, Berglund P, Demler O, et al: The epidemiology of major depressive disorder: results from the National Comorbidity Survey Replication (NCS-R). JAMA 289:3095–3105, 2003

Manji H, Drevets W, Charney D: The cellular neurobiology of depression. Nat Med 5:541–547, 2001

Stein DJ, Kupfer DJ, Schatzberg AF (eds): The American Psychiatric Publishing Textbook of Mood Disorders. Washington, DC, American Psychiatric Publishing, 2006

Online Resources

American Psychiatric Association Practice Guidelines: http://www.psych.org/psych_pract/treatg/pg/prac_guide.cfm

National Comorbidity Survey: http://www.hcp.med.harvard.edu/ncs/ncs_data.php

National Institute of Clinical Excellence, UK: http://www.nice.org.uk/page.aspx?o=mental

Texas Medication Algorithm Project: http://www.dshs.state.tx.us/mhprograms/TMAPover.shtm

References

Ahlfors UG, Baastrup PC, Dencker SJ: Flupenthixol decanoate in recurrent manic depressive illness. Acta Psychiatr Scand 64:226–237, 1981

Akiskal HS: Prevalent clinical spectrum of bipolar disorder: beyond DSM-IV. J Clin Psychopharmacol 16:4S–14S, 1996

Akiskal HS, Rosenthal RH, Rosenthal TL, et al: Differentiation of primary affective illness from situational, symptomatic, and secondary depressions. Arch Gen Psychiatry 36:635–643, 1979

American Psychiatric Association: Diagnostic and Statistical Manual of Mental Disorders, 4th Edition, Text Revision. Washington, DC, American Psychiatric Association, 2000a

American Psychiatric Association: Practice Guideline for the Treatment of Patients With Major Depressive Disorder, 2nd Edition. Washington, DC, American Psychiatric Association, 2000b

American Psychiatric Association: Practice guideline for the treatment of patients with borderline personality disorder. American Psychiatric Association. Am J Psychiatry 158 (10 suppl):1–52, 2001

American Psychiatric Association: Practice guideline for the treatment of patients with bipolar disorder (revision). Am J Psychiatry 159 (4 suppl):1–50, 2002

Amsterdam JD, Maislin G, Rosenzweig M, et al: Gonadotropin (LH and FSH) response after submaximal GnRH stimulation in depressed premenopausal women and healthy controls. Psychoneuroendocrinology 20:311–321, 1995

Andrews G, Henderson S, Hall W: Prevalence, comorbidity, disability and service utilisation. Overview of the Australian National Mental Health Survey. Br J Psychiatry 178:145–153, 2001

Angst J, Cassano G: The mood spectrum: improving the diagnosis of bipolar disorder. Bipolar Disord 7 (suppl 4): 4–12, 2005

Arango V, Underwood MD, Boldrini M, et al: Serotonin 1A receptors, serotonin transporter binding and serotonin transporter mRNA expression in the brainstem of depressed suicide victims. Neuropsychopharmacology 25:892–903, 2001

Arborelius L, Owens MJ, Plotsky PM, et al: The role of corticotropin-releasing factor in depression and anxiety disorders. J Endocrinol 160:1–12, 1999

Aronson R, Offman HJ, Joffe RT, et al: Triiodothyronine augmentation in the treatment of refractory depression: a meta-analysis. Arch Gen Psychiatry 53:842–848, 1996

Asberg M, Traskman L, Thoren P: 5-HIAA in the cerebrospinal fluid: a biochemical suicide predictor? Arch Gen Psychiatry 33:1193–1197, 1976

Avis NE, Crawford SL, McKinlay SM: Psychosocial, behavioral, and health factors related to menopause symptomatology. Womens Health 3:103–120, 1997

Ayuso-Mateos JL, Vasques-Barquero JL, Dowrick C, et al: Depressive disorders in Europe: prevalence figures from the ODIN study. Br J Psychiatry 179:308–316, 2001

Badner JA, Gershon ES: Meta-analysis of whole-genome linkage scans of bipolar disorder and schizophrenia. Mol Psychiatry 7:405–411, 2002

Baldessarini RJ, Tondo L, Hennen J: Lithium treatment and suicide risk in major affective disorders: update and new findings. J Clin Psychiatry 64 (suppl 5):44–52, 2003

Ballmaier M, Toga AW, Blanton RE: Anterior cingulate, gyrus rectus, and orbitofrontal abnormalities in elderly depressed patients: an MRI-based parcellation of the prefrontal cortex. Am J Psychiatry 161:99–108, 2004

Baraban SC, Tallent MK: Interneuron Diversity Series: Interneuronal neuropeptides—endogenous regulators of neuronal excitability. Trends Neurosci 27:135–142, 2004

Baron M, Gruen R, Anis L, et al: Schizoaffective illness, schizophrenia and affective disorders: morbidity risk and genetic transmission. Acta Psychiatr Scand 65:253–262, 1983

Bauer M, Berghofer A, Bschor T, et al: Supraphysiological doses of L-thyroxine in the maintenance treatment of prophylaxis-resistant affective disorders. Neuropsychopharmacology 27:620–628, 2002

Baumgartner A, von Stuckrad M, Muller-Oerlinghausen B, et al: The hypothalamic-pituitary-thyroid axis in patients maintained on lithium prophylaxis for years: high triiodothyronine serum concentrations are correlated to the prophylactic efficacy. J Affect Disord 34:211–218, 1995

Beck AT: Depression: Clinical, Experimental, and Theoretical Aspects. New York, Harper & Row, 1967

Beck AT: Cognitive Therapy and the Emotional Disorders. New York, International Universities Press, 1976

Beck AT, Emery G: Anxiety Disorders and Phobias: A Cognitive Perspective. New York, Basic Books, 1985

Beck AT, Rush AJ, Shaw BF, et al: Cognitive Therapy of Depression. New York, Guilford, 1979

Biederman J, Mick E, Faraone SV, et al: Pediatric mania: a developmental subtype of bipolar disorder? Biol Psychiatry 48:458–466, 2000

Bijl RV, Ravelli A, van Zessen G: Prevalence of psychiatric disorder in the general population: results of the Netherlands Mental Health Survey and Incidence Study (NEMESIS). Soc Psychiatry Psychiatr Epidemiol 33:587–595, 1998

Birmaher B, Ryan N, Williamson DE, et al: Childhood and adolescent depression: a review of the past 10 years, part I. J Am Acad Child Adolesc Psychiatry 35:1427–1439, 1996

Bittner A, Goodwin RD, Wittchen HU, et al: What characteristics of primary anxiety disorders predict subsequent major depressive disorder? J Clin Psychiatry 65:618–626, 2004

Bowden CL: Predictors of response to divalproex and lithium. J Clin Psychiatry 56 (suppl 2):25–30, 1995

Bowden CL, Brugger AM, Swann AC, et al: Efficacy of divalproex vs lithium and placebo in the treatment of mania. The Depakote Mania Study Group. JAMA 271:918–924, 1994

Bowden CL, Calabrese JR, McElroy SL, et al: Efficacy of divalproex versus lithium and placebo in maintenance treatment of bipolar disorder. Arch Gen Psychiatry 57:481–489, 2000

Bowden CL, Calabrese JR, Sachs GS, et al: A placebo-controlled 18-month trial of lamotrigine and lithium maintenance treatment in recently manic or hypomanic patients with bipolar I disorder. Arch Gen Psychiatry 60:392–400, 2003

Bowlby J: Attachment and Loss, Vol 1: Attachment. New York, Basic Books, 1969

Bowlby J: Attachment and Loss, Vol 2: Separation. New York, Basic Books, 1973

Bowlby J: Attachment and Loss, Vol 3: Loss, Sadness and Depression. New York, Basic Books, 1980

Brady KT, Sonne SC: The relationship between substance abuse and bipolar disorder. J Clin Psychiatry 56 (suppl 3): 19–24, 1995

Brown G: Life events and affective disorder: replications and limitations. Psychosom Med 55:248–259, 1993

Brown G, Eales M: Etiology of anxiety and depressive disorders in an inner-city population. Psychol Med 23:155–165, 1993

Burgess S, Geddes J, Hawton K, et al: Lithium for maintenance treatment of mood disorders. Cochrane Database Syst Rev (3):CD003013, 2001

Burnes DD, Spangler DL: Does psychotherapy homework lead to improvements in depression in cognitive-behavioral therapy or does improvement lead to increased homework compliance? J Consult Clin Psychol 68:46–56, 2000

Burt T, Lisanby SH, Sackeim HA: Neuropsychiatric applications of transcranial magnetic stimulation: a meta-analysis. Int J Neuropsychopharmacol 5:73–103, 2002

Butler AC, Chapman JE, Forman EM, et al: The empirical status of cognitive-behavioral therapy: a review of meta-analyses. Clin Psychol Rev 26:17–31, 2006

Bylund DB: Subtypes of alpha 2-adrenoceptors: pharmacological and molecular biological evidence converge. Trends Pharmacol Sci 9:356–361, 1988

Cahill L, McGaugh JL, Weinberger NM: The neurobiology of learning and memory: some reminders to remember. Trends Neurosci 24:578–581, 2001

Calabrese JR, Bowden CL, Sachs GS, et al: A double-blind placebo-controlled study of lamotrigine monotherapy in outpatients with bipolar I depression. Lamictal 602 Study Group. J Clin Psychiatry 60:79–88, 1999

Campbell S, Marriott M, Nahmias C, et al: Lower hippocampal volume in patients suffering from depression: a meta-analysis. Am J Psychiatry 161:598–607, 2004

Carlson GA, Jensen PS, Findling RL, et al: Methodological issues and controversies in clinical trials with child and adolescent patients with bipolar disorder: report of a consensus conference. J Child Adolesc Psychopharmacol 13:13–27, 2003

Caspi A, Sugden K, Moffitt TE, et al: Influence of life stress on depression: moderation by a polymorphism in the 5-htt gene. Science 301:386–389, 2003

Chen L, Zhuang X: Transgenic mouse models of dopamine deficiency. Ann Neurol 54 (suppl 6):S91–S102, 2003

Chueire VB, Silva ET, Perotta E, et al: High serum TSH levels are associated with depression in the elderly. Arch Gerontol Geriatr 36:281–288, 2003

Clarke GN, Rohde P, Lewinsohn PM, et al: Cognitive-behavioral treatment of adolescent depression: efficacy of acute group treatment and booster sessions. J Am Acad Child Adolesc Psychiatry 38:272–279, 1999

Clayton PJ: Bereavement and depression. J Clin Psychiatry 51(suppl):34–38; discussion 39–40, 1990

Copolov DL, Rubin RT, Stuart GW, et al: Specificity of the salivary cortisol dexamethasone suppression test across psychiatric diagnoses. Biol Psychiatry 25:879–893, 1989

Coryell W: Psychotic depression. J Clin Psychiatry 57 (suppl 3): 27–31; discussion 49, 1996

Coryell W, Winokur G: Course and outcome, in Handbook of Affective Disorders, 2nd Edition. Edited by Paykel ES. New York, Guilford, 1992, pp 89–108

Cotter D, Mackay D, Chana G, et al: Reduced neuronal size and glial cell density in area 9 of the dorsolateral prefrontal cortex in subjects with major depressive disorder. Cereb Cortex 12:386–394, 2002

Crismon ML, Trivedi M, Pigott TA, et al: The Texas Medication Algorithm Project: report of the Texas Consensus Conference Panel on Medication Treatment of Major Depressive Disorder. J Clin Psychiatry 60:142–156, 1999

Dardennes R, Even C, Bange F: Comparison of carbamazepine and lithium in the prophylaxis of bipolar disorders: a meta-analysis. Br J Psychiatry 166:375–381, 1995

Davis JM, Janicak PG, Sakkas P, et al: Electroconvulsive therapy in the treatment of the neuroleptic malignant syndrome. Convuls Ther 7:111–120, 1991

de Boer TH, Nefkens F, van Helvoirt A, et al: Differences in modulation of noradrenergic and serotonergic transmission by the alpha-2 adrenoceptor antagonists, mirtazapine, mianserin and idazoxan. J Pharmacol Exp Ther 277:852–860, 1996

de Graaf R, Bijl RV, Spijker J, et al: Temporal sequencing of lifetime mood disorders in relation to comorbid anxiety and substance use disorders—findings from the Netherlands Mental Health Survey and Incidence Study. Soc Psychiatry Psychiatr Epidemiol 38:1–11, 2003

Delgado PL, Price LH, Heninger GR, et al: Neurochemistry of affective disorders, in Handbook of Affective Disorders, 2nd Edition. Edited by Paykel ES. Edinburgh, UK, Churchill Livingstone, 1992, pp 219–253

Delgado PL, Miller HL, Salomon RM, et al: Monoamines and the mechanism of antidepressant action: effects of catecholamine depletion on mood of patients treated with antidepressants. Psychopharmacol Bull 29:389–396, 1993

Demet MM, Ozmen B, Deveci A, et al: Depression and anxiety in hyperthyroidism. Arch Med Res 33:552–556, 2002

Demyttenaere K, Bruffaerts R, Posada-Villa J, et al, WHO World Mental Health Survey Consortium: Prevalence, severity, and unmet need for treatment of mental disorders in the World Health Organization World Mental Health Surveys. JAMA 291:2581–2590, 2004

Di Matteo V, De Blasi A, Di Giulio C, et al: Role of 5-HT(2C) receptors in the control of central dopamine function. Trends Pharmacol Sci 22:229–232, 2001

Dimmock PW, Wyatt KM, Jones PW, et al: Efficacy of selective serotonin reuptake inhibitors in premenstrual syndrome: a systematic review. Lancet 356:1131–1136, 2000

Duman RS: Depression: a case of neuronal life and death? Biol Psychiatry 56:141–145, 2004

Ehrenreich H, Halaris A, Ruether E, et al: Psychoendocrine sequelae of chronic testosterone deficiency. J Psychiatr Res 33:379–387, 1999

Emslie GJ, Rush AJ, Weinberg WA, et al: Recurrence of major depressive disorder in hospitalized children and adolescents. J Am Acad Child Adolesc Psychiatry 36:785–792, 1997

Engum A, Bjoro T, Mykletun A, et al: An association between depression, anxiety and thyroid function—a clinical fact or an artefact? Acta Psychiatr Scand 106:27–34, 2002

Fava M, Rosenbaum JF, McGrath PJ, et al: Lithium and tricyclic augmentation of fluoxetine treatment for resistant major depression: a double-blind, controlled study. Am J Psychiatry 151:1372–1374, 1994

Fava M, Rush AJ, Trivedi MH, et al: Background and rationale for the Sequenced Treatment Alternatives to Relieve Depression (STAR*D) study. Psychiatr Clin North Am 26:457–494, 2003

Frank E, Kupfer DJ, Perel JM, et al: Three-year outcomes for maintenance therapies in recurrent depression. Arch Gen Psychiatry 47:1093–1099, 1990

Frank E, Swartz HA, Kupfer DJ: Interpersonal and social rhythm therapy: managing the chaos of bipolar disorder. Biol Psychiatry 48:593–604, 2000

Freeman MP, Freeman SA, McElroy SL: The comorbidity of bipolar and anxiety disorders: prevalence, psychobiology, and treatment issues. J Affect Disord 68:1–23, 2002

Freeman MP, Wiegand C, Gelenberg AJ: Lithium, in The American Psychiatric Publishing Textbook of Psychopharmacology, 3rd Edition. Edited by Schatzberg AF, Nemeroff CB. Washington, DC, American Psychiatric Publishing, 2004, pp 547–565

Freeman TW, Clothier JL, Pazzaglia P, et al: A double-blind comparison of valproate and lithium in the treatment of acute mania. Am J Psychiatry 149:108–111, 1992

Freud S: The ego and the id (1923), in The Standard Edition of the Complete Psychological Works of Sigmund Freud, Vol 19. Translated and edited by Strachey J. London, Hogarth Press, 1961, pp 1–66

Gabbard GO: Psychodynamic Psychotherapy in Clinical Practice, 3rd Edition. Washington, DC, American Psychiatric Press, 2000

Gallagher-Thompson D, Steffen AM: Comparative effects of cognitive-behavioral and brief psychodynamic psychotherapies for depressed family caregivers. J Consult Clin Psychol 62:543–549, 1994

Gallo JJ, Rabins PV: Depression without sadness: alternative presentations of depression in late life. Am Fam Physician 60:820–826, 1999

George MS, Sackeim HA, Marangell LB, et al: Vagus nerve stimulation: a potential therapy for resistant depression? Psychiatr Clin North Am 23:757–783, 2000

Gershon ES: Genetics, in Manic-Depressive Illness. Edited by Goodwin FK, Jamison KR. London, Oxford University Press, 1988, pp 373–401

Gershon ES, Hamovit J, Guroff JJ, et al: A family study of schizoaffective, bipolar I, bipolar II, unipolar, and normal control probands. Arch Gen Psychiatry 39:1157–1167, 1982

Goodwin GM, for the Consensus Group of the British Association for Psychopharmacology: Evidence-based guidelines for treating bipolar disorder: recommendations from the British Association for Psychopharmacology. J Psychopharmacol 17:149–173, 2003

Goodwin RD, Jacobi F, Bittner A, et al: Epidemiology of mood disorders, in The American Psychiatric Publishing Textbook of Mood Disorders. Edited by Stein DJ, Kupfer DJ, Schatzberg AF. Washington, DC, American Psychiatric Publishing, 2006, pp 33–54

Gould E, Tanapat P: Stress and hippocampal neurogenesis. Biol Psychiatry 46:1472–1479, 1999

Gould MS, Greenberg T, Velting DM, et al: Youth suicide risk and preventive interventions: a review of the past 10 years. J Am Acad Child Adolesc Psychiatry 42:386–405, 2003

Grant SJ, Redmond DE Jr: The neuroanatomy and pharmacology of the nucleus locus coeruleus. Prog Clin Biol Res 71:5–27, 1981

Gray PB, Singh AB, Woodhouse LJ, et al: Dose-dependent effects of testosterone on sexual function, mood, and visuospatial cognition in older men. J Clin Endocrinol Metab 90:3838–3846, 2005

Greenberg PE, Kessler RC, Nells TL, et al: Depression in the workplace: an economic perspective, in Selective Serotonin Reuptake Inhibitors: Advances in Basic Research and Clinical Practice. Edited by Feighner JP, Boyer WF. New York, Wiley, 1996, pp 327–363

Grey M, Whittemore R, Tamborlane W: Depression in type I diabetes in children: natural history and correlates. J Psychosom Res 53:907–911, 2002

Grof P: Selecting effective long-term treatment for bipolar patients: monotherapy and combinations. J Clin Psychiatry 64 (suppl 5):53–61, 2003

Gutierrez MA, Stimmel GL, Aiso JY: Venlafaxine: a 2003 update. Clin Ther 25:2138–2154, 2003

Halbreich U: Hormonal interventions with psychopharmacological potential: an overview. Psychopharmacol Bull 33:281–286, 1997

Halbreich U, Borenstein J, Pearlstein T, et al: The prevalence, impact, and burden of premenstrual dysphoric disorder. Psychoneuroendocrinology 28 (suppl 3):1–23, 2003

Hamilton M: A rating scale for depression. J Neurol Neurosurg Psychiatry 23:56–62, 1960

Hartlage S, Alloy LB, Vazquez C, et al: Automatic and effortful processing in depression. Psychol Bull 113:247–278, 1993

Hasler G, Drevets W, Manji H, et al: Discovering endophenotypes for major depression. Neuropsychopharmacology 29:1765–1781, 2004

Heilig M, Widerlov E: Neurobiology and clinical aspects of neuropeptide Y. Crit Rev Neurobiol 9:115–136, 1995

Hickie I, Scott E, Wilhelm K, et al: Subcortical hyperintensities on magnetic resonance imaging in patients with severe depression—a longitudinal evaluation. Biol Psychiatry 42:367–374, 1997

Hirschfeld RM, Bowden CL, Gitlin MJ, et al: Practice guideline for the treatment of patients with bipolar disorder (revision). Am J Psychiatry 159:1–50, 2002

Iqbal MM, Gunlapalli SP, Ryan WG, et al: Effects of antimanic mood-stabilizing drugs on fetuses, neonates, and nursing infants. South Med J 94:304–322, 2001

Jarrett RB, Kraft D: Prophylactic cognitive therapy for major depressive disorder. In Session: Psychotherapy in Practice 3:65–79, 1997

Jobson K: International Psychopharmacology Algorithm Project: algorithms in psychopharmacology. Int J Psychiatry Clin Pract 1 (suppl 1):S3–S4, 1997

Joffe RT: Refractory depression: treatment strategies, with particular reference to the thyroid axis. J Psychiatry Neurosci 22:327–331, 1997

Joffe RT, Marriott M: Thyroid hormone levels and recurrence of major depression. Am J Psychiatry 157:1689–1691, 2000

Joffe RT, Singer W: A comparison of triiodothyronine and thyroxine in the potentiation of tricyclic antidepressants. Psychiatry Res 32:241–251, 1990

Katon W, Von Korff M, Lin E, et al: Stepped collaborative care for primary care patients with persistent symptoms of depression: a randomized trial. Arch Gen Psychiatry 56:1109–1115, 1999

Keck PE Jr, McElroy SL: Lithium and mood stabilizers, in The American Psychiatric Publishing Textbook of Mood Disorders. Edited by Stein DJ, Kupfer DJ, Schatzberg AF. Washington, DC, American Psychiatric Publishing, 2006, pp 281–290

Keck PE Jr, McElroy SL, Strakowski SM: Anticonvulsants and antipsychotics in the treatment of bipolar disorder. J Clin Psychiatry 59 (suppl 6):74–81; discussion 82, 1998

Keck PE Jr, Strakowski SM, McElroy SL: The efficacy of atypical antipsychotics in the treatment of depressive symptoms, hostility, and suicidality in patients with schizophrenia. J Clin Psychiatry 61 (suppl 3):4–9, 2000

Keck PE Jr, Strakowski SM, Hawkins JM, et al: Rapid lithium administration in the treatment of acute mania. Bipolar Disord 3:68–72, 2001

Kellar K, Cascio C, Bergstrom D, et al: Electroconvulsive shock and reserpine: effects on beta-adrenergic receptors in rat brain. J Neurochem 37:830–836, 1981

Keller MB, Baker L: Bipolar disorder: epidemiology, course, diagnosis, and treatment. Bull Menninger Clin 55:172–181, 1991

Keller MB, McCullough JP, Klein DN, et al: A comparison of nefazodone, the cognitive behavioral-analysis system of psychotherapy, and their combination for the treatment of chronic depression. N Engl J Med 342:1462–1470, 2000

Keller MB, Ryan N, Strober M, et al: Efficacy of paroxetine in the treatment of adolescent major depression: a randomized, controlled trial. J Am Acad Child Adolesc Psychiatry 40:762–772, 2001

Kendler KS: Major depression and the environment: a psychiatric genetic perspective. Pharmacopsychiatry 31:5–9, 1998

Kendler KS, Thornton LM, Gardner CO: Stressful life events and previous episodes in the etiology of major depression in women: an evaluation of the "kindling" hypothesis. Am J Psychiatry 157:1243–1251, 2000

Kendler KS, Prescott CA, Myers JK, et al: The structure of genetic and environmental risk factors for common psychiatric and substance use disorders in men and women. Arch Gen Psychiatry 60:929–937, 2003

Kessler RC, McGonagle KA, Zhao S, et al: Lifetime and 12-month prevalence of DSM-III-R psychiatric disorders in the United States. Results from the National Comorbidity Survey. Arch Gen Psychiatry 51:8–19, 1994

Kessler RC, Walters EE: Epidemiology of DSM-III-R major depression and minor depression among adolescents and young adults in the National Comorbidity Survey. Depress Anxiety 7:3–14, 1998

Kessler RC, Berglund P, Demler O, et al: The epidemiology of major depressive disorder results from the National Comorbidity Survey Replication (NCS-R). JAMA 289:3095–3105, 2003

Ketter TA, George MS, Kimbrell TA: Functional brain imaging, limbic function, and affective disorders. Neuroscientist 2:55–65, 1996

Khantzian EJ: The self-medication hypothesis of addictive disorders: focus on heroin and cocaine dependence. Am J Psychiatry 142:1259–1264, 1985

Klein M: Mourning and its relation to manic-depressive states (1940), in Love, Guilt and Reparation and Other Works 1921–1945. New York, Free Press, 1975, pp 344–369

Kleinman A, Good B: Culture and Depression: Studies in the Anthropology and Cross-Cultural Psychiatry of Affect and Disorder. Berkeley, University of California Press, 1985

Klerman GL, Weissman MM, Rounsaville BJ, et al: Interpersonal Psychotherapy of Depression. New York, Basic Books, 1984

Klose M, Jacobi F: Can gender differences in the prevalence of mental disorders be explained by sociodemographic factors? Arch Womens Ment Health 7:133–148, 2004

Kovacs M: Presentation and course of major depressive disorder during childhood and later years of the life span. J Am Acad Child Adolesc Psychiatry 35:705–715, 1996

Kramlinger KG, Post RM: The addition of lithium to carbamazepine. Arch Gen Psychiatry 46:794–800, 1989

Kramlinger KG, Post RM: Ultra-rapid and ultradian cycling in bipolar affective illness. Br J Psychiatry 168:314–323, 1996

Kroeze WK, Kristiansen K, Roth BL: Molecular biology of serotonin receptors structure and function at the molecular level. Current Topics in Medicinal Chemistry 2:507–528, 2002

Kumar A, Jin Z, Bilker W, et al: Late-onset minor and major depression: early evidence for common neuroanatomical substrates detected by using MRI. Proc Natl Acad Sci USA 95:7654–7658, 1998

Lam DH, Watkins ER, Hayward P, et al: A randomized controlled study of cognitive therapy for relapse prevention for bipolar affective disorder: outcome of the first year. Arch Gen Psychiatry 60:145–152, 2003

Larson EW, Richelson E: Organic causes of mania. Mayo Clin Proc 63:906–912, 1988

Lauterborn JC, Poulsen FR, Stinis CT, et al: Transcript-specific effects of adrenalectomy on seizure-induced BDNF expression in rat hippocampus. Brain Res Mol Brain Res 55:81–91, 1998

Leader JB, Klein DK: Social adjustment in dysthymia, double depression and episodic major depression. J Affect Disord 37:91–101, 1996

Lewy AJ, Sack RL, Singer CM, et al: Winter depression and the phase-shift hypothesis for bright light's therapeutic effects: history, theory, and experimental evidence. J Biol Rhythms 3:121–134, 1988

Lisanby SH, Maddox JH, Prudic J, et al: The effects of electroconvulsive therapy on memory of autobiographical and public events. Arch Gen Psychiatry 57:581–590, 2000

Luborsky L: Principles of Psychoanalytic Psychotherapy: A Manual for Supportive Expressive Treatment. New York, Basic Books, 1984

Maes M, Meltzer HY: The serotonin hypothesis of major depression, in Psychopharmacology: The Fourth Generation of Progress. Edited by Bloom FE, Kupfer DJ, Bunney BS, et al. New York, Raven, 1995, pp 933–944

Maes M, Scharpe S, Meltzer HY, et al: Relationships between interleukin-6 activity, acute phase proteins, and function of the hypothalamic-pituitary-adrenal axis in severe depression. Psychiatry Res 49:11–27, 1993

Malison RT, Price LH, Berman RM, et al: Reduced midbrain serotonin transporter binding in depressed vs healthy subjects as measured by 123b-CIT SPECT. Biol Psychiatry 44:1090–1098, 1998

Mann JJ: Neurobiological correlates of the antidepressant action of electroconvulsive therapy. J ECT 14:172–180, 1998

Mann JJ, Huang Y, Underwood MD, et al: A serotonin transporter gene promoter polymorphism (5-HTTLPR) and prefrontal cortical binding in major depression and suicide. Arch Gen Psychiatry 57:729–738, 2000

Marcus R, Carson W, McQuada R, et al: Long-term efficacy of aripiprazole in the maintenance treatment of bipolar disorder. Paper presented at the 42nd annual meeting of the American College of Neuropsychopharmacology, San Juan, PR, December 7–11, 2003

Markowitz JC: Interpersonal psychotherapy for chronic depression. J Clin Psychol 59:847–858, 2003

Markowitz JC, Kocsis JH, Fishman B, et al: Treatment of HIV-positive patients with depressive symptoms. Arch Gen Psychiatry 55:452–457, 1998

Matt GE, Vazquez C, Campbell WK: Mood-congruent recall of affectively toned stimuli: a meta-analytic review. Clin Psychol Rev 12:227–255, 1992

Mayberg HS: Modulating dysfunctional limbic-cortical circuits in depression: towards development of brain-based algorithms for diagnosis and optimised treatment. Br Med Bull 65:193–207, 2003

Mayberg HS: Brain imaging, in The American Psychiatric Publishing Textbook of Mood Disorders. Edited by Stein DJ, Kupfer DJ, Schatzberg AF. Washington, DC, American Psychiatric Publishing, 2006, pp 219–234

McCullough JP: Treatment for Chronic Depression: Cognitive Behavioral Analysis System of Psychotherapy. New York, Guilford, 2000

McEwen BS: Stress and hippocampal plasticity. Annu Rev Neurosci 22:105–122, 1999

McGuffin P, Rijsdijk S, Andrew M, et al: The heritability of bipolar affective disorder and the genetic relationship to unipolar depression. Arch Gen Psychiatry 60:497–502, 2003

Mendlewicz J, Rainer JD: Adoption study supporting genetic transmission in manic-depressive illness. Nature 368:327–329, 1977

Miklowitz DJ, Hooley JM: Developing family psychoeducational treatments for patients with bipolar and other severe psychiatric disorders: a pathway from basic research to clinical trials. J Marital Fam Ther 24:419–435, 1998

Moniz E: Prefrontal leucotomy in the treatment of mental disorders. Am J Psychiatry 93:1379–1385, 1937

Monroe RRJ: Maintenance electroconvulsive therapy. Psychiatr Clin North Am 14:947–960, 1991

Moore GJ, Bebchuk JM, Hasanat K, et al: Lithium increases N-acetyl-aspartate in the human brain: in vivo evidence in support of bcl-2's neurotrophic effects? Biol Psychiatry 48:1–8, 2000

Moore JD, Bona JR: Depression and dysthymia. Med Clin North Am 85:631–644, 2001

Mufson L, Weissman MM, Moreau D, et al: Efficacy of interpersonal psychotherapy for depressed adolescents. Arch Gen Psychiatry 56:573–579, 1999

Murray CJL, Lopez AD: The Global Burden of Disease: A Comprehensive Assessment of Mortality and Disability From Diseases, Injuries and Risk Factors in 1990 and Projected to 2020. Cambridge, MA, Harvard University Press, 1996

Nelson JC, Charney DS: The symptoms of major depressive illness. Am J Psychiatry 138:1–13, 1981

Nemeroff C: The neurobiological consequences of child abuse. Paper presented at the 156th annual meeting of the American Psychiatric Association, May 19, 2003

Nesse RM: The evolution of hope and despair. J Soc Issues 66:429–469, 1999

Nesse RM: Evolutionary explanations for mood and mood disorders, in The American Psychiatric Publishing Textbook of Mood Disorders. Edited by Stein DJ, Kupfer DJ, Schatzberg AF. Washington, DC, American Psychiatric Publishing, 2006, pp 159–178

Nobler MS, Sackeim HA: Electroconvulsive therapy and transcranial magnetic stimulation, in The American Psychiatric Publishing Textbook of Mood Disorders. Edited by Stein DJ, Kupfer DJ, Schatzberg AF. Washington, DC, American Psychiatric Publishing, 2006, pp 317–336

Nobler MS, Sackeim HA, Moeller JR, et al: Quantifying the speed of symptomatic improvement with electroconvulsive therapy: comparison of alternative statistical methods. Convuls Ther 13:208–221, 1997

Oldehinkel AJ, Wittchen HU, Schuster P: Prevalence, 20-month incidence and outcome of unipolar depressive disorders in a community sample of adolescents. Psychol Med 29:655–668, 1999

Ostroff RB, Nelson JC: Risperidone augmentation of selective serotonin reuptake inhibitors in major depression. J Clin Psychiatry 60:256–259, 1999

Osuji IJ, Cullum CM: Cognition in bipolar disorder. Psychiatr Clin North Am 28:427–441, 2005

O'Toole SM, Rubin RT: Neuroendocrine aspects of primary endogenous depression, XIV: gonadotropin secretion in female patients and their matched controls. Psychoneuroendocrinology 20:603–612, 1995

Parmelee PA, Ketz IR, Lawton MP: Depression among institutionalized aged: assessment and prevalence estimation. J Gerontol 44:M22–M29, 1989

Pascual-Leone A, Houser CM, Reese K, et al: Safety of rapid-rate transcranial magnetic stimulation in normal volunteers. Electroencephalogr Clin Neurophysiol 89:120–130, 1993

Paykel ES: Correlates of a depressive typology. Arch Gen Psychiatry 27:203–210, 1972

Perlis RH, Brown E, Baker RW, et al: Clinical features of bipolar depression versus major depressive disorder in large multicenter trials. Am J Psychiatry 163:225–231, 2006

Perry A, Tarrier N, Morriss R, et al: Randomised controlled trial of efficacy of teaching patients with bipolar disorder to identify early symptoms of relapse and obtain treatment. BMJ 318:149–153, 1999

Perry PJ: Pharmacotherapy for major depression with melancholic features: relative efficacy of tricyclic versus selective serotonin reuptake inhibitor antidepressants. J Affect Disord 39:1–6, 1996

Peveler R, Carson A, Rodin G: Depression in medical patients. BMJ 325:149–152, 2002

Pezawas L, Angst J, Kasper S: Recurrent brief depression revisited. Int Rev Psychiatry 17:63–70, 2005

Plotsky PM, Owens MJ, Nemeroff CB: Psychoneuroendocrinology of depression: hypothalamic-pituitary-adrenal axis. Psychiatr Clin North Am 21:293–307, 1998

Post RM: Transduction of psychosocial stress into the neurobiology of recurrent affective disorder. Am J Psychiatry 149:999–1010, 1992

Potter WZ, Rudorfer MV, Manji H: The pharmacological treatment of depression. N Engl J Med 325:633–642, 1991

Price JS: The dominance hierarchy and the evolution of mental illness. Lancet 2:243–246, 1967

Prien RF, Kupfer DJ, Mansky PA, et al: Drug therapy in the prevention of recurrences in unipolar and bipolar affective disorders: report of the NIMH Collaborative Study Group comparing lithium carbonate, imipramine, and a lithium carbonate-imipramine combination. Arch Gen Psychiatry 41:1096–1104, 1984

Rajkowska G: Anatomical pathology, in The American Psychiatric Publishing Textbook of Mood Disorders. Edited by Stein DJ, Kupfer DJ, Schatzberg AF. Washington, DC, American Psychiatric Publishing, 2006, pp 179–198

Rajkowska G, Halaris A, Selemon LD: Reductions in neuronal and glial density characterize the dorsolateral prefrontal cortex in bipolar disorder. Biol Psychiatry 49:741–752, 2001

Regier DA, Farmer ME, Rae DS, et al: Comorbidity of mental disorders with alcohol and other drug abuse: results from the Epidemiologic Catchment Area (ECA) Study. JAMA 264:2511–2518, 1990

Rehm LP: A self-control model of depression. Behav Ther 8:787–804, 1977

Ressler KJ, Nemeroff CB: Role of norepinephrine in the pathophysiology and treatment of mood disorders. Biol Psychiatry 46:1219–1233, 1999

Robinson RG, Kubos KL, Starr LB, et al: Mood disorders in stroke patients: importance of location of lesion. Brain 107:81–93, 1984

Roose SP, Glassman AH, Siris SG, et al: Comparison of imipramine and nortriptyline induced orthostatic hypotension: a meaningful difference. J Clin Psychopharmacol 1:316–319, 1981

Rosenthal NE, Sack DA, Gillin JC, et al: Seasonal affective disorder: a description of the syndrome and preliminary findings with light therapy. Arch Gen Psychiatry 41:72–80, 1984

Rosoklija G, Toomayan G, Ellis SP, et al: Structural abnormalities of subicular dendrites in subjects with schizophrenia and mood disorders: preliminary findings. Arch Gen Psychiatry 57:349–356, 2000

Rubin RT: Pharmacoendocrinology of major depression. Eur Arch Psychiatry Neurol Sci 238:259–267, 1989

Rubinow DR, Schmidt PJ, Roca CA, et al: Gonadal hormones and behavior in women: concentrations versus context, in Hormones, Brain and Behavior. Edited by Pfaff D, Arnold AP, Etgen AM, et al. New York, Academic Press, 2002, pp 37–73

Sackeim HA: Magnetic stimulation therapy and ECT. Convuls Ther 10:255–258, 1994

Sackeim HA, Rush AJ: Melancholia and response to ECT (letter). Am J Psychiatry 152:1242–1243, 1995

Sackeim HA, Luber B, Katzman GP, et al: The effects of electroconvulsive therapy on quantitative electroencephalograms: relationship to clinical outcome. Arch Gen Psychiatry 53:814–824, 1996

Saito S, Yoshikawa D, Nishihara F, et al: The cerebral hemodynamic response to electrically induced seizures in man. Brain Res 673:93–100, 1995

Santarelli L, Saxe M, Gross C, et al: Requirement of hippocampal neurogenesis for the behavioral effects of antidepressants. Science 301:805–809, 2003

Sartorius N, Ustun TB, Korten A, et al: Progress toward achieving a common language in psychiatry, II: results from the international field trials of the ICD-10 diagnostic criteria for research for mental and behavioral disorders. Am J Psychiatry 152:1427–1437, 1995

Schatzberg AF, Rush AJ, Arnow BA, et al: Chronic depression: medication (nefazodone) or psychotherapy (CBASP) is effective when the other is not. Arch Gen Psychiatry 62:513–520, 2005

Schulberg HC, Block MR, Madonia MJ, et al: Treating major depression in primary care practice: eight-month clinical outcomes. Arch Gen Psychiatry 53:913–919, 1996

Scott J, Garland A, Moorhead S: A pilot study of cognitive therapy in bipolar disorders. Psychol Med 31:459–467, 2001

Segurado R, Detera-Wadleigh SD, Levinson DF, et al: Genome scan meta-analysis of schizophrenia and bipolar disorder, part III: bipolar disorder. Am J Hum Genet 73:49–62, 2003

Seidman SN: Psychoneuroendocrinology of mood disorders, in The American Psychiatric Publishing Textbook of Mood Disorders. Edited by Stein DJ, Kupfer DJ, Schatzberg AF. Washington, DC, American Psychiatric Publishing, 2006, pp 117–130

Sheline YI: Neuroimaging studies of mood disorder effects on the brain. Biol Psychiatry 54:338–352, 2003

Sheline YI, Gado MH, Kraemer HC: Untreated depression and hippocampal volume loss. Am J Psychiatry 161:1309–1310, 2004

Shelton RC, Tollefson GD, Tohen M, et al: A novel augmentation strategy for treating resistant major depression. Am J Psychiatry 158:131–134, 2001

Singh JB, Quiroz JA, Gould TD, et al: Molecular and cellular neurobiology of severe mood disorders, in The American Psychiatric Publishing Textbook of Mood Disorders. Edited by Stein DJ, Kupfer DJ, Schatzberg AF. Washington, DC, American Psychiatric Publishing, 2006, pp 197–218

Smith D, Dempster C, Glanville J, et al: Efficacy and tolerability of venlafaxine compared with selective serotonin reuptake inhibitors and other antidepressants: a meta-analysis. Br J Psychiatry 180:396–404, 2002

Smith S: Tryptophan in the treatment of resistant depression: a review. Pharm J 261:819–821, 1998

Soares J, Mann J: The anatomy of mood disorders—review of structural neuroimaging studies. Biol Psychiatry 41:86–106, 1997

Solomon DA, Ryan CE, Keitner GI: A pilot study of lithium carbonate plus divalproex sodium for the continuation and maintenance treatment of patients with bipolar I disorder. J Clin Psychiatry 58:95–99, 1997

Spijker J, de Graaf R, Bijl RV, et al: Duration of major depressive episodes in the general population: results from the Netherlands Mental Health Survey and Incidence Study. Br J Psychiatry 181:208–213, 2002

Squire LR, Slater PC: Electroconvulsive therapy and complaints of memory dysfunction: a prospective three-year follow-up study. Br J Psychiatry 142:1–8, 1983

Starkstein SE, Robinson RG (eds): Depression in Neurologic Diseases. Baltimore, MD, Johns Hopkins University Press, 1993

Starkstein SE, Mayberg HS, Berthier ML, et al: Mania after brain injury: neuroradiological and metabolic findings. Ann Neurol 27:652–659, 1990

Steiner M, Dunn E, Born L: Hormones and mood: from menarche to menopause and beyond. J Affect Disord 74:67–83, 2003

Stewart JW, McGrath PJ, Quitkin FM: Do age of onset and course of illness predict different treatment outcome among DSM IV depressive disorders with atypical features? Neuropsychopharmacology 26:237–245, 2002

Stewart WF, Ricci JA, Chee E, et al: Cost of lost productive work time among US workers with depression. JAMA 289:3135–3144, 2003

Stoll AL, Mayer PV, Kolbrener M, et al: Antidepressant-associated mania: a controlled comparison with spontaneous mania. Am J Psychiatry 151:1642–1645, 1994

Strakowski SM: Clinical update in bipolar disorders: second-generation antipsychotics in the maintenance therapy of bipolar disorder. Available at: http://www.medscape.com/viewprogram/2496. Release date June 26, 2003

Sullivan P, Kendler K: Genetic case-control studies in neuropsychiatry. Arch Gen Psychiatry 58:1015–1024, 2001

Suppes T, Swann AC, Dennehy EB, et al: Texas Medication Algorithm Project: development and feasibility testing of a treatment algorithm for patients with bipolar disorder. J Clin Psychiatry 62:439–447, 2001

Swann AC, Bowden CL, Calabrese JR, et al: Pattern of response to divalproex, lithium, or placebo in four naturalistic subtypes of mania. Neuropsychopharmacology 26:530–536, 2002

Teasdale JD, Barnard PJ: Affect, Cognition and Change: Re-Modelling Depressive Thought. Hove, East Sussex, UK, Lawrence Erlbaum, 1993

Thase ME: Novel transdermal delivery formulation of the monoamine oxidase inhibitor selegiline nearing release for treatment of depression. J Clin Psychiatry 67:671–672, 2006

Thase ME, Beck AT: Overview of cognitive therapy, in Cognitive Therapy With Inpatients: Developing a Cognitive Milieu. Edited by Wright JH, Thase ME, Beck AT, et al. New York, Guilford, 1993, pp 3–34

Thase ME, Simons AD, McGeary J, et al: Relapse after cognitive-behavior therapy of depression: potential implications for longer courses of treatment? Am J Psychiatry 149:1046–1052, 1992

Tohen M, Bowden CL, Calabrese JR, et al: Olanzapine versus placebo for relapse prevention in bipolar disorder. Paper presented at the annual meeting of the American Psychiatric Association, San Francisco, CA, May 17–22, 2003

Torres GE, Gainetdinov RR, Caron MG: Plasma membrane monoamine transporters: structure, regulation and function. Nat Rev Neurosci 4:13–25, 2003

Trivedi MH, Rush AJ, Crismon ML, et al: Clinical results for patients with major depressive disorder in the Texas Medication Algorithm Project. Arch Gen Psychiatry 61:669–680, 2004

Videbech P: PET measurements of brain glucose metabolism and blood flow in major depressive disorder: a critical review. Acta Psychiatr Scand 101:11–20, 2000

Wagner KD, Ambrosini PJ, Rynn M, et al: Efficacy of sertraline in the treatment of children and adolescents with major depressive disorder. JAMA 290:1033–1041, 2003

Wang C, Cunningham G, Dobs A, et al: Long-term testosterone gel (AndroGel) treatment maintains beneficial effects on sexual function and mood, lean and fat mass, and bone mineral density in hypogonadal men. J Clin Endocrinol Metab 89:2085–2098, 2004

Wang PS, Kessler RC: Global burden of mood disorders, in The American Psychiatric Publishing Textbook of Mood Disorders. Edited by Stein DJ, Kupfer DJ, Schatzberg AF. Washington, DC, American Psychiatric Publishing, 2006, pp 55–68

Wang PS, Beck A, Berglund P, et al: Chronic medical conditions and work performance in the health and work performance questionnaire calibration surveys. J Occup Environ Med 45:1303–1311, 2003

Weisler RH, Kalali AH, Ketter TA, the SPD417 Study Group: A multicenter, randomized, double-blind, placebo-controlled trial of beaded carbamazepine extended-release capsules (beaded-ERC-CBZ; SPD417) as monotherapy for bipolar patients with manic or mixed episodes. J Clin Psychiatry 65:478–484, 2004

Weissman MM, Myers J: Affective disorders in a V.S. urban community: the use of research diagnostic criteria in an epidemiological survey. Arch Gen Psychiatry 35:1304–1311, 1978

Weissman MM, Bruce LM, Leaf PJ, et al: Affective disorders, in Psychiatric Disorders in America: The Epidemiologic Catchment Area Study. Edited by Robins LN, Regier DA. New York, Free Press, 1991, pp 53–80

Weissman MM, Bland RC, Canino GJ, et al: Cross-national epidemiology of major depression and bipolar disorder. JAMA 276:293–299, 1996

Weissman MM, Markowitz JC, Klerman GL: Comprehensive Guide to Interpersonal Psychotherapy. New York, Basic Books, 2000

Wells KB, Stewart A, Hays RD, et al: The functioning and well-being of depressed patients: results from the Medical Outcomes Study. JAMA 262:914–919, 1989

Whybrow PC, Bauer MS, Gyulai L: Thyroid axis considerations in patients with rapid cycling affective disorder. Clin Neuropharmacol 15 (suppl 1, pt A):391A–392A, 1992

Williams JMG: Depression, in Science and Practice of Cognitive Behavior Therapy. Edited by Clark DM, Fairburn CG. Oxford, England, Oxford University Press, 1997, pp 259–283

World Health Organization: International Statistical Classification of Diseases and Related Health Problems, 10th Revision. Geneva, Switzerland, World Health Organization, 1992

Young RC, Meyers BS: Psychopharmacology, in Comprehensive Review of Geriatric Psychiatry. Edited by Sadavoy J, Lazarus LW, Jarvik LF. Washington, DC, American Psychiatric Press, 1992, pp 435–467

Zornberg GL, Pope HG Jr: Treatment of depression in bipolar disorder: new directions for research. J Clin Psychopharmacol 13:397–408, 1993

12

ANXIETY DISORDERS

Eric Hollander, M.D.
Daphne Simeon, M.D.

Anxiety disorders are the most common of all psychiatric illnesses and result in considerable functional impairment and distress. Recent research developments have had a broad impact on our understanding of the underlying mechanisms of illness and treatment response. Working with patients who have an anxiety disorder can be highly gratifying for the informed psychiatrist, because these patients, who are in considerable distress, often respond to proper treatment and return to a high level of functioning. The major anxiety disorders presented in this chapter are panic disorder, generalized anxiety disorder (GAD), social anxiety disorder, specific phobias, obsessive-compulsive disorder (OCD), and posttraumatic stress disorder (PTSD). Table 12–1 presents a summary overview of the prevalence, gender ratio, and comorbidities of the major anxiety disorders.

A diagnostic decision tree of the anxiety disorders is presented in Figure 12–1. If pathological anxiety is induced by either psychoactive substance use or an Axis III physical illness, it is classified in DSM-IV-TR (American Psychiatric Association 2000) under the anxiety disorders (substance-induced anxiety disorder or anxiety disorder due to a general medical condition, respectively). DSM-IV-TR specifies the subtype of organic anxiety as generalized anxiety, panic attacks, or obsessive-compulsive symptoms.

Panic Disorder

Definition

DSM-II (American Psychiatric Association 1968) described an ill-defined condition of *anxiety neurosis,* a term first coined by Freud in 1895 (Breuer and Freud 1893–1895/1955), which included any patient with chronic tension, excessive worry, frequent headaches, or recurrent anxiety attacks. However, subsequent findings suggested that discrete, spontaneous panic attacks may be qualitatively dissimilar to other chronic anxiety states. Patients with panic attacks were found, for example, to be unique in their panic-induction responsiveness to sodium lactate infusion, familial aggregation, development of agoraphobia, and treatment response to tricyclic antidepressants (TCAs). Thus, DSM-III (American Psychiatric Association 1980) and the subsequent DSM-III-R (American Psychiatric Association 1987) divided the category of anxiety neurosis into panic disorder and GAD.

The DSM-IV-TR definition of a *panic attack* is presented in Table 12–2. Panic disorder is subdivided into panic disorder with and without agoraphobia, as in DSM-III-R, depending on whether there is any secondary phobic avoidance (Table 12–3).

TABLE 12–1. Approximate lifetime prevalence, gender ratio, and common comorbidities for the major anxiety disorders

Disorder	Prevalence	Females:Males	Comorbidity
Panic disorder	2%–4%	2+:1	Depression, other anxiety disorders
Generalized anxiety disorder	5%–7%	2:1	Overall, 90%; 50%–60% for major depression or other anxiety disorder
Social phobia	13%–16%	1+:1	Twofold risk for alcohol dependence, three- to sixfold risk of mood disorders
Specific phobias	10%	2:1	Depression and somatoform disorders
Agoraphobia	6%	2:1	
Obsessive-compulsive disorder	2%–3%	1:1	Anxiety, depression, tics, hypochondriasis, eating disorder, body dysmorphic disorder (childhood-onset more common in males)
Posttraumatic stress disorder	7%–9%	2:1	Depression, obsessive-compulsive disorder, panic, phobias

DSM-IV (American Psychiatric Association 1994) clarified several issues regarding the diagnosis and differential diagnosis of panic disorder that remained obscured in DSM-III-R. Panic attacks are well known to occur not only in panic disorder but in other anxiety disorders as well (e.g., specific phobia, social phobia, and PTSD). In these other disorders, panic attacks are situationally bound or cued—that is, they occur exclusively within the context of the feared situation. DSM-IV clarified this confusion by explicitly presenting the definition of panic attacks independently of panic disorder and specifying that a panic attack can be "unexpected (uncued)," "situationally bound (cued)," or "situationally predisposed."

The differential diagnosis can sometimes become complicated when, historically, one or several unexpected panic attacks initially occur in a specific situation, consistent with a diagnosis of panic disorder, but later evolve into a chronic condition in which the attacks are cued exclusively by that situation or when avoidance of that situation develops because of fear of another attack. Is the diagnosis in such a case panic disorder with agoraphobia or social/specific phobia? DSM-IV-TR retains the distinct diagnoses of panic disorder with agoraphobia, social anxiety disorder, and specific phobia and specifies that panic attacks can occur as a feature of all three of these disorders. Therefore clinical judgment regarding the preponderant clinical pattern is called for in making the differential diagnosis in such cases.

Clinical Description

Onset

In the typical onset of a case of panic disorder, individuals are engaged in some ordinary aspect of life when suddenly their heart begins to pound, and they cannot catch their breath. They feel dizzy, light-headed, and faint and are convinced they are about to die. Panic disorder patients are usually young adults, most likely in the third decade, although onset may be as late as the sixth decade.

Although the first attack generally strikes during some routine activity, several events are often associated with the early presentation of panic disorder. Not uncommonly, the first panic attack occurs in the context of a life-threatening illness or accident, the loss of a close interpersonal relationship, or a separation from family (e.g., starting college or accepting a job out of town). Patients developing either hypo- or hyperthyroidism may get the first flurry of attacks at this time. Attacks also begin in the immediate postpartum period. Finally, many patients have reported experiencing their first attacks while taking drugs of abuse, especially marijuana, lysergic acid diethylamide (LSD), sedatives, cocaine, and amphetamines. However, even when these concomitant conditions are resolved, the attacks often continue unabated. This situation gives the impression that some stressors may act as triggers to provoke the beginning of panic attacks in patients who are already predisposed.

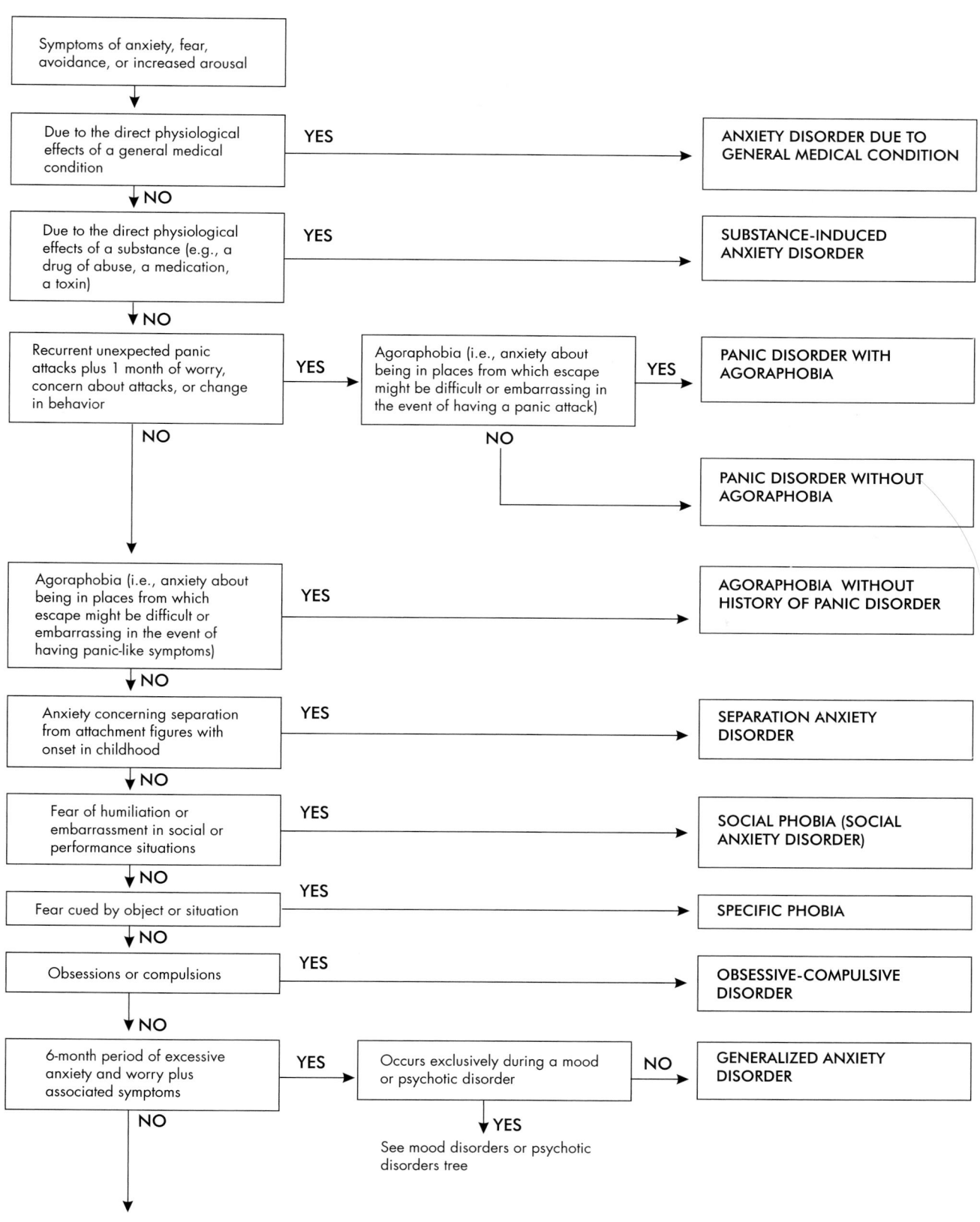

FIGURE 12–1. Diagnostic decision tree for anxiety disorders.

Patients may have more than one disorder and thus must be evaluated for each disorder.

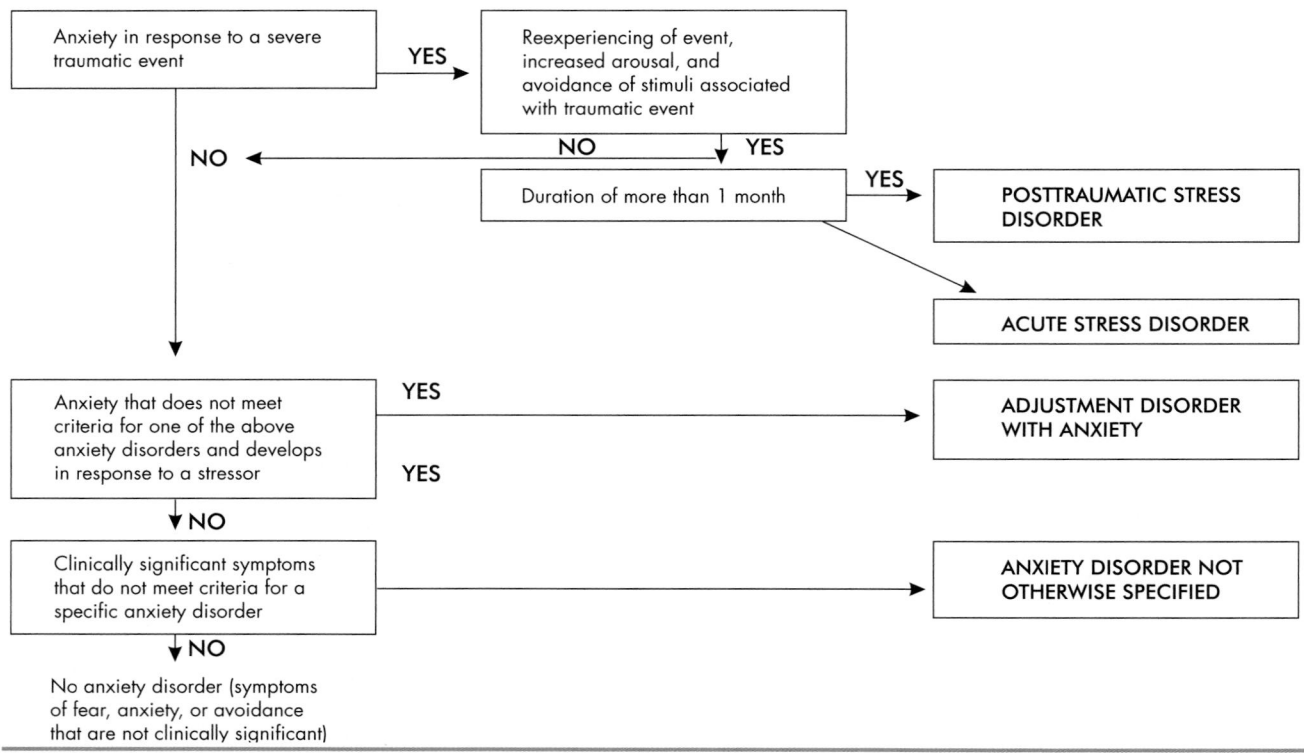

FIGURE 12–1. Diagnostic decision tree for anxiety disorders. *(continued)*

Patients may have more than one disorder and thus must be evaluated for each disorder.

TABLE 12–2. **DSM-IV-TR diagnostic criteria for panic attacks**

Note: A panic attack is not a codable disorder. Code the specific diagnosis in which the panic attack occurs (e.g., 300.21 panic disorder with agoraphobia)

A discrete period of intense fear or discomfort, in which four (or more) of the following symptoms developed abruptly and reached a peak within 10 minutes:

(1) palpitations, pounding heart, or accelerated heart rate
(2) sweating
(3) trembling or shaking
(4) sensations of shortness of breath or smothering
(5) feeling of choking
(6) chest pain or discomfort
(7) nausea or abdominal distress
(8) feeling dizzy, unsteady, light-headed, or faint
(9) derealization (feelings of unreality) or depersonalization (being detached from oneself)
(10) fear of losing control or going crazy
(11) fear of dying
(12) paresthesias (numbness or tingling sensations)
(13) chills or hot flushes

Patients experiencing their first panic attack generally fear they are having a heart attack or losing their mind. Such patients often rush to the nearest emergency department, where routine laboratory tests, electrocardiography, and physical examination are performed. All that is found is an occasional case of sinus tachycardia, and the patients are reassured and sent home. These patients may indeed feel reassured, and at this point the diagnosis of panic disorder would be premature. However, perhaps a few days or even weeks later they will again have the sudden onset of severe anxiety with all of the associated physical symptoms. Again, they seek emergency medical treatment. At this point, they may be told the problem is psychological, be given a prescription for a benzodiazepine tranquilizer, or be referred for extensive medical workup.

Symptoms

Typically, during a panic attack, a patient will be engaged in a routine activity, perhaps reading a book, eating in a restaurant, driving a car, or attending a concert, when he or she will experience the sudden onset of overwhelming fear, terror, apprehension, and a sense of impending doom. Several of a group of associated symptoms, mostly physical, are also experienced: dyspnea, palpitations, chest pain or discomfort,

TABLE 12–3. **DSM-IV-TR diagnostic criteria for panic disorder with or without agoraphobia**

Diagnostic criteria for 300.01 panic disorder without agoraphobia

A. Both (1) and (2):

    (1) recurrent unexpected panic attacks

    (2) at least one of the attacks has been followed by 1 month (or more) of one (or more) of the following:

        (a) persistent concern about having additional attacks

        (b) worry about the implications of the attack or its consequences (e.g., losing control, having a heart attack, "going crazy")

        (c) a significant change in behavior related to the attacks

B. Absence of agoraphobia.

C. The panic attacks are not due to the direct physiological effects of a substance (e.g., a drug of abuse, a medication) or a general medical condition (e.g., hyperthyroidism).

D. The panic attacks are not better accounted for by another mental disorder, such as social phobia (e.g., occurring on exposure to feared social situations), specific phobia (e.g., on exposure to a specific phobic situation), obsessive-compulsive disorder (e.g., on exposure to dirt in someone with an obsession about contamination), posttraumatic stress disorder (e.g., in response to stimuli associated with a severe stressor), or separation anxiety disorder (e.g., in response to being away from home or close relatives).

Diagnostic criteria for 300.21 panic disorder with agoraphobia

A. Both (1) and (2):

    (1) recurrent unexpected panic attacks

    (2) at least one of the attacks has been followed by 1 month (or more) of one (or more) of the following:

        (a) persistent concern about having additional attacks

        (b) worry about the implications of the attack or its consequences (e.g., losing control, having a heart attack, "going crazy")

        (c) a significant change in behavior related to the attacks

B. The presence of agoraphobia.

TABLE 12–3. **DSM-IV-TR diagnostic criteria for panic disorder with or without agoraphobia** (*continued*)

C. The panic attacks are not due to the direct physiological effects of a substance (e.g., a drug of abuse, a medication) or a general medical condition (e.g., hyperthyroidism).

D. The panic attacks are not better accounted for by another mental disorder, such as social phobia (e.g., occurring on exposure to feared social situations), specific phobia (e.g., on exposure to a specific phobic situation), obsessive-compulsive disorder (e.g., on exposure to dirt in someone with an obsession about contamination), posttraumatic stress disorder (e.g., in response to stimuli associated with a severe stressor), or separation anxiety disorder (e.g., in response to being away from home or close relatives).

choking or smothering sensations, dizziness or unsteady feelings, feelings of unreality (derealization and/or depersonalization), paresthesias, hot and cold flashes, sweating, faintness, trembling and shaking, and a fear of dying, going crazy, or losing control of oneself. It is clear that most of the physical sensations of a panic attack represent massive overstimulation of the autonomic nervous system.

Attacks usually last from 5 to 20 minutes and rarely as long as an hour. Patients who claim they have attacks that last a whole day may fall into one of four categories. Some patients continue to feel agitated and fatigued for several hours after the main portion of the attack has subsided. At times, attacks occur, subside, and occur again in a wave-like manner. Alternatively, the patient with so-called long panic attacks often has some other form of pathological anxiety, such as severe generalized anxiety, agitated depression, or obsessional tension states. Finally, in some cases, such severe anticipatory anxiety may develop with time in expectation of future panic attacks that the two may blend together in the patient's description and be difficult to distinguish.

Although many people experience an occasional unexpected attack of panic, the diagnosis of panic disorder is only made when the attacks occur with some regularity and frequency. However, patients with occasional unexpected panic attacks may be genetically similar to patients with panic disorder. A twin study found the best results for genetic linkage when patients with regular panic attacks were included together with patients who had only occasional attacks (Torgersen 1983).

Some patients do not progress in their illness beyond the point of continuing to have unexpected panic attacks. Most patients develop some degree of anticipatory anxiety consequent to the experience of repetitive panic attacks. The patient comes to dread experiencing an attack and starts worrying about doing so in the intervals between attacks. This can progress until the level of fearfulness and autonomic hyperactivity in the interval between panic attacks almost approximates the level during the actual attack itself. Such patients may be mistaken for GAD patients.

It is warranted to draw some further attention to what appears to be the cardinal symptom of panic. A number of lines of research evidence indicate that hyperventilation may be the central feature in the pathophysiology of panic attacks and panic disorder. Patients with panic disorder have been shown to be chronic hyperventilators who also acutely hyperventilate during spontaneous and induced panic (the possible etiologies of this are discussed later in this section). This hyperventilation then induces hypocapnia and alkalosis, leading to decreased cerebral blood flow and to the dizziness, confusion, and derealization characteristic of panic attacks. Indeed, signs and symptoms of hyperventilation seem to disappear once a patient with panic disorder has been successfully treated with antipanic medication. Also, behavioral breathing retraining treatments aimed at teaching the patient not to hyperventilate are successful in decreasing the frequency of panic attacks, presumably by dampening the ventilatory overreaction that may constitute the hallmark of panic.

Agoraphobia.   Agoraphobia frequently develops in response to panic attacks, leading to the DSM-IV-TR diagnosis of panic disorder with agoraphobia. The clinical picture in agoraphobia consists of multiple and varied fears and avoidance behaviors that center around three main themes: 1) fear of leaving home, 2) fear of being alone, and 3) fear of being away from home in situations where one can feel trapped, embarrassed, or helpless. According to DSM-IV-TR, the fear is one of developing distressing symptoms in such situations where escape is difficult or help is unavailable. Typical agoraphobic fears are of using public transportation (e.g., buses, trains, subways, planes); being in crowds, theaters, elevators, restaurants, supermarkets, or department stores; waiting in line; or traveling a distance from home. In severe cases, patients may be completely housebound, fearful of leaving home without a companion or even of staying home alone.

Most cases of agoraphobia begin with a series of spontaneous panic attacks. If the attacks continue, the patient usually develops a constant anticipatory anxiety characterized by continued apprehension about the possible occasion and consequences of the next attack. Agoraphobic symptoms represent a tertiary phase in the illness. Many patients will causally relate their panic attacks to the particular situation in which the attacks have occurred. They then avoid these situations in an attempt to prevent further panic attacks (Figure 12–2).

For example, a man who has had several attacks while taking the train to work may attribute the attacks to the train and, in order to avoid the train, start driving to work. If he still experiences panic attacks in the morning while driving to work rather than on the train, he interprets this as a sign that the attacks have spread to driving situations rather than as an indication that they were not, in the first place, caused by the train. Agoraphobic persons frequently fear situations in which they feel they cannot leave abruptly if an attack occurs, such as crowded rooms, front-row seats, tunnels, bridges, and airplanes. Some individuals continue to have spontaneous panic attacks throughout the course of the illness. In other cases, after the initial phase of the illness, attacks may occur rarely or exclusively when the patient ventures into the feared situation.

One interesting aspect of agoraphobia is the effect of a trusted companion on phobic behavior. Many patients who are unable to leave the house alone can travel long distances and partake in most activities if accompanied by a spouse, family member, or close friend. It is unclear whether vulnerability to panic attacks is actually decreased in this situation or whether the patient feels less helpless and isolated. In addition to panic attacks and chronic anxiety, agoraphobic patients frequently exhibit symptoms of demoralization or secondary depression, multiple somatic complaints, and alcohol or sedative drug abuse.

Character Traits

It has not been clearly established whether particular character types are correlated with panic disorder, and studies are further confounded because the presence of panic disorder may have secondary effects on personality. Noyes et al. (1991) conducted personality follow-up of panic disorder patients treated for panic over 3 years and found that the initial avoidant and dependent traits were to a large extent state related and waned with the treatment of panic. On the other hand, experience leads many clinicians to feel that patients with agoraphobia and panic are more likely to have histories of dependent character traits that antedate the onset of panic.

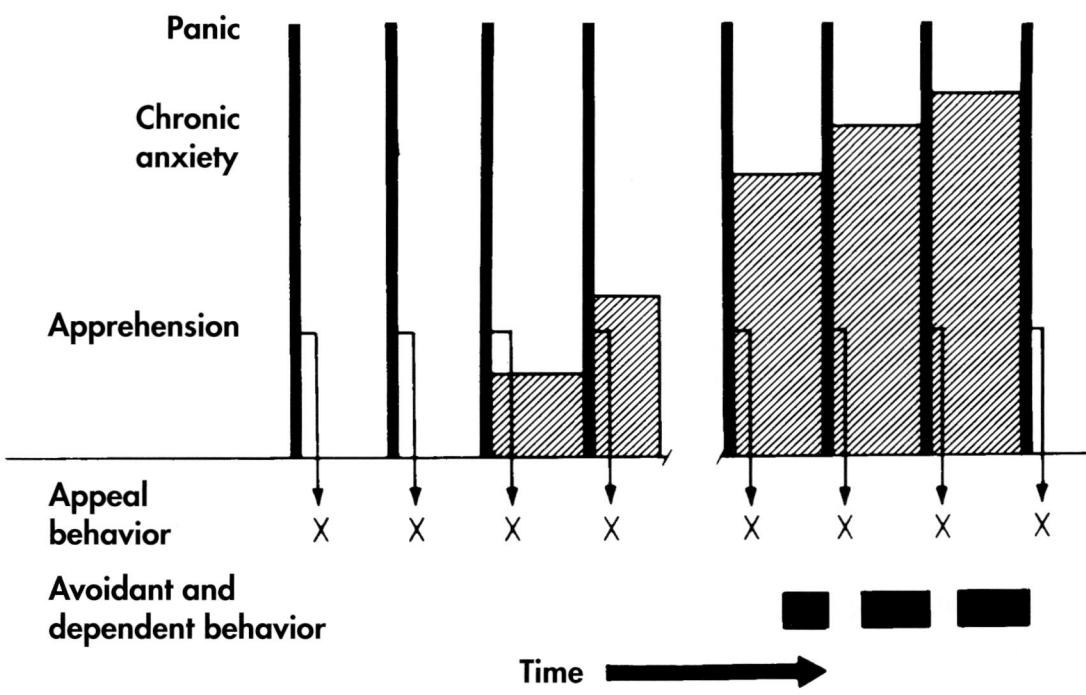

FIGURE 12–2. Development of agoraphobia.

After onset of unexpected panic attacks *(solid bars),* patient develops acute help-seeking behavior *(X),* then apprehension culminating in chronic anxiety *(shaded areas),* and finally agoraphobic behavior *(black blocks).*

Epidemiology

The National Institute of Mental Health Epidemiologic Catchment Area (ECA) study examined the population prevalence of DSM-III-diagnosed panic disorder using the Diagnostic Interview Schedule (Regier et al. 1988). The 1-month, 6-month, and lifetime prevalence rates for panic disorder at all five study sites combined were 0.5%, 0.8%, and 1.6%, respectively. Women had a 1-month prevalence rate of 0.7%, which was significantly higher than the 0.3% rate found among men; women also tended to have a greater rise in panic disorder in the age range of 25 to 44 years, and their attacks tended to continue longer into older age (Regier et al. 1988).

More recently, the 2001–2002 National Epidemiologic Survey on Alcohol and Related Conditions (NESARC), which included about 43,000 participants, revealed a 1-year and lifetime prevalence of panic disorder of 2.1% and 5.1%, respectively (Grant et al. 2006); rates for panic disorder without agoraphobia were 1.6% and 4.0%, respectively, exceeding those of panic disorder with agoraphobia (0.6% and 1.1%, respectively). Being female, Native American, middle-aged, widowed/separated/divorced, and of low income increased risk for panic disorder, whereas being Asian,

African American, or Hispanic decreased risk. Subjects with agoraphobia had an earlier age at onset, more severe symptoms, greater disability, and greater Axis I and II comorbidity compared with subjects without agoraphobia and were more likely to seek treatment early on. Thus, the overrepresentation of panic disorder with agoraphobia in treatment settings probably reflects greater treatment seeking and more severe disorder. On the other hand, agoraphobia without panic disorder was quite rare, with a 0.17% lifetime prevalence, raising questions about its standing as a distinct Axis I disorder. The National Comorbidity Survey Replication study reported highly similar findings, with a lifetime prevalence of 3.7% for panic disorder without agoraphobia and 1.1% with agoraphobia (Kessler et al. 2006), and again the presence of agoraphobia was associated with greater symptom severity, comorbidity, and impairment.

Etiology
Biological Theories

A number of biological theories of panic disorder figure prominently in the psychiatric literature; we summarize the evidence for or against some of the most promising ones. Certain agents have a powerful and specific capacity to induce panic, in contrast to other agents that produce prominent physiological changes but fail to induce panic. These findings argue strongly against the notion that panic is a reaction to nonspecific distressing stimuli and suggest more specific biological bases, even if these involve multiple neurochemicals and circuits. The various theories described in the following sections should not be viewed as mutually exclusive but rather as potentially interlocking pieces of a larger puzzle. The theories are summarized in Table 12–4; neurochemical, imaging, and genetic findings are described in the discussions that follow.

The sympathetic system.   Studies of normal subjects exposed to novel stress typically demonstrate elevations in plasma catecholamine levels. Elevated plasma levels of epinephrine are not, however, a regular accompaniment of panic attacks induced in the laboratory (Liebowitz et al. 1985a). It is not clear whether administration of catecholamines can actually provoke anxiety reactions and, if so, whether the reaction is specific only to patients with anxiety disorder. Researchers in the 1930s and 1940s did show that epinephrine infusion caused the physical, but not necessarily the emotional, symptoms of anxiety in human subjects, and for many years the possibility that panic attacks were manifestations of massive discharge from the β-adrenergic nervous system was considered. The β-adrenergic hypothesis of panic has received some support from studies claiming that β-adrenergic–blocking drugs, such as propranolol, have an ameliorative effect on panic attacks and anxiety. When the properly designed and controlled studies of β-adrenergic blockers used in specific well-diagnosed anxiety disorders are reviewed, however, only modest antianxiety effects can actually be demonstrated. No study has ever shown that β-adrenergic blockers are specifically effective in blocking spontaneous panic attacks. For example, intravenously administered propranolol, in doses sufficient to achieve full peripheral β-adrenergic blockade, was not able to block a sodium lactate–induced panic attack in patients with panic disorder (Gorman et al. 1983). Examination of various autonomic parameters seems to dispel the notion of simple autonomic dysregulation in panic (M. B. Stein and Asmundson 1994). Indeed, there does not appear to be global sympathetic activation in panic disorder patients at rest or even during panic attacks in some patients (Wilkinson et al. 1998).

The locus coeruleus has also been implicated in the pathogenesis of panic attacks. This nucleus is located in the pons and contains more than 50% of all noradrenergic neurons in the entire central nervous sys-

TABLE 12–4. **Biological models of panic disorder**
Hyperreactivity of the locus coeruleus
Dysregulated serotonergic modulation
Decreased γ-aminobutyric acid (GABA)–benzodiazepine receptor complex binding
Hypersensitive brain stem carbon dioxide (CO_2) chemoreceptors
Hypersensitive conditioned fear network centered in the amygdala
Moderate genetic component

tem. It sends afferent projections to a wide area of the brain, including the hippocampus, amygdala, limbic lobe, and cerebral cortex. Electrical stimulation of the animal locus coeruleus produces a marked fear and anxiety response, whereas ablation of the animal locus coeruleus renders an animal less susceptible to fear response in the face of threatening stimuli (Redmond 1979). In humans, drugs known to be capable of increasing locus coeruleus discharge in animals are anxiogenic, whereas many drugs that curtail locus coeruleus firing and decrease central noradrenergic turnover are antianxiety agents.

Yohimbine challenge has been reported to induce greater anxiety and a greater increase in plasma 3-methoxy-4-hydroxyphenylglycol (MHPG), a major noradrenergic metabolite, in patients who have frequent panic attacks compared with patients who have panic attacks less frequently or healthy control subjects. Such a finding is suggestive of heightened central noradrenergic activity in panic (Charney et al. 1984). The results from challenge tests with the α_2-adrenergic agonist clonidine, although difficult to interpret, have suggested noradrenergic dysregulation in panic, with hypersensitivity of some and subsensitivity of other brain α_2-adrenoreceptors. Compared with control subjects, panic disorder patients had heightened cardiovascular responses but blunted growth hormone responses to clonidine (Nutt 1989). Dysregulated noradrenergic function, in the form of markedly elevated MHPG volatility in response to clonidine challenge, has been described in panic disorder patients and normalizes after treatment with selective serotonin reuptake inhibitors (SSRIs) (Coplan et al. 1997).

However, buspirone, which is also reported to increase locus coeruleus firing, is an anxiolytic medication and has not been reported to induce panic. Examples of medications that curtail locus coeruleus firing are clonidine, propranolol, benzodiazepines, morphine, endorphin, and TCAs. These drugs range from those clearly effective in blocking human panic attacks (e.g., TCAs) to those of more dubious efficacy (e.g., clonidine, propranolol, and standard benzodiazepines). Also, controversy exists about the relevance of these animal models. Redmond (1979) and colleagues have produced abundant evidence that situations that provoke fear and anxiety in laboratory animals are associated with increases in locus coeruleus discharge and in central noradrenergic turnover. This would, of course, support the idea that the locus coeruleus is a kind of generator for anxiety attacks. However, there is no consistent pattern of increased locus coeruleus discharge associated with anxiety in animals; the locus coeruleus may be involved in arousal and response to novel stimuli rather than in anxiety (Aston-Jones et al. 1984).

The panicogen sodium lactate.

Although not without some controversy, sodium lactate provocation of panic attacks has captured a lot of attention as an experimental model for understanding the pathogenesis of spontaneous panic attacks. Lactate-provoked panic is specific to patients with prior spontaneous attacks, closely resembles such attacks, and can be blocked by the same drugs that block natural attacks (Liebowitz et al. 1984). Pitts and McClure (1967) administered intravenous infusions of sodium lactate to patients with "anxiety" disorder and found that most of the patients had an anxiety attack during the infusion. The subjects all believed that these attacks were quite typical of their naturally occurring attacks. Control subjects did not experience panic attacks during the infusion.

Having been replicated on numerous occasions under proper experimental conditions, the finding that 10 mL/kg of 0.5 molar sodium lactate infused over 20 minutes will provoke a panic attack in most patients with panic disorder but not in normal control subjects is now a well-accepted fact. The mechanism, however, that may account for the observed biochemical and physiological changes (Liebowitz et al. 1985a) has been subject to much uncertainty and controversy. Theories have included nonspecific arousal that cognitively triggers panic; induction of metabolic alkalosis; hypocalcemia; alteration of the ratio of nicotinamide-adenine dinucleotide (NAD) to the hydrogenated (reduced) form of nicotinamide-adenine dinucleotide (NADH); and transient intracerebral hypercapnia. In a recent study, subjects with panic disorder were found to have greater hypocapnia in response to hyperventilation, whereas their pH response was not altered, implicating exaggerated buffering possibly mediated by increased lactate (Friedman et al. 2006).

The GABA–benzodiazepine system.

Another area of inquiry that may relate to the biology of panic is the γ-aminobutyric acid (GABA)–benzodiazepine receptor complex; the benzodiazepine receptor is linked to a receptor for the inhibitory neurotransmitter GABA. Binding of a benzodiazepine to the benzodiazepine receptor facilitates the action of GABA, effectively slowing neural transmission. One series of compounds, the β-carbolines, which are inverse agonists of this receptor complex, produces an acute anxiety syndrome when administered to laboratory animals or to normal human volunteers. On the other hand, benzodiazepines have long been known to be a highly efficacious treatment for panic. The possibility is then raised that either aberrant production of an endogenous ligand or altered receptor sensitivity may occur in patients with panic, interfering with proper benzodiazepine receptor function and causing their symptoms.

There is support for such a theory, although findings in the literature to date have been to a degree contradictory. One study found that panic disorder patients, compared with healthy control subjects, demonstrated less reduced saccadic eye movement velocity in response to diazepam, suggesting hyposensitivity of the benzodiazepine receptor in panic (Roy-Byrne et al. 1990). The benzodiazepine antagonist flumazenil was found to be panicogenic in panic patients but not in control subjects, suggesting a deficiency in an endogenous anxiolytic ligand or altered benzodiazepine receptor sensitivity in panic (Nutt et al. 1990). However, another study of flumazenil responses in panic was negative (Strohle et al. 1999).

More recently, imaging studies have consistently revealed alterations in this system. Decreased benzodiazepine receptor binding by single photon emission computed tomography (SPECT) was found in the hippocampus of panic disorder patients, and prefrontal cortex binding was also decreased in those subjects who experienced an attack during the scanning (Bremner et al. 2000). These findings could tie in neatly to the current neurocircuitry of fear model of panic, described later, in which the amygdala, hippocampus, and prefrontal cortex play a central role in modulating conditioned fear responses. Similarly, a global decrease in benzodiazepine receptor binding has been found with positron emission tomography (PET), most prominent in the prefrontal cortex and the insula (Malizia et al. 1998). Another study reported that a 22% reduction in total occipital GABA levels was found in panic subjects compared with control subjects (Goddard et al. 2001a). In a magnetic resonance spectroscopy study that measured total occipital cortex GABA levels, panic disorder patients, compared with healthy control subjects, were found to have a deficient GABA neuronal response after acute oral benzodiazepine administration, suggesting that a trait-like abnormality in GABA function may contribute to the pathogenesis of panic (Goddard et al. 2004).

The serotonergic system. Although the serotonergic system has not been as extensively investigated in panic as other neurochemical systems, it is widely thought that it may be one of the systems that at least indirectly modulate dysregulated responses in the disorder. Indirect evidence is provided by the high efficacy of serotonin reuptake inhibitors in treating panic. It has recently been proposed that serotonergic medications may act by desensitizing the brain's fear network via projections from the raphe nuclei to the locus coeruleus, inhibiting noradrenergic activation; to the periaqueductal gray region, inhibiting freeze/flight responses; to the hypothalamus, inhibiting corticotropin-releasing factor (CRF) release; and possibly directly at the level of the amygdala, inhibiting excitatory pathways from the cortex and the thalamus (Gorman et al. 2000). In one study, depletion of tryptophan, a serotonin precursor, resulted in increased anxiety and carbon dioxide (CO_2)–induced panic attacks in panic patients but not in comparison subjects (Miller et al. 2000). A radioligand PET imaging study provided evidence for decreased distribution of serotonin (5-hydroxytryptamine) type 1A ($5-HT_{1A}$) receptor binding in the cingulate cortex and dorsal raphe in panic disorder participants compared with healthy control subjects (Neumeister et al. 2004). Another radioligand PET study reported significant decreases in serotonin transporter binding in the midbrain, temporal lobes, and thalamus in participants with current panic disorder, and this decrease correlated significantly with greater panic symptom severity (Maron et al. 2004).

Hypothalamic-pituitary-adrenal axis. The hypothalamic-pituitary-adrenal (HPA) system, which is central to an organism's response to stress, would clearly be of interest in panic disorder, in which increased early life stressful events such as separations, losses, and abuse have been described (M.B. Stein et al. 1996). However, HPA findings in panic have been very contradictory and have not consistently supported HPA axis dysregulation in the disorder. Cortisol responses in lactate-induced panic have suggested HPA axis involvement in anticipatory anxiety, as is known to occur in other anxiety and stress states, but not in the actual panic attacks (Hollander et al. 1989). There is

some evidence for uncoupling of noradrenergic and HPA axis activity in panic disorder patients (Coplan et al. 1995). In one study, adrenocorticotropic hormone and cortisol responses to CRF challenge were not clearly altered in panic patients compared with healthy subjects (Curtis et al. 1997). More recently, a metyrapone and combined metyrapone/dexamethasone challenge study failed to find any HPA axis response difference between panic disorder and control patients (Kellner et al. 2004).

Carbon dioxide hypersensitivity theory. Controlled hyperventilation and respiratory alkalosis do not routinely provoke panic attacks in most patients with panic disorder. Surprisingly, however, giving these patients a mixture of 5% CO_2 in room air to breathe causes panic almost as often as does a sodium lactate infusion (Gorman et al. 1984). This finding has been consistently replicated and appears specific to panic disorder (Kent et al. 2001). Similarly, sodium bicarbonate infusion provokes panic attacks in patients with panic disorder at a rate comparable with that induced by CO_2 inhalation (Gorman et al. 1989). Aberrant respiratory sensitivity to CO_2 may be a familial trait that comprises a risk factor for developing panic disorder, a hypothesis supported by one study (Coryell et al. 2001) but not by another (Pine et al. 2005).

By what mechanism, then, does 5% CO_2 induce panic? When CO_2 is added to inspired air, it causes a reliable dose-dependent increase in rat locus coeruleus firing. Alternatively, panic disorder patients may have hypersensitive brain stem CO_2 chemoreceptors in their medulla. Indeed, during the CO_2 induction procedure, panic disorder patients who experience panic attacks while breathing 5% CO_2 demonstrate a much faster increase in inspiratory drive than do nonpanicking patients or normal control subjects; inspiratory drive is thought to reflect most directly the brain stem component of respiratory regulation (Gorman et al. 1988). In an interesting study of CO_2 inhalation sensitivity before and after psychotherapy or medication treatment in panic disorder patients, it was found that after treatment patients exhibited diminished subjective panic responses, whereas objective respiratory physiological responses remained unchanged, suggesting that treatment strengthened higher cortical control over subcortical fear-related circuitry (Gorman et al. 2004).

Such a model is of interest because it could account for the generally well-established fact that hyperventilation does not cause panic, whereas CO_2, lactate, and bicarbonate do. Infused lactate is metabolized to bicarbonate, which is then converted in the periphery to

CO_2. In other words, CO_2 constitutes the common metabolic product of both lactate and bicarbonate. This CO_2 then selectively crosses the blood-brain barrier and produces transient cerebral hypercapnia. The hypercapnia then sets off the brain stem CO_2 chemoreceptors, leading to hyperventilation and panic. Thus, a "false suffocation alarm" theory of panic has been formulated (D. F. Klein 1993) that proposes that patients with panic are hypersensitive to CO_2 because they have an overly sensitive brain stem suffocation alarm system. This condition constitutes, in a sense, the opposite of the hyposensitive suffocation alarm seen in Ondine's curse, a rare illness in which the afflicted are at risk for suffocating in their sleep. D. F. Klein (1993) proposed that such a theory of panic could explain, for example, the tendency of panic attacks to occur during high-CO_2 states such as deep non–rapid eye movement sleep, premenstrually, and sometimes with relaxation, but not during childbirth, an event otherwise characterized by extreme hyperventilation and potentially catastrophic cognitions.

This theory may be supported by the variety of subtle respiratory dysfunctions that appear to be associated with panic, such as preexisting pulmonary disease, panic disorder patients' tendency to chronically hyperventilate, their increased variance in tidal volume during steady-state respiration, and their greater irregularities in nocturnal breathing (M. B. Stein et al. 1995b). There is some evidence that irregular breathing patterns are intrinsic to panic patients and are not influenced by induced hyperventilation or cognitive manipulation, suggesting a brain stem rather than a higher brain level dysregulation (Abelson et al. 2001). A recent study of respiratory physiology in panic disorder patients found that, compared with control subjects, patients manifested greater entropy in baseline respiratory patterns, indicating higher levels of irregularity and complexity in their respiratory function (Caldirola et al. 2004). Increased gray matter volume in the brain stem of panic patients compared with control subjects has provided preliminary structural evidence for a role of the brain stem in the neurocircuitry of panic (Protopopescu et al. 2006). On the other hand, Gorman et al. (2000) argued that brain stem respiratory centers are a secondary mechanism by which panic attack symptoms relating to respiration become manifest, as one of several pathways that become activated by central excitation of the amygdala.

Neurocircuitry of fear. The neurocircuitry of fear model integrates neurochemical, imaging, and treatment findings in the disorder coupled with human and animal studies in the neurobiology of conditioned fear

responses (Gorman et al. 2000). The model proposes that panic attacks are analogous to animal fear and avoidance responses and may be manifestations of dysregulation in the brain circuits underlying conditioned fear responses. Panic is speculated to originate in an abnormally sensitive fear network, centered in the amygdala. Input into the amygdala is modulated by both thalamic input and prefrontal cortical projections, and there are amygdalar projections to several areas involved in various aspects of the fear response, such as the locus coeruleus and arousal, the brain stem and respiratory activation, the hypothalamus and activation of the HPA stress axis, and the cortex and cognitive interpretations. This model is thought to explain why a variety of biologically diverse agents have panicogenic properties, by acting at different pathways or on neurochemical systems of this network; it is proposed that the respiratory brain stem nucleus could not be directly triggered by such a variety of agents (Gorman et al. 2000). Thus, dysregulated "cross-talk" between various neurotransmitter systems, such as serotonergic, noradrenergic, GABAergic, CRF, and others, may underlie the pathogenesis of panic.

Neuroimaging studies are implicating these and other areas in the neurocircuitry of panic. A PET functional neuroimaging study supported an amygdala-based fear network in panic, revealing significantly higher glucose uptake under resting conditions in the bilateral amygdala, hippocampus, thalamus, midbrain, caudal pons, medulla, and cerebellum in panic disorder participants compared with healthy control subjects (Sakai et al. 2005). A functional magnetic resonance imaging (fMRI) study examining the functional neural correlates of disease-related emotional stimuli reported that panic patients showed activation in the right amygdala and hippocampus while performing the panic-related emotional Stroop task (van den Heuvel et al. 2005b). A pilot PET study in panic disorder found that decreased orbitocortical frontal cortex activation predicted heightened anxiety in response to intravenous challenge with the panicogen doxapram, again supporting a model of diminished top-down inhibition by prefrontal cortical regions over hypersensitive limbic regions (Kent et al. 2005). Structural volumetric studies have reported decreased gray matter volumes bilaterally in the putamen of panic disorder participants, the magnitude of which was associated with panic severity (Yoo et al. 2005).

Genetics. Several family and twin studies of panic disorder have consistently supported the presence of a moderate genetic influence in the expression of panic disorder. Crowe et al. (1983) found a morbidity risk for panic disorder of 24.7% among relatives of patients with panic disorder compared with only 2.3% among normal control subjects. Torgersen (1983) completed a study of 32 monozygotic and 53 dizygotic twins and found panic attacks to be five times more frequent in the former. However, the absolute concordance rate in monozygotic twins was 31%, suggesting that nongenetic factors also play an important role in the development of the illness. Moderate heritability was also found in a female twin study (Kendler et al. 1992). Individuals with an early onset of the disorder appear to have a much higher familial aggregation of the disorder, possibly suggesting a stronger genetic component in a familial subtype of the disorder, which might better lend itself to molecular genetic studies (Goldstein et al. 1997). Although an earlier whole-genome scan in 23 panic pedigrees did not yield any evidence of linkage (Knowles et al. 1998), later genome scan studies have revealed links to chromosomes 7p (Crowe et al. 2001), 7q (Cheng et al. 2006), 13q (Hamilton et al. 2003), and 9q (Thorgeirsson et al. 2003).

There have been a number of preliminary positive studies of putative genetic markers and candidate genes for panic disorder, including the X-linked monoamine oxidase-A gene in females (Deckert et al. 1999), the cholecystokinin gene (Wang et al. 1998), the cholecystokinin receptor gene (Kennedy et al. 1999), and the adenosine 2A receptor gene (Deckert et al. 1998; Hamilton et al. 2004), the catechol-*O*-methyltransferase gene (Hamilton et al. 2002; Woo et al. 2002, 2004), the peripheral benzodiazepine receptor gene (Nakamura et al. 2006), and the 5-HT$_{2A}$ receptor gene (Inada et al. 2003). There is also evidence of interactions of serotonergic and noradrenergic gene variants in panic disorder (Freitlag et al. 2006). Another important strategy is to examine genetic influences on behaviorally inhibited temperament, which is a risk factor for anxiety disorders. One study found that in families with panic-disordered parents, behavioral inhibition in the offspring was associated with corticotropin-releasing hormone variants (Smoller et al. 2005). It is likely that genetic variants of several or multiple candidate genes in different neurotransmitter systems, each with minor individual effects, all contribute to panic susceptibility (Maron et al. 2005). Also, panic and agoraphobia may share some, but not all, of their susceptibility loci (J. Gelernter et al. 2001).

Psychodynamic Theories

In this subsection we present the major landmarks in the evolution of psychodynamic theories of anxiety and panic and their relationship to recent biological advances. More lengthy expositions and critiques of the psychoanalytic theories can be referred to by interested readers (see Cooper 1985; Michels et al. 1985; Nemiah 1988).

Freud's first theory of anxiety neurosis (id or impulse anxiety).　In his earliest concept of anxiety formation, Freud (1895b[1894]/1962) postulated that anxiety stems from the direct physiological transformation of libidinal energy into the somatic symptoms of anxiety, without the mediation of psychic mechanisms. He found evidence for this process in the sexual practices and experiences of patients with anxiety, which were characterized by disturbed sexual arousal and continence and coitus interruptus. He termed such anxiety an "actual neurosis" as opposed to a psychoneurosis, because of the postulated absence of psychic processes. Such anxiety, originating from overwhelming instinctual urges, would today be referred to as *id* or *impulse anxiety*.

Over the next several years, Freud started to modify his theory. Although the basic tenet that anxiety stemmed from undischarged sexual energy remained the same, this was no longer posited to be due to external constraints such as sexual dysfunctions. In accordance with Freud's developing topographic theory of the mind, anxiety resulted from forbidden sexual drives in the unconscious being repressed by the preconscious.

Structural theory and intrapsychic conflict.　By 1926, with the advent of the structural theory of the mind, Freud's theory of anxiety had undergone a major transformation (Freud 1926/1959). According to Freud, anxiety is an affect belonging to the ego and acts as a signal alerting the ego to internal danger. The danger stems from intrapsychic conflict between instinctual drives from the id, superego prohibitions, and external reality demands. Anxiety acts as a signal to the ego for the mobilization of repression and other defenses to counteract the threat to intrapsychic equilibrium. Inhibitions and neurotic symptoms develop as measures designed to avoid the dangerous situation and to allow only partial gratification of instinctual wishes, thus warding off signal anxiety. In the revised theory, then, anxiety leads to repression, instead of the reverse.

Early on, Freud (1895a[1894]/1962) also observed that in the analysis of phobias, nothing is ever found but the emotional state of anxiety. In the case of agoraphobia we often find the recollection of an anxiety attack, and what the patient actually fears is the occurrence of such an attack under the special conditions in which the patient believes he or she cannot escape it. This is a succinct description, made more than a century ago, of the development of anticipatory anxiety and agoraphobia following a panic attack. At that time, Freud did not consider phobias to be psychologically mediated. Rather, he understood them, like anxiety neurosis, to be manifestations of a physiologically induced tension state. Undischarged libidinal energy was physiologically transformed into anxiety, which became attached to and partly discharged through objects that were, by their nature or in the patient's prior experience, dangerous.

The intrapsychic conflict model of anxiety continues to constitute a major tenet of contemporary psychoanalytic theory. Psychoanalytic theorists after Freud, such as Melanie Klein (1948) and Joachim Flescher (1955), also made significant contributions to the understanding of the psychodynamic origins of anxiety. Whereas Freud concentrated on the role of sexual impulses and the oedipal conflict in the genesis of anxiety, these theorists drew attention to the role that aggressive impulses and preoedipal dynamics can also play in generating anxiety. Since Freud, the psychodynamic literature has also to a degree shifted away from formulations that primarily emphasize libidinal wishes and castration fears in understanding phobias such as agoraphobia (Michels et al. 1985). For example, the significance of a trustworthy and safe companion in individuals with agoraphobia could be understood as a simultaneous expression of aggressive impulses toward the companion and a magical wish to protect the companion from such impulses by always being together. Alternatively, excessive fear of object loss and its concomitant separation anxiety could explain both the fear of being away from home alone and the alleviation of this fear when a companion is present.

Although psychoanalytic theories are not universally accepted by psychiatrists today, they remain an invaluable tool in the understanding and treatment of at least some patients. Also, it should be pointed out that Freud's theory of anxiety formation is not incompatible with biological theories of anxiety. Although Freud's first model of anxiety was later overshadowed by the conflictual model, modern biological theories of panic are in many ways more reminiscent of his original physiological formulation. Furthermore, Freud maintained on numerous occasions that biological predispositions to psychiatric symptoms are undoubtedly operant in most conditions and that constitutional factors could play a role in the particular form that neurotic symptoms take in different patients.

Indeed, what psychoanalytic theory does not help

us with is a better understanding of the determinants of the various specific forms in which anxiety symptoms manifest themselves. Some patients have anxiety attacks, others have more chronic forms of anxiety, and still others have phobias, obsessions, or compulsions. Freud himself attempted to address this problem of choice of neurosis and partly explained it on the basis of constitutional factors—a concept essentially similar to modern biological notions. In an attempt to reconcile this unpredictability with classical psychodynamic theory, it has been postulated that patients with unconscious conflict and a neural predisposition to panic may manifest their anxiety in the form of panic attacks, whereas individuals without this neural predisposition may manifest milder forms of signal anxiety (Nemiah 1981). Along these more contemporary lines of thinking, a psychodynamic study of patients with panic disorder found that in patients who are neurophysiologically predisposed to early fearfulness, exposure to parental behaviors that augment this fearfulness may result in disturbances of object relations and persistence of conflicts surrounding dependence and catastrophic fears of helplessness, all of which are accessible in psychodynamic treatment (Shear et al. 1993).

With the broadening of psychodynamic theory over the decades, different forms of anxiety have been elaborated, such as annihilation anxiety, separation anxiety, anxiety over loss of the other's love, castration anxiety, superego anxiety, and id anxiety. In particular, greater emphasis on preoedipal dynamics and research in infant and child development has brought to the forefront attachment theories and the importance of attachment disturbances in the genesis of psychopathology. In the early 1960s, D. F. Klein proposed an etiological theory that agoraphobia with panic attacks may represent an aberrant function of the biological substrate that underlies normal human attachment and threats to it (i.e., separation anxiety). Based on Bowlby's (1973) work on attachment and separation, D. F. Klein (1981) advanced the notion that the attachment of an infant human or animal to its mother is not simply a learned response but is genetically programmed and biologically determined. Indeed, 20%–50% of adults with panic disorder and agoraphobia recall manifesting symptoms of pathological separation anxiety, often taking the form of school phobia, when they were children. Furthermore, the initial panic attack in the history of a patient who goes on to develop panic disorder is sometimes preceded by the real or threatened loss of a significant relationship. One systematic study has shown that the number and severity of recent life events, especially events related to loss, were greater in new-onset panic patients than in control subjects (Faravelli and Pallanti 1989). A blinded psychodynamic study showed separation anxiety to be a significantly more prevalent theme in the dreams and screen memories of panic patients than in normal control subjects.

Infant animals demonstrate their anxiety when separated from the mother by a series of high-pitched cries, called "distress vocalizations." Imipramine has been found to be effective in blocking distress vocalizations in mammals such as dogs and monkeys and is a highly effective antipanic drug in adult humans. Hypothesizing a link between adult panic attacks and childhood separation anxiety, Gittelman-Klein and Klein (1971) conducted a study of imipramine treatment for children with school phobia. In these children, fear of separation from their mothers was usually the basis behind refusing to go to school. The drug proved successful in getting the children to return to school. However, a more recent longitudinal study failed to find a higher risk of panic disorder and agoraphobia in adulthood in those children who had been diagnosed with separation anxiety disorder in childhood compared with those with other childhood anxiety disorders (Aschenbrand et al. 2003).

Thus, evidence suggests that the same drug that diminishes protest anxiety in higher mammals also reduces separation anxiety in children and blocks panic attacks in adults. This is further confirmation of the link between separation anxiety and panic attacks. Is early separation anxiety linked to agoraphobia and to panic attacks per se? If imipramine affects panic attacks, and separation anxiety is linked to agoraphobia, then why is imipramine effective in the treatment of school phobia? On the other hand, children with school phobia do not have spontaneous panic attacks, but this could be related to their young age. Perhaps both panic disorder and panic disorder with agoraphobia are linked to a biologically disordered separation mechanism that is responsive to imipramine. This may occur if the retrospective histories of a lesser degree of separation anxiety in patients with panic attacks alone are misremembered.

Contemporary psychoanalysts, in response, have claimed that this neurophysiological and ethological model of a disrupted separation mechanism and panic may be unnecessarily reductionistic (Michels et al. 1985). They point out an inconsistency between the conceptualization of panic attacks as spontaneous and the frequently reported histories of childhood separation anxiety in patients with panic attacks and state that psychological difficulties with separation can also play a role in subsequent vulnerability to panic. On the other hand, contemporary psychoanalysts have also given more credence to the role of biological substrates in the genesis of anxiety symptoms in at least some patients who have developed their anxious personality structure secondary to a largely contentless biological dysregulation, so that although psychological triggers for anxiety may still be found, the anxiety threshold is so low in these patients that it is no longer useful to view the psychological event as etiologically significant (Cooper 1985).

Learning Theories

Behavior or learning theorists hold that anxiety is conditioned by the fear of certain environmental stimuli. If every time a laboratory animal presses a bar it receives a noxious electric shock, the pressing of the lever becomes a conditioned stimulus that precedes the unconditioned stimulus (i.e., the shock). The conditioned stimulus releases a conditioned response in the animal, anxiety, that leads the animal to avoid contact with the lever, thereby avoiding the shock. Successful avoidance of the unconditioned stimulus, the shock, reinforces the avoidant behavior. This leads to a decrease in anxiety level.

By analogy with this animal model, we might say that anxiety attacks are conditioned responses to fearful situations. For example, an infant learns that if his or her mother is not present (i.e., the conditioned stimulus), he or she will suffer hunger (i.e., the unconditioned stimulus), and thus the infant learns to become anxious automatically whenever the mother is absent (i.e., the conditioned response). The anxiety may persist even after the child is old enough to feed him- or herself. To give another example, a life-threatening situation in someone's life (e.g., skidding in a car during a snowstorm) is paired with the experience of rapid heartbeat (i.e., the conditioned stimulus) and tremendous anxiety. Long after the accident, rapid heartbeat alone, whether during vigorous exercise or minor emotional upset, becomes capable by itself of provoking the conditioned response of an anxiety attack.

Certain problems are posed by such a theory. First, although some traumatic situations, such as thyroid disease, cocaine intoxication, or life-threatening events, such as a suffocation incident, do seem to be paired with the onset of panic disorder, for many patients no such traumatic event can ever be located. Of note, however, traumatic suffocation incidents have been found in about 20% of panic patients, significantly more than in psychiatric comparison subjects

(Bouwer and Stein 1997). Clinical experience does not support that anxiety disorder patients undergo repeated traumatic events, and therefore they should be able to extinguish their anxiety. So even though learning theories have a powerful basis in experimental animal research, they do not seem to explain adequately, in and of themselves, the pathogenesis of human anxiety disorders. However, coupled with a dysregulated biological mechanism or vulnerability that may be linked to the process of fear conditioning in panic, such as altered functioning of the amygdala and related fear circuits (discussed earlier), heightened anxiety responses could conceivably persist over time.

Traumatic Antecedents

Childhood interpersonal trauma also appears to make a contribution to the likelihood that individuals will manifest panic disorder. In a clinical cross-sectional study comparing panic disorder and psychiatrically healthy subjects, severe traumatic events during childhood and unfavorable parental attitudes were associated with panic disorder (Bandelow et al. 2002). Similarly, examination of trauma rates in the National Comorbidity Survey community sample, after disaggregating the impact of comorbid PTSD, found that 24% of females and 5% of males with panic disorder reported histories of sexual molestation, suggesting the latter could be one risk factor for developing panic disorder (Leskin and Sheikh 2002). In a large prospective birth cohort studied to the age of 21 years, exposure to childhood physical and sexual abuse was associated with increased risk of later panic attacks and disorder, even after adjusting for prospectively assessed confounding factors. Exposure to interparental violence was not a factor (Goodwin et al. 2005).

Course, Prognosis, Morbidity, and Mortality

The course of illness without treatment is highly variable and is summarized in Table 12–5.

At present, there is no reliable way to know which patient will develop, for example, agoraphobia. The illness seems to have a waxing and waning course in which spontaneous recovery occurs, only to be followed months to years later by a new outburst. At the extreme, some patients become completely housebound for decades. Treatment aimed at blocking the occurrence of the attacks, described in detail later, is appropriate at any point in the course of the illness when such attacks are occurring. Results are often dramatic. Pharmacological blockade of panic attacks early

TABLE 12–5. Course and prognosis of panic disorder

Course

Variable, typically with periods of exacerbations and remissions

Outcome

About 33% recover, 50% have limited impairment, 20% or less have major impairment

Predictors of worse prognosis

More severe initial panic attacks
More severe initial agoraphobia
Longer duration of illness
Comorbid depression
History of separation from parent (e.g., death, divorce)
High interpersonal sensitivity
Single marital status

in the illness, before phobic avoidance has become an ingrained way of life, often leads to complete remission. Even years into the illness, effective disruption of the attacks with medication can lead to resolution of anticipatory anxiety and phobias without other treatment. However, a substantial number of patients with significant phobic avoidance remain anxious and frightened of confronting feared situations even after the attacks have been blocked. Such patients require other forms of intervention, described elsewhere in this chapter. A 7-year follow-up study examined prognostic factors in naturalistically treated patients with panic disorder. Although patients had generally good outcomes, there were several predictors of poorer outcome, including greater severity of panic attacks and agoraphobia, longer duration of illness, comorbid major depression, separation from a parent by death or divorce, high interpersonal sensitivity, low social class, and single marital status (Noyes et al. 1993). Another long-term outcome study over a 5-year period had fairly optimistic findings: 34% of patients were recovered, 46% were minimally impaired, and 20% remained moderately to severely impaired; the most significant predictor of poor outcome was an anxious-fearful personality type, followed by poor response to initial treatment (O'Rourke et al. 1996). Finally, another large outcome study showed that less than 20% of panic disorder patients remained seriously agoraphobic or disabled. Panic attack frequency at baseline, initial medication, and continuous use of medication were not related to outcome, whereas longer duration of illness and more severe initial avoidance were unfavorable predictors (Katschnig et al. 1995).

The impact of comorbidity is another important consideration in assessing prognosis. A recent 5-year prospective, longitudinal, naturalistic study reported that, in contrast to GAD and social phobia, the likelihood of panic disorder remission was not affected by comorbid personality disorders (Massion et al. 2002).

An increased death rate from cardiovascular illness in panic disorder was partly supported in an epidemiological investigation by Weissman et al. (1990). In this study, panic disorder patients had a significantly higher risk for strokes than did patients with other psychiatric disorders, although several methodological limitations were identified. Of note, such medical risks are not routinely evident to clinicians in the usual status of patients undergoing treatment for panic disorder. Most such patients have normal medical workups. The one cardiovascular abnormality that has been found to occur at a higher rate in patients with panic disorder is mitral valve prolapse. This association could conceivably explain a higher incidence of cardiovascular-related death in patients with panic disorder; however, mitral valve prolapse itself is rarely a cause of premature death or major morbidity. One other possible explanation for increased cardiovascular/cerebrovascular risk in patients with panic disorder may be related to aspects of their lifestyle. Such patients tend to live relatively sedentary lives, and some report that vigorous physical exercise precipitates their panic attacks, leading them to avoid exertion of any kind. Heavy cigarette smoking, alcoholism, and poor diets could also contribute to an increased risk in panic patients. Alternatively, left ventricular enlargement and increased risk of thromboembolic events have also been contemplated to account for the association (Weissman et al. 1990).

A possible association between panic disorder and increased suicide risk has received extensive attention and does not appear to hold up based on extensive epidemiological analyses. Allgulander and Lavori (1991) conducted a large retrospective survey in Sweden and found an increased suicide risk in panic disorder in the absence of comorbid diagnoses. Epidemiological data further supported this finding in the ECA study, where the lifetime rate of suicide attempts in persons with uncomplicated panic disorder was 7%, about the same as the 7.9% rate for uncomplicated major depression (J. Johnson et al. 1990). However, in a reanalysis of the ECA data controlling for all comorbidity rather than one disorder at a time, an association between panic and suicide attempts could no longer be shown (Hornig and McNally 1995). Similarly, a 5-year prospective study concluded that there was no association

between panic and suicide risk in the absence of other risk factors (Warshaw et al. 2000). Finally, reanalysis of the National Comorbidity Survey data revealed that in the absence of comorbidity, panic disorder responders were not at heightened risk of self-reported suicide attempts (Vickers and McNally 2004).

Diagnosis

Physical Signs and Behavior

The diagnosis of panic disorder is made when a patient experiences recurrent panic attacks that are discrete and unexpected and followed by a month of persistent anticipatory anxiety or behavioral change. These panic attacks are characterized by a sudden crescendo of anxiety and fearfulness, in addition to the presence of at least four physical symptoms. Finally, these attacks are not secondary to a known organic factor or due to another mental disorder. However, these diagnoses are not always obvious, and a number of other psychiatric and medical disorders may mimic these conditions (Table 12–6).

Differential Diagnosis

Other psychiatric illnesses.   Although the medical conditions that mimic anxiety disorder are usually easily ruled out, psychiatric conditions that involve pathological anxiety can make the differential diagnosis of panic disorder difficult. By far the most problematic is the differentiation of primary anxiety disorder from depression.

Patients with depression often manifest signs of anxiety and may even have frank panic attacks. On the other hand, patients with panic disorder, if untreated for significant amounts of time, routinely become demoralized as the impact of the illness progressively restricts their ability to enjoy a normal life. Further complicating the picture is the fact that some, but not all, studies have shown that patients with anxiety disorder have increased family history of affective disorder.

Although the differentiation of anxiety from depression can at times strain even the most experienced clinician, several points are helpful. Patients with panic disorder generally do not demonstrate the full range of vegetative symptoms seen in depression. Thus, anxious patients usually have trouble falling asleep—not early morning awakening—and do not lose their appetite. Diurnal mood fluctuation is uncommon in anxiety disorder. Perhaps of greatest importance is the fact that most anxious patients do not lose the capacity to enjoy things or to be cheered up as endogenously depressed patients do.

TABLE 12–6. Differential diagnosis of panic disorder

Anxious depression

Somatization with panic-like physical complaints

Social phobia with socially cued panic attacks

Generalized anxiety with severe symptoms or during peak periods

Posttraumatic stress disorder with intense physiological response to reminders of the trauma

Agoraphobia secondary to conditions other than panic (depression, posttraumatic stress, paranoia, psychosis)

Obsessional anxiety of near-panic severity

Depersonalization disorder

Personality disorder with anxiety symptoms

Hyperthyroidism

Hypothyroidism

Mitral valve prolapse

Pheochromocytoma

The order of developing symptoms also differentiates depression from anxiety. In cases of panic disorder, anxiety symptoms usually precede any seriously altered mood. Patients can generally recall having anxiety attacks first, then becoming gradually more disgusted with life, and then feeling depressed. In depression, patients usually experience dysphoria first, with anxiety symptoms coming later. However, panic disorder can be complicated by secondary major depression and vice versa.

A few other psychiatric conditions often need to be differentiated from panic disorder. Patients with somatization disorder complain of a variety of physical ailments and discomforts, none of which are substantiated by physical or laboratory findings. Unlike panic disorder patients, somatizing patients present with physical problems that do not usually occur in episodic attacks but are virtually constant.

Patients with depersonalization disorder have episodes of derealization/depersonalization without the other symptoms of a panic attack. However, panic attacks not infrequently involve depersonalization and derealization as prominent symptoms.

Although patients with panic disorder often fear they will lose their minds or go crazy, psychotic illness is not an outcome of anxiety disorder. Reassuring the patient on this point is often the first step in a successful treatment.

Undoubtedly some patients with anxiety disorders abuse alcohol and drugs, such as sedatives, in attempts at self-medication. In one study, after successful detoxification a group of alcoholic patients with a prior history of panic disorder were treated with medication to block spontaneous panic attacks (Quitkin and Babkin 1982). These patients did not resume alcohol consumption once their panic attacks were eliminated.

With regard to the agoraphobic component of the disorder, widespread fears and avoidance of being alone or of leaving home can also be seen in paranoid and psychotic states, PTSD, and major depressive disorders. Psychotic states can be differentiated from agoraphobia by the presence of delusions, hallucinations, and thought process disorder. Although agoraphobic patients are frequently afraid that they are going crazy, they do not exhibit psychotic symptomatology. Patients with PTSD have a typical history of trauma, such as a fear of being or of traveling alone after an assault.

The distinction between depressive disorders and agoraphobia is more difficult. Both groups commonly experience spontaneous panic attacks. Patients with agoraphobia are frequently demoralized and will state that they feel depressed. Close questioning, however, usually does not reveal further vegetative symptoms or a loss of pleasure or interest in activities. Early morning awakening and pervasive anhedonia, which are common symptoms in endogenous depression, are rare in agoraphobia. Agoraphobic individuals will usually say they would love to leave home and engage in a variety of activities, if only they could be sure of not panicking. In contrast, depressed individuals usually see no point in going out because nothing gives them any pleasure, and they believe that people will be better off without them.

Patients with atypical depression (i.e., depression characterized by hypersomnia, hyperphagia, extreme low energy, and depressed but reactive mood) frequently have panic attacks but rarely have agoraphobia as part of their life history or current symptomatology. Patients with atypical depression and a history of panic attacks may respond preferentially to monoamine oxidase inhibitors (MAOIs; Liebowitz et al. 1985b).

Hyperthyroidism and hypothyroidism. Both hyper- and hypothyroidism can present with anxiety unaccompanied by other signs or symptoms. For this reason, it is imperative that all patients complaining of anxiety undergo routine thyroid function tests, including the evaluation of the level of thyroid-stimulating hormone. It should be remembered, however, that thyroid disease can act as one of the predisposing triggers to panic disorder, so that even when the apparently primary thyroid disease is corrected, panic attacks may continue until specifically treated.

Cardiac disease.   The relationship of mitral valve prolapse to panic disorder has attracted a great deal of attention over the years. This usually benign condition has been shown by a number of investigators to occur more frequently in patients with panic disorder than in normal subjects. However, screening of patients known to have mitral valve prolapse reveals no greater frequency of panic disorder than is found in the overall population.

Although patients with mitral valve prolapse occasionally complain of palpitations, chest pain, light-headedness, and fatigue, symptoms of a full-blown panic attack are rare. A comparison of symptoms in mitral valve prolapse and panic disorder is provided in Table 12–7. Panic patients with and without mitral valve prolapse are similar in several important ways. Treatment for panic attacks works regardless of the presence of the prolapsed valve, and patients with both mitral valve prolapse and panic disorder are just as sensitive to sodium lactate as are those with panic disorder alone. Some have speculated that mitral valve prolapse and panic disorder may represent manifestations of the same underlying disorder of autonomic nervous system function (Gorman et al. 1981). Others have suggested that panic disorder, by creating intermittent states of high circulating catecholamine levels and tachycardia, actually causes mitral valve prolapse (Mattes 1981). There are reports that mitral valve prolapse might go away if the panic disorder is controlled (Gorman et al. 1981). A meta-analytic study of 21 studies found that there does appear to be a significant association between panic disorder and mitral valve prolapse, although the possibility of publication bias favoring positive reports cannot be ruled out (Katerndahl 1993).

In any event, it is clear that the presence of mitral valve prolapse in patients with panic disorder has little clinical or prognostic importance in the management of spontaneous panic attacks. What it may tell us about the underlying etiology of panic disorder is a question currently under vigorous investigation.

Other medical illnesses.   Hyperparathyroidism occasionally presents as anxiety symptoms, warranting a serum calcium level before definitive diagnosis is made.

A variety of cardiac conditions can initially present as anxiety symptoms, although in most cases, the patient complains prominently of chest pain, skipped

TABLE 12–7. Comparison of symptoms of mitral valve prolapse and panic disorder

Symptoms	Mitral valve prolapse	Panic disorder
Fatigue	+	−
Dyspnea	+	++
Palpitations	++	++
Chest pain	++	+
Syncope	+	−
Choking	−	++
Dizziness	−	++
Derealization	−	++
Hot/cold flashes	−	++
Sweating	−	++
Fainting	−	++
Trembling	−	++
Fear of dying, going crazy, losing control		++

Note.   + = occasionally; ++ = often present; − = rarely present.

beats, or palpitations. Ischemic heart disease and arrhythmias, especially paroxysmal atrial tachycardia, should be ruled out by electrocardiography.

Pheochromocytoma is a rare, usually benign tumor of the adrenal medulla that secretes catecholamines in episodic bursts. During an active phase, the patient characteristically experiences flushing, tremulousness, and anxiety. Blood pressure is usually elevated during the active phase of catecholamine secretion but not at other times. Therefore, merely finding a normal blood pressure does not rule out a pheochromocytoma. If this condition is suspected, the diagnosis is made by collection of urine for 24 hours for determination of catecholamine metabolite concentration. In a study of patients with confirmed pheochromocytoma, about half met criteria for the physical symptoms of panic attacks, but none had panic disorder, because they did not experience terror during the attacks and did not develop anticipatory anxiety or agoraphobia (Starkman et al. 1990).

Disease of the vestibular nerve can cause episodic bouts of vertigo, lightheadedness, nausea, and anxiety that mimic panic attacks. Rather than merely feeling dizzy, such patients often experience true vertigo in which the room seems to spin in one direction during each attack. Otolaryngology consultation is warranted when this condition is suspected. Some panic patients primarily complain of dizziness or unsteadiness. Whether they are a distinct subgroup with definite neurological abnormalities is currently under study.

Although many patients believe that their anxiety disorder is caused by reactive hypoglycemia, there is no scientific proof at present that this is ever a cause of any psychiatric disturbance. Glucose tolerance tests are not helpful in establishing hypoglycemia as the cause of anxiety, because up to 40% of the normal population has a random low blood-sugar level during a routine glucose tolerance test. The only convincing way to establish hypoglycemia as a cause of symptoms is to document a low blood sugar level at the same time the patient is symptomatic. Studies with insulin tolerance tests in panic disorder have yielded negative results.

Treatment

Pharmacotherapy

Antidepressants. When initiating a drug regimen for a patient with panic disorder, it is crucial for the patient to understand that the drug will block the panic attacks but may not necessarily decrease the amount of intervening anticipatory anxiety and avoidance, at least initially. For patients with severe anxiety, it can be helpful to initially prescribe a concomitant benzodiazepine that can be gradually tapered and discontinued after several weeks of antidepressant treatment. Also importantly, some patients with panic disorder display an initial hypersensitivity to antidepressants, whether TCAs or serotonin reuptake inhibitors, during which they complain of jitteriness, agitation, a speedy feeling, and insomnia. Although this is usually transient, it is one of the main reasons why patients unfortunately opt to discontinue medication early on. Therefore, it is strongly recommended that patients with panic disorder be started on lower dosages of antidepressants than would be given to depressed patients. The central feature in the treatment of panic disorder is the pharmacological blockade of the spontaneous panic attacks. Several classes of medications have been shown to be effective in accomplishing this goal, and a summary of the pharmacological treatment of panic disorder is presented in Table 12–8.

Historically, the most widely studied and used medications in the past were the TCAs, especially imipramine (D. F. Klein 1964; Mavissakalian and Michelson 1986a, 1986b). Other TCAs, such as desipramine, nortriptyline, and clomipramine, have also been

---

TABLE 12–8. Pharmacological treatment of panic disorder

Selective serotonin reuptake inhibitors and serotonin–norepinephrine reuptake inhibitors

General indications: First-line, alone or in combination with benzodiazepines if needed. Also first choice with comorbid obsessive-compulsive disorder, generalized anxiety disorder, depression, and social phobia. Start with very low dosages and increase; response seen with low to moderate dosages.

Sertraline, paroxetine: FDA approved
Fluvoxamine, fluoxetine, citalopram, escitalopram: similarly efficacious
Venlafaxine extended-release: FDA approved

Tricyclic antidepressants

General indications: Established efficacy, second line if SSRIs fail or are not tolerated.

Imipramine: well studied
Clomipramine: high efficacy but not easily tolerated
Desipramine: if low tolerance to anticholinergic side effects
Nortriptyline: if prone to orthostatic hypotension, elderly

Monoamine oxidase inhibitors

General indications: Poor response or tolerance to other antidepressants; comorbid atypical depression or social phobia.

Phenelzine: most studied
Tranylcypromine: less sedation

High-potency benzodiazepines

General indications: Poor response or tolerance of antidepressants; prominent anticipatory anxiety or phobic avoidance; initial treatment phase until antidepressant begins to work.

Clonazepam: longer-acting, less frequent dosing, less withdrawal, first choice
Alprazolam: well studied but short-acting
Alprazolam extended-release: once-daily dosing

Other medications

General indications: Particularly as augmentation in patients whose illness is refractory or who are intolerant of the above medications, not well tested to date.

Pindolol: effective augmentation in one controlled trial
Valproic acid: open trials only
Inositol: open trials only
Clonidine: initial response tends to fade in open trials
Atypical antipsychotics: open trials

Note. FDA = U.S. Food and Drug Administration; SSRIs = selective serotonin reuptake inhibitors.

found effective, although they have not been studied as extensively as imipramine. The presence of depressed mood is not a predictor or requirement for this class of medications to be effective in blocking panic attacks. At present, newer antidepressants, in particular the SSRIs, have been shown to be efficacious in treating panic, and given their several advantages over TCAs they have become the first-line treatment for panic. TCAs are now reserved for patients who do not have a good response to, or do not tolerate, newer antidepressants.

A standard TCA regimen is to start the patient at a dosage of 10 mg qhs of imipramine and increase the dosage by 10 mg every other night until 50 mg is reached. The dosage can be given all at once. Because 50 mg is usually inadequate for full panic blockade, the dosage can then be raised by 25-mg increments every 3 days or by 50-mg increments weekly to as high as 300 mg. Most patients need at least 150 mg daily of TCAs, and unfortunately, underdosage commonly occurs. In some cases, a dosage of imipramine of more than 300 mg is necessary. On "high" imipramine dosing of around 200 mg/day, more than 80% of patients show a marked response in panic attacks (Mavissakalian and Perel 1989). Panic patients not responding to high dosages of imipramine should have blood TCA levels measured. Often, blood levels will be disproportionately low for the dosage, suggesting rapid metabolism or excretion, malabsorption, or noncompliance. Patients who experience excessive anticholinergic side effects to imipramine can be given desipramine instead. The elderly or patients who are otherwise very sensitive to orthostatic hypotension can be tried on nortriptyline.

A number of controlled treatment trials have now shown that the potent serotonin reuptake blockers are highly effective in the treatment of panic. Given their higher safety, tolerability, and ease of administration compared with TCAs, they comprise the first line in the treatment of panic disorder, either alone or in combination with benzodiazepine when needed. As a first-line treatment, they also offer the advantage that they are effective for several of the commonly comorbid disorders, such as depression, social phobia, GAD, and OCD. Although paroxetine and sertraline are the only U.S. Food and Drug Administration (FDA)–approved SSRIs for this indication, all SSRIs have comparable efficacy in treating panic. A head-on comparison of paroxetine (40–60 mg/day) with sertraline (50–150 mg/day) reported similar efficacy for the two medications (Bandelow et al. 2004).

Several controlled trials have documented the effi-

cacy of SSRIs in treating panic disorder. Fluvoxamine at dosages of up to 150 mg/day was reported efficacious in a large controlled trial (Asnis et al. 2001). The efficacy of paroxetine has been demonstrated at dosages of 20–60 mg daily (Oehrberg et al. 1995). In another study, only the 40-mg daily dosage of paroxetine reached statistically significant superiority over placebo during a 10-week period, whereas the 10-mg and 20-mg dosages did not, highlighting the importance of trying higher dosages if response to lower dosages is inadequate (Ballenger et al. 2000). A placebo-controlled trial of controlled-release paroxetine in about 900 patients demonstrated superiority for the active treatment at dosages ranging from 25 to 75 mg/day, and paroxetine controlled-release was well tolerated, with an 11% dropout rate due to adverse events (Sheehan et al. 2005).

The SSRI sertraline has also been found to be efficacious in treating panic disorder in large controlled trials (Londborg et al. 1998; Pohl et al. 1998). Sertraline not only markedly decreased the number of panic attacks but also led to significant improvement in life quality and had a low dropout rate (Pohl et al. 1998); there was no difference among three sertraline dosages of 50, 100, or 200 mg daily in reducing panic attacks (Londborg et al. 1998). A prior history of benzodiazepine use did not appear to affect the tolerability or response to sertraline treatment, regardless of whether the response to the benzodiazepine had been good or bad (Rapaport et al. 2001).

Another SSRI, citalopram, has been shown to be efficacious in treating panic disorder in an 8-week controlled trial in which the middle dosage of 20–30 mg/day conferred the most advantageous risk–benefit ratio compared with higher and lower dosages (Wade et al. 1997). In a 1-year controlled maintenance extension of the same study, the lowest dosage of 10–15 mg was not better than placebo, whereas the middle dosage of 20–30 mg daily again showed the best response (Lepola et al. 1998).

Fluoxetine, especially at a dosage of 20 mg/day rather than 10 mg/day, was also shown to be superior to placebo in the acute treatment of panic disorder (D. Michelson et al. 1998); this study used a wide range of measures and demonstrated that global improvement was more related to phobia, anxiety, depression, and impairment than to panic attacks per se, highlighting the importance of looking at the larger picture when assessing change. Over a 6-month maintenance treatment period, the initial responders to acute fluoxetine treatment demonstrated significant further improvement if randomized to fluoxetine and significant worsening if randomized to placebo (D. Michelson et al. 1999).

Another study showed that both escitalopram and citalopram were comparably superior to placebo in treating panic disorder symptoms and severity, and escitalopram had a low discontinuation rate of 6% (Stahl et al. 2003).

A meta-analysis of 43 treatment studies compared the short-term efficacy of SSRIs versus TCAs and reported no differences in effect sizes in reducing panic symptoms, agoraphobic avoidance, anxiety, depressive symptoms, or proportion of patients free of panic attacks at endpoint; however, dropout rate was significantly lower in those treated with SSRIs (18%) versus TCAs (31%) (Bakker et al. 2002). Like the TCAs, SSRIs can cause uncomfortable overstimulation in panic patients if started at the usual dosages. It is therefore suggested that treatment be started gingerly at 5–10 mg/day for fluoxetine, paroxetine, and citalopram and 25 mg/day for sertraline and fluvoxamine. The dosage can then be gradually increased to an average dosage through weekly adjustments. A moderate or lower daily dosage is usually adequate for most patients, as in the trials just described, and high dosages are generally not needed and less tolerated.

Venlafaxine is also effective in treating panic disorder. A large multisite placebo-controlled trial of venlafaxine extended-release in 361 adult patients, using a flexible dosage range of 75–225 mg/day for 10 weeks, reported better response and remission rates than placebo with a greater improvement in number of panic attacks, anticipatory anxiety, fear, and avoidance (Bradwejn et al. 2005). An open trial of mirtazapine administered at 30 mg/day for 3 months to 45 panic disorder patients also showed a pronounced decline in panic attacks and anticipatory anxiety, coupled with a very low 6% discontinuation rate (Sarchiapone et al. 2003). This finding has not yet been replicated in a controlled trial. Although one small open trial reported significant improvement in panic using bupropion (Simon et al. 2003), controlled data and clinical lore do not support its use.

MAOIs are equally as effective as the TCAs and the SSRIs in treating panic. Both phenelzine and tranylcypromine successfully treat panic, although phenelzine has been studied more extensively. Phenelzine can be started at 15 mg daily in the morning. The dosage is then increased by 15 mg every 4–7 days as tolerated, up to a maximum of 60–90 mg daily. If sedation or weight gain is of concern, tranylcypromine may be tried, starting at 10 mg in the morning and increasing by 10 mg every 4 days to a maximum of 80 mg daily.

TCAs and serotonin reuptake inhibitors are typically preferred over MAOIs because they are better tolerated and obviate the need for dietary restrictions and the risk of hypertensive crises. Furthermore, patients who do not respond to a TCA or a serotonin reuptake inhibitor alone may respond to a combination of the two. However, MAOIs are an option to consider for patients who fail to tolerate or to respond well to other antidepressants. In patients with concomitant atypical depression or social phobia, MAOIs may be an appropriate earlier choice for treatment if SSRIs do not confer adequate results.

Full remission of panic attacks with antidepressants usually requires 4–12 weeks of treatment. Subsequently, the duration of required treatment in order to prevent relapse is a function of the natural course of panic disorder. The disorder can probably best be characterized as chronic, with an exacerbating and remitting course. Therefore, complete agreement has not been reached regarding the recommended course of treatment. In a controlled prospective study, a very high relapse rate for panic was found when imipramine was discontinued after 6 months of acute treatment. However, half-dosage imipramine at around 80 mg/day was successful in preventing relapse during 1 year of maintenance treatment (Mavissakalian and Perel 1992). Thus, a reasonable recommendation in treating panic patients is to keep them on full-dosage medication for at least 6 months to prevent early relapse. Afterward, patients can be tapered to half-dosage medication and be followed to ensure that clinical improvement is maintained. Subsequently, the clinician may attempt gradual dosage decreases every few months, as long as the improvement is maintained, and reach a minimal dosage on which the patient is relatively symptom-free. Some patients may eventually be able to completely stop medications, whereas others will not.

Benzodiazepines. Although clinicians prefer to use antidepressants for the first-line treatment of panic, high-potency benzodiazepines are also highly effective in treating the condition. In one study, 82% of patients treated acutely with alprazolam showed at least moderate improvement in panic compared with 43% given placebo. Onset of response was rapid, with significant improvement occurring in the first couple weeks of treatment, and the mean final dosage was 5.7 mg/day. After 8 weeks of acute treatment, patients were tapered off medication over 4 weeks; 27% experienced rebound panic attacks, and 35% had withdrawal symptoms. After discontinuation, panic outcome for the alprazolam-treated group was not significantly different from that for the placebo group (Pecknold et al. 1988). Clonazepam appears equally promising in the acute treatment of panic, according to a large multi-center trial (Rosenbaum et al. 1997). In the acute treatment of panic attacks, the lowest dosage of 0.5 mg/day was least efficacious, but dosages of 1.0 mg/day or higher (2, 3, and 4 mg/day) were equally efficacious, and the lower dosages of 1–2 mg/day were better tolerated. Long-term efficacy, possible tolerance and dependency, and difficulties in discontinuing the medication are the main areas of concern when choosing benzodiazepine treatment. Naturalistic follow-up studies of long-term benzodiazepine treatment appear generally optimistic, because most patients maintain their therapeutic gains without increasing their benzodiazepine dosage over time.

These medications have fewer initial side effects than TCAs and serotonin reuptake inhibitors. However, the general treatment principle is that anxiolytics should be reserved until the different classes of antidepressants have failed, because they do pose some risk of tolerance, dependence, and withdrawal. For patients with severe acute distress and disability who may require immediate relief, it may be indicated to start with a benzodiazepine and then replace it with an antidepressant. There is evidence that benzodiazepines may be more effective, at least initially, in ameliorating the associated anticipatory anxiety and phobic avoidance, and this may be another indication for their initial use. A double-blind study that examined early coadministration of clonazepam (4 weeks, then 3-week discontinuation taper) during 12 weeks of treatment with sertraline did document more rapid stabilization of panic symptoms in the first 3 weeks of treatment in the sertraline-plus-clonazepam group, although treatment outcome and dropout rates did not differ by the end of the trial (Goddard et al. 2001b).

Clonazepam should generally be preferred as a first choice, because it is longer acting and thus has the advantage of less frequent twice-daily or even once-daily dosing and less risk of withdrawal symptoms than alprazolam. It should generally be started at 0.5 mg bid and increased only if needed, usually to a maximum dosage of 4 mg/day. Alprazolam is usually started at 0.5 mg qid and is gradually increased to an average dosage of 4 mg/day and a range of 2–10 mg/day according to the individual patient. Treatment of at least 6 months is recommended, as with the antidepressants. Patients' moods must be followed, because alprazolam may occasionally cause mania, and clonazepam may cause depression. Discontinuation must be gradual to prevent withdrawal: 15% of the total dosage weekly is generally a safe regimen, but an even slower rate may be required to prevent the recurrence of panic. In a controlled study, one-third of patients were unable to tolerate a 4-week taper off alprazolam after 8 months of maintenance treatment; the strongest predictor of taper failure was initial severity of panic attacks rather than alprazolam dosage (Rickels et al. 1993). The distinction between actual withdrawal and a simple recrudescence of the original anxiety symptom when the benzodiazepine is stopped remains controversial and can be difficult to make clinically. It has been convincingly shown that the introduction of cognitive-behavioral therapy (CBT) greatly increases the likelihood that panic patients will be able to successfully taper off benzodiazepines (Otto et al. 1993; Spiegel et al. 1994).

Although benzodiazepines are generally safe, with side effects limited mainly to sedation, there is a concern that some patients may become tolerant or even addicted to these medications. However, available data indicate that most patients are able to stop taking benzodiazepines without serious sequelae and that the problem of tolerance and dependence is overestimated and probably limited to an addiction-prone population or to patients with more refractory panic disorder who may escalate standard benzodiazepine usage in unsuccessful attempts at self-medication.

Other medications.   Buspirone is a 5-HT$_{1A}$ agonist, nonbenzodiazepine antianxiety agent and has not been found effective in treating panic. Similarly, there is no evidence that β-adrenergic–blocking drugs, such as propranolol, are effective in blocking spontaneous panic attacks. If panic attacks occur in a specific social context, such as public speaking, a trial of β-blockers would be indicated.

Clonidine, which inhibits locus coeruleus discharge, would seem for theoretical reasons to be a good antipanic drug. Although some patients may initially respond to clonidine, the therapeutic effect tends to be lost in a matter of weeks due to receptor habituation. This loss of response, plus a number of bothersome side effects, makes clonidine a poor initial choice for treatment of panic disorder. However, one controlled study found clonidine to be efficacious for both panic disorder and GAD (Hoehn-Saric et al. 1993).

When response to SSRIs and other antidepressants has been inadequate, one augmentation strategy shown to be effective in a small blinded trial may be to add pindolol at 2.5 mg three times a day (Hirschmann et al. 2000).

Valproic acid may also have some beneficial effects

in the treatment of panic attacks (Keck et al. 1993). In one open trial, all 12 patients were moderately to markedly improved after 6 weeks of treatment, and 11 continued the medication and maintained their gains after 6 months (Woodman and Noyes 1994). Controlled trials, however, have not been reported. A fairly large controlled trial of another mood stabilizer, gabapentin, at flexible dosages of 600–3,600 mg daily, showed it to be no better than placebo in treating panic disorder (Pande et al. 2000), although a post hoc analysis showed it to have some efficacy in the more severely symptomatic patients, suggesting that an augmentation study in refractory panic might be worthwhile.

Inositol, an intracellular second messenger precursor, has been reported to have some efficacy in treating panic disorder in two small double-blind, controlled 4-week trials at a dosage of 12–18 g/day (Benjamin et al. 1995; Palatnik et al. 2001).

Atypical antipsychotics have also received attention in recent years. In one study, patients who had previously not responded to SSRI monotherapy were treated openly for 12 weeks with 5 mg/day of olanzapine added to an SSRI, resulting in 82% of patients rated as responders by the end of the trial (Sepede et al. 2006). Similarly, another open trial of 10 patients with refractory panic disorder treated for 8 weeks with flexible-dose olanzapine at an average dosage of 12 mg/day resulted in an approximately 75% decrease in panic attacks and anticipatory anxiety (Hollifield et al. 2005).

Psychotherapy

Psychodynamic psychotherapy. Even after medication has blocked the actual panic attacks, a subgroup of panic patients remain wary of independence and assertiveness. In addition to supportive and behavioral treatment, traditional psychodynamic psychotherapy might be helpful for some of these patients. Significant unconscious conflict over separations during childhood sometimes appears to operate in patients with panic disorder, leading to a reemergence of anxiety symptoms in adult life each time a new separation is imagined or threatened. Furthermore, it has been found that comorbid personality disorder is the major predictor of continued social maladjustment in patients otherwise treated for panic disorder (Noyes et al. 1990), suggesting that psychodynamic therapy may be an important additional treatment for at least some patients with panic.

Systematic studies examining the efficacy of psychodynamically oriented psychotherapy in panic disorder are few but promising. Psychodynamically ori-

ented clinicians tend to agree that psychological factors do not appear to be significant in a proportion of patients with panic and emphasize the importance of conducting a psychodynamic assessment to determine whether a particular patient will benefit from a psychodynamic treatment component (Gabbard 1990). Cooper (1985) emphasized that in patients with a predominant biological component to their illness, insistence on dynamic understanding and on responsibility for one's symptoms may, in the long run, be not only useless but potentially harmful, leading to further damage in self-esteem and strengthened masochistic defenses. However, it is also clear that there are case reports of patients who were successfully treated for panic with psychodynamic therapy or psychoanalysis. A controlled study showed that a 15-session course of brief dynamic psychotherapy combined with initial clomipramine treatment led to much lower relapse rates up to 9 months after patients had been tapered off the medication (Wiborg and Dahl 1996). An open trial of psychodynamic monotherapy in panic disorder documented clear efficacy for this modality, at least in the selected sample, and emphasized the need for further and controlled studies (Milrod et al. 2000). The study included 14 patients with panic disorder who were treated for 12 weeks with twice-weekly psychodynamic psychotherapy alone. Results showed significant improvement in panic, anxiety, depression, and overall impairment. In the completed report of these open trials, there were 16 responders out of 21 patients treated with panic-focused psychodynamic psychotherapy, and symptomatic gains were maintained over a 6-month follow-up (Milrod et al. 2001).

Pharmacotherapy is in no way incompatible with behavioral or psychodynamic treatment for patients with panic disorder. The notion that reducing the symptoms of anxiety disorder with medication will disturb a successful psychotherapy has never been convincingly shown and is largely dogmatic. Indeed, successful psychotherapy often cannot take place until the more debilitating aspects of these syndromes have been eliminated pharmacologically.

Supportive psychotherapy. Despite adequate treatment of panic attacks with medication, phobic avoidance may remain. Supportive psychotherapy and education about the illness are necessary to urge the patient to confront the phobic situation. Patients who fail to respond may then need additional psychotherapy, either dynamic or behavioral. Encouragement from other patients with similar conditions is often quite helpful. Yet supportive psychotherapy alone is not an effective enough treatment for panic disorder.

Cognitive-behavioral therapy.   CBTs have long focused on phobic avoidance, but more recently the techniques have been developed and shown to be effective for panic attacks. In recent years, interest in CBT for panic has surged, and it has become firmly established as a first-line treatment for this disorder and found to be comparable in effectiveness to first-line medication treatments (Table 12–9).

The major behavioral techniques for the treatment of panic attacks are breathing retraining, to control both acute and chronic hyperventilation; exposure to somatic cues, usually involving a hierarchy of exposure to feared sensations through imaginal and behavioral exercises; and relaxation training. Cognitive treatment of panic involves cognitive restructuring, so as to give the uncomfortable affects and physical sensations associated with panic a more benign interpretation. These techniques can be administered in various combinations. The pure cognitive view is that panic attacks consist of normal physical sensations (e.g., palpitations, slight dizziness) to which panic disorder patients grossly overreact with catastrophic cognitions. A more middle-of-the-road view is that panic patients do have extreme physical sensations, such as bursts of tachycardia, but can still significantly help themselves by changing their interpretation of the event from "I am going to die of a heart attack" to "There go my heart symptoms again." Such a theory has received experimental validation: Sanderson et al. (1989) provoked panic attacks in panic disorder patients using CO_2 inhalation; it was found that when patients had an illusion of control over the inhaled mixture, they experienced significantly fewer and less severe attacks and had less catastrophic cognitions.

Several studies have shown that these various cognitive and behavioral techniques are successful in the treatment of panic disorder (Barlow et al. 1989; Beck et al. 1992; L. Michelson et al. 1990; Salkovskis et al. 1986). A study comparing CBT with in vivo exposure alone found similar efficacy for the two at the end of acute treatment and at 1-year follow-up (Ost et al. 2004). Similarly, a study comparing cognitive therapy to interoceptive exposure found similar efficacy (Arntz 2002). Another study compared in vivo exposure, interoceptive exposure, combination of the two exposures, and a control group and reported comparable high efficacy for all three active-treatment groups, with an average 60% improvement after 10 weeks of acute treatment and 77% improvement at follow-up 1 year later (Ito et al. 2001). Findings are inconsistent as to whether applied relaxation is equally efficacious or inferior to CBT for controlling panic attacks (Arntz and van den Hout 1996; Ost and Westling 1995).

TABLE 12–9. Cognitive and behavioral approaches to treating panic disorder

Interoceptive exposure (to the somatic cues of panic attacks)

Situational exposure (to the settings that are phobically avoided)

Cognitive restructuring

Breathing retraining

Applied relaxation training

Findings on long-term outcome of panic with CBT appear to be favorable, especially with combined cognitive restructuring and exposure. In a study examining the long-term outcome of panic disorder with agoraphobia in a group of 200 patients initially treated with exposure therapy, there was evidence of lasting relief for the majority of patients for up to a decade after treatment, with 23% experiencing relapse at some time during follow-up; 93% were in remission after 2 years and 62% after 10 years (Fava et al. 2001b).

In addition, there is evidence that the introduction of CBT can reduce the risk of rebound panic in patients who are tapered off antipanic medications such as benzodiazepines or antidepressants (Schmidt et al. 2002). Conversely, there is evidence that in patients who do not benefit adequately from cognitive therapy alone, the addition of adjunctive SSRI treatment can be beneficial (Kampman et al. 2002).

Treatment of the agoraphobic component of panic disorder.   There continues to be some disagreement in the literature regarding the best method of treatment for agoraphobia with panic attacks. Antipanic medication is given to block the occurrence of panic attacks, and its efficacy in this regard is well documented. However, medication alone is often not adequate treatment in patients with significant agoraphobic avoidance; it is generally accepted that some means of exposing agoraphobic patients to the feared situations is necessary for overall improvement. This may be achieved through various nonspecific methods, such as psychoeducation, reassurance, and supportive therapy. However, focused CBT is, on the whole, more successful than nonspecific techniques in reducing agoraphobic avoidance.

Some studies have not found imipramine to have a significant effect on agoraphobia when given alone or with anti-exposure instructions (Marks et al. 1983; Telch et al. 1985), whereas others have shown imipramine alone to decrease phobic avoidance (Mavissakalian and Perel 1995). Most studies, however, concur that the combination of medication and behavioral treatment (exposure) is superior to medication or behavioral treatment alone for treating phobic avoidance (de Beurs et al. 1995; Mavissakalian and Michelson 1986a; Telch et al. 1985; Zitrin et al. 1980). In a large controlled study of alprazolam plus exposure in patients with panic and agoraphobia, the improvements in attacks, anxiety, and avoidance were found to be largely independent of each other, and only early improvement in avoidance predicted global improvement after treatment (Basoglu et al. 1994).

Treatment with combined medication and psychotherapy. The relative and combined efficacy of medications and CBT for panic disorder has been the focus of numerous investigations. One controlled study found cognitive therapy, relaxation, and imipramine to be similarly effective, and cognitive therapy had more lasting effects at 9-month follow-up after treatment was discontinued (D.M. Clark et al. 1994). In another study, after the initiation of medication treatment for initial symptom control, the introduction of CBT greatly increased the likelihood that a patient would be able to successfully taper off medication (Otto et al. 1993). There is also evidence that patients who fail to adequately respond to pharmacotherapy can have significant and sustained improvements with subsequent CBT (Heldt et al. 2006). In a primary care setting, the addition of CBT resulted in statistically and clinically significant improvement in panic disorder after 3 months relative to medication treatment alone (Craske et al. 2005).

The largest study comparing medication, CBT, and combination treatment acutely and longer term (Barlow et al. 2000) was a multisite controlled study of 312 patients with panic disorder randomly assigned to five different treatments: imipramine alone, CBT alone, imipramine plus CBT, placebo alone, and CBT plus placebo. In the initial 3-month acute-treatment phase, medication and CBT had similar efficacy, with limited advantage for combined treatment. For responders treated in the 6-month maintenance phase, imipramine produced a higher quality of response than CBT alone, and there was an even more substantial advantage for combined treatment. Finally, at 6-month follow-up after termination of treatment, CBT had more durable results. This most comprehensive study to date on the issue clearly suggests that both psychotherapy and medication treatment must be seriously considered in treating a patient with panic, each having its advantages and disadvantages. In an important finding for the application of optimal treatment in nonpsychiatric primary care settings, a recent large controlled study demonstrated that delivery of evidence-based CBT and medication using a collaborative care model was significantly more effective than the usual primary care treatment for panic disorder (Roy-Byrne et al. 2005).

A recent meta-analytic study, based on 23 randomized comparisons involving about 1,700 participants, found that combined treatment was superior to antidepressant pharmacotherapy and to psychotherapy alone. However, after termination of acute-phase treatment, combination therapy was more effective than pharmacotherapy alone but as effective as psychotherapy, suggesting a more lasting effect of psychotherapy (Furukawa et al. 2006).

Generalized Anxiety Disorder

Definition and Clinical Description

DSM-IV-TR sharpened the distinction of GAD from "normal" anxiety by specifying that in GAD the worry must be clearly excessive, pervasive, difficult to control, and associated with marked distress or impairment. DSM-IV-TR also clarified that the diagnosis of GAD is excluded when occurring exclusively in relation to other major Axis I disorders, and the cumbersome somatic symptom list from the DSM-III-R was simplified (Table 12–10).

GAD is the main diagnostic category for prominent and chronic anxiety in the absence of panic disorder. The essential feature of this syndrome, according to DSM-IV-TR, is persistent anxiety lasting at least 6 months. The symptoms of this type of anxiety fall within two broad categories: apprehensive expectation and worry, and physical symptoms. Patients with GAD are constantly worried over minor matters, fearful, and anticipating the worst. Muscle tension, restlessness, a "keyed up" feeling, difficulty concentrating, insomnia, irritability, and fatigue are typical signs of GAD and have become the symptom criteria for the disorder in DSM-IV-TR after a number of studies attempted to single out the physical symptoms that are the most distinctive and characteristic of GAD. Motor tension and hypervigilance better differentiate GAD from other anxiety states than autonomic hyperactivity. The diagnosis of GAD is made when a patient experiences at least 6 months of chronic anxiety and excessive worry. At least three of six physical symp-

TABLE 12–10. DSM-IV-TR diagnostic criteria for generalized anxiety disorder

A. Excessive anxiety and worry (apprehensive expectation), occurring more days than not for at least 6 months, about a number of events or activities (such as work or school performance).

B. The person finds it difficult to control the worry.

C. The anxiety and worry are associated with three (or more) of the following six symptoms (with at least some symptoms present for more days than not for the past 6 months). **Note:** Only one item is required in children.
  (1) restlessness or feeling keyed up or on edge
  (2) being easily fatigued
  (3) difficulty concentrating or mind going blank
  (4) irritability
  (5) muscle tension
  (6) sleep disturbance (difficulty falling or staying asleep, or restless unsatisfying sleep)

D. The focus of the anxiety and worry is not confined to features of an Axis I disorder, e.g., the anxiety or worry is not about having a panic attack (as in panic disorder), being embarrassed in public (as in social phobia), being contaminated (as in obsessive-compulsive disorder), being away from home or close relatives (as in separation anxiety disorder), gaining weight (as in anorexia nervosa), having multiple physical complaints (as in somatization disorder), or having a serious illness (as in hypochondriasis), and the anxiety and worry do not occur exclusively during posttraumatic stress disorder.

E. The anxiety, worry, or physical symptoms cause clinically significant distress or impairment in social, occupational, or other important areas of functioning.

F. The disturbance is not due to the direct physiological effects of a substance (e.g., a drug of abuse, a medication) or a general medical condition (e.g., hyperthyroidism) and does not occur exclusively during a mood disorder, a psychotic disorder, or a pervasive developmental disorder.

toms must also be present. Finally, this chronic anxiety must not be secondary to another Axis I disorder or a specific organic factor.

The necessity of the "excessive worry" criterion in making the GAD diagnosis has been questioned and investigated in epidemiological samples, finding that the lifetime prevalence of GAD increases by about 40% when the excessiveness requirement is removed (Ruscio et al. 2005). Those who do have excessive worry have GAD onset earlier in life, a more chronic course, and greater symptom severity and comorbidity. However, even those without excessive worry manifest substantial persistence, impairment, comorbidity, and treatment seeking and share familial aggregation with those who do have excessive worry, questioning the validity of the excessiveness requirement and highlighting the need for more research (Ruscio et al. 2005).

Similarly, the 6-month duration criterion may be arbitrary and has come under scrutiny. The National Comorbidity Survey database has shown that a large number of people have a GAD-like syndrome of 1–5 months' duration, and they are similar to the DSM-IV-TR-defined group in onset, persistence, impairment, comorbidity, parental GAD, and sociodemographic correlates; thus the basis for excluding these individuals from the GAD diagnosis may need to be reexamined (Kessler et al. 2005). Finally, there are data that challenge the DSM-IV-TR hierarchy by which GAD cannot be diagnosed in the presence of concurrent major depression (Zimmerman and Chelminski 2003).

Epidemiology and Comorbidity

One epidemiological study using DSM-IV criteria (Carter et al. 2001) found a 1.5% 1-year prevalence for threshold GAD and a 3.6% 1-year prevalence for subthreshold GAD. Higher rates of the disorder were found in women (2.7%) and the elderly (2.2%). A high degree of comorbidity was again confirmed: 59% for major depression and 56% for other anxiety disorders. The NESARC revealed a 1-year and lifetime DSM-IV GAD prevalence of 2.1% and 4.1%, respectively, with rates higher in female, middle-aged, widowed/separated/divorced, and low-income individuals (Grant et al. 2005b).

Despite its high comorbidity with substance use and other anxiety, mood, and personality disorders (Grant et al. 2005b), GAD stands on its own as a disorder with distinct onset, course, impairment, and prognosis. GAD and depression each show their own statistically significant and independent associations with impairment, of roughly equal magnitude, which cannot be accounted for by comorbidity or sociodemographic variables (Kessler et al. 1999a). Disability and impairment in pure GAD have been found to be equivalent to those of pure mood disorders and significantly greater than those of pure substance use and other anxiety and personality disorders (Grant et al. 2005b).

On certain quality-of-life indexes, individuals with pure GAD actually fare worse than those with pure major depression (Wittchen et al. 2000).

With regard to Axis II comorbidity, the personality types of patients with GAD have not been well characterized. Although dependent and avoidant personality disorders are commonly found to co-occur with GAD, it is not clear whether such personality disorders are primary or consequent to the GAD itself.

Etiology

Biological Theories

Although the neurobiology of GAD is among the least investigated in the anxiety disorders, advances are now being made (a summary is presented in Table 12–11).

Recent work has focused on brain circuits underlying the neurobiology of fear in animal models and in humans and on how inherited and acquired vulnerabilities in these circuits might underlie a variety of anxiety disorders. It is speculated that alterations in the structure and function of the amygdala, which are central to fear-related behaviors, may be associated with GAD. This was supported in a magnetic resonance imaging volumetric study comparing children and adolescents with GAD with healthy comparison subjects matched for other general characteristics. Children with GAD were found to have larger right and total amygdala volumes (DeBellis et al. 2000). The prefrontal cortex and medial temporal lobe are involved in controlling fear and anxiety, and there is evidence for heightened cortical activity and decreased basal ganglia activity in GAD, possibly accounting for the observed arousal and hypervigilance (Buchsbaum et al. 1987; Wu et al. 1991).

Abnormalities of the GABA–benzodiazepine receptor complex have also been implicated in GAD. The benzodiazepine receptor is linked to a receptor for the inhibitory neurotransmitter GABA. Binding of a benzodiazepine to the benzodiazepine receptor facilitates the action of GABA, effectively slowing neural transmission. One series of compounds, the β-carbolines, which are inverse agonists of this receptor complex, produce an acute anxiety syndrome when administered to laboratory animals or to normal human volunteers. Accordingly, benzodiazepines are well established as an efficacious treatment of GAD. GAD subjects have been found to have decreased benzodiazepine receptor density in peripheral blood cells as well as decreased transcriptional mRNA encoding for the receptor, both of which return to normal values with treatment and reduction in anxiety levels (Fer-

TABLE 12–11. Biological models of generalized anxiety disorder

Abnormalities of the γ-aminobutyric acid (GABA)–benzodiazepine receptor

Hypersensitive conditioned fear network centered in the amygdala

Noradrenergic activation

Serotonergic dysregulation

Modest genetic component

rarese et al. 1990; Rocca et al. 1998). Similarly, benzodiazepine receptor binding has been found to be significantly decreased in the left temporal pole of GAD patients compared with healthy control subjects (Tiihonen et al. 1997b).

Evidence for noradrenergic dysregulation in GAD has yielded mixed results. Abelson et al. (1991) reported a blunted growth hormone response to clonidine in GAD compared with responses in normal control subjects. Plasma norepinephrine and its metabolite were found to be elevated, and α_2 adrenoreceptors decreased, in GAD patients compared with normal control subjects (Sevy et al. 1989). Other studies of the noradrenergic system have been negative (R.J. Mathew et al. 1981). There is also some evidence of serotonergic dysregulation in GAD, such as heightened anxiety responses to the partial serotonin agonist meta-chlorophenylpiperazine (*m*-CPP) compared with control subjects (Germine et al. 1992). Auditory evoked potentials have revealed disturbed exteroceptive sensory processing in GAD at the level of the primary auditory cortex, with increased neuronal firing in the serotonergic dorsal raphe (Senkowski et al. 2003). People with GAD do not show heightened sensitivity to 35% CO_2 inhalation as do people with panic, supporting the conceptualization of GAD and panic as two discrete disorders (Perna et al. 1999).

There appears to be a genetic component to GAD, albeit relatively modest. Kendler et al. (1992) studied GAD in female twins and determined that the familial component of the disorder was almost entirely genetic, with a modest heritability of about 30%. Twin studies have reported about 20%–33% overlap in genetic influences between GAD and neuroticism, whereas environmental influences on GAD and neuroticism were largely unshared (Hettema et al. 2004).

There have been minimal molecular genetic studies of GAD to date, requiring replication, that have suggested associations to polymorphisms of the dopamine D_2 receptor gene, the serotonin transporter gene, the dopamine transporter gene, and the monoamine oxidase-A gene.

Psychological Theories

Cognitive hypotheses regarding both the origins and maintenance of GAD have been thoroughly summarized in recent work (Aikins and Craske 2001). With regard to its origins, it has been proposed that insecure attachment relationships and ambivalence toward caregivers, as well as parental overprotection and lack of emotional warmth, may all contribute to later development of anxiety. Regarding mechanisms that may perpetuate GAD, three are summarized. First, worry is used as a strategy for avoiding intense negative affects. Second, worry about unlikely and future threat removes the need to deal with more proximal and realistic threats and limits the capacity to find solutions to more immediate conflicts. Finally, individuals with GAD engage in a certain degree of magical thinking and believe that their worry helped prevent a feared outcome, thus leading to a negative reinforcement of the process of worrying. In terms of the etiology of GAD, cognitive theory speculates a relationship to early cognitive schemas born from negative experiences of the world as a dangerous place (Barlow 1988) or insecure, anxious early attachments to important caregivers (Cassidy 1995).

There is some evidence for specificity in cognitive content in the various anxiety disorders. GAD patients demonstrate more cognitions in the categories of interpersonal confrontation, competence, acceptance, concern about others, and worry over minor matters, whereas panic disorder patients have more cognitions related to physical catastrophes (Breitholtz et al. 1999). There is also evidence that the process of meta-worry—that is, worrying about the worrying in itself—contributes to the high degree of pathological worry in GAD (Wells and Carter 1999).

In addition, certain information-processing biases may characterize GAD and permit the perpetuation of worry as the central cognitive strategy (Aikins and Craske 2001). These include a bias for threat-related information in implicit memory processes (MacLeod and McLaughlin 1995), selective attentional biases for threatening information (Mogg et al. 1989, 2000), and difficulty in decision making when faced with ambiguity (MacLeod and Cohen 1993).

An emotional dysregulation model has also been proposed for GAD, based on evidence from both nonclinical and clinical samples reporting heightened intensity of emotions, poorer understanding of emotions, greater negative reactivity to emotional experiences, diminished ability to self-soothe after negative emotions, and overall greater difficulty managing emotional reactions (Mennin et al. 2005).

Course and Prognosis

In contrast with panic disorder, no overwhelming single event prompts the patient with GAD to seek help. Such patients seem only over time to develop the recognition that their experience of chronic tension, hyperactivity, worry, and anxiety is excessive. Often they will state that there has never been a time in their lives, as long as they can remember, that they were not anxious. GAD is a more chronic condition than panic disorder, with fewer periods of spontaneous remission. Of GAD subjects followed over a 5-year period, only 18%–35% achieved full remission (Woodman et al. 1999; Yonkers et al. 1996). Patients with GAD experience substantial interference with their lives and have a high degree of professional help seeking and a high use of medications (Wittchen et al. 1994). GAD patients with an earlier onset of anxiety symptoms in the first two decades of life appear to be overall more impaired, have more severe anxiety that may not be precipitated by specific stressful events, and have histories of more childhood fears, disturbed family environments, and greater social maladjustment (Hoehn-Saric et al. 1993). In clinical samples, GAD is commonly comorbid with major depression and other anxiety disorders but still emerges as a clearly distinct entity (Wittchen et al. 2000). Abuse of alcohol, barbiturates, and antianxiety medications is also common. Comorbid avoidant and dependent personality disorders appear to lessen the likelihood of remission from GAD (Massion et al. 2002). Contrary to panic disorder, which declines with old age, GAD appears to account for a lot of the anxiety states in late life, often occurring comorbidly with medical illnesses (Flint 1994). In these elderly patients it is particularly important to differentiate GAD from other anxiety states that could be related to delirium, dementia, psychosis, and depression or could be manifestations of underlying medical illnesses.

Differential Diagnosis

The diagnosis of GAD is excluded when occurring exclusively in relation to other major Axis I disorders. We now know that clinicians must be cautious and conservative in applying this criterion, because as previously described, there are now compelling data demonstrating that even in the presence of high comorbidity of GAD with other anxiety and mood disorders, GAD is clearly a discrete disorder in terms of its onset, course, and associated impairment. Finally, the distinction between GAD and "normal" anxiety must be made; in GAD the worry must be clearly excessive, pervasive, difficult to control, and associated with marked distress or impairment. The differential diagnosis of GAD is summarized in Table 12–12.

Treatment

The pharmacological treatment of GAD is summarized in Table 12–13. Although the major changes in diagnostic criteria in consecutive editions of DSM, the presence of frequent comorbidity, and a tendency to view GAD as a secondary or minor condition hampered past treatment research, pharmacotherapy options have blossomed in recent years.

Benzodiazepines

In past years, benzodiazepines were the first-line treatment of GAD. Currently, however, newer medication choices such as buspirone, SSRIs, and serotonin and norepinephrine reuptake inhibitors (SNRIs) have replaced the benzodiazepines as first-line treatments. A number of controlled studies clearly show that chronically anxious patients respond well to benzodiazepines, and all benzodiazepines are probably similarly efficacious in treating GAD. There is some evidence that benzodiazepines may be more effective in treating the physical symptoms of anxiety, whereas antidepressants, whether TCAs or SSRIs, may be more effective in treating the psychic symptoms (Rocca et al. 1998). Although benzodiazepines are generally safe, with side effects limited mainly to sedation and slowed mentation, there is a concern that some patients may become tolerant or even addicted to these medications. However, available data indicate that the concern over benzodiazepine abuse in chronically anxious populations is overestimated, and in reality most patients continue to derive clinical benefits without developing abuse or dependence (Romach et al. 1995). Concerns over addiction are probably justified, for the most part, in individuals with histories of addiction proneness.

Buspirone

Buspirone is a 5-HT$_{1A}$ agonist, nonbenzodiazepine antianxiety agent that may have similar efficacy to the benzodiazepines in treating GAD. Its advantages are a different side-effect profile without sedation and the absence of tolerance and withdrawal. Its disadvantage is a slower rate of onset (Rickels et al. 1988), which can lead to early patient noncompliance. Rickels et al. (1988) compared the efficacy of the benzodiazepine

TABLE 12–12. **Differential diagnosis of generalized anxiety disorder**

Anxious depression

Panic attacks or anticipatory anxiety

Social anxiety

Posttraumatic stress disorder–related hyperarousal symptoms

Obsessional fearfulness

Hypochondriasis

Paranoid anxiety associated with psychosis or personality disorder

clorazepate to the nonbenzodiazepine buspirone in the acute treatment, maintenance, and discontinuation of patients with GAD. The two medications had similar efficacy by the fourth week of treatment, and benefits were maintained over a 6-month period, with an approximately 60% reduction of anxiety scores. There was no evidence of tolerance to either medication over the 6-month period. In the first 2 weeks of medication discontinuation, patients who had been on clorazepate had a transient increase of anxiety consistent with withdrawal, whereas those who received buspirone did not.

Treatment with buspirone is usually started at 5 mg tid, and the dosage can be increased until a maximum dosage of 60 mg/day is reached. A twice-daily regimen is probably as efficacious as a thrice-daily regimen and easier to comply with. There has existed a suggestion in the literature that patients previously treated with benzodiazepines may not respond successfully to buspirone. However, a controlled treatment study has refuted this, finding that patients who gradually discontinued lorazepam and were then treated with buspirone in a double-blind fashion did not exhibit benzodiazepine withdrawal or rebound anxiety and did as well with buspirone as they had done with lorazepam (Delle Chiaie et al. 1995). On the other hand, DeMartinis et al. (2000) retrospectively analyzed a large data set with respect to history of benzodiazepine use prior to a controlled clinical trial. They found that clinical response to buspirone was similar to benzodiazepine response in patients who had never used or had remotely used benzodiazepines, but patients who had used benzodiazepines within 1 month of starting the trial had a higher attrition rate and less clinical improvement if randomized to buspirone rather than to benzodiazepine. There is recent evidence, via a controlled trial (Rickels et al.

TABLE 12–13. **Pharmacological treatment of generalized anxiety disorder**

Venlafaxine extended-release

General indications: First-line treatment; approved by FDA, with proven efficacy in large controlled trials; generally well tolerated; once-daily dosing; recommended starting dosage is 75 mg/day, which may be adequate for a number of patients.

Selective serotonin reuptake inhibitors (SSRIs)

General indications: First-line treatment; paroxetine is FDA-approved; generally well tolerated; once-daily dosing; recommended starting dosage is 20 mg/day, which may be adequate for many patients; other SSRIs also efficacious.

Benzodiazepines

General indications: Well-known efficacy and widely used; all appear similarly efficacious; issues with dependence and withdrawal in certain patients; may be more effective for the physical rather than cognitive symptoms of generalized anxiety disorder.

Buspirone

General indications: Proven efficacy; well tolerated; a trial is generally indicated in all patients; compared with benzodiazepines, takes longer to take action and is not associated with a "high"; may have less efficacy and compliance with very recent benzodiazepine use.

Tricyclic antidepressants (TCAs)

General indications: Demonstrated efficacy in few trials; more side effects than benzodiazepines, buspirone, and newer antidepressants; delayed action compared with benzodiazepines; may be more effective for cognitive rather than physical symptoms of anxiety.

Imipramine: demonstrated efficacy
Trazodone: demonstrated efficacy

Other medications

Clonidine: tends to lose initial response

Propranolol: may be useful adjuvant in patients with pronounced palpitations and tremor

Atypical antipsychotics

Riluzole: open trials

Tiagabine: randomized controlled trial, mixed results

Pregabalin: not marketed in United States

Note. FDA = U.S. Food and Drug Administration.

2000), that in long-term benzodiazepine users, a successful strategy may be to start buspirone or an antidepressant for 1 month prior to undertaking a gradual 4- to 6-week taper of the benzodiazepine. Other independent predictors of successful benzodiazepine taper were lower initial dosages and less severe and chronic anxiety symptoms.

Antidepressants

Over the past few years, newer antidepressants have become established as first-line treatments for GAD, because controlled trials have documented their efficacy and because they tend to be well tolerated, require only once-daily dosing, and do not risk abuse and dependence. Several large controlled trials to date have established the efficacy of extended-release venlafaxine, an SNRI, in treating GAD (Davidson et al. 1999; Gelenberg et al. 2000; Rickels et al. 2000). Venlafaxine has been found effective in dosages ranging from 75 to 225 mg/day. Response rate is approximately 70%, with benefits appearing as early as the first 2 weeks of treatment. Venlafaxine is generally well tolerated, with nausea, somnolence, and dry mouth being the most common side effects. Studies have not revealed consistent differences in efficacy as a function of dosing, suggesting that it can be started at 75 mg/day for GAD and subsequently be increased if clinical improvement is not adequate and side effects permit. In a trial comparing venlafaxine 75–150 mg, buspirone 30 mg, and placebo in GAD without depression over an 8-week period, both medications were superior to placebo, and there was weak evidence for possible superiority of venlafaxine over buspirone by some, but not all, measures (Davidson et al. 1999).

SSRIs are also efficacious in treating GAD. The SSRI paroxetine has been studied in several controlled trials. One trial showed paroxetine at fixed dosages of both 20 mg and 40 mg daily to be superior to placebo over an 8-week treatment period, with approximately two-thirds of patients considered responders (Bellew et al. 2000). Another large flexible-dosing trial showed that paroxetine at dosages ranging from 20 to 50 mg daily was superior to placebo in treating GAD over an 8-week period (Pollack et al. 2001). It also showed that about two-thirds of patients who did not respond to the initial 20-mg dosage responded to higher dosages of 30, 40, or 50 mg daily (McCafferty et al. 2001). In a paroxetine trial using dosages of 20–40 mg/day, an approximately 65% response rate and 33% remission rate were reported (Rickels et al. 2003). In addition, a 6-month discontinuation study found that only about 10% of patients relapsed when continuing medication versus a 40% relapse rate on placebo (Stocchi et al. 2003). Sertraline has also been found to be superior to placebo in decreasing both the psychic and somatic symptoms of GAD during a 12-week treatment (Dahl et al. 2005) at flexible dosages of 50–150 mg/day (Allgulander et al. 2004), and one study showed comparable efficacy and tolerability for paroxetine and sertraline (Ball et al. 2005). Three pooled similar placebo-controlled trials of the SSRI escitalopram, administered for 8 weeks at a dosage of 10–20 mg/day, reported significant improvement in GAD with good tolerability in more than 800 patients (Goodman et al. 2005).

Several older studies have shown TCAs to be effective in treating chronically anxious patients independent of the presence of depressive symptoms, although TCA use has largely fallen out of favor recently in favor of the newer antidepressants. In one controlled study comparing imipramine and alprazolam in treating GAD, similar efficacy was found for the two medications, with imipramine acting more on negative affects and cognitions and alprazolam acting more on somatic symptoms (Hoehn-Saric et al. 1988). In another study, imipramine up to 143 mg/day, trazodone up to 255 mg/day, and diazepam up to 26 mg/day were found comparable after 8 weeks of treatment, with about two-thirds of GAD patients experiencing moderate to marked improvement in anxiety.

A recent open trial reported that mirtazapine, at a daily dosage of 30 mg for 12 weeks, resulted in at least 50% improvement in 80% of 44 patients (Gambi et al. 2005).

Other Medications

β-Adrenergic-blocking drugs such as propranolol may only be rarely indicated as an adjuvant in patients who experience significant palpitations or tremor. Clonidine, which inhibits locus coeruleus discharge, would seem for theoretical reasons to be a good antianxiety drug. A tendency to lose clinical response, plus a number of bothersome side effects, makes clonidine a poor initial choice for treatment.

In patients with refractory GAD, SSRI augmentation with the atypical antipsychotic olanzapine, at a mean dosage of 8.7 mg/day, has been tested in a double-blind design (Pollack et al. 2005) and showed modest benefit for some patients. Similarly, the effect of risperidone augmentation in patients not adequately responding to standard anxiolytic treatment was found to be marginal (Brawman-Mintzer et al. 2005). In contrast, an open monotherapy trial of ziprasidone in 13 patients with treatment-resistant illness reported more positive findings; 84% of patients responded and

46% remitted after 7 weeks of treatment with ziprasidone, 20–80 mg/day (Snyderman et al. 2005).

Riluzole, an antiglutamatergic agent, has also been studied in an open-label trial and appears promising, with 12 of 15 completers responding to the 8-week treatment (S. J. Mathew et al. 2005). A multicenter placebo-controlled study of the selective GABA reuptake inhibitor tiagabine, administered for 8 weeks at dosages of 4–16 mg/day, reported mixed results, with efficacy demonstrated by some analyses but not by the primary intent-to-treat analysis (Pollack et al. 2005). Placebo-controlled trials of the new anxiolytic pregabalin, a calcium-binding presynaptic inhibitor of excitatory neurotransmission, have reported efficacy at dosages ranging from 150 to 600 mg/day, generally demonstrating superiority to placebo, fairly rapid onset, and similar response to a benzodiazepine active control group; dizziness and sedation are reported at higher dosages, but the medication was well tolerated overall (Pohl et al. 2005; Rickels et al. 2005).

Psychotherapy

Research into the psychotherapy of GAD has not been as extensive as for other anxiety disorders. Still, a number of studies exist that clearly show that a variety of psychotherapies are helpful in treating GAD (Table 12–14).

Given the previously described cognitive profile of GAD, several aspects of the disorder can serve as the foci of psychotherapeutic interventions. These include the heightened tendency to perceive threat; the expectation of low-likelihood catastrophic outcomes; poor problem solving, especially in the face of ambivalence or ambiguity; the central feature of worry; and the physical symptoms of anxiety. A variety of treatments have been developed for GAD, including cognitive restructuring; behavioral anxiety management, such as relaxation and rebreathing techniques; exposure therapy with or without a cognitive component; and psychodynamic treatment.

CBT is superior to general nondirective or supportive therapy in treating GAD (Chambless and Gillis 1993) and possibly superior to behavior therapy alone (Borkovec and Costello 1993). Cognitive therapy alone may have an edge over behavioral therapy alone, according to some studies (Butler et al. 1991) but not others (Ost and Breitholtz 2000). In a study that compared four conditions—behavioral therapy alone, cognitive therapy alone, combined CBT, and a wait-list control group—all three active treatments were similarly efficacious and superior to the control condition during an up to 2-year follow-up period; however, the com-

TABLE 12–14. Cognitive and behavioral approaches to treating generalized anxiety disorder

| Exposure |
| Cognitive restructuring |
| Breathing retraining |
| Applied relaxation training |

bined CBT group had a much lower dropout rate than the other groups (Barlow et al. 1992). Cognitive therapy and applied relaxation were found to have similar effectiveness during a 12-week treatment and at a 6-month follow-up (Arntz 2003). Another randomized study compared cognitive, analytic, and behavioral management in treating subjects with GAD (Durham et al. 1994). Cognitive therapy emerged as superior, with some edge over behavioral management alone and a significantly better result than analytic treatment. A "well-being" component aimed at restoring overall function may be a useful addition to usual CBT (Fava et al. 2005).

Combined Pharmacotherapy and Psychotherapy

In a meta-analysis of 65 CBT and pharmacological treatment studies of GAD, overall similar efficacy was reported for the two treatment approaches, with lower attrition rates for psychotherapy (Mitte 2005). There are minimal data on the use of combined psychotherapy and medication in the treatment of GAD. In one study comparing CBT, benzodiazepine, a combination of the two, and placebo (Power et al. 1990), CBT alone or with medication tended to emerge as superior. It appears, however, that the CBT component of the study was more intensive than the medication treatment, and further studies are clearly needed in this area.

Social Phobia (Social Anxiety Disorder)

Definition and Clinical Description

The central feature of social phobia is a marked, persistent fear of social situations in which public humiliation or embarrassment is possible. DSM-IV-TR criteria for social phobia are presented in Table 12–15.

Socially phobic individuals fear and/or avoid a

TABLE 12–15. DSM-IV-TR diagnostic criteria for social phobia

A. A marked and persistent fear of one or more social or performance situations in which the person is exposed to unfamiliar people or to possible scrutiny by others. The individual fears that he or she will act in a way (or show anxiety symptoms) that will be humiliating or embarrassing. **Note:** In children, there must be evidence of the capacity for age-appropriate social relationships with familiar people and the anxiety must occur in peer settings, not just in interactions with adults.

B. Exposure to the feared social situation almost invariably provokes anxiety, which may take the form of a situationally bound or situationally predisposed panic attack. **Note:** In children, the anxiety may be expressed by crying, tantrums, freezing, or shrinking from social situations with unfamiliar people.

C. The person recognizes that the fear is excessive or unreasonable. **Note:** In children, this feature may be absent.

D. The feared social or performance situations are avoided or else are endured with intense anxiety or distress.

E. The avoidance, anxious anticipation, or distress in the feared social or performance situation(s) interferes significantly with the person's normal routine, occupational (academic) functioning, or social activities or relationships, or there is marked distress about having the phobia.

F. In individuals under age 18 years, the duration is at least 6 months.

G. The fear or avoidance is not due to the direct physiological effects of a substance (e.g., a drug of abuse, a medication) or a general medical condition and is not better accounted for by another mental disorder (e.g., panic disorder with or without agoraphobia, separation anxiety disorder, body dysmorphic disorder, a pervasive developmental disorder, or schizoid personality disorder).

H. If a general medical condition or another mental disorder is present, the fear in criterion A is unrelated to it, e.g., the fear is not of stuttering, trembling in Parkinson's disease, or exhibiting abnormal eating behavior in anorexia nervosa or bulimia nervosa.

Specify if:

   Generalized: if the fears include most social situations (also consider the additional diagnosis of avoidant personality disorder)

variety of situations in which they would be required to interact with others or to perform a task in front of other people. Typical social phobias are of speaking, eating, or writing in public; using public lavatories; and attending parties or interviews. In addition, a common fear of socially phobic individuals is that other people will detect and ridicule their anxiety in social situations. An individual may have one, limited, or numerous social fears. Social phobia is described as generalized if the social fear encompasses most social situations as opposed to being present in circumscribed ones. Generalized social phobia is overall a more serious and impairing condition. Generalized social phobia can be reliably diagnosed as a subtype; it has an earlier onset, and affected individuals are more often single and have more interactional fears and greater comorbidity with atypical depression and alcoholism (Mannuzza et al. 1995).

As in specific phobias, the anxiety in social phobia is stimulus bound. When forced or surprised into the phobic situation, the individual experiences profound anxiety accompanied by a variety of somatic symptoms. Interestingly, different anxiety disorders tend to be characterized by their own constellation of most prominent somatic symptoms. For example, palpitations and chest pain or pressure are more common in panic attacks, whereas sweating, blushing, and dry mouth are more common in social anxiety. Actual panic attacks may also occur in individuals with social phobia in response to feared social situations. Blushing is the cardinal physical symptom characteristic of social phobia, whereas commonly encountered cognitive constellations include tendencies for self-focused attention, negative self-evaluation regarding social performance, difficulty gauging nonverbal aspects of one's behavior, discounting of social competence in positive interactions, and a positive bias toward appraising others' social performance (Alden and Wallace 1995).

Individuals who have only limited social fears may be functioning well overall and be relatively asymptomatic unless confronted with the necessity of entering their phobic situation. When faced with this necessity, they are often subject to intense anticipatory anxiety. Multiple social fears, on the other hand, can lead to chronic demoralization, social isolation, and disabling vocational and interpersonal impairment. Alcohol and sedative drugs are often utilized to alleviate at least the anticipatory component of this anxiety disorder, possibly leading to abuse. In a study that systematically compared individuals with a public speaking phobia with those with generalized social phobia, the latter were found to be younger, less educated, and

have greater anxiety, depression, fears of negative social evaluation, and unemployment (Heimberg et al. 1990b).

Epidemiology and Comorbidity

In the National Comorbidity Survey (Kessler et al. 1994; Magee et al. 1996), which employed DSM-III-R criteria, social phobia had a lifetime occurrence of 13.3%, 1-year incidence of 7.9%, and 1-month incidence of 4.5% and was somewhat more common in women than in men (lifetime, 15.5% vs. 11.1%). Of those affected, about one-third reported exclusively public speaking fears, whereas the rest were characterized by at least one other social fear. About one-third had multiple fears qualifying for the generalized type of social phobia, which was found to be more persistent, impairing, and comorbid than the specific public speaking type. The NESARC found a 1-year and lifetime prevalence of DSM-IV social anxiety disorder of 2.8% and 5.0%, respectively (Grant et al. 2005a). Being Native American, being young in age, or having low income increased risk, whereas being male; being Asian, Hispanic, or African American; or living in urban settings reduced risk. Mean age at onset was 15 years. The disorder was chronic; mean age at first treatment was about 12 years later, and 80% had never received treatment. There was significant comorbidity with other psychiatric disorders, especially GAD, bipolar I, and avoidant and dependent personality disorders.

Epidemiological studies have consistently found significant comorbidity between lifetime social phobia and various mood disorders, with an approximately three- to sixfold higher risk for dysthymia, depression, and bipolar disorder (Kessler et al. 1999b). Social phobia almost always predated the mood disorder and was a predictor not only of a higher likelihood of future mood disorder but also of more severity and chronicity.

Social phobia can be associated with a variety of personality disorders, particularly avoidant personality disorder. In epidemiologically identified probands with social phobia alone, avoidant personality disorder alone, or both, a similarly elevated familial risk of social phobia has been found, suggesting that the Axis I and II disorders may represent dimensions of social anxiety rather than discrete conditions (Tillfors et al. 2001a). Indeed, a review of the literature comparing generalized social phobia, avoidant personality disorder, and shyness concluded that all three may exist on a continuum (Rettew 2000) or may even be alternative conceptualizations of the same underlying condition (Ralevski et al. 2005).

Social phobia is a highly disabling disorder whose

impact on functioning and quality of life has probably been greatly underestimated and hidden in past years. Socially phobic persons are impaired on a broad spectrum of measures, ranging from dropping out of school to experiencing significant disability in whatever their main activities are. They describe dissatisfaction with many aspects of life, and the quality of their life is rated as quite low. Importantly, comorbid depression seems to contribute only modestly to these outcomes. Even in preadolescent children, pervasive and serious functional impairment can already be found.

Etiology

Psychosocial Theories

A number of mechanisms are proposed in learning theories as contributors to the pathogenesis of social phobia (Stemberger et al. 1995), and risk factors for social anxiety are summarized in Table 12–16.

Risk factors include direct exposure to socially related traumatic events, vicarious learning through observing others engaged in such traumatic situations, and information transfer (i.e., things that one hears in various contexts regarding social interactions). There is a significant familial component to social phobia, part of which is thought to be heritable (see section "Genetics" later in this chapter) and part acquired. Parents, whether socially anxious themselves or not, might rear socially anxious children through various mechanisms, such as lack of adequate exposure to social situations and development of social skills, overprotectiveness, controlling and critical behavior, modeling of socially anxious behaviors, and fearful information conveyed about social situations (Hudson and Rapee 2000). For example, in an experimental paradigm it has been shown that socially ambiguous situations are interpreted favorably by children without socially phobic parents but avoidantly when family input is negative (Dadds et al. 1996).

Parental social phobia is a strong risk factor for social phobia among adolescent offspring, as is parental depression, any other anxiety disorder, any alcohol use disorder, and parental overprotection or rejection; overall family functioning was not predictive (Lieb et al. 2000). Other potential risk factors for social phobia identified in a large epidemiological sample include lack of a close relationship with an adult, not being firstborn for males, parental marital conflict, general parental psychiatric history, moving several times as a child, childhood abuse, running away from home, and doing poorly in school (Chartier et al. 2001). Types of family adversity also appear to affect females differently than males (DeWit et al. 2005); social anxiety dis-

TABLE 12–16. Risk factors for social anxiety
Parental psychiatric history (especially social phobia, other anxiety disorders, depression)
Parental marital conflict
Parental overprotection or rejection
Childhood abuse
Childhood lack of close relationship with an adult
Not being firstborn for males
Frequent moves in childhood
Poor school performance
Running away from home

order in males was associated with the absence of one parent or other adult confidant during childhood, while in females the disorder was associated with parental conflict and paternal physical abuse during childhood.

A number of cognitive distortions have been identified in individuals with social phobia, all centering around various manifestations of a core negative representation of one's social self. There is evidence that socially phobic individuals do not habituate to negative social information as easily as nonanxious control subjects (Amir et al. 2001); have an attentional and implicit memory bias for socially threatening information (Rinck and Becker 2005); are flexible in interpreting anxiety symptoms exhibited by others but are more judgmental of their own (Roth et al. 2001); make negative interpretations of ambiguous social events and catastrophic interpretations of mildly negative social events (Stopa and Clark 2000); have difficulty disengaging attention from threatening material (Amir et al. 2003); have persistent postevent negative self-appraisal ruminations (Abbott and Rapee 2004); have faulty learning of nonthreatening meanings (Amir et al. 2005a); have a diminished perception of control over anxiety-related symptoms (Hofmann 2005); and have a negative expectation that social success will result in greater future social demands (Wallace and Alden 1997). Children with social phobia, compared with their nonanxious peers, have been found to have social skills deficits, more negative self-talk, less competent social performance with peers, and fewer positive outcomes from peers (Spence et al. 1999).

Biological Theories

Biological theories of social phobia are summarized in Table 12–17.

TABLE 12–17.	Biological models of social anxiety disorder

Hypersensitive conditioned fear network centered in the amygdala

Abnormalities of the γ-aminobutyric acid (GABA)–benzodiazepine receptor

Noradrenergic activation

Decreased dopaminergic tone

Altered serotonin availability

Modest to moderate genetic component

Neurochemistry. Neurochemical studies of social phobia have not been as systematic or consistently replicated as those in panic disorder, but they have to date implicated a number of neurotransmitter systems, including the noradrenergic, GABAergic, dopaminergic, and serotonergic systems. Patients with social phobia exhibit a blunted growth hormone response to clonidine challenge, suggesting underlying noradrenergic dysfunction (Tancer et al. 1993), but this was not replicated in a subsequent study (Tancer et al. 1994). GABA–benzodiazepine receptor involvement is unclear. One study found that the benzodiazepine antagonist flumazenil did not induce a greater surge in anxiety in subjects with social phobia compared with control subjects (Coupland et al. 2000). However, another study showed significantly decreased peripheral benzodiazepine receptor density in subjects with generalized social phobia compared with a healthy group (M.R. Johnson et al. 1998).

Despite the now-documented efficacy of serotonin reuptake inhibitors in treating social phobia, little is directly known about serotonergic involvement in the disorder. One study found increased cortisol response to fenfluramine suggestive of altered serotonergic sensitivity (Tancer et al. 1994). However, other studies found no evidence of altered serotonin reuptake sites in platelets in social phobia (M.B. Stein et al. 1995a) and no abnormality in the prolactin response to m-CPP (Hollander et al. 1998). More recently, a tryptophan depletion protocol resulted in significant increase in anxiety during an autobiographical script in SSRI-treated social anxiety patients, suggesting that improvement in social anxiety by SSRIs is mediated via increased serotonin availability (Argyropoulos et al. 2004).

Two studies have found normal basal functioning of the HPA axis in social phobia, as measured by basal cortisol levels and the dexamethasone suppression test (Condren et al. 2002; Uhde et al. 1994). However,

under psychosocial stress socially phobic individuals did manifest a significantly more robust peak cortisol response compared with control subjects (Condren et al. 2002).

There is also evidence that social phobia may be associated with a decreased central dopaminergic tone. Individuals with comorbid panic and social phobia have been found to have decreased levels of the dopamine metabolite homovanillic acid in the cerebrospinal fluid (CSF) (M. Johnson et al. 1994). Social phobia was associated with a significant 20% decrease in dopamine transporter site density in the striatum on SPECT (Tiihonen et al. 1997a) and with decreased dopamine D_2 receptor binding potential (Schneier et al. 2000).

Neuroimaging. Provocation paradigms that evoke social anxiety have blossomed over the past several years and have consistently highlighted dysfunctional brain circuits in social phobia. Several imaging studies have demonstrated heightened brain activation in social phobia in brain regions associated with emotional processing. A model involving the neurocircuitry of fear, similar to that described for panic disorder and involving faulty conditioned fear responses, has also been implicated in other anxiety disorders, each disorder for its specific triggers, including socially threatening cues in social phobia. A study comparing socially phobic individuals with healthy control subjects demonstrated selectively higher activation in the amygdala, a center for the emotional processing of fearfulness, in response to emotionally neutral faces during fMRI (Birbaumer et al. 1998). In a PET study utilizing social anxiety–provoking scripts, individuals with social phobia showed greater blood flow in the anterior cingulate, the dorsolateral prefrontal cortex, the orbitofrontal cortex, and the insula, all areas involved in emotional processing, whereas the amygdalae were relatively deactivated (Bell et al. 1999). Along these lines, one study has found signal decreases in the amygdala and hippocampus in normal subjects presented with the conditioned stimulus of a neutral face associated with an unconditioned stimulus, whereas socially phobic subjects exhibited opposite increased activations in both regions (Schneider et al. 1999). An fMRI study found heightened amygdala activation in socially phobic persons compared with control subjects when viewing angry or disgusted faces, compared with happy faces (M.B. Stein et al. 2002). In an fMRI study examining amygdalar activation to happy versus harsh (angry, fearful, disgusted) faces, socially phobic participants showed greater amygdalar activation than control subjects in response to the harsh faces, which correlated with the severity of social anxiety symptoms (Phan et al. 2006b). In another fMRI study, socially phobic patients showed greater anterior cingulate activation than nonanxious control subjects when processing disgust versus neutral faces (Amir et al. 2005b). Magnetic resonance spectroscopy has shown significantly higher glutamate levels in the anterior cingulate of patients with social anxiety compared with control subjects, which correlates with symptom severity (Phan et al. 2005). PET imaging has shown significant deactivation in the lingual gyrus and medial frontal gyrus in socially phobic patients during exposure to public speaking, suggesting a strategy of visual avoidance employed to dampen phobic anxiety (Van Ameringen et al. 2004b). fMRI imaging has shown greater activity in the subcortical, limbic, and paralimbic regions and less cortical activity in the anterior cingulate and prefrontal cortex during anticipation of public speaking in socially phobic persons compared with healthy controls, again suggesting diminished cortical inhibition of automatic emotional processing (Lorberbaum et al. 2004). A PET imaging study reported that during a public speaking task, nonphobic subjects revealed relatively increased cortical rather than subcortical activity, whereas phobic subjects showed increased subcortical activity (Tillfors et al. 2001b).

The short allele of the serotonin transporter gene has been implicated in vulnerability to mood disorders (Hariri et al. 2005), and a recent PET study found that those with social anxiety disorder who have one or two copies of the short allele exhibited significantly elevated trait and state anxiety and enhanced right amygdala activation during a public speaking task compared with social anxiety disorder patients homozygous for the long allele (Furmark et al. 2004).

Neuroimaging, coupled with treatment interventions, has revealed findings along the same lines. A SPECT study of subjects with social phobia imaged before and after SSRI treatment showed higher baseline activity in the left temporal cortex and left midfrontal regions in nonresponders compared with responders (Van Der Linden et al. 2000). A PET study examining brain activation in response to a public speaking task found that after treatment with citalopram or CBT, brain activity was attenuated in the amygdala, hippocampus, and neighboring cortical areas, suggesting common sites of action of the two treatments (Furmark et al. 2002). Medication treatment resulted in decreased cerebral blow flow in responders during a public speaking task in the rhinal cortex, amygdala, and hippocampal-parahippocampal regions (Furmark et al. 2005).

Genetics.   A strong familial risk for social phobia has been identified that is believed to be partly heritable and partly environmental. First-degree relatives of probands with generalized social phobia have an approximately 10-fold higher risk for generalized social phobia or avoidant personality disorder. One twin study has not supported a genetic component to social and specific phobia, in contrast to panic disorder, GAD, and PTSD, suggesting environmental causation (Skre et al. 1993). An adolescent female twin study has estimated the heritability of social phobia to be 28%, with strong evidence for shared genetic vulnerability between social phobia and major depression (Nelson et al. 2000).

The personality trait of behavioral inhibition, which is believed to be largely heritable and becomes manifest and fixed in early childhood (Kagan et al. 1987), is thought to be one of the substrates onto which social phobia might develop, but it is neither necessary nor sufficient for the development of the disorder. Behavioral inhibition assessed in toddlerhood has been found, prospectively, to be a strong predictor of social anxiety in adolescence (C. Schwartz et al. 1999). Similarly, behavioral inhibition, in the form of both social avoidance and fearfulness in early high school, prospectively predicted the onset of social phobia 4 years later in adolescence (Hayward et al. 1998).

There are few genetic molecular studies in social phobia. One report found no linkage to the serotonin transporter or 5-HT$_{2A}$ receptor gene in generalized social phobia (M. B. Stein et al. 1998a). A genomewide linkage scan study reported strongest linkage to chromosome 16 in a region implicating the norepinephrine transporter gene (J. Gelernter et al. 2004). The short allele of the serotonin transporter gene (*5-HTT*) has been implicated in vulnerability to mood disorders (Hariri et al. 2005), and there is evidence that it may also be implicated in anxiety disorders such as social anxiety disorder (Furmark et al. 2004).

Course and Prognosis

Social phobia has its onset mainly in adolescence and early adulthood, earlier than with agoraphobia, and the course of illness is very chronic. Mean age at onset is around 19 years. Onset of symptoms is sometimes acute after a humiliating social experience but is usually insidious over months or years and without a clear-cut precipitant. Interestingly, in clinical studies, men are equally or even more commonly affected than women, in distinction to other anxiety disorders. This may reflect who is more likely to seek treatment under societal role demands, however, rather than prevalence rates in the population at large.

Social phobia is clearly a chronic and potentially highly impairing condition; course and prognosis are summarized in Table 12–18. It has been found that more than half of social phobia patients report significant impairment in some areas of their lives, independent of the degree of social support (Stein and Kean 2000). Predictors of good outcome in social phobia are onset after age 11 years, absence of psychiatric comorbidity, and higher educational status (Davidson et al. 1993b). Comorbid avoidant personality disorder has been found to predict a 41% lower likelihood of social phobia remission (Massion et al. 2002). In a large retrospective survey of individuals ages 15–64 years with lifetime social phobia, approximately half of the sample had recovered from their illness at the time of survey, with a median illness duration of 25 years. Significant predictors of recovery were childhood social context, such as no siblings and small-town rearing, onset after age 7 years, fewer symptoms, and absence of comorbid health problems or depression or the occurrence of comorbid illness prior to the onset of social phobia (DeWit et al. 1999). Yet another study has confirmed better prognosis with medication treatment for later disorder onset (especially adult onset) compared with earlier onset, more for symptom improvement but also for work impairment, even when accounting for severity and duration of illness (Van Ameringen et al. 2004c). In a prospective epidemiological study, social anxiety disorder in nondepressed adolescents and young adults at baseline was associated with an increased likelihood of depressive disorder during a 3- to 4-year follow-up period; moreover, comorbid social anxiety in adolescents who were already depressed was associated with a more malignant course of the depressive illness (M. B. Stein et al. 2001a).

Diagnosis and Differential Diagnosis

Differential diagnosis of social anxiety disorder is summarized in Table 12–19. Before the diagnosis of social anxiety disorder can be made, the presence of other disorders that may cause irrational fear of people and avoidance behaviors must be ruled out. Avoidance of social situations is seen as part of avoidant, schizoid, and paranoid personality disorders; agoraphobia; OCD; depressive disorders; schizophrenia; and paranoid disorders.

Persons with paranoid disorders fear that something unpleasant will be done to them by others. In contrast, those with social phobia fear that them-

TABLE 12–18. Course and prognosis of social anxiety disorder

Course

Typically early onset at or before adolescence and very chronic course

Outcome

About one-half found to be recovered after 25 years of illness

Predictors of poorer prognosis

Onset before age 8–11 years

Psychiatric comorbidity

Lower educational status

More symptoms at baseline

Comorbid health problems

TABLE 12–19. Differential diagnosis of social anxiety disorder

Personality disorder, such as avoidant, schizoid, paranoid

Axis I paranoid disorder such as paranoid schizophrenia or paranoid delusional disorder

Depression-related social withdrawal secondary to anhedonia or feelings of defectiveness

Obsessive-compulsive disorder–related fears exacerbated in social settings (e.g., contamination)

Panic disorder with phobic avoidance not limited to social situations

Deficits/impaired social skills associated with schizophrenia and related disorders

selves will act inappropriately and cause their own embarrassment or humiliation.

In avoidant personality disorder the central fear is also rejection, ridicule, or humiliation by others. The distinction between this entity and generalized social phobia may be conceptual and semantic, and its validity is a subject of dispute. Automatically labeling such patients as having avoidant personalities may lead practitioners away from potentially useful pharmacotherapy and behavioral treatment efforts.

Some agoraphobic patients say that they are afraid they will embarrass themselves by losing control if they panic while in a social situation. These patients are distinguished from patients with social phobia by the presence of panic attacks that also occur in situations not involving scrutiny or evaluation by others.

Interpersonal anxiety or fears of humiliation leading to social avoidance are not diagnosed as social phobia when occurring in the context of schizophrenia, schizophreniform or brief reactive psychoses, and major depressive disorder. Patients with psychotic vulnerabilities and massive social isolation or poor interpersonal skills may occasionally be mistaken as having social phobia if seen when they are in nonpsychotic or prepsychotic phases of illness.

Social withdrawal seen in depressive disorders is usually associated with a lack of interest or pleasure in the company of others rather than a fear of scrutiny. In contrast, individuals with social phobia generally express the wish to be able to interact appropriately with others and anticipate pleasure in this eventuality.

Treatment

Pharmacological Treatment

The pharmacological treatment of social anxiety disorder is summarized in Table 12–20. There are a number of medication options that are clearly helpful.

Beta-blockers. In performance-type social phobia, several analogue (i.e., nonclinical samples with performance or social anxiety) studies have shown β-blocker efficacy, particularly when these agents are used acutely prior to a performance. Many performing artists or public speakers find that β-blockers, taken orally a few hours before stage time, reduce palpitations, tremor, and the "butterflies feeling." Although a variety of β-blockers have been used in studies and are probably efficacious for performance anxiety, the most common ones used are propranolol, 20 mg, or atenolol, 50 mg, taken about 45 minutes before a performance. It also seems that they are more effective in controlling stage fright, with minimal or no side effects, than are benzodiazepines, which may decrease subjective anxiety but not optimize performance and may have an adverse effect on "sharpness."

Newer antidepressants. In the past decade, newer antidepressants have been tested and have shown efficacy in treating social phobia, resulting in the SSRIs becoming the first-line treatment for the disorder. They are generally well tolerated, easy to dispense and monitor, and used in standard dosages comparable with those used in depression. Paroxetine is FDA approved for treating social phobia, with efficacy shown in several controlled trials (Baldwin et al. 1999; M.B.

TABLE 12–20. Pharmacological treatment of social anxiety disorder

Selective serotonin reuptake inhibitors (SSRIs)

General indications: First-line treatment; shown efficacy; well tolerated; once-daily dosing; effective for comorbid depression, panic, generalized anxiety disorder, or obsessive-compulsive disorder.

Paroxetine: best studied in large controlled trials; FDA-approved; average dosage 40 mg/day
Other SSRIs: also efficacious
Venlafaxine: also efficacious
Mirtazapine: also efficacious, fewer data

Benzodiazepines

General indications: Clinically widely used and reportedly efficacious in open trials; generally well tolerated; concerns about dependence and withdrawal in certain patients.

Clonazepam: long-acting; efficacy demonstrated in controlled trial

Beta-blockers

General indications: Highly effective for performance anxiety, taken on an as-needed basis about 1 hour before event. For the most part not helpful in patients with generalized social phobia.

Propranolol, atenolol

Monoamine oxidase inhibitors (MAOIs)

General indications: Demonstrated high effectiveness; may be difficult to tolerate and require dietary restrictions; effective for several comorbid conditions including atypical depression, social phobia, and panic; well worth trying in patients with otherwise refractory illness.

Phenelzine: most studied
Tranylcypromine: also effective

Other medications

Gabapentin: effective in one controlled trial

Buspirone: well tolerated; effective in open but not in controlled trial

Bupropion: effective in open trial

Topiramate: open trial

Pregabalin: controlled trial

Atypical neuroleptics: open trials

D-cycloserine: used in conjunction with exposure therapy

Note. FDA=U.S. Food and Drug Administration.

Stein et al. 1998b). About one-half to two-thirds of patients studied responded to acute treatment at average dosages of about 40 mg/day. In a 12-week study comparing 20, 40, and 60 mg/day, paroxetine at a dosage of 20 mg/day was found to be efficacious compared with placebo, and clear advantages were not identified for the higher dosages in this study (Liebowitz et al. 2002a). A pooled analysis of three placebo-controlled multicenter trials of paroxetine examined predictors of treatment response and concluded that duration of treatment was the only significant predictor, with many nonresponders at week 8 achieving response by week 12 (D.J. Stein et al. 2002a, 2002b). Additionally, a 6-month double-blind, maintenance-phase treatment with paroxetine for patients who had initially responded to a 12-week acute treatment found that significantly fewer patients relapsed (14%) when maintained on paroxetine compared with placebo (39%).

Fluvoxamine, given at 150 mg/day for 12 weeks, resulted in substantial improvement in 46% of patients compared with a 7% improvement among subjects given placebo in one controlled trial (van Vliet et al. 1994), replicated in a subsequent larger study with a comparable mean dosage of 200 mg/day and a response rate of 43% (M.B. Stein et al. 1999). Efficacy for sertraline at dosages of 50–200 mg/day was shown in one placebo-controlled study (Katzelnick et al. 1995). A later large 20-week trial of sertraline versus placebo confirmed sertraline's efficacy, using flexible dosing up to 200 mg/day and a 53% response rate (Van Ameringen et al. 2001). Similarly, a 12-week large sertraline trial using dosages of 50–200 mg/day demonstrated superiority to placebo, with only 8% of patients discontinuing due to adverse events (Liebowitz et al. 2003). A 20-week treatment study with sertraline, 50–200 mg/day, reported a 53% response rate with medication compared with 29% for placebo (Van Ameringen et al. 2001). Similar responses were found in an open trial of fluoxetine (Van Ameringen et al. 1993) and an open trial of citalopram (Bouwer and Stein 1998). A 12-week placebo-controlled trial of escitalopram, 10–20 mg/day, reported efficacy with a 54% responder rate, good tolerability, and significant improvement in work and social impairment (Kasper et al. 2005). A double-blind discontinuation study examined relapse in socially phobic patients initially treated openly for 12 weeks with escitalopram, 10–20 mg/day, and found that the risk of relapse was almost three times higher in patients who discontinued active treatment (Montgomery et al. 2005).

Newer antidepressants other than SSRIs are also efficacious in treating social phobia. A 12-week extended-release venlafaxine study, using dosages of 75–225 mg/day, demonstrated significant benefit over placebo in social anxiety symptoms and social impairment, with good tolerability (Rickels et al. 2004). A 6-month placebo-controlled trial of venlafaxine extended-release at a low dosage (75 mg/day) or higher dosage (150–225 mg/day) showed similar superiority to placebo at both dosages, with a 58% response rate and a 31% remission rate (M.B. Stein et al. 2005). Similarly, a 12-week venlafaxine extended-release study using flexible dosing (75–225 mg/day) reported superiority to placebo, with a 44% response rate and a 30% remission rate (Liebowitz et al. 2005). A placebo-controlled trial of mirtazapine in 66 women with social phobia also reported efficacy (Muehlbacher et al. 2005). Bupropion is the least studied antidepressant to date, but it may have some efficacy in social phobia (Emmanuel et al. 1991).

Benzodiazepines. Benzodiazepines can also be helpful in treating generalized social phobia, despite the usual concerns about their chronic use. Several open trials have reported positive results, and in one controlled study clonazepam at dosages of 0.5–3.0 mg/day (mean dosage, 2.4 mg/day) was found to be superior to placebo, with a response rate of 78% and improvement in social anxiety, avoidance, performance, and negative self-evaluation (Davidson et al. 1993a). Alprazolam has also been found to be superior to placebo, with results comparable with those for phenelzine and CBT. However, the alprazolam group had the highest relapse rate 2 months after treatment discontinuation (C.S. Gelernter et al. 1991). Given its longer half-life, clonazepam is a better choice than alprazolam. Both have advantages, such as relatively rapid onset of action and good tolerability. Disadvantages are the potential for abuse, withdrawal, relapse, and lack of efficacy for comorbid depression. The benzodiazepines would not be considered a first-line treatment for social phobia.

Monoamine oxidase inhibitors. MAOIs were the medications proven most effective in treating generalized social phobia until recently. Liebowitz et al. (1992) conducted a controlled study comparing phenelzine, atenolol, and placebo in the treatment of patients with DSM-III social phobia. About two-thirds of patients had a marked response to phenelzine, at dosages of 45–90 mg/day, whereas atenolol was not superior to placebo. Tranylcypromine in dosages of 40–60 mg/day was also associated with significant improvement in about 80% of patients with DSM-III social phobia treated openly for 1 year (Versiani et al. 1988). One study (C.S. Gelernter et al. 1991) compared cognitive-behavioral group treatment with phenelzine, alprazolam, and placebo. Although all groups improved significantly with treatment, phenelzine tended to be superior in absolute clinical response and decreased impairment. Despite their proven efficacy in social phobia, MAOIs are no longer a first-line treatment given their dietary and medication restrictions, the potential for hypertensive crises, and the frequently not-well-tolerated side effects.

Other medication options. Although augmentations and combinations have not been systematically tested in clinical trials, in practice they are often combined in order to attain a sufficiently satisfactory response. A study combining double-blind clonazepam (1–2 mg/day) with open-label paroxetine found that the addition of clonazepam did not lead to more rapid response but did tend to be associated with a more robust global response by the end of treatment, suggesting that in some patients who do not benefit adequately from antidepressant monotherapy, benzodiazepines can lead to additional improvement (Seedat and Stein 2004).

A placebo-controlled trial of the anticonvulsant gabapentin found it superior to placebo at a mean dosage of about 2,900 mg/day, with a response rate approaching 40% of subjects (Pande et al. 1999). The anticonvulsant levetiracetam was not found to be efficacious in a pilot placebo-controlled study (Zhang et al. 2005). An open trial of topiramate, at dosages of up to 400 mg/day, reported benefit in treating social anxiety disorder (Van Ameringen et al. 2004a).

Buspirone, a 5-HT$_{1A}$ agonist anxiolytic, in dosages up to 30 mg/day, was not shown to be efficacious in a controlled study (van Vliet et al. 1997). Pregabalin at a dosage of 600 mg/day was shown to be superior to placebo in a 10-week treatment of social anxiety disorder, whereas pregabalin at a dosage of 150 mg/day was not (Pande et al. 2004). St. John's wort was no more effective than placebo in one study (Kobak et al. 2005a, 2005b). A pindolol augmentation study of SSRIs did not report additional benefit (M.B. Stein et al. 2001b). Atypical antipsychotics have also received limited attention in treating social anxiety. An open-label trial of quetiapine monotherapy in 13 patients with GAD, treated for 12 weeks at a mean dosage of 250 mg/day, reported a response rate of 70% (Schutters et al. 2005). A small placebo-controlled olanzapine trial found that olanzapine was superior to placebo (Barnett et al. 2002).

A new medication approach specifically targeting axillary hyperhydrosis in socially phobic patients with excessive sweating appears promising. Placebo-controlled administration of a one-time bilateral axillary intradermal injection of botulinum toxin coupled with 8-week open treatment with paroxetine resulted in significantly greater improvement in daily activities, work, social functioning, and overall disability (Connor et al. 2006a).

Cognitive and Behavioral Therapies

Three major cognitive-behavioral techniques are used in the treatment of social phobia: exposure, cognitive restructuring, and social skills training (Table 12–21).

Exposure treatment involves imaginal or in vivo exposure to specific feared performance and social situations. Although patients with very high levels of social anxiety may need to start out with imaginal exposure until a certain degree of habituation is attained, therapeutic results are not gained until in vivo exposure to the real-life feared situations is done. Social skills training employs modeling, rehearsal, role-playing, and assigned practice to help individuals learn appropriate behaviors and decrease anxiety in social situations, with an expectation that this will lead to more positive responses from others. This type of training is not necessary for all individuals with social phobia and is more applicable to those who have actual deficits in social interacting above and beyond their anxiety or avoidance of social situations. Cognitive restructuring focuses on poor self-concepts, the fear of negative evaluation by others, and the attribution of positive outcomes to chance or circumstance and negative outcomes to one's own shortcomings. It consists of a variety of homework identifying negative thoughts, evaluating their accuracy, and reframing them in a more realistic way.

Results of older studies of behavioral treatments for social phobia were difficult to evaluate because of heterogeneous phobic patient samples, lack of operational definitions of disorder and improvement ratings, and the presentation of outcome data in terms of mean change scores rather than level of achieved functioning. However, in the past decade or so the cognitive-behavioral treatment of social phobia has blossomed and attracted great attention, detailed treatment strategies and approaches have been delineated, and more thorough systematic studies in well-defined clinical populations have emerged.

Exposure, cognitive restructuring, and social skills training may all be of significant benefit to patients with social phobia. In addition, these techniques appear superior to nonspecific supportive therapy, as

TABLE 12–21. Cognitive and behavioral approaches to treating social anxiety disorder

Exposure (imaginal and/or in vivo)

Cognitive restructuring

Social skills training (modeling, rehearsal, role-playing, practice)

Virtual reality (VR) exposure

Exposure preceded by D-cycloserine administration

shown in a randomized, controlled study comparing supportive therapy with initial individual cognitive therapy followed by group social skills training (Cottraux et al. 2000). The success of CBTs appears to be mediated, at least in part, by a decrease in self-focused attention (Woody et al. 1997). Decreases in negative self-focused thoughts and social anxiety symptoms were significantly intercorrelated in patients treated with CBT but not with exposure, despite the comparable improvement of the two groups (Hofmann et al. 2004). Attempts to correlate patient type (social skills deficits vs. phobic anxiety/avoidance) with preferred treatment modality (social skills training vs. exposure) have not always been fruitful (Wlazlo et al. 1990). Heimberg et al. (1990a) compared cognitive-behavioral group treatment with a credible psychoeducational-supportive control intervention in patients with DSM-III social phobia; both groups got better, but the cognitive-behavioral group showed more improvement, especially in patients' self-appraisal.

It has been suggested that cognitive aspects may be of greater importance in social phobia than in other anxiety or phobic conditions, and therefore cognitive restructuring may be a necessary component to maximize treatment gains. Mattick et al. (1989) reported that combination treatment was superior to either exposure or cognitive restructuring alone in social phobia; cognitive restructuring alone was inferior to exposure alone in decreasing avoidant behavior, but exposure alone did not change self-perception and attitude.

Although long-term outcome is more difficult to assess, studies suggest that CBT leads to long-lasting gains (Turner et al. 1995) and therefore may be of particular significance in social anxiety disorder, which tends to have a chronic, often lifetime, course. One exposure study examining long-term outcome reported that even though one patient out of three was unable to complete treatment or did not benefit sufficiently from it, exposure provided lasting effects for the ma-

jority of patients over a 6-year follow-up (Fava et al. 2001a). At this point, it appears that in vivo exposure is a critical component of the treatment and that the introduction of cognitive restructuring at some point in the treatment contributes to further gains and to their long-term maintenance. Social phobia is a disorder that often starts in the early years, and it is encouraging to know that in prepubertal children, both behavioral therapy consisting of social skills training and anxiety reduction techniques (Beidel et al. 2000) and CBT alone or with the parents (Spence et al. 2000) have been found to be highly effective in controlled trials.

Very recently, virtual reality therapy techniques have surfaced as an interesting and potentially powerful alternative to standard exposure therapies in treating phobias, including social phobia. In a study of 36 social anxiety disorder participants randomly assigned to virtual reality therapy versus standard group CBT, improvement was significant and comparable in the two groups; the virtual environments recreated four situations salient to social phobia, performance, intimacy, scrutiny, and assertiveness (Klinger et al. 2005).

Other Types of Psychotherapy

The successful use of medication and/or behavioral treatments has resulted in psychodynamic therapy for phobias falling out of favor (Gabbard 1990). However, in those patients in whom underlying conflicts associated with phobic anxiety and avoidance can be identified by the clinician and lend to insightful exploration, psychodynamic therapy can be of benefit. Furthermore, a psychodynamic approach may be valuable in understanding and resolving the secondary interpersonal ramifications in which phobic patients and their partners are often caught up and that could serve as resistances to the successful implementation of medication or behavioral treatments (Gabbard 1990). A recent trial of interpersonal psychotherapy, adapted to treating social phobia, showed that seven of nine patients treated openly for 14 weeks showed significant improvement (Lipsitz et al. 1999b), suggesting that this modality does merit further study.

Combination Treatment

Combination treatment with CBT and medication has also received some attention. It appears that medication alone compared with CBT alone has comparable results in the acute treatment of social phobia (Heimberg et al. 1998; Otto et al. 2000). In a rigorous comparison with the medication "gold standard" phenelzine, group CBT was essentially found to have similar efficacy over 12 weeks, although with a longer time to reach response and some inferiority in some of the final measures (Heimberg et al. 1998). In a more recent study, treatment outcome was compared for medication alone (fluoxetine 10–60 mg/day), CBT alone, combined medication and CBT, CBT and placebo, and placebo (Davidson et al. 2004). The response rate was about 50% for both monotherapies and for combined treatment, significantly better than the 32% response rate for placebo alone, leading to the conclusion that combined treatment did not offer any advantage during the acute phase of treatment.

However, the longer-term impact of the two forms of therapy may be more relevant when selecting type of treatment or opting for combination. In a continuation of the previously described study (Heimberg et al. 1998), responders continued treatment with phenelzine or CBT for a 6-month maintenance phase and were then followed for an additional 6-month treatment-free phase (Liebowitz et al. 1999). Both treatments maintained their effectiveness for the first 6 months, with phenelzine preserving its slight superiority over CBT. However, after treatment ended, CBT was associated with a greater likelihood of maintaining a good response. Along similar lines, another study compared the benefits of sertraline alone, sertraline plus exposure therapy, and exposure alone during a 1-year follow-up randomized trial and found that the exposure alone group continued to yield further improvement 6 months after treatment cessation, in contrast to a tendency toward deterioration in the sertraline alone and the sertraline-plus-exposure groups (Haug et al. 2003). Therefore, in a newly presenting patient with social phobia who is reluctant to try medication, it is a very reasonable course to recommend CBT, and even in patients opting for medication treatment, the addition of psychotherapy may contribute to sustaining improvement down the road.

In an exciting development in the combined treatment of social phobia, exposure therapy has been combined with the prior administration of the glutamatergic N-methyl-D-aspartate (NMDA) receptor agonist D-cycloserine, which promotes extinction learning, thus enhancing the effectiveness of fear-reduction learning strategies. In a recent study of 27 participants with public speaking anxiety, four sessions involving exposure to public speech situations were preceded 1 hour prior by double-blind administration of 50 mg D-cycloserine or placebo. Those who received D-cycloserine reported robustly less social anxiety during the exposure therapy than those receiving placebo (Hofmann et al. 2006).

Specific Phobias

Definition and Clinical Description

Specific phobias are circumscribed fears of specific objects, situations, or activities. The syndrome has three components: an anticipatory anxiety that is brought on by the possibility of confrontation with the phobic stimulus, the central fear itself, and the avoidance behavior by which the individual minimizes anxiety. In specific phobia, the fear is usually not of the object itself but of some dire outcome that the individual believes may result from contact with that object. For example, persons with driving phobia are afraid of accidents; those with snake phobia, that they will be bitten; and those who are claustrophobic, that they will suffocate or be trapped in an enclosed space. These fears are excessive, unreasonable, and enduring; although most individuals with specific phobias will readily acknowledge that they know there is really nothing to be afraid of, reassuring them of this does not diminish their fear.

In DSM-IV, for the first time, types of specific phobias were adopted: natural environment (e.g., storms); animal (e.g., insects); blood-injury-injection; situational (e.g., cars, elevators, bridges); and other (e.g., choking, vomiting). The validity of such distinctions is supported by data showing that these types tend to differ with respect to age at onset, mode of onset, familial aggregation, and physiological responses to the phobic stimulus (Fyer et al. 1990). A comparable structure has been found in child and adolescent specific phobia, clustering into three subtypes (Muris et al. 1999). DSM-IV and DSM-IV-TR make the diagnosis of phobic disorder only when single or multiple phobias are the predominant aspect of the clinical picture, a source of significant distress to the individual, and not the result of another mental disorder. The diagnostic criteria for specific phobia are presented in Table 12–22.

Epidemiology

In the National Comorbidity Survey (Magee et al. 1996), which employed DSM-III-R criteria, specific phobias had the same lifetime prevalence of 11.3%, with a median age of illness onset of 15, and women were affected more than twice as often as men. In a community study of adolescents, the prevalence of specific phobias was found to be 3.5%, higher in girls than boys, and to have significant comorbidity with depressive and somatoform disorders in about one-

TABLE 12–22.   **DSM-IV-TR diagnostic criteria for specific phobia**

A.   Marked and persistent fear that is excessive or unreasonable, cued by the presence or anticipation of a specific object or situation (e.g., flying, heights, animals, receiving an injection, seeing blood).

B.   Exposure to the phobic stimulus almost invariably provokes an immediate anxiety response, which may take the form of a situationally bound or situationally predisposed panic attack.   **Note:** In children, the anxiety may be expressed by crying, tantrums, freezing, or clinging.

C.   The person recognizes that the fear is excessive or unreasonable.   **Note:** In children, this feature may be absent.

D.   The phobic situation(s) is avoided or else is endured with intense anxiety or distress.

E.   The avoidance, anxious anticipation, or distress in the feared situation(s) interferes significantly with the person's normal routine, occupational (or academic) functioning, or social activities or relationships, or there is marked distress about having the phobia.

F.   In individuals under age 18 years, the duration is at least 6 months.

G.   The anxiety, panic attacks, or phobic avoidance associated with the specific object or situation are not better accounted for by another mental disorder, such as obsessive-compulsive disorder (e.g., fear of dirt in someone with an obsession about contamination), posttraumatic stress disorder (e.g., avoidance of stimuli associated with a severe stressor), separation anxiety disorder (e.g., avoidance of school), social phobia (e.g., avoidance of social situations because of fear of embarrassment), panic disorder with agoraphobia, or agoraphobia without history of panic disorder.

Specify type:

> **Animal type**
> **Natural environment type** (e.g., heights, storms, water)
> **Blood-injection-injury type**
> **Situational type** (e.g., airplanes, elevators, enclosed places)
> **Other type** (e.g., fear of choking, vomiting, or contracting an illness; in children, fear of loud sounds or costumed characters)

third of the sample (Essau et al. 2000). It is rare for individuals to seek treatment for this disorder.

Etiology

Psychodynamic Theory

With the 1909 publication of the case of "Little Hans," Freud started to develop a psychological theory of phobic symptom formation (Freud 1909/1955). Little Hans was a 5-year-old boy who developed a phobia of horses. Through an analysis of the boy's conversations with his parents over a period of months, Freud hypothesized that Little Hans's unconscious and forbidden sexual feelings for his mother and aggressive, rivalrous feelings for his father, blocked from discharge because of repression, became physiologically transformed into anxiety, which was then displaced onto a symbolic object, in this case horses, the avoidance of which partly relieved Little Hans's anxiety. Freud later reconceptualized the case of Little Hans in the context of his evolving structural theory. Freud hypothesized that phobic symptoms occur as part of the resolution of intrapsychic conflict between instinctual impulses, superego prohibitions, and external reality constraints. Signal anxiety is experienced by the ego when such unconscious impulses threaten to break through. Such anxiety serves to mobilize not only further repression but, in the case of phobia formation, projection and displacement of the conflict onto a symbolic object, which can then be avoided as a neurotic solution to the original conflict. In the case of Little Hans, sexual feelings for his mother, aggressive feelings toward his father, and the guilty fear of retribution and castration by his father generated anxiety as a signal of oedipal conflict. The conflict became displaced and projected onto an avoidable object, horses, which Little Hans consequently feared would bite him. According to Freud, such a phobic symptom had two advantages. It avoided the ambivalence inherent in Little Hans's original conflict, because he not only hated but also loved his father. It also allowed his ego to cease generating anxiety as long as he could avoid the sight of horses. The cost of this compromise was that Little Hans had become housebound. Psychodynamic work with phobias, then, focuses on the symbolic meanings that the phobic object carries for any individual and the conflicts that it serves to avoid.

Behavioral Theories

In learning theory, phobic anxiety is thought to be a conditioned response acquired through association of the phobic object (i.e., the conditioned stimulus) with a noxious experience (i.e., the unconditioned stimulus).

Initially, the noxious experience (e.g., an electric shock) produces an unconditioned response of pain, discomfort, and fear. If the individual frequently receives an electric shock when in contact with the phobic object, then by contiguous conditioning the appearance of the phobic object alone may come to elicit an anxiety response (i.e., conditioned response). Avoidance of the phobic object prevents or reduces this conditioned anxiety and is therefore perpetuated through drive reduction. This classical learning theory model of phobias has received much reinforcement from the relative success of behavioral (i.e., deconditioning) techniques in the treatment of many patients with specific phobias. However, it has also been criticized on the grounds that it is not consistent with a number of empirically observed aspects of phobic behavior in humans.

Models of the etiology of specific phobias have recently been elaborated and critiqued by Fyer (1998). She concluded that in order to satisfactorily explain specific phobia, a modified conditioning model would be needed, on four counts. First, many phobic patients do not recall an initial aversive event, suggesting that if such an event had occurred, it must be encoded by amygdala-based emotional memory but not by hippocampal-based episodic memory, because it either occurred before age 3 years or was encoded under highly stressful conditions. Second, it turns out that a very small number of objects account for most of human phobias, suggesting that there may be an evolutionarily wired biological preparedness toward specific stimuli that would be easily conditioned but difficult to extinguish. Third, only a minority of individuals exposed to a certain stimulus develop a phobic reaction, suggesting that additional factors such as genetic vulnerabilities or previous experiences play a role. Fourth, most phobias are resistant to extinction in the absence of specific interventions, despite belief and evidence that there is nothing to fear.

Another model of specific phobias is the nonassociative learning model (Fyer 1998), which is in a sense the converse of the conditioned model just described. It proposes that each species has certain innate fears that are part of normal development and that what goes wrong in specific phobia is a failure to habituate over time to these intrinsic developmental fears. This failure could be due to various processes, such as stressful life events, constitutional vulnerabilities, or unsafe environments.

Biological Theories

Some interesting hypotheses about the origin of phobias have resulted from integration of ethological, bio-logical, and learning theory approaches. Fyer et al. (1990) found high familial transmission for specific phobias, with a roughly threefold risk for first-degree relatives of affected subjects; there was no increased risk for other comorbid phobic or anxiety disorders. However, one twin study did not support a genetic component to specific phobias, suggesting environmental causation (Skre et al. 1993). One whole-genome scan study implicated a chromosome 14 risk locus in simple phobia (J. Gelernter et al. 2003).

The neurobiology of specific phobias has been studied more in the past several years. Two studies examining response to CO_2 inhalation in subjects with specific phobia have found no differences from healthy subjects and no hypersensitivity, as is found in panic disorder (Antony et al. 1997).

The brain circuits mediating conditioned fear responses have emerged as central to the pathogenesis of a number of anxiety disorders, and there is increasing evidence that the model also applies to specific phobias. Such a model is attractive in that it may account for the occurrence of such a highly fearful response to the conditioned phobic stimulus, mediated by the amygdala, sometimes without hippocampal or cortically based knowledge or memory of why there is such fear. Studies exposing specific phobia subjects to masked stimuli—that is, very brief stimuli that can only be perceived implicitly—have lent partial support to the notion that phobic stimuli, even when not consciously registered, can elicit a subjective or objectively measured fearful response (Van Den Hout et al. 1997).

Brain imaging studies in specific phobias have begun to illuminate their neurocircuitry. Two studies reported activation of the visual associative cortex (Fredrikson et al. 1993) and of the somatosensory cortex (Rauch et al. 1995), suggesting visual and tactile imagery as one component of the phobic response. A volumetric study comparing those with an animal phobia with healthy control subjects reported increased cortical thickness in paralimbic and sensory cortical areas implicated in the processing of phobic stimuli (Rauch et al. 2004). An fMRI study examining spider phobia implicated the right amygdala in automatic stimulus processing, whereas wider circuits involving the insula, anterior cingulate, and dorsomedial prefrontal cortex were implicated in attentional processes involved in threat evaluation (Straube et al. 2004). Phobia-related stimuli elicit heightened activation in the prefrontal cortex, cingulate, and insula in spider phobic individuals but not in control subjects.

Imaging studies have been combined with treatment in order to examine the changes in brain activity that may mediate treatment response. A cerebral blood flow study examined individuals with spider phobia before and after cognitive therapy and found different brain activation patterns in two groups of phobic patients (Johanson et al. 2006). Those patients who managed to control their emotional reaction during spider exposure before treatment showed increased activation in the prefrontal cortex, whereas after successful treatment they showed a decline in activation in this region. In contrast, patients who reported panic during the initial spider exposure showed hypoactivity in the frontal cortex at that time and then showed an increase in prefrontal regional cerebral blood flow in the spider challenge after cognitive therapy. In other words, in both groups activation of the prefrontal cortex varied with the capacity to self-regulate, whether intrinsically or as a result of treatment. In another study using fMRI before and after CBT, phobic subjects before CBT showed dorsolateral prefrontal cortex activation, reflecting the use of metacognitive strategies aimed at self-regulating fear as well as parahippocampal activation related to the automatic reactivation of the contextual fear memory; after successful completion of CBT, no significant activation was found in either brain region (Paquette et al. 2003). Another fMRI study before and after CBT found significant reduction of hyperactivity in the insula and the anterior cingulate cortex of the treated group compared with the wait-list group (Straube et al. 2006).

Course and Prognosis

Animal phobias usually begin in early childhood, whereas situational phobias tend to start later in adolescence or early adulthood. Although systematic prospective studies are limited, it appears that specific phobias follow a chronic course unless treated. A recent study followed up specific phobia patients 10–16 years after an initial treatment and found that even among responders with complete initial recovery, about half were clinically symptomatic at follow-up, and none of the patients who had not improved with the initial treatment were any better at follow-up; this study suggests that specific phobias may be resistant to treatment or often do not receive treatment (Lipsitz et al. 1999a).

Treatment

The treatment of choice for specific phobias is exposure, aimed at fear extinction. The problem lies in persuading the patient that exposure is worth trying and will be beneficial. Exposure treatments may be divided into two groups depending on whether exposure to the phobic object is "in vivo" or "imaginal." In vivo exposure involves the patient in real-life contact with the phobic stimulus. Imaginal techniques confront the phobic stimulus through the therapist's descriptions and the patient's imagination.

The method of exposure in both the in vivo and imaginal techniques can be graded or ungraded. Graded exposure uses a hierarchy of anxiety-provoking events varying from least to most stressful. The patient begins at the least stressful level and gradually progresses up the hierarchy. Ungraded exposure begins with the patients confronting the most stressful items in the hierarchy. Exposure can be accompanied by varying degrees and types of cognitive interventions that decatastrophize the phobic stimulus and encourage risk taking.

Most exposure techniques have been used in both individual and group settings. In a group setting, both the example and the encouragement of other members are often particularly helpful in persuading the patient to reenter the phobic situation. Techniques may include systematic desensitization, imaginal flooding, prolonged in vivo exposure, and participant modeling and reinforced practice.

Studies thus far have not conclusively shown any one exposure technique to be superior to other techniques or to be specifically indicated for particular phobic subtypes. For those patients whose phobic symptoms include panic attacks, antipanic medication may also be indicated.

In recent years, promising computer-aided self-help exposure programs via the Internet, with brief telephone support from a therapist, have been developed for those who are unable to travel due to their phobias (Kenwright and Marks 2004). Another new and exciting development in the treatment of all phobias, including specific phobias, is the development of virtual reality exposure techniques, which permit "virtual exposure" in a clinical setting, greatly facilitating the ease of administration of many in vivo–type exposures. One virtual reality study of driving phobia reported positive results (Wald and Taylor 2003). Similarly promising results were reported in a virtual reality treatment study of spider phobia (Garcia-Palacios et al. 2002) and one of flying phobia (Banos et al. 2002).

Medications have not generally been shown to be effective in treating specific phobias. TCAs, benzodiazepines, and β-blockers generally do not appear useful for specific phobias based on the limited number of studies available to date. One recent small controlled trial, in which 11 patients were randomized to either placebo or paroxetine up to 20 mg/day for 4 weeks, reported that one out of six patients responded to placebo and three out of five to paroxetine (Benjamin et al. 2000). Similarly, dramatic success using SSRIs was reported in three cases of childhood refractory choking phobia that had not responded to other interventions (Banerjee et al. 2005).

There has been a recent surge in interest in the combination of medication and exposure therapy, traditional or virtual reality, in treating anxiety and fear, including specific phobias. In this treatment paradigm, a 50-mg dose of D-cycloserine, a glutamatergic agent which at low dosages has NMDA receptor agonist effects and facilitates new learning, is combined with exposure to further promote extinction. In a treatment study of 28 patients with acrophobia (fear of heights), all subjects received two virtual reality exposure sessions and were premedicated with either D-cycloserine or placebo. The combination treatment group manifested significantly greater improvement, which persisted at 3-month follow-up (Ressler et al. 2004).

Obsessive-Compulsive Disorder

Definition

The essential features of OCD are obsessions or compulsions. DSM-IV-TR criteria for OCD are presented in Table 12–23.

TABLE 12–23. **DSM-IV-TR diagnostic criteria for obsessive-compulsive disorder**

A. Either obsessions or compulsions:

  Obsessions as defined by (1), (2), (3), and (4):
  (1) recurrent and persistent thoughts, impulses, or images that are experienced, at some time during the disturbance, as intrusive and inappropriate and that cause marked anxiety or distress
  (2) the thoughts, impulses, or images are not simply excessive worries about real-life problems
  (3) the person attempts to ignore or suppress such thoughts, impulses, or images, or to neutralize them with some other thought or action
  (4) the person recognizes that the obsessional thoughts, impulses, or images are a product of his or her own mind (not imposed from without as in thought insertion)
  Compulsions as defined by (1) and (2):
  (1) repetitive behaviors (e.g., hand washing, ordering, checking) or mental acts (e.g., praying, counting, repeating words silently) that the person feels driven to perform in response to an obsession, or according to rules that must be applied rigidly
  (2) the behaviors or mental acts are aimed at preventing or reducing distress or preventing some dreaded event or situation; however, these behaviors or mental acts either are not connected in a realistic way with what they are designed to neutralize or prevent or are clearly excessive

B. At some point during the course of the disorder, the person has recognized that the obsessions or compulsions are excessive or unreasonable. **Note:** This does not apply to children.

C. The obsessions or compulsions cause marked distress, are time consuming (take more than 1 hour a day), or significantly interfere with the person's normal routine, occupational (or academic) functioning, or usual social activities or relationships.

D. If another Axis I disorder is present, the content of the obsessions or compulsions is not restricted to it (e.g., preoccupation with food in the presence of an eating disorder; hair pulling in the presence of trichotillomania; concern with appearance in the presence of body dysmorphic disorder; preoccupation with drugs in the presence of a substance use disorder; preoccupation with having a serious illness in the presence of hypochondriasis; preoccupation with sexual urges or fantasies in the presence of a paraphilia; or guilty ruminations in the presence of major depressive disorder).

E. The disturbance is not due to the direct physiological effects of a substance (e.g., a drug of abuse, a medication) or a general medical condition.

Specify if:

   With poor insight: if, for most of the time during the current episode, the person does not recognize that the obsessions and compulsions are excessive or unreasonable

The terminology of "obsessions" or "compulsions" is sometimes used more broadly to characterize conditions that are not true OCD. Although some activities, such as eating, sexual behavior, gambling, or drinking, when engaged in excessively may be referred to as "compulsive," these activities are distinguished from true compulsions in that they are experienced as pleasurable and ego-syntonic, although their consequences may become increasingly unpleasant and ego-dystonic over time. Obsessive brooding, ruminations, or preoccupations, typically characteristic of depression, may be unpleasant but are distinguished from true obsessions because they are not as senseless or intrusive and the individual regards them as meaningful, although possibly excessive and painful.

There are several presentations of OCD based on symptom clusters. One group includes patients with obsessions about dirt and contamination, whose rituals center around compulsive washing and avoidance of contaminated objects. A second group includes patients with pathological counting and compulsive checking. A third group includes purely obsessional patients with no compulsions. Primary obsessional slowness is evident in another group, in whom slowness is the predominant symptom. Patients may spend many hours every day washing, getting dressed, and eating breakfast, and life goes on at an extremely slow speed. Some OCD patients, called "hoarders," are unable to throw anything out for fear they might someday need something they discarded.

In DSM-IV-TR, OCD is classified among the anxiety disorders because 1) anxiety is often associated with obsessions and resistance to compulsions, 2) anxiety or tension is often immediately relieved by yielding to compulsions, and 3) OCD often occurs in association with other anxiety disorders. However, compulsions decrease anxiety only transiently, and the nature of the fears in OCD is distinct from those of other anxiety disorders.

Certain diagnostic disputes regarding OCD were investigated in the DSM-IV field trial and led to some changes in criteria and clarifications in DSM-IV. Even though obsessions are typically experienced as egodystonic, there is a wide range of insight in patients with OCD. Although most patients have some degree of insight, about 5% are convinced that their obsessions and compulsions are reasonable. Based on this, the DSM-IV specified a poor insight type if, for most of the time during the current episode, the person does not recognize that the obsessions and compulsions are excessive or unreasonable. DSM-IV also made explicit that compulsions can be either behavioral or mental.

Mental rituals are encountered in the great majority of OCD patients and, like behavioral compulsions, are intended to reduce anxiety or prevent harm. Although over 90% of patients have features of both obsessions and compulsions, 28% are bothered mainly by obsessions, 20% by compulsions, and 50% by both (Foa et al. 1995).

More recently, it has been disputed whether OCD belongs with the rest of the anxiety disorders, which are subsumed by the stress and fear circuitry, or in a separate grouping of compulsive spectrum disorders; various sources of evidence support this view, which will be grappled with in DSM-V (Bartz and Hollander 2006).

Clinical Description

Onset

OCD usually begins in adolescence or early adulthood but can begin prior to that time; 31% of first episodes occur between ages 10 and 15 years, with 75% developing OCD by age 30. In most cases, no particular stress or event precipitates the onset of OCD symptoms, and after an insidious onset there is a chronic and often progressive course. However, some patients describe a sudden onset of symptoms. This is particularly true of patients with a neurological basis for their illness. There is evidence of OCD associated with the 1920s encephalitis epidemic, abnormal birth events, and onset following head injury or seizures. Of interest are reports of new onset of OCD during pregnancy (Neziroglu et al. 1992).

Symptoms

Obsessions. Obsessive and compulsive symptoms have been recognized for centuries and were first described in the psychiatric literature by Esquirol in 1838 (Rachman and Hodgson 1980). Obsessional thoughts were defined by Karl Westphal in 1878 as ideas that in an otherwise intact intelligence, without being caused by an emotional or affect-like state, and against the will of the person come into the foreground of the consciousness (Westphal 1878).

An *obsession* is an intrusive, unwanted mental event usually evoking anxiety or discomfort. Obsessions may be thoughts, ideas, images, ruminations, convictions, fears, or impulses and are often of an aggressive, sexual, religious, disgusting, or nonsensical content. Obsessional ideas are repetitive thoughts that interrupt the normal train of thinking, whereas obsessional images are often vivid visual experiences. Much obsessive thinking involves horrific ideas. The person may think of doing the worst possible thing (e.g., blasphemy, rape, murder, child molestation). Obsessional convictions are often characterized by an element of magical thinking, such as "step on the crack, break your mother's back." Obsessional ruminations may involve prolonged, excessive, and inconclusive thinking about metaphysical questions. Obsessional fears often involve dirt or contamination and differ from phobias because they are present in the absence of the phobic stimulus. Other common obsessional fears involve harm coming to oneself or to others as a consequence of the patient's misdoings, such as one's home catching on fire because the stove was not checked or running over a pedestrian because of careless driving. Obsessional impulses may be aggressive or sexual, such as intrusive impulses of stabbing one's spouse or raping one's child.

Attributing these obsessions to an internal source, the patient resists or controls them to a variable degree, and significant impairment in functioning can result. *Resistance* is the struggle against an impulse or intrusive thought, and *control* is the patient's actual success in diverting his or her thinking. Obsessions are usually accompanied by compulsions but may also occur as the main or only symptom. Approximately 10%–25% of OCD patients are purely obsessional or predominantly experience obsessions (Akhtar et al. 1975; Rachman and Hodgson 1980).

Another hallmark of obsessive thinking involves lack of certainty or persistent doubting. In contrast to manic or psychotic patients, who manifest premature certainty, OCD patients are unable to achieve a sense of certainty between incoming sensory information and internal beliefs. Are my hands clean? Is the door locked? Is the fertilizer poisoning the water supply? Compulsive rituals such as excessive washing or checking appear to arise from this lack of certainty and consist of a misguided attempt to increase certainty.

Compulsions.   A *compulsive ritual* is a behavior that usually reduces discomfort but is carried out in a pressured or rigid fashion. Such behavior may include rituals involving washing, checking, repeating, avoiding, striving for completeness, and being meticulous. Washers represent about 25%–50% of most OCD samples (Akhtar et al. 1975; Rachman and Hodgson 1980). These individuals are concerned with dirt, contaminants, or germs and may spend many hours a day washing their hands or showering. They may also attempt to avoid contaminating themselves with feces, urine, or vaginal secretions.

"Checkers" have pathological doubt and thus compulsively check to see if they have, for example, run over someone with their car or left the door unlocked. Checking often fails to resolve the doubt and, in some cases, may actually exacerbate it. In the DSM-IV field trial, washing and checking were the two most common groups of compulsions.

Although slowness results from most rituals, it is the major feature of the rare and disabling syndrome of primary obsessional slowness. It may take several hours for the obsessionally slow individual to get dressed or get out of the house. This slowness may be a response to a lack of certainty as well. These patients may have little anxiety despite their obsessions and rituals.

Mental compulsions are also quite common and should be inquired about directly, because they could go undetected if the clinician only asks about behavioral rituals. Such patients, for example, may replay over and over in their minds past conversations with others to make sure they did not somehow incriminate themselves. In the DSM-IV OCD field trials, 80% of patients had both behavioral and mental compulsions, and mental compulsions were the third most common type after checking and washing.

Although distinct symptom clusters exist (washers, checkers, those who are purely obsessional, hoarders, and those with primary slowness), these symptoms may overlap or develop sequentially. One study examined the distribution and grouping of obsessive-compulsive symptoms in about 300 OCD patients and found that a total of four symptom dimensions accounted for more than 60% of variance: obsessions and checking, symmetry and ordering, cleanliness and washing, and hoarding (Leckman et al. 1997). Similarly, a more recent meta-analysis of several factor-analytic studies involving more than 2,000 patients identified the same four consistent "syndromes": symmetry/ordering, hoarding, contamination/cleaning, and obsessions/checking (Mataix-Cols et al. 2005). These four syndromes can coexist in any one patient and be continuous with more normative obsessive-compulsive phenomena. Therefore, these subtypes may prove useful in the future when examining possible genetic, neurobiological, or treatment-response heterogeneity in OCD.

Character Traits

Psychoanalytic theorists have suggested that there is a continuum between compulsive personality and OCD. Janet (1908) stated that all obsessional patients have a premorbid personality that is causally related to the disorder. Freud (1913/1958) noted an association between obsessional neurosis (i.e., OCD) symptoms and personality traits such as obstinacy, parsimony, punctuality, and orderliness.

However, phenomenological and epidemiological evidence suggests that OCD is frequently distinct from obsessive-compulsive personality disorder. OCD symptoms are ego-dystonic, whereas obsessive-compulsive personality traits are ego-syntonic and do not involve a sense of compulsion that must be resisted against. Epidemiological studies show that obsessive-compulsive character pathology is neither necessary nor sufficient for the development of OCD symptoms. When patients with obsessional traits decompensate, they often develop depression, paranoia, or somatization rather than OCD. Although the older literature suggested the presence of definite obsessional traits in as many as two-thirds of OCD patients, structured personality assessments were not used. In more recent standardized evaluations, only a minority of OCD patients had DSM-III-R obsessive-compulsive personality disorder, whereas other personality disorders such as avoidant or dependent were more common (Thomsen and Mikkelsen 1993). In addition, personality disorders may be more common in the presence of a longer duration of OCD, suggesting they could be secondary to the Axis I disorder, and criteria for personality disorders may no longer be met after successful treatment of the OCD (Baer and Jenike 1992). Another recent study supports that there may exist a familial spectrum of OCD and obsessive-compulsive personality disorder (Samuels et al. 2006).

Epidemiology

The ECA study (described earlier in this chapter) suggested that OCD is quite common, with a 1-month prevalence of 1.3%, a 6-month prevalence of 1.5%, and a lifetime rate of 2.5% (Regier et al. 1988). In clinical samples of adult OCD, there is a roughly equal ratio of men to women (A. Black 1974). However, in childhood-onset OCD, about 70% of patients are male (Swedo et al. 1989b). This difference seems to be accounted for by the earlier age at onset in males, and it may suggest partly differing etiologies or vulnerabilities in the two sexes.

Twin and family studies have found a greater degree of concordance for OCD (defined broadly to include obsessional features) among monozygotic twins compared with dizygotic twins (G. Carey and Gottesman 1981), suggesting that some predisposition to obsessional behavior is inherited. There have been no studies of OCD in adopted children or monozygotic twins raised apart. Studies of first-degree relatives of OCD patients show a higher-than-expected incidence

of a variety of psychiatric disorders, including obsessive-compulsive symptoms, anxiety disorders, and depression (D.W. Black et al. 1992; G. Carey and Gottesman 1981). Family studies suggest a genetic link between OCD and Tourette's syndrome (Nee et al. 1982). A recent large family study found that OCD was about fourfold more common in relatives of OCD probands than in control relatives, and the finding was more robust for obsessions. Interestingly, age at onset of OCD in probands was very strongly related to familiality; no OCD was detected in relatives of probands with onset after age 18 (Nestadt et al. 2000b). This study suggests, as does a similar one in panic disorder, that there may exist a more strongly familial subtype of OCD with an earlier onset. Family studies have also shown that OCD spectrum disorders, such as body dysmorphic disorder, hypochondriasis, eating disorder, and grooming conditions, occur more frequently than expected in the relatives of those with OCD (Bienvenu et al. 2000).

There are reports demonstrating comorbidity of OCD with schizophrenia, depression, other anxiety disorders such as panic disorder and simple and social phobia, eating disorders, autism, and Tourette's syndrome. Epidemiologically, the OCD comorbidity risk for other major psychiatric disorders was found to be fairly high but nondistinctive (Karno et al. 1988). In a clinical sample of schizophrenic and schizoaffective patients, about 8% met criteria for OCD, highlighting the importance of screening for obsessive-compulsive symptoms in such populations where detection may be more difficult (Eisen et al. 1997).

Etiology

Psychodynamic Theory

Psychodynamic theory views OCD as residing on a continuum with obsessive-compulsive character pathology and suggests that OCD develops when defense mechanisms fail to contain the obsessional character's anxiety. In this model, obsessive-compulsive pathology involves fixation and subsequent regression from the oedipal to the earlier anal developmental phase. The fixation is presumably due to excessive investment in anal eroticism resulting from excessive frustrations or gratifications in the anal phase.

Obsessive-compulsive patients are thought to utilize the defense mechanisms of isolation, undoing, reaction formation, and regression, and ambivalence to control unacceptable sexual and aggressive impulses. These defense mechanisms are unconscious and thus not readily apparent to the patient.

Isolation. Isolation is an attempt to separate the feelings or affects from the thoughts, fantasies, or impulses associated with them. An example is a patient who describes a particularly gruesome thought or fantasy but denies any feelings of anxiety or disgust associated with it.

Undoing. Undoing is an attempt to magically reverse a psychological event, such as a word, thought, or gesture. A real or imagined act can be undone by evoking its opposite, such as turning on and then turning off a light switch. A patient who feels he has spent too much money on an item for his own pleasure may attempt to undo this by returning the object or punishing himself through some other deprivation.

Reaction formation. The defense of reaction formation substitutes an unacceptable unconscious impulse with its opposite. Thus, a patient who has sadistic impulses to hurt people might behave in a passive or masochistic manner or excessively pronounce his love at moments of heightened anger.

Regression. In OCD, regression is theorized to take place from the genital oedipal phase to the earlier pregenital anal-sadistic phase, which has not been fully relinquished. This regression helps the patient avoid genital conflicts and the anxiety associated with them. Themes characteristic of the anal phase typically reflect conflicts surrounding ambivalence, control, dirt, order, and parsimony.

Ambivalence. In normal development, aggressive impulses are neutralized, and loving feelings predominate toward significant objects. In OCD, strong aggressive impulses are thought to reemerge toward love objects, resulting in displaced ambivalence and paralyzing doubts. In addition, the characteristic thought omnipotence results in magical ideation and lack of certainty, such that thoughts of harming someone become confused with action and may lead to a sense of uncertainty over actually having harmed someone.

Cognitive and Behavioral Theories

A prominent behavioral model of the acquisition and maintenance of obsessive-compulsive symptoms derives from the two-stage learning theory of Mowrer (1939). In Stage 1, anxiety is classically conditioned to a specific environmental event (i.e., classical conditioning). The person then engages in compulsive rituals (escape/avoidance responses) in order to decrease anxiety. If the individual is successful in reducing anxiety, the compulsive behavior is more likely to occur in the future (Stage 2: operant conditioning). Higher-order conditioning occurs when other neutral stimuli such as words, images, or thoughts are associated with the initial stimulus and the associated anxiety is diffused. Ritualized behavior preserves the fear response, because the person avoids the eliciting stimulus and thus avoids extinction. Likewise, anxiety reduction after the ritual preserves the compulsive behavior.

Certain types of cognitions and cognitive processes are highly characteristic of OCD and presumably contribute, if not to the genesis, then at least to the maintenance of the disorder. In particular, negative beliefs about responsibility, especially responsibility surrounding intrusive cognitions, may be a key factor influencing obsessive behavior (Salkovskis et al. 2000). Three main types of dysfunctional beliefs have been identified in OCD: responsibility and overestimation of threat, perfectionism and intolerance of uncertainty, and importance and control of thoughts (S. Taylor et al. 2005). Subjects with OCD also appear to have memory biases toward disturbing themes, for example, better memory for contaminated objects than control subjects with comparable memory (Radomsky and Rachman 1999). Individuals with OCD who "check" have been found not to have memory impairments that presumably could account for the increased checking, but rather, they have decreased confidence in their memory (MacDonald et al. 1997). People with OCD have been found to have deficits in selective attention, and it has been proposed that such deficits may relate to their diminished ability to selectively ignore intrusive cognitive stimuli (Clayton et al. 1999).

Biological Theories

Although OCD used to be viewed as having a psychological etiology, a wealth of biological findings that have emerged over the past few decades have rendered OCD one of the most elegantly elaborated psychiatric disorders from a biological standpoint (Table 12–24).

The association of OCD with a variety of neurological conditions or more subtle neurological findings has been known for some time. Such findings include the onset of OCD following head trauma or von Economo's disease; a high incidence of neurological premorbid illnesses in OCD; an association of OCD with birth trauma; abnormalities on the electroencephalogram, auditory evoked potentials, and ventricular brain ratio on computed tomography scan; an association with diabetes insipidus; and the presence of significantly more neurological soft signs in OCD patients compared with healthy control subjects. Basal

TABLE 12–24. Biological models of obsessive-compulsive disorder

Serotonergic dysregulation

Additional dopaminergic dysregulation, at least in subgroup of patients

Neuropeptide abnormalities (oxytocin, vasopressin, somatostatin)

Hyperactive orbitofrontal–limbic–basal ganglia circuitry

Autoimmune streptococcal-related component in some individuals

Genetic component, ? polymorphisms of the catechol-O-methyltransferase and serotonin transporter genes

ganglia abnormalities were particularly suspected in the pathogenesis of OCD, given that OCD is closely associated with Tourette's syndrome (Pauls et al. 1986), in which basal ganglia dysfunction results in abnormal involuntary movements, as well as with Sydenham's chorea, another disorder of the basal ganglia (Swedo et al. 1989a). Neuropsychological findings in OCD are also of some interest, although not always consistent, and have suggested abnormalities in memory, memory confidence, trial-and-error learning, and processing speed.

A certain form of OCD with childhood onset is believed to be related to an autoimmune process secondary to streptococcal infection. In such children, enlarged basal ganglia have been found on magnetic resonance imaging scans, which is consistent with an autoimmune hypothesis (Giedd et al. 2000). A particular B lymphocyte antigen, which can be identified by the monoclonal antibody D8/17, is expressed in nearly all patients with rheumatic fever and is thought to be a trait marker for susceptibility to group A streptococcal infection complications. Children with OCD and without a history of rheumatic fever or Sydenham's chorea have now been found to have significantly greater B cell D8/17 expression than control children, suggesting that D8/17 may serve as a marker for susceptibility to childhood-onset OCD (Murphy et al. 1997). More recently, such children have also been found to have elevated anti–basal ganglia antibodies compared with pediatric autoimmune, neurological, or streptococcal control subjects (Dale et al. 2005). Children with multiple streptococcal infections within the past year are threefold more likely to be newly diagnosed with OCD or tic disorder (Mell et al. 2005).

Neuroanatomy and Functional Neurocircuitry

A neuroethological model of OCD has been proposed by Rapoport, Swedo, and their group (Swedo 1989; Wise and Rapoport 1989), based on the hypothesized orbitofrontal–limbic–basal ganglia dysfunction. The basal ganglia act as a gating station that filters input from the orbitofrontal and the cingulate cortex and mediates the execution of motor patterns. Obsessions and compulsions are conceptualized as species-specific fixed action patterns that are normally adaptive but in OCD become inappropriately released, repetitive, and excessive. This could be due to a heightened internal drive state or an increased responsivity to external releasers. For example, OCD behaviors such as excessive washing or saving may be dysregulated manifestations of normal grooming or hoarding behaviors. Studies documenting significant volumetric abnormalities in treatment-naive children with OCD suggest that a developmentally mediated dysplasia of the ventral prefrontal-striatal circuitry may underlie OCD (Rosenberg and Keshavan 1998).

Along the lines of this model, a plethora of neuroimaging studies have yielded a sophisticated neuroanatomical underpinning for OCD, specifically implicating orbitofrontal–limbic–basal ganglia circuits. Volumetric imaging studies have consistently revealed abnormal volumes in the implicated circuit, including reduced orbitofrontal and amygdala volumes (Szeszko et al. 1999); smaller basal ganglia (Rosenberg et al. 1997); enlarged thalamus (Gilbert et al. 2000); increased volume of the orbitofrontal cortex and thalamus (J.J. Kim et al. 2001); smaller globus pallidus and increased anterior cingulate cortex (Szeszko et al. 2004); reduced orbitofrontal cortex gray matter, increased putamen, and reduced amygdala (Pujol et al. 2004); and increased orbitofrontal and decreased anterior cingulate gray matter (Valente et al. 2005). Baxter et al. (1987) compared OCD patients and normal control subjects using PET and found higher metabolic rates in the orbitofrontal gyri and caudate nuclei in OCD. Similarly, Swedo et al. (1989c) showed higher metabolic activity in the orbitofrontal and cingulate regions in OCD. Flor-Henry (1983) hypothesized that the fundamental symptomatology of obsessions was due to a defect in neural inhibition of dominant frontal systems, leading to the inability to inhibit unwanted verbal-ideational mental representations and their corresponding motor sequences. It has been suggested that the severity of obsessive urges correlates with orbitofrontal and basal ganglia activity, whereas the accompanying anxiety is reflected by activity in the hippocampus and cingulate cortex (McGuire et al. 1994). With fMRI, it has been possible to demonstrate that during the behavioral provocation of symptoms in OCD patients, significant increases in relative blood flow occur in "real" time in the caudate, cingulate cortex, and orbitofrontal cortex relative to the resting state (Adler et al. 2000; Breiter et al. 1996; Rauch et al. 1994). Using emotional Stroop tasks, OCD patients displayed specific neural responses to OCD-related words, with increased activation of frontostriatal and temporal regions (van den Heuvel et al. 2005b). White matter abnormalities in the anterior cingulate have also been implicated in OCD, suggesting defects in connectivity of the cingulate with other regions involved in the OCD circuitry (Szeszko et al. 2005). Deficient sensorimotor gating, as measured via the prepulse inhibition paradigm, supports the model of deficient frontostriatal circuits in OCD (Hoenig et al. 2005). Deficits in executive function planning, associated with frontostriatal dysfunction, have also been found in OCD, irrespective of state symptomatology (van den Heuvel et al. 2005a). OCD patients show greater activation of the anterior cingulate in tasks involving error processing (Fitzgerald et al. 2005). There is also some evidence that different OCD symptom dimensions (washing, checking, and hoarding) are mediated by relatively distinct components of the frontostriatothalamic circuits (Mataix-Cols et al. 2004).

Of great interest are a number of studies that have now been conducted that demonstrate not only functional but also structural brain changes after a variety of treatments for OCD. After treatment of OCD with serotonin reuptake inhibitors or behavior therapy, hyperactivity decreases in the caudate, orbitofrontal lobes, and cingulate cortex in those patients who have good treatment responses (Baxter et al. 1992; Perani et al. 1995; Swedo et al. 1992b). Also, after successful behavioral treatment the correlations in brain activity between the orbital gyri and the caudate nucleus decrease significantly, suggesting a decoupling of malfunctioning brain circuits (J.M. Schwartz et al. 1996). In children with OCD, a decrease in initially abnormally large thalamic size has been imaged after successful response to paroxetine treatment (Gilbert et al. 2000). Magnetic resonance spectroscopy has also revealed a decrease in initially elevated caudate glutamate concentration in children with OCD after successful paroxetine treatment (Rosenberg et al. 2000). In another study, after improvement of OCD with SSRI or behavioral therapy, there was decreased activation of the prefrontal and cingulate cortex under symptom provocation (Nakao

et al. 2005). A PET study showed that better SSRI treatment response was associated with lower activity in the orbitofrontal cortex and greater activity in the posterior cingulate cortex (Rauch et al. 2002). Interestingly, successful SSRI treatment of OCD or major depression resulted in cerebral activity changes that were disorder specific rather than treatment specific; only OCD treatment was associated with significant metabolic decreases in the caudate, orbitofrontal cortex, and thalamus (Saxena et al. 2002).

Neurochemistry

Parallel to the functional neuroanatomy, the neurochemistry of OCD has become extensively elaborated. Serotonin has been implicated in mediating impulsivity, suicidality, aggression, anxiety, social dominance, and learning. Dysregulation of this behaviorally inhibitory neurotransmitter possibly contributes to the repetitive obsessions and ritualistic behaviors seen in OCD patients. Despite some conflicting and nonreplicated data, extensive research has now clearly implicated the serotonergic system in the pathogenesis of OCD. Considerable indirect evidence supporting the role of serotonin in OCD stems from the well-documented antiobsessional effects of potent serotonin reuptake inhibitors, such as clomipramine, and of the SSRIs in contrast to the ineffectiveness of noradrenergic antidepressants such as desipramine. Furthermore, reduction of OCD symptoms during clomipramine treatment was shown to correlate with a decrease in platelet serotonin level (Flament et al. 1987) and in CSF 5-hydroxyindoleacetic acid (Swedo et al. 1992a).

The use of pharmacological challenge agents to stimulate or block serotonin receptors has also proved a fruitful technique in elucidating the neurochemistry of OCD. Oral *m*-CPP, a partial serotonin agonist, has been found to transiently exacerbate obsessive-compulsive symptoms in a subgroup of OCD patients (Hollander et al. 1992). After treatment of OCD with serotonin reuptake blockers such as clomipramine or fluoxetine, *m*-CPP challenge no longer induced symptom exacerbation (Hollander et al. 1991a; Zohar et al. 1988). A blunted prolactin response to *m*-CPP challenge has also been found in OCD patients by some investigators (Charney et al. 1988; Hollander et al. 1992) but not others (Zohar et al. 1988). Other serotonin agonists, such as tryptophan, fenfluramine, and ipsapirone, or antagonists, such as metergoline, have not been shown to induce consistent behavioral or neuroendocrine response abnormalities in patients with OCD.

More recently, an acute tryptophan-depletion study in SSRI-treated and remitted OCD patients failed to provoke OCD symptom exacerbation, in contrast to its mood-worsening effect, suggesting that obsessive-compulsive symptoms are not dependent on short-term presynaptic serotonin availability (Berney et al. 2006). Increased 5-HT$_{2A}$ receptor binding has been reported in the caudate nuclei of OCD patients, suggestive of diminished serotonin transmission in the corticostriatal loop (Adams et al. 2005). In summary, all studies taken together suggest that serotonergic dysregulation in OCD is complex and probably involves variations in receptor function according to brain region and receptor subtypes.

It also does not appear that serotonergic dysregulation alone can fully explain the neurochemistry of OCD. It is possible that the serotonergic system may, in part, be modulating or compensating for other dysfunctional neurotransmitter systems or neuromodulators. Various neuropeptide abnormalities have started to be elucidated in the past few years. Abnormalities in CSF vasopressin (Swedo et al. 1992a), CSF somatostatin (Altemus et al. 1993), and CSF oxytocin (Leckman et al. 1994) have been implicated in OCD. With clomipramine treatment, CSF levels of vasopressin and somatostatin tend to decrease while oxytocin increases (Altemus et al. 1994). All these neuropeptides may be implicated in arousal, memory, and the acquisition and maintenance of conditioned perseverative behaviors. The noradrenergic α2 agonist clonidine has been reported to induce a transient improvement in OCD symptoms when administered to patients intravenously (Hollander et al. 1991b) or orally (Knesevich 1982), although other noradrenergic challenge findings have been negative (Lucey et al. 1992).

Dopaminergic dysregulation has been variously implicated in OCD (Goodman et al. 1990) through the association between OCD and Tourette's syndrome; reports of exacerbation of obsessive-compulsive symptoms with chronic stimulants; an association between higher pretreatment CSF homovanillic acid and good treatment outcome (Swedo et al. 1992a); blunted growth hormone response to the dopamine agonist apomorphine (Brambilla et al. 1997); use of dopamine blockers to augment partial treatment response with serotonin reuptake blockers (McDougle et al. 1990); and decreased dopamine D$_2$ receptor binding in the caudate nucleus of OCD patients (Denys et al. 2004b). In a putative rat model of OCD, the dopamine D$_2$/D$_3$ receptor agonist quinpirole has been shown to induce compulsive checking in specific locations of an open field (Dvorkin et al. 2006).

Of late, there has been increased interest in possible glutamatergic dysregulation in OCD, and magnetic resonance spectroscopy studies have shown elevated glutamate levels in several regions involved in the hyperactive cortico-striato-limbic-thalamic circuitry (Pittenger et al. 2006). Similarly, CSF glutamate was found to be significantly elevated in medication-naive adult OCD subjects compared with control subjects (Chakrabarty et al. 2005).

Genetics

Segregation analyses have provided support for a single major gene involvement in OCD (Alsobrook et al. 1999; Nestadt et al. 2000a), and genomewide linkage studies have provided evidence for linkage on chromosome 9p (Hanna et al. 2002; Willour et al. 2004). Candidate genes that have been implicated to date include the GABA type B receptor 1 gene (Zai et al. 2005a), the 5-HT$_{1D}$ receptor gene (Mundo et al. 2000), the 5-HT$_{2A}$ receptor gene (Enoch et al. 2001; Meira-Lima et al. 2004), the catechol-O-methyltransferase (COMT) gene (Karayiorgou et al. 1997, 1999; Lochner et al. 2005), the dopamine D$_4$ receptor gene (Millet et al. 2003), the glutamate kainate receptor GRIK2 gene (Delorme et al. 2004), and the glutamate NMDA receptor gene (Arnold et al. 2004). Findings regarding the serotonin transporter gene have been both positive (Bengel et al. 1999) and negative (Billet et al. 1997; Chabane et al. 2004; Frisch et al. 2000); more recently, homozygosity for the long allele L(A) of the serotonin transporter gene was found to exert a moderate effect on risk for OCD (odds ratio = 1.8; Hu et al. 2006). No associations were shown with mutations of the 5-HT$_{2B}$ receptor gene (S. J. Kim et al. 2000), the tryptophan hydroxylase gene (Han et al. 1999), the 5-HT$_{2C}$ receptor gene (Cavallini et al. 1998; Frisch et al. 2000), the dopamine transporter and dopamine D$_4$ receptor genes (Frisch et al. 2000), or the brain-derived neurotrophic factor gene (Zai et al. 2005b). In summary, then, genes predisposing to OCD have not been consistently identified to date. The OCD Collaborative Genetics Study (OCGS) is a six-site linkage study with a National Institute of Mental Health–based cell repository awaiting findings (Samuels et al. 2006).

Course and Prognosis

Studies of the natural course of the illness suggest that 24%–33% of patients have a fluctuating course, 11%–14% have a phasic course with periods of complete remission, and 54%–61% have a constant or progressive course (A. Black 1974; Table 12–25). Although prognosis of OCD has traditionally been considered to be poor, with new developments in behavioral and pharmacological treatments this prognosis is now considerably improved. The disorder usually has a major impact on daily functioning, with some patients spending many waking hours consumed with their obsessions and rituals. Patients are often socially isolated, marry at an older age, and have high celibacy rates (particularly in males) and a low fertility rate. Compounding the situation, depression and anxiety are common complications of OCD.

A major follow-up study was reported that examined the course of patients over a 40-year period in Sweden, from approximately the 1950s to the 1990s (Skoog and Skoog 1999). Findings were more optimistic than expected, with improvement noted in 83% of individuals. Of those, about half were fully or almost fully recovered. Importantly, predictors of worse outcome were earlier onset, a more chronic course at baseline, poorer social functioning at baseline, having both obsessions and compulsions, and having magical symptoms.

In terms of acute treatment, the presence of hoarding obsessions and compulsions is associated with poorer response to both medication treatment (Mataix-Cols et al. 1999) and CBT (Rufer et al. 2006).

Diagnosis

Although a variety of biological and neuropsychiatric markers have been associated with OCD, the diagnosis rests purely on the psychiatric examination and history. DSM-IV-TR defines OCD as the presence of either obsessions or compulsions that cause marked distress, are time consuming, or interfere with social or occupational functioning. Although all other Axis I disorders are allowed to be comorbidly present, the OCD symptoms must not be just secondary to another disorder (e.g., thoughts about food in the presence of an eating disorder or guilty thoughts in the presence of major depression). The diagnosis is usually clear-cut, but occasionally it can be more difficult to distinguish OCD from depression, psychosis, phobias, or severe obsessive-compulsive personality disorder.

Differential Diagnosis

The differential diagnosis of OCD is summarized in Table 12–26.

Schizophrenia.   In some cases the course of OCD may more closely resemble that of schizophrenia, with chronic debilitation, decline, and profound impairment in social and occupational functioning. Sometimes it is difficult to distinguish between an obsession (e.g., contamination) and a delusion (e.g., being poi-

---

TABLE 12–25. Course and prognosis of obsessive-compulsive disorder

Course

   Less than 15% phasic with periods of complete remission

   One-fourth to one-third have fluctuating course

   Half (50%) have constant or progressive illness

Outcome

   80% improve over 40 years

Predictors of worse prognosis

   Early age at onset

   Longer duration of illness

   Presence of both obsessions and compulsions

   Poorer baseline social functioning

   Magical thinking

---

soned). An obsession is typically ego-dystonic, resisted, and recognized as having an internal origin. A delusion is not resisted and is believed to be external. OCD patients may, however lack insight, and obsessions in 12% of cases may become delusions. Yet longitudinal studies show that OCD patients are not at increased risk of developing schizophrenia. Both disorders may exist independently, and DSM-IV-TR allows the diagnosis of both disorders. Thus, the presence of significant obsessive-compulsive symptoms in a schizophrenic patient warrants separate treatment.

Depression.   Patients with OCD frequently have complicating depression, and these patients may be difficult to distinguish from depressed patients who have complicating obsessive symptoms. Patients with psychotic depression, agitated depression, or premorbid obsessional features prior to depression are particularly likely to develop obsessions. These "secondary" obsessions often involve aggressive themes, but the distinction between primary and secondary obsessions rests on the order of occurrence. In addition, depressive ruminations, in contrast to pure obsessions, are often focused on a past incident rather than a current or future event and are rarely resisted.

Phobic disorders.   A close connection exists between OCD and phobic and anxiety disorders. OCD patients who are compulsive cleaners appear very similar to phobic individuals and are often mislabeled "germ phobics." Both have avoidant behavior, both

TABLE 12–26. Differential diagnosis of obsessive-compulsive disorder

Eating disorder with obsessions surrounding food and weight

Body dysmorphic disorder with obsessions about body appearance other than weight

Hypochondriasis with obsessions related to feared illnesses

Panic disorder or generalized anxiety (if obsessional anxiety is severe)

Obsessive ruminations of depressions (typically mood congruent)

Severe obsessive-compulsive personality disorder

Paranoid psychosis (e.g., delusions of poisoning rather than contamination fears)

Social phobia (if avoiding social situations because they exacerbate illness)

TABLE 12–27. Pharmacological treatment of obsessive-compulsive disorder

Serotonin reuptake inhibitors

General indications: First-line treatments; moderate to high dosages.

> *Fluoxetine, fluvoxamine, sertraline:* efficacy shown in large controlled trials
> *Paroxetine, citalopram:* less studied, similar efficacy
> *Clomipramine:* efficacy shown in multiple controlled trials; may have small superiority over SSRIs, however, typically not used until at least two SSRIs have failed secondary to side-effect profile; can be used in low dosages in combination with SSRIs in patients with more refractory illness; clomipramine plus desmethylclomipramine levels must be closely followed for toxicity
> *Venlafaxine, mirtazapine:* less studied

Augmentation strategies

General indications: Partial response to serotonin reuptake inhibitors; presence of other target symptoms.

> *Atypical antipsychotics:* several studies show additional benefit
> *Pindolol:* effective in controlled trial
> *Clonazepam:* effective in controlled trial; comorbid very high anxiety
> *Buspirone:* one positive trial, three negative
> *Lithium:* ineffective in controlled trial
> *Trazodone:* ineffective in controlled trial
> *Monoamine oxidase inhibitors:* hardly any evidence; possibly phenelzine in symmetry obsessions
> *Topiramate*
> *Riluzole*

Other medications

> *Intravenous clomipramine:* efficacy in controlled trial of oral clomipramine–refractory patients
> *Plasma exchange and intravenous immunoglobulin:* effective in children with streptococcus-related obsessive-compulsive disorder

Note. SSRIs = selective serotonin reuptake inhibitors.

show intense subjective and autonomic responses to focal stimuli, and both are said to respond to similar behavioral interventions. Both have excessive fear, although disgust is prominent in OCD patients and not in phobic patients. Also, OCD patients can never entirely avoid the obsession, whereas phobic patients have more focal, external stimuli that they can successfully avoid.

Patients with OCD who experience high levels of anxiety may describe panic-like episodes, but these are secondary to obsessions and do not arise spontaneously. Unlike with panic disorder patients, there is no precipitation of anxiety attacks with lactate infusions in OCD patients (Gorman et al. 1985). OCD does, however, appear to have increased comorbidity with simple and social phobia and panic disorder (Rasmussen and Tsuang 1986).

Treatment

Pharmacotherapy

Advances in recent decades in the pharmacotherapy of OCD have been quite dramatic and have generated a great deal of excitement for successful treatment of this disorder. What was previously thought to be a rare, psychodynamically laden, and difficult-to-treat illness now appears to have a strong biological component and to respond well to potent serotonin reuptake blockers. The pharmacological approach to treatment of OCD is summarized in Table 12–27.

Serotonin reuptake inhibitors. The most extensively studied medication for the treatment of OCD is clomipramine, a potent serotonin reuptake inhibitor with weak norepinephrine reuptake blockade. A series of well-controlled, double-blind studies have undisputedly documented the efficacy of clomipramine in reducing OCD symptoms. The largest of these was a multicenter trial comparing clomipramine with placebo in more than 500 patients with OCD. On an average dosage of 200–250 mg/day of clomipramine, the average reduction in OCD symptoms was about 40%, and about 60% of all patients were clinically much or very much improved (Clomipramine Collaborative Study Group 1991). The very low placebo response rate of 2% documents that OCD is a chronic disorder with infrequent spontaneous remissions. Patients should typically be started on 25 mg of clomipramine at nighttime, and the dosage then should be gradually increased by 25 mg every 4 days or 50 mg every week until a maximum dosage of 250 mg is reached. Some patients are unable to tolerate the highest dosage and may be stabilized at 150 mg or 200 mg. Improvement with clomipramine is relatively slow, with maximal response occurring after 5–12 weeks of treatment. Some of the more common side effects reported by patients are dry mouth, tremor, sedation, nausea, and ejaculatory failure in men. The seizure risk is comparable with that of TCAs and is acceptable for dosages up to 250 mg/day in the absence of prior neurological history. Clomipramine is equally effective for OCD patients with pure obsessions and those with rituals, in contrast to behavioral treatments, which are less useful for patients who predominantly experience obsessions. Controlled studies have also demonstrated that clomipramine is effective in treating OCD when other antidepressants, such as amitriptyline, nortriptyline, desipramine, and the MAOI clorgyline, have no therapeutic effect. This finding strongly suggests that improvement in OCD symptoms is mediated through the blockade of serotonin reuptake.

Numerous controlled trials since the early 1990s have documented the efficacy of all SSRIs for OCD. Fluoxetine has been shown to be superior to placebo in treating OCD at dosages of 20–60 mg/day, with greater efficacy at higher dosages (Montgomery et al. 1993; Tollefson et al. 1994). Similarly, fluoxetine has been shown to be safe and efficacious in treating OCD in children (Liebowitz et al. 2002b).

Fluvoxamine has also been found to have a significant antiobsessional effect in several controlled studies (Hollander et al. 2003c; Jenike et al. 1990). The required daily dosage is titrated up to a maximum of 300 mg. The efficacy of fluvoxamine for OCD has also been demonstrated for children and adolescents (Apter et al. 1994). The efficacy of fluvoxamine in treating pediatric OCD for those ages 8–17 years was further confirmed in a multicenter trial using dosages of 50–200 mg/day. In this trial, 42% of subjects were responders, defined as a 25% symptomatic improvement, and the medication was well tolerated in the pediatric group;

asthenia and insomnia were the most common side effects (Riddle et al. 2001).

Sertraline is another serotonin reuptake blocker whose efficacy for OCD has been established at daily dosages ranging from 50 to 200 mg (Greist et al. 1995a; Kronig et al. 1999). Response began to appear as early as the third week of treatment and was firmly apparent by the eighth week (Kronig et al. 1999). Similarly, sertraline has been found to be effective in treating childhood OCD for those ages 6–17 years in a large multicenter trial using dosages up to 200 mg/day. Again, improvement started to appear around the third week, and 42% of children were significantly improved after 12 weeks. The medication was overall well tolerated; the most common side effects were agitation, insomnia, nausea, and tremor (March et al. 1998b).

Paroxetine and citalopram are also efficacious in treating OCD, generally at dosages of 20–60 mg/day. A multicenter trial reported that citalopram treatment, in dosages of 20, 40, and 60 mg/day, was superior to placebo, without significant differences between the three dosages, although the highest response rate of 65% occurred in the 60 mg/day group (Montgomery et al. 2001). A multicenter paroxetine trial found that the 40 mg/day and 60 mg/day groups, but not the 20 mg/day group, improved significantly more than placebo (Hollander et al. 2003a). A multicenter randomized, controlled trial demonstrated efficacy for paroxetine in children and adolescents with OCD (Geller et al. 2004).

One issue with SSRI treatment is how high to push the dosage, beyond the standard recommended OCD treatment dosage, in an attempt to get a response. One study examined this question in subjects who did not respond to 16 weeks of treatment with sertraline 200 mg/day and found that increasing to a mean dosage of 350 mg/day did result in some symptom improvement but no change in responder status (Ninan et al. 2006).

The SNRI venlafaxine also appears effective in treating OCD. One study reported comparable effectiveness for paroxetine and venlafaxine and also found that some nonresponders benefited from switching to the alternate medication (Denys et al. 2004c). An open trial of venlafaxine in 39 patients, about two-thirds of whom had not responded to SSRIs, reported that about two-thirds responded to venlafaxine at a mean dosage of about 225 mg/day (Hollander et al. 2003b). Despite its putative serotonergic properties, a 12-week placebo-controlled trial of St. John's wort monotherapy yielded negative results (Kobak et al. 2005a). Open-trial monotherapy followed by double-blind discontinuation of mirtazapine, in dosages of 30–60 mg/day, showed preliminary evidence of efficacy that awaits larger replication (Koran et al. 2005). Another study reported that the response to citalopram was accelerated with mirtazapine augmentation (Pallanti et al. 2004).

Although clomipramine appears to have an edge over SSRIs in treating OCD, satisfactory systematic comparisons of the various serotonin reuptake blockers, balancing benefits and side effects, have not been conducted. Given the similar efficacy of these five medications for OCD, an extremely large prospective study would have to be undertaken in order to demonstrate small but significant differences between the various medications. Three meta-analytic studies have addressed these questions by retrospective analyses of treatment data from past trials, and these have supported a small but significant superiority for clomipramine over the SSRIs (Greist et al. 1995b; Piccinelli et al. 1995; D.J. Stein et al. 1995). Similarly, a meta-analysis of pediatric studies found superiority for clomipramine and comparable efficacy among SSRIs (Geller et al. 2003). The clinical applicability of this finding may, however, be limited, because in clinical practice actual or expected tolerability of different medications often takes precedence over small differences in efficacy. The SSRIs are better tolerated than clomipramine by most patients, because of clomipramine's strong anticholinergic side effects, and have therefore become the well-established first line of treatment for OCD. If patients do not have a good response to an adequate trial of at least two SSRIs, augmentation with clomipramine or switching to clomipramine alone should be undertaken; the reverse is also true.

Medication combination and augmentation. It is important to keep in mind that the medication response in OCD is not as dramatic as in, for example, major depression: a considerable number of patients show a negligible or partial response to the first-line medications. As a helpful rule of thumb, it is useful to remember that approximately 40%–60% of OCD patients improve by about 30%–60% with a first-line drug. Thus, various combination and augmentation strategies are often needed to attain a satisfactory response. The most commonly used augmenting agents in OCD are buspirone, clonazepam, atypical antipsychotics, inositol, and glutamatergic agents. As these augmentation strategies are more rigorously tested, they often do not look as promising as was initially thought. Still, given the relatively limited treatment options, these strategies are worth undertaking sequentially, beginning with the most compelling ones.

In the following discussion we summarize the findings in favor of or against the various augmenting agents for OCD.

Although an initial small study reported similar efficacy for clomipramine alone versus buspirone alone in treating OCD (Pato et al. 1991), three other studies failed to show a significant benefit to buspirone augmentation in clomipramine-treated (Pigott et al. 1992a), fluoxetine-treated (Grady et al. 1993), or fluvoxamine-treated (McDougle et al. 1993b) patients. If tried, higher dosages of 30–60 mg/day should be targeted. A controlled study of lithium augmentation of clomipramine did not detect any benefit (Pigott et al. 1991). A controlled study of trazodone alone in OCD again showed no benefit compared with placebo (Pigott et al. 1992b). A controlled crossover study showed clonazepam to be effective in 40% of OCD subjects who failed to respond to clomipramine trials (Hewlett et al. 1992), and clonazepam may also be helpful with the very high anxiety levels frequently associated with OCD. Evidence in support of MAOIs is very weak despite a positive report (Vallejo et al. 1992), possibly with the exception of some benefit for symmetry obsessions from phenelzine (Jenike et al. 1997). A controlled trial of lithium augmentation was also negative (McDougle et al. 1991a), as were a trazodone controlled trial (Pigott et al. 1992b) and a desipramine controlled augmentation trial (Barr et al. 1997). In a small open trial, 10 OCD patients who had failed to respond to serotonin reuptake inhibitor trials were treated with inositol augmentation, 18 mg/day, for 6 weeks; only 3 patients reported clinically significant improvement, leaving inositol as an option of unclear efficacy (Seedat and Stein 1999). A placebo-controlled augmentation trial with eicosapentaenoic acid was not effective for OCD (Fux et al. 2004).

Antipsychotics are the main medication class used to augment partial response to serotonin reuptake blockers in OCD. McDougle et al. (1990) first reported that about 50% of OCD patients improved noticeably when pimozide was added to fluvoxamine; comorbid tic disorders or schizotypal personality predicted a good response. OCD patients with comorbid tic disorders may actually be less responsive to SSRI monotherapy (McDougle et al. 1993a) and appear to respond well to haloperidol augmentation (McDougle et al. 1994). In more recent years, atypical antipsychotics have received increasing attention as a major augmentation strategy for OCD, regardless of comorbid tics or schizotypy, and such a strategy is now supported by controlled trials.

Risperidone has been successfully used for augmentation in open trials, with good results for horrific mental imagery rather than comorbid tic disorders (Saxena et al. 1996). In another 8-week open trial in which risperidone, 3 mg/day, was added to an SSRI in 20 patients with refractory OCD, all subjects were described as showing some improvement (Pfanner et al. 2000). A 6-week controlled trial of risperidone in patients with serotonin reuptake inhibitor–refractory illness found significant improvement in half of the patients (McDougle et al. 2000), and this response was not associated with the presence of tics or schizotypy. Another placebo-controlled risperidone augmentation trial similarly showed better results than placebo, with 40% of patients rated as responders (Hollander et al. 2003a). A small brief double-blind augmentation trial showed similar improvement in obsessions with risperidone and haloperidol compared with placebo (Li et al. 2005). Four pediatric patients with refractory OCD have also been described as responsive to risperidone augmentation (Fitzgerald et al. 1999). Another placebo-controlled risperidone augmentation trial using low-dosage risperidone in 45 patients also reported modest efficacy over placebo (Erzegovesi et al. 2005).

Olanzapine has been reported beneficial in four open-label augmentation trials; however, one placebo-controlled augmentation trial found no benefit (Shapira et al. 2004), whereas another reported significant improvement compared with placebo at a mean dosage of about 10 mg/day, with 15% of patients discontinuing treatment due to side effects (Bystritsky et al. 2004). Two placebo-controlled quetiapine augmentation studies yielded negative results (P. D. Carey et al. 2005; Fineberg et al. 2005), whereas two other placebo-controlled augmentation trials reported that approximately 50%–60% of patients responded to the augmentation (Atmaca et al. 2002; Denys et al. 2004a). A small open monotherapy trial of aripiprazole, in dosages of 10–30 mg/day, reported modest results, with some improvement in three of seven participants (Connor et al. 2005). Clozapine has been reported to worsen OCD, although reports are contradictory. The general conclusion, then, regarding atypical antipsychotic augmentation is that these agents have modest efficacy but are worth trying in patients with treatment-resistant illness.

Beyond antipsychotics, other medications have been used for augmentation in those with treatment-resistant OCD. Fourteen patients with treatment-refractory OCD who had not responded to three SSRI trials received paroxetine augmentation with pindolol or placebo for 6 weeks; compared with placebo, pindolol at 2.5 mg tid was significantly superior in reducing OCD symptoms (Dannon et al. 2000). An open trial of bupropion monotherapy at 300 mg/day reported no benefit (Vulink et al. 2005). A case report of successful topiramate augmentation of paroxetine treatment has been reported (Hollander and Dell'Osso 2006). Similarly, an open series reported that 11 of 16 patients responded to topiramate augmentation at a mean dosage of 250 mg/day (Van Ameringen et al. 2006). Preliminary data on the antiglutamatergic agent riluzole appear promising (Pittenger et al. 2006). In an open trial, about half of 13 patients with treatment-resistant OCD responded to the addition of riluzole, 50 mg bid, to their ongoing regimen (Coric et al. 2005). In a single case report, augmentation of fluvoxamine with the antiglutamatergic amino acid N-acetylcysteine was reported effective (Lafleur et al. 2006).

The combination of clomipramine with an SSRI is also a commonly used strategy for treating refractory patients and is generally well tolerated, although lower dosages of clomipramine should be used with monitoring of blood levels to avoid toxicity because clomipramine levels can become markedly elevated. In one small randomized trial in patients with refractory OCD, citalopram combined with clomipramine led to significantly greater improvement than citalopram alone (Pallanti et al. 1999).

Other somatic treatment options. Although there are no definitive predictors of medication treatment response, several factors appear to be predictive of a poorer prognosis, including earlier onset, longer duration of illness, higher frequency of compulsions, washing rituals, a chronic course, prior hospitalizations, and the presence of avoidant, borderline, and schizotypal as well as multiple personality disorders. A review of 274 OCD patients found no differences between responsive and nonresponsive subjects in age, gender, age at onset, duration of illness, or symptom subtypes. Responders had a higher incidence of family history of tics, sudden onset of OCD, and an episodic course of illness. Nonresponders had more severe symptomatology, poorer insight into their OCD, and comorbid eating disorder (Hollander et al. 2001).

When oral medications fail to be successful enough in patients with highly refractory illness, other somatic treatment options can be considered. Intravenous clomipramine has met with some success in OCD refractory to oral clomipramine (Fallon et al. 1998). More recently, another study has supported the effectiveness of pulse-loaded intravenous clomipramine in treatment-resistant OCD (Koran et al. 2006).

Plasma exchange and intravenous immunoglobulin have been found to be effective in lessening symptom severity in children with streptococcal infection–triggered OCD (Perlmutter et al. 1999), but plasma exchange treatment was found not to help children whose OCD did not have streptococcus-related exacerbations (Nicolson et al. 2000).

Electroconvulsive therapy may be considered in highly refractory cases, although its efficacy is very debatable (Maletzky et al. 1994).

Recently, repetitive transcranial magnetic stimulation (TMS) has been used to treat OCD. A sham-controlled low-frequency TMS treatment of the right prefrontal cortex did not report significant benefit (Alonso et al. 2001). Another study compared right versus left prefrontal TMS in patients with treatment-refractory OCD and found a similar responder rate of 25% for both treatments, although the absence of a sham control group makes interpretation of efficacy difficult (Sachdev et al. 2001). Similarly, an open pilot trial of low-frequency TMS delivered to the supplementary motor area reported benefits (Mantovani et al. 2006).

In extreme cases of severely impaired patients with refractory OCD, neurosurgery can be considered. In a thorough retrospective analysis, Jenike et al. (1991) estimated that in at least 25%–30% of patients, cingulotomy resulted in notable improvement. This response rate was confirmed in a 2-year prospective cingulotomy study (Baer et al. 1995). Guidelines for the use of neurosurgical techniques in the treatment of severe refractory OCD, including selection, documented failed treatments, indications, contraindications, benefits, risks, and workup, have been thoroughly reviewed elsewhere (Mindus and Jenike 1992). A review of 29 patients who underwent capsulotomy between 1976 and 1989 at the Karolinska Hospital in Stockholm, Sweden, found that positive clinical outcome was associated with lesioning to the middle of the right anterior limb of the internal capsule (Lippitz et al. 1999). Another review of 44 patients who underwent single or multiple cingulotomies for refractory OCD reported that almost 3 years later 32% were classified as treatment responders and another 14% as partial responders, and there were few adverse effects (Dougherty et al. 2002). Higher cerebral metabolic activity in the posterior cingulate presurgery has been identified as a predictor of better response to cingulotomy (Rauch et al. 2001).

A new development, which if successful may gradually replace neurosurgery for refractory OCD, is deep-brain stimulation (Rauch et al. 2006). In four highly refractory OCD patients, this treatment resulted in dramatic improvement in one patient and moderate improvement in another (Abelson et al. 2005). In a long-term blinded electrical capsular stimulation study, three of four patients with refractory illness responded to the treatment (Nuttin et al. 2003).

Maintenance treatment.   OCD tends to be a chronic illness, and many patients may require indefinite drug treatment to stay well. Long-term continuation of medication treatment generally maintains a good treatment response; this is widely supported in clinical treatment and has been validated by a 1-year double-blind sertraline maintenance study at dosages of 50–200 mg/day (Greist et al. 1995c). In a subsequent study, patients who maintained their response in the earlier study were given a second year of open maintenance treatment with sertraline at the same dosages, during which they maintained or even slightly improved their gains (Rasmussen et al. 1997). Conversely, in a double-blind discontinuation study of OCD patients who had done well on clomipramine for about 1 year, 90% had substantial worsening within 7 weeks (Pato et al. 1988). Similarly, after 1-year follow-up patients who were randomly assigned to continue fluoxetine rather than be switched to placebo had much lower rates of relapse (Romano et al. 2001). At follow-up after several years, most patients remained symptomatic and required continued pharmacotherapy, with a substantial minority of 20% remaining refractory to multiple treatment regimens (Leonard et al. 1993).

Cognitive-Behavioral Therapy

Behavioral treatments of OCD (Table 12–28) can be highly effective and involve two main components: 1) exposure procedures that aim to decrease the anxiety associated with obsessions and 2) response prevention techniques that aim to decrease the frequency of rituals or obsessive thoughts. Exposure techniques range from systematic desensitization with brief imaginal exposure to flooding, in which prolonged exposure to the real-life ritual-evoking stimuli causes profound discomfort. Exposure techniques aim to ultimately decrease the discomfort associated with the eliciting stimuli through habituation. In exposure therapy, the patient is assigned homework exercises that must be adhered to, and he or she may require assistance from the therapist (in a home visit) or from family members to achieve exposure at home. Response prevention involves having patients face feared stimuli (e.g., dirt, chemicals) without excessive hand washing or tolerate doubt (e.g., "Is the door really locked?") without excessive checking. Initial work may involve delaying performance of the ritual, but ultimately the patient works to fully resist the compulsions. The psychoeducation and support of family members can be pivotal to the success of the behavioral therapy, because family dysfunction is very prevalent and the majority of parents or spouses accommodate to or are involved in the patients' rituals, possibly as a way to reduce the anxiety or anger that patients may direct at their family members.

It is generally agreed upon that combined behavioral techniques—that is, exposure and response prevention (ERP)—yield the greatest improvement. It is also generally reported that patients who primarily experience obsessions and have few rituals are the least responsive to behavioral treatment, although new behavioral techniques for obsessions may also be promising. Using the combined techniques of in vivo ERP, up to 75% of ritualizing patients willing and able to undergo the arduous treatment were reported to show significant improvement (Marks et al. 1975). Foa et al. (1984) systematically compared in vivo exposure, response prevention, and the two treatments combined (ERP). All groups improved, but the combined treatment was superior in decreasing anxiety, rituals, and overall impairment. The proportion of clinical responders, defined as those patients who showed at least 30% improvement with treatment, was 33% for response prevention, 55% for exposure, and 90% for ERP. Of interest, this study found that the majority of OCD patients successfully treated with behavior therapy had relapsed at follow-up, suggesting that, just as with medication, long-term behavioral maintenance treatment may be necessary. Predictors of poorer outcome for behavioral treatment of OCD include initial depression, initial OCD severity, longer duration, and lower motivation for treatment (Keijsers et al. 1994). ERP has also been used successfully to treat children and adolescents with OCD, with at least 50% improvement in the vast majority of participants (Franklin et al. 1998). A maintenance program can be highly effective in helping patients maintain their benefits from CBT over several years of follow-up (Marks 1997; McKay 1997).

Cognitive therapy has also been more recently advocated and is efficacious in the treatment of OCD, centering on cognitive reformulation of themes related to the perception of danger, estimation of catastrophe, expectations about anxiety and its consequences, excessive responsibility, thought–action fusion, and illogical inferences. Several studies have directly compared cognitive versus behavioral therapy for OCD in randomized trials and have reported similar efficacy

TABLE 12–28. Cognitive and behavioral approaches to treating obsessive-compulsive disorder

Graded exposure (imaginal and/or in vivo)
Flooding
Response prevention
Cognitive restructuring

(Cottraux et al. 2001; van Oppen et al. 1995; Whittal et al. 2005). A meta-analysis of cognitive versus behavioral treatment trials for OCD reported that behavioral treatment was somewhat more effective in clinically significant improvement (about 50%–60% of participants), whereas for full remission the two approaches had a similar effectiveness of about 25% (Fisher and Wells 2005).

Combination Pharmacotherapy and Psychotherapy

The relative efficacy of pharmacotherapy versus psychotherapy for OCD is an important question in deciding what first-line treatment to undertake. A meta-analytic comparison study of OCD treatments, after controlling for a number of confounding variables, found that clomipramine, SSRIs, and ERP all had comparable results (Kobak et al. 1998). Similarly in children, a study comparing behavioral treatment versus clomipramine found that both were similarly helpful, suggesting that nonpharmacological options are a reasonable first-line option in the younger population in an initial attempt to avoid medication (de Haan et al. 1998). A recent 12-week multicenter study, however, suggested that behavior therapy may have an edge over medication therapy (Foa et al. 2005b; Simpson et al. 2005). The study compared ERP alone, clomipramine alone, their combination, and a placebo pill in 122 adults with OCD and found that both ERP and combination treatment were superior to medication alone (response rates for all groups were 62%, 42%, 70%, and 8%, respectively). ERP and combination treatment had a greater edge over clomipramine alone for remission compared with response; a sizable number of patients did not achieve remission by the end of treatment regardless of the type of treatment. Similarly, a large pediatric trial found that combination treatment was superior both to CBT and to sertraline alone and therefore recommended that this age group start treatment with CBT or combined treatment (Pediatric OCD Treatment Study Team 2004). There is also evidence that in the short term (12 weeks) after treatment discontinuation, patients who were treated with ERP relapsed significantly less than those treated with medication alone (Simpson et al. 2004). However a longer-term (5-year) follow-up study has reported that long-term outcome did not differ among patients initially treated with cognitive therapy alone, ERP alone, or psychotherapy combined with medication, with an overall remission rate of about 50%; patients initially treated with medication were more likely to be taking medication at follow-up (van Oppen et al. 2005). So, in sum, medication and CBT are approximately equal first-line treatment choices.

Despite the similar efficacy of pharmacotherapy and CBT for OCD, given the common failure of either treatment to achieve a strong enough response or remission, combination therapy, either concurrent or sequential, is commonly used and recommended in the treatment of OCD. A common approach used in clinical practice, especially by psychiatrists, is to start out with medication, attain a degree of clinical improvement that will allow better utilization of CBT, and then possibly attempt some degree of medication taper once CBT has been mastered and effective. In a study testing this commonly used paradigm, it appeared quite effective. Patients who remained symptomatic with a 12-week course of an SSRI were entered into a course of exposure and ritual prevention and subsequently demonstrated a 50% decrease in their OCD symptoms (Simpson et al. 1999). In another study, patients who did respond to initial 3-month medication treatment were randomly assigned to continue medication alone or to have behavior therapy added for the next 6 months; the latter group showed significantly greater benefits (Tenneij et al. 2005). Similarly, in a wait-list controlled trial of CBT in OCD patients who had failed to adequately respond to multiple serotonin reuptake inhibitor medications, about 50% showed clinically significant improvement, and most maintained it at 6-month follow-up; poor insight and low CBT effort predicted lesser gains (Tolin et al. 2004). In brief, the conclusion is that patients who are initially treated with medication, regardless of degree of initial response, have a good likelihood of some further improvement with the introduction of CBT.

Other Psychotherapy

Patients with OCD frequently present with symptoms that appear laden with unconscious symbolism and dynamic meaning. However, OCD has generally proven refractory to psychoanalytically oriented as well as to loosely structured, nondirective, exploratory psychotherapies. In contrast to its lack of efficacy in treating chronic OCD, dynamic psychotherapy may be helpful for acute and limited symptoms in patients who are otherwise psychologically minded and motivated to explore their conflicts and for obsessive character traits of perfectionism, doubting, procrastination, and indecisiveness (Salzman 1985).

OCD patients need supportive treatment even while pharmacotherapy or behavior therapy is being applied. Because of their tendency toward excessive doubt, these patients may require a great deal of reassurance during the early phase of treatment. More active supportive therapy that encourages risk taking helps OCD patients live with their anxiety, and a focus on the present has been reported to be helpful (Salzman 1985).

Posttraumatic Stress Disorder

Definition

PTSD was first introduced in DSM-III, spurred in part by the increasing recognition of posttraumatic conditions in veterans of the Vietnam War. The current DSM-IV-TR diagnostic criteria for PTSD are presented in Table 12–29.

Beginning with DSM-III-R, the disorder is classified with the anxiety disorders, and the major criteria of an extreme precipitating stressor, intrusive recollections, emotional numbing, and hyperarousal have been maintained. The DSM-III-R descriptor of the traumatic event as one "outside the range of usual human experience" was considered rather vague and unreliable and was eliminated. New duration criteria were also established, subdividing the disorder into acute or chronic.

Not all investigators agree that PTSD belongs with the anxiety disorders. Although anxiety is a prominent symptom, so are depression and dissociation. The necessity of a precipitating stressor or trauma in diagnosing the disorder differs from other anxiety disorders and is more reminiscent of conditions such as brief reactive psychosis, acute stress disorder, pathological bereavement, and adjustment disorders. ICD-10 (World Health Organization 1992), for example, classifies all such disorders as stress related. In acknowledgment of the spectrum of disorders stemming from severe stress, DSM-IV added acute stress disorder to the anxiety disorders. Acute stress disorder is similar to PTSD in the precipitating traumatic event and in symptomatology, but it is time limited, up to 1 month after the event. In

TABLE 12–29.   DSM-IV-TR diagnostic criteria for posttraumatic stress disorder

A. The person has been exposed to a traumatic event in which both of the following were present:

    (1) the person experienced, witnessed, or was confronted with an event or events that involved actual or threatened death or serious injury, or a threat to the physical integrity of self or others

    (2) the person's response involved intense fear, helplessness, or horror.   **Note:** In children, this may be expressed instead by disorganized or agitated behavior.

B. The traumatic event is persistently reexperienced in one (or more) of the following ways:

    (1) recurrent and intrusive distressing recollections of the event, including images, thoughts, or perceptions.   **Note:** In young children, repetitive play may occur in which themes or aspects of the trauma are expressed.

    (2) recurrent distressing dreams of the event. **Note:** In children, there may be frightening dreams without recognizable content.

    (3) acting or feeling as if the traumatic event were recurring (includes a sense of reliving the experience, illusions, hallucinations, and dissociative flashback episodes, including those that occur on awakening or when intoxicated).   **Note:** In young children, trauma-specific reenactment may occur.

    (4) intense psychological distress at exposure to internal or external cues that symbolize or resemble an aspect of the traumatic event

    (5) physiological reactivity on exposure to internal or external cues that symbolize or resemble an aspect of the traumatic event

C. Persistent avoidance of stimuli associated with the trauma and numbing of general responsiveness (not present before the trauma), as indicated by three (or more) of the following:

    (1) efforts to avoid thoughts, feelings, or conversations associated with the trauma

    (2) efforts to avoid activities, places, or people that arouse recollections of the trauma

    (3) inability to recall an important aspect of the trauma

    (4) markedly diminished interest or participation in significant activities

    (5) feeling of detachment or estrangement from others

    (6) restricted range of affect (e.g., unable to have loving feelings)

    (7) sense of a foreshortened future (e.g., does not expect to have a career, marriage, children, or a normal life span)

D. Persistent symptoms of increased arousal (not present before the trauma), as indicated by two (or more) of the following:

    (1) difficulty falling or staying asleep

    (2) irritability or outbursts of anger

    (3) difficulty concentrating

    (4) hypervigilance

    (5) exaggerated startle response

E. Duration of the disturbance (symptoms in criteria B, C, and D) is more than 1 month.

F. The disturbance causes clinically significant distress or impairment in social, occupational, or other important areas of functioning.

Specify if:

    Acute: if duration of symptoms is less than 3 months

    Chronic: if duration of symptoms is 3 months or more

Specify if:

    With delayed onset: if onset of symptoms is at least 6 months after the stressor

addition, dissociative symptoms figure prominently in the definition of acute stress disorder, whereas they are not addressed in the PTSD description. It has now been well established by a number of studies, including prospective ones, that acute stress disorder is a highly reliable predictor of developing PTSD down the road; it may well be that the two should not be defined as discrete disorders. In a study of people who had mild traumatic brain injury in motor vehicle accidents, 82% of those who met acute stress disorder criteria were diagnosed with PTSD 6 months later (Bryant and Harvey 1998), as opposed to only 11% of those without acute stress, and a steady 80% were diagnosed with PTSD 2 years after the accident (Harvey and Bryant 2000).

Beyond the symptoms of PTSD per se, increasing attention has been drawn to an enduring constellation of traits that frequently develop in individuals subjected to chronic trauma as children or adults. Investigators such as Herman and van der Kolk (1987) had originally suggested that a discrete entity of complicated posttraumatic syndromes be recognized, otherwise designated as "DESNOS" (disorders of extreme stress not otherwise specified), characterized by lasting changes in identity, interpersonal relationships, and the sense of life's meaning (Herman et al. 1989; van der Kolk and Saporta 1991). Similar personality changes are recognized by the ICD-10 and classified as "enduring personality change after catastrophic experience." Increasing attention has been drawn in recent years to the concept of "trauma-spectrum" disorders, which can include admixtures of posttraumatic stress, dissociative, somatoform, and conversion symptoms, and the classification approach to trauma-related conditions is a subject of ongoing debate.

Clinical Description

A soldier participates in the torture and murder of civilians. A passenger is the sole survivor of a commercial airliner. A woman is raped and severely beaten by an unknown assailant. The characteristic features that may develop after traumatic events such as these include psychic numbing, reexperiencing of the trauma, and increased autonomic arousal. The trauma is reexperienced in recurrent painful and intrusive recollections, daydreams, or nightmares. Dissociative states may occur, lasting from minutes to days, in which there is a dreamlike, unreal state with hazy memory and a distorted sense of time. Psychic numbing or emotional anesthesia is manifest by diminished responsiveness to the external world, with feelings of being detached from other people, loss of interest in

usual activities, and inability to feel emotions such as intimacy, tenderness, or sexual interest. Symptoms of excessive autonomic arousal may include hyperactivity and irritability, an exaggerated startle response, difficulty concentrating, and sleep abnormalities. Rape or mugging victims sometimes become afraid to venture forth alone for variable periods of time. Situations reminiscent of the original trauma may be systematically avoided.

Other symptoms may include guilt about having survived, guilt about not having prevented the traumatic experience, depression, anxiety, panic attacks, shame, and rage. There may be prolonged episodes of intense affect; increased irritability; explosive, hostile behavior; and impulsive behavior. Other accompanying or complicating symptoms associated with PTSD may include substance abuse, self-injurious behavior and suicide attempts, occupational impairment, and interference with interpersonal relationships.

Epidemiology

Although there are marked individual differences in how people react to stress, when stressors become extreme, such as in concentration camp situations or in extended combat, the rate of morbidity rapidly increases. In a large randomized community survey of young adults, the lifetime prevalence of PTSD was found to be 9.2% (Breslau et al. 1991). The prevalence was higher in women (11.3%) than in men (6%). In the National Comorbidity Survey, the lifetime prevalence of PTSD was similarly found to be 7.8% and was again more common in women. The most common stressors were combat exposure in men and sexual assault in women (Kessler et al. 1995).

Symptoms of PTSD, too few in number to meet the full diagnostic criteria, are quite common in the general population. In a Canadian community survey, full PTSD was found in 2.7% of women and 1.2% of men, whereas partial PTSD was found in an additional 3.4% of women and 0.3% of men. Such individuals, seemingly women in particular, may be important to identify because they experience clinically meaningful distress and functional impairment (M.B. Stein et al. 1997). The gender difference in PTSD prevalence, higher in women, has been consistent across a number of studies. It appears that women are more likely to develop PTSD than men with comparable exposure to traumatic events, especially if exposure is before age 15 (Breslau et al. 1997a). This difference is not well understood and could involve characteristics of both the individuals and the traumatic experiences.

A high rate of comorbid disorders is found in

PTSD. In the Breslau et al. (1991) survey, a high comorbidity risk was found for OCD, agoraphobia, panic, and depression, whereas the association with drug or alcohol abuse was weaker. The comorbidity of PTSD with depression is a very consistent one, and the nature of the relationship between the two conditions is controversial. Epidemiological analyses suggest that in trauma victims the vulnerabilities for PTSD and depression are not separate, but rather the risk for depression is highly elevated in just those trauma victims who manifest PTSD (Breslau et al. 2000). On the other hand, a prospective study of a large sample of trauma survivors found depression and PTSD to be independent sequelae of trauma (Shalev et al. 1998a, 1998b). Regardless of causality, it is clear that PTSD in women increases the risk for new onset of both depression and alcohol use disorder (Breslau et al. 1997b). The Australian National Survey of Mental Health and Well-Being, of about 10,000 participants, found that about one-fourth of those with PTSD had an alcohol use disorder whereas about one-third of those with opioid use disorder had PTSD (Mills et al. 2006). Individuals with PTSD may be more likely to manifest borderline or self-defeating personality disorder, and it appears that the actual PTSD diagnosis rather than the trauma history accounts for this association (Shea et al. 2000).

Etiology

The severity of the stressor in PTSD differs in magnitude from that found in adjustment disorder, which is usually less severe and within the range of common life experience. However, this relationship between the severity of the stressor and the type of subsequent symptomatology is not always predictable. For example, studies of bereavement and divorce have found that stressors within the range of usual human experience can also produce a distinctive syndrome of reexperiencing the trauma (Horowitz et al. 1980). In effect, it has generally been underestimated that in the average community setting, common events such as sudden loss of a spouse are a much more frequent cause for PTSD than assault and violence (Breslau et al. 1998).

Nevertheless, events such as sexual assault or armed robbery, which are interpersonal insults to integrity, self-esteem, and security, are particularly likely to lead to PTSD. When stressors become extreme (e.g., rape, extended combat, torture, or concentration camp experiences), the rate of morbidity significantly increases. For example, the ECA study found that in men who had served in Vietnam, 4% of those who were in combat but were not wounded had PTSD, whereas 20% of those in combat who had been wounded developed PTSD. In even more horrendous conditions, such as those experienced by American prisoners of war held by the Japanese during World War II, extremely high PTSD incidences of 84% lifetime and 59% decades after have been reported (Engdahl et al. 1997). Variable rates have been found in individuals subjected to major noninterpersonal trauma such as in severely injured accident victims, ranging from a very low 2% (Schnyder et al. 2001) to 32% (Koren et al. 1999). After severe traumatic brain injury, a 27% PTSD incidence has been reported (Bryant et al. 2000). Childhood interpersonal trauma can often result in PTSD, as is widely known clinically and documented by numerous studies. In an inner-city child psychiatry clinic, more than half of the traumatized children had syndromal or subsyndromal PTSD, with experiencing physical abuse or witnessing domestic violence being the strongest contributors (Silva et al. 2000). In a large community sample followed prospectively into young adulthood, about one-third of the children who had experienced substantiated sexual abuse, physical abuse, or neglect had PTSD (Widom 1999). As an average, it is estimated that approximately one-fourth of all individuals who experience major trauma develop PTSD (Breslau et al. 1991). In addition, as described by McFarlane (1990), a definite dose–response relationship exists between the impact of the trauma and PTSD. Still, it is rare even for overwhelming trauma to lead to PTSD in more than half of the exposed populations, clearly suggesting that other etiological factors also play a role (McFarlane 1990). A discussion of such predictors follows.

Risk Factors and Predictors

There is agreement that a variety of premorbid risk factors predispose to the development of PTSD (Table 12–30). Although the disorder can certainly develop in people without significant preexisting psychopathology, a number of biological and psychological variables have been identified that render individuals more vulnerable to the development of PTSD. In one study of a Vietnam veteran outreach center, a prior history of good adolescent friendships was predictive of PTSD, whereas a history of poor adolescent friendships was more likely in those who did not have PTSD. In addition, this study reported a number of patients with good premorbid adjustment, low childhood trauma, and good adolescent relationships who experienced prolonged trauma in Vietnam and developed severe PTSD (Lindy et al. 1984). In general, however, previous adversity has been associated with a higher likelihood of developing PTSD.

The greater the amount of previous trauma experienced by an individual, the more likely he or she is to develop symptoms after a stressful life event (Horowitz et al. 1980). In addition, individuals with prior traumatic experiences are more likely to become exposed to future traumas, because they can be prone to behaviorally reenact the original trauma (van der Kolk 1989). In a study of Vietnam veterans, those with PTSD had higher rates of childhood physical abuse than those without PTSD, as well as a significantly higher rate of total traumatic events prior to joining the military (Bremner et al. 1993b).

McFarlane (1989) found that the severity of exposure to disaster was the major determinant of early posttraumatic morbidity, whereas preexisting psychological disorders better predicted the persistence of posttraumatic symptoms over time. An epidemiological survey identified, albeit retrospectively, different risk factors for becoming exposed to trauma and for developing PTSD after traumatic exposure (Breslau et al. 1991). Risk factors for exposure to trauma were male sex, childhood conduct problems, extraversion, and family history of substance abuse or psychiatric problems. Risk factors for developing PTSD after traumatic exposure were disrupted parental attachments, anxiety, depression, and family history of anxiety. Having an Axis II disorder also increases the risk for chronic PTSD (Ursano et al. 1999). Having a past history of PTSD increases the risk for both acute and chronic PTSD (Ursano et al. 1999). Compared with nonchronic PTSD, chronic PTSD of greater than 1 year's duration has been specifically associated with higher rates of comorbid anxiety and depressive disorders and a family history of antisocial behavior (Breslau and Davis 1992). Also, a nationally representative sample provided evidence that self-criticism and the broader personality domain of neuroticism may comprise a robust risk factor for PTSD (Cox et al. 2004).

Interestingly, parental PTSD is also a risk factor for PTSD in offspring, even in the absence of elevated trauma (Yehuda et al. 1998b). Findings with regard to gender are conflicting, in that female gender has been associated with chronic PTSD in one study (Breslau and Davis 1992) whereas only with acute PTSD in another (Ursano et al. 1999). An additional risk factor that has been associated with higher likelihood of developing PTSD is lower premorbid intelligence (Macklin et al. 1998). Neurological compromise, with increased neurological soft signs and childhood histo-

TABLE 12–30.	Risk factors for posttraumatic stress disorder (PTSD)

Past history of trauma prior to the index trauma

Past history of PTSD

Past history of depression

Past history of anxiety disorders

Comorbid Axis II disorders (predictive of greater chronicity)

Family history of anxiety (including parental PTSD)

Disrupted parental attachments

Severity of exposure to trauma (more predictive of acute symptoms)

High premorbid intelligence may be protective

ries of neurodevelopmental problems and lower intelligence, is also associated with PTSD (Gurvits et al. 2000); a recent monozygotic twin study demonstrated that the presence of neurological soft signs is a familial vulnerability factor rather a function of trauma or of the disorder itself (Gurvits et al. 2006).

Early predictors of PTSD after a traumatic event have also received great attention, because of their obvious potential significance for early intervention and prevention. As previously stated, the occurrence of acute stress disorder in the first month after trauma is a very strong predictor of later PTSD. An acute stress disorder diagnosis combined with a resting heart rate greater than 90 bpm has a surprisingly high sensitivity (88%) and specificity (85%) in predicting development of PTSD (Bryant et al. 2000). Similarly, high heart rate and decreased cortisol in the acute aftermath strongly correlate with later PTSD (Yehuda et al. 1998a). In a prospective study, initial urinary cortisol and epinephrine levels immediately after trauma predicted up to 10% of the variance in PTSD symptoms 6 weeks later (Delahanty et al. 2005). Even elevated heart rate, on its own, shortly after trauma is a significant predictor of later PTSD (Shalev et al. 1998b). A heart rate greater than 95 bpm in acutely injured patients was found to be a significant independent predictor of PTSD symptoms 1 year later, with modest specificity and sensitivity (Zatzick et al. 2005). One prospective study has also implicated lower plasma GABA levels peritraumatically in the development of later PTSD (Vaiva et al. 2004).

Other findings of great interest are that the administration of certain agents medically indicated in the acute aftermath of medical traumas (e.g., cardiac surgery, intensive care unit stays, burns) may be protective against developing later PTSD. For example, stress doses of hydrocortisone administered perioperatively to cardiac surgery patients are associated with lower intensity of chronic stress and PTSD symptoms 6 months later (Schelling et al. 2004). There is also evidence that acute morphine administration in children for the treatment of acute burns was associated with diminished PTSD 6 months later in a dose-related fashion (Saxe et al. 2001).

Increased attention to dissociative phenomena and their relationship to posttraumatic symptoms has revealed that greater dissociation around the time of the traumatic event, known as peritraumatic dissociation, is a strong predictor of the later development of PTSD (Marmar et al. 1994; Shalev et al. 1996). Although peritraumatic dissociation may serve as one "marker" helpful in identifying individuals at high risk for developing PTSD, many individuals go on to develop PTSD in the absence of pronounced peritraumatic dissociation, so peritraumatic dissociation should be viewed as one predictor in the context of other factors in the aftermath of trauma (Ozer et al. 2003).

Cognitive and Behavioral Theories

A cognitive model has been proposed for the persistence of PTSD symptoms, suggesting that PTSD becomes persistent when individuals process the trauma in a way that leads to a sense of serious and current threat. This occurs through excessively negative appraisals of the trauma or its consequences and a disturbance of autobiographical memory so that there is poor contextualization and strong associative memory (Ehlers and Clark 2000).

Behavioral theory suggests that there is a disturbance of conditioned responses in PTSD. Autonomic responses to both innocuous and aversive stimuli are elevated, with larger responses to unpaired cues and reduced extinction of conditioned responses (Peri et al. 2000). It has been proposed that PTSD individuals have higher sympathetic system arousal at the time of conditioning and therefore are more conditionable than trauma-exposed individuals without PTSD (Orr et al. 2000). Individuals with PTSD also generalize fear-related conditioned responses across stimuli, having been sensitized by stress (Grillon and Morgan 1999).

Recent studies have also revealed a number of disturbances in cognitive processes associated with PTSD. For example, the high incidence of PTSD after severe traumatic brain injury with loss of consciousness and few traumatic memories suggests that trauma can mediate PTSD in part at an implicit level (Bryant et al. 2000). Impairments in explicit memory have been associated with PTSD (Bremner et al. 1993a) and may be related to hippocampal toxicity resulting from stress-mediated elevations in norepinephrine (Bremner et al. 1995). In addition, PTSD subjects may not exhibit recall deficits for trauma-related words but rather for positive and neutral words, suggesting that avoiding the encoding of disturbing information does not occur in PTSD (McNally et al. 1998). This appears consistent with the intrusive nature of traumatic memories clinically encountered in the disorder.

Biological Theories

More than a century ago, Janet described the breakdown in normal adaptation, information processing, and action that can result from overwhelming trauma and noted the automatic emotional and physical overreaction that occurs with reexposure (van der Kolk and van der Hart 1989). Freud (1919/1955) implicated a biological basis to posttraumatic symptoms in the form of a physical fixation to the trauma. Pavlov (1927/1960) demonstrated chronic change in autonomic nervous system activity level in response to repeated traumatic exposure. Kardiner (1959) comprehensively described the phenomenology of war traumatic neurosis, identifying five cardinal features: 1) persistence of startle response, 2) fixation on the trauma, 3) atypical dream life, 4) explosive outbursts, and 5) overall constriction of the personality. He labeled this condition as a "physioneurosis," implying an interaction of psychological and biological processes, which serves as a forerunner of current psychobiological models of PTSD. Biological theories related to trauma are listed in Table 12–31.

Sympathetic System

The neurobiological response to acute stress and trauma involves the release of various stress hormones that allow the organism to respond adaptively to stress. These releases include heightened secretion of catecholamines and cortisol. When PTSD develops under severe or repeated trauma, the stress response becomes dysregulated, and chronic autonomic hyperactivity sets in. This manifests itself in the "positive" symptoms of PTSD—that is, the hyperarousal and intrusive recollections. A wide range of data supports this hypothesis. The noradrenergic system, originating in the locus coeruleus, regulates arousal. Animals

TABLE 12–31. Biological models of posttraumatic stress disorder

Limbic hyperactivity (amygdala, cingulate) and cortical hyporesponsivity (prefrontal, Broca's area) to traumatic stimuli

Hypothalamic-pituitary-adrenal axis dysregulation

Noradrenergic activation

Heightened physiological responses

Endogenous opioid dysregulation

Dysregulated serotonergic modulation

Hippocampal toxicity, decreased volumes

exposed to inescapable shock initially show evidence of increased turnover of norepinephrine, with subsequent depletion of central norepinephrine (Anisman et al. 1980). Animals that have experienced previous inescapable shock are more sensitive to norepinephrine depletion. Long-standing increases in the urinary catecholamines norepinephrine and epinephrine have been found in PTSD patients, as well as elevated plasma norepinephrine (Spivak et al. 1999). Elevated CSF norepinephrine has also been identified in men with chronic PTSD compared with control subjects (Geracioti et al. 2001). Agents that stimulate the arousal system, such as lactate (Rainey et al. 1987) and yohimbine (Southwick et al. 1997), induce flashbacks and increases in core PTSD symptoms. A decrease in the number and sensitivity of α_2-adrenergic receptors, possibly as a consequence of chronic noradrenergic hyperactivity, has been reported (Perry et al. 1987). In an epidemiological community study, PTSD was associated with significantly elevated urinary catecholamine levels (Young and Breslau 2004a, 2004b).

In patients with PTSD, heightened physiological responses to stressful stimuli such as blood pressure, heart rate, respiration, galvanic skin responses, and electromyographic activity have long been documented (Kolb 1987; Pitman et al. 1987). Studies of the startle response in PTSD have reported heightened amplitude of startle in some samples but not in others (Lipschitz et al. 2005). Heart rate variability during sleep in the first month after a life-threatening trauma is greater in those who subsequently develop PTSD compared with those who do not (Mellman et al. 2004).

Endogenous Opioid System

Although in the past affective numbing was understood primarily as a psychological defense against overwhelming emotional pain, recent research has suggested a biological component to the "negative" symptoms of PTSD. Van der Kolk et al. (1984) proposed that animal models of inescapable shock may parallel the development of PTSD in humans. Animals prevented from escaping from severe stress develop a syndrome of learned helplessness (Maier and Seligman 1976) that resembles the symptoms of constricted affect, withdrawal, amotivation, and decline in functioning associated with PTSD.

Animals exposed to prolonged or repeated inescapable stress develop analgesia, which appears to be mediated by release of endogenous opiates and is blocked by the opiate antagonist naloxone (Maier et al. 1980). Similarly, it is suggested that in humans who have sustained prolonged or repeated trauma, endogenous opiates are readily released with any stimulus that is reminiscent of the original trauma, leading to analgesia and psychic numbing (van der Kolk et al. 1984). Pitman et al. (1990) compared pain intensity with thermal stimuli in Vietnam veterans with PTSD and veterans without PTSD who were watching a war videotape. PTSD patients, but not control subjects, had a 30% analgesia when pretreated with a placebo injection; this analgesia was eliminated with naloxone pretreatment. On the basis of such findings, the concept of trauma addiction has been proposed (van der Kolk et al. 1984). After a transient opioid burst upon reexposure to traumatic stimuli, accompanied by a subjective sense of calm and control, opiate withdrawal may set in. This withdrawal may then contribute to the hyperarousal symptoms of PTSD, leading the individual to a vicious cycle of traumatic reexposures in order to gain transient symptomatic relief. The noradrenergic and opiatergic systems of the brain interact and may serve reciprocal functions.

Serotonergic System

The serotonergic system has also been implicated in the symptomatology of PTSD (van der Kolk and Saporta 1991), although such work is still in its infancy. The septohippocampal brain system contains serotonergic pathways and mediates behavioral inhibition and constraint. The role of serotonergic deficit in impulsive aggression has been studied extensively. In animals, repeated inescapable shock can lead to serotonin depletion. Thus, the irritability and outbursts seen in patients with PTSD may be related to serotonergic deficit. The partial serotonin agonist m-CPP induces an increase in PTSD symptoms suggestive of a sensitized serotonergic system, and interestingly, this appears to be a separate subgroup of PTSD subjects from the ones exhibiting noradrenergic sensitization (Southwick et al. 1997). A blunted prolactin response to fenfluramine challenge is supportive of central serotonergic dysregulation in PTSD (Davis et al. 1999). A PET study of 5-HT$_{1A}$ receptor binding found no change in PTSD (Bonne et al. 2005). The efficacy of SSRIs in PTSD is also indirectly supportive of dysregulated serotonergic modulation in PTSD.

Hypothalamic-Pituitary-Adrenal Axis

A number of findings in PTSD have implicated a chronic dysregulation of HPA axis functioning that is highly characteristic of this disorder and distinct from that seen in other psychiatric disorders such as depression. The findings include elevated CSF corticotropin-releasing hormone (Bremner et al. 1997a), low urinary cortisol (Mason et al. 1986) and an elevated urinary norepinephrine/cortisol ratio (Mason et al. 1988), a blunted adrenocorticotropic hormone response to CRF (Smith et al. 1989), enhanced suppression of cortisol after dexamethasone administration, and decrease in lymphocyte glucocorticoid receptor number. These findings are consistent with a model of a highly sensitized HPA axis that is hyperresponsive to stress and the effects of cortisol (Yehuda et al. 1995).

However, not all studies of the HPA axis in PTSD are consistent with this profile, and a number of conflicting studies suggest that the patterns of HPA axis dysregulation in PTSD may have considerable heterogeneity and depend on various factors in addition to simple diagnosis. For example, clinical and community samples have revealed absence of lower basal concentration or enhanced suppression of cortisol (Lindley et al. 2005), normal peripheral and elevated CSF cortisol levels (Baker et al. 2005), normal ambient salivary cortisol levels (Young and Breslau 2004b), and normal urinary cortisol levels (Young and Breslau 2004a).

Neuropeptides

One study found significantly elevated basal CSF substance P in PTSD patients compared with control subjects, and under traumatic symptom provocation, but not after neutral provocation, there was a marked increase in CSF substance P (Geracioti et al. 2006). Another study found that neuropeptide Y plasma concentrations were associated with degree of symptom improvement, lower combat exposure, and positive coping (Yehuda et al. 2006).

Brain Neuroanatomy and Neurocircuitry

Structural neuroimaging findings in PTSD have generally reported smaller volumes in brain structures involved in the modulation of emotion and memory. The most consistent findings relate to the hippocampus, with numerous studies reporting decreased hippocampal volume in adults with PTSD, including combat veterans (Bremner et al. 1995), adult survivors of childhood abuse (Bremner et al. 1997b), and police officers (Lindauer et al. 2004), to name a few. A meta-analysis of nine studies that examined hippocampal volume in PTSD, in a total of 133 patients, found decreased right and left volumes compared with traumatized and nontraumatized control subjects (Kitayama et al. 2005). However, one large study in children with PTSD found larger hippocampi, controlling for total brain volume, compared with matched non-PTSD control subjects (Tupler and DeBellis 2006). To further complicate matters, smaller hippocampi have been found in monozygotic twins of veterans with PTSD who were not exposed to combat. Smaller hippocampi have also been found in comparable groups exposed to the extreme stress of large burns, regardless of PTSD presence (Winter and Irle 2004). At this point, then, it remains unclear to what degree smaller hippocampi constitute a preexisting vulnerability to PTSD, what the developmental determinants are, or if smaller hippocampi are an outcome of traumatic stress or PTSD illness itself or its chronicity. Deficits in verbal memory have been correlated with decreased hippocampal volume in some (Bremner et al. 1995) but not all PTSD studies. Decreased anterior cingulate volume has also been reported in PTSD, consistent with the general model of diminished ventromedial cortical inhibition (Woodward et al. 2006).

Functional neuroimaging studies have generated a model suggestive of limbic sensitization and diminished cortical inhibition in PTSD, with specific dysfunction in brain areas involved in memory, emotion, and visuospatial processing (Bremner et al. 1999). PET imaging with PTSD symptom provocation using audiotaped traumatic scripts showed activation of the right limbic and paralimbic systems and of the visual cortex (Rauch et al. 1996). PET imaging during auditory exposure to traumatic scripts has shown that abuse memories are associated with decreased blood flow in the medial prefrontal cortex, hippocampus, and visual association cortex (Bremner et al. 1999). When mental images of combat-related pictures are generated by PTSD veterans, blood flow increases in the amygdala and anterior cingulate and decreases in Broca's area. These patterns may relate to the nonverbal emotional visual imagery involved in reexperiencing PTSD symptoms (Shin et al. 1997). Enhanced amygdala activation to general negative stimuli, as well as to traumatic stimuli, has been reported in several PTSD studies, and this amygdala hyperactivation is dissociated from higher cortical inhibitory influences as evidenced by diminished medial prefrontal cortical activation (Phan et al. 2006a; Rauch et al. 2000; Shin et al. 2004, 2005). Furthermore, a reciprocal relationship has been shown between prefrontal cortex and amygdalar activation, as well as a relationship of PTSD symptom severity to amygdala overactivation and prefrontal cortex hypoactivation (Shin et al. 2004). On the other hand, absence of ventromedial prefrontal cortex deactivation in traumatized non-PTSD control subjects may be a compensatory, protective change in brain function after trauma (Phan et al. 2006a). The exaggerated amygdalar response to emotional stimuli has also been found to be present early in the course of acute PTSD (Armony et al. 2005). Exposure of PTSD subjects to traumatic stimuli results in decreased blood flow in the medial prefrontal cortex, an area responsible for the regulation of emotional response via inhibition of the amygdala (Bremner et al. 1999). In contrast to the relative deactivation of prefrontal and cingulate regions in PTSD reported in response to threatening stimuli, anterior cingulate responses to nonthreatening stimuli may be enhanced, indicative of a generalized hypervigilance (Bryant 2005). Furthermore, it has been shown that PTSD patients who respond to traumatic scripts with dissociation versus arousal/intrusions manifest different patterns of brain activation (Lanius et al. 2005).

Imaging studies before and after treatment in PTSD are not many, but some compelling findings are emerging. The animal literature does show that antidepressants promote hippocampal neurogenesis. In adult patients with PTSD, treatment with an SSRI for 1 year resulted in a 5% increase in hippocampal volume along with a 35% improvement in declarative memory (Bremner and Vermetten 2004; Vermetten et al. 2003). There is limited evidence that successful treatment of PTSD with eye movement desensitization and reprocessing may result not in reduced limbic activity but rather in increased cingulate and prefrontal activity, which enhances the ability to differentiate real threat (Levin et al. 1999).

Genetics

A large study of Vietnam veteran twins found that genetic factors accounted for 13%–34% of the variance in liability to the various PTSD symptom clusters, whereas no etiological role was found for shared environment (True et al. 1993). Molecular genetic studies of PTSD are very few. An initial study found an as-

sociation with a polymorphism of the dopamine D_2 receptor (Comings et al. 1996), not replicated later (J. Gelernter et al. 1999). Similar to mood and other anxiety disorders, the short allele genotype of the serotonin transporter gene has been preliminarily implicated in PTSD (H.J. Lee et al. 2005).

Course and Prognosis

The course and prognosis of PTSD are summarized in Table 12–32.

Scrignar (1984) divided the clinical course of PTSD into three stages. Stage I involves the response to trauma. Nonsusceptible persons may experience an adrenergic surge of symptoms immediately after the trauma but do not dwell on the incident. Predisposed persons have higher levels of anxiety and dissociation at baseline, an exaggerated response to the trauma, and an obsessive preoccupation with it following the trauma. If symptoms persist beyond 4–6 weeks, the patient enters Stage II, or acute PTSD. Feelings of helplessness and loss of control, symptoms of increased autonomic arousal, reliving of the trauma, and somatic symptoms may occur. The patient's life becomes centered around the trauma, with subsequent changes in lifestyle, personality, and social functioning. Phobic avoidance, startle responses, and angry outbursts may occur. In Stage III, chronic PTSD develops, with disability, demoralization, and despondency. The patient's emphasis changes from preoccupation with the actual trauma to preoccupation with the physical disability resulting from the trauma. Somatic symptoms, chronic anxiety, and depression are common complications at this time, as are substance abuse, disturbed family relations, and unemployment. Some patients may focus on compensation and lawsuits.

It is important to be aware that PTSD can often be a very chronic condition. A large prospective longitudinal study of adolescents and young adults found that about half showed no significant remission of their PTSD symptoms over a 3- to 4-year period (Perkonigg et al. 2005). Factors associated with a more chronic course were comorbid anxiety and somatoform disorders, greater avoidant symptoms at baseline, and experiencing new traumatic events during the interim period. In another study, the full remission rate from chronic PTSD over a 5-year prospectively studied period was only 18%, highlighting the frequent chronicity of the illness; history of alcohol abuse and childhood trauma were associated with less remission (Zlotnick et al. 1999). Even when correcting for comorbid psychiatric or medical disorders, people with PTSD manifest significant impairment in major do-

TABLE 12–32. Course and prognosis of posttraumatic stress disorder (PTSD)

Course

80% longer than 3 months

75% longer than 6 months

50% 2 years' duration

Outcome

Minority can remain symptomatic for years or decades

Predictors of worse outcome

Greater number of PTSD symptoms

Psychiatric history of other anxiety and mood disorders

Higher numbing or hyperarousal to stressors

Comorbid medical illnesses

Female sex

Childhood trauma

Alcohol abuse

TABLE 12–33. Differential diagnosis of posttraumatic stress disorder (PTSD)

Depression after trauma (numbing and avoidance may be present, but not hyperarousal and intrusive symptoms)

Panic disorder if the panic attacks are not limited to reminders/triggers of the trauma

Generalized anxiety (may have similar symptoms to PTSD hyperarousal)

Agoraphobia (if avoidance not directly trauma related)

Specific phobia (if avoidance not directly trauma related)

Adjustment disorder (usually less severe stressor and different symptoms)

Acute stress disorder (if less than 1 month has elapsed since trauma)

Dissociative disorders (if prominent dissociative symptoms)

Factitious disorders or malingering (especially if there could be apparent secondary gain)

mains of living such as physical limitations, unemployment, poor physical health, and diminished well-being; it is therefore crucial in multiply afflicted patients to specifically identify and target PTSD (Zatzick et al. 1997).

Diagnosis

The diagnosis of PTSD is usually not difficult if there is a clear history of exposure to a traumatic event, followed by symptoms of intense anxiety lasting at least 1 month, with arousal and stimulation of the autonomic nervous system, numbing of responsiveness, and avoidance or reexperiencing of the traumatic event. However, a wide variety of anxiety, depressive, somatic, and behavioral symptoms for which the relationship between their onset and the traumatic event is less clear-cut may easily lead to misdiagnosis.

Differential Diagnosis

The differential diagnosis of PTSD is described in Table 12–33.

Organic Mental Disorders

Following acute physical traumas, head trauma, or concussion, an organic mental disorder must be ruled out, because this diagnosis has important treatment implications. Mild concussions may leave no immediate apparent neurological signs but may have residual long-term effects on mood and concentration. A careful evaluation of the nature of the head trauma, including medical records and witnesses' observations, followed by mental status evaluation, neurological examination, and, if indicated, laboratory examinations, is essential in a diagnostic workup. Malnutrition may occur during prolonged stressful periods and may also lead to organic brain syndromes. Survivors of death camps may have symptoms of an organic mental disorder such as failing memory, difficulty concentrating, emotional lability, headaches, and vertigo. Other causes of organic mental disorder may occasionally mimic PTSD if anxiety, depression, personality changes, or abnormal behaviors are present. Abnormalities of cognition, memory, altered sensorium or level of consciousness, or focal neurological signs would suggest an organic mental disorder.

Organic mental disorders that could mimic PTSD include organic personality syndrome, delirium, amnestic syndrome, organic hallucinosis, or organic intoxication and withdrawal states. In addition, patients with PTSD may cope through excessive use of alcohol, drugs, caffeine, or tobacco and thus may present with a combination of organic and psychological factors. In this case, each concomitant disorder should be diagnosed.

Mood and Anxiety Disorders

Major depression. There is much overlap between PTSD and major mood disorders. Symptoms such as psychic numbing, irritability, sleep disturbance, fatigue, anhedonia, impairments in family and social relationships, anger, concern with physical health, and pessimistic outlook may occur in both disorders. In some veteran outreach populations, 70%–80% of patients meet diagnostic criteria for both disorders. Major depression is a frequent complication of PTSD; when it occurs, it must be treated aggressively, because comorbidity carries an increased risk of suicide. If major depression develops secondary to PTSD, both disorders should be diagnosed. Dysthymic symptoms are frequently secondary to PTSD, but if of sufficient severity, the additional diagnosis of dysthymic disorder should be made.

Phobic disorders. Following a traumatic event, patients may be aversively conditioned to the surroundings of the trauma and develop a phobia of objects, surroundings, or situations that remind them of the trauma itself. Phobic patients experience anxiety in the feared situation, whereas avoidance is accompanied by anxiety reduction that reinforces the avoidant behavior. In PTSD, the phobia may be symptomatically similar to specific phobia, but the nature of the precipitant and the symptom cluster of PTSD distinguish this condition from simple phobia.

Generalized anxiety disorder. The symptoms of GAD, such as motor tension, autonomic hyperactivity, apprehensive expectation, and vigilance and scanning, are also present in PTSD. However, the onset and course of the illness differ: GAD has an insidious or gradual onset and a course that fluctuates with environmental stressors, whereas PTSD has an acute onset often followed by a chronic course. Phobic symptoms, which are absent in GAD, are often present in PTSD. DSM-IV-TR does not allow for the diagnosis of GAD if PTSD is present.

Panic disorder. Patients with PTSD may also experience panic attacks. In some patients, panic attacks predate the PTSD or do not occur exclusively in the context of stimuli reminiscent of the traumatic event. In some patients, however, panic attacks develop after the PTSD and are cued solely by traumatic stimuli.

Adjustment disorder. Adjustment disorders are maladaptive reactions to identifiable psychosocial pressures. Signs and symptoms may include a wide variety of disturbances and emerge within 3 months of the stressful event. If symptoms are of sufficient severity to meet other Axis I criteria, then the diagnosis of adjustment disorder is not made. Adjustment disorder differs from PTSD in that the stressor is usually less severe and within the range of common experience, and the characteristic symptoms of PTSD, such as reexperiencing the trauma, are absent. The prognosis of full recovery in adjustment disorder is usually excellent.

Compensation neurosis (factitious disorder and malingering). Both factitious disorder and malingering involve conscious deception and feigning of illness, although the motivation for each condition differs. Factitious disorder may present with physical or psychological symptoms; the feigning of symptoms is under voluntary control, and the motivation is to assume the "patient" role. Chronic factitious disorder with physical symptoms (i.e., Munchausen's syndrome) involves frequent doctor visits and surgical interventions. PTSD differs from this by its absence of fabricated symptoms, acute onset after a trauma, and absence of a bizarre pretraumatic medical history.

Malingering involves the conscious fabrication of an illness for the purpose of achieving a definite goal such as money, compensation, and so forth. Malingerers often reveal an inconsistent history, unexpected symptom clusters, a history of antisocial behavior and substance abuse, and chaotic lifestyle, and there is often a discrepancy between history, claimed distress, and objective data.

Postconcussion syndrome. Mental disorders secondary to head injury are influenced by physiological, psychological, and environmental factors. Psychological symptoms are extremely common after mild closed head injuries, even without loss of consciousness. The so-called postconcussion syndrome comprises the symptoms of headache, dizziness, irritability, and emotional lability after a head injury with concussion. Depression and lethargy are the affective symptoms that occur most commonly. These symptoms bear no relation to the degree of physical injury.

Treatment

Pharmacotherapy

A variety of different psychopharmacological agents have been used in the treatment of PTSD by clinicians and reported in the literature as case reports, open clinic trials, and controlled studies. These are summarized in the following sections; in recent years, SSRIs and other serotonergic agents have emerged as the first-line pharmacological treatment of PTSD (Table 12–34).

Serotonin reuptake inhibitors. SSRIs have become established as first-line medications for PTSD treatment (D.J. Stein et al. 2006). Several initial open trials of fluoxetine had reported marked improvement in PTSD symptoms at a wide range of dosages (Davidson et al. 1991; McDougle et al. 1991b; Shay 1992). Subsequently, in a double-blind trial comparing fluoxetine and placebo, fluoxetine led to a significant reduction of PTSD symptomatology, especially for arousal and numbing symptoms (van der Kolk et al. 1994). Currently, sertraline is FDA approved for the treatment of PTSD, after two large controlled trials documented its efficacy. In a 12-week multicenter placebo-controlled trial, sertraline at dosages of 50–200 mg/day resulted in significant benefits that began to manifest by week 2. The responder rate was more than 50%, and improvement in both numbing and arousal symptoms, but not reexperiencing, was significantly greater with sertraline than with placebo (Brady et al. 2000). Very similar results were reported in another large multicenter sertraline study with very similar design (Davidson et al. 2001), with a 60% responder rate. Sertraline has also been shown to prevent relapse during a double-blind 6-month discontinuation study (Davidson et al. 2001).

Open trials of fluvoxamine (De Boer et al. 1992; Neylan et al. 2001) have also reported efficacy. A randomized, controlled trial of paroxetine, 20–40 mg/day, in 186 adults with chronic PTSD showed significant improvement in all three symptom clusters compared with placebo, as well as better social and occupational functioning (R.D. Marshall et al. 2001). An open citalopram trial reported more modest efficacy, with 42% of treated patients experiencing at least a 30% symptom improvement (English et al. 2006).

Newer serotonergic antidepressants other than SSRIs may also be beneficial. A controlled comparison of venlafaxine extended-release (mean dosage, 225 mg/day), sertraline (150 mg/day), and placebo reported modest benefits, with response rates of 30%, 24%, and 20%, respectively (Davidson et al. 2006). A randomized comparison of mirtazapine (mean dosage, 34 mg/day) and sertraline (100 mg/day) reported comparable outcomes at 6 weeks, with large reductions in PTSD symptoms (Chung et al. 2004). A small double-blind trial of mirtazapine monotherapy, at

TABLE 12–34. Pharmacotherapy of posttraumatic stress disorder (PTSD)

Selective serotonin reuptake inhibitors (SSRIs)

General indications: First-line treatment; well-tolerated; once/day dosing; documented efficacy.

Sertraline: U.S. Food and Drug Administration–approved, large controlled trials
Other SSRIs: similar efficacy
Venlafaxine, mirtazapine

Other antidepressants

Tricyclic antidepressants: overall modest results when tested in double-blind fashion
Monoamine oxidase inhibitors: may be superior to tricyclics, especially for intrusive symptoms

Other medications

General indications: When response to first-line options not adequate; additional treatment of specific PTSD symptoms or comorbid disorders.

Prazosin: nightmares and daytime intrusions
Atypical antipsychotics: several studies documenting some benefit
Clonidine: some efficacy in open treatment
Lithium: improvement in intrusive symptoms and irritability in open trial
Anticonvulsants (carbamazepine, valproate, lamotrigine, tiagabine, topiramate, levetiracetam, dilantin): mostly open trials showing some efficacy
Buspirone: efficacy in an open trial
Triiodothyronine: improvement in small open trial, possibly antidepressant response
Trazodone, benzodiazepines, diphenhydramine: sleep disturbance

dosages up to 45 mg/day, reported a responder rate of 65%, significantly higher than the 20% placebo responder rate (Davidson et al. 2003).

There may also be benefit to continuing SSRI treatment beyond the initial 6-month period; one double-blind discontinuation study found that relapse on placebo was about 3.5 times greater than during continued fluoxetine treatment (Davidson et al. 2005).

Tricyclic antidepressants. A positive effect of imipramine on posttraumatic night terrors was reported by J.R. Marshall (1975). Controlled studies of TCAs in PTSD have not overall reported much success in decreasing posttraumatic symptoms. In a 4-week double-blind, crossover study of desipramine and placebo in 18 veterans with PTSD, only depressive symptoms improved; anxiety, intrusive symptoms, and avoidance did not change with desipramine therapy (Reist et al. 1989). Davidson et al. (1990) conducted a 4- to 8-week double-blind comparison of amitriptyline and placebo in 46 veterans with PTSD. Although depression and anxiety decreased, decrease in intrusive and avoidant symptoms was apparent only in a subgroup of patients who completed 8 weeks of amitriptyline and was marginal; at the end of the study, roughly two-thirds of patients in both treatment groups still met criteria for PTSD.

Monoamine oxidase inhibitors. An early study of MAOIs described five cases of "traumatic war neurosis" in whom phenelzine, in dosages of 45–75 mg/day, improved traumatic dreams, flashbacks, startle reactions, and violent outbursts (Hogben and Cornfield 1981). Positive effects of phenelzine on intrusive posttraumatic symptoms have been reported in subsequent small open trials (Davidson et al. 1987; van der Kolk 1983). Subsequently, an 8-week randomized, double-blind trial compared phenelzine (71 mg), imipramine (240 mg), and placebo in 34 veterans with PTSD (Frank et al. 1988) and found that phenelzine tended to be superior to imipramine. The most marked improvement with phenelzine was in intrusive symptoms, which showed a 60% average reduction.

Adrenergic blockers. Kolb et al. (1984) treated 12 Vietnam veterans with PTSD in an open trial of the β-blocker propranolol over a 6-month period. Dosage ranged from 120 to 160 mg daily. Eleven patients reported a positive change in self-assessment at the end of the 6-month period, with less explosiveness, fewer nightmares, improved sleep, and a decrease in intrusive thoughts, hyperalertness, and startle. Another open pilot study by this group (Kolb et al. 1984) using clonidine, a noradrenergic α_2 agonist, was conducted with nine Vietnam veterans with PTSD. Dosages of 0.2–0.4 mg/day of clonidine were administered over a 6-month period. Eight patients reported improvements in their capacity to control their emotions and lessened explosiveness, and a majority reported improvements in sleep and nightmares, as well as psychosocial improvement, and lowered startle, hyperalertness, and intrusive thinking. These findings support the role of noradrenergic hyperactivity in the maintenance of autonomic arousal symptoms in PTSD. In a retrospective treatment review of Cambodian patients with PTSD, Kinzie and Leung (1989) found that the majority of patients benefited from the combination of clonidine and a TCA as opposed to either medication taken alone.

Recently, the α_1-adrenergic antagonist prazosin has emerged as a very promising agent in the treatment of PTSD. Evidence supporting its use is mostly available for bedtime administration, but benefits can also occur for daytime symptoms. In an initial 6-week trial of prazosin in 5 patients given 1–4 mg/day, all showed moderate to marked improvement in PTSD, with at least moderate improvement of nightmares (F. B. Taylor and Raskind 2002). In a double-blind, placebo-controlled crossover trial, 10 war veterans were treated with bedtime prazosin at a mean dosage of 10 mg/day, resulting in significant improvement in nightmares, difficulty falling and staying asleep, and overall PTSD severity (Raskind et al. 2003). More recently, pilot use of prazosin during the day in an open trial revealed possible clinical benefit with decreased psychological distress to trauma cues (F.B. Taylor et al. 2006).

There is also recent interest in using β-blockers in the acute aftermath of a trauma in order to diminish the consolidation of traumatic memories and attenuate the course of posttraumatic symptoms and evolving PTSD. A small nonrandomized study provided evidence that patients who were treated with propranolol (40 mg tid for 7 days) shortly after trauma exposure fared better 2 months later with regard to PTSD symptoms than those who refused acute propranolol treatment. In a randomized study of about 40 patients, propranolol 40 mg qid or placebo was administered for 10 days within 6 hours of the trauma. PTSD symptoms were assessed 1 month posttrauma, and it appeared that propranolol may have a preventive effect, although findings were not very robust (Pitman et al. 2002).

Mood stabilizers and anticonvulsants. In a small open trial of lithium for treating PTSD, van der Kolk (1983) reported improvement in intrusive recollections and irritability in more than half of the patients treated. However, there have been no controlled trials. In an open trial of carbamazepine in 10 patients with PTSD, Lipper et al. (1986) reported moderate to great improvement in intrusive symptoms in 7 patients. Wolf et al. (1988) reported decreased impulsivity and angry outbursts in 10 veterans who were also treated with carbamazepine; all patients had normal electroencephalograms. Valproic acid was initially reported to decrease irritability and angry outbursts in two veterans with PTSD (Szymanski and Olympia 1991). An open trial of 16 patients treated openly with valproate for 8 weeks reported a significant decrease in hyperarousal and intrusion but not numbing (R.D. Clark et al. 1999b), whereas another 8-week open trial of valproate monotherapy reported no benefits (Otte et al. 2004). In a very small placebo-controlled trial of lamotrigine at dosages up to 500 mg/day, more patients appeared to respond to lamotrigine (Hertzberg et al. 1999); this finding warrants larger studies of lamotrigine. Tiagabine was also reported effective in a 12-week acute treatment trial, with increasing likelihood of remission during continuation treatment (Connor et al. 2006b), as well as in a case series at a mean dosage of 8 mg/day (F.B. Taylor 2003). Levetiracetam was reported to be an effective augmentation, with a 56% responder rate in a retrospective analysis of patients with treatment-resistant PTSD (Kinrys et al. 2006). Topiramate also looked promising in treating PTSD in one open trial of 33 civilians with chronic nonhallucinatory PTSD; at a median dosage of 50 mg/day about three-fourths of patients were rated as responders after 4 weeks, with a rapid median response interval of 9 days (Berlant 2004). Dilantin was reported effective in one open 12-week trial in 9 adult patients (Bremner and Vermetten 2004).

Other medications. A small open trial of buspirone reported that seven of eight patients experienced a significant reduction in PTSD symptoms, but there are no controlled studies (Duffy and Malloy 1994). In a small open trial, triiodothyronine was reported to result in significant clinical improvement in four of five PTSD patients who had only partial responses to SSRIs; however, it remains unclear whether this was not primarily an antidepressant response (Agid et al. 2001). Cyproheptadine has been reported to greatly decrease the nightmares characteristic of PTSD (R.D. Clark et al. 1999a; Gupta et al. 1998). An open trial of bupropion in PTSD reported global improvement secondary to decreased depression, but PTSD symptoms remained mostly unchanged (Canive et al. 1998).

Atypical antipsychotics can also be useful in treating PTSD. Quetiapine may be helpful in improving the sleep disturbance associated with the disorder (Robert et al. 2005). An open trial with risperidone, 2–4 mg/day, in veterans with psychotic PTSD led to an overall improvement of both PTSD and psychotic symptoms (Kozaric-Kovacic et al. 2005). A small 8-week placebo-controlled risperidone trial in women with PTSD related to childhood abuse reported a significant improvement in intrusive and arousal symptoms. A larger, placebo-controlled augmentation trial using risperidone to treat chronic PTSD also reported beneficial reductions in symptoms of PTSD, anxiety, and psychotic-spectrum positive symptoms (Bartzokis et al. 2005). An open quetiapine augmentation trial, using a mean dosage of 100 mg/day, resulted in an approximately 25% decline in PTSD symptom severity (Hamner et al. 2003).

Low-dosage cortisol has also been tried in treating PTSD, but not enough is known yet about guidelines and recommendations. In one study using a double-blind crossover design, three patients with chronic PTSD received cortisol 10 mg/day for 1 month. The cortisol treatment resulted in a moderate decline in traumatic memories and reexperiencing symptoms (Aerni et al. 2004).

Transcranial magnetic stimulation. TMS was found to have some transient efficacy in decreasing core PTSD symptoms in 10 patients treated openly (Grisaru et al. 1998). In a randomized and blinded study, 24 PTSD patients were assigned to high-frequency, low-frequency, or sham TMS to the right dorsolateral prefrontal cortex for a total of 10 sessions; the high-frequency group showed marked improvement in PTSD core symptoms and in anxiety (H. Cohen et al. 2004).

Psychotherapy

General principles. It is generally agreed that some form of psychotherapy is necessary in the treatment of posttraumatic pathology. Crisis intervention shortly after the traumatic event is effective in reducing immediate distress and possibly preventing chronic or delayed responses, and if the pathological response is still tentative, it may allow for briefer intervention.

Brief dynamic psychotherapy has been advocated both as an immediate treatment procedure and as a way of preventing chronic disorder. The therapist must establish a working alliance that allows the patient to work through his or her reactions.

The literature has suggested that persons with disrupted early attachments or abuse who have been traumatized earlier in their lives are more likely to develop PTSD than those with stable backgrounds. The occurrence of psychic trauma in a person's past may psychologically and biologically predispose him or her to respond excessively and maladaptively to intense experiences and affects (Herman et al. 1989; Krystal 1968; van der Kolk 1987b). Therefore, attempting to modify preexisting conflicts, developmental difficulties, and defensive styles that render the person especially vulnerable to traumatization by particular experiences is central to the treatment of traumatic syndromes.

The "phase oriented" treatment model suggested by Horowitz (1976) strikes a balance between initial supportive interventions to minimize the traumatic state and increasingly aggressive "working through" at later stages of treatment. Establishment of a safe and communicative relationship, reappraisal of the traumatic event, revision of the patient's inner model of self and world, and planning for termination with a re-experiencing of loss are all important therapeutic issues in the treatment of PTSD. Herman et al. (1989) emphasized the importance of validating the patient's traumatic experiences as a precondition for reparation of damaged self-identity.

Embry (1990) outlined seven major parameters for effective psychotherapy in war veterans with chronic PTSD: 1) initial rapport building, 2) limit setting and supportive confrontation, 3) affective modeling, 4) defocusing on stress and focusing on current life events, 5) sensitivity to transference/countertransference issues, 6) understanding of secondary gain, and 7) therapist's maintenance of a positive treatment attitude.

Group psychotherapy can also serve as an important adjunctive treatment, or as the central treatment mode, in traumatized patients (van der Kolk 1987a). Because of past experiences, such patients are often mistrustful and reluctant to depend on authority figures, whereas the identification, support, and hopefulness of peer settings can facilitate therapeutic change.

Drug treatment has been impressionistically reported to have a positive impact on psychotherapy in 70% of cases, with improvements in symptom severity leading to a more positive and motivated approach to psychotherapy and an enhancement of accessibility to uncovering and working through (Bleich et al. 1986).

Cognitive and Behavioral Therapies

A variety of cognitive and behavioral techniques have gained increasing popularity and validation in the treatment of PTSD (Table 12–35).

People involved in traumatic events such as accidents frequently develop phobias or phobic anxiety related to or associated with these situations. When a phobia or phobic anxiety is associated with PTSD, systematic desensitization or graded exposure has been found to be effective. This is based on the principle that when patients are gradually exposed to a phobic or anxiety-provoking stimulus, they will become habituated or deconditioned to the stimulus. Variations of this treatment include using imaginal techniques (i.e., imaginal desensitization) and exposure to real-life situations (i.e., in vivo desensitization). Prolonged exposure, a form of extended repeat exposure to the same traumatic memory over a series of sessions, if tolerated, is an effective technique first reported to be successful in the treatment of Vietnam veterans (Fairbank and Keane 1982) and has become established as a first-line treatment of PTSD (Foa et al. 2000). Virtual reality exposure is another computer-based exposure tech-

TABLE 12–35. Cognitive and behavioral approaches to treating posttraumatic stress disorder

Graded exposure (imaginal and/or in vivo)

Prolonged exposure

Virtual reality exposure

Cognitive reprocessing

Stress inoculation training

Hypnosis

Affect management

Eye movement desensitization and reprocessing

nique that has been piloted in Vietnam veterans and appears promising (Rothbaum et al. 2001).

Relaxation techniques produce the beneficial physiological result of reducing motor tension and lowering the activity of the autonomic nervous system, effects that may be particularly efficacious in PTSD. Progressive muscle relaxation involves contracting and relaxing various muscle groups to induce the relaxation response. This is useful for symptoms of autonomic arousal such as somatic symptoms, anxiety, and insomnia. Hypnosis has also been used to induce the relaxation response with success in PTSD. Relaxation, combined with elements of distraction, thought-stopping, and self-guided dialogue, is a technique known as stress inoculation training.

Cognitive therapy, also referred to as cognitive reprocessing or restructuring, involves various cognitive formulations and corrections of patients' traumatic recollections—that is, identifying distorted and maladaptive cognitions and replacing them with more realistic ones (Resick et al. 2002). Cognitive processing therapy was shown to be more efficacious than waitlist control in a study of women with childhood sexual abuse (Chard 2005).

Numerous studies have documented the effectiveness of all of these psychotherapies in treating PTSD. Generally speaking, exposure and cognitive processing have overall comparable effectiveness. A randomized trial comparing imaginal exposure with cognitive therapy in 72 patients with chronic PTSD (Tarrier et al. 1999) found comparable significant improvement, although not complete remission, with the two treatments. Another controlled study in 87 patients with chronic PTSD compared exposure therapy, cognitive restructuring, their combination, and simple relaxation techniques; both the behavioral and the cognitive treatment resulted in marked improvement, with gains maintained after 6 months, whereas their combination was of no additional benefit and relaxation treatment yielded only modest improvement (Marks et al. 1998). In another study, exposure therapy, stress inoculation training, their combination, and a control waiting list were compared in assaulted women with chronic PTSD; all three active treatments resulted in comparable improvement, and the gains were maintained during up to 1-year follow-up (Foa et al. 1999). In yet another treatment study of female rape victims, both prolonged exposure and cognitive processing led to comparable PTSD improvement compared with a "minimal attention" intervention, with cognitive therapy demonstrating somewhat better outcome for guilt reduction (Resick et al. 2002).

The question of whether the addition of a cognitive restructuring component further enhances prolonged exposure therapy is an issue on which not everyone agrees. A study of 58 civilians with PTSD found that both exposure alone and exposure combined with cognitive restructuring had better outcome than a supportive counseling control intervention, yet the combined treatment led to greater reduction in PTSD symptoms and in maladaptive cognitions than exposure alone (Bryant et al. 2003). However, another similar study of 171 female assault survivors compared two active treatments, prolonged exposure alone and prolonged exposure plus cognitive restructuring, with a wait-list control and found that adding cognitive restructuring did not enhance the effectiveness of the exposure (Foa et al. 2005a). Importantly for clinicians, the study also reported that CBT conducted by therapists with minimal CBT experience was just as effective as that conducted by CBT experts.

A meta-analysis of randomized, controlled psychotherapy trials for PTSD (Bisson and Andrew 2005) concluded, overall, that both trauma-focused CBT and stress management therapy were significantly more effective than non–trauma focused usual-care therapies or wait-list assignment.

CBT appears to also be highly beneficial for children and adolescents. In an open trial of CBT in 17 children with PTSD, more than half no longer met disorder criteria after treatment and were doing even better at 6-month follow-up (March et al. 1998a). A more recent large multisite randomized, controlled trial for children with sexual abuse–related PTSD compared trauma-focused CBT with standard child-centered therapy and found that the former was markedly more beneficial in treating PTSD, depression, behavior problems, shame, and abuse-related attributions (J. A. Cohen et al. 2004).

Other Psychotherapies

In addition to the more mainstream prolonged exposure, cognitive processing, and relaxation techniques, other psychotherapeutic approaches can be helpful in PTSD. Brief eclectic psychotherapy is a manualized therapy found effective in police officers in a randomized trial (Lindauer et al. 2005). Imagery rehearsal therapy, delivered over only three sessions to a very large sample of 168 women with histories of assault or sexual abuse, resulted in a marked decrease in chronic nightmares (Krakow et al. 2001). Another approach, affect management, also appears to be beneficial; in a randomized study of adult women with PTSD and childhood sexual abuse who were already receiving individual psychotherapy and pharmacotherapy, those who underwent a 3-month course of group affect-management treatment demonstrated significantly fewer PTSD and dissociative symptoms after the treatment (Zlotnick et al. 1997). A pilot open trial of interpersonal psychotherapy adapted for treating PTSD also reported benefits (Bleiberg and Markowitz 2005).

Eye movement desensitization and reprocessing (EMDR) is a technique that has been extensively applied to the treatment of trauma-related pathology. There continues to be some controversy in the literature regarding the efficacy of EMDR as well as its underlying mechanisms of action. In a 5-year follow-up study of a small group of veterans who had initially been treated with EMDR with modest benefits, all benefit was lost at follow-up (Macklin et al. 2000). EMDR was found to be superior to relaxation in treating PTSD in one study (Carlson et al. 1998). A randomized study comparing EMDR with CBT found that CBT was significantly more effective, and its superiority became even more apparent at 3-month follow-up (Devilly and Spence 1999). Comparable efficacy between EMDR and prolonged exposure with stress inoculation was found by another study (C. Lee et al. 2002). Another study comparing exposure therapy, EMDR, and relaxation training found similar reductions in anger and guilt at the end of treatment and at 3-month follow-up (Stapleton et al. 2006).

Key Points

- Anxiety disorders are prevalent in the general population, with lifetime prevalence ranging from about 2%–3% for panic disorder and OCD to 15% for social anxiety disorder.

- Anxiety disorders are highly treatable: medication and CBT constitute first-line treatments for all these disorders.

- The "neurocircuitry of fear" has been implicated in all anxiety disorders except for OCD, in which there is evidence of a hyperactive orbitofrontal-limbic-basal ganglia-thalamic circuitry.

- Serotonin reuptake inhibitors are the first-line treatment for all anxiety disorders.

- Exposure, relaxation, and cognitive restructuring are the main types of psychotherapies helpful in treating the anxiety disorders.

Suggested Readings

Barlow DH: Clinical Handbook of Psychological Disorders: A Step-by-Step Treatment Manual, 3rd Edition. New York, Guilford, 2001

Hollander E, Bakalar N: Coping With Social Anxiety: The Definitive Guide to Effective Treatment Options. New York, Henry Holt and Company, 2005

Hollander E, Simeon D: Concise Guide to the Anxiety Disorders. Washington, DC, American Psychiatric Publishing, 2003

Hollander E, Stein DJ (eds): Obsessive Compulsive Disorders. New York, Marcel Dekker, 1997

Horowitz MJ: Treatment of Stress Response Syndromes. Washington, DC, American Psychiatric Publishing, 2003

Stein DJ, Hollander E: The American Psychiatric Publishing Textbook of Anxiety Disorders. Washington, DC, American Psychiatric Publishing, 2002

Yehuda R: Treating Trauma Survivors With PTSD. Washington, DC, American Psychiatric Publishing, 2002

References

Abbott MJ, Rapee RM: Post event rumination and negative self appraisal in social phobia before and after treatment. J Abnorm Psychol 113:136–144, 2004

Abelson JL, Glitz D, Cameron OG, et al: Blunted growth hormone response to clonidine in patients with generalized anxiety disorder. Arch Gen Psychiatry 48:157–162, 1991

Abelson JL, Weg JG, Nesse RM, et al: Persistent respiratory irregularity in patients with panic disorder. Biol Psychiatry 49:588–595, 2001

Abelson JL, Curtis GC, Sagher O, et al: Deep brain stimulation for refractory obsessive-compulsive disorder. Biol Psychiatry 57:510–516, 2005

Adams KH, Hansen ES, Pinborg LH, et al: Patients with obsessive compulsive disorder have increased 5-HT2A receptor binding in the caudate nuclei. Int J Neuropsychopharmacol 8:391–401, 2005

Adler CM, McDonough-Ryan P, Sax KW, et al: fMRI of neuronal activation with symptom provocation in unmedicated patients with obsessive compulsive disorder. J Psychiatr Res 34:317–324, 2000

Aerni A, Traber R, Hock C, et al: Low dose cortisol for symptoms of posttraumatic stress disorder. Am J Psychiatry 161:1488–1490, 2004

Agid O, Shalev AY, Lerer B: Triiodothyronine augmentation of selective serotonin reuptake inhibitors in posttraumatic stress disorder. J Clin Psychiatry 62:169–173, 2001

Aikins DE, Craske MG: Cognitive theories of generalized anxiety disorder. Psychiatr Clin North Am 24:57–74, 2001

Akhtar S, Wig NN, Varma VK, et al: A phenomenological analysis of symptoms in obsessive-compulsive neurosis. Br J Psychiatry 127:342–348, 1975

Alden LE, Wallace ST: Social phobia and social appraisal in successful and unsuccessful social interactions. Behav Res Ther 33:497–505, 1995

Allgulander C, Lavori PW: Excess mortality among 3302 patients with "pure" anxiety neurosis. Arch Gen Psychiatry 48:599–602, 1991

Allgulander C, Dahl AA, Austin C, et al: Efficacy of sertraline in a 12-week trial for generalized anxiety disorder. Am J Psychiatry 161:1642–1649, 2004

Alonso P, Pujol J, Cardoner N, et al: Right prefrontal repetitive transcranial magnetic stimulation in obsessive compulsive disorder: a double blind, placebo controlled study. Am J Psychiatry 158:1143–1144, 2001

Alsobrook JP II, Leckman JF, Goodman WK, et al: Segregation analysis of obsessive-compulsive disorder using symptom-based factor scores. Am J Med Genet 88:699–675, 1999

Altemus M, Pigott T, L'Heureux F, et al: CSF somatostatin in obsessive-compulsive disorder. Am J Psychiatry 150:460–464, 1993

Altemus M, Swedo SE, Leonard HL, et al: Changes in cerebrospinal fluid neurochemistry during treatment of obsessive-compulsive disorder with clomipramine. Arch Gen Psychiatry 51:794–803, 1994

American Psychiatric Association: Diagnostic and Statistical Manual of Mental Disorders, 2nd Edition. Washington, DC, American Psychiatric Association, 1968

American Psychiatric Association: Diagnostic and Statistical Manual of Mental Disorders, 3rd Edition. Washington, DC, American Psychiatric Association, 1980

American Psychiatric Association: Diagnostic and Statistical Manual of Mental Disorders, 3rd Edition, Revised. Washington, DC, American Psychiatric Association, 1987

American Psychiatric Association: Diagnostic and Statistical Manual of Mental Disorders, 4th Edition. Washington, DC, American Psychiatric Association, 1994

American Psychiatric Association: Diagnostic and Statistical Manual of Mental Disorders, 4th Edition, Text Revision. Washington, DC, American Psychiatric Association, 2000

Amir N, Coles ME, Brigidi B, et al: The effect of practice on recall of emotional information in individuals with generalized social phobia. J Abnorm Psychol 110:76–82, 2001

Amir N, Elias J, Klumpp H, et al: Attentional bias to threat in social phobia: facilitated processing of threat of difficulty disengaging attention from threat. Behav Res Ther 41:1325–1335, 2003

Amir N, Beard C, Przeworkski A: Resolving ambiguity: the effect on interpretation of ambiguous events in generalized social phobia. J Abnorm Psychol 114:402–408, 2005a

Amir N, Klumpp H, Elias J, et al: Increased activation of the anterior cingulated cortex during processing of disgust faces in individuals with social phobia. Biol Psychiatry 57:975–981, 2005b

Anisman HL, Pizzino A, Sklar LS: Coping with stress, norepinephrine depletion and escape performance. Brain Res 191:583–588, 1980

Antony MM, Brown TA, Barlow DH: Response to hyperventilation and 5.5% carbon dioxide inhalation of subjects with types of specific phobia, panic disorder, or no mental illness. Am J Psychiatry 154:1089–1095, 1997

Apter A, Ratzoni G, King RA, et al: Fluvoxamine open-label treatment of adolescent inpatients with obsessive-compulsive disorder or depression. J Am Acad Child Adolesc Psychiatry 33:342–348, 1994

Argyropoulos SV, Hood SD, Adrover M, et al: Tryptophan depletion reverses the therapeutic effect of selective serotonin reuptake inhibitors in social anxiety disorder. Biol Psychiatry 56:503–509, 2004

Armony JL, Corbo V, Clement MH, et al: Amygdala response in patients with cute PTSD to masked and unmasked emotional facial expressions. Am J Psychiatry 162:1961–1963, 2005

Arnold PD, Rosenberg DR, Mundo E, et al: Association of a glutamate (NMDA) subunit receptor gene (GRIN2B) with obsessive compulsive disorder: a preliminary study. Psychopharmacology 174:530–538, 2004

Arntz A: Cognitive therapy versus interoceptive exposure as treatment of panic disorder without agoraphobia. Behav Res Ther 40:325–341, 2002

Arntz A: Cognitive therapy versus applied relaxation as treatment of generalized anxiety disorder. Behav Res Ther 41:633–646, 2003

Arntz A, van den Hout M: Psychological treatments of panic disorder without agoraphobia: cognitive therapy versus applied relaxation. Behav Res Ther 34:113–121, 1996

Aschenbrand SG, Kendall PC, Webb A, et al: Is childhood separation anxiety a predictor of adult panic disorder and agoraphobia? A seven-year longitudinal study. J Am Acad Child Adolesc Psychiatry 42:1476–1485, 2003

Asnis GM, Hameedi FA, Goddard AW, et al: Fluvoxamine in the treatment of panic disorder: a multi-center, double-blind, placebo-controlled study in outpatients. Psychiatry Res 103:1–14, 2001

Aston-Jones SL, Foote FE, Bloom FE: Norepinephrine, in Frontiers of Clinical Neuroscience, Vol 2. Edited by Ziegler, Lake CR. Baltimore, MD, Williams & Wilkins, 1984, pp 92–116

Atmaca M, Kuloglu M, Tezcan E, et al: Quetiapine augmentation in patients with treatment resistant obsessive compulsive disorder: a single blind, placebo controlled study. Int Clin Psychopharmacol 17:115–119, 2002

Baer L, Jenike MA: Personality disorders in obsessive-compulsive disorder. Psychiatr Clin North Am 15:803–812, 1992

Baer L, Rauch SL, Ballantine HT, et al: Cingulotomy for intractable obsessive-compulsive disorder. Prospective long-term follow-up of 18 patients. Arch Gen Psychiatry 52:384–392, 1995

Baker DG, Ekhator NN, Kasckow JW, et al: Higher levels of basal serial CSF cortisol in combat veterans with post-traumatic stress disorder. Am J Psychiatry 162:992–994, 2005

Bakker A, van Balkom AJ, Spinhoven P: SSRIs vs. TCAs in the treatment of panic disorder: a meta-analysis. Acta Psychiatr Scand 106:163–167, 2002

Baldwin D, Bobes J, Stein DJ, et al: Paroxetine in social phobia/social anxiety disorder: a randomized, double-blind, placebo-controlled study. Br J Psychiatry 175:120–126, 1999

Ball SG, Kuhn A, Wall D, et al: Selective serotonin reuptake inhibitor treatment for generalized anxiety disorder: a double-blind, prospective comparison between paroxetine and sertraline. J Clin Psychiatry 66:94–99, 2005

Ballenger JC, Wheadon DE, Steiner M, et al: Double-blind, fixed-dose, placebo-controlled study of paroxetine in the treatment of panic disorder. Am J Psychiatry 155:36–42, 2000

Bandelow B, Spath C, Tichauer GA, et al: Early traumatic life events, parental attitudes, family history, and birth risk factors in patients with panic disorder. Compr Psychiatry 43:269–278, 2002

Bandelow B, Behnke K, Lenoir S, et al: Sertraline versus paroxetine in the treatment of panic disorder: an acute, double-blind noninferiority comparison. J Clin Psychiatry 65:405–413, 2004

Banerjee SO, Bhandari RP, Rosenberg DR: Use of low dose selective serotonin reuptake inhibitors for severe, refractory choking phobia in childhood. J Dev Behav Pediatr 26:123–127, 2005

Banos RM, Botella C, Perpina C, et al: Virtual reality in treatment of flying phobia. IEEE Trans Inf Technol Biomed 6:206–212, 2002

Barlow DH: Anxiety and Its Disorders: The Nature and Treatment of Anxiety and Panic. New York, Guilford, 1988

Barlow DH, Craske MG, Cerny JA, et al: Behavioral treatment of panic disorder. Behav Ther 20:261–282, 1989

Barlow DH, Rapee RM, Brown TA: Behavioral treatment of generalized anxiety disorder. Behav Ther 23:551–570, 1992

Barlow DH, Gorman JM, Shear MK, et al: Cognitive-behavioral therapy, imipramine, or their combination for panic disorder: a randomized controlled trial. JAMA 283:2529–2536, 2000

Barnett SD, Kramer ML, Casat CD, et al: Efficacy of olanzapine in social anxiety disorder: a pilot study. J Psychopharmacol 16:365–368, 2002

Barr LC, Goodman WK, Anand A, et al: Addition of desipramine to serotonin reuptake inhibitors in treatment-resistant obsessive-compulsive disorder. Am J Psychiatry 154:1293–1295, 1997

Bartz JA, Hollander E: Is obsessive compulsive disorder an anxiety disorder? Prog Neuropsychopharmacol Biol Psychiatry 30:338–352, 2006

Bartzokis G, Lu PH, Turner J: Adjunctive risperidone in the treatment of chronic combat related posttraumatic stress disorder. Biol Psychiatry 57:474–479, 2005

Basoglu M, Marks IM, Kilic C, et al: Relationship of panic, anticipatory anxiety, agoraphobia and global improvement in panic disorder with agoraphobia treated with alprazolam and exposure. Br J Psychiatry 164:647–652, 1994

Baxter LR Jr, Phelps ME, Mazziotta JC, et al: Local cerebral glucose metabolic rates in obsessive-compulsive disorder: a comparison with rates in unipolar depression and in normal controls. Arch Gen Psychiatry 44:211–218, 1987

Baxter LR Jr, Schwartz JM, Bergman KS, et al: Caudate glucose metabolic rate changes with both drug and behavior therapy for obsessive-compulsive disorder. Arch Gen Psychiatry 49:681–689, 1992

Beck AT, Sokol L, Clark DA, et al: A crossover study of focused cognitive therapy for panic disorder. Am J Psychiatry 149:778–783, 1992

Beidel DC, Turner SM, Morris TL: Behavioral treatment of childhood social phobia. J Consult Clin Psychol 68:1072–1080, 2000

Bell CJ, Malizia AL, Nutt DJ: The neurobiology of social phobia. Eur Arch Psychiatry Clin Neurosci 249:S11–S18, 1999

Bellew KM, McCafferty JP, Iyengar M, et al: Paroxetine treatment of GAD: a double-blind, placebo-controlled trial. Presented at the annual meeting of the American Psychiatric Association, Chicago, IL, 2000

Bengel D, Greenberg BD, Cora-Locatelli G, et al: Association of the serotonin transporter promoter regulatory region polymorphism and obsessive-compulsive disorder. Mol Psychiatry 4:463–466, 1999

Benjamin J, Levine J, Fux M, et al: Double-blind, placebo-controlled, crossover trial of inositol treatment for panic disorder. Am J Psychiatry 152:1084–1086, 1995

Benjamin J, Ben-Zion IZ, Karbofsky E, et al: Double-blind, placebo-controlled study of paroxetine for specific phobia. Psychopharmacology (Berl) 149:194–196, 2000

Berlant JL: Prospective open label study of add on monotherapy topiramate in civilians with chronic nonhallucinatory posttraumatic stress disorder. BMC Psychiatry 4:24, 2004

Berney A, Sookman D, Leyton M, et al: Lack of effects on core obsessive compulsive symptoms of tryptophan depletion during symptom provocation in remitted obsessive compulsive disorder patients. Biol Psychiatry 59:853–857, 2006

Bienvenu OJ, Samuels JF, Riddle MA, et al: The relationship of obsessive-compulsive disorder to possible spectrum disorders: results from a family study. Biol Psychiatry 48:287–293, 2000

Billet EA, Richter MA, King N, et al: Obsessive compulsive disorder, response to serotonin reuptake inhibitors and the serotonin transporter gene. Mol Psychiatry 2:403–406, 1997

Birbaumer N, Grodd W, Diedrich O, et al: fMRI reveals amygdala activation to human faces in social phobics. Neuroreport 9:1223–1226, 1998

Bisson J, Andrew M: Psychological treatment of post-traumatic stress disorder. Cochrane Database Syst Rev (2):CD003388, 2005

Black A: The natural history of obsessional neurosis, in Obsessional States. Edited by Beech HK. London, England, Methuen, 1974, pp 19–54

Black DW, Noyes R, Goldstein RB, et al: A family study of obsessive-compulsive disorder. Arch Gen Psychiatry 49:362–368, 1992

Bleiberg KL, Markowitz JC: A pilot study of interpersonal psychotherapy for posttraumatic stress disorder. Am J Psychiatry 162:181–183, 2005

Bleich A, Siegel B, Garb R, et al: Post-traumatic stress disorder following combat exposure: clinical features and psychopharmacological treatment. Br J Psychiatry 149:365–369, 1986

Bonne O, Bain E, Neumeister A, et al: No change in serotonin type 1A receptor binding in patients with posttraumatic stress disorder. Am J Psychiatry 162:383–385, 2005

Borkovec TD, Costello E: Efficacy of applied relaxation and cognitive-behavioral therapy in the treatment of generalized anxiety disorder. J Consult Clin Psychol 61:611–619, 1993

Bouwer C, Stein DJ: Association of panic disorder with a history of traumatic suffocation. Am J Psychiatry 154:1566–1570, 1997

Bouwer C, Stein DJ: Use of the selective serotonin reuptake inhibitor citalopram in the treatment of generalized social phobia. J Affect Disord 49:79–82, 1998

Bowlby J: Attachment and Loss, Vol 2: Separation: Anxiety and Anger. New York, Basic Books, 1973

Bradwejn J, Ahokas A, Stein DJ, et al: Venlafaxine extended-release capsules in panic disorder: flexible-dose, double-blind, placebo-controlled study. Br J Psychiatry 187:352–359, 2005

Brady K, Pearlstein T, Asnis GM, et al: Efficacy and safety of sertraline treatment of posttraumatic stress disorder: a randomized controlled trial. JAMA 283:1837–1844, 2000

Brambilla F, Bellodi L, Perna G, et al: Dopamine function in obsessive-compulsive disorder: growth hormone response to apomorphine stimulation. Biol Psychiatry 42:889–897, 1997

Brawman-Mintzer O, Knapp RG, Nietert PJ: Adjunctive risperidone in generalized anxiety disorder: a double-blind, placebo-controlled study. J Clin Psychiatry 66:1321–1325, 2005

Breiter HC, Rauch SL, Kwong KK, et al: Functional magnetic resonance imaging of symptom provocation in obsessive-compulsive disorder. Arch Gen Psychiatry 53:595–606, 1996

Breitholtz E, Johansson B, Ost LG: Cognitions in generalized anxiety disorder and panic disorder patients. A prospective approach. Behav Res Ther 37:533–544, 1999

Bremner JD, Vermetten E: Neuroanatomical changes associated with pharmacotherapy in posttraumatic stress disorder. Ann NY Acad Sci 1032: 154–157, 2004

Bremner JD, Scott TM, Delaney RC, et al: Deficits in short-term memory in posttraumatic stress disorder. Am J Psychiatry 150:1015–1019, 1993a

Bremner JD, Southwick SM, Johnson DR, et al: Childhood physical abuse and combat-related posttraumatic stress disorder in Vietnam veterans. Am J Psychiatry 150:235–239, 1993b

Bremner JD, Randall P, Scott TM, et al: MRI-based measurement of hippocampal volume in patients with combat-related posttraumatic stress disorder. Am J Psychiatry 152:973–981, 1995

Bremner JD, Licinio J, Darnell A, et al: Elevated CSF corticotropin-releasing factor concentrations in posttraumatic stress disorder. Am J Psychiatry 154:624–629, 1997a

Bremner JD, Randall P, Vermetten E, et al: Magnetic resonance imaging-based measurement of hippocampal volume in posttraumatic stress disorder related to childhood physical and sexual abuse: a preliminary report. Biol Psychiatry 41:23–32, 1997b

Bremner JD, Narayan M, Staib LH, et al: Neural correlates of memories of childhood sexual abuse in women with and without posttraumatic stress disorder. Am J Psychiatry 156:1787–1795, 1999

Bremner JD, Innis RB, White T, et al: SPECT [I-123] iomazenil measurement of the benzodiazepine receptor in panic disorder. Biol Psychiatry 47:96–106, 2000

Breslau N, Davis GC: Posttraumatic stress disorder in an urban population of young adults: risk factors for chronicity. Am J Psychiatry 149:671–675, 1992

Breslau N, Davis GC, Andreski P, et al: Traumatic events and posttraumatic stress disorder in an urban population of young adults. Arch Gen Psychiatry 48:216–222, 1991

Breslau N, Davis GC, Andreski P, et al: Sex differences in posttraumatic stress disorder. Arch Gen Psychiatry 54:1044–1048, 1997a

Breslau N, Davis GC, Peterson EL, et al: Psychiatric sequelae of posttraumatic stress disorder in women. Arch Gen Psychiatry 54:81–87, 1997b

Breslau N, Kessler RC, Chilcoat HD, et al: Trauma and posttraumatic stress disorder in the community: the 1996 Detroit Area Survey of Trauma. Arch Gen Psychiatry 55:626–632, 1998

Breslau N, Davis GC, Peterson EL, et al: A second look at comorbidity in victims of trauma: the posttraumatic stress disorder–major depression connection. Biol Psychiatry 48:902–909, 2000

Breuer T, Freud S: Studies on hysteria (1893–1895), in The Standard Edition of the Complete Psychological Works of Sigmund Freud, Vol 2. Edited by Strachey J. London, England, Hogarth, 1955, pp 1–319

Bryant RA: Predicting posttraumatic stress disorder from acute reactions. J Trauma Dissociation 6:5–15, 2005

Bryant RA, Harvey AG: Relationship between acute stress disorder and posttraumatic stress disorder following mild traumatic brain injury. Am J Psychiatry 155:625–629, 1998

Bryant RA, Marosszeky JE, Crooks J, et al: Posttraumatic stress disorder after severe traumatic brain injury. Am J Psychiatry 157:629–631, 2000

Bryant RA, Moulds ML, Guthrie RM, et al: Imaginal exposure alone and imaginal exposure with cognitive restructuring in treatment of posttraumatic stress disorder. J Consult Clin Psychol 7:706–712, 2003

Buchsbaum MS, Wu J, Haier R, et al: Positron emission tomography assessment of effects of benzodiazepines on regional glucose metabolic rate in patients with anxiety disorder. Life Sci 40:2393–2400, 1987

Butler G, Fennell M, Robson P, et al: Comparison of behavior therapy and cognitive behavior therapy in the treatment of generalized anxiety disorder. J Consult Clin Psychol 59:167–175, 1991

Bystritsky A, Ackerman DL, Rosen RM, et al: Augmentation of serotonin reuptake inhibitors in refractory obsessive compulsive disorder using adjunctive olanzapine: a placebo controlled trial. J Clin Psychiatry 65:565–568, 2004

Caldirola D, Bellodi L, Caumo A, et al: Approximate entropy of respiratory patterns in panic disorder. Am J Psychiatry 161:79–87, 2004

Canive JM, Clark RD, Calais LA, et al: Bupropion treatment in veterans with posttraumatic stress disorder: an open study. J Clin Psychopharmacol 18:379–383, 1998

Carey G, Gottesman II: Twin and family studies of anxiety, phobic, and obsessive disorders, in Anxiety: New Research and Changing Concepts. Edited by Klein DF, Rabkin J. New York, Raven, 1981, pp 117–136

Carey PD, Vythilingum B, Seedat S, et al: Quetiapine augmentation of SRIs in treatment refractory obsessive-compulsive disorder: a double blind, randomized, placebo controlled study. BMC Psychiatry 5:44, 2005

Carlson JG, Chemtob CM, Rusnak K, et al: Eye movement desensitization and reprocessing (EMDR) treatment for combat-related posttraumatic stress disorder. J Trauma Stress 11:3–24, 1998

Carter RM, Wittchen HU, Pfister H, et al: One-year prevalence of subthreshold and threshold DSM-IV generalized anxiety disorder in a nationally representative sample. Depress Anxiety 13:78–88, 2001

Cassidy J: Attachment and generalized anxiety disorder, in Rochester Symposium on Developmental Psychopathology, Vol 6: Emotion, Cognition and Representation. Edited by Cicchetti D, Toth S. New York, University of Rochester Press, 1995, pp 343–370

Cavallini MC, Di-Bella D, Pasquale L, et al: 5HT2C CYS23/SER23 polymorphism is not associated with obsessive-compulsive disorder. Psychiatry Res 77:97–104, 1998

Chabane N, Millet B, Delorme R, et al: Lack of evidence for association between serotonin transporter gene (5-HTTLPR) and obsessive compulsive disorder by case control and family association study in humans. Neurosci Lett 363:154–156, 2004

Chakrabarty K, Bhattacharyya S, Christopher R, et al: Glutamatergic dysfunction in OCD. Neuropsychopharmacology 30:1735–1740, 2005

Chambless DL, Gillis MM: Cognitive therapy of anxiety disorders. J Consult Clin Psychol 61:248–260, 1993

Chard KM: An evaluation of cognitive processing therapy for the treatment of posttraumatic stress disorder related to childhood sexual abuse. J Consult Clin Psychol 73:965–971, 2005

Charney DS, Heninger GR, Breier A: Noradrenergic function in panic anxiety: effects of yohimbine in healthy subjects and patients with agoraphobia and panic disorder. Arch Gen Psychiatry 41:751–763, 1984

Charney DS, Goodman WK, Price LH, et al: Serotonin function in obsessive-compulsive disorder: a comparison of the effects of tryptophan and m-chlorophenylpiperazine in patients and healthy subjects. Arch Gen Psychiatry 45:177–185, 1988

Chartier MJ, Walker JR, Stein MB: Social phobia and potential childhood risk factors in a community sample. Psychol Med 31:307–315, 2001

Cheng R, Juo SH, Loth JE, et al: Genome-wide linkage scan in a large bipolar disorder sample from the National Institute of Mental Health genetics initiative suggests putative loci for bipolar disorder, psychosis, suicide, and panic disorder. Mol Psychiatry 11:252–260, 2006

Chung MY, Min KH, Jun YJ, et al: Efficacy and tolerability of mirtazapine and sertraline in Korean veterans with posttraumatic stress disorder: a randomized open label trial. Hum Psychopharmacol 19:489–494, 2004

Clark DM, Salkovskis PM, Hackmann A, et al: A comparison of cognitive therapy, applied relaxation therapy and imipramine in the treatment of panic disorder. Br J Psychiatry 164:759–769, 1994

Clark RD, Canive JM, Calais LA, et al: Cyproheptadine treatment of nightmares associated with posttraumatic stress disorder. J Clin Psychopharmacol 19:486–487, 1999a

Clark RD, Canive JM, Calais LA, et al: Divalproex in posttraumatic stress disorder: an open-label clinical trial. J Trauma Stress 12:395–401, 1999b

Clayton IC, Richards JC, Edwards CJ: Selective attention in obsessive-compulsive disorder. J Abnorm Psychol 108:171–175, 1999

Clomipramine Collaborative Study Group: Clomipramine in the treatment of patients with obsessive-compulsive disorder. Arch Gen Psychiatry 48:730–738, 1991

Cohen H, Kaplan Z, Kotler M, et al: Repetitive transcranial magnetic stimulation of the right dorsolateral prefrontal cortex in posttraumatic stress disorder: a double blind, placebo controlled study. Am J Psychiatry 161:515–524, 2004

Cohen JA, Deblinger E, Mannarino AP, et al: A multisite, randomized controlled trial for children with sexual abused related PTSD symptoms. J Am Acad Child Adolesc Psychiatry 43:393–402, 2004

Comings DE, Muhleman D, Gysin R: Dopamine D2 receptor (DRD2) gene and susceptibility to posttraumatic stress disorder: a study and replication. Biol Psychiatry 40:368–372, 1996

Condren RM, O'Neill A, Ryan MC, et al: HPA axis response to a psychological stressor in generalized social phobia. Psychoneuroendocrinology 27:693–703, 2002

Connor KM, Payne VM, Gadde KM, et al: The use of aripiprazole in obsessive compulsive disorder: preliminary observations in 8 patients. J Clin Psychiatry 66:49–51, 2005

Connor KM, Cook JL, Davidson JR: Botulinum toxin treatment of social anxiety disorder with hyperhydrosis: a placebo controlled double blind trial. J Clin Psychiatry 67:30–36, 2006a

Connor KM, Davidson JR, Weisler RH, et al: Tiagabine for posttraumatic stress disorder: effects of open label and double blind discontinuation treatment. Psychopharmacology (Berl) 184:21–25, 2006b

Cooper AM: Will neurobiology influence psychoanalysis? Am J Psychiatry 142:1395–1402, 1985

Coplan JD, Pine D, Papp L, et al: Uncoupling of the noradrenergic-hypothalamic-pituitary-adrenal axis in panic disorder patients. Neuropsychopharmacol 13:65–73, 1995

Coplan JD, Papp LA, Pine D, et al: Clinical improvement with fluoxetine therapy and noradrenergic function in patients with panic disorder. Arch Gen Psychiatry 54:643–648, 1997

Coric V, Taskiran S, Pittenger C, et al: Riluzole augmentation in treatment resistant obsessive compulsive disorder: an open label trial. Biol Psychiatry 58:424–428, 2005

Coryell W, Fyer A, Pine D, et al: Aberrant respiratory sensitivity to CO(2) as a trait of familial panic disorder. Biol Psychiatry 49:582–587, 2001

Cottraux J, Note I, Albuisson E, et al: Cognitive behavior therapy versus supportive therapy in social phobia: a randomized controlled trial. Psychother Psychosom 69:137–146, 2000

Cottraux J, Note I, Yao SN, et al: A randomized controlled trial of cognitive therapy versus intensive behavior therapy in obsessive compulsive disorder. Psychother Psychosom 70:288–297, 2001

Coupland NJ, Bell C, Potokar J, et al: Flumazenil challenge in social phobia. Anxiety 111:27–30, 2000

Cox B, MacPherson PS, Enns MW, et al: Neuroticism and self criticism associated with posttraumatic stress disorder in a nationally representative sample. Behav Res Ther 42:105–114, 2004

Craske MG, Golinelli D, Stein MB, et al: Does the addition of cognitive behavioral therapy improve panic disorder treatment outcome relative to medication alone in the primary-care setting? Psychol Med 35:1645–1654, 2005

Crowe RR, Noyes R, Pauls DL, et al: A family study of panic disorder. Arch Gen Psychiatry 40:1065–1069, 1983

Crowe RR, Goedken R, Samuelson S, et al: Genomewide survey of panic disorder. Am J Med Genet 105:105–109, 2001

Curtis GC, Abelson JL, Gold PW: Adrenocorticotropic hormone and cortisol responses to corticotropin-releasing hormone: changes in panic disorder and effects of alprazolam treatment. Biol Psychiatry 41:76–85, 1997

Dadds MR, Barrett PM, Rapee RM, et al: Family process and child anxiety and aggression: an observational analysis. J Abnorm Child Psychol 24:187–203, 1996

Dahl AA, Ravindran A, Allgulander C, et al: Sertraline in generalized anxiety disorder: efficacy in treating the psychic and somatic anxiety factors. Acta Psychiatr Scand 111:429–435, 2005

Dale RC, Heyman I, Giovannoni G, et al: Incidence of anti-brain antibodies in children with obsessive compulsive disorder. Br J Psychiatry 187:314–319, 2005

Dannon PN, Sasson Y, Hirschmann S, et al: Pindolol augmentation in treatment-resistant obsessive compulsive disorder: a double-blind placebo controlled trial. Eur Neuropsychopharmacol 10:165–169, 2000

Davidson J, Walker JI, Kilts C: A pilot study of phenelzine in the treatment of post-traumatic stress disorder. Br J Psychiatry 150:252–255, 1987

Davidson J, Kudler H, Smith R, et al: Treatment of posttraumatic stress disorder with amitriptyline and placebo. Arch Gen Psychiatry 47:259–266, 1990

Davidson J, Roth S, Newman E: Fluoxetine in post-traumatic stress disorder. J Trauma Stress 4:419–423, 1991

Davidson J, Potts N, Richichi E, et al: Treatment of social phobia with clonazepam and placebo. J Clin Psychopharmacol 13:423–428, 1993a

Davidson JR, Hughes DL, George LK, et al: The epidemiology of social phobia: findings from the Duke Epidemiological Catchment Area Study. Psychol Med 23:709–718, 1993b

Davidson JR, DuPont RL, Hedges D, et al: Efficacy, safety, and tolerability of venlafaxine extended release and buspirone in outpatients with generalized anxiety disorder. J Clin Psychiatry 60:528–535, 1999

Davidson JR, Rothbaum BO, van der Kolk BA, et al: Multicenter, double blind comparison of sertraline and placebo in the treatment of posttraumatic stress disorder. Arch Gen Psychiatry 58:485–492, 2001

Davidson JR, Weisler RH, Butterfield MI, et al: Mirtazapine vs placebo in posttraumatic stress disorder: a pilot trial. Biol Psychiatry 53:188–191, 2003

Davidson JR, Foa E, Huppert JD, et al: Fluoxetine, comprehensive cognitive behavioral therapy, and placebo in generalized social phobia. Arch Gen Psychiatry 61:1005–1013, 2004

Davidson JR, Connor KM, Hertzberg MA, et al: Maintenance therapy with fluoxetine in posttraumatic stress disorder: a placebo controlled discontinuation study. J Clin Psychopharmacol 25:166–169, 2005

Davidson JR, Rothbaum BO, Tucker P, et al: Venlafaxine extended release in posttraumatic stress disorder: a sertraline and placebo controlled study. J Clin Psychopharmacol 26:259–267, 2006

Davis LL, Clark DM, Kramer GL, et al: D-fenfluramine challenge in posttraumatic stress disorder. Biol Psychiatry 45:928–930, 1999

de Beurs E, van Balkom AJ, Lange A, et al: Treatment of panic disorder with agoraphobia: comparison of fluvoxamine, placebo and psychological panic management combined with exposure and of exposure in vivo alone. Am J Psychiatry 152:683–691, 1995

De Boer M, Op den Velde W, Falger PJ, et al: Fluvoxamine treatment for chronic PTSD: a pilot study. Psychother Psychosom 57:158–163, 1992

de Haan E, Hoogduin KA, Buitelaar JK, et al: Behavior therapy versus clomipramine for the treatment of obsessive-compulsive disorder in children and adolescents. J Am Acad Child Adolesc Psychiatry 37:1022–1029, 1998

DeBellis MD, Casey BJ, Dahl RE, et al: A pilot study of amygdala volumes in pediatric generalized anxiety disorder. Biol Psychiatry 48:51–57, 2000

Deckert J, Nothen MM, Franke P, et al: Systematic mutation screening and association study of the A1 and A2a adenosine receptor genes in panic disorder suggest a contribution of the A2a gene to the development of the disease. Mol Psychiatry 3:81–85, 1998

Deckert J, Catalano M, Syagailo YV, et al: Excess of high activity monoamine oxidase A gene promoter alleles in female patients with panic disorder. Hum Mol Genet 81:228–234, 1999

Delahanty DL, Nugent NR, Christopher NC, et al: Initial urinary epinephrine and cortisol levels predict acute PTSD symptoms in child trauma victims. Psychoneuroendocrinology 30:121–128, 2005

Delle Chiaie R, Pancheri P, Casacchia M, et al: Assessment of the efficacy of buspirone in patients affected by generalized anxiety disorder, shifting to buspirone from prior treatment with lorazepam: a placebo-controlled, double-blind study. J Clin Psychopharmacol 15:12–19, 1995

Delorme R, Krebs MO, Chabane N, et al: Frequency and transmission of glutamate receptors GRIK2 and GRIK3 polymorphisms in patients with obsessive compulsive disorder. Neuroreport 15:699–702, 2004

DeMartinis N, Rynn M, Rickels K, et al: Prior benzodiazepine use and buspirone response in the treatment of generalized anxiety disorder. J Clin Psychiatry 61:91–94, 2000

Denys D, deGeus F, van Megen HJ, et al: A double-blind, randomized, placebo-controlled trial of quetiapine addition in patients with obsessive-compulsive disorder refractory to serotonin reuptake inhibitors. J Clin Psychiatry 65:1040–1048, 2004a

Denys D, van der Wee N, Janssen J, et al: Low level of dopaminergic D2 receptor binding in obsessive-compulsive disorder. Biol Psychiatry 55:1041–1045, 2004b

Denys D, van Megen HJ, van der Wee N, et al: A double-blind switch study of paroxetine and venlafaxine in obsessive-compulsive disorder. J Clin Psychiatry 65:37–43, 2004c

Devilly GJ, Spence SH: The relative efficacy and treatment distress of EMDR and a cognitive-behavior trauma treatment protocol in the amelioration of posttraumatic stress disorder. J Anxiety Disord 13:131–157, 1999

DeWit DJ, Ogborne A, Offord DR, et al: Antecedents of the risk of recovery from DSM-III-R social phobia. Psychol Med 29:569–582, 1999

DeWit DJ, Chandler Coutts M, Offord DR, et al: Gender differences in the effects of family adversity on the risk of onset of DSM-III-R social phobia. J Anxiety Disord 19:479–502, 2005

Dougherty DD, Baer L, Cosgrove GR, et al: Prospective long term follow up of 44 patients who received cingulotomy for treatment refractory obsessive compulsive disorder. Am J Psychiatry 159:269–274, 2002

Duffy JD, Malloy PF: Efficacy of buspirone in the treatment of posttraumatic stress disorder: an open trial. Ann Clin Psychiatry 6:33–37, 1994

Durham RC, Murphy R, Allan T, et al: Cognitive therapy, analytic psychotherapy and anxiety management training for generalized anxiety disorder. Br J Psychiatry 165:315–323, 1994

Dvorkin A, Perrault ML, Szechtman H: Development and temporal organization of compulsive checking induced by repeated injections of the dopamine agonist quinpirole in an animal model of obsessive compulsive disorder. Behav Brain Res 169:303–311, 2006

Ehlers A, Clark DM: A cognitive model of posttraumatic stress disorder. Behav Res Ther 38:319–345, 2000

Eisen JL, Beer DA, Pato MT, et al: Obsessive-compulsive disorder in patients with schizophrenia or schizoaffective disorder. Am J Psychiatry 154:271–273, 1997

Embry CK: Psychotherapeutic interventions in chronic posttraumatic stress disorder, in Posttraumatic Stress Disorder: Etiology, Phenomenology, and Treatment. Edited by Wolf ME, Mosnaim AD. Washington, DC, American Psychiatric Press, 1990, pp 226–236

Emmanuel NP, Lydiard BR, Ballenger JC: Treatment of social phobia with bupropion. J Clin Psychopharmacol 1:276–277, 1991

Engdahl B, Dikel TN, Eberly R, et al: Posttraumatic stress disorder in a community group of former prisoners of war: a normative response to severe trauma. Am J Psychiatry 154:1576–1581, 1997

English BA, Jewell M, Jewell G, et al: Treatment of chronic posttraumatic stress disorder in combat veterans with citalopram: an open trial. J Clin Psychopharmacol 26:84–88, 2006

Enoch MA, Greenberg BD, Murphy DL, et al: Sexually dimorphic relationship of a 5 HT2A promoter polymorphism with obsessive compulsive disorder. Biol Psychiatry 49:385–388, 2001

Erzegovesi S, Guglielmo E, Siliprandi F, et al: Low dose risperidone augmentation of fluvoxamine treatment in obsessive compulsive disorder: a double blind, placebo controlled study. Eur Neuropsychopharmacol 15:69–74, 2005

Essau CA, Conradt J, Petermann F: Frequency, comorbidity, and psychosocial impairment of specific phobia in adolescents. J Clin Child Psychol 29:221–231, 2000

Fairbank TA, Keane TM: Flooding for combat-related stress disorders: assessment of anxiety reduction across traumatic memories. Behav Ther 13:499–510, 1982

Fallon BA, Liebowitz MR, Campeas R, et al: Intravenous clomipramine for obsessive-compulsive disorder refractory to oral clomipramine: a placebo-controlled study. Arch Gen Psychiatry 55:918–924, 1998

Faravelli C, Pallanti S: Recent life events and panic disorder. Am J Psychiatry 146:622–626, 1989

Fava GA, Grandi S, Rafanelli C, et al: Long term outcome of social phobia treated by exposure. Psychol Med 31:899–905, 2001a

Fava GA, Rafanelli C, Grandi S, et al: Long-term outcome of panic disorder with agoraphobia treated by exposure. Psychol Med 31:891–898, 2001b

Fava GA, Ruini C, Rafanelli C, et al: Well-being therapy of generalized anxiety disorder. Psychother Psychosom 74:26–30, 2005

Ferrarese C, Appollonio I, Frigo M, et al: Decreased density of benzodiazepine receptors in lymphocytes of anxious patients: reversal after chronic diazepam treatment. Acta Psychiatr Scand 82:169–173, 1990

Fineberg NA, Sivakumaran T, Roberts A, et al: Adding quetiapine to SRI in treatment resistant obsessive compulsive disorder: a randomized controlled treatment study. Int Clin Psychopharmacol 20:223–226, 2005

Fisher PL, Wells A: How effective are cognitive and behavioral treatments for obsessive compulsive disorder? A clinical significance analysis. Behav Res Ther 43:1543–1558, 2005

Fitzgerald KD, Stewart CM, Tawile V, et al: Risperidone augmentation of serotonin reuptake inhibitor treatment of pediatric obsessive compulsive disorder. J Child Adolesc Psychopharmacol 9:115–123, 1999

Fitzgerald KD, Welsh RC, Gehrig WJ, et al: Error-related hyperactivity of the anterior cingulated cortex in obsessive-compulsive disorder. Biol Psychiatry 57:287–294, 2005

Flament MF, Rapoport JL, Murphy DL, et al: Biochemical changes during clomipramine treatment of childhood obsessive-compulsive disorder. Arch Gen Psychiatry 44:219–225, 1987

Flescher J: A dualistic viewpoint on anxiety. J Am Psychoanal Assoc 3:415–446, 1955

Flint AJ: Epidemiology and comorbidity of anxiety disorders in the elderly. Am J Psychiatry 151:640–649, 1994

Flor-Henry P: The obsessive-compulsive syndrome, in Cerebral Basis of Psychopathology. Edited by Flor-Henry P. Boston, MA, John Coright, 1983, pp 301–311

Foa EB, Steketee G, Grayson JB, et al: Deliberate exposure and blocking of obsessive-compulsive rituals: immediate and long-term effects. Behav Ther 15:450–472, 1984

Foa EB, Kozak MJ, Goodman WK, et al: DSM-IV field trial: obsessive-compulsive disorder. Am J Psychiatry 152:90–96, 1995

Foa EB, Dancu CV, Hembree EA, et al: A comparison of exposure therapy, stress inoculation therapy, and their combination for reducing posttraumatic stress disorder in female assault victims. J Consult Clin Psychol 67:194–200, 1999

Foa EB, Keane TM, Friedman MJ: Effective Treatments for PTSD: Practice Guidelines From the International Society for Traumatic Stress Studies. New York, Guilford, 2000

Foa E, Hembree EA, Cahill SP, et al: Randomized trial of prolonged exposure for posttraumatic stress disorder with and without cognitive restructuring: outcome at academic and community clinics. J Consult Clin Psychol 73:953–962, 2005a

Foa EB, Liebowitz MR, Kozak MJ, et al: Randomized, placebo controlled trial of exposure and ritual prevention, clomipramine, and their combination in the treatment of obsessive compulsive disorder. Am J Psychiatry 162:151–161, 2005b

Frank JB, Kosten TR, Giller EL Jr, et al: A randomized clinical trial of phenelzine and imipramine for posttraumatic stress disorder. Am J Psychiatry 145:1289–1291, 1988

Franklin ME, Kozak MJ, Cashman L, et al: Cognitive-behavioral treatment of pediatric obsessive-compulsive disorder: an open clinical trial. J Am Acad Child Adolesc Psychiatry 37:412–419, 1998

Fredrikson M, Wik G, Greitz T, et al: Regional cerebral blood flow during experimental phobic fear. Psychophysiology 30:126–130, 1993

Friedman SD, Mathis CM, Hayes C, et al: Brain pH response to hypoventilation in panic disorder: preliminary evidence for altered acid-base regulation. Am J Psychiatry 163:710–715, 2006

Freitlag CM, Domschke K, Rothe C, et al: Interaction of serotonergic and noradrenergic gene variants in panic disorder. Psychiatr Genet 16:59–65, 2006

Freud S: Obsessions and phobias (1895a[1894]), in The Standard Edition of the Complete Psychological Works of Sigmund Freud, Vol 3. Translated and edited by Strachey J. London, England, Hogarth, 1962, pp 69–84

Freud S: On the grounds for detaching a particular syndrome from neurasthenia under the description anxiety neurosis (1895b[1894]), in The Standard Edition of the Complete Psychological Works of Sigmund Freud, Vol 3. Translated and edited by Strachey J. London, England, Hogarth, 1962, pp 85–117

Freud S: Analysis of a phobia in a five-year-old boy (1909), in The Standard Edition of the Complete Psychological Works of Sigmund Freud, Vol 10. Translated and edited by Strachey J. London, England, Hogarth, 1955, pp 1–149

Freud S: The disposition to obsessional neurosis: a contribution to the problem of choice of neurosis (1913), in The Standard Edition of the Complete Psychological Works of Sigmund Freud, Vol 12. Translated and edited by Strachey J. London, Hogarth, 1958, pp 311–326

Freud S: Introduction to Psychoanalysis and the War Neuroses (1919), in The Standard Edition of the Complete Psychological Works of Sigmund Freud, Vol 17. Translated and edited by Strachey J. London, England, Hogarth, 1955, pp 205–215

Freud S: Inhibitions, symptoms and anxiety (1926), in The Standard Edition of the Complete Psychological Works of Sigmund Freud, Vol 20. Translated and edited by Strachey J. London, England, Hogarth, 1959, pp 75–175

Frisch A, Michaelovsky E, Poyurovsky M, et al: Association between obsessive-compulsive disorder and polymorphisms of genes encoding components of the serotonergic and dopaminergic pathways. Eur Neuropsychopharmacol 10:205–209, 2000

Furmark T, Tillfors M, Marteinsdottir I, et al: Common changes in cerebral blood flow in patients with social phobia treated with citalopram or cognitive behavioral therapy. Arch Gen Psychiatry 59:425–433, 2002

Furmark T, Tillfors M, Garpenstrand H, et al: Serotonin transporter polymorphism related to amygdala excitability and symptom severity in patients with social phobia. Neurosci Lett 362:189–192, 2004

Furmark T, Appel L, Michelgard A, et al: Cerebral blood flow changes after treatment of social phobia with the neurokinin 1 antagonist GR205171, citalopram or placebo. Biol Psychiatry 58:132–142, 2005

Furukawa TA, Watanabe N, Churchill R: Psychotherapy plus antidepressant for panic disorder with and without agoraphobia: systematic review. Br J Psychiatry 188:305–312, 2006

Fux M, Benjamin J, Nemets B: A placebo controlled cross over trial of adjunctive EPA in OCD. J Psychiatr Res 38:323–325, 2004

Fyer AJ: Current approaches to etiology and pathophysiology of specific phobia. Biol Psychiatry 44:1295–1304, 1998

Fyer AJ, Mannuzza S, Gallops MS, et al: Familial transmission of simple phobias and fears: a preliminary report. Arch Gen Psychiatry 47:252–256, 1990

Gabbard GO: Psychodynamic Psychiatry in Clinical Practice. Washington, DC, American Psychiatric Press, 1990

Gambi F, De-Berardis D, Campanella D, et al: Mirtazapine treatment of generalized anxiety disorder: a fixed dose, open label study. J Psychopharmacol 19:483–487, 2005

Garcia-Palacios A, Hoffman H, Carlin A, et al: Virtual reality in the treatment of spider phobia: a controlled study. Behav Res Ther 40:983–993, 2002

Gelenberg AJ, Lydiard RB, Rudolph RL, et al: Efficacy of venlafaxine extended-release capsules in nondepressed outpatients with generalized anxiety disorder: a 6-month randomized controlled trial. JAMA 283:3082–3088, 2000

Gelernter CS, Uhde TW, Cimbolic P, et al: Cognitive-behavioral and pharmacological treatments of social phobia: a controlled study. Arch Gen Psychiatry 48:938–945, 1991

Gelernter J, Southwick S, Goodson S, et al: No association between D2 dopamine receptor (DRD2) "A" system alleles or DRD2 haplotypes and posttraumatic stress disorder. Biol Psychiatry 45:620–625, 1999

Gelernter J, Bonvicini K, Page G, et al: Linkage genome scan for loci predisposing to panic disorder or agoraphobia. Am J Med Genet 105:548–557, 2001

Gelernter J, Page GP, Bonvicini K, et al: A chromosome 24 risk locus for simple phobia: results from a genomewide linkage scan. Mol Psychiatry 8:71–82, 2003

Gelernter J, Page GP, Stein MB, Woods SW: Genome-wide linkage scan for loci predisposing to social phobia: evidence for a chromosome 16 risk locus. Am J Psychiatry 161:59–66, 2004

Geller DA, Biederman J, Stewart SE, et al: Which SSRA? A meta analysis of pharmacotherapy trials in pediatric obsessive compulsive disorder. Am J Psychiatry 160:1919–1928, 2003

Geller DA, Wagner KD, Emslie G, et al: Paroxetine treatment in children and adolescents with obsessive compulsive disorder: a randomized, multicenter, double blind, placebo controlled trial. J Am Acad Child Adolesc Psychiatr 43:1387–1396, 2004

Geracioti TD Jr, Baker DG, Ekhator NN, et al: CSF norepinephrine concentrations in posttraumatic stress disorder. Am J Psychiatry 158:1227–1230, 2001

Geracioti TD, Carpenter LL, Owens MJ, et al: Elevated cerebrospinal fluid substance P concentrations in posttraumatic stress disorder and major depression. Am J Psychiatry 163:637–643, 2006

Germine M, Goddard AW, Woods SW, et al: Anger and anxiety responses to m-chlorophenylpiperazine in generalized anxiety disorder. Biol Psychiatry 32:457–461, 1992

Giedd JN, Rapoport JL, Garvey MA, et al: MRI assessment of children with obsessive-compulsive disorder or tics associated with streptococcal infection. Am J Psychiatry 157:281–283, 2000

Gilbert AR, Moore GJ, Keshavan MS, et al: Decrease in thalamic volumes of pediatric patients with obsessive-compulsive disorder who are taking paroxetine. Arch Gen Psychiatry 57:449–456, 2000

Gittelman-Klein R, Klein DF: Controlled imipramine treatment of school phobia. Arch Gen Psychiatry 25:204–207, 1971

Goddard AW, Brouette T, Almai A, et al: Early coadministration of clonazepam with sertraline for panic disorder. Arch Gen Psychiatry 58:681–686, 2001a

Goddard AW, Mason GF, Almai A, et al: Reductions in occipital cortex GABA levels in panic disorder detected with 1H-magnetic resonance spectroscopy. Arch Gen Psychiatry 58:556–561, 2001b

Goddard AW, Mason GF, Appel M, et al: Impaired GABA neuronal response to acute benzodiazepine administration in panic disorder. Am J Psychiatry 161:2186–2193, 2004

Goldstein RB, Wickramaratne PJ, Horwath E, et al: Familial aggregation and phenomenology of "early" onset (at or before age 20 years) panic disorder. Arch Gen Psychiatry 54:271–278, 1997

Goodman WK, McDougle CJ, Price LH, et al: Beyond the serotonin hypothesis: a role for dopamine in some forms of obsessive compulsive disorder? J Clin Psychiatry 51 (suppl):36–43, 1990

Goodman WK, Bose A, Wang Q: Treatment of generalized anxiety disorder with escitalopram: pooled results from double-blind, placebo-controlled trials. J Affect Discord 87:161–167, 2005

Goodwin RD, Fergusson DM, Horwood LJ: Childhood abuse and familial violence and the risk of panic attacks and panic disorder in young adulthood. Psychol Med 35:881–890, 2005

Gorman JM, Fyer AF, Gliklich J, et al: Effect of imipramine on prolapsed mitral valves of patients with panic disorder. Am J Psychiatry 138:977–978, 1981

Gorman JM, Levy GF, Liebowitz MR, et al: Effect of acute β-adrenergic blockade on lactate-induced panic. Arch Gen Psychiatry 40:1079–1082, 1983

Gorman JM, Askanazi J, Liebowitz MR, et al: Response to hyperventilation in a group of patients with panic disorder. Am J Psychiatry 141:857–861, 1984

Gorman JM, Liebowitz MR, Fyer AJ, et al: Lactate infusions in obsessive-compulsive disorder. Am J Psychiatry 142:864–866, 1985

Gorman JM, Fyer MR, Goetz R, et al: Ventilatory physiology of patients with panic disorder. Arch Gen Psychiatry 45:31–39, 1988

Gorman JM, Battista D, Goetz RR, et al: A comparison of sodium bicarbonate and sodium lactate infusion in the induction of panic attacks. Arch Gen Psychiatry 46:145–150, 1989

Gorman JM, Kent JM, Sullivan GM, et al: Neuroanatomical hypothesis of panic disorder, revised. Am J Psychiatry 157:493–505, 2000

Gorman JM, Martinez J, Coplan JD, et al: The effect of successful treatment on the emotional and physiological response to carbon dioxide inhalation in patients with panic disorder. Biol Psychiatry 56:862–867, 2004

Grady TA, Pigott TA, L'Heureux F, et al: Double-blind study of adjuvant buspirone for fluoxetine-treated patients with obsessive-compulsive disorder. Am J Psychiatry 150:819–821, 1993

Grant BF, Hasin DS, Blanco C, et al: The epidemiology of social anxiety disorder in the United States: results from the National Epidemiologic Survey on Alcohol and Related Conditions. J Clin Psychiatry 66:1351–1361, 2005a

Grant BF, Hasin DS, Stinson FS, et al: Prevalence, correlates, comorbidity, and comparative disability of DSM-IV generalized anxiety disorder in the USA: results from the National Epidemiologic Survey on Alcohol and Related Conditions. Psychol Med 35:1747–1759, 2005b

Grant BF, Hasin DS, Stinson FS, et al: The epidemiology of DSM-IV panic disorder and agoraphobia in the United States: results from the National Epidemiologic Survey on Alcohol and Related Conditions. J Clin Psychiatry 67:363–374, 2006

Greist JH, Chouinard G, DuBoff E, et al: Double-blind parallel comparison of three dosages of sertraline and placebo in outpatients with obsessive-compulsive disorder. Arch Gen Psychiatry 52:289–295, 1995a

Greist JH, Jefferson JW, Kobak KA, et al: Efficacy and tolerability of serotonin transport inhibitors in obsessive-compulsive disorder: a meta-analysis. Arch Gen Psychiatry 52:53–60, 1995b

Greist JH, Jefferson JW, Kobak KA, et al: A 1-year double-blind placebo-controlled fixed dose study of sertraline in the treatment of obsessive-compulsive disorder. Int Clin Psychopharmacol 10:57–65, 1995c

Grillon C, Morgan CA: Fear-potentiated startle conditioning to explicit and contextual cues in Gulf War veterans with posttraumatic stress disorder. J Abnorm Psychol 108:134–142, 1999

Grisaru N, Amir M, Cohen H, et al: Effect of transcranial magnetic stimulation in posttraumatic stress disorder: a preliminary study. Biol Psychiatry 44:52–55, 1998

Gupta S, Popli A, Bathurst E, et al: Efficacy of cyproheptadine for nightmares associated with posttraumatic stress disorder. Compr Psychiatry 39:160–164, 1998

Gurvits TV, Gilbertson MW, Lasko NB, et al: Neurologic soft signs in chronic posttraumatic stress disorder. Arch Gen Psychiatry 57:181–186, 2000

Gurvits TV, Metzger LJ, Lasko NB, et al: Subtle neurologic compromise as vulnerability factor for combat related posttraumatic stress disorder: results of a twin study. Arch Gen Psychiatry 63:571–576, 2006

Hamilton SP, Slager SL, Heiman GA, et al: Evidence for a susceptibility locus for panic disorder near the catechol-O-methyltransferase gene on chromosome 22. Biol Psychiatry 51:591–601, 2002

Hamilton SP, Fyer AJ, Durner M, et al: Further genetic evidence for a panic disorder syndrome mapping to chromosome 13q. Proc Natl Acad Sci USA 100:2550–2555, 2003

Hamilton SP, Slager SL, DeLeon AB, et al: Evidence for genetic linkage between a polymorphism in the adenosine 2A receptor and panic disorder. Neuropsychopharmacol 29:558–565, 2004

Hamner MB, Deitsch SE, Brodrick PS, et al: Quetiapine treatment in patients with posttraumatic stress disorder: an open trial of adjunctive therapy. J Clin Psychopharmacol 23:15–20, 2003

Han L, Nielsen DA, Rosenthal NE, et al: No coding variant of the tryptophan hydroxylase gene detected in seasonal affective disorder, obsessive-compulsive disorder, anorexia nervosa, and alcoholism. Biol Psychiatry 45:615–619, 1999

Hanna GL, Veenstra VanderWeele J, Cox NJ, et al: Genome wide linkage analysis of families with obsessive compulsive disorder ascertained through pediatric probands. Am J Med Genet 114:541–552, 2002

Hariri AR, Drabant EM, Munoz KE, et al: A susceptibility gene for affective disorders and the response of the human amygdala. Arch Gen Psychiatry 62:146–152, 2005

Harvey AG, Bryant RA: Two-year prospective evaluation of the relationship between acute stress disorder and posttraumatic stress disorder following mild traumatic brain injury. Am J Psychiatry 157:626–628, 2000

Haug TT, Blomhoff S, Hellstrom K, et al: Exposure therapy and sertraline in social phobia: 1-year follow up of a randomized controlled trial. Br J Psychiatry 182:312–318, 2003

Hayward C, Killen JD, Draemer HC, et al: Linking self-reported childhood behavioral inhibition to adolescent social phobia. J Am Acad Child Adolesc Psychiatry 37:1308–1316, 1998

Heimberg RG, Dodge CS, Hope DA, et al: Cognitive behavioral group treatment for social phobia: comparison with a credible placebo control. Cognit Ther Res 14:1–23, 1990a

Heimberg RG, Hope DA, Dodge CS, et al: DSM-III-R subtypes of social phobia: comparison of generalized social phobics and public speaking phobics. J Nerv Ment Dis 178:172–179, 1990b

Heimberg RG, Liebowitz MR, Hope DA, et al: Cognitive behavioral group therapy vs phenelzine therapy for social phobia: a 12-week outcome. Arch Gen Psychiatry 55:1133–1141, 1998

Heldt E, Gus-Manfro G, Kipper L, et al: One-year follow-up of pharmacotherapy-resistant patients with panic disorder treated with cognitive-behavior therapy: outcome and predictors of remission. Behav Res Ther 44:657–665, 2006

Herman JL, van der Kolk BA: Traumatic antecedents of borderline personality disorder, in Psychological Trauma. Edited by van der Kolk BA. Washington, DC, American Psychiatric Press, 1987, pp 111–126

Herman JL, Perry JC, van der Kolk BA: Childhood trauma in borderline personality disorder. Am J Psychiatry 146:490–495, 1989

Hertzberg MA, Butterfield MI, Feldman ME, et al: A preliminary study of lamotrigine for the treatment of posttraumatic stress disorder. Biol Psychiatry 45:1226–1229, 1999

Hettema JM, Prescott CA, Kendler KS: Genetic and environmental sources of covariation between generalized anxiety disorder and neuroticism. Am J Psychiatry 161:1581–1587, 2004

Hewlett WA, Vinogradov S, Agras WS: Clomipramine, clonazepam, and clonidine treatment of obsessive-compulsive disorder. J Clin Psychopharmacol 12:420–430, 1992

Hirschmann S, Dannon PN, Iancu I, et al: Pindolol augmentation in patients with treatment-resistant panic disorder: a double-blind, placebo-controlled trial. J Clin Psychopharmacol 20:556–559, 2000

Hoehn-Saric R, McLeod DR, Zimmerli WD: Differential effects of alprazolam and imipramine in generalized anxiety disorder: somatic versus psychic symptoms. J Clin Psychiatry 49:293–301, 1988

Hoehn-Saric R, Hazlett RL, McLeod DR: Generalized anxiety disorder with early and late onset of anxiety symptoms. Compr Psychiatry 34:291–298, 1993

Hoenig K, Hochrein A, Quednow BB, et al: Impaired prepulse inhibition of acoustic startle in obsessive compulsive disorder. Biol Psychiatry 57:1153–1158, 2005

Hofmann SG: Perception of control over anxiety mediates the relation between catastrophic thinking and social anxiety in social phobia. Behav Res Ther 43:885–895, 2005

Hofmann SG, Moscovitch DA, Kim HJ, et al: Changes in self perception during treatment of social phobia. J Consult Clin Psychol 72:588–596, 2004

Hofmann SG, Meuret AE, Smits JA, et al: Augmentation of exposure therapy with D-cycloserine for social anxiety disorder. Arch Gen Psychiatry 63:298–304, 2006

Hogben GL, Cornfield RB: Treatment of traumatic war neurosis with phenelzine. Arch Gen Psychiatry 38:440–445, 1981

Hollander E, Dell'Osso B: Topiramate plus paroxetine in treatment resistant obsessive compulsive disorder. Int Clin Psychopharmacol 21:189–191, 2006

Hollander E, Liebowitz MR, Gorman JM, et al: Cortisol and sodium lactate-induced panic. Arch Gen Psychiatry 46:135–140, 1989

Hollander E, DeCaria C, Gully R, et al: Effects of chronic fluoxetine treatment on behavioral and neuroendocrine responses to meta-chlorophenylpiperazine in obsessive-compulsive disorder. Psychiatry Res 36:1–17, 1991a

Hollander E, DeCaria C, Nitescu A, et al: Noradrenergic function in obsessive-compulsive disorder: behavioral and neuroendocrine responses to clonidine and comparison to healthy controls. Psychiatry Res 37:161–177, 1991b

Hollander E, DeCaria CM, Nitescu A, et al: Serotonergic function in obsessive-compulsive disorder: behavioral and neuroendocrine responses to oral m-chlorophenylpiperazine and fenfluramine in patients and healthy volunteers. Arch Gen Psychiatry 49:21–28, 1992

Hollander E, Kwon J, Weiller F, et al: Serotonergic function in social phobia: comparison to normal control and obsessive-compulsive disorder subjects. Psychiatry Res 79:213–217, 1998

Hollander E, Bienstock C, Pallanti S, et al: The International Treatment Refractory OCD Consortium: preliminary findings. Presented at the 5th International OCD Conference, Sardinia, Italy, March 2001

Hollander E, Baldini Rossi N, Sood E, et al: Risperidone augmentation in treatment resistant obsessive compulsive disorder: a double blind, placebo controlled study. Int J Neuropsychopharmacol 6:397–401, 2003a

Hollander E, Friedberg J, Wasserman D, et al: Venlafaxine in treatment resistant obsessive compulsive disorder. J Clin Psychiatry 64:546–550, 2003b

Hollander E, Koran LM, Goodman WK, et al: A double blind, placebo controlled study of the efficacy and safety of controlled release fluvoxamine in patients with obsessive compulsive disorder. J Clin Psychiatry 64:640–647, 2003c

Hollifield M, Thompson PM, Ruiz JE, et al: Potential effectiveness and safety of olanzapine in refractory panic disorder. Depress Anxiety 21:33–40, 2005

Hornig CD, McNally RJ: Panic disorder and suicide attempt: a reanalysis of data from the Epidemiologic Catchment Area study. Br J Psychiatry 167:76–79, 1995

Horowitz MJ: Stress-Response Syndromes. New York, Jason Aronson, 1976

Horowitz MJ, Wilner N, Kaltreider N, et al: Signs and symptoms of posttraumatic stress disorders. Arch Gen Psychiatry 37:88–92, 1980

Hu XZ, Lipsky RH, Zhu G, et al: Serotonin transporter promoter gain of function genotypes are linked to obsessive compulsive disorder. Am J Hum Genet 78:815–826, 2006

Hudson J, Rapee R: The origins of social phobia. Behav Modif 24:102–129, 2000

Inada Y, Yoneda H, Koh J, et al: Positive association between panic disorder and polymorphism of the serotonin 2A receptor gene. Psychiatry Res 118:25–31, 2003

Ito LM, deAraujo LA, Tess VL, et al: Self-exposure therapy for panic disorder with agoraphobia: randomized controlled study of external v. interoceptive self-exposure. Br J Psychiatry 178:331–336, 2001

Janet P: Les Obsessions et la Psychasthenie, 2nd Edition. Paris, France, Bailliere, 1908

Jenike MA, Hyman S, Baer L, et al: A controlled trial of fluvoxamine in obsessive-compulsive disorder: implications for a serotonergic theory. Am J Psychiatry 147:1209–1215, 1990

Jenike MA, Baer L, Ballantine HT, et al: Cingulotomy for refractory obsessive-compulsive disorder: a long-term follow-up of 33 patients. Arch Gen Psychiatry 48:548–555, 1991

Jenike MA, Baer L, Minichiello WE, et al: Placebo-controlled trial of fluoxetine and phenelzine for obsessive-compulsive disorder. Am J Psychiatry 154:1261–1264, 1997

Johanson A, Risberg J, Tucker DM, et al: Changes in frontal lobe activity with cognitive therapy for spider phobia. Appl Neuropsychol 13:34–41, 2006

Johnson J, Weissman MM, Klerman GL: Panic disorder, comorbidity, and suicide attempts. Arch Gen Psychiatry 47:805–808, 1990

Johnson M, Lydiard R, Zealberg J, et al: Plasma and CSF HVA levels in panic patients with comorbid social phobia. Biol Psychiatry 36:425–427, 1994

Johnson MR, Marazziti D, Brawman MO, et al: Abnormal benzodiazepine receptor density associated with generalized social phobia. Biol Psychiatry 43:306–309, 1998

Kagan J, Reznick JS, Snidman N: The physiology and psychology of behavioral inhibition in children. Child Dev 58:1459–1473, 1987

Kampman M, Keijers GP, Hoogduin CA, et al: A randomized, double-blind, placebo-controlled study of the effects of adjunctive paroxetine in panic disorder patients unsuccessfully treated with cognitive-behavioral therapy alone. J Clin Psychiatry 63:772–777, 2002

Karayiorgou M, Altemus M, Galke BL, et al: Genotype determining low catechol-*O*-methyltransferase activity as a risk factor for obsessive-compulsive disorder. Proc Natl Acad Sci USA 94:4572–4575, 1997

Karayiorgou M, Sobin C, Bludell ML, et al: Family based association studies support a sexually dimorphic effect of COMT and MAOA on genetic susceptibility to obsessive-compulsive disorder. Biol Psychiatry 45:1178–1189, 1999

Kardiner A: Traumatic neurosis of war, in American Handbook of Psychiatry, Vol 201. Edited by Arieti S. New York, Basic Books, 1959, pp 245–257

Karno M, Golding JM, Sorenson SB, et al: The epidemiology of obsessive-compulsive disorder in five US communities. Arch Gen Psychiatry 45:1094–1099, 1988

Kasper S, Stein DJ, Loft H, et al: Escitalopram in the treatment of social anxiety disorder: randomized, placebo controlled, flexible dosage study. Br J Psychiatry 186:22–26, 2005

Katerndahl DA: Panic and prolapse: meta-analysis. J Nerv Ment Dis 181:539–544, 1993

Katschnig H, Amering M, Stolk JM, et al: Long-term follow-up after a drug trial for panic disorder. Br J Psychiatry 167:487–494, 1995

Katzelnick DJ, Kobak KA, Greist JH, et al: Sertraline for social phobia: a double-blind, placebo-controlled crossover study. Am J Psychiatry 152:1368–1371, 1995

Keck PE, Taylor VE, Tugrul KC, et al: Valproate treatment of panic disorder and lactate-induced panic attacks. Biol Psychiatry 33:542–546, 1993

Keijsers GP, Hoogduin CA, Schaap CP: Predictors of treatment outcome in the behavioral treatment of obsessive-compulsive disorder. Br J Psychiatry 165:781–786, 1994

Kellner M, Schick M, Yassouridis A, et al: Metyrapone tests in patients with panic disorder. Biol Psychiatry 56:898–900, 2004

Kendler KS, Neale MC, Kessler RC, et al: Generalized anxiety disorder in women: a population-based twin study. Arch Gen Psychiatry 49:267–272, 1992

Kennedy JL, Bradwejn J, Koszycki D, et al: Investigation of cholecystokinin system genes in panic disorder. Mol Psychiatry 4:284–285, 1999

Kent JM, Papp LA, Martinez JM, et al: Specificity of panic response to CO(2) inhalation in panic disorder: a comparison with major depression and premenstrual dysphoric disorder. Am J Psychiatry 158:58–67, 2001

Kent JM, Coplan JD, Mawlawi O, et al: Prediction of panic response to a respiratory stimulant by reduced orbitofrontal cerebral blood flow in panic disorder. Am J Psychiatry 162:1379–1381, 2005

Kenwright M, Marks IM: Computer aided self help for phobia/panic via internet at home: a pilot study. Br J Psychiatry 184:448–449, 2004

Kessler RC, McGonagle KA, Zhao S, et al: Lifetime and 12-month prevalence of DSM-III-R psychiatric disorders in the United States: results from the National Comorbidity Survey. Arch Gen Psychiatry 51:8–19, 1994

Kessler RC, Sonnega A, Bromet E, et al: Posttraumatic stress disorder in the National Comorbidity Survey. Arch Gen Psychiatry 52:1048–1060, 1995

Kessler RC, DuPont RL, Berglund P, et al: Impairment in pure and comorbid generalized anxiety disorder and major depression at 12 months in two national surveys. Am J Psychiatry 156:1915–1923, 1999a

Kessler RC, Stang P, Wittchen HU, et al: Lifetime comorbidities between social phobia and mood disorders in the US National Comorbidity Survey. Psychol Med 29:555–567, 1999b

Kessler RC, Brandenburg N, Lane M, et al: Rethinking the duration requirement for generalized anxiety disorder: evidence from the National Comorbidity Survey Replication. Psychol Med 35:1073–1082, 2005

Kessler RC, Chiu WT, Jin R, et al: The epidemiology of panic attacks, panic disorder, and agoraphobia in the National Comorbidity Survey Replication. Arch Gen Psychiatry 63:415–424, 2006

Kim JJ, Lee MC, Kim J, et al: Grey matter abnormalities in obsessive compulsive disorder: statistical parametric mapping of segmented magnetic resonance images. Br J Psychiatry 179:330–334, 2001

Kim SJ, Veenstra-VanderWeele J, Hanna GL, et al: Mutation screening of human 5HT(2B)receptor gene in early onset obsessive-compulsive disorder. Mol Cell Probes 14:47–52, 2000

Kinrys G, Wygant LE, Pardo TB, et al: Levetiracetam for treatment-refractory posttraumatic stress disorder. J Clin Psychiatry 67:211–214, 2006

Kinzie JD, Leung P: Clonidine in Cambodian patients with posttraumatic stress disorder. J Nerv Ment Dis 177:546–550, 1989

Kitayama N, Vaccarino C, Kutner M, et al: Magnetic resonance imaging (MRI) measurement of hippocampal volume in posttraumatic stress disorder: a meta analysis. J Affect Disord 88:79–86, 2005

Klein DF: Delineation of two drug responsive anxiety syndromes. Psychopharmacologia 5:397–408, 1964

Klein DF: Anxiety reconceptualized, in Anxiety: New Research and Changing Concepts. Edited by Klein DF, Rabkin JG. New York, Raven, 1981, pp 235–263

Klein DF: False suffocation alarms, spontaneous panics, and related conditions: an integrative hypothesis. Arch Gen Psychiatry 50:306–317, 1993

Klein M: A contribution to the theory of anxiety and guilt. Int J Psychoanal 29:114–123, 1948

Klinger E, Bouchard S, Legeron P, et al: Virtual reality therapy versus cognitive behavior therapy for social phobia: a preliminary controlled study. Cyberpsychol Behav 8:76–88, 2005

Knesevich JW: Successful treatment of obsessive-compulsive disorder with clonidine hydrochloride. Am J Psychiatry 139:364–365, 1982

Knowles JA, Fyer AJ, Vieland VJ, et al: Results of a genome-wide genetic screen for panic disorder. Am J Med Genet 28:139–147, 1998

Kobak KA, Greist JH, Jefferson JW, et al: Behavioral versus pharmacological treatments of obsessive compulsive disorder: a meta-analysis. Psychopharmacology (Berl) 136:205–216, 1998

Kobak KA, Taylor LV, Bystritsky A, et al: St. John's wort versus placebo in obsessive compulsive disorder: results from a double blind study. Int Clin Psychopharmacol 20:299–304, 2005a

Kobak KA, Taylor LV, Warner G, et al: St. John's wort versus placebo in social phobia: results from a placebo controlled pilot study. J Clin Psychopharmacol 25:51–58, 2005b

Kolb LC: A neuropsychological hypothesis explaining posttraumatic stress disorders. Am J Psychiatry 144:989–995, 1987

Kolb LC, Burris BC, Griffiths S: Propranolol and clonidine in treatment of the chronic post-traumatic stress disorders of war, in Post-Traumatic Stress Disorder: Psychological and Biological Sequelae. Edited by van der Kolk BA. Washington, DC, American Psychiatric Press, 1984, pp 97–105

Koran LM, Gamel NN, Choung HW, et al: Mirtazapine for obsessive compulsive disorder: an open trial followed by double blind discontinuation. J Clin Psychiatry 66:515–520, 2005

Koran LM, Aboujaoude E, Ward H, et al: Pulse loaded intravenous clomipramine in treatment resistant obsessive compulsive disorder. J Clin Psychopharmacol 26:79–83, 2006

Koren D, Arnon I, Klein E: Acute stress response and posttraumatic stress disorder in traffic accident victims: a one-year prospective, follow-up study. Am J Psychiatry 156:367–373, 1999

Kozaric-Kovacic D, Pivac N, Muck Seler D, et al: Risperidone in psychotic combat related posttraumatic stress disorder: an open label trial. J Clin Psychiatry 66:922–927, 2005

Krakow B, Hollifield M, Johnston L, et al: Imagery rehearsal therapy for chronic nightmares in sexual assault survivors with posttraumatic stress disorder: a randomized controlled trial. JAMA 286:537–545, 2001

Kronig MH, Apter J, Asnis G, et al: Placebo-controlled, multicenter study of sertraline treatment for obsessive-compulsive disorder. J Clin Psychopharmacol 19:172–176, 1999

Krystal H: Massive Psychic Trauma. New York, International Universities Press, 1968

Lafleur DL, Pittenger C, Kelmendi B, et al: N acetylcysteine augmentation in serotonin reuptake inhibitor refractory obsessive compulsive disorder. Psychopharmacology 284:254–256, 2006

Lanius RA, Williamson PC, Bluhm RL, et al: Functional connectivity of dissociative responses in posttraumatic stress disorder: a functional magnetic resonance imaging investigation. Biol Psychiatry 57:873–884, 2005

Leckman JF, Goodman WK, North WG, et al: Elevated cerebrospinal fluid levels of oxytocin in obsessive-compulsive disorder: comparison with Tourette's syndrome and healthy controls. Arch Gen Psychiatry 51:782–792, 1994

Leckman JF, Grice DE, Boardman J, et al: Symptoms of obsessive-compulsive disorder. Am J Psychiatry 154:911–917, 1997

Lee C, Gavriel H, Drummond P, et al: Treatment of PTSD: stress inoculation training with prolonged exposure compared to EMDR. J Clin Psychol 58:1071–1089, 2002

Lee HJ, Lee MS, Kang RH, et al: Influence of serotonin transporter promoter gene polymorphism on susceptibility to posttraumatic stress disorder. Depress Anxiety 21:1135–1139, 2005

Leonard HL, Swedo SE, Lenane MC, et al: A 2- to 7-year follow-up study of 54 obsessive compulsive children and adolescents. Arch Gen Psychiatry 50:429–439, 1993

Lepola UM, Wade AG, Leinonen EV, et al: A controlled, prospective, 1-year trial of citalopram in the treatment of panic disorder. J Clin Psychiatry 59:528–534, 1998

Leskin GA, Sheikh JI: Lifetime trauma history and panic disorder: findings from the National Comorbidity Survey. J Anxiety Disord 16:599–603, 2002

Levin P, Lazrove S, van der Kolk B: What psychological testing and neuroimaging tell us about the treatment of posttraumatic stress disorder by eye movement desensitization and reprocessing. J Anxiety Disord 13:159–172, 1999

Li X, May RS, Tolbert LC, et al: Risperidone and haloperidol augmentation of serotonin reuptake inhibitors in refractory obsessive compulsive disorder: a crossover study. J Clin Psychiatry 66:736–743, 2005

Lieb R, Wittchen HU, Hofler M, et al: Parental psychopathology, parenting styles, and the risk of social phobia in offspring: a prospective-longitudinal community study. Arch Gen Psychiatry 57:859–866, 2000

Liebowitz MR, Fyer AJ, Gorman JM, et al: Lactate provocation of panic attacks, I: clinical and behavioral findings. Arch Gen Psychiatry 41:764–770, 1984

Liebowitz MR, Gorman JM, Fyer AJ, et al: Lactate provocation of panic attacks, II: biochemical and physiological findings. Arch Gen Psychiatry 42:709–719, 1985a

Liebowitz MR, Gorman JM, Fyer AJ, et al: Social phobia: review of a neglected anxiety disorder. Arch Gen Psychiatry 42:729–736, 1985b

Liebowitz MR, Schneier F, Campeas R, et al: Phenelzine vs atenolol in social phobia: a placebo-controlled comparison. Arch Gen Psychiatry 49:290–300, 1992

Liebowitz MR, Heimberg RG, Schneier FR, et al: Cognitive-behavioral therapy versus phenelzine in social phobia: long-term outcome. Depress Anxiety 10:89–98, 1999

Liebowitz MR, Stein MB, Tancer M, et al: A randomized, double blind, fixed dose comparison of paroxetine and placebo in the treatment of generalized social anxiety disorder. J Clin Psychiatry 63:66–74, 2002a

Liebowitz MR, Turner SM, Piacentini J, et al: Fluoxetine in children and adolescents with OCD: a placebo controlled trial. J Am Acad Child Adolesc Psychiatry 41:1431–1438, 2002b

Liebowitz MR, De Martinis NA, Weihs K, et al: Efficacy of sertraline in severe generalized social anxiety disorder: results of a double blind, placebo controlled study. J Clin Psychiatry 64:785–792, 2003

Liebowitz MR, Gelenberf AJ, Munjack D: Venlafaxine extended release vs. placebo and paroxetine in social anxiety disorder. Arch Gen Psychiatry 62:190–198, 2005

Lindauer RJ, Vlieger EJ, Jalink M, et al: Smaller hippocampal volume in Dutch police officers with posttraumatic stress disorder. Biol Psychiatry 56:356–363, 2004

Lindauer RJ, Gersons BP, vanMeijel EP, et al: Effects of brief eclectic psychotherapy in patients with posttraumatic stress disorder: randomized clinical trial. J Trauma Stress 18:205–212, 2005

Lindley SEE, Carlson EB, Benoit M: Basal and dexamethasone suppressed salivary cortisol concentration in a community sample of patients with posttraumatic stress disorder. Biol Psychiatry 55:940–945, 2005

Lindy JD, Grace MC, Green BL: Building a conceptual bridge between civilian trauma and war trauma: preliminary psychological findings from a clinical sample of Vietnam veterans, in Post-Traumatic Stress Disorder: Psychological and Biological Sequelae. Edited by van der Kolk BA. Washington, DC, American Psychiatric Press, 1984, pp 44–57

Lipper S, Davidson JRT, Grady TA, et al: Preliminary study of carbamazepine in post-traumatic stress disorder. Psychosomatics 27:849–854, 1986

Lippitz BE, Mindus P, Meyerson BA, et al: Lesion topography and outcome after thermocapsulotomy or gamma knife capsulotomy for obsessive-compulsive disorder: relevance of the right hemisphere. Neurosurgery 44:452–458, 1999

Lipschitz DS, Mayes LM, Rasmussen AM, et al: Baseline and modulated acoustic startle responses in adolescent girls with posttraumatic stress disorder. J Am Acad Child Adolesc Psychiatry 44:807–814, 2005

Lipsitz JD, Mannuzza S, Klein DF, et al: Specific phobia 10–16 years after treatment. Depress Anxiety 10:105–111, 1999a

Lipsitz JD, Markowitz JC, Cherry S, et al: Open trial of interpersonal psychotherapy for the treatment of social phobia. Am J Psychiatry 156:1814–1816, 1999b

Lochner C, Kinnear CJ, Hemmings SM, et al: Hoarding in obsessive compulsive disorder: clinical and genetic correlates. J Clin Psychiatry 66:1155–1160, 2005

Londborg PD, Wolkow R, Smith WT, et al: Sertraline in the treatment of panic disorder: a multi-site, double-blind, placebo-controlled, fixed-dose investigation. Br J Psychiatry 173:54–60, 1998

Lorberbaum JP, Lose S, Johnson MR, et al: Neural correlates of speech anticipatory anxiety in generalized social phobia. Neuroreport 15:2701–2705, 2004

Lucey JV, Barry S, Webb MG, et al: The desipramine-induced hormone response and the dexamethasone suppression test in obsessive-compulsive disorder. Acta Psychiatr Scand 86:367–370, 1992

MacDonald PA, Antony MM, Macleod CM, et al: Memory and confidence in memory judgements among individuals with obsessive compulsive disorder and nonclinical controls. Behav Res Ther 35:497–505, 1997

Macklin ML, Metzger LJ, Litz BT, et al: Lower precombat intelligence is a risk factor for posttraumatic stress disorder. J Consult Clin Psychol 66:323–326, 1998

Macklin ML, Metzger LJ, Lasko NB, et al: Five-year follow-up study of eye movement desensitization and reprocessing therapy for combat-related posttraumatic stress disorder. Compr Psychiatry 41:24–27, 2000

MacLeod C, Cohen IL: Anxiety and the interpretation of ambiguity: a text comprehension study. J Abnorm Psychol 2:102, 1993

MacLeod C, McLaughlin K: Implicit and explicit memory bias in anxiety: a conceptual replication. Behav Res Ther 33:1–14, 1995

Magee WJ, Eaton WW, Wittchen HU, et al: Agoraphobia, simple phobia, and social phobia in the National Comorbidity Survey. Arch Gen Psychiatry 53:159–168, 1996

Maier SF, Seligman ME: Learned helplessness: theory and evidence. J Exp Psychol 105:3–46, 1976

Maier SF, Dovies S, Gran JW: Opiate antagonists and long-term analgesic reaction induced by inescapable shock in rats. J Comp Physiol Psychol 94:1172–1183, 1980

Maletzky B, McFarland B, Burt A: Refractory obsessive compulsive disorder and ECT. Convuls Ther 10:34–42, 1994

Malizia AL, Cunningham VJ, Bell CJ, et al: Decreased brain GABA (A)-benzodiazepine receptor binding in panic disorder: preliminary results from a quantitative PET study. Arch Gen Psychiatry 55:715–720, 1998

Mannuzza S, Schneier FR, Chapman TF, et al: Generalized social phobia: reliability and validity. Arch Gen Psychiatry 52:230–237, 1995

Mantovani A, Lisanby SH, Pieraccini F, et al: Repetitive transcranial magnetic stimulation in the treatment of obsessive compulsive disorder and Tourette's syndrome. Int J Neuropsychopharmacol 9:95–100, 2006

March JS, Amaya-Jackson L, Murray MC, et al: Cognitive-behavioral psychotherapy for children and adolescents with posttraumatic stress disorder after a single-incident stressor. J Am Acad Child Adolesc Psychiatry 37:585–593, 1998a

March JS, Biederman J, Wolkow R, et al: Sertraline in children and adolescents with obsessive-compulsive disorder: a multicenter randomized controlled trial. JAMA 280:1752–1756, 1998b

Marks I: Behaviour therapy for obsessive-compulsive disorder: a decade of progress. Can J Psychiatry 42:1021–1027, 1997

Marks IM, Hodgson R, Rachman S: Treatment of chronic obsessive-compulsive neurosis by in vivo exposure: a two-year follow-up and issues in treatment. Br J Psychiatry 127:349–364, 1975

Marks IM, Gray S, Cohen D, et al: Imipramine and brief therapist-aided exposure in agoraphobics having self-exposure homework. Arch Gen Psychiatry 40:153–162, 1983

Marks I, Lovell K, Noshirvani H, et al: Treatment of posttraumatic stress disorder by exposure and/or cognitive restructuring: a controlled study. Arch Gen Psychiatry 55:317–325, 1998

Marmar CR, Weiss DS, Schlenger WE, et al: Peritraumatic dissociation and posttraumatic stress in male Vietnam theater veterans. Am J Psychiatry 151:902–907, 1994

Maron E, Kuikka JT, Shlik J, et al: Reduced brain serotonin transporter binding in patients with panic disorder. Psychiatry Res 132:173–181, 2004

Maron E, Nikopensius T, Koks S, et al: Association study of 90 candidate gene polymorphisms in panic disorder. Psychiatr Genet 15:17–24, 2005

Marshall JR: The treatment of night terrors associated with posttraumatic syndrome. Am J Psychiatry 132:293–295, 1975

Marshall RD, Beebe KL, Oldham M, et al: Efficacy and safety of paroxetine treatment for chronic PTSD: a fixed-dose, placebo-controlled study. Am J Psychiatry 158:1982–1988, 2001

Mason JW, Giller EL, Kosten TR, et al: Urinary free-cortisol levels in posttraumatic stress disorder patients. J Nerv Ment Dis 174:145–149, 1986

Mason JW, Giller EL, Kosten TR, et al: Elevation of urinary norepinephrine/cortisol ratio in posttraumatic stress disorder. J Nerv Ment Dis 176:498–502, 1988

Massion AO, Dyck IR, Shea MT, et al: Personality disorders and time to remission in generalized anxiety disorder, social phobia, and panic disorder. Arch Gen Psychiatry 59:434–440, 2002

Mataix-Cols D, Rauch SL, Manzo PA, et al: Use of factor-analyzed symptom dimensions to predict outcome with serotonin reuptake inhibitors and placebo in the treatment of obsessive-compulsive disorder. Am J Psychiatry 156:1409–1416, 1999

Mataix-Cols D, Wooderson S, Lawrence N, et al: Distinct neural correlates of washing, checking, and hoarding symptom dimensions in obsessive compulsive disorder. Arch Gen Psychiatry 61:564–576, 2004

Mataix-Cols D, Rosario Campos MC, Leckman JF: A multi-dimensional model of obsessive compulsive disorder. Am J Psychiatry 162:228–238, 2005

Mathew RJ, Ho BT, Kralik P, et al: Catecholamines and monoamine oxidase activity in anxiety. Acta Psychiatr Scand 63:245–252, 1981

Mathew SJ, Amiel JM, Coplan JD, et al: Open-label trial of riluzole in generalized anxiety disorder. Am J Psychiatry 162:2379–2381, 2005

Mattes J: More on panic disorder and mitral valve prolapse (letter). Am J Psychiatry 138:1130, 1981

Mattick RP, Peters L, Clarke JC: Exposure and cognitive restructuring for social phobia: a controlled study. Behav Ther 20:3–23, 1989

Mavissakalian M, Michelson L: Agoraphobia: relative and combined effectiveness of therapist-assisted in vivo exposure and imipramine. J Clin Psychiatry 47:117–122, 1986a

Mavissakalian M, Michelson L: Two-year follow-up of exposure and imipramine treatment of agoraphobia. Am J Psychiatry 143:1106–1112, 1986b

Mavissakalian M, Perel JM: Imipramine dose-response relationship in panic disorder with agoraphobia: preliminary findings. Arch Gen Psychiatry 46:127–131, 1989

Mavissakalian M, Perel JM: Clinical experiments in maintenance and discontinuation of imipramine therapy in panic disorder with agoraphobia. Arch Gen Psychiatry 49:318–323, 1992

Mavissakalian M, Perel JM: Imipramine treatment of panic disorder with agoraphobia: dose ranging and plasma level-response relationships. Am J Psychiatry 152:673–682, 1995

McCafferty JP, Bellew KM, Zaninelli RM: Paroxetine treatment of GAD: an analysis of response by dose. Presented at the annual meeting of the American Psychiatric Association, New Orleans, LA, May 2001

McDougle CJ, Goodman WK, Price LH, et al: Neuroleptic addition in fluvoxamine-refractory obsessive-compulsive disorder. Am J Psychiatry 147:652–654, 1990

McDougle CJ, Price LH, Goodman WK, et al: A controlled trial of lithium augmentation in fluvoxamine-refractory obsessive-compulsive disorder: lack of efficacy. J Clin Psychopharmacol 11:175–181, 1991a

McDougle CJ, Southwick SM, Charney DS, et al: An open trial of fluoxetine in the treatment of posttraumatic stress disorder. J Clin Psychopharmacol 11:325–327, 1991b

McDougle CJ, Goodman WK, Leckman JF, et al: The efficacy of fluvoxamine in obsessive-compulsive disorder: effects of comorbid chronic tic disorder. J Clin Psychopharmacol 13:354–358, 1993a

McDougle CJ, Goodman WK, Leckman JF, et al: Limited therapeutic effect of addition of buspirone in fluvoxamine-refractory obsessive-compulsive disorder. Am J Psychiatry 150:647–649, 1993b

McDougle CJ, Goodman WK, Leckman JF, et al: Haloperidol addition in fluvoxamine-refractory obsessive-compulsive disorder: a double-blind, placebo-controlled study in patients with and without tics. Arch Gen Psychiatry 51:302–308, 1994

McDougle CJ, Epperson CN, Pelton GH, et al: A double-blind, placebo-controlled study of risperidone addition in serotonin reuptake inhibitor-refractory obsessive-compulsive disorder. Arch Gen Psychiatry 57:794–801, 2000

McFarlane AC: The aetiology of post-traumatic morbidity: predisposing, precipitating and perpetuating factors. Br J Psychiatry 154:221–228, 1989

McFarlane AC: Vulnerability to posttraumatic stress disorder, in Posttraumatic Stress Disorder: Etiology, Phenomenology, and Treatment. Edited by Wolf ME, Mosnaim AD. Washington, DC, American Psychiatric Press, 1990, pp 2–20

McGuire PK, Bench CJ, Frith CD, et al: Functional anatomy of obsessive-compulsive phenomena. Br J Psychiatry 164:459–468, 1994

McKay D: A maintenance program for obsessive-compulsive disorder using exposure with response prevention: 2-year follow-up. Behav Res Ther 35:367–369, 1997

McNally RJ, Metzger LJ, Lasko NB, et al: Directed forgetting of trauma cues in adult survivors of childhood sexual abuse with and without posttraumatic stress disorder. J Abnorm Psychol 107:596–601, 1998

Meira-Lima I, Shavitt RG, Miguita K, et al: Association analysis of the catechol-O-methyltransferase (COMT), serotonin transporter(5-HTT) and serotonin 2A receptor (5HT2A) gene polymorphisms with obsessive compulsive disorder. Genes Brain Behav 3:75–79, 2004

Mell LK, Davis RL, Owens D: Association between streptococcal infection and obsessive compulsive disorder, Tourette's syndrome and tic disorder. Pediatrics 116:56–60, 2005

Mellman TA, Knorr BR, Pigeon WR, et al: Heart rate variability during sleep and the early development of posttraumatic stress disorder. Biol Psychiatry 55:953–956, 2004

Mennin DS, Heimberg RG, Turk CL, et al: Preliminary evidence for an emotion dysregulation model of generalized anxiety disorder. Behav Res Ther 43:1281–1310, 2005

Michels R, Frances A, Shear MK: Psychodynamic models of anxiety, in Anxiety and the Anxiety Disorders. Edited by Tuma AH, Maser JD. Hillsdale, NJ, Lawrence Erlbaum, 1985, pp 595–618

Michelson D, Lydiard RB, Pollack MH, et al: Outcome assessment and clinical improvement in panic disorder: evidence from a randomized controlled trial of fluoxetine and placebo. The Fluoxetine Panic Disorder Study Group. Am J Psychiatry 155:1570–1577, 1998

Michelson D, Pollack M, Lydiard RB, et al: Continuing treatment of panic disorder after acute response: randomized, placebo-controlled trial with fluoxetine. The Fluoxetine Panic Disorder Study Group. Br J Psychiatry 174:213–218, 1999

Michelson L, Marchione K, Greenwald M, et al: Panic disorder: cognitive-behavioral treatment. Behav Res Ther 28:141–151, 1990

Miller HE, Deakin JF, Anderson IM: Effect of acute tryptophan depletion on CO_2-induced anxiety in patients with panic disorder and normal volunteers. Br J Psychiatry 176:182–188, 2000

Millet B, Chabane N, Delorme R, et al: Association between the dopamine receptor D4 (DRD4) gene and obsessive compulsive disorder. Am J Med Genet B Neuropsychiatr Genet 116:55–59, 2003

Mills KI, Teesson M, Ross J, et al: Trauma, PTSD, and substance use disorders: findings from the Australian National Survey of Mental Health and Well-Being. Am J Psychiatry 163:652–658, 2006

Milrod B, Busch F, Leon AC, et al: Open trial of psychodynamic psychotherapy for panic disorder: a pilot study. Am J Psychiatry 157:1878–1880, 2000

Milrod B, Busch F, Leon AC, et al: A pilot open trial of brief psychodynamic psychotherapy for panic disorder. J Psychother Pract Res 10:239–245, 2001

Mindus, Jenike MA: Neurosurgical treatment of malignant obsessive-compulsive disorder. Psychiatr Clin North Am 15:921–938, 1992

Mitte K: Meta-analysis of cognitive-behavioral treatments for generalized anxiety disorder: a comparison with pharmacotherapy. Psychol Bull 131:785–795, 2005

Mogg K, Mathews A, Weinman J: Selective processing of threat cues in anxiety states: a replication. Behav Res Ther 27:317–323, 1989

Mogg K, Millar N, Bradley BP: Biases in eye movements to threatening facial expressions in generalized anxiety disorder and depressive disorder. J Abnorm Psychol 109:695–704, 2000

Montgomery SA, McIntyre A, Osterheider M, et al: A double-blind, placebo-controlled study of fluoxetine in patients with DSM-III-R obsessive-compulsive disorder. The Lilly European OCD Study Group. Eur Neuropsychopharmacol 3:143–152, 1993

Montgomery SA, Kasper S, Stein DJ, et al: Citalopram 20 mg, 40 mg, 60mg are all effective and well tolerated compared with placebo in obsessive compulsive disorder. Int J Clin Psychopharmacol 16:75–86, 2001

Montgomery SA, Nil R, Durr-Pal N, et al: A 24 week randomized, double blind, placebo controlled study of escitalopram for the prevention of generalized social anxiety disorder. J Clin Psychiatry 66:1270–1278, 2005

Mowrer O: A stimulus response analysis of anxiety and its role as a reinforcing agent. Psychol Rev 46:553–565, 1939

Muehlbacher M, Nickel MK, Nickel C, et al: Mirtazapine treatment of social phobia in women: a randomized, double-blind, placebo-controlled study. J Clin Psychopharmacol 25:580–583, 2005

Mundo E, Richter MA, Sam F, et al: Is the 5-HT(1Dbeta) receptor gene implicated in the pathogenesis of obsessive-compulsive disorder? Am J Psychiatry 157:1160–1161, 2000

Muris P, Schmidt H, Meckelbach H: The structure of specific phobia symptoms among children and adolescents. Behav Res Ther 37:863–868, 1999

Murphy TK, Goodman WK, Fudge MW, et al: B lymphocyte antigen D8/17: a peripheral marker for childhood-onset obsessive-compulsive disorder and Tourette's syndrome? Am J Psychiatry 154:402–407, 1997

Nakamura K, Yamada K, Iwayama Y, et al: Evidence that variation in the peripheral benzodiazepine receptor (PBR) gene influences susceptibility to panic disorder. Am J Med Genet 141:222–226, 2006

Nakao T, Nakagawa A, Yoshiura T, et al: Brain activation of patients with obsessive compulsive disorder during neuropsychological and symptom provocation tasks before and after symptom improvement: a functional magnetic resonance imaging study. Biol Psychiatry 57:901–910, 2005

Nee LE, Caine ED, Polinsky RJ, et al: Gilles de la Tourette syndrome: clinical and family study of 50 cases. Ann Neurol 7:41–49, 1982

Nelson EC, Grant JD, Bucholz KK, et al: Social phobia in a population-based female adolescent twin sample: comorbidity and associated suicide-related symptoms. Psychol Med 30:797–804, 2000

Nemiah JC: A psychoanalytic view of phobias. Am J Psychoanal 41:115–120, 1981

Nemiah JC: The psychodynamic view of anxiety: an historical approach, in Handbook of Anxiety, Vol 1. Edited by Roth M, Noyes R, Burrows GD. Amsterdam, The Netherlands, Elsevier, 1988, pp 277–303

Nestadt G, Lan T, Samuels J, et al: Complex segregation analysis provides compelling evidence for a major gene underlying obsessive-compulsive disorder and for heterogeneity by sex. Am J Hum Genet 67:1611–1616, 2000a

Nestadt G, Samuels J, Riddle M, et al: A family study of obsessive-compulsive disorder. Arch Gen Psychiatry 57:358–363, 2000b

Neumeister A, Bain E, Nugent AC, et al: Reduced serotonin type 1A receptor binding in panic disorder. J Neurosci 24:589–591, 2004

Neylan TC, Metzler TJ, Schoenfeld FB, et al: Fluvoxamine and sleep disturbances in posttraumatic stress disorder. J Trauma Stress 14:461–467, 2001

Neziroglu F, Anemone R, Yaryura-Tobias JA: Onset of obsessive-compulsive disorder in pregnancy. Am J Psychiatry 149:947–950, 1992

Nicolson R, Swedo SE, Lenane M, et al: An open trial of plasma exchange in childhood-onset obsessive-compulsive disorder without poststreptococcal exacerbations. J Am Acad Child Adolesc Psychiatry 39:1313–1315, 2000

Ninan PT, Koran LM, Kiev A, et al: High-dose sertraline strategy for nonresponders to acute treatment for obsessive-compulsive disorder: a multicenter double-blind trial. J Clin Psychiatry 67:15–22, 2006

Noyes R Jr, Reich JH, Christiansen J, et al: Outcome of panic disorder: relationship to diagnostic subtypes and comorbidity. Arch Gen Psychiatry 47:809–818, 1990

Noyes R Jr, Reich JH, Suelzer M, et al: Personality traits associated with panic disorder: change associated with treatment. Compr Psychiatry 32:283–294, 1991

Noyes R Jr, Clancy J, Woodman C, et al: Environmental factors related to the outcome of panic disorder: a seven-year follow-up study. J Nerv Ment Dis 181:529–538, 1993

Nutt DJ: Altered central α2-adrenoreceptor sensitivity in panic disorder. Arch Gen Psychiatry 46:165–169, 1989

Nutt DJ, Glue P, Lawson C, et al: Flumazenil provocation of panic attacks: evidence for altered benzodiazepine receptor sensitivity in panic disorder. Arch Gen Psychiatry 47:917–925, 1990

Nuttin BJ, Gabriels LA, Cosyns PR, et al: Long term electrical capsular stimulation in patients with obsessive compulsive disorder. Neurosurgery 52:1263–1272, 2003

O'Rourke D, Fahy TJ, Brophy J, et al: The Galway study of panic disorder, III: outcome at 5 to 6 years. Br J Psychiatry 168:462–469, 1996

Oehrberg S, Christiansen PE, Behnke K, et al: Paroxetine in the treatment of panic disorder: a randomised, double-blind, placebo-controlled study. Br J Psychiatry 167:374–379, 1995

Orr SP, Metzger LJ, Lasko NB, et al: De novo conditioning in trauma-exposed individuals with and without post-traumatic stress disorder. J Abnorm Psychol 109:290–298, 2000

Ost LG, Breitholtz E: Applied relaxation versus cognitive therapy in the treatment of generalized anxiety disorder. Behav Res Ther 38:777–790, 2000

Ost LG, Westling BE: Applied relaxation vs. cognitive behavior therapy in the treatment of panic disorder. Behav Res Ther 33:145–158, 1995

Ost LG, Thulin U, Ramnero J: Cognitive behavior therapy vs. exposure in vivo in the treatment of panic disorder with agoraphobia. Behav Res Ther 42:1105–1127, 2004

Otte C, Wiedemann K, Yassouridis A, et al: Valproate monotherapy in the treatment of civilian patients with non combat related posttraumatic stress disorder: an open label study. J Clin Psychopharmacol 24:106–108, 2004

Otto MW, Pollack MH, Sachs GS, et al: Discontinuation of benzodiazepine treatment: efficacy of cognitive-behavioral therapy for patients with panic disorder. Am J Psychiatry 150:1485–1490, 1993

Otto MW, Pollack MH, Gould RA, et al: A comparison of the efficacy of clonazepam and cognitive-behavioral group therapy for the treatment of social phobia. J Anxiety Disord 14:345–358, 2000

Ozer EJ, Best SR, Lipsey TL, et al: Predictors of posttraumatic stress disorder and symptoms in adults: a meta analysis. Psychol Bull 129:52–72, 2003

Palatnik A, Frolov K, Fux M, et al: Double-blind, crossover trial of inositol versus fluvoxamine for the treatment of panic disorder. J Clin Psychopharmacol 21:335–339, 2001

Pallanti S, Quercioli L, Paiva RS, et al: Citalopram for treatment-resistant obsessive-compulsive disorder. Eur Psychiatry 14:101–106, 1999

Pallanti S, Quercioli L, Bruscholi M: Response acceleration with mirtazapine augmentation of citalopram in obsessive compulsive disorder patients without comorbid depression: a pilot study. J Clin Psychiatry 65:1394–1399, 2004

Pande AC, Davidson JRT, Jefferson JW, et al: Treatment of social phobia with gabapentin: a placebo-controlled study. J Clin Psychopharmacol 19:341–348, 1999

Pande AC, Pollack MH, Crockatt J, et al: Placebo-controlled study of gabapentin treatment of panic disorder. J Clin Psychopharmacol 20:467–471, 2000

Pande AC, Feltner DE, Jefferson JW, et al: Efficacy of the novel anxiolytic pregabalin in social anxiety disorder: a placebo controlled, multicenter study. J Clin Psychopharmacol 24:141–149, 2004

Paquette V, Levesque J, Mensour B, et al: "Change the mind and you change the brain": effects of cognitive behavioral therapy on the neural correlates of spider phobia. Neuroimage 18:401–409, 2003

Pato MT, Zohar-Kadouch R, Zohar J, et al: Return of symptoms after discontinuation of clomipramine in patients with obsessive-compulsive disorder. Am J Psychiatry 145:1521–1525, 1988

Pato MT, Pigott TA, Hill JL, et al: Controlled comparison of buspirone and clomipramine in obsessive-compulsive disorder. Am J Psychiatry 148:127–129, 1991

Pauls DL, Towbin KE, Leckman JF, et al: Gilles de la Tourette's and obsessive-compulsive disorder: evidence supporting a genetic relationship. Arch Gen Psychiatry 43:1180–1182, 1986

Pavlov IP: Conditional Reflexes: An Investigation of the Physiological Activity of the Cerebral Cortex (1927). Edited by Anrep GV. New York, Bover, 1960

Pecknold JC, Swinson RP, Kuch K, et al: Alprazolam in panic disorder and agoraphobia: results from a multicenter trial, III: discontinuation effects. Arch Gen Psychiatry 45:429–436, 1988

Pediatric OCD Treatment Study Team: Cognitive behavior therapy, sertraline, and their combination for children and adolescents with obsessive compulsive disorder: the Pediatric OCD Treatment Study (POTS) randomized controlled trial. JAMA 292:1969–1976, 2004

Perani D, Colombo C, Bressi S, et al: [18F] FDG PET study in obsessive-compulsive disorder: a clinical/metabolic correlation study after treatment. Br J Psychiatry 166:244–250, 1995

Peri T, Ben Shakhar G, Orr SP, et al: Psychophysiological assessment of aversive conditioning in posttraumatic stress disorder. Biol Psychiatry 47:512–519, 2000

Perkonigg A, Pfister H, Stein MB, et al: Longitudinal course of posttraumatic stress disorder and posttraumatic stress disorder symptoms in a community sample of adolescents and young adults. Am J Psychiatry 162:1320–1327, 2005

Perlmutter SJ, Leitman SF, Garvey MA, et al: Therapeutic plasma exchange and intravenous immunoglobulin for obsessive-compulsive disorder and tic disorders in childhood. Lancet 354:1153–1158, 1999

Perna G, Bussi R, Allevi L et al: Sensitivity to 35% carbon dioxide in patients with generalized anxiety disorder. J Clin Psychiatry 60:379–384, 1999

Perry BD, Giller EL Jr, Southwick SM: Altered plasma alpha2-adrenergic binding sites in posttraumatic stress disorder (letter). Am J Psychiatry 144:1511–1512, 1987

Pfanner C, Marazziti D, Dell'Osso L, et al: Risperidone augmentation in refractory obsessive-compulsive disorder: an open-label study. Int Clin Psychopharmacol 15:297–301, 2000

Phan KL, Fitzgerald DA, Cortese BM, et al: Anterior cingulated neurochemistry in social anxiety disorder: 1H-MRS at 4 Tesla. Neuroreport 16:183–186, 2005

Phan KL, Britton JC, Taylor SF, et al: Corticolimbic blood flow during nontraumatic emotional processing in posttraumatic stress disorder. Arch Gen Psychiatry 63:184–192, 2006a

Phan KL, Fitzgerald DA, Nathan PJ, et al: Association between amygdala hyperactivity to harsh faces and severity of social anxiety in generalized social phobia. Biol Psychiatry 59:424–429, 2006b

Piccinelli M, Pini S, Bellantuono C, et al: Efficacy of drug treatment in obsessive-compulsive disorder: a meta-analytic review. Br J Psychiatry 166:424–443, 1995

Pigott TA, Pato MT, L'Heureux F, et al: A controlled comparison of adjuvant lithium carbonate or thyroid hormone in clomipramine-treated patients with obsessive-compulsive disorder. J Clin Psychopharmacol 11:242–248, 1991

Pigott TA, L'Heureux F, Hill JL, et al: A double-blind study of adjuvant buspirone hydrochloride in clomipramine-treated patients with obsessive-compulsive disorder. J Clin Psychopharmacol 12:11–18, 1992a

Pigott TA, L'Heureux F, Rubenstein CS, et al: A double-blind, placebo controlled study of trazodone in patients with obsessive-compulsive disorder. J Clin Psychopharmacol 12:156–162, 1992b

Pine DS, Klein RG, Robertson Nay R, et al: Response to 5% carbon dioxide in children and adolescents: relationship to panic disorder in parents and anxiety disorders in subjects. Arch Gen Psychiatry 62:73–80, 2005

Pitman RK, Orr SP, Forgue DF, et al: Psychophysiological assessment of post-traumatic stress disorder imagery in Vietnam combat veterans. Arch Gen Psychiatry 44:970–975, 1987

Pitman RK, van der Kolk BA, Orr SP, et al: Naloxone-reversible analgesic response to combat-related stimuli in posttraumatic stress disorder: a pilot study. Arch Gen Psychiatry 47:541–544, 1990

Pitman RK, Sanders KM, Zusman RM, et al: Pilot study of secondary prevention of posttraumatic stress disorder with propranolol. Biol Psychiatry 51:189–192, 2002

Pittenger C, Krystal JH, Coric V: Glutamate-modulating drugs as novel pharmacotherapeutic agents in the treatment of obsessive compulsive disorder. NeuroRx 3:69–81, 2006

Pitts FN, McClure JN: Lactate metabolism in anxiety neurosis. N Engl J Med 277:1329–1336, 1967

Pohl RB, Wolkow RM, Clary CM: Sertraline in the treatment of panic disorder: a double-blind multicenter trial. Am J Psychiatry 155:1189–1195, 1998

Pohl RB, Feltner DE, Fieve RR, et al: Efficacy of pregabalin in the treatment of generalized anxiety disorder: double-blind, placebo-controlled comparison of BID versus TID dosing. J Clin Psychopharmacol 25:151–158, 2005

Pollack MH, Zaninelli R, Goddard A, et al: Paroxetine in the treatment of generalized anxiety disorder: results of a placebo-controlled, flexible-dosage trial. J Clin Psychiatry 62:350–357, 2001

Pollack MH, Roy-Byrne PP, Van Ameringen M, et al: The selective GABA reuptake inhibitor tiagabine for the treatment of generalized anxiety disorder: results of a placebo-controlled study. J Clin Psychiatry 66:1401–1408, 2005

Power KG, Simpson RJ, Swanson V, et al: A controlled comparison of cognitive-behaviour therapy, diazepam, and placebo, alone and in combination, for the treatment of generalized anxiety disorder. J Anxiety Disord 4:267–292, 1990

Protopopescu X, Pan H, Tuescher O, et al: Increased brainstem volume in panic disorder: a voxel-based morphometric study. Neuroreport 17:361–363, 2006

Pujol J, Soriano Mas C, Alonso P, et al: Mapping structural brain alterations in obsessive compulsive disorder. Arch Gen Psychiatry 61:720–730, 2004

Quitkin F, Babkin J: Hidden psychiatric diagnosis in the alcoholic, in Alcoholism and Clinical Psychiatry. Edited by Soloman J. New York, Plenum, 1982, pp 129–140

Rachman SJ, Hodgson RJ: Obsessions and Compulsions. Englewood Cliffs, NJ, Prentice-Hall, 1980

Radomsky AS, Rachman S: Memory bias in obsessive-compulsive disorder. Behav Res Ther 37:605–618, 1999

Rainey JM Jr, Aleem A, Ortiz A, et al: Laboratory procedure for the inducement of flashbacks. Am J Psychiatry 144:1317–1319, 1987

Ralevski E, Sanislow CA, Grilo CM, et al: Avoidant personality disorder and social phobia: distinct enough to be separate disorders? Acta Psychiatr Scand 112:208–214, 2005

Rapaport MH, Pollack MH, Clary CM, et al: Panic disorder and response to sertraline: the effect of previous treatment with benzodiazepines. J Clin Psychopharmacol 21:104–107, 2001

Raskind MA, Peskind ER, Kanter ED, et al: Reduction of nightmares and other PTSD symptoms in combat veterans by prazosin: a placebo controlled study. Am J Psychiatry 160:371–373, 2003

Rasmussen SA, Tsuang MT: Clinical characteristics and family history in DSM-III obsessive compulsive disorder. Am J Psychiatry 143:317–322, 1986

Rasmussen S, Hackett E, DuBoff E, et al: A 2-year study of sertraline in the treatment of obsessive-compulsive disorder. Int Clin Psychopharmacol 12:309–316, 1997

Rauch SL, Jenike MA, Alpert NM, et al: Regional cerebral blood flow measured during symptom provocation in obsessive-compulsive disorder using oxygen 15-labeled carbon dioxide and positron emission tomography. Arch Gen Psychiatry 51:62–70, 1994

Rauch SL, Savage CR, Alpert NM, et al: A positron emission tomographic study of simple phobic symptom provocation. Arch Gen Psychiatry 52:20–28, 1995

Rauch SL, van der Kolk BA, Fisler RE, et al: A symptom provocation study of posttraumatic stress disorder using positron emission tomography and script-driven imagery. Arch Gen Psychiatry 53:380–387, 1996

Rauch SL, Whalen PJ, Shin LM, et al: Exaggerated amygdala response to masked facial stimuli in posttraumatic stress disorder: a functional MRI study. Biol Psychiatry 47:769–776, 2000

Rauch SL, Dougherty DD, Cosgrove GR, et al: Cerebral metabolic correlates as potential predictors of response to anterior cingulotomy for obsessive compulsive disorder. Biol Psychiatry 50:659–667, 2001

Rauch SL, Jenike MA, Alpert NM, et al: Predictors of fluvoxamine response in contamination-related obsessive compulsive disorder: a PET symptom provocation study. Neuropsychopharmacology 27:782–791, 2002

Rauch SL, Wright I, Martis B, et al: A magnetic resonance imaging study of cortical thickness in animal phobia. Biol Psychiatry 55:946–952, 2004

Rauch SL, Dougherty DD, Malone D, et al: A functional neuroimaging investigation of deep brain stimulation in patients with obsessive compulsive disorder. J Neurosurg 104:558–565, 2006

Redmond DE Jr: New and old evidence for the involvement of a brain norepinephrine system in anxiety, in Phenomenology and Treatment of Anxiety. Edited by Fann WE, Karacan I, Pokorny AD, et al. New York, Spectrum, 1979, pp 153–203

Regier DA, Boyd JH, Burke JD Jr, et al: One-month prevalence of mental disorders in the United States, based on five Epidemiologic Catchment Area sites. Arch Gen Psychiatry 45:977–986, 1988

Reist C, Kauffmann CD, Haier RJ, et al: A controlled trial of desipramine in 18 men with posttraumatic stress disorder. Am J Psychiatry 146:513–516, 1989

Resick PA, Nishith P, Weaver TL, et al: A comparison of cognitive processing therapy with prolonged exposure and a waiting condition for the treatment of chronic posttraumatic stress disorder in female rape victims. J Consult Clin Psychol 70:867–879, 2002

Ressler KJ, Rothbaum BO, Tannenbaum L, et al: Cognitive enhancers as adjuncts to psychotherapy: use of D-cycloserine in phobic individuals to facilitate extinction of fear. Arch Gen Psychiatry 61:1136–1144, 2004

Rettew DC: Avoidant personality disorder, generalized social phobia, and shyness: putting the personality back into personality disorders. Harv Rev Psychiatry 8:283–297, 2000

Rickels K, Schweizer E, Csanalosi I, et al: Long-term treatment of anxiety and risk of withdrawal: prospective comparison of clorazepate and buspirone. Arch Gen Psychiatry 45:444–450, 1988

Rickels K, Downing R, Schweizer E, et al: Antidepressants for the treatment of generalized anxiety disorder: a placebo-controlled comparison of imipramine, trazodone, and diazepam. Arch Gen Psychiatry 50:884–895, 1993

Rickels K, DeMartinis N, Garcia-Espana F, et al: Imipramine and buspirone in treatment of patients with generalized anxiety disorder who are discontinuing long-term benzodiazepine therapy. Am J Psychiatry 157:1973–1979, 2000

Rickels K, Zaninelli R, McCafferty J: Paroxetine treatment of generalized anxiety disorder: a double-blind, placebo-controlled study. Am J Psychiatry 160:749–756, 2003

Rickels K, Mangano R, Khan A: A double blind placebo controlled study of a flexible dose of venlafaxine ER in adult outpatients with generalized social anxiety disorder. J Clin Psychopharmacol 24:488–496, 2004

Rickels K, Pollack MH, Feltner DE, et al: Pregabalin for treatment of generalized anxiety disorder: a 4-week, multicenter, double-blind, placebo-controlled trial of pregabalin and alprazolam. Arch Gen Psychiatry 62:1022–1033, 2005

Riddle MA, Reeve EA, Yaryura-Tobias JA, et al: Fluvoxamine for children and adolescents with obsessive-compulsive disorder: a randomized, controlled, multicenter trial. J Am Acad Child Adolesc Psychiatry 40:222–229, 2001

Rinck M, Becker ES: A comparison of attentional biases and memory biases in women with social phobia and major depression. J Abnorm Psychol 114:62–74, 2005

Robert S, Hamner MB, Kose S, et al: Quetiapine improves sleep disturbances in combat veterans with PTSD: sleep data from a prospective, open label study. J Clin Psychopharmacol 25:387–388, 2005

Rocca P, Beoni AM, Eva C, et al: Peripheral benzodiazepine receptor messenger RNA is decreased in lymphocytes of generalized anxiety disorder patients. Biol Psychiatry 43:767–773, 1998

Romach M, Busto U, Somer G, et al: Clinical aspects of chronic use of alprazolam and lorazepam. Am J Psychiatry 152:1161–1167, 1995

Romano S, Goodman W, Tamura R, et al: Long-term treatment of obsessive-compulsive disorder after an acute response: a comparison of fluoxetine versus placebo. J Clin Psychopharmacol 21:46–52, 2001

Rosenbaum JF, Moroz G, Bowden CL: Clonazepam in the treatment of panic disorder with or without agoraphobia: a dose–response study of efficacy, safety, and discontinuance. Clonazepam Panic Disorder Dose-Response Study Group. J Clin Psychopharmacol 17:390–400, 1997

Rosenberg DR, Keshavan MS: A.E. Bennett Research Award: toward a neurodevelopmental model of obsessive-compulsive disorder. Biol Psychiatry 43:623–640, 1998

Rosenberg DR, Keshavan MS, O'Hearn KM, et al: Frontostriatal measurement in treatment-naïve children with obsessive-compulsive disorder. Arch Gen Psychiatry 54:824–830, 1997

Rosenberg DR, Benazon NR, Gilbert A, et al: Thalamic volume in pediatric obsessive-compulsive disorder patients before and after cognitive behavioral therapy. Biol Psychiatry 48:294–300, 2000

Roth D, Antony MM, Swinson RP: Interpretations for anxiety symptoms in social phobia. Behav Res Ther 39:129–138, 2001

Rothbaum Bo, Hodges LF, Ready D, et al: Virtual reality exposure therapy for Vietnam veterans with posttraumatic stress disorder. J Clin Psychiatry 62:617–622, 2001

Roy-Byrne PP, Cowley DS, Greenblatt DJ, et al: Reduced benzodiazepine sensitivity in panic disorder. Arch Gen Psychiatry 47:534–538, 1990

Roy-Byrne PP, Craske MG, Stein MB, et al: A randomized effectiveness trial of cognitive-behavioral therapy and medication for primary care panic disorder. Arch Gen Psychiatry 62:290–298, 2005

Rufer M, Ricke S, Moritz S, et al: Symptom dimensions in obsessive compulsive disorder: prediction of cognitive behavior therapy outcome. Acta Psychiatr Scand 113: 440–446, 2006

Ruscio AM, Lane M, Roy-Byrne P, et al: Should excessive worry be required for a diagnoses of generalized anxiety disorder? Results from the U.S. National Comorbidity Survey replication. Psychol Med 35:1761–1772, 2005

Sachdev PS, McBrider R, Loo CK, et al: Right versus left prefrontal transcranial magnetic stimulation for obsessive compulsive disorder: a preliminary investigation. J Clin Psychiatry 62:981–984, 2001

Sakai Y, Kumano H, Nishikawa M, et al: Cerebral glucose metabolism associated with a fear network in panic disorder. Neuroreport 16:927–931, 2005

Salkovskis PM, Jones DRO, Clark DM: Respiratory control in the treatment of panic attacks: replication and extension with concurrent measurement of behaviour and pCO2. Br J Psychiatry 148:526–532, 1986

Salkovskis PM, Wroe AL, Gledhill A, et al: Responsibility attitudes and interpretations are characteristic of obsessive compulsive disorder. Behav Res Ther 38:347–372, 2000

Salzman L: Comments on the psychological treatment of obsessive-compulsive patients, in Obsessive-Compulsive Disorder: Psychological and Pharmacological Treatment. Edited by Mavissakalian M, Turner SM, Michelson L. New York, Plenum, 1985, pp 155–165

Samuels JF, Riddle MA, Greenberg BD, et al: The OCD Collaborative Genetics Study: methods and sample description. Am J Med Genet B Neuropsychiatr Genet 141:201–207, 2006

Sanderson WC, Rapee RM, Barlow DH: The influence of an illusion of control on panic attacks induced via inhalation of 5.5% carbon dioxide-enriched air. Arch Gen Psychiatry 46:157–162, 1989

Sarchiapone M, Armore M, De Risio S, et al: Mirtazapine in the treatment of panic disorder: an open-label trial. Int Clin Psychopharmacol 18:35–38, 2003

Saxe G, Stoddard F, Courtney D, et al: Relationship between acute morphine and the course of PTSD in children with burns. J Am Acad Child Adolesc Psychiatry 40:915–921, 2001

Saxena S, Wang D, Bystritsky A, et al: Risperidone augmentation of SRI treatment for refractory obsessive-compulsive disorder. J Clin Psychiatry 57:303–306, 1996

Saxena S, Brody AL, Ho ML, et al: Differential cerebral metabolic changes with paroxetine treatment of obsessive compulsive disorder vs major depression. Arch Gen Psychiatry 59:250–261, 2002

Schelling G, Kilger E, Roozendaal B, et al: Stress doses of hydrocortisone, traumatic memories, and symptoms of posttraumatic stress disorder in patients after cardiac surgery: a randomized study. Biol Psychiatry 55:627–633, 2004

Schmidt NB, Wollaway-Bickel K, Trakowski JH, et al: Antidepressant discontinuation in the context of cognitive behavioral treatment for panic disorder. Behav Res Ther 40:67–73, 2002

Schneider F, Weiss U, Kessler C, et al: Subcortical correlates of differential classical conditioning of aversive emotional reactions in social phobia. Biol Psychiatry 45:863–871, 1999

Schneier F, Liebowitz MR, Abi-Dargham A, et al: Low dopamine D2 binding potential in social phobia. Am J Psychiatry 157:457–459, 2000

Schnyder U, Moergeli H, Klaghofer R, et al: Incidence and prediction of posttraumatic stress disorder symptoms in severely injured accident victims. Am J Psychiatry 158:595–599, 2001

Schutters SI, Van Megen HJ, Westenberg HG: Efficacy of quetiapine in generalized social anxiety disorder: results from an open label study. J Clin Psychiatry 66:540–542, 2005

Schwartz C, Snidman N, Kagan J: Adolescent social anxiety as an outcome of inhibited temperament in childhood. J Am Acad Child Adolesc Psychiatry 38:1008–1015, 1999

Schwartz JM, Stoessel PW, Baxter LR, et al: Systematic changes in cerebral glucose metabolic rate after successful behavior modification treatment in obsessive-compulsive disorder. Arch Gen Psychiatry 53:109–113, 1996

Scrignar CB: Post-Traumatic Stress Disorder: Diagnosis, Treatment, and Legal Issues. New York, Praeger, 1984

Seedat S, Stein DJ: Inositol augmentation of serotonin reuptake inhibitors in treatment-refractory obsessive-compulsive disorder: an open trial. Int Clin Psychopharmacol 14:353–356, 1999

Seedat S, Stein MB: Double blind, placebo controlled assessment of combined clonazepam with paroxetine compared with paroxetine monotherapy for generalized social anxiety disorder. J Clin Psychiatry 65:244–248, 2004

Senkowski D, Linden M, Zubragel D, et al: Evidence for disturbed cortical signal processing and altered serotonergic neurotransmission in generalized anxiety disorder. Biol Psychiatry 53:304–314, 2003

Sepede G, Mancini E, Salerno RM, Ferro FM: Olanzapine augmentation in treatment-resistant panic disorder: a 12-week, fixed-dose, open-label trial. J Clin Psychopharmacol 26:45–49, 2006

Sevy S, Papadimitriou GN, Surmont DW, et al: Noradrenergic function in generalized anxiety disorder, major depressive disorder, and healthy subjects. Biol Psychiatry 15:141–152, 1989

Shalev AY, Peri T, Canetti L, et al: Predictors of PTSD in injured trauma survivors: a prospective study. Am J Psychiatry 153:2219–2225, 1996

Shalev AY, Freedman S, Peri T, et al: Prospective study of posttraumatic stress disorder and depression following trauma. Am J Psychiatry 155:630–637, 1998a

Shalev AY, Sahar T, Freedman S, et al: A prospective study of heart rate response following trauma and the subsequent development of posttraumatic stress disorder. Arch Gen Psychiatry 55:553–559, 1998b

Shapira NA, Ward HE, Mandoki M, et al: A double blind, placebo controlled trial of olanzapine addition in fluoxetine refractory obsessive compulsive disorder. Biol Psychiatry 55:553–555, 2004

Shay J: Fluoxetine reduces explosiveness and elevates mood of Vietnam combat vets with PTSD. J Trauma Stress 5:97–101, 1992

Shea MT, Zlotnick C, Dolan R, et al: Personality disorders, history of trauma, and posttraumatic stress disorder in subjects with anxiety disorders. Compr Psychiatry 41:312–325, 2000

Shear MK, Cooper AM, Klerman GL, et al: A psychodynamic model of panic disorder. Am J Psychiatry 150:859–866, 1993

Sheehan DV, Burnham DB, Iyengar MK, et al: Efficacy and tolerability of controlled-release paroxetine in the treatment of panic disorder. J Clin Psychiatry 66:34–40, 2005

Shin LM, Kosslyn SM, McNally RJ, et al: Visual imagery and perception in posttraumatic stress disorder: a positron emission tomographic investigation. Arch Gen Psychiatry 54:233–241, 1997

Shin LM, Orr SP, Carson MA, et al: Regional cerebral blood flow in the amygdala and medial prefrontal cortex during traumatic imagery in male and female Vietnam veterans with PTSD. Arch Gen Psychiatry 61:168–176, 2004

Shin LM, Wright CA, Cannstraro PA, et al: A functional magnetic resonance imaging study of amygdala and medial prefrontal cortex responses to overtly presented fearful faces in posttraumatic stress disorder. Arch Gen Psychiatry 62:273–281, 2005

Silva RR, Alpert M, Munoz DM, et al: Stress and vulnerability to posttraumatic stress disorder in children and adolescents. Am J Psychiatry 157:1229–1235, 2000

Simon NM, Emmanuel N, Ballenger J, et al: Bupropion sustained release for panic disorder. Psychopharmacol Bull 37:66–72, 2003

Simpson HB, Gorfinkle KS, Liebowitz MR: Cognitive-behavioral therapy as an adjunct to serotonin reuptake inhibitors in obsessive-compulsive disorder: an open trial. J Clin Psychiatry 60:584–590, 1999

Simpson HB, Liebowitz MR, Foa EB, et al: Post treatment effects of exposure therapy and clomipramine in obsessive compulsive disorder. Depress Anxiety 19:225–233, 2004

Simpson HB, Huppert JD, Petkova E, et al: Response versus remission in obsessive compulsive disorder. J Clin Psychiatry 67:269–276, 2005

Skoog G, Skoog I: A 40-year follow-up of patients with obsessive-compulsive disorder. Arch Gen Psychiatry 56:121–127, 1999

Skre I, Onstad S, Torgensen S, et al: A twin study of DSM-III-R anxiety disorders. Acta Psychiatr Scand 88:85–92, 1993

Smith MA, Davidson J, Ritchie JC, et al: The corticotropin releasing hormone test in patients with posttraumatic stress disorder. Biol Psychiatry 26:349–355, 1989

Smoller JW, Yamaki LH, Fagerness JA, et al: The corticotropin-releasing hormone gene and behavioral inhibition in children at risk for panic disorder. Biol Psychiatry 57:1485–1492, 2005

Snyderman SH, Rynn MA, Rickels K: Open-label pilot study of ziprasidone for refractory generalized anxiety disorder. J Clin Psychopharmacol 25:497–499, 2005

Southwick SM, Krystal JH, Bremner JD, et al: Noradrenergic and serotonergic function in posttraumatic stress disorder. Arch Gen Psychiatry 54:749–758, 1997

Spence SH, Donovan C, Brechman-Toussant M: Social skills, social outcomes, and cognitive features of childhood social phobia. J Abnorm Psychol 108:211–221, 1999

Spence SH, Donovan C, Brechman TM: The treatment of childhood social phobia: the effectiveness of a social skills training-based, cognitive-behavioural intervention, with and without parental involvement. J Child Psychol Psychiatry 41:713–762, 2000

Spiegel DA, Bruce TJ, Gregg SF, et al: Does cognitive behavior therapy assist slow-taper alprazolam discontinuation in panic disorder? Am J Psychiatry 151:876–881, 1994

Spivak B, Vered Y, Graff E, et al: Low platelet-poor plasma concentrations of serotonin in patients with combat-related posttraumatic stress disorder. Biol Psychiatry 45:840–845, 1999

Stahl SM, Gergel I, Li D: Escitalopram in the treatment of panic disorder: a randomized, double-blind, placebo-controlled trial. J Clin Psychiatry 64:1322–1327, 2003

Stapleton JA, Taylor S, Asmundson GJ: Effects of three PTSD treatments on anger and guilt: exposure therapy, eye movement desensitization and reprocessing, and relaxation training. J Trauma Stress 19:19–28, 2006

Starkman MN, Cameron OG, Nesse RM, et al: Peripheral catecholamine levels and the symptoms of anxiety: studies in patients with and without pheochromocytoma. Psychosom Med 52:129–142, 1990

Stein DJ, Spadaccine E, Hollander E: Meta-analysis of pharmacotherapy trials for obsessive-compulsive disorder. Int Clin Psychopharmacol 10:11–18, 1995

Stein DJ, Stein MB, Pitts CD, et al: Predictors of response to pharmacotherapy in social anxiety disorder: an analysis of 3 placebo controlled paroxetine trials. J Clin Psychiatry 63:152–155, 2002a

Stein DJ, Versiani M, Hair, T, et al: Efficacy of paroxetine for relapse prevention in social anxiety disorder: a 24 week study. Arch Gen Psychiatry 59:1111–1118, 2002b

Stein DJ, Ipser JC, Seedat S: Pharmacotherapy for post traumatic stress disorder. Cochrane Database Syst Rev (1):CD002795, 2006

Stein MB, Asmundson GJ: Autonomic function in panic disorder: cardiorespiratory and plasma catecholamine responsivity to multiple challenges of the autonomic nervous system. Biol Psychiatry 36:548–558, 1994

Stein MB, Kean YM: Disability and quality of life in social phobia: epidemiologic findings. Am J Psychiatry 157:1606–1613, 2000

Stein MB, Delaney SM, Chartier M, et al: 3H paroxetine binding to platelets of patients with social phobia: comparison to patients with panic disorder and healthy volunteers. Biol Psychiatry 37:224–228, 1995a

Stein MB, Millar TW, Larsen DK, et al: Irregular breathing during sleep in patients with panic disorder. Am J Psychiatry 152:1168–1173, 1995b

Stein MB, Walker JR, Anderson G, et al: Childhood physical and sexual abuse in patients with anxiety disorders and in a community sample. Am J Psychiatry 153:275–277, 1996

Stein MB, Walker JR, Hazen AL, et al: Full and partial posttraumatic stress disorder: findings from a community survey. Am J Psychiatry 154:1114–1119, 1997

Stein MB, Chartier MJ, Kozak MV, et al: Genetic linkage to the serotonin transporter protein and 5HT2A receptor genes excluded in generalized social phobia. Psychiatry Res 81:283–291, 1998a

Stein MB, Liebowitz MR, Lydiard B, et al: Paroxetine treatment of generalized social phobia (social anxiety disorder): a randomized controlled trial. JAMA 280:708–713, 1998b

Stein MB, Fyer AJ, Davidson JRT, et al: Fluvoxamine treatment of social phobia (social anxiety disorder): a double-blind, placebo-controlled study. Am J Psychiatry 156:756–760, 1999

Stein MB, Feutsch M, Muller N, et al: Social anxiety disorder and the risk of depression: a prospective community study of adolescents and young adults. Arch Gen Psychiatry 58:251–258, 2001a

Stein MB, Sareen J, Hami S, et al: Pindolol potentiation of paroxetine for generalized social phobia: a double blind, placebo controlled, crossover study. Am J Psychiatry 158:1725–1727, 2001b

Stein MB, Goldin PR, Sareen J, et al: Increased amygdala activation to angry and contemptuous faces in generalized social phobia. Arch Gen Psychiatry 59:1027–1034, 2002

Stein MB, Pollack MH, Bystritsky A, et al: Efficacy of low and higher dose extended-release venlafaxine in generalized social anxiety disorder: a 6-month randomized controlled trial. Psychopharmacol (Berl) 177:280–288, 2005

Stemberger RT, Turner SM, Beidel DC, et al: Social phobia: an analysis of possible developmental factors. J Abnorm Psychol 104:526–531, 1995

Stocchi F, Nordera G, Jokinen RH, et al: Efficacy and tolerability of paroxetine for the long-term treatment of generalized anxiety disorder. J Clin Psychiatry 64:250–258, 2003

Stopa L, Clark DM: Social phobia and interpretation of social events. Behav Res Ther 38:273–283, 2000

Straube T, Kolassa IT, Glauer M, et al: Effect of task conditions on brain responses to threatening faces in social phobics: an event-related functional magnetic resonance imaging study. Biol Psychiatry 56:921–930, 2004

Straube T, Glauer M, Dilger S, et al: Effects of cognitive behavioral therapy on brain activation in specific phobia. Neuroimage 29:125–135, 2006

Strohle A, Kellner M, Holsboer F, et al: Behavioral, neuroendocrine, and cardiovascular response to flumazenil: no evidence for an altered benzodiazepine receptor sensitivity in panic disorder. Biol Psychiatry 45:321–326, 1999

Swedo SE: Rituals and releasers: an ethological model of obsessive-compulsive disorder, in Obsessive-Compulsive Disorder in Children and Adolescents. Edited by Rapoport JL. Washington, DC, American Psychiatric Press, 1989, pp 269–288

Swedo SE, Rapoport JL, Cheslow DL, et al: Increased incidence of obsessive-compulsive symptoms in patients with Sydenham's chorea. Am J Psychiatry 146:246–249, 1989a

Swedo SE, Rapoport JL, Leonard H, et al: Obsessive-compulsive disorder in children and adolescents: clinical phenomenology of 70 consecutive cases. Arch Gen Psychiatry 46:335–341, 1989b

Swedo SE, Schapiro MB, Grady CL, et al: Cerebral glucose metabolism in childhood-onset obsessive-compulsive disorder. Arch Gen Psychiatry 46:518–523, 1989c

Swedo SE, Leonard HL, Kruesi MJP, et al: Cerebrospinal fluid neurochemistry in children and adolescents with obsessive-compulsive disorder. Arch Gen Psychiatry 49:29–36, 1992a

Swedo SE, Pietrini P, Leonard HL, et al: Cerebral glucose metabolism in childhood-onset obsessive-compulsive disorder: revisualization during pharmacotherapy. Arch Gen Psychiatry 49:690–694, 1992b

Szeszko PR, Robinson D, Alvir JM, et al: Orbital frontal and amygdala volume reductions in obsessive-compulsive disorder. Arch Gen Psychiatry 56:913–919, 1999

Szeszko PR, MacMillan S, McMeniman M, et al: Brain structural abnormalities in psychotropic drug naïve pediatric patients with obsessive compulsive disorder. Am J Psychiatry 161:1049–1056, 2004

Szeszko PR, Ardekani BA, Ashtari M, et al: White matter abnormalities in obsessive compulsive disorder: a diffusion tensor imaging study. Arch Gen Psychiatry 62:782–790, 2005

Szymanski HV, Olympia J: Divalproex in posttraumatic stress disorder (letter). Am J Psychiatry 148:1086–1087, 1991

Tancer ME, Stein MB, Uhde TW: Growth hormone response to intravenous clonidine in social phobia: comparison to patients with panic disorder and healthy volunteers. Biol Psychiatry 34:591–595, 1993

Tancer ME, Mailman RB, Stein MB, et al: Neuroendocrine responsivity to monoaminergic system probes in generalized social phobia. Anxiety 1:216–223, 1994

Tarrier N, Pilgrim H, Sommerfield C, et al: A randomized trial of cognitive therapy and imaginal exposure in the treatment of chronic posttraumatic stress disorder. J Consult Clin Psychol 67:13–18, 1999

Taylor FB: Tiagabine for posttraumatic stress disorder: a case series of 7 women. J Clin Psychiatry 64:1421–1425, 2003

Taylor FB, Raskind MA: The alpha1-adrenergic antagonist prazosin improves sleep and nightmares in civilian trauma posttraumatic stress disorder. J Clin Psychopharmacol 22:82–85, 2002

Taylor FB, Lowe K, Thompson C, et al: Daytime prazosin reduces psychological distress to trauma specific cues in civilian trauma posttraumatic stress disorder. Biol Psychiatry 59:577–581, 2006

Taylor S, McKay D, Abramowitz JS: Hierarchical structure of dysfunctional beliefs in obsessive compulsive disorder: Cogn Behav Ther 34:216–228, 2005

Telch MJ, Agras WG, Taylor CM, et al: Combined pharmacological and behavioral treatment for agoraphobia. Behav Res Ther 23:325–335, 1985

Tenneij NH, van Megen HJ, Denys DA, et al: Behavior therapy augments response of patients with obsessive compulsive disorder responding to drug treatment. J Clin Psychiatry 66:1169–1175, 2005

Thomsen PH, Mikkelsen HU: Development of personality disorders in children and adolescents with obsessive-compulsive disorder: a 6- to 22-year follow-up study. Acta Psychiatr Scand 87:456–462, 1993

Thorgeirsson TE, Oskarsson H, Desnica N, et al: Anxiety with panic disorder linked to chromosome 9q in Iceland. Am J Hum Genet 72:1221–1230, 2003

Tiihonen J, Kuikka J, Bergstrom K, et al: Dopamine reuptake site densities in patients with social phobia. Am J Psychiatry 154:239–242, 1997a

Tiihonen J, Kuikka J, Rasanen P, et al: Cerebral benzodiazepine receptor binding and distribution in generalized anxiety: a fractal analysis. Mol Psychiatry 2:463–471, 1997b

Tillfors M, Furmark T, Ekselius L, et al: Social phobia and avoidant personality disorder as related to parental history of social anxiety: a general population study. Behav Res Ther 39:289–298, 2001a

Tillfors M, Furmark T, Marteinsdottir I, et al: Cerebral blood flow in subjects with social phobia during stressful speaking tasks, a PET study. Am J Psychiatry 158:1220–1226, 2001b

Tolin DF, Maltby N, Diefenback GJ, et al: Cognitive behavioral therapy for medication nonresponders with obsessive compulsive disorder: a wait list controlled open trial. J Clin Psychiatry 65:922–931, 2004

Tollefson GD, Rampey AH, Potvin JH, et al: A multicenter investigation of fixed-dose fluoxetine in the treatment of obsessive-compulsive disorder. Arch Gen Psychiatry 51:559–567, 1994

Torgersen S: Genetic factors in anxiety disorders. Arch Gen Psychiatry 40:1085–1089, 1983

True WR, Rice J, Eisen SA, et al: A twin study of genetic and environmental contributions to liability for posttraumatic stress symptoms. Arch Gen Psychiatry 50:257–264, 1993

Tupler LA, DeBellis MD: Segmented hippocampal volume in children and adolescents with posttraumatic stress disorder. Biol Psychiatry 59:523–529, 2006

Turner SM, Beidel DC, Cooley-Quille MR: Two-year follow-up of social phobias treated with social effectiveness therapy. Behav Res Ther 33:553–555, 1995

Uhde TW, Tancer ME, Gelernter CS, et al: Normal urinary free cortisol and postdexamethasone cortisol in social phobia: comparison to normal volunteers. J Affect Disord 30:155–161, 1994

Ursano RJ, Fullerton CS, Epstein RS, et al: Acute and chronic posttraumatic stress disorder in motor vehicle accident victims. Am J Psychiatry 156:589–595, 1999

Vaiva G, Thomas P, Ducrocq F, et al: Low posttrauma GABA plasma levels as a predictive factor in the development of acute posttraumatic stress disorder. Biol Psychiatry 55:250–254, 2004

Valente AA Jr, Miguel EC, Castro CC, et al: Regional gray matter abnormalities in obsessive compulsive disorder: a voxel based morphometry study. Biol Psychiatry 58:479–487, 2005

Vallejo J, Olivares J, Marcos T, et al: Clomipramine versus phenelzine in obsessive-compulsive disorder: a controlled clinical trial. Br J Psychiatry 161:665–670, 1992

Van Ameringen M, Mancini C, Streiner DL: Fluoxetine efficacy in social phobia. J Clin Psychiatry 54:27–32, 1993

Van Ameringen MA, Lane RM, Walker JR, et al: Sertraline treatment of generalized social phobia: a 20-week, double-blind, placebo-controlled study. Am J Psychiatry 158:275–281, 2001

Van Ameringen M, Mancini C, Pipe B, et al: An open trial of topiramate in the treatment of generalized social phobia. J Clin Psychiatry 65:1674–1678, 2004a

Van Ameringen M, Mancini C, Szechtman H, et al: A PET provocation study of generalized social phobia. Psychiatry Res 132:13–18, 2004b

Van Ameringen M, Oakman J, Mancini C, et al: Predictors of response in generalized social phobia: effect of age of onset. J Clin Psychopharmacol 24:42–48, 2004c

Van Ameringen M, Mancini C, Patterson B, et al: Topiramate augmentation in treatment resistant obsessive compulsive disorder: a retrospective, open label case series. Depress Anxiety 23:1–5, 2006

van den Heuvel OA, Veltman DJ, Groenewegen HJ, et al: Disorder-specific neuroanatomical correlates of attentional bias in obsessive-compulsive disorder, panic disorder, and hypochondriasis. Arch Gen Psychiatry 62:922–933, 2005a

van den Heuvel OA, Veltman DJ, Groenewegen HJ, et al: Frontal striatal dysfunction during planning in obsessive compulsive disorder. Arch Gen Psychiatry 62:301–309, 2005b

Van Den Hout M, Tenney N, Huygens K, et al: Preconscious processing bias in specific phobia. Behav Res Ther 35:29–34, 1997

van der Kolk BA: Psychopharmacological issues in posttraumatic stress disorder. Hosp Community Psychiatry 34:683–691, 1983

van der Kolk BA: The role of the group in the origin and resolution of the trauma response, in Psychological Trauma. Edited by van der Kolk BA. Washington, DC, American Psychiatric Press, 1987a, pp 153–171

van der Kolk BA: The separation cry and the trauma response: developmental issues in the psychobiology of attachment and separation, in Psychological Trauma. Edited by van der Kolk BA. Washington, DC, American Psychiatric Press, 1987b, pp 31–62

van der Kolk BA: The compulsion to repeat the trauma: reenactment, revictimization, and masochism. Psychiatr Clin North Am 12:389–411, 1989

van der Kolk BA, Saporta J: The biological response to psychic trauma: mechanisms and treatment of intrusion and numbing. Anxiety Res 4:199–212, 1991

van der Kolk BA, van der Hart O: Pierre Janet and the breakdown of adaptation in psychological trauma. Am J Psychiatry 146:1530–1540, 1989

van der Kolk BA, Boyd H, Krystal J, et al: Post-traumatic stress disorder as a biologically based disorder: implications of the animal model of inescapable shock, in Post-Traumatic Stress Disorder: Psychological and Biological Sequelae. Edited by van der Kolk BA. Washington, DC, American Psychiatric Press, 1984, pp 123–134

van der Kolk BA, Dreyfuss D, Michaels M, et al: Fluoxetine in posttraumatic stress disorder. J Clin Psychiatry 55:517–522, 1994

Van Der Linden G, van-Heerden B, Warwick J, et al: Functional brain imaging and pharmacotherapy in social phobia: single photon emission computed tomography before and after treatment with the selective serotonin reuptake inhibitor citalopram. Prog Neuropsychopharmacol Biol Psychiatry 24:419–438, 2000

van Oppen P, de Haan E, van Balkom AJ, et al: Cognitive therapy and exposure in vivo in the treatment of obsessive compulsive disorder. Behav Res Ther 33:379–390, 1995

van Oppen P, van Balkom AJ, de Haan E, et al: Cognitive therapy and exposure in vivo alone and in combination with fluvoxamine in obsessive compulsive disorder: a 5 year follow up. J Clin Psychiatry 66:1415–1422, 2005

van Vliet IM, den Boer JA, Westenberg HG: Psychopharmacological treatment of social phobia: a double blind placebo controlled study with fluvoxamine. Psychopharmacol (Berl) 115:128–134, 1994

van Vliet IM, den Boer JA, Westenberg HGM, et al: Clinical effects of buspirone in social phobia: a double-blind placebo-controlled study. J Clin Psychiatry 58:164–168, 1997

Vermetten E, Vythilingam M, Southwick SM, et al: Long term treatment with paroxetine increases verbal declarative memory and hippocampal volume in posttraumatic stress disorder. Biol Psychiatry 54:693–702, 2003

Versiani M, Mundim FD, Nardi AE, et al: Tranylcypromine in social phobia. J Clin Psychopharmacol 8:279–283, 1988

Vickers K, McNally RJ: Panic disorder and suicide attempt in the National Comorbidity Survey. J Abnorm Psychol 113:582–591, 2004

Vulink NC, Denys D, Westenberg HG: Bupropion for patients with obsessive compulsive disorder: an open label, fixed dose study. J Clin Psychiatry 66:228–230, 2005

Wade AG, Lepola U, Koponen HJ, et al: The effect of citalopram in panic disorder. Br J Psychiatry 170:549–553, 1997

Wald J, Taylor S: Preliminary research on the efficacy of virtual reality exposure therapy to treat driving phobia. Cyberpsychol Behav 6:459–465, 2003

Wallace ST, Alden LE: Social phobia and positive social events: the price of success. J Abnorm Psychol 106:416–424, 1997

Wang Z, Valdes J, Noyes R, et al: Possible association of a cholecystokinin promoter polymorphism (CCK-36CT) with panic disorder. Am J Med Genet 81:228–234, 1998

Warshaw MG, Dolan RT, Keller MB: Suicidal behavior in patients with current or past panic disorder: five years of prospective data from the Harvard/Brown Anxiety Research Program. Am J Psychiatry 157:1876–1878, 2000

Weissman MM, Markowitz JS, Ouellette R, et al: Panic disorder and cardiovascular/cerebrovascular problems: results from a community survey. Am J Psychiatry 147:1504–1508, 1990

Wells A, Carter K: Preliminary tests of a cognitive model of generalized anxiety disorder. Behav Res Ther 37:585–594, 1999

Westphal K: Ueber Zwangsverstellungen [obsessional thoughts]. Arch Psychiatr Neurol 8:734–750, 1878

Whittal ML, Thordarson DS, McLean PD, et al: Treatment of obsessive compulsive disorder: cognitive behavior therapy vs. exposure and response prevention. Behav Res Ther 43:1559–1576, 2005

Wiborg IM, Dahl AA: Does brief dynamic psychotherapy reduce the relapse rate of panic disorder? Arch Gen Psychiatry 53:689–694, 1996

Widom CS: Posttraumatic stress disorder in abused and neglected children grown up. Am J Psychiatry 156:1223–1229, 1999

Wilkinson DJ, Thompson JM, Lambert GW, et al: Sympathetic activity in patients with panic disorder at rest, under laboratory mental stress, and during panic attacks. Arch Gen Psychiatry 55:511–520, 1998

Willour VL, Yoa Shugart Y, Samuels J, et al: Replication study supports evidence for linkage to 9p24 in obsessive compulsive disorder. Am J Hum Genet 75:508–513, 2004

Winter H, Irle E: Hippocampal volume in adult burn patients with and without posttraumatic stress disorder. Am J Psychiatry 161:2194–2200, 2004

Wise SP, Rapoport JL: Obsessive-compulsive disorder: is it a basal ganglia dysfunction? in Obsessive-Compulsive Disorder in Children and Adolescents. Edited by Rapoport JL. Washington, DC, American Psychiatric Press, 1989, pp 327–344

Wittchen HU, Zhao S, Kessler RC, et al: DSM-III-R generalized anxiety disorder in the National Comorbidity Survey. Arch Gen Psychiatry 51:355–364, 1994

Wittchen HU, Carter RM, Pfister H, et al: Disabilities and quality of life in pure and comorbid generalized anxiety disorder and major depression in a national survey. Int Clin Psychopharmacol 15:319–328, 2000

Wlazlo Z, Schroeder-Hartwig K, Hand I, et al: Exposure in vivo vs social skills training for social phobia: long-term outcome and differential effects. Behav Res Ther 28:181–193, 1990

Wolf ME, Alavi A, Mosnaim AD: Posttraumatic stress disorder in Vietnam veterans, clinical and EEG findings: possible therapeutic effects of carbamazepine. Biol Psychiatry 23:642–644, 1988

Woo JM, Yoon KS, Yu BH: Catechol-O-methyltransferase genetic polymorphism in panic disorder. Am J Psychiatry 159:1785–1787, 2002

Woo JM, Yoon KS, Choi YH, et al: The association between panic disorder and the L/L genotype of catechol-O-methyltransferase. J Psychiatr Res 38:365–370, 2004

Woodman CL, Noyes R: Panic disorder: treatment with valproate. J Clin Psychiatry 55:134–136, 1994

Woodman CL, Noyes R, Black DW, et al: A 5-year follow-up study of generalized anxiety disorder and panic disorder. J Nerv Ment Dis 187:3–9, 1999

Woodward SH, Kaloupek DG, Streeter CC, et al: Decreased anterior cingulated volume in combat related PTSD. Biol Psychiatry 59:582–587, 2006

Woody SR, Chambless DL, Glass CR: Self-focused attention in the treatment of social phobia. Behav Res Ther 35:117–129, 1997

World Health Organization: International Statistical Classification of Diseases and Related Health Problems, 10th Revision (ICD-10). Geneva, Switzerland, World Health Organization, 1992

Wu JC, Buchsbaum MS, Hershey TG, et al: PET in generalized anxiety disorder. Biol Psychiatry 29:1181–1199, 1991

Yehuda R, Boisoneau D, Lowy MT, et al: Dose-response changes in plasma cortisol and lymphocyte glucocorticoid receptors following dexamethasone administration in combat veterans with and without posttraumatic stress disorder. Arch Gen Psychiatry 52:583–593, 1995

Yehuda R, McFarlane AC, Shalev AY: Predicting the development of posttraumatic stress disorder from the acute response to a traumatic event. Biol Psychiatry 44:1305–1313, 1998a

Yehuda R, Schmeidler J, Wainberg M, et al: Vulnerability to posttraumatic stress disorder in adult offspring of Holocaust survivors. Am J Psychiatry 155:1163–1171, 1998b

Yehuda R, Brand S, Yang RK: Plasma neuropeptide Y concentration in combat exposed veterans: relationship to trauma exposure, recovery from PTSD, and coping. Biol Psychiatry 59:660–663, 2006

Yonkers KA, Warshaw MG, Massion AO, et al: Phenomenology and course of generalised anxiety disorder. Br J Psychiatry 168:308–313, 1996

Yoo HK, Kim MJ, Kim SJ, et al: Putaminal gray matter volume decrease in panic disorder: an optimized voxel-based morphometry study. Eur J Neurosci 22:2089–2094, 2005

Young EA, Breslau N: Cortisol and catecholamines in posttraumatic stress disorder: an epidemiologic community study. Arch Gen Psychiatry 61:394–401, 2004a

Young EA, Breslau N: Saliva cortisol in posttraumatic stress disorder: a community epidemiologic study. Biol Psychiatry 56:205–209, 2004b

Zai G, Arnold P, Burroughs E, et al: Evidence for the gamma-aminobutyric acid type B receptor 1 (GABBR1) gene as a susceptibility factor in obsessive compulsive disorder. Am J Med Genet B Neuropsychiatr Genet 134:25–29, 2005a

Zai G, Arnold P, Strauss J, et al: No association between brain derived neurotrophic factor gene and obsessive compulsive disorder. Psychiatr Genet 15:235, 2005b

Zatzick DF, Marmar CR, Weiss DS, et al: Posttraumatic stress disorder and functioning and quality of life outcomes in a nationally representative sample of male Vietnam veterans. Am J Psychiatry 154:1690–1695, 1997

Zatzick DF, Russo J, Pitman RK, et al: Reevaluating the association between emergency department heart rate and the development of posttraumatic stress disorder: a public health approach. Biol Psychiatry 57:91–95, 2005

Zhang W, Connor KM, Davidson JR: Levetiracetam in social phobia: a placebo controlled pilot study. J Psychopharmacol 19:551–553, 2005

Zimmerman M, Chelminski I: Generalized anxiety disorder in patients with major depression: is DSM-IV's hierarchy correct? Am J Psychiatry 160:504–512, 2003

Zitrin CM, Klein DF, Woerner MG: Treatment of agoraphobia with group exposure in vivo and imipramine. Arch Gen Psychiatry 37:63–72, 1980

Zlotnick C, Shea TM, Rosen K, et al: An affect-management group for women with posttraumatic stress disorder and histories of childhood sexual abuse. J Trauma Stress 10:425–436, 1997

Zlotnick C, Warshaw M, Shea MT, et al: Chronicity in posttraumatic stress disorder (PTSD) and predictors of course of comorbid PTSD in patients with anxiety disorders. J Trauma Stress 12:89–100, 1999

Zohar J, Insel TR, Zohar-Kadouch RC, et al: Serotonergic responsivity in obsessive-compulsive disorder: effects of chronic clomipramine treatment. Arch Gen Psychiatry 45:167–172, 1988

13

SOMATOFORM DISORDERS

Sean H. Yutzy, M.D.
Brooke S. Parish, M.D.

The somatoform disorders were first delineated as a class of psychiatric disorders in DSM-III (American Psychiatric Association 1980). The class was created to facilitate the differential diagnosis of disorders characterized primarily by "physical symptoms suggesting physical disorder (hence somatoform) for which there are no demonstrable organic findings or known physiological mechanisms and for which there is positive evidence, or a strong presumption, that the symptoms are linked to psychological factors or conflicts" (American Psychiatric Association 1980, p. 241). With minor modifications, this grouping and its underlying concept were retained in DSM-III-R (American Psychiatric Association 1987) and, after some debate (Martin 1995), in DSM-IV (American Psychiatric Association 1994) as well as DSM-IV-TR (American Psychiatric Association 2000). (Noteworthy here was that the explicit diagnostic criteria from DSM-IV remained the same in DSM-IV-TR.) In contrast to factitious disorders and malingering, somatoform disorder symptoms are not under voluntary control. The stipulation in DSM-IV-TR that symptoms are not fully accounted for by known physiological mechanisms distinguishes somatoform disorders from disorders formerly designated as psychophysiological disorders, some of which are included in DSM-IV-TR under "Psychological Factors Affecting Medical Condition." Beliefs involving preoccupations with symptoms are not of delusional intensity, except possibly for body dysmorphic disorder. Symptoms are not better accounted for by other mental disorders.

In DSM-IV-TR, the disorders included under the somatoform rubric are somatization disorder, undifferentiated somatoform disorder, conversion disorder, pain disorder, hypochondriasis, body dysmorphic disorder, and the residual category somatoform disorder not otherwise specified (NOS). DSM-IV-TR criteria for these disorders are outlined in Table 13–1. The grouping is based on the clinical utility of a shared diagnostic concern rather than assumptions regarding shared etiology or mechanism—that is, occult "physical" or "organic" pathology underlying the symptoms is excluded. In DSM-IV-TR terminology, such etiologies are referred to as "general medical conditions" or the "direct effects of a substance." General medical conditions include all conditions not included in the mental disorders section of ICD-10 (World Health Organization 1992b). As examples, all infectious and parasitic, endocrine, nutritional, metabolic, immunological, and congenital disorders affecting virtually any organ system (including the nervous system) are considered general medical conditions. This terminology was adopted to avoid the implication that mental (i.e., psychiatric) conditions do not have organic... underscore the view that psychiatric... medical conditions.

609

13–1. DSM-IV-TR somatoform disorders: a comparison

DSM-IV-TR somatoform disorder	General description	Temporal and other requirements	Exclusions by other psychiatric illness	Other exclusions
Somatization disorder	History of many physical complaints: pain in at least four different sites or functions, two nonpain gastrointestinal, one sexual or reproductive, one pseudoneurological (conversion or dissociative).	Onset before age 30 years. Occurs over a period of several years. Treatment sought, or significant impairment in social, occupational, or other important areas of functioning.	Not specified.	Not fully explained by a known general medical condition or the direct effect of a substance.
Undifferentiated somatoform disorder	One or more physical complaints.	Duration of at least 6 months. Clinically significant distress or impairment in social, occupational, or other important areas of functioning.	Not better accounted for by another mental disorder.	Not fully explained by a known general medical condition or pathophysiological mechanism (i.e., the effects of injury, medication, drugs, alcohol).
Conversion disorder	Symptoms or deficits affecting voluntary motor or sensory function suggesting a neurological or other general medical condition.	Psychological factors associated. Clinically significant distress or impairment in social, occupational, or other important areas of functioning or warrants medical evaluation.	Not limited to pain or sexual dysfunction. Not exclusively during course of somatization disorder. Not better accounted for by another mental disorder.	Not intentionally produced or feigned. Not fully explained by a neurological or other general medical condition, by the direct effect of a substance, or as a culturally sanctioned behavior or experience.
Pain disorder	Pain a predominant focus of clinical presentation. Of sufficient severity to warrant clinical attention.	Clinically significant distress or impairment in social, occupational, or other important areas of functioning. Psychological factors have an important role.	Not better accounted for by a mood, anxiety, or psychotic disorder and does not meet criteria for dyspareunia.	Not specified.

TABLE 13–1.　DSM-IV-TR somatoform disorders: a comparison *(continued)*

DSM-IV-TR somatoform disorder	General description	Temporal and other requirements	Exclusions by other psychiatric illness	Other exclusions
Hypochondriasis	Preoccupation with fears of having, or the idea that one has, a serious disease, based on the misinterpretation of bodily symptoms. Persists despite appropriate medical evaluation and reassurance.	Duration of at least 6 months. Clinically significant distress or impairment in social, occupational, or other important areas of functioning.	Not exclusively during course of generalized anxiety, obsessive-compulsive, or panic disorder; a major depressive episode; separation anxiety; or another somatoform disorder.	Not of delusional intensity. Not restricted to circumscribed concern about appearance.
Body dysmorphic disorder	Preoccupation (may be of delusional intensity) with imagined defect in appearance or markedly excessive concern with slight physical anomaly.	Clinically significant distress or impairment in social, occupational, or other important areas of functioning.	Not better accounted for by another mental disorder (e.g., dissatisfaction with body shape or size in anorexia nervosa).	Not specified.
Somatoform disorder not otherwise specified	Disorders with specified somatoform symptoms. Examples include pseudocyesis, disorders of less than 6 months' duration with fatigue or body weakness, nonpsychotic hypochondriacal symptoms, or other physical complaints.	Can be of less than 6 months' duration.	Does not meet criteria for any specific somatoform disorder.	Not specified.

Source.　Adapted with permission from Martin RL: "Somatoform Disorders in the General Hospital Setting," in *Handbook of Studies on General Psychiatry.* Edited by Judd FK, Burrows GD, Lipsitt DR. Amsterdam, The Netherlands, Elsevier, 1991, pp. 251–266. Copyright 1991 Elsevier Science Publishers.

The utility of grouping disorders on the basis of a shared clinical concern was endorsed by the symptom-driven *DSM-IV Primary Care Version* (American Psychiatric Association 1995), which included "unexplained physical symptoms" as the basis of 1 of its 10 algorithms. Likewise, the *ICD-10 Diagnostic and Management Guidelines for Mental Disorders in Primary Care* (World Health Organization 1996) was organized with a diagnostic category for "unexplained somatic complaint."

Historically, many overlapping, conflicting, and even contradictory diagnostic conventions have been used to identify and distinguish somatoform disorders. For the sake of consistency, this chapter uses DSM-IV-TR criteria and terminology, with other systems reviewed and contrasted when appropriate. Table 13–2 lists the categories best corresponding to DSM-IV-TR somatoform disorders in DSM-I (American Psychiatric Association 1952), DSM-II (American Psychiatric Association 1968), DSM-III, and DSM-III-R as well as ICD-9 (World Health Organization 1977) and ICD-10.

No general heading corresponding to "somatoform" existed in DSM-I and DSM-II. In DSM-I, with only "conversion reaction" specifically listed, conditions corresponding to the DSM-IV-TR somatoform disorders would have been diagnosed under "psychoneurotic disorders." DSM-II included "hysterical neurosis, conversion type" under "Neuroses." Both DSM-I and DSM-II included a "psychophysiological" category, encompassing syndromes involving organ systems under autonomic nervous system control. A somatoform grouping was not incorporated into the international system until ICD-10. In ICD-9, disorders corresponding to DSM-IV somatoform disorders were included under "Neurotic Disorders." The ICD-10 somatoform category is conceptualized in a manner similar to what was introduced with DSM-III, emphasizing as the main feature "physical symptoms" that are not adequately explained by physical disorders. In addition, ICD-10 includes a medical utilization specification requiring a "repeated presentation" of symptoms, "persistent requests for medical investigations," and resistance to consideration of "psychological causation" despite "repeated negative findings and reassurances by doctors that the symptoms have no physical basis" (World Health Organization 1992a, p. 161). ICD-10 somatoform disorders include somatization disorder, undifferentiated somatoform disorder, hypochondriacal disorder (which also subsumes DSM-IV-TR body dysmorphic disorder), somatoform autonomic dysfunction (a category not included in DSM-IV-TR that corresponds, in part, to the DSM-I and DSM-II

psychophysiological disorders), persistent somatoform pain disorder, other somatoform disorders, and somatoform disorder, unspecified. Conversion disorder is not included as a somatoform disorder but is subsumed under a fused dissociative (conversion) disorder. As is discussed in the section on conversion disorder later in this chapter, this option was considered carefully in the preparation of DSM-IV, but it was decided that conversion disorder would remain in the somatoform grouping on the basis that it met the essential requirement of presentation with physical symptoms suggesting a general medical condition but for which there is no adequate medical or physiological explanation (Martin 1995).

Despite inconsistencies between DSM-IV and ICD-10, sufficient overlap existed to permit generalizations regarding specific somatoform disorders, as long as the differences were kept in mind. The comparability and, by design, compatibility of DSM-IV and ICD-10 provided evidence of expanding international cooperation in developing a common language to foster better communication among clinicians and researchers worldwide.

Given the heterogeneity of the somatoform disorder class, extensive discussion of the class, in general, is not particularly useful. The specific somatoform disorders are best discussed individually. Thus, with the exception of pain disorders, which are reviewed in a separate chapter of this textbook (see Chapter 25, "Pain Disorders," by Leo), we review the somatoform disorders included in DSM-IV-TR. For convenience, the disorders are discussed in the order in which they appear in DSM-IV-TR.

Somatization Disorder

Definition and Clinical Description

The core features of somatization disorder are recurrent multiple physical complaints that are not fully explained by physical factors and that result in medical attention or significant impairment.

A patient with somatization disorder is typified by the following example:

An internist referred a married, 35-year-old woman to a psychiatrist because of the physician's inability to establish a clear longitudinal history and medical explanation for her numerous physical complaints. Physical examination and laboratory testing had been completely unrevealing. The physician had

TABLE 13–2. DSM-IV-TR somatoform disorders and corresponding categories in previous DSM and ICD diagnostic systems

DSM-I (1952)	DSM-II (1968)	ICD-9 (1977)	DSM-III (1980)	DSM-III-R (1987)	ICD-10 (1992)	DSM-IV (1994)/ DSM-IV-TR (2000)
—	—	—	Somatoform disorders	Somatoform disorders	Somatoform disorders; also dissociative (conversion) disorders	Somatoform disorders
—	—	Other neurotic disorders: somatization disorder, Briquet's disorder	Somatization disorder	Somatization disorder	Somatization disorder	Somatization disorder
—	—	—	Atypical somatoform disorder	Undifferentiated somatoform disorder	Undifferentiated somatoform disorder	Undifferentiated somatoform disorder
Conversion reaction	Hysterical neurosis, conversion type	Conversion disorder	Conversion disorder	Conversion disorder	Dissociative (conversion) disorders	Conversion disorder
—	Hysterical neurosis, conversion type	Psychalgia, psychogenic pain	Psychogenic pain disorder	Somatoform pain disorder	Persistent pain disorder	Pain disorder
Psychoneurotic reaction: other	Hypochondriacal neurosis	Hypochondriasis	Hypochondriasis	Hypochondriasis	Hypochondriasis	Hypochondriasis
—	—	—	Atypical somatoform disorder: dysmorphophobia	Body dysmorphic disorder	Included under hypochondriacal disorder	Body dysmorphic disorder
—	—	—	Atypical somatoform disorder	Somatoform disorder not otherwise specified	Other somatoform disorders	Somatoform disorder not otherwise specified

Source. Adapted with permission from Martin RL: "Somatoform Disorders in the General Hospital Setting," in *Handbook of Studies on General Psychiatry.* Edited by Judd FK, Burrows GD, Lipsitt DR. Amsterdam, The Netherlands, Elsevier, 1991, pp. 251–266. Copyright 1991 Elsevier Science Publishers.

treated her for anxiety and depressive complaints; however, the pharmacotherapy, which was initially apparently effective, subsequently failed.

On presentation to the psychiatrist, the patient offered a laundry list of physical complaints in a dramatic yet vague manner. The patient often went into elaborate and flamboyant discussions of her marital, social, and occupational problems. Careful review of the presentation identified a long history of chronic physical complaints without medical explanation. Furthermore, the physical problems appeared to be temporally associated with multiple psychosocial stressors.

Somatization disorder is the most pervasive somatoform disorder. By definition, somatization disorder is a polysymptomatic disorder affecting multiple body systems. Symptoms of other specific somatoform disorders (e.g., conversion disorder and pain disorder) are included in the diagnostic criteria for somatization disorder. Undifferentiated somatoform disorder, in essence, represents a syndrome similar to somatization disorder but with a less extensive symptomatology. From a hierarchical perspective, none of these disorders is diagnosed if symptoms occur exclusively during the course of somatization disorder.

Somatization disorder has been the most rigorously studied somatoform disorder and is the best validated in terms of diagnostic reliability, stability over time, prediction of medical utilization, and even heritability. Yet its validity as a discrete syndrome has been challenged (Bass and Murphy 1990). Vaillant (1984), noting that most of the research on this disorder has emanated from four academic centers in the midwestern United States, went so far as to state that the diagnosis "lies in the eyes of the beholder."

Diagnosis

History

The DSM-IV-TR criteria for somatization disorder are the product of a long and inconsistent approach to a syndrome characterized by multiple unexplained physical complaints (Martin 1988). Originally designated as "hysteria," the syndrome was first described at least 4,000 years ago, with its conceptualization probably originating in Egypt (Goodwin and Guze 1996). In Egyptian medicine, it was believed that physical displacement of the uterus precipitated symptoms (Veith 1965); treatment consisted of attempting to attract the "wandering womb" back to its proper site.

Freud devoted a great deal of attention to the concept of hysteria (Breuer and Freud 1893–1895/1955). In fact, many of the principles of psychoanalysis were developed through observations of hysteria. Dynamic theorists postulated the operation of the ego defense mechanism of conversion in hysteria. This mechanism was conceptualized as the converting of "psychic energy" into physical symptoms. Later, Stekel (1943) coined the term *somatization*, which he regarded as similar to Freud's concept of conversion.

Pierre Briquet (1859) described in his monograph *Traité, Clinique et Thérapeutique Y l'Hystérie* a syndrome corresponding to somatization disorder as it is conceptualized today. He described hysteria as characterized by multiple dramatic and excessive medical complaints in the absence of demonstrable organic pathology. Purtell et al. (1951) resurrected Briquet's concept, adding a quantitative perspective by providing a list of associated symptoms, which was further refined by Perley and Guze (1962).

Hysteria was included as one of the 14 "canonized" psychiatric disorders in the influential criteria described by Feighner et al. (1972). The disorders included were those considered by the authors to have been validated sufficiently. For hysteria, the Feighner criteria required a chronic or recurrent illness beginning before age 30 that included a dramatic, vague, or complicated medical history. The diagnosis required 25 "positive" medically unexplained symptoms (from a list of 59) in 9 of 10 groups (Table 13–3); 20 symptoms in the same number of groups were necessary for a probable diagnosis. To be counted as positive, a symptom had to meet one of the following: 1) have caused the patient to see a physician or other health care provider, 2) have precipitated disability that interfered with the patient's life, 3) have led the patient to take medicine on one or more occasions, or 4) have been of "clinical significance" despite not fulfilling one of the three previously mentioned criteria. An example of this fourth criterion would be a brief spell of blindness that the patient minimizes.

As is discussed in this chapter, the syndrome as defined by Feighner et al. (1972) remains the gold standard because it has been the best validated. In particular, clinical, epidemiological, and follow-up studies that used the Feighner criteria support their validity, reliability, and internal consistency (Barsky 1989). The stability of the disorder is supported by the finding that in the 6–8 years after initial diagnosis, there is a 90% probability that the clinical picture will remain essentially unchanged and that no general medical condition or new mental disorder will develop to explain the original symptoms (Barsky 1989).

Despite such validation, the construct was underused by clinicians (Cloninger 1994). This underuse has

TABLE 13–3. Feighner criteria symptom list for hysteria (somatization disorder)

Group 1

Headaches
Sickly most of life

Group 2

Blindness
Paralysis
Anesthesia
Aphonia
Fits or convulsions
Unconsciousness
Amnesia
Deafness
Hallucinations
Urinary retention
Trouble walking
Other unexplained "neurological symptoms"

Group 3

Fatigue
Lump in throat
Fainting spells
Visual blurring
Weakness
Dysuria

Group 4

Breathing difficulty
Palpitations
Anxiety attacks
Chest pain
Dizziness

Group 5

Anorexia
Weight loss
Marked fluctuations in weight
Nausea
Abdominal bloating
Food intolerances
Diarrhea
Constipation

Group 6

Abdominal pain
Vomiting

Group 7

Dysmenorrhea
Menstrual irregularity
Amenorrhea
Excessive bleeding

TABLE 13–3. Feighner criteria symptom list for hysteria (somatization disorder) (continued)

Group 8

Sexual indifference
Frigidity
Dyspareunia
Other sexual difficulties
Vomiting all 9 months of pregnancy at least once, or hospitalization for hyperemesis gravidarum

Group 9

Back pain
Joint pain
Extremity pain
Burning pains of the sexual organs, mouth, or rectum
Other bodily pains

Group 10

Nervousness
Fears
Depressed feelings
Need to quit working, or inability to carry on regular duties because of feeling sick
Crying easily
Feeling life is hopeless
Thinking a good deal about dying
Wanting to die
Thinking of suicide
Suicide attempts

Note. Twenty-five positive symptoms in nine groups required for a diagnosis of definite hysteria; 20 positive symptoms in nine groups required for a diagnosis of probable hysteria.

Source. Adapted from Perley and Guze 1962. Reprinted with permission from Cloninger CR: "Somatoform and Dissociative Disorders," in *The Medical Basis of Psychiatry,* 2nd Edition. Edited by Winokur G, Clayton P. Philadelphia, PA, WB Saunders, 1994, pp. 169–192. Copyright 1994, WB Saunders Company.

been attributed to two sources: the pejorative connotation of the term *hysteria* and the complexity of remembering the numerous symptoms divided into various groups not organized according to any obvious logic. The criteria were intended principally for a research setting in which the investigator completed his or her systematic assessment with a checklist to evaluate for the presence of the syndrome.

In addition to its definition as a syndrome characterized by many somatic complaints, hysteria was frequently confused with the dramatic and volatile hysterical personality characteristics as described by Chodoff and Lyons (1958). Guze (1970) suggested the more neutral eponym *Briquet's syndrome.* In DSM-III, the syndrome was descriptively renamed *somatization disorder.*

The criteria in DSM-III were simplified as follows:

1. The required number of symptoms was lowered to 14 for women and 12 for men, from a list of 37 commonly identified somatic complaints. The 37 symptoms listed were those that best discriminated somatization disorder from other disorders. The number of symptoms required of men was lowered in an attempt to reduce a possible sex bias because of the impossibility of menstrual and pregnancy symptoms in men.
2. The group requirement was eliminated because it seemed to add little information.
3. Depressive and panic attack symptoms were eliminated to avoid overlap with depressive and panic disorders.

The diagnostic criteria for somatization disorder also required a history of physical symptoms of several years' duration beginning before the patient was 30 years old. Conditions similar to those defined by the Feighner criteria were necessary to consider a symptom positive. Exclusion of a medical explanation was determined if the symptoms were not adequately explained by a "physical disorder or physical injury" and were "not side effects of medication, drugs, or alcohol" (American Psychiatric Association 1980, p. 243). The clinician did not need to be convinced that the symptom had actually occurred; a patient's report was sufficient.

The criteria for somatization disorder were modified only slightly for DSM-III-R. The changes included shortening the symptom list to 35 and requiring 13 symptoms for the diagnosis in both sexes. A symptom was not counted if it occurred only during a panic attack. Symptoms were to be counted as present if there was no specific pathology or pathophysiological mechanism. In addition, if organic pathology was identified, the complaint or resulting social or occupational impairment must have grossly exceeded what would be expected from the physical findings.

Unfortunately, diagnostic concordance between the simplified DSM-III somatization disorder criteria and the Feighner criteria was less than optimal. As a result, the question was raised whether the types of cases identified by DSM-III criteria constituted a valid disease entity (Cloninger et al. 1986; Guze et al. 1986). The adequacy of the criteria also was questioned when the National Institute of Mental Health's Epidemiologic Catchment Area (ECA) studies (L.N. Robins et al.

1984), which used DSM-III criteria, found a much lower lifetime prevalence rate (0.2%–0.3%) of somatization disorder for women in the general population than the 2% estimated by Woodruff et al. (1971), who used the Feighner criteria. Furthermore, and particularly noteworthy, was that many psychiatrists considered both the DSM-III and the DSM-III-R criteria too lengthy and complex for routine clinical use.

DSM-IV-TR Criteria

In an attempt to address these issues for DSM-IV, a comprehensive reassessment of the extant literature and preexisting data sets was coordinated by the American Psychiatric Association. On the basis of this review, Cloninger and Yutzy (1993) suggested a diagnostic strategy that simplified the criteria for somatization disorder and appeared useful in routine practice. Data from a sample of 500 psychiatric outpatients were reanalyzed, leading to the development of an empirically derived algorithm to diagnose somatization disorder. This algorithm required four pain symptoms, two nonpain gastrointestinal symptoms, one nonpain sexual or reproductive symptom, and one pseudoneurological (conversion or dissociative) symptom. This approach was adopted for DSM-IV (Table 13–4). The data reanalysis criteria identified nearly the same patients as did both the original Feighner criteria for hysteria and the DSM-III-R criteria for somatization disorder (κ=0.79, sensitivity = 81%, specificity = 96%) (Yutzy et al. 1992).

The new criteria were tested in a multicenter field trial designed to examine their concordance with previous diagnostic criteria. This study (Yutzy et al. 1995) found excellent agreement with the newly proposed diagnostic strategy and these earlier criteria: DSM-III-R (κ=0.84, sensitivity=84%, specificity=98%), DSM-III (κ=0.82, sensitivity=82%, specificity=98%), and the original Feighner criteria for hysteria (κ=0.79, sensitivity = 80%, specificity = 97%). These findings supported the DSM-IV diagnostic strategy for somatization disorder.

Differential Diagnosis

The symptom picture encountered in somatization disorder is frequently nonspecific and can overlap with a multitude of medical disorders. According to Cloninger (1994), three features are useful in discriminating between somatization disorder and physical illness: 1) involvement of multiple organ systems, 2) early onset and chronic course without development of physical signs of structural abnormalities, and 3) absence of characteristic laboratory abnormalities of the sug-

TABLE 13–4. DSM-IV-TR diagnostic criteria for somatization disorder

A. A history of many physical complaints beginning before age 30 years that occur over a period of several years and result in treatment being sought or significant impairment in social, occupational, or other important areas of functioning.

B. Each of the following criteria must have been met, with individual symptoms occurring at any time during the course of the disturbance:

   (1) *four pain symptoms:* a history of pain related to at least four different sites or functions (e.g., head, abdomen, back, joints, extremities, chest, rectum, during menstruation, during sexual intercourse, or during urination)

   (2) *two gastrointestinal symptoms:* a history of at least two gastrointestinal symptoms other than pain (e.g., nausea, bloating, vomiting other than during pregnancy, diarrhea, or intolerance of several different foods)

   (3) *one sexual symptom:* a history of at least one sexual or reproductive symptom other than pain (e.g., sexual indifference, erectile or ejaculatory dysfunction, irregular menses, excessive menstrual bleeding, vomiting throughout pregnancy)

   (4) *one pseudoneurological symptom:* a history of at least one symptom or deficit suggesting a neurological condition not limited to pain (conversion symptoms such as impaired coordination or balance, paralysis or localized weakness, difficulty swallowing or lump in throat, aphonia, urinary retention, hallucinations, loss of touch or pain sensation, double vision, blindness, deafness, seizures; dissociative symptoms such as amnesia; or loss of consciousness other than fainting)

C. Either (1) or (2):

   (1) after appropriate investigation, each of the symptoms in criterion B cannot be fully explained by a known general medical condition or the direct effects of a substance (e.g., a drug of abuse, a medication)

   (2) when there is a related general medical condition, the physical complaints or resulting social or occupational impairment are in excess of what would be expected from the history, physical examination, or laboratory findings

D. The symptoms are not intentionally produced or feigned (as in factitious disorder or malingering).

gested physical disorder (Table 13–5). These features should be considered in cases for which careful analysis leaves the etiology unclear. The clinician also should be aware that several medical disorders may be confused with somatization disorder (Table 13–6). Patients with multiple sclerosis or systemic lupus erythematosus (SLE) may have vague functional and sensory disturbances with unclear physical signs. Patients with acute intermittent porphyria may have a history of episodic pain and various neurological disturbances, and patients with hemochromatosis often have vague and diffuse pains that may be confused with those described by patients who have somatization disorder.

According to Cloninger (1994), three psychiatric disorders must be carefully considered in the differential diagnosis of somatization disorder: anxiety disorders (in particular, panic disorder), mood disorders, and schizophrenia. The most troublesome distinction is between anxiety disorders and somatization disorder. Individuals with generalized anxiety disorder may have a multitude of physical complaints that are also frequently found in patients with somatization disorder. Individuals with anxiety disorders also may have disease concerns and hypochondriacal complaints common to somatization disorder. Similarly, patients with somatization disorder often report panic (anxiety) attacks. Although the usual parameters of age at onset and course may be helpful in differentiating between an anxiety disorder and somatization disorder, the presence of certain traits, symptoms, and social factors can be of assistance. In particular, the presence of histrionic personality traits, conversion and dissociative symptoms, sexual and menstrual problems, and social impairment supports a diagnosis of somatization disorder (Cloninger 1994). In addition, gender should be considered because men are much more likely to have anxiety disorders than somatization disorder. Precise diagnosis, although difficult, is clinically important because the medical management of somatization disorder differs from that of anxiety disorders.

Patients with mood disorders, especially depression, may have somatic complaints. Commonly, the chief complaint may be headache, gastrointestinal disturbance, or unexplained pain. However, such symptoms resolve with successful treatment of the mood disorder, whereas in somatization disorder, the physical complaints continue. Patients with somatization disorder frequently complain of depression and often fulfill the criteria for major depression (DeSouza et al. 1988). It is not clear, however, whether these complaints truly reflect the clinical state or are simply a reflection of overreporting.

TABLE 13–5. Features useful in discriminating between somatization disorder and general medical conditions

Involvement of multiple organ systems

Early onset and chronic course without development of physical signs of structural abnormalities

Absence of characteristic laboratory abnormalities of the suggested physical disorder

TABLE 13–6. General medical conditions that may be confused with somatization disorder

Multiple sclerosis

Systemic lupus erythematosus

Acute intermittent porphyria

Hemochromatosis

Patients with schizophrenia may have unexplained somatic complaints. Careful evaluation often identifies delusions, hallucinations, and/or a formal thought disorder. Rarely will the somatic symptoms be extensive enough to meet the criteria for somatization disorder. It should be noted that occasionally a patient with extensive somatic symptomatology and no evidence of psychosis subsequently will develop clinical symptoms of schizophrenia (Goodwin and Guze 1996). As described in the section on conversion disorder later in this chapter, reports of hallucinations are common among women with somatization disorder (R.L. Martin, unpublished observations, 1998). Caution must be taken not to equate such reports with a psychotic diagnosis, which can lead to unnecessary long-term treatment with neuroleptics.

Individuals with antisocial, borderline, and/or histrionic personality disorder may have an associated somatization disorder (Cloninger et al. 1997; Hudziak et al. 1996; Stern et al. 1993). Antisocial personality disorder has been shown to cluster both within individuals and within families (Cloninger and Guze 1970; Cloninger et al. 1975) and may have a common etiology in many cases.

Patients with somatization disorder often complain of psychological or interpersonal problems in addition to somatic symptoms. Wetzel et al. (1994) summarized these as "psychoform symptoms." In this study, Minnesota Multiphasic Personality Inventory (Hathaway and McKinley 1943) profiles of somatization disorder patients mimicked multiple psychiatric disorders.

Commonly, individuals with somatization disorder are inconsistent historians, and obtaining the medical records often will be necessary to definitively establish the diagnosis.

Natural History

E. Robins and O'Neal (1953) found somatization disorder to be unusual in children younger than 9 years. In most cases, characteristic symptoms begin during adolescence, and the criteria are satisfied by the mid-20s (Guze and Perley 1963; Purtell et al. 1951).

Somatization disorder is a chronic illness with fluctuations in the frequency and diversity of symptoms, but it rarely, if ever, totally remits (Guze and Perley 1963; Guze et al. 1986). The most active symptomatic phase is usually early adulthood, but aging does not lead to total remission (Goodwin and Guze 1996). Pribor et al. (1994) found that patients with somatization disorder age 55 years and older did not differ from younger patients in terms of the number of somatization symptoms or the use of health care services. Longitudinal prospective studies have confirmed that 80%–90% of the patients diagnosed with somatization disorder maintain a consistent clinical syndrome and retain the same diagnosis over many years (Cloninger et al. 1986; Guze et al. 1986; Perley and Guze 1962).

According to Goodwin and Guze (1996), the most frequent and important complications of somatization disorder are repeated surgical operations, drug dependence, suicide attempts, and marital separation or divorce. These authors suggested that the first two complications are preventable if the disorder is recognized and the patient's symptoms are managed appropriately. Generally, because of awareness that somatization disorder is an alternative explanation for various pains and other symptoms, invasive techniques can be withheld or postponed when objective indications are absent or equivocal. There is no evidence of excess mortality in patients with somatization disorder.

Avoiding the prescribing of habit-forming or addictive substances for persistent or recurrent complaints of pain should be paramount in the mind of the treating physician. Suicide attempts are common, but completed suicide is not (Martin et al. 1985; G.E. Murphy and Wetzel 1982). It is unclear whether marital or occupational dysfunction can be minimized through psychotherapy.

Epidemiology

The lifetime risk, prevalence, and incidence of somatization disorder are unclear. The lifetime risk for somatization disorder was estimated at about 2% in women when age at onset and method of assessment were taken into account (Cloninger et al. 1975). This risk is similar to the previously noted 2% prevalence rate identified by Woodruff et al. (1971). Cloninger et al. (1984), using complete lifetime medical records, found a 3% frequency of somatization disorder in 859 Swedish women in the general population. However, the ECA study (L.N. Robins et al. 1984), using nonphysician interviewers, found a lifetime risk of somatization disorder of only 0.2%–0.3% for women. However, the prevalence of somatization disorder may be underestimated in studies relying on interviews by nonphysicians. In a study by L.N. Robins et al. (1981), nonphysicians, when compared with psychiatrists, showed high (i.e., 97%–99%) diagnostic specificity for somatization disorder. However, diagnostic sensitivity for nonphysicians was low (55% for Feighner-defined hysteria and 41% for DSM-III-defined somatization disorder). The diagnostic criteria for somatization disorder require judgments as to whether symptoms are fully explained medically. Patients with somatization disorder often attribute symptoms to various physical disorders. Nonphysicians rarely have the expertise to evaluate such statements critically and may tend to accept them. To properly assess somatic complaints relative to objective findings and the known course of disease may require that the interviewer have an adequate medical background (Cloninger 1994). Additionally, patients may be less inclined to describe physical complaints to nonphysicians. All of these factors may lead to the underdiagnosis of somatization disorder, which may account for the low prevalence of somatization disorder in large-scale population surveys that use nonphysician interviewers.

Somatization disorder is diagnosed predominantly in women and rarely in men. Some have suggested that this sex difference may be artifactual, because somatization disorder criteria are biased against making the diagnosis in men because of the inapplicability of pregnancy and menstrual complaints. Also, men tend to report fewer symptoms than do women. Some investigators have suggested an adjustment for this discrepancy (Temoshok and Attkisson 1977). DSM-III reduced the number of symptoms required to diagnose somatization disorder from 14 (in women) to 12 in men, compensating for the inapplicable gynecological symptoms but not for the response bias in the number of somatic complaints. Diagnosis of somatization disorder remains much less frequent in men than in women unless the number of somatic complaints required for diagnosis in men is reduced to half (i.e., 7) of

the 14 required in women (Cloninger 1994). The symptoms of somatization disorder were counted in a study of psychiatric outpatients and their relatives (Cloninger et al. 1986). Frequency counts were identified for probands and for the relatives of nonsomatizing subjects. The prevalence of somatization disorder was 22% in outpatient women when DSM-III criteria of 14 unexplained symptoms in women were used, compared with 2.9% in the female relatives of nonsomatizing subjects. When the DSM-III criterion of 12 unexplained symptoms in men was applied, the prevalence of somatization disorder in the male relatives of nonsomatizing subjects was only 0.3%, making the disorder more than 10 times as prevalent in women as in men. When the symptom count for men was reduced to 7 or 8 symptoms, the prevalences in men and women were about the same. However, according to Cloninger (1994), men who had from 7 to 11 somatic complaints had a mixed picture of anxiety and personality disorders and did not cluster in families with somatizing subjects of either sex.

Etiology

The etiology of somatization disorder is unknown, but it is clearly a familial disorder. In several studies, approximately 20% of the female first-degree relatives of patients with somatization disorder also met criteria for the disorder (Cloninger and Guze 1970; Guze et al. 1986; Woerner and Guze 1968). Guze et al. (1986) demonstrated the familial nature of somatization disorder in a "blind" family study and documented an association between somatization disorder and antisocial personality disorder in male and female relatives. In addition, several studies have suggested that male relatives of female patients with somatization disorder have an increased risk of antisocial personality disorder and alcoholism (Cloninger et al. 1975; Woerner and Guze 1968). Cloninger et al. (1986) found that men with multiple somatic complaints were clinically heterogeneous and did not aggregate in families with either male or female somatizing subjects. Overall, these findings suggest that somatization disorder in women shares a common etiology with antisocial personality disorder, whereas somatization disorder in men may be related more to anxiety disorders (Cloninger et al. 1984, 1986).

A relation between somatization disorder and certain personality disorders has been posited. Hudziak et al. (1996) and Cloninger et al. (1997) identified similarities and even overlap between somatization disorder and borderline personality disorder, as did Stern et al. (1993) with personality disorders broadly. These studies support interpretations that somatization disorder is more of a personality (Axis II) disorder than an Axis I disorder, considering its early onset, nonremitting nature, and pervasiveness, which in some cases results in chronic dysfunctional states.

Familial aggregation in somatization disorder could result from genetic factors, environmental influences, or both. Bohman et al. (1984) used comprehensive lifetime medical records in an adoption study in Sweden and identified two discrete types of somatoform disorders in women. One form, described as "high-frequency somatization," was characterized by frequent headaches, backaches, gastrointestinal disturbances, and gynecological complaints associated with psychiatric disability (Figure 13–1). Review of the psychiatric evaluations showed overlap with somatization disorder. Women who were adopted before age 3 years had a fivefold increase in high-frequency somatization disorder if their biological parents had alcoholism or were antisocial. Risk of somatization disorder in the adopted children varied according to the social status of the adoptive parents. In a cross-fostering analysis that considered the possible combinations of genetic background and postnatal influences, both factors contributed independently to the risk of somatization.

Experimental neuropsychological testing has indicated that individuals with somatization disorder have difficulty with information processing related to problems with attention and memory (Almgren et al. 1978; Bendefeldt et al. 1976; Ludwig 1972). Flor-Henry et al. (1981) investigated the neuropsychological functioning of patients with somatization disorder and compared it with control subjects, psychotic depressive patients, and schizophrenic patients. All comparison groups were matched to the patients with somatization disorder for sex, age, handedness, and Wechsler Adult Intelligence Scale–Revised (WAIS-R; Wechsler 1981) full-scale IQ. Compared with the control subjects, patients with somatization disorder had bilateral, symmetrical patterns of frontal lobe dysfunction. The authors also noted nondominant hemisphere dysfunction, with impairment greater in the anterior as opposed to the posterior regions. Patients with somatization disorder had greater dominant hemisphere impairment than did control subjects and psychotic depressive patients, a finding also reported for persons with antisocial personality disorder. Patients with somatization disorder had less nondominant hemisphere disorganization than did schizophrenic patients. This pattern of neuropsychological impairment permitted identification of patients with somatization disorder from control subjects and patients in the comparison groups.

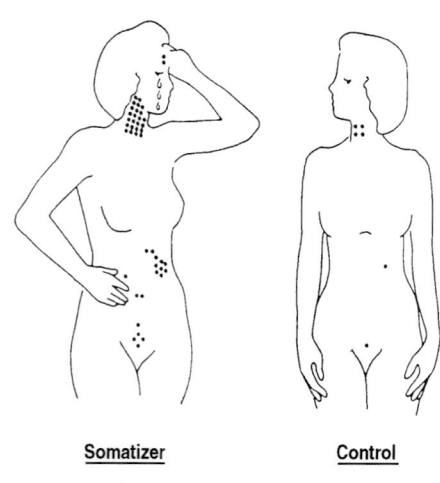

Somatizer   **Control**

• 1 Somatic sick leave/10 person-years
� 1 Psychiatric sick leave/10 person-years

FIGURE 13–1.   Distribution and number of sick leave occasions in Swedish somatizing ("high-frequency") subjects and control nonsomatizing subjects.

Source. Reprinted with permission from Cloninger CR: "Somatoform and Dissociative Disorders," in *The Medical Basis of Psychiatry,* 2nd Edition. Edited by Winokur G, Clayton PJ. Philadelphia, PA, WB Saunders, 1994, pp. 169–192. Copyright 1994, WB Saunders Company.

Other theories attempt to explain the characteristics of patients with somatization disorder. In particular, Shapiro (1965) and Horowitz (1977) suggested that "hysterical" information processing may be responsible for many of the clinical features. The information-processing deficit may be the basis for the somatic complaints, mental status findings of vagueness and circumstantiality, and many social, interpersonal, and occupational problems prominent in these patients and their biological relatives (Cloninger 1978; Flor-Henry et al. 1981; Horowitz 1977). Ford (1983) and Quill (1985) postulated a social communication model based on the theory that individuals with somatization disorder learn to somatize as a means of expressing emotion (i.e., distress) in their family constellation, evoking support and care from significant individuals. Further work needs to be done to evaluate these theories.

Treatment

Somatization disorder is difficult to treat, and there appears to be no single superior treatment approach (G. E. Murphy 1982). Primary care physicians generally can manage patients with somatization disorder adequately, but the expertise of at least a consulting psychiatrist has been shown to be useful. In a prospective, randomized, controlled study, Smith et al. (1986) found a reduction in health care costs for patients with somatization disorder who received a psychiatric consultation as opposed to those who did not receive a consultation. Reduced expenditures were largely the result of decreased rates of hospitalization. These gains were accomplished with no decrement in medical status or in patient satisfaction, suggesting that many of the evaluations and treatments otherwise provided to patients with somatization disorder are unnecessary. Smith et al. (1986) suggested that treatment include regularly scheduled visits with an appropriate physician. The frequency of visits should be determined on the basis of support for the patient, not in response to the frequency or severity of complaints.

Scallet et al. (1976) reviewed the earlier psychiatric literature on treatment of hysteria and reported the success rates of various approaches. Although most of the studies were uncontrolled and otherwise methodologically flawed, one study by Luff and Garrod (1935) noted a 51% improvement rate at 3-year follow-up in patients treated with an "eclectic approach." As summarized by Scallet et al. (1976), this treatment involved "reeducation, reassurance and suggestion." These techniques were also described by Carter (1949) as being effective in the treatment of acute conversion.

An eclectic approach accords well with the general principles of treatment recommended by Quill (1985), Cloninger (1994), and Smith et al. (1986). Three important suggestions emerge from review of these reports: 1) establish a firm therapeutic alliance with the patient, 2) educate the patient about the manifestations of somatization disorder, and 3) provide consistent reassurance (Table 13–7). Implementation of these principles, as described in more detail in the following paragraphs, may greatly facilitate clinical management of somatization disorder and prevent potentially serious complications, including the effects of unnecessary diagnostic and therapeutic procedures. The superiority of more specific treatment approaches has not yet been documented in controlled trials (Kellner 1989); this subject is discussed in greater detail later in the chapter.

First, a firm therapeutic alliance must be established. The basis of any satisfactory treatment relationship is a firm therapeutic alliance; it is particularly important in the treatment of patients with somatization disorder, but it is often difficult to attain. Generally, multiple physicians already have been consulted in an attempt to discover a physical explanation for the symptoms offered. The patient usually has received the message (overtly or covertly) that the difficulty is "mental," "psychological," or "psychiatric," and the

TABLE 13–7. Main treatment principles in approaching a patient with somatization disorder

1. Establish a firm therapeutic alliance at the outset.
2. Provide education about the illness.
3. Offer consistent reassurance.

physician is not particularly interested in continuing to provide care to him or her. That message promotes a pattern of "doctor shopping," which may lead to unnecessary diagnostic procedures and treatments. To prevent harm, a therapeutic alliance is essential. The first step in establishing such an alliance is for the physician to acknowledge the patient's pain and suffering. This acknowledgment communicates to the patient that the physician is caring, compassionate, and interested in providing assistance. The physician should then conduct an exhaustive review of the patient's medical history, including careful examination of medical records. Such a review generally will strengthen the incipient therapeutic bond by demonstrating the physician's willingness to take the time and effort to gain an understanding of the patient. In addition, this step is crucial in ruling out medical disorders that can include nonspecific motor and sensory abnormalities or transient or equivocal signs (e.g., multiple sclerosis, SLE, acute intermittent porphyria, hemochromatosis) (see Table 13–6). Also, a thorough medical knowledge of the patient initially will allow better ongoing assessment of symptomatology. After the diagnosis of somatization disorder is firmly established, elaborate diagnostic evaluations should be conducted based on objective evidence and not just subjective complaints. However, the clinician must always remain cognizant that patients with somatization disorder are not immune to developing physical illness.

Education is the second general principle. Cloninger (1994) favors informing the patient of the diagnosis and describing the various facets of somatization disorder in a positive light. The patient should be advised that he or she is not "crazy" but has a medically recognized illness. The condition will not lead to chronic mental or physical deterioration (or death). The clinician should be careful to strike a balance between painting a positive picture of the disorder and conducting a realistic discussion of prognosis, goals, and treatment.

The third principle is consistent reassurance. Patients with somatization disorder often become concerned that the physician is not performing a sufficiently thorough evaluation and may threaten to seek care from a different physician. Such challenges should be directly addressed with reassurance that the possibility of an undiscovered physical illness is being appropriately assessed on a continuing basis and that changing physicians would place decisions in the hands of someone unaware of the complexities of the patient's case. The patient should be reassured that there is no evidence of a physical cause for the complaint but that there may be a link with stress. A thorough review of complaints commonly identifies a temporal association of symptoms with interpersonal, social, or occupational problems. Discussion of such associations may help the patient gain insight that the problems may precipitate somatic or psychological symptoms. In patients for whom introspection is difficult, modification of behavior by using simple behavioral management techniques may be useful.

During the late 1990s and early 2000s, cognitive-behavioral approaches embodying some of the principles just described were applied to "somatization" patients and yielded tentatively positive results in small studies (Kroenke and Swindle 2000; Lidbeck 1997). In 2001 the National Institute of Mental Health funded a single-blind, active-control, parallel-assignment interventional study of cognitive-behavioral therapy (CBT) for somatization disorder in the primary care setting. In this study, Allen et al. (2006) found that CBT with psychiatric consultation was more effective in producing symptom improvement and functioning than psychiatric consultation alone.

In addition to these approaches, several issues merit consideration in the treatment of somatization disorder. Because patients with somatization disorder also frequently complain of anxiety and depressive symptoms, prescription medications for these complaints should be held to a minimum and carefully monitored. Wheatley (1962, 1964, 1965) found that low doses of anxiolytic drugs provided some improvement in symptoms in a series of double-blind clinical trials. Although chlordiazepoxide was recommended for reasons of safety, patient preference, and effectiveness in symptom relief, the best results were obtained by optimistic physicians using low dosages of anxiolytic medications, regardless of which drug was given (Wheatley 1965). Pharmacotherapy in the management of patients with somatization disorder must be tempered with the knowledge that these patients may take medicines inconsistently and unpredictably, may develop drug dependence, and may overdose in suicide gestures or attempts.

The clinician should develop a relationship with the patient's family. This facilitates attaining a better appreciation of the patient's social structure, which may be crucial to understanding and managing the patient's often chaotic personal lifestyle. When appropriate, the clinician must place firm limits on excessive demands, manipulations, and attention seeking (G. E. Murphy 1982; G. E. Murphy and Guze 1960).

Undifferentiated Somatoform Disorder

Definition and Clinical Description

The essential aspect of undifferentiated somatoform disorder is the presence of one or more clinically significant, medically unexplained somatic symptoms with a duration of 6 months or more that are not better accounted for by another mental disorder (Table 13–8; see also Table 13–1 for comparison with other somatoform disorders). In effect, this category serves to capture syndromes that resemble somatization disorder but do not meet the full criteria. Symptoms that may be seen include those also considered for somatization disorder.

Diagnosis

History

The category of undifferentiated somatoform disorder did not exist prior to DSM-III-R. At that time, it was added to cover those syndromes that in DSM-III simply would have been included under "atypical somatoform disorder." It is not clear whether the category *undifferentiated somatoform disorder* has been well adopted by clinicians, but several studies support its existence. Alternative terms that have been proposed include "subsyndromal," *"forme fruste,"* or "abridged" somatization disorder (Kirmayer and Robbins 1991) as well as "multisomatoform disorder" (Kroenke et al. 1997).

DSM-IV-TR Criteria

After some debate, minor changes in the category *undifferentiated somatoform disorder* were made in DSM-IV. Because of perceived low use of the undifferentiated somatoform disorder diagnosis by clinicians, which was attributed to ambiguity of the term *undifferentiated disorder,* the term *multisomatoform disorder* was suggested. However, because the scarce empirical data available seemed to indicate a variable course, with unclear boundaries with normality and other mental disorders (especially anxiety and depressive disorders),

TABLE 13–8. DSM-IV-TR diagnostic criteria for undifferentiated somatoform disorder

A. One or more physical complaints (e.g., fatigue, loss of appetite, gastrointestinal or urinary complaints).

B. Either (1) or (2):

(1) after appropriate investigation, the symptoms cannot be fully explained by a known general medical condition or the direct effects of a substance (e.g., a drug of abuse, a medication)

(2) when there is a related general medical condition, the physical complaints or resulting social or occupational impairment is in excess of what would be expected from the history, physical examination, or laboratory findings

C. The symptoms cause clinically significant distress or impairment in social, occupational, or other important areas of functioning.

D. The duration of the disturbance is at least 6 months.

E. The disturbance is not better accounted for by another mental disorder (e.g., another somatoform disorder, sexual dysfunction, mood disorder, anxiety disorder, sleep disorder, or psychotic disorder).

F. The symptom is not intentionally produced or feigned (as in factitious disorder or malingering).

this term was not adopted. As a result, the only changes involved substituting the standard "general medical condition" for DSM-III-R's "organic pathology." A threshold for diagnosis also was added, requiring clinically significant distress or impairment. Instead of excluding the diagnosis on the basis of "occurrence exclusively during the course of another mental disorder," exclusion in DSM-IV was on the basis of "not better accounted for by another mental disorder."

Kroenke et al. (1997) used improved diagnostic criteria with inclusion and exclusion criteria and found that the proposed multisomatoform disorder had a large and independent effect on impairment in a study of 1,000 patients from four primary care sites. In terms of validity of the proposed disorder, evidence of temporal stability is still lacking.

Differential Diagnosis

Principal considerations in the differential diagnosis include the question of whether, with follow-up, crite-

ria for somatization disorder will be met. Patients with somatization disorder are typically inconsistent historians. During one evaluation, they may report many symptoms and fulfill criteria for the full syndrome, whereas during another, they may report fewer symptoms, perhaps only fulfilling criteria for an abridged syndrome (Martin et al. 1979). Another consideration is whether the somatic symptoms qualifying a patient for the diagnosis of undifferentiated somatoform disorder are the manifestation of a depressive or an anxiety disorder. Indeed, high rates of major depression and anxiety disorders have been found in somatizing patients attending family medicine clinics (Kirmayer et al. 1993).

Epidemiology

Some investigators have argued that undifferentiated somatoform disorder is the most common somatoform disorder. Escobar et al. (1991) used a construct requiring six somatic symptoms for women and four for men and reported that in the United States 11% of non-Hispanic whites and Hispanics, as well as 15% of blacks, fulfilled the criteria. In Puerto Rico, 20% met the criteria. A preponderance of women was evident in all groups except the Puerto Rican sample.

Etiology

If undifferentiated somatoform disorder is simply an abridged form of somatization disorder, etiological theories reviewed under that diagnosis should also apply to undifferentiated somatoform disorder. Of theoretical interest would be the question of why the syndrome is fully expressed in some and only partially in others. Some investigators postulate theories of etiology involving primarily the concept of somatization, for which there are numerous explanations. As reviewed by Kirmayer and Robbins (1991), somatization can be viewed as a pattern of illness behavior by which bodily idioms of distress may serve as symbolic means of social regulation as well as protest or contestation. As yet, there is little, if any, empirical evidence for such theories.

Treatment

Existing data have been derived from studies fraught with methodological problems, including the use of diverse groups with only a certain number of chronic somatic complaints in common. Several studies suggested that improvement is accelerated with psychotherapy of a supportive, rather than a nondirective, type. However, a substantial proportion of patients improve or recover with no formal psychotherapy. Judicious use of pharmacotherapy appears to be beneficial, with trials of antidepressant medications indicated for patients with depressive symptoms and trials of buspirone, benzodiazepines, and propranolol for patients with anxiety symptoms. Again, definitive recommendations await a more extensive empirical database.

Conversion Disorder

Definition and Clinical Description

The essential features of conversion disorder are the nonintentionally produced symptoms or deficits affecting voluntary motor or sensory function that suggest but are not fully explained by a neurological or general medical condition, by the direct effects of a substance, or by a culturally sanctioned behavior or experience. Specific symptoms mentioned as examples in DSM-IV-TR include motor symptoms such as impaired coordination or balance, paralysis or localized weakness, difficulty swallowing or lump in throat (e.g., "globus hystericus"), aphonia, and urinary retention; sensory symptoms, including hallucinations, loss of touch or pain sensation, double vision, blindness, and deafness; and seizures or convulsions with voluntary motor or sensory components. Single episodes usually involve one symptom, but longitudinally, other conversion symptoms will be evident as well. Psychological factors generally appear to be involved, because symptoms often occur in the context of a conflictual situation that may in some way be resolved with the development of the symptom.

An example of a typical patient with conversion disorder follows:

> A woman in her early 20s was brought to the emergency department by female relatives after an argument with her husband that led to his leaving the household. She showed variable impairment in gait, at times appearing quite unstable and needing the support of another person, a piece of furniture, or the walls to ambulate. At other times, her gait was only mildly unsteady. A psychiatry consultation was requested, but before it occurred, the woman was observed to have a "seizure" during which she showed generalized shaking that seemed to wax and wane. No incontinence was noted. Following the episode, she had a questionable Babinski sign on the left side. Her eyes remained closed, and she was variably responsive to questions. When unresponsive, she

showed no spontaneous voluntary movement, but she resisted passive movement, such as when attempts were made to open her eyelids to evaluate her pupils.

> Internal medicine consultation resulted in routine laboratory work, lumbar puncture, and magnetic resonance imaging. The patient was admitted to the medical intensive care unit. No abnormalities were noted in any of the laboratory or imaging procedures.

> The next day, the patient was fully responsive, showed no impairment in gait, and had no episodes of "seizures." She had a hazy recollection of the preceding day, but when questioned, she did remember the argument with her husband. She reported unhappiness about her marital difficulties, but she did not report enough symptoms to warrant diagnosis of a depressive episode. She was not particularly interested in exploring psychological issues. She denied prior psychiatric problems or treatment, although relatives reported a similar episode 4 years previously, after a disagreement with a boyfriend. The patient had a normal neurological examination except for a questionable Babinski sign on the left side. It was concluded that her apparent neurological presentation was attributable to a mixture of conversion and dissociative symptoms. The patient and her family were cautioned to be vigilant for any symptoms suggesting neurological dysfunction.

> She was transferred to the psychiatry service, from which she was discharged 2 days later with a follow-up plan that included marital counseling.

This case illustrates several typical aspects of the presentation and course of conversion disorder to be discussed later in this section.

Diagnosis

History

Some of the major early contributions to the study of conversion disorder were by neurologists, including Charcot (Torack 1978) and Breuer and Freud (1893–1895/1955) in the late nineteenth century and early twentieth century. As shown in Table 13–2, conversion disorder was called "conversion reaction" in DSM-I and "hysterical neurosis, conversion type" in DSM-II. In both DSM-I and DSM-II, the conversion process was restricted to the production of symptoms affecting the voluntary motor and sensory nervous systems. Symptoms considered to be generally related to the autonomic nervous system were subsumed under the psychophysiological disorders.

Other terms such as "acute hysteria" also have been used. Unfortunately, "conversion disorder" or "conversion hysteria" was used by some clinicians synonymously with "hysteria," a term replaced by somatization disorder in DSM-III. Generally, hysteria was used to describe a more pervasive, chronic, and polysymptomatic disorder. Although conversion symptoms are perhaps the most dramatic symptoms of somatization disorder, the disorder is characterized by multiple unexplained symptoms in many organ systems. In conversion disorder, a single symptom, traditionally of a pseudoneurological type (i.e., suggesting neurological disease), suffices. Such inconsistency in the use of terms has resulted in a great deal of confusion, both in research and in clinical practice.

Adding to this confusion was a change introduced in DSM-III and retained in DSM-III-R, wherein the concept of conversion was expanded to include disorders characterized by symptoms involving any "loss of, or alteration in, physical functioning suggesting a physical disorder" (American Psychiatric Association 1987) as long as the mechanism of conversion was evident—that is, the symptom was "an expression of a psychological conflict or need" (American Psychiatric Association 1987). Thus, symptoms involving the autonomic or endocrine systems, such as vomiting (supposedly representing revulsion and disgust) and pseudocyesis (as a manifestation of unconscious conflict about, or the need for, pregnancy), were included as examples of conversion symptoms.

DSM-IV-TR Criteria

As defined in DSM-IV-TR, nonintentional "symptoms or deficits affecting voluntary motor or sensory function" (American Psychiatric Association 2000, p. 498) are central to conversion disorder (Table 13–9). The majority of such symptoms will suggest a neurological condition (i.e., are pseudoneurological), but other general medical conditions may be suggested as well. Pseudoneurological symptoms remain the classic symptomatology. By definition, symptoms limited to pain or disturbance in sexual functioning are not included.

In conversion disorder, as in the other somatoform disorders, the symptom cannot be fully explained by a known physical disorder. This criterion is perhaps the most imperative diagnostic consideration. In addition, the symptom is defined as not fully explained by a culturally sanctioned behavior or experience. Symptoms such as seizurelike episodes occurring in conjunction with certain religious ceremonies and culturally expected responses, such as women swooning in response to excitement, would qualify as examples.

DSM-IV-TR specifies that the symptoms in conversion disorder are not intentionally produced, thus distinguishing conversion symptoms from those of a

TABLE 13–9. DSM-IV-TR diagnostic criteria for conversion disorder

A. One or more symptoms or deficits affecting voluntary motor or sensory function that suggest a neurological or other general medical condition.

B. Psychological factors are judged to be associated with the symptom or deficit because the initiation or exacerbation of the symptom or deficit is preceded by conflicts or other stressors.

C. The symptom or deficit is not intentionally produced or feigned (as in factitious disorder or malingering).

D. The symptom or deficit cannot, after appropriate investigation, be fully explained by a general medical condition, or by the direct effects of a substance, or as a culturally sanctioned behavior or experience.

E. The symptom or deficit causes clinically significant distress or impairment in social, occupational, or other important areas of functioning or warrants medical evaluation.

F. The symptom or deficit is not limited to pain or sexual dysfunction, does not occur exclusively during the course of somatization disorder, and is not better accounted for by another mental disorder.

Specify type of symptom or deficit:

With motor symptom or deficit

With sensory symptom or deficit

With seizures or convulsions

With mixed presentation

factitious disorder or malingering. Although this judgment is difficult to make, it is an important one because the recommended management and expected outcome of factitious disorder and malingering are markedly different.

Clinical judgment also is required in determining whether psychological factors are etiologically related to the symptom. Inclusion of this criterion is perhaps a holdover from the initial conceptualization of conversion symptoms as representing the conversion of unconscious psychic conflict into a physical symptom. As reviewed by Cloninger (1987), such determination is virtually impossible except in cases in which there is a temporal relationship between a psychosocial stressor and the symptom or in cases in which similar situations led to conversion symptoms in the past.

Differential Diagnosis

Conversion symptoms suggest physical illness, and nonpsychiatrists are generally seen initially. Neurologists are frequently consulted by primary care physicians for such symptoms because most suggest neurological disease. It has been estimated that 1% of the patients admitted to the hospital for neurological problems have conversion symptoms (Marsden 1986), and up to one-third of new neurology clinic patients have medically unexplained symptoms (Carson et al. 2003; Stone et al. 2003). One major problem with conversion symptoms is that they suggest neurological or general medical conditions, and a conversion (mis-) diagnosis may be applied when a true illness is present. Some older studies found that significant proportions of patients initially diagnosed with conversion symptoms had neurological illnesses on follow-up. Slater and Glithero (1965) found a misdiagnosis rate of 50% during a 7- to 11-year follow-up; Gatfield and Guze (1962) reported a rate of 21%. In 1996 Mace and Trimble observed a rate of 15%. However, other recent studies have suggested a misdiagnosis rate of around 4%, which has been stable since 1970 (Stone et al. 2005). Also noteworthy is the fact that misdiagnosis may happen in reverse, with patients with multiple sclerosis ultimately being diagnosed with conversion disorder (Hankey and Stewart-Wynne 1987). The trend toward less misdiagnosis may reflect increasing sophistication in neurological diagnosis. Nevertheless, one needs to be tentative in making a diagnosis of conversion disorder.

Symptoms of various neurological illnesses may seem to be inconsistent with known neurophysiology or neuropathology and may suggest conversion. Diseases to be considered include multiple sclerosis (consider blindness secondary to optic neuritis with initially normal fundi), myasthenia gravis, periodic paralysis, myoglobinuric myopathy, polymyositis, other acquired myopathies (all of which may include marked weakness in the presence of normal deep tendon reflexes), and Guillain-Barré syndrome, in which early weakness of the arms and legs may be inconsistent (Cloninger 1994). As reviewed by Ford and Folks (1985), more than 13% of actual neurological cases are diagnosed as "functional" before the elucidation of a neurological illness. Initial evidence of some neurological disease is predictive of a subsequent neurological explanation (Mace and Trimble 1996).

Complicating diagnosis is the fact that physical illness and conversion (or other apparent psychiatric overlay) are not mutually exclusive. Patients with incapacitating and frightening physical illnesses may appear to exaggerate their symptoms. Patients with actual neurological illness also may have "pseudosymptoms." For example, patients with actual seizures often have pseudoseizures (Desai et al. 1982).

Considering these observations, physicians should resist an incautious diagnosis of conversion disorder when faced with difficult-to-interpret symptoms. The occurrence of apparent conversion symptoms mandates a thorough evaluation for possible underlying physical explanation. This evaluation may include physical and psychiatric examinations, X rays, and blood and urine tests as symptoms and signs indicate.

Longitudinal studies indicate the most reliable predictor that a patient with apparent conversion symptoms will not later be shown to have a physical disorder is a history of conversion or other unexplained symptoms (Cloninger 1994). Patients with somatization disorder will manifest multiple symptoms in multiple organ systems, including the voluntary motor and sensory nervous systems. Thus, apparent conversion symptoms in the context of somatization disorder should indicate that an underlying physical disorder is unlikely. Although conversion symptoms may occur at any age, vulnerability for conversion symptoms is first manifested most often in late adolescence or early adulthood (Cloninger 1994). Conversion symptoms first occurring in middle age or later should increase suspicion of an occult physical illness.

DSM-IV-TR lists hallucinations among the examples of sensory nervous system symptoms. Reports of hallucinations suggest psychosis, especially schizophrenia, or a mood disorder with psychotic features. In fact, DSM-III and DSM-III-R virtually forced this interpretation because the only contexts in which hallucinations were mentioned in conjunction with a nonpsychotic disorder were with the reexperiencing of the traumatic event in posttraumatic stress disorder (PTSD) and with the hearing, by one personality, the voice(s) of one or more of the other personalities in multiple personality disorder (dissociative identity disorder in DSM-IV). Hallucinations as conversion symptoms have long been reported (Andrade and Srinath 1986; Fitzgerald and Wells 1977; Goodwin et al. 1971; Modai and Cygielman 1986). In DSM-IV's somatization disorder field trial, one-third of a large sample of nonpsychotic women with evidence of unexplained somatic complaints reported a history of hallucinations. Among the 40% who met criteria for somatization disorder, more than half reported hallucinations (R.L. Martin, unpublished observations, 1998). Women with other conversion symptoms were more likely to report hallucinations than were those women with no other conversion symptoms, giving further support for including hallucinations as conversion symptoms.

Generally, conversion disorder hallucinations differ in several ways from hallucinations in psychotic conditions and are referred to by some as "pseudohallucinations." Conversion disorder hallucinations typically occur in the absence of other psychotic symptoms. Insight that the hallucinations are not "real" is generally retained. Conversion hallucinations often involve more than one modality, whereas hallucinations in psychoses generally involve a single sensory modality (especially auditory; secondarily, tactile). They may have a naive, fantastic, or childish content, as in a fairy tale, and are described eagerly as an interesting story (e.g., "A big green frog came in, sat down next to me, and began talking to me"). Conversion hallucinations are often psychologically meaningful (e.g., "I heard my ex-boyfriend's voice telling me that he had made a big mistake"). Because hallucinations as part of psychoses also may share some of these features, vigilance must be maintained for the emergence of other signs of psychosis. A diagnosis of conversion disorder should not be made if the hallucinations are better accounted for by PTSD or dissociative identity disorder (multiple personality disorder).

An association between conversion symptoms affecting voluntary motor and sensory functioning and dissociative symptoms affecting memory and identity should be noted. Traditionally, such symptoms have been attributed to similar psychological mechanisms. The two types of symptoms often occur in the same individual, sometimes during the same episode of illness (consider the example of the patient with conversion disorder discussed at the beginning of this section). Thus, patients with conversion disorder should be screened for dissociative symptoms, and patients with dissociative disorder should be evaluated for conversion symptoms.

Natural History

Onset of conversion disorder is generally from late childhood to early adulthood. Conversion disorder is rare before age 10 years (Maloney 1980) and seldom first presents after age 35 years, but it has been reported to begin as late as the ninth decade (Weddington 1979). When onset is in middle or late age, the possibility of a neurological or other medical condition is increased.

Onset of conversion disorder is generally acute, but it may be characterized by gradually increasing symptomatology. The typical course of individual conversion symptoms is generally short; half (Folks et al. 1984) to nearly all (Carter 1949) patients show a disappearance of symptoms by the time of hospital discharge. However, 20%–25% will relapse within 1 year. Factors traditionally associated with good prognosis include acute onset, presence of clearly identifiable stress at the time of onset, short interval between onset and institution of treatment, and good intelligence (Toone 1990). One recent study noted a better outcome for patients with affective illnesses and a poor prognosis for those with personality disorders (Mace and Trimble 1996). The study also reported that a diagnosis of somatization disorder at follow-up was especially associated with chronicity. Symptoms of blindness, aphonia, and paralysis have been noted to have a relatively good prognosis, whereas seizures and tremor were identified to be more persistent (Toone 1990). However, these findings were not supported in the Mace and Trimble (1996) study. When followed up longitudinally, some patients initially diagnosed only with conversion disorder will subsequently meet the criteria for somatization disorder (Kent et al. 1995; Mace and Trimble 1996).

Generally, individual conversion symptoms are self-limited and do not lead to physical changes or disabilities. Occasionally, physical sequelae such as atrophy may occur, but this is rare. Morbidity in terms of marital and occupational impairment appears to be less than that in somatization disorder (Kent et al. 1995; Tomasson et al. 1991). In a long-term follow-up study (up to 44 years) of a small number (*N*=28) of individuals with conversion disorder, excess mortality by unnatural causes was observed (Coryell and House 1984). None of the deaths in this study was by suicide.

Epidemiology

Conclusions regarding the epidemiology of conversion disorder are compromised by methodological differences in diagnostic boundaries as well as by ascertainment procedures from study to study. Vastly different estimates have been reported. Lifetime prevalence rates of treated conversion symptoms in general populations have ranged from 11 in 100,000 to 500 in 100,000 (Ford and Folks 1985; Toone 1990). A marked excess of women compared with men develop conversion symptoms. More than 25% of healthy postpartum and medically ill women report having had conversion symptoms sometime during their lives (Cloninger 1994).

Approximately 5%–24% of psychiatric outpatients, 5%–14% of general hospital patients, and 1%–3% of outpatient psychiatric referrals have a history of conversion symptoms (Cloninger 1994; Ford 1983; Toone 1990). Conversion is associated with lower socioeconomic status, lower education, lack of psychological sophistication, and rural setting (Folks et al. 1984; Guze and Perley 1963; Lazare 1981; Stefansson et al. 1976; Weinstein et al. 1969). Consistent with this finding, much higher rates (nearly 10%) of outpatient psychiatric referrals in developing countries are for conversion symptoms. As countries develop, there may be a declining incidence over time, which may relate to increasing levels of education and sophistication (Stefanis et al. 1976).

Conversion disorder appears to be diagnosed more often in women than in men, with ratios varying from 2:1 (Ljundberg 1957; Stefansson et al. 1976) to 10:1 (Raskin et al. 1966). In part, this variance may relate to referral patterns, but it also appears that indeed a predominance of women compared with men develop conversion symptoms.

Etiology

An etiological hypothesis is implicit in the term *conversion*. The term, in fact, is derived from the hypothesized conversion of psychological conflict into a somatic symptom. Several psychological factors have been implicated in the pathogenesis, or at least pathophysiology, of conversion disorder. However, as the following discussion will show, such etiological relationships are difficult to establish. (Refer to Table 13–10 for definitions.)

In primary gain, anxiety is theoretically reduced by keeping an internal conflict or need out of awareness by symbolic expression of an unconscious wish as a conversion symptom. However, individuals with active conversion symptoms often continue to show marked anxiety, especially on psychological tests (Lader and Sartorius 1968; Meares and Horvath 1972). Symbolism is infrequently evident, and its evaluation involves highly inferential and unreliable judgments (Raskin et al. 1966). Interpretation of symbolism in persons with occult medical disorder has been noted to contribute to misdiagnosis. Secondary gain, whereby conversion symptoms allow avoidance of noxious activities or the obtaining of otherwise unavailable support, also may occur in persons who have medical conditions, who often take advantage of such benefits (Raskin et al. 1966; Watson and Buranen 1979).

Individuals with conversion disorder may show a lack of concern, in keeping with the nature or implications of the symptom (the so-called *la belle indifférence*). However, such indifference to symptoms is not invariably present in conversion disorder (Lewis and Ber-

TABLE 13–10. **Key terms**
Conversion: Hypothesized conversion of a psychological conflict into a somatic complaint.
Primary gain: Anxiety is theoretically reduced by keeping an internal conflict or need out of conscious awareness through production of a symptom; the symptom is involuntarily produced and not under conscious control.
Secondary gain: The symptom is voluntarily produced and under conscious control; production is for the purpose of a goal, such as avoiding work, obtaining money (i.e., malingering).
La belle indifférence: The individual seems indifferent or disinterested in personal medical issues that should concern anyone.

man 1965; Sharma and Chaturvedi 1995), and it also can be seen in individuals with general medical conditions (Raskin et al. 1966), sometimes as denial or stoicism (Pincus 1982). Conversion symptoms may be revealed in a dramatic or histrionic fashion. A minority of individuals with conversion disorder fulfill criteria for histrionic personality disorder. A dramatic presentation of conversion disorder can be seen in distressed individuals with medical conditions. Even symptoms based on underlying medical conditions often respond to suggestion, at least temporarily (Gatfield and Guze 1962). Patients with conversion disorder may have a history of disturbed sexuality (Lewis 1974), with many (one-third) reporting a history of sexual abuse, especially incestuous. (Thus, two-thirds do not report such a history.) Individuals with conversion disorder are often reported to be the youngest, or else the youngest of a sex, in sibling order, but these are not consistent findings (Stephens and Kamp 1962; Ziegler et al. 1960).

Limited data suggest that conversion symptoms are more frequent in relatives of individuals with conversion disorder (Toone 1990). Rates that were 10 times greater than similarly derived general population estimates in female relatives and approximately 5 times the corresponding rate in male relatives were reported in a nonblind study (Ljundberg 1957). Accumulated data from available twin studies show 9 concordant and 33 discordant monozygotic pairs and 0 concordant and 43 discordant dizygotic pairs (Inouye 1972). Nongenetic familial factors, particularly incestuous childhood sexual abuse, also may be frequent. Nearly one-third of the individuals with medically unexplained seizures reported childhood sexual abuse, as compared with fewer than 10% of those with complex partial epilepsy (Alper et al. 1993). High rates also have been noted in overlapping dissociative conditions. Rates of reported childhood sexual abuse as high as 83% have been noted in individuals with dissociative identity disorder. Women with somatization disorder (many of whom will have conversion or dissociative symptoms) have rates of reported abuse as high as 50% (Martin 1995).

If not directly etiological, many factors have been suggested as predisposing individuals to conversion disorder. In many instances, preexisting personality disorders are diagnosable and may predispose some individuals to conversion disorder. Several psychosocial factors in addition to a history of abuse may be involved. Preliminary functional imaging studies postulate an association among conversion disorder, depression, and PTSD (Ballmaier and Schmidt 2005). Individuals from rural backgrounds and those who are psychologically and medically unsophisticated appear to be predisposed to conversion disorder, as are those with existing neurological disorders. In the last case, a tendency to conversion symptoms has been attributed to "modeling"—that is, patients with neurological disorders are likely to observe in others, as well as in themselves, various neurological symptoms that they at other times simulate as conversion symptoms.

Treatment

Generally, the initial aim in treating conversion disorder is the removal of the symptom. The pressure behind accomplishing this goal depends on the distress and disability associated with the symptom (Merskey 1989). If the patient is not in particular discomfort and the need to regain function is not great, direct attention may not be necessary. In any situation, direct confrontation is not recommended. Such a communication may cause a patient to feel even more isolated. A conservative approach of reassurance and relaxation is effective. Reassurance need not come from a psychiatrist but can be performed effectively by the primary physician. After physical illness is excluded, prognosis for conversion symptoms is good. Folks et al. (1984), for example, found that half of 50 general hospital patients with conversion symptoms showed complete remission by the time of discharge.

If symptoms do not resolve with a conservative approach and there is an immediate need for symptom resolution, several techniques, including narcoanalysis (e.g., amobarbital interview), hypnosis, and behavior therapy, may be tried (Merskey 1989). It does appear that prompt resolution of conversion symptoms

is important in that the duration of conversion symptoms is associated with greater risk of recurrence and chronic disability (Cloninger 1994).

In narcoanalysis, amobarbital or another sedative-hypnotic medication such as lorazepam is given to the patient intravenously to the point of drowsiness. Sometimes this is followed by administration of a stimulant medication such as methamphetamine. The patient is then encouraged to discuss stressors and conflicts. This technique may be effective in the short term, leading to at least temporary symptom relief and expansion of the information known about the patient. This technique has not been shown to be especially effective with more chronic conversion symptoms. In hypnotic therapy, symptoms may be removed during a hypnotic state, with the suggestion that the symptoms will gradually improve posthypnotically. Information about stressors and conflicts may be explored as well. Hypnotherapy is thought to be particularly effective with motor symptoms. Behavior therapy, including relaxation training and even aversion therapy, has been proposed and reported by some investigators to be effective.

It is evident that it may not be the particular technique that is associated with symptom relief but the influence of suggestion. Various rituals such as exorcism and other religious ceremonies undoubtedly have led to immediate "cures." Suggestion seems to play a big part in cases of mass hysteria, in which individuals exposed to a "toxin" develop similar symptoms that do not appear to have any organic basis. Often, the epidemic can be contained if affected individuals are segregated. Simple announcements that no toxin was present and that reported "symptomatology" is linked to mass hysteria have been effective.

Anecdotal reports exist of positive response to somatic treatments such as phenothiazines, lithium, and even electroconvulsive therapy (ECT). Of course, in some cases, such a response again may be attributable to suggestion. In others, it may be that symptom removal occurred because of resolution of another psychiatric disorder, especially a mood disorder. Interestingly, even without a diagnosable mood disorder, antidepressants may be helpful (Bourgeois et al. 2002; Hurwitz 2004).

Thus far, the discussion on treatment of conversion disorder has centered on acute treatment primarily for symptom removal. Longer-term approaches would include strategies that were previously discussed for somatization disorder. These involve a pragmatic, conservative approach that entails support for and exploration of various areas of conflict, particularly interpersonal relationships. Ford (1995) suggested a treatment strategy based on "three Ps," whereby predisposing factors, precipitating stressors, and perpetuating factors are identified and addressed. A certain degree of insight may be attained, at least in terms of appreciating relationships between various conflicts and stressors and the development of symptoms. More ambitious goals have been adopted by some in terms of long-term, intensive, insight-oriented psychotherapy, especially of a psychodynamic nature. Reports of such approaches date from Freud's work with Anna O. Three studies involving a series of patients treated with psychoanalytic psychotherapy have reported success (Merskey 1989).

Hypochondriasis
Definition and Clinical Description

The essential feature in hypochondriasis is preoccupation not with symptoms themselves but rather with the fear or idea of having a serious disease, based on the misinterpretation of bodily signs and sensations (see Table 13–1). The preoccupation persists despite evidence to the contrary and reassurance from physicians. Some degree of preoccupation with disease is apparently quite common. As reviewed by Kellner (1987), 10%–20% of "normal" and 45% of "neurotic" persons have intermittent, unfounded worries about illness, with 9% of patients doubting reassurances given by physicians. In another review, Kellner (1985) estimated that 50% of all patients attending physicians' offices "suffer either from primary hypochondriacal syndromes or have 'minor somatic disorders with hypochondriacal overlay'" (p. 822). How these estimates relate to hypochondriasis as a disorder is difficult to assess because they do not appear to distinguish between preoccupation with symptoms (as is present in somatization disorder) and preoccupation with the implications of the symptoms (as is the case in hypochondriasis).

Diagnosis

History

Clinical descriptions of a syndrome designated *hypochondriasis* and characterized by preoccupation with bodily function can be found in the writings of the Hippocratic era (Stoudemire 1988). The Greeks attributed the syndrome to disturbances of viscera below the xiphoid cartilage, hence the term *hypochondria*. Even

into the nineteenth century, the term *hypochondriasis*, unlike the topographically nonspecific concept of more recent usage, was used specifically for somatic complaints below the diaphragm (Cloninger et al. 1984). As reviewed by M.R. Murphy (1990), Gillespie, in 1928, encapsulated a concept of hypochondriasis that is essentially identical to modern concepts, emphasizing preoccupation with a disease conviction "far in excess of what is justified," implying "an indifference to the opinion of the environment, including irresponsiveness to persuasion" (M.R. Murphy 1990, p. 28). Gillespie considered hypochondriasis a discrete disease entity. DSM-I did not include hypochondriasis as a separate illness, only mentioning "hypochondriacal preoccupation" as one of the malignant symptoms observed in psychotic but not reactive depression. As shown in Table 13–2, the syndrome was included in DSM-II as "hypochondriacal neurosis" and in ICD-9, DSM-III, DSM-III-R, and ICD-10 as "hypochondriasis."

Throughout the modern period, there has been controversy over whether hypochondriasis represents an independent, discrete disease entity, as proposed by Gillespie. Kenyon (1976), in an often quoted but perhaps methodologically flawed study (see M.R. Murphy 1990), concluded that hypochondriasis was virtually always secondary to another psychiatric disorder, usually depression. Barsky and various colleagues (Barsky and Klerman 1983; Barsky et al. 1986, 1990) extensively studied patients with hypochondriacal complaints using a set of operational criteria derived from DSM-III. These authors concluded that of the many patients with such complaints, few will meet criteria for the full diagnosis. However, they noted no bimodality, suggesting that hypochondriasis represents a continuum rather than a discrete entity or possibly a heterogeneous disorder. There has also been an ongoing debate whether hypochondriasis should remain in the somatoform disorders section of the DSM or be moved to the anxiety disorders section as part of the "OCD spectrum." However, very early functional imaging studies with patients diagnosed with OCD compared with those with hypochondriasis appear quite different (Van den Heuvel et al. 2005).

DSM-IV-TR Criteria

Specific criteria for the diagnosis of hypochondriasis are presented in Table 13–11.

As is explained in the following discussion, hypochondriasis is not diagnosed if symptoms occur exclusively during the course of generalized anxiety disorder, anxiety disorder, obsessive-compulsive disorder (OCD), panic disorder, a major depressive episode, separation anxiety, or another somatoform disorder.

TABLE 13–11. **DSM-IV-TR diagnostic criteria for hypochondriasis**

A. Preoccupation with fears of having, or the idea that one has, a serious disease based on the person's misinterpretation of bodily symptoms.

B. The preoccupation persists despite appropriate medical evaluation and reassurance.

C. The belief in criterion A is not of delusional intensity (as in delusional disorder, somatic type) and is not restricted to a circumscribed concern about appearance (as in body dysmorphic disorder).

D. The preoccupation causes clinically significant distress or impairment in social, occupational, or other important areas of functioning.

E. The duration of the disturbance is at least 6 months.

F. The preoccupation is not better accounted for by generalized anxiety disorder, obsessive-compulsive disorder, panic disorder, a major depressive episode, separation anxiety, or another somatoform disorder.

Specify if:

With poor insight: if, for most of the time during the current episode, the person does not recognize that the concern about having a serious illness is excessive or unreasonable

---

Differential Diagnosis

The first step in evaluating patients with hypochondriasis is to assess the possibility of physical disease. The list of serious diseases associated with the type of complaints seen in hypochondriacal patients is extensive, yet certain general categories emerge (Kellner 1985, 1987). These include neurological diseases, such as myasthenia gravis and multiple sclerosis; endocrine diseases; systemic diseases, such as SLE, that affect several organ systems; and occult malignancies.

If, after appropriate assessment, the probability of physical illness appears low, the condition should be considered relative to other psychiatric disorders (i.e., whether the hypochondriacal symptoms represent a primary disorder or are secondary to another psychiatric illness). As previously mentioned, one useful criterion is whether the belief is of delusional proportions. Patients with hypochondriasis as a primary disorder, although extremely preoccupied, are generally able to acknowledge the possibility that their concerns are unfounded. Delusional patients, on the other hand, are

not. Hypochondriasis with poor insight would lie somewhere in between, with the patient not recognizing that the concern is unwarranted for most of the episode. Somatic delusions of serious illness are seen in some cases of major depressive disorder and in schizophrenia. A useful discriminator is the presence of other psychiatric symptoms. A patient with hypochondriacal concerns secondary to depression should show other symptoms of depression such as sleep and appetite disturbance, feelings of worthlessness, and self-reproach, although elderly patients particularly may deny sadness or other expressions of depressed mood. Generally, schizophrenic patients will have bizarre delusions of illness (e.g., "I have congenital Hodgkin's caused by a snail hormone imbalance") and will show other signs of schizophrenia such as looseness of associations, peculiarities of thought and behavior, hallucinations, and other delusions. A confounding feature is the fact that hypochondriacal patients often will develop anxiety or depression in association with their hypochondriacal concerns. In general, characterizing the chronology of the episode will separate such patients from those with hypochondriasis.

Treatment trials also may have diagnostic significance. Depressed patients who are hypochondriacal may respond to antidepressant medication or ECT (often necessary in reversing a depressive state of sufficient severity to lead to such profound symptoms), with resolution of the hypochondriacal as well as the depressive symptoms. In schizophrenic patients, a disease-related delusion may show improvement with neuroleptic treatment. Although if questioned carefully the patient still may report a somatic delusion, preoccupation with the delusion will have diminished.

Natural History

Traditionally, limited data suggested that approximately one-fourth of the patients with a diagnosis of hypochondriasis do poorly, two-thirds show a chronic but fluctuating course, and one-tenth recover. However, such predictions may not reflect advances in psychopharmacology. It also must be remembered that such findings pertain to the full syndrome. A much more variable course is seen in patients with some hypochondriacal concerns.

Epidemiology

Estimates of the frequency of hypochondriacal symptoms warranting a diagnosis are somewhat compromised because DSM-III-R did not provide threshold criteria, other than requiring a duration of more than 6 months. The ECA study (L.N. Robins et al. 1984) did not assess for hypochondriasis. One study reported prevalences ranging from 3% to 13% in different cultures (Kenyon 1965), but it is not clear whether this range represented the full syndrome or just hypochondriacal symptoms. More recent studies suggest a prevalence in general medical practice of 3%–9% (Barsky et al. 1990; Escobar et al. 1998; Kellner et al. 1983/1984). As previously mentioned, many patients have such symptoms as part of other psychiatric disorders, particularly depressive and anxiety disorders, whereas others develop transient hypochondriacal symptoms in response to stress, particularly serious physical illness.

Etiology

In considering hypochondriasis as an aspect of depression or anxiety disorders, it has been posited that these conditions create a state of hypervigilance to insult, including overperception of physical problems (Barsky and Klerman 1983). Hypochondriasis has been discussed extensively in the psychoanalytic literature. Freud hypothesized that it represented "the return of object libido onto the ego with cathexis to the body" (Viederman 1985, p. 13). This theory has formed the basis for a number of psychoanalytic interpretations, including disturbed object relations, repressed hostility displaced to the body so that anger can be communicated indirectly to others, and dynamics involving masochism, guilt, conflicted dependency needs, and a need to suffer and be loved at the same time (Stoudemire 1988). Such "narcissistic" mechanisms have been thought to make patients unanalyzable. Other psychological theories involve defenses against feelings of low self-esteem, inadequacy, perceptual and cognitive abnormalities, and reinforcement for assuming the sick role.

More recently, hypochondriasis has been classified by some within the posited obsessive-compulsive spectrum disorders, which include, in addition to OCD, body dysmorphic disorder, anorexia nervosa, Tourette's disorder, and certain impulsive disorders (e.g., trichotillomania and pathological gambling; Hollander 1993). This clustering is based, in part, on the phenomenological similarity of repetitive thoughts and behaviors that are difficult or impossible to delay or inhibit (Martin and Yutzy 1997).

Treatment

Patients referred early for psychiatric evaluation and treatment of hypochondriasis appear to have a better prognosis than those continuing with only medical evaluations and treatments (Kellner 1983). Psychiatric referral should be performed with sensitivity. Perhaps the best guideline to follow is for the referring physician to stress that the patient's distress is serious and that psychiatric evaluation will be a supplement to, not a replacement for, continued medical care.

Hypochondriacal symptoms secondary to depressive and anxiety disorders may improve with successful treatment of the primary disorder. However, until recently, hypochondriasis as a primary condition was not considered to be responsive to known psychopharmacological medications. Early results of placebo-controlled, double-blind studies are pending, but anecdotal case reports, open-label trials, and review of preliminary data show some promise for the selective serotonin reuptake inhibitors (SSRIs; Fallon et al. 1996). Interestingly, these medications have been shown to be effective in OCD, and preliminary data are promising for their use in other obsessive-compulsive spectrum disorders, including body dysmorphic disorder and anorexia nervosa.

Investigators have tried many psychotherapeutic approaches in treating hypochondriasis. These may be summarized as supportive, rational, ventilative, and educative (Kellner 1987).

Stoudemire (1988) suggested an approach that includes consistent treatment, generally by the same primary physician, with supportive, regularly scheduled office visits not based on the evaluation of symptoms. Hospitalization, medical tests, and medications with addictive potential are to be avoided if possible. Focus during the office visits gradually should be shifted from symptoms to social or interpersonal problems. Psychotherapeutic approaches may be enhanced greatly by the promising potential of effective pharmacotherapy. Of note, CBT has recently been found to be effective in one study in which 57% of CBT-treated patients at 12-month follow-up had a lessening of hypochondriacal beliefs (Barsky and Ahern 2004). There is increasing hope for attaining the overriding goal in treating hypochondriacal patients: preventing adoption of the sick role and chronic invalidism (Kellner 1987).

Body Dysmorphic Disorder
Definition and Clinical Description

The essential feature of body dysmorphic disorder is a preoccupation with some imagined defect in appearance or markedly excessive concern with a minor physical anomaly (Table 13–12). Such preoccupation persists even after reassurance. Common complaints include a diversity of imagined flaws of the face or head, such as various defects in the hair (too much or too little), skin, shape of the face, or facial features. However, any body part may be the focus, including genitals, breasts, buttocks, extremities, shoulders, and even overall body size. De Leon et al. (1989) stated that the nose, ears, face, and sexual organs are most often involved. It is not surprising, then, that patients with body dysmorphic disorder are found most commonly among persons seeking cosmetic surgery.

The following case example illustrates some of the diagnostic and therapeutic uncertainties surrounding body dysmorphic disorder, especially regarding overlap with depressive and obsessive-compulsive disorders.

> The patient, a male in his mid-20s, received outpatient psychiatric care after 4 years of preoccupation with facial asymmetry and a blemish, defects not evident to others. He had been treated previously with unsuccessful trials of imipramine, phenelzine, perphenazine, and haloperidol. Seeing his reflection in a mirror or shiny surface resulted in a compulsion (accompanied by "a sick, anxious feeling") to inspect the blemish; thus, the patient avoided viewing all such surfaces. He also experienced what he described as a "sinking feeling" in his chest if he touched his face, particularly in the area of the blemish. He grew a beard so that he would not have to shave himself and then went to a barber weekly for a shave. He retained insight that there was no actual defect but had once made an appointment with a plastic surgeon. He was embarrassed about his preoccupation and concealed it from others. Although diligent in his work and studies and somewhat perfectionistic in general, he had no other evident obsessions or compulsions.
>
> From the start of his current treatment, an educative approach was taken. He did extensive reading on body dysmorphic and obsessive-compulsive disorders and their therapies.
>
> The SSRIs fluoxetine, sertraline, paroxetine, and fluvoxamine were not available at the time the patient was treated. While taking clomipramine (100 mg/day; he was unable to tolerate larger dosages because of extreme dry mouth), he showed some improvement because he was less dysphoric when ruminating about the blemish, but the preoccupation remained. Similarly, alprazolam "only took the edge off."
>
> The patient became markedly dysphoric and developed suicidal ideation after a breakup with a girlfriend. He received six ECT treatments, and his depressive and body dysmorphic symptoms improved dramatically. Although the "idea" of the blemish remained, it no longer preoccupied him. For the first time in several years, he could actually look at himself in the mirror and touch his face without discomfort. Although the benefit from ECT was transient, it gave him hope that he could be free of his preoccu-

TABLE 13–12. DSM-IV-TR diagnostic criteria for body dysmorphic disorder

A. Preoccupation with an imagined defect in appearance. If a slight physical anomaly is present, the person's concern is markedly excessive.

B. The preoccupation causes clinically significant distress or impairment in social, occupational, or other important areas of functioning.

C. The preoccupation is not better accounted for by another mental disorder (e.g., dissatisfaction with body shape and size in anorexia nervosa).

pation. He continued taking clomipramine.

On his own initiative, he obtained bromazepam, a benzodiazepine available in Europe but not the United States. He reported that with this drug, his preoccupation was "more under control." This drug has been found in some, but not all, studies to be effective in treating OCD (Hewlett 1993). After fluvoxamine was introduced, he began taking this drug. He tolerated it much better than clomipramine, and the dosage was increased to 300 mg/day. Buspirone was added, and the bromazepam was discontinued.

On this regimen, he still has concerns about his face, but "it doesn't rule me the way it used to." He maintains a successful professional practice. He has never married but has had a succession of girlfriends.

Diagnosis

History

As is evident in Table 13–2, body dysmorphic disorder was not even mentioned in the official nomenclatures until DSM-III and then only parenthetically as dysmorphophobia. The syndrome, generally under the rubric of dysmorphophobia, has a long history in the European and Japanese literature, with much less attention in the U.S. literature (Phillips and Hollander 1996).

DSM-IV-TR Criteria

In DSM-IV-TR, the essential feature of body dysmorphic disorder is preoccupation with an imagined defect in appearance or markedly excessive concern for a slight anomaly (see Table 13–12). This criterion represents a slight change from that in DSM-III-R, in which the phrase "in a normal-appearing person" was included. Because a person with some defect may have a preoccupation with a different imagined or exaggerated defect, this phrase was dropped.

As in other somatoform disorders, diagnosis requires that the preoccupation causes clinically significant distress or impairment, thus excluding those individuals with trivial symptoms. As is explained in the following discussion, body dysmorphic disorder is not diagnosed if the preoccupation is better accounted for by another mental disorder. On the other hand, DSM-IV dropped the exclusion on the basis of the preoccupation being delusional.

Differential Diagnosis

By definition, body dysmorphic disorder is not diagnosed when the body preoccupation is better accounted for by another mental disorder. Anorexia nervosa, in which there is dissatisfaction with body shape and size, is specifically mentioned in the criteria as an example of such an exclusion. In DSM-III-R, transsexualism (gender identity disorder in DSM-IV-TR) also was mentioned as such a disorder. Although not specifically mentioned in DSM-IV and DSM-IV-TR, if a preoccupation is limited to discomfort or a sense of inappropriateness of one's primary and secondary sex characteristics, coupled with a strong and persistent cross-gender identification, body dysmorphic disorder would not be diagnosed. Diagnostic problems may develop when a patient has the mood-congruent ruminations of major depression (e.g., preoccupation with a perceived unattractive appearance in association with poor self-esteem). However, such concerns generally lack the focus on a particular body part that is seen in body dysmorphic disorder. Somatic obsessions and even grooming or cleaning rituals in OCD may suggest body dysmorphic disorder; however, in such cases, other obsessions and compulsions are seen as well. In body dysmorphic disorder, the preoccupations are limited to concerns with appearance. Preoccupations in body dysmorphic disorder may reach delusional proportions, and patients with this disorder may show ideas of reference regarding defects in their appearance, which may lead to consideration of the diagnosis of schizophrenia. However, bizarre delusions and hallucinations are not seen in patients with body dysmorphic disorder. From the other perspective, schizophrenic patients with somatic delusions generally do not focus on a specific defect in appearance.

Unlike the diagnostic guideline for hypochondriasis, if the preoccupation is of psychotic proportions, a diagnosis of body dysmorphic disorder still can be made. De Leon et al. (1989) pointed out the difficulties in determining whether a dysmorphophobic concern is delusional. They suggest that cases be classified as "primary dysmorphophobia" without attempting to distinguish between delusional and nondelusional concerns, as long as schizophrenia, major depression, and or-

ganic mental disorders are excluded. This point of view was adopted in DSM-IV (Phillips and Hollander 1996). In body dysmorphic disorder, it appears that a continuum exists between preoccupations and delusions, and thus it is difficult, if not impossible, to draw a discrete boundary between body dysmorphic disorder and delusional disorder, somatic type. Furthermore, individual patients seem to move along this continuum. Thus, it was decided to allow both diagnoses if a dysmorphic preoccupation was delusional. This decision was controversial, and the debate continues.

Patients with body dysmorphic disorder often isolate themselves, and social phobia may be suspected. Social phobia is often seen as a comorbid state with body dysmorphic disorder (Phillips and Stout 2005), and in some cultures body dysmorphic disorder may be conceptualized as social phobia. However, in social phobia alone the person may feel self-conscious but will not focus on a specific imagined defect. Persons with histrionic personality disorder may be vain and excessively concerned with appearance. However, in this disorder, the focus is on maintaining a good or even an exceptional appearance rather than preoccupation with a defect.

Natural History

Onset of body dysmorphic disorder usually begins in adolescence or early adulthood (Phillips 1991). The disorder is generally a chronic condition, with a waxing and waning of intensity but rarely full remission (Phillips et al. 1993). Over a lifetime, multiple preoccupations are typical. (In their study, Phillips et al. [1993] found an average of four preoccupations.) In some people, the preoccupation remains unchanged; in others, preoccupations with newly perceived defects are added to the original ones. In some individuals, symptoms remit only to be replaced by others.

Recent studies of special populations have revealed varying findings regarding outcomes, with one study finding that at 4-year follow-up, 58% of patients were in full remission and 84% were in partial remission (Phillips et al. 2005). A second study found that only 9% experienced full remission, with 21% experiencing partial remission (Phillips et al. 2006). Body dysmorphic disorder is highly incapacitating. Almost all persons with this disorder show marked impairment in social and occupational activities. About 75% will never marry, and among those who do, most will divorce (Phillips 1995). Perhaps a third become housebound. Most attribute their limitations to embarrassment concerning their "defect." The precise extent to which patients with body dysmorphic disorder receive surgery or medical treatments is unknown. Of interest, Phillips (2001) found that nearly one-half of adolescents studied had received medical or surgical treatment that was usually ineffective in relieving the symptoms of body dysmorphic disorder. Superimposed depressive episodes are common, as are suicidal ideation and suicide attempts. The estimated lifetime risk of depression is 76% (Gunstad and Phillips 2003). The lifetime suicide attempt rate has been estimated at 22%–24% (Phillips and Diaz 1997; Veale et al. 1996). The completed suicide rate is unknown.

Epidemiology

The lifetime risk of body dysmorphic disorder in the general population is unknown, but it is thought to be underdiagnosed even when patients are in psychiatric care. Often patients will not mention their concerns unless directly asked. Studies have reported prevalences varying from 0.7% to 5% in special populations (Bohne et al. 2002; Otto et al. 2001; Rief et al. 2006). Grant et al. (2001) found a prevalence rate of 13% in psychiatric inpatients. Although body dysmorphic disorder is seldom reported in psychiatric settings, Andreasen and Bardach (1977) estimated that 2% of the patients seeking corrective cosmetic surgery have this disorder. Generally, patients with body dysmorphic disorder are seen psychiatrically only after referral from plastic surgery, dermatology, and otorhinolaryngology clinics (De Leon et al. 1989). The male-to-female ratio is about 1:1 (Phillips 1995).

Etiology

Although the etiology of body dysmorphic disorder remains elusive, there has been significant nosological debate recently in several areas. First, the possibility that the label represents a spectrum of disorders as opposed to simply psychotic versus nonpsychotic variants has been raised. Although not a settled issue, the general consensus appears to support this position (Castle and Rossel 2006). The second issue is whether body dysmorphic disorder should be classified as an anxiety disorder, particularly a variant of OCD. This is problematic because patients with body dysmorphic disorder tend to be younger, more socially dysfunctional, and nonresponsive to antipsychotics. Also, one would opine that if both illnesses represented variants of the same disorder, then upon resolution of the obsessive symptoms, the body dysmorphic symptoms should subside, which is not the case. Phillips and Stout (2005) found that only 10% of patients had reso-

lution of their body dysmorphic symptoms after their OCD symptoms resolved.

Treatment

Simply recognizing that a complaint derives from body dysmorphic disorder may have therapeutic benefit by interrupting an unending procession of repeated evaluations by physicians and eliminating the possibility of needless surgery. Surgery actually has been recommended as a treatment for this disorder, but there is no clear evidence that it is helpful. There is a long history of anecdotal reports suggesting the value of diverse treatments, including behavior therapy, dynamic psychotherapy, and pharmacotherapy. Recommended medications include neuroleptics and antidepressants (De Leon et al. 1989). Response to neuroleptic treatment has been suggested as a diagnostic test to distinguish body dysmorphic disorder from delusional disorder, somatic type (Riding and Munro 1975). Delusional syndromes, in general, may respond to neuroleptics, whereas in body dysmorphic disorder, even when the bodily preoccupations are psychotic, there is less likelihood of success. Pimozide has been singled out as a neuroleptic having specific effectiveness for somatic delusions, but this drug does not appear to be any more effective than other neuroleptics in treating body dysmorphic disorder.

In earlier reports, it was not clear if reported response to antidepressant drugs or ECT was due to amelioration of dysmorphic symptoms per se or to improvement in depressive symptoms. Several studies have suggested that SSRIs, including fluoxetine, fluvoxamine, and clomipramine, have been effective in treating the disorder (Hollander et al. 1993; Phillips et al. 1993). Patients showing a partial response to the SSRI may benefit further from augmentation with buspirone. Improvement with SSRIs seems to be a primary effect in that response was not predicted on the basis of coexisting major depression or OCD. Also of note are observations that patients with somatic delusions may respond to SSRIs.

Somatoform Disorder Not Otherwise Specified

Definition and Clinical Description

Somatoform disorder NOS is the true residual category for the somatoform disorders. By definition, conditions included under this category are characterized by somatoform symptoms that do not meet the criteria for any of the specified somatoform disorders. DSM-IV-TR gives several examples, but syndromes potentially included under this category are not limited to those examples. Unlike undifferentiated somatoform disorder, no minimum duration is required. In fact, some disorders may be relegated to the NOS category because they do not meet the time requirements for a specified somatoform disorder.

Diagnosis

History

DSM-III included atypical somatoform disorder, a minimally defined residual category requiring only that the predominant disturbance of a disorder be characterized by organically or pathophysiologically unexplained physical symptoms or complaints that are apparently linked to psychological factors. The only example given was dysmorphophobia. In DSM-III-R, the atypical category was renamed and redefined, requiring only the presence of "somatoform symptoms" (implying that no organic or pathophysiological mechanism was present) and that criteria for any specific somatoform or other psychiatric disorder with physical symptoms were not present. Examples given included nonpsychotic hypochondriacal symptoms and physical complaints of less than 6 months' duration that are not related to stress.

DSM-IV-TR Criteria

The basic DSM-IV-TR requirement for a diagnosis of somatoform disorder NOS is that a disorder with somatoform symptoms does not meet criteria for a specified somatoform disorder (Table 13–13). The first example of such a disorder listed in DSM-IV-TR is pseudocyesis. In DSM-III and DSM-III-R, pseudocyesis was included as a conversion disorder under criteria broadened to include any alteration or loss of physical functioning, suggesting a physical disorder that was an expression of psychological conflict or need. After contraction of conversion disorder to voluntary motor and sensory dysfunction in DSM-IV, pseudocyesis was excluded and relegated to the NOS category. Oddly enough, pseudocyesis lends itself to a quite specific definition. The criteria for pseudocyesis were derived from a review of the existing literature. Because of its rarity, however, pseudocyesis is not listed as a specified somatoform disorder.

Two other examples given are syndromes that resemble specified somatoform syndromes, somatiza-

TABLE 13–13. DSM-IV-TR diagnostic criteria for somatoform disorder not otherwise specified

This category includes disorders with somatoform symptoms that do not meet the criteria for any specific somatoform disorder. Examples include

1. Pseudocyesis: a false belief of being pregnant that is associated with objective signs of pregnancy, which may include abdominal enlargement (although the umbilicus does not become everted), reduced menstrual flow, amenorrhea, subjective sensation of fetal movement, nausea, breast engorgement and secretions, and labor pains at the expected date of delivery. Endocrine changes may be present, but the syndrome cannot be explained by a general medical condition that causes endocrine changes (e.g., a hormone-secreting tumor).

2. A disorder involving nonpsychotic hypochondriacal symptoms of less than 6 months' duration.

3. A disorder involving unexplained physical complaints (e.g., fatigue or body weakness) of less than 6 months' duration that are not due to another mental disorder.

tion disorder, undifferentiated somatoform disorder, or hypochondriasis but have a duration of less than the required 6 months. An additional example is a condition described as involving complaints such as fatigue or body weakness not due to another mental disorder, again with a duration of less than 6 months. Such a syndrome would resemble neurasthenia, a syndrome with a long historical tradition. Included in DSM-II, ICD-9, and ICD-10, neurasthenia was considered for inclusion as a specified DSM-IV somatoform disorder. After careful review, neurasthenia was not adopted because it was difficult to delineate from depressive, anxiety, and other somatoform disorders and because there was a lack of systematic study supporting it. Finally, there was concern that neurasthenia would become a "wastebasket" category, the availability of which might promote premature closure of the diagnostic process so that other mental disorders, as well as other general medical disorders, would be overlooked.

Differential Diagnosis

As mentioned in the preceding discussion, DSM-IV-TR lists several syndromes that, if not for their short duration, would qualify for a diagnosis as the specified somatoform disorder that they resemble.

Pseudocyesis deserves further attention. Although not mentioned in DSM-II, it probably would have fit best as a psychophysiological endocrine disorder. In DSM-III and DSM-III-R, pseudocyesis was specifically listed as a conversion symptom. Its presumed mechanism was ambivalence about pregnancy, with the resulting conflict expressed somatically, leading to resolution (primary gain) and unconsciously needed environmental support (secondary gain). Pseudocyesis could have been subsumed under the heading "Psychological Factors Affecting Medical Condition." An argument can be made for its inclusion as a medical condition because, based on a literature review (Martin 1995), in most if not all cases, it appears that a neuroendocrine change accompanies, and at times may antedate, the false belief of pregnancy. However, in most instances, a discrete general medical condition (such as a hormone-secreting tumor) cannot be identified. It might have been included as a specified somatoform disorder except for its rarity; Whelan and Stewart (1990) reported six cases in 20 years of consulting to a unit delivering 2,500 women per year. Yet pseudocyesis appears as a reasonably discrete syndrome such that specific criteria derived from the literature are included in its listing as a somatoform disorder NOS (see Table 13–13).

Epidemiology, Etiology, and Treatment

Discussion of epidemiology, etiology, and treatment for a residual category such as somatoform disorder NOS would not be meaningful, given that the category represents a grouping of diverse disorders. Conditions that would warrant diagnosis of a specified somatoform disorder except for their insufficient duration (less than 6 months) are probably best considered to be in the spectrum of the resembled disorder. Thus, the epidemiological, etiological, and treatment considerations pertaining to the specified disorder should be reviewed because these may apply, at least in part, to the shorter-duration syndromes.

In a comprehensive review of pseudocyesis, Small (1986) stated: "Of all that has been written on the subject [of pseudocyesis], therapy is least discussed" (p. 456). In another report, Whelan and Stewart (1990) emphasized two principles in treating pseudocyesis. First, the patient should be clearly, yet "empathically," advised that she (or the rare he) is not pregnant. If such simple advice is not effective, objective procedures such as ultrasound are recommended to demonstrate

to the patient that there is no visible evidence of a fetus. Alternatively, menses may be induced. Remarkably, such straightforward approaches are often effective (Cohen 1982). According to Whelan and Stewart (1990), the second principle, which goes hand in hand with the first, is that the patient's expectations, fears, and fantasies should be explored to discover the reason that the false pregnancy was "needed." They also advised providing a face-saving resolution to the patient's lack of pregnancy, such as allowing the patient to take the position that a "miscarriage" has occurred. However, systematic data on the effectiveness of these and other treatment approaches are lacking. Whatever the therapy, relapses are common. According to Ford (1995), there are limited data on the prognosis for women with pseudocyesis. Concomitant disorders such as major depression should be treated in the usual manner.

Conclusion

Syndromes now subsumed under the rubric "somatoform disorders" have had a tortuous course in the evolution of psychiatric nosology and therapy. Yet they are extremely important because they are disorders that must be differentiated from conditions with identifiable, and often treatable, physical bases.

Developments in the past decade are encouraging. Coordinated effort has been made to establish a common, globally used nomenclature. Somatoform disorders as delineated in DSM-IV-TR are compatible with, although not identical to, counterparts in ICD-10. A common and more explicitly defined nosology is conducive to empirical research that is truly comparable from one investigation to the next. Initial observations on the pharmacological treatment of several of the disorders, namely hypochondriasis and body dysmorphic disorder, are promising and not only may add to our therapeutic armamentarium but also may suggest avenues for improved pathophysiological as well as etiological understanding of these two somatoform disorders.

Ultimately, it may prove possible to obtain a better understanding of the somatoform disorders, a group of complex, incapacitating disorders. Better understanding should facilitate more effective treatments. Already there has been some preliminary discussion regarding the development of practice guidelines for somatoform disorders. Consideration of guidelines would have been highly unlikely even a few years ago.

Key Points

- The somatoform disorders are grouped because they suggest a physical disorder for which there are no organic findings or known physiological mechanism or there is a strong presumption that the symptoms are linked to psychological issues.

- Somatization disorder is uncommon, but it is considered one of very few valid and reliable mental illnesses.

- Conversion disorder is a diagnosis that should be applied only after significant effort has been expended to eliminate any possible treatable organic disorder.

- Hypochondriasis is a rather uncommon disorder that usually follows a fluctuating course.

- Body dysmorphic disorder is a diagnosis in evolution, with conflicting data regarding amenability to treatment.

Suggested Readings

Castle DJ, Phillips KA: Obsessive-compulsive spectrum disorders: a defensible construct. Aust N Z J Psychiatry 40:114–120, 2006

Castle DJ, Rossell SL: An update on body dysmorphic disorder. Curr Opin Psychiatry 19:74–78, 2006

Hurwitz TA: Somatization and conversion disorder. Can J Psychiatry 49:172–178, 2004

Lamberg L: New mind/body tactics target medically unexplained physical symptoms and fears. JAMA 294:2152–2154, 2005

Phillips KA: Body dysmorphic disorder: recognizing and treating imagined ugliness. World Psychiatry 3:12–17, 2004

References

Allen L, Woolfolk R, Escobar J, et al: Cognitive-behavioral therapy for somatization disorder. Arch Intern Med 166:1512–1518, 2006

Almgren P-E, Nordgren L, Skantze H: A retrospective study of operationally defined hysterics. Br J Psychiatry 132:67–73, 1978

Alper K, Devinsky O, Vasquez B, et al: Nonepileptic seizures and childhood sexual and physical abuse. Neurology 43:1950–1953, 1993

American Psychiatric Association: Diagnostic and Statistical Manual: Mental Disorders. Washington, DC, American Psychiatric Association, 1952

American Psychiatric Association: Diagnostic and Statistical Manual of Mental Disorders, 2nd Edition. Washington, DC, American Psychiatric Association, 1968

American Psychiatric Association: Diagnostic and Statistical Manual of Mental Disorders, 3rd Edition. Washington, DC, American Psychiatric Association, 1980

American Psychiatric Association: Diagnostic and Statistical Manual of Mental Disorders, 3rd Edition, Revised. Washington, DC, American Psychiatric Association, 1987

American Psychiatric Association: Diagnostic and Statistical Manual of Mental Disorders, 4th Edition. Washington, DC, American Psychiatric Association, 1994

American Psychiatric Association: Diagnostic and Statistical Manual of Mental Disorders, 4th Edition, Primary Care Version. Washington, DC, American Psychiatric Association, 1995

American Psychiatric Association: Diagnostic and Statistical Manual of Mental Disorders, 4th Edition, Text Revision. Washington, DC, American Psychiatric Association, 2000

Andrade C, Srinath S: True auditory hallucinations as a conversion symptom. Br J Psychiatry 148:100–102, 1986

Andreasen NC, Bardach J: Dysmorphophobia: symptom or disease? Am J Psychiatry 134:673–676, 1977

Ballmaier M, Schmidt R: Conversion disorder revisited. Functional Neurology 20:105–113, 2005

Barsky AJ: Somatoform disorders, in Comprehensive Textbook of Psychiatry, 5th Edition, Vol 1. Edited by Kaplan HI, Sadock BJ. Baltimore, MD, Williams & Wilkins, 1989, pp 1009–1027

Barsky AJ, Ahern DK: Cognitive behavior therapy for hypochondriasis. JAMA 291:1464–1470, 2004

Barsky AJ, Klerman GL: Overview: hypochondriasis, bodily complaints, and somatic styles. Am J Psychiatry 140:273–283, 1983

Barsky AJ, Wyshak G, Klerman GL: Hypochondriasis: an evaluation of the DSM-III criteria in medical outpatients. Arch Gen Psychiatry 43:493–500, 1986

Barsky AJ, Wyshak G, Klerman GL, et al: The prevalence of hypochondriasis in medical outpatients. Soc Psychiatry Psychiatr Epidemiol 25:89–94, 1990

Bass CM, Murphy MR: Somatization disorder: critique of the concept and suggestions for future research, in Somatization: Physical Symptoms and Psychological Illness. Edited by Bass C. Oxford, England, Blackwell Scientific, 1990, pp 301–332

Bendefeldt F, Miller LL, Ludwig AM: Cognitive performance in conversion hysteria. Arch Gen Psychiatry 33:1250–1254, 1976

Bohman M, Cloninger CR, von Knorring A-L, et al: An adoption study of somatoform disorders, III: cross-fostering analysis and genetic relationship to alcoholism and criminality. Arch Gen Psychiatry 41:872–878, 1984

Bohne A, Wilhelm S, Keuthen N, et al: Prevalence of body dysmorphic disorder in a German college student sample. Psychiatry Res 109:101–104, 2002

Bourgeois JA, Chang CH, Hilty DM, et al: Clinical manifestations and management of conversion disorders. Curr Treat Options Neurol 4:487–497, 2002

Breuer J, Freud S: Studies on hysteria (1893–1895), in the Standard Edition of the Complete Psychological Works of Sigmund Freud, Vol 2. Translated and edited by Strachey J. London, England, Hogarth, 1955, pp 1–311

Briquet P: Traité Clinique et Thérapeutique Y l'Hystérie. Paris, France, J-B Balliere & Fils, 1859

Carson A, Best S, Postma K, et al: The outcome of neurology patients with medically unexplained symptoms: a prospective study. J Neurol Neurosurg Psychiatry 74:897–900, 2003

Carter AB: The prognosis of certain hysterical symptoms. BMJ 1:1076–1079, 1949

Castle DJ, Rossell SL: An update on body dysmorphic disorder. Curr Opin Psychiatry 19:74–78, 2006

Chodoff P, Lyons H: Hysteria, the hysterical personality and "hysterical" conversion. Am J Psychiatry 114:734–740, 1958

Cloninger CR: The link between hysteria and sociopathy: an integrative model based on clinical, genetic, and neurophysiological observations, in Psychiatric Diagnosis: Explorations of Biological Predictors. Edited by Akiskal HS, Webb WL. New York, Spectrum, 1978, pp 189–218

Cloninger CR: Diagnosis of somatoform disorders: a critique of DSM-III, in Diagnosis and Classification in Psychiatry: A Critical Appraisal of DSM-III. Edited by Tischler GL. New York, Cambridge University Press, 1987, pp 243–259

Cloninger CR: Somatoform and dissociative disorders, in The Medical Basis of Psychiatry, 2nd Edition. Edited by Winokur G, Clayton P. Philadelphia, PA, WB Saunders, 1994, pp 169–192

Cloninger CR, Guze SB: Psychiatric illness and female criminality: the role of sociopathy and hysteria in the antisocial woman. Am J Psychiatry 127:303–311, 1970

Cloninger CR, Yutzy S: Somatoform and dissociative disorders: a summary of changes for DSM-IV, in Current Psychiatric Therapy. Edited by Dunner DL. Philadelphia, PA, WB Saunders, 1993, pp 310–313

Cloninger CR, Reich T, Guze SB: The multifactorial model of disease transmission, III: familial relationship between sociopathy and hysteria (Briquet's syndrome). Br J Psychiatry 127:23–32, 1975

Cloninger CR, Sigvardsson S, von Knorring A-L, et al: An adoption study of somatoform disorders, II: identification of two discrete somatoform disorders. Arch Gen Psychiatry 41:863–871, 1984

Cloninger CR, Martin RL, Guze SB, et al: A prospective follow-up and family study of somatization in men and women. Am J Psychiatry 143:873–878, 1986

Cloninger CR, Bayon C, Przybeck TR: Epidemiology and Axis I comorbidity of antisocial personality, in Handbook of Antisocial Behavior. Edited by Stoff DM, Breiling J, Maser JD. New York, Wiley, 1997, pp 12–21

Cohen LM: A current perspective of pseudocyesis. Am J Psychiatry 139:1140–1144, 1982

Coryell W, House D: The validity of broadly defined hysteria and DSM-III conversion disorder: outcome, family history, and mortality. J Clin Psychiatry 45:252–256, 1984

De Leon J, Bott A, Simpson GM: Dysmorphophobia: body dysmorphic disorder or delusional disorder, somatic subtype? Compr Psychiatry 30:457–472, 1989

Desai BT, Porter RJ, Penry K: Psychogenic seizures: a study of 42 attacks in six patients, with intensive monitoring. Arch Neurol 39:202–209, 1982

DeSouza C, Othmer E, Gabrielli W Jr, et al: Major depression and somatization disorder: the overlooked differential diagnosis. Psychiatr Ann 18:340–348, 1988

Escobar JI, Swartz M, Rubio-Stipec M, et al: Medically unexplained symptoms: distribution, risk factors, and comorbidity, in Current Concepts of Somatization: Research and Clinical Perspectives. Edited by Kirmayer LJ, Robbins JM. Washington, DC, American Psychiatric Press, 1991, pp 63–78

Escobar JL, Gara MA, Waitzkins H, et al: DSM-IV Hypochondriasis in primary care. Gen Hosp Psychiatry 20:155–159, 1998

Fallon BA, Schneir FR, Narshall R, et al: The pharmacotherapy of hypochondriasis. Psychopharmacol Bull 32:607–611, 1996

Feighner JP, Robins E, Guze SB, et al: Diagnostic criteria for use in psychiatric research. Arch Gen Psychiatry 26:57–63, 1972

Fitzgerald BA, Wells CE: Hallucinations as a conversion reaction. Dis Nerv Syst 38:381–383, 1977

Flor-Henry P, Fromm-Auch D, Tapper M, et al: A neuropsychological study of the stable syndrome of hysteria. Biol Psychiatry 16:601–626, 1981

Folks DG, Ford CV, Regan WM: Conversion symptoms in a general hospital. Psychosomatics 25:285–295, 1984

Ford CV: The Somatizing Disorders: Illness as a Way of Life. New York, Elsevier, 1983

Ford CV: Conversion disorder and somatoform disorder not otherwise specified, in Treatment of Psychiatric Disorders, 2nd Edition. Edited by Gabbard GO. Washington, DC, American Psychiatric Press, 1995, pp 1737–1753

Ford CV, Folks DG: Conversion disorders: an overview. Psychosomatics 26:371–383, 1985

Gatfield PD, Guze SB: Prognosis and differential diagnosis of conversion reactions (a follow-up study). Dis Nerv Syst 23:623–631, 1962

Goodwin DW, Guze SB: Psychiatric Diagnosis, 5th Edition. New York, Oxford University Press, 1996

Goodwin DW, Alderson P, Rosenthal R: Clinical significance of hallucinations in psychiatric disorders. Arch Gen Psychiatry 24:76–80, 1971

Grant JE, Kim SU, Crow SJ: Prevalence and clinical features of body dysmorphic disorder in adolescents and adult psychiatric inpatients. J Clin Psychiatry 62:517–522, 2001

Gunstad J, Phillips KA: Axis I comorbidity in body dysmorphic disorder. Compr Psychiatry 44:270–276, 2003

Guze SB: The role of follow-up studies: their contribution to diagnostic classification as applied to hysteria. Semin Psychiatry 2:392–402, 1970

Guze SB, Perley MJ: Observations on the natural history of hysteria. Am J Psychiatry 119:960–965, 1963

Guze SB, Cloninger CR, Martin RL, et al: A follow-up and family study of Briquet's syndrome. Br J Psychiatry 149:17–23, 1986

Hankey GJ, Stewart-Wynne EG: Pseudo-multiple sclerosis: a clinico-epidemiological study. Clin Exp Neurol 24:11–19, 1987

Hathaway SR, McKinley JC: Minnesota Multiphasic Personality Schedule. Minneapolis, MN, University of Minnesota Press, 1943

Hewlett HA: The use of benzodiazepines in obsessive-compulsive disorder and Tourette's syndrome. Psychiatr Ann 23:309–316, 1993

Hollander E: Obsessive-compulsive spectrum disorders: an overview. Psychiatric Annals 23:355–358, 1993

Hollander E, Cohen LJ, Simeon D: Body dysmorphic disorder. Psychiatr Ann 23:359–364, 1993

Horowitz MJ: Hysterical Personality. New York, Jason Aronson, 1977

Hudziak JJ, Boffeli TJ, Kreisman JJ, et al: Clinical study of the relation of borderline personality disorder to Briquet's syndrome (hysteria), somatization disorder, antisocial personality disorder, and substance abuse disorders. Am J Psychiatry 153:1598–1606, 1996

Hurwitz TA: Somatization and conversion disorder. Can J Psychiatry 49:172–178, 2004

Inouye E: Genetic aspects of neurosis. Int J Ment Health 1:176–189, 1972

Kellner R: The prognosis of treated hypochondriasis: a clinical study. Acta Psychiatr Scand 67:69–79, 1983

Kellner R: Functional somatic symptoms and hypochondriasis: a survey of empirical studies. Arch Gen Psychiatry 42:821–833, 1985

Kellner R: Hypochondriasis and somatization. JAMA 258:2718–2722, 1987

Kellner R: Somatization disorder, in Treatments of Psychiatric Disorders: A Task Force Report of the American Psychiatric Association, Vol 3. Washington, DC, American Psychiatric Association, 1989, pp 2166–2171

Kellner R, Abbott P, Pathak D, et al: Hypochondriacal beliefs and attitudes in family practice and psychiatric patients. Int J Psychiatry Med 13:127–139, 1983/1984

Kent D, Tomasson K, Coryell W: Course and outcome of conversion and somatization disorders: a four-year follow-up. Psychosomatics 36:138–144, 1995

Kenyon FE: Hypochondriasis: a survey of some historical, clinical, and social aspects. Br J Psychiatry 138:117–133, 1965

Kenyon FE: Hypochondriacal states. Br J Psychiatry 129:1–14, 1976

Kirmayer LJ, Robbins JM: Introduction: concepts of somatization, in Current Concepts of Somatization: Research and Clinical Perspectives. Edited by Kirmayer LJ, Robbins JM. Washington, DC, American Psychiatric Press, 1991, pp 1–19

Kirmayer LJ, Robbins JM, Dworkind M, et al: Somatization and the recognition of depression and anxiety in primary care. Am J Psychiatry 150:734–741, 1993

Kroenke K, Spitzer RL, de Gruy FV, et al: Multisomatoform disorder: an alternative to undifferentiated somatoform disorder for the somatizing patient in primary care. Arch Gen Psychiatry 54:352–358, 1997

Kroenke K, Swindle R: Cognitive-behavioral therapy for somatization and symptom syndromes: a critical review of controlled clinical trials. Psychother Psychosom 9:205–215, 2000

Lader M, Sartorius N: Anxiety in patients with hysterical conversion symptoms. J Neurol Neurosurg Psychiatry 31:490–495, 1968

Lazare A: Conversion symptoms. N Engl J Med 305:745–748, 1981

Lewis WC: Hysteria: the consultant's dilemma: twentieth century demonology, pejorative epithet, or useful diagnosis? Arch Gen Psychiatry 30:145–151, 1974

Lewis WC, Berman M: Studies of conversion hysteria, I: operational study of diagnosis. Arch Gen Psychiatry 13:275–282, 1965

Lidbeck J: Group therapy for somatization disorders in general practice: effectiveness of a short cognitive-behavioral treatment model. Acta Psychiatr Scand 196:14–24, 1997

Ljundberg L: Hysteria: clinical, prognostic and genetic study. Acta Psychiatr Scand Suppl 32:1–162, 1957

Ludwig AM: Hysteria: a neurobiological theory. Arch Gen Psychiatry 27:771–777, 1972

Luff MC, Garrod M: The after-results of psychotherapy in 500 adult cases. BMJ 2:54–59, 1935

Mace CJ, Trimble MR: Ten-year prognosis of conversion disorder. Br J Psychiatry 169:282–288, 1996

Maloney MJ: Diagnosing hysterical conversion disorders in children. J Pediatr 97:1016–1020, 1980

Marsden CD: Hysteria: a neurologist's view. Psychol Med 16:277–288, 1986

Martin RL: Problems in the diagnosis of somatization disorder: effects on research and clinical practice. Psychiatr Ann 18:357–362, 1988

Martin RL: Somatoform disorders in the general hospital setting, in Handbook of Studies on General Psychiatry. Edited by Judd FK, Burrows GD, Lipsitt DR. Amsterdam, The Netherlands, Elsevier, 1991, pp 251–266

Martin RL: DSM-IV changes in the somatoform disorders. Psychiatr Ann 25:29–39, 1995

Martin RL, Yutzy SH: Somatoform disorders, in Psychiatry. Edited by Tasman A, Kay J, Lieberman JA. Philadelphia, PA, WB Saunders, 1997, pp 1119–1155

Martin RL, Cloninger CR, Guze SB: The evaluation of diagnostic concordance in follow-up studies, II: a blind prospective follow-up of female criminals. J Psychiatr Res 15:107–125, 1979

Martin RL, Cloninger CR, Guze SB, et al: Mortality in a follow-up of 500 psychiatric outpatients, II: cause-specific mortality. Arch Gen Psychiatry 42:58–66, 1985

Meares R, Horvath TB: "Acute" and "chronic" hysteria. Br J Psychiatry 121:653–657, 1972

Merskey H: Conversion disorder, in Treatments of Psychiatric Disorders: A Task Force Report of the American Psychiatric Association, Vol 3. Washington, DC, American Psychiatric Association, 1989, pp 2152–2159

Modai I, Cygielman G: Conversion hallucinations: a possible mental mechanism. Psychopathology 19:324–326, 1986

Murphy GE: The clinical management of hysteria. JAMA 247:2559–2564, 1982

Murphy GE, Guze SB: Setting limits. Am J Psychother 14:30–47, 1960

Murphy GE, Wetzel RD: Family history of suicidal behavior among suicide attempters. J Nerv Ment Dis 170:86–90, 1982

Murphy MR: Classification of the somatoform disorder, in Somatization: Physical Symptoms and Psychological Illness. Edited by Bass C. Oxford, UK, Blackwell Scientific, 1990, pp 10–39

Otto M, Wilhelm S, Cohen L, et al: Prevalence of body dysmorphic disorder in a community sample of women. Am J Psychiatry 158:2061–2063, 2001

Perley M, Guze SB: Hysteria: the stability and usefulness of clinical criteria: a quantitative study based upon a 6- to 8-year follow-up of 39 patients. N Engl J Med 266:421–426, 1962

Phillips KA: Body dysmorphic disorder: the distress of imagined ugliness. Am J Psychiatry 148:1138–1149, 1991

Phillips KA: Body dysmorphic disorder: clinical features and drug treatment. CNS Drugs 3:30–40, 1995

Phillips KA: Body dysmorphic disorder, in Somatoform and Factitious Disorders (Review of Psychiatry series, Vol 20, No 3; Oldham JM, Riba MB, series eds). Edited by Phillips KA. Washington, DC, American Psychiatric Publishing, DC, 2001, pp 67–94

Phillips KA, Diaz SF: Gender differences in body dysmorphic disorder. J Nerv Ment Dis 185:570–577, 1997

Phillips KA, Hollander E: Body dysmorphic disorder, in DSM-IV Sourcebook, Vol 2. Edited by Widiger TA, Frances AJ, Pincus HA, et al. Washington, DC, American Psychiatric Press, 1996, pp 949–960

Phillips KA, Stout RL: Associations in the longitudinal course of body dysmorphic disorder with major depression, obsessive-compulsive disorder and social phobia. J Psychiatry Res 40:360–369, 2005

Phillips KA, McElroy SL, Keck PE Jr, et al: Body dysmorphic disorder: 30 cases of imagined ugliness. Am J Psychiatry 150:302–308, 1993

Phillips KA, Grant JE, Siniscalchi JM, et al: A retrospective follow-up study of body dysmorphic disorder. Compr Psychiatry 46:315–321, 2005

Phillips KA, Pagano ME, Menard W, et al: A 12-month follow-up study of the course of body dysmorphic disorder. Am J Psychiatry 163:5:907–912, 2006

Pincus J: Hysteria presenting to a neurologist, in Hysteria. Edited by Roy A. London, England, Wiley, 1982, pp 131–144

Pribor EF, Smith DS, Yutzy SH: Somatization disorder in the elderly. Am J Geriatr Psychiatry 2:109–117, 1994

Purtell J, Robins E, Cohen M: Observations on clinical aspects of hysteria: a quantitative study of 50 hysteria patients and 156 control subjects. JAMA 146:902–909, 1951

Quill TE: Somatization disorder: one of medicine's blind spots. JAMA 254:3075–3079, 1985

Raskin M, Talbott JA, Meyerson AT: Diagnosis of conversion reactions: predictive value of psychiatric criteria. JAMA 197:530–534, 1966

Riding J, Munro A: Pimozide in the treatment of monosymptomatic hypochondriacal psychosis. Acta Psychiatr Scand 52:23–30, 1975

Rief W, Buhlmann U, Wilhelm A, et al: The prevalence of body dysmorphic disorder in a population based survey. Psychol Med 36:877–885, 2006

Robins E, O'Neal P: Clinical features of hysteria in children. The Nervous Child 10:246–271, 1953

Robins LN, Helzer JE, Croughan J, et al: National Institute of Mental Health Diagnostic Interview Schedule: its history, characteristics, and validity. Arch Gen Psychiatry 38:381–389, 1981

Robins LN, Helzer JE, Weissman MM, et al: Lifetime prevalence of specific psychiatric disorders in three sites. Arch Gen Psychiatry 41:949–958, 1984

Scallet A, Cloninger CR, Othmer E: The management of chronic hysteria: a review and double-blind trial of electrosleep and other relaxation methods. Dis Nerv Syst 37:347–353, 1976

Shapiro D: Neurotic Styles. New York, Basic Books, 1965

Sharma P, Chaturvedi SK: Conversion disorder revisited. Acta Psychiatr Scand 92:301–304, 1995

Slater ETO, Glithero C: A follow-up of patients diagnosed as suffering from "hysteria." J Psychosom Res 9:9–13, 1965

Small GW: Pseudocyesis: an overview. Can J Psychiatry 31:452–457, 1986

Smith GR Jr, Monson RA, Ray DC: Psychiatric consultation in somatization disorder: a randomized controlled study. N Engl J Med 314:1407–1413, 1986

Stefanis C, Markidis M, Christodoulou G: Observations on the evolution of the hysterical symptomatology. Br J Psychiatry 128:269–275, 1976

Stefansson JH, Messina JA, Meyerowitz S: Hysterical neurosis, conversion type: clinical and epidemiological considerations. Acta Psychiatr Scand 59:119–138, 1976

Stekel W: The Interpretation of Dreams: New Developments and Technique, Vols 1 and 2. Translated by Paul E, Paul C. New York, Liveright, 1943

Stephens JH, Kamp M: On some aspects of hysteria: a clinical study. J Nerv Ment Dis 134:305–315, 1962

Stern J, Murphy M, Bass C: Personality disorders in patients with somatization disorder: a controlled study. Br J Psychiatry 163:785–789, 1993

Stone J, Sharpe M, Rothwell PM, et al: The 12 year prognosis of unilateral functional weakness and sensory disturbance. J Neurol Neurosurg Psychiatry 74:591–596, 2003

Stone J, Smyth R, Carson A, et al: Systematic review of misdiagnosis of conversion symptoms and "hysteria." BMJ 331:989, 2005

Stoudemire GA: Somatoform disorders, factitious disorders, and malingering, in American Psychiatric Press Textbook of Psychiatry. Edited by Talbott JA, Hales RE, Yudofsky SC. Washington, DC, American Psychiatric Press, 1988, pp 533–556

Temoshok L, Attkisson CC: Epidemiology of hysterical phenomena: evidence for a psychosocial theory, in Hysterical Personality. Edited by Horowitz MJ. New York, Jason Aronson, 1977, pp 143–222

Tomasson K, Kent D, Coryell W: Somatization and conversion disorders: comorbidity and demographics at presentation. Acta Psychiatr Scand 84:288–293, 1991

Toone BK: Disorders of hysterical conversion, in Physical Symptoms and Psychological Illness. Edited by Bass C. London, England, Blackwell Scientific, 1990, pp 207–234

Torack RM: Historical overview of dementia, in The Pathological Physiology of Dementia. Edited by Torack RA. New York, Springer-Verlag, 1978, pp 1–16

Vaillant GE: The disadvantages of DSM-III outweigh its advantages. Am J Psychiatry 141:542–545, 1984

Van den Heuvel OA, Veltman DJ, Groenewegen HJ, et al: Disorder-specific neuroanatomical correlates of attention bias in obsessional-compulsive disorder, panic disorder, and hypochondriasis. Arch Gen Psychiatry 62:922–933, 2005

Veale D, Boocock A, Gournay K, et al: Body dysmorphic disorder: a survey of fifty cases. Br J Psychiatry 169:196–201, 1996

Veith I: Hysteria: The History of a Disease. Chicago, IL, University of Chicago Press, 1965

Viederman M: Somatoform and factitious disorders, in Psychiatry, Vol 1. Edited by Cavenar JO. Philadelphia, PA, JB Lippincott, 1985, pp 1–20

Watson CG, Buranen C: The frequency and identification of false positive conversion reactions. J Nerv Ment Dis 167:243–247, 1979

Wechsler D: Wechsler Adult Intelligence Scale—Revised. New York, Psychological Corporation, 1981

Weddington WW: Conversion reaction in an 82-year-old man. J Nerv Ment Dis 167:368–369, 1979

Weinstein EA, Eck RA, Lyerly OG: Conversion hysteria in Appalachia. Psychiatry 32:334–341, 1969

Wetzel RD, Guze SB, Cloninger CR, et al: Briquet's syndrome (hysteria) is both a somatoform and a "psychoform" illness: an MMPI study. Psychosom Med 56:564–569, 1994

Wheatley D: Evaluation of psychotherapeutic drugs in general practice. Psychopharmacol Bull 2:25–32, 1962

Wheatley D: General practitioner clinical trials: phenobarbitone compared with an inactive placebo in anxiety states. Practitioner 192:147–151, 1964

Wheatley D: General practitioner clinical trials: chlordiazepoxide in anxiety states, II: long-term study. Practitioner 195:692–695, 1965

Whelan CI, Stewart DE: Pseudocyesis: a review and report of six cases. Int J Psychiatry Med 20:97–108, 1990

Woerner PI, Guze SB: A family and marital study of hysteria. Br J Psychiatry 114:161–168, 1968

Woodruff RA, Clayton PJ, Guze SB: Hysteria: studies of diagnosis, outcome, and prevalence. JAMA 215:425–428, 1971

World Health Organization: The ICD-9 Classification of Mental and Behavioural Disorders, 9th Revision: Clinical Descriptions and Diagnostic Guidelines. Geneva, Switzerland, World Health Organization, 1977

World Health Organization: The ICD-10 Classification of Mental and Behavioural Disorders, 10th Revision: Clinical Descriptions and Diagnostic Guidelines. Geneva, Switzerland, World Health Organization, 1992a

World Health Organization: International Statistical Classification of Diseases and Related Health Problems, 10th Revision. Geneva, Switzerland, World Health Organization, 1992b

World Health Organization: Diagnostic and Management Guidelines for Mental Disorders in Primary Care: ICD-10 Chapter V Primary Care Version. Gottingen, Germany, Hogrefe & Huber, 1996

Yutzy SH, Pribor EF, Cloninger CR, et al: Reconsidering the criteria for somatization disorder. Hosp Community Psychiatry 43:1075–1076, 1149, 1992

Yutzy SH, Cloninger CR, Guze SB, et al: The DSM-IV field trial: somatization disorder: testing a new proposal. Am J Psychiatry 152:97–101, 1995

Ziegler FJ, Imboden JB, Meyer E: Contemporary conversion reactions: a clinical study. Am J Psychiatry 116:901–910, 1960

14

FACTITIOUS DISORDER AND MALINGERING

Barbara E. McDermott, Ph.D.
Martin H. Leamon, M.D.
Marc D. Feldman, M.D.
Charles L. Scott, M.D.

Factitious disorder and malingering are often linked, because both conditions involve the feigning or production of physical and/or psychological symptoms absent any underlying pathology. The distinction between the two is the motivation for the production of symptoms. In factitious disorder, the motivation is presumed to be unconscious and is related to the desire to assume the sick role. In contrast, malingering is viewed as the intentional production (or reporting) of symptoms for a specific purpose associated with some secondary gain, such as evading criminal prosecution or receiving financial compensation. Thus, in distinguishing the two, the treater is left to determine the underlying motivation for symptom production. Although there has been argument about the veracity of this taxonomy (Cunnien 1997; Rogers et al. 2005), reliable discrimination is important for a variety of reasons. Of primary importance is that the two conditions call for very different treatment or management approaches. The following discussion of both disorders will aid the clinician in making this crucial determination.

Factitious Disorder

Factitious disorder is characterized by a person intentionally fabricating or inducing signs or symptoms of other illnesses solely to become identified as "ill" or as a patient. Such patients have been described in medical writing throughout history (Feldman et al. 1994; Gavin 1843) and throughout the world (Bappal et al. 2001; Mizuta et al. 2000). The concept became firmly established in modern medical thinking in 1951 when Asher (1951) described what has since been classified a subtype of factitious disorder known as Munchausen syndrome. In many patients, factitious disorder remains undiagnosed, and even when recognized, it often goes untreated (Toth and Baggaley 1991). Yet factitious disorder causes significant morbidity and mortality (Baker and Major 1994; Folks 1995), consumes an astonishing amount of medical resources (Feldman 1994a), and produces significant emotional distress in the patients themselves, in their caregivers, and in their close relationships (Feldman and Smith 1996). In recent years, the medical literature about factitious disorders has continued to expand, with the publication of lay and professional books on the topic (Feldman 2004; Feldman and Eisendrath 1996; Feldman et al. 1994) and the establishment of a factitious disorder Web site (http://munchausen.com) and discussion group (http://health.groups.yahoo.com/group/cravin4care/).

Classification

DSM-IV-TR (American Psychiatric Association 2000) requires three criteria for the diagnosis of factitious disorder (Table 14–1). The first, the intentional production or feigning of physical or psychological signs or symptoms, distinguishes factitious disorder from the somatoform disorders, in which physical symptoms are viewed as unconsciously produced. The second and third criteria, that the motivation for the behavior is to assume the sick role and that external incentives for the behavior are absent, distinguish factitious disorder from malingering. DSM-IV-TR classifies the disorder based on the predominant type of factitious symptoms presented, whether physical or psychological. Individual case histories (Bauer and Boegner 1996; Craddock and Brown 1993) suggest that this categorization may be somewhat arbitrary because the same patient may have different presentations across time. Predominantly physical symptoms may be feigned at one time and predominantly psychological or a mixed picture at another. Rogers et al. (1989) also raised epistemological objections to this subtyping, arguing, in part, that factitious disorder with predominantly psychological signs and symptoms confers a psychiatric disorder to someone who, by definition, is merely pretending to have one. The fourth subtype is factitious disorder not otherwise specified (Table 14–2). This code should be used for disorders with factitious symptoms that do not meet criteria for one of the other subtypes. The sole example in DSM-IV-TR is factitious disorder by proxy (discussed in the "Factitious Disorder by Proxy" section later in this chapter).

ICD-10 (World Health Organization 1992), although slightly different, uses similarly defined operational criteria, emphasizing that the motivation for this behavior is almost always obscure and presumed internal (Freyberger and Schneider 1994). The ICD-10 criteria also highlight the prevalence of comorbid psychiatric disorders.

Other authors have used different typologies. Nadelson (1979) distinguished between factitious disorders of the Munchausen and the non-Munchausen type. This typology may have prognostic and treatment implications. Munchausen syndrome comprises

TABLE 14–1. DSM-IV-TR diagnostic criteria for factitious disorder

A. Intentional production or feigning of physical or psychological signs or symptoms.

B. The motivation for the behavior is to assume the sick role.

C. External incentives for the behavior (such as economic gain, avoiding legal responsibility, or improving physical well-being, as in malingering) are absent.

Code based on type:

300.16   with predominantly psychological signs and symptoms: if psychological signs and symptoms predominate in the clinical presentation

300.19   with predominantly physical signs and symptoms: if physical signs and symptoms predominate in the clinical presentation

300.19   with combined psychological and physical signs and symptoms: if both psychological and physical signs and symptoms are present but neither predominates in the clinical presentation

TABLE 14–2. DSM-IV-TR diagnostic criteria for factitious disorder not otherwise specified

This category includes disorders with factitious symptoms that do not meet the criteria for factitious disorder. An example is factitious disorder by proxy: the intentional production or feigning of physical or psychological signs or symptoms in another person who is under the individual's care for the purpose of indirectly assuming the sick role.

Source.   American Psychiatric Association 2000.

about 10% of patients with factitious disorders (Eisendrath 1994). The eponym remains in wide use and describes a variant of DSM-IV-TR's factitious disorder. In this subtype of factitious disorder, multiple hospitalizations with dramatic and often life-threatening presentations, wandering from hospital to hospital (peregrination), and pathological lying (*pseudologia fantastica*, the telling of dramatic tales that merge truth and falsehood and that the listener initially finds intriguing) are prominent. The Munchausen patient shows a pattern of feigning illness at numerous hospital emergency departments, often in different cities; gaining admission and sometimes undergoing invasive procedures; becoming quarrelsome with hospital staff; and often being discharged against medical advice or simply disappearing when their ruse is discovered. Asher, using the anglicized spelling, drew the term from Rudolf Erich Raspe's 1785 book, *Baron Munchausen's Narrative of His Marvelous Travels and Campaigns in Russia,* which further exaggerated the whimsical accounts of the sporting and military adventures, as well as the peregrinations, of a real-life German cavalry officer in the Russian army, Baron Karl Friedrich Hieronymous von Münchhausen (1720–1797) (Raspe 1787).

Other expressions concerning patients of this type have been quite colorful but often with derogatory overtones: peregrinating problem patients (Chapman 1957), "hospital hobos" (Clark and Melnick 1958), and hospital addicts (Barker 1962), and, for a subset of plastic surgery patients, the SHAFT syndrome (**s**ad, **h**ostile, **a**nxious, **f**rustrating, and **t**enacious; Kasdan et al. 1998).

As described, the vast majority of factitious disorder patients are of the non-Munchausen type. Characterized by several authors (Ford 1986; Freyberger et al. 1994; Guziec et al. 1994; Plassmann 1994b; Reich and Gottfried 1983), these patients are mostly young women with conforming lifestyles and more family support and involvement than Munchausen patients. These patients have been described as passive and immature, and a significant proportion have health-related jobs or training. Most are not wanderers, have single-system complaints, and generate fewer hospitalizations than do Munchausen patients, but the overall severity and morbidity of their illness may be just as great (Sutherland and Rodin 1990).

Others (Eisendrath 1996) have classified patients with factitious disorders according to the manner in which illness is simulated and by the type of simulated illness. Patients may simply report invented symptoms and false medical histories—for example, online in Internet chat rooms (Feldman 2000) or directly to clinicians, as in the case example in the following "Diagnosis" section. They may exaggerate symptoms, for example, by claiming that occasional tension headaches are continual crippling migraines. They may manipulate diagnostic instruments to give false readings, such as manipulating electrocardiogram leads to simulate arrhythmia (Ludwigs et al. 1994) or rubbing thermometers to fake fevers (Aduan et al. 1979). They also may tamper with laboratory specimens, such as adding blood to urine or sputum. They may purposefully cause actual tissue damage or biochemical abnormalities in their bodies, either inducing new injury or exacerbating existing conditions, by active methods

such as intentionally traumatic self-catheterization, self-induced infection of wounds or skin with bacteria, injection of unneeded or excessive insulin, or ingestion of thyroid hormones or anticoagulants. Finally, dissimulators temporarily avoid necessary medical treatment to exacerbate existing conditions.

Classification by type of simulated illness is most useful to the clinician who begins to suspect factitious illness and who then looks for evidence to support the suspicion. Wallach (1994) and Nordmeyer (1994) give thorough descriptions of presentations of factitious illness in the different organ systems and some suggestions for their detection. Almost any conceivable condition can be simulated, depending on the knowledge, motivation, creativity, and covert skill of the patient. An exhaustive list of the medical disorders that have been feigned or produced by patients with factitious disorder would approximate the index of a pathology textbook.

Diagnosis

Mr. A, a middle-aged, middle-ranking U.S. military officer, was stationed at what was widely held to be a desirable post in Europe. He was married with no children, by mutual decision with his attentive wife. His superiors described his military career performance as slightly better than average. He was hospitalized for evaluation when a sentry discovered him one evening walking around outside, disorganized and talking disjointedly about Vietnam.

Mr. A was psychiatrically hospitalized at a U.S. military psychiatric ward in Europe, where he described long-standing symptoms of posttraumatic stress disorder (PTSD) from his experiences as part of an elite covert operations team functioning behind enemy lines. He readily engaged in ward activities and in his treatment program. He was evaluated by experienced psychiatrists, psychologists, and nursing staff. His cognitive and affective presentations in ward activities, group psychotherapy, and individual psychotherapy were thought to be consistent with delayed-onset PTSD. When he showed no improvement after 2 weeks of intensive treatment, he was transferred to a military medical center in the United States for further treatment.

Mr. A's presentation remained unchanged, although he seemed to show some improvement. He received much support from the other military patients and was regarded as tragically courageous. The psychiatric resident responsible for Mr. A's direct care (one of the authors of this chapter) spent time reading the literature on the treatment of PTSD, and Mr. A received extra individual psychotherapy, a valued commodity on a busy inpatient service. A search of his military records detected no history of Vietnam service, and Mr. A carefully explained that his record had been officially manipulated because of the classified nature of his activities. Knowledgeable military sources confirmed that although Mr. A's explanation was unusual, it could be correct. In couples psychotherapy sessions, Mr. A gently explained to his wife that he had withheld this important part of his premarital history from her because of the pain it caused him to recall these experiences as well as because of the classified nature of his activities. She continued to be emotionally supportive, after gradually accepting that her husband had been so secretive. As time went on, it became clear that Mr. A was facing discharge from military service, which neither he nor his wife wanted. For several reasons, it also seemed unlikely that Mr. A would receive any disability payments once discharged.

After several months of hospitalization, Mr. A's mother was contacted (with his consent). She seemed to be a reliable source but expressed complete bewilderment at her son's predicament. She explained that Mr. A had not been in Vietnam or even in the military during the time he claimed but had been living with her, working in a store.

When Mr. A was presented with his mother's information, he seemed nonplussed, confirmed that his mother was correct, and acknowledged that he had fabricated the Vietnam and PTSD history. He would not engage in further discussion of his hospitalization or his story. The other patients on the ward continued to support Mr. A and were indignant that his doctors questioned the veracity of his story (despite Mr. A's public admission of its invention). His wife was confused. He continued to be superficially pleasant and cooperative on the ward until he was released from the hospital and the military. He received no disability, returned to his wife's hometown, and was lost to follow-up at that time.

Many factors can suggest a diagnosis of factitious disorder (Freyberger et al. 1994; Popli et al. 1992). There can be discrepancies between objective findings, such as pronounced differences between oral, rectal, axillary, and urine temperatures or involuntary contractions measured in "paralyzed" limbs (Ziv et al. 1998). Objective findings might be inconsistent with clinical history or symptoms, as in the preceding case example or when mixed bowel flora is isolated from "spontaneous" skin lesions. The illness course could be markedly atypical, or the condition can fail to respond as expected to usual therapies, as demonstrated by erratic blood sugars or failure of wounds to heal. A patient may be unusually acquiescent to invasive diagnostic studies or may be unusually quarrelsome and argumentative with staff, particularly when it comes to trying to obtain old records to confirm history. A patient who describes a flamboyant, fascinating life with connections to well-known people may nevertheless have no visitors or callers. Unexplained medical paraphernalia or medications may be found in the patient's hospital room.

These indicators notwithstanding, verification of the first criterion requires that the patient be feigning or intentionally producing illness. The physician becomes a detective, working against the patient's overt desires, trying to discover the ruse. This role shift destabilizes the relationship (Duffy 1993; Paar 1994). The dilemma is especially complex when patients have combinations of feigned and actual illness (Nordmeyer 1994; Sutherland and Rodin 1990) or develop an actual illness in the attempt to simulate one. An example is the ambulance attendant who repeatedly infected her surgical incision with fecal material; with worsening infections and continued antibiotic treatment, she developed kidney failure (Feldman et al. 1994). Similarly, the patient who has had multiple abdominal surgeries for factitious causes may still develop adhesions or fistulas that may require surgical intervention. Additionally, some general medical conditions may be difficult to diagnose initially, leading to an erroneous clinical impression of fabricated symptoms (Baddley et al. 1998; Koo et al. 1996). Other illnesses, such as multiple sclerosis or systemic lupus erythematosus, may have fluctuating courses or in themselves produce inconsistent findings suggestive of factitious disorder (Liebson et al. 1996).

The DSM-IV-TR criteria also require that the feigning be intentional. Psychoses, mood disorders (Roy and Roy 1995), and dissociative disorders (Toth and Baggaley 1991) need to be ruled out as alternative etiologies. The hunt for intentionality raises ethical and legal issues of informed consent, right to privacy, and malpractice (Houck 1992). Almost by definition, patients with factitious disorder deny their simulations. Rather than being proved irrefutably, intentionality is more likely to be inferred through a process of diagnostic and treatment procedures that "confirm the absence" of any naturally occurring disease process that can account for the observed physical problem (Dixon and Abbey 1995; Feldman et al. 2001).

Furthermore, the patient's specific motivation must be "to assume the sick role" (American Psychiatric Association 2000). Yet such patients often are unaware of their motivations, despite being aware of their role in producing their illness (Eisendrath 1996). Patients can be extremely resistant to psychological inquiry or may prematurely leave the hospital (Bauer and Boegner 1996), rendering psychological motivational assessment incomplete (Baker and Major 1994; Topazian and Binder 1994). Motivations may be multiple and mixed (Rogers et al. 1989), with clear secondary gains coexisting with less conscious or more subtle ones (Khan et al. 2000; Lawrie et al. 1993). Nonetheless, most authors believe attempts must be made to investigate and clarify the motivational factors operative in the patients (e.g., Feldman et al. 1994), although Turner (2006) focuses on behavior rather than motives.

The notion of the sick role (Parsons 1951) is complex. Some authors see it as a psychological position in which the patient receives overt empathic support and is subject to overtly reduced expectations—that is, the sick role is a nonpathological mode of functioning that the factitious disorder patient adopts for pathological reasons. Others see the sick role of the factitious disorder patient as inherently pathological. Plassmann (1994b) saw it in terms of the patient's "disturbed relationship to his or her own body" (p. 7) combined with a seriously disturbed doctor–patient relationship. Spivak et al. (1994) similarly described "disturbances in the sense of self and in the sense of reality" (p. 26).

Another factor complicating the diagnosis is the high prevalence of comorbid disorders (Sutherland and Rodin 1990). Substance use disorders (Bauer and Boegner 1996; Parker 1993; Popli et al. 1992), personality disorders (particularly borderline and antisocial) (Bauer and Boegner 1996; Nadelson 1979; Overholser 1990), malingering (Gorman and Winograd 1988; Harrington et al. 1990), dissociative disorders (Toth and Baggaley 1991), eating disorders (Mizuta et al. 2000), suicidality, and mood disorders (Gielder 1994; Sutherland and Rodin 1990) may coexist. The comorbidities can overwhelm the diagnostic picture, and the factitious disorder diagnosis can be ignored altogether (Toth and Baggaley 1991).

There are no valid and reliable diagnostic tests for factitious disorder. Psychological testing may reflect comorbid conditions (Babe et al. 1992) or, in cases of factitious disorder with predominantly psychological signs and symptoms, may give "fake bad" or invalid results (Zimmerman et al. 1991). Such results are not pathognomonic (Liebson et al. 1996) but of the same order as spurious thermometer readings in cases of factitious fever. Neuroimaging studies are discussed in the "Etiology" section later in this chapter.

Epidemiology

Data on incidence and prevalence rates for factitious disorder are difficult to gather, vary considerably, and must be viewed with a critical eye. The covert nature of the disorder can lead to missed diagnosis and underestimation of rates or, conversely, to the same case being counted twice (Duffy 1992; Ifudo and Friedman 1993; Ifudo et al. 1992) and inflating apparent rates.

Sutherland and Rodin (1990) diagnosed factitious disorder in 0.8% of all psychiatric consultation-liaison service referrals of medical or surgical inpatients. Bhugra (1988) found 0.5% of psychiatric admissions to have Munchausen syndrome. Ballas (1996) found that 0.9% of the patients in a sickle cell program could have factitious disorder. Bauer and Boegner (1996) diagnosed factitious disorders in 0.3% of neurological admissions. Fliege et al. (2007) found that of more than 100 clinicians with diverse specialties, the average estimate of frequency was 1.3%. Others (Eisendrath 1996) have reported rates between approximately 2% and 10%, with the higher rates in case series of fevers of unknown origin. Rates are higher in more specialized treatment settings. Most reported cases have been in patients in their 20s–40s, but it has been reported in children, adolescents, and geriatric patients (Angus et al. 2007; Libow 2000; Zimmerman et al. 1991).

Etiology

Psychodynamic explanations for these paradoxical disorders have been provided by several authors. Many have noted the apparent prevalence of histories of early childhood physical or sexual abuse, with disturbed parental relationships and emotional deprivation. Histories of early illness or extended hospitalizations also have been noted. Nadelson (1979) conceptualized factitious disorder as a manifestation of borderline character pathology rather than as an isolated clinical syndrome. The patient becomes both the "victim and the victimizer" by garnering medical attention from physicians and other health care workers while defying and devaluing them. Projection of hostility and worthlessness onto the caregiver occurs as he or she is both desired and rejected. Plassmann (1994b, 1994c) viewed the disorders as a "symptom of a psychic problem complex." Early traumas are dealt with narcissistically and through dissociation, denial, and a type of projection. The patient's body, or part of the body, becomes perceived as an external object or as a fused symbiotic combination of self and object, which then comes to represent negative affects (hate, fear, pain), the associated negative object concepts, and negative self-concepts. In the face of early deprivation and assaults, the "body self" is split off to preserve the "psychic self" (Hirsch 1994). When subsequent life events activate these affects or concepts, the result is extreme anxiety and growing derealization. Eventually, the patient acts out or involves the medical system in a type of countertransference identification, which results in manipulations of the body of the patient. The manipulation results in emotional relief, albeit transient and incomplete, in the manner of most repetitious compromises. Other intrapsychic, cognitive, social learning, and behavioral theories have been advanced as well (Feldman et al. 2001; Ford 1996b).

Neuropathological bases for the disorders also have been suggested, on the basis of abnormal single photon emission computed tomography (Mountz et al. 1996), computed tomography (Babe et al. 1992), and magnetic resonance imaging (Yang et al. 2005) scans and neuropsychological testing (Pankratz and Lezak 1987). No consistent findings have yet been reported. Intriguing, however, is the suggestion that *pseudologia fantastica* may be a syndrome related to, but distinct from, factitious disorder, with its own associated pathology (Hardie and Reed 1998; Mountz et al. 1996; Newmark et al. 1999).

Although many cases of factitious disorder are chronic, the stressor of recurrent object loss, or fear of loss, occurs over and over in the literature as an antecedent of a factitious episode (Ballard and Stoudemire 1992; Linde 1996). For example, Carney (1980) found that 74% of his patients with factitious disorder experienced severe sexual or marital stress prior to the development of factitious signs or symptoms.

Treatment

Once the diagnosis is suspected, it is essential to examine the treatment system for countertransference reactions (Crawford et al. 2005). Plassmann (1994b) saw the patient's ability to induce a countertransference identification in the physician as a core of the disorder, and several authors (Freyberger et al. 1994; Kalivas 1996) viewed the physician's countertransference feelings as partially diagnostic for the disorder. In general medical settings, the risk of nontherapeutic countertransference reactions usually calls for obtaining psychiatric consultation (Stotland 1989) that then often involves working with the entire treatment team of physicians, nurses, ethics and risk management committees, and others (Eisendrath and Feder 1996). In psychiatric settings, this step may call for some additional reflection on the case, a treatment planning conference, or a discussion with a clinical consultant or with colleagues. As Feldman and Feldman (1995) described, countertransference can lead to several adverse consequences. "Therapeutic nihilism" on the part of the treatment system may lead to an unexamined assumption that the patient cannot or should not be treated, with subsequent failure to diagnose or refer. Anger and aversion can rupture any therapeutic alliance, undermine the unity of a treatment team, or lead to punitive acting-out against the patient. Genu-

ine comorbid or concomitant illness may be overlooked. Nonemergent breaches of confidentiality may ensue in the diagnostic hunt or in the supposed effort to "warn" colleagues. Overidentification with the patient or activation of rescue fantasies can sabotage treatment efforts and, as Willenberg (1994) warns, can reinforce the patient's internal splitting and actually support continued factitious behaviors.

As discussed previously, the diagnosis must be confirmed. Erroneous diagnosis of factitious disorder can result in its own trauma and may be perpetuated in medical records (Guziec et al. 1994). Teasell and Shapiro (1994), however, argued against the necessity of a completely accurate diagnosis of factitious disorder once the contribution of general medical illness has been factored out. The patient then must be informed of a change in treatment plan, and an attempt must be made to enlist him or her in that plan. The literature generally refers to this process (perhaps alluding to its countertransference aspects) as containing an element of "confrontation." There is now general agreement that treatment begins at this point and that it is best done indirectly, with minimal expectation that the patient "confess" or acknowledge the deception. It is a delicate process, with patients frequently leaving the hospital against medical advice or otherwise leaving treatment (Baile et al. 1992; Baker and Major 1994; Ballas 1996; Songer 1995). Guziec et al. (1994) aptly likened this process to making a psychodynamic interpretation. Eisendrath (1989) described techniques for reducing confrontation, such as using inexact interpretations, therapeutic double binds, and other strategic and face-saving techniques to allow the patient tacitly to relinquish the factitious signs and symptoms.

Some authors recommend inpatient psychiatric hospitalization, often protracted and/or involuntary (Plassmann 1994a; Powell and Boast 1993). However, many (e.g., Guziec et al. 1994; Teasell and Shapiro 1994) describe treatment being initiated in the general medical inpatient setting where the factitious disorder has been diagnosed and continuing in the psychiatric outpatient setting. Although the patient with Munchausen syndrome is regarded as less likely to engage in treatment (Eisendrath 1989; Stotland 1989), and the patient with general factitious disorder is seen as more available for intervention, there are case reports of Munchausen patients responding favorably to treatment (Feldman 2006; Rothchild 1994; Spivak et al. 1994).

No comparative studies of different therapeutic approaches have been done, but several different techniques have been described. Regardless of modality, treatment must be collaborative and involve some level of communication among all of the patient's treatment providers (Eisendrath and Feder 1996). The psychodynamic approach to treatment (Plassmann 1994a; Spivak et al. 1994) generally focuses not on the factitious behaviors themselves but on the underlying dynamic issues, with the therapist taking a neutral stance toward the factitious nature of the behaviors. As indicated, strategic-behavioral approaches also have been used (Solyom and Solyom 1990; Teasell and Shapiro 1994), implementing standard behavioral techniques as well as the therapeutic double bind, in which the only way out is to abandon the target factitious behaviors. In one particularly intractable case, Schwarz et al. (1993) used a unique combination strategy involving weekly psychotherapy provided by the primary care physician and a carefully designed paradoxical unrestricted hospital admission policy to control factitious behavior. The unrestricted access to the hospital reduced the need for deception. Pharmacotherapy, when used, targets specific symptoms, such as depression or transient psychosis, or comorbid disorders. Some patients cease factitious behaviors on their own as a result of unanticipated life change (e.g., marriage or involvement in a church group that provides the requisite attention and support). Perceiving an "addictive" quality to their factitious behaviors, others have creatively evolved personal "12-Step" programs that have helped them end the deceptions.

The treatment of factitious disorder is not without its pitfalls. In addition to the challenges of diagnosis and countertransference, significant medicolegal issues must be considered, both in the malpractice and in the workers' compensation arenas. Houck (1992) provided a thorough review, and Janofsky (1994) discussed several forensic cases.

Insufficient studies have been done to address conclusively the prognostic factors in factitious disorder, but children, patients with major depression, and those without personality disorders may have better prognoses (Folks 1995; Libow 2000). The literature on this disorder is certainly ample, and it implies that the factitious disorder patient, although requiring considerable therapeutic skill, may be approached with a cautious hope for improvement.

Factitious Disorder by Proxy

In 1977, the British pediatrician Roy Meadow described another scenario involving factitious illness. He presented his observations on a number of cases in each of which a mother had intentionally induced illness in her infant, not in herself. Concealing the deception, the mother then presented the child for medical care, resulting in extensive, often invasive, evaluations and examinations of the child. Despite the outward appearance of being concerned and caring, the mother continued to fabricate illness in her child. Meadow employed the term *Munchausen syndrome by proxy* to describe such scenarios. The children in these situations may be subject to considerable and prolonged morbidity, with a mortality of 6%–10% (Rosenberg 1987; Schreier and Libow 1993b; Sheridan 2003).

As Schreier and Libow (1993a) wrote, "With the exception perhaps of incest, this simultaneously long-term, close-yet-destructive relationship between perpetrator and victim has no parallel in human psychology." There has been a continued expansion of the medical literature about this type of fabricated illness, with the publication of lay and professional books on the topic (e.g., Adshead and Brooke 2001; Eminson and Postlethwaite 2000; Lasher and Sheridan 2004; Levin and Sheridan 1995; Schreier and Libow 1993a, 1996). Gregory (2004) has written a memoir about her victimization by factitious disorder by proxy.

Classification

DSM-IV-TR provides research criteria for factitious disorder by proxy in Appendix B, "Criteria Sets and Axes Provided for Further Study" (American Psychiatric Association 2000). The criteria are similar to those for factitious disorder, with the addition of the "by proxy" specification (Table 14–3). Much of the literature, however, retains the use of the eponym *Munchausen syndrome by proxy,* and there is considerable debate about how best to use that term and the term *factitious disorder by proxy* (Fisher and Mitchell 1995; R. Meadow 1995).

TABLE 14–3. **DSM-IV-TR research criteria for factitious disorder by proxy**

A. Intentional production or feigning of physical or psychological signs or symptoms in another person who is under the individual's care.

B. The motivation for the perpetrator's behavior is to assume the sick role by proxy.

C. External incentives for the behavior (such as economic gain) are absent.

D. The behavior is not better accounted for by another mental disorder.

The debate revolves around four questions:

1. Does the syndrome require legally defined child abuse and/or neglect to have occurred?
2. Does the syndrome pertain to the diagnosis of an individual (implying some degree of homogeneous individual psychopathology), or does it pertain to a situation (without homogeneous psychopathology in the fabricator)?
3. Does the syndrome require an attribution or determination of the fabricator's primary motivation, and if so, what is the nature of that motivation?
4. Does the conferring of a psychiatric diagnosis mitigate the fabricator's responsibility for egregious behavior?

DSM-IV-TR uses factitious disorder by proxy to describe a mental disorder in an individual who is specifically motivated to attain the sick role through someone else who is under that person's care. Technically, because factitious disorder by proxy is a research diagnosis, an individual meeting factitious disorder by proxy criteria would actually be given a diagnosis of factitious disorder not otherwise specified. The proxy, if psychiatrically diagnosed, could receive different diagnoses, depending on the circumstances and the proxy's psychiatric symptoms.

R. Meadow (1995) used Munchausen syndrome by proxy to refer to a particular form of child abuse characterized by a particular behavior and attitude on the part of the perpetrator (usually the mother) and reserved factitious disorder by proxy as an individual diagnosis were one needed. Munchausen syndrome by proxy is something a person *in loco parentis* commits, not a disorder he or she has (S.R. Meadow 1995). Bools (1996) viewed the attempt to label the perpetrator of child abuse with any new diagnosis as "(pseudo) psychiatric" and reserved either term to describe a situation of child abuse. In contrast to DSM-IV-TR, ICD-10 also classifies factitious disorder by proxy not as a disorder but as a form of child abuse (World Health Organization 1992).

Schreier and Libow (1993a) applied the term *Munchausen syndrome by proxy* to describe a disorder in the fabricator who has a specific and particular primary motivation, which is "the mother's intense need to be in a relationship with doctors and/or hospitals. The child is used to gain and maintain this contact." This motivation is a true perversion in the analytical sense of the term (Schreier 1992). Schreier's (1996) later writing included perpetrators who fabricate with a proxy in order to build "a highly manipulative relationship with a powerful transferential figure," specifically

"professionals who occupy positions of power in society," not just physicians.

Another authority, Ford (1996a), argued that the fabricator should receive no syndrome-related diagnosis for the factitious behavior out of concern that diagnosis may provide a legal defense for behavior he views as predominantly criminal. Uniquely, however, he would use the diagnosis of factitious disorder not otherwise specified to apply to the proxy-victim.

DSM-IV-TR criteria allow the proxy to be other than a child and the caregiver to be other than the mother. Although the overwhelming majority of cases involve mother and child (Sheridan 2003), instances have been described in which the proxies were able-bodied adults, hospital and nursing home patients, or even pets (Milani 2006) and the perpetrators were fathers, other relatives, babysitters, partners, health care professionals, or paraprofessionals (Chantada et al. 1994; Yorker 1996a).

The earlier discussion notwithstanding, for the purposes of this chapter, we use DSM-IV-TR terminology. We also use the term *factitious disorder by proxy* and *Munchausen syndrome by proxy* interchangeably, rely primarily on DSM-IV-TR research criteria, and use the paradigm of the mother-perpetrator and the child proxy-victim.

Diagnosis

Certain clusters of warning signs (Table 14–4) can suggest a diagnosis of factitious disorder by proxy.

A proposed diagnostic indicator, described by Szajnberg et al. (1996), is a particular type of countertransference that the clinician experiences (even in cases in which the illness fabrication has been proven): "the clinician has a recurrent, uncanny, ego-dystonic, and uncomfortable sense of *disbelief* that this parent has perpetrated his or her child's symptoms and illness" (p. 230). They recommend that two clinicians be present during a diagnostic factitious disorder by proxy interview: one to conduct the interview and the other to observe the interpersonal process.

Verification of the DSM-IV-TR diagnosis is a process fraught with the same type of difficulties mentioned in the discussion of factitious disorder earlier in this chapter. The mother's principal motivation must be determined (Kahan and Yorker 1991; Morley 1995), and any motivation other than attaining the sick role by proxy must be ruled out (Bools 1996; R. Meadow 1995). Also required is the determination that the mother is intentionally fabricating or inducing the child's illness. Because child abuse is a crime, proving the fabrication becomes a forensic process rather than

---

TABLE 14–4. Warning signs for factitious disorder by proxy

- The episodes of illness occur only when the child is, or has recently been, alone with the parent.

- The parent has taken the child to numerous caregivers, resulting in multiple diagnostic evaluations but neither cure nor definitive diagnosis.

- The other parent (usually the father) is notably uninvolved despite the ostensive health crises.

- The parent is proved to have provided false information to health care professionals or others.

- The parent continually advocates for painful or risky diagnostic tests for the child.

- The child persistently fails to tolerate or respond to usual medical therapies.

- Signs and symptoms abate or do not occur when the child is separated from the parent.

- Another child in the family has had unexplained illness or childhood death.

- The parent has a personal history of factitious disorder.

Source. Data from Bools et al. 1992; Jani et al. 1992; Jureidini 1993; Libow 1995; R. Meadow 1982; Schreier and Libow 1996.

---

a clinical medical investigation (Yorker 1996b). Various techniques have been used, including covert video surveillance in the hospital (Samuels et al. 1992), searching of rooms and belongings (Ford 1996a), and special handling of laboratory specimens (Kahan and Yorker 1991). Some of these techniques raise obvious legal and ethical issues that must be resolved before their implementation (Evans 1995; Ford 1996a; Samuels et al. 1992). Once the deceptions are exposed, the intentionality usually is readily inferred, given the amount of premeditation that is required, for example, to repeatedly suffocate (Samuels et al. 1992), poison (McClure et al. 1996), or inject (Sigal et al. 1990) the proxy-victim.

The ability of the mother with factitious disorder by proxy to deceive and to appear to be a caring, concerned parent can be astounding. In one case in which the mother confessed to repeatedly poisoning two of her children with salt, the mother was "so convincing in her performance that local authorities were reported as digging up pipes in the street looking for contamination" (p. 195), presumably of the water sup-

ply (Coombe 1995). Video surveillance has clearly shown that the caring presentation is a performance and that when the mother thinks she is unobserved, she gives the child minimal attention (Samuels et al. 1992) or is abusive.

The cautions against making a false-positive diagnosis of factitious disorder apply to factitious disorder by proxy as well (R. Meadow 1995; Schreier and Libow 1994). Added to these risks is that of making false criminal accusations with adverse results on the involved family (Rand and Feldman 1999; Schreier and Libow 1993b).

Once factitious disorder by proxy has been diagnosed, it is important to assess the entire family, including the proxy. Other children may also be proxies, other family members may be participating in the factitious behavior, and the proxy him- or herself may be actively cooperating with the fabrications (Awadallah et al. 2005).

Epidemiology

The prevalence of factitious disorder by proxy is unknown, but one study that made the diagnosis very conservatively estimated 2.8 cases per 100,000 children age 1 year or younger or 0.5 cases per 100,000 children age 16 years or younger (McClure et al. 1996). Among select populations, such as in cases of fevers of unknown origin (Aduan et al. 1979), discharges against medical advice (Jani et al. 1992), or pediatric specialty registers (Schreier and Libow 1993b), the rates may be substantially higher. The child typically is 2–5 years old at diagnosis (Sheridan 2003; Yorker and Kahan 1990). Length of time from onset of symptoms in the child to diagnosis can vary widely, averaging 15 months (±14 months) in one series (Rosenberg 1987) to years in another (Libow 1995). Methods are legion, but smothering, poisoning, and fabricated history of seizures or fever are most commonly reported (McClure et al. 1996). In most cases, however, multiple methods have been used to fabricate a variety of illnesses in the child (Bools et al. 1992). Behavioral conditions and psychiatric disorders also may be feigned (Schreier 2000). In a high percentage of cases, other siblings had been proxy-victims as well (Sheridan 2003).

A substantial minority (i.e., greater than would be expected in a general population sample but still the minority) of the mothers have connections to the health professions (Ostfeld and Feldman 1996), have received prior psychiatric attention (Alexander et al. 1990; Samuels et al. 1992), or have indications of preexisting factitious disorder in themselves (R. Meadow 1982). Actual psychosis is rare (Bools 1996). No consistent profile on psychological testing has been shown (Rand 1996). The most common comorbid psychiatric disorder in factitious disorder by proxy is a personality disorder (Schreier 1992), and substance use disorders are less commonly reported.

Etiology

Although perpetrators rarely make themselves available for psychiatric or psychological study, most authors postulate that the maternal pathology arises from childhood roots, characterized by "quietly traumatic" emotional neglect and abandonment. Some descriptions of the hypothesized childhood deficits suggest that they occur later than those hypothesized to result in factitious disorder, whereas other authors see the dynamics as more similar (Schreier and Libow 1993a). Adshead and Bluglass (2005) found unresolved trauma or loss reactions in the majority of their sample. They concluded that insecure attachment is a risk factor. Others have emphasized the role of modern medicine, with its predilection for invasive and aggressive diagnostic testing, in the etiology of the syndrome (Donald and Jureidini 1996). Schreier and Libow (1993a), Parnell and Day (1998), and Rogers (2004) have written extensively on the etiological hypotheses, and the reader is referred to their work.

Treatment and Prognosis

Mothers engaging in factitious disorder by proxy are universally regarded as very resistant and difficult to treat (Schreier and Libow 1994). Some of the difficulty stems from the mother's massive use of denial and projective identification (Coombe 1995; Feldman 1994b; Schreier 1992). Another source stems from the process by which treatment is usually initiated. Experience with factitious disorder has shown that an indirect, nonconfrontational approach is most effective and that some continuing of the factitious behavior is to be expected during the course of treatment. In factitious disorder by proxy, because of the necessity to protect the proxy, an indirect approach permitting continued factitious behavior is not possible. The first stage of treatment in factitious disorder by proxy usually begins with the involvement of child protection authorities, the initiation of legal proceedings against the parent, and the removal of the child from the home.

Management of factitious disorder by proxy requires coordinated multidisciplinary, multiagency involvement (Coombe 1995; Parnell and Day 1998). Individual treatment includes long-term psychotherapy (group, individual, or combined) and focuses on helping the perpetrator express feelings and needs for support and recognition more directly, with less use of projection and with the development of empathic capacity (Coombe 1995). As with the treatment of factitious disorder, the factitious behavior is rarely the primary focus. Pharmacotherapy is used only to treat comorbid conditions.

One study (Berg and Jones 1999) followed up 13 mothers who were specifically selected "on the basis of the likelihood of successful intervention" for a mean of 27 months after an inpatient intervention. All of these perpetrators were atypical in that they freely admitted to having engaged in the abuse. Ten (77%) were reunited with their children, with only one recurrence of factitious disorder by proxy illness during the follow-up period. However, the results in more typical, unselected samples have been distinctly unfavorable; thus the overall prognosis is guarded, with a high likelihood of continued factitious disorder by proxy behavior (Bools et al. 1993, 1994; Davis et al. 1998; Libow 1995; R. Meadow 1993). Management is usually coordinated and directed through the legal system, and protection of the child is the priority (Kahan and Yorker 1991; Lasher and Sheridan 2004).

Malingering
Classification

DSM-IV-TR classifies malingering under "Additional Conditions That May Be a Focus of Clinical Attention." Malingering in this nomenclature is not considered to be a diagnosis, as by definition it is "the intentional production of false or grossly exaggerated physical or psychological symptoms motivated by external incentives" (American Psychiatric Association 2000). External incentives that may motivate a person to malinger symptoms include avoiding work, evading criminal prosecution, obtaining drugs, receiving financial compensation, avoiding military duty, or escaping other intolerable situations. Table 14–5 provides the DSM-IV-TR guidelines for when to suspect malingering. However, many experts consider these criteria overly broad and inclusive, which may in turn lead to the overidentification of patients as malingerers. For example, Rogers (1990a) noted that using these guidelines as criteria for detecting malingering—that is, requiring that an individual meet two of the four criteria—leads to the correct classification of approximately two-thirds of true malingerers. However, he determined that this strategy led to the overclassifica-

TABLE 14–5. **DSM-IV-TR warning signs for malingering**

- The individual's evaluation occurs in a medicolegal context, such as referral from an attorney.

- A marked discrepancy exists between the person's claims and objective findings.

- The individual is uncooperative during the diagnostic evaluation and in complying with the prescribed treatment regimen.

- Antisocial personality disorder is present.

tion of true psychiatric patients. Rogers concluded that persons meeting two of the four DSM-IV-TR criteria have a one in five chance of being a true malingerer. An 80% false-positive rate is inordinately high and generally considered unacceptable.

Research has been divided on whether individuals with antisocial personality disorder are more likely to malinger. For example, Gacono et al. (1995) found that individuals found "not guilty by reason of insanity" who subsequently admitted feigning mental illness were more likely to be diagnosed with antisocial personality disorder and to score higher on a measure of psychopathy (Hare Psychopathy Checklist—Revised [PCL-R]; Hare 1991) than individuals receiving the same verdict who did not admit to malingering. In contrast, Poythress et al. (2001) found that prisoners scoring high on a measure of psychopathy (Psychopathic Personality Inventory; Lilienfeld and Andrews 1996) were no more likely than other prisoners to malinger. Delain et al. (2003) found that defendants in criminal court with a diagnosis of antisocial personality disorder were more likely to malinger memory deficits (as measured by the Test of Memory Malingering; Tombaugh 1996) than defendants without this diagnosis. However, recently it has been suggested that such discrepancies may be related to the *success* of the person in malingering and that the real question is: Are individuals with antisocial personality more likely to *attempt* to malinger? Kucharski et al. (2006) found that criminal defendants scoring in the high psychopathy range (PCL-R score greater than 29) were more likely to score in the malingering range on standardized assessments. The authors concluded that their study provided some support for the DSM-IV-TR recommendation of suspecting malingering in the presence of antisocial personality disorder. Moreover, not surprisingly, the affective and interpersonal features of psychopathic persons (which include pathological lying) were best at discriminating malingerers from nonmalingerers.

Rogers (1990b) described three models to explain the underlying motivation of an individual who malingers: the pathogenic model, the criminological model, and the adaptational model. Although the pathogenic model no longer receives general support (Vitacco and Rogers 2005), it warrants a historical discussion. In this model, the malingerer's motivation is based on true psychopathology. The production of symptoms is postulated to be an effort to gain control over real symptoms. The eventual outcome is the replacement of feigned symptoms with real ones. However, research has not shown this prediction to hold true (Resnick 1997). The criminological model presumes an underlying "badness" of the malingerer and is based on the DSM suggestions for when to be suspicious of malingering. As Rogers (1997) so eloquently noted, "a bad person (APD [antisocial personality disorder]) in bad circumstances (legal difficulties) who is performing badly (uncooperative)" (p. 7) is considered highly likely to malinger. The final motivation is the adaptational model, wherein the malingerer evaluates the cost–benefit of an assessment. In this model, malingering may be more likely under three circumstances: 1) when the context is adversarial, 2) the personal stakes are high, and 3) there are no viable alternatives. It is important to note that these models only provide explanations for the behavior; they are not intended as prescriptions for the detection of malingering. Rogers has found empirical support for these models (Rogers et al. 1998a).

Diagnostic confusion between malingering and other mental disorders, particularly factitious disorder, can be traced to Asher's (1951) original description of Munchausen syndrome. He attributed several possible motives to Munchausen syndrome, including "a desire to escape from the police" and "a desire to get free board and lodgings for the night" (p. 339), motives that would now clearly classify feigned illness behavior as malingering. The tendency to include malingering within the factitious disorder spectrum was further reinforced by Spiro (1968), who recommended that in individuals with Munchausen syndrome, "malingering should only be diagnosed in the absence of psychiatric illness and the presence of behavior appropriately adaptive to a clear-cut long-term goal" (p. 569). There are, however, many examples of patients with factitious disorder who also malinger (see "Diagnosis" subsection of "Factitious Disorder" section earlier in this chapter). Other disorders to consider in the differential diagnosis of malingering include conversion disorder and/or other somatoform disorders. Although all of these diagnoses may involve physical symptoms, none involve the production of symptoms for external incentives. Individuals with conversion disorder or another somatoform disorder experience symptoms that cannot be fully explained by a medical condition and are often connected to psychological reasons of which the person is unaware. Finally, malingerers should be distinguished from individuals who confabulate, because confabulation involves unintentionally filling in missing information with what one believes to have happened, when, in fact, it did not happen at all (Newmark et al. 1999; Resnick 2000).

The term *malingering by proxy* also has been suggested (Bools 1996) for those cases in which illness is fabricated in a child for secondary gain, such as for the purpose of obtaining social assistance benefits (Cassar et al. 1996). The literature contains several case reports of parents who report or induce their children to report disability for the purpose of litigation and ultimately financial remuneration (Lu and Boone 2002; Stutts et al. 2003)

There has been increasing interest in characterizing the successful malingerer. Research has indicated that there is a technique for "falling under the radar" of the detection methods for malingering. Gold and Frueh (1999) found that extreme reports of symptoms were more likely to be identified as malingering. In support of this, as a direct evaluation of malingering methods, Edens et al. (2001) found that "successful malingerers"—that is, individuals who simulated mental illness but scored below the cut points on structured assessments of malingering—differed from unsuccessful malingerers in specific ways. Successful malingerers endorsed significantly fewer numbers of legitimate symptoms and avoided endorsing absurd or bizarre symptoms. Interestingly, although successful malingerers believed they would appear less psychologically impaired, they did not expect to be any more successful in evading detection.

Detection ("Diagnosis")

Physicians are trained to assess and treat individuals who actually have medical or mental health symptoms. A care provider's natural inclination is to accept the person's reported symptoms at face value. Rosenhan (1973) conducted a famous study that demonstrated clinicians' tendency to blindly accept reported mental health symptoms. In this study, eight non–mentally ill individuals presented to a psychiatric hospital alleging that they were hearing very atypical voices. Based on this one reported symptom, every person was admitted to the hospital and given a

schizophrenia diagnosis, even though each person ceased reporting any symptoms after admission.

The detection of malingering in the forensic arena is particularly crucial, because the avoidance of criminal prosecution is a strong motivation (Resnick 1984). The detection of malingered psychosis in particular is especially important, because psychotic symptoms often are offered as the basis for an insanity defense (Cornell and Hawk 1989). However, erroneously concluding that a defendant is malingering can have rather serious negative consequences. In addition to delaying potentially appropriate treatment, such mislabeling may lead to the inappropriate conviction of truly mentally ill individuals. Thus, the detection of malingered psychosis, and distinguishing such from true psychosis, is of paramount importance.

Cornell and Hawk (1989) contrasted the clinical presentations of two groups of criminal defendants: those diagnosed as genuinely psychotic and those diagnosed as malingering. Interestingly, they found the incidence of malingering to be relatively low: 8%, or 25 cases out of 314 evaluations. They found that defendants diagnosed as malingering presented with visual hallucinations, exaggerated behavior, and symptoms that typically do not cluster together (such as psychomotor retardation and hallucinations). In contrast, genuinely psychotic patients evidenced disturbed affect and formal thought disorders. The authors concluded that malingerers may overlook more subtle, but more common, symptoms of psychosis such as thought disorder and disturbances of affect.

Consistent with this research, Resnick (2000) noted that the better clinicians understand characteristics of a true illness, the more likely they will be able to detect feigned symptoms. Malingering is "so easy to define but so difficult to diagnose" (Resnick 1997, p. 48). When a clinician suspects that a symptom may be fabricated or exaggerated, he or she should be on alert for various inconsistencies that may appear in the individual's evaluation. First, the individual may present inconsistencies in what he or she actually reports. For example, a person may report that he or she is currently unable to talk, despite speaking eloquently throughout the interview. Second, a malingerer's observed behavior may differ significantly from the symptoms he or she reports. The person who describes active, continuous, disturbing hallucinations during the interview but shows no evidence of distraction illustrates this type of inconsistency, suggestive of malingering. Third, malingerers may behave in a dramatically different way depending on who they believe is observing them. This disparity in presentation is illustrated by a person who

TABLE 14–6. Clinical decision model for the assessment of malingering of psychosis

The evaluee's presentation meets the following criteria:

  A. Understandable motive to malinger

  B. Marked variability of presentation as observed in at least one of the following:

    1. Marked discrepancies in interview and noninterview behavior

    2. Gross inconsistencies in reported psychotic symptoms

    3. Blatant contradictions between reported prior episodes and documented psychiatric history

  C. Improbable psychiatric symptoms as evidenced by one or more of the following:

    1. Reporting elaborate psychotic symptoms that lack common paranoid, grandiose, or religious themes

    2. Sudden emergence of purported psychotic symptoms to explain antisocial behavior

    3. Atypical hallucinations or delusions (see Table 14–7)

  D. Confirmation of malingered psychosis by either

    1. Admission of malingering following confrontation

    2. Presence of strong corroborative information, such as psychometric data or history of malingering

Source. Resnick 1997.

TABLE 14–7. Threshold model for the assessment of hallucinations and delusions

Malingering should be suspected if any combination of the following is observed:

Hallucinations

  Continuous rather than intermittent hallucinations

  Vague or inaudible hallucinations

  Hallucinations not associated with delusions

  Stilted language reported in hallucinations

  Inability to state strategies to diminish voices

  Self-report that all command hallucinations were obeyed

  Visual hallucinations in black and white

Delusions

  Abrupt onset or termination

  Eagerness to call attention to delusions

  Conduct markedly inconsistent with delusions

  Bizarre content without disordered thinking

Source. Resnick 1997.

presentation of manufactured psychotic symptoms (Tyrer et al. 2001).

When evaluating possible malingering, the clinician should consider obtaining additional information from collateral sources and psychological testing to verify the person's reported symptoms. In addition to the clinical interview, sources of information that may be useful include interviews with family members, friends, co-workers, employers, clinical staff, other therapists, jail or prison personnel, and probation or parole officers. Records often relevant to the malingering assessment include past medical records, psychiatric records, educational records, work records, rap sheets, court evaluations, and prior disability claims.

Psychological testing is often used in malingering assessments and may include structured interviews to evaluate psychotic symptoms (Rogers et al. 1992), various personality inventories, and neuropsychological testing to assess cognitive deficits (Liebson et al. 1996). Witztum et al. (1996) described several military inductees who received erroneous diagnoses of malingering; diagnoses of severe psychiatric disorders were missed because of assessment problems. They also noted, as did DuAlba and Scott (1993), the important role of cross-cultural issues in the assessment of malingering.

acts in a confused, disoriented manner in the clinician's office and shortly after leaving is observed by ward staff winning a brilliant game of chess. Fourth, psychological test data may be inconsistent with the history provided by malingerers. Finally, malingerers often report symptoms that are inconsistent with how genuine symptoms normally manifest.

Table 14–6 provides a suggested clinical decision model for the assessment of malingered psychosis (Resnick 1997). In determining whether reported hallucinations or delusions are fabricated or exaggerated, the factors outlined in Table 14–7 also may prove helpful (Resnick 1997). Note that a bona fide diagnosis of a past psychotic disorder does not necessarily exclude a

Structured Assessments of Malingering

Although suggestions have been outlined for the clinical assessment of malingering (Cornell and Hawk 1989; Resnick 1997), structured assessments recently have been developed to aid in the detection of malingering. Prior to the development of these specialized assessments, subscales of standard psychological tests were used as an indicator of assessment attitudes, both for malingering and for other dissimulation. Perhaps the most common and extensively researched of these is the Minnesota Multiphasic Personality Inventory (MMPI) and its revision, the MMPI-2 (Butcher et al. 1989). In two meta-analyses of the validity scales of the MMPI (Berry et al. 1991) and the MMPI-2 (Rogers et al. 1994b), the F scale (Infrequency) and the F–K index (Dissimulation) were shown to be superior to other indices of malingering. Unfortunately, because these indices can be elevated in individuals with true psychiatric disorders, other scales have been developed in an effort to aid in this distinction. For example, Arbisi and Ben-Porath (1995) developed the Infrequency–Psychopathology scale (F(p)) using items endorsed infrequently even by psychiatric inpatients. However, recent research suggests that this scale does not improve the detection of malingerers over the F scale when used alone (Kucharski et al. 2004). Two significant drawbacks to the use of the MMPI-2 in the detection of malingering are the length of time required to complete this assessment and the required reading level (seventh grade) of the examinee. Additionally, the administration and interpretation of the MMPI-2 are not readily available to all examiners. For these reasons, screening tools have been developed to quickly assess for the possibility of malingering before more extensive evaluations are conducted. Table 14–8 provides a summary of some assessments commonly used in the detection of malingered psychiatric disturbances.

Screening Tools for Malingering

Paper and Pencil Tests

M Test.   The M Test (Beaber et al. 1985) was developed in the 1980s as a brief screen for malingered psychosis. In its original form, three types of items were developed: items that would be expected to be endorsed in one direction by all individuals, regardless of diagnosis (8 in all), items that were true indicators of schizophrenia (10), and items that were not true indicators of schizophrenia (15). Although this instrument is brief and relatively easy to administer, it evidenced

TABLE 14–8.   Standardized assessments for detecting the malingering of psychiatric disturbances

Screening tools

M Test

   33 items

   Assesses true and untrue indicators of schizophrenia

Structured Inventory of Malingered Symptomatology

   75 items, true/false

   Assesses malingering of five types: low intelligence, affective disorders, neurological impairment, psychosis, amnestic disorders

Miller Forensic Assessment of Symptoms Test

   25 items, structured interview

   Assesses malingering with seven subscales: unusual hallucinations, reported vs. observed, rare combinations, extreme symptomatology, negative image, unusual symptom course, suggestibility

Comprehensive assessments

Minnesota Multiphasic Personality Inventory, 2nd Edition

   567 items, true/false

   Assesses psychiatric disorders and personality functioning

   3 basic validity scales, 10 clinical scales

   Requires interpretation by a psychologist

Personality Assessment Inventory

   344 items, true/false

   Assesses adult personality and psychopathology

   4 validity scales, 11 clinical scales

   Requires interpretation by a psychologist

Structured Interview of Reported Symptoms

   156 items, structured interview

   Assesses malingering with eight primary scales: rare symptoms, symptom combinations, improbable or absurd symptoms, blatant symptoms, subtle symptoms, selectivity of symptoms, severity of symptoms, reported vs. observed symptoms poor discrimination in a group of male prisoners (Smith and Borum 1992).

Structured Inventory of Malingered Symptomatology.   The Structured Inventory of Malingered Symptomatology (SIMS; Smith and Burger 1997) is a 75-item true/false self-report test designed to assess malingering of a variety of types of pathology. Some items are similar to those contained in other scales, whereas others were developed specifically for this instrument. The SIMS contains five subscales: low intelligence, affective disorders, neurological impairment, psychosis, and amnestic disorders. Each subscale consists of 15 items. The advantage of the SIMS is that it screens for malingered psychiatric *and* cognitive symptomatology. The SIMS has been found to be useful as a screening test (Lewis et al. 2002), although recent research suggests that there may be a high false-positive rate in a clinical population (Edens et al. 1999).

Interview Format

Miller Forensic Assessment of Symptoms Test. The Miller Forensic Assessment of Symptoms Test (Miller 2001), which was developed as a screening instrument designed to identify malingered psychopathology, is a 25-item structured interview that can be administered in approximately 5 minutes. It consists of items rationally derived from the literature on constructs useful in identifying malingerers and yields scores relevant to seven strategies: unusual hallucinations, reported versus observed, rare combinations, extreme symptomatology, negative image, unusual symptom course, and suggestibility. Research indicates that it is effective in identifying feigning in a variety of settings (Guy and Miller 2004; Jackson et al. 2005).

Comprehensive Assessments of Malingering

In addition to the screening tools just described, several more comprehensive methods are available to detect malingering. As noted previously, the MMPI-2 is widely used as an assessment tool in the detection of malingered psychopathology. In addition, other instruments have been useful for this purpose.

Personality Assessment Inventory.   The Personality Assessment Inventory (Morey 1991) is a 344-item self-report instrument developed as an objective inventory of adult personality and psychopathology. It contains 22 scales: 4 validity scales, 11 clinical scales, 5 treatment scales, and 2 interpersonal scales. Three indices have been identified as useful in the detection

of malingering: the Negative Impression scale and the Malingering index, both of which are composite scales of the Personality Assessment Inventory, and the Rogers Discriminant Function scale (Rogers et al. 1996), which is an empirically derived combination of 20 Personality Assessment Inventory scale scores. Each of these scales have shown some utility in the detection of malingering (Bagby et al. 2002; Calhoun et al. 2000; Rogers et al. 1998b), although recent studies indicate that the Negative Impression scale has been the most effective in detecting malingering in a criminal forensic sample (Boccaccini et al. 2006; Kucharski et al. 2007).

Structured Interview of Reported Symptoms.   The Structured Interview of Reported Symptoms (SIRS; Rogers et al. 1992) was developed to assess a broad range of strategies to detect malingering. It is a 156-item structured interview that takes approximately 30–45 minutes to administer. The SIRS contains eight primary scales (rare symptoms, symptom combinations, improbable or absurd symptoms, blatant symptoms, subtle symptoms, severity of symptoms, selectivity of symptoms, reported vs. observed symptoms) and five supplementary scales (direct appraisal of honesty, defensive symptoms, overly specific symptoms, symptom onset and resolution, and inconsistency of symptoms). Responses on the primary scales are classified as honest, indeterminate, probable, or definite. An individual is considered to be feigning psychiatric symptoms if he or she scores in the definite range on at least one primary subscale or the probable range on three or more primary subscales. The SIRS has been shown to be a reliable method for detecting malingering (Hayes et al. 1998).

Epidemiology

Malingering of psychiatric symptoms is not a rare event. The reported incidence of malingering varies depending on the population in question. In a study of malingered mental illness in a metropolitan emergency department, 13% of patients were strongly suspected or considered to be malingering. Reasons identified for malingering included seeking hospitalization for food and shelter, attempting to gain medication, attempting to avoid incarceration, and seeking financial gain (Yates et al. 1996). Rogers et al. (1993) estimated that approximately half of the individuals evaluated for personal injury claims were feigning all or part of their cognitive deficits. A group of forensic psychologists estimated that malingering occurred in almost 16% of forensic patients and more than 7% of nonforensic patients (Rogers et al. 1994a). Additionally, almost 21% of defendants undergoing evaluations of criminal responsibility engaged in or were suspected of engaging in malingering (Rogers 1986). In contrast, Cornell and Hawk (1989) found the incidence of malingering in a sample of defendants referred for an evaluation of competence to stand trial and/or criminal responsibility to be 8%. Gold and Frueh (1999) found that either 14% or 22% of veterans referred for an evaluation for PTSD were classified as "extreme exaggerators" on the MMPI-2, depending on the criteria used. Clearly, the context of the evaluation bears greatly on the probability that malingering will occur.

Treatment

When a determination of malingering is made, the clinician is faced with the dilemma of how to "treat" a nondisorder. Depending on the situation, the clinician may elect to confront the individual with the assessment. Pankratz and Erickson (1990) emphasized the importance of permitting the malingerer to save face. Possible verbal interventions include statements such as "You haven't told me the whole truth" or "The type of symptoms that you are reporting are not consistent with known mental illness" (Inbau and Reid 1967). The clinician should be prepared for some individuals to react defensively and to refuse to accept this diagnosis, even when faced with strong evidence that they are faking symptoms. In contrast, when other individuals are confronted, they admit that their symptoms are faked and give up the charade. Han (1997) described a method of intervention based on cognitive-behavioral techniques that effectively reduced the likelihood of the recurrence of malingering. This intervention, termed "comprehensive management of prisoners," included family, educational, and occupational intervention designed to reduce the motivation to malinger. The management of malingering must first be based on an understanding of the motivations for symptom production (Adetunji et al. 2006). Finally, many of Houck's (1992) warnings about the medicolegal pitfalls in the assessment and treatment of a factitious disorder also apply to the assessment and disposition of the malingerer.

Key Points

- The distinction between factitious disorder and malingering lies in the underlying motivation for the production of symptoms.

- The motivation for factitious disorder is to assume the sick role and is often presumed to be unconscious.

- The motivation for malingering involves the attainment of a tangible reward.

- Factors suggestive of factitious disorder include discrepancies between objective findings, inconsistencies between objective findings and clinical history or symptoms, an atypical illness course, and conditions that fail to respond to usual therapies.

- Factors suggestive of malingering include inconsistencies between reported versus observed behavior and the reporting of improbable or absurd symptoms in the presence of an understandable motive to malinger.

- The treatment/management of both factitious disorder and malingering involves "delicate" confrontation with minimal expectations of confessions.

- The treatment for factitious disorder involves focusing on the underlying motivation for the behavior, which often can be psychodynamic in nature.

- The management of malingering involves understanding the secondary gains associated with the production of symptoms in order to address these expectations.

- Factitious disorder by proxy involves maltreatment and, when suspected, must be reported to child protection authorities.

Suggested Readings

Feldman MD: Playing Sick: Untangling the Web of Munchausen Syndrome, Munchausen by Proxy, Malingering, and Factitious Disorder. New York, Brunner-Routledge, 2004

Feldman MD, Eisendrath SJ: The Spectrum of Factitious Disorders. Washington, DC, American Psychiatric Press, 1996

Lasher LJ, Sheridan MS: Munchausen by Proxy: Identification, Intervention, and Case Management. New York, Haworth, 2004

Rogers R: Clinical Assessment of Malingering and Deception, 2nd Edition. New York, Guilford, 1997

Vitacco JM, Rogers R: Assessment of malingering in correctional settings, in Handbook of Correctional Mental Health Edited by Scott CL, Gerbasi JB. Washington, DC, American Psychiatric Publishing, 2005, pp 133–153

References

Adetunji BA, Basil B, Mathews M, et al: Detection and management of malingering in a clinical setting. Prim Psychiatry 13:61–69, 2006

Adshead G, Bluglass K: Attachment representations in mothers with abnormal illness behavior by proxy. Br J Psychiatry 187:328–333, 2005

Adshead G, Brooke D (eds): Munchausen's Syndrome by Proxy: Current Issues in Assessment, Treatment and Research. London, England, Imperial College Press, 2001

Aduan RP, Fauci AS, Dale DC, et al: Factitious fever and self-induced infection: a report of 32 cases and review of the literature. Ann Intern Med 90:230–242, 1979

Alexander R, Smith W, Stevenson R: Serial Munchausen syndrome by proxy. Pediatrics 86:581–585, 1990

American Psychiatric Association: Diagnostic and Statistical Manual of Mental Disorders, 4th Edition, Text Revision. Washington, DC, American Psychiatric Association, 2000

Angus J, Affleck AG, Croft JC, et al: Dermatitis artefacta in a 12-year-old girl mimicking cutaneous T-cell lymphoma. Pediatr Dermatol 24:327–329, 2007

Arbisi PA, Ben-Porath YS: An MMPI-2 infrequent response scale for use with psychopathological populations: The Infrequency-Psychopathology Scale, F(p). Psychol Assess 7:424–431, 1995

Asher R: Munchausen's syndrome. Lancet 1(6):339–341, 1951

Awadallah N, Vaughan A, Franco K, et al: Munchausen by proxy: a case, chart series, and literature review of older victims. Child Abuse Negl 29:931–941, 2005

Babe KS Jr, Peterson AM, Loosen PT, et al: The pathogenesis of Munchausen syndrome: a review and case report. Gen Hosp Psychiatry 14:273–276, 1992

Baddley J, Daberkow D, Hilton C: Insulinoma masquerading as factitious hypoglycemia. South Med J 91:1067–1069, 1998

Bagby RM, Nicholson RA, Bacchiochi JR, et al: The predictive capacity of the MMPI-2 and PAI validity scales and indexes to detect coached and uncoached feigning. J Pers Assess 78:69–86, 2002

Baile WF, Kuehn CV, Straker D: Factitious cancer. Psychosomatics 33:100–105, 1992

Baker CE, Major E: Munchausen's syndrome: a case presenting as asthma requiring ventilation. Anaesthesia 49:1050–1051, 1994

Ballard RS, Stoudemire A: Factitious apraxia. Int J Psychiatry Med 22:275–280, 1992

Ballas SK: Factitious sickle cell acute painful episodes: a secondary type of Munchausen syndrome. Am J Hematol 53:254–258, 1996

Bappal B, George M, Nair R, et al: Factitious hypoglycemia: a tale from the Arab World. Pediatrics 107:180–181, 2001

Barker JC: The Syndrome of hospital addiction (Munchausen syndrome): a report on the investigation of seven cases. J Men Sci 108:167–182, 1962

Bauer M, Boegner F: Neurological syndromes in factitious disorder. J Nerv Ment Dis 184:281–288, 1996

Beaber RJ, Marston A, Michelli J, et al: A brief test for measuring malingering in schizophrenic individuals. Am J Psychiatry 142:1478–1481, 1985

Berg B, Jones D: Outcome of psychiatric intervention in factitious illness by proxy (Munchausen's syndrome by proxy). Arch Dis Child 81:465–472, 1999

Berry DTR, Baer RA, Harris MJ: Detection of malingering on the MMPI: a meta-analytic review. Clin Psychol Rev 11:585–598, 1991

Bhugra D: Psychiatric Munchausen's syndrome: literature review with case reports. Acta Psychiatr Scand 77:497–503, 1988

Boccaccini MT, Murrie DC, Duncan SA: Screening for malingering in a criminal-forensic sample with the Personality Assessment Inventory. Psychol Assess 18:415–423, 2006

Bools C: Factitious illness by proxy: Munchausen syndrome by proxy. Br J Psychiatry 169:268–275, 1996

Bools CN, Neale BA, Meadow SR: Co-morbidity associated with fabricated illness (Munchausen syndrome by proxy). Arch Dis Child 67:77–79, 1992

Bools CN, Neale BA, Meadow SR: Follow up of victims of fabricated illness (Munchausen syndrome by proxy). Arch Dis Child 69:625–630, 1993

Bools C, Neale B, Meadow R: Munchausen syndrome by proxy: a study of psychopathology. Child Abuse Negl 18:773–788, 1994

Butcher JN, Dahlstrom WG, Graham JR, et al.: MMPI-2: Manual for Administration and Scoring. Minneapolis, University of Minnesota Press, 1989

Calhoun PS, Earnst KS, Tucker DD, et al: Feigning combat-related posttraumatic stress disorder on the Personality Assessment Inventory. J Pers Assess 75:338–350, 2000

Carney MW: Artefactual illness to attract medical attention. Br J Psychiatry 136:542–547, 1980

Cassar J, Hales E, Longhurst J, et al: Can disability benefits make children sicker? J Am Acad Child Adolesc Psychiatry 35:700–701, 1996

Chantada G, Casak S, Plata JD, et al: Children with fever of unknown origin in Argentina: an analysis of 113 cases. Pediatr Infect Dis J 13:260–263, 1994

Chapman JS: Peregrinating problem patients: Munchausen's syndrome. JAMA 165:927–933, 1957

Clark E, Melnick SC: The Munchausen syndrome or the problem of hospital hoboes. Am J Med 25:6–12, 1958

Coombe P: The inpatient psychotherapy of a mother and child at the Cassel Hospital: a case of Munchausen's syndrome by proxy. Br J Psychother 12:195–207, 1995

Cornell DG, Hawk GL: Clinical presentation of malingerers diagnosed by experienced forensic psychologists. Law Hum Behav 13:375–383, 1989

Craddock N, Brown N: Munchausen syndrome presenting as mental handicap. Mental Handicap Research 6:184–190, 1993

Crawford SM, Jeyasanger G, Wright M: A visitor with Munchausen's syndrome. Clin Med 5:400–401, 2005

Cunnien AJ: Psychiatric and medical syndromes associated with deception, in Clinical Assessment of Malingering and Deception, 2nd Edition. Edited by Rogers R. New York, Guilford, 1997, pp 23–46

Davis P, McClure R, Rolfe K, et al: Procedures, placement, and risks of further abuse after Munchausen syndrome by proxy, nonaccidental poisoning and nonaccidental suffocation. Arch Dis Child 78:217–221, 1998

Delain SL, Stafford KP, Ben-Porath YS: Use of the TOMM in a criminal court forensic assessment setting. Assessment 10:370–381, 2003

Dixon D, Abbey S: Cupid's arrow: an unusual presentation of factitious disorder. Psychosomatics 36:502–504, 1995

Donald T, Jureidini J: Munchausen syndrome by proxy: child abuse in the medical system. Arch Pediatr Adolesc Med 150:753–758, 1996

DuAlba L, Scott RL: Somatization and malingering for workers' compensation applicants: a cross-cultural MMPI study. J Clin Psychol 49:913–917, 1993

Duffy TP: The Red Baron. N Engl J Med 327:408–411, 1992

Duffy TP: Kidney-related Munchausen's syndrome and the Red Baron. N Engl J Med 328:61–62, 1993

Edens JF, Otto RK, Dwyer T: Utility of the Structured Inventory of Malingered Symptomatology in identifying persons motivated to malinger psychopathology. J Am Acad Psychiatry Law 27:387–396, 1999

Edens JF, Guy LS, Otto RK, et al: Factors differentiating successful versus unsuccessful malingerers. J Pers Assess 77:333–338, 2001

Eisendrath SJ: Factitious physical disorders: treatment without confrontation. Psychosomatics 30:383–387, 1989

Eisendrath SJ: Factitious physical disorders. West J Med 160:177–179, 1994

Eisendrath SJ: Current overview of factitious physical disorders, in The Spectrum of Factitious Disorders. Edited by Feldman MD, Eisendrath SJ. Washington, DC, American Psychiatric Press, 1996, pp 21–36

Eisendrath SJ, Feder A: Management of factitious disorders, in The Spectrum of Factitious Disorders. Edited by Feldman MD, Eisendrath SJ. Washington, DC, American Psychiatric Press, 1996, pp 195–213

Eminson M, Postlethwaite RJ (eds): Munchausen Syndrome by Proxy Abuse: A Practical Approach. Oxford, England, Butterworth-Heinemann, 2000

Evans D: The investigation of life-threatening child abuse and Munchausen syndrome by proxy. J Med Ethics 21:9–13, 1995

Feldman MD: The costs of factitious disorders. Psychosomatics 35:506–507, 1994a

Feldman MD: Denial in Munchausen syndrome by proxy: the consulting psychiatrist's dilemma. Int J Psychiatry Med 24:121–128, 1994b

Feldman MD: Munchausen by Internet: detecting factitious illness and crisis on the Internet. South Med J 93:669–672, 2000

Feldman MD: Playing Sick? Untangling the Web of Munchausen syndrome, Munchausen by Proxy, Malingering and Factitious Disorder. New York, Brunner-Routledge, 2004

Feldman MD: Recovery from Munchausen syndrome. South Med J 99:1398–1399, 2006

Feldman MD, Eisendrath SJ (eds): The Spectrum of Factitious Disorders. Washington, DC, American Psychiatric Press, 1996

Feldman MD, Feldman JM: Tangled in the web: countertransference in the therapy of factitious disorders. Int J Psychiatry Med 25:389–399, 1995

Feldman MD, Smith R: Personal and interpersonal toll of factitious disorders, in The Spectrum of Factitious Disorders. Edited by Feldman MD, Eisendrath SJ. Washington, DC, American Psychiatric Press, 1996, pp 175–194

Feldman MD, Ford CV, Reinhold T: Patient or Pretender: Inside the Strange World of Factitious Disorders. New York, Wiley, 1994

Feldman MD, Hamilton JC, Deemer HN: A critical analysis of factitious disorders, in Somatoform and Factitious Disorders. Edited by Phillips KA. Washington, DC, American Psychiatric Publishing, 2001, pp 129–166

Fisher GC, Mitchell I: Is Munchausen syndrome by proxy really a syndrome? Arch Dis Child 72:530–534, 1995

Fliege H, Grimm A, Eckhardt-Henn A, et al: Frequency of ICD-10 factitious disorder: survey of senior hospital consultants and physicians in private practice. Psychosomatics 48:60–64, 2007

Folks DG: Munchausen's syndrome and other factitious disorders. Neurol Clin 13:267–281, 1995

Ford CV: The somatizing disorders. Psychosomatics 27:327–331, 335–337, 1986

Ford CV: Ethical and legal issues in factitious disorders: an overview, in The Spectrum of Factitious Disorders. Edited by Feldman MD, Eisendrath SJ. Washington, DC, American Psychiatric Press, 1996a, pp 51–63

Ford CV: Lies! Lies!! Lies!!! The Psychology of Deceit. Washington, DC, American Psychiatric Press, 1996b

Freyberger HJ, Schneider W: Diagnosis and classification of factitious disorder with operational diagnostic systems. Psychother Psychosom 62:27–29, 1994

Freyberger H, Nordmeyer JP, Freyberger HJ, et al: Patients suffering from factitious disorders in the clinico-psychosomatic consultation liaison service: psychodynamic processes, psychotherapeutic initial care and clinico-interdisciplinary cooperation. Psychother Psychosom 62:108–122, 1994

Gacono CB, Meloy JR, Sheppard K, et al: A clinical investigation of malingering and psychopathy in hospitalized insanity acquittees. Bull Am Acad Psychiatry Law 23:387–397, 1995

Gavin H: On Feigned and Factitious Diseases, Chiefly of Soldiers and Seamen, on the Means Used to Simulate or Produce Them, and on the Best Mode of Discovering Imposters: Being the Prize Essay in the Class of Military Surgery, in the University of Edinburgh, Session, 1835–6, With Additions. London, England, John Churchill Princess Street Soho, 1843

Gielder U: Factitious disease in the field of dermatology. Psychother Psychosom 62:48–55, 1994

Gold PB, Frueh BC: Compensation-seeking and extreme exaggeration of psychopathology among combat veterans evaluated for posttraumatic stress disorder. J Nerv Ment Dis 187:680–684, 1999

Gorman WF, Winograd M: Crossing the border from Munchausen to malingering. J Fla Med Assoc 75:147–150, 1988

Gregory J: Sickened: The Memoir of a Munchausen by Proxy Childhood. New York, Bantam, 2004

Guy LS, Miller HA: Screening for malingered psychopathology in a correctional setting: utility of the Miller-Forensic Assessment of Symptoms Test (M-FAST). Crim Justice Behav 31:695–716, 2004

Guziec J, Lazarus A, Harding JJ: Case of a 29-year-old nurse with factitious disorder: the utility of psychiatric intervention on a general medical floor. Gen Hosp Psychiatry 16:47–53, 1994

Han S: Social rehabilitation of ex-malingerers from prison. Int Med J 4:73–75, 1997

Hardie T, Reed A: Pseudologia fantastica, factitious disorder and impostership: a deception syndrome. Med Sci Law 38:198–201, 1998

Hare RD: The Hare Psychopathy Checklist—Revised. Toronto, ON, Multi-Health System, 1991

Harrington WZ, Jackimczyk KC, Seligson RA: Thiopental-facilitated interview in respiratory Munchausen's syndrome. Ann Emerg Med 19:941–942, 1990

Hayes JS, Hale DB, Gouvier WD: Malingering detection in a mentally retarded forensic population. Appl Neuropsychol 5:33–36, 1998

Hirsch M: The body as a transitional object. Psychother Psychosom 62:78–81, 1994

Houck CA: Medicolegal aspects of factitious disorder. Psychiatr Med 10:105–116, 1992

Ifudo O, Friedman EA: Kidney-related Munchausen's syndrome and the Red Baron (letter). N Engl J Med 328:61, 1993

Ifudo O, Kolasinski SL, Friedman EA: Brief report: kidney-related Munchausen's syndrome. N Engl J Med 327:388–389, 1992

Inbau FE, Reid JE: Criminal Interrogation and Confessions. Baltimore, MD, Williams & Wilkins, 1967

Jackson RL, Rogers R, Sewell KW: Forensic applications of the Miller Forensic Assessment of Symptoms Test (MFAST): screening for feigned disorders in competency to stand trial evaluations. Law Hum Behav 29:199–210, 2005

Jani S, White M, Rosenberg LA, et al: Munchausen syndrome by proxy. Int J Psychiatry Med 22:343–349, 1992

Janofsky JS: The Munchausen syndrome in civil forensic psychiatry. Bull Am Acad Psychiatry Law 22:489–497, 1994

Jureidini J: Obstetric factitious disorder and Munchausen syndrome by proxy. J Nerv Ment Dis 181:135–137, 1993

Kahan B, Yorker BC: Munchausen syndrome by proxy: clinical review and legal issues. Behav Sci Law 9:73–83, 1991

Kalivas J: Malingering versus factitious disorder (letter). Am J Psychiatry 153:1108, 1996

Kasdan ML, Soergel TM, Johnson AL, et al: Expanded profile of the SHAFT syndrome. J Hand Surg (Am) 23:26–31, 1998

Khan I, Fayaz I, Ridgley J, et al: Factitious clock drawing and constructional apraxia. J Neurol Neurosurg Psychiatry 68:106–107, 2000

Koo J, Gambla C, Fried R: Pseudopsychodermatological disease. Dermatol Clin 14:525–530, 1996

Kucharski LT, Johnsen D, Procell S: The utility of the MMPI-2 infrequency psychopathology F(p) and the revised infrequency psychopathology scales in the detection of malingering. Am J Forensic Psychol 22:33–40, 2004

Kucharski LT, Duncan S, Egan SS, et al: Psychopathy and malingering of psychiatric disorder in criminal defendants. Behav Sci Law 24:633–644, 2006

Kucharski LT, Toomey JP, Fila K, et al: Detection of malingering of psychiatric disorder with the Personality Assessment Inventory: an investigation of criminal defendants. J Pers Assess 88:25–32, 2007

Lasher LJ, Sheridan MS: Munchausen by Proxy: Identification, Intervention, and Case Management. Binghamton, NY, Haworth Press, 2004

Lawrie SM, Goodwin G, Masterton G: Munchausen's syndrome and organic brain disorder. Br J Psychiatry 162:545–549, 1993

Levin AV, Sheridan MS (eds): Munchausen Syndrome by Proxy: Issues in Diagnosis and Treatment. New York, Lexington Books, 1995

Lewis JL, Simcox AM, Berry D: Screening for feigned psychiatric symptoms in a forensic sample by using the MMPI-2 and the Structured Inventory of Malingered Symptomatology. Psychol Assess 14:170–176, 2002

Libow J: Munchausen by proxy victims in adulthood: a first look. Child Abuse Negl 19:1131–1142, 1995

Libow J: Child and adolescent illness falsification. Pediatrics 105:336–342, 2000

Liebson E, White R, Albert M: Cognitive inconsistencies in abnormal illness behavior and neurologic disease. J Nerv Ment Dis 184:122–125, 1996

Lilienfeld SO, Andrews BP: Development and preliminary validation of a self-report measure of psychopathic personality traits in noncriminal populations. J Pers Assess 66:488–524, 1996

Linde P: A bewitching case of factitious disorder in Zimbabwe. Gen Hosp Psychiatry 18:440–443, 1996

Lu PH, Boone KB: Suspect cognitive symptoms in a 9-year-old child: malingering by proxy? Clin Neuropsychol 16:90–96, 2002

Ludwigs U, Ruiz H, Isaksson H, et al: Factitious disorder presenting with acute cardiovascular symptoms. J Intern Med 236:685–690, 1994

McClure RJ, Davis PM, Meadow SR, et al: Epidemiology of Munchausen syndrome by proxy, nonaccidental poisoning, and nonaccidental suffocation. Arch Dis Child 75:57–61, 1996

Meadow R: Munchausen syndrome by proxy: the hinterland of child abuse. Lancet 2(8033):343–345, 1977

Meadow R: Munchausen syndrome by proxy. Arch Dis Child 57:92–98, 1982

Meadow R: False allegations of abuse and Munchausen syndrome by proxy. Arch Dis Child 68:444–447, 1993

Meadow R: What is, and what is not, "Munchausen syndrome by proxy?" Arch Dis Child 72:534–538, 1995

Meadow SR: Munchausen syndrome by proxy. Med Leg J 63:89–104, 1995

Milani M: Problematic client-animal relationships: Munchausen by proxy. Can Vet J 47:1161–1164, 2006

Miller H: Miller Forensic Assessment of Symptoms Test (MFAST) Professional Manual. Odessa, FL, Psychological Assessment Resources, 2001

Mizuta I, Fukunaga T, Sato H, et al: A case report of comorbid eating disorder and factitious disorder. Psychiatry Clin Neurosci 54:603–606, 2000

Morey LC: Personality Assessment Inventory (PAI). Tampa, FL, Psychological Assessment Resources, 1991

Morley CJ: Practical concerns about the diagnosis of Munchausen syndrome by proxy. Arch Dis Child 72:528–529, 1995

Mountz JM, Parker PE, Liu HG, et al: Tc-99m HMPAO brain SPECT scanning in Munchausen syndrome. J Psychiatry Neurosci 21:49–52, 1996

Nadelson T: The Munchausen spectrum: borderline character features. Gen Hosp Psychiatry 1:11–17, 1979

Newmark N, Adityanjee, Kay J: Pseudologia fantastica and factitious disorder: review of the literature and a case report. Compr Psychiatry 40:89–95, 1999

Nordmeyer JP: An internist's view of patients with factitious disorders and factitious clinical symptomatology. Psychother Psychosom 62:30–40, 1994

Ostfeld BM, Feldman MD: Factitious disorder by proxy: clinical features, detection, and management, in The Spectrum of Factitious Disorders. Edited by Feldman MD, Eisendrath SJ. Washington, DC, American Psychiatric Press, 1996, pp 83–108

Overholser JC: Differential diagnosis of malingering and factitious disorder with physical symptoms. Special issue: malingering and deception—an update. Behav Sci Law 8:55–65, 1990

Paar GH: Factitious disorders in the field of surgery. Psychother Psychosom 62:41–47, 1994

Pankratz L, Erickson RC: Two views of malingering. Clin Neuropsychol 4:379–389, 1990

Pankratz L, Lezak MD: Cerebral dysfunction in the Munchausen syndrome. Hillside J Clin Psychiatry 9:195–206, 1987

Parker PE: A case report of Munchausen syndrome with mixed psychological features. Psychosomatics 34:360–364, 1993

Parnell TF, Day DO: Munchausen by Proxy Syndrome: Misunderstood Child Abuse. Thousand Oaks, CA, Sage Publications, 1998

Parsons T: The Social System. Glencoe, IL, Free Press, 1951

Plassmann R: Inpatient and outpatient long-term psychotherapy of patients suffering from factitious disorder. Psychother Psychosom 62:96–107, 1994a

Plassmann R: Munchausen syndromes and factitious diseases. Psychother Psychosom 62:7–26, 1994b

Plassmann R: Structural disturbances in the body self. Psychother Psychosom 62:91–95, 1994c

Popli AP, Masand PS, Dewan MJ: Factitious disorders with psychological symptoms. J Clin Psychiatry 53:315–318, 1992

Powell R, Boast N: Resource implications of Munchausen's Syndrome (letter). Br J Psychiatry 162:848, 1993

Poythress NG, Edens JF, Watkins MM: The relationship between psychopathic personality features and malingering symptoms of major mental illness. Law Hum Behav 25:567–582, 2001

Rand DC: Comprehensive psychosocial assessment in factitious disorder by proxy, in The Spectrum of Factitious Disorders. Edited by Feldman MD, Eisendrath SJ. Washington, DC, American Psychiatric Press, 1996, pp 109–133

Rand DC, Feldman MD: Misdiagnosis of Munchausen syndrome by proxy: a literature review and four new cases (review). Harv Rev Psychiatry 7:94–101, 1999

Raspe RE: Baron von Munchausen's narrative of his marvellous travels and campaigns in Russia. Oxford, UK, Smith (anonymously published), 1785

Raspe RE: Gulliver Revived, Containing Singular Travels, Campaigns, Voyages and Adventures in Russia, Iceland, Turkey, Egypt, Gibraltar, up the Mediterranean, and on the Atlantic Ocean: Also, an account of a Voyage Into the Moon, with Many Extraordinary Particulars Relative to the Cooking Animal in That Planet, Which Are Here Called the Human Species, 4th Edition. Norfolk, VA, John M'Lean, 1787

Reich P, Gottfried LA: Factitious disorders in a teaching hospital. Ann Intern Med 99:240–247, 1983

Resnick PJ: The detection of malingered mental illness. Behav Sci Law 2:20–38, 1984

Resnick PJ: Malingered psychosis, in Clinical Assessment of Malingering and Deception, 2nd Edition. Edited by Rogers R. New York, Guilford, 1997, pp 47–67

Resnick PJ: The clinical assessment of malingered mental illness, in Annual Board Review Course Syllabus. Bloomfield, CT, American Academy of Psychiatry and the Law, 2000, pp 842–866

Rogers R: Conducting Insanity Evaluations. New York, Van Nostrand Reinhold, 1986

Rogers R: Development of a new classificatory model of malingering. Bull Am Acad Psychiatry Law 18:323–333, 1990a

Rogers R: Models of feigned mental illness. Prof Psychol Res Pr 21:182–188, 1990b

Rogers R: Introduction, in Clinical Assessment of Malingering and Deception, 2nd Edition. Edited by Rogers R. New York, Guilford, 1997, pp 1–9

Rogers R: Diagnostic, explanatory, and detection models of Munchausen by proxy: extrapolations from malingering and deception. Child Abuse Negl 28:225–238, 2004

Rogers R, Bagby RM, Rector N: Diagnostic legitimacy of factitious disorder with psychological symptoms. Am J Psychiatry 146:1312–1314, 1989

Rogers R, Bagby RM, Dickens SE: Structured Interview of Reported Symptoms (SIRS) and professional manual. Odessa, FL, Psychological Assessment Resources, 1992

Rogers R, Harrell EH, Liff CD: Feigning neuropsychological impairment: a critical review of methodological and clinical considerations. Clin Psychol Rev 13:255–274, 1993

Rogers R, Sewell KW, Goldstein AM: Explanatory models of malingering: a prototypical analysis. Law Hum Behav 18:543–552, 1994a

Rogers R, Sewell KW, Salekin RT: A meta-analysis of malingering on the MMPI-2. Assessment 1:227–237, 1994b

Rogers R, Sewell KW, Morey LC, et al: Detection of feigned mental disorders on the Personality Assessment Inventory: a discriminant analysis. J Pers Assess 67:629–640, 1996

Rogers R, Salekin RT, Sewell KW, et al: A comparison of forensic and nonforensic malingerers: a prototypical analysis of explanatory models. Law Hum Behav 22:353–367, 1998a

Rogers R, Sewell KW, Cruise KR: The PAI and feigning: a cautionary note on its use in forensic-correctional settings. Assessment 5:399–405, 1998b

Rogers R, Jackson RL, Kaminski PL: Factitious psychological disorders: the overlooked response style in forensic evaluations. Journal of Forensic Psychology Practice 5:21–41, 2005

Rosenberg DA: Web of deceit: a literature review of Munchausen syndrome by proxy. Child Abuse Negl 11:547–563, 1987

Rosenhan DL: On being sane in insane places, in Down to Earth Sociology: Introductory Readings, 11th Edition. Edited by Henslin JA. New York, Free Press, 2001, pp 278–289

Rothchild E: Fictitious twins, factitious illness. Psychiatry 57:326–332, 1994

Roy M, Roy A: Factitious hypoglycemia: an 11-year follow-up. Psychosomatics 36:64–65, 1995

Samuels MP, McClaughlin W, Jacobson RR, et al: Fourteen cases of imposed upper airway obstruction. Arch Dis Child 67:162–170, 1992

Schreier HA: The perversion of mothering: Munchausen syndrome by proxy. Bull Menninger Clin 56:421–437, 1992

Schreier HA: Repeated false allegations of sexual abuse presenting to sheriffs: when is it Munchausen by proxy? Child Abuse Negl 20:985–991, 1996

Schreier H: Factitious disorder by proxy in which the presenting problem is behavioral or psychiatric. J Am Acad Child Adolesc Psychiatry 39:668–670, 2000

Schreier HA, Libow JA: Hurting for Love: Munchausen by Proxy Syndrome. New York, Guilford, 1993a

Schreier HA, Libow JA: Munchausen syndrome by proxy: diagnosis and prevalence. Am J Orthopsychiatry 63:318–321, 1993b

Schreier HA, Libow JA: Munchausen by proxy syndrome: a clinical fable for our times. J Am Acad Child Adolesc Psychiatry 33:904–905, 1994

Schreier HA, Libow JA: Munchausen by proxy: the deadly game. Saturday Evening Post 268:40–41, 1996

Schwarz K, Harding R, Harrington D, et al: Hospital management of a patient with intractable factitious disorder. Psychosomatics 34:265–267, 1993

Sheridan MS: The deceit continues: an updated literature review of Munchausen syndrome by proxy. Child Abuse Negl 27:431–451, 2003

Sigal M, Gelkopf M, Levertov G: Medical and legal aspects of the Munchausen by proxy perpetrator. Med Law 9:739–749, 1990

Smith GP, Borum R: Detection of malingering in a forensic sample: a study of the M Test. J Psychiatry Law 20:505–514, 1992

Smith GP, Burger GK: Detection of malingering: validation of the Structured Inventory of Malingered Symptomatology (SIMS). J Am Acad Psychiatry Law 25:183–189, 1997

Solyom C, Solyom L: A treatment program for functional paraplegia/Munchausen syndrome. J Behav Ther Exp Psychiatry 21:225–230, 1990

Songer DA: Factitious AIDS: a case reported and literature review. Psychosomatics 36:406–411, 1995

Spiro HR: Chronic factitious illness: Munchausen's syndrome. Arch Gen Psychiatry 18:569–579, 1968

Spivak H, Rodin G, Sutherland A: The psychology of factitious disorders: a reconsideration. Psychosomatics 35:25–34, 1994

Stotland NL: Munchausen syndrome. JAMA 261:447, 1989

Stutts JT, Hickey SE, Kasdan ML: Malingering by proxy: a form of pediatric condition falsification. J Dev Behav Pediatr 24:276–278, 2003

Sutherland AJ, Rodin GM: Factitious disorders in a general hospital setting: clinical features and a review of the literature. Psychosomatics 31:392–399, 1990

Szajnberg NM, Moilanen I, Kanerva A, et al: Munchausen-by-proxy syndrome: countertransference as a diagnostic tool. Bull Menninger Clin 60:229–237, 1996

Teasell RW, Shapiro AP: Strategic-behavioral intervention in the treatment of chronic nonorganic motor disorders. Am J Phys Med Rehabil 73:44–50, 1994

Tombaugh TN: Test of Memory Malingering (TOMM). New York, Multi-Health Systems, 1996

Topazian M, Binder HJ: Factitious diarrhea detected by measurement of stool osmolality. N Engl J Med 330:1418–1419, 1994

Toth EL, Baggaley A: Coexistence of Munchausen's syndrome and multiple personality disorder: detailed report of a case and theoretical discussion. Psychiatry 54:176–186, 1991

Turner MA: Factitious disorders: reformulating the DSM-IV criteria. Psychosomatics 47:23–32, 2006

Tyrer P, Babidge N, Emmanuel J, et al: Instrumental psychosis: the Good Soldier Svejk syndrome. J R Soc Med 94:22–25, 2001

Vitacco JM, Rogers R: Assessment of malingering in correctional settings, in Handbook of Correctional Mental Health. Edited by Scott CL, Gerbasi JB. Washington, DC, American Psychiatric Publishing, 2005, pp 133–153

Wallach J: Laboratory diagnosis of factitious disorders. Arch Intern Med 154:1690–1696, 1994

Willenberg H: Countertransference in factitious disorder. Psychother Psychosom 62:129–134, 1994

Witztum E, Grinshpoon A, Margolin J, et al: The erroneous diagnosis of malingering in a military setting. Mil Med 161:225–229, 1996

World Health Organization: The ICD-10 Classification of Mental and Behavioral Disorders. Geneva, Switzerland, World Health Organization, 1992

Yang Y, Raine A, Lencz T, et al: Prefrontal white matter in pathological liars. Br J Psychiatry 187:320–325, 2005

Yates BD, Nordquist CR, Schultz-Ross RA: Feigned psychiatric symptoms in the emergency room. Psychiatr Serv 47:998–1000, 1996

Yorker BC: Hospital epidemics of factitious disorder by proxy, in The Spectrum of Factitious Disorders. Edited by Feldman MD, Eisendrath SJ. Washington, DC, American Psychiatric Press, 1996a, pp 157–174

Yorker BC: Legal issues in factitious disorder by proxy, in The Spectrum of Factitious Disorders. Edited by Feldman MD, Eisendrath SJ. Washington, DC, American Psychiatric Press, 1996b, pp 135–156

Yorker BC, Kahan BB: Munchausen's syndrome by proxy as a form of child abuse. Arch Psychiatr Nurs 4:313–318, 1990

Zimmerman JG, Hussian RA, Tintner R, et al: Factitious Disorder in a geriatric patient. Clin Gerontol 11:3–11, 1991

Ziv I, Djaldetti R, Zoldan Y, et al: Diagnosis of "nonorganic" limb paresis by a novel objective motor assessment: the quantitative Hoover's test. J Neurol 245:797–802, 1998

15

DISSOCIATIVE DISORDERS

José R. Maldonado, M.D., F.A.P.M., F.A.C.F.E.
David Spiegel, M.D.

The dissociative disorders involve a disturbance in the integrated organization of identity, memory, perception, or consciousness. Events normally experienced on a smooth continuum are isolated from the other mental processes with which they would ordinarily be associated. This discontinuity results in a variety of dissociative disorders depending on the primary cognitive process affected. When memories are poorly integrated, the resulting disorder is *dissociative amnesia*. Fragmentation of identity results in *dissociative fugue* or *dissociative identity disorder* (DID; formerly multiple personality disorder). Disordered perception yields *depersonalization disorder*. Dissociation of aspects of consciousness produces *acute stress disorder* and various dissociative trance and possession states (Table 15–1).

These dissociative disorders are a disturbance more in the organization or structure of mental contents than in the contents themselves. Memories in dissociative amnesia are not so much distorted or bizarre as they are segregated from one another. The identity temporarily lost in dissociative fugue, or the aspects of the self that are fragmented in DID, are two-dimensional aspects of an overall personality structure. In this sense, it has been said that patients with DID suffer not from having more than one personality but rather from having less than one personality. The problem is the failure of integration, the decontextualization of information, rather than the contents of the

TABLE 15–1. DSM-IV-TR dissociative disorders
Dissociative amnesia (300.12)
Dissociative fugue (300.13)
Dissociative identity disorder (300.14; formerly multiple personality disorder)
Depersonalization disorder (300.6)
Dissociative disorder not otherwise specified (300.15)
Related disorders
Dissociative trance disorder
Acute stress disorder (308.3)

fragments. In summary, all types of dissociative disorders have in common a lack of immediate access to the entire personality structure or mental content in one form or another.

The dissociative disorders have a long history in classical psychopathology but until recently have been largely ignored. Nonetheless, the phenomena are sufficiently persistent and interesting that they have elicited growing attention from both professionals and the public. The dissociative disorders remain an area of psychopathology for which the best treatment is psychotherapy (Maldonado et al. 2000). As mental disorders, they have much to teach us about the way humans adapt to traumatic stress and about information processing in the brain.

Development of the Concept

Jean Martin Charcot (1890), the well-known French neurologist, became interested in the dissociative symptoms experienced by some of his patients who had unusual neurological symptoms. He discovered that hypnosis could reproduce and reverse some of the deficits manifested by his patients. Charcot believed that even a normal process such as hypnosis, which could be used to access dissociated mental contents, was itself evidence of pathology (*un etat nerveux artificiel ou experimentale*, "an artificial or experimental nervous state"). He thought, for example, that once patients were cured of hysteria, they would no longer be hypnotizable. We now know this not to be the case because many "normal" individuals are highly hypnotizable (Hilgard 1965; H. Spiegel and Spiegel 2004).

Nevertheless, the French physician and psychologist Pierre Janet (1920) is credited with the initial description of dissociation as a disorder, a *desagregation mentale*. The term *desagregation* carries with it a slightly different nuance than does the English translation (i.e., dissociation) because it implies a separation of certain mental contents from their general tendency to aggregate or be processed together. Janet (1920, p. 332) described hysteria as "a malady of the personal synthesis." He viewed dissociation as a purely pathological process. Janet's theory of hysteria was based on three psychological models. First, in the hierarchical model, Janet related hysterical symptoms to the activities within the lower strata of mental hierarchy (*automatisms psychologiques*), which were seen during somnambulism. The second model was based on the concept of a psychological system, hypothetically composed of ideas, images, feelings, sensations, and movements. Thus, the dissociation of psychological functions was fundamental to the mechanism of hysteria in which the loss of integration was thought to engender fixed ideas (*ideas fixes*) and to lead to the development of a system that was isolated from the whole personality system. Finally, the third model, the economic model, explained various psychiatric disorders as a loss of equilibration between psychological force and psychological tension. In this model, an unexpected emotional experience causes a consumption of reserved psychological force, which is followed by exhaustion, leading

to or associated with hysterical symptoms. Janet was probably the first to study psychological trauma as a principal cause of dissociation.

The dissociative disorders might have been studied more intensively during the twentieth century had not Janet's and Charcot's work been so thoroughly eclipsed by the psychoanalytic approach pioneered by Freud. Freud learned the use of hypnotic techniques from Charcot and applied them in the treatment of some of his first cases. In his early writings with Breuer, Freud began an exploration of dissociative phenomena, similar to those that Janet had described earlier. Cases in the *Studies on Hysteria* (Breuer and Freud 1893–1895/1955), such as that of Anna O., clearly involved dissociative phenomena. Indeed, Anna O. had many symptoms suggestive of DID (Nakdimen 1988). However, Breuer and Freud reformulated the role of the capacity to dissociate through the concept of "hypnoid states, rather than the mechanism of dissociation." Indeed, they thought that dissociative symptoms should be attributed to the capacity to enter these hypnoid states rather than the reverse (Breuer and Freud 1893–1895/1955). However, in an effort to develop a more general theory of human psychopathology, Freud went on to study other kinds of patients, such as those with "obsessive compulsive neurosis" (i.e., obsessive-compulsive disorder) and schizophrenia. This shift in the patient population studied may well account for much of Freud's waning interest in dissociation as a defense and his increasing interest in repression as a more general model for motivated forgetting in unconscious processes. Much has recently been made of the fact that Freud abandoned the seduction theory of the etiology of the neuroses. What may have happened is that he abandoned the study of individuals for whom trauma plausibly could be applied as an etiological factor in their psychiatric disorder.

Discussion of dissociation and its relation to trauma all but disappeared after Janet. However, during World War II and the postwar period, some psychiatrists began to pay attention to two emerging phenomena: 1) a high incidence of "traumatic neurosis" among combatants and 2) dissociative symptoms such as fugue and amnesia observed among ex-inmates of concentration camps. In the 1970s, interest in dissociation and trauma was revived in different areas: the feminist movement was linked with concerns about child sexual abuse, public curiosity about multiple personalities was heightened by books and movies, and posttraumatic stress disorder (PTSD) was recognized among Vietnam War veterans. Hilgard (1977) developed a neodissociation theory designed to revive interest in Janetian psychology and psychopathology. Hilgard postulated a mental structure with divisions that were horizontal rather than vertical, which had characterized Freud's archaeological model. Unlike Freud's system, Hilgard's model would allow for immediate access to consciousness of any of a variety of warded-off memories. In the dynamic unconscious model, repressed memories must first go through a process of transformation as they are accessed and lifted from the depths of the unconscious. In Hilgard's model, amnesia is a crucial mediating mechanism that provides the barriers that divide one set of mental contents from another. Thus, the flexible and reversible use of amnesia is a key defensive tool, whereas the reversal of amnesia is an important therapeutic tool.

Repression as a general model for keeping information out of conscious awareness differs from dissociation in six important ways (Table 15–2):

1. The organizational structure of mental contents in dissociation is thought of as horizontal, with subunits of information divided from one another but equally available to consciousness (Hilgard 1977). Repressed information, on the other hand, is presumed to be stored in an archaeological manner, at various depths, and therefore different components are not equally accessible (Freud 1923/1961).
2. Subunits of information are presumed to be divided by amnesic barriers in dissociation, whereas dynamic conflict, or motivated forgetting, is the mechanism underlying repression.
3. The information kept out of awareness in dissociation is often for a discrete and sharply delimited time, usually for a traumatic experience, whereas repressed information may be for a variety of experiences, fears, or wishes scattered across time. Dissociation is often elicited as a defense, especially af-

ter episodes of physical trauma, whereas repression is a response to warded-off fears and wishes or in response to other dynamic conflicts.
4. Dissociated information is stored in a discrete and untransformed manner, whereas repressed information is usually disguised and fragmented. Even when repressed information becomes available to consciousness, its meaning is hidden (e.g., in dreams, slips of the tongue).
5. Retrieval of dissociated information often can be direct. Techniques such as hypnosis can be used to access warded-off memories. In contrast, uncovering of repressed information often requires repeated recall trials through intense questioning, psychotherapy, or psychoanalysis with subsequent interpretation (i.e., of dreams).
6. The focus of psychotherapy for dissociation is integration, via control of access to dissociated states and working through of traumatic memories. The classical psychotherapy for repression involves interpretation, including working through of the transference.

There is debate about whether dissociation is a subtype of repression or vice versa. Such a dispute is probably not resolvable, but what has become clear in recent years is that given the complexity of human information processing, the accomplishment of a sense of mental unity is an achievement, not a given (Kihlstrom and Hoyt 1990; D. Spiegel 1990a). What is remarkable is not that dissociative disorders occur but rather that they do not occur more often, given the fact that information processing comprises a variety of reasonably autonomous subsystems involving perception, memory storage and retrieval, intention, and action (Baars 1988; Cohen and Servan-Schreiber 1992a, 1992b; Rumelhart and McClelland 1986; D. Spiegel 1991c).

TABLE 15–2. Differences between dissociation and repression

	Dissociation	Repression
Organizational structure	Horizontal	Vertical
Barriers	Amnesia	Dynamic conflict
Etiology	Trauma	Developmental conflict over unacceptable wishes
Contents	Untransformed: traumatic memories	Disguised primary process: dreams, slips
Means of access	Hypnosis	Interpretation
Psychotherapy	Access, control, and work through traumatic memories	Interpretation, transference

Models and Mechanisms of Dissociation

Dissociation and Information Processing

Modern information processing–based theories, including connectionist and parallel distributed processing (PDP) models (Rumelhart and McClelland 1986), take a bottom-up rather than a top-down approach to cognitive organization. Traditional models emphasize a superordinate organization in which broad categories of information structure the processing of specific examples. In the more Aristotelian PDP models, subunits or neural nets process information through computation of co-occurrence of input stimuli. The activation patterns in these neural nets allow for category recognition. For example, the category "kitchen" is built up from the frequent co-occurrence of "appliances of a certain type" rather than being the basis for recognizing its components. The output of one set of nets becomes the input to another, thereby gradually building up integrated and complex patterns of activation and inhibition. Such bottom-up processing models have the advantage of accounting for the processing of vast amounts of information and for the human ability to recognize patterns on the basis of approximate information. However, such models make the classification and integration of information problematic. In PDP models, it is theoretically likely that failures in integration of mental contents will occur. Indeed, attempts have been made to model psychopathology based on difficulties in neural net information processing, for example, in schizophrenia and bipolar disorder (Hoffman 1987), as well as in dissociative disorders (D. Li and Spiegel 1992). The idea is that when a net runs into difficulty in balancing the processing of input information (a model for traumatic input), it is more likely to have difficulty achieving a unified and balanced output. Such neural nets tend to fall into a "dissociated" situation in which they move in one direction or another but cannot reach an optimal balanced solution, and therefore they are unable to process smoothly all of the incoming information.

Such bottom-up information processing systems have more the problems of a democracy than a monarchy. The difficulty is achieving unity of representation and action. In such models, consciousness is viewed as analogous to the rostrum in a legislature where competing subunits vie for attention and the ability to broadcast their input to the system as a whole

(Baars 1988). Indeed, such information processing models have now become of considerable interest in cognitive psychology (Kihlstrom 1987), and modern memory research, as mentioned earlier in this chapter, provides other examples of structural dissociation of mental elements (Schacter 1996).

A study by Williams et al. (2006) using functional magnetic resonance imaging (fMRI) found that many of the same regions of the human brain are activated during conscious attention to signals of fear and in the absence of awareness for these signals. Through fMRI studies with connectivity analysis in healthy human subjects, they were able to demonstrate that level of awareness for signals of fear depends on mode of functional connectivity in amygdala pathways rather than discrete patterns of activation in these pathways. Awareness for fear relied on negative connectivity within both cortical and subcortical pathways to the amygdala, suggesting that reentrant feedback may be necessary to afford such awareness. In contrast, responses to fear in the absence of awareness were supported by positive connections in a direct subcortical pathway to the amygdala, consistent with the view that excitatory feed-forward connections along this pathway may be sufficient for automatic responses to "unseen" fear. These findings may explain how "dissociated or unknown" memory content may exert its effects eliciting fear, panic or triggering altered/dissociated states in victims of trauma.

From a more clinical perspective, dissociation may be explained by one of three proposed models or combinations of these: 1) the neurological model, which suggests that some underlying neurological process, such as hemispheric disconnection or epilepsy, plays a role in promoting dissociative symptoms; 2) the role enactment model or social role demand theory, which suggests that the symptoms are an artificial social construct rather than a true psychiatric disorder; and 3) the autohypnotic model, a theory that recognizes and reconciles the connection between traumatic events, dissociative experiences, and hypnotizability. These models have been described at length elsewhere (Maldonado 2007) and will not be discussed here.

Dissociation and Memory Systems

Modern research on memory shows that there are at least two broad categories of memory, variously described as *explicit* and *implicit* (Schacter 1992; Squire 1992) or *episodic* and *semantic* (Tulving 1983). These two memory systems serve different functions. *Explicit* (or *episodic*) memory involves recall of personal experience identified with the self (e.g., "I was at the ball game last week"). *Implicit* (or *semantic*) memory involves the execution of routine operations, such as riding a bicycle or typing. Such operations may be carried out with a high degree of proficiency with little conscious awareness of either their current execution or the learning episodes on which the skill is based. Indeed, these two types of memory may well have different anatomical localizations: the limbic system, especially the hippocampal formation, and mammillary bodies for episodic memory; and the basal ganglia and cortex for procedural (or semantic) memory (Mishkin 1987; Squire 1992).

Indeed, the distinction between these two types of memory may account for certain dissociative phenomena (D. Spiegel et al. 1993). The automaticity observed in certain dissociative disorders may be a reflection of the separation of self-identification in certain kinds of explicit memory from routine activity in implicit or semantic memory. It is thus not at all foreign to our mental processing to act in an automatic way devoid of explicit self-identification. Were it necessary for us to retrieve explicit memories of how and when we learned all of the activities we are required to perform, it is highly unlikely that we would be able to function with anything like the degree of efficiency we have. Many athletes report focusing on some detail of the event and allowing their bodies to do what they need to, when in fact they are performing extremely well. There is thus a fundamental model in memory research for the dissociation between identity and performance that may well find its pathological reflection in disorders such as dissociative amnesia, fugue, and identity disorder.

Meares (1999) suggested that traumatic memories are represented in a way that is qualitatively different from nontraumatic memories. His argument depends on a concept of self that is double, involving mental life and the individual's own reflection on it. If trauma is seen as causing an uncoupling, or de-doubling, of consciousness, then the traumatic diminishment of the subject–object distinction in psychic life will have several effects. First, it will change the form of conscious awareness to a state that is focused on the present and on immediate stimuli. Second, the memory system in which the traumatic events are recorded will be nonepisodic, thus lacking the reflective component, making it unconscious. Third, the traumatized–traumatizer dyad will be represented not as two persons in a relationship but more as a nearly fused unit. This fused representation will not be integrated into the system of self as the stream of consciousness but is

more likely to remain relatively sequestered. Finally, in an "uncoupled" state, the interpretation of the "meaning" of the traumatic event is impaired, and its construction will be determined by affect.

Elzinga et al. (2007) used fMRI to assess the working memory in dissociative disorder patients during performance of a parametric, verbal working-memory task and compared them with healthy control subjects. Imaging data (fMRI) showed that both groups activated brain regions typically involved in working memory (i.e., anterior, dorsolateral and ventrolateral prefrontal cortex, and parietal cortex) but the dissociative disorder patients showed more activation in these areas, particularly in the left anterior prefrontal cortex, dorsolateral prefrontal cortex, and parietal cortex. As expected given these findings, dissociative disorder patients also made fewer errors with increasing task load compared with healthy control subjects. This study replicated findings of previous studies in individuals with high (but nonpathological) levels of dissociation, thus suggesting that trait dissociation is associated with enhanced working-memory capacities. Similarly, these differences in working memory may help distinguish dissociative disorder patients from patients with PTSD, who generally show impaired working memory.

Dissociation and Trauma

An important development in the modern understanding of dissociative disorders is the exploration of the link between trauma and dissociation (D. Spiegel and Cardeña 1991). Trauma can be understood as the experience of being made into an object or a thing, the victim of someone else's rage or of nature's indifference. It is the ultimate experience of helplessness and loss of control over one's own body. There is growing clinical and some empirical evidence that dissociation may occur especially as a defense during trauma—an attempt to maintain mental control at the very moment when physical control has been lost (Bremner and Brett 1997; Butler et al. 1996; Eriksson and Lundin 1996; Kluft 1984a, 1984c; Koopman et al. 1995, 1996; Putnam 1985; D. Spiegel 1984; D. Spiegel et al. 1988; van der Hart et al. 2005b). One patient with DID reported "going to a mountain meadow full of wildflowers" when she was being sexually assaulted by her drunken father. She would concentrate on how pleasant and beautiful this imaginary scene was as a way of detaching herself from the immediate experience of terror, pain, and helplessness. Such individuals often report seeking comfort from imaginary playmates or imagined protectors or absorbing themselves in some perceptual distraction, such as the pattern of the wallpaper. Many rape victims report floating above their bodies, feeling sorry for the persons being assaulted beneath them. Evidence (Putnam 1993; Terr 1991) indicates that children exposed to multiple traumas are more likely to use dissociative defense mechanisms, which include spontaneous trance episodes and amnesia. In fact, van der Hart et al. (2005b) have postulated that traumatization essentially involves some degree of division or dissociation of psychobiological systems that constitute personality. By this theory, the dissociative parts of the personality avoid traumatic memories and perform functions in daily life, while one or more other parts remain fixated in traumatic experiences and defensive actions. Unfortunately, the dissociated memories may manifest in negative and positive dissociative symptoms that must be distinguished from alterations of consciousness.

As is noted in the discussion on DID later in this chapter, an accumulating literature suggests a connection between a history of physical and sexual abuse in childhood and the development of dissociative symptoms (Chu et al. 1999; Coons 1994; Coons and Milstein 1986; Irwin 1999; Kluft 1984c; Mulder et al. 1998; Sar et al. 1996, 2000; Scroppo et al. 1998; D. Spiegel 1984). When Mulder et al. (1998) examined the relation between childhood sexual abuse, childhood physical abuse, current psychiatric illness, and measures of dissociation in an adult population, they found that 6.3% of the abused population had three or more frequently occurring dissociative symptoms. Among these individuals, the rate of childhood sexual abuse was two and one-half times as high, the rate of physical abuse was five times as high, and the rate of current psychiatric disorder was four times as high as the respective rates for the other subjects. Similarly, a study by Collin-Vézina and Hébert (2005) found that sexual victimization significantly increases the odds of presenting with a clinical level of dissociation and PTSD symptoms by eightfold and fourfold, respectively.

Evidence is accumulating that dissociative symptoms are more prevalent in patients with Axis II disorders such as borderline personality disorder when there has been a history of childhood abuse (Brenner 1996a, 1996b; Brodsky et al. 1995; Chu and Dill 1990; Darves-Bornoz 1997; Herman et al. 1989; Spitzer et al. 2006a). Shearer (1994) studied 62 women diagnosed with borderline personality disorder and found that univariate analyses demonstrated that patients with borderline personality disorder and greater dissociative experience are related to more self-reported traumatic experiences, posttraumatic symptoms, behavioral dyscontrol, self-injurious behavior, and alcohol abuse. Their findings also suggested that scores on the Dissociative Experiences Scale (DES; Bernstein and Putnam 1986) were predicted particularly by adult sexual assault, behavioral dyscontrol, and both sexual and physical abuse in childhood. Spitzer et al. (2006a) administered the DES and the Inventory of Personality Organization (IPO) to 222 patients with borderline personality disorder. They found the Reality Testing subscale of the IPO to be the most important predictor of dissociation and suggested that dissociation may reflect a preoedipal "pretend" mode of psychic functioning. Finally, Watson et al. (2006) examined 139 borderline personality disorder patients and found that their levels of dissociation increased with levels of childhood trauma, supporting the hypothesis that traumatic childhood experiences engender dissociative symptoms later in life. More importantly, these findings suggest that emotional abuse and neglect may be at least as important as physical and sexual abuse in the development of dissociative symptoms.

However, another way to examine the connection between dissociation and trauma is to look at the link between recent trauma and dissociative symptoms (Carlier et al. 1996; Darves-Bornoz 1997; Darves-Bornoz et al. 1999; Eriksson and Lundin 1996; Koopman et al. 1994, 1995, 1996; Marmar et al. 1996; D. Spiegel 1991a, 1991b; D. Spiegel and Cardeña 1991; van der Kolk et al. 1994). If it is indeed the case that trauma seems to elicit dissociation, this should be observable in the immediate aftermath of natural disasters, combat, and physical assault.

The early literature examining responses to trauma provides hints of dissociative symptoms, but these symptoms often were not systematically assessed. In a classic article on the symptomatology and management of acute grief in the aftermath of the Coconut Grove fire, Lindemann (1944/1994) noted that those individuals who had been injured or had lost loved ones but who acted as though little or nothing had happened had an extremely poor prognosis. Indeed, it was the absence of posttraumatic symptoms in this group compared with the agitation, dysphoria, and restlessness that typified most survivors that led Lindemann to formulate the normal process of acute grief.

Researchers have observed that numbing (i.e., loss of responsiveness in the wake of trauma) is a strong predictor of later PTSD symptomatology. For example, Z. Solomon et al. (1988, 1989) observed that psychic numbing accounted for 20% of the variance in later PTSD among Israeli combat soldiers. McFarlane (1986) found that numbing in response to the Ash Wednesday bush fires in Australia was a significant predictor of later posttraumatic symptomatology. Similarly, research on hostages and survivors of other life-threatening events indicates that more than half have experienced feelings of unreality, automatic movements, lack of emotion, and a sense of detachment (Madakasira and O'Brien 1987; Sloan 1988). Symptoms of depersonalization and hyperalertness also frequently occur (Noyes and Slymen 1978–1979). Numbing, loss of interest, and an inability to feel deeply about anything were reported in about a third of the survivors of the Kansas City Hyatt Regency skywalk collapse (Wilkinson 1983) and in a similar proportion of survivors of the North Sea oil rig collapse (Holen 1993). This finding is consistent with studies of survivors of the Loma Prieta earthquake (Cardeña and Spiegel 1993), in which a quarter of a sample of healthy students reported marked depersonalization during and immediately after the earthquake. Koopman et al. (1994) discovered that a combination of acute dissociative and anxiety symptoms was a significant predictor of PTSD 7 months after the Oakland–Berkeley fires.

A study comparing psychiatric patients and a general population sample proposed a model in which alexithymic characteristics contribute to the development of pathological dissociation and stress-related disorders such as PTSD (Grabe et al. 2000). A study by D.M. Johnson et al. (2001) confirmed that peritraumatic dissociation was strongly related to later development of PTSD, dissociation, and depression in patients seeking treatment for childhood sexual abuse. Data analysis indicated that women who experienced penile penetration, believed someone or something else would be killed, or were injured as a result of the abuse had more severe peritraumatic dissociation. Regression analyses indicated that peritraumatic dissociation was the only variable to significantly predict symptom severity across symptom type or disorder. Similarly, Hetzel and McCanne (2005) found that different types of childhood abuse may lead to different adult problems. For example, the combined sexual and physical abuse and sexual abuse only groups reported significantly higher numbers of PTSD symptoms compared with the physical abuse only and the no abuse (control) groups. The combined sexual and physical abuse and physical abuse only groups also reported significantly more adult sexual and physical victimization than the sexual abuse only and control groups. The results suggest that across all four groups, higher levels of peritraumatic dissociation were associated with higher levels of PTSD and adult sexual and physical victimization. The authors concluded that peritraumatic dissociation may have a broad effect on PTSD development and adult victimization.

Finally, a follow-up study of victims of the World Trade Center disaster conducted by Simeon et al. (2005) found that baseline (peritraumatic) dissociation was the strongest predictor of dissociation at follow-up, while baseline posttraumatic stress was the strongest predictor of posttraumatic stress (PTSD) at follow-up. Of the four peritraumatic distress factors generated in the original survey, "loss of control" and "guilt/shame" were significantly related to dissociation and posttraumatic stress at follow-up, while "helplessness/anger" was associated only with posttraumatic stress at follow-up. These studies confirmed previous findings by O'Toole et al. (1999) that having been wounded was not related to lifetime or current PTSD, whereas peritraumatic dissociation was related to all diagnostic components of PTSD. Similarly, Olde et al. (2005) found a 2.1% incidence of PTSD in a population of 140 women following childbirth. In their sample, both perinatal negative emotional reactions and perinatal dissociative reactions predicted PTSD symptoms at 3 months postpartum.

Brauchle (2006) studied 135 psychosocial disaster workers (6 weeks and 6 months after the index catastrophe) using the Acute Stress Disorder Scale (ASDS), the Posttraumatic Stress Diagnostic Scale (PDS) and the German short version of the Dissociative Experience Scale (FDS-20). He found that persistent dissociation and acute stress symptoms were correlated with later acute and chronic PTSD diagnosis. His findings support the notion that persistent dissociation is a main predictor of acute and chronic posttraumatic stress symptoms, at least in disaster workers. Briere et al. (2006) evaluated peritraumatic dissociation and PTSD from a multivariate perspective. They looked at data from two cohorts: 52 local community participants and 386 participants from the general population with histories of exposure to at least one traumatic event. Subjects were assessed for the presence of PTSD and were administered measures of dissociation and peritraumatic distress. In both studies, peritraumatic dissociation, persistent dissociation, peritraumatic distress, and generalized dissociative symptoms were associated with PTSD by univariate analyses. However, multivariate analyses in both studies indicated that PTSD status was no longer related to peritraumatic dissociation once other variables (especially persistent and generalized dissociation) were taken into account. These findings suggest that it is less what happens at the time of a trauma (e.g., disrupted encoding) that predict PTSD than what occurs thereafter (i.e., persistent avoidance).

Draijer and Langeland (1999) administered the DES and the Structured Trauma Interview to 160 inpatients consecutively admitted to a general psychiatric hospital. They found that 18% of the patients had a DES score greater than 30, which is usually considered the cutoff for dissociative disorders. In their sample, 26.4% of the patients reported early separation, 30.1% had witnessed interparental violence, 23.6% reported physical abuse, 34.6% reported sexual abuse, 11.7% reported rape before age 16, and 42.1% reported sexual and/or physical abuse. In this population, the level of dissociation was primarily related to reported overwhelming childhood experiences (e.g., sexual and physical abuse). Furthermore, when sexual abuse was severe (e.g., involving penetration or several perpetrators, lasting more than 1 year), dissociative symptoms were even more prominent. The highest dissociation levels were found in patients reporting cumulative sexual trauma (e.g., intrafamilial and extrafamilial) or both sexual and physical abuse. In particular, maternal dysfunction was related to the level of dissociation. With control for gender and age, stepwise multiple regression analysis indicated that the severity of dissociative symptoms was best predicted by reported sexual abuse, physical abuse, and maternal dysfunction. More recently, Foote et al. (2006) conducted a study to assess the prevalence of DSM-IV dissociative disorders in an inner-city outpatient psychiatric population ($n=82$) using a structured interview for dissociative disorders, the Dissociative Disorders Interview Schedule. They found that 29% of the subjects met DSM-IV diagnostic criteria for a dissociative disorder. Among this group, DID was diagnosed in 6% of subjects. Compared with patients without a dissociative disorder diagnosis, dissociative disorder patients were significantly more likely to report childhood physical abuse (71% vs. 27%) and childhood sexual abuse (74% vs. 29%), even though the two groups did not differ significantly on any demographic measure, including gender. Furthermore, a chart review of identified subjects revealed that only 5% of patients in whom a dissociative disorder was identified during the study had previously received a dissociative disorder diagnosis. This is the last in a series of clinical studies confirming that dissociative disorders are highly prevalent in clinical (psychiatric) populations and that the diagnosis is often missed.

These findings echo those of Nijenhuis et al. (1998), who reported that patients with dissociative disorder experienced more severe and multifaceted traumatiza-

tion. In their study, physical and sexual trauma predicted somatoform dissociation, and sexual trauma predicted psychological dissociation as well. These results suggest that pathological dissociation was best predicted by early onset of reported intense, chronic, and multiple traumatization. Thus, physical trauma seems to elicit dissociation or compartmentalization of experience and often may become the matrix for later posttraumatic symptomatology, such as dissociative amnesia for the traumatic episode. There is evidence for a dissociative subtype of PTSD that is associated with more severe childhood maltreatment (Ginzburg et al. 2006). Indeed, more extreme dissociative disorders, such as DID, have been conceptualized as chronic PTSD (Kluft 1984b, 1991; D. Spiegel 1984, 1986a). Recollection of trauma tends to have an off–on quality involving either intrusion or avoidance (Horowitz 1976), in which victims either intensively relive the trauma as though it were recurring or have difficulty remembering it (Cardeña and Spiegel 1993; Christianson and Loftus 1987; Madakasira and O'Brien 1987).

Investigators (Dominguez et al. 2004) studied the relationship between exposure to traumatic events, posttraumatic suffering and dissociative symptoms, and the relationship between type of trauma and dissociation in a large sample of outpatient adults seeking treatment at an urban ambulatory mental health clinic in Jerusalem ($n=298$). They found that 98% of subjects reported experiencing at least one lifetime traumatic event. Eighty-three percent of subjects reported high levels of intrusion and avoidance symptoms, while 15% reported high levels of dissociative phenomena. In this sample there was an association between physical and sexual abuse and high levels of dissociation, particularly in subjects reporting a history of early childhood abuse and an increased prevalence of lifetime traumatic events.

Others (Te Wildt 2004) have theorized that the new digital media may adversely affect people's mental health, an effect that is widely underestimated. Maldonado et al. (2002) conducted a study to assess the consequences of a generic social event. The study suggested that 1) unrelated consecutive societal events may have an additive effect on the development of trauma-related symptoms; 2) physical presence at the site of the trauma may not be needed for a person to be psychologically affected; and 3) distant exposure to vicarious traumatic events (e.g., Internet, television, and media coverage) may somehow sensitize individuals to develop acute stress–like reactions when exposed to future traumatic events. Therefore, psychiatrists need to consider the potential impact of the information transmitted via the Internet and the general media and its potential impact on the general population, as well as on their patients in particular.

There is recent evidence of a possible neural basis for the difficulty integrating traumatic memory and components of identity and consciousness among those with dissociative disorders. Using magnetic resonance imaging Vermetten et al. (2006) found that hippocampal and amygdala volumes were significantly smaller (19% and 32%, respectively) in patients diagnosed with dissociative identity disorder compared with healthy volunteers (Figure 15–1). A study of women with major depressive disorder also demonstrated that smaller hippocampal volume (18% smaller) was observed only in the group of women who had a history of severe and prolonged physical and/or sexual abuse in childhood (Vythilingam et al. 2002).

This would plausibly hamper the ability to encode, store, and retrieve memories and manage associated affect (Schacter et al. 1996). The hippocampus is involved in generating context, which helps to put information into perspective. It has been shown to buffer the effects of stressful input on hypothalamic-pituitary-adrenal (HPA) axis activation (Wolf et al. 2002). Furthermore, dissociation in response to script-driven imagery is associated with decreased activity in the parahippocampal gyrus (Lanius et al. 2002). Thus, reduced hippocampal size and function hinder memory processing and the ability to comprehend context, thereby impairing the integration of memory and identity.

More recently, Lanius et al. (2005) used fMRI to assess interregional brain activity covariations during traumatic script-driven imagery in subjects with PTSD compared with non-PTSD control subjects. fMRI studies were conducted in PTSD subjects with a dissociative response, PTSD subjects with a flashback response, and healthy control subjects. The authors found greater activation of neural networks involved in representing bodily states in dissociated PTSD subjects than in non-PTSD control subjects. Specifically, comparing dissociated PTSD patients and control subjects' connectivity maps in the left ventrolateral thalamus (VLT) (–14, –16, 4) revealed that control subjects had higher covariations between activations in VLT and in the left superior frontal gyrus (Brodmann's area [BA] 10), right parahippocampal gyrus (BA 30), and right superior occipital gyrus (BA 19, 39), whereas greater covariation with VLT in dissociated PTSD subjects occurred in the right insula (BA 13, 34), left parietal lobe (BA 7), right middle frontal gyrus (BA 8), superior temporal gyrus (BA 38, 34), and right cuneus (BA 19). These results suggest interregional brain activity covariations dur-

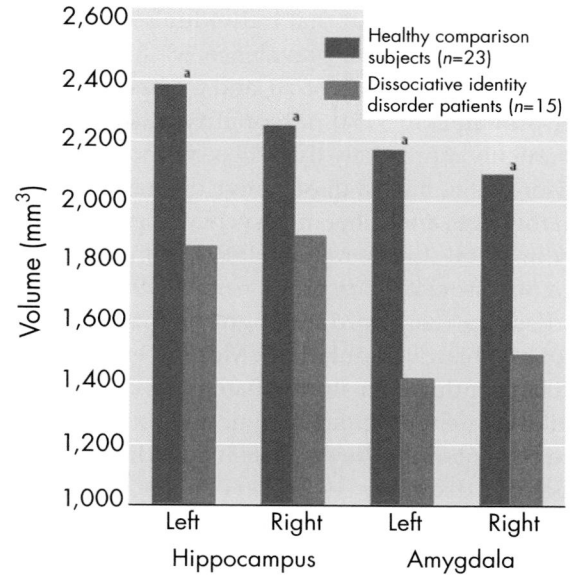

FIGURE 15–1. Hippocampal and amygdalar volumes in patients with dissociative identity disorder (DID) and healthy comparison subjects.
[a]Significant difference between groups (*P*<0.05, *t* test for nonpaired samples).
Source. Reprinted from Vermetten E, Schmahl C, Lindner S, et al: "Hippocampal and Amygdalar Volumes in Dissociative Identity Disorder." *American Journal of Psychiatry* 163:630–636, 2006. Copyright 2006. Used with permission.

ing traumatic script-driven imagery in PTSD subjects with dissociated traumatic memories, but fail to explain whether variations in interregional brain connectivity are the cause of memory defects or are themselves caused by the dissociation of memories.

Universality and Transcultural Aspects of Dissociation

In the United States, the incidence of dissociative symptoms and dissociative disorders varies according to the population under study. Dissociative symptoms also have been reported in virtually every major psychiatric disorder and, in less severe forms, even in nonpatient ("normal") populations (Giese et al. 1997). In the general population, 6.3% of adults have reported three to four dissociative symptoms (Mulder et al. 1998). Recently, Johnson et al. (2006) conducted a study among adults (*n*=658) in the community focusing on the association between dissociative disorders and co-occurring Axis I disorders. They found a 0.8% prevalence of depersonalization disorder, a 1.8% prevalence of dissociative amnesia, a 1.5% prevalence of dissociative identity disorder, and a 4.4% prevalence of dissociative disorder not otherwise specified. As expected, they also found that individuals with Cluster A (dissociative disorder prevalence: 58%), B (dissociative disorder prevalence: 68%), and C (dissociative disorder prevalence: 37%) personality disorders were substantially more likely than those without personality disorders to have a dissociative disorder.

In the acute and subacute psychiatric population of a day hospital, Lussier et al. (1997) found a 9% incidence of dissociative disorder. Coons (1998) reported that dissociative disorders might be present in 5%–10% of psychiatric populations. More recently, Foote et al. (2006) conducted a study of an inner-city hospital-based outpatient psychiatric clinic and found that 29% of the patients interviewed received a diagnosis of a dissociative disorder.

Dissociative disorders have been described in many cultures and settings. In Uganda, dissociative amnesia and depersonalization were generally recognized and seen as the result of traumatic experiences, although DID was confused with spirit possession (Van Dujil et al. 2005). An evaluation of a Turkish psychiatric inpatient population found a 10.2% incidence of dissociative disorders and a 5.4% incidence of DID (Tutkun et al. 1998). A study (Sar et al. 2000) suggested that dissociative disorders occurred in 12% of psychiatric outpatient subjects in Turkey. On the other hand, several studies of DID in the general (nonpsychiatric) population in Turkey yielded an incidence ranging from 1.1% to 1.7% (Akyuz et al. 1999; Sar et al. 2007a). Nevertheless, the highest incidence of DID in the Turkish population has been found in the context of the psychiatric emergency room, with the incidence of dissociative disorders in general, and of DID in particular, being as high as 34.9% and 14%, respectively (Sar et al. 2007b). A study of 216 Swedish adolescents revealed an 8.8% prevalence of dissociative symptoms (Svedin et al. 2004). Friedl and Draijer (2000) conducted a study of Dutch psychiatric inpatients and found that 8% had dissociative disorders and 2% presented with factitious DID. Similarly, a study of admitted Swiss psychiatric inpatients reported a 5% incidence of dissociative disorders (Mihaescu et al. 1998; Modestin et al. 1996). Middleton and Butler (1998) found that DID was not uncommon among Australian psychiatric patients. A study of the assessment of pathological dissociation in Finland (n=2,001) revealed a prevalence of 3.4% in the general population (Maaranen et al. 2005), although the prevalence of dissociative disorders among psychiatric patients has been reported as 17% (Lipsanen et al. 2004). In Ethiopia, Awas et al. (1999) described a lifetime prevalence of dissociative disorders of 6.3% among 501 subjects in a rural community. Gast et al. (2001) conducted a study of hospitalized German psychiatric patients and found a 4.4% incidence of dissociative disorders, including a 0.9% incidence of both DID and depersonalization disorder and a 2.6% incidence of DID not otherwise specified. Draijer and Langeland (1999) described an 18% incidence of dissociative disorders in patients admitted to a general psychiatric hospital in the Netherlands. The prevalence of dissociative disorders among the general population in Iran was found to be 0.77% (Mohammadi et al. 2005). Spitzer et al. (2006b) reported that the incidence of pathological dissociation among German psychiatric patients ranged from 2.2% to 5.4%, while in the nonclinical samples it ranged between 0.3% and 1.8%. Similarly, Rodewald et al. (2006) found the prevalence of DID and DID-NOS to be 5% in clinical samples among German inpatients.

Acute Stress Disorder

Although acute stress disorder is classified among the anxiety disorders in DSM-IV-TR (American Psychiatric Association 2000), mention is made of it in this chapter because half of the symptoms of this disorder are dissociative in nature (Table 15–3). The diagnostic criteria for this disorder would designate as symptomatic approximately one-fourth to one-third of individuals exposed to serious trauma. These symptoms are strongly predictive of later development of PTSD in some (Brewin et al. 1999; Butler et al. 1996; Classen et al. 1998; Koopman et al. 1994; Waelde et al. 2001) but not all (Barton et al. 1996; Harvey and Bryant 1998) studies. Similarly, the occurrence of PTSD is predicted by intrusion, avoidance, and hyperarousal symptoms in the immediate aftermath of rape (Rothbaum and Foa 1993) and combat trauma (Blank 1993; Z. Solomon and Mikulincer 1988). Although most individuals experiencing serious trauma are initially symptomatic, most will recover without developing PTSD. Most studies show that 25% or fewer of those who experience serious trauma later become symptomatic. Harvey and Bryant (1999) reported that the occurrence of full and subsyndromal acute stress disorder was approximately 13% and 21%, respectively. They found that most subjects who met criteria for subsyndromal acute stress disorder did not meet the acute stress disorder criteria for dissociation. At least 80% of the individuals who reported derealization also reported reduced awareness and depersonalization.

TABLE 15–3. DSM-IV-TR diagnostic criteria for acute stress disorder

A. The person has been exposed to a traumatic event in which both of the following were present:

    (1) the person experienced, witnessed, or was confronted with an event or events that involved actual or threatened death or serious injury, or a threat to the physical integrity of self or others

    (2) the person's response involved intense fear, helplessness, or horror

B. Either while experiencing or after experiencing the distressing event, the individual has three (or more) of the following dissociative symptoms:

    (1) a subjective sense of numbing, detachment, or absence of emotional responsiveness

    (2) a reduction in awareness of his or her surroundings (e.g., "being in a daze")

    (3) derealization

    (4) depersonalization

    (5) dissociative amnesia (i.e., inability to recall an important aspect of the trauma)

C. The traumatic event is persistently reexperienced in at least one of the following ways: recurrent images, thoughts, dreams, illusions, flashback episodes, or a sense of reliving the experience; or distress on exposure to reminders of the traumatic event.

D. Marked avoidance of stimuli that arouse recollections of the trauma (e.g., thoughts, feelings, conversations, activities, places, people).

E. Marked symptoms of anxiety or increased arousal (e.g., difficulty sleeping, irritability, poor concentration, hypervigilance, exaggerated startle response, motor restlessness).

F. The disturbance causes clinically significant distress or impairment in social, occupational, or other important areas of functioning or impairs the individual's ability to pursue some necessary task, such as obtaining necessary assistance or mobilizing personal resources by telling family members about the traumatic experience.

G. The disturbance lasts for a minimum of 2 days and a maximum of 4 weeks and occurs within 4 weeks of the traumatic event.

H. The disturbance is not due to the direct physiological effects of a substance (e.g., a drug of abuse, a medication) or a general medical condition, is not better accounted for by brief psychotic disorder, and is not merely an exacerbation of a preexisting Axis I or Axis II disorder.

This diagnostic category should be useful not only for research on the normal and abnormal processes of adjusting to trauma but also as a means of providing an important opportunity for early preventive intervention. Dissociation may work well at the time of trauma, but if the defense persists too long, it interferes with the working through (in Lindemann's terms, the "grief work" [Lindemann 1944/1994; D. Spiegel 1981]) necessary to put traumatic experience into perspective and reduce the likelihood of later PTSD or other symptomatology. Therefore, psychotherapy aimed at helping individuals acknowledge, bear, and put into perspective traumatic experience shortly after the trauma should be helpful in reducing the incidence of later PTSD.

In the following discussions, we review the diagnosis and treatment of the dissociative disorders as defined in DSM-IV-TR.

Dissociative Amnesia

The hallmark of dissociative amnesia is the inability to recall important personal information, usually of a traumatic or stressful nature, which cannot be explained by ordinary forgetfulness (American Psychiatric Association 2000) (Table 15–4). Dissociative amnesia is considered the most common of all dissociative disorders (Putnam 1985). Amnesia is a symptom commonly found in several other dissociative and anxiety disorders, including acute stress disorder, PTSD, somatization disorder, dissociative fugue, and DID (American Psychiatric Association 2000). A higher incidence of dissociative amnesia has been described in the context of war and natural and other disasters (Maldonado et al. 2000). There appears to be a direct relation between the severity of the exposure to trauma and the incidence of amnesia (G.R. Brown and Anderson 1991; Chu and Dill 1990; Putnam 1985, 1993).

Dissociative amnesia is the classical functional disorder of memory and involves difficulty in retrieving discrete components of episodic memory (see Table 15–2). It does not, however, involve a difficulty in memory storage, as in Wernicke-Korsakoff syndrome. Because the amnesia primarily involves difficulties in retrieval rather than encoding or storage, the memory deficits usually are reversible. Once the amnesia has cleared, normal memory function is resumed (Schacter et al. 1982). Dissociative amnesia has three primary characteristics:

1. The memory loss is episodic. The first-person recollection of certain events is lost, rather than knowledge of procedures.

2. The memory loss is for a discrete period of time, ranging from minutes to years. It is not vagueness or inefficient retrieval of memories, but rather a dense unavailability of memories that had been clearly accessible. Unlike in the amnestic disorders, for example, from damage to the medial temporal lobe in surgery (Squire and Zola-Morgan 1991) or in Wernicke-Korsakoff syndrome, there is usually no difficulty in learning *new* episodic information. Thus, the amnesia is typically retrograde rather than anterograde (Loewenstein 1991a), with one or more discrete periods of past information becoming unavailable. However, Kluft (1988) observed a dissociative syndrome of continuous difficulty in incorporating new information that mimics organic amnestic syndromes.

3. The memory loss is generally for events of a traumatic or stressful nature. In one study (Coons and Milstein 1986), the majority of cases involved child abuse (60%), but disavowed behaviors such as marital problems, sexual activity, suicide attempts, criminal behavior, and the death of a relative also were precipitants.

Dissociative amnesia is most common in the third and fourth decades of life (Coons and Milstein 1986). It usually involves one episode, but multiple periods of lost memory are not uncommon (Coons and Milstein 1986). Comorbidity with conversion disorder, bulimia, alcohol abuse, and depression is common, and Axis II diagnoses of histrionic, dependent, and borderline personality disorders occur in a substantial minority of such patients (Coons and Milstein 1986). Legal difficulties, such as driving under the influence of alcohol, also accompany dissociative amnesia in a minority of cases. Occasionally, there may be a history of head trauma. If that is the case, usually the trauma is too slight to have physiological consequences. In a recent study of community adults, the prevalence of dissociative amnesia was 1.8% (J.G. Johnson et al. 2006).

The typical course of dissociative amnesia is described in the following case.

> A 54-year-old man was involved in a motorcycle accident. He was wearing a helmet, which was damaged but did protect him during the accident. He was found to have suffered no significant head trauma. The patient did not lose consciousness, and he talked with a friend after the accident about it. However, he had no memory of the accident or of the 12 hours afterward. His first recollection was of a friend telling him, "You crashed my motorcycle." When he returned the next day to the hospital where he had been treated, he recognized a nurse as someone fa-

TABLE 15–4. DSM-IV-TR diagnostic criteria for dissociative amnesia

A. The predominant disturbance is one or more episodes of inability to recall important personal information, usually of a traumatic or stressful nature, that is too extensive to be explained by ordinary forgetfulness.

B. The disturbance does not occur exclusively during the course of dissociative identity disorder, dissociative fugue, posttraumatic stress disorder, acute stress disorder, or somatization disorder and is not due to the direct physiological effects of a substance (e.g., a drug of abuse, a medication) or a neurological or other general medical condition (e.g., amnestic disorder due to head trauma).

C. The symptoms cause clinically significant distress or impairment in social, occupational, or other important areas of functioning.

miliar, and she told him that he had been yelling when they treated his injured left knee. Yet this visit did not stimulate any direct recollection of his time in the hospital. The man had recovered no memory of the accident a month later.

Dissociative amnesia usually involves discrete boundaries around the period of time unavailable to consciousness. Individuals with such a disorder lose the ability to recall what happened during a specific time. They demonstrate not vagueness or spotty memory but rather a loss of any episodic memory for a finite period. Such individuals initially may not be aware of the memory loss—that is, they may not remember that they do not remember. However, they may find, for example, new purchases in their homes but have no memory of having obtained them. They report being told that they have done or said things that they cannot remember.

Dissociative amnesia most frequently occurs after an episode of trauma, and the onset may be sudden or gradual.

> A 30-year-old woman was beaten and raped by a man who drove her home from a party. She had refused to let him enter her apartment, but he returned a few minutes later, claiming that he had to make a telephone call. He then sexually assaulted her. She screamed and struggled and called the police immediately afterward. The man was arrested when he returned to retrieve some jewelry she had pulled off his neck during the struggle. Although she had not sustained a concussion, she began to lose memory of the rape in the ensuing week. By the end of the week, she

had no memory of the rape but became listless and depressed. In psychotherapy, she used hypnosis to help retrieve her memory, which she was gradually able to do.

Some individuals do experience episodes of selective amnesia, usually for specific traumatic incidents, which may be more interwoven with periods of intact memory. In these cases, the amnesia is for a type of material remembered rather than for a discrete period of time.

Despite the fact that certain information is kept out of consciousness in dissociative amnesia, such information may exert an influence on consciousness. For example, a rape victim with no conscious recollection of the assault will nonetheless behave like someone who has been sexually victimized. Such individuals often show detachment and demoralization, are unable to enjoy intimate relationships, and show hyperarousal to stimuli reminiscent of the trauma. This phenomenon is similar to priming in memory research. Individuals who have read a word in a list will complete a word stem for such a word (e.g., a partial word such as *pre* for *prepare*) minutes or hours later more quickly than they would for a word they have not recently seen. This phenomenon occurs even though they cannot consciously recall having read the word that constitutes the prime. Similarly, individuals instructed in hypnosis to forget having seen a list of words will nonetheless show priming effects from the hypnotically suppressed list. It is the essence of dissociative amnesia that material being kept out of conscious awareness is nonetheless active and may influence consciousness indirectly: out of sight does not mean out of mind.

Individuals with dissociative amnesia generally do not have disturbances of identity, except to the extent that their identity is influenced by the warded-off memory. It is not uncommon for such individuals to develop depressive symptoms as well, especially when the amnesia is in the wake of a traumatic episode.

Treatment

To date, no controlled studies have addressed the treatment of dissociative amnesia. No established pharmacological treatments are available, except for the use of benzodiazepines or barbiturates for drug-assisted interviews (Maldonado et al. 2000). Most cases of dissociative amnesia revert spontaneously, especially when the individuals are removed from stressful or threatening situations, when they feel physically and psychologically safe, and/or when

they are exposed to cues from the past (e.g., family members) (W. Brown 1918; Kardiner and Spiegel 1947; Loewenstein 1991b; Maldonado et al. 2000; Reither and Stoudemire 1988). When a safe environment is not enough to restore normal memory functioning, the amnesia sometimes can be breached using techniques such as pharmacologically mediated interviews (i.e., barbiturates and benzodiazepines) (Baron and Nagy 1988; Naples and Hackett 1978; Perry and Jacobs 1982; Wettstein and Fauman 1979).

On the other hand, most patients with dissociative disorder are highly hypnotizable on formal testing and therefore are easily able to make use of hypnotic techniques such as age regression (H. Spiegel and Spiegel 2004). Patients are hypnotized and instructed to experience a time before the onset of the amnesia as though it were the present. Then the patients are reoriented in hypnosis to experience events during the amnesic period. Hypnosis can enable such patients to reorient temporally and therefore to achieve access to otherwise dissociated memories.

If the warded-off memory has traumatic content, patients may abreact (i.e., express strong emotion) as these memories are elicited, and they will need psychotherapeutic help in integrating these memories and the associated affect into consciousness.

One technique that can help bring such memories into consciousness while modulating the affective response to them is the split screen technique (D. Spiegel 1981). In this approach, patients are taught, by using hypnosis, to relive the traumatic event as if they were watching it on an imaginary movie or television screen. This technique is often helpful for individuals who are unable to relive the event as if it were occurring in the present tense, either because that process is too emotionally taxing or because they are not sufficiently hypnotizable to be able to engage in hypnotic age regression. The screen technique also can be used to provide dissociation between the psychological and the somatic aspects of the memory retrieval. Individuals can be put into self-hypnosis and instructed to get their bodies into a state of floating comfort and safety. They are reminded that no matter what they see on the screen, their bodies will be safe and comfortable.

A victim of a violent attempted rape had developed a selective amnesia for much of the physical struggle itself. She had sustained a basilar skull fracture, but she had not been rendered unconscious. She also had a generalized seizure shortly after the assault. She initially sought help with hypnosis in an attempt to improve her recollection of the assailant's face.

The woman was instructed in the split screen technique and used it to relive the assault. She remembered two things that she had not previously re-called: 1) the assailant was surprised at how hard she was fighting with him, and 2) she recognized that he intended not merely to rape her but to kill her. She became convinced that had she let him drag her into her apartment, she likely would not have survived. She was tearful and frightened as she recalled this aspect of the assault that had been previously unavailable to consciousness.

She was then instructed to divide the imaginary screen in half, picturing on the left side an image of the viciousness and intensity of the assault on her and on the other side recognizing what she had done to protect herself. She was instructed to concentrate on these two aspects of the assault and then, when she was ready, to bring herself out of the state of self-hypnosis. She was told that she could use this as a self-hypnosis exercise several times a day if she wished, as a means of putting her memories of the rape into perspective. This cognitive and emotional restructuring of the traumatic memories made them more bearable in consciousness.

Before this psychotherapy, she had blamed herself for having fought so hard that she was seriously injured. Afterward, she recognized that she may have saved her life by fighting off the assailant so vigorously. This positive therapeutic outcome occurred despite the fact that she was unable to recall any new details about the assailant's physical appearance.

Psychotherapy for dissociative amnesia involves accessing the dissociated memories, working through affectively loaded aspects of these memories, and supporting the patient through the process of integrating these memories into consciousness.

Dissociative Fugue

Dissociative fugue combines failure of integration of certain aspects of personal memory with loss of customary identity and automatisms of motor behavior (Table 15–5). Patients appear "normal," usually showing no signs of psychopathology or cognitive deficit. Fugue involves one or more episodes of sudden, unexpected, purposeful travel away from home, coupled with an inability to recall portions or all of one's past, and a loss of identity or the assumption of a new identity. In contrast to patients who have DID, if patients with dissociative fugue develop a new identity, the old and new identities do not alternate. The onset is usually sudden, and it frequently occurs after a traumatic experience or bereavement. A single episode is not uncommon, and spontaneous remission of symptoms can occur without treatment.

It was thought that the assumption of a new identity, as in the classic case of the Reverend Ansel Bourne

TABLE 15–5. DSM-IV-TR diagnostic criteria for dissociative fugue

A. The predominant disturbance is sudden, unexpected travel away from home or one's customary place of work, with inability to recall one's past.

B. Confusion about personal identity or assumption of a new identity (partial or complete).

C. The disturbance does not occur exclusively during the course of dissociative identity disorder and is not due to the direct physiological effects of a substance (e.g., a drug of abuse, a medication) or a general medical condition (e.g., temporal lobe epilepsy).

D. The symptoms cause clinically significant distress or impairment in social, occupational, or other important areas of functioning.

(James 1890/1950), was typical of dissociative fugue. However, Reither and Stoudemire (1988), in their review of the literature, documented that in most cases, there is loss of personal identity but no clear assumption of a new identity. Glisky et al. (2004) reported on a case of psychogenic fugue in which the individual lost access not only to his autobiographical memories but also to his native German language. Neuropsychological, behavioral, electrophysiological, and functional neuroimaging tests converged on the conclusion that this individual suffered an episode of psychogenic fugue, during which he lost explicit knowledge of his personal past and his native language. At the same time, he appeared to retain implicit knowledge of autobiographical facts and of the semantic or associative structure of the German language. The patient's poor performance on tests of executive control and reduced activation of frontal compared to parietal brain regions during lexical decision were suggestive of reduced frontal function, consistent with models of psychogenic fugue proposed by Kopelman et al. (1994).

Many cases of dissociative fugue remit spontaneously. But again, hypnosis can be useful in accessing dissociated material. The following case was reported by H. Spiegel and Spiegel (2004):

A woman who appeared dazed but physically unharmed was brought into an army hospital emergency department by the base guards because she had been found wandering near the army base. She reported that she did not know who she was, where she lived, or how she happened to be there. Initially, plans were made to admit her to the hospital for a full neurological and psychiatric evaluation. She proved to be highly hypnotizable, and in hypnosis, age regression was used to take her back to an earlier year. She then reported her name and that she lived some 500 miles away. The time was changed again in hypnosis to a period just before this apparent fugue episode. She then reported having received unsigned letters from someone at the army base where her husband was stationed, reporting that her husband was having an affair. This had deeply upset her, and it turned out that her husband was indeed a soldier on the base near which she had been found wandering. They were reunited and reconciled, and the fugue episode ended.

Not infrequently, fugue episodes represent dissociated but purposeful activity, as in the following case.

A businessman found himself on several occasions on transatlantic flights from California to London without recollecting who he was or how he had gotten on the airplane. In psychotherapy exploring these fugue episodes, it was determined that he had had an extremely conflicted relationship with a successful but neglectful father. The father had recently died, leaving the patient financially well off but emotionally ambivalent, with a sense of incompleteness about his relationship with his father. The patient had spent his boyhood years in London, and he recognized in therapy that the travel to London seemed to represent an unconscious attempt to revisit his childhood years and "set his father straight"—something he had never been able to do while his father was alive.

In this case, the dissociative fugue was a form of pathological grief reaction.

Hypnosis can be helpful in accessing otherwise unavailable components of memory and identity. The approach used is similar to that for dissociative amnesia. Hypnotic age regression can be used as the framework for accessing information available at a previous time. Demonstrating to patients that such information can be made available to consciousness enhances their sense of control over the material and facilitates the therapeutic working through of emotionally laden aspects of it.

A woman in a Department of Veterans Affairs hospital had lost all memory of the preceding 10 months and insisted that she was in a different hospital from where she had been during the previous December. She proved on testing with the Hypnotic Induction Profile (H. Spiegel and Spiegel 2004) to be highly hypnotizable. She was then put into hypnosis with a simple rapid-induction technique involving the following instruction: On 1, do one thing: look up. On 2, do two things: slowly close your eyes, and take a deep breath. On 3, do three things: let the breath out,

let your eyes relax but keep them closed, and let your body float. Then let one hand or the other float up into the air like a balloon, and that is your signal to yourself that you are ready to concentrate.

When she did this, she was told that we would be changing times, that we would count backward in years, and that when her eyes opened, she would be at an earlier time in her life. We agreed that when I touched her forehead, she would close her eyes and we would change times again. We then began counting several years back. When she opened her eyes, she spoke as though she were in some different place earlier in her life. She was reoriented to the time when she really was in another psychiatric hospital in a different city, and she talked about that experience. She was then instructed to close her eyes again and count forward in months to the current month. She opened her eyes and was then properly oriented and had episodic memory for what had transpired in her life in recent months.

Once reorientation is established and the overt aspects of the fugue have been resolved, it is important to work through interpersonal or intrapsychic issues that underlie the dissociative defenses. Individuals with dissociative fugue are often relatively unaware of their reactions to stress because they so effectively can dissociate them (H. Spiegel 1974). Thus, effective psychotherapy is also anticipatory, helping patients to recognize and modify their tendency to set aside their own feelings in favor of those of others.

Patients with dissociative fugue may be helped with a psychotherapeutic approach that facilitates conscious integration of dissociated memories and motivations for behavior previously experienced as automatic and unwilled. It is often helpful to address current psychosocial stressors, such as marital conflict, with the involved individuals, as in the previously discussed case of the woman found on the army base. To the extent that current psychosocial stress triggers fugue, resolution of that stress can help resolve the fugue state and reduce the likelihood of recurrence. Highly hypnotizable individuals prone to these extreme dissociative symptoms (D. Spiegel et al. 1988; H. Spiegel 1974; H. Spiegel and Spiegel 2004) often have great difficulty in asserting their own point of view in a personal relationship. Rather, they interact with others as though they were undergoing a spontaneous trance experience. One such individual described herself as a "disciple in search of a teacher." Psychotherapy can be effective in helping such individuals recognize and modify their tendency toward unthinking compliance with others and toward extreme sensitivity to rejection and disapproval.

In the past, sodium amobarbital or other short-acting sedatives were used to reverse dissociative amnesia or fugue. More recently, Ilechukwu and Henry (2006) described the use of intravenous lorazepam for the same purpose. However, such techniques offer no advantage over hypnosis and are not especially effective (Perry and Jacobs 1982). Not infrequently, the ceremony of injecting the drug elicits spontaneous hypnotic phenomena before the pharmacological effect is felt, and sedation and other side effects can be troublesome.

There is at least one case report on the use of a locator beacon attached to a patient with dissociative fugue, which has proven effective in the curtailment of dissociative fugue episodes (Macleod 1999).

Depersonalization Disorder

The essential feature of depersonalization disorder is the occurrence of persistent feelings of unreality, detachment, or estrangement from oneself or one's body, usually with the feeling that one is an outside observer of one's own mental processes (Steinberg 1991). Thus, depersonalization disorder is primarily a disturbance in the integration of perceptual experience (Table 15–6). Individuals who have depersonalization disorder are distressed by it. Different from those with delusional disorders and other psychotic processes, those with depersonalization disorder have intact reality testing. Patients are aware of some distortion in their perceptual experience and therefore are not delusional. The symptom is often transient and may co-occur with a variety of other symptoms, especially anxiety, panic, or phobic symptoms. Indeed, the content of the anxiety may involve fears of "going crazy." Derealization frequently co-occurs with depersonalization disorder, in which affected individuals notice an altered perception of their surroundings, resulting in the world seeming unreal or dreamlike. Affected individuals often will ruminate about this alteration and be preoccupied with their own somatic and mental functioning.

Hunter et al. (2004) conducted a study using computerized databases and citation searches to assess the prevalence of symptoms of depersonalization and derealization in both clinical and nonclinical settings. They found that transient symptoms of depersonalization/derealization are common in the general population, with a lifetime prevalence rate of between 26% and 74% and a current prevalence rate of between 31% and 66% at the time of a traumatic event. Community surveys employing standardized diagnostic interviews revealed rates of between 1.2% and 1.7% for 1-month prevalence of symptoms of depersonalization/ derealization in a UK sample and a 2.4% current prev-

TABLE 15–6.	DSM-IV-TR diagnostic criteria for depersonalization disorder

A. Persistent or recurrent experiences of feeling detached from, and as if one is an outside observer of, one's mental processes or body (e.g., feeling like one is in a dream).

B. During the depersonalization experience, reality testing remains intact.

C. The depersonalization causes clinically significant distress or impairment in social, occupational, or other important areas of functioning.

D. The depersonalization experience does not occur exclusively during the course of another mental disorder, such as schizophrenia, panic disorder, acute stress disorder, or another dissociative disorder, and is not due to the direct physiological effects of a substance (e.g., a drug of abuse, a medication) or a general medical condition (e.g., temporal lobe epilepsy).

alence rate in a Canadian sample. Current prevalence rates between 1% and 16% were reported in samples of consecutive inpatient admissions, although these rates were considered to be underestimates. Prevalence rates in clinical samples of specific psychiatric disorders varied between 30% (for war veterans with PTSD) and 60% (for those with unipolar depression). There was a high prevalence of depersonalization/derealization symptoms within panic disorder samples, with rates varying from 7.8% to 82.6%.

Giesbrecht et al. (2007) studied the relationship between dissociative tendencies (as measured with the Dissociative Experiences Scale [DES] and HPA axis functioning in two samples of undergraduate students. The investigators induced acute stress by means of the Trier Social Stress Test, while monitoring subjective and physiological stress measures (i.e., cortisol). The study found that subjective stress experiences (as measured by the Tension-Anxiety subscale of the Profile of Mood States [POMS]), were positively related to trait dissociation. Regarding physiological measures, they found that subjects scoring high on the depersonalization/derealization subscale of the DES exhibited more pronounced cortisol responses, while individuals scoring high on the absorption subscale showed attenuated responses.

Depersonalization as a symptom is seen in several psychiatric and neurological disorders. Unlike other dissociative disorders, the presence of which excludes other mental disorders such as schizophrenia and substance abuse, depersonalization disorder frequently co-occurs with such disorders. It is often a symptom of anxiety disorders and PTSD. In fact, about 69% of patients with panic disorder experience depersonalization or derealization during their panic attacks (Ball et al. 1997). Episodes of depersonalization also may occur as a symptom of alcohol and drug abuse, as a side effect of prescription medication, and during stress and sensory deprivation. Depersonalization is considered a disorder when it is a persistent and predominant symptom. The phenomenology of the disorder involves both the initial symptoms themselves and the reactive anxiety caused by them. In a recent study of community adults, the prevalence of depersonalization disorder was 0.8% (J.G. Johnson et al. 2006).

Treatment

Depersonalization is most often transient and may remit without formal treatment. Recurrent or persistent depersonalization should be thought of both as a symptom in and of itself and as a component of other syndromes requiring treatment, such as anxiety disorders and schizophrenia.

The symptom itself may respond to self-hypnosis training. Often, hypnotic induction will induce transient depersonalization symptoms in patients. This is a useful exercise because by having a structure for inducing the symptoms, one provides patients with a context for understanding and controlling them. The symptoms are presented as a spontaneous form of hypnotic dissociation that can be modified. Individuals for whom this approach is effective can be taught to induce a pleasant sense of floating lightness or heaviness in place of the anxiety-related somatic detachment. Often, the use of an imaginary screen to picture problems in a way that detaches them from the typical somatic response is also helpful (H. Spiegel and Spiegel 2004).

Other treatment modalities used (Maldonado et al. 2000) include behavioral techniques such as paradoxical intention, record keeping, positive reward, flooding, psychotherapy (especially psychodynamic), cognitive-behavioral therapy, and psychoeducation. Hunter et al. (2005) reported on an open study in which 21 patients with depersonalization disorder were treated individually with cognitive-behavioral therapy. The authors reported significant improvements in patient-defined measures of depersonalization/derealization severity as well as in standardized measures of dissociation, depression, anxiety, and general functioning at the end of treatment and at 6-month follow-up.

Virtually all types of psychotropic medications, including psychostimulants, antidepressants, antipsychotics, anticonvulsants, and benzodiazepines, have been tried with modest success. Appropriate treatment of comorbid disorders is an important part of treatment. Use of antianxiety medications for generalized anxiety, panic, or phobic disorders; antidepressants for treatment of comorbid depression or anxiety; and antipsychotic medications for true psychosis should help in these conditions.

Dissociative Identity Disorder (Multiple Personality Disorder)

Prevalence

There are no convincing studies of the absolute prevalence of DID. The initial systematic report on the epidemiology of DID estimated a prevalence in the general population of 0.01% (Coons 1984). The estimated prevalence is approximately 3% of psychiatric inpatients (Ross 1991; Ross et al. 1991b). Studies conducted in the general population suggest a prevalence higher than initially reported by Coons (1984) but lower (about 1%) than the one described in psychiatric settings and specialized treatment units (Ross 1991; Vanderlinden et al. 1991). Loewenstein (1994) reported that the prevalence in North America is about 1%, compared with a prevalence of 10% for all dissociative disorders as a group. Loewenstein's findings were replicated by Rifkin et al. (1998), who studied 100 randomly selected women, ages 16–50 years, who had been admitted to an acute psychiatric hospital and found that 1% of the subjects had DID. There is evidence that dissociative disorders are often underdiagnosed (D. Spiegel 2006). Foote et al. (2006) carefully assessed 231 consecutive admissions to an inner-city mental health clinic and interviewed 82 of those willing to cooperate with the study. Twenty-nine percent of this sample met DSM-IV (American Psychiatric Association 1994) criteria for a dissociative disorder (8 with dissociative amnesia, 7 with dissociative disorder not otherwise specified, 5 with DID, and 4 with depersonalization disorder). Only 5% of this sample had previously been diagnosed with a dissociative disorder. Furthermore, the study provided additional evidence linking both physical and sexual abuse to dissociative symptoms, determining an odds ratio of 5.86 for physical abuse and 7.87 for sexual abuse. In a recent study of community adults, the prevalence of dissociative identity disorder was 1.5% (J.G. Johnson et al. 2006).

The number of reported DID cases has risen considerably in recent years. Factors that account for this increase include a more general awareness of the diagnosis among mental health professionals; the availability, starting with DSM-III (American Psychiatric Association 1980), of specific diagnostic criteria (Table 15–7); and reduced misdiagnosis of DID as schizophrenia or borderline personality disorder. Although the increase in reported cases is best documented in North America, a number of studies in Europe have shown similar phenomenology and links to trauma history (Boon and Draijer 1993a, 1993b; Gast et al. 2001; Nijenhuis et al. 1998). In fact, there are reports of DID in almost all societies and races, making it a true cross-cultural diagnosis (Coons et al. 1991). Case reports have described DID or related disorders among Asians (Putnam 1989; Yap 1960), African Americans (Coons and Milstein 1986), Europeans (Boon and Draijer 1993a, 1993b; Freyberger et al. 1998; Nijenhuis et al. 1998; Spitzer et al. 1999), Hispanics (Ronquillo 1991; R. Solomon 1983), and inhabitants of Australia and New Zealand (L. Brown et al. 1999; Gelb 1993; Middleton and Butler 1998), Canada (Horen et al. 1995; Ross et al. 1989, 1991a, 1991b), the Caribbean (Wittkower 1970), India (Adityanjee et al. 1989; Varma et al. 1981), Japan (Berger et al. 1994), the Netherlands (Boon and Draijer 1993b; Draijer and Langeland 1999; Friedl and Draijer 2000; Nijenhuis et al. 1997; Sno and Schalken 1999; van Dyck 1993), Norway (Boe et al. 1993), Sweden (Eriksson and Lundin 1996), Switzerland (Modestin et al. 1996), and Turkey (Akyuz et al. 1999; Chodoff 1997; Sar et al. 1996, 2000; Tutkun et al. 1998; Yargic et al. 1998).

Other authors attribute the increase in reported cases to hypnotic suggestion and misdiagnosis (Brenner 1994, 1996a; Frankel 1990; Ganaway 1995). Proponents of this point of view argue that individuals with DID are as a group highly hypnotizable and therefore quite suggestible and that a few specialist clinicians usually make the vast majority of diagnoses. However, it has been observed that the symptomatology of patients diagnosed by specialists in dissociation does not differ from that assessed by psychiatrists, psychologists, and physicians in more general practices, who diagnose one or two cases per year. On the other hand, Akyuz et al. (1999) examined the prevalence of DID in the general population of a rural area in Turkey. They found that 1.7% received a diagnosis of dissociative disorder according to a structured interview, and half of these fulfilled clinical criteria for DID, yielding a

TABLE 15–7. DSM-IV-TR diagnostic criteria for dissociative identity disorder

A. The presence of two or more distinct identities or personality states (each with its own relatively enduring pattern of perceiving, relating to, and thinking about the environment and self).

B. At least two of these identities or personality states recurrently take control of the person's behavior.

C. Inability to recall important personal information that is too extensive to be explained by ordinary forgetfulness.

D. The disturbance is not due to the direct physiological effects of a substance (e.g., blackouts or chaotic behavior during alcohol intoxication) or a general medical condition (e.g., complex partial seizures). **Note:** In children, the symptoms are not attributable to imaginary playmates or other fantasy play.

minimum prevalence of 0.4% for DID. Thus, their data, derived from a population with no public awareness about DID and no exposure to systematic psychotherapy (thus eliminating the possible "iatrogenic contamination factor"), suggest that DID cannot be considered simply an iatrogenic artifact, a culture-bound syndrome, or a phenomenon induced by media influences.

In a study (Chu et al. 1999) of female patients admitted to a unit specializing in the treatment of trauma-related disorders, participants reporting any type of childhood abuse had elevated levels of dissociative symptoms that were significantly higher than those in subjects not reporting abuse. Higher dissociative symptom levels were correlated with early age at onset of physical and sexual abuse and with more frequent sexual abuse. A substantial proportion of participants with all types of abuse reported partial or complete amnesia for abuse memories. For physical and sexual abuse, early age at onset was correlated with greater levels of amnesia. Participants who reported recovering memories of abuse generally recalled these experiences while at home, alone, or with family or friends. Although some participants were in treatment at the time, very few were in therapy sessions during their first memory recovery. Suggestion was generally denied as a factor in memory recovery, and most participants were able to find strong corroboration of their recovered memories.

If such patients were so suggestible and subject to directive influence by diagnosticians, then it is surprising that their presenting symptoms persisted for an average of 6.5 years before the diagnosis was made (Putnam et al. 1986). Rather, it would seem likely that such patients would accept a suggestion that they have another disorder, such as schizophrenia, dysthymia, substance use disorder, or borderline personality disorder, because they encounter many clinicians who are unaware of or not familiar with DID. Because these patients are indeed highly hypnotizable and therefore suggestible (Frischholz 1985), care must be taken in the manner in which the illness is presented to them. However, it is unlikely that the increased number of cases currently reported is accounted for by suggestion alone. Rather, a reduction in previous misdiagnoses and an increase in recognition of the prevalence and sequelae of physical and sexual abuse in childhood (Coons et al. 1988; Finkelhor 1984; Frischholz 1985; Goodwin 1982; Herman et al. 1989; Kluft 1984c, 1991; Pribor and Dinwiddie 1992; Putnam 1988; Putnam et al. 1986; Ross 1989; D. Spiegel 1984; Terr 1991) are also likely explanations. There have been reports of "definite independent confirmation of the histories of abuse" (Coons 1994; Martinez-Taboas 1996) establishing not only the association between dissociative disorders and trauma but also the occurrence of amnesia in response to traumatic experiences. Furthermore, a study among Dutch psychiatrists (Sno and Schalken 1999) reported that 40% have made the diagnosis of DID at least once. The diagnosis was made statistically significantly more frequently by female psychiatrists, by psychiatrists age 50 years or younger, and by those certified after 1982. No correlation was observed with primary theoretical orientation or the type or topography of work facility. The mean age of the selected patients was 33.2 years, and the female-to-male ratio was 9 to 1. Similar to their American counterparts, most patients were seen once a week in an outpatient setting, and individual psychotherapy and adjunctive anxiolytic or antidepressant medications were the most widely endorsed treatment modalities. Different from more typical American practice, hypnosis was rarely used. This study suggested that the diagnosis of DID should not be dismissed as a local (American) eccentricity and minimized via attributions about the roles of suggestibility, hypnosis, and culture.

The skepticism regarding the existence of DID is compounded in the case of criminals because of issues of suspected malingering. Lewis et al. (1997) reviewed the clinical records of 12 murderers with a DSM-IV–defined diagnosis of DID. Data were gathered from medical, psychiatric, social service, school, military, and prison records and from records of interviews with subjects' family members. In their sample, they were able to independently corroborate the presence of signs and symptoms of DID in childhood and adulthood from several sources in all 12 cases. Furthermore, objective evidence of severe abuse was obtained in 11 cases. Of interest, most subjects had amnesia for most of the abuse and thus underreported it. Marked changes in writing style and/or signatures were documented in 10 cases.

Course

DID is diagnosed in childhood with increasing frequency (Kluft 1984a, 1984b) but typically emerges between adolescence and the third decade of life; it rarely presents as a new disorder after an individual reaches the age of 40 years, but there is often considerable delay between initial symptom presentation and diagnosis (American Psychiatric Association 2000; Putnam et al. 1986). The female-to-male sex ratio of DID is 5 to 4 in children and adolescents and 9 to 1 in adults (Hocke and Schmidtke 1998; Sno and Schalken 1999).

Untreated, DID is a chronic and recurrent disorder. It rarely remits spontaneously, but the symptoms may not be evident for some time (Kluft 1985c). DID has been called "a pathology of hiddenness" (Gutheil, as quoted in Kluft 1988, p. 575). The dissociation itself hampers self-monitoring and accurate reporting of symptoms. Many patients with the disorder are not fully aware of the extent of their dissociative symptomatology. They may be reluctant to bring up symptoms because of having encountered frequent skepticism. Furthermore, because most patients with DID report histories of sexual and physical abuse (Coons and Milstein 1992; Coons et al. 1988; Kluft 1985b, 1988, 1991; Putnam 1988; Putnam et al. 1986; Ross 1989; Ross et al. 1990; Schultz et al. 1989; D. Spiegel 1984), the shame associated with that experience, as well as fear of retribution, may inhibit reporting of symptoms.

One last consequence of DID is the subjects' inability to be adequate parents, at least while symptomatic. In a qualitative analysis of the experience of parenting of mothers with dissociative disorders, Benjamin et al. (1998) reported that the functioning of DID mothers, as well as their subjective experience of mothering, was poorer than that of either clinical or nonclinical control mothers. All five symptom areas of dissociation (amnesia, depersonalization, derealization, identity confusion, and identity alteration) impeded their parenting efforts. Their findings highlight the need to address parenting problems in the treatment of those with dissociative disorders.

Comorbidity

It is extremely rare to see a case of DID without any additional psychiatric disorders. To find comorbid Axis I or II disorders in patients diagnosed with DID is the norm (Maldonado and Spiegel 2005). The major comorbid psychiatric illnesses of DID are the depressive disorders (Putnam et al. 1986; Ross and Norton 1989; Ross et al. 1989; Sar et al. 2007b; Yargic et al. 1998), substance use disorders (Anderson et al. 1993; Dunn et al. 1995; Ellason et al. 1996; Karadag et al. 2005; Putnam et al. 1986; Rivera 1991), and borderline personality disorder (Anderson et al. 1993; Brodsky et al. 1995; Ross 2007; Sar et al. 2007b; Shearer 1994; Yargic et al. 1998). Sexual (Brenner 1996b; van der Kolk et al. 1994), eating (Berger et al. 1994; Valdiserri and Kihlstrom 1995; van der Kolk et al. 1994), somatoform (Spitzer et al. 1999; Yargic et al. 1998), and sleep (Putnam et al. 1986) disorders occur less commonly. Patients with DID frequently engage in self-mutilative behavior (Gainer and Torem 1993; Putnam et al. 1986; Ross and Norton 1989; Zweig-Frank et al. 1994), impulsiveness, and overvaluing and devaluing of relationships that make approximately a third of DID patients fit the criteria for borderline personality disorder as well. Such individuals also show higher levels of depression (Horevitz and Braun 1984). Conversely, research shows dissociative symptoms in many patients with borderline personality disorder, especially those who report histories of physical and sexual abuse (Chu and Dill 1990; Ogata et al. 1990; Ross 2007).

In a study attempting to identify the risk factors associated with the dissociative symptomatology of borderline personality disorder patients, four risk factors were found to be significantly associated with the level of dissociation reported: 1) inconsistent treatment by a caregiver, 2) sexual abuse by a caregiver, 3) witnessing sexual violence as a child, and 4) adult rape history (Zanarini et al. 2000b). The results of this study suggested that both sexual trauma and something intrinsic to the borderline diagnosis itself are risk factors for dissociative phenomena among borderline patients. Indeed, the impulsiveness, splitting, and hostility frequently seen in some older personality states are similar to the presentations seen in many patients with borderline personality disorder. A recent study by Watson et al. (2006) suggested that patients with borderline personality disorder demonstrate levels of dissociation that increase with levels of childhood trauma, supporting the hypothesis that traumatic childhood experiences engender dissociative symptoms later in life. Their study also suggested that emotional abuse and neglect may be at least as important as physical and sexual abuse in the development of dissociative symptoms.

Wildgoose et al. (2000) suggested that the single factor mediating the main differences between borderline personality disorder and other personality disorders is the presence of dissociation. When compared with control groups, patients with borderline personality disorder have higher levels of dissociation (26% in borderline personality disorder subjects vs. 3% in control subjects), as measured by the DES (Zanarini et al. 2000a). The researchers also found a wider range of dissociative experiences in this population, including absorption, depersonalization, and amnesia. Golynkina and Ryle (1999) described how in borderline personality disorder, partial dissociation provoked by trauma and deprivation in childhood results in the persistence of separate self states, as is the case in DID. The characteristics of these and alternations between them are seen to account for the main features of the condition. As in cases of DID, patients with borderline personality disorder have difficulties in recalling specific autobiographical memories. These difficulties are related to their tendency to dissociate, and it may help patients with borderline personality disorder (as it does patients with DID) to avoid episodic information that would evoke acutely negative affects (Jones et al. 1999). Similarly, a study of patients engaging in deliberate self-injurious behavior (Low et al. 2000) found that the frequency of this behavior was primarily related to increased dissociation, and a secondary component was mediated by low self-esteem, anger, impulsivity, and a history of sexual and physical abuse.

Comorbidity is complex in that patients with concurrent diagnoses of DID and borderline personality disorder (approximately one-third) also are more likely to meet the criteria for major depressive disorder. In addition, they frequently meet the criteria for PTSD, with intrusive flashbacks, recurring dreams of physical and sexual abuse, avoidance and loss of pleasure of usually pleasurable activities, and symptoms of hyperarousal, especially when exposed to reminders of childhood trauma (Kluft 1985a, 1991; Putnam 1993; D. Spiegel 1990b; van der Kolk and Fisler 1995; van der Kolk et al. 1994, 1996). Ross (2007) studied a group of 93 inpatient subjects who met criteria for borderline personality disorder and compared them with a group ($n=108$) who did not. The two groups were then compared on dissociative symptoms and disorders. The subjects with borderline personality disorder reported significantly more dissociative symptoms and disorders on all measures. He found that 59% of the borderline patients met criteria for a dissociative disorder on the Dissociative Disorders Interview Schedule (DDIS), compared with 22% of the nonborderline patients. Furthermore, in a sample of 1,301 college students in Turkey, Sar et al. (2006) found that 8.5% met diagnostic criteria for borderline personality disorder (as measured by the Structured Clinical interview for DSM-IV Axis II Personality Disorders). Of those, a significant majority (72.5%) of the borderline personality disorder group had a comorbid dissociative disorder, compared with only 18.0% for the comparison group of students without borderline personality disorder ($P<0.001$).

Brenner (1999) postulated that dissociation may be seen as a complex defense and that DID may be thought of as a "lower level dissociative character." Furthermore, Brenner theorized that patients with DID have a unique psychic structure—the "dissociative self"—whose function is to create "alter personalities" out of disowned affects, memories, fantasies, and drives. According to his theory, this "dissociative self" must be dissolved to integrate the "alter personalities."

In addition, these patients often receive misdiagnoses of schizophrenia (Coons 1984; Ellason and Ross 1995; Kluft 1987; Putnam et al. 1986; Ross and Norton 1988; Ross et al. 1990; Steinberg et al. 1994). This diagnostic confusion is understandable given that the first-rank criterion for schizophrenia is that the patient has an apparent delusion (e.g., that his or her body is occupied by more than one person). These patients frequently have auditory hallucinations in which one personality state speaks to or comments on the activities of another (Bliss 1986; Bliss et al. 1983; Coons 1984; Kluft 1987; Peterson 1995; Putnam et al. 1986; Ross et al. 1990). When these patients receive misdiagnoses of schizophrenia, they are frequently given neuroleptics, with poor therapeutic response.

Individuals with DID report an average of 15 somatic or conversion symptoms (Anderson et al. 1993; Bowman 1993; Bowman and Markand 1996; Kaplan et al. 1995; Ross et al. 1989, 1990) and other psychosomatic symptoms such as migraine headaches (D. Spiegel 1987). Studies show that approximately one-third of these patients have complex partial seizures (Schenk and Bear 1981), although more recent studies have not found seizure rates to be that high and do not show substantial elevations in DES scores in patients with complex partial seizures compared with scores in other neurological patients (Loewenstein and Putnam 1988). There is sufficient comorbidity that patients receiving recent diagnoses of DID should be evaluated for the possibility of a seizure disorder.

Genetics

Jang et al. (1998) conducted a classic twin study to assess the relative influence of genetic and environmental influences on measures of pathological and nonpathological dissociative experience. Subjects were volunteers from the general population and included 177 monozygotic and 152 dizygotic twin pairs who completed two measures of dissociative capacity identified from the items constituting the DES. The genetic correlation between these measures was estimated at 0.91, suggesting common genetic factors underlying pathological and nonpathological dissociative capacity. Genetic and environmental correlations between the DES and measures of personality disorder traits (Dimensional Assessment of Personality Pathology—Basic Questionnaire [DAPP-BQ]; Livesley and Jackson 2002) also were estimated. Significant genetic correlations (median=0.38) were found between the DES and the DAPP-BQ measures of cognitive dysregulation, affective lability, and suspiciousness, suggesting that the genetic factors underlying particular aspects of personality disorder also influence dissociative capacity.

Psychological Testing

The diagnosis of DID can be facilitated by psychological testing (Scroppo et al. 1998). Form level on the Rorschach test usually is within the normal range, but emotionally dramatic responses are common, often involving mutilation, especially on the color cards (such responses are often seen in patients with histrionic personality disorder as well). Good form level is useful in distinguishing DID patients from schizophrenic patients, who have poor form level. Leavitt and Labott (1998) replicated these findings. Their results indicated that Rorschach signs for the Labott, Barach, and Wagner Rorschach markers were significantly better than chance at classifying patients as having DID or as not having DID. The Labott system, which performed the best, was able to accurately classify 92% of the sample. The fact that two relatively rare sets of signs (DID and Rorschach) converged in the same small sector of the psychiatric population represents evidence of linkage that is clinically meaningful and not explainable on the basis of artificial creation. That the Rorschach signs operate independent of external bias, yet correspond to the diagnoses obtained through psychiatric evaluation in an inpatient setting, argues for the validity of the DID diagnosis. Also, unlike individuals with schizophrenia, those with DID score far higher than healthy individuals on standard measures of hypnotizability, whereas schizophrenic patients tend to show lower than normal or an absence of high hypnotizability (Lavoie and Sabourin 1980; Pettinati et al. 1990; D. Spiegel and Fink 1979; D. Spiegel et al. 1982; van der Hart and Spiegel 1993). Thus, there is comparatively little overlap in the hypnotizability scores of schizophrenic patients and those of DID patients.

More recently, scales of trait dissociation have been developed (Bernstein and Putnam 1986; Ross 1989), and patients with DID score extremely high on these scales in contrast to healthy populations and other patient groups (Ross et al. 1990; Steinberg et al. 1990). These include the DES (Bernstein and Putnam 1986; Carlson et al. 1993), the Somatoform Dissociation Questionnaires (SDQ-20 and SDQ-5; Nijenhuis et al. 1996, 1997, respectively), the Clinician-Administered Dissociative States Scale (Bremner et al. 1998), the Structured Clinical Interview for DSM-IV Dissociative Disorders—Revised (Steinberg 2000), and the Adolescent Dissociative Experiences Scale (Armstrong et al. 1997).

The DES is widely used for the screening of dissociative experiences. The scale has been translated into and validated in Chinese (Xiao et al. 2006), Czech (Ptacek et al. 2007), French (Darves-Bornoz et al. 1999), German (the "Fragebogen zu dissoziativen Symptomen"; Freyberger et al. 1998; Gast et al. 2001; Spitzer et al. 1998), Spanish (Icaran et al. 1996; Martinez-Taboas and Bernal 2000), Swedish (Körlin et al. 2007; Nilsson and Svedin 2006), and Turkish (Sar et al. 1996).

Physiological Measures

A number of studies have found biological correlates to dissociative disorders. Yet, to date, it is difficult to determine whether these biological changes are the product of dissociative processes or what causes dissociative symptoms.

Miller (1989) conducted complete ophthalmological examinations to test whether DID subjects would show greater variability in visual functioning across alter personalities than would control subjects role-playing DID. The results of his analyses showed that DID subjects had significantly more variability across alter personalities than did their control counterparts on measures of visual acuity with correction, visual acuity without correction, visual fields, manifest refraction, and eye muscle balance. Regarding the clinical significance of these findings, blind ratings of the data were performed by comparing the results of the individual dependent measures across the alter personalities of individual DID and control subjects according to established ophthalmological criteria. The ratings for clinical significance showed that the DID subjects had 4.5 times the average number of changes in optical functioning between alter personalities of the control subjects ($P<0.01$).

Putnam et al. (1990) studied differential autonomic nervous system activity across subjects diagnosed with DID and control subjects who produced "alter" personality states by simulation and by hypnosis or deep relaxation. Eighty-nine percent of the DID subjects consistently manifested physiologically distinct alter personality states.

Simeon et al. (2007) found that dissociative disorder patients had significantly elevated 24-hour urinary cortisol compared with the healthy control subjects. The dissociative disorder group demonstrated significantly greater resistance to, and faster escape from, dexamethasone suppression compared with the healthy control group. The dissociative disorder group demonstrated a significantly inverse correlation between dissociation severity and cortisol reactivity, after controlling for all other symptomatology. Thus, this study suggested a distinct pattern of HPA axis dysregulation in patients suffering from dissociative disorders, emphasizing the importance of further study of stress-response systems in dissociative psychopathology. A similar study (Giesbrecht et al. 2007), this one conducted in undergraduate volunteer subjects, corroborated the findings of Simeon et al. (2007), demonstrating that subjects who scored high on the depersonalization/derealization subscale of the Dissociative Experiences Scale exhibited more pronounced cortisol responses, whereas subjects who scored high on the absorption subscale showed attenuated responses. These findings suggest that various types of dissociation (depersonalization/derealization versus absorption) are differentially related to HPA axis activity (i.e., cortisol stress responses).

Lapointe et al. (2006) used quantitative electroencephalography (EEG) to assess the intrapersonal variability of brain electrical activity of women diagnosed with DID. The findings showed that the two EEG records of a DID subject (alter 1 vs. alter 2) were more different from each other than were the two EEG records of a single control subject, but less different from each other than the EEG records of two separate control subjects.

Reinders et al. (2003, 2006) studied the different emotional mental states of core consciousness in patients with DID using functional neuroimaging. The authors believe they were able to demonstrate specific changes in localized brain activity consistent with DID patients' ability to generate at least two distinct mental states of self-awareness, each with its own access to autobiographical trauma-related memory. Their findings suggest the existence of different regional cerebral blood flow patterns for different senses of self and theorize that the medial prefrontal cortex and the posterior associative cortices to have an integral role in conscious experience.

Treatment

Psychotherapy

Therapeutic direction. It is possible to help patients with DID gain control in several ways over the dissociative process underlying their symptoms. The fundamental psychotherapeutic stance should involve meeting patients halfway in the sense of acknowledging that they experience themselves as fragmented, yet the reality is that the fundamental problem is a failure of integration of disparate memories and aspects of the self. Therefore, the goal in therapy is to facilitate integration of disparate elements. This can be done in a variety of ways.

Secrets are frequently a problem with DID patients, who attempt to use the therapist to reinforce a dissociative strategy that withholds relevant information from certain personality states. Such patients often like to confide plans or stories to the therapist with the idea that the information is to be kept from other parts of the self, for example, traumatic memories or plans for self-destructive activities. Clear limit setting and commitment on the part of the therapist to helping all portions of a patient's personality structure learn about warded-off information are important. It is wise to clarify explicitly that the therapist will not become involved in secret collusion. Furthermore, when important agreements are negotiated, such as a commitment on the part of the patient to seek medical help before acting on a thought to harm self or others, it is useful to discuss with the patient that this is an "all-points bulletin," that is, one that requires attention from all the relevant personality states. The excuse that certain personality states were "not aware" of the agreement should not be accepted.

Maldonado (2000) described a series of "rules of engagement" (Table 15–8) to be used in the treatment of DID. These rules were designed to facilitate the therapist–patient contract by establishing clear lines of communication, delineating therapeutic boundaries, eliminating splitting, and enhancing control over dissociative experiences. The rules call for free access to all pertinent old records and permission to discuss all past and current pertinent information with previous therapists; cooperation in the completion of a full organic/neurological workup; a contract for safety; the establishment of a hierarchical pattern of communication and a hierarchical pattern of responsibility; agreement for a limited exploration followed by therapeutic condensation of memories—that is, an "all details are not needed" policy rather than an endless fishing exploration; a "no secrets" policy; an increased level of communication and cooperation between patient and

TABLE 15–8. "Rules of engagement" in the treatment of dissociative identity disorder

1. Free access to all pertinent records
2. Review of all available and pertinent records
3. Freedom to discuss all past and current pertinent information with previous therapists
4. Complete organic/neurological workup
5. Contract for safety
6. Increased communication and cooperation among alters
7. "No secrets" policy
8. Establishment of hierarchical pattern of communication
9. Establishment of hierarchical pattern of responsibility
10. Limited exploration followed by therapeutic condensation of memories
11. "All details are not needed" policy
12. Rules regarding contact during hospitalizations and continued therapy after discharge
13. Videotaping
14. Ultimate goal: "full integration"
15. "One day you will make me obsolete" principle

therapist and among alters; detailed rules regarding therapist–patient contact during hospitalization and continued therapy after discharge; need for videotaping; and, finally, clear understanding of the ultimate treatment goal: "full integration."

For example, a patient with DID who had been in treatment for many years demonstrated a new alter who threatened to arrange for an apparently accidental death. The therapist told the alter that he, the therapist, would have to share this information with the other personalities. "You can't do that," the alter replied. "That would violate doctor–patient confidentiality." Suppressing a smile, the therapist explained that confidentiality did not apply between identities.

Hypnosis. Hypnosis can be helpful in therapy as well as in diagnosis (Kluft 1982, 1985a, 1985c, 1992, 1999; Maldonado and Spiegel 1995, 1998; Maldonado et al. 2000; Smith 1993; H. Spiegel and Spiegel 2004).

First, the simple structure of hypnotic induction may elicit dissociative phenomena. For example, the Hypnotic Induction Profile (H. Spiegel and Spiegel 2004) was administered to a woman who had experienced hysterical pseudoseizures. In the middle of a routine induction, her head suddenly turned to the side and she relived, with considerable affect, as if it were happening in present tense, an episode in which she had been abducted and sexually assaulted. This enabled her and the clinician to reanalyze her symptoms as spontaneous dissociation, similar to the hypnotic state she had been in. The capacity to elicit such symptoms on command provides the first hint of the ability to control these symptoms. Most of these patients have the experience of being unable to stop dissociative symptoms but are often intrigued by the possibility of starting them. This carries with it the potential for changing or stopping the symptoms as well.

Hypnosis can be helpful in facilitating access to dissociated personalities. The personalities may simply occur spontaneously during hypnotic induction. An alternative strategy is to hypnotize the patient and use age regression to help the patient reorient to a time when a different personality state was manifest. An instruction later to change times back to the present tense usually elicits a return to the other personality state. This then becomes an alternative means of teaching the patient control over the dissociation.

Alternatively, entering the state of hypnosis may make it possible to simply "call up" different identities or personality states. Patients can be taught a simple self-hypnosis exercise (as noted earlier in this chapter in the "Dissociative Fugue" section). For example, the patient can be told to count to himself or herself from 1 to 3: On 1, do one thing: look up. On 2, do two things: slowly close your eyes, and take a deep breath. On 3, do three things: let the breath out, let your eyes relax but keep them closed, and let your body float. Then let one hand float up into the air like a balloon. Develop a pleasant sense of floating throughout your body. After some formal exercises such as this, it is often possible to simply ask to speak with a given alter personality, without the formal use of hypnosis. Merely asking to talk with a given identity usually suffices after a while.

Memory retrieval.   Because loss of memory in DID is complex and chronic, its retrieval is likewise a more extended and integral part of the psychotherapeutic process. The therapy becomes an integrating experience of information sharing among disparate personality elements. In conceptualizing DID as a chronic PTSD, the psychotherapeutic strategy involves a focus on working through traumatic memories in addition to controlling the dissociation.

Controlled access to memories greatly facilitates psychotherapy. As in the treatment of dissociative amnesia, a variety of strategies can be used to help DID patients break down amnesic barriers. Use of hypnosis to go to that place in imagination and ask one or more such parts of the self to interact can be helpful.

Once these memories of earlier traumatic experiences have been brought into consciousness, it is crucial to help the patient work through the painful affect, inappropriate self-blame, and other reactions to these memories. A model of grief work is helpful, enabling the patient to acknowledge and bear the import of such memories (Lindemann 1944/1994; D. Spiegel 1981). It may be useful to have the patient visualize the memories rather than relive them as a way of making their intensity more manageable. It also can be useful to have the patient divide the memories onto two sides of an imaginary screen—for example, on one side, picturing something an abuser did to him or her, and on the other side, picturing how the patient tried to protect himself or herself from the abuse.

> A young woman with DID remembered a particularly painful episode in hypnosis. When she was 12 years old, her stepfather smoked a good deal of marijuana and then forced her to have oral sex with him. She recalled being repelled by what he was forcing her to do and then remembered that she had gagged and vomited all over him. "I spoiled his fun. He threw me up against a wall, but it did not bother me a bit because I knew I ruined it for him." She was instructed to picture on one side of the screen what he had done to her and on the other what she had done to him.

Such techniques can help make the traumatic memories more bearable by placing them in a broader perspective, one in which the trauma victim also can identify adaptive aspects of his or her response to the trauma.

This technique and similar approaches can help these individuals work through traumatic memories, enabling them to bear the memories in consciousness and therefore reducing the need for dissociation as a means of keeping such memories out of consciousness. Although these techniques can be helpful and often result in reduced fragmentation and integration (Kluft 1985a, 1985c, 1986, 1992; Maldonado and Spiegel 1995, 1998; D. Spiegel 1984, 1986a), several complications can occur in the psychotherapy of these patients as well.

The information retrieved from memory in these ways should be reviewed, traumatic memories put into perspective, and emotional expression encouraged and worked through, with the goal of sharing the information as widely as possible among various parts of the patient's personality structure. Instructing other alter personalities to "listen" while a given alter is talking, and reviewing previously dissociated material uncovered, can be helpful. The therapist conveys his or her desire to disseminate the information, without accepting responsibility for transmitting it across all personality boundaries.

The "rule of thirds."　Psychotherapy with a DID patient can be a time-consuming and emotionally taxing process. The "rule of thirds" (Kluft 1988, 1991) is a helpful guideline. The therapist should spend the first third of the psychotherapy session assessing the patient's current mental state and life problems and defining a problem area that might benefit from retrieval into conscious memory and working through. The therapist should spend the second third of the session accessing and working through this memory. The therapist should allow a final third for helping the patient assimilate the information, regulate and modulate emotional responses, and discuss any responses to the therapist and plans for the immediate future.

It is wise to use this final third of the session for debriefing and helping the patient to reorient, to attempt to integrate the new material, to transmit information across personalities, and to prepare to terminate the session. There may be resistance on the part of the therapist to doing this because the intense abreactive materials are often so compelling and interesting. There also may be resistance on the part of the patient to sharing of information across personalities.

Given the intensity of the material that often emerges involving memories of sexual and physical abuse, and the sudden shifts in mental state accompanied by amnesia, the therapist is called on to take a clear and structured role in managing the psychotherapy. Appropriate limits must be set about self-destructive or threatening behavior and agreements made regarding physical safety and treatment compliance, and other matters must be presented to the patient in such a way that dissociative ignorance is not an acceptable explanation for failure to live up to agreements.

Traumatic transference.　Transference applies with special meaning in patients who have been physically and sexually abused. These patients have had presumed caregivers who acted instead in an exploitative and sometimes sadistic fashion. These patients thus expect the same from their therapists. Although their reality testing is good enough that they can perceive genuine caring, they expect therapists either to exploit them, with the patients viewing the working through of traumatic memories as a reinflicting of the trauma and the therapists' taking sadistic pleasure in the patients' suffering, or to be excessively passive, with the patients identifying the therapists with some uncaring family figure who knew abuse was occurring but did little or nothing to stop it. It is important in managing the therapy to keep these issues in mind and make them frequent topics of discussion. Attention to these issues can diffuse, but not eliminate, such traumatic transference distortions of the therapeutic relationship (Maldonado and Spiegel 1995, 1998; D. Spiegel 1988).

Integration.　The ultimate goal of psychotherapy for patients with DID is integration of the disparate states. There can be considerable resistance to this process. Early in therapy, the patient views the dissociation as tremendous protection: "I knew my father could get some of me, but he couldn't get all of me." Indeed, he or she may experience efforts of integration as an attempt on the part of the therapist to "kill" personalities. These fears must be worked through and the patient shown how to control the degree of integration, giving the patient a sense of gradually being able to control his or her dissociative processes in the service of working through traumatic memories. The process of the psychotherapy, in emphasizing control, must alter rather than reinforce the content, which involves reexperiencing of helplessness, a symbolic reenactment of trauma (D. Spiegel 1986b).

As previously mentioned, a patient with DID often fears integration as an attempt to "kill" alter personalities and make the patient more vulnerable to mistreatment by depriving him or her of the dissociative defense. At the same time, this defense represents an internalization of the abusive person or persons in the patient's memory. Setting aside the defense also means acknowledging and bearing the discomfort of helplessness at having been victimized and working through the irrational self-blame that gave the patient a fantasy of control over events that he or she was in fact helpless to control. Yet difficult as it is, ultimately, the goal of psychotherapy is mastery over the dissociative process, controlled access to dissociative states, integration of warded-off painful memories and material, and a more integrated continuum of identity, memory, and consciousness (Maldonado and Spiegel 1995, 1998; D. Spiegel 1988). Although there have been no controlled trials of psychotherapy outcome in patients with this disorder, case series reports indicate a positive outcome in most cases (Kluft 1984c, 1986, 1991).

Cognitive-Behavioral Approaches

Fine (1999) summarized the tactical-integration model for the treatment of dissociative disorders. This consists of structured cognitive-behavioral–based treatments that foster symptom relief, followed by integration of the personalities and/or ego states into one mainstream of consciousness. This approach promotes proficiency in control over posttraumatic and dissociative symptoms, is collaborative and exploratory, and conveys a consistent message of empowerment to the patient.

In addition, both cognitive analytic therapy (CAT; Kellett 2005; Ryle and Fawkes 2007) and dialectic behavioral therapy (DBT; Braakmann et al. 2007) have been found to be helpful as adjunctive or primary treatment of patients with DID. In CAT, multiplicity is understood in terms of a range of self–other patterns (i.e., reciprocal role relationships) originating in childhood. These patterns alternate in determining experience and action according to the situation (i.e., contextual multiplicity). They may be restricted by adverse childhood experiences (i.e., diminished multiplicity), and severe deprivation or abuse may result in a structural dissociation of self-processes (i.e., pathological multiplicity). In CAT practice (Ryle and Fawkes 2007), descriptions of dysfunctional relationship patterns and of transitions between them are worked out by therapist and patient at the start of therapy and are used by both throughout its course.

In a study using DBT, Braakmann et al. (2007) found that patients with high preintervention levels of dissociation achieved the greatest relative symptom reduction. These results are explained by the DBT treatment setting, which includes specific psychoeducation and treatment concerning dissociative behavior.

Psychopharmacology

To date, no good evidence shows that medication of any type has a direct therapeutic effect on the dissociative process manifested by patients with DID (Loewenstein 1991b; Markowitz and Gill 1996; Putnam 1989). In fact, most dissociative symptoms seem relatively resistant to pharmacological intervention (Loewenstein 1991a, 1991b). Thus, pharmacological treatment has been limited to the control of signs and symptoms afflicting patients with DID or comorbid conditions rather than the treatment of dissociation per se.

Whereas in the past, short-acting barbiturates such as sodium amobarbital were used intravenously to reverse functional amnesias, this technique is no longer used, largely because of poor results (Perry and Jacobs 1982).

Benzodiazepines have at times been used to facilitate recall through controlling secondary anxiety associated with retrieval of traumatic memories. However, these effects may be nonspecific at best. Furthermore,

sudden mental state transitions induced by medications may increase rather than decrease amnesic barriers, as the recent concern about triazolam, a short-acting benzodiazepine hypnotic, indicates. Thus, inducing state changes pharmacologically could in theory add to difficulty in retrieval. The only systematic study on the use of benzodiazepines in patients with DID was conducted by Loewenstein et al. (1988). In their study, they used clonazepam successfully to control PTSD-like symptoms in a small sample (n=5) of DID patients, achieving improvement in sleep continuity and a decrease in frequency of flashbacks and nightmares.

Antidepressants are the most useful class of psychotropic agents for patients with DID. Such patients frequently have dysthymic disorder or major depression as well, and when these disorders are present, especially with somatic signs and suicidal ideation, antidepressant medication can be helpful. At least two studies report on the successful use of antidepressant medications (Barkin et al. 1986; Kluft 1984a, 1985b). The use of antidepressants should be limited to the treatment of DID patients who experience symptoms of major depression (Barkin et al. 1986). The selective serotonin reuptake inhibitors (SSRIs) are effective at reducing comorbid depressive symptoms and have the advantage of far less lethality in overdose compared with tricyclics and monoamine oxidase inhibitors (MAOIs). Medication compliance is a problem with such patients because dissociated personality states may interfere with the taking of medication by the patients' "hiding" or hoarding of pills, or patients may overdose.

Antipsychotics are rarely useful in reducing dissociative symptoms. They are used occasionally for containing impulsive behavior, with varying effect. More often, they are used with little benefit when DID patients have been given misdiagnoses of schizophrenia (Kluft 1987). In addition to the risks of side effects such as tardive dyskinesia, the neuroleptics may reduce the range of affect, thereby making patients with DID look spuriously as though they were schizophrenic. In fact, most DID researchers have reported an extremely high incidence of adverse side effects with the use of neuroleptic medications (Barkin et al. 1986; Kluft 1984a, 1988; Putnam 1989; Ross 1989).

Anticonvulsants have been used to treat seizure disorders (Mesulam 1981; Schenk and Bear 1981), which have a high rate of comorbidity with DID, mood disorders (Fichtner et al. 1990), and the impulsiveness associated with personality disorders. These agents have been used to reduce impulsive behavior but are rarely definitively helpful. The high incidence of serious side effects (Devinsky et al. 1989) and abuse or overdose potential also should be kept in mind.

DeBattista et al. (1998) reported on four cases of DID associated with severe self-destructive behavior and comorbid major depression treated with electroconvulsive therapy (ECT). In three of the patients, ECT appeared to be helpful in treating the comorbid depression without adversely affecting the DID.

Other Therapeutic Approaches

Krakauer (2006) described the "two-part film" (TPF) technique, a phase-oriented approach to treating dissociative disorders. The emphasis is on the technique's value in interdicting maladaptive interpersonal and intrapersonal patterns that perpetuate depression, anxiety, dissociation, and self-defeating behaviors. The technique is similar to the screen techniques described in the hypnotic literature. There are some clear differences, however, including a minimally directive therapist role, reliance on the inner wisdom of the client, present and future orientation, and amplification of desired affective and somatic experiences. Price (2007) described how "body therapy" for women receiving psychotherapy for childhood sexual abuse has been found to achieve reductions in dissociation, as measured by the DES. Furthermore, the author reported an incremental effect across time and a strong association between change in dissociation and health outcomes. Similarly, high levels of dissociation at baseline predicted a positive response to the intervention.

Studies of eye movement desensitization and reprocessing (EMDR) have provided mixed outcomes and little support for any specific effect of the use of structured eye movements during psychotherapy. It may well mobilize therapeutic elements common to various exposure, desensitization, hypnotic, and cathartic methods.

Legal Aspects of Memory Work and Hypnosis Recall

A major application of hypnosis in the legal setting has been for the purpose of refreshing recollection of witnesses and victims of crimes (Gravitz 1995). There have been some positive results with this technique—for example, the case involving the driver of a hijacked school bus in Chowchilla, CA (People v. Schoenfeld 1980). Under hypnosis, and not previously, the driver was able to recall the numbers and letters on the license plate of the car that overtook the bus. This led to the arrest and conviction of the kidnappers.

Nonetheless, there has been serious criticism of the use of hypnosis with witnesses and victims. Two charges are leveled at the technique. One is confabulation—that is the creation of pseudo memories that are reported as real (Laurence and Perry 1983) and become what has been called an "honest liar" (H. Spiegel 1980), someone who believes his or her misstatement out of a desire to please the hypnotist or simply as a result of being in the nonrational hypnotic state itself. The second problem is concreting—that having gone through the process of hypnosis, even if new information is not made up, the subject will emerge with an enhanced conviction (i.e., increased confidence) that his or her memories are correct and that the subject will therefore be more convincing to a jury than he or she should be (Diamond 1980; Dywan 1995; McConkey 1992; Orne 1979; D. Spiegel and Scheflin 1994; D. Spiegel and Spiegel 1987). There is evidence that under hypnosis people are more likely to make confident errors—the accuracy of the memories they produce is no better than usual but their confidence in the accuracy of their memories increases (McConkey 1992).

On the other hand, people do dissociate during trauma, often failing to recall events despite being conscious at the time (Cardeña and Spiegel 1993; Spiegel and Cardeña 1991). There is evidence that such memory gaps may persist for years or even decades after such traumatic events as physical or sexual abuse (Williams 1994). Confirming these findings, van der Hart et al. (2005a) conducted a study assessing the memory of DID patients. A systematic interview data of all patients revealed that all participants reported a history of severe childhood abuse; 93.3% reported some period of amnesia for the index traumatic event, and 33.3% reported periods of amnesia for significant nontraumatic childhood experiences. Similarly, all subjects who had been amnesic for their trauma reported that their memories were initially retrieved in the form of somatosensory flashbacks. These findings suggested that, like PTSD patients, DID patients at least initially recall their trauma-related memories not as a narrative, but as somatosensory reexperiencing. Of note, some DID subjects also recalled emotionally charged nontraumatic life events with significant somatosensory components.

Courts have been uniformly unwilling to admit the testimony of a person hypnotized while testifying. More recently, however, courts have also begun to exclude testimony of witnesses who have previously been hypnotized about the event in question. The case law has provided some examples of egregious misuses of hypnosis. For example, in *People v. Shirley* (1982), a woman whose memory of the details of a questionable sexual assault was obscured because of her having ingested a substantial amount of alcohol was hypnotized by a member of the prosecution team the night before she was to testify. Her testimony improved dramatically. The conviction was overturned by the California Supreme Court, which ruled that any witness or victim who had been hypnotized about the facts of a crime could not subsequently testify. In other words, the use of hypnosis created an issue of admissibility rather than weight given to testimony. The court excluded defendants from this prohibition. In a subsequent case, *People v. Guerra* (1984), the conviction of a rapist was likewise overturned, because critical details regarding the nature of the attack were provided by the witness only during a hypnosis session in which considerable pressure was applied for her to remember penetration by the assailant. However, in this case the California Supreme Court left open the possibility that the testimony of a witness whose story had not changed despite a hypnotic interrogation might be salvaged. The Arizona Supreme Court (State ex rel. Collins v. Superior Court 1982) retreated from its extreme position and adopted a standard that holds in New York (People v. Hughes 1983) and New Jersey (*People v. Hurd* 1980), among other states, which is that such witnesses may testify about their prehypnotic recollection of events. The United States Supreme Court, in *Rock v. Arkansas* (1987), ruled that a defendant could testify about his or her prehypnotic recollection of events, thereby rejecting a per se exclusion of testimony that could have been influenced by hypnosis.

The reason for the courts' objection to the use of hypnosis is a combination of real and exaggerated dangers of hypnosis. Nevertheless, from a practical point of view, it is wise to caution attorneys and witnesses that the use of hypnosis might leave open the possibility of challenge to witnesses' credibility or even to the inadmissibility of their testimony (Scheflin and Shapiro 1989; D. Spiegel and Scheflin 1994). Taking note of this problem, the California Legislature (1985) passed a law stating that witnesses would be allowed to testify after hypnotic interrogation if certain guidelines were followed. These guidelines include the use of an independent expert psychiatrist or psychologist as a hypnosis consultant, careful documentation of the witness's memory before hypnosis, and electronic recording of all interaction preceding, during, and after hypnosis sessions (Maldonado and Spiegel 1998; D. Spiegel and Spiegel 1987). The kind of situation in which hypnosis is most likely to be worth the risk is one in which there is a traumatic amnesia for the

events of a crime or in which all other avenues of exploration have been exhausted. Hypnosis should not be used as a replacement for routine police work. In the "FBI Guidelines for Use of Hypnosis" (Ault 1979) detailed the parameters and rules to follow in order to maximize the yield of hypnotic recollection while preserving the integrity of the process.

The Council on Scientific Affairs of the American Medical Association convened a panel of experts to examine the research evidence relevant to this problem. The report issued by the panel (Orne et al. 1985) concluded that what evidence exists indicates that the use of hypnosis tends to increase the productivity of witnesses, resulting in new memories, some of which are true and some of which are incorrect. Furthermore, some studies showed an increase in the confidence assigned by hypnotized subjects to their memories despite the fact that the percentage of correct responses had not improved. The panel noted that the analogy between the laboratory setting in which most of the studies were done and the real-life situation in the courtroom must be drawn with great caution and that situations in which extreme emotional and physical trauma have occurred differ markedly. The panel recommended that careful guidelines similar to the ones outlined in the California law be followed when hypnosis is used in the forensic setting (Bloom 1994; Maldonado and Spiegel 1998; D. Spiegel and Spiegel 1987).

Certainly, it is clear that hypnosis is no truth serum and that the courts must weigh the effects of any hypnotic induction on a witness. At the same time, hypnosis may in certain cases help a traumatized and amnesic witness to recall details not brought forward through conventional interrogation methods (D. P. Brown et al. 1998). Despite the former popularity of hypnosis as a way of "improving" eyewitness memory, many courts almost always regard the use of this testimony to be inadmissible, whereas others allow it only when strict procedural guidelines have been followed. Although the U.S. Supreme Court recognized a defendant's constitutional right to admit his own hypnotically elicited testimony, others have recognized a constitutional basis to exclude hypnotically elicited testimony in most other circumstances (Newman and Thompson 1999).

Maldonado (2000) summarized and adapted the guidelines provided by the American Medical Association (Orne et al. 1985) and the American Society of Clinical Hypnosis (Hammond et al. 1995) for the use of hypnosis as a method of memory enhancement. The guidelines suggest that when hypnosis or any other memory enhancement method is being used for forensic purposes or in the context of working out traumatic memories, especially those related to childhood physical and/or sexual abuse, the steps shown in Table 15–9 should be applied. (For an extensive review of hypnotic technique and the uses, potential side effects, and legal implications of hypnosis, see Chapter 89, "Hypnosis," in Maldonado and Spiegel [2007].)

Dissociative Trance Disorder

Cultural Context

Dissociative phenomena are ubiquitous around the world, occurring in virtually every culture (Castillo 1994a, 1994b; Kirmayer 1993; Lewis-Fernandez 1993). These phenomena seem to be more prevalent in the less heavily industrialized Second and Third World countries, although they can be found everywhere. For this reason, some scholars have argued against the inclusion of possession or dissociative trance disorder as a DSM diagnostic category (Noll 1993). There are descriptions of mediums or possession episodes in different cultures, but they all may serve a similar purpose. There are shamans among Hispanics (Alonso 1988; Pineros et al. 1998) and in Brazil (Moreira-Almeida et al. 2007; Shapiro 1992), China (Gaw et al. 1998; Kua et al. 1993), India (Moore 1993; Nuckolls 1991), Iran (Safa 1988), Israel (Bilu and Beit-Hallahmi 1989; Shirali et al. 1986), Japan (Eguchi 1991; Etsuko 1991), Madagascar (Sharp 1990, 1994), Malaysia (McLellan 1991), Nepal (van Ommeren et al. 2004); New Guinea (Schieffelin 1996), Samoa (Mageo 1996), Singapore (Kua et al. 1986), South Africa (Heap and Ramphele 1991), South Asia (Castillo 1994a), Thailand (Trangkasombat et al. 1998), Zambia (Pullela 1986), and Zanzibar (Tantam 1993). Other dissociative syndromes include demonic possession in Brazil (Heap and Ramphele 1991), Chilopa ritual sacrifices in Malawi (Machleidt and Peltzer 1991), ritual homicide in Italy (Ferracuti and DeMarco 2004), dissociative stupor and trance states in Japan (Nakanishi 2003), Zar possession in Northern Sudan (Boddy 1988) and Ethiopia (Witztum et al. 1996), and pseudohallucinations in Turkey (van der Zwaard et al. 2000).

Most scholars agree that the most common clinical features of trance states are amnesia, emotional disturbances, and loss of identity (D. Li and Spiegel 1992). In a study comparing the characteristic features of the possession trance in three different ethnic groups of Chinese, Malayans, and Indians, Kua et al. (1986)

TABLE 15–9. Guidelines for the use of hypnosis in memory work

1. Before hypnosis use, perform a thorough evaluation of the patient.

2. Explore the patient's expectations about treatment in general and hypnosis use in particular.

3. Obtain the patient's permission to consult with his or her attorney.

4. Clarify your role (i.e., therapist vs. forensic consultant) before initiating any assessment and/or treatment. Make sure the patient clearly understands your role in the case.

5. Obtain written informed consent regarding the nature of hypnotic retrieval (explain to the subject and his or her attorney about the nature of hypnotically retrieved memories) and possible side effects of memory work.

6. Clarify the patient's expectation regarding hypnotically enhanced or recovered memories.

7. Maintain neutrality throughout every interaction with the patient.

8. Make a videotape recording of the interview and hypnotic session.

9. Thoroughly document any and all prehypnosis memories.

10. Objectively measure hypnotizability.

11. Carefully document your discussion of hypnosis and memory, issues of accuracy of memory, informed consent, and the maintenance of a stance of neutrality and nonleading approach.

12. Use an expert as a hypnosis consultant.

13. Conduct the interview in a neutral tone; avoid leading or suggestive questions.

14. Demonstrate a balance between supportiveness and empathy, while assisting the patient to critically evaluate the elicited material.

15. Do not encourage patients to institute litigation or to confront alleged perpetrators based solely on information retrieved under hypnosis.

16. Carefully debrief the subject at the end of each session.

17. Carefully document and produce a report containing

    Detailed prehypnotic memories.
    Hypnotizability score.
    Hypnotic techniques used.
    Any significant behavior.
    Any confirmed or new memories and details.

found a set of similarities, including alteration in the level of consciousness, amnesia for the period of the trance, stereotyped behavior characteristic of a deity, duration of less than 1 hour, fatigue at the termination of the trance, normal behavior in the interval between trances, onset before age 25 years, low socioeconomic status, low educational attainment, and prior witnessing of a trance.

Dissociative symptoms are widely understood as an idiom of distress. In Singapore, stressors associated with the development of dissociative trance disorder include problems with military life (38%), conflicts over religious and cultural issues (38%), and domestic disharmony and marital woes (24%) (Ng and Chan 2004). In South Africa, major depression and bereavement have been described as triggers for the development of dissociative trance disorder (Szabo et al. 2005).

The major purposes served by possession and trance states include the need to gain power, prestige, and status and the desire to express aggressive and sexual impulses (Shirali et al. 1986), especially given the cultural overdetermination of women's selfhood (Boddy 1988). Spirit possession rituals may mystify the source of women's suppression and absolve them of any responsibility for an otherwise unacceptable challenge to patriarchal control (Sered 1994). They also may provide the subject with a sense of social association and ultimately attempt to make something socially useful from feelings such as aggression that were previously socially destructive (Tantam 1993), may provide a release from normative structural constraints, and may facilitate role reversal and role enhancement (McLellan 1991). Dissociative trance disorders, especially possession disorder, are probably more common than is usually thought. Ferracuti et al. (1996) reported on 10 patients undergoing exorcisms for devil trance possession state. Subjects were studied with the Dissociative Disorders Diagnostic Schedule and the Rorschach test. Subjects were found to have many traits in common with patients with DID. Despite claiming possession by a demon and various paranormal phenomena, most of them managed to maintain normal social functioning. Thus, in this sample of subjects reporting demonic possession, dissociative trance disorder appeared to be a distinct clinical manifestation of a dissociative continuum, sharing some features with dissociative disorders in general and DID in particular.

Ataque de nervios is a common self-labeled Hispanic folk diagnosis that describes dramatic episodic outbursts of negative emotion in response to a stressor, sometimes involving destructive behavior. A study among 70 Hispanic outpatients conducted by Schechter et al. (2000) found that significantly more subjects with an anxiety or a mood disorder plus ataque de nervios reported a history of physical abuse, sexual abuse, and/or a substance-abusing caregiver than did those with psychiatric disorder but no ataque de nervios. As in the case of dissociative disorders, in some Hispanic individuals, ataque de nervios may represent a culturally sanctioned expression of extreme affect dysregulation associated with antecedent childhood trauma.

In a case–control study of 32 girls ages 9–14 years afflicted with an outbreak of spirit possession in the south of Thailand, Trangkasombat et al. (1998) found that the children with spirit possession were firstborn and came from small families (e.g., 1–3 children). Compared with the control subjects, children with spirit possession had a family life characterized by more psychosocial stressors, and they had significantly higher rates of psychiatric disorders, anxious and fearful character traits, histrionic character traits, and histories of recurrent trance states. The history of traumatic experiences and exposure to spirit possession ceremonies were more frequent in spirit-possessed children than in control children.

Similarly, Gaw et al. (1998) described the clinical characteristics of 20 hospitalized psychiatric patients in the Hebei Province of China who believed that they were possessed. These patients had been given the Chinese diagnosis of *yi-ping* (hysteria) by Chinese physicians before being recruited for the study. The investigators found that among their subjects, the mean age was 37 years; most patients were women from rural areas with little education; and most reported significant events preceding the episode of possession, including interpersonal conflicts, subjectively meaningful circumstances, illness, and death of an individual or dreaming of a deceased individual. Possessing entities were thought to be spirits of deceased individuals, deities, animals, and devils. About one-fifth of their sample reported multiple possessions. In most instances, the initial experience of possession typically came on acutely and often became a chronic relapsing event. Almost all subjects manifested the loss of control over their actions, change in their usual pattern of behavior, loss of awareness of surroundings, loss of personal identity, inability to distinguish reality from fantasy, change in tone of voice, and loss of perceived sensitivity to pain. The authors suggested that their findings indicate that this type of possession syndrome is clinically similar to the DSM-IV-TR diagnosis of dissociative trance disorder under the category of dissociative disorder not otherwise specified.

Some even suggest that possession can be interpreted as historical discourse, usually containing tales of tradition (Mageo 1996), or even as an alternative method of healing—not too different from Western psychotherapy (C. Li et al. 1992; Machleidt and Peltzer 1991; Mulhern 1991; Tantam 1993)—thus performing a wider social function. In fact, "when the embodiment of an alternative identity is exercised in the cross-cultural complex of spirit possession, it provides a conduit through which subjective suffering can be transcended and through which the past, present, and future can be expressed" (Mulhern 1991, p. 770).

The trance and possession categories of dissociative trance disorder constitute by far the most common kinds of dissociative disorders around the world. Several studies of dissociative disorders in India, for example, reported that dissociative trance and possession are the most prevalent dissociative disorders (i.e., approximately 3.5% of psychiatric admissions; Adityanjee et al. 1989; Saxena and Prasad 1989). On the other hand, DID, which is relatively more common in the United States, is rarely diagnosed in India. Cultural and biological factors may account for the different content and form of dissociative symptoms. Nonetheless, the underlying dissociative mechanism inhibiting integration of perception, memory, and identity makes these syndromes an important class of dissociative disorders.

Differences in culture clearly influence almost all mental disorders, and therefore the contents of religious delusions will be different in a Hindu or Muslim person with schizophrenia than in a Christian person with the same disorder. Depression takes a very different form in China, resembling what used to be called *neurasthenia*, with a variety of somatic symptoms predominating more than the guilty ruminations seen in the West (Kleinman 1977). Likewise, the variations in form of the dissociative disorders only serve to underscore the ubiquity of the dissociative mechanism. Nonetheless, the variety of mental content is worthy of attention. The DSM-IV Task Force voted to include dissociative trance disorder in an appendix to DSM-IV to stimulate further research on the question of whether it should be a separate Axis I disorder rather than an example in the category of dissociative disorders not otherwise specified, in which it was placed in DSM-III-R (American Psychiatric Association 1987) (Table 15–10). Some suggest, and we agree, that the inclusion of trance and possession disorder in DSM-IV intends to develop a sense of cultural sensitivity and internationalization of DSM. On the other hand, designating trance and possession disorder as a formal diagnostic

---

TABLE 15–10. DSM-IV-TR research criteria for dissociative trance disorder

A. Either (1) or (2):

  (1) trance, i.e., temporary marked alteration in the state of consciousness or loss of customary sense of personal identity without replacement by an alternate identity, associated with at least one of the following:

    (a) narrowing of awareness of immediate surroundings, or unusually narrow and selective focusing on environmental stimuli

    (b) stereotyped behaviors or movements that are experienced as being beyond one's control

  (2) possession trance, a single or episodic alteration in the state of consciousness characterized by the replacement of customary sense of personal identity by a new identity. This is attributed to the influence of a spirit, power, deity, or other person, as evidenced by one (or more) of the following:

    (a) stereotyped and culturally determined behaviors or movements that are experienced as being controlled by the possessing agent

    (b) full or partial amnesia for the event

B. The trance or possession trance state is not accepted as a normal part of a collective cultural or religious practice.

C. The trance or possession trance state causes clinically significant distress or impairment in social, occupational, or other important areas of functioning.

D. The trance or possession trance state does not occur exclusively during the course of a psychotic disorder (including mood disorder with psychotic features and brief psychotic disorder) or dissociative identity disorder and is not due to the direct physiological effects of a substance or a general medical condition.

---

disorder carries with it the risks of attempting to craft a global nosological system, an impossible task. Furthermore, the composite category "dissociative trance disorder," encompassing both trance and possession phenomena, may be misinterpreted as "a single, uniform diagnostic construct and may suggest a greater degree of phenomenological uniformity than exists among indigenous syndromes, creating a hybrid nosological entity without validity" (Lewis-Fernandez 1993, p. 123).

These dissociative episodes usually are understood as an idiom of distress, yet they are not viewed as normal. That is, they are not a generally accepted part of cultural and religious practice that may often involve normal trance phenomena, such as trance dancing in the Balinese Hindu culture. Trance dancers in that culture are remarkable for being the only portion of this socially stable society able to elevate their social status. This elevation of social status is done through developing an ability to enter trance states. They are able within the social ceremony to induce an altered state of consciousness in which they dance over hot coals, hold a sword at their throat, or in other ways show exceptional powers of concentration and physical prowess. They are frequently watched by other dancers to make sure that they retain control and do not hurt themselves. This form of trance is considered socially normal and even exalted. By contrast, trance and possession disorder is viewed by the local community as a common but aberrant form of behavior that requires intervention. Although trance and possession disorder is clearly an idiom of distress (e.g., discomfort in a new family environment), most individuals use an array of alternative strategies for coping with such distress. Thus, cultural informants make it clear that persons with trance and possession trance disorders are acting abnormally, if recognizably.

It is interesting that the most common form of dissociative disorder in the West is DID—that is, the experience of fragmentation of individual identity—whereas in the East, this disorder involves possession by an outside spirit, deity, or other entity. Given the greater sociocentric organization of culture in the East, it makes sense that the dissociative problem would take the form of an intruding outside identity, whereas in the West, the disorder takes the form of competing internal identities. Nevertheless, some have proposed that possession trance and multiple personality disorders arose on the basis of similar histories of child abuse and the use of dissociation as a defense mechanism (Bourguignon 1989). Still, different cultures apply their own idiosyncratic etiological theories. The therapeutic approaches and subjects' responses may be rather similar or radically different, depending on the traditional beliefs of the culture in question.

Classification

Dissociative trance disorder has been divided into two broad categories: dissociative trance and possession trance (Table 15–11).

Dissociative Trance

Dissociative trance phenomena are characterized by a sudden alteration in consciousness not accompanied by distinct alternative identities. In this form, the dissociative symptom involves consciousness rather than identity. Also, in dissociative trance, the activities performed are rather simple, usually involving sudden collapse, immobilization, dizziness, shrieking, screaming, or crying. Memory is rarely affected, and amnesia, if any, is fragmented.

Dissociative trance phenomena frequently involve sudden extreme changes in sensory and motor control. Classic examples include *ataque de nervios*, which is prevalent throughout Latin America. This condition, for example, is estimated to have a 12% lifetime prevalence rate in Puerto Rico (Lewis-Fernandez 1993). Typically, the individual suddenly starts to shake convulsively, hyperventilate, scream, and show agitation and aggressive movements. These behaviors may be followed by collapse and loss of consciousness. Afterward, such individuals report being exhausted and may have some amnesia for the event (Lewis-Fernandez 1993).

Falling out occurs frequently among African Americans in the southern United States. Affected individuals may collapse suddenly, unable to see or speak even though they are conscious. These persons may be confused afterward but usually are not amnesic to the episode (Lewis-Fernandez 1993).

In the Malay version of trance disorder, *latah*, affected individuals may have a sudden vision of a spirit that is threatening them. These persons scream or cry, strike out physically, and may need restraints. They may report amnesia, but they do not clearly take on the identity of the offending spirit (Lewis-Fernandez 1993).

Possession Trance

In contrast to dissociative trance, possession trance involves the assumption of a distinct alternate identity, usually that of a deity, an ancestor, or a spirit. The person in this trance often engages in rather complex activities, which may take the form of expressing otherwise forbidden thoughts or needs, negotiating for change in family or social status, or engaging in aggressive behavior. Possession usually involves amnesia for a large portion of the episode during which the alternate identity was in control of the person's behavior.

In Indian possession syndrome, the affected individual suddenly begins speaking in an altered voice with an altered identity, usually that of a deity recognizable to others. Through this voice, a person may refer to himself or herself in the third person. The affected per-

TABLE 15–11. Comparison of Western and Eastern types of dissociative syndromes

Dissociative phenomena	Western	Eastern
Identity	DID: multiple internal identities	Possession trance: control by external identities
	Dissociative fugue	
Memory	Dissociative amnesia	Secondary in dissociative trance, more common in possession trance
Perception	Depersonalization disorder	Dissociative trance (e.g., *latah, ataque de nervios*)
Consciousness	Acute stress disorder	Dissociative trance

Note. DID = dissociative identity disorder.

son's "spirit" may negotiate for changes in the family environment or become agitated or aggressive. Possession syndrome typically occurs in a recently married woman who finds herself uncomfortable or unwelcome in her mother-in-law's home. Such individuals usually are unable to directly express their discomfort.

Treatment

Treatment of these disorders varies from culture to culture. Most syndromes occur within the context of acute social stress and thus serve the purpose of recruiting help from the family and other support systems or removing the subject from the immediate danger or threat. Ceremonies to remove or appease the invading spirit are commonly used (Pineros et al. 1998). The role of psychiatry should be focused on ruling out any possible organic cause for the symptoms shown, treating comorbid psychiatric conditions (if any are present), avoiding excess medication, understanding the social context and role of the syndrome, and facilitating a favorable outcome.

Dissociative Disorder— Conversion Type?

Conversion disorder has been a diagnosis in transition throughout its history in the *Diagnostic and Statistical Manual of Mental Disorders* (DSM). The original DSM (American Psychiatric Association 1952) listed the disorder as "conversion reaction." DSM-II (American Psychiatric Association 1968) listed the disorder as "hysterical neurosis (conversion type)" under the category of Dissociative Disorders. It was not until DSM-III (American Psychiatric Association 1980) that conversion disorder moved from the Dissociative Disorders to the Somatoform Disorders diagnostic cluster. Still, the

Tenth Edition of the *International Classification of Diseases* (ICD-10; World Health Organization 1992) continues to categorize conversion as "dissociative (conversion) disorder." Ever since its move in DSM-III to the Somatoform Disorders category, there have been calls to return conversion disorder to the Dissociative Disorders category. On the other hand, let us not forget that most of the syndromes now classified under Dissociative Disorders—including "psychogenic" or "functional" amnesia, fugue, dissociative identity disorder (DID; also known as multiple personality disorder), and depersonalization disorder—were once classified, along with conversion disorder, as forms of hysteria.

More recently, a number of experts have been suggesting that it is time to return conversion disorder to a more appropriate place under the dissociative disorders (Bowman 2006; R.J. Brown et al. 2007; Maldonado 2007). As expressed by Maldonado (2007, p. 596),

> The symptoms of conversion disorder may appear to serve a number of unconscious purposes, such as the expression of forbidden wishes or impulses in a masked form, the imposition of self-punishment via a disabling symptom for a forbidden wish or wrongdoing, or the removal of oneself from an overwhelming, life-threatening situation. The symptoms are theorized to be secondary to the repression or dissociation of memories and/or affects, the goal being symbolic resolution of unconscious conflicts and an attempt to keep painful memories out of consciousness. Thus, instead of "experiencing" the pain associated with certain affects, patients unconsciously "convert" painful affects into pseudo-medical symptoms, thus maintaining the dissociation of affect from memories. Therefore, patients generally perceive themselves as victims of their symptoms.

Since the beginning, scientists have described an association between conversion phenomena and hypnotizability or dissociative phenomena. Maldonado (2007) has suggested that hypnosis-facilitated techniques have a unique advantage over other treatment modalities, as they help bridge the dissociation of affect from the deficits:

> Indeed, it is likely that patients with a conversion disorder may be using their own hypnotic capacity to dissociate in order to displace uncomfortable feelings or affects into a chosen body part that then becomes dysfunctional. (p. 602)

R.J. Brown et al. (2007) have made a strong case for reclassifying conversion disorder:

> On balance, the frequent co-occurrence of dissociative and pseudo-neurological symptoms, their joint classification in ICD-10, and the theoretical and empirical arguments for common underlying mechanisms, provide a strong case for moving pseudo-neurological symptoms (i.e., Conversion Disorder) to the Dissociative Disorder category in DSM-V... grouping pseudo-neurological symptoms with the dissociative disorders would also foster a more integrated approach to theory, research, and clinical practice in relation to these conditions. (p. 375)

Conclusion

The dissociative disorders constitute a challenging component of psychiatric illness. The failure of integration of memory, identity, perception, and consciousness seen in these disorders results in symptomatology that illustrates fundamental problems in the organization of mental processes. Dissociative phenomena often occur during and after physical trauma but also may represent transient or chronic defensive patterns. Dissociative disorders are generally treatable and constitute a domain in which psychotherapy is a primary modality, although pharmacological treatment of comorbid conditions such as depression can be quite helpful. The dissociative disorders are ubiquitous around the world, although they take a variety of forms. They represent a fascinating window into the processing of identity, memory, perception, and consciousness, and they pose a variety of diagnostic, therapeutic, and research challenges.

Key Points

- Dissociative disorders are underdiagnosed.

- Dissociation is a common component of acute response to trauma, and dissociative fugue, amnesia, and identity disorders often have a traumatic etiology.

- Dissociation represents a failure of integration of identity, memory, perception, and consciousness.

- The primary treatments for dissociative disorders involve various psychotherapies, including hypnosis, trauma-related psychotherapies, and cognitive therapies.

- Common comorbid conditions requiring treatment include depression, substance use disorders, and borderline personality disorder.

- Dissociative symptoms are ubiquitous around the world, but the content of the dissociative symptoms varies, involving "possession" by external entities more often in the East, and fragmentation of individual identity in the West.

Suggested Readings

Appelbaum PS, Uyehara LA, Elin MR (eds): Trauma and Memory: Clinical and Legal Controversies. New York, Oxford Press, 1997

Bremner JD, Marmar CA (eds): Trauma, Memory, and Dissociation. Washington, DC, American Psychiatric Press, 1998

Brown D, Scheflin AW, Hammond DC: Memory, Trauma Treatment, and the Law. New York, WW Norton, 1997

Fink G (ed): Encyclopedia of Stress, 2nd Edition. Academic Press, Oxford, 2007

Foa EB (ed): Effective Treatments for PTSD: Practice Guidelines from the International Society for Traumatic Stress Studies. New York, Guilford, 2000

Cardeña E, Maldonado J, van der Hart O, et al: Hypnosis, in Effective Treatments for PTSD. Edited by Foa EB, Keane TM, Friedman MJ. New York, Guilford, 2000, pp 247–279

Hammond DC, Garver RB, Mutter CB, et al: Clinical Hypnosis and Memory: Guidelines for Clinicians and for Forensic Hypnosis. Bloomingdale, IL, American Society of Clinical Hypnosis Press, 1995

Hilgard ER: Divided Consciousness: Multiple Controls in Human Thoughts and Action. New York, Wiley, 1977

Horowitz MJ: Stress Response Syndromes. New York, Jason Aronson, 1976

Janet P: Psychological Healing: A Historical and Clinical Study. New York, Macmillan, 1925

Janet P: The Major Symptoms of Hysteria: Fifteen Lectures Given in the Medical School of Harvard University, 2nd Edition. New York, Macmillan, 1920

Kardiner A, Spiegel H: War, Stress and Neurotic Illness. New York, Hoeber, 1947

Kluft RP (ed): Childhood Antecedents of Multiple Personality. Washington, DC, American Psychiatric Press, 1985

Kluft RP: Incest-Related Syndromes of Adult Psychopathology. Washington, DC, American Psychiatric Press, 1988

Loewenstein RJ (ed): Multiple personality disorder. Psychiatr Clin North Am 14(3), 1991

Loewenstein RJ: Diagnosis, epidemiology, clinical course, treatment, and cost effectiveness of treatment of dissociative disorders and MPD: report submitted to the Clinton Administration Task Force on Health Care Financing Reform. Dissociation 7:3–11, 1994

Lynn SJ, Rhue J (eds): Dissociation: Clinical, Theoretical and Research Perspectives. New York, Guilford, 1994

Marmar R, Bremmer D (eds): Trauma, Memory, and Dissociation. Washington, DC, American Psychiatric Press, 1998

Nathan PE, Gorman JM (eds): A Guide to Treatments That Work, 2nd Edition. New York, Oxford Press, 2000, pp 463–496

Oldham JM, Skodol AE, Bender DS (eds): Textbook of Personality Disorders. Washington, DC, American Psychiatric Publishing, 2005, pp 493–521

Prince M: Dissociation of a Personality. New York, Longman, Green, 1906

Putnam FW: Diagnosis and Treatment of Multiple Personality Disorder. New York, Guilford, 1989

Ross CA: Multiple Personality Disorder: Diagnosis, Clinical Features, and Treatment. New York, Wiley, 1989

Russell DEH: The Secret Trauma: Incest in the lives of Girls and Women. New York, Basic Books, 1986

Schacter DL (ed): Searching for Memory: The Brain, the Mind, and the Past. New York, Basic Books, 1996

Sidis B, Goodhart SP: Multiple Personality. New York, Appleton-Century-Crofts, 1905

Singer JL (ed): Repression and dissociation. Chicago, IL, University of Chicago Press, 1990, pp 121–142

Spiegel D: Multiple personality as a post-traumatic stress disorder. Psychiatr Clin North Am 7:101–110, 1984

Spiegel D: Dissociating damage. Am J Clin Hypnosis 29:123–131, 1986

Spiegel D (ed): Dissociation: Culture, Mind, and Body. Washington, DC, American Psychiatric Press, 1994

Spiegel D: Recognizing traumatic dissociation. Am J Psychiatry 163:566–568, 2006

Spiegel H, Spiegel D: Trance and Treatment: Clinical Uses of Hypnosis, 2nd Edition. Washington, DC, American Psychiatric Publishing, 2004

van der Kolk BA, McFarlane AC, Weisaeth L (eds): Traumatic Stress: The Effects of Overwhelming Experience on Mind, Body, and Society. New York, Guilford, 1996

Vermetten E, Dorahy MJ, Spiegel D (eds): Traumatic Dissociation: Neurobiology and Treatment. Washington, DC, American Psychiatric Publishing, 2007

Online Resources

Sidran Traumatic Stress Foundation (http://www.sidran.org)

Stanford University Psychosocial Treatment Laboratory (http://med.stanford.edu/school/psychiatry/PSTreatLab)

Society for Clinical and Experimental Hypnosis (http://www.sceh.us)

International Society for the Study of Trauma and Dissociation (http://www.isst-d.org)

National Center for PTSD (http://www.ncptsd.va.gov/ncmain/index.jsp)

References

Adityanjee, Raju GSP, Khandelwal SK: Current status of multiple personality disorder in India. Am J Psychiatry 146:1607–1610, 1989

Akyuz G, Dogan O, Sar V, et al: Frequency of dissociative identity disorder in the general population in Turkey. Compr Psychiatry 40:151–159, 1999

Alonso L: Mental illness complicated by the santeria belief in spirit possession. Hosp Community Psychiatry 39:1188–1191, 1988

American Psychiatric Association: Diagnostic and Statistical Manual: Mental Disorders. Washington, DC, American Psychiatric Association, 1952

American Psychiatric Association: Diagnostic and Statistical Manual of Mental Disorders, 2nd Edition. Washington, DC, American Psychiatric Association, 1968

American Psychiatric Association: Diagnostic and Statistical Manual of Mental Disorders, 3rd Edition. Washington, DC, American Psychiatric Association, 1980

American Psychiatric Association: Diagnostic and Statistical Manual of Mental Disorders, 3rd Edition, Revised. Washington, DC, American Psychiatric Association, 1987

American Psychiatric Association: Diagnostic and Statistical Manual of Mental Disorders, 4th Edition. Washington, DC, American Psychiatric Association, 1994

American Psychiatric Association: Diagnostic and Statistical Manual of Mental Disorders, 4th Edition, Text Revision. Washington, DC, American Psychiatric Association, 2000

Anderson G, Yasenik L, Ross CA: Dissociative experiences and disorders among women who identify themselves as sexual abuse survivors. Child Abuse Negl 17:677–686, 1993

Armstrong JG, Putnam FW, Carlson EB, et al: Development and validation of a measure of adolescent dissociation: the Adolescent Dissociative Experiences Scale. J Nerv Ment Dis 185:491–497, 1997

Ault RL Jr: FBI guidelines for use of hypnosis. Int J Clin Exp Hypn 27:449–451, 1979

Awas M, Kebede D, Alem A: Major mental disorders in Butajira, southern Ethiopia. Acta Psychiatr Scand Suppl 397:56–64, 1999

Baars BJ: A Cognitive Theory of Consciousness. New York, Cambridge University Press, 1988

Ball S, Robinson A, Shekhar A, et al: Dissociative symptoms in panic disorder. J Nerv Ment Dis 185:755–760, 1997

Barkin R, Braun BG, Kluft RP: The dilemma of drug therapy for multiple personality disorder, in Treatment of Multiple Personality Disorder. Edited by Braun BG. Washington, DC, American Psychiatric Press, 1986, pp 107–132

Baron DA, Nagy R: The amobarbital interview in a general hospital setting, friend or foe: a case report. Gen Hosp Psychiatry 10:220–222, 1988

Barton KA, Blanchard EB, Hickling EJ: Antecedents and consequences of acute stress disorder among motor vehicle accident victims. Behav Res Ther 34:805–813, 1996

Benjamin LR, Benjamin R, Rind B: The parenting experiences of mothers with dissociative disorders. J Marital Fam Ther 24:337–354, 1998

Berger D, Saito S, Ono Y, et al: Dissociation and child abuse histories in an eating disorder cohort in Japan. Acta Psychiatr Scand 90:274–280, 1994

Bernstein EM, Putnam FW: Development, reliability, and validity of a dissociation scale. J Nerv Ment Dis 174:727–735, 1986

Bilu Y, Beit-Hallahmi B: Dybbuk-possession as a hysterical symptom: psychodynamic and socio-cultural factors. Isr J Psychiatry Relat Sci 26:138–149, 1989

Blank AS Jr: The longitudinal course of posttraumatic stress disorder, in Posttraumatic Stress Disorder: DSM-IV and Beyond. Edited by Davidson JRT, Foa EB. Washington, DC, American Psychiatric Press, 1993, pp 3–22

Bliss EL: Multiple Personality, Allied Disorders, and Hypnosis. New York, Oxford University Press, 1986

Bliss EL, Larson EM, Nakashima SR: Auditory hallucinations and schizophrenia. J Nerv Ment Dis 171:30–33, 1983

Bloom PB: Clinical guidelines in using hypnosis in uncovering memories of sexual abuse: a master class commentary. Int J Clin Exp Hypn 42:173–178, 1994

Boddy J: Spirits and selves in Northern Sudan: the cultural therapeutics of possession and trance. American Ethnologist 15:4–27, 1988

Boe T, Haslerud J, Knudsen H: Multiple personality: a phenomenon also in Norway? Tidsskr Nor Laegeforen 113:3230–3232, 1993

Boon S, Draijer N: Multiple personality disorder in the Netherlands: a clinical investigation of 71 patients. Am J Psychiatry 150:489–494, 1993a

Boon S, Draijer N: Multiple Personality Disorder in the Netherlands: A Study on Reliability and Validity of the Diagnosis. Amsterdam, The Netherlands, Swets & Zeitlinger, 1993b

Bourguignon E: Multiple personality, possession trance, and the psychic unity of mankind. Ethos 17:371–384, 1989

Bowman ES: Etiology and clinical course of pseudoseizures: relationship to trauma, depression, and dissociation. Psychosomatics 34:333–342, 1993

Bowman ES: Why conversion seizures should be classified as a dissociative disorder. Psychiatr Clin North Am 29:185–211, 2006

Bowman ES, Markand ON: Psychodynamics and psychiatric diagnoses of pseudoseizure subjects. Am J Psychiatry 153:57–63, 1996

Braakmann D, Ludewig S, Milde J, et al: Dissociative symptoms during treatment of borderline personality disorder. Psychother Psychosom Med Psychol 57(3–4):154–160, 2007

Brauchle G: Persistent dissociation as predictor of posttraumatic stress disorder in psychosocial disaster workers. Psychother Psychosom Med Psychol 56:342–346, 2006

Bremner JD, Brett E: Trauma-related dissociative states and long-term psychopathology in posttraumatic stress disorder. J Trauma Stress 10:37–49, 1997

Bremner JD, Krystal JH, Putnam FW, et al: Measurement of dissociative states with the Clinician-Administered Dissociative States Scale (CADSS). J Trauma Stress 11:125–136, 1998

Brenner I: The dissociative character: a reconsideration of "multiple personality." J Am Psychoanal Assoc 42:819–846, 1994

Brenner I: The characterological basis of multiple personality. Am J Psychother 50:154–166, 1996a

Brenner I: On trauma, perversion, and "multiple personality." J Am Psychoanal Assoc 44:785–814, 1996b

Brenner I: Deconstructing DID. Am J Psychother 53:344–360, 1999

Breuer J, Freud S: Studies on hysteria (1893–1895), in The Standard Edition of the Complete Psychological Works of Sigmund Freud, Vol 2. Translated and edited by Strachey J. London, England, Hogarth Press, 1955, pp 201–319

Brewin CR, Andrews B, Rose S, et al: Acute stress disorder and posttraumatic stress disorder in victims of violent crime [see comments]. Am J Psychiatry 156:360–366, 1999

Briere J, Scott C, Weathers F: Peritraumatic and persistent dissociation in the presumed etiology of PTSD. Am J Psychiatry 162:2295–2301, 2005

Brodsky BS, Cloitre M, Dulit RA: Relationship of dissociation to self-mutilation and childhood abuse in borderline personality disorder. Am J Psychiatry 152:1788–1792, 1995

Brown DP, Scheflin AW, Hammond DC: Memory, Trauma Treatment, and the Law. New York, WW Norton, 1998

Brown GR, Anderson B: Psychiatric morbidity in adult inpatients with childhood histories of sexual and physical abuse. Am J Psychiatry 148:55–61, 1991

Brown L, Russell J, Thornton C, et al: Dissociation, abuse and the eating disorders: evidence from an Australian population. Aust N Z J Psychiatry 33:521–528, 1999

Brown RJ, Cardeña E, Nijenhuis E, et al: Should conversion disorder be reclassified as a dissociative disorder in DSM-V? Psychosomatics 48:369–378, 2007

Brown W: The treatment of cases of shell shock in an advanced neurological centre. Lancet 2:197–200, 1918

Butler LD, Duran EFD, Jasiukatis P, et al: Hypnotizability and traumatic experience: a diathesis-stress model of dissociative symptomatology. Am J Psychiatry 153:42–63, 1996

California Legislature: AB 2669 Chapter 7, Hypnosis of Witnesses, added to Chapter 7, Division 6, of the Evidence Code, enacted January 1, 1985

Cardeña E, Spiegel D: Dissociative reactions to the San Francisco Bay Area earthquake of 1989. Am J Psychiatry 150:474–478, 1993

Carlier IV, Lamberts RD, Fouwels AJ, et al: PTSD in relation to dissociation in traumatized police officers. Am J Psychiatry 153:1325–1328, 1996

Carlson EB, Putnam FW, Ross CA, et al: Validity of the Dissociative Experiences Scale in screening for multiple personality disorder: a multicenter study. Am J Psychiatry 150:1030–1036, 1993

Castillo RJ: Spirit possession in South Asia, dissociation or hysteria? I: theoretical background. Cult Med Psychiatry 18:1–21, 1994a

Castillo RJ: Spirit possession in South Asia, dissociation or hysteria? II: case histories. Cult Med Psychiatry 18:141–162, 1994b

Charcot JM: Oeuvres Completes de J M Charcot, Tome XI. Paris, France, Lecrosnier et Babe, 1890

Chodoff P: Turkish dissociative identity disorder (letter). Am J Psychiatry 154:1179, 1997

Christianson SA, Loftus EF: Memory for traumatic events. Applied Cognitive Psychology 1:225–239, 1987

Chu JA, Dill DL: Dissociative symptoms in relation to childhood physical and sexual abuse. Am J Psychiatry 147:887–892, 1990

Chu JA, Frey LM, Ganzel BL, et al: Memories of childhood abuse: dissociation, amnesia, and corroboration. Am J Psychiatry 156:749–755, 1999

Classen C, Koopman C, Hales R, et al: Acute stress disorder as a predictor of posttraumatic stress symptoms. Am J Psychiatry 155:620–624, 1998

Cohen JD, Servan-Schreiber D: Introduction to neural network models in psychiatry. Psychiatr Ann 22:113–118, 1992a

Cohen JD, Servan-Schreiber D: A neural network model of disturbances in the processing of context in schizophrenia. Psychiatr Ann 22:131–136, 1992b

Collin-Vézina D, Hébert M: Comparing dissociation and PTSD in sexually abused school-aged girls. J Nerv Ment Dis 193:47–52, 2005

Coons PM: The differential diagnosis of multiple personality: a comprehensive review. Psychiatr Clin North Am 7:51–65, 1984

Coons PM: Confirmation of childhood abuse in child and adolescent cases of multiple personality disorder and dissociative disorder not otherwise specified. J Nerv Ment Dis 182:461–464, 1994

Coons PM: The dissociative disorders: rarely considered and underdiagnosed. Psychiatr Clin North Am 21:637–648, 1998

Coons PM, Milstein V: Psychosexual disturbances in multiple personality: characteristics, etiology, and treatment. J Clin Psychiatry 47:106–110, 1986

Coons PM, Milstein V: Psychogenic amnesia: a clinical investigation of 25 cases. Dissociation 5:73–79, 1992

Coons PM, Bowman ES, Milstein V: Multiple personality disorder: a clinical investigation of 50 cases. J Nerv Ment Dis 17:519–527, 1988

Coons PM, Bowman ES, Kluft RP, et al: The cross-cultural occurrence of MPD: additional cases from a recent survey. Dissociation 4:124–128, 1991

Darves-Bornoz JM: Rape-related psychotraumatic syndromes. Eur J Obstet Gynecol Reprod Biol 71:59–65, 1997

Darves-Bornoz JM, Degiovanni A, Gaillard P: Validation of a French version of the Dissociative Experiences Scale in a rape-victim population. Can J Psychiatry 44:271–275, 1999

DeBattista C, Solvason HB, Spiegel D: ECT in dissociative identity disorder and comorbid depression. J ECT 14:275–279, 1998

Devinsky O, Putnam F, Grafman J, et al: Dissociative states and epilepsy. Neurology 39:835–840, 1989

Diamond BL: Inherent problems in the use of pretrial hypnosis on a prospective witness. California Law Review 68:313–349, 1980

Dominguez DV, Cohen M, Brom D: Trauma and dissociation in psychiatric outpatients. Isr J Psychiatry Relat Sci 41:98–110, 2004

Draijer N, Langeland W: Childhood trauma and perceived parental dysfunction in the etiology of dissociative symptoms in psychiatric inpatients. Am J Psychiatry 156:379–385, 1999

Dunn GE, Ryan JJ, Paolo AM, et al: Comorbidity of dissociative disorders among patients with substance use disorders. Psychiatr Serv 46:153–156, 1995

Dywan J: The illusion of familiarity: an alternative to the report-criterion account of hypnotic recall. Int J Clin Exp Hypn 43:194–211, 1995

Eguchi S: Between folk concepts of illness and psychiatric diagnosis: kitsune-tsuki (fox possession) in a mountain village of western Japan. Cult Med Psychiatry 15:421–451, 1991

Ellason JW, Ross CA: Positive and negative symptoms in dissociative identity disorder and schizophrenia: a comparative analysis. J Nerv Ment Dis 183:236–241, 1995

Ellason JW, Ross CA, Sainton K, et al: Axis I and II comorbidity and childhood trauma history in chemical dependency. Bull Menninger Clin 60:39–51, 1996

Elzinga BM, Ardon AM, Heijnis MK, et al: Neural correlates of enhanced working-memory performance in dissociative disorder: a functional MRI study. Psychol Med 37:235–245, 2007

Eriksson NG, Lundin T: Early traumatic stress reactions among Swedish survivors of the Estonia disaster. Br J Psychiatry 169:713–716, 1996

Etsuko M: The interpretations of fox possession: illness as metaphor. Cult Med Psychiatry 15:453–477, 1991

Ferracuti S, DeMarco MC: Ritual homicide during dissociative trance disorder. Int J Offender Ther Comp Criminol 48:59–64, 2004

Ferracuti S, Sacco R, Lazzari R: Dissociative trance disorder: clinical and Rorschach findings in 10 persons reporting demon possession and treated by exorcism. J Pers Assess 66:525–539, 1996

Fichtner CG, Kuhlman DT, Gruenfeld MJ, et al: Decreased episodic violence and increased control of dissociation in a carbamazepine-treated case of multiple personality. Biol Psychiatry 27:1045–1052, 1990

Fine CG: The tactical-integration model for the treatment of dissociative identity disorder and allied dissociative disorders. Am J Psychother 53:361–376, 1999

Finkelhor D: Child Sexual Abuse: New Theory and Research. New York, Free Press, 1984

Foote B, Smolin Y, Kaplan M, et al: Prevalence of dissociative disorders in psychiatric outpatients. Am J Psychiatry 163:623–629, 2006

Frankel FH: Hypnotizability and dissociation. Am J Psychiatry 147:823–829, 1990

Freud S: The ego and the id (1923), in The Standard Edition of the Complete Psychological Works of Sigmund Freud, Vol 19. Translated and edited by Strachey J. London, England, Hogarth Press, 1961, pp 3–66

Freyberger HJ, Spitzer C, Stieglitz RD, et al: Questionnaire on dissociative symptoms: German adaptation, reliability and validity of the American Dissociative Experience Scale (DES). Psychother Psychosom Med Psychol 48:223–229, 1998

Friedl MC, Draijer N: Dissociative disorders in Dutch psychiatric inpatients. Am J Psychiatry 157:1012–1013, 2000

Frischholz EJ: The relationship among dissociation, hypnosis, and child abuse in the development of multiple personality disorder, in Childhood Antecedents of Multiple Personality Disorder. Edited by Kluft RP. Washington, DC, American Psychiatric Press, 1985, pp 99–126

Gainer MJ, Torem MS: Ego-state therapy for self-injurious behavior. Am J Clin Hypn 35:257–266, 1993

Ganaway GK: Hypnosis, childhood trauma, and dissociative identity disorder: toward an integrative theory. Int J Clin Exp Hypn 43:127–144, 1995

Gast U, Rodewald F, Nickel V, et al: Prevalence of dissociative disorders among psychiatric inpatients in a German university clinic. J Nerv Ment Dis 189:249–257, 2001

Gaw AC, Ding Q, Levine RE, et al: The clinical characteristics of possession disorder among 20 Chinese patients in the Hebei province of China. Psychiatr Serv 49:360–365, 1998

Gelb JL: Multiple personality disorder and satanic ritual abuse. Aust N Z J Psychiatry 27:701–708, 1993

Giesbrecht T, Smeets T, Merckelbach H, et al: Depersonalization experiences in undergraduates are related to heightened stress cortisol responses. J Nerv Ment Dis 195:282–287, 2007

Giese AA, Thomas MR, Dubovsky SL: Dissociative symptoms in psychotic mood disorders: an example of symptom nonspecificity. Psychiatry 60:60–66, 1997

Ginzburg K, Koopman C, Butler LD, et al: Evidence for a dissociative subtype of post-traumatic stress disorder among help-seeking childhood sexual abuse survivors. J Trauma Dissociation 7:7–27, 2006

Glisky EL, Ryan L, Reminger S, et al: A case of psychogenic fugue: I understand, aber ich verstehe nichts. Neuropsychologia 42:1132–1147, 2004

Golynkina K, Ryle A: The identification and characteristics of the partially dissociated states of patients with borderline personality disorder. Br J Med Psychol 72:429–445, 1999

Goodwin J: Sexual Abuse: Incest Victims and Their Families. Boston, MA, Wright/PSG, 1982

Grabe HJ, Rainermann S, Spitzer C, et al: The relationship between dimensions of alexithymia and dissociation. Psychother Psychosom 69:128–131, 2000

Gravitz MA: First admission (1846) of hypnotic testimony in court. Am J Clin Hypn 37:326–330, 1995

Hammond DC, Garver RB, Mutter CB, et al: Clinical Hypnosis and Memory: Guidelines for Clinicians and for Forensic Hypnosis. Bloomingdale, IL, American Society of Clinical Hypnosis Press, 1995

Harvey AG, Bryant RA: Relationship between acute stress disorder and posttraumatic stress disorder: a prospective evaluation of motor vehicle accident survivors. J Consult Clin Psychol 66:507–512, 1998

Harvey AG, Bryant RA: Dissociative symptoms in acute stress disorder. J Trauma Stress 12:673–680, 1999

Heap M, Ramphele M: The quest for wholeness: health care strategies among the residents of council-built hostels in Cape Town. Soc Sci Med 32:117–126, 1991

Herman JL, Perry JC, van der Kolk BA: Childhood trauma in borderline personality disorder. Am J Psychiatry 146:490–495, 1989

Hetzel MD, McCanne TR: The roles of peritraumatic dissociation, child physical abuse, and child sexual abuse in the development of posttraumatic stress disorder and adult victimization. Child Abuse Negl 29:915–930, 2005

Hilgard ER: Hypnotic Susceptibility. New York, Harcourt, Brace and World, 1965

Hilgard ER: Divided Consciousness: Multiple Controls in Human Thought and Action. New York, Wiley-Interscience, 1977

Hocke V, Schmidtke A: "Multiple personality disorder" in childhood and adolescence. Z Kinder Jugendpsychiatr Psychother 26:273–284, 1998

Hoffman RE: Computer simulations of neural information processing and the schizophrenia-mania dichotomy. Arch Gen Psychiatry 44:178–188, 1987

Holen A: Normal and pathological grief: recent views. Tidsskr Nor Laegeforen 113:2089–2091, 1993

Horen SA, Leichner PP, Lawson JS: Prevalence of dissociative symptoms and disorders in an adult psychiatric inpatient population in Canada. Can J Psychiatry 40:185–191, 1995

Horevitz RP, Braun BG: Are multiple personalities borderline? An analysis of 33 cases. Psychiatr Clin North Am 7:69–87, 1984

Horowitz MJ: Stress Response Syndromes. New York, Jason Aronson, 1976

Hunter EC, Sierra M, David AS: The epidemiology of depersonalisation and derealisation. A systematic review. Soc Psychiatry Psychiatr Epidemiol 39:9–18, 2004

Hunter EC, Baker D, Phillips ML, et al: Cognitive-behavioural therapy for depersonalization disorder: an open study. Behav Res Ther 43:1121–1130, 2005

Icaran E, Colom R, Orengo-Garcia F: Validation study of the Dissociative Experiences Scale in Spanish population sample. Actas Luso Esp Neurol Psiquiatr Cienc Afines 24:7–10, 1996

Ilechukwu ST, Henry T: Amytal interview using intravenous lorazepam in a patient with dissociative fugue. Gen Hosp Psychiatry 28:544–545, 2006

Irwin HJ: Pathological and nonpathological dissociation: the relevance of childhood trauma. J Psychol 133:157–164, 1999

James W: The Principles of Psychology (1890). New York, Dover, 1950

Janet P: The Major Symptoms of Hysteria: Fifteen Lectures Given in the Medical School of Harvard University, 2nd Edition. New York, Macmillan, 1920

Jang KL, Paris J, Zweig-Frank H, et al: Twin study of dissociative experience. J Nerv Ment Dis 186:345–351, 1998

Johnson DM, Pike JL, Chard KM: Factors predicting PTSD, depression, and dissociative severity in female treatment-seeking childhood sexual abuse survivors. Child Abuse Negl 25:179–198, 2001

Johnson JG, Cohen P, Kasen S, et al: Dissociative disorders among adults in the community, impaired functioning, and Axis I and II comorbidity. J Psychiatr Res 40:131–140, 2006

Jones B, Heard H, Startup M, et al: Autobiographical memory and dissociation in borderline personality disorder. Psychol Med 29:1397–1404, 1999

Kaplan ML, Asnis GM, Lipschitz DS, et al: Suicidal behavior and abuse in psychiatric outpatients. Compr Psychiatry 36:229–235, 1995

Karadag F, Sar V, Tamar-Gurol D, et al: Dissociative disorders among inpatients with drug or alcohol dependency. J Clin Psychiatry 66:1247–1253, 2005

Kardiner A, Spiegel H: War, Stress and Neurotic Illness. New York, Hoeber, 1947

Kellett S: The treatment of dissociative identity disorder with cognitive analytic therapy: experimental evidence of sudden gains. J Trauma Dissociation 6:55–81, 2005

Kihlstrom JF: The cognitive unconscious. Science 237:1445–1452, 1987

Kihlstrom JF, Hoyt IP: Repression, dissociation, and hypnosis, in Repression and Dissociation: Implications for Personality Theory, Psychopathology, and Health. Edited by Singer JL. Chicago, IL, University of Chicago Press, 1990, pp 181–208

Kirmayer LJ: Pacing the void: social and cultural dimensions of dissociation, in Dissociation: Culture, Mind, and Body. Edited by Spiegel D. Washington, DC, American Psychiatric Press, 1993, pp 91–122

Kleinman A: Depression, somatization and the "new cross-cultural psychiatry." Soc Sci Med 11:3–10, 1977

Kluft RP: Varieties of hypnotic intervention in the treatment of multiple personality. Am J Clin Hypn 24:230–240, 1982

Kluft RP: An introduction to multiple personality disorder. Psychiatric Annals 14:19–24, 1984a

Kluft RP: Multiple personality in childhood. Psychiatr Clin North Am 7:121–134, 1984b

Kluft RP: Treatment of multiple personality disorder: a study of 33 cases. Psychiatr Clin North Am 7:9–29, 1984c

Kluft RP: Hypnotherapy of childhood multiple personality disorder. Am J Clin Hypn 27:201–210, 1985a

Kluft RP: The natural history of multiple personality disorder, in Childhood Antecedents of Multiple Personality. Edited by Kluft RP. Washington, DC, American Psychiatric Press, 1985b, pp 197–238

Kluft RP: Using hypnotic inquiry protocols to monitor treatment progress and stability in multiple personality disorder. Am J Clin Hypn 28:63–75, 1985c

Kluft RP: Personality unification in multiple personality disorder: a follow-up study, in Treatment of Multiple Personality Disorder. Edited by Braun BG. Washington, DC, American Psychiatric Press, 1986, pp 29–60

Kluft RP: First-rank symptoms as a diagnostic clue to multiple personality disorder. Am J Psychiatry 144:293–298, 1987

Kluft RP: The dissociative disorders, in American Psychiatric Press Textbook of Psychiatry. Edited by Talbott JA, Hales RE, Yudofsky SC. Washington, DC, American Psychiatric Press, 1988, pp 557–585

Kluft RP: Multiple personality disorder, in American Psychiatric Press Review of Psychiatry, Vol 10. Edited by Tasman A, Goldfinger SM. Washington, DC, American Psychiatric Press, 1991, pp 161–188

Kluft RP: The use of hypnosis with dissociative disorders. Psychiatr Med 10:31–46, 1992

Kluft RP: An overview of the psychotherapy of dissociative identity disorder. Am J Psychother 53:289–319, 1999

Koopman C, Classen C, Spiegel D: Predictors of posttraumatic stress symptoms among survivors of the Oakland/Berkeley, Calif., firestorm. Am J Psychiatry 151:888–894, 1994

Koopman C, Classen C, Cardeña E, et al: When disaster strikes, acute stress disorder may follow. J Trauma Stress 8:29–46, 1995

Koopman C, Classen C, Spiegel D: Dissociative responses in the immediate aftermath of the Oakland/Berkeley firestorm. J Trauma Stress 9:521–540, 1996

Kopelman MD, Panayiotopoulos CP, Lewis P: Transient epileptic amnesia differentiated from psychogenic "fugue": neuropsychological, EEG, and PET findings. J Neurol Neurosurg Psychiatry 57:1002–1004, 1994

Korlin D, Edman G, Nyback H: Reliability and validity of a Swedish version of the Dissociative Experiences Scale (DES-II). Nord J Psychiatry 61:126–142, 2007

Krakauer SY: The two-part film technique: empowering dissociative clients to alter cognitive distortions and maladaptive behaviors. J Trauma Dissociation 7:39–57, 2006

Kua EH, Sim LP, Chee KT: A cross-cultural study of the possession-trance in Singapore. Aust N Z J Psychiatry 20:361–364, 1986

Kua EH, Chew PH, Ko SM: Spirit possession and healing among Chinese psychiatric patients. Acta Psychiatr Scand 88:447–450, 1993

Lanius RA, Williamson PC, Boksman K, et al: Brain activation during script-driven imagery induced dissociative responses in PTSD: a functional magnetic resonance imaging investigation. Biol Psychiatry 52:305–311, 2002

Lanius RA, Williamson PC, Bluhm RL, et al: Functional connectivity of dissociative responses in posttraumatic stress disorder: a functional magnetic resonance imaging investigation. Biol Psychiatry 57:873–884, 2005

Lapointe AR, Crayton JW, DeVito R, et al: Similar or disparate brain patterns? The intra-personal EEG variability of three women with multiple personality disorder. Clin EEG Neurosci 37:235–242, 2006

Laurence JR, Perry C: Hypnotically created memory among highly hypnotizable subjects. Science 222:523–524, 1983

Lavoie G, Sabourin M: Hypnosis and schizophrenia: a review of experimental and clinical studies, in Handbook of Hypnosis and Psychosomatic Medicine. Edited by Burrows GD, Dennerstein L. New York, Elsevier, 1980

Leavitt F, Labott SM: Rorschach indicators of dissociative identity disorders: clinical utility and theoretical implications. J Clin Psychol 54:803–810, 1998

Lewis DO, Yeager CA, Swica Y, et al: Objective documentation of child abuse and dissociation in 12 murderers with dissociative identity disorder. Am J Psychiatry 154:1703–1710, 1997

Lewis-Fernandez R: Culture and dissociation: a comparison of ataque de nervios among Puerto Ricans and "possession syndrome" in India, in Dissociation: Culture, Mind, and Body. Edited by Spiegel D. Washington, DC, American Psychiatric Press, 1993, pp 123–167

Li C, Sun Y, Fang M: Trance states, altered states of consciousness, and related issues. Chinese Mental Health Journal 6:167–170, 1992

Li D, Spiegel D: A neural network model of dissociative disorders. Psychiatr Ann 22:144–147, 1992

Lindemann E: Symptomatology and management of acute grief. 1944. Am J Psychiatry 151 (6 suppl):155–160, 1994

Lipsanen T, Korkeila J, Peltola P, et al: Dissociative disorders among psychiatric patients. Eur Psychiatry 19:53–55, 2004

Livesley WJ, Jackson DN: Manual for the Dimensional Assessment of Personality Pathology—Basic Questionnaire (DAPP-BQ). Port Huron, MI, Sigma Press, 2002

Loewenstein RJ: An official mental status examination for complex chronic dissociative symptoms and multiple personality disorder. Psychiatr Clin North Am 14:567–604, 1991a

Loewenstein RJ: Psychogenic amnesia and psychogenic fugue: a comprehensive review, in American Psychiatric Press Review of Psychiatry, Vol 10. Edited by Tasman A, Goldfinger SM. Washington, DC, American Psychiatric Press, 1991b, pp 189–222

Loewenstein RJ: Diagnosis, epidemiology, clinical course, treatment, and cost effectiveness of treatment of dissociative disorders and MPD: report submitted to the Clinton Administration Task Force on Health Care Financing Reform. Dissociation 7:3–11, 1994

Loewenstein RJ, Putnam FW: A comparative study of dissociative symptoms in patients with complex partial seizures, multiple personality disorder and posttraumatic stress disorder. Dissociation 1:17–23, 1988

Loewenstein RJ, Hornstein N, Farber B: Open trial of clonazepam in the treatment of posttraumatic stress symptoms in MPD. Dissociation 1:3–12, 1988

Low G, Jones D, MacLeod A, et al: Childhood trauma, dissociation and self-harming behaviour: a pilot study. Br J Med Psychol 73:269–278, 2000

Lussier RG, Steiner J, Grey A, et al: Prevalence of dissociative disorders in an acute care day hospital population. Psychiatr Serv 48:244–246, 1997

Maaranen P, Tanskanen A, Honkalampi K, et al: Factors associated with pathological dissociation in the general population. Aust N Z J Psychiatry 39:387–394, 2005

Machleidt W, Peltzer K: The Chilopa ceremony: a sacrificial ritual for mentally (spiritually) ill patients in a traditional healing centre in Malawi. Psychiatria Danubina 3:205–227, 1991

Macleod AD: Posttraumatic stress disorder, dissociative fugue and a locator beacon. Aust N Z J Psychiatry 33:102–104, 1999

Madakasira S, O'Brien KF: Acute posttraumatic stress disorder in victims of a natural disaster. J Nerv Ment Dis 175:286–290, 1987

Mageo JM: Spirit girls and marines: possession and ethnopsychiatry as historical discourse in Samoa. American Ethnologist 23:61–82, 1996

Maldonado JR: Diagnosis and treatment of dissociative disorders, in Manual for the Course: Advanced Hypnosis: The Use of Hypnosis in Medicine and Psychiatry. Annual meeting of the American Psychiatric Association, Chicago, IL, May 13–18, 2000

Maldonado JR: Conversion disorder, in Gabbard's Treatments of Psychiatric Disorders, 4th Edition. Edited by Gabbard GO. Washington, DC, American Psychiatric Publishing, 2007, pp 443–456

Maldonado JR: Dissociation, in Encyclopedia of Stress, 2nd Edition, Vol 1. Edited by Fink G. Oxford, UK, Academic Press, 2007, pp 828–837

Maldonado JR, Spiegel D: Using hypnosis, in Treating Women Molested in Childhood. Edited by Classen C. San Francisco, CA, Jossey-Bass, 1995, pp 163–186

Maldonado JR, Spiegel D: Trauma, dissociation, and hypnotizability, in Trauma, Memory, and Dissociation. Edited by Marmar CR, Bremmer JD. Washington, DC, American Psychiatric Press, 1998, pp 57–106

Maldonado JR, Spiegel D: Dissociative states in personality disorders, in Textbook of Personality Disorders. Edited by Oldham JM, Skodol AE, Bender DS. Washington, DC, American Psychiatric Publishing, 2005, pp 493–521

Maldonado JR, Spiegel D: Hypnosis, in Psychiatry, 2nd Edition. Edited by Tasman A, Kay J, Lieberman J. New York, Wiley, 2007

Maldonado JR, Butler LD, Spiegel D: Treatment of dissociative disorders, in Treatments That Work. Edited by Nathan P, Gorman JM. New York, Oxford University Press, 2000, pp 463–493

Maldonado JR, Page K, Koopman C, et al: Acute stress reactions following the assassination of Mexican presidential candidate Colosio. J Trauma Stress 15:401–405, 2002

Markowitz JS, Gill HS: Pharmacotherapy of dissociative identity disorder. Ann Pharmacother 30:1498–1499, 1996

Marmar CR, Weiss DS, Metzler TJ, et al: Characteristics of emergency services personnel related to peritraumatic dissociation during critical incident exposure. Am J Psychiatry 153 (suppl 7):94–102, 1996

Martinez-Taboas A: Repressed memories: some clinical data contributing toward its elucidation. Am J Psychother 50:217–230, 1996

Martinez-Taboas A, Bernal G: Dissociation, psychopathology, and abusive experiences in a nonclinical Latino university student group. Cultural Diversity and Ethnic Minority Psychology 6:32–41, 2000

McConkey KM: The effects of hypnotic procedures on remembering, in Contemporary Hypnosis Research. Edited by Fromm E, Nash MR. New York, Guilford, 1992, pp 405–426

McFarlane AC: Posttraumatic morbidity of a disaster: a study of cases presenting for psychiatric treatment. J Nerv Ment Dis 174:4–14, 1986

McLellan S: Deviant spirits in West Malaysian factories. Anthropologica 33:145–160, 1991

Meares R: The "adualistic" representation of trauma: on malignant internalization. Am J Psychother 53:392–402, 1999

Mesulam MM: Dissociative states with abnormal temporal lobe EEG: multiple personality and the illusion of possession. Arch Neurol 38:178–181, 1981

Middleton W, Butler J: Dissociative identity disorder: an Australian series. Aust N Z J Psychiatry 32:794–804, 1998

Mihaescu G, Vanderlinden J, Sechaud M, et al: The Dissociation Questionnaire DIS-Q: preliminary results with a French-speaking Swiss population. Encephale 24:334–346, 1998

Miller SD: Optical differences in cases of multiple personality disorder. J Nerv Ment Dis 177:480–486, 1989

Mishkin M, Appenzeller T: The anatomy of memory. Sci Am 256:80–89, 1987

Modestin J, Ebner G, Junghan M, et al: Dissociative experiences and dissociative disorders in acute psychiatric inpatients. Compr Psychiatry 37:355–361, 1996

Mohammadi MR, Davidian H, Noorbala AA, et al: An epidemiological survey of psychiatric disorders in Iran. Clin Pract Epidemiol Ment Health 1:16, 2005

Moore EP: Gender, power, and legal pluralism: Rajasthan, India. American Ethnologist 20:522–542, 1993

Moreira-Almeida A, Lotufo Neto F, Greyson B: Dissociative and psychotic experiences in Brazilian spiritist mediums. Psychother Psychosom 76:57–58, 2007

Mulder RT, Beautrais AL, Joyce PR, et al: Relationship between dissociation, childhood sexual abuse, childhood physical abuse, and mental illness in a general population sample. Am J Psychiatry 155:806–811, 1998

Mulhern S: Embodied alternative identities. Bearing witness to a world that might have been. Psychiatr Clin North Am 14:769–786, 1991

Nakanishi T: [Dissociative stupor, trance and possession disorders]. Ryoikibetsu Shokogun Shirizu (38):501–502, 2003

Nakdimen KA: Psychoanalysis and multiple personality. Am J Psychiatry 145:896–897, 1988

Naples M, Hackett T: The Amytal interview: history and current uses. Psychosomatics 19:98–105, 1978

Newman AW, Thompson JW Jr: Constitutional rights and hypnotically elicited testimony. J Am Acad Psychiatry Law 27:149–154, 1999

Ng BY, Chan YH: Psychosocial stressors that precipitate dissociative trance disorder in Singapore. Aust N Z J Psychiatry 38:426–432, 2004

Nijenhuis ER, Spinhoven P, van Dyck R, et al: The development and psychometric characteristics of the Somatoform Dissociation Questionnaire (SDQ-20). J Nerv Ment Dis 184:688–694, 1996

Nijenhuis ER, Spinhoven P, van Dyck R, et al: The development of the Somatoform Dissociation Questionnaire (SDQ-5) as a screening instrument for dissociative disorders. Acta Psychiatr Scand 96:311–318, 1997

Nijenhuis ER, Spinhoven P, van Dyck R, et al: Degree of somatoform and psychological dissociation in dissociative disorder is correlated with reported trauma. J Trauma Stress 11:711–730, 1998

Nilsson D, Svedin CG: Evaluation of the Swedish version of Dissociation Questionnaire (DIS-Q), DIS-Q-Sweden, among adolescents. J Trauma Dissociation 7:65–89, 2006

Noll R: Exorcism and possession: the clash of worldviews and the hubris of psychiatry. Dissociation 6 (special issue):250–253, 1993

Noyes R, Slymen DJ: The subjective response to life-threatening danger. Omega 9:313–321, 1978–1979

Nuckolls CW: Deciding how to decide: possession-mediumship in Jalari divination. Med Anthropol 13 (special issue):57–82, 1991

Ogata SN, Silk KR, Goodrich S, et al: Childhood sexual and physical abuse in adult patients with borderline personality disorder. Am J Psychiatry 147:1008–1013, 1990

Olde E, van der Hart O, Kleber RJ, et al: Peritraumatic dissociation and emotions as predictors of PTSD symptoms following childbirth. J Trauma Dissociation 6:125–142, 2005

Orne MT: The use and misuse of hypnosis in court. Int J Clin Exp Hypn 27:311–341, 1979

Orne MT, Axelrad AD, Diamond BL, et al: Scientific status of refreshing recollection by the use of hypnosis. JAMA 253:1918–1923, 1985

O'Toole BI, Marshall RP, Schureck RJ, et al: Combat, dissociation, and posttraumatic stress disorder in Australian Vietnam veterans. J Trauma Stress 12:625–640, 1999

People v Guerra, C-41916 Supreme Court, CA, Orange Co (1984)

People v Hughes, 59 NY2d 523, 466 NYS2d 255, 543 NE2d 484 (1983)

People v Hurd, Supreme Court, NJ, Somerset Co, April 2, 1980

People v Schoenfeld, 168 Cal Rptr 762, 111 CA3d 671 (1980)

People v Shirley, 31 Cal 3d 18, 641 P2d 775 (1982), modified 918a (1982)

Perry JC, Jacobs D: Overview: clinical applications of the Amytal interview in psychiatric emergency settings. Am J Psychiatry 139:552–559, 1982

Peterson G: Auditory hallucinations and dissociative identity disorder. Am J Psychiatry 152:1403–1404, 1995

Pettinati HM, Kogan LG, Evans FJ, et al: Hypnotizability of psychiatric inpatients according to two different scales. Am J Psychiatry 147:69–75, 1990

Pineros M, Rosselli D, Calderon C: An epidemic of collective conversion and dissociation disorder in an indigenous group of Colombia: its relation to cultural change. Soc Sci Med 46:1425–1428, 1998

Pribor EF, Dinwiddie SH: Psychiatric correlates of incest in childhood. Am J Psychiatry 149:52–56, 1992

Price C: Dissociation reduction in body therapy during sexual abuse recovery. Complement Ther Clin Pract 13:116–128, 2007

Ptacek R, Bob P, Paclt I, et al: Psychobiology of dissociation and its clinical assessment. Neuro Endocrinol Lett 28:191–198, 2007

Pullela S: An outbreak of epidemic hysteria: an illustrative case study. Irish Journal of Psychiatry 7:9–11, 1986

Putnam FW: Dissociation as a response to extreme trauma, in Childhood Antecedents of Multiple Personality. Edited by Kluft RP. Washington, DC, American Psychiatric Press, 1985, pp 65–97

Putnam FW: The disturbance of "self" in victims of childhood sexual abuse, in Incest-Related Syndromes of Adult Psychopathology. Edited by Kluft RP. Washington, DC, American Psychiatric Press, 1988, pp 113–132

Putnam FW: Diagnosis and Treatment of Multiple Personality Disorder. New York, Guilford, 1989

Putnam FW: Dissociative disorders in children: behavioral profiles and problems. Child Abuse Negl 17:39–45, 1993

Putnam FW, Guroff JJ, Silberman EK, et al: The clinical phenomenology of multiple personality disorder: review of 100 recent cases. J Clin Psychiatry 47:285–293, 1986

Putnam FW, Zahn TP, Post RM: Differential autonomic nervous system activity in multiple personality disorder. Psychiatry Res 31:251–260, 1990

Reinders AA, Nijenhuis ER, Paans AM, et al: One brain, two selves. Neuroimage 20:2119–2125, 2003

Reinders AA, Nijenhuis ER, Quak J, et al: Psychobiological characteristics of dissociative identity disorder: a symptom provocation study. Biol Psychiatry 60:730–740, 2006

Reither AM, Stoudemire A: Psychogenic fugue states: a review. South Med J 81:568–571, 1988

Rifkin A, Ghisalbert D, Dimatou S, et al: Dissociative identity disorder in psychiatric inpatients. Am J Psychiatry 155:844–845, 1998

Rivera M: Multiple personality disorder and the social systems: 185 cases. Dissociation 4:79–82, 1991

Rock v Arkansas, 107 S Ct 2704, 97 LEd 2d 37 (1987)

Rodewald F, Gast U, Emrich HM: Screening for major dissociative disorders with the FDS, the German version of the Dissociative Experience Scale. Psychother Psychosom Med Psychol 56:249–258, 2006

Ronquillo EB: The influence of "espiritismo" on a case of multiple personality disorder. Dissociation 4:39–45, 1991

Ross CA: Multiple Personality Disorder: Diagnosis, Clinical Features, and Treatment. New York, Wiley, 1989

Ross CA: Epidemiology of multiple personality disorder and dissociation. Psychiatr Clin North Am 14:503–518, 1991

Ross CA: Borderline personality disorder and dissociation. J Trauma Dissociation 8:71–80, 2007

Ross CA, Norton GR: Multiple personality disorder patients with a prior diagnosis of schizophrenia. Dissociation 1:39–42, 1988

Ross CA, Norton GR: Suicide and parasuicide in multiple personality disorder. Psychiatry 52:365–371, 1989

Ross CA, Norton GR, Wozney K: Multiple personality disorder: an analysis of 236 cases. Can J Psychiatry 34:413–418, 1989

Ross CA, Miller SD, Reagor P, et al: Structured interview data on 102 cases of multiple personality disorder from four centers. Am J Psychiatry 147:596–601, 1990

Ross CA, Joshi S, Currie R: Dissociative experiences in the general population: a factor analysis. Hosp Community Psychiatry 42:297–301, 1991a

Ross CA, Anderson G, Fleischer WP, et al: The frequency of multiple personality disorder among psychiatric inpatients. Am J Psychiatry 148:1717–1720, 1991b

Rothbaum BO, Foa EB: Subtypes of posttraumatic stress disorder and duration of symptoms, in Posttraumatic Stress Disorder: DSM-IV and Beyond. Edited by Davidson JRT, Foa EB. Washington, DC, American Psychiatric Press, 1993, pp 23–35

Rumelhart DE, McClelland JL: Parallel Distributed Processing: Explorations in the Microstructure of Cognition, Vols 1 and 2. Cambridge, MA, MIT Press, 1986

Ryle A, Fawkes L: Multiplicity of selves and others: cognitive analytic therapy. J Clin Psychol 63:165–174, 2007

Safa K: Reading Saedi's Ahl-e Hava: pattern and significance in spirit possession beliefs on the southern coasts of Iran. Cult Med Psychiatry 12:85–111, 1988

Sar V, Yargic LI, Tutkun H: Structured interview data on 35 cases of dissociative identity disorder in Turkey. Am J Psychiatry 153:1329–1333, 1996

Sar V, Tutkun H, Alyanak B, et al: Frequency of dissociative disorders among psychiatric outpatients in Turkey. Compr Psychiatry 41:216–222, 2000

Sar V, Akyuz G, Kugu N, et al: Axis I dissociative disorder comorbidity in borderline personality disorder and reports of childhood trauma. J Clin Psychiatry 67:1583–1590, 2006

Sar V, Akyüz G, Dogan O: Prevalence of dissociative disorders among women in the general population. Psychiatry Res 149(1–3):169–176, 2007a

Sar V, Koyuncu A, Ozturk E, et al: Dissociative disorders in the psychiatric emergency ward. Gen Hosp Psychiatry 29:45–50, 2007b

Saxena S, Prasad KVSR: DSM-III subclassification of dissociative disorders applied to psychiatric outpatients in India. Am J Psychiatry 146:261–262, 1989

Schacter DL: Understanding implicit memory: a cognitive neuroscience approach. Am Psychol 47:559–569, 1992

Schacter DL: In Search of Memory. Cambridge, MA, Harvard University Press, 1996

Schacter DL, Wang PL, Tulving E, et al: Functional retrograde amnesia: a quantitative case study. Neuropsychologia 20:523–532, 1982

Schacter DL, Koutstaal W, Norman KA: Can cognitive neuroscience illuminate the nature of traumatic childhood memories? Curr Opin Neurobiol 6:207–214, 1996

Schechter DS, Marshall R, Salman E, et al: Ataque de nervios and history of childhood trauma. J Trauma Stress 13:529–534, 2000

Scheflin AW, Shapiro JL: Trance on Trial. New York, Guilford, 1989

Schenk L, Bear D: Multiple personality and related dissociative phenomena in patients with temporal lobe epilepsy. Am J Psychiatry 138:1311–1316, 1981

Schieffelin EL: Evil spirit sickness, the Christian disease: the innovation of a new syndrome of mental derangement and redemption in Papua, New Guinea. Cult Med Psychiatry 20:1–39, 1996

Schultz R, Braun BG, Kluft RP: Multiple personality disorder: phenomenology of selected variables in comparison to major depression. Dissociation 2:45–51, 1989

Scroppo JC, Drob SL, Weinberger JL, et al: Identifying dissociative identity disorder: a self-report and projective study. J Abnorm Psychol 107:272–284, 1998

Sered SS: Ideology, autonomy, and sisterhood: an analysis of the secular consequences of women's religions. Gender and Society 8:486–506, 1994

Shapiro DJ: Symbolic fluids: the world of spirit mediums in Brazilian possession groups. Dissertation Abstracts International 53:867–868, 1992

Sharp LA: Possessed and dispossessed youth: spirit possession of school children in northwest Madagascar. Cult Med Psychiatry 14:339–364, 1990

Sharp LA: Exorcists, psychiatrists, and the problems of possession in northwest Madagascar. Soc Sci Med 38:525–542, 1994

Shearer SL: Dissociative phenomena in women with borderline personality disorder. Am J Psychiatry 151:1324–1328, 1994

Shirali P, Kishwar A, Bharti SP: Life stress, demographic variables and personality (TAT) in eleven cases of possession (trance-medium) in Shimla Tehsil. Personality Study and Group Behaviour 6:73–81, 1986

Simeon D, Greenberg J, Nelson D, et al: Dissociation and posttraumatic stress 1 year after the World Trade Center disaster: follow-up of a longitudinal survey. J Clin Psychiatry 66:231–237, 2005

Simeon D, Knutelska M, Yehuda R, et al: Hypothalamic-pituitary-adrenal axis function in dissociative disorders, post-traumatic stress disorder, and healthy volunteers. Biol Psychiatry 61:966–973, 2007

Sloan P: Posttraumatic stress in survivors of an airplane crash landing: a clinical and exploratory research intervention. J Trauma Stress 1:211–229, 1988

Smith WH: Incorporating hypnosis into the psychotherapy of patients with multiple personality disorder. Bull Menninger Clin 57:344–354, 1993

Sno HN, Schalken HF: Dissociative identity disorder: diagnosis and treatment in the Netherlands. Eur Psychiatry 14:270–277, 1999

Solomon R: The use of the MMPI with multiple personality patients. Psychol Rep 53:1004–1006, 1983

Solomon Z, Mikulincer M: Psychological sequelae of war: a 2-year follow-up study of Israeli combat stress reaction casualties. J Nerv Ment Dis 176:264–269, 1988

Solomon Z, Mikulincer M, Bleich A: Characteristic expressions of combat-related posttraumatic stress disorder among Israeli soldiers in the 1982 Lebanon war. Behav Med 14:171–178, 1988

Solomon Z, Mikulincer M, Benbenisty R: Combat stress reaction: clinical manifestations and correlates. Military Psychology 1:17–33, 1989

Spiegel D: Vietnam grief work using hypnosis. Am J Clin Hypn 24:33–40, 1981

Spiegel D: Multiple personality as a post-traumatic stress disorder. Psychiatr Clin North Am 7:101–110, 1984

Spiegel D: Dissociating damage. Am J Clin Hypn 29:123–131, 1986a

Spiegel D: Dissociation, double binds, and posttraumatic stress in multiple personality disorder, in Treatment of Multiple Personality Disorder. Edited by Braun BG. Washington, DC, American Psychiatric Press, 1986b, pp 61–77

Spiegel D: Chronic pain masks depression, multiple personality disorder. Hosp Community Psychiatry 38:933–935, 1987

Spiegel D: Dissociation and hypnosis in posttraumatic stress disorders. J Trauma Stress 1:17–33, 1988

Spiegel D: Hypnosis, dissociation, and trauma: hidden and overt observers, in Repression and Dissociation: Implications for Personality Theory, Psychopathology, and Health. Edited by Singer JL. Chicago, IL, University of Chicago Press, 1990a, pp 121–142

Spiegel D: Trauma, dissociation, and hypnosis, in Incest-Related Syndromes of Adult Psychopathology. Edited by Kluft RL. Washington, DC, American Psychiatric Press, 1990b, pp 247–261

Spiegel D: Dissociation and trauma, in American Psychiatric Press Review of Psychiatry, Vol 10. Edited by Tasman A, Goldfinger SM. Washington, DC, American Psychiatric Press, 1991a, pp 261–275

Spiegel D: Dissociative disorders: afterword, in American Psychiatric Press Review of Psychiatry, Vol 10. Edited by Tasman A, Goldfinger SM. Washington, DC, American Psychiatric Press, 1991b, p 276

Spiegel D: Dissociative disorders: foreword, in American Psychiatric Press Review of Psychiatry, Vol 10. Edited by Tasman A, Goldfinger SM. Washington, DC, American Psychiatric Press, 1991c, pp 143–144

Spiegel D: Recognizing traumatic dissociation. Am J Psychiatry 163:566–568, 2006

Spiegel D, Cardeña E: Disintegrated experience: the dissociative disorders revisited. J Abnorm Psychol 100:366–378, 1991

Spiegel D, Fink R: Hysterical psychosis and hypnotizability. Am J Psychiatry 136:777–781, 1979

Spiegel D, Scheflin AW: Dissociated or fabricated? Psychiatric aspects of repressed memory in criminal and civil cases. Int J Clin Exp Hyp 42:411–432, 1994

Spiegel D, Spiegel H: Forensic uses of hypnosis, in Handbook of Forensic Psychology. Edited by Weiner IB, Hess AK. New York, Wiley, 1987, pp 490–507

Spiegel D, Detrick D, Frischholz E: Hypnotizability and psychopathology. Am J Psychiatry 139:431–437, 1982

Spiegel D, Hunt T, Dondershine HE: Dissociation and hypnotizability in posttraumatic stress disorder. Am J Psychiatry 145:301–305, 1988

Spiegel D, Frischholz EJ, Spira J: Functional disorders of memory, in American Psychiatric Press Review of Psychiatry, Vol 12. Edited by Oldham JM, Riba MB, Tasman A. Washington, DC, American Psychiatric Press, 1993, pp 747–782

Spiegel H, Spiegel D: Trance and Treatment: Clinical Uses of Hypnosis, 2nd Edition. Washington, DC, American Psychiatric Publishing, 2004

Spiegel H: Hypnosis and evidence: help or hindrance? Ann N Y Acad Sci 347:73–85, 1980

State ex rel Collins v Superior Court, 132 Ariz 180, 644 P2d 1266 (1982), supplemental opinion filed May 4, 1982

Spiegel H: The grade 5 syndrome: the highly hypnotizable person. Int J Clin Exp Hypn 22:303–319, 1974

Spiegel H, Spiegel D: Trance and Treatment: Clinical Uses of Hypnosis, 2nd Edition. Washington, DC, American Psychiatric Publishing, 2004

Spitzer C, Freyberger HJ, Stieglitz RD, et al: Adaptation and psychometric properties of the German version of the Dissociative Experience Scale. J Trauma Stress 11:799–809, 1998

Spitzer C, Spelsberg B, Grabe HJ, et al: Dissociative experiences and psychopathology in conversion disorders. J Psychosom Res 46:291–294, 1999

Spitzer C, Barnow S, Armbruster J, et al: Borderline personality organization and dissociation. Bull Menninger Clin 70:210–221, 2006a

Spitzer C, Barnow S, Grabe HJ, et al: Frequency, clinical and demographic correlates of pathological dissociation in Europe. J Trauma Dissociation 7:51–62, 2006b

Squire LR: Memory and the hippocampus: a synthesis from findings with rats, monkeys, and humans. Psychol Rev 99:195–231, 1992

Squire LR, Zola-Morgan S: The medial temporal lobe memory system. Science 253:1380–1386, 1991

Steinberg M: The spectrum of depersonalization: assessment and treatment, in American Psychiatric Press Review of Psychiatry, Vol 10. Edited by Tasman A, Goldfinger SM. Washington, DC, American Psychiatric Press, 1991, pp 223–247

Steinberg M, Rounsaville B, Cicchetti DV: The Structured Clinical Interview for DSM-III-R Dissociative Disorders: preliminary report on a new diagnostic instrument. Am J Psychiatry 147:76–82, 1990

Steinberg M, Cicchetti D, Buchanan J, et al: Distinguishing between multiple personality disorder (dissociative identity disorder) and schizophrenia using the Structured Clinical Interview for DSM-IV Dissociative Disorders. J Nerv Ment Dis 182:495–502, 1994

Steinberg M: Advances in the clinical assessment of dissociation: the SCID-D-R. Bull Menninger Clin 64:146–163, 2000

Svedin CG, Nilsson D, Lindell C: Traumatic experiences and dissociative symptoms among Swedish adolescents. A pilot study using Dis-Q-Sweden. Nord J Psychiatry 58:349–355, 2004

Szabo CP, Jonsson G, Vorster V: Dissociative trance disorder associated with major depression and bereavement in a South African female adolescent. Aust N Z J Psychiatry 39:423, 2005

Tantam D: An exorcism in Zanzibar: insights into groups from another culture. Group Analysis 26:251–260, 1993

Terr LC: Childhood traumas: an outline and overview. Am J Psychiatry 148:10–20, 1991

Te Wildt BT: [Psychological impact of the new digital media]. Fortschr Neurol Psychiatr 72:574–585, 2004

Trangkasombat U, Su-Umpan U, Churujiporn V, et al: Risk factors for spirit possession among school girls in southern Thailand. J Med Assoc Thai 81:541–546, 1998

Tulving E: Elements of Episodic Memory. Oxford, England, Clarendon Press, 1983

Tutkun H, Sar V, Yargic LI, et al: Frequency of dissociative disorders among psychiatric inpatients in a Turkish university clinic. Am J Psychiatry 155:800–805, 1998

Valdiserri S, Kihlstrom JF: Abnormal eating and dissociative experiences. Int J Eat Disord 17:373–380, 1995

van der Hart O, Spiegel D: Hypnotic assessment and treatment of trauma-induced psychoses: the early psychotherapy of Breukink and modern views. Int J Clin Exp Hypn 41:191–209, 1993

van der Hart O, Bolt H, van der Kolk BA: Memory fragmentation in dissociative identity disorder. J Trauma Dissociation 6:55–70, 2005a

van der Hart O, Nijenhuis ER, Steele K: Dissociation: an insufficiently recognized major feature of complex posttraumatic stress disorder. J Trauma Stress 18:413–423, 2005b

van der Kolk BA, Fisler R: Dissociation and the fragmentary nature of traumatic memories: overview and exploratory study. J Trauma Stress 8:505–525, 1995

van der Kolk BA, Hostetler A, Herron N, et al: Trauma and the development of borderline personality disorder. Psychiatr Clin North Am 17:715–730, 1994

van der Kolk BA, Pelcovitz D, Roth S, et al: Dissociation, somatization, and affect dysregulation: the complexity of adaptation of trauma. Am J Psychiatry 153 (suppl 7):83–93, 1996

Vanderlinden J, Van Dyck R, Vandereycken W, et al: Dissociative experiences in the general population of the Netherlands and Belgium: a study with the Dissociative Questionnaire (DIS-Q). Dissociation 4:180–184, 1991

van der Zwaard R, Feijen RA, van der Post LF: [Perceptual disorders in a Turkish woman: hallucinations or pseudohallucinations?]. Ned Tijdschr Geneeskd 144:729–732, 2000

Van Duijl M, Cardena E, De Jong JT: The validity of DSM-IV dissociative disorders categories in south-west Uganda. Transcult Psychiatry 42:219–241, 2005

van Dyck R: Dissociation, hypnosis and multiple personality disorders. Ned Tijdschr Geneeskd 137:1863–1864, 1993

van Ommeren M, Komproe I, Cardena E, et al: Mental illness among Bhutanese shamans in Nepal. J Nerv Ment Dis 192:313–317, 2004

Varma VK, Bouri M, Wig NN: Multiple personality in India: comparison with hysterical possession state. Am J Psychother 35:113–120, 1981

Vermetten E, Schmahl C, Lindner S, et al: Hippocampal and amygdalar volumes in dissociative identity disorder. Am J Psychiatry 163:630–636, 2006

Vythilingam M, Heim C, Newport J, et al: Childhood trauma associated with smaller hippocampal volume in women with major depression. Am J Psychiatry 159:2072–2080, 2002

Waelde L, Koopman C, Rierdan J, et al: Symptoms of acute stress disorder and posttraumatic stress disorder following exposure to disastrous flooding. J Trauma Dissociation 2:37–52, 2001

Watson S, Chilton R, Fairchild H, et al: Association between childhood trauma and dissociation among patients with borderline personality disorder. Aust N Z J Psychiatry 40:478–481, 2006

Wettstein RM, Fauman BJ: The amobarbital interview. JACEP 8:272–274, 1979

Wildgoose A, Waller G, Clarke S, et al: Psychiatric symptomatology in borderline and other personality disorders: dissociation and fragmentation as mediators. J Nerv Ment Dis 188:757–763, 2000

Wilkinson CB: Aftermath of a disaster: the collapse of the Hyatt Regency hotel skywalks. Am J Psychiatry 140:1134–1139, 1983

Williams LM: Recall of childhood trauma: a prospective study of women's memories of childhood sexual abuse. J Consult Clin Psychol 62:1167–1176, 1994

Williams LM, Das P, Liddell BJ, et al: Mode of functional connectivity in amygdala pathways dissociates level of awareness for signals of fear. J Neurosci 26:9264–9271, 2006

Wittkower ED: Transcultural psychiatry in the Caribbean: past, present, and future. Am J Psychiatry 127:162–166, 1970

Witztum E, Grisaru N, Budowski D: The "Zar" possession syndrome among Ethiopian immigrants to Israel: cultural and clinical aspects. Br J Med Psychol 69:207–225, 1996

Wolf OT, Convit A, de Leon MJ, et al: Basal hypothalamo-pituitary-adrenal axis activity and corticotropin feedback in young and older men: relationships to magnetic resonance imaging-derived hippocampus and cingulate gyrus volumes. Neuroendocrinology 75:241–249, 2002

Xiao Z, Yan H, Wang Z, et al: Trauma and dissociation in China. Am J Psychiatry 163:1388–1391, 2006

Yap PM: The possession syndrome: a comparison of Hong Kong and French findings. J Ment Sci 106:114–137, 1960

Yargic LI, Sar V, Tutkun H, et al: Comparison of dissociative identity disorder with other diagnostic groups using a structured interview in Turkey. Compr Psychiatry 39:345–351, 1998

Zanarini MC, Ruser T, Frankenburg FR, et al: The dissociative experiences of borderline patients. Compr Psychiatry 41:223–227, 2000a

Zanarini MC, Ruser TF, Frankenburg FR, et al: Risk factors associated with the dissociative experiences of borderline patients. J Nerv Ment Dis 188:26–30, 2000b

Zweig-Frank H, Paris J, Guzder J: Psychological risk factors for dissociation and self-mutilation in female patients with borderline personality disorder. Can J Psychiatry 39:259–264, 1994

16

HUMAN SEXUALITY AND SEXUAL DYSFUNCTIONS

Judith V. Becker, Ph.D.
Jill D. Stinson, Ph.D.

Clinicians see patients who have a variety of sexual dysfunctions. A woman who has previously been molested or sexually assaulted may no longer be desirous of sex or may have difficulty with arousal. A man who has recently been widowed may experience difficulty achieving erections when he enters the dating scene. A woman with multiple sclerosis may no longer have orgasms. A man who is taking antihypertensive medication may have difficulty obtaining an erection. Recently postmenopausal women may find intercourse painful. Patients who are on antidepressants or antipsychotic medication may report impairment in their sexual functioning. It is important that clinicians be knowledgeable about human sexuality, the stages of sexual arousal, and sexual dysfunctions so that they can appropriately evaluate and provide treatment to their patients who present with sexual dysfunctions.

Until recently, the scientific literature has focused on sexual dysfunction as experienced by male patients. However, new research is emerging that addresses the assessment and treatment of sexual dysfunctions in female patients. Recently, an international multidisciplinary consensus development conference on female sexual dysfunction was convened to address problems with current classification systems.

Each of the experts serving on the international panel possessed research and/or clinical expertise in the area of female sexual disorders. This panel issued a consensus report describing their final classification system, which preserved the four major categories of sexual dysfunctions listed in DSM-IV-TR (American Psychiatric Association 2000) with some alterations made (Basson et al. 2001). The classifications of sexual dysfunctions discussed in this chapter are found in DSM-IV-TR and are listed in Table 16–1.

Sexual Dysfunctions

Male and Female Physiology

Human sexual functioning requires a complex interaction of the nervous, vascular, and endocrine systems to produce arousal and orgasm. Sexual arousal in men occurs in the presence of visual stimuli (e.g., a naked person), fantasies, or physical stimulation of the genitals or other areas of the body (e.g., the nipples). This stimulation leads to involuntary discharge in the parasympathetic nerves that control the diameter and valves of the penile blood vessels. Blood flow increases into the

TABLE 16–1. **DSM-IV-TR classifications of sexual dysfunctions**

Sexual desire disorders

Hypoactive sexual desire disorder

Sexual aversion disorder

Sexual arousal disorders

Female sexual arousal disorder

Male erectile disorder

Orgasmic disorders

Female orgasmic disorder

Male orgasmic disorder

Premature ejaculation

Sexual pain disorders

Dyspareunia (not due to a general medical condition)

Vaginismus (not due to a general medical condition)

Others

Sexual dysfunction due to a general medical condition

Substance-induced sexual dysfunction

Sexual dysfunction not otherwise specified

---

corpora cavernosa, two cylinders of specialized tissue in the penis that distend with blood to produce an erection. Continued stimulation leads to emission of semen and ejaculation, which are controlled through sympathetic fibers and the pudendal nerve. Dopaminergic systems in the central nervous system facilitate arousal and ejaculation, whereas serotonergic systems inhibit these functions. In addition, androgens must be present to expedite sexual arousal (and to some extent erection and ejaculation) (Figures 16–1 and 16–2).

In women, as in men, arousal depends on fantasies, visual stimuli, and physical stimulation; in general, the latter is more important for women, whereas visual cues are more important for men. Again, this stimulation leads to parasympathetic nervous discharge that increases blood flow to the female genitalia, resulting in lubrication of the vagina and some enlargement of the clitoris. Continued stimulation of the clitoris— either directly or through intercourse—results in orgasm. Estrogens and progestins play a role in female sexual functioning; however, androgens are important

in the maintenance of sexual arousal in women. As in men, dopaminergic systems facilitate female sexual arousal and orgasm, whereas serotonergic systems inhibit these functions.

It is readily apparent that normal sexual functioning and processes require intact neural and vascular connections to the genitals along with normal endocrine functioning. Any illness that interferes with these systems can lead to sexual dysfunction: neurological diseases (e.g., multiple sclerosis, lumbar or sacral spinal cord trauma, herniated disks), thrombosis of the arteries or veins of the penis, diabetes mellitus (which causes both neurological and vascular damage), endocrine disorders (e.g., hyperprolactinemia), liver disease (which leads to a buildup of estrogen), and so forth.

Similarly, drugs that affect these systems also can impair sexual functioning (Table 16–2). Thus, antihypertensives, because of their antiadrenergic effects, can impair erectile function in men and vaginal lubrication in women. Antipsychotics, tricyclic antidepressants, and monoamine oxidase inhibitors can inhibit these same functions through their anticholinergic effects. Antipsychotics can impair arousal and orgasm because of their dopamine-blocking effects, whereas serotonin reuptake inhibitors (e.g., fluoxetine, sertraline, paroxetine, fluvoxamine, citalopram) can inhibit arousal and orgasm through their serotonergic effects. Spironolactone, steroids, and estrogens can decrease sexual desire through their antiandrogenic effects.

The sexual response cycle of men and women consists of four stages: excitement, plateau, orgasm, and resolution (Masters and Johnson 1966, 1970) (Table 16–3; Figure 16–3). The *excitement stage* in both men and women is characterized by erotic feelings that lead to penile erection in men and vaginal lubrication in women. Also, both heart rate and blood pressure increase. The *plateau stage* is characterized by further sexual pleasure and increased muscle tension, heart rate, and blood flow to the genitals. During the male *orgasmic stage,* semen is ejaculated from the penis in spurts. Orgasm for women consists of reflex rhythmic contractions of the circumvaginal muscles. During *resolution,* the final stage, the sex-specific physiological responses return to a resting state. In men, there is a refractory period after orgasm during which it is not possible to have another erection. The length of this period varies between individuals and increases with age. Women are variable—some have a refractory period after orgasm, whereas others do not and can have multiple sequential orgasms.

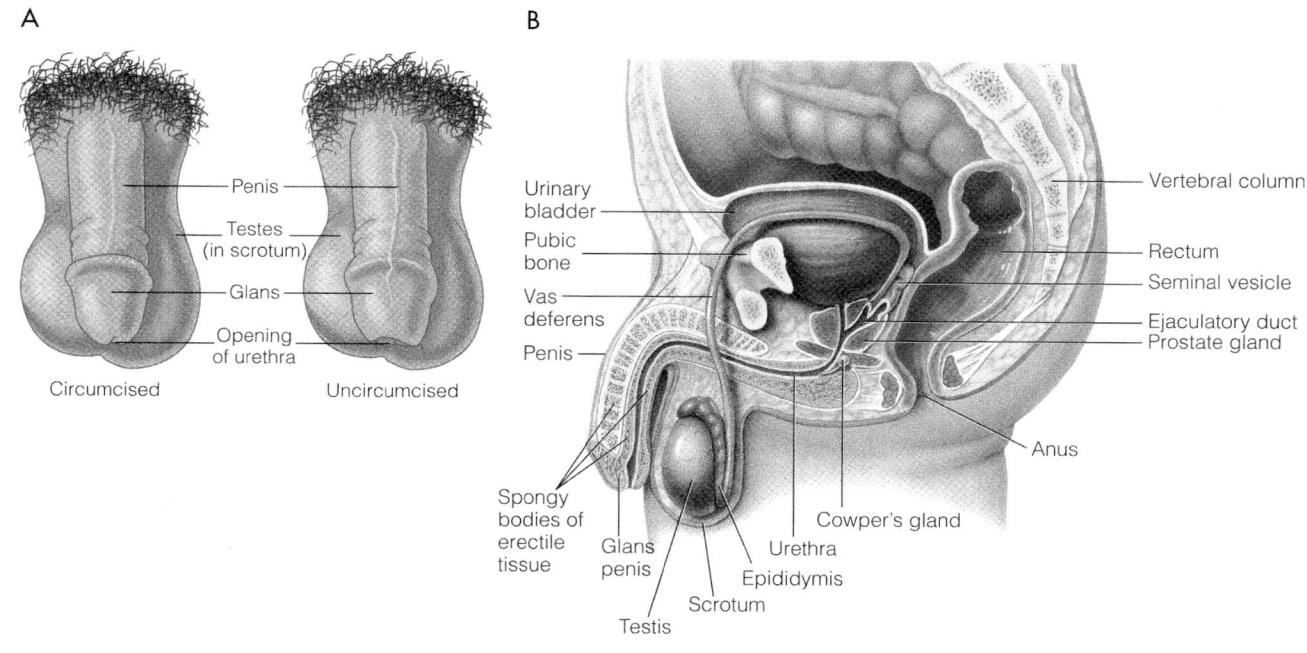

FIGURE 16–1. The male sex organs and reproductive structures.

(A) External structure. (B) Internal structure.
Source.   Reprinted from *An Invitation to Health* (with ThomsonNOW(T) and InfoTrac(R) 1-Semester Printed Access Card), 12th Edition, by Hales, Dianne. 2007. Used with permission of Brooks/Cole, a division of Thomson Learning: www.thomson-rights.com. Fax 800-730-2215.

Sexual dysfunctions occur when there are disruptions of any of the four stages of sexual response because of anatomical, physiological, or psychological factors. Sexual orientation is not a determining factor; consequently, heterosexual, homosexual, or bisexual individuals may experience a sexual dysfunction at some point in their lives.

Sexual dysfunctions may be lifelong or may develop after a period of normal sexual functioning. For example, a woman who has never achieved an orgasm would be classified as having a primary female orgasmic disorder, whereas a woman who has been orgasmic at one point in her life but is currently unable to achieve orgasm is experiencing a secondary orgasmic disorder. Sexual dysfunctions may be further characterized as to whether they are present in all sexual activities or are situational. For example, a man who has an erection during masturbation but not during sexual interaction with a partner has a situational erectile disorder. Further, when a sexual dysfunction is diagnosed, the following types should be specified: dysfunction due to psychological factors or dysfunction due to combined psychological factors and a general medical condition.

Epidemiology

The exact prevalence of sexual dysfunctions is difficult to determine. Early community studies designed to estimate prevalence found wide variation in the occurrence of sexual dysfunctions (Spector and Carey 1990). More recent findings demonstrate similar variation. A recent review of the literature suggested that among community samples, rates of sexual dysfunction were 0%–3% for male orgasmic disorder, 0%–5% for male erectile disorder, 0%–3% for male hypoactive sexual desire disorder, and 4%–5% for premature ejaculation. For female orgasmic disorder, the rates were 7%–10% (Simons and Carey 2001). However, prevalence estimates were notably higher when obtained from primary care and sexuality clinic samples, where individuals were seeking help for problematic sexual functioning.

A comprehensive survey conducted on a representative sample of the U.S. population between 19 and 59 years of age suggested the following prevalence estimates: 3% for male dyspareunia, 15% for female dyspareunia, 10% for male orgasm problems, 25% for female orgasm problems, 33% for female hypoactive

(a) External Structure

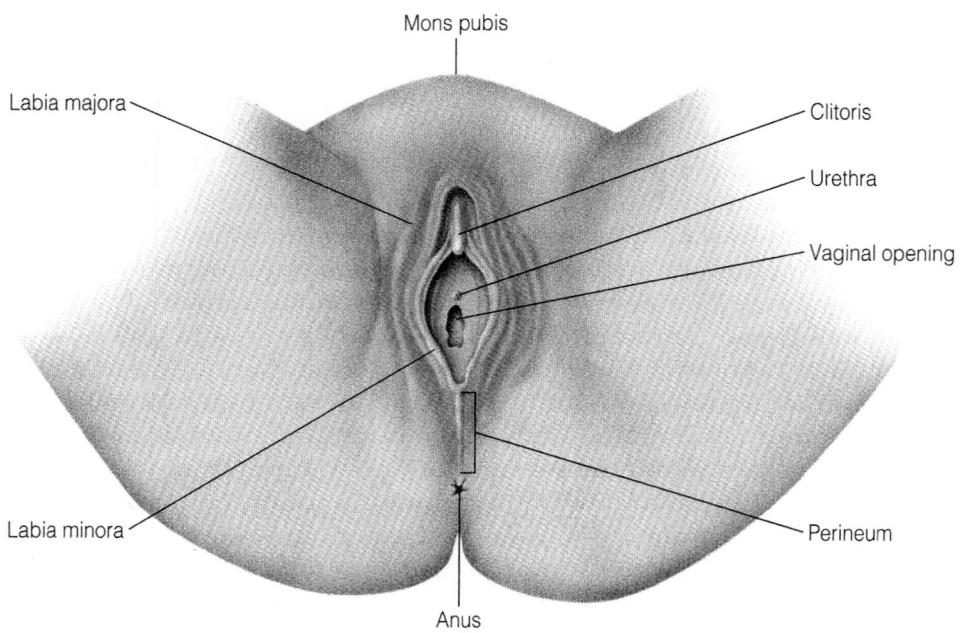

(b) Internal Structure

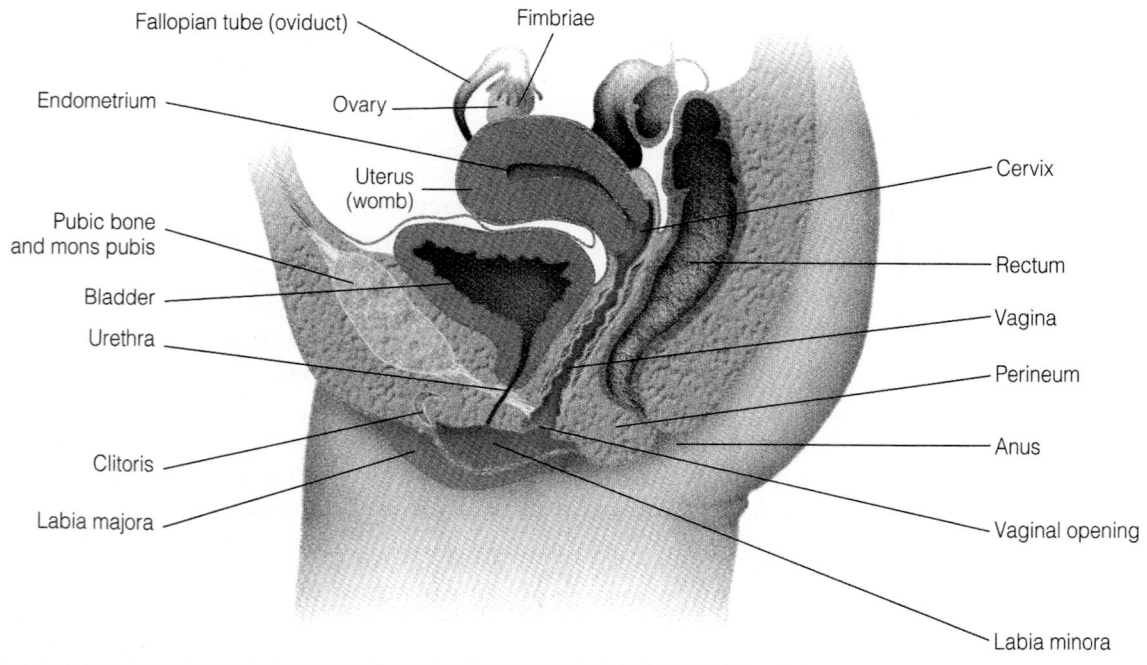

FIGURE 16–2.   The female sex organs and reproductive structures.

(A) External structure. (B) Internal structure.

Source.   Reprinted from *An Invitation to Health* (with ThomsonNOW(T) and InfoTrac(R) 1-Semester Printed Access Card), 12th Edition, by Hales, Dianne. 2007. Used with permission of Brooks/Cole, a division of Thomson Learning: www.thomson-rights.com. Fax 800-730-2215.

TABLE 16–2. Commonly used medications that may interfere with sexual functioning

Abused drugs	Antihypertensives	Antipsychotics	Antidepressants	Others
Alcohol	Diuretics	Thioridazine	Tricyclic antidepressants	Cimetidine
Marijuana	Methyldopa	Thiothixene	Mirtazapine (rare)	Estrogens
Opiates	Clonidine	Chlorpromazine	Monoamine oxidase	Steroids
Cocaine	Beta-blockers	Perphenazine	inhibitors	
Amphetamines	Guanethidine	Fluphenazine	Nefazodone (rare)	
Methylenedioxy-methamphetamine (MDMA; "Ecstasy")	Ace inhibitors	Risperidone	Serotonin reuptake	
		Olanzapine	inhibitors	
			Trazodone (priapism)	
			Venlafaxine	

TABLE 16–3. Four stages of the sexual response cycle

Excitement

- Initiated by physical or psychological erotic stimulation

- Increases in heart rate, breathing, and blood pressure; vasocongestion in the skin becomes apparent

- In males, increased blood flow to the penis and partial erection

- In females, increased blood flow to the genitals, vaginal lubrication, and nipples become stiff and erect

Plateau

- Further increases in heart rate, blood flow, and muscle tension

- Increase of sexual pleasure with additional stimulation

- In males, penis becomes more fully erect and begins to secrete seminal fluid

- In females, increased blood flow to and some swelling of the genitals; further lubrication of the vagina

Orgasm

- Both males and females experience quick muscular contractions in pelvic muscles (as well as uterine and vaginal muscles in females) and an associated euphoric sensation; males ejaculate approximately 2–5 mL of semen

Resolution

- Occurs following orgasm; relaxation of muscles and activity of parasympathetic nervous system

- Some may return to plateau phase here and experience multiple orgasms, whereas others may not respond to sexual stimulation while in this phase

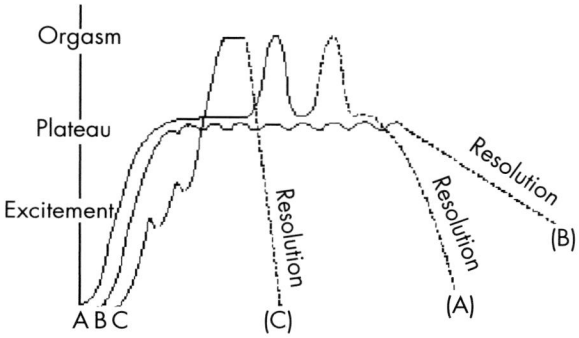

FIGURE 16–3. The human sexual response cycle, as seen in three different patients.

Source. Masters and Johnson 1966.

sexual desire, 27% for premature ejaculation, 20% for female arousal problems, and 10% for male erectile difficulties (American Psychiatric Association 2000) (Table 16–4). These findings demonstrate far higher rates of sexual dysfunction, especially among females, than was evident from the aggregate research literature.

There does appear to be some impact of age on epidemiological samples. Prevalence research for sexual dysfunctions in mature adults suggests that the rate of reported dysfunction increases with age for both men and women, with 20%–30% of men and 40%–45% of women reporting clinically significant sexual difficulties in later life (Hayes and Dennerstein 2005; Lewis et al. 2004).

Comparative studies of clinical samples over time suggest an increase in the frequency of hypoactive sexual desire disorder, male and female orgasmic disorder, and male erectile disorder and a decrease in premature ejaculation as presenting problems. These

TABLE 16–4.   Prevalence estimates for male and female sexual dysfunctions

Male sexual dysfunction	%	Female sexual dysfunction	%
Premature ejaculation	27	Female hypoactive sexual desire	33
Male orgasmic disorder	10	Female orgasmic disorder	25
Erectile dysfunction	10	Female arousal disorder	20
Male dyspareunia	3	Female dyspareunia	15

Source.   American Psychiatric Association 2000.

TABLE 16–5.   Multicausal theory of sexual dysfunctions

1. Misinformation or ignorance regarding sexual and social interaction
2. Unconscious guilt and anxiety concerning sex
3. Performance anxiety, as the most common cause of erectile and orgasmic dysfunctions
4. Partners' failure to communicate to each other their sexual feelings and those behaviors in which they want to engage

findings could be due to improvements in assessment and diagnosis, increased willingness to report such difficulties, or realistic changes in the prevalence in the general population. Clearly, a significant percentage of men and women in our society experience sexual problems at some time in their lives.

Etiology

Kaplan (1974) argued for a multicausal theory of sexual dysfunctions, combining intrapsychic, interpersonal, and behavioral characteristics into four factors that play a role in the development of these disorders (Table 16–5).

Other factors may lead to the development of a sexual dysfunction. One such etiological consideration is an unacknowledged homosexual orientation, with attempts to function sexually with a person of the opposite sex. This could lead to decreased sexual desire or arousal as well as difficulties with orgasm. Another factor to consider is the presence of other sexual dysfunctions. Some sexual dysfunctions can lead to secondary sexual problems; for example, a person who does not have erections or cannot achieve orgasm may develop a lack of sexual desire secondary to not experiencing any positive gratification from the sexual interaction. Many sexual problems may be related to sexual trauma. For example, a history of incest, child sexual abuse, or rape may place an individual at risk for developing sexual problems later (Becker et al. 1986; Leonard and Follette 2002). Sexual dysfunctions can occur as secondary to major psychiatric disorders such as schizophrenia, depression, and severe personality disorders. As previously discussed, physical, neurological, and physiological problems can lead to sexual dysfunction. The use of a single medication, or

of multiple medications, is one of the most common causes of sexual dysfunction. Medications that may affect sexual functioning are discussed later in this chapter.

Interestingly, no DSM category describes a primary disorder of increased sexual desire, but this has been reported in a few cases with the use of selective serotonin reuptake inhibitors (SSRIs) (Chollet and Andreatini 2003; Greil et al. 2001; Samuel 2006) and is correlated with several neurological syndromes (Britton 1998; Emory et al. 1995; Freymann et al. 2005; Wiseman et al. 2000). Montaldi (2002) posits that while some hypersexual behaviors are conceptualized as compulsive behaviors similar to others on Axis I, a subset of these behaviors are more accurately characterized as Axis II psychopathology. This research suggests that hypersexual activity is perhaps less like the other sexual dysfunctions described here. Relatively little research has been done on hypersexuality, and further research is clearly needed to identify the causal mechanisms behind such behavior.

Finally, many cases of dysfunction involve both organic and psychogenic factors, especially in the case of an erectile disorder. A man may have a mild degree of organic impairment, perhaps due to diabetes or vascular insufficiency; fail several times at obtaining an erection; and then become vulnerable to performance anxiety. In this case, treatment aimed at reducing the psychogenic factors may be sufficient to improve sexual functioning. Conversely, even if a man has evidence of psychological factors contributing to erectile disorder, it is still necessary to evaluate him for organic abnormalities (LoPiccolo and Stock 1986).

Differential Diagnosis

Patients with a sexual dysfunction should be medically evaluated by a gynecologist or urologist to rule out treatable organic etiologies. These organic factors may be local diseases of the genitals, vascular illnesses, neurological diseases, endocrine disorders, or systemic illnesses. Patients should always be asked about medications, including over-the-counter medicines and illegal drugs.

A number of physiological assessments are also available to supplement the information reported by the patient. Psychophysiological procedures have been developed to assess patients' erections. During rapid eye movement (REM) sleep, men experience penile erections defined as nocturnal penile tumescence (NPT). Although NPT measures can be equivocal, they can be of help in discriminating potential organic factors in a patient with self-reported erectile problems. For example, a man with "psychogenic" impotence should have erections while sleeping, whereas a man with "organic" impotence should not have an erection at any time. However, many men have both organic and psychological causes underlying their erectile problems, and thus the results of NPT testing require cautious interpretation. It is possible that men with a predominance of psychogenic factors may still lack nocturnal tumescence, whereas men with an organically based dysfunction may still have nocturnal erections. Other assessment procedures focus on penile tumescence and blood flow, including Doppler ultrasonography, penile blood pressure measurement, and arteriography. Papaverine injections of the corpora cavernosa are also used to assess vascular competence. If potential neurological etiologies are suspected, nerve root stimulation may assist in assessing the role of any neurological damage.

Typical physiological measures of arousal in females evaluate vaginal blood volume and vaginal pulse amplitude. Measures of vaginal blood volume are believed to indicate slow changes in the collection of blood in the vaginal tissue, while measures of vaginal pulse amplitude reflect changes in vaginal blood volume at the occurrence of each heartbeat. Vaginal photoplethysmography is perhaps the most commonly used physiological measurement in both research and clinical samples (Hoon et al. 1976; Laan et al. 1995; Sintchak and Geer 1975). This technique assesses both vaginal blood volume and vaginal pulse amplitude by using a light to reflect the amount and movement of blood through the vaginal tissues but has been criticized for its lack of a sound theoretical basis for deriving the interpretations of the results (Meston 2000). Other measures, such as the vaginal thermistor and heated oxygen electrode, examine heat dissipation, while newer work with measuring clitoral blood flow with duplex Doppler ultrasound also shows promise as a physiological measure of female sexual arousal (Khalifé et al. 2000; Meston 2000).

Researchers have also identified vaginal vascular changes in women during REM sleep, and physiological assessment techniques are being explored to evaluate these changes in women who have sexual dysfunctions. The use of additional techniques, such as the application of topical vasoactive agents during psychophysiological assessment, can also be successful in identifying women with sexual dysfunctions (Bechara et al. 2003).

Descriptions and Treatments of Sexual Dysfunctions

Sexual Desire Disorders

Hypoactive Sexual Desire Disorder

The DSM-IV-TR diagnostic criteria for hypoactive sexual desire disorder (also known as inhibited sexual desire) are shown in Table 16–6.

TABLE 16–6. DSM-IV-TR diagnostic criteria for hypoactive sexual desire disorder

A. Persistently or recurrently deficient (or absent) sexual fantasies and desire for sexual activity. The judgment of deficiency or absence is made by the clinician, taking into account factors that affect sexual functioning, such as age and the context of the person's life.

B. The disturbance causes marked distress or interpersonal difficulty.

C. The sexual dysfunction is not better accounted for by another Axis I disorder (except another sexual dysfunction) and is not due exclusively to the direct physiological effects of a substance (e.g., a drug of abuse, a medication) or a general medical condition.

Specify type:

> **Lifelong type**

> **Acquired type**

Specify type:

> **Situational type**

> **Generalized type**

Specify:

> **Due to psychological factors**

> **Due to combined factors**

It is also important to determine whether hypoactive sexual desire is the primary problem or the consequence of another underlying sexual problem. Frequently, a male or female who is experiencing either inhibited sexual excitement or an orgasmic problem may develop hypoactive sexual desire because sexual activity is not found to be reinforcing. It is also important to differentiate this disorder, in which there is an absence of sexual desire and fantasies, from sexual aversion, in which there is avoidance of sexual activity because of extreme anxiety. As with the other dysfunctions, this disorder may be lifelong, may occur after a period of good sexual appetite, or may occur only in a certain context (e.g., with the individual's current partner). It is important to assess whether the desire disorder is substance-induced (i.e., due to the effects of drugs or medications). The assessment of individuals with hypoactive sexual desire disorder requires a medical workup, psychological evaluation, and assessment of the relationship.

Hypoactive sexual desire disorder is perhaps the most common sexual complaint among females, but until recently, there was no validated instrument to assess its severity. The Female Sexual Function Index (FSFI; Rosen et al. 2000), the Sexual Interest and Desire Inventory—Female (SIDI-F; Sills et al. 2005), and the Sexual Desire Inventory (Spector et al. 1996) are all measures designed to assess the nature and severity of sexual dysfunction in women who have hypoactive sexual desire. Each of these instruments has shown promise in accurately and reliably identifying and describing women with clinically significant decreases in sexual desire (Clayton et al. 2006; Meston 2003; Sills et al. 2005; Wiegel et al. 2005).

Hypoactive sexual desire disorder has been the most difficult of all the dysfunctions to treat. Testosterone has been used for both males and females to treat inhibited sexual desire; however, masculinizing side effects make its use problematic in women. There is no consistent evidence to indicate its success in increasing sexual interest in men, even when initial serum testosterone levels are low (O'Carroll and Bancroft 1984). In women, there does appear to be some evidence suggestive of improvement in sexual interest and desire after application of low-dose testosterone therapy (Simpkins and Van Meter 2005; Van Anders et al. 2005), but the success of this treatment may be limited to those women who demonstrated insufficient or decreased levels of androgens at initial assessment (Simpkins and Van Meter 2005) and may not be any more effective than therapy (Dow and Gallagher 1989).

Bupropion sustained-release has also been used in the treatment of hypoactive sexual desire disorder in women. Results from an empirical study evaluating its effectiveness in nondepressed women indicated that 29% of the evaluable participants responded to the treatment (Segraves et al. 2001). Other studies have achieved similar results, with increases in sexual desire, arousal, and sexual satisfaction among the female participants after taking bupropion sustained-release (Dobkin et al. 2006; Segraves et al. 2004).

The most effective treatments involve a combination of cognitive therapy to deal with maladaptive beliefs (e.g., that partners must always want sex at the same time), behavioral treatment (e.g., exercises to enhance sexual pleasure and communication), and marital therapy (e.g., to deal with the individual's use of sex to control the relationship). When the problem is secondary to prescription medication, one could consider waiting for the patient to accommodate to the drug, lowering the dose, giving drug holidays, changing to another drug within the same therapeutic class, changing to a new therapeutic class, or adding a pharmacological antidote (although none is currently approved by the U.S. Food and Drug Administration [FDA] for this purpose) (Finger 2001). These suggestions can apply to drug-induced sexual problems, including those discussed later in this chapter.

Sexual Aversion Disorder

The DSM-IV-TR diagnostic criteria for sexual aversion disorder are shown in Table 16–7.

The major goal of treatment is to reduce the patient's fear and avoidance of sexual activity. This goal can be accomplished via systematic desensitization. First, the patient is gradually exposed to sexual scenarios in his or her imagination and then progressively moves toward in vivo exposure to the actual sexual situations that generate anxiety. The successful treatment of sexual phobias using tricyclic antidepressants as well as sex therapy has also been reported (Carey 1998; Kaplan et al. 1982).

Sexual Arousal Disorders

Female Sexual Arousal Disorder

The DSM-IV-TR diagnostic criteria for female sexual arousal disorder are shown in Table 16–8.

Treatment of impairment of sexual arousal in women often involves the reduction of anxiety associated with sexual activity. Thus, behavioral techniques such as those involving sensate focus are most often effective (Kaplan 1974). Sensate focus exercises (Masters and Johnson 1970) are techniques in which the patient

TABLE 16–7. DSM-IV-TR diagnostic criteria for sexual aversion disorder

A. Persistent or recurrent extreme aversion to, and avoidance of, all (or almost all) genital sexual contact with a sexual partner.

B. The disturbance causes marked distress or interpersonal difficulty.

C. The sexual dysfunction is not better accounted for by another Axis I disorder (except another sexual dysfunction).

Specify type:

Lifelong type

Acquired type

Specify type:

Situational type

Generalized type

Specify:

Due to psychological factors

Due to combined factors

TABLE 16–8. DSM-IV-TR diagnostic criteria for female sexual arousal disorder

A. Persistent or recurrent inability to attain, or to maintain until completion of the sexual activity, an adequate lubrication-swelling response of sexual excitement.

B. The disturbance causes marked distress or interpersonal difficulty.

C. The sexual dysfunction is not better accounted for by another Axis I disorder (except another sexual dysfunction) and is not due exclusively to the direct physiological effects of a substance (e.g., a drug of abuse, a medication) or a general medical condition.

Specify type:

Lifelong type

Acquired type

Specify type:

Situational type

Generalized type

Specify:

Due to psychological factors

Due to combined factors

engages in nongenital, nondemand caressing with a partner and concentrates on pleasurable feelings. Gradually, the patient engages in pleasurable genital sexual activities (e.g., touch, oral contact) with no penetration permitted until anxiety has been decreased sufficiently.

The pharmacological agent sildenafil also has been described as being successful in the treatment of psychotropic-induced sexual dysfunctions in females. Although not yet approved by the FDA for use in women, treatment with sildenafil citrate or other phosphodiesterase 5 inhibitors may also increase female sexual arousal, as measured by both subjective reports and objective physiological measures (Berman et al. 2001; Richardson et al. 2005; Salerian et al. 2000). However, other evidence suggests that sildenafil is not always successful in treating this disorder (Basson et al. 2002). Use of topical alprostadil cream applied to the genital area may also serve as a viable treatment method (Islam et al. 2001; Padma-Nathan et al. 2003). Before initiating medication-based treatment of this disorder, complete medical and psychosocial evaluations should be conducted, and the partner or spouse should be included in the treatment whenever possible.

Male Erectile Disorder

The DSM-IV-TR diagnostic criteria for male erectile disorder are shown in Table 16–9.

The treatment of erectile problems is generally easier if the patient has a willing sexual partner to participate in therapy. However, treatment is possible without a partner's attendance. Initially, the clinician should inform the patient with male erectile dysfunction that he is not alone in this problem and that, in fact, most men are unable to generate an erection at some time in their lives. Epidemiology research suggests that approximately one-third of men experience erectile dysfunction, affecting 20%–25% of young males under the age of 40 years and more than 50% of men age 60 years or older (Heruti et al. 2004; Jackson et al. 2006). Until recently, the most frequently used interventions have been behavioral. However, with the introduction of new pharmacological agents such as sildenafil citrate, tadalafil, and vardenafil—all phosphodiesterase 5 inhibitors that relax smooth muscles in the penis and thereby allow for increased blood flow and engorgement of penile tissues—many patients are opting for a convenient medication as treatment. Before discussing the research on pharmacological treatments, we review the behavioral interventions.

A successful treatment for arousal and erectile dis-

TABLE 16–9. DSM-IV-TR diagnostic criteria for male erectile disorder

A. Persistent or recurrent inability to attain, or to maintain until completion of the sexual activity, an adequate erection.

B. The disturbance causes marked distress or interpersonal difficulty.

C. The erectile dysfunction is not better accounted for by another Axis I disorder (other than a sexual dysfunction) and is not due exclusively to the direct physiological effects of a substance (e.g., a drug of abuse, a medication) or a general medical condition.

Specify type:

Lifelong type

Acquired type

Specify type:

Situational type

Generalized type

Specify:

Due to psychological factors

Due to combined factors

orders in patients with partners has been the use of behavioral assignments to gradually decrease performance anxiety. Sensate focus exercises, described above, are used to reduce anxiety and increase erectile functioning and show moderate success in decreasing experiences of erectile dysfunction. Group therapy, hypnotherapy, and systematic desensitization also have been used successfully in cases of erectile difficulties. Again, these treatments act to reduce anxiety associated with being sexual. Although psychoanalysis is not indicated in the treatment of simple erectile dysfunction, psychodynamic interventions may be helpful in alleviating intrapsychic conflicts contributing to performance anxiety. Couples therapy also is often helpful in treating these patients (Leiblum and Rosen 1991). Recent comparisons of behavioral and pharmacological treatments suggest that these nonmedical interventions are equally successful at reducing rates of erectile dysfunction in those patients with psychogenic causes of the disorder (Melnik and Abdo 2005).

Various somatic treatments also can be used for erectile disorders, even when these disorders are primarily due to nonorganic factors. Testosterone is often used by nonpsychiatric physicians to treat impotence; however, there is no indication for its use except when erectile problems are due to hypogonadism (O'Carroll and Bancroft 1984; Shabsigh 2005). Vasoactive injections into the corpora cavernosa can also be used to treat erectile disorders and may produce erections lasting up to several hours. Most injections consist of a combination of papaverine (a smooth-muscle relaxant) and phentolamine (an α-adrenergic blocker), although other agents (e.g., prostaglandin E_1) also can be used. Success rates for this treatment are high (about 85%), with improvements in erectile capacity, sexual satisfaction, and frequency of intercourse (Althof et al. 1991). The combination of traditional sex therapy techniques and these injections may be helpful even in those men with purely psychogenic erectile dysfunction (Weiss et al. 1991). However, side effects of the injections, including priapism (i.e., a prolonged, painful erection), fibrotic nodules in the penis, and mild alteration in liver function tests, as well as pain at the site of the injection and limitations on frequent use, often prevent men from utilizing this treatment (Cooper 1991; Levine et al. 1989). Topical medications also may play a role in the treatment of erectile dysfunction by directly relaxing arterial smooth muscle in the penis. Nitroglycerin patches have been found to improve erectile function in about 40% of patients (Meyhoff et al. 1992); the most common side effect is headache. Topical minoxidil also has been found to be helpful in some patients (Cavallini 1991); however, further evaluation of this treatment is required.

Early oral medications included yohimbine, an α-adrenergic antagonist (Witt 1998), and dopamine agonists such as bromocriptine (Lal et al. 1991), which were beneficial in treating erectile dysfunction. However, the more recent introduction of phosphodiesterase 5 inhibitors such as sildenafil sulfate, tadalafil, and vardenafil has greatly changed the way in which this dysfunction is now treated. These medications operate by releasing nitric oxide into the corpus cavernosum, which then activates the enzyme guanylate cyclase and results in increased levels of cyclic guanosine monophosphate (cGMP). This produces smooth-muscle relaxation in the corpus cavernosum and allows the inflow of blood during sexual stimulation. Numerous empirical studies have demonstrated the success of these agents (Carson 2004; Dinsmore 2004; Hatzichristou et al. 2005; Padma-Nathan et al. 2004).

A major noninvasive, nonpharmacological treatment for erectile dysfunction is an external vacuum device. The device consists of a plastic cylinder with one end open and the other end connected to a vacuum pump. A vacuum is created that draws blood into the penis. A tension ring is then slipped from the cylinder to the base of the penis for up to 30 minutes. This treatment shows high success rates among patients and has the advantages of being noninvasive, being relatively inexpensive, and having few side effects—bruising, physical discomfort, and blocked ejaculation are the most common (Turner et al. 1991). Disadvantages are that erections last only 30 minutes and the patient must interrupt sexual activity to use the device (Turner et al. 1992).

For men with pure organic or combination organic–psychogenic impotence who do not respond to other treatment measures, penile prostheses can be implanted. Two types are currently available: a bendable silicone implant and an inflatable implant. However, these should be used only after careful psychiatric, sexual, and urological evaluations. Several drawbacks must be considered before recommending this form of treatment, including the risk of surgery and postoperative infection, the destruction of natural erectile capacity, and mechanical breakdown (about 20%).

Orgasmic Disorders

Female Orgasmic Disorder

The DSM-IV-TR diagnostic criteria for female orgasmic disorder are shown in Table 16–10.

The most likely way for a woman with general anorgasmia (i.e., never having had an orgasm) to become orgasmic is through a program of directed masturbation (LoPiccolo and Stock 1986). Any discomfort that the patient may feel about exploring her own body should be discussed. Next, the patient should be instructed in a systematic program for exercising the pubococcygeal muscle, a muscle involved in orgasms. Once the patient has mastered these exercises, she should be placed on a masturbatory program that begins with a gradual visual and tactile exploration of her body and moves toward focused genital touching. Use of sexual fantasies combined with stimulation is also taught. The clinician may recommend use of a vibrator if the woman is unable to have an orgasm when engaging in focused genital touching. Once the woman is able to have an orgasm through self-stimulation, she then teaches her sexual partner (using sensate focus exercises) the type of genital stimulation she requires to have an orgasm.

For a woman with anorgasmia, it is imperative to explore the relationship and involve her partner in treatment. Couples therapy, if indicated, and graduated exposure exercises also can be used in treatment. Treatments that focus on communication and relationship skills have been found to have high success rates (Milan et al. 1988).

TABLE 16–10. **DSM-IV-TR diagnostic criteria for female orgasmic disorder**

A. Persistent or recurrent delay in, or absence of, orgasm following a normal sexual excitement phase. Women exhibit wide variability in the type or intensity of stimulation that triggers orgasm. The diagnosis of female orgasmic disorder should be based on the clinician's judgment that the woman's orgasmic capacity is less than would be reasonable for her age, sexual experience, and the adequacy of sexual stimulation she receives.

B. The disturbance causes marked distress or interpersonal difficulty.

C. The orgasmic dysfunction is not better accounted for by another Axis I disorder (except another sexual dysfunction) and is not due exclusively to the direct physiological effects of a substance (e.g., a drug of abuse, a medication) or a general medical condition.

Specify type:

> **Lifelong type**
>
> **Acquired type**

Specify type:

> **Situational type**
>
> **Generalized type**

Specify:

> **Due to psychological factors**
>
> **Due to combined factors**

Communication is vital in the process of assisting anorgasmic women to become orgasmic (Kelly et al. 2006). In a recent study, communication patterns were assessed in heterosexual couples in which the woman was experiencing female orgasmic disorder and compared to the communication patterns of two groups of control couples. Results indicated that the sexually dysfunctional couples experienced poorer communication, greater blame, and less openness than the control groups while discussing sexual topics. Similar research has additionally demonstrated that anorgasmic women and their male partners reported increased discomfort in discussing clitoral stimulation and other related sexual topics (Kelly et al. 2004).

The most frequent complaint of women experiencing an orgasmic problem is that they are not orgasmic through penile–vaginal intercourse. When becoming orgasmic through intercourse is a patient's treatment goal, the clinician should ensure that she and her partner are aware that adequate stimulation both before and during intercourse is necessary. In addition, the clinician may suggest various sexual positions that allow stimulation of the clitoris by the patient or her partner during intercourse. For women who are fearful of "letting go" during intercourse, systematic desensitization is often helpful. The therapist may wish to explore with the patient any religious concerns or personal beliefs regarding intercourse and sexual pleasure. Appropriate therapy can be offered to deal with these issues while still working within the parameters of the patient's personal beliefs and morals. Finally, the patient should be told not to expect to have an orgasm every time she has intercourse, given that only a minority of women are regularly orgasmic during intercourse.

Some medications have also been useful in increasing orgasmic responding in women. Sildenafil has been used for the treatment of low arousal and anorgasmia, with 67% of women in two studies reporting an increasing ability to achieve orgasm (Berman et al. 2001; Salerian et al. 2000). Other medications used to treat different sexual dysfunctions may also be useful in increasing orgasmic response in women (Dobkin et al. 2006).

Male Orgasmic Disorder

The DSM-IV-TR diagnostic criteria for male orgasmic disorder are shown in Table 16–11.

The treatment of male orgasmic disorder is similar to that of female orgasmic disorder. The patient should be told that when he masturbates, he should masturbate as quickly as possible to ejaculation while fantasizing that his penis is inside his partner's vagina and ejaculating. A second technique is to teach the patient and his partner sensate focus exercises. If the patient is able to masturbate in the presence of his partner, he is instructed to place his partner's hand over his so that she can see how much touching he requires. He should then place his hand over hers while she masturbates him to ejaculation. Finally, she should sit astride him and stimulate him, eventually putting his penis in her vagina when he reaches the point of ejaculatory inevitability. If a man is uncomfortable ejaculating in the presence of his partner, systematic desensitization is used to help him become more comfortable in her presence.

Much like females with orgasmic disorder or other sexual dysfunctions, males with psychotropically induced orgasmic disorder also show improvement after taking sildenafil (Salerian et al. 2000), with approximately 77% reporting increased orgasmic functioning. Imipramine has also demonstrated success in

TABLE 16–11.   DSM-IV-TR diagnostic criteria for male orgasmic disorder

A. Persistent or recurrent delay in, or absence of, orgasm following a normal sexual excitement phase during sexual activity that the clinician, taking into account the person's age, judges to be adequate in focus, intensity, and duration.

B. The disturbance causes marked distress or interpersonal difficulty.

C. The orgasmic dysfunction is not better accounted for by another Axis I disorder (except another sexual dysfunction) and is not due exclusively to the direct physiological effects of a substance (e.g., a drug of abuse, a medication) or a general medical condition.

Specify type:

   Lifelong type

   Acquired type

Specify type:

   Situational type

   Generalized type

Specify:

   Due to psychological factors

   Due to combined factors

treating psychotropically induced orgasmic dysfunction in male patients (Aizenburg et al. 1996).

Premature Ejaculation

The DSM-IV-TR diagnostic criteria for premature ejaculation are shown in Table 16–12.

Premature ejaculation is the most prevalent of all male sexual problems. The treatment of premature ejaculation can involve training the individual to tolerate high levels of excitement without ejaculating and reducing anxiety associated with sexual arousal. One successful intervention is the start–stop technique (Semans 1956). This procedure involves having the patient lie on his back while his partner strokes his penis. The patient then focuses on the pleasurable feelings resulting from the penile stimulation and the sensations that precede his urge to ejaculate. When he feels that he is about to ejaculate, he signals his partner to stop stimulation. The patient should start and stop at least four times before he allows himself to ejaculate.

A second procedure, the "squeeze" technique (Masters and Johnson 1970), can be done in conjunction with the start–stop technique. In the squeeze tech-

TABLE 16–12. DSM-IV-TR diagnostic criteria for premature ejaculation

A. Persistent or recurrent ejaculation with minimal sexual stimulation before, on, or shortly after penetration and before the person wishes it. The clinician must take into account factors that affect duration of the excitement phase, such as age, novelty of the sexual partner or situation, and recent frequency of sexual activity.

B. The disturbance causes marked distress or interpersonal difficulty.

C. The premature ejaculation is not due exclusively to the direct effects of a substance (e.g., withdrawal from opioids).

Specify type:

Lifelong type

Acquired type

Specify type:

Situational type

Generalized type

Specify:

Due to psychological factors

Due to combined factors

nique, the patient's partner is taught to place her thumb on the frenulum of the penis and her first and second fingers on the opposite sides of the head of the penis. When the patient feels that he is going to ejaculate, the partner squeezes for up to 5 seconds and then releases the penis for up to 30 seconds. This technique is continued until the individual is no longer on the verge of ejaculating, where the patient's partner then resumes penile stimulation.

Several subtypes of biogenic and psychogenic premature ejaculation have been identified (Metz and Pryor 2000). Biogenic types include 1) neurological constitution, 2) physical illness, 3) physical injury, and 4) pharmacological side effects. Medical conditions that can contribute to premature ejaculation include arteriosclerosis, benign prostatic hyperplasia, cardiovascular disease, diabetes, injury to the sympathetic nervous system, pelvic injuries, prostate cancer, prostatitis, urethritis, urinary incontinence, polycythemia, and polyneuritis (Baum and Spieler 2001). Psychogenic types consist of 1) psychological constitution or chronic psychological disorders, 2) psychological distress, and 3) psychosexual skills deficit. A fourth psy-

chogenic subtype is concomitant with another sexual dysfunction. Specific treatments for this disorder should be determined following a comprehensive assessment of the relevant subtype (Metz and Pryor 2000). Pharmacological treatment should be considered for those with severe neurological constitution. Training the patient in cognitive-behavioral arousal management also may be useful in less severe cases. Psychosexual treatment combines various strategies, including physiological relaxation, pubococcygeal muscle training, cognitive and behavioral pacing strategies, and the involvement of the partner in the therapy (Metz and Pryor 2000).

A new functional–sexological treatment for premature ejaculation has been recently introduced (de Carufel and Trudel 2006) and involves the modulation of sexual excitement through several techniques. Men are instructed in specific ways of altering their typical bodily movements and positioning during sexual intercourse, the use of positions that require less muscular tension, variations in the speed and intensity of pelvic movements, and breathing involving the diaphragm and are provided education regarding sensuality and the sexual responses of men and women. When compared with traditional behavioral treatments, including the squeeze and stop/start techniques, this functional–sexological treatment demonstrates similar effectiveness in improving subjective duration of intercourse, sexual satisfaction, and satisfaction with overall treatment results.

Somatic treatments for premature ejaculation have included intracavernous injection of papaverine and phentolamine (Fein 1990) and the use of oral medications such as the tricyclic antidepressant clomipramine (Richardson and Goldmeier 2005; Segraves et al. 1993; Strassberg et al. 1999) and SSRIs (Baum and Spieler 2001; Richardson and Goldmeier 2005; Waldinger et al. 2003), which can decrease libido and delay orgasm, as well as oral analgesics such as tramadol (Safarinejad and Hosseini 2006), which reduce penile sensation. Other potential somatic interventions include topical agents such as SS-cream, which can cause mild penile burning or pain, or anesthetic creams, which may cause penile numbness (Baum and Spieler 2001; Richardson and Goldmeier 2005). Chloraseptic mouthwash may also retard sexual stimulation and result in increased ejaculation latency (Baum and Spieler 2001). However, many of these medications and somatic interventions may lead to negative side effects that should be discussed with the patient (Althof 1995; de Carufel and Trudel 2006).

Sexual Pain Disorders

Dyspareunia

The DSM-IV-TR diagnostic criteria for dyspareunia are shown in Table 16–13.

It is imperative that a comprehensive physical and gynecological or urological examination be conducted. In the absence of organic pathology, the patient's fear and anxiety underlying sexual functioning should be investigated. Systematic desensitization has been found to be successful in the treatment of this disorder in some women. Physiotherapy has also been recommended as a potential treatment for dyspareunia and involves a number of techniques designed to decrease pelvic and vulvar pain and increase circulation and muscular mobility and flexibility in these regions (Graziottin and Brotto 2004; Rosenbaum 2005). A diagnosis incorporating medical as well as psychosexual factors is a crucial step in the effective treatment of this disorder (Graziottin 2001). Therefore, in addition to the physiological interventions described above, therapy related to the individual's or couple's psychosexual issues may also be beneficial.

Vaginismus

The DSM-IV-TR diagnostic criteria for vaginismus are shown in Table 16–14.

Vaginismus can be diagnosed with certainty only through a gynecological examination. Some women who are anxious about sex may experience muscular tightening and some pain during penetration, but these women do not have vaginismus. It is important to rule out other Axis I disorders (e.g., somatization disorder), substance-induced disorders, or a general medical condition.

Systematic desensitization has been the most effective treatment method for vaginismus. A useful procedure involves the systematic insertion of dilators of graduated sizes, either in the physician's office or in the privacy of the patient's home. Some clinicians have the patient or her partner gradually insert a tampon or fingers until penile penetration can be effected (Kaplan 1974). The clinician may suggest that the patient gently stroke her genitals, including her clitoris, during the insertion procedure. Additionally, penile penetration should be effected with the partner lying on his back and the patient controlling the actual insertion and subsequent movement during intercourse. Follow-up studies have reported maintenance of treatment gains over time for most women (Scholl 1988). As described above, physiotherapy with targeted relaxation and desensitization procedures may also be useful in the treatment of this disorder (Rosenbaum 2005).

TABLE 16–13. **DSM-IV-TR diagnostic criteria for dyspareunia**

A. Recurrent or persistent genital pain associated with sexual intercourse in either a male or a female.

B. The disturbance causes marked distress or interpersonal difficulty.

C. The disturbance is not caused exclusively by vaginismus or lack of lubrication, is not better accounted for by another Axis I disorder (except another sexual dysfunction), and is not due exclusively to the direct physiological effects of a substance (e.g., a drug of abuse, a medication) or a general medical condition.

Specify type:

> **Lifelong type**
> **Acquired type**

Specify type:

> **Situational type**
> **Generalized type**

Specify:

> **Due to psychological factors**
> **Due to combined factors**

TABLE 16–14. **DSM-IV-TR diagnostic criteria for vaginismus**

A. Recurrent or persistent involuntary spasm of the musculature of the outer third of the vagina that interferes with sexual intercourse.

B. The disturbance causes marked distress or interpersonal difficulty.

C. The disturbance is not better accounted for by another Axis I disorder (e.g., somatization disorder) and is not due exclusively to the direct physiological effects of a general medical condition.

Specify type:

> **Lifelong type**
> **Acquired type**

Specify type:

> **Situational type**
> **Generalized type**

Specify:

> **Due to psychological factors**
> **Due to combined factors**

Sexual Dysfunction Due to a General Medical Condition

The diagnosis of sexual dysfunction due to a general medical condition is made if there is evidence from the history, physical examination, or laboratory findings of a general medical condition judged to be etiologically related to the sexual dysfunction (e.g., male erectile disorder due to a general medical condition, dyspareunia due to a general medical condition). Several examples of medical conditions associated with sexual dysfunction were listed in the beginning of this chapter, including those which interfere with circulation and normative endocrine functioning.

Substance-Induced Sexual Dysfunction

The diagnosis of substance-induced sexual dysfunction is made if there is a clinically significant sexual dysfunction that results in marked distress or interpersonal difficulty and occurs only in the presence of substance or medication use. Depending on the substance involved, the dysfunction may involve impaired desire, arousal, or orgasm or sexual pain. In a community sample, it was noted that inhibited orgasm was associated with marijuana and alcohol use, and painful sexual intercourse was associated with marijuana and illicit drug use (Johnson et al. 2004). Additionally, inhibited sexual desire was also related to alcohol and illicit drug use in this sample for both males and females.

A number of substances have demonstrated an adverse impact on sexual functioning (see Table 16–2).

Alcohol, psychomotor stimulants such as cocaine or amphetamines, opiates, antipsychotic medications, antidepressants, sedatives, and marijuana may reduce sexual arousal in both males and females when used at high doses or over a long period of time. Chronic use of cocaine or amphetamines, as well as typical use of some antipsychotic medications, can impair the ejaculatory response in males.

These drugs of abuse can impair sexual functioning through various mechanisms, which were briefly discussed at the beginning of this chapter. Cocaine may impair sexual functioning because of its ability to deplete dopamine stores with chronic use. Chronic opiate and alcohol use also may interfere with endogenous dopamine and serotonin functioning, leading to impaired sexual functioning. Long-term opiate use may also reduce testosterone levels in the body, thereby decreasing normal sexual arousal. A similar but temporary effect may be seen after marijuana use. Evidence also suggests that the negative effects of methylenedioxymethamphetamine (MDMA; "Ecstasy") on the brain's serotonergic systems can lead to significant sexual dysfunction in heavy or chronic users (Parrott 2006).

Because of the complexity of the relationship between substance use and sexual functioning, careful assessment must precede any attempts at treating the sexual dysfunction. Other medical or psychiatric conditions that may also contribute to the reported sexual difficulties must be explored. Factors that might contribute to the development of both sexual dysfunction and substance use (e.g., relationship problems) should be considered as well before a final diagnosis of substance-induced sexual dysfunction is made.

Key Points

- Sexual dysfunctions are divided into four primary categories: sexual desire disorders, sexual arousal disorders, orgasmic disorders, and sexual pain disorders. DSM-IV-TR diagnostic criteria for each of these categories are outlined in this chapter.

- Sexual dysfunctions are relatively common disorders in both males and females, affecting up to 20%–30% of the population at some point in their lives. Improvements in assessment and diagnosis have increased our understanding of sexual dysfunction and its variation across the life span.

- Causes of sexual dysfunction are numerous and varied, with external influences such as disease, medication, or substance use and internal influences such as anxiety, other psychological disorders, or lack of communication regarding sexual interests or desires all playing a role.

- Treatments for sexual dysfunctions often involve a combination of psychological and behavioral interventions. Recent advances in pharmacological agents designed to affect sexual performance have also helped in the treatment of sexual dysfunctions, particularly male orgasmic disorders. Successful treatment may require addressing both psychogenic and physiological etiologies of the dysfunction.

Suggested Reading

Basson R, Berman J, Burnett A, et al: Full report from the International Development Conference on Female Sexual Dysfunction: definitions and classifications. J Sex Marital Ther 27:83–245, 2001

References

Aizenburg D, Shiloh R, Zemishlany Z, et al: Low-dose imipramine for thioridazine-induced male orgasmic disorder. J Sex Marital Ther 22:225–229, 1996

Althof SE: Pharmacological treatment for rapid ejaculation: Preliminary strategies, concerns, and questions. Sex Marital Ther 10:247–251, 1995

Althof SE, Turner LA, Levine SB, et al: Sexual, psychological, and marital impact of self-injection of papaverine and phentolamine: a long-term prospective study. J Sex Marital Ther 17:101–112, 1991

American Psychiatric Association: Diagnostic and Statistical Manual of Mental Disorders, 4th Edition, Text Revision. Washington, DC, American Psychiatric Association, 2000

Basson R, Berman J, Burnett A, et al: Report of the International Development Conference on Female Sexual Dysfunction: definitions and classifications. J Sex Marital Ther 27:83–94, 2001

Basson R, McInnes R, Smith MD, et al: Efficacy and safety of sildenafil citrate in women with sexual dysfunction associated with female sexual arousal disorder. J Womens Health Gend Based Med 11:367–377, 2002

Baum N, Spieler B: Medical management of premature ejaculation. Med Aspects Hum Sex 1:15–25, 2001

Bechara A, Bertolino MV, Cassade A, et al: Duplex Doppler ultrasound assessment of clitoral hemodynamics after topical administration of Alprostadil in women with arousal and orgasmic disorders. J Sex Marital Ther 29 (suppl 1):1–10, 2003

Becker JV, Skinner LJ, Abel GG, et al: Level of postassault sexual functioning in rape and incest victims. Arch Sex Behav 15:37–49, 1986

Berman JR, Berman LA, Lin H, et al: Effect of sildenafil on subjective and physiologic parameters of the female sexual response in women with sexual arousal disorder. J Sex Marital Ther 27:411–420, 2001

Britton KR: Medroxyprogesterone in the treatment of aggressive hypersexual behaviour in traumatic brain injury. Brain Inj 12:703–707, 1998

Carey MP: Cognitive-behavioral treatment of sexual dysfunctions, in International Handbook of Cognitive and Behavioural Treatments for Psychological Disorders. Edited by Caballo VE. Oxford, England, Pergamon/Elsevier Science, 1998, pp 251–280

Carson CC: Erectile dysfunction: Evaluation and new treatment options. Psychosom Med 66:664–671, 2004

Cavallini G: Minoxidil versus nitroglycerin: a prospective double-blind controlled trial in transcutaneous erection facilitation for organic impotence. J Urol 146:50–53, 1991

Chollet CA, Andreatini R: Effect of bupropion on sexual dysfunction induced by fluoxetine: a case report of hypersexuality. J Clin Psychiatry 64:1268–1269, 2003

Clayton AH, Segraves RT, Leiblum S, et al: Reliability and validity of the Sexual Interest and Desire Inventory—Female (SIDI-F), a scale designed to measure severity of female hypoactive sexual desire disorder. J Sex Marital Ther 32:115–135, 2006

Cooper AJ: Evaluation of I-C papaverine in patients with psychogenic and organic impotence. Can J Psychiatry 36:574–578, 1991

de Carufel F, Trudel G: Effects of a new functional-sexological treatment for premature ejaculation. J Sex Marital Ther 32:97–114, 2006

Dinsmore W: Treatment of erectile dysfunction. Int J STD AIDS 15:215–221, 2004

Dobkin RD, Menza M, Marin H, et al: Bupropion improves sexual functioning in depressed minority women: an open-label switch study. J Clin Psychopharmacol 26:21–26, 2006

Dow MGT, Gallagher J: A controlled study of combined hormonal and psychological treatment for sexual unresponsiveness in women. Br J Clin Psychol 28:201–212, 1989

Emory LE, Cole CM, Meyer WJ: Use of Depo-Provera to control sexual aggression in persons with traumatic brain injury. J Head Trauma Rehabil 10:47–58, 1995

Fein RL: Intracavernous medication for treatment of premature ejaculation. Urology 35:301–303, 1990

Finger WW: Antidepressants and sexual dysfunction: managing common treatment pitfalls. Med Aspects Hum Sex 1:12–18, 2001

Freymann N, Michael R, Dodel R, et al: Successful treatment of sexual disinhibition in dementia with carbamazepine: a case report. Pharmacopsychiatry 38:144–145, 2005

Graziottin A: Clinical approaches to dyspareunia. J Sex Marital Ther 27:489–501, 2001

Graziottin A, Brotto LA: Vulvar vestibulitis syndrome: a clinical approach. J Sex Marital Ther 30:125–139, 2004

Greil W, Horvath A, Sassim N, et al: Disinhibition of libido: an adverse effect of SSRI? J Affect Disord 62:225–228, 2001

Hatzichristou D, Cuzin B, Martin-Morales A, et al: Vardenafil improves satisfaction rates, depressive symptomatology, and self-confidence in a broad population of men with erectile dysfunction. J Sex Med 2:109–116, 2005

Hayes R, Dennerstein L: The impact of aging on sexual function and sexual dysfunction in women: a review of population-based studies. J Sex Med 2:317–330, 2005

Heruti R, Shochat T, Tekes-Manova D, et al: Prevalence of erectile dysfunction among young adults: results of a large-scale survey. J Sex Med 1:284–291, 2004

Hoon PW, Wincze JP, Hoon EF: Physiological assessment of sexual arousal in women. Psychophysiology 13:196–204, 1976

Islam A, Mitchel J, Rosen R, et al: Topical Alprostadil in the treatment of female sexual arousal disorder: a pilot study. J Sex Marital Ther 27:531–540, 2001

Jackson G, Rosen RC, Kloner RA, et al: The second Princeton consensus on sexual dysfunction and cardiac risk: new guidelines for sexual medicine. J Sex Med 3:28–36, 2006

Johnson SD, Phelps DL, Cottler LB: The association of sexual dysfunction and substance use among a community epidemiological sample. Arch Sex Behav 33:55–63, 2004

Kaplan HS: The New Sex Therapy: Active Treatment of Sexual Dysfunctions. New York, Brunner/Mazel, 1974

Kaplan HS, Fyer AJ, Novick A: The treatment of sexual phobias: the combined use of antipanic medication and sex therapy. J Sex Marital Ther 8:3–28, 1982

Kelly MP, Strassberg DS, Turner CM: Communication and associated relationship issues in female anorgasmia. J Sex Marital Ther 30:263–276, 2004

Kelly MP, Strassberg DS, Turner CM: Behavioral assessment of couples' communication in female orgasmic disorder. J Sex Marital Ther 32:81–95, 2006

Khalifé S, Binik YM, Cohen DR, et al: Evaluation of clitoral blood flow by color Doppler ultrasonography. J Sex Marital Ther 26:187–189, 2000

Laan E, Everaerd W, Evers A: Assessment of female sexual arousal: response specificity and construct validity. Psychophysiology 32:476–485, 1995

Lal S, Kiely ME, Thavundayil JX, et al: Effect of bromocriptine in patients with apomorphine-responsive erectile impotence: an open study. J Psychiatry Neurosci 16:262–266, 1991

Leiblum SR, Rosen RC: Couples therapy for erectile disorders: conceptual and clinical considerations. J Sex Marital Ther 17:147–159, 1991

Leonard LM, Follette VM: Sexual functioning in women reporting a history of child sexual abuse: review of the empirical literature and clinical implications. Annu Rev Sex Res 13:346–388, 2002

Levine SB, Althof SE, Turner LA, et al: Side effects of self-administration of intracavernous papaverine and phentolamine for the treatment of impotence. J Urol 141:54–57, 1989

Lewis RW, Fugl-Meyer KS, Bosch R, et al: Epidemiology/risk factors of sexual dysfunction. J Sexual Medicine 1:35–39, 2004

LoPiccolo J, Stock WE: Treatment of sexual dysfunction. J Consult Clin Psychol 54:158–167, 1986

Masters WH, Johnson VE: Human Sexual Response. Boston, MA, Little, Brown, 1966

Masters WH, Johnson VE: Human Sexual Inadequacy. Boston, MA, Little, Brown, 1970

Melnik T, Abdo CHN: Psychogenic erectile dysfunction: comparative study of three therapeutic approaches. J Sex Marital Ther 31:243–255, 2005

Meston CM: The psychophysiological assessment of female sexual function. J Sex Educ Ther 25:6–16, 2000

Meston CM: Validation of the Female Sexual Function Index (FSFI) in women with female orgasmic disorder and in women with hypoactive sexual desire disorder. J Sex Marital Ther 29:39–46, 2003

Metz ME, Pryor JL: Premature ejaculation: a psychophysiological approach for assessment and management. J Sex Marital Ther 26:293–320, 2000

Meyhoff HH, Rosenkilde P, Bodker A: Non-invasive management of impotence with transcutaneous nitroglycerin. Br J Urol 69:88–90, 1992

Milan RJ, Kilmann PR, Boland JP: Treatment outcome of secondary orgasmic dysfunction: a two- to six-year follow-up. Arch Sex Behav 17:463–480, 1988

Montaldi DF: Understanding hypersexuality with an Axis II model. J Psychol Human Sex 14:1–24, 2002

O'Carroll R, Bancroft J: Testosterone therapy for low sexual interest and erectile dysfunctions in men: a controlled study. Br J Psychiatry 145:146–151, 1984

Padma-Nathan H, Brown C, Fendl J, et al: Efficacy and safety of a topical Alprostadil cream for the treatment of female sexual arousal disorder (FSAD): a double-blind, multicenter, randomized, and placebo-controlled clinical trial. J Sex Marital Ther 29:329–344, 2003

Padma-Nathan H, Christ G, Adaikan G, et al: Pharmacotherapy for erectile dysfunction. J Sex Med 1:128–140, 2004

Parrott AC: MDMA in humans: factors which affect the neuropsychobiological profiles of recreational ecstasy users, the integrative role of bioenergetic stress. J Psychopharmacol 20:147–163, 2006

Richardson D, Goldmeier D: Pharmacological treatment for premature ejaculation. Int J STD AIDS 16:709–711, 2005

Richardson D, Goldmeier D, Kocsis A: PDE5 inhibitors may help some women with sexual problems. Sexual and Relationship Therapy 20:65–69, 2005

Rosen R, Brown C, Heiman J, et al: The Female Sexual Function Index (FSFI): a multidimensional self-report instrument for the assessment of female sexual function. J Sex Marital Ther 26:191–208, 2000

Rosenbaum TY: Physiotherapy treatment of sexual pain disorders. J Sex Marital Ther 31:329–240, 2005

Safarinejad MR, Hosseini SY: Pharmacotherapy for premature ejaculation. Current Drug Therapy 1:37–46, 2006

Salerian AJ, Vittone BJ, Geyer SP, et al: Sildenafil for psychotropic-induced sexual dysfunction in 31 women and 61 men. J Sex Marital Ther 26:133–140, 2000

Samuel RZ: The unusual side effect of excessive sexual desire with paroxetine use. Primary Psychiatry 13:40–42, 2006

Scholl GM: Prognostic variables in treating vaginismus. Obstetrics Gynecology 72:231–235, 1988

Segraves RT, Saran A, Segraves K, et al: Clomipramine versus placebo in the treatment of premature ejaculation: a pilot study. J Sex Marital Ther 19:198–200, 1993

Segraves RT, Croft H, Kavoussi R, et al: Bupropion sustained release (SR) for the treatment of hypoactive sexual desire (HSDD) in nondepressed women. J Sex Marital Ther 27:303–316, 2001

Segraves RT, Clayton A, Croft H, et al: Bupropion sustained release for the treatment of hypoactive sexual desire disorder in premenopausal women. J Clin Psychopharmacol 24:339–342, 2004

Semans JH: Premature ejaculation: a new approach. South Med J 9:353–357, 1956

Shabsigh R: Testosterone therapy in erectile dysfunction and hypogonadism. J Sex Med 2:785–792, 2005

Sills T, Wunderlich G, Pyke R, et al: The Sexual Interest and Desire Inventory—Female (SIDI-F): item response analyses of data from women diagnosed with hypoactive sexual desire disorder. J Sex Med 2:801–818, 2005

Simons JS, Carey M: Prevalence of sexual dysfunctions: results from a decade of research. Arch Sex Behav 30:177–219, 2001

Simpkins JW, Van Meter R: Potential testosterone therapy for hypogonadal sexual dysfunction in women. J Womens Health (Larchmt) 14:449–451, 2005

Sintchak G, Geer JH: A vaginal plethysmograph system. Psychophysiology 12:113–115, 1975

Spector IP, Carey MP: Incidence and prevalence of the sexual dysfunctions: a critical review of the empirical literature. Arch Sex Behav 19:389–408, 1990

Spector IP, Carey MP, Steinberg L: The Sexual Desire Inventory: development, factor structure, and evidence of reliability. J Sex Marital Ther 22:175–190, 1996

Strassberg DS, de Gouveia Brazao CA, Rowland DL, et al: Clomipramine in the treatment of rapid (premature) ejaculation. J Sex Marital Ther 25:89–101, 1999

Turner LA, Althof SE, Levine SB, et al: External vacuum devices in the treatment of erectile dysfunction: a one-year study of sexual and psychosocial impact. J Sex Marital Ther 17:81–93, 1991

Turner LA, Althof SE, Levine SB, et al: Twelve-month comparison of two treatments for erectile dysfunction: self-injection versus external vacuum devices. Urology 39:139–144, 1992

Van Anders SM, Chernick AB, Chernick BA, et al: Preliminary clinical experience with androgen administration for pre- and postmenopausal women with hypoactive sexual desire. J Sex Marital Ther 31:173–185, 2005

Waldinger MD, Zwinderman AH, Olivier B: Antidepressants and ejaculation: a double-blind, randomized, fixed-dose study with mirtazapine and paroxetine. J Clin Psychopharmacol 23:467–470, 2003

Weiss JN, Ravalli R, Badlani GH: Intracavernous pharmacotherapy in psychogenic impotence. Urology 37:441–443, 1991

Wiegel M, Meston C, Rosen R: The Female Sexual Function Index (FSFI): cross-validation and development of clinical cutoff scores. J Sex Marital Ther 31:1–20, 2005

Wiseman SV, McAuley JW, Freidenberg GR, et al: Hypersexuality in patients with dementia: possible response to cimetidine. Neurology 54:2024, 2000

Witt DK: Yohimbine for erectile dysfunction. J Fam Pract 46:282–283, 1998

17

GENDER IDENTITY DISORDERS AND PARAPHILIAS

Judith V. Becker, Ph.D.
Bradley R. Johnson, M.D.

Sexuality is an important part of the lives of people. Thus, it is important that students of human behavior be informed about and conversant with issues such as normative sexual development, gender roles, gender identity, sexual orientation, and the wide range of sexual behaviors individuals may fantasize about or engage in. When sexual behaviors are defined by cultures or society as being atypical, they are referred to as *paraphilias*. This chapter focuses on gender identity disorders and paraphilias.

Gender Identity Disorders

Gender and Sexual Differentiation

The genetic *sex* of an individual is determined at conception, but development from that point on is influenced by many factors. For the first few weeks of gestation, the gonads are undifferentiated. If the Y chromosome is present in the embryo, the gonads will differentiate into testes. A substance referred to as the H-Y antigen is responsible for this transformation. If the Y chromosome or H-Y antigen is not present in the developing embryo, the gonads will develop into ovaries.

Like the gonads, the internal and external genital structures are initially undifferentiated in the fetus. If the gonads differentiate into testes, fetal androgen (i.e., testosterone) is secreted, and these structures develop into male genitalia (epididymis, vas deferens, ejaculatory ducts, penis, and scrotum). In the absence of fetal androgen, these structures develop into female genitalia (fallopian tubes, uterus, clitoris, and vagina). It is important to note that the development of genitalia in utero depends on the presence or absence of fetal androgen, from whatever source. Thus, if fetal androgen is present in a genetically determined female (e.g., adrenal hyperplasia), male genitalia will develop, even in the presence of ovaries, and the child will be born with either ambiguous or male genitals. Likewise, if fetal androgen is missing (e.g., enzyme deficiency) or androgen receptors are defective (e.g., testicular feminization), female genitalia will develop even though the individual has the Y chromosome and testes.

Psychosexual development also is thought to be influenced by a complex interaction of factors, both pre- and postnatal. Before discussing these factors, however, it is important to break down psychosexual behavior into several components. *Gender identity* is an individual's perception and self-awareness of being male or female. *Gender role* is the behavior that an individual engages in that identifies him or her to others as being male or female (e.g., wearing dresses and makeup). *Sexual orientation* "refers to erotic attraction to males, females, or both" (American Psychiatric Association 2000).

Prenatal hormones play a role in the differentiation of the mammalian brain. However, their exact effect on psychosexual development in humans has not been established. Although they may contribute to the development of gender role behaviors, their effect on that development is still debated. In fact, some have proposed that hormones have little or no effect on sexual orientation (Bancroft 1994; Byne and Parsons 1993). All in all, they do not appear to play a major part in gender identity differentiation (Ehrhardt and Meyer-Bahlburg 1981).

Gender identity appears to develop in the early years of life and generally is established by age 3 years. Gender identity seems to depend on the sex in which an individual is reared, regardless of biological factors. The evidence for this comes from studies of children born with genitalia that are ambiguous or opposite from their genetic sex (Money and Ehrhardt 1974). These children have been found to develop gender identity consistent with the gender assigned to them at birth as long as their parents are unambiguous about the child's sex and surgical and hormonal corrections are made. Thus, a child with testicular feminization will grow up with a female gender identity, even though "she" has testes, if assigned and raised as a girl and the aforementioned conditions are met. Similarly, a genetic female with ambiguous genitalia caused by congenital adrenal hyperplasia, if reared as a boy, will develop a male gender identity; if reared as a girl, the individual will develop a female gender identity. In contrast, Diamond (1965) asserts that "the evidence and arguments...show, primarily owing to prenatal genic and hormonal influences, human beings are definitely predisposed at birth to a male or female gender orientation" (p. 167).

Gender identity, once it is firmly established, is extremely resistant to change. For example, if a genetic female who is reared as a boy (e.g., as a result of exposure to fetal androgens) suddenly develops breasts and other female secondary sex characteristics during puberty, his gender identity will remain male, and he will likely want to correct the changes. However, if a child's physical appearance is ambiguous, or if the caregivers are inconsistent in their view of the child as male or female, gender identity may not develop strongly, leading to possible "change" or confusion regarding gender identity at a later time in life. In contrast to this view, Cohen-Kettenis (2005) reviewed studies on gender identity outcome in individuals with 5α-reductase-2 deficiency and 17β-hydroxysteroid dehydrogenase-3 deficiency and concluded that "the number of gender role changes reported in the literature is considerable and certainly higher than in other intersex conditions" (p. 407). Cohen-Kettenis (2005) posited that various factors may determine whether individuals with these conditions raised as girls will make the switch after puberty to a male gender identity, including a biological factor, such as "the severity of the mutation in terms of the in vitro enzyme production deficiency" (p. 407), cultural factors, environmental factors, and the individuals' reaction to their genital appearance.

If gender identity develops between birth and age 3 years and depends on sex of rearing, what are the factors that contribute to its development? Several theories attempt to answer this question. Biological factors that have not yet been discovered may influence the development of gender identity, and in some instances, it has been suggested that biological factors may override sex assignment at birth (Ehrhardt and Meyer-Bahlburg 1981). According to a learning theory model, gender identity begins to develop when the child imitates or identifies with same-sex models. The child is then reinforced for having this identification and for engaging in "appropriate" sex-role behaviors. Psychoanalytic authors have stressed the emergence of gender identity disorder during the preoedipal period, and how the disorder develops in relation to attachment (Zucker and Bradley 1995). Others have emphasized that the mothers of boys with gender identity disorder have experienced a high rate of adverse events such as sexual and physical assaults, death of a child, or husbands' extramarital affairs during the sensitive period of gender identity formation (as reported in Zucker and Bradley 1995).

Criteria for Diagnosing Gender Identity Disorder

Currently, it is accepted that there are two necessary components of gender identity disorder: a strong and persistent cross-gender identification (not merely a desire for any perceived cultural advantages of being the other sex) and a persistent discomfort with one's sex or sense of inappropriateness in the gender role of that sex (Table 17–1). The diagnosis is not given if the person has a concurrent physical condition such as partial androgen insensitivity syndrome or congenital adrenal hyperplasia, and as with many other diagnoses in DSM-IV-TR, there must be evidence of clinically significant distress or impairment (American Psychiatric Association 2000).

TABLE 17–1. **DSM-IV-TR diagnostic criteria for gender identity disorder**

A. A strong and persistent cross-gender identification (not merely a desire for any perceived cultural advantages of being the other sex).

In children, the disturbance is manifested by four (or more) of the following:

(1) repeatedly stated desire to be, or insistence that he or she is, the other sex

(2) in boys, preference for cross-dressing or simulating female attire; in girls, insistence on wearing only stereotypical masculine clothing

(3) strong and persistent preferences for cross-sex roles in make-believe play or persistent fantasies of being the other sex

(4) intense desire to participate in the stereotypical games and pastimes of the other sex

(5) strong preference for playmates of the other sex

In adolescents and adults, the disturbance is manifested by symptoms such as a stated desire to be the other sex, frequent passing as the other sex, desire to live or be treated as the other sex, or the conviction that he or she has the typical feelings and reactions of the other sex.

B. Persistent discomfort with his or her sex or sense of inappropriateness in the gender role of that sex.

In children, the disturbance is manifested by any of the following: in boys, assertion that his penis or testes are disgusting or will disappear or assertion that it would be better not to have a penis, or aversion toward rough-and-tumble play and rejection of male stereotypical toys, games, and activities; in girls, rejection of urinating in a sitting position, assertion that she has or will grow a penis, or assertion that she does not want to grow breasts or menstruate, or marked aversion toward normative feminine clothing.

In adolescents and adults, the disturbance is manifested by symptoms such as preoccupation with getting rid of primary and secondary sex characteristics (e.g., request for hormones, surgery, or other procedures to physically alter sexual characteristics to simulate the other sex) or belief that he or she was born the wrong sex.

TABLE 17–1. **DSM-IV-TR diagnostic criteria for gender identity disorder** *(continued)*

C. The disturbance is not concurrent with a physical intersex condition.

D. The disturbance causes clinically significant distress or impairment in social, occupational, or other important areas of functioning.

Code based on current age:

302.6 **Gender identity disorder in children**

302.85 **Gender identity disorder in adolescents or adults**

Specify if (for sexually mature individuals):

Sexually attracted to males

Sexually attracted to females

Sexually attracted to both

Sexually attracted to neither

Zucker (2005) provided an overview of various measures pertaining to assessing gender identity, gender role, and sexual orientation that have been used in assessment studies of children and adults with gender identity disorder and/or children and adults with various physical intersex conditions. He reported that all of the measures have good psychometric properties.

Gender Identity Disorder of Adulthood

Historically, gender identity disorders were first introduced in DSM-III (American Psychiatric Association 1980) and were included in the section on psychosexual disorders. In DSM-III-R (American Psychiatric Association 1987), the gender identity disorders were moved to the section "Disorders Usually First Evident in Infancy, Childhood, or Adolescence." Additionally, in DSM-III-R, gender identity disorder of adulthood, nontranssexual type, was added. Up to this point, the essential features of the principal diagnostic categories in the subclass *transsexualism* were a persistent sense of discomfort and inappropriateness about one's anatomical sex and a persistent wish to be rid of one's genitals and to live as a member of the other sex.

The term *transsexualism* was eliminated in DSM-IV (American Psychiatric Association 1994). A single diagnostic term, *gender identity disorder*, was introduced to apply to children, adolescents, and adults. The disorder was also placed in the "Sexual and Gender Identity Disorders" section (American Psychiatric Association 1994). The term remained the same in the current DSM-IV-TR edition. The elimination of the term *transsexualism* alters the sense that it exists as a single disorder and presents it conceptually as a spectrum of disorders. However, the term still appears to describe appropriately what is now referred to as *gender identity disorder of adulthood*.

Although not considered an actual diagnosis in DSM-IV-TR, the term *gender dysphoria* has been used to characterize a person's sense of discomfort or unease about his or her status as male or female (Zucker and Green 1997). Gender dysphoria has been classified as primary or secondary as it relates to transsexualism (Person and Ovesey 1974). *Primary transsexuals* have a profound lifelong disturbance of core gender identity. They have histories of cross-dressing as children but never were aroused by wearing opposite-sex clothes. They usually have a clear history of engaging in opposite-sex gender-role behaviors. *Secondary transsexuals* also can have a long history of gender identity confusion; however, in these individuals, the identity disturbance follows other cross-gender behavior such as transvestism or effeminate homosexuality. Blanchard (2005) reviewed his prior taxonomic research, which indicated that heterosexual, asexual, and bisexual transsexuals were more similar to each other and to transvestites than any of them were to the homosexual transsexuals. He coined the term *autogynephilia* to describe those males who have "love of oneself as a woman" (Blanchard 2005).

The diagnosis of *gender identity disorder not otherwise specified* is used when there are disorders in gender identity that are not classified as a specific gender identity disorder and may include intersex conditions and the accompanying gender dysphoria, transient cross-dressing behavior that may be stress related, or persistent preoccupation with castration or penectomy without the desire to acquire the sex characteristics of the opposite sex (American Psychiatric Association 2000).

Epidemiology

Although there are no recent epidemiological studies to provide prevalence data, gender identity disorder of adulthood is still thought to be rare, with prior estimates of 30,000 cases worldwide (Lothstein 1980). Approximately 1 per 30,000 adult males and 1 per 100,000 females seek sex reassignment surgery (American Psychiatric Association 2000). Cases have been described throughout history, but only in the past few decades has scientific and media attention focused on this phe-

nomenon, and a few specialized gender identity clinics have been developed. Transsexual individuals most commonly request *sex reassignment*—that is, change in their physical appearance (usually by hormonal and surgical means) to correspond with their self-perceived gender. However, it is important to remember that not all those who seek sex reassignment are transsexual; cross-gender wishes may occur in transvestism (i.e., wearing opposite-gender clothes for erotic purposes) or effeminate homosexuality in men.

It has been concluded that three to four times as many males as females apply for sex reassignment, but approximately equal numbers of males and females are reassigned (J.K. Meyer 1982). Virtually all of the women who apply have a sexual orientation toward women. Male transsexuals are predominantly homosexual in orientation, but approximately 25% are sexually attracted to women. Some of these "heterosexual" transsexuals enter into "lesbian" relationships after they are reassigned as females. These findings provide further evidence of the separateness of gender identity and sexual orientation. Many male and female transsexuals also have been described as being hyposexual or asexual. However, both male and female patients often have a fear of homosexual attraction and thus choose to remain asexual rather than acknowledge their homosexual orientation.

Comorbidity

Among those adults who are diagnosed as having gender identity disorder, there is a high degree of concomitant psychiatric disorder, most commonly borderline, antisocial, or narcissistic personality disorder; substance abuse; and suicidal or self-destructive behavior (J.K. Meyer 1982). These individuals can be demanding and manipulative and often resist interventions other than sex reassignment. In a recent study (a Campo et al. 2003), it was reported that 61% of those with gender identity disorder had comorbid psychiatric illness.

Etiology

There are still no well-established or exhaustive explanations for the development of gender identity disorder. As noted earlier in this chapter, gender identity appears to be established and influenced by psychosocial factors during the first few years of life. However, many authors have argued that biological factors, if not causative, may predispose an individual to a gender identity disorder. It is important to realize, however, that researchers still have been unable to identify a biological anomaly or variant associated specifically with gender identity disorder.

As mentioned earlier in this section, prenatal sex hormones probably have little causal effect on gender identity and possibly sexual orientation. However, studies of females with congenital adrenal hyperplasia caused by high levels of androgens prenatally (Collaer and Hines 1995) suggest there may be a relation between such disorders and gender identity problems. This type of example leads us to realize that further research in this area needs to be done.

Some researchers have found decreased levels of testosterone in male transsexuals and abnormally high levels of testosterone in female transsexuals, but the findings have been inconsistent, and the studies from which they were obtained were not well controlled. Tests for H-Y antigen have been found to be negative in male transsexuals and positive in female transsexuals in a high percentage of cases; however, there has been a consistent failure to replicate these findings (Hoenig 1985).

Although no correlation has been made with specific temporal lobe abnormalities, there have been case reports of individuals who developed gender identity disorder following onset of temporal lobe seizures, which reverted with the use of anticonvulsive medication. Studies of electroencephalograms in male and female transsexuals have detected abnormalities in 30%–70%; however, only one of the studies used control groups, and the effect of medications, especially estrogen, was not taken into account (Hoenig 1985).

Family studies have been difficult to carry out given the low incidence of gender identity disorders. To date, no clear increase in familial incidence has been documented.

Learning theory models suggest that gender dysphoria arises from absent or inconsistent reinforcement for identification with same-sex models. Cross-gender identification and behaviors take place, and these are reinforced with either overt or covert approval from the child's caregivers.

Psychoanalytic theory argues that early deprivation of the male child by his mother leads to a symbiotic merger with the mother and lack of full individuation as a separate person. In the case of borderline personality disorder, this process leads to general identity confusion and loss of ego boundaries when the individual is under stress. In gender dysphoria, the defect is isolated to gender. However, the same ego impairment, disordered object relations, and primitive defense mechanisms (i.e., denial and splitting) are present (J.K. Meyer 1982). The same psychoanalytic theories also attempted to explain homosexuality.

Clinical studies (Green 1987; Stoller 1968, 1975a, 1975b, 1979) have reported that boys with gender identity disorder often have an overly close relationship with their mother and a distant, ambivalent relationship with their father. Stoller (1968) argued that the boy who is excessively close to his mother, in absence of the father, may have difficulty in separating himself from the female body and feminine behavior. It is important to note that not all children with gender identity disorder become adults with gender identity disorder.

Diagnosis and Evaluation

Individuals who request sex reassignment require careful evaluation by a psychiatrist or psychologist with experience in the management of gender identity disorders. They should undergo a complete psychosexual evaluation, in addition to a thorough psychiatric or psychological examination. Patients with other primary psychiatric diagnoses may present as transsexuals. Psychotic patients may have delusions centered around their genitalia (e.g., that someone has substituted the incorrect genitals, that God is telling them to change their sex). When the psychosis is treated, the cross-gender wishes usually resolve. Individuals with severe personality disorders, especially borderline, can have transient wishes to change gender as part of their overall identity diffusion during times of stress. Effeminate homosexual men may desire to change sex in order to be more attractive to men; usually this desire fluctuates with time. Transvestites (described in the "Paraphilias" section later in this chapter) are heterosexual men aroused by wearing female garments. To increase their arousal, they may progress to actually wishing to become a woman; again, however, this wish is usually not continuous over a long period, and their gender identity is male. Adolescents sometimes become gender dysphoric because of developing homosexual feelings that need to be resolved. For each of these patients, psychotherapy is indicated to deal with the appropriate issues leading to their request for sex reassignment.

Unfortunately, individuals requesting sex reassignment often hide the truth in an effort to obtain hormonal and surgical change. Therefore, it is imperative to contact significant others in the patient's life (e.g., family members, spouse, sexual partners) to confirm the pervasive and nonremitting nature of the gender identity disturbance.

Treatment

Because most gender dysphoric individuals have adamant requests for sex reassignment (many often are already taking opposite-sex hormones supplied by other physicians), it is extremely difficult to engage these patients in treatment with anything other than surgical sex reassignment as the goal. These patients see psychotherapy as a means of discouraging them from surgery. However, because surgery is irreversible, it is important to engage these patients in psychotherapy, even if surgery is indicated. The therapist should be careful to base the goals of therapy on what is desired by the patient. These goals should be identified at the beginning of therapy, including a discussion on informed consent as to the possible outcomes and complications that could arise secondary to the use of psychotherapy.

Supportive psychotherapy can serve various purposes in transsexual individuals. First, there have been reports, albeit few, of reversal of patients' gender identity disorders. Second, a trial of psychotherapy is often useful in cases in which the diagnosis is not clear. Third, dealing with patients' fears of homosexuality may sometimes change their wishes for surgical reassignments. Fourth, psychotherapy plays an important role in patients' adjustment to the process of sex reassignment. Finally, therapy is often helpful in the postsurgical adjustment of patients with gender identity disorder.

The therapist must be comfortable in treating patients who have gender identity disorders. Furthermore, the therapist must be comfortable with his or her own sexual identity and sexual issues so that countertransference does not adversely affect the treatment. For those transsexual persons with poor ego functioning, psychoanalysis is not generally indicated (J.K. Meyer 1982). Dynamic psychotherapy may be used but must involve parameters applied to borderline patients (e.g., structured therapy, limit setting, ego support, and short-term goals).

Behavior therapy has been used in ego-dystonic male transsexuals in several cases (Barlow et al. 1979). The treatment can be helpful to those who wish to alter their effeminate behaviors, including female patterns of behavior (e.g., sitting, walking, social behavior, vocal characteristics). These behaviors are then changed with videotapes and modeling of masculine behaviors in which the patients are trained to engage. Attempts had been made to change the patients' arousal pattern from homosexual to heterosexual; however, this attempt was successful in only one in three cases. The American Psychiatric Association (2000) issued a position statement asserting that it "opposes any psychiatric treatment, such as 'reparative' or conversion therapy, which is based on the assumption that homosexuality per se is a mental disorder or based on the a priori assumption that a patient should change his or her homosexual orientation."

Sexual reassignment to the opposite sex has been the most widely used and studied treatment modality for adults with gender identity disorder. Early reports of outcome were extremely positive, with dramatic changes in social functioning and satisfaction. Hormonal treatment and surgery have become more readily available for adults with gender identity disorder, often with little preparation other than a brief consultation with a psychiatrist. This approach led to an increase in the reports of poor results and realization that sex reassignment was not a panacea. Clinicians who are considering providing services to gender dysphoric patients should familiarize themselves with the *Standards of Care for Gender Identity Disorders* (M. Meyer et al. 2001), which is published by the Harry Benjamin International Gender Dysphoria Association.

Green and Fleming (1990) reviewed the literature written during 1979 through 1989 on both male-to-female and female-to-male postoperative transsexuals. Only 11 follow-up studies were located in the literature. These authors concluded that preoperative factors indicative of a favorable outcome included an absence of psychosis as well as mental and emotional stability shown prior to the surgery; a successful adaptation to the desired gender for at least 1 year; an understanding of the consequences and limitations of the surgery; and the seeking of preoperative psychotherapy. These authors reported that there was some evidence that outcome was somewhat less favorable for secondary transsexuals, even when these individuals were denied surgery. Data from this report indicated that outcomes were considered satisfactory for 97% of the female-to-male transsexuals and for 87% of the male-to-female transsexuals.

Y. Smith et al. (2001) conducted a prospective follow-up study with 20 treated adolescent transsexuals to evaluate early sex reassignment and with 21 nontreated and 6 delayed-treatment adolescents to evaluate the decisions not to allow them to start sex reassignment, especially at an early age. The treated group who received sex reassignment surgery did not continue to have gender dysphoria, and they were thought to be psychologically and socially functioning quite well 1–4 years postoperatively. None of these individuals expressed regret over their decision to have the surgery. However, although the nontreated group also showed improvement, they had a more dysfunctional psychological profile; therefore, it is important to carefully screen those who are cleared for reassignment and treatment, especially if they are too young or have made their decision too quickly and without careful thought.

DeCuypere et al. (2005) conducted a follow-up of 55 transsexual patients (both male-to-female and female-to-male) after sex reassignment surgery. The purpose of this study was to evaluate the sexual and general health of patients following surgery. Those researchers found that few and minor problems were observed in the patients, and most were reversible with appropriate treatment. Male-to-female patients experienced more general health problems. The researchers stated this might have been explained by smoking habits and older age. The patients reported that their expectations regarding the surgery were met on both a social and emotional level but not so much on a physical and sexual level. However, it is important to note that 80% reported improvement in their sexuality. One specific sexual change noted was that the female-to-male patients reported an increase in masturbation and a trend toward more sexual excitement, satisfaction, and orgasm. The majority of patients reported a more powerful change in orgasmic feeling.

Y. Smith et al. (2005) investigated whether transsexuals can be divided into subtypes based on sexual orientation and whether the subtypes are similar for male-to-female and female-to-male transsexuals. The sample consisted of 187 homosexual and nonhomosexual transsexuals. The homosexual transsexuals were younger at the time they applied for sex reassignment surgery and had stronger cross-gender identities in childhood. They were functioning psychologically at a better level than the nonhomosexual transsexuals. Fewer of the homosexual transsexuals reported ever having been married. The researchers reported that distinguishing between subtypes of transsexuals on the basis of sexual orientation was clinically meaningful. They noted that the "more vulnerable" nonhomosexual transsexuals may benefit from receiving professional guidance before and during the course of this treatment.

Sex reassignment is a long process that must be carefully monitored. Patients with other primary psychiatric diagnoses and secondary transsexuals should be screened out and given other appropriate treatment. If the patient is considered appropriate for sex reassignment, psychotherapy should be started to prepare the patient for the cross-gender role. The patient should then go out into the world and live in the cross-gender role before surgical reassignment. Males should cross-dress, have electrolysis, and practice female behaviors. They can even change their identity to female on official documents and at work. Females should cut their hair, bind or conceal their breasts, and similarly take on the identity of a man. After 1–2 years, if these measures have been successful and the patient still wishes reassignment, hormone treatment is be-

gun. Estrogens are given to the male patient, resulting in redistribution of body fat in a more "feminine" pattern and enlargement of the breasts. This treatment is not without possible medical complications, and patients should be followed up closely by a physician. Side effects of estrogen treatment may include deep vein thrombosis, thromboembolic disorders, increased blood pressure, weight gain, impaired glucose tolerance, liver abnormalities, and depression. Testosterone given to the female patient causes redistribution of fat, growth of facial and body hair, enlargement of the clitoris, and deepening of the voice. Unwanted side effects of testosterone treatment include acne, edema secondary to sodium retention, and impairment of liver function. After 1–2 years of hormone therapy, the patient may be considered for surgical reassignment if such a procedure is still desired. In the male-to-female patient, this consists of bilateral orchiectomy, penile amputation, and creation of an artificial vagina. Female-to-male patients undergo bilateral mastectomy and optional hysterectomy with removal of ovaries. Efforts to create an artificial penis have met with mixed results thus far; at this point, it is better to counsel the patient to focus on mutual body caressing, oral-genital stimulation, and other forms of sexual pleasuring that do not necessarily involve having a penis sufficient for vaginal penetration. Overall cosmetic and functional results from surgery have been variable in both male and female transsexuals. Postsurgical complications can occur and include the following: for genetic females, chest wall scars and polycystic ovary disease; for genetic males, urethral stenosis, misdirected urinary streams, vaginal strictures, and rectovaginal fistulas. The *Standards of Care for Gender Identity Disorders* states, "benefit from psychotherapy may be attained at every stage of gender evolution" including "the post-surgical period when the anatomic obstacles to gender comfort have been removed and the person continues to feel a lack of genuine comfort and skill in living in the new gender role" (M. Meyer et al. 2001).

Readers are referred to the *Standards of Care for Gender Identity Disorders* for treatment recommendations for adults (M. Meyer et al. 2001).

Gender Identity Disorder of Childhood

Because of the difficulty and turmoil involved in treating late-adolescent and adult patients who have gender identity disorder, researchers and clinicians began to evaluate and treat children with gender identity problems. Strictly speaking, this disorder is seen in a child who perceives him- or herself as being of the opposite sex.

However, it is often difficult to separate gender identity from gender-role behavior in children. Boys with normal gender identity may play with "girl" dolls. Many girls in our culture are "tomboys" and like rough and contact games. However, in this gender identity syndrome, there is a repeated pattern of opposite-gender role behavior accompanied by a disturbance in the child's perception of "being" a boy or a girl. The exact incidence of gender identity disorder in children is not known, but like adult gender dysphoria, it is a rare disorder.

Children with gender identity problems express a desire to become a member of the opposite sex. Boys wish to have a vagina and may play at breast-feeding. Girls wish to have a penis and may simulate a penis with various objects or stand to urinate. Boys cross-dress with dresses, makeup, and jewelry, whereas girls may resist wearing dresses at any cost and wear short hair. Both sexes identify with role models of the opposite sex (e.g., a boy insists that he is Supergirl in a game). In evaluating a child, it is important not to look solely at behavior; there also must be a disturbance in the child's sexual identity. As in the evaluation of adults, the child should be evaluated for other psychiatric disorders such as psychosis or adjustment disorder.

Prevalence and Etiology

One study looking at children referred to a specificity clinic for gender identity disorder from the period 1978–1995 found a boy-to-girl sex ratio of 6.6:1 (Zucker et al. 1997). As with adult gender dysphoria, the etiology of childhood gender identity disorder is unclear. The theories outlined earlier in this chapter for adults who have gender identity disorder also apply to children. Additional factors that have been suggested are parents' indifference to or encouragement of opposite-sex behavior; regular cross-dressing as a young boy by a female; lack of male playmates during a boy's first years of socialization; excessive maternal protection, with inhibition of rough-and-tumble play; or absence of or rejection by an older male early in life (Green 1974). Gender identity disorder in children has been posited as being the result of child and family pathology (Zucker and Bradley 1995).

Physical Appearance

It is interesting to note that several studies have associated gender identity disorder with greater physical attractiveness in boys when compared with the physical attractiveness of clinical control subjects who did not have the disorder (Green 1987; Zucker et al. 1993). Fridell et al. (1996) concluded that girls with gender identity disorder often were seen as less attractive than those in a control group.

Course

Retrospective studies of transsexuals (Green 1974) have shown a high incidence of childhood cross-gender behavior. There appear to be two main pathways to adult gender identity disorder, one that involves childhood gender identity disorder and one that develops in early to middle adulthood, sometimes concurrent with transvestic fetishism (American Psychiatric Association 2000). Longitudinal research with boys who demonstrate gender identity disorder and a comparison group found that a large proportion of the boys with gender identity disorder (about 68%) were bisexually or homosexually oriented, whereas none of a demographically matched comparison sample reported a bisexual or homosexual orientation (Green 1985). According to the American Psychiatric Association, "only a very small number of children with GID will continue to have symptoms that meet criteria in adolescence or adulthood" and that "by late adolescence or adulthood, about three-quarters of boys who had a childhood history of Gender Identity Disorder report a homosexual or bisexual orientation, but without concurrent Gender Identity Disorder" (American Psychiatric Association 2000, p. 580). The proportion of female children with gender identity disorder who report bisexual or homosexual orientation in adolescence and adulthood is unknown.

Treatment

A comprehensive assessment is required to provide appropriate services to a child with gender identity disorder. Hormonal or surgical therapies should not be considered for this age group. M. Meyer et al. (2001) recommend that

1. The professional recognize and accept the gender identity problem.
2. The assessment explore the nature and characteristics of the child's or adolescent's gender identity.
3. Therapy focus on ameliorating any comorbid problems in the child's life and on reducing distress the child experiences from his or her gender identity problem and other difficulties.

Not all children with childhood gender identity disorder will develop the adult disorder. Consequently, when a child presents with gender identity disorder, the clinician should assess what is in the best interest of the child, considering parental concerns and the child's wishes. Unfortunately, such children can be subject to social ostracism; therefore, support needs to be provided to the child, and parents may be given information as to how best to protect their child from harassment. Readers are referred to Zucker and Bradley (1995) for a review of treatment research on children with gender identity disorder. These authors stated that treatment has three goals: increasing peer support and acceptance, treating co-occurring mental health concerns, and reducing the likelihood of transsexualism in adulthood (Zucker and Bradley 1995). Behavior therapy has been used in the past to modify specific cross-gender behaviors in a manner similar to that described for adults as well as to enhance contingency management (e.g., reinforcing behaviors consistent with the child's phenotype sex). Analytically oriented treatment has dealt with the family dynamics (e.g., a powerful, masculine-devaluing mother; an ineffective, emotionally absent father) and individual dynamics (e.g., castration anxiety following surgery) of the child. There is a dearth of research regarding treatment of children with gender identity disorder.

In treating adolescents with gender identity disorder, clinicians should take a conservative approach, given that a hallmark of adolescence involves identity issues. As with young children, therapy may involve individual and family therapy. The adolescents also need to learn coping skills to deal with any harassment or ostracism they may experience. M. Meyer et al. (2001) indicated that adolescents may be eligible for fully and partially reversible physical interventions. The reader is referred to the *Standards of Care for Gender Identity Disorders* (M. Meyer et al. 2001) for more detailed information.

Paraphilias

Paraphilias are one of the most misunderstood categories of diagnosis in psychiatry. Frequently associated with sexual offenses, the two concepts of paraphilias and sexual offense do not necessarily or always go hand in hand. In fact, many people commit sexual offenses that do not meet the criteria for a sexual paraphilia; likewise, there are people who can be diagnosed with a paraphilia and never commit a sex crime.

The paraphilias (Table 17–2) are characterized by experiencing, over a period of at least 6 months, "recurrent, intense sexually arousing fantasies, sexual

TABLE 17–2. Paraphilias

Exhibitionism	Exposure of genitals to an unsuspecting stranger
Fetishism	Arousal to nonliving objects
Frotteurism	Touching and rubbing against a nonconsenting person
Pedophilia	Urges and fantasies involving prepubescent children
Sexual masochism	Deriving sexual excitement from being humiliated, beaten, bound, or otherwise made to suffer
Sexual sadism	Urges and fantasies of acts in which psychological and/or physical suffering of the victim is sexually exciting
Transvestic fetishism	Urges and fantasies involving cross-dressing
Voyeurism	Observing an unsuspecting person naked, disrobing, or engaged in sex
Necrophilia	Contact with corpses
Urophilia	Urine
Zoophilia	Animals
Klismaphilia	Enemas
Telephone scatalogia	Obscene telephone calls
Partialism	Exclusive focus on one part of body

urges, or behaviors" (American Psychiatric Association 2000, p. 566) generally involving nonhuman objects or nonconsenting partners. In diagnosing any of the paraphilias, a further criterion is that the person has acted on the urges or is markedly distressed by them—that is, they may have engaged in a behavior that is sexually inappropriate or even illegal, but they may only have the urges or fantasies of the paraphilia and never act upon them. The first part of this section discusses some of the more common types of paraphilias diagnosed.

Types of Paraphilias
Exhibitionism

Exhibitionism is defined as the exposure of one's genitals to an unsuspecting person or stranger. It may involve masturbation during the exposure, and in some cases the individual tries to surprise or shock the observer. The individual may hope or desire that the observer will become sexually aroused or join in the sexual activity. It is generally thought to be a disorder of males, sometimes has an early onset (before age 18 years), and is directed primarily at females (Murphy 1997). Victims can be adults, children, or adolescents (Gittleson et al. 1978; MacDonald 1973). As with many types of paraphilias, there are no good personality profiles for exhibitionists (Blair and Lanyon 1981). Few arrests occur in offenders over the age of 40, suggesting that the condition may become less common after about 40 years of age (American Psychiatric Association 2000).

Fetishism

Fetishism is sexual arousal involving the use of nonliving objects such as women's underpants, bras, stockings, shoes, boots, or other apparel (American Psychiatric Association 2000). Masturbation may accompany the person holding, rubbing, or smelling the item. In general, the person may have difficulty in getting sexually aroused in the absence of the item. Mason (1997) concluded that there is no good epidemiological data for this paraphilia, but it appears to be more common in males than females. There are a number of theories as to the etiology of this class of paraphilia (i.e., biological, conditioning, social learning, and psychoanalytic), but they are nearly impossible to test empirically.

Frotteurism

Frotteurism involves touching and rubbing against another nonconsenting person (American Psychiatric Association 2000). It frequently takes place in crowded places such as on a bus or subway, in a crowded hall, or on a busy sidewalk. Although there are many different ways that a person can engage in frotteuristic activity, it is not uncommon that a male would rub his genitals against the unsuspecting victim; however, the behavior may include touching or rubbing the genitals or sexual organs of victims without their being aware that they have been offended against. Freund et al. (1997) have concluded that this disorder is actually part of a courtship disorder, seeing it as similar in this regard to voyeurism, exhibitionism, and even rape.

Pedophilia

Pedophilia is defined as sexual attraction to, or sexual behavior involving, a prepubescent boy or girl, generally age 13 or younger. By definition, in order to give a diagnosis of pedophilia, the individual must be at least 16 years of age and at least 5 years older than the child.

Many misuse the term *pedophilia* in cases involving sexual attraction to or activity with a postpubescent boy or girl who is still under the age of 18. This situation is referred to as *hebephilia* instead. It is not uncommon for an individual with pedophilia to have a certain age range of child to which they are sexually attracted, and the attraction can be gender specific or to both male and female children. There are specifiers listed in DSM-IV-TR (American Psychiatric Association 2000), including being limited to incest, exclusive type (attracted only to children) and nonexclusive type. Those attracted to females often prefer 8- to 10-year-olds, whereas those who prefer male children are often attracted to an older age range. There is a large spectrum of inappropriate sexual activity that has been seen between adults and children, ranging from undressing and looking at the child to penetration of different forms and even to torture. There have been cases in which pedophilia started in adolescence and other cases that did not seem to begin until mid-adulthood.

Sexual Masochism

The diagnostic criteria for *sexual masochism* are intense sexually arousing fantasies, urges, or behaviors involving the act, whether real or simulated, of "being humiliated, beaten, bound, or otherwise made to suffer" (American Psychiatric Association 2000, p. 573). Such acts may include restraint, blindfolding, paddling, spanking, whipping, beating, electrical shocks, cutting, piercing, and such humiliating acts as being urinated or defecated on. A variation on this issue is *infantilism*—that is, the individual desires to be treated as an infant, even to the point of wearing diapers. *Hypoxyphilia* is a dangerous and potentially life-threatening form of sexual masochism that involves sexual arousal by oxygen deprivation through a number of possible means. This specific type of behavior works against the proposal by some (Baumeister and Butler 1997) that sexual masochism may not be pathological or is even a fairly innocuous activity.

Sexual Sadism

Sexual sadism involves real acts (not simulated) in which sexual arousal is achieved from the psychological or physical suffering of the victim (American Psychiatric Association 2000). Although it may involve a consenting partner who has sexual masochistic desires, it often involves nonconsenting victims. The sadistic acts may involve such things as controlling or dominating the victim but may also include such things as restraint, blindfolding, paddling, spanking, whipping, pinching, beating, burning, electrical shocks, rape, cutting, stabbing, strangulation, torture, mutilation, or even killing. Such fantasies may have begun in childhood but are usually present in these cases by early adulthood. Hucker (1997) discussed that sexual sadism may include a number of subcategories of paraphilia, including necrophilia (sexual attraction or behavior with a corpse), sadistic and lust murders (sexual arousal from killing), and sadistic rape. The authors believed that rape should possibly be considered a separate paraphilia in its own right, but this issue has been controversial due to the legal implication of the term *rape* versus its use from a psychiatric or psychological perspective.

Transvestic Fetishism

Identified separate from the general concept of fetishism, *transvestic fetishism* involves cross-dressing by a male in women's attire, in most cases producing sexual arousal (American Psychiatric Association 2000). The disorder has only been described in heterosexual males and is not diagnosed if it occurs exclusively in the case of gender identity disorder. It may begin in childhood or may start in adulthood, may be temporary or chronic, and may lead to gender dysphoria in some cases. It is often at this point that the person may seek treatment.

Voyeurism

Voyeurism is commonly seen as the act of becoming sexually aroused while viewing nudity or sexual activity by others when they do not realize they are been watched or have not given permission. The act of looking while another unsuspecting person is naked, is disrobing, or is engaging in sexual activity leads to sexual excitement, but generally there is no sexual activity between the voyeur and the victim. The person is usually masturbating while watching, or shortly thereafter, and in some cases, the voyeuristic behavior may be the sole form of sexual activity for the person. The onset of this type of behavior often starts in adolescence and can become chronic (American Psychiatric Association 2000).

Paraphilia Not Otherwise Specified

There are numerous other sexually deviant fantasies or behaviors that do not fit any of the paraphilic categories described here or variations that do not meet the full criteria. The diagnosis of *paraphilia not otherwise specified* can be given in these situations, including such examples as telephone scatologia (obscene phone calls), necrophilia (if not part of a sexually sadistic diagnosis), partialism (exclusive focus on part of the

body), zoophilia (animals), coprophilia (feces), klismaphilia (enemas), and urophilia (urine) (American Psychiatric Association 2000). Sometime the act of rape would fit in this category if another paraphilia such as sadism did not fit the particular case.

Epidemiology

The paraphilias rarely cause personal distress, and individuals with these disorders usually come for treatment because of pressure from their partners or the authorities. Thus, there are few data on the prevalence or course of many of these disorders. Historically, information on those paraphilias involving victims (pedophilia, exhibitionism) has been obtained from studies of incarcerated sex offenders. However, these data are limited in that many sex offenders are not arrested, and those who are tend to underreport their deviant behavior for fear of further prosecution. For example, two large studies of incarcerated sex offenders found that the offenders had committed only a small number of sexually deviant acts (Gebhard et al. 1965).

In contrast, studies of nonincarcerated pedophiles have been enlightening regarding what has been learned about paraphilias in general. Abel et al. (1987) gathered data through structured clinical interviews of 561 men with paraphilias regarding demographic characteristics, frequency and variety of deviant sexual acts, and number and characteristics of victims. The majority of their participants (all of whom who gave information under a Certificate of Confidentiality) were well educated, although there was a spread of educational backgrounds; half had formed a significant relationship with an adult partner; and 67% fell into the age range of 20–39 years. The authors reported an average number of crimes and victims that was substantially higher than had been realized before and reported that their subjects molested young boys five times more often than they did young girls.

Abel et al. (1988) shed more light on paraphilias when they further analyzed their information gleaned from this same group and discovered that most persons with paraphilias have had significant experience with as many as 10 different types of deviant sexual behavior (Figure 17–1). It is important to note that more than 50% of these individuals develop the onset of their paraphilic arousal before age 18 years.

The vast majority of individuals with these disorders are men. For example, among reported cases of sexual abuse, more than 90% of offenders are men (Finkelhor 1986). However, it is interesting to note that one study (Risin and Koss 1988) reported that 42.7% of college males who reported that they had been sexu-

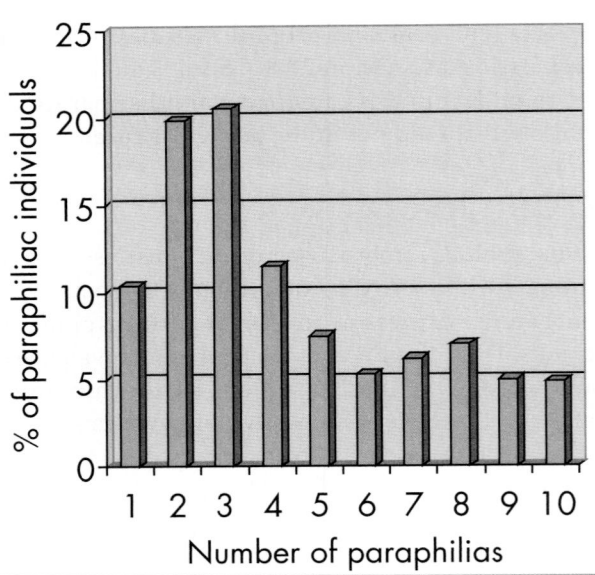

FIGURE 17–1.   Multiple paraphiliac diagnoses.

ally victimized were abused by women. Fallen (1989) reported that 5%–15% of perpetrators were females.

Etiology

Various theories have been put forth to explain the development of paraphilias. As with the gender identity disorders, biological factors have been postulated. Destruction of parts of the limbic system in animals causes hypersexual behavior (Klüver-Bucy syndrome), and temporal lobe diseases such as psychomotor seizures or temporal lobe tumors have been implicated in some persons with paraphilias. It also has been suggested that abnormal levels of androgens may contribute to inappropriate sexual arousal. Most studies, however, have dealt only with violent sex offenders and have yielded inconclusive results (Bradford and McLean 1984).

Psychoanalytic theories have postulated that severe castration anxiety during the oedipal phase of development leads to the substitution of a symbolic object (inanimate object or an anatomical part) for the mother, as in fetishism and transvestism. Similarly, anxiety over arousal to the mother can lead to the choice of "safe," inappropriate sexual partners, as in pedophilia or zoophilia, or safe sexual behaviors in which there is no sexual contact, as in exhibitionism and voyeurism. Some psychoanalytic theories have suggested that a paraphilia represents an attempt by an individual to recreate and master early childhood punishment or humiliation (Stoller 1975a, 1975b). Some view deviant sexual behavior as an alternative to neurotic develop-

ment, attributing it to ego acceptance of unrepressed infantile sexual fantasies (Abel et al. 1993).

According to learning theory, sexual arousal develops when an individual engages in a sexual behavior that is subsequently reinforced through sexual fantasies and masturbation. It is thought that there are certain vulnerable periods (e.g., puberty) when the development of sexual arousal can occur. For example, if an adolescent boy is sexual with a 7-year-old boy, and there are no negative consequences, the adolescent may continue to fantasize about having sex with the boy and masturbate to those fantasies, developing arousal to young boys (i.e., pedophilia). Similarly, if a young boy is experimenting and puts on his sister's panties or is cross-dressed by a relative and becomes aroused, he may develop arousal to wearing women's clothes (i.e., transvestism).

A number of theories have been proposed to explain the behavior of individuals who sexually abuse children. Finkelhor (1984) hypothesized that there were four underlying factors involved in child molestation. Specifically, sex offenders of children experienced emotional congruence; that is, they found sex with children to be emotionally satisfying. They also found the behavior to be sexually arousing. A third factor related to having sex with children is that these men were unable to meet their needs in a sexually and socially appropriate way (blockage). Finally, child molesters experienced disinhibition in that they are able to behave in ways contrary to social norms.

Hall and Hirschman (1992) proposed a quadripartite model of child molestation. The four components included physiological sexual arousal, cognitive distortions that justify sex with children, personality problems, and affective dyscontrol. Marshall and Barbaree (1990) proposed that individuals who engage in sexual activity with children during their own childhood experience developmentally adverse events. As those children enter adolescence, their sexual fantasies may involve sexual scripts that involve aggression and sex. These youth might lack self-regulation skills, may be lacking in social skills, and may experience negative states that increase the probability that they will engage in inappropriate sexual behavior.

The Pathways model was suggested by Ward and Siegert (2002), who proposed that there are multiple pathways that lead to behavior involving the sexual abuse of a child. Each one of the pathways involves a set of dysfunctional psychological mechanisms that constitute vulnerability factors that are influenced by distal and proximal factors including environmental, cultural, and biological events.

More recently, Ward and Beech (2006) presented an integrated theory to explain the onset, development, and maintenance of sexual offending behavior. The model is comprehensive in that they examined factors that affect the developing brain, including genetic variations, neurobiology, and evolution, as well as ecological factors, including personal circumstances and physical environment, and discuss how all of these factors affect neuropsychological functioning. The authors stated that their theory unifies a range of sexual offending theories and has the potential to "provide well grounded guidance to researchers working on different facets of sexual offending, and remind those operating purely with psychological or social models that it is ultimately necessary to cash them out in biological and neuroscientific terms" (p. 61). These authors believe that their integrated theory is an abstract framework for thinking about sex offending and that future research needs to apply it to different types of sexual crimes, including child molestation, exhibitionism, and rape.

Another theoretical model of the development of paraphilias is based on cognitive distortions. Distortions in thinking, or thinking errors, provide a way for an individual to give him- or herself permission to engage in inappropriate or deviant sexual behaviors. Examples of such faulty beliefs include the following: it is all right to have sex with a child as long as the child agrees; watching a woman through a window as she undresses does not cause her any harm; and if a child stares at my penis, he or she likes what he or she is seeing and wants to be sexual (Abel et al. 1984).

As theory and model development continues, it is important that developing theories are comprehensive and include evolutionary, neuroendocrine, and social learning factors.

Diagnosis

It is important to distinguish between paraphilias such as fetishism and transvestism and normal variations of sexual behavior. Some couples occasionally augment their usual sexual activities with activities such as bondage or cross-dressing. Transvestism, however, would be diagnosed only if a heterosexual male, over a period of at least 6 months, had recurrent, intense sexual urges and sexually arousing fantasies involving cross-dressing and if the person is distressed by the urges or has acted on them. Only when these activities are the exclusive or preferred means of achieving sexual excitement and orgasm, or when the sexual behavior is not consensual, is the paraphilia diagnosed. Obviously, nonconsensual sexual activities such as sexual

contact with children or exhibitionism never can be appropriate; children never can give consent for sexual activity with an adult.

Inappropriate sexual behavior is not always the result of a paraphilia. A psychotic patient may cross-dress because of a delusional belief that God wishes him or her to hide his or her true sex. A manic patient may expose himself to women because of his hypersexuality and belief that he will be able to "pick them up." A patient with dementia can behave in a sexually inappropriate manner (e.g., masturbate in a room full of people) because of cognitive impairment. An individual with mental retardation may engage in a sexually inappropriate behavior because of cognitive impairment, poor impulse control, and lack of sexual knowledge. Individuals with antisocial personality disorder also can commit deviant sexual acts; such behaviors usually are part of their overall disregard for societal norms and sanctions.

Clinical Evaluation

In evaluating an individual for paraphilic behavior, a careful psychiatric evaluation must be done to exclude the aforementioned possible causes of this behavior. A detailed sexual history should be taken, noting the onset and course of paraphilic and appropriate sexual fantasies and behavior and the present degree of control over the deviant behavior. In addition, the individual should be evaluated for faulty beliefs about his or her sexual behavior (i.e., cognitive distortions), social and assertive skills with appropriate adult partners, sexual dysfunctions, and sexual knowledge. Table 17–3 lists information that is important to collect during a clinical psychosexual interview, which may then be confirmed with collateral sources. Table 17–4 lists specific details that may be covered in the sexual history portion of the evaluation.

Phallometric Assessment

Phallometric assessments (i.e., measurements of penile erection) have been used to objectively assess sexual arousal in individuals who have engaged in paraphilic behavior. This finding is important because persons with paraphilias, especially those in trouble with the law, are reluctant to disclose the full extent of their deviant behavior and fantasies. A transducer (either a thin metal ring or mercury-in-rubber strain gauge) is placed around the penis, and the degree of erection is recorded while the individual is exposed to various sexual stimuli (audiotapes, slides, videotapes) depicting paraphilic and appropriate sexual scenes. This information is then

TABLE 17–3. Psychosexual assessment

- A history of present and past psychiatric illness and treatments

- A family psychiatric history

- A social history

- A medical history, including such things as past surgical procedures, chronic medical illnesses, acute traumatic injury, head trauma, history of seizures, and history of loss of consciousness

- A history of current and past medications and other medical treatments

- A developmental history, learning such things as whether the child was the product of a planned pregnancy; whether the mother was exposed to alcohol, drugs, or abuse during the pregnancy; and whether there were any complications with the delivery

- Information about the temperament of the youth as he or she was a developing infant and toddler

- A history of interactions with other children and adults while growing up

- A history of educational development, including whether he or she was referred for special education services or has learning disabilities

- An employment history

- Family history and functioning

- Future plans for employment, education, and family

- Emotional, physical, and sexual abuse history

- The current living arrangements and social and financial support

- A history of legal problems

- A history of gang involvement

- A history of violent behaviors

- Alcohol and substance use history

- A detailed sexual history

TABLE 17–4. Sexual history

- When puberty began

- When the person as an adolescent first became aware of his or her own sexuality (for a male, when he became aware of obtaining erections and when the erections correlated with sexual stimuli or fantasies)

- Personal beliefs about sex

- How the person's sexual relationships developed (such as when the person experienced his or her first crush and romantic kiss and how the person first learned about sex)

- The nature of his or her first type of sexual contact (such as prolonged kissing, touching, oral sexual contact, anal sexual contact, and actual intercourse)

- Number of sexual contacts

- Age range of sexual fantasies and contacts

- Gender of sexual fantasies and contacts

- Exposure to sexually stimulating materials (such as magazines, videos, books, Internet Web sites, sexual toll telephone calls, adult bookstores, strip clubs)

- Personal feelings about his or her body and sexual organs and any sexual dysfunctions

- Fantasies and behaviors regarding common as well as serious sexual paraphilias and related topics (such as exhibitionism, voyeurism, frotteurism, pedophilia, sexual masochism, sexual sadism, transvestism, zoophilia, necrophilia, rape, killing, torture, control)

- History of gender identity concerns or disorder

- Any other pertinent sexual issue not covered previously

recorded on a polygraph or computer, and the degree of arousal to deviant sexual scenes is compared with arousal to nonparaphilic scenes.

Phallometric assessments of sexual age and gender preferences have excellent discriminant validity with extrafamilial child molesters (Freund and Blanchard 1989). However, exclusively incestuous offenders are less likely to show inappropriate sexual age preferences in phallometric assessment as compared with extrafamilial child molesters (Barbaree and Marshall 1989). Although phallometric assessments attempt to measure the degree of sexual preference among stimulus categories, they do not detail whether someone has engaged in paraphilic behavior or has committed a sexual offense. Furthermore, some individuals are able to influence their responses in order to appear to have nonparaphilic preferences (Freund et al. 1988). Further research is indicated to standardize this form of assessment and to establish the psychometric properties.

As with the interpretation of most physiological procedures, many urge caution in interpreting plethysmograph outcomes; that is, the setting in which the data are obtained is quite different from the real world. There can be variation within subjects over time, and therefore, the interpretation must be made within the context of the offender's history, available records, and psychological characteristics (Dougher 1995).

Other Assessment Tools

Recently, there has been an effort to examine other methods to assess deviant sexual interest. The Abel Assessment for Sexual Interest is an instrument that measures the subject's viewing time of specially designed photographs of clothed models, assuming that the length of viewing time may correlate to the measure of sexual interest. Although this seems like a less invasive and simple method compared with the plethysmograph, the procedure and its reliability, sensitivity, and specificity must be corroborated (Krueger et al. 1998). Abel et al. (1998) reported, however, that data support the use of their instrument. Measuring sexual interest may not be the same as sexual arousal; thus, both the Abel Assessment for Sexual Interest and plethysmography may have their separate uses.

There are other psychosexual tests and checklists that are used at times to gain additional information (Table 17–5). One should be careful to correlate the findings on these measures to the clinical evaluation and not depend on them for diagnosis. Collateral sources of information may be quite helpful to corroborate claims from the person if an offense has been committed, reviewing such items as police reports, victim statements, prior mental health records, jail or prison records, sex offender treatment records, and school records. One may consider also interviewing family members, friends, or even victims in some cases to obtain additional information.

Therapeutic Treatment of Paraphilias

A variety of behavior therapies have been used to treat paraphilias. Various aversive conditioning methods (e.g., noxious odors) and covert sensitization have been used to decrease deviant sexual behavior. (In the latter approach, the individual pairs his or her inappropriate sexual fantasies with aversive, anxiety-provoking scenes, under the guidance of a therapist.) *Satiation* is a technique in which the individual uses his or her deviant fantasies postorgasm in a repetitive

---

TABLE 17–5. Some psychosexual tests and checklists

- *Abel and Becker Cognitions Scales:* Assesses irrational or distorted thoughts regarding inappropriate sexual behaviors (adult and adolescent versions)

- *Bumby Cognitive Distortions Scales:* Includes a Molest scale and a Rape scale to assess irrational or distorted thoughts regarding inappropriate sexual behaviors

- *Rape Myth Acceptance Scale:* A measure of the acceptance of myths about rape

- *Psychopathy Checklist—Revised (PCL-R):* Assesses degree of psychopathy

- *Multiphasic Sex Inventory—2:* A self-report questionnaire designed to assess a wide range of psychosexual characteristics (adult and adolescent versions)

- *Sexual Interest Cardsort:* A self-report measure of sexual preference or interests (adult and adolescent versions)

---

manner to the point of satiating himself or herself with the deviant stimuli, in essence making the fantasies and behavior boring (Marshall and Barbaree 1978).

Skills training and cognitive restructuring to change the individual's maladaptive beliefs are also used in behavioral treatments. Marshall et al. (1991), in a comprehensive review of the literature of treatment outcome studies for a variety of sex offenders, concluded that treatment programs that use comprehensive cognitive-behavioral interventions, as well as those that use antiandrogens in combination with psychological treatment, are the most effective.

Empathy training is routinely utilized in the treatment of sex offenders (Monto et al. 1998). Additionally, some have found that helping the offender improve self-esteem can reduce loneliness and increase intimacy (Marshall et al. 1997).

Psychoanalysis and psychodynamic therapy have been used in treating paraphilias. Identification and resolution of early conflicts, trauma, and humiliation are thought to remove the individual's anxiety toward appropriate partners and enable him or her to give up the paraphilic fantasies. Although psychodynamic psychotherapy has been useful in the treatment of some individuals, there has been disappointment with the results of this therapy as the sole form of treatment in cases of deviant sexual arousal (Crawford 1981).

Some outcome studies of sex offender programs have yielded generally optimistic results regarding recidivism outcome (Freeman-Longo and Knopp 1992; Marshall and Pithers 1994).

Hanson et al. (2002) conducted a meta-analytic review of the effectiveness of psychological treatment for sex offenders. Forty-two studies were reviewed, with a combined sample of 9,316 sex offenders. The results indicated that the sexual reoffense rate was lower for those sex offenders who received treatment (12.3%) than for those in the comparison groups (16.8%). It also indicated that the more contemporary treatment approaches—specifically those that involve cognitive-behavioral or systemic therapy—reported a reduction in sexual recidivism from 17.4% to 9.9%.

More recently Marques et al. (2005) conducted the only large-scale randomly controlled outcome study to date with incarcerated sex offenders. Those in the experimental group underwent a 3-year intensive cognitive-behavioral treatment program within a relapse prevention framework. Follow-up time, on average, was 8 years. Results indicated that those who received the cognitive-behavioral treatment did not differ from untreated volunteer control subjects in their rates of sexual recidivism (22% and 20%, respectively) or in violent recidivism (16.2% and 11.6%, respectively). In discussing the results of this clinical research project, which began 20 years earlier, the authors noted that they would have conducted the study differently now than they had designed it then. They indicated that they would make sure that the treatment intensity and content were tailored to the offenders' risk levels and specifically their treatment needs and responsivity factors. This would include regular monitoring of progress toward treatment goal, an aftercare component that was based on an individualized interdisciplinary case management model including high-risk offenders.

Kirsch and Becker (2006) recently commented on the major discrepancies between the most widely used treatments and the prevailing etiological theories of sexually deviant behavior. They noted that treatment programs to date have only resulted in modest reductions in sexual recidivism for two reasons: flaws in the etiological theory of sex offending upon which the treatment programs are established, and flaws in the theory of treatment delivery with respect to the methods that are being utilized to reduce sexual offending behavior. They noted that empirical literature on risk factors for recidivism has largely been ignored. Risk factor literature indicates that antisocial lifestyle and deviant sexual interests are the largest predictors of sexual recidivism. Thus, within treatment programs, greater attention should be paid to addressing antisocial orientation and antisocial lifestyle. Despite the re-

search findings in that area, treatment programs continue to focus on enhancing psychological adjustment and working with features of clinical presentation while devoting less attention to characteristics associated with general criminal lifestyle.

The majority of work conducted to date is focused on static risk factors, including criminal history, personality traits, and demographic characteristics, as long-term predictors of recidivism. Only recently has the focus been on dynamic risk factors, when, in fact, dynamic risk factors are probably the more appropriate target of treatment, given their amenability to change. Researchers need to determine the mechanisms of change that produce reductions in sexual recidivism. Given the heterogeneity among sex offender populations it is important to identify moderating variables. Treatment should be tailored to specific subtypes of offenders. Much of the treatment is geared toward establishing goals that involve the avoidance of behaviors, and less attention is paid to creating positive goals such as striving toward engaging in prosocial behaviors. Very little research has been directed toward what factors are related to treatment dropout and to motivation for treatment. We conclude that sex offender theory and treatment should be guided by empirical evidence, and targeted research in the field will lead to development of more optimal treatment programs.

Biological and Pharmacological Treatments of Paraphilias

Hormonal Treatments

Biological treatments traditionally have been reserved for individuals with pedophilia, sexual sadism, or exhibitionism, although occasionally individuals with other paraphilias receive treatment with medications (Bradford and Kaye 1999).

Studer et al. (2005) recently demonstrated a clear relationship between serum testosterone and sexual violence, demonstrating that men with higher testosterone tended to have committed the most invasive sexual crimes. They concluded that high testosterone levels were significantly predictive of sexual recidivism in those who did not complete treatment. Thus, there may be cases in which medically lowering of testosterone levels may be helpful in decreasing the risk of recidivism in those with paraphilias (Saleh and Guidry 2003), although one has to keep in mind that even with a lowering of pathological sexual cravings, a mere lowering of testosterone levels does not instill a conscience and sense of moral responsibility in offenders (Berlin 2003).

Hormonal treatments have been attempted for a number of years in the paraphilic population, with the initial treatments focusing on blocking or decreasing the level of circulating androgens. Surgical castration has been used widely in Europe with incarcerated sex offenders. However, some have suggested that surgical castration is not always an effective means of eliminating deviant sexual behavior and that almost one-third of castrated men can still engage in intercourse. Many view surgical castration not only as highly intrusive but also as cruel and unusual punishment. The results from this procedure are variable, unpredictable, and irreversible (Heim 1981; Wille and Beier 1989).

Interestingly, Weinberger et al. (2005) recently reviewed the relationship of surgical castration and sexual recidivism in a sexually violent predator/sexually dangerous person population, concluding that surgically castrated sex offenders had a very low incidence of sexual recidivism. However, they also pointed out that whereas orchiectomy can reduce sexual desire, it does not completely eliminate the ability to obtain an erection in response to sexually stimulating material, and the effects can be reversed by testosterone replacement. Berlin (2005) responded by saying that from a treatment standpoint, if lowering testosterone can provide a decrease in sexual appetite in this population, there seems to be little reason to use surgical castration, because the same effects can be achieved with testosterone-lowering medications.

Antiandrogenic medications have been used throughout the world since the late 1960s to treat sex offenders. As early as the 1940s, estrogens were used to treat sex offenders, but by the 1960s this practice had been discontinued due to serious side effects (Neuman and Kalmus 1991). Next, a progestin derivate, cyproterone acetate, was introduced in Europe and Canada, but it has never been made available in the United States. Medroxyprogesterone acetate is available in the United States, and now gonadotropin-releasing hormone agonists are being used, including leuprolide acetate. Each of these medications works because of its effect on sexual libido by ultimately (albeit by different mechanisms) lowering testosterone levels. For example, medroxyprogesterone acetate appears to act by blocking testosterone synthesis, whereas cyproterone acetate acts primarily by blocking central and peripheral androgen receptors. Both may be given orally or via long-acting intramuscular depot injection (to improve compliance). They do not appear to influence the direction of sexual drive toward appropriate adult partners; rather, they act to decrease libido and thus break the individual's pattern of compulsive deviant sexual behavior. These agents thus work best in those paraphilic persons with a high sexual drive and less well in those with a low sexual drive or an antisocial personality (Cooper 1986). Leuprolide acetate works by stimulating follicle-stimulating hormone and luteinizing hormone secretion initially, and then downregulating luteinizing hormone–releasing hormone receptors on follicle-stimulating hormone– and luteinizing hormone–secreting cells in the pituitary. This, in turn, decreases testosterone production.

Although some clinicians feel that these types of biological interventions are useful in treating sex offenders (Berlin 2005; Bradford 2001; Kafka 1995; Kravitz et al. 1995), there are still relatively few methodological studies with the use of the medications in this population. Some researchers have examined the effect that cyproterone acetate has on sleeping and waking penile erections in pedophiles. Cooper and Cernovovsky (1992) reported that all measures of nocturnal penile tumescence decreased while the patients were taking cyproterone acetate. Results of arousal assessment while patients were awake were somewhat more variable. While the subjects were taking cyproterone acetate, levels of serum testosterone, follicle-stimulating hormone, and luteinizing hormone also decreased, but prolactin levels did not show consistent changes.

A few researchers (Cooper et al. 1992; Hucker et al. 1988) have demonstrated that many sex offenders are reluctant to use this form of treatment, and these medications can be the cause of numerous side effects. Hormonal treatment should not be viewed as a guarantee against recidivism (Briken et al. 2004). These medications never should be used as the only form of treatment; the patient must acknowledge his or her responsibility for his or her sexual behavior and participate in individual or group psychotherapy.

The most significant long-term side effects with use of hormonal treatment are weight gain, increased blood pressure, impaired glucose tolerance, and gallbladder disease (W.J. Meyer et al. 1985). Some clinicians (Reilly et al. 2000) also warn that one should be careful of medical contraindications to the use of hormonal treatments, such as preexisting pituitary disease, liver disease, and thromboembolic disorders. These medications have also been associated with cardiac complications as well as osteoporosis, which also has been seen in surgically castrated individuals. One may want to consider consulting with an endocrinologist and/or internist before and while embarking on this type of treatment.

Treatment protocols often include monitoring of blood pressure, weight, testosterone level, follicle-stimulating hormone, luteinizing hormone, liver function tests, electrolytes, and glucose; bone scans of pelvis and long bones; and a complete blood count at baseline, with the laboratory tests being repeated about every 2–3 months until the patient is stable and then every 6 months thereafter, and the bone scan repeated annually. The patient also should receive a physical examination yearly. Phallometric testing can be done at intervals as determined helpful. One could consider baseline and follow-up electrocardiographic monitoring.

The use of antiandrogenic medications often is referred to as *chemical castration*. Although the legal issues raised concerning surgical castration are similar to those concerning chemical castration, the use of these medications is at least reversible and less invasive. These medications are not approved by the U.S. Food and Drug Administration for the treatment of paraphilias; however, their use has become a standard of care within the field. Their use may be considered with individuals who are not doing well with cognitive-behavioral treatments or who are at high risk of recidivism.

Other Pharmacological Treatments

Another promising focus of research has been on the use of other forms of pharmacological treatment for paraphilias. There have now been a number of case reports and open label studies using the selective serotonin reuptake inhibitors (SSRIs) in treating paraphilias and nonparaphilic sexual disorders (Bradford 1996; Kafka 2000; Saleh 2004). Although sexual libido may decrease as a side effect of an SSRI, one has to keep in mind that there may be multiple reasons as to these agents' possible effectiveness. SSRIs have been approved for such things as major depression, generalized anxiety disorder, panic disorder, and obsessive-compulsive disorder. However, there have been studies to show their benefit in such off-label uses as aggression, self-injurious behavior, and impulsivity. Hollander et al. (1996, 2000) proposed that sexual compulsions may overlap with impulsive disorders and obsessive-compulsive disorders. Is it possible that serotonergic agents may help improve mood, decrease impulsivity, decrease sexual obsessions, and lead to sexual dysfunction (Rothschild 2000), which in combination decreases the chance of recidivism in men with paraphilias?

To our knowledge, there have been no double-blind, placebo-controlled studies to test the efficacy of SSRIs in treating paraphilias. However, case reports and open-label studies go back to as early as 1990, concluding that SSRIs can be helpful in treating paraphilia and related disorders (Greenberg and Bradford 1997), with fluoxetine (Bianchi 1990; Coleman et al. 1992; Emmanuel et al. 1991; Kafka 1991a, 1991b; Kafka and Prentky 1992; Lorefice 1991; Perilstein et al. 1991) and sertraline (Bradford et al. 1995; Greenberg et al. 1996) having been the most studied. Other serotonergic agents such as fluvoxamine and clomipramine have also been studied (Clayton 1993; Greenberg et al. 1996; Zohar et al. 1994), as have nefazodone (Coleman et al. 2000) and even buspirone (Fedoroff 1988).

SSRIs may be useful for treating different types of sexually inappropriate behaviors. For example, fluoxetine has been used successfully in the treatment of patients with voyeurism (Emmanuel et al. 1991), exhibitionism, pedophilia (Bourgeois and Klein 1996), and frottage (Perilstein et al. 1991) and in persons who have committed rape (Kafka 1991b).

Stein et al. (1992) discussed the use of serotonergic medications (e.g., fluoxetine, clomipramine, fluvoxamine, or fenfluramine) in the treatment of sexual obsessions, addictions, and paraphilias. They hypothesized that compulsivity and impulsivity may occur on a neurobiological spectrum on which obsessions and compulsions are at the compulsive end of the spectrum and paraphilias are at the impulsive end. Kafka and Prentky (1992) reported that SSRI treatment was beneficial both for paraphilias and for nonparaphilic sexual addictions, believing that the enhancement of central serotonin neurotransmission by the SSRI may ameliorate symptoms of mood disorder, heightened sexual desire, compulsivity, and impulsivity associated with these disorders. There was suspicion in a case report, however, that an SSRI may have caused sexual obsessions in a previously nonobsessed individual (Balon 1994); this serves as a reminder that individuals treated with these agents should be monitored for outcome. Subjective reports of sexual interest, masturbatory frequency, deviant fantasy, and sexual activity can be monitored. In some cases, periodic phallometric testing could be used, but there is question as to whether such testing actually measures treatment success.

Kafka (2000) summarized data regarding the current knowledge of using SSRIs in the treatment of both paraphilias and paraphilia-related disorders. The SSRIs can be prescribed in the typical antidepressant dosages, although in our experience, higher dosages, as often are necessary in the treatment of obsessions, are sometimes necessary. It is important to realize, however, that more research is needed regarding the use of SSRIs for this purpose because the current knowledge is still based mostly on case reports and open clinical trials. As similarly discussed with hormonal agents in treating paraphilias, SSRIs are not approved in the United States for the treatment of paraphilias and thus are prescribed off-label in treating sexual disorders. Again, the use of SSRIs has become a standard of care in the field and is a less invasive treatment than the use of castration or even hormonal medications, with less potential side effects.

Kafka and Hennen (2000) described an open trial of psychostimulants added to SSRIs when treating paraphilias in men. They concluded that methylphenidate sustained-release can be cautiously and effectively combined with SSRIs in ameliorating paraphilias in some selected cases.

Although neuroleptic medications can reduce sexual drive (Olfson et al. 2005), they have not been found to be successful in treating paraphilias. Additionally, there have been case reports of use with mood stabilizers in treating single cases of paraphilia (Cesnik and Coleman 1989; Goldberg and Buongiorno 1983), but no larger studies have shown their overall effectiveness as of yet.

Because adolescents are estimated to commit as much as 20% of rapes and 50% of child molestations (Hunter 2000), some have proposed using medication treatments in this younger population in more severe cases. The use of SSRIs in the adolescent population is quite limited (Galli et al. 1998) but may be considered with informed consent from the parents or guardian. The use of hormonal agents in the adolescent population is not without controversy, because these agents can suppress androgen levels that affect physiological changes seen in puberty, including growth. It is recommended that if a trial of hormonal agents is deemed necessary in an adolescent, the drugs be prescribed for only short periods of time and only for adolescents whose sexual aggression has not responded to other treatments (Saleh and Grasswick 2005). Finally, naltrexone was used in a small open-ended prospective study (Ryback 2004), with decreased fantasies and masturbation reported in adjudicated adolescent sexual offenders. However, more research is necessary to conclude if this treatment will actually turn out to be helpful in those who struggle with paraphilias.

Paraphilias and Comorbid Psychiatric Diagnoses

In addition to using medication treatments specifically focused on treating paraphilias, psychiatrists also must focus on treating comorbid psychiatric disorders in those with paraphilias (Johnson 2005). In the adult population, studies have identified the relationship between mental illness and violent crime (Marzuk 1996; Monahan and Steadman 1994; Swanson 1993; Volavka 1995), concluding the most common diagnoses seen in the violent adult population include psychotic disorders, depression, bipolar disorder, substance abuse disorders, and antisocial personality disorder. However, these earlier studies did not break down the correlation of comorbid psychiatric illnesses and sexual offense.

Three of the earlier studies that focused on adult male sex offenders reported similar results, showing higher levels of mood disorders, substance abuse disorders, impulse-control disorders, anxiety disorders, and antisocial personality disorder (Kafka and Prentky 1994; McElroy et al. 1999; Raymond et al. 1999). However, these studies were preliminary and conducted with small groups of subjects.

More recent studies have had larger sample sizes. Kafka and Hennen (2000) studied 120 males with paraphilias or paraphilia-related disorders and found the most common Axis I disorders to be mood disorders (71.6%), substance abuse (40.8%), anxiety disorders (38.3%), and attention-deficit/hyperactivity disorder (35.8%).

Langstrom et al. (2004) studied the psychiatric disorders that occur among sex offenders ($N=1,215$) and found that alcohol abuse was the most frequent diagnosis, followed by drug abuse, personality disorder, and psychosis.

Dunsieth et al. (2004) published results of psychiatric features of 113 men convicted of sexual offenses, showing high lifetime rates of substance abuse (85%), paraphilias (74%), mood disorders (58%), impulse-control disorders (38%), and anxiety disorders (23%). They also reported that 9% of their population had an eating disorder, and 56% could be diagnosed with an antisocial personality disorder. The most common mood disorders diagnosed were bipolar disorder and depression. These percentages are much higher than the lifetime prevalence of these disorders seen in the general population (Kessler et al. 2005). Grant (2005) studied male subjects ($N=25$) diagnosed with exhibitionism, of whom 92% had an Axis I disorder (major depression or substance abuse) and 40% had an Axis II disorder. When focusing on adolescent sex offender populations, the most common comorbid psychiatric disorders may actually be substance abuse, conduct disorder, depression, impulse-control disorders, and learning disabilities (Becker et al. 1986, 1991, 1993;

Fehrenbach et al. 1986; Kavoussi et al. 1988; Mathews et al. 1997; W.R. Smith et al. 1987).

Risk Assessment of Sex Offenders

A question that mental health professionals who evaluate or treat individuals with paraphilias that involve victims are often asked to address is whether the individual is at risk to reoffend. This is also important in those states that have sexually violent predators legislation and where individuals may be petitioned for civil commitment. Sixteen states at the present time have relevant statues that allow for the civil commitment of individuals who have committed sexual offenses and remain a risk to society. Although the terminology of the statutes may vary from state to state, in general the commitment criteria involve an individual who has been convicted or adjudicated insane of a sexually violent offense and presently has a mental disorder, paraphilia, personality disorder, or conduct disorder that predisposes the person to commit sexual acts such as to render a person a danger to the health and safety of others.

Historically, individuals have used clinical judgment in determining whether a person poses a risk of either violent or sexually violent behavior. Doren (2002) noted that there are different methods that have been used to conduct risk assessments, including unguided clinical judgment, guided clinical judgment, clinical judgment based on an amnestic approach, research-guided clinical judgment, clinically adjusted actuarial approach, and purely actuarial approach. The field of risk assessment now has available a number of actuarial risk assessment instruments for use. Doren (2002) noted that when selecting what instrument to utilize, the following issues need to be addressed: statistical demonstration of reliability and validity; degree of concordance between what the instrument was designed to measure and the legally defined risk; availability of information required to employ the instrument; and availability of interpretive information. Actuarial assessment instruments include the STATIC-99, the Sex Offender Risk Appraisal Guide, the Violence Risk Appraisal Guide, the Rapid Risk Assessment for Sex Offense Recidivism, and the Minnesota Sex Offender Screening Tool—Revised, among others. When conducting a risk assessment, it is important that the assessment be comprehensive and include a review of official court documents and interview of the offender, use of a risk assessment instrument, and assessment of dynamic risk factors. See Doren (2002) for information regarding risk assessment instruments as well as information on report writing and court testimony.

Recently, Hanson and Morton-Bourgon (2005) conducted a meta-analysis assessing the characteristics of persistent sexual offenders. The meta-analysis consisted of 82 recidivism studies involving 29,450 sexual offenders. Results indicated that, on average, the recidivism rate for sexual offenders was 13.7%, the offenders' violent recidivism rate was 14.3%, and the violent nonsexual recidivism rate was 14.3%. The overall recidivism rate—that is, the commission of any crime—was 36.2%. The average follow-up time for these offenders was between 5 and 6 years. The authors noted that because not all sex offenses are detected, the recidivism figure should be considered an underestimate. Results indicated that the strongest predictors of sexual recidivism were sexual deviancy and antisocial orientation. Although significant advances have been made in risk assessment and treatment of the paraphilias, many questions remain to be answered. Only by rigorous research designs will we ultimately be able to answer some of the questions raised by Kirsch and Becker (2006). By successfully treating those individuals who have paraphilias that involve the victimization of children, adolescents, and adults, we will make our society safer.

Key Points

- Whereas the genetic sex of an individual is determined at conception, gender identity develops during the early years of life.

- Gender identity disorder requires a strong and persistent cross-gender identification and a persistent discomfort with one's sex or sense of inappropriateness in the gender role of that sex.

- The term *transsexualism* was eliminated in DSM-IV and replaced by *gender identity disorder.*

- Approximately 1 in 30,000 adult males and 1 in 100,000 females seek sex reassignment surgery. After surgery, patients report few problems and marked improvement in their sexuality.

- The paraphilias are characterized by experiencing, over a period of at least 6 months, recurrent, intense sexually arousing fantasies, sexual urges, or behaviors, generally involving nonhuman objects or nonconsenting partners.

- The most common paraphilias are exhibitionism, fetishism, frotteurism, pedophilia, sexual masochism, sexual sadism, transvestic fetishism, and voyeurism.

- The numerous other sexually deviant fantasies or behaviors are given the diagnosis of *paraphilia not otherwise specified.*

- A variety of behavioral therapies, hormonal treatments, and psychopharmacological treatments have been used to manage paraphilias.

Suggested Readings

American Psychiatric Association: Position Statement: Committee on Psychotherapy by Psychiatrists (COPP) Position Statement on Therapies Focused on Attempts to Change Sexual Orientation (Reparative or Conversion Therapies). Approved May 2000. Available at: http://www.psych.org/psych_pract/copptherapyaddendum 83100.cfm. Accessed October 15, 2007.

Freeman D: False prediction of future dangerousness: error rates and Psychopathy Checklist—Revised. J Am Acad Psychiatry Law 29:89–95, 2001

Kafka MP: A DSM-IV Axis I comorbidity study of males (n=120) with paraphilias and paraphilia-related disorders. Sex Abuse 14:349–366, 2002

Sreenivasan S, Kirkish P, Garrick T, et al: Actuarial risk assessment models: a review of critical issues related to violence and sex-offender recidivism assessments. J Am Acad Psychiatry Law 28:438–448, 2000

References

a Campo J, Nijiman H, Merckelback H, et al: Psychiatric comorbidity of gender identity disorders: a survey among Dutch psychiatrists. Am J Psychiatry 160:1332–1336, 2003

Abel GG, Becker JV, Cunningham-Rathner J: Complications, consent, and cognitions in sex between children and adults. Int J Law Psychiatry 7:89–103, 1984

Abel GG, Becker JV, Mittelman M, et al: Self-reported sex crimes of nonincarcerated paraphiliacs. J Interpers Violence 2:3–25, 1987

Abel GG, Becker JV, Cunningham-Rathner J, et al: Multiple paraphilic diagnosis among sex offenders. Bull Am Acad Psychiatry Law 16:153–168, 1988

Abel GG, Osborn CA, Twigg DA: Sexual assault through the life span: adult offenders with juvenile histories, in The Juvenile Sex Offender. Edited by Barbaree HE, Marshall WL, Hudson SM. New York, Guilford, 1993, pp 104–117

Abel GG, Huffman J, Warberg BW, et al: Visual reaction time and plethysmography as measures of sexual interest in child molesters. Sex Abuse 10:81–95, 1998

American Psychiatric Association: Diagnostic and Statistical Manual of Mental Disorders, 3rd Edition. Washington, DC, American Psychiatric Association, 1980

American Psychiatric Association: Diagnostic and Statistical Manual of Mental Disorders, 3rd Edition, Revised. Washington, DC, American Psychiatric Association, 1987

American Psychiatric Association: Diagnostic and Statistical Manual of Mental Disorders, 4th Edition. Washington, DC, American Psychiatric Association, 1994

American Psychiatric Association: Diagnostic and Statistical Manual of Mental Disorders, 4th Edition, Text Revision. Washington, DC, American Psychiatric Association, 2000

American Psychiatric Association: Position Statement: Committee on Psychotherapy by Psychiatrists (COPP) Position Statement on Therapies Focused on Attempts to Change Sexual Orientation (Reparative or Conversion Therapies). Approved May 2000. Available at: http://www.psych.org/psych_pract/copptherapyaddendum83100.cfm. Accessed October 15, 2007.

Balon R: Sexual obsessions associated with fluoxetine. J Clin Psychiatry 55:496, 1994

Bancroft J: Homosexual orientation: the search for a biological basis. Br J Psychiatry 164:437–440, 1994

Barbaree HE, Marshall WL: Erectile responses among heterosexual child molesters, father–daughter incest offenders, and matched nonoffenders: five distinct age preference profiles. Canadian Journal of Behavioral Sciences 21:70–82, 1989

Barlow DH, Abel GG, Blanchard EB: Gender identity change in transsexuals: follow-up and replications. Arch Gen Psychiatry 36:1001–1007, 1979

Baumeister RF, Butler JL: Sexual masochism: deviance without pathology, in Sexual Deviance. Edited by Laws DR, O'Donohue W. New York, Guilford, 1997, pp 225–239

Becker JV, Kaplan MS, Cunningham-Rathner J, et al: Characteristics of adolescent incest sexual perpetrators: preliminary findings. J Fam Violence 1:85–97, 1986

Becker JV, Kaplan MS, Tenke CE, et al: The incidence of depressive symptomatology in juvenile sex offenders with a history of abuse. Child Abuse Negl 15:531–536, 1991

Becker JV, Harris CD, Sales BD: Juveniles who commit sexual offenses: a critical review of research, in Sexual Aggression. Edited by Hall RG, Hinschman R, Graham J, et al. Philadelphia, PA, Taylor-Francis, 1993, pp 215–228

Berlin FS: Sex offender treatment and legislation. J Am Acad Psychiatry Law 31:510–513, 2003

Berlin FS: Commentary: the impact of surgical castration on sexual recidivism risk among civilly committed sexual offenders. J Am Acad Psychiatry Law 33:37–41, 2005

Bianchi MD: Fluoxetine treatment of exhibitionism (letter to editor). Am J Psychiatry 147:1089–1090, 1990

Blair CD, Lanyon RI: Exhibitionism: etiology and treatment. Psychol Bull 89:439–463, 1981

Blanchard R: Early history of the concept of autogynephilia. Arch Sex Behav 34:439–446, 2005

Bourgeois JA, Klein M: Risperidone and fluoxetine in the treatment of pedophilia with comorbid dysthymia. J Clin Psychopharmacol 16:257–258, 1996

Bradford J: The role of serotonin in the future of forensic psychiatry. Bull Am Acad Psychiatry Law 24:57–72, 1996

Bradford J: The neurobiology, neuropharmacology, and pharmacological treatment of paraphilias and compulsive sexual behavior. Can J Psychiatry 46:26–34, 2001

Bradford J, Kaye NS: Pharmacological treatment of sexual offenders. Newsl Am Acad Psychiatry Law 24:16–17, 1999

Bradford J, McLean D: Sexual offenders, violence, and testosterone: a clinical study. Can J Psychiatry 29:335–343, 1984

Bradford J, Greenberg DM, Gojer JJ, et al: Sertraline in the treatment of pedophilia: an open labeled study. Paper presented at the annual American Psychiatric Association Congress, Miami, FL, May 1995

Briken P, Hill A, Berner W: A relapse in pedophilic sex offending and subsequent suicide attempt during luteinizing hormone-releasing hormone treatment (letter to editor). J Clin Psychiatry 65:1429, 2004

Byne W, Parsons B: Human sexual orientation: the biological theories reappraised. Arch Gen Psychiatry 50:228–239, 1993

Cesnik JA, Coleman E: Use of lithium carbonate in the treatment of autoerotic asphyxia. Am J Psychother 43:277–285, 1989

Clayton AH: Fetishism and clomipramine. Am J Psychiatry 150:673–674, 1993

Cohen-Kettenis PT: Gender change in 46,XY persons with 5α-reductase-2 deficiency and 17β-hydroxysteroid dehydrogenase-3 deficiency. Arch Sex Behav 34:399–410, 2005

Coleman E, Cesnick J, Moore A, et al: An exploratory study of the role of psychotropic medications in the treatment of sex offenders. Journal of Offender Rehabilitation 18:75–88, 1992

Coleman E, Gratzer T, Nesvacil L, et al: Nefazodone and the treatment of nonparaphilic compulsive sexual behavior: a retrospective study. J Clin Psychiatry 61:282–284, 2000

Collaer ML, Hines M: Human behavioral sex differences: a role for gonadal hormones during early development? Psychol Bull 118:55–107, 1995

Cooper AJ: Progestogens in the treatment of male sex offenders: a review. Can J Psychiatry 31:73–79, 1986

Cooper AJ, Cernovovsky Z: The effects of cyproterone acetate on sleeping and waking penile erections in pedophiles: possible implications for treatment. Can J Psychiatry 37:33–39, 1992

Cooper AJ, Sandhu S, Losztyn S, et al: A double blind placebo controlled trial of medroxyprogesterone acetate and cyproterone acetate with seven pedophiles. Can J Psychiatry 37:687–693, 1992

Crawford D: Treatment approaches with pedophiles, in Adult Sexual Interest in Children. Edited by Cook M, Howells K. New York, Academic Press, 1981, pp 181–217

DeCuypere G, T-Sjoen G, Beerten R, et al: Sexual and physical health after sex reassignment surgery. Arch Sex Behav 34:679–690, 2005

Diamond M: A critical evaluation of the ontogeny of human sexual behavior. Q Rev Biol 40:147–175, 1965

Doren DM: Evaluating Sex Offenders: A Manual for Civil Commitment and Beyond. Thousand Oaks, CA, Sage, 2002

Dougher MJ: Clinical assessment of sex offenders, in The Sex Offender, Vol 1: Corrections, Treatment and Legal Practice. Edited by Schwartz BK, Cellini HR. Kingston, NJ, Civic Research Institute, 1995, pp 11.1–11.13

Dunsieth NW, Nelson EB, Brusman-Lovins LA, et al: Psychiatric and legal features of 113 men convicted of sexual offenses. J Clin Psychiatry 65:293–300, 2004

Ehrhardt AA, Meyer-Bahlburg HFL: Effects of prenatal sex hormones on gender-related behavior. Science 211:1312–1318, 1981

Emmanuel NP, Lydiard RB, Ballenger JC: Fluoxetine treatment of voyeurism (letter). Am J Psychiatry 148:950, 1991

Fallen KC: Characteristics of a clinical sample of sexually abused children: how boy and girl victims differ. Child Abuse Negl 13:281–291, 1989

Fedoroff JP: Buspirone hydrochloride in the treatment of transvestic fetishism. J Clin Psychiatry 49:408–409, 1988

Fehrenbach PA, Smith W, Monastersky C, et al: Adolescent sexual offenders: offender and offense characteristics. Am J Orthopsychiatry 56:225–233, 1986

Finkelhor D: Child Abuse: New Theory and Research. New York, Free Press, 1984

Finkelhor D: Source Book on Child Sex Abuse. Beverly Hills, CA, Sage, 1986

Freeman-Longo RE, Knopp FH: State-of-the-art sex offender treatment: outcome and issues. Annals of Sex Research 5:141–160, 1992

Freund K, Blanchard R: Phallometric diagnosis of pedophilia. J Consult Clin Psychol 57:100–105, 1989

Freund K, Watson R, Rienzo D: Signs of feigning in the phallometric test. Behav Res Ther 26:105–112, 1988

Freund K, Seto MC, Kuban M: Frotteurism and the theory of courtship disorder, in Sexual Deviance. Edited by Laws DR, O'Donohue W. New York, Guilford, 1997, pp 111–130

Fridell SR, Zucker KJ, Bradley SJ, et al: Physical attractiveness of girls with gender identity disorder. Arch Sex Behav 25:17–31, 1996

Galli VB, Raute NJ, McConville BJ, et al: An adolescent male with multiple paraphilias successfully treated with fluoxetine. J Child Adolesc Psychopharmacol 8:195–197, 1998

Gebhard PH, Gagnon JH, Pomeroy WB, et al: Sex Offenders. New York, Harper & Row, 1965

Gittleson NL, Eacott SE, Mehta BM: Victims if indecent exposure. Br J Psychiatry 132:61–66, 1978

Goldberg RL, Buongiorno PA: The use of carbamazepine for the treatment of paraphilias in a brain damaged patient. Intl J Psychiatry Med 12:275–279, 1983

Grant JE: Clinical characteristics and psychiatric comorbidity in males with exhibitionism. J Clin Psychiatry 66:1367–1371, 2005

Green R: Sexual Identity Conflict in Children and Adults. New York, Basic Books, 1974

Green R: Gender identity in childhood and later sexual orientation: follow-up of 78 males. Am J Psychiatry 142:339–341, 1985

Green R: The Sissy Boys Syndrome and the Development of Homosexuality. New Haven, CT, Yale University Press, 1987

Green R, Fleming DT: Transsexual surgery follow-up: status in the 1990s, in Annual Review of Sex Research, Vol 1. Edited by Bancroft J, Davis CM, Weinstein D. Lake Mills, IA, Society for the Scientific Study of Sex, 1990, pp 163–174

Greenberg DM, Bradford JM: Treatment of the paraphilic disorders: a review of the role of the selective serotonin reuptake inhibitors. Sex Abuse 9:349–360, 1997

Greenberg DM, Bradford JM, Curry S, et al: A comparison of treatment of paraphilias with tree serotonin reuptake inhibitors: a retrospective study. Bull Am Acad Psychiatry Law 24:525–532, 1996

Hall G, Hirschman R: Sexual aggression against children: a conceptual perspective of etiology. Crim Justice Behav 19:8–23, 1992

Hanson RK, Morton-Bourgon K: The characteristics of persistent sexual offenders: a meta-analysis of recidivism studies. J Consult Clin Psychol 73:1154–1163, 2005

Hanson RK, Gordon A, Harris AJR, et al: First report of the collaborative outcome data project on the effectiveness of psychological treatment for sex offenders. Sex Abuse 14:169–197, 2002

Heim N: Sexual behavior of castrated sex offenders. Arch Sex Behav 10:11–19, 1981

Hoenig J: Etiology of transsexualism, in Gender Dysphoria: Development, Research, Management. Edited by Steiner BW. New York, Plenum, 1985, pp 33–73

Hollander E, Kwon JH, Stein DJ, et al: Obsessive-compulsive and spectrum disorders: overview and quality of life issues. J Clin Psychiatry 57 (suppl):3–6, 1996

Hollander E, Twersky R, Bienstock C: The obsessive compulsive spectrum: a survey of 800 practitioners. CNS Spectr 5:61–63, 2000

Hucker SJ: Sexual sadism, in Sexual Deviance. Edited by Laws DR, O'Donohue W. New York, Guilford, 1997, pp 194–209

Hucker SJ, Langevin R, Bain J: A double-blind trial of sex-drive reducing medication in pedophiles. Annals of Sex Research 1:227–247, 1988

Hunter JA: Understanding Juvenile Sex Offending: Research Findings and Guidelines for Effective Treatment (Juvenile Justice Fact Sheet). Charlottesville, Institute of Law, Psychiatry, and Public Policy, University of Virginia, 2000

Johnson B: Comorbid diagnosis of sexually abusive youth, in Current Perspectives: Working With Sexually Aggressive Youth and Youth with Sexual Behavior Problems. Edited by Longo R, Prescott D. Holyoke, MA, NEARI Press, 2005, pp 167–192

Kafka MP: Successful antidepressant treatment of non-paraphilic sexual addictions and paraphilias in men. J Clin Psychiatry 52:60–65, 1991a

Kafka MP: Successful treatment of paraphilic coercive disorder (a rapist) with fluoxetine hydrochloride. Br J Psychiatry 158:844–847, 1991b

Kafka MP: Current concepts in the drug treatment of paraphilias and paraphilia-related disorders. CNS Drugs 3:9–21, 1995

Kafka MP: Psychopharmacological treatments for non-paraphilic compulsive sexual behaviors. CNS Spectr 5:49–59, 2000

Kafka MP, Hennen J: Psychostimulant augmentation during treatment with selective serotonin reuptake inhibitors in men with paraphilias and paraphilia-related disorders: a case series. J Clin Psychiatry 61:664–670, 2000

Kafka MP, Prentky R: Fluoxetine treatment of nonparaphilic sexual addictions and paraphilias in men. J Clin Psychiatry 53:351–358, 1992

Kafka MP, Prentky R: Preliminary observations of DSM-III-R Axis I comorbidity in men with paraphilias and paraphilia-related disorders. J Clin Psychiatry 55:481–487, 1994

Kavoussi RJ, Kaplan M, Becker JV: Psychiatric diagnoses in adolescent sex offenders. J Am Acad Child Adolesc Psychiatry 27:241–243, 1988

Kessler RC, Berglund P, Demler O, et al: Lifetime prevalence and age-of-onset distributions of DSM-IV disorders in the national comorbidity survey replication. Arch Gen Psychiatry 62:593–602, 2005

Kirsch L, Becker JV: Sexual offending: theory of problem, theory of change, and implication for treatment effectiveness. Aggress Behav 11:208–224, 2006

Kravitz HW, Haywood TW, Kelly J, et al: Medroxyprogesterone treatment for paraphiliacs. Bull Am Acad Psychiatry Law 23:19–33, 1995

Krueger RB, Bradford JW, Glancy GD: Report from the Committee on Sex Offenders: the Abel Assessment for Sexual Interest—a brief description. J Am Acad Psychiatry Law 26:277–280, 1998

Langstrom N, Sjostedt G, Grann M: Psychiatric disorders and recidivism in sexual offenders. Sex Abuse 16:139–150, 2004

Lorefice LS: Fluoxetine treatment of a fetish (letter to the editor). J Clin Psychiatry 52:41, 1991

Lothstein L: The postsurgical transsexual: empirical and theoretical considerations. Arch Sex Behav 9:547–564, 1980

MacDonald JM: Indecent Exposure. Springfield, IL, Charles C. Thomas, 1973

Marques JK, Wiederanders M, Day DM, et al: Effects of a relapse prevention program on sexual recidivism: final results from California's sex offender treatment and evaluation project (SOTEP). Sex Abuse 17:79–107, 2005

Marshall WL, Barbaree HE: The reduction of deviant arousal: satiation treatment for sexual aggressors. Crim Justice Behav 5:294–303, 1978

Marshall WL, Barbaree HE: An integrated theory of the etiology of sexual offending, in Handbook of Sexual Assault: Issues, Theories and Treatment of the Offender. Edited by Marshall WL, Laws DR, Barbaree HE. New York, Plenum, 1990, pp 257–275

Marshall WL, Pithers W: A reconsideration of treatment outcome with sex offenders. Crim Justice Behav 21:6–27, 1994

Marshall WL, Jones R, Ward T, et al: Treatment outcome with sex offenders. Clin Psychol Rev 11:465–485, 1991

Marshall WL, Champagne F, Sturgeon C, et al: Increasing the self-esteem of child molesters. Sex Abuse 9:321–333, 1997

Marzuk PM: Violence, crime, and mental illness: how strong a link? Arch Gen Psychiatry 53:481–486, 1996

Mason FL: Fetishism: psychopathology and theory, in Sexual Deviance. Edited by Laws DR, O'Donohue W. New York, Guilford, 1997, pp 75–91

Mathews R, Hunter JA, Vuz J: Juvenile female sexual offenders: clinical characteristics and treatment issues. Sex Abuse 9:187–199, 1997

McElroy S, Soutullo CA, Taylor P, et al: Psychiatric features of 36 men convicted of sexual offenses. J Clin Psychiatry 60:414–420, 1999

Meyer JK: The theory of gender identity disorders. J Am Psychoanal Assoc 30:381–418, 1982

Meyer M, Bockting WO, Cohen-Kettenis P, et al: The Harry Benjamin International Gender Dysphoria Association's Standards of Care for Gender Identity Disorders, 6th Version. Minneapolis, MN, Harry Benjamin International Gender Dysphoria Association, 2001. Available at: http://www.symposion.com/ijt/soc_2001/index.htm. Accessed October 15, 2007.

Meyer WJ, Walker PA, Emory LE, et al: Physical, metabolic, and hormonal effects on men of long-term therapy with medroxyprogesterone acetate. Fertil Steril 43:102–109, 1985

Monahan J, Steadman HJ (eds): Violence and Mental Disorder: Developments in Risk Assessment. Chicago, IL, University of Chicago Press, 1994

Money J, Ehrhardt AA: Man and Woman, Boy and Girl: The Differentiation and Dimorphism of Gender Identity From Conception to Maturity. Baltimore, MD, Johns Hopkins University Press, 1974

Monto M, Zgourides G, Harris R: Empathy, self-esteem, and the adolescent sexual offender. Sex Abuse 10:127–140, 1998

Murphy WD: Exhibitionism: psychopathology and theory, in Sexual Deviance. Edited by Laws DR, O'Donohue W. New York, Guilford, 1997, pp 22–39

Neuman F, Kalmus J: Hormonal treatment of sexual deviations. Arch Gen Psychiatry 57:1012–1032, 1991

Olfson M, Uttaro T, Carson WH, et al: Male sexual dysfunction and quality of life in schizophrenia. J Clin Psychiatry 66:331–338, 2005

Perilstein RD, Lipper S, Friedman LJ: Three cases of paraphilias responsive to fluoxetine treatment. J Clin Psychiatry 52:169–170, 1991

Person E, Ovesey L: The transsexual syndrome in males, II: secondary transsexualism. Am J Psychother 28:174–193, 1974

Raymond NC, Coleman E, Ohlerking F, et al: Psychiatric comorbidity in pedophilic sex offenders. Am J Psychiatry 156:786–788, 1999

Reilly D, Delva N, Hudson R: Protocols for the use of cyproterone, medroxyprogesterone, and leuprolide in the treatment of paraphilia. Can J Psychiatry 45:559–563, 2000

Risin LI, Koss MP: The sexual abuse of boys: childhood victimizations reported by a national survey, in Rape and Sexual Assault II. Edited by Burgess AW. New York, Garland, 1988, pp 91–104

Rothschild AJ: Sexual side effects of antidepressants. J Clin Psychiatry 61 (suppl):28–36, 2000

Ryback RS: Naltrexone in the treatment of adolescent sexual offenders. J Clin Psychiatry 65:982–986, 2004

Saleh FM: Serotonin reuptake inhibitors and the paraphilias. Newsl Am Acad Psychiatry Law 29:12–13, 2004

Saleh FM, Grasswick LJ: Juvenile Sexual Offenders. Newsl Am Acad Psychiatry Law 30:12–13, 2005

Saleh FM, Guidry LL: Psychosocial and biological treatment considerations for the paraphilic and nonparaphilic sex offender. J Am Acad Psychiatry Law 31:486–493, 2003

Smith WR, Monastersky D, Deisher RM: MMPI-based personality types among juvenile sexual offenders. J Clin Psychol 43:422–430, 1987

Smith Y, Ban Goozen S, Cohen-Kettenis PT: Adolescents with gender identity disorder who were accepted or rejected for sex reassignment surgery: a prospective follow-up study. J Am Acad Child Adolesc Psychiatry 40:472–481, 2001

Smith Y, van Goozen SH, Kupier AJ, et al: Transsexual sub types: clinical and theoretical significance. Psychiatry Res 137:151–160, 2005

Stein DJ, Hollander E, Anthony DT, et al: Serotonergic medications for sexual obsessions, sexual addictions and paraphilias. J Clin Psychiatry 53:267–271, 1992

Stoller RJ: Sex and Gender, Vol 1: The Development of Masculinity and Femininity. New York, Science House, 1968

Stoller RJ: Perversion: The Erotic Form of Hatred. New York, Pantheon, 1975a

Stoller RJ: Sex and Gender, Vol 2: The Transsexual Experiment. London, England, Hogarth, 1975b

Stoller RJ: Fathers of transsexual children. J Am Psychoanal Assoc 27:837–866, 1979

Studer LH, Aylwin AS, Reddon JR: Testosterone, sexual offense recidivism, and treatment effect among adult male sex offenders. Sex Abuse 17:171–181, 2005

Swanson JW: Alcohol abuse, mental disorder, and violent behavior: an epidemiologic inquiry. Alcohol Health Res World 17:123–132, 1993

Volavka J: Neurobiology of Violence. Washington, DC, American Psychiatric Press, 1995

Ward T, Beech A: An integrated theory of sexual offending. Aggression and Violent Behavior 11:44–63, 2006

Ward T, Siegert RJ: Toward a comprehensive theory on child sexual abuse: a theory knitting perspective. Psychology, Crime and Law 9:319–351, 2002

Weinberger LE, Sreenivasan S, Garrick T, et al: The impact of surgical castration on sexual recidivism risk among sexually violent predatory offenders. J Am Acad Psychiatry Law 33:16–36, 2005

Wille R, Beier K: Castration in Germany. Annals of Sex Research 2:103–133, 1989

Zohar J, Kaplan Z, Benjamin J: Compulsive exhibitionism successfully treated with fluvoxamine: a controlled case study. J Clin Psychiatry 55:86–88, 1994

Zucker KJ: Measurement of psychosexual differentiation. Arch Sex Behav 34:375–388, 2005

Zucker KJ, Bradley SJ: Gender Identity Disorder and Psychosexual Problems in Children and Adolescents. New York, Guilford, 1995

Zucker KJ, Green R: Gender identity and psychosexual disorders, in Textbook of Child and Adolescent Psychiatry, 2nd Edition. Edited by Wiener JM. Washington, DC, American Psychiatric Press, 1997, pp 657–676

Zucker KJ, Bradley SJ, Lowry Sullivan CB, et al: A gender identity interview for children. J Pers Assess 61:443–456, 1993

Zucker KJ, Bradley SJ, Sanikhani M: Sex differences in referral rates of children with gender identity disorder: some hypotheses. J Abnorm Child Psychol 25:217–227, 1997

18

ADJUSTMENT DISORDERS

James J. Strain, M.D.
Kimberly G. Klipstein, M.D.
Jeffrey H. Newcorn, M.D.

In the gray area of diagnosis that lies between normal behavior, problem-level issues, and major disorders reside the *subthreshold* disorders, which are often poorly defined, overlap with other diagnostic groupings, have indefinite symptomatology, and consequently present confounds for reliability and validity. DSM-IV-TR (American Psychiatric Association 2000, pp. xxx–xxi) describes these boundary categories within another conceptual framework:

> A compelling literature documents that there is much "physical" in "mental" disorders and much "mental" in "physical" disorders.... [N]o definition adequately specifies precise boundaries for the concept of "mental disorder." The concept...lacks a consistent operational definition that covers all situations. Whatever its original cause,...[a mental disorder] must currently be considered a manifestation of a behavioral, psychological, or biological dysfunction in the individual.

The issue of defining boundaries is especially problematic in the subthreshold diagnoses (e.g., the adjustment disorders), for which there are no symptom checklists, algorithms, or guidelines for the "quantification of attributes." No symptom inventory or checklist has been constructed or easily emanates from the DSM-IV-TR diagnostic criteria (Table 18–1). The diagnosis is derived from matching the patient's emotions, feelings, behaviors, and life circumstances to a conceptual framework.

Adjustment disorder—a subthreshold diagnosis—has undergone a major evolution since DSM-I, in which it was considered a "transient situational personality disorder" (American Psychiatric Association 1952) (Table 18–2).

According to DSM-IV (American Psychiatric Association 1994), "[t]he essential feature of an adjustment disorder is the development of clinically significant emotional or behavioral symptoms in response to an identifiable psychosocial stressor or stressors" (p. 623). Less phenomenological and more etiological in nature, this definition differs from most Axis I disorders in DSM-IV in that it was to remain atheoretical. In the recent DSM-IV Text Revision (DSM-IV-TR; American Psychiatric Association 2000), the term *psychosocial stressor* was changed to the broader concept of *stressor*. Emotional reactions to physical stress, such as the Chernobyl reactor incident (Havenaar et al. 1996) or cardiac surgery (Oxman et al. 1994), are well

This work was funded by The Malcolm Gibbs Foundation, Inc., New York, New York.

TABLE 18–1. DSM-IV-TR diagnostic criteria for adjustment disorders

A. The development of emotional or behavioral symptoms in response to an identifiable stressor(s) occurring within 3 months of the onset of the stressor(s).

B. These symptoms or behaviors are clinically significant as evidenced by either of the following:

   (1) marked distress that is in excess of what would be expected from exposure to the stressor

   (2) significant impairment in social or occupational (academic) functioning

C. The stress-related disturbance does not meet the criteria for another specific Axis I disorder and is not merely an exacerbation of a preexisting Axis I or Axis II disorder.

D. The symptoms do not represent bereavement.

E. Once the stressor (or its consequences) has terminated, the symptoms do not persist for more than an additional 6 months.

Specify if:

   Acute: if the disturbance lasts less than 6 months

   Chronic: if the disturbance lasts for 6 months or longer

Adjustment disorders are coded based on the subtype, which is selected according to the predominant symptoms. The specific stressor(s) can be specified on Axis IV.

309.0	**With depressed mood**
309.24	**With anxiety**
309.28	**With mixed anxiety and depressed mood**
309.3	**With disturbance of conduct**
309.4	**With mixed disturbance of emotions and conduct**
309.9	**Unspecified**

documented in the literature and suggest that a psychosocial stressor as a criterion is too restrictive.

Critics of the adjustment disorder diagnosis present a threefold argument. They state that the symptom complex is too subjective or "depends structurally on clinical judgment" as opposed to sound, operational criteria (Casey et al. 2001). Second, the idea of a "clinically significant" emotional reaction to a particular stressor is also fraught with subjectivity. Powell and McCone (2004) made this point in their case report of the treatment of a patient with adjustment disorder secondary to the September 11th terrorist attacks. Because there has never before been a large-scale terrorist attack in America, how are clinicians to know what a "normal" response to such an event would be? Finally, the concept of the "stressor" lacks quantifiable and qualifiable guidelines, thus contributing to the vague and nonspecific nature of the adjustment disorder diagnosis.

The lack of specificity in the diagnosis of adjustment disorders may alternatively be considered an advantage. It allows clinicians to "tag" early or temporary mental states when the clinical picture is vague and indistinct but the morbidity is more than expected in a normal reaction. This clinical picture may be the earliest sign of an evolving major mental disorder. Therefore, the adjustment disorders occupy an essential place in the psychiatric taxonomic spectrum. The diagnoses range from normal to problem-level diagnoses (V codes in DSM-III-R [American Psychiatric Association 1987] and DSM-IV), adjustment disorders, minor disorders, those "not otherwise specified," and finally to major mental disorders. As such, adjustment disorders would "outrank" problem-level disorders but be "outranked" by a specific diagnosis, even if it was in the minor or not-otherwise-specified category (Strain et al. 1998a). The adjustment disorder category has also been described as having "clinical appeal" to both doctors and patients. The idea of temporary emotional symptoms resulting directly from a stressful life event seems more of a normal human reaction than a pathological psychiatric state and thus is less stigmatizing. Additionally, the disorder's more benign course (especially in adults) allows a clinician to be more prognostically optimistic. This optimism is shared by medical insurance carriers, who do not consider the diagnosis to be a preexisting condition when evaluating patients' risks. Although this more *laissez-faire* application of the diagnosis could be detrimental to the purity of the diagnostic category, a too-rigid application of DSM-IV-TR criteria would equally undermine the diagnosis of adjustment disorder (Casey 2001).

DSM-IV-TR updated the "Associated Features and Disorders" section to clarify comorbidity with other disorders. For example, adjustment disorders are associated with suicide attempts, suicide, excessive substance use, and somatic complaints. Adjustment disorder has been reported in individuals with preexisting mental disorders in selected samples, such as children

TABLE 18–2. Diagnostic categories of adjustment disorder

DSM-I (1952): Transient situational personality disorder

Gross stress reaction

Adult situational reaction

Adjustment reaction of infancy

Adjustment reaction of childhood

Adjustment reaction of adolescence

Adjustment reaction of late life

Other transient situational personality disturbance

DSM-II (1968): Transient situational disturbance

Adjustment reaction of infancy

Adjustment reaction of childhood

Adjustment reaction of adolescence

Adjustment reaction of adult life

Adjustment reaction of late life

DSM-III (1980): Adjustment disorder

Adjustment disorder with depressed mood

Adjustment disorder with anxious mood

Adjustment disorder with mixed emotional features

Adjustment disorder with disturbance of conduct

Adjustment disorder with mixed disturbance of emotions and conduct

Adjustment disorder with work (or academic) inhibition

Adjustment disorder with withdrawal

Adjustment disorder with atypical features

DSM-III-R (1987): Adjustment disorder

Adjustment disorder with depressed mood

Adjustment disorder with anxious mood

Adjustment disorder with mixed emotional features

Adjustment disorder with disturbance of conduct

Adjustment disorder with mixed disturbance of emotions and conduct

Adjustment disorder with work (or academic) inhibition

Adjustment disorder with withdrawal

Adjustment disorder with physical complaints

Adjustment disorder not otherwise specified

TABLE 18–2. Diagnostic categories of adjustment disorder *(continued)*

DSM-IV (1994) and DSM-IV-TR (2000): Adjustment disorder

Adjustment disorder with depressed mood

Adjustment disorder with anxiety

Adjustment disorder with mixed anxiety and depressed mood

Adjustment disorder with disturbance of conduct

Adjustment disorder with mixed disturbance of emotions and conduct

Adjustment disorder unspecified

and adolescents and in general medical and surgical patients. The presence of an adjustment disorder may complicate the course of illness in individuals who have a general medical condition (e.g., decreased compliance with the recommended medical regimen or increased length of hospital stay).

With regard to specific culture, age, and gender issues, it is necessary to take these attributes into account when making the clinical judgment of whether the individual's response to the stressor is maladaptive or in excess of that which normally would be expected. For example, women are given the diagnosis of adjustment disorder twice as often as men. In children and adolescents, however, the gender assignment of adjustment disorder is equivalent.

In DSM-IV-TR, the section on "Prevalence" has been altered to include rates in children, adolescents, and the elderly (2%–8% in community samples). Adjustment disorder "has been diagnosed in up to 12% of general hospital inpatients who are referred for a mental health consultation, in 10%–30% of those in mental health outpatient settings, and in as many as 50% in special populations that have experienced a specific stressor (e.g., following cardiac surgery)" (American Psychiatric Association 2000, p. 681). Those populations with increased stressors (e.g., indigent patients, medically ill patients) are at higher risk for adjustment disorder.

In the "Course" section, information about progression to other disorders has been added. Adjustment disorder may progress to more severe mental disorders in children and adolescents more frequently than in adults (Andreasen and Hoenk 1982). However, this increased risk may be secondary to the co-occurrence of other mental disorders or the fact that the subthreshold presentation was an early phase of a more pernicious illness.

Regarding other diagnoses, the adjustment disorder diagnosis can be used with another Axis I diagnosis if the symptoms of that diagnosis meet criteria for a major diagnosis (e.g., major depressive disorder), even if a stressor had precipitated that major depressive disorder. The not-otherwise-specified disorders do not require a stressor. If the symptoms extant are secondary to the direct physiological effects of a general medical condition and/or its treatment, adjustment disorder should not be diagnosed. Additionally, demoralization has been suggested as another V-code category and should be distinguished from adjustment disorder and other pathological conditions (Slavney 1999). Adjustment disorder is a stress-related phenomenon in which the stressor has precipitated maladaptation and symptoms (within 3 months of the occurrence of the stressor) that are time limited until the stressor is removed or a new state of adaptation has occurred (see Table 18–1). Other acute stress disorders were described as possible diagnoses during the development of DSM-IV, for example, those stress reactions that follow a disaster or cataclysmic personal event (e.g., acute stress disorder) (Spiegel 1994).

In summary, every aspect of the diagnostic construct for the adjustment disorders constitutes a conundrum for assessment and measurement: the stressor, the maladaptive reaction to the stressor, and the time and relationship between the stressor and the psychological response. None of these three components is operationalized behaviorally to complement a diagnostic decision tree. The adjustment disorders are further characterized by heterogeneous modifiers that describe mood, behavior, emotions, or a mixture of all three. Once again, there is no guideline for assessing whether the mood, behavior, or emotion is sufficient to warrant its descriptive use. This lack of specificity obviously compromises validity and reliability. Ironically, however, it is this uncertainty regarding diagnosis that makes this genre of diagnosis so important (R.L. Spitzer, personal communication, April 1991). It permits observations of patients and interventions by psychiatrists to be catalogued within the psychiatric taxonomy for medical record keeping and billing purposes that otherwise could not be appropriately coded with the psychiatric lexicon, that is, DSM-IV-TR. The etiological and dynamic attributes of adjustment disorder make it an intriguing diagnostic category that constitutes a "linchpin" on the border between normality, problems of living, and pathology. Spitzer has used the term "wild card" for the adjustment disorders because it permits a diagnosis and psychiatric intervention for a condition that may be subthreshold

or a *form fruste* of pathology to come (R.L. Spitzer, personal communication, April 1992).

Definition and History

Wise (1988) summarized the historical evolution of the adjustment disorders since 1945. Early on, the diagnostic concept included the notion of a transient situational disturbance, initially codified by developmental epochs (see Table 18–2). It evolved to embody a disorder of adjustment characterized by mood, behavior, or work (or academic) inhibition (DSM-III; American Psychiatric Association 1980). Finally, it was defined to include physical complaints as well as other mood and behavioral disturbances (DSM-III-R).

With the opportunity to develop yet another evolutionary step—the DSM-IV initiative—the subthreshold diagnostic category of adjustment disorder was reexamined. From a review of the literature, reanalysis of existing data sets, and observations of the other pertinent diagnoses (e.g., minor depression, posttraumatic stress disorder, minor anxiety), modifications for DSM-IV and their rationale were formulated based on empirical evidence.

As a result of the review of the literature and the Western Psychiatric Institute and Clinic data reanalysis supported by a MacArthur grant, the American Psychiatric Association Task Force on Psychological System Interface Disorders recommended that specific changes be included in DSM-IV and now DSM-IV-TR:

1. Enhance the clarity of the language.
2. Describe the time of the reaction to reflect duration: acute (less than 6 months) or chronic (6 months or longer).
3. Allow for the continuation of the stressor for an indefinite period.
4. Eliminate the subtypes of mixed emotional features, work (or academic) inhibition, withdrawal, and physical complaints. (These subtypes were rarely being employed.)

Although it might be argued that the adjustment disorders could be placed in an innovative category of "stress response syndromes" or, for that matter, in several diverse locations within the DSM classification (Strain et al. 1993), the literature does not offer data to support such an alternative placement. In the extreme, adjustment disorder could be eliminated altogether, with the advantage of maintaining the atheoretical approach of DSM-III-R, DSM-IV, and DSM-IV-TR. This solution, however, did not seem beneficial in view of findings that show that adjustment disorder is a valid diagnosis (Jones et al. 1999; Kovacs et al. 1994).

The criterion and predictive validity of the diagnosis of adjustment disorder in 92 children who had new-onset type 1 diabetes mellitus were examined by Kovacs et al. (1995). DSM-III criteria plus four clinically significant signs or symptoms were used, and the time frame was extended to 6 months after the diagnosis of diabetes. Thirty-three percent of the cohort developed adjustment disorder (mean, 29 days after the medical diagnosis), and the average episode length was 3 months, with a recovery rate of 100%. The 5-year cumulative probability of a new psychiatric disorder was 0.48 in comparison with 0.16 for the non–adjustment disorder subjects. The findings support the criterion validity of the adjustment disorder diagnosis.

Construct validity also was observed in a retrospective data study comparing outpatients with single-episode major depression, recurrent major depression, dysthymia, depression not otherwise specified, and adjustment disorder with depressed mood with or without mixed anxiety (Jones et al. 1999). The Medical Outcomes Study 36-item Short Form Health Status Survey (SF-36) was completed before and 6 months after treatment. Multivariate analysis of variance, multivariate analysis of covariance, and χ^2 test were used to clarify the relations among diagnosis, sociodemographic data, and Physical Component Summary and Mental Component Summary scores on the SF-36. The diagnostic categories were significantly different at baseline but did not differ with regard to outcome at follow-up. Females were significantly more likely to be given the diagnosis of major depression or dysthymia than adjustment disorder. Females also were more likely than males to score lower on the Mental Component Summary scale at admission. Patients with adjustment disorder scored higher on all SF-36 scales, as did the other diagnostic groups at baseline and again at follow-up. No significant difference was seen among diagnostic groups with regard to treatment outcome. The authors concluded that the results support the construct validity of the adjustment disorder diagnostic category (Jones et al. 1999).

In reviewing the diagnosis of adjustment disorder for DSM-IV, two issues emerged as fundamental. First, the effect of the imprecision of this diagnosis on reliability and validity because of the lack of behavioral or operational criteria must be determined. One study (Aoki et al. 1995) found three psychological tests— Zung's Self-Rating Anxiety Scale (Zung 1971), Zung's Self-Rating Depression Scale (Zung 1965), and Profile of Mood States (McNair et al. 1971)—to be useful tools for the diagnosis of adjustment disorder among physical rehabilitation patients. Although Aoki et al. (1995) succeeded in reliably differentiating patients with adjustment disorder from healthy patients, they did not distinguish them from patients with major depression or posttraumatic stress disorder.

Second, the classification of syndromes that do not fulfill the criteria for a major mental illness but indicate serious (or incipient) symptomatology that requires intervention and/or treatment, by default, may be viewed as "subthreshold" and afforded a subthreshold interest by health care workers and third-party payers. Thus, the construct of adjustment disorder is designed as a means for classifying psychiatric conditions having a symptom profile that is as yet insufficient to meet the more specifically operationalized criteria for the major syndromes but that is 1) clinically significant and deemed to be in excess of a normal reaction to the stressor in question (taking culture into account), 2) associated with impaired vocational or interpersonal functioning, and 3) not solely the result of a psychosocial problem (V code) requiring medical attention (e.g., noncompliance, phase-of-life problem).

Attention to minor mental symptoms (and psychiatric morbidity) may forestall their evolution to more serious disorders and allow remediation before relationships, work, and functioning have been so impaired that they are disrupted or permanently sundered. In the gray area of early diagnosis, enormous salutary effects with modest therapeutic investment may occur. In the era of early diagnosis, guidelines are the most tenuous. It is the professionals at the "front door"—those involved in primary care, triage, and emergency department treatment—who must be assisted to make this most difficult call: Is there sufficient psychiatric morbidity to warrant mental health assessment and/or intervention? (See Table 18–3.)

With the lack of specificity that characterizes the adjustment disorder diagnoses, however, it is often difficult to truly distinguish them from other psychiatric syndromes. Spalletta et al. (1996) observed that assessment of suicidal behavior is an important tool in differentiating major depression, dysthymia, and adjustment disorder. Furthermore, patients with adjustment disorder were observed to be among the most common recipients of a deliberate self-harm diagnosis, with the majority involving self-poisoning (Vlachos et al. 1994). Thus, deliberate self-harm is more common in these patients (Vlachos et al. 1994), whereas the percentage of suicidal behavior was found to be higher in depressed patients (Spalletta et al. 1996). In a more

TABLE 18-3. Symptom comparisons among subtypes of adjustment disorder (AD) in 2,224 adult (ages 19–64 years) psychiatric patients

Differential symptoms	AD Axis II	AD with depression	AD with anxiety	AD with emotional features	AD with conduct disorder	AD with mixed features
Hyposomnia	1.19	1.33*	0.99	1.03	0.63	0.98
Appetite decreased	0.76	0.89*	0.41	0.58	0.35	0.66
Weight decreased	0.47	0.53*	0.22	0.33	0.23	0.40
Alcohol use	0.60	0.67	0.20	0.35	0.70	1.03*
Non-CNS depressant	0.45	0.51	0.10	0.28	0.40	0.66*
Violent behavior	0.44	0.30	0.19	0.33	1.14*	0.95
Impulsivity	0.72	0.69	0.41	0.57	1.67*	1.35
Other antisocial behavior	0.24	0.25	0.09	0.16	0.35	0.46*
Self-centered	0.12	0.08	0.15	0.17	0.09	0.28*
Undue perfectionism	0.15	0.11	0.31*	0.26	0.00	0.04
Decreased motor activity	0.39	0.48*	0.09	0.30	0.12	0.28
Increased motor activity	0.44	0.32	0.68*	0.58	0.58	0.65
Social withdrawal	0.58	0.67*	0.29	0.52	0.16	0.36
Bizarre behavior	0.03	0.03	0.01	0.02	0.21*	0.09
Hostility	0.28	0.23	0.11	0.26	0.60	0.71*
Generalized anxiety	0.63	0.49	1.52*	0.85	0.37	0.55
Panic attacks	0.11	0.08	0.32*	0.16	0.00	0.04
Situational anxiety	0.13	0.09	0.37*	0.20	0.00	0.09
Depressed mood	1.52	1.78*	0.70	1.27	0.65	1.16
Low self-esteem	0.98	1.10*	0.82	0.84	0.51	0.77
Elated mood	0.04	0.02	0.03	0.05	0.00	0.13*
Suspiciousness	0.21	0.19	0.16	0.22	0.14	0.37*
Somatic preoccupation	0.09	0.07	0.24*	0.13	0.05	0.05

TABLE 18–3. Symptom comparisons among subtypes of adjustment disorder (AD) in 2,224 adult (ages 19–64 years) psychiatric patients *(continued)*

Differential symptoms	AD Axis II	AD with depression	AD with anxiety	AD with emotional features	AD with conduct disorder	AD with mixed features
Suicidal indicators	0.87	1.04*	0.14	0.56	0.77	1.04
Homicidal ideation	0.21	0.19	0.02	0.18	0.42	0.48*
Homicidal behavior	0.07	0.05	0.02	0.05	0.40*	0.23
Developmental intellectual deficit	0.06	0.04	0.07	0.07	0.26*	0.11
Lack of insight	0.60	0.56	0.37	0.57	1.42*	0.97

Note. CNS=central nervous system.
*Group with the highest score, significantly higher than at least one other AD subtype at *P*<0.01. (Mezzich et al. 1981).

recent study, Casey et al. (2006) examined variables that might distinguish adjustment disorder from other depressive episodes. The patients were screened for depression severity with the Beck Depression Inventory (BDI) and then interviewed with Schedule for Clinical Assessment in Neuropsychiatry, which includes questions assessing the presence of adjustment disorder. The authors were unable to find any independent variables that distinguished adjustment disorder from other depressive episodes, including the severity of the BDI score at the outset.

DSM-III-R has been described as "medical illness and age unfair" (i.e., it does not sufficiently take into account the issues of age and/or medical illness) (L. George, personal communication, June 1981; Strain 1981). Eventually, to enhance reliability and validity, there needs to be a psychiatric taxonomy that considers developmental epoch (e.g., children and youth, adults, young elderly, and old elderly) and medical illness with its symptomatology. Many studies have found patients with adjustment disorder to be significantly younger compared with patients who have a major psychiatric diagnosis (Despland et al. 1995; Mok and Walter 1995). Zarb's (1996) study suggested that cognitively impaired elderly, when evaluated with individual items of the Geriatric Depression Scale (Yesavage et al. 1982–1983), had adjustment disorder rather than major depression. In addition, Despland et al. (1995) reported that the patient group with adjustment disorder with depressive or mixed symptoms included more women than men, thus resulting in a sex ratio resembling that for major depression or dysthymia. Therefore, future editions of DSM may be able to take into account the differences encountered in symptom profiles for gender, various developmental epochs, and medical and psychiatric comorbidity. (See Table 18–1 for DSM-IV-TR diagnostic criteria for adjustment disorders, and Table 18–2 for DSM-I diagnoses for adjustment disorder by developmental epoch.)

Epidemiology

Andreasen and Wasek (1980) reported that 5% of an inpatient and outpatient sample were labeled as having adjustment disorder. Fabrega et al. (1987) observed that 2.3% of a sample of patients at a walk-in clinic (diagnostic and evaluation center) met criteria for adjustment disorder, with no other diagnoses on Axis I or Axis II; 20% had the diagnosis of adjustment disorder when patients with other Axis I diagnoses (i.e., Axis I comorbidities) also were included. In general hospital

psychiatric consultation populations, adjustment disorder was diagnosed in 21.5% (Popkin et al. 1990), 18.5% (Foster and Oxman 1994), and 11.5% (Snyder and Strain 1989).

Strain et al. (1998b) examined the consultation-liaison data from seven university teaching hospitals in the United States, Canada, and Australia. The sites had all used a common computerized clinical database to examine 1,039 consecutive referrals—the MICRO-CARES software system (Strain et al. 1998b). Adjustment disorder was diagnosed in 125 patients (12.0%); it was the sole diagnosis in 81 (7.8%) and comorbid with other Axis I and II diagnoses in 44 (4.2%). It had been considered as a "rule-out" diagnosis in an additional 110 (10.6%). Adjustment disorder with depressed mood, anxious mood, or mixed emotions were the most common subcategories used. Adjustment disorder was diagnosed comorbidly most frequently with personality disorder and organic mental disorder. Sixty-seven subjects (6.4%) were assigned a V-code diagnosis only. Patients with adjustment disorder were referred significantly more often for problems of anxiety, coping, and depression; had less past psychiatric illness; and were rated as functioning better than those patients with major mental disorders—all consistent with the construct of adjustment disorder as a maladaptation to a psychosocial stressor. Interventions used for this general hospital inpatient cohort were similar to those for other Axis I and II diagnoses, in particular, the prescription of antidepressant medications. Patients with adjustment disorder required a similar amount of clinical time and resident supervision when compared with patients with other Axis I and II disorders.

Oxman et al. (1994) observed that 50.7% of elderly patients (age 55 years or older) receiving elective surgery for coronary artery disease developed adjustment disorder related to the stress of surgery. Thirty percent had symptomatic and functional impairment 6 months after surgery. Kellermann et al. (1999) reported that 27% of elderly patients examined 5–9 days after a cerebrovascular accident fulfilled the criteria for adjustment disorder. Spiegel (1996) observed that half of all cancer patients have a psychiatric disorder, usually an adjustment disorder with depression. Adjustment disorder is frequently diagnosed in patients with head and neck surgery (16.8%; Kugaya et al. 2000); patients with HIV (dementia and adjustment disorder, 73%; Pozzi et al. 1999); cancer patients from a multicenter survey of consultation-liaison psychiatry in oncology (27%; Grassi et al. 2000); dermatology patients (29% of the 9% who had psychiatric diagnoses;

Pulimood et al. 1996); and suicide attempters examined in an emergency department (22%; Schnyder and Valach 1997). Other studies include the diagnosis of adjustment disorder in more than 60% of burn inpatients (Perez-Jimenez et al. 1994), 20% of patients in early stages of multiple sclerosis (Sullivan et al. 1995), and 40% of poststroke patients (Shima et al. 1994).

D. Schafer (personal communication, April 1990) noted that up to 70% of children in the psychiatric setting may be given the diagnosis of adjustment disorder in a variety of mental health care settings. Faulstich et al. (1986) reported the prevalence (12.5%) of DSM-III adjustment disorder and conduct issues for adolescent psychiatric inpatients.

Etiology

Stress has been described as the etiological agent for adjustment disorders. However, diverse variables and modifiers are involved regarding who will experience an adjustment disorder following stress. Cohen (1981) argued that 1) acute stresses are different from chronic ones in both psychological and physiological terms, 2) the meaning of the stress is affected by "modifiers" (e.g., ego strengths, support systems, prior mastery), and 3) the manifest and latent meanings of the stressor(s) must be differentiated (e.g., loss of job may be a relief or a catastrophe). Adjustment disorder with maladaptive denial of pregnancy, for example, can be a consequence of a stressor such as separation from a partner (Brezinka et al. 1994). An objectively overwhelming stress may have little effect on one individual, whereas a minor one could be regarded as cataclysmic by another. A recent minor stress superimposed on a previous underlying (major) stress that has no observable effect on its own may have a significant additive effect (i.e., concatenation of events; B. Hamburg, personal communication, April 1990).

Andreasen and Wasek (1980) described the differences between the types of stressors found in adolescents and those found in adults: 59% and 35%, respectively, of the precipitants had been present for 1 year or more and 9% and 39% for 3 months or less. Fabrega et al. (1987) reported that their adjustment disorder group had greater registration of stressors compared with the specific-diagnosis and the non-illness cohorts. There was a significant difference in the amount of stressors reported relevant to the clinical request for evaluation: the group with adjustment disorder, compared with the specific-diagnosis and the no-illness patients, was overrepresented in the "higher stress category." Popkin et al. (1990) reported that in 68.6% of the cases in their consultation cohort, the medical illness itself was judged to be the primary psychosocial stressor. Snyder and Strain (1989) observed that stressors as assessed on Axis IV were significantly higher ($P=0.0001$) for consultation patients with adjustment disorder than for patients with other diagnostic disorders.

Although more attention has been paid to the current precipitating stressor in the diagnosis of adjustment disorders, recent research highlights the role of childhood experiences in the later development of these disorders. Several recent studies of young male soldiers with adjustment disorder secondary to conscription revealed that stress at a young age, such as abusive and overprotective parenting or adverse early family events, is a risk factor for the later development of adjustment disorder (For-Wey et al. 2002; Hansen-Schwartz et al. 2005). In a similar cohort, a history of childhood separation anxiety was found to be correlated with the later development of adjustment disorder (Giotakos and Konstantakopoulos 2002).

Clinical Features

Nine different types of adjustment disorder were listed in DSM-III-R. As in DSM-III, DSM-III-R adjustment disorder was classified according to the predominant symptoms extant. In DSM-IV-TR, adjustment disorder was reduced to six types that again are classified according to their clinical features: with depressed mood, with anxiety, with mixed anxiety and depressed mood, with disturbance of conduct, with mixed disturbance of emotions and conduct, and unspecified (Table 18–4). In their study, Despland et al. (1995) suggested reducing the subtypes even further, demonstrating identical profiles for adjustment disorder with depressed mood and adjustment disorder with mixed anxiety and depressed mood and proposing assimilation of mixed anxiety and depressed mood into the depressed mood category. These two groups represented 57% of their adjustment disorder sample; the remainder was classified as adjustment disorder with anxiety and other categories. Of note, it had been suggested by the DSM-IV Adjustment Disorder Work Group that suicide and deliberate self-harm could be subtypes of adjustment disorder, but the problem of suicidal symptomatology without another psychiatric diagnosis is placed in the F-code section in DSM-IV-TR, "Other Conditions That May Be a Focus of Clinical Attention." Clearly, what is regarded as a subthreshold diagnosis—adjustment disorder—does not necessarily imply the presence of subthreshold symptomatology.

TABLE 18–4. Types of DSM-IV-TR adjustment disorder

With depressed mood	The predominant symptoms are those of a minor depression. For example, the symptoms might be depressed mood, tearfulness, and hopelessness.
With anxiety	This type of adjustment disorder is diagnosed when anxiety symptoms are predominant, such as nervousness, worry, and jitteriness. The differential diagnosis would include anxiety disorders.
With mixed anxiety and depressed mood	This category should be used when the predominant symptoms are a combination of depression and anxiety or other emotions. An example would be an adolescent who, after moving away from home and parental supervision, reacts with ambivalence, depression, anger, and signs of increased dependence.
With disturbance of conduct	The symptomatic manifestations are those of behavioral misconduct that violate societal norms or the rights of others. Examples are fighting, truancy, vandalism, and reckless driving.
With mixed disturbance of emotions and conduct	This diagnosis is made when the disturbance combines affective and behavioral features of adjustment disorder with mixed emotional features and adjustment disorder with disturbance of conduct.
Unspecified	This is a residual diagnosis within the diagnostic category. This diagnosis can be used when a maladaptive reaction that is not classified under other adjustment disorders occurs in response to stress. An example would be a patient who, when given a diagnosis of cancer, denies the diagnosis of malignancy and is noncompliant with treatment recommendations.

Treatment

Psychotherapy

Treatment of adjustment disorder rests primarily on psychotherapeutic measures that enable reduction of the stressor, enhanced coping with the stressor that cannot be reduced or removed, and establishment of a support system to maximize adaptation. The first goal is to note significant dysfunction secondary to a stressor and to help the patient moderate this imbalance. Many stressors may be avoided or minimized (e.g., taking on more responsibility than can be managed by the individual or putting oneself at risk by having unprotected sex with an unknown partner). Other stressors may elicit an overreaction on the part of the patient (e.g., abandonment by a lover). The patient may attempt suicide or become reclusive, damaging his or her source of income. In this situation, the therapist would attempt to help the patient put his or her rage and other feelings into words rather than into destructive actions and assist more optimal adaptation and mastery of the trauma–stressor. The role of verbalization cannot be overestimated in an attempt to reduce the pressure of the stressor and enhance coping. The therapist also needs to clarify and interpret the meaning of the stressor for the patient. For example, a mastectomy may have devastated a patient's feelings

about her body and herself. It is necessary to clarify that the patient is still a woman, capable of having a fulfilling relationship, including a sexual one, and that the patient can have the cancer removed or treated and not have a recurrence. Otherwise, the patient's pernicious fantasies—"all is lost"—may take over in response to the stressor (i.e., the mastectomy) and make her dysfunctional in work and/or sex and precipitate a painful disturbance of mood that is incapacitating.

Counseling, psychotherapy, medical crisis counseling, crisis intervention, family therapy, and group treatment may be used to encourage the verbalization of fears, anxiety, rage, helplessness, and hopelessness related to the stressors imposed on a patient. The goals of treatment in each case are to expose the concerns and conflicts that the patient is experiencing, identify means to reduce the stressors, enhance the patient's coping skills, and help the patient gain perspective on the adversity and establish relationships (i.e., a support network) to assist in the management of the stressors and the self. Cognitive-behavioral therapy, for example, was successfully used in young military recruits (Nardi et al. 1994).

In terms of the DSM-III-R criteria, Sifneos (1989) stated that patients with adjustment disorders can profit most from brief psychotherapy. The psychotherapy should attempt to reframe the meaning of the stressor(s). The treatment should expose the concerns and conflicts that the patient is experiencing; identify means to reduce the stressor(s); enhance the patient's coping skills; and help the patient gain perspective on the adversity, establish relationships, attend support groups or self-help groups, and manage the stressor and the self. Although brief therapeutic interventions are usually all that are needed, ongoing stressors or enduring character pathology that may make a patient vulnerable to stress intolerance may signal the need for lengthier treatments.

Many types of therapeutic modalities have a place in the treatment of adjustment disorders. Wise (1988), drawing from military psychiatry, emphasized the treatment variables of Brevity, Immediacy, Centrality, Expectance, Proximity, and Simplicity (BICEPS principles). The treatment approach is brief, usually no more than 72 hours (True and Benway 1992). Such treatment would be similar to that prescribed for an acute stress disorder—the new diagnosis proposed by Spiegel and included in DSM-IV and DSM-IV-TR. The implication that maladaptation secondary to stressors requires immediate amelioration is important for the adjustment disorders, to avoid losses and dysfunction at work, in school, or with relationships.

Interpersonal psychotherapy was applied to depressed HIV-positive outpatients and found to be useful (Markowitz et al. 1992). Markowitz et al.'s (1992) description of the mechanisms of interpersonal psychotherapy is important in understanding psychotherapeutic approaches to the adjustment disorders. These mechanisms include psychoeducation about the sick role, a here-and-now framework, formulation of the problems from an interpersonal perspective, exploration of options for changing dysfunctional behavior patterns, identification of focused interpersonal problem areas, and the confidence that therapists gain from a systematic approach to problem formulation and treatment.

Lazarus (1992) described a seven-pronged approach to the treatment of minor depression. The procedures used included assertiveness training, a "sensate focus" of enjoyable events, coping, imagery, time projection, cognitive disputation, role-playing, desensitization, family therapy, and biological prophylaxis. The treatment was directed toward dysfunctional thoughts, behaviors, and relationships. Selmi et al. (1990) reported that patients whose symptoms met Research Diagnostic Criteria for major and minor depression were randomly assigned to computer-based cognitive-behavioral therapy, a therapist, or placebo; the two therapeutic modalities were both associated with improvement compared with the control condition.

A recent article in the geriatric literature described the use of a type of psychotherapy called "ego enhancing therapy" for the treatment of adjustment disorders in late life. Elderly patients are particularly vulnerable to the development of adjustment disorders as the stress of medical illness abounds. Additionally, life transitions such as relocating to a nursing home or losing one's driving privileges are commonly experienced as stressors in the elderly. A treatment that strengthens a patient's ego functions by helping him or her acknowledge the stressor and by promoting coping strategies can be useful in this population. An active therapeutic stance and the use of life review can help to foster a sense of mastery over the stressor (Frankel 2001).

Support groups have also been employed in patients with adjustment disorders. These groups help patients adjust and enhance their coping mechanisms (Fawzy et al. 2003; Spiegel et al. 1989). Although studies looking at the survival benefits of psychosocial group interventions have been mixed and show at most modest benefits, improvements in mood, distress level, and overall quality of life in cancer patients who attend support groups are very well documented (Goodwin et al. 2001; Newell et al. 2002). It would be important to investigate whether other stress-related disorders are improved by such systematic and carefully defined behavioral interventions.

Another therapeutic modality, eye movement desensitization and reprocessing, has been recently studied in patients with adjustment disorder. This psychotherapeutic technique, which has been shown to be effective in the treatment of posttraumatic stress disorder, was used with nine patients with adjustment disorder. Results showed significant improvement in patients with anxious or mixed features but not in those with depressed mood. Additionally, those with ongoing stressors did not show improvement (Mihelich 2000).

Akechi et al. (2004) investigated associated and predictive factors in cancer patients with adjustment disorder and major depression. Findings revealed that psychological distress in these patients was associated with a variety of factors, including social supports, physical functioning and limitations, and existential issues. Although the findings are not surprising, they do highlight the necessity of a comprehensive care plan for the treatment of adjustment disorders that includes physical, psychosocial, and existential components. Studies have yet to evaluate the potential role of family and couples therapy as well as alternative therapies such as acupuncture and yoga, but based on these findings, there may well be a role for these modalities in the future treatment of adjustment disorders.

A search of the Cochrane Database revealed only two randomized, controlled trials of specific psychotherapeutic treatment of adjustment disorders. Gonzalez-Jaimes and Turnbull-Plaza (2003) showed that "mirror psychotherapy" for patients with adjustment disorder with depressed mood secondary to a myocardial infarction was both an efficient and effective treatment. Mirror therapy is described as a type of therapy comprising psycho-corporal, cognitive, and neurolinguistic components with a holistic focus. As part of the treatment, a mirror is used to encourage patient acceptance of his or her physical condition that resulted from past self-care behaviors. In this study, mirror therapy was compared with two other treatments, Gestalt psychotherapy or medical conversation, in addition to a control group. Depressive symptoms improved in all treatment groups compared with the control group, but mirror therapy appeared significantly more effective than other treatments in decreasing symptoms of adjustment disorder at posttest evaluation.

In another randomized, controlled trial, an "activating intervention" was carried out for the treatment of adjustment disorders resulting in occupational dysfunction. In this study, 192 employees were randomized to receive either the intervention or care as usual (van der Klink and van Dijk 2003). The intervention consisted of an individual cognitive-behavioral approach to a graded activity, similar to stress inoculation training. Goals of treatment emphasized the acquisition of coping skills and the regaining of control. The treatment proved to be effective in decreasing sick leave duration and shortening long-term absenteeism when compared with the control group; both intervention and control groups, however, showed similar amounts of symptom reduction. This study formed the basis for the "Dutch Practice Guidelines for the Treatment of Adjustment Disorders in Primary and Occupational Health Care" (van der Klink et al. 2003). These guidelines were prepared by a team of 21 occupational health physicians and one psychologist and subsequently reviewed and tested by 15 experts, including several psychiatrists and psychologists and 21 practicing occupational health physicians.

Although no other randomized, controlled trials involving the psychotherapeutic treatment of pure cohorts of patients with adjustment disorders could be found, many exist that studied an array of depressive and anxiety disorders and included adjustment disorders in their cohorts. For example, a recent trial comparing brief dynamic therapy with brief supportive therapy in patients with minor depressive disorders, including adjustment disorders, was found in the Cochrane Database. Although both therapies proved efficacious in reducing symptoms, brief dynamic therapy was more effective at 6-month follow-up (Maina et al. 2005).

Pharmacotherapy

Although psychotherapy has historically been the mainstay of treatment for the adjustment disorders, Stewart et al. (1992) emphasized the importance of including psychopharmacological interventions in the treatment of minor depression. These authors argued that pharmacotherapy is generally recommended, but data do not support this contention. Despite the lack of rigorous scientific evidence, Stewart and colleagues advocated successive trials with antidepressants in any depressed patient (major or minor disorders), particularly if he or she has not benefited from psychotherapy or other supportive measures for 3 months. In a recent randomized, controlled trial in the treatment of minor depressive disorder, fluoxetine proved superior to placebo in reducing depressive symptoms, improving overall psychosocial functioning, and alleviating suffering (Judd 2000). The question remains, does this also apply to adjustment disorders with depressed mood?

As an example, the following patient did not respond to counseling and was sufficiently distressed by her mood disorder to require pharmacotherapeutic intervention:

> A 35-year-old married woman, the mother of three children, was desperate when she learned that she had cancer and would need a mastectomy followed by chemotherapy and radiation. She was convinced that she would not recover, that her body would be forever distorted and ugly, that her husband would no longer find her attractive, and that her children would be ashamed of her baldness and the fact that she had cancer. She wondered if anyone would ever want to touch her again. Her mother and sister had also experienced breast cancer, and the patient felt that she was fated to an empty future.
>
> Despite several sessions to deal with her feelings, the patient's dysphoria remained profound. She exhibited no vegetative signs indicating major depression, she was not anhedonic or guilt-ridden, and she admitted no suicidal ideation. Her clinician decided to add antidepressant pharmacotherapy (fluoxetine, 20 mg/day) to her psychotherapy sessions to decrease her continuing unpleasant mood state. Two weeks later, the patient reported that she was feeling less despondent and less concerned about the future.

As the patient came to terms with the overwhelming stressor and was assisted with antidepressant agents, her depressed mood improved, and her ability to employ more adequate coping strategies to handle her serious medical illness was mobilized.

Randomized, controlled pharmacological trials of the use of pharmacotherapy in patients with adjustment disorder are rare. As mentioned earlier, formal psychotherapy appears to be the current treatment of choice (Uhlenhuth et al. 1995), although psychotherapy combined with benzodiazepines also is used, especially for patients with severe life stress(es) and a significant anxious component (Shaner 2000; Uhlenhuth et al. 1995). Tricyclic antidepressants or buspirone was recommended in place of benzodiazepines for patients with current or past heavy alcohol use because of the greater risk of dependence in these patients (Uhlenhuth et al. 1995). In a 25-week multicenter randomized, placebo-controlled, double-blind trial, WS 1490 (a special extract from kava-kava) was reported to be effective in adjustment disorder with anxiety and did not have the tolerance issues associated with tricyclics and benzodiazepines (Volz and Kieser 1997). In a similar randomized, controlled trial, Bourin et al. (1997) randomized patients to receive either Euphytose—a preparation containing a combination of plant extracts (*Crataegus, Ballota, Passiflora,* and *Valeriana,* which have mild sedative effects, and *Cola* and *Paullinia,* which mainly act as mild stimulants)—or placebo. Patients taking the experimental drug improved significantly more than those taking placebo. In another study, tianeptine, alprazolam, and mianserin were found to be equally effective in symptom improvement in patients with adjustment disorder with anxiety (Ansseau et al. 1996). In a randomized, double-blind study, trazodone was more effective than clorazepate in cancer patients for the relief of anxious and depressed symptoms (Razavi et al. 1999). Similar findings were observed in HIV-positive patients with adjustment disorder (DeWit et al. 1999).

It is important to note that there are no randomized, controlled trials employing selective serotonin reuptake inhibitors (SSRIs), mixed SSRI atypicals (nefazodone and venlafaxine), buspirone, or mirtazapine. These newer antidepressant medications have fewer side effects and may offer symptom relief of dysphoric moods with minimal adverse reactions and interactions. The difficulty in obtaining an adjustment disorder study cohort with reliable and valid diagnoses may impede the conduct of a controlled clinical trial comparing these newer antidepressant agents against placebo and psychotherapy. Additionally, treatment outcome studies are compromised by not knowing when to examine the outcome of an intervention. In the case of the adjustment disorders, should this be when the stressors have stabilized, when the stressors have abated, or after an agreed-on time (e.g., 3 months) has elapsed? The stressor attributes a further confound obtaining a homogeneous sample because of the differences in the stressors, including nature (quality), severity (quantity), and acuteness (less than 6 months) or chronicity (more than 6 months). Psychotropic medication has been used in medically ill patients, terminally ill patients, and patients with illness refractory to verbal therapies. In a study of medically ill patients with depressive disorders (unspecified), Rosenberg et al. (1991) reported that 16 of 29 patients (55%) improved within 2 days of treatment with the maximal dosage of amphetamine derivatives. The presence of delirium was associated with a decreased response. Whether methylphenidate would be useful in adjustment disorders with depressed mood remains to be investigated.

Reynolds (1992), reviewing randomized, controlled trials, stated that bereavement-related syndromal depression also appears to respond to antidepressant medication. By definition, however, bereavement is considered not as an adjustment disorder but rather as a stress-related response disorder and as such is classified as a V code—a problem-level diagnosis—warranting the attention of a mental health professional. Ordinarily, medication is not prescribed for problem-level diagnoses; rather, counseling, psychotherapy, support, and so forth are the interventions of choice. If medication is prescribed for minor disorders (including subthreshold disorders), the predominant mood that accompanies the (adjustment) disorder is an important consideration. Schatzberg (1990) recommended that therapists consider both psychotherapy and pharmacotherapy in adjustment disorders with anxious mood and that anxiolytics should be part of psychiatrists' armamentarium. Nguyen et al. (2006), using a double-blind, randomized controlled trial, compared the efficacies of etifoxine, a nonbenzodiazepine anxiolytic drug, and lorazepam, a benzodiazepine, in the treatment of adjustment disorder with anxiety in a primary care setting. Efficacy was evaluated on days 7 and 28 using the Hamilton Rating Scale for Anxiety. The two drugs were found to be equivalent in anxiolytic efficacy on day 28. However, overall more etifoxine recipients responded to the treatment. Moreover, 1 week after stopping treatment, fewer patients taking etifoxine experienced rebound anxiety compared with lorazepam patients.

Regardless of whether psychotherapy or pharmacotherapy are used alone or in combination, a significant aspect of treatment is for the physician to keep alert to the fact that the diagnosis of adjustment disorder may indicate a patient who is in the early phase of a major mental disorder that has not yet evolved to full-blown symptoms. Therefore, if a patient continues to worsen, becomes more symptomatic, and does not respond to treatment, it is critical to review the patient's symptoms and the diagnosis for the presence of a major mental disorder. The patient in the earlier case example may have been in the early phase of a major depressive disorder, but at the time of assessment, she appeared at a subthreshold level of diagnosis.

Treatment of Adjustment Disorders in Primary Care

Primary care is regarded as an important venue for the identification and treatment of depression, including the adjustment disorders. The Agency for Health Care Policy and Research (1993) developed guidelines for the treatment of depression in primary care. It would seem that if any depressive disorders could be treated in primary care, the adjustment disorders—subthreshold—would be the most likely candidates. Schulberg et al. (1993) considered whether randomized, controlled trials are able to determine the validity of transferring treatments for major depression from the psychiatric to the primary care sector. Schulberg et al. (2002) in a more recent study reviewed the clinical and cost effectiveness of psychotherapy for treating major and minor depression in primary care practice. They concluded that when used to treat minor depression or dysthymia, the effectiveness of psychotherapy in comparison to usual care was equivocal. A randomized controlled trial was conducted at the University of Washington, Seattle, to determine the specificity and intensity of mental health training programs that are necessary to ensure the sufficient transfer of knowledge from psychiatrists to primary care physicians (Katon and Gonzales 1994). This trial included providing education to the patient and the physician as well as changing the structure of medical care delivery to enhance the primary care physician's capacity to adequately treat depressive disorders. In an editorial on the "white papers," a series of articles commissioned by the Services Research and Clinical Epidemiology Branch of the National Institute of Mental Health (NIMH) for the July 2000 14th NIMH Conference on

Mental Health Services Research, Katon and Gonzales (2002) reported that

> programs aimed at physician education have had no lasting effects on patient outcomes, whereas multimodal collaborative intervention programs that integrated a range of physician extenders such as nurses or mental health specialists to increase rates of frequency of follow-up, monitor outcomes, activate patients to become partners in their care and facilitate referral to specialists have had marked effects on improving outcomes for primary care patients. (p. 196)

Current data would indicate that informing the primary care physician that the patient has depression is not sufficient for enhancing patient outcome. Optimal therapeutic outcome in the primary care setting depends on three actions: 1) sufficient patient education, 2) conjoint sessions with the psychiatrist and the primary care physician, and 3) sufficient follow-up by the psychiatrist during the course of treatment. Although adjustment disorders were not the focus of the Katon studies just described, Katon's research group examined depression treatment issues in real-world settings, including the measurement of disability and cost; in addition, they addressed the issue of effectiveness research and its needed methodology (Katon 1999). Barrett et al. (1999) undertook a comparison of paroxetine, problem-solving therapy, and placebo for minor depression and dysthymia in primary care patients.

Strain et al. (1998b) observed in multiple settings that adjustment disorder patients seen in psychiatric consultation in the general hospital setting required just as much of the psychiatric consultant's time and were just as likely to receive medication as were patients with major psychiatric disorders. As mentioned earlier, the adjustment disorders are currently thought to require talking treatment (psychotherapy and/or counseling), which takes time and is poorly reimbursed for primary care physicians. Because talking effectively may require more skill than prescribing drugs, treatment of adjustment disorders in the primary care setting remains problematic.

Hameed et al. (2005) in a retrospective chart review sought to determine if there was a difference in antidepressant efficacy in the treatment of major depressive disorder versus adjustment disorder in a primary care setting. Patients had been prescribed mostly SSRIs. DSM-IV-TR symptoms, Patient Health Questionnaire–9 depression rating scale scores, and functional disability reports were systematically used to assess patients' response. Results showed that neither depressed nor adjustment disorder patients demonstrated a difference in clinical response to any particular antidepressant. Patients with a diagnosis of adjustment disorder, however, were twice as likely to respond to standard antidepressant treatment as depressed patients. This study suggests that antidepressants are very effective in treating depression in the primary care setting and may be even more effective in the treatment for adjustment disorder with depressed mood.

Course and Prognosis

DSM-IV-TR criterion E for adjustment disorder implies a good long-term outcome by stating "once the stressor (or its consequences) has terminated, the symptoms do not persist for more than an additional 6 months" (American Psychiatric Association 2000, p. 683). Andreasen and Hoenk's (1982) landmark study demonstrated this by showing that prognosis was favorable for adults but that in adolescents, many major psychiatric illnesses eventually occur. At 5-year follow-up, 71% of the adults were completely well, 8% had an intervening problem, and 21% had developed a major depressive disorder or alcoholism. In adolescents at 5-year follow-up, only 44% were without a psychiatric diagnosis, 13% had an intervening psychiatric illness, and 43% had gone on to develop major psychiatric morbidity (e.g., schizophrenia, schizoaffective disorder, major depression, bipolar disorder, substance abuse, personality disorders). In contrast to the predictors for major pathology in adults, the chronicity of the illness and the presence of behavioral symptoms in the adolescents were the strongest predictors for major pathology at the 5-year follow-up. The number and type of symptoms were less useful than the length of treatment and chronicity of symptoms as predictors of future outcome.

Mezzich et al. (1981) and Strain et al. (1998a) observed that many of the subtypes of adjustment disorder were infrequently used (e.g., "with mixed emotional features"), whereas "with physical complaints," a DSM-III-R category, had insufficient time to be observed. Both subtypes were deleted in DSM-IV-TR.

As Chess and Thomas (1984) reported, it is important to note that adjustment disorder with disturbance of conduct, regardless of age, has a more guarded outcome. Just as Andreasen and Wasek (1980) observed, Chess and Thomas (1984) underscored that a significant number of adjustment disorder patients either do not improve or grow worse in adolescence and early adult life. Furthermore, it is not always possible to predict the developmental course of the disorder in the early period after its identification. They suggested

that active appropriate therapeutic intervention be provided in all cases.

Despland et al. (1997) observed 52 patients with adjustment disorder at the end of treatment or after 3 years of treatment. Results showed the occurrence of psychiatric comorbidity (31%), suicide attempts (14%), development of a more serious psychiatric disorder (29%), and an unfavorable clinical state (23%). Adjustment disorder is an important disorder requiring follow-up and observation. Spalletta et al. (1996) stated that suicidal behavior and deliberate self-harm are important predictors in diagnosis of adjustment disorder. These symptoms can lead to the most distressing consequence—death. However, there was considerable discussion regarding the inclusion of a subtype of adjustment disorder for patients with suicidal thoughts and/or deliberate self-harm in the DSM-IV revision process. Consensus was that such additions to the taxonomy would raise other conflicts. None of the other diagnoses have a subcode for suicidal behavior or deliberate self-harm, although it is commonly encountered in major depression, substance abuse, and borderline personality disorders. In fact, suicidal behavior or deliberate self-harm can accompany any psychiatric diagnosis. There was concern that adjustment disorder with suicidal intent or attempt would be used as a diagnostic assignment rather than the major mental disorder that did not list the opportunity to specify suicide. The desire to specify and highlight the behavior of suicidality could co-opt the obligation for the accurate diagnosis. In effect, a behavior would trump the syndromal diagnosis of a disorder. Consequently, the behavior of suicide or self-mutilation is coded in DSM-IV-TR under an F code: "Other Conditions That May Be a Focus of Clinical Attention." Therefore, there would be two Axis I designations: the primary disorder and the condition indicated by the F code.

Kovacs et al. (1994) also examined children and youth (ages 8–13 years) for up to 8 years and found that, controlling for the effects of comorbidity, adjustment disorder does not predict later dysfunction. A more recent report by Jones et al. (2002) examined 10 years of readmission data for various psychiatric diagnoses, including the adjustment disorders. They found that admission diagnosis was a significant predictor of readmission and that adjustment disorders had the lowest readmission rates. Furthermore, initial psychological recovery from an adjustment disorder may in large part be attributable to removal of the stressor. This was found to be the case in prisoners who developed adjustment disorders after being placed in solitary confinement and whose symptoms resolved shortly after their release (Andersen et al. 2000).

Although most studies do point to a more benign prognosis for the adjustment disorders, it is important to realize that the risk of serious morbidity and mortality still exists. Many studies investigating the association between suicide and adjustment disorder underscore the importance of monitoring patients closely for suicidality. Runeson et al. (1996) observed from psychological autopsy methods that the median interval between first suicidal communication and suicide was very short in the patients with adjustment disorder (<1 month) compared with patients who have major depression (3 months), borderline personality disorder (30 months), or schizophrenia (47 months). Portzky et al. (2005) conducted psychological autopsies on adolescents with adjustment disorder who had committed suicide and found that suicidal thinking in these patients was brief and evolved rapidly and without warning. A slightly different profile was found in two other studies that looked at suicide attempters with a diagnosis of adjustment disorder. These patients were more likely to have poor overall psychosocial functioning, prior psychiatric treatment, personality disorders, substance abuse histories, and a current "mixed" symptom profile of depressed mood and behavioral disturbances (Kryzhanovskaya and Canterbury 2001; Pelkonen et al. 2005). A study of the neurochemical variables of adjustment disorder patients of all ages who had attempted suicide revealed biological correlates consistent with the more major psychiatric disorders. Attempters were found to have lower platelet monoamine oxidase activity, higher 3-methoxy-4-hydroxyphenylglycol (MHPG) activity, and higher cortisol levels than control subjects. Although these findings differ from the lower MHPG and cortisol levels found in patients with major depression and suicidality, they are similar to findings in other major stress-related conditions.

Conclusion

The etiological and dynamic attributes of the diagnosis of adjustment disorders make them a fascinating diagnostic category that constitutes a linchpin between normality and pathology, between subthreshold psychiatric morbidity and more serious mental disorders. Appropriate and timely treatment is essential for patients with adjustment disorders so that their symptoms do not worsen, their important relationships are not further impaired, or their capacity to work, study, or be active in their essential interpersonal pursuits is not compromised. In a nutshell, treatment must attempt to forestall further erosion of the patient's capacity to function, which could ultimately have grave consequences. Maladaptation may impede the patient to a point at which irreversible losses in important sectors of his or her life occur. The cost to the patient and to society as a whole in terms of disability and lost productivity is enormous. Future research should encompass systematic clinical trials aimed at pure cohorts of patients with adjustment disorders. Cost-benefit analyses of the various treatment modalities must also be undertaken. Although this diagnosis lacks rigorous specificity, its treatment is no less challenging or less important.

The issues of diagnostic rigor and clinical utility seem at odds for the adjustment disorders. Clinicians need a "wild card," and field studies need to use reliable and valid instruments (e.g., depression or anxiety rating scales, stress assessments, length of disability, treatment outcome, family patterns) to determine more exact specification of the parameters of the diagnosis. Identification of the time course, remission or evolution to another diagnosis, and evaluation of stressors (characteristics, duration, and nature of adaptation to stress) would enhance the understanding of the concept of a stress-response illness.

Studies with adequate symptom checklists rated independently from the establishment of the diagnosis would help clarify the threshold between major and minor depression and anxiety, as well as help guide an entry cutoff point for adjustment disorder. Although the upper threshold is established by the criteria for the major syndromes, the lower threshold between an adjustment disorder and problems of living/normality is bereft of operational criteria that would define an entry "boundary." The careful examination of associated demographic and treatment outcome variables also would enable clinicians to describe more specifically the boundaries between diagnoses. Associated features such as family history, biological correlates, treatment response, and long-term course are all critical to establishing the authenticity of a diagnosis—that is, construct and criterion validity. The theory and practice of medicine have documented the need for a comprehensive multidimensional formulation of multiple physiological and functional variables and mechanisms to describe an illness.

Regardless of their position on the diagnostic tree, subthreshold syndromes can encompass significant psychopathology that must be not only recognized but also treated (e.g., suicidal ideation or behavior). Cross-sectionally, adjustment disorder may appear to be the incipient phase of an emerging major syndrome. Consequently, adjustment disorder, despite its problems with reliability and validity, serves an important diagnostic function in the practice of psychiatry. Problem- and subthreshold-level diagnoses are critical to the function of any medical discipline. Because this disorder may be the initial phase, or a mild form, of a dysfunction that is not yet fully developed, the relation between the incipient and the developed and between the subthreshold and the defined must be described. This apparent chaos, lack of specificity, and questionable reliability and validity are the hallmark of interface disorders and subthreshold phenomena, whether they are in diabetes mellitus, hypertension, or depression.

Combined with the remaining problem of the certainty of the diagnosis, the question prevails: Should drugs be used in the treatment of adjustment disorders? The solution to this dilemma demands a caution with regard to pharmacological intervention; the pharmacological studies are currently inconclusive. The diagnostic uncertainty of adjustment disorder presents sufficient difficulty in and of itself, with its mixed features, frequent combination with medical comorbidity, and placement in the gray area of diagnosis (Hosaka et al. 1994; Hugo et al. 1996; Oxman et al. 1994). It is better to be cautious and delay psychotropic drug administration rather than subject the patient to the risk of unfavorable other drug–psychotropic drug interaction(s). The condition may resolve, or it may evolve into a major psychiatric illness that needs to be treated accordingly, which could include pharmacological agents.

Perhaps secondary to the subjective nature of the diagnosis, diagnostic tools to aid clinicians in identifying this condition are significantly lacking. Many widely used screening instruments (e.g., Clinical Interview Schedule—Revised, Composite International Diagnostic Interview) found in psychiatric research today fail to incorporate the diagnosis (Casey 2001; Casey et al. 2001). Although the Hospital Anxiety and Depression Scale, a commonly used self-report screen for psychological distress in hospitalized patients, does not screen for adjustment disorders specifically, a recent study of terminally ill cancer patients found it to be a useful predictor of adjustment disorders and major depression in patients who did not show clinical evidence of psychological distress at baseline (Akechi et al. 2004). Brief screening instruments have also recently been developed to help in the detection of adjustment disorders in cancer patients. The one-question interview and the impact thermometer are two such instruments that appear efficacious in identifying patients (Akizuki et al. 2003, 2005). Although they

have shown to be valid tools, they lack the ability to distinguish between adjustment disorder and other depressive disorders, thus limiting their usefulness in promoting the concept of adjustment disorder as a separate and meaningful diagnostic entity.

The characteristics of a mental disorder vary over the life cycle, and this variation is clearly illustrated by the adjustment disorders. Certain developmental epochs may be associated with a particular symptom profile, as seen with acute myocardial infarction and appendicitis. The effect of the stressor may vary, and the assessment of functioning must be "measured" according to the demands of the developmental stage (e.g., school [youth], work [adults], self-care and maintenance [elderly]). The symptom characteristics and functional assessment of other diagnoses also may vary along the developmental schema from birth to senescence. Illnesses such as major depressive disorders, organic mental disorders, sexual dysfunctions, and eating disorders need to be reformulated in another hierarchy to incorporate the vicissitudes of the stage of the life cycle extant at the time of the assessment. Considering normal variations across developmental epochs would make adjustment disorder and other DSM-IV-TR disorders much more reliable and valid and less vulnerable to being characterized as "unfair" in regard to the aged, children and youth, or the medically ill (L. George, personal communication, May 1981; Strain 1981). The result would be a taxonomy accommodating to the vicissitudes of development, gender, age, and medical illness.

Such an effort also may make adjustment disorder, and DSM-IV-TR and future editions of DSM, more useful to child psychiatrists, pediatricians, geriatricians, geriatric psychiatrists, and primary care specialists, who currently believe that too often their patients' problems do not conform to psychiatry's lexicon. In fact, a significant number of their patients remain at the problem level of diagnoses with their somatic complaints as well. It is common for a fever of unknown origin not to be diagnosed or for chest pain to remain unspecified. It is the *art* of medicine that makes it a profession, and it is a most difficult one at the interface of medicine and psychiatry, or at the interface of normality and pathology. Anna Freud (1968) emphasized the difficulty of understanding normality and pathology in her assessments of childhood. This important advice would prevail across the life cycle and be an important challenge to the developers of the subthreshold diagnoses (e.g., adjustment disorder) and future editions of DSM.

Key Points

- Adjustment disorders are of two forms: acute (6 months or less) and chronic (greater than 6 months).

- In children, adjustment disorders are predictive of more serious mental illnesses for late adolescence and adulthood.

- An adjustment disorder diagnosis can be used concurrently with another Axis I diagnosis.

- The adjustment disorders have a clear threshold for when they are supplanted by another Axis I diagnosis, because the other diagnoses have established thresholds and symptom guidelines. The point at which the patient crosses the threshold between normal behavior and an adjustment disorder is less clear, however, because the symptom guidelines for entry are less specific.

- It has been suggested that adjustment disorders could be placed with other diagnoses identified by the mood and behavior; for example, adjustment disorder with depressed mood could be positioned as an affective disorder.

Suggested Readings

Newcorn JH, Strain J: Adjustment disorder in children and adolescents, in DSM-IV Source Book, Vol 3. Washington, DC, American Psychiatric Association, 1997, pp 291–301

Sadock BJ, Sadock VA: Kaplan and Sadock's Pocket Handbook of Clinical Psychiatry, 4th Edition. Philadelphia, PA, Lippincott Williams & Wilkins, 2005, pp 2055–2062

Strain JJ, Klipstein K: Adjustment disorder, in Treatments of Psychiatric Disorders, 4th Edition (TPD-IV). Edited by Gabbard GO. Washington, DC, American Psychiatric Publishing, 2006, pp 419–426

Strain JJ, Newcorn J, Mezzich J, et al: Adjustment disorder: the MacArthur reanalysis, in DSM-IV Source Book, Vol 4. Washington, DC, American Psychiatric Association, 1998, pp 403–424

Strain JJ, Wolf D, Newcorn J, et al: Adjustment disorder, in DSM-IV Source Book, Vol 2. Washington, DC, American Psychiatric Association, 1996, pp 1033–1049

References

Agency for Health Care Policy and Research: Depression Guideline Panel: Depression in Primary Care, Vol 1: Diagnosis and Detection; Vol 2: Treatment of Major Depression. Clinical Practice Guideline no. 5 (AHCPR publications 93-0550, 93-0551). Rockville, MD, U.S. Department of Health and Human Services, Public Health Service, Agency for Health Care Policy and Research, 1993

Akechi T, Okuyama T, Sugawara Y, et al: Major depression, adjustment disorders, and post-traumatic stress disorder in terminally ill cancer patients: associated and predictive factors. J Clin Oncol 22:1957–1965, 2004

Akizuki N, Akechi T, Nakanishi T, et al: Development of a brief screening interview for adjustment disorders and major depression in patients with cancer. Cancer 97:2605–2613, 2003

Akizuki N, Yamawaki S, Akechi T, et al: Development of an impact thermometer for use in combination with the distress thermometer as a brief screening tool for adjustment disorders and/or major depression in cancer patients. J Pain Symptom Manage 29:91–99, 2005

American Psychiatric Association: Diagnostic and Statistical Manual: Mental Disorders. Washington, DC, American Psychiatric Association, 1952

American Psychiatric Association: Diagnostic and Statistical Manual of Mental Disorders, 3rd Edition. Washington, DC, American Psychiatric Association, 1980

American Psychiatric Association: Diagnostic and Statistical Manual of Mental Disorders, 3rd Edition, Revised. Washington, DC, American Psychiatric Association, 1987

American Psychiatric Association: Diagnostic and Statistical Manual of Mental Disorders, 4th Edition. Washington, DC, American Psychiatric Association, 1994

American Psychiatric Association: Diagnostic and Statistical Manual of Mental Disorders, 4th Edition, Text Revision. Washington, DC, American Psychiatric Association, 2000

Andersen HS, Sestoft D, Lillebaek T, et al: A longitudinal study of prisoners on remand: psychiatric prevalence, incidence and psychopathology in solitary vs. non-solitary confinement. Acta Psychiatr Scand 102:19–25, 2000

Andreasen NC, Wasek P: Adjustment disorders in adolescents and adults. Arch Gen Psychiatry 37:1166–1170, 1980

Andreasen NC, Hoenk PR: The predictive value of adjustment disorders: a follow-up study. Am J Psychiatry 139:584–590, 1982

Ansseau M, Bataille M, Briole G, et al: Controlled comparison of tianeptine, alprazolam and mianserin in the treatment of adjustment disorders with anxiety and depression. Hum Psychopharmacol 11:293–298, 1996

Aoki T, Hosaka T, Ishida A: Psychiatric evaluation of physical rehabilitation patients. Gen Hosp Psychiatry 17:440–443, 1995

Barrett JE, Williams JW Jr, Oxman TE, et al: The treatment effectiveness project: a comparison of the effectiveness of paroxetine, problem-solving therapy, and placebo in the treatment of minor depression and dysthymia in primary care patients: background and research plan. Gen Hosp Psychiatry 21:260–273, 1999

Bourin M, Bougerol T, Guitton B, et al: A combination of plant extracts in the treatment of outpatients with adjustment disorder with anxious mood: controlled study versus placebo. Fundam Clin Pharmacol 11:127–132, 1997

Brezinka C, Huter O, Biebl W, et al: Denial of pregnancy: obstetrical aspects. J Psychosom Obstet Gynaecol 15:1–8, 1994

Casey P: Adult adjustment disorder: a review of its current diagnostic status. J Psychiatr Pract 7:32–40, 2001

Casey P, Dowrick C, Wilkinson G: Adjustment disorders fault line in the psychiatric glossary. Br J Psychiatry 179:479–481, 2001

Casey P, Maracy M, Kelly BD, et al: Can adjustment disorder and depressive episode be distinguished? J Affect Disord 92:291–297, 2006

Chess S, Thomas A: Origins and Evolution of Behavior Disorders: From Infancy to Early Adult Life. New York, Brunner/Mazel, 1984

Cohen F: Stress and bodily illness. Psychiatr Clin North Am 4:269–286, 1981

Despland JN, Monod L, Ferrero F: Clinical relevance of adjustment disorder in DSM-III-R and DSM-IV. Compr Psychiatry 36:456–460, 1995

Despland JN, Monod L, Ferrero F: Etude clinique du trouble de l'adaptation selon le DSM-III-R. Schweiz Arch Neurol Neurochir Psychiatr 148:19–24, 1997

DeWit S, Cremers L, Hirsch D, et al: Efficacy and safety of trazodone versus clorazepate in the treatment of HIV-positive subjects with adjustment disorders: a pilot study. J Int Med Res 27:223–232, 1999

Fabrega H Jr, Mezzich JE, Mezzich AC: Adjustment disorder as a marginal or transitional illness category in DSM-III. Arch Gen Psychiatry 44:567–572, 1987

Faulstich ME, Moore JR, Carey MP, et al: Prevalence of DSM-III conduct and adjustment disorders for adolescent psychiatric inpatients, in Adolescence, Vol 21, No 82. San Diego, CA, Libra Publishers, 1986, pp 333–337

Fawzy FI, Canada AL, Fawzy NW: Malignant melanoma: effects of a brief, structured psychiatric intervention on survival and recurrence at 10-year follow-up. Arch Gen Psychiatry 60:100–103, 2003

For-Wey L, Fei-Yin L, Bih-Ching S: The relationship between life adjustment and parental bonding in military personnel with adjustment disorder in Taiwan. Mil Med 167:678–682, 2002

Foster P, Oxman T: A descriptive study of adjustment disorder diagnoses in general hospital patients. Ir J Psychol Med 11:153–157, 1994

Frankel M: Ego enhancing treatment of adjustment disorders of later life. J Geriatr Psychiatry 34:221–223, 2001

Freud A: Normality and Pathology: Assessment of Childhood. New York, International Universities Press, 1968

Giotakos O, Konstantakopoulos G: Parenting received in childhood and early separation anxiety in male conscripts with adjustment disorder. Mil Med 167:28–33, 2002

Gonzalez-Jaimes EI, Turnbull-Plaza B: Selection of psychotherapeutic treatment for adjustment disorder with depressive mood due to acute myocardial infarction. Arch Med Res 34:298–304, 2003

Goodwin PJ, Leszcz M, Ennis M, et al: The effects of group psychosocial support on survival in metastatic breast cancer. N Engl J Med 345:1719–1726, 2001

Grassi L, Gritti P, Rigatelli M, et al: Psychosocial problems secondary to cancer: an Italian multicenter survey of consultation-liaison psychiatry in oncology. Italian Consultation-Liaison Group. Eur J Cancer 36:579–585, 2000

Hameed U, Schwartz TL, Malhotra K, et al: Antidepressant treatment in the primary care office: outcomes for adjustment disorder versus major depression. Ann Clin Psychiatry 17:77–81, 2005

Hansen-Schwartz J, Kijne B, Johnsen A, et al: The course of adjustment disorder in Danish male conscripts. Nord J Psychiatry 59:193–196, 2005

Havenaar JM, Van den Brink W, Van den Bout J, et al: Mental health problems in the Gomel region (Belarus): an analysis of risk factors in an area affected by the Chernobyl disaster. Psychol Med 26:845–855, 1996

Hosaka T, Aoki T, Ichikawa Y: Emotional states of patients with hematological malignancies: preliminary study. Jpn J Clin Oncol 24:186–190, 1994

Hugo FJ, Halland AM, Spangenberg JJ, et al: DSM-III-R classification of psychiatric symptoms in systemic lupus erythematosus. Psychosomatics 37:262–269, 1996

Jones R, Yates WR, Williams S, et al: Outcome for adjustment disorder with depressed mood: comparison with other mood disorders. J Affect Disord 55:55–61, 1999

Jones R, Yates WR, Zhou MD: Readmission rates for adjustment disorders: comparison with other mood disorders. J Affect Disord 71:199–203, 2002

Judd LL: Diagnosis and treatment of minor depressive disorders. Int J Neuropsychopharmacol 3 (suppl):S66, 2000

Katon W: Treatment trials in real world settings: methodological issues and measurement of disability and costs. Gen Hosp Psychiatry 21:237–238, 1999

Katon W, Gonzales J: A review of randomized trials of psychiatric consultation-liaison studies in primary care. Psychosomatics 35:268–278, 1994

Katon W, Gonzales J: Primary care and treatment of depression: a response to the NIMH "White Papers." Gen Hosp Psychiatry 24:194–196, 2002

Kellermann M, Fekete I, Gesztelyi R, et al: Screening for depressive symptoms in the acute phase of stroke. Gen Hosp Psychiatry 21:116–121, 1999

Kovacs M, Gatsonis C, Pollock M, et al: A controlled prospective study of DSM-III adjustment disorder in childhood: short-term prognosis and long-term predictive validity. Arch Gen Psychiatry 51:535–541, 1994

Kovacs M, Ho V, Pollock MH: Criterion and predictive validity of the diagnosis of adjustment disorder: a prospective study of youths with new-onset insulin-dependent diabetes mellitus. Am J Psychiatry 152:523–528, 1995

Kryzhanovskaya L, Canterbury R: Suicidal behavior in patients with adjustment disorders. Crisis 22:125–131, 2001

Kugaya A, Akechi T, Okuyama T, et al: Prevalence, predictive factors, and screening for psychological distress in patients with newly diagnosed head and neck cancers. Cancer 88:2817–2823, 2000

Lazarus AA: The multimodal approach to the treatment of minor depression. Am J Psychother 46:50–57, 1992

Maina G, Forner F, Bogetto F: Randomized controlled trial comparing brief dynamic and supportive therapy with waiting list condition in minor depressive disorders. Psychother Psychosom 74:43–50, 2005

Markowitz JC, Klerman GL, Perry SW: Interpersonal psychotherapy of depressed HIV-positive outpatients. Hosp Community Psychiatry 43:885–890,1992

McNair DM, Lorr M, Doppelman LF (eds): Manual for the Profile of Mood States. San Diego, CA, Educational and Industrial Testing Service, 1971

Mezzich JE, Dow JT, Rich CL, et al: Developing an efficient clinical information system for a comprehensive psychiatric institute, II: initial evaluation form. Behavioral Research Methods and Instrumentation 13:464–478, 1981

Mihelich ML: Eye movement desensitization and reprocessing treatment of adjustment disorder. Dissertation Abstracts International 61:1091, 2000

Mok H, Walter C: Brief psychiatric hospitalization: preliminary experience with an urban short-stay unit. Can J Psychiatry 40:415–417, 1995

Nardi C, Lichtenberg P, Kaplan Z: Adjustment disorder of conscripts as a military phobia. Mil Med 159:612–616, 1994

Newell SA, Sanson-Fisher RW, Savolainen NJ: Systematic review of psychological therapies for cancer patients: overview and recommendations for future research. J Natl Cancer Inst 94:558–584, 2002

Nguyen N, Fakra E, Pradel V, et al: Efficacy of etifoxine compared to lorazepam monotherapy in the treatment of patients with adjustment disorders with anxiety: a double-blind controlled study in general practice. Hum Psychopharmacol 21:139–149, 2006

Oxman TE, Barrett JE, Freeman DH, et al: Frequency and correlates of adjustment disorder relates to cardiac surgery in older patients. Psychosomatics 35:557–568, 1994

Pelkonen M, Marttunen M, Henriksson M, et al: Suicidality in adjustment disorder, clinical characteristics of adolescent outpatients. Eur Child Adolesc Psychiatry 14:174–180, 2005

Perez-Jimenez JP, Gomez-Bajo GJ, Lopez-Catillo JJ, et al: Psychiatric consultation and post-traumatic stress disorder in burned patients. Burns 20:532–536, 1994

Popkin MK, Callies AL, Colon EA, et al: Adjustment disorders in medically ill patients referred for consultation in a university hospital. Psychosomatics 31:410–414, 1990

Portzky G, Audenaert K, van Heeringen K: Adjustment disorder and the course of the suicidal process in adolescents. J Affect Disord 87:265–270, 2005

Powell S, McCone D: Treatment of adjustment disorder with anxiety: a September 11, 2001, case study with a 1-year follow-up. Cogn Behav Pract 11:331–336, 2004

Pozzi G, Del Borgo C, Del Forna A, et al: Psychological discomfort and mental illness in patients with AIDS: implications for home care. AIDS Patient Care STDS 13:555–564, 1999

Pulimood S, Rajagopalan B, Rajagopalan M, et al: Psychiatric morbidity among dermatology inpatients. Natl Med J India 9:208–210, 1996

Razavi D, Kormoss N, Collard A, et al: Comparative study of the efficacy and safety of trazodone versus clorazepate in the treatment of adjustment disorders in cancer patients: a pilot study. J Int Med Res 27:264–272, 1999

Reynolds CF: Treatment of depression in special populations. J Clin Psychiatry 53 (9, suppl):45–53, 1992

Rosenberg PB, Ahmed I, Hurwitz S: Methylphenidate in depressed medically ill patients. J Clin Psychiatry 52:263-267, 1991

Runeson BS, Beskow J, Waern M: The suicidal process in suicides among young people. Acta Psychiatr Scand 93:35–42, 1996

Schatzberg AF: Anxiety and adjustment disorder: a treatment approach. J Clin Psychiatry 51 (suppl):20–24, 1990

Schnyder U, Valach L: Suicide attempters in a psychiatric emergency room population. Gen Hosp Psychiatry 19:119–129, 1997

Schulberg HC, Coulehan JL, Block MR, et al: Clinical trials of primary care treatments for major depression: issues in design, recruitment and treatment. Int J Psychiatry Med 23:29–42, 1993

Schulberg HC, Raue PJ, Rollman BL: The effectiveness of psychotherapy in treating depressive disorders in primary care practice: clinical and cost perspectives. Gen Hosp Psychiatry 24:203–212, 2002

Selmi PM, Klein MH, Greist JH, et al: Computer-administered cognitive-behavioral therapy for depression. Am J Psychiatry 147:51–56, 1990

Shaner R: Benzodiazepines in psychiatric emergency settings. Psychiatr Ann 30:268–275, 2000

Shima S, Kitagawa Y, Kitamura T, et al: Poststroke depression. Gen Hosp Psychiatry 16:286–289, 1994

Sifneos PE: Brief dynamic and crisis therapy, in Comprehensive Textbook of Psychiatry IV, 5th Edition, Vol 2. Edited by Kaplan HI, Sadock BJ. Baltimore, MD, Williams & Wilkins, 1989, pp 1562–1567

Slavney PR: Diagnosing demoralization in consultation psychiatry. Psychosomatics 40:325–329, 1999

Snyder S, Strain JJ: Differentiation of major depression and adjustment disorder with depressed mood in the medical setting. Gen Hosp Psychiatry 12:159–165, 1989

Spalletta G, Troisi A, Saracco M, et al: Symptom profile: Axis II comorbidity and suicidal behaviour in young males with DSM-III-R depressive illnesses. J Affect Disord 39:141–148, 1996

Spiegel D: DSM-IV Options Book. Washington, DC, American Psychiatric Association, 1994

Spiegel D: Cancer and depression. Br J Psychiatry 168 (suppl):109–116, 1996

Spiegel, D, Bloom JR, Kramer HJC, et al: Effect of psychosocial treatment on survival of patients with metastatic breast cancer. Lancet 14:88–89, 1989

Stewart JW, Quitkin FM, Klein DF: The pharmacotherapy of minor depression. Am J Psychother 46:23–36, 1992

Strain JJ: Diagnostic considerations in the medical setting. Psychiatr Clin North Am 4:287–300, 1981

Strain JJ, Newcorn J, Wolf D, et al: Considering changes in adjustment disorder. Hosp Community Psychiatry 44:13–15, 1993

Strain JJ, Newcorn JH, Mezzich JE, et al: Adjustment disorder: the MacArthur reanalysis, in DSM-IV Sourcebook, Vol 4. Washington, DC, American Psychiatric Association, 1998a, pp 403–424

Strain JJ, Smith GC, Hammer JS, et al: Adjustment disorder: a multisite study of its utilization and interventions in the consultation-liaison psychiatry setting. Gen Hosp Psychiatry 20:139–149, 1998b

Sullivan MJ, Winshenker B, Mikail S: Screening for major depression in the early stages of multiple sclerosis. Can J Neurol Sci 22:228–231, 1995

True PK, Benway MW: Treatment of stress reaction prior to combat using the "BICEPS" model. Mil Med 157:380–381,1992

Uhlenhuth EH, Balter MB, Ban TA, et al: International study of expert judgment on therapeutic use of benzodiazepines and other psychotherapeutic medications, III: clinical features affecting experts' therapeutic recommendations in anxiety disorders. Psychopharmacol Bull 31:289–296, 1995

van der Klink JJL, van Dijk FJH: Dutch practice guidelines for managing adjustment disorders in occupational and primary health care. Scand J Work Environ Health 29:478–487, 2003

van der Klink JJL, Blonk RWB, Schene AH, et al: Reducing long term sickness absence by an activating intervention in adjustment disorders: a cluster randomized controlled design. Occup Environ Med 60:429–437, 2003

Vlachos IO, Bouras N, Watson JP, et al: Deliberate self-harm referrals. Eur Psychiatry 8:25–28, 1994

Volz HP, Kieser M: Kava-kava extract WS 1490 versus placebo in anxiety disorders: a randomized placebo-controlled 25-week outpatient trial. Pharmacopsychiatry 30:1–5, 1997

Wise MG: Adjustment disorders and impulse disorders not otherwise classified, in American Psychiatric Press Textbook of Psychiatry. Edited by Talbot JA, Hales RE, Yudofsky SC. Washington, DC, American Psychiatric Press, 1988, pp 605–620

Yesavage JA, Brink TL, Rose TL, et al: Development and validation of geriatric depression screening scale: a preliminary report. J Psychiatry Res 17:37–49, 1982–1983

Zarb J: Correlates of depression in cognitively impaired hospitalized elderly referred for neuropsychological assessment. J Clin Exp Neuropsychol 18:713–723, 1996

Zung W: A self-rating depression scale. Arch Gen Psychiatry 12:63–70, 1965

Zung W: A rating instrument for anxiety disorders. Psychosomatics 12:371–379, 1971

19

IMPULSE-CONTROL DISORDERS NOT ELSEWHERE CLASSIFIED

Eric Hollander, M.D.

Heather A. Berlin, D.Phil., M.P.H.

Dan J. Stein, M.D., Ph.D.

Whereas impulse-control disorders (ICDs) were once conceptualized as either addictive or compulsive behaviors, they are now classified within the DSM-IV-TR (American Psychiatric Association 2000) ICD category. These include intermittent explosive disorder (IED; failure to resist aggressive impulses), kleptomania (failure to resist urges to steal items), pyromania (failure to resist urges to set fires), pathological gambling (failure to resist urges to gamble), and trichotillomania (failure to resist urges to pull one's hair) (Table 19–1). However, behaviors characteristic of these disorders may be notable in individuals as symptoms of another mental disorder. If the symptoms progress to such a point that they occur in distinct, frequent episodes and begin to interfere with the person's normal functioning, they may then be classified as a distinct ICD.

There are also a number of other disorders that are not included as a distinct category but are categorized as ICDs not otherwise specified in DSM-IV-TR. These include sexual compulsions (impulsive-compulsive sexual behavior), compulsive shopping (impulsive-compulsive buying disorder), skin picking (impulsive-compulsive psychogenic excoriation), and Internet addiction (impulsive-compulsive computer usage

disorder). One proposal for the research agenda leading up to DSM-V is to include these emerging disorders as new and unique ICDs rather than lumping them together as ICDs not otherwise specified. These disorders are unique in that they share features of both impulsivity and compulsivity and might be labeled as ICDs. Patients afflicted with these disorders engage in the behavior to increase arousal. However, there is a compulsive component in which the patient continues to engage in the behavior to decrease dysphoria. An area of discussion for DSM-V may include whether these disorders should be recognized as distinct ICDs.

In DSM-IV-TR, ICDs are characterized by five stages of symptomatic behavior (Table 19–2). First is the increased sense of tension or arousal, followed by the failure to resist the urge to act. Third, there is a heightened sense of arousal. Once the act has been completed, there is a sense of relief from the urge. Finally, the patient experiences guilt and remorse at having committed the act.

To properly conceptualize ICDs, it is helpful to understand the role of impulsivity within them. Impulsivity is a defining characteristic of many psychiatric illnesses, even those not classified as ICDs, including

TABLE 19–1. DSM-IV-TR impulse-control disorders

Impulse-control disorders not elsewhere classified

Intermittent explosive disorder

Kleptomania

Pyromania

Pathological gambling

Trichotillomania

Impulse-control disorders not otherwise specified

Impulsive-compulsive sexual disorder

Impulsive-compulsive self-injurious disorder

Impulsive-compulsive Internet usage disorder

Impulsive-compulsive buying disorder

Other disorders with impulsivity

Childhood conduct disorders

Binge-eating disorder

Bulimia nervosa

Paraphilias

  Exhibitionism

  Fetishism

  Frotteurism

  Pedophilia

  Sexual masochism

  Sexual sadism

  Transvestic fetishism

  Voyeurism

  Paraphilia not otherwise specified

Bipolar disorder

Attention-deficit/hyperactivity disorder

Substance use disorders

Cluster B personality disorders

Neurological disorder with disinhibition

Source.   American Psychiatric Association 2000.

Cluster B personality disorders such as borderline personality disorder (BPD) and antisocial personality disorder, neurological disorders characterized by disinhibited behavior, attention-deficit/hyperactivity disorder (ADHD), substance and alcohol abuse, conduct

TABLE 19–2. Core features of impulse-control disorders

Essential features	Failure to resist an impulse, drive, or temptation to perform an act that is harmful to the person or to others
Before the act	The individual feels an increasing sense of tension or arousal
At the time of committing the act	The individual experiences pleasure, gratification, or relief
After the act	The individual experiences a sense of relief from the urge The individual may or may not feel regret, self-reproach, or guilt

Source.   American Psychiatric Association 2000.

disorder, binge eating, bulimia, and paraphilias. It is important for clinicians to recognize that individuals who are prone to impulsivity and ICDs are often afflicted with a cluster of related conditions including sexual compulsions, substance use disorders, and posttraumatic stress disorder and to screen for comorbid conditions, such as bipolar spectrum disorders and ADHD, that contribute to impulsivity (Figure 19–1).

Impulsivity research has been conducted both in disorders characterized by impulsivity, such as BPD, antisocial personality disorder, and conduct disorder, and in traditional ICDs, such as IED. As such, the basic tenets of impulsivity can be applied both to the ICDs and to other related psychiatric conditions.

Impulsivity—the failure to resist an impulse, drive, or temptation that is potentially harmful to oneself or others—is both a common clinical problem and a core feature of human behavior. An impulse is rash and lacks deliberation. It may be sudden and ephemeral, or a steady rise in tension may reach a climax in an explosive expression of the impulse, which may result in careless actions without regard for self or others. Impulsivity is evidenced behaviorally as carelessness; an underestimated sense of harm; extraversion; impatience, including the inability to delay gratification; and a tendency toward risk taking, pleasure, and sensation seeking (Hollander 2002). What makes an impulse pathological is an inability to resist it and its expression. The nature of impulsivity as a core symptom domain within the ICDs allows it to be distinguished as either a symptom or a distinct disorder, much in the same way as anxiety or depression.

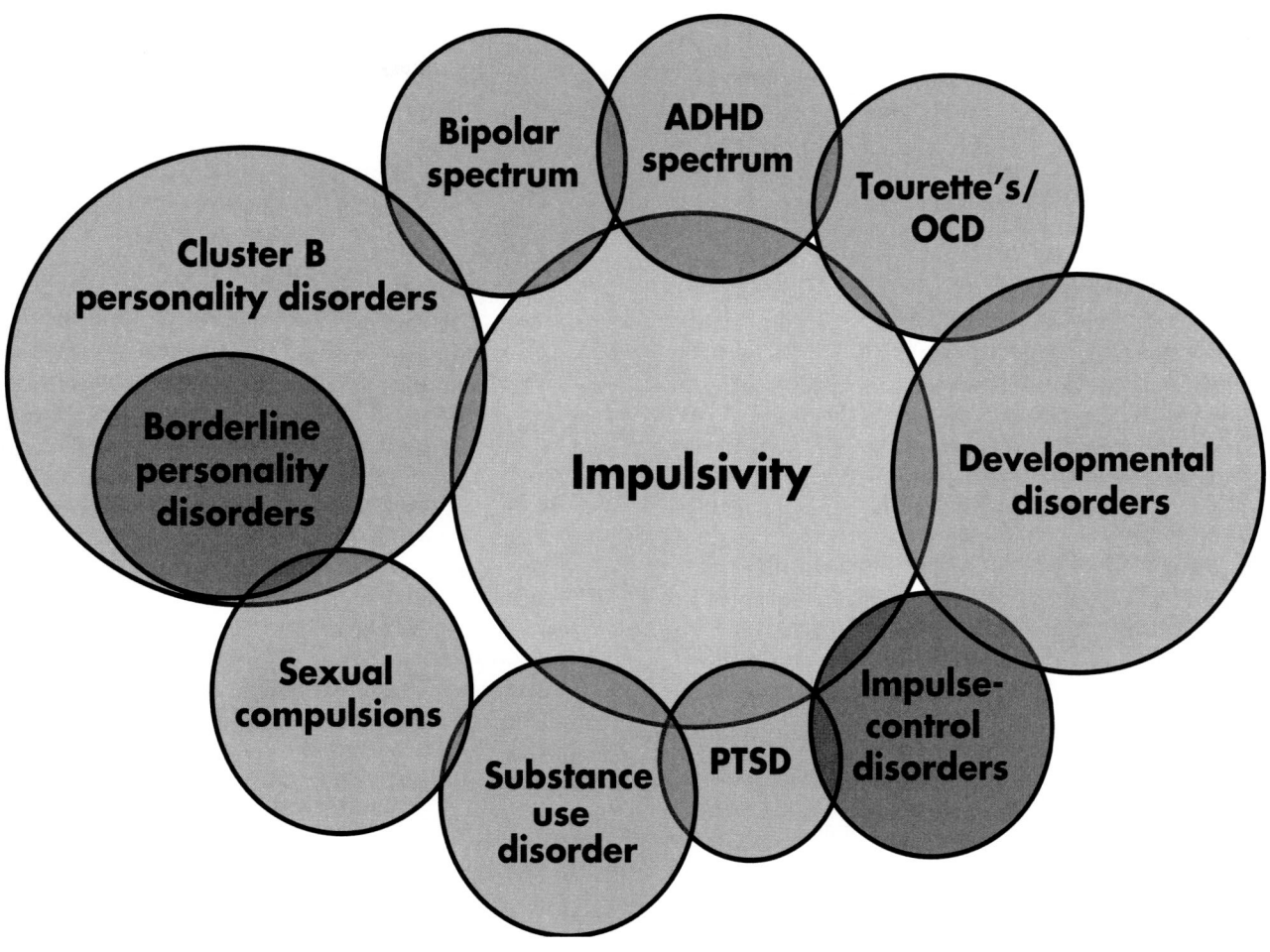

FIGURE 19–1.   Impulsive disorder spectrum.

ADHD=attention-deficit/hyperactivity disorder; OCD=obsessive-compulsive disorder; PTSD=posttraumatic stress disorder.

Source.   Reprinted from Hollander E, Baker BR, Kahn J, et al.: "Conceptualizing and Assessing," in *Clinical Manual of Impulse-Control Disorders.* Edited by Hollander E, Stein DJ. Washington, DC, American Psychiatric Publishing, 2006, pp. 1–18. Copyright 2006, American Psychiatric Publishing. Used with permission.

Intermittent Explosive Disorder

Definition and Diagnostic Criteria

IED is a DSM diagnosis used to describe people with pathological impulsive aggression. Many clinicians and researchers rarely consider this diagnosis, although impulsive aggressive behavior is relatively common. In community surveys, 12%–25% of men and women in the United States reported engaging in physical fights as adults, a frequent manifestation of impulsive aggression (Robins and Regier 1991). Impulsive aggressive behavior usually is pathological and causes substantial psychosocial distress or dysfunction (McElroy et al. 1998). Being on the receiving end of impulsive aggressive behavior can lead to similar behavior in a child who grows up in this environment (Huesmann et al. 1984).

Research Criteria for Intermittent Explosive Disorder–Revised

Due to difficulties with the DSM criteria, until recently little research was done using categorical expressions of impulsive aggression. To use an IED diagnosis in research studies, research criteria were created. The Research Criteria for Intermittent Explosive Disorder—Revised (IED-R) described five criteria for IED, emphasizing the severity, impulsive nature, frequency, and pathology of the impulsive aggressive behavior. Less severe impulsive aggressive behavior (i.e., verbal aggression or aggression toward property) was included because these forms of aggression had been shown to respond to treatment (Coccaro and Kavoussi 1997). The criteria also specified that *impulsive,* not *premeditated,* aggression would be required for this diagnosis. Prior research had shown psychosocial, biological, and treatment response findings specific to only impulsive and not premeditated aggression. A minimal frequency of aggressive acts was required to increase the reliability of the IED diagnosis and exclude those without severe symptoms. Finally, to distinguish the IED diagnosis as pathological, the criteria required the presence of subjective distress and/or social or occupational dysfunction.

IED-R and DSM-IV Criteria: Defining Integrated Research Criteria for Intermittent Explosive Disorder

Although DSM-IV (American Psychiatric Association 1994) made some changes to the IED criteria (Table 19–3), it still did not provide criteria useful for research. The "aggressive impulses" of criterion A are not specific in terms of the type or number of acts or the time frame during which the acts must occur. Apparently, no official guidelines for these items had been determined or considered by the DSM-IV subcommittee.

When the subjects from the original IED-R series were reassessed with Research Criteria for IED-R and DSM-IV IED criteria, 69% met both IED-R and DSM-IV IED diagnoses, 20% met criteria for only DSM-IV IED, and 11% met criteria for only IED-R (Coccaro 2003). Because the two criteria sets did not differentiate groups with different aggression and impulsivity levels, and each alone leaves a number of subjects undiagnosed, Integrated Research Criteria for Intermittent Explosive Disorder (IED-IR) were created to allow subjects from any or both of these groups to be identified.

Epidemiology

DSM-IV-TR describes IED as "apparently rare." However, clinical interview or survey data give a different picture. A number of studies have looked at clinical populations, and one community survey has been done to determine the prevalence of IED. Numbers range between 1.1% and 6.3%. The evaluation of studies is complicated by the variety of defining criteria used, from DSM-III (American Psychiatric Association 1980) to current research criteria and IED-IR. More re-

---

TABLE 19–3.   DSM-IV-TR diagnostic criteria for intermittent explosive disorder

A. Several discrete episodes of failure to resist aggressive impulses that result in serious assaultive acts or destruction of property.

B. The degree of aggressiveness expressed during the episodes is grossly out of proportion to any precipitating psychosocial stressors.

C. The aggressive episodes are not better accounted for by another mental disorder (e.g., antisocial personality disorder, borderline personality disorder, a psychotic disorder, a manic episode, conduct disorder, or attention-deficit/hyperactivity disorder) and are not due to the direct physiological effects of a substance (e.g., a drug of abuse, a medication) or a general medical condition (e.g., head trauma, Alzheimer's disease).

---

cently, Zimmerman et al. (1998) used the Structured Clinical Interview for DSM-IV to study current or lifetime IED in 411 outpatient psychiatric subjects. They reported a rate of 3.8% for current IED and 6.2% for lifetime IED using DSM-IV criteria. A recent reanalysis of a much larger sample from the same population revealed similar rates of IED (Coccaro et al. 2005). Further, data from a pilot community sample study revealed a community rate of lifetime IED by DSM-IV-TR criteria at 4% and by IED-IR criteria at 5.1% (Coccaro et al. 2004). Considering the rates found in these more recent studies, IED could be as common as other major psychiatric disorders such as schizophrenia or bipolar illness. Most of the limited published data on gender differences suggest that males outnumber females with IED. However, more recent data suggest that the male-to-female ratio is approximately 1 to 1 (Coccaro et al. 2005).

Comorbidity

Subjects with IED most frequently have other Axis I and II disorders. The most frequent Axis I diagnoses comorbid with IED lifetime include mood, anxiety, substance, eating, and other ICDs ranging in frequency from 7% to 89% (Coccaro et al. 1998a; McElroy et al. 1998). Such Axis I comorbidity rates raise the question of whether IED constitutes a separate disorder. However, recent data finding earlier onset of IED compared with all disorders, except for phobic-type anxiety disorders, suggest that IED is not secondary to these other disorders (Coccaro et al. 2005).

Bipolar Disorder

McElroy et al. (1998) reported that the aggressive episodes observed in their subjects resembled "microdysphoric" manic episodes. Symptoms in common with both manic and IED episodes included irritability (79%–92%), increased energy (83%–96%), racing thoughts (62%–67%), anxiety (21%–42%), and depressed (dysphoric) mood (17%–33%). However, this finding may not be surprising, because 56% of the subjects in question had a comorbid bipolar diagnosis of some type (bipolar I, 33%; bipolar II, 11%; bipolar not otherwise specified or cyclothymia, 11%). The Rhode Island Hospital Study (Coccaro et al. 2005) suggests a much lower rate of comorbid bipolar illness, with a rate of 11% (bipolar I, 5%; bipolar II, 5%; bipolar not otherwise specified, 1%). Regardless, clinicians should fully evaluate for bipolar disorder prior to determining treatment for IED because mood stabilizers, rather than selective serotonin reuptake inhibitors (SSRIs), would be the first-line treatment for IED comorbid with bipolar disorder.

Other Impulse-Control Disorders

McElroy et al. (1998) reported that up to 44% of their IED subjects had another ICD, such as compulsive buying (37%) or kleptomania (19%). However, in the Coccaro et al. (1998a) study, few IED subjects had a comorbid ICD, and in the Rhode Island Hospital Study, only 5% of IED subjects had another ICD (Coccaro et al. 2005).

Borderline and Antisocial Personality Disorders

Coccaro et al. (1998a) reported the rate of BPD and/or antisocial personality disorder in IED subjects to be 38%. However, rates of IED in subjects with BPD have been noted at 78% and in subjects with antisocial personality disorder at 58% (Coccaro et al. 1998a). A review of unpublished data from the author's (E. Hollander, unpublished, 2005) research program suggests that these rates are lower among subjects not seeking treatment and are lowest in the community (23% for BPD and/or antisocial personality disorder; see also Coccaro et al. 2004). Regardless, BPD and antisocial personality disorder subjects with a comorbid diagnosis of IED do appear to have higher scores for aggression and lower scores for general psychosocial function than do BPD/antisocial personality disorder subjects without IED (Coccaro et al. 2005).

Pathogenesis
Family and Twin Studies

Clinical observation and family history data suggest that IED is familial. Familial aggregation of temper outbursts and IED has been reported in psychiatric patients with "temper problems" (Mattes and Fink 1987), and McElroy et al. (1998) reported that nearly a third of first-degree relatives of IED probands had IED. A recent blinded, controlled family history study using IED-IR criteria (Coccaro 1999) found a morbid risk of IED of 26% in relatives of IED-IR probands compared with 8% among the relatives of control probands, a significant difference. Although twin studies have confirmed the hypothesis that both impulsivity (Seroczynski et al. 1999) and aggression (Coccaro et al. 1997a) are under substantial genetic influence, there are no twin studies of IED itself. Genetic influence for these two traits ranges from 28% to 47%, with nonshared environmental influences making up the lion's share of the remaining variance.

Molecular Genetic Studies

Studies of particular genes in aggressive populations have used the candidate gene approach. *Candidate genes* are the genes for proteins with a suspected, or proven, biological association to a disorder (e.g., serotonin [5-HT] receptors in aggression). The polymorphism HTR1B/G861C and short tandem repeat locus D6S284 are part of the gene for the 5-HT_{1B} receptor for serotonin. These genetic sites were examined in 350 Finnish sibling pairs and 305 Southwestern American Indian sibling pairs, both with a high rate of alcoholism. The diagnoses of antisocial personality disorder and IED were used to examine the traits of impulsivity and aggression. The rate of IED in relatives of antisocial personality disorder probands was 15%, and the relatives of healthy control subjects had neither IED nor antisocial personality disorder. Lappalainen et al. (1998) were able to discover that the gene predisposing to antisocial personality disorder and alcoholism resides close to the HTR1B version of the coding sequence. They concluded that impulsivity and aggression might be influenced, in part, by 5-HT_{1B} receptors. Other candidate genes include the genes for tryptophan hydroxylase and monoamine oxidase-A. Manuck et al. (1999, 2000) revealed an association of the traits of aggression, impulsivity, and serotonin activity (tested by *d,l-Fen* challenge) with variations in both the tryptophan hydroxylase and monoamine oxidase-A genes in community samples.

Biological Correlates

Serotonin and other centrally acting neurotransmitters are the most studied biological factors in aggression. Measures examining central (as well as peripheral) serotonin function correlate inversely with life history, questionnaire, and laboratory measures of aggression. This relationship has been demonstrated by cerebrospinal fluid 5-hydroxyindoleacetic acid (CSF 5-HIAA; Linnoila et al. 1983; Virkkunen et al. 1994), physiological responses to serotonin agonist probes (Coccaro et al. 1989, 1997b; Dolan et al. 2001; Manuck et al. 1998), and platelet measures of serotonin activity (Birmaher et al. 1990; Coccaro et al. 1996). The type of aggression associated with reduced central serotonin function appears to be *impulsive,* as opposed to *nonimpulsive,* aggression (Linnoila et al. 1983; Virkkunen et al. 1994). These findings suggest that impulsive aggressive behavior can be distinguished biologically from nonimpulsive aggression. Interestingly, the inverse relationship between aggression and serotonin is not observed when catecholamine system function is impaired (Coccaro et al. 1989; Wetzler et al. 1991).

There is also evidence to support the role of other nonserotonergic brain systems and modulators in impulsive aggression. These findings suggest a facilitating role for dopamine (DePue et al. 1994), norepinephrine (Coccaro et al. 1991), vasopressin (Coccaro et al. 1998b), brain-derived neurotrophic factor (Lyons et al. 1991), opiates (Post et al. 1984), and testosterone (Giammanco et al. 2005; Virkkunen et al. 1994) and an inhibitory interaction between neuronal nitric oxide synthase and testosterone in rodents (Kriegsfeld et al. 1997).

Imaging and Brain Localization

Few localization and functional studies have looked at impulsive aggression or IED. Using fluorodeoxyglucose positron emission tomography (PET), Siever et al. (1999) found blunted glucose utilization responses to serotonin stimulation in the orbitofrontal cortex (an area associated with impulsive aggression) of IED subjects with BPD. A similar finding was reported in the anterior cingulate and anteromedial orbital cortex of impulsive aggressive subjects after stimulation with the direct serotonin agonist *m*-chlorophenylpiperazine (New et al. 2002). Using PET with a $5-HT_{1A}$ antagonist in healthy volunteers, Parsey et al. (2002) found a significant inverse correlation between lifetime aggression and serotonin receptor binding in the dorsal raphe, anterior cingulate cortex, amygdala, medial prefrontal cortex (PFC), and orbital PFC. Using neuropsychological testing in impulsive aggressive subjects, Best et al.'s (2002) data supported a possible dysfunc-

tional frontal circuit. More work is needed to reveal the specific functional brain abnormalities in impulsive aggressive individuals.

Course

Limited research is available concerning the age at onset and natural course of IED. However, according to DSM-IV-TR, the onset appears to be from childhood to the early 20s. The age at onset and course of IED distinguish it as separate from its comorbid diagnoses. The course of IED is variable, with an episodic course in some and a more chronic course in others. A mean age at onset of 16 years and an average duration of about 20 years have been described (McElroy et al. 1998). Preliminary data (Coccaro et al. 2005) confirm these findings and indicate that onset of DSM-IV-TR IED occurs by the end of the first decade in 31%, by the end of the second decade in 44%, by the end of the third decade in 19%, and by the end of the fourth decade in only 6%.

The mode of onset of IED is abrupt and without a prodromal period. Episodes typically last less than 30 minutes and involve physical assault, verbal assault, and/or destruction of property. If provocation is involved, it is usually from a known person and is seemingly minor in nature (McElroy et al. 1998). Many individuals frequently have minor aggressive episodes in the interim between severely aggressive/destructive episodes. Considerable distress and social, financial, occupational, or legal consequences typically result from these episodes.

Treatment

There are few studies in which subjects with IED have been the focus of treatment. There are, however, a number of studies concerning the treatment of impulsive aggression in related subjects (Table 19–4).

Pharmacotherapy

A number of medications have been used to treat impulsive aggression, such as tricyclic antidepressants, benzodiazepines, mood stabilizers, and neuroleptics. Recently, pharmacotherapy studies of aggression have turned to SSRIs and mood stabilizers as first-line treatments. Fluoxetine and other SSRIs have been studied in impulsive aggressive subjects and IED patients. In a treatment trial of subjects meeting IED-IR criteria, impulsive aggressive behavior did respond to fluoxetine (Coccaro and Kavoussi 1997), but non-serotonin-specific antidepressants had little benefit for impulsive aggression and many side effects in treatment studies.

TABLE 19–4. **Intermittent explosive disorder: treatment summary**

Authors	Treatment	Description
Pharmacotherapy		
Coccaro and Kavoussi 1997	Fluoxetine	Double-blind, placebo-controlled; subjects meeting IED-IR criteria; reduced impulsive aggression
Soloff et al. 1986a	Amitriptyline	Double-blind, placebo-controlled; BPD and SPD inpatients; affective symptoms improved; impulsivity and aggression worsened
Cornelius et al. 1993 Soloff et al. 1993	Phenelzine vs. haloperidol	Double-blind, placebo-controlled; BPD inpatients; phenelzine produced moderate reduction in anger and hostility; only minor benefits in depression and irritability after 16 weeks
Cowdry and Gardner 1988	Alprazolam, tranylcypromine, carbamazepine, trifluoperazine	Double-blind, placebo-controlled, crossover; treatment-resistant BPD outpatients with history of impulsive aggression; improved with tranylcypromine, carbamazepine (decreased behavioral dyscontrol severity and frequency of impulsive aggression episodes; 18% had worsening of mood), and trifluoperazine (improved depression and anxiety objective, not subjective, ratings); increased severity and frequency of episodes of serious dyscontrol with alprazolam
Links et al. 1990	Lithium vs. desipramine	Placebo-controlled; BPD outpatients; objective ratings of anger and suicidality improved with lithium; no improvement in mood
Sheard et al. 1976	Lithium	Double-blind, placebo-controlled; chronically impulsive aggressive prisoners; significant reduction in objective (not subjective) aggressive behavior
Barratt et al. 1997	Phenytoin	Double-blind, placebo-controlled, crossover; impulsive aggressive prisoners; reduced impulsive aggressive acts, but not premeditated aggressive acts
Kavoussi and Coccaro 1998	Divalproex	Open-label trial; variety of personality disorders resistant to SSRIs; decreased irritability and impulsive aggression
Hollander et al. 2003	Divalproex	Double-blind, placebo-controlled; Cluster B personality disorder; decreased impulsive aggression, irritability, and global severity
Soloff et al. 1986b, 1989	Haloperidol vs. amitriptyline	Double-blind, placebo-controlled; BPD inpatients; with haloperidol, decreased symptom severity; depression, hostile depression, anxiety, hostility, impulsivity, schizotypal symptoms, paranoid ideation, psychoticism; improved global functioning

TABLE 19–4. Intermittent explosive disorder: treatment summary *(continued)*

Authors	Treatment	Description
Montgomery and Montgomery 1982	Flupenthixol	Placebo-controlled; people with history of suicidal and parasuicidal behavior; decreased suicidal and parasuicidal behavior
Zanarini and Frankenburg 2001	Olanzapine	Double-blind, placebo-controlled; BPD patients; improved anger, hostility, impulsivity, and interpersonal relationships, but not depression
Psychotherapy		
Grodnitzky and Tafrate 2000	Imaginal exposure therapy	Adult outpatients referred for anger management; decreased anger and habituated to anger-provoking scenarios
Deffenbacher et al. 2000, 2002	Relaxation training; relaxation training plus cognitive therapy	Controlled trial; college students with high driving anger; decreased trait anger and driving anger
Linehan et al. 1994	Dialectical behavior therapy vs. treatment as usual	Chronically suicidal BPD patients; improvement in anger, social adjustment, and global functioning

Note. BPD=borderline personality disorder; IED-IR=Integrated Research Criteria for Intermittent Explosive Disorder; SPD=schizotypal personality disorder; SSRI=selective serotonin reuptake inhibitor.

Soloff et al. (1986a) found that affective symptoms improved with amitriptyline in some BPD and schizotypal personality disorder inpatients, but impulsivity and aggression worsened in a set of patients, perhaps due to the noradrenergic effects of tricyclic antidepressants (Links et al. 1990). Thus, clinicians should be cautious when using the new dual-action antidepressants in these patients.

Monoamine oxidase inhibitors such as tranylcypromine and phenelzine have also been studied in impulsively aggressive subjects. In a double-blind study, Soloff et al. (1993) found that compared with placebo and haloperidol, phenelzine produced a moderate reduction in anger and hostility in BPD patients. Yet a 16-week continuation phase revealed that the subjects had experienced only minor benefits in depression and irritability and remained substantially impaired after the treatment phase (Cornelius et al. 1993; Soloff et al. 1993). In a double-blind crossover trial (Cowdry and Gardner 1988), treatment-resistant BPD patients with a history of impulsive aggression showed improvement with tranylcypromine, carbamazepine (decreased severity of behavioral dyscontrol), and trifluoperazine but had an increase in the severity and frequency of the episodes of serious dyscontrol with alprazolam. Benzodiazepine treatment might have released the subjects' control or inhibition of these episodes.

Mood stabilizers have also been used to treat aggression. Links et al. (1990) found objective ratings of anger and suicidality in BPD outpatients improved the most on lithium compared with desipramine and placebo, but subjects and their clinicians did not report any improvement in mood. Sheard et al. (1976) found an improvement using lithium versus placebo in chronically aggressive prisoners. Again, however, only objective findings supported this; no improvement was reported subjectively. Barratt et al. (1997) also reported a reduction in aggression with phenytoin in impulsive aggressive prisoners.

The other mood stabilizers studied for impulsive aggression are carbamazepine and divalproex. In the Cowdry and Gardner (1988) study, carbamazepine lessened episodes of impulsive aggression in BPD subjects, but 18% of subjects had a worsening of mood that improved once carbamazepine was stopped. Kavoussi and Coccaro (1998) and Hollander et al. (2003) reported an anti-aggressive effect of divalproex sodium in IED subjects with a Cluster B personality disorder. Given the relative adverse event profiles for SSRIs versus mood stabilizers, it is likely that clinical treatment of IED patients should start with SSRIs unless the subject is extremely aggressive or has a history of a bipolar disorder, in which case treatment with a mood stabilizer would be more appropriate.

The neuroleptics haloperidol, trifluoperazine, and depot flupenthixol have all been studied in BPD patients. Cowdry and Gardner's (1988) subjects showed significant improvement in depression and anxiety objective ratings with trifluoperazine, but subjective ratings did not support this. Trifluoperazine was seen as less useful than tranylcypromine (a monoamine oxidase inhibitor) and carbamazepine in improving behavior and affect among subjects. Soloff et al. (1986b, 1989) found that BPD inpatients improved on hostility and global function measurements with haloperidol, but considerable depression remained. Montgomery and Montgomery (1982) found that suicidal and parasuicidal behavior, in subjects with a history of such behaviors, decreased in a depot flupenthixol treatment group versus a placebo group. Zanarini and Frankenburg (2001) compared the atypical antipsychotic olanzapine with placebo in outpatients with BPD. The treatment improved anger, hostility, and other symptoms but did not improve depression, and patients remained quite ill.

Psychotherapy

Anger treatment studies focus on treatment of anger as a component of other psychiatric illnesses such as substance abuse, posttraumatic stress disorder, depression, and domestic violence and in forensic and mentally impaired populations. Therapy for anger and aggression focuses on cognitive-behavioral group therapy. In a few rare cases, anger is addressed as the primary or only problem, and a limited number of treatments have been described. Imaginal exposure therapy, used frequently in anxiety disorders, was studied in a noncontrolled pilot study of anger treatment (Grodnitzky and Tafrate 2000). Subjects habituated to anger-provoking scenarios, and the treatment was felt to be useful.

In a controlled trial of college students with high levels of driving anger, Deffenbacher et al. (2000) compared pure relaxation training with relaxation training combined with cognitive therapy and an assessment-only control. Neither treatment condition improved general trait anger, but both treatments improved driving anger. When repeated in a new population of drivers with higher anger levels, both treatments lowered trait anger (Deffenbacher et al. 2002). Because relaxation training with cognitive therapy provided little gain over pure relaxation training, relaxation training in itself may be adequate treatment for driving anger.

Other versions of cognitive-behavioral therapy (CBT), such as dialectical behavior therapy, have been studied in BPD patients. One study showed improvement in anger, social adjustment, and global function-

ing compared with a treatment-as-usual condition (Linehan et al. 1994). Improvement in anger and impulsivity has been shown with dialectical behavior therapy across many disorders. There are no published double-blind, placebo-controlled studies on IED subjects in therapy, but studies of therapy for IED subjects are ongoing.

Kleptomania
Definition and Diagnostic Criteria

Kleptomania was officially designated a psychiatric disorder in 1980 in DSM-III, and in DSM-III-R (American Psychiatric Association 1987) it was grouped under the category "disorders of impulse control not elsewhere classified." Kleptomania is currently classified in DSM-IV-TR as an ICD, but it is still poorly understood and has received very little empirical study. The DSM-IV-TR criteria for kleptomania are listed in Table 19–5.

Criterion A, which focuses on the senselessness of the items stolen, has often been considered the criterion that distinguishes kleptomania patients from ordinary shoplifters (Goldman 1991), but interpretation of this criterion is controversial. The archetype of the middle-aged female kleptomania patient who steals peculiar items may not adequately account for all people with kleptomania (Goldman 1991; McElroy et al. 1991a). Patients with kleptomania may in fact desire the items they steal and be able to use them, but they do not need them. This may be particularly the case with kleptomania patients who hoard items (Goldman 1991), for which multiple versions of the same item are usually not needed, but the item itself may be desired and may be of practical use to the patient.

Patients with kleptomania often report amnesia surrounding the act of shoplifting (Goldman 1991; Grant 2004) and deny feelings of tension or arousal prior to shoplifting and feelings of pleasure or relief after the thefts. They often recall entering and leaving a store but have no memory of events in the store, including the theft (Grant 2004). Other patients, who are not amnestic for the thefts, describe shoplifting as "automatic" or "a habit" and may also deny feelings of tension prior to a theft or pleasure after the act (DSM-IV-TR criterion B or C), although they report an inability to control their shoplifting (criterion A). Some patients report that they felt tension and pleasure when they started stealing, but it became a "habit" over time. Some speculate that patients who are amnestic for shoplifting or who shoplift "out of habit" represent two subtypes of kleptomania.

TABLE 19–5. DSM-IV-TR diagnostic criteria for kleptomania

A. Recurrent failure to resist impulses to steal objects that are not needed for personal use or for their monetary value.

B. Increasing sense of tension immediately before committing the theft.

C. Pleasure, gratification, or relief at the time of committing the theft.

D. The stealing is not committed to express anger or vengeance and is not in response to a delusion or a hallucination.

E. The stealing is not better accounted for by conduct disorder, a manic episode, or antisocial personality disorder.

Epidemiology

Although preliminary evidence suggests that the lifetime prevalence of kleptomania may be approximately 0.6% (Goldman 1991), this figure may be an underestimate. The shame and embarrassment associated with stealing prevent most people from voluntarily reporting kleptomania symptoms (Grant and Kim 2002c). No national epidemiological studies of kleptomania have been performed, but studies of kleptomania in various clinical samples suggest a higher prevalence. A recent study in the United States of 204 adult psychiatric inpatients with multiple disorders revealed that kleptomania may in fact be fairly common. The study found that 7.8% ($n=16$) endorsed current symptoms consistent with a diagnosis of kleptomania and 9.3% ($n=19$) had a lifetime diagnosis of kleptomania (Grant et al. 2005). Kleptomania appeared equally common in patients with mood, anxiety, substance use, or psychotic disorders. These findings are further supported by two French studies. One study of 107 inpatients with depression found that 4 (3.7%) had kleptomania (Lejoyeux et al. 2002); in another study of 79 inpatients with alcohol dependence, 3 patients (3.8%) reported symptoms consistent with kleptomania (Lejoyeux et al. 1999). In two studies examining comorbidity in pathological gamblers, rates of comorbid kleptomania were found to range from 2.1% to 5% (Grant and Kim 2003; Specker et al. 1995). A study of bulimia patients found that 24% met DSM-III criteria for kleptomania (Hudson et al. 1983).

The literature clearly suggests that the majority of patients with kleptomania are women (e.g., Grant and Kim 2002b; McElroy et al. 1991b; Presta et al. 2002). One explanation for this is that kleptomania occurs more frequently in women, but another reason may be that women are more likely to present for psychiatric evaluation. The courts may send male shoplifters to prison while sending female shoplifters for psychiatric evaluation (Goldman 1991). The severity of kleptomania symptoms and the clinical presentation of symptoms do not appear to differ based on gender (Grant and Kim 2002b).

Comorbidity

High rates of other psychiatric disorders have been found in patients with kleptomania and have sparked debate over the proper characterization of this disorder. Rates of lifetime comorbid affective disorders range from 59% (Grant and Kim 2002b) to 100% (McElroy et al. 1991b). The rate of lifetime comorbid bipolar disorder has been reported as ranging from 9% (Grant and Kim 2002b) to 27% (Bayle et al. 2003) to 60% (McElroy et al. 1991b). Studies have also found high lifetime rates of comorbid anxiety disorders (60%–80%; McElroy et al. 1991b, 1992), ICDs (20%–46%; Grant and Kim 2003), substance use disorders (23%–50%; Grant and Kim 2002b; McElroy et al. 1991b), and eating disorders (60%; McElroy et al. 1991b). Personality disorders have been found in 43%–55% of patients with kleptomania, the most common being paranoid personality disorder and histrionic personality disorder (Bayle et al. 2003; Grant 2004).

Pathogenesis
Biological Theories

Serotonin and inhibition.   Patients with kleptomania report significant elevations of impulsivity and risk taking compared with control subjects (Bayle et al. 2003; Grant and Kim 2002d), and diminished inhibitory mechanisms may underlie the risk-taking behavior of kleptomania. The most well-studied inhibitory pathways involve serotonin and the PFC (Chambers et al. 2003). Decreased measures of serotonin have long been associated with a variety of adult risk-taking behaviors including alcoholism, fire setting, and pathological gambling (Moreno et al. 1991; Virkkunen et al. 1994). Blunted serotonergic responses in the ventromedial PFC have been seen in people with impulsive aggression (New et al. 2002), and this region has also been implicated in poor decision making (Bechara 2003), as seen in those with kleptomania.

Although there are few biological studies of kleptomania, early evidence may support a theory of serotonergic involvement in the disorder. One study found a lower number of the platelet serotonin transporter in kleptomania patients versus healthy control subjects (Marazziti et al. 2000). Pharmacological case studies suggest that serotonin reuptake inhibitors such as clomipramine and the SSRIs (Lepkifker et al. 1999; McElroy et al. 1991b) may reduce the impulsive behavior associated with kleptomania.

Dopamine and reward deficiency.   Dopaminergic systems influencing rewarding and reinforcing behaviors have also been implicated in ICDs and may play a role in the pathogenesis of kleptomania. One proposed mechanism is "reward deficiency syndrome," a hypothesized hypodopaminergic state involving multiple genes and environmental stimuli that puts an individual at high risk for multiple addictive impulsive and compulsive behaviors (Blum et al. 2000). Alterations in dopaminergic pathways have been proposed as underlying the seeking of rewards (e.g., shoplifting) that trigger the release of dopamine and produce feelings of pleasure (Blum et al. 2000). Furthermore, dopamine release into the nucleus accumbens has been implicated in the translation of motivated drive into action, serving as a "go" signal (Chambers et al. 2003). Dopamine release into the nucleus accumbens seems maximal when reward probability is most uncertain, suggesting it plays a central role in guiding behavior during risk-taking situations (Fiorillo et al. 2003). The structure and function of dopamine neurons within the nucleus accumbens, in conjunction with glutamatergic afferent and intrinsic γ-aminobutyric acid (GABA)-ergic activities, appear to change in response to experiences that influence the function of the nucleus accumbens. Thus, future behavior may be determined in part by prior rewarding experiences via neuroplastic changes in the nucleus accumbens. This may explain why, over time, many kleptomania patients report shoplifting "out of habit" even without a pronounced urge or craving.

Opioid system, cravings, and pleasure.   Preclinical and clinical studies demonstrate that the underlying biological mechanism of urge-based disorders may involve the processing of incoming reward inputs by the ventral tegmental area–nucleus accumbens–orbitofrontal cortex (VTA-NA-OFC) circuit (Hyman 1993; Koob and Bloom 1988), which modulates animal and human motivation (e.g., urges, cravings). Dopamine may play a major role in the regulation of this region (Koob 1992).

Kleptomaniacs report frequent urges to steal that result in theft two times per week, on average (Grant and Kim 2002b). Thus, urges linked to the experienc-

ing of reward and pleasure may represent an important clinical target in treating kleptomania. Many indicate that the act of stealing reduces the urges or the tension these urges produce (McElroy et al. 1991b). Although many report the urges as intrusive, the act of stealing is often a "thrill" for some, producing a pleasurable feeling (Goldman 1991; Grant and Kim 2002b). The μ-opioid system is thought to underlie urge regulation by processing reward, pleasure, and pain at least in part via modulation of dopamine neurons in mesolimbic pathway through GABA interneurons (Potenza and Hollander 2002). Studies of naltrexone, a μ-opioid antagonist, have demonstrated its efficacy in reducing urges in those with kleptomania and other ICDs (Dannon et al. 1999; Grant and Kim 2002c; Kim et al. 2001). Naltrexone may be effective by modulating dopamine function within the VTA-NA-OFC circuit via the antagonism of opioid receptors in the ventral tegmental area (Broekkamp and Phillips 1979).

In summary, repeated kleptomanic behavior may be a result of an imbalance between a pathologically increased urge and a pathologically decreased inhibition. The repeated shoplifting may therefore be due to increased activity of the mesocorticolimbic dopamine circuitry, indirectly enhanced through the opioid system, and decreased activity in the cortical inhibitor processes, largely influenced via serotonin.

Psychological Theories

Kleptomania may result from an attempt to relieve feelings of depression through stimulation (Goldman 1991; McElroy et al. 1991a). Risk-taking behavior may produce an antidepressant effect for some patients (Fishbain 1987; Goldman 1991). Shoplifting may distract depressed patients from stressors and unpleasant cognitions. Ironically, problems resulting directly from shoplifting (e.g., embarrassment and shame from getting caught) may in turn lead to even more shoplifting as a misguided means of symptom management (Goldman 1991). The self-medication hypothesis of shoplifting is supported by reports from patients with kleptomania of high lifetime rates of depression (45%–100%; Bayle et al. 2003; McElroy et al. 1991b), which usually (60% of cases) precedes the kleptomanic behavior (McElroy et al. 1991b). Furthermore, several case studies report patients who described shoplifting as relief for their depressed moods (Fishbain 1987) and suggest that kleptomania symptoms improve with antidepressants (Lepkifker et al. 1999; McElroy et al. 1991b).

Behavioral models also provide clues as to the pathogenesis of kleptomania. From an operant viewpoint, the positive reinforcer in kleptomania is the acquisition of items for nothing, and the intermittent reinforcement (e.g., not always being able to shoplift because of store security) of kleptomanic behavior may therefore be particularly resistant to extinction. Physiological arousal related to shoplifting (Goldman 1991) may be another reinforcer that initiates and perpetuates the behavior. Negative reinforcement (i.e., involving the removal of a punishing stimulus) hypothesizes that shoplifting is performed to experience relief from the aversive arousal of urges. The self-medication theory of kleptomania may represent a negative reinforcement. This could explain why kleptomaniac behavior continues despite the offender being frequently apprehended.

There may also be specific cognitive errors that are directly linked to kleptomanic behavior: 1) belief that only shoplifting will reduce the urge or the depressive state, 2) selective memory (e.g., remembering the thrill of shoplifting and ignoring the shame and embarrassment from being apprehended), and 3) erroneous self-assessment (e.g., that one deserves to be caught stealing because one is not intrinsically worth anything). A biopsychological perspective will most likely provide the most useful understanding for the treatment and prevention of kleptomania.

Course

Kleptomania may begin in childhood, adolescence, or adulthood and sometimes in late adulthood. However, most patients have an onset of symptoms before age 21 years (i.e., by late adolescence; Goldman 1991; Grant and Kim 2002b; McElroy et al. 1991a, 1991b; Presta et al. 2002). Onset beyond 50 years of age is unusual, and in some of these cases, remote histories of past kleptomania can be elicited (Goldman 1991). Most clinical samples of kleptomania patients report shoplifting for more than 10 years prior to entering treatment (Goldman 1991; Grant and Kim 2002c; McElroy et al. 1991b).

Due to the sparse data on the course of kleptomania and the unavailability of longitudinal studies, the prognosis is not clearly known. However, without treatment the behavior may persist for decades, despite multiple convictions for shoplifting (arrest or imprisonment), with transient periods of remission. Three typical courses have been described: sporadic with brief episodes and long periods of remission; episodic with protracted periods of stealing and periods of remission; and chronic with varying intensity (American Psychiatric Association 2000). Fifteen or 16 years may pass before an individual seeks treatment (Goldman 1991; McElroy et al. 1991a). At peak frequency, McElroy et al. (1991a) found a mean of 27 episodes of theft per month, with one patient reporting as many as 4 thefts per day.

Treatment

Studies of treatment approaches for kleptomania are summarized in Table 19–6.

Pharmacotherapy

No medication is currently approved by the U.S. Food and Drug Administration for treating kleptomania, so it is important to inform patients of "off-label" uses of medications for this disorder and the empirical basis for considering medication treatment.

Only case reports, two small case series, and one open-label study of pharmacotherapy have been conducted for kleptomania. Various medications—tricyclic antidepressants, SSRIs (Lepkifker et al. 1999), mood stabilizers, and opioid antagonists—have been examined for the treatment of kleptomania (Grant and Kim 2002c; McElroy et al. 1989). McElroy et al. (1991b) reported treatment response in 10 of 20 patients with the following single agents: fluoxetine, nortriptyline, trazodone, clonazepam, valproate, and lithium. Other agents used successfully as monotherapy for kleptomania include fluvoxamine (Chong and Low 1996) and paroxetine (Kraus 1999). Combinations of medications have also been effective in case reports: lithium plus fluoxetine (Burstein 1992), fluvoxamine plus buspirone (Durst et al. 1997), fluoxetine plus lithium, fluoxetine plus imipramine (McElroy et al. 1991b), and fluvoxamine plus valproate (Kmetz et al. 1997).

The findings from case reports have not been consistent. Seven cases of fluoxetine, three of imipramine, two of lithium as monotherapy, two of lithium augmentation, four of tranylcypromine, and one of carbamazepine combined with clomipramine all failed to reduce kleptomania symptoms (McElroy et al. 1991b). Some evidence suggests that SSRIs may even induce kleptomania symptoms (Kindler et al. 1997). A case series found that kleptomania symptoms respond to topiramate (Dannon 2003). In another case series, the two subjects treated with naltrexone responded to medication (Dannon et al. 1999).

In the only open-label medication trial for kleptomania, naltrexone (mean effective dosage, 145 mg/day) resulted in a significant decline in the intensity of urges to steal, stealing thoughts, and stealing behavior (Grant and Kim 2002c). A lower dosage, possibly 50 mg/day, may be effective in younger people with kleptomania (Grant and Kim 2002a). Opioid antagonists

TABLE 19–6. **Kleptomania: treatment summary**

Authors	Treatment	Description
Pharmacotherapy		
Lepkifker et al. 1999	Fluoxetine or paroxetine plus psychotherapy	Kleptomania patients ($n=5$); successfully treated
McElroy et al. 1989	Fluoxetine, trazodone, or tranylcypromine	Kleptomania and bulimia nervosa patients ($n=3$); partial or complete response of both bulimic and kleptomanic
McElroy et al. 1991b	Fluoxetine, nortriptyline, trazodone, clonazepam, valproate, lithium	Kleptomania patients ($n=20$); 10 of 20 responded to treatment
Chong and Low 1996	Fluvoxamine	Kleptomania patient ($n=1$); successfully treated with fluvoxamine; failed to respond to psychotherapy, behavioral therapy, and pharmacotherapy with clomipramine, imipramine, and lithium
Kraus 1999	Paroxetine	Kleptomania patient ($n=1$); successfully treated
Burstein 1992	Lithium plus fluoxetine	Kleptomania patient ($n=1$); successfully treated
Durst et al. 1997	Fluvoxamine plus buspirone	Kleptomania patient ($n=1$); successfully treated
McElroy et al. 1991b	Fluoxetine plus imipramine Fluoxetine plus lithium	Kleptomania patient ($n=1$); remission with fluoxetine plus imipramine Kleptomania patient ($n=1$); partial response with fluoxetine plus lithium
Kmetz et al. 1997	Fluvoxamine plus valproate	Kleptomania patient ($n=1$); successfully treated
Kindler et al. 1997	Selective serotonin reuptake inhibitors (SSRIs)	Depressed patients ($n=3$); induced kleptomanic behavior
Dannon 2003	Topiramate (alone or plus SSRIs)	Kleptomania patients ($n=3$); responded well
Dannon et al. 1999	Naltrexone	Kleptomania patients ($n=2$); responded well
Grant and Kim 2002a	Naltrexone	Adolescent with kleptomania ($n=1$); responded to treatment
Grant and Kim 2002c	Naltrexone	Only open-label medication trial for kleptomania ($n=10$); reduced urges to steal, stealing thoughts, and stealing behavior; improved social and occupational functioning
Psychotherapy		
Fishbain 1988 Schwartz 1992	Psychoanalysis	Limited success for kleptomania symptoms, but usually with the addition of medication

TABLE 19–6. **Kleptomania: treatment summary** *(continued)*

Authors	Treatment	Description
McElroy et al. 1991b	Insight-oriented psychotherapy	Kleptomania patients (*n*=11); unsuccessful
Gauthier and Pellerin 1982 Glover 1985 Keutzer 1972	Behavioral therapy (i.e., covert sensitization, exposure and response prevention, conditioning)	Successfully treated some cases of kleptomania
McConaghy and Blaszczynski 1988	Imaginal desensitization	Compulsive shoplifting (*n*=2); complete remission
Gudjonsson 1987	Substitution of urges to steal with alternative sources of satisfaction/excitement	Kleptomania patient (*n*=1); successfully treated for 5 months; reported 2 years of symptom remission

such as naltrexone may be effective in reducing both the urges to shoplift and the shoplifting behavior by reducing the "thrill" associated with shoplifting and thus preventing the positive reinforcement of the behavior. Antidepressants, particularly those that influence serotonergic systems (e.g., serotonin reuptake inhibitors), may also be effective in reducing the symptoms of kleptomania by targeting serotonergic systems implicated in impaired impulse regulation. If kleptomania represents both impaired urge regulation and inhibition of behavior, both opioid antagonists and antidepressants may play a pivotal role in controlling this behavior.

Psychotherapy

Many different kinds of psychotherapy have been tried in the treatment of kleptomania. The success of these therapies exists only in case reports, with no published controlled trials of therapy. Psychoanalysis has resulted in some limited success for kleptomania symptoms, but usually with the addition of medication (Fishbain 1988; Schwartz 1992). Insight-oriented psychotherapy, however, has been unsuccessful in treating this disorder in 11 published cases (McElroy et al. 1991b). Behavioral therapies such as covert sensitization, exposure and response prevention, and conditioning have successfully treated some cases of kleptomania (Gauthier and Pellerin 1982; Glover 1985; Keutzer 1972).

Imaginal desensitization uses the idea of imagining the steps of stealing while maintaining a relaxed state. The patient then images the potential scene of stealing but also imagines his or her ability to not steal in that context. Undergoing fourteen 15-minute sessions over 5 days, two patients reported complete remission of symptoms for a 2-year period (McConaghy and Blaszczynski 1988). Learning to substitute alternative sources of satisfaction and excitement when urges

to steal occur was successful in a woman treated weekly for 5 months who later reported 2 years of remitted symptoms (Gudjonsson 1987).

Because few empirical studies are available, research is needed to guide the selection of which psychotherapy to utilize and to investigate the combination of medication and psychotherapy in treating patients with kleptomania.

Pyromania
Definition and Diagnostic Criteria

The essential feature of pyromania is multiple deliberate and purposeful (rather than accidental) fire setting (Table 19–7). The fire-setting behavior is primary, unrelated to another psychiatric state or to ideology, vengeance, or criminality, and does not result from impaired judgment (e.g., in dementia or mental retardation). DSM-IV-TR also excludes "communicative arson," by which some individuals with mental disorders or personality disorders use fire to communicate a desire or need.

Another important clinical feature of pyromania is the fascination of subjects with fire. People with pyromania like watching fire. They are often recognized as regular "watchers" at fires in their neighborhoods. They may like setting off false fire alarms. Their fascination with fire leads some to seek employment or to volunteer as a firefighter. Patients may be indifferent to the consequences of the fire for life or property or may get satisfaction from the resulting destruction. Their behaviors may lead to property damage, legal consequences, or injury or loss of life to themselves or others.

Recent diagnostic classifications include pyromania among the ICDs. Although the fire setting results

TABLE 19–7. DSM-IV-TR diagnostic criteria for pyromania

A. Deliberate and purposeful fire setting on more than one occasion.

B. Tension or affective arousal before the act.

C. Fascination with, interest in, curiosity about, or attraction to fire and its situational contexts (e.g., paraphernalia, uses, consequences).

D. Pleasure, gratification, or relief when setting fires, or when witnessing or participating in their aftermath.

E. The fire setting is not done for monetary gain, as an expression of sociopolitical ideology, to conceal criminal activity, to express anger or vengeance, to improve one's living circumstances, in response to a delusion or hallucination, or as a result of impaired judgment (e.g., in dementia, mental retardation, substance intoxication).

F. The fire setting is not better accounted for by conduct disorder, a manic episode, or antisocial personality disorder.

from a failure to resist an impulse, there may be important preparation of the fire (Wise and Tierney 1999). The person may leave obvious clues of his or her fire preparation. Pyromania, however, is considered an uncontrolled and most often impulsive behavior.

Epidemiology

Most epidemiological studies have not directly focused on pyromania. These studies include various populations of arsonists or fire setters. Most reveal a preponderance of males with a history of fire fascination (Barker 1994). They also suggest that true pyromania is rare. Fire setting for profit or revenge or secondary to delusions or hallucinations is more frequent than "authentic" ICD. Fire setting is frequent in children and in adolescents. "True" pyromania in childhood rarely appears. Juvenile fire setting is most often associated with conduct disorder, ADHD, or adjustment disorder.

The classic study *Pathological Fire-Setting (Pyromania)* by Lewis and Yarnell (1951) is one of the largest epidemiological studies of this topic and includes approximately 2,000 records from the National Board of Fire Underwriters and cases provided through fire departments, psychiatric clinics and institutions, and police departments near New York City. Thirty-nine

percent of the fire setters from the study received the diagnosis of pyromania. Twenty-two percent had borderline to dull normal intelligence, and 13% had between dull and low average intelligence. The authors also described the fire setter as a "pale and yellow, insignificant creature" driven by an irresistible impulse to set fires. The peak incidence of fire setting was between the ages of 16 and 18 years, but this observation has not been confirmed by more recent studies. Pyromania is found in adolescents and is also present at any age. Among females, the diversity of ages is particularly apparent (Barker 1994).

The high prevalence rates of pyromania have not been confirmed by more recent studies. Koson and Dvoskin (1982) found no cases of pyromania in a population of 26 arsonists. Ritchie and Huff (1999) identified only 3 cases of pyromania in 283 cases of arson. According to DSM-IV-TR, pyromania occurs more often in males, especially those with poorer social skills and learning difficulties. This notation confirms the Lewis and Yarnell (1951) data that only 14.8% of those with pyromania are female.

Comorbidity

Pyromania and Depression

Lejoyeux et al. (2002) assessed ICDs, using the Minnesota Impulsive Disorders Interview, in 107 depressed inpatients who met DSM-IV-TR criteria for major depressive episodes (Tables 19–8 and 19–9). Thirty-one depressed patients met criteria for ICDs: 18 had IED, 3 had pathological gambling, 4 had kleptomania, 3 had pyromania, and 3 had trichotillomania. Patients with comorbid ICDs were significantly younger (mean age, 37.7 vs. 42.8 years). Patients with pyromania had a higher number of previous depressions (3.3 vs. 1.3, $P=0.01$). Bipolar disorders were more frequent in the ICD group than in the group without ICDs (19% vs. 1.3%, $P=0.002$). Bulimia (42% vs. 10.5%, $P=0.005$) and compulsive buying (51% vs. 22%, $P=0.006$) were significantly more frequent in the ICD group. The findings of this study may suggest higher prevalence rates of ICDs than are found in a less severely ill population. There were no significant gender differences among patients presenting with ICDs, and in all cases the ICD appeared when patients no longer had mania or hypomania.

Pyromania and Alcohol Dependence

Laubichler et al. (1996) compared the files ($n=103$) of criminal fire setters and subjects with pyromania. Subjects with pyromania were younger (average age, 20 years) than criminal fire setters (average age, 30 years).

TABLE 19–8. Sociological and demographic characteristics of depressed patients without and with impulse-control disorders (ICDs)

	No ICD	Pyromania	Pathological gambling	Intermittent explosive disorder	Kleptomania	Trichotillomania	All ICDs
Patients, n (%)	76 (71.0)	3 (2.8)	3 (2.8)	18 (16.8)	4 (3.7)	3 (2.8)	31 (29.0)
Age, y (mean ± SD)	42.8 (13.9)	49.3 (6.6)	46.6 (13)	35.1 (10)[a]	39.7 (2.5)	30 (5)	37.7 (11)
Gender ratio, men:women	17:59	1:2	2:1	3:15	0:4	0:3	6:25
Married, n (%)	34 (44.7)	3 (100)	3 (100)	9 (50)	3 (75)	3 (100)	21 (67)[b]

[a]Difference statistically significant between ICD and non-ICD groups, $t=2.19$, $df=92$, $P=0.03$.
[b]Difference statistically significant between ICD and non-ICD groups, $\chi^2=4.66$, $df=1$, $P=0.03$.
Source. Adapted from Lejoyeux et al. 2002.

TABLE 19–9. Clinical characteristics of depressed patients with and without impulse-control disorders (ICDs)

	No ICD	Pyromania	Pathological gambling	Intermittent explosive disorder	Kleptomania	Trichotillomania	All ICDs
Patients, n	76	3	3	18	4	3	31
Previous depressive episodes, n (mean ± SD)	1.3 (1.3)	3.3 (1)[a]	1.3 (1.1)	1.3 (1.5)	5.7 (4)[b]	0	1.9 (2.4)
History of manic episodes (bipolar disorder), n (%)	1 (1.3)	0	0	3 (16)	3 (75)	0	6 (19)[c]
Suicide attempts, n (mean ± SD)	1.1 (2.1)	1 (1)	1 (1.7)	0.5 (0.6)	6 (4.2)[d]	0.6 (0.5)	1.3 (2.3)
Antisocial personality, n (%)	1 (1.3)	0	0	1 (5.5)	0	0	1 (3)
Borderline personality, n (%)	8 (10)	1 (33)	1 (33)	5 (27)	1 (25)	0	8 (26)
Bulimia, n (%)	8 (10.5)	0	1 (33)	5 (27)	4 (100)	3 (100)	13 (42)[e]
Compulsive buying, n (%)	17 (22)	0	3 (100)	9 (50)	1 (25)	3 (100)	16 (51)[f]

Note. Student's t test was used.
[a]Difference between non-ICD and pyromania groups, $t=2.46$, $df=77$, $P=0.01$.
[b]Difference between non-ICD and kleptomania groups, $t=5.33$, $df=78$, $P<0.0001$.
[c]Difference between non-ICD and ICD groups, $\chi^2=8.95$, $df=1$, $P=0.002$.
[d]Difference between non-ICD and kleptomania groups, $t=4.17$, $df=78$, $P<0.001$.
[e]Difference between non-ICD and ICD groups, $\chi^2=11.8$, $df=1$, $P=0.0005$.
[f]Difference between non-ICD and ICD groups, $\chi^2=7.5$, $df=1$, $P=0.006$.
Source. Adapted from Lejoyeux et al. 2002.

Seventy of the 103 subjects had consumed alcohol before setting a fire. Fifty-four presented with alcohol dependence. The authors suggested a correlation between the amount of alcohol consumed and the frequency of fire setting. Rasanen et al. (1995) found that young arsonists have frequent alcohol problems: 82% had alcoholism and 82% were intoxicated at the time of committing the crime. The excessive consumption of alcohol had a close connection with the arson committed.

Lejoyeux et al. (1999) searched for ICDs among consecutive admissions for detoxification of alcohol-dependent patients in a French department of psychiatry. They found 30 alcohol-dependent persons presenting with at least one ICD (19 with IED, 7 with pathological gambling, 3 with kleptomania, and 1 case of trichotillomania), but none of the patients presented with two or more ICDs, and no patient presented with pyromania. However, it cannot be concluded from such a limited population that pyromania is not associated with alcohol dependence. Further studies are clearly needed to corroborate or refute this preliminary result.

Fire Setting and Psychiatric Disorders

In most cases, fire-setting behavior is not directly related to pyromania. On the other hand, fire setting in subjects who do not have pyromania appears frequent and often underrecognized. Among psychiatric patients, some research found that 26% of the subjects had a history of fire-setting behavior. Sixteen percent of these patients had actually set fires (Geller and Bertsch 1985). Ritchie and Huff (1999) reviewed mental health records and prison files from 283 arsonists, 90% of whom had a recorded history of mental health problems. Thirty-six percent had schizophrenia or bipolar disorder, and 64% were misusing alcohol or drugs at the time of their fire setting.

Pathogenesis
Biological Markers

Virkkunen et al. (1987, 1994) suggested that pyromania may be associated with reactive hypoglycemia and/or lower concentrations of 3-methoxy-4-hydroxyphenylglycol (MHPG) and CSF 5-HIAA. Their results supported the hypothesis that poor impulse control in criminal offenders is associated with low levels of certain CSF monoamine metabolites and with a hypoglycemic trend.

Impulse fire setters who are violent offenders are often dependent on alcohol and have a father who is also alcohol dependent (Linnoila et al. 1989). Virkkunen et al. (1996) investigated biochemical and family variables and predictors of recidivism among forensic psychiatric patients who had set fires. Male alcoholic patients and fire setters ($n=114$) were followed for an average of 4.5 years after their release from prison. Low CSF 5-HIAA and homovanillic acid concentrations were associated with a family history of paternal alcoholism with violence. A low plasma cholesterol concentration was associated with a family history positive for paternal alcoholism without violence. Compared with nonrecidivists, the recidivists who set fires during the follow-up period had low CSF 5-HIAA and MHPG concentrations and early family environments characterized by paternal absence and the presence of brothers at home.

Psychodynamic Models

Psychodynamic models refer to the symbolism of fire, which is complemented by "normal" human interest in fire. Fire interest starts between 2 and 3 years of age and was almost universal in a study of healthy schoolboys at ages 6, 8, and 10 years (Kafry 1980). Among children, the distinction between normal interest in fire and excessive interest leading to pyromania is not always clear. Playing with matches is not a symptom of pyromania. Kolko and Kazdin (1989) showed that "future" pyromaniacs had more curiosity about fire and liked to be in contact with peers or family members involved with fire. According to Geller and Bertsch (1985), children at risk of pyromania were more often involved in fire setting, threatening to set a fire, sounding a false fire alarm, or calling the fire department with a false report of fire than were control subjects. Thus, there may be a continuum between excessive interest in fire and "pure" pyromania.

Since the first description of pyromania by M. Marc, a French psychiatrist, in 1833, the symbolic sexual dimension of pyromania has been noted. Pyromaniacs were later described as fire fetishists. Many pyromaniacs have fire fetishes. A "fire experience" may become a "fire fetish" (McGuire et al. 1965). For example, a fire fantasy, whether imagined or recalled, just before orgasm is conditioned by the positive feedback of orgasm to become more and more exciting.

Lewis and Yarnell (1951) suggested three main groups of fire setters: the accidental, the occasional, and the habitual. Motivations might include sexual gratification derived from converting a sexual impulse into substitutive excitement, or accidental or unintentional, delusional, erotic, revenge, or group effect in children and adolescents. The diverse symbolism of fire is represented in the psychoanalytic interpretations of pyromania.

Females with pyromania frequently have a history of self-harm, sexual abuse, and psychosocial traumas (Noblett and Nelson 2001). The authors suggested that pyromania could be a displacement of aggression, which is observed in people with a history of sexual trauma. Patients may be unable to directly confront people. The channeling of aggression through fire setting may be seen as an attempt to influence their environment and improve their self-esteem where other means have failed. Fire setting may be an attempt at communication by individuals with few social skills (Geller and Bertsch 1985).

The most frequent motives for arson by juveniles (Rasanen et al. 1995) are revenge on parents or other authorities, the search for heroism or excitement, self-destructiveness, the craving for sensation, and an expression of outrage. There is also a lot of self-destructive behavior by juveniles before committing arson: 74% have suicidal thoughts and 44% have tried to commit suicide before committing their crimes.

Course

According to DSM-IV-TR, there are insufficient data to establish a typical age at onset of pyromania and to predict the longitudinal course. In individuals with pyromania, fire-setting incidents are episodic and may wax and wane in frequency. Studies indicate that the recidivism rate for fire setters ranges from 4.5% (Mavromatis and Lion 1977) to 28% (Lewis and Yarnell 1951). Barnett et al. (1997, 1999) compared mentally ill and mentally "healthy" fire setters from trial records in Germany in a cross-sectional and 10-year follow-up study. Mentally disordered arsonists were more likely than those with no disorder to have a history of arson before their trial. They also were more often convicted of arson again (11% relapse compared with 4%), had fewer registrations of common offenses such as theft as well as traffic violations and alcohol-related offenses, had a higher rate of recurrence, and committed fewer common offenses other than fire setting. Among all arsonists who committed crimes other than arson, those who were found to be partly responsible for their arson committed the highest number of offenses, followed by those who were deemed not responsible for their actions and those who were fully responsible.

Treatment

Treatment for fire setters is problematic because they frequently refuse to take responsibility for their acts, are in denial, have alcoholism, and lack insight (Mavromatis and Lion 1977). Behavioral treatments such as aversive therapy have helped fire setters (Koles and Jenson 1985; McGrath and Marshall 1979). Other methods of treatment rely on positive reinforcement with threats of punishment, stimulus satiation, and operant structured fantasies (Bumpass et al. 1983). Bumpass et al. (1983) treated 29 child fire setters and used a graphing technique that sequentially correlated external stress, behavior, and feelings on graph paper. After treatment (average follow-up, 2.5 years), only 2 of the 29 children continued to set fires. Studies of treatment approaches for pyromania are summarized in Table 19–10.

TABLE 19–10. Pyromania: treatment summary

Authors	Treatment	Description
Psychotherapy		
McGrath and Marshall 1979	Behavioral therapy	Child fire setter ($n=1$); successful
Koles and Jenson 1985	Behavioral therapy	Child fire setter ($n=1$); successful
Bumpass et al. 1983	Technique that sequentially correlates external stress, behavior, and feelings on graph paper to help patients become aware of the cause–effect relationship between feelings and behavior so as to substitute an acceptable behavior	Child fire setters ($n=29$); after treatment (average follow-up, 2.5 years), only 2 of the 29 children continued to set fires
G. A. Franklin et al. 2002	Trauma Burn Outreach Prevention Program (TBOPP), 1-day, interactive program focusing on the medical, financial, legal, and societal impact of fire setting, emphasizing individual accountability and responsibility	132 juveniles (66 arsonists, 66 fire setters) in the TBOPP group; 102 juveniles (33 arsonists and 66 fire setters) in the no-TBOPP group; TBOPP participants had essentially no recidivism compared with the no-TBOPP group

G.A. Franklin et al. (2002) confirmed the positive effect of a prevention program for pyromania. In 1999, they developed the Trauma Burn Outreach Prevention Program. All subjects arrested and convicted after setting a fire received 1 day of information. The program's interactive content focused on the medical, financial, legal, and societal impacts of fire-setting behavior. The rate of recidivism was less than 1% in the group who attended the program compared with 36% in the control group.

Pathological Gambling

Definition and Diagnostic Criteria

Pathological gambling has been considered a distinct diagnostic entity since 1980, when it was first included in DSM-III and similarly in ICD-9-CM (World Health Organization 1978). DSM-IV-TR currently classifies pathological gambling as an ICD not elsewhere classified. The essential feature of pathological gambling is recurrent gambling behavior that is maladaptive (e.g., loss of judgment, excessive gambling) and in which personal, family, or vocational endeavors are disrupted (Table 19–11).

Epidemiology

Prevalence estimates for pathological gambling range from 1% to 3% of the U.S. population (American Psychiatric Association 1994) and show increasing prevalence among females (33% of pathological gambling patients are women; Lesieur 1988) and high school students (1.7%–5.7%; Ladouceur and Mireault 1988; Lesieur and Klein 1987). A U.S. national survey suggested that 68% of the general population participated in some form of gambling and that 0.77% of American adults are considered probable pathological gamblers (Commission on the Review of the National Policy Toward Gambling 1976). Prevalence estimates of probable pathological gambling from state surveys range from 1.2% to 3.4%, with increased rates in states that provide greater opportunity for legal gambling (Commission on the Review of the National Policy Toward Gambling 1976; Volberg 1990; Volberg and Steadman 1988, 1989).

A meta-analysis of 120 published studies indicated that the lifetime prevalence of serious gambling (meeting DSM criteria for pathological gambling) among adults is 1.6% (Shaffer et al. 1999). Among those younger than 18 years, the prevalence is 3.9%, with past-year rates for adults and adolescents being 1.1%

TABLE 19–11. **DSM-IV-TR diagnostic criteria for pathological gambling**

A. Persistent and recurrent maladaptive gambling behavior as indicated by five (or more) of the following:

(1) is preoccupied with gambling (e.g., preoccupied with reliving past gambling experiences, handicapping or planning the next venture, or thinking of ways to get money with which to gamble)

(2) needs to gamble with increasing amounts of money in order to achieve the desired excitement

(3) has repeated unsuccessful efforts to control, cut back, or stop gambling

(4) is restless or irritable when attempting to cut down or stop gambling

(5) gambles as a way of escaping from problems or of relieving a dysphoric mood (e.g., feelings of helplessness, guilt, anxiety, depression)

(6) after losing money gambling, often returns another day to get even ("chasing" one's losses)

(7) lies to family members, therapist, or others to conceal the extent of involvement with gambling

(8) has committed illegal acts such as forgery, fraud, theft, or embezzlement to finance gambling

(9) has jeopardized or lost a significant relationship, job, or educational or career opportunity because of gambling

(10) relies on others to provide money to relieve a desperate financial situation caused by gambling

B. The gambling behavior is not better accounted for by a manic episode.

and 5.8%, respectively (Shaffer and Hall 1996).

Prevalence estimates of pathological gambling in the general population differ from estimates in a treatment-seeking population. In a New York State epidemiological survey, relative to gamblers identified in treatment programs, there were higher rates of pathological or probable pathological gamblers who were female (36% vs. 7%, respectively), younger (less than 30 years; 38% vs. 18%, respectively), and nonwhite (43% vs. 9%, respectively) (Volberg and Steadman 1988). Female pathological gamblers clearly represent an understudied and underserved group, because they account for approximately one-third of pathological gamblers (Lesieur 1988). Prevalence estimates of pathological gambling among high school students range from 1.7% to 3.6% (Ladouceur and Mireault 1988) to 5.7% (Lesieur and Klein 1987).

Comorbidity

The literature to date strongly suggests that three Axis I disorders frequently co-occur with pathological gambling: substance abuse or dependence, affective disorders (i.e., bipolar spectrum disorders), and ADHD (Figure 19–2).

There appears to be a strong relationship between pathological gambling and substance abuse, as evidenced by the high rates of comorbid substance abuse and dependence with pathological gambling (Lesieur 1988; Lesieur et al. 1986; Linden et al. 1986; McCormick et al. 1984). Failure to treat comorbid substance use disorders in gamblers may lead to higher relapse rates (Maccallum and Blaszczynski 2002). Pathological gambling is also highly comorbid with affective disorders among inpatient (McCormick et al. 1984) and outpatient (Linden et al. 1986) samples.

Pathological gambling has been associated with ADHD (Carlton and Goldstein 1987). Interestingly, because an association between alcoholism and childhood ADHD has been found (Wood et al. 1983), as well as high co-occurrence between pathological gambling and alcohol abuse (Linden et al. 1986; McCormick et al. 1984), inadequate impulse control may be a key factor that links these three disorders dimensionally (Carlton and Manowitz 1988).

Pathological gambling has been described as being part of the obsessive-compulsive spectrum and sharing features with both obsessive-compulsive disorder (OCD) and the impulsive cluster of obsessive-compulsive spectrum disorders (Bienvenu et al. 2000; Dell'Osso et al. 2005).

Compulsive sexual behavior, compulsive buying disorder, and IED are relatively frequent, as are personality disorders. Murray (1993) found that pathological gamblers fit no particular personality profile, but several investigators have reported abnormal personality traits in pathological gamblers based on dimensional assessments (e.g., Roy et al. 1989). Taber et al. (1987) reported that 20% of 66 pathological gambling inpatients had personality disorders.

Pathogenesis

Neurobiology

There is evidence of serotonergic, noradrenergic, and dopaminergic dysfunction in pathological gambling,

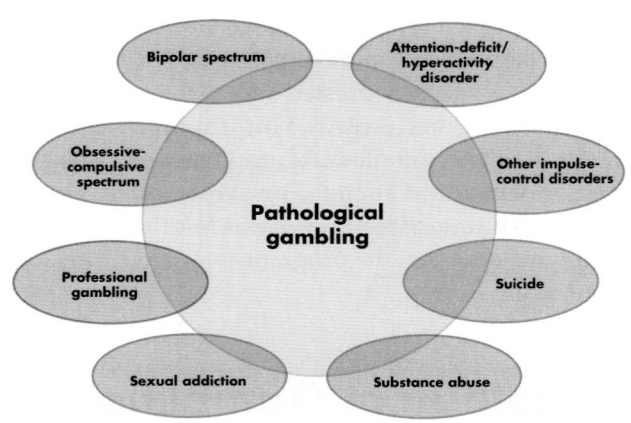

FIGURE 19–2. Pathological gambling: comorbidity and issues in classification.

Source. Reprinted from Pallanti S, Baldini Rossi N, Hollander E: "Pathological Gambling," in *Clinical Manual of Impulse-Control Disorders.* Edited by Hollander E, Stein DJ. Washington, DC, American Psychiatric Publishing, 2006, pp. 251–289. Copyright 2006, American Psychiatric Publishing. Used with permission.

and each of these neurotransmitter systems may play a unique role in the mechanisms that underlie the arousal, behavioral initiation, behavioral disinhibition, and reward or reinforcement evident in pathological gambling and other addictive disorders (Table 19–12).

Serotonergic function is linked to behavioral initiation, inhibition, and aggression. Noradrenergic function mediates arousal and detects novel or aversive stimuli. Dopaminergic function is associated with reward and reinforcement mechanisms. Thus, decreased serotonin, increased norepinephrine, and increased dopamine function facilitate addictive or impulsive behavior (Table 19–13).

Evidence of serotonergic dysfunction in pathological gamblers comes from neurobiological studies (Carrasco et al. 1994; DeCaria et al. 1998; Moreno et al. 1991). There is evidence of serotonergic dysfunction in depression (Coccaro et al. 1989), impulsivity (Linnoila et al. 1983), suicidality (Mann et al. 1992), and alcoholism (Tollefson 1991). This is of interest because pathological gambling is strongly associated with depression (Roy et al. 1988a, 1988b), impulsivity (Moreno et al. 1991), suicidality (Ciarrochi and Richardson 1989), and alcohol or drug abuse (Linden et al. 1986; McCormick et al. 1984). Thus, pathological gambling may also be associated with serotonergic dysfunction as it relates to these comorbid features.

In addition to being considered an ICD, pathological gambling has also been linked phenomenologically

TABLE 19–12. Developmental and neurobiological model of pathological gambling

Vulnerable state

Primed genetically/neurobiologically

Repeated environmental exposure

Gambling cycle: behavioral mechanisms

Stimulation readiness $\rightarrow$ norepinephrine

Behavioral initiation $\rightarrow$ serotonin

Reward/reinforcement $\rightarrow$ dopamine

Behavioral disinhibition $\rightarrow$ serotonin

Source. Reprinted from Pallanti S, Baldini Rossi N, Hollander E: "Pathological Gambling," in *Clinical Manual of Impulse-Control Disorders.* Edited by Hollander E, Stein DJ. Washington, DC, American Psychiatric Publishing, 2006, p. 262. Used with permission.

TABLE 19–13. Evidence of neurobiological dysfunction in pathological gambling

Norepinephrine dysfunction

Increased urinary norepinephrine levels

Increased cerebrospinal fluid MHPG levels

Enhanced growth hormone response to clonidine

Serotonin dysfunction

Low platelet monoamine oxidase activity

Blunted prolactin response to intravenous clomipramine and increased response to *m*-chlorophenylpiperazine

Response to serotonin reuptake inhibitors

Dopamine dysfunction

Increased prevalence of altered alleles of the genes for dopamine receptors D_1, D_2, D_3, and D_4

Note. MHPG = methoxyhydroxyphenylglycol.

Source. Reprinted from Pallanti S, Baldini Rossi N, Hollander E: "Pathological Gambling," in *Clinical Manual of Impulse-Control Disorders.* Edited by Hollander E, Stein DJ. Washington, DC, American Psychiatric Publishing, 2006, p. 263. Used with permission.

to OCD and obsessive-compulsive related/spectrum disorders (DeCaria and Hollander 1993; DeCaria et al. 1992; Hollander and Wong 1995a, 1995b), which have also shown evidence for serotonergic dysfunction (Hollander et al. 1992a). Furthermore, patients with OCD, obsessive-compulsive spectrum disorders, and pathological gambling respond well to serotonin re-

uptake blockers such as clomipramine or the SSRIs (Clomipramine Collaborative Study Group 1991; Hollander 1993; Hollander et al. 1992b).

The noradrenergic system also seems to play a role in the pathophysiology of pathological gambling. Pathological gamblers have shown significantly higher CSF MHPG levels, a metabolite of norepinephrine, and greater urinary output of norepinephrine than control subjects (Roy et al. 1988a). Measures of extraversion in pathological gamblers significantly correlate with indices of noradrenergic function (Roy et al. 1989). Furthermore, increased noradrenergic function has been associated with arousal, irritability, and risk-taking behavior (Coccaro et al. 1991), and pathological gambling has been associated with increased arousal and tonic activity of the central noradrenergic system (Brown 1986; Commission on the Review of the National Policy Toward Gambling 1976; Dickerson et al. 1987; Roy et al. 1988a). Noradrenergic mechanisms have also been associated with impulsive and compulsive behavior in other related disorders (Glassman et al. 1993; Hollander et al. 1991).

Genetics

Serotonergic, noradrenergic, and dopaminergic genes have been investigated because of the putative role of these neurotransmitters in pathological gambling, and a number of molecular genetic studies performed to date have reported findings consistent with the involvement of these neurotransmitter systems in pathological gambling (Comings et al. 1996, 1997; Ibanez et al. 2000, 2001; Perez de Castro et al. 1997, 2002). However, some of the studies performed to date have not been adequately controlled for potential differences in racial and ethnic compositions, factors that could account for differences in allelic variant distributions. As such, these studies, although promising, should be regarded as preliminary.

Studies with clinical samples of pathological gamblers suggest an incidence of about 20% of pathological gambling in first-degree relatives (Ibanez et al. 2003; Lesieur 1988), and this led to the consideration of the possible role of a genetic component in the development of pathological gambling. Gambino et al. (1993) found that patients who perceived that their parents had gambling problems were three times more likely to score as probable pathological gamblers on the South Oaks Gambling Screen (Lesieur and Blume 1987). Those who also perceived that their grandparents had gambling problems had a 12-fold increased risk compared with patients who did not perceive gambling problems in their parents and grandparents.

At present, the main source of evidence for the genetic influence in the etiology of pathological gambling derives from a study of 3,359 male twin pairs from the Vietnam Era Twin Registry cohort (Eisen et al. 1998, 2001; Slutske et al. 2000). These data suggest that gambling problems of increasing severity represent a single continuum of vulnerability rather than distinct entities (Eisen et al. 1998, 2001), a genetic susceptibility model in the pathogenesis of pathological gambling (Eisen et al. 1998), and indicate a common genetic vulnerability for pathological gambling and alcohol dependence in men (Slutske et al. 2000). In a smaller twin study, Winters and Rich (1999) found a significant heritability explaining "high action" gambling, like casinos and gambling slot machines, in 92 monozygotic and dizygotic male twin pairs, but no significant differences in heritability were found among males for "low action" games and among 63 female monozygotic and dizygotic twin pairs for either "high action" or "low action" gambling.

Neuropsychology

Clinical comorbidities, along with observations that pathological gambling involves strong motivations to engage in gambling and subjective feelings of reward, withdrawal, and craving for gambling, support the categorization of pathological gambling as "a nonpharmacological addiction" (Blanco et al. 2001; Holden 2001). This view is corroborated by neuroimaging findings that gambling-associated cognitive and motivational events, or responses of pathological gamblers to gambling-related stimuli, are associated with metabolic changes in brain regions implicated in research of substance use disorders (Breiter et al. 2001; Holden 2001; Potenza et al. 2003). Using fluorodeoxyglucose PET in unmedicated pathological gamblers without comorbid substance use disorders ($n=7$), Hollander et al. (2001) found heightened limbic and sensory activation in a gambling-for-money condition with increased emotional valence and greater risk and reward, which confirms the salience of monetary reward in the development of pathological gambling.

Data exist to support the notion that individuals with impaired impulse control exhibit abnormalities in risk–benefit decision making in both gambling and nongambling activities and that their cognitive or emotional sense of what distinguishes gambling from other decisions of daily living may be compromised (Bechara 2001; Bechara et al. 2000, 2001; Crean et al. 2000; Petry 2001a, 2001b, 2001c; Petry and Casarella 1999; Potenza 2001; Rogers and Robbins 2001). These deficits could produce an inability to inhibit motivated drives to gamble, leading to persistent gambling. Myopia for the future and insensitivity to punishment have also been shown in patients with orbitofrontal and ventromedial PFC lesions (Bechara et al. 1994; Berlin et al. 2004), using gambling tasks. Cavedini et al.'s (2002) data suggest a link between pathological gambling and other disorders (i.e., OCD and drug addiction) associated with diminished ability to evaluate future consequences, which may be explained at least in part by an abnormal functioning of the orbitofrontal cortex. Attention problems and impulsivity in pathological gamblers could reflect deficits in executive functioning that are often a consequence of minimal brain damage with orbitofrontal cortex impairment (Berlin et al. 2004; Rugle and Melamed 1993; Specker et al. 1995).

Course

The course of pathological gambling tends to be chronic, but the pattern of gambling may be regular or episodic. Chronicity is usually associated with increases in the frequency of gambling and the amount gambled. Gambling may increase during periods of increased stress. Gambling behavior frequently leads to severe personal, familial, financial, social, and occupational impairment.

Psychiatric disorders such as major depression and alcohol or substance abuse and dependence may develop from or be exacerbated by pathological gambling. There is also a mortality risk associated with pathological gambling. Estimates of suicide attempts in pathological gamblers range from 17% to 24% (Ciarrochi and Richardson 1989; Hollander et al. 2000a). One study found that the suicide rate in cities where gambling has been legalized is four times higher than the rate in cities without legal gambling (Phillips et al. 1997). Younger patients are more likely to have suicidal tendencies and major depressive disorders (McCormick et al. 1984). Because most pathological gamblers begin gambling during adolescence (Hollander et al. 2000a), early identification and intervention are critical.

Gender differences have been described in the course of pathological gambling. In males, the disorder usually begins in adolescence (Hollander et al. 2000a) and may remain undiagnosed for years; male pathological gamblers often present with a 20- to 30-year gambling history, with gradual development of dependence. In contrast, onset of pathological gambling in females is more likely to occur later in life. Prior to their seeking treatment, the duration of pathological gambling in women is approximately 3 years.

Thus, as a result of the differences in onset and duration, female pathological gamblers generally have a better prognosis than male pathological gamblers (Rosenthal 1992). Female pathological gamblers also tend to be depressed and may use gambling as an anesthetic, accompanied by excitement, to escape from life's problems (i.e., as in a dissociative state [Jacobs 1988]).

Treatment

There is a relative lack of effective treatments for pathological gambling reported in the literature. The uncontrolled and few controlled treatment studies in the literature, although helpful in providing preliminary direction, are frequently methodologically flawed. Studies of treatment approaches for pathological gambling are summarized in Table 19–14.

TABLE 19–14. **Pathological gambling: treatment summary**

Authors	Treatment	Description
Pharmacotherapy		
de la Gandara 1999 Hollander et al. 1992b, 1998, 2000a Kim et al. 2002 Zimmerman et al. 2002	Serotonin reuptake inhibitors	Positive results
Pallanti et al. 2002b	Serotonin antagonist (nefazodone)	Prospective 8-week open-label; pathological gambling outpatients ($N=14$); improvements in all gambling outcome measures and depression and anxiety ratings
Haller and Hinterhuber 1994 Hollander et al. 2002 Pallanti et al. 2002a	Mood stabilizers	Positive results
Kim et al. 2001	Opiate antagonist (naltrexone)	1-week single-blind placebo lead-in followed by an 11-week double-blind naltrexone or placebo trial; subjects with pathological gambling disorder ($N=45$); significant improvement on all three gambling symptom measures
Potenza and Chambers 2001	Atypical antipsychotics	Positive results
Psychotherapy		
Petry and Armentano 1999, review	Gamblers Anonymous (GA); cognitive-behavioral therapy	Only 8% of GA attendees achieve a year of abstinence; combining professional therapy and GA participation may improve retention and abstinence; the few studies of cognitive-behavioral treatments are promising
Russo et al. 1984 Taber 1981 Taber et al. 1987	Inpatient programs for pathological gambling with various combinations of individual and group psychotherapy and substance use treatment	Total abstinence was reported by 55%–56% of the patients 1 year later; improved interpersonal relationships, better financial status, decreased depression, and participation in professional aftercare and GA
Dickerson et al. 1990	Self-help manuals	Useful for some
Ladouceur 1990	Cognitive restructuring	Decrease in the frequency of gambling and irrational verbalizations associated with gambling

Pharmacotherapy

Currently there are only a few controlled pharmacological treatment studies of pathological gambling, although this is a recently developing area of research. Pharmacological treatment studies of pathological gambling have demonstrated some promising results with the use of serotonin reuptake inhibitors (de la Gandara 1999; Hollander et al. 1992b, 1998, 2000b; Kim et al. 2002; Zimmerman et al. 2002), serotonin antagonists (Pallanti et al. 2002a), mood stabilizers (Haller and Hinterhuber 1994; Hollander et al. 2002; Pallanti et al. 2002b), opiate antagonists (Kim et al. 2001), and atypical antipsychotics (Potenza and Chambers 2001). However, some studies have not reported significant findings, primarily due to small samples, high placebo response rates, or high rates of discontinuation (Blanco et al. 2002; Grant et al. 2003).

These data suggest the need for conducting well-designed controlled clinical trials of various pharmacological agents in the treatment of pathological gambling, according to different clinical presentations and comorbidities. Treatment should ultimately target all symptom domains within the individual patient that contribute to compulsive gambling, including common comorbid conditions such as bipolar spectrum disorder, ADHD, and substance abuse/dependence disorders.

Psychotherapy

Treatment modalities for pathological gambling are similar to those of other substance abuse disorders and were created based on the addiction model, such as self-help groups, inpatient treatment programs, and rehabilitation programs. Essential features of any therapeutic intervention for pathological gambling include the need to establish both a therapeutic alliance and network, address the underlying pathology, interrupt the behavior and maintain abstinence, problem-solve, and improve quality of life.

The most popular intervention for problem gambling is Gamblers Anonymous (GA), which is similar to Alcoholics Anonymous and Narcotics Anonymous. However, evidence suggests that GA may not be very effective when used without other treatment modalities (Petry and Armentano 1999). Retrospective studies show a dropout rate of up to 70% within the first year (Stewart and Brown 1988), and overall dropout rates range from 75% to 90% (Moody 1990). Only 8% of GA members report total abstinence at 1-year follow-up and 7% at 2-year follow-up (Brown 1985). Although participation in GA's spousal component, Gam-Anon, may be helpful for some family members,

little evidence suggests that it reduces disordered gambling (Petry and Armentano 1999).

Inpatient programs for pathological gambling have included various combinations of individual and group psychotherapy and substance use treatment (Taber 1981), and most strongly encouraged or required attendance at GA meetings. Many patients improved in all programs, and outcome studies have shown 55% of patients reporting abstinence at 1-year follow-up (Russo et al. 1984; Taber et al. 1987). Although methodologically flawed, these reports suggest that professionally delivered multimodal therapy programs, given alone or in combination with GA, may be more effective than GA alone. Self-help manuals may also be useful for some (Dickerson et al. 1990), and studies comparing their effectiveness with professionally delivered CBT are ongoing (Petry and Armentano 1999).

Early reports in the psychoanalytic literature suggest that problem gambling is regressive and representative of various pregenital and genital instincts, unconscious conflicts, or painful affects. Most studies that report good outcomes are based on single-case studies, and some authors believe that purely psychodynamic treatment of pathological gambling is difficult. Rosenthal and Rugle (1994) published a contemporary psychodynamic approach to pathological gambling treatment that integrates traditional psychodynamic psychotherapy with an addiction model.

Behavioral, cognitive, and combined cognitive-behavioral methods have been used in treating pathological gambling. Aversive therapy has been employed to reach the goal of total abstinence of gambling, as have behavior monitoring, contingency management, contingency contracting, covert sensitization, systematic desensitization, imaginal desensitization, in vivo exposure, imaginal relaxation, psychoeducation, cognitive restructuring, problem-solving skills training, social skills training, and relapse prevention. Use of cognitive restructuring facilitates a decrease in the frequency of gambling and irrational verbalizations associated with gambling (Ladouceur 1990).

Trichotillomania

Definition and Diagnostic Criteria

Trichotillomania is a chronic ICD characterized by repetitive pulling out of one's own hair, resulting in noticeable hair loss. The DSM-IV-TR criteria for trichotillomania are listed in Table 19–15.

Criteria B and C are somewhat controversial in

TABLE 19–15.	**DSM-IV-TR diagnostic criteria for trichotillomania**

A. Recurrent pulling out of one's hair resulting in noticeable hair loss.

B. An increasing sense of tension immediately before pulling out the hair or when attempting to resist the behavior.

C. Pleasure, gratification, or relief when pulling out the hair.

D. The disturbance is not better accounted for by another mental disorder and is not due to a general medical condition (e.g., a dermatological condition).

E. The disturbance causes clinically significant distress or impairment in social, occupational, or other important areas of functioning.

light of data suggesting that a significant minority of individuals who pull their hair do not report experiencing these feelings (Christenson et al. 1991a; Hanna 1997; King et al. 1995; Schlosser et al. 1994). These findings suggest that the current diagnostic classification of trichotillomania may be overly restrictive, particularly with respect to pediatric samples. As of now, it is unclear whether chronic hair pulling is best conceptualized as a single entity or as a symptom with myriad root causes yet to be identified, with little unifying these subtypes theoretically.

Approximately 75% of adult trichotillomania patients report that most of their hair-pulling behavior takes place "automatically" or outside of awareness, whereas the remaining 25% describe themselves as primarily focused on hair pulling when they pull (Christenson and Mackenzie 1994). However, some patients engage in both types of hair pulling. Compared with unfocused hair pullers, the subset who primarily engage in focused hair pulling are more likely to pull hair from the pubic area and to report shame as a result of their hair pulling (du Toit et al. 2001). Some suggest that trichotillomania patients who engage primarily in focused hair pulling are more similar to patients with OCD and may be more responsive to pharmacological interventions found effective for OCD (Christenson and O'Sullivan 1996; du Toit et al. 2001). The issue of trichotillomania subtyping is one of both considerable importance and ongoing debate, and no formal subtyping system incorporating affective correlates of pulling has been advanced.

The few published data on how trichotillomania presents in children and adolescents suggest similari-

ties to adult hair pulling. As with adults, the scalp is the most common pulling site in children and adolescents, followed by eyelashes and eyebrows (Hanna 1997; Reeve 1999). In one study, almost half of children and adolescents described having a ritual or routine involved in pulling their hair (Hanna 1997). The absence of body hair on younger children precludes pulling from certain sites, but clinical work with adolescents appears consistent with the adult data in that pulling from sites other than the face and scalp is also common. When completed, ongoing research regarding the preferred pulling sites of children and adolescents will add to this knowledge base (M.E. Franklin et al. 2002; Tolin et al. 2002).

Epidemiology

Early clinical studies suggested that trichotillomania was extremely rare; however, survey research with nonclinical samples has indicated that hair pulling is more common than originally suggested. In studies involving college samples, 10%–13% of students reported hair pulling, with the prevalence of clinically significant pulling ranging between 1% and 3.5% (Christenson et al. 1991c; Rothbaum et al. 1993). A large epidemiological study of trichotillomania and skin picking using self-report instruments is under way in a large sample of college freshmen (Hajcak et al. 2006). Epidemiological research on trichotillomania is extremely limited both in terms of the number of studies and methodology. One epidemiological survey of 17-year-old adolescents in Israel suggests a prevalence rate of 1% for current or past hair pulling, with fewer reporting noticeable hair loss or distress from these symptoms (King et al. 1995). There is a need for more epidemiological research on trichotillomania.

Comorbidity

Psychiatric comorbidity is quite common among adults with trichotillomania. Christenson et al. (1991a) found that approximately 82% of an adult sample with trichotillomania met criteria for a past or current comorbid Axis I disorder, the most common being affective, anxiety, and addictive disorders. Of the patients with comorbid disorders, there was a lifetime prevalence rate of 65% for mood disorders, 57% for anxiety disorders, 22% for substance abuse disorders, 20% for eating disorders, and 42% for personality disorders. The most frequently cited comorbid personality disorders are histrionic, borderline, and obsessive-compulsive (Christenson et al. 1992; Schlosser et al. 1994; Swedo and Leonard 1992). In a larger sample of adults seeking treatment for trichotillomania, Christenson (1995) found comorbidity rates of 57% for major depression, 27% for generalized anxiety disorder, 20% for eating disorders, 19% for alcohol abuse, and 16% for other substance abuse. In a mixed sample of children, adolescents, and adults with trichotillomania, Swedo and Leonard (1992) found comorbidity rates of 39% for unipolar depression, 32% for generalized anxiety disorder, 16% for OCD, and 15% for substance abuse.

Reeve et al. (1992) and King et al. (1995) found that 7 of 10 and 9 of 15 children with trichotillomania had at least one comorbid Axis I disorder, respectively. M.E. Franklin et al. (2002) and Tolin et al. (2002) reported little comorbidity in their pediatric treatment-seeking samples, suggesting that comorbidity may develop secondarily in the wake of trichotillomania. Sampling issues most likely underlie these observed differences. Nevertheless, if it is indeed the case that children and adolescents with trichotillomania are less comorbid than adults with trichotillomania, successful early intervention in children and adolescents with trichotillomania may help reduce the rates and severity of later adult psychiatric comorbidity and functional impairment (Keuthen et al. 2002). More longitudinal and psychopathology research is needed.

A key debate in the field is whether trichotillomania should be conceptualized as an ICD or a variant of OCD. In support of the classification as an obsessive-compulsive spectrum disorder is the apparent similarity between compulsions and the repetitive and perceived uncontrollable nature of hair pulling and accompanying anxiety relief (Swedo 1993; Swedo and Leonard 1992), the possible selective responsiveness of trichotillomania to serotonin reuptake inhibitors, and the elevated rates of OCD in patients with trichotillomania (Christenson et al. 1991a). Others argue that trichotillomania and OCD are separate diagnoses because trichotillomania is not characterized by persistent intrusive thoughts regarding hair pulling, hair pulling often occurs outside awareness, and the repetitive behavior in trichotillomania is generally limited to hair pulling whereas compulsions in OCD often consist of a variety of anxiety-relieving behaviors. Those with OCD also describe their compulsions as unpleasant but necessary to reduce negative affect (i.e., maintained by negative reinforcement), whereas most subjects with trichotillomania describe hair pulling as pleasurable or satisfying (i.e., maintained by positive reinforcement). Furthermore, OCD patients' age at onset is generally later (Himle et al. 1995; Swedo 1993; Tukel et al. 2001), they report higher levels of overall anxiety (Himle et al. 1995; Tukel et al. 2001),

and they have a more restricted range of affective states than trichotillomania patients (Stanley and Cohen 1999). The proposed difference between OCD and trichotillomania has led to the use of disparate CBT strategies for each.

Many authors (e.g., Christenson and Mansueto 1999) have noted similarities among skin picking and severe nail biting as well as common co-occurrence. If the skin picking and nail biting appear to be largely negatively reinforcing—reducing anxiety associated with specific obsessional thoughts and/or reducing the likelihood of feared outcomes—they may be better conceptualized as OCD behaviors. Clinical experience suggests these conditions are much more likely to formally resemble trichotillomania. More research is needed to determine whether they are all one entity or distinct conditions.

Pathogenesis

Figure 19–3 shows a schematic diagram of a preliminary biopsychosocial model of trichotillomania. This model is preliminary, because the available experimental and descriptive psychopathology research in trichotillomania is sparse. This model is heuristic rather than explanatory, but it is hoped it will stimulate new studies on the mechanisms of trichotillomania and be modified as new data become available.

Biological Vulnerability

Biological vulnerabilities likely increase the probability that a person will develop trichotillomania. Familial research suggests that trichotillomania may be associated with increased rates of OCD or other excessive habits among first-degree relatives (Bienvenu et al. 2000; King et al. 1995). This is consistent with the notion of a genetic basis for a spectrum of excessive grooming behaviors that include trichotillomania, but environmental factors such as social learning cannot be ruled out.

Neuroimaging has demonstrated hyperactivity in the left cerebellum and right superior parietal lobe (Swedo et al. 1991) and possible structural abnormalities in the left putamen (O'Sullivan et al. 1997), left inferior frontal gyrus, and right cuneal cortex (Grachev 1997). Trichotillomania patients have also shown errors in spatial processing (Rettew et al. 1991), divided attention (Stanley et al. 1997), nonverbal memory, and executive functioning (Keuthen et al. 1996), although in the latter study, Bonferroni correction for multiple comparisons would have made these differences nonsignificant. Studies like these do not necessarily imply that preexisting brain abnormalities cause the symp-

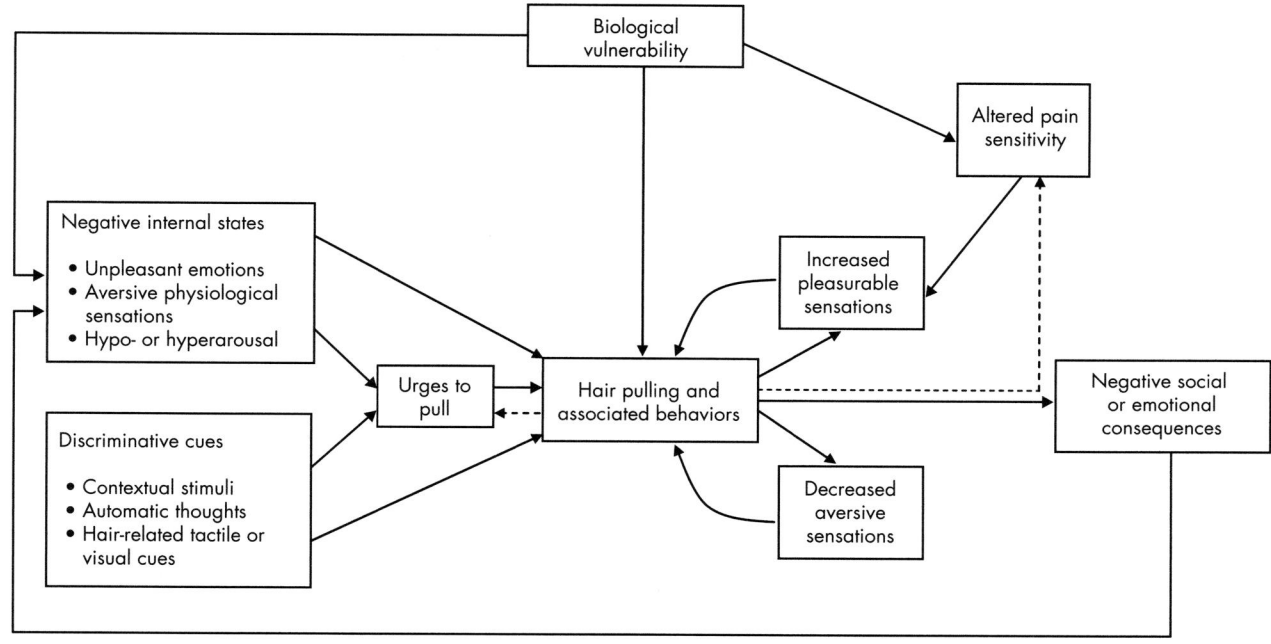

FIGURE 19–3. Schematic diagram of a preliminary biopsychosocial model of trichotillomania.

Source. Reprinted from Franklin ME, Tolin DF, Diefenbach GJ: Trichotillomania, in *Clinical Manual of Impulse-Control Disorders.* Edited by Hollander E, Stein DJ. Washington, DC, American Psychiatric Publishing, 2006, pp. 149–173. Copyright 2006, American Psychiatric Publishing. Used with permission.

toms of trichotillomania; it may be that chronic trichotillomania or its associated features lead to changes in brain structure or function or that both trichotillomania and the brain abnormalities are caused by a third, unknown, variable.

Altered Pain Sensitivity

Individuals with trichotillomania often report that hair pulling is not painful (Christenson et al. 1991c) or in many cases that it feels good or pleasurable (Stanley et al. 1992). To date, no studies have compared hair-pulling sensations between those with trichotillomania and those without, but it is suspected that those without trichotillomania generally do not derive pleasure from pulling; rather, they are likely to describe it as painful. Thus, alterations in pain sensitivity may influence the reinforcing quality of pulling behavior. One possible mechanism for such alterations is upregulation of the endogenous opioid system; this model has not been supported by challenge tasks (Frecska and Arato 2002), although some evidence suggests that pulling may decrease with administration of opiate receptor antagonists (Carrion 1995; Christenson et al. 1994a). Trichotillomania patients do not appear to show reduced pain in nonpulling areas such as the fin-

gertips (Christenson et al. 1994b), so pain sensations are not globally altered in trichotillomania but rather are diminished only at the sites of pulling. This may result from habituation of the pain response caused by repeated pulling over time, although pain absence has been noted even in young children with short pulling histories (Chang et al. 1991). To date, no studies of pain tolerance at the preferred pulling site have been conducted. For those patients who do experience pulling-related pain, the pain itself may be reinforcing because it distracts the individual from negative emotional or physiological states (Christenson and Mansueto 1999).

Hair-Pulling Cues

The behavioral model of hair pulling suggests that pulling begins as a normal response to stress but eventually becomes associated with a variety of internal and external cues through conditioning (Mansueto et al. 1997). Christenson et al. (1993) identified two facets of hair-pulling cues: negative affect (hyperarousal) and sedentary/contemplative cues (hypoarousal, e.g., boredom, fatigue, sedentary activities like reading, television). Physical sensations such as skin sensitivity, itching, irritation, pressure, and burning sensations preceding pulling episodes have also been identified as arousal cues for hair pulling (Mansueto 1990).

Cognitions may serve as cues and consequences to the behavioral sequence. Negative cognitions about the pulling habit itself, such as fear of negative evaluation or worry that the urges to pull will never go away or will get stronger until they pull, resulting in negative emotion, may also increase urges to pull. Belief in the positive effects of hair pulling (e.g., "Hair pulling will make me feel better") or pulling-facilitative thoughts (e.g., "I'll just pull one") may also cue pulling episodes (Gluhoski 1995).

Common contextual cues linked with pulling or pulling-related feelings by conditioning include visual signs that hair is misshapen or unattractive, tactile sensations like feeling a coarse hair, places or activities where pulling has previously occurred, being alone, or the presence of pulling implements like tweezers.

Reinforcement

Hair pulling is often preceded by negative internal states such as unpleasant emotions, aversive physiological sensations, or dysregulated arousal. Hair pulling appears to result in a decrease of these states. Over time, hair-pulling urges that are reinforced by pulling lead to stronger urges to pull, which perpetuates the behavioral cycle. Trichotillomania patients report retrospectively that pulling leads to reduced feelings of tension, boredom, and anxiety, and nonclinical hair pullers also report reductions in sadness and anger (Stanley et al. 1995). In these cases, hair pulling is negatively reinforced and is thus somewhat similar to the compulsive behaviors seen in OCD (Tolin and Foa 2001). However, to the extent that hair pulling evokes pleasurable sensations (Stanley et al. 1992), the habit may also be strengthened via *positive* reinforcement (Mansueto et al. 1997). Pleasure may be obtained not only through pulling but also through associated behaviors like playing with or inspecting the hair, oral stimulation, or trichophagia (Christenson and Mansueto 1999). Thus, pulling may be maintained by either negative or positive reinforcement. Some trichotillomania patients may experience one or the other form of reinforcement, or different kinds of reinforcement may be active for the same person at different times. Careful attention to hair-pulling contingencies is important in planning therapeutic interventions for trichotillomania.

Course

Age of onset usually ranges from early childhood to young adulthood. Initial onset after young adulthood is uncommon, but there have been reports of onset as early as 14 months and as late as 61 years. Peak age of onset in children is at about age 5–8 years, whereas for patients who present to clinicians in adulthood, the mean age of onset is about 13 years (Rothbaum et al. 1993; Swedo et al. 1989).

Transient periods of hair pulling in early childhood may be considered benign and usually have a self-limited course, with most cases remitting spontaneously by the teenage years. Circumscribed periods of hair pulling (weeks to months) followed by complete remission are common among children. This may be because it usually represents a "habit" without the presence of an obvious precipitant or a transient behavior in response to a psychosocial stressor.

Trichotillomania in adolescents and adults typically follows a chronic course, involves multiple hair sites, and is associated with high rates of psychiatric comorbidity (Christenson et al. 1991a). The chronic course may take one of two patterns: in one, the frequency and severity of hair pulling wax and wane over months, without any true remissions; in the other, episodes are characterized by frequent hair pulling separated by long periods of remission (Moore and Jefferson 2004). Some have continuous symptoms for decades. For others, the disorder may come and go for weeks, months, or years. Sites of hair pulling may vary over time. Progression of the condition seems to be unpredictable.

Treatment

The treatment literature for trichotillomania is generally made up of case studies, with progressively more controlled investigation in recent years. In general, knowledge about trichotillomania treatments is limited by small sample sizes, lack of specificity regarding sample characteristics, nonrandom assignment to treatment, dearth of long-term follow-up data, exclusive reliance on patient self-report measures, and lack of information regarding rates of treatment refusal and dropout. Studies of treatment approaches for trichotillomania are summarized in Table 19–16.

Pharmacotherapy

Of the six randomized controlled trials evaluating the efficacy of pharmacotherapy conducted to date, five involved serotonin reuptake inhibitors. This may reflect the previously prevailing view that trichotillomania is a variant of OCD and thus ought to be responsive to the same pharmacological agents proven successful in OCD. In sum, results from these con-

TABLE 19–16. **Trichotillomania: treatment summary**

Authors	Treatment	Description
Pharmacotherapy		
Swedo et al. 1989, 1993	Clomipramine vs. desipramine	10-week double-blind crossover; women with severe trichotillomania ($n=13$); greater improvement and reduced severity of symptoms with clomipramine vs. desipramine; patients reported that compulsion decreased in intensity, and they were more able to resist the urge to pull out their hair with clomipramine; 40% (moderate) reduction in severity of symptoms at a mean of 4.3 years of follow-up
Christenson et al. 1991c	Fluoxetine	18-week placebo-controlled, double-blind crossover; adult chronic hair pullers ($n=15$ completers); short-term efficacy of fluoxetine in the treatment of trichotillomania was not demonstrated
Streichenwein and Thornby 1995	Fluoxetine	Long-term (31-week) double-blind, placebo-controlled crossover; adult chronic hair pullers ($n=16$ completers); efficacy of fluoxetine in the treatment of trichotillomania was not demonstrated
Ninan et al. 2000	CBT vs. clomipramine	Placebo-controlled, randomized, parallel treatment; patients with trichotillomania ($n=16$ completers); CBT dramatically reduced symptoms and was significantly more effective than clomipramine or placebo; clomipramine reduced symptoms more than placebo, but the difference was not significant
van Minnen et al. 2003	Behavior therapy vs. fluoxetine vs. wait list	12-week randomized, wait list–controlled; patients with trichotillomania ($n=40$ completers); behavioral therapy was highly effective for reducing symptoms of trichotillomania in the short term, while fluoxetine was not
Epperson et al. 1999	SSRIs plus risperidone	Open-label; 3 patients with serotonin reuptake inhibitor–refractory trichotillomania; all 3 patients had a robust decrease in hair pulling measured by clinician-rated instruments
Stein and Hollander 1992	SSRIs plus pimozide	Open-label; improvement in hair pulling in 6 of 7 trichotillomania patients; response was sustained in those able to tolerate their medication
Stewart and Nejtek 2003	Olanzapine	3-month open-label; patients with trichotillomania ($n=16$ completers at 1 week); decreased hair pulling and anxiety, with global improvement

TABLE 19-16. Trichotillomania: treatment summary *(continued)*

Authors	Treatment	Description
Christenson et al. 1994b	Naltrexone	Placebo-controlled, double-blind; reducing trichotillomania symptoms in patients with trichotillomania
Pollard et al. 1991	Clomipramine	Open-label; 3 of 4 patients with trichotillomania relapsed completely at 3-month follow-up, although still taking previously effective levels of the drug; remaining patient relapsed for 2 weeks but regained initial treatment benefits
Iancu et al. 1996	Serotonergic drugs	Open-label; 12 patients with trichotillomania; treatment response not maintained at follow-up
Psychotherapy		
Ninan et al. 2000 van Minnen et al. 2003	CBT	See above
Azrin et al. 1980	Habit reversal	Habit reversal was more effective than negative practice in treating trichotillomania
Lerner et al. 1998 Keuthen et al. 2001 Mouton and Stanley 1996	CBT	Significant relapse following CBT

Note. CBT=cognitive-behavioral therapy; SSRI=selective serotonin reuptake inhibitor.

trolled studies of serotonin reuptake inhibitors are equivocal at best, although in view of the small sample sizes more controlled research should be conducted to determine their efficacy more definitively (Christenson et al. 1991b; Ninan et al. 2000; Streichenwein and Thornby 1995; Swedo et al. 1989, 1993; van Minnen et al. 2003). Perhaps important differences between OCD and trichotillomania underlie this apparent difference in treatment response. However, several case studies indicated that augmentation of SSRIs with atypical neuroleptics may be beneficial (Epperson et al. 1999; Stein and Hollander 1992), and an open trial suggested that olanzapine may be efficacious as a monotherapy for trichotillomania (Stewart and Nejtek 2003). Interestingly, naltrexone, an opioid-antagonist thought to decrease positive reinforcement, has also been found superior to placebo in reducing trichotillomania symptoms (Christenson et al. 1994a).

Although no double-blind discontinuation studies have been conducted in trichotillomania, evidence from open studies suggests that treatment response gained from pharmacotherapy may not be maintained in the long run (Iancu et al. 1996; Pollard et al. 1991). The absence of a single randomized, controlled trial in pediatric trichotillomania limits treatment recommendations for this population.

Psychotherapy

With respect to behavioral approaches and CBT, a variety of specific techniques have been applied, including awareness training, self-monitoring, aversion, covert sensitization, negative practice, relaxation training, habit reversal, competing response training, stimulus control, and overcorrection. Although the state of the CBT literature justifies only cautious recommendations, habit reversal, awareness training, and stimulus control are generally purported as the core efficacious interventions for trichotillomania.

Successful outcome has been reported with several of the aforementioned interventions. However, because the vast majority of the literature consists of uncontrolled case reports or small case series, confident conclusions cannot be drawn about the specificity of the observed reductions. This is evidenced by the three randomized trials with adults that have been conducted regarding the efficacy of CBT. Ninan et al. (2000) found CBT superior to clomipramine and placebo at posttreatment, and the same pattern was reported by van Minnen et al. (2003) in their randomized, controlled trial of CBT, fluoxetine, and a wait-list condition. Azrin et al. (1980) found that habit reversal was more effective than negative practice. The significant problem of relapse following CBT has been highlighted in several studies (Keuthen et al. 2001; Lerner et al. 1998; Mouton and Stanley 1996).

The limited and equivocal treatment literature suggests that there is neither a universal nor a complete response to any treatment for trichotillomania. Controlled studies examining the efficacy of CBT treatments involving habit reversal, pharmacotherapy, and their combination are needed.

Impulse-Control Disorders Not Otherwise Specified

As mentioned earlier, there are a number of other disorders that are not included as a distinct category but are categorized as ICDs not otherwise specified in DSM-IV-TR. These include sexual compulsions (impulsive-compulsive sexual behavior), compulsive shopping (impulsive-compulsive buying disorder), skin picking (impulsive-compulsive psychogenic excoriation), and Internet addiction (impulsive-compulsive computer usage disorder). We briefly describe the nature of each of these behaviors and discuss provisional diagnostic criteria that fall within the framework of ICDs.

Sexual Compulsions

Sexual compulsions have been conceptualized in several compelling ways, most commonly as addictive, impulsive, or compulsive disorders. There is no universal agreement on the nature, or even the definition, of sexual compulsions, but at the core are sexual thoughts, urges, and behaviors that are difficult to resist. Sexual compulsions can be categorized as either paraphilias or paraphilia-related disorders, sometimes referred to as nonparaphilic sexual addictions, with the division between the two based on whether the particular sexual compulsion is outside societal norms, although this boundary is not always easily placed. Whether looking at clinical or forensic populations, it is clear that many individuals have an inability to control their sexual thoughts, urges, and behaviors, despite negative consequences.

The paraphilias form a recognized category of disorders in DSM-IV-TR. These disorders all entail socially deviant sexual thoughts, urges, or behaviors that are generally intense and persistent and either involve nonconsenting persons or lead to distress or impairment in functioning. In contrast, paraphilia-related disorders involve sexual thoughts, urges, and behaviors that are normative but occur with such frequency

or intensity that they lead to distress or impairment in functioning (Kafka 1994, 1997). None of the paraphilia-related disorders are designated as specific disorders in DSM-IV-TR.

Sexual compulsions can be conceptualized as being on an obsessive-compulsive spectrum (Bradford 2001; Hollander and Wong 1995a) because, like OCD, sexual compulsions are characterized by obsessive preoccupations (sexual thoughts, fantasies, and urges) and compulsive repetitive behaviors (in this case, sexual behaviors). The compulsive sexual behaviors differ somewhat from OCD ritual compulsions. OCD rituals are not pleasurable activities engaged in for their own sake but rather are neutral or often irritating and unpleasant behaviors that are engaged in to reduce anxiety. Sexual behaviors generally have an element of pleasure, at least initially, although they may lose their pleasurable quality over time; in this regard, they are more similar to addictions and to ICDs such as pathological gambling.

Sexual obsessions can be a presentation of OCD. Paraphilias and paraphilia-related obsessions can be distinguished from the sexual obsessions that are part of OCD because the latter are characterized by recurrent intrusive sexual thoughts and/or images that are ego dystonic, are morally repugnant, induce anxiety, and usually lead to avoidance and nonsexual rituals rather than to sexual behaviors (Hollander and Wong 1995a). The obsessive thoughts often include the fear or belief that one may actually have somehow committed the feared sexual behavior without knowing it. Therefore, the rituals that accompany sexual obsessions in OCD are repetitive behaviors of a nonsexual nature meant somehow to avoid or undo the distressing sexual thoughts or fears. These rituals can take almost any form. For example, someone with an OCD sexual obsession may have intrusive thoughts of having sexual relations with a stranger he passed on the street and may feel compelled to confess to his wife that he may have had sexual relations with the stranger.

Compulsive Shopping

Many terms have been used for compulsive shopping, including *pathological spending, compulsive consumption, addictive compulsion, addictive shopping, uncontrolled buying, shopaholism,* and even *mall mania.* The most widely used terms are *compulsive shopping* and *compulsive buying.* There has been considerable debate in the professional literature about the appropriate classification of compulsive shopping. Some investigators have suggested that compulsive shopping is similar to drug or alcohol addiction (Glatt and Cook

1987; Krych 1989), whereas other researchers have focused on the disorder's similarity to OCD, placing it within the obsessive-compulsive spectrum (Frost et al. 1998; Hollander 1993). Hollander (1993), for example, described an impulsive-compulsive spectrum of behavior involving many disorders that he related to OCD, including compulsive shopping. Yet other investigators, following in the tradition of Kraepelin and Bleuler, have favored its classification as a disorder of impulse control similar to disorders such as pathological gambling (Black et al. 2001), whereas some have related compulsive buying to the mood and anxiety disorders (Lejoyeux et al. 1996; McElroy et al. 1995). There is currently little evidence to favor the classification of compulsive shopping as an addiction, an obsessive-compulsive spectrum disorder, or a mood disorder (Black 2000).

Currently, although DSM-IV-TR has no diagnostic category for compulsive buying, individuals with the disorder can be placed in the residual category "disorders of impulse control not otherwise specified." In DSM-IV-TR, ICDs share an inability to resist an "impulse, drive, or temptation to perform an act that is harmful to the person or to others" (p. 663). One could debate whether compulsive shopping is a harmful act, but its secondary consequences frequently are harmful to the individual.

Following the tradition of criteria-based diagnoses, McElroy et al. (1994) developed an operational definition of compulsive shopping for both clinical and research use (Table 19–17). Their definition recognizes that compulsive buying has both cognitive and behavioral components, each potentially causing impairment manifested through personal distress; social, marital, or occupational dysfunction; or financial or legal problems. They exclude from the definition persons whose excessive buying occurs in the context of mania or hypomania. The definition developed by these investigators is now widely used by psychiatric researchers.

Self-Injurious Behavior

Self-injurious behavior (SIB) can be defined as any behavior involving the deliberate infliction of direct physical harm to one's own body without any intent to die as a consequence of the behavior. DSM-IV-TR offers a few diagnoses under which many, but not all, SIBs can be "fitted": trichotillomania or ICDs not otherwise specified (both under Axis I ICDs); Axis II BPD under the criterion "recurrent suicidal behavior, gestures, or threats, or self-mutilating behavior" (p. 710); and stereotypic movement disorder with self-injurious behavior (disorders of infancy, childhood, or adolescence).

TABLE 19–17. Diagnostic criteria for compulsive buying

1. Maladaptive preoccupation with buying or shopping, or maladaptive buying or shopping impulses or behavior as indicated by at least one of the following:

    a. Frequent preoccupation with buying or impulses to buy that are experienced as irresistible, intrusive, and/or senseless

    b. Frequent buying of more than can be afforded, frequent buying of items that are not needed, or shopping for longer periods of time than intended

2. The buying preoccupations, impulses, or behaviors cause marked distress, are time-consuming, significantly interfere with social or occupational functioning, or result in financial problems (e.g., indebtedness or bankruptcy).

3. The excessive buying or shopping behavior does not occur exclusively during periods of hypomania or mania.

Source.   Reprinted from McElroy S, Keck PE Jr, Pope HG Jr, et al.: "Compulsive Buying: A Report of 20 Cases." *Journal of Clinical Psychiatry* 55:242–248, 1994. Copyright 1994, Physicians Postgraduate Press. Used with permission.

More recently, Simeon and Favazza (2001) proposed a phenomenologically based and clinically relevant comprehensive schema for the classification of all SIBs. They proposed four major categories: stereotypic, major, compulsive, and impulsive. *Stereotypic* behaviors refer to highly repetitive, monotonous, fixed, often rhythmic, seemingly highly driven, and usually content-less (i.e., devoid of thought, affect, and meaning) acts that can range widely in self-inflicted tissue injury from mild to severe or even life-threatening at times. These appear more strongly biologically driven than other types of SIB and are frequently associated with mental retardation (estimates of SIB in people with mental retardation range from 3% to 46% [Bodfish et al. 1995; Winchel and Stanley 1991]), autism, and syndromes such as Lesch-Nyhan, Cornelia de Lange's, and Prader-Willi.

Major SIBs include dramatic and often life-threatening forms of self-injury and involve major and often irreversible destruction of body tissue such as castration, eye enucleation, and amputation of extremities. They are most frequently associated with psychotic states such as schizophrenia but also with intoxications, neurological conditions, bipolar disorder, severe personality disorders, and transsexualism. Common themes involve sin, sexual temptation, punishment, and salvation. Religious delusions are quite common (Nakaya 1996).

Compulsive self-injury includes repetitive, often ritualistic behaviors that typically occur multiple times daily, such as trichotillomania (hair pulling), onychophagia (nail biting), and skin picking or skin scratching (neurotic excoriations). Of these, trichotillomania is by far the most extensively investigated and the only one diagnostically classified as a discrete disorder in DSM-IV-TR. Compulsive SIBs other than hair pulling, such as skin picking and nail biting, appear to be quite common but have received much less attention in the psychiatric literature.

Impulsive SIBs include skin cutting, skin burning, and self-hitting. These behaviors may be broadly conceptualized as acts of impulsive aggression, not unlike impulsive suicide attempts, where the target of the aggression is the self. These behaviors frequently permit those who engage in them to obtain rapid but short-lived relief from a variety of intolerable states, serving a pathological but life-sustaining function. To maximize treatment effectiveness, patients' highly complex determinants, motivations, and precipitants need to be thoroughly understood at a descriptive and motivational level on an individual basis.

Five descriptive stages have been delineated in impulsive self-injury (Leibenluft et al. 1987). The precipitating event often involves real or perceived loss, rejection, or abandonment. It is followed by the escalation of various types of intolerable affects. After failed attempts to forestall the SIB, the behavior is executed and is typically followed by short-lived emotional relief. Individuals describe various self-states and associated motivations leading up to the self-injury (Favazza 1989, 1996; Leibenluft et al. 1987).

Impulsive SIBs are at times so habitual and repetitive that they can occur on a daily basis without major precipitants, becoming in a sense "compulsions." Indeed, there is some evidence that patients with impulsive SIBs who have obsessional traits are more likely to engage in repetitive self-injury (McKay et al. 2000). Thus, it is probably more accurate to conceptualize impulsive self-injury as encompassing some obsessive-compulsive traits, just as compulsive self-injury may encompass some impulsive traits. Both types of traits facilitate the perpetuation of SIBs via the difficulty in controlling impulses and the tendency to repeat.

Problematic Internet Use

Behavioral problems associated with the Internet have been described with various terms such as *computer addiction, Internet addiction (disorder), Internetomania,* *pathological Internet use,* and *problematic Internet use.* There are few studies on problematic Internet use, and most have been conducted online and have lacked control populations (DeAngelis 2000). Given these limitations, it appears that between 6% and 14% of those who use the Internet may be problematic users (DeAngelis 2000). In a study of inappropriate Internet use in the workplace, 60% of the participating corporations reported employees engaged in various improper Internet use, and 30% of the companies reported terminating employees for their behavior (Greenfield 2000). In two online studies of Taiwanese college students, including one with more than 753 participants, more than 10% of the students were noted to be potential "Internet addicts" (Chou 2001; Tsai and Lin 2001). With the continued rapid expansion and increased availability of the Internet, the number of Internet-associated behavior problems is likely to grow.

Problematic Internet use can be typified by the Internet user's inability to limit Internet use, which leads to psychological impairment as well as social, educational, and occupational dysfunction (Shapira et al. 2000). Use of the Internet may be associated with numerous risks to the user. The Internet may be utilized by some to access areas that may be a manifestation of their psychiatric illness, for example, compulsive gambling, paraphilias, and compulsive buying. Some small psychiatric studies have demonstrated that many of the evaluated individuals with problematic Internet use have comorbid psychiatric illnesses, especially mood and anxiety disorders (Black et al. 1999; Shapira et al. 2000). These same studies revealed significant distress and daily dysfunction among problematic users. Individuals with problematic Internet use have been noted to prefer computer activities that entail large amounts of interpersonal interaction, such as E-mail, chat rooms, and interactive gaming (Black et al. 1999; Chou 2001; Griffiths 1995, 1996; Shapira et al. 2000; Young 1998). Studies demonstrate that Internet usage is gender and age dependent, with females and mature "addicts" preferring chat rooms that contain sexual material and males and younger "addicts" more tempted by pornographic and gaming sites (Mitchell 2000).

Whether these aberrant and problematic behaviors are the result of a unique disorder or are simply a manifestation of other psychiatric illnesses remains to be seen. Thus, it is imperative that suggested criteria be able to distinguish problematic Internet use from other psychiatric illnesses.

"Behavioral addiction," a variant of the classic addiction model, has been proposed as a way of conceptualizing Internet dependence (Bradley 1990; Marks 1990) as well as other disorders such as compulsive shopping, compulsive gambling, compulsive sexual behavior, kleptomania, and overeating. In a survey of 129 college students, Greenberg et al. (1999) found that students with behavioral addictions (Internet, exercise, gambling) tended to also be addicted to substances, including nicotine and alcohol. Psychological dependence is present in both substance and behavioral addictions (Bradley 1990; Marks 1990). In the early 1990s, the term "technological addiction" was coined by Griffiths (1995, 1996) to describe "nonchemical (behavioral) addictions which involve human–machine interaction" (Griffiths 1995, p. 15). Some suggest that technological addictions, like computer and Internet addiction, may be similar to drug addiction due to the presence of common components such as euphoria, tolerance, withdrawal, and relapse (Griffiths 1995). "Technological addictions" have been studied primarily in gamblers addicted to slots or "fruit machines" that use operant conditioning to train gamblers to expect a reward for their behavior (Donegan et al. 1983). Not every pull of the lever results in a reward, and thus the gamble ensues (Griffiths 1993). Griffiths (1995) proposed that two kinds of people become addicted to the Internet: those who are intrinsically attracted to the technology and those who use the technology as a diversion from life's displeasures. As the technology improves (increased speed, improved graphics), more individuals may be adversely affected by the Internet (Griffiths 1995; Griffiths and Parke 2002).

Conclusion

This chapter has focused on disorders found in the DSM-IV-TR section on ICDs not otherwise classified:

IED, kleptomania, pathological gambling, pyromania, and trichotillomania. Nevertheless, pathological impulsivity may be a crucial construct in understanding a broad range of psychiatric disorders, ranging from common psychotic disorders (e.g., bipolar disorder) to a range of conditions that have emerged together with new lifestyles and technologies (e.g., compulsive shopping, Internet addiction). The development of reliable diagnostic criteria for ICDs has been extremely useful in promoting research on these disorders and has provided a basis for epidemiological work demonstrating the prevalence of these disorders, their high comorbidity and morbidity, and their significant social costs. At the same time, advances in basic research on impulsivity and addiction, together with new methods in clinical research, have led to increased understanding of the overlapping neurocircuitry and neurochemistry that may be involved in a range of these conditions, and this in turn may ultimately lead to a revised nosology of these conditions. Developments in psychometrics and psychobiology have in turn encouraged researchers to conduct rigorous randomized clinical trials of a range of medications and psychotherapies in the ICDs, and a number of effective strategies are now available. Nevertheless, the range of clinical trials in this area remains comparatively limited, and for now clinicians are required to adopt a flexible approach that includes multiple modalities of intervention in the management of the ICDs. Although many patients can be helped by such an approach, much further work is needed to delineate fully the psychobiology of these disorders and to develop effective treatments. There is also a need to develop coordinated approaches to the prevention of disorders, such as pathological gambling, which are influenced greatly by the availability of particular facilities or technologies.

Key Points

- Pathological impulsivity is a useful construct in understanding a broad range of psychiatric symptoms and disorders, including the ICDs not otherwise specified.

- ICDs are highly prevalent and associated with significant disability and costs but receive disproportionately little attention from clinicians and researchers.

- There are now structured diagnostic instruments and standardized rating scales that allow reliable diagnosis and assessment of the ICDs.

- There have been significant advances in our understanding of the neuronal circuitry that mediates impulsivity, as well as in the delineating of the contributing genes and proteins in this circuitry.

- Ultimately, a better understanding of the psychobiological underpinnings of impulsivity, behavior addiction, and other related constructs may lead to changes in our classification of these disorders.

- Although no medication is registered for the treatment of ICDs, a number of randomized, controlled trials have demonstrated the potential value of pharmacotherapy.

- Current clinical practice also emphasizes the need for a comprehensive approach to management that includes psychotherapy and family intervention. Additional work is needed to improve efficacy.

Suggested Readings

Coccaro E (ed): Aggression: Psychiatric Assessment and Treatment. New York, Informa Healthcare, 2003

Coccaro E: Intermittent explosive disorder. Curr Psychiatry Rep 2:67–71, 2005

Dell'Osso B, Altamura AC, Allen A, et al: Epidemiologic and clinical updates on impulse control disorders: a critical review. Eur Arch Psychiatry Clin Neurosci 256:464–475, 2006

Grant JE, Potenza MN (eds): Pathological Gambling: A Clinical Guide to Treatment. Washington, DC, American Psychiatric Publishing, 2004

Grant JE, Potenza MN: Impulse-control disorders: clinical characteristics and pharmacological management. Ann Clin Psychiatry 16:27–34, 2004

Hollander E, Evers M: New developments in impulsivity. Lancet 358:949–950, 2001

Hollander E, Stein DJ (eds): Impulsivity and Aggression. Sussex, England, Wiley, 1995

Hollander E, Stein DJ (eds): Clinical Manual of Impulse-Control Disorders. Washington, DC, American Psychiatric Publishing, 2006

Stein DJ, Christenson G, Hollander E: Trichotillomania. Washington, DC, American Psychiatric Press, 1999

References

American Psychiatric Association: Diagnostic and Statistical Manual of Mental Disorders, 3rd Edition. Washington, DC, American Psychiatric Association, 1980

American Psychiatric Association: Diagnostic and Statistical Manual of Mental Disorders, 3rd Edition, Revised. Washington, DC, American Psychiatric Association, 1987

American Psychiatric Association: Diagnostic and Statistical Manual of Mental Disorders, 4th Edition. Washington, DC, American Psychiatric Association, 1994

American Psychiatric Association: Diagnostic and Statistical Manual of Mental Disorders, 4th Edition, Text Revision. Washington, DC, American Psychiatric Association, 2000

Azrin NH, Nunn RG, Frantz SE: Treatment of hair pulling (trichotillomania): a comparative study of habit reversal and negative practice training. J Behav Ther Exp Psychiatry 11:13–20, 1980

Barker AF: Arson: A Review of the Psychiatric Literature. Institute of Psychiatry, Maudsley Monographs No 35. Oxford, England, Oxford University Press, 1994

Barnett W, Richter P, Sigmund D, et al: Recidivism and concomitant criminality in pathological firesetters. J Forensic Sci 42:879–883, 1997

Barnett W, Richter P, Renneberg B: Repeated arson: data from criminal records. Forensic Sci Int 101:49–54, 1999

Barratt ES, Stanford MS, Felthous AR, et al: The effects of phenytoin on impulsive and premeditated aggression: a controlled study. J Clin Psychopharmacol 17:341–349, 1997

Bayle FJ, Caci H, Millet B, et al: Psychopathology and comorbidity of psychiatric disorders in patients with kleptomania. Am J Psychiatry 160:1509–1513, 2003

Bechara A: Neurobiology of decision-making: risk and reward. Semin Clin Neuropsychiatry 6:205–216, 2001

Bechara A: Risky business: emotion, decision-making, and addiction. J Gambling Stud 19:23–51, 2003

Bechara A, Damasio AR, Damasio H, et al: Insensitivity to future consequences following damage to human prefrontal cortex. Cognition 50:7–15, 1994

Bechara A, Damasio H, Damasio AR: Emotion, decision making and the orbitofrontal cortex. Cereb Cortex 10:295–307, 2000

Bechara A, Dolan S, Denburg N, et al: Decision-making deficits, linked to a dysfunctional ventromedial prefrontal cortex, revealed in alcohol and stimulant abusers. Neuropsychologia 39:376–389, 2001

Berlin HA, Rolls ET, Kischka U: Impulsivity, time perception, emotion and reinforcement sensitivity in patients with orbitofrontal cortex lesions. Brain 127:1108–1126, 2004

Best M, Williams JM, Coccaro EF: Evidence for a dysfunctional prefrontal circuit in patients with an impulsive aggressive disorder. Proc Natl Acad Sci U S A 99:8448–8453, 2002

Bienvenu OJ, Samuels JF, Riddle MA, et al: The relationship of obsessive-compulsive disorder to possible spectrum disorders: results from a family study. Biol Psychiatry 48:287–293, 2000

Birmaher B, Stanley M, Greenhill L, et al: Platelet imipramine binding in children and adolescents with impulsive behavior. J Am Acad Child Adolesc Psychiatry 29:914–918, 1990

Black DW: The obsessive-compulsive spectrum: fact or fancy? in Obsessive-Compulsive Disorders. Edited by Maj M, Sartorius N, Okasha A, et al. New York, Wiley, 2000, pp 233–235

Black DW, Belsare G, Schlosser S: Clinical features, psychiatric comorbidity, and health-related quality of life in persons reporting compulsive computer use behavior. J Clin Psychiatry 60:839–844, 1999

Black DW, Monahan P, Schlosser S, et al: Compulsive buying severity: an analysis of Compulsive Buying Scale results in 44 subjects. J Nerv Ment Dis 189:123–127, 2001

Blanco C, Moreyra P, Nunes EV, et al: Pathological gambling: addiction or compulsion? Semin Clin Neuropsychiatry 6:167–176, 2001

Blanco C, Petkova E, Ibanez A, et al: A pilot placebo-controlled study of fluvoxamine for pathological gambling. Ann Clin Psychiatry 14:9–15, 2002

Blum K, Braverman ER, Holder JM, et al: Reward deficiency syndrome: a biogenetic model for the diagnosis and treatment of impulsive, addictive, and compulsive behaviors. J Psychoactive Drugs 32 (suppl):1–68, 2000

Bodfish JM, Crawford TM, Powell SB, et al: Compulsions in adults with mental retardation: prevalence, phenomenology and comorbidity with stereotypy and self-injury. Am J Ment Retard 100:183–192, 1995

Bradford JM: The neurobiology, neuropharmacology, and pharmacological treatment of paraphilias and compulsive sexual behavior. Can J Psychiatry 46:26–33, 2001

Bradley BP: Behavioural addictions: common features and treatment implications. Br J Addict 85:1417–1419, 1990

Breiter HC, Aharon I, Kahneman D, et al: Functional imaging of neural responses to expectancy and experience of monetary gains and losses. Neuron 30:619–639, 2001

Broekkamp CL, Phillips AG: Facilitation of self-stimulation behavior following intracerebral microinjections of opioids into the ventral tegmental area. Pharmacol Biochem Behav 11:289–295, 1979

Brown RI: The effectiveness of Gamblers Anonymous, in The Gambling Studies: Proceedings of the 6th National Conference on Gambling and Risk-Taking. Edited by Eadington WR. Reno, University of Nevada, 1985

Brown RI: Arousal and sensation-seeking components in the general explanation of gambling and gambling addictions. Int J Addict 21:1001–1016, 1986

Bumpass ER, Fagelman FD, Brix RJ: Intervention with children who set fires. Am J Psychother 37:328–345, 1983

Burstein A: Fluoxetine-lithium treatment for kleptomania. J Clin Psychiatry 53:28–29, 1992

Carlton PL, Goldstein L: Physiological determinants of pathological gambling, in A Handbook of Pathological Gambling. Edited by Glaski T. Springfield, IL, Charles C Thomas, 1987, pp 657–663

Carlton PL, Manowitz P: Physiological factors as determinants of pathological gambling. Journal of Gambling Behavior 3:274–285, 1988

Carrasco J, Saiz-Ruiz J, Moreno I, et al: Low platelet MAO activity in pathological gambling. Acta Psychiatr Scand 90:427–431, 1994

Carrion VG: Naltrexone for the treatment of trichotillomania: a case report. J Clin Psychopharmacol 15:444–445, 1995

Cavedini P, Riboldi G, Keller R, et al: Frontal lobe dysfunction in pathological gambling patients. Biol Psychiatry 51:334–341, 2002

Chambers RA, Taylor JR, Potenza MN: Developmental neurocircuitry of motivation in adolescence: a critical period of addiction vulnerability. Am J Psychiatry 160:1041–1052, 2003

Chang CH, Lee MB, Chiang YC: Trichotillomania: a clinical study of 36 patients. J Formos Med Assoc 90:176–180, 1991

Chong SA, Low BL: Treatment of kleptomania with fluvoxamine. Acta Psychiatr Scand 93:314–315, 1996

Chou C: Internet heavy use and addiction among Taiwanese college students: an online interview study. Cyberpsychol Behav 4:573–585, 2001

Christenson GA: Trichotillomania: from prevalence to comorbidity. Psychiatric Times 12:44–48, 1995

Christenson GA, Mackenzie TB: Trichotillomania, in Handbook of Prescriptive Treatments for Adults. Edited by Hersen M, Ammerman RT. New York, Plenum, 1994, pp 217–235

Christenson GA, Mansueto CS: Trichotillomania: descriptive characteristics and phenomenology, in Trichotillomania. Edited by Stein DJ, Christenson GA, Hollander E. Washington, DC, American Psychiatric Press, 1999, pp 1–41

Christenson GA, O'Sullivan RL: Trichotillomania: rational treatment options. CNS Drugs 6:23–34, 1996

Christenson GA, Mackenzie TB, Mitchell JE: Characteristics of 60 adult chronic hair pullers. Am J Psychiatry 148:365–370, 1991a

Christenson GA, Mackenzie TB, Mitchell JE, et al: A placebo-controlled, double-blind crossover study of fluoxetine in trichotillomania. Am J Psychiatry 148:1566–1571, 1991b

Christenson GA, Pyle RL, Mitchell JE: Estimated lifetime prevalence of trichotillomania in college students. J Clin Psychol 52:415–417, 1991c

Christenson GA, Chernoff-Clementz E, Clementz BA: Personality and clinical characteristics in patients with trichotillomania. J Clin Psychiatry 53:407–413, 1992

Christenson GA, Ristvedt SL, MacKenzie TB: Identification of trichotillomania cue profiles. Behav Res Ther 31:315–320, 1993

Christenson GA, Crow SJ, Mackenzie TB: A placebo controlled double blind study of naltrexone for trichotillomania. Paper presented at the 147th annual meeting of the American Psychiatric Association, Philadelphia, PA, May 1994a

Christenson GA, Raymond NC, Faris PL, et al: Pain thresholds are not elevated in trichotillomania. Biol Psychiatry 36:347–349, 1994b

Ciarrochi J, Richardson R: Profile of compulsive gamblers in treatment: update and comparisons. Journal of Gambling Behavior 5:53–65, 1989

Clomipramine Collaborative Study Group: Clomipramine in the treatment of patients with obsessive-compulsive disorder. Arch Gen Psychiatry 48:730–738, 1991

Coccaro EF: Family history study of intermittent explosive disorder. Paper presented at the 152nd annual meeting of the American Psychiatric Association, Washington, DC, May 1999

Coccaro EF: Intermittent explosive disorder, in Aggression: Psychiatric Assessment and Treatment. Edited by Coccaro EF. New York, Marcel Dekker, 2003, pp 149–166

Coccaro EF, Kavoussi RJ: Fluoxetine and impulsive aggressive behavior in personality disordered subjects. Arch Gen Psychiatry 54:1081–1088, 1997

Coccaro EF, Siever LJ, Klar HM, et al: Serotonergic studies in patients with affective and personality disorders: correlates with suicidal and impulsive-aggressive behavior. Arch Gen Psychiatry 46:587–599, 1989

Coccaro EF, Lawrence T, Trestman R, et al: Growth hormone responses to intravenous clonidine challenge correlate with behavioral irritability in psychiatric patients and healthy volunteers. Psychiatry Res 39:129–139, 1991

Coccaro EF, Kavoussi RJ, Sheline YI, et al: Impulsive aggression in personality disorder correlates with tritiated paroxetine binding in the platelet. Arch Gen Psychiatry 53:531–536, 1996

Coccaro EF, Bergeman CS, Kavoussi RJ, et al: Heritability of aggression and irritability: a twin study of the Buss-Durkee Aggression Scales in adult male subjects. Biol Psychiatry 41:273–284, 1997a

Coccaro EF, Kavoussi RJ, Hauger RL: Serotonin function and anti-aggressive responses to fluoxetine: a pilot study. Biol Psychiatry 42:546–552, 1997b

Coccaro EF, Kavoussi RJ, Berman ME, et al: Intermittent explosive disorder-revised: development, reliability and validity of research criteria. Compr Psychiatry 39:368–376, 1998a

Coccaro EF, Kavoussi RJ, Hauger RL, et al: Cerebrospinal fluid vasopressin: correlates with aggression and serotonin function in personality disordered subjects. Arch Gen Psychiatry 55:708–714, 1998b

Coccaro EF, Schmidt CA, Samuels JF, et al: Lifetime and 1-month prevalence rates of intermittent explosive disorder in a community sample. J Clin Psychiatry 65:820–824, 2004

Coccaro EF, Posternak MA, Zimmerman M: Prevalence and features of intermittent explosive disorder in a clinical setting. J Clin Psychiatry 66:1221–1227, 2005

Comings DE, Rosenthal RJ, Lesieur HR, et al: A study of the dopamine D2 receptor gene in pathological gambling. Pharmacogenetics 6:223–234, 1996

Comings DE, Gade R, Wu S, et al: Studies of the potential role of the dopamine D1 receptor gene in addictive behaviors. Mol Psychiatry 2:44–56, 1997

Commission on the Review of the National Policy Toward Gambling: Gambling in America. Washington, DC, U.S. Government Printing Office, 1976

Cornelius JR, Soloff P, Perel JM, et al: Continuation pharmacotherapy of borderline personality disorder with haloperidol and phenelzine. Arch Gen Psychiatry 150:1843–1848, 1993

Cowdry RW, Gardner DL: Pharmacotherapy of borderline personality disorder: alprazolam, carbamazepine, trifluoperazine, and tranylcypromine. Arch Gen Psychiatry 45:111–119, 1988

Crean JP, de Wit H, Richards JB: Reward discounting as a measure of impulsive behavior in a psychiatric outpatient population. Exp Clin Psychopharmacol 8:155–162, 2000

Dannon PN: Topiramate for the treatment of kleptomania: a case series and review of the literature. Clin Neuropharmacol 26:1–4, 2003

Dannon PN, Iancu I, Grunhaus L: Naltrexone treatment in kleptomanic patients. Hum Psychopharmacol 14:583–585, 1999

de la Gandara JJ: Fluoxetine: open-trial in pathological gambling. Paper presented at the 152nd annual meeting of the American Psychiatric Association, Washington, DC, May 1999

DeAngelis T: Is Internet addiction real? APA Monitor on Psychology (serial online), Vol 31, 2000. Available at: http://www.apa.org/monitor/apr00. Accessed September 7, 2004.

DeCaria C, Hollander E: Pathological gambling, in Obsessive-Compulsive Related Disorders. Edited by Hollander E. Washington, DC, American Psychiatric Press, 1993, pp 155–178

DeCaria C, Hollander E, Frenkel M, et al: Pathological gambling: an OCD related disorder? Paper presented at the 145th annual meeting of the American Psychiatric Association, Washington, DC, May 1992

DeCaria CM, Begaz T, Hollander E: Serotonergic and noradrenergic function in pathological gambling. CNS Spectr 3:38–47, 1998

Deffenbacher JL, Lynch RS, Oetting ER, et al: Characteristics and treatment of high-anger drivers. J Couns Psychol 47:5–17, 2000

Deffenbacher JL, Filetti LB, Lynch RS, et al: Cognitive-behavioral treatment of high anger drivers. Behav Res Ther 40:895–910, 2002

Dell'Osso B, Allen A, Hollander E. Comorbidity issues in the pharmacological treatment of pathological gambling: a critical review. Clin Pract Epidemiol Ment Health 10:1–21, 2005

DePue RA, Luciana M, Arbisi P, et al: Dopamine and the structure of personality: relation of agonist-induced dopamine activity to positive emotionality. J Pers Soc Psychol 67:485–498, 1994

Dickerson M, Hinchy J, Falve J: Chasing, arousal and sensation-seeking in off-course gamblers. Br J Addict 82:673–680, 1987

Dickerson M, Hinchy J, England SL: Minimal treatments and problem gamblers: a preliminary investigation. J Gambl Stud 6:87–102, 1990

Dolan M, Anderson IM, Deakin JF: Relationship between 5-HT function and impulsivity and aggression in male offenders with personality disorders. Br J Psychiatry 178:352–359, 2001

Donegan NH, Rodin J, O'Brien CP, et al: A learning-theory approach to commonalities, in Commonalities in Substance Abuse and Habitual Behavior. Edited by Levison PK, Gerstein DR, Maloff DR. Lexington, MA, DC Heath, 1983, pp 111–156

du Toit PL, van Kradenburg J, Niehaus DHJ, et al: Characteristics and phenomenology of hair-pulling: an exploration of subtypes. Compr Psychiatry 42:247–256, 2001

Durst R, Katz G, Knobler HY: Buspirone augmentation of fluvoxamine in the treatment of kleptomania. J Nerv Ment Dis 185:586–588, 1997

Eisen SA, Lin N, Lyons MJ, et al: Familial influences on gambling behavior: an analysis of 3359 twin pairs. Addiction 93:1375–1384, 1998

Eisen SA, Slutske WS, Lyons MJ, et al: The genetics of pathological gambling. Semin Clin Neuropsychiatry 6:195–204, 2001

Epperson NC, Fasula D, Wasylink S, et al: Risperidone addition in serotonin reuptake inhibitor-resistant trichotillomania: three cases. J Child Adolesc Psychopharmacol 9:43–49, 1999

Favazza AR: Why patients mutilate themselves. Hosp Community Psychiatry 40:137–145, 1989

Favazza AR: Bodies Under Siege: Self-Mutilation and Body Modification in Culture and Psychiatry. Baltimore, MD, Johns Hopkins University Press, 1996

Fiorillo CD, Tobler PN, Schultz W: Discrete coding of reward probability and uncertainty by dopamine neurons. Science 299:1898–1902, 2003

Fishbain DA: Kleptomania as risk-taking behavior in response to depression. Am J Psychother 41:598–603, 1987

Fishbain DA: Kleptomanic behavior response to perphenazine-amitriptyline HCl combination. Can J Psychiatry 33:241–242, 1988

Franklin GA, Pucci PS, Arbabi S, et al: Decreased juvenile arson and firesetting recidivism after implementation of a multidisciplinary prevention program. J Trauma 53:260–266, 2002

Franklin ME, Keuthen NJ, Spokas ME, et al: Pediatric trichotillomania: descriptive psychopathology and comorbid symptomatology. Paper presented at the Trichotillomania: Psychopathology and Treatment Development Symposium, conducted at the 36th annual meeting of the Association for the Advancement of Behavior Therapy, Reno, NV, November 2002

Frecska E, Arato M: Opiate sensitivity test in patients with stereotypic movement disorder and trichotillomania. Prog Neuropsychopharmacol Biol Psychiatry 26:909–912, 2002

Frost RO, Kim HJ, Morris C, et al: Hoarding, compulsive buying and reasons for saving. Behav Res Ther 36:657–664, 1998

Gambino B, Fitzgerald R, Shaffer HJ, et al: Perceived family history of problem gambling and scores on SOGS. J Gambl Stud 9:169–184, 1993

Gauthier J, Pellerin D: Management of compulsive shoplifting through covert sensitization. J Behav Ther Exp Psychiatry 13:73–75, 1982

Geller J, Bertsch G: Fire-setting behavior in the histories of a state hospital population. Am J Psychiatry 142:464–468, 1985

Giammanco M, Tabacchi G, Giammanco S, et al: Testosterone and aggressiveness. Med Sci Monit 11:RA136–RA145, 2005

Glassman AH, Covey LS, Dalack GW, et al: Smoking cessation, clonidine, and vulnerability to nicotine among dependent smokers. Clin Pharmacol Ther 54:670–679, 1993

Glatt MM, Cook CC: Pathological spending as a form of psychological dependence. Br J Addict 82:1252–1258, 1987

Glover JH: A Case of kleptomania treated by covert sensitization. Br J Clin Psychol 24:213–214, 1985

Gluhoski VL: A cognitive approach for treating trichotillomania. J Psychother Pract Res 4:277–285, 1995

Goldman MJ: Kleptomania: making sense of the nonsensical. Am J Psychiatry 148:986–996, 1991

Grachev ID: MRI-based morphometric topographic parcellation of human neocortex in trichotillomania. Psychiatry Clin Neurosci 51:315–321, 1997

Grant JE: Co-occurrence of personality disorders in persons with kleptomania: a preliminary investigation. J Am Acad Law Psychiatry 34:395–398, 2004

Grant JE, Kim SW: Adolescent kleptomania treated with naltrexone: a case report. Eur Child Adolesc Psychiatry 11:92–95, 2002a

Grant JE, Kim SW: Clinical characteristics and associated psychopathology of 22 patients with kleptomania. Compr Psychiatry 43:378–384, 2002b

Grant JE, Kim SW: An open label study of naltrexone in the treatment of kleptomania. J Clin Psychiatry 63:349–356, 2002c

Grant JE, Kim SW: Temperament and early environmental influences in kleptomania. Compr Psychiatry 43:223–229, 2002d

Grant JE, Kim SW: Comorbidity of impulse-control disorders among pathological gamblers. Acta Psychiatr Scand 108:207–213, 2003

Grant JE, Kim SW, Potenza MN, et al: Paroxetine treatment of pathological gambling: a multi-centre randomized controlled trial. Int Clin Psychopharmacol 18:243–249, 2003

Grant JE, Levine L, Kim D, et al: Impulse-control disorders in adult psychiatric inpatients. Am J Psychiatry 162:2184–2188, 2005

Greenberg JL, Lewis SE, Dodd DK: Overlapping addictions and self-esteem among college men and women. Addict Behav 24:565–571, 1999

Greenfield D: Lost in cyberspace: the web @ work, 2000. Available at: http://www.virtual-addiction.com/pdf/lostincyberspace.pdf. Accessed on September 7, 2004.

Griffiths MD: Fruit machine gambling: the importance of structural characteristics. J Gambl Stud 9:101–119, 1993

Griffiths MD: Technological addictions. Clin Psychol Forum 95:14–19, 1995

Griffiths MD: Internet addiction: an issue for clinical psychology? Clin Psychol Forum 97:32–36, 1996

Griffiths MD, Parke J: The social impact of Internet gambling. Soc Sci Comput Rev 20:312–320, 2002

Grodnitzky GR, Tafrate RC: Imaginal exposure for anger reduction in adult outpatients: a pilot study. J Behav Ther Exp Psychiatry 31:259–279, 2000

Gudjonsson GH: The significance of depression in the mechanism of "compulsive" shoplifting. Med Sci Law 27:171–176, 1987

Hajcak G, Franklin ME, Simons RF, et al: Hairpulling and skin picking in relation to affective distress and obsessive-compulsive symptoms. J Psychopathol Behav Assess 28:177–185, 2006

Haller R, Hinterhuber H: Treatment of pathological gambling with carbamazepine. Pharmacopsychiatry 27:129, 1994

Hanna GL: Trichotillomania and related disorders in children and adolescents. Child Psychiatry Hum Dev 27:255–268, 1997

Himle JA, Bordnick PS, Thyer BA: A comparison of trichotillomania and obsessive-compulsive disorder. J Psychopathol Behav Assess 17:251–260, 1995

Holden C: "Behavioral" addictions: do they exist? Science 294:980–982, 2001

Hollander E (ed): Obsessive-Compulsive Related Disorders. Washington, DC, American Psychiatric Press, 1993

Hollander E: Impulsive and compulsive disorders, in Neuropsychopharmacology: The Fifth Generation in Progress. Edited by Davis K, Charney D, Coyle J, et al. New York, American College of Neuropsychopharmacology, 2002, pp 1591–1757

Hollander E, Wong CM: Body dysmorphic disorder, pathological gambling, and sexual compulsions. J Clin Psychiatry 56 (suppl):7–12, 1995a

Hollander E, Wong CM: Introduction: obsessive-compulsive spectrum disorders. J Clin Psychiatry 56 (suppl):3–6, 1995b

Hollander E, DeCaria C, Nitescu A, et al: Noradrenergic function in obsessive-compulsive disorder: behavioral and neuroendocrine responses to clonidine and comparison to healthy controls. Psychiatry Res 37:161–177, 1991

Hollander E, DeCaria C, Nitescu A, et al: Serotonergic function in obsessive-compulsive disorder: behavioral and neuroendocrine responses to oral m-CPP and fenfluramine in patients and healthy volunteers. Arch Gen Psychiatry 49:21–28, 1992a

Hollander E, Frenkel M, DeCaria C, et al: Treatment of pathological gambling with clomipramine (letter). Am J Psychiatry 149:710–711, 1992b

Hollander E, DeCaria CM, Mari E, et al: Short-term single-blind fluvoxamine treatment of pathological gambling. Am J Psychiatry 155:1781–1783, 1998

Hollander E, Buchalter AJ, DeCaria CM: Pathological gambling. Psychiatr Clin North Am 23:629–642, 2000a

Hollander E, DeCaria CM, Finkell JN, et al: A randomized double-blind fluvoxamine/placebo crossover trial in pathological gambling. Biol Psychiatry 47:813–817, 2000b

Hollander E, Pallanti S, Baldini Rossi N, et al: Sustained release lithium/placebo treatment response and FDG-PET imaging of wagering in bipolar spectrum pathological gamblers. Paper presented at the American College of Neuropsychopharmacology Annual Conference, Waikoloa Village, HI, December 2001

Hollander E, Pallanti S, Baldini Rossi N, et al: Sustained release lithium/placebo treatment response in bipolar spectrum pathological gamblers. Paper presented at the New Clinical Drug Evaluation (NCDEU) Annual Meeting, Boca Raton, FL, June 2002

Hollander E, Tracy KA, Swann AC, et al: Divalproex in the treatment of impulsive aggression: efficacy in cluster B personality disorders. Neuropsychopharmacology 28:1186–1197, 2003

Hudson JI, Pope HG, Jonas JM, et al: Phenomenological relationship of eating disorders to major affective disorder. Psychiatry Res 9:345–354, 1983

Huesmann LR, Leonard E, Lefkowitz M, et al: Stability of aggression over time and generations. Dev Psychopathol 20:1120–1134, 1984

Hyman SE: Molecular and cell biology of addiction. Curr Opin Neurol Neurosurg 6:609–613, 1993

Iancu I, Weizman A, Kindler S, et al: Serotonergic drugs in trichotillomania: treatment results in 12 patients. J Nerv Ment Dis 184:641–644, 1996

Ibanez A, de Castro IP, Fernandez-Piqueras J, et al: Pathological gambling and DNA polymorphic markers at MAO-A and MAO-B genes. Mol Psychiatry 5:105–109, 2000

Ibanez A, Blanco C, Donahue E, et al: Psychiatric comorbidity in pathological gamblers seeking treatment. Am J Psychiatry 158:1733–1735, 2001

Ibanez A, Blanco C, de Castro IP, et al: Genetics of pathological gambling. J Gambl Stud 19:11–22, 2003

Jacobs DF: Evidence for a common dissociative-like reaction among addicts. Journal of Gambling Behavior 4:27–37, 1988

Kafka MP: Paraphilia-related disorders: common, neglected and misunderstood. Harv Rev Psychiatry 2:39–40, 1994

Kafka MP: Hypersexual desire in males: an operational definition and clinical implications for males with paraphilias and paraphilia-related disorders. Arch Sex Behav 25:505–526, 1997

Kafry D: Playing with matches: children and fire, in Fires and Human Behavior. Edited by Canter D. New York, Wiley, 1980, pp 47–62

Kavoussi RK, Coccaro EF: Divalproex sodium for impulsive aggressive behavior in patients with personality disorder. J Clin Psychiatry 59:676–680, 1998

Keuthen NJ, Savage CR, O'Sullivan RL, et al: Neuropsychological functioning in trichotillomania. Biol Psychiatry 39:747–749, 1996

Keuthen NJ, Fraim C, Deckersbach TD, et al: Longitudinal follow-up of naturalistic treatment outcome in patients with trichotillomania. J Clin Psychiatry 62:101–107, 2001

Keuthen NJ, Franklin ME, Bohne A, et al: Functional impairment associated with trichotillomania and implications for treatment development. Paper presented at the Trichotillomania: Psychopathology and Treatment Development Symposium conducted at the 36th annual meeting of the Association for the Advancement of Behavior Therapy, Reno, NV, November 2002

Keutzer C: Kleptomania: a direct approach to treatment. Br J Med Psychol 45:159–163, 1972

Kim SW, Grant JE, Adson DE, et al: Double-blind naltrexone and placebo comparison study in the treatment of pathological gambling. Biol Psychiatry 49:914–921, 2001

Kim SW, Grant JE, Adson DE, et al: A double-blind placebo-controlled study of the efficacy and safety of paroxetine in the treatment of pathological gambling. J Clin Psychiatry 63:501–507, 2002

Kindler S, Dannon PN, Iancu I, et al: Emergence of kleptomania during treatment for depression with serotonin selective reuptake inhibitors. Clin Neuropharmacol 20:126–129, 1997

King RA, Scahill L, Vitulano LA, et al: Childhood trichotillomania: clinical phenomenology, comorbidity, and family genetics. J Am Acad Child Adolesc Psychiatry 34:1451–1459, 1995

Kmetz GF, McElroy SL, Collins DJ: Response of kleptomania and mixed mania to valproate. Am J Psychiatry 154:580–581, 1997

Koles MR, Jenson WR: Comprehensive treatment of chronic fire setting in a severely disordered boy. J Behav Ther Exp Psychiatry 16:81–85, 1985

Kolko D, Kazdin AE: Assessment of dimensions of childhood fire-setting among patients and nonpatients: the fire-setting risk interview. J Abnorm Child Psychol 17:157–176, 1989

Koob GF: Drugs of abuse: anatomy, pharmacology and function of reward pathways. Trends Pharmacol Sci 13:177–184, 1992

Koob GF, Bloom FE: Cellular and molecular mechanisms of drug dependence. Science 242:715–723, 1988

Koson DF, Dvoskin J: Arson: a diagnostic study. Bull Am Acad Psychiatry Law 10:39–49, 1982

Kraus JE: Treatment of kleptomania with paroxetine. J Clin Psychiatry 60:793, 1999

Kriegsfeld LJ, Dawson TM, Dawson VL, et al: Aggressive behavior in male mice lacking the gene for neuronal nitric oxide synthase requires testosterone. Brain Res 769:66–70, 1997

Krych R: Abnormal consumer behavior: a model of addictive behaviors. Adv Consum Res 16:745–748, 1989

Ladouceur R: Cognitive activities among gamblers. Paper presented at the Association for Advancement of Behavior Therapy (AABT) Convention, San Francisco, CA, November 1990

Ladouceur R, Mireault C: Gambling behavior among high school students in the Quebec area. Journal of Gambling Behavior 4:3–12, 1988

Lappalainen J, Long JC, Eggert M, et al: Linkage of antisocial alcoholism to the serotonin 5-HT1B receptor gene in 2 populations. Arch Gen Psychiatry 55:989–994, 1998

Laubichler W, Kuhberger A, Sedlmeier P: "Pyromania" and arson: a psychiatric and criminological data analysis (in German). Nervenarzt 67:774–780, 1996

Leibenluft E, Gardner DL, Cowdry RW: The inner experience of the borderline self-mutilator. J Personal Disord 1:317–324, 1987

Lejoyeux M, Andes J, Tassian V, et al: Phenomenology and psychopathology of uncontrolled buying. Am J Psychiatry 152:1524–1529, 1996

Lejoyeux M, Feuché N, Loi S, et al: Study of impulse-control disorders among alcohol-dependent patients. J Clin Psychiatry 40:302–305, 1999

Lejoyeux M, Arbaretaz M, McLoughlin M, et al: Impulse-control disorders and depression. J Nerv Ment Dis 190:310–314, 2002

Lepkifker E, Dannon PN, Ziv R, et al: The treatment of kleptomania with serotonin reuptake inhibitors. Clin Neuropharmacol 22:40–43, 1999

Lerner J, Franklin ME, Meadows EA, et al: Effectiveness of a cognitive-behavioral treatment program for trichotillomania: an uncontrolled evaluation. Behav Ther 29:157–171, 1998

Lesieur HR: The female pathological gambler, in Gambling Studies: Proceedings of the 7th International Conference on Gambling and Risk-Taking. Edited by Eadington WR. Reno, University of Nevada, 1988, pp 230–258

Lesieur H, Blume S: The South Oaks Gambling Screen (SOGS): a new instrument for the identification of pathological gamblers. Am J Psychiatry 144:1184–1188, 1987

Lesieur HR, Klein R: Pathological gambling among high school students. Addict Behav 12:129–135, 1987

Lesieur H, Blume S, Zoppa R: Alcoholism, drug abuse, and gambling. Alcohol Clin Exp Res 10:33–38, 1986

Lewis NDC, Yarnell H: Pathological Firesetting (Pyromania): Nervous and Mental Disease Monograph No 82. New York, Coolidge Foundation, 1951

Linden RD, Pope HG, Jonas JM: Pathological gambling and major affective disorders: preliminary findings. J Clin Psychiatry 47:201–203, 1986

Linehan MM, Tutek DA, Heard HL, et al: Interpersonal outcome of cognitive behavioral treatment for chronically suicidal borderline patients. Am J Psychiatry 151:1771–1776, 1994

Links PS, Steiner M, Boiago I, et al: Lithium therapy for borderline patients: preliminary findings. J Personal Disord 4:173–181, 1990

Linnoila M, Virkkunen M, Scheinin M, et al: Low cerebrospinal fluid 5-hydroxyindoleacetic acid concentration differentiates impulsive from nonimpulsive violent behavior. Life Sci 33:2609–2614, 1983

Linnoila M, De Jong J, Virkkunen M: Family history of alcoholism in violent offenders and impulsive fire setters. Arch Gen Psychiatry 46:613–616, 1989

Lyons WE, Mamounas LA, Ricaurte GA: Brain-derived neurotrophic factor-deficient mice develop aggressiveness and hyperphagia in conjunction with brain serotonergic abnormalities. Proc Natl Acad Sci U S A 96:15239–15244, 1991

Maccallum F, Blaszczynski A: Pathological gambling and comorbid substance use. Aust N Z J Psychiatry 36:411–415, 2002

Mann JJ, McBride PA, Brown RP, et al: Relationship between central and peripheral serotonin indexes in depressed and suicidal psychiatric inpatients. Arch Gen Psychiatry 49:442–446, 1992

Mansueto CS: Typography and phenomenology of trichotillomania. Paper presented at the annual convention of the Association for Advancement of Behavior Therapy, San Francisco, CA, November 1990

Mansueto CS, Stemberger RMT, Thomas AM, et al: Trichotillomania: a comprehensive behavioral model. Clin Psychol Rev 17:567–577, 1997

Manuck SB, Flory JD, McCaffery JM, et al: Aggression, impulsivity, and central nervous system serotonergic responsivity in a nonpatient sample. Neuropsychopharmacology 19:287–299, 1998

Manuck SB, Flory JD, Ferrell RE, et al: Aggression and anger-related traits associated with a polymorphism of the tryptophan hydroxylase gene. Biol Psychiatry 45:603–614, 1999

Manuck SB, Flory JD, Ferrell RE, et al: A regulatory polymorphism of the monoamine oxidase-A gene may be associated with variability in aggression, impulsivity, and central nervous system serotonergic responsivity. Psychiatry Res 95:9–23, 2000

Marazziti D, Presta S, Pfanner C, et al: The biological basis of kleptomania and compulsive buying. Paper presented at the American College of Neuropsychopharmacology 39th Annual Meeting. San Juan, Puerto Rico, December 2000

Marks I: Behavioural (nonchemical) addictions. Br J Addict 85:1389–1394, 1990

Mattes JA, Fink M: A family study of patients with temper outbursts. J Psychiatr Res 21:249–255, 1987

Mavromatis M, Lion JR: A primer on pyromania. Dis Nerv Syst 38:954–955, 1977

McConaghy N, Blaszczynski A: Imaginal desensitization: a cost-effective treatment in two shoplifters and a binge-eater resistant to previous therapy. Aust N Z J Psychiatry 22:78–82, 1988

McCormick RA, Russo AM, Ramirez LF, et al: Affective disorders among pathological gamblers seeking treatment. Am J Psychiatry 141:215–218, 1984

McElroy SL, Keck PE, Pope HG, et al: Pharmacological treatment of kleptomania and bulimia nervosa. J Clin Psychopharmacol 9:358–360, 1989

McElroy SL, Hudson JI, Pope HG, et al: Kleptomania: clinical characteristics and associated psychopathology. Psychol Med 21:93–108, 1991a

McElroy SL, Pope HG, Hudson JI, et al: Kleptomania: a report of 20 cases. Am J Psychiatry 148:652–657, 1991b

McElroy SL, Hudson JI, Pope HG, et al: The DSM-III-R impulse-control disorders not elsewhere classified: clinical characteristics and relationship to other psychiatric disorders. Am J Psychiatry 149:318–327, 1992

McElroy SL, Keck PE Jr, Pope HG Jr, et al: Compulsive buying: a report of 20 cases. J Clin Psychiatry 55:242–248, 1994

McElroy SL, Keck PE, Phillips KA: Kleptomania, compulsive buying, and binge-eating disorder. J Clin Psychiatry 56 (suppl):14–26, 1995

McElroy SL, Soutullo CA, Beckman DA, et al: DSM-IV intermittent explosive disorder: a report of 27 cases. J Clin Psychiatry 59:203–210, 1998

McGrath P, Marshall PG: A comprehensive treatment program for a fire-setting child. J Behav Ther Exp Psychiatry 10:69–72, 1979

McGuire RJ, Carlisle JM, Young BG: Sexual deviations as conditioned behaviour: a hypothesis. Behav Res Ther 2:185–190, 1965

McKay D, Kulchycky S, Danyko S: Borderline personality and obsessive-compulsive symptoms. J Personal Disord 14:57–63, 2000

Mitchell P: Internet addiction: genuine diagnosis or not? Lancet 355:632, 2000

Montgomery SA, Montgomery D: Pharmacological prevention of suicidal behavior. J Affect Disord 4:291–298, 1982

Moody G: Quit Compulsive Gambling. London, Thorsons, 1990

Moore DP, Jefferson JW: Handbook of Medical Psychiatry, 2nd Edition. St. Louis, MO, Mosby, 2004

Moreno I, Saiz-Ruiz J, Lopez-Ibor JJ: Serotonin and gambling dependence. Hum Psychopharmacol 6:9–12, 1991

Mouton SG, Stanley MA: Habit reversal training for trichotillomania: a group approach. Cogn Behav Pract 3:159–182, 1996

Murray JB: Review of research on pathological gambling. Psychol Rep 72:791–810, 1993

Nakaya M: On background factors of male genital self-mutilation. Psychopathology 29:242–248, 1996

New AS, Hazlett EA, Buchsbaum MS: Blunted prefrontal cortical ^{18}fluorodeoxyglucose positron emission tomography response to meta-chlorophenylpiperazine in impulsive aggression. Arch Gen Psychiatry 59:621–629, 2002

Ninan PT, Rothbaum BO, Marsteller FA, et al: A placebo-controlled trial of cognitive-behavioral therapy and clomipramine in trichotillomania. J Clin Psychiatry 61:47–50, 2000

Noblett S, Nelson B: A psychosocial approach to arson: a case controlled study of female offenders. Med Sci Law 41:325–330, 2001

O'Sullivan RL, Rauch SL, Breiter HC, et al: Reduced basal ganglia volumes in trichotillomania measured via morphometric magnetic resonance imaging. Biol Psychiatry 42:39–45, 1997

Pallanti S, Baldini Rossi N, Sood E, et al: Nefazodone treatment of pathological gambling: a prospective open-label controlled trial. J Clin Psychiatry 63:1034–1039, 2002a

Pallanti S, Quercioli L, Sood E, et al: Lithium and valproate treatment of pathological gambling: a randomized single-blind study. J Clin Psychiatry 63:559–564, 2002b

Parsey RV, Oquendo MA, Simpson NR, et al: Effects of sex, age, and aggressive traits in man on brain serotonin 5-HT$_{1A}$ receptor binding potential measured by PET using [C-11]WAY-100635. Brain Res 954:173–182, 2002

Perez de Castro I, Ibanez A, Torres P, et al: Genetic association study between pathological gambling and a functional DNA polymorphism at the D4 receptor gene. Pharmacogenetics 7:345–348, 1997

Perez de Castro I, Ibanez A, Saiz-Ruiz J, et al: Concurrent positive association between pathological gambling and functional DNA polymorphisms at the MAO-A and the 5-HT transporter genes. Mol Psychiatry 7:927–928, 2002

Petry NM: Delay discounting of money and alcohol in actively using alcoholics, currently abstinent alcoholics, and controls. Psychopharmacology (Berl) 154:243–250, 2001a

Petry NM: Pathological gamblers, with and without substance use disorders, discount delayed rewards at high rates. J Abnorm Psychol 110:482–487, 2001b

Petry NM: Substance abuse, pathological gambling, and impulsiveness. Drug Alcohol Depend 63:29–38, 2001c

Petry NM, Armentano C: Prevalence, assessment, and treatment of pathological gambling: a review. Psychiatr Serv 50:1021–1027, 1999

Petry NM, Casarella T: Excessive discounting of delayed rewards in substance abusers with gambling problems. Drug Alcohol Depend 56:25–32, 1999

Phillips DP, Welty WR, Smith MM: Elevated suicide levels associated with legalized gambling. Suicide Life Threat Behav 27:373–378, 1997

Pollard CA, Ibe IO, Krojanker DN, et al: Clomipramine treatment of trichotillomania: a follow-up report on four cases. J Clin Psychiatry 52:128–130, 1991

Post RM, Pickar D, Ballenger JC, et al: Endogenous opiates in cerebrospinal fluid: relationship to mood and anxiety, in Neurobiology of Mood Disorders. Edited by Post RM, Ballenger JC. Baltimore, MD, Williams & Wilkins, 1984, pp 356–368

Potenza MN: The neurobiology of pathological gambling. Semin Clin Neuropsychiatry 6:217–226, 2001

Potenza MN, Chambers RA: Schizophrenia and pathological gambling. Am J Psychiatry 158:497–498, 2001

Potenza MN, Hollander E: Pathological gambling and impulse-control disorders, in Neuropsychopharmacology: The 5th Generation of Progress. Edited by Coyle JT, Nemeroff C, Charney D, et al. Baltimore, MD, Lippincott Williams & Wilkins, 2002, pp 1725–1741

Potenza MN, Steinberg MA, Skudlarski P, et al: Gambling urges in pathological gambling: a functional magnetic resonance imaging study. Arch Gen Psychiatry 60:828–836, 2003

Presta S, Marazziti D, Dell'Osso L, et al: Kleptomania: clinical features and comorbidity in an Italian sample. Compr Psychiatry 43:7–12, 2002

Rasanen P, Hirvenoja R, Hakko H, et al: A portrait of a juvenile arsonist. Forensic Sci Int 73:41–47, 1995

Reeve E: Hair pulling in children and adolescents, in Trichotillomania. Edited by Stein DJ, Christenson GA, Hollander E. Washington, DC, American Psychiatric Press, 1999, pp 201–224

Reeve EA, Bernstein GA, Christenson GA: Clinical characteristics and psychiatric comorbidity in children with trichotillomania. J Am Acad Child Adolesc Psychiatry 31:132–138, 1992

Rettew DC, Cheslow DL, Rapoport JL, et al: Neuropsychological test performance in trichotillomania: a further link with obsessive-compulsive disorder. J Anxiety Disord 5:225–235, 1991

Ritchie EC, Huff TG: Psychiatric aspects of arsonists. J Forensic Sci 44:733–740, 1999

Robins LN, Regier DA: Psychiatric Disorders in America. New York, Free Press, 1991

Rogers RD, Robbins TW: Investigating the neurocognitive deficits associated with chronic drug misuse. Curr Opin Neurobiol 11:250–257, 2001

Rosenthal RJ: Pathological gambling. Psychiatr Ann 22:72–78, 1992

Rosenthal R, Rugle L: A psychodynamic approach to the treatment of pathological gambling, part I: achieving abstinence. J Gambl Stud 10:21–42, 1994

Rothbaum BO, Shaw L, Morris R, et al: Prevalence of trichotillomania in a college freshman population (letter to the editor). J Clin Psychiatry 54:72, 1993

Roy A, Adinoff B, Roehrich L, et al: Pathological gambling: a psychobiological study. Arch Gen Psychiatry 45:369–373, 1988a

Roy A, Custer R, Lorenz V, et al: Depressed pathological gamblers. Acta Psychol Scand 77:163–165, 1988b

Roy A, DeJong J, Linnoila M: Extroversion in pathological gamblers: correlates with indexes of noradrenergic function. Arch Gen Psychiatry 46:679–681, 1989

Rugle L, Melamed L: Neuropsychological assessment of attention problems in pathological gamblers. J Nerv Ment Dis 181:107–112, 1993

Russo AM, Taber JI, McCormick RA, et al: An outcome study of an inpatient treatment program for pathological gambling. Hosp Community Psychiatry 35:823–827, 1984

Schlosser S, Black DW, Blum N, et al: The demography, phenomenology, and family history of 22 persons with compulsive hair pulling. Ann Clin Psychiatry 6:147–152, 1994

Schwartz JH: Psychoanalytic psychotherapy for a woman with diagnoses of kleptomania and bulimia. Hosp Community Psychiatry 43:109–110, 1992

Seroczynski AD, Bergeman CS, Coccaro EF: Etiology of the impulsivity/aggression relationship: genes or environment? Psychiatry Res 86:41–57, 1999

Shaffer HJ, Hall MN: Estimating the prevalence of adolescent gambling disorders: a quantitative synthesis and guide toward standard gambling nomenclature. J Gambl Stud 12:193–214, 1996

Shaffer HJ, Hall MN, Vanderbilt J: Estimating the prevalence of disordered gambling behavior in the United States and Canada: a research synthesis. Am J Public Health 89:1369–1376, 1999

Shapira NA, Goldsmith TG, Keck PE, et al: Psychiatric features of individuals with problematic Internet use. J Affect Disord 57:267–272, 2000

Sheard M, Manini J, Bridges C, et al: The effect of lithium on impulsive aggressive behavior in man. Am J Psychiatry 133:1409–1413, 1976

Siever LJ, Buchsbaum MS, New AS, et al: d,l-Fenfluramine response in impulsive personality disorder assessed with [18F]fluorodeoxyglucose positron emission tomography. Neuropsychopharmacology 20:413–423, 1999

Simeon D, Favazza AR: Self-injurious behaviors: phenomenology and assessment, in Self-Injurious Behaviors: Assessment and Treatment. Edited by Simeon D, Hollander E. Washington, DC, American Psychiatric Publishing, 2001, pp 1–28

Slutske WS, Eisen S, True WR, et al: Common genetic vulnerability for pathological gambling and alcohol dependence in men. Arch Gen Psychiatry 57:666–673, 2000

Soloff PH, George A, Nathan RS, et al: Paradoxical effects of amitriptyline in borderline patients. Am J Psychiatry 143:1603–1605, 1986a

Soloff PH, George A, Nathan RS, et al: Progress in pharmacotherapy of borderline disorders. Arch Gen Psychiatry 43:691–697, 1986b

Soloff PH, George A, Nathan RS, et al: Amitriptyline versus haloperidol in borderlines: final outcomes and predictors of response. J Clin Psychopharmacol 9:238–246, 1989

Soloff PH, Cornelius J, Anselm G, et al: Efficacy of phenelzine and haloperidol in borderline personality disorder. Arch Gen Psychiatry 50:377–385, 1993

Specker SM, Carlson GA, Christenson GA, et al: Impulse-control disorders and attention deficit disorder in pathological gamblers. Ann Clin Psychiatry 7:175–179, 1995

Stanley MA, Cohen LJ: Trichotillomania and obsessive-compulsive disorder, in Trichotillomania. Edited by Stein DJ, Christenson GA, Hollander E. Washington, DC, American Psychiatric Press, 1999, pp 225–261

Stanley MA, Swann AC, Bowers TC, et al: A comparison of clinical features in trichotillomania and obsessive-compulsive disorder. Behav Res Ther 30:39–44, 1992

Stanley MA, Borden JW, Mouton SG, et al: Nonclinical hair-pulling: affective correlates and comparison with clinical samples. Behav Res Ther 33:179–186, 1995

Stanley MA, Hannay HJ, Breckenridge JK: The neuropsychology of trichotillomania. J Anxiety Disord 11:473–488, 1997

Stein DJ, Hollander E: Low-dose pimozide augmentation of serotonin reuptake blockers in the treatment of trichotillomania. J Clin Psychiatry 53:123–126, 1992

Stewart R, Brown RIF: An outcome study of Gamblers Anonymous. Br J Psychiatry 152:284–288, 1988

Stewart RS, Nejtek VA: An open-label, flexible-dose study of olanzapine in the treatment of trichotillomania. J Clin Psychiatry 64:49–52, 2003

Streichenwein SM, Thornby JI: A long-term, double-blind, placebo-controlled crossover trial of the efficacy of fluoxetine for trichotillomania. Am J Psychiatry 152:1192–1196, 1995

Swedo SE: Trichotillomania. Psychiatr Ann 23:402–407, 1993

Swedo SE, Leonard HL: Trichotillomania: an obsessive compulsive spectrum disorder? Psychiatr Clin North Am 15:777–790, 1992

Swedo SE, Leonard HL, Rapoport JL, et al: A double-blind comparison of clomipramine and desipramine in the treatment of trichotillomania hair pulling. N Engl J Med 321:497–501, 1989

Swedo SE, Rapoport JL, Leonard HL, et al: Regional cerebral glucose metabolism of women in trichotillomania. Arch Gen Psychiatry 48:828–833, 1991

Swedo SE, Lenane MC, Leonard HL: Long-term treatment of trichotillomania (hair pulling) (letter to the editor). N Engl J Med 329:141–142, 1993

Taber JI: Group psychotherapy with pathological gamblers. Paper presented at the 5th National Conference on Gambling and Risk-Taking. South Lake Tahoe, NV, October 1981

Taber JI, McCormick RA, Russo AM, et al: Follow-up of pathological gamblers after treatment. Am J Psychiatry 144:757–761, 1987

Tolin DF, Foa EB: Compulsions, in The Corsini Encyclopedia of Psychology and Behavioral Science, 3rd Edition. Edited by Craighead WE, Nemeroff CB. New York, Wiley, 2001, pp 338–339

Tolin D, Franklin ME, Diefenbach G, et al: CBT for pediatric trichotillomania: an open trial. Paper presented at the Trichotillomania: Psychopathology and Treatment Development Symposium conducted at the 36th annual meeting of the Association for the Advancement of Behavior Therapy, Reno, NV, November 2002

Tollefson GD: Anxiety and alcoholism: a serotonin link. Br J Psychiatry 159 (suppl):34–39, 1991

Tsai CC, Lin SS: Analysis of attitudes toward computer networks and Internet addiction of Taiwanese adolescents. Cyberpsychol Behav 4:373–376, 2001

Tukel R, Keser V, Karali NT, et al: Comparison of clinical characteristics in trichotillomania and obsessive-compulsive disorder. J Anxiety Disord 15:433–441, 2001

van Minnen A, Hoogduin KA, Keijsers GP, et al: Treatment of trichotillomania with behavioral therapy or fluoxetine. Arch Gen Psychiatry 60:517–522, 2003

Virkkunen M, Nuutila A, Goodwin FK: Cerebrospinal fluid monoamine metabolite levels in male arsonists. Arch Gen Psychiatry 44:241–247, 1987

Virkkunen M, Rawlings, Takola R: CSF biochemistries, glucose metabolism, and diurnal activity rhythms in alcoholic, violent offenders, fire setters, and healthy volunteers. Arch Gen Psychiatry 51:20–27, 1994

Virkkunen M, Eggert M, Rawlings R, et al: A prospective follow-up study of alcoholic violent offenders and fire setters. Arch Gen Psychiatry 53:523–529, 1996

Volberg RA: Estimating the prevalence of pathological gambling in the United States. Paper presented at the 8th International Conference on Risk and Gambling, London, England, August 1990

Volberg RA, Steadman HJ: Refining prevalence estimates of pathological gambling. Am J Psychiatry 145:502–505, 1988

Volberg RA, Steadman HJ: Prevalence estimates of pathological gambling in New Jersey and Maryland. Am J Psychiatry 146:1618–1619, 1989

Wetzler S, Kahn RS, Asnis GM, et al: Serotonin receptor sensitivity and aggression. Psychiatry Res 37:271–279, 1991

Winchel RM, Stanley M: Self-injurious behavior: a review of the behavior and biology of self-mutilation. Am J Psychiatry 148:306–317, 1991

Winters KC, Rich T: A twin study of adult gambling behavior. J Gambl Stud 14:213–225, 1999

Wise MG, Tierney JG: Impulse-control disorders not elsewhere classified, in The American Psychiatric Press Textbook of Psychiatry, 3rd Edition. Edited by Hales RE, Yudofsky SC, Talbott JA. Washington, DC, American Psychiatric Press, 1999, pp 773–794

Wood DR, Wender PH, Reimherr FW: The prevalence of attention deficit disorder, residual type, or minimum brain dysfunction in a population of male alcoholic patients. Am J Psychiatry 140:95–98, 1983

World Health Organization: International Classification of Diseases, 9th Revision, Clinical Modification. Ann Arbor, MI, Commission on Professional and Hospital Activities, 1978

Young KS: Caught in the Net: How to Recognize the Signs of Internet Addiction and a Winning Strategy for Recovery. New York, Wiley, 1998

Zanarini MC, Frankenburg FR: Olanzapine treatment of female borderline personality disorder patients: a double-blind, placebo-controlled pilot study. J Clin Psychiatry 62:849–854, 2001

Zimmerman M, Mattia J, Younken S, et al: The prevalence of DSM-IV impulse-control disorders in psychiatric outpatients (NR265), in 1998 New Research Program and Abstracts, American Psychiatric Association 151st Annual Meeting, Toronto, ON, May 30–June 4, 1998

Zimmerman M, Breen RB, Posternak MA: An open-label study of citalopram in the treatment of pathological gambling. J Clin Psychiatry 63:44–48, 2002

20

PERSONALITY DISORDERS

Andrew E. Skodol, M.D.
John G. Gunderson, M.D.

Clinicians frequently encounter patients with personality disorders in both outpatient and inpatient settings. Studies indicate that at least 50% of patients evaluated in clinical settings have a personality disorder (Zimmerman et al. 2005), often comorbid with an Axis I disorder, making personality disorders among the most frequently seen by mental health professionals. Personality disorders are also common in the general population, with an estimated prevalence of about 12% (Torgersen 2005).

Patients with personality disorders are among the most complex and clinically challenging. Some patients intensely desire relationships with others but fearfully avoid them because they anticipate rejection. Others endlessly seek admiration and are engrossed with grandiose fantasies of limitless power, brilliance, or ideal love. Still others have self-concepts so disturbed that they feel they embody evil or do not exist and, consequently, engage in self-mutilation or attempt suicide.

General Considerations

What Is a Personality Disorder?

According to DSM-IV-TR (American Psychiatric Association 2000), personality disorders are patterns of inflexible and maladaptive personality traits and be-

haviors that cause subjective distress, significant impairment in social or occupational functioning, or both. These patterns deviate markedly from the culturally expected and accepted range and are manifest in two or more of the following areas: cognition, affectivity, control over impulses and need gratification, and ways of relating to others. The maladaptive traits and behaviors are pervasive—that is, they are exhibited across a broad range of contexts and situations rather than in only one specific triggering situation or in response to a particular stimulus or person. Finally, the patterns must have been stably present and enduring since adolescence or early adulthood.

Although useful for identifying the prototypic personality disorder, this definition has ambiguities and limitations. It can be difficult, for example, to determine whether personality traits are inflexible or to differentiate deviance from normality or sickness from health. Inflexibility of personality is a key feature that helps to distinguish normal personality traits or styles from personality disorders. Inflexibility is indicated by a narrow repertoire of responses that are repeated even when the situation calls for an alternate behavior or in the face of clear evidence that a behavior is inappropriate or not working. For example, an obsessive-compulsive person rigidly adheres to rules and organization even in recreation and loses enjoyment as a consequence. An avoidant person is so fearful of being scrutinized or criticized, even in group situations in which he or she could hardly be the focus of such attention, that life becomes painfully lonely. In addition, whether dependence on others, compulsive work habits, or extreme self-confidence is considered excessive or problematic depends to some extent on the personal, social, and cultural context in which each occurs.

Some personality disorders, by their nature, may not be accompanied by obvious subjective distress on the part of the patient. Examples would include schizoid personality disorder, in which a patient is ostensibly satisfied with his or her social isolation and does not seem to need or desire the companionship of others, and antisocial personality disorder, in which the patient has utter disdain and disregard for social norms and will not experience distress unless his or her activities are thwarted. On the other side of the coin are patients with borderline personality disorder, who are likely to experience and express considerable distress, especially when disappointed in a significant other, or patients with avoidant personality disorder, who, in contrast with schizoid patients, are usually very uncomfortable and unhappy with their lack of close friends and companions. All personality disorders are maladaptive, however, and are accompanied by functional impairment in school or at work, in social relationships, or at leisure.

Furthermore, the stability of personality disorders has recently been called into question (Skodol et al. 2005a; Zanarini et al. 2005). Personality and personality disorders have traditionally been assumed to reflect stable descriptions of a person, at least after a certain age. Thus, the patterns of inner experience and behaviors described are called "enduring." These concepts persist as integral to the definition of personality disorder despite a growing body of empirical evidence that suggests that personality disorder psychopathology is not as stable as the DSM definition would indicate. Longitudinal studies indicate that personality disorders tend to improve over time, at least from the point of view of their overt clinical signs and symptoms. Furthermore, personality disorder criteria sets consist of combinations of pathological personality traits and symptomatic behaviors (McGlashan et al. 2005). Some behaviors, such as "self-mutilating behavior" (borderline personality disorder), may manifest much less frequently than traits such as "views self as socially inept, personally unappealing, or inferior to others" (avoidant personality disorder) (American Psychiatric Association 2000). How stable individual manifestations of personality disorders actually are or what the stable components of personality disorders

are have become areas of active empirical research. It may be that some features of personality psychopathology, in fact, wax and wane depending on the circumstances of a person's life.

History of Personality Disorders

Personality types and disorders have been described for thousands of years, as evidenced by Hippocrates' description of four temperaments: the pessimistic melancholic, the overly optimistic sanguine, the irritable choleric, and the apathetic phlegmatic. Notably, the early Greeks' theory that these temperaments were determined by the relative proportion of the four bodily humors (black bile, blood, yellow bile, and phlegm, respectively) is reflected in current attempts to discover biogenetic bases of personality.

In the early 1800s, psychiatrists such as Pinel, Esquirol, Rush, and Pritchard wrote about socially maladaptive personality types seen in clinical settings. More specific personality types were then described at the turn of the twentieth century, when, for example, Janet (1901) and Freud (Breuer and Freud 1893–1895/1957) delineated the psychological traits associated with hysteria, the forerunner of histrionic personality disorder. Subsequently, within the framework of early psychoanalytic instinct theory, Abraham proposed that arrests at the three psychosexual stages of childhood development—the oral, anal, and phallic phases—led to the development of the dependent, obsessive-compulsive, and hysterical character types, respectively. However, this view changed as early instinct theory and the subsequent ego-psychological theoretical model were gradually supplanted by object relations theory, which proposes that personality is shaped largely by the child's early relationships with parents. In this framework, dependent personality traits derive from parental deprivation, obsessive-compulsive traits from control struggles with parental figures, and hysterical traits, in part, from parental eroticization and competition. The borderline and narcissistic personality disorder concepts also developed out of the object relations framework.

From a quite different perspective, in the 1920s the German phenomenologists Kraepelin (1921) and Kretschmer (1925) described personality types in terms of the spectrum concept—the theory that personality types are biogenetically related variants of the paranoid and affective psychoses (which would now be considered Axis I disorders). These early spectrum personality types were forerunners of the current paranoid, schizotypal, cyclothymic, and depressive personality disorders. In contrast, Schneider (1958), another German phenomenologist, did not subscribe to the spectrum concept but considered personality disorders to represent socially deviant and extreme variants of normally occurring personality traits. He developed the first comprehensive system of personality disorder categories, which provided the template for many of those contained in the *International Statistical Classification of Diseases and Related Health Problems,* 10th Revision (ICD-10; World Health Organization 1992) and DSM-IV-TR. Both the spectrum concept of personality disorders (Krueger et al. 2005) and the relationships of personality disorders to normal personality traits are currently experiencing revivals in current research efforts to reconceptualize personality disorders for DSM-V (Clark 2005).

Personality disorders have been included in every version of DSM, but only paranoid, obsessive-compulsive, and antisocial personality disorders have been consistent DSM "members" (Figure 20–1). Some current categories (e.g., borderline personality disorder) were added to later editions, whereas others (e.g., inadequate personality) were dropped. The theoretical underpinnings of the DSM personality disorder categories have also changed over the years.

DSM-I (American Psychiatric Association 1952) defined personality disorders not as stable and enduring patterns but as traits that malfunction under stressful circumstances, leading to inflexible and maladaptive behavior. DSM-II (American Psychiatric Association 1968) emphasized that personality disorders involve distress and impairment in functioning, not merely socially deviant behavior. In DSM-III (American Psychiatric Association 1980), several major changes in personality disorder conceptualization and classification were made. There was a shift away from a psychoanalytic orientation toward an atheoretical, descriptive approach. Specific diagnostic criteria were added, and the personality disorders were placed on a separate axis, which highlighted their importance.

The changes made in DSM-III-R (American Psychiatric Association 1987) and DSM-IV (American Psychiatric Association 1994) attempted to increase the reliability and validity of the personality disorder categories by incorporating findings from the growing empirical literature (Widiger et al. 1996). Although current DSM descriptions attempt to represent an optimal synthesis of clinical tradition and research findings, such descriptions are certain to continue to evolve in anticipation of DSM-V and beyond as our understanding of these disorders increases.

Classification Issues

Since DSM-III, the personality disorders have been grouped into three clusters: the *odd or eccentric Cluster A* (paranoid, schizoid, and schizotypal); the *dramatic, emotional, or erratic Cluster B* (borderline, histrionic, narcissistic, and antisocial); and the *anxious or fearful Cluster C* (avoidant, dependent, and obsessive-compulsive) (Table 20–1). Although these clusters were originally based on face validity alone, they have since received some empirical support (Sanislow et al. 2002). Nonetheless, these clusters are limited because they are based on descriptive similarities rather than on similarities in etiology or external validators such as family history or treatment response. Recently, interest in personality disorders in Cluster A has increased because neurobiological abnormalities found in patients with schizotypal personality disorder and in patients with chronic schizophrenia suggest common vulnerabilities as well as factors that protect vulnerable patients from developing frank psychosis (Siever and Davis 2004).

A pressing issue is whether the personality disorders are best classified as dimensions or categories (Widiger and Samuel 2005). Do personality disorders exist along dimensions that reflect extreme variants of general personality functioning, or are they distinct categories that are qualitatively different, and clearly demarcated, from normal personality traits and one another? Categorical diagnoses of personality disorders have been increasingly criticized for a number of reasons. First, excessive diagnostic co-occurrence between personality disorders has been observed in many studies: most patients with personality disorders meet criteria for more than one disorder. Second, there is considerable heterogeneity of features among patients receiving the same diagnosis. For example, given that a diagnosis of borderline personality disorder requires any 5 of 9 criteria from its polythetic criteria set, there are 256 different ways to meet the criteria for the disorder. The thresholds for making personality disorder diagnoses are arbitrary in that they were decided on the basis of expert consensus and not on the basis of empirical research. How different is a patient who meets 5 of 8 criteria for dependent personality disorder, the diagnostic threshold, from one who meets 4 of 8 (subthreshold)? Finally, despite listing 10 specific personality disorder types in DSM-IV-TR, the residual category of personality disorder not otherwise specified may be the most common in clinical practice (Verheul and Widiger 2004), suggesting inadequate coverage of personality psychopathology by the DSM.

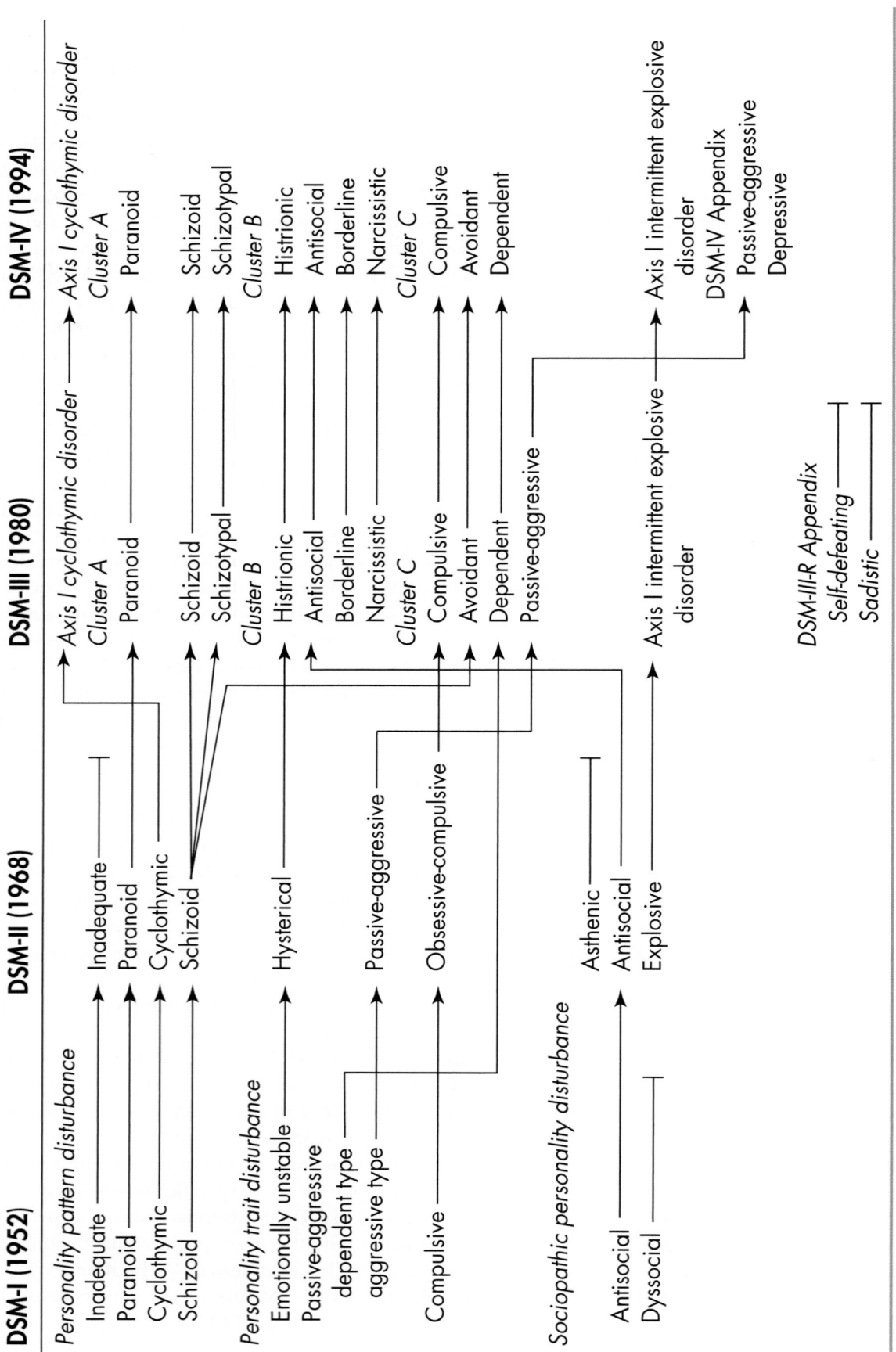

FIGURE 20–1. Ontogeny of personality disorder classification.

Note. "——|" indicates that category was discontinued.
Source. Reprinted from Skodol AE: "Classification, Assessment, and Differential Diagnosis of Personality Disorders." *Journal of Practical Psychiatry and Behavioral Health* 3:261–274, 1997. Copyright 1997, Lippincott Williams & Wilkins. Used with permission.

TABLE 20–1. DSM-IV-TR personality clusters, specific types, and their defining clinical features

Cluster	Type	Characteristic features
A (odd or eccentric)		
	Paranoid	Pervasive distrust and suspiciousness of others such that their motives are interpreted as malevolent
	Schizoid	Pervasive pattern of detachment from social relationships and restricted range of expression of emotions in interpersonal settings
	Schizotypal	Pervasive pattern of social and interpersonal deficits marked by acute discomfort with, and reduced capacity for, close relationships as well as by cognitive or perceptual distortions and eccentricities of behavior
B (dramatic, emotional, or erratic)		
	Antisocial	History of conduct disorder before age 15 years; pervasive pattern of disregard for and violation of the rights of others; current age at least 18 years
	Borderline	Pervasive pattern of instability of interpersonal relationships, self-image, and affects and marked impulsivity
	Histrionic	Pervasive pattern of excessive emotionality and attention seeking
	Narcissistic	Pervasive pattern of grandiosity (in fantasy or behavior), need for admiration, and lack of empathy
C (anxious or fearful)		
	Avoidant	Pervasive pattern of social inhibition, feelings of inadequacy, and hypersensitivity to negative evaluation
	Dependent	Pervasive and excessive need to be taken care of that leads to submissive and clinging behavior and fears of separation
	Obsessive-compulsive	Pervasive pattern of preoccupation with orderliness, perfectionism, and mental and interpersonal control at the expense of flexibility, openness, and efficiency

Source. Adapted from American Psychiatric Association 2000.

Many different dimensional approaches to personality disorder assessment have been proposed as alternatives to DSM-IV-TR categories (Widiger and Simonsen 2005). The simplest has been to simply transform the categories into dimensions by counting criteria or rating the degree to which patients meet criteria on a continuous scale (Oldham and Skodol 2000). This approach has been shown to increase the strength of the relationship of personality disorder representations with external validators such as functional impairment (Skodol et al. 2005b). Another "person-centered" dimensional approach is the prototype matching approach proposed by Westen et al. (2006). Using this approach, clinicians rate the degree to which patients meet written descriptions of a prototypical patient with each personality disorder on continuous scales.

This approach has also been shown to have clinical utility and is very "clinician friendly." Other dimensional approaches rate pathological personality traits on scales of severity (Clark 1993; Livesley and Jackson 2000), whereas still other "spectrum" models attempt to bring together Axis I and Axis II disorders that seem to share fundamental underlying dimensions of psychopathology, such as internalization versus externalization (Krueger et al. 2005) or cognitive/perceptual versus affective disturbances (Siever and Davis 1991).

The most widely used dimensional approaches describe personality according to a number of broad factors and more narrow trait dimensions and assess the degree to which traits are present for a given patient. These may more comprehensively cover both normal and pathological personality traits. Indeed, one of the

TABLE 20–2. The five-factor model of personality

Factor domains	Facets (primary adjective correlates)
Neuroticism	Anxiety (anxious, fearful, worrying)
	Angry hostility (angry, irritable, impatient)
	Depression (worrying, –contented, –confident)
	Self-consciousness (shy, –self-confident, timid)
	Impulsiveness (moody, irritable, sarcastic)
	Vulnerability (–clear-thinking, –self-confident, –confident)
Extraversion	Warmth (friendly, warm, sociable)
	Gregariousness (sociable, outgoing, pleasure-seeking)
	Assertiveness (aggressive, –shy, assertive)
	Activity (energetic, hurried, quick)
	Excitement-seeking (pleasure-seeking, daring, adventurous)
	Positive emotions (enthusiastic, humorous, praising)
Openness	Fantasy (dreamy, imaginative, humorous)
	Aesthetics (imaginative, artistic, original)
	Feelings (excitable, hurried, quick)
	Actions (interests wide, imaginative, adventurous)
	Ideas (idealistic, interests wide, inventive)
	Values (–conservative, unconventional, –cautious)
Agreeableness	Trust (forgiving, trusting, –suspicious)
	Straightforwardness (–complicated, –demanding, –clever)
	Altruism (warm, soft-hearted, gentle)
	Compliance (–stubborn, –demanding, –headstrong)
	Modesty (–show-off, –clever, –assertive)
	Tender-mindedness (friendly, warm, sympathetic)
Conscientiousness	Competence (efficient, self-confident, thorough)
	Order (organized, thorough, efficient)
	Dutifulness (–defensive, –distractible, –careless)
	Achievement-striving (thorough, ambitious, industrious)
	Self-disciplined (organized, –lazy, efficient)
	Deliberation (–hasty, –impulsive, –careless)

Note.   Minus signs before adjectives indicate negative correlations with the facet scale.

Source.   Adapted from McCrae RR, Costa PT Jr: "Discriminant Validity of NEO PI-R Facet Scales," in *Education and Psychological Measurement* 52:229–237, 1992. Copyright 1992, Sage Publications. Used with permission.

recent large-scale efforts in personality research has been to describe DSM personality disorder types in terms of dimensions of general personality functioning (Widiger 2000). Of special significance are the widely heralded "Big Five" dimensions of the Five-Factor Model of Personality: neuroticism, extraversion, openness, agreeableness, and conscientiousness (Table 20–2; Costa and McCrae 1990). Cloninger's seven-dimension psychobiological model of temperament and character (Table 20–3; Cloninger et al. 1993), which was theoretically linked to abnormalities in specific neurotransmitter systems, has generated a large body of research, but the data have generally not supported these neurobiological hypotheses (Paris 2005b).

Dimensional models vary in the empirical support each has received. Fortunately, the broad domains of most trait-based models can be integrated into a common structure consisting of four basic personality dimensions: 1) extraversion versus introversion, 2) antagonism versus compliance, 3) constraint versus impulsivity, and 4) emotional dysregulation versus emotional stability (Markon et al. 2005; Widiger and Mullins-Sweatt 2005). Furthermore, the genetic and phenotypic structure of the basic traits delineating personality disorders has been shown to be consistent (Livesley et al. 1998). Dimensional approaches are, however, unfamiliar to those trained in a medical model of diagnosis; are complex to use (up to 30 dimensions to

TABLE 20–3. The seven-factor model of personality: temperament and character inventory

Temperament	Descriptors of extreme variants		Character	Descriptors of extreme variants	
	High	Low		High	Low
Harm avoidance	Pessimistic Fearful Shy Fatigable	Optimistic Daring Outgoing Energetic	Self-directedness	Responsible Purposeful Resourceful Self-accepting Disciplined	Blaming Aimless Inept Vain Undisciplined
Novelty seeking	Exploratory Impulsive Extravagant Irritable	Reserved Rigid Frugal Stoic	Cooperative	Tender-hearted Empathic Helpful Compassionate Principled	Intolerant Insensitive Hostile Revengeful Opportunistic
Reward dependence	Sentimental Open Warm Sympathetic	Critical Aloof Detached Independent	Self-transcendent	Self-forgetful Transpersonal Spiritual Enlightened Idealistic	Unimaginative Controlling Materialistic Possessive Practical
Persistence	Industrious Determined Ambitious Perfectionistic	Lazy Spoiled Underachieving Pragmatic			

Source. Adapted from Cloninger CR: "The Genetics and Psychobiology of the Seven-Factor Model of Personality," in *Biology of Personality Disorders*. Edited by Silk KR. Washington, DC, American Psychiatric Press, 1998, pp. 63–92. Copyright 1998, American Psychiatric Press. Used with permission.

describe personality by the facets of the Five-Factor Model); and have sparse empirical data to support their utility for clinical decision making (First et al. 2004; Verheul 2005). Given that clinicians already overlook personality disorders in their diagnostic assessments (Zimmerman and Mattia 1999), it seems unlikely that they would embrace a more demanding assessment model.

The categorical model, in contrast, better reflects how clinicians think—that is, in terms of pathological syndromes that a person either has or does not have. The use of categories also makes it possible for clinicians to summarize patients' difficulties succinctly and facilitates communication about them. Although DSM-IV-TR is based primarily on the categorical model, it also incorporates a dimensional approach to a limited extent in that it encourages clinicians to identify problematic personality traits that are subthreshold for any particular diagnosis. Classification models that incorporate both a dimensional and a categorical approach may ultimately prove most useful to clinicians, and several such models have been proposed (Gunderson 1992).

These and other classification issues are currently being debated and researched, which is likely to lead

to changes in the future classification of personality disorders. Whatever system is used, it is important that it be useful to clinicians and, ultimately, reflect what is known about the etiology of these disorders.

Assessment Issues and Methods

The assessment of Axis II disorders is in some ways more complex than that of Axis I disorders. It can be difficult to assess multiple domains of experience and behavior (i.e., cognition, affect, impulse control, and interpersonal interactions) and to determine that traits are distressing or impairing, of early onset, pervasive, and sufficiently enduring (Skodol 2005). Nonetheless, a personality disorder assessment is essential to the comprehensive evaluation and adequate treatment of all patients.

Comprehensiveness of Evaluation

A skilled clinical interview is the mainstay of personality disorder diagnosis and requires the clinician to be familiar with DSM criteria, take a longitudinal view, and use multiple sources of information. A psychodynamic perspective may contribute depth to the assessment through its attention to defenses, attitudes, and development. However, because an open-ended approach may provide insufficient information to assess all Axis II disorders, the addition of a self-report or semistructured (i.e., interviewer-administered) personality disorder assessment instrument may be used to augment a clinical interview (Table 20–4) (Kaye and Shea 2000; McDermut and Zimmerman 2005). Such instruments systematically assess each personality disorder criterion with standard questions or probes. Although self-report instruments have the advantage of saving interviewer time and being free of interviewer bias, they often yield false-positive diagnoses and allow contamination of Axis II traits by Axis I states. Semistructured interviews—which require the interviewer to use certain questions, but allow further probing—facilitate accurate diagnosis in several ways: they ensure coverage of relevant domains of personality psychopathology, allow the interviewer to attempt to differentiate Axis II traits from Axis I states, encourage clarification of contradictions or ambiguities in the patient's response, and provide the opportunity to determine that traits are pervasive (i.e., by eliciting multiple examples of trait expression) rather than limited to a specific situation.

Nonetheless, even with the use of a semistructured interview, the interviewer must use his or her judgment. For example, is a given trait present in enough situations to be considered pervasive? How much distress or impairment is necessary to consider the criterion present? Is a given characteristic a personality trait or a symptom of an Axis I disorder (i.e., a state)? Other limitations are that agreement among existing instruments is fairly low, and the instruments do not indicate which disorder in any given patient is most severe or should be the focus of treatment.

TABLE 20–4.   Features of interviews and self-report instruments for the assessment of personality disorders

Interview or instrument	Author	Type	Special features
Structured Interview for DSM-IV Personality Disorders (SIDP-IV)	Pfohl et al. 1997	Interview	Patient and informant questions
International Personality Disorders Examination (IPDE)	Loranger 1999	Interview	Detailed instruction manual; translated into several languages
Structured Clinical Interview for DSM-IV Axis II Personality Disorders (SCID-II)	First et al. 1997	Interview	Axis I section; Axis II screening questionnaire
Diagnostic Interview for DSM-IV Personality Disorders (DIPD-IV)	Zanarini et al. 1996	Interview	Good test–retest reliability
Personality Disorder Interview–IV (PDI-IV)	Widiger et al. 1995	Interview	Detailed instruction manual; categorical and dimensional assessments
Personality Diagnostic Questionnaire–4 (PDQ-4)	Hyler 1994	Self-report	Face-valid items; useful for screening
Millon Clinical Multiaxial Inventory–III (MCMI-III)	Millon et al. 1997	Self-report	Dimensions of Axis I and Axis II psychopathology
Wisconsin Personality Inventory–IV (WPI-IV)	M. Klein 1993	Self-report	Integrated structural analysis of social behavior model[a]
Schedule for Nonadaptive and Adaptive Personality (SNAP)	Clark 1993	Self-report	Normal and abnormal personality trait measures; DSM-IV diagnoses

Note.   All instruments listed assess the full range of personality disorders. Other instruments are available to assess certain individual personality disorders.
[a]See L.S. Benjamin 1974.

Source.   Adapted from Skodol and Oldham 1991.

Ego-Syntonic Traits

As noted earlier, some patients are unaware of the traits that reflect their disorder or may not perceive them as problematic. This limited self-awareness can interfere with personality disorder assessment, especially if the questions asked have negative or unflattering implications. This problem can be reduced by the use of multiple sources of information (e.g., medical records and informants who know the patient well). Still, because studies have shown low concordance rates between patient-based and informant-based interviews (Klonsky et al. 2002), interviewers will also need to rely on their personal experience with the patient to reach a conclusion (Westen 1997). Which source of information—the patient, the informant, or the interviewer's firsthand experience with the patient—is most useful for a specific clinical purpose, such as choosing a treatment or predicting outcome, has yet to be definitively determined. In practice, clinicians value and use all perspectives in their diagnostic appraisals, but treatment plans always need to begin with problems that the patient can acknowledge.

State Versus Trait

The presence of an Axis I disorder can complicate the assessment of Axis II traits. For example, a person with social withdrawal, low self-esteem, and lack of motivation or energy due to major depression might appear to have avoidant or dependent personality disorder, when in fact these features reflect the Axis I condition. A hypomanic person with symptoms of grandiosity or hypersexuality might appear narcissistic or histrionic. In some cases, assessment of Axis II disorders may need to wait until the Axis I condition, such as severe depression or a manic episode, has subsided. However, the clinician can often differentiate personality traits from Axis I states during an Axis I episode by asking the patient to describe his or her usual personality at times not in an Axis I episode; the use of informants who have observed the patient over time with and without an Axis I disorder can also be helpful. Systematic assessment of Axis I conditions before turning attention to Axis II is invaluable in alerting the clinician to which Axis II traits will need particularly careful assessment. This task can be very difficult, however, in patients with Axis I conditions that are chronic and of early onset.

Medical Illness Versus Trait

Similarly, the interviewer must ascertain that apparent personality traits are not symptoms of a medical illness. For example, aggressive outbursts caused by a seizure disorder should not be attributed to borderline or antisocial personality disorder, nor should the unusual perceptual experiences that can accompany temporal lobe epilepsy be attributed to schizotypal personality disorder. A medical evaluation should be included if a medical causation is suspected.

Situation Versus Trait

The interviewer should also determine that personality disorder features are pervasive—that is, not limited to only one situation or occurring in response to only one specific trigger or person. Similarly, personality traits should be relatively enduring rather than transient. Asking the patient for behavioral examples of the expression of traits can help determine that the trait is indeed present in a wide variety of situations and is expressed in many relationships. Specific behaviors, such as suicidal or other self-destructive behaviors, may only be evident in specific situations, but the trait of impulsivity should be more persistent.

Sex and Cultural Bias

Although most research suggests that existing personality disorder criteria are relatively free of sex bias (Morey et al. 2005), interviewers can unknowingly allow such bias to affect their assessments. It is important, for example, that histrionic, borderline, and dependent personality disorders be assessed as carefully in men as in women and that obsessive-compulsive, antisocial, and narcissistic personality disorders be assessed as carefully in women as in men. Interviewers should also be careful to avoid cultural bias when diagnosing personality disorders, especially when evaluating such traits as diffidence, passivity, emotionality, suspiciousness, or recklessness; emphasis on work and productivity; or unusual beliefs and rituals that may reflect different norms in different cultures (Alarcon 2005).

Diagnosis of Personality Disorders in Children and Adolescents

Because the personalities of children and adolescents are still developing, personality disorders should be diagnosed with care in this age group. Although children and early adolescents frequently manifest significant personality disorder characteristics (Johnson et al. 2000), it is often preferable to defer diagnoses until early adulthood, at which time a personality disorder diagnosis may be appropriate if the features appear to be pervasive, stable, and likely to be enduring. Early diagnosis may prove to be wrong as stage-specific difficulties of adolescence resolve and as the person matures (Cohen and Crawford 2005). A meta-analysis of

152 longitudinal studies of personality traits showed that change was the rule up until about the age of 22 (Roberts and DelVecchio 2000). Nonetheless, adolescents with high levels of personality psychopathology are at greater risk for developing personality disorders in early adulthood (Kasen et al. 1999).

Clinical Significance of Personality Disorders

By definition, personality disorders cause significant problems for those who have them. Persons with these disorders often suffer, and their relationships with others are typically problematic. They have difficulty responding flexibly and adaptively to the environment and to the changes and demands of life, and they lack resilience when under stress. Instead, their usual ways of responding tend to perpetuate and intensify their difficulties. However, these individuals are often oblivious to the fact that their personality causes them problems, and they may instead blame others for their difficulties or even deny that they have any problems at all.

A number of studies have compared patients with personality disorders with patients with no personality disorder or with Axis I disorders and have found that patients with personality disorders were more likely to be separated, divorced, or never married and to have had more unemployment, frequent job changes, or periods of disability. Patients with personality disorders only rarely have been found to be less well educated, however. Studies that have examined quality of functioning found poorer social functioning or interpersonal relationships and poorer work functioning or occupational achievement and satisfaction. Among the different personality disorders, those with severe types, such as schizotypal and borderline, have been found to have significantly more impairment at work, in social relationships, and at leisure than patients with less severe types, such as obsessive-compulsive disorder, or with an impairing Axis I disorder, such as major depressive disorder in the absence of personality disorder. Even the less impaired patients with personality disorders (e.g., obsessive-compulsive), however, have moderate to severe impairment in at least one area of functioning (or a Global Assessment of Functioning rating of 60 or less) (Skodol et al. 2002). Thus, patients with specific personality disorders differ from each other not only in the degree of associated functional impairment but also in the breadth of impairment across functional domains.

Impairment in functioning in patients with personality disorders tends to be persistent even beyond apparent improvement in personality disorder psychopathology itself (Seivewright et al. 2004; Skodol et al.

2005c). The persistence of impairment is understandable because personality disorder psychopathology has usually been relatively long-standing and therefore has disrupted a person's work and social development over a period of time (Roberts et al. 2003). The "scars" or residua of personality disorder pathology may take time to heal or be overcome. With time (and treatment), however, improvements in functioning can occur.

Personality disorders also often cause problems for others and are costly to society. They are associated with elevated rates of separation, divorce, conflict with family members and romantic partners, child custody proceedings, homelessness, high-risk sexual behavior, and perpetration of child abuse. Those with personality disorders also have increased rates of accidents; police contacts; emergency department visits; medical hospitalization and treatment utilization; violence and criminal behavior, including homicide; self-injurious behavior; attempted suicide; and completed suicide. A high percentage of individuals with criminal convictions (70%–85% in some studies), 60%–70% of individuals with alcoholism, and 70%–90% of persons who abuse drugs have a personality disorder.

Finally, personality disorders should be identified because of their treatment implications. Personality disorders often need to be a focus of treatment or, at the very least, need to be taken into account when comorbid Axis I disorders are treated, because their presence often affects an Axis I disorder's prognosis and treatment response. For example, patients with depressive disorders, bipolar disorder, panic disorder, obsessive-compulsive disorder, and substance abuse often respond less well to pharmacotherapy when they have a comorbid personality disorder. The presence of a comorbid personality disorder is also associated with poor compliance with pharmacotherapy. Furthermore, personality disorders have been shown to predict the development and relapse of major depression (Johnson et al. 2005b), and individuals with a personality disorder are less likely to remit from major depression (Grilo et al. 2005), bipolar disorder (Dunayevich et al. 2000), and generalized anxiety disorder (Yonkers et al. 2000). As most clinicians are well aware, the characteristics of patients with personality disorders are likely to be manifested in the treatment relationship regardless of whether the personality disorder is the focus of treatment. For example, some patients may be overly dependent on the clinician, others may not follow treatment recommendations, and still others may experience significant conflict about getting well. Although individuals with personality disorders tend to use psychiatric services extensively (Bender et al. 2001), they are more likely to be dissatisfied with the treatment they receive (Kent et al. 1995).

Etiology and Pathogenesis

What causes personality disorders is the most enigmatic and challenging question relevant to this group of complex disorders. As was described in the section on the history of personality disorders, various hypotheses have been formulated over the years. Psychoanalytic theory has tended to emphasize the contribution of developmental and environmental factors, such as pathological or inadequate parenting, whereas neurobiological perspectives have emphasized genetic, constitutional, or biological factors.

As is the case with other psychiatric disorders, the answer is not likely to be simple. All available data suggest that personality disorders (as well as normal personality traits) result from a complex combination of, and interaction between, temperament (genetic and other biological factors) and psychological (developmental or environmental) factors (Paris 2005a). Although the degree to which genetic and environmental factors contribute to etiology may vary for different personality disorders, the first major twin study indicates that both factors are important in all of these disorders (Torgersen et al. 2000). Of relevance, too, are studies showing that approximately half the observed variance in personality traits such as neuroticism, introversion, and submissiveness can be traced to genetic variation (Carey and DiLalla 1994).

Investigation of the underlying neurobiology of personality disorders is rapidly increasing. A growing body of evidence supports the importance of various neurobiological abnormalities in persons with schizotypal personality disorder: increased dopaminergic activity, particularly in the striatum, has been shown to be related to psychotic-like symptoms, and decreased dopaminergic activity, particularly in prefrontal regions, to deficit-like symptoms (Siever and Davis 2004). Temporal cortex volume reductions comparable with those of patients with schizophrenia have also been found; however, frontal volumes are preserved, perhaps serving as a buffer against severe cognitive or social deterioration. Striatal volumes are reduced in schizotypal patients, consistent with reduced dopaminergic activity, in comparison with patients with schizophrenia (Shihabuddin et al. 2001). Abnormalities in the serotonin system, which appears to mediate behavioral inhibition, have been found in impulsive/aggressive individuals with borderline and antisocial personality disorders (Coccaro et al. 1996). Molecular genetic analyses have suggested associations of neu-

roticism and the short allele of the serotonin transporter gene (5-HTTLPR) (Lesch et al. 1996) and between novelty seeking and the long allele of the dopamine receptor gene (DRD4) (J. Benjamin et al. 1996). Although these studies have opened up a new frontier in research on personality traits and disorders, early results have generally not been replicated or the gene polymorphisms in question have been found to be less specific than originally thought (Kluger et al. 2002; Munafo et al. 2003).

Increasing numbers of studies of environmental antecedents of personality disorders, such as family environment and sexual and physical abuse, are substantiating a likely role for such factors in the development of certain disorders, particularly borderline personality disorder (Zanarini 1997). In addition, defense mechanisms appear to play an important role in the expression of personality disorders, which are characterized by less mature defense mechanisms such as projection and acting out (Perry and Bond 2005). Research in these areas is expected to continue to increase rapidly. In addition to providing information about the origins of the personality disorders, such findings are expected to open new avenues for treating these often difficult-to-treat patients.

Treatment

Because personality disorders have been thought to consist of deeply ingrained attitudes and behavior patterns that consolidate during development and have endured since early adulthood, they have traditionally been believed to be very resistant to change. Moreover, as noted previously, treatment efforts are further confounded by the degree to which patients with personality disorders do not recognize their maladaptive personality traits as undesirable or in need of change. Despite this general wariness about the treatability of patients with personality disorders, increasing evidence has accumulated from longitudinal studies that personality disorders are quite variable in their course (Grilo and McGlashan 2005) and much more malleable and treatable than had been thought (Leichsenring and Leibing 2003).

Psychoanalysts pioneered the notion that persons with personality disorders could respond to treatment (Gabbard 2005). The original conception of neurosis as a specific set of symptoms related to a discrete developmental phase or to discrete conflicts was gradually replaced by the idea that more enduring defensive styles and identification processes were the building blocks of character traits. From this perspective, Wilhelm Reich (1949) and others developed the concepts of *character analysis* and *defense analysis*. These processes refer to an analyst's efforts to address the ways in which a person resists learning and the confrontations by which the analyst draws attention to the maladaptive effects of the patient's character traits. A parallel development in technique evolved from group therapy experience. Maxwell Jones (1953) identified the value of confrontations delivered within group settings in which peer pressure made it difficult for patients to ignore feedback or to leave the group (Piper and Ogrodniczuk 2005). Here, too, a primary goal of treatment was to render more dystonic the ego-syntonic, but maladaptive, aspects of the patient's interpersonal and behavioral style. This general principle was subsequently adopted by other forms of sociotherapy, notably those within hospital milieus and in family therapies.

Families or couples may present complications because the designated patient's disordered interpersonal and behavioral patterns may serve functions for, or be complementary to, the disordered patterns of persons with whom the patient is closely associated. For example, a dependent person is apt to bond with an overly authoritarian partner, or an emotionally constricted and obsessional person may find an emotionally expressive, hysterical person particularly attractive. Under these circumstances, treatment is primarily directed not at confronting the maladaptive aspects of one person's character traits but rather at identifying the ways in which these aspects may be welcomed and reinforced in one relationship but maladaptive and impairing in others (Sholevar 2005).

Significant developments in the treatment of personality disorders include the use of multiple modalities, the growth of an empirical base of the results of treatment studies, and greater optimism about treatment effectiveness. Reviews of psychotherapy outcome studies, including psychodynamic/interpersonal, cognitive-behavioral, mixed, and supportive therapies, have found that psychotherapy was associated with a significantly faster rate of recovery compared with the natural course of personality disorders (Leichsenring and Leibing 2003; Perry et al. 1999). Therapeutic nihilism has yielded to widespread but very inconsistent use of the spectrum of potentially valuable treatment modalities. However, each personality disorder's particular problematic interpersonal style of relating to others will necessarily affect the alliance with the therapist, on which the success of treatment will depend (Bender 2005).

A significant development has been the application of cognitive-behavioral strategies to personality disorders. These strategies generally are more focused and structured than psychodynamic therapies. Cognitive strategies involve identifying specific internal mental schemes by which patients typically misunderstand certain situations or misrepresent themselves and then learning how to modify those internal schemes (Beck et al. 2004). Cognitive therapy for personality disorders is more complicated than for most Axis I disorders because of the unique challenges (e.g., cognitive and affective avoidance, lack of psychological flexibility, pervasiveness of problems, and ambivalence about having problems and getting treatment for them) that character pathology presents. Behavioral strategies involve efforts to diminish traits such as impulsivity or to increase assertiveness by using relaxation techniques, role-playing exercises, and other behavioral techniques. A specific type of cognitive-behavioral therapy called dialectical behavior therapy (Linehan 1993), developed for suicidal and self-injuring patients with borderline personality disorder, has recently come into broad use (Stanley and Brodsky 2005).

Although psychotherapy remains the mainstay of the treatment of personality disorders, in the past two decades the use of pharmacotherapy has begun to be explored as biological dimensions of personality psychopathology that may respond to different medication classes have been identified. For example, research has increasingly suggested that impulsivity and aggression may respond to serotonergic medications; mood instability and lability may respond to serotonergic medications, other antidepressants, and mood stabilizers; and psychotic-like experiences may respond to antipsychotics (Soloff 2005). These principles have been incorporated into the *Practice Guideline for Borderline Personality Disorder* (American Psychiatric Association 2001).

An overview of our knowledge about the potential usefulness of the three major types of psychiatric treatment—psychotherapies, sociotherapies, and pharmacotherapies—is provided in Table 20–5. It is expected that use of these therapies will increasingly be guided by more specific and empirically based information on which modalities, in what sequence, are most effective for the treatment of each personality disorder.

A clinically oriented overview of each DSM-IV-TR personality disorder follows. These descriptions, although based on clinical tradition, have also been informed by the recent explosion of empirical research on personality disorders—a development facilitated by their placement on a separate Axis II in DSM-III. This research has focused on many different aspects of personality disorders, such as their descriptive features,

TABLE 20–5. **Evidence of treatment effectiveness for personality disorders**

	ST	SZ	P	B	AS	H	N	OC	D	AV
Psychotherapies	–	+	–	++	–	+	++	++	++	++
Sociotherapies[a]	±	+	–	++	+	–	–	–	+	+
Pharmacotherapies	+	–	±	+	–	–	–	–	–	±

Note. –=no support; ±=uncertain support; +=modestly helpful; ++=significantly helpful. ST=schizotypal; SZ=schizoid; P=paranoid; B=borderline; AS=antisocial; H=histrionic; N=narcissistic; OC=obsessive-compulsive; D=dependent; AV=avoidant.
[a]Includes group, family, and milieu therapies.

family history, course, treatment response, and etiology, including their psychodynamic, biogenetic, and sociocultural roots. Ongoing research is gradually enhancing our understanding of these complex disorders.

Specific Personality Disorders

Paranoid Personality Disorder

History

Paranoid personality disorder has been richly and consistently represented in the descriptive psychiatric literature. It was described by Mayer, Koch, Kraepelin, Bleuler, Kretschmer, and Schneider under such rubrics as the "pseudoquerulent type" and the "fanatic psychopath" (Millon 1981). This disorder has, however, received less attention in the psychoanalytic literature than have many other personality disorders.

Paranoid personality disorder is one of the four personality disorders to have been included in every version of DSM, and its description has consistently focused on the disorder's central feature of a pervasive and unwarranted mistrust of others.

Epidemiology

Paranoid personality disorder is estimated to occur in 1.25%–1.5% of the general population (Torgersen 2005). It has been found to be more common among men than women (Zimmerman and Coryell 1990).

Clinical Features

Persons with paranoid personality disorder have a pervasive, persistent, and inappropriate mistrust of others (Table 20–6). They are suspicious of others' motives and assume that others intend to exploit, harm, or deceive them. Thus, they may question, without justifica-

tion, the loyalty or trustworthiness of friends or romantic partners, and they are reluctant to confide in others for fear the information will be used against them. Persons with paranoid personality disorder appear guarded, tense, and hypervigilant, and they frequently scan their environments for clues of possible attack, deception, or betrayal. They often find "evidence" of such malevolence by misinterpreting benign events (such as a glance in their direction) as demeaning or threatening. In response to perceived or actual insults or betrayals, these individuals overreact quickly, becoming excessively angry and responding with counterattacking behavior. They are unable to forgive or forget such incidents and instead bear long-term grudges against their supposed betrayers; some persons with paranoid personality disorder are extremely litigious. Whereas individuals with this disorder can appear quietly and tensely aloof and hostile, others are overtly angry and combative. Persons with this disorder are usually socially isolated and, because of their paranoia, often have difficulties with bosses and co-workers.

Differential Diagnosis

Unlike paranoid personality disorder, the Axis I disorders *paranoid schizophrenia* and *delusional disorder, persecutory type,* are both characterized by prominent and persistent paranoid delusions of psychotic proportions; paranoid schizophrenia is also accompanied by hallucinations and other core symptoms of schizophrenia. Although paranoid and schizotypal personality disorders both involve suspiciousness, paranoid personality disorder does not include magical thinking, perceptual distortions, or odd thinking or speech. People who are extremely self-conscious may fear that others are watching them or have negative or critical thoughts about them. They are projecting their negative ideas about themselves onto others, whereas paranoid people project malevolent thoughts and feelings onto others.

TABLE 20–6. DSM-IV-TR diagnostic criteria for paranoid personality disorder

A. A pervasive distrust and suspiciousness of others such that their motives are interpreted as malevolent, beginning by early adulthood and present in a variety of contexts, as indicated by four (or more) of the following:

    (1) suspects, without sufficient basis, that others are exploiting, harming, or deceiving him or her

    (2) is preoccupied with unjustified doubts about the loyalty or trustworthiness of friends or associates

    (3) is reluctant to confide in others because of unwarranted fear that the information will be used maliciously against him or her

    (4) reads hidden demeaning or threatening meanings into benign remarks or events

    (5) persistently bears grudges, i.e., is unforgiving of insults, injuries, or slights

    (6) perceives attacks on his or her character or reputation that are not apparent to others and is quick to react angrily or to counterattack

    (7) has recurrent suspicions, without justification, regarding fidelity of spouse or sexual partner

B. Does not occur exclusively during the course of schizophrenia, a mood disorder with psychotic features, or another psychotic disorder and is not due to the direct physiological effects of a general medical condition.

Note: If criteria are met prior to the onset of schizophrenia, add "premorbid," e.g., "paranoid personality disorder (premorbid)."

Etiology

Some psychological theories suggest that paranoid personality disorder originates from having been the object of excessive parental rage or from having been repeatedly humiliated by others. Either type of experience could lead to feelings of inadequacy and vulnerability, followed by projection onto others of hostility and rage, as well as a tendency to blame others for one's shortcomings and problems. The defense mechanism of projection is generally assumed to be involved in the expression of this disorder's features.

It seems likely that paranoid personality disorder has neurobiological contributions. Early in the twentieth century, Kraepelin (1921) theorized that this personality disorder was the premorbid character type of persons predisposed to paranoia (now known as Axis I delusional disorder). An association between these two disorders has received some support from family history studies that found a greater morbid risk of paranoid personality disorder in the first-degree relatives of delusional disorder probands than in relatives of probands with schizophrenia or medical illness (Kendler and Gruenberg 1982). Several studies have found paranoid personality disorder in the relatives of probands with schizophrenia, but others have not (Webb and Levinson 1993). Links to full-blown psychotic disorders implicate the involvement of both environmental and constitutional factors in the etiology of paranoid personality disorder.

Treatment

Because they mistrust others, persons with paranoid personality disorder usually avoid psychiatric treatment. If they do seek treatment, the therapist immediately encounters the challenge of engaging them and keeping them in treatment. This can best be accomplished by maintaining an unusually respectful, straightforward, and unintrusive style aimed at building trust. If a rupture develops in the treatment relationship—for example, the patient accuses the therapist of some fault—it is best simply to offer a straightforward apology, if warranted, rather than to respond evasively or defensively. It is also best to avoid an overly warm style, because excessive warmth and expression of interest can intensify the patient's thoughts about the therapist's motives (Appelbaum 2005). A supportive individual psychotherapy that incorporates such approaches may be the best treatment for these patients (Gabbard 2000).

Although group treatment or cognitive-behavioral treatment aimed at anxiety management and the development of social skills can occasionally be of benefit, these patients tend to resist such approaches because of their suspiciousness, hypersensitivity to criticism, and misinterpretation of others' comments (Piper and Ogrodniczuk 2005).

Although seldom studied, antipsychotic medications may be sometimes useful in the treatment of paranoid personality disorder. Patients may view such treatment with mistrust; however, these medications are more clearly indicated in the treatment of the overtly psychotic decompensations that these patients sometimes experience (Table 20–7).

TABLE 20–7. Treatment of paranoid personality disorder

Supportive individual psychotherapy

Antipsychotic medications for psychotic decompensation

Schizoid Personality Disorder

History

Schizoid personality disorder was originally thought to be the personality type associated with schizophrenia—a role now largely assumed by schizotypal personality disorder. As a trait-like variant of schizophrenia, schizoid personality disorder was described by Hoch (1910) as the "shut-in personality," by Bleuler (1922) as "schizoidie," and by Kraepelin (1919) as "autistic personality." A similar personality type could also be found in the psychoanalytic literature in writings by the object relations theorists Fairbairn (1940/1952) and Guntrip (1971), who used the term in a broader fashion to describe socially withdrawn patients who had difficulties with intimacy and some of the behavioral peculiarities now subsumed by schizotypal personality disorder.

Schizoid personality disorder has been included in every version of DSM, but its meaning has varied significantly in the different DSM editions. Broadly defined in DSM-I and DSM-II, the category was divided in DSM-III into the schizoid, avoidant, and schizotypal types of personality disorder.

Epidemiology

Schizoid personality disorder is one of the rarest personality disorders, occurring in less than 1% of the general population (Torgersen 2005). Like paranoid personality disorder, schizoid personality disorder is more common among men than women (Torgersen et al. 2001; Zimmerman and Coryell 1990).

Clinical Features

Schizoid personality disorder is characterized by a profound defect in the ability to relate to others in a meaningful way (Table 20–8). Persons with this disorder have little or no desire for relationships with others and, as a result, are extremely socially isolated. They prefer to engage in solitary, often intellectual, activities, such as computer games or puzzles, and they often create an elaborate fantasy world that they retreat into and that substitutes for relationships with real people. As a result of their lack of interest in relationships, they have few or no close friends or confidants. They date infrequently, seldom marry, and have little interest in sex, and they often work at jobs requiring little interpersonal interaction (e.g., as a night watchman). These individuals are also notable for their lack of emotional expression or affect. They usually appear cold, detached, aloof, and constricted, and they have particular discomfort with warm feelings. Few, if any,

TABLE 20–8. DSM-IV-TR diagnostic criteria for schizoid personality disorder

A. A pervasive pattern of detachment from social relationships and a restricted range of expression of emotions in interpersonal settings, beginning by early adulthood and present in a variety of contexts, as indicated by four (or more) of the following:

  (1) neither desires nor enjoys close relationships, including being part of a family
  (2) almost always chooses solitary activities
  (3) has little, if any, interest in having sexual experiences with another person
  (4) takes pleasure in few, if any, activities
  (5) lacks close friends or confidants other than first-degree relatives
  (6) appears indifferent to the praise or criticism of others
  (7) shows emotional coldness, detachment, or flattened affectivity

B. Does not occur exclusively during the course of schizophrenia, a mood disorder with psychotic features, another psychotic disorder, or a pervasive developmental disorder and is not due to the direct physiological effects of a general medical condition.

Note: If criteria are met prior to the onset of schizophrenia, add "premorbid," e.g., "schizoid personality disorder (premorbid)."

activities or experiences give them pleasure, resulting in chronic anhedonia.

Differential Diagnosis

Schizoid personality disorder shares the features of social isolation and restricted emotional expression with schizotypal personality disorder, but it lacks the latter disorder's characteristic cognitive and perceptual distortions. Unlike individuals with avoidant personality disorder, who intensely desire relationships but avoid them because of exaggerated fears of rejection, persons with schizoid personality disorder have little or no apparent interest in developing relationships with others. Schizoid individuals can be distinguished from those with paranoid personality disorder by the lack of suspiciousness and mistrust. They can be differentiated from milder forms of autistic disorder or Asperger's disorder by the more severely impaired social interactions and stereotyped behavior and interests seen in the latter.

Etiology

Clinicians have noted that schizoid personality disorder occurs in adults who experienced cold, neglectful, and ungratifying relationships in early childhood, which presumably had led these persons to assume that relationships are not valuable or worth pursuing. There is reason to believe that constitutional factors contribute to the childhood pattern of shyness that often precedes the disorder. Introversion (intimacy problems, inhibition), which characterizes schizoid (as well as avoidant and schizotypal) personality disorder, appears to be substantially heritable (DiLalla et al. 1996). Prenatal exposure to famine has also been shown to increase the risk for schizoid personality disorder, suggesting a role for environmental factors very early in development (Hoek et al. 1996).

Treatment

Persons with schizoid personality disorder, like those with paranoid personality disorder, rarely seek treatment. They do not perceive the formation of any relationship—including a therapeutic relationship—as potentially valuable or beneficial. They may, however, occasionally seek treatment for an associated problem, such as depression, or they may be brought for treatment by others. Whereas some patients can tolerate only a supportive therapy or treatment aimed at the resolution of a crisis or associated Axis I disorder, others may actually do well with insight-oriented psychotherapy aimed at effecting a basic shift in their comfort with intimacy and affects.

Development of a therapeutic alliance may be difficult and can be facilitated by an interested and caring attitude to address the possibility of underlying neediness (Bender 2005) and by avoidance of early interpretation or confrontation. Some authors have suggested the use of so-called inanimate bridges, such as writing and artistic productions, to ease the patient into a therapy relationship. Incorporation of cognitive-behavioral approaches that encourage gradually increasing social involvement may be of value (Beck et al. 2004). Although many patients may be unwilling to participate in a group, group therapy may also facilitate the development of social skills and relationships (Piper and Ogrodniczuk 2005) (Table 20–9).

Schizotypal Personality Disorder

History

Even the precursors of modern-day schizotypal personality disorder were linked theoretically to schizo-

TABLE 20–9. Treatment of schizoid personality disorder

Supportive individual psychotherapy

Psychodynamic individual psychotherapy

Cognitive-behavioral psychotherapy

Group psychotherapy

phrenia. Bleuler's (1922) concept of *latent schizophrenia*, which consisted of mild or attenuated symptoms of schizophrenia without deterioration into psychosis, was one of the major clinical forerunners of schizotypal personality disorder. The term *schizotype*, coined by Rado (1956), denoted a presumed nonpsychotic phenotypic variant of the schizophrenia genome. This term was later used to refer to the "borderline schizophrenia" syndrome identified in the Danish adoption studies, which was a milder schizophrenia-like disorder found in the biological relatives of probands with schizophrenia (Kety et al. 1968).

Schizotypal personality disorder was new to DSM-III; its criteria were based on the characteristics of the relatives (i.e., the "schizotypes") identified in the Danish adoption studies (Spitzer et al. 1979). Conceptualizing a nonpsychotic variant of schizophrenia as a personality disorder called attention to the different prognostic and treatment implications of these diagnoses.

Epidemiology

Schizotypal personality disorder occurs in 0.7%–1.2% of the general population (Torgersen 2005). Unlike the other two Cluster A personality disorders, no gender difference in prevalence has been found for this disorder (Torgersen et al. 2001; Zimmerman and Coryell 1990).

Clinical Features

Schizotypal personality disorder, like schizophrenia, is characterized by positive, psychotic-like symptoms and negative, deficit-like symptoms (Table 20–10). Persons with schizotypal personality disorder experience cognitive or perceptual distortions (positive), behave in an eccentric manner, and are socially withdrawn and anxious (negative). Common cognitive and perceptual distortions include ideas of reference, bodily illusions, and unusual telepathic and clairvoyant experiences. These distortions, which are inconsistent with subcultural norms, occur frequently and are an important and pervasive component of the person's experience. They help explain the odd and eccentric

TABLE 20–10. DSM-IV-TR diagnostic criteria for schizotypal personality disorder

A. A pervasive pattern of social and interpersonal deficits marked by acute discomfort with, and reduced capacity for, close relationships as well as by cognitive or perceptual distortions and eccentricities of behavior, beginning by early adulthood and present in a variety of contexts, as indicated by five (or more) of the following:

(1) ideas of reference (excluding delusions of reference)

(2) odd beliefs or magical thinking that influences behavior and is inconsistent with subcultural norms (e.g., superstitiousness, belief in clairvoyance, telepathy, or "sixth sense"; in children and adolescents, bizarre fantasies or preoccupations)

(3) unusual perceptual experiences, including bodily illusions

(4) odd thinking and speech (e.g., vague, circumstantial, metaphorical, overelaborate, or stereotyped)

(5) suspiciousness or paranoid ideation

(6) inappropriate or constricted affect

(7) behavior or appearance that is odd, eccentric, or peculiar

(8) lack of close friends or confidants other than first-degree relatives

(9) excessive social anxiety that does not diminish with familiarity and tends to be associated with paranoid fears rather than negative judgments about self

B. Does not occur exclusively during the course of schizophrenia, a mood disorder with psychotic features, another psychotic disorder, or a pervasive developmental disorder.

Note: If criteria are met prior to the onset of schizophrenia, add "premorbid," e.g., "schizoid personality disorder (premorbid)."

behavior characteristic of this disorder. Individuals with schizotypal personality disorder may, for example, talk to themselves in public, gesture for no apparent reason, or dress in a peculiar or unkempt fashion. Their speech is often odd and idiosyncratic—for example, unusually circumstantial, metaphorical, or vague—and their affect is constricted or inappropriate. Such a person may, for example, laugh inappropriately when discussing his or her problems.

Persons with schizotypal personality disorder are socially uncomfortable and isolated, with few friends. This isolation is often due to their eccentric cognitions and behavior, as well as their lack of desire for relationships, which stems in part from their suspiciousness of others. If they develop relationships, they tend to remain distant or may end them because of their persistent social anxiety and paranoia.

Differential Diagnosis

Schizotypal personality disorder shares the feature of suspiciousness with paranoid personality disorder and that of social isolation with schizoid personality disorder, but the latter two disorders lack the markedly peculiar behavior and significant cognitive and perceptual distortions typical of schizotypal personality disorder. The symptoms of schizotypal personality disorder appear to be attenuated versions of the symptoms of schizophrenia, but enduring periods of overt psychosis and social deterioration over time are not characteristic.

Etiology

Schizotypal personality disorder is considered a schizophrenia spectrum disorder—that is, related to Axis I schizophrenia (Siever and Davis 2004). Phenomenological as well as genetic, biological, treatment, and outcome data support this link. For example, family history studies show an increased risk for schizophrenia-related disorders in relatives of schizotypal probands and, conversely, an increased risk for schizotypal personality disorder in relatives of probands with schizophrenia (Kendler et al. 1993; Torgersen et al. 1993). Both the positive and the negative components of schizotypal personality are moderately heritable (Linney et al. 2003), although only the deficit symptoms may be genetically related to schizophrenia (Fanous et al. 2001; Torgersen et al. 2002). In addition, at least some forms of schizotypal personality disorder involve abnormalities of brain structure, physiology, chemistry, and functioning characteristic of schizophrenia, for example, increased cerebrospinal fluid and reduced cortical volume; temporal lobe volume reductions and dysfunctions; abnormalities of brain physiological functions that modulate attention and inhibit sensory input, such as P50 suppression, prepulse inhibition, impaired smooth-pursuit eye movements, and poor performance on the continuous performance task. Higher cerebrospinal fluid and plasma homovanillic acid concentrations correlated to psychotic-like symptoms and lower concentrations correlated with deficit-like symptoms have been found in patients with schizotypal personality disorder as well as in patients with schizophrenia. Patients with schizotypal personalities have also been shown to have impaired performance on tests of executive function and other tests of visual or auditory attention, such as the Wisconsin Card Sorting Test and the backward masking task, and deficits on verbal learning and working memory tasks, attention-orienting tasks, and instrumental motor tasks. Because of this evidence, schizotypal personality disorder is classified in ICD-10 with schizophrenia rather than with the personality disorders. Differences between the disorders also exist, however, particularly with respect to frontal lobe structure and functioning, which may account for the absence of overt psychosis in schizotypal patients (Suzuki et al. 2005). Genetic or environmental factors that promote greater frontal lobe capacity and reduced striatal dopaminergic reactivity might protect persons with schizotypal personality disorder from developing psychosis and the severe social and cognitive deterioration of chronic schizophrenia (Siever and Davis 2004). It is not clear whether there is a subtype of schizotypal personality disorder that represents a milder trait-like, nonpsychotic variant of schizophrenia and another that represents schizophrenia's prodrome, which might progress to the more florid psychotic episodes of true schizophrenia.

Treatment

Because they are socially anxious and somewhat paranoid, persons with schizotypal personality disorder usually avoid psychiatric treatment. They may, however, seek such treatment—or be brought for treatment by concerned family members—when they become depressed or overtly psychotic. As with patients with paranoid personality disorder, it is difficult to establish an alliance with schizotypal patients, and they are unlikely to tolerate exploratory techniques that emphasize interpretation or confrontation. A supportive relationship that counters cognitive distortions and ego-boundary problems may be useful (Stone 1985). This may involve an educational approach that fosters the development of social skills or encourages risk-taking behavior in social situations or, if these efforts fail, encourages the development of activities with less social involvement. If the patient is willing to participate, cognitive-behavioral therapy and highly structured educational groups with a social skills focus may also be helpful.

Several studies support the usefulness of low-dosage antipsychotic medications in the treatment of schizotypal personality disorder, including atypical antipsychotics such as risperidone (double-blind, placebo-controlled study; Koenigsberg et al. 2003) and olanzapine (Keshavan et al. 2004). These medications may ameliorate the anxiety and psychotic-like features associated with this disorder, and they are particularly

TABLE 20–11. **Treatment of schizotypal personality disorder**

Supportive individual psychotherapy

Cognitive-behavioral psychotherapy

Psychoeducational, social skills group therapy

Low-dosage antipsychotic medications

indicated in the treatment of the more overt psychotic decompensations that these patients can experience (Table 20–11).

Antisocial Personality Disorder
History

Pritchard (1835) used the term *moral insanity* to describe people with a pattern of repeated immoral behaviors for which they were not fully responsible. The disorder he characterized has been described by many other psychiatric luminaries using a variety of labels (Millon 1981). Even as psychiatry has decried the use of this diagnosis for excusing antisocial acts, it has been steadfast in recognizing that such persons have significant psychological impairment.

By the late nineteenth century, the term *psychopathic personality* had become a broadly applicable descriptor for persons with socially maladaptive character traits. Harvey Cleckley's 1941 definition of the psychopath (Cleckley 1964) heavily influenced the DSM-I and DSM-II definitions of antisocial personality, whereas the definitions of antisocial personality in DSM-III and DSM-III-R rested on the empirical work of Robins (1966). The DSM-III and DSM-III-R definitions consisted of an established pattern of conduct disorder in childhood as well as a set of socially noxious behaviors (e.g., law-breaking, assaults, deceits) occurring in adulthood. These definitions had the assets of being explicitly behavioral and of enhancing reliable assessment but had the liability of focusing too much on criminal acts. In DSM-IV, the Robins behaviorally based manifestations were combined with Cleckley's psychopathic traits, such as lack of empathy and remorse, to bring the disorder's definition back in line with clinical observations and with personality trait–based descriptions.

Epidemiology

Antisocial personality disorder occurs in about 1.7% of the general population (Torgersen 2005). It is much more common among men than women (Torgersen et al. 2001; Zimmerman and Coryell 1989).

Clinical Features

The central feature of antisocial personality disorder is a long-standing pattern of socially irresponsible behaviors that reflects a disregard for the rights of others (Table 20–12). Many persons with this disorder engage in repeated unlawful acts. The more prevailing personality characteristics include a lack of interest in or concern for the feelings of others, deceitfulness, and, most notably, a lack of remorse for the harm they may cause others. These characteristics generally make antisocial individuals fail in roles requiring fidelity (e.g., as a spouse), honesty (e.g., as an employee), or reliability (e.g., as a parent). Some antisocial persons possess a glibness and charm that can be used to seduce, outwit, and exploit others. Although most antisocial persons are indifferent to their effects on others, a notable subgroup takes sadistic pleasure in doing harm (Stone 2005). Recent research has demonstrated that psychopathy is multidimensional and that each dimension may have distinct developmental trajectories (Edens et al. 2006) and may be variants of normal personality traits and behaviors (Hare and Neumann 2005). Antisocial personality syndromes are associated with high rates of substance abuse (Compton et al. 2005), which may contribute to the persistence of antisocial behavior over time (Malone et al. 2004).

Differential Diagnosis

The primary differential diagnostic issue involves narcissistic personality disorder. Indeed, these two disorders may be variants of the same basic type of psychopathology (Hare et al. 1991). However, the antisocial person, unlike the narcissistic person, is likely to be reckless and impulsive. In addition, narcissistic individuals' exploitiveness and disregard for others are attributable to their sense of uniqueness and superiority rather than to a desire for materialistic gains.

Etiology

Twin and adoption studies indicate that genetic factors predispose to the development of antisocial personality disorder (Grove et al. 1990; Lyons et al. 1995). Nonetheless, it is unclear how much variance is accounted for by genetic factors and whether the nature of the predisposition is relatively specific or is best conceptualized in terms of relatively nonspecific traits such as impulsivity, excitability, or hostility. Conduct problems (56%), stimulus seeking (40%), and callousness (56%) are antisocial traits that have substantial heritability (Jang et al. 1996). Psychopathic traits of fearless dominance and impulsive antisociality also show significant genetic influences (Blonigen et al. 2005).

TABLE 20–12. DSM-IV-TR diagnostic criteria for antisocial personality disorder

A. There is a pervasive pattern of disregard for and violation of the rights of others occurring since age 15 years, as indicated by three (or more) of the following:

   (1) failure to conform to social norms with respect to lawful behaviors as indicated by repeatedly performing acts that are grounds for arrest

   (2) deceitfulness, as indicated by repeated lying, use of aliases, or conning others for personal profit or pleasure

   (3) impulsivity or failure to plan ahead

   (4) irritability and aggressiveness, as indicated by repeated physical fights or assaults

   (5) reckless disregard for safety of self or others

   (6) consistent irresponsibility, as indicated by repeated failure to sustain consistent work behavior or honor financial obligations

   (7) lack of remorse, as indicated by being indifferent to or rationalizing having hurt, mistreated, or stolen from another

B. The individual is at least age 18 years.

C. There is evidence of conduct disorder (see DSM-IV-TR p. 98) with onset before age 15 years.

D. The occurrence of antisocial behavior is not exclusively during the course of schizophrenia or a manic episode.

Growing evidence indicates that the impulsive and aggressive behaviors may be mediated by abnormal serotonin transporter functioning in the brain (Coccaro et al. 1996). Different psychophysiological patterns may characterize aggression, psychopathy, and antisocial behavior, however (Lorber 2004). Persons with antisocial personality disorder have reductions in whole brain volumes and in the volume of the temporal lobe in particular (Barkataki et al. 2006). Brain activation in the limbic-prefrontal circuit of the brain during fear conditioning has been shown to be deficient in psychopathic criminal offenders (Birbaumer et al. 2005). Neurocognitive impairments in spatial and memory functions have been found in adolescents with persistent antisocial behavior (Raine et al. 2005).

In addition to biological factors, it is also clear that the early family lives of these persons often pose severe environmental handicaps in the form of absent, inconsistent, or abusive parenting. Indeed, many family members also have significant action-oriented psychopathology, such as substance abuse or antisocial personality disorder itself. Modern behavioral genetic research is focusing on interactions between genes and the environment to explain the genesis of antisocial behavior (Moffitt 2005; Reiss et al. 1995).

Treatment

It is clinically important to recognize antisocial personality disorder, because an uncritical acceptance of these individuals' glib or shallow statements of good intentions and collaboration can permit them to have disruptive influences on treatment teams and other patients. However, there is little evidence to suggest that this disorder can be successfully treated by usual psychiatric interventions. Of interest, nonetheless, are reports suggesting that in confined settings, such as the military or prisons, depressive and introspective concerns may surface. Under these circumstances, confrontation by peers may bring about changes in the antisocial person's social behaviors (Table 20–13). It is also notable that some antisocial patients demonstrate an ability to form a therapeutic alliance with psychotherapists, which augurs well for these patients' future course (Woody et al. 1985). These findings contrast with the clinical tradition that emphasizes such persons' inability to learn from harmful consequences. Yet longitudinal follow-up studies have shown that the prevalence of this disorder diminishes with age as these individuals become more aware of the social and interpersonal maladaptiveness of their most harmful social behaviors.

TABLE 20–13. **Treatment of antisocial personality disorder**

Peer group, milieu therapy

Borderline Personality Disorder

History

The borderline personality disorder (BPD) construct originated from the observations of psychoanalytic psychotherapists who were impressed by these patients' demanding search for nurturance, their disregard for the usual boundaries of therapy, and their tendency to regress in unstructured situations. Impelled by the clinical importance of foreseeing such problems and by a new wave of psychotherapeutic optimism, empirical work was initiated to better define this disorder. Early research raised the question of whether such patients had an atypical form of mood disorder rather than an atypical form of schizophrenia, as had been thought, and more importantly led to inclusion of BPD in DSM-III.

The development of diagnostic criteria provoked an effusion of further empirical research that has led to revisions of this disorder's construct and informed its treatment (Gunderson et al. 1991). BPD has become the most widely studied personality disorder. Evidence for its validity is growing, and the disorder is now recognized as the most prevalent Axis II disorder in most clinical settings.

Epidemiology

BPD occurs in 1%–1.5% of the general population (Torgersen 2005). Although it has been shown to be more common among women than men in clinical settings (Morey et al. 2005), this difference may be largely the result of sampling bias (i.e., more women seek treatment), because no gender difference in prevalence has been found in community-based studies (Torgersen et al. 2001; Zimmerman and Coryell 1990).

Clinical Features

BPD is characterized by instability and dysfunction in affective, behavioral, and interpersonal domains. Central to the psychopathology of this disorder are a severely impaired capacity for attachment (Levy et al. 2005) and predictably maladaptive behavior patterns related to separation (Gunderson 1996). When borderline patients feel cared for, held on to, and supported, depressive features (notably loneliness and emptiness) are most evident (Table 20–14). When the threat of losing such a sustaining relationship arises, the idealized image of a beneficent caregiver is replaced by a devalued image of a cruel persecutor. This shift between idealization and devaluation is called *splitting*. An impending separation also evokes intense abandonment fears. To minimize these fears and to prevent the separation, rageful accusations of mistreatment and cruelty and angry self-destructive behaviors may occur. These behaviors often elicit a guilty or fearful protective response from others.

Another central feature of this disorder is extreme affective instability that often leads to impulsive and self-destructive behaviors. These episodes are usually brief and reactive and involve extreme alternations between angry and depressed states. The experience and expression of anger can be particularly difficult for the borderline patient. During periods of unusual stress, dissociative experiences, ideas of reference, or desperate impulsive acts (including substance abuse and promiscuity) commonly occur.

Roughly half of borderline patients have significant remissions of their overt psychopathology within 2 years. Levels of social dysfunction, severity of child-

TABLE 20–14. **DSM-IV-TR diagnostic criteria for borderline personality disorder**

A pervasive pattern of instability of interpersonal relationships, self-image, and affects, and marked impulsivity beginning by early adulthood and present in a variety of contexts, as indicated by five (or more) of the following:

(1) frantic efforts to avoid real or imagined abandonment. **Note:** Do not include suicidal or self-mutilating behavior covered in criterion 5.

(2) a pattern of unstable and intense interpersonal relationships characterized by alternating between extremes of idealization and devaluation

(3) identity disturbance: markedly and persistently unstable self-image or sense of self

(4) impulsivity in at least two areas that are potentially self-damaging (e.g., spending, sex, substance abuse, reckless driving, binge eating). **Note:** Do not include suicidal or self-mutilating behavior covered in criterion 5.

(5) recurrent suicidal behavior, gestures, or threats, or self-mutilating behavior

(6) affective instability due to a marked reactivity of mood (e.g., intense episodic dysphoria, irritability, or anxiety usually lasting a few hours and only rarely more than a few days)

(7) chronic feelings of emptiness

(8) inappropriate, intense anger or difficulty controlling anger (e.g., frequent displays of temper, constant anger, recurrent physical fights)

(9) transient, stress-related paranoid ideation or severe dissociative symptoms

hood trauma, and persistence of substance abuse are predictive of a worse prognosis (Gunderson et al. 2006). Overall, the longer-term course of BPD may be more benign than previously thought and may be predicted from historical, clinical, functional, and personality features (Zanarini et al. 2006). About 10% of patients with the disorder commit suicide, however (Oldham 2006).

Differential Diagnosis

The most common differential diagnosis involves the interface of BPD with bipolar disorder—particularly bipolar II. The major distinctions are that bipolar patients have periods of elation and borderline patients have abandonment fears and repeated episodes of self-harm when alone.

Borderline patients' intense feelings of being bad or evil are distinctly different from the idealized self-image of narcissistic persons. Patients with BPD differ from those with antisocial personality disorder in that the impulsive behaviors of borderline patients are pri-

marily interpersonally oriented and aimed toward obtaining support rather than materialistic gains. Paranoid ideas may also occur in patients with schizotypal or paranoid personality disorders, but these symptoms are more transient, interpersonally reactive, and responsive to external structuring in borderline patients. Patients with dependent personality disorder are characterized by fear of abandonment, but they react to such threats by efforts at appeasement and submissiveness rather than with feelings of emptiness and rage.

Etiology

Psychoanalytic theories have emphasized the importance of early parent–child relationships in the etiology of BPD. These theories have emphasized 1) maternal mismanagement of the 2- to 3-year-old child's efforts to become autonomous (Masterson 1972), 2) exaggerated maternal frustration that aggravates the child's anger (Kernberg 1975), or 3) inattention to the child's emotions and attitudes (Adler 1985). A considerable body of empirical research has embellished these theories by documenting a high frequency of traumatic early abandonment, physical abuse, and sexual abuse (Johnson et al. 2005a). These traumatic experiences appear to occur within a context of sustained neglect from which the pre-borderline child develops enduring rage and self-hatred. The lack of reliably involved attachment to caretakers during development is a source of borderline patients' inability to maintain stable senses of themselves or of others without ongoing contact (i.e., their defects of object constancy or lack of stable introjects) (Gunderson 1996).

Zanarini and Frankenburg (1997) proposed a tripartite causative model of BPD consisting of a traumatic childhood, a vulnerable temperament, and triggering events. Linehan's biosocial theory suggests that a biological disposition toward emotional vulnerability, exposure to invalidating environments, and deficits in emotion-regulation skills are key etiological factors (Linehan 1993). Joyce et al. (2003) proposed a distinctive combination of risk factors consisting of a temperament characterized by high novelty seeking and high harm avoidance, childhood abuse and/or neglect, and childhood or adolescent psychopathology in the affective, conduct, and substance abuse domains. Posner et al. (2003) included a combination of high negative emotionality and a deficit in an executive attentional control network in their proposed model.

Twin study evidence of 69% overall heritability for BPD (Torgersen et al. 2000) has mobilized efforts to identify genetic contributions to the etiology of specific borderline traits. Siever and Davis (1991) posited fundamental dimensions of affective instability and impulsive aggression underlying BPD. Livesley et al. (1993) found heritability of about 50% for borderline traits such as affective lability and insecure attachment and later for the broader domains of emotional dysregulation and dissocial behavior (Livesley et al. 1998). There is evidence of serotonergic dysfunction in the borderline trait of impulsivity. Structural and functional neuroimaging studies have shown reductions in frontal and orbitofrontal lobe volumes, altered metabolism in prefrontal brain regions, and failure of activation of these brain regions under stress. Because these brain regions are important in serotonergic function and mediate affective control, the observed deficits may be the source of the disinhibited impulses and affects characteristic of patients with BPD. Other studies have shown hyperactivity of the amygdala, which also plays a central role in emotion regulation. Patients with BPD perform poorly in multiple neurocognitive domains, particularly on functions lateralized to the right hemisphere. It is unknown, however, whether neurobiological dysfunctions are due to genetics, pre- or postnatal factors, or adverse events during childhood or are the consequences of the disorder (Lieb et al. 2004). Thus, although the etiology of BPD has yet to be determined, it is undoubtedly complex and multifactorial.

Treatment

Borderline patients are high utilizers of psychiatric outpatient, inpatient, and psychopharmacological treatment (Table 20–15). The extensive literature on the treatment of BPD universally notes the extreme difficulties that clinicians encounter with these patients. These problems derive from the patients' appeal to their treaters' nurturing qualities and their rageful accusations in response to their treaters' perceived failures. Often therapists develop intense countertransference reactions that lead them to attempt to re-parent or, conversely, to reject borderline patients. As a consequence, regardless of the treatment approach used, personal maturity and considerable clinical experience are important assets.

Much of the early treatment literature focused on the value of intensive exploratory psychotherapies directed at modifying borderline patients' basic character structure. However, this literature has increasingly suggested that improvement may be related not to the acquisition of insight but to the corrective experience of developing a stable, trusting relationship with a therapist who fails to retaliate in response to these patients' angry and disruptive behaviors. Paralleling this development has been the suggestion that supportive

TABLE 20–15. Treatment of borderline personality disorder

Psychodynamic individual psychotherapy

Supportive individual psychotherapy

Cognitive-behavioral or schema-focused psychotherapy

Dialectical behavior therapy

Interpersonal psychotherapy

Family psychoeducation

Selective serotonin reuptake inhibitor antidepressant medications

Atypical antipsychotic medications

Anticonvulsant medications

psychotherapies or group therapies may bring about similar changes (Appelbaum 2005; Piper and Ogrodniczuk 2005). Evidence has provided support for the effectiveness of an 18-month psychoanalytic treatment called "mentalization-based treatment" that took place in a partial hospital setting (Bateman and Fonagy 1999). In addition, a long-term phased model of psychodynamic therapy that combined hospital-based and community-based strategies was reported to be more effective than hospital-based treatment alone (Chiesa and Fonagy 2000).

At present, treatment of borderline patients typically includes cognitive-behavioral and pharmacological interventions (American Psychiatric Association 2001). Linehan et al. (2006) have shown that behavioral treatment consisting of a once-weekly individual and twice-weekly group regimen can effectively diminish the self-destructive behaviors and hospitalizations of borderline patients. The success and cost benefits of this treatment, called *dialectical behavior therapy,* have led to its widespread adoption and to modifications that can be used in a variety of settings. *Schema-focused therapy* is a newer cognitive therapy that has also been shown to be efficacious (Giesen-Bloo et al. 2006).

Although no one medication has been found to have dramatic or predictable effects, studies indicate that many medications may diminish specific problems such as impulsivity, affective lability, or intermittent cognitive and perceptual disturbances (Table 20–16), as well as irritability and aggressive behavior (Soloff 2005). Most recently, studies have shown efficacy for atypical antipsychotics for dysphoria and aggression (Soler et al. 2005) and anticonvulsants for anger and aggression (Hollander et al. 2005). In general, the

TABLE 20–16. Medication efficacy in borderline personality disorder

Medication	Affective dysregulation	Impulsivity	Psychotic-like features
Monoamine oxidase inhibitors	+	+	?
Serotonin reuptake inhibitors[a]	++	++	?
Tricyclic antidepressants	±	±	±
Typical antipsychotics	+	+	++
Atypical antipsychotics	+	+	++
Mood stabilizers	+	+	+
Benzodiazepines	±	−	?

Note. ++=clear improvement; +=modest improvement; ±=variable improvement or worsening; −=some worsening. The information in this table should be considered tentative; some medications have received relatively little investigation, many medication trials have been small and open, and few of the medications listed have been directly compared with one another.
[a]Most published studies of serotonin reuptake inhibitors have used fluoxetine.

profusion of treatment modalities and the introduction of empiricism point toward the increasing use of more focused treatment strategies.

Histrionic Personality Disorder

History

An early conceptualization of histrionic personality disorder can be found in accounts of hysteria written by Pierre Janet and Sigmund Freud. Janet was impressed with the role of actual seduction (or other trauma) in childhood, whereas Freud focused on the unconscious elaboration of the child's sexual drive (i.e., libido). Subsequent psychoanalytic observers noted that hysterical symptoms were often associated with a particular set of character traits, which led to the designation of a hysterical type of personality disorder in DSM-II.

The initial empirical examination of hysterical personality traits used factor-analytic methods, which helped consolidate this syndrome's components and also led to a broad definition. Indeed, this disorder's early definitions were so broad that they rendered the diagnosis meaningless to some.

The label *hysterical* was changed to *histrionic* in DSM-III in an effort to use a term that was more theoretically neutral and more in line with psychiatry's descriptive tradition. Whereas the term *hysterical personality* still connotes the conflicted eroticization of parental figures, the term *histrionic* reflects the diagnostician's concern with the observable features of emotional instability and attention seeking. The DSM-III version of the criteria of this disorder, however, largely captured its more severe "oral" and manipula-

tive elements and thereby unintentionally magnified its overlap with other categories, such as BPD.

The modifications of DSM-III-R and DSM-IV helped distinguish histrionic personality disorder from others and placed it within the range of less severe personality disorders that can be conceptualized as maladaptive variants of normally occurring traits. This view was reflected by Chodoff's (1982) suggestion that this disorder represents a caricature of stereotypic femininity.

Epidemiology

Histrionic personality disorder is one of the most frequently occurring personality disorders; it occurs in almost 2% of the general population (Torgersen 2005). Those with histrionic personality disorder are more often women (Torgersen et al. 2001; Zimmerman and Coryell 1990).

Clinical Features

Central to histrionic personality disorder is an overconcern with attention and appearance (Table 20–17). Persons with this disorder spend an excessive amount of time seeking attention and making themselves attractive. The desire to be found attractive may lead to inappropriately seductive or provocative dress and flirtatious behavior, and the desire for attention may lead to other flamboyant acts or self-dramatizing behavior. All of these features reflect these persons' underlying insecurity about their value as anything other than fetching companions. Persons with histrionic personality disorder also display an effusive, but labile

TABLE 20–17. DSM-IV-TR diagnostic criteria for histrionic personality disorder

A pervasive pattern of excessive emotionality and attention seeking, beginning by early adulthood and present in a variety of contexts, as indicated by five (or more) of the following:

(1) is uncomfortable in situations in which he or she is not the center of attention
(2) interaction with others is often characterized by inappropriate sexually seductive or provocative behavior
(3) displays rapidly shifting and shallow expression of emotions
(4) consistently uses physical appearance to draw attention to self
(5) has a style of speech that is excessively impressionistic and lacking in detail
(6) shows self-dramatization, theatricality, and exaggerated expression of emotion
(7) is suggestible, i.e., easily influenced by others or circumstances
(8) considers relationships to be more intimate than they actually are

and shallow, range of feelings. They are often overly impressionistic and given to hyperbolic descriptions of others (e.g., "She's wonderful" or "She's horrible"). More generally, these persons do not attend to detail or facts, and they are reluctant or unable to make reasoned critical analyses of problems or situations. Persons with this disorder often present with complaints of depression, somatic problems of unclear origin, and a history of disappointing romantic relationships.

Differential Diagnosis

Histrionic personality disorder can be confused with dependent, borderline, and narcissistic personality disorders. Histrionic individuals are often willing, even eager, to have others make decisions and organize their activities for them. However, unlike persons with dependent personality disorder, histrionic persons are uninhibited and lively companions who willfully forgo appearing autonomous because they believe that this attracts others. Unlike persons with BPD, those with histrionic personality do not perceive themselves as bad, and they lack ongoing problems with rage or willful self-destructiveness. Persons with narcissistic personality disorder also seek attention to sustain their self-esteem but differ in that their self-esteem is characterized by grandiosity, and the attention they crave must be admiring.

Etiology

Psychoanalytic theory proposes that histrionic personality disorder originates in the oedipal phase of development (i.e., 3–5 years of age), when an overly eroticized relationship with the opposite-sex parent is unduly encouraged and the child fears that the consequences of this excitement will be the loss of, or retaliation by, the same-sex parent. This conflict results in lasting character formations of exaggerated fantasy and exhibitionistic promise with inhibited factual analysis and diminished actual productivity. Research suggests that qualities such as emotional expressiveness (Jang et al. 1996) and egocentricity (Torgersen et al. 1993) are heritable temperaments. From this perspective, histrionic personality disorder would consist of extreme variants of temperamental dispositions, the environmental contributions of which may be less specific than those of the aforementioned theories.

Treatment

Individual psychodynamic psychotherapy, including psychoanalysis (Table 20–18), remains the cornerstone of most treatment for persons with histrionic personality disorder (Gabbard 2005). This treatment is directed at increasing patients' awareness of 1) how their self-esteem is maladaptively tied to their ability to attract attention at the expense of developing other skills, and 2) how their shallow relationships and emotional experience reflect unconscious fears of real commitments. Much of this increase in awareness occurs through analysis of the here-and-now doctor–patient relationship rather than through the reconstruction of childhood experiences. Therapists should be aware that the typical idealization and eroticization that such patients bring into treatment are the material for exploration, and thus therapists should be aware of countertransferential gratification.

TABLE 20–18. Treatment of histrionic personality disorder

Psychodynamic individual psychotherapy

Psychoanalysis

Narcissistic Personality Disorder
History

Havelock Ellis (1898) introduced the term *narcissism* in 1898 to describe a type of sexual perversion involving treating oneself as a sexual object. Freud then adopted the term to describe a more general attitude of self-absorption and self-love. Later, analysts moved the concept toward excessive self-love and grandiosity that develop in response to injured self-esteem (Morrison 1989). The concept of a narcissistic type of personality disorder developed only during the 1980s and was inspired largely by the enormous attention given to pathological narcissism in the psychoanalytic community (Gunderson et al. 1991). Ironically, this attention was largely an outgrowth of Heinz Kohut's (1971) theoretical and clinical contributions, many of which focused on nonpathological narcissism.

Epidemiology

Narcissistic personality disorder is among the rarest disorders found in community studies, with a prevalence of only about 0.5% (Torgersen 2005). It appears to be more common among men (Torgersen et al. 2001; Zimmerman and Coryell 1990).

Clinical Features

Because persons with narcissistic personality disorder have grandiose self-esteem, fantasies of unlimited potential, a sense of entitlement, and needs for admiration, they are vulnerable to intense reactions when their self-image is damaged (Table 20–19). They respond with strong feelings of hurt or anger to even small slights, rejections, defeats, or criticisms. As a result, persons with narcissistic personality disorder usually go to great lengths to avoid exposure to such experiences, and when that fails, they react by becoming devaluative or rageful. Serious depression can ensue, which is the usual precipitant for their seeking clinical help. In relationships, narcissistic persons are often quite distant and try to sustain "an illusion of self-sufficiency" (Modell 1975). They lack empathy for others, are often envious, and may exploit others for self-serving ends. They are likely to feel that those with whom they associate need to be special and unique because they see themselves in these terms; thus, they usually wish to be associated only with persons, institutions, or possessions that will confirm their sense of superiority. The DSM-IV-TR criteria are most accurate in identifying the arrogant, socially conspicuous forms of narcissistic personality disorder; however, there are other forms in which a conviction of personal superiority is hidden behind social withdrawal and a facade of self-sacrifice and even humility.

Differential Diagnosis

Narcissistic personality disorder can be most readily confused with antisocial and histrionic personality disorders. Like persons with antisocial personality disor-

---

TABLE 20–19. DSM-IV-TR diagnostic criteria for narcissistic personality disorder

A pervasive pattern of grandiosity (in fantasy or behavior), need for admiration, and lack of empathy, beginning by early adulthood and present in a variety of contexts, as indicated by five (or more) of the following:

(1) has a grandiose sense of self-importance (e.g., exaggerates achievements and talents, expects to be recognized as superior without commensurate achievements)

(2) is preoccupied with fantasies of unlimited success, power, brilliance, beauty, or ideal love

(3) believes that he or she is "special" and unique and can only be understood by, or should associate with, other special or high-status people (or institutions)

(4) requires excessive admiration

(5) has a sense of entitlement, i.e., unreasonable expectations of especially favorable treatment or automatic compliance with his or her expectations

(6) is interpersonally exploitative, i.e., takes advantage of others to achieve his or her own ends

(7) lacks empathy: is unwilling to recognize or identify with the feelings and needs of others

(8) is often envious of others or believes that others are envious of him or her

(9) shows arrogant, haughty behaviors or attitudes

---

der, those with narcissistic personality disorder are capable of exploiting others, but narcissistic persons usually rationalize their behavior on the basis of the specialness of their goals or their personal virtue. In contrast, antisocial persons' goals are materialistic, and their rationalizations, if offered, are based on a view that others would do the same to them. The narcissistic person's excessive pride in achievements, relative constraint in expression of feelings, and disregard for other people's rights and sensitivities help distinguish him or her from persons with histrionic personality disorder. Perhaps the most difficult differential diagnostic problem is whether a person who meets criteria for narcissistic personality disorder has a stable personality disorder or is in an episode of an Axis I disorder, such as an adjustment reaction. If the emergence of narcissistic traits has been defensively triggered by experiences of failure or rejection, these traits may diminish radically and self-esteem may be restored when new relationships or successes occur. When manic, patients with bipolar disorder can appear quite similar to those with narcissistic personality disorder.

Etiology

Little scientific evidence is available about the pathogenesis of narcissistic personality disorder. Reconstructions based on developmental history and observations in psychoanalytic treatment indicate that this disorder develops in persons who have had their fears, failures, or dependency responded to with criticism, disdain, or neglect during their childhood years. Such experiences leave them contemptuous of such reactions in themselves and others and inexperienced in viewing others as sources of comfort and support. They develop a veneer of invulnerability and self-sufficiency that masks their underlying emptiness and constricts their capacity to feel deeply.

Treatment

Individual psychodynamic psychotherapy, including psychoanalysis (Table 20–20), is the cornerstone of treatment for persons with narcissistic personality disorder (Gabbard 2005). Following Kohut's lead, some therapists believe that the vulnerability to narcissistic injury indicates that intervention should be directed at conveying empathy for the patient's sensitivities and disappointments. This approach, in theory, allows a positive idealized transference to develop that will then be gradually disillusioned by the inevitable frustrations encountered in therapy—disillusionment that will clarify the excessive nature of the patient's reactions to frustrations and disappointments. An alternative view, explicated by Kernberg (1975), is that the vulnerability should be addressed earlier and more directly by interpretations and confrontations through which these persons will come to recognize their grandiosity and its maladaptive consequences. With either approach, the psychotherapeutic process usually requires a relatively intensive schedule over a period of years in which the narcissistic patient's hypersensitivity to slights and tendency to treat the therapist almost exclusively as an object for gratifying his or her needs must be foremost in the therapist's mind and interventions.

TABLE 20–20. **Treatment of narcissistic personality disorder**

Psychodynamic individual psychotherapy

Avoidant Personality Disorder

History

Avoidant personality disorder, which was new to DSM-III, was theoretically derived from Millon's (1981) typology of personality disorders (corresponding to his active–detached pattern). The disorder has some historical antecedents, including Kretschmer's (1925) hyperaesthetic type, Schneider's (1959) sensitive type, Horney's (1945) detached type, and Fenichel's (1945) phobic character. In DSM-III-R, the avoidant personality disorder construct was brought closer to the psychoanalytic construct of the phobic character. The changes of DSM-IV focused on better differentiating this disorder from the Axis I condition of generalized social phobia (Millon 1981).

Epidemiology

Estimates of the prevalence of avoidant personality disorder based on epidemiological studies vary widely, resulting in a mean prevalence of 1.35% but a pooled prevalence of almost 3% (Torgersen 2005). This is in part due to the frequency with which it was found in a Scandinavian study (Torgersen et al. 2001), which illustrates how culture may contribute to the form a personality disorder may take. Avoidant personality disorder may be more common among women (Zimmerman and Coryell 1989, 1990).

Clinical Features

Persons with avoidant personality disorder experience excessive and pervasive anxiety and discomfort in social situations and in intimate relationships (Table 20–21). Although strongly desiring relationships, they avoid them because they fear being ridiculed, criticized, rejected, or humiliated. These fears reflect their low self-esteem and hypersensitivity to negative evaluation by others. When they do enter into social situations or relationships, they feel inept and are self-conscious, shy, awkward, and preoccupied with being criticized or rejected. Their lives are constricted in that they tend to avoid not only relationships but also any new activities because they fear that they will embarrass or humiliate themselves. Patients with avoidant personality disorder may engage in deliberate self-harm (Klonsky et al. 2003) and experience disability in social, educational, and physical realms (Kessler 2003).

Differential Diagnosis

Schizoid personality disorder also involves social isolation, but the schizoid person does not desire relationships, whereas the avoidant person desires them but avoids them because of anxiety and fears of humiliation and rejection. Whereas avoidant personality disorder is characterized by avoidance of situations and relationships involving possible rejection, disappointment, ridicule, or shame, Axis I social phobia usually

TABLE 20–21. DSM-IV-TR diagnostic criteria for avoidant personality disorder

A pervasive pattern of social inhibition, feelings of inadequacy, and hypersensitivity to negative evaluation, beginning by early adulthood and present in a variety of contexts, as indicated by four (or more) of the following:

(1) avoids occupational activities that involve significant interpersonal contact, because of fears of criticism, disapproval, or rejection
(2) is unwilling to get involved with people unless certain of being liked
(3) shows restraint within intimate relationships because of the fear of being shamed or ridiculed
(4) is preoccupied with being criticized or rejected in social situations
(5) is inhibited in new interpersonal situations because of feelings of inadequacy
(6) views self as socially inept, personally unappealing, or inferior to others
(7) is unusually reluctant to take personal risks or to engage in any new activities because they may prove embarrassing

consists of specific fears related to social performance (e.g., a fear of saying something inappropriate or of being unable to answer questions in front of other people). Furthermore, patterns of avoidance in persons with avoidant personality disorder often extend beyond social situations to include emotional and novelty avoidance (Taylor et al. 2004). Some avoidant persons are actually vulnerable subtypes of narcissistic character styles (Dickinson and Pincus 2003).

Etiology

Millon (1981) suggested that avoidant personality disorder develops from parental rejection and censure, which may be reinforced by rejecting peers. Psychodynamic theory suggests that avoidant behavior may derive from early life experiences that lead to an exaggerated desire for acceptance or an intolerance of criticism. Research on childhood experiences of avoidant persons reveals negative childhood memories (e.g., of isolation, rejection) (Meyer and Carver 2000); poorer athletic performance, less involvement in hobbies, and less popularity (Rettew et al. 2003); and parental neglect (Joyce et al. 2003). Research in the biological sphere has implicated the importance of inborn temperament in the development of avoidant behavior. Kagan (1989) found that some children as young as 21 months manifest increased physiological arousal and avoidant traits in social situations (e.g., retreat from

the unfamiliar and avoidance of interaction with strangers) and that this social inhibition tends to persist for many years. Family studies have demonstrated elevated rates of trait and social anxiety, as well as personality traits such as harm avoidance, in the first-degree relatives of patients with generalized social phobia, suggesting that social anxiety lies on a continuum that may be influenced by familial factors (Stein et al. 2001).

Treatment

Because of their excessive fear of rejection and criticism and their reluctance to form relationships, individuals with avoidant personality disorder may be difficult to engage in treatment. Engagement in psychotherapy may be facilitated by the therapist's use of supportive techniques, sensitivity to the patient's hypersensitivity, and gentle interpretation of the defensive use of avoidance. Although early in treatment these patients may tolerate only supportive techniques, they may eventually respond well to all kinds of psychotherapy (Gabbard 2005). Clinicians should be aware of the potential for countertransference reactions such as overprotectiveness, hesitancy to adequately challenge the patient, or excessive expectations for change.

Although few data exist, it seems likely that assertiveness and social skills training may increase patients' confidence and willingness to take risks in social situations. Cognitive techniques that gently challenge patients' pathological assumptions about their sense of ineptness may also be useful (Beck et al. 2004). Group experiences—perhaps, in particular, homogeneous supportive groups that emphasize the development of social skills—may prove useful for avoidant patients (Piper and Ogrodniczuk 2005).

Promising preliminary data suggest that avoidant personality disorder may improve with treatment with monoamine oxidase inhibitors or serotonin reuptake inhibitors. Anxiolytics sometimes help patients better manage anxiety (especially severe anxiety) caused by facing previously avoided situations or trying new behaviors (Table 20–22).

Dependent Personality Disorder

History

Abraham's (1927) "oral" character was the major clinical predecessor of dependent personality disorder (DPD). This character type was thought to result from fixation at the first, or oral, stage of psychosexual development—a theory that was reflected in Fenichel's

TABLE 20–22.   Treatment of avoidant personality disorder

Supportive individual psychotherapy

Psychodynamic individual psychotherapy

Cognitive-behavioral psychotherapy

Assertiveness and social skills training

Group psychotherapy

Monoamine oxidase inhibitor and selective serotonin reuptake inhibitor antidepressant medications

Antianxiety medications

TABLE 20–23.   DSM-IV-TR diagnostic criteria for dependent personality disorder

A pervasive and excessive need to be taken care of that leads to submissive and clinging behavior and fears of separation, beginning by early adulthood and present in a variety of contexts, as indicated by five (or more) of the following:

(1) has difficulty making everyday decisions without an excessive amount of advice and reassurance from others
(2) needs others to assume responsibility for most major areas of his or her life
(3) has difficulty expressing disagreement with others because of fear of loss of support or approval.   **Note:** Do not include realistic fears of retribution.
(4) has difficulty initiating projects or doing things on his or her own (because of a lack of self-confidence in judgment or abilities rather than a lack of motivation or energy)
(5) goes to excessive lengths to obtain nurturance and support from others, to the point of volunteering to do things that are unpleasant
(6) feels uncomfortable or helpless when alone because of exaggerated fears of being unable to care for himself or herself
(7) urgently seeks another relationship as a source of care and support when a close relationship ends
(8) is unrealistically preoccupied with fears of being left to take care of himself or herself

(1945) observation that "certain persons act as nursing mothers in all their object relationships" (p. 489). This personality type was similar to Horney's "compliant" type (Millon 1981).

DPD was a subtype of passive-aggressive personality disorder in DSM-I and did not become a separate disorder until DSM-III. The changes of DSM-IV put greater emphasis on the disorder's central features and attempted to diminish its overlap with other personality disorders.

Epidemiology

DPD occurs in about 1.25% of the general population (Torgersen 2005) and is much more common among women (Torgersen et al. 2001; Zimmerman and Coryell 1989, 1990).

Clinical Features

Dependent personality is characterized by an excessive need to be cared for by others, which leads to submissive and clinging behavior and excessive fears of separation (Table 20–23). Although these individuals are able to care for themselves, they doubt their abilities and judgment, and they view others as much stronger and more capable than they are. These persons excessively rely on "powerful" others to initiate and do things for them, make their decisions, assume responsibility for their actions, and guide them through life. Low self-esteem and doubts about their effectiveness lead them to avoid positions of responsibility. Because they feel unable to function without excessive guidance, they go to great lengths to maintain dependent relationships. They may, for example, always agree with those on whom they depend, and they tend to be excessively passive and self-sacrificing. Because they feel incapable of caring for themselves

when relationships end, these individuals feel helpless and fearful. They may indiscriminately begin another relationship so that they can be provided with direction and nurturance—an unfulfilling or even abusive relationship may seem better than being on their own.

Differential Diagnosis

Although persons with BPD also dread being alone and need ongoing support, dependent persons want others to assume a controlling function that would frighten the borderline patient. Moreover, persons with DPD become appeasing rather than rageful or self-destructive when threatened with separation. Although both avoidant and dependent personality disorders are characterized by low self-esteem, rejection sensitivity, and an excessive need for reassurance, persons with DPD seek out rather than avoid relationships, and they quickly and indiscriminately replace ended relationships instead of further withdrawing from others.

Etiology

Abraham (1927) suggested that the dependent character derives from either overindulgence or underindulgence during the oral phase of development (i.e., birth to age 2 years). Subsequent empirical data have given more support to the underindulgence hypothesis. However, studies of adults have not supported a specific association between feeding or other oral habits in childhood and dependency in adulthood. Caretaking patterns unrelated to the oral phase, per se—for example, in the care of a child with chronic physical illness or parenting that punishes independent behaviors—are probably more important to this disorder's development. Genetic or constitutional factors, such as innate submissiveness, may also contribute to this disorder's etiology; a twin study found heritability of 45% on a scale measuring submissiveness (Jang et al. 1996). Another twin study found no heritability for submissiveness, based on DSM-III-R criteria, 4% for insecurity, and 63% for self-effacing behavior (Torgersen et al. 1993). These studies raise complex questions about the heritable components of personality traits and their assessment.

Cultural and social factors may also play a role in the development of DPD. Dependency is considered not only normative but desirable in certain cultures, including our own. Thus, DPD may represent an exaggerated and maladaptive variant of normal dependency; that is, it may—along with histrionic, obsessive-compulsive, and avoidant personality disorders—best be conceptualized as a "trait" disorder (i.e., occurring on a continuum with normal personality traits). It is important to recognize that to qualify for a diagnosis of DPD, dependent traits should be so extreme that they cause significant distress or impairment in functioning.

Treatment

Patients with DPD often enter therapy with complaints of depression or anxiety that may be precipitated by the threatened or actual loss of a dependent relationship. They often respond well to various types of individual psychotherapy. Treatment may be particularly helpful if it explores the patients' fears of independence; uses the transference to explore their dependency; and is directed toward increasing patients' self-esteem, sense of effectiveness, assertiveness, and independent functioning. These patients often seek an excessively dependent relationship with the therapist, which can lead to countertransference problems that may actually reinforce their dependence. The therapist may, for example, overprotect or be overly directive

with the patient, give inappropriate reassurance and support, or prolong the treatment unnecessarily. He or she may also have excessive expectations for change or withdraw from a patient who is perceived as too needy.

Group therapy (Piper and Ogrodniczuk 2005) and cognitive-behavioral therapy (Beck et al. 2004) aimed at increasing independent functioning, including assertiveness and social skills training, may be useful for some patients. If the patient is in a relationship that is maintaining and reinforcing his or her excessive dependence, couples or family therapy may be helpful (Table 20–24).

TABLE 20–24. Treatment of dependent personality disorder

Psychodynamic individual psychotherapy

Cognitive-behavioral psychotherapy

Group psychotherapy

Assertiveness and social skills training

Couples therapy

Family therapy

Obsessive-Compulsive Personality Disorder

History

In the early 1900s, Freud (1908/1924) made his often-cited observation that persons with obsessive-compulsive personality disorder (OCPD) were characterized by the three "peculiarities" of orderliness (which included cleanliness and conscientiousness), parsimony, and obstinacy. Similarly, in 1918, Ernest Jones (1918/1938) described these individuals as being preoccupied with cleanliness, money, and time. These observations were repeatedly cited and amplified in the subsequent psychoanalytic literature—the disorder often being referred to as *anal character*—and in the descriptive literature (Millon 1981).

This disorder's DSM description has closely mirrored these earlier clinical observations. In addition, in keeping with its consistent representation in the clinical literature, OCPD is one of four personality disorders that have been included in every version of DSM. In European psychiatry, this disorder has been referred to as *anancastic personality disorder,* a term used by Kretschmer and Schneider in the 1920s and still used in ICD-10.

Epidemiology

OCPD, like histrionic personality disorder, is one of the most common in the general population, with a prevalence of about 2% (Torgersen 2005). Unlike histrionic personality, however, OCPD is more common in men than in women (Torgersen et al. 2001; Zimmerman and Coryell 1989, 1990).

Clinical Features

As Freud noted, and as DSM-IV-TR criteria reflect, persons with OCPD are excessively orderly (Table 20–25). They are neat, punctual, overly organized, and overly conscientious. Although these traits might be considered virtues, especially in cultures that subscribe to the Puritan work ethic, to qualify as OCPD the traits must be so extreme that they cause significant distress or impairment in functioning. As Abraham (1923) noted, these individuals' perseverance is unproductive. For example, attention to detail is so excessive or time-consuming that the point of the activity is lost, conscientiousness is so extreme that it causes rigidity and inflexibility, and perfectionism interferes with task completion. Although these individuals tend to work extremely hard, they do so at the expense of leisure activities and relationships. As Shapiro (1965) pointed out, the most characteristic thought of persons with OCPD is "I should"—a phrase that aptly reflects their severe superego and captures their overly high standards, drivenness, conscientiousness, perfectionism, rigidity, and devotion to work and duties.

These individuals also tend to be overly concerned with control—not only over the details of their own lives but also over their emotions and other people. They have difficulty expressing warm and tender feelings, often using stilted, distant phrasing that reveals little of their inner experience. They may be obstinate and reluctant to delegate tasks or to work with others unless others submit exactly to their ways of doing things, which reflects their needs for interpersonal control as well as their fears of making mistakes. Their tendency to doubt and worry also manifests itself in their inability to discard worn-out or worthless objects that might be needed in the future, and as Freud and Jones noted, persons with OCPD are miserly toward themselves and others. A caricatured description of such persons is conveyed by Rado's (1959) phrase "living machines."

Differential Diagnosis

OCPD differs from Axis I obsessive-compulsive disorder in that the latter disorder is characterized by specific repetitive thoughts and ritualistic behaviors rather

TABLE 20–25. DSM-IV-TR diagnostic criteria for obsessive-compulsive personality disorder

A pervasive pattern of preoccupation with orderliness, perfectionism, and mental and interpersonal control, at the expense of flexibility, openness, and efficiency, beginning by early adulthood and present in a variety of contexts, as indicated by four (or more) of the following:

(1) is preoccupied with details, rules, lists, order, organization, or schedules to the extent that the major point of the activity is lost

(2) shows perfectionism that interferes with task completion (e.g., is unable to complete a project because his or her own overly strict standards are not met)

(3) is excessively devoted to work and productivity to the exclusion of leisure activities and friendships (not accounted for by obvious economic necessity)

(4) is overconscientious, scrupulous, and inflexible about matters of morality, ethics, or values (not accounted for by cultural or religious identification)

(5) is unable to discard worn-out or worthless objects even when they have no sentimental value

(6) is reluctant to delegate tasks or to work with others unless they submit to exactly his or her way of doing things

(7) adopts a miserly spending style toward both self and others; money is viewed as something to be hoarded for future catastrophes

(8) shows rigidity and stubbornness

than the personality traits of orderliness, perfectionism, and control. In addition, the symptoms of obsessive-compulsive disorder have traditionally been considered ego-dystonic, whereas the traits and behaviors of OCPD have been considered ego-syntonic. These two disorders are sometimes, but not often, comorbid.

Etiology

Freud's view that OCPD derives from difficulties occurring during the anal stage of psychosexual development (age 2–4 years) was echoed and elaborated on by subsequent psychoanalytic thinkers such as Karl Abraham and Wilhelm Reich (Reich 1933). According to this theory, children's infantile anal–erotic libidinal impulses conflict with parental attempts to socialize them—in particular, to toilet train them. Although these theories emphasize the importance of children's perceptions of parental disapproval during toilet training, and of ensuing parent–child control struggles—what

Rado (1959) referred to as "the battle of the chamber pot"—these factors are not currently considered central to this disorder's etiology. It may be, however, that conflicts arising during toilet training—such as those characteristic of Erikson's (1950) stage of autonomy versus shame—and continuing during other developmental stages do play a role. In particular, excessive parental control, criticism, and shaming may result in an insecurity that is defended against with perfectionism, orderliness, and an attempt to maintain self-control.

Freud believed that constitutional factors also play an important role in the formation of OCPD; similarly, Rado postulated the etiological importance of constitutionally excessive rage that leads to power struggles with others. Compulsivity (37%), oppositionality (46%), restricted expression of emotion (50%; Jang et al. 1996), and perfectionism (30%; Torgersen et al. 1993) have all been shown to be moderately heritable. An increase in serotonin activity has been associated with perfectionism and compulsivity. As is the case with other personality disorders, more empirical studies are needed to clarify this disorder's sources.

Treatment

Persons with OCPD may seem difficult to treat because of their excessive intellectualization and difficulty expressing emotion. However, these patients often respond well to psychoanalytic psychotherapy or psychoanalysis (Gabbard 2005). Therapists usually need to be relatively active in treatment. They should also avoid being drawn into interesting but affectless discussions that are unlikely to have therapeutic benefit. In other words, rather than intellectualizing with patients, therapists should focus on the feelings these patients usually avoid. Other defenses common in this disorder, such as rationalization, isolation, undoing, and reaction formation, should also be identified and clarified. Power struggles that may occur in treatment offer opportunities to address the patient's excessive need for control.

Cognitive techniques may also be used to diminish the patient's excessive need for control and perfection (Beck et al. 2004). Although patients may resist group treatment because of their need for control, dynamically oriented groups that focus on feelings may provide insight and increase patients' comfort with exploring and expressing new affects (Table 20–26).

Other Personality Disorders

The following three personality disorders were considered for inclusion on DSM-IV Axis II on the basis of

TABLE 20–26. Treatment of obsessive-compulsive personality disorder

Psychodynamic individual psychotherapy

Psychoanalysis

Cognitive-behavioral therapy

Psychodynamic group psychotherapy

their historical tradition, clinical utility, and/or empirical support. However, they were thought to require further study. Of note, all three disorders involve chronically morose people who have problems with direct expression of their aggression.

Depressive Personality Disorder

Of all the personality disorders, depressive personality disorder may have the longest clinical tradition, having been recognized 2,000 years ago by Hippocrates in his description of the "black gall," or melancholic temperament. Kraepelin (1921) also described this temperament and, like Hippocrates, considered it a depressive-spectrum disorder—a constitutional trait-like variant of the more severe depressive disorders and one predisposing to them. Schneider's (1959) description of this personality type led to its inclusion in ICD-9 (World Health Organization 1977) as an affective personality disorder. Kernberg (1988), who drew from the writings of Laughlin, emphasized this personality type's psychodynamic features, which include a severe superego, the inhibited expression of aggression, and an excessive dependence that is defended against with counterdependence. Because of the strength of this disorder's historical tradition, its inclusion in ICD-9, and some empirical evidence in its support, depressive personality disorder was added to an appendix in DSM-IV.

Persons with depressive personality disorder are persistently gloomy, burdened, worried, serious, pessimistic, and incapable of enjoyment or relaxation (Table 20–27). They also tend to be guilty, moralistic, self-denying, passive, unassertive, and introverted. They have low self-esteem and are excessively sensitive to criticism and rejection. Although they may be critical of others, they have difficulty directing criticism or any form of aggression toward others and find it easier to criticize themselves. They are also overly dependent on the love and acceptance of others, but they inhibit the expression of this dependency and may instead appear counterdependent.

Although concern has been expressed that this personality disorder may overlap excessively with Axis I

TABLE 20–27.	DSM-IV-TR research criteria for depressive personality disorder

A. A pervasive pattern of depressive cognitions and behaviors beginning by early adulthood and present in a variety of contexts, as indicated by five (or more) of the following:

   (1) usual mood is dominated by dejection, gloominess, cheerlessness, joylessness, unhappiness

   (2) self-concept centers around beliefs of inadequacy, worthlessness, and low self-esteem

   (3) is critical, blaming, and derogatory toward self

   (4) is brooding and given to worry

   (5) is negativistic, critical, and judgmental toward others

   (6) is pessimistic

   (7) is prone to feeling guilty or remorseful

B. Does not occur exclusively during major depressive episodes and is not better accounted for by dysthymic disorder.

TABLE 20–28.	DSM-IV-TR research criteria for passive-aggressive personality disorder (negativistic personality disorder)

A. A pervasive pattern of negativistic attitudes and passive resistance to demands for adequate performance, beginning by early adulthood and present in a variety of contexts, as indicated by four (or more) of the following:

   (1) passively resists fulfilling routine social and occupational tasks

   (2) complains of being misunderstood and unappreciated by others

   (3) is sullen and argumentative

   (4) unreasonably criticizes and scorns authority

   (5) expresses envy and resentment toward those apparently more fortunate

   (6) voices exaggerated and persistent complaints of personal misfortune

   (7) alternates between hostile defiance and contrition

B. Does not occur exclusively during major depressive episodes and is not better accounted for by dysthymic disorder.

depressive disorders—in particular, dysthymia—available data suggest that its overlap with dysthymia, major depression, and other personality disorders is far from complete and that depressive personality disorder appears to be a separate construct (D.N. Klein and Shih 1998). This disorder should not be diagnosed, however, if it occurs only during major depressive episodes. Although depressive personality disorder appears distinct from Axis I depressive disorders, family history and other data suggest that it may be related to these disorders, giving support to Kraepelin's spectrum concept.

Depressive personality disorder is thought to respond well to psychoanalytic psychotherapy and psychoanalysis.

Negativistic Personality Disorder

Negativistic personality disorder entered the appendix in DSM-IV as a replacement for passive-aggressive personality disorder, which was thought to be excessively narrow, representing a single behavior or defense mechanism rather than an extensive pattern of traits and behaviors characteristic of a personality disorder. Other limitations of passive-aggressive personality disorder in previous versions of DSM were its scant empirical support and the fact that passive-aggressive behavior can be normative, even laudable, in certain situations. Negativistic personality disorder is a broader construct that has some historical prece-

dents, including Schneider's (1923) "ill-tempered depressives."

Negativistic personality disorder, like passive-aggressive personality disorder, describes a pervasive pattern of passive resistance to demands for social and occupational performance (Table 20–28). However, it also encompasses a wide range of negativistic attitudes and behaviors, such as anger, pessimism, and cynicism; sullenness and argumentativeness; criticism of others; and envy of those who are perceived as more fortunate. In addition, these individuals tend to alternate between hostile self-assertion and contrite submission. A factor-analytic study found that negativistic personality disorder is a unidimensional construct that is associated with narcissistic personality disorder (Fossati et al. 2000). The clinical features of this disorder and its distinctiveness from other personality disorders remain to be empirically confirmed.

Self-Defeating Personality Disorder

Self-defeating personality disorder has been the subject of much controversy. This personality type has a significant historical and clinical tradition, beginning with Kraft-Ebbing's nineteenth-century description of sexual masochism (which is classified as a paraphilia in DSM) and Freud's subsequent description of moral masochism, a pattern of nonsexual submissive behavior that leads to psychological pain and mistreatment.

Nonetheless, concerns have been raised about the misuse of the diagnosis—in particular, that it may be misapplied to women who are actually being abused and thereby be used to blame the victim. In part due to these concerns, self-defeating personality disorder has never been an official psychiatric diagnosis. It was included in the DSM-III-R appendix but was not included in DSM-IV or DSM-IV-TR. However, this disorder's proponents argue that its features are distinctive, predict the occurrence of impairment and distress, and apply to men as well as to women and that the disorder is a clinically useful concept with important treatment implications (Cruz et al. 2000).

Self-defeating personality disorder applies to persons who exhibit a pervasive pattern of self-defeating behavior that does not occur only in response to, or in anticipation of, physical, sexual, or psychological abuse. Persons with this disorder feel unworthy of being treated well and, as a result, treat themselves poorly and unwittingly encourage others to make them suffer. They may, for example, reject opportunities for pleasure, choose people or situations that lead to mistreatment or failure, and incite others to become angry with them or reject them. If things do go well for them, they attempt to undermine themselves by, for example, becoming depressed or causing themselves pain.

The treatment of the disorder is complicated by the patient's self-defeating tendencies; patients may unknowingly sabotage the treatment and their progress because they feel undeserving of improvement or happiness. Exploring the patient's need to be victimized and making his or her investment in suffering ego-dystonic may allow a successful outcome with insight-oriented psychotherapy or psychoanalysis (Gabbard 2005).

Conclusion

Clinical interest and research in the personality disorders have grown enormously since 1980, when these disorders were put on a separate axis in DSM-III. The ensuing period has brought to light more specific and effective treatment strategies and a better understanding of these disorders' prognosis and etiology. Even more dramatic than the knowledge gained is the heightened awareness of the clinical impact and potential research significance of personality disorders and the new and more informed questions that this awareness has generated. Remaining challenges include a resolution of the boundaries between personality disorders and both normal personality and Axis I conditions, the discovery of biogenetic bases for personality traits underlying disorders, and the development of even more effective treatments. There is good reason to believe that with continued inquiry by clinical and basic-science investigators, the classification of personality disorders will continue to change so that it becomes even more tightly linked to etiology, treatment, and outcome.

Key Points

- Personality disorders are common in clinical settings and in the community.

- Personality disorders can be challenging to diagnose.

- Personality disorders cause significant problems for those who have them and for others and are costly to society.

- Personality disorders often complicate the treatment of other mental disorders.

- Personality disorders result from an interaction between temperamental (genetic/biological) and psychological (developmental/environmental) factors.

Suggested Readings

Beck AT, Freeman A, Davis DD, et al: Cognitive Therapy of Personality Disorders, 2nd Edition. New York, Guilford, 2004

Cloninger CR (ed): Personality and Psychopathology. Washington, DC, American Psychiatric Press, 1999

Costa PT, Widiger TA: (eds): Personality Disorders and the Five-Factor Model of Personality, 2nd Edition. Washington, DC, American Psychological Association, 2001

Gunderson JG: Borderline Personality Disorder: A Clinical Guide. Washington, DC, American Psychiatric Press, 2001

Livesley WJ (ed): Handbook of Personality Disorders: Theory, Research, and Treatment. New York, Guilford, 2001

Oldham JM, Skodol AE, Bender DS (eds): American Psychiatric Publishing Textbook of Personality Disorders. Washington, DC, American Psychiatric Publishing, 2005

Paris J: Personality Disorders Over Time: Precursors, Course, and Outcome. Washington, DC, American Psychiatric Publishing, 2003

Pervin L, John O (eds): Handbook of Personality: Theory and Research, 2nd Edition. New York, Guilford, 1999

Plomin R, Caspi A: Behavioral Genetics and Personality. New York, Guilford, 1999

Stone MH: Personality-Disordered Patients: Treatable and Untreatable. Washington, DC, American Psychiatric Publishing, 2006

References

Abraham K: Contributions to the theory of the anal character. Int J Psychoanal 4:400–418, 1923

Abraham K: The influence of oral eroticism on character formation, in Selected Papers on Psychoanalysis. Edited by Jones E. London, England, Hogarth Press, 1927, pp 393–406

Adler G: Borderline Psychopathology and Its Treatment. New York, Jason Aronson, 1985

Alarcon RD: Cross-cultural issues, in The American Psychiatric Publishing Textbook of Personality Disorders. Edited by Oldham JM, Skodol AE, Bender DS. Washington, DC, American Psychiatric Publishing, 2005, pp 561–578

American Psychiatric Association: Diagnostic and Statistical Manual: Mental Disorders. Washington, DC, American Psychiatric Association, 1952

American Psychiatric Association: Diagnostic and Statistical Manual of Mental Disorders, 2nd Edition. Washington, DC, American Psychiatric Association, 1968

American Psychiatric Association: Diagnostic and Statistical Manual of Mental Disorders, 3rd Edition. Washington, DC, American Psychiatric Association, 1980

American Psychiatric Association: Diagnostic and Statistical Manual of Mental Disorders, 3rd Edition, Revised. Washington, DC, American Psychiatric Association, 1987

American Psychiatric Association: Diagnostic and Statistical Manual of Mental Disorders, 4th Edition. Washington, DC, American Psychiatric Association, 1994

American Psychiatric Association: Diagnostic and Statistical Manual of Mental Disorders, 4th Edition, Text Revision. Washington, DC, American Psychiatric Association, 2000

American Psychiatric Association: Practice guideline for the treatment of patients with borderline personality disorder. Am J Psychiatry 158 (suppl):1–52, 2001

Appelbaum AH: Supportive therapy, in The American Psychiatric Publishing Textbook of Personality Disorders. Edited by Oldham JM, Skodol AE, Bender DS. Washington, DC, American Psychiatric Publishing, 2005, pp 335–346

Barkataki I, Kumari V, Das M, et al: Volumetric structural brain abnormalities in men with schizophrenia or antisocial personality disorder. Behav Brain Res 169:239–247, 2006

Bateman A, Fonagy P: Effectiveness of partial hospitalization in the treatment of borderline personality disorder: a randomized controlled trial. Am J Psychiatry 156:1563–1569, 1999

Beck AT, Freeman A, Davis DD, et al: Cognitive Therapy of Personality Disorders, 2nd Edition. New York, Guilford, 2004

Bender DS: Therapeutic alliance, in The American Psychiatric Publishing Textbook of Personality Disorders. Edited by Oldham JM, Skodol AE, Bender DS. Washington, DC, American Psychiatric Publishing, 2005, pp 405–420

Bender DS, Dolan RT, Skodol AE, et al: Treatment utilization by patients with personality disorders. Am J Psychiatry 158:295–302, 2001

Benjamin J, Patterson C, Greenberg BD, et al: Population and familial association between D4 receptor gene and measures of novelty seeking. Nat Genet 12:81–84, 1996

Benjamin LS: Structural analysis of social behavior. Psychol Rev 81:392–425, 1974

Birbaumer N, Veit R, Lotze M, et al: Deficient fear conditioning in psychopathy: a functional magnetic resonance imaging study. Arch Gen Psychiatry 62:799–805, 2005

Bleuler E: Die Probleme der Schizoidie und der Syntonie. Zeitschrift fur die gesamte Neurologie und Psychiatrie 78:373–388, 1922

Blonigen DM, Hicks BM, Krueger RF, et al: Psychopathic personality traits: heritability and genetic overlap with internalizing and externalizing psychopathology. Psychol Med 35:637–648, 2005

Breuer J, Freud S: Studies on Hysteria (1893–1895). Translated and edited by Strachey J. New York, Basic Books, 1957

Carey G, DiLalla DL: Personality and psychopathology: genetic perspectives. J Abnorm Psychol 103:32–43, 1994

Chiesa M, Fonagy P: Cassel personality disorder study. Br J Psychiatry 176:485–491, 2000

Chodoff P: Hysteria and women. Am J Psychiatry 139:545–551, 1982

Clark LA: Schedule for Nonadaptive and Adaptive Personality (SNAP). Minneapolis, University of Minnesota Press, 1993

Clark LA: Temperament as a unifying basis for personality and psychopathology. J Abnorm Psychol 114:505–521, 2005

Cleckley H: The Mask of Sanity, 4th Edition. St Louis, MO, CV Mosby, 1964

Cloninger CR, Svrakic DM, Przybeck TR: A psychobiological model of temperament and character. Arch Gen Psychiatry 50:975–990, 1993

Coccaro EF, Kavoussi RJ, Sheline YI, et al: Impulsive aggression in personality disorder: correlates with tritiated paroxetine binding in the platelet. Arch Gen Psychiatry 53:531–536, 1996

Cohen P, Crawford T: Developmental issues, in The American Psychiatric Publishing Textbook of Personality Disorders. Edited by Oldham JM, Skodol AE, Bender DS. Washington, DC, American Psychiatric Publishing, 2005, pp 171–185

Compton WM, Conway KP, Stinson FS, et al: Prevalence, correlates, and comorbidity of DSM-IV antisocial personality syndromes and alcohol and specific drug use disorders in the United States: results from the national epidemiologic study on alcohol and related conditions. J Clin Psychiatry 66:677–685, 2005

Costa P, McCrae R: Personality disorders and the five-factor model of personality. J Personal Disord 4:362–371, 1990

Cruz J, Joiner TE, Johnson JG, et al: Self-defeating personality disorder reconsidered. J Personal Disord 14:64–71, 2000

Dickinson KA, Pincus AL: Interpersonal analysis of grandiose and vulnerable narcissism. J Personal Disord 17:188–207, 2003

DiLalla DL, Carey G, Gottesman II, et al: Heritability of MMPI personality indicators of psychopathology in twins reared apart. J Abnorm Psychol 105:491–499, 1996

Dunayevich E, Sax KW, Keck PE Jr, et al: Twelve-month outcome in bipolar patients with and without personality disorders. J Clin Psychiatry 61:134–139, 2000

Edens JF, Marcus DK, Lillienfeld SO, et al: Psychopathic, not psychopath: taxometric evidence for the dimensional structure of psychopathy. J Abnorm Psychol 115:131–144, 2006

Ellis H: Auto-erotism: a psychological study. Alienist and Neurologist 19:260–299, 1898

Erikson EH: Childhood and Society. New York, WW Norton, 1950

Fairbairn WRD: Schizoid factors in the personality (1940), in Psychoanalytic Studies of the Personality. London, England, Tavistock, 1952, pp 3–27

Fanous A, Gardner C, Walsh D, et al: Relationship between positive and negative symptoms of schizophrenia and schizotypal symptoms in nonpsychotic relatives. Arch Gen Psychiatry 58:669–673, 2001

Fenichel O: The Psychoanalytic Theory of the Neurosis. New York, WW Norton, 1945

First MB, Gibbon M, Spitzer RL, et al: Structured Clinical Interview for DSM-IV Axis II Personality Disorders (SCID-II). Washington, DC, American Psychiatric Press, 1997

First M, Pincus H, Levine J, et al: Clinical utility as a criterion for revising psychiatric diagnoses. Am J Psychiatry 161:949–954, 2004

Fossati A, Maffei C, Bagnato M, et al: A psychometric study of DSM-IV passive-aggressive (negativistic) personality disorder criteria. J Personal Disord 14:72–83, 2000

Freud S: Character and anal erotism (1908), in Collected Papers, Vol 2. London, England, Hogarth, 1924, pp 45–50

Gabbard GO: Psychodynamic Psychiatry in Clinical Practice, 3rd Edition. Washington, DC, American Psychiatric Publishing, 2000

Gabbard GO: Psychoanalysis, in The American Psychiatric Publishing Textbook of Personality Disorders. Edited by Oldham JM, Skodol AE, Bender DS. Washington, DC, American Psychiatric Publishing, 2005, pp 257–273

Giesen-Bloo J, van Dyck R, Spinhoven P, et al: Outpatient psychotherapy for borderline personality disorder: randomized trial of schema-focused therapy vs. transference-focused psychotherapy. Arch Gen Psychiatry 63:649–658, 2006

Grilo CM, McGlashan TH: Course and outcome of personality disorders, in The American Psychiatric Publishing Textbook of Personality Disorders. Edited by Oldham JM, Skodol AE, Bender DS. Washington, DC, American Psychiatric Publishing, 2005, pp 103–115

Grilo CM, Sanislow CA, Shea MT, et al: Two-year prospective naturalistic study of remission from major depressive disorder as a function of personality disorder comorbidity. J Consult Clin Psychol 73:78–85, 2005

Grove WM, Eckert ED, Heston L, et al: Heritability of substance abuse and antisocial behavior: a study of monozygotic twins reared apart. Biol Psychiatry 27:1293–1304, 1990

Gunderson JG: Diagnostic controversies, in American Psychiatric Press Review of Psychiatry, Vol 11. Edited by Tasman A, Riba M. Washington, DC, American Psychiatric Press, 1992, pp 9–24

Gunderson JG: The borderline patient's intolerance of aloneness: insecure attachment and therapist availability. Am J Psychiatry 153:752–758, 1996

Gunderson JG, Ronningstam E, Smith LE: Narcissistic personality disorder: a review of data on DSM-III-R descriptions. J Personal Disord 5:167–177, 1991

Gunderson JG, Daversa MT, Grilo CM, et al: Predictors of 2-year outcome for patients with borderline personality disorder. Am J Psychiatry 163:822–826, 2006

Guntrip HJ: The schizoid problem, in Psychoanalytic Theory, Therapy, and the Self. New York, Basic Books, 1971, pp 145–174

Hare RD, Neumann CS: Structural models of psychopathy. Curr Psychiatry Rep 7:57–64, 2005

Hare RD, Hart SD, Harpur TJ: Psychopathy and the DSM-IV criteria for antisocial personality disorder. J Abnorm Psychol 100:391–398, 1991

Hoch A: Constitutional factors in the dementia praecox group. Review of Neurology and Psychiatry 8:463–475, 1910

Hoek HW, Susser E, Buck KA, et al: Schizoid personality disorder after prenatal exposure to famine. Am J Psychiatry 153:1637–1639, 1996

Hollander E, Swann AC, Coccaro EF, et al: Impact of trait impulsivity and state aggression on divalproex versus placebo response in borderline personality disorder. Am J Psychiatry 162:621–624, 2005

Horney K: Our Inner Conflicts: A Constructive Theory of Neurosis. New York, WW Norton, 1945

Hyler SE: Personality Diagnostic Questionnaire–4 (PDQ-4). New York, New York State Psychiatric Institute, 1994

Janet P: The Mental State of Hystericals: A Study of Mental Stigmata and Mental Accidents. Translated by Corson CR. New York, GP Putnam's Sons, 1901

Jang KL, Livesley WJ, Vernon PA, et al: Heritability of personality disorder traits: a twin study. Acta Psychiatr Scand 94:438–444, 1996

Johnson JG, Cohen P, Kasen S, et al: Age-related change in personality disorder trait levels between early adolescence and adulthood: a community-based longitudinal investigation. Acta Psychiatr Scand 102:265–275, 2000

Johnson JG, Bromley E, McGeoch PG: Role of childhood experiences in the development of maladaptive and adaptive personality traits, in The American Psychiatric Publishing Textbook of Personality Disorders. Edited by Oldham JM, Skodol AE, Bender DS. Washington, DC, American Psychiatric Publishing, 2005a, pp 209–221

Johnson JG, First MB, Cohen P, et al: Adverse outcomes associated with personality disorder not otherwise specified in a community sample. Am J Psychiatry 162:1926–1932, 2005b

Jones E: Anal-erotic character traits (1918), in Papers on Psychoanalysis. London, England, Balliere, Tindall & Cox, 1938, pp 531–555

Jones M: The Therapeutic Community: A New Treatment in Psychiatry. New York, Basic Books, 1953

Joyce PR, McKenzie JM, Luty SE, et al: Temperament, childhood environment and psychopathology as risk factors for avoidant and borderline personality disorders. Aust N Z J Psychiatry 37:756–764, 2003

Kagan J: Temperamental influences on the preservation of styles of social behavior. McLean Hospital Journal 14:23– 34, 1989

Kasen S, Cohen P, Skodol AE, et al: The influence of child and adolescent psychiatric disorders on young adult personality disorder. Am J Psychiatry 156:1529–1535, 1999

Kaye AL, Shea MT: Personality disorders, personality traits, and defense mechanisms measures, in Handbook of Psychiatric Measures. Edited by Task Force for the Handbook of Psychiatric Measures. Washington, DC, American Psychiatric Association, 2000, pp 713–749

Kendler KS, Gruenberg AM: Genetic relationship between paranoid personality disorder and the "schizophrenic spectrum" disorders. Am J Psychiatry 139:1185–1186, 1982

Kendler KS, McGuire M, Gruenberg AM, et al: The Roscommon family study, III: schizophrenia-related personality disorders in relatives. Arch Gen Psychiatry 50:781–788, 1993

Kent S, Fogarty M, Yellowlees P: A review of studies of heavy users of psychiatric services. Psychiatr Serv 46:1247–1253, 1995

Kernberg OF: Borderline Conditions and Pathological Narcissism. New York, Jason Aronson, 1975

Kernberg OF: Clinical dimensions of masochism. J Am Psychoanal Assoc 36:1005–1029, 1988

Keshavan M, Shad M, Soloff P, et al: Efficacy and tolerability of olanzapine in the treatment of schizotypal personality disorder. Schizophr Res 71:97–101, 2004

Kessler RC: The impairments caused by social phobia in the general population: implications for intervention. Acta Psychiatr Scand Suppl (417):19–27, 2003

Kety SS, Rosenthal D, Wender PH, et al: The types and prevalence of mental illness in the biological and adoptive families of adopted schizophrenics, in The Transmission of Schizophrenia. Edited by Rosenthal D, Kety SS. Oxford, England, Pergamon, 1968, pp 345–362

Klein DN, Shih JH: Depressive personality: associations with DSM-III-R mood and personality disorders and negative and positive affectivity, 30-month stability, and prediction of course of Axis I depressive disorders. J Abnorm Psychol 107:319–327, 1998

Klein M: Wisconsin Personality Inventory-IV (WPI-IV). Madison, University of Wisconsin, 1993

Klonsky ED, Oltmanns TF, Turkheimer E: Informant-reports of personality disorder: relation to self-reports and future directions. Clin Psychol Sci Pract 9:300–311, 2002

Klonsky ED, Oltmanns TF, Turkheimer E: Deliberate self-harm in a nonclinical population: prevalence and psychological correlates. Am J Psychiatry 160:1501–1508, 2003

Kluger AN, Siegfried Z, Ebstein RP: A meta-analysis of the association between DRD4 polymorphism and novelty seeking. Mol Psychiatry 7:712–717, 2002

Koenigsberg HW, Reynolds D, Goodman M, et al: Risperidone in the treatment of schizotypal personality disorder. J Clin Psychiatry 64:628–634, 2003

Kohut H: The Analysis of the Self: A Systematic Approach to the Psychoanalytic Treatment of Narcissistic Personality Disorders. New York, International Universities Press, 1971

Kraepelin E: Dementia Praecox and Paraphrenia. Edinburgh, Scotland, E & S Livingstone, 1919

Kraepelin E: Manic-Depressive Insanity and Paranoia. Translated by Barclay RM. Edited by Robertson GM. Edinburgh, Scotland, E & S Livingstone, 1921

Kretschmer E: Physique and Character. New York, Harcourt, Brace, 1925

Krueger RF, Markon KE, Patrick CJ, et al: Externalizing psychopathology in adulthood: a dimensional-spectrum conceptualization and its implications for DSM-V. J Abnorm Psychol 114:537–550, 2005

Leichsenring F, Leibing E: The effectiveness of psychodynamic therapy and cognitive behavior therapy in the treatment of personality disorders: a meta-analysis. Am J Psychiatry 160:1223–1232, 2003

Lesch KP, Bengel D, Heils A: Association of anxiety-related traits with a polymorphism in the serotonin transporter gene regulatory region. Science 274:1527–1531, 1996

Levy KN, Meehan KB, Weber M, et al: Attachment and borderline personality disorder: implications for psychotherapy. Psychopathology 38:64–74, 2005

Lieb K, Zanarini MC, Schmahl C, et al: Borderline personality disorder. Lancet 364:453–461, 2004

Linehan MM: Cognitive-Behavioral Treatment of Borderline Personality Disorder. New York, Guilford, 1993

Linehan MM, Comtois KA, Murray AM, et al: Two-year randomized controlled trial and follow-up of dialectical behavior therapy vs. therapy by experts for suicidal behaviors and borderline personality disorder. Arch Gen Psychiatry 63:757–766, 2006

Linney YM, Murray RM, Peters ER, et al: A quantitative genetic analysis of schizotypal personality traits. Psychol Med 33:803–816, 2003

Livesley J, Jackson D: Dimensional Assessment of Personality Pathology. Port Huron, MI, Sigma, 2000

Livesley WJ, Jang KL, Jackson DN, et al: Genetic and environmental contributions to dimensions of personality disorder. Am J Psychiatry 150:1826–1831, 1993

Livesley WJ, Jang KL, Vernon PA: Phenotypic and genetic structure of traits delineating personality disorder. Arch Gen Psychiatry 55:941–948, 1998

Loranger AW: International Personality Disorders Examination (IPDE) Manual. Odessa, FL, Psychological Assessment Resources, 1999

Lorber MF: Psychophysiology of aggression, psychopathy, and conduct problems: a meta-analysis. Psychol Bull 130:531–552, 2004

Lyons MJ, True WR, Eisen SA, et al: Differential heritability of adult and juvenile antisocial traits. Arch Gen Psychiatry 52:906–915, 1995

Malone SM, Taylor J, Marmorstein NR, et al: Genetic and environmental influences on antisocial behavior and alcohol dependence from adolescence to early adulthood. Dev Psychopathol 16:943–966, 2004

Markon KE, Krueger RF, Watson D: Delineating the structure of normal and abnormal personality: an integrative hierarchical approach. J Personal Soc Psychol 88:139–157, 2005

Masterson JF: Treatment of the Borderline Adolescent: A Developmental Approach. New York, Wiley-Interscience, 1972

McDermut W, Zimmerman M: Assessment Instruments and standardized evaluation, in The American Psychiatric Publishing Textbook of Personality Disorders. Edited by Oldham JM, Skodol AE, Bender DS. Washington, DC, American Psychiatric Publishing, 2005, pp 89–101

McGlashan TH, Grilo CM, Sanislow CA, et al: Two-year prevalence and stability of individual criteria for schizotypal, borderline, avoidant, and obsessive-compulsive personality disorders: toward a hybrid model of Axis II disorders. Am J Psychiatry 162:883–889, 2005

Meyer B, Carver CS: Negative childhood accounts, sensitivity, and pessimism: a study of avoidant personality disorder features in college students. J Personal Disord 14:233–248, 2000

Millon T: Disorders of Personality—DSM-III: Axis II. New York, Wiley, 1981

Millon T, Davis R, Millon C: Manual for the MCMI-III. Minneapolis, MN, National Computer Systems, 1997

Modell AH: A narcissistic defense against affects and the illusion of self-sufficiency. Int J Psychoanal 56:275–282, 1975

Moffitt TE: The new look of behavioral genetics in developmental psychopathology: gene-environment interplay in antisocial behaviors. Psychol Bull 131:533–554, 2005

Morey LC, Alexander GM, Boggs C: Gender, in The American Psychiatric Publishing Textbook of Personality Disorders. Edited by Oldham JM, Skodol AE, Bender DS. Washington, DC, American Psychiatric Publishing, 2005, pp 541–559

Morrison AP: Introduction, in Essential Papers on Narcissism. Edited by Morrison AP. New York, New York University Press, 1989, pp 1–11

Munafo MR, Clark TG, Moore LR, et al: Genetic polymorphisms and personality in healthy adults: a systematic review and meta-analysis. Mol Psychiatry 8:471–484, 2003

Oldham J: Borderline personality disorder and suicidality. Am J Psychiatry 163:20–26, 2006

Oldham JM, Skodol AE: Charting the future of Axis II. J Personal Disord 14:17–29, 2000

Paris J: A current integrative perspective on personality disorders, in The American Psychiatric Publishing Textbook of Personality Disorders. Edited by Oldham JM, Skodol AE, Bender DS. Washington, DC, American Psychiatric Publishing, 2005a, pp 119–128

Paris J: Neurobiological dimensional models of personality: a review of the models of Cloninger, Depue, and Siever. J Personal Disord 19:156–170, 2005b

Perry JC, Bond M: Defensive functioning, in The American Psychiatric Publishing Textbook of Personality Disorders. Edited by Oldham JM, Skodol AE, Bender DS. Washington, DC, American Psychiatric Publishing, 2005, pp 523–540

Perry JC, Banon E, Ianni F: Effectiveness of psychotherapy for personality disorders. Am J Psychiatry 156:1312–1321, 1999

Pfohl B, Blum N, Zimmerman M: Structured Interview for DSM-IV Personality. Washington, DC, American Psychiatric Press, 1997

Piper WE, Ogrodniczuk JS: Group treatment, in The American Psychiatric Publishing Textbook of Personality Disorders. Edited by Oldham JM, Skodol AE, Bender DS. Washington, DC, American Psychiatric Publishing, 2005, pp 347–357

Posner MI, Rothbart MK, Vizueta N, et al: An approach to the psychobiology of personality disorders. Dev Psychopathol 15:1093–1106, 2003

Pritchard JC: A Treatise on Insanity. London, England, Sherwood, Gilbert & Piper, 1835

Rado S: Schizotypal organization: preliminary report on a clinical study of schizophrenia, in Psychoanalysis and Behavior. New York, Grune & Stratton, 1956, pp 1–10

Rado S: Obsessive behavior, in American Handbook of Psychiatry, Vol 1. Edited by Arieti S. New York, Basic Books, 1959, pp 324–344

Raine A, Moffit TE, Caspi A, et al: Neurocognitive impairments in boys on the life-course persistent antisocial path. J Abnorm Psychol 114:38–49, 2005

Reich W: Charakteranalyse: Technik und Grundlagen fur studierende und praktizierende Analytiker. Leipzig, Germany, IM Selbstverlage des Verfassers, 1933

Reich W: On the technique of character analysis, in Character Analysis, 3rd Edition. New York, Simon & Schuster, 1949, pp 39–113

Reiss D, Hetherington EM, Plomin R, et al: Genetic questions for environmental studies: differential parenting and psychopathology in adolescence. Arch Gen Psychiatry 52:925–936, 1995

Rettew DC, Zanarini MC, Yen S, et al: Childhood antecedents of avoidant personality disorder: a retrospective study. J Am Acad Child Adolesc Psychiatry 42:1122–1130, 2003

Roberts BW, DelVecchio WF: The rank-order consistency of personality traits from childhood to old age: a quantitative review of longitudinal studies. Psychol Bull 126:3–25, 2000

Roberts BW, Caspi A, Moffitt TE: Work experiences and personality development in young adulthood. J Personal Soc Psychol 84:582–593, 2003

Robins LN: Deviant Children Grown Up: A Sociological and Psychiatric Study of Sociopathic Personality. Baltimore, MD, Williams & Wilkins, 1966

Sanislow CA, Morey LC, Grilo CM, et al: Confirmatory factor analysis of DSM-IV borderline, schizotypal, avoidant, and obsessive-compulsive personality disorders: findings from the Collaborative Longitudinal Personality Study. Acta Psychiatr Scand 105:28–36, 2002

Schneider K: Die psychopathischen Personlichkeiten. Vienna, Austria, Deuticke, 1923

Schneider K: Psychopathic Personalities. Springfield, IL, Charles C Thomas, 1958

Schneider K: Clinical Psychopathology. Translated by Hamilton MW. London, England, Grune & Stratton, 1959

Seivewright H, Tyrer P, Johnson T: Persistent social dysfunction in anxious and depressed patients with personality disorder. Acta Psychiatr Scand 109:104–109, 2004

Shapiro D: Neurotic Styles. New York, Basic Books, 1965

Shihabuddin L, Buchsbaum MS, Hazlett EA, et al: Striatal size and relative glucose metabolic rate in schizotypal personality disorder and schizophrenia. Arch Gen Psychiatry 58:877–884, 2001

Sholevar GP: Family therapy, in The American Psychiatric Publishing Textbook of Personality Disorders. Edited by Oldham JM, Skodol AE, Bender DS. Washington, DC, American Psychiatric Publishing, 2005, pp 359–373

Siever LJ, Davis KL: A psychobiological perspective on the personality disorders. Am J Psychiatry 148:1647–1658, 1991

Siever LJ, Davis KL: The pathophysiology of schizophrenia disorders: perspectives from the spectrum. Am J Psychiatry 161:398–413, 2004

Skodol AE: Manifestations, clinical diagnosis, and comorbidity, in The American Psychiatric Publishing Textbook of Personality Disorders. Edited by Oldham JM, Skodol AE, Bender DS. Washington, DC, American Psychiatric Publishing, 2005, pp 57–87

Skodol AE, Oldham JM: Assessment and diagnosis of borderline personality disorder. Hosp Community Psychiatry 42:1021–1028, 1991

Skodol AE, Gunderson JG, McGlashan TH, et al: Functional impairment in patients with schizotypal, borderline, avoidant, or obsessive-compulsive personality disorder. Am J Psychiatry 159:276–283, 2002

Skodol AE, Gunderson JG, Shea MT, et al: The Collaborative Longitudinal Personality Disorders Study (CLPS): overview and implications. J Personal Disord 19:487–504, 2005a

Skodol AE, Oldham JM, Bender DS, et al: Dimensional representations of DSM-IV personality disorders: relationships to functional impairment. Am J Psychiatry 162:1919–1925, 2005b

Skodol AE, Pagano MP, Bender DS, et al: Stability of functional impairment in patients with schizotypal, borderline, avoidant, or obsessive-compulsive personality disorder over two years. Psychol Med 35:443–451, 2005c

Soler J, Pascual JC, Carlos J, et al: Double-blind, placebo-controlled study of dialectical behavior therapy plus olanzapine for borderline personality disorder. Am J Psychiatry 162:1221–1224, 2005

Soloff PH: Somatic treatments, in The American Psychiatric Publishing Textbook of Personality Disorders. Edited by Oldham JM, Skodol AE, Bender DS. Washington, DC, American Psychiatric Publishing, 2005, pp 387–403

Spitzer RL, Endicott J, Gibbon M: Crossing the border into borderline personality and borderline schizophrenia: the development of criteria. Arch Gen Psychiatry 36:17–24, 1979

Stanley B, Brodsky BS: Dialectical behavior therapy, in The American Psychiatric Publishing Textbook of Personality Disorders. Edited by Oldham JM, Skodol AE, Bender DS. Washington, DC, American Psychiatric Publishing, 2005, pp 307–320

Stein MB, Chartier MJ, Lizak MV, et al: Familial aggregation of anxiety-related quantitative traits in generalized social phobia: clues to understanding "disorder" heritability? Am J Med Genet 105:79–83, 2001

Stone M: Schizotypal personality: psychotherapeutic aspects. Schizophr Bull 11:576–589, 1985

Stone M: Violence, in The American Psychiatric Publishing Textbook of Personality Disorders. Edited by Oldham JM, Skodol AE, Bender DS. Washington, DC, American Psychiatric Publishing, 2005, pp 477–491

Suzuki M, Zhou S-Y, Takahashi T, et al: Differential contributions of prefrontal and temporolimbic pathology to mechanisms of psychosis. Brain 128:2109–2122, 2005

Taylor CT, Laposa JM, Alden LE: Is avoidant personality disorder more than just social avoidance? J Personal Disord 18:571–594, 2004

Torgersen S: Epidemiology, in The American Psychiatric Publishing Textbook of Personality Disorders. Edited by Oldham JM, Skodol AE, Bender DS. Washington, DC, American Psychiatric Publishing, 2005, pp 129–141

Torgersen S, Onstad S, Skre I, et al: "True" schizotypal personality disorder: a study of co-twins and relatives of schizophrenic probands. Am J Psychiatry 150:1661–1667, 1993

Torgersen S, Lygren S, Øien PA, et al: A twin study of personality disorders. Compr Psychiatry 41:416–425, 2000

Torgersen S, Kringlen E, Cramer V: The prevalence of personality disorders in a community sample. Arch Gen Psychiatry 58:590–596, 2001

Torgersen S, Edvardsen J, Øien PA, et al: Schizotypal personality disorder inside and outside the schizophrenia spectrum. Schizophr Res 54:33–38, 2002

Verheul R: Clinical utility of dimensional models for personality pathology. J Personal Disord 19:283–302, 2005

Verheul R, Widiger TA: A meta-analysis of the prevalence and usage of the personality disorder not otherwise specified (PDNOS) diagnosis. J Personal Disord 18:309–319, 2004

Webb CT, Levinson DF: Schizotypal and paranoid personality disorder in the relatives of patients with schizophrenia and affective disorders: a review. Schizophr Res 11:81–92, 1993

Westen D: Divergences between clinical and research methods for assessing personality disorders: implications for research and the evolution of Axis II. Am J Psychiatry 154:895–903, 1997

Westen D, Shedler J, Bradley R: A prototype approach to personality disorder diagnosis. Am J Psychiatry 163:846–856, 2006

Widiger TA: Personality disorders in the 21st century. J Personal Disord 14:3–16, 2000

Widiger TA, Mullins-Sweatt SN: Categorical and dimensional models of personality disorders, in The American Psychiatric Publishing Textbook of Personality Disorders. Edited by Oldham JO, Skodol, AE, Bender DS. Washington, DC, American Psychiatric Publishing, 2005, pp 35–53

Widiger TA, Samuel DB: Diagnostic categories or dimensions? A question for the Diagnostic and Statistical Manual of Mental Disorders—Fifth Edition. J Abnorm Psychol 114:494–504, 2005

Widiger TA Simonsen E: Alternative dimensional models of personality disorder: finding a common ground. J Personal Disord 19:110–130, 2005

Widiger TA, Mangine S, Corbitt EM, et al: Personality Disorder Interview-IV (PDI-IV): A Semi-structured Interview for the Assessment of Personality Disorders. Professional Manual. Odessa, FL, Psychological Assessment Resources, 1995

Widiger TA, Frances AJ, Pincus HA, et al: DSM-IV Sourcebook, Vol 2. Washington, DC, American Psychiatric Association, 1996

Woody GE, McLellan AT, Luborsky L, et al: Sociopathy and psychotherapy outcome. Arch Gen Psychiatry 42:1081–1086, 1985

World Health Organization: International Classification of Diseases, 9th Revision. Geneva, World Health Organization, 1977

World Health Organization: International Statistical Classification of Diseases and Related Health Problems, 10th Revision. Geneva, Switzerland, World Health Organization, 1992

Yonkers KA, Dyck IR, Warshaw M, et al: Factors predicting the clinical course of generalised anxiety disorder. Br J Psychiatry 176:544–549, 2000

Zanarini M: Role of Sexual Abuse in the Etiology of Borderline Personality Disorder. Washington, DC, American Psychiatric Press, 1997

Zanarini M, Frankenburg FR: Pathways to the development of borderline personality disorder. J Personal Disord 11:93–104, 1997

Zanarini MC, Frankenburg FR, Chauncey DL, et al: The Diagnostic Interview for DSM-IV Personality Disorders. Belmont, MA, McLean Hospital, Laboratory for the Study of Adult Development, 1996

Zanarini MC, Frankenberg FR, Hennen J, et al: The McLean Study of Adult Development (MSAD): overview and implications of the first six years of prospective follow-up. J Personal Disord 19:505–523, 2005

Zanarini MC, Frankenberg FR, Hennen J, et al: Prediction of the 10-year course of borderline personality disorder. Am J Psychiatry 163:827–832, 2006

Zimmerman M, Coryell W: DSM-III personality disorder diagnoses in a nonpatient sample: demographic correlates and comorbidity. Arch Gen Psychiatry 46:682–689, 1989

Zimmerman M, Coryell W: Diagnosing personality disorders in the community: a comparison of self-report and interview measures. Arch Gen Psychiatry 47:527–531, 1990

Zimmerman M, Mattia JI: Differences between clinical and research practices in diagnosing borderline personality disorder. Am J Psychiatry 156:1570–1574, 1999

Zimmerman M, Rothchild L, Chelminski I: The prevalence of DSM-IV personality disorders in psychiatric outpatients. Am J Psychiatry 162:1911–1918, 2005

DISORDERS USUALLY FIRST DIAGNOSED IN INFANCY, CHILDHOOD, OR ADOLESCENCE

Amy M. Ursano, M.D.

Paul H. Kartheiser, M.D.

L. Jarrett Barnhill, M.D.

In recent years, it has become increasingly recognized that many psychiatric disorders have their onset in youth. Like many experiences of childhood, these disorders can have enduring effects, and they may affect an individual's sense of satisfaction with relationships, occupation, or self and ultimately play a significant role in the development of adult psychopathology. Variations in the presentation of psychiatric diagnoses can often be attributed to an individual's developmental stage. In fact, disorders such as separation anxiety or elimination disorder represent normal behavior at an early age, although continued symptoms inappropriate to a patient's developmental level become diagnosable and thereby a focus of treatment. Despite limited research, we have effective treatments for many childhood psychiatric illnesses. Child development and child psychiatric treatment are discussed elsewhere in this volume (see Chapter 7, "Normal Child and Adolescent Development," by Gemelli, and Chapter 36, "Treatment of Children and Adolescents," by Crawford et al.).

This chapter focuses on the DSM-IV-TR (American Psychiatric Association 2000) category "Disorders Usually First Diagnosed in Infancy, Childhood, or Adolescence," which includes conditions that not only begin in childhood but also are typically diagnosed during childhood (Table 21–1). Disorders such as those of mood and anxiety, psychosis, substance use, and eating may also have an onset of symptoms during childhood, although they may not be fully recognized or diagnosed for some time. These disorders are discussed in other chapters in this volume. With a strong understanding of child development, child psychopathology, and treatment, we are better able to treat patients of all ages.

TABLE 21–1. DSM-IV-TR disorders usually first diagnosed in infancy, childhood, or adolescence

Mental retardation
  Mild mental retardation
  Moderate mental retardation
  Severe mental retardation
  Profound mental retardation
  Mental retardation, severity unspecified

Learning disorders
  Reading disorder
  Mathematics disorder
  Disorder of written expression
  Learning disorder not otherwise specified

Motor skills disorder
  Developmental coordination disorder

Pervasive developmental disorders
  Autistic disorder
  Rett's disorder
  Childhood disintegrative disorder
  Asperger's disorder
  Pervasive developmental disorder not otherwise specified

Attention-deficit and disruptive behavior disorders
  Attention-deficit/hyperactivity disorder
    Predominantly inattentive type
    Predominantly hyperactive–impulsive type
    Combined type
    Not otherwise specified
  Conduct disorder
  Oppositional defiant disorder
  Disruptive behavior disorder not otherwise specified

Feeding and eating disorders of infancy or early childhood
  Pica
  Rumination disorder of infancy
  Feeding disorder of infancy or early childhood

Tic disorders
  Tourette's disorder
  Chronic motor or vocal tic disorder
  Transient tic disorder
  Tic disorder not otherwise specified

Communication disorders
  Expressive language disorder
  Mixed receptive–expressive language disorder
  Phonological disorder
  Stuttering
  Communication disorder not otherwise specified

TABLE 21–1. DSM-IV-TR disorders usually first diagnosed in infancy, childhood, or adolescence *(continued)*

Elimination disorders
  Encopresis
  Enuresis

Other disorders of infancy, childhood, or adolescence
  Separation anxiety disorder
  Selective mutism
  Reactive attachment disorder of infancy or early childhood
  Stereotypic movement disorder
  Disorder of infancy, childhood, or adolescence not otherwise specified

Source.   American Psychiatric Association 2000.

Mental Retardation
Clinical Description

Intellectual disability (previously termed *mental retardation*) is a developmental disorder with onset prior to age 18 years characterized by impairments in measured intellectual performance and adaptive skills across multiple domains (Table 21–2). DSM-IV-TR classifies mental retardation as an Axis II disorder, segregated from most primary psychiatric disorders. The separation of developmental disorders from mental disorders is an attempt to establish and maintain the boundary between these conditions, and to remind clinicians that intellectual disability is not synonymous with psychiatric illness (Harris 2006).

The clinical reality is more complex. It is often difficult to differentiate severe behavioral disorders from primary psychiatric diagnosis in patients with intellectual disability. Aggression, self-injurious behavior (SIB), social withdrawal, stereotypies, and mannerisms are the most frequent reasons for referrals. Yet even when these challenging behaviors are accompanied by affective disturbances or impulse dyscontrol, many individuals fail to meet the diagnostic criteria for major psychiatric disorders. To complicate matters further, these challenging behaviors can represent state-related changes signaling the onset of another psychiatric disorder. For example, escalating irritability during a manic episode may also be associated with increased aggressive behavior. For patients with intellectual disability and major depressive disorder, the emergence of anhedonia can decrease the effectiveness of previously effective reinforcers and undermine alternate reinforcement strategies (Aman et al. 2003).

TABLE 21–2. DSM-IV-TR diagnostic criteria for mental retardation

A. Significantly subaverage intellectual functioning: an IQ of approximately 70 or below on an individually administered IQ test (for infants, a clinical judgment of significantly subaverage intellectual functioning).

B. Concurrent deficits or impairments in present adaptive functioning (i.e., the person's effectiveness in meeting the standards expected for his or her age by his or her cultural group) in at least two of the following areas: communication, self-care, home living, social/interpersonal skills, use of community resources, self-direction, functional academic skills, work, leisure, health, and safety.

C. The onset is before age 18 years.

Code based on degree of severity reflecting level of intellectual impairment:

317	**Mild mental retardation:**	IQ level 50–55 to approximately 70
318.0	**Moderate mental retardation:**	IQ level 35–40 to 50–55
318.1	**Severe mental retardation:**	IQ level 20–25 to 35–40
318.2	**Profound mental retardation:**	IQ level below 20 or 25
319	**Mental retardation, severity unspecified:**	when there is strong presumption of mental retardation but the person's intelligence is untestable by standard tests

In many clinical settings, the boundary between challenging behaviors in individuals with intellectual disability and psychiatric disorders is difficult to establish. These issues can be especially confusing for individuals with severe to profound intellectual disability. This is in part due to higher rates of brain disorders such as complex forms of epilepsy and cerebral palsy. Affective disturbances, psychotic symptoms, and impulsive-disruptive behaviors as well as internalizing symptoms are more likely to occur in these neurologically compromised patients. These factors not only increase the risk for psychiatric disorders but also exert a profound influence on the clinical expression, differential diagnosis, treatment, and long-term prognosis for many psychiatric disorders (Barnhill 1999).

To cope with the complexity of patients with intellectual disabilities, psychiatrists and other mental health professionals need to develop a systematic approach. It is important to think in terms of a transactional model: the interaction between environmental influences, social ecology, anomalous brain development, behavioral phenotypes, and challenging behaviors or mental disorders. For each patient there is a life story filled with learning and experiences within a social context. In order to understand intellectual disability, we need to look at development as an ever-changing epigenetic progression, more of a mosaic than a linear process (Barnhill 2003).

Society, Culture, and Intellectual Disability

Clinicians making the diagnosis of intellectual disability must cope with a range of sociocultural issues and circumstances. IQ tests in general were designed to measure specific learning that is predictive of academic performance. As a result, questions may reflect cultural or technological experiences that are not universal. At best, standardized instruments sample a limited range of cognitive abilities when compared with the scope of human adaptability and skills. Much of human intelligence is linked to the capacity to adapt to ecological challenges and complex social relationships—mastering calculus and Shakespeare were much later steps.

The definition of disability is also intertwined with social experiences and culture. As education and the knowledge base in a culture become more specialized, the need for more specific learning replaces traditional knowledge, with a growing emphasis on academic performance. This frequently disproportionately marginalizes individuals with intellectual disability. In less technologically advanced cultures, social and occupational roles remain available that are no longer relevant or valued in industrialized societies. These opportunities allow people with intellectual disability to participate in more significant social and occupational roles, which allows for greater integration into the community.

Epidemiology

Intellectual disability is operationally defined by scores on tests of measured intelligence that are 2 standard deviations below the mean (with the mean equal to 100 IQ points and each standard deviation equal to 15 points). According to a symmetrical bell-shape curve, 3% of the population should be intellectually disabled. Yet prevalence studies from community samples consistently report rates of 1.5%. This discrepancy may be due to age and socioeconomic status of the population surveyed; early loss of infants with severe illness; unexplained death in individuals with epilepsy, congenital abnormalities, or associated diseases; and "disappearance" of individuals with mild disability and good adaptive skills once their school careers are over (Aman et al. 2003).

Across the spectrum of intellectual disability, there is a 1.4 to 1.0 male-to-female ratio. The preponderance of males is also observed in many developmental disorders, including attention-deficit/hyperactivity disorder (ADHD) and some learning disorders (LDs), autism spectrum disorders, and Tourette's disorder. Sources of this gender bias include vulnerability to chromosomal and genetic aberrances (X-linked disorders) and increased susceptibility to prenatal and perinatal insults among males. For some genetic disorders and autism, affected females may have more severe subtypes of the disorder (Guthrie et al. 1999; Joy et al. 2003).

Individuals classified as having mild intellectual disability comprise nearly 89%, those with moderate disability comprise 7%, and those with severe to profound disability approximately 3%–4% of those identified (Table 21–3). Community surveys may be skewed in favor of identifying individuals capable of living and working in their home communities (i.e., mild to moderate) with a lower intensity of challenging behaviors and infrequently co-occurring neuropsychiatric disorders. Surveys of state-run residential centers tend to be subject to the opposite trend, identifying more individuals with severe to profound intellectual disability who have posed significant challenges to community-based programs (Vaccarino and Leckman 2003).

The patterns of residential placement also reflect sociocultural, economic, and traditional patterns of dealing with people with intellectual disability. The availability of quality care is frequently the factor that results in placement, especially for individuals with complex medical and neurological needs. The lack of clinicians skilled in functional analysis and behavioral interventions and the limited availability of crisis services and early treatment intervention programs restrict the carrying capacity of many communities, especially in the cases of people with severe or challenging behaviors and comorbid psychiatric disorders (Aman et al. 2003; Coccaro and Siever 2002).

Etiology

The more common biological causes of intellectual disability include prenatal exposure to toxins or infectious agents, genetic and chromosomal abnormalities, disturbances in normal brain development, nutritional factors, and early postnatal insults. The most common sources of prenatal neurotoxicity are alcohol and other substances of abuse. The adverse effects of these neurotoxins on development are further influenced by general maternal health and nutritional status; the timing, dose, and duration of exposure; number of previous pregnancies; and intrauterine growth relative to gestational age (Harris 2006; Vaccarino and Leckman 2003). A similar pattern of risk factors exists for most infectious disease: type of infection, inherent neurotropism of the virus or bacteria, timing of exposure (e.g., first trimester in rubella), and time of recognition and treatment. Postnatal exposures tend to be most devastating to infants and very young children (Joy et al. 2003). In the developing world, exposure to pre- and postnatal infectious diseases and environmental neurotoxins (e.g., HIV and water-borne pollutants) remains a major etiology of developmental disabilities in children (Harris 2006). Starvation and malnutrition have a profound impact on brain development.

Postnatal injuries, including shaken baby syndrome, neonatal meningitis, and intracranial vascular events, can have catastrophic consequences. As with toxic exposure, the timing of the insults is crucial to the impact and prognosis. Severe brain trauma during infancy can produce severe intellectual disability due to adverse effects on basic skill acquisition. This observation may appear counterintuitive in light of the greater plasticity and capacity for functional reorganization in infants and young children. However, outcome studies suggest limits to neuroplasticity. In addition to their neurocognitive deficits, many of these children are affected by deficient cognitive stimulation; parental psychopathology; and disorganized, chaotic settings (Goldstein and Reynolds 1999).

For many years, the risk for and increased prevalence of mild intellectual disability were attributed to parental intelligence, psychosocial and educational factors, and the influence of multiple unknown genes on intelligence. An errant extension of the polygenetic model offered that less intelligent parents tended to produce less intelligent children—the mistaken ideology behind eugenics, sterilization programs, and exterminations of the twentieth century. The effects of genes on intelligence are far more complex than this simple understanding and are themselves subject to social influences. Children from chaotic and understimulating environments are at greater risk for cognitive and educational deficits. Academic performance is also adversely affected by poverty, parental atti-

TABLE 21–3. **Clinical features of mental retardation**

	Mild	Moderate	Severe	Profound
IQ	50–55 to approximately 70	35–40 to 50–55	20–25 to 35–40	<20 or 25
Age at death (years)	50s	50s	40s	About 20
Percentage of mentally retarded population	89	7	3	1
Socioeconomic class	Low	Less low	No skew	No skew
Academic level achieved by adulthood	Sixth grade	Second grade	Below first-grade level in general	Below first-grade level in general
Education	Educable	Trainable (self-care)	Untrainable	Untrainable
Residence	Community	Sheltered	Mostly living in highly structured and closely supervised settings	Mostly living in highly structured and closely supervised settings
Economic	Makes change; manages a job; budgets money with effort or assistance	Makes small change; is usually able to manage change well	Can use coin machines; can take notes to shop owner	Is dependent on others for money management

Source. Reprinted from American Psychiatric Association: *Diagnostic and Statistical Manual of Mental Disorders,* 4th Edition, Text Revision. Washington, DC, American Psychiatric Association, 2000. Used with permission.

tudes, substance abuse, psychopathology, and neglect or abuse (Harris 2006).

Individuals with severe intellectual disability have greater prevalence rates for genetic disorders, severe prenatal insults, complicated and medically refractory forms of symptomatic epilepsies, and serious developmental brain anomalies. The confluence of both genetic and developmental anomalies, motor disorders, sensory impairments, and language communication deficits further limit adaptive skills in this population (Joy et al. 2003).

Finally, many individuals with intellectual disability are more sensitive to environmental challenges, illness, or physiological stresses. Lacking efficient communication strategies, these individuals may display disruptive or challenging behaviors that often correlate with the course of a particular ailment (Barnhill 2003).

Diagnostic Evaluation

The diagnosis of intellectual disability often begins with parent or teacher concerns. Formal diagnosis re-

quires a multidisciplinary process that incorporates familial, genetic, developmental, and educational history into a thorough medical neurological examination. To accurately assess adaptive skills, it is essential to collect data from multiple sources. Medical and neurological evaluations should be comprehensive and look specifically for treatable conditions. Detailed neuroimaging and neurophysiological, genetic, and metabolic studies are needed if there is a high index of suspicion for structural anomalies, seizures, or genetic-metabolic disorders (Joy et al. 2003).

Children with mild disability may not be diagnosed until they have poor academic performance. Early recognition can also be delayed by sociocultural factors such as disruptive behaviors, diminished suspicion among teachers, relatively high levels of social and adaptive skills, and preconceived biases about individuals with mild intellectual disability. Workup includes an assessment of psychosocial factors and adaptive skills, measures of intellectual abilities, and psychoeducational testing. If questions arise, referrals should be made for more extensive medical and neurological evaluations (Harris 2006).

Detailed genetic testing is often not practical, but children from families with histories of developmental disorders, mental retardation, or specific syndromes such as fragile X syndrome warrant a more extensive workup (Harris 2002). Specifically, such a workup should be pursued in the presence of significant dysmorphology, multiorgan or multisystem involvement, and other comorbid medical or neurological conditions, including poorly controlled mixtures of complex and simple partial or myoclonic seizures (Guthrie et al. 1999). A combination of multiple dysmorphic features, anatomical (often cardiac or gastrointestinal) abnormalities, growth delays, endocrine problems, and intellectual disability suggests chromosomal abnormalities (Guthrie et al. 1999). Severe intellectual disability, progression of symptoms, biochemical abnormalities (e.g., elevated ammonia levels, elevated amino or organic acids), liver abnormalities, growth and maturational delays, abnormal neuroimaging studies, and seizures may indicate an underlying metabolic abnormality (Joy et al. 2003).

The pattern of inheritance is also helpful when considering a more extensive workup. Parents of children with autosomal recessive disorders may not be affected themselves or (as heterozygotes or carriers) may have only mild symptoms. Twenty-five percent of siblings may also be affected. Autosomal dominant disorders appear in up to 50% of siblings and family members (except for new mutations) but display variable expression (penetrance) or severity. Affected males suggest X-linked disorders or possible mitochondrial disorders, and further genetic testing would be indicated (Guthrie et al. 1999).

Due to significant delays in sensorimotor and language development, children with severe to profound intellectual disability are often recognized at a younger age. They are more likely to have prenatal developmental motor disorders, perinatal trauma, congenital infections, and genetic or chromosomal disorders. Syndromal diagnoses can help define treatment approaches and alert clinicians to the presence of associated behavioral and cognitive phenotypes (Moldavsky et al. 2001).

Degenerative disorders may also cause intellectual disability. Disintegrative disorder of childhood presents with a period of normal development followed by accelerated regression of cognitive and socioemotional adaptive skills. It may be a matter of time before the degenerative course of the disorder is recognized. Some leukodystrophies may present with behavioral or cognitive decline in childhood or, in the case of mild enzyme deficiencies, during early adulthood. Although the individual may not test in the range of in-tellectual disability initially, the progressive nature of the neurological disorder will become apparent as old skills are lost and new skills are not acquired. Unfortunately, the longitudinal progression or temporal profile of these losses may not be appreciated during a single interview or a one-time evaluation (Joy et al. 2003).

Behavioral Phenotypes

In recent years, there has been growing interest in the behavioral phenotypes associated with specific genetic syndromes. Behavioral phenotypes are patterns of cognition and behavior that have a greater probability of expression within a specific disorder (Harris 2002). For example, social anxiety or gaze aversion is a signature trait in fragile X syndrome. Another, more dramatic example is the compulsive and relentless SIB associated with Lesch-Nyhan syndrome (Goldstein and Reynolds 1999). In both examples, the likelihood of specific emotional responses and behaviors occurring in these syndromes is greater than in the general population of individuals with intellectual disability. Although patients with specific behavioral phenotypes do not meet the criteria for major psychiatric disorders, and the boundary between known behavioral phenotypes and psychiatric disorders is still unsettled, behavioral phenotypes do provide clues about the complex nature of gene–behavior interactions. For example, nearly one-third of children with velocardiofacial syndrome (22q deletions) develop symptoms consistent with adolescent-onset bipolar disorder and psychosis (Goldstein and Reynolds 1999; Harris 2002).

Comorbid Psychiatric Disorders

All psychiatric diagnoses may co-occur with intellectual disability. Comorbid diagnoses include depression, bipolar and anxiety disorders, autistic spectrum disorders, LDs, and psychotic disorders. These individuals may have disruptive behavior disorders, and up to 50% may have ADHD.

The accurate diagnosis of primary psychiatric disorders in individuals with intellectual disability requires an understanding of the degree of their intellectual disability and of their verbal and communicative abilities, as well as a knowledge of comorbid medical or neurological conditions. The clinician must also appreciate that severe behavioral disorganization may be a response to environmental challenges. It is difficult for many clinicians to reliably diagnose comorbid disorders because psychiatrists generally depend on an individual's self-report of mental or emotional states. Nonverbal patients require additional tools, including instruments standardized for patients with intellectual disability. It is important for the clinician to directly examine or observe the individual and to review reports from multiple sources familiar with the person as well as objective behavioral data (Aman et al. 2003; Einfield and Aman 1995).

Once adequate information is obtained, it may still be difficult to distinguish symptoms related to intellectual disability (e.g., baseline aggression) from those secondary to a psychiatric disorder (e.g., increase in baseline aggression in an individual with comorbid bipolar disorder). Diagnosis is further complicated in patients with moderate to severe intellectual disability because they may present with atypical or subsyndromal symptoms of mood or anxiety disorders, phobias, or even prodromal schizophrenia. These complexities partly explain the reason so many patients with intellectual disability are classified with "not otherwise specified" diagnoses (Barnhill 2003; Harris 2006).

Treatment

There is no cure for intellectual disability. Prevention and early intervention remain the most effective treatments. This includes bypassing of enzymatic defects in metabolic disorders, better prenatal care, treatments for infectious diseases, and early recognition and treatment of seizure disorders (Aman et al. 2003). The most effective early intervention strategies employ child-specific ecological modifications (e.g., environmental enrichment) and developmentally focused education and behavioral interventions. For example, there is growing evidence that the severity of intellectual disability in children with trisomy 21 can be modified with early, intensive enrichment experiences. In addition, focused efforts directed at temperamental vulnerabilities or behavioral phenotypes may impact the emergence of challenging behaviors. These intervention strategies allow for accommodation and skill training that are specific to the individual neurobiological, cognitive, or emotional needs and vulnerabilities of the child (Harris 2006).

Setting

Most treatment plans involve some form of habilitation that enhances adaptive or social skills or provides training for specific vocational or educational niches. These programs usually include school-based training, assisted employment, communication enhancement, and daily living skill training. Other community-based programs focus on enhancing family supports, respite services, and developmental centers (Griffiths et al. 1998).

Complicated medical and neurological problems, challenging behaviors, and comorbid psychiatric disorders create service delivery problems. In fact, aggression, property destruction, severe self-injury, and other disruptive behaviors are the most common causes for out-of-home placement. In the past, many of these individuals lived in larger residential facilities or custodial programs. Advocates for humane and humanizing treatment have changed this referral pattern dramatically (Coccaro and Siever 2002; Stein et al. 2002). Improvements in behavioral and psychopharmacological strategies for severe challenging behaviors have also made a significant contribution to the community placement movement. Access and utilization of services and the availability of qualified trained personnel vary across demographic, economic, and social settings. Advances in technology (e.g., telemedicine) are expanding service delivery to remote or sparsely populated regions. The unequal distribution of services and providers remains an issue in many settings and negatively impacts the carrying capacity of many community programs.

Many individuals with intellectual disability do well in either family or community settings as opposed to institutional placement. These individuals tend to have few problematic behaviors and minimal neurological or psychiatric symptoms. Those with mild intellectual disabilities and no significant behavioral or psychiatric disorders may rarely come to attention once their school careers end. These individuals may use clinical services when crises emerge, but rates of challenging behaviors and psychiatric disorders are at most moderately elevated. Those with histories of abuse, childhood behavioral or emotional problems, and family histories of addiction or major psychiatric disorders may require higher levels of care (Griffiths et al. 1998; Harris 2006).

Psychotherapy

Psychotherapy can be an important part of the treatment plan. For individuals with mild intellectual disability, verbal and cognitive skills may be adequate for modified forms of several psychotherapies. There is growing evidence that modified forms of traditional supportive, dynamic, cognitive, and dialectic behavioral therapy can be extremely effective. The availability of qualified or skilled therapists is frequently the limiting factor to their use (Harris 2006). In individuals with severe intellectual disability, impaired or absent language and communication skills and severe cognitive deficits prevent the use of many forms of psychotherapy. Behavioral interventions remain the most common form of therapy. The goal of behavioral therapy is to reduce unwanted behaviors by modifying environmental or antecedent factors or by changing the contingencies of maladaptive behaviors. Successful strategies can range from extinction procedures, differential reinforcement of alternative or incompatible behaviors, or skill building through shaping techniques. (See Chapter 31 in this volume, "Cognitive Therapy," by Wright et al. for further discussion of behavioral therapy.)

Pharmacotherapy

Pharmacotherapy has a complicated history in the management of individuals with intellectual disability. In the past, medications were used to effect behavioral control or to compensate for overcrowding and lack of programming in custodial institutions. In contrast to the pharmacological revolution that largely depopulated mental institutions and propelled the community mental health movement, many of the same drugs allowed for a paradoxical increase in the size of many residential programs for individuals with intellectual disability. More effective tranquilization or behavioral controls allowed for higher population densities. In some community settings, there is a shortage of qualified personnel, and facilities may have inadequate behavioral or habilitation programs. Under these circumstances, unfortunately, psychotropics are often used in lieu of effective behavioral programs, and polypharmacy has become the new form of maintaining community-based "behavioral management" (Harris 2006).

Even with effective behavioral programming, many individuals with intellectual disability continue to show challenging behaviors. In order to maintain or preserve a least restrictive placement, there is a frequent need for well-monitored pharmacotherapy. The decision to proceed with medication management is the result of a careful review of the neurobiology and etiology of intellectual disability, the presence of a specific behavioral phenotype, the history of past treatment, and a medical-neurological workup. The clinician needs to integrate available behavioral data and consult with all members of the treatment team about special environmental or interpersonal factors (Aman et al. 2003).

It is not uncommon to see individuals with severe intellectual disability taking extremely high dosages of multiple medications. There seems to be a growing trend toward polypharmacy based on treatment models extrapolated from basic research or inaccurately diagnosed psychiatric disorders. At the root of this trend is a preference for selecting pharmacological agents based on a single symptom (e.g., a patient who is crying or appears sad must be depressed) or hypothetical neurotransmitter abnormality (e.g., all aggression is related to reductions in serotonin activity). The basic problem with this approach is the failure to recognize the heterogeneity of challenging behaviors (Barnhill 2003).

Even the treatment of clearly defined psychiatric disorders is confounded by comorbidities in individuals as well as possible drug-related or iatrogenic symptoms in patients who may be prescribed medications by several physicians. Much of our limited evidence base for the use of pharmacological agents does not account for these comorbid conditions. A full understanding of a patient's presentation comes from integrating this information with knowledge of the patient's developmental, neurological, and medical history (Aman et al. 2003; Harris 2006).

There has been an explosion in the use of second- and third-generation antipsychotic drugs, antidepressant or antianxiety drugs (e.g., selective serotonin reuptake inhibitors [SSRIs], serotonin–norepinephrine reuptake inhibitors (SNRIs), atypical antidepressants), and antiepileptic mood stabilizers. These medications are used to treat primary psychiatric disorders as well as challenging behaviors. When compared with previous approaches, these newer agents appear to reduce some of the intolerable side effects of older agents (e.g., extrapyramidal symptoms, risk of tardive dyskinesia, sedation, and anticholinergic side effects). However, the new treatments are not without side effects. Dermatological, hematological, endocrinological, and cardiac side effects are still problematic. In every situation, the clinician must use a limited evidence base for individuals with intellectual disability to make risk–benefit judgments. Unfortunately many treatment approaches are "off-label" or extrapolated from data in typical children or adults (Aman et al. 2003; Joy et al. 2003; see Chapter 36 in this volume, "Treatment of Children and Adolescents," by Crawford et al.).

Clinicians face three basic issues when considering pharmacotherapy in individuals with intellectual disability. The first involves the focus of treatment. Typically, symptoms (as opposed to syndromes or disorders) are the target of medication interventions. The goal is to establish accurate psychiatric diagnoses and direct treatment at the problematic symptoms. Response can be monitored through available assessment and treatment instruments. Those designed for or adapted to people with intellectual disability are preferred. If there is no diagnosable disorder but challenging behaviors remain resistant to behavioral interventions, then pharmacotherapy should proceed based on the best available evidence-based data. If such evidence is lacking, the best practices or expert consensus data can help with clinical decision making.

The second issue relates to the difficulty in making reliable psychiatric diagnoses in patients with intellectual disability. These disorders may affect the clinical course, prognosis, and treatment of the presenting syndrome. There is also the degree of heterogeneity within diagnostic categories, such as differences in sleep disturbance within mood disorders. This heterogeneity is compounded among patients with severe intellectual disability, who often have additional neurological, developmental, metabolic, and neurophysiological disorders (Barnhill 2003).

The third issue involves the heterogeneity of intellectual disability itself. There are many subgroups of intellectual disability based on severity, comorbid neurological disorders, genetic etiology, and underlying developmental brain abnormalities. For example, individual patients with fragile X syndrome vary from the lengths of CGG repeats and degree of DNA methylation to such epigenetic phenomena as intellectual ability and presence and severity of stereotypies or self-injury. Individuals with trisomy 21 and mood disorders need to be evaluated for thyroid dysfunction, basal ganglia abnormalities, or the emergence of apathy and seizures in conjunction with the cognitive decline of evolving dementia. The clinician must account for these variables in order to match treatment to psychiatric diagnosis and to determine and monitor the pre-illness baseline (and assess recovery or remission) as well as anticipate potential adverse drug effects (Joy et al. 2003).

There is no single drug effective against all forms of aggression or SIB, so clinicians should make every effort to define subtypes of challenging behaviors based on etiological differences. Starting low and going slow with medication is the most reasonable strategy. The clinician will need to establish dosage- or serum-level response curves based on behavioral data; monitor for side effects such as akathisia, irritability, or disinhibition; and make adjustments in medications as indicated. The decision to eventually reduce or discontinue the medication should be based on a risk–benefit analysis that includes risk of long-term side effects, past history of regression at lower dosages, and the inherent severity or dangerousness of the behavior. Every decision should be made in conjunction with the behavioral therapist and direct-care staff or family. Polypharmacy should be the exception rather than the rule (Aman et al. 2003).

Intellectual Disability Summary

Intellectual disability is a complex, heterogeneous collection of disorders characterized by deficits in measured intelligence and adaptive abilities and onset during the developmental period. Depending on the severity of the intellectual disability, there is a considerable range of comorbid neurological, metabolic, and genetic disorders that can confound psychiatric care. Challenging behaviors emerge in the context of medical, neurological, and ecological variables that are manifestations of a mismatch between the individual's needs and abilities and his or her living environment. These individuals challenge our understanding of the relationships between brain development and behavior. In essence, the understanding of intellectual disability requires a thorough working knowledge of developmental neuropsychiatry and an appreciation of the multiple factors that influence human behavior.

The treatment of challenging behaviors and neuropsychiatric disorders requires a team. There is probably no single treatment modality that fits each individual. Combined treatments often are needed. The ultimate goal of treatment is to maximize the quality of life for individuals with intellectual disability. Many individuals with intellectual disability are subject to daily stressors that seriously tax their capacity to adapt. In order to be helpful, clinicians need to approach each individual from a biopsychosocial frame of reference.

Learning Disorders and Motor Skills Disorder

Clinical Description

LDs involve deficits in acquiring and performing basic academic skills. Currently, LDs are categorized into disorders of reading, mathematics, and written expression (Tables 21–4, 21–5, and 21–6). Developmental coordination disorder (DCD), the only motor skills disorder in DSM, is defined in DSM-IV-TR by significant impairment in gross or fine motor coordination, including delays in motor milestones or difficulty with other expected motor tasks during development (Table 21–7). It is often co-occurring and closely related to LD of written expression. The presence of neurological soft signs in individuals with LD of written expression is evidence of problems in the regulation of sensorimotor functions that may lie on a continuum with motor skill disorders (Rourke et al. 2003).

TABLE 21–4. DSM-IV-TR diagnostic criteria for reading disorder

A. Reading achievement, as measured by individually administered standardized tests of reading accuracy or comprehension, is substantially below that expected given the person's chronological age, measured intelligence, and age-appropriate education.

B. The disturbance in criterion A significantly interferes with academic achievement or activities of daily living that require reading skills.

C. If a sensory deficit is present, the reading difficulties are in excess of those usually associated with it.

Coding note: If a general medical (e.g., neurological) condition or sensory deficit is present, code the condition on Axis III.

TABLE 21–5. DSM-IV-TR diagnostic criteria for mathematics disorder

A. Mathematical ability, as measured by individually administered standardized tests, is substantially below that expected given the person's chronological age, measured intelligence, and age-appropriate education.

B. The disturbance in criterion A significantly interferes with academic achievement or activities of daily living that require mathematical ability.

C. If a sensory deficit is present, the difficulties in mathematical ability are in excess of those usually associated with it.

Coding note: If a general medical (e.g., neurological) condition or sensory deficit is present, code the condition on Axis III.

TABLE 21–6. DSM-IV-TR diagnostic criteria for disorder of written expression

A. Writing skills, as measured by individually administered standardized tests (or functional assessments of writing skills), are substantially below those expected given the person's chronological age, measured intelligence, and age-appropriate education.

B. The disturbance in criterion A significantly interferes with academic achievement or activities of daily living that require the composition of written texts (e.g., writing grammatically correct sentences and organized paragraphs).

C. If a sensory deficit is present, the difficulties in writing skills are in excess of those usually associated with it.

Coding note: If a general medical (e.g., neurological) condition or sensory deficit is present, code the condition on Axis III.

TABLE 21–7. DSM-IV-TR diagnostic criteria for developmental coordination disorder

A. Performance in daily activities that require motor coordination is substantially below that expected given the person's chronological age and measured intelligence. This may be manifested by marked delays in achieving motor milestones (e.g., walking, crawling, sitting), dropping things, "clumsiness," poor performance in sports, or poor handwriting.

B. The disturbance in criterion A significantly interferes with academic achievement or activities of daily living.

C. The disturbance is not due to a general medical condition (e.g., cerebral palsy, hemiplegia, or muscular dystrophy) and does not meet criteria for a pervasive developmental disorder.

D. If mental retardation is present, the motor difficulties are in excess of those usually associated with it.

Coding note: If a general medical (e.g., neurological) condition or sensory deficit is present, code the condition on Axis III.

The current diagnostic criteria for LD emphasize lags in academic performance. From a practical standpoint, most state and federal guidelines use a definition that relies on a discrepancy of 1.5 to 2 standard deviations between expected performance on standardized tests and measured intellectual abilities. These current diagnostic criteria do not address the underlying neuropsychological diversity of LD and therefore may have limited value for educational planning and interventions (Rourke et al. 2003).

There have been efforts to subdivide specific LDs based on neuropsychological profiles in order to better focus compensatory or remediation efforts (Connors and Schulte 2002). A broader approach to LD classification distinguishes language-based from nonverbal problems (Fletcher 2005; Forrest 2004). Another model subdivides LDs into the following functional categories: problems with 1) input, 2) processing, or 3) output of information. These categorizations demonstrate the suitability of including DCD with DSM-IV-TR's LDs.

Reading Disorder

Reading is crucial to academic performance and functioning in societies with significant education-based social stratification. Historically, reading disorders were considered perceptual disorders. In recent years the focus has shifted to the relationship between reading speed and accuracy and morpheme–phoneme and visual grapheme processing speed and factors related to reading comprehension. Currently the literature supports the idea that reading is hierarchically organized and requires the functional integrity of multiple interconnected brain circuits (Ramus et al. 2003).

Developmentally, reading progresses from sight recognition of words and the use of contextual cues (e.g., pictures) to increased use of rapid phonetic analysis and syntactical cues. Clinically, reading correlates with the speed and efficiency of processing and responding to phonemes (i.e., speed and accuracy of processing).

Written Expression and Motor Skills Disorders

Although distinct disorders, disorder of written expression and DCD are interrelated. Writing is a motor skill, and some problems described in disorders of written language are shared with other motor dyspraxias. Writing, however, involves combining these motor skills with reading language. Handwriting and motor dyscoordination are commonly problematic in nonverbal LDs, tic disorders, and other developmental disorders. For many of these children, the quality of oral presentations, richness of language, and complexity of ideas that emerge in oral presentations differ considerably from those in written assignments. Written work often appears telegraphic and in some respects resembles that produced by persons with acquired lesions associated with nonfluent or Broca's aphasia (Ardila and Surloff 2006).

Writing provides graphic evidence of the maturation of the complex motor-cognitive pathways. The development of writing skills begins with grasp and motor skill, fluency of rapid movements, organization and connection with cognition, and ultimately the capacity to switch modalities (e.g., use a word processor). Delays in written language may co-occur with other motor skill disorders but are often recognized later, when demands for written expression increase (Peters et al. 2001). Recent federal education statutes require writing proficiency and may increase the pressure on children with these disabilities.

In some respects, written language is a subset of motor skill disorders, which are disorders of planning, organization, and implementation of motor programs. They differ from paralysis or paresis based on the level of motor impairment. Clumsiness is one example of DCD. It may involve deficits in learning new motor skills, automatization, and implementation of fine motor skills. Aside from writing and sports performance, motor skills disorders may not be as devastating for children in electronically advanced societies as for those in cultures that still require manual dexterity for trades or artisanship (Peters et al. 2001; Rourke et al. 2003).

Mathematics Disorders

Like writing disorders, math disabilities represent a mixture of hierarchically organized cognitive operations. Early risk factors involve difficulty with spatial concepts (e.g., "above," "under") and other features of nonverbal LD (Mazzocco 2001; Rourke et al. 2003). The problems range from failing to recognize the differences between "1+2" and "1×2" or being unable to maintain the spatial integrity of figure columns to being unequal to the demands of multistep sequenced tasks such as long division (Fletcher 2005; Marshall et al. 1999). In short, math disorder represents a derailment of the progression of skills, a failure to move from counting to basic math operations (arithmetic) and then on to advanced mathematics that require sequential reasoning, significant verbal skills, and abstract reasoning (Fletcher 2005). Mathematical reasoning may be deficient. An interesting deficit involves poor estimating ability or a difficulty recognizing math errors or the validity of answers. Even more intriguing are math savants. Those with autism can sometimes perform unbelievable arithmetic computations but are unable to use these skills in making change or to enhance occupational functioning (Lachiewicz et al. 2006).

Epidemiology

LDs are the most prevalent developmental disorders of childhood. Although standardized definitions exist, the prevalence rates vary. The inconsistency among reported prevalence rates may be due to the clinical heterogeneity and the evolving nature of these diagnoses. For example, the age of recognition for LD and DCD is influenced by the type and severity of demands placed on the child. Additional factors affecting identification include the threshold for recognition (e.g., the index of suspicion by teachers or parents), quality and availability of referral resources, instability of the diagnosis over time, impact of changing sociocultural or medical factors, state-related behavioral changes or disruptive behaviors, and variations in standards used by communities to qualify for services (Ingalls and Goldstein 1999).

The most common LD, reading disorder, is thought to occur in 2%–10% of all children. It accounts for up to 80% of children diagnosed with an LD (Shaywitz et al. 2000). Reading disorders tend to have the greatest impact on education levels and occupational achievement, but many children learn to compensate to some degree. Mathematics disorders are thought to occur in 1%–6%, and disorders of written expression have a prevalence of 2%–8% (American Academy of Child and Adolescent Psychiatry 1998). DCD is estimated to occur in up to 6% of children 5–11 years old (American Psychiatric Association 2000). Perhaps the most devastating LD involves a combination of academic skill deficits. The global disabilities overlap and are frequently confused with intellectual disability or pervasive developmental disorder (PDD) (Lachiewicz et al. 2006; Rourke et al. 2003).

There are gender differences in the prevalence rates for LD and DCD. As is the case for many developmental disorders, males are most often affected by DCD and LDs, except for mathematics disorder, which affects more girls than boys. There are also gender differences in the types of comorbid psychiatric disorders that may affect LDs. Males more frequently present with disruptive behaviors such as ADHD, oppositional defiant disorder (ODD), and conduct disorder (CD; Connors and Schulte 2002). Females with LD more typically demonstrate internalizing disorders.

The rate of comorbid psychiatric disorders may be as high as 50% in children and adolescents with LD. Language disorders frequently co-occur, and 20% of individuals with LD may also have ADHD. In adolescents, conduct problems and LDs may co-occur. Additionally, those with LD are at increased risk for substance use disorders (Klein and Mannuzza 2000). These comorbid psychiatric disorders may delay the recognition of reading disorders and affect access to and utilization of compensatory interventions (Connors and Schulte 2002). DCD is commonly associated with LDs, communication disorders, and ADHD (American Psychiatric Association 2000).

Etiology

Although most LDs are either language or nonverbally based, the differences in functional neuroimaging studies make clear that no single area represents the reading or mathematics "center." Instead, a network that integrates both hemispheres and multiple regions and subcortical circuitries develops. This degree of coherence and integration follows a developmental trajectory that changes with neuronal maturation, myelinization of key interconnecting pathways, and prefrontal/executive supervision (Litt et al. 2005; Rourke et al. 2003). These processes appear to be disrupted in children with LD.

Controversial but interesting findings have demonstrated acalculia in children with a dysfunctional left angular gyrus, suggesting that math abilities are linked to integrative centers because this same area is associated with finger recognition and right–left orientation as well as reading skills (Forrest 2004; Marshall et al. 1999).

Reading disorder seems to be characterized by a distortion in the integration and functional coherence between diverse regions within the central nervous system. From this perspective, reading disability is a persistent expression of a developmental disruption of brain maturation and skill acquisition (Online Mendelian Inheritance in Man Database 2003).

Multiple genes may be implicated in reading disorder. Specifically, a marker gene on chromosome 6 appears to underlie phonological and syntactical analysis (Online Mendelian Inheritance in Man Database 2003). Several other chromosomal abnormalities involving genetic duplication are associated with language and reading difficulties (e.g., XYY and XXY in males) (Ingalls and Goldstein 1999). Neurodevelopmental disorders such as epilepsy, phakomatoses, and neuronal migration and maturation disorders affect learning and play a role in many cases of LD (Ramus et al. 2003).

Written language involves both morpheme–phoneme processing and motor planning. In some respects, written language may be a highly specialized subset of motor skills disorder, in which the deficits involve motor planning, sequencing, fine motor skills, automatization of the linkages between thought and ideas, word finding, syntax, editing, and output (writing). With practice, these skills become automatic. Slowed output may interrupt this transformation, requiring the child to "think" about subprocesses (how to make a "d") rather than the topic at hand. The praxis and higher-order planning of written expression involves an additional complex network that includes the cerebellum, basal ganglia, and multiple cortical centers (Ardila and Surloff 2006; Ramus et al. 2003).

Course and Prognosis

There is considerable variability in the developmental course of LD. A subset of children presents with delays in skill acquisition that suggest an aberrant trajectory for brain maturation that improves with maturity. Others appear to have a developmental deficit or functional "lesion" that requires more extensive remedial training or habilitation. Many of these children may have lifelong problems or display only partial compensation (Litt et al. 2005).

DCD is first typically diagnosed when parents notice a delay in motor skill development. These children are frequently teased by peers because of their clumsiness. This often leads to low self-esteem, feelings of inadequacy, and social withdrawal. There is variable course with this disorder, with some individuals fully remitting and others retaining some deficit throughout their lifetimes.

Diagnostic Evaluation

The diagnosis of LD requires a discrepancy between a child's age, general intellectual ability, and performance on tests of academic ability. The child's chronological age is commonly linked to grade placement and incremental increases in the complexity of academic expectations and demands. The capacity of a child to master grade-level materials is dependent on proper classroom instruction and extraclassroom exposure to learning environments as well as general intellectual ability. Problems with many of these areas may contribute to academic difficulty and lead to an assessment of LD (Ingalls and Goldstein 1999; Rourke et al. 2003; Weinberg and McLean 1986).

Determining a child's intellectual capacity is essential to an evaluation of LD. An analysis of the subtest scores on current intelligence tests provides clues about subtypes of learning problems, but these are by no means the definitive test instruments for LD (Lachiewicz et al. 2006; Stengel-Rutkowski and Anderlik 2005). The assessment instruments for LD are developmental tests designed and standardized based on a child's age and intelligence level. There are general tests of academic skills (e.g., Wide Range Achievement Test, Woodcock Johnson Test of Educational Abilities) that provide an overview of major areas of academic performance. More specialized instruments focus on specific domains such as written expression, mathematical abilities, or subtypes of reading disorders. Neuropsychological assessments help define functional domains that underlie learning and can be quite helpful in planning cognitive remediation (Connors and Schulte 2002; Rourke et al. 2003; Weinberg and McLean 1986). Each subtest provides a piece of the puzzle but may not entirely explain an individual's struggles in school. It is important to listen to the life story of each child because determination, motivation,

talents, and passions all affect learning (Rourke et al. 2003).

A key feature of the current criteria for LD requires exposure to age-appropriate learning experiences. Children need a safe and enriching environment that provides basic learning experiences. Extreme forms of childhood deprivation and abuse seriously disrupt the epigenesis of brain maturation, learning, and mental health. Less dramatic examples include high rates of both cognitive deficits and poor academic performance in many children of families with low levels of parental interest and educational achievement, poor prenatal care, intrauterine exposure to toxins, high levels of chaos, violence and abuse, mental illness, and substance use (Litt et al. 2005).

General intelligence and emerging specialized academic skills are sensitive to environmental factors. In addition, these same factors influence academic motivation, school attendance, peer attitudes toward school, dropout rates, disruptive behavior, and risk of major psychiatric and substance use disorders. These in turn affect academic performance (Fletcher 2005; Forrest 2004).

In the evaluation of DCD, one must obtain a careful history, including prenatal and perinatal history, as well as a review of developmental milestones and specific behaviors such as grasping, drawing, and dressing (Denckla and Roeltgen 1992). DCD requires a medical evaluation to rule out neurological conditions or PDDs. If mental retardation is present, the motor difficulties must be greater than those usually associated with the level of retardation. Consultation with an occupational therapist may be appropriate.

Treatment

Like other chronic illnesses in children, LDs are probably not curable. Treatment consists primarily of compensatory techniques or technologies to minimize the impact of these disorders on educational and social function. The importance of an individualized education plan with tailored treatment by communicative providers supported by involved, interested parents cannot be overstressed. Behavioral techniques attempt to develop effective strategies to assist learning and ultimately promote self-esteem. Even with compensatory techniques and functional improvement, the underlying neurocognitive substrates may continue to influence brain development and increase the risk for comorbid behavioral and psychiatric disorders (Fletcher 2005; Litt et al. 2005).

There are no pharmacological cures for LD. At best, medications may help reduce the impact of co-occurring disorders, such as ADHD or mood disorders, that can have profound effects on symptom manifestation. Medications, notably anticonvulsant drugs, may impede learning in complex ways. For example, anticonvulsants may reduce the disruptive effects of seizures, but at high serum levels they also disrupt learning and attention. Over the past 25 years, various alternative medication strategies have evolved to supplement classroom interventions, but support and objective randomized studies have not substantiated their efficacy. The use of piracetam, vitamin supplements, and traditional psychotropic medications, including cholinesterase inhibitors, is currently enjoying increased popularity. The treatment effects of these novel strategies are modest (Connors and Schulte 2002; Rourke et al. 2003).

As with LD, the most significant intervention for a child with DCD who meets criteria for special education in the public school is the implementation of an individualized education plan with annual goals for improvement. The primary treatment for DCD is occupational therapy either individually or with a group.

Communication Disorders

Communication disorders, as defined in DSM-IV-TR, are characterized by delays in expressive or receptive language in excess of the difficulties expected given an individual's intelligence and that result in significant scholastic, work, or social interference. These disorders have an enormous impact on concurrent and subsequent developmental modalities, social functioning, and psychiatric outcomes.

Expressive Language Disorder and Mixed Receptive–Expressive Language Disorder

Clinical Description

In expressive language disorder, language understanding is intact, but the individual cannot express him- or herself adequately. This impairment often results in brief verbal responses and incorrect sentences and use of words. Seemingly regressive or immature speech is common and is consistent with the slow acquisition of skills (Table 21–8). In mixed receptive–expressive language disorder, the impaired expressive communication is compounded by deficits in comprehension of aspects of language (Table 21–9). Given the disparate abilities between intellect and expressive

---

TABLE 21–8. DSM-IV-TR diagnostic criteria for expressive language disorder

A. The scores obtained from standardized individually administered measures of expressive language development are substantially below those obtained from standardized measures of both nonverbal intellectual capacity and receptive language development. The disturbance may be manifest clinically by symptoms that include having a markedly limited vocabulary, making errors in tense, or having difficulty recalling words or producing sentences with developmentally appropriate length or complexity.

B. The difficulties with expressive language interfere with academic or occupational achievement or with social communication.

C. Criteria are not met for mixed receptive–expressive language disorder or a pervasive developmental disorder.

D. If mental retardation, a speech–motor or sensory deficit, or environmental deprivation is present, the language difficulties are in excess of those usually associated with these problems.

Coding note: If a speech–motor or sensory deficit or a neurological condition is present, code the condition on Axis III.

---

skills, significant frustration is common and can be conceptualized as an etiology for the social difficulties and dysphoria individuals with these disorders often experience.

Epidemiology

Prevalences for the communication disorders are difficult to determine given the variable definitions that have been, and continue to be, used. The U.S. Department of Education reported that 18.9% of the nearly 5.8 million children in the public schools receiving special education are treated for "speech and language impairments" (U.S. Department of Education 2002), although this number may be limited by the availability of services. Male predominance of 3–4 to 1 is evident.

Etiology

Etiologies for communication disorders are often found in combination and appear to be cumulative. Biological factors such as prenatal exposures, perinatal adversity, early childhood illness (e.g., otitis media), and known genetic or metabolic disorders have been

TABLE 21-9. **DSM-IV-TR diagnostic criteria for mixed receptive–expressive language disorder**

A. The scores obtained from a battery of standardized individually administered measures of both receptive and expressive language development are substantially below those obtained from standardized measures of nonverbal intellectual capacity. Symptoms include those for expressive language disorder as well as difficulty understanding words, sentences, or specific types of words, such as spatial terms.

B. The difficulties with receptive and expressive language significantly interfere with academic or occupational achievement or with social communication.

C. Criteria are not met for a pervasive developmental disorder.

D. If mental retardation, a speech–motor or sensory deficit, or environmental deprivation is present, the language difficulties are in excess of those usually associated with these problems.

Coding note: If a speech–motor or sensory deficit or a neurological condition is present, code the condition on Axis III.

shown to be important. Environmental risk factors such as abuse, neglect, and poverty have also been implicated.

Psychiatric comorbidity is common. The possibility of a common etiology between the language disorders and ADHD has been proposed. Disruptive behavior disorders, anxiety disorders, and substance use disorders are frequently comorbid in these individuals.

Course and Prognosis

Approximately one-half of young children with expressive and mixed receptive–expressive language disorders develop normal language abilities by adolescence. Those with persistent disorders typically demonstrate greater severity of symptoms at the time of initial presentation. A diagnosis of mixed receptive–expressive language disorder may have a poorer prognosis than that of expressive language disorder.

Diagnostic Evaluation

In addition to documenting the developmental history, careful assessment of language can occur in the context of a clinical examination. Rutter (1987) proposed special attention to inner language (the use of symbolization), language production, phonation, and

pragmatic communication. Should concerns arise, a referral for further assessment involving cognitive and language testing should be made.

Treatment

Specialized treatment for children identified as having a communication disorder is available through special education services in the public school system. The interventions available vary from system to system but should follow from an individualized assessment and plan. Specific approaches are roughly categorized as behavioral, child-centered, or a combination of these approaches (Paul 2001).

Phonological Disorder

Clinical Description and Symptoms

Very common in pediatric populations, phonological disorder is characterized by impairment in the ability to produce and use developmentally appropriate speech sounds. Typically, this results in poor intelligibility or gives the appearance of persistent "baby talk" (Table 21–10). Most children do grow out of their symptoms; however, especially in moderate to severe cases, difficulties persist.

Epidemiology

Occurring in nearly 20% of preschool and approximately 6% of school-age children, phonological disorder's prevalence decreases with advancing age. Milder forms are more common than moderate and severe cases. Phonological disorder affects males more frequently than females and is associated with LDs, enuresis, neurological soft signs, DCD, and scholastic difficulty (American Psychiatric Association 2000).

Etiology

Speech production impairments due solely to intellectual disability, hearing impairment, or problems with the speech mechanism are excluded from the diagnosis. As in the other communication disorders, biological and environmental factors are likely.

Diagnostic Evaluation

Again, as in the other communication disorders, screening can occur during initial interviews, paying special attention to developmental history and school difficulties. Given the high rates of comorbidity with additional communication disorders and LDs, assessments of intelligence and hearing and a full speech language assessment are often warranted.

TABLE 21–10. DSM-IV-TR diagnostic criteria for phonological disorder

A. Failure to use developmentally expected speech sounds that are appropriate for age and dialect (e.g., errors in sound production, use, representation, or organization such as, but not limited to, substitutions of one sound for another [use of /t/ for target /k/ sound] or omissions of sounds such as final consonants).

B. The difficulties in speech sound production interfere with academic or occupational achievement or with social communication.

C. If mental retardation, a speech–motor or sensory deficit, or environmental deprivation is present, the speech difficulties are in excess of those usually associated with these problems.

Coding note: If a speech–motor or sensory deficit or a neurological condition is present, code the condition on Axis III.

Treatment

Amelioration of symptoms can be gained through the use of speech therapy. Appropriate treatment of associated difficulties is important.

Stuttering

Clinical Description

Stuttering is the interruption of normal flow of speech. It is characterized by frequent repetitions or prolongations of sounds or syllables, involuntary and irregular hesitation, broken words, and silent or audible blocking (Table 21–11). Stuttering typically begins between 2 and 7 years of age, with a peak onset at age 5 years. Stuttering must be distinguished from normal dysfluencies that occur frequently in young children but generally last less than 6 months. The onset is typically insidious, and the child is usually unaware. Anxiety commonly aggravates the disturbance. About two-thirds of individuals who stutter ultimately are able to make effective use of treatment techniques and overcome the difficulty. Some individuals recover spontaneously, typically before the age of 16 years.

Epidemiology

Approximately 1% of young children stutter, and increased rates of comorbid communication disorders such as phonological disorder are often found. The male-to-female ratio is approximately 3 to 1 (American Psychiatric Association 2000). This may be secondary

TABLE 21–11. DSM-IV-TR diagnostic criteria for stuttering

A. Disturbance in the normal fluency and time patterning of speech (inappropriate for the individual's age), characterized by frequent occurrences of one or more of the following:

(1) sound and syllable repetitions

(2) sound prolongations

(3) interjections

(4) broken words (e.g., pauses within a word)

(5) audible or silent blocking (filled or unfilled pauses in speech)

(6) circumlocutions (word substitutions to avoid problematic words)

(7) words produced with an excess of physical tension

(8) monosyllabic whole-word repetitions (e.g., "I-I-I-I see him")

B. The disturbance in fluency interferes with academic or occupational achievement or with social communication.

C. If a speech–motor or sensory deficit is present, the speech difficulties are in excess of those usually associated with these problems.

Coding note: If a speech–motor or sensory deficit or a neurological condition is present, code the condition on Axis III.

to the fact that females demonstrate higher rates of recovery compared with males. The effect of stuttering on self-esteem may be linked with increased impairments in social functioning as well as academic and occupational difficulties.

Etiology

Genetic mechanisms for stuttering are strongly implicated given the strong familial association and high rates of affected first-degree relatives. Stuttering may also be acquired by stroke or degenerative disorder located in the cerebellum, basal ganglia, or cortex.

Diagnostic Evaluation

In addition to the comprehensive interview that is appropriate when concern for a communication disorder is raised, potential organic (i.e., brain-based) causes of stuttering need to be considered and ruled out. Assessments of speech, language, and hearing are needed, and referral to speech language specialist is typically made.

Treatment

Behavioral interventions are the cornerstone of treatment for stuttering. These include specific speech therapy as well as elements of relaxation, rhythm control, feedback, modification of environmental triggers, role-playing, and assertiveness training. Pharmacotherapy and psychotherapy can be considered for associated amenable symptoms (e.g., performance anxiety, self-esteem).

Pervasive Developmental Disorders

The PDDs are a heterogeneous group of neuropsychiatric disorders characterized by recognizable patterns of deviation in typical development during the first years of life. These deviations typically arise in the areas of 1) social understanding and interest, 2) communication, and 3) cognitive abilities; however, additional domains of development are frequently involved. Assessment of the affected individual is often complicated by the nonuniform degree of disruption within specific areas of development, and highly individualized profiles of abilities, interests, and difficulties are typical.

Autistic Disorder

Clinical Description

First formally described by Kanner (1943), "early infantile autism" was characterized by autistic disinterest in the social environment and obsessive insistence on sameness. Additional features included speech delay, echolalia and pronoun reversal, and unusual repetitive motor behaviors (or stereotypies). Kanner's use of the word *autism* may have unintentionally contributed to an unfortunate and long-lasting association with Bleuler's description of schizophrenia, and for decades, autism was considered by many to be the first manifestation of schizophrenia. Various terms (e.g., childhood schizophrenia, infantile or symbiotic psychosis) were used in response to prominent theories regarding autism's etiology, and numerous diagnostic criteria were put forth. In 1968, Rutter proposed four essential characteristics that emanated from the existing evidence and were present in nearly all children with autism: 1) lack of social interest and responsiveness, 2) impaired language, 3) bizarre motor behavior, and 4) onset prior to the age of 30 months. In 1980, with the development of DSM-III (American Psychiatric

Association 1980), Rutter's basic criteria predominated, and the diagnosis of infantile autism was included with the new class of "pervasive developmental disorders." In DSM-IV (American Psychiatric Association 1994), the diagnosis of autistic disorder was established via a large multisite study (Volkmar et al. 1994), and emphasis was placed on developmental aspects of the disorder. Minor adjustments to the diagnostic criteria were made in DSM-IV-TR in an attempt to facilitate clinical use (Table 21–12).

Individuals with autistic disorder may present at any age although most often in the first few years of life. Widely varying levels of relative strengths and weaknesses in specific areas of functioning are typical, and when the diagnosis co-occurs with intellectual disability (mental retardation), this intellectual profile can help to distinguish the diagnosis from the often uniform pattern of difficulties seen in intellectual disability alone. Studies have validated the diagnosis of autism in children younger than 3 years (Baird et al. 2000; Lord 1995), and (in a sample of 82 consecutive referrals) the mean child age at which parents became concerned was 19.1 months and at which they first sought professional advice was 24.1 months (DeGiacomo and Fombonne 1998). A subset of children diagnosed with autism appears to develop the characteristics after an apparently typical initial 2 years of development, although it is difficult to clarify whether these cases demonstrated subtle or unnoticed findings prior to the initial concern.

Although frequently associated with intellectual disability, the diagnoses of autistic disorder and mental retardation are distinct. Approximately two-thirds to three-fourths of individuals with autism also have intellectual disability. Clinicians should be aware that individuals with autism seem to be especially disadvantaged when it comes to performance on standardized assessments of cognitive ability due to the condition's inherent difficulties in verbal and reading comprehension, sequencing, feature extraction, and executive function. The presence of extraordinary abilities or savant skills is rare.

Social Interaction

Individuals with autistic disorder demonstrate wide ranges of interest and ability in social interaction. Kanner's (1943) original description of infantile autism, which described an aloof disinterest in others and avoidance of eye contact, represents only a portion of the autistic population. Many accurately diagnosed individuals with autistic disorder demonstrate social interest but lack the understanding necessary for typical

TABLE 21–12. DSM-IV-TR diagnostic criteria for autistic disorder

A. A total of six (or more) items from (1), (2), and (3), with at least two from (1), and one each from (2) and (3):

  (1) qualitative impairment in social interaction, as manifested by at least two of the following:

    (a) marked impairment in the use of multiple nonverbal behaviors such as eye-to-eye gaze, facial expression, body postures, and gestures to regulate social interaction

    (b) failure to develop peer relationships appropriate to developmental level

    (c) a lack of spontaneous seeking to share enjoyment, interests, or achievements with other people (e.g., by a lack of showing, bringing, or pointing out objects of interest)

    (d) lack of social or emotional reciprocity

  (2) qualitative impairments in communication as manifested by at least one of the following:

    (a) delay in, or total lack of, the development of spoken language (not accompanied by an attempt to compensate through alternative modes of communication such as gesture or mime)

    (b) in individuals with adequate speech, marked impairment in the ability to initiate or sustain a conversation with others

    (c) stereotyped and repetitive use of language or idiosyncratic language

    (d) lack of varied, spontaneous make-believe play or social imitative play appropriate to developmental level

  (3) restricted repetitive and stereotyped patterns of behavior, interests, and activities, as manifested by at least one of the following:

    (a) encompassing preoccupation with one or more stereotyped and restricted patterns of interest that is abnormal either in intensity or focus

    (b) apparently inflexible adherence to specific, nonfunctional routines or rituals

    (c) stereotyped and repetitive motor mannerisms (e.g., hand or finger flapping or twisting, or complex whole-body movements)

    (d) persistent preoccupation with parts of objects

B. Delays or abnormal functioning in at least one of the following areas, with onset prior to age 3 years: (1) social interaction, (2) language as used in social communication, or (3) symbolic or imaginative play.

C. The disturbance is not better accounted for by Rett's disorder or childhood disintegrative disorder.

reciprocal interaction. Early on there is often a lack of social referencing, and others exist solely as objects. Attachment to unusual things may be evident, whereas attachment to and affection for others typically demonstrate significant delay. Social interest may grow with time; however, a lack of reciprocity and an inability to appreciate others' perceptions may cause increasing problems with maturing peers, and frustration over friendships is common.

Communication Impairment

Individuals with autism typically demonstrate impaired verbal comprehension, delayed and unusual speech, and limited nonverbal communication. Mutism is very common among people with autism, and even in bright individuals, speech can be slow to develop (or appear to explode fully developed after a period of delay). Gestures are infrequently used. Echola-

lia, pronoun reversals, and abnormal or absent intonation can make the speech of individuals with autism difficult to understand. The subtleties of humor and imaginative or abstract thought typically remain elusive. Topics of discussion tend to be limited to areas of special interest. Often, high-functioning people with autism develop and rely on scripted bits of dialogue, which can prove surprisingly effective during superficial or initial interactions.

Patterns of Behavior

People with autism are uncommonly resistant to change, and seemingly minor alterations to an expected pattern can provoke significant distress and anxiety. This often results in the routinization of activities. Ritualized compulsive thoughts and behavior are commonplace and may be manifest in preoccupations, repetitive questioning, and physical mannerisms (e.g., hand flapping, spinning). Unusual responses to sensory stimuli are commonplace, with many people with autism becoming "overwhelmed" by sounds, smells, or levels of light that are tolerable for others or in turn tolerating (even enjoying) stimuli that nonautistic individuals find noxious. Associated physical observations often include poor motor imitation, gait and tone abnormalities, and neurological soft signs and may include hyperactivity and SIB. "Impulsivity," upon careful assessment, frequently becomes explicable in light of an understanding of the individual's special interests or anxieties.

Epidemiology

Autism appears to occur in approximately 10–20 per 10,000 births (Fombonne et al. 2006; Gillberg and Wing 1999), although widely varying prevalences have been reported (0.15–34.00 per 10,000; see Tsai 2004). Prevalences have consistently increased since the mid-1990s, and this has raised public concern. It is difficult to ascertain whether a true increase in incidence exists or whether it is a reflection of expanding awareness and ascertainment. A male predominance of approximately 4 to 1 exists, although females tend to be more severely affected and may have greater cognitive impairment. Approximately 70% have intellectual disability, although this percentage has declined in recent years, likely due to increased popular awareness of autism as well as the widening acceptance of the concept of a spectrum of dysfunction in the disorder. Early suggestions that autism is associated with higher socioeconomic class were the result of ascertainment bias.

Psychiatric comorbidities have been difficult to quantify given the significant symptom overlap between autism, mental retardation, and other psychiatric disorders. Careful consideration and, ideally, comparison with a large population of individuals with autism are necessary to distinguish, for example, the anxiety, obsessive and compulsive behaviors, or impulsivity common in autism from anxiety disorders, obsessive-compulsive disorder (OCD), and impulse-control disorders, respectively. Psychiatric diagnoses should not accumulate unless the symptoms are beyond those expected given the presence of autism and the condition warrants intervention beyond that which might be considered for autism alone. Complicating this is the necessity of recognizing nonclassical psychiatric presentations in patients with communication and/or cognitive difficulties.

Seizure disorder is more common in individuals with autism and demonstrates an apparent bimodal distribution of onset, with new seizures appearing more frequently in the first year of life and again during adolescence.

Severe environmental deprivation can result in a presentation that demonstrates many features consistent with the diagnosis; however, the extent of the presentation's reversibility and modification with appropriate intervention often distinguish this from autism.

Etiology

Certain medical conditions are associated with autism; tuberous sclerosis, fragile X syndrome, maternal rubella, congenital hypothyroidism, phenylketonuria, Down syndrome, neurofibromatosis, and Angelman's syndrome are some of the conditions that have been identified. In the vast majority of cases (likely greater than 90%), there is no readily identifiable cause for autism.

A growing body of evidence from family, twin, and chromosomal studies supports the genetic basis of autism. First-degree family members of individuals with autism have been shown to have greater-than-expected incidences of anxiety disorders, major depression, and motor tics. Additionally, parents of children with autism have been shown to have higher rates of rigidity, aloofness, anxiety, and limited friendships, part of a constellation of characteristics that has been called the "broad autism phenotype" (Piven et al. 1997). Multiple studies have shown that 2%–7% of siblings of people with autism have autism themselves. Studies have shown very high concordance for autism in monozygotic twins and relatively low concordance for dizygotic twins. Studies that have implicated chromosomal abnormalities (most frequently 7q and 15q) and numerous candidate genes require replication. These promising genetic findings have been effective in eradicating the errant belief that autism arose from deviant parenting. A rapidly expanding body of information from functional imaging studies (e.g., functional magnetic resonance imaging [fMRI]) may unite neuropsychological profiles with the neuroanatomical abnormalities that imaging studies have identified. New techniques such as diffusion tensor imaging may provide support for the "impaired neural connectivity" theory of autism. Findings that have implicated prenatal, immunological, and biochemical (e.g., serotonin, catecholamines) factors await replication or additional work to assess their significance. Despite popular concern regarding the implication of the measles-mumps-rubella vaccine or thimerosal exposure in the etiology of autism, this is not supported by the current evidence (Fombonne et al. 2006).

Course and Prognosis

Although autism is a chronic condition, most individuals demonstrate gradual improvement in their symptoms due to further maturation and understanding a need to modify their behavior. Improvement is consistently maximized when people with autism are provided adequate support, education (which can draw on individual strengths), and management of problematic symptoms or comorbidities. The amount of improvement is closely tied to symptom severity, cognitive and language ability, and the establishment of realistic expectations given the specific areas of difficulty.

Diagnostic Evaluation

Accurate diagnosis is predicated on a complete psychiatric and medical evaluation. Given the rare but recognizable medical conditions associated with autism, close attention to maternal and prenatal histories is necessary. Assessment of the person's early development requires an informed historian. Sensory evaluations (hearing, including brain-stem auditory evoked responses [if necessary] and visual screening) are often necessary. The use of standardized diagnostic assessments is not indicated for the clinical diagnosis of autistic disorder but may prove useful along with cognitive and language testing for subsequent treatment decisions. Additional clinically informed laboratory data are often gathered, often based on the age at presentation. Genetic screening for metabolic disorders, chromosome analysis, and genetic counseling in cases of intellectual disability and potentially identifiable syndromes are warranted. Heavy metal screening is appropriate if a possible history of ingestion is identified. Neurological consultation may be warranted secondary to clinical concerns regarding the presence of seizures, and electroencephalograms are often obtained. In most idiopathic cases of autism, neuroimaging is neither warranted nor currently clinically useful.

Treatment

The foundations of effective treatment in autistic disorder comprise parental counseling, child educational interventions that are tailored to an individual student's strengths and difficulties, and behavior (e.g., skill acquisition and practice in a social group) and environmental modification (e.g., the use of schedules, visual cueing, and highly structured settings). Although historically psychotherapy—even for high-functioning individuals—was discouraged, cognitive-behavioral approaches may be beneficial given the level of some individuals' interest and insight as compared with often disparate successes and facility.

There are no pharmacological treatments for autistic disorder. However, psychopharmacological interventions often play a supportive role in the treatment of some individuals. The careful selection and surveillance of appropriate target symptoms are of the utmost importance and demand close contact with families and care providers. Additionally, given the level of rigidity and resistance to change that most individuals with autism demonstrate, the seemingly inconsequential addition of a medication into a morning routine, for example, can be enough to induce significant distress. Thus, extended medication trial durations are often appropriate to ensure that the clinician is measuring a medication effect. Perhaps related to this is the clinical belief that individuals with autism often are responsive to seemingly trivial dosages of psychoactive medication. All of this serves to remind the clinician of the importance of "starting low and going slow" with medications in a population that is often limited or unusual in its ability to report benefit and side effects.

Recently, we have witnessed an increase in the amount of psychopharmacological research in developmentally disordered populations. Although a treatment for autism remains unlikely, we have the benefit of a few small studies (and ongoing active larger ones) assessing the value of certain treatments for various associated symptoms. The SSRIs, especially fluoxetine, sertraline, and citalopram, seem to be beneficial in the reduction of compulsive and repetitive behaviors, behavioral rigidity, and aggression (Posey et al. 2006). The atypical antipsychotic risperidone reduces self-injury and aggression (McCracken et al. 2002) and repetitive behaviors (McDougle et al. 2005), but caution is urged, given this drug class's characteristic weight gain and other potential and serious side effects. Other commonly prescribed medications from pediatric formulary include α-agonists targeting impulsivity and hyperactivity, stimulants for hyperactivity and poor concentration (although there are especially polarizing views regarding a role for stimulants in individuals with PDD), and anticonvulsants for serious aggression.

The value of various nutritional, dietary, and "nutriceutical" reports of benefit in autism is difficult to assess. Melatonin is often used to facilitate sleep; however, at the present time no specific interventions from these generally unscrutinized reports can be recommended.

Rett's Disorder

Clinical Description

Originally described in 1966, Rett's disorder is characterized by a period of decelerated head growth, loss of purposeful hand movements, midline upper extremity stereotypies (e.g., hand-wringing), severe psychomotor retardation, gait and truncal apraxia, impaired language, and social withdrawal. Typically diagnosed after age 3 years, the disorder exists almost exclusively in females. Associated findings include respiratory symptoms (e.g., breath holding, wakeful apnea, hyperventilation), seizures, spasticity, muscle wasting and dystonia, scoliosis, and growth retardation. Evidence of intrauterine growth retardation, perinatal brain damage, or metabolic or progressive neurological disorder excludes the diagnosis (Table 21–13).

Symptoms

Children with Rett's disorder often also have unusual sleep architecture and increased daytime, decreased nighttime, and increased total sleep. Thyroid problems, increased risk of osteoporosis, and feeding problems due to oropharyngeal abnormalities warrant clinical vigilance.

Epidemiology

Estimates of prevalence of Rett's disorder range from 0.44 to 2.10 per 10,000 females. A handful of cases in males have been reported and usually demonstrate an atypical presentation.

Etiology

Multiple different mutations in the gene encoding MECP2 at Xq28 have been identified in a large number of individuals with typical and atypical Rett's disorder (Amir et al. 1999), and nearly all appear to be spontaneous mutations.

Course and Prognosis

A four-stage model of this progressive disorder has been proposed (Hagberg and Witt-Engerström 1986):

1. Early-onset stagnation stage from age 6 months to 1.5 years, with decelerated head growth, hypotonia, and loss of interest in play
2. Rapid developmental regression stage from age 1–2 years and lasting 13–19 months, with the onset of autistic symptoms and often seizures
3. Pseudostationary stage typically occurring at age 3–4 years but may be delayed and persists for years

TABLE 21–13. DSM-IV-TR diagnostic criteria for Rett's disorder

A. All of the following:

  (1) apparently normal prenatal and perinatal development

  (2) apparently normal psychomotor development through the first 5 months after birth

  (3) normal head circumference at birth

B. Onset of all of the following after the period of normal development:

  (1) deceleration of head growth between ages 5 and 48 months

  (2) loss of previously acquired purposeful hand skills between ages 5 and 30 months with the subsequent development of stereotyped hand movements (e.g., hand-wringing or hand washing)

  (3) loss of social engagement early in the course (although often social interaction develops later)

  (4) appearance of poorly coordinated gait or trunk movements

  (5) severely impaired expressive and receptive language development with severe psychomotor retardation

to decades, with the development of characteristic respiratory abnormalities

4. Late motor deterioration stage often occurring during school age or early adolescence, with muscle wasting, weakness, scoliosis, and limb distortion; most individuals with Rett's disorder live well into adulthood (summarized from Tsai 2004)

Diagnostic Evaluation

Clinical diagnosis of Rett's disorder can be supported by molecular analysis of the gene encoding MECP2 at Xq28, although an absence of recognizable gene abnormality at this site does not refute the diagnosis.

Treatment

As is indicated for other PDDs, supportive treatment for families and individuals with Rett's disorder is indicated. Additional education modification is warranted in light of the accompanying intellectual disability. Preparation for the typically worsening physical limitations is appropriate.

Childhood Disintegrative Disorder

Clinical Description

In 1908, Heller described a series of cases of pediatric dementia with onset after age 3–4 years, during which time development had been entirely normal. Originally called *dementia infantilis,* this relatively rare syndrome consists of cognitive decline that usually stabilizes and remains static or improves minimally over time. Additional researchers have described similar presentations and developed the diagnostic term *disintegrative psychosis of childhood.* This has become childhood disintegrative disorder (Table 21–14). The validity of this diagnosis has been well demonstrated (Volkmar and Rutter 1995).

The loss of communication abilities and social functioning in these individuals mimics the presentation in autism. Initial behavioral symptoms (such as tantrums, anxiety, or irritability, sometimes appearing after a neurological illness) are sometimes present, and cognitive symptoms develop abruptly (over days to weeks) or gradually (over weeks to months) and ultimately progress to loss of cognitive ability, speech and language, and social skills. Typically individuals with childhood disintegrative disorder have higher incidences of new-onset seizures (when compared with individuals with intellectual disability alone).

Epidemiology

An incidence of 1 per 100,000 is commonly accepted, with a significant male predominance.

Etiology

No underlying cause of childhood disintegrative disorder has been identified.

Course and Prognosis

The progressive loss of abilities over days to months appears to be very consistent, with a minority of individuals experiencing persistent decline and usually death. Most experience stabilization of symptoms (with or without minimal improvement), and the prognosis becomes a product of the person's ultimate level of cognitive ability and adaptive functioning.

Diagnostic Evaluation

The diagnostic workup of childhood disintegrative disorder is similar to that in autistic disorder; however, the extent of neurological evaluation is appropriately intensified.

TABLE 21–14.   DSM-IV-TR diagnostic criteria for childhood disintegrative disorder

A. Apparently normal development for at least the first 2 years after birth as manifested by the presence of age-appropriate verbal and nonverbal communication, social relationships, play, and adaptive behavior.

B. Clinically significant loss of previously acquired skills (before age 10 years) in at least two of the following areas:

  (1) expressive or receptive language

  (2) social skills or adaptive behavior

  (3) bowel or bladder control

  (4) play

  (5) motor skills

C. Abnormalities of functioning in at least two of the following areas:

  (1) qualitative impairment in social interaction (e.g., impairment in nonverbal behaviors, failure to develop peer relationships, lack of social or emotional reciprocity)

  (2) qualitative impairments in communication (e.g., delay or lack of spoken language, inability to initiate or sustain a conversation, stereotyped and repetitive use of language, lack of varied make-believe play)

  (3) restricted, repetitive, and stereotyped patterns of behavior, interests, and activities, including motor stereotypies and mannerisms

D. The disturbance is not better accounted for by another specific pervasive developmental disorder or by schizophrenia.

Treatment

Support for families and adaptation of the psychosocial intervention recommended in autistic disorder are appropriate. A role for medications targeting specific problematic symptoms can be envisioned as being useful; however, there are few data to support this.

Asperger's Disorder

Clinical Description

While Kanner was describing early infantile autism in the United States, Asperger reported on a series of patients who demonstrated similar presentations. Similar to those with Kanner's *infantile autism,* these boys demonstrated poor social understanding and skills, intense special interests, and clumsiness but lacked language delay. Asperger referred to these patients as "little professors" (Asperger 1944/1991). The diagnosis of Asperger's disorder came to increased prominence (especially in the United States) during the 1980s. The clinical picture of individuals with Asperger's disorder is notable for the lack of intellectual disability, but as with autistic disorder, variable presentations are common (Table 21–15). The differentiation of Asperger's disorder from autism (especially in individuals with normal intelligence) can be quite difficult, and controversy exists as to whether Asperger's disorder represents a PDD subtype or the highest-functioning portion of an autistic disorder spectrum (South et al. 2005).

Impairments in social interaction and restricted and repetitive interests and behaviors are hallmarks of the disorder. Unusual communication is common, often characterized by pedantic speech, intense preoccupations, and poor or nonexistent nonverbal communication, although in distinction from autistic disorder, "clinically significant general delay in language" and "cognitive delay" are exclusionary criteria. In addition, it is commonly held that individuals with Asperger's disorder are clumsy.

Epidemiology

Prevalence rates of 0.6–10.0 per 10,000 have been published, although some of these studies lack the application of consistent diagnostic criteria. Investigation of associated psychiatric comorbidities has implicated similar diagnoses to those associated with autistic disorder; affective illness, Tourette's disorder, ADHD, anxiety disorders, and schizophrenia have all been associated with Asperger's disorder.

Etiology

The specific etiology of Asperger's disorder is unknown, although most agree that similarities to autistic disorder imply similar etiologies.

Course and Prognosis

Although the characteristics of Asperger's disorder appear to be lifelong in their duration, more recent research seems to suggest that individuals with the disorder demonstrate higher rates of employment and education and greater levels of self-sufficiency than those with autistic disorder.

TABLE 21–15. DSM-IV-TR diagnostic criteria for Asperger's disorder

A. Qualitative impairment in social interaction, as manifested by at least two of the following:
 (1) marked impairment in the use of multiple nonverbal behaviors such as eye-to-eye gaze, facial expression, body postures, and gestures to regulate social interaction
 (2) failure to develop peer relationships appropriate to developmental level
 (3) a lack of spontaneous seeking to share enjoyment, interests, or achievements with other people (e.g., by a lack of showing, bringing, or pointing out objects of interest to other people)
 (4) lack of social or emotional reciprocity

B. Restricted repetitive and stereotyped patterns of behavior, interests, and activities, as manifested by at least one of the following:
 (1) encompassing preoccupation with one or more stereotyped and restricted patterns of interest that is abnormal in either intensity or focus
 (2) apparently inflexible adherence to specific, nonfunctional routines or rituals
 (3) stereotyped and repetitive motor mannerisms (e.g., hand or finger flapping or twisting, or complex whole-body movements)
 (4) persistent preoccupation with parts of objects

C. The disturbance causes clinically significant impairment in social, occupational, or other important areas of functioning.

D. There is no clinically significant general delay in language (e.g., single words used by age 2 years, communicative phrases used by age 3 years).

E. There is no clinically significant delay in cognitive development or in the development of age-appropriate self-help skills, adaptive behavior (other than in social interaction), and curiosity about the environment in childhood.

F. Criteria are not met for another specific pervasive developmental disorder or schizophrenia.

Diagnostic Evaluation

The evaluation does not differ significantly from that recommended in autistic disorder. Given the exclusionary criteria of the diagnosis, careful attention to the individual's history of cognitive and language development is necessary.

Treatment

As in autistic disorder, appropriate recognition of the profile of the individual's strengths and difficulties will guide intervention. Cognitive approaches in individual therapy can be beneficial for interested and motivated people. Pharmacological interventions target similar behavioral symptoms to those described for autism.

Attention-Deficit/ Hyperactivity Disorder

Clinical Description

ADHD is defined by three core symptom clusters: inattention, hyperactivity, and impulsivity (Table 21–16). DSM-IV-TR divides ADHD into three types according to the presence or absence of six symptoms in each category. These are primarily inattentive type, primarily hyperactive–impulsive type, and combined type (for those with symptoms in both categories). Some symptoms must be present prior to age 7 years and must occur for at least 6 months in more than one setting. They must cause clinically significant impairment in social, academic, or occupational functioning and be inconsistent for developmental age and intellectual ability (American Psychiatric Association 2000).

Individuals with ADHD have poorer academic performance and higher rates of LDs than other children. As a result of their academic struggles, they often need tutoring or special classroom placement. They may also need to repeat a grade. They have difficulties in executive functioning as demonstrated by poor planning and deficits in working memory, verbal fluency, and motor sequencing. Additional impairments of executive functioning include an inability to attend, encode, and manipulate information as well as an inability to organize and manage a sequence of actions. These children are often rejected by peers as a result of their impulsive and hyperactive behaviors. This rejection has a strong relationship with poor outcomes such as conduct disturbance, substance abuse, and school failure.

The inattentive subtype shows deficits in focused and selective attention. These children tend to be less active and may have more anxiety and somatic complaints than those with the combined or hyperactive–impulsive type. They have higher rates of LDs as well. On the other hand, children with the combined type have deficits in sustained attention and distractibility. They frequently have more externalizing behaviors, show increased aggression and delinquency, and are more likely to be diagnosed with a comorbid disruptive behavior disorder.

Epidemiology

DSM-IV-TR estimates rates of ADHD to be between 3% and 7% in school-age children, although it has been reported to range from 1.9% to 14.4% (Scahill and Schwab-Stone 2000). Its prevalence varies with different treatment settings and is most common in school-age children. Higher IQ can often compensate for the impairments of ADHD and may lead to a later diagnosis. ADHD accounts for 30%–50% of referrals for mental health services for children (Multimodal Treatment of ADHD Cooperative Group 1999).

Teachers identify fewer girls than boys with ADHD symptoms, and the combined type is the most common subtype in both girls and boys. The disorder is more common in males than females, at a ratio of 4 to 1 (Gershorn 2002), although this decreases to 2 to 1 for the predominantly inattentive type (Wolraich et al. 1996). Interestingly, even among children meeting criteria for any subtype of ADHD, fewer girls than boys receive an ADHD diagnosis or stimulant treatment.

Approximately 4% of college-age students and adults have ADHD, with a gender ratio of 1 to 1 (Wilens and Dodson 2004). Anywhere from 4% to 75% of cases persist to adulthood (Fischer 1997; Hechtman 1993). This wide range is likely secondary to methodological differences in the studies. Family history of ADHD, psychosocial adversity, and comorbidity with conduct, mood, and anxiety disorders increase the risk of persistence of ADHD symptoms (Biederman et al. 1996). The gender ratio in adults is approximately 1 to 1. Rates of the disorder may vary across cultures, countries, and settings (urban, suburban, or rural) (Shen et al. 1985; Verhulst et al. 1993; Zahner et al. 1993).

ADHD is highly comorbid with other psychiatric disorders (Table 21–17). Up to two-thirds of individuals with ADHD have another comorbid psychiatric disorder such as disruptive behavior disorders, mood or anxiety disorders, LDs, language disorders, mental retardation, borderline intellectual functioning, PDDs, and psychotic disorders. Other disruptive behaviors occur with high frequency—50% with ODD and 30%–50% with CD. Additionally, 15%–20% may have a mood disorder, and another 20–25% may have a co-occurring anxiety disorder that may affect the overall degree of impairment (Biederman et al. 1991; Jensen et al. 1993; Newcorn and Halperin 1994). Children with both ADHD and CD often have greater disability and a longer persistence of symptoms than children with either disorder alone. A high frequency of tic disorders and ADHD has led to the question of possible genetic relationship between these disorders (Comings and Comings 1990). Speech and language delays are com-

TABLE 21–16. **DSM-IV-TR diagnostic criteria for attention-deficit/hyperactivity disorder**

A. Either (1) or (2):

(1) six (or more) of the following symptoms of **inattention** have persisted for at least 6 months to a degree that is maladaptive and inconsistent with developmental level:

Inattention

(a) often fails to give close attention to details or makes careless mistakes in schoolwork, work, or other activities

(b) often has difficulty sustaining attention in tasks or play activities

(c) often does not seem to listen when spoken to directly

(d) often does not follow through on instructions and fails to finish schoolwork, chores, or duties in the workplace (not due to oppositional behavior or failure to understand instructions)

(e) often has difficulty organizing tasks and activities

(f) often avoids, dislikes, or is reluctant to engage in tasks that require sustained mental effort (such as schoolwork or homework)

(g) often loses things necessary for tasks or activities (e.g., toys, school assignments, pencils, books, or tools)

(h) is often easily distracted by extraneous stimuli

(i) is often forgetful in daily activities

(2) six (or more) of the following symptoms of **hyperactivity-impulsivity** have persisted for at least 6 months to a degree that is maladaptive and inconsistent with developmental level:

Hyperactivity

(a) often fidgets with hands or feet or squirms in seat

(b) often leaves seat in classroom or in other situations in which remaining seated is expected

(c) often runs about or climbs excessively in situations in which it is inappropriate (in adolescents or adults, may be limited to subjective feelings of restlessness)

(d) often has difficulty playing or engaging in leisure activities quietly

(e) is often "on the go" or often acts as if "driven by a motor"

(f) often talks excessively

Impulsivity

(g) often blurts out answers before questions have been completed

(h) often has difficulty awaiting turn

(i) often interrupts or intrudes on others (e.g., butts into conversations or games)

B. Some hyperactive–impulsive or inattentive symptoms that caused impairment were present before age 7 years.

C. Some impairment from the symptoms is present in two or more settings (e.g., at school [or work] and at home).

D. There must be clear evidence of clinically significant impairment in social, academic, or occupational functioning.

E. The symptoms do not occur exclusively during the course of a pervasive developmental disorder, schizophrenia, or other psychotic disorder and are not better accounted for by another mental disorder (e.g., mood disorder, anxiety disorder, dissociative disorder, or a personality disorder).

Code based on type:

314.01   Attention-deficit/hyperactivity disorder, combined type: if both criteria A1 and A2 are met for the past 6 months

314.00   Attention-deficit/hyperactivity disorder, predominantly inattentive type: if criterion A1 is met but criterion A2 is not met for the past 6 months

314.01   Attention-deficit/hyperactivity disorder, predominantly hyperactive–impulsive type: if criterion A2 is met but criterion A1 is not met for the past 6 months

Coding note: For individuals (especially adolescents and adults) who currently have symptoms that no longer meet full criteria, "in partial remission" should be specified.

TABLE 21–17. Psychiatric disorders often associated with attention-deficit/hyperactivity disorder

Conduct disorder

Oppositional defiant disorder

Anxiety disorders

Learning disorders

Motor skills disorder

Substance use disorders

Communication disorders

Bipolar disorder

Major depression

Posttraumatic stress disorder

Obsessive-compulsive disorder

Tourette's disorder

Schizophrenia

Mental retardation

Pervasive developmental disorders, including autistic disorder

Note. Various psychiatric states should be assessed clinically in individuals with attention-deficit/hyperactivity disorder, even though strong statistical associations have not been shown for each of these conditions.

Source. American Psychiatric Association 2000.

mon in children with ADHD. LDs may occur in 10%–25% of those with ADHD, although in general children with ADHD with or without a formal LD perform more poorly academically than those without ADHD (Faraone et al. 1993). In adolescents, ADHD may also be associated with substance use disorders, CDs, and mood and anxiety disorders. Adults with ADHD are most commonly at risk for comorbid depression, anxiety, and substance use disorders (Spencer et al. 1999).

It is important to remember that symptoms of inattention and impulsivity are not equivalent to a diagnosis of ADHD. A variety of disorders can be mistaken for ADHD (Table 21–18). Additionally, other medical disorders can present with the symptoms of inattention, hyperactivity, or impulsivity. It is essential that the clinician be vigilant and rule out any underlying causes of illness. Physical causes of inattention include impaired vision or hearing, sequelae of head trauma, seizures, acute or chronic medical illness, poor sleep, and poor nutrition. Various drugs, including pseudoephedrine, carbamazepine, benzodiazepines, and theophylline, may cause symptoms of ADHD.

Differentiating ADHD from bipolar disorder in children may be particularly challenging. There is significant symptom overlap (distractibility, impulsivity, hyperactivity, mood swings, irritability), and it is imperative the clinician make every effort to differentiate these disorders (Table 21–19). Distinguishing characteristics of bipolar disorder include grandiosity, elevated mood, and a decreased need for sleep. A true family history of bipolar disorder aids in this diagnosis. Helpful distinguishing characteristics of ADHD may be younger age at onset, sustained clinical course, and family history. The presence of both ADHD and bipolar disorder signals a very serious prognosis with high risk for hospitalization, suicide, and chronic psychosocial and psychiatric disability.

Etiology

ADHD is a heterogeneous behavioral disorder with multiple possible etiologies. A number of biological and environmental factors have been implicated.

Genetics

ADHD is a highly familial disorder, with 25%–50% of cases occurring in families. Among first-degree relatives of children with ADHD, 15%–25% have the disorder, and up to 50% of children whose parents have the disorder also have ADHD (Wilens and Dodson 2004). Adoption studies confirm the greater frequency of ADHD in first-degree biological relatives of adopted probands than in adoptive families (Hechtman 1994). Concordance is higher in first-degree relatives than in half-siblings and higher in monozygotic than in dizygotic twins. There may be several genes involved in ADHD, and their effects are cumulative. Abnormalities in genes coding for proteins in the central nervous dopamine function have been implicated (Gainetdinov and Caron 2001). The specific genes associated with ADHD include the dopamine receptor gene, the dopamine transporter gene, and the dopamine-beta-hydroxylase gene (Wilens and Dodson 2004).

Neuroanatomical and Neurochemical Factors

Although the specific pathophysiology of ADHD remains unclear, recent research on the neural circuits of the prefrontal cortex and striatum, as well as on the brain-stem catecholamine systems that innervate these circuits, has advanced our understanding of the possible underlying mechanisms of this disorder. Neuroimaging studies have suggested that impair-

TABLE 21–18. Differential diagnosis of attention-deficit/hyperactivity disorder (ADHD)

Psychiatric

Conduct disorder
Oppositional defiant disorder
Major depression
Anxiety (situational, developmental)
Separation anxiety disorder
Posttraumatic stress disorder
Panic disorder
Phobic disorder
Dissociative disorders
Bipolar disorder
Early schizophrenia
Psychotic agitation
Substance use disorders (intoxication or withdrawal)
Attention-seeking or manipulative behavior

Psychosocial

Physical or sexual abuse
Neglect
Boredom
Overstimulation
Sociocultural deprivation

Medical

Thyroid disorders
Drug-induced agitation
Recreational stimulants
Medical stimulants: pseudoephedrine
Barbiturates, benzodiazepines
Carbamazepine
Theophylline

Extreme prenatal or perinatal problem (rare)

Brain damage (following trauma or infection)
Lead poisoning (postnatal toxicity)
Teratogenic effect of exposure to alcohol, cocaine, lead, probably cigarette smoke

Dietary

Excessive caffeine

Hunger

Constipation

Minor persistent pain

Normal behavior

Note. Various etiological factors give rise to ADHD or to conditions that look like ADHD. ADHD look-alike disorders may be more clinically appropriate diagnoses for individual patients than ADHD, and some look-alikes may be better diagnosed as comorbid conditions with ADHD. Because of the common co-occurrence of ADHD and ADHD look-alike conditions, all of these disorders and some etiological conditions that give rise to them must be considered in the differential diagnosis of ADHD. In clinical practice, all of the factors listed in the table (disorders, symptoms, situations, and states) should be considered—either identified or ruled out—before a firm diagnosis of ADHD is made. In effect, ADHD is a "diagnosis of exclusion"—a diagnosis that is made by the exclusion of other factors.

Source. Reprinted from American Psychiatric Association: *Diagnostic and Statistical Manual of Mental Disorders,* 4th Edition, Text Revision. Washington, DC, American Psychiatric Association, 2000. Used with permission.

TABLE 21–19. Differentiating attention-deficit/hyperactivity disorder (ADHD) from bipolar affective disorder

ADHD	Shared characteristics	Bipolar affective disorder
Family history of ADHD	Distractibility	Grandiosity
Younger age at onset	Impulsivity	Decreased need for sleep
Sustained clinical course	Hyperactivity	Elevated mood
	Mood swings	Family history
	Irritability	Episodic clinical course

ments in prefrontal-striatal regions play a central role in the pathophysiology of ADHD. Structural imaging studies using magnetic resonance imaging (MRI) have revealed subtle but unique anomalies in the prefrontal cortex and basal ganglia of children with ADHD. Other anomalies found in children with ADHD include smaller right prefrontal cortex, caudate nucleus, and globus pallidus (Castellanos et al. 2003) as well as a smaller anterior genu of the corpus callosum (Hynd et al. 1991), reduced white matter in the parietal-occip-

ital region (Filipek et al. 1997), and a smaller posterior vermis of the cerebellum (Motofsky et al. 1998). Functional imaging, including fMRI, single photon emission computed tomography, and positron emission tomography, has supported lower basal activity in prefrontal cortex and striatum in children and adults with ADHD (Rubia et al. 1999), although not in adolescents (Zametkin et al. 1993). These areas of the brain are highly sensitive to catecholamine input, including norepinephrine and dopamine, and therefore these catecholamines may play a central role in the patho-physiology of ADHD. Although no clear evidence of noradrenergic dysfunction has been reported to date, findings have suggested that children with ADHD may show abnormalities in dopamine function in the central nervous system (Ernst et al. 1999).

Other Medical Illness

Although an increased risk of ADHD has been reported in a rare genetic disorder of generalized resistance to thyroid hormone (Hauser et al. 1993), the rate of thyroid abnormalities in children with ADHD is very low (Elia et al. 1994). There is no evidence to support routine screening of thyroid function in children with ADHD without other indicators of thyroid disease. There may be increased rates of ADHD in children with a history of recurrent ear infections and acquired sensorineural hearing loss (Elia et al. 1994; Kelly et al. 1993). However, there does not appear to be evidence to support the idea that children with allergies or allergic-type illness such as asthma or eczema have higher rates of ADHD (Biederman et al. 1994; McGee et al. 1993).

Prenatal and Perinatal Factors

Exposure to toxins during pregnancy may contribute to the development of ADHD. Maternal smoking during pregnancy is associated with higher rates of ADHD in offspring, possibly linked to increased fetal testosterone (Rizwan et al. 2007). Children exposed to lead and alcohol during pregnancy can manifest many symptoms of inattention, hyperactivity, and impulsivity. Perinatal complications may also play a role in the development of ADHD. Retrospective studies comparing human subjects with ADHD and those without the disorder found higher rates of antepartum hemorrhage, prolonged labor, and low Apgar scores (Chandola et al. 1992). Children with low birth weight and white matter injury may be at increased risk for development of ADHD as well (Whitaker et al. 1997). Animal model studies have found that asphyxiation at or near birth leads to overactivity and attentional problems (Sechzer et al. 1973; Speiser et al. 1983), although the correlation to human behavior is not certain.

Diet

The role of preservatives, artificial dyes, or food allergies on hyperactivity and impulsivity remains controversial, with studies both supporting and refuting their importance (Barling and Bullen 1985; Egger et al. 1992; K.S. Rowe and Rowe 1994).

Diagnostic Evaluation

The clinical evaluation of ADHD requires multiple sources and types of diagnostic information. Parent and child interviews are supplemented with information from school reports, teacher and parent rating scales, neuropsychological data as indicated, and direct clinical observation. Although there is no simple physical finding or laboratory test that will aid in the diagnosis of ADHD, it is important to rule out other medical causes of inattention and impulsivity.

Interviews and Rating Scales

Diagnosing ADHD in children and adolescents is complicated by the fact that signs may not be directly observable. In a highly structured or novel setting or in a setting with one-to-one supervision or frequent rewards for positive behavior, a child with ADHD may not appear to be inattentive or hyperactive–impulsive. Some children and most adolescents are able to maintain attention in an office setting. Conversely, symptoms of this disorder typically worsen in situations that are unstructured or minimally supervised (American Psychiatric Association 2000). Therefore, multiple sources are necessary for diagnosis. The child interview is best done with a flexible approach that allows for exploration of presenting symptoms. Additional, more structured questioning may be necessary to review symptoms of ADHD and its common comorbidities. Many children lack insight into their behavioral problems or are unable or unwilling to report their symptoms. It is generally held that parents are better reporters of externalizing behaviors, and children are better reporters of internalizing symptoms (American Academy of Child and Adolescent Psychiatry 1997).

The parent interview is the core of the diagnostic assessment, and the diagnosis is more valid when based on parental report (Pelham et al. 1992). Parental report may, however, be influenced by parental psychopathology, the presence of comorbid CD in children, and/or cultural factors (Abikoff et al. 1993; Fergusson et al. 1993). Parent and teacher reports of child behavioral problems and individual child self-report are very different. Although teachers and parents generally agree if a child is at risk, the correlation between their reports is low, likely due to the different environments in which they observe the child. The most commonly used scales are also the best normed and validated. They include the Child Behavior Checklist, the Teacher Report Form of the Child Behavior Checklist, the Conners Parent and Teacher Forms, the Attention Deficit With Hyperactivity Comprehensive Teacher

Rating Scale, and the Barkley Home Situations. Identification of behavioral disorders in children is significantly correlated between structured interviews and dimensional scales (Jensen et al. 1993). Structured interviews such as the Diagnostic Interview Schedule for Children continue to be used mainly in research. Although these measures are less useful in identifying ADHD symptoms, they may be helpful in identifying comorbid or alternative diagnoses. Additional scales such as the Conners abbreviated form and the Child Attention Problems Rating Scale are commonly used to assess the patient's response to medication.

Testing

Although there is no specific neuropsychological test for ADHD, testing may provide additional information helpful in establishing a diagnosis and treatment plan. Information from cognitive or educational testing may assist the examiner in providing perspective on level of cognitive or attentional functioning as well as assessing for mental retardation or LDs. This information is essential for developing a treatment plan.

Language disorders may present with inattention, restlessness, or motor hyperactivity. Partial loss of vision or hearing may present similarly. Therefore, screening for these impairments is warranted. In special circumstances, occupational or recreational evaluations may provide supplementary information regarding motor clumsiness or adaptive skills (American Academy of Child and Adolescent Psychiatry 1997).

Medical Evaluation

Children with ADHD should have a complete medical evaluation and physical examination. Originally termed *minimal brain dysfunction,* ADHD has been associated with subtle signs of abnormal brain function such as neurological soft signs (asymmetric reflexes, inability to perform rapid alternating movements, minor choreoathetoid movements) and poor motor coordination (Ornoy et al. 1993; Vitiello et al. 1990). However, these soft neurological signs do not aid in diagnosing ADHD and may be more often associated with anxiety disorders. Although there is evidence both supporting and refuting psychostimulants' effects on growth, height and weight should be measured prior to initiating treatment with a psychostimulant and periodically during the course of treatment (Charach et al. 2006; Spencer et al. 2006; Zachor et al. 2006). These medications may cause a temporary delay in weight gain. Baseline blood pressure and pulse should be obtained, especially if considering treatment with a psychostimulant (see Chapter 36 in this volume, "Treatment of Children and Adolescents," by Crawford et al.). Thyroid function tests are indicated only in the presence of clinical findings of hyperthyroidism or hypothyroidism, goiter, family history of thyroid disease, or decreased growth velocity. There are no clear data to support the routine measurement of zinc levels in these children (Arnold and DiSilvestro 2005). Although lead poisoning has been associated with cognitive and behavioral disturbances, it only accounted for 1% of the variance once psychosocial factors were controlled for. As a result, lead levels should be obtained only as clinically indicated. Routine electroencephalogram, computed tomography, or MRI scanning is not warranted as part of the diagnostic workup for ADHD unless there is clinical concern for seizures or other neurological disorders.

Course and Prognosis

Some behaviors characteristic of ADHD are observable by the preschool years. Hyperactive and impulsive behaviors usually predate reports of inattention, although inattention frequently is not noted until the child faces the increased demands of elementary school. ADHD is a chronic and enduring disorder, with most of those referred for treatment as children experiencing impairment through adolescence. Up to 65% of children continue to have features of ADHD into adulthood (American Academy of Child and Adolescent Psychiatry 1997). Several studies have found that most hyperactive and impulsive symptoms remit by the time patients reach adulthood, although symptoms of inattention tend to remain. A family history of ADHD, psychosocial adversity, and comorbidity with conduct, mood, and anxiety disorders increase the risk for persistence of ADHD symptoms.

Complications of the disorder include lower academic and professional achievement and increased risk of antisocial behaviors and substance abuse. Some studies indicate those with inattention more often have educational difficulties, and those with hyperactivity and impulsivity have a greater risk for the development of conduct problems. People with ADHD have an increased risk of injury because of their decreased perception of danger. Impairment in adults is most often the result of inattention, disorganization (poor executive functioning), and impulsivity. Additionally, ADHD may affect sexual behavior, with studies showing adults with ADHD having more children at a young age but with only half of them retaining custody of these children. High levels of impulsivity lead to increased risk for sexually transmitted diseases (Table 21–20).

TABLE 21–20. Secondary effects of attention-deficit/hyperactivity disorder

Low self-esteem

Compromised social skills

More school failure

More changes in residence

More cigarette, marijuana, and alcohol use

More traffic violations and car accidents

More court appearances and felony convictions

Increased risk of sexually transmitted disease

Source.   Spencer et al. 1999; Wilens and Dodson 2004.

TABLE 21–21. Positive effects of psychostimulant treatment

Reduced core symptoms of hyperactivity, impulsivity, inattention

Improved parent–child interactions

Improved on-task behaviors

Improved short-term memory

Improved reaction time

Improved math computation and problem solving

Source.   American Academy of Child and Adolescent Psychiatry 2002.

Treatment

Treatment of ADHD includes both nonpharmacological and pharmacological interventions. The central role of medication for treatment of ADHD was described in the landmark National Institute of Mental Health–funded Multimodal Treatment of ADHD study (Multimodal Treatment of ADHD Cooperative Group 1999). In this study, children ages 7–9 years with ADHD, combined type, were randomized to receive medication (primarily psychostimulants), psychosocial interventions (parent training, intensive summer treatment program, and school consultation), the combined medication and psychosocial treatments, or standard community care. This study suggests that subjects receiving the combination of medication and psychosocial intervention fared only slightly better than those receiving medication alone.

Medication

Psychostimulants.   The psychostimulants are one of the oldest and most established psychopharmacological treatments of ADHD. They have demonstrated efficacy in numerous double-blind, placebo-controlled trials of children and adults. Psychostimulants reduce symptoms of ADHD, including inattention, impulsivity, and hyperactivity. Psychostimulants have been shown to improve symptoms of ADHD in the presence of other comorbid psychiatric disorders. They may also improve symptoms of CD and anxiety disorder. Additionally, the psychostimulants are thought to improve parent–child interactions, on-task behaviors, and compliance. Other positive effects include improved peer nomination rankings of social standing and increased attention during sports activities. Psy-

chostimulants improve short-term memory, reaction time, math computation, problem solving, and sustained attention (American Academy of Child and Adolescent Psychiatry 2002; Table 21–21).

Most hyperactive children improve with psychostimulant medication, although this response is not diagnostic of the disorder. Although most data come primarily from studies of hyperactive boys, the core symptoms of ADHD in girls appear to respond similarly to this class of medication. Psychostimulant medication generally remains effective over many years; however, a small subset of patients may develop tolerance to a medication after several months of treatment. These patients who do not have additional psychiatric or medical illness to account for the diminished therapeutic effect of the psychostimulant will frequently respond to an alternate psychostimulant.

Some individuals with ADHD do not respond to psychostimulants. In some cases, symptoms of a comorbid disorder such as an anxiety disorder, bipolar disorder, or psychotic disorder may be exacerbated by these medications. Patients with neurodevelopmental or other neurological disorders may be particularly sensitive to treatment and may have adverse or paradoxical effects even at low dosages.

Methylphenidate is a short-acting agent that generally requires several daily doses. It is approved by the U.S. Food and Drug Administration (FDA) for children to age 6 years, although there are several published reports finding methylphenidate effective in younger children. Dexmethylphenidate hydrochloride (Focalin) is the *d-threo*-enantiomer of short-acting racemic methylphenidate and is currently approved for treatment of ADHD (Wigal et al. 2004). The development of long-acting methylphenidate agents such as Concerta, Metadate CD, and Ritalin LA has allowed for improved benefit from once-daily dosing and eliminated the need for midday dosing at school. It also seems to have decreased the incidence of rebound—a phenomenon often seen in shorter-acting preparations in which symptom exacerbation occurs prior to administration of the next dose.

Dextroamphetamine and mixed amphetamine salts (Adderall) are additional psychostimulants used in the treatment of ADHD. The short-acting amphetamines have a slightly longer half-life than methylphenidate but still require multiple daily doses. The dextroamphetamine preparations are FDA-approved for ADHD treatment in children as young as 3 years. Longer-acting preparations include dextroamphetamine spansules and Adderall XR. Like the longer-acting methylphenidate formulations, these allow for once-daily dosing and a decrease in rebound effects.

Magnesium pemoline, although effective, has been associated with potential life-threatening hepatic failure and is no longer recommended even for second- or third-line treatment of ADHD.

The mechanism of action of psychostimulants is not entirely clear but likely augments dopaminergic and adrenergic activity in the central nervous system. Side effects of the psychostimulants are generally mild and may include delayed sleep, decreased appetite, weight loss, stomachache, headache, minor increases in blood pressure and heart rate, tremor, cognitive overfocus, and irritability. In healthy people, the most serious adverse effects of psychostimulants include psychosis and the development or exacerbation of tics. Although psychostimulants have been known to decrease the seizure threshold, there is no evidence to show increased seizure activity with their use. Psychostimulants do not cause addiction, and in fact, children with ADHD treated with stimulants are less likely to abuse substances than other children with ADHD. Psychostimulants may cause reduced or slowed height and weight gain, although no long-term adverse effects on final adult height are apparent. The decrease in weight gain is small, and the effects on height may be minimized through the use of "drug holidays" on weekends or school holidays.

Atomoxetine. Atomoxetine (Strattera) is the first nonstimulant medication FDA-approved for the treatment of ADHD in children and adolescents. It is used as the first line and in treatment-refractory cases. Sometimes it is chosen for treatment of individuals with substance use disorders because of its low potential for abuse. Isolated cases of reversible liver failure have been reported, although these have not affected practice recommendations.

Tricyclic antidepressants. Tricyclic antidepressants (TCAs) can treat core symptoms of ADHD, although they are less effective than psychostimulants in addressing inattention. Low dosages are effective for once-daily administration. However, sudden cardiac death reported in five children and adolescents treated with desipramine (Popper and Elliott 1990; Riddle et al. 1991) has led to concern about use of TCAs in nonlethal disorders such as ADHD. Several of the patients who died had preexisting cardiovascular risks. TCAs may be considered for those who do not respond to psychostimulants, those who develop depression, or those who have a tic disorder.

Alpha-agonists. α-Adrenergic agonists such as clonidine and guanfacine have some evidence to support their use in the treatment of ADHD. However, they remain third-line agents due to a lack of replicated double-blind, placebo-controlled trials. In general, α-agonists are able to treat the core symptoms of impulsivity and hyperactivity but are typically less effective than psychostimulants in treating inattention. They may be especially helpful in treating patients with ADHD and comorbid tic or Tourette's disorder (Chappell et al. 1995; Scahill et al. 2001). Additionally, they have been used to treat associated aggression or insomnia. Side effects include drowsiness, hypotension, and bradycardia. Clonidine should be tapered, because sudden discontinuation may cause rebound hypertension and tachycardia.

Other medications. Bupropion has been helpful in treatment of ADHD in children and adults, although it may worsen tics in children with tic disorders (Spencer et al. 1993). Monoamine oxidase inhibitors have also been effective, although the risk of hypertensive crisis with dietary noncompliance limits their use. Antipsychotics appear to be effective in treating symptoms of ADHD, but the risks of neurological and metabolic side effects make this class of medicines best suited for treatment of patients with severe illness that has been refractory to other interventions. A recent double-blind, placebo-controlled trial found modafinil to be effective and well tolerated in the treatment of ADHD in children (Biederman et al. 2006).

Psychosocial Interventions

For accurate diagnosis and effective treatment, the physician must coordinate all aspects of treatment. Medication; psychoeducation of patients, families, and teachers; and consistent communication with families and schools comprise the core aspects of treatment for ADHD. More intensive psychosocial interventions are commonly used, although their efficacy remains to be validated and their use may be of greater benefit to patients with comorbid disorders or those whose symptoms do not normalize with medication treatment alone. Although medications address the core symptoms of inattention, hyperactivity, and impulsivity, it may be helpful in some cases to include environmental modifications at home and school to treat the behavioral symptoms of the disorder. Disabilities in academic and social spheres may benefit from specific skill development. Adjunctive psychotherapy can address relationship or peer difficulties that are often seen in this population (American Academy of Child and Adolescent Psychiatry 1997; Swanson et al. 1993).

ADHD Summary

ADHD is a common disorder that is well studied, particularly in children. There is strong evidence to support that ADHD has biological underpinnings as well as important environmental influences that affect its presentation and course of illness. Core symptoms of inattention, impulsivity, and hyperactivity often result in poor academic or work performance as well as relational difficulties and low self-esteem. Hyperactivity and impulsivity frequently remit by adulthood, although inattentive symptoms tend to remain. ADHD is highly comorbid and appears to be an enduring condition in some patients. Effective treatments are available with medication as the central component. Psychostimulants are safe and well tolerated in most individuals. In uncomplicated cases, research has shown little benefit of the addition of psychosocial interventions to treatment with psychostimulants. In the future, research will describe the underlying pathophysiology of the disorder and perhaps better define its subtypes. Greater understanding of this complex disorder will allow for better treatment interventions and outcomes for patients.

Disruptive Behavior Disorders

The classification of CD and ODD together within the disruptive behavior disorders is controversial due to the wide range of possible etiologies and presentations and the unclear relationship between these two diagnoses.

Conduct Disorder

Clinical Description

CD is among the most frequently made and probably overused diagnoses in child psychiatry. Despite this, many individuals with this disorder are probably undertreated. *Conduct disorder* describes a pattern of behavior that demonstrates disregard for societal norms and the rights of others. Subtyping based on the individual's age of initial symptom presentation helps determine prognosis. Severity is based on the number of symptoms and the amount of harm induced. Numerous questionably related symptoms are listed in the diagnostic schema and range in gravity from curfew violations to rape (Table 21–22).

The importance of differentiating CD from other delinquent behavior is underappreciated. Recognizing adaptive or subcultural delinquency in specific sociocultural environments is important for accurate diagnosis (Popper et al. 2003). The absence of impulsivity is a hallmark of the diagnosis (Halperin et al. 1995); its presence likely indicates comorbid psychiatric disorder.

Epidemiology

The prevalence of CD has been estimated to be between 1% and 10%, with variable reports attributable to differing detection methods and diagnostic criteria (e.g., clinical interviews vs. arrests) and varying populations. A male predominance is accepted and ranges from 2 to 1 to 4 to 1, with the child-onset subtype demonstrating especially greater male predominance.

In most cases CD is comorbid with additional psychiatric disorders, and this contributes to the lack of clear epidemiological evidence for the disorder. ADHD is frequently present and contributes to more severe aggression and antisocial behavior (J.L. Walker et al. 1987). Major and minor mood symptoms and cognitive difficulties, including LDs and substance use disorders, are frequently comorbid, and prevalence rates in excess of 50% have been reported for all these conditions in individuals with CD.

Etiology

The interplay of biological, psychological, and social factors contributes to the development of the disruptive behavior disorders. It has been suggested that the common co-occurrence of CD, ODD, and ADHD results from shared genetic influences, although each distinct disorder maintains unique genetic factors (Dick et al. 2005). Genetic factors have also been strongly associated with aspects of antisocial person-

TABLE 21–22. DSM-IV-TR diagnostic criteria for conduct disorder

A. A repetitive and persistent pattern of behavior in which the basic rights of others or major age-appropriate societal norms or rules are violated, as manifested by the presence of three (or more) of the following criteria in the past 12 months, with at least one criterion present in the past 6 months:

Aggression to people and animals

(1) often bullies, threatens, or intimidates others

(2) often initiates physical fights

(3) has used a weapon that can cause serious physical harm to others (e.g., a bat, brick, broken bottle, knife, gun)

(4) has been physically cruel to people

(5) has been physically cruel to animals

(6) has stolen while confronting a victim (e.g., mugging, purse snatching, extortion, armed robbery)

(7) has forced someone into sexual activity

Destruction of property

(8) has deliberately engaged in fire setting with the intention of causing serious damage

(9) has deliberately destroyed others' property (other than by fire setting)

Deceitfulness or theft

(10) has broken into someone else's house, building, or car

(11) often lies to obtain goods or favors or to avoid obligations (i.e., "cons" others)

(12) has stolen items of nontrivial value without confronting a victim (e.g., shoplifting, but without breaking and entering; forgery)

Serious violations of rules

(13) often stays out at night despite parental prohibitions, beginning before age 13 years

(14) has run away from home overnight at least twice while living in parental or parental surrogate home (or once without returning for a lengthy period)

(15) is often truant from school, beginning before age 13 years

B. The disturbance in behavior causes clinically significant impairment in social, academic, or occupational functioning.

C. If the individual is age 18 years or older, criteria are not met for antisocial personality disorder.

Code based on age at onset:

312.81 **Conduct disorder, childhood-onset type:** onset of at least one criterion characteristic of conduct disorder prior to age 10 years

312.82 **Conduct disorder, adolescent-onset type:** absence of any criteria characteristic of conduct disorder prior to age 10 years

312.89 **Conduct disorder, unspecified onset:** age at onset is not known

Specify severity:

Mild: few if any conduct problems in excess of those required to make the diagnosis **and** conduct problems cause only minor harm to others

Moderate: number of conduct problems and effect on others intermediate between "mild" and "severe"

Severe: many conduct problems in excess of those required to make the diagnosis **or** conduct problems cause considerable harm to others

ality and traits that likely contribute to CD, such as aggressiveness, novelty seeking, and inattention (Hendren and Mullen 2006). Specific genes responsible for the serotonin transporter (Seeger et al. 2001), the 5-HT_{1B} receptor (Soyka et al. 2004), and adrenergic func-

tion (Comings et al. 2000) have been associated with conduct problems in children. Despite common assumptions about the role of hormones in adolescent behavioral changes, relatively few studies have examined this relationship. Interestingly, although elevated levels of testosterone have been associated with increased aggression in boys with deviant peer groups, similar elevations have been noted in other boys who demonstrate greater degrees of leadership among their nondeviant peers (R. Rowe et al. 2004). Varying degrees and components of serotonin function are frequently noted among individuals having difficulty with aggression and impulsivity.

Neuropsychological associations include relatively low IQ, even in prospective studies, independent of social class. Cognitively, children with conduct problems demonstrate more immature styles of problem solving and social interaction. The importance of parental psychopathology and impoverished home environments is striking, although the linkage is not very clear. The degree of parental discord distinct from actual divorce and separation (Hetherington and Stanley-Hagan 1999), larger family size, absent fathers, and fewer cultural or ethnic interests all correlate with increased risk of behavioral dysfunction.

Course and Prognosis

The course of CD is highly variable. Increased severity correlates with greater likelihood for chronicity (American Psychiatric Association 2000). Younger age at symptom appearance and the presence of aggression are both associated with poorer prognosis. As many as 40% of children with CD become antisocial adults, especially those with drug use prior to age 15 years, those with a history of out-of-home placement, and those who live in extreme poverty (Robins and Ratcliff 1979). "Resilient" children appear to be highly intelligent firstborn children of small, low-discord families (Werner 1989).

Diagnostic Evaluation

Accurate diagnosis of the disruptive behavior disorders requires accurate information. The necessity of accessing multiple sources of information, often in various agencies, is of paramount importance for making a diagnosis, recommending treatment, and predicting prognosis. The difficulty encountered in this process can have significant effects on the effort expended by individuals performing the evaluation.

Treatment

The lack of specificity in the diagnosis of CD contributes to the wide range of interventions that have been proposed as treatment. Several types of treatment have been shown to be beneficial. An appreciation of the psychosocial components of the disorder and clear understanding of the community's resources will aid the clinician in the selection of treatment with the highest likelihood for success. It is especially important to recognize and initiate treatment for any comorbid psychiatric disorders. Evidence supports three major types of interventions for CD: parent management training, problem-solving skills training, and multisystemic therapy (Brestan and Eyberg 1998; Farmer et al. 2002).

Parent management training teaches appropriate means of interacting that promote positive and discourage antisocial behaviors. It uses positive reinforcements and negative consequences and teaches negotiation skills. The reliance on parental efforts can be a liability of this treatment in this population. Problem-solving skills training consists of cognitive-based approaches and uses modeling and role-playing to help individuals identify and better handle potentially difficult situations. Targeting these difficulties in a population with executive function deficits and commonly co-occurring ADHD can be difficult and reinforces the need for accurate assessment and treatment of comorbidities. Not surprisingly, greater successes have been noted in older children.

Multisystemic therapy is based on making use of available systems within the child's world and maximizing positive interactions and effects. Peers, families, schools, and other communities are all involved. It is then customized for the individual. This strength of the therapy makes it expensive and difficult to replicate, but effective.

Pharmacological interventions for CD are directed at troublesome symptoms and behaviors, but given the lack of specificity of symptoms of this diagnosis, it is not surprising that clear replicable findings are lacking. The most appropriate targets of medication intervention are aggression, impulsivity, hyperactivity, and mood symptoms. Antipsychotics, antidepressants, mood stabilizers, anticonvulsants, stimulants, and adrenergic agents have all been shown to be effective (Tcheremissine and Lieving 2006); however, it remains difficult to differentiate benefit in CD itself from psychiatric comorbidity. (See Chapter 36 in this volume, "Treatment of Children and Adolescents" by Crawford et al. for a discussion of treatment.)

Oppositional Defiant Disorder
Clinical Description

ODD recognizes a persistent pathological pattern of interaction, which for briefer periods of time and during well-recognized periods of development is appropriate and typical. Anger and temper management are frequently at the core of the disorder. Authority figures are usually the recipients of often brief tantrums. As in

CD, impulsivity is usually absent, and the arguments take on an importance all their own. Many children with ODD would rather win the battle and lose the war. Recognition of societal rules and personal rights distinguishes children with ODD from those with CD. Most children with ODD do not progress to CD; those with earlier onset of symptoms, physical aggression, low socioeconomic status, and parental substance abuse are more likely to develop CD (Loeber et al. 1995; Table 21–23).

Epidemiology

Prevalence estimates for ODD range from 2% to 12%, with a male predominance of approximately 2 to 1 (American Psychiatric Association 2000). Comorbid psychiatric diagnoses are similar to those for CD and include ADHD and anxiety and mood disorders. Careful attention to elements of the history and presentation is necessary to discern ODD from reactive symptoms secondary to covert psychiatric difficulties.

TABLE 21–23. DSM-IV-TR diagnostic criteria for oppositional defiant disorder

A. A pattern of negativistic, hostile, and defiant behavior lasting at least 6 months, during which four (or more) of the following are present:

   (1) often loses temper

   (2) often argues with adults

   (3) often actively defies or refuses to comply with adults' requests or rules

   (4) often deliberately annoys people

   (5) often blames others for his or her mistakes or misbehavior

   (6) is often touchy or easily annoyed by others

   (7) is often angry and resentful

   (8) is often spiteful or vindictive

   Note: Consider a criterion met only if the behavior occurs more frequently than is typically observed in individuals of comparable age and developmental level.

B. The disturbance in behavior causes clinically significant impairment in social, academic, or occupational functioning.

C. The behaviors do not occur exclusively during the course of a psychotic or mood disorder.

D. Criteria are not met for conduct disorder, and, if the individual is age 18 years or older, criteria are not met for antisocial personality disorder.

Etiology

The etiology of ODD is unknown, although it appears to be multifactorial. Familial factors are often cited and include inadequate parenting, violence, and attachment issues. (See further discussion in "Conduct Disorder.")

Course and Prognosis

Although the diagnosis has been shown to persist for at least 4 years, most children with ODD do not go on to demonstrate antisocial behaviors as adults.

Diagnostic Evaluation

Given the high incidence of comorbidity and potential etiologies of oppositional behavior, careful interviewing of the individual and family is necessary. Special attention to common sources of family conflict and individual frustration is worthwhile.

Treatment

Treatment typically consists of psychotherapeutic interventions, including individual behaviorally focused therapy and family work. Parent training involvement appears key for successful intervention. Pharmacotherapy is typically not indicated.

Feeding and Eating Disorders of Infancy or Early Childhood

Pica

Clinical Description

Pica is the persistent eating of nonnutritive substances that is inappropriate to the developmental level of the individual. The mouthing and eating of nonnutritive substances are commonly observed and developmentally appropriate in a significant number of typically developing 12- to 36-month-old children (Table 21–24). Such eating may also be seen in pregnant women and individuals with severe or profound mental retardation. In some cultures, the eating of nonnutritive substances such as clay is thought to be of value.

Epidemiology

Prevalence of pica is not clearly established, although it is estimated that 10%–20% of children display pica-like behavior. Spontaneous remission, often after just a few months, is common. Intellectual disability is commonly associated with pica, and 20%–40% of institutionalized individuals with severe to profound mental

TABLE 21–24. DSM-IV-TR diagnostic criteria for pica

A. Persistent eating of nonnutritive substances for a period of at least 1 month.

B. The eating of nonnutritive substances is inappropriate to the developmental level.

C. The eating behavior is not part of a culturally sanctioned practice.

D. If the eating behavior occurs exclusively during the course of another mental disorder (e.g., mental retardation, pervasive developmental disorder, schizophrenia), it is sufficiently severe to warrant independent clinical attention.

retardation have pica. The prevalence of pica in pregnant women has been reported to be from 0% to 70%.

Etiology

Many children with pica have parents who demonstrated the disorder, and a multifactorial etiology is likely. Psychosocial stress, deprivation, family psychopathology, and disruption to parent–child nurturance can be involved in the etiology. Many children with pica also exhibit other excessive oral activities (e.g., thumb sucking, nail biting). In intellectual disability, self-stimulation is the likely etiology. Eating of ice in pregnant women has been associated with iron deficiency, and prescription of iron supplements has improved the anemia and decreased the consumption of ice.

Course and Prognosis

Pica usually starts in the second year of life and remits prior to age 6 years; however, in intellectual disability, pica may be lifelong. The risk of toxic ingestion or complication of specific ingestion is significant. Complications of pica may include constipation, fecal impaction, malabsorption, intestinal obstruction, and anemia. Ingestion of lead-containing items may lead to toxic encephalopathy or learning impairments.

Diagnostic Evaluation

Evaluation of the child should include detailed developmental and parental histories and an assessment of the home environment, including the parent–child relationship. The diagnosis should be considered in cases of accidental ingestion, anemia, chronic constipation, or other results of nonnutritive ingestion. Children with pica should have a zinc protoporphyrin and lead level taken to assess possibility of lead intoxication.

Treatment

Behavioral therapies that reward appropriate eating or negatively reinforce nonfood ingestion have been successful, notably in individuals with intellectual disability. Reducing the availability of potentially ingestible nonfood items in the home can be beneficial. Psychosocial interventions have not been evaluated but include improving parent–child interactions and increasing supervision and stimulation of the child. Improvements in personal and household hygiene appear to be helpful. Public health efforts focused on decreasing exposure to lead have been very effective.

Rumination Disorder

Clinical Description

Rumination disorder is the repeated regurgitation and rechewing of food. It is commonly seen in infants and is frequently accompanied by rhythmic movements and relaxation. Other self-soothing behaviors are often observed in children with rumination disorder, such as thumb sucking, head banging, and body rocking. The behaviors are particularly prominent when the infant is alone (Table 21–25).

Epidemiology

No prevalence rates for rumination disorder exist, but it appears to be rare and declining in populations of individuals without intellectual disability. It may occur more often in males than in females. In individuals with intellectual disability, it is fairly common, with 10% of institutionalized individuals with intellectual disability showing the symptoms of the disorder.

Etiology

Both environmental and biological causes have been suggested. Frequently inadequacy of the parent–child relationship is cited as a cause of rumination disorder, forcing the child to seek gratification internally; however, no clear evidence to support this theory exists. Predisposing factors for rumination disorder may also include other psychosocial stressors such as lack of stimulation or neglect. Exploration of the relationship between rumination disorder and gastroesophageal reflux may prove fruitful. Genetic factors in the disorder are unknown.

Course and Prognosis

Typically appearing between the ages of 3 and 12 months, rumination disorder frequently spontaneously remits by age 3 years. Individuals with intellec-

TABLE 21–25.	DSM-IV-TR diagnostic criteria for rumination disorder

A. Repeated regurgitation and rechewing of food for a period of at least 1 month following a period of normal functioning.

B. The behavior is not due to an associated gastrointestinal or other general medical condition (e.g., esophageal reflux).

C. The behavior does not occur exclusively during the course of anorexia nervosa or bulimia nervosa. If the symptoms occur exclusively during the course of mental retardation or a pervasive developmental disorder, they are sufficiently severe to warrant independent clinical attention.

tual disability frequently demonstrate longer duration or chronicity. Risks associated with the disorder include aspiration and malnutrition. A major complication is the parental reaction to the symptoms, including anxiety, frustration, distress, and disgust, all of which may contribute to disrupted attachment and understimulation of the child.

Diagnostic Evaluation

Evaluation for rumination disorder should include a full psychiatric and behavioral assessment of parent and child. Observation of parent–child interactions is also informative. Evaluation of potential medical etiologies or resultant effects of rumination may be necessary, including workup for gastroesophageal reflux or physiological abnormalities.

Treatment

No specific treatments for rumination disorder have been developed, although behavioral interventions that attempt to reward nonrumination with parental attention and negatively reinforce further rumination have been shown to be effective (Lavigne et al. 1981). Medications, including sedatives and antispasmodics, have been tried. Hospitalization can provide a new feeding environment for the child and a brief respite for the parents.

Feeding Disorder of Infancy or Early Childhood

Clinical Description

Approximately 80% of cases of failure to thrive are attributed to nonorganic causes. The diagnosis of feeding disorder of infancy or early childhood attempts to de-

scribe these cases and is characterized by the failure to eat and gain or maintain weight in the presence of adequate food. Infants may refuse to eat or eat inadequately. Young children's consumption may be limited by behavioral or developmental problems, or they may restrict themselves to excessively narrow choices (Table 21–26). Further subtyping is likely appropriate, and additional diagnoses such as feeding disorder of state regulation, feeding disorder of caregiver–infant reciprocity, infantile anorexia, sensory food aversions, posttraumatic feeding disorder, and feeding disorder associated with concurrent medical illness may better clarify potential etiologies and guide treatment (Chatoor 2004).

Epidemiology

Community-based estimates of nonorganic failure to thrive are 1%–4%. These represent 1%–5% of pediatric hospital admissions (Popper et al. 2003).

Etiology

Various specific and combined factors are typically involved. Chatoor's diagnostic subdivisions make clear some of the more common etiologies. There may be difficulties with infant regulation of sleep and calmness that interfere with feeding. The infant may refuse to eat or may be unable to communicate hunger signals to the caregiver. Aversion to certain tastes, textures, or smells may cause individuals to refuse to eat. Impairments in social reciprocity or infant–caregiver attachment may also contribute to this clinical picture. Food refusal may follow a traumatic event or repeated traumatic insult to the oropharynx or gastrointestinal tract. In these situations, the infant may show anticipatory distress or intense resistance to feedings (Chatoor 2004). Early childhood separation individuation may include power struggles about food that may lead to picky eating or food refusal.

Course and Prognosis

Onset is typically within the first year of life, although it may be somewhat later in individuals with intellectual disability. A full range of outcomes is possible, from spontaneous remission to severe malnutrition and death. Mortality rates have been reported as high as 25%. Feeding disorders of infancy are associated with lower IQ, short stature, hyperactivity, and an increased risk for eating disorders (Marchi and Cohen 1990).

Diagnostic Evaluation

Careful elimination of medical causes of failure to thrive; attention to parental and developmental history and the parent–child relationship, including tempera-

TABLE 21–26.   DSM-IV-TR diagnostic criteria for feeding disorder of infancy or early childhood

A. Feeding disturbance as manifested by persistent failure to eat adequately with significant failure to gain weight or significant loss of weight over at least 1 month.

B. The disturbance is not due to an associated gastrointestinal or other general medical condition (e.g., esophageal reflux).

C. The disturbance is not better accounted for by another mental disorder (e.g., rumination disorder) or by lack of available food.

D. The onset is before age 6 years.

TABLE 21–27.   Some common tics

Simple motor tics	Simple vocal tics
Eye blinking	Throat clearing
Shoulder shrugging	Grunting
Mouth opening	Yelling/screaming
Flicking hair out of one's eyes	Sniffing
Arm extending	Barking
Facial grimacing	Snorting
Lip licking	Coughing
Eye rolling	Spitting
Squinting/opening eyes	Humming

Source.   From Eapen et al. 2002.

ment; evaluation of the home or feeding environment; and elements of behavioral analysis are necessary to clarify the diagnosis.

Treatment

Appropriate treatment targets the specific or suspected etiology of the disorder. At the time of diagnosis, hospitalization is frequently encouraged to completely evaluate the child, control the environment, and alleviate some of the stress incumbent on the parent. Parent education and training are typically important. Specific interventions are then clarified based on the characteristic and supposed etiology.

Tic Disorders

Clinical Description

A *tic* is a rapid, involuntary, and apparently meaningless movement or vocalization. Most simple tics go unnoticed or fail to reach a level of conscious awareness. Many children are not bothered by their motor tics and frequently display some indifference toward them. Vocal tics are frequently disruptive and distressing. Often these are inaccurately described as disruptive habits. In general, tics are sensitive to stress and fatigue. They wax and wane in severity, but for most children, they are not progressive (Walkup et al. 2006; Table 21–27).

Tics belong to the class of hyperkinetic movement disorders, which includes chorea, choreoathetoid movements, myoclonus, tremors, and some dystonias. Hyperkinetic movement disorders represent abnormalities in the complex interconnections between the premotor and motor cortex, basal ganglia, limbic system, thalamus, and selected cerebellar nuclei. Because of the complex neurobiology of these networks, it may not be surprising that tics are associated with a range of cognitive, behavioral, and emotional symptoms. The assessment and treatment of tics and tic disorders must include consideration of their frequent but variable associations with other psychiatric and medical disorders (Swerdlow and Leckman 2002).

Tic disorders are differentiated by the duration, frequency, severity, and anatomical location of the abnormal movements or vocalization (Table 21–28). All tic disorders share the common features of a waxing and waning course, an exacerbation by stress and fatigue, and an increased risk of mood-related symptoms. Tourette's disorder is further distinguished by the development of more complex tics over time and the presence of prodromal sensations or urges to perform the tic (Robertson 2000).

Epidemiology

Tics are exceedingly common. Transient tics occur in 10%–25% of early school-age males and in somewhat fewer similarly aged females. Most often tics disappear over a period of weeks to months. Tic disorders demonstrate a greater male predominance than transient tics, with males presenting with tics two to four times more frequently than females. Affected females are more likely to present with more severe tics and higher rates of obsessive-compulsive symptoms. This gender bias may be related to a higher genetic threshold or family loading for tic disorders in affected females (Leckman et al. 2003; Santangelo et al. 1994; Saxena et al. 2001).

Tic disorders are frequently associated with additional psychiatric disorders such as ADHD, OCD, mood and anxiety disorders, ODD, or CD. The presence of these disorders has a profound influence on the clinical presentation and course of the tic disorder. LDs, including disorders of written expression, and speech and language disorders, such as stuttering and

TABLE 21–28. DSM-IV-TR diagnostic criteria for tic disorders

Criteria	Tic disorder not otherwise specified	Transient tic disorder	Chronic vocal tic disorder	Chronic motor tic disorder	Tourette's disorder
Typology of tics	Motor or vocal tics	Motor or vocal tics	Vocal tics	Motor tics	Motor and phonic tics
Age at onset	>18 years	<18 years	<18 years	<18 years	<18 years
Duration	<4 weeks	<1 year >4 weeks	>1 year	>1 year	>1 year
Frequency	No pattern required	No pattern required	Multiple tics per day	Multiple tics per day	Multiple tics per day
Exclusion	Fails to meet criteria for other tic disorder	Drug effects (stimulants) General medical conditions	Presence of motor tics Medication induced General medical condition	Presence of vocal tics Medication induced General medical conditions	Medication induced General medical conditions

other forms of speech dysfluency, are additional comorbidities (Robertson 2000; Saint-Cyr et al. 1995).

SIB is more common in this population than previously appreciated. The prevalence rates for potentially tissue-damaging self-injury in individuals with tic disorders may be as high as 15%–30%. It is apparent that there are several subtypes of self-injury involved in this statistic. One subtype consists of high-frequency, low-intensity behaviors (e.g., rubbing, nail biting, nose picking, and trichotillomania). Injury occurs as a result of repetition. Many of these behaviors occur during periods of decreased attention or periods of minimal demand or activity (Barnhill and Horrigan 2002). More severe SIB is often directed at areas of pain or the perceived location of associated sensory phenomena and is often terminated only when it "feels right." Individuals with severe SIB may have more severe tics and accompanying compulsive behaviors. The presence of dystonia or chorea, older age at onset, cognitive changes, or biting with severe tissue damage requires a more extensive diagnostic assessment.

Etiology

Tic disorders represent dysfunction within a complex network involving the limbic system, prefrontal cortex, and basal ganglia. Analogously, the neurobehavioral symptoms associated with tic disorders involve circuits related to attention, sensory gating, impulse control, capacity for automatization of motor skills (written language), and prepotent inhibition of automatic repetitive behaviors (Leckman et al. 2003; Potenza and Hollander 2002; Robertson 2000).

Early studies of the functional neuroanatomy and neurochemical substrates of tic disorders supported a dopamine-centric view. This model was derived from research examining dopamine receptors, dopamine transporter protein transport, and dopamine synthesis pathways as well as the presence of changes in tic severity after administration of dopamine agonists and the observation of clinical benefit during treatment with dopamine antagonists such as haloperidol or pimozide. Subsequent research has implicated many other neurotransmitters, peptide neuromodulators, and second messenger systems, and it is becoming increasingly apparent that differences in the type and topography of tics and co-occurring neuropsychiatric disorders reflect neurochemical heterogeneity. Although dopamine and serotonin remain key players, the full story is increasingly complicated (Jankovic and DeLeon 2002; Walkup et al. 2006).

A great deal of effort has gone into determining and defining the genetic risk for tic disorders. There are several promising approaches, although a definitive marker gene remains elusive. Pedigree studies suggest familial clusters of affected probands. These same studies also reveal significant diversity of phenotypic expression. Monozygotic twins yield markedly elevated rates of concordance and similar types and severity of tics when compared with dizygotic twins. It is also apparent that not only are monozygotic twins more likely to have Tourette's disorder (greater than 50% versus 20% for dizygotic twins), but this gap widens when the presence of obsessive-compulsive symptoms is included in the comparison (Leckman et al. 2003).

The precise mode of transmission is unknown. It has been postulated that Tourette's disorder is an autosomal dominant disorder with variable penetrance and phenotypic variability resulting from environmental influences. Other evidence suggests polygenic influences or even a single gene with multiple effects. Most comorbid conditions appear to be inherited independently. Variation in dimensions such as tic type, severity, and course may be secondary to environmental factors such as exposure to neurotoxins, prenatal complications (e.g., hyperemesis gravidarum), or the product of medication side effects (Walkup et al. 2006).

Additional insight into the causes of tic disorders may be gained by examining what is known about abnormal movements in general. Abnormal movements may be caused by neuroendocrine or autoimmune disorders, infectious disease, trauma, or exposure to a range of neurotoxins with a predilection for the basal ganglia and related systems. Additionally, a wide range of abnormalities can accompany tics: high levels of thyroid hormones, low calcium, high antistreptolysin antibodies or antistreptococcal DNA-ase B titers, or elevated antinuclear antibody, low ceruloplasmin, and high urinary copper levels. For example, immunological or postinfectious hyperkinetic movement disorders such as Sydenham's chorea or pediatric autoimmune neuropsychiatric disorders associated with streptococcal infections link an immune response (e.g., plasma cell production of antibodies) and antibody specificity with reversible changes in basal ganglia structures. The associated emotional, cognitive, and behavioral sequelae of these secondary tic disorders may provide insight into the role of fronto-striatal-limbic-cerebellar networks in the etiology of tic and other neuropsychiatric disorders (Edwards et al. 2004; Walkup et al. 2006).

Clinically, Tourette's disorder may represent a final common pathway for several overlapping developmental movement disorders. This is supported by the wide variability of abnormal movements (e.g., simple tics versus dystonic tics) as well as their sensitivity and response to pharmacological intervention. In this model, an insult at various points in cortical, limbic, and subcortical pathways could produce different clinical symptoms and associated comorbid conditions. This model may also account for some of the difficulties in identifying marker genes on human genome surveys (Leckman et al. 2003; Swerdlow and Leckman 2002).

Course and Prognosis

The severity and intensity of tics tend to wax and wane over time. Many resolve spontaneously and, although being worrisome to many parents, rarely result in a referral for treatment. The short duration of transient tic disorders suggests that duration may be related to maturational vulnerabilities and environmental factors. It is likely that transient tics represent a lower genetic loading for movement disorders and more likely that they represent a mild developmental delay in the normal maturation of inhibitory mechanisms. The emergence of commonly co-occurring conditions among preschoolers and early elementary school–age children (e.g., nightmares, parasomnias, migraine headaches, and symptoms associated with ADHD) supports a developmental model (King et al. 2003; Robertson 2000).

Over a period of months, simple tics may develop into persistent motor or phonic tics. By definition, chronic motor tic disorder, phonic tic disorder, and Tourette's disorder persist longer than 1 year. For children with chronic tic disorder, the appearance of either vocalizations or movements tends to remain stable. In contrast, Tourette's disorder often begins with a simple motor tic (e.g., blinking) and progresses over a period of months to years into more complex motor and (often later) phonic tics.

Tic disorders follow a similar trajectory as other nonprogressive hyperkinetic movement disorders. For some, tics reach their peak intensity 4–5 years after onset and then begin to decline in severity. Others experience an increase in severity during the surge in androgen activity present in early puberty. Of course, tics beginning at age 7 years are reaching a natural peak in intensity during early puberty, and the associated androgen surge may be less relevant than previously thought (Bruun and Budman 1994). By late adolescence, most children with tics will experience a gradual decline in tic frequency.

Other patients experience increasingly severe tics and repetitive motion injury, self-injury, or complications from long-term treatment (e.g., tardive dyskinesia) (Robertson 2000).

Complex tics, sensory tics, and prodromal sensations frequently generate more psychological and social distress. Patients with complex motor tics often complain about prodromal urges and the presence of sensory tics. Movements may transiently diffuse the urges or sensations, making these tics (or movements) appear volitional. Movements can be confused with compulsions, stereotypies, or annoying deliberate behaviors in the classroom setting. The associated urge to move can be confused with akathisia or restless legs syndrome.

The persistence of tics during sleep warrants further workup to evaluate for periodic limb movements or nocturnal seizures. Complex tics, especially those with visual imagery or prodromal sensory phenomena, also blur the boundaries between primary psychiatric and neurological disorders (Eapen et al. 2002; Robertson 2000).

A second developmental subtype includes people whose tics diminish and are subsequently replaced by obsessive-compulsive symptoms (e.g., a need for symmetry; counting, ordering, and hoarding behaviors) (de Groot and Bornstein 1994; Eapen et al. 2002). For these patients, obsessions may be intrusive images or violent or sexual thoughts. This group includes a larger proportion of females. Compulsive behaviors associated with previous tic disorders frequently differ from compulsions in children with OCD. Many of these tic-associated compulsive behaviors require a sense of "feeling right" (rather than alleviating associated anxiety) in order to terminate the repetitive behavior. In general, these patients can be less responsive to SSRIs and cognitive-behavioral therapies than individuals with OCD (Baer 1994; Iiada et al. 1996).

Pallilalia (the need to repeat your own thoughts or sounds), echolalia and echopraxia (the need to repeat another's words or movements), coprolalia and copropraxia (the production of obscene language or movements), compulsive self-injury, and suggestibility are frequently reported in patients with more complicated or severe tic disorders. In the past, these odd behaviors were misattributed to psychosis, conversion disorders, or other primary psychiatric disorders. Clinical evidence suggests that these phenomena are also observed in neurological disorders that involve frontostriatal and medial prefrontal lesions. Similar symptoms are observed in later-onset frontotemporal degenerative disorders and other movement disorders. A mixture of apathy and explosive aggressive behaviors, property destruction, and changes in emotional reactivity may accompany these disorders (Eapen et al. 2002; Jankovic and DeLeon 2002).

The persistence of Tourette's or chronic tic disorder

into adulthood suggests that there are likely both genetic and environmental factors that contribute to the disorder's persistence. One factor may be the severity of the tic disorder during development. A second may relate to bilineal inheritance, suggesting the impact of genetic loading. Psychosocial factors such as a history of traumatic exposure may also increase a child's vulnerability. Finally, the treatment of tics during childhood can contribute to a prolongation or aberration in the natural course of subclinical tics (e.g., the development of tardive Tourette's disorder following prolonged antipsychotic drug exposure) (King et al. 2003).

Diagnostic Evaluation

Tics are differentiated from chorea, athetosis, dystonia, myoclonus, and tremors through careful assessment of the age of the patient at symptom onset, distribution, duration, capacity for suppression, provocative agents or events, and the natural course of movements and vocalizations (which can be well characterized through video recording).

It is important to differentiate tics from other hyperkinetic movements and neurological disorders, such as myoclonic epilepsy, and repetitive behaviors associated with perseveration or frontotemporal disorders. In contrast to myoclonic seizures and some nocturnal paroxysmal movements, tics tend to diminish in intensity during sleep. Unfortunately, comorbidity with restless legs syndrome, periodic limb movements during sleep, and some parasomnias complicates the sleep–tic relationship. In contrast to many other basal ganglia movements, tics are not directly related to the initiation of voluntary movements and can be suppressed for periods of time (Jankovic and DeLeon 2002; Walkup et al. 2006). It can be difficult to differentiate some complex tics from stereotypies, mannerisms, and other compulsive or ritualistic behaviors seen in autistic disorders (Barnhill and Horrigan 2002).

The purpose of a detailed neurological examination of children with tic disorders is to characterize the nature of the movement disorder and eliminate more serious developmental neuropsychiatric disorders. In general, tics are not accompanied by lateralizing neurological symptoms such as hemiparesis, severe rigidity, akinesia, or seizures. Many children with tics do have nonspecific developmental soft signs that are also present in ADHD, LDs, and PDDs. Findings such as unilateral rigidity, movement dysfluency, or overflow/synkinesias suggest lateralization within the basal ganglia, whereas perceptual motor skills and executive deficits suggest a more complex brain region relationship. In general, most of these findings may

have greater educational than neurological significance (Walkup et al. 2006).

In many settings, an MRI or computed tomography scan is routinely ordered, although lacking other abnormal physical findings or laboratory evidence, the yield from these studies is typically low. An electroencephalogram may show nonspecific findings in the absence of clear-cut myoclonic or paroxysmal events (either nocturnal or daytime). For example, hyperekplexia (excessive startle response) and physiological symptoms associated with acute stress can be confused with tics. The persistence of abnormal movements during sleep or in relation to specific stimuli is helpful in clarifying the differential diagnosis (Jankovic and DeLeon 2002; see Table 21–29).

Treatment

It is essential to assess the impact of the tic disorder on the person's quality of life and overall psychological adjustment. For most children, the decision to treat tic disorders is not related to tic severity. Treatment is more often related to psychosocial disruptions, peer reactions, or the emotional sensitivity of the affected child. For adults with persistent tics, treatment decisions are often based on the severity of the persistent tics, psychiatric comorbidity, and the degree of interference with work or social interaction (King et al. 2003). It is essential to evaluate the level of discomfort and distress experienced by the patient and the family.

Treatment planning requires a thorough understanding of the tic disorder's natural course; relationship to the person's developmental, psychosocial, and academic needs and stressors; severity of the abnormal movements and vocalizations; disruptive symptoms (e.g., coprolalia, copropraxia); psychiatric comorbidity; and the risk–benefit ratio of available treatments.

The treatment of tics proceeds algorithmically in most situations. For simple tics with few indicators of significant distress, a watch-and-wait strategy is often appropriate. On the other hand, individuals with severe tics and highly disruptive comorbid symptoms can require more immediate treatment. Many children with severe tics are resistant to or intolerant of standard treatments outlined in evidence-based protocols. Treatment of these severe cases may require appropriation of neuropharmacological treatments of non-tic-related movement disorders such as dystonia or myoclonic disorders (Walkup et al. 2006).

Treatment risks and benefits must correlate with the severity of symptoms. Exposing a child to the risks of haloperidol for isolated eye blinking and sniffing is as inappropriate as treating a child with severe dys-

TABLE 21–29. Differential diagnosis of tics

Inherited forms of movement disorders	Causes of secondary tic disorders
Huntington's disease	Autoimmune disorders
Neuroacanthocytosis	Cerebrovascular events
Torsion dystonias	Chromosomal disorders
Tourette's disorder	Degenerative disorders
Wilson's disease	Metabolic disorders
	Neurocutaneous syndromes
	Neurotoxins
	Pediatric autoimmune neuropsychiatric disorders associated with streptococcal infections (PANDAS)
	Stimulant- or medication-induced (immediate or tardive responses)
	Sydenham's chorea
	Tourette's disorder
	Traumatic brain injury

Source. Jankovic and DeLeon 2002; Robertson 2000; Walkup et al. 2006.

tonic tics with low-dosage clonidine. The waxing and waning course of tic disorders can make it difficult to assess the effectiveness of treatments. Naturally waning tics may create the illusion of a positive treatment response (King et al. 2003).

For most children, tics are stable, generally mild, nonprogressive, and rarely treated. However, watchful waiting may not be an appropriate strategy when severe ADHD or obsessive-compulsive symptoms are present. Because rates of ADHD exceed 40% in many children with tics, the chance of a child having both disorders is quite likely. The presence of ADHD raises several questions. Until relatively recently, the stimulant drugs were considered a causative factor in the development of tic disorders, and this class of drugs was contraindicated in children with abnormal movements. Although there are children for whom stimulants play a key role in the onset and evolution of their tic disorder, subsequent research has failed to support a categorical assumption. In most children, stimulant drugs have minimal or no impact on the course of tics. In some severe tic disorders, both direct and indirect dopamine agonists have palliative effects (Walkup et al. 2006). The severity of the core symptoms of ADHD, coupled with family attitudes, often determines the role of stimulants in treatment. For those disinclined to

use stimulants, clonidine, guanfacine, TCAs, modafinil, atomoxetine, SSRIs, SNRIs, and mecamylamine (Inversine) are available as treatments for tics and ADHD-related symptoms. If nonstimulant treatments of comorbid tic disorder and ADHD are not useful, stimulants should be considered after careful review of the potential risks and benefits with the family and child (King et al. 2003). α-Agonists (e.g., clonidine, guanfacine) may be helpful for tics, ADHD, and explosive behaviors.

Comorbid obsessive-compulsive symptoms can also pose significant diagnostic and treatment difficulties. It can be difficult to differentiate OCD from complex tics and repetitive behaviors common to tic disorders (e.g., arranging, need for symmetry, arithmomania, and "just right" sensations). One approach may be to address phenomenological differences in core symptoms. A second may involve a pharmacological dissection of treatment response (Eapen et al. 2002; Santangelo et al. 1994).

Many patients with obsessive-compulsive spectrum disorders are less responsive to SSRIs. In addition, some exhibit a form of behavioral disinhibition. For these children, compulsive behaviors in the context of significant impulsivity, fewer anxiety-related complaints, and the presence of a growing urge can predict a less complete response to SSRIs and cognitive and behavioral therapies. In these circumstances, the addition of a low dosage of a second-generation antipsychotic drug, anticonvulsant, or naltrexone can be helpful (Potenza and Hollander 2002).

The high prevalence rates for co-occurring tic disorders, ADHD, and explosive behaviors further complicate treatment decision making. α-Agonists, mood stabilizers, or newer antipsychotic drugs appear to be the most common add-on choices for clinicians (King et al. 2003). Subsequent stimulant, atomoxetine, or mecamylamine trials may be warranted.

In general, mood disorders are common in patients with movement disorders. Mood changes associated with basal ganglia disorders can affect the intensity of abnormal movements. For many, the intensity of movements worsens with depression, and in bipolar patients, it improves with hypomania. The waxing and waning of tics and explosive aggressive behaviors may be confused with hyperthymia or the mixed state or noncyclical form of bipolar disorder (Robertson 2000).

Tic Disorders Summary

Tic disorders, like other hyperkinetic movement disorders, are frequently comorbid with disorders such as OCD, ADHD, LDs (often of written expression), and deficits in executive function. These comorbidities also implicate the basal ganglia and pre-motor pathways, limbic system, and prefrontal regions in the pathophysiology of the disorder. Development affects the course of illness.

Although tic disorders can intensify as they evolve in some individuals, there is no evidence of neurodegenerative changes in cognition or motor skills. Clinicians need to be aware of the differences between transient, primary, and secondary tics as well as causes of abnormal movements acquired later in life.

The appearance of tics and co-occurring conditions early in life can affect subsequent psychological or cognitive development, especially the acquisition of specific skills. Most children with tic disorders have few adverse consequences, but some, especially those with severe tics, comorbid neuropsychiatric symptoms, or psychiatric disorders, have problems that affect a broad range of psychosocial dimensions. Treatment attempts to minimize (and often not completely eliminate) tics and should include both pharmacotherapy and psychotherapy.

Elimination Disorders

Encopresis

Clinical Description

Encopresis is defined by DSM-IV-TR as the repeated involuntary and intentional passage of feces into inappropriate places by children older than 4 years or with an equivalent developmental level (Table 21–30). It is subdivided into primary and secondary types. In primary encopresis, a period of fecal continence has never developed and is typically associated with developmental delay or fixation. Secondary encopresis, found in slightly more than one-half of cases, follows at least 1 year of fecal continence and is associated with conduct problems. Behavioral problems, found in approximately one-third of individuals afflicted, often resolve with the improvement of encopresis.

Encopresis with constipation and overflow incontinence (or "retentive" encopresis) describes 75%–95% of cases and is typically accompanied by pain and embarrassment. Chronic constipation and infrequent bowel movements result in frequent (up to several times per day) passage of liquid stool and staining of undergarments. Encopresis without constipation and overflow incontinence can be intentional (and associated with fecal smearing and other behavioral problems) or due to inadequate sensation, concern, or training.

TABLE 21–30. DSM-IV-TR diagnostic criteria for encopresis

A. Repeated passage of feces into inappropriate places (e.g., clothing or floor) whether involuntary or intentional.

B. At least one such event a month for at least 3 months.

C. Chronological age is at least 4 years (or equivalent developmental level).

D. The behavior is not due exclusively to the direct physiological effects of a substance (e.g., laxatives) or a general medical condition except through a mechanism involving constipation.

Code as follows:

787.6 With constipation and overflow incontinence

307.7 Without constipation and overflow incontinence

Epidemiology

Encopresis is likely individually underreported. Prevalences of 1.5%–7.5% have been reported, with a 3 to 1 to 4 to 1 male predominance (C.E. Walker et al. 1988). Some studies have suggested an association with lower socioeconomic status. Psychiatric comorbidity accompanies 35% of children with encopresis (Popper et al. 2003). Associated disorders include mental retardation, CD, ODD, psychotic disorders, and mood disorders.

Etiology

The diagnosis of encopresis should exclude any medically explained causes of fecal incontinence, such as hypercalcemia, hypothyroidism, lactase deficiency, anal fissure or malformation, aganglionic megacolon, rectal stenosis, and trauma. Altered motility and abnormal secretion of gastrointestinal hormones may also cause encopresis. Encopresis with constipation and overflow incontinence can be due to any nonmedical cause of chronic constipation, inadequate training, or avoidance of toileting. The causes of nonretentive encopresis can include diminished sensory appreciation or lack of appropriate planning, training, or interest.

Course and Prognosis

Most individuals with encopresis get better. Treatment results in recovery rates of 30%–50% after 1 year and 48%–75% after 5 years (Loening-Baucke 2002). Poor prognostic indicators include soiling at night or as an expression of anger, a nonchalant attitude, and conduct problems (Landman and Rappaport 1985).

Diagnostic Evaluation

It is important to rule out medical reasons for fecal incontinence, such as endocrinological sequelae, aganglionic megacolon (Hirschsprung's disease), and anal fissure, although extensive workup is not often necessary (Loening-Baucke 2002). An abdominal roentgenogram can aid diagnosis and management of encopresis (Rockney et al. 1995). Careful attention to developmental history, history of toilet training. and observation of family interactions is important to fully assess this often unpleasant and distressing problem.

Treatment

Treatment typically consists of a combination of medical, behavioral, and psychotherapeutic interventions. Education of the patient and family about the disorder, workup, and etiologies can help to alleviate the stresses associated with this problem. For individuals with impaction, laxatives or enemas are frequently required. Subsequently, high-fiber diets and increased water consumption are recommended. A "sitting schedule" is established and compliance is rewarded; sometimes aversive consequences, such as bathing and washing soiled linens, are useful for noncompliance. Psychotherapeutic intervention can target self-esteem in individuals or utilize family work focusing on possible etiologies or results of the disorder.

Enuresis

Clinical Description

Although the term is frequently used to describe urinary incontinence regardless of its cause, more accurately, *enuresis* is the persistence of medically unexplained urinary incontinence after the typical age of bladder control. Subtyping occurs according to the time of day it occurs. Nocturnal enuresis is more common, and children with diurnal enuresis usually have nocturnal symptoms as well. Approximately 80% of children have primary enuresis, where bladder control has never been attained. The remaining children have previously achieved bladder control, and the term *secondary enuresis* is often used. The relationship between primary and secondary distinction and the incidence and severity of associated psychopathology are not clear (Table 21–31).

Epidemiology

Reported prevalence rates vary wildly, with estimates as high as 25% for occasional nocturnal enuresis. More

TABLE 21–31. DSM-IV-TR diagnostic criteria for enuresis

A. Repeated voiding of urine into bed or clothes (whether involuntary or intentional).

B. The behavior is clinically significant as manifested by either a frequency of twice a week for at least 3 consecutive months or the presence of clinically significant distress or impairment in social, academic (occupational), or other important areas of functioning.

C. Chronological age is at least 5 years (or equivalent developmental level).

D. The behavior is not due exclusively to the direct physiological effect of a substance (e.g., a diuretic) or a general medical condition (e.g., diabetes, spina bifida, a seizure disorder).

Specify type:

Nocturnal only

Diurnal only

Nocturnal and diurnal

significant enuresis in children older than 5 years is 7%–10% for males and 3% of females. Associated psychiatric diagnoses include ADHD, anxiety disorders, encopresis, and developmental delays.

Etiology

No clear etiology for enuresis is known, although genetic transmission appears likely. Sleep stages do not appear to be related to the occurrence of enuresis. The role of individual diurnal variations of endogenous antidiuretic hormone is not clear. Abnormalities of bladder anatomy, function, and size have been implicated in a minority of cases. Secondary enuresis in young children has been associated with stressful environments or events.

Course and Prognosis

Left untreated, enuresis abates at a rate of about 10%–20% per year. Approximately 1% of adults have enuresis. Adolescent-onset enuresis appears to have more associated psychopathology and poorer prognosis. Individuals with enuresis often feel embarrassment and anger. The secondary effects include punishment from caregivers, teasing from peers, and social withdrawal.

Diagnostic Evaluation

The elimination of possible medical etiologies may require urological evaluation, because approximately 20% of children with nocturnal enuresis are found to have urological abnormalities. Urinary infections and seizure disorders are often suspected, and urinary analysis is warranted, but electroencephalograms are likely to have a low yield.

Treatment

Behavioral and pharmacological interventions are both effective in treating enuresis; however, behavioral interventions likely have greater safety. The most successful and commonly used behavioral interventions are the bell and pad or a simple alarm clock set to the time of night when bladders are typically full. These awaken the child upon, or at the time most likely for, enuresis. Both of these methods show success rates of approximately 75%.

Imipramine initiated at 25 mg and titrated every 4–7 days to a maximum of 5 mg/kg is effective for enuresis. Most children respond in the 75–125 mg range, and electrocardiograms should be obtained and followed at dosages above 3.5 mg/kg (Mikkelsen and Rapoport 1980). Desmopressin acetate is widely used and approximately as effective as the bell and pad method. Reductions in frequency of enuresis ranging from 10%–91% have been reported; however, continued use of desmopressin acetate is required for continuing bladder control (Moffat et al. 1993). Given the high rate of spontaneous remission in enuresis, long-term continuous treatment with medication is inappropriate (see Chapter 36 in this volume, "Treatment of Children and Adolescents," by Crawford et al.).

Other Disorders of Infancy, Childhood, or Adolescence

Separation Anxiety Disorder

Clinical Description

Separation anxiety is a normal developmental phenomenon typically beginning around 6 or 7 months, peaking around 18 months, and decreasing after 30 months (see Chapter 7 in this volume, "Normal Child and Adolescent Development," by Gemelli). Some features of separation anxiety may persist subclinically into childhood and early adolescence. Separation anxiety disorder, however, is characterized by an overwhelming fear of separation or loss of an attachment figure, typically a parent or caregiver. This anxiety response may include cognitive distortions, affective arousal, and behavioral and somatic symptoms. Associated with intense sympathetic arousal, separation distress produces exaggerated proximity-seeking (clinging) and is subject to a rapid expansion of anticipatory triggers and generalization that include enhanced sensitivity to future separations, fears of catastrophic separation, disruption of sleep initiation, and increased frequency of anxiety dreams (nightmares; Table 21–32). As expected, fear conditioning to both specific (separation) and context-dependent (setting) conditions can become paired with anticipatory experiences (e.g., the ride to school triggers the anxiety response) (Swedo and Pine 2005).

Intense fear often limits an individual's exposure to typical child and adolescent experiences. As a result, separation anxiety disorder can affect academic achievement, peer relationships, and overall growth and development. School refusal is often thought to be a behavioral manifestation of the disorder; however, this behavior can be associated with a number of diagnoses, including generalized anxiety disorder, specific phobia, thought disorders, and depression, in addition to separation anxiety disorder.

Epidemiology

DSM-IV-TR reports a prevalence of about 4%; however, a recent large-scale study of children ages 9–13 years found an overall rate of 1% for males and females (Costello et al. 2003). The prevalence of separation anxiety disorder declines with increasing age (American Psychiatric Association 2000). The disorder may be slightly more prevalent in females. It is more common in first-degree relatives and occurs relatively frequently in children of mothers with panic disorder. Separation anxiety frequently accompanies generalized anxiety disorder, although the former often has its onset at an earlier age. Individuals with separation anxiety disorder may be at increased risk for the development of other anxiety disorders, including panic disorder with agoraphobia and depressive disorders.

Etiology

A complicated interaction among genetic factors, temperament, attachment, parental anxiety, parenting style, and life experiences is the generally accepted etiology of anxiety in children. Increased risk factors include high reactivity in novel situations, insecure attachment patterns, parents with anxiety disorders, and parents who are more intrusive and controlling of their children.

Course and Prognosis

Separation anxiety disorder may develop after some life stress, loss, or trauma. Onset may be as young as preschool and may occur any time prior to age 18 years;

TABLE 21–32. **DSM-IV-TR diagnostic criteria for separation anxiety disorder**

A. Developmentally inappropriate and excessive anxiety concerning separation from home or from those to whom the individual is attached, as evidenced by three (or more) of the following:

(1) recurrent excessive distress when separation from home or major attachment figures occurs or is anticipated

(2) persistent and excessive worry about losing, or about possible harm befalling, major attachment figures

(3) persistent and excessive worry that an untoward event will lead to separation from a major attachment figure (e.g., getting lost or being kidnapped)

(4) persistent reluctance or refusal to go to school or elsewhere because of fear of separation

(5) persistently and excessively fearful or reluctant to be alone or without major attachment figures at home or without significant adults in other settings

(6) persistent reluctance or refusal to go to sleep without being near a major attachment figure or to sleep away from home

(7) repeated nightmares involving the theme of separation

(8) repeated complaints of physical symptoms (such as headaches, stomachaches, nausea, or vomiting) when separation from major attachment figures occurs or is anticipated

B. The duration of the disturbance is at least 4 weeks.

C. The onset is before age 18 years.

D. The disturbance causes clinically significant distress or impairment in social, academic (occupational), or other important areas of functioning.

E. The disturbance does not occur exclusively during the course of a pervasive developmental disorder, schizophrenia, or other psychotic disorder and, in adolescents and adults, is not better accounted for by panic disorder with agoraphobia.

Specify if:

Early onset: if onset occurs before age 6 years

however, adolescent onset is rare and can have ominous overtones, because it can be an early expression of severe mood disorder or schizophrenia. Left untreated, as many as 80%–95% of children with separation anxiety disorder experience remission; however, continued exposure may intensify the severity of affective response (sensitization) or refusal behaviors (avoiding separation) and expand from specific foci (e.g., the mother) to anticipatory triggers (e.g., school). Unfortunately, tantrums and "clinging" (proximity-seeking behaviors), along with refusals to leave home or attend school, can be reinforced by equally anxious family members. Because parents can be overwhelmed by a sense of helplessness in the face of protest behaviors, separation anxiety and avoidance behaviors readily become a multigenerational defense against leaving home or a familiar community.

Diagnostic Evaluation

Evaluation of separation anxiety disorder requires interviewing the child and parents together and individ-ually. In addition, it should include a systematic review of the classroom environment, the context of the emergence of symptoms, previous interventions, family reactions to these behaviors, and functions of the behavior within the existing structure of the family system. The age at onset of school refusal should be considered. Transient separation anxiety is not uncommon in preschool or day-care settings. Onset among school-age children may represent true separation anxiety disorder or emerging mood or panic disorders (Labellarte and Ginsburg 2003).

Treatment

The treatment of childhood separation anxiety includes cognitive-behavioral therapy. There is some evidence to support adjunctive parent therapy and parental anxiety management for children (Cobham et al. 1998; Mendlowitz et al. 1999). In conjunction with these therapies, pharmacological interventions include SSRIs, TCAs, and, in some circumstances, short trials of high-potency benzodiazepines (i.e., clonazepam or alprazolam) (Barnett and Riddle 2003; see Chapter 36 in this volume, "Treatment of Children and Adolescents," by Crawford et al.).

Selective Mutism

Clinical Description

Selective mutism is not classified as either a primary communication or anxiety disorder. Although current diagnostic criteria require exclusion of communication and other psychiatric disorders, it is apparent that there is a considerable overlap between these conditions. As such, selective mutism includes a spectrum of potential communication problems that range from articulation and dysfluency (stuttering) issues and expressive language weakness to concerns about communicating in a second language. However, the key component to the disorder is a form of avoidant behavior: the refusal to speak in public settings despite speaking with minimal difficulty in other situations such as with family, close associates, or members of the primary language community (Table 21–33). Typically, these individuals refuse to speak in certain social settings, although they may use gestures, nods, whispers, or written words to communicate. Associated features include excessive shyness, clinging, compulsive traits, fear of embarrassment, social isolation, controlling behaviors, and temper tantrums (American Psychiatric Association 2000).

TABLE 21–33. **DSM-IV-TR diagnostic criteria for selective mutism**

A. Consistent failure to speak in specific social situations (in which there is an expectation for speaking, e.g., at school) despite speaking in other situations.

B. The disturbance interferes with educational or occupational achievement or with social communication.

C. The duration of the disturbance is at least 1 month (not limited to the first month of school).

D. The failure to speak is not due to a lack of knowledge of, or comfort with, the spoken language required in the social situation.

E. The disturbance is not better accounted for by a communication disorder (e.g., stuttering) and does not occur exclusively during the course of a pervasive developmental disorder, schizophrenia, or other psychotic disorder.

Epidemiology

Prevalence estimates range from 0.03% to 2.00%, with the variability likely secondary to differences in ages and threshold for diagnosis. There is a slight female predominance. Comorbid disorders may include language or speech disorders, neurological disorders, and mental retardation. Studies have found high prevalence of comorbid avoidant personality disorder or social phobia. Other anxiety disorders are also often present in these patients (Black and Uhde 1995).

Etiology

Originally selective mutism was understood psychodynamically as a primitive assertion of autonomy. More recently, a posttraumatic etiology is thought to be possible in light of the high prevalence of physical and sexual abuse in these children. Additionally, cerebellar lesions and genetic involvement have been postulated as possible etiologies.

Course and Prognosis

Selective mutism may present between the ages of 3 and 5 years, although diagnosis is often delayed until elementary school. The disorder may persist for a few weeks or months or for several years. Some cases do not emerge until adolescence, although these individuals often show passive-aggressive or antisocial features and generally have a poorer prognosis. Complications include academic difficulties and poor peer relationships.

Diagnostic Evaluation

Diagnostic evaluations generally focus on ruling out comorbid psychiatric disorders such as mood and anxiety disorders as well as other causes of decreased language use such as PDD, autism spectrum disorder, mental retardation, expressive language disorder, or deafness. It is helpful to rule out a primary neurological disorder. It is important to evaluate the familial patterns of communication as well as look at the possibility of physical or sexual abuse.

Treatment

Treatment of selective mutism includes both pharmacological and psychotherapeutic interventions. SSRIs have been shown to improve selective mutism and general level of functioning (Black and Uhde 1994). Fluoxetine specifically has been shown beneficial in case studies, one open trial, and one double-blind, placebo-controlled trial. Monoamine oxidase inhibitors have been described as helpful in single case studies and for use in refractory cases. Anxiolytics and atypical antipsychotics may be used adjunctively. Psychotherapeutic treatment of selective mutism focuses mainly on desensitization procedures. The patient is paired with both an "outsider" and a family member (whom the patient is comfortable speaking around). Decreasing the presence of the family member ideally leads to secondary generalization in which the patient can talk with the "outsider." Contingency management, exposure-based techniques, and self-modeling are also frequently used. The pairing of this behavioral protocol with antianxiety medication serves to desensitize and reduce high levels of anxiety. Medications are eventually tapered and discontinued if possible (Koda et al. 2003). Individual psychodynamically oriented psychotherapy, play therapy, and family therapy are commonly used, although there is limited evidence to support these treatments.

Reactive Attachment Disorder of Infancy or Early Childhood

Clinical Description

Attachment is a central component of social and emotional development, and disordered attachment is defined by specific patterns of abnormal behavior in the context of pathogenic care beginning before age 5 years (American Academy of Child and Adolescent Psychiatry 2005; see Chapter 7 in this volume, "Normal Child and Adolescent Development," by Gemelli). *Reactive attachment disorder* (RAD) encompasses manifestations of two outcomes of prolonged neglect or physical or emotional abuse: children who are hypervigilant and aloof (inhibited subtype) or children who are indiscriminant in their attachments (disinhibited subtype) (Table 21–34). Inhibited children maintain a degree of wariness and may appear hypoactive or lethargic. As infants, they have little interaction with their environment and often resist being held. Conversely, disinhibited children demonstrate exaggerated, although emotionally empty, attachments and may show inappropriate clinging or hugging. These children fail to discriminate between attachment figures and often seek and are apparently willing to accept comfort from anyone, even strangers. In both types of RAD, disturbances in relatedness, emotional reactivity, and cognition are thought to arise from disordered development of early interpersonal attachment.

TABLE 21–34. **DSM-IV-TR diagnostic criteria for reactive attachment disorder**

A. Markedly disturbed and developmentally inappropriate social relatedness in most contexts, beginning before age 5 years, as evidenced by either (1) or (2):

  (1) persistent failure to initiate or respond in a developmentally appropriate fashion to most social interactions, as manifest by excessively inhibited, hypervigilant, or highly ambivalent and contradictory responses (e.g., the child may respond to caregivers with a mixture of approach, avoidance, and resistance to comforting, or may exhibit frozen watchfulness)

  (2) diffuse attachments as manifest by indiscriminate sociability with marked inability to exhibit appropriate selective attachments (e.g., excessive familiarity with relative strangers or lack of selectivity in choice of attachment figures)

B. The disturbance in criterion A is not accounted for solely by developmental delay (as in mental retardation) and does not meet criteria for a pervasive developmental disorder.

C. Pathogenic care as evidenced by at least one of the following:

  (1) persistent disregard of the child's basic emotional needs for comfort, stimulation, and affection

  (2) persistent disregard of the child's basic physical needs

  (3) repeated changes of primary caregiver that prevent formation of stable attachments (e.g., frequent changes in foster care)

D. There is a presumption that the care in criterion C is responsible for the disturbed behavior in criterion A (e.g., the disturbances in criterion A began following the pathogenic care in criterion C).

Specify type:

  Inhibited type: if criterion A1 predominates in the clinical presentation

  Disinhibited type: if criterion A2 predominates in the clinical presentation

Epidemiology

Very few data exist describing the prevalence of RAD, although the disorder is considered to be "rare." In the few available studies of high-risk children in foster care or institutional settings, 30%–40% had signs of RAD (Smyke et al. 2002; Zeanah et al. 2002, 2005). Associated disorders include mental retardation, developmental delay, language disorder, and posttraumatic stress disorder.

Etiology

By definition, RAD results from pathogenic care that includes a persistent disregard for the basic emotional or physical needs of a child or multiple changes in caregivers that do not allow for the development of a stable attachment. However, our understanding of its etiology has evolved from one of faulty parenting to a transactional model in which a developmental deficit in attachment signaling or behavior may play a role (Zeanah et al. 2002). Infants who have chronic illness or handicaps or those who are unwanted may be unable to elicit attachment behaviors from early caregivers. Many parental factors contribute to a disrupted attachment and may include depression, psychosis, mental retardation, or substance abuse as well as poverty, poor education, or chaotic life. Although PDD is excluded from the differential diagnosis of RAD, a study of the core features of autism may provide clues to the origins of detachment and unusual or aberrant forms of attachment behaviors, because children with autism form attachments but do so in an idiosyncratic or peculiar fashion (Sund and Wichstrom 2002). RAD is not the universal outcome of neglectful and abusive parenting. The factors that contribute to resiliency are unknown.

Course and Prognosis

The course and prognosis of untreated RAD range from spontaneous remission to death and other sequelae of pathological parenting. Children from deprived backgrounds may go on to have low IQ, short stature, and hyperactivity. The persistence of the inhibited type of RAD is exceedingly rare in children adopted out of institutions into more normal environments, although the quality of subsequent attachments may still be compromised. Some children with RAD, disinhibited type, retain a pattern of indiscriminate sociability even after adoption. The quality of the new setting is a significant factor in determining the extent of subsequent behavioral and emotional problems (Zeanah 2000).

Diagnostic Evaluation

In addition to a full psychiatric examination of the child, observation of mother–child interactions and a psychiatric examination of the parents are essential to the diagnosis of RAD. A home visit, if the parents are willing, may provide a more complete picture of the relationship with parents. Physical examination may reveal growth delay, neurological disorder, evidence of physical abuse, vitamin deficiencies, malnutrition, or infectious diseases.

Treatment

The primary intervention in the treatment of RAD is to provide a safe environment and basic medical care. One of the most important interventions for children with RAD who lack an attachment to a discriminated caregiver is for the clinician to advocate for an emotionally available attachment figure for the child (American Academy of Child and Adolescent Psychiatry 2005). This caregiver must be sensitive to and invested in the child. Once the child is in a secure and stable placement, initial therapy should focus on fostering positive interactions with the caregiver. Sometimes, individual treatment for the parent is in order. Dyadic interactive therapy can help promote positive interactions, greater mutual understanding, and a rebuilding of trust. Individual therapy with the child may also be helpful. Therapy designed to improve the quality of attachment through a process of regression and corrective reexperiencing ("therapeutic holding" or "rebirthing therapy") has no empirical support and has been associated with serious injury and death.

No psychopharmacological intervention trials for RAD have been conducted. We can treat comorbid psychiatric disorders, but successful behavioral or pharmacological interventions directed at the core features of disordered attachment may prove more challenging (Zeanah et al. 2002). Recent research indicates that during social contact, reward pathways are activated and communicate with regions processing social, facial, and affective information. These findings suggest that several peptide neuromodulators (endorphins, oxytocin, neuropeptide Y) and neurotransmitters are involved in attachment behaviors and may be the foci of future treatment interventions (Davidson 2003).

Stereotypic Movement Disorder

Clinical Description

The diagnostic criteria for stereotypic movement disorder (SMD) include repetitive and purposeless behaviors, such as hand flapping and body rocking, as well as many forms of self-injury, such as head banging. The combination of both stereotypy and SIB creates a heterogeneous condition that encompasses a range of repetitive behaviors in which there is considerable variability of typology, severity, motivational or functional states, and treatment approaches (Rapp and Vollmer 2005a). Additional diversity is the result of the changing nature of SMD during child development, the co-occurrence of intellectual disability, and the relationship of symptom severity to other childhood neuropsychiatric disorders (De Raeymaecker 2006; Table 21–35).

In the general population, SMD mainly affects infants, toddlers, and young children. Persistence beyond this age group suggests other factors such as intellectual disability, PDD, sensory deficit (deafness, blindness), or possibly psychosis. When compared with typically developing children and adults, persistent stereotypies and SIB are far more common in those with severe intellectual disability. Several stereotypies may occur at once, and their frequency may increase with stress, frustration, and boredom.

In addition to differences between subtypes of stereotypies and SIB, there are also major variations in motivation (function), trigger factors, intensity, severity of behaviors, and, in the case of SIB, pain thresholds and termination events (Richman and Lindauer 2005; Robertson 2000). For example, pain may serve as a triggering event, but it can also function to terminate self-injury. In some disorders, such as Lesch-Nyhan syndrome, SIB is severe and extremely painful yet continues until interrupted. Affected individuals may use self-imposed restraints to prevent the binges of mutilating injury (Barnhill 2003).

The current criteria for SMD exclude tics and other movement disorders, OCD, PDDs, and neurodegenerative disorders characterized by perseveration of motor responses (Owley et al. 2005; Robertson 2000). For most children with these disorders, the boundaries between stereotypies, self-injury, tics, and obsessive-compulsive symptoms and autistic spectrum disorders are often difficult to determine (Richman and Lindauer 2005).

Epidemiology

Transient stereotypies during early development occur in 15%–20% of the general population. These are thought to affect men and women equally, although there are indications that head banging is more prevalent in males, with a 3 to 1 ratio, and self-biting may be more common in women (American Psychiatric Asso-

TABLE 21–35. DSM-IV-TR diagnostic criteria for stereotypic movement disorder
A. Repetitive, seemingly driven, and nonfunctional motor behavior (e.g., hand shaking or waving, body rocking, head banging, mouthing of objects, self-biting, hitting own body).
B. The behavior markedly interferes with normal activities or results in self-inflicted bodily injury that requires medical treatment (or would result in an injury if preventive measures were not used).
C. If mental retardation is present, the stereotypic or self-injurious behavior is of sufficient severity to become a focus of treatment.
D. The behavior is not better accounted for by a compulsion (as in obsessive-compulsive disorder), a tic (as in tic disorder), a stereotypy that is part of a pervasive developmental disorder, or hair pulling (as in trichotillomania).
E. The behavior is not due to the direct physiological effects of a substance or a general medical condition.
F. The behavior persists for 4 weeks or longer.
Specify if:
With self-injurious behavior: if the behavior results in bodily damage that requires specific treatment (or that would result in bodily damage if protective measures were not used)

ciation 2000). The prevalence of SIB is higher in children and adults living in large residential treatment facilities (Barnhill 2003; Symons et al. 2005). SIB resulting in tissue damage affects 15%–20% of adults with severe intellectual disability.

The prevalence, severity, and typology of SIB are affected by comorbid medical conditions (e.g., headaches, constipation, or neurodegenerative disorders such as neuroacanthocytosis), behavioral phenotypes (Lesch-Nyhan, Prader-Willi, fragile X, or Smith-Magenis syndrome), drug side effects (akathisia), and comorbid psychiatric disorders (Barnhill 2006; Rapp and Vollmer 2005b). Psychiatric disorders can affect the frequencies of premorbid stereotypies and SIB. For example, there can be a dramatic rise in stereotypic behaviors with the onset of mania or in SIB with major depression. For others, SIB may be a core part of the psychiatric disorder. Patients with borderline personality disorder, schizophrenia, suicidal behavior in major depressive disorder, and posttraumatic stress disorder may engage in SIB. These forms of SIB differ considerably. It is thought that SMD may be the final common pathway for multiple neurobiological substrates (Barnhill 2003; Rapp and Vollmer 2005a).

Etiology

SMDs serve multiple functions and are maintained by many different forms of reinforcement (Kennedy et al. 2000). The most common presentations of SMD in those referred for assessment are behavioral responses to significant overarousal or distress. Stereotypies that emerge during periods of increased environmental demands or uncomfortable affect are frequently anxiety reducing and allow the individual to temporarily escape the stressful circumstances (De Raeymaecker 2006). This may lead to an increased frequency of these behaviors and ultimately may interfere with school performance, occupational functioning, and social interaction. This is more likely to occur with intellectual disability, neurodevelopmental disorders, autism, and behavioral phenotypes such as fragile X syndrome (Symons et al. 2005; Troster 1994).

Some repetitive behaviors appear enjoyable and are thought to be intrinsically reinforcing. This self-stimulation often occurs during boredom or isolation. Other behaviors emerge in understimulating environments (vacuous behaviors) but seem to provide little evidence of intrinsic reinforcement or relief from observable distress (Barnhill 2003, 2006). Some individuals experience a compulsive need to self-injure regardless of pain or other adverse consequences. The forces driving these progressive forms of SIB are unknown but share features with compulsive behaviors and addiction (Barnhill 2003).

In the past, a relative dopamine excess and serotonin deficiency were seen as the major factors in repetitive and self-injurious behaviors. More recently, γ-aminobutyric acid, glutamate, endorphins, vasopressin, oxytocin, corticotropin-releasing hormone, neurosteroids, and other neuropeptides have been thought to play a role. Other factors include phenotypic differences in enzyme systems, transporter proteins, second messenger systems, differences in stress responses, and pain sensitivity (Edwards et al. 2004; Rapp and Vollmer 2005b).

Course and Prognosis

Between 6 and 12 months of age, repetitive behaviors arise as part of normal development during periods of increased arousal or focused attention and are manifestations of neurodevelopmental reflexes. By early childhood, these reflexes have largely disappeared, and there is a growing divergence between normal childhood repetitive behaviors and those associated with OCD. Emerging OCD differs both quantitatively (frequency) and qualitatively from developmental ritualistic behaviors. Qualitative differences of OCD include a relatively narrow range of anxieties and rituals; a decreased association with social behaviors; a motivational state coupled to internal distress, urges, fears, and obsessions; and typically a sense that the behaviors are dystonic to the individual (Richman and Lindauer 2005; Symons et al. 2005).

Once diagnosed, children with SMD follow a variable developmental course. For some, SIB or repetitive behaviors appear during early childhood but then abate with age. For others, SMD progresses from low-intensity stereotypic behaviors (rocking or nail biting) to more severe behaviors (SIBs). This developmental transformation toward self-injury during childhood is accompanied by changes in typology and severity or a shift from intrinsically motivated repetitive behavior toward escape-motivated SMD (Rapp and Vollmer 2005b; Symons et al. 2005).

Diagnostic Evaluation

In the diagnostic evaluation for SMD, the clinician must acquire a detailed description and behavioral analysis of the behaviors and evaluate for genetic, neurological, psychiatric, and psychosocial variables (Rapp and Vollmer 2005b). In early childhood SMD, one must rule out intellectual disability or PDD. Later-onset SMD requires further evaluation for anxiety, mood, or psychotic disorders. Additionally, the clinician must look carefully for medication side effects that may cause or confound these repetitive movements, particularly with dopamine agonists such as stimulants.

Many stereotypic or repetitive behaviors associated with SMD are also observed in patients with tics, OCD, and autistic spectrum disorders. It can be difficult to distinguish SMD from these disorders (Owley et al. 2005). Additionally, with increasingly severe intellectual disability, many children present with persistent repetitive behaviors that defy easy classification (Troster 1994).

Treatment

SMD is often treatment resistant. Behavioral interventions as well as pharmacotherapy may be indicated. Although typically part of behavioral treatments, positive reinforcement has generally not been effective when used alone in SMD. Overcorrection has the most empirical support, although efforts to reduce anxiety and block the pleasurable effects of self-stimulation can also be useful. In non-SIB, ignoring behaviors can be an effective part of a treatment plan, whereas mildly aversive stimuli in SIB can be helpful.

Young children engaged in SMD need to be evaluated for the inappropriateness of the repetitive behaviors. If these behaviors are developmentally appropriate for chronological age, then no treatment is necessary unless parental anxiety is sufficient to disrupt their normal time-limited course. Overprotectiveness, inadvertent reinforcement, and a family dynamic that "pathologizes" these behaviors may require intervention. Psychotherapy, family therapy, and behavioral interventions may be helpful in these situations. Behavioral modification techniques include antecedent (e.g., environmental enrichment) and consequent (differential reinforcement of alternate behaviors) interventions (see Chapter 31 in this volume, "Cognitive Therapy," by Wright et al.).

Behaviors that meet criteria for OCD or comorbid tic disorders may require psychotherapy and, depending on severity, perhaps pharmacotherapy. SSRIs can be helpful but should be used in conjunction with cognitive-behavioral therapy or response prevention therapies (Rapp and Vollmer 2005a, 2005b). Patients with genetic syndromes or specific behavioral phenotypes may require a more comprehensive assessment and referral to clinicians familiar with these syndromes. For patients with SMD and intellectual disability, SSRIs, mood-stabilizing antiepileptic agents, opiate blockers such as naltrexone, and second-generation antipsychotic drugs can be helpful, but the clinician needs to be aware that adverse drug reactions can contribute to an escalation in SMD and SIB (Rapp and Vollmer 2005a; see Chapter 36 in this volume, "Treatment of Children and Adolescents," by Crawford et al.).

Stereotypic Movement Disorder Summary

SMD is a developmental disorder characterized by repetitive behaviors and, in some situations, SIBs. The clinician must distinguish between normal developmental repetitive behaviors and those that represent significant risk for psychopathology. Although excluded from the diagnosis, tic disorders, OCD, and autistic spectrum disorders may overlap with SMD, and their exclusion can be difficult. Because intellectual disability is also a risk factor for persistent or progressive forms of SMD, the clinician may need to request help from individuals skilled in working with this population. The hasty and injudicious use of medication protocols can become counterproductive and expose children to risks that might be avoided by careful assessment and behavioral interventions.

Conclusion

Many psychiatric disorders have their onset in childhood or adolescence. These disorders can influence development and continue into adulthood, exerting significant and long-lasting effects on a person's self-esteem and sense of satisfaction with relationships or jobs. Variations in presentation may depend on the individual's developmental level. Research in child psychiatric disorders is continuing to increase, and effective treatments are now available for many childhood psychiatric disorders.

Key Points

- Pervasive developmental disorders are neuropsychiatric disorders of development characterized by social, communication, and behavioral symptoms that vary in presentation and severity among individuals.

- Conduct disorder and oppositional defiant disorder are heterogeneous, nonspecific diagnoses with likely multifactorial etiologies. Comorbid psychiatric diagnoses are common and require attention. Effective treatments incorporate cognitive skill development, parental training, and involvement of appropriate community systems.

- Attention-deficit/hyperactivity disorder is a highly comorbid disorder and appears to be an enduring condition in some patients.

- Current diagnostic criteria for learning disorders emphasize a lag in academic performance. Most state and federal guidelines define learning disorders as a discrepancy of 1.5 to 2.0 standard deviations between expected performance on standardized tests and measured intellectual abilities.

- Stereotypic or repetitive behaviors may arise as part of normal development between 6 and 12 months of age.

- A complete psychiatric examination of a child should include a complete medical evaluation and physical examination to assess for organic etiologies of presenting symptoms.

Suggested Readings

Dulcan MK: Helping Parents, Youth, and Teachers Understand Medications for Behavioral and Emotional Problems: A Resource Book of Medication Information Handouts. Washington, DC, American Psychiatric Publishing, 2007

Dulcan MK, Wiener JM: Essentials of Child and Adolescent Psychiatry. Washington, DC, American Psychiatric Publishing, 2006

Dulcan MK, Martini R, Lake M: Concise Guide to Child and Adolescent Psychiatry, 3rd Edition. Washington, DC, American Psychiatric Publishing, 2003

Gemelli R: Normal Child and Adolescent Development. Washington, DC, American Psychiatric Publishing, 1996

Green WH: Child and Adolescent Clinical Psychopharmacology. Philadelphia, PA, Lippincott Williams & Wilkins, 2006

Lewis M: Child and Adolescent Psychiatry: A Comprehensive Textbook, 3rd Edition. Philadelphia, PA, Lippincott Williams & Wilkins, 2002

Online Resources

American Academy of Child and Adolescent Psychiatry (www.aacap.org)

Children and Adults with Attention Deficit/Hyperactivity Disorder (www.chadd.org)

Learning Disabilities Association of America (www.ldaamerica.org)

National Institutes of Mental Health (www.nimh.nih.gov)

National Mental Health Association (www.nmha.org)

Online Mendelian Inheritance in Man (www.ncbi.nlm.nih.gov/sites/entrez?db=OMIM)

Tourette Syndrome Association, Inc. (www.tsa-usa.org)

References

Abikoff H, Courtney M, Pelham WEJ, et al: Teacher's ratings of disruptive behaviors: the influence of halo effects. J Abnorm Child Psychol 21:519–533, 1993

Aman MG, Lindsay RL, Nash PL, et al: Individuals with mental retardation, in Pediatric Psychopharmacology. Edited by Martin A, Scahill L, Charney DS, et al. New York, Oxford University Press, 2003, pp 617–630

American Academy of Child and Adolescent Psychiatry: Practice parameters for the assessment and treatment of children, adolescents, and adults with attention deficit/hyperactivity disorder. J Am Acad Child Adolesc Psychiatry 36 (suppl):85S–121S, 1997

American Academy of Child and Adolescent Psychiatry: Practice parameters for the assessment and treatment of children and adolescents with language and learning disorders. J Am Acad Child Adolesc Psychiatry 37:46S–62S, 1998

American Academy of Child and Adolescent Psychiatry: Practice parameters for the use of stimulant medications in the treatment of children, adolescents, and adults. J Am Acad Child Adolesc Psychiatry 41 (suppl):26S–49S, 2002

American Academy of Child and Adolescent Psychiatry: Practice parameters for the assessment and treatment of children and adolescents with reactive attachment disorder of infancy and early childhood. J Am Acad Child Adolesc Psychiatry 44:1206–1219, 2005

American Psychiatric Association: Diagnostic and Statistical Manual of Mental Disorders, 3rd Edition. Washington, DC, American Psychiatric Association, 1980

American Psychiatric Association: Diagnostic and Statistical Manual of Mental Disorders, 4th Edition. Washington, DC, American Psychiatric Association, 1994

American Psychiatric Association: Diagnostic and Statistical Manual of Mental Disorders, 4th Edition, Text Revision. Washington, DC, American Psychiatric Association, 2000

Amir RE, Van den Veyver IB, Wan M, et al: Rett syndrome is caused by mutation in X-linked MECP2, encoding methyl-CpG-binding protein 2. Nat Genet 23:185–188, 1999

Ardila S, Surloff C: Dysexecutive agraphia: a major executive dysfunction sign. Int J Neuroscience 116:653–663, 2006

Arnold LE, DiSilvestro RA: Zinc in attention-deficit/hyperactivity disorder. J Child Adolesc Psychopharmacol 15:619–627, 2005

Asperger H: "Autistic psychopathy" in childhood (1944), in Autism and Asperger Syndrome. Translated and annotated by Frith U. Cambridge, UK, Cambridge University Press, 1991, pp 37–92

Baer L: Factor analysis of symptom subtypes of obsessive-compulsive disorders and their relationship to personality and tic disorders. J Clin Psychiatry 53 (suppl):18–23, 1994

Baird G, Charman T, Baron-Cohen S, et al: A screening instrument for autism at 18 months of age: a 6-year follow-up study. J Am Acad Child Adolesc Psychiatry 39:694–702, 2000

Barling J, Bullen G: Dietary factors and hyperactivity: a failure to replicate. J Genet Psychol 146:117–123, 1985

Barnhill LJ: Can the DSM-IV be salvaged? Ment Health Aspects Dev Disabil 6:85–99, 1999

Barnhill LJ: Neurobiology of self-injurious behavior: is there a relationship to addictions? Nat Assoc Dual Diag Bull 6:29–37, 2003

Barnhill LJ: Stereotypic movement disorder. Nat Assoc Dual Diag Bull 9:23–26, 2006

Barnhill LJ, Horrigan JP: Tourette's syndrome and autism: a search for common ground. Ment Health Aspects Dev Disabil 5:7–15, 2002

Barnett SR, Riddle MA: Anxiolytics, buspirone, and others, in Pediatric Psychopharmacology. Edited by Martin A, Scahill L, Charney DS, et al. New York, Oxford University Press, 2003, pp 341–352

Biederman J, Newcorn J, Sprich S: Comorbidity of attention deficit hyperactivity disorder with conduct, depressive, anxiety, and other disorders. Am J Psychiatry 148:564–577, 1991

Biederman J, Milberger S, Faraone SV, et al: Associations between childhood asthma and ADHD: issues of psychiatric comorbidity and familiality. J Am Acad Child Adolesc Psychiatry 33:842–848, 1994

Biederman J, Faraone SV, Milberger S, et al: Predictors of persistence and remission of ADHD into adolescence: results from a four-year prospective follow-up study. J Am Acad Child Adolesc Psychiatry 35:343–351, 1996

Biederman J, Swanson JM, Wigal SB, et al: A comparison of once-daily and divided doses of modafinil in children with attention-deficit/hyperactivity disorder: a randomized, double blind, and placebo-controlled study. J Clin Psychiatry 67:727–735, 2006

Black B, Uhde TW: Treatment of elective mutism with fluoxetine: a double blind, placebo-controlled study. J Am Acad Child Adolesc Psychiatry 33:1000–1106, 1994

Black B, Uhde TW: Psychiatric characteristics of children with selective mutism: a pilot study. J Acad Child Adolesc Psychiatry 34:847–856, 1995

Brestan EV, Eyberg SM: Effective psychosocial treatment of conduct-disordered children and adolescents: 29 years, 82 studies, 5275 children. J Clin Child Psychol 27:180–189, 1998

Bruun RD, Budman CL: Natural history of Gilles de la Tourette's syndrome, in Handbook of Tourette's Syndrome and Related Tic Behavioral Disorders. Edited by Kurlan R. New York, Marcel-Dekker, 1994, pp 27–43

Castellanos FX, Sharp WS, Gottesman RF, et al: Anatomic brain abnormalities in monozygotic twins discordant for attention deficit hyperactivity disorder. Am J Psychiatry 160:1693–1696, 2003

Chandola CA, Robling MR, Peters TJ, et al: Pre and perinatal factors and the risk of subsequent referral for hyperactivity. J Child Psychol Psychiatry 33:1077–1090, 1992

Chappell PB, Riddle MA, Scahill L, et al: Guanfacine treatment of comorbid attention-deficit hyperactivity disorder and Tourette's syndrome: preliminary clinical experience. J Am Acad Child Adolesc Psychiatry 34:1140–1146, 1995

Charach A, Figueroa M, Chen S, et al: Stimulant treatment over 5 years: effects on growth. J Am Acad Child Adolesc Psychiatry 45:415–421, 2006

Chatoor I: Feeding and eating disorders of infancy and early childhood, in The American Psychiatric Publishing Textbook of Child and Adolescent Psychiatry. Edited by Wiener JM, Dulcan MK. Washington, DC, American Psychiatric Publishing, 2004, pp 639–657

Cobham VE, Dadds MR, Spence SH: The role of parental anxiety in the treatment of childhood anxiety. J Consult Clin Psychol 66:893–905, 1998

Coccaro EF, Siever LJ: Pathophysiology and treatment of aggression, in Neuropsychopharmacology: Fifth Generation of Progress. Edited by Davis KL, Charney DS, Coyle JT, et al. Baltimore, MD, Lippincott Williams & Wilkins, 2002, pp 1709–1724

Comings DE, Comings BG: A controlled family history of Tourette's syndrome, I: attention-deficit hyperactivity disorder and learning disorders. J Clin Psychiatry 51:275–280, 1990

Comings DE, Gade-Andovalu R, Gonzales N, et al: Comparison of the role of dopamine, serotonin and noradrenaline genes in ADHD, ODD, and conduct disorder: multivariate regression analysis of 20 genes. Clin Genet 57:178–196, 2000

Connors CK, Schulte AC: Learning disorders, in Neuropsychopharmacology: The Fifth Generation of Progress. Edited by Davis KL, Charney D, Coyle JT, et al. Baltimore, MD, Lippincott Williams & Wilkins, 2002, pp 597–610

Costello EJ, Mustillo S, Erkanli A, et al: Prevalence and development of psychiatric disorders in childhood and adolescence. Arch Gen Psychiatry 60:837–844, 2003

Davidson RJ: Emotion and disorders of emotion: perspectives from affective neuroscience, in Neuropsychiatry, 2nd Edition. Edited by Schiffer RB, Rao SM, Fogel BS. Baltimore, MD, Lippincott Williams & Wilkins, 2003, pp 467–480

de Groot CM, Bornstein RA: Obsessive characteristics in subjects with Tourette's syndrome are related to characteristics in their parents. Compr Psychiatry 35:248–251, 1994

De Raeymaecker DM: Psychomotor development and psychopathology in childhood. Int Rev Neurobiology 72:83–101, 2006

DeGiacomo A, Fombonne E: Parental recognition of developmental abnormalities in autism. Eur Child Adolesc Psychiatry 7:131–136, 1998

Denckla MB, Roeltgen DP: Disorders of motor function and control, in Handbook of Neuropsychology, Vol 6. Edited by Rapin I, Segalowitz SJ. Amsterdam, The Netherlands, Elsevier, 1992, pp 455–476

Dick DM, Viken RJ, Kaprio J, et al: Understanding the covariation among childhood externalizing symptoms: genetic and environmental influences on conduct disorder, attention deficit hyperactivity disorder, and oppositional defiant disorder symptoms. J Abnorm Child Psychol 33:219–229, 2005

Eapen V, Yakeley JW, Robertson MM: Gilles de la Tourette's syndrome and obsessive-compulsive disorder, in Neuropsychiatry, 2nd Edition. Edited by Schiffer RL, Rao SM, Fogel BS. Baltimore, MD, Lippincott Williams & Wilkins, 2002, pp 947–990

Edwards MJ, Dale RC, Church AJ, et al: Adult-onset tic disorders, motor stereotypies, and behavioral disturbances associated with antibasal ganglia antibodies. Mov Disord 19:1190–1196, 2004

Egger J, Stolla A, McEwen LM: Controlled trial of hyposensitization in children with food-induced hyperkinetic syndrome. Lancet 339:1150–1153, 1992

Elia J, Gulotta C, Rose SR, et al: Thyroid function and attention deficit hyperactivity disorder. J Am Acad Child Adolesc Psychiatry 33:169–172, 1994

Einfield SL, Aman M: Issues in the taxonomy of psychopathology in mental retardation. J Autism Dev Disord 25:143–167, 1995

Ernst M, Zametkin AJ, Matochik JA, et al: High midbrain [18F]DOPA accumulation in children with attention deficit hyperactivity disorder. Am J Psychiatry 156:1209–1215, 1999

Farmer EM, Compton SN, Bums BJ, et al: Review of the evidence base for treatment of childhood psychopathology: externalizing disorders. J Consult Clin Psychol 70:1267–1302, 2002

Faraone SV, Biederman J, Lehman BK, et al: Intellectual performance and school failure in children with attention deficit hyperactivity disorder and their siblings. J Abnorm Psychol 102:616–623, 1993

Fergusson DM, Lynskey MT, Horwood LJ: The effect of maternal depression on maternal ratings of child behavior. J Abnorm Child Psychol 21:245–269, 1993

Filipek PA, Semrud-Clikeman M, Steingard RJ, et al: Volumetric MRI analysis comparing subjects having attention deficit hyperactivity disorder with normal controls. Neurology 48:589–601, 1997

Fischer M: Persistence of ADHD into adulthood: it depends on whom you ask. ADHD Rep 5:8–10, 1997

Fletcher JM: Predicting math outcomes: reading predictors and comorbidity. J Learn Disabil 38:308–312, 2005

Fombonne E, Zakarian R, Bennett A, et al: Pervasive developmental disorders in Montreal, Quebec, Canada: prevalence and links with immunizations. Pediatrics 118:e139–e150, 2006

Forrest BJ: The utility of math difficulties, internalized psychopathology, and visual spatial deficits to identify children with nonverbal learning disability syndrome: evidence for visual spatial disability. Child Neuropsychol 10:129–146, 2004

Gainetdinov RR, Caron MG: Genetics of childhood disorders: XXIV, ADHD, part 8: hyperdopaminergic mice as an animal model of ADHD. J Am Acad Child Adolesc Psychiatry 40:380–382, 2001

Gershorn J: A meta-analytic review of gender differences in ADHD. J Atten Disord 5:143–154, 2002

Gillberg C, Wing L: Autism: not an extremely rare disorder. Acta Psychiatr Scand 99:399–406, 1999

Goldstein S, Reynolds CR: Handbook of Neurodevelopmental and Genetic Disorders in Children. New York, Guilford, 1999

Griffiths DM, Gardner WI, Nugent JA: Behavioral Supports and Community Living. Kingston, NY, NADD Press, 1998

Guthrie E, Mast J, Engel M: Diagnosing genetic anomalies by inspection. Child Adolesc Psychiatr Clin N Am 8:777–790, 1999

Hagberg BA, Witt-Engerström I: Rett syndrome: a suggested staging system for describing impairment profile with increasing age toward adolescence. Am J Med Genet 24:47–59, 1986

Halperin JM, Newcorn JH, Matier K, et al: Impulsivity and the initiation of fights in children with disruptive behavior disorders. J Child Psychol Psychiatry 36:1199–1211, 1995

Harris JC: Behavioral phenotypes of neurodevelopmental disorders: portals into the developing brain, in Neuropsychopharmacology: Fifth Generation of Progress. Edited by Davis KM, Charney D, Coyle JT, et al. Baltimore, MD, Lippincott Williams & Wilkins, 2002, pp 625–638

Harris JC: Intellectual Disability: Understanding Its Development, Causes, Classification, Evaluation and Treatment. New York, Oxford University Press, 2006

Hauser P, Zametkin AJ, Martinez P, et al: Attention deficit hyperactivity disorder in people with generalized resistance to thyroid hormone. N Engl J Med 328:997–1001, 1993

Hechtman L: Long-term outcome in attention-deficit hyperactivity disorder. Psychiatr Clin North Am 1:553–565, 1993

Hechtman L: Genetic and neurobiological aspects of attention deficit hyperactivity disorder: a review. J Psychiatry Neurosci 19:193–201, 1994

Hendren RL, Mullen DJ: Conduct disorder and oppositional defiant disorder, in Essentials of Child and Adolescent Psychiatry. Edited by Dulcan MK, Wiener JM. Washington, DC, American Psychiatric Publishing, 2006

Hetherington EM, Stanley-Hagan M: The adjustment of children with divorced parents: a risk and resiliency perspective. J Child Psychol Psychiatry 40:129–140, 1999

Hynd GW, Semrud-Clikeman M, Lorys AR, et al: Corpus callosum morphology in attention deficit-hyperactivity disorder: morphometric analysis of MRI. J Learn Disabil 24:141–146, 1991

Iiada J, Sakiyama S, Iwasaka H, et al. The clinical features of Tourette's disorders and obsessive-compulsive disorders. J Psychiatry Clin Neurosci 50:185–189, 1996

Ingalls S, Goldstein S: Learning disabilities, in Handbook of Neurodevelopmental and Genetic Disorders in Children. Edited by Goldstein S, Reynolds CR. New York, Guilford, 1999, pp 101–154

Jankovic J, DeLeon ML: Basal ganglia and behavioral disorders, in Neuropsychiatry, 2nd Edition. Edited by Schiffer RL, Rao SM, Fogel BS. Baltimore, MD, Lippincott Williams & Wilkins, 2002, pp 934–945

Jensen PS, Shervette RE, Xenakis SN, et al: Anxiety and depressive disorders in attention deficit disorder with hyperactivity: new findings. Am J Psychiatry 150:1203–1209, 1993

Joy SP, Lord JS, Green L, et al: Mental retardation and developmental disabilities, in Neuropsychiatry, 2nd Edition. Edited by Schiffer RS, Rao SM, Fogel BS. Baltimore, MD, Lippincott Williams & Wilkins, 2003, pp 552–604

Kanner L: Autistic disturbances of affective contact. Nervous Child 2:217–250, 1943

Kelly DP, Kelly BJ, Jones MI, et al: Attention deficits in children and adolescents with hearing loss: a survey. Am J Dis Child 147:737–741, 1993

Kennedy CH, Meyer KA, Knowles T, et al: Analyzing the multiple functions of stereotypical behavior for students with autism: implications for assessment and treatment. J Appl Behav Anal 33:559–571, 2000

King RA, Scahill L, Lombroso P, et al: Tourette's syndrome and other tic disorders, in Pediatric Psychopharmacology. Edited by Martin A, Scahill L, Charney DS, et al. New York, Oxford University Press, 2003, pp 526–542

Klein RG, Mannuzza S: Children with uncomplicated reading disorders grown up: a prospective follow-up into adulthood, in Learning Disabilities: Implications for Psychiatric Treatment (Review of Psychiatry series, Vol 19, No 5; Oldham JO, Riba MB, series eds.). Edited by Greenhill LL. Washington, DC, American Psychiatric Press, 2000, pp 1–31

Koda V, Charney DS, Pine D: Neurobiology of early onset anxiety disorders, in Pediatric Psychopharmacology. Edited by Martin A, Scahill L, Charney DS, et al. New York, Oxford University Press, 2003, pp 138–149

Labellarte M, Ginsburg G: Anxiety disorders, in Pediatric Psychopharmacology. Edited by Martin A, Scahill L, Charney DS, et al. New York, Oxford University Press, 2003, pp 497–510

Lachiewicz AM, Dawson DV, Spirigidiollozzi GA, et al: Arithmetic difficulties in females with the fragile X premutation. Am J Med Genet 140:665–672, 2006

Landman GB, Rappaport L: Pediatric management of severe treatment-resistant encopresis. J Dev Behav Pediatr 6:349–351, 1985

Lavigne JV, Burns WJ, Cotter PD: Rumination in infancy: recent behavioral approaches. Int J Eat Disord 1:70–82, 1981

Leckman JF, Yeh C-B, Lombroso PJ: Neurobiology of tic disorders, in Pediatric Psychopharmacology. Edited by Martin A, Scahill L, Charney DS, et al. New York, Oxford University Press, 2003, pp 164–174

Litt J, Taylor HG, Klein N, et al: Learning disabilities in children with very low birthweight: prevalence, neuropsychological correlations, educational interventions. J Learn Disabil 38:13–41, 2005

Loeber R, Green SM, Keenan K, et al: Which boys will fare worse? Early predictors for the onset of conduct disorder in a six-year longitudinal study. J Am Acad Child Adolesc Psychiatry 34:499–509, 1995

Loening-Baucke V: Encopresis. Curr Opin Pediatr 14:570–575, 2002

Lord C: Follow-up of two-year-olds referred for possible autism. J Child Psychol Psychiatry 36:1365–1382, 1995

Marchi M, Cohen P: Early childhood eating behaviors and adolescent eating disorders. J Am Acad Child Adolesc Psychiatry 29:112–117, 1990

Marshall RM, Schafer VA, O'Donnell L, et al: Arithmetic disabilities and ADD subtypes: implications for the DSM-IV. J Learn Disabil 32:239–247, 1999

Mazzocco MM: Math learning disability and math LD subtypes: evidence from studies of turner syndrome, fragile X, and neurofibromatosis type I. J Learn Disabil 34:520–533, 2001

McCracken JT, McGough J, Shah B, et al: Risperidone in children with autism and serious behavioral problems. N Engl J Med 347:314–321, 2002

McDougle CJ, Scahill L, Aman MG, et al: Risperidone for the core symptom domains of autism: results from the study by the autism network of the research units on pediatric psychopharmacology. Am J Psychiatry 162:1142–1148, 2005

McGee R, Stanton WR, Sears MR: Allergic disorders and attention deficit disorder in children. J Abnorm Child Psychol 21:79–88, 1993

Mendlowitz SL, Manassis K, Bradley S, et al: Cognitive-behavioral group treatments in childhood anxiety disorders: the role of parental involvement. J Am Acad Child Adolesc Psychiatry 38:1223–1229, 1999

Mikkelsen EJ, Rapoport JL: Enuresis: psychopathology, sleep stage and drug response. Urol Clin North Am 7:361–377, 1980

Moffat ME, Harlos S, Kirshen AJ, et al: Desmopressin acetate and nocturnal enuresis: how much do we know? Pediatrics 92:420–425, 1993

Moldavsky M, Lev D, Lerman-Sagie T: Behavioral phenotypes of genetic syndromes: a reference guide for psychiatrists. J Am Acad Child Adolesc Psychiatry 40:749–760, 2001

Motofsky SH, Reiss AL, Lockhart P, et al: Evaluation of cerebellar size in attention-deficit hyperactivity disorder. J Child Neurol 13:434–439, 1998

Multimodal Treatment of ADHD Cooperative Group: A 14-month randomized clinical trial of treatment strategies for attention-deficit/hyperactivity disorder. The Multimodal Treatment of ADHD Cooperative Group: Multimodal Treatment Study of Children with ADHD. Arch Gen Psychiatry 56:1073–1086, 1999

Newcorn JH, Halperin JM: Comorbidity among disruptive behavior disorders: impact on severity, impairment, and response to treatment. Child Adolesc Psychiatr Clin N Am 3:227–252, 1994

Online Mendelian Inheritance in Man Database: Reading Disability. Bethesda, MD, National Institutes of Health and Johns Hopkins University, 2003

Ornoy A, Uriel L, Tennenbaum A: Inattention, hyperactivity and speech delay at 2–4 years of age as a predictor for ADD-ADHD syndrome. Isr J Psychiatry Relat Sci 30:155–163, 1993

Owley T, Leventhal B, Cook E: EPS or stereotypies? J Child Adolesc Psychopharmacol 15:150–151, 2005

Paul R: Language Disorders From Infancy Through Adolescence: Assessment and Intervention, 2nd Edition. St. Louis, MO, Mosby, 2001

Pelham WEJ, Gnagy EM, Greenslade KE, et al: Teacher ratings of DSM-III-R symptoms for the disruptive behavior disorders. J Am Acad Child Adolesc Psychiatry 31:210–218, 1992

Peters JM, Barnett AL, Henderson SE: Clumsiness, dyspraxia, and developmental coordination disorder. Child Care Health Dev 27:399–412, 2001

Piven J, Palmer P, Landa R, et al: Personality and language characteristics in parents from multiple-incidence autism families. Am J Med Genet 74:398–411, 1997

Popper CW, Elliot GR: Sudden death and tricyclic antidepressants: clinical considerations for children. J Child Adolesc Psychopharmacol 1:125–132, 1990

Popper CW, Gammon GD, West SA, et al: Disorders usually first diagnosed in infancy, childhood, or adolescence, in The American Psychiatric Publishing Textbook of Clinical Psychiatry. Edited by Hales RE, Yudofsky SC. Washington, DC, American Psychiatric Publishing, 2003, pp 833–974

Posey DJ, Erickson CA, Stigler KA, et al: The use of selective serotonin reuptake inhibitors in autism and related disorders. J Child Adolesc Psychopharmacol 16:181–186, 2006

Potenza MN, Hollander E: Pathological gambling and impulse control disorders, in Neuropsychopharmacology: Fifth Generation of Progress. Edited by Davis KL, Charney DS, Coyle JT, et al. Baltimore, MD, Lippincott Williams & Wilkins, 2002, pp 1725–1742

Ramus F, Rosen S, Dakin SC, et al: Theories of developmental dyslexia: insights from multiple case study of dyslexic adults. Brain 126:841–865, 2003

Rapp JT, Vollmer TR: Stereotypy I: a review of behavioral assessment and treatment. Res Dev Disabil 26:527–547, 2005a

Rapp JT, Vollmer TR: Stereotypy II: a review of the neurobiological interpretations and suggestions for integration with behavioral methods. Res Dev Disabil 26:548–564, 2005b

Richman DM, Lindauer SE: Longitudinal assessment of stereotypic, proto-injurious, and self-injurious behavior exhibited by young children with developmental delays. Am J Ment Retard 110:439–450, 2005

Riddle MA, Nelson JC, Kleinman CS, et al: Sudden death in children receiving Norpramin: a review of three reported cases and commentary. J Am Acad Child Adolesc Psychiatry 30:104–108, 1991

Rizwan S, Manning JT, Brabin BJ: Maternal smoking during pregnancy and possible effects of in utero testosterone: evidence from the 2D:4D finger length ratio. Early Hum Dev 83:87–90, 2007

Robertson MM: Tourette's syndrome, associated conditions, and the complexities of treatment. Brain 23:425–463, 2000

Robins LN, Ratcliff KS: Risk factors in the continuation of childhood antisocial behavior into adulthood. Int J Ment Health 7:96–111, 1979

Rockney RM, McQuade WH, Days AL: The plain abdominal roentgenogram in the management of encopresis. Arch Pediatr Adolesc Med 149:623–627, 1995

Rourke BP, Hayman-Abello BA, Collins DW: Learning disabilities: a neuropsychological perspective, in Neuropsychiatry, 2nd Edition. Edited by Schiffer RB, Rao SM, Fogel BS. Baltimore, MD, Lippincott Williams & Wilkins, 2003, pp 630–659

Rowe KS, Rowe KJ: Synthetic food coloring and behavior: a dose response effect in a double-blind, placebo-controlled, repeated-measures study. J Pediatr 125:691–698, 1994

Rowe R, Maughan B, Worthman CM, et al: Testosterone, antisocial behavior and social dominance in boys: pubertal development and biosocial interaction. Biol Psychiatry 55:546–552, 2004

Rubia K, Overmeyer S, Taylor E, et al: Hypofrontality in attention-deficit hyperactivity disorder during high-order motor control: a study with functional MRI. Am J Psychiatr 156:891–896, 1999

Rutter M: Concepts of autism: a review of research. J Child Psychol Psychiatry 9:1–25, 1968

Rutter M: Assessment objectives and principles, in Language Development and Disorders. Edited by Yule W, Rutter M. Philadelphia, PA, JB Lippincott, 1987, pp 295–311

Saint-Cyr JA, Taylor AE, Nicholson K: Behavior and the basal ganglia. Adv Neurol 28:273–281, 1995

Santangelo SI, Pauls DL, Goldstein JM, et al: Tourette's syndrome: what are the influences of gender and comorbid obsessive-compulsive disorders? J Am Acad Child Adolesc Psychiatry 33:785–804, 1994

Saxena S, Bota RG, Brody AI: Brain behavior relationships in obsessive-compulsive disorders. Semin Clin Neuropsychiatry 6:82–101, 2001

Scahill L, Schwab-Stone M: Epidemiology of ADHD in school-age children. Child Adolesc Psychiatr Clin N Am 9:541–555, 2000

Scahill L, Chappell PB, Kim YS, et al: A placebo-controlled study of guanfacine in the treatment of children with tic disorders and attention deficit hyperactivity disorder. Am J Psychiatry 158:1067–1074, 2001

Sechzer JA, Faro MD, Windle WF: Studies of monkeys asphyxiated at birth: implications for minimal cerebral dysfunction. Semin Psychiatry 5:19–34, 1973

Seeger G, Schloss P, Schmidt MH: Functional polymorphism within the promoter of the serotonin transporter gene is associated with severe hyperkinetic disorders. Mol Psychiatry 6:235–238, 2001

Shaywitz BA, Pugh KR, Fletcher JM, et al: What cognitive and neurobiological studies have taught us about dyslexia, in Learning Disabilities: Implications for Psychiatric Treatment (Review of Psychiatry series, Vol 19, No 5; Oldham JM and Riba MB, series eds.). Edited by Greenhill LL. Washington, DC, American Psychiatric Press, 2000, pp 59–96

Shen YC, Wang YF, Yang XL: An epidemiological investigation of minimal brain dysfunction in six elementary schools in Beijing. J Child Psychol Psychiatry 26:777–787, 1985

Smyke AT, Dumitrescu A, Zeanah CH: Attachment disturbances in young children, I: the continuum of caretaking casualty. J Am Acad Child Adolesc Psychiatry 41:972–982, 2002

South M, Ozonoff S, McMahon WM: Repetitive behavioral profile in Asperger's syndrome and high functioning autism. J Autism Dev Disord 35:145–158, 2005

Soyka M, Preuss UW, Koller G, et al: Association of the 5-HT$_{1B}$ receptor gene and antisocial behavior and alcoholism. J Neural Transm 111:101–109, 2004

Speiser Z, Korczyn AD, Teplitzky I, et al: Hyperactivity in rats following postnatal anoxia. Behav Brain Res 7:379–382, 1983

Spencer TJ, Biederman J, Steingard R, et al: Bupropion exacerbates tics in children with attention-deficit hyperactivity disorder and Tourette's syndrome. J Am Acad Child Adolesc Psychiatry 32:211–214, 1993

Spencer TJ, Biederman J, Wilens TE: Attention-deficit/hyperactivity disorder and comorbidity. Pediatr Clin North Am 46:915–927, 1999

Spencer TJ, Faraone SV, Biederman J, et al: Does prolonged therapy with a long-acting stimulant suppress growth in children with ADHD? J Am Acad Child Adolesc Psychiatry 45:527–537, 2006

Stein DJ, Zohar J, Simeon D: Compulsive and impulsive aspects of self-injurious behavior, in Neuropsychopharmacology: Fifth Generation of Progress. Edited by Davis KL, Charney D, Coyle JT, et al. Baltimore, MD, Lippincott Williams & Wilkins, 2002, pp 1743–1758

Stengel-Rutkowski S, Anderlik L: Abilities and needs of children with genetic syndromes. Genet Couns 16:383–391, 2005

Sund AM, Wichstrom L: Insecure attachment as a risk factor for future depressive symptoms in early adolescence. J Am Acad Child Adolesc Psychiatry 41:1478–1485, 2002

Swanson JM, McBurnett K, Wigal T, et al: Effect of stimulant medication on children with attention deficit disorder: "a review of reviews." Except Child 60:154–162, 1993

Swedo SE, Pine DS (eds): Anxiety disorders. Child Adolesc Psychiatr Clin N Am 14:xv–xviii, 2005

Swerdlow NR, Leckman JF: Tourette's syndrome and related disorders, in Neuropsychopharmacology: Fifth Generation of Progress. Edited by Davis KL, Charney DS, Coyle JT, et al. Baltimore, MD, Lippincott Williams & Wilkins, 2002, pp 1685–1698

Symons FJ, Sperry LA, Dropik PL, et al: The early development of stereotypy and self-injury: a review of research methods. J Intel Disabil Res 49:144–158, 2005

Tcheremissine OV, Lieving LM: Pharmacological aspects of the treatment of conduct disorder in children and adolescents. CNS Drugs 20:549–565, 2006

Troster H: Prevalence and functions of stereotyped behaviors in nonhandicapped children in residential care. J Abnorm Child Psychol 22:79–97, 1994

Tsai LY: Autistic disorder, in The American Psychiatric Publishing Textbook of Child and Adolescent Psychiatry, 3rd Edition. Edited by Weiner JM, Dulcan MK. Washington, DC, American Psychiatric Publishing, 2004, pp 261–315

U.S. Department of Education: Twenty-Fourth Annual Report to Congress on the Implementation of the Individuals With Disabilities Education Act. Washington, DC, U.S. Office of Special Education Programs, 2002

Vaccarino FM, Leckman JF: Overview of brain development, in Pediatric Psychopharmacology. Edited by Martin A, Scahill L, Charney DS, et al. New York, Oxford University Press, 2003, pp 3–19

Verhulst FC, Achenbach TM, Ferdinand RF, et al: Epidemiological comparisons of American and Dutch adolescents' self-reports. J Am Acad Child Adolesc Psychiatry 32:1135–1144, 1993

Vitiello B, Stoff D, Atkins M, et al: Soft neurological signs and impulsivity in children. J Dev Behav Pediatr 11:112–115, 1990

Volkmar FR, Rutter M: Childhood disintegrative disorder: results of the DSM-IV field trial. J Am Acad Child Adolesc Psychiatry 34:1092–1095, 1995

Volkmar FR, Klin A, Siegel B, et al: Field trial for autistic disorder in DSM-IV. Am J Psychiatry 151:1361–1367, 1994

Walker CE, Miller L, Bonner B: Incontinence disorders: enuresis and encopresis, in Handbook of Pediatric Psychology. Edited by Routh D. New York, Guilford, 1988, pp 263–298

Walker JL, Lahey BB, Hynd GW, et al: Comparison of specific patterns of antisocial behavior in children with conduct disorder with or without coexisting hyperactivity. J Consult Clin Psychol 55:910–913, 1987

Walkup JT, Mink JW, Hollenbeck PJ: Advances in Neurology, Vol 99. Baltimore, MD, Lippincott Williams & Wilkins, 2006

Weinberg WA, McLean A: A diagnostic approach to developmental specific learning disorders. J Child Neurol 2:158–172, 1986

Werner EE: High risk children in young adulthood: a longitudinal study from birth to 32 years. Am J Orthopsychiatry 59:72–81, 1989

Whitaker AH, Van Rossen R, Feldman JF, et al: Psychiatric outcomes in low-birth-weight children at age 6 years: relation to neonatal cranial ultrasound abnormalities. Arch Gen Psychiatry 54:847–856, 1997

Wigal S, Swanson JM, Feifel D, et al: A double-blind, placebo-controlled trial of dexmethylphenidate hydrochloride and D,L-threomethylphenidate hydrochloride in children with attention-deficit/hyperactivity disorder. J Am Acad Child Adolesc Psychiatry 43:1406–1414, 2004

Wilens TE, Dodson W: A clinical perspective of attention-deficit/hyperactivity disorder into adulthood. J Clin Psychiatry 65:1301–1313, 2004

Wolraich M, Hannah J, Pinnock T, et al: Comparison of diagnostic criteria for attention-deficit/hyperactivity disorder in a country-wide sample. J Am Acad Child Adolesc Psychiatry 35:319–324, 1996

Zachor DA, Roberts AW, Hodgens JB, et al: Effects of long-term psychostimulant medication on growth of children with ADHD. Res Dev Disabil 27:162–174, 2006

Zahner GE, Jacobs JH, Freeman DHJ, et al: Rural-urban child psychopathology in a northeastern US state: 1986–1989. J Am Acad Child Adolesc Psychiatry 32:378–387, 1993

Zametkin AJ, Liebenauer LL, Fitzgerald GA, et al: Brain metabolism in teenagers with attention-deficit hyperactivity disorder. Arch Gen Psychiatry 50:333–340, 1993

Zeanah CH: Disturbances of attachment in young children adopted from institutions. J Dev Behav Pediatr 21:230–236, 2000

Zeanah CH, Smyke AT, Dumitrescu A: Attachment disturbances in young children, II: indiscriminant behavior and institutional care. J Am Acad Child Adolesc Psychiatry 41:983–989, 2002

Zeanah CH, Smyke AT, Koga S, et al: Attachment in institutionalized and noninstitutionalized Romanian children. Child Development 75:1015–1028, 2005

22

SLEEP DISORDERS

Daniel J. Buysse, M.D.
Patrick J. Strollo Jr., M.D.
Jed E. Black, M.D.
Phyllis G. Zee, M.D., Ph.D.
John W. Winkelman, M.D., Ph.D.

Sleep and wakefulness are fundamental behavioral-neurobiological states present in all animals, including human beings. Although the function of sleep and sleep–wake rhythms has long been debated, it is unlikely that such a fundamental process will ever be equated with a single function. Theories of the function of sleep focus on several possibilities:

- *Ecological or environmental advantage:* Sleep provides a regular period of behavioral inactivity that matches animals to their ideal temporal environmental within the light–dark cycle.
- *Physical restoration:* Sleep deprivation is associated with impaired glucose metabolism and relative insulin insensitivity (Spiegel et al. 1999) and altered immune function. Conversely, sleep may help to restore these functions.
- *Optimizing of waking neurocognitive and emotional function:* Sleep deprivation is associated with clear decrements in subjective alertness, vigilance, and decision making (Belenky et al. 2003; Harrison and Horne 2000; VanDongen et al. 2003) and with adverse effects on mood (Pilcher and Huffcutt 1996).
- *Learning:* Beyond simple performance, visual and other forms of learning are enhanced by sleep and

impaired by sleep loss (Stickgold et al. 2000). Rapid eye movement (REM) sleep is associated with activation of limbic system structures, suggesting a role in emotional processing (Nofzinger et al. 1997).
- *Health and survival:* Studies in rats show that death is the inevitable consequence of prolonged sleep deprivation (Rechtschaffen et al. 1989). In human beings, epidemiological studies show an association between both short (<5 hours) and long (>9 hours) sleep durations and increased mortality risk (Kripke et al. 2002). Similar studies demonstrate relationships between sleep duration and obesity, weight gain, and cardiovascular disease (Hasler et al. 2004). As discussed later, specific sleep disorders also have clear adverse consequences on health outcomes.

Sleep and its disorders are particularly relevant to psychiatric practice. Virtually every psychiatric disorder can be associated with disturbances of sleep–wake function or circadian rhythms. Growing evidence suggests that sleep disturbances are associated with increased risk of subsequent psychiatric disorders, and persistent sleep symptoms adversely affect the outcome of psychiatric disorders. Primary sleep disorders often include neuropsychiatric symptoms, which can make differential diagnoses challenging. Finally, many of the treatments used for sleep disorders, including behavioral and pharmacological treatments, fall within the purview of psychiatric practice. Detailed information on the topics in this chapter can be found in more specialized references (Chokroverty 1999; Kryger et al. 2005). Information on pediatric sleep disorders is not presented in this chapter but can be found elsewhere (Sheldon et al. 2005).

Neurobiology of Circadian Rhythms and Sleep

Most physiological and psychological functions in humans demonstrate endogenous rhythms. These rhythms differ in *period,* or the time to complete one cycle, ranging from very short (e.g., electroencephalographic and cardiac rhythms) to very long (e.g., menstrual cycle). *Circadian rhythms* are those with a period length of approximately 24 hours. Humans have a circadian rhythm period of just over 24 hours (Czeisler et al. 1999). The sleep–wake cycle is the most obvious circadian rhythm, but virtually all other physiological systems also show circadian variation, including hormone secretion (e.g., cortisol, melatonin), core body temperature, cardiovascular function, sleepiness/alertness, and cognitive and psychomotor function (Czeisler et al. 2005). The *amplitude* of a rhythm is a measure of the "size" of oscillation from peak to trough, and *phase* refers to the timing of a rhythm.

Circadian rhythms are *endogenous*—that is, inherent properties of the organism—and not the result of the environmental light–dark cycle. Although circadian rhythms can be synchronized *(entrained)* to external time cues, they are expressed even in temporal and environmental isolation. Environmental time cues are also called *zeitgebers,* or "time givers." In humans and most animals, bright light is the strongest zeitgeber for entraining circadian rhythms, although light of lower light intensity, such as ordinary room light, also affects circadian rhythm timing (Zeitzer et al. 2000). Light-induced phase shifts are most sensitive to short wavelength light of approximately 460 nanometers (nm; blue-green range) (Lockley et al. 2003). The effect of zeitgebers on the timing of rhythms is time dependent. For instance, bright light given toward the end of the usual sleep period causes circadian rhythms to move to an earlier time ("phase advance"), whereas light given near usual bedtime causes circadian rhythms to move to a later time ("phase delay"). The pattern of phase-shifting effects as a function of circadian time is

called the *phase response curve.* Melatonin, a pineal hormone secreted during hours of darkness, is an important endogenous modulator of circadian rhythms and sleep. *Exogenous* melatonin administration in the early evening produces phase advances, and administration in the early morning produces phase delays (Cajochen et al. 2003).

Circadian rhythms are generated and controlled within the central nervous system (CNS). The major pacemakers of the circadian system are the paired suprachiasmatic nuclei (SCN) of the hypothalamus (Moore 1997). Specialized melanopsin-containing retinal ganglion cells project through the retino-hypothalamic tract to the SCN, providing light input independent of vision (Bellingham and Foster 2002). The SCN has efferent pathways to the hypothalamus and thalamus through which it transmits timing information to the rest of the CNS, including sleep–wake systems (Czeisler et al. 2005; Pace-Schott and Hobson 2002). Rhythmic activity of the SCN in turn results from a transcription–translation feedback loop involving a set of circadian rhythm genes (King and Takahashi 2000). These genes code for protein products that have feedback control over their own production, cycling on a near 24-hour rhythm. Mutations in these genes are associated with lengthening or shortening of the free-running period.

Sleep is a rapidly reversible neurobehavioral state characterized by almost simultaneous change in the activity patterns and mode of firing of CNS neurons and circuits. Periodicity (i.e., a circadian rhythm) is the most dominant feature of human circadian rhythms, and rapid reversibility distinguishes it from pathological states such as coma and unconsciousness. Sleep onset is an involuntary process that occurs only when neurobiological and environmental circumstances permit.

In humans, the electrophysiological characteristics of sleep can be characterized by polysomnography, an adaptation of electroencephalography. Polysomnography typically includes electroencephalography to measure brain electrical activity, electrooculography to measure eye movements, and submental surface electromyography to measure muscle tone (Figure 22–1). Patterns of electroencephalographic activity, eye movements, and muscle tone reveal clear differences between wakefulness and sleep, which is further divided into two states, REM sleep and non–rapid eye movement (NREM) sleep (Carskadon and Rechtschaffen 2005). These three states are distinguished by characteristic patterns of environmental responsiveness, general physiology, electroencephalographic waveforms, muscle tone, and mental activity (Table 22–1). NREM sleep

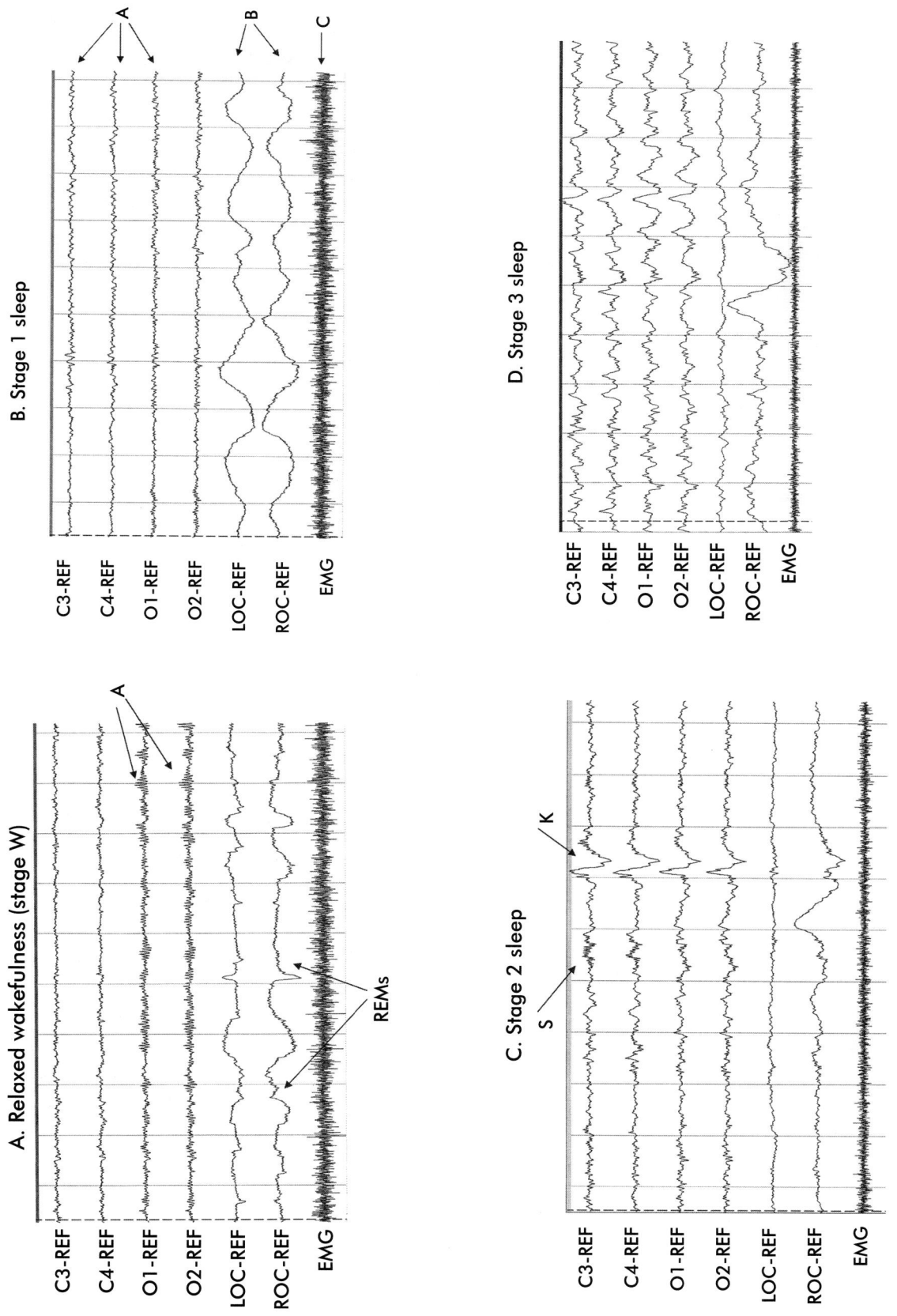

A. Relaxed wakefulness (stage W)

B. Stage 1 sleep

C. Stage 2 sleep

D. Stage 3 sleep

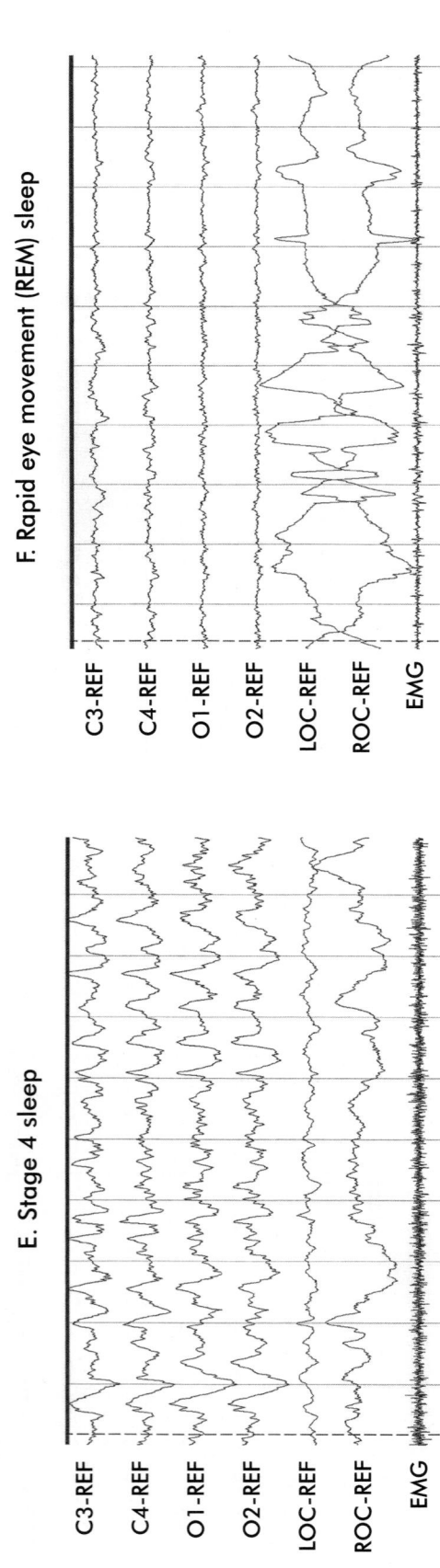

FIGURE 22–1. Polysomnography in different sleep stages.

The six panels show activity in the electroencephalogram (EEG), electrooculogram (EOG), and electromyogram (EMG) during wakefulness and the different sleep stages. Each tracing shows 30 seconds. The EEG segments marked "A" show alpha rhythm, which is characteristic of relaxed wakefulness with eyes closed. The arrows marked "REMs" show rapid eye movements. The channels are labeled on the left side: C3, C4, O1, and O2 are EEG leads; LOC and ROC are leads at the left and right outer canthus of the eye. **B,** Stage 1 non–REM (NREM) sleep is characterized by a slight increase in EEG amplitude and slowing of EEG frequencies (*A*), slow rolling eye movements (indicated by reciprocal "hills and valleys" in the EOG channels, [*B*]) and lower muscle tone (*C*). **C,** Stage 2 NREM sleep is characterized by further slowing of the EEG, together with an increase in amplitude. Phasic events include "K complexes," isolated large-amplitude slow EEG waves (*K*) and "sleep spindles," episodic bursts of fast EEG activity lasting approximately 0.5 seconds (*S*). EOG shows underlying brain electrical activity, and therefore resembles the EEG. Muscle tone is further reduced. **D,** Stage 3 sleep is characterized by large-amplitude, slow (0.5–4.0 Hz) EEG activity, also known as "delta" or "slow-wave sleep" activity, that constitutes 20%–50% of the 30-second epoch. EOG mirrors EEG activity, and muscle tone is low. **E,** Stage 4 sleep is identical to Stage 3, except that delta activity occupies greater than 50% of the epoch. **F,** REM sleep is characterized by the return of faster-frequency, mixed-voltage EEG, similar to Stage 1 NREM sleep. The hallmark of REM is the appearance of phasic rapid eye movements, which present as large-amplitude "spiky" waveforms that clearly differ from the slower eye movements of Stage 1 NREM. Muscle tone is essentially absent, except for the intermittent occurrence of phasic muscle twitches, which often accompany eye movements.

Source. Reprinted from Buysse DJ (ed): *Sleep Disorders and Psychiatry* (Review of Psychiatry Series, Volume 24, Number 2; Oldham JM and Riba MB, series editors). Washington, DC, American Psychiatric Publishing, 2005, pp. 7–9. Copyright 2005, American Psychiatric Publishing. Used with permission.

TABLE 22–1. **Physiological characteristics of sleep–wake states**

	Wake	**NREM**	**REM**
Electroencephalogram	Fast, low voltage	Slow, high voltage	Fast, low voltage
Eye movement	Vision-related	Slow, irregular	Rapid
Muscle tone	++	+	0
Neuronal activity in LDT/PPT	+	0	++
Neuronal activity in LC/DR/TMN	++	+	0
Neuronal activity in VLPO (cluster)	0	++	+?
Neuronal activity in VLPO (extended)	0	+?	++
Neuronal activity in hypocretin neurons	++	0?	0?
Heart rate, blood pressure, respiratory rate	Variable	Slow/low, regular	Variable, higher than NREM
Responses to hypoxia and hypercarbia	Active	Reduced responsiveness	Lowest responsiveness
Thermoregulation	Behavioral and physiological regulation	Physiological regulation only	Reduced physiological regulation
Mental activity	Full	None or limited	Story-like dreams

Note. +=activity level; 0=inactive; DR=dorsal raphe; LC=locus coeruleus; LDT=laterodorsal pontine tegmentum; NREM=non–rapid eye movement sleep; PPT=pedunculopontine tegmentum; REM=rapid eye movement sleep; TMN=tuberomammillary nucleus; VLPO (cluster)=central portion of ventrolateral preoptic nucleus; VLPO (extended) = peripheral portion of ventrolateral preoptic nucleus.

Source. Adapted from Saper et al. 2001.

is subdivided into four stages of increasing "depth," which correlate with decreasing arousability. NREM and REM sleep cycle periodically across the night (Figure 22–2). Most Stage 3–4 NREM sleep ("deep" or "delta" sleep) occurs in the first half of the night. NREM and REM sleep alternate approximately every 90–100 minutes during the sleep period. REM sleep episodes become longer and more intense toward the morning hours, as measured by the number of eye movements and complexity of dream mentation.

Sleep stages are affected by a number of individual and environmental factors. Age is the most important of these (Ohayon et al. 2004). Newborns spend nearly 50% of sleep in a form of sleep resembling REM, but this decreases rapidly in the first year of life. Sleep duration also dramatically decreases from infancy through childhood and then increases slightly in adolescence. Across the adult life span, Stage 3–4 sleep gradually diminishes from its peak in late adolescence. In later adulthood, the number and duration of awakenings and the amount of Stage 1 sleep increase, whereas Stage 2 NREM and REM sleep are relatively consistent. In addition, the entire sleep period tends to

phase delay during adolescence and then phase advance during later adulthood.

Physiologically, human sleep is regulated by two processes, a homeostatic factor and a circadian factor (Figure 22–3). The homeostatic factor represents an increase in sleep "drive" as a function of prior wakefulness and can be measured in the time course of electroencephalographic slow-wave activity across a sleep period. Homeostatic sleep drive builds up during waking hours and then decreases during subsequent sleep. The second regulatory factor is the circadian rhythm of sleep and wakefulness. In humans, the circadian drive for sleep is highest in the second half of the usual sleep period. Homeostatic and circadian sleep factors typically function interactively. Homeostatic sleep drive builds up near the approaching usual sleep time at night and ensures rapid entry into deep NREM sleep. As homeostatic sleep drive weakens during the middle of the night, circadian sleep drive increases, maintaining sleep for the second half of the sleep period.

Sleep and wakefulness are controlled by a number of widely distributed brain systems (Pace-Schott and Hobson 2002). No single region of the brain is neces-

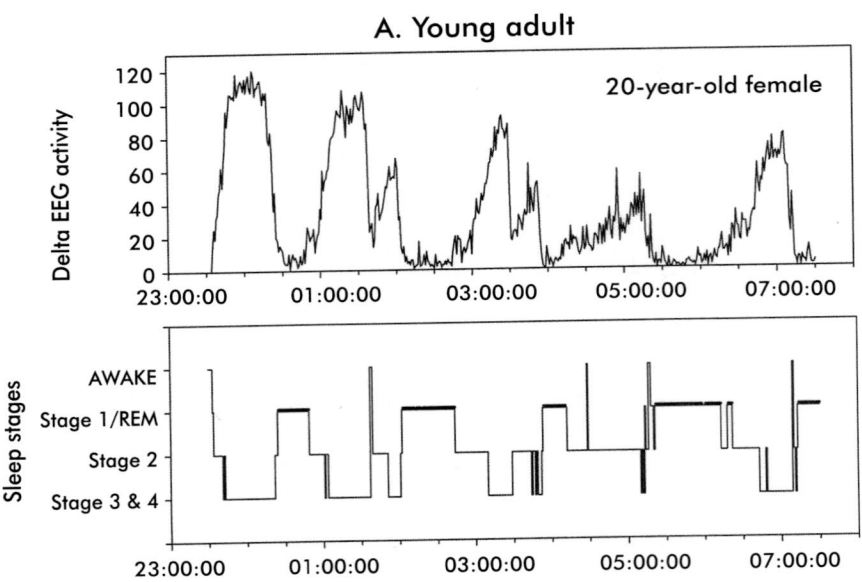

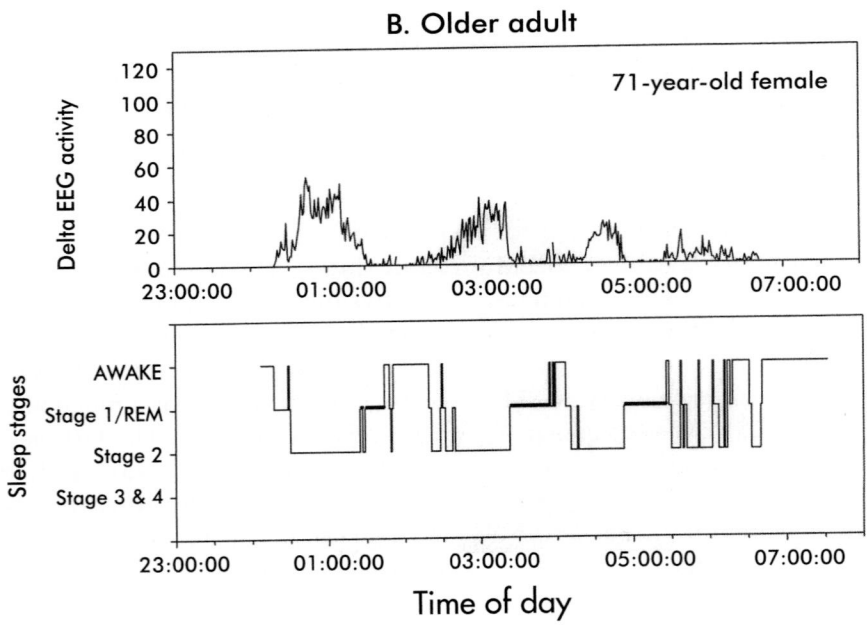

FIGURE 22–2. Hypnograms of sleep stages in healthy subjects.

Each 20- to 30-second epoch of sleep for an entire night is assigned a sleep stage by a human "scorer." These epoch scores can then be displayed graphically in a "hypnogram," to display the progression of sleep stages across the night. **A,** Hypnogram for an entire night of sleep in a healthy young adult. Sleep stages are indicated by increasing "depth" on the vertical axis, with REM sleep represented by heavy horizontal lines. Time is indicated on the horizontal axis. Note that most Stage 3–4 NREM sleep occurs in the early part of the night, and REM periods get longer toward the end of the night. **B,** Hypnogram for an older adult. Note the absence of Stage 3–4 NREM sleep and the greater amount of wakefulness during the sleep period.

Source. Reprinted from Buysse DJ (ed): *Sleep Disorders and Psychiatry* (Review of Psychiatry Series, Volume 24, Number 2; Oldham JM and Riba MB, series editors). Washington, DC, American Psychiatric Publishing, 2005, p. 10. Copyright 2005, American Psychiatric Publishing. Used with permission.

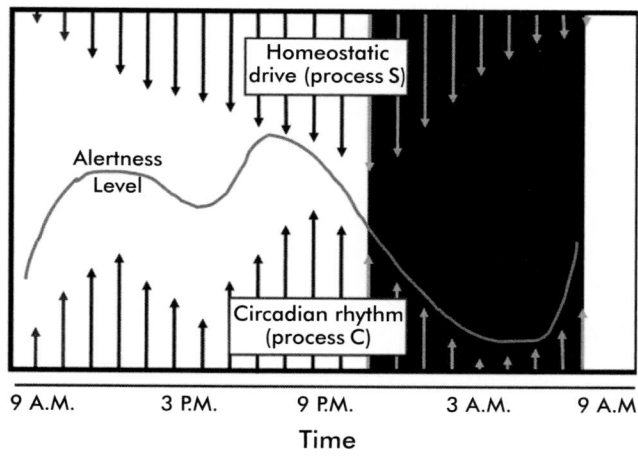

FIGURE 22–3. The two-process model.

Alertness level is determined by the interaction between two processes. The sleep homeostatic drive (Process S) promotes sleep and builds up during wake, reaching a maximum in the late evening (near the usual sleep time). The circadian rhythm system (Process C) promotes wakefulness during the day. It is biphasic and tends to dip in the mid-afternoon. Process C also reaches its peak in the evening to counterbalance the accumulation of homeostatic drive that has built up throughout the day and it begins to fall just before the usual bedtime. This system promotes wakefulness during the day and consolidates sleep at night.

Source. Reprinted from Buysse DJ (ed): *Sleep Disorders and Psychiatry* (Review of Psychiatry Series, Vol 24, No 2; Oldham JM and Riba MB, series editors). Washington, DC, American Psychiatric Publishing, 2005, p. 191. Copyright 2005, American Psychiatric Publishing. Used with permission.

sary or sufficient for the generation of sleep or wakefulness. The brain regions critical for normal wakefulness include the histaminergic nuclei of the posterior hypothalamus, the cholinergic nuclei of the basal forebrain, and the noradrenergic and serotonergic nuclei of the ascending reticular activating system and the midbrain and pontine tegmentum. In addition, a more recently discovered system promotes wakefulness through the activity of a peptide neurotransmitter called hypocretin or orexin. The hypocretin system stabilizes wakefulness through its innervation of cholinergic, aminergic, and histaminergic brain systems. Regions critical for the generation of NREM sleep include the solitary tract, which projects ventrally through the basal forebrain and dorsally through the thalamus to the cortex. Progressive hyperpolarization of corticothalamic circuits during NREM sleep underlies the characteristic rhythmic waveforms of this state. The ventrolateral preoptic area of the hypothalamus, one of the few brain regions that becomes more

active during sleep than wakefulness, acts as a "sleep switch" through reciprocal interactions with wake-promoting centers described earlier (Saper et al. 2001). In addition, homeostatic sleep regulation may involve activity of extracellular adenosine in the basal forebrain. Finally, REM sleep results from reciprocal interactions between brain stem cholinergic "REM on" nuclei and noradrenergic/serotonergic "REM off" nuclei in the pontine tegmentum.

Although numerous neurotransmitters are involved in sleep–wake state regulation, their activities are complicated and often apparently contradictory (Zoltoski et al. 1999). In general, the neurotransmitters acetylcholine, histamine, serotonin, norepinephrine, and hypocretin promote wakefulness. The inhibitory neurotransmitters γ-aminobutyric acid (GABA) and galanin are associated with inhibitory influences that promote NREM sleep. Other substances including cytokines, prostaglandins, and various hormones also influence sleep–wake states.

Clinical Assessment of Sleep and Sleep Disorders

Clinical Evaluation

The diagnosis and management of patients with sleep complaints rest on an accurate clinical history. Important elements of the history include the nature, severity, and frequency of the symptoms; duration of the complaint; associated impairments; and exacerbating and alleviating factors. The following aspects of the clinical evaluation are particularly relevant to sleep and circadian rhythm disorders:

- *24-hour history.* Because sleep affects wakefulness and vice versa, it is important to assess both nighttime and daytime symptoms. Following the chronology of a "typical" night and day is essential for assessing sleep problems and daytime sleepiness.
- *Regularity of sleep–wake patterns.* Many patients with sleep disorders develop highly irregular schedules, seeking to "catch" sleep whenever they can. This pattern can itself contribute to further sleep difficulties.
- *Bed partner history.* Certain symptoms, including snoring and sleep-related behaviors, may not be evident to the person with the disorder itself.
- *Medical, neurological, and psychiatric disorders.* Sleep problems are associated with a wide variety of other disorders that may exacerbate symptoms (Table 22–2).

TABLE 22–2. Medical and psychiatric disorders and conditions associated with insomnia

System	Examples
Cardiovascular	Congestive heart failure
Pulmonary	Chronic obstructive pulmonary disease, asthma
Renal and genitourinary	Chronic renal failure, prostatic hypertrophy
Gastrointestinal	Gastroesophageal reflux disease
Musculoskeletal	Fibromyalgia, osteoarthritis, rheumatoid arthritis
Endocrine	Hyperthyroidism, diabetes
Neurological	Parkinson's disease, cerebrovascular disease
Other	Menopause
Mood disorders	Major depression, dysthymic disorder, bipolar affective disorder
Anxiety disorders	Generalized anxiety disorder, panic disorder, posttraumatic stress disorder
Psychotic disorders	Schizophrenia
Substance use disorders	Alcohol, sedatives

TABLE 22–3. Medications and substances associated with insomnia

Alcohol (acute use, withdrawal)

Caffeine

Nicotine

Antidepressants (selective serotonin reuptake inhibitor, serotonin–norepinephrine reuptake inhibitor)

Corticosteroids

Decongestants (phenylpropanolamine, pseudoephedrine)

β agonists, theophylline derivatives

β antagonists

Statins

Stimulants

Dopamine agonists

- *Medications and substances.* All drugs affecting control of nervous system function, and many used for medical disorders, can affect sleep (Table 22–3).
- *Physical examination.* Although most sleep disorders have no specific physical findings, sleep apnea syndromes often do. Thus it is useful to evaluate the following minimal features in patients presenting with sleep–wake complaints: height, weight, and body mass index; neck circumference; patency or oral and nasal airways; and craniofacial abnormalities, including retrognathia. Cardiopulmonary and neurological examinations can reveal associated heart failure in sleep apnea or neuropathies that may contribute to restless legs syndrome (RLS).
- *Questionnaires.* Sleep–wake diaries may give a more complete picture of the individual's sleep patterns and day-to-day variability and may even help the individual identify patterns that are contributing to sleep problems (Figure 22–4). The Epworth Sleepiness Scale (Johns 1991) assesses daytime sleepiness by asking the likelihood of falling asleep in specific behavioral situations. Scores range from 0 (no sleepiness) to 24 (extreme sleepiness). The Pittsburgh Sleep Quality Index is a 19-item self-rated scale that assesses global sleep quality, with scores ranging from 0 (good sleep quality) to 21 (poor sleep quality) (Buysse et al. 1989). A score greater than 5 is associated with significant sleep problems.
- *Actigraphy.* Actigraphy measures body movement patterns during sleep through a small accelerometer worn on the wrist. Patterns of motor activity correspond reasonably well to sleep and wakefulness and may be useful for assessing sleep–wake patterns over time.
- *Polysomnography.* In addition to electroencephalography, electrooculography, and electromyography, clinical polysomnography typically includes measurements of nasal–oral airflow, nasal pressure, and chest and abdominal movements to assess breathing; oximetry to measure desaturation events; electrocardiography; and anterior tibialis electromyography to assess leg movements during sleep (Figure 22–5). Polysomnography is indicated for the evaluation of patients with suspected sleep apnea and narcolepsy and may be useful to correctly diagnose parasomnias. It is not routinely indicated for the assessment of insomnia, circadian rhythm sleep disorders (CRSDs), or RLS but is reserved for atypical or treatment-resistant cases (Chesson et al.

A. Graphic sleep diary

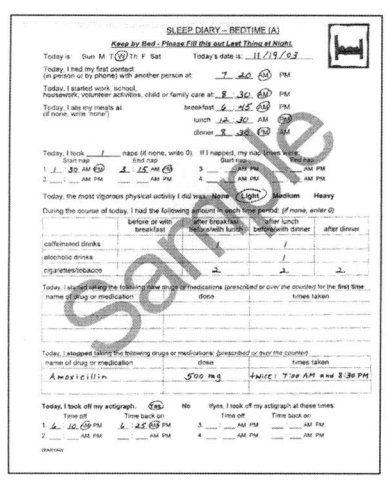

B. Text sleep diary

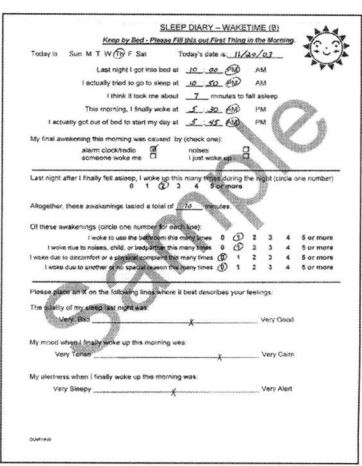

FIGURE 22–4. **Sleep–wake diaries.**

A, In a graphic sleep diary, the subject "blocks out" the times he or she was actually asleep. In this example, the subject had very irregular sleep timing with some very long sleep episodes. **B,** In a text sleep diary, the subject writes in the times of going to bed, waking up, napping, and so on.

Source. Reprinted from Buysse DJ (ed): *Sleep Disorders and Psychiatry* (Review of Psychiatry Series, Volume 24, Number 2; Oldham JM and Riba MB, series editors). Washington, DC, American Psychiatric Publishing, 2005, p. 16. Copyright 2005, American Psychiatric Publishing. Used with permission.

1997). Objective daytime sleepiness is assessed with a variant of polysomnography called the multiple sleep latency test (MSLT). After a night of polysomnographically monitored sleep, the patient is permitted to nap four or five times at 2-hour intervals during the day. Mean sleep latency serves as an overall measure of daytime sleepiness, with values greater than 10 minutes generally considered normal, values of 8 or fewer minutes indicating clinically significant sleepiness, and values of 5 or fewer minutes indicating severe sleepiness. REM sleep in two or more naps suggests narcolepsy.

Classification of Sleep–Wake Disorders

Sleep disorders involve a variety of conditions with physiological, neurological, or behavioral origins. Classification systems for sleep disorders include DSM-IV-TR (American Psychiatric Association 2000), the International Classification of Sleep Disorders, 2nd Edition (ICSD-2; American Academy of Sleep Medicine 2005), and ICD-9 and ICD-10 (World Health Organization 1992). An outline of the ICSD-2 classifications is shown in Table 22–4. DSM-IV-TR classifies sleep dis-

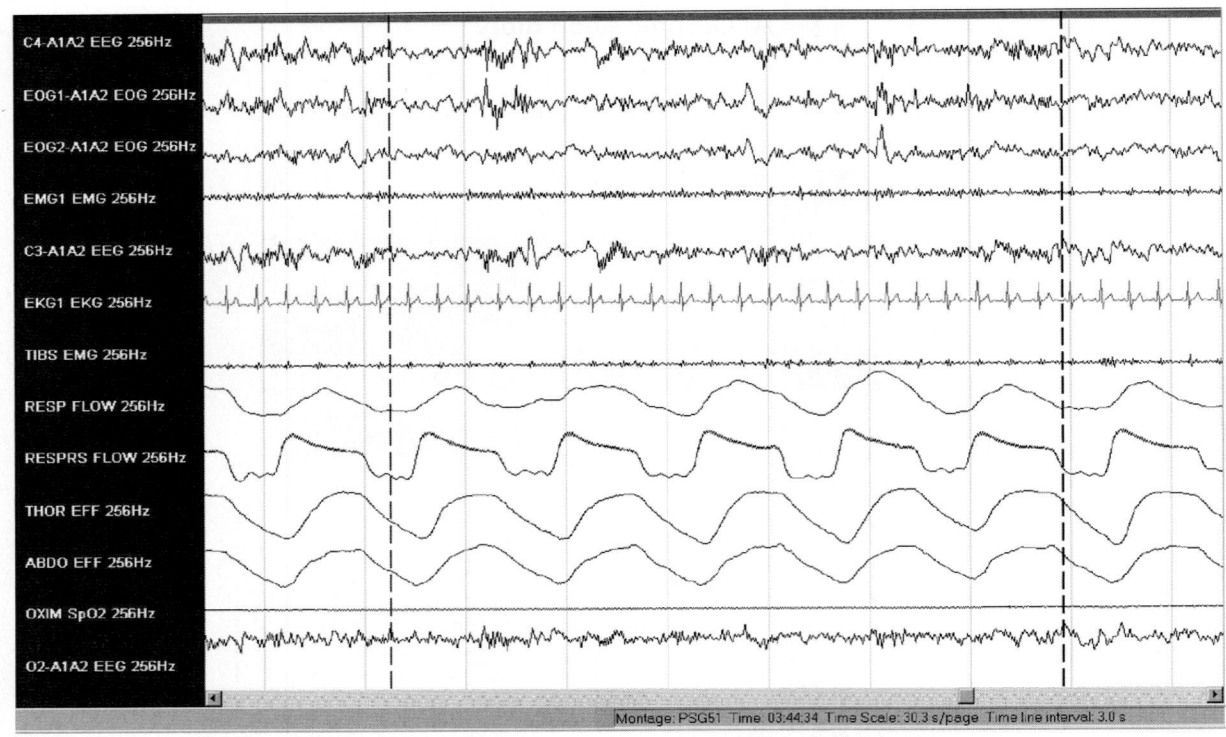

FIGURE 22–5. A 30-second epoch of a typical clinical polysomnogram (PSG).

In addition to an electroencephalogram (EEG [C4-A1A2, C3-A1A2, O2-A1A2]), electrooculogram (EOG [EOG1-A1A2, EOG2-A1A2]), and electromyogram (EMG [EMG1]), a clinical PSG includes additional channels for monitoring leg movements (anterior tibialis leads [TIBS EMG]), breathing patterns (nasal pressure [RESPRS], oral–nasal thermistors [RESP]), chest and abdominal wall movements (THOR EFF, ABDO EFF), oximetry (OXIM), and electrocardiogram (ECG [ECG1]).

Source. Reprinted from Buysse DJ (ed): *Sleep Disorders and Psychiatry* (Review of Psychiatry Series, Volume 24, Number 2; Oldham JM and Riba MB, series editors). Washington, DC, American Psychiatric Publishing, 2005, p. 18. Copyright 2005, American Psychiatric Publishing. Used with permission.

orders into dyssomnias (insomnias, hypersomnias, and CRSDs), parasomnias, and secondary sleep disorders. ICSD-2 categorizes sleep disorders into six groups: insomnias, sleep-related breathing disorders, hypersomnias not due to a sleep-related breathing disorder, CRSDs, parasomnias, and sleep-related movement disorders. The remainder of this chapter follows the ICSD-2 classification.

Insomnia Disorders
Definition and Description

Insomnia refers to the complaint of difficulty falling asleep, frequent or prolonged awakenings, inadequate sleep quality, or short overall sleep duration in an individual who has adequate time available for sleep. Insomnia is not defined by polysomnography or a specific sleep duration. Because insomnia occurs only when there is adequate opportunity for sleep, it must be distinguished from sleep deprivation, in which the individual has relatively normal sleep ability but inadequate opportunity for sleep. An *insomnia disorder* is a syndrome consisting of the insomnia complaint together with significant impairment or distress. Common daytime impairments associated with insomnia include mood disturbances (irritability, mild dysphoria, or difficulty tolerating stress), impaired cognitive function (difficulty concentrating, completing tasks, or performing complex, abstract, or creative tasks), and daytime fatigue (Moul et al. 2002). Clinicians are often taught that insomnia is a symptom rather than a disorder and that it is almost always "secondary." However, based on consistencies in clinical features, course, and response to treatment, a recent National Institutes of Health conference suggested that "comorbid" insomnia may be a more appropriate term than "secondary" (National Institutes of Health 2005).

TABLE 22–4. ICSD-2 sleep disorder classifications

I. Insomnias

Adjustment insomnia

Psychophysiological insomnia

Paradoxical insomnia

Idiopathic insomnia

Insomnia due to mental disorder

Inadequate sleep hygiene

Behavioral insomnia of childhood

Insomnia due to drug or substance

Insomnia due to alcohol

Insomnia due to medical condition

II. Sleep-related breathing disorders

Central sleep apnea syndromes

Obstructive sleep apnea syndromes (obstructive sleep apnea, adult; obstructive sleep apnea, pediatric)

Sleep-related hypoventilation/hypoxemic syndromes

Other sleep-related breathing disorders

III. Hypersomnias of central origin (not due to a circadian rhythm sleep disorder, sleep-related breathing disorder, or other cause of disturbed nocturnal sleep)

Narcolepsy with cataplexy

Narcolepsy without cataplexy

Narcolepsy due to medical condition

Recurrent hypersomnia

Idiopathic hypersomnia with long sleep time

Idiopathic hypersomnia without long sleep time

Behaviorally induced insufficient sleep syndrome

Hypersomnia due to medical condition

Hypersomnia due to drug or substance

IV. Circadian rhythm sleep disorders

Circadian rhythm sleep disorder, delayed sleep phase type

Circadian rhythm sleep disorder, advanced sleep phase type

Circadian rhythm sleep disorder, irregular sleep–wake type

Circadian rhythm sleep disorder, nonentrained type

Circadian rhythm sleep disorder due to medical condition

TABLE 22–4. ICSD-2 sleep disorder classifications *(continued)*

V. Parasomnias

Disorders of arousal from non-REM sleep (confusional arousals, sleepwalking, sleep terrors)

Parasomnias usually associated with REM sleep (REM sleep behavior disorder, recurrent isolated sleep paralysis, nightmare disorder)

Other parasomnias (e.g., sleep-related enuresis, sleep-related groaning [catathrenia], exploding head syndrome, sleep-related hallucinations, sleep-related eating disorder)

VI. Sleep-related movement disorders

Restless legs syndrome

Periodic limb movement sleep disorder

Sleep-related leg cramps

Sleep-related bruxism

Sleep-related rhythmic movement disorder

Sleep-related movement disorder due to drug or substance

Sleep-related movement disorder due to medical condition

Note. Selected ICSD-2 categories have been collapsed in table to simplify presentation. ICSD-2 = International Classification of Sleep Disorders, 2nd Edition (American Academy of Sleep Medicine 2005); REM = rapid eye movement.

Epidemiology and Consequences

The 1-year prevalence of insomnia symptoms is approximately 30%–40% in the general population and up to 66% in primary care and psychiatric settings. The prevalence of primary insomnia as a specific disorder is in the range of 5%–10% of the general population (Ohayon 2002). Established risk factors for insomnia include older age, female sex, being divorced or separated, unemployment, and comorbid medical and psychiatric illness. Factors that commonly initiate or maintain insomnia include psychosocial stresses such as moves, relationship difficulties, occupational and financial problems, and caregiving responsibilities. The natural history of insomnia determined from population-based studies has not been well described. However, longitudinal studies of clinical patients and population samples indicate that insomnia is a chronic or recurring condition in approximately 50%–85% of affected individuals. Remission does occur, even in older adults (Foley et al. 1999), particularly when comorbid medical and psychiatric conditions are effectively treated (Katz and McHorney 1998).

The consequences of insomnia include increased risk for the later development of depressive, anxiety, and substance use disorders (Breslau et al. 1996; Riemann and Voderholzer 2003). Comorbid insomnia is associated with more severe symptoms and worse treatment outcomes in patients with major depressive disorder and alcohol dependence. Insomnia is also associated with increased health care utilization, absenteeism, direct and indirect medical costs, motor vehicle and other accidents, falls in the elderly, and reduced quality of life (reviewed in Buysse 2005).

Pathophysiology and Etiology

Insomnia is often thought to result from increased arousal. *Arousal* refers to the individual's state of CNS activity and reactivity, ranging from sleep to wakefulness with excitement or panic. *Hyperarousal* is characterized by a high level of alertness either tonically or in response to specific situations such as the sleep environment. Hyperarousal in insomnia is suggested by evidence from psychophysiological, metabolic, electrophysiological, neuroendocrine, and functional neuroanatomical evidence (reviewed in Perlis et al. 2005). Functional imaging studies demonstrate increased glucose metabolic rates during wakefulness and sleep and attenuation of the usual NREM sleep–related decline in metabolism in brain-stem arousal centers in subjects with insomnia compared with healthy control subjects. Self-reported wakefulness during sleep is related to increased metabolic activity in the same regions (Nofzinger 2006; Nofzinger et al. 2004).

Psychological and behavioral theories may also help to explain the development and persistence of insomnia. In Spielman et al.'s (1987) behavioral model (Figure 22–6), individual predisposing factors such as heightened physiological or cognitive arousal interact with external precipitating factors or stressors to produce acute insomnia. Perpetuating factors—that is, maladaptive coping strategies such as spending more time in bed—maintain and reinforce insomnia even after the original precipitants recede. In Morin's (1993) model, cognitive hyperarousal is indicated by sleep-focused, ruminative thoughts, particularly around bedtime. A vicious cycle of cognitive arousal, physiological arousal, sleep disturbance, and daytime consequences ensues, leading to the adoption of maladaptive coping strategies. Perlis et al. (1997) proposed a neurocognitive model of insomnia emphasizing the central role of cortical arousal. This model suggests that cortical arousal, as measured by beta electroencephalographic activity, leads to both physiological and cognitive arousal. Harvey (2002) proposed that cognitive strategies employed by people with insomnia maintain sleep disturbances by producing selective attention and monitoring toward autonomic symptoms and environmental cues associated with sleeplessness. Psychological and behavioral theories of insomnia are important not only for their heuristic value but also for the interventions they have generated.

Assessment and Diagnosis

The assessment of patients with insomnia rests on a detailed clinical history focusing on specific symptoms, chronology, exacerbating and alleviating factors, and response to previous treatments. The insomnia history should cover the patient's usual sleep and wake periods, specifically considering behaviors, cognitions, and environmental factors related to bedtime and sleep and variability of sleep from day to day. Symptoms of RLS, snoring or breathing problems, and pain or limitations to mobility during sleep should also be assessed. Other important elements of the history include exercise routines, regularity of work and daytime activities, limitations in these activities, and daytime sleepiness and napping.

Polysomnography is not routinely recommended for the evaluation of chronic insomnia (Sateia et al. 2000) because in most cases it simply confirms the patient's subjective report without indicating a cause for awakenings. It may be useful in specific situations, however, including patients with additional symptoms of sleep apnea, periodic limb movements, or parasomnias.

Symptom-based classifications of insomnia (i.e., sleep-onset, sleep maintenance, or mixed-type insomnia) are of limited value because the specific type of sleep complaint often varies within an individual over time (Hohagen et al. 1994), and a majority of patients actually complain of more than one type of sleep disturbance. Duration-based classifications (e.g., acute, short-term, and chronic insomnia) are also of limited value due to the high rate of chronicity or recurrence in insomnia symptoms. The DSM-IV-TR and ICSD-2 classifications of specific diagnoses are preferred because they include specific criteria.

Behavioral and Psychological Treatment

Behavioral and psychological treatments aim to reduce sleep latency and improve sleep consolidation by changing behaviors, habits, and cognitions that interfere with sleep. Table 22–5 summarizes the major components of behavioral and psychological treatments

Sleep disturbance
(arbitrary units)

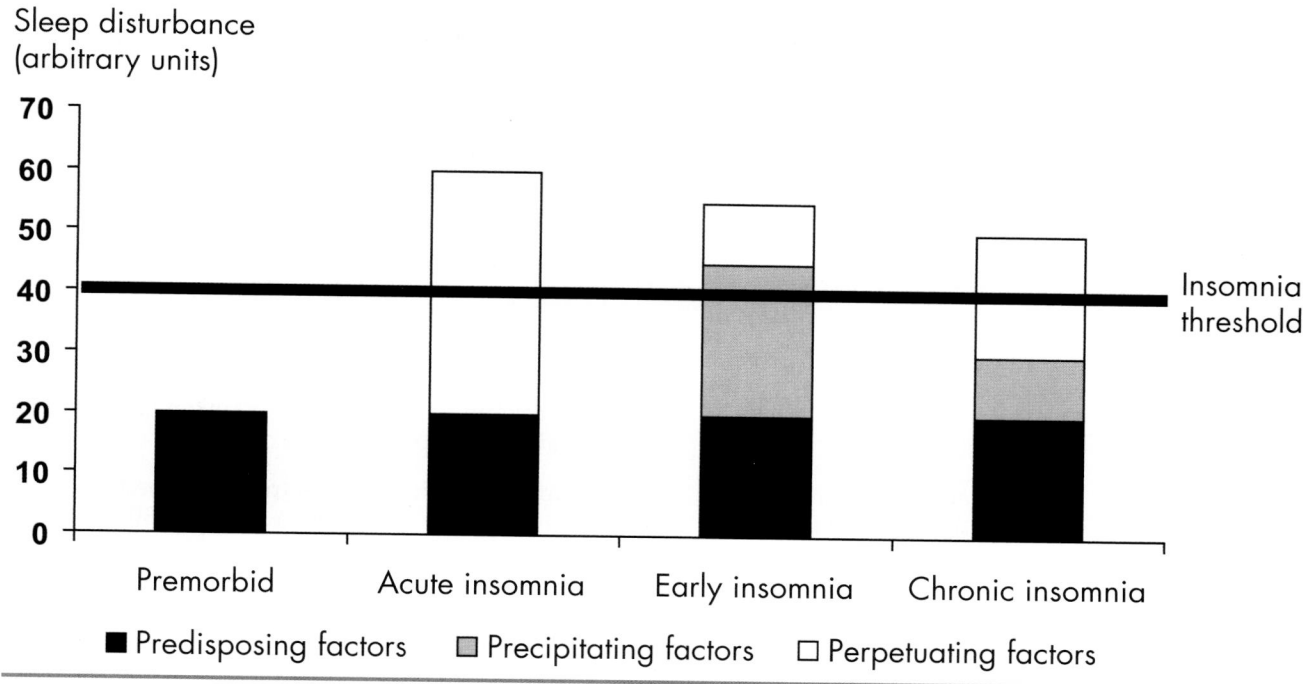

FIGURE 22–6. Heuristic model of the development of insomnia.

This behavioral model of insomnia proposes that individuals have varying predisposition for insomnia and that specific precipitating factors will lead vulnerable individuals to cross the insomnia "threshold." Behavioral factors lead to perpetuation of the insomnia after the original precipitants have receded. The y axis indicates sleep disturbance (higher numbers = worse), and the x axis represents successive stages of insomnia.

Source. Adapted from Spielman AJ: "Assessment of Insomnia." *Clinical Psychology Review* 6:11–25, 1986.

for insomnia, which can be administered in individual or group format.

Meta-analyses have demonstrated that behavioral interventions for insomnia significantly reduce sleep-onset latency, reduce wake time after sleep onset, and improve total sleep time (Irwin et al. 2006; Morin et al. 2006). These effects are comparable in magnitude with those achieved with hypnotic medications (Smith et al. 2002). Approximately 70%–80% of insomnia patients benefit from behavioral interventions, and improvements are maintained or enhanced at follow-up. Stimulus control, sleep restriction, and multicomponent cognitive-behavioral interventions show the most robust effects. In general, behavioral interventions have somewhat smaller effects in older adults than in middle-aged subjects. Cognitive-behavioral interventions for insomnia are also effective at improving sleep quality in patients with comorbid medical and psychiatric illnesses and specific conditions such as cancer and chronic pain (Lichstein et al. 2005). A growing number of studies also show that cognitive-behavioral treatments delivered in the primary and psychiatric care settings are also efficacious (Edinger and Sampson 2003; Espie et al. 2001). New treatment modalities such

as home-based treatment (Espie et al. 2001), telephone interventions, Internet-based interventions (Strom et al. 2004), and self-help material (Mimeault and Morin 1999) are being investigated to disseminate these treatments and reduce patient burden and costs. Most behavioral treatments share basic principles that can be used effectively in a variety of clinical settings (Germain et al. 2006). These specific interventions are reasonably straightforward and rely on principles of the two-process model of sleep regulation described earlier. They include restricting time in bed to match actual sleep time; setting a regular wakeup time, regardless of sleep duration the night before; not going to bed unless sleepy; and not staying in bed during prolonged awakenings.

Pharmacological Treatment

Drugs approved for the treatment of insomnia include benzodiazepine receptor agonists (BzRAs) and a melatonin receptor agonist (Walsh et al. 2005b). However, physicians frequently use other off-label medications for insomnia, despite the lack of efficacy and safety data (Buysse et al. 2005b; Walsh 2004).

TABLE 22–5. Cognitive-behavioral interventions for insomnia

Intervention	General description	Specific techniques
Stimulus control	A set of behaviors that promote associative conditioning between the sleep environment and sleepiness	Go to bed only when feeling sleepy and intending to fall asleep. If unable to fall asleep within 10–20 minutes (without watching the clock, 10–20 minutes is equivalent to repositioning yourself twice to try to fall asleep), leave the bed and the bedroom. Return only when feeling sleepy again. Use the bed and bedroom for sleep only. Do not read, watch television, talk on the phone, worry, or plan activities in the bedroom. Set the alarm and wake up at a regular time every day. Do not snooze or nap during the day.
Sleep restriction therapy	Sleep practices that increase "sleep drive" and facilitate the ability to sleep	Restrict time awake in bed by setting strict bedtime and rising schedules limited to the average number of hours of actual sleep reported in one night. Increase time in bed by advancing bedtime by 15–30 minutes when the time spent asleep is at least 85% of the allowed time in bed. Keep a fixed wakeup time, regardless of actual sleep duration. If after 10 days sleep efficiency is lower than 85%, delay bedtime by 15–30 minutes.
Relaxation training	Training in techniques that decrease waking arousal and facilitate sleep at night (muscular tension and cognitive arousal are incompatible with sleep).	Practice muscle relaxation daily, using progressive relaxation training. Use guided imagery to decrease rumination at bedtime by replacing arousing mental content with soothing images and deliberately avoiding intrusive thoughts.
Cognitive restructuring of irrational sleep-related beliefs	Identification, challenge, and replacement of dysfunctional beliefs and attitudes regarding sleep and sleep loss. These beliefs increase arousal and tension, which in turn impede sleep and reinforce the dysfunctional beliefs.	Address irrational beliefs and fears about sleep, including • Overestimation of numbers of hours of sleep necessary to be rested. • Overall apprehensive expectation that sleep cannot be controlled. • Fear of getting out of bed when awake for fear of the time when sleep will come.
Sleep hygiene	Promote behaviors that improve sleep; limit behaviors that harm sleep	Avoid naps. Get regular exercise, at least 6 hours before sleep. Maintain a regular sleep schedule 7 nights a week. Avoid stimulants (caffeine, nicotine). Limit alcohol intake. Do not look at the clock when awake in bed.

Benzodiazepine Receptor Agonists

BzRAs are indicated for the treatment of acute insomnia and chronic primary insomnia. They are useful as adjunctive therapies for secondary insomnia related to certain medical conditions, psychiatric disorders, and other primary sleep disorders such as RLS and CRSDs.

These agents bind at specific recognition sites on the $GABA_A$ receptor. $GABA_A$ receptors are widely distributed in the CNS, including the cortex, basal ganglia, and cerebellum. The $GABA_A$ receptor comprises five protein subunits; BzRAs bind at the interface of α and γ subunits (Bateson 2004). Some of these drugs, such as zolpidem and zaleplon, bind relatively selectively at $GABA_A$ receptors containing α_1 subunits. The clinical significance of this selectivity is not clear, although such agents may be relatively more specific for hypnotic effects and have lower abuse liability. $GABA_A$ receptors with α_1 subunits mediate the sedative, amnestic, and anticonvulsant effects of BzRAs, whereas those containing α_2 and α_3 subunits mediate anxiolytic and myorelaxant effects (Mohler et al. 2002).

The BzRAs have different clinical effects primarily as a result of their different pharmacokinetic properties, including rate of absorption, extent of distribution, and terminal elimination half-life (Table 22–6). Pharmacokinetic properties and dosage determine a drug's duration of action. Pharmacokinetic properties are important in selecting a particular agent for a particular patient. For instance, a very short-acting drug such as zaleplon may be helpful for patients with sleep onset problems, whereas longer-acting drugs such as temazepam may be more useful for frequent awakenings.

As a class, BzRAs decrease sleep latency; those with longer duration of action also decrease the number and duration of awakenings from sleep and increase sleep duration. Most decrease Stage 3–4 NREM sleep and REM sleep by small amounts, but the clinical significance of these changes is unclear. Meta-analyses have demonstrated these agents to be efficacious in the treatment of chronic insomnia (Holbrook et al. 2000; Nowell et al. 1997; Soldatos et al. 1999) on self-reported outcomes of sleep latency, sleep duration, number of awakenings, and sleep quality. Effects are comparable in magnitude with those of cognitive-behavioral therapies (Smith et al. 2002).

Most studies of BzRAs have been conducted for short durations, which limits their clinical utility, because the majority of patients treated with these drugs have chronic insomnia. In one randomized placebo-controlled study, the efficacy of eszopiclone was demonstrated over 6 months of continued nightly use, with better eszopiclone outcomes on subjective sleep and daytime functioning measures (Krystal et al. 2003). Other studies have demonstrated efficacy for zolpidem, zaleplon, and eszopiclone over 4–5 weeks of nightly use, suggesting that BzRAs may be efficacious over longer periods in at least some patients. These agents are also efficacious when used intermittently (i.e., 3–5 times per week) (Perlis et al. 2004; Walsh et al. 2000).

Agents in this class have similar side effects that differ only according to their pharmacokinetic properties. Effects include sedation, impaired psychomotor

performance (Vermeeren 2004), falls and hip fractures in the elderly (Cumming and Le Couteur 2003), motor vehicle accidents (Thomas 1998), and respiratory depression of minimal clinical significance in most patients (Camacho and Morin 1995).

Although tolerance has long been a concern with BzRAs, evidence presented here shows no general loss of efficacy with nightly or intermittent treatment. Epidemiological studies show that up to two-thirds of patients taking hypnotics chronically report substantial ongoing benefit (Ohayon and Guilleminault 1999). In many placebo-controlled BzRA trials, placebo-treated groups show gradual improvements over time, which may also account for some of the apparent loss of efficacy with BzRA treatment. Discontinuance effects include *rebound insomnia,* defined as an increase in sleep problems to a level greater than the baseline level upon discontinuation of the drug. A meta-analysis suggests that rebound insomnia is a short-lived, dosage-dependent phenomenon (Soldatos et al. 1999). Nevertheless, abrupt discontinuation of BzRAs does lead to worsening of symptoms compared with the treatment period. BzRAs have marginal tendency for self-administration in animals, which is often used as a model of abuse potential in humans (Woods and Winger 1995), and they are rarely the drug of choice in humans who abuse drugs. Nevertheless, individuals with a past history of substance abuse, particularly of sedatives or alcohol, should be treated cautiously (Griffiths and Weerts 1997).

Limited evidence suggests that BzRAs are an efficacious adjunctive treatment in patients with insomnia comorbid with medical and psychiatric disorders. For instance, zolpidem improved sleep time and wakefulness after sleep onset in depressed patients treated with selective serotonin reuptake inhibitors (SSRIs; Asnis et al. 1999), and eszopiclone coadministered with fluoxetine improved both sleep and depressive symptoms relative to placebo (Fava et al. 2006).

Melatonin and Melatonin Receptor Agonists

As described earlier, melatonin is a pineal hormone secreted exclusively at night in a strong circadian rhythm. Exogenous melatonin has been studied as a hypnotic. It is rapidly absorbed, with peak levels occurring in 20–30 minutes, and has an elimination half-life of 40–60 minutes. Studies of subjective effects in healthy young adults given melatonin during the daytime, when activity of the SCN is greatest, support its hypnotic efficacy (Cajochen et al. 2003). When given at night, melatonin can decrease subjective sleep latency, although other effects are less consistent (Brzezinski et

TABLE 22–6. Benzodiazepine receptor agonists: pharmacokinetics

Drug	Onset of action, min	Elimination half-life, h	Typical adult dosage, mg
Zaleplon	10–20	1.0	5–20
Zolpidem	10–20	1.5–2.4	5–10 (IR) 5–10 (MR)
Eszopiclone	10–30	5–6	1–3
Triazolam	10–20	1.5–5	0.125–0.25
Temazepam	45–60	8–20	7.5–30
Estazolam*	15–30	20–30	0.5–2
Quazepam*	15–30	15–120	7.5–15
Flurazepam*	15–30	36–120	15–30

Note. IR = immediate release; MR = modified release.
*Has active metabolite.

al. 2005), and its efficacy on polysomnographic measures is not well documented. Ramelteon is a synthetic agonist of melatonin MT_1 and MT_2 receptors, with much higher affinity than endogenous melatonin. Controlled clinical trials have demonstrated its efficacy for reducing sleep latency, but with variable effects on sleep duration (Buysse et al. 2005a; Erman et al. 2006).

Other Agents

Other drugs and compounds are often used to treat insomnia, despite the lack of a U.S. Food and Drug Administration indication and the small amount of efficacy and safety data supporting their use (reviewed in Buysse et al. 2005b). The use of sedating antidepressants may be related to their lack of abuse potential as well as the perception that they may help subsyndromal depression. Small placebo-controlled clinical trials in primary insomnia support the efficacy of trazodone, doxepin, and trimipramine. Mirtazapine has been evaluated in small studies of healthy adults and patients with depression that documented improvements in sleep latency, awakenings, Stage 1 NREM sleep, and Stage 3–4 NREM sleep (Winokur et al. 2000). Effects of sedating antidepressants are summarized in Table 22–7.

Other drugs used to treat insomnia include antihistamines, alcohol, valerian, gabapentin and pregabalin, and sedating antipsychotic drugs. As stated earlier, there is generally very little empirical evidence supporting the efficacy and safety of these drugs for treating insomnia. In some cases, potential adverse effects are substantial.

Sleep-Related Breathing Disorders

Several different types of sleep-related breathing disorders have been described, including central sleep apnea syndromes, obstructive sleep apnea (OSA) syndromes, and sleep-related hypoventilation/hypoxemic syndromes (American Academy of Sleep Medicine 2005). This chapter focuses on OSA syndrome in adults, which is the most prevalent and best studied of these conditions.

Obstructive Sleep Apnea

Definition and Description

OSA is characterized by repetitive episodes of complete (apnea) or partial (hypopnea) upper airway obstruction during sleep that often result in oxygen desaturation and terminate with brief arousals. By definition, apnea and hypopnea events last for 10 seconds or longer and are accompanied by continued efforts to breathe. Obstructive hypopneas are typically defined by a decrease in airflow of 30% or more with desaturation of 4% or more (Strollo and Rogers 1996; Figure 22–7). Because the neurocognitive and cardiovascular outcomes are similar for apneas and hypopneas, these events are typically counted together in providing an overall index of severity, the apnea–hypopnea index (AHI; number of apneas and hypopneas per hour of sleep) (Gottlieb et al. 1999). Mild OSA is defined as an AHI between 5 and 15, moderate OSA as an AHI of 15–30, and severe OSA as an AHI of

TABLE 22–7. Summary of other drugs used to treat insomnia[a]

Drug	Sleep latency	Sleep continuity[b]	Stage 3/4 NREM sleep amount, %	REM sleep	Other
Trazodone	↓	↔ to ↑	↑	↔ Amount, % (↓ to ↑ in individual studies)	Infrequent side effect of priapism
Doxepin	↓	↑	↔	↓ Amount, % of REM; ↑ phasic eye movements (REM density)	↓ Sleep apnea (minor effect); ↔ or ↑ periodic limb movements; ↑ restless legs symptoms; may induce eye movements during NREM sleep; anticholinergic effects
Amitriptyline	↓	↑	↔	↓ Amount, % of REM; ↑ phasic eye movements (REM density)	
Trimipramine	↓	↑	↔	↔ Amount, %	
Mirtazapine	↓	↑	↔	↔	May cause weight gain
Melatonin	↓	↔ to ↑	↔	↔	
Diphenhydramine	↓	↔ to ↑	↔ to ↑	↓	Anticholinergic effects
Valerian	↓	↔ to ↑	↔ to ↑	↔ to ↑	Inconsistent effects on sleep continuity, Stage 3/4
Gabapentin	↔	↔ to ↑	↑	↔	↓ Periodic limb movements
Tiagabine	↔	↑	↑	↔	Infrequent side effect of seizures
Olanzapine, quetiapine	↔ to ↓	↑	↑	↔ to ↓	Reports of increased periodic limb movements, sleep-related eating
γ-Hydroxybutyrate	↔ to ↓	↑	↑	↔ to ↓	Side effects of sleepwalking, enuresis; abuse potential
Chloral hydrate	↓	↑	↔	↔ to ↓	Rapid tolerance; hepatotoxicity

[a]Reported effects are based on preponderance of evidence from published studies (see text for details). Many effects are inconsistent between individual studies. "↑" indicates increase from pretreatment baseline; "↓" indicates decrease from pretreatment baseline; "↔" indicates no change from pretreatment baseline.

[b]*Sleep continuity* refers to the proportion of sleep relative to wakefulness after sleep onset as reflected by measures such as sleep efficiency. Other indicators of sleep continuity, such as wakefulness after sleep onset or number of awakenings, would have opposite signs. Thus, "↑" indicates improvement in overall sleep continuity.

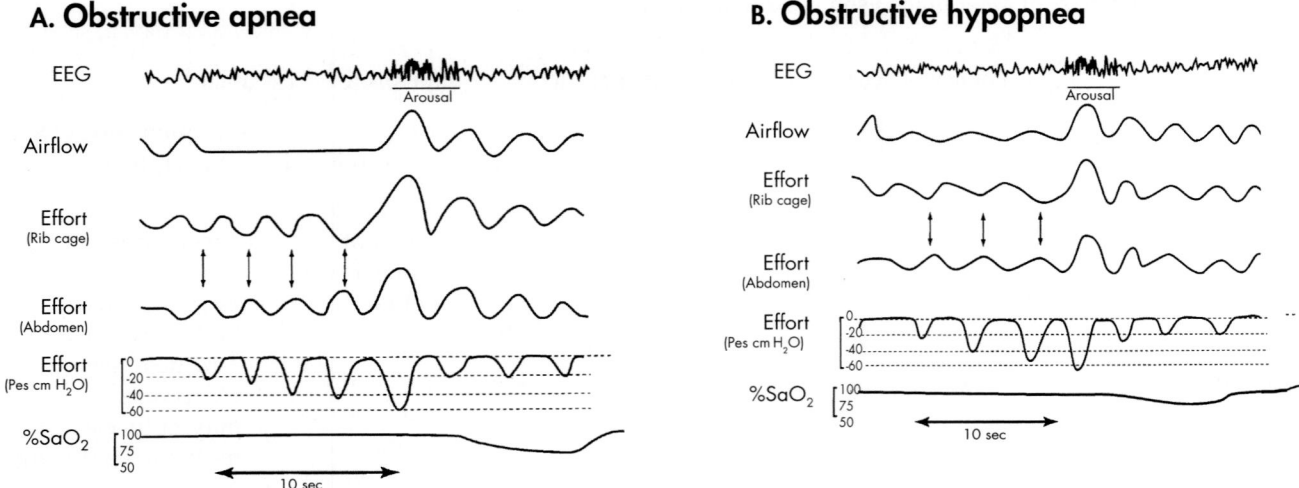

FIGURE 22–7. Obstructive apnea and obstructive hypopnea.

A, Diagrammatic representation of obstructive apnea. Increasing ventilatory effort is seen in the rib cage, the abdomen, and the level of esophageal pressure (measured with an esophageal balloon), despite lack of oronasal airflow. Arousal on the electroencephalogram (EEG) is associated with increasing ventilatory effort, as indicated by the esophageal pressure. Oxyhemoglobin desaturation follows the termination of apnea. Note that during apnea, the movements of the rib cage and the abdomen (Effort) are in opposite directions *(arrows)* as a result of attempts to breathe against a closed airway. Once the airway opens in response to arousal, rib-cage and abdominal movements become synchronous. **B,** Diagrammatic representation of obstructive hypopnea. Decreased airflow is associated with increasing ventilatory effort (reflected by the esophageal pressure) and subsequent arousal on the EEG. Rib-cage and abdominal movements are in opposite directions during hypopnea *(arrows)*, reflecting increasingly difficult breathing against a partially closed airway. Rib-cage and abdominal movements become synchronous after arousal produces airway opening. Oxyhemoglobin desaturation follows the termination of hypopnea.

Source. Adapted from Strollo PJ, Rogers RM: "Obstructive Sleep Apnea." *New England Journal of Medicine* 334:99–104, 1996.

greater than 30. In addition to apneas and hypopneas, the OSA syndrome includes a complaint of daytime sleepiness or insomnia, loud snoring, and/or episodes of breath holding, gasping, or choking during sleep. Other findings include complaints of fatigue, memory and cognitive difficulty, obesity, and hypertension or other cardiovascular disease.

Epidemiology and Consequences

In predominately white middle-aged cohorts, the prevalence of the OSA defined as AHI of 10 or greater with daytime sleepiness and/or hypertension is approximately 5% (Young et al. 2002). In a longitudinal family study, the 5-year incidence of mild OSA (AHI 10–15) was 7.5% and of moderate to severe OSA (AHI ≥ 15) was 16% (Tishler et al. 2003). Clinical studies indicate an increased risk in men, with a male-to-female prevalence ratio of 3.3 to 1 (Bixler et al. 2001; Young et al. 1993). Increasing weight and advancing age also increase the risk of OSA (Young et al. 2002), although the age effect plateaus after age 65 years (Young et al. 1993). Menopause increases risk in women; OSA prevalence is 2.7% in postmenopausal women without hormone replacement therapy versus 0.6% in the pre-

menopausal population (Bixler et al. 2001). The prevalence of OSA appears to be higher among African Americans compared with European Americans (Ancoli-Israel et al. 1995).

OSA is associated with significant cardiovascular, metabolic, and neurocognitive consequences (Table 22–8). Normal cardiovascular responses to sleep, including decreased blood pressure and heart rate, are negatively affected by OSA (discussed later). AHI is related in a dosage-dependent manner with cardiovascular complications (Shahar et al. 2001) including nocturnal and diurnal systemic hypertension, diurnal pulmonary hypertension, atrial dysrhythmias, heart failure, myocardial infarction, and stroke. Nocturnal hypoxemia associated with OSA and the respiratory mechanical consequences associated with obesity have been linked with pulmonary hypertension and right-sided heart failure (Bady et al. 2000). Treatment of OSA with continuous positive airway pressure (CPAP) is associated with improvement in pulmonary hypertension and right heart failure, suggesting a causal relationship (Sajkov et al. 2002). AHI is also related in a dosage-dependent manner with biomarkers of the metabolic syndrome (e.g., serum glucose and in-

TABLE 22–8. Comorbidities and consequences associated with obstructive sleep apnea syndrome

Cardiovascular complications	Metabolic complications	Neurocognitive complications
Nocturnal dysrhythmias	Leptin resistance	Daytime sleepiness
Bradydysrhythmias	Insulin resistance	Motor vehicle accidents
Atrial fibrillation		Work-related accidents
Nocturnal hypertension		Impaired neuropsychological function
Diurnal hypertension		Impaired quality of life
Pulmonary hypertension		
Congestive heart failure		
Myocardial infarction		
Stroke		

sulin sensitivity), even after controlling for concomitant obesity (Punjabi et al. 2003). Leptin, an adipokine that regulates metabolic and ventilatory control, is elevated in patients with OSA compared with matched obese control subjects (Ip et al. 2000).

OSA also shows dose–response relationships with neurocognitive consequences including daytime sleepiness (Gottlieb et al. 1999) and motor vehicle and occupational accidents (Lindberg et al. 2001; Teran-Santos et al. 1999), even after adjusting for body mass index, alcohol consumption, eyesight, medications, driving experience, and sleep schedule. Untreated OSA is also associated with significant deficits in neuropsychological functions such as vigilance, executive functioning, and coordination (Beebe et al. 2003). Analysis of a large managed-care database identified a significant increase in the odds ratio for OSA in patients prescribed antidepressant medication (Farney et al. 2004). Persistent fatigue after adequate treatment for OSA may indicate concomitant untreated depression (Bardwell et al. 2003) or possibly residual daytime sleepiness related to OSA. However, given the high prevalence of both depressive disorders and OSA in the population, true co-occurrence of these conditions is likely to be common.

OSA and its consequences ultimately affect quality of life, as measured by both generic and disease-specific measures. Conversely, treatment of OSA improves sleepiness, cognitive function, and quality of life (Engleman and Douglas 2004).

Pathophysiology

The human upper airway lacks rigid support from bone or cartilage in the retropalatal and retrolingual airway (Figure 22–8). During inspiration, negative in-

trathoracic pressure results in a suction force applied to this small, compliant upper airway, and narrowing (hypopnea) or closure (apnea) may occur. Vibration of these structures produces snoring. Thus, the primary cause for apnea is small functional airway diameter. Craniofacial structure and function and obesity are the major determinants of small airway diameter in adults. During the transition from wakefulness to sleep, muscle tone decreases and snoring and airway narrowing occur in vulnerable individuals. Arousal from sleep, precipitated by increased airway resistance, hypopnea, or apnea, stimulates resumption of breathing (Gleeson et al. 1990).

Attempting to breathe against a partially or completely obstructed airway leads to increased intrathoracic pressure, hypoventilation, and increased vagal tone; subsequent arousals are accompanied by increased sympathetic tone. Repeated episodes of bradycardia-tachycardia and increased sympathetic tone (Somers et al. 1995) lead to the cardiovascular effects described earlier. The ischemia–reperfusion associated with intermittent hypoxemia also results in oxidative stress and subsequent endothelial dysfunction (Lavie 2003). Biomarkers of oxidative stress such as C-reactive protein and interleukin 6 increase the risk for, and progression of, cardiovascular and metabolic disease.

Assessment and Diagnosis

The history and physical examination can identify patients at high risk for OSA, which is then confirmed with polysomnography. Nightly loud snoring, breathing pauses during sleep, snorting, choking, and subjective daytime sleepiness all suggest the diagnosis of OSA. Obesity (particularly upper-body obesity) and systemic hypertension are often present. In some indi-

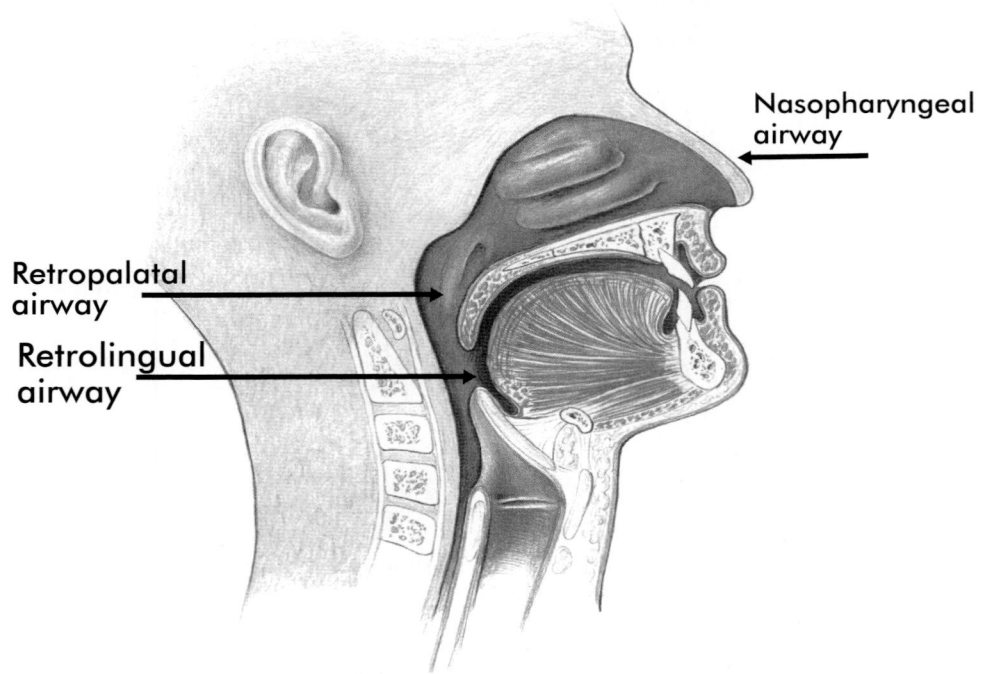

FIGURE 22–8.   Potential sites of airway instability.

Cross-sectional view of the upper airway depicting the potential sites of airway instability *(arrows)*.

Source.   Reprinted from Buysse DJ (ed): *Sleep Disorders and Psychiatry* (Review of Psychiatry Series, Volume 24, Number 2; Oldham JM and Riba MB, series editors). Washington, DC, American Psychiatric Publishing, 2005, p. 82. Copyright 2005, American Psychiatric Publishing. Used with permission.

viduals, craniofacial abnormalities (retrognathia or micrognathia) and/or soft tissue abnormalities, such as enlarged tonsils, lateral narrowing of the airway, or an elongated soft palate, place the patient at risk for OSA (Schellenberg et al. 2000; Zonato et al. 2003). Signs of right-sided heart failure in the absence of established heart disease may suggest occult OSA. However, clinical findings alone are not sufficiently precise to confirm a diagnosis of OSA (Schellenberg et al. 2000). Objective measurement and quantification of sleep and breathing with polysomnography are the current standard for diagnosing OSA.

Treatment

Behavioral treatments play a minor role in treatment of OSA. Because obesity is a major risk factor for OSA, weight loss improves both sleep and breathing (Peppard et al. 2000). Sleep deprivation increases the severity of daytime sleepiness and decreases upper airway muscle tone and should therefore be avoided. Alcohol and BzRA hypnotics also reduce upper airway muscle tone. If the patient clearly has positional OSA (typically worse in the supine position), lateral sleep position or elevation of the head of bed may be helpful.

Positive pressure delivered via nasal or nasal–oral mask reliably treats airway closure during sleep and is the first-line treatment for OSA. Positive pressure therapy works by pneumatically "splinting" the airway open during sleep (Figure 22–9). The treatment effect is virtually immediate when proper positive pressure titration is performed. Positive pressure can be applied as CPAP or as bilevel positive airway pressure (BPAP). With BPAP, the pressure setting is higher during inspiration than expiration, accounting for normal variation in pressure during the respiratory cycle. Both CPAP and BPAP machines are electrically operated and highly portable. Placebo-controlled, randomized clinical trials of positive pressure therapy have documented a favorable effect on quality of life, objective daytime function, and blood pressure. Emerging data indicate that CPAP also improves insulin sensitivity, left ventricular function, pulmonary hypertension, endothelial function, and cardiovascular and overall mortality (Punjabi and Beamer 2005; Strollo et al. 2005; Weaver and George 2005).

Objective adherence to positive pressure therapy is similar to most medical regimens, approximately 50% (Grunstein 2005). Acceptance and adherence can be improved with patient education and attention to patient–machine interface problems. CPAP and BPAP

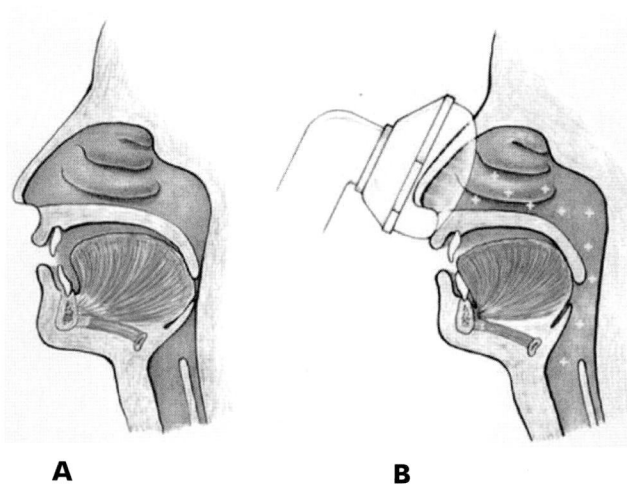

A   **B**

FIGURE 22–9.   Upper airway in obstructive sleep apnea, without treatment and with CPAP treatment.
Cross-sectional view of the upper airway, illustrating closure at the level of the palate and base of tongue typically seen in obstructive sleep apnea **(A)** and when the airway is pneumatically splinted open with continuous positive airway pressure (CPAP) **(B)**.
Source.   Reprinted from Buysse DJ (ed): *Sleep Disorders and Psychiatry* (Review of Psychiatry Series, Vol 24, No 2; Oldham JM and Riba MB, series editors). Washington, DC, American Psychiatric Publishing, 2005, p. 93. Copyright 2005, American Psychiatric Publishing. Used with permission.

are usually delivered via a nasal interface, and proper fit is essential. Patients with OSA frequently report nasal congestion prior to treatment, which can be exacerbated by positive pressure therapy and compounded by nasal dryness. Heated humidifiers for the CPAP/BPAP unit frequently improve nasal dryness and subsequent congestion. Occasionally, a mask that covers both the nose and mouth can be helpful. In patients who are claustrophobic, desensitization may be helpful.

Oral appliance therapy (OAP) modifies the position of the mandible and tongue to increase the upper airway size and reduce collapsibility. OAP is regarded as second-line therapy for OSA because it requires multiple adjustments over weeks to months, it is not 100% effective, and objective adherence is difficult to measure. Methodologically rigorous studies on the effectiveness of OAP are limited but suggest that approximately 33% of patients achieve optimal therapy (Lim et al. 2003). Patients who respond best have mild supine positional OSA and snoring (Marklund et al. 2004). OAP favorably affects subjective sleepiness, sleep-disordered breathing, and blood pressure compared with control interventions (Gotsopoulos et al. 2004).

Two basic types of OAP are commonly used: tongue-retaining devices and mandibular advancement devices. A patent nasal airway is essential for both types. Patients with mild to moderate OSA who do not accept (or cannot tolerate) positive pressure therapy are reasonable candidates for OAP. Side effects are usually mild and infrequently require intervention but can include mucosal dryness, tooth discomfort, and hypersalivation (Fritsch et al. 2001). Mandibular devices change occlusion over time; regular dental follow-up is mandatory in patients using these devices long term.

Surgical therapy has a small but important role in the management of adult OSA and can be broadly divided into two categories: tracheostomy (bypass of the upper airway) and reconstruction of the upper airway, which can involve multiple sites from the nasopharynx to the epiglottis (Figure 22–10). Tracheostomy was the original treatment for severe OSA but is now reserved for the small group of patients with severe and potentially life-threatening OSA who are intolerant of CPAP/BPAP. There are few well-designed studies to definitively evaluate the effect of simple reconstructive upper airway surgery on OSA (Bridgman and Dunn 2000), but case series provide support for surgery as a treatment option in some patients (Riley et al. 2000). The most common procedure is uvulopalatopharyngoplasty, which involves altering the size and the stiffness of the soft palate. This procedure is highly effective in treating loud snoring, but its impact on OSA is less certain, with reported success ranging from 7% to 60% (Sher 1995). The traditional uvulopalatopharyngoplasty approach involves trimming the palate with a scalpel and performing a tonsillectomy. It can also be performed using a laser to cut palatal tissue, which can be performed under local anesthesia and titrated to effect (elimination of snoring) in the outpatient clinic (Littner et al. 2001). Finally, radiofrequency ablation can be used to "stiffen" the palate. This approach produces less pain, but its effects are less robust and persistent (Blumen et al. 2002).

Reconstruction surgery is associated with less certain results than tracheostomy or positive pressure therapy because airway closure in OSA may occur at more than one site. Therefore, a phased approach to upper airway reconstruction has been described (Morrison et al. 1993). Phase I generally involves a palatoplasty and genioglossal advancement (Powell et al. 2005); phase II involves maxillomandibular advancement. Upper airway reconstruction for obstructive sleep hypopnea or apnea should be considered only after CPAP/BPAP trials. In individuals with retrogna-

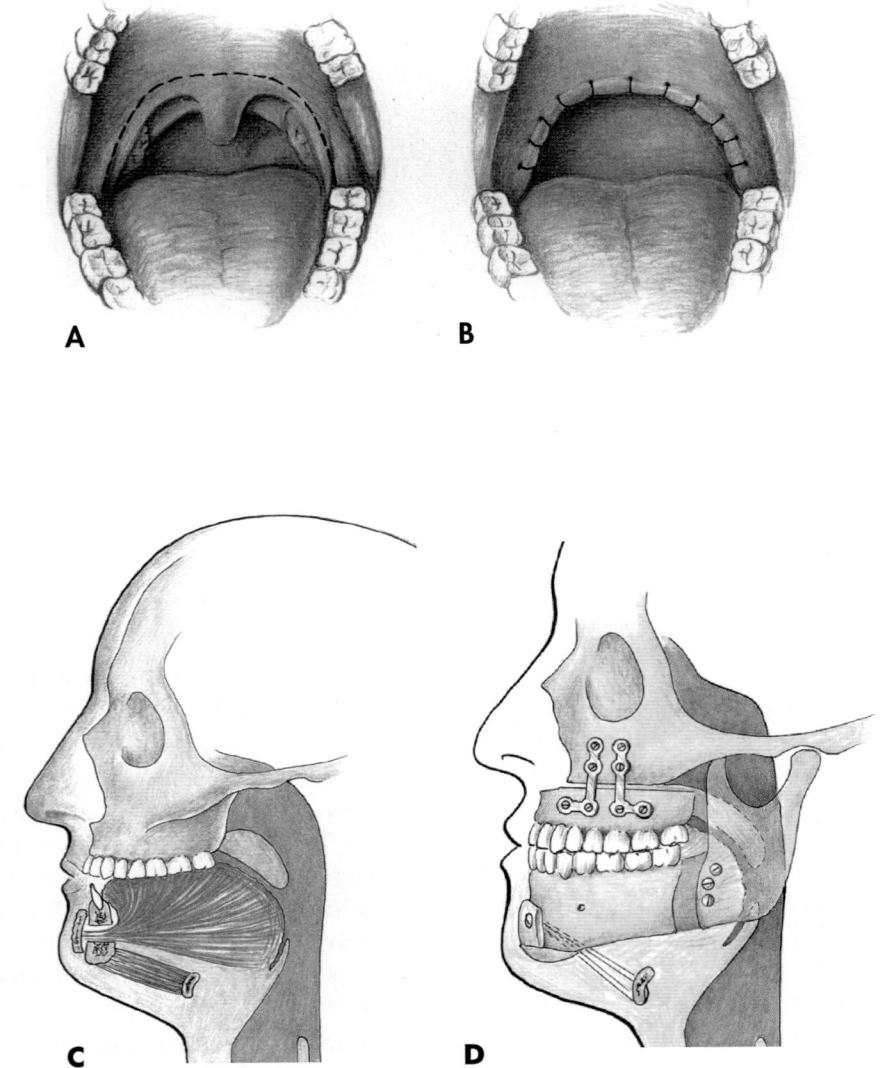

FIGURE 22–10. Surgical treatment for adult obstructive sleep apnea.

A, Appearance of the oropharynx prior to uvulopalatopharyngoplasty (UPP), with *dotted line* identifying site of incision. **B,** Postoperatively, with sutures in place. **C,** Phase I, UPP and genioglossal advancement. **D,** Phase II, maxillomandibular advancement.

Source. Reprinted from Buysse DJ (ed): *Sleep Disorders and Psychiatry* (Review of Psychiatry Series, Volume 24, Number 2; Oldham JM and Riba MB, series editors). Washington, DC, American Psychiatric Publishing, 2005, pp. 98–99. Copyright 2005, American Psychiatric Publishing. Used with permission.

thia or micrognathia, particularly young adults, surgical treatment may be reasonable at an earlier stage. Postoperative polysomnography should be performed to document changes in the AHI and sleep quality.

Medication plays no role in the treatment of obstructed breathing, per se, but may be important for treating concomitant depression and residual daytime sleepiness after adequate treatment. Residual daytime sleepiness in OSA may be related to the disorder itself (Pack et al. 2001), which is associated with gray matter loss in the frontal, parietal, and temporal cortex, anterior cingulate, hippocampus, and cerebellum (Macey et al. 2002). Long-term intermittent hypoxia may lead to significant oxidative injuries in the wake-promoting regions of the basal forebrain and brain stem and lead to sleepiness (Veasey et al. 2004). Modafinil (discussed later) is an efficacious adjunctive therapy for OSA patients with residual daytime sleepiness despite adequate treatment with CPAP (Pack et al. 2001). Insomnia can also be encountered in OSA, although its true prevalence is unknown. Some reports have suggested improvement of insomnia with positive pressure treatment (Guilleminault et al. 2002a, 2002b). BzRAs should generally be avoided in patients with OSA or suspected OSA unless they have been diagnosed and treated.

Hypersomnias of Central Origin

Hypersomnias are sleep disorders characterized by severe sleepiness due to dysfunction of CNS mechanisms regulating sleep–wake states. This distinguishes the hypersomnias from other sleep disorders marked by sleepiness, such as OSA and circadian rhythm disorders, whose etiology relates instead to sleep disruption or abnormal timing of the alertness–sleepiness rhythm.

Narcolepsy

Definition and Description

Narcolepsy is a syndrome characterized by profound excessive daytime sleepiness (EDS), which often occurs in association with cataplexy, hypnagogic or hypnopompic hallucinations, sleep paralysis, automatic behavior, and disrupted nocturnal sleep (American Academy of Sleep Medicine 2005). It is subdivided into two types: narcolepsy with cataplexy and narcolepsy without cataplexy. EDS is manifest as an increased propensity to fall asleep in relaxed or sedentary situations or a struggle to avoid sleeping in these situations. EDS may be so severe as to be irresistible, leading to sleep in inappropriate or dangerous situations. Brief naps temporarily relieve the sleepiness in many patients. EDS can lead to related symptoms, including "automatic behavior" (behavior that the individual does not recall), irritability, and poor memory, concentration, and attention. The overall amount of sleep per 24 hours is not increased in narcolepsy. In fact, many patients report fragmented nocturnal sleep, suggesting that the underlying disorder is an inability to maintain any stable sleep–wake state (Guilleminault and Fromherz 2005).

Cataplexy is the partial or complete loss of bilateral voluntary muscle tone in response to strong emotion and occurs in 60%–100% of patients with narcolepsy. The atonia may be minimal, occurring in a few muscle groups and causing subtle symptoms (ptosis, head drooping, slurred speech, dropping objects) or severe, resulting in complete collapse. Cataplectic episodes

usually last from a few seconds to a minute or two (Honda 1988). The patient is awake and oriented during these episodes, thus distinguishing cataplexy from sleep episodes. Cataplexy is most often triggered by positive emotional experiences, such as laughter, but can be triggered by other strong emotions (Gelb et al. 1994) and is exacerbated by stress, fatigue, or sleepiness. The onset of cataplexy typically occurs within a few months of the onset of EDS but may be delayed by years (Honda 1988). *Hypnagogic* and *hypnopompic hallucinations* are visual, tactile, auditory, or multisensory events lasting up to a few minutes during the transition from wakefulness to sleep (hypnagogic) or from sleep to wakefulness (hypnopompic). Hallucinations may combine elements of dream sleep and consciousness and are often bizarre or disturbing to patients. *Sleep paralysis* is the inability to move for a few seconds to a few minutes during wake–sleep or sleep–wake transitions. Sleep paralysis can be frightening, particularly when accompanied by hallucinations or the sensation of being unable to breathe. Hypnagogic hallucinations, sleep paralysis, and automatic behavior are not specific to narcolepsy and may occur in other sleep disorders as well as in healthy individuals. However, their co-occurrence with EDS strongly suggests narcolepsy.

Epidemiology

EDS occurring 3 or more days per week and interfering with daily activities has been reported in approximately 15% of the adult population in Western countries (Ohayon et al. 2002). The prevalence of narcolepsy in the United States, Western Europe, the Middle East, and Japan is approximately 0.05%, with a range of 0.002%–0.160% (Mignot 1998). Symptoms of narcolepsy most often begin during adolescence or young adulthood but can occur at any age. The usual course of symptoms is stable in the absence of treatment. Narcolepsy is associated with complications including depression, motor vehicle and other accidents, and significant occupational impairment due to sleepiness.

Pathophysiology

Narcolepsy results from dysfunction of the hypothalamic peptide neuromodulator hypocretin (orexin). Using gene-targeting and positional cloning strategies, narcolepsy was identified in mice with a knockout of the pre-pro-hypocretin gene (Chemelli et al. 1999), and canine narcolepsy was associated with mutations in the hypocretin receptor 2 gene (Lin et al. 1999). Although mutations in hypocretin-related genes are extremely rare in humans, the majority (85%–90%) of patients with narcolepsy–cataplexy have low or undetectable levels of hypocretin 1 in their cerebrospinal fluid (Nishino et al. 2000), a finding specific for this disorder (Mignot 2005). Postmortem studies in narcoleptic patients have confirmed deficiency of the hypocretin 1 and 2 ligand (Thannickal et al. 2000). Human narcolepsy demonstrates familial aggregation but no simple genetic mechanism. Narcolepsy shows a strong association with specific human leukocyte antigen (HLA) haplotypes, particularly DQB1*0602, which is present in approximately 90% of individuals with unequivocal cataplexy and only approximately 40% of those without cataplexy (Mignot 2005). Hypocretin deficiency is tightly associated with occurrence of cataplexy and the DQB1*0602 haplotype. The strong association between HLA type and narcolepsy with cataplexy raises the possibility that narcolepsy is an autoimmune disease, but there is no convincing evidence of typical autoimmune markers in narcolepsy (Fredrikson et al. 1990; Matsuki et al. 1988; Mignot 2005).

Assessment and Diagnosis

Clinical assessment of individuals presenting with EDS should focus on the severity, frequency, and situations in which sleepiness occurs. The relationship between EDS and nighttime sleep is also important; individuals with narcolepsy frequently report no strong relationship, which distinguishes narcolepsy from sleep deprivation. A clinical history of severe EDS coupled with cataplexy and/or sleep-related hallucinations or sleep paralysis is virtually diagnostic of narcolepsy. Polysomnography is also an important part of the evaluation and differential diagnosis. It can identify OSA, periodic limb movement disorder (PLMD), and REM sleep behavior disorder that may contribute to EDS and nocturnal sleep disruption (Overeem et al. 2001). Individuals with narcolepsy may also demonstrate sleep-onset REM periods during nocturnal polysomnography testing. The MSLT demonstrates reduced sleep latency (≤ 8 minutes) coupled with two or more sleep-onset REM periods. *Sleep-onset REM periods* are not specific for narcolepsy and may be due to sleep deprivation, rebound from REM-suppressing medication, altered sleep schedules, OSA, and delayed sleep phase syndrome. However, when these conditions are ruled out, these periods are highly suggestive of narcolepsy (Guilleminault and Fromherz 2005).

Treatment

The effective treatment of EDS requires regular, structured nocturnal sleep and planned daytime naps. A nocturnal sleep period of 8 hours or more should be encouraged, with consistent bedtimes and awakening times. Shift work in any form is usually problematic for individuals with narcolepsy. Scheduling two or more brief naps at regular times during the day is almost always necessary to further enhance daytime function in patients with narcolepsy.

Stimulants are indicated for the treatment of EDS in narcolepsy (Guilleminault and Fromherz 2005; Mitler et al. 1994; Table 22–9). These drugs produce substantial improvement but do not restore daytime alertness to normal levels. Traditional stimulants include methylphenidate, dextroamphetamine, and methamphetamine, which are available as immediate-release and delayed-release preparations. Patients may experience negative effects with any alerting agent, including nervousness, anorexia, weight loss, and sleep disruption. Some patients report rebound hypersomnia (exacerbation of sleepiness) as the dose wears off, and/or tolerance to the alerting effect may occur with time in some patients. In cases of tolerance, switching to a different class of medication or providing a "drug holiday" can be useful. Dosages of 20–80 mg/day are typical for most stimulants (10–40 mg for methamphetamine). Modafinil is a wake-promoting agent that is somewhat less potent than traditional agents, but with greater tolerability. The mechanism of action of modafinil appears to be mediated through inhibition of the dopamine transporter (Wisor and Eriksson 2005). The duration of effect of modafinil is relatively long as a result of its half-life of 12–15 hours. The efficacy of modafinil has been evaluated extensively in EDS due to narcolepsy, idiopathic hypersomnia, and sleep apnea (U.S. Modafinil in Narcolepsy Multicenter Study Group 1998). An agent unrelated to the traditional stimulants that also enhances alertness in narcolepsy is sodium oxybate (γ-hydroxybutyrate) (Mamelak et al. 2004). The mechanism of action of this agent is unknown. Sodium oxybate has similar efficacy as other agents, and its effect may be additive with other stimulants (U.S. Xyrem Multicenter Study Group 2002). Combining two alerting agents of different chemical classes may be necessary when a single agent is insufficient.

Medications used to treat cataplexy also improve hallucinations and sleep paralysis. In addition to its effect on EDS, sodium oxybate reduces cataplexy, reduces nocturnal sleep disruptions, and consolidates sleep (U.S. Xyrem Multicenter Study Group 2002). Low dosages of tricyclic antidepressants and typical antidepressant dosages of SSRIs and serotonin–norepinephrine reuptake inhibitors are also useful in treating cataplexy (Guilleminault and Fromherz 2005). Tolerance to cataplexy medications can occur, requiring a medication switch or drug holiday.

TABLE 22–9. Common alerting agents for the treatment of excessive daytime sleepiness

Agent	Receptor	Elimination half-life (h)	Time to maximal plasma concentration (h)	Usual dosage	Side effects
Modafinil	Unknown	15	2–4	100–400 mg + once daily or divided	Headache, nausea, anxiety, irritability
Amphetamines	Dopamine agonist	10 (SR: 15+)	2 (SR: 8–10)	5–60 mg divided	Both amphetamines and methylphenidate: headache, anxiety/ irritability, increased blood pressure, palpitation, appetite suppression, tremor, insomnia
Methylphenidate	Dopamine agonist	4 (SR: 8–10)	2 (SR: 5)	5–60 mg divided	
Pemoline*	Dopamine agonist	12	2–4	18.75–112.5 mg daily or divided	As above, but milder
γ-Hydroxybutyrate	Inadequately characterized	2	1	6–9 g + liquid solution divided nightly	Sedation, nausea, confusional arousals, sleepwalking

Note. SR = sustained-release.
*Potentially hepatotoxic—frequent liver function monitoring required.

Idiopathic Hypersomnia

Idiopathic hypersomnia is characterized by EDS without the specific features of narcolepsy or other sleep disorders. It occurs in two variants, one with long nocturnal sleep time and difficulty awakening and one without long nocturnal sleep time, but it can be quite heterogeneous in presentation (Bassetti et al. 2005). It is believed to be less common than narcolepsy, but its precise prevalence is uncertain due to the lack of strict diagnostic criteria and specific biological markers. Onset typically occurs in adolescence or early adulthood, and symptoms generally persist throughout adulthood. Distinguishing idiopathic hypersomnia from narcolepsy can be difficult, but patients with idiopathic hypersomnia do not have cataplexy or significant nocturnal sleep disruption. In the subtype with long nighttime sleep, patients are usually difficult to awaken in the morning, becoming confused, disoriented, uncoordinated, irritable, or even abusive in response to the efforts of others to rouse them. Patients often take long naps, which, in contrast to naps in narcolepsy, do not improve alertness. "Microsleeps," with or without automatic behavior, may occur throughout the day. Polysomnography in idio-

pathic hypersomnia usually reveals short sleep latency, increased total sleep time, and normal sleep continuity. Sleep latency on MSLT is usually short (8–10 minutes or less), but in contrast to narcolepsy, sleep-onset REM periods are not typically seen. The etiology and pathophysiology of idiopathic hypersomnia are unknown, but viral illnesses, including Guillain-Barré syndrome, hepatitis, mononucleosis, and atypical viral pneumonia, may precipitate sleepiness in a subset of patients. Familial cases have been described, with increased frequency of HLA-Cw2 and HLA-DR11 (Montplaisir and Poirier 1988). Some of these patients have associated symptoms suggesting autonomic nervous system dysfunction, including orthostatic hypotension, syncope, vascular headaches, and peripheral vascular complaints. However, most patients have neither a family history nor an obvious associated viral illness. Neurochemical studies using cerebrospinal fluid have suggested that patients with idiopathic hypersomnia may have altered noradrenergic system function (Bassetti et al. 2005). Treatment includes adequate nocturnal sleep time, scheduled daytime naps, and stimulant medications as described earlier for narcolepsy, but these interventions are less consistently helpful in this condition.

Recurrent Hypersomnia

Two types of recurrent hypersomnia have been described. *Kleine-Levin syndrome* is an uncommon disorder that occurs primarily in adolescents (Critchley 1967), with a male preponderance. It is characterized by repeated episodes of EDS that are often accompanied by hyperphagia, aggressiveness, and hypersexuality. These episodes last for days to weeks and are separated by asymptomatic periods of weeks or months. During symptomatic periods, individuals sleep up to 18 hours per day and are usually drowsy (often to the degree of stupor), confused, and irritable. During symptomatic episodes, polysomnographic studies show long total sleep time with high sleep efficiency and decreased slow-wave sleep. MSLT studies demonstrate short sleep latencies and sleep-onset REM periods (Rosenow et al. 2000). The etiology of this syndrome remains unknown, although structural brain lesions have been reported in some cases.

In *menstrual-related hypersomnia*, EDS occurs during the several days prior to menstruation (Billiard et al. 1975). The prevalence of this syndrome has not been well characterized. The etiology also is not known, but presumably the symptoms are related to hormonal changes. Some cases of menstrual-related hypersomnia have responded to the blocking of ovulation with estrogen and progesterone (oral contraceptives) (Bamford 1993).

Behaviorally Induced Insufficient Sleep Syndrome (Sleep Deprivation)

Sleep deprivation and sleep restriction are endemic in Western societies. Recent data show that American adults on average get approximately 6.5 hours of sleep at night, which contrasts with the 7–8 hours they typically obtain under conditions of time isolation and self-selected bedtimes. This also represents a decrease in sleep time over the past 100 years (Walsh et al. 2005a). Insufficient sleep syndrome is characterized by complaints of EDS, sometimes quite severe, which is related to curtailed sleep duration at night. The EDS may lead to occupational or motor vehicle accidents as well as use of over-the-counter or illicit substances to promote wakefulness. Other symptoms of sleep restriction include mood lability, poor concentration, and impaired interpersonal function. When their schedule permits, affected individuals sleep longer and report reduced daytime symptoms (American Academy of Sleep Medicine 2005). However, recovery from sleep restriction does not occur immediately and may require several days to a week for full recovery. A careful history and sleep diary are usually adequate to identify insufficient sleep. However, "treatment" may be quite difficult, because it requires a commitment to behavioral change and acceptance of fewer waking hours.

Hypersomnia Due to Other Conditions

EDS can be a symptom of many medical and psychiatric conditions as well as an effect of medications and/or substances. EDS is often associated with neurological disorders, including structural, vascular, traumatic, toxic, infectious, and metabolic encephalopathic processes. EDS may result either from direct involvement of discrete brain regions (especially the brain-stem reticular formation or midline diencephalic structures) or from the effects of disrupted sleep continuity. Patients with neuromuscular disorders or peripheral neuropathies may also develop EDS because of associated central or obstructive sleep apnea, pain, or PLMD (George 2000). Patients with myotonic dystrophy often have EDS, even in the absence of sleep-disordered breathing (Gibbs et al. 2002). Sleepiness may occur with acute infectious illness even without direct CNS involvement and may be mediated by cytokines, including interferon, interleukins, and tumor necrosis factor (Toth and Opp 2002). Psychiatric disorders, especially depression, are often accompanied by complaints of EDS. Indeed, tiredness, fatigue, and lack of energy are reported by a large majority of patients with major depression. However, rating scales and MSLT findings suggest that actual EDS is much less common than complaints of fatigue or lack of energy (Nofzinger et al. 1991).

Circadian Rhythm Sleep Disorders

Alterations in the regulation of the circadian timing system, or a misalignment between the endogenous circadian rhythm and the external physical or social environment, can affect the timing or duration of sleep and give rise to CRSD (Reid and Zee 2005). Several distinct subtypes of CRSD have been described (Figure 22–11). The approach to assessment and diagnosis is described first, because this is similar across all subtypes.

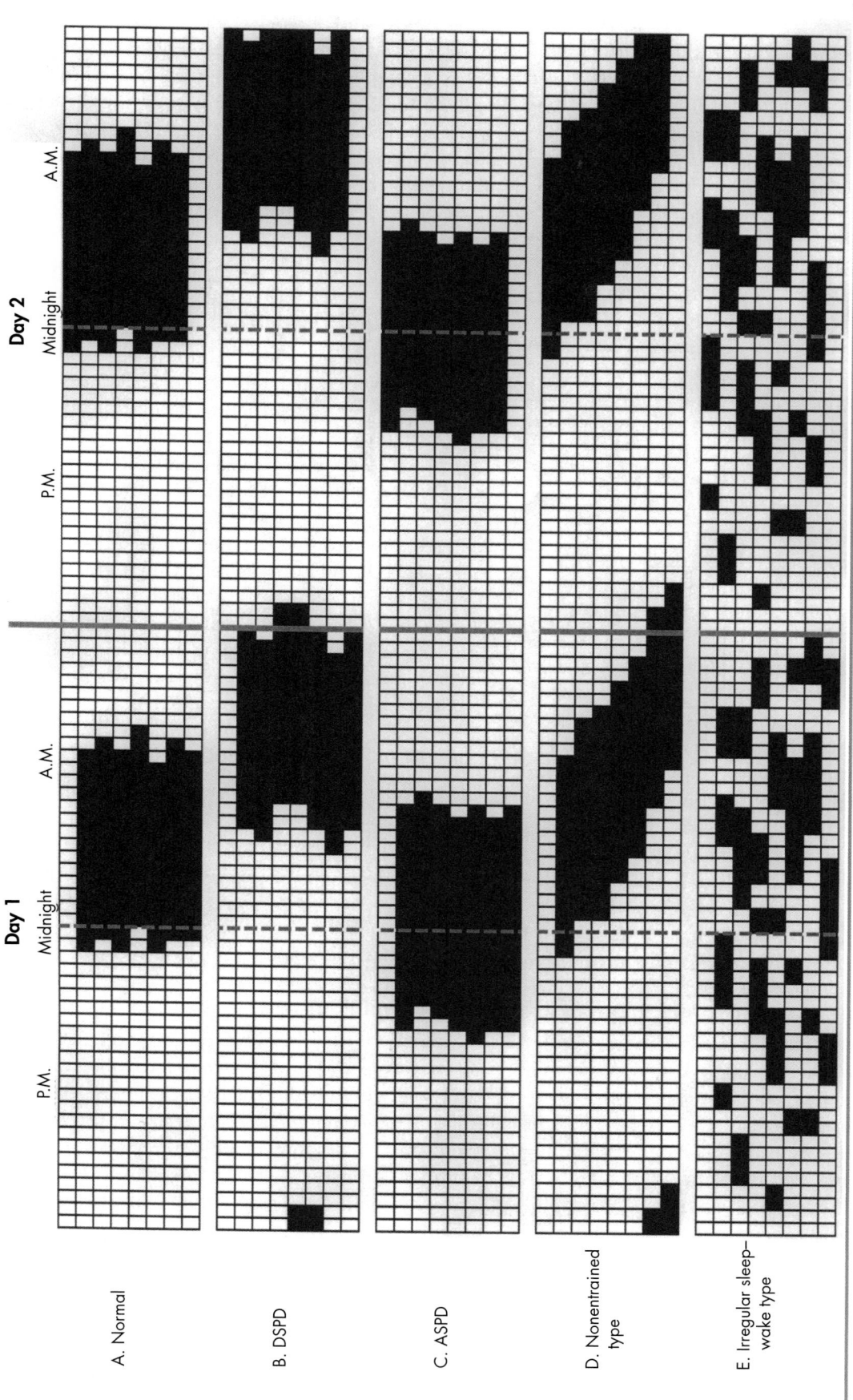

FIGURE 22–11. Schematic representations of normal sleep and circadian rhythm sleep disorders.

Data are shown for 7 days and nights for each condition. *Black bars:* Sleep; *Open rectangles:* Wakefulness. For each hypothetical condition, sleep–wake data are "double plotted" (i.e., each day's data are shown both to the right of and below the previous day) to facilitate viewing the pattern across days. Each *horizontal line* shows 2 days; the *heavy vertical line* separates successive days. The *dashed vertical line* indicates midnight. For comparative purposes, each condition is shown with a total sleep time of approximately 8 hours. **A,** Normal sleep. Sleep hours across successive days fall at about midnight to 7:00 A.M. **B,** Delayed sleep phase disorder (DSPD). Sleep hours are consistently delayed, with average sleep times of approximately 4:00 A.M. to noon. **C,** Advanced sleep phase disorder (ASPD). Sleep hours are consistently advanced, with average sleep times of approximately 8:00 P.M. to 4:00 A.M. **D,** Nonentrained type. Sleep hours are progressively later each day, following an underlying circadian rhythm period closer to 25 hours than 24. **E,** Irregular sleep–wake type. Sleep–wake hours occur irregularly over the 24-hour day, with no discernible circadian pattern.

Assessment and Diagnosis

The diagnosis of CRSD rests on clinical history. CRSDs are distinguished from subclinical symptoms or circadian preferences by impairment in social, occupational, or other areas of functioning. Sleep–wake diaries are useful for confirming abnormalities of sleep–wake timing, and actigraphy provides objective verification of rest–activity patterns. Sleep diaries and actigraphy should be obtained for 1–2 weeks in order to capture the individual's typical schedule variations, such as work and nonwork days. Physiological markers of circadian phase, such as melatonin or core body temperature rhythms, can confirm abnormal circadian phase but are rarely used in clinical practice. Although polysomnography is not required for the diagnosis of CRSD, it may be useful to exclude other sleep disorders such as OSA or RLS. Polysomnographic findings in individuals with CRSD may vary depending on the time of the sleep recording in relation to the individual's usual sleep–wake schedule. When objective evaluation of sleepiness is needed, such as in shift work disorder when safety is of significant concern, the MSLT should be conducted during usual work hours.

Medical history is an important aspect of assessment in CRSD. Shift work disorder is associated with increased prevalence of medical disorders such as cardiovascular and gastrointestinal disorders, sleep apnea, obesity, and miscarriage (Scott 2000; Wagner 1996). Neurological disorders affecting the structure of the circadian pacemaker, its afferents, or its efferents (e.g., visual impairment, tumors, dementia, stroke) should be considered in individuals with irregular sleep–wake pattern and nonentrained type.

Evaluation of CRSD should routinely include screening for psychiatric disorders and psychoactive medications. The prevalence of affective and personality disorders is high in patients with CRSDs such as delayed sleep phase disorder (DSPD) and irregular sleep–wake pattern (Dagan 2002). Affective and personality disorders may contribute to social withdrawal, which can lead to a decrease in light exposure, physical activity, and social cues, thereby perpetuating abnormal sleep timing. Because depressed patients often complain of early-morning awakening, it is important to distinguish advanced sleep phase disorder (ASPD) from major depression and other affective disorders (Wagner 1996). Individuals with CRSD may use alcohol, sedative-hypnotics, and stimulants to alleviate symptoms, which may lead to substance dependence.

The role of voluntary behavior often poses a problem in the evaluation of CRSD. For instance, some adolescents and young adults prefer delayed sleep–wake schedules and are not strongly motivated to change this pattern; socially withdrawn or cognitively impaired individuals may not see an irregular sleep–wake pattern as undesirable. In such cases, altered timing of light exposure can lead to a self-perpetuating cycle of sleep–wake disturbance.

Delayed Sleep Phase Disorder

Definition and Description

DSPD is characterized by habitual sleep–wake times that are substantially later than societal norms, resulting in complaints of difficulty falling asleep at night and difficulty waking up in the morning (Regestein and Monk 1995). Individuals with DSPD typically fall asleep between 2:00 and 6:00 A.M. and wake up between 10:00 A.M. and 1:00 P.M. (Weitzman et al. 1981). When allowed to sleep at their preferred sleep–wake times, DSPD patients have relatively normal sleep architecture and quality. The preference for delayed sleep–wake times remains stable over a long period of time, is not the result of external time demands, and is accompanied by greater than usual difficulty adjusting sleep–wake times (Dagan 2002).

Epidemiology and Consequences

The prevalence of DSPD in the general population has been estimated to be less than 1% (Wagner 1996). However, DSPD is more common among adolescents, with a reported prevalence of 7%–16% (Pelayo et al. 1988). Approximately 7% of patients with chronic insomnia presenting to a sleep clinic may have DSPD (Weitzman et al. 1981).

Pathophysiology

Evidence for genetic contributions to DSPD comes from studies of family history (Ancoli-Israel et al. 2001) and polymorphisms in circadian rhythm genes (*Per3, Arylalkylamine N-acetyltransferase, HLA,* and *Clock*) and circadian gene polymorphisms in affected kindreds (Archer et al. 2003; Hohjoh et al. 2003). Circadian physiological dysregulation may also contribute to DSPD through factors including 1) long endogenous circadian period (Regestein and Monk 1995); 2) alteration of circadian entrainment by light, as might result from decreased phase advances to morning light or increased delays to evening light (Weitzman et al. 1981); 3) alteration in light sensitivity, and in particular, increased sensitivity to nighttime light (Aoki et al. 2001); and 4) behavioral factors, such as increased exposure to evening light and decreased exposure to morning light, that may help to perpetuate the phase delay (Ozaki et al. 1996). Finally, alterations in homeostatic sleep regulatory processes may also contribute to DSPD. Although sleep architecture is usually described as normal (Uchiyama et al. 1992; Weitzman et al. 1981), individuals with DSPD may have decreased ability to compensate for sleep loss during wakefulness (Uchiyama et al. 2000).

Treatment

Treatment success depends on many variables including severity of the disorder, comorbid psychopathology, ability and willingness of the patient to comply with treatment, school or work schedules, and social pressures (Regestein and Monk 1995; Thorpy et al. 1988). Chronotherapy is a behavioral treatment in which bedtime is delayed (i.e., moved to a later clock time) by approximately 3 hours every 2 days until the desired sleep time is achieved (Weitzman et al. 1981). Patients need to be free of social and work requirements for at least 1 week and adhere to a strict sleep–wake schedule. In addition, light exposure needs to be carefully controlled (discussed later). The strict protocol and length of treatment may limit its acceptability for some patients, but in adolescents, for whom behavioral factors are important, strict sleep–wake schedules are often useful. Bright-light exposure during the early morning hours is an accepted and effective treatment for DSPD (Chesson et al. 1999). Although the optimal timing, intensity, and duration of light treatment are not well defined, typical regimens include exposure to broad-spectrum light of 2,000–10,000 lux for approximately 1–2 hours shortly after awakening. Compliance with daily or chronic intermittent exposure to light may be difficult. One important factor that affects compliance is the inability of patients to wake up in the morning for light exposure (Thorpy et al. 1988). Blue wavelength light may enhance compliance by permitting shorter-duration, lower-intensity light exposure. Melatonin has both circadian phase shifting effects and mild hypnotic effects. Melatonin, 1–5 mg administered in the evening, advances both sleep onset and wake times and improves quality of life of DSPD patients (Dahlitz et al. 1991; Mundey et al. 2005), but definitive clinical guidelines for the use of melatonin have not been developed. Hypnotic medications and stimulants are commonly prescribed for patients with DSPD, but there is little evidence documenting their efficacy and no established guidelines for their use.

Advanced Sleep Phase Disorder

Definition and Description

ASPD is characterized by habitual sleep–wake times that are substantially earlier than societal norms, resulting in complaints of sleepiness in the late afternoon and evening and sleep maintenance insomnia or waking up too early in the morning. Individuals with ASPD typically report sleep onset between 6:00 and 9:00 P.M. and wake times between 2:00 and 5:00 A.M. (Kamei et al. 1998). When allowed to follow their usual schedule, ASPD patients have normal sleep architecture and quality for age.

Epidemiology

The actual prevalence of ASPD in the general population is unknown, but it has been estimated to be about 1% in middle-age and older adults. Because circadian rhythms tend to advance with age, only a few case reports have described ASPD *not* associated with aging (Jones et al. 1999; Reid et al. 2001).

Pathophysiology

Genetic factors appear to play an important role in the pathogenesis of ASPD. Several families with ASPD have been identified (Jones et al. 1999; Reid et al. 2001), and the phenotype segregates with an autosomal dominant mode of inheritance. Mutations in the circadian clock *hPer2* and *CK1 delt*a genes have been linked to ASPD, indicating genetic heterogeneity (Toh et al. 2001; Xu et al. 2005). As with DSPD, physiological dysregulation may also play a role. Specifically, ASPD may be related to an unusually short endogenous circadian period or alterations in the entrainment process of the circadian system (Jones et al. 1999). Similar to DSPD, the interaction between circadian timing and sleep homeostatic regulation may be altered in individuals with ASPD and in older adults with nonpathologically advanced sleep phase (Duffy and Czeisler 2002).

Treatment

Treatment principles for ASPD are similar to those for DSPD, except for the timing of interventions. Chronotherapy for ASPD requires progressively advancing sleep time (i.e., moving it to an earlier clock time) by 2 hours every 2 days until the desired sleep time is achieved (Moldofsky et al. 1986). Exposure to evening bright light (7:00–9:00 P.M.) delays circadian rhythms and improves sleep efficiency, but patients may have difficulty maintaining the treatment regimen (Suhner et al. 2002). Concurrently, patients should avoid bright light in the early morning hours, because morning light exposure further advances circadian rhythms. Theoretically, melatonin given in the morning could delay circadian rhythms in ASPD, but there are few empirical data documenting its efficacy, and residual sedating effects may limit its utility. As with DSPD, the appropriate role of hypnotic and stimulant medications in ASPD is uncertain.

Nonentrained Type

Definition and Description

CRSD, nonentrained type, is characterized by a progressive delay of the sleep period across days, corresponding to the endogenous period of the circadian clock. In nonentrained type the circadian clock is not entrained or only weakly entrained to the physical and social 24-hour cycle. When sleep–wake timing is in phase with the environment, sleep quality and duration are typically normal. However, because the endogenous period of the human circadian clock is slightly longer than 24 hours (Czeisler et al. 1999), sleep–wake times gradually delay across days and are eventually out of phase with desired or conventional times. Complaints of insomnia or excessive sleepiness arise when the individual attempts to keep conventional hours, but these complaints vary from week to week.

Epidemiology

Nonentrained-type CRSD was originally described in blind people, with an estimated prevalence of 50% (Sack et al. 1992). There have been only a few reports of this condition in sighted individuals (McArthur et al. 1996).

Pathophysiology

CRSD nonentrained type in blind individuals most likely results from a lack of photic entrainment due to damage of photoreceptors. However, scheduled social or physical activities serve as sufficiently powerful synchronizing agents to maintain entrainment in many of these individuals. In blind individuals with intact retinal ganglion cells and retinohypothalamic pathways, the circadian system can still be entrained to light (Czeisler et al. 1995). The pathophysiology of nonentrained type in sighted individuals is less clear. These individuals may have very long endogenous circadian periods outside of the range of entrainment to the 24-hour day (Uchiyama et al. 2002), as suggested by reports of DSPD patients who develop a nonentrained type during phase delay chronotherapy (Oren

and Wehr 1992). As with DSPD, alterations in the response of the circadian system to synchronizing agents such as light could result in weakened entrainment or lack of entrainment of the circadian rhythms.

Treatment

Behavioral strategies such as timed, regular schedules of sleep, social, and work activities may help to entrain circadian rhythms in blind individuals with nonentrained type. When structured activity alone is insufficient to maintain entrainment, melatonin 10 mg, taken 1 hour before bedtime, can entrain the timing of sleep (Sack et al. 2000), and as little as 0.5 of melatonin may be sufficient to maintain entrainment (Lewy et al. 2001). Based on available data in blind people, melatonin in the evening and bright-light exposure during the day are reasonable approaches to reinforce entrainment in sighted persons.

Irregular Sleep–Wake Type (Irregular Sleep–Wake Rhythm)

Definition and Description

CRSD irregular sleep–wake type is characterized by the absence of clearly identifiable major sleep or wake periods during the 24-hour day. Patients with this disorder may complain of insomnia and/or excessive sleepiness, typically associated with three or more irregular sleep periods per day, each lasting a few hours.

Epidemiology

The prevalence of irregular sleep–wake type in the general population is unknown. It was originally described in cognitively intact, physically ill patients who had spent years bedridden and isolated, but it is most commonly seen in patients with underlying neurological dysfunction, such as mental retardation, traumatic brain injury, and dementia (Hoogendijk et al. 1996; Witting et al. 1990).

Pathophysiology

Although its pathophysiology is unknown, irregular sleep–wake type may reflect low-amplitude or irregular circadian rhythms due to dysfunction of the circadian system. Structural changes in the hypothalamus and SCN have been implicated in patients with Alzheimer's disease (Hoogendijk et al. 1996). Irregular sleep–wake type is most common in populations who have decreased exposure to synchronizing agents such as light and activity (Pollak and Stokes 1997; Van Someren et al. 1996). Therefore, both circadian dysfunction and decreased exposure to environmental zeitgebers may lead to development and maintenance of irregular or arrhythmic sleep and wake patterns.

Treatment

Treatment of irregular sleep–wake type is aimed at consolidating nocturnal sleep by strengthening exposure to zeitgebers and by promoting wakefulness during the day. Specific methods include structuring of social and physical activities, increasing exposure to morning bright light, and minimizing light and noise at night (Ancoli-Israel et al. 2002; Naylor et al. 2000; Van Someren et al. 1999). Other treatments may include vitamin B_{12} and hypnotics.

Shift Work Type (Shift Work Disorder)

Definition and Description

Shift work disorder is characterized by excessive sleepiness during work hours that are scheduled during the usual sleep period (when circadian alertness is low) and insomnia when attempting to sleep during the usual wake period (when circadian alertness is high). Shift work disorder is most commonly seen in association with night and early-morning shift schedules. Patients report decreased total sleep time, poor sleep quality, and impaired performance at work (Akerstedt 2003; Knauth et al. 1980). Safety at work and during the morning commute is a major concern due to decreased alertness.

Epidemiology

Shift work disorder is likely to be very common, but the actual prevalence is unknown. Approximately 20% of the workforce in industrialized countries has nonstandard work schedules (Presser 1999). Based on data available for night shift workers, approximately 5% of the population is likely to be affected by shift work disorder (Akerstedt 2003). As discussed earlier, shift work disorder is associated with medical and psychiatric morbidity. Mood symptoms and disorders are associated with current and former shift work (Scott 2000). Because irregular schedules and sleep deprivation can exacerbate mania, patients with bipolar disorder may be at particular risk for adverse consequences of shift work.

Pathophysiology

Shift work disorder results from misalignment between scheduled work and sleep times and the endogenous circadian rhythm of alertness and sleep propensity. Even among permanent night workers, internal circadian rhythms are usually out of phase with the desired sleep–wake times (Dumont et al. 2001). Chronic cumulative sleep loss may also contribute to excessive sleepiness.

Treatment

The goal of clinical management is to align the circadian propensity for sleep and wakefulness with the work schedule as well as to employ behavioral approaches to improve sleep quality and work performance. For rotating shifts, a clockwise rotation, in which the schedule is delayed from day to evening to night is recommended. Because disturbances in sleep and wakefulness are most common among night shift workers, most treatment strategies have focused on this group. Family, social, and environmental factors are critical in the management of shift work disorder. Family responsibilities can limit time available for sleep, and family dynamics can affect coping ability with shift work. Adherence to good sleep habits and practices is important for all patients and includes protecting sleep time, decreasing daytime noise, and providing a dark and comfortable room. Educating the individual, family members, and employers regarding the disorder is essential for effective management.

Timed bright light (1,200–10,000 lux for 3–6 hours) and melatonin accelerate circadian adaptation to night shift (Burgess et al. 2002; Sharkey et al. 2001). A regimen of intermittent exposure to bright light (20-minute blocks per hour) during the night shift may also improve adaptation (Boivin and James 2002). Intermittent or continuous light exposure should begin early in the shift and terminate approximately 2 hours before the end of the shift to avoid the potential advancing effects of early-morning bright light (Crowley et al. 2003). Bright-light exposure during the morning commute may also prevent the desired phase delay and should be avoided (Boivin and James 2002; Crowley et al. 2003). Melatonin given at bedtime after a night shift may increase sleep duration but has limited effects on alertness (Burgess et al. 2002) and questionable additive benefit when combined with intermittent bright-light therapy and morning light avoidance (Crowley et al. 2003).

Pharmacological treatment may target both sleep and alertness. Hypnotics treat insomnia but do not necessarily address circadian misalignment and therefore are often insufficient therapy by themselves. Caffeine alleviates sleepiness, one of the most debilitating symptoms of this disorder (Babkoff et al. 2002). Modafinil is approved for the treatment of excessive sleepiness and neurobehavioral deficits associated with shift work disorder (Walsh et al. 2004).

Jet Lag Disorder

Definition and Description

Jet lag disorder refers to sleep–wake disturbances associated with rapid travel across time zones, resulting from a transient mismatch between the external physical/social environment and the timing of the individual's endogenous circadian rhythm. Symptoms include difficulty falling asleep at night, daytime sleepiness, general malaise, gastrointestinal upset, and mood changes (Winget et al. 1984). Symptoms of jet lag are transient, with resolution as the traveler adjusts physiologically and socially to the destination time zone. The severity and duration of symptoms are related to the number of time zones crossed. Eastward travel, in which adjustment requires an advance shift of circadian rhythms, is usually more difficult than westward travel and affects up to 80% of business travelers (Wagner 1996). Sleep-onset difficulties are more common with eastward travel, and evening sleepiness and sleep maintenance problems are more prominent with westward travel (Boulos et al. 1995). Factors such as anxiety, air quality, lack of physical activity, and dehydration also contribute to the sleep loss and malaise that often accompany jet travel.

Pathophysiology

The pathophysiology of jet lag disorder is similar to that of shift work disorder. An important difference is that, in jet lag disorder, social and environmental time cues favor adaptation to a new circadian phase and eventual resolution of symptoms.

Treatment

Treatment of jet lag disorder must address both reentrainment of the circadian clock and sleep loss. Travelers should be encouraged to wear loose, comfortable clothing; use ear plugs and eyeshades; increase fluid intake; and avoid alcohol and caffeine during flight. On arrival, jet lag symptoms and sleep disturbance can be ameliorated by eating meals at local times, getting exercise and light exposure at times appropriate to the new environment, and maintaining good sleep habits (Waterhouse et al. 1997). Entrainment to the new time zone can be accelerated by appropriately timed bright-light exposure and light avoidance and use of melatonin (Beaumont et al. 2004; Burgess et al. 2003). Appropriate timing of light exposure depends on the direction of travel. For example, upon arrival after eastward flights, travelers should stay awake but avoid bright light in the early morning, and then try to get light in the afternoon (Herxheimer and Waterhouse 2003). Melatonin 2–5 mg taken close to local bedtime for up to approximately 4 days prior to and after travel can alleviate jet lag (Herxheimer and Petrie 2002; Herxheimer and Waterhouse 2003). Short-term use of short-acting hypnotics may be useful in the management of insomnia symptoms (Jamieson et al. 2001). Although not approved for this use, stimulant medications such as modafinil may improve alertness at appropriate times in the new time zone.

Parasomnias

The term *parasomnia* derives from the Latin *para* (next to) and *somnus* (sleep). Parasomnias are defined as undesirable physical or experiential events that accompany sleep (American Academy of Sleep Medicine 2005) and are generally divided into those arising from NREM sleep and those arising from REM sleep. These types of parasomnias can often be distinguished by their clinical features, time of occurrence, and associated autonomic activation (Table 22–10).

NREM Parasomnias

Clinical Features, Epidemiology, and Pathophysiology

Arousal from sleep is not an all-or-none phenomenon, but rather a continuum of reestablishing alertness, judgment, and control over behavior (Mahowald and Schenck 2001). Behaviors or mood states can be expressed during such partial arousals, which may be partially or completely divorced from awareness. Most commonly, such behaviors involve dissociated motor activities (walking, eating, sexual activity) or emotional responses (fear, anger, sexual excitement) (Schenck and Mahowald 2000). They are distinguished from waking behavior by the absence of complex mentation and sound judgment and by reduced response to environmental feedback. The relationship between sleep-related behaviors and emotional states and waking motivations, psychological states, or psychopathology is unclear. NREM parasomnias show clear familial aggregation (Mahowald and Cramer Bornemann 2005). Specific NREM parasomnias share many features that may provide insight into their pathophysiology. For example, episodes occur most frequently in children and are typically brief, are associated with amnesia, occur in the

TABLE 22–10. **Overview of parasomnias**

	NREM parasomnias			REM parasomnias	
	Confusional arousals	**Sleepwalking**	**Sleep terrors**	**REM sleep behavior disorder**	**Nightmare disorder**
Stage of arousal	NREM 2–4	NREM 3–4	NREM 3–4	REM	REM
Time of night	Anytime	First 2 hours	First 2 hours	Anytime	Anytime
EEG with event	NA	Mixed	Mixed	Characteristic of REM	NA
EMG with event	Low	Low	Low	High, variable	NA
Relative unresponsiveness during event	Yes	Yes	Yes	Yes	Yes
Autonomic activity	Low	Low	High	High	High
Amnesia	Yes	Yes	Yes	No	No
Confusion following episode	Yes	Yes	Yes	No	No
Family history of parasomnias	Yes	Yes	Yes	No	No

Note. EEG=electroencephalogram; EMG=electromyogram; NA=not available; NREM=non–rapid eye movement; RBD=REM sleep behavior disorder; REM=rapid eye movement.

first 1–2 hours of sleep, and arise from slow-wave sleep. Several subtypes, defined by clinical features, have been described.

Confusional arousals are brief, simple motor behaviors that usually occur without strong affective expression during partial arousals from NREM sleep. Confusional arousals may occur during daytime naps. Mental confusion with automatic behavior, indistinct speech, and relative unresponsiveness to the environment are hallmarks (Mahowald and Cramer Bornemann 2005). Amnesia for events is dense; without an observer's report, they may go unnoticed. Individuals do not report dreams upon achieving full alertness, but rather simple mentation. Electroencephalographic recordings at the time of confusional arousals may show delta waves (characteristic of slow-wave sleep), theta, or alpha activity or alternation between sleep and waking activity (Gaudreau et al. 2000). Epidemiological information is unreliable, but roughly 10%–20% of children and 2%–5% of adults report a history of confusional arousals (Ohayon et al. 1999). The expression of confusional arousals depends upon a genetic predisposition combined with a precipitating event, which may be endogenous (e.g., OSA, pain, leg movements) or exogenous (e.g., forced awakening or

environmental disruption) (Hublin et al. 2001). In predisposed individuals, sleep deprivation, medications, sleep disorders, stress, and circadian misalignment may aggravate or precipitate NREM parasomnia.

Variants of confusional arousals include excessive sleep inertia ("sleep drunkenness"; Mahowald and Cramer Bornemann 2005), sleep-related abnormal sexual behavior ("sexsomnia"; Shapiro et al. 2003), and sleep-related violence (Cartwright 2004). Unlike confusional arousals, sleep drunkenness arises from final awakenings in the morning, but in other respects it is similar to confusional episodes arising from slow-wave sleep. Sleep-related abnormal sexual behavior is usually distinct from the individual's typical behavior in terms of partner or sexual act. Sleep-related violence is also generally distinct from the individual's waking behavior and occurs with anger or fear as the dominant emotion, agitated resistance to the environment, a slow return to normal levels of alertness following the event, and subsequent amnesia. The majority of cases occur in young or middle-aged males with a prior history of sleepwalking (Bonkalo 1974).

Sleepwalking also occurs within the first 1 or 2 hours of sleep without substantial affective activity, but it involves more elaborate behavior than confusional arousals. Actions are typically simple, such as attempts to use the bathroom, go to the kitchen, or leave the home. Although the sleepwalker's eyes are open, behavior is often clumsy (Crisp 1996). Dreaming is usually not present or consists of only simple mentation (e.g., "had to find my ring"). If the episode is interrupted, responses may be absent, incomplete, or inappropriate. If left alone, sleepwalkers usually return to sleep, at times in unusual places; if attempts are made to arouse them, they may take a prolonged period of time to become fully alert. Individuals may become violent or agitated if sleepwalking episodes are interrupted. As in other NREM parasomnias, full or partial amnesia is typical.

Sleepwalking occurs in 10%–20% of children and 1%–4% of adults (Ohayon et al. 1999). It is most common in children between 5 and 10 years of age and becomes less and less prevalent with increasing age. There are no gender or racial differences in prevalence. Genetic factors appear to play an important role in sleepwalking, as evidenced by epidemiological and twin studies (Hublin et al. 2001). Risk of sleepwalking roughly doubles when one parent has a positive history and triples when both parents have a history. Genetic factors account for approximately 60%–80% of the variance in sleepwalking.

Approximately 80% of adults with sleepwalking report a continuous history from childhood, although many will not come to medical attention until their 20s or 30s as a result of bed-partner concerns. The frequency of sleepwalking is quite variable, but it usually occurs infrequently—that is, once or twice a month.

The relationship between psychiatric disorders and sleepwalking is controversial (Schenck and Mahowald 2000). Although childhood sleepwalking does not appear to be associated with psychiatric disorder, a variety of psychiatric disorders may increase the risk of sleepwalking persisting into adulthood (Ohayon et al. 1999). Sleepwalking is not thought to represent latent psychopathology or the underlying "true" motivations of the sufferer (Hartman et al. 2001). Stress, sleep deprivation (Joncas et al. 2002), and chaotic sleep schedules may also increase the risk of sleepwalking.

Documentation of sleepwalking in a sleep laboratory is often difficult because of the irregular occurrence of episodes (Broughton et al. 1986). Most polysomnography studies have demonstrated an increase in brief arousals from slow-wave sleep, with preservation of a sleeping electroencephalogram accompanied by autonomic activation (increased heart rate and respiration) following the arousal (Gaudreau et al. 2000).

Polysomnography may be useful to identify precipitants to the episodes, such as OSA, periodic leg movements, or nocturnal seizures.

Sleep terrors share many features with sleepwalking but are characterized by more intense motor, autonomic, and affective activity and experience. Sleepwalking and sleep terrors may occur in the same individual. In children, sleep terrors are heralded by a piercing scream, with apparent extreme fear, crying, and inconsolability (Mahowald and Cramer Bornemann 2005). In adults, agitation is common, with the perception of an imminent threat requiring escape or defense (Schenck et al. 1997). For this reason, persons with sleep terrors may cause injury to themselves, others, or property. Dreams are usually not reported, but simple thoughts are sometimes present ("The room is on fire," or "I am being attacked") that can be difficult to dispel, even after awakening. The individual may incorporate bed partners or family members into the threatening scenario, potentially harming them. For this reason, individuals having a sleep terror should be gently redirected. Recollection of the event afterward is limited.

Sleep terrors are less common than sleepwalking, with roughly 5% of children and 1%–2% of adults reporting a history of such events (Ohayon et al. 1999). As with sleepwalking, genetic factors appear to increase susceptibility to sleep terrors, and precipitating factors can be either endogenous or exogenous. Polysomnography may not capture episodes, although multiple brief arousals from slow-wave sleep with heightened autonomic activity may be observed (Gaudreau et al. 2000).

Assessment and Diagnosis

The differential diagnosis of patients with abnormal sleep-related motor or affective behaviors includes nocturnal panic attacks, nocturnal dissociative episodes, frontal lobe seizures, delirium associated with medical or neurological disorders, and REM sleep behavior disorder. A daytime history of behaviors similar to the nocturnal behaviors (e.g., panic or dissociative episode) suggests a diagnosis other than NREM parasomnia. Similarly, overnight polysomnographic monitoring may confirm REM sleep behavior disorder or a seizure disorder.

Treatment

The decision to treat NREM parasomnias is based upon the frequency of events, risk of injury to self or others, and distress the behaviors cause the patient or family members (Schenck and Mahowald 2000). Parasomnias typically occur infrequently but unpredictably, raising the question of whether chronic treatment of episodic events is warranted.

For most children, parasomnias do not require treatment, because there is little risk of harm and the child is unaware of the events. Regulating the sleep–wake schedule and avoiding sleep deprivation can reduce the frequency of events. For sleepwalking, the sleeping environment must be made safe by locking doors and windows and keeping hallways and stairs well lit.

Treatment of sleepwalking or sleep terrors in adults involves three steps: modification of predisposing and precipitating factors; enhancing safety of the sleeping environment; and when these are not successful, pharmacotherapy. Sleep disorders, medical disorders (pain, nocturia, dyspnea), and sleep-disrupting medications should be addressed when possible. If the parasomnia occurs within the first half of the sleep period, short-acting BzRAs such as triazolam (0.125–0.25 mg hs) or zolpidem (5–10 mg hs) are recommended. Clonazepam (0.5–1.0 mg qhs) is the most commonly used BzRA for parasomnias and has been used successfully for extended periods without the development of tolerance (Schenck and Mahowald 1996). These medications may suppress arousals or decrease slow-wave sleep. However, no controlled efficacy trials have been performed for NREM parasomnias.

Sleep-Related Eating Disorder

Sleep-related eating disorder is a recently described disorder, and information regarding its description, course, prevalence, and treatment is more limited. It combines features of a sleep disorder (sleepwalking) with that of an eating disorder (binge-eating disorder) (Schenck et al. 1991; Winkelman 2006). The behavior consists of repeated partial arousals from sleep with eating in a compulsive or driven manner, although the persons may later report that they were not hungry. Preferred foods are typically high in carbohydrates. In distinction to sleepwalking, sleep-related eating disorder usually occurs every night or multiple times per night. Level of awareness varies, but recollection of events is usually incomplete, and individuals often report that they were half-awake, half-asleep during episodes. Individuals are often ashamed of the behavior, gain weight, and alter daytime food consumption in order to limit 24-hour calorie consumption.

The prevalence of this disorder is estimated at 1%–5% of adults and is two to four times more common in women. It most often begins in late adolescence or early adulthood and runs a chronic course without

treatment (Winkelman et al. 1999). Eating disorders increase the risk of sleep-related eating disorder, but only a minority of those with the disorder have anorexia, bulimia, or daytime binge-eating disorder (Schenck et al. 1993). A history of sleepwalking is also common, but once nocturnal eating becomes established, typical sleepwalking behaviors are usually not observed. RLS is also commonly observed in those with sleep-related eating disorder, and treatment of the former can eliminate the latter. BzRAs may also be associated with the disorder (Morgenthaler and Silber 2002). Roughly one-third of patients have a first-degree family member with sleep-related eating disorder as well, consistent with the familial patterns observed in both sleepwalking (Hublin et al. 2001) and daytime eating disorders.

In distinction to the other NREM parasomnias, eating episodes in sleep-related eating disorder can occur at any time of the night and from all stages of NREM sleep (Winkelman 2006). Polysomnographic features characteristic of sleepwalking, such as frequent arousals from slow-wave sleep, are commonly observed (Schenck et al. 1991). The underlying pathophysiology is unclear. Abnormalities in the expression of peptides regulating both appetite and the sleep–wake cycle have been described (Birketvedt et al. 1999), but it is unclear whether these are a cause or a consequence of the disordered eating and sleep–wake cycle.

The major differential diagnosis for sleep-related eating disorder is nocturnal eating syndrome. In the latter, the individual eats an excessive amount of food either before bed or during nocturnal awakenings while maintaining full consciousness (Schenck et al. 1993). Thus, these two diagnoses represent ends of a continuum of related nocturnal eating disorders distinguished by level of awareness.

Treatment of sleep-related eating disorder is targeted at the underlying causes of abnormal arousals and/or disordered eating. As with other NREM parasomnias, behavioral measures are essential and include ensuring the safety of the sleeping environment, avoiding sleep deprivation and irregular sleep schedules, and normalizing the daytime eating schedule. Individuals with a history of sleepwalking can be treated with short- to intermediate-acting BzRAs or other sedating medications such as trazodone. However, such medications can also aggravate the dissociated eating and amnesia. Agents that suppress or normalize eating disorders, such as SSRIs or topiramate, have been effective in some case series (Winkelman 2003). Dopamine agonists may also be useful, particularly for patients with RLS (Schenck et al. 1993).

REM-Related Parasomnias

REM Sleep Behavior Disorder

In REM sleep behavior disorder (RBD), the usual atonia of REM sleep is absent, allowing the sleeper to enact dreams that, when agitated or violent, can result in injury to the sleeper or bed partner (Mahowald and Schenck 2005). During such episodes, the sleeper has his or her eyes closed and is completely unresponsive to the environment until awakened, at which point he or she will achieve rapid and full alertness and report a dream that usually corresponds to the exhibited behavior. Fully expressed episodes of the disorder are intermittent, but talking, shouting, and fragmentary motor activity often occur between such events.

RBD is chronic and usually observed in males older than 50 years. It is strongly associated with neurological disorders characterized by accumulation of α-synuclein protein (Parkinson's disease, dementia with Lewy bodies, and multiple system atrophy) and may serve as an early marker of these disorders (Boeve et al. 2003). Up to two-thirds of patients followed for 10 years developed Parkinson's disease (Schenck et al. 1996). Although the site of pathology in RBD is not clear, dopamine transporter abnormalities in the nigrostriatal system and a reduction in peri-locus coeruleus neurons have been reported (Turner et al. 2000). More widespread CNS dysfunction is suggested by slowing of the electroencephalogram during wakefulness as well as subtle neuropsychological dysfunction (Gagnon et al. 2004). The discovery of RBD was anticipated by animal studies in which lesions around the locus coeruleus produced "REM sleep without atonia," thus implicating these brain-stem areas in the control of motor activity during REM sleep (Hendricks et al. 1981).

REM-suppressing antidepressants, including SSRIs and monoamine oxidase inhibitors, are an important risk factor for RBD (Mahowald and Schenck 2005). Acute and chronic administration of serotonergic antidepressants can produce subclinical illness, in which motor tone disinhibited during REM has been demonstrated with both acute and chronic administration of serotonergic antidepressants (Winkelman and James 2004).

The diagnosis of RBD is made by polysomnography, which demonstrates elevated muscle tone or excessive phasic muscle activity during REM sleep (American Academy of Sleep Medicine 2005). Large body movements and REM-related behaviors may also appear during the polysomnogram. Periodic limb movements of sleep may be observed during both REM and NREM sleep.

First-line treatment consists of BzRAs. The most commonly used agent is clonazepam (0.5–1.0 mg), which decreases the number and extent of pathological dream-enacting behaviors (Mahowald and Schenck 2005). Although clonazepam is generally well tolerated, its long half-life and the age of most patients with the disorder may lead to daytime sleepiness and/or cognitive impairment. In this case, shorter-acting benzodiazepines (e.g., lorazepam 1–2 mg) may be preferable. Melatonin (3–15 mg qhs) and pramipexole (0.5–1.0 mg qhs) have also been used with some success. Discontinuing medications such as antidepressants should be attempted if clinically possible. As with the NREM parasomnias, ensuring the safety of the sleeping environment for both the patient and bed partner is essential (Mahowald and Schenck 2005).

Nightmare Disorder

Nightmare disorder is characterized by recurrent distressing dreams that usually arise from REM sleep and are followed by an awakening, with full recall. The dominant emotion is usually fear, although anger, sadness, and embarrassment may also be present. Nightmares may occur at any time of night but are more common in the final third of the night when REM is most prominent (American Academy of Sleep Medicine 2005; Nielsen and Zadra 2005). In distinction to sleep terrors, return to sleep after a nightmare is usually delayed, and frequent nightmares may lead to a fear of going to sleep. Nightmares are not associated with complex acting out of dreams as in RBD.

Occasional nightmares are common in both children and adults (Nielsen and Zadra 2005). Approximately 5% of adults report frequent nightmares (Ohayon et al. 1997). The prevalence is higher in women than men. Nightmare distress is associated with psychiatric illness and psychopathology (Nielsen and Zadra 2005). Polysomnography is generally of little diagnostic value for frequent nightmares, except to rule out RBD or NREM parasomnias.

Nightmares occur in more than 50% of individuals with posttraumatic stress disorder and are a diagnostic feature of this disorder (Neylan et al. 1998). In posttraumatic stress disorder the nightmare often has a thematic or literal association with the traumatic event (Harvey et al. 2003). Such nightmares are rarely observed in the sleep laboratory but have been seen originating from both REM and NREM sleep.

Nightmare treatment includes pharmacological and behavioral/psychological approaches. Prazosin (4–12 mg qhs; Raskind et al. 2003), cyproheptadine (Gupta et al. 1998), anticonvulsants (Berlant and Van

Kammen 2002), and antipsychotic medications (Labbate and Douglas 2000) have all been efficacious in placebo-controlled trials and/or uncontrolled case series. Imagery rehearsal, in which new versions (with better outcomes) of nightmares are rehearsed during the day, has demonstrated consistent benefit for trauma-related and non-trauma-related nightmares (Krakow et al. 2001).

Sleep-Related Movement Disorders: Restless Legs Syndrome and Periodic Limb Movement Disorder

Although a variety of sleep-related movement disorders are seen in clinical practices, including sleep-related bruxism and rhythmic movement disorder, the most prevalent and clinically significant is RLS. Because this disorder is frequently accompanied by PLMD, the two are described together.

Definition and Description

RLS is a sensory-motor disorder characterized by an urge to move the legs, accompanied by uncomfortable or unpleasant sensations (Allen et al. 2003; Montplaisir et al. 2005; Walters 1995). The restlessness and dysesthesias of RLS are variously described as "achy," "creepy-crawly," "electric," "like a coiled spring," "something running down my veins," "itchy," and "painful." The urge to move and unpleasant leg sensations worsen during periods of rest or inactivity such as lying, sitting, and attempting to sleep. Symptoms are temporarily relieved by movement, such as walking or stretching. Persons with RLS often move excessively in bed or interrupt activities requiring immobility in order to relieve the sensations. Such movement has both voluntary and involuntary aspects. The movement is described as irrepressible but can be delayed or avoided by distraction. While the person is asleep, characteristic periodic movements of the legs appear, with a distinctive pattern and distribution. Finally, the urge to move or unpleasant sensations are typically worse, or occur exclusively, in the evening or night between 8 P.M. and 4 A.M. RLS symptoms demonstrate a true circadian rhythm, in phase with body temperature and melatonin rhythms (Michaud et al. 2004).

The majority of individuals with RLS have symptoms infrequently (up to four times per month), but approximately 25% describe daily or near-daily symptoms. RLS is strongly associated with sleep-onset and sleep-maintenance insomnia. Due to the circadian rhythm of RLS symptoms, some patients adopt atypical sleep–wake schedules. Despite the sleep disruption caused by RLS, excessive daytime sleepiness is not typical, and the ability to nap is often impaired by RLS symptoms.

Approximately 80% of RLS patients have periodic limb movements of sleep (PLMS), which are brief (0.5–5.0 seconds) repetitive, stereotyped movements of the foot and leg appearing at roughly 20-second intervals (Montplaisir et al. 2005; Figure 22–12). The magnitude of these movements may vary from barely discernible to very large. They can be associated with arousal from sleep and elevated heart rate and blood pressure (Winkelman 1999). More than 5 such movements with arousal per hour of sleep is considered abnormal; RLS patients frequently have more than 40 per hour. However, given the high prevalence of PLMS in the general population, polysomnographic findings are not specific for PLMS (Montplaisir et al. 2005). Involuntary periodic leg movements can also be observed during periods of immobility in wakefulness.

Epidemiology and Consequences

The prevalence of RLS is approximately 3%–5% in adult populations of northern European descent, rising roughly linearly with age to 10% of those older than 65 years (Montplaisir et al. 2005; Ohayon and Roth 2002). Prevalence rates appear to be lower in other ethnic groups and are approximately 50% higher in women than men. RLS is more common in individuals with medical disorders including end-stage renal disease (15%–30%; Unruh et al. 2004; Winkelman et al. 1996), iron deficiency anemia (Berger et al. 2002), and rheumatoid arthritis (Reynolds et al. 1986). It is also common in pregnant women, affecting up to 33% of those in the third trimester (Suzuki et al. 2003). RLS is associated with impaired quality of life (Hening et al. 2004) and with a substantial risk of depression, even when controlling for confounding disorders (Ulfberg et al. 2001).

The onset of RLS can occur at any age: 10%–20% of patients reported onset before the age of 10 years and 40% by the age of 20 years (Montplaisir et al. 2005). Early onset is associated with a family history of RLS (Winkelmann et al. 2000), whereas late-onset RLS suggests secondary causes. The longitudinal course of RLS is not well defined, although it has been traditionally thought that the severity progresses over time.

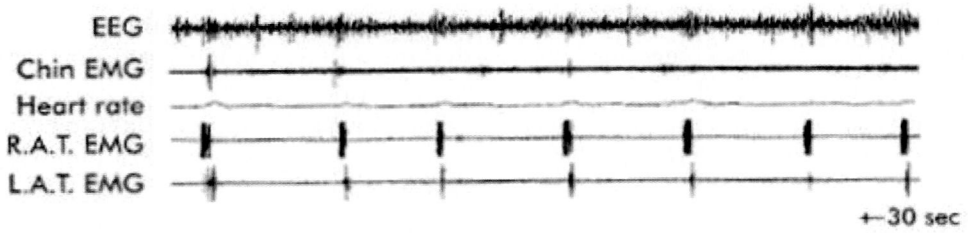

FIGURE 22–12.   Polysomnographic recording of periodic limb movements of sleep.

EEG=electroencephalogram; EMG=electromyogram; R.A.T.=right anterior tibialis; L.A.T.=left anterior tibialis.

Source.   Reprinted from Czeisler CA, Winkelman JW, Richardson GS: "Sleep Disorders," in *Harrison's Principles of Internal Medicine,* 16th Edition. Edited by Kasper DL, Braunwald E, Fauci A, et al. New York, McGraw-Hill Professional, 2004, pp. 153–162. Copyright 2004, The McGraw-Hill Co. Used with permission.

Pathophysiology

Approximately 30%–50% of individuals with RLS report an affected first-degree family member (Winkelmann et al. 2000). In two recent genomewide association studies, three distinct sequence variants were identified in patients with RLS (Stefansson et al. 2007; Winkelmann et al. 2007). The variant found in both of the studies—a sequence variant in an intron on chromosome 6p—predicted the presence of both PLMS and iron deficiency in patients with RLS and their families. Significant linkages to chromosomes 14q, 12q, and 9p have also been reported (Montplaisir et al. 2005).

Several lines of evidence suggest a role for abnormal CNS iron transport and/or utilization in RLS. The prevalence of iron deficiency is increased in RLS, and iron repletion can relieve RLS (O'Keeffe et al. 1994). Likewise, reductions in cerebrospinal fluid ferritin (the protein storage form of iron) have been observed, even when serum iron is normal (Connor et al. 2003). Iron is also required for dopamine synthesis and dopamine receptor regulation (Allen 2004). Successful treatment of RLS with dopaminergic precursors and agonists has also focused attention on the dopaminergic system. However, studies examining dopamine system structure and function have yielded inconsistent findings, including D_2 dopamine receptor density, response to dopaminergic antagonists, and physiological responses to L-dopa challenge at different times of day (Montplaisir et al. 2005). The A11 dopaminergic system, which originates in the thalamus and descends to the spinal cord, may also be relevant to RLS, as suggested by abnormal responses to tibial nerve stimulation (Bara-Jimenez et al. 2000) and the presence of PLMS in patients with cord transections (de Mello et al. 1996).

Assessment and Diagnosis

RLS is a clinical diagnosis based on the presence of consistent symptoms. Physical examination yields no specific findings for idiopathic RLS, but individuals with comorbid disorders (e.g., end-stage renal disease) will have findings consistent with that disorder. Polysomnography may be useful to rule out other sleep disorders, including sleep apnea, and for documenting the presence and severity of PLMS. The dysesthesias of RLS are often difficult to distinguish from those of peripheral neuropathies (e.g., diabetes, toxic, idiopathic), particularly when RLS is described as "painful." Given the age distribution of neuropathies and RLS, these two disorders commonly co-occur. Furthermore, painful peripheral neuropathy, like RLS, often worsens at night. However, neuropathic symptoms generally do not improve with movement. Nocturnal leg cramps, which do occur at night and do improve with movement, may also be difficult to distinguish from RLS. However, leg cramps arise precipitously from sleep and are not associated with feelings of motor restlessness.

The distinction between RLS and akathisia related to antipsychotic or serotonergic antidepressant drugs can be difficult. It is particularly difficult to determine whether symptoms represent akathisia or medication-related RLS. Both are clinical diagnoses, and both may produce periodic leg movements of sleep. A history of RLS prior to antidepressant administration, the presence of a sensory component, nocturnal worsening of symptoms, and a therapeutic response to dopaminergic agonists all suggest a diagnosis of RLS. Anxiety associated with bedtime and sleep onset can also manifest with "an inability to get comfortable," restlessness, and vague sensory complaints. However, the lack of localization to the legs, the strict localization of the experience to the bed, and the anxiety regarding sleeplessness all suggest anxiety rather than RLS.

Treatment

Patients should first be evaluated and treated for reversible causes of RLS, such as iron deficiency, antidepressant use, or opiate withdrawal (Montplaisir et al. 2005; Silber et al. 2004). If underlying causes cannot be identified or modified, treatment of primary and secondary RLS is nearly identical. Behavioral measures include avoidance of caffeine, alcohol, and sleep deprivation. Individuals with RLS should also avoid unnecessary immobility. In addition, individuals with RLS are encouraged to aim for 80%–90% (rather than 100%) control of symptoms outside of the sleep setting, which will also limit the dosage and duration of treatment. In individuals with intermittent symptoms, medications may be used on an as-needed basis.

Dopaminergic agents are considered first-line treatments for RLS (Montplaisir et al. 2005; Silber et al. 2004). L-dopa, the first dopaminergic agent used for RLS, can dramatically improve RLS symptoms and sleep latency (Trenkwalder et al. 1995). Its short duration of action is often associated with "rebound" RLS symptoms several hours later, which can be mitigated with use of longer-acting preparations (Collado-Seidel et al. 1999). Although extremely effective, two additional problems are often seen with L-dopa: augmentation and tolerance. *Augmentation,* the appearance of RLS symptoms progressively earlier during the day, is observed in roughly two-thirds of individuals treated with L-dopa (Allen and Earley 1996). Treatment with additional doses of the drug earlier in the day only exacerbates this problem and may lead to severe symptoms throughout the day. Other manifestations of augmentation include extension of RLS symptoms to other body parts and shorter duration of treatment effectiveness after a dose. *Tolerance* to L-dopa is manifested by reduced effectiveness of the medication over time (Allen and Earley 1996).

The long-acting dopamine receptor agonists pramipexole and ropinirole are now considered first-line therapy for RLS and are approved by the U.S. Food and Drug Administration for this indication. The binding profiles of these dopaminergic agonists to dopamine receptor subtypes (D_1–D_5) remain in dispute, but it appears that pramipexole has a higher affinity for the D_3 receptor than ropinirole (Piercey 1998). The importance of this distinction for the treatment of RLS is unclear, although D_3 receptors in the limbic system may be relevant to the psychiatric effects of these medications (Goldberg et al. 2004).

The efficacy of both pramipexole and ropinirole in RLS have been demonstrated in numerous double-blind, placebo-controlled trials with durations ranging from 3 to 12 weeks (Trenkwalder et al. 2004; Winkelman et al. 2006). Both agents dramatically reduce the number of periodic leg movements in sleep and improve subjective sleep quality. Long-term placebo-controlled trials of these agents have not been performed. However, longitudinal naturalistic studies suggest that one-third of patients develop augmentation (i.e., the appearance of RLS symptoms progressively earlier during the day) after 8–12 months on dopaminergic agents (Winkelman and Johnston 2004). Augmentation developing with dopamine agonists can usually be managed by earlier dosing of medication, unlike the case for the severe augmentation observed with L-dopa. No randomized studies have examined the comparative efficacy of different dopaminergic agents. The ergot-derived dopaminergic agonist pergolide is avoided for use in RLS due to its potential to produce cardiac valve regurgitation (Zanettini et al. 2007).

Most individuals with RLS obtain substantial relief with dopaminergic therapies, but for more severely afflicted individuals, adjunctive treatment may be required. Second-line agents for RLS include short-acting opiates such as oxycodone and codeine. In severely affected individuals who report refractory distressing symptoms throughout the day, sustained-release forms of oxycodone, morphine, or methadone may be necessary. Caution is warranted when prescribing opiates, given their potential for abuse and respiratory suppression.

Anticonvulsants are also considered second-line agents for RLS and may be used as adjuncts to dopaminergic agonists or as alternatives for patients who cannot tolerate these drugs or have contraindications to these drugs. Controlled trials have demonstrated efficacy for both gabapentin (Garcia-Borreguero et al. 2002) and carbamazepine (Telstad et al. 1984) compared with placebo. Although gabapentin is not as effective as dopaminergic agonists in reducing periodic limb movements, it is sometimes used as an adjunctive treatment for its sedative effect.

Dopaminergic agonists are extremely effective for the sensory and motor symptoms of RLS, but clinical trials have demonstrated only modest improvements in polysomnographically recorded sleep efficiency. Short- to intermediate-acting benzodiazepines can treat mild RLS and persistent sleep disturbance (Silber et al. 2004). Approximately 33%–60% of patients taking pramipexole for RLS also take hypnotics such as benzodiazepines, sedating antidepressants, or anticonvulsants to assist with sleep (Winkelman and Johnston 2004).

Conclusion

Sleep and wakefulness are fundamental neurobiological states that promote physical and mental health and functioning. Sleep disturbances are commonly seen in patients with psychiatric disorders. Conversely, psychiatric symptoms and disorders are common among patients with sleep disorders. Sleep disorders represent a heterogeneous group of conditions characterized by dysfunction in neurobiological and systemic physiological systems. Major categories of sleep disorders include insomnias, sleep-related breathing disorders, hypersomnias, circadian rhythm sleep disorders, parasomnias, and sleep-related movement disorders. Evaluation of sleep disorders rests on an accurate history of sleep and wake symptoms, comorbid psychiatric and medical conditions, and medication and substance use in some cases supplemented by polysomnographic (PSG) sleep studies and other specialized techniques. Treatments of sleep disorders vary considerably among the specific categories of disorders, and may include psychological and behavioral interventions, medications, somatic treatments, and surgery. Mental health practitioners are well positioned to contribute to the evaluation and management of sleep disorder patients within the multidisciplinary field of sleep medicine.

Key Points

- Human sleep is regulated physiologically by the interaction of homeostatic sleep drive and the circadian timing system. Dysregulation of these factors can contribute to insomnia, hypersomnia, and circadian rhythm sleep disorders. Behavioral treatments of sleep disorders work in part by reinforcing the activity of these regulatory processes.

- Insomnia is a complaint of poor sleep and impaired daytime function in an individual with adequate sleep opportunity. Efficacy has been well demonstrated for behavioral treatments and BzRAs.

- OSA should be suspected in overweight patients with daytime sleepiness, loud snoring, and neurocognitive symptoms including depression. Continuous positive pressure applied via nasal mask is an efficacious first-line treatment.

- Narcolepsy, a disorder characterized by extreme sleepiness, cataplexy, and sleep-related hallucinations and paralysis, is caused by dysfunction of hypocretin-containing neurons in the hypothalamus. Treatment includes stimulants for improving daytime sleepiness and agents such as antidepressants or sodium oxybate to control cataplexy.

- CRSDs result from misalignment of the individual's circadian timing system with the light–dark cycle of the work, social, or physical environment. Behavioral interventions, appropriately timed exposure to light and darkness, and exogenous melatonin may all improve circadian alignment.

- RLS is characterized by unpleasant feelings in the legs and an urge to move, which are temporarily relieved by movement. Efficacious treatments include dopamine receptor agonists, BzRAs, antiepileptic drugs, and opiate analgesics.

- Parasomnias are abnormal behavioral or affective events that occur in association with sleep or arousals from sleep. Distinctive clinical features characterize those occurring in association with NREM sleep and those occurring in association with REM sleep.

Suggested Readings

American Academy of Sleep Medicine: The International Classification of Sleep Disorders, 2nd Edition (ICSD-2): Diagnostic and Coding Manual. Westchester, IL, American Academy of Sleep Medicine, 2005

Buysse DJ (ed): Sleep Disorders and Psychiatry (Review of Psychiatry Series Vol 24, No 1. Oldham JM, Riba MB, series eds). Washington, DC, American Psychiatric Publishing, 2005

Chokroverty S: Sleep Disorders Medicine, 3rd Edition. Boston, MA, Butterworth Heinemann, 2007

Kryger MH, Roth T, Dement W (eds): Principles and Practice of Sleep Medicine, 4th Edition. Philadelphia, PA, Elsevier, 2005

Sheldon SH, Kryger MH, Ferber R: Principles and Practice of Pediatric Sleep Medicine. Philadelphia, PA, Elsevier, 2005

Online Resources

American Academy of Sleep Medicine: http://aasmnet.org

National Center on Sleep Disorders Research: http://www.nhlbi.nih.gov/about/ncsdr/index.htm

National Sleep Foundation: http://www.sleepfoundation.org

Sleep Research Society: http://www.sleepresearchsociety.org

References

Akerstedt T: Shift work and disturbed sleep/wakefulness. Occup Med 53:88–94, 2003

Allen R: Dopamine and iron in the pathophysiology of restless legs syndrome (RLS). Sleep Med 5:385–391, 2004

Allen R, Earley CJ: Augmentation of the restless legs syndrome with carbidopa/levodopa. Sleep 19:205–213, 1996

Allen R, Picchietti D, Hening WA, et al: Restless legs syndrome: diagnostic criteria, special considerations, and epidemiology: a report from the restless legs syndrome diagnosis and epidemiology workshop at the National Institutes of Health. Sleep Med 4:101–119, 2003

American Academy of Sleep Medicine: The International Classification of Sleep Disorders, 2nd Edition (ICSD-2): Diagnostic and Coding Manual. Westchester, IL, American Academy of Sleep Medicine, 2005

American Psychiatric Association: Diagnostic and Statistical Manual of Mental Disorders, 4th Edition, Text Revision. Washington, DC, American Psychiatric Association, 2000

Ancoli-Israel S, Klauber MR, Stepnowsky C, et al: Sleep-disordered breathing in African-American elderly. Am J Respir Crit Care Med 152:1946–1949, 1995

Ancoli-Israel S, Schnierow B, Kelsoe J, et al: A pedigree of one family with delayed sleep phase syndrome. Chronobiol Int 18:831–840, 2001

Ancoli-Israel S, Martin JL, Kripke DF, et al: Effect of light treatment on sleep and circadian rhythms in demented nursing patients. J Am Geriatr Soc 50:282–289, 2002

Aoki H, Ozeki Y, Yamada N: Hypersensitivity of melatonin suppression in response to light in patients with delayed sleep phase syndrome. Chronobiol Int 18:263–271, 2001

Archer SN, Robilliard DL, Skene DJ, et al: A length polymorphism in the circadian clock gene Per3 is linked to delayed sleep phase syndrome and extreme diurnal preference. Sleep 26:413–415, 2003

Asnis GM, Chakraburtty A, DuBoff EA, et al: Zolpidem for persistent insomnia in SSRI-treated depressed patients. J Clin Psychiatry 60:668–676, 1999

Babkoff H, French J, Whitmore J, et al: Single-dose bright light and/or caffeine effect on nocturnal performance. Aviat Space Environ Med 73:341–350, 2002

Bady E, Achkar A, Pascal S, et al: Pulmonary arterial hypertension in patients with sleep apnea syndrome. Thorax 55:934–939, 2000

Bamford CR: Menstrual-associated sleep disorder: an unusual hypersomniac variant associated with both menstruation and amenorrhea with a possible link to prolactin and metoclopramide. Sleep 16:484–486, 1993

Bara-Jimenez W, Aksu M, Graham B, et al: Periodic limb movements in sleep: state-dependent excitability of the spinal flexor reflex. Neurology 54:1609–1616, 2000

Bardwell WA, Moore P, Ancoli-Israel S, et al: Fatigue in obstructive sleep apnea: driven by depressive symptoms instead of apnea severity? Am J Psychiatry 160:350–355, 2003

Bassetti C, Pelayo R, Guilleminault C: Idiopathic hypersomnia, in Principles and Practices of Sleep Medicine, 4th Edition. Edited by Kryger MH, Roth T, Dement WC. Philadelphia, PA, Elsevier, 2005, pp 791–800

Bateson AN: The benzodiazepine site of the $GABA_A$ receptor: an old target with new potential? Sleep Med 5 (suppl 1):S9–S15, 2004

Beaumont M, Batejat D, Pierard C, et al: Caffeine or melatonin effects on sleep and sleepiness after rapid eastward transmeridian travel. J Appl Physiol 96:50–58, 2004

Beebe DW, Groesz L, Wells C, et al: The neuropsychological effects of obstructive sleep apnea: a meta-analysis of norm-referenced and case-controlled data. Sleep 26:298–307, 2003

Belenky G, Wesensten NJ, Thorne DR, et al: Patterns of performance degradation and restoration during sleep restriction and subsequent recovery: a sleep dose-response study. J Sleep Res 12:1–12, 2003

Bellingham J, Foster RG: Opsins and mammalian photoentrainment. Cell Tissue Res 309:57–71, 2002

Berger K, von Eckardstein A, Trenkwalder C, et al: Iron metabolism and the risk of restless legs syndrome in an elderly general population: the MEMO-Study. J Neurol 249:1195–1199, 2002

Berlant J, Van Kammen DP: Open-label topiramate as primary or adjunctive therapy in chronic civilian posttraumatic stress disorder: a preliminary report. J Clin Psychiatry 63:15–20, 2002

Billiard M, Guilleminault C, Dement WC: A menstruation-linked periodic hypersomnia: Kleine-Levin syndrome or new clinical entity? Neurology 25:436–443, 1975

Birketvedt GS, Florholmen J, Sundsfjord J, et al: Behavioral and neuroendocrine characteristics of the night-eating syndrome. JAMA 282:657–663, 1999

Bixler EO, Vgontzas AN, Lin HM, et al: Prevalence of sleep-disordered breathing in women: effects of gender. Am J Respir Crit Care Med 163:608–613, 2001

Blumen MB, Dahan S, Fleury B, et al: Radiofrequency ablation for the treatment of mild to moderate obstructive sleep apnea. Laryngoscope 112:2086–2092, 2002

Boeve BF, Silber MH, Parisi JE, et al: Synucleinopathy pathology and REM sleep behavior disorder plus dementia or parkinsonism. Neurology 61:40–45, 2003

Boivin DB, James FO: Circadian adaptation to night-shift work by judicious light and darkness exposure. J Biol Rhythms 17:556–567, 2002

Bonkalo A: Impulsive acts and confusional states during incomplete arousal from sleep: criminological and forensic implications. Psychiatr Q 48:400–409, 1974

Boulos Z, Campbell SS, Lewy AJ, et al: Light treatment for sleep disorders, consensus report, VII: jet lag. J Biol Rhythms 10:167–176, 1995

Breslau N, Roth T, Rosenthal L, et al: Sleep disturbance and psychiatric disorders: a longitudinal epidemiological study of young adults. Biol Psychiatry 39:411–418, 1996

Bridgman SA, Dunn KM: Surgery for obstructive sleep apnea. Cochrane Database Syst Rev (2):CD001004, 2000

Broughton R, Valley V, Aguirre M, et al: Excessive daytime sleepiness and the pathophysiology of narcolepsy-cataplexy: a laboratory perspective. Sleep 9:205–215, 1986

Brzezinski A, Vangel MG, Wurtman RJ, et al: Effects of exogenous melatonin on sleep: a meta-analysis. Sleep Med Rev 9:41–50, 2005

Burgess HJ, Sharkey KM, Eastman CI: Bright light, dark and melatonin can promote circadian adaptation in night shift workers. Sleep Med Rev 6:407–420, 2002

Burgess HJ, Crowley SJ, Gazda CJ, et al: Preflight adjustment to eastward travel: 3 days of advancing sleep with and without morning bright light. J Biol Rhythms 18:318–328, 2003

Buysse DJ (ed): Sleep Disorders and Psychiatry (Review of Psychiatry Series Vol 24, No 1. Oldham JM, Riba MB, series eds). Washington, DC, American Psychiatric Publishing, 2005

Buysse DJ, Reynolds CF, Monk TH, et al: The Pittsburgh Sleep Quality Index: a new instrument for psychiatric practice and research. Psychiatry Res 28:193–213, 1989

Buysse D, Bate G, Kirkpatrick P: Fresh from the pipeline: Ramelteon. Nat Rev Drug Discov 4:881–882, 2005a

Buysse DJ, Schweitzer PK, Moul DE: Clinical pharmacology of other drugs used as hypnotics, in Principles and Practices of Sleep Medicine, 4th Edition. Edited by Kryger MH, Roth T, Dement WC. Philadelphia, PA, Elsevier, 2005b, pp 452–467

Cajochen C, Kräuchi K, Wirz-Justice A: Role of melatonin in the regulation of human circadian rhythms and sleep. J Neuroendocrinol 15:432–437, 2003

Camacho ME, Morin CM: The effect of temazepam on respiration in elderly insomniacs with mild sleep apnea. Sleep 18:644–645, 1995

Carskadon MA, Rechtschaffen A: Monitoring and staging human sleep, in Principles and Practice of Sleep Medicine, 4th Edition. Edited by Kryger MH, Roth T, Dement WC. Philadelphia, PA, Elsevier, 2005, pp 1359–1377

Cartwright R: Sleepwalking violence: a sleep disorder, a legal dilemma, and a psychological challenge. Am J Psychiatry 161:1149–1158, 2004

Chemelli RM, Willie JT, Sinton CM, et al: Narcolepsy in orexin knockout mice: molecular genetics of sleep regulation. Cell 98:437–451, 1999

Chesson AL, Ferber RA, Fry JM, et al: The indications for polysomnography and related procedures. Sleep 20:423–487, 1997

Chesson AL, Littner M, Davila D, et al: Practice parameters for the use of light therapy in the treatment of sleep disorders. Standards of Practice Committee, American Academy of Sleep Medicine. Sleep 22:641–660, 1999

Chokroverty S: Sleep Disorders Medicine, 2nd Edition. Boston, MA, Butterworth Heinemann, 1999

Collado-Seidel V, Kazenwadel J, Wetter TC, et al: A controlled study of additional sustained-release L-dopa in L-dopa-responsive restless legs syndrome with late-night symptoms. Neurology 52:285–290, 1999

Connor JR, Boyer PJ, Menzies SL, et al: Neuropathological examination suggests impaired brain iron acquisition in restless legs syndrome. Neurology 61:304–309, 2003

Crisp AH: The sleepwalking/night terrors syndrome in adults. Postgrad Med J 72:599–604, 1996

Critchley M: The syndrome of hypersomnia and periodical megaphagia in the adult male (Kleine-Levin): what is its natural course? Rev Neurol (Paris) 116:647–650, 1967

Crowley SJ, Lee C, Tseng CY, et al: Combinations of bright light, scheduled dark, sunglasses, and melatonin to facilitate circadian entrainment to night shift work. J Biol Rhythms 18:513–523, 2003

Cumming RG, Le Couteur DG: Benzodiazepines and risk of hip fractures in older people: a review of the evidence. CNS Drugs 17:825–837, 2003

Czeisler CA, Shanahan TL, Klerman EB, et al: Suppression of melatonin secretion in some blind patients by exposure to bright light. N Engl J Med 332:6–11, 1995

Czeisler CA, Duffy JF, Shanahan TL, et al: Stability, precision, and near-24-hour period of the human circadian pacemaker. Science 284:2177–2181, 1999

Czeisler CA, Buxton OM, Sinngh Khasla SB: Human circadian timing system and sleep–wake regulation, in Principles and Practices in Sleep Medicine, 4th Edition. Edited by Kryger MH, Roth T, Dement WC. Philadelphia, PA, Elsevier, 2005, pp 375–394

Dagan Y: Circadian rhythm sleep disorders (CRSD). Sleep Med Rev 6:45–54, 2002

Dahlitz M, Alvarez B, Vignau J, et al: Delayed sleep phase syndrome response to melatonin. Lancet 337:1121–1124, 1991

Danoff SK, Grasso ME, Terry PB, et al: Pleuropulmonary disease due to pergolide use for restless legs syndrome. Chest 120:313–316, 2001

de Mello MT, Lauro FA, Silva AC, et al: Incidence of periodic leg movements and of the restless legs syndrome during sleep following acute physical activity in spinal cord injury subjects. Spinal Cord 34:294–296, 1996

Duffy JF, Czeisler CA: Age-related change in the relationship between circadian period, circadian phase, and diurnal preference in humans. Neurosci Lett 318:117–120, 2002

Dumont M, Benhaberou-Brun D, Paquet J: Profile of 24-h light exposure and circadian phase of melatonin secretion in night workers. J Biol Rhythms 16:502–511, 2001

Edinger JD, Sampson WS: A primary care "friendly" cognitive behavior insomnia therapy. Sleep 26:177–182, 2003

Engleman HM, Douglas NJ: Sleep, 4: sleepiness, cognitive function, and quality of life in obstructive sleep apnea/hypopnea syndrome. Thorax 59:618–622, 2004

Erman M, Seiden D, Zammit G, et al: An efficacy, safety, and dose-response study of Ramelteon in patients with chronic primary insomnia. Sleep Med 7:17–24, 2006

Espie CA, Inglis SJ, Tessier S: The clinical effectiveness of cognitive behaviour therapy for chronic insomnia: implementation and evaluation of a sleep clinic in general medical practice. Behav Res Ther 39:60, 2001

Farney RJ, Lugo A, Jensen RL, et al: Simultaneous use of antidepressant and antihypertensive medications increases likelihood of diagnosis of obstructive sleep apnea syndrome. Chest, 125:1279–1285, 2004

Fava M, McCall WV, Krystal A, et al: Eszopiclone co-administered with fluoxetine in patients with insomnia coexisting with major depressive disorder. Biol Psychiatry 59:1052–1060, 2006

Foley DJ, Monjan A, Simonsick EM, et al: Incidence and remission of insomnia among elderly adults: an epidemiologic study of 6,800 persons over three years. Sleep 22:S366–S372, 1999

Fredrikson S, Carlander B, Billiard M, et al: CSF immune variables in patients with narcolepsy. Acta Neurol Scand 81:253–254, 1990

Fritsch KM, Iseli A, Russi EW, et al: Side effects of mandibular advancement devices for sleep apnea treatment. Am J Respir Crit Care Med 164:813–818, 2001

Gagnon JF, Fantini ML, Bedard MA, et al: Association between waking EEG slowing and REM sleep behavior disorder in PD without dementia. Neurology 62:401–406, 2004

Garcia-Borreguero D, Larrosa O, de la Llave Y, et al: Treatment of restless legs syndrome with gabapentin: a double-blind, cross-over study. Neurology 59:1573–1579, 2002

Gaudreau H, Joncas S, Zadra A, et al: Dynamics of slow-wave activity during the NREM sleep of sleepwalkers and control subjects. Sleep 23:755–760, 2000

Gelb M, Guilleminault C, Kraemer H, et al: Stability of cataplexy over several months: information for the design of therapeutic trials. Sleep 17:265–273, 1994

George CFP: Neuromuscular disorders, in Principles and Practice of Sleep Medicine, 3rd Edition. Edited by Kryger MH, Roth T, Dement WC. Philadelphia, PA, WB Saunders, 2000, pp 1087–1092

Germain A, Moul DE, Franzen PL, et al: Effects of a brief behavioral treatment for late-life insomnia: preliminary findings. J Clin Sleep Med 2:403–406, 2006

Gibbs JW, III, Ciafaloni E, Radtke RA: Excessive daytime somnolence and increased rapid eye movement pressure in myotonic dystrophy. Sleep 25:662–665, 2002

Gleeson K, Zwillich CW, White DP: The influence of increasing ventilatory effort on arousal from sleep. Am Rev Respir Dis 142:295–300, 1990

Goldberg JF, Burdick KE, Endick CJ: Preliminary randomized, double-blind, placebo-controlled trial of pramipexole added to mood stabilizers for treatment-resistant bipolar depression. Am J Psychiatry 161:564–566, 2004

Gotsopoulos H, Kelly JJ, Cistulli PA: Oral appliance therapy reduces blood pressure in obstructive sleep apnea: a randomized, controlled trial. Sleep 27:934–941, 2004

Gottlieb DJ, Whitney CW, Bonekat WH, et al: Relation of sleepiness to respiratory disturbance index: the Sleep Heart Health Study. Am J Respir Crit Care Med 159:502–507, 1999

Griffiths RR, Weerts EM: Benzodiazepine self-administration in humans and laboratory animals: implications for problems of long-term use and abuse. Psychopharmacology 134:1–37, 1997

Grunstein R: Continuous positive airway pressure treatment for obstructive sleep apnea-hypopnea syndrome, in Principles and Practices of Sleep Medicine, 4th Edition. Edited by Kryger MH, Roth T, Dement WC. Philadelphia, PA, Elsevier, 2005, pp 1066–1080

Guilleminault C, Fromherz S: Narcolepsy: diagnosis and management, in Principles and Practices of Sleep Medicine, 4th Edition. Edited by Kryger MH, Roth T, Dement WC. Philadelphia, PA, Elsevier, 2005, pp 780–790

Guilleminault C, Palombini L, Poyares D, et al: Chronic insomnia, premenopausal women and sleep disordered breathing: part 1. J Psychosom Res 53:611–615, 2002a

Guilleminault C, Palombini L, Poyares D, et al: Chronic insomnia, premenopausal women and sleep disordered breathing: part 2. J Psychosom Res 53:617–623, 2002b

Gupta S, Popli A, Bathurst E, et al: Efficacy of cyproheptadine for nightmares associated with posttraumatic stress disorder. Compr Psychiatry 39:160–164, 1998

Harrison Y, Horne JA: The impact of sleep deprivation on decision making: a review. J Exp Psychol Appl 6:236–249, 2000

Hartman D, Crisp AH, Sedgwick P: Is there a dissociative process in sleepwalking and night terrors? Postgrad Med J 77:244–249, 2001

Harvey AG: A cognitive model of insomnia. Behav Res Ther 40:869–893, 2002

Harvey AG, Jones C, Schmidt DA: Sleep and posttraumatic stress disorder: a review. Clin Psychol Rev 23:377–407, 2003

Hasler G, Buysse DJ, Klaghofer R, et al: The association between short sleep duration and obesity in young adults: a 13-year prospective study. Sleep 27:661–666, 2004

Hendricks JC, Morrison AR, Farnbach GL, et al: A disorder of rapid eye movement sleep in a cat. J Am Vet Med Assoc 178:55–57, 1981

Hening W, Walters AS, Allen RP, et al: Impact, diagnosis and treatment of restless legs syndrome (RLS) in a primary care population: the REST (RLS epidemiology, symptoms, and treatment) primary care study. Sleep Med 5:237–246, 2004

Herxheimer A, Petrie KJ: Melatonin for the prevention and treatment of jet lag. Cochrane Database Syst Rev CD001520, 2002

Herxheimer A, Waterhouse J: The prevention and treatment of jet lag. BMJ 326:296–297, 2003

Hohagen F, Kappler C, Schramm E, et al: Sleep onset insomnia, sleep maintaining insomnia and insomnia with early morning awakening: temporal stability of subtypes in a longitudinal study on general practice attenders. Sleep 17:551–554, 1994

Hohjoh H, Takasu M, Shishikura K, et al: Significant association of the arylalkylamine N-acetyltransferase (AA-NAT) gene with delayed sleep phase syndrome. Neurogenetics 4:151–153, 2003

Holbrook AM, Crowther R, Lotter A, et al: Meta-analysis of benzodiazepine use in the treatment of insomnia. Can Med Assoc J 162:225–233, 2000

Honda Y: Clinical features of narcolepsy: Japanese experiences, in HLA in Narcolepsy. Edited by Honda Y, Juti T. Berlin, Germany, Springer-Verlag, 1988, pp 24–57

Hoogendijk WJ, Van Someren EJ, Mirmiran M, et al: Circadian rhythm-related behavioral disturbances and structural hypothalamic changes in Alzheimer's disease. Int Psychogeriatr 8 (suppl):245–252, 1996

Hublin C, Kaprio J, Partinen M, et al: Parasomnias: co-occurrence and genetics. Psychiatr Genet 11:65–70, 2001

Ip MS, Lam KS, Ho C, et al: Serum leptin and vascular risk factors in obstructive sleep apnea. Chest 118:580–586, 2000

Irwin MR, Cole JC, Nicassio PM: Comparative meta-analysis of behavioral interventions for insomnia and their efficacy in middle-aged adults and in older adults 55+ years of age. Health Psychol 25:3–14, 2006

Jamieson AO, Zammit GK, Rosenberg RS, et al: Zolpidem reduces the sleep disturbance of jet lag. Sleep Med 2:423–430, 2001

Johns MW: A new method for measuring daytime sleepiness: the Epworth Sleepiness Scale. Sleep 14:540–545, 1991

Joncas S, Zadra A, Paquet J, et al: The value of sleep deprivation as a diagnostic tool in adult sleepwalkers. Neurology 58:936–940, 2002

Jones CR, Campbell SS, Zone SE, et al: Familial advanced sleep-phase syndrome: a short-period circadian rhythm variant in humans. Nat Med 5:1062–1065, 1999

Kamei Y, Urata J, Uchiyaya M, et al: Clinical characteristics of circadian rhythm sleep disorders. Psychiatry Clin Neurosci 52:234–235, 1998

Katz DA, McHorney CA: Clinical correlates of insomnia in patients with chronic illness. Arch Intern Med 158:1099–1107, 1998

King DP, Takahashi JS: Molecular genetics of circadian rhythms in mammals. Annu Rev Neurosci 23:713–742, 2000

Knauth P, Landau K, Droge C, et al: Duration of sleep depending on the type of shift work. Int Arch Occup Environ Health 46:167–177, 1980

Krakow B, Hollifield M, Johnston L, et al: Imagery rehearsal therapy for chronic nightmares in sexual assault survivors with posttraumatic stress disorder: a randomized controlled trial. JAMA 286:537–545, 2001

Kripke DF, Garfinkel L, Wingard DL, et al: Mortality associated with sleep duration and insomnia. Arch Gen Psychiatry 59:131–136, 2002

Kryger MH, Roth T, Dement WC: Principles and Practice of Sleep Medicine, 4th Edition. Philadelphia, PA, Elsevier, 2005

Krystal AD, Walsh JK, Laska E, et al: Sustained efficacy of eszopiclone over 6 months of nightly treatment: results of a randomized, double-blind, placebo-controlled study in adults with chronic insomnia. Sleep 26:793–799, 2003

Labbate LA, Douglas S: Olanzapine for nightmares and sleep disturbance in posttraumatic stress disorder (PTSD). Can J Psychiatry 45:667–668, 2000

Lavie L: Obstructive sleep apnea syndrome: an oxidative stress disorder. Sleep Med Rev 7:35–51, 2003

Lewy AJ, Bauer VK, Hasler BP, et al: Capturing the circadian rhythms of free-running blind people with 0.5 mg melatonin. Brain Res 918:96–100, 2001

Lichstein KL, Nau SD, McCrae CS, et al: Psychological and behavioral treatments for secondary insomnias, in Principles and Practices of Sleep Medicine, 4th Edition. Edited by Kryger MH, Roth T, Dement WC. Philadelphia, PA, Elsevier, 2005, pp 738–748

Lim J, Lasserson TJ, Fleetham J, et al: Oral appliances for obstructive sleep apnea. Cochrane Database Syst Rev CD004435, 2003

Lin L, Faraco J, Li R, et al: The sleep disorder canine narcolepsy is caused by a mutation in the hypocretin (orexin) receptor 2 gene. Cell 98:365–376, 1999

Lindberg E, Carter N, Gislason T, et al: Role of snoring and daytime sleepiness in occupational accidents. Am J Respir Crit Care Med 164:2031–2035, 2001

Littner M, Kushida CA, Hartse K, et al: Practice parameters for the use of laser-assisted uvulopalatoplasty: an update for 2000. Sleep 24:603–619, 2001

Lockley SW, Brainard GC, Czeisler CA: High sensitivity of the human circadian melatonin rhythm to resetting by short wavelength light. J Clin Endocrinol Metab 88:4502–4505, 2003

Macey PM, Henderson LA, Macey KE, et al: Brain morphology associated with obstructive sleep apnea. Am J Respir Crit Care Med 166:1382–1387, 2002

Mahowald MW, Cramer Bornemann MA: NREM sleep-arousal parasomnias, in Principles and Practices of Sleep Medicine, 4th Edition. Edited by Kryger MH, Roth T, Dement WC. Philadelphia, PA, Elsevier, 2005, pp 889–896

Mahowald MW, Schenck CH: Evolving concepts of human state dissociation. Arch Ital Biol 139:269–300, 2001

Mahowald MW, Schenck CH: REM sleep parasomnias, in Principles and Practices of Sleep Medicine, 4th Edition. Edited by Kryger MH, Roth T, Dement WC. Philadelphia, PA, Elsevier, 2005, pp 897–916

Mamelak M, Black J, Montplaisir J, et al: A pilot study on the effects of sodium oxybate on sleep architecture and daytime alertness in narcolepsy. Sleep 27:1327–1334, 2004

Marklund M, Stenlund H, Franklin KA: Mandibular advancement devices in 630 men and women with obstructive sleep apnea and snoring: tolerability and predictors of treatment success. Chest 125:1270–1278, 2004

Matsuki K, Juji T, Honda Y: Immunological features of narcolepsy in Japan, in HLA in Narcolepsy. Edited by Honda Y, Juti T. Berlin, Germany, Springer-Verlag, 1988, pp 150–157

McArthur AJ, Lewy AJ, Sack RL: Non-24-hour sleep–wake syndrome in a sighted man: circadian rhythm studies and efficacy of melatonin treatment. Sleep 19:544–553, 1996

Michaud M, Dumont M, Selmaoui B, et al: Circadian rhythm of restless legs syndrome: relationship with biological markers. Ann Neurol 55:372–380, 2004

Mignot E: Genetic and familial aspects of narcolepsy. Neurology 50:S16–S22, 1998

Mignot E: Narcolepsy: Pharmacology, pathophysiology, and genetics, in Principles and Practices of Sleep Medicine, 4th Edition. Edited by Kryger MH, Roth T, Dement WC. Philadelphia, PA, Elsevier, 2005, pp 761–779

Mimeault V, Morin CM: Self-help treatment for insomnia: bibliotherapy with and without professional guidance. J Consult Clin Psychol 67:511–519, 1999

Mitler MM, Aldrich MS, Koob GF, et al: Narcolepsy and its treatment with stimulants: ASDA standards of practice. Sleep 17:352–371, 1994

Mohler H, Fritschy J, Rudolph U: A new benzodiazepine pharmacology. J Pharmacol Exp Ther 300:2–8, 2002

Moldofsky H, Musisi S, Phillipson EA: Treatment of a case of advanced sleep phase syndrome by phase advance chronotherapy. Sleep 9:61–65, 1986

Montplaisir J, Poirier G: HLA in disorders of excessive sleepiness without cataplexy in Canada, in HLA in Narcolepsy. Edited by Honda Y, Juti T. Berlin, Germany, Springer-Verlag, 1988, pp 186–190

Montplaisir J, Nicolas A, Denesle R, et al: Restless legs syndrome improved by pramipexole: a double-blind randomized trial. Neurology 52:938–943, 1999

Montplaisir J, Allen RP, Walters AS, et al: Restless legs syndrome and periodic limb movements during sleep, in Principles and Practices of Sleep Medicine, 4th Edition. Edited by Kryger MH, Roth T, Dement WC. Philadelphia, PA, Elsevier, 2005, pp 839–852

Moore RY: Circadian rhythms: basic neurobiology and clinical applications. Annu Rev Med 48:253–266, 1997

Morgenthaler TI, Silber MH: Amnestic sleep-related eating disorder associated with zolpidem. Sleep Med 3:323–327, 2002

Morin CM: Insomnia: Psychological Assessment and Management, 17th Edition. New York, Guilford, 1993

Morin CM, Bootzin RR, Buysse DJ, et al: Psychological and behavioral treatment of insomnia: an update of recent evidence (1998–2004). Sleep 29:1398–1414, 2006

Morrison DL, Launois SH, Isono S, et al: Pharyngeal narrowing and closing pressures in patients with obstructive sleep apnea. Am Rev Respir Dis 148:606–611, 1993

Moul DE, Buysse DJ, Nofzinger EA, et al: Symptoms reports in severe chronic insomnia. Sleep 25:553–563, 2002

Mundey K, Benloucif S, Harsanyi K, et al: Phase-dependent treatment of delayed sleep phase syndrome with melatonin. Sleep 28:1271–1278, 2005

National Institutes of Health: NIH State-of-the-Science Conference Statement on Manifestations and Management of Chronic Insomnia in Adults. Bethesda, MD, National Institutes of Health, 2005

Naylor E, Penev PD, Orbeta L, et al: Daily social and physical activity increases slow-wave sleep and daytime neuropsychological performance in the elderly. Sleep 23:87–95, 2000

Neylan TC, Marmar CR, Metzler TJ, et al: Sleep disturbances in the Vietnam generation: findings from a nationally representative sample of male Vietnam veterans. Am J Psychiatry 155:929–933, 1998

Nielsen TA, Zadra A: Nightmares and other common dream disturbances, in Principles and Practices of Sleep Medicine, 4th Edition. Edited by Kryger MH, Roth T, Dement WC. Philadelphia, PA, Elsevier, 2005, pp 926–935

Nishino S, Ripley B, Overeem S, et al: Hypocretin (orexin) deficiency in human narcolepsy. Lancet 355:39–40, 2000

Nofzinger EA: Neuroimaging of sleep and sleep disorders. Curr Neurol Neurosci Rep 6:149–155, 2006

Nofzinger EA, Thase ME, Reynolds CF, et al: Hypersomnia in bipolar depression: a comparison with narcolepsy using the multiple sleep latency test. Am J Psychiatry 148:1177–1181, 1991

Nofzinger EA, Mintun MA, Wiseman MB, et al: Forebrain activation in REM sleep: an FDG PET study. Brain Res 770:192–201, 1997

Nofzinger EA, Buysse DJ, Germain A, et al: Functional neuroimaging evidence for hyperarousal in insomnia. Am J Psychiatry 161:2126–2131, 2004

Nowell PD, Mazumdar S, Buysse DJ, et al: Benzodiazepines and zolpidem for chronic insomnia: a meta-analysis of treatment efficacy. JAMA 278:2170–2177, 1997

O'Keeffe ST, Gavin K, Lavan JN: Iron status and restless legs syndrome in the elderly. Age Ageing 23:200–203, 1994

Ohayon MM: Epidemiology of insomnia: What we know and what we still need to learn. Sleep Med Rev 6:97–111, 2002

Ohayon MM, Guilleminault C: Epidemiology of sleep disorders, in Sleep Disorders Medicine: Basic Science, Technical Considerations and Clinical Aspects. Edited by Chokroverty S. Boston, MA, Butterworth-Heinemann, 1999, pp 301–316

Ohayon MM, Roth T: Prevalence of restless legs syndrome and periodic limb movement disorder in the general population. J Psychosom Res 53:547–554, 2002

Ohayon MM, Morselli PL, Guilleminault C: Prevalence of nightmares and their relationship to psychopathology and daytime functioning in insomnia subjects. Sleep 20:340–348, 1997

Ohayon MM, Guilleminault C, Priest RG: Night terrors, sleepwalking, and confusional arousals in the general population: their frequency and relationship to other sleep and mental disorders. J Clin Psychiatry 60:268–276, 1999

Ohayon MM, Priest RG, Zulley J, et al: Prevalence of narcolepsy symptomatology and diagnosis in the European general population. Neurology 58:1826–1833, 2002

Ohayon MM, Carskadon MA, Guilleminault C, et al: Meta-analysis of quantitative sleep parameters from childhood to old age in healthy individuals: developing normative sleep values across the human life span. Sleep 27:1255–1273, 2004

Oren DA, Wehr TA: Hypernyctohemeral syndrome after chronotherapy for delayed sleep phase syndrome. N Engl J Med 327:1762, 1992

Overeem S, Mignot E, Van Dijk JG, et al: Clinical features, new pathophysiological insights, and future perspectives. J Clin Neurophysiol 18:78–105, 2001

Ozaki S, Uchiyama M, Shirakawa S, et al: Prolonged interval from body temperature nadir to sleep offset in patients with delayed sleep phase syndrome. Sleep 19:36–40, 1996

Pace-Schott EF, Hobson JA: The neurobiology of sleep: genetics, cellular physiology and subcortical networks. Nat Rev Neurosci 3:591–605, 2002

Pack AI, Black JE, Schwartz JR, et al: Modafinil as adjunct therapy for daytime sleepiness in obstructive sleep apnea. Am J Respir Crit Care Med 164:1675–1681, 2001

Pelayo R, Thorpy MJ, Glovinsky P: Prevalence of delayed sleep phase syndrome among adolescents. Sleep Res 17:392, 1988

Peppard PE, Young T, Palta M, et al: Longitudinal study of moderate weight change and sleep-disordered breathing. JAMA 284:3015–3021, 2000

Perlis ML, Giles DE, Mendelson WB, et al: Psychophysiological insomnia: the behavioural model and a neurocognitive perspective. J Sleep Res 6:179–188, 1997

Perlis ML, McCall WV, Krystal AD, et al: Long-term, non-nightly administration of zolpidem in the treatment of patients with primary insomnia. J Clin Psychiatry 65:1128–1137, 2004

Perlis ML, Smith MT, Pigeon WR: Etiology and pathophysiology of insomnia, in Principles and Practices of Sleep Medicine, 4th Edition. Edited by Kryger MH, Roth T, Dement WC. Philadelphia, PA, Elsevier, 2005, pp 714–725

Piercey MF: Pharmacology of pramipexole, a dopamine D3-preferring agonist useful in treating Parkinson's disease. Clin Neuropharmacol 21:141–151, 1998

Pilcher JJ, Huffcutt AI: Effects of sleep deprivation on performance: a meta-analysis. Sleep 19:318–326, 1996

Pollak CP, Stokes PE: Circadian rest-activity rhythms in demented and nondemented older community residents and their caregivers. J Am Geriatr Soc 45:446–452, 1997

Powell NB, Riley RW, Guilleminault C: Surgical management of sleep-disordered breathing, in Principles and Practices of Sleep Medicine, 4th Edition. Edited by Kryger MH, Roth T, Dement WC. Philadelphia, PA, Elsevier, 2005, pp 1081–1097

Presser HB: Towards a 24 hour economy. Science 284:1778–1779, 1999

Punjabi NM, Beamer BA: Sleep apnea and metabolic dysfunction, in Principles and Practices of Sleep Medicine, 4th Edition. Edited by Kryger MH, Roth T, Dement WC. Philadelphia, PA, Elsevier, 2005, pp 1034–1042

Punjabi NM, Ahmed MM, Polotsky VY, et al: Sleep-disordered breathing, glucose intolerance, and insulin resistance. Respir Physiol Neurobiol 136:167–178, 2003

Raskind MA, Peskind ER, Kanter ED, et al: Reduction of nightmares and other PTSD symptoms in combat veterans by prazosin: a placebo-controlled study. Am J Psychiatry 160:371–373, 2003

Rechtschaffen A, Bergmann BM, Everson CE, et al: Sleep deprivation in the rat, X: integration and discussion of findings. Sleep 12:68–87, 1989

Regestein QR, Monk TH: Delayed sleep phase syndrome: a review of its clinical aspects. Am J Psychiatry 152:602–608, 1995

Reid KJ, Chang AM, Dubocovich ML, et al: Familial advanced sleep phase syndrome. Arch Neurol 58:1089–1094, 2001

Reid KJ, Zee PC: Circadian disorders of the sleep–wake cycle, in Principles and Practices of Sleep Medicine, 4th Edition. Edited by Kryger MH, Roth T, Dement WC. Philadelphia, PA, Elsevier, 2005, pp 691–701

Reynolds G, Blake DR, Pall HS, et al: Restless leg syndrome and rheumatoid arthritis. Br Med J 292:659–660, 1986

Riemann D, Voderholzer U: Primary insomnia: a risk factor to develop depression? J Affect Disord 76:255–259, 2003

Riley RW, Powell NB, Li KK, et al: Surgery and obstructive sleep apnea: long-term clinical outcomes. Otolaryngol Head Neck Surg 122:415–421, 2000

Rosenow F, Kotagal P, Cohen BH, et al: Multiple sleep latency test and polysomnography in diagnosing Kleine-Levin syndrome and periodic hypersomnia. J Clin Neurophysiol 17:519–522, 2000

Sack RL, Lewy AJ, Blood ML, et al: Circadian rhythm abnormalities in totally blind people: incidence and clinical significance. J Clin Endocrinol Metab 75:127–134, 1992

Sack RL, Brandes RW, Kendall AR, et al: Entrainment of free-running circadian rhythms by melatonin in blind people. N Engl J Med 343:1070–1077, 2000

Sajkov D, Wang T, Saunders NA, et al: Continuous positive airway pressure treatment improves pulmonary hemodynamics in patients with obstructive sleep apnea. Am J Respir Crit Care Med 165:152–158, 2002

Saper CB, Chou TC, Scammell TE: The sleep switch: hypothalamic control of sleep and wakefulness. Trends Neurosci 24:726–731, 2001

Sateia MJ, Doghramji K, Hauri PJ, et al: Evaluation of chronic insomnia: an American Academy of Sleep Medicine review. Sleep 23:243–308, 2000

Schellenberg JB, Maislin G, Schwab RJ: Physical findings and the risk for obstructive sleep apnea: the importance of oropharyngeal structures. Am J Respir Crit Care Med 162:740–748, 2000

Schenck CH, Mahowald MW: Long-term, nightly benzodiazepine treatment of injurious parasomnias and other disorders of disrupted nocturnal sleep in 170 adults. Am J Med 100:333–337, 1996

Schenck CH, Mahowald MW: Parasomnias: managing bizarre sleep-related behavior disorders. Postgrad Med 107:145–156, 2000

Schenck CH, Hurwitz TD, Bundlie SR, et al: Sleep-related eating disorders: polysomnographic correlates of a heterogeneous syndrome distinct from daytime eating disorders. Sleep 14:419–431, 1991

Schenck CH, Hurwitz TD, O'Connor KA, et al: Additional categories of sleep-related eating disorders and the current status of treatment. Sleep 16:457–466, 1993

Schenck CH, Bundlie SR, Mahowald MW: Delayed emergence of a parkinsonian disorder in 38% of 29 older men initially diagnosed with idiopathic rapid eye movement sleep behaviour disorder. Neurology 46:388–393, 1996

Schenck CH, Boyd JL, Mahowald MW: A parasomnia overlap disorder involving sleepwalking, sleep terrors, and REM sleep behavior disorder in 33 polysomnographically confirmed cases. Sleep 20:972–981, 1997

Scott AJ: Shift work and health. Prim Care 27:1057–1079, 2000

Shahar DR, Schulz R, Shahar A, et al: The effect of widowhood on weight change, dietary intake and eating behavior in the elderly population. J Aging Health 13:186–199, 2001

Shapiro CM, Trajanovic NN, Fedoroff JP: Sexsomnia: a new parasomnia? Can J Psychiatry 48:311–317, 2003

Sharkey KM, Fogg LF, Eastman CI: Effects of melatonin administration on daytime sleep after simulated night shift work. J Sleep Res 10:181–192, 2001

Sheldon SH, Kryger MH, Ferber R: Principles and Practice of Pediatric Sleep Medicine. Philadelphia, PA, Elsevier, 2005

Sher AE: Update on upper airway surgery for obstructive sleep apnea. Curr Opin Pulm Med 1:504–511, 1995

Silber MH, Ehrenberg BL, Allen RP, et al: An algorithm for the management of restless legs syndrome. Mayo Clin Proc 79:916–922, 2004

Smith MT, Perlis ML, Park A, et al: Comparative meta-analysis of pharmacotherapy and behavior therapy for persistent insomnia. Am J Psychiatry 159:5–11, 2002

Soldatos CR, Dikeos DG, Whitehead A: Tolerance and rebound insomnia with rapidly eliminated hypnotics: a meta-analysis of sleep laboratory studies. Int Clin Psychopharmacol 14:287–303, 1999

Somers VK, Dyken ME, Clary MP, et al: Sympathetic neural mechanisms in obstructive sleep apnea. J Clin Invest 96:1897–1904, 1995

Spiegel K, Leproult R, Van Cauter E: Impact of sleep debt on metabolic and endocrine function. Lancet 354:1435–1439, 1999

Spielman AJ: Assessment of insomnia. Clin Psychol Rev 6:11–25, 1986

Spielman AJ, Caruso LS, Glovinsky PB: A behavioral perspective on insomnia treatment. Psychiatr Clin North Am 10:541–553, 1987

Stefansson H, Rye DB, Hicks A, et al: A genetic risk factor for periodic limb movements in sleep. N Engl J Med 357:639–647, 2007

Stickgold R, Whidbee D, Schirmer B, et al: Visual discrimination task improvement: a multi-step process occurring during sleep. J Cogn Neurosci 12:246–254, 2000

Strollo PJ, Rogers RM: Obstructive sleep apnea. N Engl J Med 334:99–104, 1996

Strollo PJ, Atwood CW, Sanders MH: Medical therapy for obstructive sleep apnea-hypopnea syndrome, in Principles and Practices of Sleep Medicine, 4th Edition. Edited by Kryger MH, Roth T, Dement WC. Philadelphia, PA, Elsevier, 2005, pp 1053–1065

Strom L, Pettersson R, Andersson G: Internet-based treatment for insomnia: a controlled evaluation. J Consult Clin Psychol 72:113–120, 2004

Suhner AG, Murphy PJ, Campbell SS: Failure of timed bright light exposure to alleviate age-related sleep maintenance insomnia. J Am Geriatr Soc 50:617–623, 2002

Suzuki K, Ohida T, Sone T, et al: The prevalence of restless legs syndrome among pregnant women in Japan and the relationship between restless legs syndrome and sleep problems. Sleep 26:673–677, 2003

Telstad W, Sorensen O, Larsen S, et al: Treatment of the restless legs syndrome with carbamazepine: a double blind study. Br Med J 288:444–446, 1984

Teran-Santos J, Jimenez-Gomez A, Cordero-Guevara J: The association between sleep apnea and the risk of traffic accidents. N Engl J Med 340:847–851, 1999

Thannickal TC, Moore RY, Nienhuis R, et al: Reduced number of hypocretin neurons in human narcolepsy. Neuron 27:469–474, 2000

Thomas RE: Benzodiazepine use and motor vehicle accidents: systematic review of reported association. Can Fam Physician 44:799–808, 1998

Thorpy MJ, Korman E, Spielman AJ, et al: Delayed sleep phase syndrome in adolescents. J Adolesc Health 9:22–27, 1988

Tishler PV, Larkin EK, Schluchter MD, et al: Incidence of sleep-disordered breathing in an urban adult population: the relative importance of risk factors in the development of sleep-disordered breathing. JAMA 289:2230–2237, 2003

Toh KL, Jones CR, He Y, et al: An hPer2 phosphorylation site mutation in familial advanced sleep phase syndrome. Science 291:1040–1043, 2001

Toth LA, Opp MR: Sleep and infection, in Sleep Medicine. Edited by Lee-Chiong TL, Sateia MJ, Carskadon MA. Philadelphia, PA, Hanley & Belfus, 2002, pp 77–83

Trenkwalder C, Stiasny K, Pollmacher T, et al: L-dopa therapy of uremic and idiopathic restless legs syndrome: a double-blind, crossover trial. Sleep 18:681–688, 1995

Trenkwalder C, Garcia-Borreguero D, Montagna P, et al: Ropinirole in the treatment of restless legs syndrome: results from the TREAT RLS 1 study, a 12 week, randomised, placebo controlled study in 10 European countries. J Neurol Neurosurg Psychiatry 75:92–97, 2004

Turner RS, D'Amato CJ, Chervin RD, et al: The pathology of REM sleep behavior disorder with comorbid Lewy body dementia. Neurology 55:1730–1732, 2000

U.S. Modafinil in Narcolepsy Multicenter Study Group: Randomized trial of modafinil for the treatment of pathological somnolence in narcolepsy. U.S. Modafinil in Narcolepsy Multicenter Study Group. Ann Neurol 43:88–97, 1998

U.S. Modafinil in Narcolepsy Multicenter Study Group: Randomized trial of modafinil as a treatment for the excessive daytime somnolence of narcolepsy. U.S. Modafinil in Narcolepsy Multicenter Study Group. Neurology 54:1166–1175, 2000

U.S. Xyrem Multicenter Study Group: A randomized, double-blind, placebo-controlled multicenter trial comparing effects of three doses of orally administered sodium oxybate with placebo for the treatment of narcolepsy. Sleep 25:42–49, 2002

Uchiyama M, Okawa M, Shirakawa S, et al: A polysomnographic study on patients with delayed sleep phase syndrome (DSPS). Jpn J Psychiatry Neurol 46:219–221, 1992

Uchiyama M, Okawa M, Shibui K, et al: Poor compensatory function for sleep loss as a pathogenic factor in patients with delayed sleep phase syndrome. Sleep 23:553–558, 2000

Uchiyama M, Shibui K, Hayakawa T, et al: Larger phase angle between sleep propensity and melatonin rhythms in sighted humans with non-24-hour sleep–wake syndrome. Sleep 25:83–88, 2002

Ulfberg J, Nystrom B, Carter N, et al: Prevalence of restless legs syndrome among men aged 18 to 64 years: an association with somatic disease and neuropsychiatric symptoms. Mov Disord 16:1159–1163, 2001

Unruh ML, Levey AS, D'Ambrosio C, et al: Restless legs symptoms among incident dialysis patients: association with lower quality of life and shorter survival. Am J Kidney Dis 43:900–909, 2004

Van Someren EJ, Hagebeuk EE, Lijzenga C, et al: Circadian rest-activity rhythm disturbances in Alzheimer's disease. Biol Psychiatry 40:259–270, 1996

Van Someren EJ, Swaab DF, Colenda CC, et al: Bright light therapy: improved sensitivity to its effects on rest-activity rhythms in Alzheimer patients by application of nonparametric methods. Chronobiol Int 16:505–518, 1999

VanDongen HA, Maislin G, Mullington JM, et al: The cumulative cost of additional wakefulness: dose-response effects on neurobehavioral functions and sleep physiology from chronic sleep restriction and total sleep deprivation. Sleep 26:117–126, 2003

Veasey SC, Davis CW, Fenik P, et al: Long-term intermittent hypoxia in mice: protracted hypersomnolence with oxidative injury to sleep–wake brain regions. Sleep 27:194–201, 2004

Vermeeren A: Residual effects of hypnotics: epidemiology and clinical implications. CNS Drugs 18:297–328, 2004

Wagner DR: Disorders of the circadian sleep–wake cycle. Neurol Clin 14:651–670, 1996

Walsh JK: Pharmacological management of insomnia. J Clin Psychiatry 65 (suppl):41–45, 2004

Walsh JK, Roth T, Randazzo A, et al: Eight weeks of non-nightly use of zolpidem for primary insomnia. Sleep 23:1087–1096, 2000

Walsh JK, Randazzo AC, Stone KL, et al: Modafinil improves alertness, vigilance, and executive function during simulated night shifts. Sleep 27:434–439, 2004

Walsh JK, Dement WC, Dinges DF: Sleep medicine, public policy, and public health, in Principles and Practices of Sleep Medicine, 4th Edition. Edited by Kryger MH, Roth T, Dement WC. Philadelphia, PA, Elsevier, 2005a, pp 648–656

Walsh JK, Roehrs T, Roth T: Pharmacological treatment of primary insomnia, in Principles and Practices of Sleep Medicine, 4th Edition. Edited by Kryger MH, Roth T, Dement WC. Philadelphia, PA, Elsevier, 2005b, pp 749–760

Walters AS: Toward a better definition of the restless legs syndrome. The International Restless Legs Syndrome Study Group. Mov Disord 10:634–642, 1995

Waterhouse J, Reilly T, Atkinson G: Jet-lag. Lancet 350:1611–1616, 1997

Weaver TE, George CFP: Cognition and performance in patients with obstructive sleep apnea, in Principles and Practices of Sleep Medicine, 4th Edition. Edited by Kryger MH, Roth T, Dement WC. Philadelphia, PA, Elsevier, 2005, pp 1023–1033

Weitzman ED, Czeisler CA, Coleman RM, et al: Delayed sleep phase syndrome: a chronobiological disorder with sleep-onset insomnia. Arch Gen Psychiatry 38:737–746, 1981

Wetter TC, Stiasny K, Winkelmann J, et al: A randomized controlled study of pergolide in patients with restless legs syndrome. Neurology 52:944–950, 1999

Winget CM, DeRoshia CW, Markley CL, et al: A review of human physiological and performance changes associated with desynchronosis of biological rhythms. Aviat Space Environ Med 55:1085–1096, 1984

Winkelman JW: The evoked heart rate response to periodic leg movements of sleep. Sleep 22:575–580, 1999

Winkelman JW: Treatment of nocturnal eating syndrome and sleep-related eating disorder with topiramate. Sleep Med 4:243–246, 2003

Winkelman JW: Efficacy and tolerability of topiramate in the treatment of sleep-related eating disorder: a retrospective case series. J Clin Psychiatry 67:1729–1734, 2006

Winkelman JW, James L: Serotonergic antidepressants are associated with REM sleep without atonia. Sleep 27:317–321, 2004

Winkelman JW, Johnston L: Augmentation and tolerance with long-term pramipexole treatment of restless legs syndrome (RLS). Sleep Med 5:9–14, 2004

Winkelman JW, Chertow GM, Lazarus JM: Restless legs syndrome in end-stage renal disease. Am J Kidney Dis 28:372–378, 1996

Winkelman JW, Herzog DB, Fava M: The prevalence of sleep-related eating disorder in psychiatric and nonpsychiatric populations. Psychol Med 29:1461–1466, 1999

Winkelmann J, Wetter TC, Collado-Seidel V, et al: Clinical characteristics and frequency of the hereditary restless legs syndrome in a population of 300 patients. Sleep 23:597–602, 2000

Winkelmann J, Muller-Myhsok B, Wittchen HU, et al: Complex segregation analysis of restless legs syndrome provides evidence for an autosomal dominant mode of inheritance in early age at onset families. Ann Neurol 52:297–302, 2002

Winkelman JW, Sethi KD, Kushida CA, et al: Efficacy and safety of pramipexole in restless legs syndrome. Neurology 67:1034–1039, 2006

Winkelmann J, Schormair B, Lichtner P, et al: Genome-wide association study of restless legs syndrome identifies common variants in three genomic regions. Nat Genet 39:1000–1006, 2007

Winokur A, Sateia MJ, Hayes JB, et al: Acute effects of mirtazapine on sleep continuity and sleep architecture in depressed patients: a pilot study. Biol Psychiatry 48:75–78, 2000

Wisor JP, Eriksson KS: Dopaminergic-adrenergic interactions in the wake-promoting mechanism of modafinil. Neuroscience 132:1027–1034, 2005

Witting W, Kwa IH, Eikelenboom P, et al: Alterations in the circadian rest-activity rhythm in aging and Alzheimer's Disease. Biol Psychiatry 27:563–572, 1990

Woods J, Winger G: Current benzodiazepine issues. Psychopharmacology 118:107–115; discussion 118, 1995

World Health Organization: International Statistical Classification of Diseases and Related Health Problems, 10th Edition. Geneva, Switzerland, World Health Organization, 1992

Xu Y, Padiath QS, Shapiro RE, et al: Functional consequences of a CKIdelta mutation causing familial advanced sleep phase syndrome. Nature 434:640–644, 2005

Young T, Palta M, Dempsey J, et al: The occurrence of sleep-disordered breathing among middle-aged adults. N Engl J Med 328:1230–1235, 1993

Young T, Peppard PE, Gottlieb DJ: Epidemiology of obstructive sleep apnea: a population health perspective. Am J Respir Crit Care Med 165:1217–1239, 2002

Zanettini R, Antonini A, Gatto G, et al: Valvular heart disease and the use of dopamine agonists for Parkinson's disease. N Engl J Med 356:39–46, 2007

Zeitzer JM, Dijk DJ, Kronauer R, et al: Sensitivity of the human circadian pacemaker to nocturnal light: melatonin phase resetting and suppression. J Physiol 526:695–702, 2000

Zoltoski RK, de Jesus Cabeza R, Gillin JC: Biochemical pharmacology of sleep, in Sleep Disorders Medicine. Edited by Chokroverty S. Boston, MA, Butterworth-Heinemann, 1999, pp 63–94

Zonato AI, Bittencourt LR, Martinho FL, et al: Association of systematic head and neck physical examination with severity of obstructive sleep apnea-hypopnea syndrome. Laryngoscope 113:973–980, 2003

23

EATING DISORDERS

Anorexia Nervosa, Bulimia Nervosa, and Obesity

Katherine A. Halmi, M.D.

The eating disorders *anorexia nervosa* and *bulimia nervosa* and the condition of *obesity* have been known since earliest times in Western civilization. Well-documented case reports of anorexia nervosa are found in literature describing early Christian saints. Bell (1985) reported the severe starving behavior and bingeing episodes of Saint Catherine of Siena, described the kind of reed she used to induce vomiting, and listed the herbal cathartics that she used for purging. Although binge eating and purging behavior are certainly described in Roman civilization, the disorder of bulimia nervosa as we define it today has not been so well documented.

The eating disorders are entities or syndromes and not specific diseases with a common cause, common course, and common pathology. They are best conceptualized as syndromes and are therefore classified on the basis of the clusters of symptoms they present.

Because an important interaction exists between psychology and physiology in the eating disorders, this chapter begins with a brief section on the physiology of eating. Following this, the characteristics of anorexia nervosa, bulimia nervosa, and obesity are reviewed, with emphasis on the distinctive clinical features, medical complications, epidemiology, course, prognosis, pathogenic development, treatment, and theories of etiology.

Physiology and Behavioral Pharmacology of Eating
A Systems Conceptualization

A major conceptual revision for understanding the physiology and behavior of eating has expanded the dual-center theory of hypothalamic facilitatory and inhibitory centers for eating. The sensitive hypothalamic eating centers are part of a broad complex of neuroregulator interactions that includes a peripheral satiety system (gastrointestinal and pancreatic hormones released by food passing through the gastrointestinal tract) and a broad neural network affecting feeding, within the brain. Eating behavior is now known to reflect an interaction between an organism's physiological state and environmental conditions. Salient physiological variables include the balance of various neuropeptides and neurotransmitters, metabolic state, metabolic rate, condition of the gastrointestinal tract, amount of storage tissue, and sensory receptors for taste and smell. Environmental conditions include features of the food such as taste, texture, novelty, accessibility, and nutritional composition as well as other external conditions such as ambient temperature, presence of other people, and stress (Blundell and Hill 1986).

To understand eating behavior, it is also important to recognize the role of conditioned (learned) components in the initiation and termination of nutrient ingestion. Because of methodological complexities, this area has received little study. Booth (1985) provided the best discussion of conditioned appetites and satieties because he focused attention on the interaction between psychological and physiological phenomena.

It is important to remember that when an exogenous agent such as a drug or peptide is given to an animal or a human, it does not simply activate a specific set of receptors that induce specific responses; it intervenes in a complex transactional fabric as well (Blundell and Hill 1986).

Neurotransmitters

Biogenic Amines

The study of catecholaminergic pathways in the hypothalamus by Leibowitz (1980) led to the discovery of the role of α_2-adrenergic receptors in the paraventricular nucleus (PVN) and the β_2-adrenergic receptors in the perifornical hypothalamus (PFH) in feeding. Microinjection of α_2 agonists to the PVN produces hyperphagia and causes a preferential ingestion of carbohydrate. This adrenergic β_2-responsive circuit in the PFH inhibits feeding. Underweight anorexia nervosa patients and persons without eating disorders in times of dieting have reduced central and peripheral norepinephrine activity (Pirke 1996). This is confirmed by hypothermia, bradycardia, and hypotension.

Serotonin, an indoleamine, has been shown to facilitate satiety (Hoebel 1977) and may at least in part control the intake of carbohydrate (Wurtman and Wurtman 1979). Serotonin injected peripherally and centrally into the PVN suppresses deprivation-induced and norepinephrine-induced eating (Leibowitz 1980).

The serotonin type 2A (5-HT$_{2A}$) receptor is a G protein–coupled receptor that controls signal transduction by activating phospholipase C (Eison and Mullins 1996). Properties of the 5-HT$_{2A}$ receptor such as ligand affinity receptor downregulation or signal transduction could be affected by any disturbance or alteration in a genetic coding variant for this receptor. Such an aberration may contribute to the disturbed and disor-

dered eating behavior in anorexia nervosa and bulimia nervosa.

Some evidence indicates that serotonin neuronal activity is involved in behavioral inhibition (Soubrie 1986), obsessive-compulsive disorder (OCD; Barr et al. 1992), anxiety and fear (Charney et al. 1990), and depression (Grahame-Smith 1992); serotonin neuronal activity also has well-established involvement with satiety for food intake. Anorexia nervosa has comorbid or coexisting disturbances of behavioral inhibition, obsessive-compulsive problems, excessive anxiety and fear, and depression. Bulimia nervosa is frequently characterized by behavioral disinhibition and depression.

Dopamine seems to play a more complicated role in eating behavior. Low doses of dopamine and dopamine agonist stimulate feeding, whereas higher doses inhibit feeding (Leibowitz 1980). Glucose administration suppresses firing in substantia nigra dopamine neurons. There is evidence of increased hypothalamic dopamine turnover during feeding. This finding suggests that central dopamine mechanisms mediate the rewarding effects of food as they mediate the rewarding effects of intracranial self-stimulation and the self-stimulation of psychoactive drugs. The dopamine antagonist pimozide suppresses sham feeding intake of sucrose. This may be due to the inhibition of the rewarding effect of glucose (Gibbs and Smith 1984). In free-feeding rats, however, pimozide causes an increase in meal size.

Peptides and Opioids

Corticotropin-releasing factor (CRF) acts within the PVN to inhibit feeding. Norepinephrine seems to inhibit the CRF inhibitory feeding effect. The pancreatic polypeptide neuropeptide Y increases both food and water intake when injected into the PVN. Another pancreatic polypeptide, peptide YY, is a more potent stimulator of feeding than neuropeptide Y (Morley and Levine 1985).

Opioid antagonism decreases feeding in many species but has no effect in reducing food intake in other species. Under some physiological conditions, such as starving or insulin-induced hypoglycemia, naloxone fails to inhibit feeding. Stress-induced eating is probably driven by activation of the opioid system. Dynorphin, an endogenous κ opioid receptor ligand, enhances feeding. Again, the major site of action for dynorphin appears to be the PVN (Morley and Levine 1985).

Vasopressin and oxytocin are neuropeptides distributed in the brain and function as long-acting neuromodulators with complex behavioral effects that are often reciprocal. Oxytocin antagonizes vasopressin's consolidation of learning acquired during aversive conditioning (Bohus et al. 1978). The dysregulation of secretion of these hormones in anorexia nervosa (Demitrack et al. 1992) may enhance the retention of cognitive distortions of the aversive consequences of eating.

Peripheral Satiety Network

Several peptides are released by ingested food from the gastrointestinal tract. Some of these inhibit feeding by activating ascending vagal fibers. Cholecystokinin is the most extensively studied of these peptides. Its effects, mediated by vagal fibers, have been traced to the PVN of the hypothalamus, where lesions abolish its effect on feeding. Low doses of cholecystokinin infused into the PVN attenuate feeding, and central infusions of cholecystokinin antibodies enhance feeding. The potency of the satiety effect of cholecystokinin varies across animal species. Other peptides that appear to inhibit feeding via vagal fibers are glucagon, somatostatin, and thyrotropin-releasing hormone.

Bombesin is a gastric peptide that inhibits feeding, independent of vagal fibers. Gastrin-releasing peptide and calcitonin also inhibit feeding (Gibbs and Smith 1984). Some of these peptides, such as cholecystokinin, bombesin, and glucagon, when administered parenterally to humans, have produced satiety. However, their usefulness as therapeutic agents at present is limited because of their restricted absorption from the gut and the high doses required induce adverse effects such as nausea.

Leptin is a protein hormone secreted by adipose tissue cells and believed to act as an afferent signal and regulator of body fat stores (Zhang et al. 1994). Leptin activates receptors and is coded by the *DB* gene in the hypothalamus and OB receptors in the choroid plexus (Tartaglia et al. 1995). Defects in the leptin coding sequence in rodents result in leptin deficiency and defects in leptin receptors, which are associated with obesity (Chen et al. 1996). Leptin is positively correlated with fat mass in humans in all weight ranges (Considine et al. 1996). Underweight patients with anorexia nervosa have significantly reduced plasma and cerebrospinal fluid (CSF) leptin concentrations compared with normal-weight control subjects (Mantzoros et al. 1997). These levels reach normal values with weight restoration. Because acute fasting-induced weight loss provokes a decline in leptin concentration that is disproportionate to the amount of fat loss (Boden et al. 1996), it has been hypothesized that leptin is a protecting regulator against starvation. Reduced leptin concentrations induce a variety of neuroendo-

crine responses, including decreased thyroid thermogenesis, increased secretion of stress steroid, and decreased procreation (Ahima et al. 1996).

Ghrelin is a gastrointestinal peptide secreted in the stomach that indirectly stimulates hunger. Ghrelin levels increase with food restriction (Gualillo et al. 2002). Ghrelin levels peak prior to mealtime and decline with feeding and thus seem to have a role in short-term feeding (Cummings et al. 2001). Ghrelin levels are elevated in underweight anorexia nervosa patients and decrease with weight gain; ghrelin levels are negatively correlated with body mass index (BMI) (Le Roux et al. 2005).

Melanocortin receptor activity and Agouti-related protein may also be involved in regulating food intake and weight. Kas et al. (2003) induced physical hyperactivity and self-starvation in rats by restricting food in the presence of running wheels. They found that the increased melanocortin receptors in the ventral medial hypothalamus were suppressed with a central infusion of Agouti-related protein; thus, the survival rate in these rats was increased because of the decreased physical hyperactivity and increased food intake.

Anorexia Nervosa

Definition

Anorexia nervosa is a disorder characterized by preoccupation with body weight and food, behavior directed toward losing weight, peculiar patterns of handling food, weight loss, intense fear of gaining weight, disturbance of body image, and amenorrhea. DSM-IV-TR (American Psychiatric Association 2000a) criteria for anorexia nervosa are included in Table 23–1.

Clinical Features

Individuals with anorexia nervosa typically express an intense fear of gaining weight, tend to be preoccupied with thoughts of food, and worry irrationally about fatness. Denial of their own clearly observable symptoms is characteristic of anorexic patients. They frequently look in mirrors to make sure they are thin, and they incessantly express concern about looking fat and feeling flabby. Collecting recipes and preparing elaborate meals for their families are other behaviors that reflect their preoccupation with food. Peculiar handling of food is frequent in individuals with anorexia. They will hide carbohydrate-rich foods and hoard large quantities of candies, carrying them in their pockets and purses. Often, they will try to dispose of their food

TABLE 23–1. DSM-IV-TR diagnostic criteria for anorexia nervosa

A. Refusal to maintain body weight at or above a minimally normal weight for age and height (e.g., weight loss leading to maintenance of body weight less than 85% of that expected; or failure to make expected weight gain during period of growth, leading to body weight less than 85% of that expected).

B. Intense fear of gaining weight or becoming fat, even though underweight.

C. Disturbance in the way in which one's body weight or shape is experienced, undue influence of body weight or shape on self-evaluation, or denial of the seriousness of the current low body weight.

D. In postmenarcheal females, amenorrhea, i.e., the absence of at least three consecutive menstrual cycles. (A woman is considered to have amenorrhea if her periods occur only following hormone, e.g., estrogen, administration.)

Specify type:

Restricting type: during the current episode of anorexia nervosa, the person has not regularly engaged in binge-eating or purging behavior (i.e., self-induced vomiting or the misuse of laxatives, diuretics, or enemas)

Binge-eating/purging type: during the current episode of anorexia nervosa, the person has regularly engaged in binge-eating or purging behavior (i.e., self-induced vomiting or the misuse of laxatives, diuretics, or enemas)

surreptitiously to avoid eating. Anorexic persons will spend a great deal of time cutting food into small pieces and rearranging the food on their plates.

Anorexic patients' fear that they are gaining weight exists even in the face of increasing cachexia, and they characteristically show disinterest in and even resistance to treatment. Persons with this disorder lose weight by drastically reducing their total food intake and disproportionately decreasing the intake of high-carbohydrate and fatty foods. Some individuals with anorexia will develop rigorous exercise programs, and others simply will be as active as possible at all times. Self-induced vomiting and laxative and diuretic abuse are other purging behaviors by which anorexic persons attempt to lose weight. Weight loss and a refusal to maintain body weight over a minimal normal weight for age and height are the most characteristic features of this disorder. Anorexic individuals have a

disturbance in the way in which they experience their body weight and shape. They often fail to recognize that their degree of emaciation is dangerous. Their cognition is so distorted that they judge their self-worth predominantly by body shape and weight.

Obsessive-compulsive behavior often develops after the onset of anorexia nervosa. An obsession with cleanliness, an increase in housecleaning activities, and a more compulsive approach to studying are not uncommonly observed in these patients.

Amenorrhea can appear before noticeable weight loss has occurred. Poor sexual adjustment is frequently present in patients with anorexia. Many adolescent patients with anorexia have delayed psychosocial sexual development, and adults often have a markedly decreased interest in sex with the onset of anorexia nervosa.

Patients with anorexia nervosa can be divided into two groups: those who binge eat and purge and those who merely restrict food intake to lose weight. There is a relatively frequent association with impulsive behavior such as suicide attempts, self-mutilation, stealing, and substance abuse (including alcohol abuse) among bulimic anorexic individuals, who are also less likely to be regressed in their sexual activity and may in fact be promiscuous. Bulimic anorexic patients are more likely to have discrete personality disorder diagnoses (Halmi 1987).

Medical Complications

Most of the physiological and metabolic changes in anorexia nervosa are secondary to the starvation state or purging behavior and are reversed with nutritional rehabilitation (Table 23–2). We often find abnormalities in hematopoiesis, such as leukopenia and relative lymphocytosis, in acutely emaciated anorexic patients. Individuals with anorexia nervosa who engage in self-induced vomiting or who abuse laxatives and diuretics are liable to develop hypokalemic alkalosis. These patients often have elevated serum bicarbonate levels, hypochloremia, and hypokalemia. Patients with electrolyte disturbances have physical symptoms of weakness and lethargy and, at times, have cardiac arrhythmias. The latter condition may threaten sudden cardiac arrest, a frequent cause of death in patients who purge. Other complications of bingeing and purging are discussed in the section on bulimia nervosa.

Elevation of serum enzymes reflects fatty degeneration of the liver and is observed both in the emaciated anorexic phase and during refeeding. Elevated serum cholesterol levels tend to occur more frequently in younger patients. Carotenemia is often observed in

TABLE 23–2. Medical complications of anorexia nervosa

Cardiovascular
  Bradycardia
  Orthostatic hypotension
  Arrhythmias
  Electrocardiogram changes—QTc prolongation
  ST–T wave abnormalities
Central nervous system
  Peripheral neuropathy
  Enlarged ventricles
  Decreased gray and white matter
  Cognitive impairment
Endocrine/metabolic
  Hypothermia
  Amenorrhea
  Hypokalemia
  Electrolyte abnormalities
  Hypercholesterolemia
Gastrointestinal
  Vomiting
  Constipation
  Diarrhea
  Parotid hyperplasia
  Increased serum amylase
  Abnormal liver function tests
Renal
  Hypokalemic nephropathy
Hematological
  Anemia
  Leukopenia with relative lymphocytosis
Integument
  Lanugo
  Carotenoderma
Muscular
  Muscle wasting
  Creative kinase abnormalities
Pulmonary
  Decreased pulmonary capacity
Reproductive
  Amenorrhea, secondary or primary
  Decreased serum estrogen in females
  Decreased serum testosterone in males
  Loss of libido
Skeletal
  Osteopenia
  Osteoporosis
  Pathological stress fractures

malnourished anorexic patients. All of these physiological changes reverse themselves with nutritional rehabilitation (Halmi and Falk 1981). Amenorrhea, which is a major diagnostic criterion for anorexia nervosa, is not related simply to weight loss and is discussed in the section "Etiology and Pathogenesis" later in this chapter.

Epidemiology, Course, and Prognosis

The incidence of anorexia nervosa has increased since the mid–twentieth century, both in the United States and in Western Europe. In Monroe County, New York, the average annual incidence rate of 0.35 per 100,000 population in the 1960s increased to 0.64 per 100,000 in the 1970s (Jones et al. 1980). In London, the prevalence of anorexia nervosa was 1 severe case in approximately 200 girls ages 12–18 years in the 1970s (Crisp et al. 1976). An incidence study in northeastern Scotland in the 1980s found 4 cases of anorexia nervosa per 100,000 population per annum (Szmukler 1985). A more recent incidence study conducted in northeastern Scotland (Eagles et al. 1995) reported that between 1965 and 1991, the incidence of anorexia nervosa increased nearly sixfold (from 3 per 100,000 to 17 cases per 100,000 population). These studies probably underestimate the true incidence, because not all cases come to the attention of health care providers. Hoek (1991) found the incidence of anorexia nervosa at the primary care level in Holland to be 6.3 cases per 100,000 population per year during the period 1985–1986 and 8.1 per 100,000 during the period 1987–1989. Rooney et al. (1995) surveyed patients recruited for study from the level of primary care in England. The prevalence of anorexia nervosa was 20.2 cases per 100,000 population (0.02% of the total population). The prevalence among female patients ages 15–29 years was 115.4 cases per 100,000 population (0.1%). In Rochester, Minnesota, Lucas et al. (1991) recorded a point prevalence of anorexia nervosa of 0.2% for females and 0.02% for males on January 1, 1980. Five years later, their survey showed that the point prevalence of anorexia nervosa had increased to 0.48% among female adolescents ages 15–19 years. A more recent survey that followed high school students to age 24 years found the incidence of eating disorders to be 2.8% by age 18 years and 1.3% for ages 19–23 years. The lifetime prevalence of anorexia nervosa was 0.6% (Lewinsohn et al. 2000). Only 4%–6% of the anorexic population is male (Halmi 1974).

In a community epidemiological survey in Canada, Woodside et al. (2001) found that men with eating disorders were very similar to women with the same diagnoses. The pattern of familial aggregation of eating disorders in males with anorexia nervosa was found to be highly similar to that observed in recent family studies of affected females (Strober et al. 2001).

The course of anorexia nervosa varies from a single episode with weight and psychological recovery, to nutritional rehabilitation with relapses, to an unremitting course resulting in death. Two of the most methodologically satisfying long-term follow-up studies have shown a mortality rate of 6.6% at 10 years after a well-defined treatment program (Halmi et al. 1991) and a mortality rate of 18% at 30-year follow-up (Theander 1985).

These studies, in addition to a follow-up study by Hsu et al. (1979), found that many patients with anorexia may show considerable improvement in their medical condition, but most still had the characteristic psychological set of the illness. Fewer than one-fourth of these patients could be considered to have made a good psychological adjustment when they were followed up to ages 20–50 years. At the end of his 30-year follow-up study, Theander (1985) found that 75% of his patients could be classified as being in a psychologically stable state. This was not true at the time of earlier follow-up examinations. Generally speaking, poor outcome in the studies mentioned earlier was associated with longer duration of illness, older age at onset, previous admissions to psychiatric hospitals, poor childhood social adjustment, premorbid personality difficulties, and disturbed relationships between patients and other family members.

A prospective 5-year study of 95 patients with anorexia nervosa in Australia found that 3 patients had died, 56 had no eating disorder diagnosis, and the remainder had a continuation of their illness with psychosocial difficulties (Ben-Tovin et al. 2001). All of these outcome studies indicate that anorexia nervosa is a serious chronic disorder.

Etiology and Pathogenesis

A specific etiology and pathogenesis leading to the development of anorexia nervosa are unknown. Anorexia nervosa begins after a period of severe food deprivation (Tables 23–3 and 23–4).

Previous periods of severe food restriction are often reported, and a history of earlier dieting is not unusual. The question is, what is unique about the individual who goes on to develop anorexia nervosa?

The psychological theories concerning the causes of anorexia have centered mostly on phobic mecha-

TABLE 23–3. Common reasons for severe food deprivation

Willful dieting for the purpose of being more attractive
Willful dieting for the purpose of being more professionally competent (e.g., ballet dancers, gymnasts, jockeys)
Food restriction secondary to severe stress
Food restriction secondary to severe illness and/or surgery
Involuntary starvation

TABLE 23–4. Satiety peptides

Hypothalamic neuropeptides
Corticotropin-releasing hormone
Thyrotropin-releasing hormone
α-Melanocyte-stimulating hormone
Neurotensin
Somatostatin
Leptin
Gut-related peptides
Cholecystokinin
Peptide YY
Bombesin
Gastrin-releasing peptide

nisms and psychodynamic formulations. Crisp (1976) postulated that anorexia nervosa constitutes a phobic avoidance response to food resulting from the sexual and social tension generated by the physical changes associated with puberty.

Psychodynamic theories have focused on fantasies of oral impregnation and dependent seductive relationships with warm, passive fathers and guilt over aggression toward ambivalently regarded mothers.

A cognitive and perceptual developmental defect was postulated by Bruch (1962) as the cause of anorexia nervosa. She described the disturbances of body image (denial of emaciation), disturbances in perception (lack of recognition or denial of fatigue, weakness, hunger), and a sense of ineffectiveness as being caused by untoward learning experiences.

Russell (1969) suggested that the amenorrhea may be caused by a primary disturbance of hypothalamic function and that the full expression of this disturbance is induced by psychological stress. He thought that the malnutrition of anorexia nervosa perpetuates the amenorrhea but is not primarily responsible for the endocrine disorder. This hypothesis is supported by the fact that the return of normal menstrual cycles lags behind the return to a normal body weight; the resumption of menses in anorexia nervosa is associated with marked psychological improvement (Falk and Halmi 1982).

Further support for the theory of disturbed hypothalamic function in anorexia nervosa comes from neurotransmitter studies. The increased cortisol production present in anorexia nervosa has been traced to the hypothalamus. Two groups of investigators (Gold et al. 1986; Hotta et al. 1986) showed that patients with anorexia have increased CRF in their CSF, which probably means that increased CRF production from the hypothalamus is causing the cortisol changes observed in anorexia. Because central neurotransmitters such as dopamine, serotonin, and norepinephrine all influence appetite, satiety, and eating behavior, it is reasonable to study these neurotransmitters in patients with anorexia.

Although assessment of neurotransmitter function in the brain in humans has serious methodological problems, preliminary indirect studies indicate that a dysregulation of all three of these neurotransmitters probably occurs. Kaye et al. (1984a) showed a decreased serotonin turnover in bulimic anorexic patients compared with restricting anorexic patients. In addition, Kaye et al. (1984b) showed low CSF norepinephrine levels in long-term anorexic patients who had attained a weight within at least 15% of their normal weight range. Owen et al. (1983) showed that individuals with anorexia have a blunted growth hormone response to L-dopa, indicating a defect at the postsynaptic dopamine receptor sites. More recently, Brambilla et al. (2001) reported a blunted growth hormone response to postsynaptic D_2 receptor stimulation with apomorphine in underweight anorexic patients. They suggested that the postsynaptic D_2 receptors are downregulated in anorexia nervosa because of a peripheral negative feedback linked to a hyperfunctioning somatotropic axis or to a hypothalamic presynaptic dopamine hypersecretion and/or reduced dopamine reuptake. In this study, growth hormone responses did not correlate with BMI but did correlate negatively with scores on the Eating Disorder Inventory Scale. Thus, dopamine alteration in anorexia nervosa may be linked to psychopathological parameters.

The serotonin 1A ($5-HT_{1A}$) receptor is associated with anxiety and feeding behavior. A study using positron emission tomography (PET) imaging and a specific $5-HT_{1A}$ receptor antagonist, [carbonyl-^{11}C] WAY-100635, found that women who had recovered from the bulimic type of anorexia nervosa had significantly increased binding potential in the cingulate, lateral mesial temporal, lateral medial orbital frontal, parietal, and prefrontal cortical regions and in the dorsal raphe compared with controlled women. No differences were found for women recovered from restricting-type anorexia nervosa relative to control subjects. In women with the restricting type of anorexia, the $5-HT_{1A}$ postsynaptic receptor binding in the mesial temporal and subgenual cingulate regions was positively correlated with harm avoidance (Bailer et al. 2005). This altered serotonergic function may be related to the anxiety symptoms that persist after recovery from anorexia nervosa. Another study using PET showed that women recovered from anorexia nervosa had significantly higher [^{11}C] raclopride binding potential in the anteroventral striatum compared with control women. The binding potential was positively related to harm avoidance in the dorsal raphe and dorsal putamen. The authors postulated that individuals with anorexia nervosa may have a dopamine-related disturbance of reward mechanisms contributing to their altered hedonics of eating and their ascetic, anhedonic temperament (Frank et al. 2005).

Neuropeptide Y, a powerful endogenous stimulant of eating behavior in the central nervous system, was found to be significantly elevated in the CSF of emaciated patients with anorexia (Kaye et al. 1990). The neuropeptide Y levels generally returned to a normal range with long-term weight restoration. A reduction of food intake may produce a homeostatic increase in neuropeptide Y secretion that should serve to stimulate feeding, but this mechanism seems to be ineffective in the patient with anorexia nervosa. The relation between neuropeptide Y and CRF and luteinizing hormone secretion in anorexia nervosa is an area that needs further investigation (Table 23–5).

There is increasing evidence for genetic influences in the development of anorexia nervosa. Family studies have shown significantly increased prevalence of eating disorders in relatives of patients with anorexia nervosa compared with relatives of control persons (Lilenfeld et al. 1998; Strober et al. 1985). Twin studies of anorexia nervosa have shown concordance rates for monozygotic twins to be 52%–56%, whereas concordance rates for dizygotic twins were estimated to be 5%–11% (Holland et al. 1988; Wade et al. 2000). The first genomewide linkage analysis of families in which at least two affected relatives had the diagnosis of re-

TABLE 23–5. Neurotransmitters and neuropeptides in anorexia nervosa

Hormone	Effect on eating behavior	Functional status in anorexia nervosa	Clinical manifestations
Norepinephrine	Inhibits the CRF-inhibiting feeding effect	↓	Decreased food intake
Serotonin	Facilitates satiety	↑	Feeling full after a minimal intake of food
Dopamine	Mediates rewarding effects of food	↓	?
Corticotropin-releasing factor (CRF)	Inhibits feeding; stimulates motor activity	↑	Decreased food intake; increased motor activity
Neuropeptide Y	Increases food intake	↑	Should stimulate feeding, but ineffective in anorexia nervosa
Cholecystokinin	Attenuates feeding	↑	Decreased meal size

Note.   This table is, of course, oversimplified; actual phenomena are more complex.

stricting anorexia nervosa without binge eating or purging behavior showed a peak multipoint nonparametric linkage score of 3.45, suggesting evidence for the presence of an anorexia nervosa susceptibility locus on chromosome 1p (Grice et al. 2002). To further explore the genetic contributions to anorexia nervosa, the psychiatric, personality, and temperament phenotypes of individuals diagnosed with eating disorders, all obtained through a participant with anorexia nervosa, were analyzed with a multipoint affected-sibling-pair linkage analysis using a novel method that incorporated covariates. Drive for thinness and obsessionality were the covariates used in this analysis, because they identified an extreme cluster of affected sibling pairs who had high and concordant values on these traits and other clusters of affected sibling pairs who had lower scores on these traits. The linkage analysis of these covariates showed several regions of suggestive linkage: one on chromosome 1, another on chromosome 2, and a third region on chromosome 13 (Devlin et al. 2002). Finding suggestive linkage sites is of interest because these regions may harbor excellent candidate genes for liability for eating disorders. A subsequent study in this same eating disorder population showed serotonin 1D (5-HT_{1D}) and delta opioid receptor loci in the first chromosome linkage region described earlier to exhibit significant association to anorexia nervosa (Bergen et al. 2003). Dopaminergic neuronal function modulates feeding behavior, motor activity, and reward-motivated behavior. For this rea-

son the authors of this study examined in the same eating disorder population the presence of functional polymorphisms or changes at the dopamine D_2 receptor. Polymorphisms or changes in the D_2 receptor were significantly associated (exhibited significant linkage and association) to the anorexia nervosa diagnosis. Thus individuals with a diagnosis of anorexia nervosa and these D_2 receptor changes should exhibit altered D_2 receptor availability in neuroimaging studies compared with individuals without a diagnosis of anorexia nervosa and without these receptor changes. This is a necessary area for future investigation.

In a study comparing the mothers of 57 anorexic patients with those of age- and sex-matched control subjects, Halmi et al. (1991) found a significantly greater prevalence of OCD in the mothers of the anorexic patients. Serotonin dysregulation may be a link between the OCD of the mothers and the anorexia nervosa in their daughters.

Treatment

A multifaceted treatment endeavor with medical management and behavioral, individual, cognitive, and family therapy is necessary to treat anorexia nervosa (Table 23–6). The first step in treatment is to obtain the anorexic patient's cooperation in a treatment program. Most patients with anorexia nervosa are disinterested and even resistant to treatment and are brought to the therapist's office unwillingly by relatives or friends.

TABLE 23–6. Treatment of anorexia nervosa

Type of treatment	Key elements	Measurements	Indications
Medical management	Weight restoration	Weight (outpatient— weekly; inpatient—daily)	Below normal weight for age and height by ≥10%
	Rehydration and correction of serum electrolytes	Serum electrolytes	History of vomiting, laxative abuse, severe restriction of food and fluids
Behavior therapy	Positive reinforcements for weight gain	Weight (outpatient— weekly; inpatient—daily)	Underweight
	Response prevention for binge eating and purging	Serum electrolytes and serum amylase	Weakness, puffy cheeks— parotid enlargement, scars on dorsum of hands, fainting spells
Cognitive therapy	Operationalizing beliefs, evaluating automatic thoughts, prospective hypothesis testing, examination of underlying assumptions	Assessment of distorted cognitions (e.g., all-or-none/black-or-white thinking), feeling fat, self-worth measured solely by body image, pervasive sense of ineffectiveness except in losing weight	Disturbance in way one's body weight or shape is experienced; denial of seriousness of low body weight; relentless pursuit of thinness for control of environment
Family therapy	Family counseling or therapy format based on needs of specific family	Analysis of family functioning, roles, and interactions	If patient is living with family, some type of family counseling or therapy is essential
Pharmacotherapy			
Chlorpromazine	Liquid form, start low doses, such as 10 mg tid, and gradually increase	Complete blood count, lying and standing blood pressure	Severely delusional, overactive, hospitalized patients
Cyproheptadine	Liquid form, start 4 mg bid and increase to 8 mg tid if necessary	Complete blood count with platelets	Severely overactive anorexic patient who does not binge and purge
Fluoxetine	Preferable to use after weight restoration because of tendency to induce arousal	Complete blood count, observation of total sleep and activity	Severely obsessive-compulsive behaviors related or unrelated to eating disorders, severe depression
Clomipramine	Necessary to start in very low doses because of hypotension side effects; preferable to use after weight restoration	Complete blood count, lying and standing blood pressure, electrocardiogram	Severely obsessive-compulsive behaviors
Tricyclic antidepressants	Necessary to start in very low doses because of hypotension side effects; preferable to use after weight restoration	Complete blood count, lying and standing blood pressure, electrocardiogram	Severe depression

For these patients, it is important to emphasize the benefits of treatment and to reassure them that treatment can bring about a relief of insomnia and depressive symptoms, a decrease in the obsessive thoughts about food and body weight that interfere with the ability to concentrate on other matters, an increase in physical well-being and energy, and an improvement in peer relationships.

The immediate aim of treatment should be to restore the patient's nutritional state to normal. Mere emaciation or the state of being mildly underweight (15%–25% below normal weight) can cause irritability, depression, preoccupation with food, and sleep disturbance. It is exceedingly difficult to achieve behavioral change with psychotherapy in a patient who is experiencing the psychological effects of emaciation. Outpatient therapy as an initial approach has the best chance for success in patients with anorexia who 1) have had the illness for less than 6 months, 2) are not bingeing and vomiting, and 3) have parents who are likely to cooperate and effectively participate in family therapy.

The more severely ill patient with anorexia may present an extremely difficult medical-management challenge and should be hospitalized and undergo daily monitoring of weight, food and calorie intake, and urine output. In the patient who is vomiting, frequent assessment of serum electrolytes is necessary. Behavior therapy is most effective in the medical management and nutritional rehabilitation of the patient with anorexia, although there are times when other target behaviors can be changed with this approach. Behavior therapy can be used in both outpatient and inpatient settings.

The operant conditioning paradigm has been the most effective form of behavior therapy for the treatment of anorexia nervosa. This can be used both in the context of a structured ward setting and in an individualized treatment program set up after a behavioral analysis of the patient has been completed. Positive reinforcements are used and consist of increased physical activity, visiting privileges, and social activities contingent on weight gain. An individual behavioral analysis may show other positive reinforcements to be more clinically relevant in the particular cases. The timing of reinforcement is important in behavior therapy. An adolescent patient needs at least a daily reinforcement for weight increase, which should be approximately 0.5 lb or 0.1 kg per day. Making positive reinforcements contingent only on weight gain is helpful in reducing the staff–patient arguments and stressful interactions concerning how and what the patient is eating, because

weight is an objective measure. In addition to being used to induce weight gain, behavior therapy can be used to stop vomiting. A response-prevention technique is used when bingeing and purging patients are required to stay in an observed dayroom area for 2–3 hours after every meal. Very few patients vomit in front of other people, and thus the emesis response is prevented and, eventually, stopped completely.

Cognitive therapy techniques for treating anorexia nervosa were developed by Garner and Bemis (1982). The assessment of cognition is a first step in cognitive therapy. Patients are asked to write down their thoughts on an assessment form so that cognitions can be examined for systematic distortions in the processing and interpretation of events. Cognitive techniques include operationalizing beliefs, decentering, using the "what if" technique, evaluating autonomic thoughts, testing prospective hypotheses, reinterpreting body image misperception, examining underlying assumptions, and modifying basic assumptions.

Cognitive-behavioral therapy (CBT) for prevention of relapse of anorexia nervosa was further developed by Kleifield et al. (1996), who created an easy-to-use treatment manual. The CBT is based on two core assumptions about the disorder. The first assumption is that anorexia nervosa has a significant positive functioning in the patient's life and develops as a way of coping with adverse experiences often associated with developmental transitions and distressing life events. The anorexic patient's deficient coping abilities produce anxiety and fear, and the patient is distracted from these anxieties by an overwhelming preoccupation with food and weight. The anorexic condition is also a reinforcing one in that the patient experiences a surge of confidence and a sense of competence and control after being successful in dieting. The second assumption is that food restriction and ritualistic food avoidance behaviors become independent of the events or issues provoking them. The anorexic patient's extreme anxiety about gaining weight and becoming fat is alleviated by not eating. The relief of anxiety about gaining weight—the anxiety being alleviated through avoidance of food—is another strong reinforcement and thus a key factor in the persistence with which these patients pursue food restriction.

On the basis of the aforementioned assumptions, two separate pathways are taken in treatment. First, the dietary restriction is regarded as a food phobia, and change in eating behavior is a primary objective. Behavioral methods such as monitoring food intake and the details surrounding food intake, along with techniques such as increasing exposure, are used to increase the patient's food intake gradually. Cognitive-behavioral methods are used to reduce the anxiety associated with behavioral change. Cognitive techniques such as cognitive restructuring and problem solving help the patient deal with distorted and overvalued beliefs about food and thinness and cope with life's stresses.

A family analysis should be done on all patients with anorexia who are living with their families. On the basis of this analysis, a clinical judgment should be made regarding what type of family therapy or counseling is clinically advisable. In some cases, family therapy will not be possible. However, in those cases, issues of family relationships must be dealt with in individual therapy and, in some cases, in brief counseling sessions with immediate family members. A controlled family therapy study by Russell et al. (1987) showed that patients with anorexia younger than 18 years benefited from family therapy and patients older than 18 years did worse in family therapy compared with the control therapy. A subsequent study by LeGrange et al. (1992) compared conjoint family therapy in which the whole family was treated together and a family counseling in which parents were treated separately from their daughter. Both treatments were brief, with an average of nine sessions over a 6-month period. The patients were adolescents, ages 12–17 years. A 32-week assessment showed that the two groups did not differ in their weight, which was in the normal range. A subsequent study with 40 patients replicated these results (Dare and Eisler 2002). Drugs can be useful adjuncts in the treatment of anorexia nervosa. The first drug used in treating anorexia was chlorpromazine. This medication is especially effective in patients with anorexia who are severely obsessive-compulsive. No controlled, double-blind study has been done to prove definitely the efficacy of chlorpromazine in inducing weight gain in persons with anorexia. This is surprising, given that it was the first drug used and was the preferred drug for most severely ill anorexic patients for many years, especially in Europe. More recently atypical antipsychotics have been studied in acutely ill anorexia nervosa patients. A 10-week open-label trial evaluating olanzapine showed 18 patients with anorexia nervosa received 10 mg/day. Four of the 18 patients dropped out, and 10 of the 14 patients who completed the study gained an average of 8.75 pounds; the other 4 lost a mean of 2.25 pounds. Olanzapine plasma levels showed that compliance seemed to affect outcome of weight gain. Those patients who lost weight had negligible levels of olanzapine (Powers et al. 2002). Case reports for risperidone show a positive outcome on weight gain.

Another category of drugs frequently used in the treatment of anorexia nervosa is the antidepressants. A double-blind study in which 72 patients with anorexia were randomly assigned to amitriptyline, cyproheptadine (an antihistaminic drug), and placebo therapy showed that both cyproheptadine and amitriptyline had a marginal effect in decreasing the number of days necessary to achieve a normal weight. Cyproheptadine had an unexpected antidepressant effect demonstrated by a significant decrease in scores on the Hamilton Rating Scale for Depression (Halmi et al. 1986). In the bulimic subgroups of patients with anorexia, cyproheptadine had a negative effect compared with both placebo and amitriptyline. This differential effect within the bulimic anorexic subgroups indicates a real medical distinction and appears to justify this subgrouping. Cyproheptadine has the advantage of not having the tricyclic antidepressant side effects of reducing blood pressure and increasing heart rate. This makes it especially attractive for use in emaciated individuals with anorexia.

Other drugs have been tested in patients with anorexia but have not had much of an effect. The results of small studies exploring the efficacy of fluoxetine and clomipramine suggest that both of these medications warrant further study (Crisp et al. 1987; Gwirtsman et al. 1990). Both fluoxetine and clomipramine are potent inhibitors of serotonin reuptake, and both have proven effective in OCD as well as depression. These medications may be effective in preventing relapse in anorexia nervosa. Because of certain side effects (anorexia and hyperactivity in fluoxetine therapy; hypotension and tachycardia in clomipramine therapy), special caution is necessary when these medications are given to underweight anorexic patients. At a 6- to 18-month follow-up of 31 patients who had been taking fluoxetine after inpatient weight restoration, 29 patients were found to have maintained their weight at or above 85% of average body weight (Kaye et al. 2001). In this study, restricting anorexic patients responded significantly better than did bulimic and purging-type anorexic patients. The authors judged the overall response to be good in 10 patients, partial in 17 patients, and poor in 4 patients.

Acceptance of treatment and relatively high dropout rates pose a major problem for research in the treatment of anorexia nervosa. In a study of 122 anorexia nervosa patients randomized to CBT, fluoxetine, or their combination for a 1-year treatment, the overall dropout rate was 46%. Treatment acceptance defined as staying in treatment for at least 5 weeks occurred in 73% of the randomized cases. Of the 41 patients assigned to medication alone, acceptance occurred in 56% and in the other two groups the acceptance rate was 81%. This study showed that anorexia nervosa patients will not accept medication unless it is combined with psychotherapy. Among patients who accepted treatment, those with high self-esteem were more likely than those with low self-esteem to complete treatment (Halmi et al. 2005).

A multifaceted treatment approach is necessary for effective care of patients with anorexia nervosa. As medical rehabilitation proceeds, an associated improvement in psychological state occurs. Behavioral contingencies are useful for inducing weight gain and changing the medical condition of the patient. Cyproheptadine may be helpful in facilitating weight gain and decreasing depressive symptomatology in the restricting anorexic patient. If an anorexic patient has a predominance of depressive symptoms and is within 80% of a normal weight range, fluoxetine should be useful for treating the depression.

Severely obsessive-compulsive, anxious, and agitated anorexic patients are likely to require chlorpromazine or an atypical antipsychotic medication such as risperidone or olanzapine. All patients need individual cognitive psychotherapy. The more severely ill patients need hospitalization initially, followed by a well-planned continued outpatient treatment program (Garner and Garfinkel 1985). Prevention of relapse is a major part of the treatment of anorexia nervosa. Family therapy is essential for children younger than 18 years of age and is equally effective in conjoint or separated format. Effectively treating adolescents before the age of 18 years is the best way to prevent chronic anorexia nervosa.

It is obvious that treating patients with chronic anorexia nervosa involves high rates of morbidity and mortality. Preventing the chronicity of anorexia nervosa should be a major aim. Focusing on early diagnosis and adequate treatment of the younger anorectic patient would be the best strategy to prevent chronic anorexia nervosa.

Bulimia Nervosa

Definition

Bulimia is a term that means "binge eating." This behavior has become a common practice among female students in universities and, more recently, in high schools. Not all persons who engage in binge eating require a psychiatric diagnosis. Bulimia can occur in anorexia nervosa; when this happens, the patient, under

---

TABLE 23–7. DSM-IV-TR diagnostic criteria for bulimia nervosa

A. Recurrent episodes of binge eating. An episode of binge eating is characterized by both of the following:

  (1) eating, in a discrete period of time (e.g., within any 2-hour period), an amount of food that is definitely larger than most people would eat during a similar period of time and under similar circumstances

  (2) a sense of lack of control over eating during the episode (e.g., a feeling that one cannot stop eating or control what or how much one is eating)

B. Recurrent inappropriate compensatory behavior in order to prevent weight gain, such as self-induced vomiting; misuse of laxatives, diuretics, enemas, or other medications; fasting; or excessive exercise.

C. The binge eating and inappropriate compensatory behaviors both occur, on average, at least twice a week for 3 months.

D. Self-evaluation is unduly influenced by body shape and weight.

E. The disturbance does not occur exclusively during episodes of anorexia nervosa.

Specify type:

  Purging type: during the current episode of bulimia nervosa, the person has regularly engaged in self-induced vomiting or the misuse of laxatives, diuretics, or enemas

  Nonpurging type: during the current episode of bulimia nervosa, the person has used other inappropriate compensatory behaviors, such as fasting or excessive exercise, but has not regularly engaged in self-induced vomiting or the misuse of laxatives, diuretics, or enemas

---

the DSM-IV-TR system, should have a diagnosis of *anorexia nervosa, binge-eating/purging type.* Bulimia also can occur in a normal-weight condition associated with psychological symptomatology. In that case, a diagnosis of *bulimia nervosa* applies (Table 23–7). Normal-weight bingeing and purging patients can fall into two categories: 1) normal-weight bulimic patients who have never had a history of anorexia nervosa and 2) those who have had a history of anorexia nervosa. Unfortunately, the DSM-IV-TR classification system does not separate these two subgroups of bulimic patients. The term *bulimia nervosa* implies a psychiatric impairment and therefore is a better label than simply *bulimia*.

Bulimia nervosa is a disorder in which the behavior of bulimia or binge eating is the predominant behavior. *Binge eating* is defined as an episodic, uncontrolled, rapid ingestion of large quantities of food over a short period. Abdominal pain or discomfort, self-induced vomiting, sleep, or social interruption terminates the bulimic episode. Feelings of guilt, depression, or self-disgust follow. Bulimic patients often use cathartics for weight control and have an eating pattern of alternate binges and fasts. Bulimic patients have a fear of not being able to stop eating voluntarily. The food consumed during a binge usually has a highly dense calorie content and a texture that facilitates rapid eating. Frequent weight fluctuations occur, but without the severity of weight loss present in anorexia nervosa.

Bulimia is also encountered in DSM-IV-TR *binge-eating disorder* (BED), which did not exist in DSM-III-R (American Psychiatric Association 1987). This disorder is listed as an example under the category "Eating Disorder Not Otherwise Specified" (Tables 23–8 and 23–9). Insufficient data are currently available to make BED a distinct Axis I diagnosis. Preliminary field studies show that most persons who meet criteria for BED are obese. In the next 5 years, epidemiological studies will determine whether BED is a distinct disorder or merely the nonpurging type of bulimia.

Clinical Features

Bulimia nervosa usually begins after a period of dieting of a few weeks to a year or longer. The dieting may or may not have been successful in achieving weight loss. Most binge-eating episodes are followed by self-induced vomiting. Episodes are less frequently followed by use of laxatives. A minority of bulimic patients use diuretics for weight control. The average length of a bingeing episode is about 1 hour. Most patients learn to vomit by sticking their fingers down their throat, and after a short time they learn to vomit on a reflex basis. Some patients have abrasions and scars on the backs of their hands (called *Russell's sign*) from their persistent efforts to induce vomiting. Most bulimic patients do not eat regular meals and have difficulty feeling satiety at the end of a normal meal. Bulimic patients usually prefer to eat alone and at their homes. Approximately one-third to one-fifth of bulimic patients will choose a weight within a normal weight range as their ideal body weight. About one-fourth to one-third of the patients with bulimia nervosa have had a history of anorexia nervosa.

Most bulimic patients have depressive signs and symptoms. They have problems with interpersonal re-

TABLE 23–8. DSM-IV-TR diagnostic criteria for eating disorder not otherwise specified

The eating disorder not otherwise specified category is for disorders of eating that do not meet the criteria for any specific eating disorder. Examples include

1. For females, all of the criteria for anorexia nervosa are met except that the individual has regular menses.

2. All of the criteria for anorexia nervosa are met except that, despite significant weight loss, the individual's current weight is in the normal range.

3. All of the criteria for bulimia nervosa are met except that the binge eating and inappropriate compensatory mechanisms occur at a frequency of less than twice a week or for a duration of less than 3 months.

4. The regular use of inappropriate compensatory behavior by an individual of normal body weight after eating small amounts of food (e.g., self-induced vomiting after the consumption of two cookies).

5. Repeatedly chewing and spitting out, but not swallowing, large amounts of food.

6. Binge-eating disorder: recurrent episodes of binge eating in the absence of the regular use of inappropriate compensatory behaviors characteristic of bulimia nervosa (see Table 23–9 for suggested research criteria).

lationships, self-concept, and impulsive behaviors and show high levels of anxiety and compulsivity. Chemical dependency is not unusual in this disorder, alcohol abuse being the most common. Bulimic persons will abuse amphetamines to reduce their appetite and to lose weight. Impulsive stealing usually occurs after the onset of binge eating; however, about one-fourth of patients actually begin stealing before the onset of bulimia. Food, clothing, and jewelry are the items most commonly stolen.

Medical Complications

Patients with bulimia nervosa who engage in self-induced vomiting and abuse purgatives or diuretics are susceptible to hypokalemic alkalosis. These patients have electrolyte abnormalities, including elevated serum bicarbonate levels, hypochloremia, hypokalemia, and, in a few cases, low serum bicarbonate levels indicating a metabolic acidosis. The latter is particularly true among individuals who abuse laxatives.

TABLE 23–9. DSM-IV-TR research criteria for binge-eating disorder

A. Recurrent episodes of binge eating. An episode of binge eating is characterized by both of the following:

    (1) eating, in a discrete period of time (e.g., within any 2-hour period), an amount of food that is definitely larger than most people would eat in a similar period of time under similar circumstances

    (2) a sense of lack of control over eating during the episode (e.g., a feeling that one cannot stop eating or control what or how much one is eating)

B. The binge-eating episodes are associated with three (or more) of the following:

    (1) eating much more rapidly than normal

    (2) eating until feeling uncomfortably full

    (3) eating large amounts of food when not feeling physically hungry

    (4) eating alone because of being embarrassed by how much one is eating

    (5) feeling disgusted with oneself, depressed, or very guilty after overeating

C. Marked distress regarding binge eating is present.

D. The binge eating occurs, on average, at least 2 days a week for 6 months.

    Note: The method of determining frequency differs from that used for bulimia nervosa; future research should address whether the preferred method of setting a frequency threshold is counting the number of days on which binges occur or counting the number of episodes of binge eating.

E. The binge eating is not associated with the regular use of inappropriate compensatory behaviors (e.g., purging, fasting, excessive exercise) and does not occur exclusively during the course of anorexia nervosa or bulimia nervosa.

It is important to remember that fasting can promote dehydration, which results in volume depletion. This can promote generation of aldosterone, which promotes further potassium excretion from the kidneys. Thus, there can be an indirect renal loss of potassium as well as a direct loss through self-induced vomiting. Patients with electrolyte disturbances have physical symptoms of weakness and lethargy and at times have cardiac arrhythmias. The latter, of course, can lead to a sudden cardiac arrest. Patients with bulimia nervosa can have severe attrition and erosion of the teeth, causing an irritating sensitivity, pathological pulp exposures, loss of integrity of the dental arches, diminished masticatory ability, and an unaesthetic appearance.

Parotid gland enlargement associated with elevated serum amylase levels is commonly observed in patients who binge and vomit. In fact, the serum amylase level is an excellent way to follow reduction of vomiting in patients with eating disorders who deny purging episodes. Acute dilatation of the stomach is a rare emergency condition for patients who binge. Esophageal tears also can occur through the process of self-induced vomiting. A complication of shock can result subsequent to the esophageal tear and should be treated by experienced medical and surgical personnel. Severe abdominal pain in the patient with bulimia nervosa should alert the physician to a diagnosis of gastric dilatation and the need for nasogastric suction, X-rays, and surgical consultation.

Cardiac failure caused by cardiomyopathy from ipecac intoxication is a medical emergency that is being reported more frequently and that usually results in death. Symptoms of precardial pain, dyspnea, and generalized muscle weakness associated with hypotension, tachycardia, and abnormalities on the electrocardiogram should alert one to possible ipecac intoxication. Other laboratory findings may include elevated liver enzymes and an increased erythrocyte sedimentation rate. Obviously, at this point the patient should be under a cardiologist's care. An echocardiogram will show a cardiomyopathy contraction pattern associated with congestive heart failure.

Other mechanisms for cardiac arrhythmias and sudden death in bulimic patients probably exist. The arrhythmias noted here are associated with electrolyte disturbances and ipecac intoxication. More recent studies have shown arrhythmias associated with bingeing behavior even when serum electrolytes are within normal limits.

A summary of medical complications of bulimia nervosa is presented in Table 23–10.

Epidemiology, Course, and Prognosis

There have been only a few incidence studies of bulimia nervosa. This is not surprising, given the fact that this disorder emerged only in 1980 as the distinct diagnostic entity presented in DSM-III (American Psychiatric Association 1980). The following studies have had an adequate sample size. Soundy et al. (1995) screened all medical records of health care providers, general

TABLE 23–10. Medical complications of bulimia nervosa

Behavioral and physical aberrations	Physiological disturbances
Binge eating	Acute dilatation of stomach—shock
Self-induced vomiting	Esophageal tears—shock; dehydration Metabolic alkalosis—hypochloremia, hypokalemia, weakness, lethargy Cardiac arrhythmias—cardiac arrest Erosion of dental enamel—caries, exposure of pulp
Parotid gland enlargement (self-induced vomiting or excessive gum chewing)	Elevated serum amylase
Ipecac use	Hypotension, tachycardia, electrocardiographic abnormalities, elevated liver enzymes

practitioners, and specialists in Rochester, Minnesota, over the period 1980–1990 for a clinical diagnosis of bulimia nervosa and found an annual incidence of 3.5 cases per 100,000 population. Hoek et al. (1995), using DSM-III-R criteria, examined a large general practice study representative of the population covering the period 1985–1989 in the Netherlands and found an annual incidence of 11.5 cases per 100,000 population. Turnbull et al. (1996) screened the United Kingdom general practice research database covering a large representative sample of English and Welsh population for bulimia nervosa in 1993 and found an annual incidence of 12.2 cases per 100,000 population. In DSM-III, bulimia nervosa was referred to as "bulimia," and the criteria did not allow one to distinguish between occasional binge-eating episodes and the truly incapacitating disorder of bulimia nervosa. The bulimia nervosa diagnostic criteria have been revised every few years, and this may account for the disparity in reported prevalence rates for this disorder. Studies that used strict criteria found prevalence rates between 1 and 3.8 per 100 females (Hart and Ollendick 1985; Schotte and Stunkard 1987). In a study combining surveys and in-

terviews of women in the first year of college, Kurth et al. (1995) found the prevalence of bulimia nervosa to be 2%. In a Canadian community sample in which a structured interview was used, prevalence rates of this disorder were 1% (Garfinkel et al. 1995). Hoek (1991) found a 1-year prevalence rate of bulimia nervosa of 0.17% among adolescent girls and young women 15–29 years of age in a primary care health delivery system. The prevalence of males in the bulimia nervosa population varies between 10% and 15%. In most studies, the average age at onset of bulimia nervosa is 18 years (range: 12–35 years). These studies have shown a much higher representation of the social classes IV and V (includes workers with low personal incomes and no college degrees and persons who drift in and out of poverty) in patients with bulimia nervosa compared with patients with anorexia nervosa.

Intervention studies on the prevention of eating disorders to date have not produced impressive results. Most studies have been designed to target and measure change on the individual level. Austin (2000) suggested that expecting children to develop resilience to unhealthy pressures may be a less successful strategy than making significant changes in the social environment. An example would be "a model of proactive primary prevention targeted at environmental change and cross-disciplinary collaboration with coronary heart disease, cancer and obesity prevention intervention research" (Austin 2000, p. 1252).

Combining the results of meta-analyses by Keel and Mitchell (1997) and Nielsen (2001) yields a corrected mortality rate for bulimia nervosa of 0.4% (11 deaths in 2,692 patients), which indicates that persons with bulimia nervosa have a 1.5 increase in mortality risk. Thus, little information is available on the natural course of this disorder and on outcome predictors.

Etiology and Pathogenesis

Fairburn and Cooper (1984) found that a rigid diet was the most commonly reported precipitant of binge-eating behavior and that a gross bingeing bout was the most common precipitant for vomiting behavior. This finding may shed some light on the physiological mechanisms involved in binge eating and purging. For example, the period of strict dieting may influence peptide and neurotransmitter secretion, which may in turn affect appetite and satiety mechanisms. Studies of satiety responses in patients with eating disorders have shown that the perceptions of hunger and satiety are disturbed in patients who binge and purge (Halmi and Sunday 1991). Another study showed distinct differences in taste preferences for sweetness and "fattiness" in restricting anorexic patients, bulimic anorexic patients, normal-weight bulimic patients, and control subjects (Sunday and Halmi 1990). Further identification of disturbances in the psychological processes of hunger, satiety, and taste could provide important clues concerning impaired central mechanisms. Evidence for dysregulation of serotonergic neurotransmission in bulimia nervosa consists of blunted prolactin response to the serotonin receptor agonist *meta*-chlorophenylpiperazine (*m*-CPP), 5-hydroxytryptophan, and *dl*-fenfluramine and enhanced migraine-like headache response to *m*-CPP challenge. Low levels of CSF 5-hydroxyindoleacetic acid are associated with impulsive and aggressive behaviors and are also present in bulimia nervosa patients (Jimerson et al. 1997; Levitan et al. 1997). In a large interview study by Braun et al. (1994), 31% of the bulimic subgroups had a Cluster B (impulsive) disorder. Borderline personality disorder was present in 25% of the bulimic subgroups and was the most common Cluster B condition.

Studies of recovered bulimia nervosa women (Kaye et al. 2001), using PET [^{18}F] altanserin, a specific 5-HT$_{2A}$ receptor antagonist, found a significant reduction in bilateral medial orbital frontal cortex 5-HT$_{2A}$ binding. These data provide further evidence for serotonergic dysregulation in bulimia nervosa.

In a study of clinical features, Hatsukami et al. (1984) found that 43.5% of a sample of 108 women with bulimia nervosa had an affective disorder at some time in their lives, and 18.5% had a history of alcohol or drug abuse. Although there is a high association of mood disorder with bulimia nervosa, insufficient current evidence is available to support describing bulimia nervosa as a mere *forme fruste* of mood disorder. Bulimia nervosa theoretically fits well into an addictive model (Szmukler and Tantam 1984).

A study that used the Minnesota Multiphasic Personality Inventory to compare women with bulimia nervosa with women who abused alcohol and drugs found that the two groups had similar profiles. They had elevations on the scales denoting depression, impulsivity, anger, rebelliousness, anxiety, rumination, social withdrawal, and idiosyncratic thinking (Hatsukami et al. 1982). Two studies that used the Social Adjustment Scale found that women with bulimia nervosa were significantly worse in all areas of adjustment (work, social, and leisure activities; relationship with extended family; role as spouse; role as parent; and membership in a family unit) than were women in a control sample (Johnson and Berndt 1983; Norman and Herzog 1984). These findings remained stable after 1 year. These latter studies indicate that one might

expect to find a higher prevalence of Axis II DSM-IV-TR diagnoses in the patients with bulimia nervosa than in a normal population.

The percentage of individuals with DSM-III-R bulimia (including anorexic bulimic individuals) who have at least one personality disorder has been reported to be 77% (Powers et al. 1988), 69% (Wonderlich et al. 1990), 62% (Gartner et al. 1989), 61% (Schmidt and Telch 1990), 33% (Ames-Frankel et al. 1992), and 23% (Herzog et al. 1992). All of these studies used established diagnostic interviews, but the findings are not in agreement. This is probably a result of several factors: 1) some of the studies with very small numbers of patients may represent a biased sample; 2) studies used different criteria, ranging from DSM-III to DSM-III-R, for both eating disorders and personality disorders; and 3) some of the Axis II interviewers lacked information about the patients' Axis I diagnosis, which may have led to false-positive personality disorder diagnoses. Nonetheless, substantial evidence indicates that personality disorders are commonly associated with bulimia nervosa.

A study determining coherent groupings of personality profiles of bulimia and anorexia patients was conducted by psychiatrists and psychologists who used a Q-sort procedure. With a cluster-analytic procedure, three categories of patients emerged: 1) a high functioning–perfectionistic group, 2) a constricted-overcontrolled group, and 3) an emotionally dysregulated–undercontrolled group. These categorizations were significantly effective in predicting eating disorder symptoms (Westen and Harden-Fischer 2001). Thus, personality patterns may account for meaningful variations within eating disorder diagnoses.

There is substantial literature that shows bulimia nervosa is strongly familial (Lilenfeld et al. 1998; Strober et al. 2000) and that this familiality is due largely to the additive effects of genes (Bulik et al. 2000). A linkage study of multiplex families with eating disorders that were identified through a proband with bulimia nervosa showed the highest multipoint logarithm of odds score observed (3.39) was on chromosome 10. This is evidence of the presence of a susceptibility locus for bulimia nervosa on chromosome 10p (Bulik et al. 2002). The next stage of research indicated will be to explore likely candidate genes under the observed linkage peak.

Treatment

Treatment studies of bulimia nervosa have proliferated in the past 15 years, in contrast to the relatively few treatment studies of anorexia nervosa. This is probably because of the greater prevalence of bulimia nervosa and the fact that this disorder usually can be treated on an outpatient basis. Specific therapy techniques such as behavior therapy, cognitive therapy, psychodynamic therapy, and "psychoeducation therapy" have been conducted in both individual and group formats (Table 23–11). There are no controlled studies in which patients were randomly assigned to individual or group therapy for any of these techniques. Multiple controlled drug treatment studies also have been conducted in the past decade. Often a variety of therapy techniques such as cognitive therapy, behavior therapy, and drug treatment may be used together in either individual or group therapy. Unfortunately, there is no way to predict at present what bulimic patient will respond to what type of therapy or treatment. The American Psychiatric Association (2000b) revised practice guideline for the treatment of patients with eating disorders has a helpful section on developing a treatment plan for the individual patient. Factors that need to be considered are level of care (outpatient, intensive outpatient, partial hospitalization, residential treatment center, or inpatient hospitalization), site of treatment (availability of medical care), and family assessment and treatment.

Psychodynamic Therapy

Lacey (1983) described the use of psychodynamic therapy with cognitive and behavioral techniques in both individual and group therapy formats. Common themes that need to be dealt with are poor self-esteem, dependency problems, and a sense of ineffectiveness.

Cognitive-Behavioral Therapy

Fourteen published controlled studies have examined the efficacy of CBT in bulimia nervosa. One of the first and best descriptions of CBT was by Fairburn (1981). All of the subjects in these 14 studies were outpatients, with the exception of one study of the effectiveness of CBT in individual therapy that involved inpatients. Nearly all of the studies used a psychoeducational component that included information on the social-cultural emphasis on thinness; set point theory; the physical effects and medical complications of bingeing, purging, and abuse of laxatives and diuretics; and how dieting and fasting precipitate binge–purge cycles. Self-monitoring was an important part of all of these studies and usually consisted of a daily record of the times and durations of meals and a record of binge-eating and purging episodes as well as descriptions of moods and circumstances surrounding binge–purge episodes. The

studies stressed the importance of eating regular meals.

Cognitive restructuring is the basis of all the CBT programs. The first step in cognitive therapy is the assessment of cognition. Patients are asked to write their thoughts on an assessment form so that cognitions can be examined for systematic distortions in the processing and interpretation of events. Two reviews of controlled studies of CBT for bulimia nervosa concluded that CBT benefits most patients (Fairburn et al. 1992a; Gotestam and Agras 1989). CBT was more effective than treatment with antidepressants alone, self-monitoring plus supportive psychotherapy, and behavioral treatment without the cognitive treatment component. One-year follow-up studies with CBT have shown a good maintenance of change superior to that following treatment with antidepressants.

Behavior therapy is used specifically to stop the binge-eating/purging behaviors. Behavioral approaches include restricting exposure to cues that trigger a binge–purge episode, developing a strategy of alternative behaviors, and delaying the vomiting response to eating. Response prevention is a technique used specifically to prevent vomiting. After eating, a patient is placed in a situation in which it is very difficult for him or her comfortably to vomit. Adding exposure (i.e., requiring the patient to binge) did not seem to enhance the effects of response prevention (Rosen 1982).

The combined effects of CBT and antidepressant medication for bulimia nervosa were examined in three studies. Mitchell et al. (1990) found that group CBT was superior to imipramine therapy for decreasing binge eating and purging, and the combined treatment showed no additive effects for those treated with group CBT alone. Agras et al. (1992) had similar results comparing individual CBT, desipramine therapy, and the combination at 16 weeks. However, at 32 weeks, only the combined treatment given for 24 weeks was superior to medication given for 16 weeks. In a third study, CBT plus medication (desipramine, followed by fluoxetine in nonresponders) was superior to medication alone, but supportive psychotherapy plus medication was not. CBT plus medication was superior to CBT alone.

A study of interpersonal therapy (IPT), which targets interpersonal functioning, showed that IPT was equivalent to CBT in reducing bulimic symptoms and psychopathology; at follow-up, it was actually superior to CBT (Fairburn et al. 1992b). This was the first study to show that bulimia nervosa may be treated successfully without focusing directly on the patient's eating habits and attitudes toward shape and weight. In a multisite study comparing CBT with IPT, bulimic pa-

TABLE 23–11. Treatment of bulimia nervosa

Type of treatment	Indications	Measurements	Key elements
Cognitive-behavioral therapy (CBT)			
Group	Outpatients—young adults	Psychiatric and medical evaluations before entering therapy	Psychoeducational component on all aspects of the bulimic disorder
Individual	Inpatients; outpatients—adolescents and adults with severe character disorders	Self-recording of medical consultations available throughout treatment	Self-monitoring, cognitive restructuring
Behavior therapy	Usually used in conjunction with computed tomography	Same as for CBT	Restricting exposure to cues, developing alternative behaviors, response prevention to stop vomiting
Interpersonal therapy	Outpatients—young adults	Psychiatric and medical evaluations before entering therapy and consultation available during treatment	Focuses on interpersonal relationships
Pharmacotherapy			
Antidepressants Fluoxetine Desipramine Imipramine Nortriptyline	Binge-eating behavior, depression, unwillingness to enter CBT	Initial evaluation: complete blood count, serum electrolytes and amylase, electrocardiogram, blood pressure; repeat above after 1 week and then as often as clinically indicated	Antidepressant drugs affect catecholamine and indoleamine function, which modulates eating behavior

tients had 19 sessions of treatment over a 20-week period and were evaluated for 1 year after treatment. CBT was significantly superior to IPT at the end of treatment for the number of participants recovered (29% vs. 6%). At a 1-year follow-up, no significant difference was found between the two treatments. However, CBT was significantly more rapid in initiating improvement in patients with bulimia nervosa compared with IPT. Therefore, the authors suggested that CBT should be considered the preferred psychotherapeutic treatment for bulimia nervosa (Agras et al. 2000).

A multicenter treatment study that used a sequential design, which more realistically represents the practice of treating bulimia nervosa by primary care physicians, showed those patients who failed to respond to CBT and were randomized to either IPT or fluoxetine improved equally in both treatments. However, only 20% of these patients in each form of treatment became abstinent, which is not a very impressive figure (Mitchell et al. 2002). One study showed that in-dividuals with bulimia nervosa who did not respond to or had relapsed following CBT or IPT had a significantly better response to fluoxetine compared with placebo (Walsh et al. 2000). In the next 3–4 years, these studies will yield some very useful data to aid in the decisions about what kind of therapy should be given to which patients.

Drug Therapy

Studies of antidepressant medications have consistently shown some efficacy in the treatment of bulimia nervosa. These studies were prompted by observations that patients with bulimia nervosa also had significant mood disturbances. Since 1980, more than a dozen double-blind, placebo-controlled trials of various antidepressants were conducted in normal-weight outpatients with bulimia nervosa. (For a review of these studies, see Fairburn et al. 1992a.) All of these trials found a significantly greater reduction in binge eating when antidepressant medication was administered than when placebo was given. Antidepressants improved mood and reduced psychopathological symptoms such as preoccupation with shape and weight. These studies provide evidence for the short-term efficacy of antidepressant medication, but long-term efficacy remains unknown. The average rate of abstinence from bingeing and purging in these studies was 22%, indicating that most patients remain symptomatic at the end of treatment with antidepressants. Both of the systematic studies conducted to evaluate maintenance of change in bulimic symptomatology yielded disappointing results: most subjects did not maintain improvement (Pyle et al. 1990; Walsh et al. 1991). The dosage of antidepressant medication to treat bulimia nervosa was similar to that used in the treatment of depression. The antidepressants used in the controlled-treatment studies of bulimia nervosa included desipramine, imipramine, amitriptyline, nortriptyline, phenelzine, and fluoxetine. It should be noted that bulimic patients are impulsive and cannot follow diets; therefore, the drug phenelzine should not be used to treat binge eating in bulimia nervosa patients. There have been several deaths in bulimic patients who were treated with this drug. Topiramate, an antiepileptic agent, was shown in a placebo-controlled, double-blind trial to be effective in reducing binge–purge behavior in BED (McElroy et al. 2003), and more recently studies have been under way with topiramate in treating bulimia nervosa.

The current data suggest that the treatment of choice for bulimia nervosa should be CBT and that a single antidepressant administered in the absence of psychotherapy cannot be considered an adequate treatment.

Obesity

Definition

In contrast to anorexia nervosa and bulimia nervosa, obesity is classified not as a psychiatric disorder but as a medical disorder. Obesity is an excessive accumulation of body fat and operationally is defined as overweight. The BMI, defined as weight (kg)/height (m²), has the highest correlation, 0.8, with body fat measured by other, more precise laboratory methods. *Mild overweight* is defined as a BMI of 25–30 or body weight between the upper limit of normal and 20% above that limit on standard height–weight charts. *Obesity* is defined as a BMI greater than 30 or body weight greater than 20% above the upper limit for height (Bray 1978; see Figure 23–1).

Clinical Features

The most obvious clinical features of obesity are physical; these features are discussed in the section on "Medical Complications" that follows. The psychological and behavioral aspects of obesity are best considered grouped in two categories: *eating behavior* and *emotional disturbance.* There is considerable heterogeneity in eating patterns. Most commonly, obese persons complain that they cannot restrain their eating and that they have difficulty achieving satiety. Some obese persons cannot distinguish hunger from other dysphoric states and will eat when they are emotionally upset.

The most methodologically satisfying studies have shown that there is no distinct or excess psychopathology in obesity. In one study of severely obese patients who had gastric bypass surgery, the most prevalent psychiatric diagnosis was major depressive disorder. However, this diagnosis was no more prevalent in the obese patients than in the general population. Self-disparagement of body image is especially present in those who have been obese since childhood. This may be due to the continual bombardment of social prejudice against obese people. The stigmatization and prejudice against obese types are well documented in studies of educational disadvantages and of employment prejudices against obese persons. Many obese individuals develop anxiety and depression when they attempt to diet (Halmi et al. 1980). Because health risks and mortality vary with degree of adiposity, Bray (1986) proposed a classification into low-risk (BMI = 25–30), moderate-risk (BMI = 31–40), and high-risk (BMI > 40) individuals.

Medical Complications

Obesity affects a great variety of physiological functions (Table 23–12). Blood circulation may be overtaxed as body weight increases, and congestive heart failure may occur in grossly obese individuals. Hypertension is strongly associated with obesity, and the prevalence of carbohydrate intolerance in grossly obese subjects is approximately 50%. Increased body fat in the upper region of the body as opposed to the lower region is more likely to be associated with the onset of diabetes mellitus. The impairment of pulmonary function becomes extreme in severe obesity and involves hypoventilation, hypercapnia, hypoxia, and somnolence (i.e., pickwickian syndrome). The latter syndrome has a high mortality rate. Obesity may accelerate the development of osteoarthritis and of dermatological problems from stretching of the skin, intertrigo, and acanthosis nigricans. Obese women are

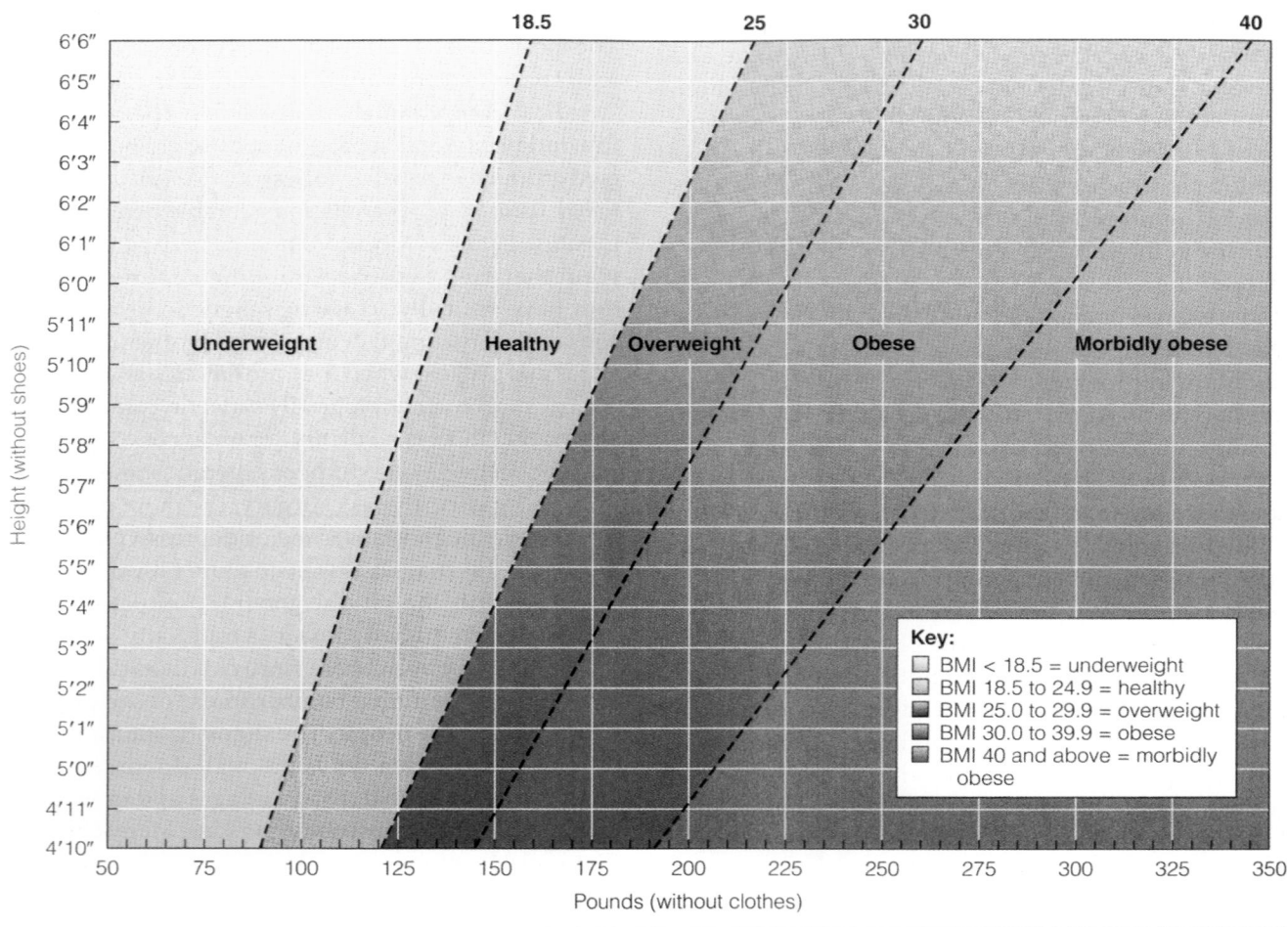

FIGURE 23–1. Body mass index values used to assess weight for adults.

Source. Reprinted from *An Invitation to Health* (with ThomsonNOW(T) and InfoTrac(R) 1-Semester Printed Access Card), 12th Edition, by Hales, Dianne. 2007. Used with permission of Brooks/Cole, a division of Thomson Learning: www.thomson-rights.com. Fax 800-730-2215.

TABLE 23–12. **Medical complications of obesity**

Insulin resistance

Glucose intolerance

Type 2 diabetes

Low high-density lipoprotein cholesterol

High triglycerides

Elevated blood pressure

Inflammation

Endothelial dysfunction

Susceptibility to thrombosis

Increased incidence of cardiovascular disease

Increased mortality

an obstetrical risk, being susceptible to toxemia and hypertension.

Obesity has been associated with several types of cancer. Obese males have a higher rate of prostate and colorectal cancer, and obese females have increased incidences of gallbladder, breast, cervical, endometrial, uterine, and ovarian cancer. Most studies on the topic suggest that obesity influences the development and progression of both endometrial and breast cancer through influences on estrogen production. Low-density lipoprotein levels are increased in obesity, and levels of high-density lipoproteins (high-density lipoprotein cholesterol) are reduced. The low levels of high-density lipoproteins may be one mechanism by which obesity is associated with an increased risk for cardiovascular disease.

Epidemiology, Course, and Prognosis

If obesity is defined as the state of being 20% above ideal weight, then nearly a quarter of the U.S. population would be considered obese (VanItallie 1985). Socioeconomic status is highly correlated with obesity: the condition is much more common among women (less so among men) of low status. This relationship is also present in obese children. Increasing age and obesity are associated until age 50 years. The prevalence of obesity is higher in women compared with men; in those older than 50 years, this may be due to the increased mortality rate among obese men with advancing age.

Unfortunately, life expectancy and obesity studies are restricted to life insurance studies and therefore do not represent a random American population. Despite these limitations, studies have shown a progressive increase in "excess mortality" as BMI increased (Society of Actuaries 1992). Another study of grossly obese persons showed that excess mortality was greatly increased in younger men (ages 25–34 years) and gradually declined with age (Stevens et al. 1998).

Etiology and Pathogenesis

It is unlikely that obesity has a single etiology. In the first section of this chapter, the complex neural mechanisms involved in the control of feeding behavior were discussed. Lipid, amino acid, and glucose metabolism all seem to affect, in some way, central neural regulatory mechanisms that influence eating behavior. Obesity is regarded today by most investigators as a disorder of energy balance, a disorder with a strong genetic component that is modulated by cultural and environmental influences (Flegal et al. 2002).

Obesity has a definite familial aspect. Eighty percent of the offspring of two obese parents are obese, compared with 40% of the offspring of one obese parent and only 10% of the offspring of lean parents. Findings of twin and adoption studies suggest that genetic factors play a strong role in the development of obesity.

The cloning and sequencing of the mouse obese (*Ob*) gene and its human homologue in 1994 (Zhang et al. 1994) provided the basis for further research into the pathways that regulate adiposity and body weight. Leptin, the gene product of the *Ob* gene, was shown to be a 16-kd protein that is present in mouse and human plasma (Halaas et al. 1995). Intraperitoneal injections of recombinant leptin decrease food intake and increase energy expenditure in wild-type mice. Leptin reduces body fat in mice, and its absence in mice with the *Ob* gene leads to a massive increase in body fat. In both humans and rodents, leptin is highly correlated with BMI and amount of body fat (Maffei et al. 1995). Weight loss due to food restriction was associated with a decrease in plasma leptin concentrations in mice and obese humans. These data suggest that leptin serves an endocrine function, regulating body weight and stores of body fat.

Obese persons have larger and more numerous fat cells. Cellular proliferation tends to occur early in life but also will occur in adult life when the existing fat cells are greatly enlarged. The regulation of fat cell proliferation and size is not well understood. The relation of physical activity to obesity is complex. It is known that obese people are less active than people of normal weight. The increase in caloric expenditure by physical activity is small. Animal studies show that physical activity actually decreases food intake and may actually prevent the decline in metabolic rate that usually accompanies dieting.

Treatment

For mild obesity (20%–40% overweight), the most efficient treatment to date is behavioral modification in groups, a balanced diet, and exercise. This is usually done by both commercial and nonprofit large organizations. For moderate obesity (41%–100% overweight), a medically supervised protein-sparing modified fast (400–700 calories per day) is often necessary. This diet may or may not be combined with behavioral modification techniques. A behavior analysis is necessary to set up a sensible behavioral modification program. Antecedents of eating behavior, the eating behavior itself, the consequences of the behavior, and the acceptable rewards for carrying out various prescribed behaviors are all analyzed. Behavioral treatment programs include self-monitoring, nutrition education, physical activity, and cognitive restructuring.

The use of medication such as phenylpropanolamine or fenfluramine was popular in the past. The problem with these drugs is that on withdrawal, a rebound ballooning up of weight occurs; some patients have concomitant lethargy and depression. In 1997, fenfluramine was removed from the market by the U.S. Food and Drug Administration for treatment of obesity because of the adverse effects of pulmonary hypertension and mitral valve impairment.

Only one long-term (5 years) controlled study has documented the safety and efficacy of the fenfluramine–phentermine combination (Weintraub 1992). The National Task Force on the Prevention and Treatment of Obesity (1996) reviewed all English-language reports of studies in which human obesity was treated with medication that was given for at least 24 weeks. The task force found that the net weight loss attributable to medication use was modest, ranging from 2 kg to 10 kg. The weight loss tended to reach a plateau by 6 months. Most adverse effects were mild and self-limited, but rare serious outcomes such as pulmonary hypertension have been reported. The task force's conclusion was that pharmacotherapy for obesity, when combined with appropriate behavioral approaches to change diet and amount of physical activity, helps some obese patients lose weight and maintain weight loss for at least 1 year (National Task Force on the Prevention and Treatment of Obesity 1996). The task force also stated that until more data are available, pharmacotherapy cannot be recommended for routine use in obese individuals. They did acknowledge that it may be helpful in carefully selected patients.

Severe obesity (more than 100% above a normal weight) is the least common form of obesity and is most effectively treated by surgical procedures that reduce the size of the stomach. These procedures produce a large weight loss and show a good record of weight loss maintenance.

Behavioral modification is the treatment of choice for overweight children and should include involvement of the parents and the schools. Psychotherapy is not recommended as a treatment per se for obesity, although some patients may have particular problems that may be effectively treated or helped with psychotherapy. For excellent discussions on the treatment of obesity, see Brownell (1984), Lasagna (1987), and Stunkard (1984).

Conclusion

The eating disorders are complex syndromes in which the interactions among environmental, psychological, and physiological factors both create and maintain the disturbed eating behavior. The more precise an understanding we obtain of the connectedness of basic physiological changes, psychological changes, and eating behavior, the better we will be able to design effective treatment interventions.

Many questions remain to be asked about our current treatment interventions. For example, how long should the bulimic patient be treated with antidepressants? Would periodic follow-up behavioral sessions prevent relapse in bulimic patients treated with behavior therapy? How can we identify the most likely effective treatment for a patient?

Continued prospective longitudinal studies are necessary for bulimia nervosa, because no information is available on what happens to this addictive-like bingeing–purging behavior over the course of a lifetime. Although disturbed eating behavior has been present throughout the history of humankind, it has been systematically studied with scientific methodology only in the past few decades. There is a continued need for further study of eating disorders.

Key Points

- Chronic anorexia nervosa is best prevented by early diagnosis and early intensive treatment.

- Adolescents with anorexia nervosa are most effectively treated with family therapy, either conjoint or with separate parental counseling.

- CBT specific for bulimia is the most effective treatment for bulimia nervosa.

- Serotonin reuptake inhibitors are effective in reducing bingeing episodes and have a more benign side-effect profile compared with tricyclic antidepressants.

- Obesity is a complex medical disorder with no single etiology. There is no guaranteed effective treatment over time. Behavioral modification is the treatment of choice for overweight children.

Suggested Readings

Bailer UF, Kaye WH: A review of neuropeptide and neuroendocrine dysregulation in anorexia and bulimia nervosa. Curr Drug Targets CNS Neurol Disord 2:53–59, 2003

Bensimhon DR, Kraus WE, Donahue MP: Obesity and physical activity: a review. Am Heart J 151:598–603, 2006

Halmi KA, Agras S, Crow S, et al: Predictors of treatment acceptance and completion in anorexia nervosa. Arch Gen Psychiatry 62:1–6, 2005

Kaye W, Strober M, Jimmerson D: The neurobiology of eating disorders, in The Neurobiology of Mental Illness. Edited by Charney DF, Nestler EJ. New York, Oxford University Press, 2004, pp 1112–1128

Maj M, Halmi K, Lopez-Ibor JJ, et al (eds): Eating Disorders. Chichester, England, Wiley, 2003

References

Agras WS, Rossiter EM, Arnow B, et al: Pharmacological and cognitive-behavioral treatment for bulimia nervosa: a controlled comparison. Am J Psychiatry 149:82–87, 1992

Agras WS, Walsh BT, Fairburn CG: A multicenter comparison of cognitive-behavioral therapy and interpersonal psychotherapy for bulimia nervosa. Arch Gen Psychiatry 57:459–466, 2000

Ahima RS, Prabakarn D, Mantzoros C, et al: Role of leptin in the neuroendocrine response to fasting. Nature 382:250–252, 1996

American Psychiatric Association: Diagnostic and Statistical Manual of Mental Disorders, 3rd Edition. Washington, DC, American Psychiatric Association, 1980

American Psychiatric Association: Diagnostic and Statistical Manual of Mental Disorders, 3rd Edition, Revised. Washington, DC, American Psychiatric Association, 1987

American Psychiatric Association: Diagnostic and Statistical Manual of Mental Disorders, 4th Edition, Text Revision. Washington, DC, American Psychiatric Association, 2000a

American Psychiatric Association: Practice guideline for the treatment of patients with eating disorders (revision). Am J Psychiatry 157 (suppl):1–39, 2000b

Ames-Frankel J, Devlin MJ, Walsh BT, et al: Personality disorders and eating disorders. J Clin Psychiatry 53:90–96, 1992

Austin B: Prevention research in eating disorders: theory and new directions. Psychol Med 30:1249–1262, 2000

Bailer U, Frank G, Henry S, et al: Altered brain serotonin $5HT_{1A}$ receptor binding after recovery from anorexia nervosa measured by positron emission tomography and [carbonyl^{11}C] WAY-100635. Arch Gen Psychiatry 62:1032–1041, 2005

Barr LC, Goodman WK, Price LH, et al: The serotonin hypothesis of obsessive compulsive disorder: implications of pharmacological challenge studies. Clin Psychiatry 53:17–28, 1992

Bell RM: Holy Anorexia. Chicago, IL, University of Chicago Press, 1985

Ben-Tovin D, Walker K, Gilchrist P: Outcome in patients with eating disorders: a 5 year study. Lancet 357:1254–1257, 2001

Bergen AW, van Den Bree M, Yeager M, et al: Candidate genes for anorexia nervosa in the 1p33–36 linkage region: serotonin 1D and delta opioid receptor loci exhibit significant association to anorexia nervosa. Mol Psychiatry 8:397–406, 2003

Blundell JE, Hill A: Behavioral pharmacology of feeding: relevance of animal experiments for studies in man, in Pharmacology of Eating Disorders. Edited by Carruba M, Blundell J. New York, Raven, 1986, pp 51–70

Boden G, Chen X, Mazzoli M, et al: Effect of fasting on serum leptin in normal subjects. J Clin Endocrinol Metab 81:3419–3423, 1996

Bohus B, Kovacs GL, de Wied D: Oxytocin, vasopressin and memory: opposite effects on consolidation and retrieval processes. Brain Res 157:414–417, 1978

Booth DA: Food-conditioned eating preferences and aversions with interceptive elements: conditioned appetite and satieties. Ann N Y Acad Sci 443:22–41, 1985

Brambilla F, Bellodi L, Arancio C, et al: Central dopaminergic function in anorexia and bulimia nervosa: a psychoneuroendocrine approach. Psychoneuroendocrinology 26:393–409, 2001

Braun DL, Sunday SR, Halmi KA: Psychiatric comorbidity in patients with eating disorders. Psychol Med 24:859–867, 1994

Bray GA: Definition, measurement and classification of the syndromes of obesity. Int J Obesity 2:99–112, 1978

Bray GA: Effects of obesity on health and happiness, in Handbook of Eating Disorders: Physiology, Psychology, and Treatment. Edited by Brownell KD, Foreyt JP. New York, Basic Books, 1986, pp 3–44

Brownell KD: New developments in the treatment of obese children and adolescents, in Eating and Its Disorders. Edited by Stunkard AJ, Stellar E. New York, Raven, 1984, pp 175–184

Bruch H: Perceptual and conceptual disturbance in anorexia nervosa. Psychosom Med 24:187–195, 1962

Bulik C, Sullivan PE, Wade T: Twin studies of eating disorders: a review. Int J Eat Disord 27:1–20, 2000

Bulik C, Devlin B, Bacanu S, et al: Significant linkage on chromosome 10p in families with bulimia nervosa. Am J Hum Gent 72:200–207, 2002

Charney DS, Wood SW, Krystal JH, et al: Serotonin function and human anxiety disorders. Ann NY Acad Sci 600:558–573, 1990

Chen H, Charlat O, Tartaglia LA, et al: Evidence that the diabetes gene encodes the leptin receptor: identification of a mutation in the leptin receptor gene in the DB/DB mice. Cell 84:491–495, 1996

Considine RV, Sinha MK, Heiman ML, et al: Serum immunoreactive-leptin concentrations in normal-weight and obese humans. N Engl J Med 334:292–295, 1996

Crisp AH: The possible significance of some behavioral correlates of weight and carbohydrate intake. J Psychosom Res 11:117–123, 1976

Crisp AH, Palmer RL, Kalucy RS, et al: How common is anorexia nervosa? A prevalence study. Br J Psychiatry 128:549–552, 1976

Crisp AH, Lacey JH, Crutchfield M: Clomipramine and "drive" in people with anorexia nervosa: an inpatient study. Br J Psychiatry 150:355–358, 1987

Cummings DE, Purnell JQ, Frayo RS, et al: A preprandial rise in plasma ghrelin levels suggest a role in meal initiation in humans. Diabetes 50:1714–1719, 2001

Dare C, Eisler I: Family therapy and eating disorders, in Eating Disorders and Obesity. Edited by Fairburn CG, Bronell KD. New York, Guilford, 2002, pp 314–319

Demitrack MA, Kalogeras KT, Altemus M, et al: Plasma and cerebrospinal fluid measures of arginine vasopressin secretion in patients with bulimia nervosa and in healthy subjects. J Clin Endocrinol Metab 74:1277–1283, 1992

Devlin B, Bacanu SA, Klump K et al: Linkage analysis of anorexia nervosa incorporating behavioral covariates. Hum Mol Genet 11:689–696, 2002

Eagles T, Johnston M, Hunter D, et al: Increasing incidence of anorexia nervosa in the female population of northeast Scotland. Am J Psychiatry 152:1266–1271, 1995

Eison AS, Mullins UL: Regulation of central 5-HT$_{2A}$ receptors: a review of in vivo studies. Behav Brain Res 73:177–181, 1996

Fairburn C: A cognitive behavioral approach to the treatment of bulimia. Psychol Med 11:707–711, 1981

Fairburn CG, Cooper PJ: The clinical features of bulimia nervosa. Br J Psychiatry 144:238–246, 1984

Fairburn CG, Agra WS, Wilson GT: The research on the treatment of bulimia nervosa: practical and theoretical implications, in Biology of Feast and Famine: Relevance to Eating Disorders. Edited by Anderson GH, Kennedy SH. New York, Academic Press, 1992a, pp 318–340

Fairburn CG, Jones R, Pevelar RC, et al: Three psychological treatments for bulimia nervosa: a comparative trial. Arch Gen Psychiatry 48:463–469, 1992b

Falk JR, Halmi KA: Amenorrhea in anorexia nervosa: examination of the critical body hypothesis. Biol Psychiatry 17:799–806, 1982

Flegal KM, Carroll MD, Ogden CL, et al: Prevalence and trends in obesity among U.S. adults. JAMA 288:1723–1727, 2002

Frank G, Bailer U, Henry S, et al: Increased dopamine D2/D3 receptor binding after recovery from anorexia nervosa measured by positron emission tomography and [11C] raclopride. Biol Psychiatry 5:1–5, 2005

Garfinkel P, Goering L, Spegg C, et al: Bulimia nervosa in a Canadian community sample: prevalence and comparison of subgroups. Am J Psychiatry 52:1052–1058, 1995

Garner DM, Bemis KM: A cognitive-behavioral approach to anorexia nervosa. Cognit Ther Res 6:1223–1250, 1982

Garner DM, Garfinkel PE: Handbook of Psychotherapy for Anorexia Nervosa. New York, Guilford, 1985

Gartner AF, Marcus RN, Halmi KA, et al: DSM-III-R personality disorders in patients with eating disorders. Am J Psychiatry 146:1585–1591, 1989

Gibbs J, Smith GP: Satiety hormones, in Frontiers in Neuroendocrinology, Vol 8. Edited by Martini L, Gonong W. New York, Raven, 1984, pp 98–132

Gold PW, Gwirtsman H, Kaye W, et al: Pathophysiological mechanisms in underweight and weight corrected patients. N Engl J Med 314:335–342, 1986

Gotestam KA, Agras WS: Bulimia nervosa: pharmacological and psychological approaches to treatment. Nordisk Psykiatrisk Tidsskrift 43:543–551, 1989

Grahame-Smith DG: Serotonin in affective disorders. Int Clin Psychopharmacol 6 (suppl):5–13, 1992

Grice D, Halmi KA, Fichter MM, et al: Evidence for a susceptibility gene for anorexia nervosa on chromosome 1. Am J Hum Gent 70:787–792, 2002

Gualillo O, Caminos JE, Nogueiras R, et al: Effective food restriction on ghrelin in normal-cycling female rats and in pregnancy. Obes Res 10:682–687, 2002

Gwirtsman HE, Guze BH, Yager J, et al: Fluoxetine treatment of anorexia nervosa: an open trial. J Clin Psychiatry 51:378–382, 1990

Halaas J, Gajiwala K, Maffei M, et al: Weight-reducing effects of the protein encoded by the obese gene. Science 269:543–546, 1995

Halmi KA: Anorexia nervosa: demographic and clinical features in 94 cases. Psychosom Med 36:18–26, 1974

Halmi KA: Anorexia nervosa and bulimia, in Handbook of Adolescent Psychology. Edited by Hersen M, Van Hasselt T. New York, Pergamon, 1987, pp 265–287

Halmi KA, Falk JR: Common physiological changes in anorexia nervosa. Int J Eat Disord 1:16–27, 1981

Halmi KA, Sunday SR: Temporal patterns of hunger and satiety ratings and related cognitions in anorexia and bulimia. Appetite 16:219–237, 1991

Halmi KA, Stunkard AJ, Mason EE: Emotional responses to weight reduction by three methods: gastric bypass, jejunoileal bypass, diet. Am J Clin Nutr 33:446–451, 1980

Halmi KA, Eckert E, LaDu T, et al: Anorexia nervosa: treatment efficacy of cyproheptadine and amitriptyline. Arch Gen Psychiatry 43:177–181, 1986

Halmi KA, Eckert E, Marchi P, et al: Comorbidity of psychiatric diagnoses in anorexia nervosa. Arch Gen Psychiatry 48:712–718, 1991

Halmi KA, Agras S, Crow S, et al: Predictors of treatment acceptance and completion in anorexia nervosa. Arch Gen Psychiatry 62:1–6, 2005

Hart K, Ollendick TH: Prevalence of bulimia in working and university women. Am J Psychiatry 142:851–854, 1985

Hatsukami J, Mitchell J, Eckert E: Similarities and differences on the MMPI between women with bulimia and women with alcohol and drug abuse problems. Addict Behav 7:435–439, 1982

Hatsukami J, Mitchell J, Eckert E, et al: Affective disorder and substance abuse in women with bulimia. Psychol Med 14:704–710, 1984

Herzog DB, Keller MB, Lavori PW, et al: The prevalence of personality disorders in 210 women with eating disorders. J Clin Psychiatry 53:147–152, 1992

Hoebel BG: Pharmacological control of feeding. Annu Rev Pharmacol Toxicol 17:605–621, 1977

Hoek H: The incidence and prevalence of anorexia nervosa and bulimia nervosa in primary care. Psychol Med 21:455–460, 1991

Hoek HW, Bartelds A, Bosveld J, et al: Impact of urbanization on detection rates of eating disorders. Am J Psychiatry 152:1272–1278, 1995

Holland AJ, Sicotte N, Tresure J: Anorexia nervosa: evidence for a genetic basis. J Psychosom Res 32:561–571, 1988

Hotta M, Chibasaki T, Masuda A, et al: The responses of plasma adrenal corticotropin and cortisol to corticotropin-releasing hormone and cerebral spinal fluid immunoreactive CRH in anorexia nervosa patients. J Clin Endocrinol Metab 62:319–321, 1986

Hsu LK, Crisp AH, Harding B: Outcome of anorexia nervosa. Lancet 1(8107):61–65, 1979

Jimerson DC, Wolfe BE, Metzger ED, et al: Decrease serotonin function in bulimia nervosa. Arch Gen Psychiatry 54:529–534, 1997

Johnson C, Berndt DJ: Preliminary investigation of bulimia and life adjustment. Am J Psychiatry 140:774–777, 1983

Jones D, Fox MM, Babigian HM, et al: Epidemiology of anorexia nervosa in Monroe County, NY, 1960–1976. Psychosom Med 42:551–558, 1980

Kas MJ, Van Elburg A, Engeland HV, et al: Refinement of behavioral traits in animals for the genetic dissection of eating disorders. Eur J Pharmacol 480:13–20, 2003

Kaye WH, Ebert M, Gwirtsman H, et al: Differences in brain serotonergic metabolism between nonbulimic and bulimic patients with anorexia nervosa. Am J Psychiatry 141:1598–1601, 1984a

Kaye WH, Ebert MH, Raleigh M, et al: Abnormalities in CNS monoamine metabolism in anorexia nervosa. Arch Gen Psychiatry 41:350–355, 1984b

Kaye WH, Berrettini W, Gwirtsman HE, et al: Altered cerebrospinal fluid neuropeptide Y and peptide YY immunoreactivity in anorexia and bulimia nervosa. Arch Gen Psychiatry 47:548–556, 1990

Kaye WH, Nagata T, Weltzin T, et al: Double-blind placebo-controlled administration of fluoxetine in restricting and restricting-purging type anorexia nervosa. Biol Psychiatry 49:644–652, 2001

Keel PK, Mitchell JE: Outcome in bulimia nervosa. Am J Psychiatry 154:313–321, 1997

Kleifield E, Wagner S, Halmi K: Cognitive-behavioral treatment of anorexia nervosa. Psychiatr Clin North Am 19:715–734, 1996

Kurth C, Krahn D, Nairn K, et al: The severity of dieting and bingeing behaviors in college women: interview validation of survey data. J Psychiatry Res 29:211–225, 1995

Lacey JH: An outpatient treatment program for bulimia nervosa. Int J Eat Disord 2:209–241, 1983

Lasagna L: The pharmacotherapy of obesity, in Psychopharmacology: The Third Generation of Progress. Edited by Meltzer HY. New York, Raven, 1987, pp 1281–1284

Le Roux CW, Patterson M, Vincent RP, et al: Postprandial plasma ghrelin is suppressed proportional to meal calorie content in normal-weight but not obese subjects. J Clin Endocrinol Metab 90:1068–1071, 2005

LeGrange D, Eisler I, Dare C, et al: Evaluation of family treatment in adolescent anorexia nervosa: a pilot study. Int J Eat Disord 12:347–358, 1992

Leibowitz SF: Neurochemical systems of the hypothalamus: control of feeding and drinking behavior and water electrolyte excretion, in Handbook of the Hypothalamus, Vol 3. Edited by Morgane PJ, Panksepp J. New York, Raven, 1980, pp 299–347

Levitan RD, Kaplan AS, Joffe RT, et al: Hormonal and subjective responses to intravenous meta-chlorophenylpiperazine in bulimia nervosa. Arch Gen Psychiatry 54:521–527, 1997

Lewinsohn PM, Striegel-Moore RH, Seeley JR: Epidemiology and natural course of eating disorders in young women from adolescence to young adulthood. J Am Acad Child Adolesc Psychiatry 39:1284–1292, 2000

Lilenfeld LR, Kaye WH, Greeno CG, et al: A controlled family study of anorexia nervosa and bulimia nervosa: psychiatric disorders in first-degree relatives and effects of proband comorbidity. Arch Gen Psychiatry 55:603–610, 1998

Lucas A, Beard C, O'Fallon W, et al: Fifty year trends in the incidence of anorexia nervosa in Rochester, Minnesota: a population-based study. Am J Psychiatry 148:917–922, 1991

Maffei M, Halaas J, Ravussin E, et al: Leptin levels in human and rodent: measurement of plasma leptin and OB RNA in obese and weight-reduced subjects. Nat Med 1:1155–1161, 1995

Mantzoros C, Flier JS, Lesem MD, et al: Cerebrospinal fluid leptin in anorexia nervosa: correlation with nutritional status and potential role in resistance to weight gain. J Clin Endocrinol Metab 82:1845–1851, 1997

McElroy SL, Arnold LM, Shapira N: Topiramate in the treatment of binge eating disorder associated with obesity: a randomized, placebo-controlled trial. Am J Psychiatry 160:255–261, 2003

Mitchell JE, Pyle RL, Eckert ED, et al: A comparison study of antidepressants and structured intensive group therapy in the treatment of bulimia nervosa. Arch Gen Psychiatry 47:149–157, 1990

Mitchell JE, Halmi K, Wilson GT, et al: A randomized secondary treatment study of women with bulimia nervosa who failed to respond to CBT. Int J Eat Disord 32:271–278, 2002

Morley J, Levine AS: Pharmacology of eating behavior. Annu Rev Pharmacol Toxicol 25:127–146, 1985

National Task Force on the Prevention and Treatment of Obesity: Long-term pharmacotherapy in the management of obesity. JAMA 276:1907–1915, 1996

Nielsen S: Epidemiology and mortality of eating disorders. Psychiatr Clin North Am 24:201–214, 2001

Norman KA, Herzog DB: Persistent social maladjustment in bulimia: one year follow-up. Am J Psychiatry 141:444–446, 1984

Owen WP, Halmi KA, Lasley E, et al: Dopamine regulation in anorexia nervosa. Psychopharmacol Bull 19:578–580, 1983

Pirke KM: Central and peripheral noradrenaline regulation in eating disorders. Psychiatry Res 62:43–49, 1996

Powers PS, Covert DL, Brightwell DR, et al: Other psychiatric disorders among bulimic patients. Compr Psychiatry 29:503–508, 1988

Powers PS, Santana CA, Bannon YS: Olanzapine in the treatment of anorexia nervosa: an open label trial. Int J Eat Disord 32:146–154, 2002

Pyle RL, Mitchell JE, Eckert ED, et al: Maintenance treatment and 6 month outcome for bulimia patients who respond to initial treatment. Am J Psychiatry 147:871–875, 1990

Rooney B, McClelland L, Crisp AH, et al: The incidence and prevalence of anorexia nervosa in three suburban health districts in southwest London, UK. Int J Eat Disord 18:299–307, 1995

Rosen J: Bulimia nervosa: treatment with exposure and response prevention. Behav Ther 13:117–124, 1982

Russell GFM: Metabolic, endocrine and psychiatric aspects of anorexia nervosa. Scientific Basis of Medicine Annual Review 14:236–255, 1969

Russell GFM, Szmukler JI, Dare C, et al: An evaluation of family therapy in anorexia nervosa and bulimia nervosa. Arch Gen Psychiatry 44:1047–1056, 1987

Schmidt ND, Telch MJ: Prevalence of personality disorders among bulimics, non-bulimic binge eaters and normal controls. J Psychopathol Behav Assess 12:170–185, 1990

Schotte D, Stunkard A: Bulimia vs. bulimic behaviors on a college campus. JAMA 9:1213–1215, 1987

Society of Actuaries: Life Tables for the United States Social Security Area 1900–2080: Actuarial Study No 107, August 1992 (SSA Publ No 11-11536). Washington, DC, U.S. Department of Health and Human Services, 1992

Soubrie P: Reconciling the role of central serotonin neurosis in human and animal behavior. Behav Brain Sci 9:319–363, 1986

Soundy TJ, Lucas AR, Suman VJ: Bulimia nervosa in Rochester, Minnesota from 1980 to 1990. Psychol Med 25:1065–1071, 1995

Stevens J, Ooi J, Pamuk E, et al: The effect of age on the association between body mass index and mortality. N Engl J Med 338:1–7, 1998

Strober M, Morell W, Burroughs J, et al: A controlled family study of anorexia nervosa. Psychiatry Res 19:329–346, 1985

Strober M, Freeman R, Lampert C, et al: Control family study of anorexia nervosa and bulimia nervosa: evidence of shared liability and transmission of partial syndromes. Am J Psychiatry 157:393–401, 2000

Strober M, Freeman R, Lampert C, et al: Males with anorexia nervosa: a controlled study of eating disorders in first-degree relatives. Int J Eat Disord 29:263–269, 2001

Stunkard AJ: The current status of treatment for obesity in adults, in Eating and Its Disorders. Edited by Stunkard AJ, Stellar E. New York, Raven, 1984, pp 157–174

Sunday SR, Halmi KA: Taste perceptions and hedonics in eating disorders. Physiol Behav 48:587–594, 1990

Szmukler JI: The epidemiology of anorexia nervosa and bulimia. J Psychiatry Res 19:1243–1253, 1985

Szmukler JI, Tantam D: Anorexia nervosa: starvation dependence. Br J Med Psychol 57:305–310, 1984

Tartaglia LA, Dembski M, Weng X, et al: Identification and expression cloning of a leptin receptor, OB-R. Cell 83:1263–1271, 1995

Theander S: Outcome and prognosis in anorexia nervosa and bulimia, in Anorexia Nervosa and Bulimic Disorders. Edited by Szmukler GI, Slade PD, Harris P, et al. London, Pergamon, 1985, pp 493–508

Turnbull S, Ward A, Treasure J, et al: The demand for eating disorder care an epidemiological study using the general practice research database. Br J Psychiatry 169:705–712, 1996

VanItallie TB: Health implications of overweight and obesity in the United States. Ann Intern Med 103:983–988, 1985

Wade TD, Bulik CM, Neal EMC, et al: Anorexia and major depression: shared genetic and environmental risk factors. Am J Psychiatry 157:469–471, 2000

Walsh BT, Hadigan CM, Devlin MJ, et al: Long-term outcome of antidepressant treatment for bulimia nervosa. Am J Psychiatry 148:1206–1212, 1991

Walsh BT, Agras WS, Devlin MJ, et al: Fluoxetine in bulimia nervosa following poor response to psychotherapy. Am J Psychiatry 157:1332–1334, 2000

Weintraub M: Long-term weight control: the National Heart, Lung and Blood Institute funded multi-modal intervention study. Clin Pharmacol Ther 51:581–585, 1992

Westen D, Harden-Fischer J: Personality profiles in eating disorders: rethinking the distinction between Axis I and Axis II. Am J Psychiatry 158:547–562, 2001

Wonderlich SA, Swift WJ, Slotnick HB, et al: DSM-III-R personality disorders and eating disorder subtypes. Int J Eat Disord 9:607–616, 1990

Woodside DB, Garfinkel PE, Lin E, et al: Comparisons of men with full or partial eating disorders, men without eating disorders, and women with eating disorders in the community. Am J Psychiatry 158:570–574, 2001

Wurtman JJ, Wurtman RJ: Drugs that enhance central serotonergic transmission diminished elective carbohydrate consumption by rats. Life Sci 24:895–904, 1979

Zhang Y, Prenca R, Maffei M, et al: Positional cloning of the mouse obese gene and its human homologue. Nature 372:425–432, 1994

PSYCHOLOGICAL FACTORS AFFECTING MEDICAL CONDITIONS

James L. Levenson, M.D.

The fact that psychological factors and psychiatric disorders may affect the clinical course of medical illness is incontrovertible and is no longer the topic of serious debate. For example, psychiatric disorders may negatively affect outcome, increasing adverse events, length of stay in general hospital patients, and health care costs (Daumit et al. 2006; Walker et al. 2003). A striking example is the increased morbidity and mortality associated with major depression in patients with coronary artery disease (Frasure-Smith et al. 1993). Although most of the consultation-liaison literature has focused on interrelations between comorbid psychiatric and medical disorders, a wealth of epidemiological research has identified behavioral risk factors for the development of medical illness. Behavioral factors such as cigarette smoking, obesity, alcohol and substance dependence, and hazardous sexual practices are major causes of premature death and medical morbidity both in the United States and worldwide. A description of areas of investigation for classifying the psychological, behavioral, and social factors that may affect physical health is presented in Table 24–1.

This chapter originally grew out of the work of the committee that examined the diagnostic category "psychological factors affecting a medical condition" in DSM-IV (American Psychiatric Association 1994; Table 24–2). An expanded version of the committee's examination of the relation among psychiatric, behavioral, and psychological factors and the onset, precipitation, and exacerbation of medical disorders was published more than a decade ago (Stoudemire 1995). Their reviews were summarized in previous editions of this book and have been updated, with special emphasis on the implications for clinical practice, selectively focusing on oncology, endocrinology, cardiology, pulmonology, gastroenterology, rheumatology, dermatology, and end-stage renal disease. Fuller review of the effects of psychological factors and psychiatric disorders on medical illnesses can be found elsewhere (Levenson 2005). With a few exceptions, I do not address social factors that also have important effects on the incidence and course of medical disorders, such as social support, education, class, employment, and neighborhood (Isaacs and Schroeder 2004; Kawachi and Berkman 2003).

TABLE 24–1. Psychological and behavioral factors affecting medical conditions

I. Psychophysiology
  A. Physiological reactions to psychological and behavioral variables
  B. Biological regulatory mechanisms associated with behavioral and psychological variables
    1. Psychoneurophysiology
    2. Psychoneuroendocrinology
    3. Psychoneuroimmunology
    4. Psychocardiology

II. Effects of concurrent psychiatric illness on the course and outcome of medical disorders

III. Behavioral risk factors for disease and injury
  A. Personality variables
  B. Cigarette smoking
  C. Dietary habits
  D. Alcohol and substance abuse
  E. Hazardous sexual behavior
  F. Risk-taking behaviors (accidents, injury)
  G. Noncompliance with medical treatment
  H. Violence, suicide, homicide
  I. Stressful or disruptive life change

Source. Reprinted with permission from Stoudemire A, Hales RE: "Psychological and Behavioral Factors Affecting Medical Conditions and DSM-IV: An Overview." *Psychosomatics* 32:5–13, 1991. Copyright 1991, Academy of Psychosomatic Medicine.

Psychological Factors in Cancer

The relation between psychological factors and the onset and course of neoplastic disease serves as a prototype in examining the literature on this topic because many health care professionals and laypersons believe that psychological factors play a major role in cancer onset and progression. This belief has been strengthened, in part, by a rapidly growing literature, both scientific and popular, examining the role of psychological factors in cancer. Enthusiasm for therapeutic interventions based on "psychosomatic" relations in oncology should be tempered by the recognition that the scientific evidence of such relations has yielded few confirmed conclusions and has many methodological limitations. In this section, I critically summarize the literature on cancer and its potential connections to affective states, coping/defensive style and personality traits, interpersonal relationships, stressful life events, and psychosocial interventions.

Affective States and Cancer

The relationship between depression and cancer has been the focus of extensive study from several perspectives. The large epidemiological Western Electric study reported that depressive symptoms were associated with twice as high a risk of death from cancer 17 years later and with a higher-than-normal incidence of cancer for the first 10 years (Shekelle et al. 1991). This finding persisted at 20-year follow-up (Persky et al. 1987). The Western Electric study has been cited for many years as supporting the association between depressive symptoms and increased cancer risk. Other studies, however, have reported negative findings (for review, see Levenson and McDonald 2002). Studies with 10- and 15-year follow-up found no significant depressive symptoms that could be seen as predictors of cancer morbidity or mortality (Levenson and McDonald 2002). A meta-analysis of studies relating depression to cancer development reported a small but significant association but of a magnitude of little practical significance (McGee et al. 1994). Recent large prospective cohort studies found no effect of depression on breast cancer risk in Finnish women (Aro et al. 2005) or on any cancer risk in Danish people (Bergelt et al. 2005).

Besides epidemiological studies, other studies have examined the effect of depression on outcome in cancer patients, most often examining survival with breast cancer. In the year after the diagnosis of breast cancer, half of the women in the cohort studied by Burgess et al. (2005) had clinically significant depression, anxiety, or both. Breast cancer patients who had a "fighting spirit" or who used denial had a higher survival rate than did those with stoic acceptance or who expressed hopelessness and helplessness (Greer et al. 1979). Subsequent studies have provided positive, negative, or mixed associations between depression and mortality in cancer patients (Levenson and McDonald 2002). Outcome variables other than mortality are worthy of investigation because depression could be reasonably expected to result in poorer pain control, less adherence to treatment, and decreased desire for life-sustaining therapy.

Other affective states have received much less attention. Emotional distress in general appeared to lead to decreased survival in patients with lung cancer (Faller et al. 1999), as did anger in patients with metastatic melanoma (Butow et al. 1999). Bereavement has been recognized as a significant stressor and often has been assumed to be a risk factor in cancer onset and progression. McKenna et al. (1999), in a meta-analysis of 46 studies of breast cancer, found only a modest

TABLE 24–2. **DSM-IV-TR diagnostic criteria for specified psychological factor affecting general medical condition**

A. A general medical condition (coded on Axis III) is present.

B. Psychological factors adversely affect the general medical condition in one of the following ways:

   (1) the factors have influenced the course of the general medical condition as shown by a close temporal association between the psychological factors and the development or exacerbation of, or delayed recovery from, the general medical condition

   (2) the factors interfere with the treatment of the general medical condition

   (3) the factors constitute additional health risks for the individual

   (4) stress-related physiological responses precipitate or exacerbate symptoms of the general medical condition

Choose name based on the nature of the psychological factors (if more than one factor is present, indicate the most prominent):

   Mental disorder affecting... *[indicate the general medical condition]* (e.g., an Axis I disorder such as major depressive disorder delaying recovery from a myocardial infarction)

   Psychological symptoms affecting... *[indicate the general medical condition]* (e.g., depressive symptoms delaying recovery from surgery; anxiety exacerbating asthma)

   Personality traits or coping style affecting... *[indicate the general medical condition]* (e.g., pathological denial of the need for surgery in a patient with cancer; hostile, pressured behavior contributing to cardiovascular disease)

   Maladaptive health behaviors affecting... *[indicate the general medical condition]* (e.g., overeating; lack of exercise; unsafe sex)

   Stress-related physiological response affecting... *[indicate the general medical condition]* (e.g., stress-related exacerbations of ulcer, hypertension, arrhythmia, or tension headache)

   Other or unspecified psychological factors affecting... *[indicate the general medical condition]* (e.g., interpersonal, cultural, or religious factors)

association between separation or loss experiences and development of cancer. A large Danish prospective cohort study comparing cancer patients who had lost a child prior to diagnosis of cancer with other cancer patients found no evidence that the death of a child influenced survival (Li et al. 2003). Considering retrospective and prospective, clinical and population-based studies, bereavement has not to date been convincingly shown to influence cancer onset or progression (Levenson and McDonald 2002).

Coping Styles, Personality Traits, and Cancer

A large body of literature has described the cancer patient's degree of emotional expressiveness versus repressiveness and its purported effect on prognosis. Temoshok et al. (1985) described a "type C behavior pattern," typified as a cooperative, unassertive patient who suppresses negative emotions, particularly anger, and who accepts and complies with external authorities. The Melbourne Colorectal Cancer Study found that cancer patients were more likely to have certain

personality traits (similar to the type C pattern) than were control subjects (Kune et al. 1991). Research over the past 25 years has both supported and refuted the belief that cancer development or mortality is influenced by coping, defensive style, or personality traits (Levenson and McDonald 2002).

Cassileth et al. (1988) found that none of the multiple psychosocial factors thought to be predictive of health predicted cancer survival. No differences in coping styles were found between breast cancer patients and control subjects (Buddeberg et al. 1991) or head and neck cancer patients and control subjects (Yamagiwa et al. 1991), and no relation was seen between coping style and breast cancer course (Soler-Vila et al. 2003). Kreitler et al. (1993) found that repression and defensiveness increased in patients *after* the cancer was diagnosed, which highlights one of the flaws in retrospective studies. Epidemiological studies have not supported a relation between "emotional repression" and cancer incidence or mortality (Bleiker et al. 1996). The meta-analysis by McKenna et al. (1999) found only a modest association between denial or repression coping and breast cancer onset.

Stressful Life Events and Cancer

Both retrospective clinical and prospective epidemiological human studies have shown an increased incidence of stressful life events preceding the onset of breast, colorectal, cervical, pancreatic, gastric, and lung cancer, but many other studies have failed to find such associations (Levenson and McDonald 2002). Some early studies linked stressful life events to progression or recurrence of cancer, but later reports found no effect of stressful life events on relapse or progression. Most of the studies used aggregate measures of stressful life events rather than examining specific types of stress. Some investigators have implicated work stress or loss of employment as increasing the risk of lung cancer (Lynge and Anderson 1997) and colorectal cancer (Courtney et al. 1993). However, a more recent large Danish prospective study found that women with high stress at baseline had a *reduced* risk of developing breast cancer (Nielsen et al. 2005). In a review of human and animal studies, Fox (1983) concluded that if stressful events do have an effect on cancer incidence, it is small—a conclusion that still appears appropriate today.

Psychosocial Intervention and Cancer Outcome

In contrast to the lack of convincing support for an etiological relation between psychological factors and cancer, most studies of group therapy in cancer patients have shown improvement in mood, pain, and quality of life (P.J. Goodwin et al. 2001; Spiegel et al. 1989), although some have not (Bordeleau et al. 2003). Relaxation training and cognitive-behavioral therapy also have reduced anxiety and depression in cancer patients (for review, see Holland et al. 1998).

Spiegel et al. (1989) performed a small randomized controlled trial of supportive group therapy with training in self-hypnosis for pain control in women with metastatic breast cancer. The psychotherapy treatment group had less mood disturbance, fewer phobic responses, and less pain, as well as increased survival compared with the control group (34.8 months vs. 18.9 months). The possibility that a psychological intervention might improve longevity in metastatic breast cancer patients was exciting; this finding was supported by some other studies but not by the definitive replication study (P.J. Goodwin et al. 2001) and some others. Lower mortality has been reported with structured psychiatric group intervention in other cancers as well (Fawzy et al. 1993), but far more evidence shows improvements in indices of quality of life such as mood, energy, and pain control. Patients can be told that group therapy contributes to living better, not necessarily longer.

Mechanisms

The question of *how* psychological factors might influence cancer onset and progression has many potential answers. The immune system is probably important for some, but not all, cancer surveillance, and much research has focused on the influence of psychological factors on immune function relevant to cancer.

Various behavioral explanations that may account for the effects of psychological factors on cancer development and course also have been examined. The effect of some psychological factors (e.g., cynicism) on mortality may be mediated by smoking and alcohol. Psychological factors also affect how patients seek medical attention for their initial cancer symptoms and their self-care and treatment preferences (Greimel et al. 1997). Cancer prevention also is influenced by psychological factors, which affect, for example, use of Papanicolaou tests and mammography (Leiferman and Pheley 2006) and genetic testing (Case et al. 2005). Some relations between psychological factors, behavior, and cancer may be cancer-type specific (e.g., sexual behavior and cervical cancer).

In summary, several studies have lent some support to the relation among a variety of psychological factors and the onset, exacerbation, or outcome of neoplastic disease. Currently, no clear associations (let alone causal relations) have been proven, both because of methodological limitations in the positive studies and because of the failure of other studies of comparable methodology to find such relations. Compared with other known risk factors, psychological factors alone (other than cigarette smoking and alcoholism) make a small contribution to cancer onset.

Clinical Implications

Depression and anxiety remain common but still relatively underdiagnosed and undertreated in cancer patients. Whether mood disorders affect the incidence, course, or clinical outcomes of cancer has not yet been definitively answered by systematic research. Nevertheless, depression and anxiety warrant clinical attention because of their clearly adverse effects on quality of life. Behaviors with obviously harmful effects on patients with cancer (e.g., smoking, alcohol abuse, noncompliance with treatment) also should be targeted for intervention. The current literature on coping and personality style does not support the conclusions that any particular type of coping style is superior for all patients. Popular literature may lead some patients to feel responsible for their disease (or relapse) because they were unable to develop the "right attitude" or personality characteristics to "beat" cancer. Psychiatrists have a responsibility not only to avoid contributing to such simplistic, guilt-generating views but also to help patients (and some other physicians) understand the value of a range of individualized approaches to adaptation.

Psychotherapeutic interventions may be of great benefit to cancer patients. Studies show that psychotherapy can reduce anxiety, depression, and traumatic stress in patients with cancer (e.g., P.J. Goodwin et al. 2001) and enhance meaning and spirituality (Breitbart et al. 2004), although benefits may not accrue for all patients (Vos et al. 2004). The few studies that appeared to show reduced mortality in patients receiving such interventions led some to suggest overly optimistic benefits of psychological therapies toward cure or remission, which creates a risk of deeply disappointing patients and their families and distracting them from the direct benefits of psychiatric treatment for quality of life. Psychiatrists should keep in mind that psychosocial interventions are more likely to contribute to *quality* than to *quantity* of life in cancer patients. There is much enthusiasm among many professionals and laypersons for treatments promising to overcome cancer through "mind over body," but current scientific evidence supports a more cautious view. Psychiatric interventions are primarily justified if they reduce distress and dysfunction, such as when depressive or anxiety disorders are diagnosed in the context of illness with cancer. Randomized controlled trials have shown the benefits of antianxiety and antidepressant medications in cancer patients (e.g., Roscoe et al. 2005). The diagnosis and treatment of psychiatric disorders in these patients are discussed in detail elsewhere (Holland et al. 1998; Massie and Greenberg 2005). Several of the most important findings in the relation between psychological factors and cancer, including several sentinel outcome studies, are highlighted in Table 24–3.

Psychological Factors and Endocrine Disease

Although there is a considerable amount of literature on psychoneuroendocrinology, particularly regarding the biology of mood disorders, little methodologically sound research exists regarding the clinical aspects of psychological factors and how these factors potentially influence endocrine diseases, with the exception of diabetes mellitus. In the following section, I review psychological factors affecting diabetes mellitus, Graves' disease, and Cushing's disease. The subject of psychiatric symptoms caused or exacerbated by endocrine disorders is reviewed elsewhere (Goebel-Fabbri et al. 2005).

Diabetes Mellitus

There has long been speculation about the role of psychological factors and the onset of diabetes mellitus. Several early studies showed a relation between stressful life events and the onset of diabetes mellitus, but they were retrospective, were significantly flawed, and yielded inconclusive findings regarding the causal relation between stress and disease onset (Stoudemire 1995).

One group avoided recall bias by assessing the number of stressful life events in community residents without any history of diabetes before administering a glucose tolerance test. Diabetes was newly diagnosed in 5% and positively associated with the number of stressful life events (Mooy et al. 2000). Wales (1995) reviewed a number of conflicting study results and suggested that, in general, psychological stress may produce a deterioration in glycemic control in the as-yet-undiagnosed asymptomatic patient, which precipitates symptoms and makes the diagnosis evident.

Other investigations have examined the role of psychological factors in affecting the course of diabetes mellitus. Early studies were flawed primarily because of difficulties in accurately measuring glucose control, whereas more recent studies measure hemoglobin A_{1c} (HbA1c), a reliable measure of metabolic control. Studies in clinical samples generally have found an association between perceived stress and poorer metabolic control whether assessed by blood glucose (Garay-Sevilla et al. 2000) or HbA1c (Lloyd et al. 1999), but such studies were typically cross-sectional, limiting any conclusions about causality. More persuasive are prospective within-subject analyses showing that poorer metabolic control is caused by standardized laboratory stress (Goetsch et al. 1993) or normal life stress (Kramer et al. 2000), although these studies used relatively small numbers of subjects.

Depression (symptoms or diagnosis) may adversely affect glycemic control and increase the risk for diabetic complications, but study findings have been variable. As assessed by HbA1c, metabolic control has been found to be poorer in depressed children (Lernmark et al. 1999), in depressed men but not women (Lloyd et al. 2000), and in depressed type 1 but not type 2 diabetic persons (de Groot et al. 1999). In a compre-

TABLE 24–3.   Illustrative classic studies supporting the effects of psychological factors on cancer

Psychological factor	Study type	Cancer type	Findings	Reference(s)
Depression	Epidemiological	Mixed	2× risk of death from cancer at 20-year follow-up	Persky et al. 1987
Personality traits	Case control	Colorectal	Cancer patients less likely to have expressive personality traits	Kune et al. 1991
Stressful life events	Case control	Breast	Increased stressful life events preceding cancer onset	Geyer 1991
Group therapy with training in self-hypnosis	Randomized controlled trial	Breast	Reductions in distress and pain and increased survival in treatment group	Spiegel et al. 1989

hensive meta-analytic review, Lustman et al. (2000) concluded that a consistently strong association was found between elevated HbA1c values (indicating chronic hyperglycemia) and depression. This relation appears to be bidirectional, with depression provoking hyperglycemia and poor diabetic control contributing to depression. One potential explanation is that depression, anxiety, and stress are often associated with increases in cortisol and other counterregulatory hormones opposing the action of insulin. It is also logical to suspect that poorer compliance might account for depression's effects on diabetic management. Ciechanowski et al. (2000) found that depressive symptom severity was associated with poorer adherence to diet and medications as well as more functional impairment. They also found that adherence in diabetes is lacking in patients with a "dismissing attachment" style of relating, who also had poorer doctor–patient communication (Ciechanowski et al. 2001). Depressed patients with diabetes have more severe diabetic symptoms (Ludman et al. 2004), more disability (Von Korff et al. 2005), greater mortality (Katon et al. 2005), and higher health care costs (Simon et al. 2005).

As with other medical illnesses, the role of personality characteristics and coping strategies also has been studied in relation to the course of diabetes mellitus in both children and adults, but no clear conclusions have emerged. For example, one study found poorer glycemic control only in patients with a "Cluster B dependent profile" (Orlandini et al. 1997), another found poorer glycemic control only in those who are more altruistic (Lane et al. 2000), and a third found no correlation with any personality variables (Perros et al. 1998). Similarly, studies in children have provided mixed and counterintuitive associations between personality and glucose control.

Although several studies have reported the effects

of behavioral or psychosocial interventions on glucose control in diabetic patients, results have not been consistent. However, randomized controlled trials have found that cognitive-behavioral therapy, relaxation training, or coping skills training can improve glucose control in diabetes (Grey et al. 2000; Lustman et al. 1998). Antidepressant treatment of depression in diabetes is effective and produces an early trend toward better glycemic control, although some antidepressants can cause moderate hyperglycemia or hypoglycemia (Goebel-Fabbri et al. 2005). The Pathways Study, the most comprehensive clinical trial of enhanced treatment for depression in diabetic patients, reported that it improved the quality of care and outcomes for depression but did not result in improved glycemic control (Katon et al. 2004).

Deterioration in glucose tolerance in schizophrenic and bipolar patients undergoing treatment is likely to be caused by most of the newer antipsychotic drugs. However, diabetes was a major problem for schizophrenic and bipolar patients even before the widespread use of atypical antipsychotic drugs, presumably because of obesity (a side effect of conventional antipsychotics), unhealthy diets, and poorer health care (Ruzickova et al. 2003). Optimal management of diabetes requires patients to be organized, precise, meticulous, and consistent, which is very difficult to attain for most patients who also have severe mental illness.

Further studies evaluating the role of psychological factors in the onset and course of diabetes mellitus are needed to clarify the current conflicting data regarding stress and this disease. Clarifying this relation will improve our understanding of the potential role of behavioral interventions as mediators in the effects of stress on diabetic patients. Examples of key findings in the relation between psychological factors and diabetes are shown in Table 24–4.

TABLE 24–4. Illustrative studies supporting the effects of psychological factors on diabetes mellitus

Psychological factor	Study type	Findings	Reference(s)
Stressful life events	Prospective epidemiological	New-onset diabetes associated with number of stressful events	Mooy et al. 2000
Perceived stress	Cross-sectional	Poor metabolic control	Lloyd et al. 1999
Depression	Cross-sectional	Poor adherence, more impairment, higher costs, poor doctor–patient relationships	Ciechanowski et al. 2000, 2001
Cognitive-behavioral therapy	Randomized controlled trial	Improved glucose control	Lustman et al. 1998

Graves' Disease

Weiner (1977) provided the classic review of psychological factors in Graves' disease in his textbook *Psychobiology and Human Disease*. It is apparent from Weiner's review that numerous methodological flaws have made early studies difficult to interpret. Complicating the studies of Graves' disease are the variable onset and course of the disease itself, making it difficult to measure changes in onset and course related to psychological factors. Furthermore, hyperthyroidism itself produces psychological, behavioral, and neuropsychiatric signs and symptoms (Goebel-Fabbri et al. 2005).

Minimal evidence suggests that psychological characteristics of patients predispose them to develop Graves' disease or any thyroid disorder, for that matter (Weiner 1977). However, stressful life events have been identified as risk factors for Graves' disease (Santos et al. 2002). Japanese investigators found that stressful life events and smoking were associated with Graves' disease in women but not in men (Yoshiuchi et al. 1998b). However, as with other diseases, such studies of stressful life events preceding disease onset are nonspecific and subject to recall bias, and they do not shed light on etiology. A study of patients with chronic stress due to panic disorder found no evidence that previous or current Graves' hyperthyroidism occurred more frequently in the patients with panic disorder than in the control subjects (Chiovato et al. 1998). Two prospective studies in patients newly diagnosed with Graves' disease found that after the investigators adjusted for confounding variables, psychological stress adversely affected the response to treatment and prognosis (Fukao et al. 2003; Yoshiuchi et al. 1998a). More prospective studies are needed to better establish the effects of psychological factors on Graves' disease.

Cushing's Disease

Dr. Cushing himself argued that emotional stress contributed to the development of the disease that bears his name. As is the case for Graves' disease, although some evidence suggests that preceding stressful life events are more common than in control subjects, compelling evidence that psychological factors affect Cushing's disease is lacking. Although it is clearly known that stressful stimuli may lead to acute increased secretion of corticosteroids, the magnitude of such physiological hypercortisolism is much lower than that occurring in Cushing's disease. However, it is well recognized that significant hypercortisolism of any etiology, including Cushing's disease, can cause a wide range of neuropsychiatric phenomena (Goebel-Fabbri et al. 2005). Much more research is needed to illuminate these issues and other questions pertaining to the effects of psychological factors on endocrine disorders.

Psychological Factors and Cardiac Disorders

Coronary Artery Disease

The effects of psychological, social, and behavioral factors on cardiovascular disease have garnered considerable clinical attention and have been a primary focus of epidemiological and psychosomatic medicine research for the past 30 years. Patients with severe mental disorders have about twice the prevalence of the classic risk factors for coronary artery disease (CAD) (Birkenaes et al. 2006). Evidence from methodologically rigorous studies of a strong association between CAD and depressive disorders is especially compelling (Shapiro 2005). The prevalence of major depression in patients with CAD is much higher, especially after myocardial infarction, than in the general population. Depression not only commonly occurs alongside CAD but also negatively affects outcome in CAD. The magnitude of the effects of depression on morbidity and mortality in CAD is on a par with the effects of the recognized medical risk factors. Major depression is a significant predictor of mortality after an acute myocardial infarction, equal to the effect of predictors such as history of myocardial infarction or indexes of cardiac function (Carney et al. 2003; Frasure-Smith et al. 1993, 1995a). In an epidemiological study that followed a cohort of 3,000 individuals ages 55–85 for 4 years, major depression tripled the relative risk of cardiac mortality in those without heart disease and quadrupled it in those who did have cardiac disease (Penninx et al. 2001). Patients hospitalized for unstable angina who also had depressive symptoms were four times more likely to have myocardial infarction or die the following year than were those without depression (after adjusting for other factors) (Lesperance et al. 2000).

In addition to its effects on morbidity and mortality in CAD, depression can profoundly affect patients' quality of life and functioning. The severity of depressive symptoms has a greater effect on functional disability in CAD than does the number of stenosed coronary arteries. In the Heart and Soul Study of more than 1,000 outpatients with stable CAD, depressive symptoms strongly (negatively) contributed to health status, including symptom burden, physical limitation, quality of life, and overall health, but measures of ischemia and ejection fraction did not contribute (Ruo et al. 2003).

Several candidate explanations exist for the effects of depression on clinical outcome in CAD (Shapiro 2005). As discussed later in this chapter (see "Lifestyle Risk Factors"), depression is closely associated with nicotine addiction, but depression still adversely affects CAD outcome even after controlling for smoking. Depression may interfere with compliance with recommended lifestyle modification, medication, and cardiac rehabilitation (Carney et al. 1995). Evidence is accumulating that depressed patients may have alterations in platelet aggregation mediated by alterations in plasma serotonin. Another potential mechanism contributing to the diminished survival of depressed patients with CAD is reduced heart rate variability (Shapiro 2005). Also, some of the adverse effects of depression may be mediated through the cardiac effects of stress, as described later in this section. Depression's effects on heart rate variability and resting heart rate may explain the increased risk of ventricular arrhythmias and sudden death in depressed cardiac patients

(Shapiro 2005). Proinflammatory mediators associated with depression also may contribute to CAD (Parissis et al. 2004).

Anxiety is also extremely common in patients with CAD, and it too adversely affects outcome in CAD. Some evidence indicates that anxiety after myocardial infarction leads to more frequent readmission for unstable angina and more recurrences of myocardial infarction, after controlling for many confounding factors including comorbid depression (Frasure-Smith et al. 1995b). In a large clinical trial, patients who had a high level of anxiety after myocardial infarction had almost five times the risk for serious ischemic events or death compared with those without anxiety, making post–myocardial infarction anxiety one of the strongest predictors of in-hospital complications (Moser and Dracup 1996). Anxiety's adverse effects on outcome in CAD may be mediated via effects on heart rate variability, QT interval prolongation, or other abnormalities in autonomic nervous responses (Januzzi et al. 2000). As with depression, some of anxiety's effects may be related to the effects of stress on the heart (described in the following paragraph).

There are many forms of stress, and many studies report the adverse effects of stress on patients with preexisting heart disease (Krantz et al. 2000). The INTERHEART study of more than 11,000 patients with first myocardial infarction, compared with more than 13,000 control subjects, from 52 countries found that higher rates of stress factors (work, home, financial, and major life events) were associated with increased risk of myocardial infarction (Rosengren et al. 2004). Psychological stress has been considered to play an important role in precipitating cardiac events and sudden death in such patients. Psychological stress lowers the threshold for life-threatening ventricular arrhythmias. Experimental standardized mental stressors provoke ischemia in many patients with CAD, usually silent (asymptomatic). Such experimental stress-induced silent ischemia is clinically significant. Those who experience it are twice as likely to later have fatal and nonfatal cardiac events compared with those who do not (Jiang et al. 1996). Mental tension, frustration, and sadness double the risk for regular ischemia in CAD (Gullette et al. 1997).

Studies that document increases in myocardial infarction and/or sudden death after missile attacks, earthquakes, and other disasters confirm the effects of stress on heart disease (Krantz et al. 2000). A prospective study of middle-aged women who had been hospitalized for myocardial infarction or unstable angina found that after adjusting for other psychosocial and cardiac variables, women with severe marital stress had triple the risks of recurrent coronary events than did those women without marital stress (Orth-Gomér et al. 2000).

The relation between type A behavior and CAD has been controversial. Type A is a complex construct of multiple traits, including impatience, hostility, intense achievement drive, and time urgency. Many studies have supported type A behavior as a risk factor for the development of CAD and a predictor of worse outcome, but an equal number of studies have had negative results. Although there is support for the proposition that type A behavior is associated with an increased risk of developing heart disease, type A behavior does not appear to cause increased morbidity or mortality in those who have already developed CAD (Shapiro 2005). Because of the conflicting findings across many studies, investigators have attempted to identify a particular component of the type A syndrome that might be more significantly predictive. Of the type A traits, hostility has been the most consistently associated with increased cardiac events and mortality (Boyle et al. 2004). Anger, which is related but not identical to the concept of hostility, appears to be an especially potent trigger of ischemia (Ironson et al. 1992). How hostility or other elements of type A behavior might lead to CAD, or worsen its outcome, is unknown. Mechanisms considered have included alterations in the balance between sympathetic and parasympathetic nervous system activity and related changes in blood pressure and heart rate control.

Sudden cardiac death after acute psychological stress has long been reported anecdotally but is difficult to study empirically. Evidence suggests that a variety of psychological stressors may sometimes play an important role in precipitating serious ventricular arrhythmias. The incidence of life-threatening ventricular arrhythmias increased in New York City after the attacks on the World Trade Center (Steinberg et al. 2005).

Fewer studies of the effects of psychological factors on cardiac conditions other than CAD have been done, but in congestive heart failure, depression appears to increase the mortality risk (Jiang et al. 2001) and is a strong predictor of poor quality of life (Rumsfeld et al. 2003). Many studies have linked depression and other negative psychological states to increased cardiovascular risk, but some evidence also indicates that positive factors such as optimism may be protective (Giltay et al. 2004). Some illustrative studies supporting the effects of various psychological factors on CAD are shown in Table 24–5.

Hypertension

Because about 85% of hypertension cases are classified as primary (essential) hypertension, in which the etiology cannot be specified, psychological factors have been intensively studied as potential contributors to its pathogenesis (Shapiro 2005). The magnitude of blood pressure reactivity to stress has received some support as a factor in the development of hypertension and its progression. Many investigators have examined the relations between personality, coping style, blood pressure reactivity, and hypertension, but conclusions remain controversial. Findings regarding blood pressure reactivity in response to stress in normotensive individuals are not necessarily relevant to clinical hypertension. In some, but not all, studies, a high level of anxiety has been a strong prospective predictor for the development of hypertension, as has job strain. A large prospective population-based study found a dose–response relation between the type A behavior factors of time urgency/impatience and hostility and increasing risk for hypertension (Yan et al. 2003). Studies of psychological treatments for hypertension, primarily relaxation techniques and biofeedback, have sometimes found modest but clinically significant sustained reductions in blood pressure. However, such techniques are less effective than drug therapy.

Overall, the evidence for an important role for psychological factors affecting hypertension is equivocal compared with the evidence relating depression and mental stress to CAD (Friedman et al. 2001).

Clinical Implications

The role of psychological factors in cardiac disease is one of the most investigated categories of psychosomatic medicine, but as noted earlier, ambiguity and controversy regarding the importance of specific factors remain. Nevertheless, sufficient replicated evidence indicates that significant psychiatric disorders, especially major depression, have adverse effects on clinical outcome after myocardial infarction. Patients with mental disorders also may fare poorly because they are less likely to receive definitive interventions such as cardiac catheterization and angioplasty. Druss et al. (2000) found that patients with schizophrenia who had had myocardial infarctions were only 41% as likely to undergo catheterization as were those without mental disorders. Because of the weight of the evidence implicating psychological factors, especially depression, in the development and outcome of CAD, there are strong arguments for psychological and psychiatric intervention for prevention of heart disease

TABLE 24–5.   Illustrative studies supporting the effects of psychological factors on coronary artery disease

Psychological factor	Study type	Findings	Reference(s)
Depression	Prospective	Higher mortality after myocardial infarction	Frasure-Smith et al. 1993, 1995a
Anxiety	Prospective clinical trial	More ischemic events and death after myocardial infarction	Moser and Dracup 1996
Mental stress	Epidemiological studies after disasters	More sudden deaths and more myocardial infarctions	Krantz et al. 2000
Schizophrenia	Retrospective	Less likely to receive catheterization	Druss et al. 2000
Optimism	Prospective epidemiological	Lower cardiovascular mortality	Giltay et al. 2004

(Rozanski et al. 1999). There have been several clinical trials of psychological and psychopharmacological interventions, some of which have been successful in both reducing emotional distress and improving medical outcomes—the Sertraline Antidepressant Heart Attack Randomized Trial (SADHART; Glassman et al. 2002) and a trial of a psychological intervention, the Enhancing Recovery in Coronary Heart Disease (EN-RICHD) study (Writing Committee for the ENRICHD Investigators 2003). The diagnosis and treatment of psychiatric disorders in patients with heart disease are discussed in detail elsewhere (Shapiro 2005).

Lifestyle Risk Factors

As emphasized in the introduction to this chapter, it is now well established that lifestyle behaviors are risk factors that significantly contribute to the mortality rate in the United States (see Table 24–1). The most widely studied risk factors are cigarette smoking, obesity, and alcohol consumption, all of which affect the development, perpetuation, and exacerbation of medical illnesses.

Cigarette Smoking

Cigarette smoking remains the single most important modifiable risk factor for illness and the greatest single cause of preventable premature deaths. Cigarette smoking is a powerful independent contributor to myocardial infarction, sudden death, peripheral vascular disease, and stroke. It acts synergistically with other traditional risk factors such as hypertension and high blood cholesterol to increase the risk of CAD. Smoking

accounts for about 80% of the deaths related to chronic obstructive pulmonary disease (COPD). Tobacco's role in causing lung cancer has long been established, but its use increases the risk of many other types of cancer. Psychological factors affect initiation of, continuation of, withdrawal from, and relapse into smoking. Best studied has been the complex interactive relations among depression, smoking, and medical illness that complicate smoking cessation in those who have a history of depression (Wilhelm et al. 2004). Overall, persons with mental illness are about twice as likely to smoke as others are, and the increased risk is found with all the major anxiety, mood, and psychotic disorders (Lasser et al. 2000).

Unfortunately, smoking cessation is a difficult intervention. The difficulty is compounded by the physical dependence on nicotine in chronic smokers. Effective treatments are now available, especially when behavioral and pharmacological approaches are combined, but abstinence is maintained at 1 year in only about one-third of the research subjects receiving the most effective intervention (bupropion plus cessation counseling). On the positive side, mentally ill smokers can have substantial quit rates (about 37%) with or without smoking cessation treatment (Lasser et al. 2000).

Obesity

After cigarette smoking, obesity is the second most widely studied risk factor associated with increased morbidity and mortality. A strong association exists between obesity and hypertension, hypercholesterolemia, and diabetes mellitus as risk factors for cardiovascular disease. Obesity also may increase the risk of prostate, colon, and rectal cancer in men and endometrial, cervical, ovarian, breast, and gallbladder cancer in women. For those individuals with morbid obesity (more than 100 pounds overweight), sudden death, lung disease, sleep apnea, cardiomyopathy, congestive heart failure, liver dysfunction, gastroesophageal reflux, osteoarthritis, chronic pain, and thromboembolic disease are common complications. Functional limitations and negative psychosocial sequelae also are well-documented outcomes in individuals with morbid obesity.

Achieving weight reduction is complicated by psychological, social, and cultural factors. Psychological factors such as anxiety, depression, and stress contribute to overeating in some individuals. Obesity is more common in some psychiatric disorders, but most overweight and obese persons in the community do not have mental disorders (McElroy et al. 2004). Overall, only modest evidence shows that psychological and behavioral factors play a role in the development of obesity (Power and Parsons 2000). However, the evidence to date supports the use of behavioral and cognitive-behavioral strategies for weight loss in mild to moderate obesity, mainly useful when combined with dietary change and exercise (Shaw et al. 2005).

Alcohol Consumption

Alcohol consumption is associated with increased morbidity and mortality from accidents, violence, suicide, gastrointestinal ulcers and bleeding, cirrhosis, and several cancers, but regular modest intake is associated with reductions in coronary heart disease and thrombotic stroke (Hill 2005). Other lifestyle factors that have been associated with negative health outcomes include sedentary lifestyle; diet high in cholesterol and fats and low in fiber; sexual practices known to increase the risk of infection with HIV, hepatitis B, and other transmissible organisms; overexposure to sun and other ultraviolet light; lack of use of safety restraints when riding in motor vehicles; and other psychoactive substance use and abuse.

Clinical Implications

With the currently established evidence of the morbidity and mortality associated with lifestyle risk factors, psychiatrists have a responsibility to collaborate with other health care professionals in assisting patients with behavior changes. This is especially true for patients with psychotic disorders, who have high rates of smoking and obesity (de Leon and Diaz 2005). With cigarette smoking being the single most important modifiable risk factor for illness in the United States, treatment of nicotine dependence should play a central role in the treatment plans of those patients who continue to abuse tobacco, with special attention to any comorbid depressive or anxiety disorders. Similarly, interventions for preventing or reducing obesity are of central importance in treating conditions such as heart disease, diabetes, pulmonary disease, and chronic pain. Lifestyle risk factors may be only one part of the explanation of how psychological factors can affect the development and outcome of medical disorders, but they are identifiable and at least potentially modifiable.

Psychological Factors and Pulmonary Diseases

Asthma

Asthma historically was considered a classic "psychosomatic" illness; that is, it was believed that specific personality types and/or particular unconscious conflicts created vulnerability to asthma and could precipitate asthmatic attacks. Research over the ensuing decades has discredited this view that asthma can be understood and treated via psychoanalytic theory and treatment but also has documented that psychological factors do greatly affect the course of asthma. The evidence to date indicates that no specific "asthmatic personality" exists and that psychopathology does not account for asthma's etiology. However, symptoms of anxiety and depression are common in asthma. In a population-based sample of more than 13,000 Germans, asthma was associated with significantly increased likelihood of anxiety disorders (especially panic, generalized anxiety disorder, and phobias) and mood disorders (R.D. Goodwin et al. 2003).

Psychological factors can have profound effects on the symptoms and course of asthma. Rimington et al. (2001) found that anxiety and depression helped to explain asthma symptom scores, even after they controlled for lung function and treatment. Asthma symptom severity increased 27% in patients in New York City following the terrorist attacks on September 11, 2001 (Centers for Disease Control and Prevention 2002), and posttraumatic stress disorder was a significant predictor of the increase (Fagan et al. 2003). A multicenter European study of 715 community-dwelling young adults found that anxiety and depression scores independently predicted more wheezing, breathlessness, and nocturnal chest tightness but not a diagnosis of asthma (Janson et al. 1994). Rietveld et al. (1999) provided additional support for this relation in a controlled experiment comparing adolescents with asthma and nonasthmatic control subjects exposed to a standardized stressor (a frustrating computer task). Breathlessness increased in all the patients with asthma after the stressor, but no changes occurred in any objective pulmonary functions. Thus, psychological stress and distress make patients with asthma feel physically worse, despite no actual change in lung function in these studies. However, the theory that psychological factors might adversely affect pulmonary function in asthma remains quite possible. Le Son and Gershwin (1996) analyzed a retrospective cohort of 550 young adult hospitalized patients with asthma to determine risk factors for intubation. Psychological factors and psychosocial problems were more powerful predictors for intubation (odds ratio = 25.0; 95% confidence interval = 12.4–50.8) than any other examined variable (e.g., smoking, infection, prior hospitalization). Although impressive, this finding does not shed light on how psychological factors' effects on outcome in asthma are mediated, but other studies do. Psychological morbidity is associated with high levels of denial and delays in seeking medical attention in severe asthma, which may be life-threatening (Miles et al. 1997). Overuse of sympathomimetic drugs, especially over-the-counter agents or herbal remedies containing ephedrine, contributes to asthma mortality, as does underuse of inhaled corticosteroids. Psychological morbidity is associated with less adherence to prescribed inhaled steroids and consequently poorer control of asthma (Cluley and Cochrane 2001). In particular, noncompliant patients with asthma are more depressed than are compliant patients. Perhaps as a consequence, psychiatric symptoms in patients with severe asthma are associated with increased health care use (independent of severity of asthma), including more frequent visits to primary care physicians, emergency department visits, exacerbations, and hospitalizations (ten Brinke et al. 2001).

Chronic Obstructive Pulmonary Disease

COPD encompasses emphysema and chronic bronchitis, which are most often caused by cigarette smoking. Although patients with COPD differ from those with asthma in demographics, pathophysiology, treatment, and prognosis, there are similarities in the effects of psychological factors on each. Depression and anxiety are common in COPD patients (Aydin and Ulusahin 2001), although this in part reflects the frequency of depression and anxiety disorders in past or current smokers. Psychological distress amplifies perceived dyspnea, or breathlessness, without necessarily causing changes in measured pulmonary functions. Depression and anxiety appear to result in lower exercise tolerance (Withers et al. 1999), less adherence to treatment, poorer health status (Gudmundsson et al. 2006), and more disability (Aydin and Ulusahin 2001). Anxious COPD patients are more likely to be hospitalized and rehospitalized (Gudmundsson et al. 2005). Depression in outpatients with COPD may even be an independent predictor of mortality (Stage et al. 2005). Both pulmonary rehabilitation and cognitive-behavioral psychotherapy may improve exercise tolerance in anxious patients with COPD (Eiser et al. 1997; Withers et al. 1999).

COPD itself, through adverse effects on arterial oxygen and/or carbon dioxide concentrations, can cause cognitive dysfunction that impairs compliance. Chronic hypoxemia may result in irreversible hypoxic brain injury. Memory and concentration disturbances are especially common. Patients on chronic ventilation present some diagnostic and therapeutic problems, and psychological factors can affect weaning.

Clinical Implications

A history that suggests a connection between stressful events and aggravation of asthmatic symptoms should lead to psychiatric consultation. A specific aim of the consultation would include helping the patient develop heightened awareness of the typical stressors that appear to trigger dyspnea so that the patient can develop coping strategies for dealing with them. The psychiatrist also can evaluate the role of anxiolytics or antidepressants in those asthmatic patients for whom pharmacotherapy is indicated. Generally, asthmatic patients do not chronically retain carbon dioxide unless they also have COPD; thus, the judicious use of low-dose benzodiazepines is not necessarily contraindicated. Panic attacks may be difficult to distinguish from acute asthmatic attacks or may occur intertwined with each other. Patients may inappropriately use bronchodilator medications for the treatment of such anxiety, which may then sympathomimetically exacerbate anxiety symptoms. Benzodiazepines are appropriate acutely in such situations, and antidepressants should be considered for prophylactic management.

As noted, adverse effects of psychological morbidity, such as poorer adherence, exacerbation of subjective dyspnea, and more emergency department visits and hospitalizations, are also seen in patients with asthma or COPD. The appropriate treatment of anxiety disorders or major depression thus forms an essential part of the medical management of patients with chronic or recurrent pulmonary disease. Pathological avoidance or denial, whether by the patient or, in the case of pediatric patients with asthma, the family, also calls for intervention. Nothing is more critical in the management of asthma or COPD than smoking cessation. Failure to treat a comorbid mood or anxiety disorder will undermine the success of interventions to help the patient stop smoking. Some of the key findings regarding psychological factors and pulmonary disease are shown in Table 24–6.

Psychological Factors and Rheumatological Disease

Psychiatric aspects of the full array of rheumatological diseases can be found elsewhere (Dickens et al. 2005). Here the focus is on rheumatoid arthritis. Among patients and physicians, there is widespread anecdotal agreement that emotional factors affect the clinical course of rheumatoid arthritis. Since the work of Alexander (1950) and others, there has been interest in the personality profiles of rheumatoid arthritis patients, although the theory that certain neurotic conflicts or personality types were specific to rheumatoid arthritis has been disproven. The loss of mobility, jobs, and relationships contributes to depression and withdrawal, eroding support systems that are so important for patients with chronic illness. Certain "personality traits" and an increased incidence of psychiatric disturbance should be considered complications of rheumatoid arthritis and not causes of the disease.

Some earlier research suggested that stressful life events play a role in the development or onset of rheumatoid arthritis, but recent studies have not supported any significant relation between the two (Dickens et al.

2005). As with other chronic diseases, psychological factors do exert significant effects on symptoms, disability, and treatment in rheumatoid arthritis. Depression is very common and is associated with more pain and greater disability independent of objective indexes of rheumatoid arthritis disease severity. Depressed rheumatoid arthritis patients perceive their illness as more serious and are more pessimistic about treatment compared with nondepressed rheumatoid arthritis patients (Murphy et al. 1999). Even a history of major depression predicts higher levels of pain in rheumatoid arthritis patients years later (Fifield et al. 1998). A recent large longitudinal study found depression to be an independent risk factor for mortality in patients with rheumatoid arthritis (Ang et al. 2005). Randomized controlled trials of antidepressants in depressed rheumatoid arthritis patients show both the efficacy of treatment and the improvement in pain, morning stiffness, and disability scores (Bird and Broggini 2000). However, causal relations should not be understood simplistically; for example, some antidepressants have analgesic effects independent of their antidepressant effects. In children with juvenile rheumatoid arthritis, maternal emotional distress and the child's emotional distress are associated with higher reported pain after adjusting for disease characteristics (Ross et al. 1993).

The mechanisms by which psychological factors affect the course of rheumatoid arthritis have not been well characterized. Psychoneuroimmunological explanations appear less fitting than psychological effects on pain perception, energy, exercise tolerance, analgesic use, and treatment compliance (Dickens et al. 2005). Although the early view of rheumatoid arthritis as a classic psychosomatic disorder has been discarded, the consensus in the rheumatological literature is that psychological factors are important, but their relations with illness in rheumatoid arthritis are complex in both adults and children.

TABLE 24–6. Illustrative studies supporting the effects of psychological factors on pulmonary disease

Psychological factor	Study type	Findings	Reference(s)
Stress	Standardized experimental stressor	Increased breathlessness in asthmatic patients	Rietveld et al. 1999
Psychopathology	Clinical cohort	More asthma exacerbations, more health care use	ten Brinke et al. 2001
Depression and anxiety	Varied	Lower exercise tolerance, less compliance, more disability	Aydin and Ulusahin 2001; Withers et al. 1999

Clinical Implications

Psychological morbidity in rheumatoid arthritis patients, as noted, results in higher levels of pain, but it also leads to poorer quality of life, more work disability, more joint surgery, use of more resources, and lower compliance (Dickens et al. 2005). A randomized controlled trial found that group cognitive-behavioral therapy improved psychological and physical symptoms (Sharpe et al. 2001). Psychiatrists should be especially alert to the existence of mood disorders because depressive symptoms may be falsely attributed to rheumatoid arthritis itself.

Assessment of the support system is an early step in the total evaluation of a patient, and active attempts should be made to maintain the involvement of the patient's family and friends. Depression and demoralization can easily lead to a downward spiral of inactivity, social withdrawal, and nonparticipation in physical therapy, with associated deconditioning, loss of muscle mass, and distancing or even abandonment by the patient's support system. The amplification of pain by depression or other emotional distress often leads to overuse of analgesics and their chronic risks of toxicity.

Psychological Factors and Gastrointestinal Disorders

Peptic Ulcer Disease

Early investigators of psychosomatic illnesses focused on duodenal ulcer, for which psychological factors were thought to play a larger role than in gastric ulcer. Alexander (1950) suggested that duodenal ulcer occurred after an increase in responsibility or frustration in individuals with unmet wishes to be cared for ("oral dependency"). In a classic study testing this hypothesis, Weiner et al. (1957) combined preexisting individual psychological characteristics and a biological trait (high pepsinogen secretion) to predict successfully when men undergoing the stress of army draft would develop duodenal ulcer.

Understanding the pathogenesis of peptic ulcers has been revolutionized by the discovery of the central role of the bacterium *Helicobacter pylori*. Consequently, many physicians have concluded that peptic ulcer is an infectious disease, except when attributable to nonsteroidal anti-inflammatory drugs (NSAIDs), and that psychological factors are irrelevant. However, only a fraction of the people colonized by *H. pylori* or taking NSAIDs develop peptic ulcers, leaving open the possi-

TABLE 24–7. Factors affecting the development and progression of peptic ulcer disease

Primary	Secondary
Helicobacter pylori Nonsteroidal anti-inflammatory drugs	Disasters Occupational or family conflict Psychological distress (anxiety, depression) Smoking Alcohol abuse Poor diet Insomnia

bility of other contributing factors. A substantial body of research shows that psychosocial factors contribute to 30%–65% of ulcers (Levenstein 2000), summarized in Table 24–7. Psychological factors are most likely to be present in patients with duodenal ulcer who have few conventional medical risk factors (especially *H. pylori*) (Levenstein 2000). Psychological stress is an independent risk factor for the development (Rosenstock et al. 2003) and recurrence (Levenstein 2000) of duodenal ulcer. It has been repeatedly shown that peptic ulcer has been triggered by stress after experiencing a disaster, such as bombardment, earthquake, economic crises, being a prisoner of war, or being one of the "boat people" refugees. Job or wage conflicts and family problems also increase the risk of developing peptic ulcer. Depression, maladjustment, and hostility also are prospectively associated with peptic ulcer (Levenstein 2000). Stress, anxiety, and depression retard healing of ulcers and worsen the prognosis.

Whether specific emotions or character traits are pathogenic for peptic ulcer disease remains controversial, with very limited empirical support, and some "neurotic" traits may be the consequence rather than the cause of ulcer. Psychological factors appear to influence peptic ulcer development or course through both health risk behaviors and psychophysiological mechanisms. The former include smoking, alcohol abuse, overuse of NSAIDs, poor diet, and insomnia. The latter include pepsinogen and acid secretion, altered blood flow, impairment of mucosal defenses, and cortisol's slowing of healing (Levenstein 2000).

Irritable Bowel Syndrome

Psychopathology is extremely common in patients with irritable bowel syndrome (IBS), including anxiety (especially panic attacks), depression, and somatization, but there is no unique pattern of psychological characteristics (Walker et al. 1990). Patients with IBS are more likely to have a history of childhood sexual abuse compared with patients who have other gastrointestinal disorders (Walker et al. 1993), but this finding is most characteristic of those patients seeking care at tertiary referral centers. There does not appear to be any increased incidence of childhood sexual abuse in individuals in the community with symptoms of IBS who have not sought treatment. Indeed, almost all of the psychological traits or symptoms that are more common in IBS are differentially increased only in those who have sought medical care for their symptoms (Herschbach et al. 1999). Although both patients with IBS and their physicians observe that their gastrointestinal symptoms seem aggravated by stress, no clear evidence shows that stress causes a gastrointestinal smooth muscle response different from that in control subjects without IBS. Thus, the predominant effect of psychological factors in IBS appears to be on pain and other symptom sensitivity and perception and health care–seeking behaviors. For example, Gwee et al. (1999) prospectively followed up a cohort of patients who had an episode of infectious gastroenteritis to determine which factors might predict those patients who would go on to develop IBS. They found that those who had more stressful life events and those with higher hypochondriasis scores were more likely to develop IBS, even though there were no differences in intestinal physiological measures between those who did and did not develop IBS. In patients with severe IBS, concurrent psychiatric disorders are associated with significant impairment in health-related quality of life and higher health care costs (Creed et al. 2005).

Inflammatory Bowel Disease

Ulcerative colitis was described in early literature as a psychosomatic disease, but no specific psychological factor has ever been shown to contribute to the cause of ulcerative colitis or Crohn's disease. Psychological distress is common in both types of inflammatory bowel disease (IBD), but it may be a consequence of the chronic disease and its complications or a contributing stressor. Depression may predict relapse in IBD (Mittermaier et al. 2004). Anxiety (state, not trait) and depression are correlated with more physical morbidity and malnutrition in IBD, but the direction of causation is not clear (Addolorato et al. 1997). However, psychological stress does affect symptom complaints and may aggravate mucosal disease activity in ulcerative colitis (Levenstein et al. 1994). The presence of a concurrent psychiatric disorder contributes substantially to disability and distress in patients with IBD. In-

deed, depression and a depressive style of coping are better predictors of subjective impairment in IBD than is inflammatory activity (Cuntz et al. 1999).

Clinical Implications

Patients with peptic ulcer whose condition is refractory to treatment should be screened for high state and trait anxiety characteristics. Cognitive-behavioral therapy can help patients feel a greater sense of mastery over feared calamities and less helpless and overwhelmed. One randomized trial found no benefits in preventing recurrence, but other benefits were found (Wilhelmsen et al. 1994). Psychiatrists also can evaluate patients for appropriate use of anxiolytics. Clinicians also should identify depression, overuse of NSAIDs, alcohol abuse, smoking, job stress, and other psychosocial factors that may aggravate peptic ulcer for appropriate therapeutic intervention.

Patients with IBS should be evaluated for the presence of anxiety, mood, and somatoform disorders. Many patients seem to benefit from antianxiety and antidepressant drugs, but the benefits sometimes may be unrelated to the psychotropic effects (e.g., tricyclics' anticholinergic effects may reduce some IBS symptoms) (Creed and Olden 2005). Cognitive therapy also may be helpful for IBS, as shown in controlled trials (Creed et al. 2003).

Psychotherapy can significantly aid patients who are struggling to cope with ulcerative colitis or Crohn's disease (Maunder and Esplen 2001). A European prospective multicenter controlled trial of psychotherapy in Crohn's disease did not find statistically significant differences, but the trends were toward fewer episodes of IBD and less surgery resulting from failure of drug treatment in patients who received standard treatment plus psychotherapy (Jantschek et al. 1998). Pharmacological treatment of concurrent mood or anxiety disorders also can be very helpful.

The treatment of psychiatric disorders in patients with gastroenterological disease is examined in detail elsewhere (Creed and Olden 2005).

Psychological Factors and Dermatological Disorders

By way of its appearance and sensory capacities, the skin serves as a major interface for emotional expression in the interpersonal world. The range of normal emotions affects the appearance of the skin (e.g., flushing, sweating, blanching). Psychophysiological reactions are more easily observed in the skin than in any other organ through, for example, changes in skin conductance and blood flow. Although understudied empirically, the effects of psychological factors on skin have long been recognized by clinicians. Angioedema for many years was called angioneurotic edema. Pathological behavioral processes also come into play, including neglect of normal skin care and compulsive scratching and picking. It has long been believed that stressful life events trigger or exacerbate skin diseases. Some empirical support exists for this theory in psoriasis, alopecia areata, atopic dermatitis, and urticaria, but less evidence exists for this theory in vitiligo, lichen planus, acne, pemphigus, and seborrheic dermatitis (Arnold 2005). Because of the central social and psychological role played by the skin and its appearance, skin diseases can produce a host of psychological reactions, including depressive reactions, shame, social withdrawal, obsessive-compulsive behaviors, and rage (Stoudemire 1995). Psychiatric consultation is thus an important part of the treatment approach for many dermatological patients.

Psoriasis

Psoriasis produces hyperproliferative dry patches that require chronic treatment with topical preparations. It is a common illness, affecting up to 3 million individuals in the United States. Psychological factors are stronger determinants of disability in patients with psoriasis than are objective indexes of disease severity (Richards et al. 2001). The anxiety and shame associated with the disorder combine to exact a tremendous psychological toll, with intense anticipation of rejection, a sense of defectiveness, and social withdrawal. Patients with psoriasis (and many other skin diseases) feel very stigmatized because others avoid touching them. Bleeding psoriatic lesions are especially strongly correlated with feelings of stigma. Stigmatization and deprivation of social touching result in depression, despair, isolation, and noncompliance (Gupta et al. 1998). Stress- and depression-related neuropeptides may have a role in the pathogenesis of psoriasis (Panconesi and Hautmann 1996). More than half of all patients with the disease never enter remission and may be at greatest risk for social isolation. Defensive maneuvers such as social isolation contribute to the lack of potentially helpful relationships that could provide the regulation of painful affects. In a longitudinal study, Scharloo et al. (2000) found that patients with psoriasis who more actively coped, expressed more emotion, and sought more social support had better physical health, were less anxious and depressed, and needed

less treatment 1 year later. Excessive worrying has significant detrimental effects on treatment outcome in patients with psoriasis treated with photochemotherapy (Fortune et al. 2003).

Atopic Dermatitis

Stressful life events appear to precipitate and aggravate atopic dermatitis, and adults with atopic dermatitis have more anxiety and depression than do clinical and disease-free control groups (Arnold 2005). The mechanism for the effect of psychological distress may be through perturbation of epidermal permeability barrier homeostasis (Garg et al. 2001). A vicious cycle of itching, scratching, and aggravation of lesions is common, and a variety of cognitive and behavioral interventions have been helpful in reduction of symptoms and secondary anxiety and depressive symptoms (Arnold 2005).

Acne

Many psychological studies of patients with acne show a high prevalence of emotional symptoms, with anxiety and depression, especially poor self-esteem and negative self-image, being the most common (Arnold 2005). Acute stress aggravates the severity of acne (Chiu et al. 2003). Successful treatment of severe acne tends to reverse symptoms such as depressive affect and anxiety but produces little change in personality structure (Van der Meeren et al. 1985). Although adherence to treatment regimens constitutes an important variable in outcome, few studies have examined the psychological factors involved. Self-excoriative behavior is an important aggravating factor in acne, and it is more strongly correlated with psychological factors (poor self-concept, perfectionistic and compulsive personality traits) than with dermatological indexes of acne severity (Gupta et al. 1996). The use of isotretinoin for severe acne has been reported to cause depression, suicidal ideation, and other psychiatric symptoms sometimes, but not all studies have shown such adverse effects (Arnold 2005).

Urticaria

Urticaria is a common dermatological syndrome, producing wheal and flare "hives" that disappear within 24 hours. Lesions lasting longer should raise the suspicion of a vasculitic process and provoke a focus on etiologies other than the drugs and psychological causes common in transient urticaria. Evidence indicates an association between stressful life events and the onset of urticaria, and depression and anxiety are common in patients with chronic idiopathic urticaria (Arnold 2005). Neurophysiological mechanisms in anxiety-induced urticaria are similar to those in systemic anaphylaxis. Treatment generally involves antihistamines and reassurance about the transience of the lesions, but antidepressants also may be helpful (Arnold 2005).

Clinical Implications

The psychological sequelae of dermatological illnesses may be as important as the antecedents, and as noted earlier, they have erosive effects on support systems and compliance. Active psychiatric intervention in collaboration with dermatologists can interrupt this downward spiral. For many patients with skin diseases characterized by chronic pruritus, psychosocial stressors have a direct exacerbating effect, and psychotherapy, with or without anxiolytics, may help immensely in mitigating the adverse effects of such stressors. Patients with idiopathic urticaria commonly experience flares caused by anxiety. Anxiolytics and antidepressants may be quite helpful. Dermatologists often prescribe doxepin, although its efficacy against pruritus may derive primarily from its potent antihistaminic effects.

Psychological Factors and End-Stage Renal Disease

As treatment for end-stage renal disease (ESRD) has evolved, there has been extensive interest in the psychiatric and psychosocial aspects of dialysis and transplantation (Cohen et al. 2005, Kimmel 2000). In the following sections, I discuss the literature regarding quality of life and different treatment modalities, the effects of depression and noncompliance on outcome, and the case of patients who wish to withdraw from dialysis.

Quality of Life and Treatment Modality

Several studies have compared psychosocial quality of life for patients who have dialysis compared with renal transplantation. Of the studies in the United States and in other countries, most have found better psychosocial functioning in transplant patients (Cohen et al. 2005). Similar results have been found in children with renal failure. Other studies have shown no difference

in the psychological adjustment of patients receiving either of the two treatment modalities. Investigators also have compared the quality of life among patients receiving different dialysis modalities. Some have found continuous ambulatory peritoneal dialysis to be associated with better psychological outcome. Others have found mixed results or no differences in psychosocial outcomes. Home dialysis is preferred over center dialysis by those patients capable of handling it. All of these quality-of-life studies must be interpreted cautiously because patients are never randomly assigned to receive a particular form of dialysis or transplantation. Thus, outcome differences may be related to pretreatment differences in medical, psychosocial, or other variables. Nevertheless, most studies continue to show that patients receiving peritoneal dialysis rate their care higher than those receiving hemodialysis (Cohen et al. 2005; Rubin et al. 2004).

Effects of Depression on Outcome

Depressive symptoms predict overall quality of life more than does adequacy of biochemical dialysis, even after adjusting for other variables (Steele et al. 1996). A Canadian research group (Burton et al. 1986) found that *depression* was a better predictor of shorter survival than was age or a composite physiological index of clinical variables. Several other investigators have noted that depression in patients with ERSD is associated with higher mortality and morbidity (Shulman et al. 1989). Other studies have found no effects of depression on survival (Kutner et al. 1994). A fundamental weakness of most early studies was that no attempt was made to measure or to control for disease severity, a major confounding factor in studies relating psychopathology to outcome in the medically ill. Later studies have controlled for illness severity and other potential confounds, and depression still predicts higher mortality (Kimmel et al. 2000). For example, a prospective study in peritoneal dialysis patients found higher depressive symptoms associated with a greater risk for peritonitis, after the investigators controlled for other risk factors (Troidle et al. 2003).

Effects of Compliance on Outcome

From a clinical standpoint, compliance is an important factor in the management of dialysis patients. Noncompliance may appear as skipped or shortened dialysis sessions, excessive interdialytic weight gain, and medication or dietary noncompliance. Psychosocial factors with demonstrated effects on compliance in ESRD include patients' beliefs about their health behaviors, "locus of control" and self-efficacy, family problems, social support, and daily stress (Stoudemire 1995). Compliance also varies between cultures. Bleyer et al. (1999) found rates of missed hemodialysis treatments of 28.1 per 100 patient months in the United States, compared with no missed treatments in any of the Japanese or Swedish patients. Compliance is a complex multidimensional array of behaviors, and the relation between compliance and health outcomes in dialysis patients is not a simple one (Kaveh and Kimmel 2001). Different forms of compliance usually are intercorrelated but not always (Leggat et al. 1998). Cluster analysis was used to identify three distinct profiles of noncompliance among renal transplant recipients: accidental noncompliers, invulnerables, and decisive noncompliers (Greenstein and Siegal 1998).

The multiple dimensions and types of noncompliance in dialysis patients, as well as confounding factors such as culture and substance abuse, make it unsurprising that the literature to date does not show that noncompliance clearly predicts higher morbidity and mortality. Nevertheless, clinicians' experience that noncompliance leads to worse outcomes, including higher risk of death, is supported by large multicenter studies (Leggat et al. 1998). After heart disease, noncompliance is the most common "medical contraindication" excluding patients from renal transplantation (Holley et al. 1998).

Small studies of kidney transplant patients have shown that pretransplant noncompliance predicts posttransplant noncompliance and graft failure (Rodriguez et al. 1991). Noncompliant kidney transplant patients are more likely to be depressed and have other psychosocial problems than are compliant patients (Rodriguez et al. 1991). Overall, although the effects of noncompliance on dialysis and renal transplant patients are well recognized by clinicians, compliance should be regarded as a complex set of behaviors that requires more detailed investigation.

Withdrawal From Dialysis

Psychiatric consultation may be requested when long-term dialysis patients wish to discontinue treatment, raising clinical, liaison, and ethical issues (Cohen et al. 2005). In a large study of dialysis patients (Neu and Kjellstrand 1986), dialysis was discontinued in 9%, accounting for 22% of all deaths. Half of the patients withdrawn were incompetent and required surrogate decision making. Similar studies have been done in other countries (Catalano et al. 1996). Early studies that had pointed to a high rate of suicide in dialysis patients overestimated suicide prevalence by not distinguishing rational treatment withdrawal from suicide. A more recent study reported a suicide rate of 4% of those withdrawing from dialysis (Catalano et al. 1996). The true rate of suicide in dialysis has not been established systematically, nor has there been sufficient empirical characterization of the psychological factors that may affect the decision to withdraw from treatment. Although only a small fraction of those withdrawing from dialysis are suicidal, depressive symptoms appear to contribute to the decision in many patients (McDade-Montez et al. 2006). Consensus guidelines for withholding or withdrawing from dialysis, including psychiatric and behavioral reasons, have been developed in the United States and other countries (Cohen et al. 2005).

Several of the major studies examining psychological factors and outcome in renal disease are summarized in Table 24–8.

TABLE 24–8. Illustrative studies supporting the effects of psychological factors on end-stage renal disease

Psychological factor	Study type	Treatment modality	Findings	Reference(s)
Depression	Cohort	Hemodialysis	Depression predicts shorter survival	Burton et al. 1986; Kimmel et al. 2000
Cultural differences	Survey	Hemodialysis	28.1 missed treatments per 100 patient months in United States versus none in Japan and Sweden	Bleyer et al. 1999
Noncompliance	Cohort	Renal transplantation	Pretransplant noncompliance predicts posttransplant noncompliance and graft failure	Rodriguez et al. 1991

Mechanisms

The current state of research allows for informed speculation on how psychological factors such as depression might influence outcome in ESRD. Clinical experience is that depressed ESRD patients are more likely to evidence poor self-care, noncompliance, and poor medical follow-up. Noncompliance may be the key intervening mechanism for the effects of depression and other psychological factors. Depression also has been associated in other populations with increased use of analgesics, which have been shown to have a role in the etiology and exacerbation of chronic renal failure. Depression is associated with smoking, alcoholism, and other forms of substance abuse that are highly prevalent in patients with ESRD (Hegde et al. 2000) and are major causes of increased morbidity and mortality themselves. Depression may adversely affect outcome in ESRD by serving as a risk factor for other medical comorbidity—for example, myocardial infarction or malnutrition.

Clinical Implications

Psychiatrists are sometimes asked to participate in decision making about which ESRD treatment modality best suits a particular patient. Current research sheds some light on this question, but it still must be answered according to the preferences and needs of the particular patient. Which modality is most appealing to the patient (e.g., regarding lifestyle, body image, and demands of the treatment)? With which treatment will the patient be most compliant?

Depression is the most common psychiatric disorder in ESRD patients, and the symptoms may be difficult to distinguish from uremia or other comorbid medical conditions. Careful differential diagnosis will identify those patients who should receive treatment for depression, with subsequent expectable improvement in quality of life and functional capacity. Details of the treatment of psychiatric disorders in renal failure and dialysis patients may be found elsewhere (Cohen et al. 2005).

Noncompliance remains the reason that psychiatrists are most often consulted by nephrologists. The psychiatrist should help the ESRD treatment team avoid simplistic thinking about noncompliance and be aware of the risk of scapegoating the patient. Noncompliance, as previously noted, represents a complex set of behaviors and interpersonal relationships (patient, family, physician, nurse) with important cultural and ethical considerations. Behavioral interventions have been shown to improve compliance with fluid restrictions (Sagawa et al. 2003). The most extreme form of noncompliance is refusal to accept, or withdrawal from, treatment for ESRD. Some clinicians err in regarding such patients as always depressed and suicidal, whereas others err in the opposite direction, too often accepting such a decision at face value as rational. Psychiatrists have a crucial role in what can be a difficult distinction between autonomous rational decision making and irrational suicidal giving up, symptomatic of a treatable depression (Cohen et al. 2005).

Conclusion

The DSM-IV-TR (American Psychiatric Association 2000) diagnostic criteria for psychological factors affecting a medical condition are shown in Table 24–2. In this chapter, I have attempted to recognize and illustrate the complexity of the myriad relations between psychological factors and medical conditions, including onset, course, and outcome of illness. Psychological factors appear to be independent risk factors for some medical diseases, although confounding with other risk factors is typical. Psychological factors may physiologically affect somatic symptoms but more often affect patients' perception of their symptoms. The importance of such "subjective" effects should not be underestimated; as noted in this chapter, cardinal symptoms of many diseases are more closely correlated with psychological factors than with objective indexes of disease severity. The mechanisms by which psychological factors affect medical conditions are still being worked out and require much more research. The range of possible mechanisms is wide, including effects via psychophysiology (e.g., psychoneuroimmunology), the doctor–patient relationship, compliance, and health care use. Although controlled trials now support the value of timely psychiatric and psychotherapeutic interventions in many medical illnesses, much work remains to determine the most effective applications of mental health services in medically ill patients.

Key Points

- Psychological factors have profound adverse effects on many medical conditions, including

  1. Decreasing functional capacity and quality of life

  2. Increasing risk for developing the medical disorder

  3. Increasing morbidity and mortality

  4. Increasing health care costs

- The mechanisms by which psychological factors affect medical conditions include

  1. Promotion of other risk factors

  2. Amplification of somatic symptoms

  3. Interference with access to health care

  4. Decreased motivation and compliance

  5. Effects on the doctor–patient relationship

  6. Effects on pathophysiology

Suggested Readings

Levenson JL (ed): The American Psychiatric Publishing Textbook of Psychosomatic Medicine. Arlington, VA, American Psychiatric Publishing, 2005

Levenson JL (ed): Essentials of Psychosomatic Medicine. Arlington, VA, American Psychiatric Publishing, 2007

Stoudemire A (ed): Psychological Factors Affecting Medical Conditions. Washington, DC, American Psychiatric Press, 1995

References

Addolorato G, Capristo E, Stefanini GF, et al: Inflammatory bowel disease: a study of the association between anxiety and depression, physical morbidity, and nutritional status. Scand J Gastroenterol 32:1013–1021, 1997

Alexander F: Psychosomatic Medicine: Its Principles and Applications. New York, WW Norton, 1950

American Psychiatric Association: Diagnostic and Statistical Manual of Mental Disorders, 4th Edition. Washington, DC, American Psychiatric Association, 1994

American Psychiatric Association: Diagnostic and Statistical Manual of Mental Disorders, 4th Edition, Text Revision. Washington, DC, American Psychiatric Association, 2000

Ang DC, Choi H, Kroenke K, et al: Comorbid depression in an independent risk factor for mortality in patients with rheumatoid arthritis. J Rheumatol 32:1013–1019, 2005

Arnold LM: Dermatology, in The American Psychiatric Publishing Textbook of Psychosomatic Medicine. Edited by Levenson JL. Washington, DC, American Psychiatric Publishing, 2005, pp 629–646

Aro AR, De Koning HJ, Schreck M, et al: Psychological risk factors of incidence of breast cancer: a prospective cohort study in Finland. Psychol Med 35:1515–1521, 2005

Aydin IO, Ulusahin A: Depression, anxiety comorbidity, and disability in tuberculosis and chronic obstructive pulmonary disease patients: applicability of GHQ-12. Gen Hosp Psychiatry 23:77–83, 2001

Bergelt C, Christensen J, Prescott E, et al: Vital exhaustion and risk for cancer: a prospective cohort study on the association between depressive feelings, fatigue, and risk of cancer. Cancer 104:1288–1295, 2005

Bird H, Broggini M: Paroxetine versus amitriptyline for treatment of depression associated with rheumatoid arthritis: a randomized, double blind, parallel group study. J Rheumatol 27:2791–2797, 2000

Birkenaes AB, Søgaard AJ, Engh JA, et al: Sociodemographic characteristics and cardiovascular risk factors in patients with severe mental disorders compared with the general population. J Clin Psychiatry 67:425–433, 2006

Bleiker EM, van der Ploeg HM, Hendriks JH, et al: Personality factors and breast cancer development: a prospective longitudinal study. J Natl Cancer Inst 88:1478–1482, 1996

Bleyer AJ, Hylander B, Sudo H, et al: An international study of patient compliance with hemodialysis. JAMA 281:1211–1213, 1999

Bordeleau L, Szalai JP, Ennis, M, et al: Quality of life in a randomized trial of group psychosocial support in metastatic breast cancer: overall effects of the intervention and an exploration of missing data. J Clin Oncol 21:1944–1951, 2003

Boyle SH, Williams RB, Mark DB, et al: Hostility as a predictor of survival in patients with coronary artery disease. Psychosom Med 66:629–632, 2004

Breitbart W, Gibson C, Poppito SR, et al: Psychotherapeutic interventions at the end of life: a focus on meaning and spirituality. Can J Psychiatry 49:366–372, 2004

Buddeberg C, Wolf C, Sieber M, et al: Coping strategies and course of disease of breast cancer patients: results of a 3-year longitudinal study. Psychother Psychosom 55:151–157, 1991

Burgess C, Cornelius V, Love S, et al: Depression and anxiety in women with early breast cancer: five year observational cohort study. BMJ 330:702, 2005

Burton JJ, Kline SA, Lindsay RM, et al: Relationship of depression to survival in chronic renal failure. Psychosom Med 48:261–269, 1986

Butow PN, Coates AS, Dunn SM: Psychosocial predictors of survival in metastatic melanoma. J Clin Oncol 17:2256–2263, 1999

Carney RM, Freeland KE, Eisen SA, et al: Major depression and medication adherence in elderly patients with coronary artery disease. Health Psychol 14:88–90, 1995

Carney RM, Blumenthal JA, Catellier D, et al: Depression as a risk factor for mortality after acute myocardial infarction. Am J Cardiol 92:1277–1281, 2003

Case DO, Andrews JE, Johnson JD, et al: Avoiding versus seeking: the relationship of information seeking to avoidance, blunting, coping, dissonance, and related concepts. J Med Libr Assoc 93:353–362, 2005

Cassileth BR, Walsh WP, Lusk EJ: Psychosocial correlates of cancer survival: a subsequent report 3 to 8 years after cancer diagnosis. J Clin Oncol 6:1753–1759, 1988

Catalano C, Goodship TH, Graham KA, et al: Withdrawal of renal replacement therapy in Newcastle Upon Tyne. Nephrol Dial Transplant 11:133–139, 1996

Centers for Disease Control and Prevention: Self-reported increase in asthma severity after the September 11 attacks on the World Trade Center—Manhattan—New York, 2001. MMWR Morb Mortal Wkly Rep 51:781–784, 2002

Chiovato L, Marino M, Perugi G, et al: Chronic recurrent stress due to panic disorder does not precipitate Graves' disease. J Endocrinol Invest 21:758–764, 1998

Chiu A, Chon SY, Kimball AB: The response of skin disease to stress: changes in the severity of acne vulgaris as affected by examination stress. Arch Dermatol 139:897–900, 2003

Ciechanowski PS, Katon WJ, Russo JE: Depression and diabetes: impact of depressive symptoms on adherence, function, and costs. Arch Intern Med 160:3278–3285, 2000

Ciechanowski PS, Katon WJ, Russo JE, et al: The patient–provider relationship: attachment theory and adherence to treatment in diabetes. Am J Psychiatry 158:29–35, 2001

Cluley S, Cochrane GM: Psychological disorder in asthma is associated with poor control and poor adherences to inhaled steroids. Respir Med 95:37–39, 2001

Cohen LM, Levy NB, Tessier EG, et al: Renal disease, in The American Psychiatric Publishing Textbook of Psychosomatic Medicine. Edited by Levenson JL. Washington, DC, American Psychiatric Publishing, 2005, pp 483–493

Courtney JG, Longnecker MP, Theorell T, et al: Stressful life events and the risk of colorectal cancer. Epidemiology 4:407–414, 1993

Creed F, Olden KW: Gastrointestinal disorders, in The American Psychiatric Publishing Textbook of Psychosomatic Medicine. Edited by Levenson JL. Washington, DC, American Psychiatric Publishing, 2005, pp 465–481

Creed F, Fernandes L, Guthrie E, et al: The cost-effectiveness of psychotherapy and paroxetine for severe irritable bowel syndrome. Gastroenterology 124:303–317, 2003

Creed F, Ratcliffe J, Fernandes L, et al: Outcome in severe irritable bowel syndrome with and without accompanying depressive, panic and neurasthenic disorders. Br J Psychiatry 186:507–515, 2005

Cuntz U, Welt J, Ruppert E, et al: Determination of subjective burden from chronic inflammatory bowel disease and its psychosocial consequences: results from a study of 200 patients. Psychother Psychosom Med Psychol 49:494–500, 1999

Daumit GL, Pronovost PJ, Anthony CB, et al: Adverse events during medical and surgical hospitalizations for persons with schizophrenia. Arch Gen Psychiatry 63:267–272, 2006

de Groot M, Jacobson AM, Samson JA, et al: Glycemic control and major depression in patients with type 1 and type 2 diabetes mellitus. J Psychosom Res 46:425–435, 1999

de Leon J, Diaz FJ: A meta-analysis of worldwide studies demonstrates an association between schizophrenia and tobacco smoking behaviors. Schizophr Res 76:135–157, 2005

Dickens C, Levenson JL, Cohen W: Rheumatology, in The American Psychiatric Publishing Textbook of Psychosomatic Medicine. Edited by Levenson JL. Washington, DC, American Psychiatric Publishing, 2005, pp 535–554

Druss BG, Bradford DW, Rosenheck RA, et al: Mental disorders and use of cardiovascular procedures after myocardial infarction. JAMA 283:506–511, 2000

Eiser N, West C, Evans S, et al: Effects of psychotherapy in moderately severe COPD: a pilot study. Eur Respir J 10:1581–1584, 1997

Fagan J, Galea S, Ahern J, et al: Relationship of self-reported asthma severity and urgent health care utilization to psychological sequelae of the September 11, 2001 terrorist attacks on the World Trade Center among New York City area residents. Psychosom Med 65:993–996, 2003

Faller H, Bulzebruck H, Drungs P, et al: Coping, distress, and survival among patients with lung cancer. Arch Gen Psychiatry 56:756–762, 1999

Fawzy FI, Fawzy NW, Hyun CS, et al: Malignant melanoma: effects of an early structured psychiatric intervention, coping, and affective state on recurrence and survival 6 years later. Arch Gen Psychiatry 50:681–689, 1993

Fifield J, Tennen H, Reisine S, et al: Depression and the long-term risk of pain, fatigue, and disability in patients with rheumatoid arthritis. Arthritis Rheum 41:1851–1857, 1998

Fortune DG, Richards HL, Kirby B, et al: Psychological distress impairs clearance of psoriasis in patients treated with photochemotherapy. Arch Dermatol 139:752–756, 2003

Fox BH: Current theory of psychogenic effects on cancer incidence and prognosis. J Psychosoc Oncol 1:17–31, 1983

Frasure-Smith N, Lesperance F, Talajic M: Depression following myocardial infarction: impact on 6-month survival. JAMA 270:1819–1825, 1993

Frasure-Smith N, Lesperance F, Talajic M: Depression and 18-month prognosis after myocardial infarction. Circulation 91:999–1005, 1995a

Frasure-Smith N, Lesperance F, Talajic M: The impact of negative emotions on prognosis following myocardial infarction: is it more than depression? Health Psychol 14:388–398, 1995b

Friedman R, Schwartz JE, Schnall PL, et al: Psychological variables in hypertension: relationship to casual or ambulatory blood pressure in men. Psychosom Med 63:19–31, 2001

Fukao A, Takamatsu J, Murakami Y, et al: The relationship of psychological factors to the prognosis of hyperthyroidism in antithyroid drug-treated patients with Grave's disease. Clin Endocrinol 58:550–555, 2003

Garay-Sevilla ME, Malacara JM, Gonzalez-Contreras E, et al: Perceived psychological stress in diabetes mellitus type 2. Rev Invest Clin 52:241–245, 2000

Garg A, Chren MM, Sands LP, et al: Psychological stress perturbs epidermal permeability barrier homeostasis: implications for the pathogenesis of stress-associated skin disorders. Arch Dermatol 137:53–59, 2001

Geyer S: Life events prior to manifestation of breast cancer: a limited prospective study covering eight years before diagnosis. J Psychosom Res 35:355–363, 1991

Giltay EJ, Geleijnse JM, Zitman FG, et al: Dispositional optimism and all-cause and cardiovascular mortality in a prospective cohort of elderly Dutch men and women. Arch Gen Psychiatry 61:1126–1135, 2004

Glassman AH, O'Connor CM, Califf RM, et al: Sertraline treatment of major depression in patients with acute MI or unstable angina. JAMA 288:701–709, 2002

Goebel-Fabbri A, Musen G, Sparks CR, et al: Endocrine and metabolic disorders, in The American Psychiatric Publishing Textbook of Psychosomatic Medicine. Edited by Levenson JL. Washington, DC, American Psychiatric Publishing, 2005, pp 495–516

Goetsch VL, VanDorsten B, Pbert LA, et al: Acute effects of laboratory stress on blood glucose in non-insulin-dependent diabetes. Psychosom Med 55:492–496, 1993

Goodwin PJ, Leszcz M, Ennis M, et al: The effect of group psychological support on survival in metastatic breast cancer. N Engl J Med 345:1719–1726, 2001

Goodwin RD, Jacobi F, Thefeld W: Mental disorders and asthma in the community. Arch Gen Psychiatry 60:1125–1130, 2003

Greenstein S, Siegal B: Compliance and noncompliance in patients with a functioning renal transplant: a multicenter study. Transplantation 66:1718–1726, 1998

Greer S, Morris T, Pettingale KW: Psychological response to breast cancer: effect on outcome. Lancet 2:785–787, 1979

Greimel ER, Padilla GV, Grant MM: Self-care response to illness of patients with various cancer diagnoses. Acta Oncol 36:141–150, 1997

Grey M, Boland EA, Davidson M, et al: Coping skills training for youth with diabetes mellitus has long-lasting effects on metabolic control and quality of life. J Pediatr 137:107–113, 2000

Gudmundsson G, Gislason T, Janson C, et al: Risk factors for rehospitalisation in COPD: role of health status, anxiety and depression. Eur Respir J 26:414–419, 2005

Gudmundsson G, Gislason T, Janson C, et al: Depression, anxiety and health status after hospitalisation for COPD: a multicentre study in the Nordic countries. Respir Med 100:87–93, 2006

Gullette ECD, Blumenthal JA, Babyak M, et al: Effects of mental stress on myocardial ischemia during daily life. JAMA 277:1521–1525, 1997

Gupta MA, Gupta AK, Schork NJ: Psychological factors affecting self-excoriative behavior in women with mild-to-moderate facial acne vulgaris. Psychosomatics 37:127–130, 1996

Gupta MA, Gupta AK, Watteel GN: Perceived deprivation of social touch in psoriasis is associated with greater psychological morbidity: an index of the stigma experience in dermatological disorders. Cutis 61:339–342, 1998

Gwee KA, Leong YL, Graham C, et al: The role of psychological and biological factors in postinfective gut dysfunction. Gut 44:400–406, 1999

Hegde A, Veis JH, Seidman A, et al: High prevalence of alcoholism in dialysis patients. Am J Kidney Dis 35:1039–1043, 2000

Herschbach P, Henrich G, von Rad M: Psychological factors in functional gastrointestinal disorders: characteristics of the disorder or of the illness behavior? Psychosom Med 61:148–153, 1999

Hill JA: In vino veritas: alcohol and heart disease. Am J Med Sci 329:124–135, 2005

Holland JC, Romano SJ, Heiligenstein JH, et al: A controlled trial of fluoxetine and desipramine in depressed women with advanced cancer. Psychooncology 7:291–300, 1998

Holley JL, Monaghan J, Byer B, et al: An examination of the renal transplant evaluation process focusing on cost and the reasons for patient exclusion. Am J Kidney Dis 32:567–574, 1998

Ironson G, Taylor CB, Boltwood M, et al: Effects of anger on left ventricular ejection fraction in coronary artery disease. Am J Cardiol 70:281–285, 1992

Isaacs SL, Schroeder SA: Class—the ignored determinant of the nation's health. N Engl J Med 351:1137–1142, 2004

Janson C, Bjornsson E, Hetta J, et al: Anxiety and depression in relation to respiratory symptoms and asthma. Am J Respir Crit Care Med 149:930–934, 1994

Jantschek G, Zeitz M, Pritsch M, et al: Effect of psychotherapy on the course of Crohn's disease: result of the German prospective multicenter psychotherapy treatment study of Crohn's disease. German Study Group on Psychosocial Intervention in Crohn's Disease. Scand J Gastroenterol 33:1289–1296, 1998

Januzzi JL, Stern TA, Pasternak RC, et al: The influence of anxiety and depression on outcomes of patients with coronary artery disease. Arch Intern Med 160:1913–1921, 2000

Jiang W, Babyak M, Krantz DS, et al: Mental stress-induced myocardial ischemia and cardiac events. JAMA 275:1651–1656, 1996

Jiang W, Alexander J, Christopher E, et al: Relationship of depression to increased risk of mortality and rehospitalization in patients with congestive heart failure. Arch Intern Med 161:1849–1856, 2001

Katon WJ, Von Korff M, Lin EH, et al: The Pathways Study: a randomized trial of collaborative care in patients with diabetes and depression. Arch Gen Psychiatry 61:1042–1049, 2004

Katon WJ, Rutter C, Simon G, et al: The association of comorbid depression with mortality in patients with type 2 diabetes. Diabetes Care 28:2668–2772, 2005

Kaveh K, Kimmel PL: Compliance in hemodialysis patients: multidimensional measures in search of a gold measure. Am J Kidney Dis 37:244–266, 2001

Kawachi I, Berkman LF (eds): Neighborhoods and Health. New York, Oxford University Press, 2003

Kimmel PL: Psychosocial factors in adult end-stage renal disease patients treated with hemodialysis: correlates and outcomes. Am J Kidney Dis 35:S132–S140, 2000

Kimmel PL, Peterson RA, Weihs KL, et al: Multiple measurements of depression predict mortality in a longitudinal study of chronic hemodialysis outpatients. Kidney Int 57:2093–2098, 2000

Kramer JR, Ledolter J, Manos GN, et al: Stress and metabolic control in diabetes mellitus: methodological issues and an illustrative analysis. Ann Behav Med 22:17–28, 2000

Krantz DS, Sheps DS, Carney RM, et al: Effects of mental stress in patients with coronary artery disease: evidence and clinical implications. JAMA 283:1800–1802, 2000

Kreitler S, Chaitchik S, Kreitler H: Repressiveness: cause or result of cancer? Psychooncology 2:43–54, 1993

Kune GA, Kune S, Watson LF, et al: Personality as a risk factor in large bowel cancer: data from the Melbourne Colorectal Cancer Study. Psychol Med 21:29–41, 1991

Kutner NG, Lin LS, Fielding B, et al: Continued survival of older hemodialysis patients: investigation of psychosocial predictors. Am J Kidney Dis 24:42–49, 1994

Lane JD, McCaskill CC, Williams PG, et al: Personality correlates of glycemic control in type 2 diabetes. Diabetes Care 23:1321–1325, 2000

Lasser K, Boyd JW, Woolhandler S, et al: Smoking and mental illness: a population-based prevalence study. JAMA 284:2606–2610, 2000

Leggat JE Jr, Orzol SM, Hulbert-Shearin TE, et al: Noncompliance in hemodialysis: predictors and survival analysis. Am J Kidney Dis 32:139–145, 1998

Leiferman JA, Pheley AM: The effect of mental distress on women's preventive health behaviors. Am J Health Promot 20:196–199, 2006

Lernmark B, Persson B, Fisher L, et al: Symptoms of depression are important to psychological adaptation and metabolic control in children with diabetes mellitus. Diabet Med 16:14–22, 1999

Le Son S, Gershwin ME: Risk factors for asthmatic patients requiring intubation, III: observations in young adults. J Asthma 33:27–35, 1996

Lesperance F, Frasure-Smith N, Juneau M, et al: Depression and 1-year prognosis in unstable angina. Arch Intern Med 160:1354–1360, 2000

Levenson JL (ed): The American Psychiatric Publishing Textbook of Psychosomatic Medicine. Washington, DC, American Psychiatric Publishing, 2005

Levenson JL, McDonald MK: The role of psychological factors in cancer onset and progression: a critical appraisal, in The Psychoimmunology of Cancer, 2nd Edition. Edited by Lewis CE, O'Brien R, Barraclough J. New York, Oxford University Press, 2002, pp 149–163

Levenstein S: The very model of a modern etiology: a biopsychosocial view of peptic ulcer. Psychosom Med 62:176–185, 2000

Levenstein S, Prantera C, Varvo V, et al: Psychological stress and distress activity in ulcerative colitis: a multidimensional cross-sectional study. Am J Gastroenterol 89:1219–1225, 1994

Li J, Johansen C, Olsen J: Cancer survival in parents who lost a child: a nationwide study in Denmark. Br J Cancer 88:1698–1701, 2003

Lloyd CE, Dyer PH, Lancashire RJ, et al: Association between stress and glycemic control in adults with type 1 (insulin-dependent) diabetes. Diabetes Care 22:1278–1283, 1999

Lloyd CE, Dyer PH, Barnett AH: Prevalence of symptoms of depression and anxiety in a diabetes clinic population. Diabet Med 17:198–202, 2000

Ludman EJ, Katon W, Russo J, et al: Depression and diabetes symptom burden. Gen Hosp Psychiatry 26:430–436, 2004

Lustman PJ, Freedland KE, Griffith LS, et al: Predicting response to cognitive behavior therapy of depression in type 2 diabetes. Gen Hosp Psychiatry 20:302–306, 1998

Lustman PJ, Anderson RJ, Freedland KE, et al: Depression and poor glycemic control: a meta-analytic review of the literature. Diabetes Care 23:934–942, 2000

Lynge E, Anderson O: Unemployment and cancer in Denmark, 1970–1975 and 1986–1990. IARC Sci Publ 138:353–359, 1997

Massie MJ, Greenberg DB: Oncology, in The American Psychiatric Publishing Textbook of Psychosomatic Medicine. Edited by Levenson JL. Washington, DC, American Psychiatric Publishing, 2005, pp 517–534

Maunder RG, Esplen MJ: Supportive-expressive group psychotherapy for persons with anti-inflammatory bowel disease. Can J Psychiatry 46:622–626, 2001

McDade-Montez EA, Christensen AJ, Cvengros JA, et al: The role of depression symptoms in dialysis withdrawal. Health Psychol 25:198–204, 2006

McElroy SL, Kotwal R, Malhotra S, et al: Are mood disorders and obesity related? A review for the mental health professional. J Clin Psychiatry 65:634–651, 2004

McGee R, Williams S, Elwood M: Depression and the development of cancer: a meta-analysis. Soc Sci Med 38:187–192, 1994

McKenna MC, Zevon MA, Corn B, et al: Psychosocial factors and the development of breast cancer: a meta-analysis. Health Psychol 18:520–531, 1999

Miles JF, Garden GM, Tunnicliffe WS, et al: Psychological morbidity and coping skills in patients with brittle and non-brittle asthma: a case-control study. Clin Exp Allergy 27:1151–1159, 1997

Mittermaier C, Dejaco C, Waldhoer T, et al: Impact of depressive mood on relapse in patients with inflammatory bowel disease: a prospective 18-month follow-up study. Psychosom Med 66:79–84, 2004

Mooy JM, deVries H, Grootenhuis PA, et al: Major stressful life events in relation to prevalence of undetected type 2 diabetes: the Hoorn Study. Diabetes Care 23:197–201, 2000

Moser DK, Dracup K: Is anxiety early after myocardial infarction associated with subsequent ischemic and arrhythmic events? Psychosom Med 58:395–401, 1996

Murphy H, Dickens C, Creed F, et al: Depression, illness perception and coping in rheumatoid arthritis. J Psychosom Res 46:155–164, 1999

Neu S, Kjellstrand CM: Stopping long-term dialysis: an empirical study of withdrawal of life-supporting treatment. N Engl J Med 314:14–20, 1986

Nielsen NR, Zhang ZF, Kristensen TS, et al: Self reported stress and risk of breast cancer: prospective cohort study. BMJ 331:548, 2005

Orlandini A, Pastore MR, Fossati A, et al: Personality traits and metabolic control: a study in insulin-dependent diabetes mellitus patients. Psychother Psychosom 66:307–313, 1997

Orth-Gomér K, Wamala SP, Horsten M, et al: Marital stress worsens prognosis in women with coronary heart disease: the Stockholm Female Coronary Risk Study. JAMA 284:3008–3014, 2000

Panconesi E, Hautmann G: Psychophysiology of stress in dermatology: the psychobiological pattern of psychosomatics. Dermatol Clin 14:399–421, 1996

Parissis JT, Adamopoulos S, Rigas A, et al: Comparison of circulating proinflammatory cytokines and soluble apoptosis mediators in patients with chronic heart failure with versus without symptoms of depression. Am J Cardiol 94:1326–1328, 2004

Penninx BWJH, Beekman ATF, Honig A, et al: Depression and cardiac mortality. Arch Gen Psychiatry 58:221–227, 2001

Perros P, Deary IJ, Frier BM: Factors influencing preference of insulin regimen in people with type 1 (insulin-dependent) diabetes. Diabetes Res Clin Pract 39:23–29, 1998

Persky VW, Kempthorne-Rawson J, Shekelle RB: Personality and risk of cancer: 20-year follow-up of the Western Electric Study. Psychosom Med 49:435–449, 1987

Power C, Parsons T: Nutritional and other influences in childhood as predictors of adult obesity. Proc Nutr Soc 59:267–272, 2000

Richards HL, Fortune DG, Griffiths CE, et al: The contribution of perceptions of stigmatization to disability in patients with psoriasis. Psychosom Res 50:11–15, 2001

Rietveld S, van Beest I, Everaerd W: Stress-induced breathlessness in asthma. Psychol Med 29:1359–1366, 1999

Rimington LD, Davies DH, Lowe D, et al: Relationship between anxiety, depression, and morbidity in adult asthma patients. Thorax 56:266–271, 2001

Rodriguez A, Diaz M, Colon A, et al: Psychosocial profile of noncompliant transplant patients. Transplant Proc 23:1807–1809, 1991

Roscoe JA, Morrow GR, Hickok, JT, et al: Effect of paroxetine hydrochloride (Paxil) on fatigue and depression in breast cancer patients receiving chemotherapy. Breast Cancer Res Treat 89:243–249, 2005

Rosengren A, Hawken S, Ounpuu S, et al: Association of psychosocial risk factors with risk of acute myocardial infarction in 11,119 cases and 13,648 controls from 52 countries (the INTERHEART study): case-control study. Lancet 364:953–962, 2004

Rosenstock S, Jorgensen T, Bonnevie O, et al: Risk factors for peptic ulcer disease: a population based prospective cohort study comprising 2416 Danish adults. Gut 52:186–193, 2003

Ross CK, Lavigne JV, Hayford JR, et al: Psychological factors affecting reported pain in juvenile rheumatoid arthritis. J Pediatr Psychol 18:561–573, 1993

Rozanski A, Blumenthal JA, Kaplan J: Impact of psychological factors on the pathogenesis of cardiovascular disease and implications for therapy. Circulation 99:2192–2217, 1999

Rubin HR, Fink NE, Plantinga LC, et al: Patients' ratings of dialysis care with peritoneal dialysis vs. hemodialysis. JAMA 291:697–703, 2004

Rumsfeld JS, Havranek E, Masoudi FA, et al: Depressive symptoms are the strongest predictors of short-term declines in health status in patients with heart failure. J Am Coll Cardiol 42:1811–1817, 2003

Ruo B, Rumsfeld JS, Hlatky MA, et al: Depressive symptoms and health-related quality of life. JAMA 290:215–221, 2003

Ruzickova M, Slaney C, Garnham J, et al: Clinical features of bipolar disorder with and without comorbid diabetes mellitus. Can J Psychiatry 48:458–461, 2003

Sagawa M, Oka M, Chabeyer W: The utility of cognitive behavioural therapy on chronic hemodialysis patients' fluid intake: a preliminary examination. Int J Nurs Stud 40:367–373, 2003

Santos AM, Nobre EL, Garcia e Costa J, et al: Grave's disease and stress. Acta Med Port 15:423–427, 2002

Scharloo M, Kaptein AA, Weinman J, et al: Patients' illness perceptions and coping as predictors of functional status in psoriasis: a 1-year follow-up. Br J Dermatol 142:899–907, 2000

Shapiro PA: Cardiology, in The American Psychiatric Publishing Textbook of Psychosomatic Medicine. Edited by Levenson JL. Washington, DC, American Psychiatric Publishing, 2005, pp 423–444

Sharpe L, Sensky T, Timberlake N, et al: A blind, randomized, controlled trial of cognitive-behavioural intervention for patients with recent onset rheumatoid arthritis: preventing psychological and physical morbidity. Pain 89:275–283, 2001

Shaw K, O'Rourke P, Del Mar C, et al: Psychological interventions for overweight or obesity. Cochrane Database Syst Rev (2):CD003818, 2005

Shekelle RB, Rossof AH, Stamler J: Dietary cholesterol and incidence of lung cancer: the Western Electric Study. Am J Epidemiol 134:480–484; discussion 543–544, 1991

Shulman R, Price JD, Spinelli J: Biopsychosocial aspects of long-term survival on end-stage renal failure therapy. Psychol Med 19:945–954, 1989

Simon GE, Katon WJ, Lin EH, et al: Diabetes complications and depression as predictors of health service costs. Gen Hosp Psychiatry 27:344–351, 2005

Soler-Vila H, Kasl SV, Jones BA: Prognostic significance of psychosocial factors in African American and white breast cancer patients: a population-based study. Cancer 98:1299–1308, 2003

Spiegel D, Bloom JR, Kraemer HC, et al: Effect of psychosocial treatment on survival of patients with metastatic breast cancer. Lancet 2:888–891, 1989

Stage KB, Middelboe T, Pisinger C: Depression and chronic obstructive pulmonary disease (COPD): impact on survival. Acta Psychiatr Scand 111:320–323, 2005

Steele TE, Baltimore D, Finkelstein SH, et al: Quality of life in peritoneal dialysis patients. J Nerv Ment Dis 184:368–374, 1996

Steinberg JS, Arshad A, Kowalski M, et al: Increased incidence of life-threatening ventricular arrhythmias in implantable defibrillator patients after World Trade Center attack. J Am Coll Cardiol 45:1732–1733, 2005

Stoudemire A (ed): Psychological Factors Affecting Medical Conditions. Washington, DC, American Psychiatric Press, 1995

Stoudemire A, Hales RE: Psychological and behavioral factors affecting medical conditions and DSM-IV: an overview. Psychosomatics 32:5–13, 1991

Temoshok L, Heller BW, Sageviel RW, et al: The relationship of psychological factors of prognostic indicators in cutaneous malignant melanoma. J Psychosom Res 29:139–153, 1985

ten Brinke A, Ouwerkerk ME, Zwinderman AH, et al: Psychopathology in patients with severe asthma is associated with increased health care utilization. Am J Respir Crit Care Med 163:1093–1096, 2001

Troidle L, Watnick S, Wuerth DB, et al: Depression and its association with peritonitis in long-term peritoneal dialysis patients. Am J Kidney Dis 42:350–354, 2003

Van der Meeren HLM, Van der Schaar WW, Van den Hurk CMAM: The psychological impact of severe acne. Cutis 36:84–86, 1985

Von Korff M, Katon W, Lin EH, et al: Potentially modifiable factors associated with disability among people with diabetes. Psychosom Med 67:233–240, 2005

Vos PJ, Garssen B, Visser AP, et al: Psychosocial intervention for women with primary, nonmetastatic breast cancer: a comparison between participants and non-participants. Psychother Psychosom 73:276–285, 2004

Wales JK: Does psychological distress cause diabetes? Diabet Med 12:109–112, 1995

Walker EA, Roy-Byrne RP, Katon WJ: Irritable bowel syndrome and psychiatric illness. Am J Psychiatry 174:565–572, 1990

Walker EA, Katon WJ, Roy-Byrne RP, et al: Histories of sexual victimization in patients with irritable bowel syndrome or inflammatory bowel disease. Am J Psychiatry 150:1502–1506, 1993

Walker EA, Katon W, Russo J, et al: Health care costs associated with posttraumatic stress disorder symptoms in women. Arch Gen Psychiatry 60:369–374, 2003

Weiner H: Psychobiology and Human Disease. New York, Elsevier, 1977

Weiner H, Thaler M, Reiser MF, et al: Etiology of duodenal ulcer, I: relation of specific psychological characteristics to rate of gastric secretion (serum pepsinogen). Psychosom Med 19:1–10, 1957

Wilhelm K, Arnold K, Niven H, et al: Grey lungs and blue moods: smoking cessation in the context of lifetime depression history. Aust N Z J Psychiatry 38:896–905, 2004

Wilhelmsen I, Haug TT, Ursin H, et al: Effect of short-term cognitive psychotherapy on recurrence of duodenal ulcer: a prospective randomized trial. Psychosom Med 56:440–448, 1994

Withers NJ, Rudkin ST, White RJ: Anxiety and depression in severe chronic obstructive pulmonary disease: the effects of pulmonary rehabilitation. J Cardiopulm Rehabil 19:362–365, 1999

Writing Committee for the ENRICHD Investigators: Effects of treating depression and low perceived social support on clinical events after myocardial infarction: the Enhancing Recovery in Coronary Heart Disease Patients (ENRICHD) randomized trial. JAMA 289:3106–3116, 2003

Yamagiwa M, Harada T, Kubo M, et al: [Psychological states and personality as factors in the morbidity of head and neck malignant tumors] (in Japanese). Nippon Jibiinkoka Gakkai Kaiho 94:767–773, 1991

Yan LL, Liu K, Matthews K, et al: Psychosocial factors and risk of hypertension: the Coronary Artery Risk Development in Young Adults (CARDIA) study. JAMA 290:2138–2148, 2003

Yoshiuchi K, Kumano H, Nomura S, et al: Psychological factors influencing the short-term outcome of antithyroid drug therapy in Graves' disease. Psychosom Med 60:592–596, 1998a

Yoshiuchi K, Kumano H, Nomura S, et al: Stressful life events and smoking were associated with Graves' disease in women, but not in men. Psychosom Med 60:182–185, 1998b

25

PAIN DISORDERS

Raphael J. Leo, M.D.

Complaints of pain are the most common reason for patient presentations to ambulatory medical settings (Schappert 1992), accounting for approximately 35 million office visits annually (Knapp and Koch 1984). Most of these remit spontaneously or respond to simple treatment interventions; however, as many as one-fourth of these symptoms remain chronic (Schappert 1992). Chronic pain is pervasive; clinicians in a variety of specialties are likely to encounter patients with pain who present treatment challenges. The costs of chronic pain are monumental when health care, absenteeism, lost wages, and disability are considered (Fishman et al. 1997; Loeser 1999; Stewart et al. 2003). The pervasiveness, refractoriness, and costs associated with chronic pain have rendered chronic pain management a public health priority, spurring multiple efforts directed at understanding the pathophysiological processes underlying pain and at refining treatment strategies. Because of the complexities involved in the experience of pain, its management requires a comprehensive assessment and the implementation of multimodal treatment strategies, incorporating both psychopharmacological and psychosocial interventions.

Pain Disorder

Extensive effort has been devoted to defining pain and its associated features in psychiatric and nonpsychiat-

ric circles. According to the International Association for the Study of Pain, *pain* is broadly defined as "an unpleasant sensory and emotional experience associated with actual or potential tissue damage, or described in terms of such damage" (Merskey and Bogduk 1994, p. 210). Conceptualized in this way, pain is not only a physical or sensory phenomenon but also a complex perception incorporating emotional and psychological processes (Osterweis et al. 1987).

The *Diagnostic and Statistical Manual of Mental Disorders* (DSM) has undergone modifications over the years to better conceptualize the psychological disturbances related to the experience of pain. In early versions, clinicians were required to infer whether psychological underpinnings or conflicts precipitated pain complaints. If physical examination and diagnostic evaluation failed to uncover a medical cause for the pain, psychiatric labels were invoked reflecting the psychological origins of the pain—for example, *psychogenic pain disorder* from DSM-III (American Psychiatric Association 1980) and *somatoform pain disorder* from DSM-III-R (American Psychiatric Association 1987). The criteria outlined in previous versions of DSM perpetuated a dualistic conceptualization of pain, definable in terms of physical versus psychological origins.

Physical pain is often accompanied by emotional distress and cognitive disturbances and has significant social and interpersonal ramifications. Thus, given the inherent blurring of physical and psychological components in the experience of pain, distinguishing physically from psychologically based pain was subjectively determined. Thus, it is unsurprising that rates of diagnosis of pain disorder varied tremendously across a number of clinical studies from 0.3% (Fishbain et al. 1986) to 100% (Owen-Salters et al. 1996), raising questions about the reliability of the diagnostic taxonomy at the time.

There was a transition in the diagnostic criteria for pain disorder in DSM-IV and DSM-IV-TR (American Psychiatric Association 1994, 2000). There is no longer a requirement for exclusion of a physical cause for the pain, and the primacy of psychological factors (i.e., conflicts, defenses, and emotional states) underlying and accounting for pain was deemphasized. DSM-IV-TR leaves open the possibility that psychological factors can contribute to the pain experience by precipitating, exacerbating, or maintaining pain but do not necessarily have to fully account for it. This approach is more consistent with current views of the interrelationship between pain and psychological factors, as in the aforementioned International Association for the Study of Pain definition. The diagnostic criteria for pain disorder are summarized in Table 25–1.

TABLE 25–1. DSM-IV-TR diagnostic criteria for pain disorder

A. Pain in one or more anatomical sites is the predominant focus of the clinical presentation and is of sufficient severity to warrant clinical attention.

B. The pain causes clinically significant distress or impairment in social, occupational, or other important areas of functioning.

C. Psychological factors are judged to have an important role in the onset, severity, exacerbation, or maintenance of the pain.

D. The symptom or deficit is not intentionally produced or feigned (as in factitious disorder or malingering).

E. The pain is not better accounted for by a mood, anxiety, or psychotic disorder and does not meet criteria for dyspareunia.

Code as follows:

    307.80 Pain disorder associated with psychological factors: psychological factors are judged to have the major role in the onset, severity, exacerbation, or maintenance of the pain. (If a general medical condition is present, it does not have a major role in the onset, severity, exacerbation, or maintenance of the pain.) This type of pain disorder is not diagnosed if criteria are also met for somatization disorder.

    Specify if:

        Acute: duration of less than 6 months

        Chronic: duration of 6 months or longer

    307.89 Pain disorder associated with both psychological factors and a general medical condition: both psychological factors and a general medical condition are judged to have important roles in the onset, severity, exacerbation, or maintenance of the pain. The associated general medical condition or anatomical site of the pain (see below) is coded on Axis III.

    Specify if:

        Acute: duration of less than 6 months

        Chronic: duration of 6 months or longer

Note: The following is not considered to be a mental disorder and is included here to facilitate differential diagnosis.

    Pain disorder associated with a general medical condition: a general medical condition has a major role in the onset, severity, exacerbation, or maintenance of the pain. (If psychological factors are present, they are not judged to have a major role in the onset, severity, exacerbation, or maintenance of the pain.) The diagnostic code for the pain is selected based on the associated general medical condition if one has been established (see Appendix G) or on the anatomical location of the pain if the underlying general medical condition is not yet clearly established—for example, low back (724.2), sciatic (724.3), pelvic (625.9), headache (784.0), facial (784.0), chest (786.50), joint (719.40), bone (733.90), abdominal (789.0), breast (611.71), renal (788.0), ear (388.70), eye (379.91), throat (784.1), tooth (525.9), and urinary (788.0).

In contrast to many other psychiatric disorders, the criteria for pain disorder often are perceived as insufficiently operationalized, lacking a checklist of symptoms that collectively define the syndrome. There are no guidelines that allow one to ascertain whether psychological factors "have an important role" in pain (criterion C) or determine when pain is "not better accounted for" by a mood disorder (criterion E) (M.D. Sullivan 2000); in fact, this can be quite undecipherable given the high comorbidity of mood disturbances with pain (Dersh et al. 2002; Fishbain 1999a).

In DSM-IV-TR, there is an acknowledgment that pain can be associated with a general medical condition, psychological factors, or both. Pain disorder associated with a general medical condition is recorded solely on Axis III, because psychological factors are thought to have minimal or no involvement in the pain experience. When psychological factors are implicated and believed to have a significant contributory role in the pain, one of the two other types of pain disorder would be encoded on Axis I. However, the distinctions often can be ambiguous. Furthermore, questions arise as to whether the subtypes represent clinically useful subclassifications; for example, Aigner and Bach (1999) determined that pain disorder with psychological features could not be distinguished from pain disorder with both psychological and general medical features in terms of pain severity or disability measures.

Although improved over previous versions, the DSM-IV-TR taxonomy has been criticized on several counts (Table 25–2). First, the intent in the recent revision of pain disorder nosology was to deviate from dualistic conceptualizations of pain. Ironically, the current subtyping in DSM-IV-TR still compels the clinician to infer whether, and to what extent, psychological factors are involved in the patient's pain, reflecting the vestiges of mind–body dualism (Boland 2002). Additionally, by being grouped under the rubric of somatoform disorders, pain disorder may still connote the implied dualism of other somatoform disorders—that is, somatic preoccupation occurring in the absence of—or in excess of what would be expected from—objective findings. In anticipation of DSM-V, it has been suggested that pain disorder be removed from the somatoform disorder classification altogether and instead be confined to Axis III (Mayou et al. 2005).

Second, the nosology of pain disorder is likely to be misunderstood by nonpsychiatric clinicians (Mayou et al. 2003); the potential pejorative implication may be that the patient is disingenuous, exaggerating, or faking. When utilized, therefore, psychiatrists may need to be explicit about the intended meaning of the clinical terminology and specify that it in no way implies that the patient's complaints are imaginary.

Third, the characteristics of patients with pain disorder can overlap considerably with those of patients with other somatoform disorders, obscuring distinction (Hiller et al. 2000). For example, in somatization disorder, patients seek out medical attention for unexplained symptoms, some of which are pain related. There are many pain conditions that defy clear etiological explanation. Similarly, it may be well within the repertoire of pain patients to become preoccupied with fears of having a dreaded medical condition based on misinterpretation of common, and perhaps innocuous, bodily sensations. Convinced of illness, such individuals may vigorously pursue medical attention and display hypochondriacal-like symptoms (Barsky 1979). Somatoform disorders are discussed elsewhere in this volume (see Chapter 13, "Somatoform Disorders," by Yutzy and Parish). Additionally, even though it is not a psychiatric disorder, malingering can also be quite difficult to decipher from pain disorder. Lacking a sophisticated or practical means of communicating their distress, pain patients who experience frustration related to inadequate relief or who perceive treating sources as inattentive may be driven to engage in seemingly manipulative behaviors in order to enlist others to provide care (Boland 2002).

TABLE 25–2. Criticisms of the DSM-IV-TR nosology of pain disorder

The current subcategories of pain disorder in DSM-IV-TR still compel clinicians to infer whether, and to what extent, psychological factors are involved in the patient's pain.

The nosology of pain disorder is likely to be misunderstood by nonpsychiatric clinicians; the potential pejorative implication may be that the pain is imaginary.

The characteristics of pain patients with pain disorder can overlap considerably with those of other somatoform disorders.

The current diagnostic criteria of pain disorder are not useful with regard to assisting in the planning and coordination of treatment.

Last, questions arise as to the usefulness of the current diagnostic criteria in terms of assisting in the planning and coordination of treatment. Significant modifications in the nosology of pain disorder still appear to be warranted.

Biopsychosocial Perspective

Although pain disorder lacks rigorous diagnostic criteria, the current conceptualization lends itself to understanding the pain patient and approaching treatment holistically. Rather than dichotomizing between physical versus psychological origins, the biopsychosocial perspective maintains that the experience of pain and the patient's presentation and response to treatment are determined by the interaction of biological factors, the patient's psychological makeup, the presence of psychological comorbidities, and the extent of social support and extenuating environmental circumstances (Gallagher 1999; Leo 2007).

The spectrum of biopsychosocial issues pertinent to a particular patient can vary as his or her condition proceeds through successive phases (Gatchel 1991). Following tissue injury, trauma, and inflammation, there is an acute pain phase in which treatment is focused on pain relief, identification, and if possible, remediation of the underlying medical condition. Patients are likely to experience fear and anxiety initially, such as alarm, fear about what the pain means, and concerns over having access to measures to alleviate it. Psychological and social covariates have a limited role in the precipitation, maintenance, or exacerbation of the pain during this phase; consequently, psychiatric involvement may not be required or, at most, would be limited. At times, focused psychopharmacological and psychotherapeutic interventions may be required briefly to address mood disturbances, adjustment disorders, ineffective coping with stress, and so on until relief is achieved and the condition improves. Generally, most patients recover as expected.

However, for those in whom pain persists (i.e., subacute and subsequent chronic phases), psychological and social covariates begin to take on a greater role in the overall pain experience, influenced by premorbid, semidormant characteristics and personality traits that become activated by the stress of unremitting pain (Dersh et al. 2002). Eventually, patients are likely to manifest preoccupation with pain and perceived disability. The long duration of the pain has multiple ef-

fects, with commensurate changes in mood, thought patterns, perceptions, coping abilities, and personality. Activities may be forestalled for fear that pain will be elicited; there may be a decline in the patient's interests and profound effects on social and interpersonal capabilities. Psychological vulnerabilities may take a foothold, manifesting as psychiatric disorders. The patient may show impatience with treatment measures, intolerance for adverse effects, and impersistence with rehabilitative measures. Beset with multiple psychosocial stressors, the needs of the chronic pain patient can overwhelm the solo practitioner. A psychiatrist is likely to be enlisted, working in a coordinated fashion with practitioners in other disciplines to assist the afflicted individual in managing pain and improving adaptive function.

Comprehensive Pain Assessment

In order to yield optimal functional improvements, the treatment of pain with all of its ramifications requires a comprehensive pain assessment that follows a general biopsychosocial approach. A detailed history of the events leading to the pain and its course, duration, and associated features is the foundation for establishing management strategies. A historical perspective of the pain history may be useful to evaluate the patient's early pain complaints, history of medical interventions, and response to treatment. This may serve as a backdrop against which the current pain experiences can be compared. Prior treatment experiences may shape the patient's relationships with treatment providers, influence his or her expectations about participating in rehabilitative approaches, and influence perceived treatment efficacy.

Assessment can be greatly enriched by examining the psychological, social, and functional aspects of the pain experience and illuminating those factors that may predispose, activate, and perpetuate pain and disability. Issues warranting clinical attention are listed in Table 25–3. It is essential to assess for psychiatric comorbidities accompanying the pain (Fishbain 1999a). Failure to recognize and treat coexisting psychiatric disorders can impede efforts at effective pain management.

Several pain scales are available, including the Visual Analogue Scale and the Numerical Rating Scales, which serve to provide an index of pain severity (Jensen et al. 1986). Repeated use of such scales by the

TABLE 25–3. **Components of a comprehensive biopsychosocial assessment of chronic pain patients**

Somatic component

Features of the pain (characteristics, severity, location, radiation, duration, precipitating and mitigating factors)

Elements of treatment ameliorating or exacerbating pain

Psychological component

Comorbid psychiatric disorders

Subsyndromal psychological states influencing pain severity:

Mood/affective states (sadness, fear, anger)

Cognitions (beliefs about the meaning of the pain, ineffective cognitive appraisals, perceived disability, expectations about the future)

Coping repertoire (capacity to employ measures to address physical and emotional distress, despair, suicidal ideation)

Social component

Social support network (the accessibility and availability of significant persons in the patient's life; impact of pain on relationships; capacity for intimacy, sexuality, mutuality)

Adaptational/functional component (activities of daily living, recreation, life satisfaction)

Effect on vocational/academic pursuits

Legal issues (litigation related to injuries, workers' compensation)

Health insurance/disability (costs of medical care)

TABLE 25–4. **Psychometric scales used in assessing chronic pain**

Coping Strategies Questionnaire: Assessment of coping strategies in one's repertoire to deal with chronic pain; may predict the level of activity, physical impairment, and psychological functioning associated with pain (Rosenstiel and Keefe 1983).

Fear-Avoidance Beliefs Questionnaire: Assesses beliefs characterized by danger, threat, or harm associated with pain; the degree to which patients assign threat to activities may limit their participation in, and lead to avoidance of, activities related to work (Waddell et al. 1993).

McGill Pain Questionnaire: Assesses the features of pain severity and intensity; allows patients to qualify pain in emotional, cognitive/evaluative, and sensory terms (Melzack 1975).

Minnesota Multiphasic Personality Inventory: Personality profiles and pathological assessment of patients with chronic pain (Hathaway et al. 1989).

Multidimensional Pain Inventory: Assessment of one's appraisals of pain, its impact on functioning, and perceived responses of others in response to pain (Kerns et al. 1985).

Patient Outcome Questionnaire: Assesses patient satisfaction with pain treatment, how the patient perceived clinician responsiveness to pain complaints, and disclosure to patients of instructions regarding use of pain medications (American Pain Society Quality of Care Committee 1995).

Quality of Life: Assesses the impact of chronic pain states on various aspects of one's life: activity, recreation, and leisure time activities; social interactions; work; and adaptive self-care.

Source. Reprinted from Leo RJ: *Clinical Manual of Pain Management in Psychiatry.* Washington, DC, American Psychiatric Publishing, 2007, p. 49. Used with permission.

patient can offer the clinician an index of treatment efficacy and can serve to identify areas that require further attention. In addition, multidimensional pain assessments can also be employed that expand the clinical focus beyond pain intensity to other domains, such as the affective components of pain and the impact of pain on the patient's quality of life. Several of these assessment instruments are listed and described in Table 25–4. Use of such assessments may complement the information gathered from the clinical interview and may serve to enhance development of comprehensive treatment programs contoured to the individual's specific needs.

Comorbid Psychiatric Conditions

Depression

Depression prevalence rates among patients with chronic pain are substantially higher than those in the general population, with estimates varying from 30% to 54% (Banks and Kerns 1996). Depression, therefore, constitutes a common psychiatric comorbidity (Fishbain 1999a; Koenig and Clark 1996). Estimates vary depending on the variety of pain conditions examined, whether patients were sampled from clinical or community settings, and the methodologies employed.

Although much of the data suggest that chronic pain predisposes patients to depression (Fishbain et al. 1997), there are some data that suggest depression can predict future pain. For example, in a 10-year longitudinal study of industrial workers, depression predicted the development of low back pain and other musculoskeletal impairments (Leino and Magni 1993). Subjective assessments of depression predicted the development of fibromyalgia in 25% of women in a 5-year follow-up survey (Forseth et al. 1999).

Emerging evidence suggests several theoretical physiological substrates linking depression, and perhaps anxiety, with pain (Table 25–5). Given these potential common underlying mediators, it is likely that depression and pain have reciprocal influences. With persisting pain, there is increased substance P and cytokine activity along with reduced catecholamine activity, predisposing one to depression. As depression progresses, substance P activity is augmented while catecholamine descending inhibition of peripheral pain transmission is reduced, leading to enhanced pain perception and severity. Thus, depressed patients may see themselves as having more pain and disability as compared with nondepressed counterparts (Dworkin et al. 1990; Greden 2003; Kroenke et al. 1994). Similarly, patients with depression and medical illness tend to report more somatic symptoms and concerns than those medically ill persons without depression (Katon et al. 2001). Depression may result in perpetuation of pain, increasing the number, severity, and duration of physical symptoms and enhancing subjective assessments of pain-related disability (e.g., higher unemployment rates) (Bair et al. 2003; Burns et al. 1998b).

Depression is associated with poor prognosis among patients with pain (Bair et al. 2003), influencing both adaptation to illness and quality of life. Health-risk behaviors are often associated with depression, such as cigarette smoking, overeating, and decreased physical activity, complicating the functional disability of patients with pain. Furthermore, depressed patients are associated with higher nonadherence rates than are nondepressed patients, which undermines rehabilitative efforts and increases health care utilization (DiMatteo et al. 2000). Treatment of depression, therefore, is a necessary component to multimodal treatment approaches to address pain; when effectively treated, patients experience dramatically less interference from pain (Lin et al. 2003).

Anxiety

Research findings suggest a relationship between anxiety states and arthritic conditions (McWilliams et al. 2003), migraine (Swartz et al. 2000), back pain (McWilliams et al. 2004), and fibromyalgia (H. Cohen et al. 2002). In a cross-sectional study of chronic pain patients, a tendency to worry was significantly associated with long-term suffering related to pain (Lackner and Quigley 2005). The presence of comorbid anxiety may lead to hyperarousal and increased vigilance for pain and somatic concerns. Anxiety may influence the emotional valence associated with somatic sensations and increase proclivity to misinterpret somatic experiences (Derakshan and Eysenck 1997; van der Kolk et al. 1996).

Fears related to precipitating pain can lead to restriction of movement and avoidance of activity, undermining rehabilitative measures such as physical therapy and thereby contributing to deconditioning and muscle weakness (Vlaeyen et al. 1995). Hence, once activity is undertaken, the patient will be more likely to experience fatigue, reduced exercise tolerance, and an increased tendency toward further pain (Asmundson et al. 1999). The treatment of comorbid anxiety may serve to supplement preventive pain treatment measures (e.g., with migraine; Breslau and Davis 1993) and enhance rehabilitative measures and is, therefore, a necessary component of comprehensive pain treatment.

It should be recognized that patients with painful terminal conditions, such as those related to cancer, may experience existential anxiety related to life meaning and productivity, unachieved aspirations, and concerns over leaving a legacy (Leo 2007). Addressing existential issues openly may be an essential component of end-of-life care.

Sleep Disorders

Sleep disturbances are common among patients with a variety of pain disorders (Moldofsky 2001). The etiology is likely to be multifactorial, including disruptions due to pain itself, comorbid psychiatric disturbances, effects of pain medications, lack of aerobic exercise, and behavioral conditioning due to protracted reclining and daytime napping (M.J.M. Cohen et al. 2000). As a consequence, patients may report difficulty falling asleep, frequent awakenings and disrupted sleep, decreased total sleep time, and daytime fatigue. Measures to address these difficulties require that patients be educated about development of appropriate sleep hygiene techniques. Dosing of pain medications may

TABLE 25–5. Biological substrates common to pain and depression

Biological substrates	Pain	Depression	Relationship
Catecholamines	Rostral ventromedial medulla (5-HT) and dorsolateral pontine tegmentum (NE) inhibit pain transmission from spinal dorsal horn (Fields and Basbaum 1999)	Locus coeruleus (NE) and raphe nucleus (5-HT) project to limbic system and other brain areas (Blier and Abbott 2001)	Decreased catecholamines increases pain and depression
Substance P	Binding to neurokinin receptors centrally and peripherally increases pain transmission (Doyle and Hunt 1999)	Central substance P increased in animal paradigms of stress; inhibits activity of locus coeruleus and raphe nucleus (Mantyh 2002; Santarelli et al. 2002)	Increased central substance P activity increases pain and depression
Opioid receptor	Modulates pain transmission centrally and peripherally	Present in limbic structures; deactivation of μ-receptors associated with dysphoria (Zubieta et al. 2003)	Decreased opioid receptor activity can augment pain and depression
Cytokines	Proinflammatory agents promote pain	Interferon-α administered to patients induces depression (Capuron et al. 2002)	Increased cytokine activity augments pain and depression

Note.   5-HT = 5-hydroxytryptamine (serotonin); NE = norepinephrine.

Source.   Reprinted from Leo RJ: "Chronic Pain and Comorbid Depression." *Current Treatment Options in Neurology* 7:403–412, 2005. Used with permission from Current Science, Inc.

need to be adjusted to reduce sleep-interfering effects. Nonbenzodiazepine sedatives, such as zolpidem, may be indicated to facilitate sleep. In conjunction, antidepressants and anticonvulsants required for certain pain states can be useful in augmenting sleep potential due to their sedating effects. Stimulants may be required to reduce excess daytime sedation associated with opiate analgesic use.

Substance Abuse and Dependence

Rates of substance abuse or dependence among patients with chronic pain have been reportedly higher than those in the general population (Brown et al. 1996). For most, the substance use disorder preceded the onset of the pain disorder (Brown et al. 1996). In fact, a preexisting substance use disorder may predispose the individual to accidents and injuries, some of which may evolve into chronic pain syndromes (Polatin et al. 1993).

Although chronic pain patients may be vulnerable to developing new substance use disorders in the course of treatment (Brown et al. 1996; Dersh et al. 2002;

Dunbar and Katz 1996), some contend that this is an extraordinarily rare event (Zenz et al. 1992). Risk factors include a prior history of substance abuse, prior physical or sexual abuse, major depression, anxiety disorders, and personality disorders (Dersh et al. 2002; Fishbain et al. 1998). Although opiates have been a predominant focus, several other agents used in pain treatment are likewise prone to abuse and dependence, including the muscle relaxant carisoprodol (Soma), ketamine, ergot alkaloids, and barbiturates employed in migraine treatment, and benzodiazepines.

Although challenging, effective pain management should never be withheld because of an abuse or addiction history. Effective treatment may require use of an array of pain-reducing approaches—such as the use of adjunctive agents or those with low abuse potential and physical and psychological therapies—as well as participation in concurrent substance abuse treatment programs. In some cases, detoxification may be required before treatment can be initiated. The substances abused may have appeal as a means of controlling psychological distress (e.g., cannabis and benzodiazepine abuse to reduce underlying anxiety or address ineffective coping). Thus, psychological interventions, along with prudent psychopharmacological interventions for underlying psychiatric disorders, may also be required to effect optimal pain control.

Treatment Approaches

Given the inherent complexities involved in the pain experience, it is essential to keep in mind that the goals of treatment include providing pain relief and maximizing functioning and quality of life while at the same time keeping risk of iatrogenic harm to a minimum. The issues discussed here focus on the psychiatrist's role in pain management strategies.

Psychotherapy

In addition to the comorbid psychiatric conditions described previously, there are a number of subsyndromal psychological factors—such as troubling affective states, problematic cognitive styles, and ineffective coping strategies and interpersonal factors—that can accompany the experience of pain. If unattended, such factors can heighten pain awareness, interfere with adaptation to illness, and compromise rehabilitative measures.

Pain severity is likely to be temporally related to particular affective states. For example, among inpatients with chronic pain, pain ratings were linearly correlated with anger, fear (or anxiety), and depression. On the other hand, the presence of joy, interest, and surprise were predictive of lower pain severity (Fernandez and Milburn 1994). Ineffective expression of anger and hostility may serve to enhance pain intensity and perceived disability (Burns et al. 1996, 1998a; Fernandez and Turk 1995). It is speculated that under such circumstances, activation of the autonomic nervous system and endocrine systems (e.g., cortisol) brought on by ineffective management of unpleasant emotional states may contribute to physiological changes that enhance pain (Huyser and Parker 1999). Psychotherapeutic endeavors that enhance one's ability to more effectively modulate day-to-day emotions might reduce the distress experienced by patients with chronic or recurrent pain.

The experience of the pain goes beyond mere sensory phenomena. It can shape the manner in which patients make sense about events in their lives. In addition, it can alter how patients perceive themselves and the world. Thus, problematic beliefs about the self (e.g., inadequacy, helplessness, and undesirability), the world (e.g., dangerousness), and the future (e.g., hopelessness) can emerge, producing significant distress.

An individual harboring such beliefs may experience a loss of self-esteem and self-efficacy, loss of connections with others, and marked disappointment and disillusionment in addition to physical discomfort. Such beliefs may lead to unhealthy behaviors such as substance abuse, nonadherence with treatment, withdrawal from support systems, and incapacitating emotional states (e.g., marked dysphoria, anger, anxiety) warranting psychotherapeutic intervention. In fact, low self-efficacy is a predictor of perceived disability resulting from persisting pain (Arnstein 2000).

The patient's cognitive style and propensity toward distorted appraisal of life events can impair functioning (Jensen et al. 1991b). For example, the pain experience can be aggravated by catastrophizing (M.J. Sullivan et al. 1998), in which there is a tendency to exaggerate pain and related threatening information, thus interfering with the patient's ability to attend to those matters within his or her control and to pursue productive activities (Crombez et al. 1998). Catastrophizing has been associated with increased pain and perceived disability, poor adjustment to pain, and marked emotional distress (Hasenbring et al. 2001; M.J. Sullivan et al. 2001). Other examples of problematic cognitive styles interfering with the adjustment to pain are listed in Table 25–6. Such beliefs can hamper the development of effective coping strategies and exasperate treating sources along with other social supports.

The distress related to pain, unpleasant emotional states, and negative cognitions may be difficult for patients to tolerate. The strategies employed by the individual to self-soothe, reduce distress, and modulate unpleasant physical and emotional states can be quite diverse. Patients who employ passive coping by hoping for relief, praying, avoiding activity, and so on may be at a distinct disadvantage compared with those individuals who employ more proactive coping strategies such as distracting oneself with other activities or engaging in self-statements that can produce relief (Jensen et al. 1991b; Rosenstiel and Keefe 1983). Perceived self-efficacy may be a major determinant of the patient's ability to utilize proactive coping strategies (Jensen et al. 1991a). Evidence of ineffective coping (e.g., a tendency to embellish or magnify somatic complaints; self-medicating inappropriately or abusing substances so as to assuage distress) warrants intervention, because such behaviors can undermine treatment endeavors. Emotion-focused coping strategies can be quite effective and easily taught to patients to facilitate stress management. Those with a limited repertoire of coping abilities may experience despair and

TABLE 25–6. Problematic cognitive patterns in pain

Catastrophizing: The tendency to view and expect the worst (e.g., "I am doomed to have pain and misery forever!")

Helplessness: The belief that nothing that one does matters, that there is no benefit despite one's best efforts (e.g., "My doctor says that I should exercise to improve my osteoarthritis. I know it won't help!")

Help-rejecting: Rejecting efforts of well-meaning others as a means of expressing anger, securing ongoing "support" or attention, and even manipulating others (e.g., "I had problems with the last four medicines you gave me.")

Labeling: Ascribing a behavior of an individual to a characteristic or nature of the individual (e.g., the patient who is disappointed with the ineffectiveness of a medication may need to discount the qualifications of the clinician: "The medication the doctor gave me didn't help. What a quack!")

Magnification: The exaggeration of the significance of a negative event (e.g., "My pain got worse at work yesterday. I had to leave an hour early. I might as well come to grips with the fact that I am totally disabled!")

Overgeneralization: Expanding one adverse event or setback to many or all aspects of his or her life (e.g., "If this medication doesn't help me, nothing will!")

Personalization: The interpretation that an event or situation is indicative of something about oneself (e.g., "Because of the pain, I am a worthless failure!")

Selective abstraction: The propensity to attend selectively to negative aspects of one's life while ignoring satisfying and rewarding aspects (e.g., "Everything that happens in my life is bad!")

Source. Reprinted from Leo RJ: *Clinical Manual of Pain Management in Psychiatry.* Washington, DC, American Psychiatric Publishing, 2003, p. 43. Used with permission.

even suicidal ideation. Suicide rates are quite high among patients with chronic pain (Chochinov et al. 1998; Fishbain 1999b), necessitating the recognition of lethality and appropriate intervention.

It is pertinent to consider significant persons in the patient's life and how those relationships have been influenced by the pain. Changes in role responsibilities in the home as a result of pain may cause marked distress, accompanied by resentment and anger. There may be little emotional reserve to invest in other relationships and loss of intimacy and sexual satisfaction.

How pain is communicated, what responses are generated from others, and how the patient perceives those responses may suggest areas warranting intervention. For example, for some patients there may be much to be gained interpersonally by focusing on their complaints, such as avoiding conflicts or communicating displeasure with others (Fishbain 1994; Ford 1986). An inability to negotiate interpersonal difficulties, such as through a tendency toward a lack of assertiveness (Lackner and Gurtman 2005) or an inability of the patient's support system to adapt appropriately to the patient's needs, may foster isolation and impair the patient's abilities to cope effectively.

Psychotherapy Modalities

There has been a tendency to emphasize time-limited psychotherapy and focused adjunctive therapeutic techniques in pain management. Cognitive-behavioral therapy (CBT) has dominated the literature in terms of its applicability to pain treatment. However, it should be recognized that other therapeutic approaches have promise in pain management as well (Table 25–7). For example, the individual experiencing marked difficulties in role transitions or relationship difficulties with spouse or other family members as a result of illness may benefit from interpersonal psychotherapy (M.M. Weissman et al. 2000) or marital and family therapies. Operant conditioning techniques may be employed to modify disruptive, pain-associated behaviors that have become incorporated into the patient's customary repertoire through prior environmental contingencies. Excess reclining, avoidance of activity, and immobility may be modifiable with graded exposure, pacing of activities, and judicious implementation of social/environmental reinforcements (Sanders 2003). The selection of psychotherapy modality would therefore depend on the particular patient's needs, the commitment to pursue psychotherapy, and the training and skills of the psychiatrists and other available mental health practitioners.

CBT involves a collaborative process between the therapist and patient. Initial sessions involve elicitation of the patient's perception of the pain; appraisals of current life situations; beliefs about life, relationships, and the future; and current coping measures. The focus shifts in subsequent sessions to empirically assess the accuracy and overall usefulness of the patient's beliefs and coping strategies, replacing those that are maladaptive with alternative approaches. In so doing, it is expected that there will be resultant improvements in the patient's mood, ability to interpret day-to-day events, and adaptation.

TABLE 25–7. Psychotherapeutic modalities employed in pain management

Modality	Techniques	Uses
Behavioral	Activity scheduling; pacing and graded activity; desensitization	Increase exercise/activity levels; overcome fear–avoidance
Cognitive-behavioral	Collaborative process identifying cognitive appraisals; cognitive restructuring; assess utility of coping strategies; coping skills training	Reduce depression and anxiety associated with pain; develop effective coping strategies; reduce problematic cognitive styles
Interpersonal	Role-playing, analysis of communication patterns	Address role transitions due to pain; relationship difficulties/conflicts
Adjunctive techniques		
Biofeedback	Physiological parameters are measured and fed back to patient to facilitate mastery over them	Muscle relaxation; control of physiological parameters contributing to pain (e.g., headache)
Guided imagery	Talking patient through pleasant scenarios to produce vivid distracting and relaxing images	Relaxation; distraction from pain
Hypnosis	Focused attention and dissociation directed at altering pain experiences	Relaxation; pain severity reduction; distraction
Progressive muscle relaxation	Sequential muscle tightening and subsequent relaxation	Muscle relaxation; distraction from pain

In a meta-analysis of randomized, controlled trials comparing patients treated with CBT with wait-list control patients with chronic low back pain, rheumatoid arthritis, osteoarthritis, fibromyalgia, and unspecified somatic pains, CBT was found to be significantly more effective in reducing pain severity ratings and expression of pain, and it improved coping strategies (Morley et al. 1999; Sharpe et al. 2001). Unfortunately, sample sizes were significantly underpowered because it is often difficult to retain patients in complex, multicomponent treatment approaches for prolonged periods (Morley et al. 1999). In addition, measures of health care utilization, analgesic use, and resumption of occupational capacity after treatment were notably sparse in several studies.

Adjunctive therapeutic techniques such as relaxation training, biofeedback, and hypnosis can be useful in the armamentarium of acute and chronic pain states (Orne 1976; Turk et al. 1979; Turner and Chapman 1982a, 1982b). In general, such measures facilitate relaxation, can reduce physiological parameters linked with the genesis and perpetuation of pain, and, in the case of hypnosis, can lead to dissociative states resulting in modifications of the experience of pain. However, these measures can be limited in their utility among highly distressed and distracted patients (Leo

2007). Interventions to mitigate co-occurring depression or anxiety may be required initially, so as to render patients amenable to participating in and practicing these interventions for reduction of pain severity.

There is modest evidence for the utility of adjunctive measures in the treatment of pain (Blanchard et al. 1990; Carroll and Seers 1998; Keel et al. 1998; Sarnoch et al. 1997). Some practitioners question the utility of biofeedback and the necessity of the instrumentation required to effectively provide biofeedback training, arguing that other modalities, such as relaxation training, are equally efficacious (Silver and Blanchard 1978). On the other hand, the efficacy of hypnosis has been largely anecdotal. Interestingly, imaging technology has suggested that hypnosis can alter signal changes in areas of the brain involved with perception and integration of sensory information (e.g., the sensory cortex and thalamus), and it may be through such mechanisms that painful experiences are altered (Raz and Shapiro 2002).

Pharmacological Approaches

An array of agents is currently available for pain treatment (Table 25–8). Although an exhaustive review is beyond the scope of this chapter, the types of treatment modalities and issues pertaining mostly to the practice

TABLE 25–8. **Adjuvant medications for pain management**

Class of medication	Indication	Limitations
Antidepressants	Neuropathic pain, tension and migraine headaches, fibromyalgia, functional gastrointestinal disorders, comorbid depression/anxiety	Analgesia is best with agents possessing NE/5-HT reuptake influences Side effects: TCAs are perhaps least tolerable; drug interactions
Anticonvulsants	Neuropathic pain, migraine headache, central pain, phantom limb pain	Side effects: sedation, motor and gastrointestinal adverse effects, rash, drug interactions
Benzodiazepines	Muscle relaxation, anxiety associated with acute pain and procedures/interventions, insomnia	Abuse/dependence potential; sedation
Lithium	Cluster headache prophylaxis	Not effective for episodic cluster headache; risk of toxicity if dehydration occurs or with certain drug combinations
Stimulants	Opiate analgesia augmentation, opiate-induced fatigue and sedation	Abuse/dependence potential; overstimulation, anorexia, insomnia
NMDA antagonists	Opiate analgesia augmentation, neuropathic pain	Side effects: hallucinations with ketamine
Muscle relaxants	Acute muscle pain, muscle spasticity, fibromyalgia	Abuse/dependence potential with some agents; delirium from abrupt baclofen withdrawal; questionable utility in long-term use

Note. 5-HT=5-hydroxytryptamine (serotonin); NE=norepinephrine; NMDA=*N*-methyl-D-aspartate; TCAs=tricyclic antidepressants.

of psychiatry are emphasized. Selection of pharmacological approaches will need to be individualized, taking into account such factors as cost, ease of use, tolerability of side effects, drug interactions with co-administered medications, and clinical comorbidities.

Nonsteroidal Anti-Inflammatory Drugs and Acetaminophen

Effective for mild to moderate acute and chronic pain, nonsteroidal anti-inflammatory drugs (NSAIDs; including aspirin) act by interfering with prostaglandin synthesis and pain-inducing inflammatory processes (Table 25–9). The exact mechanism of acetaminophen analgesic activity is unclear, but it is thought to be a weak inhibitor of prostaglandin synthesis (Lucas et al. 2005). However, these agents are limited by a ceiling effect—that is, a dosage limit beyond which the analgesic effect is no longer appreciated. Adverse effects associated with NSAIDs include gastric irritation and ulceration, renal dysfunction, and bleeding due to decreased platelet aggregation. The cyclooxygenase-2 inhibitors have a lower incidence of gastrointestinal side

effects; however, the risks associated with stroke and cardiovascular complications have resulted in the withdrawal of the commercial availability of two of these agents, rofecoxib and valdecoxib. At the time of this writing, only celecoxib (Celebrex) is still available for use. For acetaminophen, there are concerns over hepatotoxicity in dosages beyond 4,000 mg daily.

There are a few noteworthy psychiatric considerations associated with the use of these agents. Co-administration of NSAIDs and lithium can lead to lithium toxicity and should be avoided. Anecdotally, NSAIDs can induce or exacerbate mood disturbances and psychosis in older patients and those with preexisting psychiatric conditions (Browning 1996; Jiang and Chang 1999). Caution is advised when co-administering medications with acetaminophen that may enhance the risk of liver toxicity, for example, nefazodone or chlorzoxazone.

Opioids

Opioids are recommended for the management of moderate to severe acute pain and cancer pain (World

TABLE 25–9. Pharmacological approaches for mild to moderate pain

Class of medication	Mechanism	Indication	Limitations
NSAIDs	Prostaglandin synthesis inhibitor	Bone pain, inflammatory pain	Ceiling effect; gastrointestinal and renal effects; increased bleeding
Acetaminophen	Prostaglandin synthesis inhibitor	Headache, inflammatory pain	Ceiling effect; hepatotoxic effects
Celecoxib	Cyclooxygenase-2 inhibitor	Rheumatoid arthritis and osteoarthritis	High doses may be associated with gastrointestinal effects; patients with cardiovascular risk factors may require aspirin supplementation
Tramadol	Weak opiate agonist; NE and 5-HT reuptake inhibitor	Acute and chronic pain, cancer pain	Seizure risk; potential for serotonin syndrome; abuse potential

Note. 5-HT=5-hydroxytryptamine (serotonin); NE=norepinephrine; NSAIDs=nonsteroidal anti-inflammatory drugs.

Health Organization 1990). Increasingly, opioids are employed for management of moderate to severe non-malignant pain (Clark 2002; Zenz et al. 1992). As a class, these agents stimulate mu, kappa, and delta opiate receptors, resulting in inhibition of pain transmission in the peripheral and central nervous systems.

Generally, opioids are effective when administered on a scheduled basis rather than "as needed" (Portenoy 1996). However, the need for supplemental opioids should be anticipated to address breakthrough pain emerging between scheduled doses (Portenoy and Hagen 1990). Ideally, opioids should be administered in the least invasive route possible; oral administration would be preferable over intramuscular. Transmucosal or transdermal applications may be alternatives for patients who are incapable of swallowing orally administered agents. Adverse effects associated with opioid analgesia need to be addressed in order to facilitate patient comfort (McQuay 1997); common interventions are summarized in Table 25–10.

Although accompanied by fewer gastrointestinal and other adverse effects, opiate agonist–antagonists such as butorphanol and nalbuphine have ceiling effects limiting their utility in regard to analgesia for severe pain. Some adverse effects can be avoided with the use of transdermal fentanyl.

There are several noteworthy drug interactions involving opioids and concurrently administered medications (K.C. Jackson and Lipman 2001). Opiates may produce excess sedation when co-administered with benzodiazepines, tricyclic antidepressants, or other sedative-hypnotics. Adjustments in co-administered

TABLE 25–10. Management strategies for opioid adverse effects

Adverse effect	Strategy
Delirium	Antipsychotics (e.g., haloperidol)
Dysphoria	Stimulants, antidepressants
Gastrointestinal	
Constipation	Stool softeners (e.g., bisacodyl)
Nausea	Antiemetics (e.g., metoclopramide)
Hypogonadism	Testosterone
Pruritis	Antihistamines (e.g., diphenhydramine)
Respiratory depression	Naloxone (acutely); lowered opioid doses; use of alternative agonists–antagonists
Sedation	Stimulants (e.g., methylphenidate)

medications may be required. Concomitant administration of carbamazepine or phenytoin with many opioids can cause heightened opioid metabolism, resulting in inadvertent undermining of analgesia and, in some cases, withdrawal. Paroxetine administration can interfere with the metabolism of codeine, which is necessary for its conversion to morphine, thus compromising its analgesic effects. Co-administration of meperidine and monoamine oxidase inhibitors (MAOIs) can precipitate serotonin syndrome and severe potentially life-threatening sequelae.

Fear of addiction is often offered as an explanation of why clinicians are inclined to suboptimally manage pain. Such concerns are moot in the context of pain treatment for patients with terminal conditions. Addiction to opiate analgesics is unlikely in the treatment of acute pain and cancer pain, particularly in those patients without a personal or familial history of substance abuse/dependence or those without premorbid psychopathology (Passik and Weinreb 2000). However, addiction concerns are particularly heightened when long-term treatment of chronic, nonmalignant pain is encountered. Psychiatrists may be enlisted in the care of the patient who is perceived to be medication seeking or to address issues pertaining to opioid abuse and dependence.

The presence of substance dependence is suggested by a desire for acquisition of opioids for something other than pain relief (e.g., its psychological effects). The patient who is addicted to analgesics experiences a loss of control over the use of the agent; compulsively consuming or misusing medication that impedes the patient's adaptive function and role responsibilities undermines interpersonal relationships and interferes with rehabilitation. Aberrant drug use behaviors suggestive of abuse or dependence include multiple calls to clinicians requesting additional medications for "lost" or "stolen" prescriptions; multiple unsanctioned dosage escalations without clinical consultation; acquisition of additional opiates "off the street," from friends and family, or from multiple treating sources unknown to the patient's primary treatment provider; concurrent abuse of illicit substances; and adulteration of use of prescribed medications, such as injecting crushed medications intended solely for oral use (Miotto et al. 1996).

Clinicians may be apt to misinterpret some behaviors of pain patients as being indicative of an underlying substance disorder. Predictably, patients requiring long-term opiates will develop tolerance, but tolerance alone does not constitute dependence. Such patients may find previously effective analgesic dosages to be ineffective over time and may, as a result, solicit higher dosages or additional medications for breakthrough pain. Opiate rotation—that is, sequential trials of analgesics—can be helpful in optimizing analgesic effects when tolerance develops (Quang-Cantagrel et al. 2000). However, switching to an agonist–antagonist in a patient who had been receiving full agonists can exacerbate pain and should be avoided. Co-administration of adjunctive agents such as antidepressants, N-methyl-D-aspartate (NMDA) antagonists, or calcium channel antagonists may also be helpful in augmenting pain relief.

Bear in mind that new injuries or illness, disease progression, and the addition of concomitant medications that enhance opiate metabolism may be factors to consider when patients report that previous analgesic regimens become suddenly ineffective. Careful reassessment of such patients is required.

Patients may engage in behaviors that appear seemingly manipulative or addiction-like if pain is inadequately treated, as with inadequate dosing or inordinately spaced dosing. This is referred to as *pseudoaddiction* (D. E. Weissman and Haddox 1989), and such patients may embellish symptoms or use up prescribed medications in excess of the intended rates. Not surprisingly, deciphering between addiction and pseudoaddiction can be somewhat difficult. Opioid therapy should offer a true difference in the quality of life of the patient through improved pain relief and functioning. If, after optimizing analgesic treatment, the manipulative behaviors cease and participation in treatment and adaptive functioning are both enhanced, the presumption is that the behavior is indeed a reflection of pseudoaddiction. On the other hand, in a patient who is abusing his or her medication, increasing accessibility to opioids will impair adherence and exacerbate maladaptive functioning.

Patients with recent or current opiate addictions can pose particular challenges in the context of pain management (Prater et al. 2002). Due to their tolerance for narcotics, these patients' opioid requirements can be quite high, beyond customary dosages. Use of opiate agonists-antagonists should be avoided in the context of recent opiate abuse, because these can precipitate withdrawal, enhancing distress and discomfort. Use of long-acting preparations such as transdermal fentanyl (Duragesic) or controlled-release oral morphine sulfate (MS Contin), among others, and analgesics with less potential of inducing euphoria (e.g., methadone) may be preferable. Despite morphine's long half-life, its analgesic effects appear to be short-lived; thus, morphine should be administered in multiple divided daily doses on a scheduled basis so as to mitigate pain. Detoxification from opiates should be addressed once pain management is no longer indicated. To do so in the acute pain treatment context would add inordinately to patient suffering and may compromise treatment alliances. It may be prudent to implement a treatment contract (Dunbar and Katz 1996) stipulating the patient's and clinician's responsibilities regarding ongoing care. Such contracts may specify parameters of therapy, for example, making opiates contingent upon verifiable participation in substance abuse treatment and other pain-related treatment modalities (e.g., regular attendance at scheduled medical appointments, participation in physical therapy or psychiatric treatment).

Tramadol

Tramadol (Ultram) is useful in the treatment of mild to moderate acute and chronic pain (see Table 25–9). It is unique in that it possesses dual pharmacological effects: weak opiate agonist effects along with reuptake inhibition of norepinephrine and serotonin. A variant that combines the anti-inflammatory effects of acetaminophen with tramadol (i.e., Ultracet) is available that is effective in moderate to severe pain (Schnitzer 2003). Risks associated with tramadol use include seizures (especially in those with epilepsy), head trauma, alcohol withdrawal (Gardner et al. 2000), and serotonin syndrome, especially when co-administered with serotonergic antidepressants or MAOIs (Lange-Asschenfeldt et al. 2002).

The abuse and dependence liability of tramadol was thought to be quite low. However, reports have emerged indicating that tramadol is an agent on which patients can become quite dependent, particularly patients with preexisting drug or alcohol dependence (Leo et al. 2000).

Antidepressants

The analgesic properties of antidepressants are often underappreciated by many clinicians. Although antidepressants would be a consideration for patients with pain and comorbid depression or anxiety, evidence suggests that antidepressants have analgesic effects independent of influences on mood. Specifically, analgesic effects of antidepressants can be achieved earlier than, and at dosages far lower than, their antidepressant effects; such analgesic effects have been demonstrated in patients with chronic pain who are not depressed (Ansari 2000; Egbunike and Chaffee 1990; Fishbain 2000). Therefore, antidepressants may be appropriately utilized for patients with chronic pain, regardless of whether the patient is depressed.

Antidepressants can be useful to address pain associated with neuropathy (e.g., postherpetic, diabetic, and poststroke pain), headache (e.g., tension, migraine), oral–facial pain, fibromyalgia, and functional gastrointestinal disorders (Ansari 2000; Collins et al. 2000; J. L. Jackson et al. 2000; Magni 1991; Onghena and Van Houdenhove 1992; Rowbotham et al. 2005). The pain-mitigating effects of antidepressants remain a subject of intensive investigation and are thought to involve a number of supraspinal, spinal, and peripheral processes (Table 25–11). In addition, when concur-

rently administered, some antidepressants may augment opiate analgesia (Schreiber et al. 2002).

Although controversies arise as to the validity of the monoamine hypothesis of pain modulation (Jasmin et al. 2003), evidence gathered from clinical trials and meta-analyses suggests that antidepressants influencing both noradrenergic and serotonergic transmission exert analgesic effects that are greater than those antidepressants with more specific effects, such as influencing either serotonin or norepinephrine reuptake alone (Lynch 2001; Max 1994; Max et al. 1992; McQuay et al. 1996; Mochizucki 2004; Sussman 2003). Much of the data on analgesic efficacy of antidepressants has largely focused on tricyclic antidepressants (TCAs). For example, in a review of randomized controlled trials in which TCAs and anticonvulsants were employed to treat pain associated with diabetic and postherpetic neuropathies, it was found that one-third of patients achieved at least 50% pain relief with either antidepressants or anticonvulsants (Collins et al. 2000; McQuay 2002). However, the side effects of the TCAs (e.g., anticholinergic and α-adrenergic influences) limit their utility in pain treatment. When compared with anticonvulsants, adverse effects were slightly more common with TCAs (Collins et al. 2000; McQuay 2002).

The serotonin and norepinephrine reuptake inhibitors (SNRIs) venlafaxine and duloxetine have demonstrated utility as analgesic agents and bypass several of the untoward effects commonly associated with the TCAs. Both agents have been demonstrated to have pain-mitigating effects in randomized, controlled trials of patients with neuropathy (Goldstein et al. 2005; Rowbotham et al. 2004; Sindrup et al. 2003) and fibromyalgia (Arnold et al. 2004; Zijlstra et al. 2002), with and without comorbid depression. Duloxetine has received U.S. Food and Drug Administration (FDA) approval for treatment of diabetic neuropathy. Simultaneous norepinephrine and serotonin influences are achieved at low dosages with duloxetine; dosages as low as 20 mg/day may be sufficient (Goldstein et al. 2005). The serotonin effects predominate at low dosages for venlafaxine. To achieve pain-mitigating effects, antidepressant-level dosing may be required (Zijlstra et al. 2002). Adverse effects of SNRIs can include nausea, dry mouth, nervousness, constipation, and somnolence.

The utility of selective serotonin reuptake inhibitors (SSRIs) in pain is limited by the relatively small sample sizes and low dosage ranges employed in various studies (Ansari 2000). Generally, these agents are not as consistently analgesic as the TCAs or SNRIs (Lynch 2001; Sindrup and Jensen 1999). For example,

TABLE 25–11. Analgesic effects of antidepressants

	Site of action	Mechanism	Effect
Supraspinal[a]	Descending inhibitory fibers from raphe nucleus and locus coeruleus	Increases 5-HT and NE	Enhanced pain modulation through heightened activity of descending fibers extending to the dorsal horn
Spinal	Pain-inhibiting interneurons[b]	Stimulation of α_1 receptors	Increased GABA and glycine release inhibiting pain transmission
	Pain-promoting interneurons[c]	Stimulation of α_2 receptors	Decreased glutamate release preventing further pain augmentation
Periphery	Peripheral neurons[d]	Voltage-gated sodium channel blockade	Decreased firing of neurons, reduced input to the dorsal horn
	Inflammation[e]	5-HT$_2$ antagonism	Reduced pain in formalin models of pain

Note. 5-HT=5-hydroxytryptamine (serotonin); GABA=γ-aminobutyric acid; NE=norepinephrine.
[a]Fields and Basbaum 1999; Sindrup and Jensen 1999.
[b]Baba et al. 2000.
[c]Kawasaki et al. 2003.
[d]Gerner et al. 2001.
[e]Abbott et al. 1997.

Source. Reprinted from Leo RJ: *Clinical Manual of Pain Management in Psychiatry.* Washington, DC, American Psychiatric Publishing, 2003, p. 100. Used with permission.

clinical trials assessing efficacy of SSRIs for addressing pain associated with neuropathy and fibromyalgia have yielded conflicting results (Anderberg et al. 2000; Arnold et al. 2002; Collins et al. 2000; Lynch 2001; Max 1994; Max et al. 1992; McQuay 2002; McQuay et al. 1996; Norregaard et al. 1995; Sindrup and Jensen 1999; Sussman 2003); there are limited data suggesting that paroxetine and citalopram may be effective in alleviating symptoms of diabetic neuropathy (Sindrup et al. 1990, 1992) and that fluoxetine is useful in fibromyalgia (Arnold et al. 2002). Use of SSRIs is associated with, and may potentially exacerbate, restless legs syndrome (Ohayon and Roth 2002).

Treatment should be initiated early in the course of illness for optimal results. For example, when amitriptyline is initiated within 3 months of developing the rash of herpes zoster infection, patients are less likely to develop the complications of postherpetic neuralgia (Bowsher 1997). Restriction of and delays in the efficacy of TCAs in producing analgesia would be expected if administered after significant peripheral and central pathophysiological mechanisms have set in. It is best to initiate treatment at low dosages; gradual dosage in-

creases are possible approximately every 3–7 days. If pain relief is inadequate, optimization of dosages should be undertaken unless side effects supervene.

The presence of certain medical comorbidities may preclude the use of selected antidepressant agents. The presence of heart block, arrhythmias, or severe cardiac disease precludes use of TCAs. In the event of renal dysfunction, dosages of venlafaxine would need to reduced, and if the dysfunction is severe enough, use of this agent would be precluded. For patients with hepatic disease, TCAs can conceivably exacerbate encephalopathy risk.

Although less extensively studied than the previously mentioned antidepressants, there are some data suggesting the utility of bupropion and nefazodone for selected pain states, such as neuropathy and headache (Saper et al. 2001; Semenchuk and Davis 2000; Semenchuk et al. 2001). Nefazodone use has been linked with hepatic dysfunction, and its use should be avoided in patients taking concurrent medications with potential hepatotoxic effects (e.g., acetaminophen). Trazodone has not been found to have significant analgesic properties. Mirtazapine for pain has been essentially understudied. Although not currently available in the United States, emerging antidepressant therapies potentially useful for pain include milnacipran (Ixel), an SNRI, and reboxetine, a norepinephrine reuptake inhibitor (Krell et al. 2005; Leo and Brooks 2006; Vitton et al. 2004).

Anticonvulsants

Anticonvulsant drugs historically have demonstrated efficacy in neuropathic pain, including trigeminal neuralgia and phantom limb pain (McQuay et al. 1995), as well as migraine (Pappagallo 2003; Snow et al. 2002). Carbamazepine is FDA approved for treatment of trigeminal neuralgia; gabapentin for treatment of postherpetic neuralgia; pregabalin for postherpetic neuralgia, diabetic neuropathy, and fibromyalgia; and divalproex sodium for migraine prophylaxis. Emerging evidence suggests potential analgesic roles for newer anticonvulsant drugs, such as lamotrigine (Lamictal), oxcarbazepine (Trileptal), tiagabine (Gabitril), and topiramate (Topamax) (Galer 1995; Khoromi et al. 2005; Novak et al. 2001; Pappagallo 2003), which offer greater tolerability than some of the older anticonvulsant drugs.

Analgesia produced by anticonvulsant drugs can be quite varied (Table 25–12). Analgesia produced by carbamazepine, lamotrigine, and oxcarbazepine is presumed to be related to inhibition of voltage-gated sodium channels, which slows peripheral nerve conduction of primary afferent fibers and dampens the painful sensory information relayed to the central nervous system (Pappagallo 2003). In addition, some anticonvulsant drugs such as pregabalin and gabapentin may have a role in influencing central proneuropathic pain mechanisms mediated through calcium antagonism and γ-aminobutyric acid (GABA)-ergic mechanisms responsible for inhibiting pain processes within the central nervous system (Guay 2003; Vinik 2005).

Because of the differences in presumed mechanisms of action between anticonvulsant drugs and antidepressants, it is plausible that anticonvulsant drugs would be viable alternatives for patients who have persisting pain despite optimal antidepressant use or those for whom antidepressant use proved intolerable. Alternatively, simultaneous administration of antidepressants and anticonvulsant drugs may be employed, capitalizing on complementary mechanisms of action. When co-administered, lower dosages of either or both agents may be sufficiently analgesic, perhaps making it possible to avoid dosages that produce adverse effects.

As with most psychopharmacological agents, low dosages should be initiated and increased gradually while the patient is monitored for any intolerance or adverse events. Pain-mitigating dosages are comparable with those employed for anticonvulsant efficacy. Some data suggest that anticonvulsant drugs, such as pregabalin and gabapentin, may have a preemptive analgesic role (Dahl et al. 2004). Therefore, treatment efficacy may be best if initiated early in the course of illness.

Selection of anticonvulsant drugs for pain would require careful consideration of the risks and benefits for any given patient. Anticonvulsant drugs have mood-stabilizing effects and may be ideal for patients with bipolar disorder (Chandramouli 2002). On the other hand, certain medical comorbidities may limit use of selected anticonvulsant drugs. In the event of renal dysfunction, dosages of carbamazepine, oxcarbazepine, gabapentin, pregabalin, and topiramate would need to be reduced, and if the condition is severe enough, use of these agents may be precluded. For patients with hepatic disease, dosages of carbamazepine, oxcarbazepine, and lamotrigine should be reduced.

Adverse effects common to anticonvulsant drugs include sedation, fatigue, and gastrointestinal and motor effects (e.g., tremor, ataxia, and nystagmus). Rash and Stevens-Johnson syndrome are possible with carbamazepine and lamotrigine (Pappagallo 2003). Anticonvulsant drugs can accentuate sedative effects when combined with alcohol, benzodiazepines, or barbiturates. Carbamazepine, oxcarbazepine, phenytoin, and topiramate can reduce the efficacy of contraceptives, increasing the risk of pregnancy. Fetal malformations are associated with carbamazepine, valproate, and phenytoin use during pregnancy (Yerby 2000).

Other Psychopharmacological Agents

Benzodiazepines. Short-term use of benzodiazepines has been employed to mitigate pain arising from muscle spasm (e.g., fibromyalgia), phantom limb pain, restless legs syndrome, tension headache, trigeminal neuralgia, and neuropathic pain (Bartusch et al. 1996; Bouckoms and Litman 1985; Dellemijn and Fields 1994). However, protracted benzodiazepine use may be counterproductive. In a study of chronic pain patients referred to a tertiary pain center, regression analysis revealed that long-term benzodiazepine use predicted low activity levels, high utilization of ambulatory medical services, and high disability levels (Ciccone et al. 2000). In addition, benzodiazepines acting through GABA receptor systems influence serotonin neurotransmitter release, attenuating opioid analgesia (Nemmani and Mogil 2003). Other concerns related to long-term benzodiazepine use in chronic pain include dependence and the potential for secondary depression (King and Strain 1990). Use of

TABLE 25–12. Anticonvulsant mechanisms of action

Drug	Decrease in sodium channel activity	Increase in CNS GABA activity	Modulation of Ca^{2+} channels	Reduction of excitatory amino acid activity
Carbamazepine	+			
Phenytoin	+			
Valproate	+	+	+	
Gabapentin	+	+	+ (?)	
Lamotrigine	+		+	
Oxcarbazepine	+			
Topiramate	+	+		+
Pregabalin		+	+	
Levetiracetam			+	
Tiagabine		+		
Zonisamide	+		+	

Note. Ca^{2+}=calcium; CNS=central nervous system; GABA=γ-aminobutyric acid.
Source. Adapted from Leo 2006 and Massie 2000.

benzodiazepines has to be undertaken cautiously, because these agents can contribute to excess sedation, gait instability, and memory impairments.

Buspirone (BuSpar) may be useful to treat comorbid anxiety accompanying pain. However, direct pain-mitigating efficacy for buspirone has not been substantiated (Kishore-Kumar et al. 1989).

Stimulants. For purposes of pain management, the use of stimulants has been twofold. Although the mechanism of action remains unclear, stimulants (e.g., dextroamphetamine, methylphenidate) have been employed to augment opioid analgesia (Forrest et al. 1977). Additionally, they are employed to reduce the sedation, dysphoria, and cognitive inefficiency that can accompany opiate use. However, use of stimulants may be limited by intervening adverse effects, including overstimulation (e.g., anxiety, insomnia), appetite suppression, confusion, and even paranoia. Taken in overdose, arrhythmias, seizures, hallucinations (e.g., formication), delirium, and death can occur. Contraindications for stimulant use include glaucoma, poorly controlled hypertension, arrhythmias and cardiovascular disorders, anorexia, seizure disorders, and hyperthyroidism. Because of concerns of abuse liability, caution is advised in patients with current or preexisting substance use disorders, especially prior stimulant abuse (e.g., cocaine).

Lithium. Lithium has been employed in the prophylaxis of chronic cluster headache; the effective dosage is approximately 600–900 mg/day (Ekbom and Hardebo 2002). However, a double-blind, placebo-controlled trial found that lithium was not effective for prophylaxis of episodic cluster headache (Steiner et al. 1997). In such cases, calcium channel blockers or corticosteroids may be better alternatives.

N-Methyl-D-Aspartate Receptor Antagonists

Although the mechanisms of action have as yet to be fully elucidated, some evidence suggests that NMDA antagonists, such as dextromethorphan (Sang et al. 2002), ketamine (Eide et al. 1994), memantine (Sang et al. 2002), and amantadine (Symmetrel), may have a role in mitigating chronic pain, including neuropathy, chronic phantom pain, fibromyalgia, and pain associated with spinal cord injury. However, the analgesic effects have demonstrated inconsistent results in various trials (Eisenberg et al. 1998; Enarson et al. 1999). The side effects associated with the NMDA antagonists include sedation, dry mouth, headache, and constipation; in some cases these effects can be prohibitively severe, limiting the agents' usefulness (Eide et al. 1994); for example, ketamine can produce dissociation and delirium, and its hallucinogenic properties have rendered it a popularly abused club drug ("special K") (Dillon et al. 2003). Dextromethorphan augments serotonin in the central nervous system; combinations with serotonergic antidepressants may predispose the patient to serotonin syndrome.

Muscle Relaxants

Generally, antispasmodics are employed for acute pain arising from muscle strain or injury, such as low back pain. Included in this category are true muscle relaxants (dantrolene), GABA$_B$ agonists (baclofen [Lioresal]), GABA$_A$ agonists (diazepam), α_2 agonists (tizanidine [Zanaflex]), and centrally acting agents that are thought to suppress polysynaptic reflexes, such as carisoprodol (Soma), cyclobenzaprine (Flexeril), methocarbamol (Robaxin), and orphenadrine (Norflex), among others. Baclofen may be indicated for more chronic pain arising from muscle spasticity, such as after stroke or severe spinal cord injury. The utility of these agents over long-term use is unclear; some have been effectively employed in patients with fibromyalgia (Tofferi et al. 2004). There may be abuse potential associated with carisoprodol and methocarbamol; abrupt discontinuation of these muscle relaxants may precipitate withdrawal, including abdominal cramps, insomnia, nausea, headache, and anxiety. Severe psychiatric disturbances such as psychotic depression have been reported in association with baclofen use (Sommer and Petrides 1992), and delirium may result from its abrupt discontinuation (Leo and Baer 2005).

The side effects often associated with these agents include somnolence and anticholinergic effects. Combinations with other agents, such as alcohol, sedative-hypnotics, benzodiazepines, or barbiturates, may produce additive sedative effects. Concomitant use of TCAs can add substantially to potential anticholinergic toxicity, especially if combined with cyclobenzaprine. Combination of cyclobenzaprine with MAOIs can result in toxic reactions, including hyperthermia.

Herbal Agents

Herbal agents are commonly employed (Kaufman et al. 2002); those agents utilized for a variety of pain complaints are listed in Table 25–13. Sometimes invoked as "natural remedies," herbal agents are often believed to be safe and devoid of adverse effects, and therefore their use by patients may go unreported. It is important to make inquiries into the patient's use of herbs because these can be associated with significant adverse effects and drug interactions when unknowingly combined with prescribed medications (Ernst 2000).

Other Treatment Interventions

There are a number of therapeutic modalities and interventions available for management of acute and chronic pain (Loeser et al. 2001). The appropriateness of an intervention depends in part on the etiology and nature of the pain, the potential risks of the procedure, and the likelihood of yielding beneficial effects. Generally, conservative modalities are employed first. Certain procedures such as acupuncture, transcutaneous electrical nerve stimulation, and physical therapy carry relatively fewer risks than more aggressive interventions such as neurosurgery. However, if less invasive measures fail, treatment may advance through a number of concurrently applied modalities and eventually, perhaps, to interventions that carry more risk (Table 25–14). An emerging therapy, transcranial magnetic stimulation, has potential utility in treating neuropathic pain (e.g., poststroke pain, brachial plexus lesions) (Lefaucheur 2001; Leo and Latif 2007). Although the adverse effects of this therapy are minimal, its practical application and efficacy for pain treatment has yet to be determined.

Psychiatrists may be asked to assess the patient's suitability for various treatment interventions, such as identifying whether psychiatric conditions would interfere with outcome (Trief et al. 2000). In addition, the patient's preparedness for the risks or untoward effects and capacity to provide informed consent to undergo a procedure may warrant psychiatric evaluation.

Multidisciplinary Pain Treatment

Multidisciplinary treatment approaches are often required for complex and disabling pain conditions. Encompassing specialists in the field of anesthesiology, neurology, psychiatry, psychology, and rehabilitation medicine, such programs are directed at implementing measures whereby the patient gains mastery over pain and refines cognitive styles and coping strategies (Hoffman et al. 2007; Jensen et al. 1994, 2001). Multidisciplinary treatment programs are effective in producing symptomatic pain relief, reducing affective distress, improving adaptive functioning and quality of life (Flor et al. 1992; Jensen et al. 2001; Skevington et al. 2001). The duration of effects appears to be sustained over time, reducing disability and health care utilization (Flor et al. 1992). Unfortunately, attrition rates can be quite high (Jensen et al. 1994). Factors predisposing to attrition include a long history of pretreatment pain,

TABLE 25–13. Herbal agents used for pain

Herb	Use	Comment
Black cohosh	Menstrual pain	Can produce adverse gastrointestinal effects and abdominal, headache, and joint pain; can increase intensity of contraceptives
Chamomile	Anti-inflammatory	Acts as emetic; may interfere with anticoagulants
Evening primrose oil	Anti-inflammatory; rheumatoid arthritis, migraine	May trigger temporal lobe epilepsy; unsafe in patients taking phenothiazine antipsychotics
Feverfew	Anti-inflammatory; migraine	Interacts with antithrombotic agents
Ginkgo biloba	Claudication-related pain	Can produce gastrointestinal distress, headache
Goldenseal	Anti-inflammatory	Can produce seizure, B-vitamin deficiencies; induces abortion in pregnancy
Kava	Antispasmodic	Can potentiate sedation from barbiturates and alcohol
Topical St. John's wort	Anti-inflammatory	Can cause gastrointestinal distress; can produce serotonin syndrome if combined with selective serotonin reuptake inhibitors (it is uncertain whether this is a risk with topical applications)
Valerian	Migraine headache	Gastrointestinal distress, insomnia; interferes with anticonvulsants and anxiolytics

Source. Reprinted from Leo RJ: *Clinical Manual of Pain Management in Psychiatry.* Washington, DC, American Psychiatric Publishing, 2003, p. 121. Used with permission.

TABLE 25–14. Treatment interventions for management of acute and chronic pain conditions

Least invasive	Moderately invasive	Most invasive
Physical therapy	Trigger point injection	Neurostimulation
Massage	Peripheral nerve blocks	Implantable drug pumps
Chiropractic manipulation	Epidural blocks	Neuroablation/neurolysis
Transcutaneous electrical nerve stimulation	Thermal procedures	Surgical interventions
Acupuncture	Prolotherapy	
Transcranial magnetic stimulation[a]		

[a]Preliminary evidence only.

Source. Reprinted from Leo RJ: *Clinical Manual of Pain Management in Psychiatry.* Washington, DC, American Psychiatric Publishing, 2003, p. 162. Used with permission.

dependence on medications, multiple prior surgeries related to pain, and perceived social support for maintaining participation in treatment (King and Snow 1989; Maruta et al. 1979).

General psychiatric training renders the psychiatrist particularly well suited for the treatment of pain (Leo et al. 2003). Given that a significant number of psychosocial stressors and psychological comorbidities complicate the experience of chronic pain, there is wide acceptance for the necessity of psychiatric and other mental health practitioners in the comprehensive assessment and treatment of patients with pain. In 1998, the American Board of Psychiatry and Neurology (ABPN) and the American Board of Physical Medicine and Rehabilitation joined the American Board of Anesthesiology in recognizing pain management as an interdisciplinary subspecialty; since 2000, ABPN diplomates have been eligible to sit for the pain management subspecialty certification examination. Subspecialty certification is appropriate for psychiatrists whose practices are largely devoted to pain medicine. Invariably, given the pervasiveness of pain complaints, general psychiatrists will nonetheless encounter—and will need to be familiar with—pain management issues pertinent to the care of their patients (Leo 2007).

Key Points

- Pain is a complex perception involving sensory as well as psychological components.

- The diagnostic taxonomy of pain disorder in DSM-IV-TR recognizes that psychological factors can contribute to the experience of pain; however, critics contend that the criteria are insufficiently operationalized to distinguish pain disorder from other psychiatric conditions and that the nosology still retains vestiges of mind–body dualism.

- Common psychiatric comorbidities that accompany chronic pain include depression, anxiety, substance abuse, and sleep disorders. Treatment of comorbidities is required as part of comprehensive pain management.

- A complex array of adjuvant agents with different mechanisms of action can be employed for chronic pain treatment, including antidepressants and anticonvulsants, among other agents.

- Antidepressants have direct pain-mitigating effects apart from influences on mood. Those agents with simultaneous norepinephrine and serotonin effects appear to be most efficacious.

- Psychotherapeutic measures can be useful in the comprehensive management of pain to address comorbid psychiatric conditions and subsyndromal psychological states interfering with rehabilitation as well as to reduce the adversity produced by the pain itself.

- Multidisciplinary treatment approaches can be useful in reducing perceived pain, enhancing rehabilitative measures, reducing disability, and addressing the psychological comorbidities accompanying chronic and enduring pain.

Suggested Readings

Derby S, Chin J, Portenoy RK: Systemic opioid therapy for chronic cancer pain: practical guidelines for converting drugs and routes of administration. CNS Drugs 9:99–109, 1998

Leo RJ: Clinical Manual of Pain Management in Psychiatry. Washington, DC, American Psychiatric Publishing, 2007

Loeser JD, Butler SH, Chapman CR, et al: Bonica's Management of Pain, 3rd Edition. Philadelphia, PA, Lippincott Williams & Wilkins, 2001

Massie MJ: Pain: What Psychiatrists Need to Know (Review of Psychiatry Series, Vol 19, No 2; Oldham JM and Riba MB, series eds.). Washington, DC, American Psychiatric Press, 2000

Wall PD, Melzack R: Textbook of Pain, 4th Edition. Edinburgh, Scotland, Churchill Livingstone, 1999

Winterowd C, Beck AT, Gruener D: Cognitive Therapy With Chronic Pain Patients. New York, Springer, 2003

References

Abbott FV, Hong Y, Blier P: Persisting sensitization of the behavioural response to formalin-induced injury through activation of serotonin 2A receptors. Neuroscience 77:575–584, 1997

Aigner M, Bach M: Clinical utility of DSM-IV pain disorder. Compr Psychiatry 40:353–357, 1999

American Pain Society Quality of Care Committee: Quality improvement guidelines for the treatment of acute pain and cancer pain. JAMA 274:1874–1880, 1995

American Psychiatric Association: Diagnostic and Statistical Manual of Mental Disorders, 3rd Edition. Washington, DC, American Psychiatric Association, 1980

American Psychiatric Association: Diagnostic and Statistical Manual of Mental Disorders, 3rd Edition Revised. Washington, DC, American Psychiatric Association, 1987

American Psychiatric Association: Diagnostic and Statistical Manual of Mental Disorders, 4th Edition. Washington, DC, American Psychiatric Association, 1994

American Psychiatric Association: Diagnostic and Statistical Manual of Mental Disorders, 4th Edition, Text Revision. Washington, DC, American Psychiatric Association, 2000

Anderberg UM, Marteinsdottir I, von Knorring L: Citalopram in patients with fibromyalgia: a randomized, double-blind, placebo-controlled study. Eur J Pain 4:27–35, 2000

Ansari A: The efficacy of newer antidepressants in the treatment of chronic pain: a review of current literature. Harv Rev Psychiatry 7:257–277, 2000

Arnold LM, Hess EV, Hudson JI, et al: A randomized, placebo-controlled, double-blind, flexible-dose study of fluoxetine in the treatment of women with fibromyalgia. Am J Med 112:191–197, 2002

Arnold LM, Lu Y, Crofford LJ, et al: A double-blind, multicenter trial comparing duloxetine with placebo in the treatment of fibromyalgia patients with or without major depressive disorder. Arthritis Rheum 50:2974–2984, 2004

Arnstein P: The mediation of disability by self efficacy in different samples of chronic pain patients. Disabil Rehabil 22:794–801, 2000

Asmundson GJG, Norton PJ, Norton GR: Beyond pain: the role of fear and avoidance in chronicity. Clin Psychol Rev 19:97–119, 1999

Baba H, Shimoji K, Yoshimura M: Norepinephrine facilitates inhibitory transmission in substantia gelatinosa of adult rat spinal cord (part 1): effects on axon terminals of GABAergic and glycinergic neurons. Anesthesiology 92:473–484, 2000

Bair MJ, Robinson RL, Katon W, et al: Depression and pain comorbidity: a literature review. Arch Intern Med 163:2433–2445, 2003

Banks SM, Kerns RD: Explaining high rates of depression in chronic pain: a diathesis-stress framework. Psychol Bull 119:95–110, 1996

Barsky AJ: Patients who amplify bodily sensations. Ann Intern Med 91:63–70, 1979

Bartusch SL, Sanders BJ, D'Alessio JG, et al: Clonazepam for the treatment of lancinating phantom limb pain. Clin J Pain 12:59–62, 1996

Blanchard EB, Appelbaum KA, Radnitz CL, et al: A controlled evaluation of thermal biofeedback and thermal biofeedback combined with cognitive therapy in the treatment of vascular headache. J Consult Clin Psychol 58:216–224, 1990

Blier P, Abbott FV: Putative mechanisms of action of antidepressant drugs in affective and anxiety disorders and pain. J Psychiatry Neurosci 26:37–43, 2001

Boland RJ: How could the validity of the DSM-IV pain disorder be improved in reference to the concept that it is supposed to identify? Curr Pain Headache Rep 6:23–29, 2002

Bouckoms AJ, Litman RE: Clonazepam in the treatment of neuralgic pain syndrome. Psychosomatics 26:933–936, 1985

Bowsher D: The effects of preemptive treatment of postherpetic neuralgia with amitriptyline: a randomized, double-blind, placebo-controlled trial. J Pain Symptom Manage 13:327–331, 1997

Breslau N, Davis GC: Migraine, physical health and psychiatric disorder: a prospective epidemiology study in young adults. J Psychiatr Res 27:211–221, 1993

Brown RL, Patterson JJ, Rounds LA, et al: Substance abuse among patients with chronic back pain. J Fam Pract 43:152–160, 1996

Browning CH: Nonsteroidal anti-inflammatory drugs and severe psychiatric side effects. Int J Psychiatry Med 26:25–34, 1996

Burns JW, Johnson BJ, Mahoney N, et al: Anger management style, hostility and spouse responses: gender differences in predictors of adjustment among chronic pain patients. Pain 64:445–453, 1996

Burns JW, Johnson BJ, Devine J, et al: Anger management style and the prediction of treatment outcome among male and female chronic pain patients. Behav Res Ther 36:1051–1062, 1998a

Burns JW, Johnson BJ, Mahoney N, et al: Cognitive and physical capacity process variables predict long-term outcome after treatment of chronic pain. J Consult Clin Psychol 66:434–439, 1998b

Capuron L, Gumnick JF, Musselman DL, et al: Neurobehavioral effects of interferon-alpha in cancer patients: phenomenology and paroxetine responsiveness of symptom dimensions. Neuropsychopharmacology 26:643–652, 2002

Carroll D, Seers K: Relaxation for the relief of chronic pain: a systematic review. J Adv Nurs 27:476–487, 1998

Chandramouli J: Newer anticonvulsant drugs in neuropathic pain and bipolar disorder. J Pain Palliat Care Pharmacother 16:19–37, 2002

Chochinov HM, Wilson KG, Enns M, et al: Depression, hopelessness, and suicidal ideation in the terminally ill. Psychosomatics 39:366–370, 1998

Ciccone DS, Just N, Bandilla EB, et al: Psychological correlates of opioid use in patients with chronic nonmalignant pain: a preliminary test of the downhill spiral hypothesis. J Pain Symptom Manage 20:180–192, 2000

Clark JD: Chronic pain prevalence and analgesic prescribing in a general medical population. J Pain Symptom Manage 23:131–137, 2002

Cohen H, Neumann L, Haiman Y, et al: Prevalence of post-traumatic stress disorder in fibromyalgia patients: overlapping syndromes or post-traumatic fibromyalgia syndrome? Semin Arthritis Rheum 32:38–50, 2002

Cohen MJM, Menefee LA, Doghramji K, et al: Sleep in chronic pain: problems and treatments. Int Rev Psychiatry 12:115–126, 2000

Collins SL, Moore RA, McQuay HJ, et al: Antidepressants and anticonvulsants for diabetic neuropathy and postherpetic neuralgia: a quantitative systematic review. J Pain Symptom Manage 20:449–458, 2000

Crombez G, Eccleston C, Baeyens F, et al: When somatic information threatens, catastrophic thinking enhances attentional interference. Pain 75:187–198, 1998

Dahl JB, Mathiesen 0, Moiniche S: "Protective premedication": an option with gabapentin and related drugs? A review of gabapentin and pregabalin in the treatment of post-operative pain. Acta Anaesthesiol Scand 48:1130–1136, 2004

Dellemijn PL, Fields HL: Do benzodiazepines have a role in chronic pain management? Pain 57:137–152, 1994

Derakshan N, Eysenck MW: Interpretive biases for one's own behavior and physiology in high-trait-anxious individuals and repressors. J Pers Soc Psychol 73:816–825, 1997

Dersh J, Polatin PB, Gatchel RJ: Chronic pain and psychopathology: research findings and theoretical considerations. Psychosom Med 64:773–786, 2002

Dillon P, Copeland J, Jansen K: Patterns of use and harms associated with non-medical ketamine use. Drug Alcohol Depend 69:23–28, 2003

DiMatteo MR, Lepper HS, Croghan TW: Depression is a risk factor for noncompliance with medical treatment: meta-analysis of the effects of anxiety and depression on patient adherence. Arch Intern Med 160:2101–2107, 2000

Doyle CA, Hunt SP: Substance P receptor (neurokinin-1)-expressing neurons in lamina I of the spinal cord encode for the intensity of noxious stimulation: a c-fos study in rat. Neuroscience 89:17–28, 1999

Dunbar SA, Katz NP: Chronic opioid therapy for nonmalignant pain in patients with a history of substance abuse: report of 20 cases. J Pain Symptom Manage 11:163–171, 1996

Dworkin SF, Von Korff M, LeResche L: Multiple pains and psychiatric disturbance: an epidemiologic investigation. Arch Gen Psychiatry 47:239–244, 1990

Egbunike IG, Chaffee BJ: Antidepressants in the management of chronic pain syndromes. Pharmacotherapy 10:262–270, 1990

Eide PK, Jorum E, Stubhaug A, et al: Relief of post-herpetic neuralgia with the N-methyl-aspartic acid receptor antagonist ketamine: a double-blind cross-over comparison with morphine and placebo. Pain 58:347–354, 1994

Eisenberg E, Kleiser A, Dotort A, et al: The NMDA (N-methyl-D-aspartate) receptor antagonist memantine in the treatment of postherpetic neuralgia: a double-blind, placebo-controlled study. Eur J Pain 2:321–327, 1998

Ekbom K, Hardebo JE: Cluster headache: aetiology, diagnosis and management. Drugs 62:61–69, 2002

Enarson MC, Hays H, Woodroffe MA: Clinical experience with oral ketamine. J Pain Symptom Manage 17:384–386, 1999

Ernst E: Herb–drug interactions: potentially important but woefully under-researched. Eur J Clin Pharmacol 56:523–524, 2000

Fernandez E, Milburn TW: Sensory and affective predictors of overall pain and emotions associated with affective pain. Clin J Pain 10:3–9, 1994

Fernandez E, Turk DC: The scope and significance of anger in the experience of chronic pain. Pain 61:165–175, 1995

Fields HL, Basbaum AI: Central nervous system mechanisms of pain modulation, in Textbook of Pain, 4th Edition. Edited by Wall PD, Melzack R. Edinburgh, Scotland, Churchill Livingstone, 1999, pp 309–329

Fishbain DA: Secondary gain concept: definition, problems and its abuse in medical practice. J Pain 3:264–273, 1994

Fishbain DA: Approaches to treatment decisions for psychiatric comorbidity in the management of the chronic pain patient. Med Clin North Am 83:737–760, 1999a

Fishbain DA: The association of chronic pain and suicide. Semin Clin Neuropsychiatry 4:221–227, 1999b

Fishbain DA: Evidence-based data on pain relief with antidepressants. Ann Med 32:305–316, 2000

Fishbain DA, Goldberg M, Meagher BR, et al: Male and female chronic pain patients categorized by DSM-III psychiatric diagnostic criteria. Pain 26:181–197, 1986

Fishbain DA, Cutler R, Rosomoff HL, et al: Chronic pain-associated depression: antecedent or consequence of chronic pain? A review. Clin J Pain 13:116–137, 1997

Fishbain DA, Cutler R, Rosomoff H: Comorbid psychiatric disorders in chronic pain patients with psychoactive substance use disorders. Pain Clinic 11:79–87, 1998

Fishman P, Von Korff M, Lozano P, et al: Chronic care costs in managed care. Health Aff 16:239–247, 1997

Flor H, Fydrich T, Turk DC: Efficacy of multidisciplinary pain treatment centers: a meta-analytic review. Pain 49:221–230, 1992

Ford CU: Somatizing disorders. Psychosomatics 27:327–337, 1986

Forrest WH, Brown BW, Brown CR, et al: Dextroamphetamine with morphine for the treatment of postoperative pain. N Engl J Med 296:712–715, 1977

Forseth KO, Husby G, Gran IT, et al: Prognostic factors for the development of fibromyalgia in women with self-reported musculoskeletal pain: a prospective study. J Rheumatol 26:2458–2467, 1999

Galer BS: Neuropathic pain of peripheral origin: advances in pharmacological treatment. Neurology 45 (suppl):17–25, 1995

Gallagher RM: Treatment planning in pain medicine: integrating medical, physical, and behavioral therapies. Med Clin North Am 83:823–849, 1999

Gardner JS, Blough D, Drinkard CR, et al: Tramadol and seizures: a surveillance study in a managed care population. Pharmacotherapy 20:1423–1431, 2000

Gatchel RJ: Early development of physical and mental deconditioning in painful spinal disorders, in Contemporary Conservative Care for Painful Spinal Disorders. Edited by Mayer TG, Mooney V, Gatchel RJ. Philadelphia, PA, Lea & Febiger, 1991

Gerner P, Mujtaba M, Sinnott CJ, et al: Amitriptyline versus bupivacaine in rat sciatic nerve blockade. Anesthesiology 94:661–667, 2001

Goldstein DJ, Lu Y, Detke MJ, et al: Duloxetine vs. placebo in patients with painful diabetic neuropathy. Pain 116:109–118, 2005

Greden JF: Physical symptoms of depression: unmet needs. J Clin Psychiatry 64 (suppl):5–11, 2003

Guay DR: Oxcarbazepine, topiramate, zonisamide, and levetiracetam: potential use in neuropathic pain. Am J Geriatr Pharmacother 1:18–37, 2003

Hasenbring M, Hallner D, Klasen B: Psychological mechanisms in the transition from acute to chronic pain: over- or underrated? Schmerz 15:442–447, 2001

Hathaway SR, McKinley JC, Butcher JN, et al: Minnesota Multiphasic Personality Inventory—2: Manual for Administration. Minneapolis, University of Minnesota Press, 1989

Hiller W, Heuser J, Fichter MM: The DSM-IV nosology of chronic pain: a comparison of pain disorder and multiple somatization syndrome. Eur J Pain 4:45–55, 2000

Hoffman BM, Papas RK, Chatkoff DK, et al: Meta-analysis of psychological interventions for chronic low back pain. Health Psychology 26:1–9, 2007

Huyser BA, Parker JC: Negative affect and pain in arthritis. Rheum Dis Clin North Am 25:105–121, 1999

Jackson JL, O'Malley PG, Tomkins G, et al: Treatment of functional gastrointestinal disorders with antidepressant medications: a meta-analysis. Am J Med 108:65–72, 2000

Jackson KC, Lipman AG: Opioid analgesics, in Practical Pain Management, 3rd Edition. Edited by Tollison CD, Satterwaite JR, Tollison JW. Philadelphia, PA, Lippincott Williams & Wilkins, 2001, pp 216–231

Jasmin L, Tien D, Janni G, et al: Is noradrenaline a significant factor in the analgesic effect of antidepressants? Pain 106:3–8, 2003

Jensen MP, Karoly P, Braver S: The measurement of clinical pain intensity: a comparison of six methods. Pain 27:117–126, 1986

Jensen MP, Turner JA, Romano JM: Self-efficacy and outcome expectancies: relationship to chronic pain coping strategies and adjustment. Pain 44:263–269, 1991a

Jensen MP, Turner JA, Romano JM, et al: Coping with chronic pain: a critical review of the literature. Pain 47:249–283, 1991b

Jensen MP, Turner JA, Romano JM: Correlates of improvement in multidisciplinary treatment of chronic pain. J Consult Clin Psychol 62:172–179, 1994

Jensen MP, Turner JA, Romano JM: Changes in beliefs, catastrophizing, and coping are associated with improvement in multidisciplinary pain treatment. J Consult Clin Psychol 69:655–662, 2001

Jiang HK, Chang DM: Nonsteroidal anti-inflammatory drugs with adverse psychiatric reactions: five case reports. Clin Rheumatol 18:339–345, 1999

Katon W, Sullivan M, Walker E: Medical symptoms without identified pathology: relationship to psychiatric disorders, childhood and adult trauma, and personality traits. Ann Intern Med 134:917–925, 2001

Kaufman DW, Kelly JP, Rosenberg L, et al: Recent patterns of medication use in the ambulatory adult population of the United States: the Slone Survey. JAMA 287:337–344, 2002

Kawasaki Y, Kumamoto E, Furue H, et al: α2 adrenoceptor-mediated presynaptic inhibition of primary afferent glutamatergic transmission in rat substantia gelatinosa neurons. Anesthesiology 98:682–689, 2003

Keel PJ, Bodoky C, Gerhard U, et al: Comparison of integrated group therapy and group relaxation training for fibromyalgia. Clin J Pain 14:232–238, 1998

Kerns RD, Turk DC, Rudy TE: The West Haven-Yale Multidimensional Pain Inventory (WHYMPI). Pain 23:345–356, 1985

Khoromi S, Patsalides A, Parada S, et al: Topiramate in chronic lumbar radicular pain. J Pain 6:829–836, 2005

King SA, Snow BR: Factors for predicting premature termination from a multidisciplinary inpatient chronic pain program. Pain 39:281–287, 1989

King SA, Strain JJ: Benzodiazepine use by chronic pain patients. Clin J Pain 6:143–147, 1990

Kishore-Kumar R, Schafer SC, Lawlor BA, et al: Single doses of the serotonin agonists buspirone and m-chlorophenylpiperazine do not relieve neuropathic pain. Pain 37:223–227, 1989

Knapp DA, Koch H: The management of new pain in office-based ambulatory care: National Ambulatory Medical Care Survey, 1980 and 1981. Adv Data 97:1–9, 1984

Koenig TW, Clark MR: Advances in comprehensive pain management. Psychiatr Clin North Am 19:589–611, 1996

Krell HV, Leuchter AF, Cook IA, et al: Evaluation of reboxetine, a noradrenergic antidepressant, for the treatment of fibromyalgia and chronic low back pain. Psychosomatics 46:379–384, 2005

Kroenke K, Spitzer RL, Williams JB, et al: Physical symptoms in primary care: predictors of psychiatric disorders and functional impairment. Arch Fam Med 3:774–779, 1994

Lackner JM, Gurtman MB: Patterns of interpersonal problems in irritable bowel syndrome patients: a circumplex analysis. J Psychosom Res 58:523–532, 2005

Lackner JM, Quigley BM: Pain catastrophizing mediates the relationship between worry and pain suffering in patients with irritable bowel syndrome. Behav Res Ther 43:943–957, 2005

Lange-Asschenfeldt C, Weigmann H, Hiemke C, et al: Serotonin syndrome as a result of fluoxetine in a patient with tramadol abuse: plasma level-correlated symptomatology. J Clin Psychopharmacol 22:440–441, 2002

Lefaucheur JP, Drouot X, Keravel Y, et al: Pain relief induced by repetitive transcranial magnetic stimulation of precentral cortex. NeuroReport 12:2963–2965, 2001

Leino P, Magni G: Depressive and distress symptoms as predictors of low back pain, neck-shoulder pain, and other musculoskeletal morbidity: a 10-year follow-up of metal industry employees. Pain 53:89–94, 1993

Leo RJ: Treatment considerations in neuropathic pain. Curr Treat Options Neurol 8:389–400, 2006

Leo RJ: Clinical Manual of Pain Management in Psychiatry. Washington, DC, American Psychiatric Publishing, 2007

Leo RJ, Baer D: Delirium associated with baclofen withdrawal: a review of common presentations and management strategies. Psychosomatics 46:503–507, 2005

Leo RJ, Brooks V: Clinical Potential of milnacipran, a serotonin and norepinephrine reuptake inhibitor, in pain. Curr Opin Investig Drugs 7:637–642, 2006

Leo RJ, Latif T: Repetitive transcranial magnetic stimulation (rTMS) in experimentally induced and chronic neuropathic pain: a review. J Pain 8:453–459, 2007

Leo RJ, Narendran R, DeGuiseppe B: Methadone detoxification of tramadol dependence. J Subst Abuse Treat 19:297–299, 2000

Leo RJ, Pristach C, Streltzer J: A curriculum in pain management for psychiatry residents. Acad Psychiatry 27:1–11, 2003

Lin EHB, Katon W, Von Korff M, et al: Effect of improving depression care on pain and functional outcomes among older adults with arthritis: a randomized controlled trial. JAMA 290:2428–2434, 2003

Loeser JD: Economic implications of pain management. Acta Anaesthesiol Scand 43:957–959, 1999

Loeser JD, Butler SH, Chapman CR, et al: Bonica's Management of Pain, 3rd Edition. Philadelphia, PA, Lippincott Williams & Wilkins, 2001

Lucas R, Warner TD, Vojnovic I, et al: Cellular mechanisms of acetaminophen: role of cyclo-oxygenase. FASEB J 19:635–637, 2005

Lynch ME: Antidepressants as analgesics: a review of randomized controlled trials. J Psychiatry Neurosci 26:30–36, 2001

Magni G: The use of antidepressants in the treatment of chronic pain: a review of the current evidence. Drugs 42:730–748, 1991

Mantyh PW: Neurobiology of substance P and the NK1 receptor. J Clin Psychiatry 63 (suppl):6–10, 2002

Maruta T, Swanson DW, Swenson WM: Chronic pain: which patients may a pain-management program help? Pain 7:321–329, 1979

Massie MJ: Pain: What Psychiatrists Need to Know (Review of Psychiatry Series, Vol 19, No 2; Oldham JM and Riba MB, series eds). Washington, DC, American Psychiatric Press, 2000

Max MB: Treatment of post-herpetic neuralgia: antidepressants. Ann Neurol 35 (suppl):50–53, 1994

Max MB, Lynch SA, Muir J, et al: Effects of desipramine, amitriptyline, and fluoxetine on pain in diabetic neuropathy. N Engl J Med 326:1250–1256, 1992

Mayou R, Levenson J, Sharpe M: Somatoform disorders in DSM-V. Psychosomatics 44:449–451, 2003

Mayou R, Kirmayer LJ, Simon G, et al: Somatoform disorders: time for a new approach in DSM-V. Am J Psychiatry 162:847–855, 2005

McQuay HJ: Opioid use in chronic pain. Acta Anaesthesiol Scand 41:175–183, 1997

McQuay HJ: Neuropathic pain: evidence matters. Eur J Pain 6 (suppl):11–18, 2002

McQuay H, Carroll D, Jadad AR, et al: Anticonvulsant drugs for management of pain: a systematic review. BMJ 311:1047–1052, 1995

McQuay HJ, Tramer M, Nye BA, et al: A systematic review of antidepressants in neuropathic pain. Pain 68:217–227, 1996

McWilliams LA, Cox BJ, Enns MW: Mood and anxiety disorders associated with chronic pain: an examination in a nationally representative sample. Pain 106:127–133, 2003

McWilliams LA, Goodwin RD, Cox BJ: Depression and anxiety associated with three pain conditions: results from a nationally representative sample. Pain 111:77–83, 2004

Melzack R: The McGill Pain Questionnaire: major properties and scoring methods. Pain 1:277–299, 1975

Merskey H, Bogduk N: Classification of Chronic Pain: Descriptions of Chronic Pain Syndromes and Definitions of Pain Terms, 2nd Edition. Seattle, WA, International Association for the Study of Pain, 1994

Miotto K, Compton P, Ling W, et al: Diagnosing addictive disease in chronic pain patients. Psychosomatics 37:223–235, 1996

Mochizuki D: Serotonin and noradrenaline reuptake inhibitors in animal models of pain. Hum Psychopharmacol 19 (suppl):15–19, 2004

Moldofsky H: Sleep and pain. Sleep Med Rev 5:387–398, 2001

Morley S, Eccleston C, Williams A: Systematic review and meta-analysis of randomized controlled trials of cognitive behaviour therapy and behaviour therapy for chronic pain in adults, excluding headache. Pain 80:1–13, 1999

Nemmani KVS, Mogil JS: Serotonin-GABA interactions in the modulation of mu- and kappa-opioid analgesia. Neuropharmacology 44:304–310, 2003

Norregaard J, Volkmann H, Danneskiold-Samsoe B: A randomized controlled trial of citalopram in the treatment of fibromyalgia. Pain 61:445–449, 1995

Novak V, Kanard R, Kissel JT, et al: Treatment of painful sensory neuropathy with tiagabine: a pilot study. Clin Auton Res 11:357–361, 2001

Ohayon MM, Roth T: Prevalence of restless legs syndrome and periodic movement disorder in the general population. J Psychosom Res 53:547–554, 2002

Onghena P, Van Houdenhove B: Antidepressant-induced analgesia in chronic non-malignant pain: a meta-analysis of 39 placebo-controlled studies. Pain 49:205–219, 1992

Orne MT: Mechanisms of hypnotic pain control, in Advances in Pain Research and Therapy, Vol 1. Edited by Bonica JJ, Ale-Fessard D. New York, Raven, 1976, pp 717–726

Osterweis M, Kleinman A, Mechanic D (eds): Pain and Disability: Clinical, Behavioral, and Public Policy Perspectives. Washington, DC, National Academy Press, 1987

Owen-Salters E, Gatchel RJ, Polatin PB, et al: Changes in psychopathology following functional restoration of chronic low back pain patients: a prospective study. J Occup Rehabil 6:215–223, 1996

Pappagallo M: Newer antiepileptic drugs: possible uses in the treatment of neuropathic pain and migraine. Clin Ther 25:2506–2538, 2003

Passik SD, Weinreb HJ: Managing chronic nonmalignant pain: overcoming obstacles to the use of opioids. Adv Ther 17:70–83, 2000

Polatin PB, Kinney RK, Gatchel RJ, et al: Psychiatric illness and chronic low-back pain. The mind and the spine: which goes first? Spine 18:66–71, 1993

Portenoy RK: Opioid therapy for chronic nonmalignant pain: a review of the critical issues. J Pain Symptom Manage 11:203–217, 1996

Portenoy RK, Hagen NA: Breakthrough pain: definition, prevalence and characteristics. Pain 41:273–281, 1990

Prater CD, Zylstra RG, Miller KE: Successful pain management for the recovering addicted patient. Prim Care Companion J Clin Psychiatry 4:125–131, 2002

Quang-Cantagrel ND, Wallace MS, Magnuson SK: Opioid substitution to improve the effectiveness of chronic noncancer pain control: a chart review. Anesth Analg 90:933–937, 2000

Raz A, Shapiro T: Hypnosis and neuroscience: a cross talk between clinical and cognitive research. Arch Gen Psychiatry 59:85–90, 2002

Rosenstiel AK, Keefe FJ: The use of coping strategies in chronic low back pain patients: relationship to patient characteristics and current adjustment. Pain 17:33–44, 1983

Rowbotham MC, Goli V, Kunz NR, et al: Venlafaxine extended release in the treatment of painful diabetic neuropathy: a double-blind, placebo-controlled study. Pain 110:697–706, 2004

Rowbotham MC, Reisner LA, Davies PS, et al: Treatment response in antidepressant-naïve postherpetic neuralgia patients: double-blind, randomized trial. J Pain 6:741–746, 2005

Sanders SH: Operant therapy with pain patients: evidence for its effectiveness, in Seminars in Pain Medicine I. Edited by Lebovits AH. Philadelphia, PA, WB Saunders, 2003, pp 90–98

Sang CN, Booher S, Gilron I, et al: Dextromethorphan and memantine in painful diabetic neuropathy and postherpetic neuralgia: efficacy and dose-response trials. Anesthesiology 96:1053–1061, 2002

Santarelli L, Gobbi G, Blier P, et al: Behavioral and physiologic effects of genetic or pharmacological inactivation of the substance P receptor (NK1). J Clin Psychiatry 63 (suppl):11–17, 2002

Saper JR Lake AE, Tepper SJ: Nefazodone for chronic daily headache prophylaxis: an open-label study. Headache 41:465–474, 2001

Sarnoch H, Adler F, Scholtz OB: Relevance of muscular sensitivity, muscular activity, and cognitive variables for pain reduction associated with EMG biofeedback in fibromyalgia. Percept Mot Skills 84:1043–1050, 1997

Schappert SM: National Ambulatory Medical Care Survey: 1989 summary. Natl Vital Stat Rep 13:1–80, 1992

Schnitzer T: The new analgesic combination tramadol/acetaminophen. Eur J Anaesthesiol 20 (suppl):13–18, 2003

Schreiber S, Bleich A, Pick CG: Venlafaxine and mirtazapine: different mechanisms of antidepressant action, common opioid-mediated anti nociceptive effects: a possible opioid involvement in severe depression? J Mol Neurosci 18:143–149, 2002

Semenchuk MR, Davis B: Efficacy of sustained-release bupropion in neuropathic pain: an open-label study. Clin J Pain 16:6–11, 2000

Semenchuk MR, Sherman S, Davis B: Double-blind, randomized trial of bupropion SR for the treatment of neuropathic pain. Neurology 57:1583–1588, 2001

Sharpe L, Sensky T, Timberlake N, et al: A blind, randomized, controlled trial of cognitive-behavioural intervention for patients with recent onset rheumatoid arthritis: preventing psychological and physical morbidity. Pain 89:275–283, 2001

Silver BV, Blanchard EB: Biofeedback and relaxation training in the treatment of psychophysiological disorders: or are the machines really necessary? J Behav Med 1:217–239, 1978

Sindrup SH, Jensen TS: Efficacy of pharmacological treatments of neuropathic pain: an update and effect related to mechanism of drug action. Pain 83:389–400, 1999

Sindrup SH, Gram LF, Brosen K, et al: The selective serotonin reuptake inhibitor paroxetine is effective in the treatment of diabetic neuropathy symptoms. Pain 42:135–144, 1990

Sindrup SH, Bjerre U, Dejgaard A, et al: The selective serotonin reuptake inhibitor citalopram relieves the symptoms of diabetic neuropathy. Clin Pharmacol Ther 52:547–552, 1992

Sindrup SH, Bach FW, Madsen C, et al: Venlafaxine versus imipramine in painful polyneuropathy: a randomized, controlled trial. Neurology 60:1284–1289, 2003

Skevington SM, Carse MS, Williams AC: Validation of the WHOQOL-100: pain management improves quality of life for chronic pain patients. Clin J Pain 17:264–275, 2001

Snow V, Weiss K, Wall EM, et al: Pharmacological management of acute attacks of migraine and prevention of migraine headache. Ann Intern Med 137:840–849, 2002

Sommer BR, Petrides G: A case of baclofen-induced psychotic depression. J Clin Psychiatry 53:211–212, 1992

Steiner TJ, Hering R, Couturier EG, et al: Double-blind placebo-controlled trial of lithium in episodic cluster headache. Cephalalgia 17:673–675, 1997

Stewart WF, Ricci JA, Chee E, et al: Lost productive time and cost due to common pain complaints in the US workforce. JAMA 290:2443–2454, 2003

Sullivan MD: DSM-IV pain disorder: a case against the diagnosis. International Review of Psychiatry 12:91–98, 2000

Sullivan MJ, Stanish W, Waite H, et al: Catastrophizing, pain, and disability in patients with soft-tissue injuries. Pain 77:253–260, 1998

Sullivan MJ, Thorn B, Haythornthwaite JA, et al: Theoretical perspectives on the relation between catastrophizing and pain. Clin J Pain 17:52–64, 2001

Sussman N: SNRIs versus SSRIs: mechanisms of action in treating depression and painful physical symptoms. Prim Care Companion J Clin Psychiatry 5 (suppl):19–26, 2003

Swartz KL, Pratt LA, Armenian HK, et al: Mental disorders and the incidence of migraine headaches in a community sample: results from the Baltimore Epidemiologic Catchment Area follow-up study. Arch Gen Psychiatry 57:945–950, 2000

Tofferi JK, Jackson JL, O'Malley PG: Treatment of fibromyalgia with cyclobenzaprine: a meta-analysis. Arthritis Rheum 51:9–13, 2004

Trief PM, Grant W, Fredrickson B: A prospective study of psychological predictors of lumbar surgery outcome. Spine 25:2616–2621, 2000

Turk DC, Meichenbaum DH, Berman WH: Application of biofeedback for the regulation of pain: a critical review. Psychol Bull 86:1322–1338, 1979

Turner JA, Chapman CR: Psychological interventions for chronic pain: a critical review, I: relaxation training and biofeedback. Pain 12:1–21, 1982a

Turner JA, Chapman CR: Psychological interventions for chronic pain: a critical review, II: operant conditioning, hypnosis, and cognitive-behavioral therapy. Pain 12:23–46, 1982b

van der Kolk BA, Pelcovitz D, Roth S, et al: Dissociation, somatization, and affect dysregulation: the complexity of adaptation to trauma. Am J Psychiatry 153:83–93, 1996

Vinik A: Use of antiepileptic drugs in the treatment of chronic painful diabetic neuropathy. J Clin Endocrinol Metab 90:4936–4945, 2005

Vitton O, Gendreau M, Kranzler J, et al: Double-blind placebo controlled trial of milnacipran in the treatment of fibromyalgia. Hum Psychopharmacol 19 (suppl):27–35, 2004

Vlaeyen JWS, Kole-Snijders AMJ, Boeren RGB, et al: Fear of movement/(re)injury in chronic low back pain and its relation to behavioral performance. Pain 62:363–372, 1995

Waddell G, Newton M, Henderson I, et al: A Fear-Avoidance Beliefs Questionnaire (FABQ) and the role of fear-avoidance beliefs in chronic low back pain and disability. Pain 52:157–168, 1993

Weissman DE, Haddox JD: Opioid pseudoaddiction: an iatrogenic syndrome. Pain 36:363–366, 1989

Weissman MM, Markowitz JC, Klerman GL: Comprehensive Guide to Interpersonal Psychotherapy. New York, Basic Books, 2000

World Health Organization: Cancer pain relief and palliative care: report of a WHO expert committee. World Health Organ Tech Rep Ser 804:1–75, 1990

Yerby MS: Special considerations for women with epilepsy. Pharmacotherapy 20 (suppl):159–170, 2000

Zenz M, Strumpf M, Tryba M: Long-term oral opioid therapy in patients with chronic nonmalignant pain. J Pain Symptom Manage 7:69–77, 1992

Zijlstra TR, Barendregt PJ, van de Laar MAF: Venlafaxine in fibromyalgia: results of a randomized, placebo-controlled, double-blind trial (abstract). Arthritis Rheum 46 (suppl):105, 2002

Zubieta JK, Ketter TA, Bueller JA, et al: Regulation of human affective responses by anterior cingulate and limbic mu-opioid neurotransmission. Arch Gen Psychiatry 60:1145–1153, 2003

PSYCHIATRIC TREATMENTS

26

PSYCHOPHARMACOLOGY

Melissa Martinez, M.D.

Lauren B. Marangell, M.D.

James M. Martinez, M.D.

The pharmacological armamentarium for the treatment of psychiatric illnesses is rapidly expanding with the addition of new medications, innovative formulations of drug delivery, and the identification of potential biological treatment targets. As the psychotropic medication pharmacopoeia grows, clinicians are faced with the daunting task of incorporating an expanded knowledge base of pharmacology and medicine to prescribe these medications safely and effectively.

This chapter was designed to provide clinicians with an overview of major psychotropic medications. This chapter is not an exhaustive review; we begin with an overview of some general principles that are relevant to the safe and effective prescribing of psychotropic medications, followed by specific discussions of major classes of psychotropic medication classes, including antidepressants, anxiolytics, antipsychotics, and mood stabilizers. Stimulants and cognitive enhancers are discussed elsewhere in this volume (see

Chapter 21, "Disorders Usually First Diagnosed in Infancy, Childhood, or Adolescence," by Ursano et al., and Chapter 8, "Delirium, Dementia, and Amnestic and Other Cognitive Disorders," by Bourgeois et al.).

General Principles

Initial Evaluation

The art and skillful practice of psychopharmacology have multiple facets, including establishing proper diagnoses, identifying medication-responsive target symptoms, ruling out nonpsychiatric causes of a patient's symptomatology, noting the presence of other medical problems that will influence drug selection, evaluating concomitant medications that may cause drug–drug interactions, and evaluating personal and family histories of medication response.

The text, tables, and figures in this chapter were derived, in part, from Marangell LB, Martinez JM: *Concise Guide to Psychopharmacology*, 2nd Edition, which had its genesis in the previous edition of this chapter.

The authors wish to express sincere gratitude and acknowledgment to Stuart C. Yudofsky, M.D., Donald C. Goff, M.D., and Jonathan M. Silver, M.D., who were coauthors on the previous version of this chapter, and to Dr. Yudofsky and Dr. Silver, who also were coauthors on the first edition of the *Concise Guide to Psychopharmacology*. The "Drug Interactions" sections contain material developed over many years by Lauren B. Marangell, M.D., in collaboration with Ann Callahan, M.D., and Terence Ketter, M.D.

Target Symptoms

A key component in arriving at a well-informed treatment decision is the identification of target symptoms. Once the physician determines the proper diagnosis, he or she should identify the specific symptoms that are targets for treatment and monitor the response of these symptoms during the course of treatment. Standard rating scales are useful for monitoring target symptom changes with treatment. In the absence of formal rating scales, target symptoms can be rated on a clinician-determined scale that can be tracked over time. It is also important for the clinician to monitor the patient's functional status because major goals of treatment include both symptomatic and functional recovery.

Use of Multiple Medications

A frequent clinical error is to treat specific symptoms of a disorder with multiple drugs rather than to treat the underlying disorder itself. For example, one may see a patient who has been prescribed two different benzodiazepines (one for anxiety and one for insomnia), an analgesic for pain complaints, a stimulant medication for lethargy and impaired concentration, and a subtherapeutic dose of an antidepressant for other depressive symptoms. In some instances, the cluster of symptoms described in this example may be components of an underlying depression, which may be aggravated by the polypharmaceutical approach inherent in symptomatic treatment. Additionally, this polypharmacy approach may expose the patient to a greater side-effect burden and the potential for significant drug–drug interactions.

However, some patients may require the rational concomitant use of two or more psychotropic agents to manage their illness effectively. For example, in a patient with major depression who has had a partial, but inadequate, response to antidepressant monotherapy despite optimizing the dose, the addition of a second medication as an evidence-based augmentation strategy merits consideration.

Medication Selection

Fortunately, clinicians today are practicing psychiatry in an era that affords them numerous medication options. Because so many medication options exist, a clinician must consider numerous factors when selecting a specific psychotropic medication for a given patient. These factors include the presence of comorbid medical conditions (which may preclude the use of certain medications); the presence of comorbid psychiatric disorders (which may be exacerbated by certain medications but effectively treated by others); the use of concomitant psychotropic and nonpsychotropic medications (which may pose a risk for significant drug–drug interactions); history of response and tolerability to medication; family history of medication responses; patient-specific life circumstances that may be affected by particular side effects; patient concerns regarding the avoidance of particular side effects; and treatment costs.

For example, when a patient has both major depressive disorder and generalized anxiety disorder, a clinician initially may choose a single medication that may effectively treat both illnesses. For a patient who presents with a history of cardiovascular disease, the clinician would avoid medications with known cardiovascular risks. For patients who express concern about the potential for weight gain, the clinician may select a medication with a lower propensity for causing weight gain relative to other treatment options. In patients who are taking a complicated regimen of medications, the clinician must evaluate the potential risk for significant drug–drug interactions and avoid introducing a psychotropic medication with a known or potential risk for interactions.

Generic Substitution

Generic drugs are less expensive alternatives to original proprietary (brand-name) formulations. Some patients may favor the use of a generic medication, if available, so that they may benefit from the cost savings. However, some caution is warranted with respect to generic drugs because generic "equivalents" are not always truly equivalent. The current U.S. Food and Drug Administration (FDA) requirements center around the concept of *bioequivalence*. Products are bioequivalent if they have no significant difference in the rate at which or extent to which the active ingredient becomes available at the site of action, given the same dose and conditions. In some cases, even small differences between a proprietary formulation and a generic preparation may have clinically meaningful consequences. For example, a patient may have an allergic reaction to one generic preparation but not another of the same drug because of differences in the dye used to color the pills. Thus, the clinician should be aware of the potential for problems when patients receive generic medications and, in the event of an unexpected reaction, should ask the patient if the medication has changed in appearance. A change in size, shape, or color, for example, should alert the clinician to a probable change in generic formulation.

Drug Interactions

A drug interaction occurs when the pharmacological action of a medication is altered by a concurrently administered drug (or exogenous substance). With the increased use of psychotropic medications, the importance of drug interactions in psychopharmacology is increasingly apparent. Also, the characterization of specific cytochrome P450 (CYP) enzymes has made it possible to understand and predict many drug–drug interactions. In the following subsections, we briefly review some key types of drug interactions. For a more extensive review of the topic, we refer the reader to the excellent work by Cozza et al. (2003).

The three main types of drug interactions are *pharmacokinetic interactions, pharmacodynamic interactions,* and *idiosyncratic interactions.* Pharmacokinetic interactions occur when one medication alters the pharmacokinetics (absorption, distribution, metabolism, or excretion) of another drug. Pharmacodynamic interactions occur when the action of a drug changes at a receptor or biologically active site, which alters the pharmacological effect of a given plasma concentration of the drug. Idiosyncratic interactions occur unpredictably in a small number of patients; they are unexpected, given the known pharmacological actions of the individual drugs.

Cytochrome P450 Enzymes

Most psychotropic medications, except for lithium, are metabolized by cytochrome P450 enzymes. These enzymes are classified by families and subfamilies on the basis of similarities in amino acid sequence. Enzymes within subfamilies have relatively specific affinities for various drugs and other substances. The enzymes primarily involved in drug metabolism include CYP1A2, CYP2C9, CYP2C10, CYP2C19, CYP2D6, CYP3A3, and CYP3A4.

One important drug interaction that may involve cytochrome P450 enzymes is *enzyme inhibition.* Some medications, including several psychotropic medications, can cause clinically meaningful inhibition of one or more cytochrome P450 enzymes. If a cytochrome P450 enzyme is inhibited by a medication, then the plasma levels of concurrently administered drugs that rely on that enzyme for metabolism may increase. For example, CYP2D6 is essential for the usual metabolism of tricyclic antidepressants (TCAs). If a patient is taking a TCA and a medication that inhibits the CYP2D6 enzyme is introduced, or vice versa, plasma TCA levels increase, which may result in increased TCA-related side effects or TCA toxicity. A clinician who is

aware of the potential for this reaction might choose to use a lower dose of the TCA. This example illustrates a key clinical principle of prescribing enzyme inhibitors: in many cases, the concomitant administration of an enzyme inhibitor and a medication that is a substrate for that enzyme is not contraindicated, but the patient should be monitored for signs and symptoms related to increased substrate levels, and the substrate dose should be decreased if necessary.

With regard to many medications, the specific cytochrome P450 enzymes responsible for metabolism are not yet known, but information about the role of cytochrome P450 enzymes in drug metabolism is rapidly accumulating. A partial list of clinically important substrates for and inhibitors of the cytochrome P450 enzymes most commonly involved in drug metabolism is presented in Table 26–1.

The effects of inhibitors occur relatively rapidly (in minutes to hours) and are reversible within a time frame that depends on the half-life of the inhibitor. Additionally, there is a large amount of interindividual variation in drug metabolism and the propensity for enzyme inhibition to alter metabolism. Part of this variation is the result of genetic polymorphism, which is a heritable alteration of the enzyme. Persons who have a genetic polymorphism that causes a large reduction in the amount of active enzyme are referred to as *poor metabolizers* and are at risk for increased drug levels, which may lead to toxicity. In contrast, some people have increased amounts of an enzyme. These individuals, referred to as *ultrarapid metabolizers,* may have reduced levels of drugs that are metabolized by the enzyme, resulting in decreased efficacy.

Another important interaction that may occur with cytochrome P450 enzymes is *enzyme induction.* Induction occurs when the liver produces a greater amount of the enzyme. This increase in enzyme availability can increase elimination and reduce plasma levels of a drug (or metabolite) that is a substrate for that enzyme. One risk inherent with this interaction is a potential loss of efficacy for drugs metabolized by the induced enzyme. Indeed, if a drug's clinical effectiveness is diminished as a result of this interaction, the dose of the affected drug should be increased to achieve the same serum concentration that was previously therapeutically effective.

The effects of inducers tend to be delayed for days to weeks because this process involves enzyme synthesis. St. John's wort has been reported to decrease levels and the effectiveness of cyclosporine (Ahmed et al. 2001; Breidenbach et al. 2000; Karliova et al. 2000) and protease inhibitors (Durr et al. 2000). Examples of psy-

TABLE 26–1. Partial list of cytochrome P450 (CYP) substrates and inhibitors

	CYP1A2	CYP2D6	CYP3A3/4
Substrates[a]	Aminophylline	Most antipsychotics	Acetaminophen
	Amitriptyline	Amphetamine	Alprazolam
	Caffeine	Codeine	Amiodarone
	Clozapine (in part)	Donepezil	Antiarrhythmics
	Cyclobenzaprine	Encainide	Calcium channel blockers
	Flutamide	Flecainide	Carbamazepine
	Imipramine	Galantamine	Cyclosporine
	Riluzole	Lipophilic β-blockers	Donepezil
	Ramelteon	Mexiletine	Eszopiclone
	Theophylline	Oxycodone	Ethosuximide
		Tricyclic antidepressants[b]	Galantamine
		Tramadol	HMG-CoA reductase inhibitors
		Trazodone	Lamotrigine
		Type Ic antiarrhythmics	Lidocaine
		Venlafaxine	Midazolam
			Most antineoplastics
			Oral contraceptives
			Oxcarbazepine
			Phosphodiesterase inhibitors
			Pimozide
			Propafenone
			Protease inhibitors
			Quinidine
			Steroids
			Zaleplon
			Zolpidem
	CYP1A2	**CYP2D6**	**CYP3A3/4**
Inhibitors[c]	Cimetidine	Bupropion	Diltiazem
	Ciprofloxacin	Cimetidine	Fluvoxamine
	Enoxacin	Duloxetine	Grapefruit juice
	Flutamide	Fluoxetine	Imidazole antifungal agents
	Fluvoxamine	Paroxetine	Some macrolides
	Grapefruit juice	Quinidine	Nefazodone
	Ketoconazole	Ritonavir	Protease inhibitors
	Lomefloxacin	Sertraline	Verapamil
	Norfloxacin		

Note. HMG-CoA=3-hydroxy-3-methylglutaryl coenzyme A.
[a]Medications and substances metabolized by a given enzyme.
[b]The 2D6 enzyme is the final common pathway for the metabolism of tricyclic antidepressants.
[c]May increase levels of substrates.

Source. Callahan et al. 1996; Cozza et al. 2003; Greenblatt et al. 1998, 1999; Michalets 1998. Adapted from Marangell LB, Martinez JM: *Concise Guide to Psychopharmacology,* 2nd Edition. Arlington, VA, American Psychiatric Publishing, 2006. Used with permission.

chotropic medications with enzyme-inducing properties include carbamazepine, oxcarbazepine, and modafinil (see review by Cozza et al. 2003). Additionally, topiramate may decrease the efficacy of oral contraceptives containing ethinyl estradiol (Cozza et al. 2003).

Protein Binding

Another potential drug–drug interaction may occur when drugs compete for protein-binding sites. In short, medications are distributed to their various sites of action through the circulatory system. In the bloodstream, most psychotropic medications (except lithium) are bound to plasma proteins to different degrees. For drugs that are protein bound, the unbound fraction of the drug is pharmacologically active, whereas the bound fraction is not. When two drugs that bind to plasma proteins are present in plasma simultaneously, competition for protein-binding sites occurs. This competition for protein-binding sites can cause displacement of a previously protein-bound drug, which in the free state becomes pharmacologically active. These interactions are often referred to as *protein-binding interactions.* This type of interaction may be clinically significant if the drugs involved are highly protein bound (which results in a large change in plasma concentration of free drug from a small amount of drug displacement) and have a low therapeutic index or narrow therapeutic window (in which case small changes in plasma levels can result in toxicity or loss of efficacy) (Callahan et al. 1996).

Absorption and Excretion

Changes in plasma levels as a result of alterations in absorption or excretion are less common with psychiatric medications. Changes in plasma concentrations as a result of changes in excretion are most frequent with lithium, which is dependent on renal excretion (see "Mood Stabilizers" section later in this chapter).

Pharmacodynamic Interactions

In *pharmacodynamic interactions,* the pharmacological effect of a drug is changed by the action of a second drug at a common receptor or bioactive site. For example, the concomitant administration of two medications with anticholinergic and antihistaminergic actions can result in additive sedation, constipation, and other anticholinergic effects. To avoid these interactions to the extent possible, the clinician must be aware of all medications that a patient is taking, including over-the-counter medications, and be knowledgeable about each medication's various mechanisms of action and receptor effects.

Antidepressant Medications

Overview

One of the most rapidly expanding areas in psychopharmacology is the development of antidepressant medications. Indeed, the antidepressant class contains several different types of medications, categorized largely by their actions on neurotransmission. To date, all antidepressants appear to be similarly effective for treating major depression, but individual patients may respond preferentially to one agent or another. In addition, these medications are significantly different from one another with regard to side effects, lethality in overdose, pharmacokinetics, drug–drug interaction potential, and the ability to treat comorbid disorders. In this section, we review the pharmacological properties of the various medications within the antidepressant class and discuss some of their clinical uses.

Mechanisms of Action

All currently available antidepressant drugs affect serotonergic and/or noradrenergic neurotransmission. The effects of antidepressants on monoamine availability are immediate, but the clinical response is typically delayed for several weeks. Downregulation of receptors more closely parallels the time course of clinical response. This downregulation can be conceptualized as a marker of antidepressant-induced neuronal adaptation. Therapeutic effects are most likely related to modulation of G proteins, second-messenger systems, and gene expression, particularly genes involved in neuronal growth and regeneration (for a review, see Nestler et al. 2002). As the understanding of the neurobiology of depression progresses, we may gain a better understanding of the mechanisms of action of available antidepressants, as well as identify new targets for drug development.

Indications and Efficacy

All antidepressants are effective in the treatment of major depression. Additionally, some antidepressants are effective in obsessive-compulsive disorder (OCD; selective serotonin reuptake inhibitors [SSRIs] and clomipramine), panic disorder (TCAs and SSRIs), generalized anxiety disorder (venlafaxine and SSRIs), bulimia (TCAs, SSRIs, and monoamine oxidase inhibitors [MAOIs]), dysthymia (SSRIs), bipolar depression (with treatment with a mood stabilizer), social phobia (SSRIs, venlafaxine, MAOIs), posttraumatic stress disorder (SSRIs), irritable bowel syndrome (TCAs), enuresis (TCAs), neuropathic pain (TCAs, duloxetine), migraine headaches (TCAs), attention-deficit/hyperactivity disorder (bupropion), autism (SSRIs), late luteal phase dysphoric disorder (SSRIs), borderline personality disorder (SSRIs), and smoking cessation (bupropion). However, the FDA has not evaluated or approved the use of antidepressants to treat many of these conditions. We refer the reader to current product labeling to determine the indications for use approved by the FDA for a specific medication.

Clinical Use

In the following subsections, clinically relevant information is presented for each commonly used class of antidepressant individually. The pharmacological treatment of depression is also discussed. Information on doses and half-lives is summarized in Table 26–2, and a list of key features and side effects is presented in Table 26–3. The antidepressants currently available are classified according to their effects on neurotransmitter receptors or catabolic enzymes. All antidepressants are effective against depression when administered in therapeutic doses. The choice of a specific antidepressant medication is based on several factors, including the patient's psychiatric symptoms, history of previous treatment response and tolerability, family members' history of response, medication side-effect profiles, drug–drug interaction potentials, and the presence of comorbid disorders that may respond to (or preclude the use of) specific antidepressants. In general, SSRIs and other newer antidepressants are preferred as initial treatment options because they are better tolerated and safer than TCAs and MAOIs, although many patients benefit from treatment with the older drugs. The use of antidepressants to treat anxiety disorders is addressed in the "Pharmacotherapy for Generalized Anxiety Disorder" subsection later in this chapter.

Antidepressants and Suicide

Patients with depression and other psychiatric disorders have an increased risk for suicide and suicidal behavior. Long-term pharmacological treatment is associated with a decreased suicide rate (Angst et al. 2002), but the acute phases of treatment with antidepressants have been associated with increased risks of suicidal thoughts and behaviors. This is of particular concern in children and adolescents. A pooled analysis conducted by the U.S. Food and Drug Administration (2004) of 24 short-term placebo-controlled clinical trials among children and adolescents taking antidepressants found a risk of suicidal thinking or behavior in 4% of the patients who received antidepressants, compared with 2% of the patients who received placebo. Fortunately, no suicides were completed in these studies.

At this time, warnings apply to all antidepressant medications. Although data from adult placebo-controlled trials have not been evaluated in the same systematic manner, some adult patients might be at risk for suicide in the initial weeks of treatment. Thus, it is imperative that clinicians monitor all patients, including adults, for the emergence or worsening of suicidal thoughts or behavior during treatment with antidepressants. These warnings also underscore the need for thoughtful patient education. Specifically, the patient should be educated to call the clinician immediately if he or she experiences an increase in suicidal impulses, agitation, or severe restlessness. Family education is also warranted, particularly for pediatric patients or those with cognitive impairment.

Selective Serotonin Reuptake Inhibitors

Background

SSRIs inhibit serotonin reuptake and are largely devoid of four other major pharmacological properties inherent to other antidepressants (e.g., TCAs)—namely, muscarinic receptor blockade, histamine type 1 (H_1) receptor blockade, α_1-adrenergic receptor blockade, and norepinephrine reuptake inhibition. This pharmacological selectivity has several advantages, including a reduction in dangerous side effects. SSRIs are unlikely to affect the seizure threshold or cardiac conduction, and are relatively safe in overdose. Despite their highly selective pharmacological activity, SSRIs have a broad spectrum of action. They are efficacious in the treatment of depression and of many other psychiatric disorders, including many major anxiety disorders.

All the SSRIs have similar spectrums of efficacy and similar side-effect profiles. However, they are structurally and, in some instances, clinically distinct. For example, allergy to one SSRI does not predict allergy to another. Similarly, response or nonresponse to one SSRI does not necessarily predict a similar reaction to another SSRI. Importantly, SSRIs also have distinct pharmacokinetic properties, including differences in half-life (see Table 26–2) and drug–drug interaction potential (see Table 26–1).

Clinical Use

Although all patients with depression should undergo a thorough medical evaluation, no specific tests are re-

TABLE 26–2. **Antidepressant medications: dosing and half-life information**

Generic drug name	Proprietary drug name	Usual starting dose (mg)[a]	Usual daily dose (mg)	Available oral doses (mg)	Mean half-life, hours (active metabolites)[b]
Monoamine oxidase inhibitors					
Irreversible, nonselective monoamine oxidase inhibitors					
Isocarboxazid	Marplan	10	20–60	10	2
Phenelzine	Nardil	15	15–90	15	2
Tranylcypromine	Parnate	10	30–60	10	2
Transdermal monoamine oxidase inhibitors					
Transdermal selegiline	EMSAM	6	6	None Transdermal doses: 6 mg/24 hours 9 mg/24 hours 12 mg/24 hours	18–25
Reversible inhibitors of monoamine oxidase A					
Moclobemide[c]	Aurorix, Manerix	150	300–600	100, 150	2
Tricyclic antidepressants					
Tertiary-amine tricyclic antidepressants					
Amitriptyline	Elavil	25–50	100–300	10, 25, 50, 75, 100, 150	16 (27)
Clomipramine	Anafranil	25	100–250	25, 50, 75	32 (69)
Doxepin	Sinequan	25–50	100–300	10, 25, 50, 75, 100, 150, L	17
Imipramine	Tofranil	25–50	100–300	10, 25, 50, 75, 100, 125, 150	8 (17)
Trimipramine	Surmontil	25–50	100–300	25, 50, 100	24
Secondary-amine tricyclic antidepressants					
Desipramine	Norpramin	25–50	100–300	10, 25, 50, 75, 100, 150	17
Nortriptyline	Pamelor, Aventyl	25	50–150	10, 25, 50, 75, L	27
Protriptyline	Vivactil	10	15–60	5, 10	79
Tetracyclic antidepressants					
Amoxapine	Asendin	50	100–400	25, 50, 100, 150	8
Maprotiline	Ludiomil	50	100–225	25, 50, 75	43

TABLE 26–2. **Antidepressant medications: dosing and half-life information** *(continued)*

Generic drug name	Proprietary drug name	Usual starting dose (mg)[a]	Usual daily dose (mg)	Available oral doses (mg)	Mean half-life, hours (active metabolites)[b]
Selective serotonin reuptake inhibitors					
Citalopram	Celexa	20	20–40[d]	10, 20, 40, L	35
Escitalopram	Lexapro	10	10–20	5, 10, 20, L	27–32
Fluoxetine	Prozac	20	20–60[d]	10, 20, 40, L	72 (216)
Fluoxetine Weekly	Prozac Weekly	90	NA	90	—
Fluvoxamine[e]	Luvox	50	50–300[d]	25, 50, 100	15
Paroxetine	Paxil	20	20–60[d]	10, 20, 30, 40, L	20
Paroxetine CR	Paxil CR	25	25–62.5	12.5, 25, 37.5	15–20
Sertraline	Zoloft	50	50–200[d]	25, 50, 100	26 (66)
Serotonin–norepinephrine reuptake inhibitors					
Duloxetine	Cymbalta	30	60–90	20, 30, 60	12
Venlafaxine	Effexor	37.5	75–225	25, 37.5, 50, 75, 100	5 (11)
Venlafaxine XR	Effexor XR	37.5	75–225	37.5, 75, 150	5 (11)
Serotonin modulators					
Nefazodone[e]	Serzone	50	150–300	100, 150, 200, 250	4
Trazodone	Desyrel	50	75–300	50, 100, 150, 300	7
Norepinephrine–serotonin modulators					
Mirtazapine	Remeron	15	15–45	7.5, 15, 30, 45, soltab	20
Norepinephrine–dopamine reuptake inhibitors					
Bupropion	Wellbutrin	150	300	75, 100	14
Bupropion SR	Wellbutrin SR	150	300	100, 150	21
Bupropion XL	Wellbutrin XL	300	300	100, 150	21

Note. L=liquid; NA=not applicable; CR=controlled release; XL or XR=extended release; soltab=orally disintegrating tablets; SR=sustained release.

[a]Lower starting doses are recommended for elderly patients and patients with panic disorder, significant anxiety, or hepatic disease.

[b]Mean half-lives of active metabolites are given in parentheses.

[c]Not available in the United States.

[d]Dose varies with diagnosis. See text for specific guidelines.

[e]Generic only.

Source. Dosing information from American Psychiatric Association 2000b. Half-life data from *Physicians' Desk Reference* 2005. Dosing and half-life information for transdermal selegiline system from EMSAM 2006. Adapted from Marangell LB, Martinez JM: *Concise Guide to Psychopharmacology,* 2nd Edition. Arlington, VA, American Psychiatric Publishing, 2006, pp. 13–16. Used with permission.

TABLE 26–3. **Key side effects of major antidepressant drugs**

Medications	Sedation	Weight gain	Sexual dysfunction	Other key side effects
Tricyclic antidepressants (TCAs)	Most, yes	Yes	Yes	Anticholinergic effects, orthostasis, quinidine-like effects on cardiac conduction; lethal in overdose
Selective serotonin reuptake inhibitors (SSRIs)	Minimal	Rare	Yes	Initial: nausea, loose bowel movements, headache, insomnia
Bupropion XL	Rare	Rare	Rare	Initial: nausea, headache, insomnia, anxiety or agitation; seizure risk
Venlafaxine XR	Minimal	Rare	Yes	Similar to SSRI side effects; dose-dependent hypertension
Duloxetine	Minimal	Rare	Some	Initial: nausea; similar to SSRI side effects; avoid in patients with substantial alcohol use, hepatic insufficiency, chronic liver disease, or severe renal impairment
Trazodone	Yes	Rare	Rare	Sedation, priapism, dizziness, orthostasis
Mirtazapine	Yes	Yes	Rare	Anticholinergic effects; may increase serum lipid levels; rare: orthostasis, hypertension, peripheral edema, agranulocytosis
Monoamine oxidase inhibitors (MAOIs)	Rare	Yes	Yes	Orthostatic hypotension, insomnia, peripheral edema; avoid in patients with CHF; avoid phenelzine in patients with hepatic impairment; potentially life-threatening drug interactions; dietary restrictions

Note. XR = extended release; CHF = congestive heart failure.

Source. Adapted from Marangell LB, Martinez JM: *Concise Guide to Psychopharmacology,* 2nd Edition. Arlington, VA, American Psychiatric Publishing, 2006, pp. 18–20. Used with permission.

quired before SSRI therapy is initiated. The usual starting doses of SSRIs are summarized in Table 26–2. These standard doses generally should be decreased by 50% in patients with hepatic disease and in elderly persons (see current product labeling for specific information about dosage adjustments in special populations). In addition, patients with significant anxiety symptoms, or those who are generally sensitive to medication side effects, may experience better tolerability if lower initial doses are used; however, it is important to titrate the dose to a potentially effective dose once tolerability is achieved.

In patients with depression, SSRIs have a flat dose–response curve, meaning that higher doses tend not to be more effective than standard doses, although some patients may respond better to higher doses. Prema-

ture escalation of the SSRI dose may result in increased side effects without necessarily improving antidepressant efficacy. Therefore, we recommend maintaining the usual therapeutic dose for at least 4 weeks. If no improvement is seen after 4 weeks, a trial of a higher dose may be warranted. If a partial response is evident after 4 weeks of therapy, the dose should remain constant for an additional 2 weeks because further improvement at the initial dose may occur.

Treatment of OCD requires a longer duration and higher doses to assess efficacy. A therapeutic trial for OCD should last 8–12 weeks. Treatment of anxiety disorders is discussed in more detail later in this chapter (see subsection titled "Pharmacotherapy for Generalized Anxiety Disorder"). Late luteal phase dysphoric disorder is more responsive to serotonergic agents than to noradrenergic agents. Interestingly, late luteal phase dysphoric disorder can be treated with medication administered only during the symptomatic period before menses or on a continuous basis (Pearlstein et al. 2000; Wikander et al. 1998; Yonkers et al. 1997).

Risks, Side Effects, and Their Management

Common side effects.   Nausea, loose bowel movements, anxiety, headache, insomnia, and increased sweating are frequent initial side effects of SSRIs. They are usually dose related and may be minimized with low initial dosing and gradual titration. These early adverse effects almost always attenuate after the first few weeks of treatment. Sexual dysfunction (see "Sexual Dysfunction" subsection later in this section) is a common long-term side effect of SSRIs.

Gastrointestinal symptoms.   Nausea is a common early, and typically transient, side effect of SSRIs. Some patients report less nausea if they take the medication with food.

Sexual dysfunction.   Decreased libido, anorgasmia, and delayed ejaculation are common side effects of SSRIs. When significant sexual dysfunction persists despite a positive response to treatment, a reduction in the dose may be considered. However, the clinician must balance efficacy and tolerability; for some patients, a lower dose may improve tolerability without compromising the therapeutic benefits, whereas others may not have an adequate therapeutic response to the medication at lower doses. Importantly, some patients may experience sexual side effects throughout the medication dose range. If sexual side effects remain problematic, two main strategies are available: the antidepressant can be replaced with an alternative, or other drugs can be prescribed concomitantly to counteract the side effects. In our experience, switching from one SSRI to another does not tend to decrease sexual side effects. Antidepressants that do not commonly cause sexual dysfunction include bupropion and mirtazapine.

Several medications have been suggested as antidotes for the sexual side effects associated with antidepressant therapy. Bupropion, 75 or 150 mg/day, has been added to an SSRI regimen with some success in terms of improving libido (Labbate and Pollack 1994). Sildenafil has been used on an as-needed basis before sexual activity (Fava et al. 1998).

Stimulation and insomnia.   Some patients taking an SSRI may experience jitteriness, restlessness, muscle tension, and disturbed sleep, particularly during the early course of treatment. Patients should be informed of the possibility of the emergence of these side effects and be reassured that if they develop, they tend to be transient. In patients with prominent anxiety, SSRI therapy should be started at low doses, with subsequent titration as tolerated. Additionally, the short-term use of a benzodiazepine (if otherwise safe) may help the patient cope with overstimulation in the early stages of treatment. Despite these transient stimulating effects, SSRIs are effective in patients with anxiety or agitated depression. Similarly, insomnia may occur early in treatment, and short-term, symptomatic treatment with a hypnotic at bedtime is reasonable if necessary.

Sedation.   SSRIs may induce sedation in some patients. Altering the time of administration (e.g., having the patient take the medication in the evening rather than the morning) often is not successful.

Vivid dreams.   Reports of vivid dreams (not nightmares) are common with SSRI therapy. The mechanism of this effect is unknown.

Bleeding.   SSRIs affect serotonin systems throughout the body, including serotonin in platelets. Because platelets cannot synthesize serotonin, this effect tends to decrease platelet aggregation, which may lead to abnormal bleeding. Two large studies have reported an association between use of SSRIs and increased risk of upper gastrointestinal bleeding or other abnormal bleeding (Dalton et al. 2003; de Abajo et al. 1999). This is most commonly manifested as bruising. Therefore, it is prudent for clinicians to be cautious about prescribing SSRIs for patients with other risk factors for bleeding and to educate patients to inform them if they notice any abnormal bleeding or bruising.

Neurological effects.   Headaches are common early in treatment and usually can be managed with over-the-counter pain relief preparations. SSRIs may initially worsen migraine headaches but are often effective in reducing the severity and frequency of these headaches.

Tremor and akathisia also may occur, and they can be managed with dose reduction or the addition of a β-blocker such as propranolol (10–40 mg). There are isolated case reports of SSRI-related dystonia and increasing reports of SSRI-related exacerbation of Parkinson's disease (Di Rocco et al. 1998; Linazasoro 2000).

Weight change.   All SSRIs have the potential to cause weight gain in some individuals. In a controlled study, Fava et al. (2000) found that paroxetine was associated with greater weight gain than were fluoxetine and sertraline.

Rash. As with other medications, some patients taking an SSRI may experience a rash during the course of treatment. Severe rashes warrant treatment medication discontinuation.

Syndrome of inappropriate secretion of antidiuretic hormone. Some patients taking SSRIs may develop the syndrome of inappropriate secretion of antidiuretic hormone (SIADH), although the incidence of SIADH in the context of SSRI treatment is not known. Symptoms include lethargy, headache, hyponatremia, increased urinary sodium excretion, and hyperosmotic urine. Acute treatment of this syndrome should consist of discontinuation of the drug as well as restriction of fluid intake. Patients experiencing severe confusion, convulsions, or coma should receive intravenous sodium chloride.

Apathy syndrome. We and others have noted an apathy syndrome in some patients after months or years of successful treatment with SSRIs. The syndrome is characterized by a loss of motivation, increased passivity, and feelings of lethargy and "flatness." However, sadness, tearfulness, emotional angst, decreased concentration, feelings of hopelessness or worthlessness, and thoughts of suicide are not associated with this syndrome. If specifically asked, patients often remark that the symptoms are not experientially similar to their original depressive symptoms. This syndrome has not been adequately studied, and the pathophysiology is not known. However, there is speculation that subchronic stimulation of central serotonin attenuates dopamine functioning in several areas of the brain, including the frontal cortex. The apathy syndrome appears to be dose dependent and reversible.

It is important to distinguish the apathy syndrome from a relapse or recurrence of depressive symptoms because treatment approaches for these two scenarios are different. For instance, if an apathy syndrome is mistaken for a depressive relapse, the clinician may increase the dose of the antidepressant, thereby potentially leading to a worsening of symptoms. If dosage reduction is not effective, adding a stimulant may be beneficial. Other agents that increase dopamine also may be effective. Olanzapine, which increases frontal lobe dopamine, also has been reported to be effective in the treatment of apathy in patients taking SSRIs (Marangell et al. 2002).

Serotonin syndrome. The serotonin syndrome results from excess serotonergic stimulation and can range in severity from mild to life-threatening. The most common symptoms are confusion, flushing, diaphoresis, tremor, and myoclonic jerks. The patient may have symptoms of the serotonin syndrome in the context of monotherapy with a serotonergic medication, but this scenario is less common than symptoms resulting from use of two or more serotonergic drugs simultaneously. Discontinuation of the serotonergic medications is the first step in treatment, followed by emergency medical treatment. The serotonin type 2A (5-HT$_{2A}$) receptor antagonist cyproheptadine can be used if further treatment is warranted, beginning with an oral dose of 12 mg and then administering 2 mg every 2 hours. Although cyproheptadine is available only in oral form, tablets may be crushed, mixed in a suspension, and administered via a nasogastric tube. However, efficacy for this presumed antidote has not been established.

Discontinuation syndrome. Some patients may experience a series of symptoms after discontinuation or dose reduction of serotonergic antidepressant medications, including dizziness, headache, paresthesia, nausea, diarrhea, insomnia, and irritability. These symptoms also may be seen when a patient misses doses of a serotonergic antidepressant. A prospective double-blind, placebo-substitution study confirmed that discontinuation symptoms are most common with short-half-life antidepressants, such as paroxetine (Rosenbaum et al. 1998). To avoid a discontinuation syndrome, clinicians should slowly taper antidepressant medications on discontinuation of the drug, particularly medications with short half-lives.

Teratogenicity

Managing major depression, or any psychiatric disorder, in the context of pregnancy is challenging. Although minimizing the risk to the fetus is a clear goal, many patients, families, and even some practitioners need to be reminded that the illness of depression can have adverse effects on the fetus and neonate. Each woman who is facing pregnancy and related psychiatric treatment decisions needs to be approached and advised in the context of her unique circumstances. Some data indicate that the incidence of congenital abnormalities associated with the SSRIs is comparable to that associated with placebo, but other reports note an increased risk of congenital abnormalities, including septal heart defects, with first-trimester exposure and that this risk may be greater with paroxetine and clomipramine (Källen et al. 2006). These data have resulted in a new FDA Category D pregnancy classification for paroxetine. Other data indicate that antidepressants may increase the risk of pulmonary hypertension by about sixfold with exposure after week 20 (Chambers et al. 2006). These risks must be balanced against the risks of exacerbating mood and anxiety disorders because women who discontinue medications during pregnancy most often relapse.

Drug Interactions

Several deaths have been reported among patients taking a combination of serotonergic antidepressants and MAOIs (Hodgman et al. 1997; Kolecki 1997). Because of the potential lethality of this interaction, a patient who needs to switch from an SSRI to an MAOI must not begin taking the MAOI until the SSRI has been fully eliminated from his or her body. Thus, a period equivalent to at least five times the half-life of the SSRI is required after stopping the SSRI before an MAOI can be initiated. For example, a waiting period of at least 5 weeks is required between discontinuation of fluoxetine and institution of MAOI therapy. A 2-week waiting period is required after stopping an MAOI before an SSRI can be initiated to allow resynthesis of the monoamine oxidase enzyme in the absence of the MAOI.

The concurrent use of SSRIs and triptans (e.g., sumatriptan) has been reported to result in symptoms consistent with mild to moderate serotonin syndrome, but most patients tolerate this combination. Medications within the SSRI class also may inhibit one or more cytochrome P450 enzymes, and the SSRIs vary with regard to inhibition of specific enzymes (see Table 26–1 and extensive review in Cozza et al. 2003).

Serotonin–Norepinephrine Reuptake Inhibitors

Background

Although the SSRIs have major advantages over the TCAs, particularly with respect to safety and tolerability, a medication that has actions not only on serotonin but also on norepinephrine may have some advantages. For example, some authors have suggested that dual reuptake inhibitors may be more likely to lead to remission (Thase et al. 2001). Serotonin–norepinephrine reuptake inhibitors (SNRIs) are dual reuptake inhibitors that affect serotonin and norepinephrine but have little effect on muscarinic, H_1, or α_1-adrenergic receptors. Thus, these medications share many of the tolerability and safety benefits of the SSRIs but add an additional pharmacological action compared with SSRIs—namely, norepinephrine reuptake inhibition. Two SNRIs are currently available in the United States: venlafaxine and duloxetine.

Venlafaxine

Background. Venlafaxine is a dual reuptake inhibitor for both serotonin and norepinephrine; serotonin reuptake inhibition is prominent at lower doses, whereas norepinephrine reuptake inhibition becomes more significant at higher doses.

Clinical use. The recommended dosage range of venlafaxine is 75–225 mg/day. The extended-release (XL) preparation, which allows for once-daily dosing in most patients, is preferred over the short-acting preparation. The usual starting dosage is 37.5–75 mg/day. Dosages up to 375 mg/day have been used in patients who were otherwise nonresponsive to treatment. Blood pressure monitoring during therapy is recommended because of a dose-dependent risk of increases in mean diastolic blood pressure in some patients.

Unlike SSRIs, venlafaxine shows a positive dose–response relation: patients with mild depression may respond to lower doses, whereas patients with more severe or recurrent depression may respond better to higher doses.

Risks, side effects, and their management. The side-effect profile of venlafaxine is similar to that of SSRIs and includes gastrointestinal symptoms, sexual dysfunction, and transient discontinuation symptoms. Like the SSRIs, venlafaxine does not affect cardiac conduction or lower the seizure threshold. In most patients, venlafaxine is not associated with sedation or weight gain. Side effects that differ from those of SSRIs are hypothesized to be related to the increased noradrenergic activity of this drug at higher doses; these side effects include dose-dependent anxiety (in some patients) and dose-dependent hypertension.

Dose-dependent increases in blood pressure may occur with venlafaxine treatment. A meta-analysis found that the magnitude of change in blood pressure associated with venlafaxine use is statistically significant but is unlikely to be of clinical significance at dosages less than 300 mg/day. However, the incidence of hypertension is 13% at dosages greater than 300 mg/day. If clinically significant treatment-emergent hypertension occurs, dose reduction or treatment discontinuation should be considered.

Overdose. Few data are available regarding venlafaxine in overdose, but the drug's pharmacological profile suggests that it is safer than TCAs. In most of the reported cases to date, symptoms were not present. In other cases, somnolence, mild sinus tachycardia, and generalized convulsions were noted. Recommended treatment includes general supportive and symptomatic measures. In severe cases, dialysis should be considered.

Drug interactions. Venlafaxine does not appear to inhibit cytochrome P450 enzymes significantly and is not highly protein bound; thus, venlafaxine is less likely to contribute to protein-binding interactions than most other antidepressants. However, venlafaxine should not be combined with MAOIs because of the risk for serotonin syndrome.

Duloxetine

Background. Duloxetine hydrochloride is an SNRI that is approved by the FDA for the treatment of both major depression and the pain associated with diabetic peripheral neuropathy. Interestingly, it does not appear to induce sustained treatment-emergent hypertension compared with placebo, although rare cases are possible. Its half-life is approximately 12 hours, and it is highly protein bound. The most frequent side effect is early nausea, which is dose dependent and typically transient. Like venlafaxine, duloxetine typically is not associated with significant changes in weight.

Clinical use. The recommended dosage for the treatment of major depression is 60 mg/day, whereas in diabetic neuropathy, a dosage of up to 120 mg/day is recommended. Nausea in the early phases of treatment is dose dependent, so treatment-naive patients might benefit from starting at 30 mg/day for the first week and then increasing to the target dose of 60 mg. At present, duloxetine is not recommended for use in patients with end-stage renal disease, severe renal impairment, or any hepatic insufficiency (Cymbalta 2006).

Risks, side effects, and their management. The side-effect profile of duloxetine is similar to that of SSRIs. Like the SSRIs, duloxetine does not affect cardiac conduction or lower the seizure threshold. In most patients, duloxetine is not associated with sedation. Nausea may occur during treatment initiation, but it is generally transient.

Duloxetine has been associated with increases in serum transaminase levels. In controlled trials in major depressive disorder, elevations of alanine aminotransferase (ALT) to greater than three times the upper limit of normal occurred in 0.9% (8 of 930) of the duloxetine-treated patients and in 0.3% (2 of 652) of the placebo-treated patients (Cymbalta 2006). Additionally, postmarketing reports have indicated occur-

rences of hepatitis, hepatomegaly with liver enzyme elevation, severe hepatic enzyme elevation, and cholestatic jaundice (Cymbalta 2006). Current labeling advises that duloxetine should not be prescribed to patients with significant alcohol use (because duloxetine may interact with alcohol to produce liver injury) or evidence of chronic liver disease (Cymbalta 2006).

Duloxetine use is associated with an increased risk of mydriasis; therefore, it should not be used in patients with uncontrolled narrow-angle glaucoma.

The controlled clinical trials of duloxetine in the treatment of major depression used a rating scale to assess prospectively treatment-emergent sexual dysfunction. As with SSRIs and venlafaxine, males who received duloxetine experienced more difficulty with ability to reach orgasm than did males who received placebo. However, females taking duloxetine did not experience more sexual dysfunction than did those taking placebo (Cymbalta 2006). The reason for fewer sexual side effects in females is not clear, and some females will experience treatment-emergent anorgasmia or decreased libido.

Overdose. Few data are available regarding duloxetine in overdose. Recommended treatment includes general supportive and symptomatic measures. Dialysis is not recommended because the drug is highly protein bound.

Drug interactions. Duloxetine is a moderate inhibitor of the CYP2D6 enzyme and may increase the levels of other medications that use this enzyme. Because of the risk of serotonin syndrome, duloxetine should not be combined with MAOIs. Because duloxetine is highly bound to plasma protein, combination with another drug that is highly protein bound may cause increased free concentrations of the other drug, potentially resulting in adverse events.

Bupropion

Background

Bupropion facilitates dopamine transmission; thus, many clinicians preferentially use this agent for depressed patients with Parkinson's disease. The fact that dopamine is integrally related to the brain's reward mechanisms, which are stimulated by nicotine and other addictive substances, has provided the theoretical underpinning for recent research indicating that bupropion is an effective aid in smoking cessation. Placebo-controlled trials involving nondepressed, chronic cigarette smokers found a dose-dependent increase in the percentage of patients able to achieve abstinence.

Individuals receiving 300 mg/day of bupropion were able to sustain abstinence longer than those receiving 150 mg/day, and results achieved by patients given bupropion were superior to those achieved in the placebo groups. Bupropion is being marketed under the name Zyban as a tool for smoking cessation (Zyban 2005).

Overall, bupropion has a favorable side-effect profile. The drug is associated with little or no weight gain, has few effects on cardiac conduction, and has minimal sexual side effects. Disadvantages include an increased risk of medication-induced seizures at higher-than-recommended doses.

Clinical Use

Use of the XL preparation is preferred because of increased tolerability, decreased seizure risk, and the convenience of once-daily dosing. Treatment with the sustained-release (SR) or XL preparation is initiated at a dose of 150 mg, preferably taken in the morning. After 4 days, the dosage may be increased to 150 mg twice a day (SR) or 300 mg once daily in the morning (XL).

Contraindications

Patients with seizure disorders should not take bupropion. Similarly, an alternative treatment should be considered in patients with a history of significant head trauma, a central nervous system (CNS) tumor, or an active eating disorder.

Risks, Side Effects, and Their Management

The most common side effects of bupropion are initial headache, anxiety, insomnia, increased sweating, and gastrointestinal upset. Tremor and akathisia also may occur. Management is the same as for SSRI side effects. Bupropion is not associated with anticholinergic side effects, orthostatic hypotension, weight gain, or cardiac conduction changes.

Seizures. The incidence of seizures with the immediate-release preparation is 0.4% at doses less than 450 mg/day, provided no single dose of the short-acting preparation exceeds 150 mg. The incidence increases to 5% at dosages between 450 and 600 mg/day. The SR preparation is associated with seizure incidences of 0.1% at dosages less than 300 mg/day and 0.4% at dosages between 300 and 400 mg/day. Higher doses of the SR preparation have not been evaluated. No single dose of greater than 200 mg is recommended for the SR preparation, whereas up to 450 mg in a single dose may be given with the XL preparation. Bupropion should be used with caution in patients who are taking concomitant medications that lower the seizure threshold.

Psychosis. Reports of delusions, hallucinations, and paranoia are consistent with bupropion-mediated increases in central dopamine. Bupropion should be used with caution in patients with psychotic disorders.

Overdose

Much more is known about overdose with the immediate-release formulation of bupropion than with the newer SR and XL formulations. Reported reactions to overdose with the immediate-release form include seizures, hallucinations, loss of consciousness, and sinus tachycardia. Treatment of overdose should include induction of vomiting, administration of activated charcoal, and electrocardiographic and electroencephalographic monitoring. For seizures, an intravenous benzodiazepine preparation is recommended.

One danger associated with bupropion overdose is a risk of seizures. However, seizures are seldom life-threatening unless they result in motor vehicle accidents, falls, or other trauma-related events.

Drug Interactions

The combination of bupropion with an MAOI is potentially dangerous but less so than the combination of serotonergic drugs and MAOIs. Although the practice is not recommended, MAOIs and bupropion have been combined in some patients with refractory depression.

Data to date suggest that bupropion is metabolized by CYP2B6 (Faucette et al. 2000). Bupropion inhibits CYP2D6. Because of the risk of dose-dependent seizures, caution is warranted when bupropion is combined with other medications that might inhibit its metabolism.

Nefazodone

Nefazodone is primarily a postsynaptic 5-HT$_2$ antagonist. The branded product was removed from the market in 2003 after reports of hepatotoxicity. The reported rate of liver failure resulting in death or transplant in the United States is approximately 1 case per 250,000–300,000 patient-years of exposure (Serzone 2002). Nefazodone is available in generic formulations, mostly for patients who have been stabilized previously while taking this medication and need ongoing treatment. Individuals who develop increased serum transaminase levels of three times the upper limits of the normal range or higher should be withdrawn from nefazodone and not be considered for nefazodone rechallenge.

Trazodone

Background

Trazodone is an antidepressant that is associated with significant sedation. Currently, trazodone is not recommended as a first-line antidepressant because of an increased risk of orthostatic hypotension, arrhythmias, and priapism. However, trazodone may be useful in some patients with insomnia (although the use of trazodone specifically for insomnia is not approved by the FDA).

Clinical Use

The recommended dose range for trazodone is 200–400 mg/day in divided doses. Initial dosing should begin at 50 mg/day. For many patients, even low doses of trazodone may be associated with significant sedation; thus, most of the daily dose should be administered at night.

Risks, Side Effects, and Their Management

Excessive sedation is the most commonly encountered side effect of trazodone. Although trazodone has virtually no anticholinergic side effects, dry mouth and blurred vision occur more frequently with trazodone treatment than with placebo.

Trazodone can cause orthostatic hypotension and dizziness. Additionally, there have been reports of increased ventricular irritability among patients with conduction defects and preexisting ventricular arrhythmias (Aronson and Hafez 1986; Jankowsky et al. 1983; Vitullo et al. 1990).

Trazodone has been associated with priapism (Scher et al. 1983), which may be irreversible and require surgical intervention.

Overdose

Trazodone overdose carries a risk of myocardial irritation in patients with preexisting ventricular conduction abnormalities.

Mirtazapine

Background

Mirtazapine has been shown to reduce anxiety symptoms and sleep disturbances associated with depression as early as 1 week after the start of treatment. Other advantages are minimal sexual dysfunction, minimal nausea, and once-daily dosing. In addition, mirtazapine is unlikely to be associated with cytochrome P450–mediated drug interactions.

Mechanism of Action

Mirtazapine facilitates central serotonergic and noradrenergic transmission by antagonizing α_2-noradrenergic autoreceptors and heteroreceptors (De Boer 1996). In addition, mirtazapine antagonizes postsynaptic 5-HT_{2A}, 5-HT_3, and H_1 receptors and has moderate activity at α_1-adrenergic and muscarinic receptors.

Clinical Use

Mirtazapine treatment is initiated at a dosage of 15 mg at bedtime. The maximum recommended daily dose is 45 mg. Elderly patients and individuals with renal or hepatic disease may require lower doses.

Risks, Side Effects, and Their Management

Common side effects. The most common side effects associated with mirtazapine are sedation, weight gain, and dizziness. Somnolence occurs in more than 50% of the patients taking mirtazapine (Bremner 1995; Smith et al. 1990). Tolerance to this side effect generally develops after the first few weeks of treatment. Weight gain also may be associated with mirtazapine treatment. A mean increase of 3.7 kg over the first 28 weeks of treatment has been reported in several controlled studies (Bremner 1995; Smith et al. 1990). A relapse-prevention study with 410 depressed patients taking mirtazapine reported a mean increase in body weight of 2.5 kg after 12 weeks and a mean increase in body weight of 3.3 kg after 40 weeks (Thase et al. 2000).

Agranulocytosis. In preliminary clinical trials, 2 of 2,796 mirtazapine-treated patients developed agranulocytosis, and 1 developed severe neutropenia. All 3 patients recovered after medication discontinuation, and other possible etiologies were present in at least 1 of these individuals. Thirteen patients with pretreatment neutropenia did develop more severe neutropenia or agranulocytosis. Postmarketing evaluation to date has not established a causal relation between mirtazapine and agranulocytosis. Routine laboratory monitoring is not currently recommended.

Anticholinergic effects. Mirtazapine is associated with modest anticholinergic side effects, including dry mouth and constipation. Anticholinergic side effects and their management are discussed in the "Tricyclic and Heterocyclic Antidepressants" subsection later in this chapter.

Cardiovascular effects. Hypertension, orthostatic hypotension, dizziness, and vasodilation with peripheral edema may occur with mirtazapine treatment.

Overdose

Little is known about mirtazapine overdose. To date, patients who have overdosed have fully recovered. Warning signs include drowsiness, impaired memory, and tachycardia. Recommended treatment includes gastric lavage, cardiac monitoring, and supportive measures.

Drug Interactions

Mirtazapine does not significantly inhibit hepatic cytochrome P450 enzymes. Additive effects may occur when mirtazapine is combined with other drugs with sedative or vascular effects. Mirtazapine should not be used in combination with an MAOI or within 14 days of discontinuing treatment with an MAOI. When it is combined with fluvoxamine, a potent inhibitor of P450 enzymes—including 1A2, 2D6, and 3A4—that metabolizes mirtazapine, the plasma concentration of mirtazapine may be increased up to fourfold.

Tricyclic and Heterocyclic Antidepressants

Background

All TCAs have a three-ring nucleus. Most clinicians do not use TCAs as first-line antidepressants because, relative to the newer antidepressants, TCAs tend to have more side effects, require gradual titration, and can be lethal in overdose. Some data suggest that TCAs may be more effective than SSRIs in the treatment of major depression with melancholic features (Danish University Antidepressant Group 1990). However, many clinicians prefer the newer antidepressants because of their safety and tolerability compared with TCAs.

Imipramine, amitriptyline, clomipramine, trimipramine, and doxepin are tertiary-amine TCAs. Desipramine, nortriptyline, and protriptyline are secondary-amine TCAs. Tertiary-amine tricyclics have more potent serotonin reuptake inhibition, and secondary-amine tricyclics have more potent noradrenergic reuptake inhibition. Tertiary-amine TCAs tend to have more side effects than do secondary-amine TCAs. Desipramine and protriptyline tend to be activating. Among the TCAs, nortriptyline is the least likely to produce orthostatic hypotension. Because amoxapine has an active metabolite that antagonizes dopamine type 2 (D_2) receptors, it can cause treatment-emergent extrapyramidal side effects (EPS).

Mechanism of Action

TCAs inhibit norepinephrine, serotonin, and (to a lesser degree) dopamine reuptake. Additionally, they exert inhibitory effects on H_1, muscarinic, and α_1-adrenergic receptors.

Clinical Use

Because of potential cardiovascular effects and risks associated with TCAs, the clinician should obtain a cardiovascular history before initiating TCA therapy. In patients with preexisting heart disease and patients older than 40 years, an electrocardiogram (ECG) should be obtained before TCA treatment. TCAs should not be used in patients with bundle branch block unless all other options have failed. Additionally, other treatment options should be considered for patients with ischemic heart disease. Because orthostatic hypotension can occur with TCA treatment, other potential risk factors for hypotension should be explored.

The following dose guidelines are for healthy adults with minimal anxiety. Patients with significant anxiety, panic, or a tendency to be sensitive to side effects should receive initial doses that are 50% lower. Similarly, elderly patients and patients with cardiovascular or hepatic disease should receive lower initial doses.

Imipramine, amitriptyline, doxepin, desipramine, clomipramine, and trimipramine therapy can be initiated at 25–50 mg/day. Divided dosing may be used at first to minimize side effects, but eventually the entire dose can be given at bedtime. The dosage can be increased to 150 mg/day the second week, 225 mg/day the third week, and 300 mg/day the fourth week. The clomipramine dosage should not exceed 250 mg/day because of an increased risk of seizures at higher doses.

Nortriptyline therapy should be initiated at 25 mg/day, and the dosage should be increased to 75 mg/day over 1–2 weeks depending on tolerability and clinical response. Some patients require dosages of up to 150 mg/day. Amoxapine should be started at 50 mg/day, and the dosage should be titrated to 400 mg/day. Amoxapine has a short half-life and should be given in divided doses. Treatment with protriptyline can be started at 10 mg/day, and the dosage can be increased to 60 mg/day. Maprotiline therapy should be started at 50 mg/day, and that dosage should be maintained for 2 weeks; the risk of seizure increases if the dosage is raised too quickly. The dosage can be increased over 4 weeks to 225 mg/day.

TCA Plasma Levels and Therapeutic Monitoring

Clinically meaningful plasma levels are available for imipramine, desipramine, and nortriptyline. For imipramine, the sum of the plasma levels of imipramine and the desmethyl metabolite (desipramine) should be greater than 200 ng/mL. Desipramine levels should be greater than 125 ng/mL. A therapeutic window has been noted for nortriptyline, with optimal response between 50 and 150 ng/mL. These therapeutic levels are based on steady-state concentrations, which are reached after 5–7 days of administration of these medications. Blood should be drawn approximately 10–14 hours after the last dose of medication.

Risks, Side Effects, and Their Management

Anticholinergic effects.   Common anticholinergic side effects include dry mouth, constipation, urinary retention, blurred vision, and tachycardia. Additionally, anticholinergic medications may cause cognitive impairment and confusion. Because the tertiary-amine TCAs and protriptyline have a particularly high affinity for muscarinic receptors, these medications are more likely than others within the TCA class to have anticholinergic side effects.

Cholinergic medications have been reported to relieve some of the anticholinergic side effects (Everett 1976; Yager 1986). The addition of a medication to treat side effects should be considered only after dose reduction and alternative antidepressants with fewer anticholinergic side effects have been tried. One must proceed with great caution when using antidepressants with anticholinergic side effects in treating patients with prostatic hypertrophy, narrow-angle glaucoma, or cognitive impairment. Newer antidepressant drugs that are devoid of significant anticholinergic effects may be preferable for patients with these disorders.

Sedation.   Many TCAs can be associated with sedation. The sedative properties of TCAs appear to parallel their respective histamine receptor binding affinities.

Cardiovascular effects.   Cardiovascular effects include orthostatic hypotension, tachycardia, and cardiac conduction delays. These side effects may be clinically significant for many patients, particularly those with preexisting heart disease. Although TCAs at toxic levels can cause life-threatening arrhythmias, TCAs are potent antiarrhythmic agents, possessing quinidine-like properties. Because prolongation of PR and QRS intervals can occur with TCA use, these drugs should not be used in patients with preexisting heart block (especially right bundle branch block and left bundle branch block). In such patients, treatment with TCAs may lead to second- or third-degree heart block, both life-threatening conditions (Roose et al. 1987).

Weight gain.   Weight gain is a common side effect of TCA treatment.

Seizures.   A dose-related risk of seizures has been found with clomipramine, which has led to the recommendation that the total daily dose of this drug not exceed 250 mg. Overdoses of TCAs, particularly amoxapine and desipramine, also are associated with seizures.

Extrapyramidal side effects (amoxapine only). Amoxapine, which has a mild neuroleptic effect, can cause EPS, akathisia, and even tardive dyskinesias.

Overdose

Complications of TCA overdose may include neuropsychiatric impairment, hypotension, cardiac arrhythmias, and seizures. Anticholinergic delirium may occur, as well as other complications of anticholinergic overdose, including agitation, supraventricular arrhythmias, hallucinations, severe hypertension, and seizures. Patients with anticholinergic delirium have hot, dry skin; tachycardia; dilated pupils; dry mucous membranes; and absent bowel sounds. Anticholinergic delirium is a medical emergency and requires emergent care. Physostigmine, a centrally and peripherally acting reversible acetylcholinesterase inhibitor, may be used as a diagnostic agent in cases of suspected anticholinergic toxicity. This agent is administered intramuscularly at a dose of 1–2 mg or intravenously at a slow, controlled rate of no more than 1 mg/minute. Physostigmine should not be used to maintain reversal of the toxicity, however, because a cholinergic crisis may result. A cholinergic crisis is characterized by nausea, vomiting, bradycardia, and seizures. This reaction can be reversed by administering a potent anticholinergic drug such as atropine.

Hypotension, which may result from norepinephrine depletion or have other causes related to peripheral and central effects of TCAs, should be treated with vigorous fluid replacement. Seizures and cardiac complications also may occur with TCA overdose. When the QRS interval is less than 0.10 second, the likelihood of seizures or ventricular arrhythmias decreases. Ventricular arrhythmias that occur secondary to overdose are typical of arrhythmias resulting from high doses of quinidine-like agents and begin within the first 24 hours after hospital admission. Ventricular arrhythmias should be treated with lidocaine, propranolol, or phenytoin. Prophylactic treatment with phenytoin and insertion of a temporary pacemaker should be considered in patients with prolonged QRS intervals (i.e., longer than 120 ms).

Drug Interactions

Drugs that induce hepatic microsomal enzymes or inhibit hepatic enzymes (particularly CYP2D6 inhibitors) may alter plasma tricyclic levels. The coadministration of a TCA and a potent CYP2D6 inhibitor may result in dangerously high levels of the TCA.

Although several medications may affect TCA levels, TCAs rarely affect the metabolism of other drugs. A notable exception is valproate sodium, levels of which may decrease when a TCA is administered concurrently (Preskorn and Burke 1992). By a different mode of action, TCAs also may interfere with the mechanism of action of two antihypertensive drugs. Both guanethidine and clonidine lose effectiveness if administered concomitantly with drugs (such as TCAs) that block reuptake of catecholamines into adrenergic neurons.

Monoamine Oxidase Inhibitors

Background

Oral MAOIs are not currently used as first-line agents in the treatment of major depression, largely because newer antidepressants are generally safer and better tolerated. However, these medications remain excellent medications for patients who do not respond to the newer antidepressant drugs. Patients with atypical depression, characterized by oversleeping and overeating, show a preferential response to MAOI therapy (Quitkin et al. 1979). Recently, a patch containing the MAOI selegiline has become available, as discussed later in this section.

Mechanism of Action

The enzyme monoamine oxidase A (MAO-A) acts selectively on norepinephrine and serotonin, whereas monoamine oxidase B (MAO-B) preferentially affects phenylethylamine. Both MAO-A and MAO-B oxidize dopamine and tyramine. MAO-A inhibition appears to be most relevant to the antidepressant effects of these drugs. Drugs that inhibit both MAO-A and MAO-B are called *nonselective*. Because tyramine can be metabolized by either MAO-A or MAO-B, drugs that selectively inhibit one of these enzymes but not the other do not require dietary restrictions. MAO-A–selective drugs, such as moclobemide, are available in other countries (e.g., Canada) for the treatment of depression. MAO-B–selective drugs, such as pargyline, are marketed for other indications. Selegiline is an irreversible MAOI that is selective for MAO-B at lower doses—namely, those doses typically used in the treatment of Parkinson's disease, but selegiline inhibits both MAO-A and MAO-B at antidepressant doses.

In addition to potential selectivity for MAO-A or MAO-B, MAOIs may produce either reversible or irreversible enzyme inhibition. An *irreversible inhibitor* permanently disables the enzyme, and the enzyme must be resynthesized in the absence of the drug before the activity of the enzyme can be reestablished. MAO enzyme resynthesis may take up to 2 weeks in the absence of an MAOI; thus, an interval of approximately 14 days is required after discontinuing an irreversible MAOI before instituting treatment with other antidepressants, permitting the use of contraindicated drugs, or permitting the consumption of contraindicated foods. On the other hand, a *reversible inhibitor* can move away from the active site of the enzyme, making the enzyme available to metabolize other substances. The reversibility and selectivity of the currently available MAOIs are summarized in Table 26–4.

Clinical Use

The physician should discuss the risks associated with MAOI use with the patient and should review and discuss the need to adhere to the appropriate dietary restrictions and avoid medications that may lead to potentially dangerous interactions (Table 26–5). The patient should also be given written instructions that include a list of restricted foods and drugs, a list of safe concomitant medications, common side effects and precautions, signs and symptoms of potentially serious adverse events and instructions for action if they occur, and the importance of letting other health care providers, including dentists, know that he or she is taking an MAOI before any other treatments are prescribed or used, including anesthetic agents. Additionally, patients should be advised not to start any new medications without first informing their physician. Indeed, many patients assume that over-the-counter medications and herbal supplements are safe and pose no risk; thus, patients may hastily begin taking one of these agents without discussing it with their physician, potentially putting themselves at risk for serious drug interactions.

Phenelzine therapy is initiated at a dose of 15 mg in the morning, and the dose is increased by 15 mg every other day until a total daily dose of 60 mg is reached. If no response occurs within 2 weeks, the dose may be increased in 15-mg increments to a usual maximum of 90 mg/day. Higher doses are sometimes used, if tolerated, in patients with severe refractory depression. Treatment with tranylcypromine is initiated at a dose of 10 mg, and the dose is then increased every other day to 30 mg/day. As with phenelzine, higher doses

TABLE 26–4. **Monoamine oxidase inhibitor reversibility and selectivity**

Generic drug (proprietary names)	Monoamine oxidase enzyme inhibition	
	Inhibition type	Enzyme selectivity
Isocarboxazid (Marplan)	Irreversible	MAO-A+B
Phenelzine (Nardil)	Irreversible	MAO-A+B
Tranylcypromine (Parnate)	Irreversible	MAO-A+B
Selegiline (Eldepryl; EMSAM)	Irreversible	MAO-B[a]
Moclobemide[b] (Aurorix; Manerix)	Reversible	MAO-A

Note.   MAO=monoamine oxidase.
[a]Selective at lower doses, nonselective at higher doses. Transdermal selegiline system allows for selegiline inhibition of both MAO-A and MAO-B. Oral selegiline is not indicated for the treatment of depression.
[b]Not available in the United States.

Source.   Adapted from Marangell LB, Martinez JM: *Concise Guide to Psychopharmacology,* 2nd Edition. Arlington, VA, American Psychiatric Publishing, 2006, p. 47. Used with permission.

may be necessary when the condition is refractory to treatment (Amsterdam and Berwish 1989). After tolerance to the hypotensive side effects has developed, usually after 1 or 2 weeks, the patient may take the medication in a single daily dose in the morning. Morning dosing is preferred because these medications tend to be activating; this is especially true of tranylcypromine, which is related to amphetamine.

Selegiline is an irreversible MAOI that is selective for MAO-B at lower doses and, when administered orally, undergoes extensive first-pass metabolism to amphetamine and methamphetamine metabolites (Karoum et al. 1982). Transdermal selegiline (EMSAM), which allows selegiline to be absorbed directly into the bloodstream, avoids first-pass metabolism (Rohatagi et al. 1997) and selectively targets MAO-A and MAO-B enzymes in the brain relative to those in the gastrointestinal tract (Wecker et al. 2003). Transdermal selegiline has been shown to be effective in the short-term treatment of depression in controlled trials (Amsterdam 2003; Bodkin and Amsterdam 2002). Transdermal selegiline is applied to dry skin on the upper torso, upper thigh, or outer surface of the upper arm once every 24 hours and not applied to the same site on consecutive days (EMSAM 2006). Patients should be advised to wash their hands after applying the transdermal system and also to avoid exposing the transdermal selegiline patch to external sources of heat.

Currently, transdermal selegiline is available in three dosages: 6 mg/24 hours (20 mg/20 cm^2), 9 mg/ 24 hours (30 mg/30 cm^2), and 12 mg/24 hours (40 mg/ 40 cm^2). The recommended starting and target dose is 6 mg/24 hours, and dose increases in increments of 3 mg/24 hours should occur at intervals of at least

2 weeks. The maximum recommended daily dosage is 12 mg/24 hours. At present, no dose adjustment is required for mild to moderate renal or hepatic impairment. Additionally, current product labeling does not require dietary restrictions for the 6-mg/24-hour dosing but does require dietary restrictions for the 9-mg/ 24-hour and 12-mg/24-hour dosing (EMSAM 2006). However, the concomitant medication warnings and restrictions apply across all transdermal selegiline dosages. A medication guide with safety information, dietary restrictions, drug interaction information, and instructions for use is available for patients.

Risks, Side Effects, and Their Management

The following side effects apply to the irreversible, nonselective MAOI antidepressants (phenelzine and tranylcypromine). The most common side effects are orthostatic hypotension, headache, insomnia, weight gain, sexual dysfunction, peripheral edema, and afternoon somnolence. Although MAOIs do not have significant affinity for muscarinic receptors, anticholinergic-like side effects are present at the beginning of treatment. Dry mouth is common but not as marked as in TCA therapy. Fortunately, the more serious side effects, such as hypertensive crisis and serotonin syndrome, are not common.

Transdermal selegiline was generally well tolerated in controlled trials; common adverse events included headache, insomnia, diarrhea, dry mouth, dyspepsia, and rash (EMSAM 2006). The most commonly reported treatment-emergent adverse event was application site reaction, which was generally mild to moderate in most cases. The rates of most adverse

TABLE 26–5.   Dietary and medication restrictions for patients taking nonselective monoamine oxidase inhibitors (MAOIs)

Foods to avoid while taking an MAOI and for 2 weeks after discontinuing the medication[a]	
Aged cheeses	Sauerkraut
Aged or fermented meats (e.g., sausage, salami, pepperoni)	Soy sauce
	Tap beer, including nonalcoholic tap beer
All foods that may be spoiled	Yeast extracts (e.g., Marmite)
Fava beans and broad bean pods	
Meat extracts (e.g., Bovril)	

Safe foods	
Alcohol (but not tap beer), in moderation	Fresh yogurt
Fresh cheeses (e.g., cream cheese, cottage cheese, ricotta cheese, American cheese, moderate amounts of mozzarella)	Smoked salmon and whitefish
	Yeast and baked goods containing yeast

Drugs to avoid while taking an MAOI and for 2 weeks after discontinuing the medication[b]

All sympathomimetic and stimulant drugs

Amphetamines	Local anesthetic drugs containing epinephrine or cocaine
Buspirone	
Diet medications	Meperidine
Ephedrine	Methylphenidate
Fenfluramine and dexfenfluramine	Other antidepressant medications
Isoproterenol	Phenylephrine
Levodopa and dopamine	Phenylpropanolamine

Over-the-counter nasal decongestants; cold, sinus, and allergy medications containing pseudoephedrine, phenylephrine, or phenylpropanolamine; and supplements

Actifed	NyQuil
Alka-Seltzer Plus	Robitussin PE, DM, CF, Night Relief
Allerest	Sine-Aid
Contac	Sine-Off
Coricidin D	Sinex
CoTylenol	St. John's wort
Dristan	Triaminic
L-Tryptophan	Tylenol
Neo-Synephrine	Vicks 44M, 44D

Other medications

Carbamazepine	Oxcarbazepine

Safe cold and allergy medications	
Alka-Seltzer (plain)	Robitussin (plain)
Chlor-Trimeton Allergy (without decongestant)	Tylenol (plain)

Other safe medications	
Antibiotics	Local anesthetics without epinephrine or cocaine
Codeine	Morphine
Laxatives and stool softeners	Nonsteroidal anti-inflammatory drugs

[a]Food restrictions based on tyramine content data from Walker et al. 1996.

[b]It is strongly advised that the reader consult the current *Physicians' Desk Reference* before prescribing any medication in combination with an MAOI.

Source.   EMSAM 2006; Feinberg and Holzer 1997, 2000; Gardner et al. 1996; *Physicians' Desk Reference* 2006; Shulman and Walker 1999, 2000; Shulman et al. 1997; Walker et al. 1996, 1997; Wing and Chen 1997. Adapted from Marangell LB, Martinez JM: *Concise Guide to Psychopharmacology,* 2nd Edition. Arlington, VA, American Psychiatric Publishing, 2006, pp. 48–50. Used with permission.

events were similar between transdermal selegiline and placebo, with a local skin site reaction occurring significantly more frequently with the transdermal selegiline compared with placebo (Bodkin and Amsterdam 2002).

Hypertensive crisis. Inactivation of intestinal MAO impairs the metabolism of tyramine. Tyramine can act as a false transmitter and displace norepinephrine from presynaptic storage granules. Therefore, large amounts of dietary tyramine can result in a hypertensive crisis in patients taking MAOIs because increased amounts of norepinephrine are displaced from adrenergic terminals, resulting in profound α-adrenergic activation. This reaction has also been called the "cheese reaction" because tyramine is present in relatively high concentrations in aged cheeses.

Tyramine is formed in foods by the decarboxylation of tyrosine during the aging, ripening, or decaying process of foods. Patients receiving MAOIs should be instructed to avoid the foods listed in Table 26–5. The key foods to avoid are aged cheeses, fermented sausage, sauerkraut, soy sauce, yeast extracts such as Marmite, fava beans and broad beans (which contain dopamine), and any foods that are overripe or spoiled. Fresh unaged cheeses—such as cottage cheese, ricotta, and cream cheese—are safe. Several foods that were formerly considered dangerous are no longer on the list of prohibited substances. For example, domestic bottled or canned beer is now considered safe when consumed in moderation (Gardner et al. 1996). However, tap beer, including nonalcoholic tap beer, continues to be considered dangerous. Most wines and liquors are also considered safe when drunk in moderation. Caffeine and chocolate are of concern when consumed in large amounts.

Some drugs with sympathomimetic activity, including certain decongestants and cough syrups, should be avoided because they may precipitate a hypertensive crisis (see Table 26–5). However, pure antihistaminic drugs, such as diphenhydramine, and pure expectorants without dextromethorphan, such as guaifenesin, are permissible.

Unfortunately, even perfect compliance with dietary and other restrictions does not guarantee complete protection from MAOI-induced hypertensive crises, because spontaneous hypertension with MAOI use can also occur. These reactions range from mild to severe. A patient with a mild reaction may complain of sweating, palpitations, and a slight headache. The most severe reaction manifests as a hypertensive crisis, with severe headache, increased blood pressure, and possible intracerebral hemorrhage. If a patient taking an MAOI experiences a severe headache, he or she should seek immediate medical evaluation.

If a patient's blood pressure is greatly increased, pharmacological treatment should be instituted. A common treatment for MAOI-induced hypertension is the calcium channel blocker nifedipine. Medications with α-adrenergic–blocking properties, such as phentolamine, also may be useful. However, treatment with phentolamine may be associated with cardiac arrhythmias or severe hypotension; thus, this approach should be carried out only in an emergency department setting (Tollefson 1983).

Patients taking MAOIs are advised to carry identification cards that indicate that they are taking MAOIs. Before accepting any medication or anesthetic, patients should notify their physicians that they are taking MAOIs. When patients undergo dental procedures, local anesthetics without vasoconstrictors (e.g., epinephrine) must be used. Additionally, patients may want to have a home blood pressure cuff.

Serotonin syndrome. The combination of serotonergic drugs, such as SSRIs, with MAOIs can result in a potentially fatal hypermetabolic reaction, often referred to as the *serotonin syndrome.* Affected individuals may experience lethargy, restlessness, confusion, flushing, diaphoresis, tremor, and myoclonic jerks. As the condition progresses, hyperthermia, hypertonicity, myoclonus, and death may occur. The syndrome must be identified as rapidly as possible. Discontinuation of the serotonergic medications is the first step in treatment, followed by emergency medical treatment as required.

The combination of MAOIs with meperidine, and perhaps with other phenylpiperidine analgesics, also has been implicated in fatal reactions attributed to the serotonin syndrome. Aspirin, nonsteroidal anti-inflammatory drugs, and acetaminophen should be used for mild to moderate pain. Of the narcotic agents, codeine and morphine are safe in combination with MAOIs, although doses may need to be lower than usual.

Cardiovascular effects. The MAOIs cause significant hypotension, which is often their dose-limiting side effect. Expansion of intravascular volume through administration of salt tablets or fludrocortisone may be an effective treatment.

Weight gain. MAOIs are associated with a risk of significant weight gain during treatment.

Sexual dysfunction. MAOIs are commonly associated with treatment-emergent sexual dysfunction, including decreased libido, delayed ejaculation, anorgasmia, and impotence. Some patients become tolerant to this side effect over time, but more often the problem persists unless the dose is reduced or another medication is used to counter the sexual side effects.

CNS effects. Headache and insomnia are common initial side effects that usually disappear after the first few weeks of treatment. A brief nap may help restore alertness.

Overdose

Most complications related to MAOI overdose arise from the drugs' stimulation of the sympathetic nervous system. MAOIs are most dangerous when patients experience hypertensive crises as the result of ingesting foods with high tyramine content.

Drug Interactions

Inhibition of MAO can cause severe interactions with other drugs, as detailed in the "Hypertensive Crisis" and "Serotonin Syndrome" subsections earlier in this section. A list of some drugs that interact with the nonselective MAOIs is provided in Table 26–5.

Treatment of Specific Disorders

Pharmacotherapy for Acute Major Depression

In patients receiving antidepressants for acute major depression, the initial therapeutic response is often delayed by several weeks. Clinicians should discuss the potential delay of symptomatic improvement with their patients when prescribing antidepressants so that patients will enter treatment with informed and realistic treatment expectations; otherwise, patients may become frustrated or discouraged if they do not see immediate improvement in symptoms and may prematurely discontinue the medication or not return for further care.

Patients with severe anxiety or insomnia may benefit from the concurrent time-limited use of a benzodiazepine or short-acting hypnotic. A patient may initially experience a return of energy and motivation while still having feelings of hopelessness and excessive guilt. Among such patients, there may be an increased risk of suicide because a return of energy in an extremely dysphoric individual may provide the impetus and means for an act of self-destruction.

It is a clinical challenge to distinguish symptoms of the illness from medication side effects. Many symptoms that patients attribute to antidepressant treatment may actually be symptoms of their underlying depressive illness. Clinicians should encourage their patients to continue treatment despite their perceptions of early medication side effects (provided that the side effects are tolerable), particularly if the side effects that arise are known to be generally transient in nature.

An adequate trial of antidepressant medication is defined as treatment with therapeutic doses of a drug for a total of at least 4 weeks. After 4 weeks of antidepressant treatment, patients can be divided into three groups: 1) those who have achieved a full response, 2) those who have achieved a partial response, and 3) those who have not responded. In patients who achieve full remission, treatment should continue for a minimum of 4 months; for patients with a history of recurrent depression, treatment should continue for an even longer period (see "Maintenance Treatment of Major Depression" later in this section). If a partial response has been achieved by 4 weeks, a full response may be evident within an additional 2 weeks without further intervention. If the patient has no response at all, the dose should be increased, a different antidepressant should be used, or the therapy should be augmented with another medication (see "Treatment-Resistant Depression" later in this section).

Pharmacotherapy for Depression With Psychotic Features

Psychotic depression has been reported to respond to combined treatment with antidepressants and antipsychotics (Nelson and Bowers 1978). Patients with psychotic depression also may show a significant response to electroconvulsive therapy (ECT), which is often the treatment of choice for this disorder. Long-term treatment with antipsychotic medications is generally not warranted, but prophylactic antidepressant medication must be continued as in nonpsychotic depression.

Pharmacotherapy for Bipolar Depression

A history of episodes of mania or hypomania suggests the diagnosis of bipolar disorder. Because antidepressants can precipitate manic episodes and increase cycling in bipolar patients (Wehr and Goodwin 1979), use of mood stabilizers (e.g., lithium, lamotrigine, or quetiapine) is the appropriate first step in the treatment of bipolar depression (see "Mood Stabilizers" section later in this chapter).

Maintenance Treatment of Major Depression

Results of a National Institute of Mental Health (NIMH) collaborative study indicated that antidepressant therapy should not be discontinued before 4–5 symptom-free months have passed (Prien and Kupfer 1986). Most clinicians treat single episodes of depression for a minimum of 6 months. In most cases, antidepressant medication should be continued at the same dose that resulted in remission.

Unfortunately, depression is often recurrent. After one episode of depression, there is a 50% chance that the patient will have a second episode; after three episodes, there is a 90% chance of recurrence (American Psychiatric Association 2000a). Therefore, longer periods of antidepressant treatment, often called *maintenance treatment,* are warranted to protect against recurrence (American Psychiatric Association 2000b). The value of maintenance antidepressant treatment, with and without psychotherapy, for patients with recurrent depression was confirmed by Frank et al. (1990) in a four-arm, double-blind, placebo-controlled trial. Current World Health Organization guidelines recommend maintenance treatment for patients who have had two or more episodes of major depression within a 5-year period (Coppen et al. 1986). For patients with recurrent depression, prophylaxis is recommended for at least 5 years (Kupfer 1993). Maintenance therapy should be considered for patients with three or more episodes of major depression or those with two or more episodes and a family history of mood disorder, as well as those with a rapid recurrence of depressive episodes, an older age at onset, or severe episodes (Keller 2001). The maintenance regimen should consist of the same dose of the same drug to which the patient's symptoms initially responded and should last as long as two episode cycles, which can be up to 4 or 5 years (Keller 2001). Some patients may require lifelong antidepressant maintenance treatment.

Treatment-Resistant Depression

Patients whose depression has apparently been resistant to standard antidepressant treatment often have had inadequate trials of antidepressants or have been noncompliant with drug therapy. Depression in a patient who has failed to complete an adequate trial of an antidepressant drug does not constitute treatment-resistant depression. For patients whose condition truly is nonresponsive to treatment, or for those in whom only a partial response has occurred, treatment options include switching to another antidepressant, combining two antidepressants with different proposed mechanisms of action, or using an augmentation strategy. Augmentation involves adding another agent that is not an antidepressant, such as lithium, a thyroid hormone, or a psychostimulant. Whether to switch, augment, or combine medications depends on many factors, including the severity of the illness, side effects of the current medication, and the patient's willingness to take more than one medication.

The best data on antidepressant treatment options come from the NIH-sponsored Sequenced Treatment Alternatives to Relieve Depression (STAR*D) study. STAR*D was conducted in both psychiatric and medical outpatient settings. Researchers evaluated treatment combination, treatment augmentation, and treatment switch strategies after treatment failure with up to 14 weeks of SSRI (citalopram) monotherapy (Trivedi et al. 2006b). Initial STAR*D findings showed that 28%–33% of the patients receiving citalopram for up to 14 weeks achieved remission (Trivedi et al. 2006b). Participants who did not achieve remission with the initial citalopram trial could enter one of two steps of treatment: 1) an antidepressant switch step (from citalopram to sertraline, bupropion SR, venlafaxine XR, or cognitive therapy), or 2) an antidepressant augmentation step (bupropion SR, buspirone, or cognitive therapy) (Rush et al. 2006; Trivedi et al. 2006a).

Response and remission rates were similar across the groups opting to switch treatments and across the groups opting to augment treatment (Rush et al. 2006). Results also indicated that the likelihood of remission decreased after each treatment step (37%, 31%, 14%, and 13% remission rates after Steps 1, 2, 3, and 4, respectively) (Rush et al. 2006). Initial follow-up findings indicated that patients who showed remission at Step 1 had lower relapse rates compared with those who did not show remission at Step 1 (Rush 2007). This finding highlights the importance of achieving remission in patients who struggle with depression. Results from STAR*D also suggest that a dosage increase at 6 weeks or a longer trial on the medication (i.e., up to 10 weeks) may benefit some patients (Rush 2007; Trivedi et al. 2006b).

Additional augmentation strategies include the use of lithium (De Montigny et al. 1981; Dinan and Barry 1989; Ontiveros et al. 1991; Thase et al. 1989), triiodothyronine (Goodwin et al. 1982; R.T. Joffe 1988; R.T. Joffe and Singer 1990; R.T. Joffe et al. 1993), and stimulants (Fava et al. 2005; Fawcett et al. 1991), although these strategies are not as well supported in randomized controlled trials with the newer antidepressants. The use of more than one antidepressant in patients with treatment-resistant depression is potentially beneficial, although few systematic data are available. The key to combining two antidepressants is to choose agents that have different proposed mechanisms of action. When combining antidepressants, it is important both to ensure that the patient has had an adequate trial of a single agent and to be aware of possible drug interactions or additive side effects. Nonpharmacological options (e.g., ECT, vagus nerve stimulation, and psychotherapy) also should be considered in cases of inadequate response to treatment.

Pharmacotherapy for Borderline Personality Disorder

Numerous studies have investigated the treatment of borderline personality disorder with various antidepressants, including TCAs, MAOIs, SSRIs, and venlafaxine (American Psychiatric Association 2001; Soloff 2000). The American Psychiatric Association (2001) *Practice Guideline for the Treatment of Patients With Borderline Personality Disorder* recommends the use of SSRIs and venlafaxine (at usual antidepressant doses) for treating mood lability, depressed mood, rejection sensitivity, disinhibited anger, impulsivity, and self-damaging behaviors. The positive effects of these antidepressants on impulsive aggression and anger in placebo-controlled studies appeared to be independent of changes in affective symptoms (Salzman et al. 1995). Lithium augmentation is recommended for patients who have a partial response to an SSRI, whereas a switch to another SSRI is recommended for patients who have no response to an initial SSRI. Atypical antipsychotic agents may be useful but have been less well studied to date (Zanarini et al. 2004). MAOIs also may be effective, particularly in patients with atypical depressive symptoms, but are not recommended as first-line agents because of side effects and the need for dietary restrictions.

Discontinuation of Antidepressants

Discontinuation of antidepressant medication should be concordant with the guidelines for treatment duration (see "Pharmacotherapy for Acute Major Depression" subsection earlier in this chapter). It is advisable to taper the dose while monitoring for signs and symptoms of relapse. Abrupt discontinuation is also more likely to lead to antidepressant discontinuation symptoms, often referred to as *withdrawal symptoms*. The occurrence of these symptoms after medication discontinuation does not imply that antidepressants are addictive.

Discontinuation symptoms appear to occur most commonly after discontinuation of short-half-life serotonergic drugs (Coupland et al. 1996), such as fluvoxamine, paroxetine, and venlafaxine. Patients describe symptoms as "flulike," including nausea, diarrhea, insomnia, malaise, muscle aches, anxiety, irritability, dizziness, vertigo, and vivid dreams (Coupland et al. 1996). Patients also may experience transient "electric shock" sensations. This unique symptom is diagnostically useful and strongly suggests to the clinician that the patient is experiencing antidepressant discontinuation symptoms because the symptom rarely occurs in other conditions or as a side effect of a new medication.

Discontinuation symptoms usually occur within 1–2 days after abrupt discontinuation of a medication and subside within 7–10 days. In some instances, symptoms also may occur during tapering and dose reduction, and they may persist for up to 3 weeks. Restarting treatment with the medication and then tapering more slowly may be necessary, although it is often possible to attenuate withdrawal symptoms produced by short-half-life SSRIs by administering one dose of fluoxetine (which has a longer half-life).

Abrupt discontinuation of TCAs commonly results in diarrhea, increased sweating, anxiety, and dizziness. These symptoms were previously attributed to cholinergic rebound, but the occurrence of similar symptoms after the discontinuation of many of the newer serotonergic antidepressants suggests that the pathophysiology may be more closely related to changes in serotonin.

Antidepressant Switching

Particular care must be exercised when switching from an MAOI to other antidepressant classes. In patients who have completed an MAOI trial without achieving a therapeutic response, treatment with other antidepressants should not be started until 14 days after discontinuation of the original MAOI. Equal care is required when switching from most other antidepressants to an MAOI. An interval equal to five times the half-life of the drug, including active metabolites, is required between stopping treatment with other antidepressant medications and starting MAOI therapy. A 2-week interval is also recommended when switching from phenelzine to tranylcypromine because tranylcypromine is an amphetamine derivative.

Switching between other antidepressants is less problematic. Often, clinicians choose to discontinue the first medication before introducing the second one. In most instances, however, a medication-free period is not critical if neither medication is an MAOI. In many instances, it is possible to start administering the new drug while tapering the dose of the first. This overlapping of medications is sometimes helpful to minimize patient discomfort but must be weighed against the risk of increased side effects and drug interactions (Marangell 2001). Considerations to be taken into account when switching antidepressants include half-life and the potential for drug–drug interactions.

Switching from one SSRI or SNRI to another can be accomplished by a direct switch from one medication to the next. Although abrupt discontinuation of SSRIs or SNRIs, particularly those with short half-lives, may be associated with discontinuation effects (Rosenbaum et al. 1998), such effects generally are not seen if another medication is substituted that also inhibits the serotonin reuptake pump. Although both agents will be present until a time equal to five times the half-life of the first medication, this is not usually a problem in practice. Similarly, higher levels of either medication may occur if one or both medications inhibit cytochrome P450 enzymes (e.g., paroxetine or fluoxetine). This may lead to transient side effects, but it is not usually a safety issue. In most cases, a direct switch from one medication to another is better tolerated than a washing out of the first agent. Although cross-tapering may be useful when medications with different receptor effects are used (e.g., an SSRI and bupropion or mirtazapine), this strategy is not useful when both medications are SSRIs.

Anxiolytics, Sedatives, and Hypnotics

Overview

Anxiety and insomnia are prevalent symptoms with multiple etiologies. Effective treatments are available, but they vary by diagnosis. In most instances, the best course of action is to treat the underlying disorder rather than reflexively instituting treatment with a nonspecific anxiolytic.

In some cases, anxiolytics serve a transitional purpose. For example, for a patient with acute-onset panic disorder, severe anticipatory anxiety, and a family history of depression, administration of an antidepressant medication that also has antipanic effects may be the optimal treatment, but this will not help the patient for several weeks, during which time there is a risk of progression to agoraphobia. For this patient, starting antidepressant therapy and also attempting to obtain acute symptom relief with a benzodiazepine may be helpful. After 4 weeks, the benzodiazepine dose should be slowly tapered so that the patient's condition is controlled with the antidepressant alone.

TABLE 26–6. **Medications for the treatment of major anxiety disorders**

Anxiety disorder	Medication options
Generalized anxiety disorder	Buspirone, benzodiazepines, venlafaxine, SSRIs[a]
Obsessive-compulsive disorder	Clomipramine, SSRIs[b]
Panic disorder	SSRIs,[c] TCAs, MAOIs, benzodiazepines
Performance anxiety	β-Blockers, benzodiazepines
Social phobia	SSRIs,[d] venlafaxine, MAOIs, benzodiazepines, buspirone, venlafaxine

Note. SSRIs=selective serotonin reuptake inhibitors; TCAs=tricyclic antidepressants; MAOIs=monoamine oxidase inhibitors.
[a]SSRIs currently approved by the U.S. Food and Drug Administration (FDA) for the treatment of generalized anxiety disorder include paroxetine and escitalopram.
[b]SSRIs currently approved by the FDA for the treatment of obsessive-compulsive disorder include paroxetine, sertraline, and fluoxetine.
[c]SSRIs currently approved by the FDA for the treatment of panic disorder include paroxetine, sertraline, and fluoxetine.
[d]SSRIs currently approved by the FDA for the treatment of social phobia include paroxetine and sertraline.
Source. Adapted from Marangell LB, Martinez JM: *Concise Guide to Psychopharmacology*, 2nd Edition. Arlington, VA, American Psychiatric Publishing, 2006, p. 70. Used with permission.

In this section, we review the pharmacology of medications that are primarily classified as anxiolytic, sedative, or hypnotic agents. Diagnosis-specific treatment guidelines are outlined in Table 26–6. Common anxiolytics and hypnotics are shown in Table 26–7.

Benzodiazepines

Mechanisms of Action

Benzodiazepines facilitate inhibition by γ-aminobutyric acid (GABA), a major inhibitory neurotransmitter in the brain (reviewed by Tallman et al. 1980). The benzodiazepine receptor is a subtype of the $GABA_A$ receptor. Activation of the benzodiazepine receptor facilitates the action of endogenous GABA, which results in the opening of chloride ion channels and a decrease in neuronal excitability.

TABLE 26–7. Commonly used anxiolytic and hypnotic agents

Generic drug	Proprietary name	Dose equivalence (mg)	Typical starting dose in adults[a] (mg)	Typical daily dosage range in adults[a] (mg/day)
Anxiolytic medications				
Benzodiazepines used as anxiolytics				
Alprazolam	Xanax	0.5	0.25–0.5 tid (0.5 tid for panic)	0.75–4 (divided) (1–6 for panic)
Alprazolam extended-release	Xanax XR	NA	0.5–1	3–6
Chlordiazepoxide	Librium	10	5–25 tid or qid	15–100 (divided tid or qid)
Clonazepam	Klonopin	0.25	0.25 bid	1–4
Clorazepate	Tranxene	7.5	15 (T-tab)	T-tab: 15–60 (divided) SD: 22.5 qd to replace T-tab 7.5 tid
Diazepam	Valium	5	2–10 bid–qid	4–40 (divided)
Lorazepam	Ativan	1	0.5–2 tid–qid	2–4 (divided)
Oxazepam	Serax	15	10–30 tid–qid	30–120 (divided)
Nonbenzodiazepines used as anxiolytics				
Buspirone	BuSpar	NA	10–30 (divided)	30–60 (divided)
Hypnotic medications				
Benzodiazepines used as anxiolytics				
Estazolam	ProSom	—	1	1–2
Flurazepam	Dalmane	—	15–30	15–30
Quazepam	Doral	—	7.5–15	7.5–15
Temazepam	Restoril	—	15	15–30
Triazolam	Halcion	—	0.125	0.125–0.25
Nonbenzodiazepine GABA–benzodiazepine receptor agonists used as hypnotics				
Eszopiclone	Lunesta	NA	2	2–3
Zaleplon	Sonata	NA	5–10	5–10
Zolpidem	Ambien	NA	5–10	5–10
Zolpidem extended-release	Ambien CR	NA	12.5	6.25–12.5
Nonbenzodiazepine melatonin MT_1 and MT_2 receptor agonists used as hypnotics				
Ramelteon	Rozerem	NA	8	8

Note. tid=three-times-per-day dosing; NA=not applicable; qid=four-times-per-day dosing; bid=twice-daily dosing; qd=once-daily dosing; CR=extended release; SD=single dose; T-tab=T-shaped tablet; GABA=γ-aminobutyric acid.
[a]The typical starting doses are for healthy adults. Special populations, such as the elderly, debilitated, or hepatically or renally impaired, may require lower doses or may preclude the use of certain agents.

Source. Drug Facts and Comparisons 2002; Fuller and Sajatovic 2004b; Jenkins et al. 2001; Nishino et al. 2004; *Physicians' Desk Reference* 2006; Pies 1998; Shader and Greenblatt 2003.

Indications and Efficacy

Benzodiazepines are highly effective anxiolytics and sedatives. They also have muscle relaxant, amnestic, and anticonvulsant properties. Benzodiazepines effectively treat acute and chronic generalized anxiety and panic disorder. The high-potency benzodiazepines alprazolam and clonazepam have received more attention as antipanic agents, but double-blind studies also have confirmed the efficacy of diazepam and lorazepam in the treatment of panic disorder. Although only a few benzodiazepines are specifically approved by the FDA for the treatment of insomnia, almost all benzodiazepines may be used for this purpose. Benzodiazepines are most clearly valuable as hypnotics in the hospital setting, where high levels of sensory stimulation, pain, and acute stress may interfere with sleep. The safe, effective, and time-limited use of benzodiazepine hypnotics may, in fact, prevent chronic sleep difficulties (NIMH/NIH Consensus Development Conference Statement 1985). Benzodiazepines are also used to treat akathisia and catatonia and as adjuncts in the treatment of acute mania.

Because alcohol and barbiturates also act, in part, via the GABA$_A$ receptor–mediated chloride ion channel, benzodiazepines show cross-tolerance with these substances. Thus, benzodiazepines are used frequently for treating alcohol or barbiturate withdrawal and detoxification. Alcohol and barbiturates are more dangerous than benzodiazepines because they can act directly at the chloride ion channel at higher doses. In contrast, benzodiazepines have no direct effect on the ion channel; the effects of benzodiazepines are limited by the amount of endogenous GABA.

Benzodiazepine Selection

At equipotent doses, all benzodiazepines have similar effects. The choice of benzodiazepine is generally based on half-life, rapidity of onset, metabolism, and potency. In patients with moderate to severe hepatic dysfunction, it may be useful to avoid benzodiazepines. All benzodiazepines are metabolized at various levels by the liver, which leads to an increased risk of sedation and confusion in patients with hepatic failure. If it is necessary to prescribe this class of medication, lorazepam and oxazepam are reasonable choices because their elimination will not be significantly affected (Abernethy et al. 1984).

Risks, Side Effects, and Their Management

Sedation and impairment of performance. Benzodiazepine-induced sedation may be considered either a therapeutic action or a side effect. When a patient takes a benzodiazepine at night, particularly an agent with a long half-life, residual sedation may be present on awakening. Additionally, any benzodiazepine has the potential to cause sedation.

Impairment of performance on sensitive psychomotor tests has been well documented after the administration of benzodiazepines. Patients must be warned that driving, engaging in dangerous physical activities, and using hazardous machinery should be avoided during treatment with benzodiazepines, particularly during the early course of treatment.

Dependence, withdrawal, and rebound effects. Many patients and clinicians are concerned about the abuse and dependence potential of benzodiazepines. Most benzodiazepines have a low abuse potential when they are properly prescribed and their use is supervised (American Psychiatric Association 1990). However, physical dependence often occurs when benzodiazepines are taken at higher-than-usual doses or for prolonged periods.

If benzodiazepines are discontinued precipitously, withdrawal effects (including hyperpyrexia, seizures, psychosis, and even death) may occur. Signs and symptoms of withdrawal may include tachycardia, increased blood pressure, muscle cramps, anxiety, insomnia, panic attacks, impairment of memory and concentration, perceptual disturbances, and delirium. In addition, withdrawal-related derealization, hallucinations, and other psychotic symptoms may occur. These withdrawal symptoms may begin as early as the day after discontinuation of the benzodiazepine, and they may continue for weeks to months. Evidence indicates that withdrawal reactions associated with shorter-half-life benzodiazepines peak more rapidly and more intensely. These withdrawal symptoms may be alleviated by reintroducing the withdrawn benzodiazepine.

Rebound anxiety and insomnia also may occur when benzodiazepines are abruptly discontinued. As a general rule, most psychoactive medications should be discontinued gradually, not abruptly. For patients who have been taking benzodiazepines for longer than 2–3 months, the benzodiazepine dose should be decreased by approximately 10% per week. Therefore, in the case of a patient receiving alprazolam 4 mg/day, the dose should be tapered by 0.5 mg/week for 8 weeks.

Memory impairment. Benzodiazepines are associated with anterograde amnesia, especially when they are administered intravenously and in high doses (Dixon et al. 1984; Lucki et al. 1986; Reitan et al. 1986). Amnesia may be a desirable effect of benzodiazepines when they are used for surgical procedures, but memory impairment in other instances may be a serious liability. Clinicians should warn patients about the potential risk for amnesia when prescribing all benzodiazepines.

Disinhibition and dyscontrol. Anecdotal reports suggest that benzodiazepines may occasionally cause paradoxical anger and behavioral disinhibition (see review by Rothschild 1992). A history of hostility, impulsivity, or borderline or antisocial personality disorder is a potential predictor of this reaction. Some caution should be exercised when benzodiazepines are prescribed to patients with a history of poor impulse control and aggression.

Overdose

Benzodiazepines are remarkably safe in overdose when taken alone. Dangerous effects occur when the overdose includes several sedative drugs, especially alcohol, because of synergistic effects at the chloride ion site and resultant membrane hyperpolarization.

In an emergency setting, the benzodiazepine antagonist flumazenil may be given intravenously to reverse the effects of a potential overdose of a benzodiazepine. Caution in use of flumazenil in a mixed overdose with TCAs is warranted, however. Its use may precipitate TCA-induced arrhythmias and seizures that were suppressed by benzodiazepines.

Drug Interactions

Most sedative drugs, including narcotics and alcohol, potentiate the sedative effects of benzodiazepines. In addition, medications that inhibit hepatic CYP3A3/4 increase blood levels and hence side effects of clonazepam, alprazolam, midazolam, and triazolam. Lorazepam, oxazepam, and temazepam are not dependent on hepatic enzymes for metabolism; thus, cytochrome P450 enzyme inhibition should not significantly affect these particular benzodiazepines.

Use in Pregnancy

Anxiolytics, like most medications, should be avoided during pregnancy and breast-feeding when possible. There have been concerns that benzodiazepines, when administered during the first trimester of pregnancy, may increase the risk of malformations, particularly cleft palate. Pooled data from cohort studies do not support an increased risk, but data from case–control studies do suggest a risk (Rosenberg et al. 1983). Until further data are available, a high-quality ultrasound should be considered for women who have used benzodiazepines in the first trimester (Dolovich et al. 1998). Some reports have noted that use of benzodiazepines at close proximity to labor may lead to discontinuation symptoms in the neonate such as hypotonia, apnea, and temperature dysregulation.

Buspirone

Background

Buspirone is a partial agonist at 5-HT_{1A} receptors. It is important to note that buspirone does not interact with the GABA receptor or chloride ion channels. Therefore, it does not produce sedation, interact with alcohol, impair psychomotor performance, or pose a risk of abuse. Importantly, there is no cross-tolerance between benzodiazepines and buspirone, so benzodiazepines cannot be abruptly replaced with buspirone. Likewise, buspirone cannot be used to treat alcohol or barbiturate withdrawal and detoxification. Like the antidepressants, buspirone has a relatively slow onset of action.

Indications and Efficacy

Buspirone is effective in the treatment of generalized anxiety. Although the onset of therapeutic action is less rapid, buspirone's efficacy is not statistically different from that of benzodiazepines (Cohn and Wilcox 1986; Goldberg and Finnerty 1979). Despite its success in the treatment of generalized anxiety disorder, buspirone does not appear to be effective against panic disorder (Sheehan et al. 1990). Buspirone is also used as an augmenting agent in the treatment of OCD (Harvey and Balon 1995; Laird 1996) and depression (Sramek et al. 1996; Trivedi et al. 2006a), and some evidence suggests that buspirone therapy may be an effective treatment for social phobia (Munjack et al. 1991; Schneier et al. 1992).

Clinical Use

Buspirone is available for oral administration in a variety of dosage forms. The usual initial dosage is 7.5 mg twice a day, increased after 1 week to 15 mg twice a day. The dose may then be increased as needed to achieve optimal therapeutic response. The usual recommended maximum daily dose is 60 mg. Because buspirone is metabolized by the liver and excreted by the kidneys, it should not be administered to patients with severe hepatic or renal impairment.

Side Effects

The side effects that are more common with buspirone therapy than with benzodiazepine therapy are nausea, headache, nervousness, insomnia, dizziness, and light-headedness (Rakel 1990). Restlessness also has been reported.

Overdose

No fatal outcomes of buspirone overdose have been reported. However, overdose of buspirone with other drugs may result in more serious outcomes.

Drug Interactions

Buspirone is metabolized by CYP3A3/4. Therefore, the initial dose should be lower in patients who are also taking medications known to inhibit this enzyme. Additionally, buspirone should not be administered in combination with an MAOI.

Zolpidem and Zaleplon

Zolpidem and zaleplon are hypnotics that act at the omega-1 receptor of the central $GABA_A$ receptor complex. This selectivity is hypothesized to be associated with a lower risk of dependence. Unlike benzodiazepines, zolpidem and zaleplon do not appear to have significant anxiolytic, muscle relaxant, or anticonvulsant properties. However, amnestic effects may occur.

Indications and Efficacy

Zolpidem is a short-acting hypnotic with established efficacy in inducing and maintaining sleep. Because of the short half-life of this drug, most patients taking zolpidem report minimal daytime sedation. Zaleplon is an ultra-short-acting hypnotic; minimal residual sedative effects are seen after 4 hours of administration.

Clinical Use

Both zolpidem and zaleplon are available in 5- and 10-mg tablets for oral administration. The maximum recommended dosages for adults are 10 mg/day and 20 mg/day, respectively, administered at night. The initial dose for elderly persons should not exceed 5 mg. Caution is advised in patients with hepatic dysfunction. In general, hypnotics should be limited to short-term use, with reevaluation for more extended therapy. Zolpidem XL is available in 6.25- and 12.5-mg tablets. The recommended dose for adults is 12.5 mg before sleep (6.25 mg for elderly patients).

Side Effects

In general, side effects of zolpidem and zaleplon are similar to those of short-acting benzodiazepines. These agents should not be considered free of abuse potential.

Overdose

Both zolpidem and zaleplon appear to be nonfatal in overdose. However, overdoses in combination with other CNS depressant agents pose a greater risk. Recommended treatment consists of general symptomatic and supportive measures, including gastric lavage. Use of flumazenil may be helpful.

Drug Interactions

Research on drug interactions is limited, but any drug with CNS depressant effects could potentially enhance the CNS depressant effects of zolpidem and zaleplon through pharmacodynamic interactions. In addition, zolpidem is primarily metabolized by CYP3A3/4, and zaleplon is partially metabolized by CYP3A3/4. Thus, inhibitors of these enzymes may increase blood levels and the toxicity of zolpidem.

Ramelteon

Ramelteon is a hypnotic medication with melatonin receptor agonist activity targeting melatonin MT_1 and MT_2 receptors. It has not been proven to induce dependence. No appreciable activity on serotonin, dopamine, GABA, or acetylcholine occurs with the parent compound, but in vitro studies report that ramelteon's primary metabolite, M-II, has weak $5\text{-}HT_{2B}$ receptor agonist activity.

Indications and Efficacy

Ramelteon is indicated for the treatment of insomnia. Because its half-life is 1–2.6 hours, this medication is not thought to be associated with daytime sedation.

Clinical Use

Ramelteon is available in 8-mg tablets for oral administration. The current maximum dosage is 8 mg administered at night. Ramelteon should be used with caution in elderly patients because plasma levels were twice those in healthy adults in clinical trials. Ramelteon should not be used by patients with severe hepatic impairment. This medication has been evaluated in moderate sleep apnea and chronic obstructive pulmonary disease but not in subjects with severe sleep apnea or severe chronic obstructive pulmonary disease and is not recommended for use in these patients.

Side Effects

Common side effects include somnolence, dizziness, and fatigue. Additionally, ramelteon has been associated with decreased testosterone levels and increased prolactin levels. To date, trials of ramelteon have not indicated high abuse potential with this medication.

Overdose

Supportive measures are recommended if overdose occurs. Gastric lavage also should be considered.

Drug Interactions

Ramelteon is metabolized by hepatic metabolism; CYP1A2 is the major isoenzyme involved. Caution is recommended with other inhibitory agents such as fluvoxamine. Ramelteon is also metabolized, to a lesser extent, by CYP2C9 and CYP3A4; thus, additional caution is warranted with medications that affect these cytochrome P450 enzymes.

Eszopiclone

Eszopiclone is a hypnotic agent that is thought to act on GABA receptor complexes close to benzodiazepine receptors.

Indications and Efficacy

Eszopiclone has a half-life of approximately 6 hours and is indicated for the treatment of insomnia.

Clinical Use

Eszopiclone is available in 1-, 2-, and 3-mg tablets for oral administration. The maximum recommended dose is 3 mg/night. In the elderly, this dose is reduced to a maximum of 2 mg. No evidence of tolerance or dependence has been reported, but long-term use should be approached with caution. In addition, eszopiclone should be used cautiously in patients with substance abuse because clinical trials have shown euphoric effects at high doses.

Side Effects

Eszopiclone has side effects similar to those of short-acting benzodiazepines. Dizziness, headache, and unpleasant taste were the most commonly reported side effects in patients taking eszopiclone in clinical trials (Lunesta 2005).

Overdose

Limited information on overdose with eszopiclone is available at this time. No fatalities have been reported with up to 36 mg being taken in overdose. Overdose symptoms include impairment in consciousness, including somnolence or coma. Treatment is symptom-driven and supportive. Flumazenil may be beneficial.

Drug Interactions

Eszopiclone is metabolized in the liver by CYP3A4. Eszopiclone should not be used in patients with severe hepatic impairment. Dose adjustment and caution are recommended when prescribing eszopiclone to patients taking enzyme inhibitors such as ketoconazole, ciprofloxacin, erythromycin, isoniazid, and nefazo-

done. The use of other sedative-hypnotics is not recommended with administration of this medication.

Treatment of Specific Conditions

Pharmacotherapy for Generalized Anxiety Disorder

Generalized anxiety disorder can be treated with benzodiazepines, buspirone, and certain antidepressants (see Tables 26–6 and 26–7). Table 26–8 presents a comparison of benzodiazepines and antidepressants for the treatment of anxiety.

Benzodiazepines are rapidly effective, but they also carry the risks for abuse and sedation. Tolerance to the sedative effects of benzodiazepines often develops, but tolerance to anxiolytic effects generally does not. All benzodiazepines indicated for the treatment of anxiety are equally efficacious. The choice of a specific agent usually depends on the pharmacokinetics and pharmacodynamics of the drug. Although some patients respond to low dosages, mean doses for many patients are typically higher. When benzodiazepines are used to treat anxiety, the clinician should start with alprazolam, 0.25 mg two or three times a day, or an equivalent dosage of another benzodiazepine (see Table 26–7). The dosage should then be titrated to achieve maximal anxiolytic effect and minimal sedation. Benzodiazepines should be avoided in patients with a history of recent and/or significant substance abuse, and all patients should be advised to take the first dose at home in a situation that would not be dangerous in the event of greater-than-expected sedation.

Unlike benzodiazepines, buspirone is not associated with significant sedation, motor performance impairment, or abuse problems. However, unlike the rapid onset of action associated with benzodiazepines, response to buspirone typically occurs only after several weeks of treatment.

Buspirone does not show cross-tolerance with benzodiazepines and other sedative-hypnotic drugs such as alcohol, barbiturates, and chloral hydrate. Therefore, buspirone does not suppress benzodiazepine withdrawal symptoms. For anxious patients who are taking a benzodiazepine and require a switch to buspirone, the benzodiazepine must be tapered gradually to avoid withdrawal symptoms.

Generalized anxiety disorder also responds to antidepressant treatment. As with buspirone, response to antidepressants typically occurs after several weeks of treatment, and maximal response may take months. Venlafaxine, escitalopram, and paroxetine have received FDA approval for this indication, although the

TABLE 26–8. Comparison of benzodiazepines and antidepressants for the treatment of anxiety

Characteristic	Benzodiazepines	Antidepressants
Therapeutic effect after single dose	Yes	No
Time to full therapeutic action	Days	Weeks
Sedation	Yes	Varies
Dependence liability	Yes	No
Impaired performance	Yes	No
Suppression of sedative withdrawal symptoms	Yes	No
Once-daily dosing	No	Yes
Treatment of comorbid depression	No	Yes
Side effects	Sedation, memory impairment	Gastrointestinal effects, sexual dysfunction

Source. Adapted from Marangell LB, Martinez JM: *Concise Guide to Psychopharmacology,* 2nd Edition. Arlington, VA, American Psychiatric Publishing, 2006, p. 82. Used with permission.

other SSRIs are likely effective as well.

The duration of pharmacotherapy for generalized anxiety disorder is controversial. Psychotherapy is recommended for most patients with this disorder, and it may facilitate the tapering of doses of medication. However, generalized anxiety is often a chronic condition, and some patients require long-term pharmacotherapy. As in other anxiety disorders, the need for ongoing treatment should be reassessed every 6–12 months.

Pharmacotherapy for Panic Disorder

Benzodiazepines, TCAs, MAOIs, and SSRIs are all effective in the treatment of panic disorder. Among the benzodiazepines, the high-potency agents alprazolam and clonazepam are preferred because they are well tolerated at the higher doses often required to treat panic disorder. For the treatment of panic disorder, clonazepam therapy is started at 0.5 mg twice a day, and the dosage is often increased to a total of 2–4 mg/day in divided doses. Higher dosage levels may be necessary for complete relief of symptoms. The starting dosage of alprazolam is usually 0.25 or 0.5 mg three times a day.

Because long-term exposure to high-dose benzodiazepines may place some patients at risk for dependence, the use of antidepressants for the treatment of panic disorder should be considered. Antidepressant choices include TCAs, MAOIs, and SSRIs. For many patients, SSRIs may be considered first-line agents. MAOIs are usually reserved for patients whose symptoms have not responded to SSRIs and TCAs. Standard or high-standard antidepressant doses generally are used for the treatment of panic disorder, although some patients may be particularly sensitive to the initial stimulating effects of antidepressants. For these patients, treatment may be initiated with clonazepam or alprazolam and an antidepressant at a low dose. The antidepressant dose can then be titrated as tolerated to the effective dose range. The benzodiazepine may provide the patient with immediate anxiety relief until the antidepressant becomes effective. When panic symptoms have been absent for several weeks, the benzodiazepine dose should then be slowly tapered if possible.

The duration of pharmacotherapy for patients with panic disorder is unknown. The clinician should consider attempting a gradual medication discontinuation every 6–12 months if the patient has been relatively symptom free. However, many patients may require longer-term pharmacotherapy.

Pharmacotherapy for Social Phobia

Social phobia responds to a variety of medications, including SSRIs, MAOIs, benzodiazepines, and buspirone. Dosages for the treatment of social phobia are similar to dosages of these medications for other disorders. Although the MAOIs are highly effective, these drugs are not considered first-line agents because of the better safety and tolerability profiles of other treatment options.

Pharmacotherapy for Performance Anxiety

β-Blockers can be effective in the treatment of performance anxiety. Taken within 2 hours of the stressor, propranolol, in doses ranging from 20 to 80 mg, may reduce anxiety symptoms and improve performance on examinations (Drew et al. 1985), in public speaking (Hertley et al. 1983), and in musical performances (Brantigan et al. 1982). A trial dose of 20–40 mg of propranolol should be administered first to make sure it is well tolerated before it is used in a critical situation. Subsequently, doses of propranolol should be administered approximately 2 hours before the performance situation.

Pharmacotherapy for OCD

Currently, clomipramine and the SSRIs provide the foundation of pharmacological treatment of OCD. However, it is important to note that many patients with OCD experience only a 60% or lower improvement in symptoms (Jenike 1990). Additionally, medication responses may not be apparent until treatment has been given for 10 weeks, and some patients may require doses of SSRIs that are higher than those typically used for the treatment of major depression. Cognitive-behavioral therapy should be combined with pharmacological approaches.

The typical dose range for clomipramine in the treatment of OCD is between 150 and 200 mg/day. Before initiating clomipramine treatment, the clinician must heed all the precautions and dosing guidelines associated with the use of any TCA. Additionally, clinicians should monitor patients for the emergence of anticholinergic, antihistaminic, and α_2-adrenergic side effects.

Currently, the SSRIs paroxetine, fluoxetine, fluvoxamine, and sertraline have been approved by the FDA for the treatment of OCD. Fluoxetine has shown approximately equivalent antiobsessional effects compared with clomipramine (Pigott et al. 1990). As noted earlier, SSRI doses may need to be higher in some patients with OCD compared with doses typically used for the treatment of major depression. For fluoxetine, the recommended dosage range for the treatment of OCD is 20–60 mg/day, although some clinicians target a daily dose of up to 80 mg. Therapeutic dosages of fluvoxamine range from 100 to 300 mg/day in divided doses. The recommended dosage range of paroxetine for the treatment of OCD is 40–60 mg/day. The recommended dosage range of sertraline for the treatment of OCD is 50–200 mg/day.

The exact required duration of pharmacotherapy for OCD has not been established. OCD is often a lifelong disorder, with a waxing and waning course, for which many patients require prolonged pharmacotherapy.

Pharmacotherapy for Insomnia

Although benzodiazepines, zolpidem, zaleplon, and eszopiclone are the mainstay of pharmacotherapy for insomnia, other sedating drugs, such as trazodone, diphenhydramine, and chloral hydrate, also may be used. Medications commonly prescribed for insomnia, along with their recommended doses, are shown in Table 26–7.

Insomnia first should be addressed diagnostically, and in most cases, nonpharmacological interventions should be attempted before treatment with a hypnotic is instituted. Indeed, sleep hygiene techniques may help many patients improve their sleep without the need for hypnotic medications. When hypnotic agents are used, they should be administered in the lowest effective dose and for brief periods. If the patient has a history of substance abuse or dependence, the clinician should consider the use of nonbenzodiazepine medications to reduce the risk for abuse.

Pharmacotherapy for Alcohol Withdrawal

One potential strategy for treating alcohol withdrawal is the benzodiazepine loading-dose technique (Sellers et al. 1983). This technique takes advantage of the long half-lives of benzodiazepines such as diazepam and chlordiazepoxide. For example, patients receive 100-mg doses of chlordiazepoxide (or 20-mg doses of diazepam) every hour until no signs or symptoms of alcohol withdrawal are observed. This state is usually accompanied by mild to moderate sedation. Thereafter, no further doses of the benzodiazepine are administered. Healthy patients should receive at least 300 mg of chlordiazepoxide (or 60 mg of diazepam) in the initial loading-dose regimen (Sullivan and Seller 1986). For patients with hepatic disease, the use of lorazepam or oxazepam should be considered.

Antipsychotic Medications

Background

Antipsychotic medications, previously referred to as *major tranquilizers* or *neuroleptics*, are effective for the treatment of a variety of psychotic symptoms. Antipsychotics can be classified in several ways. One classification system is based on chemical structure; for example, phenothiazines and butyrophenones make up two chemical classes. We use the term *conventional* to signify older or first-generation antipsychotic drugs—to differentiate them from newer *atypical* or second-generation antipsychotics. Among the conventional antipsychotics, we distinguish between high- and low-potency agents because the level of potency predicts side effects. Although the term *atypical antipsychotic* lacks a single consistent definition, it generally refers to the newer antipsychotic medications that affect both 5-HT$_2$ and D$_2$ receptors. Atypical antipsychotics available in the United States include clozapine, olanzapine, risperidone, quetiapine, ziprasidone, and aripiprazole.

The favorable neurological side-effect profile of atypical antipsychotics led to their use as first-line agents for the treatment of psychosis. Additionally, atypical antipsychotics as a class were often considered to be more effective than conventional antipsychotics. As discussed later in this section, superior efficacy has clearly been documented for clozapine but not necessarily for all agents in the class (Lieberman et al. 2005). Although neurological side effects are less frequent with atypical antipsychotics compared with conventional agents, atypical antipsychotics may place some patients at risk for medical morbidity resulting from weight gain and adverse metabolic effects. Therefore, medication choices must be individualized. In this section, we first discuss properties common to most of the antipsychotic medications and then describe each of the atypical antipsychotics and treatment recommendations.

Mechanisms of Action

All available antipsychotics antagonize D$_2$ receptors in vitro. However, the theory that psychosis results from hyperdopaminergia is overly simplistic. Underactivity of dopamine in mesocortical pathways, specifically those projecting to the frontal lobes, may account for the negative symptoms of schizophrenia (e.g., anergia, apathy, lack of spontaneity) (K.L. Davis et al. 1991; Goff and Evins 1998). In addition, this underactivity in the frontal lobes may serve to disinhibit mesolimbic dopamine activity via a corticolimbic feedback loop. Overactivity of mesolimbic dopamine is the result, which manifests as the positive symptoms of schizophrenia (e.g., hallucinations, delusions).

The atypical antipsychotics have other physiological properties as well, some of which appear to relate to antagonism of the 5-HT$_2$ receptor, which may modify dopamine activity in a regionally specific manner. This dual 5-HT$_2$/D$_2$ antagonism is believed to account, at least in part, for the unique properties of this group of medications. An additional hypothesis is that the atypical antipsychotic medications have a lower liability for EPS because they have looser binding to the D$_2$ receptor (Kapur and Seeman 2001).

Indications and Efficacy

The most common indications for antipsychotic drugs are the treatment of acute psychosis and the maintenance of psychotic symptom remission in patients with schizophrenia. All conventional antipsychotics have comparable efficacy in schizophrenia when given in equivalent doses (Table 26–9) but differ somewhat in their propensity for some side effects. The atypical antipsychotics appear to be at least as effective as the conventional antipsychotics in the treatment of schizophrenia (Glick and Marder 2005; Goff et al. 1998), but they differ with respect to their tolerability profiles. Clozapine has shown efficacy in patients with schizophrenia after nonresponse to one or more antipsychotic medication trials, including other atypical antipsychotics (Kane 1996; Lewis et al. 2006; McEvoy et al. 2006).

Atypical antipsychotics also have become a key part of the pharmacological armamentarium to treat bipolar disorder. Indeed, all atypical antipsychotics (except clozapine) are approved by the FDA for the treatment of acute mania. Additionally, olanzapine and aripiprazole are approved as maintenance treatments for bipolar disorder. As of September 2007, olanzapine/fluoxetine combination therapy (marketed in the United States under the trade name Symbyax) and quetiapine are the only medications approved by the FDA specifically for the treatment of acute bipolar depressive episodes. The potential use of other atypical antipsychotics in acute bipolar depression is an area of current research interest. The use of these agents in the treatment of bipolar disorder is discussed in the "Mood Stabilizers" section later in this chapter.

Antipsychotic drugs also effectively target psychotic symptoms associated with drug intoxications, delusional disorders, and nonspecific agitation, although the data supporting their use in these conditions are limited. In addition, low doses of antipsychotics may be effective in some patients with borderline or schizotypal personality disorders, particularly when psychotic ideation is targeted (Oldham 2005). In patients with severe OCD, antipsychotics have been used to augment treatment with antiobsessional agents. Antipsychotics and other drugs with dopamine receptor–blocking action (e.g., metoclopramide) are also used for their antiemetic effect. Gilles de la Tourette's syndrome also may be controlled with antipsychotic agents.

Because of the sedating properties of some antipsychotics, these agents may be misused in certain clinical situations, such as for their use solely as hypnotic agents for patients with insomnia or as anxiolytics for

TABLE 26–9. Commonly used atypical and conventional antipsychotic drugs

Generic drug name	Trade name	Usual adult daily dose (mg)	Formulations for administration	Available oral doses (mg)	Approximate oral dose equivalents (mg)
Atypical antipsychotics					
Aripiprazole	Abilify	15–30	po, L, ODT	5, 10, 15, 20, 30; 1 mg/mL	4
Clozapine	Clozaril	250–500	po, ODT	25, 100	100
Olanzapine	Zyprexa	10–20	po, ODT, im	2.5, 5, 7.5, 10, 15, 20	4
Paliperidone	Invega	3–12	po	3, 6, 9	—
Quetiapine	Seroquel	300–600	po	25, 100, 200, 300	125
Quetiapine extended-release	Seroquel XR	400–800	po	200, 300, 400	125
Risperidone	Risperdal	4–6	po, L, ODT, D	0.25, 0.5, 1, 2, 3, 4; 1 mg/mL	1
Ziprasidone	Geodon	80–160	po, im	20, 40, 60, 80	40
Conventional antipsychotics					
Butyrophenones					
Droperidol	Inapsine	2.5–10	im	2.5 mg/mL	—
Haloperidol	Haldol	5–15	po, im, D	0.5, 1, 2, 5, 10, 20	2
Dibenzoxazepines					
Loxapine	Loxitane	45–90	po	5, 10, 25, 50	10
Dihydroindolones					
Molindone	Moban	30–60	po	5, 10, 25, 50	15
Phenothiazines					
Aliphatics					
Chlorpromazine	Thorazine	300–600	po, L, im	10, 25, 50, 100, 200; 100 mg/mL	100
Piperazines					
Fluphenazine	Prolixin	5–15	po, L, im, D	1, 2.5, 5, 10	2
Perphenazine	Trilafon, Etrafon	32–64	po, L	2, 4, 8, 16; 16 mg/mL	10
Trifluoperazine	Stelazine	15–30	po	1, 2, 5, 10	5
Piperidines					
Mesoridazine	Serentil	150–300	po	10, 25, 50, 100	50
Thioridazine	Mellaril	300–600	po, im	10, 15, 25, 50, 100	100
Diphenylbutylpiperidine					
Pimozide	Orap	2–6	po	1, 2	2
Thioxanthenes					
Thiothixene	Navane	15–30	po, L	1, 2, 5, 10, 20; 5 mg/mL	4

Note.   po=oral tablets or capsules; L=liquid; ODT=oral disintegrating tablets; im=intramuscular injections; D=decanoate.

Source.   Equivalent doses from Fuller and Sajatovic 2004a. Adapted from Marangell LB, Martinez JM: *Concise Guide to Psychopharmacology*, 2nd Edition. Arlington, VA, American Psychiatric Publishing, 2006, pp. 92–93. Used with permission.

patients with anxiety. Because of both short- and long-term adverse event risks associated with antipsychotic medications (such as neuroleptic malignant syndrome [NMS] and tardive dyskinesias, which are reviewed later in this section), antipsychotic medications should not be used solely as hypnotic or anxiolytic agents.

Clinical Use

Medication Selection

The choice of antipsychotic medication is often determined, in part, by their safety and tolerability profiles. The prescribing clinician should engage the patient in a discussion of available treatment options and their potential for both short- and long-term side effects. Clozapine is generally reserved for patients with refractory illness, particularly for patients whose symptoms have failed to respond to two or more antipsychotic medication trials (Lewis et al. 2006), because of the risk of agranulocytosis.

A useful construct for conceptualizing differences in side-effect profiles for the conventional antipsychotics is the concept of "high potency" versus "low potency." Drug potency refers to the milligram equivalence of drugs. For example, although haloperidol is more potent than chlorpromazine (haloperidol 2 mg = chlorpromazine 100 mg), therapeutically equivalent doses are equally effective (haloperidol 12 mg = chlorpromazine 600 mg). As a rule, for conventional antipsychotics only, the high-potency antipsychotic drugs have an equivalent dose of less than 5 mg (see Table 26–9). Compared with low-potency conventional antipsychotics, the high-potency agents generally have a higher degree of EPS but less sedation, fewer anticholinergic side effects, and less hypotension. Low-potency conventional antipsychotic drugs have an equivalent dose of greater than 40 mg. These drugs have a high level of sedation, anticholinergic side effects, and hypotension but a lower degree of acute EPS. Importantly, tardive dyskinesia rates do not differ between high- and low-potency conventional antipsychotics. Antipsychotic drugs with intermediate potency (i.e., equivalent dose between 5 and 40 mg) have a side-effect profile that lies between the profiles of these two groups.

The atypical antipsychotics produce fewer EPS than do conventional antipsychotics, particularly clozapine and quetiapine. Additionally, evidence to date suggests that the atypical agents are associated with lower rates of tardive dyskinesia than are the conventional agents. With the exception of risperidone, the atypical antipsychotics also produce substantially less hyperprolactinemia than do the conventional agents.

However, several safety and tolerability issues are associated with atypical antipsychotic medications, including the potential for weight gain and metabolic abnormalities. Weight gain is an important side effect associated to varying degrees with all atypical agents, with less weight gain propensity associated with ziprasidone and aripiprazole.

Optimal Dosages

An optimal dosage or therapeutic range of blood levels has not been identified for most of the antipsychotics. High-dosage strategies are no longer recommended because controlled studies found that modest dosages of conventional antipsychotic drugs are as effective as higher dosages and are better tolerated. Several reviews of controlled trials of conventional antipsychotics concluded that the optimal dosage for most patients is between 300 and 600 mg/day of chlorpromazine equivalents, with some patients responding to lower doses and with little benefit at doses greater than 700 mg/day (Appleton and Davis 1980; Baldessarini et al. 1988; J.M. Davis 1985).

It is important to note that reversal of psychosis is generally not an immediate effect of antipsychotic treatment; instead, improvement in psychosis is often gradual and may occur over several weeks to several months. Thus, clinicians should avoid premature antipsychotic dose escalations during the early phase of treatment if psychotic symptoms do not immediately respond to treatment. Typical dosing for antipsychotic medications is outlined in Table 26–9, and general guidelines for the acute use of antipsychotics are shown in Table 26–10.

Risks, Side Effects, and Their Management

Many side effects of antipsychotic drugs can be understood in terms of the drugs' receptor-blocking properties. When antipsychotics reduce dopamine activity in the nigrostriatal pathway (via dopamine receptor blockade), extrapyramidal signs and symptoms similar to those of Parkinson's disease result. Another locus of dopamine receptors is in the pituitary and hypothalamus (the tuberoinfundibular system), where dopamine is synonymous with prolactin-inhibiting factor. Blockade of dopamine in this system results in hyperprolactinemia. Similarly, antagonism of acetylcholine receptors produces symptoms such as dry mouth, blurred vision, and constipation. Antagonism of α_1-adrenergic receptors results in hypotension, and antagonism of histamine receptors is associated with sedation.

TABLE 26-10. **Guidelines for the acute use of antipsychotic drugs**

- Prior to treatment, obtain a medical and psychiatric history. Baseline laboratory studies are also indicated as part of the initial evaluation. An evaluation for the presence of any abnormal movements is also advisable. An electrocardiogram should be considered for patients with a history of cardiac problems.

- After discussion with the patient and family about the risks and benefits of treatment, select the appropriate antipsychotic agent on the basis of the patient's physical status, the side-effect profile of the drug, and the patient's previous responses to medication, if known.

- Educate the patient and family about the risks of developing metabolic syndrome, diabetes, obesity, dyslipidemia, neuroleptic malignant syndrome, and tardive dyskinesia. Document this discussion in the patient's chart.

- Initiate treatment with antipsychotic medication at low to moderate doses, depending on the patient's history and clinical presentation. Titrate as tolerated to the target dose.

- If possible, administer the antipsychotic medication at bedtime to increase adherence and minimize daytime side effects.

- If the patient has been compliant with treatment and side effects are minimal but no or minimal response to treatment occurs, increase the dose gradually (e.g., every 2–4 weeks). Full response may be delayed for 6 months or longer.

- If the patient still has no response, is taking an adequate dose, and is compliant with treatment, consider another antipsychotic medication.

Source. Lehman et al. 2004. Adapted from Marangell LB, Martinez JM: *Concise Guide to Psychopharmacology*, 2nd Edition. Arlington, VA, American Psychiatric Publishing, 2006, p. 96. Used with permission.

Extrapyramidal Side Effects

EPS include acute dystonic reactions, parkinsonian syndrome, akathisia, tardive dyskinesia, and NMS. Although high-potency conventional antipsychotics are more likely than low-potency conventional antipsychotics to cause EPS, all first-generation antipsychotic drugs are equally likely to cause tardive dyskinesia. The atypical antipsychotics cause substantially fewer EPS, although careful titration of risperidone is necessary to avoid neurological side effects. Although the use of anticholinergic agents or amantadine may prevent or ameliorate EPS, the use of atypical agents is increasingly recommended to avoid these side effects without introducing additional medications. Long-term use of anticholinergic medications should be minimized because these agents can produce significant side effects, including impairments of memory and attention. Clozapine appears to be the only agent that does not cause tardive dyskinesia, and data suggest that a reduced risk with the atypical agents is possible (Correll et al. 2004; Jeste et al. 1999; Margolese et al. 2005; Tarsy and Baldessarini 2006; Tollefson et al. 1997).

Acute dystonic reactions are among the most disturbing and acutely disabling adverse reactions that can occur with the administration of antipsychotic drugs. These reactions occur within hours or days of initiation of treatment with a high-potency conventional antipsychotic medication. The uncontrollable tightening of muscles typically involves spasms of the neck, back (opisthotonos), tongue, or muscles that control lateral eye movement (oculogyric crisis). Laryngeal involvement may compromise the airway and result in ventilatory difficulties (stridor). These reactions are often terrifying to the patient and may seriously jeopardize compliance with medications. Intravenous or intramuscular administration of anticholinergic medication is a rapid and effective treatment for acute dystonia. The drugs and dosages used to treat dystonic reactions are listed in Table 26–11. The effects of the anticholinergic drug given to reverse the dystonia wear off after several hours. Because antipsychotic drugs have long half-lives and durations of action, additional oral anticholinergic drugs should be prescribed for several days after an acute dystonic reaction or longer if treatment with the antipsychotic drug is continued unchanged. Amantadine, 100 mg twice a day, should be considered for treatment of EPS in elderly patients who are highly sensitive to anticholinergic activity, particularly if a switch to an atypical agent is not appropriate.

Acute dystonic reactions may be treated prophylactically with anticholinergic medications, such as benztropine 1–2 mg twice a day. Young patients taking high-potency antipsychotic drugs are at particularly high risk for the development of acute dystonia. We suggest that prophylactic treatment be considered for patients for whom the risk of developing extrapyramidal reactions is high, especially patients younger than 40 years starting high-potency conventional agents. Anticholinergic medication can be tapered and stopped after 10 days.

Parkinsonian syndrome has many of the features

TABLE 26–11. Drugs used to treat extrapyramidal side effects

Generic drug name	Trade name	Drug type (mechanism)	Usual adult dosage	Indications for extrapyramidal side effects
Amantadine	Symmetrel	Dopaminergic agent	100 mg po bid	Parkinsonian syndrome
Benztropine	Cogentin	Anticholinergic agent	1–2 mg po bid	Dystonia, parkinsonian syndrome
			2 mg iv[a]	Acute dystonia
Diphenhydramine	Benadryl	Anticholinergic agent	25–50 mg po tid	Dystonia, parkinsonian syndrome
			25 mg im or iv[a]	Acute dystonia
Propranolol	Inderal	β-Blocker	20 mg po tid 1 mg iv	Akathisia
Trihexyphenidyl	Artane	Anticholinergic agent	5–10 mg po bid	Dystonia, parkinsonian syndrome

Note. po=oral administration of tablets or capsules; bid=twice daily; iv=intravenous; tid=three times a day; im=intramuscular.
[a]Follow with oral medication.

Source. Adapted from Marangell LB, Martinez JM: *Concise Guide to Psychopharmacology,* 2nd Edition. Arlington, VA, American Psychiatric Publishing, 2006, p. 98. Used with permission.

of classic idiopathic Parkinson's disease, including a diminished range of facial expression, cogwheel rigidity, slowed movements, drooling, small handwriting (micrographia), and pill-rolling tremor. This side effect may appear weeks after the initiation of the antipsychotic medication. The most common treatments for idiopathic Parkinson's disease restore the dopamine–acetylcholine balance by increasing dopamine availability. The treatment of antipsychotic medication–related parkinsonism most often involves decreasing the level of acetylcholine (although amantadine, a dopaminergic drug, often effectively attenuates parkinsonian side effects without exacerbating the underlying psychotic illness). Drugs used in the treatment of the parkinsonian side effects of antipsychotic agents are listed in Table 26–11.

The rabbit syndrome, consisting of fine, rapid movements of the lips that resemble the chewing movements of a rabbit, is often considered a subset of parkinsonian side effects. This side effect occurs after more prolonged treatment and may be confused with buccolingual tardive dyskinesia. It has been found in approximately 4% of patients receiving antipsychotics without concomitant anticholinergics (Yassa and Lal 1986). Like parkinsonian side effects, the rabbit syndrome is treated effectively with anticholinergic drugs.

Akinesia is a behavioral state of diminished spontaneity characterized by decreased gestures, unspontaneous speech, apathy, and difficulty with initiating usual activities. Akinesia may appear after several weeks of therapy and is often an element of the parkinsonism syndrome. This drug-induced syndrome may be mistaken for depression or for negative symptoms of schizophrenia.

Akathisia is an extrapyramidal disorder consisting of a subjective feeling of restlessness in the lower extremities, often manifested as an inability to sit still. It is a common reaction that most often occurs shortly after initiation of treatment with a conventional antipsychotic medication or aripiprazole. After a single oral dose of 5 mg of haloperidol, 40% of patients in one study experienced akathisia; this rate increased to 75% after receiving a 10-mg nighttime dose for 1 week (van Putten et al. 1984).

Akathisia is among the most treatment resistant of the acute EPS. Benzodiazepines are helpful in some cases. The current treatment of choice for akathisia is either a switch to an atypical agent (with the exception of aripiprazole) or the addition of a β-adrenergic–blocking drug, particularly propranolol. Several well-controlled studies have documented that propranolol, in dosages up to 120 mg/day, is an effective treatment for akathisia (Adler et al. 1985, 1989; Lipinski et al. 1984). In general, the lipophilic β-blockers are more effective in treating akathisia than the hydrophilic ones. At present, controversy remains as to whether β-selective drugs effectively treat akathisia, with some negative findings (Zubenko et al. 1984b) and some positive reports (Dumon et al. 1992; Dupuis et al. 1987).

Tardive Disorders

Tardive dyskinesia is a disorder characterized by involuntary choreoathetoid movements of the face, trunk, or extremities. The syndrome is usually associated with prolonged exposure to dopamine receptor–blocking agents—most frequently, antipsychotic drugs. However, the antidepressant amoxapine and the antiemetic agents metoclopramide and prochlorperazine can also cause tardive dyskinesia. The American Psychiatric Association Task Force on Tardive Dyskinesia estimated a cumulative incidence of 5% per year of exposure among young adults and a prevalence of 30% after 1 year of treatment with conventional antipsychotics among elderly patients (American Psychiatric Association 1992). Clozapine seems to carry little or no risk of inducing tardive dyskinesia. The incidence of tardive dyskinesia associated with other atypical antipsychotics is higher than that associated with clozapine and lower than that associated with conventional antipsychotics (Correll et al. 2004; Jeste et al. 1999; Tollefson et al. 1997). Elderly patients taking antipsychotics are at increased risk for tardive dyskinesia.

Clinicians can use the Abnormal Involuntary Movement Scale (AIMS) to examine patients for the presence or emergence of tardive dyskinesia (Guy 1976). An evaluation for abnormal movements should be conducted before treatment begins and every 6 or 12 months thereafter. In typical cases, the patient is unaware of mild involuntary movements. Severe dyskinetic movements are less common, which can be disfiguring or even disabling as a result of affecting the muscles involved in the production of speech or swallowing. Although the most common form of tardive disorder is the dyskinetic variety (nonrhythmic, quick choreiform movements), other types have been identified. These include tardive akathisia, tardive dystonia, and tardive tics.

The most commonly accepted hypothesis of the mechanism for the development of tardive dyskinesia is that postsynaptic dopamine receptors develop supersensitivity to dopamine after prolonged dopamine receptor blockade. This model does not account for the time course of tardive dyskinesia onset or for the persistence of tardive dyskinesia after medication has been discontinued. Research has implicated an interaction between oxidative load (free radicals) and glutamatergic neurotoxicity in the disorder (Tsai et al. 1998).

The most significant and consistently documented risk factor for the development of tardive dyskinesia is increasing age of the patient (Branchey and Branchey 1984; Jeste and Wyatt 1982; Kane and Smith 1982). The duration of exposure to a conventional antipsychotic is also an important factor because the cumulative incidence has been shown to remain constant at about 5% for the first 8 years in nonelderly patients. Women have been found to be at greater risk for severe tardive dyskinesia, although the evidence suggests that this finding is limited to geriatric populations (Kennedy et al. 1971; Seide and Muller 1967). Other risk factors may include EPS early in the course of treatment, a history of drug holidays (a greater number of drug-free periods is associated with an increased risk), the presence of brain damage, diabetes mellitus, and a diagnosis of a mood disorder.

The issue of informed consent with respect to the risk of tardive dyskinesia has been extensively reviewed (Munetz and Roth 1985; Roth 1983). In many circumstances, full informed consent may not be obtainable for several weeks from a patient with acute psychosis. A general guideline is to inform and educate the family of the patient about the risks of tardive dyskinesia before starting the antipsychotic and to inform and educate the patient about this disorder as soon as possible. Although the evidence for reduced risk of tardive dyskinesia with atypical agents is not yet conclusive, patients and families should be informed that treatment with a conventional agent may increase the likelihood of irreversible movements compared with treatment with an atypical agent. All such discussions with patients and their families should be documented in the patients' records.

Because antipsychotic medications are the most effective treatment for most patients with schizophrenia, the situation often arises in which a patient develops tardive dyskinesia but still requires an antipsychotic medication to function. If discontinuation of the antipsychotic drug is clinically possible, tardive dyskinesia may gradually diminish; however, involuntary movements often worsen initially with tapering of the antipsychotic dose, a phenomenon referred to as *withdrawal-emergent dyskinesia* (Glazer et al. 1984). Withdrawal-emergent dyskinesia also may occur when a conventional antipsychotic is replaced with an atypical antipsychotic.

Withdrawal-emergent dyskinesia typically resolves within 6 weeks; however, suppressed or latent tardive dyskinesia that has been suppressed by D_2 receptor blockade may not resolve once it has appeared.

Conversely, movements may be masked temporarily by increasing the dosage of the antipsychotic medication, but the symptoms eventually reemerge, often in a more severe form. Anticholinergic drugs may reversibly worsen dyskinetic movements (Reunanen et al. 1982; Yassa 1985), whereas anticholinergic drugs in high doses may improve tardive dystonia (Burke et al. 1982; Fahn 1985).

No definitive treatment for tardive dyskinesias has been identified to date. α-Tocopherol (vitamin E) was shown to be of some benefit in several small studies (Adler et al. 1993; Akhtar et al. 1993; Dabiri et al. 1994; Egan et al. 1992; Elkashef et al. 1990; Lohr and Caligiuri 1996; Lohr et al. 1987), but no benefit was discerned with vitamin E in a Department of Veterans Affairs trial (Adler et al. 1998). Still, vitamin E is a relatively benign antioxidant that may protect neurons from the damaging effects of free radicals, which have been implicated in the etiology of tardive dyskinesia. Despite inconsistent evidence for efficacy, prophylaxis with vitamin E has been recommended. The typical dose of vitamin E is 1,600 IU/day.

Clozapine may be useful for certain patients with tardive dyskinesia who need an antipsychotic medication. In a clinical study by Lieberman et al. (1991), 30 patients with severe tardive dyskinesia were given clozapine at a mean dosage of 486 mg/day for 36 months. On follow-up at 100 weeks, 16 of the 30 patients showed a greater than 50% reduction in their tardive dyskinesia symptoms on the Simpson Dyskinesia Scale, and 10 patients had complete remission. According to the investigators, symptoms did not reemerge over the follow-up period, suggesting that clozapine has a therapeutic effect on tardive dyskinesia that is distinct from the effect of neuroleptics, which only mask the pathology. The study by Lieberman and colleagues seems to confirm the benefits of clozapine on tardive dyskinesia reported in an earlier study by Gerbino et al. (1980).

Neuroleptic Malignant Syndrome

In rare instances, patients taking antipsychotic medications develop a potentially life-threatening disorder known as NMS. Although it occurs most frequently with the use of high-potency conventional antipsychotic drugs, this condition may appear during treatment with any antipsychotic agent, including atypical antipsychotics. Patients with NMS typically have marked muscle rigidity, although this feature may be absent in patients taking atypical antipsychotics. Other features include fever, autonomic instability, increased white blood cell (WBC) counts (>15,000/ mm^3), increased creatine kinase levels (>300 U/mL), and delirium. The increased creatine kinase concentrations are the result of muscle breakdown, which can lead to myoglobinuria and acute renal failure.

In a large prospective study, Rosebush and Stewart (1989) found that NMS was associated most often with the initiation or increase of antipsychotic medication, and in every case it occurred within 1 month of admission to a psychiatric unit. Episodes that occurred in patients taking stable dosages of antipsychotic medications were almost always associated with antecedent dehydration. Lithium use increases the risk appreciably, as does the presence of a mood disorder. Higher dosages, rapid escalation of dosage, and intramuscular injections of antipsychotics are all associated with the development of NMS (Keck et al. 1989).

Treatment of NMS includes discontinuation of the antipsychotic medication, a thorough medical evaluation, administration of intravenous fluids and antipyretic agents, and the use of cooling blankets. Rosebush et al. (1989) reviewed 20 cases of patients who developed NMS while taking conventional agents and found that delaying reinitiation of an antipsychotic by at least 2 weeks after resolution of symptoms was associated with a markedly decreased risk of relapse. Dantrolene and bromocriptine have been reported to improve symptoms of NMS, but their efficacy over supportive care has not been proven and is controversial (Rosebush et al. 1991). Bromocriptine is a centrally active dopamine agonist that has been used successfully in some cases of NMS (Guze and Baxter 1985). Bromocriptine is administered at an initial dosage of 1.25–2.5 mg twice daily, and the dosage may be increased to 10 mg three times a day. Rigidity may respond rapidly, but the temperature elevation, blood pressure instability, and creatinine kinase level may not normalize for several days. Dantrolene sodium, a drug that is also used to treat malignant hyperthermia, is a muscle relaxant that may reduce the thermogenesis of NMS caused by the tonic contraction of skeletal muscles. The manufacturer's recommendation for administration of dantrolene for acute malignant hyperthermia is 1 mg/kg by rapid intravenous push. Administration of the drug should be continued until the symptoms are reversed or until a maximum dose of 10 mg/kg has been given. The oral dosage of dantrolene after a malignant hyperthermic crisis is 4–8 mg/ kg/day in four divided doses. This regimen should be continued until all symptoms resolve. The potential for hepatotoxicity is significant with dantrolene therapy; thus, the drug should not be administered to patients with liver dysfunction.

Anticholinergic Side Effects

Anticholinergic side effects are categorized as peripheral effects or central effects. The most common peripheral side effects are dry mouth, decreased sweating, decreased bronchial secretions, blurred vision, difficulty with urination, constipation, and tachycardia. Bethanechol chloride, a cholinergic drug that does not cross the blood-brain barrier, may effectively treat these side effects at a dosage of 25–50 mg three times a day. Central side effects of anticholinergic drugs include impairment in concentration, attention, and memory. In cases of toxicity, anticholinergic delirium—which includes hot and dry skin, dry mucous membranes, dilated pupils, absent bowel sounds, tachycardia, and confusion—may occur. Anticholinergic delirium is a medical emergency, and full supportive medical care is required. Physostigmine, a centrally and peripherally acting reversible acetylcholinesterase, may be used as a diagnostic agent in cases of suspected anticholinergic toxicity. This agent is administered intramuscularly at a dose of 1–2 mg or intravenously at a slow controlled rate of no more than 1 mg/minute. Physostigmine should not be used to maintain reversal of the toxicity, however, because a cholinergic crisis may result, characterized by nausea, vomiting, bradycardia, and seizures. This reaction can be reversed by administering a potent anticholinergic drug such as atropine.

Adrenergic Side Effects

Antipsychotics block α_1-adrenergic receptors, which can result in orthostatic hypotension and dizziness. Orthostatic hypotension is commonly associated with low-potency conventional agents. Among the atypical agents, clozapine, quetiapine, risperidone, and ziprasidone require initial dose titration, particularly in the elderly, to avoid orthostatic hypotension. Administration of epinephrine, which stimulates both α- and β-adrenergic receptors, will result in a paradoxical drop in blood pressure as a result of the stimulation of β-adrenergic receptors in the presence of α-receptor blockade. In asthmatic patients who require treatment with antipsychotics as well as episodic treatment with β-adrenergic drugs, specific warnings are necessary regarding the dangers associated with the use of epinephrine in the treatment of an acute asthmatic attack.

Endocrine Effects

Numerous studies have suggested a relation between the use of atypical antipsychotic medications and the development of hyperglycemia, dyslipidemia, and metabolic syndrome (American Diabetes Association et al. 2004; review by Citrome et al. 2005). The metabolic syndrome comprises several metabolic risk factors that may be associated with an increased cardiovascular risk. One definition of the metabolic syndrome specifies the presence of three or more of the following five clinical or laboratory features: 1) elevated plasma triglyceride levels ($\geq$150 mg/dL); 2) decreased plasma high-density lipoprotein levels (<50 mg/dL in women or <40 mg/dL in men); 3) elevated fasting glucose levels ($\geq$110 mg/dL); 4) waist circumference greater than 35 inches in women or greater than 40 inches in men; 5) elevated blood pressure ($\geq$130/85 mm Hg) (Citrome et al. 2005; Expert Panel on the Detection, Evaluation, and Treatment of High Blood Cholesterol in Adults 2001).

Hyperglycemia can develop independent of or secondary to weight gain and, in some cases, resolves after discontinuation of the medication. Patients taking clozapine and olanzapine have a higher risk of developing diabetes compared with patients taking other conventional and atypical antipsychotics (see American Diabetes Association et al. 2004). Data indicate that alterations in serum lipids are concordant with changes in body weight. Clozapine and olanzapine are associated with the greatest increases in total cholesterol, low-density lipoprotein, and triglycerides, as well as decreases in high-density lipoprotein. Aripiprazole and ziprasidone do not appear to be associated with dyslipidemia. However, monitoring should be considered for all patients taking an antipsychotic medication.

The NIMH-funded Clinical Antipsychotic Trials of Intervention Effectiveness (CATIE) randomly assigned patients with schizophrenia to treatment with perphenazine, olanzapine, risperidone, quetiapine, or ziprasidone for up to 18 months (Lieberman et al. 2005). With respect to metabolic outcomes, olanzapine-treated patients had a higher discontinuation rate as a result of weight gain or metabolic effects, whereas ziprasidone was the only medication associated with improvements in metabolic parameters (Lieberman et al. 2005).

At present, it appears appropriate to monitor all patients taking atypical antipsychotics for metabolic changes. Published guidelines recommend monitoring patients taking atypical antipsychotics for several metabolic risk factors, including personal and family history of metabolic risks (baseline and annually), waist circumference (baseline and annually), body mass index (baseline, week 4, week 8, week 12, and quarterly), blood pressure and fasting glucose levels (baseline, week 12, and annually), and lipid panel (baseline, week 12, and every 5 years) (American Diabetes Association et al. 2004).

All conventional antipsychotic medications and risperidone may cause hyperprolactinemia. Clinical signs and symptoms of hyperprolactinemia may include gynecomastia, galactorrhea, amenorrhea, and decreased libido. Although such side effects were frequently associated with hyperprolactinemia resulting from conventional antipsychotics, a review of clinical experience with risperidone found relatively low rates of side effects despite markedly elevated prolactin levels (Kleinberg et al. 1997). Hyperprolactinemia secondarily can lower estrogen levels, resulting in amenorrhea and theoretically placing patients at risk for osteoporosis and pathological fractures (Klibanski et al. 1981).

Weight Gain

Both conventional and atypical antipsychotic medications can be associated with weight gain. Antipsychotics associated with weight gain include risperidone, quetiapine, chlorpromazine, thioridazine, olanzapine, and clozapine (Allison et al. 1999; American Diabetes Association et al. 2004); however, all patients taking an antipsychotic medication should be monitored for weight gain throughout treatment. Allison et al. (1999) analyzed results from all published controlled trials of antipsychotic agents and estimated the mean weight change after 10 weeks of treatment for each agent. The effect of conventional antipsychotics ranged from a mean loss of 0.4 kg with molindone to a mean gain of 3.2 kg with thioridazine. Haloperidol produced a mean 1.1-kg weight gain. Among atypical agents, only ziprasidone produced no change in weight; the other atypical agents were associated with the following estimates of weight gain at 10 weeks: risperidone 2.1 kg, olanzapine 4.15 kg, and clozapine 4.45 kg.

Sexual Effects

A combination of anticholinergic effects, α-adrenergic receptor blockade, and hormonal effects may lead to several types of sexual difficulty. In men, inability to achieve or maintain erections, decreased ability to achieve orgasm, and changes in the pleasurable quality of orgasm have been reported with conventional agents (Ghadirian et al. 1982). Thioridazine may cause painful retrograde ejaculation, in which semen is ejected into the bladder. Priapism, which necessitates immediate urological consultation, has been reported, especially with thioridazine and chlorpromazine, although atypical agents also have been linked to priapism. Women may experience changes in the quality of orgasm as well as decreased ability to achieve orgasm with use of antipsychotics. Because sexual side effects are troubling to patients and often interfere with adherence to treatment, regular assessment by the clinician of sexual side effects is important.

Ocular Effects

Antipsychotics may cause pigmentary changes in the lens and retina, especially if the drugs are administered for long periods. Pigment deposition in the lens of the eye does not affect vision; however, pigmentary retinopathy, which can lead to irreversible blindness, has been associated specifically with the use of thioridazine. Although pigmentary retinopathy has been reported most often in patients taking more than 800 mg/day of thioridazine (the maximum recommended dose), this condition also has occurred at usual clinical doses (Ball and Caroff 1986; Hamilton 1985).

Quetiapine was associated with cataracts in preclinical safety studies conducted in beagles (Seroquel Package Insert 2001). Subsequent studies involving nonhuman primates did not detect an increased risk of cataracts; postmarketing surveys have not detected an increased risk of cataracts in patients taking quetiapine compared with patients taking other antipsychotics (Laties et al. 2000). In the CATIE trial, no significant differences were noted in the occurrence of new cataracts among the treatment groups (Lieberman et al. 2005).

Dermatological Effects

Patients taking antipsychotics, especially the aliphatic phenothiazines (e.g., chlorpromazine), may become more sensitive to sunlight, which can lead to severe sunburn.

Cardiac Effects

In materials submitted to the Psychopharmacological Drugs Advisory Committee of the FDA, Pfizer, Inc., reported results from a trial designed to examine the ECG effects of atypical agents and thioridazine at maximum therapeutic serum concentrations and at the potentially higher concentrations that might occur in clinical practice if these agents were co-prescribed with metabolic inhibitors. After correcting the QT interval for heart rate, thioridazine produced the greatest mean delay in QTc (35.6 ms), followed by ziprasidone (20.6 ms), quetiapine (9.1 ms), olanzapine (6.8 ms), and haloperidol (4.7 ms). Quetiapine produced the greatest increase in heart rate (11 beats/minute). Addition of metabolic inhibitors only produced further increases in QTc when added to quetiapine (19.7 ms) and haloperidol (8.9 ms). Although the mean 39% increase in serum ziprasidone concentrations produced by ketoconazole coadministration did not result in an increase in the mean QTc duration, ziprasidone serum concentrations weakly correlated with QTc duration. In 8 cases of overdose reported by the manufacturer and 1 published case (Burton et al. 2000), ziprasidone did not produce significant cardiac toxicity. Only 2 of 3,095 subjects (0.06%) in premarketing trials developed QTc intervals longer than 500 ms; however, participants in these trials were screened to exclude cardiac disease. In 2 reports of overdose with quetiapine, prolongation of the QT interval was observed (Gajwani et al. 2000; Hustey 1999), whereas most reported cases of overdose with risperidone and olanzapine have described relatively benign ECG findings. In the CATIE trial, ziprasidone was not associated with a greater rate of occurrences of prolonged QTc intervals compared with the other antipsychotics studied, and no instances of torsades de pointes were reported (Lieberman et al. 2005).

In several studies, sudden death attributed to thioridazine or chlorpromazine therapy in young, healthy patients has been reported (Aherwadkar et al. 1974; Giles and Modlin 1968). Thioridazine slows atrial and ventricular conduction and prolongs refractory periods. Thus, thioridazine can be quite dangerous if taken in overdose or in combination with quinidine-like drugs. Chlorpromazine also prolongs QT intervals and atrioventricular conduction, even at relatively low doses (150 mg/day). Pimozide also may produce significant changes in cardiac conduction as a result of its calcium channel–blocking properties. It is recommended that serial ECGs be performed when treatment with pimozide is started, and the drug should be discontinued if the QT interval exceeds 520 ms (in adults) or 470 ms (in children). This strategy should be considered for patients taking thioridazine and ziprasidone, but it is not mandatory in healthy patients. Extremely high doses of intravenous haloperidol have been administered safely in patients with cardiac disease, although rare cases of torsades de pointes have been reported at these doses (Metzger and Friedman 1993).

Hepatic Effects

Increased levels on liver function tests have been associated with antipsychotic treatment. If abnormalities suggest obstructive liver disease, with increases in bilirubin and alkaline phosphatase, the drug must be immediately discontinued. This reaction appears to be more common with low-potency conventional antipsychotics. Transient elevations in hepatic enzymes have been observed with olanzapine and quetiapine, but these laboratory findings have not been linked to liver injury.

Hematological Effects

Transient leukopenia and, in rare cases, agranulocytosis have been associated with neuroleptic treatment. Although agranulocytosis is strictly defined as a complete absence of all granulocytes in the blood, it also may refer to severe neutropenia, with a neutrophil count of less than 500/mL. This idiosyncratic reaction usually occurs within the first 3–4 weeks after the initiation of treatment with an antipsychotic drug. However, this risk continues for 2–3 months during therapy. A higher risk of agranulocytosis is associated with low-potency conventional antipsychotic drugs and, most significantly, clozapine.

Signs and symptoms of this reaction include high fever, stomatitis, severe pharyngitis, lymphadenopathy, and malaise. Patients should be educated about the signs and symptoms of agranulocytosis and instructed to contact their physician immediately should these symptoms develop. Treatment of this reaction requires immediate discontinuation of all medications, immediate medical evaluation and treatment, and vigorous treatment of any infections that develop. Agranulocytosis usually resolves after discontinuation of the causative agent.

Lowered Seizure Threshold

Most conventional antipsychotics are associated with a dose-dependent risk of a lowered seizure threshold, although the incidence of seizures with most of these drugs is quite small. Of all the conventional antipsychotics, molindone and fluphenazine have been shown most consistently to have the lowest potential for this side effect (Itil and Soldatos 1980; Oliver et al. 1982). The atypical antipsychotic clozapine is associated with a dose-dependent risk of seizure and has been estimated to produce seizures in as many 10% of the patients receiving the drug for 3.8 years.

Suppressed Temperature Regulation

Antipsychotic drugs directly affect the hypothalamus and suppress temperature regulation. In combination with the α-adrenergic receptor antagonism and cholinergic receptor antagonism of antipsychotics, this effect becomes particularly serious in hot, humid weather. Severe hyperthermia, rhabdomyolysis, renal failure, and death may result. This potentially life-threatening condition requires immediate medical intervention and supportive treatment. A cool environment and adequate amounts of fluids are mandatory for patients taking antipsychotic agents.

Risks in Elderly Patients With Dementia

Treatment with atypical antipsychotics recently has been associated with an almost twofold increased mortality rate when used in elderly patients with dementia. It is important to note that these medications are often used in clinical practice, but they are not approved by the FDA for the treatment of dementia-related psychosis (Herrmann and Lanctot 2005). The risk associated with atypical antipsychotics is not statistically different from the risk associated with treatment with conventional antipsychotics (Gill et al. 2005).

Use in Pregnancy

Like most other drugs, antipsychotic agents should be avoided, if possible, during pregnancy and during lactation periods for breast-feeding mothers. The use of low-potency phenothiazine antipsychotics during the first trimester of pregnancy may increase the baseline risk of congenital anomalies by 0.4%, or 4 cases per 1,000 pregnancies (Altshuler et al. 1996). Infants born to mothers who were first exposed to antipsychotic drugs during the sixth to tenth week of gestation may have an increase in birth defects (Edlund and Craig 1984).

Less is known about the risks for teratogenicity, perinatal complications, and neurobehavioral problems associated with atypical antipsychotic medications. Data from a prospective comparative study indicated that treatment with olanzapine, risperidone, quetiapine, and clozapine was not associated with a significantly higher risk of major malformations; however, treatment with these agents was associated with a lower birthrate ($P=0.05$) and higher rate of therapeutic abortions ($P=0.003$) (McKenna et al. 2005). Data related to the use of aripiprazole and ziprasidone are still limited (see review by Gentile 2004). One case of agenesis of the corpus callosum was reported with risperidone use (*Physicians' Desk Reference* 2001). A possible case of a meningocele and ankyloblepharon associated with olanzapine was reported (Arora and Praharaj 2006).

The use of medications in a woman who is pregnant is always a difficult decision. For example, Edlund and Craig (1984) pointed out that because the risk of fetal death is increased in psychotic mothers, the small risk of neuroleptic-induced teratogenesis must be assessed carefully and balanced against the risks involved in withholding treatment. These important issues have been reviewed in detail elsewhere (Altshuler et al. 1996). Additionally, the risk for the development of hyperglycemia in conjunction with the use of atypical antipsychotic medications during pregnancy must be considered.

In addition, antipsychotic agents should be prescribed with great caution in the peripartum period. Extrapyramidal symptoms and neonatal jaundice have been reported in infants following in utero exposure to conventional antipsychotic drugs. Also, neonates may be exposed to small amounts of antipsychotics in breast milk (Stewart et al. 1980). It is therefore necessary to reassess the potential risks and benefits of antipsychotic treatment as the pregnancy comes to term. As a general guideline, antipsychotic drugs should be used in pregnant patients only if absolutely necessary, at the minimal dose required, and for the briefest possible time. Documentation of informed consent from both the mother and the father is necessary. Use of ECT to treat acute psychosis in pregnant mothers should be considered.

Drug Interactions

Antipsychotic drugs have profound effects on multiple CNS receptors, and these effects are compounded when other medications are added. For example, the α-adrenergic receptor blockade of antipsychotics may affect the efficacy of the antihypertensive drug guanethidine. The sedative and anticholinergic effects of antipsychotic drugs are increased with the addition of other sedating or anticholinergic drugs. As mentioned previously, patients taking drugs with potentially serious adverse effects should be monitored through plasma level determinations when other medications are used concurrently.

Pharmacokinetic interactions with antipsychotic drugs are common and have been reviewed elsewhere (Goff and Baldessarini 1995). Most antipsychotics are metabolized by the hepatic CYP2D6 isoenzyme. Exceptions include ziprasidone and quetiapine, which are metabolized mainly by the CYP3A4 enzyme. The activity of the CYP2D6 enzyme varies greatly (on the basis of genetic polymorphisms) among individuals and can be inhibited by certain drugs, such as SSRIs. For example, the addition of fluoxetine increased serum haloperidol concentrations by 20% and serum fluphenazine concentrations by 65% in one study (Goff et al. 1995). Two categories of potential drug–drug interactions are of particular concern. The first includes interactions that can increase serum concentrations of antipsychotics to dangerous levels. For example, clozapine is metabolized by the CYP2D6, CYP3A4, and CYP1A2 isoenzymes. When taken with CYP3A4 and CYP1A2 inhibitors, such as erythromycin and fluvoxamine, serum clozapine concentrations can rise to toxic levels (L.G. Cohen et al. 1996; Wetzel et al. 1998). The other category of potentially serious interactions includes those that induce metabolism of antipsychotic agents, thereby lowering serum concentrations below a therapeutic threshold. Large reductions in serum clozapine and haloperidol concentrations have been reported with the addition of carbamazepine, phenobarbital, and phenytoin (Arana et al. 1986; Byerly and DeVane 1996). Notably, cigarette smoking can affect antipsychotic metabolism; serum concentrations of clozapine in particular are reduced with smoking and increased after smoking cessation (Byerly and DeVane 1996; Haring et al. 1989).

Atypical Antipsychotics

The atypical antipsychotics are referred to as *atypical* (compared with conventional antipsychotics) for several reasons, including their receptor binding profiles, improved side-effect profile, and spectrum of efficacy in patients with schizophrenia. In general, the atypical antipsychotic drugs provide superior efficacy for the treatment of negative symptoms, produce fewer acute motor side effects, and may reduce the risk of tardive dyskinesia compared with conventional antipsychotic drugs. These drugs also may improve cognitive function in patients with schizophrenia (Green et al. 1997; Hagger et al. 1993; Purdon et al. 2000; Rossi et al. 1997). In this subsection, we review the atypical antipsychotic medications currently available in the United States: clozapine, olanzapine, risperidone, quetiapine, ziprasidone, aripiprazole, and paliperidone.

Clozapine

Clozapine, the first of the class of atypical antipsychotic drugs, was a landmark in the treatment of schizophrenia for several reasons. It was the first medication shown to be efficacious in otherwise nonresponsive patients. In addition, clozapine was the first agent to attenuate significantly the negative symptoms of schizophrenia, such as marked social withdrawal and apathy, thereby helping many patients return to meaningful and productive lives. Also, clozapine rarely produces EPS, and to date it is the only antipsychotic drug that is not associated with treatment-emergent tardive dyskinesia. This important clinical property is concordant with the observation that chronic administration of clozapine results in selective inhibition of dopamine neurons in the mesolimbic pathways, with little functional effect on striatal dopamine tracts. Finally, clozapine has minimal effects on the tuberoinfundibular system, and therefore it does not cause hyperprolactinemia.

Clozapine is the prototype for the atypical antipsy-chotic medication class. However, because it is associated with a risk for agranulocytosis, clozapine use is restricted to patients who have not adequately responded to or tolerated treatment with two other antipsychotics (Lewis et al. 2006). Several studies have confirmed its efficacy in patients with a history of nonresponse to previous antipsychotic treatment (Kane et al. 1988; Lewis et al. 2006; McEvoy et al. 2006). Kane et al. (1988) studied patients with chronic schizophrenia whose symptoms had failed to improve after at least three adequate trials of conventional antipsychotics. Data from this large multicenter, double-blind prospective study indicated a significant improvement in 30% of the patients taking clozapine, compared with only 4% of those taking chlorpromazine. McEvoy et al. (2006) randomly assigned patients with schizophrenia who had prospectively not responded to an atypical antipsychotic medication in the CATIE trial to open treatment with clozapine or blinded treatment with olanzapine, risperidone, or quetiapine. They reported that switching to clozapine was more effective in atypical antipsychotic nonresponders than switching to a different atypical agent. Similarly, Lewis et al. (2006) randomly assigned patients with a primary psychotic disorder (schizophrenia, schizoaffective disorder, or delusional disorder) who had previously failed to respond to two or more antipsychotic medications to treatment with clozapine or a different atypical antipsychotic medication (risperidone, olanzapine, quetiapine, or amisulpride). In this trial, clozapine was associated with greater symptomatic improvement compared with the other atypical antipsychotics (Lewis et al. 2006).

Less rigorous data suggest that clozapine also may be effective in refractory schizoaffective disorder, psychotic mood disorders, and rapid-cycling bipolar disorder, even in the absence of psychosis (Calabrese et al. 1996; Keck et al. 1996; McElroy et al. 1991; Suppes et al. 1992; Zarate et al. 1995). Because clozapine appears to be devoid of parkinsonian side effects, it is also useful in low dosages (25 mg/day) for patients with Parkinson's disease and psychosis induced by dopamine agonists. Other indications require higher dosages, as discussed later, and an extended period of titration to achieve therapeutic dosages and clinical response.

Clozapine is a difficult drug for both patient and physician, but when other treatments have failed, there is no doubt that the potential benefits of this remarkable medication are worth the risks for many patients with severe psychotic illnesses.

Mechanism of action. Clozapine has a wide range of physiological actions. A great deal of research has focused on clozapine's relatively greater 5-HT$_2$ than D$_2$ antagonism, and this property has been the predominant focus of new drug development in the atypical antipsychotic medication class.

Clozapine shows high in vitro receptor affinities for the D$_4$, 5-HT$_2$, α_1-adrenergic, muscarinic, and H$_1$ receptors and a relatively weak affinity for D$_1$, D$_2$, and D$_3$ receptors. The high 5-HT$_2$-to-D$_2$ ratio is hypothesized to be responsible for many of clozapine's advantages over typical antipsychotic drugs, either directly or indirectly (Meltzer 1991). Other investigators have suggested that clozapine's superior efficacy may be related to the drug's ability to increase norepinephrine outflow (Breier et al. 1994) or may be a result of indirect effects on glutamatergic systems (Goff and Coyle 2001). Unlike conventional agents, clozapine reverses several effects produced by blockade of glutamatergic N-methyl-D-aspartate (NMDA) receptors in animal models thought to be predictive of therapeutic response in schizophrenia (Goff and Coyle 2001).

Clinical use. Because of prominent sedation and orthostatic hypotension, clozapine therapy is initiated at a dosage of 12.5 mg/day, with a rapid increase to 12.5 mg twice a day. The dose is then increased as tolerated, generally in 25- or 50-mg increments every day or every other day. Clozapine is usually added to the previous antipsychotic agent in a cross-titration in which the dose of the previous drug is tapered once a clozapine dosage of approximately 100 mg/day has been achieved. This strategy should be used with caution if the existing medication is a low-potency conventional antipsychotic because of the possibility of additive α-adrenergic and anticholinergic side effects. Clozapine doses can be increased much more rapidly in an inpatient setting, with monitoring of vital signs, than in an outpatient setting. The typical target dose is 300–500 mg/day in divided doses. Although routine blood level monitoring is not recommended, a serum level greater than 350 ng/mL is associated with a higher response rate (Perry et al. 1991). Serum levels should be ascertained in nonresponders. The duration of treatment required to assess response is longer than for most medications—that is, typically 3–6 months (Meltzer 1994). If patients are nonresponsive after 6 months of continuous clozapine treatment, the dosage may be gradually increased to a maximum of 900 mg/day.

Risks, side effects, and their management. *Agranulocytosis.* Agranulocytosis was previously estimated to occur in 0.8% of the patients receiving clozapine during the first year of treatment, with a peak inci-

dence at 3 months. However, a system of hematological monitoring has reduced agranulocytosis-related fatalities to extremely low levels (Honigfeld et al. 1998). The dispensing of clozapine in the United States is linked to weekly WBC counts during the first 6 months of treatment and biweekly counts thereafter. Strict guidelines based on WBC and absolute neutrophil counts have been set (Table 26–12). Since the implementation of the Clozaril National Registry in the United States, the rate of agranulocytosis has been estimated to be 0.38% on the basis of data collected from February 1990 to December 1994 (Honigfeld 1996; Honigfeld et al. 1998).

TABLE 26–12. Hematological monitoring guidelines for patients taking clozapine

- Initial white blood cell (WBC) count must be greater than 3,500/mm^3, and absolute neutrophil count (ANC) must be greater than 2,000/mm^3.

- Weekly WBC count and ANC are required for the first 6 months of treatment and for 4 weeks after discontinuation of clozapine. After 6 months, monitoring is required every 2 weeks; and after 12 months, monitoring is required every 4 weeks.

- If WBC count is 2,000–3,000/mm^3 or ANC is 1,000–1,500/mm^3, interrupt therapy and monitor for signs of infection. Perform WBC and differential counts daily. If no symptoms of infection are seen, if WBC count returns to greater than 3,000/mm^3, and if ANC is greater than 1,500/mm^3, resume clozapine therapy with twice-weekly WBC and differential counts until total WBC count returns to more than 3,500/mm^3 and ANC is greater than 2,000/mm^3.

- If WBC count is less than 2,000/mm^3 or ANC is less than 1,000/mm^3, discontinue clozapine and do not rechallenge. Perform WBC and differential counts daily until WBC count is greater than 3,000/mm^3 and ANC is greater than 1,500/mm^3. Then monitor twice weekly until WBC count returns to more than 3,500/mm^3 and ANC is greater than 2,000/mm^3. Then monitor weekly for 4 weeks. Treat any infection with antibiotics. Consider bone marrow aspiration to ascertain granulopoietic status. If granulopoiesis is deficient, consider protective isolation.

Source. Adapted from Marangell LB, Martinez JM: *Concise Guide to Psychopharmacology,* 2nd Edition. Arlington, VA, American Psychiatric Publishing, 2006, p. 112. Used with permission.

If agranulocytosis develops, prompt consultation with a hematologist is indicated. Reverse isolation and prophylactic antibiotics may be used to prevent infection. Granulocyte colony–stimulating factors may be used to shorten the duration and reduce the morbidity of agranulocytosis (Barnas et al. 1992; Gerson et al. 1992; Nielsen 1993). Although lithium often causes leukocytosis, it does not appear to treat or prevent clozapine-induced agranulocytosis. Once a patient has developed agranulocytosis while taking clozapine, he or she should not be rechallenged with this medication.

Clozapine is contraindicated in patients who have myeloproliferative disorders or who are immunocompromised as a result of diseases such as active tuberculosis or human immunodeficiency virus infection because of their increased risk for agranulocytosis. Concomitant administration of medications that are associated with bone marrow suppression, such as carbamazepine, is also contraindicated.

Extrapyramidal side effects. EPS are uncommon with any dose of clozapine, although some patients experience akathisia or hand tremors. Note that a risk for NMS exists; indeed, NMS has been reported in patients medicated with clozapine alone (Anderson and Powers 1991; DasGupta and Young 1991; Miller et al. 1991).

Sedation. Sedation is the most common side effect of clozapine, and it is particularly prominent early in treatment. Sedation generally attenuates when the dose is reduced, when tolerance to this side effect develops, or when a disproportionate amount is given at bedtime.

Cardiovascular effects. Hypotension and tachycardia occur in most patients taking clozapine. Additionally, cases of potentially fatal myocarditis and dilated cardiomyopathy have been reported (Kilian et al. 1999). Myocarditis typically occurs within 3 weeks of starting clozapine, but cardiomyopathy may not be apparent for several years. Although rare, treatment-emergent myocarditis and cardiomyopathy occur at a reportedly higher incidence rate with clozapine than with other antipsychotics.

Weight gain. Weight gain is a common side effect of clozapine. Body weight increases by 10% or more in many patients. One naturalistic study found that weight gain did not plateau with clozapine therapy until year 4, and the weight gain was not dose related (Henderson et al. 2000).

Endocrine effects. As noted earlier, numerous studies suggested a relation between the use of atypical antipsychotic medications and the development of hyperglycemia, dyslipidemia, and metabolic syndrome (American Diabetes Association et al. 2004; review by Citrome et al. 2005). Patients should receive nutritional counseling at the initiation of treatment with clozapine, and weight and other metabolic parameters should be monitored, as noted earlier in this section.

Hypersalivation. Hypersalivation occurs in one-third of the patients taking clozapine. However, because clozapine has potent anticholinergic properties, addition of an anticholinergic agent is not recommended for control of hypersalivation.

Fever. Clozapine is associated with benign, transient temperature increases, generally within the first 3 weeks of treatment. Patients taking clozapine who develop fevers should be evaluated for infections, agranulocytosis, and NMS.

Seizures. Clozapine is associated with a dose-dependent risk of seizures. The vast majority of clozapine-induced seizures are tonic-clonic, but myoclonic seizures also occur. Doses less than 300 mg/day are associated with a 1%–3% risk of seizures. Doses of 300–600 mg/day carry a 2.7% risk, and doses greater than 600 mg/day are associated with a 4.4% risk (Devinsky et al. 1991). Because of this risk, clozapine doses greater than 600 mg/day are not recommended unless the patient's symptoms have not responded at lower doses. Once a seizure has occurred, determining whether to continue using clozapine requires clinical judgment. Carbamazepine use must be avoided in patients taking clozapine because of the additive risk of bone marrow suppression. At present, valproate appears to be the safest anticonvulsant for patients taking clozapine.

Anticholinergic side effects. Anticholinergic effects, such as dry mouth, blurred vision, constipation, and urinary retention, are common early side effects.

Obsessive-compulsive symptoms. Clozapine has been reported to exacerbate symptoms of OCD, probably because of 5-HT$_2$ antagonism (Ghaemi et al. 1995). If this effect occurs, symptoms are usually controlled with the addition of an SSRI.

Drug interactions. Clozapine should not be combined with any drugs that have the potential to suppress bone marrow function, such as carbamazepine. There have been isolated reports of respiratory arrest in patients taking both clozapine and a high-potency benzodiazepine. Thus, benzodiazepines (particularly in high doses) should not be administered to patients taking clozapine.

Clozapine is metabolized by hepatic CYP1A2 and, to a lesser degree, CYP3A3/4; therefore, the drug is subject to changes in serum concentration when combined with medications that inhibit or induce these enzymes. Serum clozapine levels increase with coadministration of fluvoxamine or erythromycin and decrease with coadministration of phenobarbital or phenytoin and with cigarette smoking (Byerly and DeVane 1996). These pharmacokinetic interactions are particularly important because of the dose-dependent risk of seizures.

Olanzapine

Olanzapine represents a modification of the clozapine molecule. Like risperidone, olanzapine is a monoaminergic antagonist with high-affinity binding at the 5-HT$_2$ and D$_1$, D$_2$, D$_3$, and D$_4$ receptors. Compared with clozapine, olanzapine has greater D$_2$ and weaker D$_4$ and α-adrenergic affinity. Despite its structural similarity to clozapine, olanzapine is not associated with higher-than-expected rates of agranulocytosis. Although in vitro binding studies have indicated a high affinity for M$_1$ receptors, anticholinergic side effects are not as prominent as these data would predict.

In the CATIE trial, which randomly assigned 1,493 patients with chronic schizophrenia to treatment for up to 18 months with olanzapine (range=7.5–30 mg/day; mean modal dose=20.1 mg/day), quetiapine (range= 200–800 mg/day; mean modal dose=543.4 mg/day), risperidone (range=1.5–6.0 mg/day; mean modal dose=3.9 mg/day), ziprasidone (range=40–160 mg/ day; mean modal dose=112.8 mg/day), or perphenazine (range = 8–32 mg/day; mean modal dose = 20.8 mg/day), olanzapine showed better effectiveness (lower rates of discontinuation, shorter duration of successful treatment, and lower rates of hospitalizations) compared with other agents (Lieberman et al. 2005).

Acute dystonia is uncommon. Akathisia may occur, but it is significantly less common than with the conventional antipsychotic drugs. In prospective double-blind studies, treatment-emergent tardive dyskinesia was reported to occur in 1% of the olanzapine group compared with 4.6% of the haloperidol group (Tollefson et al. 1997). Olanzapine is associated with modest dose-dependent elevations in serum prolactin levels, but most often these elevations are transient and within the normal reference range (Tollefson et al. 1997).

Clinical use. The recommended starting dosage of olanzapine is 10 mg at bedtime for patients with

schizophrenia and 10–15 mg at bedtime for acutely manic patients. The clinically effective dosage range is 7.5–20 mg/day (5–20 mg/day in mania). Olanzapine can be administered in a single daily dose at bedtime. It is important to note that meaningful improvement may not be evident for the first several weeks after initiation of treatment. Usual dosages for maintenance treatment in patients with bipolar disorder range from 5 to 20 mg/day. Although no systematic data are available regarding switching from other antipsychotic drugs to olanzapine, early clinical experience favors a gradual cross-titration. Commonly, olanzapine is added to the existing antipsychotic medication, whose dose is tapered after 1–2 weeks.

Olanzapine is available in a short-acting intramuscular injectable form, providing clinicians with another option for treating acute agitation associated with psychosis or mania. A double-blind, placebo-controlled comparison of intramuscular olanzapine and intramuscular haloperidol in the treatment of acute agitation in patients with schizophrenia indicated that treatment with olanzapine was superior to intramuscular placebo injections for decreasing agitation; this reduction in agitation was dose dependent. No significant difference in response was seen between the haloperidol and the olanzapine groups. Olanzapine was well tolerated (Breier et al. 2002). Peak plasma concentrations are achieved within 15–45 minutes. It is available in vials containing 10 mg of olanzapine for administration.

Risks, side effects, and their management. *Somnolence.* Somnolence is a common, dose-dependent side effect of olanzapine. Patients often become tolerant to this side effect over time.

Anticholinergic side effects. Anticholinergic side effects are clinically less significant than would be predicted on the basis of in vitro muscarinic receptor–binding affinity. However, dry mouth has been reported in association with olanzapine treatment (Beasley et al. 1996).

Seizures. Treatment-emergent seizures are rare in the absence of concomitant medical disorders. Premarketing studies reported a 0.9% incidence of seizures, some of which were attributed to concomitant medical disorders (Zyprexa Package Insert 2007). Olanzapine should be used with caution in patients with a history of seizures and in patients with conditions that may lower the seizure threshold, such as dementia.

Hepatic effects. Transaminase levels were increased in approximately 2% of the patients taking olanzapine in premarketing evaluation. In many cases, these levels normalized without medication discontinuation. Routine laboratory monitoring is not recommended, but olanzapine should be used with caution in patients with hepatic disease or with additional risk factors for hepatic toxicity. In this group of patients, serum transaminase levels must be monitored if olanzapine is prescribed.

Weight gain. Treatment-emergent weight gain is common with olanzapine therapy and averages about 4.15 kg after 10 weeks of treatment (Allison et al. 1999). By 39 weeks, weight gain tends to plateau (Kinon et al. 2001), and approximately 20% of patients may not gain weight. Patients with higher body mass indices (>27.6 kg/m^2) tend to gain less weight than do those with lower body mass indices. Weight gain is independent of dose (Kinon et al. 2001). In the CATIE trial, significantly more olanzapine-treated patients gained 7% or more of their baseline body weight compared with those receiving other agents (Lieberman et al. 2005). Nutritional education should be provided to patients, along with monitoring of caloric intake by diet diaries, and exercise should be strongly encouraged. Weight reduction groups are often helpful in providing instructional materials and offering support.

Drug interactions.   Olanzapine is metabolized by several pathways and is unlikely to be affected by concurrent administration of other medications. Additionally, olanzapine does not appear to inhibit any cytochrome P450 enzymes. However, additive pharmacodynamic effects are expected if olanzapine is combined with medications that also have anticholinergic, antihistaminic, or α_1-adrenergic side effects.

Risperidone

Risperidone is an atypical antipsychotic medication that combines D_2 receptor antagonism with potent $5-HT_2$ receptor antagonism. Risperidone has a higher affinity for D_2 receptors than does clozapine. Risperidone also antagonizes D_1 and D_4 receptors, α_1- and α_2-adrenergic receptors, and H_1 receptors. Risperidone was more effective than haloperidol 20 mg/day against both the positive and the negative symptoms of chronic schizophrenia (Chouinard et al. 1993; Marder and Meibach 1994). The optimal dosage of risperidone in the North American trials was 6 mg/day, but subsequent clinical experience has indicated that most patients do well on lower dosages of 3–6 mg/

day, and the elderly may require dosages as low as 0.5 mg/day. Clinicians should titrate the dose of risperidone to avoid EPS. Unlike the other atypical agents, risperidone elevates prolactin levels.

Bondolfi et al. (1996) reported that risperidone was comparable to clozapine in treatment-refractory schizophrenia; however, in their study, the patients' symptoms were not as highly refractory as were the symptoms in the earlier studies of clozapine in refractory schizophrenia, and the dose of clozapine administered to the comparison group was quite low (Kane et al. 1988). Although clinical experience suggests that risperidone is unlikely to be as effective as clozapine in highly refractory cases, Marder and Meibach (1994) found that schizophrenic patients presumed to be treatment resistant because they had been hospitalized for 6 months or longer at the time of study entry did not respond to haloperidol 20 mg/day but significantly improved with risperidone 6 or 16 mg/day compared with placebo.

Clinical use.   Risperidone is most effective at total daily doses of 4–6 mg. For initial treatment, we recommend using divided doses, starting at 1 mg twice a day and quickly increasing to 2 mg twice a day. For elderly persons, the initial dose should be much lower (0.25–0.5 mg/day). After the first week of treatment, the entire dose can be given at bedtime. This approach usually helps the patient sleep and reduces daytime side effects. However, we do not suggest this practice for elderly persons because of an increased risk of falling.

Risperidone is the only atypical antipsychotic currently available in a long-acting injectable form (Risperdal Consta). Results from a 12-week multicenter double-blind study indicated that long-acting risperidone is more effective than placebo for improving the positive and negative symptoms associated with schizophrenia (Kane et al. 2003). The medication is typically well tolerated.

Risks, side effects, and their management.   Insomnia, hypotension, agitation, headache, and rhinitis are the most common side effects of risperidone. These tend to lessen with time. Overall, the drug tends to be well tolerated. Risperidone does not have significant anticholinergic side effects. Hyperprolactinemia is common.

Extrapyramidal side effects. In comparison with relatively high dosages of haloperidol (20 mg/day), risperidone is associated with a lower prevalence of acute extrapyramidal effects and akathisia. EPS occurs in a dose-dependent manner, with more frequent occurrence when the dosage is greater than 6 mg/day. Thus, clinicians are advised to titrate the dose of risperidone in a manner that maximizes its clinical benefits and minimizes EPS.

Cardiovascular effects. Brief hypotension may occur, as may be expected with α-adrenergic receptor blockade. Tachycardia is also common.

Tardive disorders. Risperidone at low doses produces few parkinsonian side effects. The incidence of risperidone-induced tardive dyskinesia is not known, but it is assumed to be between that of clozapine and the conventional antipsychotics. In one 9-month study of elderly patients, risperidone produced very low rates of tardive dyskinesia compared with haloperidol (Jeste et al. 1999).

Weight gain. Weight gain associated with risperidone treatment is quite variable and is generally less than weight gain associated with olanzapine and clozapine (Allison et al. 1999). The mean weight gain after 10 weeks of exposure to risperidone is approximately 2.1 kg. All patients taking atypical antipsychotics should be monitored for weight gain, particularly during the early course of treatment.

Drug interactions. Risperidone is metabolized primarily by CYP2D6 (Byerly and DeVane 1996). Medications that inhibit this enzyme, such as many of the SSRIs, cause increases in plasma risperidone levels. However, there does not appear to be an increase in side effects resulting from such an interaction, possibly because the primary metabolite of risperidone, 9-OH risperidone, is fully active and is excreted unchanged by the kidneys (Shelton and Stahl 2004). Inhibition of the CYP2D6 enzyme may merely alter the balance between parent drug and metabolite without significantly altering total D_2 occupancy. Pharmacodynamic interactions may occur when risperidone is combined with medications that share a similar physiological effect, such as orthostatic hypotension.

Quetiapine

Quetiapine is a dibenzothiazepine derivative with weak affinity for 5-HT_{1A}, 5-HT_2, D_1, D_2, H_1, α_1, and α_2 receptors. Quetiapine has very "loose" binding to D_2 receptors. For example, D_2 receptor occupancy may decline from approximately 57% when measured 3 hours after an oral quetiapine dose of 400 mg to 20% after 9 hours. In a fixed-dose comparison of quetiapine to haloperidol (12 mg/day) and placebo, quetiapine

was superior to placebo at doses of 150–750 mg on most measures but superior to placebo for the treatment of negative symptoms only at the 300-mg dose (Arvanitis and Miller 1997). A comparison of high-dose quetiapine (approximately 500 mg/day) and low-dose quetiapine (approximately 250 mg/day) found significantly greater efficacy with the higher dose (Small et al. 1997). Quetiapine's relatively high $5\text{-HT}_2\text{-to-}D_2$ ratio is consistent with the hypothesized advantageous properties of the atypical antipsychotics. Antagonism of H_1 receptors is associated with sedative side effects, and α_1 antagonism is associated with orthostatic hypotension.

Clinical use. Quetiapine is indicated for the treatment of schizophrenia, acute mania, and bipolar depression. Quetiapine therapy is initiated at a dose of 25 mg twice a day for patients with schizophrenia, with increases to 50 mg twice a day on day 2, 100 mg twice a day on day 3, and 100 mg in the morning and 200 mg in the evening on day 4. The optimal dosage for most patients appears to range between 400 and 600 mg/day, although the drug is safe and efficacious for some patients within a dose range of 150–750 mg. Slower titration and lower daily doses may be warranted in patients with hepatic disease and in elderly patients. Because of its relatively short half-life of 6–8 hours, quetiapine is usually administered twice daily. A new formulation of quetiapine, quetiapine XR (extended-release tablets), is administered once daily, usually in the evening. The recommended initial dosage is 300 mg/day, and the effective dosage range is 400–800 mg/day. The dose can be increased by up to 300 mg/day, and increases can occur at 1-day intervals.

For patients who have acute mania, treatment should be initiated with twice-daily doses totaling 100 mg on day 1, 200 mg on day 2, 300 mg on day 3, and 400 mg on day 4. Additional adjustments up to 800 mg/day by day 6 can be made. Doses should not be increased by more than 200 mg/day on days 5 and 6. Most patients respond to dosages between 400 and 800 mg/day. Some clinicians use lower starting doses and slower titrations for less ill outpatients; however, this practice is not supported by controlled data.

For patients struggling with bipolar depression, the recommended starting dosage for quetiapine is 50 mg/day. This dosage can be increased to 100 mg on day 2, 200 mg on day 3, and 300 mg on day 4. Although no additional benefit has been observed for dosages higher than 300 mg/day, the dosage can be titrated upward to 400 mg on day 5 and 600 mg on day 8.

Risks, side effects, and their management. Quetiapine was no different from placebo in dosages to 750 mg/day regarding EPS and changes in serum prolactin levels (Arvanitis and Miller 1997).

Somnolence. Somnolence is one of the most common side effects of quetiapine. Somnolence and psychomotor slowing are dose dependent, and patients often become tolerant to these side effects over time.

Ocular changes. As noted earlier, the development of cataracts was observed in association with quetiapine treatment in preclinical studies of beagles, but a causal relation has not been established in humans. No differences in the rates of new cataracts were noted between treatment groups (including quetiapine) in the CATIE trial (Lieberman et al. 2005).

Cardiovascular effects. Given α_1-adrenergic receptor antagonism, quetiapine may induce orthostatic hypotension and concomitant symptoms of dizziness, tachycardia, and syncope. The risk of symptomatic hypotension is particularly pronounced during initial dose titration. Quetiapine should be used with caution in patients with cardiovascular disease, cerebrovascular disease, or other illnesses predisposing to hypotension.

Hepatic effects. In premarketing trials, increased transaminase levels were noted in 6% of the patients taking quetiapine. These changes usually occur during the first weeks of treatment. Routine laboratory monitoring currently is not recommended, but quetiapine should be used with caution in patients with hepatic disease or with additional risk factors for hepatic toxicity.

Weight gain. Quetiapine is associated with weight gain. In premarketing placebo-controlled studies, a weight gain of at least 7% of body weight was observed in 23% of the quetiapine-treated patients with schizophrenia, compared with 6% of the control subjects given placebo. Thus, patients should be educated about the potential risk for weight gain, and weight should be monitored periodically throughout treatment.

Drug interactions. Quetiapine is metabolized by hepatic CYP3A3/4. Concurrent administration of cytochrome P450–inducing drugs, such as carbamazepine, decreases blood levels of quetiapine. In such circumstances, increased doses of quetiapine are appropriate. Quetiapine does not appreciably affect the pharmacokinetics of other medications. Pharmacodynamic effects are expected if quetiapine is combined with medications that also have antihistaminic or α-adrenergic side effects. Because of its potential for inducing hypotension, quetiapine also may enhance the effects of certain antihypertensive agents.

Ziprasidone

Ziprasidone is the only atypical antipsychotic available in capsule form. This medication combines a high affinity for 5-HT$_2$ receptors with an intermediate affinity for D$_2$, resulting in a very high 5-HT$_2$-to-D$_2$ affinity ratio.

Clinical use. Ziprasidone is approved for the treatment of schizophrenia and acute mania. For patients with schizophrenia, ziprasidone is usually started at a dosage of 20–40 mg twice a day. In medically healthy nonelderly patients, the dose can be rapidly titrated over 2–4 days to a typical therapeutic dosage of 60–80 mg twice a day. For patients with acute mania, treatment should be initiated at 40 mg twice a day. This dose should be increased to 60 or 80 mg twice a day on day 2 and subsequently adjusted on the basis of individual tolerance and symptoms to between 40 and 80 mg twice a day. Ziprasidone has a half-life of 5–10 hours and is usually administered twice daily with meals. Food increases absorption by approximately 100%. Ziprasidone at a dosage of 80 mg twice a day was comparable to haloperidol 15 mg/day in overall efficacy, and substantially fewer patients receiving ziprasidone required antiparkinsonian medication compared with those receiving haloperidol (10% vs. 53%) (Goff et al. 1998). Ziprasidone also has shown efficacy for negative symptoms in placebo-controlled trials (Daniel et al. 1999; Keck et al. 1998).

Because safety data regarding ziprasidone are largely derived from studies that excluded subjects with cardiac disease, clinicians should screen patients (preferably with a baseline ECG and measurement of serum electrolyte levels) for cardiac risk factors before initiating ziprasidone therapy. Patients with QTc prolongation at baseline must be monitored very closely; a cardiology consultation is recommended.

Ziprasidone is also available for intramuscular administration. The recommended dose for intramuscular injection (for the treatment of acute agitation associated with schizophrenia) is 10–20 mg, with a maximum dosage of 40 mg/day. The 10-mg doses can be administered every 2 hours, whereas the 20-mg doses can be administered every 4 hours. Peak plasma concentrations are achieved by 60 minutes.

Risks, side effects, and their management. In general, ziprasidone is well tolerated. The most common side effects are headache, dyspepsia, nausea, constipation, abdominal pain, somnolence, and EPS. Ratings of parkinsonism and akathisia with ziprasidone, 120 mg/day, did not differ from those with placebo. Although dizziness has been reported, rates of orthostatic hypotension have not differed from rates associated with placebo in controlled clinical trials. Ziprasidone produces transient hyperprolactinemia, which returns to predrug baseline levels after 12 hours; prolactin levels are significantly lower with ziprasidone than with haloperidol (Goff et al. 1998).

Cardiovascular effects. The FDA delayed approval of ziprasidone until additional safety data could be obtained regarding effects on cardiac conduction. Ziprasidone delays the QTc interval at maximum therapeutic blood levels by approximately 20 ms, on average, which is a larger effect than with other atypical agents but less than with thioridazine. As noted earlier in this section, ziprasidone was not associated with greater effects on QTc intervals in the CATIE trial compared with other agents (Lieberman et al. 2005). Although monitoring of ECGs is not routinely required, clinicians should consider the relative risk of cardiac conduction delay compared with the benefits of ziprasidone (which include tolerability and minimal weight gain) when selecting a medication.

Weight gain. Ziprasidone is associated with less weight gain than are other atypical antipsychotic agents. Allison et al. (1999) calculated a mean weight gain of less than 1 kg after 10 weeks of ziprasidone treatment.

Drug interactions. Drugs that inhibit CYP3A4 reduce metabolism of ziprasidone: concurrent treatment with ketoconazole increased blood levels of ziprasidone by approximately 40%. Carbamazepine (and possibly other enzyme inducers) may decrease ziprasidone levels by approximately 35%. Effects of ziprasidone on metabolism of other drugs have not been reported. Ziprasidone is contraindicated for use in patients taking other medications that can prolong the QT interval, including quinidine, class Ia and II antiarrhythmics, sotalol, dofetilide, dolasetron mesylate, probucol, tacrolimus, certain antibiotics (sparfloxacin, gatifloxacin, moxifloxacin), halofantrine, mefloquine, pentamidine, arsenic trioxide, certain antipsychotics (chlorpromazine, thioridazine, mesoridazine, pimozide), droperidol, and levomethadyl acetate (Geodon 2005).

Aripiprazole

Aripiprazole has a high affinity for D_2 and D_3 receptors, as well as 5-HT_{1a} and 5-HT_{2a} receptors. Aripiprazole has partial agonist activity at the D_2 and 5-HT_{1a} receptors and antagonist activity at the 5-HT_{2a} receptor.

Clinical use. Aripiprazole has been approved for treatment of schizophrenia, treatment of acute manic or mixed episodes in bipolar disorder, and maintenance treatment of bipolar disorder. The recommended starting and target dosage for aripiprazole in patients with schizophrenia is 10 or 15 mg/day. The recommended starting dose for treatment of an acute manic or mixed episode is 30 mg; the recommended dosage for maintenance treatment in stable patients is 15 mg/day. The elimination half-life is 75 hours, and steady-state concentrations are reached within 2 weeks. Therefore, dosage adjustments are recommended every 2 weeks, to allow time for clinical assessments of the medication's effects to be observed at steady-state concentrations.

Risks, side effects, and their management. The most common side effects associated with aripiprazole include headache, nausea, dyspepsia, agitation, anxiety, insomnia, somnolence, and akathisia. Aripiprazole is not associated with significant sedation, anticholinergic side effects, weight gain, or cardiovascular side effects. As with all other antipsychotic medications, aripiprazole is associated with a risk for NMS and tardive dyskinesias.

As noted earlier, elderly patients with dementia-related psychosis treated with atypical antipsychotics are at an increased risk for death compared with those receiving placebo. This warning applies across all atypical antipsychotic medications. Additionally, in controlled trials of dementia-related psychosis, aripiprazole-treated patients had an increased incidence of cerebrovascular adverse events, including deaths, with one study showing a dose-dependent relation for these adverse events (Abilify 2005).

Drug interactions. Aripiprazole is hepatically metabolized, mainly by two cytochrome P450 enzymes: CYP2D6 and CYP3A4. Therefore, dosage adjustments are necessary when this medication is given with other medications that either inhibit or induce these enzymes. For example, the dose of aripiprazole should be halved when this medication is given with ketoconazole, a CYP3A4 inhibitor, or at least decreased when given with fluoxetine, a CYP2D6 inhibitor. When aripiprazole is given with CYP3A4 inducers such as carbamazepine, the dose should be doubled.

Paliperidone

Paliperidone, a benzisoxazole derivative, is the major active metabolite of risperidone. This medication functions as an antagonist at the D_2, 5-HT_{2A}, α_1, α_2, and H_1 receptors. Whereas risperidone reaches peak plasma concentrations approximately 1 hour following a single oral dose, paliperidone reaches peak plasma concentrations 24 hours following a single oral dose, allowing for once-daily dosing rather than twice-daily dosing.

Clinical use.   Paliperidone is approved for the acute and maintenance treatment of schizophrenia. Clinical efficacy for acute treatment was established in several randomized controlled trials (Davidson et al. 2007; Kane et al. 2007; Marder et al. 2007). Effective doses, as measured by a significant decrease in PANSS scores compared with placebo, included 3–12 mg/day. In a randomized double-blind, placebo-controlled trial, Kramer et al. (2007) found that treatment with paliperidone (3–15 mg/day) significantly delayed time to relapse compared with placebo. At dosages of 3 and 6 mg/day, the rate of adverse events was similar for paliperidone and placebo. In some studies, at dosages greater than 6 mg/day, the rate of adverse events was significantly higher in the paliperidone group.

The recommended dose for paliperidone is 6 mg/day. No initial titration is necessary. If a dosage greater than 6 mg/day is required, increases in 3-mg increments every 5 days are recommended. The minimum and maximum dosages are 3 mg/day and 6 mg/day, respectively.

Risks, side effects, and their management.   The risks associated with paliperidone use are similar to those for other atypical antipsychotics. The most common adverse events, which were reported significantly more often with paliperidone than with placebo, included tachycardia (12%–14%), headache (11%–14%), somnolence (6%–11%), and anxiety (6%–9%). Extrapyramidal symptoms, including parkinsonism (3%–14%), akathisia (4%–9%), dyskinesias (3%–9%), and tremor (3%–5%), also occurred. Treatment of extrapyramidal side effects and symptoms was discussed earlier in this chapter (see "Risks, Side Effects, and Their Management" subsection under "Antipsychotic Medications").

Drug interactions.   Paliperidone is not expected to interact significantly with drugs metabolized by cytochrome P450 enzymes. However, an additive effect may occur when this medication is administered with other agents that cause orthostatic hypotension.

Long-Acting Injectable Antipsychotics

For patients with chronic psychotic symptoms who are not compliant with antipsychotic medication, a long-acting depot preparation should be considered after stabilization with oral medication. Fluphenazine, haloperidol, and risperidone are the only long-acting injectable antipsychotic medications currently available in the United States.

Conversion to a decanoate preparation is complicated by the highly variable individual pharmacokinetics of the oral and long-term depot agents. Most patients respond to a fluphenazine decanoate dose of 10–30 mg given every 2 weeks. A loading dose strategy has been established for haloperidol decanoate, in which patients receive an initial dose that is 20 times the oral maintenance dose (Ereshefsky et al. 1993). The maximum volume per injection of haloperidol decanoate should not exceed 3 mL, and the maximum dose per injection should not exceed 100 mg. If 20 times the oral dose is greater than 100 mg, the dose is given in divided injections spaced 3–7 days apart. Subsequent doses are decreased monthly, to about 10 times the oral dose by the third or fourth month. Ten times the oral dose, administered every 4 weeks, is a typical maintenance dose for haloperidol decanoate. For elderly or debilitated patients, the initial dose is 10–15 times the previous oral daily dose. Many clinicians prefer to continue giving oral medication at approximately half the previous maintenance dose during the first few months of depot antipsychotic administration rather than administer a loading dose of depot medication. This approach allows greater flexibility with regard to initial dose titration. In either approach, breakthrough psychotic symptoms are treated with supplemental oral medication, and the dose of the next scheduled depot injection can be increased accordingly. Steady-state serum concentrations are achieved after approximately 10 weeks (five injection intervals) with fluphenazine decanoate and after approximately 20 weeks with haloperidol decanoate. Side effects may take months to subside, and withdrawal dyskinesia may not appear for months after discontinuation of the decanoate formulation.

The recommended starting dose for the risperidone long-acting injection is 25 mg. Although an initial release of medication occurs, the amount released is small, and the main release of the drug begins 3 weeks after the injection. This release is maintained from 4 to 6 weeks and subsides by 7 weeks. Because not much drug is released for the first 3 weeks after the injection, oral antipsychotic supplementation is recommended. Injections are given every 2 weeks, and steady-state plasma concentrations are achieved after four injections. Dosing adjustments should not be made more often than once a month; the maximum dose is 50 mg every 2 weeks. Doses of 25, 37.5, and 50 mg are available, and different dosage strengths should not be combined. Dose titration depends on clinical symptoms. If the patient has not taken risperidone before, a trial of oral risperidone is recommended to determine whether the patient has a hypersensitivity reaction to the medication.

Treatment of Schizophrenia

General Principles

Evidence indicates that the long-term outcome for a patient with schizophrenia is better when treatment of the acute episode is initiated rapidly. After a patient's first psychotic episode, treatment with the antipsychotic medication should be continued for at least 1 year after a full remission of psychotic symptoms. A trial period without medication may then be considered, except for patients with a history of serious suicide attempts or violent, aggressive behavior (Lehman et al. 2004). The patient and his or her family should be informed about the early signs and symptoms of relapse, and they should be warned that risk for relapse is high. Some evidence shows that first-episode psychosis may be more responsive to treatment and require lower doses of antipsychotic medications compared with patients with multiple prior psychotic episodes (Lieberman et al. 1996, 1998; McEvoy et al. 1991; Schooler et al. 1997; Zhang-Wong et al. 1999), although the time to response may be longer (Lieberman et al. 1993). Additionally, a longer duration of illness prior to treatment may be a predictor of poorer treatment response and a longer time to remission (Loebel et al. 1992). These data suggest that initiating treatment early, starting with low antipsychotic doses, and allowing adequate time (e.g., 2–4 weeks) for response may be the preferred approach with these patients.

For patients with a chronic relapsing form of schizophrenia, antipsychotic medication should be continued for up to 5 symptom-free years before discontinuation (Johnson 1985) and probably indefinitely. The 2004 "Practice Guideline for the Treatment of Patients With Schizophrenia" recommends indefinite maintenance treatment for patients who have had at least two episodes of psychosis within 5 years or who have had multiple previous episodes (Lehman et al.

2004). Maintenance therapy should involve the lowest possible doses of antipsychotic drugs, and patients should be monitored closely for symptoms of relapse. If the patient is compliant with treatment, oral medications are usually sufficient. However, if the patient's treatment history suggests that the patient may not reliably take daily oral medication, a long-acting depot preparation may be indicated.

Treatment-Resistant Schizophrenia

If symptoms are not responding to the indicated treatment, if the patient is experiencing minimal side effects (e.g., EPS, hypotension, sedation), and if poor treatment adherence is not the cause, the physician can gradually increase the dose until mild side effects are noted. If no further improvement is seen after an additional 2–4 weeks at this dose, a different antipsychotic should be started. Inadequate treatment outcomes following an initial antipsychotic medication trial appear to be common; in the CATIE trial, 74% of the patients discontinued their initial randomly assigned antipsychotic medication within 18 months (Lieberman et al. 2005).

A trial of clozapine should be considered for patients who continue to have positive symptoms, frequent relapses, or aggression despite an adequate trial of at least two other antipsychotic medications, as well as for patients with intolerable side effects caused by at least two different antipsychotic medications from different classes (American Psychiatric Association 1997; Lewis et al. 2006; McEvoy et al. 2006). ECT may be considered for patients with catatonia, suicidal ideation or behavior, or persistent severe psychosis or for whom previous treatments, including clozapine, have not been effective (Lehman et al. 2004).

An additional strategy to use in nonresponsive patients is to add another medication to augment the therapeutic effects of the antipsychotic. Current augmentation strategies include adding lithium (Cole et al. 1984; Delva and Letemedni 1982), valproate (Casey et al. 2003; Citrome 2003; Linnoila et al. 1976), a benzodiazepine (Csernansky et al. 1988; Douyon et al. 1989; Nestoros et al. 1982), another antipsychotic, or a cholinergic agent (Lehman et al. 2004). Two recent controlled trials examined the usefulness of lamotrigine as adjunctive therapy in treatment-resistant schizophrenia (Kremer et al. 2004; Tiihonen et al. 2003). In a randomized, placebo-controlled crossover trial in 34 hospitalized patients with clozapine-resistant schizophrenia, lamotrigine augmentation (200 mg/day) more effectively improved positive symptoms compared with clozapine plus placebo (Tiihonen et al. 2003). In a randomized, placebo-controlled trial in 38 hospitalized schizophrenic patients receiving conventional and atypical antipsychotics, adjunctive treatment with lamotrigine (titrated to 400 mg/day) resulted in significantly greater improvements in positive symptoms in patients who completed the trial (but not in last observation carry-forward [LOCF] analysis) compared with adjunctive treatment with placebo (Kremer et al. 2004). Augmentation of antipsychotics with the omega-3 fatty acid ethyl-eicosapentaenoic acid also has been studied (Emsley et al. 2002; Fenton et al. 2001; Peet and Horrobin 2002). However, with the current availability of the atypical antipsychotics, particularly clozapine, the use of these augmenting strategies in patients with antipsychotic-resistant schizophrenia should be reserved for patients who cannot take clozapine or who have not fully responded to clozapine (American Psychiatric Association 1997). Because of the potential side effects and added cost, combination therapy should be attempted only after an adequate trial of monotherapy. If clear benefit is not apparent after 6 weeks of combination therapy, the augmenting agent should be discontinued (Lehman et al. 2004). Work with cognitive-behavioral therapy has shown considerable promise when combined with medication in refractory schizophrenia (Gould et al. 2001).

The CATIE trial (discussed earlier) examined treatment switch options when a patient with chronic schizophrenia had an inadequate response to treatment with an antipsychotic medication. Specifically, patients with schizophrenia who discontinued an atypical antipsychotic medication in phase I of CATIE ($n=444$) were randomly assigned to double-blind treatment with a different atypical antipsychotic (olanzapine, risperidone, quetiapine, or ziprasidone) (Stroup et al. 2006). Risperidone and olanzapine were associated with a longer time to discontinuation (7 months and 6.3 months, respectively) compared with quetiapine and ziprasidone (Stroup et al. 2006).

The CATIE trial also examined switching from one atypical antipsychotic to another atypical antipsychotic compared with switching to clozapine (McEvoy et al. 2006). In this phase of the trial, patients with schizophrenia ($n=99$) who discontinued treatment with an atypical antipsychotic during phase I or Ib of CATIE, mostly because of poor efficacy, were randomly assigned to blinded treatment with a different atypical antipsychotic or open treatment with clozapine (McEvoy et al. 2006). The results showed that time to treatment discontinuation as a result of poor efficacy was longer

for clozapine than for the other agents; importantly, clozapine also was associated with one case each of agranulocytosis and eosinophilia (McEvoy et al. 2006).

Mood Stabilizers

The term *mood stabilizer* is used to refer to a group of medications that are effective in the treatment of bipolar disorder. These treatments serve as the foundation for the psychopharmacological treatment of bipolar illnesses. Currently, lithium, valproate, carbamazepine, lamotrigine, and most of the atypical antipsychotic medications are approved by the FDA for the treatment of one or more phases of bipolar disorder.

In order to prescribe mood stabilizers skillfully, the clinician must have a strong knowledge of the pharmacology of each medication and appreciate the differences in efficacy as well as side effects. Compared with most other classes of psychotropic medications, the group referred to as mood stabilizers are much more diverse with respect to their pharmacokinetic and pharmacodynamic properties, side-effect profiles, and potential for drug interactions.

In this section, we review the clinical use of lithium and the anticonvulsants that are definite or probable mood stabilizers, review the use of atypical antipsychotic medications for the treatment of bipolar disorder, and conclude with a discussion of the treatment of each phase of bipolar disorder.

Lithium

Mechanism of Action

Lithium is a cation that inhibits several steps in phosphoinositide metabolism, as well as many second and third messengers, including G proteins and protein kinases (Bitran et al. 1995; Lenox et al. 1992; Manji et al. 1993, 1995, 1999). Recent evidence suggests that lithium ultimately stimulates neurite growth, regeneration, and neurogenesis, which is likely related to its therapeutic effect (Coyle and Duman 2003; Kim et al. 2004).

Indications and Efficacy

Lithium has been proven effective for acute and prophylactic treatment of both manic and depressive episodes in patients with bipolar disorder (American Psychiatric Association 2002), although patients with rapid-cycling bipolar disorder have been reported to respond less well to lithium treatment (Dunner and Fieve 1974). Lithium is also effective in prevention of future depressive episodes in patients with recurrent unipolar depressive disorder (American Psychiatric Association 2002) and as an adjunct to antidepressant therapy in depressed patients whose illness is partially refractory to treatment with antidepressants alone (discussed earlier in this chapter in the "Antidepressant Medications" section). Furthermore, lithium may be useful in maintaining remission of depressive disorders after ECT (Sackeim et al. 2001), as well as in the management of some cases of aggression and behavioral dyscontrol.

Clinical Use

Lithium carbonate is completely absorbed by the gastrointestinal tract and reaches peak plasma levels in 1–2 hours. The elimination half-life is approximately 24 hours. Steady-state lithium levels are achieved in approximately 5 days. Therapeutic plasma levels for the treatment of bipolar disorder range from 0.5 to 1.2 mEq/L. Although lower plasma levels are associated with less troubling side effects, many clinicians target lithium levels of 0.8 mEq/L or more when treating acute manic episodes. Therefore, treatment of acute mania with lithium should not be considered a failure until the treatment has been tried throughout the therapeutic plasma level range (provided that the treatment is tolerated). Additionally, more severely acutely ill patients may require combination treatment.

Serum concentrations required for prophylaxis are not as well determined. One controlled trial of patients randomly assigned to a low lithium level (0.4–0.6 mEq/L) compared with a standard-dose lithium group (0.8–1.0 mEq/L) found fewer recurrences in the standard-dose group (Gelenberg et al. 1989); however, a reanalysis of these data indicated that an abrupt decrease in serum lithium level may be a more powerful predictor of recurrence of bipolar disorder than is the absolute assignment to a low or a standard dose of lithium (Perlis et al. 2002).

Lithium dosing is based on achieving therapeutic blood levels, targeting clinical response, and minimizing side effects if possible. Lithium can be administered either as a single daily dose or in divided doses. Divided daily dosing with lithium carbonate results in several peak lithium levels a day, whereas a single daily dose is associated with a single, but higher, peak level. Some clinicians prefer evening dosing because some side effects are associated with peak blood levels. Lithium levels should be determined 12 hours after the last lithium dose. After therapeutic lithium levels have been established, levels should be measured every month for the first 3 months and every 3 months

thereafter. In patients who have remained stable and who are aware of early signs of both relapse and lithium toxicity, lithium levels may be measured less frequently. In addition, serum urea nitrogen and creatinine levels should be measured before lithium therapy has commenced and every 3–6 months during therapy, with more frequent testing if there are specific complaints or signs of renal dysfunction. As with any treatment, patients should be informed of the potential benefits and risks of lithium treatment and also should be educated about other treatment alternatives.

Contraindications and Pretreatment Medical Evaluation

Lithium should not be administered to patients with unstable renal function. Because lithium may affect functioning of the cardiac sinus node, patients with sinus node dysfunction (e.g., sick sinus syndrome) should not receive lithium. Although lithium also has acute and chronic effects on the thyroid, patients with hypothyroidism may receive lithium if the thyroid disease is adequately treated and monitored. Laboratory tests that should be performed before initiation of lithium treatment are listed in Table 26–13.

Lithium treatment during pregnancy has been associated with teratogenic effects. The risk of Ebstein's anomaly in infants exposed to lithium in utero is 0.1%–0.7%, compared with 0.01% in the general population. The overall risk of major congenital anomalies associated with lithium exposure is 4%–12%, compared with 2%–4% in comparison groups (L.S. Cohen et al. 1994). The increased risk of malformations must be weighed against the risk of harm to both mother and fetus if lithium discontinuation results in a manic relapse. Treatment decisions during pregnancy can be difficult for both the clinician and the patient, and more detailed reviews regarding treatment of bipolar disorder during pregnancy have been published elsewhere (Burt and Rasgon 2004; Freeman and Gelenberg 2005; Viguera et al. 2002; Yonkers et al. 2004).

Risks, Side Effects, and Their Management

Renal effects. In the absence of toxicity, most of the effects of lithium on the kidneys are largely reversible after discontinuation of the drug (although permanent morphological changes in renal structure may occur in some patients). However, lithium inhibits vasopressin and may result in an impairment in renal concentrating ability, called *nephrogenic diabetes insipidus* (NDI). This condition results in polyuria for up to 60% of patients taking lithium. NDI may result in serious com-

TABLE 26–13. Key characteristics of mood stabilizers[a]

	Lithium	Valproate	Carbamazepine	Lamotrigine
Available preparations	Lithium carbonate (Eskalith, Lithonate, Lithotabs; 150, 300, 600-mg tablets, capsules) Lithium citrate liquid (8 mEq/5 mL) Extended-release lithium (Eskalith CR, 450 mg; Lithobid, 300 mg)	Divalproex sodium (Depakote, 125-, 250-, 500-mg tablets; 125-mg sprinkle capsules) Valproate sodium injection (Depacon) Valproic acid (Depakene, 250-mg capsules; 250 mg/5 mL syrup) Extended-release divalproex sodium (Depakote ER, 250, 500 mg)	Carbamazepine (Tegretol; 100-mg chewable tablets; 200-mg tablets) Extended-release carbamazepine capsules (Equetro, 100, 200, 300 mg; Carbatrol, 200, 300 mg) Carbamazepine suspension (100 mg/5 mL) Extended-release carbamazepine tablets (Tegretol XR, 100, 200, 400 mg)	Lamotrigine (Lamictal, 25-, 100-, 150-, 200-mg tablets; Lamictal CD [chewable dispersible], 2-, 5-, 25-mg tablets)
Half-life (hours)	24	96	Initially, 25–65; decreases to 12–17 because of autoinduction	25–33[b]
Starting dosage	300 mg twice daily	250 mg three times a day or 20 mg/kg[c]	Tablets/capsules: 200 mg twice daily[d]; suspension: 100 mg four times a day	25 mg/day[b]
Blood level	0.8–1.2 mEq/L	45–125 µg/mL	Not helpful; monitor for signs or symptoms of toxicity	Not monitored; target dose of lamotrigine is 200 mg/day
Metabolism	Renal	Hepatic	Hepatic	Hepatic
Contraindications[e]	Unstable renal function	Hepatic dysfunction	Hepatic dysfunction, bone marrow suppression	Previous hypersensitivity to lamotrigine

TABLE 26–13. Key characteristics of mood stabilizers[a] *(continued)*

	Lithium	Valproate	Carbamazepine	Lamotrigine
Key side effects, risks, and features	Nephrogenic diabetes insipidus Reversible hypothyroidism Tremor Benign leukocytosis Weight gain Narrow therapeutic index Potentially fatal toxicity Risk of Ebstein's anomaly with first-trimester exposure	Titration or loading dose strategies Rare hepatotoxicity Rare pancreatitis Polycystic ovarian syndrome Weight gain Tremor Alopecia Rare blood cell dyscrasias Risk of neural tube defects with first-trimester exposure	Cytochrome P450 inducer (oral contraceptive failure) Autoinduction Rare blood cell dyscrasias: aplastic anemia, agranulocytosis Hepatotoxicity Rash risk, including Stevens-Johnson syndrome Risk for SIADH Teratogenicity risk: neural tube defects, craniofacial defects	Rash risk in 5%–10% Rarely, life-threatening rash (including Stevens-Johnson syndrome) Risk minimized by low starting dose and slow titration Metabolism inhibited by valproate Metabolism induced by carbamazepine
Pretreatment laboratory evaluation	Chem 20,[f] CBC, TSH level determination, ECG (if patient is 40 years of age or older or has cardiac disease); pregnancy test	AST and ALT level determination, pregnancy test	AST, ALT, CBC, sodium level; pregnancy test	None; might consider a pregnancy test

Note. SIADH=syndrome of inappropriate secretion of antidiuretic hormone; CBC=complete blood count; TSH=thyroid-stimulating hormone; ECG=electrocardiogram; AST=aspartate aminotransaminase; ALT=alanine aminotransaminase.
[a]The atypical antipsychotics are not included in this table. Please refer to the antipsychotics section of this chapter for information about their characteristics.
[b]The effective half-life of lamotrigine approximately doubles with valproate and decreases by approximately half with carbamazepine, primidone, phenytoin, phenobarbital, and rifampin; therefore, initial doses may vary depending on concomitant medications. The reader should refer to current product labeling for specific information regarding drug–drug interactions, their effects on lamotrigine, and lamotrigine dosing guidelines.
[c]Increase dose by 10%–20% when converting from valproate, divalproex, or valproic acid to the extended-release formulation of divalproex sodium.
[d]100 mg twice daily if given in combination with a neuroleptic or lithium.
[e]Lithium, valproate, and carbamazepine should be avoided in pregnancy, if possible; see text for discussion. Recent reports also have noted cases of oral clefts with lamotrigine use; see text for discussion.
[f]Especially serum urea nitrogen, creatinine, sodium, and calcium levels.

Source. Adapted from Marangell LB, Martinez JM: *Concise Guide to Psychopharmacology,* 2nd Edition. Arlington, VA, American Psychiatric Publishing, 2006, pp. 138–141. Used with permission.

plications, including dehydration, lithium toxicity, and electrolyte imbalance. Clinically significant polyuria usually reverses itself after discontinuation of lithium therapy, but it may persist for many months. However, less serious increases in urine volume may persist indefinitely, an effect that some investigators believe is a consequence of renal tubular atrophy (Hetmar et al. 1991).

Preventive and management strategies for NDI include increasing the patient's fluid intake and decreasing the amount of lithium given to the lowest effective dosage. Once-daily dosing also results in lower urinary output than the multiple-dosing schedule (Hetmar et al. 1991; Plenge et al. 1982). For some patients, potassium supplementation, 10–20 mEq/day, may be effective. The nonthiazide diuretic amiloride also may treat lithium-induced NDI. For lithium-induced NDI, amiloride is prescribed in a dosage of 5 mg twice a day and increased to 10 mg twice a day if necessary. Even though amiloride does not appear to increase plasma lithium levels, it is prudent to continue to monitor serum lithium levels with greater frequency (at least every 2 months) when amiloride is combined with lithium.

Interstitial nephritis has been reported to be a consequence of long-term lithium therapy. Hetmar et al. (1987) performed renal biopsies on 46 bipolar patients with a mean of 8 years of lithium therapy and found that the proportion of sclerotic glomeruli, atrophic tubules, and interstitial fibrosis was significantly greater in patients who had received a multiple daily dosing schedule, compared with patients with a history of once-daily dosing and with a control group with no history of lithium exposure. Lokkegaard et al. (1985) reported that decreases in the glomerular filtration rate (GFR) are detectable only after many years of lithium therapy; however, most investigators have found no clinically significant effect on the GFR (Hetmar et al. 1991; Schou 1989). Proteinuria has been reported as a rare side effect and is thought to be the consequence of either glomerular leakage or the inhibition of tubular resorption. Permanent morphological changes in renal structure have been reported in patients who have experienced lithium toxicity (Markowitz et al. 2000). To minimize the risk of renal complications, we recommend frequent patient education about the risks of renal toxicity. Nephrology consultation is warranted if routine laboratory monitoring detects a pattern of rising creatinine levels.

Thyroid dysfunction.   Reversible hypothyroidism may occur in as many as 20% of the patients receiving lithium. Therefore, thyroid function should be evaluated every 6–12 months during lithium treatment or if symptoms develop that might be attributable to thyroid dysfunction, including depression or rapid cycling. If laboratory studies indicate the development of hypothyroidism, the patient should be referred to an endocrinologist for further evaluation and management. The psychiatrist and endocrinologist can also collaborate on the appropriate treatment for the patient's bipolar illness, including whether to continue lithium treatment or switch to another medication.

Parathyroid dysfunction.   The effects of lithium on calcium metabolism may be related to lithium-induced hyperparathyroidism (Anath and Dubin 1983; Mallette and Eichhorn 1986). Clinically significant effects of hypercalcemia associated with lithium have been reported, including back pain, kyphoscoliosis, osteoporosis, hypertension, cardiomegaly, and impaired renal function. Potential neuropsychiatric sequelae include affective changes, anxiety, aggressiveness, sleep disturbance, apathy, psychosis, delirium, dementia, and seizures. Symptoms of hyperparathyroidism may be misdiagnosed as lithium toxicity or the effects of the underlying mood disorder. When signs or symptoms that might be related to hyperparathyroidism develop, serum calcium ion levels should be checked, and if they are abnormal, parathyroid hormone levels should be measured and an endocrinologist consulted.

Neurotoxicity.   Several types of neurological adverse events may occur with lithium treatment. A fine resting tremor is a common side effect of lithium. β-Blockers, such as propranolol (<80 mg/day in divided doses), may effectively treat this tremor (Zubenko et al. 1984a). Additionally, subjective memory impairment commonly occurs (Goodwin and Jamison 1990).

Cardiac effects.   Benign flattening of the T wave on the ECG occurs in 20%–30% of patients taking lithium (Bucht et al. 1984). In addition, lithium may suppress the function of the sinus node and result in sinoatrial block. Thus, an ECG should be obtained before initiating lithium treatment in patients older than 40 years or in those with a history or symptoms of cardiac disease.

Weight gain.   Weight gain is a frequent side effect of lithium treatment. Indeed, weight gain can be problematic with numerous psychotropic medications and is a potential cause for treatment noncompliance. Therefore, patients should be informed of the risk for weight gain before initiating lithium therapy and counseled regarding weight management strategies, such as dietary habits and regular exercise. If weight gain occurs during treatment and weight management interventions fail, the clinician should discuss further treatment options with the patient.

Dermatological effects.   Dermatological reactions to lithium include acne, follicular eruptions, and psoriasis. Hair loss and thinning also have been reported. Except for cases of exacerbation of psoriasis, these reactions are usually benign. Lithium-induced acne responds to topical treatment with retinoid acid, such as tretinoin (Retin-A).

Gastrointestinal symptoms.   Gastrointestinal side effects, particularly nausea and diarrhea, are common and occur early during treatment. These side effects may be alleviated by decreasing the lithium dose (must balance this strategy against the risk for reduced efficacy) or instructing the patient to take lithium with meals. In general, the slow-release formulations of lithium are more often associated with nausea, whereas the immediate-release preparations are more commonly associated with diarrhea.

Hematological effects.   The most frequent hematological change associated with lithium therapy is leukocytosis (approximately 15,000 WBCs/mm^3). This change is generally benign and typically reversible on lithium discontinuation.

Overdose and Toxicity

There is a narrow margin between therapeutic and toxic plasma lithium levels. Thus, the physician should educate the patient about the risks for lithium toxicity, the signs and symptoms of lithium toxicity, and the importance of preventing lithium toxicity by ensuring adequate salt and water intake, taking the lithium as prescribed, and following through with recommended laboratory monitoring. The signs and symptoms of lithium toxicity, as well as the recommended management of lithium toxicity, are outlined in Table 26–14.

Drug Interactions

Because lithium treatment is associated with a narrow therapeutic range, it is crucial that clinicians have good knowledge about the potential drug–drug interactions that may be associated with the concomitant administration of lithium and other drugs. Because lithium is excreted by the kidneys, any medication that alters renal function can affect lithium levels. Thiazide diuretics and nonsteroidal anti-inflammatory agents may increase lithium levels by decreasing renal clearance of lithium. Other medications that may increase lithium levels include angiotensin-converting enzyme inhibitors and cyclooxygenase-2 inhibitors (e.g., celecoxib, rofecoxib). Drugs that may decrease lithium levels include theophylline and aminophylline. Lithium may potentiate the effects of succinylcholine-like muscle relaxants.

Valproate

Divalproex sodium is approved by the FDA for the treatment of acute mania. It is commonly used for all phases of bipolar disorder, but its major body of evidence in bipolar disorder to date is in its efficacy in acute mania.

Mechanism of Action

Although many mechanisms of action have been proposed, the basis for the mood-stabilizing effects of valproate is most likely concordant with lithium's mechanism of action—specifically, attenuation of the activity of protein kinase C and other steps in the signal transduction pathway, leading to neuronal adaptation and changes in gene expression (Chen et al. 1994; Manji et al. 1996), including neurotrophic effects (Coyle and Duman 2003).

Clinical Use

Before starting treatment with valproate, patients should be told that they might experience nausea, sedation, and a fine hand tremor. These effects are often transient, but in some patients they persist. Several valproate preparations are available in the United States, including valproic acid, sodium valproate, divalproex sodium, and an XL preparation of divalproex sodium. Divalproex sodium is a dimer of sodium valproate and valproic acid with an enteric coating, and it is much better tolerated than other oral valproate preparations. The half-life of valproate is 9–16 hours.

Most clinicians use two general dosing strategies when treating acute mania: 1) a gradual dose titration or 2) a more rapid "loading dose" strategy. Most commonly, treatment with valproate is initiated with a gradual titration strategy in which it is started at a dosage of 250 mg three times a day, with subsequent increases of 250 mg every 3 days. Most patients require a daily dosage of 1,250–2,000 mg. Although valproate has a relatively short half-life, moderate doses may be given once a day at bedtime to reduce daytime sedation in patients with bipolar disorder (this strategy should not be used when the drug is being used to treat seizure disorders).

When an acutely manic patient requires rapid stabilization, valproate treatment can be initiated at a

TABLE 26–14.   Signs, symptoms, and management of lithium toxicity

Signs and symptoms of lithium toxicity

Mild to moderate intoxication (lithium level = 1.5–2.0 mEq/L)

Gastrointestinal symptoms

Vomiting

Abdominal pain

Dryness of mouth

Neurological symptoms

Ataxia

Dizziness

Slurred speech

Nystagmus

Lethargy or excitement

Muscle weakness

Moderate to severe intoxication (lithium level=2.1–2.5 mEq/L)

Gastrointestinal symptoms

Anorexia

Persistent nausea and vomiting

Neurological symptoms

Blurred vision

Muscle fasciculations

Clonic limb movements

Hyperactive deep tendon reflexes

Choreoathetoid movements

Convulsions

Delirium

Syncope

Electroencephalographic changes

Stupor

Coma

Circulatory failure (decreased blood pressure, cardiac arrhythmias, conduction abnormalities)

Severe intoxication (lithium level>2.5 mEq/L)

Generalized convulsions

Oliguria and renal failure

Death

TABLE 26–14.   Signs, symptoms, and management of lithium toxicity *(continued)*

Management of lithium toxicity

1. The patient should immediately contact his or her personal physician or go to a hospital emergency department.

2. Lithium should be discontinued, and the patient should ingest fluids if possible.

3. A physical examination (including checking of vital signs) and a neurological examination (including a complete formal mental status examination) should be performed.

4. As soon as possible, lithium and serum electrolyte levels should be measured, renal function tests performed, and an electrocardiogram obtained.

5. In cases of significant acute ingestion, residual gastric contents should be removed by induction of emesis, gastric lavage, and absorption with activated charcoal.[a]

6. Vigorous hydration and maintenance of electrolyte balance are essential.

7. In a patient with a serum lithium level greater than 4.0 mEq/L or with serious manifestations of lithium toxicity, hemodialysis should be initiated.[a]

8. Repeat dialysis may be required every 6–10 hours, until the lithium level is within nontoxic range and the patient has no signs or symptoms of lithium toxicity.

[a]Information from Goldfrank et al. 1986.

Source.   Adapted from Marangell LB, Martinez JM: *Concise Guide to Psychopharmacology,* 2nd Edition. Arlington, VA, American Psychiatric Publishing, 2006, pp. 146–147. Used with permission.

dose of 20 mg per kilogram of body weight (Keck et al. 1993). Plasma levels of 45–100 µg/mL are recommended for the treatment of acute mania (Bowden et al. 1996); however, dosing should be based on the balance between clinical response and side effects rather than on absolute blood level alone. Patients with less severe disorders, such as bipolar II disorder or cyclothymia, often respond at lower doses and blood levels (Jacobsen 1993). The XL preparation of divalproex sodium has 80%–90% of the bioavailability of the initial divalproex sodium, so doses may need to be slightly higher when this preparation is used.

Contraindications

Valproate is relatively contraindicated in patients with hepatitis or liver disease. If a patient has significant liver disease, alternative medications to treat his or her bipolar illness should be considered. Valproate should be used in such cases only as a last resort and only with the approval and continuous involvement of a gastroenterologist. Valproate has been linked to spina bifida and other neural tube defects in the offspring of patients exposed to this medication in the first trimester of pregnancy (Lammer et al. 1987; Robert and Guibaud 1982). Thus, the risks of continuing valproate therapy during pregnancy must be balanced against the risk of relapse. Abrupt discontinuation of medication in a woman with severe illness who is otherwise stable while taking valproate in the second or third trimester of pregnancy may be more harmful than helpful.

Risks, Side Effects, and Their Management

Hepatotoxicity. Although it is estimated that 1 in 118,000 patients dies from non-dose-related hepatic failure, no cases have occurred in patients older than 10 years who were receiving valproate monotherapy. Nonetheless, baseline liver function tests are indicated. If baseline test results are normal, monitoring for clinical signs of hepatotoxicity is more important than routine monitoring of liver enzyme levels, which has little predictive value and may be less effective than clinical monitoring (Pellock and Willmore 1991).

Transient mild increases in liver enzyme levels, up to three times the upper limit of normal, do not necessitate discontinuation of valproate. Although γ-glutamyltransferase levels are often checked by clinicians, these levels are often increased, without clinical significance, in patients receiving valproate and carbamazepine (Dean and Penry 1992). Likewise, plasma ammonia levels are often increased transiently during valproate treatment, but this finding does not necessitate interruption of treatment (Jaeken et al. 1980). Increases in transaminase levels are often dose dependent. If no suitable alternative treatment is available, dose reduction (with careful monitoring) may be attempted.

Hematological effects. Valproate has been associated with changes in platelet counts, but clinically significant thrombocytopenia has rarely been documented (Dean and Penry 1992). Coagulation defects also have been reported. Overall, the risk of inducing a coagulation disturbance in an otherwise healthy adult is extremely low. However, in patients in whom anticoagulation is strictly contraindicated and in patients who are already receiving anticoagulation therapy, monitoring of the coagulation profile is required at baseline, after 1 month of therapy, and then at least every 3 months.

Gastrointestinal symptoms. Multiple gastrointestinal side effects may be associated with valproate, including indigestion, nausea, and heartburn. Use of the divalproex sodium preparation and administration of the medication with food may alleviate these effects. Pancreatitis is a rare occurrence in patients receiving relatively high doses of valproate (Murphy et al. 1981). If vomiting and severe abdominal pain develop during valproate therapy, serum amylase levels should be determined immediately.

Weight gain. Weight gain is a common side effect of valproate treatment that does not appear to be dose dependent. Isojarvi et al. (1996) reported significant weight gain with associated hyperinsulinemia in approximately 50% of a cohort of women taking valproate. Given the risk of weight gain, diet and exercise should be recommended early in treatment.

Neurological effects. A benign essential tremor is a common side effect of valproate therapy. Drowsiness is another common side effect, but tolerance often develops once a steady-state level of the drug is reached.

Alopecia. Both transient and persistent hair loss have been associated with valproate use. Patients with valproate-induced alopecia may benefit from zinc supplementation, at a dose of 22.5 mg/day (Hurd et al. 1984).

Polycystic ovarian syndrome. Polycystic ovarian syndrome is characterized by menstrual irregularity, hyperandrogenism, and the exclusion of other etiologies. Isojarvi et al. (1993) reported an association between polycystic ovarian syndrome and valproate in women receiving long-term valproate treatment for epilepsy, especially those who were younger than 20 years. Recent data from the Systematic Treatment Enhancement Program for Bipolar Disorders indicated that women taking valproate had a 10.5% rate of oligomenorrhea with hyperandrogenism, compared with 1.4% of the women with bipolar disorder who were taking lithium or a different anticonvulsant (H. Joffe et al. 2006). Given these data, clinicians should document menstrual irregularities and observe for signs of hyperandrogenism, such as hirsutism.

Overdose

Valproate overdose results in increasing sedation, confusion, and ultimately coma. The patient also may manifest hyperreflexia or hyporeflexia, seizures, respiratory suppression, and supraventricular tachycardia. Treatment should include gastric lavage, electrocardiographic monitoring, treatment of emergent seizures, and respiratory support.

Drug Interactions

Valproate can inhibit hepatic enzymes, resulting in increased levels of other medications. Valproate is also highly bound to plasma proteins and may displace other highly bound drugs from protein-binding sites. Therefore, coadministered drugs that are either highly protein bound or reliant on hepatic metabolism may require dose adjustment. Drugs that may increase valproate levels include cimetidine, macrolide antibiotics (e.g., erythromycin), and felbamate. Valproate may increase concentrations of phenobarbital, ethosuximide, and the active 10,11-epoxide metabolite of carbamazepine, increasing the risk of toxicity. Valproate also may raise lamotrigine levels, increasing the risk of rash (current lamotrigine product labeling provides specific lamotrigine dosing guidelines for patients who are taking valproate). Valproate metabolism may be induced by other anticonvulsants, including carbamazepine, phenytoin, primidone, and phenobarbital, resulting in an increased total clearance of valproate and perhaps decreased efficacy.

Carbamazepine

Carbamazepine is effective in both acute and prophylactic treatment of mania (Gerner and Stanton 1992; Keck et al. 1992; Weisler et al. 2004, 2005). An XL formulation of carbamazepine, marketed in the United States under the brand name Equetro, is approved by the FDA for the treatment of acute mania. XL preparations of carbamazepine are preferred because the simplified dosage schedules may facilitate patient adherence. Other XL carbamazepine preparations include Tegretol XR and Carbatrol, although neither has been specifically indicated for the treatment of bipolar disorder.

Clinical Use

Carbamazepine should be initiated at a dosage of 200 mg twice a day, with increments of 200 mg/day every 3–5 days. Cited plasma levels of 8–12 µg/mL are based on clinical use in patients with seizure disorders and do not correlate with clinical response in patients with psychiatric disorders. We recommend a dose titration strategy that emphasizes achieving a clinical response and minimizes side effects. During the titration phase, patients may be particularly prone to side effects such as sedation, dizziness, and ataxia; if these occur, titration should be more gradual (the dosage might be 100 mg twice a day, for example). Because carbamazepine induces its own metabolism (autoinduction), dosage adjustments may be required for weeks or months after initiation of treatment to maintain therapeutic plasma levels.

Contraindications

Because of the potential for hematological and hepatic toxicity, carbamazepine should not be administered to patients with liver disease or thrombocytopenia or to those at risk for agranulocytosis. For this reason, carbamazepine is strictly contraindicated in patients receiving clozapine. Because of reports of teratogenicity, including increased risks of spina bifida (Rosa 1991), microcephaly (Bertollini et al. 1987), and craniofacial defects (Jones et al. 1989), carbamazepine is relatively contraindicated in pregnant women. Additionally, because carbamazepine has a tricyclic structure, there are concerns about concomitant use of carbamazepine and MAOIs.

Pretreatment evaluation should include a complete blood count and determination of ALT and aspartate aminotransferase (AST) levels. Because of the risk for teratogenicity, a pregnancy test also should be obtained in women of childbearing potential (see Table 26–13).

Risks, Side Effects, and Their Management

Hematological effects.   The most serious toxic hematological side effects of carbamazepine are agranulocytosis and aplastic anemia, which can be fatal. Whereas carbamazepine-induced agranulocytosis or aplastic anemia is extremely rare (Pellock 1987), other hematological effects, such as leukopenia (total WBC count <3,000 cells/mm^3), thrombocytopenia, and mild anemia, may occur more frequently. Although it is important to assess hematological function and risk factors before initiating treatment, there appears to be no benefit to ongoing monitoring in the absence of clinical indicators. When carbamazepine-induced agranulocytosis occurs, the onset is rapid. Thus, a normal complete blood count one day does not mean that agranulocytosis will not develop the next day. Therefore, it is more important to educate the patient to early signs and symptoms of agranulocytosis and thrombocytopenia and to tell the patient to inform the psychiatrist immediately if these signs and symptoms develop.

If significant leukopenia develops, such as an absolute neutrophil count of less than 1,000, carbamazepine therapy should be discontinued, and a hematologist should be consulted.

Hepatotoxicity. Carbamazepine therapy is occasionally associated with hepatic toxicity (Gram and Bentsen 1983), usually a hypersensitivity hepatitis that appears after a latency period of several weeks and involves increases in ALT, AST, and lactate dehydrogenase levels. Cholestasis is also possible, with increases in bilirubin and alkaline phosphatase concentrations. Mild transient increases in transaminase levels generally do not necessitate discontinuation of carbamazepine. If ALT or AST levels increase more than three times the upper limit of normal, carbamazepine should be discontinued.

Dermatological effects. Rash is a common side effect of carbamazepine, occurring in 3%–17% of patients (Warnock and Knesevich 1988) and typically occurring within 2–20 weeks after treatment initiation. Carbamazepine is generally discontinued if a rash develops because of the risk of progression to an exfoliative dermatitis or Stevens-Johnson syndrome, a severe bullous form of erythema multiforme (Patterson 1985).

Endocrine disorders. Carbamazepine may cause reductions in circulating thyroid hormones (Bentsen et al. 1983; Yeo et al. 1978). SIADH, with resultant hyponatremia, may be induced by carbamazepine treatment. Alcoholic patients may be at greater risk for hyponatremia. Patients taking carbamazepine who develop signs or symptoms of hyponatremia should have their serum sodium level measured.

Gastrointestinal symptoms. Nausea and occasional vomiting are common side effects of carbamazepine.

Neurological effects. Patients taking carbamazepine may develop dizziness, drowsiness, or ataxia, particularly during the early phases of treatment. If this occurs, the carbamazepine dose should be reduced and a slower titration schedule implemented.

Overdose

Carbamazepine overdose may initially present with neuromuscular disturbances, such as nystagmus, myoclonus, and hyperreflexia, which may then progress to seizures and coma. Cardiac conduction changes, nausea, vomiting, and urinary retention also may occur. Treatment of carbamazepine overdose should include induction of vomiting, gastric lavage, and supportive care. After a serious overdose, blood pressure and respiratory and kidney function should be monitored for several days.

Drug Interactions

Carbamazepine induces hepatic cytochrome P450 enzymes, which may reduce levels of other medications. Importantly, carbamazepine therapy can lead to oral contraceptive failure (Coulam and Annegers 1979). Therefore, women who are planning to initiate therapy with carbamazepine should be advised to consider alternative forms of birth control while taking carbamazepine. Use of medications or substances that inhibit CYP3A3/4 may result in significant increases in plasma carbamazepine levels (Brodie and MacPhee 1986; Cozza et al. 2003; Ketter et al. 1995).

Lamotrigine

Lamotrigine is an anticonvulsant medication that decreases sustained high-frequency repetitive firing of the voltage-dependent sodium channel, which may then decrease glutamate release (Leach et al. 1991; Macdonald and Kelly 1995). Lamotrigine is approved by the FDA for the prevention of mania and depression in patients with bipolar disorder. Two randomized controlled trials showed a greater time to intervention for any mood episode for both lamotrigine and lithium compared with placebo (Bowden et al. 2003; Calabrese et al. 2003). However, lamotrigine has not shown efficacy as a monotherapy treatment for acute mania. Lamotrigine has shown efficacy in a double-blind, placebo-controlled trial for the treatment of bipolar depression (Calabrese et al. 1999). Although lamotrigine is frequently used for the acute and longer-term control of the depressed phase of bipolar disorder (American Psychiatric Association 2002; Marangell et al. 2004), its use as a treatment for acute bipolar depression has not been approved by the FDA.

Clinical Use

Lamotrigine treatment is usually initiated at 25 mg once a day. Because the risk of a serious rash increases with rapid titration, it is essential to follow the recommended titration schedule. After 2 weeks, the dosage is increased to 50 mg/day for another 2 weeks. At week 5, the dosage can be increased to 100 mg/day and at week 6 to 200 mg/day. In patients who are taking valproate or other medications that decrease the clearance of lamotrigine, the dosing schedule and target dose are halved. Conversely, the titration schedule and dose are increased in those taking carbamazepine.

In the absence of carbamazepine or other enzyme inducers, doses higher than 200 mg are typically not recommended in the treatment of bipolar disorder.

Risks, Side Effects, and Their Management

Lamotrigine is well tolerated and is not associated with hepatotoxicity, weight gain, or significant sedation. Common early side effects include headache, dizziness, gastrointestinal distress, and blurred or double vision.

Rash.   Lamotrigine has been associated with both benign and severe rashes. A maculopapular rash develops in 5%–10% of patients taking lamotrigine, usually in the first 8 weeks of treatment. Calabrese et al. (2002) analyzed data from 12 multicenter trials of lamotrigine in patients with mood disorders and reported an 8.3% rate of benign rashes with lamotrigine therapy. Lamotrigine also has been associated with serious rashes requiring hospitalization and discontinuation of treatment. The incidence of these rashes, which have included Stevens-Johnson syndrome, is approximately 0.3% in adults receiving adjunctive treatment for epilepsy, 0.13% in adults receiving adjunctive therapy in mood disorders clinical trials, and 0.08% in adults receiving lamotrigine as initial monotherapy in mood disorders clinical trials (Lamictal 2005). It is important to note that Stevens-Johnson syndrome is potentially fatal. Before initiating lamotrigine therapy, the patient must be advised of the potential risk of developing a serious rash and the necessity to call the clinician immediately if a rash emerges. Development of a rash with concomitant systemic symptoms is a particularly ominous sign, and the patient should be evaluated immediately.

To minimize the risk of a rash, the clinician must prescribe lamotrigine in accordance with the current product labeling's recommended starting dose and titration schedule (noting that the titration schedules vary depending on the presence or absence of concomitant medications, particularly valproate). Additionally, Ketter et al. (2005) reported a decreased incidence of treatment-emergent rash by advising patients who are starting lamotrigine to avoid other new medicines and new foods, cosmetics, conditioners, deodorants, detergents, and fabric softeners, as well as sunburn and exposure to poison ivy and poison oak.

Teratogenicity.   Data published from the North American Antiepileptic Drug Registry reported 3 cases of cleft palate and 2 cases of cleft lip in infants from a total of 564 infants exposed in the first trimester to lamotrigine monotherapy (8.9 per 1,000) (Holmes et al. 2006). Data are still being collected in this and other pregnancy registries. At present, clinicians should discuss the possibility of these risks with their patients and consider treatment alternatives for patients who are contemplating pregnancy.

Drug Interactions

Several important potential drug–drug interactions may occur with lamotrigine. Of particular importance to patients with bipolar disorders, valproate will increase lamotrigine levels, and carbamazepine will decrease lamotrigine levels. These two interactions are of particular importance to psychiatrists because both drugs are commonly prescribed as mood stabilizers for patients with bipolar disorder. Many other anticonvulsants interact with lamotrigine as well. Oral contraceptives can result in decreases in lamotrigine concentrations, but lamotrigine does not affect the availability of oral contraceptives.

Oxcarbazepine

Oxcarbazepine is a keto derivative of carbamazepine but offers several advantages over carbamazepine. Specifically, oxcarbazepine does not require blood cell count, hepatic, or serum drug level monitoring; causes less cytochrome P450 enzyme induction than does carbamazepine (but may decrease effectiveness of oral contraceptives containing ethinyl estradiol and levonorgestrel); and does not induce its own metabolism. These properties, combined with its similarity to carbamazepine, led many clinicians to use this medication for the treatment of bipolar disorder. However, it is important to note that oxcarbazepine has not been approved by the FDA for the acute or long-term treatment of bipolar disorder. To date, small controlled trials have suggested efficacy in the treatment of acute mania compared with lithium and haloperidol (Emrich 1990).

Oxcarbazepine has been associated with hyponatremia (Pendlebury et al. 1989; Trileptal 2006); thus, serum sodium levels should be monitored in patients at risk. Additionally, Stevens-Johnson syndrome and toxic epidermal necrolysis may occur at rates 3- to 10-fold higher than background incidence rates (Trileptal 2006).

Other Anticonvulsants

There is considerable interest in the potential usefulness of newer anticonvulsants for the treatment of bipolar disorder. However, positive data from well-designed controlled monotherapy trials to date are lacking for these agents.

TABLE 26–15. Atypical antipsychotic dosing in the treatment of acute mania

Generic drug	Trade name	Dosing in acute mania (mg/day)[a]		
		Starting dose	Dose titration	Target dose
Olanzapine	Zyprexa	10–15	5 mg/day increments	5–20
Risperidone	Risperdal	2–3	1 mg/day increments	1–6
Aripiprazole	Abilify	15–30	15 mg increments	30
Quetiapine	Seroquel	100	50–100 mg/day increments	600
Ziprasidone	Geodon	80 (divided twice daily)	40–80 mg/day increments	120–160

[a]Lower doses and slower dose titrations are indicated for the elderly. The reader is referred to current product labeling for specific information regarding approved indications for use and dosing in special populations.

Source. Adapted from Marangell LB, Martinez JM: *Concise Guide to Psychopharmacology,* 2nd Edition. Arlington, VA, American Psychiatric Publishing, 2006, p. 161. Used with permission.

Atypical Antipsychotics

All of the atypical antipsychotic medications (olanzapine, risperidone, quetiapine, ziprasidone, and aripiprazole), except clozapine, are approved by the FDA for the treatment of acute mania. Across randomized controlled trials, atypical antipsychotics have shown efficacy in treating the core symptoms of mania. General dosing guidelines for acute mania are shown in Table 26–15. It is common clinical practice to use lower starting dosages for patients who are less ill, particularly those patients receiving treatment in outpatient settings, but this practice has not been studied in randomized controlled trials. At present, only two of the atypical antipsychotics—olanzapine and aripiprazole—have been approved by the FDA as maintenance-phase treatments for bipolar disorder, although studies are under way with the other agents. The use of these agents for the depressed phase of bipolar disorder is an area of active clinical investigation. Clozapine has not received FDA approval for use in bipolar disorder, but it is a valuable option for patients whose symptoms are otherwise resistant to treatment (Suppes et al. 1999).

Olanzapine–Fluoxetine Combination

The olanzapine–fluoxetine combination is currently the only medication approved by the FDA specifically for the treatment of depression in patients with bipolar disorder. This indication was based on data from a double-blind, randomized study in which the combi-

nation was superior to both olanzapine monotherapy and placebo (Tohen et al. 2003). Treatment-emergent mania or hypomania did not occur more frequently in the olanzapine–fluoxetine combination group than in the placebo group during the acute trial.

Clinical Use

The olanzapine–fluoxetine combination is available in four dosing preparations (6 mg/25 mg, 12 mg/25 mg, 6 mg/50 mg, 12 mg/50 mg) that allow clinicians to tailor treatment individually to provide greater or lesser amounts of each medication component. The typical starting dose for most patients is 6 mg/25 mg. Common side effects include somnolence, weight gain, increased appetite, asthenia, peripheral edema, and tremor. As one might expect, warnings and precautions that apply to either olanzapine or fluoxetine also apply to this combination treatment. For example, concomitant use of MAOIs is contraindicated given the fluoxetine component. Similarly, warnings and precautions regarding the potential association between olanzapine and hyperglycemia also apply. Additionally, clinicians should be aware of the potential drug–drug interactions that apply to either olanzapine or fluoxetine alone, such as the potential for clinically relevant CYP2D6 isoenzyme inhibition by the fluoxetine component.

Pharmacotherapy for Acute Mania

The first step in the treatment of an acute manic episode is to initiate treatment with one or two mood stabilizers with acute antimanic properties (American Psychiatric Association 2002). Lithium, valproate, carbamazepine, olanzapine, risperidone, aripiprazole, quetiapine, and ziprasidone are all indicated as single agents for the treatment of mania. Olanzapine and ziprasidone are also available in an injectable preparation. In patients who are severely ill or who have manic or mixed states with psychotic features, the American Psychiatric Association (2002) practice guideline recommends initial treatment with the combination of lithium or valproate and an atypical antipsychotic. For less severely ill patients, monotherapy is the first step in treatment if the patient is not taking a mood stabilizer. If the patient is already taking a mood stabilizer, the dose of the current medication should be optimized.

The choice of antimanic medications is based on prior response, comorbid illnesses, and the various side-effect profiles of the available medications. Importantly, the clinical response to antimanic agents may not be apparent for 1–2 weeks; thus, additional medications, such as lorazepam or clonazepam, may be effective adjuncts acutely if certain symptoms, such as severe agitation, warrant immediate control. Antidepressants exacerbate mania and should be tapered and discontinued in patients who are manic or in a mixed state.

If the manic episode is not effectively treated with monotherapy, the next step is to combine medications. After the patient is stabilized, it may be reasonable to consider tapering the dose of the first agent, although it is not unusual for patients with bipolar disorder to require long-term treatment with a combination of medications. ECT is an effective treatment for acute mania and is especially useful for patients who cannot safely wait until medication becomes effective.

Pharmacotherapy for Bipolar Depression

A common mistake is to treat bipolar depression in the same manner that one treats unipolar depression, overlooking the need for a mood stabilizer. In bipolar depression, the first pharmacological intervention should be to start or optimize treatment with a mood stabilizer rather than to start administering an antidepressant medication. In addition, thyroid function should be evaluated, particularly if the patient is taking lithium. Subclinical hypothyroidism, manifested as an increased thyroid-stimulating hormone level

and normal triiodothyronine and thyroxine levels, may present as depression in affectively predisposed individuals. In such cases, the addition of thyroid hormones may be beneficial, even if the patient has no other evidence of hypothyroidism.

Lithium, lamotrigine, quetiapine, and olanzapine–fluoxetine combination therapy are first-line treatments for bipolar depression. The response rate to lithium in bipolar depression is 79% (Zornberg and Pope 1993). In a double-blind, placebo-controlled trial, lamotrigine was shown to be effective in patients with bipolar depression (Calabrese et al. 1999). Lamotrigine can be combined with other mood stabilizers, but it is important to remember that lamotrigine therapy is started at lower doses and that dosage titration is more gradual when this medication is added to valproate therapy, given that valproate is a cytochrome P450 inhibitor and interferes with the metabolism of lamotrigine. Quetiapine monotherapy also was shown to be effective in two positive placebo-controlled trials of bipolar depression (Calabrese et al. 2005). In both trials, antidepressant efficacy was noted with both the 300-mg/day and the 600-mg/day dosage. The olanzapine–fluoxetine combination is particularly useful in patients who are not currently taking other psychiatric medications and who would benefit from taking a single pill rather than more traditional combined treatments.

Results from a recent double-blind, placebo-controlled trial indicated that adjunctive antidepressant therapy was no more effective for bipolar depression than treatment with a mood stabilizer plus placebo (Sachs et al. 2007). In addition, there were no significant differences in treatment-emergent affective switches between groups. However, some patients with bipolar disorder need antidepressant treatment. Although their propensity to cause a switch into mania or to induce rapid cycling is controversial, antidepressants do appear to present a risk for some patients. Therefore, patients with bipolar disorder should take antidepressants only in combination with a medication that has established antimanic properties. TCAs should be avoided when other viable treatment options exist. ECT should be considered in severe cases. In a 1-year randomized controlled trial, Miklowitz et al. (2007) found that specific, intensive, adjunctive psychotherapy (i.e., family-focused therapy, interpersonal and social rhythm therapy, and cognitive-behavioral therapy) was associated with higher year-end recovery rates and shorter times to recovery compared with brief therapy.

Maintenance Treatment in Bipolar Disorder

Patients with bipolar disorder require lifelong prophylaxis with a mood stabilizer, both to prevent new episodes and to decrease the likelihood that the illness will become more severe. Ninety percent of bipolar patients relapse after stopping lithium therapy, most within 6 months (Suppes et al. 1991). In addition to the single episode that may occur, each episode may further kindle the illness, thereby inducing a more malignant course with decreased treatment responsiveness. The more episodes a patient has had, the less likely the disorder is to respond to treatment (Gelenberg et al. 1989).

An additional reason for continuing effective prophylactic treatment is the possibility of discontinuation-induced refractoriness (Post et al. 1992). Some patients whose symptoms were previously treated with lithium successfully and who then have another episode after lithium has been discontinued fail to respond to retreatment with lithium. Moreover, these individuals tend to respond poorly to other treatments. Although discontinuation-induced refractoriness has been reported only with lithium, it is feasible that the phenomenon may occur with other agents. However, if tolerance develops, a period without the ineffective medication, along with institution of treatment with a different agent, is indicated. In most situations in which it is necessary to discontinue a mood stabilizer, tapering should be as slow as possible. Abruptly stopping lithium therapy is associated with a substantially higher rate of relapse than is tapering (Faedda et al. 1993).

Conclusion

The pharmacological armamentarium for treatment of psychiatric illnesses continues to expand. Results from multisite effectiveness and efficacy trials, such as CATIE and STAR*D, inform treatment and help define areas where improvement is needed. Current medications often have limited efficacy, and side effects decrease tolerability and compliance. More research is needed to address these hurdles that interfere with achieving remission.

Key Points

- Accurate diagnosis is the key to a well-informed treatment decision; whenever possible, treat the primary diagnosis and not the symptoms.

- Several factors are important when selecting an appropriate medication, including identifying medication-responsive target symptoms, ruling out nonpsychiatric causes of a patient's symptomatology, noting the presence of other medical problems that will influence drug selection, evaluating concomitant medications that may cause drug–drug interactions, and evaluating personal and family histories of medication response.

- Whenever possible, the clinician should involve the patient in medication decisions and educate the patient and significant others about the illness and potential benefits, risks, and side effects of any medication being prescribed.

- Patients must be educated about the typical time to response for the medication being prescribed and the need for strict adherence to the treatment regimen to ensure an optimal chance for treatment success.

- In addition to pharmacotherapy, other interventions such as disease-specific psychotherapies should be considered.

- When evaluating a patient with a history of treatment failures, a detailed treatment history should include a review of the dose, duration, tolerability, adherence, and reason for discontinuation for each prior treatment; many prior medication failures may be a result of inadequate dosing, inadequate treatment duration, noncompliance, or poor tolerability.

- Ongoing psychiatric and medical monitoring during treatment should be individualized to each patient according to several factors, including the severity of the illness, the current clinical status of the patient (e.g., acutely ill, partially remitted), and the specific medication(s) being prescribed.

- The clinician should evaluate response to each prescribed treatment by monitoring symptomatic and functional improvement and strive for complete symptomatic and functional recovery.

- Clinicians should be mindful of the response to each medication and consider discontinuing any treatment that has provided no benefit despite an adequate dose and duration of treatment.

Suggested Readings

Books

Cozza KL, Armstrong SC, Oesterheld JR: Concise Guide to Drug Interaction Principles for Medical Practice: Cytochrome P450s, UGTs, P-Glycoproteins, 2nd Edition. Washington, DC, American Psychiatric Publishing, 2003

Marangell LB, Martinez JM: Concise Guide to Psychopharmacology, 2nd Edition. Washington, DC, American Psychiatric Publishing, 2006

Schatzberg AF, Nemeroff CB: The American Psychiatric Publishing Textbook of Psychopharmacology, 3rd Edition. Washington, DC, American Psychiatric Publishing, 2004

Articles

Lieberman JA, Stroup TS, McEvoy JP, et al: Effectiveness of antipsychotic drugs in patients with chronic schizophrenia. N Engl J Med 353:1209–1223, 2005

McEvoy JP, Lieberman JA, Stroup TS, et al: Effectiveness of clozapine versus olanzapine, quetiapine, and risperidone in patients with chronic schizophrenia who did not respond to prior atypical antipsychotic treatment. Am J Psychiatry 163:600–610, 2006

Rush AJ, Trivedi MH, Wisniewski SR, et al: Bupropion-SR, sertraline, or venlafaxine-XR after failure of SSRIs for depression. N Engl J Med 354:1231–1242, 2006

Stroup TS, Lieberman JA, McEvoy JP, et al: Effectiveness of olanzapine, quetiapine, risperidone, and ziprasidone in patients with chronic schizophrenia following discontinuation of a previous atypical antipsychotic. Am J Psychiatry 163:611–622, 2006

Trivedi MH, Fava M, Wisniewski SR, et al: Medication augmentation after the failure of SSRIs for depression. N Engl J Med 354:1243–1252, 2006

Trivedi MH, Rush AJ, Wisniewski SR, et al: Evaluation of outcomes with citalopram for depression using measurement-based care in STAR*D: implications for clinical practice. Am J Psychiatry 163:28–40, 2006

Web Sites

American Psychiatric Association: http://www.psych.org

MedScape® Psychiatry & Mental Health: http://www.medscape.com/psychiatry

References

Abernethy DR, Greenblatt DJ, Ochs HR, et al: Benzodiazepine drug-drug interactions commonly occurring in clinical practice. Curr Med Res Opin 8 (suppl 4):80–93, 1984

Abilify (product information). Princeton, NJ, Bristol-Myers Squibb, 2005

Adler LA, Angrist B, Peselow E, et al: Efficacy of propranolol in neuroleptic-induced akathisia. J Clin Psychopharmacol 5:164–166, 1985

Adler LA, Angrist B, Reiter S, et al: Neuroleptic-induced akathisia: a review. Psychopharmacology (Berl) 97:1–11, 1989

Adler LA, Peselow E, Rotrosen J, et al: Vitamin E in the treatment of tardive dyskinesia. Am J Psychiatry 150:1405–1407, 1993

Adler LA, Edson R, Lavori P, et al: Long-term treatment effects of vitamin E for tardive dyskinesia. Biol Psychiatry 43:868–872, 1998

Aherwadkar SJ, Efendigil MC, Coulshed N: Chlorpromazine therapy and associated acute disturbances of cardiac rhythm. Br Heart J 36:1251–1252, 1974

Ahmed SM, Banner NR, Dubrey SW: Low cyclosporin-A level due to Saint-John's-wort in heart transplant patients (letter). J Heart Lung Transplant 20:795, 2001

Akhtar S, Jajor TR, Kumar S: Vitamin E in the treatment of tardive dyskinesia. J Postgrad Med 39:124–126, 1993

Allison DB, Mentore JL, Heo M, et al: Antipsychotic-induced weight gain: a comprehensive research synthesis. Am J Psychiatry 156:1686–1696, 1999

Altshuler LL, Cohen L, Szuba MP, et al: Pharmacological management of psychiatric illness during pregnancy: dilemmas and guidelines. Am J Psychiatry 153:592–606, 1996

American Diabetes Association, American Psychiatric Association, American Association of Clinical Endocrinologists, North American Association for the Study of Obesity: Consensus development conference on antipsychotic drugs and obesity and diabetes. Diabetes Care 27:596–601, 2004

American Psychiatric Association: Benzodiazepine Dependence, Toxicity, and Abuse: A Task Force Report of the American Psychiatric Association. Washington, DC, American Psychiatric Association, 1990

American Psychiatric Association: Tardive Dyskinesia: A Task Force Report of the American Psychiatric Association. Washington, DC, American Psychiatric Association, 1992

American Psychiatric Association: Practice guideline for the treatment of patients with schizophrenia. Am J Psychiatry 154 (suppl):1–63, 1997

American Psychiatric Association: Diagnostic and Statistical Manual of Mental Disorders, 4th Edition, Text Revision. Washington, DC, American Psychiatric Association, 2000a, p 372

American Psychiatric Association: Practice Guideline for the Treatment of Patients With Major Depressive Disorder, 2nd Edition. Washington, DC, American Psychiatric Association, 2000b

American Psychiatric Association: Practice Guideline for the Treatment of Patients With Borderline Personality Disorder. Washington, DC, American Psychiatric Association, 2001

American Psychiatric Association: Practice guideline for the treatment of patients with bipolar disorder (revision). Am J Psychiatry 159 (4 suppl):1–50, 2002

Amsterdam J: A double-blind, placebo-controlled trial of the safety and efficacy of selegiline transdermal system without dietary restrictions in patients with major depressive disorder. J Clin Psychiatry 64:208–214, 2003

Amsterdam J, Berwish NJ: High dose tranylcypromine therapy for refractory depression. Pharmacopsychiatry 22:21–25, 1989

Anath J, Dubin SE: Lithium and symptomatic hyperparathyroidism. J R Soc Med 96:1026–1029, 1983

Anderson ES, Powers PS: Neuroleptic malignant syndrome associated with clozapine use. J Clin Psychiatry 52:102–104, 1991

Angst F, Stassen HH, Clayton PJ, et al: Mortality of patients with mood disorders: follow-up over 34–38 years. J Affect Disord 68:167–181, 2002

Appleton WS, Davis JM: Practical Clinical Psychopharmacology, 2nd Edition. Baltimore, MD, Williams & Wilkins, 1980

Arana GW, Goff DC, Friedman H, et al: Does carbamazepine-induced reduction of plasma haloperidol levels worsen psychotic symptoms? Am J Psychiatry 143:650–651, 1986

Aronson MD, Hafez H: A case of trazodone-induced ventricular tachycardia. J Clin Psychiatry 47:388–389, 1986

Arora M, Praharaj SK: Meningocele and ankyloblepharon following in utero exposure to olanzapine. Eur Psychiatry 21:345–346, 2006

Arvanitis LA, Miller BG: Multiple fixed doses of "Seroquel" (quetiapine) in patients with acute exacerbation of schizophrenia: a comparison with haloperidol and placebo. The Seroquel Trial 13 Study Group. Biol Psychiatry 42:233–246, 1997

Baldessarini RJ, Cohen BM, Teicher MH: Significance of neuroleptic dose and plasma level in the pharmacological treatment of psychoses. Arch Gen Psychiatry 45:79–91, 1988

Ball WA, Caroff SN: Retinopathy, tardive dyskinesia, and low-dose thioridazine (letter). Am J Psychiatry 143:256–257, 1986

Barnas C, Zwierzina H, Hummer M, et al: Granulocyte-macrophage colony-stimulating factor (GM-CSF) treatment of clozapine-induced agranulocytosis: a case report. J Clin Psychiatry 53:245–247, 1992

Beasley CM, Tollefson G, Tran P, et al: Olanzapine versus placebo and haloperidol: acute phase results of the Northern American double-blind olanzapine trial. Neuropsychopharmacology 14:111–123, 1996

Bentsen KD, Gram L, Veje A: Serum thyroid hormones and blood folic acid during monotherapy with carbamazepine or valproate: a controlled study. Acta Neurol Scand 67:235–241, 1983

Bertollini R, Kallen B, Mastroiacovo P, et al: Anticonvulsant drugs in monotherapy: effect on fetus. Eur J Epidemiol 3:164–171, 1987

Bitran JA, Manji HK, Potter WZ, et al: Downregulation of PKC alpha by lithium in vitro. Psychopharmacol Bull 31:449–452, 1995

Bodkin J, Amsterdam JD: Transdermal selegiline in major depression: a double-blind, placebo-controlled, parallel-group study in outpatients. Am J Psychiatry 159:1869–1875, 2002

Bondolfi G, Baumann P, Dufour H: Treatment-resistant schizophrenia: clinical experience with new antipsychotics. Eur Neuropsychopharmacol 6 (suppl 2):S21–S25, 1996

Bowden CL, Janicak PG, Orsulak P, et al: Relation of serum valproate concentration to response in mania. Am J Psychiatry 153:765–770, 1996

Bowden CL, Calabrese JR, Sachs G, et al: A placebo-controlled 18-month trial of lamotrigine and lithium maintenance treatment in recently manic or hypomanic patients with bipolar I disorder. Lamictal 606 Study Group. Arch Gen Psychiatry 60:392–400, 2003

Branchey M, Branchey L: Patterns of psychotropic drug use and tardive dyskinesia. J Clin Psychopharmacol 4:41–45, 1984

Brantigan CO, Brantigan TA, Joseph N: Effect of beta blockade and beta stimulation on stage fright. Am J Med 72:88–94, 1982

Breidenbach T, Hoffmann MW, Becker T, et al: Drug interaction of St John's wort with cyclosporin (letter). Lancet 355:1912, 2000

Breier A, Buchanan RW, Waltrip RW II, et al: The effect of clozapine on plasma norepinephrine: relationship to clinical efficacy. Neuropsychopharmacology 10:1–7, 1994

Breier A, Meehan K, Birkett M, et al: A double-blind, placebo-controlled dose-response comparison of intramuscular olanzapine and haloperidol in the treatment of acute agitation in schizophrenia. Arch Gen Psychiatry 59:441–448, 2002

Bremner JD: A double-blind comparison of Org 3770, amitriptyline, and placebo in major depression. J Clin Psychiatry 56:519–525, 1995

Brodie MJ, MacPhee GJ: Carbamazepine neurotoxicity precipitated by diltiazem. BMJ 292:1170–1171, 1986

Bucht G, Smigan L, Wahlin A, et al: ECG changes during lithium therapy: a prospective study. Acta Med Scand 216:101–104, 1984

Burke RE, Fahn S, Jankovic J, et al: Tardive dyskinesia: late-onset and persistent dystonia caused by antipsychotic drugs. Neurology 32:1335–1346, 1982

Burt VK, Rasgon N: Special considerations in treating bipolar disorder in women. Bipolar Disord 6:2–13, 2004

Burton S, Heslop K, Harrison K, et al: Ziprasidone overdose (letter). Am J Psychiatry 157:835, 2000

Byerly MJ, DeVane CL: Pharmacokinetics of clozapine and risperidone: a review of recent literature. J Clin Psychopharmacol 16:177–187, 1996

Calabrese JR, Kimmel SE, Woyshville MJ, et al: Clozapine for treatment-refractory mania. Am J Psychiatry 153:759–764, 1996

Calabrese JR, Bowden CL, Sachs GS, et al: A double-blind placebo-controlled study of lamotrigine monotherapy in outpatients with bipolar I depression. Lamictal 602 Study Group. J Clin Psychiatry 60:79–88, 1999

Calabrese JR, Sullivan JR, Bowden CL, et al: Rash in multicenter trials of lamotrigine in mood disorders: clinical relevance and management. J Clin Psychiatry 63:1012–1019, 2002

Calabrese JR, Bowden CL, Sachs GS, et al: A placebo-controlled 18-month trial of lamotrigine and lithium maintenance treatment in recently depressed patients with bipolar I disorder. Lamictal 605 Study Group. J Clin Psychiatry 64:1013–1024, 2003

Calabrese JR, Keck PE, Macfadden W, et al: A randomized, double-blind, placebo-controlled trial of quetiapine in the treatment of bipolar I or II depression. Am J Psychiatry 162:1351–1360, 2005

Callahan AM, Marangell LB, Ketter TA: Evaluating the clinical significance of drug interactions: a systematic approach. Harv Rev Psychiatry 4:153–158, 1996

Casey DE, Daniel DG, Wassef AA, et al: Effect of divalproex combined with olanzapine or risperidone in patients with an acute exacerbation of schizophrenia. Neuropsychopharmacology 28:182–192, 2003

Chambers CD, Hernandez-Diaz S, Van Marter LJ, et al: Selective serotonin-reuptake inhibitors and risk of persistent pulmonary hypertension of the newborn. N Engl J Med 354:579–587, 2006

Chen G, Manji HK, Hawver DB, et al: Chronic sodium valproate selectively decreases protein kinase C alpha and epsilon in vitro. J Neurochem 63:2361–2364, 1994

Chouinard G, Jones BD, Remington G, et al: A Canadian multicenter, placebo-controlled study of fixed doses of risperidone and haloperidol in the treatment of chronic schizophrenic patients. J Clin Psychopharmacol 13:25–40, 1993

Citrome L: Schizophrenia and valproate. Psychopharmacol Bull 37 (suppl 2):74–88, 2003

Citrome L, Blonde L, Damatarca C: Metabolic issues in patients with severe mental illness. South Med J 98:714–720, 2005

Cohen LG, Chesley S, Eugenio L, et al: Erythromycin-induced clozapine toxic reaction. Arch Intern Med 156:675–677, 1996

Cohen LS, Friedman JM, Jefferson JW, et al: A reevaluation of risk of in utero exposure to lithium [published erratum appears in JAMA 271:1485, 1994]. JAMA 271:146–150, 1994

Cohn JB, Wilcox CS: Low-sedation potential of buspirone compared with alprazolam and lorazepam in the treatment of anxious patients: a double-blind study. J Clin Psychiatry 47:409–412, 1986

Cole JO, Gardos G, Rapkin R, et al: Lithium carbonate in tardive dyskinesia and schizophrenia, in Tardive Dyskinesia and Affective Disorders. Edited by Gardos G, Casey D. Washington, DC, American Psychiatric Press, 1984, pp 50–73

Coppen A, Mendelwicz J, Kielholz P: Pharmacotherapy of Depressive Disorders: A Consensus Statement. Geneva, Switzerland, World Health Organization, 1986

Correll CU, Leucht S, Kane JM: Lower risk for tardive dyskinesia associated with second generation antipsychotics: a systematic review of 1-year studies. Am J Psychiatry 161:414–425, 2004

Coulam CB, Annegers JF: Do anticonvulsants reduce the efficacy of oral contraceptives? Epilepsia 20:519–525, 1979

Coupland NJ, Bell CJ, Potokar JP: Serotonin reuptake inhibitor withdrawal. J Clin Psychopharmacol 16:356–362, 1996

Coyle JT, Duman RS: Finding the intracellular signaling pathways affected by mood disorder treatments. Neuron 38:157–160, 2003

Cozza KL, Armstrong SC, Oesterheld JR: Concise Guide to Drug Interaction Principles for Medical Practice: Cytochrome P450s, UGTs, P-Glycoproteins, 2nd Edition. Washington, DC, American Psychiatric Publishing, 2003

Csernansky JC, Riney SJ, Lombrozo L: Double-blind comparison of alprazolam, diazepam, and placebo for the treatment of negative schizophrenic symptoms. Arch Gen Psychiatry 45:655–659, 1988

Cymbalta (package insert). Indianapolis, IN, Eli Lilly & Co, 2006

Dabiri LM, Pasta D, Darby JK, et al: Effectiveness of vitamin E for the treatment of long-term tardive dyskinesia. Am J Psychiatry 151:925–926, 1994

Dalton SO, Johansen C, Mellemkjaer L, et al: Use of selective serotonin reuptake inhibitors and risk of upper gastrointestinal tract bleeding: a population-based cohort study. Arch Intern Med 163:59–64, 2003

Daniel DG, Zimbroff DL, Potkin SG, et al: Ziprasidone 80 mg/day and 160 mg/day in the acute exacerbation of schizophrenia and schizoaffective disorder: a 6-week placebo-controlled trial. Neuropsychopharmacology 20:491–505, 1999

Danish University Antidepressant Group: Paroxetine: a selective serotonin reuptake inhibitor showing better tolerance, but weaker antidepressant effect than clomipramine in a controlled multicenter study. J Affect Disord 18:289–299, 1990

DasGupta K, Young A: Clozapine-induced neuroleptic malignant syndrome. J Clin Psychiatry 52:105–107, 1991

Davidson M, Emsley R, Kramer M, et al: Efficacy, safety and early response of paliperidone extended-release tablets (paliperidone ER): results of a 6-week, randomized, placebo-controlled study. Schizophr Res 93:117–130, 2007

Davis JM: Maintenance therapy and the natural course of schizophrenia. J Clin Psychiatry 46:18–21, 1985

Davis KL, Kahn RS, Ko G, et al: Dopamine in schizophrenia: a review and reconceptualization. Am J Psychiatry 148:1474–1486, 1991 de Abajo FJ, Rodriguez LA, Montero D: Association between selective serotonin reuptake inhibitors and upper gastrointestinal bleeding: population based case-control study. BMJ 319:1106–1109, 1999

De Boer T: The pharmacological profile of mirtazapine. J Clin Psychiatry 57 (suppl 4):19–25, 1996

De Montigny C, Gunberg S, Mayer A, et al: Lithium induces rapid relief of depression in tricyclic antidepressant nonresponders. Br J Psychiatry 138:252–256, 1981

Dean JC, Penry JK: Valproate, in The Medical Treatment of Epilepsy. Edited by Resor SR Jr, Kutt H. New York, Marcel Dekker, 1992, pp 265–278

Delva NJ, Letemednia FJJ: Lithium treatment in schizophrenia and schizoaffective disorders. Br J Psychiatry 141:387–400, 1982

Devinsky O, Honigfeld G, Patin J: Clozapine-related seizures. Neurology 41:369–371, 1991

Di Rocco A, Brannan T, Prikhojan A, et al: Sertraline induced parkinsonism: a case report and an in-vivo study of the effect of sertraline on dopamine metabolism. J Neural Transm 105:247–251, 1998

Dinan TG, Barry S: A comparison of electroconvulsive therapy with a combined lithium and tricyclic combination among depressed tricyclic nonresponders. Acta Psychiatr Scand 80:97–100, 1989

Dixon J, Power SJ, Grundy EM, et al: Sedation for local anaesthesia: comparison of intravenous midazolam and diazepam. Anaesthesia 39:372–378, 1984

Dolovich LR, Addis A, Vaillancourt JM, et al: Benzodiazepine use in pregnancy and major malformations or oral cleft: meta-analysis of cohort and case-control studies. BMJ 317:839–843, 1998

Douyon R, Angrist B, Peselow E, et al: Neuroleptic augmentation with alprazolam: clinical effects and pharmacokinetic correlates (comment). Am J Psychiatry 146:1087–1088, 1989

Drew PJ, Barnes JN, Evans SJ: The effect of acute beta-adrenoceptor blockade on examination performance. Br J Clin Pharmacol 19:783–786, 1985

Drug Facts and Comparisons, 56th Edition. St. Louis, MO, Facts & Comparisons, A Wolters Kluwer Company, 2002, pp 915–921, 1012–1014

Dumon J-P, Catteau J, Lanvin F, et al: Randomized, double-blind, crossover, placebo-controlled comparison of propranolol and betaxolol in the treatment of neuroleptic-induced akathisia. Am J Psychiatry 149:647–650, 1992

Dunner DL, Fieve RR: Clinical factors in lithium carbonate prophylaxis failure. Arch Gen Psychiatry 30:229–233, 1974

Dupuis B, Catteau J, Dumon J-P, et al: Comparison of propranolol, sotalol, and betaxolol in the treatment of neuroleptic-induced akathisia. Am J Psychiatry 144:802–805, 1987

Durr D, Stieger B, Kullak-Ublick GA, et al: St John's wort induces intestinal P-glycoprotein/MDR1 and intestinal and hepatic CYP3A4. Clin Pharmacol Ther 68:598–604, 2000

Edlund MJ, Craig TJ: Antipsychotic drug use and birth defects: an epidemiologic reassessment. Compr Psychiatry 25:32–37, 1984

Egan MF, Hyde TM, Albers GW, et al: Treatment of tardive dyskinesia with vitamin E. Am J Psychiatry 149:773–777, 1992

Elkashef AM, Ruskin PE, Bacher N, et al: Vitamin E in the treatment of tardive dyskinesia. Am J Psychiatry 147:505–506, 1990

Emrich HM: Studies with oxcarbazepine (Trileptal) in acute mania. Int Clin Psychopharmacol 5:83–88, 1990

EMSAM (product information). Princeton, NJ, Bristol-Myers Squibb Co, 2006

Emsley R, Myburgh C, Oosthuizen P, et al: Randomized, placebo-controlled study of ethyl-eicosapentaenoic acid as supplemental treatment in schizophrenia. Am J Psychiatry 159:1596–1598, 2002

Ereshefsky L, Toney G, Saklad SR, et al: A loading-dose strategy for converting from oral to depot haloperidol. Hosp Community Psychiatry 44:1155–1161, 1993

Everett HC: The use of bethanechol chloride with tricyclic antidepressants. Am J Psychiatry 132:1202–1204, 1976

Expert Panel on the Detection, Evaluation, and Treatment of High Blood Cholesterol in Adults: Executive summary of the third report of the National Cholesterol Education Program (NCEP) expert panel on detection, evaluation, and treatment of high blood cholesterol in adults (Adult Treatment Panel III). JAMA 285:2486–2497, 2001

Faedda GL, Tondo L, Baldessarini RJ, et al: Outcome after rapid vs gradual discontinuation of lithium treatment in bipolar disorders. Arch Gen Psychiatry 50:448–455, 1993

Fahn S: A therapeutic approach to tardive dyskinesia. J Clin Psychiatry 46:19–24, 1985

Faucette SR, Hawke RL, Lecluyse EL, et al: Validation of bupropion hydroxylation as a selective marker for human cytochrome P450 2B6 catalytic activity. Drug Metab Dispos 28:1222–1230, 2000

Fava M, Rankin MA, Alpert JE, et al: An open trial of oral sildenafil in antidepressant-induced sexual dysfunction. Psychother Psychosom 67:328–331, 1998

Fava M, Judge R, Hoog SL, et al: Fluoxetine versus sertraline and paroxetine in major depressive disorder: changes in weight with long-term treatment. J Clin Psychiatry 61:863–867, 2000

Fava M, Thase ME, DeBattista C: A multicenter, placebo-controlled study of modafinil augmentation in partial responders to selective serotonin reuptake inhibitors with persistent fatigue and sleepiness. J Clin Psychiatry 66:85–93, 2005

Fawcett J, Kravitz HM, Zajecka JM, et al: CNS stimulant potentiation of monoamine oxidase inhibitors in treatment-refractory depression. J Clin Psychopharmacol 11:127–132, 1991

Feinberg SS, Holzer B: The monoamine oxidase inhibitor (MAOI) diet and kosher pizza (letter). J Clin Psychopharmacol 17:227–228, 1997

Feinberg SS, Holzer B: Clarifying the safety of the MAOI diet and pizza (letter). J Clin Psychiatry 61:145, 2000

Fenton WS, Dickerson F, Boronow J, et al: A placebo-controlled trial of omega-3 fatty acid (ethyl eicosapentaenoic acid) supplementation for residual symptoms and cognitive impairment in schizophrenia. Am J Psychiatry 158:2071–2074, 2001

Frank E, Kupfer DJ, Perel JM, et al: Three-year outcomes for maintenance therapies in recurrent depression. Arch Gen Psychiatry 47:1093–1099, 1990

Freeman MP, Gelenberg AJ: Bipolar disorder in women: reproductive events and treatment considerations. Acta Psychiatr Scand 112:88–96, 2005

Fuller MA, Sajatovic M: Lexi-Comp's Drug Information Handbook for Psychiatry, 4th Edition. Hudson, OH, Lexi-Comp, 2004a, pp 1440–1441

Fuller MA, Sajatovic M: Lexi-Comp's Drug Information Handbook for Psychiatry, 4th Edition. Hudson, OH, Lexi-Comp, 2004b, p 1420

Gajwani P, Pozuelo L, Tesar GE: QT interval prolongation with quetiapine (Seroquel) overdose. Psychosomatics 41:63–65, 2000

Gardner DM, Shulman KI, Walker SE, et al: The making of a user friendly MAOI diet. J Clin Psychiatry 57:99–104, 1996

Gelenberg AJ, Kane JM, Keller MB, et al: Comparison of standard and low serum levels of lithium for maintenance treatment of bipolar disorder. N Engl J Med 321:1489–1493, 1989

Gentile S: Clinical utilization of atypical antipsychotics in pregnancy and lactation. Ann Pharmacother 38:1265–1271, 2004

Geodon (product information). New York, Pfizer, 2005

Gerbino L, Shopsin B, Collora M: Clozapine in the treatment of tardive dyskinesia: an interim report, in Tardive Dyskinesia, Research and Treatment. Edited by Fann WE, Smith RC, Davis JM, et al. New York, SP Medical & Scientific Books, 1980, pp 475–489

Gerner RH, Stanton A: Algorithm for patient management of acute manic states: lithium, valproate, or carbamazepine? J Clin Psychopharmacol 12 (suppl):57S–63S, 1992

Gerson SL, Gullion G, Yeh HS, et al: Granulocyte colony-stimulating factor for clozapine-induced agranulocytosis (letter). Lancet 340:1097, 1992

Ghadirian AM, Chouinard G, Annable L: Sexual dysfunction and plasma prolactin levels in neuroleptic-treated schizophrenic outpatients. J Nerv Ment Dis 170:463–467, 1982

Ghaemi SN, Zarate CA Jr, Popli AP, et al: Is there a relationship between clozapine and obsessive-compulsive disorder? A retrospective chart review. Compr Psychiatry 36:267–270, 1995

Giles TD, Modlin RK: Death associated with ventricular arrhythmia and thioridazine hydrochloride. JAMA 205:108–110, 1968

Gill SS, Rochon PA, Herrmann N, et al: Atypical antipsychotic drugs and risk of ischaemic stroke: population based retrospective cohort study. BMJ 330:445, 2005

Glazer WM, Moore DC, Schooler NR, et al: Tardive dyskinesia: a discontinuation study. Arch Gen Psychiatry 41:623–627, 1984

Glick ID, Marder SR: Long term maintenance therapy with quetiapine versus haloperidol decanoate in patients with schizophrenia or schizoaffective disorder. J Clin Psychiatry 66:638–641, 2005

Goff DC, Baldessarini R: Antipsychotics, in Drug Interactions in Psychiatry, 2nd Edition. Edited by Ciraulo D, Shader R, Greenblatt D, et al. Baltimore, MD, Williams & Wilkins, 1995, pp 129–174

Goff DC, Coyle JT: The emerging role of glutamate in the pathophysiology and treatment of schizophrenia. Am J Psychiatry 158:1366–1377, 2001

Goff DC, Evins AE: Negative symptoms in schizophrenia: neurobiological models and treatment response. Harv Rev Psychiatry 6:59–77, 1998

Goff DC, Midha KK, Sarid-Segal O, et al: A placebo-controlled trial of fluoxetine added to neuroleptic in patients with schizophrenia. Psychopharmacology (Berl) 117:417–423, 1995

Goff D, Posever T, Herz L, et al: An exploratory haloperidol-controlled dose-finding study of ziprasidone in hospitalized patients with schizophrenia or schizoaffective disorder. J Clin Psychopharmacol 18:296–304, 1998

Goldberg HL, Finnerty RJ: The comparative efficacy of buspirone and diazepam in the treatment of anxiety. Am J Psychiatry 136:1184–1187, 1979

Goldfrank LR, Lewin NA, Flomenbaum NE, et al: Antidepressants: tricyclics, tetracyclics, monoamine oxidase inhibitors, and others, in Goldfrank's Toxicologic Emergencies, 3rd Edition. Edited by Goldfrank LR, Flomenbaum ME, Lewis NA, et al. Norwalk, CT, Appleton-Century-Crofts, 1986, pp 351–363

Goodwin FK, Jamison R: Manic-Depressive Illness. New York, Oxford University Press, 1990

Goodwin FK, Prange AJ, Post RM, et al: Potentiation of antidepressant effects by L-triiodothyronine in tricyclic nonresponders. Am J Psychiatry 139:34–38, 1982

Gould RA, Mueser KT, Bolton E, et al: Cognitive therapy for psychosis in schizophrenia: an effect size analysis. Schizophr Res 48:335–342, 2001

Gram LM, Bentsen KD: Hepatic toxicity of antiepileptic drugs: a review. Acta Neurol Scand Suppl 97:81–90, 1983

Green MF, Marshall BD Jr, Wirshing WC, et al: Does risperidone improve verbal working memory in treatment-resistant schizophrenia? Am J Psychiatry 154:799–804, 1997

Greenblatt DJ, von Moltke LL, Harmatz JS, et al: Drug interactions with newer antidepressants: role of human cytochromes P450. J Clin Psychiatry 59 (suppl 15):19–27, 1998

Greenblatt DJ, von Moltke LL, Harmatz JS, et al: Human cytochromes and some newer antidepressants: kinetics, metabolism, and drug interactions. J Clin Psychopharmacol 19:23S–35S, 1999

Guy W: Abnormal Involuntary Movement Scale (AIMS), in ECDEU Assessment Manual for Psychopharmacology, Revised. Washington, DC, U.S. Department of Health, Welfare, and Education, 1976, pp 534–537

Guze BH, Baxter LR: Current concepts: neuroleptic malignant syndrome. N Engl J Med 313:163–166, 1985

Hagger C, Buckley P, Kenny JT, et al: Improvement in cognitive functions and psychiatric symptoms in treatment-refractory schizophrenic patients receiving clozapine. Biol Psychiatry 34:702–712, 1993

Hamilton JD: Thioridazine retinopathy within the upper dosage limit. Psychosomatics 26:823–824, 1985

Haring C, Barnas C, Saria A, et al: Dose-related plasma levels of clozapine. J Clin Psychopharmacol 9:71–72, 1989

Harvey KV, Balon R: Augmentation with buspirone: a review. Ann Clin Psychiatry 7:143–147, 1995

Henderson DC, Cagliero E, Gray C, et al: Clozapine, diabetes mellitus, weight gain, and lipid abnormalities: a 5-year naturalistic study. Am J Psychiatry 157:975–981, 2000

Herrmann N, Lanctot KL: Do atypical antipsychotics cause stroke? CNS Drugs 19:91–103, 2005

Hertley LR, Ungapen S, Davie I, et al: The effect of beta-adrenergic blocking drugs on speakers' performance and memory. Br J Psychiatry 142:512–517, 1983

Hetmar O, Bren C, Clemmesen L, et al: Lithium: long-term effects on the kidney, II: structural changes. J Psychiatr Res 21:279–288, 1987

Hetmar O, Poulsen UJ, Ladefoged J, et al: Lithium: long-term effects on the kidney: a prospective follow-up study ten years after kidney biopsy. Br J Psychiatry 158:53–58, 1991

Hodgman MJ, Martin TG, Krenzelok EP: Serotonin syndrome due to venlafaxine and maintenance tranylcypromine therapy. Hum Exp Toxicol 16:14–17, 1997

Holmes LB, Wyszynski DF, Baldwin EJ, et al: Increased risk for non-syndromic cleft palate among infants exposed to lamotrigine during pregnancy (abstract). Birth Defects Res A Clin Mol Teratol 76:318, 2006

Honigfeld G: The Clozapine National Registry System: forty years of risk management. J Clin Psychiatry Monogr 14:29–32, 1996

Honigfeld G, Arellano F, Sethi J, et al: Reducing clozapine-related morbidity and mortality: 5 years of experience with the Clozaril National Registry. J Clin Psychiatry 59 (suppl 3):3–7, 1998

Hurd RW, Van Rinsvelt HA, Wilder BJ, et al: Selenium, zinc, and copper changes with valproic acid: possible relation to drug side effects. Neurology 34:1393–1395, 1984

Hustey FM: Acute quetiapine poisoning. J Emerg Med 17:995–997, 1999

Isojarvi JIT, Laatikainen TJ, Pakarinen AJ, et al: Polycystic ovaries and hyperandrogenism in women taking valproate for epilepsy. N Engl J Med 39:579–584, 1993

Isojarvi JI, Laatikainen TJ, Knip M, et al: Obesity and endocrine disorders in women taking valproate for epilepsy. Ann Neurol 39:579–584, 1996

Itil TM, Soldatos C: Epileptogenic side effects of psychotropic drugs: practical recommendations. JAMA 244:1460–1463, 1980

Jacobsen FM: Low-dose valproate: a new treatment for cyclothymia, mild rapid cycling disorders, and premenstrual syndrome. J Clin Psychiatry 54:229–234, 1993

Jaeken J, Casaer P, Corbeel L: Valproate, hyperammonaemia, and hyperglycinaemia (letter). Lancet 2(8188):260, 1980

Jankowsky D, Curtis G, Zisook S, et al: Trazodone-aggravated ventricular arrhythmias. J Clin Psychopharmacol 3:372–376, 1983

Jenike MA: Approaches to the patient with treatment-refractory obsessive-compulsive disorder. J Clin Psychiatry 51 (suppl):15–21, 1990

Jenkins SC, Tinsley JA, Van Loon JA: A Pocket Reference for Psychiatrists, 3rd Edition. Washington, DC, American Psychiatric Publishing, 2001, pp 133–134

Jeste DV, Wyatt RJ: Understanding and Treating Tardive Dyskinesia. New York, Guilford, 1982

Jeste DV, Lacro JP, Bailey A, et al: Lower incidence of tardive dyskinesia with risperidone compared to haloperidol in older patients. J Am Geriatr Soc 47:716–719, 1999

Joffe H, Cohen LS, Suppes T, et al: Valproate is associated with new-onset oligomenorrhea with hyperandrogenism in women with bipolar disorder. Biol Psychiatry 59:1078–1086, 2006

Joffe RT: T3 and lithium potentiation of tricyclic antidepressants. Am J Psychiatry 145:1317–1318, 1988

Joffe RT, Singer W: A comparison of triiodothyronine and thyroxine in the potentiation of tricyclic antidepressants. Psychiatry Res 32:241–251, 1990

Joffe RT, Singer W, Levitt AJ, et al: A placebo-controlled comparison of lithium and triiodothyronine augmentation of tricyclic antidepressants in unipolar refractory depression. Arch Gen Psychiatry 50:387–393, 1993

Johnson DAW: Antipsychotic medication: clinical guidelines for maintenance therapy. J Clin Psychiatry 46:6–15, 1985

Jones KL, Lacro RV, Johnson KA, et al: Pattern of malformations in the children of women treated with carbamazepine during pregnancy. N Engl J Med 320:1661–1666, 1989

Källén B, Otterblad Olausson P: Antidepressant drugs during pregnancy and infant congenital heart defect. Reprod Toxicol 21:221–222, 2006

Kane JM: Treatment-resistant schizophrenic patients. J Clin Psychiatry 57:35–40, 1996

Kane JM, Smith JM: Tardive dyskinesia: prevalence and risk factors, 1959 to 1979. Arch Gen Psychiatry 39:473–481, 1982

Kane JM, Honigfeld G, Singer J, et al: Clozapine for the treatment-resistant schizophrenic: a double-blind comparison vs chlorpromazine/benztropine. Arch Gen Psychiatry 45:789–796, 1988

Kane JM, Eerdekens M, Lindenmayer JP, et al: Long-acting injectable risperidone: efficacy and safety of the first long-acting atypical antipsychotic. Am J Psychiatry 160:1125–1132, 2003

Kane J, Canas F, Kramer M, et al: Treatment of schizophrenia with paliperidone extended-release tablets: a 6-week placebo-controlled trial. Schizophr Res 90:147–161, 2007

Kapur S, Seeman P: Does fast dissociation from the dopamine D2 receptor explain the action of atypical antipsychotics? A new hypothesis. Am J Psychiatry 158:360–369, 2001

Karliova M, Treichel U, Malago M, et al: Interaction of *Hypericum perforatum* (St. John's wort) with cyclosporin A metabolism in a patient after liver transplantation. J Hepatol 33:853–855, 2000

Karoum F, Chuang LW, Eisler T, et al: Metabolism of (-)deprenyl to amphetamine and methamphetamine may be responsible for deprenyl's therapeutic benefit: a biochemical assessment. Neurology 32:503–509, 1982

Keck PE Jr, Pope HG Jr, Cohen BM, et al: Risk factor for neuroleptic malignant syndrome. Arch Gen Psychiatry 46:914–918, 1989

Keck PE Jr, McElroy SL, Nemeroff CB: Anticonvulsants in the treatment of bipolar disorder. J Neuropsychiatry Clin Neurosci 4:395–405, 1992

Keck PE Jr, McElroy SL, Tugrul KC, et al: Valproate oral loading in the treatment of acute mania. J Clin Psychiatry 54:305–308, 1993

Keck PE Jr, McElroy SL, Strakowski SM: New developments in the pharmacological treatment of schizoaffective disorder. J Clin Psychiatry 57 (suppl 9):41–48, 1996

Keck P Jr, Buffenstein A, Ferguson J, et al: Ziprasidone 40 and 120 mg/day in the acute exacerbation of schizophrenia and schizoaffective disorder: a 4-week placebo-controlled trial. Psychopharmacology 140:173–184, 1998

Keller MB: Long-term treatment of recurrent and chronic depression. J Clin Psychiatry 62 (suppl 24):3–5, 2001

Kennedy PF, Hershon HI, McGuire RJ: Extrapyramidal disorders after prolonged phenothiazine therapy. Br J Psychiatry 118:509–518, 1971

Ketter TA, Flockhart DA, Post RM, et al: The emerging role of cytochrome P450 3A in psychopharmacology. J Clin Psychopharmacol 15:387–398, 1995

Ketter TA, Wang PW, Chandler RA, et al: Dermatology precautions and slower titration yield low incidence of lamotrigine treatment-emergent rash. J Clin Psychiatry 66:642–645, 2005

Kilian JG, Kerr K, Lawrence C, et al: Myocarditis and cardiomyopathy associated with clozapine. Lancet 354:1841–1845, 1999

Kim JS, Chang MY, Yu IT, et al: Lithium selectivity increases neuronal differentiation of hippocampal neural progenitor cells both in vitro and in vivo. J Neurochem 89:324–336, 2004

Kinon BJ, Basson BR, Gilmore JA, et al: Long-term olanzapine treatment: weight change and weight-related health factors in schizophrenia. J Clin Psychiatry 62:92–100, 2001

Kleinberg D, Brecher M, Davis J: Prolactin levels and adverse events in patients treated with risperidone. Paper presented at the 150th annual meeting of the American Psychiatric Association, San Diego, CA, May 17–22, 1997

Klibanski A, Neer R, Beitins I: Decreased bone density in hyperprolactinemic women. N Engl J Med 303:1511–1514, 1981

Kolecki P: Venlafaxine induced serotonin syndrome occurring after abstinence from phenelzine for more than two weeks (letter). J Toxicol Clin Toxicol 35:211–212, 1997

Kramer M, Simpson G, Maciulis V, et al: Paliperidone extended-release tablets for prevention of symptom recurrence in patients with schizophrenia: a randomized, double-blind, placebo-controlled study. J Clin Psychopharmacol 27:6–14, 2007

Kremer I, Vass A, Gorelik I, et al: Placebo-controlled trial of lamotrigine added to conventional and atypical antipsychotics in schizophrenia. Biol Psychiatry 56:441–446, 2004

Kupfer DJ: Management of recurrent depression. J Clin Psychiatry 54 (suppl):29–33, 1993

Labbate LA, Pollack MH: Treatment of fluoxetine-induced sexual dysfunction with bupropion: a case report. Ann Clin Psychiatry 6:13–15, 1994

Laird LK: Issues in the monopharmacotherapy and polypharmacotherapy of obsessive-compulsive disorder. Psychopharmacol Bull 32:569–578, 1996

Lamictal (product information). Research Triangle Park, NC, GlaxoSmithKline, 2005

Lammer EJ, Sever LE, Oakley GP Jr: Teratogen update: valproic acid. Teratology 35:465–473, 1987

Laties AM, Dev V, Geller W, et al: Safety update on lenticular opacities: benign experience with 620,000 US patient exposures to quetiapine (p 354), in Abstracts of the 39th Annual Meeting of the American College of Neuropharmacology. Nashville, TN, American College of Neuropharmacology, 2000

Leach MJ, Baxter MG, Critchley MA: Neurochemical and behavioral aspects of lamotrigine. Epilepsia 32 (suppl 2):S4–S8, 1991

Lehman AF, Lieberman JA, Dixon LB, et al: Practice guideline for the treatment of patients with schizophrenia, 2nd Edition. Am J Psychiatry 161 (suppl 2):1–56, 2004

Lenox RH, Watson DG, Patel J, et al: Chronic lithium administration alters a prominent PKC substrate in rat hippocampus. Brain Res 570:333–340, 1992

Lewis SW, Barnes TR, Davies L, et al: Randomized controlled trial of effect of prescription of clozapine versus other second-generation antipsychotic drugs in resistant schizophrenia. Schizophr Bull 32:715–723, 2006

Lieberman JA, Saltz BL, Johns CA, et al: The effects of clozapine on tardive dyskinesia. Br J Psychiatry 158:503–510, 1991

Lieberman J, Jody D, Geisler S, et al: Time course and biologic correlates of treatment response in first-episode schizophrenia. Arch Gen Psychiatry 50:369–376, 1993

Lieberman JA, Koreen AR, Chakos M, et al: Factors influencing treatment response and outcome of first-episode schizophrenia: implications for understanding the pathophysiology of schizophrenia. J Clin Psychiatry 57 (suppl 9):5–9, 1996

Lieberman JA, Sheitman B, Chakos M, et al: The development of treatment resistance in patients with schizophrenia: a clinical and pathophysiological perspective. J Clin Psychopharmacol 18 (2, suppl 1):20S–24S, 1998

Lieberman JA, Stroup TS, McEvoy JP, et al: Effectiveness of antipsychotic drugs in patients with chronic schizophrenia. N Engl J Med 353:1209–1223, 2005

Linazasoro G: Worsening of Parkinson's disease by citalopram. Parkinsonism Relat Disord 6:111–113, 2000

Linnoila M, Vinkar M, Hiertala O: Effect of sodium valproate on tardive dyskinesia. Br J Psychiatry 129:114–119, 1976

Lipinski JF, Zubenko GS, Cohen BM, et al: Propranolol in the treatment of neuroleptic induced akathisia. Am J Psychiatry 141:412–415, 1984

Loebel AD, Lieberman JA, Alvir JMJ, et al: Duration of psychosis and outcome in first-episode schizophrenia. Am J Psychiatry 149:1183–1188, 1992

Lohr JB, Caligiuri MP: A double-blind placebo-controlled study of vitamin E treatment of tardive dyskinesia. J Clin Psychiatry 57:167–173, 1996

Lohr JB, Cadet JL, Lohr MA, et al: Alpha-tocopherol in tardive dyskinesia. Lancet 1:913–914, 1987

Lokkegaard H, Andersen NF, Henriksen E: Renal function in 153 manic-depressive patients treated with lithium for more than five years. Acta Psychiatr Scand 71:347–355, 1985

Lucki I, Rickels K, Geller AM: Chronic use of benzodiazepines and psychomotor and cognitive test performance. Psychopharmacology (Berl) 88:426–433, 1986

Lunesta (product information). Marlborough, MA, Sepracor, 2005

Macdonald RL, Kelly KM: Antiepileptic drug mechanisms of action. Epilepsia 36:S2–S12, 1995

Mallette LE, Eichhorn E: Effects of lithium carbonate on human calcium metabolism. Arch Intern Med 146:770–776, 1986

Manji HK, Bebchuk JM, Moore GJ, et al: Modulation of CNS signal transduction pathways and gene expression by mood-stabilizing agents: therapeutic implications. J Clin Psychiatry 60 (suppl 2):27–39, 1993

Manji HK, Chen G, Shimon H, et al: Guanine nucleotide-binding proteins in bipolar affective disorder: effects of long-term lithium treatment. Arch Gen Psychiatry 52:135–144, 1995

Manji HK, Chen G, Hsiao JK, et al: Regulation of signal transduction pathways by mood-stabilizing agents: implications for the delayed onset of therapeutic efficacy. J Clin Psychiatry 57 (suppl 13):34–46, 1996

Manji HK, Chen G, Hsiao JK, et al: Regulation of signal transduction pathways by mood-stabilizing agents: implications for the delayed onset of therapeutic efficacy. J Clin Psychiatry 57:34–46, 1999

Marangell LB: Switching antidepressants for treatment-resistant major depression. J Clin Psychiatry 62 (suppl 18):12–17, 2001

Marangell LB, Martinez JM: Concise Guide to Psychopharmacology, 2nd Edition. Washington, DC, American Psychiatric Publishing, 2006

Marangell LB, Johnson CR, Kertz B, et al: Olanzapine in the treatment of apathy in previously depressed participants maintained on SSRIs: an open label, flexible-dose study. J Clin Psychiatry 63:391–395, 2002

Marangell LB, Martinez JM, Ketter TA, et al: Lamotrigine treatment of bipolar disorder: data from the first 500 patients in STEP-BD. Bipolar Disord 6:139–143, 2004

Marder SR, Meibach RC: Risperidone in the treatment of schizophrenia. Am J Psychiatry 151:825–835, 1994

Marder SR, Kramer M, Ford L, et al: Efficacy and safety of paliperidone extended-release tablets: results of a 6-week, randomized, placebo-controlled study. Biol Psychiatry [Epub ahead of print], 2007

Margolese HC, Chouinard G, Kolivakis TT, et al: Tardive dyskinesia in the era of typical and atypical antipsychotics, part 2: incidence and management strategies in patients with schizophrenia. Can J Psychiatry 50:703–714, 2005

Markowitz GS, Radhakrishnan J, Kambham N, et al: Lithium nephrotoxicity: a progressive combined glomerular and tubulointerstitial nephropathy. J Am Soc Nephrol 11:1439–1448, 2000

McElroy SL, Dessain EC, Pope HG Jr, et al: Clozapine in the treatment of psychotic mood disorders, schizoaffective disorder, and schizophrenia. J Clin Psychiatry 52:411–414, 1991

McEvoy JP, Hogarty GE, Steingard S: Optimal dose of neuroleptic in acute schizophrenia: a controlled study of the neuroleptic threshold and higher haloperidol dose. Arch Gen Psychiatry 48:739–745, 1991

McEvoy JP, Lieberman JA, Stroup TS, et al: Effectiveness of clozapine versus olanzapine, quetiapine, and risperidone in patients with chronic schizophrenia who did not respond to prior atypical antipsychotic treatment. Am J Psychiatry 163:600–610, 2006

McKenna K, Koren G, Tetelbaum M, et al: Pregnancy outcome of women using atypical antipsychotic drugs: a prospective comparative study. J Clin Psychiatry 66:444–449, 2005

Meltzer HY: The mechanism of action of novel antipsychotic drugs. Schizophr Bull 17:265–287, 1991

Meltzer HY: An overview of the mechanism of action of clozapine. J Clin Psychiatry 55 (suppl B):47–52, 1994

Metzger E, Friedman R: Prolongation of the corrected QT and torsades de pointes cardiac arrhythmia associated with intravenous haloperidol in the medically ill. J Clin Psychopharmacol 13:128–132, 1993

Michalets EL: Update: clinically significant cytochrome P450 drug interactions. Pharmacotherapy 18:84–112, 1998

Miklowitz DJ, Otto MW, Frank E, et al: Intensive psychosocial intervention enhances functioning in patients with bipolar depression: results from a 9-month randomized controlled trial. Am J Psychiatry 164:1340–1347, 2007

Miller DD, Sharafuddin MJ, Kathol RG: A case of clozapine-induced neuroleptic malignant syndrome. J Clin Psychiatry 52:99–101, 1991

Munetz MR, Roth LH: Informing patients about tardive dyskinesia. Arch Gen Psychiatry 42:866–871, 1985

Munjack DJ, Bruns J, Baltazar PL, et al: A pilot study of buspirone in the treatment of social phobia. J Anxiety Disord 5:87–98, 1991

Murphy MJ, Lyon IW, Taylor JW, et al: Valproic acid associated pancreatitis in an adult (letter). Lancet 1(8210):41–42, 1981

Nelson JC, Bowers MB: Delusional unipolar depression: description and drug response. Arch Gen Psychiatry 35:1321–1328, 1978

Nestler EJ, Barrot M, DiLeone RJ, et al: Neurobiology of depression. Neuron 34:13–25, 2002

Nestoros J, Suranyi B, Spees R, et al: Diazepam in high doses is effective in schizophrenia. Prog Neuropsychopharmacol Biol Psychiatry 6:513–518, 1982

Nielsen H: Recombinant human granulocyte colony-stimulating factor (rhG-CSF; filgrastim) treatment of clozapine-induced agranulocytosis. J Intern Med 234:529–531, 1993

NIMH/NIH Consensus Development Conference Statement: Mood disorders: pharmacological prevention of recurrences. Consensus Development Panel. Am J Psychiatry 142:469–476, 1985

Nishino S, Mishima K, Mignot E, et al: Sedative-hypnotics, in The American Psychiatric Publishing Textbook of Psychopharmacology, 3rd Edition. Edited by Schatzberg AF, Nemeroff CB. Washington, DC, American Psychiatric Publishing, 2004, pp 651–670

Oldham JM: Guideline Watch: Practice Guidelines for the Treatment of Patients With Borderline Personality Disorder. Arlington, VA, American Psychiatric Association, 2005

Oliver AP, Luchins DJ, Wyatt RJ: Neuroleptic-induced seizures: an in vitro technique for assessing relative risk. Arch Gen Psychiatry 39:206–209, 1982

Ontiveros A, Fontaine R, Elie PL, et al: Refractory depression: the addition of lithium to fluoxetine or desipramine. Acta Psychiatr Scand 83:188–192, 1991

Patterson JF: Stevens-Johnson syndrome associated with carbamazepine therapy. J Clin Psychopharmacol 5:185, 1985

Pearlstein TB, Halbreich U, Batzar ED, et al: Psychosocial functioning in women with premenstrual dysphoric disorder before and after treatment with sertraline or placebo. J Clin Psychiatry 61:101–109, 2000

Peet M, Horrobin DF: A dose-ranging exploratory study of the effects of ethyl-eicosapentaenoate in patients with persistent schizophrenic symptoms. J Psychiatr Res 36:7–18, 2002

Pellock JM: Carbamazepine side effects in children and adults. Epilepsia 28:S64–S70, 1987

Pellock JM, Willmore LJ: A rational guide to routine blood monitoring in patients receiving antiepileptic drugs. Neurology 41:961–964, 1991

Pendlebury SC, Moses DK, Eadie MJ: Hyponatremia during oxcarbazepine therapy. Hum Toxicol 8:337–344, 1989

Perlis RH, Sachs GS, Lafer B, et al: Effect of abrupt change from standard to low serum levels of lithium: a reanalysis of double-blind lithium maintenance data. Am J Psychiatry 159:1155–1159, 2002

Perry PJ, Miller DD, Arndt SV, et al: Clozapine and norclozapine plasma concentrations and clinical response of treatment-refractory schizophrenic patients. Am J Psychiatry 148:231–235, 1991

Physicians' Desk Reference, 51st Edition. Montvale, NJ, Medical Economics, 2001

Physicians' Desk Reference, 59th Edition. Montvale, NJ, Thompson PDR, 2005

Physicians' Desk Reference, 60th Edition. Montvale, NJ, Thompson PDR, 2006

Pies RW: Handbook of Essential Psychopharmacology. Washington, DC, American Psychiatric Press, 1998

Pigott TA, Pato MT, Bernstein SE, et al: Controlled comparisons of clomipramine and fluoxetine in the treatment of obsessive-compulsive disorders: behavioral and biological results. Arch Gen Psychiatry 47:926–932, 1990

Plenge P, Mellerup ET, Bolwig C, et al: Lithium treatment: does the kidney prefer one daily dose instead of two? Acta Psychiatr Scand 66:121–128, 1982

Post RM, Leverich GS, Altshuler L, et al: Lithium-discontinuation-induced refractoriness: preliminary observations. Am J Psychiatry 149:1727–1729, 1992

Preskorn SH, Burke M: Somatic therapy for major depressive disorder: selection of an antidepressant. J Clin Psychiatry 53 (suppl):5–18, 1992

Prien RF, Kupfer DJ: Continuation drug therapy for major depression episodes: how long should it be maintained? Am J Psychiatry 143:18–23, 1986

Purdon SE, Jones BDW, Stip E, et al: Neuropsychological change in early phase schizophrenia during 12 months of treatment with olanzapine, risperidone, or haloperidol. Arch Gen Psychiatry 57:249–258, 2000

Quitkin FM, Rifkin A, Klein DF: Monoamine oxidase inhibitors: a review of antidepressant effectiveness. Arch Gen Psychiatry 36:749–760, 1979

Rakel RE: Long-term buspirone therapy for chronic anxiety: a multicenter international study to determine safety. South Med J 83:194–198, 1990

Reitan JA, Porter W, Braunstein M: Comparison of psychomotor skills and amnesia after induction of anesthesia with midazolam or thiopental. Anesth Analg 65:933–937, 1986

Reunanen M, Kaarnen P, Vaisanen E: The influence of anticholinergic treatment on tardive dyskinesia caused by neuroleptic drugs. Acta Neurol Scand 65 (suppl 90): 278–279, 1982

Robert E, Guibaud P: Maternal valproic acid and congenital neural tube defects (letter). Lancet 2(8304):937, 1982

Rohatagi S, Barrett JS, DeWitt KE, et al: Integrated pharmacokinetic and metabolic modeling of selegiline and metabolites after transdermal administration. Biopharm Drug Dispos 18:567–584, 1997

Roose SP, Glassman AH, Giardina EGV, et al: Tricyclic antidepressants in depressed patients with cardiac conduction disease. Arch Gen Psychiatry 44:273–275, 1987

Rosa FW: Spina bifida in infants of women treated with carbamazepine during pregnancy. N Engl J Med 324:674–677, 1991

Rosebush P, Stewart T: A prospective analysis of 24 episodes of neuroleptic malignant syndrome. Am J Psychiatry 146:717–725, 1989

Rosebush PI, Stewart TD, Gelenberg AJ: Twenty neuroleptic rechallenges after neuroleptic malignant syndrome in 15 patients. J Clin Psychiatry 50:295–298, 1989

Rosebush PI, Stewart T, Mazurek MF: The treatment of neuroleptic malignant syndrome: are dantrolene and bromocriptine useful adjuncts to supportive care? Br J Psychiatry 159:709–712, 1991

Rosenbaum JF, Fava M, Hoog SL, et al: Selective serotonin reuptake inhibitor discontinuation syndrome: a randomized clinical trial. Biol Psychiatry 44:77–87, 1998

Rosenberg L, Mitchell AA, Parsells JL, et al: Lack of relation of oral clefts to diazepam use during pregnancy. N Engl J Med 309:1282–1285, 1983

Rossi A, Mancini F, Stratta P, et al: Risperidone, negative symptoms, and cognitive deficit in schizophrenia: an open study. Acta Psychiatr Scand 95:40–43, 1997

Roth LH: Question the experts. J Clin Psychopharmacol 3:206–207, 1983

Rothschild AJ: Disinhibition, amnestic reactions, and other adverse reactions secondary to triazolam: a review of the literature. J Clin Psychiatry 53 (suppl):69–79, 1992

Rush AJ: STAR*D: What have we learned? Am J Psychiatry 164:201–204, 2007

Rush AJ, Trivedi MH, Wisniewski SR, et al: Bupropion-SR, sertraline, or venlafaxine-XR after failure of SSRIs for depression. N Engl J Med 354:1231–1242, 2006

Sachs GS, Nierenberg AA, Calabrese JR, et al: Effectiveness of adjunctive antidepressant treatment for bipolar depression. N Engl J Med 356:1711–1722, 2007

Sackeim HA, Haskett RF, Mulsant BH, et al: Continuation pharmacotherapy in the prevention of relapse following electroconvulsive therapy: a randomized controlled trial. JAMA 285:1299–1307, 2001

Salzman C, Wolfson AN, Schatzberg A, et al: Effect of fluoxetine on anger in symptomatic volunteers with borderline personality disorder. J Clin Psychopharmacol 15:23–29, 1995

Scher M, Krieger JN, Juergens S: Trazodone and priapism. Am J Psychiatry 140:1362–1363, 1983

Schneier FR, Saoud JB, Campeas RC, et al: Buspirone in social phobia. J Clin Psychopharmacol 13:251–256, 1992

Schooler NR, Keith SJ, Severe JB, et al: Relapse and rehospitalization during maintenance treatment of schizophrenia: the effects of dose reduction and family treatment. Arch Gen Psychiatry 54:453–463, 1997

Schou M: Lithium prophylaxis: myths and realities. Am J Psychiatry 146:573–576, 1989

Seide H, Muller HR: Choreiform movements as side effects of phenothiazine medication in elderly patients. J Am Geriatr Soc 15:517–522, 1967

Sellers EM, Naranjo CA, Harrison M, et al: Oral diazepam loading: simplified treatment of alcohol withdrawal. Clin Pharmacol Ther 34:822–826, 1983

Serzone (package insert). Princeton, NJ, Bristol-Myers Squibb Co, 2002

Seroquel (package insert). Wilmington, DE, Zeneca Pharmaceuticals, 2001

Shader RI, Greenblatt DJ: Approaches to the treatment of anxiety states, in Manual of Psychiatric Therapeutics, 3rd Edition. Edited by Shader RI. Philadelphia, PA, Lippincott Williams & Wilkins, 2003, pp 199–200

Sheehan DV, Raj AB, Sheehan KH, et al: Is buspirone effective for panic disorder? J Clin Psychopharmacol 10:3–11, 1990

Shelton RC, Stahl SM: Risperidone and paroxetine given singly and in combination for bipolar depression. J Clin Psychiatry 65:1715–1719, 2004

Shulman KI, Walker SE: Refining the MAOI diet: tyramine content of pizzas and soy products. J Clin Psychiatry 60:191–193, 1999

Shulman KI, Walker SE: Reply: clarifying the safety of the MAOI diet and pizza (letter). J Clin Psychiatry 61:145–146, 2000

Shulman KI, Tailor SA, Walker SE, et al: Tap (draft) beer and monoamine oxidase inhibitor dietary restrictions. Can J Psychiatry 42:310–312, 1997

Small J, Hirsch S, Arvanitis L, et al: Quetiapine in patients with schizophrenia. Arch Gen Psychiatry 54:549–557, 1997

Smith WT, Glaudin V, Panagides J, et al: Mirtazapine vs. amitriptyline vs. placebo in the treatment of major depressive disorder. Psychopharmacol Bull 26:191–196, 1990

Soloff PH: Psychopharmacology of borderline personality disorder. Psychiatr Clin North Am 23:169–192, 2000

Sramek JJ, Tansman M, Suri A, et al: Efficacy of buspirone in generalized anxiety disorder with coexisting mild depressive symptoms. J Clin Psychiatry 57:287–291, 1996

Stewart RB, Karas B, Springer PK: Haloperidol excretion in human milk. Am J Psychiatry 137:849–850, 1980

Stroup TS, Lieberman JA, McEvoy JP, et al: Effectiveness of olanzapine, quetiapine, risperidone, and ziprasidone in patients with chronic schizophrenia following discontinuation of a previous atypical antipsychotic. Am J Psychiatry 163:611–622, 2006

Sullivan JT, Seller EM: Treating alcohol, barbiturate, and benzodiazepine withdrawal. Ration Drug Ther 20:1–9, 1986

Suppes T, Baldessarini RJ, Faedda GL, et al: Risk of recurrence following discontinuation of lithium treatment in bipolar disorder. Arch Gen Psychiatry 48:1082–1088, 1991

Suppes T, McElroy SL, Gilbert J, et al: Clozapine in the treatment of dysphoric mania. Biol Psychiatry 32:270–280, 1992

Suppes T, Webb A, Paul B, et al: Clinical outcome in a randomized 1-year trial of clozapine versus treatment as usual for patients with treatment-resistant illness and a history of mania. Am J Psychiatry 156:1164–1169, 1999

Tallman JF, Paul SM, Skolnick P, et al: Receptors for the age of anxiety: pharmacology of the benzodiazepines. Science 207:274–281, 1980

Tarsy D, Baldessarini RJ: Epidemiology of tardive dyskinesia: is risk declining with modern antipsychotics? Mov Disord 21:589–598, 2006

Thase ME, Kupfer DJ, Frank E, et al: Treatment of imipramine-resistant depressant, II: an open clinical trial of lithium augmentation. J Clin Psychiatry 50:413–417, 1989

Thase ME, Nierenberg AA, Keller MB: Mirtazapine in relapse prevention: a double-blind placebo-controlled study in depressed outpatients. Eur Neuropsychopharmacol 10 (suppl 3):265–266, 2000

Thase ME, Entsuah AR, Rudolph RL: Remission rates during treatment with venlafaxine or selective serotonin reuptake inhibitors. Br J Psychiatry 178:234–241, 2001

Tiihonen J, Hallikainen T, Ryynanen OP, et al: Lamotrigine in treatment-resistant schizophrenia: a randomized placebo-controlled crossover trial. Biol Psychiatry 54:1241–1248, 2003

Tohen M, Vieta E, Calabrese J, et al: Efficacy of olanzapine-fluoxetine combination in the treatment of bipolar I depression. Arch Gen Psychiatry 60:1079–1088, 2003

Tollefson GD: Monoamine oxidase inhibitors: a review. J Clin Psychiatry 44:280–288, 1983

Tollefson GD, Beasley CM Jr, Tamura RN: Blind, controlled long-term study of the comparative incidence of treatment-emergent tardive dyskinesia with olanzapine or haloperidol. Am J Psychiatry 154:1248–1254, 1997

Trileptal (product information). East Hanover, NJ, Novartis Pharmaceuticals Corp, 2006

Trivedi MH, Fava M, Wisniewski SR, et al: Medication augmentation after the failure of SSRIs for depression. N Engl J Med 354:1243–1252, 2006a

Trivedi MH, Rush AJ, Wisniewski SR, et al: Evaluation of outcomes with citalopram for depression using measurement-based care in STAR*D: implications for clinical practice. Am J Psychiatry 163:28–40, 2006b

Tsai G, Goff D, Chang R, et al: Markers of glutamatergic neurotransmission and oxidative stress associated with tardive dyskinesia. Am J Psychiatry 9:1207–1213, 1998

U.S. Food and Drug Administration Public Health Advisory: Suicidality in children and adolescents being treated with antidepressant medications, October 15, 2004. Available at: http://www.fda.gov/cder/drug/antidepressants/SSRIPHA200410.htm. Accessed December 7, 2005

van Putten T, May PRA, Marder SR: Akathisia with haloperidol and thiothixene. Arch Gen Psychiatry 31:67–72, 1984

Viguera AC, Cohen LS, Baldessarini RJ, et al: Managing bipolar disorder during pregnancy: weighing the risks and benefits. Can J Psychiatry 47:426–436, 2002

Vitullo RN, Wharton JM, Allen NB, et al: Trazodone-related exercise-induced nonsustained ventricular tachycardia. Chest 98:247–248, 1990

Walker SE, Shulman KI, Tailor SAN, et al: Tyramine content of previously restricted foods in monoamine oxidase inhibitor diets. J Clin Psychopharmacol 16:383–388, 1996

Walker SE, Shulman KE, Tailor SAN: Reply: tyramine content in Chinese food. J Clin Psychopharmacol 17:227–228, 1997

Warnock JK, Knesevich J: Adverse cutaneous reactions to antidepressants. Am J Psychiatry 145:425–430, 1988

Wecker L, James S, Copeland N, et al: Transdermal selegiline: targeted effects on monoamine oxidases in the brain. Biol Psychiatry 54:1099–1104, 2003

Wehr TA, Goodwin FK: Rapid-cycling in manic depressives induced by tricyclic antidepressants. Arch Gen Psychiatry 36:555–559, 1979

Weisler RH, Kalali AH, Ketter TA, et al: A multicenter, randomized, double-blind, placebo-controlled trial of extended-release carbamazepine capsules as monotherapy for bipolar disorder patients with manic or mixed episodes. J Clin Psychiatry 65:478–484, 2004

Weisler RH, Keck PE Jr, Swann AC, et al: Extended-release carbamazepine capsules as monotherapy for acute mania in bipolar disorder: a multicenter, randomized, double-blind, placebo-controlled trial. J Clin Psychiatry 66:323–330, 2005

Wetzel H, Anghelescu I, Szegedi A, et al: Pharmacokinetic interactions of clozapine with selective serotonin reuptake inhibitors: differential effects of fluvoxamine and paroxetine in a prospective study. J Clin Psychopharmacol 18:2–9, 1998

Wikander I, Sundblad C, Andersch B, et al: Citalopram in premenstrual dysphoria: is intermittent treatment during luteal phases more effective than continuous medication throughout the menstrual cycle? J Clin Psychopharmacol 18:390–398, 1998

Wing YK, Chen CN: Tyramine content in Chinese food (letter). J Clin Psychopharmacol 17:227, 1997

Yager J: Bethanechol chloride can reverse erectile and ejaculatory dysfunction induced by tricyclic antidepressants and mazindol: case report. J Clin Psychiatry 47:210–211, 1986

Yassa R: Antiparkinsonian medication withdrawal in the treatment of tardive dyskinesia: a report of three cases. Can J Psychiatry 30:440–442, 1985

Yassa R, Lal S: Prevalence of the rabbit syndrome. Am J Psychiatry 143:656–657, 1986

Yeo PP, Bates D, Howe JG, et al: Anticonvulsants and thyroid function. BMJ 1:1581–1583, 1978

Yonkers KA, Halbreich U, Freeman E, et al: Symptomatic improvement of premenstrual dysphoric disorder with sertraline treatment: a randomized controlled trial. Sertraline Premenstrual Dysphoric Collaborative Study Group. JAMA 278:983–988, 1997

Yonkers KA, Wisner KL, Stowe Z, et al: Management of bipolar disorder during pregnancy and the postpartum period. Am J Psychiatry 161:608–620, 2004

Zanarini MC, Frankenburg FR, Parachini EA: A preliminary, randomized trial of fluoxetine, olanzapine, and the olanzapine-fluoxetine combination in women with borderline personality disorder. J Clin Psychiatry 65:903–907, 2004

Zarate CA Jr, Tohen M, Baldessarini RJ: Clozapine in severe mood disorders. J Clin Psychiatry 56:411–417, 1995

Zhang-Wong J, Zipursky RB, Beiser M, et al: Optimal haloperidol dosage in first-episode psychosis. Can J Psychiatry 44:164–167, 1999

Zornberg GL, Pope HG Jr: Treatment of depression in bipolar disorder: new directions for research. J Clin Psychopharmacol 13:397–408, 1993

Zubenko GS, Cohen BM, Lipinski JF: Comparison of metoprolol and propranolol in the treatment of lithium tremor. Psychiatry Res 11:163–164, 1984a

Zubenko GS, Lipinski JF, Cohen M, et al: Comparison of metoprolol and propranolol in the treatment of akathisia. Psychiatry Res 11:143–149, 1984b

Zyban (package insert). Research Triangle Park, NC, GlaxoSmithKline, 2005

Zyprexa (package insert). Indianapolis, IN, Eli Lilly & Company, 2007

27

NONPHARMACOLOGICAL SOMATIC TREATMENTS

Mark S. George, M.D.
Ziad H. Nahas, M.D., M.S.C.R.
Jeffrey J. Borckardt, Ph.D.
Berry Anderson, B.S.N., R.N.
Milton J. Foust Jr., M.D.

Psychiatry is now developing a third realm of treatment modalities, complementing the well-established realms of psychopharmacology (medications) and psychotherapy. Various names are used to describe these treatments—ranging from "neuromodulation" to "brain stimulation techniques" to the hard-to-understand and cumbersome "nonpharmacological somatic treatments." As a class, these methods involve focal electrical brain stimulation of some sort and vary widely in their invasiveness and methods of delivery.

Table 27–1 lists the current methods. In this chapter we review only those treatments that are U.S. Food and Drug Administration (FDA) approved for treatment of traditionally defined psychiatric disorders, such as electroconvulsive therapy (ECT) and vagus nerve stimulation (VNS), or treatments that have substantial Class I randomized controlled trial (RCT) data supporting their use, such as transcranial magnetic stimulation (TMS). These techniques are also being used in traditionally defined neurological disorders (e.g., deep

The authors' work with brain stimulation treatments has been supported over the past 5 years in part by research grants from NARSAD, the Stanley Foundation, the Borderline Personality Disorders Research Foundation (BPDRF), and the Dana Foundation; by National Institute of Neurological Disorders and Stroke (NINDS) grant RO1 AG40956 (George); by National Institutes of Health (NIH) grants RO1 AG409565R01MH069887-02 (George), 1 RO1 MH069887-01 (George), and 1K08MH070915-01A1 (Nahas); and by the Defense Advanced Research Projects Agency (DARPA). The Brain Stimulation Laboratory at the Medical University of South Carolina, Charleston, has also received grant funding from GlaxoSmithKline, Jazz, Cyberonics, Neuronetics, and NeuroPace. Dr. George holds several transcranial magnetic stimulation (TMS)–related patents. These are not in the area of TMS therapeutics, but rather are for new TMS machine designs as well as for combining TMS with magnetic resonance imaging (MRI). Dr. George serves or has served as a paid consultant to several device and pharmaceutical companies (see full list).

brain stimulation [DBS] in dystonia or Parkinson's disease). We will mention their uses where appropriate, but a complete review of these treatments is found in the references listed in "Suggested Readings."

In considering these techniques, it is important to note that the brain is an electrochemical organ. All neurons transmit information and communicate with other cells through an electrical impulse (depolarization) traveling from a dendrite through the cell body out to the synapse. In our fascination with events happening chemically between neurons (psychopharmacology), we have neglected or forgotten an important principle: The entire communication and action between neurons begins with an electrical impulse.

This renaissance in brain stimulation techniques would not be nearly as successful as it is without the revolution that has occurred in brain imaging over the past 20 years. Fundamentally, one must hypothesize about where to stimulate. Therefore, the results of brain imaging studies provide the basis of knowledge necessary to hypothesize about where to apply the techniques. With some of the techniques, brain imaging also allows one to guide the individual placement (e.g., DBS). Although the regional neuroanatomy of the many kinds of depression, anxiety disorders, or schizophrenias is not as well defined as, for example, Parkinson's disease, we have a much better understanding of the regions involved in mood regulation or hallucinations than we did 20 years ago. Brain stimulation techniques largely build on this body of knowledge in terms of where they are applied.

Finally, it is rare to use any of the brain stimulation methods alone in treatment settings. Most commonly, these treatments are used in combination with medication or psychotherapy. In fact, a most interesting area of future research is the investigation of how to combine the different stimulation techniques with medications or even talking therapy. It seems likely that some medications, more than others, will work in synergy with a brain stimulation treatment for a particular disorder. It is also likely that what a person is doing or thinking while being stimulated will ultimately matter in terms of clinical response.

Electroconvulsive Therapy

ECT is the grandfather of this new family of treatments and involves the deliberate induction of a generalized tonic-clonic seizure by electrical means. Contemporary ECT devices typically deliver bidirectional (alternating current), brief-pulse, square-wave stimulation through a pair of electrodes, which are applied externally on the patient's scalp. Because of the risk of bodily harm from the convulsion, ECT is performed under general anesthesia, with the body paralyzed. As with other convulsive therapies that historically preceded ECT, the goal is to produce a seizure. The presence of seizure activity appears to be essential; stimuli that are below the seizure threshold appear to be clinically ineffective. And although the production of a seizure appears to be necessary, a seizure alone is not sufficient. Some forms of seizure induction are in fact clinically ineffective (Sackeim et al. 1993). A variety of psychiatric and neurological conditions respond favorably to ECT, particularly if they are severe or accompanied by psychotic symptoms, although the majority of patients treated with ECT have mood disorders, such as unipolar or bipolar depression. Other conditions, such as mania, schizoaffective disorder, catatonia, neuroleptic malignant syndrome, Parkinson's disease, and intractable seizures, may respond to ECT as well. Schizophrenia has also been treated with ECT, but the results tend to be less favorable than those obtained in patients with mood disorders. Patients with schizophrenia who also have a prominent disturbance of mood are likely to respond best to ECT. For a typical series or course of ECT, treatments are usually given two to three times per week for six to eight treatments. This may then be followed by maintenance treatment in the form of medication, additional ECT given at less frequent intervals, or both. A number of questions remain regarding the most effective methods for performing ECT and its mechanism or mechanisms of action. New data have suggested that shorter pulse widths are less toxic than the fatter pulse widths used in traditional ECT (Sackeim et al. 2000). (Applying electricity after the neuron has depolarized is not necessary and is perhaps cognitively harmful.) Also, ECT as practiced in the general community has lower response rates (20%–50%) than historical response rates (60%–80%) in the literature published in academic medical settings (Prudic et al. 2004). ECT is unfortunately associated with acute and sometimes chronic memory loss (Lisanby et al. 2000; Sackeim 2000). Because of these limitations, it is underused.

Transcranial Magnetic Stimulation

TMS is perhaps the most interesting of all the new techniques because the skull does not need to be opened in order to focally stimulate with TMS, no seizure is needed, and, to date, there appear to be only limited

TABLE 27–1. Overview of somatic nonpharmacological treatments

Acronym (full name)	Convulsive?	Stimulation site	Psychiatric disorders	Clinical use status
ECT (electroconvulsive therapy)	Yes	Cortical	Depression, mania, catatonia	Grandfathered FDA approval
rTMS (repetitive transcranial magnetic stimulation)		Cortical	Depression	Pivotal trial in depression complete; FDA review under way; some psychiatrists already use rTMS off-label
VNS (vagus nerve stimulation)		Cervical cranial nerve	Depression	FDA approved for treatment-resistant depression
MST (magnetic seizure therapy)	Yes	Cortical	Depression	Experimental for all conditions
DBS (deep brain stimulation)		Subcortical	Depression	FDA approved for Parkinson's disease; pivotal trials in depression under way
tDCS (transcranial direct current stimulation)		Cortical	Substance abuse, depression	Experimental for all conditions
TENS (transcutaneous electrical nerve stimulation)		Peripheral nerve	Pain	FDA approved for pain conditions
EPI-fMRI (echoplanar imaging–functional magnetic resonance imaging)		Unknown; possibly subcortical	Depression	Experimental for all conditions
FEAT (focal electrical alternating current therapy); also known as tACS (transcranial alternating current stimulation)		Cortical	Depression	Experimental for all conditions
FEAST (focal electrical alternating current seizure therapy)	Yes	Cortical	Depression	Experimental for all conditions

Note. FDA = U.S. Food and Drug Administration.

side effects (George 2002; George et al. 2000, 2002). TMS involves creating a powerful electrical current near the scalp. The electricity flowing in an electromagnetic coil on the scalp creates an extremely potent (near 1.5 Tesla) but brief (microseconds) magnetic field. The TMS magnetic field performs the neat trick of entering the surface of the brain without interference. Although skin and bone act as resistors to impede electrical currents, magnetic fields pass unimpeded through the skull and soft tissue. In the brain, the magnetic pulse encounters nerve cells with resting potentials and induces electrical current to flow (Figure 27–1). Thus, electrical energy is converted to magnetic fields, which are then con-

verted back into electrical currents in the brain (Bohning 2000). TMS is thus sometimes called "electrodeless electrical stimulation."

The magnetic field performs the trick of bridging the skull. Although magnetic fields do have biological effects on tissue, the vast majority of TMS effects most likely derive from the induced electrical currents generated in the brain rather than from the magnetic fields. TMS, with powerful but extremely brief magnetic fields, differs from the current U.S. craze of wearing (or sleeping on) constant low-field magnets. TMS directly tickles the brain electrically, while constant weak magnets do not induce currents.

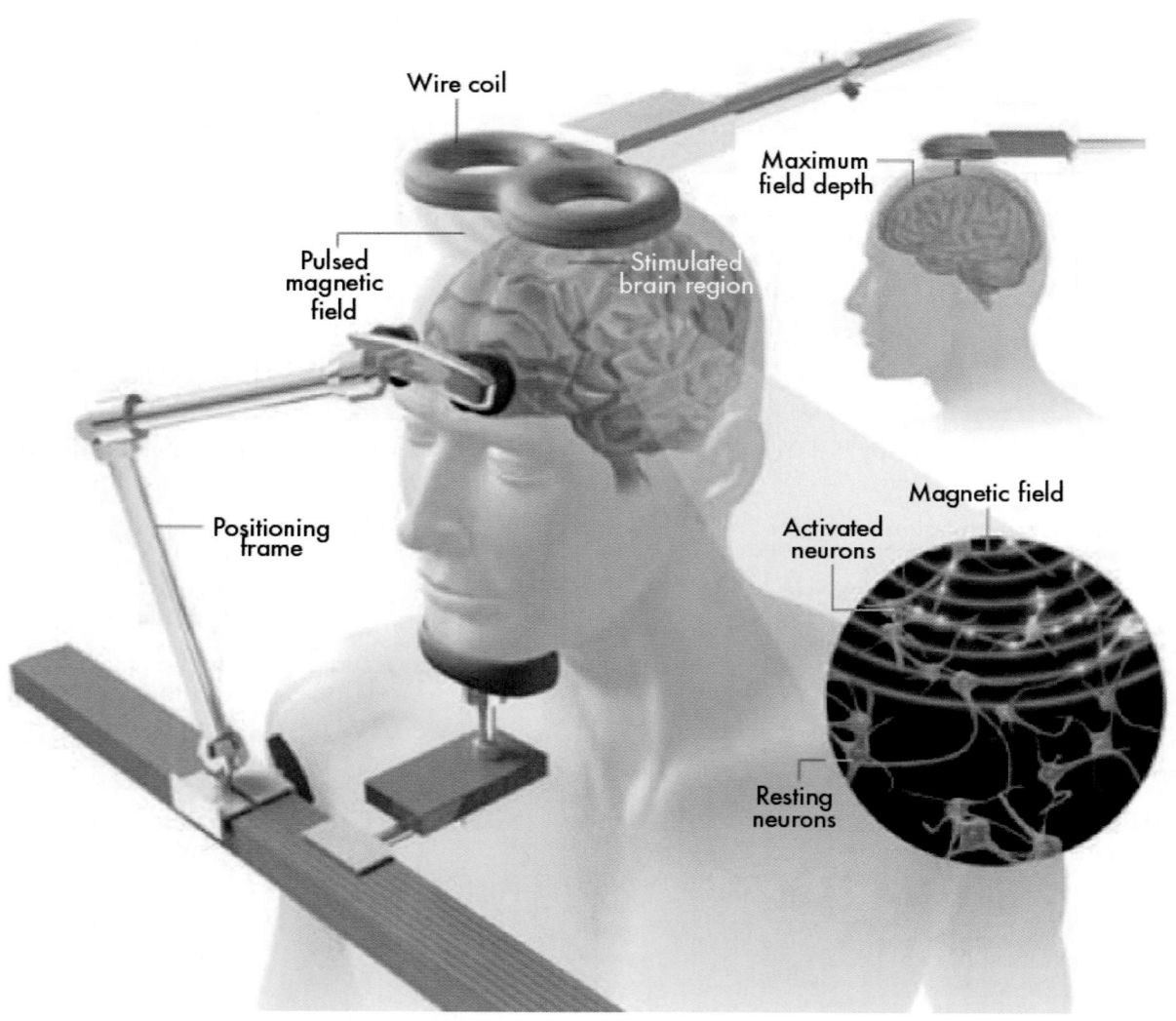

FIGURE 27–1.   Transcranial magnetic stimulation (TMS).

TMS works by first passing a powerful electrical current through a coil, which creates a transient magnetic field. The current passes unimpeded through the skull, causing electrical current to flow in neurons.

Source.   Reprinted from George MS: "Stimulating the Brain." *Scientific American* 289:66–73, 2003. Copyright 2003, Bryan Christie Design, Maplewood, New Jersey. Used with permission.

Brief History

The idea of using TMS, or something like it, to alter neural function goes back at least to the early 1900s. In 1902, Adrian Pollacsek and Berthold Beer, psychiatrists working down the street from Sigmund Freud in Vienna, filed a patent to treat depression and neuroses with an electromagnetic device that looked surprisingly like today's TMS machines (Beer 1902). The modern TMS era began in 1985 when Tony Barker and colleagues, working in Sheffield, England, created a focal electromagnetic device with sufficient power to

induce currents in the spine (Barker et al. 1985, 1987). They quickly realized that their device could also directly and noninvasively stimulate the human brain. Their apparatus could only stimulate the surface of the brain because the magnetic field weakened as distance from the coil increased. Several researchers are working on creating more powerful TMS devices that might stimulate more deeply (Roth et al. 2002).

A single pulse of TMS, applied over the motor cortex, produces a jerk-like movement in the hand, arm, face, or leg, depending on where the coil is positioned. A single pulse applied over the back of the brain can produce a phosphene. However, that is about the extent of the immediate positive effects that single-pulse TMS can produce. TMS pulses applied in rhythmic succession are referred to as repetitive TMS, or rTMS. rTMS can create behaviors not seen with single pulses, including the potential risk of causing an unintended seizure. About 20 seizures have occurred in the history of TMS use, 12 of them unintended, from well over 10,000 sessions (the total number of people stimulated is unclear). All seizures occurred during, rather than after, stimulation and were self-limited with no sequelae. rTMS seizures are more likely to occur with certain combinations of TMS intensity, frequency, duration, and interstimulus interval (Wassermann 1998; Wassermann et al. 1996).

Research

Much research is under way to determine exactly which neurons TMS affects and what the cascade of neurobiological events that follow stimulation involves. We do know that factors such as gyral anatomy (how the brain is shaped), the distance from the skull to the brain (brain atrophy), and the orientation of nerve fibers relative to coil are all important.

One of the intriguing effects of rTMS is that for brief periods of time during stimulation, rTMS can block or inhibit a brain function—that is, pulsed over the motor area that controls speech, rTMS can *temporarily* leave the patient speechless (motor aphasia), but only while the device is firing. Cognitive neuroscientists have used this knockout aspect or "temporary lesioning" ability of TMS to re-explore and test the large body of information gleaned from years of studying stroke patients. Additionally, two pulses of TMS in quick succession can provide information about the underlying excitability of a specific region of cortex. This diagnostic technique, called paired-pulse TMS, can demonstrate the behavior of local interneurons in the motor cortex and serve as indirect measures of γ-aminobutyric acid (GABA) or glutamate (Heide et al. 2006; Ziemann and Hallett 2000).

Single nerve cells develop into functioning circuits over time through repeated discharges. External low-frequency stimulation of a single nerve cell can cause *long-term depression* (LTD), wherein the efficiency of links between cells diminishes. High-frequency stimulation over time can cause the opposite effect, called *long-term potentiation* (LTP). These behaviors are thought to be involved in learning, memory, and dynamic brain changes associated with networks. An exciting aspect of research on TMS and other brain stimulation techniques has been the focus on whether

external brain stimulation can be used to change brain circuits over time in a manner analogous to the way it is used to induce LTD or LTP. Although still controversial and not fully resolved, there are a number of TMS studies showing inhibition or excitation lasting for up to several hours beyond the time of stimulation (Di Lazzaro et al. 2005; Pal et al. 2005; Wassermann et al. 1998). The clinical implications would be profound if TMS or other techniques could begin being used to change learning and memory or to resculpt brain circuits. Some basic physiological studies indicate that a circuit can only be changed while the behavior is ongoing and the cells involved in the various neural pathways are acting as a circuit (Barnes et al. 1994; Bartsch and van Hemmen 2001; Stanton and Sejnowsky 1989). An important question is whether TMS should be delivered while patients are thinking about important topics, or "abreacting." Thus, in the near future, one might combine TMS with modified forms of talking or cognitive-behavioral therapy. Much research is needed in this area.

Animal Studies With TMS

Animal and cellular studies with TMS reinforce that it is a powerful technique capable of altering neuronal function. A stumbling block encountered in using TMS in animals is the difficulty of making TMS coils that are the same relative size to humans; coils that are too small simply explode. Thus, most animal TMS studies, especially those involving small animals, have not used focal TMS as it has been used in humans. Nevertheless, studies have shown that rTMS enhances apomorphine-induced stereotypy, reduces immobility in the Porsolt swim test (Fleischmann et al. 1996), and induces electroconvulsive shock (ECS)–like changes in rodent brain monoamines, β-adrenergic receptor binding, and immediate-early gene induction (Ben-Sachar et al. 1997). Most recently, researchers have found that TMS can induce neurogenesis (Jennum and Klintgaard 1996; Post and Keck 2001; Weissman et al. 1992).

Combining TMS With Functional Imaging

A critically important area that will ultimately guide clinical parameters is combining TMS with functional imaging to directly monitor TMS effects on the brain. This will facilitate understanding of the effects of various TMS-use parameters on brain function. Because it appears that TMS at different frequencies has divergent effects on brain activity, combining TMS with functional brain imaging will better delineate not only the behavioral neuropsychology of various psychiatric syndromes but also some of the pathophysiological circuits in the brain. In contrast to imaging studies with ECT, which have revealed that ECT shuts off global and regional activity (Nobler et al. 2001), most studies using serial scans in depressed patients undergoing TMS have found increased activity in the cingulate and other limbic regions (Shajahan et al. 2002; Teneback et al. 1999). However, two studies have now shown divergent effects of TMS on regional activity in depressed patients, determined both by the frequency of stimulation and by the baseline state of the patient (Loo et al. 2003; Speer et al. 2000). That is, for patients with global or focal hypometabolism, high-frequency prefrontal stimulation increases brain activity over time. Conversely, patients with focal hyperactivity have reduced activity over time following chronic daily low-frequency stimulation. However, these two small-sample studies have numerous flaws. They simultaneously show the potential and the complexity surrounding the issue of how to use TMS to change activity in defined circuits. The studies also point out an obvious difference between TMS and ECT, in which the net effect of the ECT seizure is to decrease prefrontal and global activity (Nobler et al. 2001).

Surprisingly, TMS can be performed within a magnetic resonance imaging (MRI) scanner, which is itself a huge magnet and is constantly on (Baudewig et al. 2001; Bohning et al. 1998, 1999, 2000a, 2000b; Shastri et al. 1999). This technology has shown that prefrontal TMS at 80% motor threshold (MT) produces much less local and remote blood flow change than does 120% MT TMS (Nahas et al. 2001). Strafella et al. (2001) used positron emission tomography (PET) to show that prefrontal cortex TMS causes dopamine release in the caudate nucleus and has reciprocal activity with the anterior cingulate gyrus (Paus et al. 2001). Our group in the United States at the Medical University of South Carolina (Teneback et al. 1999), as well as others in Scotland (Shajahan et al. 2002) and Australia (Loo et al. 2003), have all shown that lateral prefrontal TMS can cause changes in the anterior cingulate gyrus and other limbic regions in depressed patients (Figure 27–2). It is thus clear that TMS delivered over the prefrontal cortex has immediate effects on important subcortical limbic regions. The initial TMS effect on cortex and the secondary synaptic changes in other regions likely differ as a function of mood state, cortical excitability, and other factors that would change resting brain activity. Combining TMS with functional imaging is likely to continue to be an important method for understand-ing TMS mechanisms of action. Combinational TMS/imaging is also likely to evolve into an important neuroscience tool for researching brain connectivity (George and Bohning 2002; Paus et al. 1997).

Therapeutic Uses of TMS

Depression

Although there is controversy, and more work is needed, certain brain regions have consistently been implicated in the pathogenesis of depression and mood regulation (George 1994; George et al. 1994a, 1994b, 1995a, 1996, 1997b, 1998; Ketter et al. 1996; Kimbrell et al. 2002). These include the medial and dorsolateral prefrontal cortex, the cingulate gyrus, and other regions commonly referred to as limbic (amygdala, hippocampus, parahippocampus, septum, hypothalamus, limbic thalamus, insula) and paralimbic (anterior temporal pole, orbitofrontal cortex). A widely held theory over the last decade has been that depression results from a dysregulation of these prefrontal cortical and limbic regions (George et al. 1994b, 1995b, 1996; Mayberg et al. 1999). The very first uses of TMS as an antidepressant were not influenced by this regional neuroanatomical literature, and stimulation was applied over the vertex (Beer 1902; Grisaru et al. 1994; Kolbinger et al. 1995). However, working within the prefrontal cortical limbic dysregulation framework outlined above, and given that theories of ECT action emphasize the role of prefrontal cortex effects (Nobler et al. 1994), in 1995 I performed the first open trial of prefrontal TMS as an antidepressant (George et al. 1995c), followed immediately by a crossover double-blind study (George et al. 1997b). My reasoning was that chronic, frequent subconvulsive stimulation of the prefrontal cortex over several weeks might initiate a therapeutic cascade of events both in the prefrontal cortex and in connected limbic regions, thereby causing the dysregulated circuits to rebalance and normalize, thus alleviating depression symptoms (George and Wassermann 1994a). The imaging evidence previously discussed now shows that this hunch was largely correct—prefrontal TMS sends direct information to important mood-regulating regions like the cingulate gyrus, orbitofrontal cortex, insula, and hippocampus. Thus, beginning with these prefrontal studies, modern TMS was specifically designed as a focal nonconvulsive, circuit-based approach to therapy.

Since the initial studies, there has been continued high interest in TMS as an antidepressant treatment. There are now more than 29 published RCTs evaluating the efficacy of TMS as an antidepressant (these are

Interleaved TMS/ BOLD fMRI
$P < 0.001$, $n = 14$ patients with depression

Left prefrontal 1-Hz TMS causes significant **secondary** activation in limbic regions
- Left dorsolateral prefrontal
- Right orbitofrontal cortex
- Insula
- Hippocampus
- Bilateral thalamus
- Bilateral midtemporal lobes (auditory cortex due to noise of discharge)

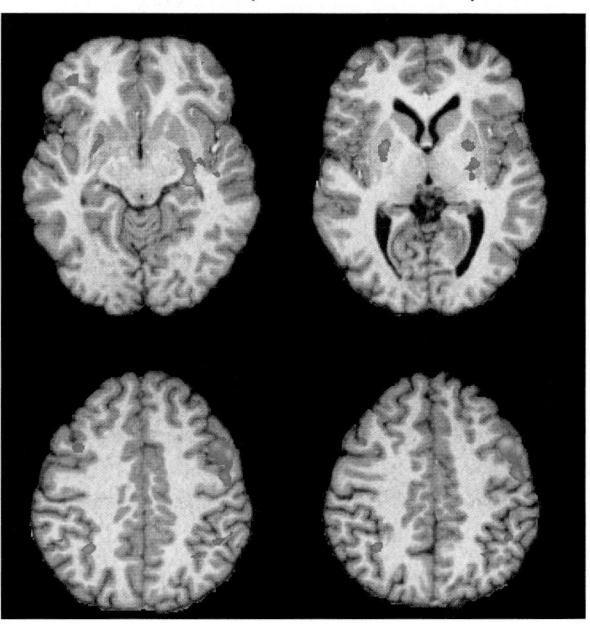

FIGURE 27–2.   Significant secondary effects of TMS (direct cortical stimulation), as seen on interleaved TMS/ BOLD fMRI.

Interleaved transcranial magnetic stimulation (TMS)/blood oxygen level–dependent (BOLD) functional magnetic resonance imaging (fMRI) reveals that left prefrontal TMS produces deeper transsynaptic effects. Shown are images from different slices of a common brain, where results from 14 medication-free depressed patients have been pooled. The areas in *red* are regions that have more blood flow when TMS is applied over the prefrontal cortex than when it is off. Note that although TMS directly stimulates only the left prefrontal cortex, there is also increased activity in many limbic and paralimbic regions connected to the frontal cortex.

Source.   Reprinted from Li X, Nahas Z, Kozel FA, et al.: "Acute Left Prefrontal Transcranial Magnetic Stimulation in Depressed Patients Is Associated With Immediately Increased Activity in Prefrontal Cortical as Well as Subcortical Regions." *Biological Psychiatry* 55:882–890, 2004. Copyright 2004, Society of Biological Psychiatry. Used with permission.

catalogued on the Web site http://www.ists.unibe.ch/TMSAvery. htm). Because initially there was no large TMS company promoting TMS as a treatment, until recently all of these studies were government or foundation sponsored, and all were conducted at a single site. As in any new field, not all findings from TMS antidepressant treatment studies have been positive (Loo et al. 1999). Five independent meta-analyses of the published or public TMS antidepressant literature, each differing in the articles included and the statistics used (Burt et al. 2002; Holtzheimer et al. 2001; Kozel and George 2002; Martin et al. 2002; McNamara et al. 2001), largely concluded that daily prefrontal TMS delivered over several weeks has antidepressant effects greater than sham treatment. Several small-sample studies have compared TMS with ECT without finding differences in efficacy. TMS was clearly more easily

tolerated than ECT, with no cognitive side effects and no need for repeated general anesthesia. Saxby Pridmore, a TMS pioneer in this area, in 2000 compared the antidepressant effects of standard ECT (three times per week) and a regimen consisting of one ECT per week followed by TMS on the other 4 weekdays (Pridmore 2000). At 3 weeks, both regimens had produced similar antidepressant effects. Relapse rates in the 6 months following ECT or rTMS were similar (Dannon et al. 2002). In sum, the studies to date suggest that TMS clinical antidepressant effects are in the range of other antidepressants and persist as long as the clinical effects following ECT.

O'Reardon et al. (2007) recently reported results from a multisite industry-sponsored RCT of 301 medication-free patients with major depression. TMS was delivered five times per week at 10-Hz frequency and

120% of motor threshold, for a duration of 4–6 weeks. Active TMS was significantly superior to sham TMS. TMS was well tolerated, with a low dropout rate for adverse events (4.5%). The adverse events observed were mild and limited to transient scalp discomfort or pain. There were no seizures. These data are under review by the FDA at the time of filing this chapter (panel hearing January 2007). TMS may be FDA approved as a treatment for depression soon. A few U.S., Canadian, and European psychiatrists are using TMS in clinical practice to treat depression under their general license to practice.

Unresolved issues.   Although the literature suggests that daily prefrontal TMS has an antidepressant effect greater than sham and that the magnitude of this effect is in the range of other antidepressants, many issues remain unresolved. Research has shown substantial evidence that prefrontal TMS produces immediate (George et al. 1999; Li et al. 2002; Nahas et al. 2001; Paus et al. 2001; Strafella et al. 2001) and longer-term (Teneback et al. 1999) changes in mood-regulating circuits. Thus, the original hypothesis about its antidepressant mechanism of action is still most likely valid. What remains unclear is which specific prefrontal or other brain locations might be best for treating depression, and whether the optimal locations can be determined with a group algorithm or with individual imaging guidance. For the most part, to find the prefrontal cortex, the coil has been positioned using the rule-based algorithm that I employed in the early studies (George et al. 1995c). However, this method was shown to be imprecise in that the particular prefrontal regions stimulated directly underneath the coil depend largely on the subject's head size (Herwig et al. 2001). Additionally, most studies have stimulated patients with the intensity needed to cause movement in the thumb (called the *motor threshold*). There is now increasing recognition that higher intensities of stimulation are needed to reach the prefrontal cortex, especially in elderly patients, where prefrontal atrophy may outpace that of the motor cortex, where the motor threshold is measured (Kozel et al. 2000; McConnell et al. 2001; Mosimann et al. 2002; Padberg et al. 2002). We are currently conducting a multisite National Institutes of Health–sponsored trial to address many of these important issues and potentially improve the way TMS is used as a treatment. There are a few case series suggesting that one can use weekly or monthly rTMS as a maintenance treatment after a patient has responded acutely (Li et al. 2004a; Nahas et al. 2000; O'Reardon et al. 2005).

Other Psychiatric Conditions

TMS has also been investigated as a possible treatment for a variety of neuropsychiatric disorders. In general, the published literature on these conditions is much less extensive than for TMS as an antidepressant. Therefore, conclusions about the clinical significance of effects must remain tentative until large-sample studies are conducted.

Schizophrenia.   *Diagnosis.*   Several studies have used TMS to investigate corticospinal conductivity in schizophrenia (Feinsod et al. 1998). In the first study of motor function in schizophrenia using TMS, Puri et al. (1996) detected a significantly shorter latency of motor-evoked potentials in nine unmedicated patients with schizophrenia compared with nine healthy subjects. Two other studies measuring motor evoked potential latency did not find a difference between medicated schizophrenia patients and healthy control subjects (Davey et al. 1997; Puri et al. 1996).

Treatment.   Hoffman et al. (1999) have used repeated daily sessions of low-frequency TMS over the temporal lobes to treat hallucinations in patients with schizophrenia. Some but not all groups have replicated these effects (d'Alfonso et al. 2002; Fitzgerald et al. 2006; Hoffman et al. 2000; Jin et al. 2006; Rollnik et al. 2000). Other investigators have studied whether TMS might be effective in treating the negative symptoms of schizophrenia (Cohen et al. 1999). Further studies are needed.

Anxiety disorders.   Several studies have shown promising results in using TMS to treat obsessive-compulsive disorder (OCD). In the initial study in the field, Greenberg et al. (1997) found that a single session of right prefrontal rTMS decreased compulsive urges for 8 hours. Mood was also transiently improved, but there was no effect on anxiety or obsessions. Two other studies have examined possible therapeutic effects of rTMS in OCD. A double-blind study using right prefrontal slow (1 Hz) rTMS and a less focal coil failed to show statistically significant effects greater than sham (Alonso et al. 2001). In contrast, in an open study of a group of 12 OCD patients refractory to standard treatments who were randomly assigned to right or left prefrontal fast rTMS, it was found that clinically significant and sustained improvement could be observed in one-third of patients (Sachdev et al. 2001). Finally, in a recent study, clinical improvements in OCD and Tourette syndrome were found in a group of patients stimulated in the supplemental motor area (Mantovani et al. 2006). Clearly, more work is warranted in examining TMS as a potential treatment for OCD.

There is also intense interest in using TMS to treat anxiety, particularly PTSD. McCann et al. (1998) reported that 2 patients with PTSD improved during open treatment with 1 Hz rTMS over the right frontal cortex. Grisaru et al. (1998) similarly stimulated 10 PTSD patients over motor cortex and found decreased anxiety. Further study is needed, particularly concerning whether to have PTSD patients remember their trauma during stimulation.

Pain. Mood-regulating centers in the brain overlap significantly with the neural pathways involved in pain regulation, especially the regions that determine whether a pain is really bothersome. Thus, some researchers have begun exploring whether TMS might have a therapeutic role in treating acute or chronic pain. There are exciting reports that TMS over either prefrontal cortex or motor cortex can acutely decrease pain in healthy adults or patients with chronic pain (Andre-Obadia et al. 2006; Johnson et al. 2006; Lefaucheur 2004; Lefaucheur et al. 2001; Pridmore and Oberoi 2000; Rollnik et al. 2002). The results of recent RCT indicate that a single 20-minute session of left prefrontal rTMS given to patients in the recovery room following surgery reduced self-administered morphine use by 40% (Borckardt et al. 2006b).

Summary of TMS

Overall, TMS is a promising new therapy, as well as a useful research tool. The bulk of clinical work to date has focused on TMS as a treatment for depression for which it is now being considered for FDA approval. It also shows some promise as a treatment for several other psychiatric disorders.

Vagus Nerve Stimulation

TMS is noninvasive, focal, largely limited to different cortical sites, and intermittent. VNS is in some sense the opposite of TMS, as it is invasive and requires surgical implantation of a device in the chest wall and a wire in the neck. The brain region stimulated always follows the same initial route—the vagus nerve in the neck. It is also a permanent implant that cannot be removed without surgery. Finally, although TMS has not been FDA approved to treat any disorder, VNS has been approved for almost 10 years as a treatment for epilepsy (Ben-Menachem et al. 1994; George et al. 1994c; Salinsky et al. 1996; Uthman et al. 1993; Vagus Nerve Stimulation Study Group 1995) and was FDA

approved in 2005 for chronic use in patients with treatment-resistant depression.

Brief History

Throughout the past century, researchers have investigated whether and to what extent stimulation of cranial nerves (CN) might have observable effects on brain function. Of all the cranial nerves, with the exception of CN I for olfaction, the vagus nerve (CN X) has been the most intriguing and arguably the most misunderstood (Ammons et al. 1983; Bailey and Bremer 1938; Duffin et al. 1994; Foley and DuBois 1937; Otterson 1981; Ter Horst and Streetland 1994). The vagus nerve helps regulate the body's autonomic functions, which are important in a variety of emotional tasks. For reasons that are unclear, most people are more familiar with the vagus nerve's efferent functions, where it serves as the messenger for signals from the brain to the viscera. Traditionally, the vagus nerve has been considered a parasympathetic efferent nerve (controlling and regulating autonomic functions such as heart rate and gastric tone). The afferent role of the vagus has been underemphasized in the traditional literature. The vagus is actually a mixed nerve composed of about 80% afferent sensory fibers carrying information to the brain from the head, neck, thorax, and abdomen (Foley and DuBois 1937) (Figure 27–3).

Over the past 100 years, several researchers have convincingly demonstrated the extensive projections of the vagus nerve via its sensory afferent connections in the nucleus tractus solitarius to diverse brain regions (Ammons et al. 1983; Bailey and Bremer 1938; Otterson 1981; Rutecki 1990; Zardetto-Smith and Gray 1990). Reasoning in part from this body of literature, Jake Zabara discovered an anticonvulsant action of VNS on experimental seizures in dogs (Zabara 1985a, 1985b, 1992). Zabara hypothesized that VNS could prevent or control the motor and autonomic components of epilepsy. Penry and others ushered in the modern clinical application of VNS in 1988 using an implanted device to treat epilepsy (Penry and Dean 1990; Uthman et al. 1993).

Although the route of entry into the brain is constrained, VNS offers the potential for modulating and modifying function in many brain regions, through transsynaptic connections (George et al. 2000; Henry 2002; Nemeroff et al. 2006). The incoming sensory (afferent) connections of the vagus nerve provide direct projections to many of the brain regions implicated in neuropsychiatric disorders. These connections provide a basis for understanding how VNS might be a portal to the brain stem and connected limbic and cor-

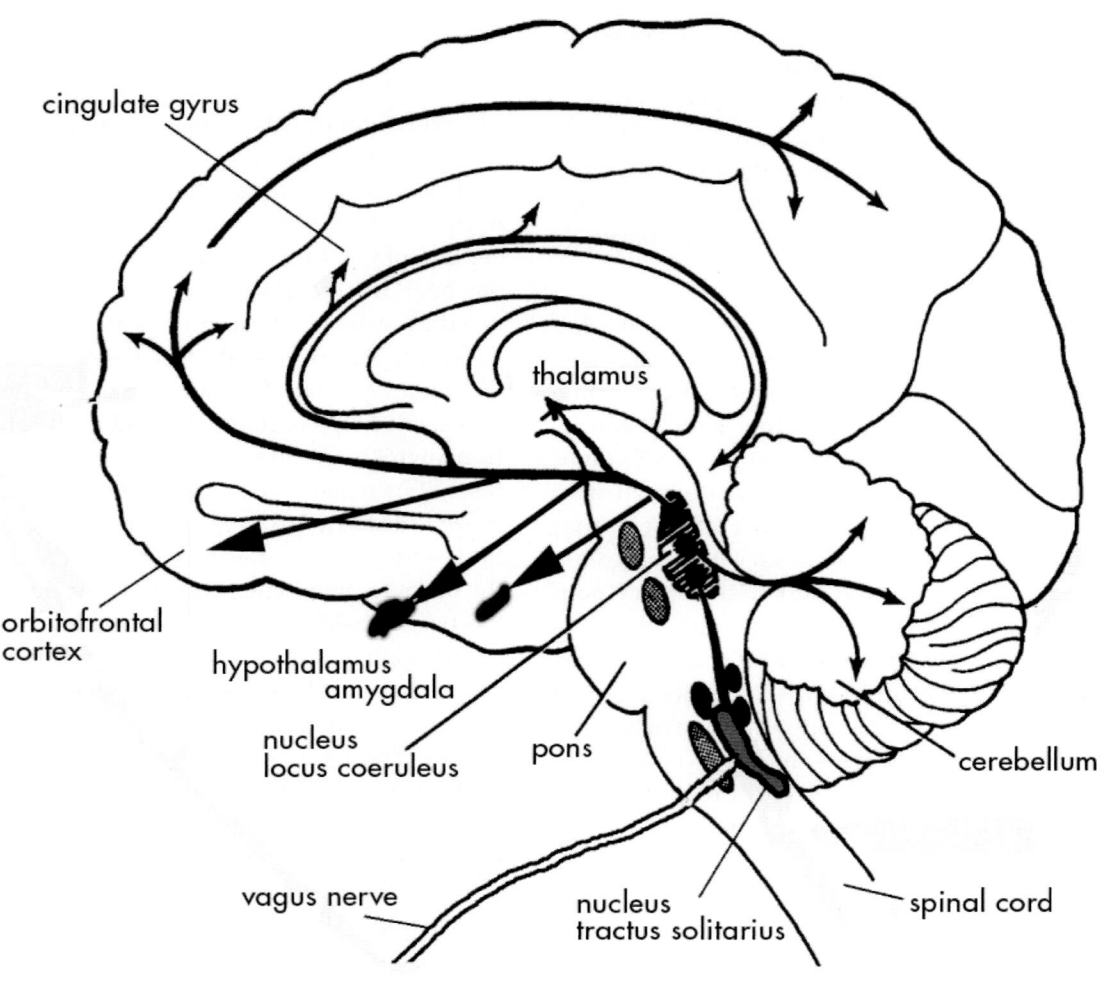

FIGURE 27–3.   **Vagus nerve anatomy.**

Drawing depicts the brain split sagittally. Note that vagus nerve afferents enter the brain stem and then travel to the locus coeruleus, as well as to other important mood- and anxiety-regulating regions.

Source.   Reprinted from George MS, Sackeim HA, Rush AJ, et al.: "Vagus Nerve Stimulation: A New Tool for Brain Research and Therapy." *Biological Psychiatry* 47:287–295, 2000. Copyright 2000, Society of Biological Psychiatry. Used with permission.

tical regions. These pathways are likely to account for the neuropsychiatric effects of VNS, and they invite additional theoretical considerations for potential research and clinical applications. Functional imaging studies in patients with implanted VNS stimulators have largely confirmed this important aspect of the neuroanatomy of the vagus (Bohning et al. 2001; Chae et al. 2003; Conway et al. 2006; Henry et al. 1998, 1999; Lomarev et al. 2002; Mu et al. 2004).

VNS Methods

The broad term *vagus nerve stimulation* refers to any technique used to stimulate the vagus nerve, includ-

ing animal studies in which the vagus was accessed through the abdomen and diaphragm. However, for virtually all human studies, *VNS* refers to stimulation of the left cervical vagus nerve using a commercial device (Figure 27–4).

VNS has been commercially available for the treatment of resistant partial-onset seizures in Europe since 1994, and in the United States since 1997. VNS resembles the implantation of a cardiac pacemaker. In both VNS and cardiac pacemakers, a subcutaneous generator sends an electrical signal to an organ through an implanted electrode. With VNS, the electrical stimulation is delivered through the generator, an implantable, multiprogrammable, bipolar pulse generator

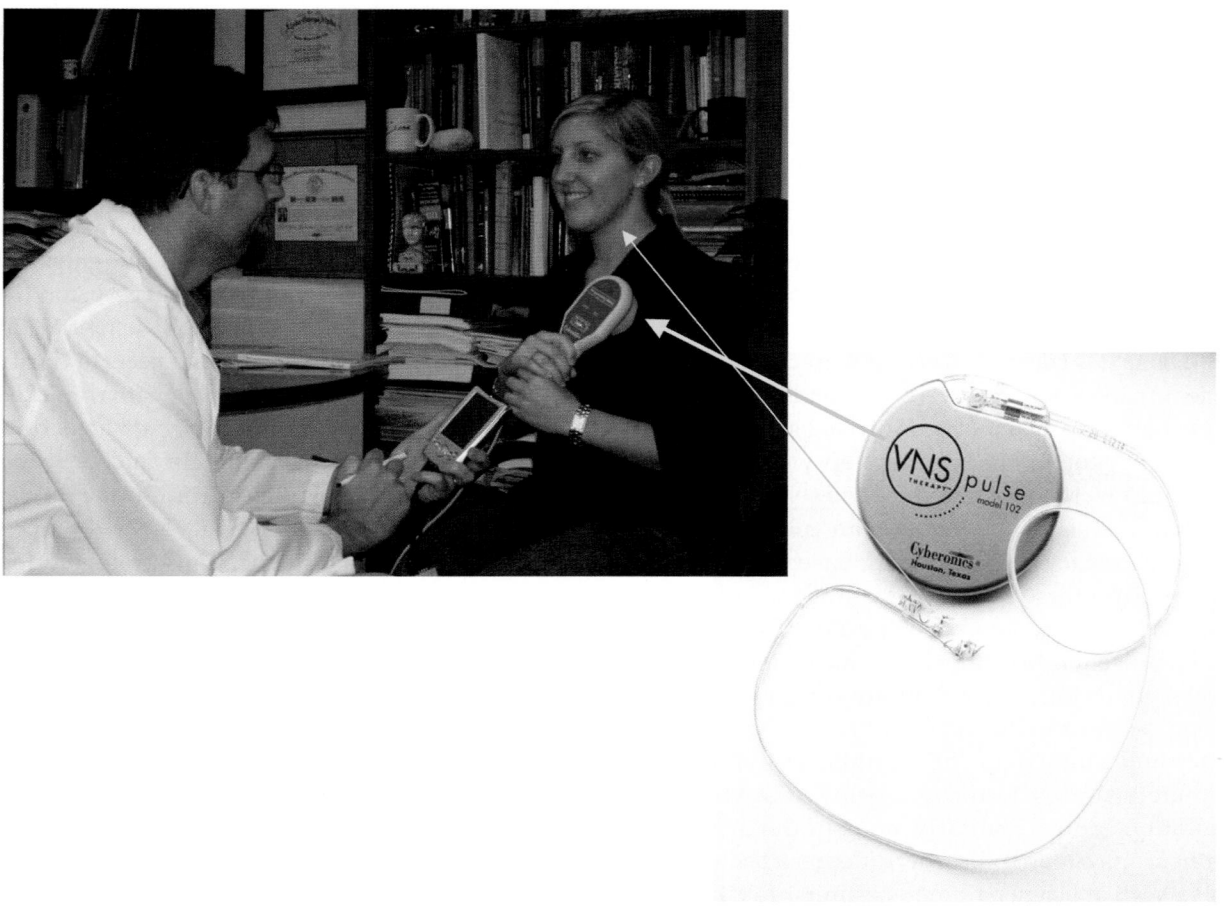

FIGURE 27–4. Dosing and delivery of vagus nerve stimulation (VNS).

Nurse Berry Anderson, left, holds the programming PDA, which is connected to an infrared wand positioned over the left chest wall of research assistant Lauren Forster (not an actual VNS patient). The VNS patient holds the wand over the generator, which is typically implanted in the left chest wall and connected by a wire to the lead wrapped under the vagus nerve in the left neck. The treating clinician can then adjust the VNS device stimulation parameters.

Source. Photo courtesy of Dr. Mark George, Medical University of South Carolina (MUSC) Brain Stimulation Laboratory.

(about the size of a pocket watch) that is implanted in the left chest wall to deliver electrical signals to the left vagus nerve through a bipolar lead. The electrode is wrapped around the vagus nerve in the neck and is connected to the generator subcutaneously.

VNS implantation surgery is typically an outpatient procedure and is most commonly, but not exclusively, performed by neurosurgeons. The VNS generator can be controlled by a personal computer or personal digital assistant (PDA) connected to an infrared wand. As a safety feature, the VNS generator is designed to shut off in the presence of a constant magnetic field. Each patient is thus given a magnet that, when held over the pulse generator, turns off stimulation. When the magnet is removed, normal programmed stimulation resumes. This allows patients to control and temporarily eliminate stimulation-related side effects during im-

portant behaviors such as public speaking (voice tremor) or heavy exercising (mild shortness of breath).

Therapeutic Uses of VNS

Epilepsy

VNS has been most extensively studied as a treatment for epilepsy. Two double-blind studies have been conducted in patients with epilepsy, with a total of 313 treatment-resistant completers (Ben-Menachem et al. 1994; Handforth et al. 1998). Among subjects with this difficult-to-treat condition, the average decline in seizure frequency was between 25% and 30% compared with baseline.

Most epilepsy patients with VNS have not been able to reduce or withdraw antiepileptic medications. Therefore, VNS, as now delivered, has not been shown to be a substitute for anticonvulsant medications. However, in some patients the dosage levels or numbers of antiepileptic medications have been decreased with the addition of VNS. VNS is increasingly being used in children with epilepsy, in part because of its lack of negative cognitive effects, which are common to other anticonvulsants (Helmers et al. 2001).

Several different programmable variables determine how to deliver VNS. These "usage parameters" include the pulse width of the electrical signal (130, 250, 500, 750, 1,000 microseconds) and the intensity (0.25–4.00 mA is clinically tolerated), frequency (1–145 Hz), length of stimulation (7–270 seconds), and length of time between trains of stimuli (0.2 second to 180 minutes). In general, the initial epilepsy usage parameter settings were those found to stop seizures acutely in animal models. The initial human epilepsy studies compared efficacy in two groups, based on different usage parameters. There was a high-stimulation group (30 Hz, 30 seconds on, 5 minutes off, 500 microseconds pulse width) and a low-stimulation group (1 Hz, 30 seconds on, 90–180 minutes off, 130 microseconds pulse width). The majority of the VNS epilepsy efficacy and safety data come from trials with usage parameters similar to those employed in the high-stimulation group. Similarly, most of the data from other neuropsychiatric disorders (depression, anxiety) involve VNS at usage parameters similar to those employed in the initial epilepsy studies. It is difficult to imagine that these usage parameters are the maximally effective choices or that the same parameters work equally well in all conditions and with all patients. Epilepsy physicians commonly switch nonresponding patients to usage parameter settings that are different from their already established settings. However, there has been no clear demonstration that changing settings improves efficacy. Understanding the translational neurobiology of these usage parameter choices and how they relate to clinical symptoms is a key area for future growth of the field.

Depression

Psychiatric research has a long history of demonstrating that anticonvulsant medications (e.g., carbamazepine) or devices (e.g., ECT) have mood-stabilizing or antidepressant effects. In early 1998, several lines of evidence suggested that VNS might have antidepressant effects. Anecdotal reports of mood improvement in VNS-implanted epilepsy patients, knowledge of vagus function and neuroanatomy, brain imaging studies, work in animals, and cerebrospinal fluid studies all supported an initial pilot clinical trial in treatment-resistant depression (George et al. 2000).

In June 1998, the first patient ever treated with VNS for the indication of depression was implanted at the Medical University of South Carolina (MUSC) in Charleston, launching an open study of VNS for the treatment of chronic or recurrent treatment-resistant depression. This study involved four sites (MUSC–Charleston; New York State Psychiatric Institute; University of Texas Southwestern Medical Center in Dallas; and Baylor College of Medicine in Houston, Texas) and initially involved 30 subjects (Rush et al. 2000), with a later extension of 30 more subjects to clarify the effect size and identify response predictors (Sackeim et al. 2001b). The study design involved selecting patients with treatment-resistant, chronic, or recurrent major depressive episode (unipolar or non-rapid-cycling bipolar) and then adding VNS to a stable regimen of antidepressant medications or no antidepressant medications. No stimulation was given for the first 2 weeks following implantation, creating a single-blind placebo phase and allowing for surgical recovery. All patients met eligibility criteria by failing to respond to at least two adequate-treatment trials in the current episode.

Ten weeks of VNS therapy were provided with medications held constant. Of 59 completers (1 patient improved during the surgical recovery period), the response rates were 30.5% for the primary Hamilton Rating Scale for Depression (HRSD28) measure, 34.0% for the Montgomery-Åsberg Depression Rating Scale, and 37.3% for the Clinical Global Impression—Improvement score (CGI-I of 1 or 2). VNS was well tolerated in this group, with side effects similar to those encountered by epilepsy patients. The most common side effect was voice alteration or hoarseness, 60.0% (36/60), which was generally mild and related to the intensity of the output current. There were no adverse cognitive effects (Sackeim et al. 2001a). The only response predictor was prior antidepressant treatment resistance. VNS as used in this open study was more effective in depressed patients who were less treatment resistant.

These encouraging initial results served as the basis for a recently completed U.S. multisite double-blind trial of VNS for chronic or recurrent treatment-resistant depression. In this trial, active VNS failed to show a statistically significant difference in acute response from the sham group (Rush et al. 2005). The sham response rate was 10%, and the active response rate was 15%.

The longer-term response rates for depression patients treated with VNS implantation are encouraging (Nahas et al. 2005) and appear to be better than what would be expected in this population (Rush et al. 2006). A parallel but nonrandomized comparison found that patients with VNS implantation had better outcomes at 1 year compared with patients receiving treatment as usual (George et al. 2005). These data served as the basis for FDA approval of VNS for the long-term (not acute) treatment of chronic recurrent depression. Thus, VNS is FDA approved, although there is no double-blind, randomized controlled evidence for the efficacy of VNS as an antidepressant in patients with depression. There are, however, open (Harden et al. 2000) and double-blind (Elger et al. 2000) studies showing that VNS has antidepressant effects in epilepsy patients with comorbid depression.

Other Potential Applications for VNS

Anxiety. As reviewed above, the sensory-afferent nerve fibers that VNS stimulates in the vagus travel to the brain and terminate in the nucleus solitary tract. These fibers are the primary means by which the brain receives information from the organs within the gut and diaphragm. From there, information travels to the locus coeruleus, the primary site of all norepinephrine fibers in the brain. Norepinephrine has long been considered to be a critical neurotransmitter system involved in the pathogenesis and regulation of anxiety. A device that directly stimulates this norepinephrine control site would likely have important effects on anxiety. Figure 27–5 shows how VNS causes activation in the orbitofrontal cortex and insula, as well as near the amygdala and hypothalamus.

The historical importance of this pathway that VNS modulates can be seen in the oldest theory about the brain origins of fear—the James-Lange theory of emotions. William James (1884) offered the radical argument that all emotion actually resided in the body and that it was the brain's interpretation of this signal through the vagus nerve that caused someone to be anxious. A device that directly affects this information flow could be a powerful way to alter anxiety. In a multisite open-treatment trial of VNS in 10 patients with treatment-resistant anxiety disorder (7 of the 10 had OCD), 30% were acute-phase responders as assessed on the Hamilton Anxiety Scale, and 3 of the 7 patients with OCD were responders as assessed on the Yale-Brown Obsessive Compulsive Scale (George et al., in press).

Obesity. Information about hunger and satiety from the stomach and small intestine travels through the vagus nerve to the brain. It seems plausible to ask whether vagus stimulation might change eating pat-

terns and other forms of craving. To investigate this, Roslin and colleagues in New York implanted bilateral subdiaphragmatic vagus stimulators in several normal-weight mongrel dogs. Over several months, chronic intermittent VNS delivered in this manner resulted in substantial weight loss. Interestingly, there was no change in the dogs' metabolism. Rather, they took much longer to consume their food, and they even left food on their plate—something mongrel dogs rarely, if ever, do (Roslin and Kurian 2001). Although VNS had no overall effect on weight in the RCT in epilepsy and depression, it is still possible that VNS might be used for the treatment of obesity. A recent laboratory study on VNS treatment in depressed patients found that the subjects had different food cravings in response to pictures of food when the device was firing compared with when it was turned off (Bodenlos et al. 2007).

Pain. Some information about pain, especially visceral pain, travels through the vagus nerve. A recent study showing changes in pain perception as a function of varying VNS settings hints at the promise of using VNS for some form of pain modulation (Borckardt et al. 2005, 2006a).

In conclusion, VNS has an important role in the treatment of epilepsy. However, the only clinical effects that have been shown with double-blind studies are in epilepsy for seizure control and in depression occurring in the setting of epilepsy. Yet, it is FDA approved for depression. There are many areas where more information would facilitate its adoption. Compared with talking therapy, medications, and even ECT, VNS requires a different approach to treating depression. Whereas other treatments can be begun, sampled, and then easily abandoned if not effective, VNS, with the installation of an implant, requires careful consideration prior to initiating therapy. Currently, there is no noninvasive method of VNS that could be tried prior to a permanent implant. Thus, it is crucial to determine from available data who is likely to respond (or not). Additionally, because of the relatively large initial capital costs of implanting a VNS generator, data are needed to convince payers that VNS is cost-effective. An initial implantation fee of around $20,000 (device and surgery) is about equal to 1 week of hospitalization or a course of outpatient ECT. VNS would thus be cost-effective for those recurrent, chronically ill patients whose implantations result in clinical improvements that eliminate the need for hospitalization, ECT, or more frequent and aggressive outpatient medication management.

Another radical difference between VNS and medication treatments is that VNS facilitates almost 100%

Within-task increases

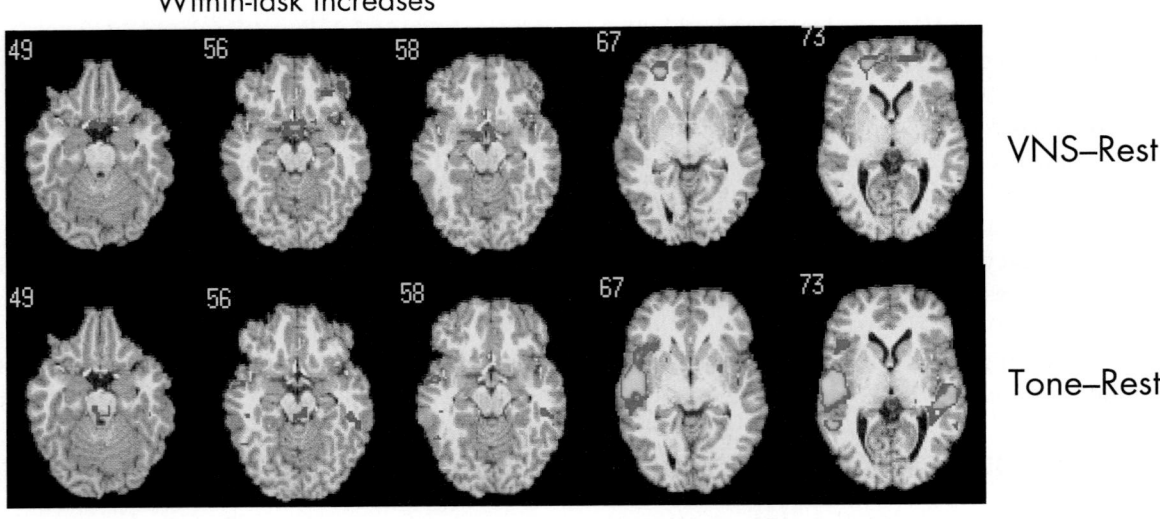

Nine subjects, Talairach space, $P < 0.001$, extent $P < 0.05$

FIGURE 27–5.   Vagus nerve stimulation (VNS) efferents in the brain.

Shown are images from representative slices of a common brain, where results from nine depressed patients have been pooled. **Top row:** The activated areas (displayed in color) are regions showing increased blood flow while the device was actively delivering stimulation, compared with the few seconds before, when it was silent. Note the activation in the hypothalamus, orbitofrontal and prefrontal cortex, and insula. **Bottom row:** The colored areas are the brain regions activated when subjects heard a tone (largely auditory cortex). VNS activates the "gut-sensory" system.

Source.   Reprinted from Lomarev M, Denslow S, Nahas Z, et al: "Vagus Nerve Stimulation (VNS) Synchronized BOLD fMRI Suggests That VNS in Depressed Adults Has Frequency/Dose Dependent Effects." *Journal of Psychiatric Research* 36:219–227, 2002. Copyright 2002, Elsevier LTD. Used with permission.

adherence. The device, once implanted, cycles on and off without problems for several years. Several studies have shown that even the best patients skip and forget medications, with resultant problems in their clinical course. VNS is thus a most interesting new approach to treating depression, but more information is critically needed.

Other Somatic Treatments

This is a fertile and rapidly growing field, with many additional brain stimulation techniques emerging almost monthly. In general, it is best to adopt an open but skeptical approach to these treatments. That is, they might work, but rigorous RCTs are needed before adoption. In addition to acupuncture, there are several small, portable stimulation methods, such as transcutaneous electrical nerve stimulation (TENS) units, that stimulate peripherally and purport to change brain function. These stimulation methods use biphasic low-voltage current and selectable parameters, such as pulse rate and pulse width to stimulate sensory nerves to block pain signals and theoretically alter brain func-

tion. As a class, there are broad neuropsychiatric therapeutic claims bandied about on the Internet and in advertisements that are not based on rigorous RCT data. Some devices in this group are designed to stimulate the earlobe, which has complex afferent fibers (including branches of the vagus nerve).

Harold Sackeim has worked for many years to build supercharged TMS devices capable of reliably producing seizures in humans, reasoning that a TMS-induced seizure would be more focal and efficient than an ECT seizure and would spare much of the brain from receiving unneeded electricity (George and Wassermann 1994b; Sackeim 1994). Magnetic seizure therapy (MST) has been shown to be feasible, first in animals and now in patients (Lisanby et al. 2003a, 2003b, 2003c). Patients have markedly less acute cognitive disruption from MST seizures than from traditional ECT. Whether MST works (i.e., has clinical antidepressant efficacy) is still not clear, and a multisite study is under way.

The most invasive of all the techniques is DBS, in which an electrode is implanted deep within the brain and connected to a generator located in the chest wall, which then sends constant electrical current into the brain. Theoretically, DBS electrodes can be removed without destroying large parts of the brain: DBS therefore has less morbidity and mortality than resective brain surgery. DBS of the internal globus pallidus or subthalamic nucleus is now an accepted treatment for Parkinson's disease, especially for those patients who are medication intolerant or medication resistant (Kumar et al. 1998; Limousin et al. 1995, 1998). It also is used in patients with dystonia. There is one small open series of DBS of the anterior cingulate for treatment-resistant depression (Mayberg et al. 2005). Because the functional neuroanatomy of depression is not nearly as well known as that for Parkinson's disease or dystonia, a great deal of caution is warranted in this area. Psychiatrists should not re-create the mistakes of the lobotomy years, when overenthusiastic adoption of an invasive technology ruined many lives and damaged the reputation of the field.

Conclusion

Psychiatry is developing an entirely new area of therapeutics involving electrical brain stimulation. This fertile field bridges neuroimaging, neuroanatomy, basic neuroscience, and engineering. The techniques are slowly being refined and tested, with a few already FDA approved and in use in clinical practice. This area will undoubtedly continue to grow as the technology develops and the knowledge base expands.

Key Points

- The brain is fundamentally an electrochemical organ, where electrical impulses serve as the basis for information flow and then cause neurotransmitter release.

- Electrical stimulation of the brain can theoretically cause focal neuropsychopharmacological changes without the side effects of systemic medications.

- Brain stimulation therapies as a class share several common concepts and principles and can be understood by identifying which procedures produce seizures on purpose (ECT, MST, focal electrical alternating current seizure therapy [FEAST]) and which do not (TMS, VNS, DBS).

- ECT is our most effective treatment for acute major depression.

- TMS is an exciting research tool.

- Repeated daily prefrontal TMS has acute antidepressant effects similar to those of medications or ECT, with few side effects.

- VNS is FDA approved for the treatment of epilepsy and treatment-resistant depression.

- VNS is best reserved for patients with a long history of depression (chronic) who cannot be given most other treatment options.

- More research on the fundamental neurobiological effects of brain electrical stimulation will help these new techniques continue to improve and evolve.

Suggested Readings

George MS: Stimulating the brain. Sci Am 289:66–73, 2003

George MS, Belmaker RH: Transcranial Magnetic Stimulation in Neuropsychiatry. Washington, DC, American Psychiatric Press, 2000

George MS, Nahas Z, Li X, et al: Novel treatments of mood disorders based on brain circuitry (ECT, MST, TMS, VNS, DBS). Semin Clin Neuropsychiatry 7:293–304, 2002

George MS, Nahas Z, Lomarev M, et al: How knowledge of regional brain dysfunction in depression will enable new somatic treatments in the new millennium. CNS Spectr 4:53–61, 1999

Henry TR: Therapeutic mechanisms of vagus nerve stimulation. Neurology 59 (6 suppl 4):S3–S14, 2002

Zangen A, Roth Y, Voller B, et al: Transcranial magnetic stimulation of deep brain regions: evidence for efficacy of the H-coil. Clin Neurophysiology 116:775–779, 2005

Online Resources

The Avery-George-Holtzheimer Database of rTMS Depression Studies: http://www.ists.unibe.ch/TMSAvery.htm

The MUSC Brain Stimulation Laboratory: Medical University of South Carolina (MUSC) Department of Psychiatry and Behavioral Sciences, Brain Stimulation Laboratory: http://www.musc.edu/fnrd/dbs.html

Optimization of Transcranial Magnetic Stimulation (TMS) for the Treatment of Depression: the National Institute of Mental Health OPT-TMS Depression Trial: http://home-page.mac.com/opttmsmusc/TEST/OPTTMSweb050908msg.htm

References

Alonso P, Pujol J, Cardoner N, et al: Right prefrontal transcranial magnetic stimulation in obsessive-compulsive disorder: a double-blind, placebo-controlled study. Am J Psychiatry 158:1143–1145, 2001

Ammons WS, Blair RW, Foreman RD: Vagal afferent inhibition of primate thoracic spinothalamic neurons. J Neurophysiol 50:926–940, 1983

Andre-Obadia N, Peyron R, Mertens P, et al: Transcranial magnetic stimulation for pain control. Double-blind study of different frequencies against placebo, and correlation with motor cortex stimulation efficacy. Clin Neurophysiol 117:1536–1544, 2006

Bailey P, Bremer F: A sensory cortical representation of the vagus nerve. With a note on the effects of low blood pressure on the cortical electrogram. J Neurophysiol 1:405–412, 1938

Barker AT, Jalinous R, Freeston IL: Non-invasive magnetic stimulation of the human motor cortex. Lancet 1(8437):1106–1107, 1985

Barker AT, Freeston IL, Jalinous R, et al: Magnetic stimulation of the human brain and peripheral nervous system: an introduction and the results of an initial clinical evaluation. Neurosurgery 20:100–109, 1987

Barnes CA, Jung MW, McNaughton BL, et al: LTP saturation and spatial learning disruption: effects of task variables and saturation levels. J Neurosci 14:5793–5806, 1994

Bartsch AP, van Hemmen JL: Combined Hebbian development of geniculocortical and lateral connectivity in a model of primary visual cortex. Biol Cybern 84:41–55, 2001

Baudewig J, Siebner HR, Bestmann S, et al: Functional MRI of cortical activations induced by transcranial magnetic stimulation (TMS). Neuroreport 12:3543–3548, 2001

Beer B: Uber das Auftreten einer objektiven Lichtempfindung in magnetischen Felde. Klinische Wochenzeitschrift 15:108–109, 1902

Ben-Menachem E, Manon-Espaillat R, Ristanovic R, et al: Vagus nerve stimulation for treatment of partial seizures, I: a controlled study of effect on seizures. Epilepsia 35:616–626, 1994

Ben-Sachar D, Belmaker RH, Grisaru N, et al: Transcranial magnetic stimulation induces alterations in brain monoamines. J Neural Transm 104:191–197, 1997

Bodenlos JS, Kose S, Borckardt JJ, et al: Vagus nerve stimulation acutely alters food craving in adults with depression. Appetite 48:145–153, 2007

Bohning DE, Shastri A, Nahas Z, et al: Echoplanar BOLD fMRI of brain activation induced by concurrent transcranial magnetic stimulation. Invest Radiol 33:336–340, 1998

Bohning DE, Shastri A, McConnell K, et al: A combined TMS/fMRI study of intensity-dependent TMS over motor cortex. Biol Psychiatry 45:385–394, 1999

Bohning DE: Introduction and overview of TMS physics, in Transcranial Magnetic Stimulation in Neuropsychiatry. Edited by George MS, Belmaker RH. Washington, DC, American Psychiatric Press, 2000, pp 13–44

Bohning DE, Shastri A, McGavin L, et al: Motor cortex brain activity induced by 1-Hz transcranial magnetic stimulation is similar in location and level to that for volitional movement. Invest Radiol 35:676–683, 2000a

Bohning DE, Shastri A, Wassermann EM, et al: BOLD-fMRI response to single-pulse transcranial magnetic stimulation (TMS). J Magn Reson Imaging 11:569–574, 2000b

Bohning DE, Lomarev MP, Denslow S, et al: Feasibility of vagus nerve stimulation-synchronized blood oxygenation level-dependent functional MRI. Invest Radiol 36:470–479, 2001

Borckardt JJ, Kozel FA, Anderson B, et al: Vagus nerve stimulation affects pain perception in depressed adults. Pain Res Manag 10:9–14, 2005

Borckardt JJ, Anderson B, Kozel FA, et al: Acute and long-term VNS effects on pain perception in a case of treatment-resistant depression. Neurocase 12:216–220, 2006a

Borckardt JJ, Weinstein M, Reeves ST, et al: Postoperative left prefrontal repetitive transcranial magnetic stimulation (rTMS) reduces patient-controlled analgesia use. Anesthesiology 105:557–562, 2006b

Burt T, Lisanby SH, Sackeim HA: Neuropsychiatric applications of transcranial magnetic stimulation. Int J Neuropsychopharmacol 5:73–103, 2002

Chae JH, Nahas Z, Lomarev M, et al: A review of functional neuroimaging studies of vagus nerve stimulation (VNS). J Psychiatr Res 37:443–455, 2003

Cohen E, Bernardo M, Masana J, et al: Repetitive transcranial magnetic stimulation in the treatment of chronic negative schizophrenia: a pilot study. J Neurol Neurosurg Psychiatry 67:129–130, 1999

Conway CR, Sheline YI, Chibnall JT, et al: Cerebral blood flow changes during vagus nerve stimulation for depression. Psychiatry Res 146:179–184, 2006

d'Alfonso AA, Aleman A, Kessels RP, et al: Transcranial magnetic stimulation of left auditory cortex in patients with schizophrenia: effects on hallucinations and neurocognition. J Neuropsychiatry Clin Neurosci 14:77–79, 2002

Dannon PN, Dolberg OT, Schreiber S, et al: Three- and six-month outcome following courses of either ECT or rTMS in a population of severely depressed individuals—preliminary report. Biol Psychiatry 51:687–690, 2002

Davey NJ, Puri BK, Lewis HS, et al: Effects of antipsychotic medication on electromyographic responses to transcranial magnetic stimulation of the motor cortex in schizophrenia. J Neurol Neurosurg Psychiatry 63:468–473, 1997

Di Lazzaro V, Pilato F, Saturno E, et al: Theta-burst repetitive transcranial magnetic stimulation suppresses specific excitatory circuits in the human motor cortex. J Physiol 565:945–950, 2005

Duffin J, Douse MA, van Alphen J: Excitation of upper cervical inspiratory neurones by vagal stimulation in the cat. Neuroreport 5:1133–1136, 1994

Elger G, Hoppe C, Falkai P, et al: Vagus nerve stimulation is associated with mood improvements in epilepsy patients. Epilepsy Res 42:203–210, 2000

Feinsod M, Kreinin B, Chistyakov A, et al: Preliminary evidence for a beneficial effect of low-frequency, repetitive transcranial magnetic stimulation in patients with major depression and schizophrenia. Depress Anxiety 7:65–68, 1998

Fitzgerald PB, Benitez J, Daskalakis JZ, et al: The treatment of recurring auditory hallucinations in schizophrenia with rTMS. World J Biol Psychiatry 7:119–122, 2006

Fleischmann A, Sternheim A, Etgen AM, et al: Transcranial magnetic stimulation downregulates beta-adrenoreceptors in rat cortex. J Neural Transm 103:1361–1366, 1996

Foley JO, DuBois F: Quantitative studies of the vagus nerve in the cat, I: the ratio of sensory and motor studies. J Comp Neurol 67:49–67, 1937

George MS: An introduction to the emerging neuroanatomy of depression. Psychiatr Ann 24:635–636, 1994

George MS: Advances in brain stimulation. Guest editorial. J ECT 18:169, 2002

George MS: Stimulating the brain. Sci Am 289:66–73, 2003

George MS, Belmaker RH: Transcranial Magnetic Stimulation in Neuropsychiatry. Washington, DC, American Psychiatric Press, 2000

George MS, Bohning DE: Measuring brain connectivity with functional imaging and transcranial magnetic stimulation (TMS), in Neuropsychopharmacology: Fifth Generation of Progress. Edited by Desimone B. New York, Lippincott Williams & Wilkins, 2002, pp 393–410

George MS, Wassermann EM: Rapid-rate transcranial magnetic stimulation and ECT. Convuls Ther 10:251–254; discussion 255–258, 1994a

George MS, Wassermann EM: Rapid-rate transcranial magnetic stimulation (rTMS) and ECT. Convuls Ther 10:251–253, 1994b

George MS, Ketter TA, Parekh PI, et al: Regional brain activity when selecting a response despite interference: an $H_2^{15}O$ PET study of the Stroop and an emotional Stroop. Hum Brain Mapp 1:194–209, 1994a

George MS, Ketter TA, Post RM: Prefrontal cortex dysfunction in clinical depression. Depression 2:59–72, 1994b

George R, Salinsky M, Kuzniecky R, et al: Vagus nerve stimulation for treatment of partial seizures, 3: long-term follow-up on first 67 patients exiting a controlled study. First International Vagus Nerve Stimulation Study Group. Epilepsia 35:637–643, 1994c

George MS, Ketter TA, Parekh PI, et al: Brain activity during transient sadness and happiness in healthy women. Am J Psychiatry 152:341–351, 1995a

George MS, Post RM, Ketter TA, et al: Neural mechanisms of mood disorders, in Current Review of Mood Disorders. Edited by Rush AJ. Philadelphia, PA, Current Medicine, 1995b, pp 20–25

George MS, Wassermann EM, Williams WA, et al: Daily repetitive transcranial magnetic stimulation (rTMS) improves mood in depression. Neuroreport 6:1853–1856, 1995c

George MS, Ketter TA, Post RM: What functional imaging studies have revealed about the brain basis of mood and emotion, in Advances in Biological Psychiatry. Edited by Panksepp J. Greenwich, CT, JAI Press, 1996, pp 63–113

George MS, Ketter TA, Parekh PI, et al: Blunted left cingulate activation in mood disorder subjects during a response interference task (the Stroop). J Neuropsychiatry Clin Neurosci 9:55–63, 1997a

George MS, Wassermann EM, Kimbrell TA, et al: Mood improvements following daily left prefrontal repetitive transcranial magnetic stimulation in patients with depression: a placebo-controlled crossover trial. Am J Psychiatry 154:1752–1756, 1997b

George MS, Huggins T, McDermut W, et al: Abnormal facial emotion recognition in depression: serial testing in an ultra-rapid-cycling patient. Behavior Modification 22:192–204, 1998

George MS, Stallings LE, Speer AM, et al: Prefrontal repetitive transcranial magnetic stimulation (rTMS) changes relative perfusion locally and remotely. Hum Psychopharmacol 14:161–170, 1999

George MS, Sackeim HA, Rush AJ, et al: Vagus nerve stimulation: a new tool for brain research and therapy. Biol Psychiatry 47:287–295, 2000

George MS, Nahas Z, Kozel FA, et al: Mechanisms and state of the art of transcranial magnetic stimulation. J ECT 18:170–181, 2002

George MS, Rush AJ, Marangell LB, et al: A one-year comparison of vagus nerve stimulation with treatment as usual for treatment-resistant depression. Biol Psychiatry 58:364–373, 2005

George MS, Ward H, Ninan PT, et al: An open-label pilot study of vagus nerve stimulation (VNS) for treatment-resistant anxiety. Brain Stimulation: Basic, Translational, and Clinical Research in Neuromodulation (in press)

Greenberg BD, George MS, Martin JD, et al: Effect of prefrontal repetitive transcranial magnetic stimulation (rTMS) in obsessive-compulsive disorder: a preliminary study. Am J Psychiatry 154:867–869, 1997

Grisaru N, Yarovslavsky U, Abarbanel J, et al: Transcranial magnetic stimulation in depression and schizophrenia. European Neuropsychopharmacology 4:287–288, 1994

Grisaru N, Amir M, Cohen H, et al: Effect of transcranial magnetic stimulation in posttraumatic stress disorder: a preliminary study. Biol Psychiatry 44:52–55, 1998

Handforth A, DeGiorgio CM, Schachter SC, et al: Vagus nerve stimulation therapy for partial-onset seizures: a randomized active-control trial. Neurology 51:48–55, 1998

Harden CL, Pulver MC, Ravdin LD, et al: A pilot study of mood in epilepsy patients treated with vagus nerve stimulation. Epilepsy Behav 1:93–99, 2000

Heide G, Witte OW, Ziemann U: Physiology of modulation of motor cortex excitability by low-frequency suprathreshold repetitive transcranial magnetic stimulation. Exp Brain Res 171:26–34, 2006

Helmers SL, Wheless JW, Frost M, et al: Vagus nerve stimulation therapy in pediatric patients with refractory epilepsy: retrospective study. J Child Neurol 16:843–848, 2001

Henry TR: Therapeutic mechanisms of vagus nerve stimulation. Neurology 59 (6 suppl 4):S3–S14, 2002

Henry TR, Bakay RA, Votaw JR, et al: Brain blood flow alterations induced by therapeutic vagus nerve stimulation in partial epilepsy, I: acute effects at high and low levels of stimulation. Epilepsia 39:983–990, 1998

Henry TR, Votaw JR, Pennell PB, et al: Acute blood flow changes and efficacy of vagus nerve stimulation in partial epilepsy. Neurology 52:1166–1173, 1999

Herwig U, Padberg F, Unger J, et al: Transcranial magnetic stimulation in therapy studies: examination of the reliability of "standard" coil positioning by neuronavigation. Biol Psychiatry 50:58–61, 2001

Hoffman RE, Boutros NN, Berman RM, et al: Transcranial magnetic stimulation of left temporoparietal cortex in three patients reporting hallucinated "voices." Biol Psychiatry 46:130–132, 1999

Hoffman RE, Boutros NN, Hu S, et al: Transcranial magnetic stimulation and auditory hallucinations in schizophrenia. Lancet 355:1073–1075, 2000

Holtzheimer PE, Russo J, Avery DH: A meta-analysis of repetitive transcranial magnetic stimulation in the treatment of depression. Psychopharmacol Bull 35:149–169, 2001

James W: What is an emotion? Mind 9:188–205, 1884

Jennum P, Klitgaard H: Repetitive transcranial magnetic stimulations of the rat. Effect of acute and chronic stimulations on pentylenetetrazole-induced clonic seizures. Epilepsy Res 23:115–122, 1996

Jin Y, Potkin SG, Kemp AS, et al: Therapeutic effects of individualized alpha frequency transcranial magnetic stimulation (alphaTMS) on the negative symptoms of schizophrenia. Schizophr Bull 32:556–561, 2006

Johnson S, Summers J, Pridmore S: Changes to somatosensory detection and pain thresholds following high frequency repetitive TMS of the motor cortex in individuals suffering from chronic pain. Pain 123:187–192, 2006

Ketter TA, Andreason PJ, George MS, et al: Anterior paralimbic mediation of procaine-induced emotional and psychosensory experiences. Arch Gen Psychiatry 53:59–69, 1996

Kimbrell TA, Ketter TA, George MS, et al: Regional cerebral glucose utilization in patients with a range of severities of unipolar depression. Biol Psychiatry 51:237–252, 2002

Kolbinger HM, Hoflich G, Hufnagel A, et al: Transcranial magnetic stimulation (TMS) in the treatment of major depression—a pilot study. Human Psychopharmacology: Clinical and Experimental 10:305–310, 1995

Kozel FA, George MS: Meta-analysis of left prefrontal repetitive transcranial magnetic stimulation (rTMS) to treat depression. J Psychiatr Pract 8:270–275, 2002

Kozel FA, Nahas Z, DeBrux C, et al: How coil- cortex distance relates to age, motor threshold, and antidepressant response to repetitive transcranial magnetic stimulation. J Neuropsychiatry Clin Neurosci 12:376–384, 2000

Kumar R, Lozano AM, Kim YJ, et al: Double-blind evaluation of subthalamic nucleus deep brain stimulation in advanced Parkinson's disease. Neurology 51:850–855, 1998

Lefaucheur JP: Transcranial magnetic stimulation in the management of pain. Suppl Clin Neurophysiol 57:737–748, 2004

Lefaucheur JP, Drouot X, Nguyen JP: Interventional neurophysiology for pain control: duration of pain relief following repetitive transcranial magnetic stimulation of the motor cortex. Neurophysiol Clin 31:247–252, 2001

Li X, Teneback CC, Nahas Z, et al: Lamotrigine inhibits the functional magnetic resonance imaging response to transcranial magnetic stimulation in healthy adults (abstract). Society of Biological Psychiatry 57th Annual Convention, Philadelphia, PA, May 16–18, 2002. Biol Psychiatry 51 (8 suppl):S67, 2002

Li X, Nahas Z, Anderson B, et al: Can left prefrontal rTMS be used as a maintenance treatment for bipolar depression? Depress Anxiety 20:98–100, 2004a

Li X, Nahas Z, Kozel FA, et al: Acute left prefrontal transcranial magnetic stimulation in depressed patients is associated with immediately increased activity in prefrontal cortical as well as subcortical regions. Biol Psychiatry 55:882–890, 2004b

Limousin P, Pollak P, Benazzouz A, et al: Effect of parkinsonian signs and symptoms of bilateral subthalamic nucleus stimulation. Lancet 345:91–95, 1995

Limousin P, Krack P, Pollak P, et al: Electrical stimulation of the subthalamic nucleus in advanced Parkinson's disease. N Engl J Med 339:1105–1111, 1998

Lisanby SH, Maddox JH, Prudic J, et al: The effects of electroconvulsive therapy on memory of autobiographical and public events. Arch Gen Psychiatry 57:581–590, 2000

Lisanby SH, Luber B, Schlaepfer TE, et al: Safety and feasibility of magnetic seizure therapy (MST) in major depression: randomized within-subject comparison with electroconvulsive therapy. Neuropsychopharmacology 28:1852–1865, 2003a

Lisanby SH, Morales O, Payne N, et al: New developments in electroconvulsive therapy and magnetic seizure therapy. CNS Spectr 8:529–536, 2003b

Lisanby SH, Moscrip T, Morales O, et al: Neurophysiological characterization of magnetic seizure therapy (MST) in non-human primates. Suppl Clin Neurophysiol 56:81–99, 2003c

Lomarev M, Denslow S, Nahas Z, et al: Vagus nerve stimulation (VNS) synchronized BOLD fMRI suggests that VNS in depressed adults has frequency/dose dependent effects. J Psychiatr Res 36:219–227, 2002

Loo C, Mitchell P, Sachdev P, et al: A double-blind controlled investigation of transcranial magnetic stimulation for the treatment of resistant major depression. Am J Psychiatry 156:946–948, 1999

Loo CK, Sachdev PS, Haindl W, et al: High (15 Hz) and low (1 Hz) frequency transcranial magnetic stimulation have different acute effects on regional cerebral blood flow in depressed patients. Psychol Med 33:997–1006, 2003

Mantovani A, Lisanby SH, Pieraccini F, et al: Repetitive transcranial magnetic stimulation (rTMS) in the treatment of obsessive-compulsive disorder (OCD) and Tourette's syndrome (TS). Int J Neuropsychopharmacol 9:95–100, 2006

Martin JLR, Barbanoj MJ, Schlaepfer TE, et al: Transcranial magnetic stimulation for treating depression. Cochrane Database Syst Rev (2):CD003493, 2002

Mayberg HS, Liotti M, Brannan SK, et al: Reciprocal limbic-cortical function and negative mood: converging PET findings in depression and normal sadness. Am J Psychiatry 156:675–682, 1999

Mayberg HS, Lozano AM, Voon V, et al: Deep brain stimulation for treatment-resistant depression. Neuron 45:651–660, 2005

McCann UD, Kimbrell TA, Morgan CM, et al: Repetitive transcranial magnetic stimulation for posttraumatic stress disorder (letter). Arch Gen Psychiatry 55:276–279, 1998

McConnell KA, Nahas Z, Shastri A, et al: The transcranial magnetic stimulation motor threshold depends on the distance from coil to underlying cortex: a replication in healthy adults comparing two methods of assessing the distance to cortex. Biol Psychiatry 49:454–459, 2001

McNamara B, Ray JL, Arthurs OJ, et al: Transcranial magnetic stimulation for depression and other psychiatric disorders. Psychol Med 31:1141–1146, 2001

Mosimann UP, Marre SC, Werlen S, et al: Antidepressant effects of repetitive transcranial magnetic stimulation in the elderly: correlation between effect size and coil-cortex distance. Arch Gen Psychiatry 59:560–561, 2002

Mu Q, Bohning DE, Nahas Z, et al: Acute vagus nerve stimulation using different pulse widths produces varying brain effects. Biol Psychiatry 55:816–825, 2004

Nahas Z, Oliver NC, Johnson M, et al: Feasibility and efficacy of left prefrontal rTMS as a maintenance antidepressant (abstract). Biol Psychiatry 47 (8 suppl):S156–S157, 2000

Nahas Z, Lomarev M, Roberts DR, et al: Unilateral left prefrontal transcranial magnetic stimulation (TMS) produces intensity-dependent bilateral effects as measured by interleaved BOLD fMRI. Biol Psychiatry 50:712–720, 2001

Nahas Z, Marangell LB, Husain MM, et al: Two-year outcome of vagus nerve stimulation (VNS) therapy for major depressive episodes. J Clin Psychiatry 66:1097–1104, 2005

Nemeroff CB, Mayberg HS, Krahl SE, et al: VNS therapy in treatment-resistant depression: clinical evidence and putative neurobiological mechanisms. Neuropsychopharmacology 31:1345–1355, 2006

Nobler MS, Sackeim HA, Prohovnik I, et al: Regional cerebral blood flow in mood disorders, III: treatment and clinical response. Arch Gen Psychiatry 51:884–897, 1994

Nobler MS, Oquendo MA, Kegeles LS, et al: Decreased regional brain metabolism after ECT. Am J Psychiatry 158:305–308, 2001

O'Reardon JP, Blumner KH, Peshek AD, et al: Long-term maintenance therapy for major depressive disorder with rTMS. J Clin Psychiatry 66:1524–1528, 2005

O'Reardon JP, Solvason HB, Janicak PG, et al: Efficacy and safety of transcranial magnetic stimulation in the acute treatment of major depression: a multisite randomized controlled trial. Biol Psychiatry [Epub ahead of print], 2007

Otterson OP: Afferent connection to the amygdaloid complex of the rat with some observations in the cat, III: afferents from lower brainstem. J Comp Neurol 202:335, 1981

Padberg F, Zwanzger P, Keck ME, et al: Repetitive transcranial magnetic stimulation (rTMS) in major depression: relation between efficacy and stimulation intensity. Neuropsychopharmacology 27:638–645, 2002

Pal PK, Hanajima R, Gunraj CA, et al: Effect of low-frequency repetitive transcranial magnetic stimulation on interhemispheric inhibition. J Neurophysiol 94:1668–1675, 2005

Paus T, Jech R, Thompson CJ, et al: Transcranial magnetic stimulation during positron emission tomography: a new method for studying connectivity of the human cerebral cortex. J Neuroscience 17:3178–3184, 1997

Paus T, Castro-Alamancos MA, Petrides M: Cortico-cortical connectivity of the human mid-dorsolateral frontal cortex and its modulation by repetitive transcranial magnetic stimulation. Eur J Neurosci 14:1405–1411, 2001

Penry JK, Dean JC: Prevention of intractable partial seizures by intermittent vagal nerve stimulation in humans: preliminary results. Epilepsy 31:S40–S43, 1990

Post A, Keck ME: TMS as a therapeutic tool in psychiatry: what do we know about neurobiological mechanisms? J Psychiatr Res 35:193–215, 2001

Pridmore S: Substitution of rapid transcranial magnetic stimulation treatments for electroconvulsive therapy treatments in a course of electroconvulsive therapy. Depress Anxiety 12:118–123, 2000

Pridmore S, Oberoi G: Transcranial magnetic stimulation applications and potential use in chronic pain: studies in waiting. J Neurol Sci 182:1–4, 2000

Prudic J, Olfson M, Marcus SC, et al: Effectiveness of electroconvulsive therapy in community settings. Biol Psychiatry 55:301–312, 2004

Puri BK, Davey NJ, Ellaway PH, et al: An investigation of motor function in schizophrenia using transcranial magnetic stimulation of the motor cortex. Br J Psychiatry 169:690–695, 1996

Rollnik JD, Huber TJ, Mogk H, et al: High frequency repetitive transcranial magnetic stimulation (rTMS) of the dorsolateral prefrontal cortex in schizophrenic patients. Neuroreport 11:4013–4015, 2000

Rollnik JD, Wustefeld S, Dauper J, et al: Repetitive transcranial magnetic stimulation for the treatment of chronic pain—a pilot study. Eur Neurol 48:6–10, 2002

Roslin M, Kurian M: The use of electrical stimulation of the vagus nerve to treat morbid obesity. Epilepsy and Behavior 2:S11–S16, 2001

Roth Y, Zangen A, Hallett M: A coil design for transcranial magnetic stimulation of deep brain regions. J Clin Neurophysiol 19:361–370, 2002

Rush AJ, George MS, Sackeim HA, et al: Vagus nerve stimulation (VNS) for treatment-resistant depressions: a multicenter study. Biol Psychiatry 47:276–286, 2000

Rush AJ, Marangell LB, Sackeim HA, et al: Vagus nerve stimulation for treatment-resistant depression: a randomized, controlled acute phase trial. Biol Psychiatry 58:347–354, 2005

Rush AJ, Trivedi MH, Wisniewski SR, et al: Bupropion-SR, sertraline, or venlafaxine-XR after failure of SSRIs for depression. N Engl J Med 354:1231–1242, 2006

Rutecki P: Anatomical, physiological, and theoretical basis for the antiepileptic effect of vagus nerve stimulation. Epilepsia 31:S1-S36, 1990

Sachdev PS, McBride R, Loo CK, et al: Right versus left prefrontal transcranial magnetic stimulation for obsessive-compulsive disorder: a preliminary investigation. J Clin Psychiatry 62:981–984, 2001

Sackeim HA: Magnetic stimulation therapy and ECT. Convuls Ther 10:255–258, 1994

Sackeim HA: Memory and ECT: from polarization to reconciliation. J ECT 16:87–96, 2000

Sackeim HA, Prudic J, Devanand DP, et al: Effects of stimulus intensity and electrode placement on the efficacy and cognitive effects of electroconvulsive therapy. N Engl J Med 328:839–846, 1993

Sackeim HA, Prudic J, Devanand DP, et al: A prospective, randomized, double-blind comparison of bilateral and right unilateral electroconvulsive therapy at different stimulus intensities. Arch Gen Psychiatry 57:425–434, 2000

Sackeim HA, Keilp JG, Rush AJ, et al: The effects of vagus nerve stimulation on cognitive performance in patients with treatment-resistant depression. Neuropsychiatry Neuropsychol Behav Neurol 14:53–62, 2001a

Sackeim HA, Rush AJ, George MS, et al: Vagus nerve stimulation (VNS) for treatment-resistant depression: efficacy, side effects, and predictors of outcome. Neuropsychopharmacology 25:713–728, 2001b

Salinsky MC, Uthman BM, Ristanovic RK, et al: Vagus nerve stimulation for the treatment of medically intractable seizures: results of a 1-year open-extension trial. The Vagus Nerve Stimulation Study Group. Arch Neurol 53:1176–1180, 1996

Shajahan PM, Glabus MF, Steele JD, et al: Left dorsolateral repetitive transcranial magnetic stimulation affects cortical excitability and functional connectivity, but does not impair cognition in major depression. Prog Neuropsychopharmacol Biol Psychiatry 26:945–954 2002

Shastri A, George MS, Bohning DE: Performance of a system for interleaving transcranial magnetic stimulation with steady-state magnetic resonance imaging. Electroencephalogr Clin Neurophysiol Suppl 51:55–64, 1999

Speer AM, Kimbrell TA, Wasserman EM, et al: Opposite effects of high and low frequency rTMS on regional brain activity in depressed patients. Biol Psychiatry 48:1133–1141, 2000

Stanton PK, Sejnowsky TJ: Associative long-term depression in the hippocampus induced by hebbian covariance. Nature 339:215–218, 1989

Strafella AP, Paus T, Barrett J, et al: Repetitive transcranial magnetic stimulation of the human prefrontal cortex induces dopamine release in the caudate nucleus. J Neurosci 21:RC157, 2001

Teneback CC, Nahas Z, Speer AM, et al: Changes in prefrontal cortex and paralimbic activity in depression following two weeks of daily left prefrontal TMS. J Neuropsychiatry Clin Neurosci 11:426–435, 1999

Ter Horst GJ, Streefland C: Ascending projections of the solitary tract nucleus, in Nucleus of the Solitary Tract. Edited by Robin I, Barraco A. Boca Raton, FL, CRC Press, 1994, pp 93–103

Uthman BM, Wilder BJ, Penry JK, et al: Treatment of epilepsy by stimulation of the vagus nerve. Neurology 43:1338–1345, 1993

Vagus Nerve Stimulation Study Group: A randomized controlled trial of chronic vagus nerve stimulation for treatment of medically intractable seizures. Neurology 45:224–230, 1995

Wassermann EM: Risk and safety of repetitive transcranial magnetic stimulation (rTMS): report and suggested guidelines from the International Workshop on the Safety of Repetitive Transcranial Magnetic Stimulation, June 5–7, 1996. Electroencephalogr Clin Neurophysiol 108:1–16, 1998

Wassermann EM, Cohen LG, Flitman SS, et al: Seizures in healthy people with repeated safe trains of transcranial magnetic stimuli. Lancet 347:825–826, 1996

Wassermann EM, Wedegaertner FR, Ziemann U, et al: Crossed reduction of human motor cortex excitability by 1-Hz transcranial magnetic stimulation. Neurosci Lett 250:141–144, 1998

Weissman JD, Epstein CM, Davey KR: Magnetic brain stimulation and brain size: relevance to animal studies. Electroencephalogr Clin Neurophysiol 85:215–219, 1992

Zabara J: Peripheral control of hypersynchronous discharge in epilepsy. Electroencephalogr Clin Neurophysiol 61 (suppl):162S, 1985a

Zabara J: Time course of seizure control to brief repetitive stimuli. Epilepsia 26:518, 1985b

Zabara J: Inhibition of experimental seizures in canines by repetitive vagal stimulation. Epilepsia 33:1005–1012, 1992

Zardetto-Smith AM, Gray TS: Organization of peptidergic and catecholaminergic efferents from the nucleus of the solitary tract to the rat amygdala. Brain Res Bull 25:875, 1990

Ziemann U, Hallett M: Basic neurophysiological studies with TMS, in Transcranial Magnetic Stimulation in Neuropsychiatry. Edited by George MS, Belmaker RH. Washington, DC, American Psychiatric Press, 2000, pp 45–98

28

BRIEF PSYCHOTHERAPIES

Mantosh J. Dewan, M.D.
Brett N. Steenbarger, Ph.D.
Roger P. Greenberg, Ph.D.

Brief therapy is a generic term referring to a class of psychotherapies that seek to accelerate change through the active, focused interventions of therapists and enhanced patient involvement in treatment. In the past several decades, various brief approaches to therapy have evolved, ranging from single-session treatments and strategic interventions of several sessions to short-term psychodynamic modalities that frequently exceed 20 sessions. At the same time, a wealth of outcome studies have informed the practice of brief therapy by identifying patients and presenting concerns likely to benefit from these approaches. The overarching message from this research is that the value of short-term work is significant but also highly dependent on the characteristics of patients and their therapists.

Brief Therapy: A Short Background

Surprisingly, Freud's own cases showed that psychoanalytic therapy was frequently of brief duration. For example, in *Studies on Hysteria* (Breuer and Freud 1893–1895/1955), Freud described three of his patients as having treatments that lasted for 9 weeks (Lucie R.),

7 weeks (Emmy Von N.), and one session (Katharina)! However, he tended not to focus on treatment outcome in his writing. Instead, he emphasized that having a neutral therapist, who was not overly involved in how treatment would turn out, could lead to important discoveries about the development of psychopathology (Fisher and Greenberg 1985).

Although Freud saw short-term cases, brief therapy arguably dates back to the publication of Alexander and French's (1946) classic work *Psychoanalytic Therapy: Principles and Applications.* They were the first to formally place the therapist in the active role of promoting patient health. Change, they argued, was not primarily a function of insight, but of experience. The therapist's role was to foster "corrective emotional experiences" within the helping relationship. This reformulation took therapists out of their historic role as "blank screens" and cast them as active treatment agents who could use their relationships with patients to catalyze needed developmental experiences. Research has gone on to support the usefulness of this more active approach. Lengthy treatment interactions, associating gains primarily with the attainment of patient insights, have not turned out to be as central to change as many psychoanalysts assumed (Fisher and Greenberg 1996). With the writings of Peter Sifneos (1972), James Mann (1973), David Malan (1976), and

Habib Davanloo (1980), brevity has become an accepted part of the psychoanalytic lexicon.

The rise of behavior therapies contributed significantly to the prominence of brief work. Behavioral treatments cast the therapist in the role of teacher. No longer was therapy about self-exploration. Rather, it was intended to teach coping skills and alter learned action patterns. This permitted therapy to be highly circumscribed, emphasizing directive teaching and structured homework assignments between sessions. Behavior therapy found its first formal exposition in the writings of B. F. Skinner in the 1950s, along with the influential *Psychotherapy by Reciprocal Inhibition* (Wolpe 1958). By the 1970s, behavior therapy had become part of the therapeutic mainstream (Skinner 1974).

Albert Ellis applied the learning paradigm to cognition with rational-emotive therapy in the 1950s. This blended the psychodynamic interest in the patient's inner life with hands-on behavioral methods. The cognitive method of teaching patients to unlearn dysfunctional thought patterns and acquire new, constructive ones continued with Aaron Beck's writings in the 1960s and the influential *Cognitive Therapy and the Emotional Disorders* (A.T. Beck 1976). The combination of a tight treatment focus and structured patient involvement between sessions ensured that cognitive therapy, like its behavioral sibling, possessed core ingredients of brevity.

Yet a third type of brief therapy emerged with the writings of Jay Haley (1963, 1976), whose *Strategies of Psychotherapy* and *Problem-Solving Therapy* drew heavily on the clinical practices of Milton Erickson (Erickson and Haley 1967). Erickson viewed the presenting concerns of patients as failed efforts to solve normal life problems. These lead to cycles in which attempted solutions reinforce initial problems, much as an insomniac patient's active efforts to sleep sustain wakefulness. The role of the therapist, Erickson held, is neither as significant other (as in brief psychodynamic work) nor as cognitive-behavioral teacher. Rather, the therapist is a problem solver who interrupts and redirects these self-reinforcing cycles. This frequently could be accomplished in a matter of several sessions through the prescription of directed tasks. With the publication of Watzlawick, Weakland, and Fisch's (1974) classic work on change processes, the strategic approach became a therapeutic staple, notably in the family therapy literature.

As rising health care costs brought attempts to manage health care in the 1980s, brief therapy found an economic and a practice rationale. Budman and Gurman (1988) found that therapy could be conducted in a time-effective manner. Research suggesting that brief modalities were effective for a variety of patients and problems (Steenbarger 1992) supported the adoption of short-term work among clinicians and managed health care organizations. The movement toward evidence-based medicine spurred the development of manualized psychotherapeutic treatments, which, by their very nature, are highly structured and limited in duration (Huppert et al. 2006). With such popularity, however, also emerged concerns about the limitations of such treatments, especially for severe and persistent emotional disorders and conditions with high relapse rates (Reed and Eisman 2006). It is fair to say that by the twenty-first century, brief therapies had become the practice rule rather than the exception among psychotherapists.

Current Models of Brief Psychotherapy

The various brief therapies make different assumptions about the causes of presenting problems and the procedures necessary to alter them. These approaches cluster within three broad models: relational, learning, and contextual (Steenbarger 2002). Because of their distinctive assumptions and practice patterns, each of these models defines brevity differently. As we emphasize later in this chapter, however, many features are common to the models, several of which are central to their efficacy.

Relational Therapies

Relational modalities include short-term psychodynamic treatments and interpersonal therapy (IPT). The key assumption of these approaches is that the presenting problems of patients reflect difficulties in significant relationships. Several important differences are evident between short-term dynamic therapies and IPT, chief among them being the focus on the therapeutic relationship as a vehicle for change.

Psychodynamic Therapy

Psychodynamic brief therapies share the premise of all psychodynamic therapies that the presenting problems of patients result from an internalization of conflicts from earlier significant relationships. The anxiety from these conflicts is controlled through defenses that aid short-term coping but forestall the conscious assimilation and working through of core relational issues. As a result, these issues resurface in future relationships whenever similar anxiety and conflict are experienced, triggering old patterns of defense. These coping efforts are no longer appropriate to present-day relationship contexts, yielding secondary conflict and the consequences that typically bring people to therapy. Thus, the psychodynamic therapist views presenting problems as more than symptoms of an underlying disorder. They are the result of outmoded, currently maladaptive (defensive) efforts in the face of repeated interpersonal conflict.

Traditional psychodynamic therapy works backward from presenting complaints to underlying core conflicts. The chief therapeutic strategy in this process is interpretation, as therapists promote insight into outmoded defenses and repeated interpersonal struggles. The therapeutic relationship becomes the locus for such insight as those struggles are reenacted in the transference relationship. As patients replay their maladaptive defensive patterns and interpersonal struggles within sessions, the dynamically oriented therapist engages the real relationship—the mature alliance between the self-observing patient and the therapist—to help the patient become aware of what is happening and why. With this insight into repetitive patterns and their consequences, patients can then attempt to rework the ways in which they handle interpersonal threats within the safe confines of the helping relationship.

Because traditional psychodynamic work requires an unfolding of historical patterns within the therapeutic relationship, it cannot be an abbreviated treatment. The focus on interpretation as a chief therapeutic tool and insight as a goal—with in-session work and an exhaustive exploration of the past as the primary context for change efforts—ensures that such therapy spans months, if not years, of analysis.

Several features of short-term psychodynamic therapy enable it to accelerate this change curve:

- *Circumscribed, here-and-now focus*—Brief dynamic work focuses on "core conflictual relationship themes" (Luborsky and Mark 1991) that represent "cyclical maladaptive patterns" (Binder and Strupp 1991) linking current, past, and therapeutic relationships. Although an understanding of the role of the past in the genesis of these themes is relevant, it is not the primary focus of short-term dynamic therapy. Rather, brief dynamic work actively focuses on highly salient present-day manifestations of the cyclical patterns.
- *Patient selection criteria*—Most short-term psychodynamic practitioners acknowledge that brief treatment is not appropriate for all patients and disor-

ders. By limiting such work to patients who are experiencing emotional discomfort, able to readily form a trusting relationship, and willing to view problems in an interpersonal context, therapists help ensure that treatment will progress quickly (Levenson 2004).

- *Active provision of positive relationship experiences within the therapy*—Following Alexander and French's (1946) early formulations, brief dynamic therapists do not rely primarily on interpretation as a source of change. Rather, change is catalyzed by the involvement of the therapist in the core relationship patterns, breaking the cycles of repetition by providing responses different from those anticipated by patients (Levenson 1995). Moreover, countertransference is not viewed merely as something for the therapist to guard against but as an inevitable and potentially useful experience that allows therapists to detect and counteract the emotional pulls of their patients.
- *Creation of heightened emotional contexts for change*—The work of Sifneos (1972) and Davanloo (1980) suggests that change can be accelerated by fostering an enhanced state of experiencing among patients. Such anxiety-provoking therapies seek to challenge and break through patterns of defense and resistance rather than relying solely on interpretation. Under these emotionally charged conditions, patients can more readily gain access to memories, impulses, and feelings associated with core conflictual patterns, facilitating an accelerated working through of these experiences within therapy.

In short, brief dynamic therapists, unlike their traditional counterparts, take an active role in the helping process, fostering and sustaining a treatment focus and initiating interventions within this focus to challenge maladaptive defensive patterns and provide new, corrective relationship experiences (Table 28–1). Although such short-term work may not be brief by managed care standards, extending to 20 or more sessions, it significantly abbreviates the traditional treatment course of psychoanalytically oriented psychotherapy. The idea that an abbreviated form of psychoanalytic therapy can achieve good results for many patients has been bolstered by research observations that (even in traditional psychoanalysis) relationship factors, persuasion, suggestion, catharsis, and the therapist as a model are much more pivotal to the change process than was previously recognized (Eisenstein et al. 1994; Fisher and Greenberg 1996; Wallerstein 1986, 1989).

TABLE 28–1. Differences between short-term psychodynamic and traditional therapies

	Short-term dynamic therapies	Traditional dynamic therapies
Therapeutic focus	Focal relationship patterns	Personality change
Therapist role	Active significant other	Blank screen
Emphasized change mechanism	Corrective relationship experiences	Insight
Mechanism for dealing with resistances	Challenge and confrontation	Interpretation

Interpersonal Therapy

IPT also sustains a focus on relationship issues but abbreviates treatment even further by not making the therapeutic relationship a primary focus. Indeed, unlike short-term psychodynamic therapy, IPT began in 1984 as a brief manualized treatment that has been successfully applied to a variety of presenting problems and interpersonal concerns (Stuart and Robertson 2003).

Central to IPT and its brevity is the establishment of a treatment focus on the interpersonal life of the patient. IPT generally focuses on difficulties and changes that patients are experiencing in relationships. Much of the work of IPT emphasizes changing patterns of communication, altering expectations within relationships, and using social supports to help patients deal with interpersonal crises (Stuart 2004; Weissman et al. 2000). Because this focus stresses current relationship concerns and how these can be handled, lengthy explorations of past relationship conflicts are not a core ingredient of IPT. Similarly, the IPT therapist does not focus on transference relationships with patients and a reenactment of past interpersonal patterns. As a result, IPT tends to be briefer than most short-term psychodynamic therapies, with treatment for depression ranging from 12 to 20 sessions (Stuart 2004).

Specific targets for IPT work include grief, interpersonal disputes, role transitions, and interpersonal sensitivity. Within these areas, more specific targets for change involve patterns of communication and patterns of attachment. The therapist takes an active role in treatment, sustaining the focus on these issues. As in short-term dynamic work, IPT achieves brevity in part by limiting its application to patients who meet specific assessment criteria. In general, IPT has been found to be efficacious for patients with mood and anxiety disorders and may not be appropriate for patients with personality disorders who have difficulty forming and sustaining therapeutic alliances (Stuart 2004).

After a period of assessment and establishment of a focus through a therapeutic contract, IPT explores current interpersonal concerns and brainstorms ways of handling them (Table 28–2). These potential solutions form the basis for between-session efforts by patients, securing their active involvement in treatment. Subsequent sessions review and refine these efforts, casting the therapist in the role of collaborative problem solver. Resistances to change are dealt with in a straightforward manner by the therapist, not as pattern reenactments to be interpreted and worked through. The goal of therapy is to promote independent functioning on the part of the patient, as well as symptom relief. As Stuart and Robertson (2003) emphasized, IPT, unlike other therapies, does not presume a complete termination of therapy at the end of treatment. Rather, therapists assume that future sessions may be necessary to maintain gains and prevent relapse.

TABLE 28–2. Differences between interpersonal therapy and short-term psychodynamic therapy

	Interpersonal therapy	Short-term psychodynamic therapy
Therapeutic focus	Current patterns in interpersonal communications and attachments	Patterns repeated in past, present, and therapeutic relationships
Therapist role	Problem solver	Transference object
Emphasized change mechanism	Attempting new patterns of communication and altered expectations in extratherapeutic relationships	Corrective relationship experiences within therapy
Structure	Brief; manualized	Time-effective; open-ended

Comparison and Summary

In summary, the relational model of therapy achieves brevity by creating a circumscribed focus on the patient's interpersonal patterns and by limiting treatment to patient groups able to sustain this focus. Whereas the role of the therapist is different in short-term dynamic therapy (a significant other) compared with IPT (a collaborative problem solver), the ultimate goal is similar: altering problem patterns by generating new, constructive relational experiences.

Learning Therapies

The learning model of treatment, which includes a wide range of cognitive-behavioral therapies, starts from a different set of premises from those in the relational model. The presenting concerns of patients are viewed as learned maladaptive patterns that can be unlearned. Moreover, patients are seen as capable of acquiring new, adaptive patterns of thought and action through skill development. As a result, the learning therapies feature the therapist in an active, directive teaching mode and the patient as a student. This structuring of the helping relationship lends itself to active skill rehearsal within sessions and directed homework between meetings. The combination of tight learning focus and active practice of techniques ensures that most learning therapies are short term by their very nature.

For purposes of exposition, it is helpful to distinguish between primarily *behavioral treatments* that emphasize exposure as a central therapeutic ingredient and *cognitive approaches* that more broadly target dysfunctional patterns of information processing for restructuring. Although these approaches have elements that overlap (e.g., patients exposed to traumatic cues may rehearse thoughts that emphasize self-control), the relative degree of emphasis is different, which affects the conduct and brevity of treatment.

Behavior Therapy

Learning therapies that use *exposure* as a core therapeutic ingredient include the work of Edna Foa and colleagues (Hembree et al. 2004) in the treatment of posttraumatic stress disorder and obsessive-compulsive disorder and David Barlow's (2002) work on panic disorder. Treatment typically begins with a period of assessment and psychosocial education. During this time, patients may keep detailed logs that track the appearance of symptoms and the circumstances surrounding these. Examination of these logs during the early sessions helps to generate a focus on the specific triggers for symptom appearance. Concurrently, therapists educate patients about the learning model, explaining how and why symptoms appear. This can be highly reassuring for patients with disorders such as panic, who may be bewildered by their symptoms.

Also early in treatment, exposure-based learning therapies introduce specific skills designed to help control symptoms. These can include efforts at relaxation, thought stopping, self-reassurance, and seeking social support. The skills are typically introduced one at a time, explained in detail as part of the aforementioned psychosocial education, modeled in session by the therapist, and rehearsed in session by patients. Only after patients understand and master skills in session do they rehearse the skills as part of between-session homework.

An important component of the brevity of these therapies stems from the subsequent employment of these skills. Once triggers for presenting symptoms have been identified, they are deliberately introduced into therapy sessions via imagery and in vivo exercises. Patients are thus required to actively use their coping skills while they are exposed to the very stimuli that have provoked symptoms. For example, a patient with a hand-washing compulsion might be exposed to dirt and then prevented from washing his hands (i.e., response prevention). A patient experiencing panic might simulate panic experiences by spinning in a chair and then using cognitive and relaxation skills to maintain composure. This in vivo exposure provides patients with firsthand emotional experiences of mastery, which appear to accelerate the pace of symptom resolution. Once initial gains are achieved, efforts at generalization commence, and the skills are used across a variety of symptom-related cues (Table 28–3). Variations in technique—and the specific needs of patients—dictate whether the exposure is attempted in a gradual way or in a more rapid, intensive fashion. Interestingly, research suggests that a significant immersion into anxiety-arousing situations often may be therapeutic because patients benefit from extended sessions of exposure (Hembree et al. 2004). As Shapiro's (2001) work suggests, exposure appears to be effective because of the opportunity it affords patients to reprocess cues associated with distress.

Cognitive Therapy

Whereas the exposure therapies have found their greatest application in the treatment of anxiety disorders, *cognitive reprocessing therapies* have been applied to depression, anxiety, eating disorders, and child and adolescent disorders (Hollon and Beck 2004). Symptoms, according to this approach, can be traced to

TABLE 28–3. Comparison of learning and relational models of brief therapy

	Learning models	Relational models
View of presenting problems	Learned maladaptive patterns of behavior and thought	Internalized relationship conflicts and patterns
Goal of therapy	Unlearning old dysfunctional patterns; acquiring new constructive ones	Novel interpersonal experiences that can be internalized
Therapist role	Directive teacher	Facilitator of exploration
Emphasized change mechanism	Rehearsal of skills and experiences of mastery during problematic situations	Changing interpersonal patterns in current relationships
Structure	Brief, often manualized or highly structured	Sometimes brief and manualized (interpersonal therapy); sometimes not (short-term dynamic)

automatic thought patterns that distort information processing about self, others, and the future. The goal of therapy is to identify these thought patterns, challenge them, and replace them with more constructive alternatives (J.S. Beck 1995). The combination of in-session rehearsal and out-of-session homework targeting core patterns of automatic thought ensures that the cognitive work is time efficient.

Like the exposure-based learning therapies, cognitive restructuring treatments begin with a period of assessment and psychosocial education. The education in the cognitive model helps patients understand the relation between thoughts and feelings and the ways in which automatic thought patterns can sustain unwanted patterns of emotion and action. Throughout cognitive therapy, therapists engage patients in a highly collaborative manner, minimizing resistances and sustaining the helping alliance.

This collaboration continues with the maintenance of a dysfunctional thought record in which patients track events, reactions to those events, and mediating beliefs. Most of these beliefs pertain to the sense of being helpless or unlovable (J.S. Beck and Bieling 2004); patients then form schemas that filter and color future perception, which creates cognitive distortions. The dysfunctional thought record enables therapists to create cognitive conceptualizations of patients, linking core beliefs to automatic thoughts, emotions, and behaviors. The record also helps patients observe their distortions as they are occurring and realize their role in maintaining presenting symptoms. From the observations of patients and therapists, a focus for intervention emerges that targets specific cognitive distortions.

Central to the cognitive restructuring therapies is a Socratic process of guided discovery between thera-

pist and patient that questions these distortions and encourages a consideration of alternative explanations (J.S. Beck and Bieling 2004). This process also occurs between sessions because therapists encourage patients to use thought records to evaluate their own degree of belief in the distortions. Each dysfunctional thought pattern is viewed by therapist and patient as a hypothesis to be questioned and tested. Behavioral experiments devised during sessions are carried out between meetings to provide direct experiential tests of patient assumptions. The goal of this "collaborative empiricism" (J.S. Beck 1995) is to create vivid experiences of disconfirmation for patients, which aid the building of new, accurate schemas (Table 28–4).

Comparison and Summary

Whereas the exposure therapies target specific conditioned responses for extinction, the cognitive restructuring therapies entail a comprehensive collaborative relationship between therapists and patients that evaluates and restructures a range of cognitive patterns. For this reason, as well as the differences between the therapies in the range of problems that they typically address, the exposure treatments tend to be briefer than the restructuring therapies, with the former frequently lasting fewer than 10 sessions and the latter typically ranging between 10 and 20 visits. Despite the differences in their specific methods, many similarities link these learning therapies. They are highly structured and focused, with active assignments during and between sessions. They seek to challenge directly and undercut the patterns that bring patients to therapy, achieving brevity by replacing verbal exploration with experiences of mastery.

TABLE 28–4. **Differences between exposure and cognitive restructuring brief therapies**

	Exposure therapies	Cognitive restructuring therapies
View of presenting problems	Conditioned patterns of emotion and behavior triggered by internal and environmental cues	The result of information processing distortions arising from dysfunctional schemas
Goal of therapy	Deconditioning of patterns through skill enactment during exposure to symptom triggers	Challenging and replacing cognitive distortions with realistic, constructive alternatives
Therapist role	Directive teacher	Collaborative empiricist
Emphasized change mechanism	Firsthand experiences of mastery	Altered cognitive schemas
Structure	Brief, with circumscribed symptom focus; often manualized or highly structured	More extended, with broader focus; often manualized or highly structured

Contextual Therapies

The aforementioned relational and learning therapies begin with a common premise—that the presenting concerns of patients are acquired over the life span as the result of problematic experience: faulty relationships or faulty learning. Both, in that sense, place the locus of problems within the patient. Contextual brief therapies, on the other hand, do not view problems as intrinsic to patients. Rather, they are seen as artifacts of person–situation interactions, which, once identified, can be rapidly modified. Short-term couples therapies, for instance, view problem patterns as sustained by the reciprocal contributions of each partner (Baucom et al. 2004). Because difficulties are seen as situational, targeted problem-solving interventions to alter these situations make the contextual therapies among the briefest of therapies.

Strategic Therapy

Strategic therapies, including single-session treatments (Hoyt et al. 1992), view presenting concerns as the result of attempts at solutions that unwittingly reinforce the very problems patients are attempting to address (Rosenbaum 1990). A person concerned about rejection in relationships, for instance, might interact in guarded ways, leading others to avoid future interaction. The problem, from the vantage point of the strategic therapist, is a function of the patient's construal of the situation. It can be resolved through skillful reframing that opens the door to new action alternatives (Fisch et al. 1982) and the creation of directed tasks (Levy and Shelton 1990) that disconfirm existing understandings. The goal of treatment is to catalyze initial change that patients can then sustain on their own, not to effect fundamental changes of personality. For this reason, strategic therapies are intentionally brief.

The initial interview of strategic therapy is designed to identify current complaints of patients and their attempts at resolution. The therapist's conceptualization is neither a diagnosis nor a formulation of personality, but a description of the current situational factors that help to maintain the patient's presenting concerns. This description includes the people involved in the patient's concerns and the roles they take, the patient's view of the situation, the sequence of behaviors that result in the patient's complaints, and the specific contexts in which these complaints arise (Rosenbaum 1990). From this conceptualization, therapists gain an appreciation of the ways in which patients feel stuck in their attempts at resolution and can begin to generate ways of becoming unstuck.

As Rosenbaum (1990) emphasized, the goal of the therapy is not to find a solution for a patient's problem but to create a situation that lends itself to spontaneous goal attainment. Many times, fresh construals and solutions will result simply when patients behave in new and unpredictable ways. The patient who is afraid of social interaction, for instance, will not interact with others if rejection is anticipated. That same patient, however, may view himself to be a kind, sensitive person and will initiate interactions to help others. Such interactions offer the possibility of positive feedback and fresh incentives to seek out further social contact. By changing the patient's context—from being stuck in a pattern to enacting a strength—the therapist allows naturally occurring growth processes to take their own course. In that sense, strategic therapy is a process for removing barriers to change and not a self-contained change process in itself (Table 28–5).

TABLE 28–5. Contextual models of brief therapy

- Presenting complaints are the result of self-reinforcing problem–solution cycles.

- Problems are a function of patients and their context, not internal to patients.

- Goal of therapy is initiating change, not seeing it to completion.

- Role of therapist is to structure experiences that undermine the stuck behavior of patients.

- Therapy is highly abbreviated.

Solution-Focused Therapy

An offshoot of strategic therapy, solution-focused brief therapy (SFBT), provides a somewhat different contextual approach to short-term change. Solution-focused brief therapists start from the premise that people are changing all the time, enacting solution patterns as well as problem ones. Indeed, there is an important sense in SFBT in which problems do not exist at all. When patients cannot reach their goals, they at some point identify that they have a problem. This reification becomes self-fulfilling: the more patients focus on their problems, the more troubled they feel and act. Equally important, such a problem focus blinds patients to the occasions in which they do, in fact, reach their goals.

The aim of SFBT is to break this self-fulfilling conceptualization. The therapist accomplishes this by focusing on solution patterns rather than on problems. Thus, the initial assessment in SFBT asks patients to identify positive presession changes and occasions during which problems either do not occur or occur less often or less intensely (Walter and Peller 1992). Enacting these exceptions to problem patterns—doing more of what is already working (de Shazer 1988; O'Hanlon and Weiner-Davis 1989)—is the focus of therapy, not an analysis of core conflicts or a teaching of skills to remediate deficits. Because the therapy is not initiating new behavior and thought patterns but instead is building on existing ones, it tends to be highly targeted, lasting several sessions on average (Steenbarger 2004).

Several other factors contribute to the brevity of SFBT, including working within patient goals to minimize resistance; maintaining a tight solution focus; involving patients in between-session efforts to enact solution patterns; and having a high degree of therapist activity (Steenbarger 2004). The emphasis on patient strength undercuts the cycle of problem-based thinking and stuck emotion and behavior. The focus on constructive change also paves the way for therapists and patients to frame goals in positive, action terms that can be supported by directed homework tasks extending the solution patterns. Such goals can be formulated with minimal historical exploration, which further contributes to brevity.

Comparison and Summary

One way SFBT differs from strategic brief therapies is that SFBT lends itself to manualization. SFBT manuals (de Shazer 1988; Walter and Peller 1992) view therapy as a series of steps involving the identification of presession change, the formulation of solution-based goals, the use of the miracle question and scaling questions to elicit exceptions to patient complaints, the provision of feedback to support change, and the assignment of tasks to extend solution patterns (Table 28–6). Like strategic therapies, SFBT relies less on verbal exploration and more on direct experience to break circular patterns that interfere with the achievement of patient goals. The goal of both therapies is not so much to resolve a problem as it is to help patients see that what they thought was a problem was in fact a function of their punctuation of experience, their ways of construing themselves and the world.

Differences and Similarities Among the Brief Therapies

The foregoing discussion has focused on describing the major schools of brief therapy and highlighted the differences among these models. Therapists approaching patients from relational, learning, and contextual vantage points differ in their conceptualization of presenting problems and the procedures necessary to address these. These therapeutic modalities differ in other ways as well:

- *Scope*—Some of the brief therapies define a relatively wide set of goals; others are much more targeted. Short-term dynamic therapies, for instance, tackle broader relationship goals than does IPT; exposure therapies and the contextual variants are more tightly focused than are cognitive restructuring therapies. As might be expected, the treatments that are most narrowly gauged tend to be the briefest; the most ambitious therapies tend to be of longer duration.
- *Degree of structure*—A subset of the brief therapies, including short-term dynamic therapy and strategic therapy, stress in-session experience as central to change. These therapies tend to feature deft use of

TABLE 28–6. Differences between strategic and solution-focused brief therapies

	Strategic therapies	Solution-focused therapies
View of presenting problems	Attempted solutions to problems further reinforce those problems	De-emphasis of problems and emphasis on exceptions to problem patterns
Goal of therapy	Interruption of problem cycles and attempts to initiate new action patterns	Creating solution patterns out of exceptions to problem patterns
Therapist role	Facilitator of change through structured tasks and experiences	Facilitator of change through construction of solution patterns
Emphasized change mechanism	Reframing of problems and direct experiences of novel action patterns	Undermining of problem focus through enactment of solutions
Structure	Highly abbreviated, but not highly structured	Highly abbreviated; often manualized or highly structured

the helping relationship and are difficult to capture in therapy manuals. Other short-term treatments, such as exposure work, cognitive restructuring therapy, and SFBT, rely heavily on between-session tasks as change elements. These tasks are relatively easy to standardize and codify in manuals.

- *Use of time in treatment*—A few of the brief treatments, such as IPT and the contextual therapies, are very explicitly brief and are frequently conducted in a time-limited mode, setting limits on the number of sessions at the outset. Other brief therapies, such as short-term psychodynamic work and cognitive restructuring, are time effective (Budman and Gurman 1988) but do not typically set upward bounds on the number of available sessions.
- *Nature of therapist activity*—Exposure therapy and the contextual therapies make extensive use of assigned tasks, placing the therapist in a directive role. The relational therapies feature a relative emphasis on exploration between therapist and patient, with less use of structured homework assignments.

Because of the foregoing differences, we can conceptualize the brief therapies along a continuum, ranging from highly abbreviated and highly structured contextual therapies to more exploratory relational treatments. The briefest treatments emphasize that the patient's presenting complaints are artifacts of self-construal and can be addressed in the here and now through experiences that undermine those construals. These highly abbreviated therapies view patients as capable of growth and change and seek only to catalyze these naturally occurring processes. The more extended short-term therapies place presenting problems into a historical context and stress insight and

corrective emotional experiences in a developed relationship as essential to change. Patients are viewed as caught in maladaptive relational patterns that are replayed across a variety of situations and, hence, need more than a change catalyst. Between these extremes, the learning therapies emphasize here-and-now unlearning of overlearned dysfunctional patterns and the acquisition of constructive alternatives through structured learning experiences (Figure 28–1).

Despite these evident differences, many underlying similarities among the brief therapies help to account for their brevity. It is not surprising that the brief therapies embody common ingredients (Greenberg 2004); a wealth of research (Lambert and Ogles 2004; Wampold 2001) has found that factors shared by the various psychotherapies account for a significant proportion of the variance in patient change. A list of common factors across all psychotherapy models (both brief and longer term) typically would include the creation of a strong therapist–patient alliance, opportunities to confront and face problems, the development of patient mastery experiences, and the facilitation of patient hope and positive expectations about the future. Specific ingredients found across the short-term treatments include the following:

- *Brevity by design*—As Budman and Gurman (1988) first noted, brief therapies are brief by design, not by default. Time is an integral part of the treatment plan, regardless of whether the therapies are explicitly time limited or simply efficient in their use of time. Increasingly, this brevity by design is accomplished through the creation and use of treatment manuals that standardize helping approaches.
- *Creation and maintenance of a therapeutic focus*— Some of the short-term modalities are briefer than

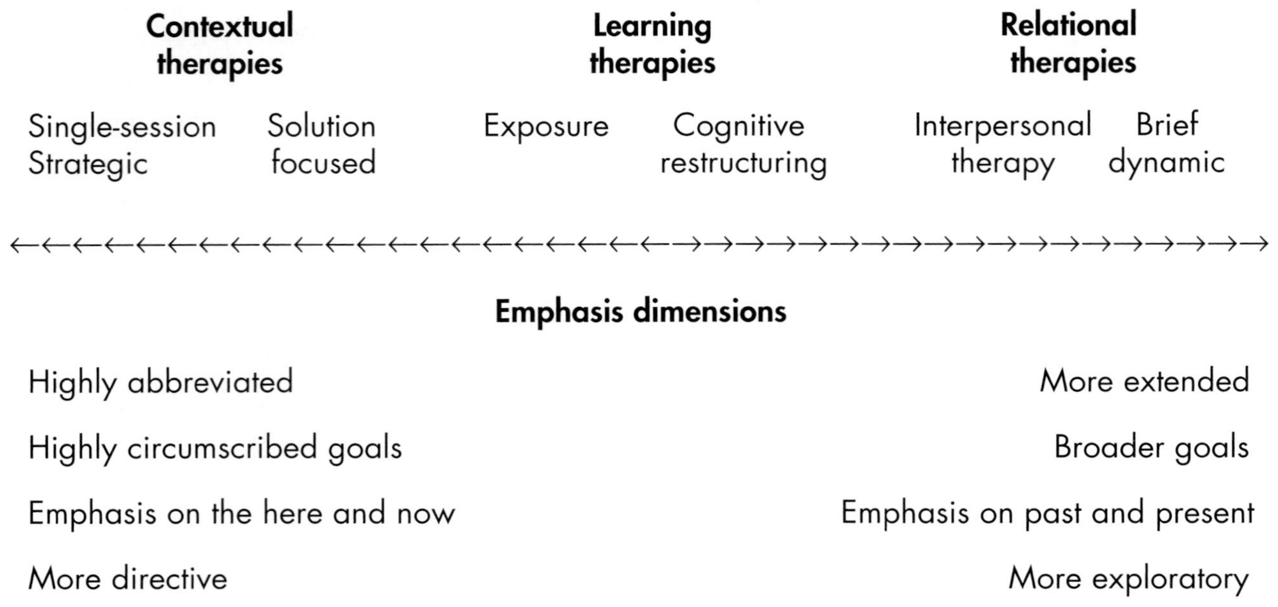

Contextual therapies		Learning therapies		Relational therapies	
Single-session Strategic	Solution focused	Exposure	Cognitive restructuring	Interpersonal therapy	Brief dynamic

←←←←←←←←←←←←←←←←←←←←←←←←←→→→→→→→→→→→→→→→→→→→→→→→

Emphasis dimensions

Highly abbreviated	More extended
Highly circumscribed goals	Broader goals
Emphasis on the here and now	Emphasis on past and present
More directive	More exploratory

FIGURE 28–1. Differences among brief therapy models.

others, but all of them target focal patient patterns rather than attempt broader personality reconstruction. A major role of the therapist is to maintain this focus from session to session by guiding discussion and facilitating between-session efforts.

- *Selectivity*—To achieve brevity, therapists need to establish a rapid rapport with patients, which means that they must work with patients capable of forming a quick alliance. Most brief therapies incorporate inclusion and exclusion criteria because patients with chronic and severe problem patterns frequently need more ongoing support than can be provided in short-term treatment.
- *Avoidance of resistance*—Many of the brief therapies include procedures designed to elicit the understanding and cooperation of patients, such as explicit efforts at education, the use of the patient's own language in framing goals, and the collaborative formulation of treatment goals. They aim to minimize resistance to change and sustain favorable expectations for outcome.
- *Activity*—Across the brief therapies, therapists take responsibility for initiating change efforts by providing new relationship experiences, teaching skills, and fostering contexts for new patterns of behavior. Patients in brief therapy are expected to explore problem patterns but also to tackle these actively through in-session experiences and between-session tasks and homework.

- *Enhanced patient experiencing*—The brief therapies emphasize the provision of new experiences, in and out of session, as facilitators of change. They supplement verbal explorations of presenting concerns with emotionally charged interventions.

Steenbarger (2002) suggested that the brief therapies have structural similarities, characterized by a series of change stages (Table 28–7). Treatment begins with a period of engagement, in which patient and therapist forge a working alliance that engages the patient's desire for change and mutually creates targets for change efforts. Central to the formation of this alliance is a translation of patients' presenting complaints into the language of a particular therapeutic approach, enabling patients to perceive their problems in a new light and fashion fresh possibilities for change. Therapy then draws on the procedures of the particular approach to create discrepant experiences that challenge old patterns of thought and behavior, facilitating new understandings and action patterns. The final phase of therapy seeks to consolidate these new understandings and skills by generalizing them to a variety of situations, thus cementing an internalization of new patterns and helping to prevent relapse. The brief therapies, from this vantage point, may be viewed as devices for generating novel experiences in the context of enhanced experiencing (Steenbarger 2006), accelerating learning processes that occur in all psychotherapies.

TABLE 28–7.	Structural elements common to the brief therapies

Engagement

Rapid formation of a therapeutic alliance and translation of presenting problems into focal goals

Discrepancy

Provision of novel skills, insights, and experiences that challenge patient patterns and facilitate new understandings and actions

Consolidation

Rehearsal of new patterns in varied contexts, accompanied by feedback, to ensure internalization and relapse prevention

Research Pertaining to Brief Therapy and Its Effectiveness

An impressive body of research documents the effectiveness of psychotherapy across a variety of presenting problems (Roth and Fonagy 2006). This is relevant to brief therapy because most treatments that have been tested for efficacy—including the manualized therapies commonly used in controlled, double-blind outcome studies—are short term. Indeed, it would not be an exaggeration to say that most of the studies on psychotherapy outcomes are investigations of the effectiveness of short-term therapies. This is partly because cognitive and behavioral therapies dominate the outcome literature (Roth and Fonagy 2006), although a sizable body of studies does support the effectiveness of short-term dynamic therapy, IPT, and SFBT (Dewan et al. 2004).

Research on Time and Outcome in Psychotherapy

A review of duration and outcome in therapy (Steenbarger 1994) observes that this relation is complicated by several factors:

- *The patient population*—If we plotted change in psychotherapy as a function of time, the curve would look different for patients with personality disorders and chronic, severe presenting problems than for those with more recent and less severe Axis I concerns (Howard et al. 1986; Lambert and Ogles

2004). In general, outcomes are more slowly achieved among patients with significant psychiatric disorders than among less impaired individuals (Lambert and Ogles 2004).

- *The outcome measures used*—Measures of patient well-being and symptom relief typically show change before measures of functional improvement do (Steenbarger 1994); as Lambert and Ogles (2004) observed in their review, the dosage of therapy needed to reach a level of success depends on the success criterion chosen. It is quite possible that brief therapies differ in their time–outcome curves simply as a function of selecting different targets for change. The relational therapies, in particular, tend to focus on functional change as a criterion of improvement, whereas behavioral therapies are more likely to emphasize symptom change.

- *The time at which change is measured*—The goal of psychotherapy, brief and otherwise, is to foster lasting change, not just improvement from the beginning of treatment to the end. The duration–outcome equation looks far more favorable for all therapies when outcomes are measured at termination than at longer-term follow-up periods. This is particularly the case for disorders that have high known rates of relapse, such as major depressive disorder and substance use disorders (Roth and Fonagy 2006). Although several studies support the long-term effectiveness of IPT and cognitive-behavioral therapies (Lambert and Ogles 2004), data also suggest that highly abbreviated treatments may run an enhanced risk of patient relapse (Steenbarger 1994) and that ongoing maintenance sessions can be effective in reducing relapse rates (Lambert and Ogles 2004) and improving long-term outcome.

Early investigations of the dose–effect relation in psychotherapy found that approximately 50% of patients have significant improvement within 8 sessions of therapy; 75% reach such improvement within 26 sessions (Howard et al. 1986). This curvilinear relation suggests that much of therapy's effect occurs in a brief period for a large proportion of patients. It also indicates that some patients benefit from more extended treatment. Lambert and Ogles (2004), in a comprehensive review, reported that the dose–effect curve is more modestly sloped than those early findings suggested. Specifically, 50% of the patients who begin treatment at lower levels of psychological functioning reach clinically significant levels of improvement within 21 sessions. This same improvement is reached within 7 sessions among patients who begin treatment at higher levels of psychological functioning when more modest symptom change criteria are used. No single dose–effect curve describes the relation between time and change across all patients. It is safe to say, however, that if the goal of treatment is sustained functional change, most individuals meeting DSM diagnostic criteria will require more time for change than is typically afforded by the briefest treatment models.

Patient Selection Criteria

These findings highlight the importance of patient selection in the conduct of brief therapy. The dose–effect research suggests some of the following inclusion criteria:

- *Duration of presenting problems*—Chronic emotional and behavioral patterns are likely to have been overlearned and thus are more likely to require ongoing intervention than are problems of more recent origin (Steenbarger 2002).
- *Interpersonal functioning*—Given the importance of the therapeutic alliance to change across all psychotherapies (Lambert and Barley 2002), it is unlikely that patients with poor interpersonal functioning and difficulties sustaining relationships will benefit from brief intervention. Indeed, they may need many sessions before they can even forge a trusting relationship.
- *Severity of presenting problems*—As noted earlier, most patients with severe presenting concerns do not achieve clinically significant outcomes in a brief time frame. This is particularly the case when the severity of presenting symptoms prevents patients from actively engaging in within-session and between-session change efforts. When presenting problems are not overwhelming, patients are more likely to be able to tolerate the added discomfort of change efforts.
- *Complexity of presenting problems*—Some problems brought to therapy, such as phobias, are relatively simple, manifesting themselves in limited ways in limited situations. Other problems, such as eating disorders, are highly complex, with manifestations cutting across mood, interpersonal functioning, and self-concept. A perusal of the outcome literature (Roth and Fonagy 2006) suggests that therapeutic outcomes are more favorable for less complex concerns, probably because targets for treatment can be more narrowly circumscribed. Many complex concerns, such as eating and substance use disorders, have high relapse rates that, in themselves, might require ongoing maintenance therapy and other extensions of treatment duration.

- *Understanding of the need for change*—Prochaska and Norcross (2002) found that the course of therapy is different for patients who have a clear understanding and acceptance of their problems and the need for change than for patients who lack such understanding. Patients in an action phase of readiness for change are much more likely to embrace the change techniques of brief treatment than are patients in precontemplative or contemplative modes. These latter groups, in fact, may require numerous sessions of problem exploration before they even acknowledge a need for change, and then targeted goals for treatment can be formulated.
- *Social supports*—When patients have weak or nonexistent social supports, they may look to therapy for support as well as for targeted change. In those cases, they are unlikely to embrace time limits on treatment. Brief therapy is most likely to proceed smoothly and without resistance if it is conducted with patients whose goals include rapid and targeted change.

The foregoing criteria, which form the acronym *DISCUS* (Table 28–8), can be useful during initial interviews in determining the likelihood that treatment changes will be achieved briefly. This can be useful in settings such as community mental health centers, managed health care plans, and college and university counseling centers, which must rationally allocate scarce treatment resources to the treatment needs of a population. The criteria also suggest that firm, brief time limits on treatment for all patients are likely to prove ineffective for a significant proportion of the population. Patients with chronic, severe, and complex presenting concerns are much more likely to require extended intervention than are patients with recent, nonsevere, and simple presentations. Similarly, brief treatments are likely to be most relevant to patients with a high readiness for change and problems with low rates of relapse.

Nevertheless, brief therapy techniques may still prove useful in the conduct of ongoing psychotherapy. Cummings and Sayama (1995) made a compelling case for intermittent brief therapy throughout the life cycle, so that the benefits of focused change are blended with the benefits of longer-term assistance. Marsha Linehan's dialectical behavior therapy (DBT; Linehan 1993), which uses sequential short-term behavioral interventions in the treatment of personality disorders, illustrates one way in which brevity may be compatible with longer-term assistance. Roth and Fonagy (2006) reported that DBT has been more effective in reducing

TABLE 28–8. Patient selection criteria predictive of success in brief therapy (DISCUS)

- Duration of presenting problems: brief
- Interpersonal functioning: good, able to quickly form a trusting relationship
- Severity of presenting problems: mild to moderate
- Complexity of presenting problems: limited, circumscribed, with low relapse potential
- Understanding of the need for change: and ready to take action
- Social supports: strong and easily accessible

the impulsive behaviors associated with borderline personality disorder than in changing facets such as interpersonal functioning. More research is needed to determine the promise and limits of sequential short-term interventions in the treatment of pervasive psychiatric disorders, particularly in light of findings that outcomes for many disorders are enhanced by the combination of brief therapies with psychopharmacological intervention (Thase and Jindal 2004).

What Works in Brief Therapy?

As mentioned earlier, a large body of research suggests that the ingredients common to the psychotherapies are more important than their specific interventions in generating clinical outcomes (Asay and Lambert 1999; Greenberg 2004; Wampold 2001). These common effective ingredients include the quality of the therapeutic relationship (Lambert and Barley 2002); patient expectations, readiness for change, and capacity for attachment (Clarkin and Levy 2004; Greenberg et al. 2006); and therapist ability to engage patients in a constructive manner (Beutler et al. 2004). A vexing finding in the psychotherapy literature is that researchers who champion specific treatment approaches consistently report more favorable results from their approaches than do researchers who do not champion specific approaches (Wampold 2001). This allegiance effect likely speaks to the role of the therapist's, as well as the patient's, expectations in generating outcomes. Indeed, when outcome studies have sought to eliminate allegiance as an outcome factor and limit outcome variance to specific treatment effects by requiring strict adherence to therapy manuals, the benefits of psychotherapy were greatly reduced or eliminated (Wampold 2001).

Given these findings, the brief therapies likely achieve their results by 1) intensifying the change ingredients found among all therapies, including longer-term ones (Steenbarger 2002), and 2) limiting application of short-term methods to patient populations most likely to benefit from psychosocial interventions. Lambert and Archer (2006) reported that patients who benefited from the initial sessions of therapy were most likely to have favorable outcomes by the end of treatment and at follow-up periods. This is significant because it suggests that the course and outcome are determined before most of the procedures that distinguish the various therapeutic schools have been initiated.

Among the brief therapies, therapists' skill factors—their ability to facilitate and sustain a treatment focus and their ability to provide novel experiences for patients—may be more important than the specific methods they use. Lambert and Archer (2006) observed that therapists who are given feedback about the progress of their poor-prognosis patients early in treatment have more favorable outcomes than do therapists who are not given feedback. This points to skill factors among therapists as potential mediators of outcome. A detailed analysis by Wampold (2001) indicated that therapist competence accounts for greater treatment variance than do specific treatments themselves. Indeed, when outcome studies assigned therapists to multiple treatments, competent therapists tended to have significantly better outcomes than did less competent ones, regardless of the treatment modality.

Finally, all this research suggests that the factors that make therapy efficient are not entirely separable from those that make therapy effective. It may not be far wrong to assert that therapy is most likely to be brief when it is performed skillfully with patients most open to, and likely to benefit from, psychosocial intervention. The skills that make for successful treatment—the ability to foster novel experiences of self and others in an emotionally charged context via the medium of a supportive alliance—appear to be equally essential to brevity.

Conclusion

Seeking to make psychotherapy treatment more efficient, innovative psychoanalysts originally presented the key components of brief therapy. They stressed narrowed patient inclusion criteria, narrowed treatment focus, an active therapist, a limit on time and/or number of sessions, and facilitation of corrective emotional experiences. Building on dynamic tradition, behaviorists, cognitive therapists, and strategic therapists went on to develop three broad models of brief therapy based on their understanding about the causes of presenting problems and the techniques necessary to alter them. *Relational therapies,* which assume that presenting symptoms are a result of problems with significant relationships, include brief psychodynamic therapies and interpersonal therapy. *Learning therapies,* such as behavior therapies and cognitive therapy, view symptoms as arising from maladaptive learned behavior patterns that can be unlearned. *Contextual therapies* place the emphasis on ways in which presenting problems are situated within—and sustained by—their psychosocial contexts. Strategic therapies and solution-focused therapy are major models of contextual therapy.

Brief therapies vary from single-session approaches and very brief strategic treatments to dynamic interventions that often exceed 20 sessions. Behavioral and cognitive therapies are of intermediate duration. Manuals developed by several treatment schools have made it easier to practice these techniques with fidelity and to conduct research. Indeed, most psychotherapy research is focused on brief therapy and clearly supports the efficacy of brief therapy approaches for a broad range of patients. As a result of the growth of brief therapy models, manuals, and research evidence, in association with fiscal constraints and demonstrated positive patient outcomes, brief therapy has become the norm for the majority of today's patients.

Key Points

- Brief therapy consists of a group of approaches to psychotherapy that include short-term psychodynamic, interpersonal, behavioral, cognitive, strategic, and solution-focused modalities.

- The various brief therapies differ in their average treatment duration, their targets for change, and their assumptions regarding change processes.

- Several common ingredients link the brief therapies, including a circumscribed treatment focus, increased therapist and patient activity, an emphasis on generating novel experiences, and patient inclusion criteria.

- Brief therapies overall are effective but are most likely to benefit patients who are ready for change and who present concerns that are recent, nonsevere, and simple, not patients with severe, chronic disorders.

- Although a sizable proportion of patients can benefit from short-term treatment, the relation between time and change is complex, mediated by the nature of the outcomes measured, the time at which progress is assessed, and the degree of patient impairment.

- Brief therapies appear to be effective to the degree that they intensify the common factors that account for change across all therapies.

Suggested Readings

Barlow DH: Clinical Handbook of Psychological Disorders, 3rd Edition. New York, Guilford, 2001

Beck JS: Cognitive Therapy: Basics and Beyond. New York, Guilford, 1995

Dewan MJ, Steenbarger BN, Greenberg RP: The Art and Science of Brief Psychotherapies: A Practitioner's Guide. Washington, DC, American Psychiatric Publishing, 2004

Levenson H: Time-Limited Dynamic Psychotherapy: A Guide to Clinical Practice. New York, Basic Books, 1995

Stuart S, Robertson M: Interpersonal Psychotherapy: A Clinician's Guide. London, Edward Arnold, 2003

Walter JL, Peller JE: Becoming Solution-Focused in Brief Therapy. New York, Brunner/Mazel, 1992

Online Resources

Academy of Cognitive Therapy: www.academyofct.org

Association of Advancement of Behavior Therapy (AABT)/Association for Behavioral and Cognitive Therapies (ABCT): www.aabt.org

International Society for Interpersonal Psychotherapy: www.interpersonalpsychotherapy.org

Society for Psychotherapy Research: www.psychotherapy-research.org

Solution Focused Brief Therapy Association: www.sfbta.org

References

Alexander F, French TM: Psychoanalytic Therapy: Principles and Applications. New York, Ronald Press, 1946

Asay TP, Lambert MJ: The empirical case for the common factors in therapy: quantitative findings, in The Heart and Soul of Change: What Works in Therapy. Edited by Hubble MA, Duncan BL, Miller SD. Washington, DC, American Psychological Association, 1999, pp 33–56

Barlow D: Anxiety and Its Disorders: The Nature and Treatment of Anxiety and Panic, 2nd Edition. New York, Guilford, 2002

Baucom DH, Epstein NB, Sullivan LJ: Brief couple therapy, in The Art and Science of Brief Psychotherapies: A Practitioner's Guide. Edited by Dewan MJ, Steenbarger BN, Greenberg RP. Washington, DC, American Psychiatric Publishing, 2004, pp 189–230

Beck AT: Cognitive Therapy and the Emotional Disorders. New York, International Universities Press, 1976

Beck JS: Cognitive Therapy: Basics and Beyond. New York, Guilford, 1995

Beck JS, Bieling PJ: Cognitive therapy: introduction to theory and practice, in The Art and Science of Brief Psychotherapies: A Practitioner's Guide. Edited by Dewan MJ, Steenbarger BN, Greenberg RP. Washington, DC, American Psychiatric Publishing, 2004, pp 15–50

Beutler LE, Malik M, Alimohamed S, et al: Therapist variables, in Bergin and Garfield's Handbook of Psychotherapy and Behavior Change, 5th Edition. Edited by Lambert MJ. New York, Wiley, 2004, pp 227–306

Binder JL, Strupp HH: The Vanderbilt approach to time-limited dynamic psychotherapy, in Handbook of Short-Term Dynamic Psychotherapy. Edited by Crits-Christoph P, Barber JP. New York, Basic Books, 1991, pp 137–165

Breuer J, Freud S: Studies in hysteria (1893–1895), in The Standard Edition of the Complete Psychological Works of Sigmund Freud, Vol 2. Translated and edited by Strachey J (in collaboration with Freud A). London, Hogarth Press, 1955, pp 1–311

Budman SH, Gurman AS: Theory and Practice of Brief Therapy. New York, Guilford, 1988

Clarkin JF, Levy KN: The influence of client variables on psychotherapy, in Bergin and Garfield's Handbook of Psychotherapy and Behavior Change, 5th Edition. Edited by Lambert MJ. New York, Wiley, 2004, pp 194–226

Cummings N, Sayama M: Focused Psychotherapy: A Casebook of Brief, Intermittent Psychotherapy Throughout the Life Cycle. New York, Brunner/Mazel, 1995

Davanloo H: Short-Term Dynamic Psychotherapy. New York, Jason Aronson, 1980

de Shazer S: Clues: Investigating Solutions in Brief Therapy. New York, WW Norton, 1988

Dewan MJ, Steenbarger BN, Greenberg RP (eds): The Art and Science of Brief Psychotherapies: A Practitioner's Guide. Washington, DC, American Psychiatric Publishing, 2004

Eisenstein S, Levy NA, Marmor J: The Dyadic Transaction: An Investigation Into the Nature of the Psycho-therapeutic Process. New Brunswick, NJ, Transaction, 1994

Erickson M, Haley J: Advanced Techniques of Hypnosis and Therapy: Selected Papers of Milton Erickson, M.D. New York, Grune & Stratton, 1967

Fisch R, Weakland JH, Segal L: The Tactics of Change. San Francisco, CA, Jossey-Bass, 1982

Fisher S, Greenberg RP: The Scientific Credibility of Freud's Theories and Therapy. New York, Columbia University Press, 1985

Fisher S, Greenberg RP: Freud Scientifically Reappraised: Testing the Theories and Therapy. New York, Wiley, 1996

Greenberg RP: Essential ingredients for successful psychotherapy: effect of common factors, in The Art and Science of Brief Psychotherapies: A Practitioner's Guide. Edited by Dewan MJ, Steenbarger BN, Greenberg RP. Washington, DC, American Psychiatric Publishing, 2004, pp 231–242

Greenberg RP, Constantino MJ, Bruce N: Are patient expectations still relevant for psychotherapy process and outcome? Clin Psychol Rev 26:657–678, 2006

Haley J: Strategies of Psychotherapy, 2nd Edition. New York, Grune & Stratton, 1963

Haley J: Problem-Solving Therapy. San Francisco, CA, Jossey-Bass, 1976

Hembree EA, Roth D, Bux DA Jr, et al: Brief behavior therapy, in The Art and Science of Brief Psychotherapies: A Practitioner's Guide. Edited by Dewan MJ, Steenbarger BN, Greenberg RP. Washington, DC, American Psychiatric Publishing, 2004, pp 51–84

Hollon SD, Beck AT: Cognitive and cognitive-behavioral therapies, in Bergin and Garfield's Handbook of Psychotherapy and Behavior Change, 5th Edition. Edited by Lambert MJ. New York, Wiley, 2004, pp 447–492

Howard KI, Kopta SM, Krause MJ, et al: The dose-effect relationship in psychotherapy. Am Psychol 41:159–164, 1986

Hoyt MF, Rosenbaum R, Talmon M: Planned single-session therapy, in The First Session in Brief Therapy. Edited by Budman SH, Hoyt MF, Friedman S. New York, Guilford, 1992, pp 59–86

Huppert JD, Fabbro A, Barlow DH: Evidence-based practice and psychological treatments, in Evidence-Based Psychotherapy: Where Practice and Research Meet. Edited by Goodheart CD, Kazdin AE, Sternberg RJ. Washington, DC, American Psychological Association, 2006, pp 131–152

Lambert MJ, Archer A: Research findings on the effects of psychotherapy and their implications for practice, in Evidence-Based Psychotherapy: Where Practice and Research Meet. Edited by Goodheart CD, Kazdin AE, Sternberg RJ. Washington, DC, American Psychological Association, 2006, pp 111–130

Lambert MJ, Barley DE: Research summary on the therapeutic relationship and psychotherapy outcome, in Psychotherapy Relationships That Work: Therapist Contributions and Responsiveness to Patients. Edited by Norcross JC. New York, Oxford University Press, 2002, pp 17–36

Lambert MJ, Ogles BM: The efficacy and effectiveness of psychotherapy, in Bergin and Garfield's Handbook of Psychotherapy and Behavior Change, 5th Edition. Edited by Lambert MJ. New York, Wiley, 2004, pp 139–193

Levenson H: Time-Limited Dynamic Psychotherapy: A Guide to Clinical Practice. New York, Basic Books, 1995

Levenson H: Time-limited dynamic psychotherapy: formulation and intervention, in The Art and Science of Brief Psychotherapies: A Practitioner's Guide. Edited by Dewan MJ, Steenbarger BN, Greenberg RP. Washington, DC, American Psychiatric Publishing, 2004, pp 157–188

Levy RL, Shelton JL: Tasks in brief therapy, in Handbook of Brief Therapies. Edited by Wells RA, Giannetti VJ. New York, Plenum, 1990, pp 145–164

Linehan MM: Cognitive-Behavioral Treatment of Borderline Personality Disorder. New York, Guilford, 1993

Luborsky L, Mark D: Short-term supportive-expressive psychoanalytic psychotherapy, in Handbook of Short-Term Dynamic Psychotherapy. Edited by Crits-Christoph P, Barber JP. New York, Basic Books, 1991, pp 110–136

Malan DH: The Frontier of Brief Psychotherapy. New York, Plenum, 1976

Mann J: Time-Limited Psychotherapy. Cambridge, MA, Harvard University Press, 1973

O'Hanlon W, Weiner-Davis J: In Search of Solution: A New Direction in Psychotherapy. New York, WW Norton, 1989

Prochaska JO, Norcross JC: Stages of change, in Psychotherapy Relationships That Work: Therapist Contributions and Responsiveness to Patients. Edited by Norcross JC. New York, Oxford University Press, 2002, pp 303–314

Reed GM, Eisman EJ: Uses and misuses of evidence: managed care, treatment guidelines, and outcomes measurement in professional practice, in Evidence-Based Psychotherapy: Where Practice and Research Meet. Edited by Goodheart CD, Kazdin AE, Sternberg RJ. Washington, DC, American Psychological Association, 2006, pp 13–36

Rosenbaum R: Strategic psychotherapy, in Handbook of the Brief Psychotherapies. Edited by Wells RA, Giannetti VJ. New York, Plenum, 1990, pp 351–404

Roth A, Fonagy P: What Works for Whom? A Critical Review of Psychotherapy Research, 2nd Edition. New York, Guilford, 2006

Shapiro F: Eye Movement Desensitization and Reprocessing: Basic Principles, Protocols, and Procedures, 2nd Edition. New York, Guilford, 2001

Sifneos PE: Short-Term Psychotherapy and Emotional Crisis. Cambridge, MA, Harvard University Press, 1972

Skinner BF: About Behaviorism. New York, Random House, 1974

Steenbarger BN: Toward science-practice integration in brief counseling and therapy. Couns Psychol 20:403–450, 1992

Steenbarger BN: Duration and outcome in psychotherapy: an integrative review. Prof Psychol Res Pr 25:111–119, 1994

Steenbarger BN: Brief therapy, in Encyclopedia of Psychotherapy, Vol 1. Edited by Hersen M, Sledge W. New York, Elsevier, 2002, pp 349–358

Steenbarger BN: Solution-focused brief therapy: doing what works, in The Art and Science of Brief Psychotherapies: A Practitioner's Guide. Edited by Dewan MJ, Steenbarger BN, Greenberg RP. Washington, DC, American Psychiatric Publishing, 2004, pp 85–118

Steenbarger BN: The importance of novelty in psychotherapy, in Clinical Strategies for Becoming a Master Psychotherapist. Edited by O'Donohue W, Cummings NA, Cummings JL. New York, Academic Press, 2006, pp 278–293

Stuart S: Brief interpersonal psychotherapy, in The Art and Science of Brief Psychotherapies: A Practitioner's Guide. Edited by Dewan MJ, Steenbarger BN, Greenberg RP. Washington, DC, American Psychiatric Publishing, 2004, pp 119–156

Stuart S, Robertson M: Interpersonal Psychotherapy: A Clinician's Guide. London, England, Edward Arnold, 2003

Thase ME, Jindal RD: Combining psychotherapy and psychopharmacology for treatment of mental disorders, in Bergin and Garfield's Handbook of Psychotherapy and Behavior Change, 5th Edition. Edited by Lambert MJ. New York, Wiley, 2004, pp 743–766

Wallerstein RS: Forty-Lives in Treatment: A Study of Psychoanalysis and Psychotherapy. New York, Guilford, 1986

Wallerstein RS: The psychotherapy research project of the Menninger Foundation: an overview. J Consult Clin Psychol 57:195–205, 1989

Walter JL, Peller JE: Becoming Solution-Focused in Brief Therapy. New York, Brunner/Mazel, 1992

Wampold BE: The Great Psychotherapy Debate: Models, Methods, and Findings. Mahwah, NJ, Lawrence Erlbaum, 2001

Watzlawick P, Weakland H, Fisch R: Change: Principles of Problem Formation and Problem Resolution. New York, WW Norton, 1974

Weissman MM, Markowitz JW, Klerman GL: Comprehensive Guide to Interpersonal Psychotherapy. New York, Basic Books, 2000

Wolpe J: Psychotherapy by Reciprocal Inhibition. Stanford, CA, Stanford University Press, 1958

29

PSYCHODYNAMIC PSYCHOTHERAPY

Robert J. Ursano, M.D.

Stephen M. Sonnenberg, M.D

Susan G. Lazar, M.D.

The beginning therapist often does not have an extensive psychoanalytic background as was the case in previous years. There may be limited opportunity during training to learn a particular psychotherapy in detail. Yet, as a clinician, he or she may want to understand and use psychodynamic psychotherapy as a part of the therapeutic armamentarium and also use psychodynamic techniques in the evaluation and treatment of patients for whom a full psychotherapy may not be appropriate or may not be possible.

Developing skill in psychodynamic psychotherapy and its techniques is a lifetime endeavor. This treatment modality provides the clinician a window on the meaning of behaviors that are inexplicable from other vantage points. Psychodynamic psychotherapy may be brief, long-term, or intermittent. The principles and techniques are similar, but each form of therapy has its advantages and limitations. Psychodynamic psychotherapy requires the therapist to recognize patterns of interpersonal interaction without engaging in the "drama." In this process the psychotherapist comes to recognize and understand his or her own reactions as early indicators of events transpiring in the treatment

and as potential roadblocks to a successful treatment. This knowledge and this skill are also applicable to other psychiatric treatment modalities, including the other psychotherapies, medication management, consultation-liaison psychiatry, outpatient and emergency room assessment and evaluation, and inpatient treatment.

In this chapter we introduce the concepts and techniques of psychoanalytic psychotherapy. The efficacy and cost-effectiveness of psychotherapy in general, and of psychodynamic psychotherapy in particular, are of special concern to evidence-based practice of medicine and mental health care (Gabbard et al. 2002). "Why psychotherapy?" is a question often asked in the cost-conscious world of present psychiatric care. In addition, it is increasingly important to recognize the basic skills and techniques of psychodynamic intervention that are used in treatments other than psychotherapy. Psychodynamic listening and psychodynamic evaluation are two such techniques that are best learned in the context of learning psychodynamic psychotherapy but are applied in many other psychiatric diagnostic, treatment, and prediction methods.

Why Psychotherapy?

Psychotherapy has long been a part of the treatment of psychiatric patients. Clinical experience and empirical research have shown psychotherapy to be both efficacious and cost-effective. The effectiveness of psychotherapy can be presented in several ways. A reevaluation of a classic study by Eysenck indicates that psychotherapy accomplishes in 15 sessions what spontaneous remission takes 2 years to do (McNeilly and Howard 1991). Smith et al. (1980) found an average effect size of 0.68; this means that after treatment, the average treated person was better off than 75% of the untreated sample (Sonnenberg et al. 1996, 2003). The effect size found by Smith and colleagues is larger than the effect sizes for some other medical treatment trials; these trials were stopped before completion because the data indicated the treatment was efficacious enough that it would be unethical to withhold treatment (Rosenthal 1990). Similarly, such effect sizes are the equivalent of a surgeon's saying that with the surgery, 66% will survive, and without it, only 34% will survive (Rosenthal and Rubin 1982). Is there any question about whether to have such a surgery? Similar effect sizes have been found for psychodynamic psychotherapy in particular (Bond and Perry 2004; Crits-Christoph 1992; Leichsenring et al. 2004).

Psychiatric illness is not uncommon. There are psychiatric "common colds" as well as psychiatric "cancers." Often we forget the range of psychiatric illnesses and therefore the range of interventions—including psychotherapy—that are needed when one considers community health needs as a whole. Because of this range of psychiatric disorders and their effects on health, there appears to be substantial economic advantage in including psychotherapy benefits in all health insurance plans, not only for those with primary psychiatric illness but also for those with medical illness and accompanying psychiatric problems.

The Contribution of Psychotherapy

Psychotherapy is essential to the care of many diagnostic groups of psychiatric patients. It can be crucial for many depressed patients, especially for those who cannot take antidepressant medication, such as pregnant and nursing mothers, some elderly depressed patients, and some depressed patients with concomitant medical illnesses. Approximately 3% of the U.S. pop-

ulation receives psychotherapy each year (Weissman et al. 2006). From 1987 to 1997, access to psychotherapy remained constant in the United States, but the number of visits per patient decreased. In 1997, 10.3% of patients had 20 visits or more, compared with 15.7% in 1987. In 1997, nearly 10 million Americans spent $5.7 billion on outpatient psychotherapy (Olfson et al. 2002).

Psychotherapy in general, and psychodynamic psychotherapy in particular, improves interpersonal and self-esteem symptoms (DiMascio et al. 1979; Klerman et al. 1974). Studies have indicated that extended dynamic psychotherapy may be more efficacious for perfectionistic depressed patients than are other treatment approaches, including medication (Blatt et al. 1995; Leichsenring and Leibing 2003; Milrod et al. 2000). One year of dynamic psychotherapy has been shown to ameliorate nausea, pain, depression, and anxiety in metastatic breast cancer patients and has been reported to lead to a substantially increased survival rate (Spiegel et al. 1989). The use of psychodynamic psychotherapy in patients with borderline personality disorder also has a growing evidence base, both of treatment and of cost–benefit (Clarkin et al. 2001; Hall et al. 2001). Briefer psychotherapy has been related to increased survival in malignant melanoma patients (Fawzy et al. 1990, 1993). Similarly, diabetic children given psychotherapy have a more stable medical course and better diabetic control than do control-group patients not given psychotherapy (Moran et al. 1991; Winkley et al. 2006).

A study of patients with unresponsive mental health problems showed significant improvement in psychological distress and social function 6 months after a trial of psychodynamic interpersonal psychotherapy. The cost of psychotherapy was recouped in 6 months from decreased health care use (Guthrie et al. 1999).

Data on the specific and differential effects of various types of psychotherapy are generally limited, with most empirical studies being of cognitive-behavioral psychotherapies. Given the complicated nature of studies of psychodynamic psychotherapy in particular, such studies may remain limited for some time. However, available data on long-term psychodynamic psychotherapy with some diagnostic groups, on brief psychodynamic psychotherapy, on interpersonal psychotherapy derived from psychodynamic psychotherapy, and on supportive psychotherapy derived from the application of psychodynamic principles indicate that psychodynamic psychotherapy is an important, valuable, and cost-effective part of the clinician's armamentarium (Lazar 1997; Leichsenring 2005; Malan 1980). Skills in this modality should be an important part of every clinician's training.

Basic Principles

Behavior, which includes thoughts, feelings, fantasies, and actions, has both direct and indirect effects on health. Psychiatric illnesses are behavioral disturbances that result in increased levels of morbidity and mortality. Psychopathology usually limits the individual's ability to see options and exercise choice. Feelings, thoughts, and actions are frequently restricted, painful, and repetitive. Psychotherapy, the "talking cure," is the medical treatment directed to changing behavior through verbal means. Through talk, psychotherapy provides understanding, support, and new experiences that can result in learning. The goal of all psychotherapies is to increase the range of behaviors available to the patient and, in this way, to relieve symptoms and alter patterns that have created increased morbidity and potential mortality.

A broad and comprehensive view of health and disease is needed in order to understand the relationship between behavior and health. The target organ of psychotherapeutic treatment is the brain. Feelings, thoughts, and behavior are basic brain functions. Therefore, if psychotherapy is to change behavior, it must at some basic level alter brain function and organization (Kandel 1999; Meany 2001). If a particular behavior is the result of neuron A firing to neuron B, then if change is to occur, neuron A must now fire to neuron C. This simplistic example underscores the importance of recognizing the complex biological results of psychotherapeutic work (Etking et al. 2005).

Behavioral change can be the result of direct biological effects at the brain level (e.g., toxins, tumors), the unfolding of biology in maturation, or the effect of past and present life experiences interacting with biological givens. Psychotherapy itself is a life experience and can become a means by which what is "outside" changes what is "inside." Our understanding of the basic sciences of this process—how what is outside affects what is inside—is only now emerging (Huttenlocher 2002; McEwen 2001; Ursano and Fullerton 1991).

Recall, for example, when you last looked at a gestalt diagram, such as the one of the beautiful woman–ugly witch. At first, perhaps the beautiful woman was the only clear image, but after certain shaded areas were pointed out, it was possible to discern the chin of a witch rather than the face of the beautiful woman. Nothing had changed in the amount of visual informa-

tion that was reaching your brain; rather, what changed was how it was organized, allowing a fuller range of meanings to be experienced and behaviors to be expressed.

A wide array of infant systems (activity level, arousal, and brain neurochemistry) are regulated by the mother–infant interaction and can be profoundly affected by it (Hofer 1984; Meany 2001). In adults, as well, the extent of social relatedness has been repeatedly shown to affect behavior as well as morbidity and mortality (House et al. 1988). For example, it is a common observation that the phobic patient will frequently approach the phobic object when with a supportive other. Why? How has the presence of another person altered brain function to allow this profound yet everyday change in behavior? Mental, symbolic, and representational events—including hopes, fears, memories, expectations, and fantasies—also serve as important biological regulators in the same way as do actual life events.

Our understanding of how the outside world (psychotherapy) can change the inside world (biology) is growing but is still in its infancy. Our basic sciences of psychotherapy have changed the question from *whether* organization, meaning, memory, expectations, and interpersonal contact influence health and behavior to *how* they influence them and to what extent.

The Focus of Psychodynamic Psychotherapy

The different psychotherapies target different aspects of psychological functioning for change. Psychodynamic (psychoanalytically oriented) psychotherapy focuses primarily on the effects of past experience on molding patterns of behavior and expectations through particular cognitions (defenses) and interpersonal styles of interaction and perception (transference) that have become repetitive and that interfere with health (Table 29–1).

An individual's past exists in the present through memory and biology. Expectations—the anticipated present and future—are formed by one's past experiences and biology. Likewise, the way in which language is used metaphorically by a patient may reflect a particular organization (cluster of feelings, thoughts, and behaviors) formed in the past and affecting present perception and behavior. By exploring the past and present meaning of events and their context, the psy-

TABLE 29–1. Psychodynamic psychotherapy

Focus

Effects of past experience on present behaviors (cognitions, affects, fantasies and actions)

Goal

Understanding the defense mechanisms and the transference responses of the patient, particularly as they appear in the doctor–patient relationship

Technique

Therapeutic alliance

Free association

Defense and transference interpretation

Frequent meetings

Duration of treatment

Months to years

chodynamic psychotherapist aims to alter the organizers of behavior, restructuring how information and experience are organized.

Psychodynamic psychotherapy (also called *psychoanalytic psychotherapy, exploratory psychotherapy,* or *insight-oriented psychotherapy*) is a method of treatment for psychiatric disorders that uses words exchanged between two people to effect changes in behavior. Psychodynamic psychotherapy shares with the other psychotherapies a general definition: a two-person interaction, primarily verbal, in which one person is designated the help giver and the other the help receiver. The goal is to elucidate the patient's characteristic problems of living; the hope is to achieve behavioral change. Psychodynamic psychotherapy uses specific techniques and a particular understanding of mental functioning to guide and direct the treatment and the therapist's interventions. As in other medical treatments, there are both indications and contraindications to this form of treatment.

Although the strategic goals of a psychodynamic treatment are to alter symptoms and change behavior to alleviate pain and suffering and decrease morbidity and mortality, the moment-to-moment objective is very different. As in surgery, in which the strategic goal is to remove disease, stop bleeding, and eliminate pain, it is not the strategic goals that direct the actual operation itself. The surgeon sometimes causes bleeding and pain and is directed by technical procedures to accomplish the overall goal. Similarly, in psychodynamic psychotherapy it is the therapist's understanding of what is causing the disease process, and of how a particular intervention will affect the recovery in the

long run, that directs the tactical moment-to-moment process of treatment.

Psychodynamic psychotherapy is based on the principles of mental functioning and the psychotherapeutic techniques originally developed by Sigmund Freud. Freud began his work by using hypnosis; he later turned to free association as the method by which to understand the unrecognized (unconscious) conflicts that arose from development and continued into adult life. Such conflicts are patterns of behavior—that is, patterns of feelings, thoughts, and behaviors laid down in the brain during childhood. These patterns are the result of the individual's developmental history and biological givens.

Typically, these unconscious conflicts are between libidinal or aggressive desires (wishes) and the fear of loss, the fear of retaliation, the limits imposed by the real world, or the opposition of conflicting desires. *Libidinal wishes* are best thought of as longings for sexual and emotional gratification. *Aggressive wishes,* on the other hand, are destructive wishes that either are primary or are the result of perceived frustration or deprivation (Ursano et al. 1990). The beginning therapist frequently confuses the old terminology of libidinal wishes with the idea of specifically genital feelings. *Sexual gratification* in psychodynamic work refers to the broad concept of bodily pleasure—the states of excitement and pleasure experienced since infancy. The patient talking about happiness, excitement, pleasure, anticipation, love, or longing is describing libidinal wishes. The desire to destroy or the experience of pleasure in anger, hate, and pain is usually the expression of aggressive wishes.

Neurotic conflict (i.e., conflicted feelings/ambivalence derived from past [usually childhood] experiences and usually out of awareness) can result in anxiety, depression, and somatic symptoms; work, social, or sexual inhibitions; or maladaptive interpersonal relations. These unconscious neurotic conflicts are evident as patterns of behavior: feelings, thoughts, fantasies, and actions. These patterns, learned in childhood, may at one time have been appropriate to the patient's childhood view of the world and may have been adaptive or even necessary for survival. Even though these behaviors are not evident to the patient initially, through the psychotherapeutic work they become clear, and their many ramifications for the patient's life become evident.

Psychodynamic psychotherapy is more focused than psychoanalysis, per se, and somewhat more oriented to the here and now. However, both these techniques share the goal of understanding the nature of the patient's conflicts—maladaptive patterns of behavior derived from childhood (also called the *infantile neurosis*)—and their effects in adult life.

The Setting of Psychodynamic Psychotherapy

Psychodynamic psychotherapy may be brief (see Chapter 28, "Brief Psychotherapies," by Dewan et al.), intermittent, or long-term. Intermittent psychotherapy is often the norm. This is the result of episodes of brief or time-limited psychodynamic psychotherapy being given to a patient over a longer period of time. Intermittent psychotherapy may also be necessary due to resources of time, money, or the patient's unwillingness to undertake longer-term treatment. Intermittent psychotherapy can also be planned after the initial evaluation as a joint plan of the therapist and patient to unfold over time, often with medication as a part of the treatment (see Chapter 33, "Combining Psychotherapy and Pharmacotherapy," by Riba and Balon). This type of psychotherapy requires study, because it has become quite common and yet is not often considered as offering both unique opportunities and limitations.

Psychodynamic psychotherapy may take months or years. Typically, a longer-term treatment is open ended; no termination date is set in the beginning of treatment. The length of treatment depends on the number of conflict areas to be addressed and the course of the treatment. Psychotherapy sessions are usually held one, two, or three times a week, although in brief treatments once a week is the norm. The frequent meetings permit a more detailed exploration of the patient's inner life and a fuller development of the transference. The frequent meetings also support the patient during the treatment process.

Medications are used as needed with patients in psychodynamic psychotherapy (see Chapter 33, "Combining Psychotherapy and Pharmacotherapy," by Riba and Balon). Medications may relieve biological symptoms or regulation disruptions that evidence shows do not respond to psychotherapy. In addition, medication may alleviate persistent and impairing symptoms, which can allow the patient to participate in psychotherapy to learn new behaviors and avoid old impairing behaviors while experiencing a fuller range of affect. In some disorders, medication may be alleviating a primary disease process so that the psychotherapy can address the illness-onset conditions and facilitate the

patient's avoidance of relapse, readjustment, recovery, and integration into family and community, thus decreasing the risk of morbidity and mortality. The meaning to the patient of the medication he or she may be taking is an important area for exploration during the psychotherapy, particularly when it is time to discontinue use of the medication.

The Technique of Psychodynamic Psychotherapy

Behavioral change occurs in psychodynamic psychotherapy primarily through two processes of treatment: understanding the cognitive and affective patterns derived from childhood (defense mechanisms) and understanding the conflicted relationship(s) one had with one's childhood significant figures as they are reexperienced in the doctor–patient relationship (transference). The recovery and understanding of these feelings and perceptions are the focus of treatment. The treatment setting is designed to facilitate the emergence of these patterns in a way that allows them to be analyzed rather than being confused with the reality of the doctor–patient relationship or being dismissed as trivial.

Primary to the success of psychoanalytically oriented psychotherapy is the need for the patient to feel engaged in the work and to trust the relationship with the therapist. This therapeutic alliance is built on the reality-based elements of the treatment, such as the mutual working together toward a common goal and the consistency and reliability of the therapist (Bruch 1974). Only in contrast to a good therapeutic alliance can the patient view the transference feelings and experience the distortion that the transference reveals.

The clinician empathically hears what the patient says in order to understand what an experience means to the patient (Fromm-Reichman 1950). What the patient is able to bring into focus is what is dealt with in the treatment (Coleman 1968). The depth of interpretation and exploration is always at the point of urgency for the patient, not ahead of or behind the patient's thoughts and feelings. Beginning therapists often think that as soon as they see something, it is time to tell the patient. The timing of when to tell the patient is the essence of the skill of the therapist; careful thought and planning are needed to determine the appropriate time. Although the actual event of interpreting—explaining a piece of behavior in the context of the present and past and in relation to transference elements—is spontaneous, it is "spontaneous" after much preparation. When to tell the patient a new piece of information is determined by when the patient can hear and understand what the therapist has to say.

The patient's free association—that is, speaking without censoring or inhibiting his or her thoughts—is encouraged. This encouragement can be as simple as telling a patient that she is free to talk about whatever she wishes. The therapist's main task is to listen to the undercurrents of the patient's associations. Frequently this involves wondering about the connection between one vignette and the next or listening for how the patient is experiencing a particular person she describes or a particular interaction with the therapist. Often, listening to the ambiguity in a patient's associations may open the door to the unconscious conflict and the person from the past to which it relates.

For example, one patient came into a psychotherapy session shortly after breaking up with his girlfriend, saying, "I want to get her back." If one hears the double meaning in the sentence—to be back with her or to take revenge on her—it will not be surprising to learn that although the patient thought he was only talking about wanting to get back together with his girlfriend, by the end of the session he was describing his particular revenge fantasy. (This patient's fantasy derived from an old movie. He fantasized about "smushing" a grapefruit in his girlfriend's face.) The conflicted feelings—longing for and hating—were foretold in the opening of the session. This long-held pattern of response to rejections matched his early experiences with a mother who would alternately see him as having exactly the same feelings as she did and later chase him with a knife. He was not yet ready to hear this connection, but it was already becoming evident. The pattern could now be watched, and the patient's awareness of it slowly increased.

The transference may be experienced by the therapist as a pressure to act in a certain way toward the patient. More often than not, for the beginning therapist it is identified, as in learning to ski, by noticing the direction in which one is about to fall! The transference is a specific example of the tendency of the brain to see the past in the present, to make use of old patterns of perception and response, and to exclude new information. When the transference is alive, it is very real to the patient, and contradictory information is disregarded. For the new therapist it is often difficult to see the irrational elements in the patient's feelings and perceptions about the therapist. Often the transference is built on a seed of accurate perception about the therapist. It is the elaboration of this seed that makes the unconscious evident. The therapist may experience the accuracy of the patient's perceptions and fail to listen to the elements of the past that may be appearing.

Exploring the transference is just a special case of the ongoing work of examining the patterns of relationships that the patient experiences. This is all part of the attempt to understand the inner world of the patient—the world of how the patient sees and experiences people and events, the world of psychic reality. Transference is not unique to the psychotherapeutic setting. It occurs throughout life and in medical treatments of all kinds. In fact, asking someone to come into a hospital (an unfamiliar setting) and take off his clothes, have no one know who he is, and be required to eat when told and go where told is a very powerful way to induce transferences! What is unique is the attempt to understand the transference and to examine it when it occurs rather than to try to undo it (Gabbard 2000; Luborsky and Crits-Christoph 1998).

The therapist may also experience feelings toward the patient that come from the therapist's past. This is called the *countertransference*. The countertransference is increased during times of stressful events and unresolved conflicts in the life of the therapist. The countertransference can be a friend, guiding one to see subtle aspects of the doctor–patient relationship that may have gone unnoticed. It can also be a block to a successful treatment, causing the therapist to misperceive and mishear the patient.

Evaluation

Assessment, Diagnosis, and Prescription of Brief, Intermittent, or Long-Term Psychodynamic Psychotherapy

Psychiatric evaluation is critical to the assessment of a patient for psychotherapy, just as for the patient who is to be seen for medication management (Ursano and Silberman 1988). The prescription of psychotherapy can be the outcome of the psychiatric evaluation. The therapist must consider the advantages, disadvantages, target symptoms, course of treatment, and contraindications for psychodynamic psychotherapy as with any other prescription.

Psychodynamic psychotherapy may be short term (brief; see Chapter 28, "Brief Psychotherapies," by Dewan et al.), long term, or intermittent. The structure of each of these requires consideration and planning of goals and targets of treatment. At present it is not uncommon for a patient to have a brief psychodynamic psychotherapy as his or her first psychotherapy. If that is not sufficient, the patient may be seen in a longer-term treatment or an additional brief treatment, or intermittently to work on focused areas that may have become evident during the first treatment. The choice of brief, intermittent, or long-term treatment is determined by the patient, type of problems (recent precipitant versus character related), degree of social supports to aid treatment responsiveness, extent of the disorder (multifocal versus unifocal conflict), and practical issues of patient availability and preferences.

As part of the evaluation for psychodynamic psychotherapy, the clinician must assess the presence or absence of organic causes for the patient's psychiatric disturbance, the need for medication, the risk of untoward outcomes (suicide, homicide, divorce, work disruption), and the possibility that the patient's condition will worsen. At times, the beginning therapist starting work in a busy outpatient service may neglect to consider the option that the patient assigned for psychotherapy was evaluated incorrectly and that individual psychodynamic psychotherapy is not the appropriate treatment or that no treatment is indicated.

The psychiatric assessment for psychodynamic psychotherapy includes the use of two important techniques: psychodynamic listening (Chessick 2000) and the psychodynamic assessment or evaluation. Both are important to distinguish as techniques because they are applicable to many types of treatment and intervention, not just to psychodynamic psychotherapy. The use of psychodynamic listening and evaluation can be critical in medication management, consultation-liaison evaluation, and inpatient treatment, to name a few.

Psychodynamic listening (Mohl 2003; Sonnenberg 1995) puts the psychiatrist in an attitude of curious inquiry, listening to the meanings, metaphors, developmental sequencing, and interpersonal nuances of the patient's story and of the doctor–patient interaction (Edelson 1993) (Table 29–2). Particular attention is paid to stories, present and past, about 1) feelings and wishes; 2) the management of various feelings through the life cycle (e.g., defense mechanisms and cognitive style) and areas of healthy interaction with the world; 3) self-esteem regulation; and 4) interpersonal relationships. These four areas reflect the four psychodynamic perspectives on psychopathology: drives, ego function, self psychology, and object relationships (Pine 1988; Table 29–3).

The psychodynamic assessment or evaluation uses

TABLE 29–2. Psychodynamic listening

I. Wishes/desires

What is the patient wishing for?

What in the patient's developmental history caused this wish to be prominent?

Are the wishes developmentally appropriate?

II. Defenses

What in the patient's developmental history disrupted his or her wishes and desires?

How does the patient keep wishes out of awareness?

III. Self-esteem

Does the patient like him- or herself?

Does he or she feel valued, admired, recognized by others?

How does the patient respond to events in life that decrease self-esteem or the feeling of being valued?

IV. Interpersonal relations—present and in memory/fantasy

Who are the important people in the patient's past and present?

How are they recalled and spoken of at the different phases of the patient's life and development?

Whom from the past does the patient behave and feel and think like (even if the patient is not aware of it)?

Whom does the patient miss and long for?

Who was lost from the patient's life at an early age (by death, moving, illness, conflict, or absence/ neglect)?

---

the data obtained from questioning and from psychodynamic listening (MacKinnon et al. 2006; Sullivan 1954; Table 29–4). The evaluation aims to integrate the patient's chief complaint; history of present illness; past history; family history; developmental history, including any traumatic events or deviations from usual developmental patterns; mental status examination; style of doctor–patient interaction; and transference and the psychiatrist's countertransference feelings. The outcome of this evaluation is a psychodynamic understanding of the patient's past and present experiences from the patient's subjective viewpoint. This psychodynamic formulation provides an integrated understanding through the patient's life cycle from the four psychodynamic perspectives on the past and

TABLE 29–3. Psychodynamic perspectives

Theory	Focus
Drive theory	Wishes and feelings
Ego function	Defense mechanisms, cognitive style, and areas of health in the personality
Self psychology	Regulation of self-esteem
Object relations	Internalized memories of interpersonal relationships
Intersubjectivity and relational theory	Subjective experience and interpersonal relations
Attachment theory	Infant–caregiver attachment

TABLE 29–4. Guidelines for psychodynamic assessment

Listen to and explore:
  The precipitants of the symptoms, of the illness, and of seeking help
  The history of significant events from childhood to the present

Identify the significant people in the patient's history from childhood to present

Ask for the patient's earliest memory

Explore any recurrent or recent dreams and the context of when they were dreamed

Observe how the patient relates to the therapist

Discuss the patient's previous treatments and therapists

Give a trial interpretation

Invite collaboration in "understanding"

present experiences of the patient, and it makes predictions of potential doctor–patient interactions and the patient's patterns of defense mechanisms and interpersonal interactions.

In this way, the evaluation phase provides information for the assessment of the type and degree of psychiatric illness and impairment, the selection of treatment modality, and the conduct of psychotherapy itself. After a well-conducted evaluation, the patient feels respected and safe, believes that his or her best interests are the primary concern of the clinician, and feels that any topic can be talked about (Levinson et al. 1967).

The therapist's asking about medical signs and symptoms and suicidal and homicidal thoughts and actions frequently relieves the patient of the feeling that he or she is the only one worried about these areas. Often the patient is wondering whether the doctor will ask about these issues. Whether the therapist inquires about these particular areas may be used by the patient as a way to assess whether the therapist is serious about listening and being concerned about the patient or whether these are topics that the clinician feels are irrelevant or too dangerous to talk about. "VIP" and physician patients in particular are alert to whether the therapist is thorough in the evaluation. The patient who feels that all areas—medical as well as behavioral—and all risks and concerns have been forthrightly and empathically explored will feel the beginning of a working relationship centered on trust and mutual respect. The beginning of the psychotherapy in the evaluation phase is critical to the psycho-

therapeutic work to follow that can include many distortions of the doctor–patient relationship. Commonly, long after a therapy has started—and frequently in its termination phase—a patient may reveal, for example, the one question the therapist asked, or the particular way in which the therapist greeted him or her at the door, that led to the feeling that working together would be possible.

Beginning the Evaluation

The evaluation begins when the therapist meets the patient (Lazare and Eisenthal 1989a, 1989b). In the outpatient setting, it is best for the therapist to introduce him- or herself and explain to the patient what the therapist knows about the patient's problems. One should not assume that a patient knows that a session is an evaluation. Rather, the therapist should set the context of the meeting, explaining that he or she, the therapist, would like to spend some time getting to know the nature of the patient's difficulties and inviting the patient to tell more (Table 29–5).

The number of evaluation sessions usually ranges from one to four, but more sessions may be needed. The length of the evaluation is determined by the amount of time required to collect the information for the diagnostic and psychodynamic assessment and to address the practical issues of beginning treatment. Usually, the beginning therapist errs on the side of short evaluations and an incomplete assessment (Table 29–6).

The clinician uses two methods for data collection during the evaluation: asking questions and listening

TABLE 29–5. **The evaluation**
Goal
Educate the patient about the evaluation process
Establish an atmosphere of safety and inquiry
Assess for the appropriate treatment
Tasks
Assess for life-threatening behaviors
Assess for organic causes of the patient's illness
Determine the diagnosis
Identify areas of conflict across the life cycle
Duration
Meet for one to four sessions
Techniques
Use questioning and listening
Listen for the patient's fears about starting treatment
Attend to the precipitants of the illness and of seeking treatment

TABLE 29–6. **Helpful hints for the evaluation**
When the clinician is only doing the evaluation and the patient will be referred to another therapist for treatment, it is most helpful to the evaluation and to its successful termination that the patient know this plan at the beginning.
Infrequently, it may be advantageous and important to have the initial evaluation done by a clinician who will not be the treating therapist. In the case where the patient needs a very firm, direct, confrontational approach to enter a much-needed treatment, the evaluating clinician who is not expecting to treat the patient may feel freer to be blunt, in a tactful manner, with the patient.
Patients must be given the time and space in which to paint a picture of their world without the therapist choosing the colors! Being either too intrusive or too silent can lead to missed information and can needlessly confuse the patient.
All therapists also experience certain therapist–patient differences that they cannot bridge, and in such cases they refer the patient to another clinician.
Early termination may be due to defenses against seeking help, a transference reaction, a decision that this is not the right treatment, or, at times, a relief of symptoms as a result of the evaluation.

unobtrusively (Silberman and Certa 2003). Both styles must be used to collect the needed information. A patient complaining of depression should not leave the first evaluation session without the clinician's knowing the severity of the depression and the risk of suicide. This usually requires at least some direct questioning. Life-threatening issues must be dealt with early in order to gather the needed diagnostic information. However, other historical information can be collected as part of the patient's story (Horowitz et al. 1995; Perry et al. 1987).

Frequently, the skill of the therapist lies in how the history and diagnostic information are collected. The more skilled the therapist, the more able he or she is to understand—to reach—and therefore to work with a wider range of patients. The skilled therapist can establish a rapport across a wide array of socioeconomic classes and sexual, racial, religious, cultural, and emotional differences.

In the first session the therapist should listen for the patient's fears of starting psychotherapy. These fears should be explored early, as they appear and are articulated by the patient. The patient will feel safer and be more interested in continuing the evaluation and the treatment when these fears have been heard, respected, and explored by the therapist. In addition, airing these

fears will leave the therapist in a better position to interpret any precipitous stopping of the treatment. It is not unusual for a patient to drop out during the evaluation phase before beginning treatment. That is one reason to view this phase as the candidacy stage. (In clinic settings, about 50% of patients stop before the fifth session [Malan et al. 1973; Table 29–7].)

TABLE 29–7. **First session**
By the end of the first session, the clinician should know the answers to these questions:
What further organic workup is needed?
Is psychosis in the differential diagnosis?
Are there any life-threatening issues, either now or possibly in the future?
How many (if any) more sessions will be taken for the evaluation?

Indications and Selection Criteria

Psychodynamic psychotherapy has its best outcomes with what have been called "neurotic-level disorders." These individuals have conflicts that are primarily oedipal in nature (e.g., competition, guilt, independence, adult sexuality and intimacy, parental loss and identification) and that are experienced as internal by the patient. Although the diagnoses in DSM-IV-TR (American Psychiatric Association 2000) are not organized by their developmental conflict level (or level of maturity of defenses), some of the disorders are more likely than others to present with a primarily neurotic-level conflict. DSM-IV-TR disorders that frequently involve a primarily neurotic conflict include obsessive-compulsive disorder, anxiety disorders (Bond and Perry 2004), conversion disorder, psychological factors affecting physical disease, dysthymic disorder, mild to moderate mood disorders (Bond 2006), adjustment disorders, and mild to moderate personality disorders (Gabbard et al. 2002; Leichsenring 2005; Leichsenring and Leibing 2003). Patients who are psychologically minded, who are able to observe feelings without acting on them, and who can obtain symptom relief through understanding may benefit from psychodynamic psychotherapy. The patient who has a supportive environment—family, friends, work—usually does better because he or she is able to use the therapy in a more intensive manner. Such a patient does not need the therapist to be a primary reality support in order to weather the stresses of life or the treatment.

When not in the acute phase of illness and when dealing with rehabilitation, adjustment, and recovery, more seriously disturbed patients—those with major depression, schizophrenia, or borderline personality disorder—can also be treated in psychodynamically informed psychotherapy, with the addition of psychosocial supports and interventions as needed (Blatt and Shahar 2004; Fonagy et al. 2005). For these patients, the treatment is usually directed toward modifying the illness-onset conditions and facilitating readjustment, recovery, and integration into the community. Supportive treatment, derived from many principles of psychodynamic psychotherapy, is the primary treatment in the acute phase of these illnesses (see Chapter 32, "Supportive Psychotherapy," by Winston). The regressive tendencies of such patients are managed in psychodynamic psychotherapy with the use of medication and with greater support and reality feedback through face-to-face meetings with the therapist (Gabbard 2005).

Patients with severe preoedipal pathology are not good candidates for psychodynamic psychotherapy. This type of pathology is manifested by an inability to form a supportive dyadic relationship, the presence of severely exploitative relationships, a chaotic lifestyle, or substantial (or dangerous) acting out. The basic requirements of psychodynamic psychotherapy—for the patient to have a strong observing ego and an ability to form a supportive therapeutic relationship—are very difficult tasks for these patients.

Although psychological mindedness is important, intelligence per se is not a selection criterion; in fact, it can reflect a highly organized obsessional character structure that may be very difficult to treat. Socioeconomic class is also not a good predictor of success in treatment. Rather, the ability to work with patients from diverse socioeconomic classes is usually a part of the therapist's task and skill: to span a range of life experiences and accurately empathize with the patient's world. The patient–therapist match is therefore very important, especially to the opening phase of treatment and the establishment of the therapeutic alliance.

In general, patients who like their therapists, who have had a shorter duration of symptoms, and who are seeking understanding of their problems as well as symptom relief have the best outcomes. The use of a trial interpretation during the evaluation phase can provide much useful information on how the patient makes use of understanding to modify symptoms and to what extent the patient experiences understanding provided through interpretation as supportive and helpful (Malan 1980).

Treatment

Psychodynamic psychotherapy is usually not a familiar form of medical treatment to the patient who is about to begin psychotherapy. At the end of the evaluation, the clinician discusses with the patient alternative forms of treatment that might in various ways be of benefit. In addition, the clinician must discuss with the patient how each of these treatments works. This approach is also true for psychodynamic psychotherapy. Psychodynamic psychotherapy can be explained to the patient as a process for learning a new method of problem solving based on an understanding of the personal life history, the workings of the mind that are outside conscious awareness, and the personal view of the world—one's psychic reality. The individual's psychic reality hinges on the way in which past experience is used as an unconscious template for present behaviors—feelings, thoughts, fantasies, and actions.

Teaching the patient about the goals and process of psychodynamic psychotherapy is very important to the successful beginning of the psychotherapy. One way to conceptualize this phase of treatment is that an atmosphere of safety must be established. Although this may seem an imposing task, it is similar to the physician's task in many situations. For example, when the family practitioner finds that an otherwise healthy patient has a high cholesterol level, he or she must educate the patient and develop a cooperative working relationship so that together they can begin a treatment to counteract the potential ill effects of this silent condition.

In the opening phase of the treatment, the patient learns that psychodynamic psychotherapy will work because in the relationship with the therapist, the patient will reexperience the past in the present through the transference relationship. By examining feelings in the therapy setting, the patient develops an understanding of how the personal past is continually reexperienced in life. The patient will then begin to understand that psychological pain can result from symbolically reliving the past in the here and now, causing the reawakening of the conflicted feelings and anxieties of childhood. The patient also learns by experience that through recognizing these unconscious processes, the painful feelings diminish and new behaviors are possible.

The patient is educated directly both through teaching and explanation and through example. At times, the clinician should explain very directly and supportively to the patient the process of the treatment. When this has been done, it is best not to continue to repeat the explanations but instead to change into a mode of understanding rather than teaching, listening to the patient's possible emotional blocks to understanding. The skilled clinician is always making decisions early in treatment about whether this is a time to educate or a time to listen to more material from the patient, delaying any further instructive comments. Generally, the new therapist struggles with how much to educate and how much to listen in the opening sessions. Later in treatment, after explanations have been given clearly, the therapist can assume that cognitive education is not the difficulty the patient is having. However, the therapist cannot assume this in the opening phase, particularly with the naïve patient. Understanding the goals and processes of treatment is important to the patient's feeling safe and comfortable enough to explore and tolerate the anxiety that arises in the treatment setting (Sonnenberg et al. 1996, 2003).

Abstinence, Neutrality, and Free Association

After the patient has begun to understand the process of treatment, the therapist will, over time, become somewhat less verbally active in order to hear more about how the patient organizes his or her psychological world. Technically this is called being abstinent. Again the therapist may need to explain this to the patient if he or she asks about the therapist's silence. The therapist might say, "I am listening to you very closely. I want to be able to best understand how you see the world and not interfere with what you are telling me." The therapist also encourages the patient to speak as freely as possible and to suspend judgment about the accuracy or logic of what is said. This may be explained to the patient in the following manner: "You are free to say whatever you would like. In fact, it is most helpful if you say whatever comes to mind. I know that is difficult to do." The therapist helps the patient say whatever comes to mind—to speak without editing thoughts—even though the patient may say things that he or she fears would be untrue or hurtful to the therapist or to loved ones.

This method of communication is known as *free association*. It is characteristic of the mode of thinking and talking used by the patient in classical psychoanalysis, although free association in classical psychoanalysis is much freer because of the other elements of the psychoanalytic treatment. However, the psychodynamic psychotherapy patient will come fairly close to that same mode of expression (S. Freud 1917/1963).

Inevitably, free association is only relative, and the unconscious conflicts the patient experiences are the major forces that block the free expression of thoughts, feelings, and fantasies. The therapist, in collaboration with the patient, listens for clues to what may be outside the patient's awareness and may appear as a block to the free expression of thoughts. These ways of thinking that block uncomfortable feelings and conflicts from being experienced are called *defense mechanisms*. The therapist carefully observes, and at the right time shares with the patient, the patterns the patient shows in his or her thoughts and feelings and the blocks to these thoughts and feelings. The therapist observes the changes in the patient's thoughts and feelings and any movement away from the treatment. The therapist experiences the patient's defense mechanisms as a resistance to the work. Through the process of understanding how the resistances—the patient's defense mechanisms—operate, the transference emerges later in treatment.

The clinician and patient work together to recognize the patterns of the patient's thoughts and feelings. This collaborative work allows the patient to experience this task as one he or she can eventually assume, rather than as something magical. This task—the analysis of defenses—forms the basis on which the patient can eventually choose alternative behaviors. At times the enthusiasm of the new therapist can lead to wanting to tell the patient a pattern without working together with the patient to identify it. This can lead to the therapist's being seen as very powerful by the patient and often will create problems later in treatment.

The patient at times experiences feelings of frustration because of the clinician's relative silence. However, the patient should, overall, experience the therapist as standing with him or her, as an ally with whom the patient can master the forces that keep so much outside consciousness (Schafer 1983). Helping the patient understand this during the opening phase of treatment is essential.

In therapy, what the patient says is met with an effort to understand, not with judgment or criticism. The therapist maintains neutrality. The job of the psychodynamic psychotherapist does not involve managing the patient's life (one reason why patient selection is so important) or judging its worth or the value of the way in which it is conducted (Poland 1984).

The therapist's abstinent, neutral demeanor in the therapeutic setting is, in part, a technique, a special form of behavior designed to offer the patient the opportunity to experience his or her own feelings, thoughts, and fantasies. Partly as a result of this unique aspect of the psychotherapeutic setting and partly because of the normal course of life, the patient is able to think in a less well-organized, less structured fashion, giving access to more unconscious feelings and thoughts and thereby acting on the psychotherapeutic stage. Over time, the therapy becomes a laboratory in which the patient can examine in detail the feelings, thoughts, and fantasies he or she experiences toward another person (the therapist) within the safety of the therapeutic alliance (Bender 2005).

Although this goal requires the therapist to be relatively passive and silent, this technical stance is not meant to be harsh or depriving. The collaboration develops in part through the clinician's appropriate concern and through explanations of the special kind of team effort and working together that are a part of the therapy. The therapist and the patient work together to understand the patient's experience, which in turn leads to the amelioration of the patient's psychic pain. The therapist and the patient are more accurately described as trying to develop a working (Greenson 1965) or therapeutic alliance (Curtis 1979; Zetzel 1956).

The psychiatrist doing this form of therapy works from the perspective of the concerned physician, with gentleness and an awareness of the patient's pain (Schafer 1983; Stone 1981). Over and over again, through working together, the physician conveys the awareness that the patient is experiencing psychological pain not only in life outside the therapy but, because of reexperiencing the past, in life inside the therapy as well. The psychiatrist conveys respect for the patient's efforts to understand him- or herself and to keep going in therapy in spite of the pain.

Transference, Defense Mechanisms, and Resistance

Transference

Transference is at the core of how psychodynamic psychotherapy works, but it is never easily understood by the patient. Freud developed the idea that all human relationships are transference relationships. By this he meant that all human beings experience others by superimposing their perceptions of figures from the past on new individuals. Today, although within psychoanalysis there exists a range of views on the nature of transference, it is generally felt that memories of the past are activated in all relationships. To some extent, each individual unconsciously plays out in current relationships certain aspects of important past relationships (Table 29–8).

TABLE 29–8.   Transference

Transference...

Is part of all relationships

Is a primary focus of psychodynamic psychotherapy

Brings the past alive to the patient in the doctor–patient relationship

Aids in remembering the past

Provides examples of patterns of interpersonal behaviors, fantasies, feelings, and thoughts that influence the patient's present relationships

Can be felt by the therapist as "role pressure"—a pressure to respond in a particular way to the patient

Because the psychodynamic psychotherapist is abstinent and does not share details of his or her personal life with the patient, the therapist creates a kind of blank screen on which the patient may paint a transference picture of his or her own design. Early in the therapy this becomes apparent. By pointing it out, the therapist and the patient create a common focus of attention. In this way the patient's understanding of how therapy works is also deepened.

People form transferences in all relationships. This is because we use the past as a pattern for understanding the present and because there seems to be in all people a psychological need to repeat the past in an effort to master that which was difficult or emotionally painful. Therefore, not just in psychoanalysis and psychodynamic psychotherapy but everywhere, people construct their relationships in the present by reproducing emotionally important aspects of their past relationships (S. Freud 1912/1958; McLaughlin 1981).

One way to vividly imagine the impact of transference is to imagine a series of transparent plastic pages in an anatomy text. When the book is first opened, the reader sees the surface of the body. When the first page is turned, the muscles are seen, with the major blood vessels barely visible beneath them. As the reader turns to the next page, the blood vessels and the major nerves are seen. The bones are visible beneath. Finally, when the last page is turned, the bones come into full view. Transference is much the same in that memories of various relationships are superimposed one on another and what we observe on the surface is determined by the subtleties beneath the surface, out of conscious awareness.

Thus, another way of conceptualizing transference is to think of the human mind as made up, in part, of sets of memories of important individuals from a person's past. These organized sets of memories are called *object representations*. Whenever a person meets someone new, he or she begins to form a new object representation. Obviously, this process proceeds to a significant extent only when the new person is of some importance to the observer; but whenever the process takes place, the observer, in an effort to understand a new acquaintance, scans his or her memories for standards against which to measure and compare the new individual. Soon, new and old object representations are psychologically connected in response to the observer's need for familiarity and to other psychological needs (explained later). The newcomer is on the receiving end of ideas, thoughts, and feelings that were originally directed toward the old friend, relative, loved one, or enemy.

What we see when we observe individuals and talk with them about their present life or current relationships is the surface of their psychological life. Beneath that surface are the memories of their important past relationships, which—like the muscles, nerves, and bones beneath the skin—constitute vital parts of the organic whole of their interpersonal world, present as well as past (Goldstein and Goldberg 2003; Sandler et al. 1973). The individual, however, perceives his or her current relationship as the whole. The connections of the current relationship to an old relationship and the way in which the present is serving as a vehicle for working out old relationships remain outside conscious awareness. Therefore, the therapist may experience the transference in the therapy as pressure to behave in a certain way toward the patient that is reminiscent of a previous relationship the patient had in childhood.

In psychodynamic psychotherapy, the therapist, through his or her neutrality, abstinence, and encouraging of free association, creates an environment in which conscious transference responses are relatively more intense than in typical relationships (although they are less intense than in a classical psychoanalysis). The development and understanding of the transference is one of the therapist's most important tools. It is the vehicle for bringing alive—in the consulting room—the patient's difficulties and for examining these in depth in an existentially meaningful environment. In fact, it is this process that, more than anything else, distinguishes psychodynamic psychotherapy from other forms of treatment.

From another perspective, the transference is the way the patient remembers what he or she has forgotten—what is unconscious and the source of psychological pain. In popular caricatures of psychiatric treatment, the patient remembers dramatic childhood events in a melodramatic fashion. In reality, this remembering occurs as a result of detailed effort to dissect the frequently small memories of long-forgotten, sometimes repetitively experienced parts of the past as they present in the transference relationship. Through the transference the patient develops an understanding of what was experienced in the past and how that experience lives on in the here and now. To help the patient understand transference and begin to develop the ability to work with it, the psychiatrist must direct the patient's attention to this dimension of his or her thoughts. Thus, the therapist may ask the patient to describe what he or she is thinking or feeling about the therapist when it appears that may be in the patient's near awareness (Halpert 1994; Ogden 1995).

Defense Mechanisms and Resistance

The psychotherapist attempts to clarify the patient's feelings and the meaning of what the patient is trying to say. At other times, the therapist may supportively confront the patient with attitudes the patient has disavowed but clearly demonstrates. In both cases the therapist is hoping to point out the kinds of thoughts and feelings that the patient obscures and the ways they are obscured, defended against, and kept unconscious. Throughout this process the patient's defensive ways of thinking are elucidated.

In the opening phase the therapist will have the opportunity to identify patterns of defense and resistance and must orient the patient to how awareness of these patterns can be used to advance the patient's knowledge of him- or herself (Loewald 1960).

Resistance is a general term referring to all the forces in the patient that oppose the painful work of therapy. There are many different categories of resistance, including general fear of any change, an overly harsh conscience that punishes a patient with the continuation of suffering, and the insistence on the gratification of childish impulses that forms part of an emotional illness. All people, including patients in therapy, employ mechanisms of defense to keep painful feelings and memories outside conscious awareness. These defense mechanisms are specific, discrete maneuvers or ways of thinking that the mind employs to avoid painful emotional material (Nemiah 1961; Shapiro 1965).

Whenever a patient is manifesting resistance, in whatever form, it is because the patient is protecting him- or herself from experiencing, including remembering or reliving, the old dangers and fears associated with the childhood conflicts and developmental difficulties of his or her life. Character (the set of expectable responses from a person in a given setting) is in great part a result of the defense mechanisms each person characteristically uses. Defenses are our cognitive mechanisms of structuring mental and emotional experience to keep psychic pain at a minimum and bring our interpersonal and intrapsychic functioning and relationships into some congruence with external reality.

The patient's defense mechanisms are an important source of resistance in psychotherapy. In 1936, Anna Freud, in *The Ego and the Mechanisms of Defense* (A. Freud 1966), outlined the functioning of many of these defense maneuvers. Since that time, the list has grown and been elaborated upon (Table 29–9). Several common and important mechanisms of defense are defined in Table 29–10. There are also more primitive mechanisms of defense—splitting, projection, projec-

TABLE 29–9. Defense mechanisms

Common defense mechanisms	Primitive defense mechanisms
Repression	Splitting
Denial	Projection
Reaction formation	Projective identification
Displacement	Omnipotence
Identification	Devaluing
Identification with the aggressor	Primitive identification
Intellectualization	
Isolation of affect	
Sublimation	

tive identification, omnipotence, devaluing, and primitive idealization—that are seen in severe personality disorders such as borderline personality disorder and psychotic disorders (Kernberg 1975).

In psychotherapy the therapist strives to help the patient understand the origins and functions of his or her defenses (i.e., the therapist interprets the defenses) so that the patient can become aware of the feelings, thoughts, and fantasies that the patient fears from the conflicts of long ago.

Use of Dreams

The therapist also attends to the dream life of the patient (Brenner 1976; S. Freud 1900/1953). Not all patients in psychotherapy work extensively with dreams, but many do, and for those who can, the work is an important tool. Every patient should be given the opportunity to work with dreams. It is in the opening phase that this road to understanding is introduced and learned. Frequently, dreams reported early in treatment are particularly revealing of the core conflicts of the patient. They can also serve to educate the patient about unconscious processes (Sharpe 1961). Dreams can be presented to the patient as thoughts and concerns the patient is having while asleep, although the rules for how these thoughts and concerns are created are different (i.e., primary process thinking) than during waking life (i.e., secondary process thinking) (Reiser 1994).

Countertransference

Countertransference is the emotional reaction of the therapist to the patient. Historically, countertransference was limited in meaning to the therapist's transfer-

TABLE 29–10.   Definitions of common mechanisms of defense

Repression	Among the first mechanisms of defense described by Sigmund Freud, this refers to the active pushing out of awareness of painful memories, feelings, and impulses.
Denial	Similar to repression, denial averts a patient's attention from painful ideas or feelings without making them completely unavailable to consciousness. A patient using denial simply ignores painful realities and acts as though they do not exist.
Reaction formation	Reaction formation consists of exaggerating one emotional trend to help repress the opposite emotion. The obsessional patient may manifest punctuality, parsimony, and cleanliness to defend against wishes to be tardy, extravagant, and messy.
Displacement	Displacement is changing the object of one's feelings to a safer one. The worker who is enraged by his boss and comes home, abuses his dog, and shouts at his family is a familiar example.
Identification with the aggressor	This is the tendency to imitate what the patient perceives as the aggressive and intimidating manner of someone toward him or her. Children who have been abused may become abusers themselves in adulthood, using identification with the aggressor as a defense.
Intellectualization	Intellectualization is the excessively factual, detailed, and cognitive way of talking about and experiencing emotionally charged topics without the feelings and associated affects.
Isolation of affect	Related to intellectualization, this is the repression of the feelings connected with a particular thought. Both intellectualization and isolation of affect are typical of obsessional patients in particular.
Sublimation	A mature mechanism of defense, sublimation is the hoped-for, healthy, nonconflicted evolution of primitive childhood impulses into a mature level of expression.

ence onto the patient. This was felt to be a response to the patient's transference. Like all transferences, the therapist's countertransference was the result of unconscious conflicts; however, these unresolved conflicts were those of the therapist rather than those of the patient. This countertransference was thought to obscure the therapist's judgment in conducting the therapy (Gabbard 1995; Gabbard and Wilkinson 2001).

Countertransferences are many and varied. Often they are the result of events occurring in the therapist's life that may make him or her more sensitive to certain themes in the patient's associations. The developmental period of the therapist's life—involving issues of intimacy, achievement, or old age, for example—may also affect how the therapist hears the patient. Intense transferences of all kinds—erotic, aggressive, devaluing, idealizing, and others—are ripe for serving as the stimulus to awaken in the therapist elements of his or her own past (Mitchell and Aron 1999).

When all one's patients seem to be talking about feeling overworked, or angry, or sad, the therapist can reflect on these feelings and wonder whether this theme is being selected by him or her rather than being the central issue for all of his or her patients. Finally, a common countertransference issue in training occurs at the end of training when both the therapist and the patient are dealing with termination. For the patient it is the end of treatment; for the therapist it is both the end of a treatment and the end of a stage of life, usually accompanied by a move and loss of colleagues and friends as well as a sense of new achievement.

The clinician may first note a patient's core conflictual issue through observing subtle emotional reactions stirred in him- or herself (Kernberg 1976; Searles 1979). The clinician can then explore these feelings, through self-analysis, as possible reverberations from the unconscious but also as emerging concerns of the patient that may be hidden in the patient's language, behavior, or fantasies.

The psychodynamic psychotherapist observes his or her own emotional reactions and values and processes them as possible windows on the patient's experience. Frequently, the more intense and even embarrassing the therapist's responses, the more likely they are to reflect a crucial, hidden, conflicted state residing within the patient. There are generally two types of countertransference reactions: concordant and complementary (Racker 1968; Table 29–11).

TABLE 29–11. Countertransference

Concordant countertransference

The therapist experiences and empathizes with the patient's emotional position (e.g., therapist thinks: "Boy, my patient is right! His boss sounds like a terrible person!").

Complementary countertransference

The therapist experiences and empathizes with the feelings of an important person from the patient's life (e.g., therapist thinks: "My patient is infuriating—I certainly see why his boss gets so angry at him!").

Termination

Often, psychodynamic psychotherapy is conducted in an open-ended fashion regardless of whether it is to be short or longer term. At the beginning of the treatment, the therapist explained to the patient that the treatment would take as long as required to discover and resolve the patient's unconscious core conflicts and for the patient to understand the workings of his or her mind.

There comes a time, however, when the patient and the psychiatrist agree that it is time to end the treatment. At this juncture the troublesome areas of the patient's personality seem to be separate from the core of the patient's sense of self (Alexander 1941). What was once central to the patient's presenting difficulties is now experienced as alien. The patient has learned to use intellect and perception in an affectively rich manner in the service of self-awareness (Dewald 1982).

The therapist must remember and the patient must come to realize that treatment goals are related to, but different from, the patient's life goals (Ticho 1972). Treatment goals are always dependent to some extent on life's demands and possibilities—what is possible at a given time of life and in a given context. Termination does not mean a patient has realized all of his or her hopes and wishes. Rather, the patient entering the end phase of treatment after a successful treatment has experienced substantial relief of psychological suffering, and this relief is evident to both the patient and the therapist. In addition, the internal conflicts of the patient, as well as the presenting symptoms, have been resolved, and reasonably permanent changes in behavior have occurred.

The patient shows a detailed understanding of the working of his or her mind and is beginning to use self-inquiry as a method of problem solving. Often there have been gains in most of these areas, although

not necessarily all. The gains are observed by the therapist and shared with the patient as part of the patient's increasing awareness of new areas of strength and conflict resolution (Table 29–12). The termination phase has its own tasks to consolidate the treatment and facilitate leave taking while maintaining the therapeutic relationship (Table 29–13).

TABLE 29–12. Criteria for termination

The patient…

Experiences relief of symptoms.

Experiences symptoms as alien.

Understands his or her characteristic defenses.

Is able to understand and recognize his or her characteristic transference responses.

Engages in ongoing self-inquiry as a method of resolving internal conflicts.

TABLE 29–13. Tasks of the termination phase

Review the treatment

The patient reviews the treatment, reconsidering his or her history and conflicts and placing in perspective what has been learned. Frequently the patient experiences a feeling of pride, strength, and gratitude to the therapist in this process while refreshing the "table of contents" of the patient's knowledge about him- or herself.

Experience the loss of the psychotherapy and the therapist

In termination, the patient experiences what is an essential and poignant aspect of the human condition: the experience of separation—the loss of a relationship with a person who has been very helpful and who often is perceived as kind and understanding. This loss may reawaken the conflicts of previous losses.

Reexperience and remaster the transference

Very often, in the context of termination, there is a recrudescence of the patient's symptoms and a return of old transference patterns and styles of interacting with the therapist.

Increase skills in self-inquiry as a method of problem solving

The patient now begins to take over the functions of the therapist. The patient increasingly exercises a greater degree of self-inquiry to resolve now well-known and well-understood internal conflicts.

Conclusion

Psychodynamic psychotherapy is now more than 100 years old. What began as "studies on hysteria" has broadened into the investigation and treatment of emotional illness throughout the human life cycle. Psychodynamic psychotherapy explores the subtleties of the effect of the mind–body connection. It examines the interaction of our neurobiology with our experiences across the life cycle and the effects on behavior and our internal as well as interpersonal lives. These patterns of early childhood—laid down on the basis of our biological givens, our early familial experiences, and our interpersonal world—form the lenses through which we view the world throughout our lives and give meaning to our adult experiences. Psychodynamic psychotherapy looks to change current mal-adaptive patterns of behavior through understanding the relationship of present symptomatic behaviors to past experiences that have provided the templates for these behaviors and for adult cognitive and emotional perception.

Further research is needed to develop the evidence base for better understanding the role of psychodynamic psychotherapy in the psychotherapy treatment armamentarium. In addition, the core concepts of psychodynamic psychotherapy—the role of conflict in our feelings, thoughts, and behaviors; the interaction of our neurobiology with our experiences throughout development and particularly in childhood; and the fact that we have feelings and thoughts outside of our awareness—require study across a wide array of health-related behaviors to identify new psychodynamically informed interventions and treatments.

Key Points

- Transference occurs in all interpersonal relationships.

- *Defense mechanisms* are cognitive mechanisms to decrease anxiety and other distressing feelings.

- Early childhood development structures brain development and leaves patterns of feelings, thoughts, behaviors, and interpersonal relating.

- Psychotherapy is an effective form of treatment, as effective as many other medical interventions.

- The working, reality-based relationship with the patient is called the *therapeutic alliance*.

- Psychodynamic psychotherapy may be brief, intermittent, or longer term.

- The principles of psychodynamic psychotherapy are used in many doctor–patient interactions other than psychodynamic psychotherapy.

Suggested Readings

Ellenberger HF: The Discovery of the Unconscious: The History and Evolution of Dynamic Psychiatry. New York, Basic Books, 1970

Foelsch PA, Levy KN, Hull JW, et al: The development of a psychodynamic treatment for patients with borderline personality disorder: a preliminary study of behavioral change. J Personal Disord 15:487–495, 2001

Freud S: The interpretation of dreams (1900), in The Standard Edition of the Complete Psychological Works of Sigmund Freud, Vols 4 and 5. Translated and edited by Strachey J. London, Hogarth Press, 1953

Freud S: The psychopathology of everyday life (1901), in The Standard Edition of the Complete Psychological Works of Sigmund Freud, Vol 6. Translated and edited by Strachey J. London, Hogarth Press, 1960

Gabbard GO: Long-Term Psychodynamic Psychotherapy: A Basic Text. Arlington, VA, American Psychiatric Publishing, 2004

Gabbard GO, Gabbard K: Psychiatry and the Cinema. Washington, DC, American Psychiatric Press, 1999

Kohut H: The Analysis of the Self: A Systematic Approach to the Psychoanalytic Treatment of Narcissistic Personality Disorders. New York, International Universities Press, 1971

Meissner WW: Freud and Psychoanalysis. Notre Dame, IN, University of Notre Dame Press, 2000

Stern DN: The Interpersonal World of the Infant: A View From Psychoanalysis and Developmental Psychology. New York, Basic Books, 2000

Ursano RJ, Sonnenberg SM, Lazar SG: Concise Guide to Psychodynamic Psychotherapy: Principles and Techniques of Brief, Intermittent, and Long-Term Psychodynamic Psychotherapy. Arlington, VA, American Psychiatric Publishing, 2004

References

Alexander F: The voice of the intellect is soft. Psychoanal Rev 28:12–29, 1941

American Psychiatric Association: Diagnostic and Statistical Manual of Mental Disorders, 4th Edition, Text Revision. Washington, DC, American Psychiatric Association, 2000

Bender DS: The therapeutic alliance in the treatment of personality disorders. J Psychiatr Pract 11:73–87, 2005

Blatt S, Shahar G: Psychoanalysis-with whom, for what and how? Comparisons with psychotherapy. J Am Psychoanal Assoc 52:393–447, 2004

Blatt S, Quinlan D, Pilkonis P, et al: Impact of perfectionism and need for approval on the brief treatment of depression: the National Institute of Mental Health Treatment of Depression Collaborative Research Program revisited. J Consult Clin Psychol 63:125–132, 1995

Bond M: Psychodynamic psychotherapy in the treatment of mood disorders. Curr Opin Psychiatry 19:40–43, 2006

Bond M, Perry C: Long-term changes in defense styles with psychodynamic psychotherapy for depressive, anxiety and personality disorders. Am J Psychiatry 161:1665–1671, 2004

Brenner C: Psychoanalytic Technique and Psychic Conflicts. New York, International Universities Press, 1976

Bruch H: Learning Psychotherapy: Rationale and Ground Rules. Cambridge, MA, Harvard University Press, 1974

Chessick RD: Psychoanalysis: clinical and theoretical. Am J Psychiatry 157:846–848, 2000

Clarkin JF, Foelsch PA, Levy KN, et al: The development of psychodynamic treatment for patients with borderline personality disorder: a preliminary study of behavioral change. J Personality Disord 15:487–495, 2001

Coleman JV: Aims and conduct of psychotherapy. Arch Gen Psychiatry 18:1–6, 1968

Crits-Christoph P: The efficacy of brief dynamic psychotherapy: a meta-analysis. Am J Psychiatry 149:151–158, 1992

Curtis HC: The concept of therapeutic alliance: implications for the "widening scope." J Am Psychoanal Assoc 27 (suppl):159–192, 1979

Dewald PA: The clinical importance of the termination phase. Psychoanal Inq 2:441–461, 1982

DiMascio A, Weissman M, Prusoff B, et al: Differential symptom reduction by drugs and psychotherapy in acute depression. Arch Gen Psychiatry 36:1450–1456, 1979

Edelson M: Telling and enacting stories in psychoanalysis and psychodynamic psychotherapy. Psychoanal Study Child 48:293–325, 1993

Etking A, Pittenger, C, Polan HJ, et al: Toward a neurobiology of psychotherapy: basic research and clinical applications. J Neuropsychiatry Clin Neurosci 17:145–158, 2005

Fawzy F, Kemeny M, Fawzy N, et al: A structured psychiatric intervention for cancer patients, II: changes over time in immunological measures. Arch Gen Psychiatry 47:729–735, 1990

Fawzy F, Fawzy N, Hyun C, et al: Malignant melanoma. Arch Gen Psychiatry 50:681–689, 1993

Fonagy P, Roth A, Higgitt A: Psychodynamic psychotherapies: evidence-based practice and clinical wisdom. Bull Menninger Clin 69:1–58, 2005

Freud A: The Ego and the Mechanisms of Defense, Revised Edition. New York, International Universities Press, 1966

Freud S: The interpretation of dreams (1900), in The Standard Edition of the Complete Psychological Works of Sigmund Freud, Vols 4 and 5. Translated and edited by Strachey J. London, England, Hogarth, 1953

Freud S: The dynamics of transference (1912), in The Standard Edition of the Complete Psychological Works of Sigmund Freud, Vol 12. Translated and edited by Strachey J. London, England, Hogarth, 1958, pp 97–108

Freud S: Resistance and repression (1917), in The Standard Edition of the Complete Psychological Works of Sigmund Freud, Vol 16. Translated and edited by Strachey J. London, England, Hogarth, 1963, pp 286–302

Fromm-Reichmann F: Principles of Intensive Psychotherapy. Chicago, IL, University of Chicago Press, 1950

Gabbard GO: Countertransference: the emerging common ground. Int J Psychoanal 76:475–485, 1995

Gabbard GO: Psychodynamic Psychiatry in Clinical Practice, 3rd Edition. Washington, DC, American Psychiatric Press, 2000

Gabbard GO: Psychodynamic Psychiatry in Clinical Practice, 4th Edition. Washington, DC, American Psychiatric Publishing, 2005

Gabbard GO, Wilkinson SM: Management of Countertransference With Borderline Patients. Washington, DC, American Psychiatric Publishing, 2001

Gabbard GO, Gunderson JG, Fonagy P: The place of psychoanalytic treatments within psychiatry. Arch Gen Psychiatry 59:505–510, 2002

Goldstein WN, Goldberg ST: The Transference in Psychotherapy. Northvale, NJ, Jason Aronson, 2003

Greenson RR: The working alliance and the transference neurosis. Psychoanal Q 34:155–181, 1965

Guthrie E, Moorey J, Margison F, et al: Cost effectiveness of brief psychodynamic-interpersonal therapy in high utilizers of psychiatric services Arch Gen Psychiatry 56:519–526, 1999

Hall J, Caleo S, Stevenson J, et al: An economic analysis of psychotherapy for borderline personality disorder patients. J Ment Health Policy Econ 4:3–8, 2001

Halpert E: Asclepius: magic in transference to physicians. Psychoanal Q 63:733–755, 1994

Hofer MA: Relationships as regulators: psychobiological perspective on bereavement. Psychosom Med 46:183–197, 1984

Horowitz MJ, Eells T, Singer J, et al: Role-relationship models for case formulation. Arch Gen Psychiatry 52:625–633, 1995

House JS, Landis KR, Umberson D: Social relationships and health. Science 241:540–545, 1988

Huttenlocher PR: Neural Plasticity. Cambridge, MA, Harvard University Press, 2002

Kandel ER: Biology and the future of psychoanalysis: a new framework for psychiatry revisited. Am J Psychiatry 156:505–524, 1999

Kernberg OF: Borderline Conditions and Pathological Narcissism. New York, Jason Aronson, 1975

Kernberg OF: Transference and countertransference in the treatment of borderline patients, in Object-Relations Theory and Clinical Psychoanalysis. New York, Jason Aronson, 1976, pp 161–184

Klerman G, DiMascio A, Weissman M, et al: Treatment of depression by drugs and psychotherapy. Am J Psychiatry 131:186–191, 1974

Lazar SG (ed): Extended dynamic psychotherapy: making the case in an era of managed care. Psychoanal Inq (special supplement):1–110, 1997

Lazare A, Eisenthal S: Clinician/patient relations, I: attending to the patient's perspective, in Outpatient Psychiatry. Edited by Lazare A. Baltimore, MD, Williams & Wilkins, 1989a, pp 125–136

Lazare A, Eisenthal S, Frank A: Clinician/Patient relations, II: conflict and negotiation, in Outpatient Psychiatry. Edited by Lazare A. Baltimore, MD, Williams & Wilkins, 1989b, pp 137–157

Leichsenring F: Are psychodynamic and psychoanalytic therapies effective? A review of empirical data. Int J Psychoanal 86:841–868, 2005

Leichsenring F, Leibing E: The effectiveness of psychodynamic therapy and cognitive behavior therapy in the treatment of personality disorders: a meta analysis. Am J Psychiatry 160:1223–1232, 2003

Leichsenring F, Rabung S, Leibing E: The efficacy of short-term psychodynamic psychotherapy in specific psychiatric disorders: a meta analysis. Arch Gen Psychiatry 61:1208–1216, 2004

Levinson D, Merrifield J, Berg K: Becoming a patient. Arch Gen Psychiatry 17:385–406, 1967

Loewald HW: On the therapeutic action of psycho-analysis. Int J Psychoanal 41:16–33, 1960

Luborsky L, Crits-Christoph P: Understanding Transference: The CCRT Method, 2nd Edition. Washington, DC, American Psychological Association Press, 1998

MacKinnon RA, Michels R, Buckley PJ (eds): The Psychiatric Interview in Clinical Practice, 2nd Edition. Washington, DC, American Psychiatric Publishing, 2006

Malan DH: Toward the Validation of Dynamic Psychotherapy. New York, Plenum, 1980

Malan DH, Heath ES, Baral HA, et al: Psychodynamic changes in untreated neurotic patients, II: apparently genuine improvement. Arch Gen Psychiatry 32:110–126, 1973

McEwen BS: Plasticity of the hippocampus: adaptation to chronic stress and allostatic load. Ann NY Acad Sci 933:265–277, 2001

McLaughlin JT: Transference, psychic reality, and countertransference. Psychoanal Q 50:639–664, 1981

McNeilly CL, Howard KI: The effects of psychotherapy: a re-evaluation based on dosage. Psychother Res 1:74–78, 1991

Meany MK: Maternal care, gene expression and the transmission of individual differences in stress reactivity across generations Annu Rev Neurosci 24:1161–1192, 2001

Milrod B, Busch F, Leon AC, et al: Open trial of psychodynamic psychotherapy for panic disorder: a pilot study. Am J Psychiatry 157:1878–1880, 2000

Mitchell S, Aron L (eds): Relational Psychoanalysis the Emergence of a Tradition. Hillsdale, NJ, Analytic Press, 1999

Mohl PC: Listening to the patient, in Psychiatry, 2nd Edition. Edited by Tasman A, Kaye J, Lieberman J. New York, Wiley, 2003, pp 3–18

Moran G, Fonagy P, Kurt A, et al: A controlled study of the psychoanalytic treatment of brittle diabetes. J Am Acad Child Adolesc Psychiatry 30:926–935, 1991

Nemiah JC: Foundations of Psychopathology. New York, Oxford University Press, 1961

Ogden TH: Analysing forms of aliveness and deadness of the transference-countertransference. Int J Psychoanal 76:695–709, 1995

Olfson M, Marcus SC, Druss B, et al: National trends in the use of outpatient psychotherapy. Am J Psychiatry 159:1914–1920, 2002

Perry S, Cooper AM, Michels R: The psychodynamic formulation: its purpose, structure and clinical application. Am J Psychiatry 144:543–550, 1987

Pine F: The four psychologies of psychoanalysis and their place in clinical work. J Am Psychoanal Assoc 36:571–596, 1988

Poland WS: On the analyst's neutrality. J Am Psychoanal Assoc 32:283–299, 1984

Racker H: Transference and Countertransference. New York, International Universities Press, 1968

Reiser MF: Memory in Mind and Brain: What Dream Imagery Reveals. New Haven, CT, Yale University Press, 1994

Rosenthal R: How are we doing in soft psychology? Am Psychol 45:775–777, 1990

Rosenthal R, Rubin DB: A simple, general-purpose display of magnitude of experimental effect. J Educ Psychol 74:166–169, 1982

Sandler J, Dare C, Holder A: The Patient and the Analyst: The Basis of the Psychoanalytic Process. New York, International Universities Press, 1973

Schafer R: The atmosphere of safety: Freud's "Papers on Technique" (1911–1915), in The Analytic Attitude. New York, Basic Books, 1983, pp 14–33

Searles HF: Countertransference and Related Subjects. New York, International Universities Press, 1979

Shapiro D: Neurotic Styles. New York, Basic Books, 1965

Sharpe EF: Dream Analysis. London, England, Hogarth Press, 1961

Silberman EK, Certa K: The psychiatric interview: settings and techniques, in Psychiatry, 2nd Edition. Edited by Tasman A, Kaye J, Lieberman J. New York, Wiley, 2003, pp 30–51

Smith ML, Glass GV, Miller TI: The Benefits of Psychotherapy. Baltimore, MD, Johns Hopkins University Press, 1980

Sonnenberg SM: Analytic listening and the analyst's self-analysis. Int J Psychoanal 76:335–342, 1995

Sonnenberg SM, Sutton L, Ursano RJ: Physician–patient relationship, in Psychiatry. Edited by Tasman A, Kaye J, Lieberman J. Philadelphia, PA, WB Saunders, 1996, pp 41–49

Sonnenberg SM, Ursano AM, Ursano RJ: Physician–patient relationship, in Psychiatry, 2nd Edition. Edited by Tasman A, Kay J, Lieberman JA. New York, Wiley, 2003, pp 52–63

Spiegel D, Bloom J, Kraemer H, et al: Effect of psychosocial treatment on survival of patients with metastatic breast cancer. Lancet 2:888–891, 1989

Stone L: Notes on the noninterpretive elements in the psychoanalytic situation and process. J Am Psychoanal Assoc 29:89–118, 1981

Sullivan HS: The Psychiatric Interview. New York, WW Norton, 1954

Ticho E: Termination of psychoanalysis: treatment goals, life goals. Psychoanal Q 41:315–333, 1972

Ursano RJ, Fullerton CS: Psychotherapy: medical intervention and the concept of normality, in Normality: Context and Theory. Edited by Offer D, Sabshin M. New York, Basic Books, 1991, pp 39–59

Ursano RJ, Silberman EK: Individual psychotherapies, in The American Psychiatric Press Textbook of Psychiatry. Edited by Talbott JA, Hales RE, Yudofsky SC. Washington, DC, American Psychiatric Press, 1988, pp 855–889

Ursano RJ, Silberman EK, Diaz A Jr: The psychotherapies: basic theoretical principles, techniques and indications, in Clinical Psychiatry for Medical Students. Edited by Stoudemire A. Philadelphia, PA, JB Lippincott, 1990, pp 855–890

Weissman MM, Verdell H, Gameroff JM, et al: National survey of psychotherapy training psychiatry, psychology and social work. Arch Gen Psychiatry 63:925–934, 2006

Winkley K, Ismail K, Landau S, et al: Psychological interventions to improve glycaemic control in patients with type 1 diabetes: systematic review and meta-analysis of randomized controlled trials. BMJ 333:55–56, 2006

Zetzel ER: Current concepts of transference. Int J Psychoanal 37:369–376, 1956

30

INTERPERSONAL PSYCHOTHERAPY

John C. Markowitz, M.D.

Interpersonal psychotherapy (IPT) is a time-limited treatment developed in the 1970s for adult outpatients with major depression by the late Gerald L. Klerman, M.D., and Myrna M. Weissman, Ph.D. IPT is well known as a research intervention, having been tested in numerous randomized, controlled clinical trials. In recent years it has begun to spread into clinical practice. In this chapter I review the research-defined indications and outline the general conduct of this relatively simple yet potent psychotherapy.

IPT is a straightforward, manual-based, focused, pragmatic, and optimistic time-limited treatment that targets particular psychiatric disorders. It was first devised and has been best tested as a treatment of major depressive episodes. IPT has two basic premises (Table 30–1): first, that depression is a medical illness that is treatable and not the patient's fault; and second, that the disorder does not occur in a vacuum but rather is influenced by and itself affects the patient's psychosocial environment. The goal of treatment is to help the patient solve a difficulty in his or her role functioning or social environment. Doing so helps the patient gain a sense of mastery over his or her functioning and relieves depressive symptoms.

IPT was defined in a manual (Klerman et al. 1984; updated by Weissman et al. 2000) and tested in randomized clinical trials. Evidence for efficacy in research trials for patients with major depressive disorder led to its adaptation and testing for other mood disorders, including modifications for adolescent and geriatric de-

TABLE 30–1. **Premises and goals of interpersonal therapy**

Axioms

1. Depression is a medical illness that is treatable and not the patient's fault.

2. Depression is influenced by and affects the patient's psychosocial environment.

Goals

The primary goal of treatment is to help the patient solve a difficulty in role functioning or social environment. This

1. Relieves symptoms.

2. Improves the patient's environment.

3. Builds social skills.

4. Fosters a sense of mastery over the environment.

pressed patients, patients with bipolar and dysthymic disorders, depressed HIV-positive or pregnant patients, and depressed primary care patients. It has also been tested and modified for nonmood disorders, including bulimia, substance abuse, and, increasingly, anxiety disorders. IPT has also been adapted for use as a maintenance treatment to forestall relapse and recurrence of depressive episodes, for couples and group formats, for use as a telephone intervention, and for a patient self-help guide (Weissman et al. 2000, 2007).

Begun as a research intervention, IPT has lately begun to spread among clinicians and in residency training programs. There have been increasing requests for training in IPT following the publication of efficacy data and the promulgation of practice guidelines that embrace IPT among antidepressant treatments. Managed care and economic pressures have also aroused interest in defined, time-limited, empirically supported treatments like IPT. Practice guidelines for mental health professionals (Karasu et al. 1993) and primary care practitioners (Agency for Health Care Policy and Research 1993a, 1993b, 1993c, 1993d) each discussed IPT as an acute and maintenance treatment for depression, used alone and in combination with medication.

The American Psychiatric Association practice guidelines for adults with major depression included IPT among the few recommended psychotherapies. The guidelines did not require efficacy data from controlled clinical trials as an inclusion criterion. IPT was deemed useful for patients in the "midst of recent conflicts with significant others and for those having difficulty adjusting to an altered career or social role or other life transition" (Karasu et al. 1993, p. 6)—that is, for depression associated with life events or interpersonal conflicts. Although many patients do present with such recent life changes, the empirical support for IPT among depressed patients generally—some of which is documented here—makes these appear to be minimal, conservative indications.

Primary care guidelines for depression are composed of four volumes (Agency for Health Care Policy and Research 1993a, 1993b, 1993c, 1993d). Both the physician and the patient guides list IPT, as well as cognitive-behavioral therapy (CBT; Beck et al. 1979), behavioral therapy, brief dynamic therapy, and marital therapy, as treatments for depression. IPT is recommended as an acute treatment for nonpsychotic depression to remove symptoms, prevent relapse and recurrence, correct provoking psychological problems with secondary symptom resolution, and address secondary consequences of depression. The guidelines state that medication alone may suffice to prevent relapse or recurrence and to maintain remitted patients with recurrent depression (E. Frank et al. 1990, 1991). These guidelines consider IPT, CBT, and behavioral treatments "effective in most cases of mild-to-moderate depression" (Agency for Health Care Policy and Research 1993b, p. 12), but indications "for continuation phase psychotherapy are unclear" (p. 18) even

though "two studies are suggestive that continuation psychotherapy may reduce the relapse rate" (p. 18). The patient guidelines list behavioral therapy, cognitive therapy, and IPT as the "most well-studied [sic] for their effectiveness in reducing symptoms of major depressive disorder" (Agency for Health Care Policy and Research 1993d, p. 23).

IPT is spreading from its initial research base in the United States. The IPT manual has been translated into Italian, German, Japanese, and Spanish and is being used more widely around the world. Descriptions of IPT have appeared in Spanish (Puig 1995) and Dutch (Blom et al. 1996) journals. The International Society for Interpersonal Psychotherapy (www.interpersonalpsychotherapy.org), established at the American Psychiatric Association Annual Meeting in May 2000 in Chicago, Illinois, has been meeting regularly. (For a complete description of IPT technique, see Weissman et al. 2000; for the patient guide, see Weissman 1995; for the group adaptation, see Wilfley et al. 2000; for the adaptation for depressed adolescents, see Mufson et al. 2004a; for dysthymic disorder, see Markowitz 1998; for bipolar disorder, see E. Frank 2005.)

Background: Theoretical and Empirical Sources

IPT is based on interpersonal theory deriving from the post–World War II work of Adolph Meyer, Harry Stack Sullivan (1953), and later John Bowlby (1973) and others. The principle abstracted from these theories is that life events occurring after the early childhood years influence psychopathology. Social supports protect against psychopathology, whereas social losses may trigger symptoms in vulnerable individuals. IPT uses this principle for practical, not etiological, purposes. It does not presume to discern the *cause* of a depressive episode—the etiology of depression being multifactorial—but pragmatically uses the connection between current life events and the onset of depressive symptoms to help the patient understand and combat his or her episode of illness. IPT is also based on psychosocial and life events research of depression, which bolstered these theories by demonstrating relationships between depression and complicated bereavement, role disputes (e.g., bad marriages), role transitions (and meaningful life changes), and interpersonal deficits (Table 30–2).

TABLE 30–2. Theoretical and empirical sources of interpersonal psychotherapy

I. **Interpersonal theory**

    A. Importance of current life events to psychopathology (Meyer, Sullivan, and others)

    B. Attachment theory (Bowlby)

II. **Empirical support: association of depressive episodes with**

    A. Complicated bereavement (grief)

    B. Marital and other interpersonal disputes (role disputes)

    C. Life events (role transitions)

    D. Isolation and lack of social support (interpersonal deficits)

Conducting IPT

General Principles

IPT therapists define depression as a *medical illness,* a treatable condition that is not the patient's fault. This definition displaces the burdensome guilt of the depressed patient from the patient him- or herself to the illness, making the symptoms ego-dystonic and discrete. It also provides hope for a response to treatment. The therapist uses DSM-IV-TR (American Psychiatric Association 2000) to make a diagnosis and rating scales such as the Hamilton Rating Scale for Depression (HRSD; Hamilton 1960) or Beck Depression Inventory (BDI; Beck 1978) to assess and explain the depressive symptoms. This helps the patient to recognize that he or she is dealing with a common mood disorder with a predictable set of symptoms and not the personal failure, weakness, or character flaw that the depressed patient often believes to be the problem. To underscore this approach, IPT therapists give depressed patients the "sick role" (Parsons 1951), excusing them from what their illness prevents them from doing while obliging them to work as patients in order to recover the healthy role they have lost.

By solving an interpersonal problem—a complicated bereavement, a role dispute or transition, or an interpersonal deficit—the IPT patient has an opportunity to both improve his or her life situation and simultaneously relieve the symptoms of the depressive episode. This coupled formula has been validated by randomized, controlled trials in which IPT has been tested and thus can be offered with confidence and

optimism. Symptomatic relief may correlate with the degree to which the patient solves his or her interpersonal crisis (Markowitz et al. 2006a). This therapeutic optimism, although hardly specific to IPT, very likely provides part of its power in re-moralizing the patient.

An eclectic therapy, IPT uses techniques seen in other treatment approaches. For example, IPT employs a medical model of depressive illness consistent with pharmacotherapy (making it highly compatible in combination with medication). It shares role-playing and a "here and now" focus with CBT and addresses interpersonal issues in a manner familiar to marital therapists. It is not the specific techniques but rather the overall strategies that make IPT a unique and coherent approach. Although IPT overlaps to some degree with psychodynamic psychotherapies and many of its early research therapists came from psychodynamic backgrounds, IPT also meaningfully differs from them in its focus on the present, not the past; its focus on real-life change rather than self-understanding; its medical model; and its avoidance of the transference and of genetic and dream interpretations (Markowitz et al. 1998b). Although, like CBT, it is a time-limited treatment targeting a syndromal constellation (e.g., major depression), IPT is considerably less structured, assigns no explicit homework, and focuses on interpersonal problem areas rather than automatic thoughts. Each of the four IPT interpersonal problem areas has discrete—if to some degree overlapping—goals for therapist and patient to pursue.

IPT techniques aid the patient's pursuit of these interpersonal goals. The therapist repeatedly helps the patient relate life events to mood and other symptoms. Techniques include an *opening question* that elicits an interval history of mood and events; a *communication analysis,* which is a reconstruction and evaluation of recent affectively charged life circumstances; an *exploration of the patient's wishes and options* in order to pursue those wishes in particular interpersonal situations; a *decision analysis* to help the patient choose which options to employ; and *role playing* to help patients prepare tactics for real life.

IPT deals with current rather than past interpersonal relationships, focusing on the patient's immediate social context. The IPT therapist attempts to intervene in symptom formation and social dysfunction associated with depression rather than addressing enduring aspects of personality. Personality is, in any case, difficult to accurately assess during an episode of an Axis I disorder such as depression (Hirschfeld et al. 1983). IPT does build new social skills (Weissman et al. 1981), which may be as valuable as changing personality traits. One study found that maintenance IPT for recurrent depression reduced Axis II Cluster C symptoms over time (Cyranowski et al. 2004).

Phases of Treatment

As an acute treatment, IPT has three phases (Table 30–3). The *early phase,* which usually lasts for one to three sessions, includes a diagnostic evaluation, psychiatric anamnesis, and setting the framework for the treatment. The therapist reviews symptoms, diagnoses the patient as depressed by standard criteria (American Psychiatric Association 2000), and gives the patient the sick role (Parsons 1951). The psychiatric history includes the "interpersonal inventory," a careful review of the patient's past and current social functioning and close relationships, and the patterns in and mutual expectations within those relationships. (The interpersonal inventory is not a structured instrument.) This evaluatory interview elucidates changes in relationships proximal to the onset of symptoms, such as death of a loved one, children leaving home, worsening marital strife, or isolation from a confidant. This review provides a framework for understanding the social and interpersonal context of the onset of depressive symptoms and provides the basis for a treatment focus.

Having assessed the need for medication based on symptom severity, past history and treatment response, and patient preference, the therapist educates the patient about depression by discussing the constellation of symptoms that define major depression, their psychosocial concomitants, and what the patient may expect from treatment. The therapist next links the depressive syndrome to the patient's interpersonal situation in a formulation (Markowitz and Swartz 1997) centered on one of four interpersonal problem areas: 1) *grief,* 2) interpersonal *role disputes,* 3) *role transitions,* or 4) *interpersonal deficits* (Table 30–4). If the patient explicitly accepts this formulation as a focus for subsequent treatment, therapy enters the middle phase.

It is important to keep treatment focused on a simple theme that even a highly distractible depressed patient can grasp. Any formulation necessarily simplifies a patient's complex situation. Although some patients may present with multiple interpersonal problems, the goal of the formulation is to isolate one or, at most, two salient problems related to the patient's mood disorder (whether as precipitant or consequence). More than two foci would mean no focus at all. The choice of focal problem area depends on clinical acumen, although research has shown that IPT therapists do agree in choosing such areas (Markowitz et al. 2000), and patients find the foci credible.

In the *middle phase,* the IPT therapist pursues strategies specific to the chosen interpersonal problem area. For *grief*—complicated bereavement following the death of a loved one—the therapist facilitates the catharsis of mourning and helps the patient find new activities and relationships to compensate for the loss. *Role disputes* are conflicts with significant others, such as a spouse, other family member, coworker, or close friend. The therapist helps the patient explore the relationship, the nature of the dispute, whether it has reached an impasse, and available options to negotiate its resolution. If these options fail, therapist and patient may conclude that the relationship has reached an impasse and consider ways to change the impasse or to end the relationship. *Role transition* includes change in life status, for example, beginning or ending a relationship or career, moving, receiving a promotion, retiring, graduating, or receiving a diagnosis of a(nother) medical illness. The patient learns to manage the change by mourning the loss of the old role while recognizing positive and negative aspects of the new role he or she is assuming and taking steps to gain mastery over the new role. *Interpersonal deficits,* the poorly named residual fourth IPT problem area, is used for patients who lack one of the first three problem areas—that is, patients who report no recent life events. This focus defines the patient as isolated and lacking social skills, including having problems in initiating or sustaining relationships; the goal is to help the patient to develop new relationships and skills. Some patients who might seem to fall into this category may in fact have dysthymic disorder, for which separate strategies have been developed (Markowitz 1998).

IPT sessions address present "here and now" problems rather than childhood or developmental issues. Sessions open with the question: "How have things been since we last met?" This focuses the patient on recent interpersonal events and recent mood, which the therapist helps the patient to link. Therapists take an active, nonneutral, supportive, and hopeful stance to counter the depressed patient's pessimism. They elicit and emphasize the options that exist for change in the patient's life, options that the depressive episode may have kept the patient from seeing or exploring fully. Understanding the situation does not suffice: therapists stress the need for patients to test these options in order to improve their lives and simultaneously treat their depressive episodes. Over the course of therapy, the IPT therapist repeats measurements such as the HRSD to gauge for both the therapist and the patient the latter's progress.

The *termination phase* of IPT, occupying the last

TABLE 30–3. Phases of interpersonal psychotherapy (IPT)

I. Early phase

  A. Deal with the depression

    1. Review depressive symptoms

    2. Name the syndrome: formal diagnosis

    3. Provide psychoeducation about depression and its treatment

    4. Give patient the "sick role"

    5. Evaluate need for medication

  B. Relate depression to interpersonal context: interpersonal inventory

    1. Nature of interaction with significant persons

    2. Reciprocal expectations of patient and significant others, and whether these were fulfilled

    3. Satisfying and unsatisfying aspects of relationships

    4. Recent changes in key relationships

    5. Changes patient desires in relationships

  C. Identify the major problem area

    1. Determine problem area related to current episode and set treatment goals.

    2. Which relationship is related to the episode? What might change in it?

  D. Explain IPT concepts and contract

    1. Outline understanding of the problem: formulation

    2. Agree on treatment goals (focal problem area)

      a. brief treatment (time limit)

      b. target is depression (not character)

    3. Describe IPT procedures: "here and now" focus, need to discuss important concerns; review of current interpersonal relations; discussion of practical aspects of treatment

II. Middle phase

Specific strategies for treating grief, role dispute, role transition, or interpersonal deficits

III. Termination phase

  A. Consolidate gains

  B. Foster independence

  C. Address guilt (and blame therapy) if nonresponder

  D. Review risk of relapse and recurrence

  E. Recontract for continuation and maintenance treatment if appropriate

---

TABLE 30–4. Interpersonal psychotherapy problem areas

Grief (complicated bereavement)

Role dispute

Role transition

Interpersonal deficits (only if none of above appropriate)

---

few sessions of acute treatment or last months of maintenance treatment, builds on the patient's newly regained sense of independence and competence by recognizing and consolidating therapeutic gains. The therapist secures self-esteem by underscoring that the patient's depressive episode has improved because of his or her actions in changing a life situation—and this at a time when the patient had felt weak and impotent. The therapist also helps the patient to anticipate triggers for and responses to depressive symptoms that might arise in the future. Compared with psychodynamic psychotherapy, IPT deemphasizes termination: it is a graduation from successful treatment. The sadness of parting from the therapist is distinguished from depressive feelings. If the patient has not improved, the therapist emphasizes that the *treatment* has failed, not the patient, and that alternative effective treatment options exist. Patients with multiple prior major depressive episodes or significant residual symptoms who successfully complete acute treatment but remain at high risk for recurrence may contract for maintenance therapy as acute treatment draws to a close.

Case Example

Ms. A, a 37-year-old married Roman Catholic Latina businesswoman, presented with a 4-month history of major depression. Her presenting 24-item HRSD score was 28. Symptoms included a depressed and anxious mood with diurnal variation, exhaustion due to insomnia, difficulty concentrating at work, and moments of passive suicidal ideation. Although she initially felt that her symptoms had arisen out of the blue, her therapist's history taking connected this depressive episode to recent life events. She had recently been promoted at work, an achievement that pleased her but also meant greater responsibilities and more time spent away from home. Her 4-year-old daughter complained about this, and her husband intensified pressure to have a second child. She felt that her husband misunderstood her difficult role as a "modern mother."

Ms. A had had one prior episode of depression 14 years before, shortly after her college graduation and on the brink of her marriage. That episode had been milder and had resolved with a course of antidepressant medication. She had no history of substance abuse, suicide attempts, or previous psychotherapy. Her family history was notable for maternal depression and for a brother's alcohol abuse. Her interpersonal inventory revealed that she had a few close friends in whom she was more likely to confide than her husband. She also counted on her family of origin for support. Her marriage had many positive aspects but was limited by her lawyer husband's "macho," authoritarian attitude. She felt she was supposed to defer to him, and thus she resentfully complied.

Ms. A was reluctant to take antidepressant medication. Her therapist diagnosed her as having a recurrent major depressive episode, explained her HRSD score, and suggested that the episode was related to an ongoing role dispute with her husband that had been exacerbated by her promotion. (Because her work was going well and she felt less conflicted about this aspect of her life, the therapist focused on the role dispute rather than the role transition.) Ms. A agreed to a 12-week course of IPT and was given the sick role.

Sessions focused on marital communication. Ms. A was fearful of her husband's anger. After role-playing what she wanted to say, and in what tone of voice, she risked confronting him. Ms. A explained to her husband how important her new job was to her and asked him for support in building her career and in caring for their daughter. They discussed compromises about work hours. She was initially discouraged when her husband reacted angrily in one of these discussions. Ms. A and her therapist then reviewed the encounter and explored options for how she could broach the topic at a calmer time of the week than previously. They role-played this interaction, with Ms. A testing different expressions of her feeling and different tones of voice. The next encounter, after the fourth week, was more successful, and in the following week she and her husband had two more productive talks and planned their first family vacation in some time. Ms. A was already feeling much better (her HRSD score at this time was 10) and on better terms with her husband. Their daughter was happier as the result of more attention from both parents. On the subsequent vacation they agreed that it would probably make more sense for them not to have another child.

By week 9 Ms. A was euthymic, functioning well both at work and at home. Her HRSD score was 5. During the termination phase, the IPT therapist emphasized that Ms. A's improvement was due to her own actions, to her finding more effective ways to communicate with her husband in resolving their role dispute. Although they were terminating acute treatment, the therapist pointed out that Ms. A had now had two episodes of major depression and was at significant risk for a third. Accordingly, they agreed to continuation treatment with monthly sessions of IPT.

IPT for Mood Disorders: Efficacy and Adaptations

The steady growth in IPT outcome research precludes description of all such studies. What follows is a selection of key research on IPT for mood and other disorders (Table 30–5).

Acute Treatment of Major Depression

IPT was first tested as an acute antidepressant treatment in a 16-week four-cell randomized trial. This compared IPT, amitriptyline, their combination, and a nonscheduled control treatment for 81 outpatients with major depression (DiMascio et al. 1979; Weissman et al. 1979). Amitriptyline alleviated symptoms more quickly, but no significant difference appeared between IPT and amitriptyline in symptom reduction at the end of treatment. Each active treatment reduced

TABLE 30–5. **Empirically based indications for interpersonal psychotherapy**

Major depression

    Acute

    Recurrent (prophylaxis)

    Geriatric patients

    Adolescent patients

    HIV-positive patients

    Primary care patients

    Conjoint therapy for depressed married women

    Postpartum and antepartum patients

Dysthymic disorder[a]

Bipolar disorder (adjunctive treatment)

Interpersonal counseling for **subsyndromal depression**

Bulimia (individual or group format)

Social phobia[b]

Posttraumatic stress disorder[b]

[a]Limited efficacy.
[b]Preliminary results encouraging.

symptoms more efficaciously than the nonscheduled control, and combined amitriptyline–IPT was more efficacious than either active monotherapy. Patients with psychotic depression did poorly on IPT alone. Naturalistic follow-up at 1 year found that many patients sustained improvement from the brief IPT intervention and that IPT patients had developed significantly better psychosocial functioning regardless of whether they received medication. This effect on social function was not found for amitriptyline alone, nor had it been evident for IPT immediately after the 16-week trial (Weissman et al. 1981).

In the landmark multisite National Institute of Mental Health Treatment of Depression Collaborative Research Program (TDCRP; Elkin et al. 1989), investigators randomly assigned 250 outpatients with major depression to 16 weeks of IPT, CBT, or either imipramine or placebo plus clinical management. Most subjects completed at least 15 weeks or 12 treatment sessions. Patients with milder depression (17-item HRSD score <20) improved equally in all four treatments. Among the more severely depressed patients (HRSD score ≥20), imipramine worked fastest and most consistently outperformed placebo. IPT was comparable to imipramine on several outcome measures, including HRSD score, and was superior to placebo for more severely depressed patients. CBT was not superior to

placebo among the more depressed patients.

Klein and Ross (1993), reanalyzing the TDCRP study data using the Johnson-Neyman technique, found an ordering for treatment efficacy with "medication superior to psychotherapy, [and] the psychotherapies somewhat superior to placebo...particularly among the symptomatic and impaired patients" (Klein and Ross 1993, p. 241). The authors found CBT "relatively inferior to IPT for patients with BDI scores greater than approximately 30, generally considered the boundary between moderate and severe depression" (p. 247). The reanalysis does not contradict the report of Elkin et al. (1989) but rather sharpens the differences among treatments.

In an 18-month naturalistic follow-up study of the TDCRP study subjects, Shea et al. (1992) found no significant difference in recovery among remitters (who had minimal or no symptoms after the end of treatment, sustained during follow-up) among the four treatments. Thirty percent of CBT, 26% of IPT, 19% of imipramine, and 20% of placebo subjects who had acutely remitted remained in remission during that time span. Among acute remitters, relapse over the 18-month follow-up was 36% for CBT, 33% for IPT, 50% for imipramine (medication having been stopped at 16 weeks), and 33% for placebo. The authors concluded that, for many patients, 16 weeks of specific treatments were insufficient to achieve full and lasting recovery.

A research group in the Netherlands compared IPT, nefazodone, IPT plus nefazodone, and placebo plus nefazodone in a randomized controlled trial for 193 patients with major depressive disorder. On the MADRS (although not on the primary outcome instrument, the HRSD), the combination of IPT and nefazodone more effectively reduced symptoms than did nefazodone alone, although it was not more effective than IPT alone or IPT plus placebo (Blom et al. 2007).

Maintenance Treatment

IPT was initially developed for and tested in an 8-month six-cell trial (Paykel et al. 1975; Weissman et al. 1974). Today this study would be considered a "continuation" treatment, because the concept of long-term maintenance antidepressant treatment has lengthened. Acutely depressed outpatient women ($N=150$) who had responded (≥50% symptom reduction rated by a clinical interviewer) to a 4- to 6-week acute phase of amitriptyline were randomly assigned to receive 8 months of weekly IPT alone, amitriptyline alone, placebo alone, combined IPT–amitriptyline or IPT–placebo, or no pill. Randomization to IPT or a low-contact psychotherapy condition occurred at entry into the continuation phase, whereas randomization to medication, placebo, or no pill occurred at the end of the second month of continuation. Maintenance pharmacotherapy prevented relapse and symptom exacerbation, whereas IPT improved social functioning (Weissman et al. 1974). The effects of IPT on social functioning did not appear for 6–8 months. Combined psychotherapy–pharmacotherapy had the best outcome.

Longer antidepressant maintenance trials of IPT have been conducted in Pittsburgh. E. Frank et al. (1990, 1991) studied 128 outpatients with multiply and rapidly recurrent depression. Patients were initially treated with combined high-dosage (>200 mg/day) imipramine and weekly IPT. Responders remained on high-dosage medication while IPT was tapered to a monthly frequency during a 4-month continuation phase. Patients who remained in remission were then randomly assigned to 3 years of either 1) ongoing high-dosage imipramine plus clinical management; 2) high-dosage imipramine plus monthly IPT; 3) monthly IPT alone; 4) monthly IPT plus placebo; or 5) placebo plus clinical management. The investigators found high-dosage imipramine to be the most efficacious treatment, protecting more than 80% of patients over 3 years. In contrast, most patients given placebo relapsed within the first few months. Once-monthly IPT, although less efficacious than medication, was statistically and clinically superior to the placebo condition in this high-risk patient population. Reynolds et al. (1999) essentially replicated these maintenance findings in a study of geriatric patients with major depression.

Women of childbearing age are the modal patients with depression. The study finding of an 82-week survival time without recurrence with IPT alone would suffice to protect many women with recurrent depression through pregnancy and nursing without medication. Further study is required to determine the efficacy of IPT relative to newer medications (e.g., selective serotonin reuptake inhibitors) and the efficacy of more-frequent-than-monthly doses of maintenance IPT. In a study of differing doses of maintenance IPT for 233 recurrently depressed women, E. Frank et al. (2007) found no differences in outcome based on frequency of sessions. Perhaps optimal dosing of maintenance IPT depends on individual patients' needs.

Geriatric Depressed Patients

IPT was first used with geriatric depressed patients as an addition to a 6-week pharmacotherapy trial in order to enhance compliance and to provide some treatment for the placebo control group (Rothblum et al. 1982; Sholomskas et al. 1983). The investigators noted that

grief and role transition specific to life changes were the prime focus of treatment. They suggested modifications of IPT, including more flexible duration of sessions, greater use of practical advice and support (e.g., arranging transportation, calling the physician), and recognition that major role changes may be impractical and detrimental (e.g., divorce at age 75 years). The 6-week trial compared standard IPT with nortriptyline treatment in 30 geriatric depressed patients. Results showed some advantages for IPT, largely because of higher attrition in the medication group due to nortriptyline side effects (Sloane et al. 1985).

Reynolds et al. (1999) conducted a 3-year maintenance study for geriatric patients with recurrent depression in Pittsburgh, Pennsylvania, using IPT and nortriptyline in a design similar to that of the E. Frank et al. (1990) study. The IPT manual was modified to allow more flexible lengths of sessions, under the assumption that some elderly patients might not tolerate 50-minute sessions. The authors found that older patients needed to address early life relationships in their psychotherapy, a distinction from the typical "here and now" focus of IPT. Like Sholomskas et al. (1983), they felt that therapists needed to help patients solve practical problems and to acknowledge that some problems may not be amenable to resolutions, such as existential late-life issues or lifelong psychopathology (Rothblum et al. 1982). Elderly depressed patients whose sleep quality normalized by early continuation phase had an 80% chance of remaining well during the first year of maintenance treatment. The response rate was similar for patients who subsequently received either nortriptyline or IPT.

Reynolds et al. (1999) acutely treated 187 geriatric patients (60 years and older) with recurrent major depression using the combination of IPT and nortriptyline. One hundred seven patients remitted and then reached recovery after continuation therapy. They were randomly assigned to one of four 3-year maintenance conditions: 1) medication clinic with nortriptyline alone, with steady-state nortriptyline plasma levels maintained in a therapeutic window of 80–120 ng/mL; 2) medication clinic with placebo; 3) monthly maintenance IPT with placebo; or 4) monthly maintenance IPT plus nortriptyline. Recurrence rates were 43% for nortriptyline alone, 90% for placebo, 64% for IPT with placebo, and 20% for combined treatment. Each monotherapy was statistically superior to placebo, whereas combined therapy showed superiority to IPT alone and a trend for superiority over medication alone.

Patients in their 70s were more likely to have recurrence and to do so more quickly than patients in their 60s. This study corroborated the maintenance findings of E. Frank and colleagues, with the difference that combined treatment had advantages over pharmacotherapy alone for the geriatric population. In a follow-up study, Reynolds et al. (2006) again found that once-monthly maintenance IPT was not efficacious in preventing relapse of depressed patients 70 years or older who had responded to the combination of IPT and paroxetine.

The comparison of high-dosage tricyclic antidepressants with low-dose maintenance IPT in both the E. Frank et al. (1990, 1991) and the Reynolds et al. (1999) studies is easy to misinterpret. Had the tricyclics been lowered comparably with the reduced psychotherapy dosage, recurrence in the medication groups might well have been greater. Yet because there were no precedents for this research, the choice of a monthly dosing interval for maintenance IPT was reasonable and indeed showed some benefit.

Depressed Adolescents

Mufson et al. (1999) modified IPT to incorporate adolescent developmental issues (IPT-A). They conducted an open feasibility and follow-up trial and then a controlled 12-week clinical trial comparing IPT-A with clinical monitoring in 48 clinic-referred adolescents ages 12–18 years who met DSM-III-R (American Psychiatric Association 1987) criteria for major depressive disorder. Patients were seen biweekly by a blind independent evaluator to assess symptomatology, social functioning, and social problem-solving skills. Thirty-two of the 48 patients completed the protocol (21 IPT-A, 11 control).

Patients who received IPT-A reported significantly greater improvement of depressive symptoms and overall social functioning, including functioning with friends and problem-solving skills. In the intent-to-treat sample, 75% of IPT-A patients met the criterion for recovery (HRSD score ≤ 6), compared with 46% of control patients. The findings support the feasibility, patient acceptance, and efficacy of 12 weeks of IPT-A with acutely depressed adolescents in reducing depressive symptomatology and improving social functioning and interpersonal problem-solving skills (Mufson et al. 1999). Mufson et al. (2004b) then tested IPT-A in an effectiveness study in school-based clinics, where they found it markedly superior to treatment as usual. The same group is now studying IPT-A in a group format for depressed adolescents (Mufson et al. 2004c).

Rosello, Bernal, and Rivera at the University of Puerto Rico compared 12 weeks of randomly assigned IPT (*n*=22), CBT (*n*=25), and a wait-list control condition (*n*=24) for adolescents ages 13–18 who met DSM-III-R criteria for major depression, dysthymia, or both. The investigators did not use Mufson's IPT-A modification. They found both IPT and CBT more efficacious than the control condition in reducing adolescents' self-ratings of depressive symptoms. IPT was more effective than CBT in increasing self-esteem and social adaptation. The effect size for IPT was 0.73 and for CBT was 0.43 (Rossello and Bernal 1999).

Depressed HIV-Positive Patients

Markowitz et al. (1992) modified IPT for depressed HIV patients (IPT-HIV), emphasizing common issues among this population including concerns about illness and death, grief, and role transitions. In a pilot open trial, 21 of the 24 depressed patients responded with symptom reduction. A 16-week study randomized 101 subjects to IPT-HIV, CBT, supportive psychotherapy, or imipramine plus supportive psychotherapy (Markowitz et al. 1998a). Echoing the results of the more severely depressed subjects in the TDCRP study (Elkin et al. 1989), all treatments were associated with symptom reduction, but IPT and the imipramine–psychotherapy combination produced significantly greater symptomatic and functional improvement than CBT or supportive psychotherapy alone. Many patients reported improvement in depressive physical symptoms that they had mistakenly attributed to HIV infection.

Depressed Primary Care Patients

Schulberg and colleagues compared IPT with pharmacotherapy for depressed ambulatory medical patients in a primary care setting (Schulberg and Scott 1991; Schulberg et al. 1993). They did not modify the IPT manual, but IPT was integrated into the routine of the primary care center; for example, nurses took vital signs before each session. If patients were medically hospitalized, IPT was continued in the hospital when possible.

Patients with current major depression (N=276) were randomly assigned to IPT, nortriptyline, or primary care physicians' usual care. They were seen weekly for 16 weeks and monthly thereafter for 4 months in IPT (Schulberg et al. 1996). Depressive symptom severity declined more rapidly with either nortriptyline or IPT than with usual care. Approximately 70% of treatment completers receiving nortriptyline or IPT, but only 20% of those in usual care, had recovered after 8 months. Brown et al. (1996) found that subjects with a lifetime history of comorbid panic disorder had a poorer response across treatments compared with those with major depression alone. These pilot findings on comorbid panic disorder are corroborated by E. Frank et al. (2000a).

These studies in depressed medical patients suggest that the life event of medical illness may provide a useful role transition focus for IPT treatment (Koszycki et al. 2004).

Conjoint IPT for Depressed Patients With Marital Disputes

Marital conflict, separation, and divorce can precipitate or complicate depressive episodes (Rounsaville et al. 1979). Some clinicians believe that individual psychotherapy for depressed patients in marital disputes may lead to premature rupture of marriages (Gurman and Kniskern 1978). Thus, a manual was developed for conjoint therapy of depressed patients with marital disputes (IPT-CM; Klerman and Weissman 1993). IPT-CM includes the spouse in all sessions and focuses on the current marital dispute. Eighteen patients with major depression linked to the onset or exacerbation of marital disputes were randomly assigned to 16 weeks of either individual IPT or IPT-CM. Patients in both treatments showed similar reductions in depressive symptoms, but patients receiving IPT-CM reported significantly better marital adjustment, marital affection, and sexual relations than did individual IPT patients (Foley et al. 1989). These pilot findings require replication with a larger sample and other control groups.

Antepartum/Postpartum Depression

Pregnancy and its aftermath are a time of heightened depressive risk when women may wish to avoid antidepressant medication; they also provide a natural role transition as an IPT focus. Spinelli at Columbia University used IPT to treat women with antepartum depression. Examination of this role transition addresses the depressed pregnant woman's self-evaluation as a parent, the physiological changes of pregnancy, and altered relationships with the spouse or significant other and with other children. Spinelli added "complicated pregnancy" as a fifth interpersonal problem area. Timing and duration of sessions are adjusted in response to bedrest, delivery, obstetrical complications, and child care. Postpartum mothers may bring children to sessions. As with depressed HIV-positive patients, telephone sessions and hospital visits are sometimes necessary (Spinelli 1997). A con-

trolled clinical trial comparing IPT with a didactic parent education group in depressed pregnant women over 16 weeks of acute treatment showed advantages for IPT (Spinelli and Endicott 2003).

O'Hara et al. (2000) compared IPT with a wait-list control condition in 120 women with postpartum depression. The 12-week trial had an 18-month follow-up. The investigators assessed both the mothers' symptom states and their interactions with their infants (Stuart and O'Hara 1995). Of the IPT group, 38% met HRSD and 44% met BDI remission criteria compared with 14% on each measure for the wait-list group. Sixty percent of IPT patients, versus 16% of control subjects, reported a greater than 50% reduction on the BDI. Women receiving IPT also showed significant improvement in social adjustment relative to the control group.

Klier et al. (2001) treated 17 women with postpartum depression in nine weekly 90-minute group sessions plus an hour-long individual termination session. Scores on the 21-item HRSD fell from 19.7 to 8.0, suggesting the efficacy of this approach. Zlotnick et al. (2001) treated 37 women at risk for postpartum depression with either four 60-minute sessions of a group based on IPT principles or usual treatment. Among the 35 subjects who completed treatment, 6 of 18 women in the control condition versus none of 17 in the interpersonal group developed depression 3 months postpartum. This preventive application of what sounds like a group form of interpersonal counseling (IPC; Klerman et al. 1987) needs replication but is exciting.

Dysthymic Disorder

A modification of IPT for dysthymic disorder (IPT-D) encourages patients to reconceptualize what they have considered to be their lifelong character flaws as egodystonic, chronic mood-dependent symptoms—as chronic but treatable "states" rather than immutable "traits." Therapy itself was defined as an "iatrogenic role transition" from believing oneself flawed in personality to recognizing and treating the mood disorder. Markowitz (1994, 1998) openly treated 17 pilot subjects with 16 sessions of IPT-D: none worsened, and 11 remitted. Medication benefits roughly half of dysthymic patients (Kocsis et al. 1988; Thase et al. 1996), but nonresponders may need psychotherapy, and even medication responders may benefit from combined treatment (Markowitz 1994). Based on these pilot results, a comparative study was conducted at Cornell Medical College in Ithaca, NY, of 16 weeks of IPT-D alone, supportive psychotherapy, sertraline plus clinical management, and a combination of IPT and sertraline. All groups improved, but IPT appeared no better than supportive psychotherapy, and overall pharmacotherapy appeared more efficacious than either psychotherapy (Markowitz et al. 2005).

Browne, Steiner, and others at McMaster University in Hamilton, Ontario, treated more than 700 dysthymic patients in the community with 12 sessions of standard IPT over 4 months, sertraline for 2 years, or a combination of the two. Patients were followed for 2 years. Although results have not yet been published, preliminary findings have been presented at several conferences (e.g., World Psychiatric Association Thematic Conference, Jerusalem, Israel, 1997; American Psychiatric Association Annual Meeting, Chicago, IL, May 2000). Using the criterion of a 40% reduction in score of the Montgomery-Åsberg Depression Rating Scale (MADRS) at 1-year follow-up, 51% of IPT-alone subjects improved, significantly fewer than the 63% taking sertraline and 62% in combined treatment who improved. On follow-up, however, IPT was associated with significant economic savings in use of health care and social services. Thus combined treatment was as efficacious as but less expensive than sertraline alone.

Feijò de Mello et al. (2001) randomly assigned 35 dysthymic outpatients to receive moclobemide with or without 16 weekly sessions of IPT. Both groups improved, but there was a nonsignificant trend for greater improvement on the HRSD and MADRS in the combined treatment group. Similarly, Hellerstein et al. (2001) found that combining interpersonal and cognitive elements improved outcome over fluoxetine alone among dysthymic patients responding to fluoxetine.

Bipolar Disorder

Frank and colleagues in Pittsburgh (E. Frank 1991; E. Frank et al. 2000a) assessed the benefits of adjunctive IPT modified by social zeitgeber theory—behavioral scheduling of daily and sleep patterns (Ehlers et al. 1988; Malkoff-Schwartz et al. 2000—as maintenance treatment in 175 lithium-stabilized bipolar patients, comparing interpersonal social rhythms therapy (IPSRT) with medication alone. The behavioral component helps to protect sleep patterns and limit the disruptions that may provoke mania; the IPT approach to depression remains largely the same. Acutely ill bipolar patients were treated with medication and randomly assigned to IPSRT or clinical management. After achieving 4 weeks of stabilization, patients were again randomized to either IPSRT or clinical management for 3 years of maintenance treatment while continuing pharmacotherapy.

A preliminary report comparing IPSRT as adjunctive treatment with conventional medication clinic treatment found no statistically significant differences in acute treatment, although median time to remission was 21 weeks with IPSRT compared with 40 weeks with clinical management (n=22). Of the first 82 subjects to enter the maintenance phase, patients who received the same treatment in both phases had lower recurrence rates and symptom scores over the following 52 weeks than those who were reassigned from one treatment to the other (E. Frank et al. 1999). In subsequent analyses it appeared that the switch from acute IPSRT to maintenance clinical management increased the risk of depressive recurrence (E. Frank et al. 2000b). Furthermore, patients who received maintenance IPSRT had fewer depressive symptoms than clinical management patients but had a similar rate of manic episodes (E. Frank et al. 1999). However, overall results in this complicated trial indicated that although there was no difference in time to initial stabilization of symptoms, IPSRT with medication was superior to the comparison condition in delaying recurrence of depressive and manic episodes (E. Frank et al. 2005).

Subsyndromally Depressed Hospitalized Elderly Patients

Mossey et al. (1996) noted that even depressive symptoms that did not reach threshold for major depression impeded recovery of hospitalized elderly patients. They conducted a 10-session trial of a modification of IPT, administered by nonpsychiatric nurses, called *interpersonal counseling* (Klerman et al. 1987) for elderly hospitalized medical patients with minor depressive symptoms. Patients were seen for 1-hour sessions on a flexible schedule that accommodated the patients' medical status. Seventy-six hospitalized patients older than 60 years who did not meet criteria for major depression but had depressive symptoms on two consecutive assessments were randomly assigned to either IPC or usual care. Researchers also followed a euthymic untreated control group. Patients found IPC feasible and tolerable. Assessment after 3 months showed nonsignificantly greater improvement in depressive symptoms and on all outcome variables for IPC relative to usual care, whereas control subjects showed a slight symptomatic worsening. Rehospitalization in the IPC and euthymic control groups was virtually identical (11%–15%) and significantly less than the subsyndromally depressed group receiving usual care (50%). Differences between IPC and usual-care groups reached statistical significance at 6 months on depressive symptom reduction and self-rated health but not physical or social functioning. The investigators felt that 10 sessions was an insufficient period for some patients and that a maintenance phase might have been useful.

IPT for Nonmood Disorders

The efficacy of IPT as a treatment for depression has led to its adaptation as a treatment for other psychiatric disorders. Life events are ubiquitous, but when is it useful to focus treatment on them? Research is beginning to answer such questions.

Substance Abuse

IPT has failed to demonstrate efficacy in two clinical trials for patients with substance abuse. Rounsaville et al. (1983) studied 72 methadone-maintained opiate abusers and found that adding adjunctive IPT to standard substance abuse care had no additional benefit in reducing psychopathology. Both treatment groups improved. The same research group found 12 weeks of IPT were ineffective and marginally worse than a behavioral control for 42 subjects with cocaine abuse who were attempting to achieve abstinence (Carroll et al. 1991). The two negative studies suggest limits to the range of utility of IPT but do not necessarily preclude its use for substance abuse. IPT might be useful, for example, as a treatment for newly abstinent alcohol-dependent patients who face psychosocial stressors that have been shown to precipitate relapse.

Eating Disorders

Fairburn et al. (1993) altered IPT for bulimic patients, eliminating the use of the sick role and of role-playing so that relatively distinct strategies could be contrasted in a comparison of IPT and CBT. Initial trials showed that although CBT worked faster, IPT had longer-term benefits comparable with CBT and superior to a behavioral control condition. In a subsequent multisite trial, however, CBT was superior to IPT (Agras et al. 2000).

Wilfley et al. (1993, 2000) modified IPT in a 16-week, 90-minute session group format. The initial IPT phase, in which the therapist identifies problem areas, presents IPT concepts, and offers a treatment contract, is conducted individually; confusion was avoided among IPT problem areas by giving almost all subjects a focus on "interpersonal deficits." They compared group IPT with group CBT and a wait-list control for 56 women with nonpurging bulimia. At termination, binge eating decreased in the IPT and CBT groups but

not in the wait-list condition. Results persisted at 1-year follow-up. A randomized clinical trial of 162 women comparing group IPT and group CBT for 20 sessions over 20 weeks yielded similar results (Wilfley et al. 2002).

A research group in Christchurch, New Zealand, studied the application of IPT to anorexia nervosa. In their trial, neither IPT nor CBT showed efficacy as an outpatient treatment, a finding unfortunately consonant with anorexia outcome literature generally (McIntosh et al. 2005).

Social Phobia

IPT has not yet been tested in controlled studies as a treatment for anxiety disorders. IPT has been modified for social phobia independently by two research groups. Lipsitz et al. (1999) at Columbia University in New York treated nine IPT pilot cases and found promising results for social phobia. They found that such standard IPT ingredients as the medical model, provision of the sick role, and the supportive therapeutic stance appear to benefit most patients. A small controlled trial has not yet been published. Weissman and Jacobson, also at Columbia, have adapted IPT in a 10-session group format for shy patients with social phobia in unstructured interpersonal situations, for example, at parties or in intimate discussions with significant others but not in defined work situations.

Panic Disorder

Arzt and van Rijsoort in Maastricht, the Netherlands, are studying IPT as a treatment for panic disorder. Lipsitz et al. (2006) reported promise for IPT in a small open trial.

Posttraumatic Stress Disorder

Posttraumatic stress disorder (PTSD) is an anxiety disorder defined by a life event, which might suggest the utility of IPT in its treatment. Krupnick and colleagues are assessing a group form of IPT for multiply victimized women in public-sector gynecology clinics in Virginia. My colleagues at Cornell University and I have modified IPT as an alternative to exposure-based psychotherapies for PTSD and have found excellent outcomes in a small pilot trial (Bleiberg and Markowitz 2005); we now plan to make a controlled comparison.

Other Applications

Research groups are testing the applicability of IPT for patients with body dysmorphic disorder, primary care patients with chronic somatization, patients with post–myocardial infarction depression (Stuart and Cole 1996), depressed cancer patients, borderline personality disorder patients (Markowitz et al. 2006b), insomnia patients, and patients with other disorders (Weissman et al. 2000). The IPT focus on life events suggests its potential applicability to patients with medical illness. Swartz et al. (2004) produced preliminary findings suggesting that IPT can be effective in a briefer eight-session form.

Interpersonal Counseling

Distress

Many patients presenting to primary care practices report psychiatric symptoms yet do not meet full criteria for a psychiatric disorder. Their symptoms can be debilitating and may result in high wasted utilization of medical procedures (Wells et al. 1989). IPC, based on IPT, was designed to treat distressed primary care patients who do not meet full syndromal criteria for psychiatric disorders. IPC is administered for a maximum of six sessions by health care professionals who lack formal psychiatric training, usually nurse practitioners. The first session can last up to 30 minutes, with subsequent shorter sessions.

In IPC, therapists assess the patient's current functioning, recent life events, occupational and familial stressors, and changes in interpersonal relationships. They assume that such events provide the context in which emotional and bodily symptoms occur. Klerman et al. (1987) studied 128 patients in a primary care clinic who scored 6 or higher on the Goldberg General Health Questionnaire (GHQ), randomizing them to IPC or to usual care without psychological treatment (Klerman et al. 1987). Over an average of 3 months, often receiving only one or two IPC sessions, IPC subjects showed significantly greater symptom relief on the GHQ than control subjects, especially mood improvement. IPC subjects were more likely to subsequently make use of mental health services, suggesting a new awareness of the psychological aspect of their symptoms.

In a dramatic study demonstrating the transplantability of IPT to a very different culture, a group variant of IPC was tested in randomly assigned villages in a poverty- and AIDS-stricken region of Uganda where depression rates are high. IPT was chosen as an intervention because antidepressant medication was unaffordable and other psychotherapies seemed incompatible with the local outlook. Researchers made adjustments for cultural differences but applied the usual IPT paradigm. In that study, the group IPC intervention was impressively more effective than treatment as usual (Bolton et al. 2003).

IPT and IPC by Telephone

Because many patients avoid or have difficulty reaching an office for face-to-face treatment, IPC is being tested as a telephone treatment. Miller and Weissman (2002) at Columbia University conducted a successful pilot feasibility trial comparing IPT by telephone with no treatment in 30 patients with recurrent major depression who had not received regular treatment. Neugebauer et al. (2006) found telephone IPC helpful as an intervention for women with minor depression postmiscarriage.

IPT Patient Guide

Weissman (1995) developed a user-friendly IPT patient guide with worksheets for depressed readers who want information about or are receiving IPT. Worksheets can be used to facilitate sessions or to monitor problem areas after treatment. The utility of the patient book in enhancing treatment has not been studied.

Summary

IPT has demonstrated efficacy as an acute and maintenance monotherapy and as a component of combined treatment for major depressive disorder. It also appears to have utility for other mood and nonmood syndromes, although the evidence for these is more sparse. Because monotherapy with either IPT or pharmacotherapy is likely to suffice for most depressed patients, combined treatment is probably best reserved for severely or chronically ill patients (Rush and Thase 1999). How best to combine time-limited psychotherapy with pharmacotherapy—for which patients, in what sequence, and so on—is an exciting area for future research.

When is one treatment likely to have a better outcome than another (Table 30–6)? Comparative trials are beginning to reveal moderating factors or predictors of treatment outcome. Studies such as the TDCRP, which compared IPT with CBT, have suggested factors that might predict better outcome with either treatment. Sotsky et al. (1991) found that depressed patients with a low baseline level of social dysfunction responded well to IPT, whereas those with severe so-

TABLE 30–6. Prescribing interpersonal therapy (IPT) and cognitive-behavioral therapy (CBT)

I. Points in common

   A. Common factors of psychotherapy

      1. Helping patient feel understood (**R**elationship)

      2. Framework for understanding (**R**ationale)

      3. Providing hope and optimism

      4. Psychoeducation

      5. Technique for getting better (**R**itual)

      6. Success experiences

   B. Common features of brief antidepressant psychotherapies

      1. Manualized

      2. Active

      3. Time limited (with comparable time courses)

      4. Structured (CBT>IPT)

      5. "Here and now" current focus

      6. Can be combined with antidepressant medication

      7. Goals of self-assertion, mastery

      8. Ultimate goal of new skills for prophylaxis

   C. Technical similarities

      1. Mobilizing patient to greater activity

      2. Linking mood to activities and reactions to events, albeit with different emphases

      3. Problem solving: "exploring options" vs. "empirical hypothesis testing"

      4. Addressing "expectations" vs. "assumptions" about others

      5. Role playing

II. Differences

   A. IPT: medical model

   B. CBT: homework

   C. Focus on affect (IPT) vs. thoughts (→ affect) (CBT), hence more external vs. more intrapsychic approach

III. Differential therapeutics of major depression: Which works better for whom?

Predictor	IPT	CBT
Life events	Present	Absent
Social dysfunction (baseline)	Low	Very high ("Interpersonal deficits")
Symptom severity (baseline)	Higher	Lower
Personality disorder	Obsessive	Avoidant

cial deficits (probably equivalent to the "interpersonal deficits" problem area) responded less well. Patients with greater symptom severity and difficulty in concentrating responded poorly to CBT. Initial severity of major depression and of impaired functioning predicted superior response to IPT and to imipramine. Imipramine also worked most efficaciously for patients with difficulty functioning at work, likely reflecting its faster onset of action. Patients with atypical depression responded better to either IPT or CBT than to imipramine or placebo (Shea et al. 1999).

Barber and Muenz (1996), looking only at TDCRP completers, found IPT more efficacious than CBT for patients with obsessive personality disorder, whereas CBT fared better for avoidant personality disorder. Biological factors such as abnormal sleep profiles on electroencephalograms predicted significantly poorer response to IPT than for patients with normal sleep parameters (Thase et al. 1997). E. Frank et al. (1991) found that psychotherapist adherence to a focused IPT approach may enhance outcome. The replication and further elaboration of these predictive factors deserve ongoing study.

Training

Until recently, IPT practitioners were few and almost exclusively limited to therapists in research studies. In response to clinical demand for this empirically supported treatment, IPT training is now increasingly included in professional workshops and conferences, with training courses conducted at university centers in Canada, the United Kingdom, continental Europe, Asia, New Zealand, and Australia. IPT is taught in a still small but growing number of psychiatric residency training programs in the United States (Lichtmacher et al. 2006; Markowitz 1995) and has been included in some family practice and primary care training programs.

Although the principles and practice of IPT are straightforward, any psychotherapy requires some innate therapeutic ability, as well as comfort with the so-called common factors of psychotherapy (J. Frank 1971): tolerating and exploring affect, helping the patient to feel understood, engendering hope, and so on. IPT training requires more than reading the manual (Rounsaville et al. 1988; Weissman et al. 1981): psychotherapy is learned by doing. Most IPT training programs are designed to help experienced therapists refocus their treatment by learning new techniques, not to teach novices psychotherapy. Candidates should have a graduate clinical degree (M.D., Ph.D., M.S.W., R.N.), several years of experience conducting psychotherapy, and clinical familiarity with the diagnoses of patients they plan to treat.

The training used in the TDCRP (Elkin et al. 1989) became the model for subsequent research studies. It included a brief didactic program, review of the manual, and a longer practicum in which the therapist treated two or three patients under close supervision monitored by videotapes of the sessions (Chevron and Rounsaville 1983). Rounsaville et al. (1986) found that psychotherapists who performed well on an initial supervised IPT case often did not require further intensive supervision and that experienced therapists committed to the approach required less supervision than others (Rounsaville et al. 1988). Some clinicians have taught themselves IPT using as guides the IPT manual (Klerman et al. 1984) and peer supervision. For research certification, we continue to recommend at least two or three successfully treated cases with hour-for-hour supervision of taped sessions (Markowitz 2001).

Although there is now a loose IPT organization, the International Society for Interpersonal Psychotherapy (ISIPT), there is no formal certificate for IPT proficiency and no accrediting board. When the practice of IPT was restricted to research settings, this was not a problem: one research group taught another in the manner just described. As IPT spreads into clinical practice, however, issues arise about standards for clinical training, and questions of competence and accreditation gain greater urgency. Training programs in IPT are still not widely available, as one U.S. Surgeon General's report noted (Satcher 1999). Many psychiatry residency and psychology training programs still focus on long-term psychodynamic psychotherapy or on cognitive therapy; in these programs, as well, the lack of exposure to time-limited treatment has been noted (Sanderson and Woody 1995–1996). Psychiatric residency and other mental health care treatment training programs should include clinical instruction in the time-limited psychotherapies described in manuals in addition to providing exposure to long-term psychotherapy. To our knowledge, no accepted model psychotherapy curriculum is available.

The educational process for IPT in clinical practice requires further study. We do not know, for example, what levels of education and experience are required to learn IPT or how much supervision an already experienced psychotherapist is likely to require.

The Future

The history of IPT has been its testing in a succession of outcome trials. These studies have helped to define diagnostic indications for this treatment. Because psychotherapy is underfunded relative to pharmacotherapy, we know far less about the dosage and indications of IPT than about antidepressant medication. Future outcome trials may continue to define the territory of IPT's utility. These should include both tests for different diagnoses, such as the anxiety disorders, and testing of dosage, including the optimal frequency and duration of IPT sessions, as well as studies of the sequencing of IPT with other treatments. For example, when and for whom is IPT best combined with pharmacotherapy? Is it best to start with pharmacotherapy and then add IPT? If so, at what interval and with what frequency? When should IPT be used as augmentation for pharmacotherapy, and vice versa? Other research may help to determine the cost-effectiveness and potential cost offset of IPT as a treatment that improves both symptoms and social functioning.

IPT is also anomalous among psychotherapies in its nearly pure focus to date on outcome studies. Until recent decades, almost all psychotherapy research consisted of process research, an analysis of what occurred between patient and therapist in sessions. The late Gerald L. Klerman emphasized the primacy of outcome research, emphasizing that if the therapy had no actual clinical benefit, its mechanism would hold little interest. Now that it is clear that IPT helps many patients, process research seems warranted to try to identify its active, mediating factors. Little is known about the specific value of many IPT interventions. It is even unclear, for example, whether focusing on a role transition rather than a role dispute makes a difference for patients or whether particular sorts of life events are helpful or unhelpful foci. Patient and therapist characteristics may also potentially influence treatment outcome.

Clinical training in IPT is likely to grow. How it spreads will be a function of training programs. Training will probably need to be formalized and accredited, both to ensure clinical competence and to satisfy managed care organizations. Research is needed on how best to teach and disseminate IPT.

In summary, IPT is a time-limited, forward-looking, pragmatically focused psychotherapy that defines psychiatric disorders as treatable medical illnesses and links them to the patient's current social situation. This strategy has proved efficacious for patients with major depression and bulimia and shows promise for other mood and nonmood disorders.

Key Points

- The interpersonal environment affects psychopathology, and vice versa.

- Depression (and other psychiatric diagnoses) can be usefully defined to the patient as a medical illness.

- Solving interpersonal problems builds social skills and relieves symptoms.

- A time limit intensifies treatment.

- IPT should be considered a first-line treatment for acute treatment of major depressive disorder and prevention of relapse.

- Sharing its medical model, IPT can be neatly combined with pharmacotherapy.

Suggested Readings

Weissman MM, Markowitz JC, Klerman GL: Comprehensive Guide to Interpersonal Psychotherapy. New York, Basic Books, 2000

Weissman MM, Markowitz JC, Klerman GL: A Clinician's Quick Guide to Interpersonal Psychotherapy. New York, Oxford University Press, 2007

Online Resource

The International Society for Interpersonal Psychotherapy: www.interpersonalpsychotherapy.org

References

Agency for Health Care Policy and Research: Depression in Primary Care, Vol 1: Detection and Diagnosis (Clinical Guideline Number 5; AHCPR Publ No 93-0550). Rockville, MD, Agency for Health Care Policy and Research, 1993a

Agency for Health Care Policy and Research: Depression in Primary Care, Vol 2: Treatment of Major Depression (Clinical Practice Guideline Number 5; AHCPR Publ No 93-0551). Rockville, MD, Agency for Health Care Policy and Research, 1993b

Agency for Health Care Policy and Research: Depression in Primary Care, Vol 3: Detection, Diagnosis, and Treatment (Quick Reference Guideline Number 5; AHCPR Publ No 93-0552). Rockville, MD, Agency for Health Care Policy and Research, 1993c

Agency for Health Care Policy and Research: Depression in Primary Care, Vol 4. Depression Is a Treatable Illness: A Patient's Guide (Consumer Guideline Number 5; AHCPR Publ No 93-0553). Rockville, MD, Agency for Health Care Policy and Research, 1993d

Agras WS, Walsh BT, Fairburn CG, et al: A multicenter comparison of cognitive-behavioral therapy and interpersonal psychotherapy for bulimia nervosa. Arch Gen Psychiatry 57:459–466, 2000

American Psychiatric Association: Diagnostic and Statistical Manual of Mental Disorders, 3rd Edition, Revised. Washington, DC, American Psychiatric Association, 1987

American Psychiatric Association: Diagnostic and Statistical Manual of Mental Disorders, 4th Edition, Text Revision. Washington, DC, American Psychiatric Association, 2000

Barber JP, Muenz LR: The role of avoidance and obsessiveness in matching patients to cognitive and interpersonal psychotherapy: empirical findings from the Treatment for Depression Collaborative Research Program. J Consult Clin Psychol 64:951–958, 1996

Beck AT: Depression Inventory. Philadelphia, PA, Center for Cognitive Therapy, 1978

Beck AT, Rush AJ, Shaw BF, et al: Cognitive Therapy of Depression. New York, Guilford, 1979

Bleiberg KL, Markowitz JC: Interpersonal psychotherapy for posttraumatic stress disorder. Am J Psychiatry 162:181–183, 2005

Blom MB, Hoencamp E, Zwaan T: Interpersoonlijke psychotherapie voor depressie: Een pilot-onderzoek. Tijdschrift voor Psychiatr 38:398–402, 1996

Blom MB, Jonker K, Dusseldorp E, et al: Combination treatment for acute depression is superior only when psychotherapy is added to medication. Psychother Psychosom 76:289–297, 2007

Bolton P, Bass J, Neugebauer R, et al: Group interpersonal psychotherapy for depression in rural Uganda: a randomized controlled trial. JAMA 289:3117–3124, 2003

Bowlby J: Attachment and Loss. New York, Basic Books, 1973

Brown C, Schulberg HC, Madonia MJ, et al: Treatment outcomes for primary care patients with major depression and lifetime anxiety disorders. Am J Psychiatry 153:1293–1300, 1996

Carroll KM, Rounsaville BJ, Gawin FH: A comparative trial of psychotherapies for ambulatory cocaine abusers: relapse prevention and interpersonal psychotherapy. Am J Drug Alcohol Abuse 17:229–247, 1991

Chevron ES, Rounsaville BJ: Evaluating the clinical skills of psychotherapists: a comparison of techniques. Arch Gen Psychiatry 40:1129–1132, 1983

Cyranowski JM, Frank E, Winter E, et al: Personality pathology and outcome in recurrently depressed women over 2 years of maintenance interpersonal psychotherapy. Psychol Med 34:659–669, 2004

DiMascio A, Weissman MM, Prusoff BA, et al: Differential symptom reduction by drugs and psychotherapy in acute depression. Arch Gen Psychiatry 36:1450–1456, 1979

Ehlers CL, Frank E, Kupfer DJ: Social zeitgebers and biological rhythms: a unified approach to understanding the etiology of depression. Arch Gen Psychiatry 45:948–952, 1988

Elkin I, Shea MT, Watkins JT, et al: National Institute of Mental Health Treatment of Depression Collaborative Research Program: general effectiveness of treatments. Arch Gen Psychiatry 46:971–982, 1989

Fairburn CG, Jones R, Peveler RC, et al: Psychotherapy and bulimia nervosa: longer-term effects of interpersonal psychotherapy, behavior therapy, and cognitive behavior therapy. Arch Gen Psychiatry 50:419–428, 1993

Feijò de Mello M, Myczowisk LM, Menezes PR: A randomized controlled trial comparing moclobemide and moclobemide plus interpersonal psychotherapy in the treatment of dysthymic disorder. J Psychother Pract Res 10:117–123, 2001

Foley SH, Rounsaville BJ, Weissman MM, et al: Individual versus conjoint interpersonal psychotherapy for depressed patients with marital disputes. International Journal of Family Psychiatry 10:29–42, 1989

Frank E: Biological order and bipolar disorder. Paper presented at the meeting of the American Psychosomatic Society, Santa Fe, NM, March 1991

Frank E: Treating Bipolar Disorder: A Clinician's Guide to Interpersonal and Social Rhythm Therapy. New York, Guilford, 2005

Frank E, Kupfer DJ, Perel JM, et al: Three-year outcomes for maintenance therapies in recurrent depression. Arch Gen Psychiatry 47:1093–1099, 1990

Frank E, Kupfer DJ, Wagner EF, et al: Efficacy of interpersonal psychotherapy as a maintenance treatment of recurrent depression. Arch Gen Psychiatry 48:1053–1059, 1991

Frank E, Swartz HA, Mallinger AG, et al: Adjunctive psychotherapy for bipolar disorder: effects of changing treatment modality. J Abnormal Psychol 108:579–587, 1999

Frank E, Shear MK, Rucci P, et al: Influence of panic-agoraphobic spectrum symptoms on treatment response in patients with recurrent major depression. Am J Psychiatry 157:1101–1107, 2000a

Frank E, Swartz HA, Kupfer DJ: Interpersonal and social rhythm therapy: managing the chaos of bipolar disorder. Biol Psychiatry 48:593–604, 2000b

Frank E, Kupfer DJ, Thase ME, et al: Two year outcomes for interpersonal and social rhythm therapy in individuals with bipolar I disorder. Arch Gen Psychiatry 62:996–1004, 2005

Frank E, Kupfer DJ, Buysse DJ, et al: Randomized trial of weekly, twice monthly, and monthly interpersonal psychotherapy as maintenance treatment for women with recurrent depression. Am J Psychiatry 164:761–767, 2007

Frank J: Therapeutic factors in psychotherapy. Am J Psychother 25:350–361, 1971

Gurman AS, Kniskern DP: Research on marital and family therapy: progress, perspective, and prospect, in Handbook of Psychotherapy and Behavior Change. Edited by Garfield SB, Bergen AB. New York, Wiley, 1978, pp 817–902

Hamilton M: A rating scale for depression. J Neurol Neurosurg Psychiatr 25:56–62, 1960

Hellerstein DJ, Little SAS, Samstag LW, et al: Adding group psychotherapy to medication treatment in dysthymia. J Psychother Pract Res 10:93–103, 2001

Hirschfeld RMA, Klerman GL, Clayton PJ, et al: Assessing personality: effects of the depressive state on trait measurement. Am J Psychiatry 140:695–699, 1983

Karasu TB, Docherty JP, Gelenberg A, et al: Practice guideline for major depressive disorder in adults. Am J Psychiatry 150 (suppl):1–26, 1993

Klein DF, Ross DC: Reanalysis of the National Institute of Mental Health Treatment of Depression Collaborative Research Program general effectiveness report. Neuropsychopharmacology 8:241–251, 1993

Klerman GL, Weissman MM: New Applications of Interpersonal Psychotherapy. Washington, DC, American Psychiatric Press, 1993

Klerman GL, Weissman MM, Rounsaville BJ, et al: Interpersonal Psychotherapy of Depression. New York, Basic Books, 1984

Klerman GL, Budman S, Berwick D, et al: Efficacy of a brief psychosocial intervention for symptoms of stress and distress among patients in primary care. Med Care 25:1078–1088, 1987

Klier CM, Muzik M, Rosenblum KL, et al: Interpersonal psychotherapy adapted for the group setting in the treatment of postpartum depression. J Psychother Pract Res 10:124–131, 2001

Kocsis JH, Frances AJ, Voss C, et al: Imipramine treatment for chronic depression. Arch Gen Psychiatry 45:253–257, 1988

Koszycki D, Lafontaine S, Frasure-Smith N, et al: An open-label trial of interpersonal psychotherapy in depressed patients with coronary disease. Psychosomatics 45:319–324, 2004

Lichtmacher J, Eisendrath SJ, Haller E: Implementing interpersonal psychotherapy in a psychiatric residency training program. Acad Psychiatry 30:385–391, 2006

Lipsitz JD, Fyer AJ, Markowitz JC, et al: An open trial of interpersonal psychotherapy for social phobia. Am J Psychiatry 156:1814–1816, 1999

Lipsitz JD, Gur M, Miller NL, et al: An open pilot study of interpersonal psychotherapy for panic disorder (IPT-PD). J Nerv Ment Dis 194:440–445, 2006

Malkoff-Schwartz S, Frank E, Anderson BP, et al: Social rhythm disruption and stressful life events in the onset of bipolar and unipolar episodes. Psychol Med 30:1005–1016, 2000

Markowitz JC: Psychotherapy of dysthymia. Am J Psychiatry 151:1114–1121, 1994

Markowitz JC: Teaching interpersonal psychotherapy to psychiatric residents. Acad Psychiatry 19:167–173, 1995

Markowitz JC: Interpersonal Psychotherapy for Dysthymic Disorder. Washington, DC, American Psychiatric Press, 1998

Markowitz JC: Learning the new psychotherapies, in Treatment of Depression: Bridging the 21st Century. Edited by Weissman MM. Washington, DC, American Psychiatric Press, 2001, pp 281–300

Markowitz JC, Swartz HA: Case formulation in interpersonal psychotherapy of depression, in Handbook of Psychotherapy Case Formulation. Edited by Eels TD. New York, Guilford, 1997, pp 192–222

Markowitz JC, Klerman GL, Perry SW, et al: Interpersonal therapy of depressed HIV-seropositive patients. Hosp Community Psychiatry 43:885–890, 1992

Markowitz JC, Kocsis JH, Fishman B, et al: Treatment of HIV-positive patients with depressive symptoms. Arch Gen Psychiatry 55:452–457, 1998a

Markowitz JC, Svartberg M, Swartz HA: Is IPT time-limited psychodynamic psychotherapy? J Psychother Pract Res 7:185–195, 1998b

Markowitz JC, Leon AC, Miller NL, et al: Rater agreement on interpersonal psychotherapy problem areas. J Psychother Pract Res 9:131–135, 2000

Markowitz JC, Kocsis JH, Bleiberg KL, et al: A comparative trial of psychotherapy and pharmacotherapy for "pure" dysthymic patients. J Affect Disord 89:167–175, 2005

Markowitz JC, Bleiberg KL, Christos P, et al: Solving interpersonal problems correlates with symptom improvement in interpersonal psychotherapy: preliminary findings. J Nerv Ment Dis 194:15–20, 2006a

Markowitz JC, Skodol AE, Bleiberg K: Interpersonal psychotherapy for borderline personality disorder: possible mechanisms of change. J Clin Psychol 62:431–444, 2006b

McIntosh VV, Jordan J, Carter FA, et al: Three psychotherapies for anorexia nervosa: a randomized, controlled trial. Am J Psychiatry 162:741–747, 2005

Miller L, Weissman M: Interpersonal psychotherapy delivered over the telephone to recurrent depressives: a pilot study. Depress Anxiety 16:114–117, 2002

Mossey JM, Knott KA, Higgins M, et al: Effectiveness of a psychosocial intervention, interpersonal counseling, for subdysthymic depression in medically ill elderly. J Gerontol 51A(4):M172–M178, 1996

Mufson L, Weissman MM, Moreau D, et al: Efficacy of interpersonal psychotherapy for depressed adolescents. Arch Gen Psychiatry 56:573–579, 1999

Mufson L, Dorta KP, Moreau D, et al: Interpersonal Therapy for Depressed Adolescents, 2nd Edition. New York, Guilford, 2004a

Mufson L, Dorta KP, Wickramaratne P, et al: A randomized effectiveness trial of interpersonal psychotherapy for depressed adolescents. Arch Gen Psychiatry 61:577–584, 2004b

Mufson L, Gallagher T, Dorta KP, et al: Interpersonal psychotherapy for adolescent depression: adaptation for group therapy. Am J Psychother 58:220–237, 2004c

Neugebauer R, Kline J, Markowitz JC, et al: Pilot randomized controlled trial of interpersonal counseling for subsyndromal depression following miscarriage. J Clin Psychiatry 67:1299–1304, 2006

O'Hara MW, Stuart S, Gorman LL, et al: Efficacy of interpersonal psychotherapy for postpartum depression. Arch Gen Psychiatry 57:1039–1045, 2000

Parsons T: Illness and the role of the physician: a sociological perspective. Am J Orthopsychiatry 21:452–460, 1951

Paykel ES, DiMascio A, Haskell D, et al: Effects of maintenance amitriptyline and psychotherapy on symptoms of depression. Psychol Med 5:67–77, 1975

Puig JS: Psicoterapia interpersonal (1). Rev Psiquiatría Fac Med Barna 22:91–99, 1995

Reynolds CF III, Frank E, Perel JM, et al: Nortriptyline and interpersonal psychotherapy as maintenance therapies for recurrent major depression: a randomized controlled trial in patients older than fifty-nine years. JAMA 281:39–45, 1999

Reynolds CF III, Dew MA, Pollock BG, et al: Maintenance treatment of major depression in old age. N Engl J Med 354:1130–1138, 2006

Rossello J, Bernal G: The efficacy of cognitive-behavioral and interpersonal treatments for depression in Puerto Rican adolescents. J Consult Clin Psychol 67:734–745, 1999

Rothblum ED, Sholomskas AJ, Berry C, et al: Issues in clinical trials with the depressed elderly. J Am Geriatr Soc 30:694–699, 1982

Rounsaville BJ, Weissman MM, Prusoff BA, et al: Marital disputes and treatment outcome in depressed women. Compr Psychiatry 20:483–490, 1979

Rounsaville BJ, Glazer W, Wilber CH, et al: Short-term interpersonal psychotherapy in methadone-maintained opiate addicts. Arch Gen Psychiatry 40:629–636, 1983

Rounsaville BJ, Chevron ES, Weissman MM, et al: Training therapists to perform interpersonal psychotherapy in clinical trials. Compr Psychiatry 27:364–371, 1986

Rounsaville BJ, O'Malley SS, Foley SH, et al: The role of manual-guided training in the conduct and efficacy of interpersonal psychotherapy for depression. J Consult Clin Psychol 56:681–688, 1988

Rush AJ, Thase ME: Psychotherapies for depressive disorders: a review, in Depressive Disorders: WPA Series Evidence and Experience in Psychiatry. Edited by Maj M, Sartorius N. Chichester, UK, Wiley, 1999, pp 161–206

Sanderson WC, Woody S: Manuals for Empirically Validated Treatments: A Project of the Task Force on Psychological Interventions. Division of Clinical Psychology. Washington, DC, American Psychological Association, 1995–1996

Satcher D: Surgeon General's Reference. Mental Health: A Report of the Surgeon General. Rockville, MD, U.S. Department of Health and Human Services, 1999

Schulberg HC, Scott CP: Depression in primary care: treating depression with interpersonal psychotherapy, in Psychotherapy in Managed Health Care: The Optimal Use of Time and Resources. Edited by Austad CS, Berman WH. Washington, DC, American Psychological Association, 1991, pp 153–170

Schulberg HC, Scott CP, Madonia MJ, et al: Applications of interpersonal psychotherapy to depression in primary care practice, in New Applications of Interpersonal Psychotherapy. Edited by Klerman GL, Weissman MM. Washington, DC, American Psychiatric Press, 1993, pp 265–291

Schulberg HC, Block MR, Madonia MJ, et al: Treating major depression in primary care practice. Arch Gen Psychiatry 53:913–919, 1996

Shea MT, Elkin I, Imber SD, et al: Course of depressive symptoms over follow-up: findings from the National Institute of Mental Health Treatment for Depression Collaborative Research Program. Arch Gen Psychiatry 49:782–794, 1992

Shea MT, Elkin I, Sotsky SM: Patient characteristics associated with successful treatment: outcome findings from the NIMH Treatment of Depression Collaborative Research Program, in Psychotherapy Indications and Outcomes. Edited by Janowsky DS. Washington, DC, American Psychiatric Press, 1999, pp 71–90

Sholomskas AJ, Chevron ES, Prusoff BA, et al: Short-term interpersonal therapy (IPT) with the depressed elderly: case reports and discussion. Am J Psychother 36:552–566, 1983

Sloane RB, Stapes FR, Schneider LS: Interpersonal therapy versus nortriptyline for depression in the elderly, in Clinical and Pharmacological Studies in Psychiatric Disorders. Edited by Burrows GD, Norman TR, Dennerstein L. London, England, John Libbey, 1985, pp 344–346

Sotsky SM, Glass DR, Shea MT, et al: Patient predictors of response to psychotherapy and pharmacotherapy: findings in the NIMH Treatment of Depression Collaborative Research Program. Am J Psychiatry 148:997–1008, 1991

Spinelli MG: Interpersonal psychotherapy for depressed antepartum women: a pilot study. Am J Psychiatry 154:1028–1030, 1997

Spinelli MG, Endicott J: Controlled clinical trial of interpersonal psychotherapy versus parenting education program for depressed pregnant women. Am J Psychiatry 160:555–562, 2003

Stuart S, Cole V: Treatment of depression following myocardial infarction with interpersonal psychotherapy. Ann Clin Psychiatry 8:203–206, 1996

Stuart S, O'Hara MW: IPT for postpartum depression. J Psychother Pract Res 4:18–29, 1995

Sullivan HS (ed): The Interpersonal Theory of Psychiatry. New York, WW Norton, 1953

Swartz HA, Frank E, Shear MK, et al: A pilot study of brief interpersonal psychotherapy for depression in women. Psychiatr Serv 55:448–450, 2004

Thase ME, Fava M, Halbreich U, et al: A placebo-controlled, randomized clinical trial comparing sertraline and imipramine for the treatment of dysthymia. Arch Gen Psychiatry 53:777–784, 1996

Thase ME, Buysse DJ, Frank E, et al: Which depressed patients will respond to interpersonal psychotherapy? The role of abnormal EEG profiles. Am J Psychiatry 154:502–509, 1997

Weissman MM: Mastering Depression: A Patient Guide to Interpersonal Psychotherapy. Albany, NY, Graywind, 1995

Weissman MM, Klerman GL, Paykel ES, et al: Treatment effects on the social adjustment of depressed patients. Arch Gen Psychiatry 30:771–778, 1974

Weissman MM, Prusoff BA, DiMascio A, et al: The efficacy of drugs and psychotherapy in the treatment of acute depressive episodes. Am J Psychiatry 136:555–558, 1979

Weissman MM, Klerman GL, Prusoff BA, et al: Depressed outpatients: results one year after treatment with drugs and/or interpersonal psychotherapy. Arch Gen Psychiatry 38:52–55, 1981

Weissman MM, Markowitz JC, Klerman GL: Comprehensive Guide to Interpersonal Psychotherapy. New York, Basic Books, 2000

Weissman MM, Markowitz JC, Klerman GL: Clinician's Quick Guide to Interpersonal Psychotherapy. New York, Oxford University Press, 2007

Wilfley DE, Agras WS, Telch CF, et al: Group cognitive-behavioral therapy and group interpersonal psychotherapy for the nonpurging bulimic individual: a controlled comparison. J Consult Clin Psychol 61:296–305, 1993

Wilfley DE, MacKenzie RK, Welch RR, et al: Interpersonal Psychotherapy for Group. New York, Basic Books, 2000

Wilfley DE, Welch RR, Stein RI, et al: A randomized comparison of group cognitive-behavioral therapy and group interpersonal psychotherapy for the treatment of overweight individuals with binge-eating disorder. Arch Gen Psychiatry 59:713–721, 2002

Wells KB, Stewart A, Hayes RD, et al: The functioning and well-being of depressed patients: results of the medical outcomes study. JAMA 262:914–919, 1989

Zlotnick C, Johnson SL, Miller IW, et al: Postpartum depression in women receiving public assistance: pilot study of an interpersonal-therapy-oriented group intervention. Am J Psychiatry 158:638–640, 2001

31

COGNITIVE THERAPY

Jesse H. Wright, M.D., Ph.D.
Michael E. Thase, M.D.
Aaron T. Beck, M.D.

Cognitive therapy (CT) is a system of psychotherapy based on theories of pathological information processing in mental disorders. Treatment is directed primarily at modifying distorted or maladaptive cognitions and related behavioral dysfunction. Therapeutic interventions are usually focused and problem oriented. Although the use of specific techniques is a major feature of this approach, there can be considerable flexibility and creativity in the clinical application of CT.

In this chapter we trace the historical origins of CT, explain basic theories, discuss experimental findings on cognitive pathology, and detail commonly used CT techniques. The main focus is on the treatment of depression and anxiety disorders in adults; CT procedures for eating disorders, psychosis, characterological problems, and other psychiatric conditions also are described. Finally, the extensive research on the effectiveness of CT is reviewed and summarized. Methods have been developed for using CT with children and adolescents, but these applications are not discussed in this chapter. Readers who wish to learn about CT for younger persons are referred to the excellent books on this topic, including those by Reinecke et al. (2003), Albano and Kearney (2000), and March and Mulle (1998).

Historical Background

The CT approach to depression was first proposed by Beck in the early 1960s (Beck 1963, 1964). He had begun to study depression from a psychoanalytical perspective several years earlier but had been struck by incongruities between the "retroflexed hostility" concept of psychoanalysis and his observations that depressed individuals usually hold negatively biased constructions of themselves and their environment (Beck 1963, 1964). Subsequently, a comprehensive CT for depression was articulated, and the treatment model was extended to a variety of other conditions, including anxiety disorders (Beck 1967, 1976). CT was described in a fully developed form in *Cognitive Therapy of Depression* (Beck et al. 1979). This volume was the culmination of a series of treatment manuals developed at the Center for Cognitive Therapy at the University of Pennsylvania. The therapy interventions were designed to be compatible with the cognitive model of depression and were drawn from several sources including the clinical experiences of Beck and colleagues and the writings of behaviorists and post-

Drs. Wright and Beck receive a portion of profits from sales of the "Good Days Ahead" software for computer-assisted cognitive therapy discussed in this chapter.

Freudian analysts (Beck et al. 1979; Wright et al. 2006).

CT is linked philosophically to the concepts of the Greek Stoic philosophers and Eastern schools of thought such as Taoism and Buddhism (Beck et al. 1979). The writing of Epictetus in the *Enchiridion* ("Men are disturbed not by things which happen, but by the opinions about the things") captures the essence of the perspective that our ideas or thoughts are a controlling factor in our emotional lives. Modern philosophers also have endorsed the concept that conscious ideas are at the center of human experience and that the meanings attached to events are a primary source of our actions. The phenomenological approach to philosophy, as exemplified in the writings of Kant, Jaspers, Binswanger, and others, has significantly influenced the development of CT (Beck et al. 1979). Frankl's (1985) logotherapy and Mahoney's (1985) and Guidano and Liotti's (1983) theories on constructivism also have played a role in formulating cognitively oriented treatment models. These authors have emphasized the importance of cognitive factors in finding meaning in life and in promoting personal growth.

There have been a number of developments in the field of psychotherapy during the twentieth century that have contributed to the formulation of the CT approach. The neo-Freudians, such as Adler, Horney, Alexander, and Sullivan, focused on the importance of perceptions of the self and on the salience of conscious experience. Other contributions came from the field of developmental psychology and from Kelly's (1955) theory of personal constructs. These writers stressed the significance of schemas (cognitive templates) in perceiving, assimilating, and acting on information from the environment.

CT also incorporates theories and treatment methods of behavior therapy. Procedures such as activity scheduling, graded task assignments, exposure, and social skills training play a fundamental role in CT (Beck et al. 1979; Meichenbaum 1977). In addition, Ellis's rational emotive therapy (Ellis 1962) has helped promulgate CT and related treatments.

Investigations in the field of cognitive psychology have solidified the concepts originally proposed by Beck and have led to a refinement of the CT approach (e.g., Alford and Beck 1997; D.A. Clark et al. 1999; Dobson and Shaw 1986; Hollon and Kendall 1980). Also, the utility of the cognitive model has been demonstrated in a number of outcome trials reviewed later in this chapter. Other developments have included the description of cognitive and behavioral techniques for personality disorders (Beck and Freeman 1990), substance abuse (Beck et al. 1992), geriatric patients (Beut-

ler et al. 1987), eating disorders (Agras et al. 1992; Fairburn et al. 1991), and bipolar disorder (Basco and Rush 2005). Also, theories and procedures have been developed for combining CT and pharmacotherapy (Wright 2004; Wright and Thase 1992), applying CT principles in the treatment of psychotic patients (Kingdon and Turkington 2005), implementing cognitively oriented inpatient treatment (Stuart et al. 1997; Wright et al. 1993), using CT in behavioral medicine (Sensky 2004), and employing computer-assisted CT to improve the efficiency of treatment (Selmi et al. 1990; Wright and Wright 1997; Wright et al. 2005).

In a review of the evolution of CT, Beck (1993) observed that intensive efforts have been made to have CT fulfill the criteria for a system of psychotherapy (Table 31–1). These criteria include 1) a comprehensive theory, 2) empirical data to support this theory, 3) an operationalized therapy that interlocks with theoretical concepts, and 4) demonstrated efficacy of the treatment (Beck 1993). The remainder of this chapter is devoted to describing basic cognitive-behavioral theories and their experimental basis, the translation of theoretical constructs into clinical practice, and the validation of CT in controlled research.

TABLE 31–1. Criteria for a system of psychotherapy

A comprehensive theory

Empirical support for the theory

An operationalized therapy based on theoretical principles

Empirical evidence for effectiveness of the psychotherapy

Basic Concepts
The Cognitive Model

The cognitive model for psychotherapy is grounded on the theory that there are characteristic errors in information processing in psychiatric disorders, and that these alterations in thought processes are closely linked to emotional reactions and dysfunctional behavior patterns (Beck 1976; Wright et al. 2006). For example, Beck and co-workers (Beck 1976) have proposed that there are three major areas of cognitive distortion in depression (the negative cognitive triad of self, world, and future) and that patients with anxiety disorders habitually overestimate the danger or risk in situations. Cognitive distortions such as misperceptions, errors in logic, or misattributions are thought to lead to dysphoric moods and maladaptive behavior. Furthermore, a vicious cycle is perpetuated when the behavioral response confirms and amplifies negatively distorted cognitions (Wright et al. 2006).

> This point is illustrated by the case of Mr. S, a 45-year-old recently divorced, depressed man. After being rebuffed on his first attempt to ask a woman for a date, Mr. S had a series of dysfunctional cognitions such as, "You should have known better.... You're a loser.... There's no use trying." His subsequent behavioral pattern was consistent with these cognitions—he made no further social contacts and became more lonely and isolated. The negative behavior led to additional maladaptive cognitions (e.g., "No one will want me.... I'll be alone the rest of my life.... What's the use of going on?").

The CT perspective can be summarized in a working model (Figure 31–1) that expands on the well-known stimulus–response paradigm (Wright 1988; Wright et al. 2006). Cognitive mediation is given the central role in this model. However, an interactive relationship between environmental influences, cognition, emotion, and behavior is also recognized. It should be emphasized that this working model does not presume that cognitive pathology is the cause of specific syndromes or that other factors such as genetic predisposition, biochemical alterations, or interpersonal conflicts are not involved in the etiology of psychiatric illnesses. Instead, the model is used simply as a guide for the actions of the cognitive therapist in clinical practice. It is assumed that most forms of psychopathology have complex etiologies involving cognitive, biological, social, and interpersonal influences, and that there are multiple, potentially useful, approaches to treatment. In addition, it is assumed that cognitive changes are accomplished through biological processes and that psychopharmacological treatments can alter cognitions (Wright and Thase 1992). This position is consistent with outcome research on CT and pharmacotherapy (Blackburn et al. 1981) and with other studies that have documented neurobiological changes associated with conditioning in animals (Kandel and Schwarz 1982; Mohl 1987) or psychotherapy in humans (Baxter et al. 1992; Goldapple et al. 2004).

The working model in Figure 31–1 posits a close relationship between cognition and emotion. The general thrust of CT is that emotional responses are largely dependent upon cognitive appraisals of the significance of environmental cues. For example, sadness is likely when an event (or memory of an event) is perceived in a negative way (such as a loss, a defeat, or

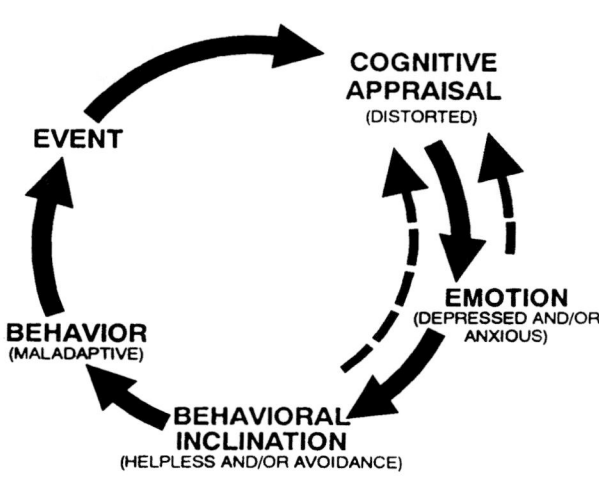

FIGURE 31–1. A working model for cognitive therapy.

Source. Adapted from Wright 1988.

a rejection), and anger is common when it is judged that there are threats to one's self or loved ones. The cognitive model also incorporates the effects of emotion on cognitive processing. Heightened emotion can stimulate and intensify cognitive distortion (Greenberg and Safran 1984). Therapeutic procedures in CT involve interventions at all points in the working model diagrammed in Figure 31–1. However, most of the effort is directed at stimulating either cognitive or behavioral change.

Levels of Dysfunctional Cognitions

Beck and colleagues (Beck 1976; Beck et al. 1979; Dobson and Shaw 1986) have suggested that there are two major levels of dysfunctional information processing: 1) automatic thoughts and 2) basic beliefs incorporated in schemas. Automatic thoughts are the cognitions that occur rapidly while a person is in a situation (or recalling an event). These automatic thoughts usually are not subjected to rational analysis and often are based on erroneous logic. Although the individual may be only subliminally aware of these cognitions, automatic thoughts are accessible through questioning techniques used in CT (Beck et al. 1979; Wright and Beck 1983). The different types of faulty logic in automatic thinking have been termed *cognitive errors* (Beck et al. 1979). Descriptions of typical cognitive errors, such as selective abstraction, arbitrary inference, and absolutistic thinking, are provided in Table 31–2.

TABLE 31–2. Cognitive errors

Selective abstraction (sometimes termed "mental filter")	Drawing a conclusion based on only a small portion of the available data
Arbitrary inference	Coming to a conclusion without adequate supporting evidence or despite contradictory evidence
Absolutistic thinking ("all or none" thinking)	Categorizing oneself or personal experiences into rigid dichotomies (e.g., all good or all bad, perfect or completely flawed, success or total failure)
Magnification and minimization	Over- or undervaluing the significance of a personal attribute, a life event, or a future possibility
Personalization	Linking external occurrences to oneself (e.g., taking blame, assuming responsibility, criticizing oneself) when there is little or no basis for making these associations
Catastrophic thinking	Predicting the worst possible outcome while ignoring more likely eventualities

Source.   Adapted from Beck AT, Rush AJ, Shaw BF, Emery G: *Cognitive Therapy of Depression.* New York, Guilford Press, 1979. Used with permission.

Schemas are deeper cognitive structures that contain the basic rules for screening, filtering, and coding information from the environment (Beck et al. 1979; D. A. Clark et al. 1999; Wright and Beck 1983). These organizing constructs are developed through early childhood experiences and subsequent formative influences. Schemas can play a highly adaptive role in allowing rapid assimilation of data and appropriate decision making. However, in psychiatric disorders there are clusters of maladaptive schemas that perpetuate dysphoric mood and ineffective or self-defeating behavior (Beck 1976; Beck and Freeman 1990). Examples of adaptive and maladaptive schemas are presented in Table 31–3.

D. A. Clark et al. (1999) have suggested that schemas can be grouped into three levels: 1) simple schemas (e.g., rules about objects in the environment) that may have little or no influence on psychopathology; 2) intermediary beliefs, rules, and assumptions (e.g., conditional rules, "if–then" statements such as "to be accepted, I must always please others"); and 3) core beliefs about the self (e.g., fundamental rules such as "I am unlovable") that often have a global and absolute quality. Schemas can vary in their degree of flexibility, permeability (i.e., the degree to which they can be modified by contradictory information), concreteness, valence, and breadth (D. A. Clark et al. 1999). It has been suggested that clusters of interrelated schemas (termed *modes*) help humans to organize and deal with the demands that are placed upon them (D. A. Clark et al. 1999).

TABLE 31–3. Adaptive and maladaptive schemas

Adaptive	Maladaptive
No matter what happens, I can manage somehow.	I must be perfect to be accepted.
If I work at something, I can master it.	If I choose to do something, I must succeed.
I'm a survivor.	I'm a fake.
Others can trust me.	Without a woman [man], I'm nothing.
I'm lovable.	I'm stupid.
People respect me.	No matter what I do, I won't succeed.
I can figure things out.	Others can't be trusted.
If I prepare in advance, I usually do better.	I can never be comfortable around others.
I like to be challenged.	If I make one mistake, I'll lose everything.
There's not much that can scare me.	The world is too frightening for me.

One of the basic tenets of CT is that maladaptive schemas often lie dormant until they are triggered by stressful life events (Beck et al. 1979; D. A. Clark et al. 1999). The newly emerged schema then influences the more superficial level of cognitive processing so that automatic thoughts are consistent with the rules of the schema. This theory applies primarily to episodic disorders such as depression. In chronic conditions (e.g., personality disturbances and eating disorders), schemas that pertain to the self may be present consistently and may be more resistant to change than in depression or anxiety disorders (Beck and Freeman 1990).

An example of the relationship between schemas and automatic thoughts can be found in the case of Mrs. C, a 39-year-old schoolteacher, married for the second time, who was functioning well until her husband made an unwise financial investment. When the family's economic situation changed, Mrs. C became depressed and started to have crying spells in her classroom. During the course of CT, several important schemas were uncovered. One of these was the maladaptive belief: "You'll fail, no matter how hard you try." This schema was associated with a host of negative automatic thoughts (e.g., "I messed up again…. We'll lose everything…. It's not worth the effort"). Although there had been a significant financial loss, and the marriage was stressed because of the situation, the emergence of Mrs. C's underlying schema led to an overgeneralization of the significance of the problem and a perpetuation of dysfunctional automatic thoughts.

Cognitive Pathology in Depression and Anxiety Disorders

The role of cognitive functioning in depression and anxiety disorders has been studied extensively. Information processing also has been examined in eating disorders, characterological problems, and other psychiatric conditions. In general, the results of this investigative effort have confirmed Beck's hypotheses (Beck 1963, 1964, 1976; Beck et al. 1979; D. A. Clark et al. 1999; Wright and Beck 1983). A full review of this research is not attempted here. However, a synthesis of results of significant studies on depression and anxiety is provided. These findings have played an important role in both confirming and shaping the treatment procedures used in CT. Cognitive pathology in eating disturbances, personality disorders, and psychoses is described in the section on CT applications.

Reviews of the voluminous research on cognitive processes in depression have found strong evidence for a negative cognitive bias in this disorder (D. A. Clark et

al. 1999). For example, distorted automatic thoughts and cognitive errors have been found to be much more frequent in depressed persons than in control subjects (Blackburn et al. 1986; Dobson and Shaw 1986; Hollon et al. 1986; LeFebvre 1981). A selective recall bias also has been described. Depressed individuals are more likely to remember negative than positive self-referent information (D. M. Clark and Teasdale 1982).

Substantial evidence has been collected to support the concept of the negative cognitive triad (D. A. Clark et al. 1999). A particularly well-designed study in this area of research was performed by Blackburn et al. (1986), who used the Cognitive Bias Questionnaire to test distortions in the three areas of the negative cognitive triad (self, world, and future). Depressed individuals scored more than twice as high on this scale as nondepressed control subjects. A large group of investigations has established that one of the elements of the negative cognitive triad, hopelessness, is highly associated with suicide risk (Beck et al. 1975, 1985b; Fawcett et al. 1987). Beck et al. (1985b) found that hopelessness was the strongest predictor of ultimate suicide in a sample of depressed inpatients followed 10 years after discharge. CT has been demonstrated to be an effective treatment approach for reducing hopelessness and suicide attempts (Brown et al. 2005).

Research on schemas has been limited by problems in measuring these underlying cognitive structures (D. A. Clark et al. 1999). The most commonly used instrument, the Dysfunctional Attitude Scale (DAS; Weissman 1979) has been criticized because it appears to tap a general tendency for negatively biased thinking and may not directly assess schemas (D. A. Clark et al. 1999). Furthermore, Beck's theories indicate that schemas become dormant during remissions; therefore, these core beliefs would not be expected to be readily accessible with a self-rating instrument such as the DAS. Nevertheless, several investigations have found high DAS scores during periods of depression and marked reductions with symptomatic improvement (e.g., Blackburn et al. 1986; DeRubeis et al. 1990; Wright et al. 2005). It has been suggested that small residual elevations in DAS scores after recovery from depression may indicate that this scale detects underlying schemas that are a marker for vulnerability to relapse (Blackburn et al. 1986).

Abramson et al. (1978) have proposed that attributions to life events are negatively distorted in depression and that misattributions can play a role in the development of this disorder. The relevance of early research on attributions has been questioned because most investigations were performed with nonclinical experimental subjects (D.A. Clark et al. 1999; Peterson et al. 1985). Also, some studies of carefully diagnosed depressed patients found little or no evidence for attributional distortions (Hargreaves 1985; Miller et al. 1982). Nevertheless, the overall results of research on attributions indicate that clinically depressed individuals are prone to blame themselves for adverse life events, give global meaning to circumscribed occurrences, and believe that negative situations will last indefinitely. In contrast, individuals who do not have depression commonly view noxious events as being due to external forces (e.g., fate, bad luck), as having isolated significance (limited only to the specific events), and being transient situations (Deutscher and Cimbolic 1990; Zimmerman et al. 1986).

Studies of responses to feedback have provided another perspective on dysfunctional information processing. Depressed individuals usually underestimate the amount of positive feedback that they receive (D.A. Clark et al. 1999; Rizley 1978; Wenzloff and Grozier 1988). In analogue experiments, depressed subjects have expended decreased effort on subsequent trials after concluding that they have performed poorly on a task (Klein et al. 1976). Interestingly, a "positive self-serving bias" has been described in nondepressed control subjects (Rizley 1978). The tendency for nondepressed individuals to hear more positive and/or less negative feedback than they actually receive and to expend extra effort after being told they have not done well may be an adaptive trait (Rizley 1978).

Studies of information processing in anxiety disorders have provided additional confirmation for the cognitive model of psychopathology. Anxious patients have been found to have an attentional bias in responding to potentially threatening stimuli (Mathews and MacLeod 1987). Individuals with significant levels of anxiety are more likely than nonanxious persons to have a facilitated intake of information about potential threat; furthermore, those with anxiety disorders are prone to interpret environmental situations as being unrealistically dangerous or risky and to underestimate their ability to cope with these situations (Mathews and MacLeod 1987). Anxious patients also have been shown to have an enhanced recall for memories associated with threatening situations or past anxiety states (Cloitre and Liebowitz 1991; Ingram et al. 1987). Thus, dysfunctional thinking in anxiety disorders spans over several phases of information processing, including attention, elaboration and inference, and retrieval from memory.

Automatic thoughts associated with themes of danger, threat, uncontrollability, or anticipated incom-

petence have been observed at much higher rates in patients with elevated levels of anxiety than those with low anxiety (Ingram et al. 1987; Kendall and Hollon 1989). In other studies of cognitive biasing in anxiety disorders, investigators have noted high frequencies of negative self-statements (Glass and Furlong 1990), beliefs that social behavior is inadequate or standards of others cannot be met (Wallace and Alden 1991), misinterpretations of bodily stimuli (McNally and Foa 1987), and overestimates of future misfortune (Mizes et al. 1987).

Comparisons of depressed and anxious patients have revealed differences between the two groups and common features of the disorders (D.A. Clark et al. 1990; Ingram et al. 1987). In depression, cognitions about hopelessness, low self-worth, and failure are more frequent, whereas in anxiety, cognitive themes are usually related to anticipated harm or danger (D.A. Clark et al. 1990). Also, depressed patients are more likely to have absolute thoughts about negative themes, whereas those with anxiety disorders tend to have questioning thoughts concerning the uncertainty of future events (D.A. Clark et al. 1990; Ingram et al. 1987). Although the content of thoughts may be different, depressed and anxious patients both have demoralization, self-absorption, a predominance of automatic information processing, and a reduction in the cognitive capacity needed for problem solving and task performance (D.A. Clark et al. 1990; Ingram et al. 1987). Findings of studies on cognitive pathology in depression and anxiety disorders are summarized in Table 31–4.

Therapeutic Principles

General Procedures

CT is usually a short-term treatment, lasting from 5 to 20 sessions. In some instances, very brief treatment courses are used for patients with mild or circumscribed problems, or longer series of CT sessions are used for those with chronic or especially severe conditions. However, the typical patient with major depression or an anxiety disorder can be treated successfully within the short-term format. After completion of the initial course of treatment, intermittent booster sessions may be useful in some cases, particularly for individuals with a history of recurrent illness or incomplete remission (Jarrett et al. 2001). Booster sessions can help maintain gains, solidify what has been learned in CT, and decrease the chances of relapse (Thase 1992).

TABLE 31–4. Pathological information processing in depression and anxiety disorders

Predominant in depression	Predominant in anxiety disorders	Common to both depression and anxiety disorders
Hopelessness	Fears of harm or danger	Demoralization
Low self-esteem	High sensitivity to information about potential threat	Self-absorption
Negative view of environment		Heightened automatic information processing
Automatic thoughts with negative themes	Automatic thoughts associated with danger, risk, uncontrollability, incapacity	Maladaptive schemas
Misattributions		Reduced cognitive capacity for problem solving
Overestimates of negative feedback	Overestimates of risk in situations	
Enhanced recall of negative memories	Enhanced recall of memories for threatening situations	
Impaired performance on cognitive tasks requiring effort, abstract thinking		

Although CT is primarily directed at the "here and now," knowledge of the patient's family background, developmental experiences, social network, and medical history helps guide the course of therapy. Collecting a thorough history is an essential component of the early phase of treatment. History taking can be augmented in CT by asking the patient to write a brief "autobiography" as one of the early homework assignments. This material is then reviewed during a subsequent therapy session.

The bulk of the therapeutic effort in CT is devoted to working on specific problems or issues in the patient's present life. The problem-oriented approach is emphasized for several reasons. First, directing the patient's attention to current problems stimulates the development of action plans that can help reverse helplessness, hopelessness, avoidance, or other dysfunctional symptoms. Second, data on cognitive responses to recent life events are more readily accessible and verifiable than for events that happened years in the past. Third, practical work on present problems helps to prevent the development of excessive dependency or regression in the therapeutic relationship. Finally, current problems usually provide ample opportunity to understand and explore the impact of past experiences.

The Therapeutic Relationship

The therapeutic relationship in CT is characterized by a high degree of collaboration between patient and therapist and an empirical tone to the work of therapy. The therapist and patient function much like an investigative team. They develop hypotheses about the validity of automatic thoughts and schemas or alternately about the effectiveness of patterns of behavior. A series of exercises or experiments is then designed to test the validity of the hypotheses and, subsequently, to modify cognitions or behavior. Beck et al. (1979) have termed this form of therapeutic relationship *collaborative empiricism*. Methods of building a collaborative and empirical relationship are listed in Table 31–5.

The therapist usually is more active in CT than in most other psychotherapies. The degree of therapist activity varies with the stage of treatment and the severity of the illness. Generally, a more directive and structured approach is emphasized early in treatment, when symptoms are severe. For example, a markedly depressed patient who is beginning treatment may benefit from considerable direction and structure because of symptoms such as helplessness, hopelessness, low energy, and impaired concentration. As the patient improves and understands more about the methods of CT, the therapist can become somewhat less active. By the end of treatment, the patient should be able to use self-monitoring and self-help techniques with little reinforcement from the therapist.

Collaborative empiricism is fostered throughout the therapy, even when directive work is required. Although the therapist may suggest specific strategies or give homework assignments designed to combat severe depression or anxiety, the patient's input is always solicited and the self-help component of CT is emphasized from the outset of treatment. Also, it is made clear that CT is not an attempt to convert all negative thoughts to positive ones. In fact, bad things do occur to people, and some individuals have behaviors that are ineffective or self-defeating. It is emphasized that in CT one seeks to obtain an accurate assessment

TABLE 31–5. Methods of enhancing collaborative empiricism

Work together as an investigative team.

Adjust therapist activity level to match the severity of illness and phase of treatment.

Encourage self-monitoring and self-help.

Obtain accurate assessment of validity of cognitions and efficacy of behavior.

Develop coping strategies for real losses and actual deficits.

Promote essential "nonspecific" therapist variables (e.g., kindness, empathy, equanimity, positive general attitude).

Provide and request feedback on regular basis.

Recognize and manage transference.

Customize therapy interventions.

Use gentle humor.

of 1) the validity of cognitions, and 2) the adaptive versus maladaptive nature of behavior. If cognitive distortions have occurred, then the patient and therapist will work together to develop a more rational perspective. On the other hand, if actual negative experiences or characteristics are identified, they will attempt to find ways to cope or to change.

The development of a collaborative working relationship is dependent on a number of therapist and patient characteristics. The "nonspecific" therapist variables that are important components of all effective psychotherapies (Davis and Wright 1994; Wright et al. 2006) are equally significant in CT (see Table 31–5). Professionals who are kind and understanding and can convey appropriate empathy make good cognitive therapists. Other factors of significance are the ability of the therapist to generate trust, to demonstrate a high level of competence, and to exhibit equanimity under pressure (Wright et al. 2006). Cognitive therapists also must be able to maintain an energetic pace and to sustain their concentration throughout the treatment sessions.

Another characteristic that can influence the therapeutic relationship is the therapist's general attitude. Clinicians with a reasonably positive outlook on life and a belief that individual efforts can lead to significant change are likely to form more adaptive therapeutic relationships than those who may be overly discouraged or pessimistic. If the latter features are present, the therapist may require personal therapy to be able to forge the collaborative and empirical relationships that are necessary for effective CT.

Additional procedures that cognitive therapists use to encourage collaborative empiricism are 1) providing feedback throughout sessions, 2) recognizing and managing transference, 3) customizing therapy interventions, and 4) using gentle humor. The therapist gives feedback to keep the therapeutic relationship anchored in the "here and now" and to reinforce the working aspect of the therapy process. Comments are made frequently throughout the session to summarize major points, to give direction, and to keep the session on target. Also, questions are asked at several intervals in each session to determine how well the patient has understood a concept or has grasped the essence of a therapeutic intervention. Because CT is highly psychoeducational, the therapist functions to some degree as a teacher. Thus, discreet positive feedback is given to help stimulate and reward the patient's efforts to learn. On a cautionary note, however, the cognitive therapist needs to avoid overzealous coaching or providing inaccurate or overdone positive feedback. Such actions will usually undermine the development of a good collaborative relationship.

Patients also are encouraged to give feedback throughout the sessions. In the beginning of treatment, patients are told that the therapist will want to hear from them regularly about how the sessions are going. What are the patient's reactions to the therapist? What things are going well? What would the patient like to change? What points are clear and make sense? What seems confusing?

A collaborative therapeutic relationship with frequent opportunities for two-way feedback generally discourages the formation of a transference neurosis. CT methodology and the short-term nature of treatment promote pragmatic working relationships as opposed to recapitulations of dysfunctional early relationships. Nevertheless, significant transference reactions can occur. These are more likely with patients who have personality disorders or other chronic illnesses that require longer-term treatment. The formation of negative or problematic transference reactions is rare in conventional short-term CT of persons with uncomplicated depression or anxiety disorders. When transference reactions occur, the cognitive therapist applies CT procedures to understand the phenomenon and to intervene. Typically, automatic thoughts and schemas that pertain to the therapeutic relationship are identified, explored, and modified if possible. Another feature of CT that increases the collaborative nature of the therapeutic relationship is the customization of therapy interventions to meet the level of the patient's cognitive and social functioning. A profoundly depressed or anxious individual of low average intelligence may require a primarily behavioral approach, with limited efforts at understanding concepts such as automatic thoughts and schemas, especially in the beginning of treatment. Conversely, a less symptomatic patient with higher intelligence and ability to grasp abstract concepts may be able to profit from schema assessment early in therapy. If treatment procedures are pitched at a proper level, the patient is more likely to understand the material of therapy and to form a collaborative relationship with the therapist who is directing the treatment.

The therapeutic relationship also can be enhanced by using gentle humor during CT sessions. For example, the therapist may encourage the patient's sense of humor by providing opportunities to laugh together at some improbable situation or humorously distorted cognition. On occasion, the therapist may use hyperbole in a discreet manner to point out an inconsistency or an illogical conclusion. Humor needs to be injected carefully into the therapeutic relationship. Some patients respond quite well to humor. Others may be limited in their ability to use this feature of therapy. However, appropriate use of humor can strengthen the therapeutic relationship in CT if patient and therapist are able to laugh with one another and to use humor to deflate exaggerated or distorted cognitions.

Assessment and Case Conceptualization

Assessment for CT begins with completion of a standard history and mental status examination. Although special attention is paid to cognitive and behavioral elements, a full biopsychosocial evaluation is completed and used in formulating the treatment plan. The Academy of Cognitive Therapy, a certifying organization for cognitive therapists, has outlined a method for assessment and case conceptualization, which involves consideration of developmental influences, family history, social and interpersonal issues, genetic and biological contributions, and strengths and assets, in addition to key automatic thoughts, schemas, and behavioral patterns (Figure 31–2). The book *Learning Cognitive-Behavior Therapy: An Illustrated Guide* (Wright et al. 2006) provides detailed methods, worksheets, and examples of use of the Academy of Cognitive Therapy formulation methods. Worksheets from this book can be downloaded from the American

Psychiatric Publishing Inc. Web site (www.appi.org). Also, the Academy of Cognitive Therapy Web site (www.academyofct.org) supplies illustrations of how to complete case conceptualizations.

The key elements of the case conceptualization are 1) an outline of the most salient aspects of the history and mental status examination; 2) detailing of at least three examples from the patient's life of the relationship between events, automatic thoughts, emotions, and behaviors (specific illustrations of the cognitive model as it pertains to this patient); 3) identification of important schemas; 4) listing of strengths; 5) a working hypothesis that weaves together all of the information in numbers 1–4 with the cognitive and behavioral theories that most closely fit the patient's diagnosis and symptoms (e.g., models for anxiety disorders, depression, eating disorders, personality disorders, and other conditions; and 6) a treatment plan (including choices for specific CT methods) that is based on the working hypothesis. The conceptualization is continually developed throughout therapy and may be augmented or revised as new information is collected and treatment methods are tested.

One of the common myths about CT is that it is a "manualized" therapy that follows a "cookbook" approach. While it is true that CT has been distinguished by clear descriptions of theory and methods, this treatment is guided by an individualized case conceptualization. Experienced therapists typically use considerable creativity in matching CT interventions to the unique attributes, cultural background, life stresses, and strengths of each patient (Table 31–6).

Structuring Therapy

Several of the structuring procedures commonly employed in CT are listed in Table 31–7. One of the most important techniques for CT is the use of a therapy agenda. At the beginning of each session, the therapist and patient work together to derive a short list of topics, usually consisting of two to four items. Generally, it is advisable to shape an agenda that 1) can be managed within the time frame of an individual session, 2) follows up on material from earlier sessions, 3) reviews any homework from the previous session and provides an opportunity for new homework assignments, and 4) contains specific items that are highly relevant to the patient but are not too global or abstract.

Agenda setting helps to counteract hopelessness and helplessness by reducing seemingly overwhelming problems down into workable segments. The agenda-setting process also encourages patients to

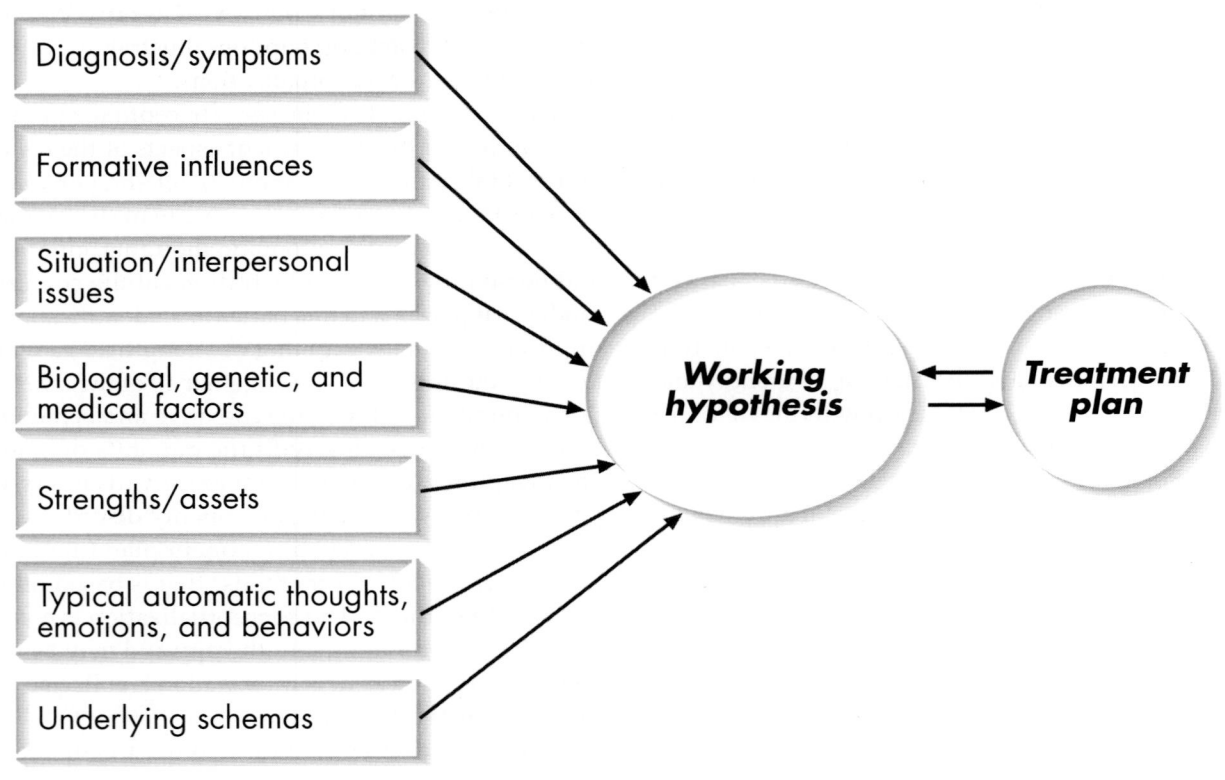

FIGURE 31–2. Case conceptualization flow chart.

Source. Reprinted from Wright JH, Basco MR, Thase ME: *Learning Cognitive-Behavior Therapy: An Illustrated Guide* (Core Competencies in Psychotherapy Series, Glen O. Gabbard, series ed.). Arlington, VA, American Psychiatric Publishing, 2006, p. 51. Copyright 2006, American Psychiatric Publishing. Used with permission.

TABLE 31–6. Key elements of cognitive therapy case conceptualization
History and mental status examination
Examples of cognitive-behavioral model from patient's life
Identification of major schemas
List of strengths
Working hypothesis
Treatment plan

TABLE 31–7. Structuring procedures for cognitive therapy
Set agenda for therapy sessions.
Give constructive feedback to direct the course of therapy.
Employ common cognitive therapy techniques on a regular basis.
Assign homework to link sessions together.

take a problem-oriented approach to their difficulties. Simply articulating a problem in a specific manner often can initiate the process of change. In addition, the agenda keeps the patient focused on salient issues and encourages efficient use of the therapy time.

The agenda is set in a collaborative manner, and decisions to depart from the agenda are made jointly between therapist and patient. When work on an agenda item generates important information on a topic that was not foreseen at the beginning of the session, the therapist and patient discuss the merits of diverting or modifying the agenda. An excessively rigid approach to using a therapy agenda is not advocated. There must be sufficient flexibility to investigate promising new leads or to allow the patient to express significant thoughts or feelings that were unexpected at the beginning of the session. However, an overall commitment to setting and following the therapy agenda gives needed structure to patients who are unable to define problems clearly or think of ways to cope with them.

Feedback procedures described earlier are also used in structuring CT sessions. For example, the therapist may observe that the patient is drifting from the established agenda or is spending time discussing a topic of questionable relevance. In situations such as these, constructive feedback is given to direct the patient back to a more profitable area of inquiry. Heavy-handed, negatively oriented feedback is avoided. Instead, the therapist tends to give encouraging remarks that point the patient to issues that provide significant opportunities for change.

Commonly used CT techniques add an additional structural element to the therapy. Examples include activity scheduling, thought recording, and graded task assignments. These interventions, and others of similar nature, provide a clear and understandable method for reducing symptoms. Repeated use of procedures such as recording, labeling, and modifying automatic thoughts helps to link sessions together, especially if they are introduced in therapy and then assigned as homework.

Psychoeducation

Psychoeducational procedures are a routine component of CT. One of the major goals of the treatment approach is to teach patients a new way of thinking and behaving that can be applied in resolving their current symptoms and in managing problems that will be encountered in the future. The psychoeducational effort usually begins with the process of socializing the patient to therapy. In the opening phase of treatment, the therapist explains the basic concepts of CT and introduces the patient to the format of CT sessions. The therapist also devotes time early in treatment to discussing the therapeutic relationship in CT and the expectations for both patient and therapist. Psychoeducational work during a course of CT often involves brief explanations or illustrations coupled with homework assignments. These activities are woven into treatment sessions in a manner that emphasizes a collaborative, active learning approach. Some cognitive therapists have described the use of "mini-lectures," but a heavily didactic approach is generally avoided.

Psychoeducation can be facilitated with reading assignments and computer programs that reinforce learning, deepen the patient's understanding of CT principles, and promote the use of self-help methods. Table 31–8 contains a list of useful psychoeducational tools, including a pamphlet, books, and a computer program, that teach the CT model and encourage self-help. Most cognitive therapists liberally use psychoeducational tools as a basic part of the therapy process.

TABLE 31–8. Psychoeducational materials and programs for cognitive therapy

Title	Authors	Description
"Coping With Anxiety"	A.T. Beck et al. 1985a	Appendix to book
"Coping With Depression"	A.T. Beck et al. 1995	Brief pamphlet
Feeling Good	Burns 1980, 1999	Book with self-help program
Getting Your Life Back: The Complete Guide to Recovery From Depression	Wright and Basco 2002	Book with self-help program; integrates cognitive therapy and biological approaches
Good Days Ahead: The Multimedia Program for Cognitive Therapy	Wright et al. 2004	Computer-assisted therapy and self-help program
Mastery of Your Anxiety and Panic	Barlow and Craske 1999	Self-help for anxiety
Mind Over Mood	Greenberger and Padesky 1995	Self-help workbook
Never Good Enough	Basco 1999	Book on perfectionism
Stop Obsessing! How to Overcome Your Obsessions and Compulsions	Foa and Wilson 2001	Self-help for OCD

Cognitive Techniques

Identifying Automatic Thoughts

Much of the work of CT is devoted to recognizing and then modifying negatively distorted or illogical automatic thoughts (Table 31–9). The most powerful way of introducing the patient to the effects of automatic thoughts is to find an in vivo example of how automatic thoughts can influence emotional responses. Mood shifts during the therapy session are almost always good places to pause to identify automatic thoughts. The therapist observes that a strong emotion such as sadness, anxiety, or anger has appeared and then asks the patient to describe the thoughts that "went through your head" just prior to the mood shift. This technique is illustrated in the example of Mr. B, a 50-year-old depressed man who had suffered several recent losses and had developed extremely low self-esteem.

> Therapist: "How did you react to your wife's criticism?"
>
> Mr. B: (Suddenly appears much more sad and anxious) "It was just too much to take."
>
> Therapist: "I can see this really upsets you. Can you think back to what went through your mind right after I asked you the last question? Just try to tell me all the thoughts that popped into your head."
>
> Mr. B: (Pause, then recounts) "I'm always making mistakes. I can't do anything right. There's no way to please her. I might as well give up."
>
> Therapist: "I can see why you felt so sad. When these kinds of thoughts just automatically pop into your mind, you don't stop to think if they are accurate or not. That's why we call them automatic thoughts."
>
> Mr. B: "I guess you're right. I hardly realized I was having those thoughts until you asked me to say them out loud."
>
> Therapist: "Recognizing that you're having automatic thoughts is one of the first steps in therapy. Now let's see what we can do to help you with your thinking and with the situation with your wife."

Beck has described emotion as the "royal road to cognition" (Beck 1989). The patient usually is most accessible during periods of affective arousal, and cognitions such as automatic thoughts and schemas generally are more potent when they are associated with strong emotional responses. Hence, the cognitive therapist capitalizes on spontaneously occurring affective states during the interview and also pursues lines of questioning that are likely to produce an intense affect. One of the misconceptions about CT is that it is an

TABLE 31–9. Methods for identifying and modifying automatic thoughts

Socratic questioning (guided discovery)
Use of mood shifts to demonstrate automatic thoughts in vivo
Imagery exercises
Role-play
Thought recording
Generating alternatives
Examining the evidence
Decatastrophizing
Reattribution
Cognitive rehearsal

overly intellectualized form of therapy. In fact, CT, as formulated by Beck et al. (1979), involves efforts to increase affect and to use emotional responses as a core ingredient of therapy.

One of the most frequently used procedures in CT is Socratic questioning. There is no set format or protocol for this technique. Instead, the therapist must rely on his or her experience and ingenuity to formulate questions that will help patients move from having a "closed mind" to a state of inquisitiveness and curiosity. Socratic questioning stimulates recognition of dysfunctional cognitions and development of a sense of dissonance about the validity of strongly held assumptions.

Socratic questioning usually involves a series of inductive questions that are likely to reveal dysfunctional thought patterns. The use of this technique to identify automatic thoughts is illustrated in the case of Ms. W, a 42-year-old woman with an anxiety disorder.

> Therapist: "What things seem to trigger your anxiety?"
>
> Ms. W: "Everything. It seems like no matter what I do, I'm nervous all the time."
>
> Therapist: "I suppose that 'everything' could trigger your anxiety and that you have no control over it. But let's stop for a moment and see if there are any other possibilities. Is that okay?"
>
> Ms. W: "Sure."
>
> Therapist: "Then try to think of a situation where your anxiety is very high and one where it's much lower."
>
> Ms. W: "Well, a high-anxiety time would be whenever I try to go out in public, like to go shopping or to a party. And a low anxiety time would be sitting at home watching TV."
>
> Therapist: "So there's some variation depending on what you are doing at the time."

Ms. W: "I guess that's right."

Therapist: "Would you like to find out what's behind the variation?"

Ms. W: "I guess. But I suppose it's just because being out with people makes me nervous and being at home feels safe."

Therapist: "That's one explanation. I wonder if there might be any others—ones that would give you some clues on how to get over the problem."

Ms. W: "I'm willing to look."

Therapist: "Well then, let's try to find out something about the different thoughts that you have about these two situations. When you think of going out to a party, what comes to mind?"

Ms. W: "I'll be embarrassed. I won't have any idea what to say or do. I'll probably panic and run out the door."

This example depicts the typical use of Socratic questions early in the therapy process. Further questioning would be required to help the patient fully understand how dysfunctional cognitions are involved in her anxiety responses and how changing these cognitions could dampen her anxiety and promote a higher level of functioning.

Imagery and role-play are used as alternate methods of uncovering cognitions when direct questions are unsuccessful in generating suspected automatic thinking (Beck et al. 1979). These techniques also are selected when only a limited amount of automatic thoughts can be brought out through Socratic questioning, and the therapist expects that more important automatic thoughts are present. Some patients may be able to use imagery procedures with few prompts or directions. In this case, the clinician only may need to ask the patient to imagine himself or herself back in a particularly troubling or emotion-provoking situation and then to describe the thoughts that occurred. However, most patients, particularly in the early phases of therapy, can benefit from "setting the scene" for the use of imagery. The patient is asked to describe the details of the setting. When and where did it take place? What happened immediately before the incident? How did the characters in the scene appear? What were the main physical features of the setting? Questions such as these help bring the scene alive in the patient's mind and facilitate recall of cognitive responses to the situation.

Role-play is a related technique for evoking automatic thoughts. When this procedure is used, the therapist first asks a series of questions to try to understand a vignette involving an interpersonal relationship or other social interchange that is likely to stimulate dysfunctional automatic thinking. Then, with the permission of the patient, the therapist briefly steps into the role of the individual in the scene and facilitates the playing out of a typical response set. Role-play is used less frequently than Socratic questioning or imagery and is best suited to therapeutic situations in which there is an excellent collaborative relationship and the patient is unlikely to respond to the role-play exercise with a negative or distorted transference reaction.

Thought recording is one of the most frequently used CT procedures for identifying automatic thoughts (J. Beck 1995; Wright et al. 2006). Patients can be asked to log their thoughts in a number of different ways. The simplest method is the two-column technique—a procedure that often is used when the patient is just beginning to learn how to recognize automatic thoughts. The two-column technique is illustrated in Table 31–10. In this case, the patient was asked to write down automatic thoughts that occurred in stressful or upsetting situations. Alternately, the patient could try to identify emotional reactions in one column and automatic thoughts in the other. A three-column exercise could include a description of the situation, a list of automatic thoughts, and a notation of the emotional response. Thought recording helps the patient to recognize the effects of underlying automatic thoughts and to understand how the basic cognitive model (i.e., relationship between situations, thoughts, feelings, and behaviors) applies to his or her own experiences. This procedure also initiates the process of modifying dysfunctional cognitions.

Thought recording is usually explained and illustrated in a therapy session and then additional exercises are assigned for homework. Depending on the case conceptualization, the therapist may suggest that the patient pay special attention to certain situations or issues (e.g., panic-inducing environmental cues, recurrent interpersonal problems, or dysfunctional behavioral responses). Also, specific assignments may be made to set up an in vivo experience that is likely to generate automatic thoughts. Examples might include discussing a troubling situation with a family member or attempting to engage in an anxiety-provoking situation or behavior that is usually avoided. Automatic thoughts that are recorded during these homework assignments are brought to the next session for review and discussion.

Modifying Automatic Thoughts

There usually is no sharp division in CT between the phases of eliciting and modifying automatic thoughts. In fact, the processes involved in identifying automatic thoughts often are enough to initiate substantive

TABLE 31–10. **Two-column thought recording**

Situation	Automatic thoughts
Call from boss to submit a report	I can't do this. I don't know what to do. It won't be acceptable.
My wife asks me to help more around the house	Nothing I do is ever enough. She thinks I don't try.
Car won't start	I was stupid to buy this car. Nothing works right anymore. This is the last straw.

change. As the patient begins to recognize the nature of his or her dysfunctional thinking, there typically is an increased degree of skepticism regarding the validity of automatic thoughts. Although patients can start to revise their cognitive distortions without specific additional therapeutic interventions, modification of automatic thoughts can be accelerated if the therapist applies Socratic questioning and other basic CT procedures to the change process (see Table 31–9).

Techniques used for revising automatic thoughts include 1) generating alternatives, 2) examining the evidence, 3) decatastrophizing, 4) reattribution, 5) thought recording, and 6) cognitive rehearsal (Beck et al. 1979; J. Beck 1995; Wright et al. 2006). Socratic questioning is used in all of these procedures. *Generating alternatives* is illustrated in the case of Ms. D, a 32-year-old woman with major depression. The therapist's questions were pointed toward helping Ms. D to see a broader range of possibilities than she had originally considered.

> Ms. D: "Every time I think of going back to school, I panic."
> Therapist: "And when you start to think of going to school, what thoughts come to mind?"
> Ms. D: "I'll botch it up. I won't be able to make it. I'll feel so ashamed when I have to drop out."
> Therapist: "What else could happen? Anything even worse, or are there any better possibilities?"
> Ms. D: "Well, it couldn't get much worse unless I never even tried at all."
> Therapist: "How would that be so bad?"
> Ms. D: "Then I'd just be the same—stuck in a rut, not going anywhere."
> Therapist: "We can take a look at that conclusion later—that not going to school would mean that you would stay in a rut; but for now let's look at the other possibilities if you do try to go to school again."

> Ms. D: "Okay. I guess there's some chance that it would go pretty well, but it'll be hard for me to manage school, the house, and all my family responsibilities."
> Therapist: "When you try to step back from the situation and not listen to your automatic thoughts, what's the most likely outcome of your going back to school?"
> Ms. D: "It will be a difficult adjustment, but it's something I want to do. I have the intelligence to do it if I apply myself."

Examining the evidence is a major component of the collaborative empirical experience in CT. Specific automatic thoughts or clusters of related automatic thoughts are set forth as hypotheses, and the patient and therapist then search for evidence both for and against the hypothesis. In the case of Ms. D, the thought "If I don't go to school, I'd just be the same—stuck in a rut, not going anywhere" was selected for an examining the evidence exercise. The therapist believed that returning to school was probably an adaptive action for the patient to take. However, it also was thought that seeing further education as the only route to change would excessively load this activity with a "make or break" mentality and would promote a disregard for other modifications that might increase self-esteem and self-efficacy.

Decatastrophizing involves efforts to reconceptualize feared outcomes in a manner that encourages coping and problem solving. This technique can be effective even if there is a reasonably high likelihood that a negative prediction will actually occur. For example, a man might correctly judge his marriage to be so troubled that his wife may ask for a divorce. In this instance, the therapist would help the patient to recognize distorted cognitions about his ability to manage a possible breakup of the marriage. The patient might think, "I couldn't make it without her" or "I'd lose everything." The decatastrophizing procedure would involve examining negative automatic thoughts for their validity; looking for previously unrecognized attributes, interests, or coping mechanisms; reviewing the ways that the patient had managed losses in the past; and stimulating the patient to think beyond the immediate situation. The use of *reattribution techniques* is based on findings of studies on the attributional process in depression explained earlier in this chapter. Depressed individuals have been found to have negatively biased attributions in three dimensions: global versus specific, internal versus external, and fixed versus variable (Abramson et al. 1978). Several different types of reattribution procedures are employed, including psychoeducation about the attributional process, Socratic questioning to stimulate reattribution, written exercises to recognize and reinforce alternate attributions, and homework assignments to test the accuracy of attributions.

Five-column Thought Change Records (TCRs; Beck et al. 1979) or other similar thought-recording devices are standard tools used in modification of automatic thoughts. The five-column TCR is used to encourage both identification and change of dysfunctional cognitions. A fourth (rational thoughts) and fifth (outcome) column are added to the three-column thought record (events, automatic thoughts, and emotions) typically used to identify automatic thoughts. The patient is instructed to use this form to capture and change automatic thoughts. Either a stressful event or a memory of an event or situation is noted in the first column. Automatic thoughts are recorded in the second column and are rated for degree of belief (how much the patient believes them to be true at the moment they occur) on a 0–100 scale. The third column is used to observe the emotional response to the automatic thoughts. The intensity of emotion is rated on a 1–100 scale. The fourth column, rational thoughts, is the most critical part of the TCR. The patient is asked to stand back from the automatic thoughts, assess their validity, and then write out a more rational or realistic set of cognitions. There are a wide variety of procedures that can be used to facilitate the development of rational thoughts for the TCR.

Most patients can learn about cognitive errors and can start to label specific instances of erroneous logic in their automatic thoughts. This is often the first step in generating a more rational pattern of cognitive responses to life events. This process is illustrated in the case of Mr. E, a 58-year-old man with major depression, who completed a TCR during the middle phase of CT (Table 31–11). He had learned how to use the TCR during prior therapy sessions and had been acquainted with the concept of cognitive errors through therapy experiences and from reading self-help materials (see Table 31–8). Mr. E noted the particular cognitive errors involved with each of his automatic thoughts and wrote out a more rational set of cognitions.

Previously described techniques such as generating alternatives, examining the evidence, and using reattribution also are used by the patient in a self-help format when the TCR is assigned for homework. In addition, the therapist often is able to help the patient refine or add to the list of rational thoughts when the TCR is reviewed at a subsequent therapy session. Repeated attention to generating rational thoughts on the TCR is usually quite helpful in breaking maladaptive patterns of automatic and negatively distorted thinking.

The fifth column of the TCR, outcome, is used to record any changes that have occurred as a result of revising and modifying automatic thoughts. In the case of Mr. E, there was a significant decrease in dysphoric affect. Although the use of the TCR will usually lead to the development of a more adaptive set of cognitions and a reduction in painful affect, on some occasions the initial automatic thoughts will prove to be accurate. In such situations, the therapist helps the patient take a problem-solving approach, including the development of an action plan, to manage the stressful or upsetting event.

Cognitive rehearsal is used to help uncover potential negative automatic thoughts in advance and to coach the patient in ways of developing more adaptive cognitions. First, the patient is asked to use imagery or role-play to identify possible distorted cognitions that could occur in a stressful situation. Second, the patient and therapist work together to modify the dysfunctional cognitions. Third, imagery or role-play is used again, this time to practice the more adaptive pattern of thinking. Finally, for a homework assignment, the patient is asked to try out the newly acquired cognitive patterns in vivo.

Identifying and Modifying Schemas

The process of identifying and modifying schemas is somewhat more difficult than changing negative automatic thoughts because these core beliefs are more deeply embedded, may be largely out of the patient's awareness, and usually have been reinforced through years of life experience. However, many of the same techniques described for automatic thoughts are employed successfully in therapeutic work at the schema level (Beck et al. 1979; Wright et al. 2006). Procedures such as Socratic questioning, imagery, role-play, and thought recording are used to uncover maladaptive schemas (Table 31–12).

As the patient gains experience in recognizing automatic thoughts, repetitive patterns begin to emerge that may suggest the presence of underlying schemas. Therapists have several options at this point. A psychoeducational approach can be used to explain the concept of schemas (may be alternately termed *core beliefs* or *basic assumptions*) and their linkage to more superficial automatic thoughts. Patients may then start to recognize schemas on their own. However, when the patient first starts to learn about basic assumptions, the therapist may need to suggest that certain schemas might be operative and then engage the patient in collaborative exercises that test these hypotheses.

TABLE 31–11. Thought Change Record—an example

Situation	Automatic thought(s)	Emotion(s)	Rational response	Outcome
Describe: a. Actual event leading to unpleasant emotion; or b. Stream of thoughts, daydream, or recollection leading to unpleasant emotion; or c. Unpleasant physiological sensations	a. Write automatic thought(s) that preceded emotion(s). b. Rate belief in automatic thought(s), 0%–100%.	a. Specify sad, anxious, angry, etc. b. Rate degree of emotion, 1%–100%.	a. Identify cognitive errors. b. Write rational response to automatic thought(s). c. Rate belief in rational response, 0%–100%.	a. Once again, rate belief in automatic thought(s), 0%–100%. b. Specify and rate subsequent emotion(s), 0%–100%.
Date: 4/15/98				
I wake up and I'm immediately troubled. I start to worry about work.	1. I can't face another day. (90%)	Sad: 90% Anxious: 80%	1. Magnification. Even though it has been rough, I have been able to get to work every day. Get a shower and make breakfast—that will get things started. (80%)	Sad: 30% Anxious: 40%
	2. The big project is due in 2 weeks; I'll never get it done. (100%)		2. Catastrophizing, all-or-none thinking. About half of the work is done. Don't panic. Break it down into pieces. Taking one step at a time helps. (95%)	
	3. Everybody knows I'm ready to fall apart. (90%)		3. Overgeneralization, magnification. Some people know I've been in trouble, but they haven't gotten down on me. I'm the one who puts me down. (95%)	
	4. It's hopeless. (85%)		4. Magnification. I know my job well and have a good track record. If I stick with this, I can probably make it. (90%)	

Source.   Adapted from Beck AT, Rush AJ, Shaw BF, Emery G: *Cognitive Therapy of Depression.* New York, Guilford Press, 1979. Used with permission.

TABLE 31–12. Methods for identifying and modifying schemas

Socratic questioning

Imagery and role-play

Thought recording

Identifying repetitive patterns of automatic thoughts

Psychoeducation

Listing schemas in therapy notebook

Examining the evidence

Listing advantages and disadvantages

Generating alternatives

Cognitive rehearsal

TABLE 31–13. Schema modification through examining the evidence

Schema: "I must be perfect to be accepted."

Evidence for	Evidence against
The better I do, the more people seem to like me.	Others who aren't "perfect" seem to be to be loved and accepted. Why should I be different?
Women who have a perfect figure are most attractive to men.	You don't have to have a perfect figure. Hardly anybody has one—just the models on television.
My parents have the highest standards; they are always pushing me to do better.	My parents want me to do well. But they'll probably accept me as long as I try to do my best, even if I don't meet all of their expectations. This statement is absolute and sets me up for failure, because no one can be perfect all the time.

Modification of schemas may require repeated attention, both in and out of therapy sessions. One commonly used procedure is to ask the patient to keep a list in a therapy notebook of all the schemas that have been identified to date. The schema list can be reviewed before each session. This technique promotes a high level of awareness of schemas and usually encourages the patient to place issues pertaining to schemas on the agenda for therapy.

CT interventions that are particularly helpful in modifying schemas include examining the evidence, listing advantages and disadvantages, generating alternatives, and using cognitive rehearsal. After a schema has been identified, the therapist may ask the patient to do a pro/con analysis (examining the evidence) using a double-column procedure. This technique usually induces the patient to doubt the validity of the schema and to start to think of alternate explanations. An examining-the-evidence intervention is illustrated in the case of Ms. R, a 24-year-old woman with depression and bulimia (Table 31–13). During the course of her CT, Ms. R identified an important schema that was affecting both the depression and the eating disorder ("I must be perfect to be accepted"). By examining the evidence, she was able to see that her schema was based at least in part on faulty logic.

Ms. R also used the listing advantages and disadvantages technique as part of the strategy to modify this maladaptive schema (Table 31–14). Some schemas appear to have few, if any, advantages (e.g., "I'm stupid"; "I'll always lose in the end"), but many schemas have both positive and negative features (e.g., "If I decide to do something, I must succeed"; "I always have

to work harder than others or I'll fail"). The latter group of schemas may be maintained even in the face of their dysfunctional aspects because they encourage hard work, perseverance, or other behaviors that are adaptive. Yet the absolute and demanding nature of the schemas ultimately leads to excessive stress, failed expectations, low self-esteem, or other deleterious results. Listing advantages and disadvantages helps the patient to examine the full range of effects of the schema and often encourages modifications that can make the schema both more adaptive and less damaging. In Ms. R's case, this exercise set the stage for another step of schema modification, generating alternatives (Table 31–15).

The list of alternative schemas will usually include several different options, ranging from rather minor adjustments to extensive revisions in the schema. The therapist uses Socratic questioning and other CT techniques such as imagery and role-play to help the patient recognize potential alternative schemas. A "brainstorming" attitude is encouraged. Instead of trying to be sure that a revised schema is entirely accurate at first glance, the therapist usually suggests that they try to

TABLE 31–14. Schema modification through listing advantages and disadvantages

Schema: "I must be perfect to be accepted."	
Advantages	**Disadvantages**
I've tried very hard to be the best.	I never really feel accepted because I've never reached perfection.
I've received top marks in school.	I'm always down on myself. I've developed bulimia. I'm obsessed with my body size.
I'm in lots of activities, and I've won dancing competitions.	I have trouble accepting my successes. I drive myself too hard and can't enjoy ordinary things.

TABLE 31–15. Schema modification through generating alternatives

Schema: "I must be perfect to be accepted."
Possible alternatives
People who are successful are more likely to be accepted.
If I try to do my best (even if it's not perfect), others are likely to accept me.
I would like to be perfect, but that's an impossible goal. I'll choose certain areas to try to excel (school, work, and career) and not demand perfection everywhere.
You don't need to be perfect to be accepted.
I'm worthy of love and acceptance without trying to be perfect.

generate a variety of modified schemas without initially considering their validity or practicality. This stimulates creativity and gives the patient further encouragement to step aside from long-standing rigid schemas.

After alternatives are generated and discussed, the therapy turns toward examining the potential consequences of changing basic attitudes. Cognitive rehearsal can be used in the therapy session to test a schema modification. This may be followed by a homework assignment to try out the revised schema in vivo. Therapist and patient work together to choose the most reasonable modifications for underlying schemas and to reinforce learning these new con-

TABLE 31–16. Behavioral procedures used in cognitive therapy

Questioning to identify behavioral patterns
Activity scheduling with mastery and pleasure recording
Self-monitoring
Graded task assignments
Behavioral rehearsal
Exposure and response prevention
Coping cards
Distraction
Relaxation exercises
Respiratory control
Assertiveness training
Modeling
Social skills training

structs through multiple practice sessions in therapy sessions and in real-life experiences.

Behavioral Procedures

Behavioral interventions are used in CT to 1) change dysfunctional patterns of behavior (e.g., helplessness, isolation, phobic avoidance, inertia, bingeing and purging); 2) reduce troubling symptoms (e.g., tension, somatic and psychic anxiety, intrusive thoughts); and 3) assist in identifying and modifying maladaptive cognitions. Table 31–16 presents a listing of behavioral techniques. As discussed earlier in this chapter, the cognitive model for therapy (see Figure 31–1) suggests that there is an interactive relationship between cognition and behavior. Thus, behavioral initiatives should influence cognition, and cognitive interventions should have an impact on behavior.

The Socratic questions used in cognitively oriented procedures have a direct parallel when the emphasis is on behavioral change. The therapist asks a series of questions that help differentiate actual behavioral deficits from negatively distorted accounts of behavior. Depressed and anxious patients usually overreport their symptomatic distress or the difficulties they have in managing situations. Often, well-framed questions can reveal cognitive distortions and also stimulate change as the patient considers the negative impact of dysfunctional behavior. Four specific behavioral techniques—

activity scheduling, graded task assignments, exposure, and coping cards—are explained below. A more detailed description of behavioral methods is available in Wright et al. (2006) or Meichenbaum (1977).

Activity scheduling is a structured method of learning about the patient's behavioral patterns, encouraging self-monitoring, increasing positive mood, and designing strategies for change (Beck et al. 1979; Wright et al. 2006). A daily or weekly activity log is employed in which the patient is asked to record what he or she does during each hour of the day and then to rate each activity for mastery and pleasure on a 0–10 scale. When the activity record is first introduced, the patient usually is asked to make a record of baseline activities without attempting to make any changes. The data are then reviewed in the next therapy session.

Almost invariably, the patient rates some activities higher than others on mastery and/or pleasure.

> For example, Mr. G, a 48-year-old depressed man who had told his therapist that "I don't enjoy anything anymore," described several activities on his daily activity log that contradicted this statement. Reading while sitting alone was rated as a 6 on mastery and 8 on pleasure, and attending his son's choir concert was rated as 7 on mastery and 10 on pleasure. Conversely, attempting to work in his home office was rated as a 1 on mastery and a 0 on pleasure. Discussion of the activity scheduling assignment with Mr. G helped him to see that he was still capable of performing reasonably well in certain activities and also that he was able to derive considerable enjoyment from some of his actions. In addition, the schedule was used to target problem areas (e.g., working in his home office) that would require further work in therapy. Finally, the activity schedule provided data that could be used in adjusting Mr. G's daily routine to promote a heightened sense of mastery and greater enjoyment.

Another behavioral procedure, the graded task assignment, can be used when the patient is facing a situation that seems excessively difficult or overwhelming. A challenging behavioral goal is broken down into small steps that can be taken one at a time. The graded task assignment is somewhat similar to the systematic desensitization protocols that are used in traditional behavior therapy (Wolpe 1969). However, a cognitive component is added to the methodology. There is an added emphasis placed on improving self-esteem and self-efficacy, countering hopelessness and helplessness, and using the graded task assignment to disprove maladaptive thoughts and schemas. With depressed individuals, the graded task assignment typically is used as a problem-solving technique. This stepwise approach, coupled with cognitive techniques

such as Socratic questioning and thought recording, can reactivate the patient and focus his or her energy in a productive manner.

An example of the use of a graded task assignment can be found in the case of Mr. G, the 48-year-old man described in the section on activity scheduling. One of the particularly troublesome items uncovered with activity scheduling was the patient's difficulty in getting to work at his home office. Socratic questioning revealed that Mr. G had been unable to work in his home office for over 6 weeks. Mail, bills, and correspondence with friends were piled up to the point that he saw the situation as impossible. Cognitions related to this problem included automatic thoughts such as "It's too much…. I've procrastinated too long this time…. I'm totally swamped…. I can't handle it."

The therapist and patient constructed a series of steps that encouraged Mr. G to approach the task and eventually master the problem. The graded task assignment included the following steps: 1) walk into the office and sit down at the desk for at least 15 minutes; 2) spend at least 20 minutes sorting mail into categories; 3) open and discard any junk mail; 4) open and read any personal letters and write list of responses required; 5) open and stack all bills; 6) clean office; 7) respond in writing to at least one letter; 8) balance checkbook; 9) pay all current or overdue bills; 10) respond to additional letters if necessary. Reasonable goals for specific time intervals were discussed, and the therapist used coaching, Socratic questioning, and other cognitive techniques to help Mr. G accomplish the task.

Exposure techniques are a central part of cognitive-behavioral approaches to anxiety disorders. For example, a phobia can be conceptualized as an unrealistic fear of an object or a situation coupled with a conditioned pattern of avoidance. Treatment can proceed along two complementary lines: cognitive restructuring to modify the dysfunctional thoughts and exposure therapy to break the pattern of avoidance. Typically, a hierarchy of feared stimuli is developed with the patient. The hierarchy should contain a number of different stimuli that cause varying degrees of distress. Usually the items are ranked by degree of distress. One commonly used system involves rating each item on a scale from 0 to 100, with 100 representing the maximum distress possible. After the hierarchy is established, the therapist and patient work collaboratively to set goals for gradual exposure, starting with the items that are ranked lower on the distress scale. Breathing training, relaxation exercises, and other behavioral methods (see Table 31–16) may be used to enhance the patient's ability to carry out the exposure protocol.

Exposure can be done with imagery in treatment sessions or in vivo. Also, innovative virtual-reality methods have been developed for exposure therapy (Rothbaum et al. 1995). Virtual-reality exposure techniques have been shown to be effective in empirical trials, but they are expensive and are not yet widely available. Clinician-administered exposure therapy is frequently used as part of the cognitive-behavioral approach to simple phobias, panic disorder with agoraphobia, social phobia, and obsessive-compulsive disorder (OCD).

Coping cards are another commonly used method to achieve behavioral change. The therapist helps the patient to identify specific actions that are likely to help her or him cope with an anticipated problem or put CT skills into action. These ideas are then written down on a small card, which the patient carries with her or him as a reminder and as a tool to help in solving problems. Coping cards often contain both cognitive and behavioral interventions, as illustrated in Figure 31–3.

Other behavioral techniques used in CT include behavior rehearsal (a procedure that is usually combined with cognitive rehearsal, described earlier), response prevention (a collaborative exercise in which the patient agrees to stop a dysfunctional behavior, such as prolonged crying spells, and to monitor cognitive responses), distraction (scheduling alternate activities that can temporarily divert a patient from intrusive thoughts, depressive ruminations, or other dysfunctional cognitions), relaxation exercises, respiratory control, assertiveness training, modeling, and social skills training (D.M. Clark et al. 1985; Meichenbaum 1977; Wright et al. 2006).

Computer-Assisted Cognitive Therapy

Newer forms of computer-assisted CT may offer significant potential for increasing the efficiency of cognitive-behavioral interventions and improving access to treatment (Pull 2005; Wright 2004; Wright and Wright 1997). An early prototype for computerized therapy was developed by Selmi et al. (1990). Their text-based program teaches patients how to use CT to cope with depression. An outcome study demonstrated that patients with mild to moderate depression responded well to the computer program (Selmi et al. 1990). Subjects who received the computerized therapy improved as much as those who were treated with standard CT, and both active treatments were superior to a wait-list control.

More recently developed computer programs have used multimedia, virtual reality, and palm-top technology to produce therapy experiences that are efficacious and appealing to patients. For example, Wright et al. (1995, 2002, 2004) have introduced a multimedia form of computer-assisted CT that is designed to be "user friendly" and to be suitable for a wide range of patients, including those with no previous computer or keyboard experience. This program ("Good Days Ahead: The Multimedia Program for Cognitive Therapy") uses a DVD-ROM format and features large amounts of video and audio, along with interactive self-help exercises. A randomized controlled trial of computer-assisted CT for depression conducted with a prototype of the Wright et al. program found that computer-assisted CT was equivalent to standard CT, even though the total therapist time in computer-assisted CT was reduced to about 4 hours (Wright et al. 2005). Subjects in this study were drug free. Computer-assisted CT and standard CT were both highly effective in relieving symptoms of depression, and both were superior to a delayed-treatment control condition. Another multimedia cognitive-behavioral therapy program, "Beating the Blues," was found to be effective in a controlled trial with primary care patients (Proudfoot et al. 2004). Persons with depression and anxiety who received treatment with this computer program had significantly greater improvement in depression than those who received treatment as usual. Both of these multimedia programs ("Good Days Ahead" and "Beating the Blues") have been well accepted by patients (Proudfoot et al. 2004; Wright et al. 2002).

Virtual reality applications for computer-assisted therapy have been directed primarily at phobias and other anxiety disorders. The virtual environment is used to simulate feared situations and to promote exposure therapy. Controlled research has supported the efficacy of virtual reality as part of a CT treatment package for fear of flying, height phobia, and other phobias (Krijn et al. 2004; Pull 2005; Rothbaum et al. 2000). This method is also showing promise in the treatment of social anxiety, posttraumatic stress disorder (PTSD), and panic disorder with agoraphobia (Pull 2005). For these conditions, the virtual environment may include simulations of other people or places such as crowded public spaces, public speaking experiences, and scenes from war zones.

Palm-top computers have been used to assist in delivering various components of CT for anxiety disorders such as relaxation instructions, spotting cognitive distortions, breathing retraining, and cognitive restructuring (Anderson et al. 2004). Typically, the palm-top computer is used between sessions with a clinician

> **Situation:** My girlfriend comes in late or does something else that makes me think she doesn't care.
>
> **Coping Strategies:**
>
> • Spot my extreme thinking, especially when I use words like <u>never</u> or <u>always</u>.
>
> • Stand back from the situation and check my thinking before I start yelling.
>
> • Think of the positive parts of our relationship.
>
> • Take a "time-out" if I start getting into a rage.
>
> • Tell her that I need to take a break to calm down.
>
> • Take a brief walk or go to another room.

FIGURE 31–3. Mr. W's coping card.

This example shows how Mr. W, a middle-aged man with bipolar disorder, developed an effective coping strategy for managing anger in situations with his girlfriend.

Source. Wright et al. 2006.

to reduce reliance on the human therapist. Although palm-top applications have been shown to be useful, there is some evidence that shortened therapy with this form of computer-assisted treatment may not always be as effective as a full course of clinician-administered therapy. Newman et al. (1997) found that immediately posttreatment, computer-assisted therapy (including four sessions with a clinician) led to significant improvement. However, the response was not as robust as standard treatment with 12 sessions with a clinician. At the follow-up evaluation both treatments were equally effective.

Possible contributions of computer-assisted CT may include decreased cost of treatment, increased access to therapy, more rapid socialization to treatment procedures and techniques, and lowered burden on therapists to teach basic CT concepts (Wright and Wright 1997). Opportunities for improved efficiency of treatment, advances in the design of computer programs, and the proliferation of computers in society may promote greater use of computer tools for CT.

Selecting Patients for Cognitive Therapy

CT procedures have been described for a large number of diagnostic categories (Beck 1993). Although there

are no contraindications to using this treatment approach, CT is usually not attempted with patients who have marked brain disease. CT can be considered a primary treatment for 1) disorders in which it has been proven to be effective in controlled research (e.g., unipolar depression [nonpsychotic], anxiety disorders, eating disorders, and psychophysiological disorders), and 2) other conditions for which a clearly detailed treatment method has been developed (e.g., personality disorders, substance abuse) and there is some evidence for CT's effectiveness. CT should be considered an adjunctive therapy for disorders such as major depression with psychotic features, bipolar illness, and schizophrenia, in which there is clear evidence for the effectiveness of biological treatments and the effects of CT alone compared with pharmacotherapy have not been studied.

Several studies have examined possible predictors for outcome in CT. Simons et al. (1985) observed that high scores on a test of self-control predicted an enhanced response to CT compared with a tricyclic antidepressant. Although several later studies (Jarrett et al. 1991; Wetzel et al. 1992) failed to replicate this finding, one other study (Burns et al. 1994) partially replicated it. Miller et al. (1989) found that high levels of cognitive dysfunction in depressed inpatients were associated with a superior response to combined treatment with

CT and pharmacotherapy as compared with pharmacotherapy alone. Chronicity and symptom severity have been associated with poorer response to CT (e.g., Thase et al. 1993, 1994), although these findings may reflect the more negative prognostic impact of these variables. When CT has been compared directly with pharmacotherapy, most studies have found little relationship between severity or endogenous subtype and differential treatment outcome (see "Effectiveness of Cognitive Therapy" section later in this chapter).

Investigations of biological predictors have yielded suggestive results. Dexamethasone nonsuppression was associated with a poorer response to both CT and pharmacotherapy in one study (McKnight et al. 1992). Thase et al. (1996) found that poorer response to an intensive inpatient CT program was associated with high levels of urinary free cortisol levels. In a large ($n=90$) outpatient study, an abnormal sleep profile (defined by multiple disturbances of electroencephalographic sleep recordings) was associated with a lower recovery rate and higher risk for relapse (Thase et al. 1996). More recently, a specific alteration in cortical activation (as measured by functional magnetic resonance imaging scanning) was strongly associated with short-term CT response (Siegle et al. 2006). Although these studies suggest that various biological markers of depression may be associated with response/nonresponse to CT, research to date does not justify the use of laboratory tests to select patients for CT.

Clinical experience has suggested that patients who do not have severe character pathology (especially borderline or antisocial features), have previously formed trusting relationships with significant others, have a belief in the importance of self-reliance, and have a curious or inquisitive nature are especially suitable for CT (Wright et al. 2006). Above-average intelligence is not associated with better outcome, and CT procedures can be simplified for those with subnormal intellectual skills or impaired learning and memory functioning. Of course, most patients do not have a full combination of the ideal features noted above. A flexible approach can be employed in which CT procedures are customized to match the special characteristics of the patient's social background, intellectual level, personality structure, and clinical disorder (Wright et al. 2006).

Cognitive Therapy Applications

The basic procedures described in this chapter are used in all CT applications. However, the targets for change,

selection of techniques, and timing of interventions may vary depending on the condition being treated and the format for therapy. A full discussion of the multiple applications and formats for CT is beyond the scope of this chapter. The reader is referred to comprehensive books on CT for a more detailed accounting of the modifications of this treatment approach for different clinical disorders (see "Suggested Readings" at end of chapter). CT methods have been outlined for a number of clinical problems not covered here, including conditions such as substance abuse (Wright et al. 1993), chronic depression (McCullough 2000), hypochondriasis (Warwick and Salkovskis 1990), body dysmorphic disorder (N.B. Schmidt and Harrington 1995), gambling addiction (Bujold et al. 1994), and psychophysiological disorders (Sensky 2004). Group CT techniques have been described by Covi and Primakoff (1988) and Freeman et al. (1992); procedures for marital and family CT have been set forth by Beck (1988), Epstein et al. (1988), and others. Also, strategies have been developed for using CT as a comprehensive model for inpatient treatment (Wright et al. 1993). In this portion of the chapter, we briefly examine the distinctive features of CT for six common psychiatric illnesses—depression, anxiety disorders, eating disorders, personality disorders, psychosis, and bipolar disorder.

Depression

In the opening phase of treatment of depression, the cognitive therapist focuses on establishing a collaborative relationship and introduces the patient to the cognitive model. Agendas, feedback, and psychoeducational procedures are used to structure sessions. The emphasis is placed on two major forms of cognitive dysfunction: negatively distorted thinking and deficits in learning and memory functioning. Early in therapy, a special effort may be placed on relieving hopelessness because of the close link between this element of the negative cognitive triad and suicide risk. Also, reduction in hopelessness can be an important step in reactivating and reenergizing the depressed patient.

Problems with learning and memory functioning are countered with the aforementioned structuring procedures and with learning reinforcement techniques such as written therapy notes, diagrams, and homework assignments. The clinician carefully matches the therapeutic work to the patient's level of cognitive functioning so that learning is encouraged and the patient is not overwhelmed with the material of therapy. Behavioral techniques, such as activity scheduling and graded task assignments, often are a major component of the opening phase of CT of depression.

The middle portion of treatment is usually devoted to eliciting and modifying negatively distorted automatic thoughts. Behavioral techniques continue to be used in most cases. By this point in the therapy, patients should understand the cognitive model and be able to employ thought monitoring techniques to reverse all three elements of the negative cognitive triad (self, world, and future). Typically, the patient is taught to identify cognitive errors (e.g., selective abstraction, arbitrary inference, absolutistic thinking) and to use procedures such as generating alternatives and examining the evidence to alter negatively distorted thinking.

Work on eliciting and testing automatic thoughts continues during the latter portion of treatment. However, if there have been gains in functioning and the patient has grasped the basic principles of CT, therapy can turn primarily to identifying and altering maladaptive schemas. The concept of schemas usually has been introduced earlier in therapy, but the principal efforts at changing these underlying structures are reserved for the late phase of treatment when the patient is more likely to grasp and retain complex therapeutic initiatives. Before therapy concludes, the therapist helps the patient review what has been learned during the course of treatment and also suggests thinking ahead to possible circumstances that could trigger a return of depression. The potential for relapse is recognized, and problem-solving strategies are developed that can be employed in future stressful situations.

Anxiety Disorders

Although the techniques used in CT for anxiety disorders are similar to those employed in the treatment of depression, treatment efforts are directed toward altering four major types of dysfunctional anxiety-producing cognitions: 1) overestimates of the likelihood of a feared event, 2) exaggerated estimates of the severity of a feared event, 3) underestimation of personal coping abilities, and 4) unrealistically low estimates of the help that others can offer. Most authors have recommended that a mixture of cognitive and behavioral measures be used in patients who have anxiety disorders (Barlow and Cerney 1988; Beck et al. 1985a).

In panic disorder, the emphasis is placed on helping the patient to recognize and change grossly exaggerated estimates of the significance of physiological responses or fears of imminent psychological disaster (Beck et al. 1985a, 1992; D.M. Clark 1986). For example, an individual with panic disorder may begin to perspire or breathe more rapidly, after which cognitions such as "I can't catch my breath.... I'll pass out.... I'll

have a stroke" increase the intensity of the autonomic nervous system activity. The vicious cycle interaction between catastrophic cognitions and physiological arousal can be broken in two complementary ways: 1) altering the dysfunctional cognitions and 2) interrupting the cascading autonomic hyperactivity. Commonly used cognitive interventions include Socratic questioning, imagery, thought recording, generating alternatives, and examining the evidence. Behavioral measures such as relaxation training and respiratory control are used to dampen the physiological arousal associated with panic (D.M. Clark et al. 1985). Also, when panic attacks are stimulated by specific situations (e.g., driving, public speaking, crowds), graded exposure may be particularly useful in helping patients to both master a feared task and overcome their panic symptoms.

CT of phobic disorders centers on modifying unrealistic estimates of risk or danger in situations and engaging the patient in a series of graded exposure assignments. Generally, cognitive and behavioral procedures are used simultaneously. For example, a graded task assignment for an individual with agoraphobia might include a stepwise increase in experiences in a social setting accompanied by use of a TCR to record and revise maladaptive automatic thinking. Patients with generalized anxiety disorder (GAD) usually have diffuse cognitive distortions about many circumstances in their lives (e.g., physical health, finances, loss of control, family issues) coupled with persistent autonomic overarousal (Beck et al. 1985a). The CT approach to GAD is closely related to methods used for panic disorder and phobias. However, special attention is paid to defining the stimuli that are associated with increased anxiety. Breaking down the generalized state of anxiety into workable segments can help the patient gain mastery over what initially appears to be an uncontrollable situation.

Behavioral techniques such as exposure and response prevention are used together with cognitive restructuring for patients with OCD (Salkovskis 1985). Cognitive interventions include challenging the validity of obsessional thoughts, attempting to replace dysfunctional cognitions with positive self-statements, and modifying negative automatic thoughts. Salkovskis and Warwick (1985) have noted that cognitive procedures may be needed in some cases to help the patient engage in exposure and response prevention. A combined approach of cognitive techniques to modify maladaptive thought patterns and behavioral interventions to counter patterns of avoidance is also used in CT for PTSD (Harvey et al. 2003).

Eating Disorders

CT is a well-established first-line treatment for bulimia nervosa and binge-eating disorder. CT for both conditions was given a grade A rating by the United Kingdom's National Institute for Clinical Excellence (NICE), indicating that there is strong support for efficacy from empirical trials (Wilson and Shafran 2005). Although methods have been described and tested for anorexia nervosa, NICE made no specific recommendations for this more severe form of eating disorder (Wilson and Shafran 2005). Considerably less research has been conducted on CT for anorexia nervosa than for other eating disorders. However, cognitive and behavioral interventions can be included in comprehensive treatment programs for this difficult-to-treat condition.

Individuals with eating disorders may have many of the same cognitive distortions that are seen in depression. However, they have an additional cluster of cognitive biases about body image, eating behavior, and weight (D. A. Clark et al. 1989). Patients with eating disorders usually place inordinate value on body shape as a measure of self-worth and as a condition for acceptance (e.g., "I must be thin to be accepted"; "If I'm overweight, nobody will want me"; "Fat people are weak"). They also may believe that any variance from their excessive standards means a total loss of control.

CT interventions are used to subject these maladaptive cognitions to empirical testing. Commonly used procedures include eliciting and testing automatic thoughts, examining the evidence, using reattribution, and giving in vivo homework assignments). In addition, behavioral techniques are used to stimulate more adaptive eating behavior and to uncover significant cognitions related to eating. As in treatment of other disorders, the relative emphasis on cognitive procedures compared with behavioral measures is dictated by the severity of the illness and the phase of treatment. An individual with anorexia nervosa who is malnourished and has an electrolyte imbalance may require hospitalization during the initial part of treatment for a contingency management program. Patients with this level of illness may have a significant impairment in learning and memory functioning and therefore have limited capacity to understand thought recording or other cognitive interventions. In contrast, a patient with uncomplicated bulimia nervosa may be able to benefit from relatively demanding cognitively oriented procedures early in treatment.

One of the critical factors in treating patients with eating disorders is the development of an effective working relationship. Compared with individuals with depression or anxiety disorders, those with eating disturbances often are reluctant to fully engage in therapy. Frequently, they have long-standing patterns of hiding their behavior from others and have developed elaborate methods of maintaining their dysfunctional approach to meals, body weight, and exercise. Thus, the patient with an eating disorder poses a special problem for the cognitive therapist. A thorough psychoeducational effort and considerable patience are usually required for the formation of a collaborative empirical relationship. Also, if the therapist focuses in the beginning on problem areas that the patient clearly wants to change (e.g., low self-esteem, hopelessness, loss of interest), struggles over control of eating disorders can be avoided until there have been successful experiences in working together in therapy.

Personality Disorders

Beck and Freeman (1990) articulated a CT approach to personality disorders that is based on a cognitive conceptualization of characterological disturbances. They suggest that the different personality types have idiosyncratic cognitions in four main areas: basic beliefs, view of self, view of others, and strategies for social interaction. For example, an individual with a narcissistic personality might believe, "I'm special.... I'm better than the rest.... Ordinary rules don't apply to me." This cognitive set leads to behavioral strategies such as manipulation, breaking rules, and exploiting others (Beck and Freeman 1990). In contrast, a person with a dependent personality disorder might have core beliefs such as, "I need others to survive.... I can't manage on my own.... I can't be happy if I'm alone." The interpersonal strategies associated with these beliefs would include efforts to cling to or entrap others (Beck and Freeman 1990).

CT methods typically employed in treatment of affective disorders may not be successful with characterological problems (Beck and Freeman 1990). Recommendations that have been made for modifying CT for treatment of personality disorders are summarized in Table 31–17 (Beck and Freeman 1990; Linehan 1993). The problem-oriented, structured, and collaborative empirical characteristics of CT are retained in therapeutic work with patients who have personality disturbances, but there is an added emphasis on the therapeutic relationship. Treatment of personality disorders with CT may take considerably longer than therapy of more circumscribed problems such as depression or anxiety. Patients with personality disturbances have deeply ingrained schemas that are unlikely to change within the short-term format used for

TABLE 31–17. Modifications of cognitive therapy for personality disorders

Pay special attention to the therapeutic relationship.

Attend to one's own (the therapist's) cognitive responses and emotional reactions.

Develop an individualized case conceptualization (including an assessment of the impact of developmental experiences, significant traumas, and environmental stresses).

Place an initial focus on increasing self-efficacy.

Use behavioral techniques, such as rehearsal and social skills training, to reverse actual deficits in interpersonal functioning.

Set firm, reasonable limits.

Set realistic goals.

Anticipate adherence problems.

Review and repeat treatment interventions.

other disorders (Brown et al. 2004). When the course of therapy lengthens, there is a greater chance for development of transference and countertransference reactions. In CT, transference is viewed as a manifestation of underlying schemas. Therefore, transferential phenomena are recognized as opportunities for examining and modifying core beliefs.

An individualized case conceptualization is used. This formulation includes hypotheses on the role of maladaptive schemas in symptom production. Consideration also is given to the influences of parent–child conflicts, traumatic experiences, and the current social network on cognitive and behavioral pathology. Patients with personality disorders often have significant real-life problems, including severely disturbed interpersonal relationships and pronounced social skills deficits.

Although an ultimate goal of treatment is to modulate ineffective or maladaptive schemas, initial efforts (using procedures such as behavioral techniques or thought recording) may be directed at more readily accessible targets such as increasing self-efficacy or decreasing dysphoric mood. Self-monitoring, self-help exercises, and the structuring procedures used in CT help prevent excessive dependency. However, patients with character disorders (especially those with borderline, narcissistic, or dependent personalities) are prone to have excessive expectations, to be overly demanding, or to exhibit manipulative behavior. Thus, the cognitive therapist needs to set firm but rea-

sonable limits and to help the patient articulate realistic treatment goals (Beck and Freeman 1990).

Adherence to treatment recommendations can be another problem in CT of personality disorders. The therapist can use procedures such as Socratic questioning or schema identification to uncover the reasons for nonadherence and help the patient follow through with homework assignments or other therapeutic work. Reviewing and repeating treatment interventions is another important component of CT for personality disorders. Considerable patience and persistence are required from the therapist as efforts are made to help the patient reverse chronic, deeply imbedded psychopathology.

Dialectical behavior therapy (DBT) is a specialized form of cognitive-behavioral therapy (CBT) developed by Marsha Linehan (1993) for treatment of borderline personality disorder. DBT employs cognitive and behavioral methods in addition to acceptance strategies derived from Zen teaching and practice. Therapy with DBT is long term and involves repeated behavioral analysis, behavioral skills instruction, contingency management, cognitive restructuring, exposure interventions to reduce avoidance and dysfunctional emotions, and mindfulness training. DBT has been used successfully in borderline patients with suicidal behavior and substance abuse (Linehan et al. 1991, 1993, 1994, 2006).

Psychosis

Psychotic illnesses are one of the indications for adjunctive CT. Although biological treatments are the accepted form of therapy for psychotic patients, several randomized controlled trials have demonstrated that CT can reduce symptoms in patients who have residual symptomatology after stabilization on medication. It has also been observed that cognitive psychotherapy can help psychotic individuals understand their disorders, adhere to treatment recommendations, and develop more effective psychosocial functioning (Cochran 1986; Kingdon and Turkington 2005).

In CT of patients who have psychotic symptoms, the therapist conveys that maladaptive cognitions and reactions to life stress may interact with biological factors in the expression of the illness. Therefore, attempts to develop more adaptive cognitions or to learn how to cope better with environmental pressures can assist with efforts toward managing the disorder. During the early part of therapy with a psychotic patient, there is a strong emphasis on building a therapeutic alliance (Kingdon and Turkington 2005). The therapist tries to normalize and destigmatize the condition

(Kingdon and Turkington 2005), and the rationale for antipsychotic medication in combination with CT is explained. Attempts may be made to stimulate hope by modifying intensely negative cognitions about the illness or its treatment (e.g., "I'm to blame.... Nothing will help.... Drugs don't work"). Usually, work on challenging hallucinations or delusions directly is delayed until a solid therapeutic relationship has been established. However, efforts are made to reverse delusional self-destructive cognitions as early as possible in the treatment process.

Reality testing is performed in a gentle, nonconfrontational manner (Kingdon and Turkington 2005). Usually delusions with lowest level of conviction are targeted first. The therapist uses guided discovery as a major intervention, but also may help the patient to record and change distorted automatic thoughts or perform examining the evidence exercises. Behavioral techniques such as activity scheduling, graded task assignments, and social skills training also are used with psychotic patients. These procedures can be used to provide needed structure or to teach adaptive behaviors. Negative symptoms are typically approached slowly in a manner that gives consideration to the difficulty of changing this manifestation of psychotic disorders (Kingdon and Turkington 2005). Other components of the CT approach to psychotic disorders may include 1) use of CT techniques that enhance medication adherence (see, e.g., Lecompte 1995), 2) identification of potential triggers for symptom exacerbation, 3) development of cognitive and behavioral strategies to manage stressful life events, and 4) implementation of family and/or group therapy applications of cognitive therapy (Wykes et al. 2005).

Bipolar Disorder

CT methods for bipolar disorder focus primarily on attempts to help persons understand and cope with a disease that is thought to have strong genetic and biological influences. For example, Basco and Rush (2005) recommend extensive psychoeducation, in addition to techniques such as mood graphing and symptom summary worksheets. The latter interventions are used to assist patients in recognizing early signs of a mood swing and then devising methods to reduce the risk of cycling into a full depression or mania. To illustrate, a person who notes that decreased sleep typically heralds the onset of a manic episode might be coached on cognitive-behavioral strategies for improving sleep patterns, or a patient who recognizes that pressured activity and distractibility often progress to more severe symptoms of mania may practice

cognitive-behavioral methods for slowing down and staying focused on productive task completion. Medication adherence is another important goal of CT for bipolar disorder (Basco and Rush 2005; Cochran 1986). Dysfunctional cognitions about medication can be modified with CT, and behavioral interventions, such as reminder systems and behavioral plans to overcome obstacles to adherence, can be used.

Treatment of depressive episodes in bipolar disorder utilizes many of the same interventions described for CT of major depression. Typically, CT is not used as a mainstay of treatment for severe mania when persons are markedly agitated or grossly psychotic. Instead, the CT effort is greater when symptoms are less extreme and the patient can concentrate on the work of therapy. The overall goals of CT for bipolar disorder are to lower symptoms of both depression and mania, improve psychosocial functioning, gain stress management skills, and reduce the risk for relapse.

Learning Cognitive Therapy

Psychiatry residents are now required to achieve competency in CT before completing their training, and many other mental health disciplines are emphasizing CT training in their educational programs. Also, clinicians who have previously completed their training without special emphasis on CT may be interested in gaining expertise in this approach. Although there are many ways to receive training in CT and to achieve competency, typical programs include at least a year of educational experiences with a series of didactic presentations, readings, video and role-play illustrations, and supervision.

The Beck Institute (www.beckinstitute.org) offers an extramural fellowship for clinicians who do not have CT training available locally and wish to enter an intensive CT educational program. A number of other centers for cognitive therapy have been established throughout the world to provide clinical service and training (listed in Wright et al. 2006). Workshops on CT are offered at annual meetings of the American Psychiatric Association, the American Psychological Association, the Association for the Advancement of Behavioral and Cognitive Therapies, and others.

Basic textbooks used for training in CT include *Learning Cognitive-Behavior Therapy: An Illustrated Guide* (Wright et al. 2006), which includes a DVD with demonstrations of CT methods; *Cognitive Therapy: Basics and Beyond* (J. Beck 1995); and *Cognitive Behavioral*

Therapy for Clinicians (Sudak 2006). Other recommended readings and Web sites are provided at the end of this chapter. The Academy of Cognitive Therapy has an especially useful Web site (www.academyofct.org) with a "training corner" for those interested in learning CT.

Effectiveness of Cognitive Therapy

CT has been investigated in many carefully designed outcome trials that have documented the effectiveness of this treatment approach. The most intensive research has been directed at CT of depression and anxiety disorders. However, there has been a steady increase in investigations of CT for eating disorders, psychosis, bipolar disorder, and other conditions. More than 350 randomized controlled trials of CT have been completed (Butler et al. 2006). Our focus here is on providing an overview of outcome research. Representative or especially important studies are discussed briefly to illustrate investigative work on CT.

Depression

Acute-Treatment-Phase Studies

Meta-analyses of the numerous outcome studies of CT for depression have found that this form of therapy compares well with other treatments for depression (Dobson 1989; Gaffan et al. 1995; Robinson et al. 1990). For example, Dobson (1989) concluded that CT was at least as effective as pharmacotherapy for depression and that there was some evidence for superiority of CT when all studies were considered together. In a subsequent review, Hollon et al. (1991) argued that some studies have been biased toward either CT or pharmacotherapy and thus suggested that firm conclusions on the relative efficacy of these treatments were still premature. One meta-analysis of 65 studies of CT for depression attempted to control for potential bias of the investigator by rating all studies on a researcher allegiance scale (Gaffan et al. 1995). Although researcher allegiance significantly predicted study outcomes, the results of Dobson's (1989) original meta-analysis were upheld.

Studies of CT for depression have been the subject of a detailed review by Thase (2001). Several of the more important investigations are noted here. The first major comparison of CT and pharmacotherapy was performed at the Center for Cognitive Therapy at the University of Pennsylvania (Rush et al. 1977). In this study, CT was found to be superior to imipramine in the treatment of depressed outpatients. However, results of this study have been questioned because of the "Lourdes effect" and because imipramine was tapered and stopped before the end of the trial. Two subsequent studies performed in the United Kingdom also found CT to be an effective treatment for depression in comparison with pharmacotherapy (Blackburn et al. 1981) or treatment as usual (Teasdale et al. 1984).

Subsequent to the original study of Rush et al. (1977), four of five major investigations in the United States have found CT and pharmacotherapy to be comparably effective. Murphy et al. (1984) at Washington University in St. Louis, Missouri, randomly assigned depressed outpatients to treatment with CT alone, nortriptyline alone, CT plus placebo, or combined CT and nortriptyline. The results of this study indicated that all treatments were effective for short-term symptom reduction. Similar findings were obtained in studies completed at the University of Minnesota (Hollon et al. 1992) and the Southwestern Medical School of the University of Texas (Jarrett et al. 1999), as well as in a two-center study conducted at the University of Pennsylvania and Vanderbilt University (DeRubeis et al. 2005). The latter study—the first to utilize a selective serotonin reuptake inhibitor—is of particular interest, because the study was limited to patients with moderate to severe depressive symptoms. Of note, although the treatments were equally effective overall, CT was somewhat more effective at the University of Pennsylvania site and pharmacotherapy was more effective at the Vanderbilt University site.

To date, only the results of the National Institute of Mental Health (NIMH) Treatment of Depression Collaborative Research Program (TDCRP; Elkin et al. 1989, 1995) have not fully supported the relative efficacy of CT as compared with pharmacotherapy. Although the difference between therapies was not significant in the primary analyses (Elkin et al. 1989), a secondary analysis suggested that CT—but not interpersonal psychotherapy (IPT)—was less effective than imipramine in more severely depressed patients (Elkin et al. 1995). However, this finding was not confirmed in a meta-analysis of individual patient data from four comparative studies (DeRubeis et al. 1999) and, consistent with the more recent findings of DeRubeis et al. (2005), may be explained by site differences in CT response (Jacobson and Hollon 1996).

Interestingly, whereas severity was associated with somewhat poorer CT response (relative to imipramine) in one secondary analysis of the TDCRP; in another secondary analysis, Stewart et al. (1998) found that CT was superior to imipramine among a subset of patients with atypical depressive symptoms. In a relatively large (*n*=108) placebo-controlled study, Jarrett et al. (1999) found that CT was as effective as a monoamine oxidase inhibitor for atypical depression.

Further evidence for the effectiveness of CT for depression has come in studies of group CT (Covi and Lipman 1987; Free et al. 1991; Zettle and Rains 1989), geriatric depressed patients (Beutler et al. 1987), and hospitalized patients (Bowers 1990; Miller et al. 1989, 2005; Thase et al. 1991). The overall results of CT outcome studies indicate that CT is an effective treatment for depression and is comparable to antidepressants in producing acute symptomatic relief across 10–12 weeks of treatment.

Long-Term Outcome Studies

Several of the investigations reviewed above have studied the durability of treatment effects across 1 and 2 years of follow-up. With one exception, results of these studies have supported the hypothesis that short-term CT is associated with a relatively low risk of subsequent relapse. For example, Kovacs et al. (1981) found that patients treated with CT in the Rush et al. (1977) study had a 31% relapse rate at 1 year, compared with a 65% relapse rate for those who had been treated with imipramine. A 2-year naturalistic follow-up investigation of patients treated in the Blackburn et al. (1981) study found a substantially lower relapse rate in patients treated with CT alone (23%) or with combined therapy (21%), as compared with those who had received pharmacotherapy alone (78%). Simons et al. (1986), who followed patients 1 year after their study, found the lowest relapse rates in patients who received CT alone (20%) or CT plus placebo (18%). Combined treatment was associated with a 43% rate of relapse after pharmacotherapy was withdrawn. The group treated with pharmacotherapy alone had the highest rate of relapse (67%). Patients in the Hollon et al. (1992) study showed the same pattern of long-term response to treatment (Evans et al. 1992). The relapse rate for those treated with pharmacotherapy (without continuation-phase pharmacotherapy) was over twice the rate for patients who received CT or combined treatment. This finding was fully replicated in the more recent University of Pennsylvania–Vanderbilt University collaboration (Hollon et al. 2005): time-limited CT has sustained efficacy comparable to continuation pharmacotherapy.

The only investigation that did not find clear-cut evidence that CT has an enduring effect was the NIMH Treatment of Depression Collaborative Research Program. However, as CT was not a particularly effective acute-phase therapy in this study (Elkin et al. 1995), it would not be expected to have an enduring effect (Thase 2001).

Two studies examined the usefulness of CT in treating residual symptoms of depression in patients who did not respond fully to antidepressants (Fava et al. 1996; Paykel et al. 1999). In the study by Fava et al. (1996), the relapse rate was 40% for CT and 90% for routine clinical management across a 6-year follow-up (Fava et al. 2004). Paykel et al. (1999) similarly observed a significant relapse-prevention effect in a two-center study of incompletely remitted patients receiving continuation pharmacotherapy. Treatment with CT reduced the hazard of relapse from 47% to 29% across 68 weeks of follow-up. Taken together, results of these investigations of the long-term effects of CT support the use of this modality to help reduce relapse and recurrence.

Perhaps the most intriguing results pertaining to longer-term outcomes come from the studies of Fava et al. (1998) and Jarrett et al. (2001). Fava et al. (1998) randomly assigned 45 remitted patients with recurrent depression to receive either 10 every-other-week sessions of CT (in addition to pharmacotherapy) or pharmacotherapy alone prior to medication discontinuation. Whereas 80% of the control group had recurrent depressive episodes across the next 24 months, 75% of the CT-treated group remained well after withdrawal of medication.

Jarrett et al. (2001) examined the role of ongoing continuation-phase CT sessions after response to acute-phase therapy. Previously, Thase et al. (1992) had suggested that CT could be terminated after 12–16 weeks of treatment *if* the initial response was brisk and complete. By contrast, incompletely remitted patients were at high (50%) risk of relapse following discontinuation of acute-phase therapy. Jarrett et al. (2001) confirmed this "at risk" assessment and demonstrated that incompletely remitted patients were "protected" from relapse by continuation-phase CT. By contrast, patients in the lower-risk (fully remitted) stratum gained no benefit from additional CT sessions. The durable relapse-prevention effects of CT may be linked to changes in affectively primed information processing (Teasdale et al. 2000).

Anxiety Disorders

CT also has been found to be an effective therapy for anxiety disorders. Especially strong evidence has been collected to support the utility of CT and related therapies in treatment of panic disorder. Two major forms of therapy have been developed: *panic control treatment* (PCT)—a combination of relaxation training, cognitive restructuring—and exposure (Barlow and Cerney 1988), and *focused cognitive therapy*—a more cognitively oriented treatment that uses exposure but places less emphasis on behavioral interventions than PCT (Beck et al. 1985a).

Barlow et al. (1989) reported that 87% of patients who completed a course of PCT were panic free after treatment and that PCT was significantly more effective than either relaxation training alone or a wait-list control condition. In a related investigation that compared PCT and alprazolam for panic disorder, this research group observed that PCT was superior to a wait-list control or placebo (Klosko et al. 1990). Of those completing the study, 87% who received PCT were free of panic attacks compared with 50% for alprazolam, 33% for the wait-list control, and 36% for placebo. The treatment protocol designed by Barlow and Cerney (1988) also was efficacious in an open trial of therapy administered by pharmacologically oriented clinicians who received training in this approach (Welkowitz et al. 1991). Shear et al. (1991a) noted that a cognitive and behavioral treatment package closely related to PCT was highly effective in clinical practice and, in addition, was capable of reversing vulnerability to sodium lactate–induced panic (Shear et al. 1991b).

In the largest study of PCT conducted to date, Barlow et al. (2000) found its short-term effects comparable to those of imipramine; both active interventions were significantly more effective than a double-blind pill placebo–clinical management condition. The combination of CT and imipramine demonstrated a modest advantage over the monotherapies. Following termination of treatment, patients treated with PCT had more durable responses than those withdrawn from imipramine.

Focused CT, as described by A.T. Beck et al. (1985a), also has fared well in outcome studies. Sokol et al. (1989) reported dramatic reductions in panic frequency (mean of 4.5 panic attacks per week before treatment to zero attacks per week after treatment) in an uncontrolled study of patients treated at the University of Pennsylvania Center for Cognitive Therapy. Subsequently, Beck et al. (1992) studied panic disorder patients who were randomly assigned to CT or supportive psychotherapy. Results strongly favored CT. After 8 weeks, almost three times as many patients who received CT (versus those who received supportive therapy) were panic free. An additional study compared focused CT, relaxation training, imipramine,

and a wait-list control in the treatment of panic disorder (D.M. Clark et al. 1994). All three active treatments were superior to the control condition, but CT led to greater reductions in anxiety levels, catastrophic cognitions, and frequency of panic attacks.

Other investigators also have documented the effectiveness of cognitive and behavioral treatment programs for panic disorder with or without agoraphobia (J.G. Beck et al. 1994; Craske et al. 1995; Heldt et al. 2006; Ost et al. 1993; Pollack et al. 1994). Otto et al. (1993) have demonstrated that CT is more effective than standard clinical management in helping panic disorder patients discontinue benzodiazepines. Also, cognitive-behavioral therapy has been shown to be an effective treatment for patients who have failed to respond to medication for panic disorder (Heldt et al. 2006). Studies that have examined the long-term effects of treatment for panic disorder have found significant relapse prevention effects for CT (Otto and Whittal 1995).

One potential criticism of the CT model for panic disorder is that some persons with this condition experience nocturnal panic in which they awaken suddenly from sleep in a panic attack. It has been reasoned that cognitive pathways for triggering or accelerating a panic attack would not be involved, or would be less salient, in nocturnal panic. However, Craske et al. (2005) demonstrated that CT is effective for nocturnal panic and that positive treatment results were maintained over a 9-month follow-up period.

Although early trials of CT for GAD reported evidence for treatment effectiveness, differences were not always found between CT and supportive or more traditional behavioral approaches (Hollon and Beck 1994). Initial studies of CT for generalized anxiety were marred by design problems such as lack of specificity in the treatment approaches, use of unsophisticated or truncated forms of CT, and selection of cognitive therapists with limited training or experience. Nevertheless, most studies of CT (or combined CT and behavior therapy) for GAD have found CT to be efficacious (Hollon and Beck 1994).

Later trials of CT for generalized anxiety used more precise research designs. Power et al. (1990) randomly assigned patients with GAD to diazepam, placebo, CT, diazepam plus CT, or placebo plus CT. Individuals treated in any of the three CT conditions were substantially improved by the end of the study. Diazepam alone also showed significant treatment effects as compared with placebo, but this was less marked than for CT.

Butler et al. (1991) performed a carefully designed

study of CT for generalized anxiety. This research group had extensive previous experience in behavior therapy practice and research. In addition, they received intensive training in CT (including supervision at the University of Pennsylvania Center for Cognitive Therapy). Adherence to the treatment models (both CT and behavior therapy) was monitored by independent raters. Results of this study indicated that CT was clearly superior to behavior therapy or a wait-list control condition. Furthermore, patients treated with CT had significantly more change in measures of dysfunctional cognition, including anxious thoughts and maladaptive beliefs. Another well-designed study compared CT with analytic psychotherapy and anxiety management training (a psychoeducation-based therapy that teaches anxiety coping strategies) for treatment of 110 patients with GAD (Durham et al. 1994). CT was clearly superior to the other treatments. The differential response between CT and analytic psychotherapy was so dramatic that the authors questioned whether analytic therapy was suitable for persons with GAD. Additional support for use of CT for GAD was reported by a German research group, which found that the mean reduction in Hamilton Anxiety Rating Scale scores was much greater with CT (35.4%) than with a wait-list control condition (6.4%) (Linden et al. 2005).

Several well-executed studies have found evidence for the effectiveness of CT for social phobia (Davidson et al. 2004; Gelernter et al. 1991; Heimberg et al. 1990; Hope et al. 1995). Heimberg's group cognitive and behavioral method has been the most widely studied (Juster and Heimberg 1995). In a large trial of 295 persons with social phobia, no differences were found between group CT and fluoxetine in producing a treatment response (51.7% versus 50.9%) (Davidson et al. 2004). This investigation also found that there was no advantage to combining treatments (54.2% response rate). All active treatments led to significantly greater response rates than a pill placebo (31.7%). However, a research group in the United Kingdom found that individual CT was superior to fluoxetine plus self-exposure and placebo plus self-exposure in relieving symptoms of social phobia (D.M. Clark et al. 2003). When individual CT was directly compared with group CT, treatment with individual format was found to be superior (Stangier et al. 2003). Thus, the possible cost advantages of group CT may be outweighed by the greater efficacy of individual therapy.

Exposure and response prevention (ERP), a treatment that is primarily behavioral in focus, has been studied widely for OCD. Although ERP is typically combined with CT in comprehensive treatment packages (James and Blackburn 1995), there has been limited research on comparing a full CT treatment method with ERP alone. Van Oppen et al. (1995) randomly assigned 71 patients with OCD who were not taking antidepressants to Beck's form of CT or ERP. Both treatments led to statistically significant improvement, but CT was superior to ERP in reducing symptoms of OCD. In contrast, Whittal et al. (2005) found that CT and ERP were equally effective in treating OCD.

A number of trials have demonstrated that ERP is an effective treatment for OCD (James and Blackburn 1995; Salkovskis and Westbrook 1989; Simpson et al. 2006). In a study of 122 patients who were treated with ERP, clomipramine, a combination of ERP and clomipramine, or a pill placebo, ERP or combination treatment was superior to pharmacotherapy in achieving remission (ERP = 52%; ERP + clomipramine = 58%; clomipramine = 25%; placebo = 0%) (Simpson et al. 2006). This research group also found that ERP was substantially better at preventing relapse than clomipramine after treatment was discontinued (Simpson et al. 2004).

PTSD has also been shown to be responsive to CT. For example, McDonagh et al. (2005) found that CT was an effective treatment for PTSD in women who had suffered childhood sexual abuse. Foa et al. (2005) compared CT with ERP in a large study ($n = 171$) of women who suffered from chronic PTSD after sexual abuse. Both treatments were significantly better than a wait-list control condition in relieving symptoms of PTSD, and treatment gains were maintained at the follow-up assessment. Another trial of CT for abused women confirmed the usefulness of this treatment method. Kubany et al. (2004) reported that a full remission of PTSD was achieved in 87% of the women treated with CT. Treatment with cognitive-behavior therapy was compared with supportive therapy and a wait-list control group in 78 persons who experienced chronic PTSD symptoms after motor vehicle accidents (Blanchard et al. 2003). Results of this study indicated that CT was more effective than supportive therapy, which in turn was more effective than the wait-list condition.

A novel approach to using CT for PTSD was reported by Bisson et al. (2004), who developed a brief four-session form of CT which they used to treat persons who had recently experienced a physical injury and who reported psychological distress. In comparison with a no-treatment control group, individuals who were treated with the CT intervention had significantly lower symptoms of PTSD. Results of this study appear to indicate that CT could be a valuable treatment very early in the course of PTSD and could have preventative effects in forestalling the full evolution of this disorder.

Eating Disorders

A large number of experimental trials have found that CT significantly improves the symptoms of bulimia nervosa (Agras et al. 1992, 2000; Banasiak et al. 2005; Carter et al. 2003; Cooper et al. 1996; Fairburn et al. 1991, 1993, 1995; Grilo and Masheb 2005; Goldbloom et al. 1997; Leitenberg et al. 1994; Thackwray et al. 1993; Walsh et al. 1997). Reviews of controlled studies of CT for bulimia nervosa have concluded that there is convincing evidence for the efficacy of cognitive-behavioral treatment (Mitchell et al. 1996; Ricca et al. 2000; Wilson 1999; Wilson and Shafran 2005). Typically, CT reduces the frequency of binge behaviors from 73% to 93% (Fairburn et al. 1992) and leads to a complete remission of bulimic symptoms in 51%–84% of cases (Carter et al. 2003; Ricca et al. 2000).

Examples of major studies of CT for bulimia nervosa include the work of Fairburn et al. (1991, 1993) and Agras et al. (2000). Fairburn et al. (1991, 1993) compared CT with behavioral treatment and interpersonal psychotherapy (IPT) and found that all three psychological treatments used by Fairburn led to improvement in bulimic symptoms. However, CT and IPT were superior to behavior therapy, and CT was the most effective in modifying extreme dieting, emesis, and dysfunctional attitudes (Fairburn et al. 1991, 1993). In another important investigation of psychological therapies for bulimia nervosa, Agras et al. (2000) involved 220 patients who were randomly assigned to either CT or IPT. CT was found to be significantly superior to IPT at the end of treatment. A 48% remission and a 29% recovery rate were observed for CT, whereas the remission rate (28%) and recovery rate (6%) were much lower for IPT.

The use of a full package of cognitive and behavioral methods (the most commonly used CT method for bulimia nervosa in clinical practice) was compared with use of behavior therapy alone by Thackwray et al. (1993). Six months after treatment, 69% of the subjects who were treated with CT were abstinent from binge eating and purging. The abstinence rates for those receiving behavior therapy alone and those in an attention placebo group were 38% and 15%, respectively. Thus, combined cognitive and behavior therapy appears to offer advantages over a purely behavioral approach to bulimia nervosa.

The relative efficacy of CT, pharmacotherapy, and combined CT and pharmacotherapy has been examined in several randomized controlled trials. Agras et al. (1992) found that CT and CT combined with desipramine were superior to desipramine alone in treatment of bulimia nervosa. Similar findings were reported by Jacobi et al. (2002), who noted that CT alone led to better outcomes than fluoxetine in the treatment of bulimia nervosa. There was no advantage to using a combination of CT and fluoxetine in this study. Reviews of investigations of combined CT and pharmacotherapy for bulimia have concluded that CT has a significant positive effect when added to antidepressant therapy (Ricca et al. 2000; Wilson 1999). However, adding medication to CT appears to offer little benefit over treatment with CT alone. The extensive evaluation conducted by the United Kingdom's NICE concluded that CT is more effective than antidepressant medication for bulimia nervosa (Wilson and Shafran 2005).

Because there are not enough trained therapists to administer CT to the large number of persons who suffer from eating disorders, several groups of investigators have examined the utility of self-help therapy tools in reducing symptoms. U. Schmidt et al. (1993) gave 28 bulimic patients a CT handbook and no other treatment. Twenty of the subjects were judged to be much improved ($n=12$) or somewhat improved ($n=8$) after using the workbook for 4–6 weeks. Another research group reported that a CT program of 8 sessions of 20–30 minutes with a social worker plus use of a self-help manual led to an 80% reduction in the frequency of bulimic episodes (Cooper et al. 1996). In a randomized controlled trial, Banasiak et al. (2005) examined the efficacy of a "guided self-help" program for bulimia nervosa. "Guided self-help" included use of the manual *Bulimia Nervosa and Binge Eating: A Guide to Recovery* (Cooper 1995) and 10 sessions with a primary care physician (one 30- to 60-minute session followed by 9 follow-up meetings lasting 20–30 minutes each). The investigators found that guided self-help led to a 60% reduction in binge eating versus 6% in a delayed-treatment control group. Similar results were reported by Grilo and Masheb (2005), who noted that guided self-help produced a 48% remission rate for binge-eating disorder (BED), whereas the control treatment had a 13% remission rate. A novel study of successful use of a CD-ROM self-help program was reviewed in the "Computer-Assisted Cognitive Therapy" section earlier in this chapter.

BED has been studied less intensively than has bulimia nervosa. Nevertheless, there is growing evidence that CT is also effective for this form of eating disorder

(Agras et al. 1994; Grilo et al. 2005; Ricca et al. 2000; Wilfley et al. 1993, 2002; Wilson 1999). In reviews of studies of CT for BED, Wilson (1999) and Ricca et al. (2000) noted that CT has been shown to be beneficial in reducing bingeing but has not been consistently helpful in promoting weight loss in persons with BED. The individual therapy format is typically used for CT or BED, but Wilfley et al. (2002) found that the recovery rate (79%) after group CT was high. One of the most influential trials of CT for BED was conducted by Grilo et al. (2005), who found the highest remission rates in patients treated with either CBT plus placebo (73%) or CBT plus fluoxetine (55%). Remission rates were significantly lower in those treated with fluoxetine alone (29%) or placebo (30%).

Psychosis

There has been a growing interest in studying the use of CT and related therapies for psychotic disorders. In early uncontrolled studies, CT was reported to reduce symptoms of schizophrenia (Garety et al. 1994; Tarrier et al. 1993). Randomized controlled studies have also documented the efficacy of CT for psychosis. A meta-analysis of 14 investigations completed between 1990 and 2004 found that CBT was significantly better than adjunctive measures in lowering psychotic symptoms (Zimmerman et al. 2005). However, the strength and durability of the effects of CT varied from study to study.

Drury et al. (1996a, 1996b) found substantial improvement in positive symptoms and reduced time required for recovery in a group of inpatients treated with CT. Forty patients with nonaffective psychosis were randomly assigned to CT plus standard clinical management or treatment as usual. CT was more effective than standard therapy in reducing positive symptoms and delusional conviction. The percentages of patients who had moderate to severe residual symptoms after treatment were 5% for those who received the added CT compared with 56% for subjects who were treated with standard therapy. In another randomized controlled trial, Kuipers et al. (1997) found superior reduction in Brief Psychiatric Rating Scale scores in patients with nonaffective psychosis treated with CT compared with routine care. But there were no significant differences observed between the treatment groups for other measures of change. Tarrier et al. (1998) studied 87 persons with schizophrenia who had persistent symptoms despite adequate medication. Subjects were randomly assigned to CT plus routine care, supportive therapy plus routine care, or routine care alone. After completion of treatment, patients who received CT had significantly lower scores on measures of positive symptoms compared with patients treated with supportive therapy or routine care alone. Changes in negative symptoms were equivalent in all three treatment groups.

One of the most carefully controlled studies of CT for psychosis reported to date was conducted by Sensky et al. (2000). Ninety persons who met DSM-IV (American Psychiatric Association 1994) criteria for schizophrenia who had persistent, drug-resistant symptoms were randomly assigned to CT or "befriending" (supportive therapy) plus routine care. Treatment manuals and taped sessions were used to ensure fidelity to the treatment method. Medication was equivalent in both treatment groups. At the end of the 9-month course of therapy, there were no differences found between the treatments. Therapy with CT and befriending were both associated with substantial improvements in positive and negative symptoms. However, at the 9-month follow-up examination, patients treated with CT had significantly lower scores on measures of both positive and negative symptoms. For example, the change in Scale for the Assessment of Negative Symptoms mean scores from baseline to 9-month follow-up was 49.3% for CT and 19.0% for befriending. Depressive symptoms were also reduced to a greater extent in patients who received CT.

Other studies of CT for psychotic disorders have also typically described positive benefits of adding psychotherapy to medication. For example, Turkington et al. (2002) observed that community nurses could be trained to deliver a form of CT that was more effective than treatment as usual in improving overall symptomatology, depression, and insight. Also, Cather et al. (2005), in a study completed in the USA, noted that a manualized version of CT showed greater benefit on within-group effect sizes than a psychoeducational approach. More modest results were described by Tarrier et al. (2004) in a large study of CT for schizophrenia and related conditions. Although Tarrier et al. found faster improvement in patients treated with CT as compared with supportive counseling, the active therapies were equivalent by 6 weeks of treatment. Both CT and supportive counseling were better than a control condition in reducing symptoms after 18 months of follow-up. Yet, neither psychotherapy had a significant effect on reducing relapse. In another study with modest effects, Rector et al. (2003) observed that CBT improved both positive and negative symptoms to no greater extent than an "enriched" form of treatment as usual. At follow-up, CT was superior to the control condition in reducing negative symptoms. In contrast to studies that showed sustained gains or further improvement at follow-up, Valmaggia et al. (2005) found that CT was superior to supportive counseling at the end of treatment but not 6 months later.

The overall results of studies of CT for nonaffective psychosis suggest that CT can add to the effects of medication and routine care in the treatment of individuals who have persistent symptoms. Nevertheless, results of studies have varied, and some studies have found only short-term benefit or partial impact on various symptoms of psychosis. The reasons for variability in outcome are unknown, but it is possible that differences in treatment methods, chronicity and severity of symptoms, control of concomitant medication use, and experience and skill of therapists may have influenced results. For example, a study by Wykes et al. (2005) observed that hallucinations were reduced significantly by group CT led by highly skilled therapists, but not by CT group therapy performed by less experienced clinicians.

Treatment protocols in most studies have focused primarily on methods of reducing delusions and hallucinations. Further research on the application of CT for positive symptoms is clearly needed. However, development and testing of specific methods for negative symptoms would be especially welcome because of the frequent resistance of these problems to pharmacotherapy. Treatment adherence is an another important target for CT of severe and chronic mental disorders. CT has been shown to improve adherence to lithium carbonate regimens in patients with bipolar disorder (Cochran 1986), and CT appeared to enhance medication use in an uncontrolled study of schizophrenic patients treated in small group homes (Perris and Skagerlind 1994). A relatively brief CT intervention was studied in a randomized controlled trial by Kemp et al. (1996, 1998), who found long-term benefits including improved medication adherence and prevention of rehospitalization. Additional research is clearly needed on the use of CT for treatment adherence.

Bipolar Disorder

Only a few randomized controlled trials have been completed on CT for bipolar disorder. A preliminary trial of 42 subjects was reported by Scott et al. (2001), who noted that relapse rates were reduced by 60% in those who received CT. Also, persons treated with CT had significantly greater improvement in ratings on the Beck Depression Inventory and the Global Assessment of Functioning Scale. Despite these encouraging findings, a subsequent study of 253 subjects by the same research group found no overall benefit of CT, as compared with treatment as usual, in reducing relapse rates (Scott et al. 2006). However, CT was more effective in forestalling relapse in persons who had fewer than 12 previous bipolar episodes.

Lam et al. (2003) found a very strong effect of CT in lowering the relapse rate for bipolar disorder patients. Subjects ($n=103$) who were having frequent relapses were randomly assigned to CT or a control group. During the first 12 months after treatment, the CT group had significantly fewer episodes of bipolar disorder, less mood symptoms, and higher social functioning. CT was less effective in subjects who had a "sense of hyperpositive self"—presumably because these individuals did not believe they needed therapy (Lam et al. 2005). A 30-month follow-up of the subjects in the Lam et al. study found that CT subjects had an overall reduction in rate of relapse compared with controls, but most of the benefit occurred in the first year. Thus, they suggested that booster sessions or maintenance therapy should be considered.

Another study of CT for bipolar disorder, conducted by Ball et al. (2006), observed that 6 months of therapy had clinical benefit in reducing depression, dysfunctional attitudes, and global ratings of symptom severity. There was a trend ($P=0.06$) for lower relapse rates in patients treated with CT. Ball et al. also noted that short-term effects were greater than long-term benefits and suggested that maintenance therapy may be needed for sustaining the benefits of CT for bipolar disorder.

The possibility that CT could improve symptoms and lower relapse rates in bipolar disorder is enticing, because many persons with this condition do not have a full response to pharmacotherapy. However, considerably more research is needed to determine the overall value of this approach and to delineate patient characteristics that may predict a favorable outcome to CT.

Outcome Research for Other Disorders

The majority of CT outcome research has been concerned with depression, anxiety disorders, eating disorders, and psychosis. However, a substantial amount of investigative work has been completed on the efficacy of CT for other conditions such as psychophysiological disorders, substance abuse, and personality disorders. A broad range of studies have examined the utility of CT in behavioral medicine (Sensky 2004). For example, multiple sclerosis patients treated with CT have been found to have significantly improved psychological and physical functioning (Rodgers et al. 1996). In another study, CT was shown to be significantly better than routine care in reducing depression and improving glucose control in persons with type 2 diabetes (Lustman et al. 1998). CT has also been demonstrated to be effective in reducing medication requirements in persons with hypertension (Shapiro et al. 1997).

Several groups have reported that CT can be a helpful approach in the management of chronic pain (Linton and Nordin 2006; Linton and Ryberg 2001; Moore et al. 2000). A meta-analysis of 25 studies of CT for pain (excluding headache) found that this approach was effective when compared with a wait-list control group and with alternative active treatments (Morley et al. 1999). The cognitive treatment model for chronic pain has been described in detail by Turk et al. (1983).

Other investigators have observed that CT can be useful in the treatment of skin disorders (Horne et al. 1989), epilepsy (Goldstein 1990), asthma (Maes and Schlosser 1988), inflammatory and irritable bowel syndromes (Kennedy et al. 2006; Payne and Blanchard 1995), temporomandibular disorders (Mishra et al. 2000; Turner et al. 2006), fibromyalgia (White and Nielson 1995), chronic fatigue syndrome (Deale et al. 2001; Stulemeijer et al. 2005), and medically unexplained physical symptoms (Kroenke and Swindle 2000). CT also has been shown to be effective in reducing the risk of disability from medical illness. In a randomized study of programs for prevention of disability from spine pain, Linton and Andersson (2000) found that a six-session cognitive-behavioral group intervention led to a ninefold lowering of the risk for long-term work absence.

One particularly useful application for CT is in the treatment of insomnia. CT has fared well in outcome studies when compared with pharmacotherapy. For example, Sivertsen et al. (2006) found that CT was superior to zopiclone in improving sleep efficiency, promoting slow-wave sleep, and reducing awake time. Similar results were reported by Wu et al. (2006), who observed long-term benefits of cognitive-behavioral therapy compared with medication for sleep. In another investigation, Jacobs et al. (2004) observed that CT was more effective than pharmacotherapy in improving sleep latency and efficiency in young and middle-aged adults, and that addition of pharmacotherapy to CT yielded no additional benefit. These studies suggest that CT offers significant advantages over sleeping medication in the treatment of insomnia.

Applications of the full CT models for substance abuse have not yet been studied extensively under controlled conditions. However, for alcoholism and other substance abuse disorders, more broadly defined cognitive-behavioral therapies have become one of the treatments of first choice (Carroll and Onkin 2005). An early investigation for substance abuse suggested that CT (plus paraprofessional drug counseling) may be superior to drug counseling alone in treatment of heroin addicts (Woody et al. 1983). In a large study of treatment for cocaine abuse, Wells et al. (1994) found that a relapse prevention program based in part on cognitive-behavioral methods and a 12-Step approach were equally effective in decreasing both cocaine and alcohol use. The patients who received relapse prevention had a lower use of alcohol than those treated with the 12-Step approach at the follow-up assessment.

Another study of CT-based relapse prevention programs found cognitive-behavioral therapy to be more effective than desipramine or clinical management in reducing cocaine use and fostering abstinence (Carroll et al. 1995). Carroll et al. (1995) observed no differences immediately after treatment in subjects with cocaine dependence who received CT (relapse prevention), desipramine, or placebo. However, the CT subjects had a significantly improved response at the 1-year follow-up. The authors concluded that this effect was likely due to "implementation of the generalizable coping skills conveyed through that treatment."

In contrast, a multicenter trial sponsored by the National Institute on Drug Abuse found that neither CT nor supportive-expressive psychotherapy was as effective as the combination of individual and group drug counseling for cocaine-dependent patients (Crits-Christoph et al. 1999). In fact, neither of the psychotherapies added to group drug counseling was any more effective than group counseling alone, despite 8–10 additional hours of one-to-one intervention. One potential explanation for this negative outcome is that many of the psychotherapists were relatively inexperienced in the treatment of chemically dependent patients.

More favorable results have been reported in studies of more broadly defined models of cognitive-behavior therapy (Carroll and Onkin 2005). For example, in two studies of patients with schizophrenia and substance abuse disorders, the combination of cognitive behavior therapy and pharmacotherapy significantly improved outcomes compared with pharmacotherapy and clinical management (Barrowclough et al. 2001; Naeem et al. 2005). Cognitive-behavior therapy also may be combined with other behavioral interventions. In one study, cognitive-behavior therapy alone was less effective than a voucher-based contingency management approach in reducing heavy marijuana use, but the combination of strategies was associated with significantly better long-term outcomes after the voucher program ended (Budney et al. 2006).

Limited research has been completed on CT for alcohol abuse, but preliminary studies have shown that alcoholic individuals, even those with significant Axis II pathology, can respond well to a CT approach (Fisher and Bentley 1996; Longabaugh et al. 1994; Schonfeld and Dupree 1995; Sitharthan et al. 1996). In combination with naltrexone therapy of alcoholism, cognitive-behavior therapy significantly reduced the likelihood of alcohol relapse and improved longer-term outcomes (Anton et al. 2005).

Outcome research on CT for personality disorders is at an early stage of development. It has been suggested that the presence of an Axis II disorder may complicate the treatment of depression, anxiety disorders, or eating disorders with CT (Persons et al. 1988; Rush and Shaw 1983). Personality disorders did not, however, predict poorer CT response in the multi-center NIMH Treatment of Depression Collaborative Research Program (Shea et al. 1990) or in a single-center study conducted by the Pittsburgh group (Stuart et al. 1992). A large randomized trial of CT for treatment of alcohol abuse similarly found that patients who had antisocial personality disorder responded well to treatment and in some cases actually did better than subjects without personality disorder (Longabaugh et al. 1994). Also, patients with body dysmorphic disorder and comorbid Axis II disorders were observed to have highly significant and substantial improvement after treatment with CT (Neziroglu et al. 1996).

The most notable research on a cognitive-behavioral approach to personality disorders has been conducted by Linehan and colleagues (Bohus et al. 2000; Linehan 1993; Linehan et al. 1991, 1993, 1994, 1999, 2006). In a randomized trial of 44 borderline patients treated with DBT or treatment as usual, significant reductions in suicidal acts and the medical risk for suicide were observed in those who received DBT (Linehan et al. 1991). At the 6-month posttreatment assessment, DBT was still superior to treatment as usual, but these differences had disappeared by the time of the 12-month assessment (Linehan et al. 1993). Subjects treated with DBT had fewer days of inpatient hospitalization than control subjects during the year after completion of therapy. In the most recent study, 101 women with borderline personality disorder were randomly assigned to 1 year of treatment with either DBT or psychodynamic psychotherapy, conducted by expert "true believers" (Linehan et al. 2006). At the end

of treatment and across a 1-year follow-up, the DBT group experienced significantly better outcomes on most measures, including a 50% greater reduction in suicidal behavior and significantly fewer psychiatric hospitalizations.

Another analysis of data from Linehan's studies indicated that DBT had mixed effects on social and interpersonal functioning (Linehan et al. 1994). In a group of 26 patients with borderline personality and chronic suicidal activities treated with DBT or treatment as usual, DBT was found to significantly improve measures of anger and interviewer-rated social adjustment. Global life satisfaction was not different in the two experimental groups.

In a study of inpatients with a variety of Axis II diagnoses, group DBT was no more effective than supportive group therapy (Springer et al. 1996). The treatment program was quite short compared with the DBT described by Linehan, and a variety of other treatments were used for this inpatient sample. Thus, the study by Springer et al. (1996) does not appear to be an adequate test of DBT. In a later uncontrolled study, Bohus et al. (2000) reported significant improvements in depression, dissociation, anxiety, and global stress after a 3-month inpatient DBT program.

Beck's model for CT of personality disorders has received only a limited amount of research. Two case series have been reported in which CT appeared to be useful for treatment of people with personality disorders (Davidson and Tyrer 1996; Nelson-Gray et al. 1996). In a meta-analysis of early studies, Leichsenring and Leibing (2003) concluded that CT and psychodynamic psychotherapy were probably comparably effective, although they pointed out the need for larger prospective studies. In the only subsequent study to specifically focus on patients with personality disorders, Svartberg et al. (2004) randomly allocated 50 patients with Cluster C personality disorders to receive 40 weeks of treatment with either CT or psychodynamic psychotherapy. Although trends favored the psychodynamic psychotherapy on several measures at the end of treatment, there were no significant differences in outcomes, both at the end of therapy and across a 2-year follow-up. In a large practical trial of 480 patients with a history of recent deliberate self-injury, the impact of personality disorder was examined in relation to response to manual-assisted CT or treatment as usual (Tyrer et al. 2004). Overall, CT conveyed a modest advantage over usual treatment. However, among a subset with borderline personality disorder, CT appeared to increase the cost of care without improving outcomes.

Outcome research has been extremely limited for any type of psychotherapy of personality disorders. These conditions are notoriously difficult to treat under controlled conditions because of pervasive interpersonal and skills deficits and a frequent need for long-term therapy. Linehan's groundbreaking research, and the work of other investigators on DBT and CT, has stimulated hope that additional studies will help elucidate the most effective methods of treating this challenging group of patients.

Conclusion

CT is a recently developed system of psychotherapy that is linked philosophically with a long tradition of viewing cognition as a primary determinant of emotion and behavior. The theoretical constructs of CT are supported by a large body of experimental findings regarding dysfunctional information processing in psychiatric disorders. In clinical practice, CT is usually short term, problem oriented, and highly collaborative. Therapists and patients work together in an empirical style, seeking to identify and modify maladaptive patterns of thinking. Behavioral techniques are used to uncover distorted cognitions and to promote more effective functioning. Also, psychoeducational procedures and homework assignments help reinforce concepts learned in therapy sessions. The goals of CT include both immediate symptom relief and the acquisition of cognitive and behavioral skills that will decrease the risk for relapse.

The efficacy of CT for depression, GAD, panic disorder, eating disorders, and other conditions has been established in a wide range of outcome studies. Newer applications for CT, such as personality disorders, substance abuse, and psychosis are beginning to receive attention from investigators. Detailed treatment manuals or other guidelines for therapy have been described for most psychiatric illnesses.

CT has rapidly evolved into one of the major psychotherapeutic orientations in modern psychiatric treatment. Future challenges for this therapy model include study of the relative importance of treatment components, detailed examination of predictors for outcome, elucidation of the interface between biological and cognitive processes, and incorporation of new developments in computer-assisted learning. The empirical nature of CT should promote further exploration of the potential uses for this treatment approach.

Key Points

- Studies of information processing in mental disorders have found characteristic patterns of cognitions that are linked with dysphoric emotions and maladaptive behavior.

- Treatment with cognitive therapy involves modification of dysfunctional cognitions and associated behaviors.

- Cognitive therapy is an active treatment characterized by a highly collaborative therapeutic relationship.

- Structure, psychoeducation, and homework are important components of treatment.

- Cognitive therapists help patients identify and change automatic thoughts and core beliefs (schemas).

- Behavioral methods are used to reverse helplessness, anhedonia, avoidance, and other core symptoms of mental disorders.

- Cognitive therapy has been extensively researched. There is strong empirical support for the efficacy of this treatment approach.

- Cognitive therapy methods have been developed for many conditions including mood and anxiety disorders, schizophrenia, eating disorders, substance abuse, and personality disorders.

Suggested Readings

Barlow DH, Cerney JA: Psychological Treatment of Panic. New York, Guilford, 1988

Basco MR, Rush AJ: Cognitive-Behavioral Therapy for Bipolar Disorder. New York, Guilford, 2005

Beck AT, Freeman A: Cognitive Therapy of Personality Disorders. New York, Guilford, 1990

Beck AT, Rush AJ, Shaw BF, et al: Cognitive Therapy of Depression. New York, Guilford, 1979

Beck AT, Emery GD, Greenberg RL: Anxiety Disorders and Phobias: A Cognitive Perspective. New York, Basic Books, 1985

Beck AT, Wright FD, Newman CF, et al: Cognitive Therapy of Substance Abuse. New York, Guilford, 1993

Beck J: Cognitive Therapy: Basics and Beyond. New York, Guilford, 1995

Clark DA, Beck AT, Alford BA: Scientific Foundations of Cognitive Theory and Therapy of Depression. New York, Wiley, 1999

Clark DM, Fairburn CG (eds): Science and Practice of Cognitive Behavior Therapy. New York, Oxford University Press, 1997

Fairburn C, Brownell K (eds): Eating Disorders and Obesity: A Comprehensive Handbook, 2nd Edition. New York, Guilford, 2002

Kingdon D, Turkington D: Cognitive Therapy for Schizophrenia. New York, Guilford, 2005

Leahy RL: Contemporary Cognitive Therapy: Theory, Research, and Practice. New York, Guilford, 2004

Linehan MM: Cognitive-Behavioral Treatment of Borderline Personality Disorder. New York, Guilford, 1993

Mahoney MJ, Freeman A (eds): Cognition and Psychotherapy. New York, Plenum, 1985

Meichenbaum DB: Cognitive-Behavior Modification: An Integrative Approach. New York, Plenum, 1977

Reinecke MA, Dattilio FM, Freeman A (eds): Cognitive Therapy With Children and Adolescents: A Casebook for Clinical Practice, 2nd Edition. New York, Guilford, 2003

Salkovskis PM (ed): Frontiers of Cognitive Therapy. New York, Guilford, 1996

Wilkes TCR, Belsher G, Rush AJ, et al: Cognitive Therapy for Depressed Adolescents. New York, Guilford, 1994

Wright JH, Basco MR, Thase ME: Learning Cognitive-Behavior Therapy: An Illustrated Guide (Core Competencies in Psychotherapy Series, Glen O. Gabbard, series ed). Arlington, VA, American Psychiatric Publishing, 2006

Online Resources

Academy of Cognitive Therapy: http://www.academyofCT.org

American Psychiatric Publishing, Inc. (for downloading of worksheets from *Learning Cognitive-Behavior Therapy: An Illustrated Guide,* by J.H. Wright, M.R. Basco, and M.E. Thase): http://www.appi.org

Association for Behavioral and Cognitive Therapies: http://www.aabt.org

Beck Institute: http://www.beckinstitute.org

British Association for Cognitive and Behavioral Psychotherapy: http://www.babcp.com

International Association for Cognitive Psychotherapy (IACP): http://www.cognitivetherapyassociation.org

mindstreet (for computer-assisted CT software): http://www.mindstreet.com

References

Abramson LY, Seligman MEP, Teasdale J: Learned helplessness in humans: critique and reformulation. J Abnorm Psychol 87:49–74, 1978

Agras WS, Rossiter EM, Arnow B, et al: Pharmacological and cognitive-behavioral treatment for bulimia nervosa: a controlled comparison. Am J Psychiatry 149:82–87, 1992

Agras WS, Telch CF, Arnow B, et al: Weight loss, cognitive-behavioral, and desipramine treatments in binge eating disorder: an additive design. Behav Ther 25:225–238, 1994

Agras WS, Walsh BT, Fairburn CG, et al: A multicenter comparison of cognitive-behavioral therapy and interpersonal psychotherapy for bulimia nervosa. Arch Gen Psychiatry 57:459–466, 2000

Albano AM, Kearney CA: When Children Refuse School: A Cognitive Behavioral Therapy Approach (Therapist Guide). San Antonio, TX, Psychological Corporation, 2000

Alford BA, Beck AT: The Integrative Power of Cognitive Therapy. New York, Guilford, 1997

American Psychiatric Association: Diagnostic and Statistical Manual of Mental Disorders, 4th Edition. Washington, DC, American Psychiatric Association, 1994

Anderson P, Jacobs C, Rothbaum BO: Computer-supported cognitive behavioral treatment of anxiety disorders. J Clin Psychol 60:253–267, 2004

Anton RF, Moak DH, Latham P, et al: Naltrexone combined with either cognitive behavioral or motivational enhancement therapy for alcohol dependence. J Clin Psychopharmacol 25:349–357, 2005

Ball JR, Mitchell PB, Corry JC, et al: A randomized controlled trial of cognitive therapy for bipolar disorder: focus on long-term change. J Clin Psychiatry 67:277–286, 2006

Banasiak SJ, Paxton SJ, Hay P: Guided self-help for bulimia nervosa in primary care: a randomized controlled trial. Psychol Med 35:1283–1294, 2005

Barlow DH, Cerney JA: Psychological Treatment of Panic. New York, Guilford, 1988

Barlow DH, Craske MG: Mastery of Your Anxiety and Panic (MAP3). Boston, MA, Graywind Publications, 1999

Barlow DH, Craske MG, Cerney JA, et al: Behavioral treatment of panic disorder. Behav Ther 20:261–268, 1989

Barlow DH, Gorman JM, Shear MK, et al: Cognitive-behavioral therapy, imipramine, or their combination for panic disorder: a randomized controlled trial. JAMA 283:2529–2536, 2000

Barrowclough C, Haddock G, Tarrier N, et al: Randomized controlled trial of motivational interviewing, cognitive behavior therapy, and family intervention for patients with comorbid schizophrenia and substance use disorders. Am J Psychiatry 158:1706–1713, 2001

Basco MR: Never Good Enough. New York, Free Press, 1999

Basco MR, Rush AJ: Cognitive-Behavioral Therapy for Bipolar Disorder. New York, Guilford, 2005

Baxter LR Jr, Schwartz JM, Bergman KS, et al: Caudate glucose metabolic rate changes with both drug and behavior therapy for obsessive-compulsive disorder. Arch Gen Psychiatry 49:681–689, 1992

Beck AT: Thinking and depression. Arch Gen Psychiatry 9:324–333, 1963

Beck AT: Thinking and depression, II: theory and therapy. Arch Gen Psychiatry 10:561–571, 1964

Beck AT: Depression: Clinical, Experimental, and Theoretical Aspects. New York, Harper & Row, 1967

Beck AT: Cognitive Therapy and the Emotional Disorders. New York, International Universities Press, 1976

Beck AT: Love Is Never Enough. New York, Harper & Row, 1988

Beck AT: Cognitive therapy and research: a 25-year retrospective. Presented at the World Congress of Cognitive Therapy. Oxford, England, 1989

Beck AT: Cognitive therapy: past, present, and future. J Consult Clin Psychol 61:194–198, 1993

Beck AT, Freeman A: Cognitive Therapy of Personality Disorders. New York, Guilford, 1990

Beck AT, Kovacs M, Weissman A: Hopelessness and suicidal behavior—an overview. JAMA 234:1146–1149, 1975

Beck AT, Rush AJ, Shaw BF, et al: Cognitive Therapy of Depression. New York, Guilford, 1979

Beck AT, Emery GD, Greenberg RL: Anxiety Disorders and Phobias: A Cognitive Perspective. New York, Basic Books, 1985a

Beck AT, Steer RA, Kovacs M, et al: Hopelessness and eventual suicide: a 10-year prospective study of patients hospitalized with suicidal ideation. Am J Psychiatry 142:559–563, 1985b

Beck AT, Sokol L, Clark DA, et al: A cross-over study of focused cognitive therapy for panic disorder. Am J Psychiatry 149:778–783, 1992

Beck AT, Greenberg RL, Beck J: Coping with depression (a booklet). Bala Cynwyd, PA, The Beck Institute, 1995

Beck J: Cognitive Therapy: Basics and Beyond. New York, Guilford, 1995

Beck JG, Stanley MA, Baldwin LE, et al: Comparison of cognitive therapy and relaxation training for panic disorder. J Consult Clin Psychol 62:818–826, 1994

Beutler LE, Scogin F, Kinkish P, et al: Group cognitive therapy and alprazolam in the treatment of depression in older adults. J Consult Clin Psychol 55:550–556, 1987

Bisson JI, Shepherd JP, Joy D, et al: Early cognitive-behavioural therapy for posttraumatic stress symptoms after physical injury. Randomised controlled trial. Br J Psychiatry 184:63–69, 2004

Blackburn IM, Bishop S, Glen AIM, et al: The efficacy of cognitive therapy in depression: a treatment trial using cognitive therapy and pharmacotherapy, each alone and in combination. Br J Psychiatry 139:181–189, 1981

Blackburn IM, Jones S, Lewin RJP: Cognitive style in depression. Br J Clin Psychol 25:241–251, 1986

Blanchard EB, Hickling EJ, Devineni T, et al: A controlled evaluation of cognitive behavioral therapy for posttraumatic stress in motor vehicle accident survivors. Behav Res Ther 41:79–96, 2003

Bohus M, Haaf B, Stiglmayr C, et al: Evaluation of inpatient dialectical-behavior therapy for borderline personality disorder—a prospective study. Behav Res Ther 38:875–887, 2000

Bowers WA: Treatment of depressed inpatients: cognitive therapy plus medication, relaxation plus medication, and medication alone. Br J Psychiatry 156:73–78, 1990

Brown GK, Newman CF, Charlesworth SE, et al: An open clinical trial of cognitive therapy for borderline personality disorder. J Personal Disord 18:257–271, 2004

Brown GK, Ten Have T, Henriques GR, et al: Cognitive therapy for the prevention of suicide attempts: a randomized controlled trial. JAMA 294:563–570, 2005

Budney AJ, Moore BA, Rocha HL, et al: Clinical trial of abstinence-based vouchers and cognitive-behavioral therapy for cannabis dependence. J Consult Clin Psychol 74:307–316, 2006

Bujold A, Ladouceur R, Sylvain C, et al: Treatment of pathological gamblers: an experimental study. J Behav Ther Exp Psychiatry 25:275–282, 1994

Burns DD: Feeling Good. New York, William Morrow, 1980

Burns DD: Feeling Good: The New Mood Therapy. New York, HarperCollins, 1999

Burns DD, Rude S, Simons AD, et al: Does learned resourcefulness predict the response to cognitive behavioral therapy for depression? Cognit Ther Res 18:277–291, 1994

Butler G, Fennell M, Robson P, et al: Comparison of behavior therapy and cognitive behavior therapy in the treatment of generalized anxiety disorder. J Consult Clin Psychol 59:167–175, 1991

Butler AC, Chapman JE, Forman EM, et al: The empirical status of cognitive-behavioral therapy: a review of meta-analyses. Clin Psychol Rev 26:17–31, 2006

Carroll KM, Onken LS: Behavioral therapies for drug abuse. Am J Psychiatry 162:1452–1460, 2005

Carroll KM, Nich C, Rounsaville BJ: Differential symptom reduction in depressed cocaine abusers treated with psychotherapy and pharmacotherapy. J Nerv Ment Dis 183:251–259, 1995

Carter FA, McIntosh VVW, Joyce PR, et al: Role of exposure with response prevention in cognitive-behavioral therapy for bulimia nervosa: three-year follow-up results. Int J Eat Disord 33:127–135, 2003

Cather C, Penn D, Otto MW, et al: A pilot study of functional cognitive behavioral therapy for schizophrenia. Schizophr Res 74:201–209, 2005

Clark DA, Feldman J, Channon S: Dysfunctional thinking in anorexia and bulimia nervosa. Cognit Ther Res 13:377–387, 1989

Clark DA, Beck AT, Stewart B: Cognitive specificity and positive-negative affectivity: complementary or contradictory views on anxiety and depression? J Abnorm Psychol 99:148–155, 1990

Clark DA, Beck AT, Alford BA: Scientific Foundations of Cognitive Theory and Therapy of Depression. New York, Wiley, 1999

Clark DM: A cognitive approach to panic. Behav Res Ther 24:461–470, 1986

Clark DM, Teasdale JD: Diurnal variation in clinical depression and the accessibility of memories of positive and negative experiences. J Abnorm Psychol 91:87–95, 1982

Clark DM, Salkovskis PM, Chalkley AJ: Respiratory control as a treatment for panic attacks. J Behav Ther Exp Psychiatry 16:23–30, 1985

Clark DM, Salkovskis PM, Hackmann A, et al: A comparison of cognitive therapy, applied relaxation and imipramine in the treatment of panic disorder. Br J Psychiatry 164:759–769, 1994

Clark DM, Ehlers A, McManus F, et al: Cognitive therapy versus fluoxetine in generalized social phobia: a randomized placebo-controlled trial. J Consult Clin Psychol 71:1058–1067, 2003

Cloitre M, Liebowitz MR: Memory bias in panic disorder: an investigation of the cognitive avoidance hypothesis. Cognit Ther Res 15:371–386, 1991

Cochran SD: Compliance with lithium regimens in the outpatient treatment of bipolar affective disorders. J Compliance Health Care 1:151–169, 1986

Cooper PJ: Bulimia Nervosa and Binge-Eating: A Guide to Recovery. New York, New York University Press, 1995

Cooper PJ, Coker S, Fleming C: An evaluation of the efficacy of supervised cognitive behavioral self-help for bulimia nervosa. J Psychosom Res 40:281–287, 1996

Covi L, Lipman RS: Cognitive behavioral group psychotherapy combined with imipramine in major depression. Psychopharmacol Bull 23:173–176, 1987

Covi L, Primakoff L: Cognitive group therapy, in The American Psychiatric Press Review of Psychiatry. Edited by Frances AJ, Hales RE. Washington, DC, American Psychiatric Press, 1988, pp 608–616

Craske MG, Maidenberg E, Bystritsky A: Brief cognitive-behavioral versus nondirective therapy for panic disorder. J Behav Ther Exp Psychiatry 26:113–120, 1995

Craske MG, Lang AJ, Aikins D, et al: Cognitive behavioral therapy for nocturnal panic. Behav Ther 36:43–54, 2005

Crits-Christoph P, Siqueland L, Blaine J, et al: Psychosocial treatments for cocaine dependence. National Institute on Drug Abuse Collaborative Cocaine Treatment Study. Arch Gen Psychiatry 56:493–502, 1999

Davidson JR, Foa EB, Huppert JD, et al: Fluoxetine, comprehensive cognitive behavioral therapy, and placebo in generalized social phobia. Arch Gen Psychiatry 61:1005–1013, 2004

Davidson KM, Tyrer P: Cognitive therapy for antisocial and borderline personality disorders: single case study series. Br J Clin Psychol 35:413–429, 1996

Davis D, Wright JH: The therapeutic relationship in cognitive-behavioral therapy: patient perceptions and therapist responses. Cogn Behav Pract 1:25–45, 1994

Deale A, Husain K, Chalder T, et al: Long-term outcome of cognitive behavior therapy versus relaxation therapy for chronic fatigue syndrome: a 5-year follow-up study. Am J Psychiatry 158:2038–2042, 2001

DeRubeis RJ, Evans MD, Hollon SD, et al: How does cognitive therapy work? Cognitive change and symptom change in cognitive therapy and pharmacotherapy for depression. J Consult Clin Psychol 58:862–869, 1990

DeRubeis RJ, Gelfand LA, Tang TZ, et al: Medication versus cognitive behavior therapy for severely depressed outpatients: mega-analysis of four randomized comparisons. Am J Psychiatry 156:1007–1013, 1999

DeRubeis RJ, Hollon SD, Amsterdam JD, et al: Cognitive therapy vs medications in the treatment of moderate to severe depression. Arch Gen Psychiatry 62:409–416, 2005

Deutscher S, Cimbolic P: Cognitive process and their relationship to endogenous and reactive components of depression. J Nerv Ment Dis 178:351–359, 1990

Dobson KS: A meta-analysis of the efficacy of cognitive therapy for depression. J Consult Clin Psychol 57:414–419, 1989

Dobson KS, Shaw BF: Cognitive assessment with major depressive disorders. Cognit Ther Res 10:13–29, 1986

Drury V, Birchwood M, Cochrane R, et al: Cognitive therapy and recovery from acute psychosis: a controlled trial, I: impact on psychotic symptoms. Br J Psychiatry 169:593–601, 1996a

Drury V, Birchwood M, Cochrane R, et al: Cognitive therapy and recovery from acute psychosis: a controlled trial, II: impact on recovery time. Br J Psychiatry 169:602–607, 1996b

Durham RC, Murphy T, Allan T, et al: Cognitive therapy, analytic psychotherapy and anxiety management training for generalized anxiety disorder. Br J Psychiatry 165:315–323, 1994

Elkin I, Shea MT, Watkins JT, et al: NIMH Treatment of Depression Collaborative Research Program, I: general effectiveness of treatments. Arch Gen Psychiatry 46:971–982, 1989

Elkin I, Gibbons RD, Shea MT, et al: Initial severity and differential treatment outcome in the National Institute of Mental Health Treatment of Depression Collaborative Research Program. J Consult Clin Psychol 63:841–847, 1995

Ellis A: Reason and Emotion in Psychotherapy. New York, Lyle Stuart, 1962

Epstein N, Schlesinger SE, Dryden W: Cognitive-Behavioral Therapy With Families. New York, Brunner/Mazel, 1988

Evans MD, Hollon SD, DeRubeis RJ, et al: Differential relapse following cognitive therapy and pharmacotherapy for depression. Arch Gen Psychiatry 49:802–808, 1992

Fairburn CG, Jones R, Peveler RC, et al: Three psychological treatments for bulimia nervosa. Arch Gen Psychiatry 48:463–469, 1991

Fairburn CG, Agras WS, Wilson GT: The research on treatment of bulimia nervosa: practical and theoretical implications, in The Biology of Feast and Famine: Relevance to Eating Disorders. Edited by Anderson GH, Kennedy SH. San Diego, CA, Academic Press, 1992, pp 318–340

Fairburn CG, Jones R, Peveler RC, et al: Psychotherapy and bulimia nervosa. Arch Gen Psychiatry 50:419–428, 1993

Fairburn CG, Norman PA, Welch SL, et al: A prospective study of outcome in bulimia nervosa and the long-term effects of three psychological treatments. Arch Gen Psychiatry 52:304–312, 1995

Fava GA, Grandi S, Zielezny M, et al: Four-year outcome for cognitive behavioral treatment of residual symptoms in major depression. Am J Psychiatry 153:945–947, 1996

Fava GA, Rafanelli C, Grandi S, et al: Prevention of recurrent depression with cognitive behavioral therapy. Arch Gen Psychiatry 55:816–820, 1998

Fava GA, Ruini C, Rafanelli C, et al: Six-year outcome of cognitive behavior therapy for prevention of recurrent depression. Am J Psychiatry 161:1872–1876, 2004

Fawcett J, Scheftner W, Clark D, et al: Clinical predictors of suicide in patients with major affective disorders: a controlled prospective study. Am J Psychiatry 144:35–40, 1987

Fisher MS, Bentley KJ: Two group therapy models for clients with a dual diagnosis of substance abuse and personality disorder. Psychiatr Serv 47:1244–1250, 1996

Foa E, Wilson R: Stop Obsessing! How to Overcome Your Obsessions and Compulsions, Revised Edition. New York, Bantam Books, 2001

Foa EB, Hembree EA, Cahill SP, et al: Randomized trial of prolonged exposure for posttraumatic stress disorder with and without cognitive restructuring: outcome at academic and community clinics. J Consult Clin Psychol 73:953–964, 2005

Frankl VE: Logos, paradox, and the search for meaning, in Cognition and Psychotherapy. Edited by Mahoney MJ, Freeman A. New York, Plenum, 1985, pp 3–49

Free ML, Oei TPS, Sanders MR: Treatment outcome of a group cognitive therapy program for depression. Int J Group Psychother 41:533–547, 1991

Freeman A, Schrodt GR, Gilson M, et al: Cognitive group therapy with inpatients, in Cognitive Therapy With Inpatients: Developing a Cognitive Milieu. Edited by Wright JH, Thase ME, Beck AT, et al. New York, Guilford, 1992, pp 121–153

Gaffan EA, Tsaousis I, Kemp-Wheeler SM: Researcher allegiance and meta-analysis: the case of cognitive therapy for depression. J Consult Clin Psychol 63:966–980, 1995

Garety PA, Kuipers L, Fowler D, et al: Cognitive behavioral therapy for drug-resistant psychosis. Br J Med Psychol 67:259–271, 1994

Gelernter CS, Uhde TW, Cimbolic P, et al: Cognitive-behavioral and pharmacological treatments of social phobia: a controlled study. Arch Gen Psychiatry 48:938–945, 1991

Glass CR, Furlong M: Cognitive assessment of social anxiety: affective and behavioral correlates. Cognit Ther Res 14:365–384, 1990

Goldapple K, Segal Z, Garson C, et al: Modulation of cortical-limbic pathways in major depression: treatment-specific effects of cognitive behavior therapy. Arch Gen Psychiatry 61:34–41, 2004

Goldbloom DS, Olmsted M, Davis R, et al: A randomized controlled trial of fluoxetine and cognitive behavioral therapy for bulimia nervosa: short-term outcome. Behav Res Ther 35:803–811, 1997

Goldstein LH: Behavioral and cognitive-behavioral treatments for epilepsy: a progress review. Br J Clin Psychol 29:257–269, 1990

Greenberg LS, Safran JD: Integrating affect and cognition: a perspective on the process of therapeutic change. Cognit Ther Res 8:559–578, 1984

Greenberger D, Padesky CA: Mind Over Mood. New York, Guilford, 1995

Grilo CM, Masheb RM: A randomized controlled comparison of guided self-help cognitive behavioral therapy and behavioral weight loss for binge eating disorder. Behav Res Ther 43:1509–1525, 2005

Grilo CM, Masheb RM, Wilson GT: Efficacy of cognitive behavioral therapy and fluoxetine for the treatment of binge eating disorder: a randomized double-blind placebo-controlled comparison. Biol Psychiatry 57:301–309, 2005

Guidano VF, Liotti G: Cognitive Processes and Emotional Disorders: A Structural Approach to Psychotherapy. New York, Guilford, 1983

Hargreaves IR: Attributional style and depression. Br J Clin Psychol 24:65–66, 1985

Harvey AG, Bryant RA, Tarrier N: Cognitive behaviour therapy for posttraumatic stress disorder. Clin Psychol Rev 23:501–522, 2003

Heimberg RG, Dodge CS, Hope DA, et al: Cognitive behavioral group treatment for social phobia: comparison with a credible placebo control. Cognit Ther Res 14:1–23, 1990

Heldt E, Gus Manfro G, Kipper L, et al: One-year follow-up of pharmacotherapy-resistant patients with panic disorder treated with cognitive-behavior therapy: outcome and predictors of remission. Behav Res Ther 44:657–665, 2006

Hollon SD, Beck AT: Cognitive and cognitive-behavioral therapies, in Handbook of Psychotherapy and Behavior Change: An Empirical Analysis, 4th Edition. Edited by Garfield SL, Bergin AE. New York, Wiley, 1994, pp 428–466

Hollon SD, Kendall PC: Cognitive self-statements in depression: development of an automatic thought questionnaire. Cognit Ther Res 4:383–395, 1980

Hollon SD, Kendall PC, Lumry A: Specificity of depressotypic cognitions in clinical depression. J Abnorm Psychol 95:52–59, 1986

Hollon SD, Shelton RC, Loosen PT: Cognitive therapy and pharmacotherapy for depression. J Consult Clin Psychol 59:88–99, 1991

Hollon SD, DeRubeis RJ, Evans MD, et al: Cognitive therapy and pharmacotherapy for depression: singly and in combination. Arch Gen Psychiatry 49:774–782, 1992

Hollon SD, DeRubeis RJ, Shelton RC, et al: Prevention of relapse following cognitive therapy vs medications in moderate to severe depression. Arch Gen Psychiatry 62:417–422, 2005

Hope DA, Heimberg RG, Bruch MA: Dismantling cognitive-behavioral group therapy for social phobia. Behav Res Ther 33:637–650, 1995

Horne DJ, White AW, Varigos GA: A preliminary study of psychological therapy in the management of atopic eczema. Br J Med Psychol 62:241–248, 1989

Ingram RE, Kendall PC, Smith TW, et al: Cognitive specificity in emotional distress. J Pers Soc Psychol 53:734–742, 1987

Jacobi C, Dahme B, Dittmann R: Cognitive-behavioural, fluoxetine and combined treatment for bulimia nervosa: short- and long-term results. European Eating Disorders Review 10:179–198, 2002

Jacobs GD, Pace-Schott EF, Stickgold R, et al: Cognitive behavior therapy and pharmacotherapy for insomnia: a randomized controlled trial and direct comparison. Arch Intern Med 164:1888–1897, 2004

Jacobson NS, Hollon SD: Prospects for future comparisons between drugs and psychotherapy: lessons from the CBT-versus-pharmacotherapy exchange. J Consult Clin Psychol 64:104–108, 1996

James IA, Blackburn IM: Cognitive therapy with obsessive-compulsive disorder. Br J Psychiatry 166:444–450, 1995

Jarrett R, Giles D, Gullion C, et al: Does learned resourcefulness predict response to cognitive therapy in depressed outpatient? J Affect Disord 23:223–229, 1991

Jarrett RB, Schaffer M, McIntire D, et al: Treatment of atypical depression with cognitive therapy or phenelzine: a double-blind, placebo-controlled trial. Arch Gen Psychiatry 56:431–437, 1999

Jarrett RB, Kraft D, Doyle J, et al: Preventing recurrent depression using cognitive therapy with and without a continuation phase: a randomized clinical trial. Arch Gen Psychiatry 58:381–388, 2001

Juster HR, Heimberg RG: Social phobia: longitudinal course and long-term outcome of cognitive-behavioral treatment. Psychiatr Clin North Am 18:821–842, 1995

Kandel ER, Schwartz JH: Molecular biology of learning: modulation of transmitter release. Science 218:433–443, 1982

Kemp R, Hayward P, Applewhaite G, et al: Compliance therapy in psychotic patients: randomised controlled trial. BMJ 312:345–349, 1996

Kemp R, Kirov G, Everitt B, et al: Randomised controlled trial of compliance therapy: 18-month follow-up. Br J Psychiatry, 172:413–419, 1998

Kelly G: The Psychology of Personal Constructs. New York, WW Norton, 1955

Kendall PC, Hollon SD: Anxious self-talk: development of the Anxious Self-Statements Questionnaire (ASSQ). Cognit Ther Res 13:81–93, 1989

Kennedy TM, Chalder T, McCrone P, et al: Cognitive behavioural therapy in addition to antispasmodic therapy for irritable bowel syndrome in primary care: randomised controlled trial. Health Technology Assessment (Winchester, England) 10:1–84, 2006

Kingdon D, Turkington D: Cognitive Therapy for Schizophrenia. New York, Guilford, 2005

Klein DC, Fencil-Morse E, Seligman MEP: Learned helplessness, depression, and the attribution of failure. J Pers Soc Psychol 33:508–516, 1976

Klosko JS, Barlow DH, Tassinari R, et al: A comparison of alprazolam and behavior therapy in treatment of panic disorder. J Consult Clin Psychol 58:77–84, 1990

Kovacs M, Rush AJ, Beck AT, et al: Depressed outpatients treated with cognitive therapy or pharmacotherapy. Arch Gen Psychiatry 38:33–39, 1981

Krijn M, Emmelkamp PMG, Olafsson RP, et al: Virtual reality exposure therapy of anxiety disorders: a review. Clin Psychol Rev 24:259–281, 2004

Kroenke K, Swindle R: Cognitive-behavioral therapy for somatization and symptom syndromes: a critical review of controlled clinical trials. Psychother Psychosom 69:205–215, 2000

Kubany ES, Hill EE, Owens JA, et al: Cognitive trauma therapy for battered women with PTSD (CTT-BW). J Consult Clin Psychol 72:3–18, 2004

Kuipers E, Garety P, Fowler D: London–East Anglia randomized controlled trial of cognitive-behavioral therapy for psychosis, I: effects of the treatment phase. Br J Psychiatry 171:319–327, 1997

Lam DH, Watkins ER, Hayward P, et al: A randomized controlled study of cognitive therapy for relapse prevention for bipolar affective disorder: outcome of the first year. Arch Gen Psychiatry 60:145–152, 2003

Lam DH, McCrone P, Wright K, et al: Cost-effectiveness of relapse-prevention cognitive therapy for bipolar disorder: 30-month study. Br J Psychiatry 186:500–506, 2005

Lecompte D: Drug compliance and cognitive-behavioral therapy in schizophrenia. Acta Psychiatr Belg 95:91–100, 1995

LeFebvre MF: Cognitive distortion and cognitive errors in depressed psychiatric and low back pain patients. J Consult Clin Psychol 49:517–525, 1981

Leichsenring F, Leibing E: The effectiveness of psychodynamic therapy and cognitive behavior therapy in the treatment of personality disorders: a meta-analysis. Am J Psychiatry 160:1223–1232, 2003

Leitenberg H, Rosen J, Wolf R, et al: Comparison of cognitive-behavioral therapy and desipramine in the treatment of bulimia nervosa. Behav Res Ther 32:37–45, 1994

Linden M, Zubraegel D, Baer T, et al: Efficacy of cognitive behaviour therapy in generalized anxiety disorders. Results of a controlled clinical trial (Berlin CBT–GAD Study). Psychother Psychosom 74:36–42, 2005

Linehan MM: Cognitive-Behavioral Treatment of Borderline Personality Disorder. New York, Guilford, 1993

Linehan MM, Armstrong HE, Suarez A, et al: Cognitive-behavioral treatment of chronically parasuicidal borderline patients. Arch Gen Psychiatry 48:1060–1064, 1991

Linehan MM, Heard HL, Armstrong HE: Naturalistic follow-up of a behavioral treatment for chronically parasuicidal borderline patients. Arch Gen Psychiatry 50:971–974, 1993

Linehan MM, Tutek DA, Heard HL, et al: Interpersonal outcome of cognitive behavioral treatment for chronically suicidal borderline patients. Am J Psychiatry 151:1771–1776, 1994

Linehan MM, Schmidt H, Dimeff, L, et al: Dialectical behavior therapy for patients with borderline personality disorder and drug-dependence. Am J Addict 8:279–292, 1999

Linehan MM, Comtois KA, Murray AM, et al: Two-year randomized controlled trial and follow-up of dialectical behavior therapy vs therapy by experts for suicidal behaviors and borderline personality disorder. Arch Gen Psychiatry 63:757–766, 2006

Linton SJ, Andersson T: Can chronic disability be prevented? A randomized trial of cognitive-behavior intervention and two forms of information for patients with spinal pain. Spine 25:2825–2831, 2000

Linton SJ, Nordin E: A 5-year follow-up evaluation of the health and economic consequences of an early cognitive behavioral intervention for back pain: a randomized controlled trial. Spine 31:853–858, 2006

Linton SJ, Ryberg M: A cognitive-behavioral group intervention as prevention for persistent neck and back pain in a nonpatient population: a randomized controlled trial. Pain 90:83–90, 2001

Longabaugh R, Rubin A, Malloy P, et al: Drinking outcomes of alcohol abusers diagnosed as antisocial personality disorder. Alcohol Clin Exp Res 18:778–785, 1994

Lustman PJ, Griffith LS, Freedland KE, et al: Cognitive behavior therapy for depression in type 2 diabetes mellitus: a randomized, controlled trial. Ann Intern Med 129:613–621, 1998

Maes S, Schlosser M: Changing health behavior outcomes in asthmatic patients: a pilot study. Soc Sci Med 26:359–364, 1988

Mahoney MJ: Psychotherapy and human change processes, in Cognition and Psychotherapy. Edited by Mahoney MJ, Freeman A. New York, Plenum, 1985, pp 3–48

March JS, Mulle K: OCD in Children and Adolescents: A Cognitive-Behavioral Treatment Manual. New York, Guilford, 1998

Mathews A, MacLeod C: An information-processing approach to anxiety. Journal of Cognitive Psychotherapy: An International Quarterly 1:105–115, 1987

McCullough JP Jr: Treatment for Chronic Depression: Cognitive Behavioral Analysis System of Psychotherapy. New York, Guilford, 2000

McDonagh A, Friedman M, McHugo G, et al: Randomized trial of cognitive-behavioral therapy for chronic post-traumatic stress disorder in adult female survivors of childhood sexual abuse. J Consult Clin Psychol 73:515–524, 2005

McKnight DL, Nelson-Gray RO, Barnhill J: Dexamethasone suppression test and response to cognitive therapy and antidepressant medication. Behav Ther 1:99–111, 1992

McNally RJ, Foa EB: Cognition and agoraphobia: bias in the interpretation of threat. Cognit Ther Res 11:567–581, 1987

Meichenbaum DB: Cognitive-Behavior Modification: An Integrative Approach. New York, Plenum, 1977

Miller IW, Klee SH, Norman WH: Depressed and nondepressed inpatients' cognitions of hypothetical events, experimental tasks, and stressful life events. J Abnorm Psychol 91:78–81, 1982

Miller IW, Norman WH, Keitner GI, et al: Cognitive-behavioral treatment of depressed inpatients. Behav Ther 20:25–47, 1989

Miller IW, Keitner GI, Ryan CE, et al: Treatment matching in the posthospital care of depressed patients. Am J Psychiatry 162:2131–2138, 2005

Mishra KD, Gatchel RJ, Gardea MA: The relative efficacy of three cognitive-behavioral treatment approaches to temporomandibular disorders. J Behav Med 23:293–309, 2000

Mitchell JE, Hoberman HN, Peterson CB, et al: Research on the psychotherapy of bulimia nervosa: half empty or half full. Int J Eat Disord 20:219–229, 1996

Mizes JS, Landolf-Fritsche B, Grossman-McKee D: Patterns of distorted cognitions in phobic disorders: an investigation of clinically severe simple phobics, social phobics, and agoraphobics. Cognit Ther Res 11:583–592, 1987

Mohl PC: Should psychotherapy be considered a biological treatment? Psychosomatics 28:320–326, 1987

Moore JE, Von Korff M, Cherkin D, et al: A randomized trial of a cognitive-behavioral program for enhancing back pain self care in a primary care setting. Pain 88:145–153, 2000

Morley S, Eccleston C, Williams A: Systematic review and meta-analysis of randomized controlled trials of cognitive behaviour therapy and behaviour therapy for chronic pain in adults, excluding headache. Pain 80:1–13, 1999

Murphy GE, Simons AD, Wetzel RD, et al: Cognitive therapy and pharmacotherapy, singly and together in the treatment of depression. Arch Gen Psychiatry 41:33–41, 1984

Naeem F, Kingdon D, Turkington D: Cognitive behavior therapy for schizophrenia in patients with mild to moderate substance misuse problems. Cogn Behav Ther 35:207–215, 2005

Nelson-Gray RO, Johnson D, Foyle LW, et al: The effectiveness of cognitive therapy tailored to depressives with personality disorders. J Personal Disord 10:132–152, 1996

Newman MG, Kenardy J, Herman S, et al: Comparison of cognitive-behavioral treatment of panic disorder with computer assisted brief cognitive behavioral treatment. J Consult Clin Psychol 65:178–183, 1997

Neziroglu F, McKay D, Todaro J, et al: Effect of cognitive behavior therapy on persons with body dysmorphic disorder and comorbid Axis II diagnoses. Behav Ther 27:67–77, 1996

Ost LG, Westling BE, Hellstrom K: Applied relaxation, exposure in vivo and cognitive methods in the treatment of panic disorder with agoraphobia. Behav Res Ther 31:383–394, 1993

Otto MW, Whittal ML: Cognitive-behavior therapy and the longitudinal course of panic disorder. Psychiatr Clin North Am 18:803–820, 1995

Otto MW, Pollack MH, Sachs GS, et al: Discontinuation of benzodiazepine treatment: efficacy of cognitive-behavioral therapy for patients with panic disorder. Am J Psychiatry 150:1485–1490, 1993

Paykel ES, Scott J, Teasdale JD, et al: Prevention of relapse in residual depression by cognitive therapy. Arch Gen Psychiatry 56:829–835, 1999

Payne A, Blanchard EB: A controlled comparison of cognitive therapy and self-help support groups in the treatment of irritable bowel syndrome. J Consult Clin Psychol 63:779–786, 1995

Perris C, Skagerlind L: Cognitive therapy with schizophrenic patients. Acta Psychiatr Scand 89 (suppl 382):65–70, 1994

Persons JB, Burns BD, Perhoff JM: Predictors of drop-out and outcome in cognitive therapy for depression in a private practice setting. Cognit Ther Res 12:557–575, 1988

Peterson C, Villanova P, Raps CS: Depression and attributions: factors responsible for inconsistent results in the published literature. J Abnorm Psychol 94:165–168, 1985

Pollack MH, Otto MW, Kaspi SP, et al: Cognitive behavior therapy for treatment-refractory panic disorder. J Clin Psychiatry 55:200–205, 1994

Power KG, Simpson RJ, Swanson V, et al: Controlled comparison of pharmacological and psychological treatment of generalized anxiety disorder in primary care. Br J Gen Pract 40:289–294, 1990

Proudfoot J, Ryden C, Everitt B, et al: Clinical efficacy of computerised cognitive-behavioural therapy for anxiety and depression in primary care: randomised controlled trial. Br J Psychiatry 185:46–54, 2004

Pull CB: Current status of virtual reality exposure therapy in anxiety disorders. Curr Opin Psychiatry 18:7–14, 2005

Rector NA, Seeman MV, Segal ZV: Cognitive therapy for schizophrenia: a preliminary randomized controlled trial. Schizophr Res 63:1–11, 2003

Reinecke MA, Dattilio FM, Freeman A (eds): Cognitive Therapy With Children and Adolescents: A Casebook for Clinical Practice, 2nd Edition. New York, Guilford, 2003

Ricca V, Mannucci E, Zucchi T, et al: Cognitive-behavioural therapy for bulimia nervosa and binge eating disorder: a review. Psychother Psychosom 69:287–295, 2000

Rizley R: Depression and distortion in the attribution of causality. J Abnorm Psychol 87:32–48, 1978

Robinson LA, Berman JS, Neimeyer RA: Psychotherapy for the treatment of depression: a comprehensive review of controlled outcome research. Psychol Bull 108:30–49, 1990

Rodgers D, Khoo K, MacEachen M, et al: Cognitive therapy for multiple sclerosis: a preliminary study. Altern Ther Health Med 2:70–74, 1996

Rothbaum BO, Hodges LF, Kooper R, et al: Effectiveness of computer-generated (virtual reality) graded exposure in the treatment of acrophobia. Am J Psychiatry 152:626–628, 1995

Rothbaum BO, Hodges L, Smith S, et al: A controlled study of virtual reality exposure therapy for the fear of flying. J Consult Clin Psychol 60:1020–1026, 2000

Rush AJ, Shaw BF: Failure in treating depression by cognitive therapy, in Failures in Behavior Therapy. Edited by Foa EB, Emmelkamp PGM. New York, Wiley, 1983, pp 213–224

Rush AJ, Beck AT, Kovacs M, et al: Comparative efficacy of cognitive therapy and pharmacotherapy in the treatment of depressed outpatients. Cognit Ther Res 1:17–37, 1977

Salkovskis PM: Obsessional-compulsive problems: a cognitive-behavioral analysis. Behav Res Ther 25:571–583, 1985

Salkovskis PM, Warwick HM: Cognitive therapy of obsessive-compulsive disorder: treating treatment failures. Behavioural Psychotherapy 13:243–255, 1985

Salkovskis PM, Westbrook D: Behavior therapy and obsessional ruminations: can failure be turned into success? Behav Res Ther 27:149–160, 1989

Schmidt NB, Harrington P: Cognitive-behavioral treatment of body dysmorphic disorder: a case report. J Behav Ther Exp Psychiatry 26:161–167, 1995

Schmidt U, Tiller J, Treasure J: Self-treatment of bulimia nervosa: a pilot study. Int J Eat Disord 13:273–277, 1993

Schonfeld L, Dupree LW: Treatment approaches for older problem drinkers. Int J Addict 30:1819–1842, 1995

Scott J, Garland A, Moorhead S: A pilot study of cognitive therapy in bipolar disorders. Psychol Med 31:459–467, 2001

Scott J, Paykel E, Morriss R, et al: Cognitive-behavioural therapy for severe and recurrent bipolar disorders: randomized controlled trial. Br J Psychiatry 188:313–320, 2006

Selmi PM, Klein MH, Greist JH, et al: Computer-administered therapy for depression. Am J Psychiatry 147:51–56, 1990

Sensky T: Cognitive-behavior therapy for patients with physical illnesses, in Cognitive-Behavior Therapy. Edited by Wright JH. Arlington, VA, American Psychiatric Publishing, 2004, pp 83–121

Sensky T, Turkington D, Kingdon D, et al: A randomized controlled trial of cognitive-behavioral therapy for persistent symptoms in schizophrenia resistant to medication. Arch Gen Psychiatry 57:165–172, 2000

Shapiro D, Hui KK, Oakley ME, et al: Reduction in drug requirements for hypertension by means of a cognitive-behavioral intervention. Am J Hypertens 10:9–17, 1997

Shea MT, Pilkonis PA, Beckham E, et al: Personality disorders and treatment outcome in the NIMH treatment of depression collaborative research program. Am J Psychiatry 147:711–718, 1990

Shear MK, Ball G, Fitzpatrick M, et al: Cognitive-behavioral therapy for panic: an open study. J Nerv Ment Dis 179:468–472, 1991a

Shear MK, Fyer AJ, Ball G, et al: Vulnerability to sodium lactate in panic disorder patients given cognitive-behavioral therapy. Am J Psychiatry 148:195–197, 1991b

Siegle GJ, Carter CS, Thase ME: Use of fMRI to predict recovery from unipolar depression with cognitive behavior therapy. Am J Psychiatry 163:735–738, 2006

Simons AD, Lustman PJ, Wetzel RD, et al: Predicting response to cognitive therapy of depression: the role of learned resourcefulness. Cognit Ther Res 9:79–89, 1985

Simons AD, Murphy GE, Levine JE, et al: Cognitive therapy and pharmacotherapy for depression: sustained improvement over one year. Arch Gen Psychiatry 43:43–49, 1986

Simpson HB, Liebowitz MR, Foa EB, et al: Post-treatment effects of exposure therapy and clomipramine in obsessive-compulsive disorder. Depress Anxiety 19:225–233, 2004

Simpson HB, Huppert JD, Petkova E, et al: Response versus remission in obsessive-compulsive disorder. J Clin Psychiatry 67:269–276, 2006

Sitharthan T, Kavanagh DJ, Sayer G: Moderating drinking by correspondence: an evaluation of a new method of intervention. Addiction 91:345–355, 1996

Sivertsen B, Omvik S, Pallesen S, et al: Cognitive behavioral therapy vs zopiclone for treatment of chronic primary insomnia in older adults: a randomized controlled trial. JAMA 295:2851–1858, 2006

Sokol L, Beck AT, Greenberg RL, et al: Cognitive therapy of panic disorder: a nonpharmacological alternative. J Nerv Ment Dis 177:711–716, 1989

Springer T, Lohr NE, Buchtel HA, et al: A preliminary report of short-term cognitive-behavioral group therapy for inpatients with personality disorders. J Psychother Pract Res 5:57–71, 1996

Stangier U, Heidenreich T, Peitz M, et al: Cognitive therapy for social phobia: individual versus group treatment. Behav Res Ther 41:991–1007, 2003

Stewart JW, Garfinkel R, Nunes EV, et al: Atypical features and treatment response in the National Institute of Mental Health Treatment of Depression Collaborative Research Program. J Clin Psychopharmacol 18:429–434, 1998

Stuart S, Simons AD, Thase ME, et al: Are personality assessments valid in acute major depression? J Affect Disord 24:281–290, 1992

Stuart S, Wright JH, Thase ME, et al: Cognitive therapy with inpatients. Gen Hosp Psychiatry 19:42–50, 1997

Stulemeijer M, de Jong LW, Fiselier TJ, et al: Cognitive behaviour therapy for adolescents with chronic fatigue syndrome: randomised controlled trial. BMJ 330:14, 2005

Sudak D: Cognitive Behavioral Therapy for Clinicians. Baltimore, MD, Lippincott Williams & Wilkins, 2006

Svartberg M, Stiles TC, Seltzer MH: Randomized, controlled trial of the effectiveness of short-term dynamic psychotherapy and cognitive therapy for cluster C personality disorders. Am J Psychiatry 161:810–817, 2004

Tarrier N, Beckett R, Harwoods S, et al: A trial of two cognitive-behavioral methods of treating drug-resistant residual psychotic symptoms in schizophrenic patients, I: outcome. Br J Psychiatry 162:524–532, 1993

Tarrier N, Yusupoff L, Kinney C, et al: Randomized controlled trial of intensive cognitive behavior therapy for patients with chronic schizophrenia. BMJ 317:303–307, 1998

Tarrier N, Lewis S, Haddock G, et al: Cognitive-behavioural therapy in first-episode and early schizophrenia: 18-month follow-up of a randomized controlled trial. Br J Psychiatry 184:231–239, 2004

Teasdale JD, Fennell MJV, Hibbert GA, et al: Cognitive therapy for major depressive disorder in primary care. Br J Psychiatry 144:400–406, 1984

Teasdale JD, Segal ZV, Williams JM, et al: Prevention of relapse/recurrence in major depression by mindfulness-based cognitive therapy. J Consult Clin Psychol 68:615–623, 2000

Thackwray DE, Smith MC, Bodfish JW, et al: A comparison of behavioral and cognitive-behavioral interventions for bulimia nervosa. J Consult Clin Psychol 61:639–645, 1993

Thase ME: Transition and aftercare, in Cognitive Therapy with Inpatients: Developing a Cognitive Milieu. Edited by Wright JH, Thase ME, Beck AT, et al. New York, Guilford, 1992, pp 414–435

Thase ME: Depression-focused psychotherapies, in Treatments of Psychiatric Disorders, 3rd Edition, Vol 2. Edited by Gabbard GO. Washington, DC, American Psychiatric Publishing, 2001, pp 1181–1227

Thase ME, Bowler K, Harden T: Cognitive behavior therapy of endogenous depression, part 2: preliminary findings in 16 unmedicated inpatients. Behav Ther 22:469–477, 1991

Thase ME, Simmons AD, McGreary J, et al: Relapse after cognitive behavior therapy of depression: potential implications for longer courses of treatment? Am J Psychiatry 149:1046–1052, 1992

Thase ME, Simons AD, Reynolds CF III: Psychobiological correlates of poor response to cognitive behavior therapy: potential indications for antidepressant pharmacotherapy. Psychopharmacol Bull 29:293–301, 1993

Thase ME, Reynolds CF III, Frank E, et al: Response to cognitive-behavioral therapy in chronic depression. J Psychother Pract Res 3:204–214, 1994

Thase ME, Simons AD, Reynolds CF III: Abnormal electroencephalographic sleep profiles in major depression. Arch Gen Psychiatry 53:99–108, 1996

Turk DC, Meichenbaum D, Genest M: Pain and Behavioral Medicine: A Cognitive-Behavioral Perspective. New York, Guilford, 1983

Turkington D, Kingdon D, Turner T: Effectiveness of a brief cognitive-behavioural therapy intervention in the treatment of schizophrenia. Br J Psychiatry 180:523–527, 2002

Turner JA, Manci L, Aaron LA: Short- and long-term efficacy of brief cognitive-behavioral therapy for patients with chronic temporomandibular disorder pain: a randomized, controlled trial. Pain 121:181–194, 2006

Tyrer P, Tom B, Byford S, et al: Differential effects of manual assisted cognitive behavior therapy in the treatment of recurrent deliberate self-harm and personality disturbance: the POPMACT study. J Personal Disord 18:102–116, 2004

Valmaggia LR, van der Gaag M, Tarrier N, et al: Cognitive-behavioural therapy for refractory psychotic symptoms of schizophrenia resistant to atypical antipsychotic medication: randomised controlled trial. Br J Psychiatry 186:324–330, 2005

Van Oppen P, De Haan E, Van Balkom AJLM, et al: Cognitive therapy and exposure in vivo in the treatment of obsessive compulsive disorder. Behav Res Ther 33:379–390, 1995

Wallace ST, Alden LE: A comparison of social standards and perceived ability in anxious and nonanxious men. Cognit Ther Res 15:237–254, 1991

Walsh BT, Wilson GT, Loeb KL, et al: Medication and psychotherapy in the treatment of bulimia nervosa. Am J Psychiatry 154:523–531, 1997

Warwick HM, Salkovskis PM: Hypochondriasis. Behav Res Ther 28:105–117, 1990

Weissman AN: The Dysfunctional Attitude Scale: a validation study. Dissertation Abstracts International 40:1389B–1390B, 1979

Welkowitz LA, Papp LA, Cloitre M, et al: Cognitive-behavior therapy for panic disorder delivered by psychopharmacologically oriented clinicians. J Nerv Ment Dis 179:473–477, 1991

Wells EA, Peterson PL, Gainey RR, et al: Outpatient treatment for cocaine abuse: a controlled comparison of relapse prevention and twelve-step approaches. Am J Drug Alcohol Abuse 20:1–17, 1994

Wenzloff RM, Grozier SA: Depression and the magnification of failure. J Abnorm Psychol 97:90–93, 1988

Wetzel R, Murphy G, Carney R, et al: Prescribing therapy for depression: the role of learned resourcefulness, a failure to replicate. Psychol Rep 70:803–807, 1992

White KP, Nielson WR: Cognitive behavioral treatment of fibromyalgia syndrome: a follow-up assessment. J Rheumatol 22:717–721, 1995

Whittal ML, Thordarson DS, McLean PD: Treatment of obsessive-compulsive disorder: cognitive behavior therapy vs. exposure and response prevention. Behav Res Ther 43(12):1559–1576, 2005

Wilfley DE, Agras WS, Telch CF, et al: Group cognitive-behavioral therapy and group interpersonal psychotherapy for the nonpurging bulimic individual: a controlled comparison. J Consult Clin Psychol 61:296–305, 1993

Wilfley DE, Welch RR, Stein RI, et al: A randomized comparison of group cognitive-behavioral therapy and group interpersonal psychotherapy for the treatment of overweight individuals with binge-eating disorder. Arch Gen Psychiatry 59:713–721, 2002

Wilson GT: Cognitive behavior therapy for eating disorders: progress and problems. Behav Res Ther 37:S79–S95, 1999

Wilson GT, Shafran R: Eating disorders guidelines from NICE. Lancet 365:79–81, 2005

Wolpe J: The Practice of Behavior Therapy. New York, Pergamon, 1969

Woody GE, Luborsky L, McLellan AT, et al: Psychotherapy for opiate addicts: does it help? Arch Gen Psychiatry 40:639–645, 1983

Wright JH: Cognitive therapy of depression, in The American Psychiatric Press Review of Psychiatry, Vol 7. Edited by Frances AJ, Hales RE. Washington, DC, American Psychiatric Press, 1988, pp 554–590

Wright JH: Combined cognitive therapy and pharmacotherapy, in Contemporary Cognitive Therapy. Edited by Leahy R. New York, Guilford, 2004, pp 341–366

Wright JH, Basco MR: Getting Your Life Back: The Complete Guide to Recovery From Depression (Paperback Edition). New York, Touchstone, 2002

Wright JH, Beck AT: Cognitive therapy of depression: theory and practice. Hosp Community Psychiatry 34:1119–1127, 1983

Wright JH, Thase ME: Cognitive and biological therapies: a synthesis. Psychiatr Ann 22:451–458, 1992

Wright JH, Wright AS: Computer-assisted psychotherapy. J Psychother Pract Res 6:315–329, 1997

Wright JH, Thase ME, Beck AT, et al (eds): Cognitive Therapy With Inpatients: Developing a Cognitive Milieu. New York, Guilford, 1993

Wright JH, Salmon P, Wright AS, et al: Cognitive Therapy: A Multimedia Learning Program. Louisville, KY, MindStreet, 1995

Wright JH, Wright AS, Salmon P, et al: Development and initial testing of a multimedia program for computer-assisted cognitive therapy. Am J Psychother 56:76–86, 2002

Wright JH, Wright AS, Beck AT: Good Days Ahead: The Multimedia Program for Cognitive Therapy. Louisville, KY, MindStreet, 2004

Wright JH, Wright AS, Albano AM, et al: Computer-assisted cognitive therapy for depression: maintaining efficacy while reducing therapist time. Am J Psychiatry 162:1158–1164, 2005

Wright JH, Basco MR, Thase ME: Learning Cognitive-Behavior Therapy: An Illustrated Guide (Core Competencies in Psychotherapy Series, Glen O. Gabbard, series ed). Arlington, VA, American Psychiatric Publishing, 2006

Wu R, Bao J, Zhang C, et al: Comparison of sleep condition and sleep-related psychological activity after cognitive-behavior and pharmacological therapy for chronic insomnia. Psychother Psychosom 75:2202–2228, 2006

Wykes T, Hayward P, Thomas N, et al: What are the effects of group cognitive behaviour therapy for voices: a randomised control trial. Schizophr Res 77:201–210, 2005

Zettle RD, Rains JC: Group cognitive and contextual therapies in treatment of depression. J Clin Psychol 45:436–445, 1989

Zimmerman G, Favrod J, Trieu VH, et al: The effect of cognitive behavioral treatment on the positive symptoms of schizophrenia spectrum disorders: a meta-analysis. Schizophr Res 77:1–9, 2005

Zimmerman M, Coryell W, Corenthal C, et al: Dysfunctional attitudes and attribution style in healthy controls and patients with schizophrenia, psychotic depression, and nonpsychotic depression. J Abnorm Psychol 95:403–405, 1986

32

SUPPORTIVE PSYCHOTHERAPY

Arnold Winston, M.D.

Supportive psychotherapy is a broadly defined approach with wide applicability and is the most extensively practiced form of individual psychotherapy. In fact, research studies agree with clinical observations that supportive psychotherapy is effective for a broad range of conditions and may be as efficacious as expressive psychotherapy (Conte 1994; Hellerstein et al. 1998; Winston and Winston 2002).

The concept of supportive psychotherapy was developed early in the twentieth century to describe a treatment approach with objectives more limited than the goals of expressive psychotherapy. The objective of supportive psychotherapy was not to change the patient's personality but to help the patient cope with symptoms, prevent relapse of serious mental illness, or help a relatively healthy person deal with a crisis or transient problem. As defined in earlier years, supportive psychotherapy is a body of techniques, such as praise, advice, exhortation, and encouragement, embedded in psychodynamic understanding and used to treat severely impaired patients. Based on this definition, early papers on psychotherapy denigrated supportive psychotherapy as the "copper" of direct suggestion compared with the "pure gold" of psychoanalysis (Freud 1919/1955). Anything other than psychoanalysis was "nothing but suggestion" (Glover 1931). Even more recently, Stewart (1985) came to the disparaging conclusion that "the highly trained psychiatrist may be tempted to delve too deeply in supportive psychotherapy and often is not as effective as someone less extensively trained" (p. 1360).

Supportive psychotherapy can now be defined as a dyadic treatment that uses direct measures to ameliorate symptoms and maintain, restore, or improve self-esteem, ego function, and adaptive skills (Pinsker 1997; Pinsker et al. 1991; Winston et al. 2004). To accomplish these objectives, treatment may involve examination of relationships, real or transferential, and examination of both past and current patterns of emotional response or behavior. Self-esteem involves the patient's sense of efficacy, confidence, hope, and self-regard. Ego or structural functions include relation to reality, thinking, defenses, object relations, regulation of affect, synthetic function, and others (Bellak 1958; Beres 1956; Winston et al. 2004). Ego functions are alternatively called psychological functions by cognitive-behavioral therapists whose formulations do not include the ego as a component of a mental apparatus. Adaptive skills are actions associated with effective functioning in multiple spheres. It should be noted that the boundary between ego functions and adaptive skills is not sharply defined. The patient's assessment of events is an ego function; the action he or she takes in response to the assessment is an adaptive skill.

The term *supportive therapy,* in settings other than formal psychotherapy, may mean nothing more than the expression of interest, attention to concrete services, encouragement, and optimism. Such expression is a supportive relationship, not supportive psychotherapy. Supportive psychotherapy is based on diagnostic evaluation; the therapist's actions are deliberate and are designed to achieve specified objectives. However, supportive relationships that do not qualify as psychotherapy may indeed be useful and sustaining.

Theory

Supportive psychotherapy is based on a number of theoretical approaches (Table 32–1), which must be integrated by the therapist in the treatment of individual patients (Winston and Winston 2002).

Psychoanalytic theory is generally viewed as the basis for supportive psychotherapy, with an emphasis on ego psychology and development (Hartmann 1958; Jacobson 1964; Mahler et al. 1975), object relations theory (Fairbairn 1952; Winnicott 1965), self psychology issues (Kohut 1971), interpersonal and relational approaches (Levenson 1983; Mitchell 1988; H.S. Sullivan 1953), and attachment theory (Bowlby 1969, 1988). The emphasis in supportive psychotherapy is on relational/interpersonal issues and the self within the reality of the present everyday world, as opposed to working on conflict and instinctual issues and focusing on the past. A supportive patient–therapist relationship provides the patient the safety to access and acknowledge painful experiences and beliefs. The therapist serves as an attachment figure providing a secure base for the patient. A major outgrowth of the psychoanalytic/dynamic approach is the conceptualization of the psychopathology–psychotherapy continuum, which matches the patient's psychopathology to the appropriate treatment (see section "The Psychopathology–Psychotherapy Continuum" below).

Supportive psychotherapy also utilizes many ideas and techniques derived from cognitive-behavioral therapy (CBT). Cognitive-behavioral techniques are an indispensable part of supportive psychotherapy and can be used for targeted problems such as panic, depression, phobias, obsessive-compulsive symptoms, and dysfunctional thinking (Pinsker 1997; Winston and Winston 2002).

Learning theory can also contribute to the techniques of supportive psychotherapy, but unfortunately learning theory has not been incorporated into most forms of psychotherapy in a systematic fashion. A great deal of supportive psychotherapy can be conceptualized as helping patients learn about their illness and helping patients learn how to behave in a more adaptive manner. Critical reflection is an important concept of learning theory. It is the process by which a person questions and then replaces or reframes an assumption and the process through which alternative perspectives are formed on previously

TABLE 32–1. Theoretical approaches

- Psychoanalytic, including
  - ego psychology and development
  - object relations
  - self psychology
  - interpersonal and relational
  - attachment
- Cognitive-behavioral
- Learning theory

taken for granted ideas, actions, and forms of reasoning. Supportive psychotherapy and other psychotherapy approaches use reframing and attempt to provide patients with alternative ways of thinking about the world, relating to others, and solving problems.

The Psychopathology–Psychotherapy Continuum

Human beings are endowed with complex psychological structures and, as a group, function along a sickness–health continuum according to their level of psychopathology, adaptive capacity, self-concept, and ability to relate to others (Figure 32–1; Winston et al. 2004).

The continuum is conceptualized as extending from the most impaired patients to the most intact and well-put-together individuals. Impairments consist of behaviors that interfere with an individual's ability to function in everyday life, form relationships, think clearly and realistically, and behave in a relatively adaptive and mature fashion. Those individuals at the far right side of the continuum tend to function well, have good relationships, and lead productive lives and are able to enjoy a wide range of activities relatively free of conflict. In the middle of the continuum are people whose adaptation and behavior are uneven, so that they have significant problems in maintaining consistent functioning and stable relationships. An individual's position on the continuum can vary over time, depending on a number of factors. These factors include response to environmental stressors, physical illness, maturational growth, and psychotherapy and/or pharmacotherapy.

Placement of individuals on the continuum is associated with diagnosis. For example, patients with

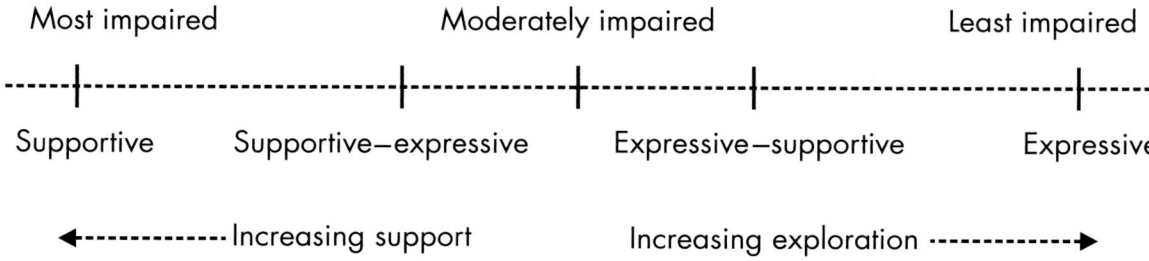

FIGURE 32–1. The psychopathology–psychotherapy continuum.

major mental disorders, pervasive developmental disorder, and severe borderline personality disorder generally lie on the left side of the psychopathology continuum. Limited intelligence and education may also place patients on the left side of the continuum. In meetings with this type of patient, the therapist focuses on the patient's daily activities, medications, and the use of resources for social rehabilitation. Patients with better adaptation are on the right side and include those individuals with Cluster C personality disorders (avoidant, dependent, obsessional), dysthymia, panic disorder, or adjustment disorders. In the middle of the continuum are individuals with conditions such as narcissistic personality disorder or nonpsychotic depressions. Substance abuse problems occur across the continuum. Although diagnosis can provide a general idea of where a person might reside on the continuum, the actual placement will depend on the individual's level of psychopathology and adaptation.

Matching psychotherapy technique to patient locus on the psychopathology continuum is of crucial importance. Individual psychotherapies are conceptualized as a spectrum or continuum that extends from supportive psychotherapy to expressive or exploratory psychotherapy, as shown in Figure 32–1. From left to right, the psychotherapy continuum begins with supportive psychotherapy, traverses through supportive–expressive psychotherapy and expressive–supportive psychotherapy, and finally ends at expressive psychotherapy. Supportive psychotherapy uses supportive approaches, including cognitive-behavioral interventions, directed toward building psychological structure, stability, a sense of self, relationships, and self-esteem. Expressive psychotherapy is indicated for patients with relatively intact structures. Expressive psychotherapy explores relational and conflict issues, seeking personality change through analysis of the relationship between therapist and patient and through development of insight into previously unrecognized feelings, thoughts, and needs.

In practice, most individuals lie at neither end of the psychopathology continuum but instead have both conflict and structural problems. Many patients will require work in both areas, generally beginning with relationship problems and structure building and then perhaps going on to address conflict issues. Therefore, the psychotherapeutic approach will often be a combined supportive–expressive psychotherapy (Luborsky 1984). "As one approaches the midpoint of this spectrum, the distinctions become blurred and less well differentiated. And even the most exploratory and expressive forms of therapy include some supportive components and experiences; and supportive forms of psychotherapy may include an expansion of patients' awareness of their own mental processes, and thus involve elements of exploratory techniques" (Dewald 1994, p. 505). The treatment of most patients involves supportive psychotherapy with some expressive elements, which should be used in a coherent, integrated fashion.

The most impaired patients require direct interventions aimed at improving ego functions, day-to-day coping, and self-esteem. Psychotherapy that is primarily expressive is contraindicated for these patients. The least impaired patients, with good relationships, who function well in everyday life, have traditionally been treated with expressive psychotherapy. However, more recent research and clinical papers indicate that patients respond equally well to supportive or expressive psychotherapy (Hellerstein et al. 1994, 1998; Rosenthal et al. 1999) and that shifting to more expressive techniques should be done only when there are positive indicators for another approach.

Indications

Because there has been a paucity of data to support the assignment of patients to a given psychotherapy, supportive psychotherapy was previously described as the treatment for individuals not suitable for expressive psychotherapy. These individuals are the so-called difficult patients (Horowitz and Marmar 1985) who generally are not thought to be suitable for expressive psychotherapy and are not likely to be amenable to change (Rosenthal et al. 1999; Winston et al. 1986). However, the Menninger psychotherapy study found that patients treated with supportive psychotherapy did as well as patients treated with psychoanalysis or expressive psychotherapy (Wallerstein 1989). More recent studies (Hellerstein et al. 1998; Piper et al. 1998) have found that higher-functioning patients respond as well to supportive psychotherapy as compared to expressive therapy (see section "Efficacy Research" later in this chapter). These findings suggest that supportive psychotherapy can be used with a wide spectrum of problems and with higher-functioning patients. Luborsky (1984) developed a supportive–expressive psychotherapy that was used in numerous clinical trials for a wide variety of diagnoses and produced positive results.

In the past (Winston et al. 1986), supportive psychotherapy was generally considered the therapy of choice for patients on the left side of the sickness–health continuum, who have higher levels of psychopathology, chronic illness, and impaired adaptive skills. Generally, patients with severe and chronic illness cannot tolerate expressive psychotherapy with its emphasis on exploration of feelings, interpersonal relationships, conflicts, and fantasies. These individuals have significant deficits in ego or psychological functioning (Table 32–2), including the following:

- *Poor reality testing and primitive defenses:* These individuals use defenses such as projection and denial, which are often maladaptive. They have great difficulty in separating self from other and may have hallucinations, delusions, thought broadcasting, and other psychotic symptoms.
- *Object relations/interpersonal relations:* These individuals have less capacity for mutuality and reciprocity and are unable to maintain stable relationships or sustained levels of intimacy or trust. This can lead to major problems in the patient–therapist relationship. In addition, such individuals cannot engage in self-observation and exploration, which limits their ability to introspect and develop insight.
- *Inadequate affect regulation and poor impulse control:* These patients have great difficulty containing aggression and tend to engage in destructive behavior.

TABLE 32–2.   Traditional selection criteria for impaired patients

- Poor reality testing
- Primitive and immature defenses
- Significantly impaired object/interpersonal relations
- Inadequate affect regulation
- Poor impulse control
- Overwhelming anxiety

- *Overwhelming anxiety:* Issues of separation or individuation can lead to severe anxiety, rendering these individuals incapable of exploring their feelings (Buckley 1986; Werman 1984).

At the other end of the sickness–health continuum are relatively healthy individuals who have become symptomatic as a result of a severe and often overwhelming traumatic event. In other circumstances, persons in this group might be referred for expressive treatment, because they have good reality testing, high-level object/interpersonal relations with an ability to form a working alliance, a capacity to tolerate and contain affects and impulses, and a capacity for introspection (Table 32–3).

In crisis situations, supportive psychotherapy is usually delivered in an acute-care or episode-of-care model.

> For example, an otherwise healthy, well-compensated man lost his wife in an automobile accident and became depressed, with a negative attitude toward work and social relationships and diminished self-esteem. He entered into a supportive psychotherapy/crisis intervention that enabled him to begin a "normal" grieving process, ultimately recover his self-esteem, and begin to plan for changes in his life.

An acute crisis is not a diagnosis but rather a general syndromal description for patients whose customary coping skills and defenses have been overwhelmed by an often-unexpected event, resulting in intense anxiety and other symptoms (Dewald 1994). Crisis is the state that people experience when faced with actual or impending loss (see section "Crisis Intervention" later in this chapter). People in crisis may meet criteria for an adjustment disorder, which tends to be time limited. Supportive psychotherapy can help these patients to manage uncomfortable feeling states and enhance their coping strategies as this disorder resolves.

TABLE 32–3. Traditional selection criteria for patients in crisis

- Relatively healthy and well functioning before crisis
- Good reality testing
- High level object/interpersonal relations
- Ability to form working alliance
- Ability to tolerate and contain affects and impulses
- Capacity for introspection
- Good social supports

The focus of the treatment is to reassure the patient that symptoms generally are time limited, reduce stress by clarifying and providing information about what the patient is having difficulty adjusting to, and support novel coping and problem-solving methods, including environmental change (Misch 2000).

Other indications for supportive psychotherapy include medical illness, substance use disorder, acute bereavement, and alexithymia. For a large number of medical conditions, supportive psychotherapy is the only treatment recommended. An understanding of an individual's defensive, cognitive, and interpersonal styles enables the therapist to assist the patient in developing better coping strategies (Bronheim et al. 1998). Supportive psychotherapy has been successfully used in patients with breast cancer (Classen et al. 2001; Hunter et al. 1996), HIV-positive patients with depression (Markowitz et al. 1995), patients with pancreatic cancer (Alter 1996), cancer patients with depression (Massie and Holland 1990), patients with chronic pain (Thomas and Weiss 2000), patients with HIV-related neuropathic pain (Evans et al. 2003), and patients with somatization disorder (Quality Assurance Project 1985). In substance use disorders, the therapist focuses first on the development of a therapeutic alliance, to enhance treatment retention and to create an environment within which the patient can begin cognitive and motivational work (O'Malley et al. 1992). In patients with poor ego strength, acute bereavement will overwhelm coping skills and produce symptoms such as self-reproach, social withdrawal, an inability to mourn, and depressive and anxiety symptoms (Horowitz et al. 1984). Supportive psychotherapy affords the patient an empathic holding environment in which the work of mourning can safely take place. In addition, healthy defenses are strengthened,

concrete assistance for routine activities is offered when needed, and the patient is helped to avoid becoming socially withdrawn (Novalis et al. 1993). Patients with alexithymia with severe restriction of affect, a seeming lack of capacity for introspection, an inability to articulate feeling states, and a diminished or absent fantasy life (Sifneos 1973, 1975) may become symptomatic in stressful situations. They tend to develop somatic preoccupations and become increasingly dysfunctional but are unable to communicate the effect of the stressful situation on their affective experience. Supportive psychotherapy, through directly working on somatic experiences and personal metaphors, can help the patient recognize, acknowledge, and identify emotions, thereby leading to an increased sense of mastery and self-esteem (Misch 2000).

There are few circumstances in which supportive psychotherapy is contraindicated (Frank 1975; Pinsker et al. 1996). It is contraindicated only when psychotherapy itself is contraindicated, in such instances as deliria, drug intoxication, late stages of dementia, malingering, psychopathy, and help-rejecting complainers.

CBT has been shown to be more effective than supportive psychotherapy for some conditions in a few studies. These disorders include panic disorder (Barlow and Craske 1989; Beck et al. 1992), obsessive-compulsive disorder (Foa and Franklin 2002; Greist 1990), bulimia nervosa (Walsh et al. 1997), and posttraumatic stress disorder (Foa 1997). However, as mentioned earlier, supportive psychotherapy uses many of the techniques of CBT, and the two approaches can be successfully integrated (Winston and Winston 2002).

Strategies

Supportive psychotherapy relies on direct measures rather than insight (Pinsker 1997). A major tenet of traditional psychoanalytic psychotherapy was that unconscious conflict that produced the symptom or personality problem would become conscious, be explored, and be worked through. As a result, the symptom or personality problem would improve, since it was no longer psychologically necessary. The working-through process involves exploring the patient's past history, particularly early relationships, in order to understand the genesis of the problems. In supportive psychotherapy, the therapist should understand many of the patient's dynamic issues and unconscious conflicts. However, conflicts generally are not explored with patients on the sicker side of the continuum. These patients are not able to contain or explore feelings and impulses and may become overwhelmed by anxiety. Instead, conscious problems and conflicts in the patient's current life are addressed (Dewald 1964/1971) (Table 32–4).

Defenses

From the point of view of psychoanalytic theory, supportive psychotherapy supports the patient's defenses. When therapy is primarily expressive, defenses are challenged and explored so that underlying conflicts, wishes, and feelings that were being defended against become available for exploration and resolution. In supportive psychotherapy, defenses are questioned or confronted only when they are maladaptive and interfere with functioning. However, in practice, one does not work directly with a defense but rather works on the attitude or behavior it expresses (Gill 1951; Winston et al. 2004). For example, the defense of projection can be harmful when a patient projects hostile feelings onto his boss and begins to argue with him. This problematic behavior at work needs to be addressed so that the patient does not lose his job.

Therapeutic Relationship

The relationship between patient and therapist is a professional one with the therapist providing a service that the patient needs. The therapist, as in all forms of psychotherapy, must maintain proper boundaries between himself or herself and the patient. The patient may need love or friendship, but the therapist does not become a lover or friend. The therapist does not advise the patient about what to invest in, how to vote, or where to vacation. These are products of his or her private, not professional, opinion. In traditional psychoanalytic psychotherapy, the therapist maintains neutrality and abstinence to further the exploratory process so that when the patient describes his or her perceptions or feelings about the therapist, these can be analyzed as products of projection onto the therapist of the feelings the patient has about important figures in his or her past or current life. These projections onto the therapist are called transference. In supportive psychotherapy, the therapist is active and conversational, takes positions, answers questions, and self-discloses. The relationship between patient and therapist is supportive, providing security and safety for the patient. The therapist serves more as a model of identification rather than a transference figure (Winston et al. 2004), thus avoiding the chilling effect that

TABLE 32–4. Strategies

- Strengthening and supporting defenses
- Maintaining and repairing the therapeutic relationship
- Promoting patient self-esteem
- Employing therapeutic self-disclosure and modeling
- Working primarily in the present

abstinence can have on patients (Pinsker 1997). A positive patient–therapist relationship is always actively fostered by the therapist and addressed and repaired when a misalliance develops (Winston and Winston 2002).

Self-Disclosure

Self-disclosure by the therapist should have a therapeutic rationale—that is, be in the interest of the patient (Winston and Winston 2002). If self-disclosure is in the therapist's interest and takes the form of bragging, complaining, seductiveness, and so on, it is a boundary violation and exploitative. Simon (1988) observed that therapist's decisions about self-disclosure are generally related to modeling and educating, promoting the therapeutic alliance, validating reality, and fostering the patient's sense of autonomy. Such disclosure enables patients with ego deficits to build a more stable and cohesive sense of self and other. Straightforward answers to personal questions from the patient can be given within appropriate social conventions of privacy and reticence. Self-disclosure does have transference implications, but the therapist need not mention this to the patient (Winston and Winston 2002).

Self-Esteem

Improvement in self-esteem is an important goal of supportive psychotherapy. The therapist's positive regard, approval, acceptance, interest, respect, genuineness, and admiration help to further the patient's self-esteem. A patient who cannot form relationships with others finds in the therapist a person who is accepting and interested. The therapist communicates his or her interest in the patient by making it evident that he or she remembers their conversations and is aware of the patient's likes, dislikes, attitudes, and general sensibility. Acceptance is communicated by the avoidance of arguing, denigrating, and criticizing verbal interactions or therapist defensiveness.

Assessment and Case Formulation

The process of evaluation and case formulation is an essential element of all psychotherapeutic approaches. A central objective of the assessment process is to diagnose the patient's illness and describe the problems so that the patient can be treated appropriately. Another important objective of the evaluation process is to establish a therapeutic relationship, which can further the patient's interest in and commitment to psychotherapy. A thorough evaluation should help the clinician to select the appropriate treatment approach. The treatment plan should be individualized to meet the needs and goals of the patient.

The organizing treatment approach for each patient should be based on the central issues emerging from the assessment and case formulation. When a therapist meets a patient for the first time, the therapist generally does not know the extent of the patient's impairment, psychopathology, or strengths. Therefore, the initial interview should begin with the therapist's attempting to understand why the patient has come for treatment. All patients should have a thorough evaluation of both current problems and past history. At the end of the evaluation, the therapist should understand the patient's problems, interpersonal relationships, everyday functioning, and psychological or executive structure. The evaluation should not be simply a series of questions and answers, but more of an exploration of the patient's life. The interview should be therapeutic, to help motivate the patient for treatment and promote the therapeutic alliance. The evaluation should promote the objectives of supportive psychotherapy: to ameliorate symptoms and to maintain, restore, or improve self-esteem, adaptive skills, and ego or psychological functions (Pinsker et al. 1991). In a supportive approach, making an evaluation therapeutic generally involves the use of supportive psychotherapy interventions, such as praise, reassurance, encouragement, clarification, and confrontation (Winston et al. 2004).

Case formulation depends on an accurate and thorough assessment of the patient. The case formulation is an explanation of the patient's symptoms and psychosocial functioning. The therapist's formulation governs his or her interventions as well as which issues in the patient's life are selected for attention. Having a sense of the underlying issues at the start of treatment enhances the therapist's ability to respond empathically. At the same time, empathy for the pa-

tient helps the therapist to guide and plan therapy effectively. The initial formulation is tentative and must be modified as more is learned about the patient during the course of psychotherapy. The DSM diagnosis is an important part of case formulation but by no means the whole story. It does not illuminate an individual's adaptive or maladaptive characteristics or explain the unique life history of an individual.

The following case formulation approaches (Winston et al. 2004) are derived from psychoanalytic (ego–interpersonal and relational psychology) and cognitive-behavioral (including learning theory) approaches (Table 32–5). Supportive therapy uses elements of all these approaches but differs in how the elements are used.

TABLE 32–5. **Types of case formulation**

- Structural
- Genetic
- Dynamic
- Cognitive-behavioral

For example, a patient's underlying or hidden conflict may be clearly understood and formulated by the therapist, but never or only partially explored in supportive psychotherapy. Although these case formulation approaches have always been described separately, a great deal of overlap exists, so there is some repetition in the descriptions.

A structural case formulation (Bellak 1958; Beres 1956; Freud 1923/1961; Winston et al. 2004) attempts to capture the relatively fixed characteristics of an individual's personality, which is understood within a functional context (in contrast to dynamic and genetic approaches, which are more content based). The structural approach is also an assessment of psychopathology and enables the clinician, with some degree of accuracy, to place the patient on the psychopathology continuum.

The major components of the structural approach are relation to reality, object relations, affect, impulse control, defenses, thought processes, and autonomous functions (perception, intention, intelligence, language, and motor development) and synthetic functions (ability to form a cohesive whole), as well as conscience, morals, and ideals (Table 32–6).

The genetic area of case formulation involves exploration of early development and life events that may help to explain an individual's current situation.

TABLE 32–6. Components of the structural approach
• Relation to reality
• Object relations
• Affect
• Impulse control
• Defenses
• Thought processes
• Autonomous functions (perception, intention, intelligence, language and motor development)
• Synthetic functions (ability to form a cohesive whole or gestalt)
• Conscience, morals, and ideals

TABLE 32–7. Goals
• Ameliorate symptoms
• Improve adaptation
• Enhance self-esteem
• Improve functioning

Life presents many challenges, conflicts, and crises. These can be traumatic, depending on their severity, the developmental stage of the child, and the quality of his or her support system. An example of a persistent difficulty or traumatic situation is the experience of a young child growing up with a violent alcoholic father who is demeaning and at times physically abusive.

The dynamic approach concerns itself with mental and/or emotional tensions that may be conscious or unconscious. The approach focuses on conflicting wishes, needs, or feelings and on their meanings. The dynamic approach focuses on current conflicts, whereas the genetic approach highlights a person's childhood traumas and conflicts and their possible meanings. In supportive psychotherapy, the most important strategic approach is the structural (and to some extent, the dynamic) formulation, since mapping out current areas of difficulty and ameliorating them are more important than understanding the genetic basis or cause of the difficulty (Rosenthal 1991; Winston et al. 2004).

The cognitive-behavioral approach addresses an individual's underlying psychological structure and the content of his or her thoughts (Winston et al. 2004). The cognitive-behavioral case formulation model has been described by Tomkins (1996) as encompassing a number of components, including the problem list, followed by core beliefs, origins, precipitants, and predicted obstacles to treatment. (For a more complete description of CBT, see Chapter 31 in this volume, "Cognitive Therapy," by Wright et al.)

A well-thought-out and comprehensive treatment plan should emerge from the case formulation (Winston et al. 2004). Generally, this plan will include treatment goals, the types of interventions to be used, and the frequency of sessions. In supportive psychother-

apy the frequency of visits should be flexible, depending on the needs of the patient. In crisis situations, patients may be seen frequently, while more stable patients may be seen less often. However, setting a specific repeated time to meet tends to reduce anxiety, which is an important objective of supportive psychotherapy.

Goals

For patients requiring supportive psychotherapy, organizing goals as stated by most authors are amelioration of symptoms and improvement and enhancement of adaptation, self-esteem, and overall functioning (Dewald 1994; Holmes 1995; Munich 1997; Winston et al. 2004). These goals are quite different from the goals of expressive psychotherapy, but similar to the goals of CBT. In expressive psychotherapy, the goals are both symptom and personality change through analysis of the patient–therapist relationship and through development of insight into previously unrecognized feeling, thoughts, needs, and conflicts (Table 32–7).

Until recently it has been assumed that long-term changes in symptoms, self-esteem, conflicts, and adaptation cannot occur in supportive psychotherapy, since supportive psychotherapy does not aim at change in personality or ego structure. However, more recent studies have suggested that supportive psychotherapy can produce personality change in patients on the healthier side of the sickness–health continuum (Rosenthal et al. 1999; Winston et al. 2001).

Setting treatment goals in psychotherapy is important in guiding the treatment, because both therapist and patient must agree on the objectives of treatment. The goals set within the first few sessions should be viewed as preliminary and open to change. Both immediate objectives for each session and ultimate goals for treatment should be considered (Parloff 1967). An example of an immediate goal in a patient who has left work would be to return to work within a week or so. An ultimate goal would be to promote job stability and improve relationships with co-workers.

Clearly outlined goals help motivate patients and

promote the therapeutic alliance as patient and therapist work toward a common end. The goals of therapy should generally be the patient's and should be realistic. In the event of disagreement on goals, the therapist enters into an exploration of the problem. For example, many patients with chronic psychiatric illness often discontinue their medications. In these cases a major goal of treatment is to help patients remain on medications. Therefore, exploring the reasons for discontinuation and educating patients about the risks of discontinuing are in order.

Finally, treatment goals should never be regarded as fixed and unchangeable. If a patient improves, goals can be expanded or changed.

Interventions

Supportive psychotherapy depends on clearly defined techniques designed to achieve the goals of maintaining or improving the patient's self-esteem, psychological (ego) functioning, and adaptation to the environment (Pinsker et al. 1991). In supportive treatment, the objectives include reduction of anxiety, promotion of stability, and relief of symptoms. These goals are accomplished by working in the here and now rather than in the past. The therapeutic relationship becomes a focus in a real as opposed to a transferential manner. Generally, resistance is not addressed, and adaptive defenses are strengthened and supported (Winston and Winston 2002).

Conversational Style of Communication

The style of communication in supportive psychotherapy tends to be more conversational than in expressive psychotherapy (Winston et al. 2004). Silences are avoided, because they can raise the individual's level of anxiety. There is a give-and-take exchange, and challenging questions are not asked. Questions beginning with "Why" are avoided, since they can increase anxiety and threaten self-esteem (Pinsker 1997).

Praise, Reassurance, and Encouragement

Praise, reassurance, and encouragement are considered useful techniques for promoting patient self-esteem, especially if the therapist is genuine when using these techniques (Lewis 1978). Patients quickly pick up on comments that are patronizing or gratu-

itous and may feel misunderstood. Praise, when offered, tends to be reality based and to support more adaptive behaviors—for example, "It's good that you can be so considerate of other people" or "It's terrific that you got yourself to go to that lecture."

Words spoken in an attempt to reassure a patient must not be empty or without basis, and the patient must believe that the reassurance is based on an understanding of his or her unique situation. Furthermore, the therapist must limit reassurance to areas in which he or she has expert knowledge or dependable common information (Winston et al. 2004). Many patients ask their therapist if they will get better. A response of "Yes, you will get better" may be misleading and false. A more appropriate response would be "Most people with your condition improve."

Encouragement has a major role in general medicine and rehabilitation. Patients with chronic schizophrenia, depression, or a passive-dependent style are often inactive, mentally and physically. The psychiatrist encourages the patient to maintain hygiene, to get exercise, to interact with other people, sometimes to be more independent, and sometimes to accept the care and concern of others. It is useful to think about encouragement as a form of coaching to help patients engage in different behaviors and activities (Pinsker 1997). For example, a patient complained that she was inept because she was unable to write a cover letter for a job application. The therapist said, "You just need to get started. Let's see what we can do now to help you get started."

Advice

Advice is an important tactic of supportive psychotherapy and should be based on the therapist's knowledge and expertise in the field of psychiatry. While early psychoanalytic authorities disparaged giving advice, P. R. Sullivan (1971) has pointed out that the value of advice giving is often underrated. In contrast to the more abstinent therapeutic stance employed in expressive psychotherapy, the therapist conducting supportive psychotherapy can be direct and take an active role with patients. Teaching and advice generally go hand in hand. In the supportive psychotherapy literature, the term *lending ego* has been used to convey that the therapist models reasonable, controlled behavior in addition to teaching about it. The therapist gives advice about or teaches about the supportive psychotherapy objectives of improving ego functions or adaptive skills, as in the following example: "You tend to put up with things until you become furious, as you did with your friend who always keeps you waiting; then you lose it and scream at people. Dealing with the problem earlier, before it becomes so upsetting and extreme, is usually a better approach." When a therapist is telephoned by a patient who becomes disorganized in response to minimal stress, the therapist tells her to first get dressed, then have breakfast, and then straighten up the house; here the therapist is not giving advice but rather providing help with routine, helping provide structure, and possibly encouraging the use of compulsive defenses.

Rationalizing and Reframing

Rationalizing and reframing provide the patient with an alternative way of looking at an event that was previously perceived as painful or negative. The challenge in using rationalization and reframing is to avoid sounding fatuous or arguing with and contradicting a patient. An example is that of a young mother who complained that her toddler had started to run away from her and expressed her belief that the child was losing interest in her. A reframing of this painful and negative perception might be "She feels secure enough with you so that she's free to explore the world."

Rehearsal or Anticipatory Guidance

Rehearsal or anticipatory guidance is a technique as useful in supportive psychotherapy as in CBT. Anticipatory guidance is a useful technique for helping patients prepare for future encounters with situations perceived as potentially problematic. Preparation for a difficult event can be likened to studying for an examination or rehearsing for a performance. The objective is to consider in advance what the obstacles might be to a proposed course of action and then to prepare strategies for dealing with them. Gaining mastery over an anticipated situation diminishes anxiety and enhances self-esteem. An example of anticipatory guidance would be taking a patient through an initial phone call to a prospective employer. The patient expects a cold reception and rejection. Rehearsal provides the patient with a number of scenarios and responses so that he or she will be equipped to cope with the anxiety engendered by making the phone call and will have a repertoire of responses ready.

Confrontation, Clarification, and Interpretation

Confrontation addresses a patient's defensive behavior by bringing to the patient's attention a pattern of behaviors, ideas, or feelings he or she has not recognized

or has avoided. In supportive psychotherapy, confrontations generally are empathically framed and are used to address maladaptive defenses; adaptive defenses are encouraged. Confrontation in a supportive mode is illustrated below:

> Patient: I went to my parents' home to speak with them about borrowing some money to pay for several unexpected bills that I have to pay, but I got into a silly argument with them and never had a chance to ask them.
> Therapist: We know that it's hard for you to ask them for anything, so could it be that you got into the argument with them to avoid asking them for money?

Clarification is summarizing, paraphrasing, or organizing without elaboration or inference. It is central to the style of communication between patient and therapist and is the most frequently used intervention in supportive–expressive psychotherapy. It demonstrates that the therapist is attentive and is processing what he or she hears. Clarification frames a communication so that both parties agree on what is being discussed. Summarizing and restating help organize the patient's thinking and provide structure. In the example below, the therapist clarifies through summarizing:

> Patient: I can't seem to concentrate on anything. My house is costing too much, so I have to sell it, but I have to fix some things in it first…I can't seem to get started. Collection agencies are after me, and my ex-wife keeps calling about child support—and now my car got hit, so I can't use it.
> Therapist: It sounds like a lot of things are troubling you and you're experiencing being overwhelmed. Let's examine these things one at a time and see what we can come up with.

An *interpretation* is an explanation that brings meaning to the patient's behavior or thinking (Othmer and Othmer 1994). Generally it makes the individual aware of something that was not previously conscious (Greenson 1967). An interpretation can link thoughts, feelings, and behaviors toward people in the patient's current life to people from the past and/or to the therapist. In supportive psychotherapy, interpretation is generally more limited in scope. Present rather than past relationships are emphasized; affects and impulses are rarely interpreted. Incomplete or inexact interpretations (Glover 1931) offer explanations that are plausible and help the patient make sense of his or her experience but do not contain material that might disturb the patient. Table 32–8 presents a list of interventions used in supportive–expressive psychotherapy.

TABLE 32–8.　**Interventions**

- Conversational style
- Praise, reassurance, and encouragement
- Advice
- Rationalizing and reframing
- Rehearsal or anticipatory guidance
- Clarification and confrontation

The Therapeutic Relationship

The components of the therapeutic relationship are considered to be the transference–countertransference configuration, the real relationship, and the therapeutic alliance (Greenson 1967). Although these three components are intimately related and form a cohesive whole, discussion of each component separately provides more clarity. Transference and real relationship issues play a role in every transaction within the therapeutic relationship. At certain times transference aspects may be more important, while at other times real relationship issues may predominate. From this point of view, a continuum exists between transference issues and real issues that corresponds to the supportive–expressive psychotherapy continuum. Expressive therapy places more emphasis on the transference, whereas supportive psychotherapy focuses more on the real relationship.

Pinsker (1997) and others (e.g., Misch 2000; Novalis et al. 1993) have described general principles that address the relationship of supportive psychotherapy and the therapeutic relationship. These principles are listed in Table 32–9.

Transference and the Real Relationship

Classically, transference has been described as a special type of object relationship consisting of behaviors, thoughts, feelings, wishes, and attitudes directed at the therapist that are related to important people in the patient's past. Most commonly displaced onto the therapist are attitudes toward significant people such as parents, siblings, grandparents, or teachers. Essentially, the past is revived in the present. The real relationship underlies all psychotherapy. It exists in the here and now of the therapeutic interaction between

TABLE 32–9.　**The patient–therapist relationship**

- Positive feelings and thoughts about the therapist are generally not focused upon in order to maintain the therapeutic alliance.

- The therapist is alert to distancing and negative patient behaviors, so as to anticipate and avoid a disruption in treatment.

- When a patient–therapist problem is not resolved through practical discussion, the therapist moves to discussion of the therapeutic relationship.

- The therapist attempts to modify the patient's distorted perceptions using clarification and confrontation, but usually not interpretation.

- If indirect means fail to address negative transference or therapeutic impasses, explicit discussion about the therapeutic relationship may be warranted.

- The therapist uses only the amount of expressive technique necessary to address negative issues in the patient–therapist relationship.

- A positive therapeutic alliance may allow the patient to listen to the therapist present material that the patient would not accept from anyone else.

- When making a statement that the patient might experience as criticism, the therapist may have to frame the statement in a supportive, empathic manner or first offer anticipatory guidance.

patient and therapist, encompassing a genuine mutual liking for each other that is authentic, trusting, and realistic, without the distortions that are characteristic of transference (Greenson 1967, 1971). The real relationship includes the patient's hopes and aspirations for help, care, understanding, and love, as well as the everyday interactions that take place on a social level between individuals.

In psychotherapy at the supportive end of the psychotherapy continuum, transference can be used to guide therapeutic interventions. However, transference is not generally discussed unless negative transference threatens to disrupt treatment. In supportive psychotherapy, positive transference reactions generally are not explored but rather are simply accepted. Negative reactions must always be investigated, however, because they may compromise the treatment (Winston and Winston 2002). In supportive psychotherapy, the real relationship is paramount and based on overt mutuality in the conduct of therapy.

In expressive psychotherapy, both positive and negative transference phenomena are of pivotal importance for identifying intrapsychic conflict; therapeutic gain is ascribed to the emotional working-through of these relationships. Transference clarification and interpretation are important interventions. The real relationship serves as more of a backdrop and the emphasis is on the transference.

Therefore, transference is increasingly worked with as one moves across the psychotherapy continuum from supportive to expressive psychotherapy, while the emphasis on the real relationship increases as one moves from expressive to supportive psychotherapy. In the middle of the continuum, where most psychotherapy takes place, a mixture of supportive and expressive approaches to transference takes place. In supportive psychotherapy, the therapist clarifies often, confronts at intervals, but interprets infrequently. The therapist's interventions assist the patient in recognizing and addressing maladaptive behavior and cognitive problems that are reflected in behavior with the therapist and are illustrative of the patient's behavior with others. The goal of these interventions is in keeping with the goals of supportive psychotherapy: to increase self-esteem and adaptive functioning.

The following vignette illustrates some of the strategies employed to address positive transference reactions at different points along the psychotherapy continuum.

> John, a 54-year-old man, tells his therapist how much his relationship with his wife has improved since he started therapy. He attributes this to the therapist's interest in him.

In supportive psychotherapy, the therapist would not explore this but would accept the compliment, conceptualizing John's statement as a reflection of the real relationship, and might say: "I'm glad to be of help to you." This opportunity also might be used to bolster the patient's self-esteem by adding, "Since our work has been a joint effort, you have to take some of the credit, too."

Countertransference

Classically, countertransference is the therapist's transference to the patient (Greenson 1967). It includes behaviors, thoughts, wishes, attitudes, and conflicts derived from the therapist's past and displaced onto the patient. A broader definition of countertransference includes the real relationship, consisting of reactions most people would have to the patient, determined by moment-to-moment interactions in the therapeutic relationship, which is a transactional construct, affected by what the therapist brings to the situation as well as by what the patient projects (Gabbard 2001; Kiesler 2001; Winston and Winston 2002). The therapist's countertransference reactions can lead to misunderstanding of the patient and can result in inappropriate behavior toward the patient. Countertransference reactions can also be a powerful tool for understanding and empathizing with the patient (Gabbard 2001). To accomplish this, the therapist must monitor his or her own feelings toward the patient to help gain access to the patient's inner world and unconscious.

The use of empathy is important in facilitating, impeding, or distorting countertransference awareness. Empathy can be defined as "feeling oneself into" something or someone (Wolf 1983). Therefore empathy is a method of gathering data about the mental life of another person. The ability to empathize by accurately sensing and understanding what a person is experiencing will enable the therapist to attend to countertransference reactions. The following is an example of the use of countertransference in supportive psychotherapy.

> A middle-aged man began to describe how people at work tend to avoid him, even when he thought he was being friendly. The therapist responded empathically by remarking "That must be hard for you." The patient reacted in an angry manner. The therapist responded by saying, "I'm finding my temperature rising with your criticisms of me, and I can't help wondering if you get your co-workers feeling the same way. However, I won't act on my feelings the way they do. I'll continue to sit and talk with you; I won't make excuses and leave."

From the vantage point of interpersonal communication theory, Kiesler (2001) described effective feedback of countertransference feelings as applying the principle that disclosing metaphors of fantasies has the least threatening effect, compared with direct feelings or tendencies toward action. This principle is highly consistent with supportive psychotherapy approaches, in which it is safer, more respectful, and more protective of the therapeutic alliance to say "I'm finding my temperature rising" rather than "I'm very angry with you." The therapist's modulated expression of countertransference feeling not only offers disconfirmation of the patient's maladaptive construal style but also models adult restraint and containment, not denial of affect. The therapist who responds to the patient's hostility in a complementarily hostile manner is arguing. Arguing not only is poor technique but also is predictive of poor outcome (Henry et al. 1986, 1990).

The Therapeutic Alliance

The therapeutic alliance is a component of the real relationship and forms an essential part of the foundation upon which all psychotherapy stands. Zetzel (1956) first used the term *therapeutic alliance* for the "unobjectionable positive transference," which was seen as an essential element in the success of psychotherapy. She believed that the capacity to form an alliance is based on an individual's early experiences with the primary caregiver. In the absence of this capacity, the task of the therapist, early in treatment, is to provide a supportive relationship to foster development of a therapeutic relationship.

Greenson (1967) emphasized the collaborative nature of the alliance, in which the patient and therapist work together to promote therapeutic change. Bordin (1979) operationalized the therapeutic alliance concept as the degree of agreement between patient and therapist concerning the tasks and goals of psychotherapy and the quality of the bond between them. He conceptualized the alliance as evolving and changing as the result of a dynamic interactive process occurring between patient and therapist. Outcome research in psychotherapy supports the idea that the quality of the therapeutic alliance is the best predictor of treatment outcome (Gaston 1990; Horvath and Symonds 1991). There is evidence that in brief supportive and supportive–expressive psychotherapies, an early and strong therapeutic alliance is predictive of positive outcome (Hellerstein et al. 1998; Luborsky 1984; Pollack et al. 1991).

The therapeutic alliance is most likely the therapeutic foundation for change in supportive psychotherapy rather than the vehicle for change as in more expressive psychotherapies (Gaston 1990; Hellerstein et al. 1998; Horvath and Symonds 1991; Westerman et al. 1995). Therefore, the therapist fosters the alliance through active measures, acting as a good parental role model, by being tolerant and nonjudgmental (Misch 2000). Direct measures that support the self-esteem of the patient support the therapeutic alliance.

Alliance Ruptures

The stability of the therapeutic alliance appears to be related to the psychotherapy continuum. The alliance tends to be more stable on the supportive psychotherapy side of the continuum than on the expressive end,

because it is not threatened by challenging confrontations or interpretations, which may heighten patient anxiety (Hellerstein et al. 1998).

Patients vary in their capacity to establish a positive alliance with a therapist. Those on the sickness side of the psychopathology continuum, with structural deficits, especially in object relations, may have problems developing a positive relationship with the therapist. The inability to establish "basic trust" (Erikson 1950) interferes with the establishment of a therapeutic bond. With these patients, a major therapeutic task, especially early in treatment, is building a trusting relationship.

Breaks in the therapeutic alliance are not unusual (Safran and Segal 1990; Safran et al.1994; Winston and Muran 1996). In fact, misunderstandings between therapist and patient occur for a number of reasons. Over the course of psychotherapy, the patient may at various times experience the therapist as critical, insensitive, distant, withholding, untrustworthy, intrusive, unempathic, and so on, which will contribute to a misalliance. In supportive psychotherapy there is ample opportunity and breadth of strategy to intervene effectively when problems in the alliance occur. Less constraint is placed on the therapist about communicating his or her sincere regret at having unwittingly impugned or patronized the patient or having raised a subject that the patient found intrusive, anxiety provoking, or simply unpalatable. Generally when the therapist anticipates or notices a misalliance, supportive techniques are used as the first line of repair of alliance ruptures (Bond et al. 1998). The therapist attempts to address the problem in a practical manner, staying within the current situation, before moving to symbolic or transference issues. The following is an example of a problem in this area.

> A patient in supportive psychotherapy, who regularly kept appointments, failed to appear at a session. The therapist did not attempt to contact the patient. In the next session, the patient began by angrily asking the therapist why there had been no attempt to contact her. The patient explained that she had been ill and taken to the hospital.

In any psychotherapy, but particularly supportive treatment, the patient should have been called. Doing so would have conveyed respect for and interest in the patient and prevented a rupture in the alliance. However, once the misalliance has occurred, the therapist must quickly move to repair the alliance by encouraging the patient to express her feelings about not being called, and then acknowledging and accepting her criticism, as well as offering an apology.

Special Populations

The psychiatric disorders on the sickness side of the psychopathology continuum, for which supportive psychotherapy is indicated, include schizophrenia, bipolar disorder, severe personality disorders, substance use disorder, and co-occurring mental illness and substance use disorders. All of these disorders may benefit from specialized approaches integrated into a supportive psychotherapy framework that is combined with cognitive-behavioral techniques. A full discussion of this topic is beyond the scope of this chapter. Therefore, only a brief summary of this work, using two disorders as illustrations, will be presented here. For a more comprehensive review, the reader is directed to Chapter 8, "Applicability to Special Populations," in the book *Introduction to Supportive Psychotherapy* (Winston et al. 2004).

For severely impaired individuals, such as patients with schizophrenia, a broader approach of social skills training (Benton and Schroeder 1990) and psychoeducation (Goldman and Quinn 1988) is indicated. Combining these approaches with supportive psychotherapy would include the following: providing education about the illness, facilitating reality testing, promoting medication compliance, helping the patient with problem solving, and reinforcing adaptive behaviors with praise (Lamberti and Herz 1995). In addition, the therapist uses supportive techniques such as behavioral goal setting, encouragement, modeling, shaping, and praise to teach interpersonal skills (Glynn et al. 2002). Studies have demonstrated the utility of these interventions in improving social competence (Heinssen et al. 2000; Lauriello et al. 1999).

Patients with substance use disorders can benefit from supportive psychotherapy, which can help develop coping strategies to control or reduce substance use and diminish anxiety and dysphoria. The therapist must actively strive to maintain a positive therapeutic alliance so that the patient can remain in treatment and actively contribute to the work of therapy. Newer evidence-based strategies such as psychoeducation, relapse prevention (Marlatt and Gordon 1985), and motivational interviewing (Rollnick and Miller 1995) should be integrated into supportive psychotherapy, along with 12-Step programs and group psychotherapy.

Crisis Intervention

Crisis intervention began during World War II when soldiers with traumatic stress disorders were treated at or near the front lines with crisis intervention techniques and quickly returned to their combat units (Glass 1954). At about the same time, Lindemann (1944) began working with survivors and relatives of survivors of the Coconut Grove night club fire in Boston. These individuals suffered from acute grief and were unable to cope with their bereavement. In his seminal article, Lindemann (1944) described normal and morbid grief and contrasted the two. The survivors and their families were helped to do the necessary "grief work," which involved going through the mourning process and experiencing the loss.

Parad and Parad (1990) defined *crisis* as an "upset in a steady state, a turning point leading to better or worse, a disruption or breakdown in a person's or family's normal or usual pattern of functioning" (pp. 3–4). A crisis occurs when an individual encounters a situation that leads to a breakdown in functioning, creating disequilibrium. Generally, a crisis is precipitated by a hazardous event or stressor, such as a catastrophe or disaster (e.g., earthquake, fire, war, terrorism), a relationship rupture or loss, rape, or abuse. A crisis may also result from a series of difficult events or mishaps rather than from one major occurrence. During crises, individuals perceive their lives, needs, security, relationships, and sense of well-being to be at risk. An individual's reaction to stress is the result of a number of factors, including age, health, personality issues, prior experience with stressful events, support and belief systems, and underlying biological or genetic vulnerability. Crises tend to be time limited, generally lasting no more than a few months; the duration depends on the stressor and on the individual's perception of and response to the stressor.

Crisis intervention is a therapeutic process aimed at restoring homeostatic balance and diminishing vulnerability to the stressor (Parad and Parad 1990; Winston et al. 2004). Homeostasis is accomplished by the therapist's helping to mobilize the individual's abilities and social network and to promote adaptive coping mechanisms to reestablish equilibrium. Crisis intervention is a short-term approach that focuses on solving the immediate problem and includes the entire therapeutic repertoire for helping patients deal with the challenges and threats of overwhelming stress (Table 32–10).

TABLE 32–10. Crisis interventions

Crisis—a situation that can lead to a breakdown in functioning, creating disequilibrium

Crisis intervention—a brief therapeutic process aimed at restoring homeostatic balance and promoting adaptive coping mechanisms

The distinction between crisis intervention and psychotherapy is often blurred, because the two approaches may overlap with regard to technique and length of treatment (Marmor 1979). Crisis intervention is generally expected to involve 1–3 sessions, whereas the duration of brief psychotherapy can extend from a few visits to 20 or more sessions. However, in recent years, crisis intervention has included treatments lasting longer than just a few sessions (Parad and Parad 1990). This more inclusive form of crisis therapy is based on a number of different treatments, including supportive–expressive, cognitive-behavioral, humanistic, family, and systems approaches, as well as the use of medication when indicated (Winston et al. 2004). Systems approaches can be broad and can encompass actions such as working with and referral to social service agencies, mobile crisis units, suicide hotlines, and law enforcement agencies. More recently, an additional focus of crisis intervention has been on emergency management and prevention through the use of various forms of debriefing (Everly and Mitchell 1999).

A thorough evaluation of a patient in crisis, including an ego assessment (Caplan 1961), is critical. The evaluation consists of assessing the individual's capacity to deal with stress, maintain ego structure and equilibrium, and deal with reality as well as assessing problem-solving and coping abilities. The evaluation session should be therapeutic as well as diagnostic since the patient is in crisis and is seeking relief from suffering.

Suicidal thoughts and behaviors are so common in patients in crisis that it is essential to ask patients about suicidal ideas and attempts. A careful and thorough assessment of the suicidal patient is critical to determine the diagnosis and the proper treatment approach. Crisis intervention approaches, generally accompanied by the use of medication, often play an important role in the treatment of suicidal individuals (Winston et al. 2004). (For a more complete description of suicide, see Chapter 43 in this volume, "Suicide," by Simon.)

Treatment approaches used vary depending on the needs of the patient but generally include supportive interventions, exposure therapy, and cognitive restructuring. Therapists must pay particular attention to establishing and maintaining a positive therapeutic alliance. The terrorist attacks of September 11, 2001, in New York City and Washington, DC, have made the general public and mental health professionals more aware of these issues and of the need for crisis intervention services.

Efficacy Research

There have been a limited number of controlled clinical trials of supportive psychotherapy. However, there are some early uncontrolled studies and some more recent controlled trials that bear on the efficacy of supportive psychotherapy. Unfortunately, there are no studies comparing supportive psychotherapy with a placebo approach or minimal therapy.

The psychotherapy research project of the Menninger Foundation was an important early study comparing supportive and expressive psychotherapy with psychoanalysis. Wallerstein and colleagues (Wallerstein 1986, 1989) studied the treatment, clinical course, and posttreatment follow-up of 42 inpatients at the Menninger Foundation. Findings included the following: psychoanalysis produced more limited outcomes than predicted, whereas psychotherapy, including supportive psychotherapy, often achieved more than predicted; all of the treatments became more supportive during the course of therapy; and supportive interventions accounted for more of the change in outcome. This study took a naturalistic approach, without control subjects or random assignment of subjects, but was noteworthy in calling attention to the possible efficacy of supportive psychotherapy.

Schizophrenia Studies

In a National Institute of Mental Health study involving schizophrenic patients treated for 2 years with either exploratory insight-oriented psychotherapy three times per week or reality-adaptive supportive psychotherapy once per week, there was clear evidence of a better outcome for patients treated with supportive psychotherapy (Gunderson et al. 1984; Stanton et al. 1984). All patients were maintained on their usual medications throughout the study. In another study, schizophrenic patients were randomly assigned to supportive psychotherapy or family therapy (Rea et al. 1991). Patients were treated for 9 months and followed for 2 years. Supportive psychotherapy patients had significant improvement in coping and interpersonal style compared with patients in family therapy. However, the data analysis in this study did not take into account the difference in coping skills between the two treatment groups. The Danish National Schizophrenia Project study of first-episode psychosis (Rosenbaum et al. 2005) found a nonsignificant tendency towards greater improvement in social functioning in patients treated with supportive psychotherapy or integrated therapy compared with treatment as usual. All patients received antipsychotic medication, and the treatment-as-usual group were given various therapies based on the needs of patients and the available resources of the clinic.

Hogarty et al. (1997) stated that supportive psychotherapy fares less well compared with other psychosocial approaches, such as family psychoeducation, skills training, or role therapy. However, defining supportive psychotherapy as not including psychoeducation, skills training, or role therapy approaches is problematic, given that these techniques are generally considered to be among the interventions used in supportive psychotherapy. This highlights the importance of describing the interventions used in psychotherapy clinical trials. More recent psychotherapy approaches with schizophrenic patients include social skills training, which may be enhanced with amplified skills training in the community (Glynn et al. 2002; Liberman et al. 1998).

Depressive Disorder Studies

Studies of patients with depressive disorders have also demonstrated the efficacy of supportive psychotherapy. In the National Institute of Mental Health Treatment of Depression Collaborative Research Program, two psychotherapies (CBT and interpersonal therapy) were compared with an antidepressant (imipramine)–clinical management condition and a control condition consisting of drug placebo and clinical management (Elkin 1994; Elkin et al. 1989; Imber et al. 1990). The clinical management was a low-level supportive psychotherapy approach. All three psychotherapies, including the low-level supportive psychotherapy, were found to be efficacious and similar on measures of depressive symptoms and overall functioning. In another study (Thompson and Gallagher 1985), 30 elderly outpatients were randomly assigned to a 16-week treatment with cognitive therapy, behavior therapy or supportive psychotherapy. Improvement was similar across the three treatment conditions at termination, but at 1-year follow-up, more of the patients in supportive psychotherapy received a diagnosis of depression. However, the small number of patients studied, as well as the type of supportive psychotherapy used, makes these findings of limited value. In a randomized clinical trial involving 100 depressed adolescents, Renaud et al. (1998) found that rapid responders to therapy had better outcomes at 1-year follow-up and better scores on some measures at 2-year follow-up. The investigators concluded that patients with milder forms of depression may benefit from initial supportive psychotherapy or short trials of more specialized

types of treatment. In another study (Maina et al. 2005), patients with minor depressions were randomly assigned to brief dynamic therapy, supportive psychotherapy, or a wait-list condition. Patients treated with brief dynamic or supportive psychotherapy showed a significant improvement after treatment compared to nontreated controls, but brief dynamic therapy was more effective at 6-month follow-up.

Anxiety Disorder Studies

Systematic hierarchical desensitization was compared with supportive psychotherapy in a 26-week treatment trial involving patients with various types of phobias (Klein et al. 1983). Both treatments performed well, and there was no difference between the two approaches. The authors speculated that for phobic individuals, psychotherapy serves as an instigator of corrective activity outside the formal session by maintaining exposure in vivo. In another study, patients with phobias and panic attacks received either imipramine plus behavior therapy or imipramine plus supportive psychotherapy (Zitrin et al. 1978). The majority of patients improved, and there was no difference in improvement rates between the two treatments. In a study of social anxiety, Alstrom et al. (1984) found that supportive psychotherapy and prolonged exposure therapy were equally effective. Shear et al. (2001) reported that emotion-focused psychotherapy, a form of supportive psychotherapy that involves empathic listening and supportive strategies, has low efficacy for the treatment of panic disorder, compared with CBT or imipramine. However, this form of supportive psychotherapy was unusual since it attempted to identify and process emotions, which is generally not done in supportive psychotherapy. The work with emotions was based on the notion that unrecognized emotions trigger panic attacks and contribute to the maintenance of the disorder.

Personality Disorder Studies

In a study comparing supportive with interpretive (expressive) psychotherapy, Piper et al. (1998) found no outcome differences between the two treatments. Patients presented with anxiety or depressive disorders, and 60.4% of subjects had a comorbid personality disorder. Hellerstein et al. (1998), in a study of patients primarily with Cluster C personality disorder and "not otherwise specified" Cluster C–type patients, compared brief supportive psychotherapy with short-term dynamic psychotherapy. They found that both therapies performed equally well on measures of symptomatology, presenting complaints, and interpersonal functioning. The majority of the patients had comorbid Axis I disorders, such as depression or anxiety. These changes were found not only at termination but also at 6-month follow-up. In a substudy of the Hellerstein et al. (1998) study, the authors used the interpersonal circumplex model and graphically demonstrated lasting positive change in interpersonal functioning in subjects treated with supportive psychotherapy (Rosenthal et al. 1999; Winston et al. 2001).

Anorexia Nervosa Studies

A recent randomized, controlled clinical trial of three psychotherapies for anorexia nervosa found that supportive psychotherapy was superior to CBT and interpersonal therapy (McIntosh et al. 2005). The supportive psychotherapy used in this study combined education, care, and support to foster a therapeutic relationship that promoted adherence to treatment together with supportive psychotherapy techniques such as praise, reassurance, and advice.

Medical Disorder Studies

Mumford et al. (1982) reviewed controlled studies of supportive psychotherapy—including education about illness and treatments, cognitive-behavioral techniques, and ventilation and reassurance in a supportive relationship—in patients recovering from myocardial infarctions and surgery. The authors found better patient experiences with pain and increased patient compliance and speed of recovery, as well as fewer complications and fewer days in the hospital.

It is clear that more research on supportive psychotherapy is needed to clarify the indications for supportive psychotherapy and its overall efficacy, as well as explicating how this treatment should be integrated with other psychotherapy and psychopharmacology approaches. However, it does appear that supportive psychotherapy is useful across a broad spectrum of psychiatric and medical disorders.

Education

It is essential for clinical psychiatrists to have a working knowledge of supportive psychotherapy, because it is the most commonly employed psychotherapy. In all forms of psychiatric practice—outpatient, inpatient, consultation-liaison, medication management, and so on—the strategies and techniques of support-

ive psychotherapy are invaluable. Every psychiatrist should be able to perform a thorough patient evaluation and diagnostic interview and be able to formulate a comprehensive treatment plan that can encompass a variety of possible approaches, including psychopharmacological and psychosocial treatments. In addition, psychiatrists should have an understanding of the therapeutic relationship and how to establish a therapeutic alliance. Concepts such as transference and countertransference, defenses, adaptive styles, and self-esteem issues all need to be understood and worked with in an effective manner.

Psychiatrists engaged primarily in the practice of psychopharmacology should have a good working knowledge of supportive psychotherapy, since this is the approach that seems to be effective with most patients and utilizes psychoeducation in a major way. Psychoeducation involves imparting information to patients, in a give-and-take manner, about psychiatric disorders, medication actions and side effects, interpersonal and family issues, and problems of everyday living.

Unfortunately, supportive psychotherapy has not been taught in any kind of systematic fashion in residency training programs. However, the new requirements of the Residency Review Committee for Psychiatry now mandate that psychiatry residents must be certified as competent by their training programs in five types of psychotherapy, one of which is supportive psychotherapy. These new requirements may help to foster the teaching and supervision of supportive psychotherapy in residency training programs.

Conclusion

Supportive psychotherapy is a broad-based treatment that is effective for many different types of patients and psychiatric disorders. Despite being the most widely used psychotherapy, it remains undervalued and is rarely taught in a systematic fashion. However, this appears to be changing because of the new requirements for the teaching of supportive psychotherapy in residency training programs. It is clear that more research in supportive psychotherapy is needed to help define and distinguish which strategies and techniques are useful with what type of patient. In addition, we need to develop a better understanding of the mechanism of change and a more comprehensive and integrated theoretical foundation for supportive psychotherapy.

Key Points

- Supportive therapy can be defined as a treatment that uses direct measures to ameliorate symptoms and to maintain, restore, or improve self-esteem, ego functions, and adaptive skills.

- Psychoanalytic theory is generally viewed as the basis for supportive psychotherapy.

- Matching psychotherapy technique to patient locus on the psychopathology continuum is of crucial importance.

- There are few circumstances in which supportive psychotherapy is contraindicated. In general, supportive psychotherapy is contraindicated only when psychotherapy itself is contraindicated (e.g., in deliria, drug intoxication, late stages of dementia, malingering, or psychopathy).

- Major strategies include strengthening defenses, maintaining and repairing the therapeutic alliance, enhancing self-esteem, and using therapeutic modeling and self-disclosure.

- Major interventions include use of a conversational communication style, praise, reassurance, encouragement, advice, rationalizing, reframing, rehearsal, clarification, and confrontation.

- Supportive psychotherapy focuses on the real relationship and less so on transference.

- A supportive relationship is not supportive psychotherapy.

- Clinical trials indicate that supportive psychotherapy is efficacious for many psychiatric disorders.

Suggested Readings

Dewald PA: Principles of supportive psychotherapy. Am J Psychother 48:505–518, 1994
Misch DA: Basic strategies of dynamic supportive therapy. J Psychother Pract Res 9:173–189, 2000
Pinsker H: A Primer of Supportive Psychotherapy. Hillsdale, NJ, Analytic Press, 1997
Winston A, Winston B: Handbook of Integrated Short-Term Psychotherapy. Arlington, VA, American Psychiatric Publishing, 2002
Winston A, Rosenthal RN, Pinsker H: Introduction to Supportive Psychotherapy. Arlington, VA, American Psychiatric Publishing, 2004

References

Alstrom JE, Nordlund CL, Persson G, et al: Effects of four treatment methods on social phobia patients not suitable for insight-oriented psychotherapy. Acta Psychiatr Scand 70:1–17, 1984
Alter CL: Palliative and supportive care of patients with pancreatic cancer. Semin Oncol 23:229–240, 1996
Barlow D, Craske M: Mastery of Your Anxiety and Panic. Albany, NY, Center for Stress and Anxiety Disorders, State University of New York, 1989
Beck AT, Sokol K, Clark DA, et al: A crossover study of focused cognitive therapy for panic disorders. Am J Psychiatry 149:778–783, 1992
Bellak L: The schizophrenic syndrome: a further elaboration of the unified theory of schizophrenia, in Schizophrenia: A Review of the Syndrome. Edited by Bellak L. New York, Logos, 1958, pp 3–63
Benton MK, Schroeder HE: Social skills training with schizophrenics: a meta-analytic evaluation. J Consult Clin Psychol 58:741–747, 1990
Beres D: Ego deviation and the concept of schizophrenia, in The Psychoanalytic Study of the Child, Vol 11. New York, International Universities Press, 1956, pp 164–235
Bond M, Banon E, Grenier M: Differential effects of interventions on the therapeutic alliance with patients with personality disorders. J Psychother Pract Res 7:301–318, 1998
Bordin ES: The generalizability of the psychoanalytic concept of the working alliance. Psychotherapy: Theory, Research, and Practice 16:252–260, 1979
Bowlby J: Attachment and Loss, Vol 1: Attachment. New York, Basic Books, 1969
Bowlby J: A Secure Base. New York, Basic Books, 1988
Bronheim HE, Fulop G, Kunkel EJ, et al: The Academy of Psychosomatic Medicine practice guidelines for psychiatric consultation in the general medical setting. The Academy of Psychosomatic Medicine. Psychosomatics 39:S8–S30, 1998
Buckley P: Supportive therapy: a neglected treatment. Psychiatr Ann 16:515–521, 1986
Caplan G: An Approach to Community Mental Health. New York, Grune & Stratton, 1961
Classen C, Butler LD, Koopman, C, et al: Supportive expressive group therapy and distress in patients with metastatic breast cancer: a randomized clinical intervention trial. Arch Gen Psychiatry 58:494–501, 2001
Conte HR: Review of research in supportive psychotherapy: an update. Am J Psychother 48:495–504, 1994
Dewald PA: Psychotherapy: A Dynamic Approach (1964). New York, Basic Books, 1971
Dewald PA: Principles of supportive psychotherapy. Am J Psychother 48:505–518, 1994

Elkin I: The NIMH Treatment of Depression Collaborative Research Program: where we began and where we are, in Handbook of Psychotherapy and Behavioral Change. Edited by Bergin AE, Garfield SL. New York, Wiley, 1994, pp 114–139

Elkin I, Shea MT, Watkins JT, et al: National Institute of Mental Health Treatment of Depression Collaborative Research Program: general effectiveness of treatments. Arch Gen Psychiatry 46:971–982, 1989

Erikson EH: Childhood and Society. New York, WW Norton, 1950

Evans S, Fishman B, Spielman L, et al: Randomized trial of cognitive behavior therapy versus supportive psychotherapy for HIV-related peripheral neuropathic pain. Psychosomatics 44:44–50, 2003

Everly GS Jr, Mitchell JT: Critical Incident Stress Management (CISM): A New Era and Standard of Care in Crisis Intervention, 2nd Edition. Ellicott City, MD, Chevron Publishing, 1999

Fairbairn WRD: An Object-Relations Theory of the Personality. New York, Basic Books, 1952

Foa EB: Trauma and women: course, predictors, and treatment. J Clin Psychiatry 58:25–28, 1997

Foa EB, Franklin ME: Psychotherapies for obsessive compulsive disorder: a review, in Obsessive Compulsive Disorder, 2nd Edition. Edited by Maj M, Sartorius N, Okasha A, et al. Chichester, England, Wiley, 2002, pp 93–115

Frank JD: General psychotherapy: the restoration of morale, in American Handbook of Psychiatry, 2nd Edition, Vol 5: Treatment. Edited by Freedman DX, Dyrud JE. New York, Basic Books, 1975, pp 117–132

Freud S: Lines of advance in psycho-analytic therapy (1919), in The Standard Edition of the Complete Psychological Works of Sigmund Freud, Vol 17. Edited by Strachey J. London, England, Hogarth Press, 1955, pp 157–168

Freud S: The ego and the id (1923), in The Standard Edition of the Complete Psychological Works of Sigmund Freud. Vol 19. Edited by Strachey J. London, England, Hogarth Press, 1961, pp 12–66

Gabbard GO: A contemporary psychoanalytic model of countertransference. J Clin Psychol 57:983–991, 2001

Gaston L: The concept of the alliance and its role in psychotherapy: theoretical and empirical considerations. Psychotherapy 27:143–153, 1990

Gill M: Ego psychology and psychotherapy. Psychoanalytic Q 20:62–71, 1951

Glass A: Psychotherapy in the combat zone. Am J Psychiatry 110:725–731, 1954

Glover E: The therapeutic effect of inexact interpretation: a contributing to the theory of suggestion. Int J Psychoanal 12:397–411, 1931

Glynn SM, Marder SR, Liberman RP, et al: Supplementing clinic-based skills training and manual-based community support sessions: effects on social adjustment of patients with schizophrenia. Am J Psychiatry 159:829–837, 2002

Goldman CR, Quinn FL: Effects of a patient education program in the treatment of schizophrenia. Hosp Community Psychiatry 39:282–286, 1988

Greenson RR: The Technique and Practice of Psychoanalysis. New York, International Universities Press, 1967

Greenson RR: The real relationship between the patient and the psychoanalyst, in The Unconscious Today. Edited by Kanzer M. New York, International Universities Press, 1971, pp 213–232

Greist JH: Treatment of obsessive-compulsiveness disorder: psychotherapies, drugs, and other somatic treatments. J Clin Psychiatry 51 (suppl):44–50, 1990

Gunderson JG, Frank AF, Katz HM, et al: Effects of psychotherapy in schizophrenia, II: comparative outcome of two forms of treatment. Schizophr Bull 10:564–598, 1984

Hartmann H: Ego Psychology and the Problem of Adaptation (1939). Translated by Rapaport D. New York, International Universities Press, 1958

Heinssen RK, Liberman RP, Kopelowicz A: Psychosocial skills training for schizophrenia: lessons from the laboratory. Schizophr Bull 26:21–46, 2000

Hellerstein DJ, Pinsker H, Rosenthal RN, et al: Supportive psychotherapy as the treatment model of choice. J Psychother Pract Res 3:300–306, 1994

Hellerstein DJ, Rosenthal RN, Pinsker H, et al: A randomized prospective study comparing supportive and dynamic therapies: outcome and alliance. J Psychother Pract Res 7:261–271, 1998

Henry WP, Schacht TE, Strupp HH: Structural analysis of social behavior: application to a study of interpersonal process in differential psychotherapeutic outcome. J Consult Clin Psychol 44:27–31, 1986

Henry WP, Schacht TE, Strupp HH: Patient and therapist introject, interpersonal process, and differential psychotherapy outcome. J Consult Clin Psychol 58:768–774, 1990

Hogarty GE, Kornblith SJ, Greenwald D, et al: Three-year trials of personal therapy among schizophrenia patients living with or independent of family, I: description of study and effects on relapse rates. Am J Psychiatry 154:1504–1513, 1997

Holmes J: Supportive psychotherapy: the search for positive meanings. Br J Psychiatry 167:439–445, 1995

Horowitz MJ, Marmar C: The therapeutic alliance with difficult patients, in Psychiatry Update: The American Psychiatric Association Annual Review, Vol 4. Edited by Hales RE, Frances AJ. Washington, DC, American Psychiatric Press, 1985, pp 573–585

Horowitz MJ, Marmar C, Weiss DS, et al: Brief psychotherapy of bereavement reactions: the relationship of process to outcome. Arch Gen Psychiatry 41:438–448, 1984

Horvath AO, Symonds BD: Relation between working alliance and outcome in psychotherapy: a meta-analysis. J Couns Psychol 38:139–149, 1991

Hunter J, Leszcz M, McLachlan SA, et al: Psychological stress response in breast cancer. Psychooncology 5:4–14, 1996

Imber SD, Pilkonis PA, Sotsky SM, et al: Mode-specific effects among three treatments for depression. J Consult Clin Psychol 58:352–359, 1990

Jacobson E: The Self and the Object World. New York, International Universities Press, 1964

Kiesler HD: Therapist countertransference: in search of common themes and empirical referents. J Clin Psychol 57:1053–1063, 2001

Klein DF, Zitrin CM, Woerner MG, et al: Treatment of phobias, II: behavior therapy and supportive psychotherapy: are there any specific ingredients? Arch Gen Psychiatry 40:139–145, 1983

Kohut H: The Analysis of the Self. New York, International Universities Press, 1971

Lamberti JS, Herz MI: Psychotherapy, social skills training, and vocational rehabilitation in schizophrenia, in Contemporary Issues in the Treatment of Schizophrenia. Edited by Shriqui CL, Nasrallah HA. Washington, DC, American Psychiatric Press, 1995, pp 713–734

Lauriello J, Bustillo J, Keith SJ: A critical review of research on psychosocial treatment of schizophrenia. Biol Psychiatry 46:1409–1417, 1999

Levenson E: The Ambiguity of Change: An Inquiry Into the Nature of Psychoanalytic Reality. New York, Basic Books, 1983

Lewis J: To Be a Therapist: The Teaching and Learning. New York, Brunner/Mazel, 1978

Liberman RP, Wallace CJ, Blackwell G, et al: Skills training versus psychosocial occupational therapy for persons with persistent schizophrenia. Am J Psychiatry 155:1087–1091, 1998

Lindemann E: Symptomatology and management of acute grief. Am J Psychiatry 101:141–148, 1944

Luborsky L: Principles of Psychoanalytic Psychotherapy: A Manual for Supportive-Expressive Treatment. New York, Basic Books, 1984

Mahler MS, Pine F, Bergman A: The Psychological Birth of the Human Infant. New York, Basic Books, 1975

Maina G, Forner F, Bogetto F: Randomized controlled trial comparing brief dynamic and supportive therapy with waiting list condition in minor depressive disorders. Psychother Psychosom 74:43–50, 2005

Markowitz JC, Klerman GL, Clougherty KE, et al: Individual psychotherapies for depressed HIV-positive patients. Am J Psychiatry 152:1504–1509, 1995

Marlatt GA, Gordon JR: Relapse Prevention: Maintenance Strategies in the Treatment of Addictive Behaviors. New York, Guilford, 1985

Marmor J: Short-term dynamic psychotherapy. Am J Psychiatry 136:149–155, 1979

Massie MJ, Holland JC: Depression and the cancer patient. J Clin Psychiatry 51 (suppl):12–19, 1990

McIntosh VW, Jordan J, Carter FA, et al: Three psychotherapies for anorexia nervosa: a randomized, controlled trial. Am J Psychiatry 162:741–747, 2005

Misch DA: Basic strategies of dynamic supportive therapy. J Psychother Pract Res 9:173–189, 2000

Mitchell S: Relational Concepts in Psychoanalysis: An Integration. Cambridge, MA, Harvard University Press, 1988

Mumford E, Schlesinger HJ, Glass CV: The effect of psychological intervention on recovery from surgery and heart attacks: an analysis of the literature. Am J Public Health 72:141–151, 1982

Munich RL: Contemporary treatment of schizophrenia. Bull Menninger Clin 61:189–221, 1997

Novalis PN, Rojcewicz SJ, Peele R: Clinical Manual of Supportive Psychotherapy. Washington, DC, American Psychiatric Press, 1993

O'Malley SS, Jaffe AJ, Chang G, et al: Naltrexone and coping skills therapy for alcohol dependence: a controlled study. Arch Gen Psychiatry 49:881–887, 1992

Othmer E, Othmer S: The Clinical Interview Using DSM-IV, Vol 1. Washington, DC, American Psychiatric Press, 1994, pp 87–97

Parad HJ, Parad LG: Crisis Intervention, Book 2: The Practitioner's Sourcebook for Brief Therapy. Milwaukee, WI, Family Service America, 1990

Parloff MB: Goals in psychotherapy: mediating and ultimate, in Goals of Psychotherapy. Edited by Mahrer AR. New York, Appleton-Century-Crofts, 1967, pp 5–19

Pinsker H: A Primer of Supportive Psychotherapy. Hillsdale, NJ, Analytic Press, 1997

Pinsker H, Rosenthal RN, McCullough L: Dynamic supportive psychotherapy, in Handbook of Short-Term Dynamic Psychotherapy. Edited by Crits-Christoph P, Barber JP. New York, Basic Books, 1991, pp 220–247

Pinsker H, Hellerstein DJ, Rosenthal RN, et al: Supportive therapy, common factors and eclecticism. Paper presented at the annual meeting of the American Psychiatric Association, New York, May 1996

Piper WE, Joyce AS, McCallum M, et al: Interpretive and supportive forms of psychotherapy and patient personality variables. J Consult Clin Psychol 66:558–567, 1998

Pollack J, Flegenheimer W, Winston A: Brief adaptive psychotherapy, in Handbook of Short-Term Dynamic Psychotherapy. Edited by Crits-Christoph P, Barber JP. New York, Basic Books, 1991, pp 199–219

Quality Assurance Project: Treatment outlines for the management of the somatoform disorders. Aust N Z J Psychiatry 19:397–407, 1985

Rea MM, Strachan AM, Goldstein MJ, et al: Changes in coping style following individual and family treatment for schizophrenia. Br J Psychiatry 158:642–647, 1991

Renaud J, Brent DA, Baugher M, et al: Rapid response to psychosocial treatment for adolescent depression: a two-year follow-up. J Am Acad Child Adolesc Psychiatry 37:1184–1190, 1998

Rollnick S, Miller WR: What is motivational interviewing? Behavioral and Cognitive Psychotherapy 23:325–334, 1995

Rosenbaum B, Valbak K, Harder S, et al: The Danish National Schizophrenia Project: prospective, comparative longitudinal treatment study of first-episode psychosis. Br J Psychiatry 186:394–399, 2005

Rosenthal RN: Identification of dual diagnoses in drug abusers, in NIDA National Conference on Drug Abuse Research and Practice: An Alliance for the 21st Century (January 12–15, 1991): Conference Highlights. Washington, DC, National Institute on Drug Abuse, 1991, pp 63–64

Rosenthal RN, Muran JC, Pinsker H, et al: Interpersonal change in brief supportive psychotherapy. J Psychother Pract Res 8:55–63, 1999

Safran JD, Segal ZV: Interpersonal Process in Cognitive Therapy. New York, Basic Books, 1990

Safran JD, Muran JC, Samstag LW: Resolving therapeutic alliance ruptures: a task analytic investigation, in The Working Alliance: Theory, Research and Practice. Edited by Horvath AO, Greenberg LS. New York, Wiley, 1994, pp 225–255

Shear KM, Houck P, Greeno C, et al: Emotion-focused psychotherapy for patients with panic disorder. Am J Psychiatry 158:1993–1998, 2001

Sifneos PE: The prevalence of "alexithymic" characteristics in psychosomatic patients. Psychother Psychosom 22:255–262, 1973

Sifneos PE: Problems of psychotherapy of patients with alexithymic characteristics and physical disease. Psychother Psychosom 26:65–70, 1975

Simon JC: Criteria for therapist self-disclosure. Am J Psychother 42:404–415, 1988

Stanton AH, Gunderson JG, Knapp PH, et al: Effects of psychotherapy in schizophrenia, I: design and implementation of a controlled study. Schizophr Bull 10:520–563, 1984

Stewart RL: Psychoanalysis and psychoanalytic psychotherapy, in Comprehensive Textbook of Psychiatry, 4th Edition. Edited by Kaplan HI, Sadock BJ. Baltimore, MD, Williams & Wilkins, 1985

Sullivan HS: Conception of Modern Psychiatry. New York, WW Norton, 1953

Sullivan PR: Learning theories and supportive psychotherapy. Am J Psychiatry 128:119–122, 1971

Thomas EM, Weiss SM: Nonpharmacological interventions with chronic cancer pain in adults. Cancer Control 7:157–164, 2000

Thompson LW, Gallagher D: Depression and its treatment. Aging (Milano) 348:14–18, 1985

Tomkins MA: Cognitive-behavioral case formulation: the case of Jim. Journal of Psychotherapy Integration 6:97–105, 1996

Wallerstein RS: Forty-two Lives in Treatment: A Study of Psychoanalysis and Psychotherapy. New York, Guilford, 1986

Wallerstein RS: The psychotherapy research project of the Menninger Foundation: an overview. J Consult Clin Psychol 57:195–205, 1989

Walsh BJ, Wilson GT, Terence G, et al: Medication and psychotherapy in the treatment of bulimia nervosa. Am J Psychiatry 154:523–531, 1997

Werman DS: The Practice of Supportive Psychotherapy. New York, Brunner/Mazel, 1984

Westerman MA, Foote JP, Winston A: Change in coordination across phases of psychotherapy and outcome: two mechanisms for the role played by patients' contribution to the alliance. J Consult Clin Psychol 24:190–195, 1995

Winnicott DW: The Maturational Process and the Facilitating Environment: Studies in the Theory of Emotional Development. London, England, Hogarth Press, 1965

Winston A, Muran JC: Common factors in the time-limited psychotherapies, in The American Psychiatric Press Review of Psychiatry, Vol 15. Edited by Dickstein LJ, Riba MB, Oldham JM. Washington, DC, American Psychiatric Press, 1996, pp 43–68

Winston A, Winston B: Handbook of Integrated Short-Term Psychotherapy. Arlington, VA, American Psychiatric Publishing, 2002

Winston A, Pinsker H, McCullough L: A review of supportive psychotherapy. Hosp Community Psychiatry 37:1105–1114, 1986

Winston A, Rosenthal RN, Muran JC: Supportive psychotherapy, in Handbook of Personality Disorders: Theory, Research, and Treatment. Edited by Livesley WJ. New York, Guilford, 2001, pp 344–358

Winston A, Rosenthal RN, Pinsker H: Introduction to Supportive Psychotherapy. Arlington, VA, American Psychiatric Publishing, 2004

Wolf ES: Empathy and countertransference, in The Future of Psychoanalysis. Edited by Goldberg A. New York, International Universities Press, 1983, pp 309–326

Zetzel E: Current concepts of transference. International Journal of Psychoanalysis 37:369–375, 1956

Zitrin CM, Klein DF, Woerner MG, et al: Behavior therapy, supportive psychotherapy, imipramine, and phobias. Arch Gen Psychiatry 35:307–316, 1978

COMBINING PSYCHOTHERAPY AND PHARMACOTHERAPY

Michelle B. Riba, M.D., M.S.
Richard Balon, M.D.

The past 50 years of psychiatric practice have seen a burgeoning of new types and classes of psychotropic agents for major and minor psychiatric disorders (Olfson et al. 1999, 2002; West et al. 2003). Along with new pharmacological modalities, there is increased understanding to support and recommend that psychotherapy be provided along with pharmacological treatments for disorders including schizophrenia, bipolar disorder, and major depression (American Psychiatric Association 1994, 1997, 2000a). In addition, guidelines and position papers have been provided by the American Psychiatric Association to assist its members and mental health professionals in understanding the complexities of providing combined treatments in the form of both psychotherapy and pharmacotherapy (American Psychiatric Association 1980, 2002a).

Evidence is accumulating that combination psychopharmacology and psychotherapy treatment affords improved outcomes for patients with major depression (Frank et al. 2000; Keller et al. 2000; Lenze et al. 2002), anxiety (Barlow et al. 2000; Mavissakalian 1993), bipolar disorder (Clarkin et al. 1998; G. A. Fava et al. 2001; Frank et al. 2005), dysthymia (Dunner et al. 1996), bulimia nervosa (Walsh et al. 1997), and nicotine dependence (U.S. Department of Health and Human Services 2000), among others. The literature abounds with recommendations for combining pharmacotherapy and psychotherapy to treat disorders as diverse as somatoform disorders (Lipsitt and Starcevic 2006), borderline personality disorder (Oldham 2006), and erectile dysfunction (Banner and Anderson 2007).

With recognition of the desirability of providing both types of treatments has come awareness of new and developing needs to address within our field. The most important is availability of clinicians who are capable of providing an appropriate and efficacious combination of pharmacotherapy *and* psychotherapy. Central to this issue is ensuring that skills and competency in combining pharmacotherapy and psychotherapy are acquired during psychiatry training—that is, assessing and documenting the competency of psychiatry residents to deliver the appropriate type of treatments, based on the appropriate diagnosis, at various levels of training (Epstein and Hundert 2002). Residents must be able to provide psychotherapy and pharmacotherapy, either in collaboration with other mental health professionals or by provision of both treatments themselves, first under supervision, and later independently. To address this important psychotherapy competency, psychiatry residency programs have again begun to emphasize the psychotherapeutic aspects of training. What might not be so clear is how training programs are helping residents learn the difficult and complex aspects of collaboration and the training stages at which different tasks need to be negotiated and mastered.

Another aspect of the discussion is the increased role that primary care plays in providing psychopharmacological treatment, often with no concomitant psychotherapy treatment or with inadequate and poorly supervised arrangements for collaboration with nonmedical therapists. Furthermore, arranging for patients to receive psychotherapy continues to be very difficult because of such factors as insurance carve-outs, lack of insurance for mental illness, complex referral patterns, shortages of psychiatrists in general and of child and adolescent psychiatrists in particular, difficulties in diagnosis of psychiatric conditions in medical settings, stigma, and so forth. Some of the difficulties relate to geography; for example, it is hard to find certain types of mental health professionals in rural areas. Innovative ways of providing psychopharmacological and psychotherapeutic treatment using telemedicine and other Web-based technologies have been introduced (Gibson et al. 2002; Stofle 2002).

Psychologists and psychiatrists continue to battle over scope of practice. Understanding of the need to provide comprehensive care for mental illness, which includes both pharmacotherapy and psychotherapy, has led psychologists to fight for prescribing privileges. At the time of this writing, two states, New Mexico and Louisiana, allow psychologists to prescribe psychotropic medications under various guidelines and algorithms. An appreciation of the need to be able to provide both pharmacology and psychotherapy has also led to the creation of various programs to teach psychopharmacological principles to psychologists.

Another important yet confusing aspect of providing psychotherapy and psychopharmacology treatment relates to how patients are triaged within the mental health system. This process is a complex patchwork that often has very little to do with the specific diagnosis or the needs of the patient, and much more to do with preferences and practices of insurance, managed care, and provider networks. How do the patient, the triager, and/or the clinician decide whether the patient will start receiving psychotherapy, or pharmacotherapy, or both? Sequencing—which treatment is started first—and who provides the care are important factors that can influence both the type of care provided and the outcome. Table 33–1 highlights some of the perplexing issues often associated with the starting point for care in the mental health system.

Combined treatments (psychotherapy and pharmacotherapy) are generally viewed as helpful and im-

portant by patients (Seligman 1995). There are various aspects, however, that are important to highlight. It is generally more costly, for example, to provide combined treatment for the first 6–12 weeks than to use psychotherapy or pharmacotherapy alone, although long-term studies, examining a variety of disorders, are needed to really understand this issue (Dewan 1999; Goldman et al. 1998; Thase 2003). Besides the cost, it would be difficult logistically to arrange for all patients receiving mental health care to be treated by two different clinicians, or by psychiatrists. Such a requirement would overwhelm the already fragmented and understaffed mental health system in this country. There is also a lack of evidence (so far) for the efficacy of combined pharmacotherapy and psychotherapy treatment for many psychiatric conditions.

There has been much debate about the role of medication in psychiatric treatment. Some clinicians have been concerned that alleviating symptoms with medication might reduce a patient's desire to make needed changes or gain insight into ongoing problems (Klerman et al. 1994). Others have noted the effect of prescribing medication on the doctor–patient relationship (Tasman et al. 2000). The prescribing clinician may be viewed as authoritarian or dictatorial, while the nonprescribing clinician may be viewed as more gentle and dynamic.

The transference and countertransference issues abound in the ways patients and clinicians interact regarding this practice. *Transference* refers to the patient's feelings toward the psychiatrist, but also, by extension, may relate to the prescribed medications, psychotherapy, other types of treatment, the clinic, or other aspects of the setting. Transference can be either positive or negative. *Countertransference* refers to the psychiatrist's feelings toward the patient, but also, by extension, may relate to general issues such as patient diagnosis, medication, clinic setting, and so forth. Because more than one clinician may be involved in combined treatment (one prescribing, one nonprescribing), there are many aspects of the transference that can develop early in treatment (Table 33–2), and a variety of diagnostic possibilities to be considered in response to the countertransference feelings (Table 33–3) (Jibson 2000). Kay (2005) and others have also pointed out that during combined pharmacotherapy and psychotherapy, patients may mistakenly attribute their improvement to the medication rather than to the active steps they have taken within the psychotherapy.

Over the past half-century, the efficacy of pharmacotherapy has been demonstrated for severe mental disorders such as schizophrenia, psychotic depression, bipo-

TABLE 33–1. Patient triaging issues associated with pharmacotherapy/psychotherapy decisions

- No recognized guidelines are available for determining the best types of care based on symptoms, specific diagnosis, or factors such as age, gender, and comorbid psychiatric or medical disorders.

- Triage is often based on insurance benefits or ability to pay.

- Many managed behavioral care intermediaries are judged according to the number of days that elapse before patients are seen by a clinician after the initial call for help. This system encourages assignment of a patient to the first available clinician rather than to the best clinician for that particular patient.

- Most insurance plans impose limits on the total number of psychotherapy or psychopharmacology encounters in a certain time period. Some insurance companies complicate the process even more by not allowing patients to schedule a psychotherapy session and a medication-review session on the same day.

- Patients do not necessarily get what they want. They may ask to see a psychiatrist; however, on the basis of the symptoms for which they are presenting, they will not be assigned to a psychiatrist, at least initially, or one may not be available.

- Much of the mental health system's triaging is conducted via telephone by workers with a variety of backgrounds, not necessarily by licensed mental health practitioners.

- Little outcomes research has examined the above-mentioned nonstandardized procedures.

- Often there is little collaboration between the professions (psychiatry, psychology, social work, primary care) on the best ways to triage and manage the issues of combined pharmacotherapy and psychotherapy. Systems of collaboration often evolve in an improvisational manner, and their stability and permanence depend primarily on payment/reimbursement factors.

- Issues related to combined pharmacotherapy and psychotherapy (e.g., sequencing) have been more extensively studied in outpatient settings, with much less attention given to psychiatry inpatient services.

- The role of the primary care provider as gatekeeper in diagnosing and triaging patients for psychotherapy and pharmacotherapy continues to be a major and important area of study. It is difficult for primary care clinicians to sort out psychiatric symptoms in the short amount of time they have with patients.

Source.   Adapted from Riba MB, Balon R: "Introduction to Integrated and Split Treatment," in *Competency in Combining Pharmacotherapy and Psychotherapy: Integrated and Split Treatment.* Arlington, VA, American Psychiatric Publishing, 2005, pp. 3–4.

TABLE 33–2. Interaction of external and internal factors in positive and negative transference feelings experienced by the patient toward the psychiatrist and the medication early in treatment

External issues	Positive factors	Transference feelings
Psychiatrist	Professional appearance	Confidence and trust
	Observance of social conventions	Validation of symptoms and distress
	Empathic listening	Nurtured
	Patient education	Cared for
	Patient involvement in decision making	Educated
	Adherence to scheduled appointment times	
	Prompt, focused response to telephone calls	
	Courteous, efficient support staff	
Medication	Highly effective	Benevolent gift
	Favorable side-effect profile	Healing remedy
	Easy to use	Useful tool
	Rapid response	Validation of suffering
		Source of hope
		Transitional object

(continued)

TABLE 33–2. Interaction of external and internal factors in positive and negative transference feelings experienced by the patient toward the psychiatrist and the medication early in treatment *(continued)*

Internal issues	Negative factors	Transference feelings
Psychiatrist	Disorganized	Distrust
	Odd behavior, grooming, or dress	Lack of confidence
	Rude interactions	Dismissed symptoms and distress
	Uninterested in patient	Disregarded
	Careless	Demeaned
	Dismissive of complaints	Confused
Medication	Limited effectiveness	Crutch
	Unfavorable side effects	Artificial treatment
	Difficult to remember	Poison
	Gradual response	Deny or avoid real issues
		Minimize interaction with therapist

Source. Reprinted from Tasman T, Riba MB, Silk KR (eds): *The Doctor–Patient Relationship in Pharmacotherapy: Improving Treatment Effectiveness.* New York, Guilford, 2000, p. 100. Copyright 2000, The Guilford Press. Used with permission.

TABLE 33–3. Diagnostic possibilities to be considered in response to countertransference feelings

Countertransference feeling	Possible patient symptom
Anger	Manipulation
Boredom	Personal disconnection
Defensiveness	Anger, hostility
Fear	Paranoia, aggression
Hopelessness	Hopelessness
Narcissism	Idealization
Rescue fantasies	Dependency
Sexual arousal	Seductiveness

Source. Reprinted from Tasman T, Riba MB, Silk KR (eds): *The Doctor–Patient Relationship in Pharmacotherapy: Improving Treatment Effectiveness.* New York, Guilford, 2000, p. 112. Copyright 2000, The Guilford Press. Used with permission.

lar disorder, and obsessive-compulsive disorder (Klerman et al. 1994). However, although the medications are effective for target symptoms, patients often have persistent psychosocial and interpersonal difficulties as well as vocational and problem-solving issues—issues not addressed by medication. As noted by Thase (2003), combined treatments came to be viewed as a means of lessening psychosocial dysfunction and improving quality of life over and above what medication can do alone. In addition, it was hoped that psychotherapy could improve adherence to medication regimens. Some therapies, such as cognitive-behavioral treatment, have been found useful as adjunctive treatment even for disorders such as schizophrenia (Turkington et al. 2004). Evidence also indicated that some forms of psychother-

apy by themselves were useful for anxiety and nonpsychotic depressive disorders. Many researchers and clinicians have tried to study combined psychotherapy and pharmacotherapy with the view that the two modalities work by nonoverlapping mechanisms—which might permit additive effects—or at least by synergistic effects. Thase (2000) and Keller et al. (2000) have shown that although there may be some synergistic and additive effects in combined treatments, it is difficult to control for and appreciate all of the nonspecific effects that occur in such complex treatment arrangements.

Wright and Hollifield (2006), discussing Gabbard (2006), noted that "genetic and biological effects of psychotherapy research strongly support an integrative model for treatment (an integrative model means combining pharmacotherapy and psychotherapy in any way) and undercut dualistic theories that separate mind and body" (p. 143). They also hypothesize some possible interactions between treatments, which are summarized in Table 33–4. Gabbard (2006), citing Hollon and Fawcett (2007), pointed out that combining treatments may enhance the magnitude of the response, the probability of response, the breadth of response, and the acceptability of treatment.

The combination of pharmacotherapy and psychotherapy frequently seems to provide various advantages and benefits over pharmacotherapy or psychotherapy alone. It is hoped that future research will provide more evidence for the advantages of combined treatment in various, if not all, mental disorders.

In this chapter we highlight some of the major aspects of combined treatment, including the choice of integrated versus split treatment; the disorders for which evidence supports the efficacy of combined

TABLE 33–4. Some hypothesized interactions between pharmacotherapy and psychotherapy

	Positive	Negative
Medication	Medication could improve concentration and thus improve memory and ability to participate in and learn from psychotherapy. Medication could reduce distorted or irrational thinking and thus promote salutary effects of psychotherapy. Medication could decrease anxiety, physiological arousal, or other painful mood states and thereby influence the patient's ability to gain from psychotherapy.	Medication could interfere with learning and impair the ability of the patient to recall or use lessons learned in therapy. Pharmacotherapy could cause a heightened risk for relapse after medication is discontinued, which might negatively affect the long-term relapse prevention effects of certain therapies. Dependency on benzodiazepines could have deleterious effects on the influence of psychotherapy. Medication could lead to premature relief of symptoms, which might reduce motivation to continue in psychotherapy.
Psychotherapy	Psychotherapy could improve medication adherence. Psychotherapy could help patients better understand and manage their illnesses. Psychotherapy could assist patients in dealing with stress, interpersonal issues, and other psychosocial influences. Psychotherapy could improve the relapse prevention effect of medication. Psychotherapy could have biological effects that work together with medication to reverse biological abnormalities.	Psychotherapy could place undue stress on patients' biologically driven illnesses.

Source. Adapted from Wright JH, Hollifield M: "Combining Pharmacotherapy and Psychotherapy. Guest Editorial." *Psychiatric Annals* 36:302–305, 2006.

treatment, and the considerations in selecting specific medications and psychotherapies for integrated- and split-treatment arrangements.

Definition of Integrated and Split Treatment

Many terms have been used in the literature to describe split and integrated treatment (Table 33–5) (Riba and Balon 2001).

We define *integrated treatment* as treatment in which pharmacotherapy and psychotherapy are provided by a single clinician, and *split treatment* as treatment in which pharmacotherapy and psychotherapy are provided by at least two different clinicians. Table 33–6 lists some examples of the types of clinicians who may be involved in the delivery of split and integrated treatment.

TABLE 33–5. Terms used to describe split and integrated treatment

Collaborative treatment

Combined treatment

Concurrent care

Co-treatment

Divided treatment

Integrated care

Conjoint treatment

Medical backup

Medication check

Medication management

Shared treatment

Split treatment

Triangular (or triangulated) treatment

TABLE 33–6. Integrated versus split treatment: professionals involved

A—Integrated treatment	B—Split treatment
Psychotherapy and pharmacotherapy provided by:	Psychotherapy and pharmacotherapy provided by a combination of clinicians from columns A and B
Psychiatrist	Psychiatrist
Internist/specialist	Psychologist
Family physician	Social worker
Psychiatric nurse practitioner or physician's assistant	Clergy
	Nurse
	Counselor (substance abuse)
Psychologist (in states allowing prescribing privileges)	
Osteopathic physician	

These definitions carry some nuances. For example, Kay (2001, p. xv) wrote: "Integrated or combined treatment is the simultaneous prescription of psychotherapy and pharmacotherapy in the treatment of a patient's mental illness." Whether medication and psychotherapy are given simultaneously or sequenced and which comes first are very interesting and complex issues. Even the very question of whether providing medication is really a psychological and/or biological treatment begs the overall issue of whether providing medication "alone" is really "integrated treatment." Steven Roose (2001) has offered a very cogent historical review of this topic, noting that when psychotropic medication first became available for psychiatric disorders, the analytic literature reflected a treatment hierarchy in which psychological treatment, specifically analytic treatment, was viewed as deep, curative, and to be left undisturbed when possible. Medication was provided to relieve symptoms without affecting the underlying psychic conflicts that were viewed as the etiology of psychological illness. From work by Gorman et al. (2000) and Kandel (1979), we have come to understand that effective treatments are not exclusively psychological or biological and that psychiatric disorders themselves are both psychological and biological. The literature addressing concepts of "mind–brain dichotomy" has noted that psychotherapy influences brain function and pharmacotherapy in turn influences the mind (Beitman 2003).

The research on combining psychotherapy and pharmacotherapy has been reviewed by Thase (2000)

and others, yielding some general conclusions. These conclusions are summarized in Table 33–7.

Integrated Treatment

Some of the difficulties surrounding the choice of integrated versus split treatment relate to the following:

1. How patients are triaged
2. Who conducts the evaluation and makes the diagnosis
3. The experience and skill level of the clinician in various types of psychotherapy
4. The goals, commitment, and resources of the patient
5. What the clinician(s) can reasonably hope to accomplish

Regardless of whether the patient is recommended for integrated treatment or split treatment, questions about the type of psychotherapy and the use of medication (whether or not to use it, when to administer it, and what type to use) clearly are relevant factors.

The first contact and the doctor–patient relationship begin with the telephone call for the initial appointment, and whoever speaks with the patient to schedule the appointment acts as an extension of the physician (Simon 2004). When a patient calls to schedule an appointment with a clinician, he or she is having a problem. The patient may have some expectations or views about what he or she might need based on his or her history, the experiences of his or her friends or family members with similar (or different) problems, portrayals in the media, or something that was said by another clinician if a clinician recommended that the patient make the call. As another explanation, perhaps the patient has no expectations and just wants help.

As described by Bender and Messner (2003), the initial call may be challenging for the novice therapist and also for the patient. It should be approached with the patient's privacy and concerns in mind (Bender and Messner 2003). The focus of the initial call is usually scheduling the initial session and determining whether insurance will cover costs. A realistic time frame for the initial session should be provided (the time should be suitable for both the patient and the clinician without the necessity of rushing in and out), and the length and cost of the session should be specified.

The first moments of the session are very important and can be anxiety provoking for the patient. The patient may analyze the way the clinician greets him or her (addressing the patient in the waiting area should be done in a way that preserves the patient's confidential-

TABLE 33–7. Conclusions from research in combined psychotherapy–pharmacotherapy

- Compared with either pharmacotherapy or psychotherapy alone, combined treatments do not uniformly provide additive benefits.

- Psychotherapy can take many forms; thus, when trying to determine whether a combination of pharmacotherapy and psychotherapy is more beneficial than either alone, it is important to be specific about what we mean. Cognitive therapy, couples therapy, and interpersonal therapies are all different, and we need to be clear about what we are specifically recommending. Furthermore, it is important to understand what measures will be used to assess response. Examples would be decreases in symptoms, rehospitalization rates, and relapse rates after treatment.

- During the process of psychotherapy, pharmacotherapy can be viewed as another psychotherapeutic intervention, making the distinction between split versus integrated care somewhat artificial (Beitman et al. 2003). Pharmacotherapy can be viewed as providing not only the active drug but also the "placebo" response, and the action of offering, prescribing, and changing medications.

- One of the basic maxims of therapeutics is to try one treatment at a time—that is, either psychotherapy or pharmacotherapy. However, there are many factors on which clinicians must base their decisions, such as patient preference, diagnosis, family history, symptom severity, previous response to treatment, family dynamics, expense, availability of clinician or type of recommended care, medical comorbidities, and substance use history. Some have suggested that both pharmacotherapy and psychotherapy should be tried from the beginning (M. Fava and Rush 2006).

- Research in the area of pharmacotherapy versus psychotherapy versus the combination is very expensive and difficult. There are many subjective aspects—even if clinicians are using manuals to provide psychotherapy, there are differences in manner, style, warmth of clinicians, and the relationship between patient and clinician. Furthermore, the order of sequencing of medication and psychotherapy probably matters for individual patients. Patient preference, patient and family psychiatric and medical history, and diagnoses are variables that affect outcome, and it is difficult, perhaps impossible, to control for these aspects in research designs.

Source. Adapted from Thase ME: "Psychopharmacology in Conjunction With Psychotherapy," in *Handbook of Psychological Change: Psychotherapy Process and Practices for the 21st Century.* Edited by Ingram R, Snyder RC. New York, Wiley, 2000, pp. 474–497.

ity), what the clinician looks like, whether and how the clinician shakes the patient's hand, and how the waiting room and office are decorated (e.g., the presence of any personal items in the office). First impressions count in almost every situation, and this is certainly true of the interaction between doctor and patient.

Patients often come in with biases, and it is helpful to understand these as well as patients' belief systems (Carli 1999) regarding medication and psychotherapy. For example, some patients have had positive experiences and been helped by psychotropic medication or other types of medication (e.g., antibiotics) in the past and therefore might be quite open to thinking about medication. If patients have had adverse drug reactions, allergic reactions, or serious side effects from medications, it would be important to discuss these issues.

Patients may be quite frightened about their psychiatric symptoms and what they imagine or fear about seeing a psychiatrist. There are many stigmatizing portrayals in movies, television, and other media in which seeing a psychiatrist is represented as a po-

tentially scary event with frightening consequences such as being locked up, being placed in a straitjacket, being immediately administered electroconvulsive therapy, or being put in a diabetic coma. Although most patients would probably not be worried about such things, it certainly would behoove the clinician to try to assess these issues and begin to allay the patient's fears and worries.

It is also important for the clinician to ask the patient about what led him or her to make the call for the appointment; how that process went; whether there was any difficulty in getting in to see the clinician; and then, as part of the history taking, what beliefs and issues the patient has that will need to be sorted out between the patient and the clinician.

Several questions to consider asking a potential patient during the initial telephone contact are listed in Table 33–8. These are open-ended questions that might help elicit issues, thoughts, and feelings that would be important to understand. If these questions are not asked early on, it is sometimes difficult to go back and retrieve important information.

TABLE 33–8. Questions to ask a patient in the initial telephone call for an appointment

- Approach the phone call with the patient's privacy and concerns in mind.

- Focus on scheduling the first session and discussing insurance coverage.

- Provide a realistic time for the initial session (i.e., a time suitable for both the patient and the clinician without the necessity of rushing in and out).

- Specify the length of the session and the cost of the session

Source.   Adapted from Bender S, Messner E: *Becoming a Therapist. What Do I Say, and Why?* New York, Guilford Press, 2003.

From the patient's point of view, the objective of the first session is often to establish comfort with and trust in the doctor. The patient wants to know if the physician has the ability, empathy, skill, and experience to be able to help him or her with the presenting symptoms and any future symptoms. Does this doctor understand what has brought the patient to the clinic? Does the doctor seem interested in the patient? And if there is some feeling that the clinician does understand, what is the hook or draw that will bring the patient back to be seen for follow-up?

The questions that the patient asks during the initial session may be about psychotherapy: Will a couch be used? Will the patient be hypnotized or hospitalized? Will the patient's significant other be asked to join in the sessions? How much will the patient be asked to reveal? How often will the patient need to come to sessions, and for how long—months or years? What is the doctor's availability, and will the patient even be seeing the doctor for follow-up? The questions may be about medication: Will the patient be forced to take medication? Will it be something like what the patient's sibling or friend has taken? What are the side effects? Will the medication have an impact on sexuality? How long will the patient need to take the medication? How much will it cost?

During the initial interview, the psychiatrist is engaged in psychotherapy: establishing and evolving the doctor–patient relationship; forming an alliance with the patient; learning to understand the resources, coping mechanisms, strengths, and weaknesses of the patient; and setting an agenda for future sessions. Whether the focus of this session is on medication, diagnosis, or other issues, the doctor must show competence, confidence, and the ability to gauge the pa-

tient's capacity for self-reflection and goal setting and must determine whether the patient is ready for the next steps. The patient's safety must always be assessed and evaluated. Although the first session contains open-ended questions, the time restriction will not allow for the entire session to be open ended, so the psychiatrist needs to become more directive. The note writing should not be extensive and should be explained to the patient in a positive fashion.

Prior to talking about medication, a diagnosis must be made. For example, one cannot talk about prescribing an antidepressant medication without talking with the patient about mood disorders. Thus, the doctor needs to determine whether the patient is ready to listen to and accept this type of discussion. Similarly, if there is a mood disorder and interpersonal psychotherapy would also be part of the treatment, the psychiatrist needs to decide whether to discuss what this type of psychotherapy entails, how many visits are required, what the goals of treatment are, and how the psychotherapy relates to taking medication. The psychiatrist also needs to find a way to gauge the patient's readiness for change (Beitman et al. 2003). Furthermore, if there is a comorbid personality disorder, it needs to be assessed and factored into the treatment plan. Without a good history, it is almost impossible to diagnose a personality disorder.

The key ingredients of the first session of combined psychotherapy–psychopharmacology treatment are summarized in Table 33–9.

Medication: General Issues to Be Addressed

If medication is one of the treatments that may be of benefit to the patient, the psychiatrist must determine and address the issues listed in Table 33–10.

The psychiatrist needs to provide a fair amount of education to the patient (and possibly to family members) when medication is prescribed. In some states, consent forms for administering medications must be signed by patients, and fact sheets about the medication and side effects must be provided and noted in the chart. These matters all take time, and the psychiatrist must gauge how much time there is in the session and decide how much time to use for all of these issues.

Patients and families cannot be hurried. As an example, it might be wise for the psychiatrist to begin the discussion about medication but delay the actual prescribing of medication until the next visit. Information on the medication could be sent home with the patient, as well as information on the diagnosis (e.g., depres-

TABLE 33–9. Key ingredients of the first session of combined treatment

1. Forging a doctor–patient alliance

2. Inquiring about how the patient got to the first session

3. Asking about and listening to belief systems about medication and psychotherapy

4. Assessing the patient's capacity for discussion of the diagnosis, treatment plan, and types of therapy

5. Assessing the psychiatrist's own capacity to deliver the recommended type of treatments

6. Reassuring the patient about the confidential nature of the treatment but also discussing reasons why the confidentiality might need to be broken (e.g., posing a danger to oneself, posing a danger to others, engaging in child abuse)

Source.   Adapted from Riba MB, Balon R: *Competency in Combining Pharmacotherapy and Psychotherapy: Integrated and Split Treatment.* Arlington, VA, American Psychiatric Publishing, 2005, p. 21.

TABLE 33–10. Medication issues to be addressed

1. Is the patient motivated to use medication? If not, what are the factors? Denial? Externalization?

2. Which are the target symptoms for the medication? Which ones are most distressing or important to the patient?

3. What are the comorbid medical or other diagnoses that might interact or relate to the use of psychotropic medication?

4. Which side effects of the medication might be most distressing to the patient? To the patient's family members?

5. What might be the obstacles to taking the medication? (Examples include scheduling of doses, the need for blood assays and laboratory visits, general problems with adherence to taking daily medication, difficulty swallowing pills, difficulty remembering to take medications, costs of medication, problems with work- or school-related functions [e.g., driving].)

6. What beliefs does the patient have about the medication? (For example, does the patient believe that psychotropic medication is addictive or causes brain damage?)

Source.   Adapted from Riba MB, Balon R: *Competency in Combining Pharmacotherapy and Psychotherapy: Integrated and Split Treatment.* Arlington, VA, American Psychiatric Publishing, 2005, pp. 21–22.

sion). Some patients might also benefit from being informed of good Web sites where additional information might be gleaned. Clinicians might want to be prepared to direct patients to such Internet sites (Hsiung 2002).

Factors Affecting the Prescribing of Medication

Most important, psychiatrists need to assess their working alliance with the patient to make the use of medications and psychotherapy successful. In addition, the clinician's skill set and the setting—inpatient versus outpatient—are important factors.

Inpatient Setting

Starting medications is easier in the inpatient setting than in the outpatient setting for several reasons: the patient can be watched continuously for side effects; the medication is provided by a nurse on a regular schedule, and thus adherence is reinforced and possibly assured; and the cost of the medication is factored into the hospital stay. Often there are groups for discussing medications; many patients are taking medication, so individual patients do not feel singled out; and because patients are not in their usual environments (e.g., home, the workplace), certain issues do not arise, such as the need to drive or to have quick reflexes. There are attending psychiatrists, nurses, and other professionals who can speak with the patient and the family to reinforce the diagnosis and the need for medication with certain types of disorders. On inpatient units, sleep patterns are monitored; appetite changes are evaluated by daily weighing and by noting food remaining on trays; and gastrointestinal side effects are noted. Medications tend to be given in somewhat higher dosages than in the outpatient setting, because the dosages can be readjusted quickly.

In addition, clinicians can arrange consultations with other physicians should there be worries about interactions with patients' other medical problems. Family meetings are usually organized to discuss a range of issues, and medications can be an item for discussion if the family and patient so choose. In addition, the hospital usually has medications available in a wide range of preparations (e.g., pill, liquid, injection), so there are options if the patient has difficulty with one type. The pharmacists in the hospital are usually very helpful with cutting pills and making it as easy as possible for patients to receive medications that are ordered.

Outpatient Setting

The outpatient setting is more difficult with regard to prescribing medications. As opposed to inpatient units, where there is a steady and constant monitoring of medication issues, there is usually a time interval between when the patient is first prescribed the medication and when the clinician next sees the patient. The clinician must inquire about the patient's form of payment for medication to make sure, for example, that the proposed medication will be on the patient's pharmacy formulary. Copayments are an issue, especially for many patients who take a number of medications. This is also a matter for discussion.

The physician might want to ask the patient to call and discuss how he or she is doing with the medication before the next appointment, especially if the follow-up appointment is not for a few weeks. The practice of scheduling a follow-up appointment for a new patient several weeks after the initial meeting should be discouraged; rather, the patient should be seen for follow-up promptly (e.g., within 1 or 2 weeks). Frequent follow-up is especially important in view of the new governmental recommendations for starting antidepressant therapy in youth, which suggest, ideally, at least weekly face-to-face contact with patients or their family members or caregivers during the first 4 weeks of medication treatment, then visits every other week for the next 4 weeks, then a visit at 12 weeks, and as clinically indicated beyond 12 weeks; additional contact by telephone may also be appropriate between face-to-face visits. During the initial phase of any treatment, it is important to help dispel anxieties about the treatment, side effects, and other issues and to foster the doctor–patient relationship. This approach to scheduling helps ensure that the physician learns about any negative side effects or problems that the patient might be having with the medication; it also offers the opportunity to discuss the dosage (and change it if necessary) and, most importantly, enables the patient to feel that the physician cares about the impact of the medication and that patient and physician are in a partnership regarding medication.

Some patients wish to use e-mail to communicate with the clinician, but we urge that communication regarding medication be conducted over the telephone and/or in person and that such conversations be documented in the patient's chart. There are various problems with e-mail communication (e.g., confidentiality, lack of nonverbal cues, time delays), and because there are so many potential problems with medication, we suggest that the telephone be used rather than e-mail (Yager 2003).

Because patients are usually working and are engaged in treatment in the outpatient setting, it is important to find out the impact of taking medications while on the job. For example, if the patient is driving as part of his or her job, does the psychotropic medication affect the patient's ability to drive or to have quick reflexes? If so, there may be a need to modify either the medication or the time of day it is taken or to try to have the patient's work responsibilities modified.

Most psychotropic medications affect libido or cause other sexual side effects, so it is important for the clinician to ask the patient questions about these effects. Patients often are too embarrassed to raise such issues and feel more secure when the physician asks about these important matters. The same is true for weight gain, sleep problems, and constipation, so these must all be routine questions.

Sometimes patients will note that their significant other or various family members are concerned about the medication they are taking. It is helpful for the physician to understand this concern, because it could be a deterrent to the patient's adherence to the medication regimen. It could be useful, for example, to have the concerned family member attend part of or a full session with the patient to discuss any problems.

Medication should be kept away from young children. It is important for the psychiatrist to ascertain who at home might have access to the patient's medication and to make sure that the medication is kept in a safe and secure location. If the patient does not want his or her children to know about the psychiatric problems or the medication, the psychiatrist should discuss this matter with the patient.

It is also very important to ascertain the patient's suicidality, homicidality, and potential for violence at every session, particularly when the patient is taking psychotropic medication—and, as noted, especially during the initial phase of antidepressant therapy.

Comorbid Medical Conditions and Substance Abuse/Dependence

Medical conditions.   Psychiatrists must be knowledgeable about patients' medical conditions, what medications patients are taking, and patients' medical and surgical histories. Allergies to medications must be noted. Especially in the outpatient setting, the psychiatrist must let the patient know that changes in medical condition or medications during the interval between appointments need to be reported to the clinician.

Communication between the psychiatrist and the primary care providers or specialists needs to be done with the patient's written consent. It is imperative that the psychiatrist let the other providers know when psychotropic medications are added or changed, again with the patient's written approval. Most patients are very appreciative that such communication occurs. Some patients may be embarrassed or say that they will feel stigmatized if their primary care provider or other doctors know about their need for psychotropic medication. In such cases, there must be frank and open discussion between the psychiatrist and the patient, and the psychiatrist should point out that he or she cannot provide good care to the patient if such information is not communicated to the other clinicians. Serious harm to the patient could result if the other clinicians do not know about the patient's use of psychotropic medication. For example, there could be problems with interactions between medications; changes in blood concentrations of medications could occur if the various prescribers are unaware of all the medications the patient is taking. If patients prohibit such communication, the psychiatrist must seriously question whether proper care can be provided to the patient, and alternatives must be discussed.

The patient (and all physician and clinician providers) should be clear about who is in charge of which medications. Primary care physicians should not, for example, prescribe psychotropic medication or change dosages without letting the psychiatrist and other mental health clinicians know, and vice versa—the psychiatrist should not prescribe medications other than psychotropic medications (although there are emergency or other exceptions for both parties). If there is no electronic medical record or if the patient is not being seen in a closed system, the caregivers should discuss ahead of time how to transmit such information in a timely fashion (e.g., telephone, e-mail, fax, letter). It should not be the responsibility of the patient to be the provider of such information.

Substance abuse/dependence. Substance abuse and dependence are the subject of another important discussion, especially in the outpatient setting, where patients have greater access to substances of abuse. Patients often do not like to admit their dependence and use of such substances as nicotine, alcohol, marijuana, and other drugs. In addition, many patients have dependences on prescribed drugs such as hydrocodone bitartrate and oxycodone hydrochloride. It is important for the physician to refrain from making assumptions about such problems and to ask questions, offer appropriate referrals for substance abuse treatment (possibly to a dual-diagnosis program), and watch carefully to determine whether prescriptions for benzodiazepines, for example, are used up too quickly. If

patients are not doing as well as expected with a certain medication over a certain period of time, the psychiatrist should consider whether there may be a confounding substance problem. Substance abuse might also be suspected in patients who ask for medical leave that is not commensurate with the primary psychiatric diagnosis. It is important to obtain a good history of substance abuse or dependence issues when starting treatment and before prescribing psychotropic medication and to continually assess for ongoing problems.

It is also important to consider the role and influence of Alcoholics Anonymous (AA). Frequently, AA participants and sponsors (particularly those who are less experienced) discourage patients from using psychotropic medications. While they may be right about benzodiazepines, it is important to clarify the role of antidepressants and other classes of psychotropic medications.

Patient Preferences and Beliefs

Some patients or their family members may be resistant to medication in general or to specific medications in particular (e.g., "I will not take lithium; that is heavy stuff"). Their preferences may also be colored by previous experiences with medications and side effects. Patients and families may be also influenced by various media reports and by direct-to-consumer advertising.

Psychiatrist Experience, Training, and Preferences

Clinical psychopharmacology has developed significantly and became quite complex over the past two decades. Psychiatrists may not be familiar with all of the new medications that have appeared on the market since they received their psychiatric training. They may have learned to use one or two medications from each class. They may be also influenced by advertising and by sales representatives.

Factors Affecting Psychotherapy Treatment Planning in Integrated Treatment

Developing a biopsychosocial formulation is the key to understanding a patient's diagnosis and devising a treatment plan. It is almost impossible to recommend a certain modality of psychotherapy without having provided it oneself. This is an area where training and abundant clinical experience are very important.

Formulating a Problem List

Although the psychiatric diagnosis is determined by using the DSM classification system, psychiatrists function under the medical model whereby they need to address the patient's issues in terms of a problem summary list. The patient's presenting problems are added to the list that already exists in the patient's file or electronic medical record. For psychiatrists, there are issues of confidentiality, privacy, and other matters that must be addressed in all systems of care.

Prioritizing Problems

It is important for the clinician to compile a list of the patient's problems and then to determine, with the patient's help, how these should be prioritized and sequenced. This is difficult work, because it often involves discussing issues that are not necessarily clear to the patient (or to the clinician) at the time. Sometimes it means waiting for further information or insight from other family members; it could mean waiting for a new job, a change in marital structure, or results of medical tests before determining the next steps. It is important for the psychiatrist to exercise patience and provide guidance without being intrusive or too directive and without moving too far ahead of the patient.

Determining Treatment Aims

One of the major tasks for the psychiatrist and the patient is to determine the aims—both pharmacological and psychotherapeutic—of the treatment. Once established, the aims should be constantly evaluated and reevaluated and may need to be modified or changed. Few assumptions should be made in the process. This undertaking is challenging, and combining medication and psychotherapy makes it difficult to tease apart cause and effect. Nevertheless, this is a major task to be addressed at every session.

Outlining the Time Frame

One of the questions most frequently asked by patients and their families is how long the process is going to take—how long will they need to take medication, and how long and how often do they need to receive psychotherapy? Most important, they want to know how soon they will begin to feel better, how long it will take for their symptoms to improve, when they can go back to work, and when they can expect to start doing better at school.

Diagnosis

As discussed earlier, evidence for the efficacy of psychotherapy in general, or of a certain type of psychotherapy in particular, in the treatment of various mental illnesses is still insufficient. Nonetheless, the diagnosis may influence the choice of psychotherapy (assuming that the psychiatrist is fairly skilled in the indicated modality). For instance, interpersonal and social rhythm therapy (Frank 2005) may be the treatment of choice for maintenance of bipolar disorder, whereas assertiveness training, role-playing, and behavioral modeling may be selected for nonmelancholic depression with features of rejection sensitivity (Parker and Manicavasagar 2005). Some personality disorders—for example, borderline personality disorder—may respond best to psychotherapy specifically in an integrated treatment model, to allow more focus on integration rather than splitting.

Patient Beliefs and Preferences

Some patients (or their family members) may not be willing to start therapy, as they may wish for a "quick fix with medication." Patients may have had a negative experience with psychotherapy previously (e.g., the course was not successful, their interaction with the therapist was not positive), or they may already be enrolled in psychotherapy elsewhere (here, the physician must decide whether to enter into a split-treatment arrangement with the existing therapist).

Psychiatrist/Physician Skills and Experience

Psychiatrists have historically been trained mostly in psychodynamic psychotherapy and in some variants of brief psychotherapy. The new Accreditation Council of Graduate Medical Education (ACGME) Residency Review Committee in Psychiatry competency requirements also include acquisition of skills and experience in cognitive-behavioral therapy and supportive therapy. Most psychiatrists, however, probably do not maintain skills in and practice *all* major psychotherapy modalities, and thus may not always be prepared to use the most appropriate psychotherapeutic modality for a specific patient (here, again, the physician must decide whether to enter into a split-treatment arrangement).

Sequence of Treatment Modalities

Sequencing of treatment modalities in integrated treatment means either starting with pharmacotherapy and later adding psychotherapy or vice versa. Psychiatrists usually start with one modality, see how it works, and then add the other one. G. A. Fava (1999) has proposed that treatment of acute major depression be started with antidepressant medication and that cognitive-behavioral therapy be reserved for the continuation phase. However, sequencing may be quite complex, and we need to learn more about it. Some may argue that clinicians considering integrated treatment should adopt a variant of the approach suggested by M. Fava and Rush (2006) for pharmacotherapy: use of augmentation or combination strategies in pharmacotherapy from the outset of treatment. It remains to be explored whether an analogous approach to integrated treatment—that is, starting medication and psychotherapy at the same time—is the best one.

Referrals and Complexity

As pointed out by Kay (2005), some patients who require medication and suffer from various severe conditions may do better in the integrated model. Some patients may be referred to a psychiatrist by a therapist who feels that a more complex approach is required, or by another physician-specialist who prefers collaboration with just one mental health professional. Once the initial evaluation is completed and some or all of the issues affecting the selection of medication and psychotherapy are addressed, the decision about sequencing has to be made, and treatment starts.

The issue of sequencing may also come into consideration at the time of treatment termination. Pharmacotherapy may be terminated first, with some form of psychotherapy continuing, either to maintain the level achieved or to address various dynamic and other issues. Psychotherapy may also be terminated first, with continuation of medication as a maintenance therapy (e.g., lithium in bipolar illness). Rarely, both modalities could be terminated simultaneously (e.g., the patient leaves town). As we have suggested elsewhere (Riba and Balon 2005), termination must be carefully planned, either from the beginning in the case of short-term treatment, or several months in advance in the case of long-term treatment. Patient worries about termination and transference must be addressed regularly. In cases where psychotherapy is terminated first, patients should be offered several intermittent sessions. Medication may need to be adjusted when psychotherapy is being terminated first. Patients should be warned to avoid stressors during the termination.

Split Treatment

As mentioned earlier, we define split treatment as pharmacotherapy and psychotherapy that are divided or shared by at least two different clinicians. There are several ways in which a psychiatrist can find himself or herself providing split treatment for a patient. Possible scenarios include the following:

A. A patient is seen by a psychiatrist for an evaluation. In the course of the evaluation, the psychiatrist determines that it would be best for the patient to see another clinician (usually a social worker or psychologist) for psychotherapy, and for the psychiatrist to see the patient for medication and medical issues related to the treatment.

B. A patient is seen by a psychiatrist for an evaluation. In the course of the evaluation, the patient tells the physician that he or she is already seeing a therapist and was referred for medication. The psychiatrist, assuming that he or she feels that medication is warranted, agrees to be the provider of the psychotropic medication and other pertinent medical management.

C. A patient is already being seen by a therapist. A primary care physician or other physician has been treating the patient with psychotropic medication, but the patient is not improving, so the physician (or the therapist) refers the patient to a clinic/psychiatrist for more expert evaluation and treatment.

D. A patient is seeing a psychiatrist for integrated treatment (psychotherapy and medication), but the psychotherapy part of the integrated care will be ending soon for some reason (e.g., psychotherapy in the frame of integrated treatment met an impasse; insurance benefits changed; patient can no longer afford to see the psychiatrist for psychotherapy and medication). The psychiatrist decides to continue to see the patient for medication and medical management while the patient is seeing another therapist.

In all of the situations outlined above, there are specific decisions that the psychiatrist must make in determining the proper care for the patient; what the psychiatrist is able and competent to provide; the timing of the combination and sequencing of medication and psychotherapy; and to whom the psychiatrist should refer the patient, based on the need for a certain type of psychotherapy.

The issues and tasks noted are some of the most difficult for even seasoned clinicians. The psychiatrist must often make these assessments in a single evaluation while also trying to formulate a diagnosis and a treatment plan, assess strengths and weaknesses of the treatment plan and obstacles to its implementation, and ascertain the patient's access to care.

The initial issues to be addressed in split treatment are similar to the issues previously described as important to address at the beginning of split treatment. These are listed in Table 33–11.

TABLE 33–11. Issues that need to be addressed at the beginning of split treatment

1. Forge a doctor–patient alliance (which, due to the nature of split treatment, is usually more difficult to forge).

2. Inquire about the referral for medication and how the patient feels about it.

3. Ask about the patient's belief systems about medication and psychotherapy, and medication versus psychotherapy.

4. Assess the patient's capacity for discussion of the diagnosis, treatment plan, combining medication and therapy, and risk and benefits of medication.

5. Assess the psychiatrist's own capacity to participate in split treatment.

6. Reassure the patient about the confidential nature of the treatment, but also discuss reasons why the confidentiality might be broken (e.g., posing a danger to oneself or to others, engaging in child abuse) and whether and how there will be communication between the physician and the patient's therapist. The physician must ask the patient explicitly for permission to communicate whether all issues that may arise may be communicated with the therapist or whether some issues should not and if so, why not.

Source. Adapted from Riba MB, Balon R: *Competency in Combining Pharmacotherapy and Psychotherapy: Integrated and Split Treatment.* Arlington, VA, American Psychiatric Publishing, 2005, p. 21.

As is true for integrated treatment, the prescribing physician must also address the patient's motivation to take medication, target symptoms, comorbidity issues, possible side effects, obstacles (blood levels, multiple doses), and patient beliefs. In addition, the prescribing physician must be prepared to address the therapist's feelings and beliefs about medication and what has been communicated about the medication between the patient and his or her therapist.

Split treatment has its positive and negative aspects (Balon 1999, 2001; Goldsmith et al. 1999). Potentially positive aspects include capitalizing on the special skills and talents of the therapist and psychiatrist, cost-effective utilization of available resources, the opportunity for the patient to select a therapist of the same gender or similar ethnic background, increased time and resources available for the patient, increased amount of clinical information, enhanced compliance, and professional and emotional support for both therapist and psychiatrist. Negative aspects of split treatment include splitting; misperceptions by therapist, patient, and/or

psychiatrist; inappropriate prescribing of medication by psychiatrist when he or she is not aware of what is going on in therapy; various legal and ethical issues (addressed later); competition between therapist and psychiatrist (Kay 2005); and various other issues.

Kay (2005) provided some useful guidelines for avoiding or managing some of the potential pitfalls that may reduce the effectiveness of split treatment. He suggested that split cases should be carefully selected; that psychiatrist and therapist should agree on the boundaries and responsibilities of the case; and that they should agree on communication between themselves and with the patient and family on issues of coverage when one of the treating parties is out of town, as well as on discussions with insurance companies. Kay also recommended obtaining informed consent for all aspects of split treatment. Further recommendations included psychoeducation of the patient and his or her family, educating the therapist about decisions regarding medication, and avoiding using the patient to convey information that would be more appropriately conveyed in a direct discussion between the therapist and psychiatrist (Kay 2005).

Factors Affecting the Prescribing of Medication in Split Treatment

Previously, we discussed factors affecting the prescribing of medication. These issues certainly also affect prescribing of medication in split treatment. We list these and additional factors in Table 33–12, with discussion of the additional factors to follow.

TABLE 33–12. Factors affecting the prescribing of medication in split treatment

Primary factors

1. Inpatient versus outpatient setting

2. Comorbid medical conditions

3. Substance abuse/dependence

4. Patient's preferences/beliefs

5. Psychiatrist's experience, training, and preferences

Additional factors

6. Therapist's experience, training, and preferences

7. Psychiatrist's experience, training, and preferences regarding split treatment

8. Patient's beliefs, preferences, and fantasies about split treatment

9. Communication between prescribing psychiatrist and therapist

Other factors that may affect the prescribing of medication in split treatment include the following:

1. *Therapist experience, training, and preferences.* Some therapists may (consciously or unconsciously) have negative feelings/attitudes toward medication (as some physicians may have toward psychotherapy). Thus, they may have consciously or unconsciously, and obviously or less obviously, communicated these feelings/attitudes to the patient. Therapists may also not be properly trained in split treatment and may not communicate properly with the treating physician about issues surrounding medication that come to light during psychotherapy sessions (e.g., subtle side effects not mentioned or explored during medication review due to lack of time, overestimation of side effects, lack of improvement not properly communicated by the patient to the physician due to fear of disappointing the physician). The therapist may also feel forced to agree to split treatment (e.g., by circumstances, patient, family members, insurance companies looking for quick fix) despite preferring to address the illness and related issues without medication. Finally, the therapist may have had a negative experience with a split-treatment arrangement in the past that may influence his or her current willingness to participate in these arrangements.

2. *Physician experience, training, and preferences regarding split treatment.* Some physicians may have had negative (real or perceived) experiences with split treatment. Some physicians (especially nonpsychiatric ones) may not be properly trained in collaboration with therapists. Finally, some psychiatrists may be forced to participate in split treatment by economic circumstances (e.g., patient inability to pay, lack of insurance coverage) despite preferring to provide both treatment modalities themselves, in an integrated model.

3. *Patient beliefs, preferences, and fantasies about split treatment.* Patients may also feel forced to participate in this arrangement by various circumstances (ability to pay, insurance) despite preferring to see just the physician or to not see a physician at all. These issues need to be explored and addressed by both the physician and the therapist.

4. *Communication between prescribing physician and therapist.* Open, respectful, and frequent communication between the prescribing physician and the therapist is the *sine qua non* for well-executed split treatment. The channels of communication should be open at all times, and especially during crisis.

Factors Affecting Psychotherapy Treatment Planning in Split Treatment

The factors affecting psychotherapy treatment planning in split treatment are similar to those in integrated treatment—formulating the problem list, prioritizing problems, determining treatment aims, outlining the treatment frame, diagnosis, patient beliefs and preferences, therapist skills and experience, sequencing, referrals, and complexity of the case. These factors are usually dealt with by the therapist; however, the physician should be involved in dealing with some of them, if not all of them. Take the example of diagnosis. Should the treating psychiatrist always accept the diagnosis established by the therapist? Definitely not. Both clinicians, physician and therapist, should always conduct their own thorough evaluation and arrive at a diagnosis on their own, and then compare that with the diagnosis of the other party. Some diagnoses (e.g., borderline personality disorder) may not be suitable for split treatment but rather should be referred for integrated treatment. Further factors that may affect psychotherapy treatment planning in split treatment include the psychiatrist's education, experience, and preferences, and communication between physician and therapist.

Sequencing of split treatment—that is, the issue of whether to start with medication, psychotherapy, or both—may be determined by circumstances and referrals. Starting both treatment modalities at the same time is probably very rare. Frequently, the patient may be referred for medication while being already enrolled in therapy, to enhance the treatment effect or to address the lack of improvement. The patient may be referred for therapy while being treated with medication by a physician, to address psychological issues that may or may not be related to the focus of medication treatment, in order to enhance adherence.

Similar to integrated treatment, the issue of sequencing may also come into consideration at the time of treatment termination. Pharmacotherapy may be terminated first, with some form of psychotherapy continuing, either to maintain the level achieved or to address various dynamic and other issues. Psychotherapy may also be terminated first, with continuation of medication as a maintenance therapy (e.g., lithium in bipolar illness). Rarely, both modalities might be terminated simultaneously (e.g., if the patient leaves town). As we suggested earlier (Riba and Balon 2005), termination must be carefully planned, either from the beginning, in the case of short-term treatment, or several months in advance, in the case of long-term treatment.

Both the psychiatrist and the therapist should be aware of each other's plans regarding termination, and their efforts should be coordinated. The patient could be offered a few extra or longer medication-review appointments in cases where therapy is terminated first, or vice versa when medication is terminated first.

Ethical, Legal, and Managerial Issues

Both integrated and split treatment may involve a myriad of complex ethical and legal issues. Lazarus (1999) described examples of ethical problems that may be encountered in split treatment, such as aiding and abetting of an unlicensed person in practicing medicine (e.g., signed blank prescriptions to be filled by a therapist), lack of independent decision-making regarding treatment by a psychiatrist in a managed care setting (i.e., being just a figurehead), acceptance of an evaluation and its conclusions by another mental health professional without conducting one's own patient evaluation, unethical fee splitting, inadequate time spent with a patient due to management pressures, and collaboration with an inadequately trained or licensed professional. The ethical issues involved in integrated treatment have received relatively little attention. Examples of such dilemmas include inadequate time spent by a clinician with a patient considering the fact that a single clinician provides and bills for both treatments (e.g., 15 minutes spent for both a medication review and a half-session of therapy is clearly not enough) and inadequate focus on one treatment modality while disproportionately emphasizing the other.

MacBeth (1999, 2001) outlined some of the legal challenges of split treatment as follows:

1. The relationship with and responsibility for nonmedical therapists (e.g., the problem of "sue every deep pocket," the joint and several liability problem, the "sink or swim together" issue, the "captain of the ship" problem, and the managed care contract problem).
2. Patient population and practice characteristics (e.g., the prescription of psychiatric medication to all or most patients is associated with an increased risk of mistakes related to medications; the provision of divided treatment involves predominantly severe mood and anxiety disorders with a higher chance of suicide; and this practice involves treatment of several hundred patients a year, which increases the chance of a mistake and legal action against the physician).

3. Financial profile of psychiatrist (e.g., psychiatrist may become the target and/or deep pocket; psychiatrists may be practicing in a system with a sovereign or charitable immunity; psychiatrists may be collaborating with underinsured or uninsured therapists; or psychiatrists may be assuming additional liability by contract).
4. System inflexibilities (e.g., there may be restrictions on the patient's access to a treating psychiatrist).
5. Physician–patient relationship (e.g., there may be a lack of strong therapeutic and/or family relationships).
6. Other professionals (e.g., there may be dependence on a therapist with inadequate education, licensure, and/or experience or dependence on unknown professionals).
7. Treatment without adequate information (e.g., there may be prescription of medication, approval of treatment, or acceptance of responsibility without patient assessment; systemic information failures; lack of authority; system disorganization).

MacBeth (1999) suggested that to protect oneself from some, if not all, of these issues, one should be involved in risk management and follow principles such as exercising continuing care and judgment in all practice circumstances; understanding operations and routines of every practice setting; weeding out or avoiding problematic practice settings; coordinating care with professionals with whom patient responsibility will be shared; understanding and using system reviews and appeal processes (managed care); setting a supervision schedule based on patient's condition and need; setting a schedule for personal assessment of the patient with regard to condition, status, and treatment; and not issuing an insurance policy to a managed care or other system.

As with ethical issues, the legal issues of integrated treatment have been less explored and are less clear. Kerber (1999) outlined issues in split treatment inherent to managed care, and Rand (1999) discussed how to maximize the effectiveness of split treatment in various settings.

Training Issues

As the practice of combining pharmacotherapy and psychotherapy has become the most frequently used approach to the treatment of mental disorders, questions have been raised about the competency of physicians and therapists to practice and participate in combining pharmacotherapy and psychotherapy. Previously, the apprenticeship model or the classic "see one, do one, teach one" approach was deemed appropriate. Recently, however, the Residency Review Committee for Psychiatry decided that adequate structured training and competency in various psychotherapy modalities, including combining pharmacotherapy and psychotherapy, are necessary and included that in its requirements. American Psychiatric Publishing recently published a series of texts on acquiring competency in various psychotherapies and also a text on competency in combining pharmacotherapy and psychotherapy (Riba and Balon 2005). This text outlines some crucial issues on training and supervising the competency in combining pharmacotherapy and psychotherapy; what it means to be competent; standards and domains of competency in this modality; guidelines on how to evaluate a resident's skills, knowledge, and attitudes in combining pharmacotherapy and psychotherapy; and the requirements and optimal experience in training. We believe that residents should be supervised, monitored, and evaluated in handling several cases of both integrated and split treatment during their training. We hope that other disciplines will get beyond introducing courses in very basic psychopharmacology and also require and develop training in split treatment.

Combined Treatment: General Clinical Applications[1]

There are several potential benefits to providing combined treatment not fully addressed previously. Using psychotherapy in a psychopharmacological treatment helps decrease the incidence of illness relapse (Hogarty et al. 1986) and diminishes symptom relapse upon medication discontinuation (Spiegel et al. 1994; Wiborg and Dahl 1996). The combination helps to foster the patient's ability to use healthy coping strategies, address issues that are not typically targeted by psychopharmacological treatments such as dysfunctional relationship patterns or negative self-appraisals due to traumatic past events, and enhances psychotropic compliance (Cochran 1984; Paykel 1995).

Similarly, there are positive aspects in using pharmacotherapy within a psychotherapeutic relationship

(Kay 2001; Klerman 1991). Ameliorating anxiety and other acute symptoms may help the patient to more easily participate in psychotherapy, enhance the patient's self esteem, improve the general environment of the doctor–patient relationship, improve cognition, and allow the medication to be viewed as a transitional object during intervening times in therapy.

Various sequencing patterns may be used when combining pharmacotherapy and psychotherapy. G. A. Fava (1999) summarized common patterns as follows:

1. Using a second type of psychotherapy when the first psychotherapy has not achieved full remission or treatment goals
2. Introducing a second type of pharmacotherapy when the first medication has not achieved adequate illness remission or symptom relief
3. Introducing psychotherapy when initial pharmacotherapy has not been adequately effective
4. Introducing pharmacotherapy when initial psychotherapy has not been fully effective

The complexity of combining medication and psychotherapy and sequencing the treatment is further intensified by the fact that patients ascribe different meanings to medication, to psychotherapy, to the sequence, and to themselves (Beck 2001; Carli 1999). Once a patient is in a combined treatment, especially in a split treatment, transference and countertransference usually become more prominent. Smith (1989, p. 79) noted that "in contemporary treatment situations that include a patient, a therapist, a pharmacotherapist, and a pill, the transference issues can become more complex than the landing patterns of airplanes at an overcrowded airport." Clinicians must be aware of this, and the prescribing psychiatrist must especially attend to the patient's feelings, experiences, and reactions. Patients must be given the opportunity to talk about their symptoms, problems with adherence to medication, side effects, and issues concerning their overall care. As suggested by Jibson (2000), psychiatrists can organize medication visits to address the various treatment aspects and questions that require attention (Table 33–13).

Furthermore, to help with the very complicated transference issues that percolate in combined treatments, Jibson (2000) offers a numbers of steps to handle these issues (Table 33–14).

---

[1] This section is adapted from Riba MB, Miller RR: Combined therapies: psychotherapy and pharmacotherapy, in *Psychiatry*, 2nd Edition. Edited by Tasman A, Kay J, Lieberman JF. Chichester, England, John Wiley & Sons, 2003, pp. 2184–2201.

TABLE 33–13. Suggested schedules for 15- to 30-minute medication visits

Activity	15-minute session	30-minute session
Open-ended questions	5 minutes	15 minutes
Follow-up questions	2 minutes	5 minutes
Specific questions regarding treatment response	2 minutes	3 minutes
Specific questions and discussion of side effects	2 minutes	2 minutes
Discussion of treatment plan	2 minutes	2 minutes
Patient education	1 minute	2 minutes
Prescriptions	1 minute	1 minute

Source. Reprinted from Tasman T, Riba MB, Silk KR (eds): *The Doctor–Patient Relationship in Pharmacotherapy: Improving Treatment Effectiveness.* New York, Guilford, 2000, p. 119. Copyright 2000, The Guilford Press. Used with permission.

TABLE 33–14. Steps in dealing with transference issues

Initial steps
- Determine patient preferences
- State physician preferences
- Educate the patient about diagnosis and treatment
- Discuss treatment options
- Emphasize the unique value and risks of each treatment option
- Consider the real situation
- Maintain a neutral stance regarding treatment choice

Follow-up steps
- Maintain open communication
- Listen for patterns and meanings
- Assess patient compliance
- Assess patient response
- Assess side effects
- Consider the real situation
- Review patient education
- State recommendations and their justifications clearly
- Keep other treatment options open

Source. Reprinted from Tasman T, Riba MB, Silk KR (eds): *The Doctor–Patient Relationship in Pharmacotherapy: Improving Treatment Effectiveness.* New York, Guilford, 2000, p. 117. Copyright 2000, The Guilford Press. Used with permission.

There are growing numbers of psychiatric disorders for which randomized controlled trials have evaluated combined treatments and demonstrated their efficacy. Unipolar depressive disorders, bipolar disorders, psychotic disorders, eating disorders, substance use disorders, and borderline personality disorder have well-developed American Psychiatric Association guidelines and evidence from other large studies for the efficacy of combined treatments (American Psychiatric Association 2000b, 2002b; Keller et al. 2000). Table 33–15 lists examples of some of the work done in investigating combined treatment, using unipolar depression as an example (Riba and Miller 2003).

Conclusion

Combination of pharmacotherapy and psychotherapy, involving either integrated or split approach, has become the most frequent approach to the treatment of mental disorders. Numerous studies have demonstrated the superiority of pharmacotherapy combined with psychotherapy over each modality alone. It is not clear which of the two approaches, integrated or split treatment, is more efficacious and cost-effective. An integrated approach, or one-person model, may be preferable for the treatment of severe mental disorders and for some personality disorders (e.g., borderline). The practice of split treatment has been considered to be cost-effective; however, the work of Dewan (1999) and Goldman et al. (1998) has raised questions about this assumption. Both approaches have their advantages and disadvantages. Both approaches are quite complex and require attention to multiple issues, including patients' feelings and beliefs about medication and psychotherapy, clinician experience and training, insurance coverage, and ethical and legal aspects. Numerous aspects of combined pharmacotherapy–psychotherapy treatment need to be addressed in future research. Examples of such aspects include whether an integrated or a split approach is better for certain disorders; whether both pharmacotherapy and psychotherapy should be started together or whether they should be sequenced—and, if sequenced, then in what order and for which disorders; and what factors in integrated or split treatment are critical to improving patient outcome (Kay 2005). The issue of which model—integrated or split—is more cost-effective remains a crucial one in today's increasingly cost-minded health care market that needs to be examined and researched more broadly and thoroughly.

TABLE 33–15. Trials of combined treatment in unipolar depression

Study	Combination used	Age/gender	Diagnosis/severity	Outcome measure	Result
Frank et al. 1990	IPT Imipramine	21–65 years, 38%–78% female	MDD, recurrent	3-year relapse rate	Combined treatment not superior
Thase et al. 1997	IPT Imipramine	Mean 44 years, 69% female	MDD, severe, recurrent MDD, less severe	Response rate Response rate	Combined treatment superior No advantage for combined treatment
Reynolds et al. 1999	IPT Nortriptyline	>59 years	MDD, recurrent	Response/recurrent rates	Combined treatment superior
Ravindran et al. 1999	Cognitive group therapy Sertraline	21–54 years, 60% female	Dysthymia DO	Variety	Combined treatment superior on measures of functional impairment
Keller et al. 2000	CBASP Nefazodone	18–75 years, 65% female	MDD, chronic	Response/remission rates	Combined treatment superior to CBT alone or medication alone
Frank et al. 2000	IPT SSRI or imipramine	21–65 years, all female	MDD, recurrent	Remission	Combined treatment superior in IPT nonresponders given medication
de Jonghe et al. 2001	SPSP Fluoxetine, amitriptyline, or moclobemide	Mean 34 years, 62% female	MDD, ambulatory	Response rate	Combined treatment superior, fewer dropouts
Lenze et al. 2002	IPT Nortriptyline	>60 years	MDD, recurrent	Social adjustment	Combined treatment superior
Hirschfeld et al. 2002	CBASP Nefazodone	18–75 years, 65% female	MDD, chronic	Psychosocial functioning	Combined treatment superior

Note. SPSP=short psychodynamic supportive psychotherapy; CBASP=cognitive–behavioral analysis system of psychotherapy; SSRI=selective serotonin reuptake inhibitor; TCA=tricyclic antidepressant; IPT=interpersonal psychotherapy.

Source. Adapted from Riba MB, Miller RR: "Combined Therapies: Psychotherapy and Pharmacotherapy," in *Psychiatry*, 2nd Edition. Edited by Tasman A, Kay J, Lieberman JF. England, John Wiley & Sons Ltd, 2003, pp. 2184–2201.

Key Points

- Combined treatment involving the combination of pharmacotherapy and psychotherapy has become the most common approach to the treatment of mental disorders.

- Numerous studies have demonstrated that combined treatment is frequently superior to pharmacotherapy or psychotherapy alone in the treatment of disorders such as major depression, anxiety, bipolar disorder, nicotine dependence, and others.

- Compared with pharmacotherapy or psychotherapy alone, combination treatment does not uniformly provide additive benefits.

- Combined treatment may be practiced in either an integrated or a split manner.

- Integrated treatment (one-person model) is a treatment approach in which pharmacotherapy and psychotherapy are provided by a single provider—preferably a physician.

- Split treatment (or two-person model) is a treatment approach in which pharmacotherapy and psychotherapy are divided up or shared by at least two different clinicians, psychiatrist and therapist.

- The predominant belief that split treatment is more cost-effective than integrated treatment has been questioned by some studies.

- Both integrated and split treatment involve complex clinical, ethical, legal, and managerial issues.

- Both integrated and split treatment require proper training, skills, and knowledge.

- Split treatment involves more complicated clinical, legal, ethical, and managerial issues.

- Patients should be involved in the decision of which treatment approach will be used and how treatment will be conducted and terminated. Informed consent should be obtained regarding the choice of treatment and arrangements for its conduct.

- Good communication between the prescribing physician and the therapist is the *sine qua non* for successful split treatment.

Suggested Readings

Beitman BD, Blinder BJ, Thase ME, et al. (eds): Integrating Psychotherapy and Pharmacotherapy: Dissolving the Mind–Brain Barrier. New York, WW Norton, 2003

Bender S, Messner E: Becoming a Therapist. What Do I Say, and Why? New York, Guilford, 2003

Kay J (ed): Integrated Treatment of Psychiatric Disorders (Review of Psychiatry Series; Oldham JM and Riba MB, series eds). Washington, DC, American Psychiatric Publishing, 2001

Riba MB, Balon R (eds): Psychopharmacology and Psychotherapy: A Collaborative Approach. Washington, DC, American Psychiatric Press, 1999

Riba MB, Balon R: Competency in Combining Pharmacotherapy and Psychotherapy: Integrated and Split Treatment (Core Competencies in Psychotherapy Series, Glen O. Gabbard, series ed). Arlington, VA, American Psychiatric Publishing, 2005

References

American Psychiatric Association: Guidelines for psychiatrists in consultative, supervisory, or collaborative relationships with nonmedical therapists. Am J Psychiatry 137:1489–1491, 1980

American Psychiatric Association: Practice guideline for the treatment of patients with bipolar disorder. Am J Psychiatry 151 (12 suppl):1–36, 1994

American Psychiatric Association: Practice guideline for the treatment of patients with schizophrenia. Am J Psychiatry 154 (4 suppl):1–63, 1997

American Psychiatric Association: American Psychiatric Association Practice Guideline for the Treatment of Patients With Major Depressive Disorder, 2nd Edition. Washington, DC, American Psychiatric Publishing, 2000a

American Psychiatric Association: Practice Guidelines for the Treatment of Patients With Eating Disorders, Revised Edition. Washington, DC, American Psychiatric Association, 2000b

American Psychiatric Association: Access to Comprehensive Psychiatric Assessment and Integrated Treatment: A Position Statement. Washington, DC, American Psychiatric Association, 2002a

American Psychiatric Association: Practice Guidelines for the Treatment of Patients With Bipolar Disorder, Revised Edition. Washington, DC, American Psychiatric Association, 2002b

Balon R: Positive aspects of collaborative treatment, in Psychopharmacology and Psychotherapy: A Collaborative Approach. Edited by Riba MB, Balon R. Washington, DC, American Psychiatric Press, 1999, pp 1–31

Balon R: Positive and negative aspects of split treatment. Psychiatr Ann 31:598–603, 2001

Banner LL, Anderson RU: Integrated sildenafil and cognitive-behavior sex therapy for psychogenic erectile dysfunction: a pilot study. J Sex Med 4(4 Pt 2):1117–1125, 2007

Barlow DH, Gorman JM, Shear MK, et al: Cognitive-behavioral therapy, imipramine, or their combination for panic disorder: a randomized controlled trial. JAMA 283:2529–2536, 2000

Beck JS: A cognitive therapy approach to medication compliance, in Integrated Treatment of Psychiatric Disorders. Edited by Kay J (Review of Psychiatry Series, Vol 20; Oldham JM and Riba MB, series eds). Washington, DC, American Psychiatric Publishing, 2001, pp 113–141

Beitman BD: Introduction, in Integrating Psychotherapy and Pharmacotherapy: Dissolving the Mind–Brain Barrier. Edited by Beitman BD, Blinder BJ, Thase ME, et al. New York, WW Norton, 2003, pp xv

Beitman BD, Blinder BJ, Thase ME, et al. (eds): Integrating Psychotherapy and Pharmacotherapy: Dissolving the Mind–Brain Barrier. New York, WW Norton, 2003

Bender S, Messner E: Becoming a Therapist: What Do I Say, and Why? New York, Guilford, 2003

Carli T: The psychologically informed psychopharmacologist, in Psychopharmacology and Psychotherapy: A Collaborative Approach. Edited by Riba MB, Balon R. Washington, DC, American Psychiatric Press, 1999, pp 179–196

Clarkin JF, Carpenter D, Hull J, et al: Effects of psychoeducational intervention for married patients with bipolar disorder and their spouses. Psychiatr Serv 49:531–533, 1998

Cochran SD: Preventing medical noncompliance in the outpatient treatment of bipolar affective disorder. J Consult Clin Psychol 52:873–878, 1984

de Jonghe F, Kool S, van Aalst G, et al: Combining psychotherapy and antidepressants in the treatment of depression. J Affect Disord 64(2–3):217–229, 2001

Dewan M: Are psychiatrists cost-effective? An analysis of integrated versus split treatment. Am J Psychiatry 156:324–326, 1999

Dunner DL, Schmaling KB, Hendrickson H, et al: Cognitive therapy versus fluoxetine in the treatment of dysthymic disorder. Depression 4:34–41, 1996

Epstein RM, Hundert EM: Defining and assessing professional competence. JAMA 287:226–235, 2002

Fava GA: Sequential treatment: a new way of integrating pharmacotherapy and psychotherapy. Psychother Psychosom 68:227–229, 1999

Fava GA, Bartolucci G, Rafanelli C, et al: Cognitive-behavioral management of patients with bipolar disorder who relapsed while on lithium prophylaxis. J Clin Psychiatry 62:556–559, 2001

Fava M, Rush AJ: Current status of augmentation and combination treatments for major depressive disorder: a literature review and a proposal for a novel approach to improve practice. Psychother Psychosom 75:139–153, 2006

Frank E: Treating Bipolar Disorder. A Clinician's Guide to Interpersonal and Social Rhythm Therapy. New York, Guilford, 2005

Frank E, Kupfer DJ, Perel JM, et al: Three-year outcomes for maintenance therapies in recurrent depression. Arch Gen Psychiatry 47:1093–1099, 1990

Frank E, Grochocinski VJ, Spanier CA, et al: Interpersonal psychotherapy and antidepressant medication: evaluation of a sequential treatment strategy in women with recurrent major depression. J Clin Psychiatry 61:51–57, 2000

Frank E, Kupfer DJ, Thase ME, et al: Two-year outcomes for interpersonal and social rhythm therapy in individual with bipolar I disorder. Arch Gen Psychiatry 62:996–1004, 2005

Gabbard GO: The rationale for combining medication and psychotherapy. Psychiatr Ann 36:315–319, 2006

Gibson SF, Morley S, Romeo-Wolff CP: A model community telepsychiatry program in rural Arizona, in E-Therapy: Case Studies, Guiding Principles, and the Clinical Potential of the Internet. Edited by Hsiung RC. New York, WW Norton, 2002, pp 69–91

Goldman W, McCulloch J, Cuffel B, et al: Outpatient utilization patterns of integrated and split psychotherapy and pharmacotherapy for depression. Psychiatr Serv 49:477–482, 1998

Goldsmith RJ, Paris M, Riba MB: Negative aspects of collaborative treatment, in Psychopharmacology and Psychotherapy: A Collaborative Approach. Edited by Riba MB, Balon R. Washington, DC, American Psychiatric Press, 1999, pp 33–63

Gorman JM, Kent JM, Sullivan GM, et al: Neuroanatomical hypothesis of panic disorder, revised. Am J Psychiatry 157:493–505, 2000

Hirschfeld RM, Dunner DL, Keitner G, et al: Does psychosocial functioning improve independent of depressive symptoms? A comparison of nefazodone, psychotherapy, and their combination. Biol Psychiatry 51:123–133, 2002

Hogarty G, Anderson CM, Reiss DJ, et al: Family psychoeducation, social skills training, and maintenance chemotherapy in the aftercare of schizophrenia. Arch Gen Psychiatry 43:633–642, 1986

Hollon SD, Fawcett J: Combined medication and psychotherapy for mood disorders, in Gabbard's Treatments of Psychiatric Disorders, 4th Edition. Edited by Gabbard GO. Arlington, VA, American Psychiatric Publishing, 2007, pp 439–448

Hsiung RC (ed): E-Therapy: Case Studies, Guiding Principles, and the Clinical Potential of the Internet. New York, WW Norton, 2002

Jibson MD: Transference and countertransference, in The Doctor–Patient Relationship in Pharmacotherapy. Edited by Tasman A, Riba MB, Silk KR. New York, Guilford, 2000, pp 95–126

Kandel E: Psychotherapy and the single synapse. N Engl J Med 308:1028–1037, 1979

Kay J: Integrated treatment: an overview, in Integrated Treatment of Psychiatric Disorders. Edited by Kay J (Review of Psychiatry Series, Vol 20; Oldham JM and Riba MB, series eds). Washington, DC, American Psychiatric Publishing, 2001, pp 1–29

Kay J: Psychotherapy and medication, in Oxford Textbook of Psychotherapy. Edited by Gabbard GO, Beck JS, Holmes J. New York, Oxford University Press, 2005, pp 463–475

Keller MB, McCullough JP, Klein DN, et al: A comparison of nefazodone, the cognitive behavioral-analysis system of psychotherapy, and their combination for the treatment of chronic depression. N Engl J Med 342:1462–1470, 2000

Kerber KB: Collaborative treatment in managed care, in Psychopharmacology and Psychotherapy: A Collaborative Approach. Edited by Riba MB, Balon R. Washington, DC, American Psychiatric Press, 1999, pp 307–324

Klerman GL: Ideologic conflicts, in Integrating Pharmacotherapy and Psychotherapy. Edited by Beitman BB, Klerman G. Washington, DC, American Psychiatric Press, 1991, pp 3–20

Klerman GL, Weissman MM, Markowitz J, et al: Medication and psychotherapy, in Handbook of Psychotherapy and Behavior Change. Edited by Bergin AE, Garfield SL. New York, Raven, 1994, pp 734–782

Lazarus J: Ethical issues in collaborative or divided treatment, in Psychopharmacology and Psychotherapy: A Collaborative Approach. Edited by Riba MB, Balon R. Washington, DC, American Psychiatric Press, 1999, pp 159–177

Lenze EJ, Dew MA, Mazumdar S, et al: Combined pharmacotherapy and psychotherapy as maintenance treatment for late-life depression: effect on social adjustment. Am J Psychiatry 159:466–468, 2002

Lipsitt DR, Starcevic V: Psychotherapy and pharmacotherapy in the treatment of somatoform disorders. Psychiatr Ann 36:341–348, 2006

MacBeth JE: Divided treatment: legal implications and risks, in Psychopharmacology and Psychotherapy: A Collaborative Approach. Edited by Riba MB, Balon R. Washington, DC, American Psychiatric Press, 1999, pp 111–158

MacBeth JE: Legal aspects of split treatment: how to audit and manage risk. Psychiatr Ann 31:605–610, 2001

Mavissakalian M: Combined behavioral therapy and pharmacotherapy of agoraphobia. J Psychiatr Res 27 (suppl 1):179–191, 1993

Oldham JM: Integrated treatment for borderline personality disorder. Psychiatr Ann 36:361–369, 2006

Olfson M, Marcus SC, Pincus HA: Trends in office-based psychiatric practice. Am J Psychiatry 156:451–457, 1999

Olfson M, Marcus SC, Druss B, et al: National trends in the use of outpatient psychotherapy. Am J Psychiatry 159:1914–1920, 2002

Parker G, Manicavasagar V: Modelling and Managing the Depressive Disorders: A Clinical Guide. Cambridge, UK, Cambridge University Press, 2005

Paykel ES: Psychotherapy, medication combinations, and compliance. J Clin Psychiatry 56 (suppl 1):24–30, 1995

Rand EH: Guidelines to maximize the process of collaborative treatment, in Psychopharmacology and Psychotherapy: A Collaborative Approach. Edited by Riba MB, Balon R. Washington, DC, American Psychiatric Press, 1999, pp 353–380

Ravindran AV, Anisman H, Merali Z, et al: Treatment of primary dysthymia with group cognitive therapy and pharmacotherapy: clinical symptoms and functional impairments. Am J Psychiatry 156:1608–1617, 1999

Reynolds CF 3rd, Miller MD, Pasternak RE, et al: Treatment of bereavement-related major depressive episodes in later life: a controlled study of acute and continuation treatment with nortriptyline and interpersonal psychotherapy. Am J Psychiatry 156:202–208, 1999

Riba M, Balon R: The challenges of split treatment, in Integrated Treatment of Psychiatric Disorders. Edited by Kay J (Review of Psychiatry Series, Vol 20; Oldham JM and Riba MB, series eds). Washington, DC, American Psychiatric Publishing, 2001, pp 143–162

Riba MB, Balon R: Competency in Combining Pharmacotherapy and Psychotherapy: Integrated and Split Treatment (Core Competencies in Psychotherapy Series, Glen O. Gabbard, series ed). Arlington, VA, American Psychiatric Publishing, 2005

Riba MB, Miller RR: Combined therapies: psychotherapy and pharmacotherapy, in Psychiatry, 2nd Edition. Edited by Tasman A, Kay J, Lieberman JF. Chichester, England, Wiley, 2003, pp 2184–2201

Roose SP: Psychodynamic therapy and medication, in Integrated Treatment of Psychiatric Disorders. Edited by Kay J (Review of Psychiatry Series, Vol 20; Oldham JM and Riba MB, series eds). Washington, DC, American Psychiatric Publishing, 2001, pp 31–50

Seligman MEP: The effectiveness of psychotherapy. The Consumer Reports study. Am Psychol 50:965–973, 1995

Simon R: Unilateral treatment termination: "You're fired." Psychiatric Times (July):25–26, 2004

Smith JM: Some dimensions of transference in combined treatment, in The Psychotherapist's Guide to Pharmacotherapy. Edited by Ellison JM. Chicago, IL, Year Book Medical, 1989, pp 79–94

Spiegel DA, Bruce TJ, Gregg SF, et al: Does cognitive-behavior therapy assist slow-taper alprazolam discontinuation in panic disorder? Am J Psychiatry 151:876–881, 1994

Stofle GS: Chat room therapy, in E-Therapy. Case Studies, Guiding Principles, and the Clinical Potential of the Internet. Edited by Hsiung RC. New York, WW Norton, 2002, pp 92–91, 135

Tasman A, Riba MB, Silk KR (eds): The Doctor–Patient Relationship in Pharmacotherapy: Improving Treatment Effectiveness. New York, Guilford, 2000

Thase ME: Psychopharmacology in conjunction with psychotherapy, in Handbook of Psychological Change: Psychotherapy Process and Practices for the 21st Century. Edited by Ingram R, Snyder RC. New York, Wiley, 2000, pp 474–497

Thase ME: Conceptual and empirical basis for integrating psychotherapy and pharmacotherapy, in Integrating Psychotherapy and Pharmacotherapy: Dissolving the Mind–Brain Barrier. Edited by Beitman BD, Blinder BJ, Thase ME, et al. New York, WW Norton, 2003, pp 111–139

Thase ME, Greenhouse JB, Frank E, et al: Treatment of major depression with psychotherapy or psychotherapy-pharmacotherapy combinations. Arch Gen Psychiatry 54:1009–1015, 1997

Turkington D, Dudley R, Warman DM, et al: Cognitive-behavioral therapy for schizophrenia. J Psychiatr Pract 10:5–16, 2004

U.S. Department of Health and Human Services: Reducing Tobacco Use: A Report of the Surgeon General. Atlanta, GA, Centers for Disease Control and Prevention, 2000

Walsh TB, Wilson GT, Loeb KL, et al: Medication and psychotherapy in the treatment of bulimia nervosa. Am J Psychiatry 154:523–531, 1997

West JC, Wilk JE, Rae DS, et al: Economic grand rounds: financial disincentives for the provision of psychotherapy. Psychiatr Serv 54:1582–1588, 2003

Wiborg IM, Dahl AA: Does brief dynamic psychotherapy reduce the relapse rate of panic disorder? Arch Gen Psychiatry 53:689–694, 1996

Wright JH, Hollifield M: Combining pharmacotherapy and psychotherapy. Guest editorial. Psychiatr Ann 36:302–305, 2006

Yager J: Suggested guidelines for e-mail communication in psychiatric practice. J Clin Psychiatry 64:799–806, 2003

34

COUPLES AND FAMILY THERAPY

Eva C. Ritvo, M.D.

Ilan Melnick, M.D.

Ira D. Glick, M.D.

"Research in many medical fields shows that families have powerful influences on health that are equal to or surpass other risk factors and that brief family interventions increase health and decrease the risk of relapse in chronic illnesses. Research in psychiatry affirms that family interventions reduce the rate of relapse, improve recovery, and increase family well-being."

Heru 2006

The structure of couples and families has changed dramatically in the past century, and the demand for couples and family therapy continues to rise. The twentieth century witnessed families being pulled apart as people spread across the globe. This century has witnessed a radical change in how individuals and families communicate with one another. Instant-messaging each other to come for dinner, text messaging during the day, and constantly changing plans thanks to the ease of cell phones are just some examples of how communication patterns have been altered. Family members who are apart can communicate better, and distances and time delays are collapsing as more and more people use IMing (instant messaging) and e-mailing.

Just as popular culture changes over time, so, too, does the nature of "love" change as society is transformed. And, some would argue, it is more difficult to connect or stay connected. Two and three centuries ago,

men and women lived together for only short periods of time (e.g., 3–4 years) because of wars, epidemics, deaths in childbirth, and the like. The average woman had two or three "significant relationships" over her lifetime; most couples never lived together for long periods. Today's couples and families face many new challenges, problems, freedoms, and expectations. In this new century, couples are finding new versions of "love and happiness" with divergent family configurations and relationship patterns (e.g., serial relationships).

Relationships are no longer defined by geographical constraints. Dating practices have dramatically changed. People can go online to one of hundreds of Web sites and "order" what they are looking for—an age range of 25–30 years, the correct religion, "must love dogs," and so forth. Even making new friends or reconnecting with old friends is as easy as jumping on the Internet. Web sites that connect people on a multitude of different levels are popping up every day. Not only styles of communication but also topics of communication are changing. Free expression of a wide range of emotions is now acceptable not only in public but also on prime-time television. Legalized marriage for homosexual couples is on the national agenda. In vitro fertilization, egg donation, conception and adoption for gay couples, and many more issues are now being openly discussed not just within families but online and on television. As the nature of communication changes, how are our relationships affected?

Some of these changes and advances are creating new issues that today's family therapist must be prepared to deal with. The Internet has made it easy for spouses to cheat. There are Web sites specifically designed for married people looking to "have some fun" on the side. There are even gender-specific Web sites to aid in the cheating process—married men seeking girlfriends and vice versa, men seeking men, and so forth. The Internet has also facilitated access to child pornography and enabled sexual predators to have easy access to children via chatrooms and sites such as "Myspace.com." Sexual addiction to Internet pornography is an issue that family therapists need to be able to diagnose and treat or refer to a skilled professional.

In this chapter, we present an introduction to couples and family therapy. The intent is to provide some of the basics—that is, the core competencies—of the family model. Many of these core capabilities are analogous to those of the individual psychotherapy model. To achieve these competencies, it is our opinion that the family model needs to be moved from the margins of training to a more central position among the various psychotherapy models. We strongly believe that the clinician who uses a broad family model will have more flexibility (and presumably greater effectiveness) in managing the broad array of psychiatric problems now seen in practice.

The chapter is divided into two sections. We discuss family therapy first, followed by couples therapy.

Family Therapy

Definition and Overview

Family therapy is a psychotherapeutic intervention in which individuals beyond the primary husband–wife dyad are involved—that is, parents, children, and even members of the extended family (broadly defined), if they share in or are part of the pathology. Major emphasis is placed on understanding how the system as a whole remains functional and on understanding individual behavior patterns as arising from and inevitably feeding back into the complex interactions within the family system. A person's thoughts, feelings, and behaviors are seen as multiply determined and as partly a product of significant interpersonal relationships. Any psychotherapeutic approach that attempts to understand or to intervene in a family system might fittingly be called family therapy. Family therapy may be thought of as any type of psychosocial intervention using a conceptual framework that gives primary emphasis to the family system and aims to affect the entire family structure.

Family therapy can be distinguished from other psychotherapies by its fundamental paradigm shift, which assumes that people are best understood as operating in systems and that treatment must include, either in person or in theoretical understanding, conceptualization of all relevant parts of the system. From this assumption comes different goals, foci, participants, and so on. Family therapy connotes a format of intervention that attempts to include the relevant system members. The presence of family members is crucial to addressing the goal of family treatment, which is the improved functioning of the family as an interlocking system and network of individuals.

The goal of family therapy is to assist the family in more successfully achieving their goals and establishing gratifying ways of living and interacting as a family unit. The family constitutes one of the most important relationships people have. The family dynamic directly affects psychological development, communication with others, emotional interactions, and self-esteem issues and can influence the course of psychiatric and general medical conditions (Heru 2006). Just as one member of a team can affect the outcomes of the group, the group may also affect the members, especially in the case of the family. Family members are usually bound together by intense and long-lasting ties of past experiences, social roles, mutual support and needs, and expectations. When the equilibrium of the family is disrupted or changes due to either internal or external factors, the family unit can become dysfunctional. Family therapy strives to help families reestablish equilibrium and function in more harmonious and productive ways (Ritvo and Glick 2002). The family therapist is especially sensitive to and trained in those aspects relating specifically to the family system—both its individual characteristics and the larger social matrix.

Functional Families

Families can be viewed as laboratories for the social, psychological, and biological development and maintenance of family members. In providing this function, couples and families must accomplish vital tasks, including the provision of basic physical needs (food, shelter, and clothing), the development of a marital coalition and the socialization of children, and the resolution of crises that can arise in relation to illness and other extra-familial life changes. Therefore, not only do families have a given structure that expresses the family's underlying belief system, but they serve to fulfill essential functions as well.

When working with a family, it is essential to understand the basics of what makes a "healthy" or functional family system. Certain characteristics can be seen in families that function well. Walsh (1993) has identified 10 processes that characterize functional—that is, "healthy" or "normal"—families (Table 34–1).

Dysfunctional Families

A functional family is like an orchestra playing a beautiful symphony: each of its members plays a different instrument, but together they add up to an overall configuration of harmony that is effective and fulfilling. Conversely, in a dysfunctional family there is a lack of such harmony, as well as a pervasive negative mood of unrelatedness. A dysfunctional family is like a poker game in which each player holds certain cards, yet no one will put them on the table. Therefore, the same old game keeps being played. No one will risk losing (or winning) by playing a new card, so in effect no one wins and no one loses, and the game becomes a pointless exercise; or else one player may win the same hollow victory repeatedly and another may always be identified as the loser.

A dysfunctional family seldom has the internal resources to change, given the unwritten rules by which it operates. If it had those resources, then it could change, and the family would therefore not be dysfunctional. A member of the family may ask for external help for him- or herself or for another family member or may try to harm him- or herself or someone else and thus come to the attention of an external agency. To take the "identified patient" at face value and to deal only with that person, without seeing the rest of the family, would represent a very distorted and limited perspective of the dysfunction inherent in the family.

Serial Relationships

Before 1960, the typical life cycle included a long courtship and long-term marriage begun in the couple's early 20s. This pattern is based on a belief that the best way to self-fulfillment is through marriage. It is still the pattern toward which most people strive. Some

---

TABLE 34–1. Characteristics of functional families

1. Connectedness and commitment of members as a caring, mutually supportive relationship unit

2. Respect for individual differences, autonomy, and separate needs, fostering the development and well-being of members of each generation, from youngest to eldest

3. For couples, a relationship characterized by mutual respect, support, and equitable sharing of power and responsibilities

4. For nurturance, protection, and socialization of children and caretaking of other vulnerable family members, effective parental/executive leadership and authority

5. Organizational stability, characterized by clarity, consistency, and predictability in patterns of interaction

6. Adaptability and flexibility to meet internal or external demands for change, to cope effectively with stress and problems that arise, and to master normative and nonnormative challenges and transitions across the life cycle

7. Open communication, characterized by clarity of rules and expectations, pleasurable interaction, and a range of emotional expression and empathic responsiveness

8. Effective problem-solving and conflict-resolution processes

9. A shared belief system that enables mutual trust, problem mastery, connectedness with past and future generations, ethical values, and concern for the larger human community

10. Adequate resources for basic economic security and psychosocial support in extended kin and friendship networks and from community and larger social systems

---

people develop a life pattern of sequential relationships that includes several long-term serious relationships and may include several marriages with the creation of two or three family units. It is often difficult to tell whether this model indicates emotional problems and fear of commitment or represents personal growth for the persons involved. A person who picks the same type of partner several times, or who goes directly from one partner to another without an effort to understand himself or herself or what happened to the earlier relationship, is more likely to choose this model of dysfunction.

Cohabitation

In the United States, couples living together as unmarried lovers has gone from being scandalous to normative in less than a generation. In other parts of the world, such consensual unions have been common for centuries. Couples cohabit for many reasons, ranging from convenience to a trial marriage to a permanently committed relationship that for emotional or economic reasons is not formalized in a legal marriage contract. Cohabiting couples have both the advantages and the disadvantages of a looser relational contract, including a sense of freedom, aliveness, and uncertainty. Although the basic tasks of couple coalition—dealing with intimacy, power, boundaries, and sexuality—are present, by definition cohabitation implies less agreement on beliefs about permanence (e.g., what the couple's status means) and also implies more permeable boundaries with the outside world than are found among married people.

Early research on cohabiting couples suggested that those who married after cohabiting were more likely to divorce (Messinger 1976). The reasons for the finding were never quite clear, although in the 1960s and 1970s one common explanation was that people who were unconventional enough to cohabit were also more willing to behave in other unconventional ways—for example, by seeking divorce. In more recent cohorts, in which cohabitation is more frequent, the differential in dissolution rates has been declining and has even reversed slightly (Schoen 1992).

Approximately 40% of cohabiting couples live with children from one or both partners. Research (e.g., Isaacs and Leon 1988) suggests that living with a biological parent and the parent's lover is an extremely difficult situation for children, who are asked to relate to a person who may leave them and who has no real rights to discipline or parent them, yet who cannot be ignored. Evidence suggests that both physical and sexual abuse are more likely with a biologically unrelated adult in the house. While children from former relationships are in the house, cohabitation should be limited to permanent or soon-to-be-married couples, whenever possible.

Marital Separation

Separation is a relatively common crisis of marital life. Although it is emotionally traumatic for the individuals involved, it can serve as an opportunity to reassess the marital contract and individual goals and sometimes can lead to a renewed and more functional marriage. Different precipitants may have brought about the separation; therefore, different issues may need to be addressed. For some couples, differences in adult development lead to a situation in which partners no longer have much in common. Spouses whose children are grown and have left home may not easily become accustomed to living alone together as a couple. With the parental role diminished or absent, there may be little emotional or functional viability left in the marriage.

Although it is natural to think of marital separation as an unfortunate event, it can also be viewed as symptomatic of marital-system problems that need attention. In this sense, separation and its subsequent resolution may offer the potential for growth and change for the better. Trial separations can be useful to provide a cooling-off period for couples whose difficulties seem insurmountable. It offers the partners the opportunity to examine their relationship more objectively. At the same time, the individuals can test their ability to adapt to living alone. This separation, together with new life experiences of various sorts (which may not have taken place had the couple stayed together), will often enable partners to change their behavior and feelings toward each other by the time they attempt reconciliation. Sometimes one spouse may use separation to manipulate the other spouse, or the separating partner may move immediately into a new relationship. If the partners are unable to communicate with each other or learn about themselves, the separation will not be much help, regardless of whether the couple reconciles. Clinical experience suggests that about half of couples that separate get back together; of those couples, about half will eventually divorce.

Divorce

The divorce rate in most developing countries has been rising, although since the mid-1980s it has shown signs of leveling off. If the relationship has been of sufficient duration for true attachment to take place (about 2 years is considered long enough), divorce can be one of the most painful experiences in anyone's life.

Divorce is a process, not an event, with its own developmental path. It usually represents one in a series of transitions that began with marital dissatisfaction and may or may not end with remarriage. A number of authors (Kessler 1975; Salts 1979) have delineated stages of the divorce process, which can be summarized as follows:

1. A predivorce phase of growing disillusionment and dissatisfaction with the marriage and arrival at some consideration of divorce.
2. The separation itself, including moving out of the house and dealing with immediate grief. For many people, this is a period of great emotional distress, confusion, and grief—a so-called crazy time.

3. A period of 1–2 years during which the couple deals with parenting issues, financial and family reorganization, community status, and legal issues. Negative life stresses are most marked during the first 2 years following divorce. Children are most likely to experience diminished parenting during this period because of the parents' preoccupation with divorce issues. Children are likely to respond with noncompliant, angry, demanding, or depressed behavior.

4. For each spouse, reforming of an identity from being part of a couple to being a single person occurs next. Because this phase occurs during the latter part of the process, issues with children also settle down unless partners continue to use children as weapons in the divorce proceedings. The legal aspects of the divorce itself may take from 3 months (in some states with an uncontested divorce) to several years, depending on the laws and the amount of anger, but the psychological issues have their own timetable. If the couple has children, they must find ways to remain connected as parents while separating as partners.

Evaluation of the Family

The family unit is more difficult to assess than the couple unit, due to the intertwining and interconnecting relationships between and among its members. Family functioning may be assessed by means of a modified version of the McMaster Model of Family Functioning (Epstein and Bishop 1981), which addresses seven dimensions of family functioning: 1) communication, 2) problem solving, 3) roles and coalition, 4) affective responsiveness, 5) affective involvement, 6) behavior control, and 7) operative family beliefs and stories.

The therapist must also elicit family members' beliefs about themselves and about the problem. The family's cultural beliefs, values, and traditions must also be evaluated, as well as the role these elements play in their interactions. Ritvo and Glick (2002) have noted the importance of understanding the following issues:

- What is the chief complaint or concern that has brought the family to therapy?
- Why has the family found it necessary to seek help at this time?
- What is the history of the presenting problem?
- What is the history of previous attempts at solving the problem, if any?
- What are the goals at this point regarding the problem?
- What are the motivators, resistances, or consequences to solving the problem?

The answers to these questions will afford insight into the family's dynamics and help the therapist begin to formulate a treatment plan (Table 34–2). A comprehensive evaluation and diagnosis should include both a functional and a descriptive formulation for both the family and the individual (Glick et al. 2000, p. 176). And, of course, diagnosis always precedes goals of therapy.

The data gathered should permit the therapist to pinpoint particular dimensions or aspects of functioning of the family and its individual members that may require special attention. As data are gathered, the therapist notes areas of health and dysfunction and creates a priority list for addressing problems. Prioritizing a family's problems allows the therapist to focus on the relative severity of the issues, establishing which should be dealt with first. These data also enable the clinician to have greater clarity about therapeutic strategies and tactics indicated for the particular phases and goals of treatment.

Strategies for Beginning Family Therapy

The skills necessary to begin working with a family are basic, assumed by all orientations, and crucial to master to enable the therapist to achieve the final goals of family intervention (Table 34–3).

It is important for therapists to obtain an extensive history during the opening sessions. However, some therapy models place less emphasis on diagnosis and extensive history and more emphasis on the here and now, working more with what happens during the session and gathering longitudinal data on an as-needed basis.

The therapist may decide to hear from each family member in turn on certain important issues, or may let the verbal interaction take its own course. Therapists should allow at least a few minutes of unguided conversation among the family members so as to witness their patterns of interaction. A decision can be made to call one parent in first, then the other, and then the children in descending order of age. Or it may appear more advantageous to call in the more easily intimidated, weaker, or passive parent first, or to allow the family to decide who speaks first. The therapist may decide to use first names for all family members, to help put everyone on an equal footing; or the therapist may prefer to be more formal in addressing the parents, to strengthen weak generational boundaries and parental functioning. Some therapists may encourage family members to communicate largely through the

TABLE 34–2. Outline for family evaluation

I. Current phase of family life cycle and identifying data

II. Explicit interview date

    A. What is the current family problem?

    B. Why does the family come for treatment at the present time?

    C. What is the background of the family problem?

    D. What is the history of past treatment attempts or other attempts at problem solving in the family?

    E. What are the family's goals and expectations of the treatment? What are their motivations and resistances?

III. Formulation of family problem areas

    A. Rating important dimensions of family functioning:

        1. Communication

        2. Problem solving

        3. Roles and coalitions

        4. Affective responsiveness and involvement

        5. Behavioral control

        6. Operative family beliefs

    B. Family classification and "diagnosis"

IV. Planning the therapeutic approach and establishing the treatment contract

TABLE 34–3. Strategies for beginning family therapy

1. **Accommodating to and joining the family.** The therapist must join the group by letting the family members know that he or she understands them and wants to work with them for their better good. The therapist must use his or her own personality traits, combined with sensitivity and warmth, to join a family in distress.

2. **Interviewing subgroups, extended family, and other networks.** The therapist must understand the tremendous power and influence of the individual's social environment. The therapist must also decide which parts of the social environment to include directly in treatment and which parts can be included for assessment only.

3. **Negotiating the goals of treatment.** The family usually comes to therapy with their own treatment goals in mind, with some individuals having specific goals for other people to change, but not themselves, and with some individuals not wanting to be there at all.

therapist, or to talk primarily to one another, at least during the first sessions or at times of stress or chaos.

The therapist must decide which path to take, based on the history of the presenting problem and the way the family members interact with one another. There is no "cookbook" layout for therapy, as family therapy is a fluid interaction that is always changing, depending on circumstances, but the therapist should always have a guiding plan of treatment in mind.

Genograms for Organizing Family Historical Data

The therapist can collect and organize historical data through the use of a genogram, the three-generational family tree depicting the family's patterns related to specific problems or to general family functioning (Figure 34–1). The genogram technique can suggest possible connections between present family events and the

prior experiences family members have shared (e.g., regarding the management of serious illnesses, losses, and other critical transitions), thereby placing the presenting problem in a historical context (McGoldrick and Gerson 1985; Shorter 1977). Constructing a genogram early on in treatment can provide a wealth of data that frequently offers clues about pressures, expectations, and hopes regarding the marriage.

Goals of Family Therapy

One convenient way to conceptualize treatment goals is to distinguish the final goals (the ultimate results desired) from the mediating (or intermediate) goals that must precede the final results. Whereas a therapist would set unique and specific goals for each individual family, certain general mediating and final goals are commonly addressed in family therapy (Tables 34–4 and 34–5). These represent relatively broad areas that allow for considerable flexibility according to the specifics of each particular family or marital unit, and they are not mutually exclusive but are often intertwined.

Treatment Strategies

The problems of families and the goals to be addressed, both mediating and final, should determine the strategies of the therapy (Table 34–6). There are various ways to conceptualize overall strategies of family intervention. We describe these strategies below.

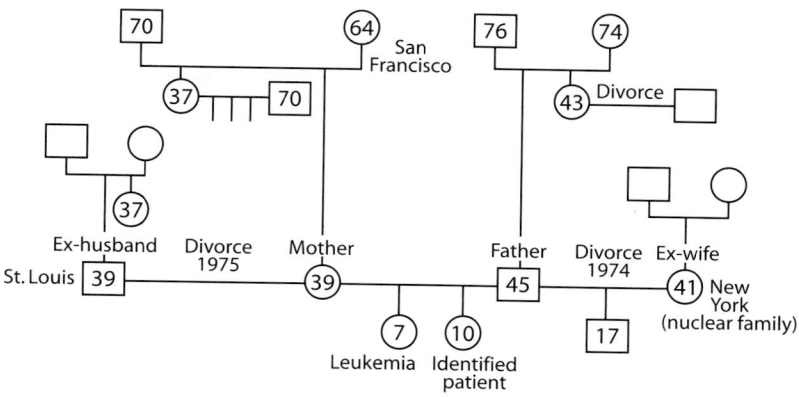

FIGURE 34–1. Genogram.

In the sample genogram shown, an overall family map has been constructed to graphically describe the identified patient, identify the other members of the family (including age, gender, and relationship to identified patient) and where they live, and highlight important and/or stressful family events (here, "divorce" of both parents).

Supporting Adaptive Mechanisms

There are a number of ways to assist families in utilizing existing strategies and developing new strategies for coping. An important focus is provision of information (psychoeducation) to the family—for example, about psychiatric illness in family members or about parenting skills. Supportive advice and encouragement of existing coping mechanisms are also effective ways to help families. The strategy of "bearing witness"—that is, the acknowledgment and understanding of the family's experience or emotional pain or trauma—can be of critical importance in a family that is attempting to recover from or cope with ongoing challenges or trauma.

Expanding Emotional Experience

To help families expand their ability to respond to emotional experiences, the therapist uses the techniques of listening, labeling, and encouraging supportive family responses to feelings shared by members. The therapist must first encourage a family member to share his or her painful experience. The therapist can then provide a model of an appropriate response by making a specific comment such as "That must be a very difficult situation for you" or by making a more generalizing comment such as "Most people would feel great pain in that situation." By validating and encouraging the open expression of feelings in family members, the therapist helps establish new ways for the family to communicate and opens the door for family members to support one another. Depending on their training and orientation, therapists may at times employ fantasy, humor and irony, direct confrontation, family sculpting, and choreography to open up new areas of immediate emotional experiencing for the family.

Developing Interpersonal Skills

Through a multitude of therapeutic techniques—including modeling of intent, listening to others, insisting that only one person speak at a time, questioning the exact meaning of what others are saying and wishing to communicate, and giving explicit instruction in communication skills—the family will learn to communication more effectively over time. This improvement in communication skills can be an end in itself or can be used to solve the specific interpersonal problems that brought the family to treatment in the first place.

Reorganizing the Family Structure

Reframing of the problems as presented by the family, reenacting the family problems with their attendant interactional sequences, reestablishing boundaries, and other restructuring moves can be used to change the structured family behaviors that are judged to be causing or contributing to the family's distress. Strategies such as insisting within sessions that parents make joint decisions about the children rather than leaving the mother in charge and the father passive, insisting that parents take charge of children rather than allowing children to control the session, and delineating responsibilities of grandparents and other adult relatives allow family members to experience new types of structure. Homework assignments that encourage clear boundaries, such as making sure that the parents' bedroom door is closed at night, help to reinforce these messages.

TABLE 34–4.   Mediating goals of family therapy

1. **Establish a working alliance.** Patients and families size up therapists very quickly, and those early attitudes are likely to persist. Thus, the early connection between the family therapist and each family member is quite crucial to the ultimate outcome of the work. Establishing such an alliance in individual therapy seems relatively simple in comparison to doing so with multiple members of a family who themselves often do not get along with each other. The therapist also must find a way to connect with each person rather than favoring certain family members.

2. **Specify problem(s).** This would include a detailed delineation of family members' feelings and behaviors around the symptoms or problems that brought the family to treatment.

3. **Clarify attempted solutions.** It is very likely that family members have attempted solutions to their problems before coming to the conclusion that they need outside intervention. Almost by definition, these are solutions that failed, so the therapist should determine what did not work (as, indeed, some would say that many problems are simply ordinary situations to which poor solutions were applied).

4. **Clarify and specify individual desires and needs as they are expressed, mediated, and met in the total family/marital environment and network of relationships.** It is the lack of clarity about—and the conflict (either overt or covert) around—such needs and desires that leads to or constitutes family pathology itself.

5. **Modify individual expectations or needs.**

6. **Recognize mutual contribution to the problem(s).** Although therapists differ in whether they believe such recognition must come early in the therapy and in how explicit it must be, the very acceptance of the family intervention format (i.e., most or all family members coming to most sessions) implies some recognition of mutual contribution to the problem, or at least to solutions.

7. **Redefine the problem(s).** Redefining a problem completely and redefining it into various parts, some of which are problematic and others not, are all steps toward finding possible solutions. For example, the therapist might say, "You are not 'bad' people; you are responding to stress with anxiety or anger."

8. **Foster improvement in communication skills.** These include listening and expressive skills, diminution of coercive and blaming behavior with increase in reciprocity, and effective problem-solving and conflict resolution behaviors.

9. **Facilitate a shift in disturbed, inflexible roles and coalitions.** This may include helping to improve family members' autonomy and individualization, promoting a more flexible assumption of leadership by particular family members as circumstances require, and facilitating general task performance by one or more family members.

10. **Educate the family about serious psychiatric illness.** In families that have one or more members with serious Axis I pathology (e.g., schizophrenia, recurrent affective illness), a common mediating goal is to increase family information about the illness, its course, and its responsiveness to environmental (including familial) stresses.

11. **Promote insight into historical factors related to current problems or current interaction patterns.** This mediating goal may be relatively important in psychodynamically oriented family or marital work but be absent from other orientations. However, other orientations may reframe particular stories about the family's history as a way of changing interactions.

Increasing Insight

Traditional techniques of psychodynamic psychotherapy, such as clarification, confrontation, and interpretation (either in the here and now or of genetic material), can be employed in the marital and family treatment formats to bring underlying conflicts to the fore and reduce conflict-laden interactions. Insight here must be relational in terms of how each person's past affects the present and the responses of others. Direct questioning of the parents and analysis of current relationships through family-of-origin work are other useful ways of developing insight and helping families to function more effectively.

TABLE 34–5. **Final goals of family therapy**

1. Reduction or elimination of symptoms, or symptomatic behavior, in one or more family members. These symptoms may include major or minor symptoms of mood and affect (anxiety and depression), thought disorder, disruptive behaviors in children and adolescents, marital conflict and fighting, and sexual disorders.

2. Resolution of the problem(s) as originally presented by the family.

3. Clear, efficient, and satisfying communication.

4. Role flexibility and adaptability within the family matrix.

5. Toleration of uniqueness and differentiation appropriate to age and developmental level.

6. Balance of power within the marital dyad, with appropriate sharing of input and autonomy for the children.

7. Increased self-esteem for individual family members.

8. Increased family/marital intimacy.

9. Resolution of neurotic conflict, inappropriate projective identification, and marital transference phenomena.

TABLE 34–6. **Strategies for attaining mediating goals of family therapy**

Mediating goals	Strategies
Increasing knowledge, decreasing guilt, redefining problems, increasing the use of adaptive coping mechanisms	Support adaptive mechanisms
Fostering appropriate emotional experience and communication	Expand emotional experience
Improving communication skills, problem-solving skills, parenting skills	Develop interpersonal skills
Clarifying boundaries, setting appropriate boundaries between familial subsystems and family of origin	Reorganize the family structure
Facilitating insight regarding current transactions and historical factors; decreasing conflict	Increase insight
Exploring family-of-origin issues	Construct an alternative reality or story

Helping the Family Understand and Modify Its Narrative

Narrative-focused strategies involve helping the family tell its story and find alternative and less problem-saturated narratives that can offer novel solutions. Both the therapist and the family members look for redefinitions (enthusiastic rather than noisy, survivor rather than victim), understandings (fear of failure rather than laziness), and novel outcomes (What about the times it doesn't fail—What happens then?).

Case Vignette

A.S., a 12-year-old girl who was the second of two children, was having problems getting along with one student in her class. A.S. and her friends would "gang up" on this one student. Her actions mostly involved name calling and poking fun at this student's awkwardness but did not get physical at any point.

The school excused the other children for their actions, but because A.S. refused to apologize, serious actions were taken against her. A.S.'s parents allowed the school to punish her in whatever manner they saw fit, and they followed the school's suggestion that she be punished at home as well. A.S. did not understand why she was punished so severely for making fun of someone, and she attempted suicide by ingesting an entire bottle of Tylenol. Her 15-year-old sister, P.S., was able to talk A.S. into going to the hospital for treatment after about 1 hour of negotiating with her through the locked bedroom door.

Soon after this incident, the family entered into therapy. The therapist saw the four family members together for an initial evaluation and history. The therapist then suggested that the father and the mother simultaneously enter couples therapy with a therapist colleague in the same building. Sessions were handled in several formats and used multiple strategies (see Table 34–6). In some sessions, the four members of the family would see the family therapist for 20 minutes together, after which the father and mother would depart for couples therapy while the children stayed together with the family therapist for the next 40 minutes. In other sessions, the therapist would see the parents for 20 minutes alone, then for 20 minutes with the children present, and then recap with everyone present for the remaining 20 minutes. The format would continually change.

The family members were able to share their individual experiences and feelings about the events that led them to seek therapy. A primary focus was issues related to why A.S. was making fun of this student to empower herself (due to her low self-esteem). As the years went on, the valuable lessons learned in family therapy helped A.S. to adjust and cope with the world.

Efficacy of Family Therapy

Marital and family therapy have been shown in controlled studies to be more efficacious than no psychotherapy across countless conditions, and family therapy is the preferred mode of treatment (compared with other types of psychotherapy) in the following conditions: couple distress or problems, sexual difficulties, mood disorders in women who have couple or marital problems, families with out-of-control children or adolescents, and families in which one member has schizophrenia or a mood disorder.

Dropouts

The dropout rate in the early stage of family therapy is relatively high. In one study, about 30% of all families referred for family treatment failed to appear for the first session ("defected"), and another 30% terminated within the first three sessions, leaving about 40% who continued (Shapiro and Budman 1973). The main reason families gave for termination was a lack of activity on the part of the therapist, whereas defectors in general had a "change of heart" and denied that a problem existed. The motivation of the husband/father appeared to play a crucial role—the more motivated he was, the more likely the family was to continue treatment.

The idea that dropping out represents "denying a problem" may or may not be true. Because the process of entering therapy is frightening for many people and because the therapist must meet the needs of several people, it is unsurprising that the process of engagement is rocky.

Couples Therapy
Definition and Overview

Marital or couples therapy can be defined as a format of intervention involving both members of a dyad, in which the focus of intervention is the problematic interactional patterns of the couple. The focus of couples therapy is on the dyad and its intimate emotional and sexual aspects. In this chapter, we use *marital therapy* and *couples therapy* interchangeably, as the majority of the issues are the same. A couple may represent man–woman, man–man, or woman–woman relationships.

The divorce rate in the United States remains fairly constant, at approximately 50%; therefore, it is not surprising that relationship distress is a common presenting complaint in most psychotherapy practices. There can be no single model to describe a functional couple, just as no single therapeutic treatment modality can be universally applied. The task of the therapist is to understand the needs of a particular couple at the time they come for treatment and to help them function as effectively as possible in the many domains that couples must navigate. Integrative treatment approaches are often the most effective. Not all marriages or relationships can or should be held together, and at times it becomes the role of the therapist to facilitate a separation in as constructive a manner as possible.

Functional Couples

The marital relationship in all societies is a peculiar combination—It represents both the most idiosyncratic and intimate and the most culturally patterned of relationships. Each society varies in its emphasis on the external aspects of the marriage (e.g., the mechanisms for transfer of property and privilege and for management of paternity) and the intimate aspects (e.g., the friendship, love, and sexual issues binding the couple). In general, the more Westernized the culture, the more free the marital choice, and the more emphasis placed on issues of love and intimacy. However, there are still strong cultural sanctions within individual races or classes.

Currently, Westernized marriages are characterized by freedom to choose a spouse, equality in terms of marriage vows (though not in terms of situation or exchange of property), emancipation from family of origin, and an increased emphasis on intimacy. Marriage, among all family relationships, is most distinguished by its peculiar power differential, which often is dictated by gender. In an emotional sense, at the level of intimacy and connection, the spouses are equal partners. The issue of power inequality in relationships bound by love is complex (Goldner et al. 1990). Reasons include men's greater power in the culture, the male's greater physical strength, and the fact that marital choice usually involves women marrying men who are older and more financially successful. Marriage is also distinguished among family relationships by its voluntary nature—Whereas one can never truly be an "ex-parent" or an "ex-child," it is possible to be an ex-spouse, to choose to truly sever a marital relationship. This vulnerability lends the relationship a particular complexity that may become central to treatment.

In Western culture today, marriage is extended to include not only the union of a man and a woman but also the union of two men or two women. Homosexual unions or life partners are becoming more common and accepted; legalization of such unions is being discussed in the legislation of several states and is a reality in some countries.

A couple's ability to communicate clearly, to solve problems, and to have a relationship free of projection and incompatible agendas is based on the intrapsychic needs of the individuals, the reflexive behaviors they bring from their families of origin, the evolving marital dynamics, and the state of marital development. A central issue in marriage is the meshing of individual needs with relationship needs. The behaviors and beliefs of dysfunctional couples tend to be more rigid than those of well-adapted couples.

Dysfunctional Couples

Periods of dysfunction are inevitable in any long-term relationship. The burden of carrying intimate, social, and parenting roles means that people will inevitably clash over some aspects of life. It is common for marriages to undergo periodic stages of crisis and reorganization. Problems occur when couples lose faith in the marriage or lose a sense of respect and warmth for each other. Partners who have had poor role models, who have had childhood experiences of loss or violence, or who are poorly suited to each other by style or inclination may have increasing problems as time goes by.

There are a number of classic theories, not mutually exclusive, that attempt to explain how marriages become conflicted to the point of impairment. Individuals come to marriage with the legacy of their multigenerational family-of-origin issues plus the beliefs and role models of their parents. This means that they carry with them firm ideas about what marriage should be like, how men and women should behave, and what behaviors signify love and respect.

In the process of mate selection, the partner is attractive partly because he or she promises rediscovery of an important lost aspect of the subject's own personality, or because he or she offers a chance to "redo" an unfinished conflict with a parent. When partners join as a couple, they make a marital "contract" in which each assumes that he or she, and the other partner, will

do certain things (Sager 1976). Some of these assumptions are conscious and shared ("You will care for the children, and I will work"), some are not shared, and some are secret even from the self. For example, a person may marry to get away from home, or may believe that as long as he acts like a "good child," his spouse will act like a good mother. Mate selection, of course, is also determined by less psychodynamic reasons, such as physical attractiveness, family demands, financial considerations, timing, and luck.

As Lewis (1998) pointed out, relationships fail when "either the person who is more powerful feels unrewarded for that responsibility, or the person with lesser power feels that they've had enough of that relatively powerless situation."

Evaluation of the Couple

Evaluation of a couple involves obtaining data on the current point in the marital and/or family life cycle, determining why the couple came for assistance at this particular time, and eliciting each partner's view of the marital or relationship problem (Table 34–7). Often, the couples therapist will hold one individual session with each partner after the first or second conjoint session. This gives each partner an opportunity to divulge information that he or she might not otherwise discuss. Issues of confidentially need to be carefully addressed.

In formulating an understanding of the marital difficulties, the evaluator will want to consider the couple's communication, problem solving, roles, affective expression and involvement, and behavioral expression, especially in the areas of sex and aggression. The clinician will also want to evaluate gender roles, cultural and racial issues, and power inequities resulting from gender, class, age, or financial status. It is critical to ask about alcohol or drug use, health (especially reproductive) issues, and verbal or physical abuse.

Even if the partners do not mention their children as a problem, the therapist should spend some time acquiring a sense of how the children are doing. It is wise to explore whether there is a favored child or a problem with any of the children, and whether the children are being pulled into marital conflicts. At times children can be the source of a couple's conflict, and at other times they may function as the glue that keeps the relationship together. If a large part of the couple's difficulty centers around issues with the children, family therapy may be the preferred treatment modality, depending on the ages of the children and the family configuration. The clinician should always ask how having a child has changed the nature of the relationship.

The clinician must always ascertain whether there

TABLE 34–7. Guidelines for interviewing couples

Questions	Rationale
Can you tell me about yourself? As individuals? As a couple?	Joining, forming an alliance with each member and the couple, creating a safe place
What brings you here? How do you understand the problem? What feelings does it elicit for each of you?	Developing an interactional problem focus
How does the problematic pattern actually work? Can you show me how it works?	Observing by staging an enactment
How did the pattern originate? How did you create it?	Placing the problem in context of their relationship, families of origin, and individual development
How have you maintained this pattern? What have you done to keep it going?	Placing the pattern or problem under their joint control
Tell me about what you believe should be happening.	Revealing myths, stories, ideas, and expectations about love, sexuality, marriage, and closeness
In what other ways is the pattern currently reinforced? What do your family and friends believe is the problem?	Reflecting how jobs, extended family members, and friends contribute to the pattern's resilience
Is this pattern always occurring, or are there exceptions?	Demonstrating how pervasive the pattern is (i.e., whether it is chronic or related to a life transition)
What have you done to try to change the pattern?	Trying to avoid redundancy by inquiring about solution behavior
Have your efforts to change the pattern made things better or worse?	Looking at the problem as attempted solutions
What has been the influence of this problem in your lives?	Looking for the influence of the problem over their lives
How motivated are you to change the pattern now?	Assessing individual's and couple's motivation
What would happen if you succeeded in changing the pattern?	Anticipating possible consequences of change, both positive and negative
What patterns of relating have you created that you want to keep?	Identifying and honoring assets and resources
Are you ready to make a change? How about trying something different?	Preparing the couple for exploring new patterns of interaction

is a concomitant psychiatric condition, especially an Axis I disorder. If one is present, the impact of the condition on each member of the couple must be explored.

Other areas deserving special attention include each spouse's commitment to the marital union and the couple's sexual life. Assessment is complicated when one spouse is keeping commitment doubts or extramarital sex a secret. Conjoint and individual sessions with each partner may be needed. When infidelity or serious commitment questions arise, the therapist and couple must address whether or not the couple should stay together.

Evaluation of Sexual Disorders

It has been estimated that about half of American marriages have some sexual problems. These can be divided into "difficulties" (e.g., inability to agree on frequency), which are clearly dyadic issues, and *dysfunctions*, which are specific problems with desire, arousal, and orgasm as categorized in DSM-IV-TR (American Psychiatric Association 2000). Dysfunctions may be organic or psychological at base, and may be lifelong or acquired, generalized or situational. They may be deeply embedded in relational power or intimacy struggles, or may be the only problem in an otherwise well-functioning relationship.

Most family therapists have believed that there is no uninvolved partner when one member of a couple presents with sexual dysfunction, which is different from saying that the relationship itself is the cause of the dysfunction. The therapist must ascertain as accurately as possible the etiology of the problem and choose the most effective therapy, whether medical, individual, or relational or a combination thereof. It is also within the therapist's purview to determine whether the couple would like to improve a technically functional but relatively unsatisfying sexual relationship, in the same way that a therapist can offer treatment focused on increasing intimacy for a couple that wishes to pursue personal growth.

A careful evaluation of the couple's total interactions must be done by the therapist, as well as a physical assessment when dysfunction is present. When it appears that the marriage is basically sound but that the couple suffers from specific sexual difficulties (which may also lead to various secondary marital consequences), the primary focus may be sex therapy. In many cases, however, specific sex therapy cannot be carried out until the relationship between the two partners improves in other respects; indeed, the sexual problems may clearly be an outgrowth of the marital difficulties. When marital problems are addressed, the sexual problems may readily resolve. It may be difficult to disentangle marital from sexual problems or to decide which came first. The priorities for therapy may not always be clear.

DSM-IV-TR (American Psychiatric Association 2000) recognizes the following sexual dysfunctions:

- *Sexual desire disorders*—hypoactive sexual desire disorder (HSDD), sexual aversion disorder
- *Sexual arousal disorders*—female sexual arousal disorder, male erectile disorder
- *Orgasmic disorders*—female orgasmic disorder, male orgasmic disorder, premature ejaculation
- *Sexual pain disorders*—dyspareunia (not due to a general medical condition), vaginismus (not due to a general medical condition) (Sexual pain disorders are coded separately if they are due to a general medical condition or are substance induced.)

Many people have more than one dysfunction (e.g., HSDD plus orgasmic disorder), and frequently each member of a couple will have a dysfunction (e.g., premature ejaculation in the man and hypoactive desire in the woman). It is important to elicit the sequencing of the onset of the dysfunctions to understand how they influence each other. As we have said, many sexual problems are not dysfunctions but rather relationally based dissatisfactions.

Specific techniques have been devised for eliciting a sexual history and for evaluating sexual functioning. The marital therapist should become familiar with these methods and obtain experience in their use. The basic components of a systemic assessment of sexual difficulties are listed in Table 34–8.

In addition, in couples where there is any possibility that the problems have an organic component, it is crucial to insist on a medical workup. This is particularly important for men, for whom small physiological changes in potency may produce anxiety that exacerbates the problem.

TABLE 34–8. Assessment of sexual problems

I. Definition of the problem

   A. How does the couple describe the problem? What are their theories about its etiology? How do they generally relate to their sexuality, as reflected in their language, attitudes toward sexuality, comfort level, and permission system?

   B. How is the problem a problem for them? What is the function of the problem in their relationship system? Is the relationship problem the central problem? Why now?

II. Relationship history

   A. Current partner

   B. Previous relationship history

   C. Psychosexual history, including information about early childhood experiences, nature of sexual encounters prior to the relationship, sexual orientation, feelings about masculinity and femininity

   D. Description of current sexual functioning, focusing on conditions for satisfactory sex, positive behaviors, specific technique, and so on. Who initiates sex, who leads, or do both? How does the couple's sexual pattern of intimacy and control reflect or compensate for other aspects of their relationship?

III. Developmental life-cycle issues (births, deaths, transitions)

IV. Medical history, focusing on current physical status, medications, and medical care, especially endocrine, vascular, metabolic

V. Goals (patient and therapist viewpoints), focusing on examining whether goals are realistic and what previous attempted solutions have yielded

The taking of an intimate sexual history of husband and wife should, of course, be done without children present. The process of taking a sexual history should be handled with care and regard for each person's level of comfort. Individuals almost always have more interesting sexual lives than one imagines, and most will be more likely to discuss these details in individual sessions than with their spouse or partner present.

When discussing sexual topics, it is important that the therapist not use terms that would be offensive or uncomfortable for him- or herself or for the couple. At the same time, care must be taken to avoid using bland generalities that fail to elicit specific sexual information. Frankness is encouraged and can be modeled by the therapist. When the partners are being vague, the therapist can follow up with more specific questions.

The therapist should use simple language or use the simplest technical sexual terms that the patient is comfortable with. Some patients will misunderstand technical terms. For others, the use of the vernacular by the therapist may be inappropriate. The problem faced in the choice of language is itself an indication of our general cultural discomfort with sexuality. The therapist's own use of a particular sexual vocabulary can be a model to help the marital partners feel comfortable in communicating with each other more openly.

Taking a sexual history of lesbian and gay couples may be particularly difficult for a heterosexual therapist, either because of discomfort with homosexuality or because of a lack of knowledge about homosexual norms and mores. In addition, the couple may have a wider or different set of sexual practices than the therapist is used to (of course, this may be true with heterosexual couples as well). The therapist has the option of educating himself or herself about homosexual sexuality (the number of books available in mainstream bookstores about gay and lesbian life has risen dramatically in the past few years, as has information available on the Internet) and/or asking the couple about their own and other common practices. If a therapist is very anxious about treating a homosexual couple, the couple may be better served by another therapist, and the appropriate referral should be made. Gay and lesbian couples may present with any of the dysfunctions or dissatisfactions of a heterosexual couple.

Identifying goals of treatment will help determine which modalities will be most effective and in what order they need to be applied. Mediating and final goals commonly addressed in couples therapy are listed in Tables 34–9 and 34–10, respectively.

TABLE 34–9. Mediating goals of couples therapy

1. Specifying the interactional problem
2. Recognizing mutual contribution to problems
3. Clarifying marital boundaries
4. Clarifying and specifying each spouse's needs and desires in the relationship
5. Increasing communication skills
6. Decreasing coercion and blame
7. Increasing differentiation
8. Resolving marital transference distortions

TABLE 34–10. Final goals of couples therapy

1. Resolving presenting problems
2. Reducing symptoms
3. Increasing intimacy
4. Increasing role flexibility and adaptability
5. Improving tolerance of differences
6. Addressing balance of power
7. Fostering clear communication
8. Resolving conflictual interaction
9. Improving relationships with children and families of origin
10. Improving psychosexual functioning

Treatment Approach

The strongest predictor of overall life satisfaction is the quality of the person's central relationship. In addition, "a good and stable relationship buffers against the genetic vulnerability to both medical and psychiatric disorder." Thus, helping a couple achieve a more satisfying relationship can have widespread and profound influence on their life and the lives of those with whom they interact.

The treatment of each couple is unique and may require a combination of couples therapy, individual therapy, group therapy (particularly self-help groups such as Alcoholics Anonymous), family therapy, and medication management. By using an integrative approach with each couple, the therapist maximizes the chances for success.

The treatment of a couple is often conceptualized as relatively brief therapy (although it need not be), usually meeting once weekly, with a focus on the marital or couple interaction. The major indication for couples therapy is the presence of relational conflict; other indications include symptomatic behaviors that affect both partners, such as depression, anxiety disorders, substance abuse, and illness in a child, partner, or other family member. The average length of treatment is six sessions.

Strategies and Techniques

Couples therapy utilizes strategies for imparting new information, strategies for opening up new and expanded individual and marital experiences, psychodynamic strategies for individual and interactional insight, communication and problem-solving strategies, and strategies for restructuring the repetitive interactions between the spouses.

As the divisive spirit of the era of the earlier schools of psychotherapy recedes and is replaced with a growing pluralism and clinical pragmatism, clinicians will attempt to integrate the various strategies into a coherent treatment approach that can be adapted to the individual case. We advocate an integrative marital therapy model that utilizes psychodynamic, behavioral, and structural-strategic strategies of intervention (see below).

For couples in which one member has an Axis I disorder, data suggest that the diagnosis and symptom picture of the affected spouse and characteristics of the other spouse stand in complex relationship to the issues in the marital interaction and should, therefore, influence the planning of intervention (i.e., the goals). For example, if one spouse has a nonendogenous unipolar depression with no clear precipitating stressful life event, the marital interaction could be a chronic stressor and contributor to the condition. Marital therapy in this situation could well be a preferred mode of intervention. On the other hand, if the spouse is suffering from bipolar illness, manic episode, and the marital interaction has been good prior to the episode, psychoeducational intervention with the couple may be in order, with little or no attention to the ongoing marital interaction.

Some couples present with chronic histories of unresolved and unrelenting conflict. Other couples are in a state of transition, perhaps moving from the initial so-called expansion stage of their marriage to the inevitable crisis related to reevaluation of the contraction stage (meaning nothing changes). In either case, clarifying the couple's process and evaluating their recurrent patterns of behavior represent the starting place for couples therapy.

TABLE 34–11. Therapist strategies in focused, active treatment of marital discord

1. Interrupt collusive processes between the partners. The interaction may involve failure on the part of one partner to perceive positive or negative aspects of the other that are clear to an outsider (e.g., cruelty or, alternatively, generosity) or buffering behavior enacted by one partner aimed at protecting the other partner from experiences that are inconsistent with that partner's self-perception (e.g., a husband working part-time views himself as breadwinner; the wife works full-time and manages checkbook to shield husband from reality of family's income and finances).

2. Link individual experiences, including past experiences and inner thoughts, to the couple relationship.

3. Create and assign tasks designed to

   • encourage the partners to differentiate between the impact of the other's behavior versus (the other's) intent.

   • bring into awareness concrete behavior of the partner that contradicts (anachronistic) past perceptions of that partner.

   • encourage both partner to acknowledge their own behavior changes that are incompatible with the maladaptive ways each has seen him- or herself and has been seen by the partner.

   These tasks also help to reconstruct the couple's narrative to make it more positive.

In treatment of marital discord, the primary focus should be the interpersonal distortions between partners, not the couple–therapist transference. However, negative transference distortions toward the therapist must be addressed quickly and overtly (Table 34–11).

The third strategy in Table 34–11 is the most important. In fact, in the initial stage of marital treatment, we ask that each partner focus on what he or she wants to change in him- or herself, *not* on how each partner wants the other partner to be different.

In this integrative model, the focus is on three related domains: the functional relationships between the antecedents and consequences of discrete interactional sequences; the recurrent patterns of interaction, including their implicit rules; and each spouse's individual schemata for intimate relationships. In the initial stage, alliances must be developed early between the therapist and each marital partner, with the therapist offering empathy, warmth, and understanding. The therapist must also ally with the couple as a unit and learn their shared language as well as their different problem-solving styles and attitudes.

Behavioral techniques, including assigning between-session homework and in-session tasks, communication skills, and problem-solving training, can facilitate the process of helping marital partners reintegrate denied aspects of themselves and of each other. However, the focus is not on behavioral change alone, given that overt behavior is seen as reflecting the interlocking feelings and perceptions of each spouse. Ideally, the treatment process should provide a secure framework in which each partner can consider what he or she wants to change in him- or herself, as opposed to how each wants the other spouse to be different; and safely explore new beliefs, feelings, and behaviors, including experimenting with new patterns of interaction that may be unfamiliar and even anxiety provoking.

Treatment of Sexual Dysfunction in Couples

Sexual dysfunction or dissatisfaction may be caused by a primary psychiatric disorder; it may also be a consequence of ignorance of sexual anatomy and physiology, negative attitudes and self-defeating behavior, anger, power or intimacy issues between the partners, medical/physiological problems, or past sexual trauma. Medication side effects are a very common cause of sexual dysfunction in our patients, many of whom are taking selective serotonin reuptake inhibitors (SSRIs). Male erection problems are proving increasingly amenable to medical forms of treatment. It is also important to remember that people vary enormously in the importance they place on the sexual or erotic aspect of their lives. According to survey results reported in *The Social Organization of Sexuality: Sexual Practices in the United States* (Laumann et al. 1994), approximately one-third of people in a relationship have sex at least twice a week, another one-third have sex a few times a month, and the remaining one-third have sex a few times a year or not at all. In general, when sex is not part of a marriage over a long period of time, the relationship has less vitality and life. However, even well-functioning marriages may have periods in which sexuality is much a less part of partners' lives (e.g., after the birth of a first child, during a family or health crisis). Different people have vastly different tolerance for such periods.

Healthy sexual functioning can be thought of as resulting from relatively nonconflicted and self-confi-

dent attitudes about sex and the belief that the partner is pleased by one's performance. Under such circumstances, a reinforcing positive cycle can be activated.

However, when either partner has doubts about his or her sexual attractiveness or ability to please the other, that partner's sexual performance may suffer. Such self-absorption and anxiety will characteristically produce a decline in sexual performance and enjoyment and can lead to impotency and orgasmic difficulties. Couple and individual difficulties of various sorts might then follow. A vicious cycle may be activated, with heightened worries leading to increasingly poor sexual performance.

Because sex involves each person being vulnerable to the other, it is difficult to have sex when one is angry or not in a mood to be close (although some people can block out other feelings and keep the sexual area more separate). In addition, a person who feels abused, mistreated, or ignored in a relationship is less likely to want to please his or her spouse. For those who feel that they have no voice in their relationship, lack of desire is sometimes the only way to manifest displeasure.

Couples who continue in marital or individual treatment for long periods of time may resolve some of their marital problems but still suffer from specific sexual difficulties in their marriage. It is also true that certain sexual problems can be dramatically reversed after relatively brief periods of sex therapy, even though such problems may have proven unresponsive to long periods of customary psychotherapy. However, sexual functioning that is suffering because the partners do not want to be close is not likely to respond to sex therapy unless other issues are also addressed.

Usually, when a couple has a generally satisfactory relationship, any minor sexual problems will be only temporary. Resolution of sexual problems in a relationship, however, will not inevitably produce positive effects in other facets of a relationship.

Marital and sexual problems can interact in various ways:

1. The sexual dysfunction *produces or contributes to* secondary marital discord. Specific strategies focused on the sexual dysfunctions would usually be considered the treatment of choice in these situations, especially if the same sexual dysfunction occurred in the person's other relationships.
2. The sexual dysfunction *is secondary to* marital discord. In such situations, general strategies of marital treatment might be considered the treatment of choice. If the marital relationship is not too severely disrupted, a trial of sex therapy might be

attempted, because a relatively rapid relief of symptoms could produce beneficial effects on the couple's interest in pursuing other marital issues.

3. Marital discord *co-occurs with* sexual problems. This situation would probably not be amenable to sex therapy, given the partners' hostility toward each other. Marital therapy would usually be attempted first, with later attention given to sexual dysfunction.

4. Sexual dysfunction *occurs without* marital discord. This combination might be found in instances where one partner's medical illness has affected his or her sexual functioning, forcing the couple to learn new ways to manage their changed circumstances. Another example might be when one partner has a history of sexual abuse or experiences a sexual assault that creates anxiety related to the sexual experience. Although individual therapy can be helpful in both of these cases, couples therapy can be especially useful in creating a safe place to address painful feelings and anxious expectations, and to provide education and guidance for couples undergoing these transitions.

Treatment of psychosexual disorders, in the model developed by Masters and Johnson (1966), consisted of a thorough assessment of the partners and the relationship, education about sexual functioning, and a series of behavioral exercises. This model was based on three fundamental postulates: 1) a parallel sequence of physiological and subjective arousal in both genders; 2) the primacy of psychogenic factors, particularly learning deficits and performance anxiety; and 3) the amenability of most sexual disorders to a brief, problem-focused treatment approach (i.e., sensate focus). Sensate-focus exercises were designed predominantly for behavioral desensitization, but also functioned to teach the partners about their own and the other's sexual desires and additionally served to elicit relationship problems. In these exercises, the couple pleasures each other, alternating in the role of giver and receiver, first in nongenital areas, then genitally, then with intercourse. In the traditional form of these exercises, intercourse is prohibited during the early stages to remove performance anxiety. There are also specific exercises for each of the sexual dysfunctions. Different authors have developed different exercises and ways of approaching them. For a complete description of sensate-focus exercises, we recommend Kaplan (1995), LoPiccolo and Stock (1996), and Zilbergeld (1992). This approach works best when the sexual problem is caused by ignorance, shame, or a specific dysfunction such as premature ejaculation. Exercises are difficult to complete if the partners feel angry or unloving toward each other.

Many of the patients treated by Masters and Johnson in the 1970s had issues related to sexual ignorance and inexperience. Two decades later, the increase in premarital sex and the proliferation of easily available articles and books on sexuality have reduced sexual ignorance and allowed some couples with sexual dysfunction to work on their issues at home. Recent studies of couples requesting sex therapy have shown a higher proportion of couples with concomitant complicated marital problems.

Other theorists in the field, particularly Schnarch (1997), have focused on cognitive/emotional issues in sexuality—in particular, the meanings attached to specific sexual acts and the level of intimacy involved. Having learned a great deal about the more mechanical and organic issues related to arousal and orgasm, it is important to rethink other aspects of sex—such as eroticism, passion, mystery, and dominance/submission—that make the act itself meaningful. This is particularly true in areas of sexual boredom or situational lack of desire. Therapists of this orientation do not use rigidly staged exercises, but instead focus on the couple's relatedness during sex; they may, however, suggest specific homework to help a couple focus on a particular aspect of their sexuality.

Although not mentioned in DSM-IV, sexual compulsions or addictions may be seen in couples. In these cases, one partner's unceasing compulsion to think about, talk about, and have sex may be very wearing to the other partner, especially since a key component of this problem is that such persons become extremely anxious if sex is denied. They may engage in multiple affairs or place constant demands on their partners. Most people who have affairs do not have a sexual compulsion.

Treatment for sexual addictions is still controversial. Some therapists use a 12-Step addiction model and group therapy; others treat it as a compulsion with individual therapy and medication (particularly SSRIs such as fluoxetine). Couples therapy is still a critical component, to educate the couple and, if multiple affairs have taken place, to discuss the viability of the marriage.

In recent years, emphasis has shifted to the role of biomedical and organic factors in the etiology of sexual dysfunction, leading to the growing use of medical and surgical treatment interventions. Particular focus has been given to the role of vascular disorders and neuroendocrine problems, as well as the tendency for many medications to affect sexual functioning. It is critical for each patient to have a thorough physical workup. For a good review on the interaction of medication and sexuality, see Abramowicz (1992).

A variety of medical approaches to the treatment of erectile disorders in men have been developed in recent years. These include, but are not limited to, surgical prostheses or penile implants (seldom used in the past few years), intracorporeal injection of vasoactive drugs such as papaverine, constriction rings and vacuum pump devices, and urethral suppositories. In 1998, oral medications for the treatment of impotence were introduced (e.g., sildenafil [Viagra]). These medications appear to be changing some of our fundamental perceptions about sexuality and treatment. That is, up to now, most sex therapists believed that introduction of a "medication" would not, or could not, change a couple's ongoing sexual relationship. It appears that this assumption is not as "true" as was once believed. Because our understanding and treatment of impotence are developing so rapidly, it is important for therapists to stay current on new research in the field. Surgical treatments are available for the correction of arterial insufficiency or venous leakage problems. These methods may be more or less acceptable both to the man and to his partner. The partner's response to the treatment is often a key element in its success. There has been some success in treating premature ejaculation with SSRIs and clomipramine; however, because these medications may also decrease sexual desire, caution and careful monitoring are indicated (Abramowicz 1992). In one study of patients on long-term SSRIs, sildenafil significantly improved erectile function, arousal, ejaculation, orgasm, and overall satisfaction domain measures compared with placebo (Nurnberg et al. 2003).

In women, most medical interventions have been for dyspareunia. Female dyspareunia secondary to the decreased vaginal lubrication of aging can be treated with topical estrogen cream or lubricant jelly. Even when an organic cause of dyspareunia is found and treated, the conditioned anxiety and lack of arousal that have become associated with sex usually require an additional course of couples therapy with a sexual focus. Hormone treatment for lack of desire has not been proven effective (Rosen and Leiblum 1995).

Efficacy of Couples Therapy

Couple Distress or Problems

Data accumulated over three decades suggest that couples therapy is superior to individual therapy for marital conflict situations. The strongest effects are in increasing marital satisfaction and reducing conflict. (It should be pointed out that these are not synonymous—some people who have high marital conflict still report high marital satisfaction, and some couples have low conflict because the marriages are "dead.") Not surprisingly, couples who are less distressed show more improvement. Some of these effects wash out over time, as is common in chronic conditions.

Sexual Difficulties

Twenty-five years of experience in treating sexual difficulties with some combination of sex therapy and couples therapy have shown such combination to be consistently superior to individual therapy in the treatment of sexual dysfunction. Although Masters and Johnson's (1970) original success rates were not repeated in later studies, 60%–95% of sexual dysfunctions can be treated, depending on the type of sexual problem. Recent advances in sex therapy have included a movement from mostly behavioral to more integrative treatment models, with more attention to cognitive and systemic factors and greater focus on organic causes and medical treatment for male dysfunction, especially erectile dysfunction (Rosen and Leiblum 1995).

Mood Disorders in Women Who Have Couples or Marital Problems

Prince and Jacobson's (1995) review of marital and family therapies for affective disorders suggested that medication plus marital therapy is more beneficial than individual therapy alone for depressed, maritally distressed women. In these cases, individual therapy does little to moderate the "toxic" marital problems that increase the depression. Drugs alone are also ineffective for this type of problem. Most treatment outcome studies have involved couples in which the wife was the depressed spouse, so we have little information to guide work with depressed married men. However, some men are deeply troubled by the experience of talking about problems, preferring to work on them in private. In addition, some depressed men have wives who are very angry about the effects of living with a depressed partner, and discussion of this anger in therapy might increase these men's depression. Parenthetically, there is some evidence that women with comorbid Axis I conditions respond better to couples therapy than do men with comorbid Axis I conditions.

What Happens If the Outcome of Marital Treatment Is Separation or Divorce?

One might automatically assume that such an outcome is deleterious and that marital and family therapy should be designed to hold the families together. On reflection, however, experience seems to indicate otherwise. Marital therapy allows the partners to examine whether or not it is to their advantage to stay together, and it gives them permission to separate if that is what they need to do.

Indications for Couples Therapy

The process of choosing a type of therapy is complex, and research is just beginning to develop guidelines for such decisions. The therapist often must base his or her judgment on clinical intuition, general clinical opinion, and the wishes and judgments of the people involved.

Marital Versus Individual Therapy

One of the most common questions for clinicians who are fluent in both therapies is the decision about type and timing of therapy. The basic theoretical premise of couples or family therapy is that many problems are purely relational, that individual symptoms in one person can be viewed as interpersonal in terms of etiology or problem maintenance, and that such symptoms or problems can be changed by altering the system. By contrast, the basic premise of individual therapy is that problems or symptoms develop because of the genes or dynamics within an individual and that change occurs in the individual (either behaviorally or through cognitive understanding of the problems) in the presence of an intense and exclusive relationship with a therapist. In truth, for many people, both forms of therapy may be useful or necessary. Self-knowledge does not always help a person understand a complex family system and how one's behavior affects and is affected by family members. In addition, family therapy does not allow for intense exploration of psychodynamic issues. Individual therapy also does not allow the clinician to see how the problems of other family members may be affecting the system. For example, a woman who requested individual treatment for "depression" was found, on family evaluation, to have a husband with untreated bipolar illness (i.e., manic symptoms). Much of what was assumed to be depression in this woman was in fact a response to the husband's behavior in manic or hypomanic states. One of the key factors in treating this woman's depression was treating the husband's symptoms and helping him acknowledge the validity of his wife's concerns about him. On the other hand, for many people symptoms occur independently of the different systems around them over time (i.e., *not* stress related).

Because people tend to select partners whose stage of differentiation is similar to their own, it is not unusual for individuals with psychological difficulties to have spouses with similar or with complementary but equally severe problems. In addition to the need to evaluate the partner, it must be recognized that such couples create problems in maintaining the family systems that need to be addressed directly. Children in such families often suffer either from genetically based similar illnesses (e.g., depression) or from symptoms that evolve as a result of dealing with parental problems. These illnesses or symptoms are often best treated with family therapy, but this does not rule out individual treatment. For many people, both types of therapy are helpful, allowing for increased pleasure with the partner and also a context for personal and private growth.

The choice of timing of therapy is always of interest. If the person is highly symptomatic and has a problem that is usually amenable to medications, it is often helpful to begin medication and family therapy first, in order to reduce the symptoms and educate the family, as well as to eliminate family sources of stress.

In general, one tries to deal with the most acute problems first. If it is possible in terms of timing and finances, it is easily possible to do individual and couples therapy at the same time. It is often recommended that the therapies be done by different therapists; however, in this strategy it is imperative that the therapists remain in contact to avoid splitting or conflicting treatment. Others, including ourselves on occasion, have treated both the couple and one member of the couple individually, although this can present some additional challenges to the therapist to remain neutral and unbiased. Our decisions about who should be treated and by whom depend more on the characteristics of the couple and how they function than on the particular diagnosis or problem area. The bias of the couple or individual must also be taken into account.

Individual, Couples, or Sex Therapy for Sexual Problems

The distinctions among individual, couples, and sex therapy were clearer a decade ago, when sex therapy primarily involved a specific and highly detailed behavioral protocol. Over the past few years, however, sex therapy has moved in the direction of further understanding of the physiological causes of sexual dysfunction on the one hand, and a focus on cognitive-behavioral issues on the other. It is clear at this point that sexual problems rarely disappear with couples therapy alone unless specific attention is paid to the nature and quality of the sexual problems. In general, it is most effective to deal with severe couple conflict before beginning to deal with sexual issues directly. Sex therapy includes education, a focus on the intimacy and power aspects of sex, and usually homework assignments that in some way deal with sexual anxiety and expansion of sexual options. Individual therapy is indicated if the problems are clearly related to the partner's history (e.g., sexual abuse, hatred of women), have occurred in multiple relationships, and are not amenable to being worked on in a couples context. Individual therapy is not an efficient way of dealing with most couple-centered sexual problems. It is also important to consider the possible role of organic problems in any dysfunction (Table 34–12).

Research has demonstrated that no one school of therapy is definitively superior to another (Shadish et al. 1993). In general the trend has been toward a more integrative approach, drawing from a variety of models and allowing for a more fluid type of work (Lebow 1997). Integrative models are likely to combine some form of here-and-now work (cognitive or behavioral) with some type of focus on historical understanding of the patterns that led to the current problem.

Contraindications to Couples Therapy

Couples therapy is not indicated for every couple in distress. In fact, at times it may even be contraindicated. If one partner is keeping an important secret (e.g., an HIV-positive man who refuses to share this information with his wife), an attempt to work with both partners as a pair may fail, and the therapist will have to take a strong stand and refuse to treat the couple. At times, one member of a couple may be too ill to benefit from couples therapy (e.g., one partner has bipolar disorder or schizophrenia and is acutely psychotic).

Other couples feel more comfortable when each partner sees his or her own therapist. At times it can be more effective to have each partner receive individual therapy, with good coordination between the two therapists. Finally, cases may be encountered in which seeing both members of a couple together may place one of the members in physical danger. When one partner has a history of violence toward the other partner, the therapist must see each party alone to ensure the safety of the individual. Discussing areas of conflict together may risk increasing the violent behavior of one partner.

Sex therapy may be contraindicated in the same situations as above. In addition, many couples do not feel comfortable in a therapy focused exclusively on sex. These couples may make more progress if the sex therapy is carefully integrated within the overall treatment of the couple. When referring a couple to a sex therapist, it is particularly important to be familiar with the skills and credentials of the therapist.

Special Issues in Couples Therapy
Homosexuality and Bisexuality

We believe that family therapists should be adequately educated in the area of human sexual orientation and sexual identity. The terms themselves are confusing. *Sexual orientation* is another way of indicating an individual's tendency to be attracted to one or both sexes. Sexual orientation, like most psychological phenomena, is not an absolute or mutually exclusive trait. One may be sexually attracted to the opposite sex, the same sex, or both. Sexual orientation falls along a continuum, with completely homosexual and completely heterosexual preferences falling at the extreme ends, and many gradations in between. Sexual orientation may also change over time. Some persons change from heterosexual to homosexual or the reverse in their 30s, 40s, or 50s. Some remain bisexual throughout their adult lives.

TABLE 34–12. Indications for sex and marital therapy	
Sex therapy	**Marital therapy**
The marital problem is clearly focused on sexual dysfunction.	Sexuality either is not an issue or is one of many issues in the marital dysfunction.
Enabling factors	**Enabling factors**
The couple is willing and able to carry out sexual-functioning tasks assigned by the therapist.	Anger and resistance are too intense for the couple to carry out extrasession tasks around sexual functioning.
The partners are strongly attached to each other; both partners are interested in reversing the sexual dysfunction.	The couple is not committed to each other; covert or overt behaviors are occurring to dissolve the marriage.

Observations of human sexual behavior, affectionate attachments, erotic fantasies, arousal, and erotic preference have suggested that sexual orientation and sexual identity are not static. *In fact, both may fluctuate over a person's lifetime.* Sometimes changes in sexuality are "just phases"; sometimes they become the predominant disposition of sexual relating. Regardless, deviation from heterosexuality in Western society is frequently accompanied by rejection, not only by one's immediate family but also by one's peers and, in some cases, society in general. Accusations of discrimination and violence, such as "gay bashing," have been a continual topic in news headlines. Bisexual individuals may experience additional nonacceptance by gay and lesbian friends or associates, who may accuse them of "fence sitting," "sleeping with the enemy," or being deviant because they are unable to choose to be hetero- or homosexual. For the therapist, countertransferential issues should be centered on understanding and listening to others' experiences even if they are quite different from our own.

Infidelity, communication, and substance abuse are issues that are common to all couples, including homosexual or bisexual couples. However, homosexual and bisexual couples must deal with additional issues, including the effects of internalized homophobia, gender role themes, societal oppression, and "coming out" (Connolly 2004).

Internalized homophobia exists when homosexual or bisexual individuals experience negative feelings and emotions toward themselves when recognizing their own sexuality (Herek 1997). This can bring about feelings of guilt, self-hatred, and negativity regarding the durability of long-term relationships (Ossana 2000). Difficulties in identity formation, identity management, and the "coming out" process can all emanate from internalized homophobia (Connolly 2004).

Societal oppression comes in two forms: homophobia and heterosexism. Homophobia is defined as any negative belief, reaction, attitude, or action toward homosexuals (Bernat 2001). Homophobia can be hostile due to its inherent discriminatory and prejudicial nature (Connolly 2004). Heterosexism is the belief that heterosexual relationships are preferable and superior to homosexual or bisexual relationships. This belief in and of itself is oppressive (Connolly 2004).

Ethical Issues in Couples and Family Therapy

The fundamental ethical dilemmas inherent in psychotherapy—confidentiality, limits of control, duty to warn/reporting of abuse, and therapist–patient boundaries—become more complex when the treatment involves more than one person. *The therapist has an ethical responsibility to everyone in the family. In some cases, individual needs and system needs may be in conflict.* For example, a husband may wish to conceal from his wife a brief episode of unprotected sex with another woman, whereas his wife is better protected, for health reasons as well as psychological reasons, if she knows about it. A wife's wish to be divorced from a psychiatrically ill and demanding husband may conflict with his need for her care. Such clinical situations provide a set of ethical dilemmas for the therapist.

The therapist must be clear that in most cases (e.g., impending divorce), his or her job is to help the partners sort out their values, obligations, and options rather than to make a decision for them. In other cases, however (e.g., the reporting of child abuse), the ethical decision *must* be the therapist's. And in still other cases, the therapist faces difficult gray areas that must be decided on a case-by-case basis. The therapist also has certain unalterable ethical obligations, such as refraining from engaging in "dual relationships" (see below) with patients or exploiting patients for the therapist's own benefit.

Although the operative concept is "First, do no harm," the issues of how one defines harm and how one determines who will or will not be harmed by a certain action are complex and difficult questions, especially when treating a couple or family. These issues are addressed in the American Association of Marital and Family Therapy (AAMFT) Code of Ethics (2006).

Conflicting Interests of Family Members

It is not unusual for the interests of each member of the couple to conflict at some point. Boszormenyi-Nagy and Spark (1973) emphasized the contractual obligations and accountability that exist between persons in the multigenerational family. *Relational ethics* is concerned with the balance of equitable fairness between people. To gauge the balance of fairness in the here and now, and across time and generations, each member must consider both his or her own interests and the interests of the other family members. The basic issue is one of *equitability*—that is, each family member is entitled to have his or her welfare and interests considered in a way that is fair to the related interests of the other family members.

There may be times when it is difficult to decide whether a recommended therapeutic action or suggested approach may be helpful for one individual but unhelpful or even temporarily harmful for the other individual. In their concern for the healthy functioning of the system as a whole, therapists may inadvertently ignore what is best for one individual. How such decisions are made is an ethical issue. Is balancing the needs and interests of both partners the therapist's concern alone, or should these decisions be shared with the couple? How much information should clients be given on the pros and cons of therapeutic modalities? Our preference is to negotiate with and give the couple all of the relevant information so that they can make the most informed decision possible. (For further discussion of ethics, see also Hare-Mustin et al. 1979 and Hare-Mustin 1980.)

Secrets and Confidentiality

Unless a therapist sees both partners together at all times, he or she will eventually face a situation in which family secrets are disclosed in individual sessions. Secrets are a common source of dysfunction, and discovering and dealing with them are a frequent focus of therapy. As Imber-Black (1993) has noted,

> Secrets, decisions about secrecy and openness, and the management of information are woven into the fabric of our society. The paradox[es] of what is to be kept secret and what is to be shared and with whom are all around us and are embedded in each encounter between family and therapist.

The therapist needs to make a distinction between secrecy and privacy. *Privacy* is usually considered to mean information held by one person that he or she would prefer not to share but that does not directly affect the relationship in question. Privacy usually implies a zone of comfort free from intrusion. *Secrets* are usually considered to be feelings or information that directly affects the relevant relationship. Secrets are most often connected to fear, anxiety, and shame and are often jointly held—that is, some people in the system know, whereas others do not. There is also a gray area in which different people may have different ideas about whether certain information is important and should be shared with a spouse or other family members. (For example, would an affair that occurred during the marriage but that ended 10 years ago be considered private or secret?)

Secrets define hierarchy and relationship, leaving the unaware mystified and out of alliance. Some are about the past (e.g., an affair that occurred many years ago) and some about the present (e.g., an ongoing affair, an impending bankruptcy). The majority of toxic secrets are in some way related to sex (including abortions and illegitimate birth), money, or betrayal.

In general, the best rule of thumb is that a secret should be disclosed if it is seriously affecting connections between people, poses danger to a family member (sexual abuse), or shapes family coalitions and alliances. In general, secrets represent such a serious barrier that it is better to disclose them, even if doing so is painful—because otherwise the sense of mystification and isolation in the unaware is very strong. (This seems to be true in many areas affecting children that were formerly always kept secret, such as adoption, out-of-wedlock birth, and artificial insemination.) However, such issues are very dependent on the situation. For example, a husband who is bisexual or homosexual but has not disclosed this to his wife and who engages in unprotected (or even protected) intercourse with men may be placing his wife in serious danger. Because the husband's sexuality is definitely the wife's concern, not telling her this secret represents a serious threat to the relationship.

The therapist must carefully consider the timing and consequences of disclosure. Premature disclosure of a family secret, before the therapist has formed an alliance with the family, can cause the family to leave therapy precipitately, with no place to deal with potentially explosive materials. The therapist must be particularly careful when there has been a history of violence or abuse. It is generally believed that if a family member refuses to divulge a secret so serious that therapy will be derailed, the therapist may terminate therapy but should not disclose that secret him- or herself. An exception is in cases of potential violence to another, especially in child abuse or threats to murder, where the therapist is required to report such knowledge to the authorities and to the potential victim, so the secret will have to be disclosed. The confusion felt by therapists faced with the requirement for reporting and knowing this may end their relationship with the family is difficult to manage, and these cases must be discussed with a supervisor or mentor. Issues around disclosure also arise in cases where one partner is HIV positive but has not disclosed this to the other partner. Legally the therapist is not obliged to do so; ethically it is extraordinarily hard not to. The patient should be strongly urged to do so. Currently, this issue of disclosure is being extensively discussed in the legal system.

Therapist–Patient Boundaries

The issue of boundaries and *dual relationships* is a critical one in all forms of psychotherapy. Because couples therapy involves more than one patient in the consulting room, there is less likelihood of inappropriate sexual contact between therapist and patient. However, there have been cases in which a therapist working with a couple began an affair with one of the spouses, either during couples therapy or after the couple left treatment.

Countertransference Issues

The fact that the issues faced by couples are the same issues that therapists face in their own lives makes it very likely that at some point countertransference issues may become ethical ones. For example, seeing a couple going through a separation at the same time one is also going through early stages of a divorce is extremely difficult to do, and the likelihood of remaining neutral to both parties is not great. Although it is obviously impossible for therapists to stop treating patients while they themselves are going through a divorce, therapists could certainly choose not to accept new patients whose situations are very similar to their own or who remind them of their departing spouse.

Substance Abuse

Substance abuse and alcoholism can put a serious strain on a couple or family. Behavioral couples therapy (BCT) has been shown to be efficacious in helping couples deal with one partner's drug or alcohol abuse. Fals-Stewart et al. (2005) reported improved functioning among couples who received such therapy, with fewer drug- or alcohol-related arrests, decreased use of alcohol or drugs, fewer hospitalizations due to drugs or alcohol, more satisfaction in the relationship, and fewer instances of violence toward the partner or family members throughout a 12-month posttreatment evaluation period. Substance abuse groups are of course helpful.

Financial Issues

Who pays the bill is a relatively simple decision in individual treatment with adult patients but is not necessarily so in couples or family therapy. The ethical issue of who pays the bill becomes especially tense in marital treatment of spouses in conflict. For example, if both spouses have insurance coverage from their respective employers, whose insurance should be used?

This becomes most delicate when the spouses have conflicting views of the matter for any number of reasons (e.g., "I don't want my secretary seeing the insurance forms"; "Using my insurance makes me the patient"). As with many concrete issues of conflict, the family therapist should approach the matter with a sense of fairness. The symbolic meanings of who pays should be thoroughly explored. When both partners have separate incomes and separate financial arrangements, they should each pay half of the bill.

Other financial questions involve sudden changes of fortune; for example, if a woman married to a well-to-do man divorces and her income drops severely and suddenly, is the therapist willing to continue treatment even if the husband refuses to pay?

For many therapists and many clients, money is the most taboo subject, even more so than sex. It is the job of therapists to clarify their own understandings and feelings about money so that they can support discussions with patients.

Conclusion

Couples, family, and sex therapy are important forms of psychotherapy. There is little question that developing the skills needed to successfully work with couples and families presenting with a wide range of difficulties requires an understanding of how relationships change over time, how problems emerge and are maintained, and how focused marital treatment can alleviate distress and dysfunction. The rewards are great when therapists can assist couples and families in recognizing and shifting the patterns that inhibit their abilities to live rich, intimate lives together. As family patterns change, so also must family therapy techniques. It is our belief that the family model should be moved from the margins to the center of psychotherapy training and practice in order to help not only families and couples but also individuals in these systems as well.

Key Points

- Couples therapy can be defined as a format of intervention involving both members of a dyad in which the focus of intervention is the problematic interactional patterns of the couple. The focus of couples therapy is on the dyad and its intimate emotional and sexual aspects.

- Family therapy is a psychotherapeutic intervention in which family members beyond the primary dyad are involved, including parents, children, and even extended family members, if they share in or are part of the pathology. The goal of family therapy is to assist the family in more successfully achieving their goals and establish gratifying ways of living and interacting as a family unit.

- Family therapists need, and should use, an integrated model.

- In this chapter we encourage the integration of a variety of techniques, depending on the particular problem and personalities of the family or couple.

- Periods of dysfunction are inevitable in any long-term marital relationship. The clinician should always ask how having a child has changed the nature of the relationship.

- The therapist must teach intimate communication (focusing on how to explore difficult issues and increase empathy).

- Gender differences in needs and communication often make marital problems more complex.

- The job of the therapist is to ascertain as well as possible the etiology of the problem and to choose the most effective therapy, whether medical, individual, or relational.

- Individuals almost always have more interesting sexual lives than one imagines; they will be more likely to discuss them in individual sessions than with their spouse or partner present.

- In general, when sex is not part of a marriage over a long period of time, the relationship has less vitality and life.

- Prince and Jacobson's (1995) review suggested that medication plus marital therapy is better than individual therapy alone.

- Our decisions about who should be treated and by whom depend more on the characteristics of the couple and how they function than on the particular diagnosis or problem area. The bias of the couple or individual must also be taken into account.

- In general, a family secret should be disclosed if it is seriously affecting connections between people, poses danger to a family member (e.g., sexual abuse), or shapes family coalitions and alliances.

- The therapist can collect and organize historical data through the use of a genogram, a three-generational family tree depicting the family's patterns regarding either specific problems or general family functioning.

Suggested Readings

Glick ID, Berman E, Clarkin JK, et al: Marital and Family Therapy, 4th Edition. Washington, DC, American Psychiatric Press, 2000

Ritvo EC, Glick ID: Concise Guide to Marital and Family Therapy. Washington, DC, American Psychiatric Press, 2002

Online Resources

www.marsvenus.com—Expert relationship advice from relationship experts on the web

www.healthyminds.org—American Psychiatric Association–sponsored web site about healthy living

www.aamft.org—The American Association for Marriage and Family Therapy web site

References

Abramowicz ME: Drugs that cause sexual dysfunction: an update. The Medical Letter 34:95–111, 1992

American Association for Marriage and Family Therapists: AAMFT Code of Ethics. Washington, DC, American Association for Marriage and Family Therapists, 2006

American Psychiatric Association: Diagnostic and Statistical Manual of Mental Disorders, 4th Edition, Text Revision. Washington, DC, American Psychiatric Association, 2000

Bernat JA, Calhoun KS, Adams HE, et al: Homophobia and physical aggression toward homosexual and heterosexual individuals. J Abnorm Psychol 110:179–187, 2001

Boszormenyi-Nagy I, Spark G: Invisible Loyalties: Reciprocity in Intergenerational Family Therapy. New York, Harper & Row, 1973

Connolly C: Clinical issues with same-sex couples: a review of the literature, in Relationship Therapy with Same-Sex Couples. Edited by Bigner JJ, Wetchler JL. New York, Haworth, 2004, pp 3–12

Epstein NB, Bishop DS: Problem-centered systems therapy of the family, in Handbook of Family Therapy. Edited by Gurman S, Kniskern DP. New York, Brunner/Mazel, 1981, pp 444–482

Fals-Stewart W, Klosterman K, Yates B, et al: Brief relationship therapy for alcoholism: a randomized clinical trial examining clinical efficacy and cost-effectiveness. Psychol Addict Behav 19:363–371, 2005

Goldner V, Penn P, Sheinberg M, et al: Love and violence: gender paradoxes in volatile attachments. Fam Process 29:343–364, 1990

Hare-Mustin R: Family therapy may be dangerous to your health. Prof Psychol 11:935–938, 1980

Hare-Mustin R, Marecek J, Caplan K, et al: Rights of clients, responsibilities of therapists. Am Psychol 34:3–16, 1979

Herek GM, Cogan JC, Gillis JR, et al: Correlates of internalized homophobia in a community sample of lesbians and gay men. J Gay Lesbian Med Assoc 2:17–25, 1997

Heru AM: Family psychiatry: from research to practice. Am J Psychiatry 163:962–968, 2006

Imber-Black E: Secrets in Families and Family Therapy. New York, WW Norton, 1993

Issacs M, Leon G: Remarriage and its alternatives following divorce: mother and child adjustment. J Marital Fam Ther 14:163–173, 1988

Kessler S: The American Way of Divorce: Prescription for Change. Chicago, IL, Nelson-Hall, 1975

Kaplan HS: The Sexual Desire Disorders: Dysfunctional Regulation of Sexual Motivation. New York, Brunner/Mazel, 1995

Laumann E, Gagnon JH, Michael RT, et al: The Social Organization of Sexuality: Sexual Practices in the United States. Chicago, IL, University of Chicago Press, 1994

Lebow J: The integrative revolution in couple and family therapy. Fam Process 36:1–17, 1997

Lewis JM: For better or worse: interpersonal relationship and individual outcome. Am J Psychiatry 155:582–589, 1998

LoPiccolo J, Stock W: Treatment of sexual dysfunction. J Consult Clin Psychol 54:158–167, 1996

Masters WH, Johnson VE: Human Sexual Response. Boston, MA, Little, Brown, 1966

Masters WH, Johnson VE: Human Sexual Inadequacy. Boston, MA, Little, Brown, 1970

McGoldrick M, Gerson R: Genograms in Family Assessment. New York, WW Norton, 1985

Messinger L: Remarriage between divorced people with children from previous marriages: a proposal for preparation for remarriage. J Marriage Fam Couns 2:193–200, 1976

Nurnberg HG, Hensley PL, Gelenberg AJ, et al: Treatment of antidepressant-associated sexual dysfunction with sildenafil: a randomized controlled trial. JAMA 289:56–64, 2003

Ossana SM: Relationship and couples counseling, in Handbook of Counseling and Psychotherapy With Lesbian, Gay, and Bisexual Clients. Edited by RM Perez, DeBord KA, Bieschke KJ. Washington, DC, American Psychological Association, 2000, pp 275–302

Prince SE, Jacobson NS: A review and evaluation of marital and family therapies for affective disorders. J Marital Fam Ther 21:377–401, 1995

Ritvo EC, Glick ID: Concise Guide to Marital and Family Therapy. Washington, DC, American Psychiatric Press, 2002

Rosen R, Leiblum S: Treatment of sexual disorders in the 1990s: an integrated approach. J Consult Clin Psychol 63:877–890, 1995

Sager C: Marriage Contracts and Couple Therapy: Hidden Forces in Intimate Relationships. New York, Brunner/Mazel, 1976

Salts CJ: Divorce process: integration of theory. J Divorce 2:233–240, 1979

Schnarch D: Passionate Marriage. New York, WW Norton, 1997

Schoen R: First unions and the stability of first marriages. J Marriage Family 54:281–84, 1992

Shadish, WR, Montgomery LM, Wilson P, et al: Effects of family and marital psychotherapies: a meta-analysis. J Consult Clin Psychol 61:992–1002, 1993

Shapiro R, Budman S: Defection, termination and continuation in family and individual therapy. Fam Process 12:55–67, 1973

Shorter E: The Making of the Modern Family. New York, Basic Books, 1977

Walsh F: Conceptualizations of normal family processes, in Normal Family Processes, 2nd Edition. Edited by Walsh F. New York, Guilford, 1993, pp 1–25

Zilbergeld B: The New Male Sexuality. New York, Bantam Books, 1992

35

GROUP THERAPY

Paul D. Cox, M.D.
Sophia Vinogradov, M.D.
Irvin D. Yalom, M.D.

Interpersonal relationships are of crucial importance to human psychological development (Siegel 1999). There are many psychiatric and therapeutic implications to this simple premise. Personality and patterns of behavior can be seen as the result of early interactions with other significant human beings. Modern schools of dynamic psychotherapy underscore the link between psychopathology and distorted interpersonal relationships and emphasize that psychiatric treatment must be directed toward understanding and correcting these distortions. Although this can of course take place in the context of the therapist–patient dyad, it is self-evident that a group of people can serve as an immensely specific therapeutic tool. In such a group setting, patients are provided with a varied array of interpersonal relationships that, with proper guidance, will permit them to identify, explore, and alter maladaptive interpersonal behavior.

Furthermore, the group setting is at once a ubiquitous and elusive phenomenon in our society. After all, groups are everywhere around us throughout our lives, from our early family units to the classroom and our classmates to the persons we surround ourselves with at work, at play, and at home. At the same time, we hear complaints about increasing interpersonal

alienation in modern life—a sense of isolation, anonymity, and even social fragmentation. Perhaps because of this factor, and because a group can provide such a powerful and unique therapeutic experience, the group setting is being used more and more not only by mental health professionals but by laypersons. Alcoholics Anonymous, Parents Without Partners, Recovery, Inc., Overeaters Anonymous, Mended Hearts, and Compassionate Friends are but a few of the current specialized and self-help groups available in the lay setting.

A number of specialized groups have been developed to function in a supportive and occasionally highly therapeutic mode in nonpsychiatric medical settings as well. The groundbreaking work of Spiegel et al. (1989) demonstrated a twofold increase in survival rate for patients with metastatic breast carcinoma who participated in a long-term psychodynamically oriented support group. Fawzy et al. (1993) found an improvement both in use of coping strategies and in immune function in patients with malignant melanoma who participated in a short-term group intervention. Group therapy enhances the quality of life of cancer patients (Blake-Mortimer 1999; Greenstein and Breitbart 2000).

Clinical Relevance of Group Therapy

Although the general principles of group therapy are increasingly being employed by the self-help group movement and by other mental health professions, mainstream psychiatric education has deemphasized the teaching and practice of group therapy. Perhaps the remedicalization of psychiatry, with its emphasis on biological modes of treatment for mental illness, accounts for this trend. Also, some psychiatrists may be alienated by the fact that the group treatment modality is being used so often by laypersons in settings that are, strictly speaking, nonpsychiatric. However, a meta-analysis by Barlow et al. (2000) suggested that many self-help groups involve professionals. These authors also noted that the effectiveness of self-help groups is an important new area of research.

Nonetheless, the estrangement of psychiatrists from group work is of some concern; after all, group therapy is a widely practiced mode of psychotherapy that is employed in a vast number of clinical settings with a proven degree of clinical effectiveness (Montgomery 2002). The advent of widespread managed care and population-based care systems is expanding the role of groups. Studies are demonstrating that when primary care doctors can refer patients to group therapy, many of the patients improve markedly (Kanas 2005).

Efficacy

First and foremost, group therapy is effective treatment. Numerous outcome studies of varying sophistication and methodological design have been performed since the early 1960s. Considerable clinical consensus and research evidence have accumulated indicating that various forms of group therapy are beneficial to their participants (Dies 1979, 1993; Hoag and Burlingame 1997; Kaul and Bednar 1986; MacKenzie 1997a; Orlinsky and Howard 1986; Piper et al. 1992; Smith et al. 1980; Yalom 1983, 1985). Investigators over the years have concluded that group treatment is as effective as individual therapy in treating psychological disorders (Shapiro and Shapiro 1982; Smith et al. 1980). Forty-eight studies that directly contrasted individual and group treatments were analyzed (McDermut et al. 2001; Truax 2001); in 43 studies, there were statistically significant reductions in depressive symptoms following group psychotherapy; 9 showed no difference between group and individual therapy.

Many previous meta-analyses have also found no major differences between the two modalities (Budman et al. 1998; McRoberts et al. 1998; Tillitski 1990; Toseland and Siporin 1986). More recent studies are beginning to delineate the specific aspects of group treatments that work with particular populations (Kanas 2005).

Numbers of Group Therapy Patients

Enormous numbers of psychiatric patients receive their sole or primary treatment in groups. This is particularly true in institutional settings and for chronically mentally ill persons. At least one-half of all psychiatric hospitals and one-quarter of all correctional institutions, not to mention the vast majority of community mental health centers, use group treatments (Shapiro 1978). Many health maintenance organizations make substantial use of group therapy as well (Cheifetz and Salloway 1984; MacKenzie 1997b, 2001a; Spitz 1997; Taylor et al. 2001). Altogether, hundreds of thousands of patients undergo group therapy. Furthermore, patients most often found in institutional settings—the chronically ill—represent one of the greatest current challenges to the psychiatric profession and to social policy regarding the mentally ill. When compared with these populations, patients receiving routine individual therapy are a relatively insignificant subset, in terms of both large-scale mental health policy and sheer numbers.

Nonpsychiatric Groups

New orders of magnitude occur when we consider the staggering number of nonpsychiatric clients who receive treatment in specialized therapy groups or in one of the vast number of self-help groups. For example, the use of groups for patients with particular medical conditions—such as cancer support groups, post–myocardial infarction groups, and diabetes education groups—is burgeoning in the health care setting (Fawzy et al. 1995; Stern 1993). In 1983, perhaps 12 million to 14 million individuals attended some form of self-help group (e.g., Alcoholics Anonymous, Compassionate Friends, Recovery, Inc.) (Lieberman 1990). Goodman and Jacobs (1994) suggested that self-help groups may become the treatment of choice for many psychopathologies and nonpsychiatric life predicaments by the year 2010 or 2020. Inevitably, the practicing therapist of nearly every persuasion will encounter clients who have had contact with some form of group experience.

Practical Aspects of Group Therapy: Cost-Effectiveness and Efficiency

At its inception, group therapy was grounded in practical aspects. To facilitate the treatment of large numbers of tuberculosis patients at the turn of the twentieth century, a Boston internist named Joseph Pratt developed a workable, efficient treatment format: group meetings. Many of Dr. Pratt's patients were indigent and could not afford private care; many were debilitated, despondent, and ostracized in the healthy community. Needing to work with many different individuals in a highly efficient manner, Dr. Pratt began organizing groups of 20 or 30 patients and lecturing them once or twice a week (Pratt 1922). Even today, of course, group therapy retains this advantageous feature of expediency. Large numbers of patients can be treated and efficient use can be made of time and other resources. For example, group therapy is at the core of effective therapeutic community treatment of homelessness (McCracken and Black 2005).

Cost-effectiveness played an important role in the early development of group therapy as well. As noted in the previous paragraph, Pratt himself worked with indigent patients, and several other early pioneers in the group lecture approach treated psychotic individuals who could afford only institutional care. Alfred Adler, an Austrian psychiatrist who became interested in theories of group behavior and of social interest, also spoke of "bringing psychology to the people" (Ansbacher 1980). In England during and after World War II, the overwhelming number of psychiatric casualties and the limited hospital staff available made group treatment the most practical modality and led to an explosion in group therapy practice and research, which included the work of Wilfred Bion and the Tavistock model of group behavior and of S.H. Foulkes and group analysis (Pines and Hutchinson 1993). The same situation holds true today in many understaffed community agencies or institutional settings: treatment groups permit more efficient use of limited staff. Leadership in managed care supports the use of groups in large part for reasons of expediency.

Fortunately, the rationale for group therapy goes well beyond economics and savings in staff time. In examining nine studies comparing the differential efficiency of individual and group therapy, Toseland and Siporin (1986) concluded that group treatment is

more consistently efficient and/or cost-effective. As efforts to maintain or improve outcomes while containing costs continue, these practical considerations of expediency and cost and staff efficiency will undoubtedly take on more weight. In fact, more than one group therapist has suggested that clinicians soon may need to justify individual therapy and defend their decision not to use the more cost-effective group therapy (Dies 1986; MacKenzie 1997b). However, although group therapy is more cost-efficient, its advantages transcend simple economic considerations: it is a form of treatment that makes use of unique therapeutic properties not shared by other psychotherapies.

Scope of Current Group Therapy Practice

Current group therapy practice encompasses a wide spectrum, ranging from the long-term interactional outpatient group and the medication support group to the time-limited psychoeducational group to the acute crisis drop-in group (MacKenzie 1997a; Vinogradov and Yalom 1989). Therapy groups can be categorized by means of four interrelated characteristics (Table 35–1): the setting of the group, its duration, its goals, and its techniques.

Setting

One distinguishing feature among groups is their clinical setting. A particularly clear distinction can be made between psychiatric inpatient and outpatient groups. Inpatient groups on a psychiatric ward tend to meet daily, are usually composed of individuals with acute psychiatric problems, and often involve mandatory participation; turnover is great, with membership fluctuating widely because of the short duration of hospitalization. Psychiatric outpatient groups, in contrast, meet once weekly, consist of individuals who show more similar and more stable levels of functioning, and involve voluntary participation; membership tends to be more stable. There can be exceptions, of course. Some inpatient wards attempt to form more homogeneous groups that are based on level of functioning, although their membership will still vary widely. And psychiatric outpatient groups encompass many variations, ranging from the monthly drop-in group for chronically ill patients in a medication clinic to the twice-weekly interactional group run in a private practitioner's office.

Inpatient versus outpatient is but one distinction. Group therapy is also practiced in myriad other clinical

TABLE 35–1. Scope of current group therapy practice

Type of group	Life of group	Attendance	Average length of stay in group	Goals	Major therapeutic factors/ techniques	Membership criteria
Prototypical interactionally oriented groups	Indefinite; as permitted by professional schedule of group leaders	Voluntary, but regular attendance essential	1–2 years	Character change; symptom relief	Interpersonal learning; corrective recapitulation of primary family group	Higher-functioning patients; interpersonal pathology; desire to change, able to tolerate interpersonal focus; able to attend all sessions
Acute inpatient groups	Indefinite; usually an integral part of ward program	Generally mandatory during hospitalization; higher turnover	1–2 days up to several weeks, depending on length of hospitalization	Restoration of function	Instillation of hope; socialization techniques; altruism; existential factors	Patients may be placed in different groups by level of functioning; membership will fluctuate widely
Follow-up or aftercare groups; discharge planning groups; day hospital groups; probation groups	Indefinite; usually associated with a specific program	Often mandatory	Usually a fixed number of sessions	Deinstitutionalization	Instillation of hope; imparting of information; imitative behavior; socializing techniques	Patients require follow-up care or aftercare; able to tolerate group setting and attend required sessions
Medication or clinic groups	Indefinite; usually part of clinic program	Voluntary; often occurring on a drop-in basis	Indefinite; based on patient's enrollment in clinic	Support; education; maintaining functions	Universality; imparting of information; socializing techniques; altruism	Patients on long-term psychiatric medication; able to tolerate group setting
Behaviorally oriented groups (e.g., eating disorders group)	Time limited, often 6–12 sessions; some ongoing	Voluntary, but regular attendance generally prerequisite for participation	Life of group	Discrete behavior change	Techniques of behavior modification; universality; imitative behavior	Patients with a specific behavioral problem; desire to change
Specialized groups for medical disorders (e.g., diabetes, heart disease)	Time limited, often 6–12 sessions; some ongoing	Voluntary; often drop-in basis	Life of group or fixed number of sessions	Education; support; socialization	Universality; cohesiveness; imparting of information; imitative behavior; altruism; existential factors	Patients with specific medical problems; desire for further education and support
Specialized groups for life events (e.g., bereavement, divorce)	Tend to be time limited, 8–12 sessions	Voluntary; often flexible	Life of group	Support; catharsis; socialization	Cohesiveness; altruism; existential factors	Patients who have undergone a life event; desire for group experience

TABLE 35–1. Scope of current group therapy practice *(continued)*

Type of group	Life of group	Attendance	Average length of stay in group	Goals	Major therapeutic factors/ techniques	Membership criteria
Specialized support groups (e.g., Vietnam veterans outreach, rape crisis, student center drop-in, professional support or professional retreat)	Indefinite; ongoing for professional retreats, which usually last 1–3 days	Usually drop-in basis; for staff support groups, especially during retreats, attendance should be mandatory for all staff members	Variable	Support; catharsis	Cohesiveness; altruism; occasional interpersonal learning	Patients/clients who belong to specialized situation; desire for support

settings, extending from the daily small groups in a psychiatric day hospital to weekly probation groups to staff retreats or support groups. Specialized groups for medical syndromes (e.g., diabetes education groups or lupus support groups) often meet in a hospital or clinic setting, whereas other types of specialized groups (e.g., rape crisis group, Vietnam veterans group) may be associated with a center that offers counseling services (e.g., rape trauma center, veterans' outreach center).

Duration

A second consideration for any therapy group is its duration. Most inpatient groups are an integral part of the treatment program and are thus indefinitely self-sustaining; the ward census may change and different kinds of patients may be hospitalized, but the group meets every day. Outpatient groups have more latitude with regard to duration. They can exist for one session only (e.g., a drop-in crisis group that meets as needed at a student health center), or they can be open-ended and long-term in nature and periodically renew their membership over the years. In an interactionally oriented outpatient group, members will usually stay in therapy for 1–3 years, and "graduating" members are replaced as they leave, so that the size of the group remains approximately constant. A substantial number of groups in the outpatient setting, however, choose a time-limited format, especially if they are focusing on a specific problem. For example, an educational–behavioral group for patients with eating disorders may be designed to meet for six sessions. At the other end of the spectrum, long-term groups for personality disorders last years and are also effective (Kanas 2005).

Goals

A third factor that can be used to characterize the different kinds of group therapy pertains to the goals of the group, which may be conceptualized as existing along a spectrum. At one end of this spectrum are the ambitious goals of long-term interactional groups: symptom relief and character change. At the other end, there is the more limited but crucial goal of restoration of function: the deinstitutionalizing role of acute inpatient therapy groups. Between these two extremes lie the goals of the large majority of therapy groups. For some, such as medication clinic groups or inpatient and outpatient groups for chronically mentally ill persons, the most important goal will be maintenance of appropriate psychosocial functioning. Numerous others, including social skills training groups and spe-

cialized and self-help groups, attempt to provide education, socialization, and support. Many symptom-oriented short-term groups that are behaviorally focused (e.g., groups centered on bulimia, agoraphobia, or smoking cessation) have the goal of discrete behavior change.

Theoretical Orientation and Techniques

A fourth aspect of any therapy group is its theoretical orientation and the techniques employed by the therapist. This aspect is closely entwined with the goals of the group. An eating disorders group with the goal of discrete behavior change, for example, may have a cognitive-behavioral orientation and may focus on identifying cognitive distortions and triggers to behavioral responses. An analytic therapy group that has the goal of improving patients' ego functioning, on the other hand, may focus on the analysis of transference and resistance.

A wide range of theories and techniques inform the current practice of group therapy (Alonso and Swiller 1993). In this chapter, we will for the most part describe an understanding and an application of group therapy that are based on an interpersonal model of psychological functioning. This interpersonal orientation has a sound clinical and empirical foundation and translates into a set of clear and coherent tasks and techniques for the group therapist.

Membership Criteria

As can be seen from Table 35–1, the specific membership criteria for a given therapy group can vary widely from one type of group to another and are intimately linked to the goals of the group. In a behaviorally oriented group for patients with obsessive-compulsive disorder, for example, inclusion criteria are obsessive-compulsive symptomatology and a desire to change. The exclusion criterion is simply an inability to partake in a group experience (an extremely paranoid and obsessive individual would be excluded, for example). In contrast, a prototypical interactionally oriented group has much more stringent inclusion criteria: a member must admit to some interpersonal pathology, must have the ego strength and functioning necessary to tolerate an interpersonal focus, and must commit to regular attendance.

From these examples, the underlying principle for membership is made clear: whatever the specific nature of the group, a member must be able to perform the group task as the group works toward its goals. A member must therefore have problem areas that are compatible with the goals of the group and must have some motivation to change. Exclusion criteria include any factors that may interfere with the group task, such as marked incompatibility with group norms or with one or more group members, inability to tolerate the group setting, or a tendency to assume a deviant role in the group. These general criteria are outlined in Table 35–2 and are discussed further in the section on selecting patients and composing a therapy group.

In sum, the scope of current group therapy practice is wide indeed; those persons receiving treatment range from severely ill hospitalized psychiatric patients to high-functioning outpatients to persons with specific nonpsychiatric problems. Group therapy is a highly flexible psychotherapeutic modality, one that can be adapted to a variety of settings, time constraints, goals, and techniques.

Therapeutic Factors in Group Therapy: The Interpersonal Focus

Consider for a moment a hypothetical therapy group—let us say an outpatient group with eight members. Psychotherapy with one individual patient is a complex enough undertaking, but a group of patients is a potential Tower of Babel! Eight individuals intensively interact together, each with a different presenting complaint, varying psychological needs, unique problems in living, and, of course, a distinct character structure. Certain theorists would even argue that a new entity, with its own personality and characteristics, has been formed: the group itself.

TABLE 35–2. **General membership criteria for group therapy**

Inclusion criteria

  Ability to perform group task

  Problem areas compatible with group goals

  Motivation to change

Exclusion criteria

  Marked incompatibility with group norms for acceptable behavior

  Inability to tolerate group setting

  Severe incompatibility with one or more members

  Tendency to assume deviant role

The complexity of understanding and making sense of this enterprise often seems overwhelming to the neophyte therapist. What is needed is some simplifying principle, some mode of distinguishing between the truly essential, mutative aspects of the therapy group experience and those elements that represent the accessory characteristics of conscious and unconscious interaction in the group. We need to ask this question: Of all the dizzying, complex events in a group's transactions, which truly help the patient to change? We must identify the actual mechanisms of change in group therapy.

Identifying the Therapeutic Factors in Group Therapy

Group therapy was practiced for nearly half a century before researchers took steps to determine which factors actually help patients to change. Since the 1950s, a variety of research approaches have been used, including the interview and testing of group therapy patients with successful outcomes, as well as questionnaires directed at experienced group therapists and trained observers. Using these methods, researchers have identified a number of mechanisms of change in group therapy, that is, the curative or therapeutic factors.

There is usually a high degree of overlap among the various classification systems proposed by different investigators (Bloch 1986; Bloch and Crouch 1985; Butler and Fuhriman 1983; Corsini and Rosenberg 1955; Dies 1993; Fuhriman and Burlingame 1990; Yalom 1970). Yalom (1995) derived an 11-factor atheoretical inventory of the therapeutic mechanisms operating in group therapy (Table 35–3): 1) instillation of hope, 2) universality, 3) imparting of information, 4) altruism, 5) development of socializing techniques, 6) imitative behavior, 7) catharsis, 8) corrective recapitulation of the primary family group, 9) existential factors, 10) group cohesiveness, and 11) interpersonal learning. Yalom suggested that these primary factors, derived from extensive clinical and research evidence, serve as provisional guidelines for determining how group therapy helps patients to change. Furthermore, these factors can constitute the basis for an effective technical approach to therapy. In his comprehensive text on group therapy, *The Theory and Practice of Group Psychotherapy,* Yalom (1995) utilized these therapeutic factors as a central organizing principle.

Let us define and briefly discuss each of these factors. The last factor—the powerful but often misunderstood mechanism of interpersonal learning—will be discussed in greater detail.

TABLE 35–3. Yalom's inventory of the therapeutic factors in group therapy

Instillation of hope

Universality

Imparting of information

Altruism

Development of socializing techniques

Imitative behavior

Catharsis

Corrective recapitulation of the primary family group

Existential factors

Group cohesiveness

Interpersonal learning

Instillation of Hope

Instilling and maintaining hope are crucial in all psychotherapies and play a unique role in group therapy. Clinical sentiment and research evidence alike indicate that faith in the treatment mode can in itself be therapeutically effective, both when the patient has a high expectation of help and when the therapist believes in the efficacy of the treatment (Bloch and Crouch 1985). In therapy groups of every ilk, there will be patients who have improved as well as members who are at a low ebb; patients will often remark at the end of therapy how important it was for them to observe the improvement of others and thus to hope for their own improvement. Many of the self-help groups that emerged in the 1970s and 1980s, such as Compassionate Friends for bereaved parents or Mended Hearts for cardiac surgery patients, also place a heavy emphasis on the instillation of hope. Groups such as Alcoholics Anonymous that are aimed at substance abuse often use the testimonials of former alcoholic or recovered addicted persons to inspire hope in new members.

Universality

Many patients go through life with a sense of isolation. Secretly convinced that they are unique in their loneliness or their wretchedness, that they alone have certain unacceptable problems or impulses, these persons remain socially isolated and have few opportunities for frank and candid consensual validation. In a therapy group, especially in its early stages, the disconfirmation of a patient's sense of uniqueness comes as a powerful sense of relief. Some specialized groups, in fact, are focused on helping individuals for whom se-

crecy has been an especially important and isolating part of life. For example, short-term structured groups for bulimic patients require open disclosure about attitudes toward body image and detailed accounts about bingeing and purging behavior. As a rule, patients experience a great sense of relief when they discover that they are not alone, that some of their problems are "universal," and that other group members share the same dilemmas. Often, the degree of relief is directly related to the degree of reluctance to disclose.

Imparting of Information

The imparting of information occurs in a group whenever a therapist gives didactic instruction to patients about mental functioning or whenever advice or direct guidance about life problems is offered either by the leader or by other group members. Although long-term interactional groups generally do not value the use of didactic education or advice, other types of groups rely more or less heavily on these two manners of imparting information. Let us briefly examine each of them in turn.

Many self-help groups such as Recovery, Inc. (for psychological problems), Make Today Count (for cancer patients), and Gamblers Anonymous emphasize *didactic instruction.* Experts are often invited to address the group, and members are strongly encouraged to exchange information among themselves. Most, if not all, specialized groups led by professionals rely heavily on this procedure as well; groups aimed at patients with a specific disorder or facing a specific life crisis (e.g., obesity, trauma such as rape, epilepsy, chronic pain) build in a teaching component and offer explicit instruction about the specific illness or life situation. Many day-treatment groups or social skills training groups for chronically mentally ill persons also use teaching and instruction.

Unlike explicit didactic instruction from the therapist, *direct advice* from other members occurs without exception in every kind of therapy group. In dynamic interactional therapy groups, it is invariably part of the early life of the group but is generally of limited value to members. Later, when the group has moved beyond an initial "problem solving" stage and has begun to engage in true interactional work, the reappearance of advice seeking or advice giving around a given issue is an important clue to resistance in the group. In contrast, noninteractionally focused groups often make explicit and effective use of direct suggestions and guidance. For example, members of behavior-shaping groups, discharge groups (those that prepare patients for discharge from the hospital), Recovery, Inc., and

Alcoholics Anonymous offer one another considerable direct advice. Discharge groups may discuss the events of a patient's trial home visit and offer suggestions for alternative behavior, whereas Alcoholics Anonymous and Recovery, Inc., use guidance and directive slogans. Research on a behavior-shaping group of male sex offenders found that the most effective form of guidance was either systematic operationalized instructions or alternative suggestions from peers about how to reach a desired goal (Flowers 1979).

Altruism

In a therapy group, patients become enormously helpful to one another: they share similar problems and offer one another support, reassurance, suggestions, and insight. To the patient starting therapy who is demoralized and who feels that he or she has nothing of value to offer anyone, the experience of being helpful to other members of the group can be surprisingly rewarding. Not only does the altruistic act boost self-esteem, it also distracts patients who spend much of their psychic energy immersed in morbid self-absorption. By its very structure, the therapy group fosters the act of being helpful to others and counters overly solipsistic preoccupation.

Development of Socializing Techniques

Social learning—the development of basic social skills—is a therapeutic factor that operates in all therapy groups, although the nature of the skills taught and the explicitness of the process vary greatly according to the type of group therapy. In some groups, such as those preparing long-term hospitalized patients for discharge or those for adolescents with behavioral problems, there may be explicit emphasis on the development of social skills. Role-playing is often employed, in which patients learn to approach prospective employers for a job or adolescent boys learn to invite a girl to a dance. In groups that are more interactionally oriented, patients often learn about maladaptive social behavior from the open feedback they offer one another. A patient may, for example, learn about a disconcerting tendency to avoid eye contact during conversation, or about the effect that his or her whispery voice and constantly folded arms have on others, or about a host of other social habits that, unbeknownst to the patient, have been undermining his or her social relationships.

Imitative Behavior

The importance of imitative behavior as a therapeutic factor in groups is difficult to gauge, but there is some evidence from social psychological research that therapists may underestimate its importance. Bandura et al. (1969), for example, experimentally demonstrated nearly 40 years ago that imitation of healthy behavior is an effective therapeutic force in the treatment of certain phobias. In group therapy we often observe patients who benefit by observing the therapy of another patient with a similar problem constellation, a phenomenon of "vicarious learning" (Bandura 1986). A timid, somewhat repressed female member might observe another woman in the group begin to improve as the woman experiments with more engaging behavior and perhaps a more attractive appearance; the timid patient may then try new ways of presenting herself as well.

Catharsis

Catharsis, or the ventilation of emotions, is a complex therapeutic factor that is linked to other processes in the group, particularly universality and cohesiveness. The sheer act of ventilation, by itself, although often accompanied by a sense of emotional arousal and relief, rarely promotes lasting change for a patient. It is the affective sharing of one's inner world, and then the acceptance by others, that is of paramount importance. Being accepted by others after expressing strong emotions brings into question one's belief that one is basically repugnant, unacceptable, or unlovable. Therapy is both an emotional and a corrective experience; for change to take place, a patient must experience something strongly in the group setting and then understand the implications of that emotional experience. We will return to this fundamental premise later when we discuss the here-and-now focus of group therapy.

Corrective Recapitulation of the Primary Family Group

Patients often enter group therapy with a history of unsatisfactory experiences in their first and most important group experience, the primary family. Because group therapy offers such a vast array of recapitulative possibilities, patients may begin to interact with leaders or other members as they once interacted with parents and siblings (Baker and Baker 1993). A helplessly dependent patient may ascribe unrealistic knowledge and power to the leader. A rebellious and defiant individual may see the therapist as someone who blocks autonomy in the group or who strips members of their individuality. The "primitive" or chaotic patient might attempt to split the co-therapists or even the entire group, igniting fires of bitter disagreement and rivalry. The competitive patient will compete with other members for the therapist's attention or perhaps seek allies in an effort to topple the therapist(s). And a self-effacing individual or one with poor self-esteem may neglect his or her own interests in a seemingly selfless effort to placate or provide for other members. All of these patterns of behavior can represent a recapitulation of early family experiences.

What is of capital importance in interactional group therapy (and to a lesser degree in other group settings that make use of psychological insight) is not only that these kinds of early familial conflicts are reenacted but that they are understood and corrected. The group leader must not permit these growth-inhibiting relationships to freeze into the rigid, impenetrable system that characterizes many family structures. Instead, the leader must constantly explore and challenge fixed roles in the group and must constantly encourage members to test new behaviors. By exploring and altering ingrained patterns of behavior with leaders and other group members, the patient is liberated from the yoke of unfinished business from the past.

Existential Factors

An existential approach to the understanding of patients' concerns posits that a human being's paramount struggle is with the givens of existence: death, isolation, freedom, and meaninglessness (Yalom 1980). In certain kinds of therapy groups, particularly those centered around patients with cancer or chronic and life-threatening medical illnesses, or in bereavement groups, members will often begin to confront some of these existential issues. They will realize that there is a limit to the guidance and support they can receive from others. They may find that the ultimate responsibility for the conduct of their lives is their own. They will often learn that although one can be close to others, there is nonetheless a basic aloneness to existence that cannot be avoided. As they accept some of these issues, many patients who are confronting death learn to face their limitations and their mortality with greater candor and courage. In group therapy, the sound and trusting relationships among members—the basic intimate encounter—have an intrinsic value in that they provide presence and a "being with" in the face of these harsh existential realities (Benioff and Vinogradov 1993; Yalom and Vinogradov 1988).

Group Cohesiveness

Although it is discussed near the end of this brief description of therapeutic factors, group cohesiveness is one of the more complex and absolutely integral features of a successful therapy group (Dies 1993). Cohe-

siveness in a group context refers to the affinity that members have for their group and for the other members. The members of a cohesive group are accepting of one another, supportive, and inclined to form meaningful relationships in the group; they are ready to perform the group task. As such, cohesiveness can be conceptualized as a necessary precondition for change rather than a true mechanism of change. And yet, many if not most psychiatric patients have had an impoverished history of belonging; never before have they been a valuable, integral, participating member of any kind of group, and the successful negotiation of a group therapy experience may in itself be curative. For these patients, group cohesiveness appears to be a true therapeutic factor. Furthermore, the social behavior required for members to be esteemed by a cohesive group tends also to be adaptive for the individual in his or her social life outside the group.

How else does group cohesiveness set the stage for change? Quite simply, by providing conditions of acceptance and understanding. Under cohesive conditions, patients are more inclined to express and explore themselves, to become aware of and integrate hitherto unacceptable aspects of themselves, and to relate more deeply to others. Cohesiveness in a group thus favors self-disclosure, risk taking, and the constructive expression of confrontation and conflict—all phenomena that facilitate successful therapy.

Highly cohesive groups are stable groups with better attendance, more active patient commitment and participation, and less membership turnover than groups that have not cohered. Some groups in certain settings, such as those specializing in a particular problem or disorder (e.g., a cancer support group or a group for women law students that is run by a university health center), will by their very nature develop a great deal of cohesiveness. In other kinds of groups, especially those in which membership changes frequently, the leader may need to actively facilitate the development of this important therapeutic factor. We will discuss means of fostering cohesiveness in the sections exploring the group therapist's tasks and techniques (Table 35–4).

Interpersonal Learning

Group therapy may make use of any number of the therapeutic factors described here, but its cardinal feature is that it draws together a number of different individuals who wish to change something about themselves or their situations. This provides each member in the group with a unique ensemble of interpersonal interactions to explore. R. D. Laing (1967) suggested,

TABLE 35–4. Group cohesiveness

Group cohesiveness is

a necessary precondition.

inherently therapeutic.

Members are

accepting of one another.

supportive.

inclined to form meaningful relationships in the group.

ready to perform the group task.

Group cohesiveness encourages

member self-disclosure.

therapeutic risk taking.

constructive expression of confrontation.

better attendance.

Group cohesiveness is facilitated by

homogeneity of membership (e.g., same presenting problem, demographic similarity).

the therapist's technique (e.g., attuning to the group's prevailing affective tone, noting similarities between members in order to emphasize potential links between members).

"My experience and my action occur in a social field of reciprocal influence and interaction. I experience myself…as experienced by and acted upon by others." Surprisingly, this potent mechanism for change in group therapy—interpersonal learning—is often overlooked, misapplied, or misunderstood by leaders, perhaps because the encouragement of interpersonal exploration requires considerable therapist skill and experience. To place the use of interpersonal learning into its full context, we will examine three underlying concepts: the importance of interpersonal relationships, the group as a social microcosm, and learning from behavioral patterns in the social microcosm.

Importance of interpersonal relationships. Humans are gregarious creatures committed for life to a social existence based on interpersonal communication through language. Harry Stack Sullivan (1953) contended that the need for interpersonal acceptance and security is basic and, given the prolonged period of helplessness during infancy, may be as crucial to survival as any biological need. To ensure and promote this interpersonal acceptance, a developing child will accentuate those aspects of behavior that meet with approval or obtain desired ends and will suppress those aspects that engender punishment or disapproval. The human personality can thus be seen as shaped almost entirely by interaction with other significant beings. Goffman (1961) noted: "There seems to be no agent more effective than another person in bringing a world for oneself alive, or, by a glance, a gesture, or a remark, shriveling up the reality in which one is lodged." Psychopathology arises when these interactions have resulted in distortions in how one perceives others and in how one reacts to them.

Psychotherapists who use an interpersonal frame of reference—and what psychotherapist does not do so at one time or another?—concentrate on the interpersonal pathology that underlies or arises from a particular symptom complex. The therapist translates symptoms into interpersonal language. For example, the psychotherapist rarely addresses "depression" per se. The typical symptom cluster of dysphoric mood and neurovegetative signs does not in and of itself offer a handhold for beginning the process of character change. Instead, the clinician forms a relationship with the person who is depressed and ascertains the underlying interpersonal problems that arise from the depression and that most certainly also exacerbate it (problems such as dependency, obsequiousness, inability to express rage, and hypersensitivity to rejection). Once these maladaptive interpersonal themes have been identified, the therapist and the patient can undertake the work of understanding and altering them.

The group as a social microcosm. Sooner or later, given enough time and freedom, each person in the group will begin to interact with other group members in the same way that he or she interacts with persons outside the group. In other words, participants create in the group the same type of interpersonal world they inhabit on the outside. The group becomes a laboratory experiment in which interpersonal strengths and weaknesses unfold "in miniature." Slowly but predictably, each individual's interpersonal pathology comes to be displayed in the group. Arrogance, impatience, narcissism, grandiosity, sexualization—all such traits eventually surface. There is hardly any need for members to describe their past or to report present difficulties with relationships in their outside life. Group behavior provides far more accurate and immediate data. Members act out their interpersonal problems before the eyes of everyone in the group, and a freely interacting group will, in time, develop into a social microcosm of each of the members of that group. The following vignettes illustrate this principle:

John, a busy and successful dentist, had serious marital problems and was "coerced" into group therapy by his wife and marriage counselor. His wife complained that he was detached and uninvolved and that she had to throw a "tantrum" to get him to respond. John believed that his wife was always angry and critical toward him for no reason. Although John was polite and ingratiating, his participation in the group remained at a superficial level even after several months. He felt distant and a bit disdainful of the group that he was "forced" to attend. Soon the female members were prodding him, complaining that he wasn't engaged in the group work, asking, "Where is John really at?" They grew angry and more shrill in their interactions with John (just like his wife) in order to elicit a response, any response, from him—a reflection in miniature of the problems in his marriage.

Elizabeth was an attractive woman who, after her husband's job promotion and transfer, had left a high-powered career and had a baby; she soon entered a severe depression and felt overwhelmed by pain she could not express. She found her life lacking in intimacy, and her outside relationships, as well as her marriage, felt superficial and inauthentic to her. In the group, Elizabeth was very popular. She was charming, sensitive, and concerned about everyone. However, she rarely let the group glimpse behind her composed facade and into the depths of her pain and despair. Her great shame about her depression (after all, she "had it so good") and even deeper shame about the childhood of poverty and abuse from which she had risen resulted in her re-creating in the group the same type of cordial but distant and unnourishing relationships she had established in her social life and marriage.

Mark joined the group after his divorce and a string of unsuccessful romantic encounters. He had no close friends, male or female. He was sexually compulsive and competitive, and although he dated frequently, the thrill of the initial sexual conquest would inevitably pall, leaving him with a feeling of emptiness. Mark soon re-created this behavior in the therapy group. Although an active and involved member, he devoted himself almost exclusively to courting the attractive women in the group, including the female co-therapist. The female members began to feel sexualized and withdrew from him. Because he had also adopted an exceedingly competitive stance with the men in the group (especially powerful men, such as the male co-therapist), Mark quickly succeeded in isolating himself from all fulfilling relationships in the social microcosm of the group.

Learning from behavioral patterns in the social microcosm.   These preceding concepts interrelate in the process of group therapy to provide the therapist with an extremely powerful tool for change: interpersonal learning. In this process, psychopathology emerges from and is embodied in distorted interpersonal interactions, in which the group becomes a social microcosm as each member displays his or her interpersonal pathology, and in which feedback allows members to identify and change their interpersonal behavior. This process is described here and is schematically outlined in Figure 35–1 (Yalom 1985, 1986, 1995).

Interpersonal learning is the primary mechanism for change in longer-term unstructured, high-functioning interaction groups; in these settings, in fact, the elements of interpersonal learning are typically ranked by members as being the most helpful aspect of the group therapy experience (Butler and Fuhriman 1980; Freedman and Hurley 1980; Lieberman et al. 1973; Yalom and Leszcz 2005). Of course, not all therapy groups concentrate in an explicit manner on interpersonal learning. However, interpersonal interaction, with its rich potential for learning and change, does occur any time a group assembles.

Forces That Modify the Therapeutic Factors in Group Therapy

We have applied a simplifying principle to the group therapeutic process and have identified a comprehensive set of therapeutic factors that operate in group therapy. And yet, group therapy is obviously a forum for change whose form, content, and process vary considerably both across groups and within the same group at any given time. In other words, different types of groups will make use of different clusters of therapeutic factors (see Table 35–1), and, furthermore, as a group evolves, different sets of factors come into play (Dies 1993). Thus, we need to be aware that three modifying forces can influence the therapeutic mechanisms at work in any given group: the type of group, the stage of therapy, and individual differences among patients.

Type of Group

Research on long-term interactional outpatient group therapy indicates that group members consistently select a constellation of three factors—interpersonal learning, catharsis, and self-understanding—as those elements of group therapy most helpful to them (Yalom and Leszcz 2005). Inpatients, in contrast, tend to identify other mechanisms: the instillation of hope and the existential factor of assumption of responsibility (Leszcz et al. 1985; Yalom 1983). This difference in emphasis is due to the fact that inpatient groups have high member turnover and are heterogeneous in clinical composition (i.e., patients with greatly differing ego strength, motivation, goals, and psychopathology meet in the same group for varying lengths of time). Furthermore, psychiatric patients usually enter the hospital in a

Displaying interpersonal pathology

Members display their characteristic interpersonally distorted behavior.

Providing feedback and self-observation

Members share observations of each other and discover some of their own blind spots.

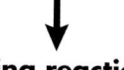

Sharing reactions

Members point out one another's blind spots and point out how each member's behavior makes them feel.

Examining results of sharing reactions

Each member begins to have a more objective picture of his or her own behavior and of the impact it has on others.

Understanding one's opinion of oneself

Each member becomes aware of how one's own behavior influences the opinions of others and, hence, one's opinions of oneself.

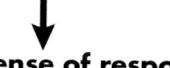

Developing a sense of responsibility

As a result of understanding how one's behavior influences one's sense of self-worth, one becomes more fully aware of responsibility for one's interpersonal life.

Realizing one's power to effect change

With the acceptance of responsibility for life's interpersonal dilemmas, each member begins to realize that one can change what one has created.

Potentiating change through high affect

The more emotionally laden are the events of this sequence, the greater is the potential for change.

FIGURE 35–1.   Learning from behavioral patterns in the social microcosm of the therapy.

state of despair, after they have exhausted other available resources. Groups that are centered around self-help concepts, such as Alcoholics Anonymous, Recovery, Inc., and support groups for bereaved parents, rely on the mechanisms of universality, guidance, altruism, and cohesiveness (Lieberman and Borman 1979).

Stage of Therapy

Patients' needs and goals change during the course of therapy and so, too, do the therapeutic factors that are

most helpful to them. In its early stages, an outpatient group is most concerned with establishing boundaries and maintaining membership, and factors such as instillation of hope, guidance, and universality loom most important. Other factors, such as altruism and group cohesiveness, will operate throughout the duration of therapy, but their nature changes with the stage of the group. In the case of altruism, for example, early in the group, patients will offer suggestions to each other, ask appropriate questions, and show concern and attention. Later, they will be able to express a deeper caring and greater support for each other and exhibit a true sharing of emotion.

Initially, group cohesiveness occurs through group support and acceptance, whereas later in the life of the group it facilitates self-disclosure. Ultimately, group cohesiveness makes it possible for members to explore issues of confrontation and conflict, issues so essential to interpersonal learning (Figure 35–2). The longer patients participate in a group, the more they value the therapeutic factors of cohesiveness, self-understanding, and interpersonal interaction (Butler and Fuhriman 1983).

Differences Among Patients

As mentioned at the beginning of this section, each patient in group therapy is different, and patients with different levels of functioning will find different therapeutic factors beneficial. Higher-functioning patients tend to value interpersonal learning more than do lower-functioning patients in the same group. In one study of inpatient groups, both types of patients chose awareness of responsibility and catharsis as helpful elements of group therapy; however, the lower-functioning patients also valued the instillation of hope, and higher-functioning patients selected universality, vicarious learning, and interpersonal learning as additional useful experiences (Leszcz et al. 1985). A group experience is something of a therapeutic cafeteria: many different mechanisms of change are available, but each individual patient will make the most use out of those particular factors that are most suited to his or her needs and problems. A passive, repressed individual may benefit from experiencing and expressing strong affect, through catharsis, for example; someone with impulse dyscontrol may profit from self-restraint and an intellectual structuring of the affective experience through imitative behavior. Some patients need to develop very basic social skills through the development of socializing techniques, whereas others benefit from the identification and exploration of much subtler interpersonal issues—for example, the patient who exaggerates helplessness and irrationality as a means of controlling other persons.

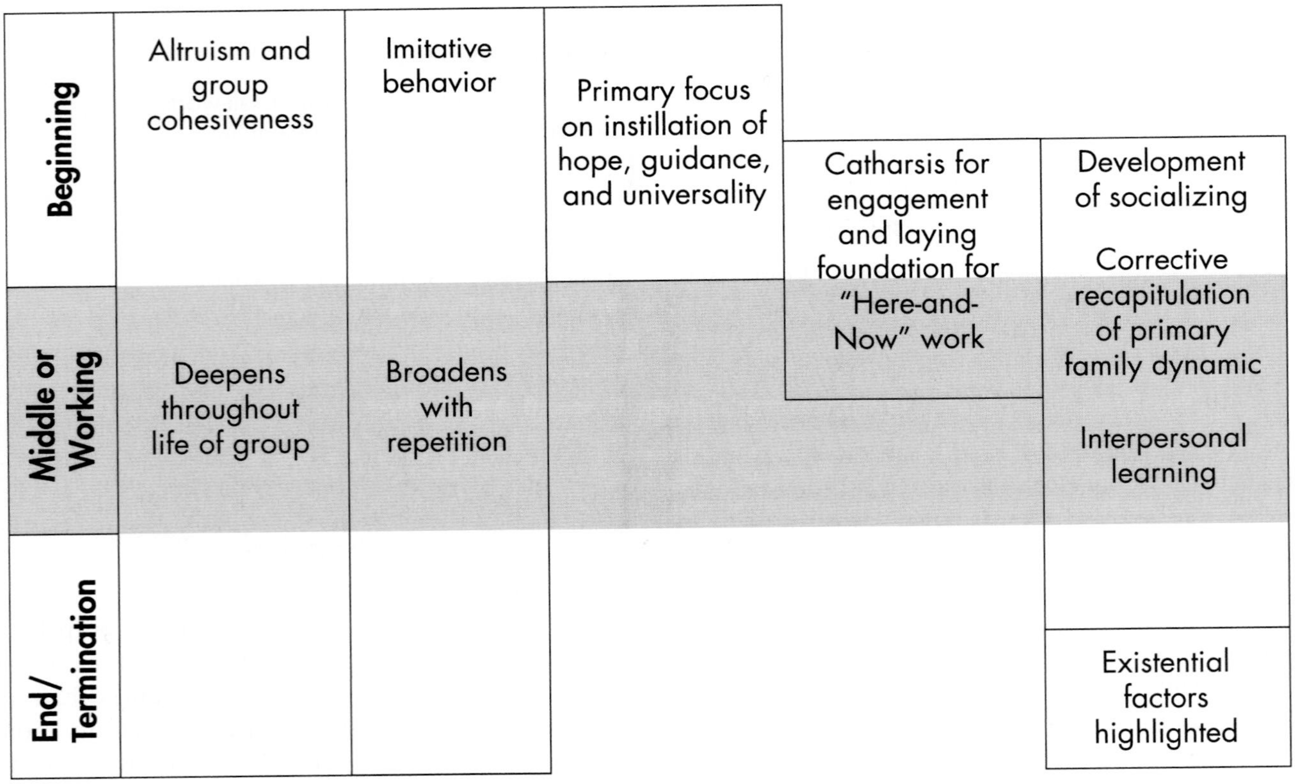

Beginning	Altruism and group cohesiveness	Imitative behavior	Primary focus on instillation of hope, guidance, and universality	Catharsis for engagement and laying foundation for "Here-and-Now" work	Development of socializing Corrective recapitulation of primary family dynamic Interpersonal learning
Middle or Working	Deepens throughout life of group	Broadens with repetition			
End/ Termination					Existential factors highlighted

FIGURE 35–2.   Group development and therapeutic factors.

Therapeutic Factors: Summary

In sum, the comparative usefulness and potency of these simplified therapeutic factors are complex and change across groups, across members of the same group, and across time. Research indicates that different types of groups make use of different therapeutic factors, and therapists who are leading groups must have a firm grasp of those factors that are most compatible with the needs and capacities of their group members. An emphasis on interpersonal learning is not appropriate for a behaviorally oriented group for persons with bulimia nervosa, just as time taken for didactic education would frustrate the members of a long-term intensive interactional group. The therapist thus has the basic task not only of understanding the appropriate mechanisms and goals for change in any given group, but also—as we shall explore in the next section—of establishing and maintaining the group within the setting of those goals.

The Therapist's Basic Tasks in Group Therapy

When a therapist begins individual psychotherapy with a new client, the therapist–patient dyad exists ipso facto, and the initial work of therapy unfolds from this point. But when a therapist starts a therapy group, the process is quite different. Long before the first meeting, the leader will have been hard at work, for the group therapist's initial task is to create a physical entity where none existed. The leader assembles a group and offers the professional help that is the initial raison d'être for the group. The leader selects the members and sets the time, place, and tone for the meetings. In sum, the therapist has the basic tasks of establishing and maintaining the group and resolving the problems typically encountered in the group setting (Table 35–5).

Let us explore some of these general principles of group format, composition, and maintenance, keeping in mind that these basic tasks can be modified to suit the needs of particular kinds of therapy groups. Optimally, the decision to start a therapy group reflects a synergy of patients' needs, therapist's skills and willingness and the necessary administrative resources. As such, all are essential: no space, no group; no patients, no group. A new group should be started with a clear idea of where the patients will come from and why they will be referred and join the new group.

TABLE 35–5. The therapist's basic tasks in group therapy

1. The decision to establish a therapy group (Needs assessment: what group will be supported by the setting and succeed?):

    a. Determine setting and size of the group.

    b. Choose frequency and length of group sessions.

    c. Decide on open versus closed group.

    d. Select a co-therapist for the group.

2. The act of creating a therapy group:

    a. Formulate appropriate goals.

    b. Select patients who can perform the group task.

    c. Prepare patients for group therapy.

3. The construction and maintenance of a therapeutic environment:

    a. Build the culture of the group explicitly and implicitly.

    b. Identify and resolve common problems (membership turnover, subgrouping, conflict).

    c. Use procedural aids as appropriate.

Establishing a Therapy Group

Determining Setting and Size

Before the first group meeting takes place, the therapist makes certain decisions about its circumstances. The most pragmatic of these involves choosing an appropriate meeting place. A setting that provides privacy and freedom from distraction is essential, of course, but a group meeting room should also be consistently available and of adequate size and have comfortable seating. A circular seating arrangement is necessary: all of the members must be able to see one another. The use of inpatient wards with long sofas does not permit good interaction. If three or four members sit in a row, they cannot see one another, and consequently most remarks in such groups are directed to the therapist, the one person visible to all. Furniture in the center of the room may hide nuances of body behavior; a table, for example, might mask the clenched fists of a member with a stoic facial expression. Some therapists provide coffee and tea at the meeting place; one effect of this is to increase the sociability of the setting, at least before the actual session.

The optimal size of a group is a function of its therapeutic goals. Organizations such as Alcoholics Anonymous and Recovery, Inc., which operate with group settings of up to 80 members, rely heavily on inspiration, guidance, and suppression to change members' behavior. However, leaders working in a large therapeutic community (e.g., in a residential halfway house) might wish to make use of a different set of factors, such as group pressure and interdependence, to foster reality testing or to instill a sense of individual responsibility to the social community. In this setting, groups of 15 or so members may be more appropriate.

The ideal size for a prototypical interactional group is 7 or 8 members, and certainly no more than 10. Too few members will not provide the critical mass necessary for interpersonal interactions. In a group that is too small, there will not be enough opportunities for broad consensual validation, and patients will tend to interact one at a time with the therapist rather than with one another. Anyone who has ever tried to conduct a group with only 2 or 3 patients knows the frustration of this enterprise. In a group with more than 10 members, however, there may be ample fruitful interaction, but some members will be left out. There will simply be insufficient time to examine and understand all of the interactions.

When the therapist is working with inpatients or leading specialized outpatient groups, his or her focus may not be as explicitly interpersonally oriented as in the prototypical interaction group, but the therapist will still want to aim for a lively and engaging group, one that encourages active participation by as many members as possible. In our clinical experience, the optimal group size that allows members to share experiences with one another ranges from a minimum of 4 or 5 to a maximum of 12; groups of 6–8 members seem to offer the greatest opportunity for verbal exchange among all patients.

Establishing Time Constraints and Selecting Open Versus Closed Groups

The late 1960s and early 1970s saw a great deal of experimentation with the time variable in group therapy. Weekly 4- to 8-hour groups were not unheard of, and marathon weekend sessions were common. Research has failed to demonstrate any superiority of the time-extended meeting, and today there is a clinical consensus that the optimal duration for a session in ongoing group therapy is between 60 and 120 minutes (Yalom and Leszcz 2005). Usually, 20–30 minutes are required for the group to warm up, and at least 60 minutes are needed to work through the major themes of the session. After about 2 hours, most therapists find they begin to fatigue and the group becomes weary and repetitious. Groups that meet frequently, such as daily inpatient groups, or groups that consist of lower-functioning patients who can tolerate only limited social stimuli do well with briefer sessions. Groups that meet less often or that are centered on higher-functioning interactional work require at least 90 minutes per session in order to be fruitful.

The frequency of meetings can vary from once a day—typically in the inpatient setting, where therapy groups meet from three to six times a week—to once every 3–12 weeks, as in clinic medication–support groups. A once-weekly schedule is most common in outpatient group work and seems well suited to supportive or specialized groups. Long-term interactional groups also tend to meet once per week, although clinical experience suggests that twice-weekly sessions, when feasible, increase the intensity and productivity of this kind of group.

The decision to make a group open or closed is related to the goals of the group and its identified life span. A closed group meets for a predetermined number of sessions, begins with a fixed number of members, and, as of the first session, closes its doors and accepts no new members. For example, therapists working with a specialized group of bereaved spouses or of patients with eating disorders may take in a fixed number of patients for a preset number of sessions, usually 8–12 meetings. In such time-limited groups, each session may follow a predetermined protocol. External time constraints can also influence the format of a group. For example, in a university health center, a support group for graduate students having trouble with their dissertations may be set up to run the length of an academic semester.

In contrast, open groups either are more flexible about size—consider the ongoing inpatient group on a psychiatric ward, which reflects ward census—or may maintain a consistent size by replacing members as they leave the group. Open groups usually have a broader set of therapeutic goals and generally meet indefinitely; although members come and go, the group has a life of its own. Such ongoing outpatient groups at psychiatric teaching centers have been known to continue for more than 20 years and to have been the training ground for generations of residents!

Using a Co-Therapist

Most group therapists prefer to work with a co-therapist. Co-therapists complement and support each other. As the therapists share points of view and examine hunches together, each therapist's observational range is broadened. There is much agreement among clinicians that a male–female co-therapist team has unique advantages. It re-creates the parental configuration of the primary family, which for many members increases the affective charge of the group. Many patients can benefit from observing a male therapist and a female therapist working together with mutual respect and without the derogation, exploitation, or sexualizing that the patients too often take for granted in male–female relationships. Moreover, the group is provided with a wider array of transferential possibilities, for patients will differ in their reactions to each of the co-therapists and to the co-therapists' relationship. In a group led by a male–female co-therapist team, for example, a somewhat histrionic female member may pander to the male leader and ignore his female counterpart, a pattern that would not emerge as clearly in a group led by one therapist. Other members may have fantasies about the relationship between the two co-therapists.

The co-therapy format seems particularly helpful for beginning therapists and for experienced therapists working with an especially difficult patient population. In addition to clarifying transference distortions of each other's presentation in the group, co-therapists can support each other in maintaining objectivity in the face of massive group pressure. We had occasion to work at one point with a lonely female member of a group, a hospital volunteer who became romantically involved with one of her psychiatric patients; she discussed this in a group session and then verbally flagellated herself. In an effort to be supportive, the other members unanimously and vociferously condoned her behavior and attempted to pressure the leaders into a noncritical stance as well. As co-therapists, we were better able to resist the powerful group pressure and maintain our professional objectivity about this woman's behavior.

Similarly, co-therapists are invaluable in helping each other constructively weather an attack from group members. A therapist under the gun may be too threatened either to clarify the attack or to encourage further exploration without appearing defensive or condescending. There is nothing more squelching than when a leader under fire says, "It's really great that you're expressing your feelings and attacking me. Keep it going!" It is usually the co-therapist who can best help members channel and express their anger in an appropriate manner and who can then lead members to examine the source and the meaning of that anger.

There is some question whether co-therapists should openly reveal their differences of opinion during the group session. Two factors to consider are the level of functioning of the group and the maturity of the group. Patients who are lower functioning and who are more fragile or unstable overall should generally not be exposed to conflict between the co-therapists, no matter how gently it is expressed. Likewise, co-therapist disagreement is not helpful early in the work with even higher-functioning patients, for a beginning group usually is not stable or cohesive enough to tolerate divisiveness in leadership. Later in such a group, however, the therapists' honesty about disagreement can contribute substantially to the potency and honesty of the group. Members observe the leaders they respect disagreeing openly and resolving their differences with honesty and tact. Members also experience the therapists not as infallible authority figures but as humans with imperfections, and they thus learn to differentiate others according to individual attributes rather than stereotyped roles.

The major disadvantages of the co-therapy format flow from problems in the co-therapy relationship itself (Table 35–6). If co-leaders are uncomfortable with each other, closed and competitive, or in wide disagreement about style and strategy, there is little chance that their group will be able to work effectively. Research has demonstrated that the major causes of failure are co-therapists' embracing vastly different ideological positions (Paulson et al. 1976) and failing to address the developmental tasks of the co-therapy relationship as these reflect the developmental tasks of the group (Dugo and Beck 1997). Therefore, when choosing a co-leader, it is important to select someone who is different enough in personal style to be complementary but who is similar in theoretical orientation and with whom you can discuss your relationship, especially as it pertains to the group's development.

Whenever two therapists of vastly different levels of experience lead a group together, it is important that they be open-minded and mature, comfortable with each other, and comfortable in their roles as co-workers or as teacher and apprentice. Splitting is a phenomenon that often occurs in groups led by co-therapists, and some patients are very perceptive about tensions in the co-therapists' relationship. For example, if a neophyte therapist feels jealous of a senior co-therapist's clinical experience and wisdom, a member might marvel at everything the older therapist says and denigrate the younger therapist's interventions. Occasionally the entire group can become split into two factions, with each co-therapist having a "team" of patients aligned with him or her; this may

TABLE 35–6. Co-leading group psychotherapy

Advantages	Disadvantages
Complementary roles	Less efficient (fee split between two therapists)
Observational range broadened	Coordination of two therapists' schedules
One holds transference while other explores patient's experience	Problems arising from ideological differences related to theoretical orientation
Inherent potential for support	
Re-creation of parental configuration	
Modeling of healthy adult relating	
Wider array of transferential possibilities	
Mentorship of less experienced therapists	

occur because the patients believe they have a special relationship with one or the other of the therapists or because they believe that one of the therapists is more intelligent, more senior, or more attractive or has a similar ethnic background. Splitting, like the problem of subgrouping that we will discuss later, should always be noted and openly interpreted in the group.

Combining Group Therapy With Other Therapeutic Modalities

The standard group therapy format, in which one therapist meets with six to eight patients, is often combined with other therapeutic modalities. For example, some or all of the patients in a given group may also be involved in concurrent individual psychotherapy with other therapists; this is often described as *conjoint therapy* and is one of the more preferable means for combining psychotherapies. Occasionally, all or some of the members in a group are in concurrent individual therapy with the group therapist in what is known as *combined therapy*. This latter therapy usually arises when a psychotherapist in solo private practice forms a group from the ranks of his or her individual patients. Both conjoint and combined therapies are frequently encountered by therapists who run groups in clinics or on inpatient wards. Amaranto and Benden (1990) are developing models to incorporate the advantages of both.

When is it useful to combine psychotherapeutic modalities? Some patients may go through a life crisis

so severe that they require temporary individual support in addition to group therapy. Others may be so chronically disabled by fear, anxiety, or aggression that they require individual therapy to participate effectively in the group and avoid becoming locked into a stereotyped role. At times, active individual intervention is necessary simply to explore the patient's conflicts in group therapy and thus prevent him or her from having an unprofitable experience or from dropping out of the group. Individual or group therapy approaches complement each other most effectively when the individual and group therapists support each other and are in frequent contact and when the individual therapy is interpersonally oriented and explores feelings and incidents related to current group meetings.

Concurrent individual therapy can hinder group therapy in several ways. When there is a marked difference in approach between the individual therapist and the group therapist, patients may become confused and the two therapies may work at cross-purposes. The patient who is used to the support and narcissistic gratification of individual therapy—who is accustomed to exploring fantasies, dreams, associations, and memories and to being the exclusive center of attention of a therapist—may become frustrated by initial group meetings. Early sessions usually offer less personal support and may be dedicated more to building a cohesive unit and to examining here-and-now interactions than to deep exploration of each member's life. Individual therapy and group therapy can also interfere with each other if patients use their individual therapy to drain off affect from the group, reacting to emotionally laden events in the group only later in the sanctum of their individual therapy hour.

Another combination is the use of group therapy with medication clinics, a practical and humane combination of modalities most often, but not exclusively, used with chronic psychiatric patients (Brook 1993, 2001). In this approach, patients who attend biweekly or monthly medication clinics, usually to receive prescriptions for antipsychotic medication or for mood stabilizers, also participate in a group meeting associated with the clinic. Sessions are generally highly structured and focus on educating patients about their medications, on solving practical problems, and on sharing a difficult plight. A chronically psychotic patient who lives in relative social isolation can use these groups to practice some basic social skills and to receive support for his or her efforts. Group therapy is used to personalize, enhance, and reinforce the patient's experience in a medication clinic.

Creating a Therapy Group
Formulating Goals

As a first step to creating a therapy group, the therapist must carefully examine all of the clinical facts of life that will bear on the group. The *intrinsic* factors (e.g., mandatory attendance for patients on legal probation, duration of treatment in a ward group of hospitalized patients with cancer) are built into the clinical situation and cannot be changed; the group leader must adapt to them. The *extrinsic* factors are those that have become tradition or policy in a given setting—an example might be an inpatient ward's fixed program of daily community meetings. Extrinsic factors are arbitrary and within the power of the therapist to change.

Once a clear view of the clinical facts of life has been obtained, the leader's second step is to construct a reasonable set of clinical goals for the group. This is the most important step in creating a therapy group, for the selection of inappropriate or vaguely defined goals is sure to result in failure. The goals of a long-term outpatient group are ambitious: to offer symptomatic relief and to change character structure. An attempt to apply these same goals to an aftercare group of patients with chronic schizophrenia would result in therapeutic nihilism.

Goals must be shaped that are appropriate to the clinical situation and achievable in the amount of time available. In time-limited specialized groups, the goals must be focused, achievable, and tailored to the capacity and potential of the group members. It is important that the therapy group be a success experience; patients enter therapy feeling defeated and demoralized, and the last thing they need is another failure.

Selecting Patients and Composing a Therapy Group

Once the therapist has a clear idea of the goals of the group—in other words, a clear idea of the group task—he or she must select members who can achieve these goals and perform the group task. The leader's expertise in the selection and preparation of members will greatly affect the group's fate. The therapist must create a group that coheres, and because nothing threatens a group's cohesiveness more than the presence of a grossly deviant member, the selection of members must be guided by the notion of group integrity and the avoidance of deviancy. A group of board-and-care-home residents with chronic schizophrenia cannot cohere effectively in the presence of an exploitative and manipulative member with a personality disorder, nor can a high-functioning group of outpa-

tients function well together in the presence of a patient who frequently goes into dissociative states.

The single most important criterion for member selection, no matter what the group, is an ability to perform the group task. Study of group failures reveals that deviancy (i.e., an inability or refusal to engage in the group task) is negatively related to outcome. An individual who considers himself or herself (or is considered by other members) to be "out of the group" or a deviant or mascot has little likelihood of profiting from the group and there is a fair chance of negative outcome for that person (Lieberman et al. 1973). Therefore, selection for a specific therapy group is, in practice, often conducted by the process of elimination. Group therapists exclude certain patients from consideration (most often because the therapist predicts the patient will assume a deviant role or because the patient lacks motivation for change) and accept remaining patients. Comprehensive group programs offer an array of groups with an array of potential tasks. A deviant from one group may benefit from participation in a different group where the membership and task fit his or her needs and abilities.

Once a leader determines that a patient could benefit from group therapy, how does he or she go about actually composing a group? How is it decided which patients will work well together? Above all, the therapist must be concerned about the group's *integrity*. Members selected must be committed to the task of therapy and to regular attendance in the group. To attempt to refine the process of composition even more—to form a group ideally composed to interact therapeutically—is every group therapist's dream, yet we lack the knowledge and instruments necessary to permit us to realize this dream. Perhaps the key concept is group cohesiveness. An effective rule of thumb for longer-term outpatient groups is "homogeneity in ego strength, heterogeneity in problem areas" (Whitaker and Lieberman 1964). In other words, patients profit from a mixture of personality styles, ages, and problem areas—all factors that enrich the broth of the ensuing group interaction—but the group coheres best if all members possess the ego strength necessary to participate equally in the group task.

The situation is different in specialized or symptom-oriented groups; in these cases, members always share at least one major problem area (e.g., an eating disorder, bereavement, chronic pain), but they may be heterogeneous in terms of ego strength. Whenever possible, the therapist aims for similar levels of motivation and psychological mindedness in the composition of the group. Having one or two members who are fragile, brittle, or work avoidant impedes the work of a fast-paced, highly motivated group. Likewise, a stolid group of more concrete chronically ill psychiatric patients can become destabilized if pushed too hard too fast by a confrontational, agitated, or manic individual (Kahn 1984; Kanas 1985, 1986). Beyond this, leaders may wish to try to balance the group composition along various parameters, such as by composing a group with an equal number of men and women, a wide age range, or varied interpersonal activity levels.

Often (as in, for example, mandatory inpatient groups or a group in a correctional institution) the therapist has minimal influence over group membership. At the very least, he or she must exercise the group therapist's prerogative and exclude those patients who are markedly incompatible with the prevailing group norms for acceptable behavior. Examples might include the physically agitated patient or the manic patient. Patients who cannot tolerate the stress of a group setting, such as extremely paranoid individuals, and patients who are absolutely incompatible with at least one other member also should not be included in the group. Group member screening is even more complicated in managed care settings. On the one hand, therapists often feel pressure from administration to fit patients into a group, and a higher risk of poor fit is tolerated. On the other hand, large institutional settings with large group programs are more likely to have a group that is suitable for any given patient. Unfortunately, the former situation is more common early in group program development.

One reason it is so difficult to compose an ideal group is that it is extremely difficult to predict subsequent group behavior from information available at the time of the screening procedure. An important source of information is the candidate's previous experience in groups. Another important source is the screening procedure itself. In the one or two intake interviews, the therapist should focus on the candidate's interpersonal functioning: past, present, and in the interview itself. The therapist must assess the individual's ability to tolerate interpersonal interactions and to reflect on them. Suitable questions might include the following: "How has the interview been for you so far today?" "Were there any parts that made you uncomfortable?" "What is it like for you to reveal things about yourself to a relative stranger?"

Preparing Patients for Group Therapy

Preparation of the patient for group therapy is another one of the therapist's essential tasks. A great deal of powerful research evidence has demonstrated that pregroup preparation decreases the number of dropouts, increases cohesiveness, and accelerates the work of therapy (Piper and Perrault 1989; Piper et al. 1982; Yalom 1966, 1995). In some settings, such as an inpatient ward or a medication support group, this preparation will of necessity be minimal and will consist mainly of orienting the patient to the time, location, composition, procedure, and goals of the group. But even this brief preparation helps to orient patients to the group experience and provides guidelines about how to benefit from the group.

For most outpatient groups, preparation is best accomplished during one or two individual sessions with each patient before he or she begins group therapy. After deciding during an intake interview that the patient is a suitable candidate for group therapy, the therapist may then proceed to prepare the patient for the group. Patients have ample amounts of primary anxiety, and therapists must avoid adding yet more—the secondary anxiety that arises from being thrown into an ambiguous, intrinsically threatening situation. Therefore, providing clarity is the chief aim of the pregroup preparatory procedure. The therapist provides patients with a cognitive structure that enables them to participate more effectively in the group from the start.

Many patients hold misconceptions about the worth and efficacy of group therapy; they believe that it is cheaper or diluted therapy and therefore not as worthwhile as individual therapy. These negative expectations must be addressed openly and corrected so that patients will engage fully in treatment. Other patients express concerns about procedure and process: the size of the group, the type of members, the amount of negative confrontation, confidentiality. One of the most pervasive fears is the fear of having to reveal oneself and confess shameful transgressions to an audience of hostile strangers. Another common worry is a fear of mental contagion, of being made sicker through association with other psychiatric patients. Often this fear is a preoccupation of schizophrenic or borderline patients, although the fear may also be observed in patients who project their own feelings of self-contempt or hostility onto others.

The importance of alliance with the therapist(s) has been widely appreciated as relevant to outcomes in most treatments. Piper et al. (2005) demonstrated that not only does level of alliance help predict outcome but that pattern of changes in alliance also predict outcome in short-term groups.

A cognitive approach to group therapy preparation has several goals (Table 35–7).

Underlying everything the therapist says is a pro-

TABLE 35–7. Rationales behind group therapy preparation

Provide a rational explanation to the patient about the group therapy process.

Describe the behavior expected of patients in the group.

Establish a treatment contract.

Raise expectations about the effects of the group.

Predict some of the common problems and discouragement that may be encountered in early meetings.

cess of demystification and the establishment of a therapeutic alliance. This comprehensive preparation enables the patient to make an informed decision to enter the therapy group and enhances commitment to the group from the beginning.

Constructing and Maintaining a Therapeutic Environment

Building the Culture of the Group

Once the group is a physical reality and the first meeting is under way, the leader must establish behavioral norms that will guide the interactions of the newly formed group. In individual therapy the therapist is the sole designated agent of direct change, but in group therapy the situation is more complex. Ideally, *all* of the members of the group will provide support, a sense of universality, and interpersonal feedback—in other words, the members themselves will be important agents of change. Any time a group of people assembles, be it in a professional, social, or even family setting, it will develop a "culture," a set of unwritten rules or norms that determine the acceptable behavioral procedure of the group. In group therapy, it is the leader's task to create a group culture maximally conducive to effective group interaction and to the development of the various therapeutic factors.

Norms constructed early in the group are important. They are shaped both by the expectations of the members as they start the group and by the behavior of the therapist during the early sessions. The therapist influences this process of norm setting in two different ways. First, the leader, in the role of technical expert, can *explicitly* shape the group norms. During early preparation of patients for group therapy, for example, patients can be given explicit instructions about the rules for appropriate behavior in the group, such as sharing concerns about body image in an eating disor-

ders group. Once a group gets under way, the leader may reward desirable behavior through social reinforcement. If a usually shy member begins to participate, or if members start to offer one another spontaneous and honest feedback, this new behavior may be shaped and rewarded verbally or nonverbally through changes in the therapist's body language, eye contact, and facial expression.

The second way the therapist shapes therapeutic norms in the group is through model setting. In an acute inpatient therapy group, for example, leaders offer a model of nonjudgmental acceptance and appreciation of members' strengths as well as problem areas, helping to shape a group that is health oriented. In a social skills training group for schizophrenic patients, the leader might choose to model simple, direct, socially rewarding conversation. No matter what the level and functioning of the group, the effective leader sets a model of interpersonal honesty and spontaneity for his or her group members. But the therapist's honesty must take place in the service of his or her background responsibility; nothing takes precedence over the goal of being helpful to the patient.

There are several basic therapeutic group norms that should be encouraged in any group setting, regardless of its orientation. The first of these is the norm of the *self-monitoring group*, in which the group itself learns to assume responsibility for its own functioning. Any therapist who has ever worked in a group in which the members are completely dependent on the leader for direction knows firsthand the signs of the passive group. The patients seem to be an audience at a play; they appear to be waiting for the leader to make the curtain rise and the action begin. The group begins to feel stilted, heavy, and forced. After every meeting, the leader feels fatigued, powerless, and irritated by the burden of making it all work.

How can the therapist build a culture that encourages the development of a self-monitoring group? This can be accomplished by keeping in mind that initially only the leader knows when a group has been productive. The therapist must start to share this knowledge with the patients at the very inception of a group and slowly educate them to recognize a good session. The therapist might say, "This was an exciting meeting today and everyone shared a lot. I hate to see it end." The evaluative function can then be shifted to the patients by the therapist's saying, "How is the group going so far today? What's been the most satisfying part?" And, finally, members can be taught that they have the ability to influence the course of a session; the therapist could say, "Things have been slow today. What could we do to make it different?" Understanding dynamics that challenge a healthy group culture is essential. Experience leading groups, supervision by experienced clinicians, and thoughtful reflection all help group therapists develop strategies to address such difficulties (Large 2005).

There are several other basic norms that influence the therapy. *General procedural norms* must always be actively shaped by the leader. Ideally, the most therapeutic procedural format of a group is one that is unstructured, unrehearsed, and freely flowing. The therapist must intervene actively to preclude the development of a nontherapeutic procedure, for example, a "taking turns" format in which members figuratively line up to discuss specific problems or life crises one after another by rote. In such an instance, the therapist might interrupt and ask how the practice got started or what effect it has on the group. The leader could also indicate that the group has many other procedural options from which to choose.

When *members consider the group important,* group therapy becomes more effective, and the leader who reinforces this norm increases the therapeutic potency of his or her group. Likewise, the therapist augments the power of the group by increasing the *continuity between meetings.* It is the task of the therapist, as the group "time-binder," to call attention to behavioral patterns developing over several meetings. Finally, a group functions best when it sees its *members as agents of help and support;* a truly therapeutic culture implies, both explicitly and implicitly, that members will learn the most and receive the most help from one another.

Identifying and Resolving Common Problems in Group Therapy

Membership problems. The early developmental sequence and potency of a therapy group are strongly affected by membership problems. Turnover in membership, tardiness, and absence are facts of life in all groups, yet these events will threaten a group's stability and integrity. Considerable absenteeism will redirect an outpatient group's attention and energy from its developmental tasks to the problem of maintaining membership, whereas continual turnover in inpatient groups powerfully affects group cohesiveness. Tardiness and irregular attendance must be discouraged in all group settings and should be regarded in the same way in which one regards these phenomena in individual therapy.

Leaders of long-term outpatient therapy groups should keep in mind that in the normal course of such groups, 10%–35% of the members will drop out in the

first 12–20 meetings (Yalom 1966, 1995). In an open group it is the therapist's task to replace dropouts by adding new members. Dropouts are threatening to the group's stability for two reasons: they impede the development of cohesiveness, and they implicitly (and sometimes explicitly) devalue the group. Dropouts are also threatening to the leader, especially to the neophyte, and the therapist may unwittingly adopt a seductive posture in an effort to keep a patient in the group. The dropout rate can be reduced through vigorous pretherapy selection and preparation (Connelly et al. 1986; McCallum et al. 1992; Orlinsky and Howard 1986; Piper and Perrault 1989). If predictions of the general problems and frustrations that can arise early in a group are made to new members ahead of time, there is less likelihood that dropping out will occur.

Subgrouping. A second problem commonly encountered in group therapy is subgrouping—the splitting off of smaller units. A subgroup usually arises from the belief by two or more members that these members can derive more gratification from a relationship with one another than from one with the entire group. Extragroup socializing, which often occurs in outpatient groups (and almost invariably in inpatient groups), is often the first stage of subgrouping. A clique of three or four members will begin to have telephone conversations, to have coffee or dinner, and to share separate observations and interactions with one another. Occasionally, two members will become sexually involved. A subgroup may also coalesce completely within the confines of the group therapy room, as members who perceive themselves to be similar form coalitions based on age, similar values, comparable education, and the like. Remaining group members, excluded from the clique, generally do not possess effective social skills and do not usually coalesce into a second subgroup. This phenomenon of "ingroup" versus "outgroup" can often be strikingly observed in inpatient settings.

The members of a subgroup can be recognized by a code of behavior: they agree with one another regardless of the issue and they avoid confrontations among their own membership; they exchange knowing glances when a member who is not in the clique speaks; they arrive and depart from the meeting together. Complications arise for all members of the therapy group, whether they belong to the subgroup or not. If a member belongs, loyalty to the subgroup is a major issue, secrets begin to be kept, and the free and honest discussion of feelings becomes inhibited. If a member has been excluded from the subgroup, complex feelings of envy, competition, and inferiority are aroused. Unfortunately, as these emotions and the anxiety associated with earlier exclusion experiences are evoked, it becomes exceptionally difficult for members to comment on their feelings of exclusion.

It is not the extragroup socializing that is crippling to a group per se; rather, it is the conspiracy of silence around it that becomes dangerous. The primary task in the group is to examine in depth the interpersonal relationships among all of the members, and extragroup socializing inhibits this examination. Important material—the relationship between members who are interacting outside the group, feelings of exclusion in patients who are not part of this interaction—remains covert, and the task of the group is sabotaged. Patients who violate group norms through the pursuit of subgrouping or through secret extragroup liaisons are opting for immediate need gratification rather than for involvement in interpersonal learning and change. Subgrouping or extragroup behavior that remains covert—that is not examined in the group session—becomes a potent form of resistance. It hobbles the therapist and makes a travesty of other members' efforts to be revealing, to give honest feedback, and to participate fully and authentically in the group process.

Subgrouping represents a situation that contains both high risk and high gain. In pregroup preparation, the therapist attempts to prevent its occurrence by actively encouraging the development of group norms whereby all extragroup behavior is subsequently brought back into the group for discussion. When it does take place, subgrouping must be explicitly identified—usually by the leader—and explored in the light of the group task, which is the in-depth examination of the interpersonal relationships among all members. When the powerful issues that give rise to subgrouping are confronted by the group, discussed openly, and worked through, they can prove to be of considerable therapeutic import in the very group they were hampering.

In fact, deliberate use of subgrouping is part of the conceptual heart of systems-centered therapy. Agazarian (1997) utilized systems theory and directed therapeutic efforts mostly toward subgroups. The group-as-a-whole is a supra-entity (it contains the subgroup) and the individual members are part of subgroups (subgroups of the subgroup). Changes occurring at the level of the subgroup influence the nature of the group-as-a-whole as well as the participating individuals. Such parsimony of effort is further enhanced by the deliberate addressing of details of subgrouping. Noting changes in the "boundaries" between subgroups (e.g., splits, containing and integrating differences) and the direction of the system's or subsystem's energy (vec-

tors) can be the basis for interventions. These interventions, placed in a framework that Agazarian (1997) called "defense modification," appear to quickly move forward the work of the group-as-a-whole as well as that of the individuals. Subgrouping, like any powerful phenomenon, can be destructive if unaddressed. However, it is also potentially instructive and productive. Agazarian enhanced group therapists' ability to use subgrouping effectively.

Conflict. Conflict, a third common problem, is inevitable in the course of a group's development. The task of the therapist is to identify conflict as it arises and to harness it in the service of the group task. Conflict resolution is virtually impossible in the presence of off-target or oblique hostility, and, once again, it is the therapist's task to identify and render overt that which has been covert. For example, he or she might say, "Bob, I've noticed that you've cut off Mary a couple of times today. I wonder if you're feeling a little angry because of the feedback the women in the group gave you last week" (Figure 35–3).

How can the therapist harness conflict in the group and use it in the service of interpersonal growth? One important step is finding the right level for the group at hand. Too much conflict is threatening and counterproductive for just about any group of individuals, but too little conflict—especially with higher-functioning patients—leaves the group stagnant, excessively cautious, and superficial. Here, a judicious amount of confrontation, anger, and conflict resolution can provide an affectively charged learning experience for group members.

Group cohesiveness is the prime prerequisite for the successful management of conflict. Members must have developed a feeling of mutual respect and trust and must value the group sufficiently to be able to tolerate confrontational or uncomfortable interactions. The leader will need to emphasize that open communication must be maintained if the group is to survive; all members must continue to deal directly with one another, no matter how angry they become. Norms must be established in which it is made clear that group members are there to understand themselves, not to outdo, defeat, or ridicule one another. Furthermore, every member is to be taken seriously. When a group begins to treat one person as someone whose opinions and anger are to be lightly regarded, the hope of effective treatment for that patient has all but officially been abandoned.

Not all groups tolerate the same level of conflict. The open conflictual confrontation that might take place between two members of a long-term outpatient

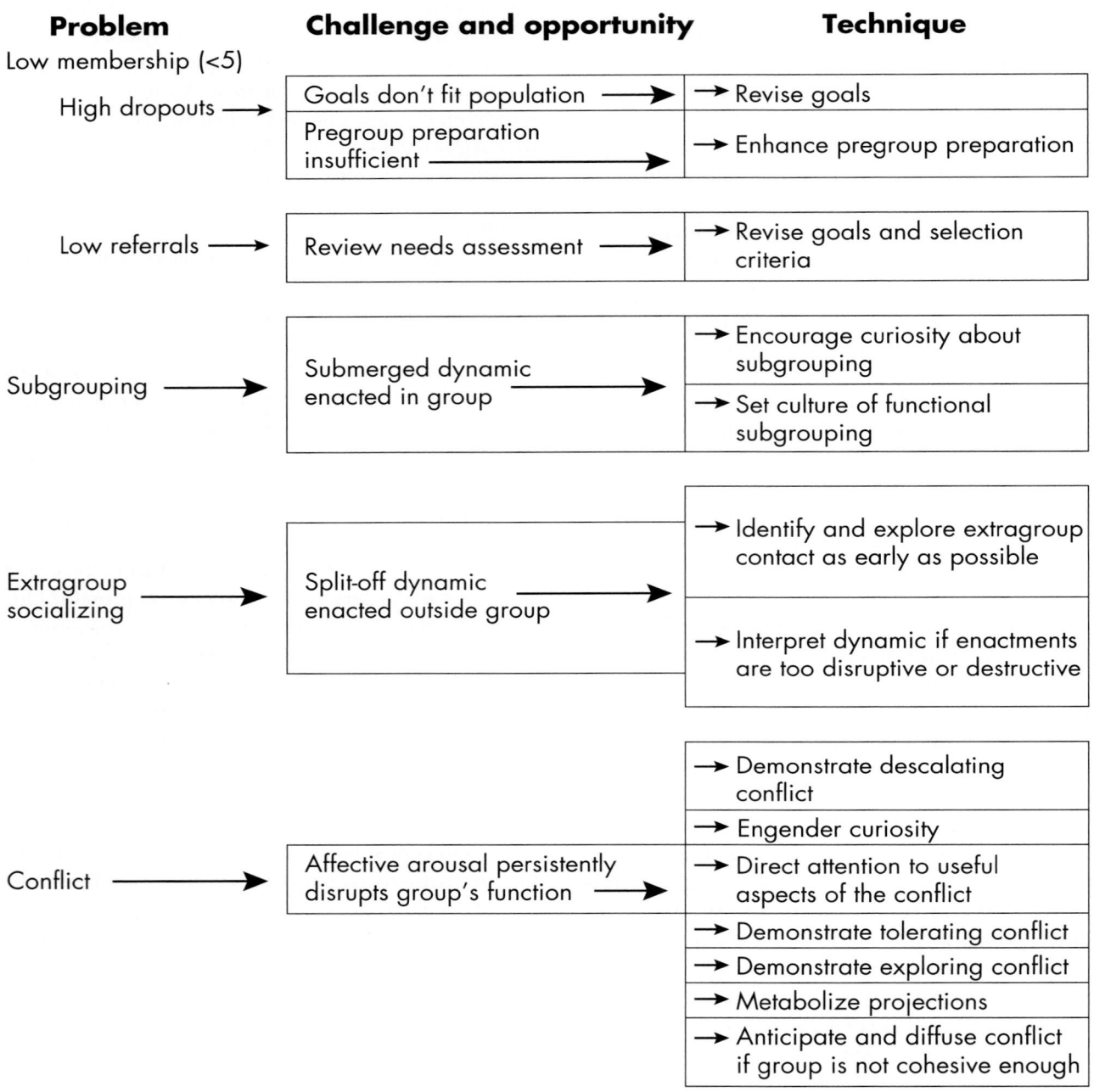

FIGURE 35–3. Common problems in group therapy.

group would be devastating in a group for schizophrenic patients (Kanas 1985, 1996). Gentle, cautious disagreement would be appropriate in a time-limited group for patients with panic disorder, whereas such disagreement would be seen as an avoidance of the real issues in a long-term outpatient group. Furthermore, even the same group may not tolerate the same level of conflict at different points in its development.

Early on, a prototypical group needs to invest its energy in the development of cohesiveness, trust, and support. In its middle phases, such a group will begin the constructive exploration of disagreement and confrontation. Much later, as members are terminating therapy, they may wish to focus again on the positive, more intimate aspects of the group experience rather than the divisive ones.

Finally, therapists should remember that conflict easily gets out of hand, no matter what the group setting. Leaders will often have to intervene vigorously to keep conflict within constructive bounds. Most often, this will include helping patients to express anger more directly and more fairly and ensuring that everyone gets a turn to respond to the anger. As with any affectively charged experience in the group, the therapist will need to encourage active feedback and consensual validation from all of the group members and, more than ever, will need to help patients process the meaning of that experience within the context of the group.

Techniques of the Group Therapist

Although individual and group therapists often use similar psychotherapeutic techniques, a number of interventions are unique to group therapy. These interventions include working in the here and now, using therapist transparency, and employing various procedural aids that can enhance the group work. We shall briefly examine each of these group therapy techniques and then describe how fundamental group therapy technology can be modified to suit a specialized group setting.

Work in the Here and Now

Even in the absence of direct leadership—for example, in a self-help group with no designated leader—an environment can develop in which nearly all of the therapeutic factors, from universality to altruism, will operate. The one important exception is the factor of interpersonal learning. In group therapy, interpersonal learning requires the presence of a leader, one who is well versed in the specific therapeutic techniques of working in the here and now. The principles of working in the here and now and the use of interpersonal learning are of most consequence in prototypic interactional groups, but these fundamental concepts can be modified to suit the needs of other kinds of groups and form an essential part of any group therapist's armamentarium (Dies 1993; Kahn 1984; Rothke 1986).

Goals

The primary goal of the long-term outpatient therapy group, and, to a lesser extent, of many other kinds of groups, is to help each individual understand as much as possible about his or her interactions with the other members of the group, therapists included. To accom-

plish this, members must learn to focus on the immediate interpersonal transactions occurring in the group. For the therapist, this means that the most fundamental principle of technique is to focus on the present, on what takes place in the therapy room in the here and now of the group interaction. By directly focusing on the here and now, the leader solicits and engages the active participation of all the members and maximizes the power and efficiency of the group. In other words, the therapy group focus is most powerful if it is basically ahistorical—that is, if it deemphasizes the historical past and even the current outside life of the individual members in favor of the here-and-now events in the group. Deemphasis does not imply that history is unimportant; rather, it implies that groups work most efficiently on the interactions occurring in the immediate present.

If it is to be therapeutically effective, a group experience must contain both an affective and a cognitive component. That is, the group members must be involved with one another in an affective matrix: they must interact freely, they must reveal a great deal of themselves, and they must experience and express important emotions. But they must also step outside that experience and examine, understand, and integrate the meaning of the emotional experience they have just undergone (Yalom and Vinogradov 1993). Thus, a here-and-now focus consists of a rotating sequence of affect evocation and affect examination (Figure 35–4).

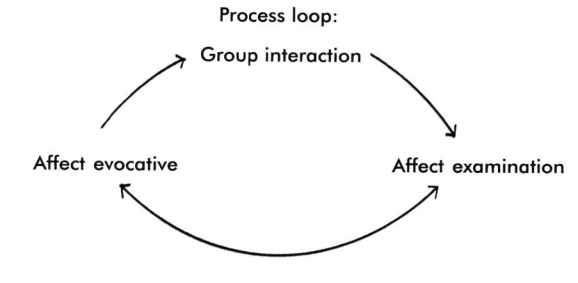

FIGURE 35–4. Schematic representation of the here-and-now technique in group therapy.

The absence of either the affective or the cognitive components of the here-and-now experience jeopardizes therapy. Encounter groups were often powerful and exciting events in the 1960s and 1970s, but many participants found that a strong emotional occurrence without subsequent examination promoted little real learning. No real therapeutic change occurs unless group members can integrate what they have learned in the here and now and then transfer that learning to their real-life situation. Likewise, leaders who focus exclusively on explanations and intellectual integration can end up squelching all expression of spontaneous affect and create a lifeless, sterile group.

Techniques

These two stages of the here-and-now focus—affect evocation followed by affect examination—are different in character and demand two very distinct sets of techniques. For the first stage, the stage of emotional experience, the therapist needs a set of techniques that will plunge the group into the immediate interpersonal interactions. For the second stage, clarification and understanding of the emotional experience, the therapist needs a set of techniques that will help the group transcend itself to examine and interpret its own experience. Let us consider each of these stages in turn.

Plunging the group into the here and now.   The starting place for shaping a group focused on the here and now is the pregroup preparation. The leader can offer the patient a rationale of the here-and-now approach through a brief, simplified discussion of the interpersonal approach to therapy. Patients benefit from an explicit description of how various kinds of psychological problems arise from (and are manifested in) patients' relationships with others and how group therapy is an ideal setting to take a close look at interpersonal relationships. Without this preparation, patients may be confused by the here-and-now focus of the group. After all, they sought therapy to deal with painful feelings such as anxiety, anger, or depression; how can they not be puzzled to find themselves in a group in which the therapist is asking them to reveal their feelings toward seven strangers? To alleviate this kind of confusion and to ensure that patients participate fully, the therapist must provide a cognitive bridge for incoming members.

After laying these foundations for the here-and-now focus in the pregroup preparation, the leader continues to reinforce this focus throughout therapy. Experienced group therapists think "here and now" at all times and consider themselves as shepherds keeping the group at work grazing on current interactions. All strays into the past, into outside life, or into intellectualization must be headed off or gently nudged back into the present. Whenever the group engages in some "there and then" discussion, for example, the group leader must think, "How can I bring this back into the here and now?"

The therapist must begin to steer the group into the here and now in its very first session. Consider for a moment the beginning of any therapy group. Typically, some member will get things started by sharing with the group a major life problem or concern and the reasons why he or she is now in this therapy group. Usually this disclosure begets both some support and some similar disclosure from others, and in a short period the group members have begun to share a great deal.

To plunge the group into the here and now, the interactionally oriented therapist may intervene with a comment such as "This group has made a good start, and many of you have shared some important things about yourselves. However, I have a hunch that something else has been happening here today as well. *[It is of course more than a hunch. The therapist knows perfectly well that what he or she is about to say has occurred.]* Each of you has found himself or herself thrown together with a group of strangers. No doubt you've been observing and sizing up one another and making first impressions." By this time, some persons in the group will be nodding in agreement, and the therapist may then set the task of the group: "Perhaps we could spend the rest of the meeting today discussing what each of you has come up with so far." Or, in a more fragile, lower-functioning group in which members might find this open-ended task threatening, an alternative suggestion could be, "Perhaps we could share what we liked the most about each other's participation so far." Now, this is no subtle intervention. It is a heavy-handed, explicit instruction to begin the process of here-and-now interaction. And yet the vast majority of groups, no matter what their composition or orientation, respond favorably to this intervention. Even groups of hospitalized patients, if proper boundaries are placed, accomplish this task with considerable ease and reward.

Group therapists must be active and continue diligently from session to session to bring the group discussion into the here and now. They must shift the content of the material from outside the group to inside the group, from abstract reflections on problems to specific revelations, from generic statements to personal disclosure. When a patient states that he or she is embarrassed to talk about certain things in the group, the therapist might ask what the patient anticipates happening if he or she were to take the risk and talk about something "embarrassing." If the patient supposes that people might laugh or be judgmental, the leader could then ask, "Who here in the group do you feel would laugh at you?" Once the group member reveals his or her guesses about others' reactions, the door is open to good interactional work. Other group members can confirm or, as is more often the case, disconfirm those guesses.

A useful technique for activating the here and now is to identify an in-group analogue for some outgroup problem and then to work on the in-group analogue rather than the out-group situation. If, for example, a male patient brings in an account of an argument he had with his wife in which she accused him of being unfeeling, it is incumbent on the group leader to search for some type of here-and-now manifestation of that conflict. The therapist might reflect on recent interactions in the group in which members wondered whether this patient was really empathic to their problems. Or the therapist might ask some of the female members of the group to picture being married to this patient. In what degree of close emotional contact could they imagine being with him? Without an intervention of this sort, the group will spend its energies on helping the patient solve the problems that led to the argument with his wife—an inefficient use of a group's time. Generally presented with incomplete or biased data, groups are almost always destined to fail to solve outside problems, and members end up feeling frustrated or discouraged.

The therapist who is experienced in working in the here and now is able to use almost every incident as a springboard for interactional exploration. If a patient monopolizes the group with a long 20-minute convoluted account of some painful period that occurred earlier in his life, the leader should start to reflect, "What are the interactional aspects of this behavior?" The leader may recall that in the first session, this patient said he often feels others don't listen to him. "Is it possible," the therapist could ask aloud, "that this is one of those times?" Another tack might be to ask why the patient chose to deliver this monologue today in the group. "What do the rest of you think? Could it be related to a feeling of being misunderstood in last week's meeting?" Or the patient could be encouraged to guess how the rest of the group is reacting to what he has been saying. Any one of these approaches has the same effect: it moves the group members away from a content-oriented monologue in which they cannot participate to a discussion of the relationships among members.

Individuals do not engage naturally and easily in the here and now. The experience is new and frightening, especially for the many patients who have not previously had close and honest relationships or who have spent their lives keeping certain thoughts and feelings—anger, pain, intimacy—covert. The therapist must offer much support, reinforcement, and explicit training. A first step is to help patients understand that the here-and-now focus is not synonymous with confrontation and conflict. In fact, many patients have problems not with anger or rage but with closeness and the honest and nondemanding or nonmanipulative expression of positive sentiments. Accordingly, it is important early in the group to encourage the expression of positive feelings as well as critical ones (Yalom and Vinogradov 1993).

The leader must teach group members how to request and how to offer feedback that is centered within the group's interactions and that is specific and personal. Observations or requests that have to do with there-and-then problems or that are global and abstract—such as "What should I do about my fights with my boyfriend?" or "You're really nice" or "Am I a boring person?"—are always unhelpful. The more specific the question or feedback, the more useful and potent it is. Much more fruitful are requests such as "I'd like to explore why I keep locking horns with the men in this group," and feedback such as "I feel closest to you when you share your pain with me, but I get turned off when you present yourself as having it all together and needing very little from the group."

Understanding the here and now. The second stage of the here-and-now focus requires an entirely different set of functions and techniques from the therapist. If the first stage demands activation and plunging of the group into the present affective experience, the second stage demands reflection, explanation, and interpretation. Often this latter phase of the group work is referred to as *group process*. If several individuals engage in a discussion, the content of their discussion is obvious; the discussion consists of the actual words spoken and the substantive issues addressed. But the process of the discussion is entirely different. The process refers to how this content was expressed and what it reveals about the nature of the relationship of the individuals holding the discussion.

The group therapist must always attend to the process of the communication in the group—that is, he or she must examine how the words exchanged shed light on the relationships among the participants. Consider, for example, the patient who suddenly reveals in a meeting that as a child she was sexually molested by her stepfather. The group members will probably probe for more "vertical disclosure," for more details such as how long the abuse lasted, what role her mother played, and whether the abuse affected the patient's relationship with men. A process-oriented therapist is more concerned about "horizontal disclosure" (i.e., disclosure about the disclosure) and, accordingly, will attend to the relational aspects of the patient's disclosure (Vinogradov and Yalom 1989). The leader may then pose questions such as "Why is Betty revealing this to us today rather than some other day?" or "What has permitted her to take this risk today?" or "What prevented her from telling us this earlier?" or "How does she anticipate the group will respond?"

The recognition of process is part of the art of psychotherapy and often requires a long apprenticeship. To understand process, one needs to register continually all of the available data. Who chooses which seat? Who is always late? At whom do members look when talking with each other? Who meets with whom at the end of the group? How does the group change when a particular member is absent? Some of the most valuable data are the therapist's own reactions. Feelings of impatience, frustration, or boredom in a group session represent valuable information and should be put to use. Likewise, when the leader feels engaged or excited by the group interactions, this is often the sign of a potent, hardworking meeting.

To recognize and understand the process in the here and now, it is helpful to keep in mind that certain tensions and processes will be present to some degree in every therapy group. One of the most fundamental of these is the struggle for dominance. Others include basic group conflicts faced by each member: the conflicts between sibling rivalry and the need for mutual support, between self-interest and the desire to help another person, and between the wish to immerse oneself in the comforting body of the group, on the one hand, and the fear of losing one's precious autonomy, on the other. Certain theoretical models of group behavior have been developed, by Bion (1959) and others, to describe and explain these basic conflicts.

The therapist who recognizes and identifies these fundamental tensions when they manifest themselves in the group will have illuminated an important part of the here-and-now process. As an example, we once had occasion to work with an articulate and provocative young man who had long enjoyed the role of dominant member of a group. When an older, very successful and aggressive man joined as a new member, the younger man gradually became withdrawn and depressed and soon announced his intention of leaving the group. It was not until the therapist called attention to the struggle for dominance that the patient began to explore some of his feelings about competition and envy.

Use of Transference and Therapist Transparency

Transference

Group members regard group therapists in an unrealistic light for many reasons. True transference or displacement of affect from some prior object, such as an early parental figure, is one reason. Conflicted attitudes toward authority as represented by the leader (e.g., dependency, autonomy, rebellion) are another. And still another reason is the patient's tendency to ascribe superhuman features to therapists so that the patient can use the therapists as a shield against existential anxiety. One realistic source of strong feelings lies in the members' explicit or intuitive appreciation of the great power that group therapists wield. The therapists' consistent presence and impartiality are essential for group survival and stability. Group therapists cannot be exposed; they can add new members, expel old members, and mobilize enormous group pressure around any issue they wish.

True transference does, of course, occur in therapy groups; indeed, it is powerful and radically influences the nature of the group discourse. But just as there will be, in any group, patients whose therapy hinges on the resolution of transference distortion, so there will also be many others whose improvement depends on interpersonal learning stemming not from transferential work with the therapist but from peer-oriented work with another member around such issues as competition, exploitation, or sexual and intimacy conflicts. Thus, if leaders ignore transference considerations, they may seriously misunderstand some important transactions; if, on the other hand, they see only the transference aspects of the group, they will fail to encourage the exploration of many other important interactions and may also fail to relate authentically to many of the group members. The cardinal rule is to maintain flexibility. Group therapists have a variety of tasks: they must make good use of any irrational attitudes toward them without at the same time neglecting a leader's many other functions in the group.

To work effectively with transference in the therapy group, leaders must help patients recognize, understand, and change their distorted attitudes. Two major approaches or techniques facilitate transference resolution in the therapy group. The first of these involves consensual validation (or, as is more often the case, consensual invalidation) by other group members of the patient's distorted views. The second, which shall be discussed separately, makes use of increased therapist transparency.

In consensual validation, a group leader encourages a patient to validate his or her impressions against those of other members. If many or all of the group members concur in the patient's view of and feelings toward the leader (say, that the leader is "too autocratic"), it can be concluded either that the patient's reaction to the therapist stems from global group forces related to the leader's role or that the reaction is not an unrealistic one at all and the patient is perceiving the leader accurately. Therapists, too, have blind spots. If, on the other hand, one member alone possesses a particular view of the therapist, then this member may be helped to examine the possibility that he or she sees the group leader, and perhaps other persons too, through an internal distorting prism.

Therapist Transparency

Group therapists can also allow a patient to confirm or disconfirm irrational impressions by gradually revealing more of themselves, reacting to the patient as a real person in the here and now. Leaders can thus respond to their patients authentically, share their feelings in a judicious and responsible manner, and acknowledge or refute motives and feelings attributed to them. In this approach, they look at their own blind spots and demonstrate respect for the feedback members offer them. In the face of mounting reality-based data about the therapist, it becomes increasingly difficult for members to maintain their fictitious beliefs about the group leader (Vinogradov and Yalom 1990).

One fear that therapists sometimes have concerning personal self-disclosure is the fear of escalation—the fear that once they reveal themselves, the insatiable group will demand even more. But strong forces in the group oppose this trend. Although members are enormously curious about their group leader, they also wish the therapist to remain unknown and all-powerful. Although they appreciate the responsible and growth-promoting use of interpersonal feedback from their leader, few want the therapist to discuss his or her personal problems (Table 35–8).

TABLE 35–8. **Qualities of self-disclosure in the group**

1. Is always member-focused and consonant with group task
2. Facilitates transference resolution
3. Models therapeutic norms
4. Participates in a member's interpersonal learning with the leader
5. Demonstrates acceptance and respect of members

There are many different approaches to therapist transparency, depending on the therapist's personal style and the goals in the group at a particular time. It is helpful to ask oneself what the purpose of self-disclosure is at any given point in the group: "Am I trying to facilitate transference resolution? Am I providing a model in an effort to create therapeutic norms? Am I attempting to assist the interpersonal learning of members by working on their relationship with me? Am I attempting to support and demonstrate my acceptance of members by saying, in effect, 'I value and respect you and demonstrate this by giving of myself'?" At all times, the therapist must consider whether transparency is consonant with other group therapy tasks (Vinogradov and Yalom 1990).

Although therapist self-disclosure generally facilitates group interaction, it is important to keep in mind that the group therapist's primary raison d'être is not to be fully self-disclosing. Furthermore, leader self-revelation must be guided by the different needs of each group member. Not all patients need the same thing, either from the therapist or from the group. Some patients need to relax controls and to learn how to express their emotions in an honest and responsible manner, whether they be anger, love, tenderness, envy, or other emotions. Other patients need the opposite, in that they need to gain impulse control and to accept limits to the expression of their emotions; their lifestyles may already be characterized by labile and immediately acted-on affect. Even the transparent and authentically self-disclosing therapist must provide some cognitive structuring—some intellectual integration to the group experience. Only in this manner can patients learn to generalize their experiences to outside life.

The leader's role undergoes a gradual metamorphosis during the life of any relatively stable interactional group. In the beginning, therapists busy themselves with the many functions necessary for the creation of the group, the development of a social system in which the many therapeutic factors may operate, and the activation and illumination of the here and now. Gradually, the leader begins to interact with each of the members, and the members' early stereotypes of the therapist become more difficult to maintain. This process between the therapist and each of the members is not qualitatively different from the interpersonal learning that ensues as a result of each member's relationship with other members. After all, therapists have no monopoly on authority, dominance, sagacity, or aloofness, and many members work out their conflicts in these areas not only with the leader but also with other members who have these attributes.

Procedural Aids

A group leader's therapeutic armamentarium can be expanded through the use of procedural aids—specialized techniques that are not essential but may facilitate the course of therapy. We discuss three such approaches: written summaries, videotaping, and structured exercises.

Written Summaries

The course of most outpatient therapy groups, especially interactionally oriented groups, is facilitated by the use of written summaries (Yalom and Leszcz 2005; Yalom et al. 1975). The most useful procedure is for the group leader to dictate a candid, concise description of the group session after each meeting and to have a transcription (of approximately two to three single-spaced pages) sent out to the group members the following day. These summaries serve to extend the effect of the group's here-and-now interactions during the week between meetings. Patients have been unanimous in their positive evaluation of this technique. Most await the arrival of the weekly summary with anticipation and read and consider it seriously. Many members reread the summaries several times, and almost all file them for future review. The patients' therapeutic perspectives and commitment are deepened, and the patient–therapist relationship is strengthened. No serious transference complications, breaks in confidentiality, or other adverse consequences have been noted to occur by practitioners of this method.

Weekly summaries are most valuable if they are honest and straightforward about the process of therapy in the group. They are virtually identical to the summaries therapists make for their own files and are based on the assumption that each patient is a full collaborator in the therapeutic process—that psychotherapy is strengthened and not weakened by demystification. The orientation of the material in the summary reflects the therapeutic orientation of the group. In a long-term interaction group, the summary focuses on the interpersonal transactions that occurred in the meeting and the therapist's reflections on some of the dynamics and implications of those transactions. In a time-limited outpatient group for bereaved spouses, the summaries are more descriptive in nature and underline some of the members' modes of coping with bereavement: loneliness, change in social role, disposition of the effects of the dead spouse, and confrontation with existential issues such as death, aloneness, meaning in life, and regret (Yalom and Vinogradov 1988).

The summary serves several functions (Table 35–9). It provides an understanding of the here-and-now events of the session and facilitates the integration of powerful affective experiences. It labels sessions as good or resistive, notes and rewards patient gains in the group, and predicts undesirable developments in the group, thus minimizing their impact. It increases group cohesiveness by emphasizing similarities among members, by underscoring the expressing of caring or other positive emotions, and by providing continuity from one meeting to another. The summary is also an ideal forum for interpretations, either for interpretations made during the session (which may have fallen on deaf ears if delivered in the midst of a heated discussion) or for new interpretations that have occurred to the therapist after the meeting. Finally, the summary provides hope to the patients by helping them realize that the group is an orderly process and that the therapist has some coherent sense of the group's long-term development.

Videotaping

Modern scientific technology has no doubt contributed to the dehumanization of present-day society; to the deconstitution of stable, support-giving social, work, and kinship groups; and, consequently, to the necessity for group therapy. However, it has also created an instrument, the videotape recorder, that has considerable potential benefit for the teaching, practice, and understanding of group therapy. Some therapists make the videotape recording a central feature of therapy; they may arrange for immediate playback of certain segments during a meeting or set up regularly scheduled playback sessions. Other therapists, ourselves included, find the technique of value but prefer to use it as a teaching device or occasionally as an auxiliary aid in the therapeutic process.

Although feedback from others about one's behavior is important, it is never as convincing as information one discovers for oneself, and videotape provides feedback that is not mediated through a second person. Often a patient's cherished self-image is radically challenged by a videotape playback. It is not unusual for a patient suddenly to recall and to accept previous feedback he or she has received from other members. The patient realizes that the group has been honest and, if anything, overprotective in previous confrontations.

Often profound realizations occur: for the first time, patients observe with their own eyes their full behavior and its impact on others. Many initial playback reactions are concerned with physical attractiveness and mannerisms, whereas in subsequent playback sessions patients begin to make more careful note

TABLE 35–9. Benefits of weekly written summary of group therapy session

1. Provides a further understanding of the here-and-now events of the session
2. Helps integrate powerful affective experiences
3. Labels the session as good or resistive
4. Notes and rewards patient gains
5. Predicts undesirable developments
6. Increases group cohesiveness by emphasizing similarities among members
7. Underscores caring or positive emotions
8. Provides continuity from meeting to meeting
9. Allows interpretations
10. Provides a view of the group's long-term development

Note. Weekly written summaries are sent to all members between sessions.

of their interactions with others, their withdrawal or timidity, and their self-preoccupation or aloofness or their hostility.

Patients who will be able to view the playback are usually receptive to the suggestion of videotaping. Often, however, they are concerned about confidentiality and need reassurance on this issue. If the videotape is to be viewed by anyone other than group members (e.g., students, researchers, supervisors), the therapist must be explicit about the purpose of the viewing and the identity of the viewers and must obtain written permission from all of the members.

Structured Exercises

The term *structured exercises* refers to the many group activities in which members follow some specific set of orders, generally prescribed by the leader. These kinds of exercises play an important role in many specialized therapy groups but may be counterproductive in long-term general outpatient groups (Lieberman et al. 1973; McKay and Paleg 1992; Yalom 1985; Yalom et al. 1975). The precise rationale of the procedures varies, but in general, structured exercises are meant to modify the pace of the group and direct group members' attention to factors deemed relevant to the group's goals. In brief interpersonal group therapy, structured exercises (warm-up procedures) permit a bypassing of hesitant, uneasy first steps of the group; others speed up interaction through assignment to individuals of interactional tasks that circumvent cautious, ritualized social behavior; still others speed up individual work by

helping members get in touch with suppressed emotions, with unknown or hidden parts of themselves, and with their physical bodies. In a medication support group or cognitive-behavioral group, a structured check-in procedure focuses attention on specific therapeutic issues and aspects of treatment.

A structured exercise may require only a few minutes, or it may consume an entire meeting. Although the exercise may be predominantly nonverbal in nature, there is always a verbal component in that the exercise generates data that subsequently can be discussed by the group. The exercise can involve the group as a whole; for example, a group of chronically mentally ill day-treatment patients may be asked to plan an outing. Or it can involve one member vis-à-vis the group: in a trust exercise, used in an encounter-type group, one member stands, with eyes closed, in the center of the group circle and then falls, allowing the group to support him or her. Exercises can include each individual within the group, such as a "go-around," in which each member is asked to give initial impressions of everyone else. In another type of go-around that is useful in the early life of a group, each member shares some background history. In working with bereaved spouses, we ask members during an early session to bring in a wedding photograph to share with the rest of the group.

Many of the therapist tasks and techniques for interactive, interpersonal group therapy—norm setting, here-and-now activation, understanding the here and now—involve approaches that have a prescriptive quality (approaches in the form of questions such as "Whose opinion in the group especially matters to you?" or "Can you look at Mary as you talk to her?" or "What has it been like for you to share that with us?" or "On a risk-taking scale of 1 to 10, how much have you risked with us today?"). Every experienced group leader uses some structured exercises, at times in a subtle and spontaneous manner. For example, if a group is tense and blocked and experiences a silence of a minute or two (a minute's silence feels very long in a group!), the leader might ask for a quick go-around in which each member says briefly what he or she had been feeling or had thought of saying, but did not, in that silence. Such an exercise usually generates much valuable data.

Although the judicious use of structured exercises can facilitate the course of group therapy, excessive use of such exercises may be counterproductive, depending on the goals of the group. In long-term interpersonal or psychodynamic group therapy, members make more therapeutic headway if the leaders encourage them to experience their timidity or suspiciousness and to understand the underlying dynamics rather than if the leaders prescribe an exercise that plunges members willy-nilly into deep disclosure or expression (Flowers and Booraem 1990). In acute or short-term settings such as inpatient groups and certain specialized outpatient groups, the situation is more complex. Faced with a limited amount of time in which to be helpful to many different patients, therapists may find that structured exercises are extremely useful: the exercises increase patient participation; provide a discrete, appropriate group task; and increase group efficiency. But there is a pitfall to be avoided. Whenever therapists prescribe structured tasks for a group, even during a single meeting, they run the risk of infantilizing members and establishing norms that block the group from developing into a potent therapeutic force. Members of a highly structured, leader-centered group begin to feel that all help emanates from the leader. They passively await their turn to work with the therapist. They de-skill themselves from an interpersonal point of view and cease to avail themselves of the help and resources that other group members can provide. Therapists leading such groups should deliberately and directly address this dynamic by encouraging task-focused member interactions. For example, in a medication support group, the therapist might encourage discussion among members on managing medication side effects. Although it is useful to impose structure judiciously when working with certain groups, it is essential to use that structure in a way that furthers the group's goals and enhances each member's functioning.

Modification of Basic Techniques for a Specialized Clinical Setting

The Acute Inpatient Therapy Group

The therapist faced with the task of organizing a therapy group in a specialized clinical situation must learn to modify fundamental group principles and techniques. We suggest these three basic steps:

- *Assessment of the clinical setting:* Determine the immutable clinical restraints surrounding the group.
- *Formulation of goals:* Develop goals that are appropriate and achievable within the existing clinical restraints.
- *Modification of traditional techniques:* Retain the basic principles of group therapy but alter techniques to adapt them to the clinical setting and to achieve the specified goals.

We shall illustrate these steps by discussing two highly specialized group settings: the acute inpatient therapy group and the outpatient medication support group. We have chosen the first setting for two reasons. First, the *clinical challenge* of inpatient group therapy is severe, and radical modifications of technique and strategy are required in order to lead effective groups in this setting (Kibel 1993). Second, the inpatient group is the most commonly encountered specialized group and is found on virtually every acute psychiatric ward in the country. Medication support groups, on the other hand, are used with less acutely ill patients and are examples of attempts to face the *fiscal challenges* of today's managed care environment. In general, specialized groups provide added value in resource-sensitive environments but require modification of group therapy technique.

Assessment of the clinical setting. The clinical setting facing the inpatient therapist appears highly inhospitable to the practice of traditional group therapy. Intrinsic limitations over which the therapist has no control include the rapid turnover of patients (patients will often be present for only a single group meeting) and the severity and heterogeneity of psychopathology among hospitalized patients. Extrinsic constraints that affect the formation of an inpatient group are represented by such matters as ward policy, staffing, and administrative support (or lack thereof) for group therapy.

The therapist must carefully delineate both the intrinsic and extrinsic limitations of the clinical setting and then take steps to change those extrinsic factors that might hinder the group. On an inpatient ward, for example, the therapist can enlist the support of administrative and clinical staff to ensure that group therapy is a part of the ward program, that group time is set aside and protected for all patients, and that there are adequate group meeting facilities.

Formulation of goals. Taking into account the clinical facts of life or constraints of the inpatient setting, the therapist must proceed to formulate appropriate goals for an inpatient therapy group (Table 35–10). Six achievable goals for the inpatient setting have been highlighted (Yalom 1983):

- *Engage patients in the therapeutic process:* Patients are helped to become involved in a process that they find constructive and supportive and will wish to continue after discharge from the hospital.
- *Teach patients that talking helps:* Patients are exposed to the benefits of psychotherapy and of improved communication skills.

- *Spot problems:* Patients are helped to learn to identify their maladaptive interpersonal behavior.
- *Decrease patients' sense of isolation:* Patients are encouraged to develop satisfying social contacts.
- *Allow patients to be helpful to others:* Patients are allowed to see that they can contribute to the lives of people around them.
- *Alleviate hospital-related anxiety:* Patients are encouraged to share concerns about the stigma of psychiatric hospitalization, to discuss distressing events on the ward (e.g., bizarre behavior of other patients, staff tensions, acutely disturbed patients), and to achieve reassurance from other group members.

Modification of traditional techniques. Once appropriate goals have been established, therapists must modify their standard group therapy techniques in order to lead effective groups on the acute psychiatric inpatient ward (Table 35–11). Four essential modifications that we will discuss are 1) the shortening of the time frame, 2) the use of direct support, 3) emphasis on the here and now, and 4) the provision of structure.

Shortening of time frame. The first and most fundamental modification the inpatient group leader makes is to shorten the time frame radically. The therapist in an acute inpatient group must consider the life of the group to be only a single session and must strive to offer something useful for as many patients as possible during that session. Naturally, a single-session time frame demands efficiency. There is no time to waste: the leader has only a single opportunity to engage each patient and must not squander that opportunity. This need for efficiency demands heightened therapist activity. The therapist must be prepared to activate the group, to call on members, to support them, and to interact personally with them.

Use of direct support. Inpatient group therapists must also learn to offer support quickly and directly. The most direct manner of offering support is simply to acknowledge openly each patient's efforts, intentions, strengths, positive contributions, and risks. If, for example, a member states that he finds a woman in the group very attractive, the leader must judiciously support this patient for the risk he has taken. The leader may wonder whether the group member has previously been able to express his admiration of another person so openly or may note that his openness encourages other members to take risks and reveal important feelings. Inpatient group therapists must try to emphasize the positive rather than the negative aspects of a person's behavior or defense. For example,

TABLE 35–10.	**Goals for acute inpatient therapy groups**
Engage patients in the therapeutic process.	
Teach patients that talking helps.	
Spot problems.	
Decrease isolation.	
Allow patients to be helpful.	
Alleviate hospital-related anxiety.	

TABLE 35–11.	**Modifications of basic techniques for acute inpatient therapy groups**
Shortening of the time frame	
Use of direct support	
Emphasis on the here and now	
Provision of structure	

rather than confront the patient who insists on playing "assistant therapist," the therapist may instead make positive comments on how helpful this patient has been to others. The stage is then set for a gentle remark on the patient's selflessness and reluctance to ask for something personal from the group.

The supportive therapist also makes it a point to help patients—especially objectionable or irritating patients—obtain support from the group. A self-centered patient who incessantly complains about a health condition or an insoluble situational problem will quickly alienate any group. When the therapist identifies such behavior, he or she must intervene quickly to circumvent the development of group animosity and rejection. The therapist may, for example, assign the patient the task of introducing new members into the group, giving positive feedback to other members, or attempting to guess and express what each member's evaluation of the group is that day. Or the leader may reframe the patient's irritating behavior: "Perhaps you have needs, too, but have trouble expressing them. I wonder if your preoccupation with your health [finances, spouse] isn't a way of asking for something from the group." Helping the patient to formulate a specific request for attention from the group often generates a positive response from the other members.

Another approach is to focus on making the group safe. Whereas some conflict and tension are necessary to the therapeutic work in a long-term outpatient group, inpatients are much too vulnerable to tolerate the additional anxiety of group conflict. The group therapist must anticipate and avoid confrontation and conflict whenever possible. If patients are irritable or critical, the leader can channel that work onto himself or herself. If two patients are locked into an adversarial position, the leader can remind them that sparks often fly between two persons who have similarities or who have envious feelings toward each other. Then each of the patients can be invited to talk about those aspects of the other that he or she admires or envies or to discuss the ways that he or she resembles the other.

When the therapist leads a group of severely regressed patients, he or she must provide even more support, in an even more direct fashion. The patients' behavior must be examined and then reframed in some positive way. The therapist can, for example, support the mute patient for staying the whole session, compliment the patient who leaves early for having stayed 20 minutes, or support inactive patients for having paid attention throughout the meeting. At times the therapist must even label inappropriate or bizarre statements as attempts to communicate with the group.

Emphasis on the here and now. These foregoing considerations of therapist efficiency, activity, and support in the inpatient setting do not make the here-and-now focus any less important than in outpatient therapy. Such a focus helps inpatients learn many important interpersonal skills: communicating more clearly, getting closer to others, expressing positive feelings, noticing personal mannerisms that push people away, listening, offering support, revealing oneself, and forming friendships. However, the clinical conditions of extremely brief treatment duration and more severe pathology demand modifications in basic technique. There is insufficient time to work through interpersonal issues. Instead, the therapist simply helps patients to spot major interpersonal problems and to reinforce interpersonal strengths. Explicit instruction must be provided about the relevance of the here and now by, for example, explaining that group therapy focuses on the way people relate to one another because that is what group therapy does best; and that, furthermore, groups do this most effectively by examining the relationships between members of the group. The group leader must emphasize that even though patients may enter the hospital for many different reasons, everyone can benefit from learning how to get more out of their relationships with others.

Provision of structure. Finally, work with the acute inpatient group requires structure, and just as there is no place in acute inpatient group work for the inactive

therapist, there is also no place for the nondirective therapist. Group leaders provide structure for the inpatient group in several ways: by instructing patients about and orienting them to the nature and purpose of the meeting, by establishing clear spatial and temporal boundaries for the group, and by using a lucid and confident personal style that reassures confused or anxious patients and contributes to a sense of structure. One of the most potent ways of providing structure is to build into each session a consistent, explicit sequence. Although different group sessions will have different sequences depending on the composition and task of the group, the following are natural lines of division:

- *The first few minutes:* The therapist provides explicit structure for the group. If there are new members (and there usually are in the acute inpatient group), this is the time to orient them to therapy.
- *Defining the task:* The therapist determines the most profitable direction for the group to take in a particular session. The leader may, for example, listen to get a sense of the urgent issues on the ward that day. Or the leader may provide a structured exercise, such as having each patient formulate (with the leader's help) an agenda to follow during that session (Yalom 1983). For example, an agenda of a shy and inhibited young depressed woman might be to try to express some positive feelings in the group.
- *Accomplishing the task:* The therapist helps the group to address the broad issues raised at the start of the session and, in the process, attempts to have as many patients participate as possible. If the group uses an agenda format, this is the "agenda filling" stage: the shy patient is helped to identify the members toward whom she feels positively and to express those feelings.
- *The final few minutes:* The leader indicates that the work phase is over and the remaining time is devoted to review and analysis of the meeting. This is the summing-up period and the self-reflective loop of the here-and-now process, in which the therapist attempts to clarify the group interaction that occurred in the session. How, for example, did the group respond when a usually shy and inhibited member openly expressed some positive sentiments?

The Medication Support Group

Therapists often work in clinical settings with significant fiscal limitations. Clinic directors often expect psychiatrists to rely on medication alone and to limit psychotherapy referrals. Insurance plans may reimburse psychiatrists only for medication visits. Patients needing prolonged medication management are often referred back to their primary care doctor. In summary, many psychiatrists face fiscal constraints that preclude leading traditional therapy groups.

Nevertheless, psychiatrists and therapists strive to provide the best treatment with the resources available. Many patients benefit from medication support groups. Here they can access the expertise of psychiatrists and therapists and the support of their peers. However, as in the case of any specialized medical treatment, some patients may need additional services. Specialized groups work best when they are part of a comprehensive treatment program.

Formulation of goals. The goals of the medication support group are modest but important. Some are similar to those for inpatient groups. Five achievable goals for medication support groups can be pursued:

- *Provide a flexible treatment setting:* Patients can attend groups more frequently when in crisis and can easily schedule early appointments with their providers.
- *Teach patients that talking in therapy groups helps:* Patients are exposed to some of the benefits of group psychotherapy.
- *Spot problems:* Group leaders can observe patients in a more complex and challenging interpersonal environment and can identify undertreated conditions and maladaptive interpersonal behavior.
- *Decrease patients' sense of isolation:* For example, each patient finds out that he or she is not the only person taking psychiatric medications.
- *Allow patients to be helpful to others:* Patients share their stories about taking medications and recovering from mental illness and thereby contribute to the lives of people around them.

Modification of traditional techniques. Three essential modifications that we will discuss are 1) the flexibility of the treatment frame, 2) the management of anxiety, and 3) the provision of structure.

Flexibility of treatment frame. In contrast to attendance at psychotherapy groups, members attend medication support groups irregularly. Similar to the inpatient unit, each meeting has a different membership, and the life of the group lasts only a single session. Therapists are active and structure meetings to achieve the group's goals and to maximize group time. Group membership changes even more than

that of inpatient groups. People managing minor crises may attend weekly. Those undergoing changes in medication may attend every 2–4 weeks. Those who are stable may attend every 4–12 weeks.

There are many benefits to this flexibility. Over the course of a long treatment, patients can use the group in different ways and can participate as members of different subgroups. Patients whose illnesses are acute, resolving, or in remission form three different subgroups. Each has something to offer the others. The stable patient can offer support to the patient undergoing medication changes and can feel justifiably proud and relieved to be stable. Members undergoing medication changes offer those in crisis a model of working with the doctor to optimize treatment. A great deal can be accomplished in medication support groups.

Management of anxiety. Despite their treatment setting and relatively high-functioning membership, medication support groups are more like inpatient than outpatient groups. Therapists must offer support quickly and directly help objectionable or irritating patients. Unlike therapists who work in settings that provide a framework for interpersonal work, medication support group therapists must intervene quickly to maintain group cohesion in the service of the group's modest goals. Work in the here and now is extraordinarily powerful, and like any potent tool, it must be wielded thoughtfully and in the appropriate setting and circumstance. If group development and group cohesion are limited by irregular attendance, then anxiety-inducing here-and-now work may also be limited. Although members are not as ill as those on an inpatient unit, the group's leaders do not have the luxury of returning group members to the inpatient unit, where they can be observed after the session. Anxiety management in medication support groups is paramount.

Provision of structure. Similar to the acute inpatient group, medication support groups require structure. Group leaders should introduce every meeting with a brief statement on the purposes and structure of the meeting. To provide appropriate medication management, medication support groups must cover specific content areas for each patient. A comprehensive check-in procedure for each patient is one way to provide a predictable structure. Although the sequential check-in process consumes most of the group time and cannot be characterized as encouraging intermember interaction, check-ins can represent opportunities for tapping therapeutic factors such as instillation of hope, universality, imparting of information, and altruism. Catharsis and existential factors are also occasionally addressed. Many patients find written check-in instructions helpful. The following instructions exemplify those often used in a check-in process:

- Please tell us your name, medications, dosages, and how you take them (compliance).
- Tell us how the medications help you. (What are your target symptoms?)
- Tell us any problems that the medications cause for you. (What are the side effects?)
- Tell us about recent or upcoming "big events." (What are the current stresses around which you might need support?)

Group Therapy Programs and Managed Care Systems

The importance of group therapy is growing in today's managed care environment. Community mental health programs, the military, and the Department of Veterans Affairs use systematic approaches to the delivery of mental health care. Group therapy is moving beyond the public sector and the private office to the private-sector institution. Health care companies are increasingly careful about allocating resources and tracking outcomes. As health care delivery systems grow, group therapy programs must become more sophisticated.

The most obvious economic reason for increased utilization of group therapy is efficient use of staff time (number of patients per staff hour). However, group therapy as a labor-saving strategy is prone to being misused. Leaders in managed care face significant challenges to expand the use of group therapy to better serve large populations. Therapists, administrators, and staff must change the institutional culture and develop protocols to implement group therapy programs. Developing such programs is similar to applying any other new strategic approach (e.g., preauthorization and concurrent utilization review). New requirements and policies may feel heavy-handed at first, but eventually the techniques useful for initiating change will be refined (Bennett 1993) and become routine. Starting a group therapy program and shifting utilization patterns are huge changes. Despite the obvious economic advantages of group therapy, institutions still face substantial internal resistance and an extraordinarily complicated evolving marketplace.

Managed care brings clinical and business activi-

ties together in complex ways. Economic risk threatens to replace clinical scope of practice as the primary paradigm for dividing up responsibility. The importance of being able to predict one's costs necessitates the use of actuarial assessments. Covering large populations enables managed care companies to predict and plan for infrequent but costly illnesses. Many costly illnesses can be prevented, and a large group therapy program can facilitate provision of preventive care for large populations, thus decreasing morbidity through secondary prevention.

Development of a Group Program

Group therapy coordination is an essential function. Someone must oversee a new program's development. Each stage entails different challenges and requires its own blend of strategies. Facilitating and reinforcing clinician behavior change are important throughout. The group program coordinator should carefully plan which groups to start first in order to maximize usefulness to patients and clinicians. There are two basic strategies. One can start several groups that will have heterogeneous memberships (i.e., demographics, diagnoses, and problems)—for example, cycles of brief interpersonal therapy groups and ongoing medication support groups. Alternatively, one can start focused groups for problems, illnesses, or stage-related difficulties that are common in one's treatment setting—for example, cognitive-behavioral group therapy for posttraumatic stress disorder or a relapse-prevention group for alcoholism. Not everyone can be effectively treated in the same type of group therapy, and the process of deciding which patient belongs in which group is still being refined (Harwood 1996). Nevertheless, the group program coordinator should prioritize the organizing of new groups based on discussions with referring staff (Table 35–12).

Starting a group program is challenging. The coordinator must maintain the support of the referring staff and attend to numerous practical matters. With each early referral, there are risks of refusal by the patient, the receiving clinician or group therapist, or the group, and a delicate balancing of priorities is required. Referral failures and dropouts discourage both the referring clinician and the group therapist. Initially, the effort put into making decisions such as those concerning which groups to start, when to start them, and how to match patients and groups will be out of proportion to the savings that a small group program produces. As a group program enlarges, fit-and-matching issues be-

TABLE 35–12. Essentials for starting a group program and seamless integration with other clinical services

1. Group therapy coordinator
2. Administrative sanction
   a. Start-up resources: clinician time and administrative support staff time
   b. Ongoing resources: space and administrative support
3. Needs assessment
4. Effective leadership

come less problematic but still require a coherent, thoughtful approach. Group program coordinators perform or oversee the many essential executive, clerical, and educational tasks necessary to develop, enlarge, and maintain a group program.

The group program should fit as seamlessly as possible with other clinical functions such as intake, crisis stabilization, individual treatment, and referral to extraclinic resources. Evaluations and crisis stabilization are almost always performed individually. After that, group or individual approaches may be used for secondary prevention—either time-limited or maintenance treatments. Preventive efforts, although historically underemphasized, are gaining in esteem as their value in capitated systems becomes apparent. Given the absence of a litmus test for likelihood to fail in group therapy, one could argue that referral to a group should always be a part of the initial treatment plan. Rather than "Who will fail in group treatment?" the question may be "How can we prepare everyone to benefit from some form of group treatment?"

Long-term groups with highly impaired populations often provide the greatest savings because of their prolonged nature and because they obviate the need for more expensive levels of care (Gabbard et al. 1997; MacKenzie 1997a). Time-limited groups focus on less impaired patients and therefore draw from a larger population. They offer increased flexibility by allowing providers additional treatment options with little impact on clinician time. Clinical benefit is essentially equivalent in a five-person versus an eight-person group, and therapist time is equal.

In settings where the shift to using group therapy is well under way, clinicians and administrators must continue their efforts. Wherever group therapy is not being used, staff members should encourage each other to ask the question "Why not group therapy?"

rather than "Why group therapy?" This is an important shift in perspective and lays the basis for changes in the institutional culture.

Delivery Systems and Group Therapy

The penetration of group psychotherapy into clinical services has always been dependent on social and political trends related to access (MacKenzie 1997a).

As noted earlier, the first therapy group is credited to the internist Joseph Pratt. At a time when tuberculosis was common, Pratt brought his sanitarium patients together for classes. Soon other practitioners, including early psychoanalysts, began seeing patients in group settings. Over the course of the next several decades, changes in the need for mental health care led to creative work and change in group therapy practice. During World War II, Wilfred Bion, a British psychoanalyst, used group process to care for patients with psychiatric problems brought about by the war. His ideas (as described earlier in this chapter) continue to influence understanding of institutional dynamics, basic group therapy, and organizational change.

During the 1970s, there was a shift from care in locked institutions to community mental health care, and T-groups and encounter groups were created. Although this was a productive period in many ways, many programs were inadequately funded. Poorly formulated systems often used group gatherings as a panacea. Thus, the psychotic symptoms of some patients suffering from schizophrenia became worse with the use of overly stimulating and anxiety-producing forms of group therapy. Poorly trained group leaders led risky endeavors that resulted in boundary violations and other negative outcomes. During this period, Yalom's empirical research (described earlier in this chapter) led to the creation of a list of therapeutic factors as well as interpersonal group psychotherapy. Group therapy, popularized and overextended during the free-love 1960s, reentered the health care arena in the 1970s.

Since the 1990s, the incentive for developing groups has been increasing. As in the past, we face the challenge of applying group therapy in thoughtful new ways and run the risk of inappropriately using group therapy as a panacea. What can we expect to be different from the past?

Changes inside and outside the field of group therapy will stimulate further development. Bion and Yalom were able to outline truths of group behavior in institutional and small group settings. Their theories are valid for patient treatment groups but are not enough in the case of group program development for primary and secondary prevention. Furthermore, treating brain disease requires integration of group behavior theory and the latest treatments (e.g., therapy with new medication, cognitive therapy for drug abuse, interpersonal therapy for eating disorders) (Verhulst 1996). Changes in the health care delivery system will likely stimulate new inquiries into overlooked or underdeveloped applications of group behavior (e.g., psychoeducational groups, medication support groups).

Health services researchers use improved information systems to analyze treatments in real clinical settings rather than just research settings. Even the modest systems currently in place will allow thoughtful planning while protecting against the most egregious misuses and overuses of group therapy. For instance, in larger populations, infrequently occurring illnesses turn up at predictable rates. Knowing this allows large managed care organizations to develop more detailed plans for systems of care, including the formation of specialized therapy groups.

There are many different ways to use group process to enhance patients' treatment. Group analysis focuses on treatment through the group. This approach continues to influence other forms of group therapy. Yalom's therapeutic factors provide a framework for therapists to enhance the efficacy of cognitive, behavioral, and psychoeducational approaches. In group therapy, universality, altruism, increased opportunity for positive modeling, and lending of hope all can amplify the impact that other approaches rely on to help patients. Increasing pressure to provide efficient care changes the direction of development and innovation. For example, homogeneous groups cohere more rapidly. This contributed to the development of symptom-specific, illness-specific, and developmental stage–specific groups. The need for resource-sensitive methods has led to the development of different types of time-limited groups. The need for a new way to incorporate group therapy will undoubtedly influence what aspects of group therapy receive the most attention in research and development circles.

Utilization of Group Programs

Despite the advantage of having multiple groups from which to choose, rarely do group therapists combine forces. With adequate communication, a better match between patient and group is possible. One of the challenges inherent in having many patients and many groups is matching patients to groups.

Unfortunately, there is still no widely applied triage system for such matching. Attaining the best

match possible depends on good communication between referring clinicians and group therapists. Every effort should be made to convey to all clinicians and staff information on the type and nature of the groups available (Crosby and Sabin 1995). Patient–treatment matching is an important research topic. Collecting outcome data and improving information systems are two important pieces of the groundwork needed to provide feedback for group therapy programs.

New information systems are allowing and patterns of reimbursement are encouraging more thoughtful utilization of group therapists. Administrative staff use larger, more sophisticated information systems to track the clinical needs of larger and larger populations. Managed care payers reward clinicians for keeping people healthy and intervening more quickly in chronic illnesses by maintaining a framework of regular contact. Although developments in group theory have been substantial and influential, the recent changes outside the field are at least as important.

The Current Response

In 1996, the American Group Psychotherapy Association (AGPA) established the National Registry of Certified Group Psychotherapists. The certification process requires high levels of training including formal didactics with specified content as well as extensive clinical experience and supervision. AGPA proactively addressed the excesses and misapplications that plagued earlier periods of group therapy expansion. Nevertheless, there is still a great deal of work to do.

Treatment–patient matching, pregroup preparation, and group program development are still underdeveloped. Many clinicians and academicians focus on developing manualized treatments for specific illnesses (Spitz 1996). Others study "group process," or how the manner in which group members relate to each other changes as a function of time. Basic scientific research on group therapy is essential. However, developing systems of care based on group therapies is a different type of challenge. One would expect managed care to be eager to meet the challenge of figuring out how best to deploy research-tested, clinically effective, and resource-sensitive treatments. However, the fluidity of people's insurance status makes large provider organizations understandably wary of long-term projects. Businesses do not have time to develop and refine innovative group therapy programs.

Established staff-model health maintenance organizations lead the effort to identify which types of groups are most useful in providing care for large capitated populations. Group coordinators focus on time-limited groups, especially psychoeducational groups, that help prevent the development of full-blown illness. In the past, groups for chronically, persistently, and severely mentally ill patients were almost exclusively the province of public mental health programs. In the past decade, several books were written on treating such patients in groups. Bauer and McBride (1996) and Stone (1996) wrote on group therapy for severely mentally ill patients (bipolar affective disorder and chronic mental illness, respectively). Development of group therapy models for psychotic disorders has been even more robust, with books by Kanas (1996), Schermer and Pines (1999), and Martindale et al. (2000). Linehan (1993), MacKenzie (2001b), and Budman et al. (1996), among others, developed or wrote about models for treating severe personality disorders in groups and empirically tested these models for efficacy.

Several approaches to time-limited group treatment for common nonpsychotic disorders are well developed and have been published in both book and workbook form. Many utilize tenets of cognitive or behavioral group therapy (e.g., Padesky on depression, Zueker-White on panic disorder). The theoretical basis and layout of the books lend themselves to a structured, focused approach. Many books provide readers with pretreatment and posttreatment assessments. Adding tests to assess parameters such as locus of control, motivation, social competence, learned resourcefulness, ego strength, coping style (Piper and Joyce 1996), psychological mindedness (McCallum and Piper 1996), and psychological defenses (Tasca et al. 1994) to the pretest may facilitate the matching of patients and groups. Paleg and Jongsma (2000) made an important contribution to comprehensive approaches to program development by compiling a book on group therapy formats for 28 different presenting problems (Figure 35–5).

Unlike time-limited cognitive or behavioral group therapy, medication support groups are less often the focus of research but are, nonetheless, common. Psychiatrists can provide secondary prevention with medication support groups. Such groups offer members regular contact with highly trained mental health professionals. Because they are more efficient in terms of numbers of patients seen, visits can be more frequent than individual medication checks. However, they need not meet weekly, because the task is different from that in a therapy group. In a medication support group, the clinician can observe the patient's level of function in an environment that is probably more like the outside world than the environment of dyadic interactions and is not limited by the patient's descrip-

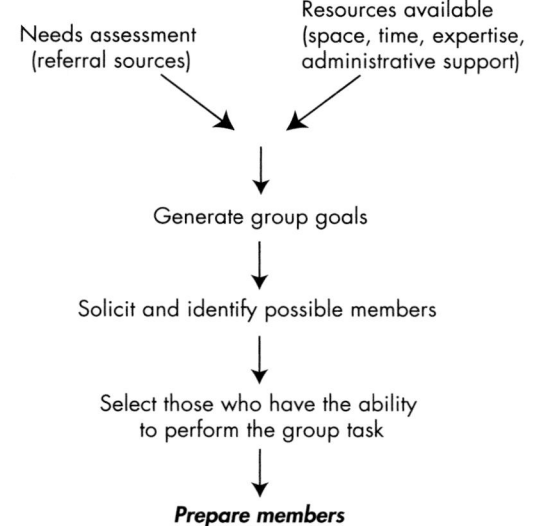

Needs assessment (referral sources)

Resources available (space, time, expertise, administrative support)

Generate group goals

Solicit and identify possible members

Select those who have the ability to perform the group task

Prepare members

1) Foster alliance with therapist(s)
2) Anticipate member pairings in group
3) Refine member goals
4) Monitor any outliers (a member substantially different from others in group; e.g., age, ethnicity)
5) Review previous experience in group settings
6) Provide cognitive structure and/or emotional containment
7) Address myths/fears

FIGURE 35–5.   Creation of a treatment group.

tions of outside events. Additionally, group therapy offers the patient the opportunity to benefit from Yalom's therapeutic factors: universality, altruism, and sharing of information.

Time-limited interpersonal group psychotherapy (TLIGP) is similar to medication support groups in that it is widely used and not commonly the subject of research. Therapists can treat interpersonal difficulties that stem either from an episode of mental illness or from relationships—problems that lead to exacerbations of one's illness. One member may focus on adjusting to the interpersonal stresses of the workplace after a serious depressive episode. Such adjustment might be especially difficult if the depression had been prolonged and modified his or her interpersonal style in an unhealthy way—for example, if the patient tended to withdraw when depressed rather than seeking help. Another patient might have a history of interpersonal difficulties that make him or her susceptible to dismissing the concerns of his or her partner regarding signs of incipient mania. In a sense, TLIGP is generic and requires less effort by the referring providers. Matching of the patient's illness and the group's purpose does not need to be as careful. Likewise, the group therapist focuses on helping the patient conceptualize his or her illness in an interpersonal framework rather than focusing on exclusionary or inclusionary criteria. Membership is heterogeneous, and the group therapists can cast a wide net. They can start groups more often simply because there are more eligible patients who can learn to conceptualize their mental illness in an interpersonal framework.

Groups in general lend themselves to more forgiving referral relationships. By *forgiving,* I mean that the referring party can err on the side of referral without worrying about unduly burdening the group therapist. Unlike a patient referred for individual treatment, who will take up a time slot all to him- or herself, a referral to a group takes up a seat rather than a time slot. TLIGP is equally effective for each member when membership is between five and eight or nine persons. Thus, referral to such a group does not need to be as rigorously assessed for its resource utilization. One could even argue that providing a time-limited group after using the patient's crisis benefit should be the standard of care because it may decrease the likelihood and severity of subsequent episodes. TLIGP may be one way to provide benefit to the patient as well as secondary prevention, all at little additional cost.

Resistance

Clinicians are responsible for overcoming not only their patients' reservations but also their own. Prospective group therapists worry about being overwhelmed. They need time before groups to prepare, after them to document the visit for all group members, and at other times during the day to return group members' phone calls. Administrators can plan for this in the clinician's schedule and/or provide additional clerical support (Cox et al. 2000). Some would argue that providing further free time for group therapists is an appropriate reward for being innovative and hard working. After all, the clinic is benefiting in that more patients receive better secondary prevention each day (Dick and Wooff 1986). Perhaps the group therapist will feel sufficiently encouraged by such a reward to start another group.

Clinicians must educate their patients about mental illness, treatment, and group therapy. The fact that group therapy is as effective as individual therapy is not widely known, even among mental health professionals. It is essential that clinicians communicate a sense of certainty about the effectiveness of group therapy to patients. In addition, one must address the patients' fear that the group will reject them. Inexperienced group therapists—even if they are experienced clinicians—are like their patients in that they, too, fear

public exposure of and shame about their mistakes. Neophyte group therapists face learning (or at least adapting to) a new set of treatment parameters. Both patients and therapists must learn how group psychotherapy can help them so that they can overcome their initial sense of intimidation.

Group members and therapists alike often feel anxious when starting a group for the first time. In addition to the specter of meeting new people, members may fear sharing shameful experiences and revealing painful feelings. Ironically, the extent to which patients expect humiliation often predicts the degree of relief they feel when they discover that other people have similar problems and fears. Similarly, therapists who are awed by the complexity of running a group and intimidated by the power of the group process may be more likely to recognize opportunities that can influence the group process. At the very least, such therapists may make better use of clinical supervision.

Just like an anxious and eager new group member, a new group therapist should be both excited and daunted by the task ahead. Treatment manuals written by experts and used in their research often focus on specific illnesses or issues and employ a wide variety of theoretical frameworks. Manuals need not be limited to research, and developing such a manual not only permits the outlining of what works well in particular situations but also reduces the neophyte group therapist's anxiety.

The Future

There continue to be large numbers of health services studies looking at the economic efficiency of different treatment systems. University researchers and managed care companies alike are seeking to clarify which treatments work under which circumstances. Clinic directors, group coordinators, and outpatient clinicians working together will better delineate the benefits of different types of group therapy and patterns of implementation for patients with various disorders. To answer the many remaining questions about helping patients by using group therapy, researchers, clinic administrators, and clinicians will need to collaborate.

Even before the ascent of managed care, several prominent authors had written books and articles on developing and maintaining group therapy training programs. Administrative sanction, effective leadership of the group program, and effective coordination of multiple practitioners are some of the essential factors of a successful group therapy training program (Lonergan 1991, 1995, 2000).

Conclusion

Group therapy is a widely practiced mode of treatment that is used effectively in a vast number of clinical settings. It involves a host of therapeutic factors or mechanisms of change, many of which are unique to group therapy. These mechanisms range from the therapeutic factors widely encountered in many different kinds of groups (such as universality, altruism, catharsis, and the imparting of information) to the potent but often misunderstood factor of interpersonal learning, which requires a skilled and experienced therapist working in a specialized interactional setting. Various constellations of these therapeutic factors operate in different types of groups at any given time. Therapists must understand the particular mechanisms of change at work in different kinds of groups and employ appropriate techniques to facilitate such mechanisms and complete the group task.

Group leaders make use of specific techniques and interventions, and all clinicians should be familiar with the technology used in group therapy. Some of these unique interventions include working in the here and now, therapist transparency, and the use of various procedural aids. These fundamental techniques can be modified to suit any specialized group setting, from the acute inpatient group to the symptom-oriented outpatient group. Indeed, the power of group therapy lies in its adaptability. Highly flexible and efficient, it may be the only mode of psychotherapy that can accommodate an almost infinite variety of settings, goals, and patients.

Key Points

- The goals of a treatment group should inform the therapist's techniques and theoretical approach and the group's structure.

- Group cohesiveness refers to the affinity that members have for their group and for the other members. A cohesive group is ready to perform the group task.

- One of the therapist's essential tasks is to prepare the patient for group therapy by demystifying the group and establishing a therapeutic alliance.

- The leader must establish behavioral norms that will guide the interactions of the newly formed group; the members themselves will be important agents of change, and a "culture"—a set of unwritten rules or norms that determine the acceptable behavioral procedures of the group—should be shaped to create an atmosphere maximally conducive to effective group interaction and to the development of the various therapeutic factors.

- Cliques forming within a group (subgrouping) and conflict between members are examples of dynamics that, if mismanaged, are destructive in the earliest stages of group development but are important therapeutic opportunities when thoughtfully negotiated in later stages.

- By directly focusing on the here and now, de-emphasizing history and life outside the group, the leader solicits and engages the active participation of all the members and maximizes the power and efficiency of the group.

- Phrases like "in-group analogue" and "social microcosm" are useful for explaining a here-and-now focus and should be explained repeatedly prior to referral, during referral, and after referral in pregroup preparation.

- *Group process* provides additional information above and beyond content. The content consists of the actual words spoken and the substantive issues addressed. The process of the discussion is entirely different and refers to how this content was expressed and what it reveals about the nature of the relationship of the individuals holding the discussion.

- Group therapy coordination is an essential function. Group program coordinators perform or oversee the many essential executive, clerical, and educational tasks necessary to develop, enlarge, and maintain a group program.

- The key question is: "How we can prepare everyone to benefit from some form of group treatment?"

Suggested Readings

Alonso A, Swiller HI (eds): Group Therapy in Clinical Practice. Washington, DC, American Psychiatric Press, 1993

Aronson S, Scheidlinger S (eds): Group Treatment of Adolescents in Context: Outpatient, Inpatient and School. Madison, CT: International Universities Press, 2002, pp 220

Bandura A: Social Foundations of Thought and Action: A Social Cognitive Theory. Englewood Cliffs, NJ, Prentice-Hall, 1986

Bauer MS, McBride L: Structured Group Psychotherapy for Bipolar Disorder: The Life Goals Program. New York, Springer, 1996

Kanas N: Group Therapy for Schizophrenic Patients. Washington, DC, American Psychiatric Press, 1996

Linehan MM: Cognitive-Behavioral Treatment of Borderline Personality Disorder. New York, Guilford, 1993

MacKenzie KR: Time-Managed Group Psychotherapy: Effective Clinical Applications. Washington, DC, American Psychiatric Press, 1997b

Paleg K, Jongsma AE Jr: The Group Therapy Treatment Planner. New York, Wiley, 2000

Piper WE, McCallum M, Azim HFA: Adaptation to Loss Through Short-Term Group Psychotherapy. New York, Guilford, 1992

Spitz HI: Group Psychotherapy and Managed Mental Health Care: A Clinical Guide for Providers. New York, Brunner/Mazel, 1996

Stone W: Group Psychotherapy for People With Chronic Mental Illness. New York, Guilford, 1996

Vinogradov S, Yalom ID: Concise Guide to Group Psychotherapy. Washington, DC, American Psychiatric Press, 1989

Yalom ID, Leszcz M: The Theory and Practice of Group Psychotherapy, 5th Edition. New York, Basic Books, 2005

Online Resources

American Group Psychotherapy Association (AGPA; http://www.AGPA.org)

Association for Specialists in Group Work (ASGW; http://www.asgw.org)—The ASGW was founded to promote quality in group work training, practice, and research both nationally and internationally. A division of the American Counseling Association (ACA), ASGW numbers among its members more than 5,800 group workers and group work educators.

Haim Weinberg's Group Psychotherapy Resource Guide (http://www.group-psychotherapy.com)—Information on group psychotherapy for the professional and the layman; includes information about the excellent group psychotherapy discussion list and a basic on group psychotherapy.

International Association of Group Psychotherapy (IAGP; http://www.iagp.com)—The purpose of the IAGP is to serve the development of group psychotherapy, as a field of practice, training, and scientific study, by means of international conferences, publications, and other forms of communication.

Children's Group Therapy Association (CGTA; http://www.cgta.net)—See the Resources section for useful links to other sites.

References

Agazarian YM: Systems-Centered Therapy for Groups. New York, Guilford, 1997

Alonso A, Swiller HI: Introduction: the case for group therapy, in Group Therapy in Clinical Practice. Edited by Alonso A, Swiller HI. Washington, DC, American Psychiatric Press, 1993, pp xxi–xxv

Amaranto EA, Benden S: Individual psychotherapy as an adjunct to group psychotherapy. Int J Group Psychother 40:91–101, 1990

Ansbacher HL: Alfred Adler, in Comprehensive Textbook of Psychiatry/III, 3rd Edition, Vol 1. Edited by Kaplan HI, Freedman AM, Sadock BJ. Baltimore, MD, Williams & Wilkins, 1980, pp 729–740

Baker MN, Baker HS: Self psychological contributions to the theory and practice of group psychotherapy, in Group Therapy in Clinical Practice. Edited by Alonso A, Swiller HI. Washington, DC, American Psychiatric Press, 1993, pp 49–68

Bandura A, Blanchard EB, Ritter B: Relative efficacy of desensitization and modeling approaches for inducing behavioral, affective, and attitudinal changes. J Pers Soc Psychol 13:173–199, 1969

Bandura A: Social Foundations of Thought and Action: A Social Cognitive Theory. Englewood Cliffs, NJ, Prentice-Hall, 1986

Barlow SH, Burlingame GM, Nebeker RS, et al: Meta-analysis of medical self-help groups. Int J Group Psychother 50:53–69, 2000

Bauer MS, McBride L: Structured Group Psychotherapy for Bipolar Disorder: The Life Goals Program. New York, Springer, 1996

Benioff L, Vinogradov S: Group psychotherapy with cancer patients and the terminally ill, in Comprehensive Textbook of Group Psychotherapy, 3rd Edition. Edited by Kaplan HI, Sadock BJ. Baltimore, MD, Williams & Wilkins, 1993, pp 477–489

Bennett MJ: View from the bridge: reflections of a recovering staff model HMO psychiatrist. Psychiatr Q 64:45–75, 1993

Bion WR: Experience in Groups. New York, Basic Books, 1959

Blake-Mortimer J, Gore-Felton C, Kimerling R, et al: Improving the quality and quantity of life among patients with cancer: a review of the effectiveness of group psychotherapy. Eur J Cancer 35:1581–1586, 1999

Bloch S: Therapeutic factors in group psychotherapy, in Psychiatry Update: American Psychiatric Association Annual Review, Vol 5. Edited by Frances AJ, Hales RE. Washington, DC, American Psychiatric Press, 1986, pp 678–698

Bloch S, Crouch E: Therapeutic Factors in Group Psychotherapy. Oxford, UK, Oxford University Press, 1985

Brook DW: Medication groups, in Group Therapy in Clinical Practice. Edited by Alonso A, Swiller HI. Washington, DC, American Psychiatric Press, 1993, pp 155–170

Brook DW: The use of medication groups for the treatment of patients with major mental illness. Funzione Gamma Journal (a bilingual [Italian and English] telematic journal of Group Psychotherapy; edited by University of Rome "La Sapienza") 2(4), 2001

Budman SH, Cooley S, Demby A, et al: A model of time-effective group psychotherapy for patients with personality disorders: the clinical model. Int J Group Psychother 46:329–355, 1996

Budman SH, Demby A, Redondon JP, et al: Comparative outcome in time-limited individual and group psychotherapy. Int J Group Psychother 48:38–63, 1998

Butler T, Fuhriman A: Patient perspective on the curative process: a comparison of day treatment and outpatient psychotherapy groups. Small Group Behavior 11:371–388, 1980

Butler T, Fuhriman A: Curative factors in group therapy: a review of the recent literature. Small Group Behavior 14:131–142, 1983

Cheifetz DI, Salloway JC: Patterns of mental health services provided by HMOs. Am Psychol 39:495–502, 1984

Connelly JL, Piper WE, De Carufel FL, et al: Premature termination in group psychotherapy: pretherapy and early therapy predictors. Int J Group Psychother 36:145–152, 1986

Corsini R, Rosenberg B: Mechanisms of group psychotherapy: processes and dynamics. J Abnorm Soc Psychol 51:406–411, 1955

Cox PD, Ilfeld F Jr, Ilfeld BS, et al: Group therapy program development: clinician-administrator collaboration in new practice settings. Int J Group Psychother 50:3–24, 2000

Crosby G, Sabin J: Developing and marketing time-limited therapy groups. Psychiatr Serv 46:7–8, 1995

Dick BM, Wooff K: An evaluation of a time-limited programme of dynamic group psychotherapy. Br J Psychiatry 148:159–164, 1986

Dies RR: Group psychotherapy: reflections on three decades of research. J Appl Behav Anal 15:361–373, 1979

Dies RR: Practical, theoretical, and empirical foundations for group psychotherapy, in Psychiatry Update: American Psychiatric Association Annual Review, Vol 5. Edited by Frances AJ, Hales RE. Washington, DC, American Psychiatric Press, 1986, pp 659–667

Dies RR: Research on group psychotherapy: overview and clinical applications, in Group Therapy in Clinical Practice. Edited by Alonso A, Swiller HI. Washington, DC, American Psychiatric Press, 1993, pp 473–518

Dugo JM, Beck AP: Significance and complexity of early phases in the development of the co-therapy relationship. Group Dynamics 1:294–305, 1997

Fawzy FI, Fawzy NW, Hyun CS, et al: Malignant melanoma: effects of an early structured psychiatric intervention, coping, and affective state on recurrence and survival 6 years later. Arch Gen Psychiatry 50:681–689, 1993

Fawzy FI, Fawzy NW, Arndt LA, et al: Critical review of psychosocial interventions in cancer care. Arch Gen Psychiatry 52:100–113, 1995

Flowers JV: The differential outcome effects of simple advice, alternatives and instructions in group psychotherapy. Int J Group Psychother 29:305–316, 1979

Flowers JV, Booraem CD: The frequency and effect on outcome of different types of interpretation in psychodynamic and cognitive-behavioral group psychotherapy. Int J Group Psychother 40:203–214, 1990

Freedman S, Hurley J: Perceptions of helpfulness and behavior in groups. Group 4:51–58, 1980

Fuhriman A, Burlingame GM: Consistency of matter: a comparative analysis of individual and group process variables. The Counseling Psychologist 18:60–63, 1990

Gabbard GO, Lazar SG, Hornberger J, et al: The economic impact of psychotherapy: a review. Am J Psychiatry 154:147–155, 1997

Goffman E: Encounters: Two Studies in the Sociology of Interaction. Indianapolis, IN, Bobbs-Merrill, 1961

Goodman G, Jacobs M: The self-help, mutual support group, in Handbook of Group Psychotherapy: An Empirical and Clinical Synthesis. Edited by Fuhriman A, Burlingame G. New York, Wiley, 1994, pp 489–526

Greenstein M, Breitbart W: Cancer and the experience of meaning: a group psychotherapy program for people with cancer. Am J Psychother 54:486–500, 2000

Harwood I: Towards optimum group placement from the perspective of self and group experience. Group Analysis 29:199–218, 1996

Hoag MJ, Burlingame GM: Evaluating the effectiveness of child and adolescent group treatment: a meta-analytic review. J Clin Child Psychol 26:234–246, 1997

Kahn EM: Group treatment interventions for schizophrenics. Int J Group Psychother 34:149–153, 1984

Kanas N: Inpatient and outpatient group therapy for schizophrenic patients. Am J Psychother 39:431–439, 1985

Kanas N: Group therapy with schizophrenics: a review of controlled studies. Int J Group Psychother 36:339–351, 1986

Kanas N: Group Therapy for Schizophrenic Patients. Washington, DC, American Psychiatric Press, 1996

Kanas N: Long-term psychodynamic group therapy for patients with personality disorders. Int J Group Psychother 56:245–250, 2005

Kaul TJ, Bednar RL: Experiential group research: results, questions, and suggestions, in Handbook of Psychotherapy and Behavior Change, 3rd Edition. Edited by Garfield SL, Bergin AE. New York, Wiley, 1986, pp 671–714

Kibel HD: Inpatient group psychotherapy, in Group Therapy in Clinical Practice. Edited by Alonso A, Swiller HI. Washington, DC, American Psychiatric Press, 1993, pp 93–111

Laing RD: The Politics of Experience. New York, Pantheon, 1967

Large TR: Resistance in long-term cancer support groups. Int J Group Psychother 55:551–573, 2005

Leszcz M, Yalom ID, Norden M: The value of inpatient group psychotherapy: patients' perceptions. Int J Group Psychother 35:411–433, 1985

Lieberman MA: A group therapist perspective on self-help groups. Int J Group Psychother 40:251–278, 1990

Lieberman MA, Borman L: Self-help groups for coping with crisis. San Francisco, CA, Jossey-Bass, 1979

Lieberman MA, Yalom ID, Miles MB: Encounter Groups: First Facts. New York, Basic Books, 1973

Linehan MM: Cognitive-Behavioral Treatment of Borderline Personality Disorder. New York, Guilford, 1993

Lonergan E[C]: Keeping a group psychotherapy program alive and well within a psychiatry residency. Group 15:168–180, 1991

Lonergan EC: Discussion. Group 19:100–107, 1995

Lonergan EC: Discussion of "group therapy program development." Int J Group Psychother 50:43–45, 2000

MacKenzie KR: Time-limited group psychotherapy: has Cinderella found her prince? Group 20:95–111, 1997a

MacKenzie KR: Time-Managed Group Psychotherapy: Effective Clinical Applications. Washington, DC, American Psychiatric Press, 1997b

Mackenzie KR: An Expectation of Radical Changes in the Future of Group Psychotherapy. Int J Group Psychother 51:243–263, 2001a

MacKenzie KR: Personality assessment in clinical practice, in Handbook of Personality Disorders: Theory, Research, and Treatment. Edited by Livesley WJ. New York, Guilford, 2001b, pp 307–320

Martindale B, Bateman A, Margison F: Psychosis: Psychological Approaches and Their Effectiveness. London, England, Gaskell/Royal College of Psychiatrists, 2000

McCallum M, Piper WE: Psychological mindedness. Psychiatry: Interpersonal and Biological Processes 59:48–64, 1996

McCallum M, Piper WE, Joyce AS: Dropping out from short-term group therapy. Psychotherapy 29:206–252, 1992

McCracken LM, Black MP: Psychiatric treatment of the homeless in a group-based therapeutic community: a preliminary field investigation. Int J Group Psychother 55:595–604, 2005

McDermut W, Miller IW, Brown RA: The efficacy of group psychotherapy for depression: a meta-analysis and review of the empirical research. Clin Psychol 8:98–116, 2001

McKay M, Paleg K: Focal Group Psychotherapy. Oakland, CA, New Harbinger, 1992

McRoberts C, Burlingame GM, Hoag MJ: Comparative efficacy of individual and group psychotherapy: a meta-analytic perspective. Group Dynamics: Theory, Research and Practice 2:101–178, 1998

Montgomery C: Role of dynamic group therapy in psychiatry. Advances in Psychiatric Treatment 8:34–41, 2002

Orlinsky DE, Howard KI: Process and outcome in psychotherapy, in Handbook of Psychotherapy and Behavior Change, 3rd Edition. Edited by Garfield SL, Bergin AE. New York, Wiley, 1986, pp 311–381

Paleg K, Jongsma AE Jr: The Group Therapy Treatment Planner. New York, Wiley, 2000

Paulson I, Burroughs JC, Gelb CB: Cotherapy: what is the crux of the relationship? Int J Group Psychother 26:213–224, 1976

Pines M, Hutchinson S: Group analysis, in Group Therapy in Clinical Practice. Edited by Alonso A, Swiller HI. Washington, DC, American Psychiatric Press, 1993, pp 29–47

Piper W[E], Joyce A: A consideration of factors influencing the utilization of time-limited, short-term group therapy. Int J Group Psychother 46:311–328, 1996

Piper WE, Perrault EL: Pretherapy preparation for group members. Int J Group Psychother 39:17–34, 1989

Piper WE, Debbane EG, Bienvenu J-P, et al: A study of group pretraining for group psychotherapy. Int J Group Psychother 32:309–325, 1982

Piper WE, McCallum M, Azim HFA: Adaptation to Loss Through Short-Term Group Psychotherapy. New York, Guilford, 1992

Piper WE, Ogrodniczuk JS, Lamarche C, et al: Level of alliance, pattern of alliance, and outcome in short-term group therapy. Int J Group Psychother 55:527–550, 2005

Pratt JH: The principles of class treatment and their application to various chronic diseases. Hospital Social Service 6:404, 1922

Rothke S: The role of interpersonal feedback in group psychotherapy. Int J Group Psychother 36:225–240, 1986

Schermer VL, Pines M: Group Psychotherapy of the Psychoses: Concepts, Interventions and Contexts. Bristol, PA, Jessica Kingsley, 1999

Shapiro DA, Shapiro D: Meta-analysis of comparative therapy outcome studies: a replication and refinement. Psychol Bull 92:581–604, 1982

Shapiro JL: Methods of Group Psychotherapy and Encounter. Itasca, IL, Peacock, 1978

Siegel DJ: Developing Mind: How Relationships and the Brain Interact to Shape Who We Are. New York, Guilford, 1999

Smith ML, Glass GV, Miller TI: The Benefits of Psychotherapy. Baltimore, MD, Johns Hopkins University Press, 1980

Spiegel D, Bloom JR, Kraemer HL, et al: Effect of psychosocial treatment on survival of patients with metastatic breast cancer. Lancet 2:888–891, 1989

Spitz HI: Group Psychotherapy and Managed Mental Health Care: A Clinical Guide for Providers. New York, Brunner/Mazel, 1996

Spitz HI: The effect of managed mental health care and group psychotherapy: treatment, training, and therapist-morale issues. Int J Group Psychother 47:23–30, 1997

Stern MJ: Group therapy with medically ill patients, in Group Therapy in Clinical Practice. Edited by Alonso A, Swiller HI. Washington, DC, American Psychiatric Press, 1993, pp 185–199

Stone W: Group Psychotherapy for People With Chronic Mental Illness. New York, Guilford, 1996

Sullivan HS: The Interpersonal Theory of Psychiatry. New York, WW Norton, 1953

Tasca GA, Russell V, Busby K: Characteristics of patients who choose between two types of group psychotherapy. Int J Group Psychother 44:499–508, 1994

Taylor NT, Burlingame GM, Kristensen KB, et al: A survey of mental health care provider's and managed care organization attitudes toward, familiarity with, and use of group interventions. Int J Group Psychother 51:243–263, 2001

Tillitski CJ: A meta-analysis of estimated effect sizes for group versus individual control treatments. Int J Group Psychother 40:215–224, 1990

Toseland RW, Siporin M: When to recommend group treatment: a review of the clinical and the research literature. Int J Group Psychother 36:171–201, 1986

Truax P: Review: group psychotherapy is effective for depression. Evidence-Based Mental Health. 4:82, 2001

Verhulst J: The role of the psychiatrist: defining methods, theories, and practice in the time of managed care. Acad Psychiatry 20:195–204, 1996

Vinogradov S, Yalom ID: Concise Guide to Group Psychotherapy. Washington, DC, American Psychiatric Press, 1989

Vinogradov S, Yalom ID: Self-disclosure in group psychotherapy, in Self-Disclosure in the Therapeutic Relationship. Edited by Stricker G, Fisher N. New York, Plenum, 1990, pp 191–203

Whitaker DS, Lieberman MAL: Psychotherapy Through the Group Process. New York, Atherton, 1964

Yalom ID: A study of group therapy dropouts. Arch Gen Psychiatry 14:393–414, 1966

Yalom ID: The Theory and Practice of Group Psychotherapy. New York, Basic Books, 1970

Yalom ID: Existential Psychotherapy. New York, Basic Books, 1980

Yalom ID: Inpatient Group Psychotherapy. New York, Basic Books, 1983

Yalom ID: The Theory and Practice of Group Psychotherapy, 3rd Edition. New York, Basic Books, 1985

Yalom ID: Interpersonal learning, in Psychiatry Update: American Psychiatric Association Annual Review, Vol 5. Edited by Frances AJ, Hales RE. Washington, DC, American Psychiatric Press, 1986, pp 699–713

Yalom ID: The Theory and Practice of Group Psychotherapy, 4th Edition. New York, Basic Books, 1995

Yalom ID, Leszcz M: The Theory and Practice of Group Psychotherapy, 5th Edition. New York, Basic Books, 2005

Yalom ID, Vinogradov S: Bereavement groups: techniques and themes. Int J Group Psychother 38:419–457, 1988

Yalom ID, Vinogradov S: Interpersonal group psychotherapy, in Comprehensive Textbook of Group Psychotherapy, 3rd Edition. Edited by Kaplan HI, Sadock BJ. Baltimore, MD, Williams & Wilkins, 1993, pp 185–195

Yalom I[D], Brown S, Bloch S: The written summary as a group psychotherapy technique. Arch Gen Psychiatry 32:605–613, 1975

SPECIAL PATIENT POPULATIONS

36

TREATMENT OF CHILDREN AND ADOLESCENTS

Glen C. Crawford, M.D.

Stephen J. Cozza, M.D.

Mina K. Dulcan, M.D.

This chapter provides an overview of and an orientation to the psychiatric treatment of children and adolescents. Treatment modalities as they apply to adults are covered in the other chapters in Part III of this textbook. In this chapter we focus on aspects of treatment that are different for children and adolescents than for adults. Childhood psychopathology and the treatment methods used for each disorder are discussed elsewhere in this volume (see Chapter 21, "Disorders Usually First Diagnosed in Infancy, Childhood, or Adolescence," by Ursano et al.). Throughout this chapter, the terms *child* and *children* refer to children of all ages, to include adolescents, unless otherwise stated.

Techniques used in the treatment of child psychiatric conditions have developed from two different sources: the traditions of understanding and treating children that were based on developmental uniqueness, and treatments that were originally designed for adults and were then applied to children and adolescents. Increasingly, more rigorous evaluation and diagnostic procedures have allowed greater specificity in the application of treatments to our younger patients. In addition, expanding research on the efficacy of specific therapeutic approaches continues to enlarge our armamentarium of empirically tested interventions.

The goals of all treatments are to reduce symptoms, to improve emotional and behavioral functioning, to remedy skill deficits, and to remove obstacles to normal development. In contrast to the treatment of adults, a child is usually brought by someone else, and in each case there are at least two clients, the parent and the child, whose needs and desires may conflict. Compared with adults, children are more dependent on others for meeting their basic needs, they have fewer choices of residence or activities, and they are required to attend school.

Evaluation

The psychiatric treatment of children should be preceded by a comprehensive clinical evaluation, the purpose of which is similar to the assessment of adults: to determine the presence of one or more psychiatric disorders and to recommend a well-formulated treatment plan that addresses the disorder. Special considerations for children make evaluation different from that for adult patients. Practitioners must have a clear understanding of normal development and the differences that may exist among children at the same or different ages, in order to distinguish normal from pathological behaviors. Also, practitioners must be able to apply developmental understanding in the diagnostic interview of the child, using approaches like imaginative play with younger children or with those less skilled in verbal communication.

Information from the school is always useful and is essential when there is concern about learning or behavior in school or peer functioning. With parental consent, the clinician talks with the teacher; obtains records of testing, grades, and attendance; and requests completion of a standardized checklist, such as the Teacher Report Form of the Child Behavior Checklist (Achenbach 1991) or the Vanderbilt ADHD Rating Scale (Wolraich et al. 1998). Even better, though less convenient, is a visit to the school to observe the youngster with peers in the classroom and on the playground and to talk with teachers and counselors.

A referral to another provider such as a pediatrician, pediatric neurologist, child psychologist, or speech and language specialist may be necessary to complete the assessment. Psychological evaluation, including an intelligence test and achievement tests, should be obtained when there is any question about learning or IQ, with additional testing as indicated.

In an emergency situation, treatment may have to be initiated following an expedited assessment of the child's medical and psychological status. A more thorough evaluation should be accomplished as soon as possible. True emergencies are, fortunately, uncommon, and in most cases the evaluation will be completed before treatment is begun. Of course, the process of assessment does not end with the initiation of treatment but continues throughout.

The American Academy of Child and Adolescent Psychiatry (AACAP) has developed practice parameters as guides to the evaluation and treatment of specific disorders. Completed practice parameters are available on the AACAP Web site (www.aacap.org) and are listed in Table 36–1.

Treatment Planning

Treatment planning takes into consideration psychiatric diagnosis, target emotional and behavioral symptoms, and the strengths and weaknesses of the patient and family. Resources and risks in the school, neighborhood, and social support network and any religious group affiliation also influence the selection of treatment strategies.

In making a plan, the clinician should consider any modality or a combination of the modalities presented in this chapter. The practice of offering a single treatment to all patients, chosen because of the clinician's own training and theoretical beliefs or because that is what the facility offers, is to be avoided, whether that modality is individual therapy, family therapy, pharmacotherapy, hospitalization, or any other form of treatment. Treatments not in the repertoire of the clinician or those requiring additional staff and/or structure should be arranged by referral. Unfortunately, the practical realities of the quality and availability of community resources and the family's ability to pay for treatment often force the clinician to make compromises to an ideal plan.

The clinician must decide which treatment is likely to be the most efficient or to have the highest benefit–risk ratio and whether treatments should be administered simultaneously or in sequence. Unfortunately, few systematic prospective studies have been conducted comparing well-defined treatments for carefully described groups of child patients.

Parents are best included in the choice of treatment strategies, with the strength of the clinician's recommendation depending on the clarity of the indications. The skilled clinician presents the probable course of the disorder if untreated, as well as the best estimate of benefits and risks of all available treatments for a particular child. The child patient is included in decision making as appropriate. The motivation and ability of the responsible adults to carry out the treatment should be considered because the best treatment has little chance of success without the cooperation of the family.

Treatment planning is an ongoing process, with reevaluations done as interventions are attempted and their results observed and as additional information about the child and family comes to light.

Informed Consent

The implementation of any treatment plan requires carefully obtained informed consent from parents before the plan is initiated. The concept of informed consent is more complicated with children because of their lack of legal competency. Although parents provide informed consent for children, clinicians should strive to obtain assent from child patients before initiating any treatment. In obtaining such assent, the clinician should be mindful of the cognitive capacities and developmental level of the patient. Such consent should include a general discussion of the selected therapeutic modality, its intended purpose, the avail-

TABLE 36–1. Practice parameters published by the American Academy of Child and Adolescent Psychiatry (AACAP)

Topic	Publication date
Aggressive Behavior in Child and Adolescent Psychiatric Institutions, With Special Reference to Seclusion and Restraint	2002
Anxiety Disorders	2007
Assessment of Children and Adolescents	1997
Assessment of the Family	2007
Assessment of Infants and Toddlers	1997
Attention-Deficit Hyperactivity Disorder	2007
Autism	1999
Bipolar Disorder	2007
Child and Adolescent Mental Health Care in Community Systems	2007
Child Custody Evaluations	1997
Conduct Disorder	1997
Consultation to Schools	2005
Depressive Disorders	2007
Electroconvulsive Therapy	2004
Enuresis	2004
Forensic Evaluations of Physical or Sexual Abuse	1997
Language and Learning Disorders	1998
Mental Retardation and Comorbid Mental Disorders	1999
Obsessive-Compulsive Disorder	1998
Oppositional Defiant Disorder	2007
Posttraumatic Stress Disorder	1998
Reactive Attachment Disorder	2005
Schizophrenia	2001
Sexually Abusive Youth	1999
Stimulant Medications	2002
Substance Use Disorders	2005
Suicidal Behavior	2001
Youth in Juvenile Detention and Correctional Facilities	2005

Source. American Academy of Child and Adolescent Psychiatry (http://www.jaacap.com). Individual AACAP practice parameters are available on the AACAP Web site.

ability of any alternative treatments (to include a choice of no treatment), and the nature of any adverse reactions that could result. An open discussion of any questions or concerns not only meets the legal obligations of practice, but also can safeguard the therapeutic alliance should undesirable side effects occur. Although not always necessary, parents' written consent may be useful in some situations. Printed materials to supplement discussion with the physician in educating parents and children regarding a variety of treatments are now available (Dulcan 2006). In addition, the Internet has become an important source of information about medications and treatments for health care consumers. Because the quality of information available on the World Wide Web is inconsistent, patients and their families benefit from guidance as to the best sources of information about mental health issues. Clinicians should also be prepared to respond to questions or concerns about treatments that may arise from a patient's or parent's "surfing" of the Internet. Some potentially useful child mental health Web sites are listed in Table 36–2.

Confidentiality

It is essential that the guidelines for confidentiality and for sharing information between parent and child be clear. Adolescents are usually more sensitive to this issue than younger children. Parents may have concerns about a therapist's keeping vital information about their child from them or indiscriminately revealing information to the child that was disclosed in confidence to the therapist. Therefore, an early and frank discussion of the importance of confidentiality, as well as its limitations, can be reassuring to both patients and their parents and can be an important first step in fostering trust in the therapeutic relationship. As a general rule, either party should be told when information from one party's session will be relayed to the other. In some situations, parents and children may participate in the decision. When children are engaged in potentially dangerous activities or have serious thoughts of harming themselves or others, parents must be informed. Carefully planned family sessions in which the therapist coaches and supports a parent or child in sharing information may be more useful than secondhand reports.

An area of increasing concern for clinicians is the impingement of insurance practices on their ability to maintain confidentiality. Clinicians should ensure that they inform children and parents of the possible need to share some information with third-party entities and make prudent choices as to the nature and quantity of information that are appropriate to pass on.

Psychopharmacology

This necessarily brief and relatively superficial section focuses on how medication treatment of children is different from that of adults. Pediatric psychopharmacology has received considerable attention in the past few years, especially as the use of psychotropic medications in children has increased. Olfson et al. (2002) reported

an almost threefold increase in overall psychotropic medication use in children and adolescents in the period from 1987 to 1996, most notably in antidepressant and stimulant use, while Zito et al. (2000) reported a trebling of stimulant use in preschool-age children in the early 1990s. Concerning increases in psychotropic polypharmacy in children and adolescents have also been described (Olfson et al. 2002). These increases have occurred despite the fact that, with the exception of the stimulant medications, there is limited empirical evidence to support the safe and effective use of these medications in the pediatric age group.

In December 2003, the British Medicines and Healthcare Regulatory Agency (MHRA) issued a notice stating that use of selective serotonin reuptake inhibitors, with the exception of fluoxetine, was contraindicated for the treatment of pediatric depression. In late 2004, the U.S. Food and Drug Administration (FDA) mandated that its strongest caution, a "black box" warning, be included in the product labeling of all antidepressants marketed in the United States to warn against the potential for increased suicidality in children taking these medications. Although controversial, these actions focused the attention of patients, parents, and prescribers on the potential risks of the use of such medications in children. Two important general principles of pediatric psychopharmacology are worth repeating: polypharmacy should be minimized, and medication should virtually never be used as the only treatment.

Most disorders of children and adolescents that require medication are either chronic (e.g., attention-deficit/hyperactivity disorder [ADHD], autistic disorder, Tourette's disorder) or likely to have recurrent episodes (e.g., mood disorders), and a long-term relationship with the physician is crucial. It is important to educate the family regarding the disorder, its treatment, and the different needs at each developmental stage. The physician must consider the meaning of the prescription and administration of a medication to the child, the family, the school, and the child's peer group.

Special Issues for Children and Adolescents

Pharmacokinetics, Pharmacodynamics, and Pharmacogenetics

Pharmacokinetics is the study of the movement of drugs into, around, and out of the body by the processes of absorption, distribution, metabolism, and elimination. Although children share some similarities in the physiological processing of medications with adults,

TABLE 36–2. Useful child mental health Web sites

About Our Kids	www.aboutourkids.org
ADD Resources	www.addresources.org
American Academy of Pediatrics	www.aap.org
American Association of Suicidology	www.suicidology.org
American Foundation for Suicide Prevention	www.afsp.org
American Medical Association	www.ama-assn.org
American Psychiatric Association	www.psych.org
American Psychological Association	www.apa.org
American Society of Adolescent Psychiatry	www.adolpsych.org
Anxiety Disorders Association of America	www.adaa.org
Autism Society of America	www.autism-society.org
Canadian Academy of Child and Adolescent Psychiatry	www.canacad.org
Canadian Mental Health Association	www.cmha.ca
Canadian Paediatric Society	www.cps.ca
Canadian Psychiatric Association	www.cpa-apc.org
Caring for Kids	www.caringforkids.cps.ca
Center for Mental Health Services	www.mentalhealth.org
Child Advocate	www.childadvocate.net
Child and Adolescent Bipolar Foundation	www.bpkids.org
Children and Adults with Attention Deficit Disorder	www.chadd.org
Connect for Kids	www.connectforkids.org
Depression and Bipolar Support Alliance	www.dbsalliance.org
Families for Depression Awareness	www.familyaware.org
Federation of Families for Children's Mental Health	www.ffcmh.org
Health Canada Mental Health Web site	www.hc-sc.gc.ca/dc-ma/mental/index_e.html
MentalHealthSites	www.mentalhealthsites.org
National Alliance for the Mentally Ill	www.nami.org
National Association of Psychiatric Health Systems	www.naphs.org
National Center for Children Exposed to Violence	www.nccev.org
National Center for Learning Disabilities	www.ncld.org
National Center for Missing and Exploited Children	www.ncmec.org
National Child Traumatic Stress Network	www.nctsnet.org
National Clearinghouse for Alcohol and Drug Information	www.health.org
National Initiative for Children's Healthcare Quality	www.nichq.org
National Institute of Child Health and Human Development	www.nichd.nih.gov
National Institute of Mental Health	www.nimh.nih.gov
National Institute on Drug Abuse	www.nida.nih.gov
National Mental Health Association	www.nmha.org

TABLE 36–2. **Useful child mental health Web sites** *(continued)*

Parents Anonymous	www.parentsanonymous.org
ParentsMedGuide	www.parentsmedguide.org
Report of the U.S. Surgeon General on Children's Mental Health	www.surgeongeneral.gov/topics/cmh
Suicide Awareness Voices of Education	www.save.org
Tourette's Syndrome Association	www.tsa-usa.org
U.S. Department of Health and Human Services Administration for Children and Families	www.hhs.gov/children

developmental differences are clinically relevant, particularly in regard to drug distribution and metabolism.

Factors that most greatly affect the developmental differences of distribution of drugs in children are differences in proportion of extracellular water volume and body fat. Extracellular water volume decreases substantially from birth through early adolescence. This decrease results in a larger distribution volume for water-soluble drugs in younger children, requiring a relatively higher dose to achieve a comparable plasma concentration (Clein and Riddle 1995).

In general, children have lower proportional body fat than adults, thus reducing the distribution volume for lipid-soluble medications. Although this would result in an expected increase in plasma concentrations of such medications in children compared with adults using weight-adjusted dosages, lower plasma levels in children have been reported. This finding indicates that other pharmacokinetic differences, presumably increased metabolism in children, offset this effect (Clein and Riddle 1995).

By late infancy to early childhood, hepatic metabolic activity is at its peak. This substantially greater metabolic rate is related to the proportionally larger liver size of children compared with adults. Relative to body weight, the liver of a toddler is 40%–50% greater and that of a 6-year-old is 30% greater than the liver of an adult. This greater metabolic rate has been postulated as the principal factor contributing to decreased drug plasma concentration levels and decreased drug half-lives in children compared with adults (Clein and Riddle 1995).

An understanding of the cytochrome P450 (CYP) enzyme system is becoming increasingly important for those clinicians who prescribe psychiatric medications to children and adolescents. Many medications either are substrates of or inhibit or induce one or more of the CYP isoenzymes. Potentially toxic interactions can result from inappropriate combinations of medications that inhibit CYP enzymes. An excellent source of information on this topic is the work by Cozza et al. (2003).

Medication dosage also is determined by pharmacodynamics, or how the biological system responds to the drug. For example, interaction with receptors is determined by receptor number, distribution, structure, function, sensitivity, and mechanism of action. Little is known about the influence of growth and development on these variables.

Pharmacogenetics is the study of how genetics influences the physiological effect of and response to drugs. Genetic variations in the CYP 2D6 isoenzyme, for example, may enhance the metabolism of medications frequently used in child and adolescent psychiatry. Polymorphisms that have been identified in certain isoenzymes of uridine 5'-diphospho-glucuronosyltransferase (UDP-glucuronosyltransferase) may affect the metabolism of almost all psychotherapeutic agents except lithium. Research is ongoing into genetic variations in drug and neurotransmitter receptor sites important to the field of psychiatry, such as serotonin, norepinephrine, and acetylcholine (G.M. Anderson and Cook 2000).

Ideally, medication doses in children should be derived from studies of children rather than adults, but studies of children often are not possible. Protocols using healthy children are not permitted, and few dosage studies have been done in symptomatic children. Dosage may be determined empirically or by weight or surface area. Generally, children are anticipated to require a higher weight-adjusted dose to achieve the same blood levels and therapeutic effects as adults. However, clinicians should remain alert to the possibility that such practice occasionally results in toxicity.

Side Effects

Side effects are common in children being treated with psychiatric medications. Clinicians must actively look for adverse reactions, as children often will not report them and parents may not notice. Occasionally, children will develop an uncharacteristic or paradoxical response to a particular medication. Such a response may be extremely individual in its manifestation, affecting one child but not another. *Behavioral toxicity* is a term that is used to describe a response to medication in which a child demonstrates behavioral or symptomatic aggravation caused by a particular medication (Van Putten and Marder 1987).

Measurement of Outcome

Effective medication management in children requires the identification of clear target symptoms that are monitored during the course of a medication trial. The physician must obtain emotional, behavioral, and physical data at baseline, periodically during treatment, and posttreatment. Therapeutic effects can be assessed by interviews and rating scales, direct observation, collection of data from outside sources (e.g., teachers), or specific tests evaluating attention or learning. A list of some clinically useful symptom rating scales is presented in Table 36–3.

In reading the psychopharmacology literature, it is important to distinguish between *statistically* significant effects and *clinically* significant ones and to know whether the target symptoms are reduced to near-normal levels or merely changed, and the clinical meaning of the change. The percentage of patients who improve may be more important than the mean change in a group. Some patients may improve and others worsen, resulting in nonsignificant group data. On the other hand, statistically significant group changes may translate into only modest changes in individual patient functioning that may not be worth the risk of medication.

Developmentally Disabled Patients

Medication effects are even more difficult to assess in children and adolescents with mental retardation or pervasive developmental disorders (PDDs). Their impaired ability to verbalize symptoms is relevant to diagnosis, measurement of efficacy, and detection of side effects. These individuals are prone to physical side effects and are at risk for idiosyncratic behavioral effects or simply less prominent therapeutic effects.

Heterogeneity of samples of autistic children in language development, motor activity, severity of stereotypies, affective range and lability, chronological age, and IQ may lead to variable drug effects. Autistic children are even more likely to react differently to specific drugs than do children with other psychiatric disorders, even when the target symptoms seem similar.

Adherence to Medication Regimen

Taking medication as directed can be particularly problematic for children, because the cooperation of two people, parent and child, and often school personnel as well, is required. In general pediatric practice, adherence to medication regimens is associated with degree of parental concern about the seriousness of the child's illness, the severity of the child's symptoms, and prior adherence to treatment (Lewis 1995). Adherence appears to be inversely related to the complexity of the medication regimen (including the number of medicines used and the frequency of dosing). Although experiences in general pediatrics and adult psychiatry indicate that educational efforts may improve compliance, administration of psychotropic medications in children is more complex. Bastiaens (1992) found no correlation between knowledge of medications and compliance in a group of inpatient children and adolescents. In a later study, he found that compliance in a group of inpatient adolescents correlated better with attitudes than with knowledge of pharmacotherapy, indicating a need to examine and explore a child's feelings about taking medication (Bastiaens 1995).

Ethical Issues

Those physicians who treat children with pharmacotherapy face significant ethical challenges (Coffey 1995). The practice of pharmacotherapy of children is often modeled on adult treatments, because rigorously controlled double-blind studies in children are relatively few. Pharmaceutical companies often do not go to the expense and trouble of testing drugs in children and adolescents, although a federal (U.S) law was passed in 1997 to encourage such testing by extending patent protection for 6 months on drugs studied in children. Additionally, the FDA released guidelines in December 2000 to encourage the clinical investigation of drugs for use in the pediatric population. Because few psychotropic medications have an approved FDA indication for children, most drugs are used "off label" in this patient group. While FDA guidelines as published in the *Physicians' Desk Reference* (PDR) are not meant to restrict the clinical practice of physicians, the clinician must be responsible for the careful use of these medications in the child population, basing decisions on a thorough understanding of the scientific literature. The lack of knowledge of the potential impact of medications on the neural development of children further complicates the issue. A clinician must balance multiple factors: the risks of the untreated disorder, the relative efficacy of medications, and the potential adverse outcomes or unknowns of medication use.

The interaction between pharmacotherapy and the environment is an issue for adult patients but even more so for children and adolescents because their im-

TABLE 36–3. Some clinically useful symptom rating scales in child and adolescent psychiatry

Scales for measuring overall symptomatology

Clinical Global Impressions (CGI) Scale

Child Behavior Checklist (CBCL)

Brief Psychiatric Rating Scale for Children (BPRS-C)

Scales for measuring specific disorders

Depression

Children's Depression Inventory (CDI)

Children's Depression Rating Scale—Revised (CDRS-R)

Beck Depression Inventory

Depression Self-Rating Scale

School Age Depression Listed Inventory

Hamilton Rating Scale for Depression

Mania

Parent–Young Mania Rating Scale (P-YMRS)

Parent–General Behavior Inventory (P-GBI)

Anxiety disorders

Multidimensional Anxiety Scale for Children (MASC)

Children's Yale-Brown Obsessive Compulsive Scale (CY-BOCS)

Pediatric Anxiety Rating Scale (PARS)

Social Phobia Anxiety Inventory for Children (SPAI-C)

Screen for Child Anxiety-Related Emotional Disorders (SCARED)

Attention-deficit/hyperactivity disorder (ADHD)

Attention Deficit Disorder Evaluation Scale— Second Edition (ADDES-2)

ADHD Symptom Rating Scale (ADHD-SRS)

Brown Attention Deficit Disorder Scales for Children and Adolescents (BADDS)

Conners Rating Scales—Revised (CRS-R)

Swanson, Kotkin, Agler, M-Flynn, and Pelham (SKAMP) Rating Scale

SNAP-IV Rating Scale

Vanderbilt ADHD Parent and Teacher Rating Scales (VADPRS/VADTRS)

Autism and mental retardation

Aberrant Behavior Checklist

Behavior Problems Inventory

Childhood Autism Rating Scale

Nisonger Child Behavior Rating Form

TABLE 36–3. Some clinically useful symptom rating scales in child and adolescent psychiatry

Tourette's disorder

Hopkins Motor and Vocal Tic Scale

Tourette's Syndrome Severity Scale

Yale Global Tic Severity Scale

Aggression and externalizing behaviors

Overt Aggression Scale

Children's Aggression Scale (Parent and Teacher Versions) (CAS-P/CAS-T)

Eyeberg Child Behavior Inventory (ECBI)

Sutter-Eyeberg Student Behavior Inventory— Revised (SESBI-R)

New York Teacher Rating Scale (NYTRS)

Note. See also the following: Ten-Year Review of Rating Scales, I–VII. *Journal of the American Academy of Child and Adolescent Psychiatry* 41(2, 6, 10, 12), 2002; 42(9, 10), 2003; and 44(4), 2005. (Individual articles from this review are listed in the Suggested Readings at the end of this chapter.)

mature developmental status places them in the care of adults, whether parents, teachers, or staff in an inpatient unit or residential treatment setting. There is a danger of misinterpreting the youngster's response to the family, school, or institutional milieu as an exacerbation requiring medication or as improvement due to a medication. Many adults seek to use drugs to control or eliminate troublesome behavior rather than instituting more time-consuming and difficult therapeutic or behavioral management strategies. The physician must therefore evaluate and monitor the environment as well as the patient, using all available information to make therapeutic decisions.

Stimulants

This category of medications is the most studied and most used in pediatric psychopharmacology and is most often prescribed by non–child psychiatrists such as pediatricians and general practitioners. Methylphenidate and dextroamphetamine, the "gold standard" medications used to treat ADHD in children, have been enhanced over the past few years by the introduction of a racemic salt formulation of amphetamine (Adderall), innovative delivery systems for methylphenidate (Concerta and Daytrana), an isomeric form of methylphenidate (Focalin), and a prodrug of dextroamphetamine (Vyvanse).

Contrary to prevailing mythology, hyperactive boys, healthy boys, and healthy adults have similar cognitive and behavioral responses to comparable doses of stimulants. Although it is clear that stimulants do *not* have a "paradoxical" effect in ADHD, the actual mechanism of action remains unclear. It is currently postulated that the therapeutic effect of stimulants is related to augmentation of dopaminergic and noradrenergic activity in the central nervous system (CNS). Stimulants reduce the performance decrement seen as patients with ADHD perform tasks, perhaps by improving motivation and focusing effort.

Indications and Efficacy

The most established indication for stimulant use is in the treatment of ADHD. There is extensive empirical support of the short-term efficacy and safety of stimulant medications (American Academy of Child and Adolescent Psychiatry 2002). The majority of the study subjects have been school-age white males. There is no evidence that efficacy or side effects differ in girls, however. In his review of nine placebo-controlled studies of the use of stimulants in preschool ADHD, Connor (2002) identified positive treatment response in eight of the nine studies. Side effects of medication in this age group were considered mild and varied with the age of the child. For example, while insomnia may be a dose-dependent side effect of methylphenidate in older children, insomnia actually improved in preschool children who received methylphenidate relative to placebo. More recently, the Preschool ADHD Treatment Study (PATS) (Greenhill et al. 2006a) found methylphenidate to be safe and effective in preschool children, although improvement was less, and side effects were somewhat greater, in comparison with school-age children. A review of studies of stimulant treatment in adolescents (Spencer et al. 1996) concluded that stimulants are just as effective in adolescents as they are in school-age children.

A study using a wide range of doses of methylphenidate and dextroamphetamine found that 96% of the sample improved behaviorally in response to one or both drugs, although some children did not continue on medication because of adverse effects (Elia et al. 1991). Stimulant effects on various domains (cognitive, behavioral, and social) are highly variable within and among individuals. A dose that produces improvement in one domain may have no effect or may even lead to worsening in another. The response may differ between measures (e.g., math and reading), even in the same domain. Specific effects documented in groups of ADHD stimulant responders are listed in Table 36–4.

The long-term therapeutic effect of stimulant med-

TABLE 36–4. Therapeutic effects of stimulant medications in attention-deficit/hyperactivity disorder responders

Cognitive effects
  Improve sustained attention
  Improve reaction time
  Reduce impulsivity
  Enhance sensitivity and style of cognitive response
  Improve short-term memory
Motor effects
  Reduce excessive motor behavior
Classroom effects
  Decrease off-task behavior
  Decrease inappropriate verbalizations
  Improve on-task seat work
  Improve academic performance
  Improve compliance
Effects on aggressivity
  Reduce physical aggression
  Reduce verbal aggression
Effects on mother/family–child interaction
  Increase maternal warmth
  Decrease maternal criticism
  Increase verbal interactions
  Enhance positive family interactions
Effects on peer relationships
  Improve peer cooperation
  Partially "normalize" peer interaction

ication remains unclear. Most studies to date have been of short duration. The National Institute of Mental Health Collaborative Multisite Multimodal Treatment Study of ADHD (MTA) was designed to address deficits in prior studies. Analysis of MTA 14-month treatment outcomes has suggested that combined medication and behavioral treatments provide no more clinical benefit in treating core ADHD symptoms than carefully managed medication alone but may offer some added benefit in other areas of social skills and academic performance (Jensen 2000). In contrast to the positive response observed in the medication group at 14 months, the follow-up of the MTA study showed no significant difference among the treatment groups (medication, behavior therapy, the combination of the two, or community care) at the 3-year mark (Jensen et al. 2007), although all groups were noted to be improved from baseline. The reasons for this change are unclear and are likely multifactorial. In a follow-up study of 79 children who completed an initial 12-month randomized controlled study of a combined methylphenidate and parent-treatment program, Charach et al. (2004) showed a greater improvement in teacher-reported symptoms of ADHD at both the 2- and 5-year points for children who remained on stimulant medication compared with those off medication. Side effects of stimulant medication did not decrease over time.

Stimulants have been found to be effective in treating ADHD symptoms in children with mental retardation. This population may be prone to more serious side effects, however (Handen et al. 1999). In their analysis of a pooled sample of 90 children from three aggregated studies of the use of methylphenidate in children with ADHD and an IQ lower than 90, Aman et al. (2003) showed that methylphenidate is effective when given as a single 0.40-mg/kg dose in the morning, although the treatment response is not as robust as it is in children with normal IQ and ADHD. In a small double-blind, controlled study of methylphenidate in children with ADHD and mild to moderate mental retardation by Pearson et al. (2003), the best response to symptoms of ADHD was seen in children treated with a 0.60-mg/kg bid regimen. As might be expected, an increase in methylphenidate-associated side effects (such as insomnia and appetite suppression) was noted as the dosage increased. Children with fragile X syndrome also have been shown to benefit significantly from stimulant treatment of ADHD symptoms (Hagerman et al. 1988).

The benefit of stimulant medication in the treatment of inattention and hyperactivity in children with PDDs remains unclear. Despite previous concern about treating children with PDDs with stimulants, small studies have described the effective use of these medications in this patient group. More recently, a multicenter double-blind, placebo-controlled crossover study of children with autism and hyperactivity conducted by the Research Units on Pediatric Psychopharmacology (RUPP) Autism Network (Aman et al. 2005) demonstrated the superiority of methylphenidate over placebo. Of note, the favorable response observed in the RUPP study was less vigorous than that seen in children with ADHD who do not have a PDD, and the incidence of side effects was greater. Clearly, more studies are needed to determine the role, if any, of stimulant medication in the treatment of the symptoms of ADHD in children with PDDs.

The use of stimulants in patients with tics or Tourette's disorder is supported by several clinical trials (Tourette's Syndrome Study Group 2002). Previously, the greatest concern about using stimulants in this population has been precipitating new tics. Often, however, patients with Tourette's disorder are far more disabled by their inattention, impulsivity, low frustration tolerance, and oppositional behavior than by the tics. The Tourette's Syndrome Study Group (2002) trial comparing methylphenidate, clonidine, and the combination of methylphenidate and clonidine to placebo in 136 children with ADHD and a chronic tic disorder showed that the frequency of tics was no more increased with methylphenidate than it was with clonidine or placebo. These studies suggest that the apparent increase in tics, previously attributed to stimulant treatment in children with ADHD and a tic disorder, may instead be a function of the natural waxing and waning nature of tics. Nevertheless, monitoring for tics during stimulant use is advised.

Stimulants have been demonstrated to have no effect on learning disabilities in the absence of an attention deficit (Gittelman et al. 1983). The use of stimulants in populations with comorbid ADHD and learning disorders appears to have a role in treating the underlying ADHD-related attentional and behavioral symptoms (Gadow 1983).

Initiation and Maintenance

The decision to medicate a child or adolescent with a stimulant is based on the presence of persistent target symptoms that are sufficiently severe to cause functional impairment at school and usually also at home and with peers. Parents must be willing to monitor medication and to attend appointments. In preschool children, other interventions are generally implemented first, unless severe impulsivity and noncompliance create an emergency situation.

Multiple outcome measures, determined by using more than one source, setting, and method of gathering data and including premedication baseline school data on behavior and academic performance, are essential. Education for the child, family, and teacher is helpful before the start of medication (see Dulcan et al. 2003). The physician should explicitly debunk common myths about stimulant treatment—for example, that stimulants have a paradoxical sedative action, that they lead to drug abuse, and that they are not needed or are ineffective after puberty. The physician should work closely with parents on dose adjustments and obtain annual academic testing and more frequent reports from teachers.

The myriad of available preparations of stimulant medication gives great flexibility in addressing the clinical needs of an individual child. Although methylphenidate is the most commonly used and best studied, no patient characteristics are helpful in suggesting which stimulant drug is best for a particular child. Twenty-five percent of a sample of boys with ADHD taking both methylphenidate and dextroamphetamine were behaviorally positive responders to one of the drugs but not the other. Of the nonresponders to each drug, the majority responded to the other drug (Elia et al. 1991). Several longer-acting preparations of stimulants are now available that allow for once- or twice-daily dosing. These particular medications are appealing for children who experience a brief duration of action of the standard formulations (2–3 hours) or severe rebound or when administering medication every 4 hours is inconvenient, stigmatizing, or impossible.

The recently published revision of the Texas Children's Medication Algorithm for ADHD (Pliszka et al. 2006) provides useful guidance to clinicians in approaching the pharmacological management of ADHD, as well as the treatment of ADHD with other comorbid disorders. In brief, the revised algorithm recommends initiating the treatment of ADHD with a stimulant medication. If the treatment response is suboptimal, or if side effects or other circumstances warrant, the next step would be the use of a different stimulant. For example, if methylphenidate (or one of its formulations) is tried first, then the next step would be the use of an amphetamine preparation, or vice versa.

Adderall, a racemic mixture of four amphetamine salts (*d*-amphetamine saccarate, *d*-amphetamine sulfate, *d,l*-amphetamine sulfate, and *d,l*-amphetamine aspartate) has been shown in several randomized double-blind, placebo-controlled studies to be of equal efficacy to methylphenidate in treating the behavioral symptoms of ADHD (Pliszka 2000). No significant difference in side effects with methylphenidate was noted. Adderall XR (extended release) incorporates immediate-release and delayed-release formulations of Adderall in a 50:50 ratio within a single capsule to provide a more extended period of action. The efficacy of Adderall XR in improving attention and classroom behavior has been demonstrated in controlled trials (McCracken et al. 2003). The long-term effectiveness and tolerability of Adderall XR has been suggested by a 24-month open-label extension study by McGough et al. (2005).

In February 2005, Health Canada (the Canadian federal department whose responsibilities include functions comparable to the U.S. FDA) suspended the sale of Adderall XR in the Canadian market after it reviewed worldwide reports of 20 instances of sudden death and 12 instances of stroke in patients taking this medication, which included 14 and 2 children, respectively (Health Canada 2005a). The non–extended-release formulation of Adderall has never been available in Canada. After an independent review of the data, Health Canada (2005b) authorized the resumption of the use of Adderall XR in August 2005, contingent upon stronger product labeling warning against the use of Adderall XR in patients with structural heart defects, as well as the potential dangers resulting from the misuse of amphetamines. The current U.S. product labeling contains similar cautions for both Adderall and Adderall XR.

Concerta is a long-acting single-daily-dose methylphenidate preparation that provides an immediate dose of methylphenidate followed by gradual release of methylphenidate over several hours by means of an osmotic release system. It has been found comparable to three-times-daily dosing of methylphenidate, and superior to placebo, in a within-subject double-blind trial and in randomized double-blind trials (Swanson et al. 2002). No significant increases in side effects were reported in the active treatment groups. An open-label multicenter study of Concerta by Wilens et al. (2005) suggested that Concerta remains effective and well tolerated in long-term treatment, although modest increases in dose may be required.

Metadate CD (controlled delivery) is a modified-release preparation of methylphenidate that incorporates immediate-release and extended-release preparations of methylphenidate to extend its length of action. In a blinded, placebo-controlled multicenter study, Greenhill et al. (2002) found Metadate CD to be safe and effective in controlling ADHD symptoms. Ritalin LA (long acting), which uses the proprietary Spheroidal Oral Drug Absorption System (SODAS) to deliver immediate- and delayed-release doses of medication, was also shown to be superior to placebo in a brief (2-week) randomized, controlled multicenter trial (Biederman et al. 2003).

Daytrana is a transdermal patch preparation of methylphenidate that has been shown to be effective in treating the symptoms of ADHD in randomized controlled trials (McGough et al. 2006). This method of administering methylphenidate is particularly useful for children who have difficulty swallowing tablets or capsules. The patch should be applied 2 hours before medication effect is needed, and it may remain in place for up to 9 hours. Although erythema at the site of application of the patch is common, use of the patch should be discontinued if contact sensitization occurs (Shire U.S. Inc.). Several dosage strengths are available, allowing for titration of dose.

Focalin (dexmethylphenidate) is the *d*-enantiomer of racemic *d,l-threo*-methylphenidate. Dexmethylphenidate was found to be significantly superior to placebo, and as effective as racemic methylphenidate, on several measures of behavior and performance in a randomized controlled trial (Wigal et al. 2004). Although a slightly longer duration of action of dexmethylphenidate compared with methylphenidate was observed, further studies are needed to determine whether dexmethylphenidate offers any other distinct clinical advantages over racemic methylphenidate. An extended-release preparation of dexmethylphenidate (Focalin XR), recently introduced into the U.S. market, has been shown to be superior to placebo in controlling ADHD symptoms in a randomized controlled trial (Greenhill et al. 2006b).

Vyvanse (lisdexamfetamine dimesylate) is a prodrug of dextroamphetamine. A therapeutically inactive molecule consisting of dextroamphetamine bound to L-lysine, lisdexamfetamine releases dextroamphetamine after ingestion. Dosed once a day, lisdexamfetamine was superior to placebo in treating symptoms of ADHD in a randomized controlled crossover study (Biederman et al. 2007a) and a randomized controlled parallel-group study (Biederman et al. 2007b).

Magnesium pemoline (previously marketed under the brand name Cylert) is a longer-acting CNS stimulant that is structurally dissimilar to methylphenidate and dextroamphetamine. Since its first use in the United States in 1975, 15 cases of acute hepatic failure have been reported to the FDA, 12 of which resulted in death or the need for liver transplantation. Pemoline was withdrawn from the U.S. market in October 2005.

Stimulant medication should be initiated with a low dose and titrated within the recommended range every week or two according to response and side effects, with body weight as a rough guide. When children reach 3 years of age, their absorption, distribution, protein binding, and metabolism of stimulants are similar to those of an adult (Coffey et al. 1983), although adults have more side effects than children do at the same mg/kg dose. Giving medication after meals minimizes anorexia. Preschool-age children or patients with ADHD, predominantly inattentive type; mental retardation; or PDDs may benefit from (and have fewer side effects with) doses lower than are used in patients with ADHD with prominent symptoms of hyperactivity or impulsivity. Starting with only a morning dose may be useful in assessing drug effect by comparing morning and afternoon school performance. The need for an after-school dose or medication on weekends should be individually determined. Whereas some children who experience sleep or appetite disturbance but a good clinical response to stimulants may benefit from a suspension of treatment on weekends and school holidays, those who are actively involved in weekend sports or extracurricular activities may require treatment during the weekends. Results from the MTA study suggest that most children continue to benefit from maintenance medication doses that are similar to the initial titration dose. However, adjustments to dose were often required in children, indicating the need for ongoing monitoring of treatment response and active medication management (Vitiello et al. 2001). MTA study results support the superiority of full-day, 7-day-per-week stimulant coverage in children with combined-type ADHD.

Behavioral checklists such as the revised versions of the Conners Teacher and Parent Rating Scales (Conners et al. 1998a, 1998b), and the parent and teacher versions of the Vanderbilt ADHD Rating Scales (Wolraich et al. 1998, 2003) are useful in assessing the severity of inattentive and hyperactive symptoms in a variety of settings prior to initiating treatment, as well as monitoring the efficacy of medication during treatment.

If symptoms are not severe outside of the school setting, children may have an annual drug-free trial in the summer, at least 2 weeks' duration but longer if possible. If school behavior and academic performance are stable, a carefully monitored trial off medication during the school year (but *not* at the beginning) will provide data on whether medication is still needed.

Tolerance is reported anecdotally, but adherence is often irregular and should be the first possibility considered when medication appears ineffective. Children should not be responsible for their medication because youngsters are impulsive and forgetful at best, and most dislike the idea of taking medication, even when they can verbalize its positive effects and cannot identify any side effects. They will often avoid, "forget," or simply refuse medication. Lower efficacy of a generic preparation may be another possibility. Decreased drug effect also may be due to a reaction to a change at home or school. Greenhill (1995) used the term *pseudotolerance* to define circumstances in which increased symptomatology is inaccurately ascribed to decreased medication efficacy (e.g., when symptoms are exacerbated due to changes in a child's life rather than changes in response to medication). True tolerance may be more likely with the long-acting formulations (Birmaher et al. 1989); if it occurs, another of the stimulants may be substituted.

Table 36–5 lists the currently available stimulant medications, their formulations, and dose ranges.

Risks and Side Effects

Most side effects are similar for all stimulants (Table 36–6). Insomnia may be due to drug effect, to rebound, or to a preexisting sleep problem. Stimulants may worsen or improve irritable mood (Gadow 1992). Black male adolescents who take stimulants may be at higher risk for elevated blood pressure (Brown and Sexson 1989).

The issue of stimulant-induced growth retardation remains a significant concern. The magnitude is dose related and appears to be greater with dextroamphetamine than with methylphenidate. In a review of 22 studies examining the effect of stimulant medication on children's growth, Poulton (2005) found 11 studies that identified height attenuation with stimulant treatment. Those studies that showed no significant effect were considered to have important design or statistical limitations. A significant stimulant-related retardation in growth rate in children treated with stimulant medication was also observed in a 3-year MTA follow-up study (Swanson et al. 2007). However, the possible mechanisms of stimulant use on growth interference and the long-term implications for final stature remain to be clearly elucidated. Although some authors have suggested that growth delays in ADHD children may be related to dysmaturity inherent in the disorder itself rather than to medication effects (Spencer et al. 1996), the findings by Swanson et al. (2007) suggest just the opposite: compared with age-matched children without ADHD, medication-naive children with ADHD had greater-than-expected initial height and weight, and those who remained unmedicated throughout the study experienced a greater growth rate. In light of these findings, measurement of height and weight at the initiation of treatment and at regular intervals throughout is recommended.

Rebound effects, consisting of increased excitability, activity, talkativeness, irritability, and insomnia, beginning 4–15 hours after a dose, may be seen as the last dose of the day wears off or for up to several days after sudden withdrawal of high daily doses of stimulants. This effect may resemble a worsening of the original symptoms (Zahn et al. 1980).

Although psychosis is a well-known side effect of all stimulant medications, psychotic symptoms have not been rigorously studied within the child and adolescent population being treated for ADHD. On chart review, one retrospective study noted that 6% of 98 children being treated with methylphenidate had demonstrated psychotic symptoms, most often hallucinations, although delusions were reported as well (Cherland and Fitzpatrick 1999). These symptoms usually abated after cessation of stimulant medication. While preliminary, these data suggest that psychotic side effects may not be an uncommon side effect among ADHD children treated with stimulant medication.

Attention is required to avoid possible emanative effects of medication—that is, indirect and inadvertent cognitive and social consequences, such as lower self-esteem and self-efficacy; attribution by child, parents, and teachers of both success and failure to the medication rather than to the child's effort; stigmatization by peers; and dependence by parents and teachers on medication rather than making needed changes in the environment (Whalen and Henker 1991). Both patients and relevant adults can be instructed that medication enables the patients to accomplish what they wish to do; it does not *make* them do anything. Children and adolescents should be given full credit for improvement and helped to take an appropriate amount of responsibility for problems.

Although there is a commonly held notion that stimulants lower the seizure threshold, there is no evidence that stimulants produce an increase in seizure activity. Addiction has *not* been found to result from the prescription of stimulants for ADHD.

Alpha$_2$-Noradrenergic Agonists

Clonidine and guanfacine are α-noradrenergic agonists approved for the treatment of hypertension.

Indications and Efficacy

Attention-deficit/hyperactivity disorder. Clonidine is useful in modulating mood and activity level and in improving cooperation and frustration tolerance in a subgroup of children with ADHD, especially those who are highly aroused, hyperactive, impulsive, defiant, and labile (Hunt et al. 1990). Steingard et al. (1993) report that children with ADHD and comorbid tics may have a more positive response to clonidine than children who have ADHD without tics. A randomized controlled trial of 136 children with ADHD and a chronic tic disorder conducted by the Tourette's Syndrome Study Group (2002) noted significant improvements in all treatment groups (clonidine, methyl-

TABLE 36–5. Clinical use of stimulant medications in pediatric patients

Generic name	Duration of action	Proprietary name	How supplied	Starting dose	Maximum daily dose	Remarks
Methylphenidate	≤6 hours	Methylin	5-, 10-, 20-mg tablets 2.5-, 5-, 10-mg chewable tablets 5 mg/5 mL oral solution 10 mg/5 mL oral solution	5 mg bid	60 mg	Give doses 3–5 hours apart. Consider a smaller starting dose for children <6 years of age.
		Ritalin	5-, 10-, 20-mg tablets			
		Generic	5-, 10-, 20-mg tablets			
Dexmethylphenidate	≤6 hours	Focalin	2.5-, 5-, 10-mg tablets	2.5 mg bid	20 mg	Start with 2.5 mg bid for children not previously treated with racemic methylphenidate. If converting from methylphenidate, start with half of daily dose of methylphenidate (maximum 20 mg/day divided bid).
Dextroamphetamine	≤6 hours	Dexedrine	5-mg tablets	<6 years: 2.5 mg/day	40 mg	**Possesses "black box" warning.** Give doses 4–6 hours apart.
		Dextrostat	5-, 10-mg tablets	≥6 years: 5 mg/day		
		Generic	5-, 10- mg tablets			
Mixed amphetamine salts	≤6 hours	Adderall	5-, 7.5-, 10-, 12.5-, 15-, 20-, 30-mg tablets	<6 years: 2.5 mg/day	40 mg	**Possesses "black box" warning.** Start with once-daily dosing; may dose twice daily if necessary.
		Generic	5-, 7.5-, 10-, 12.5-, 15-, 20-, 30-mg tablets	≥6 years: 5 mg/day		

TABLE 36–5. Clinical use of stimulant medications in pediatric patients (*continued*)

Generic name	Duration of action	Proprietary name	How supplied	Starting dose	Maximum daily dose	Remarks
Methylphenidate	≤8 hours	Metadate ER	10-, 20-mg tablets	10 mg/day	60 mg	Do not cut, crush, or chew tablets.
		Metadate CD	10-, 20-, 30-, 40-, 50-, 60-mg capsules	20 mg/day		Capsule may be swallowed whole or opened and sprinkled on applesauce. Do not crush or chew capsules.
		Methylin ER	10-, 20-mg tablets	10 mg/day		Do not cut, crush, or chew tablets.
		Ritalin SR	20-mg tablets	20 mg/day		Do not cut, crush, or chew tablets.
		Ritalin LA	10-, 20-, 30-, 40-mg capsules	20 mg/day		Capsule may be swallowed whole or opened and sprinkled on applesauce. Do not crush or chew capsules.
		Generic	20-mg tablets	20 mg/day		Do not cut, crush, or chew tablets.
Dextroamphetamine	≤8 hours	Dexedrine Spansule	5-, 10-, 15-mg capsules	5 mg/day	40 mg	**Possesses "black box" warning.** Start with once-daily dosing; may dose twice daily if necessary.
		Generic	5-, 10-, 15-mg capsules			
Methylphenidate	≤12 hours	Concerta	18-, 27-, 36-, 54-mg tablets	18 mg/day	<13 years: 54 mg/day ≥13 years: 72 mg/day or 2 mg/kg	MUST swallow whole. OROS® tablet is passed in stool.
		Daytrana	10-, 15-, 20-, 30-mg transdermal patches (nominal dose delivered over 9 hours)	10 mg/day	30 mg/day	Start with 10-mg patch applied to the hip; increase dosage weekly as necessary. Apply 2 hours before medication effect is needed. Remove patch after 9 hours' use. Erythema is a common side effect at the site of application. Alternate application site daily. More severe skin reactions may necessitate discontinuation of use.

TABLE 36–5. Clinical use of stimulant medications in pediatric patients *(continued)*

Generic name	Duration of action	Proprietary name	How supplied	Starting dose	Maximum daily dose	Remarks
Dexmethylphenidate	≤12 hours	Focalin XR	5-, 10-, 20-mg capsules	5 mg/day	20 mg/day	Start with 5 mg/day for children not previously treated with racemic methylphenidate. If converting from methylphenidate, start with half of daily dose of methylphenidate (maximum 20 mg/day divided bid). Capsule may be swallowed whole or opened and sprinkled on applesauce. Do not crush or chew capsule.
Mixed amphetamine salts	≤12 hours	Adderall XR	5-, 10-, 15-, 20-, 25-, 30-mg capsules	10 mg/day	30 mg/day	**Possesses "black box" warning.** Capsule may be swallowed whole or opened and sprinkled on applesauce. Do not crush or chew capsule.
Lisdexamfetamine	≤12 hours	Vyvanse	30-, 50-, 70-mg capsules	30 mg/day	70 mg/day	**Possesses "black box" warning.** Capsule may be swallowed whole or opened and dissolved in water. Not studied in children younger than 6 years or older than 12 years of age.

Note. Amphetamine preparations carry a "black box" warning regarding their potential for abuse and the possibility of sudden death and serious cardiovascular events if misused. They should also be avoided in patients with structural cardiac defects. All of the above medications are Drug Enforcement Administration Schedule II controlled substances. Many generic preparations of the above medications are available. Proprietary names are included for informational purposes only and do not imply endorsement of a particular preparation. Please consult chapter text and manufacturers' product inserts for further prescribing information.
Source. Adapted from product labeling and information available from Drugs@FDA (http://www.fda.gov/cder).

TABLE 36–6. Side effects of stimulant medications

Common initial side effects (try dosage reduction)

Anorexia

Weight loss

Irritability

Abdominal pain

Headaches

Emotional oversensitivity; easy crying

Less common side effects

Insomnia

Dysphoria (especially at higher doses)

Decreased social interest

Less than expected weight gain

Rebound overactivity and irritability (as dose wears off)

Anxiety

Nervous habits (e.g., picking at skin; pulling hair)

Hypersensitivity rash, conjunctivitis, or hives

Withdrawal effects

Rebound ADHD symptoms

Depression (rare)

Rare but potentially serious side effects

Motor or vocal tics

Tourette's disorder

Depression

Growth retardation

Tachycardia

Hypertension

Hallucinations

Stereotyped activities or compulsions

phenidate, and the combination of the two). The greatest benefit compared with placebo was noted in the group of children taking both clonidine and methylphenidate. While clonidine and methylphenidate individually were noted to be effective for ADHD, methylphenidate appeared more beneficial for the inattentive symptoms of ADHD, while clonidine appeared more beneficial for the impulsive and inattentive symptoms of ADHD.

A meta-analysis of the literature from 1980 to 1999 by Connor et al. (1999) demonstrated an effect size of clonidine on symptoms of ADHD that was intermediate between a higher stimulant medication response

and a lower tricyclic antidepressant medication response. A small controlled study by Connor et al. (2000) of 24 ADHD patients with comorbid aggressive oppositional defiant disorder or conduct disorder randomized into three treatment groups (clonidine, methylphenidate, or the combination) demonstrated similar treatment response of clonidine to methylphenidate in this population. No added benefit of combination treatment was noted. A more recent double-blind, randomized study by Hazell and Stuart (2003) examined the addition of either clonidine or placebo to the treatment regimen of 67 children with ADHD and comorbid conduct disorder or oppositional defiant disorder already taking either methylphenidate or dextroamphetamine. Although more children in the treatment group (clonidine plus stimulant) demonstrated improvement compared with the placebo plus stimulant group, statistically significant differences were only noted after about 5 weeks of treatment. As a result of this finding, the authors suggested that 4–6 weeks of treatment with clonidine may be necessary before its benefits can be adequately assessed.

Guanfacine has been shown effective in open trials of children with ADHD and comorbid ADHD and Tourette's disorder. A placebo-controlled study further demonstrated guanfacine's effectiveness in treating children with comorbid ADHD and tic disorders (Scahill et al. 2001), and an open-label trial (Scahill et al. 2006) supports a possible role for guanfacine in the treatment of the hyperactivity associated with pervasive developmental disorders in children, although further study is required.

Tic disorders. In one double-blind study, clonidine was found to modestly decrease complex motor and vocal tics (Leckman et al. 1991), although another study (Singer and Brown 1995) did not support this finding. Clonidine appears to be most useful in reducing subjective distress and the behavioral symptoms of hyperactivity and impulsivity that often accompany Tourette's disorder. As mentioned above, some evidence suggests that guanfacine is a useful agent in treating tics as well (Scahill et al. 2001).

Initiation and Maintenance

Because clonidine and guanfacine have similar pharmacological profiles, blood pressure and pulse should be measured before treatment and at regular intervals throughout treatment. An electrocardiogram (ECG) and baseline laboratory blood studies (especially fasting glucose) may be considered. Clonidine is initiated at a low dose of 0.05 mg (one-half of the smallest manufactured tablet) at bedtime. This low dose converts the side effect of initial sedation into a benefit. An alternate strategy is to begin with 0.025 mg qid. Either way, the dosage is then titrated gradually over several weeks to 0.15–0.30 mg/day (0.003–0.01 mg/kg/day) in three or four divided doses. Young children (ages 5–7 years) may require lower initial and maintenance doses. The transdermal form (skin patch) may be useful to improve compliance and reduce variability in blood levels. It lasts only 5 days in children (compared with 7 days in adults) (Hunt et al. 1990). Once the daily dose has been determined using pills, an equivalent-size patch may be substituted (0.1, 0.2, 0.3 mg/day). Patches should not be cut to adjust the dose, as this may damage the delivery membrane, potentially causing an increase in the delivered dose of clonidine (Broderick-Cantwell 1999). Unfortunately, patches do not adhere well in hot, humid climates. For guanfacine, dosages range from 0.5 to 4.0 mg/day, in three divided doses, and a recommended starting regimen is 0.5 mg once or twice daily in children and 1 mg once or twice daily in adolescents, to be increased every 3 or 4 days until therapeutic effect is noted (Silver 1999). When clonidine or guanfacine is discontinued, it should be tapered over several days to a week, rather than stopped suddenly, to avoid a withdrawal syndrome consisting of increased motor restlessness, headache, agitation, elevated blood pressure and pulse rate, and (in patients with Tourette's disorder) exacerbation of tics (Leckman et al. 1986).

Risks and Side Effects

Sedation and irritability are troublesome side effects of clonidine therapy, although these tend to decrease after several weeks. Dry mouth, nausea, and photophobia have been reported, with hypotension and dizziness possible at high doses. The clonidine skin patch often causes local pruritic dermatitis; daily rotation of the patch site or use of a steroid cream may minimize this. Depression may occur, often in patients with a personal or family history of depressive symptoms (Hunt et al. 1991). Glucose tolerance may decrease, especially in those patients at risk for diabetes. Although guanfacine is less sedating and less hypotensive than clonidine, it shares many of the side effects of this class of medication.

Reports of serious adverse drug reactions (including sudden death) in children treated with clonidine, alone or in combination with methylphenidate, have raised concerns about the safety of this medication in the pediatric population. In several cases, the presence of polypharmacy or other medical conditions made it more difficult to implicate clonidine in these adverse events (Wilens et al. 1999). More recent studies (Hazell and Stuart 2003; Tourette's Syndrome Study Group 2002) have demonstrated the benefits and safety of combination clonidine and methylphenidate therapy in select patient groups. Cardiovascular screening and monitoring of children treated with clonidine or guanfacine are still recommended, however, as well as gradual titration and tapering of dose to reduce cardiovascular side effects.

Horrigan and Barnhill (1999) described manic symptoms appearing in 5 children out of a group of 95 treated with guanfacine that resolved upon medication discontinuation. Prior treatment with clonidine in 4 of these 5 children did not result in manic symptoms. Further study is needed to understand the implications of this finding.

Atomoxetine

Atomoxetine, a norepinephrine reuptake inhibitor, is a nonstimulant medication approved for the treatment of ADHD in children and adults.

Indications and Efficacy

The efficacy of atomoxetine in the treatment of ADHD in the pediatric age group has been demonstrated in several controlled clinical trials (M. Weiss et al. 2005). A meta-analysis of 13 studies of the long-term use of atomoxetine in 6- and 7-year-old children concluded that atomoxetine maintained its efficacy and tolerability for up to 2 years in this patient population (Kratochvil et al. 2006). Atomoxetine was shown to be beneficial in children with comorbid ADHD and oppositional defiant disorder in a randomized controlled trial by Newcorn et al. (2005), although higher doses (1.8 mg/kg/day) were required. A small controlled pilot trial by Arnold et al. (2006) demonstrated the efficacy and safety of atomoxetine in the treatment of ADHD symptoms in children with a comorbid autism spectrum disorder.

Studies comparing the efficacy of atomoxetine with that of stimulant medications are limited. Published and unpublished comparisons of atomoxetine with stimulants suggest a smaller effect size for atomoxetine (Wigal et al. 2005). Although a prospective open-label trial by Kratochvil et al. (2002) suggested no statistically significant difference between atomoxetine and methylphenidate, important design considerations limit the conclusions that can be drawn from the study. More studies are needed to determine atomoxetine's efficacy relative to stimulant medication for the treatment of ADHD. In the meantime, atomoxetine should be considered a second-line treatment for ADHD. The revised Texas Children's Medication Algorithm (Pliszka et al. 2006) recommends the use of atomoxetine only after trials of two different stimulants, unless severe side effects from stimulants or contraindications to their use require that atomoxetine be used preferentially. Information on the concomitant use of atomoxetine and stimulants is limited to case reports and a small short-term pilot study that showed no ill effects from the combination of atomoxetine and long-acting methylphenidate, although there was no apparent clinical benefit from the combined treatment (Carlson et al. 2007). Further study of the efficacy and safety of combined atomoxetine and stimulant therapy is needed.

Initiation and Maintenance

Based on clinical studies and current drug labeling, atomoxetine may be started at a dose of 0.5 mg/kg/day. The dose can be given once a day, or in equal divided doses in the morning and evening. The dose may then be incrementally increased every few days, as tolerated, to 1.2 mg/kg/day. The total daily dose in children and adolescents weighing less than 70 kg should not exceed 1.4 mg/kg/day or 100 mg, whichever is less. For children and adults who weigh over 70 kg, the maximum daily dose is 100 mg.

Risks and Side Effects

The product labeling of atomoxetine currently includes a "black box" warning about the possibility of increased suicidal ideation in children and adolescents taking this medication. Similar to the recommendations for the use of antidepressants in the pediatric population, this risk should be discussed with parents before initiating treatment. Patients should be closely monitored for increases in anxiety, irritability, aggressiveness, or mood disturbance or the presence of suicidal thoughts. Atomoxetine should be used with caution in children with a history of bipolar disorder or who have a family history of bipolar disorder or suicide.

There have been two reported cases of hepatic injury in patients taking atomoxetine. Both patients recovered without need of a liver transplant. Although such injury is rare, patients and their caregivers should be advised of this risk and directed to immediately report to their health care providers the development of signs and symptoms that may indicate liver dysfunction.

Atomoxetine is metabolized primarily through the hepatic CYP 2D6 pathway, although it is not itself an inhibitor of this enzyme. Because adverse effects may be dose-related, atomoxetine should be used with caution, and a decreased dose may be necessary in patients who are poor metabolizers or who are taking other medications that inhibit this enzymatic pathway (Caballero and Nahata 2003).

Atomoxetine is generally well tolerated. The most common side effects include abdominal pain, headache, irritability or mood lability, dizziness, somnolence or fatigue, decreased appetite, and nausea and vomiting. Modest dose-related increases in pulse and blood pressure have also been noted. Most side effects appear to subside over time and only rarely result in discontinuation of treatment. A meta-analysis of the effect of atomoxetine on growth over a 2-year treatment period by Spencer et al. (2005) showed only minimal effects on height and weight compared with expected growth rates based on extrapolated baseline measurements and comparison to growth charts from the U.S. Centers for Disease Control and Prevention (CDC), with relative decreases of height and weight of less than 0.5 cm and 1 kg, respectively.

Modafinil

Modafinil is approved for the treatment of hypersomnolence related to narcolepsy and other sleep disorders in patients 16 years of age and older. Pharmacologically distinct from stimulant medications, its mechanism of action is not well understood. Several randomized controlled trials have shown modafinil to be effective in the treatment of ADHD in children and adolescents (Swanson et al. 2006).

In all of the aforementioned studies, modafinil was well tolerated, with insomnia, headache, stomachache, and decreased appetite being the most common side effects. Doses of modafinil in the studies varied widely, from 100 to 425 mg/day. Modafinil currently possesses no approved indication for use in ADHD. An application to the FDA to market a formulation of modafinil for the treatment of ADHD was rejected, due to concerns about severe skin rashes. Comparison studies with stimulant medication are needed to determine whether modafinil possesses any distinct advantages over currently approved therapies. Modafinil might be considered as an alternative treatment in ADHD when all standard treatments are ineffective or are poorly tolerated.

Selective Serotonin Reuptake Inhibitors

Six selective serotonin reuptake inhibitors (SSRIs) are currently approved by the FDA for use in the United

States: citalopram, escitalopram, fluoxetine, fluvox-amine, paroxetine, and sertraline. Fluoxetine is approved for the treatment of depression in children 8–17 years of age and obsessive-compulsive disorder (OCD) in children ages 7–17 years. Fluvoxamine is approved for the treatment of OCD in children 8 years of age and older, and sertraline is approved for the treatment of OCD in children 6 years of age and older. However, all of the SSRIs have been used to treat a wide variety of disorders in children and adolescents. The use of SSRIs in children has become more controversial over the past few years as the results of clinical trials, some unpublished, have called into question the efficacy of this class of medication in the treatment of pediatric depression. More importantly, concerns have been raised that antidepressants in general, and the SSRI class of antidepressants in particular, may actually induce suicidal thinking or behavior in susceptible individuals.

Controversy Surrounding SSRI Use in Children

The concern over SSRI use in children began in June 2003, when the British MHRA, which performs a function similar to that of the U.S. FDA, issued a statement to health care providers reporting the receipt of new data from clinical trials of paroxetine that did not demonstrate efficacy in depressive illness in children. Moreover, the studies also showed an increase in suicidality and potentially suicidal behavior in children taking paroxetine, relative to placebo (Duff 2003a). The MHRA advised that paroxetine not be used in children to treat depressive illness. A similar warning was issued in September 2003 for venlafaxine (Duff 2003b). In December 2003, the MHRA issued an advisory stating that, with the exception of fluoxetine, the use of any SSRI for the treatment of depression in children is contraindicated (Duff 2003c).

In the United States, the FDA monitored the MHRA developments closely. Less than 10 days after the first MHRA action, the FDA issued its own advisory to clinicians recommending that paroxetine not be used in children for the treatment of depression, pending the outcome of a review of the available clinical data (U.S. Food and Drug Administration 2003a). After conducting an initial review, the FDA issued a Public Health Advisory in October 2003 alerting clinicians to reports of suicidal thinking in children taking antidepressants (U.S. Food and Drug Administration 2003b). The Advisory further stated that while "the data do not clearly establish an association between the use of these drugs and increased suicidal thoughts or actions by pediatric patients," such an association

could not be ruled out. The FDA commissioned a team of experts from Columbia University to take a critical look at the available data and report back to the FDA as to whether the adverse events described in the studies represented suicidality. Some of the difficulty in interpreting the data arose from the differences among the various studies in defining behaviors or thoughts that could be classified under the broad rubric of "suicidality," different definitions of response among the studies, a lack of monitoring for compliance, and high rates of subject dropout in some studies (Brent and Birmaher 2004).

In their meta-analysis of published and unpublished studies on the use of SSRIs for pediatric depression, Whittington et al. (2004) concluded that only fluoxetine had a favorable risk–benefit profile for the treatment of pediatric depression. They went on to report that while published studies on the use of paroxetine and sertraline suggested a slightly favorable risk–benefit profile, adding these data to the data from unpublished studies showed that these medications were not efficacious for pediatric depression. Although Whittington and colleagues emphasized that the studies analyzed were not designed to specifically examine rare events such as suicide, the absence of evidence of efficacy in pediatric depression caused them to conclude that the risks of treatment with SSRIs (except for fluoxetine) were greater than the potential benefits to be derived from treatment (Whittington et al. 2004).

Columbia University reported its findings to the FDA in July 2004 (U.S. Food and Drug Administration 2004a). The FDA also held public meetings of its Psychopharmacological Drugs and Pediatric Advisory Committees in September 2004, during which input from the public was considered along with a review of the information to date. With incorporation of the Columbia University findings into an FDA meta-analysis of the data from published and unpublished studies, the rate of "definite or possible" suicidality among children in the treatment group was determined to be twice that of the placebo group (Newman 2004). The FDA stopped short of contraindicating the use of antidepressants in this age group but required a "black box" caution on all antidepressants, warning of the increased risk of suicidality in pediatric patients (U.S. Food and Drug Administration 2004c).

These actions on the part of the FDA have not ended the debate over SSRI use in children. No suicides actually occurred in the more than 4,000 children included in the studies of SSRI use in the pediatric population (U.S. Food and Drug Administration

2004b). The controlled studies analyzed by the FDA excluded children who had suicidal thoughts or behavior. As such, it is possible that SSRIs may reduce suicidality in medicated depressed children more than they induce it in nonsuicidal depressed children who initiate treatment (Riddle 2004). Some studies suggest that suicide rates have decreased in areas of the country where SSRI use has increased (Gibbons et al. 2005). Despite the ongoing controversy, many health care providers continue to believe, based on their own experience and the results of clinical studies, that SSRIs can be beneficial for children suffering from depression, anxiety, and other disorders.

Indications and Efficacy

Depressive disorders. Fluoxetine is currently the only SSRI that has an FDA indication for the treatment of depression in children. The efficacy of fluoxetine in treating pediatric depression has been demonstrated in two rigorous randomized, controlled trials (Emslie et al. 2002). Emslie et al. (2004) also reported on the findings of a 32-week placebo-controlled relapse prevention study, which was an extension of their 2002 study. In this trial, the mean time to relapse was greater for the fluoxetine continuation group than for the fluoxetine–placebo group ($P=0.046$), suggesting benefit from medication continuation. Study limitations included small sample size and significant withdrawal of study subjects.

The Treatment for Adolescents with Depression Study (March et al. 2006), a randomized controlled trial of 439 patients ages 12–17 years with major depressive disorder, compared the efficacy of fluoxetine (10–40 mg/day) and cognitive-behavioral therapy (CBT), either alone or in combination, with placebo over a 12-week period. At the conclusion of the study, fluoxetine with CBT and fluoxetine alone were superior to both placebo and CBT alone, as measured by the Children's Depression Rating Scale—Revised (CDRS-R).

Keller et al. (2001) undertook a double-blind, placebo-controlled study of paroxetine in which 275 adolescents with major depression were randomized to paroxetine (20–40 mg/day), imipramine (200–300 mg/day), or placebo. Although paroxetine demonstrated superiority to placebo as determined by a Hamilton Rating Scale for Depression (HAM-D) total score of 8 or less at the conclusion of the 8-week study, paroxetine did not differ significantly from placebo in its primary outcome measures. Of note, imipramine did not demonstrate a statistically significant improvement in any measurement instrument compared

with placebo. A multicenter randomized controlled trial of paroxetine in children and adolescents with major depressive disorder by Emslie et al. (2006) also failed to demonstrate paroxetine's superiority over placebo.

Wagner et al. (2003) pooled the data from two randomized, placebo-controlled trials of sertraline demonstrating that sertraline was superior to placebo as measured by overall mean change, as well as total score, on the CDRS-R. An examination of the sertraline group showed that 7 children developed agitation, compared with 2 children in the placebo group. Data from the individual studies were not separately analyzed.

Another study by Wagner et al. (2004a) examined the efficacy of citalopram compared with placebo in a randomized controlled trial of 174 children with major depression over an 8-week period. Citalopram was superior to placebo, as early as week 1 of treatment, as measured by mean change from baseline on the CDRS-R. Citalopram was also superior to placebo on the study's primary outcome measure, a score of 28 or less on the CDRS-R. The average dosage of citalopram was 24 mg/day, which was generally well tolerated.

Wagner et al. (2006a) also undertook a randomized, controlled 8-week study of escitalopram for the treatment of depression in 264 children 6–17 years of age. Escitalopram is the therapeutically active S-enantiomer of citalopram. At the conclusion of the study, escitalopram was not superior to placebo either in the primary outcome measure (mean decrease from baseline in CDRS-R total score) or in the secondary measures of outcome. Further analysis of the data suggested that escitalopram might be superior to placebo in the adolescent patient group, although the study was not designed to detect response differences in subgroups of the cohort. Additional studies are required to determine whether escitalopram is superior to placebo for adolescent depression.

Obsessive-compulsive disorder. Evidence supporting the use of SSRIs in OCD is more consistent. A meta-analysis of randomized controlled trials of medications used in the treatment of pediatric OCD by Geller et al. (2003) showed that SSRIs are superior to placebo in the treatment of OCD in the pediatric population. The four SSRIs studied in the analysis (fluoxetine, fluvoxamine, paroxetine, and sertraline) were considered to be equal in efficacy.

In 2004, the Pediatric OCD Treatment Study (POTS) (March et al. 2004) examined the use of sertraline, CBT, and the combination of the two in a 12-week randomized controlled study of 112 children and adolescents with OCD. All treatment modalities were found to be significantly superior to placebo. The combination of CBT and sertraline was superior to either CBT or sertraline monotherapy. Sertraline monotherapy was not superior to CBT monotherapy in treating pediatric OCD. Indeed, the effect size of CBT monotherapy was greater than sertraline monotherapy, with more children achieving remission from CBT monotherapy, although the benefit over sertraline monotherapy did not reach statistical significance.

A 52-week open follow-up study of 120 children and adolescents diagnosed with OCD by Cook et al. (2001) suggests that sertraline may be effective in the long-term treatment of OCD symptoms.

Other disorders. SSRIs have been shown to be effective in the treatment of anxiety disorders other than OCD in the pediatric age group. In a multicenter double-blind, placebo-controlled study, the RUPP Anxiety Study Group (Walkup et al. 2001) demonstrated superiority of fluvoxamine over placebo in treating social phobia, separation anxiety disorder, or generalized anxiety disorder in children and adolescents ages 6–17 years. Over the 8 weeks of the study, the patients who received fluvoxamine had a significantly greater decrease in their Pediatric Anxiety Rating Scale score compared with those who received placebo. As well, the fluvoxamine group showed a greater response to treatment overall as measured by the Clinical Global Impressions (CGI)—Improvement scale. Fluoxetine was found to be significantly more efficacious than placebo in treating generalized anxiety disorder, separation anxiety disorder, or social phobia in a randomized controlled trial of 74 children by Birmaher et al. (2003). Other controlled studies have demonstrated the efficacy of sertraline in the treatment of generalized anxiety disorder (Rynn et al. 2001) and paroxetine in social anxiety disorder (Wagner et al. 2004b).

Masi et al. (2001a) conducted a naturalistic study of 18 children with panic disorder treated with paroxetine at dosages of up to 40 mg/day. The results of their study suggest a possible role for this medication in the treatment of pediatric panic disorder, with over 80% of children determined to be responders based on improvements in the Clinical Global Impressions (CGI)—Severity scale. Seedat et al. (2002) compared the response of pediatric and adult patients with posttraumatic stress disorder (PTSD) to treatment with citalopram in an 8-week open trial at doses of up to 40 mg/day. At the conclusion of the study, there were no significant differences in outcome between the pediatric and adult treatment groups as measured by the CGI scale and the Clinician-Administered PTSD Scale,

with both groups showing significant improvement in symptoms of PTSD. Although these initial reports are encouraging, randomized controlled trials are needed.

A double blind, placebo-controlled study examining the effectiveness of fluoxetine in the treatment of elective mutism in a small group of children showed mixed results (Black and Uhde 1994). However, in an open trial with fluoxetine in 21 children with selective mutism conducted by Dummit et al. (1996), 76% of children were considered improved, with decreased anxiety and increased speech in public settings, during the 9-week trial. Dosages of fluoxetine ranged from 10 to 60 mg/day.

Dosage and Administration

All of the SSRIs possess a "black box" warning about the potential for increased suicidality in patients taking these medications, and patients and parents should be cautioned accordingly. While the FDA recommends weekly monitoring of children during the first 4 weeks of treatment, with additional monitoring at weeks 6, 8, and 12, the American Psychiatric Association and the American Academy of Child and Adolescent Psychiatry suggest a monitoring schedule tailored to the individual needs of the patient and his or her family (PhysiciansMedGuide). A well-written monograph on the most common complications of SSRI treatment in children and adolescents by Walkup and Labellarte (2001) may further guide clinicians in providing informed consent about SSRIs to parents and patients.

The following dosing guidelines, summarized in Table 36–7, should be considered in light of the current evidence regarding the efficacy of SSRIs in pediatric psychiatric disorders. The recently updated guidelines from the Texas Children's Medication Algorithm Project (Hughes et al. 2007) recommend the first use of either fluoxetine, sertraline, or citalopram for the treatment of pediatric major depressive disorder, based on the availability of at least one randomized controlled trial demonstrating efficacy in this age group. Fluoxetine remains the consensus conference panel's first choice, with sertraline and citalopram recommended as alternate choices. Fluoxetine, citalopram, and paroxetine may be started at dosages of 5–10 mg/day. These dosages may be increased as needed to 20 mg/day. Although most children will obtain an adequate response to 20 mg/day or less of these medications, some children may require dosages in excess of 20 mg/day. All of the above medications are available in a liquid formulation that may facilitate medication administration or dosage titration in small children. Escitalopram is generally dosed at half the usual dose for citalopram.

TABLE 36–7. Clinical use of selective serotonin reuptake inhibitors (SSRIs) in pediatric patients

Generic name	How supplied	Indications	Customary daily dosage	Remarks
Citalopram	10-, 20-, 40-mg tablets[1] 10 mg/5 mL solution	Depression*	20 mg/day	Consider a small starting dose if used in children.
Escitalopram	5-, 10-, 20-mg tablets 5 mg/5 mL solution	Depression* Generalized anxiety disorder*	10 mg/day	Consider a small starting dose if used in children. Allow 1 week between dosage increases. Dosages above 20 mg/day have not been shown to be of benefit in adult studies. A recent RCT failed to show superiority over placebo in pediatric-age patients.[2]
Fluoxetine	10-, 20-, 40-mg tablets	Depression	20 mg/day	Consider a starting dosage of 10 mg/day in smaller children.
	10-, 20-, 40-mg capsules	Obsessive-compulsive disorder	20–60 mg/day	Medication may be discontinued without tapering.
	20 mg/5 mL oral solution	Bulimia nervosa*	60 mg/day	
	90-mg capsules (for weekly administration)	Panic disorder*	20 mg/day	
Fluvoxamine	25-, 50-, 100-mg tablets	Obsessive-compulsive disorder	25 mg/day	Maximum daily dose for children 8–17 years of age is 200 mg.
Paroxetine		Depression*	20 mg/day	Indications and dosages apply only to the regular-release formulation.
	10-, 20-, 30-, 40-mg tablets	Obsessive-compulsive disorder*	40 mg/day	All indications and dosages are those for adult patients. Maximum recommended daily dosage is 60 mg.
		Panic disorder*	40 mg/day	
	10 mg/5 mL oral solution	Generalized anxiety disorder*	20 mg/day	
	12.5-, 25-, 37.5-mg controlled-release tablets[3]	Social anxiety disorder*	20 mg/day	
		Posttraumatic stress disorder*	20 mg/day	

TABLE 36–7. Clinical use of selective serotonin reuptake inhibitors (SSRIs) in pediatric patients *(continued)*

Generic name	How supplied	Indications	Customary daily dosage	Remarks
Sertraline	25-, 50-, 100-mg tablets	Obsessive-compulsive disorder	50 mg/day	Start with 25 mg/day in children and 50 mg/day in adolescents. Maximum recommended daily dosage is 200 mg.
		Depression*	50 mg/day	
		Panic disorder*	25 mg/day	
	20 mg/mL oral concentrate	Posttraumatic stress disorder*	25 mg/day	
		Premenstrual dysphoric disorder*	50 mg/day	
		Social anxiety disorder*	25 mg/day	

Note. All antidepressants carry a "black box" warning about the potential for increased suicidality in pediatric patients. All SSRIs have the potential to inhibit cytochrome P450 (CYP) 2D6 and other CYP isoenzymes. Use with caution in combination with other medications that are metabolized through these pathways. Please consult chapter text and manufacturers' product inserts for further prescribing information.
*Not an approved pediatric indication.
[1]Also available in orally disintegrating preparation.
[2]Wagner et al. 2006a.
[3]The controlled-release preparation of paroxetine (Paxil-CR) is indicated only for the treatment of depression, panic disorder, social anxiety disorder, and premenstrual dysphoric disorder in adults. It is not approved for use in children.
Source. Adapted from product labeling and information available from Drugs@FDA (http://www.fda.gov/cder).

For sertraline and fluvoxamine, dosages may be started at 25 mg/day, and increased as necessary to a dosage of 100–150 mg/day. Doses may be increased every few days as tolerated. Sertraline is also available in a liquid preparation.

Although children and adolescents as well as adults usually tolerate this class of medication well, children may experience the same constellation of side effects as seen in adults, such as gastrointestinal complaints or headache. In addition, patients may experience a discontinuation syndrome if the medication is stopped abruptly. Symptoms include malaise, myalgias, headache, and anxiety, and these may occur even if only one dose is missed. It is therefore preferable to taper the dose of medication over several days rather than discontinue the medication abruptly. This discontinuation syndrome is not usually noted with fluoxetine, because of its active metabolites and long half-life. In a patient who has a recurrence of symptoms after an initial good response, gentle inquiry about medication compliance should be made prior to making a change in dose.

Adverse Effects

Several cases of "behavioral activation" and manic symptoms, presumed to be caused by treatment with SSRIs, have been reported in pediatric patients. In many of these cases, the manic symptoms appeared within days to weeks of initiating treatment with an SSRI. Symptoms usually resolved within a few days of the reduction in dose or cessation of medication. In some cases, treatment with a mood stabilizer was necessary. In many of the cases, there was no premorbid or family history of a cyclical mood disorder. In their systematic chart review of 82 children and adolescents treated with SSRIs for depression or OCD, Wilens et al. (2003) found that 22% experienced a "psychiatric adverse event," most commonly a disturbance in mood.

Garland and Baerg (2001) reported on 5 cases of "frontal lobe syndrome," defined as apathy, disinhibition, or lack of motivation in children being treated with an SSRI. The symptoms typically developed 6–8 weeks after initiation of treatment with an SSRI, or with an increase in dose, and subsided with a decrease in dose. Sporadic reports of decreased growth, presumably due to SSRI therapy, have also been reported. Nilsson et al. (2004) analyzed the effects of fluoxetine on the growth of 96 children who were participants in the 19-week acute and continuation phases of the study on the use of fluoxetine in the treatment of pediatric depression by Emslie et al. (2002) described earlier in this chapter. Compared with children treated with placebo, children treated with fluoxetine experienced significantly less growth (1 cm ± 2.4 vs. 2.1 cm ± 2.6) and less weight gain (1.2 kg ± 2.7 vs. 2.3 kg ± 2.6) compared with placebo. These findings must be interpreted with caution, as the measurements were not collected in a standardized fashion, and there were inaccuracies in the height measurements, as suggested by some children appearing to lose height. Although no conclusions can be drawn from these reports until more definitive studies are performed, it may be prudent to monitor patients' growth during the course of their treatment.

Adolescents, like adults, may experience sexual dysfunction from SSRI therapy. Scharko (2004) published the results of his review of the literature for reports of sexual dysfunction in adolescents taking SSRIs. Despite similar rates of nonsexual adverse effects from SSRI treatment in the pediatric and adult age groups, there is very little information on SSRI-induced sexual dysfunction in adolescents compared with adults. Although many explanations are possible, Scharko (2004) speculated that the most likely reasons are that research studies have not consistently examined this side effect in the adolescent population and that clinicians do not inquire about their adolescent patients' sexual functioning. Given the potential for SSRI-induced sexual dysfunction to affect treatment adherence and quality of life, clinicians should be sensitive to the potential presence of this adverse effect in their adolescent patients.

Movement disorders (acute dystonic reactions, akathisia, and tic-like movements) have also been noted in children taking SSRIs (Sokolski et al. 2004). As SSRI-induced movement disorders are postulated to be due to serotonin-mediated inhibition of dopaminergic transmission (Lipinski et al. 1989), they may potentially occur with any of the SSRIs.

Serotonin syndrome is a potentially fatal reaction to serotonergic agents. It is more likely to occur when serotonergic agents are used in combination. Several signs characterize this syndrome: mental status changes, fever, tremor, diaphoresis, and agitation. While uncommon, there are several case reports of serotonin syndrome in the pediatric population. The syndrome may arise after only one dose of a serotonergic agent. Clinicians should be alert to the possibility of serotonin syndrome occurring in their pediatric patients and counsel patients and parents as appropriate.

Other Antidepressants

Several other antidepressants are used to treat depression and other psychiatric conditions in the pediatric population, although none have an FDA indication for their use in children. All possess a "black box" warning because of their perceived potential to induce suicidality. Studies demonstrating efficacy of these agents in the pediatric age group are limited, and in some cases studies have failed to demonstrate efficacy in children. Most of these agents would be considered second- or third-line treatments, if considered at all.

Venlafaxine

Few studies have examined the use of venlafaxine in children. In a double-blind, placebo-controlled study, Mandoki et al. (1997) compared a low dose of venlafaxine plus therapy to placebo and therapy in the treatment of 33 children ages 8–17 years with diagnoses of major depression. The study showed no significant difference between the two groups. More recently, Emslie et al. (2007) reported on two placebo-controlled trials of the use of venlafaxine in children and adolescents with depression. In children ages 7–11 years, venlafaxine was not superior to placebo on any outcome measure. And although the adolescent treatment group showed significant improvement in some outcome measures, the effect size was small and of questionable clinical significance. Moreover, more patients in the treatment group (10%) compared with the placebo group (3%) left the study due to adverse effects. In light of the current literature, the use of venlafaxine in the treatment of pediatric depression is unsupported.

Duloxetine

Duloxetine, like venlafaxine, is a selective serotonin and norepinephrine reuptake inhibitor (SSNRI), recently approved for the treatment of depression in adults. There are no open-label or randomized controlled trials of duloxetine's use in children to date.

Bupropion

Small controlled studies have demonstrated the superiority of bupropion to placebo in the treatment of ADHD in children. Conners et al. (1996) reported the findings of a multisite double-blind, placebo-controlled study corroborating these previous results, confirming that bupropion can be beneficial in the treatment of ADHD and possibly conduct disorder. Another study found the efficacy of bupropion in treating ADHD to not be significantly different from methylphenidate (Barrickman et al. 1995). Bupropion has been reported to exacerbate tics in children with comorbid ADHD and Tourette's disorder and may not be suitable for use in this population (Spencer et al. 1993).

Although bupropion is marketed in the United States as an antidepressant and as an aid in smoking cessation, the literature on its use in treating childhood depression is limited to small open-label studies. There are no controlled trials supporting the use of bupropion in pediatric depression.

Bupropion is available in three formulations. Regular-release bupropion is administered in two or three daily doses, beginning with a low dose (37.5 or 50 mg bid), with titration over 2 weeks to a usual maximum of 250 mg/day (300–400 mg/day in adolescents). A sustained-release preparation of this medication is available in generic form, allowing for once- or twice-daily dosing. An extended-release preparation of bupropion (Wellbutrin XL) permits once-daily dosing. The most serious side effect is a decrease in the seizure threshold, seen most frequently in patients with an eating disorder. Bupropion is contraindicated in this population. Other side effects in children include skin rash, perioral edema, nausea, increased appetite, agitation, and exacerbation of tics.

Mirtazapine

Mirtazapine is indicated for the treatment of depression in adults. Its pharmacological profile results in anxiolytic and antidepressant effects with less gastrointestinal upset and sexual dysfunction than SSRIs. However, somnolence and weight gain are common side effects. Although one open-label study has suggested a possible role for mirtazapine in the treatment of adolescent depression (Haapasalo-Pesu et al. 2004), randomized controlled trials are needed to determine the potential benefit of mirtazapine in the treatment of pediatric depression.

Monoamine Oxidase Inhibitors

The nonselective monoamine oxidase inhibitors (MAOIs) phenelzine, tranylcypromine, and isocarboxazid are infrequently prescribed in adults nowadays and their use in the pediatric age group is almost unheard of, given the availability of other safe and effective treatments.

However, some studies have suggested a possible role for selegiline in the treatment of children with ADHD. Selegiline, unlike the nonselective MAOIs, selectively inhibits MAO-B in therapeutic doses and is therefore much less likely to induce potentially fatal hypertensive crises due to the ingestion of tyramine-rich foods. Selegiline is metabolized to amphetamine and methamphetamine (Standaert and Young 2006), which may in part account for its usefulness in treating ADHD.

Mohammadi et al. (2004) found no significant differences in either the teachers' reports or the parents' reports on the Attention Deficit Hyperactivity Scale in their double-blind trial of 40 children who were randomized to treatment with either methylphenidate (up to 40 mg/day) or selegiline (up to 10 mg/day). A similarly designed but briefer study by Akhondzadeh et al. (2003) produced similar results. However, a small double-blind, controlled crossover study by Feigin et al. (1996) that examined the use of deprenyl (selegiline is L-deprenyl) in 24 children with both ADHD and Tourette's disorder failed to demonstrate a statistically significant benefit from deprenyl compared with placebo. While benefit was noted during the first 8-week treatment period, no benefit was noted in the second treatment period. Further study of selegiline is needed before its use can be routinely considered in pediatric ADHD.

A transdermal formulation of selegiline was recently approved in the United States for the treatment of depression. Studies of the safety and efficacy of this preparation in pediatric patients are required. The authors identified no studies of the use of selegiline in pediatric depressive disorders.

Tricyclic Antidepressants

Until the introduction of the SSRIs into the U.S. market in the late 1980s, tricyclic antidepressants (TCAs) were a mainstay in the pharmacological treatment of a wide variety of disorders in children and adolescents. However, the paucity of clinical studies demonstrating the efficacy of TCAs in children, an increased awareness of the potential cardiac effects of this class of medication, and the availability of alternative medications have resulted in a shift away from using tricyclic agents as first-line treatment (Safer 1997). Since the last edition of this textbook was published, little has been added to the medical literature regarding the use of TCAs in children.

Indications and Efficacy

Depression.   TCAs have consistently failed to show superiority over placebo in treating pediatric depression (Geller et al. 1999). Several hypotheses have been forwarded to explain this poor response including suboptimal dosing, an increase in hormone levels in adolescents, a difference in the maturation of the noradrenergic and serotonergic neurotransmitter systems, and speculation that some of the youths studied may have been in the early phase of bipolar disorder (Ambrosini 2000). Given the absence of empirical data demonstrating efficacy and the unfavorable side-effect and risk profile, TCAs appear to have no place in the treatment of pediatric depression.

Attention-deficit/hyperactivity disorder. TCAs may be indicated for those patients who do not respond to stimulants. TCAs may also be useful for the treatment of ADHD symptoms in patients with tics or Tourette's disorder (Spencer et al. 2002). Efficacy in improving cognitive symptoms does not appear to be as great as for stimulants. The revised Texas Children's Medication Algorithm (Pliszka et al. 2006) describes TCAs as a fourth-line medication in the treatment of ADHD.

Obsessive-compulsive disorder. Clomipramine, a TCA that inhibits serotonin reuptake, is indicated for the treatment of OCD in children older than 10 years of age. In their meta-analysis of pharmacological treatments for pediatric OCD, Geller et al. (2003) found clomipramine to be more effective than SSRIs. As in depression, the more favorable side-effect and safety profile of the SSRIs makes clomipramine a second- or third-line treatment of OCD in children.

Autistic disorder. Gordon et al. (1993) reported a double-blind study in which clomipramine was significantly more effective than either placebo or desipramine in improving several autistic symptoms (obsessive-compulsive symptoms, reciprocal social interactions, stereotypies, and self-injury). No difference between desipramine and placebo was noted. In an open study examining the use of clomipramine in treating young children (ages 3.5–8.7 years), Sanchez et al. (1996) reported no therapeutic effect, and significant adverse reactions were noted (urinary retention).

Enuresis. All of the TCAs have been found to be effective in the treatment of nocturnal enuresis. In 80% of patients, within the first week, TCAs reduce the frequency of bed-wetting. Total remission, however, occurs in relatively few cases. Wetting invariably returns when the drug is discontinued. Behavioral treatments that avoid drug side effects and have higher remission rates are the best first choice. Should pharmacological intervention be necessary, desmopressin (1-deamino-8-D-arginine vasopressin [DDAVP]) is a first-line treatment and is preferred over TCAs due to its greater efficacy and more favorable safety profile (Hjalmas et al. 2004). A trial with imipramine may be useful if other interventions are unsuccessful (Gepertz and Nevéus 2004).

Anxiety disorders. The majority of the work has examined the use of TCAs for separation anxiety disorder and school absenteeism. The efficacy of imipramine in patients with anxiety disorders is controversial (Klein et al. 1992), and other medications are now available. Medication may be useful as an adjunct if psychosocial treatment is ineffective. In a randomized, double-blind trial comparing imipramine plus CBT in the treatment of school refusal, imipramine plus CBT was shown to be more effective than CBT plus placebo in decreasing depressive symptoms and improving school attendance (Bernstein et al. 2000).

Initiation and Maintenance

Pharmacokinetics for TCAs are different in children than in adolescents or adults. The smaller fat-to-muscle ratio in children leads to a decreased volume of distribution, and children are not protected from excessive dosage by a large volume of fat in which the drug can be stored. Children have larger livers relative to body size, leading to faster metabolism (Sallee et al. 1986), more rapid absorption, and lower protein binding than in adults (Winsberg et al. 1974). As a result, children are likely to need a higher weight-corrected dose of TCAs than adults. Prepubertal children are prone to rapid dramatic swings in blood levels from toxic to ineffective and should have divided doses to produce more stable levels (Ryan 1992). Parents must be reminded to supervise closely the administration of medication and to keep pills in a safe place. Wilens et al. (1996) recommend guidelines for monitoring the cardiovascular effects of TCAs.

The usefulness of plasma levels is limited by the relative rarity of laboratories able to perform them satisfactorily. Medication cannot be safely titrated by plasma level, as there is no known level below which toxicity can be ensured not to occur. Plasma levels (drawn 9–11 hours after the last dose) can identify rapid and slow metabolizers. Determination of levels is recommended for patients who fail to respond to usual doses (possibly low levels) or those who have severe side effects at usual doses (possibly very high levels). If the patient's history suggests head trauma or seizures, an electroencephalogram (EEG) is indicated before starting treatment. Dosing guidelines for tricyclic agents in pediatric-age patients may be found in Table 36–8.

Attention-deficit/hyperactivity disorder. Imipramine is begun at a dosage of 10 or 25 mg/day and increased weekly. The maximum dosage is 5 mg/kg/day (given in three divided doses in children). Plasma levels do not predict efficacy. Some patients respond to a daily dose as low as 2 mg/kg. Nortriptyline is given at 25–75 mg/day in two divided doses (Saul 1985).

TABLE 36–8. Clinical use of tricyclic antidepressants in pediatric patients

Generic name	Indications	Pediatric dosing range	Remarks
Amitriptyline	Depression*	30–150 mg/day	Not recommended for use in patients <12 years of age. Does not possess a pediatric indication. Start with lower doses in adolescents.
Clomipramine	Obsessive-compulsive disorder	25–200 mg/day	Start with 25 mg/day. May increase over 2 weeks to the lesser of 100 mg/day or 3 mg/kg/day. Maximum dosage is the lesser of 200 mg/day or 3 mg/kg/day.
Desipramine	Depression*	25–100 mg/day	Not recommended for use in children. Does not possess a pediatric indication. Dosages above 150 mg/day are not recommended in adolescents. Consider ECG monitoring at initiation of treatment and at regular intervals throughout. See chapter text for further comments on the use of desipramine in pediatric patients.
Imipramine	Depression* Nocturnal enuresis	25–75 mg/day	Start with 10–25 mg/day. May increase to 50 mg/day in children <12 years of age and 75 mg in children ≥12 years of age. Dosages in excess of 2.5 mg/kg/day are not recommended in pediatric patients.
Nortriptyline	Depression*	30–50 mg/day (adolescents)	Does not possess a pediatric indication.

Note. All antidepressants carry a "black box" warning about the potential for increased suicidality in pediatric patients. Use with caution in combination with medications that inhibit cytochrome P450 (CYP) 2D6 or other CYP isoenzymes. Please consult chapter text and manufacturers' product inserts for further prescribing information.
*Not an approved pediatric indication.
Source. Adapted from product labeling and information available from Drugs@FDA (http://www.fda.gov/cder).

Obsessive-compulsive disorder.   Doses of clomipramine used to treat OCD are generally lower than TCA doses used for depression. Response is delayed for 10–14 days, as in the treatment of depression, and is unlike the immediate response seen in the treatment of ADHD or enuresis (Rapoport 1986). Clomipramine is started at 25 mg/day (or every other day) and gradually increased over 2 weeks to a maximum of 100 mg/day or 3 mg/kg/day, whichever is less. If necessary, the dosage in children and adolescents may be gradually increased up to a maximum of 200 mg/day or 3 mg/kg/day, whichever is less. Divided doses are preferable during dosage titration. Chronic treatment may be required.

Enuresis.   Daily charting of wet and dry nights is used before starting medication to obtain a baseline and subsequently to monitor progress. Much lower doses are needed than for the treatment of depression. Imipramine is started at 10–25 mg at bedtime and increased by 10- to 25-mg increments weekly to 50 mg (75 mg in preadolescents), if necessary. The maximum dosage is 2.5 mg/kg/day (Ryan 1990). Tolerance may develop, requiring a dose increase. For some children, TCAs lose their effect entirely. If medication is used chronically, the child or adolescent should have a drug-free trial at least every 6 months because enuresis has a high spontaneous remission rate.

Anxiety disorders.   In separation anxiety disorder and school nonattendance, psychological interventions such as family therapy, work with school personnel, and desensitization should be used before and along with medication. For children with school phobia, McDaniel (1986) recommends 125 mg as the maximum dose of imipramine. The starting dosage for children ages 6–8 years is 10 mg at bedtime and for older children, 25 mg at bedtime. The dosage may be increased by 10–50 mg/day, but those with school avoidance require at least 75 mg/day. Some patients require a higher dose for complete response, but if there is no detectable positive response at 125 mg/day, improvement at higher doses is unlikely. After clinical response (6–8 weeks), medication is continued at least another 8 weeks and then gradually withdrawn.

Risks and Side Effects

As with other antidepressants, TCAs are considered to have the potential to induce suicidal thoughts or behavior, regardless of the condition for which they are being used, and subsequently carry a "black box" warning to this effect. Patients and their caregivers should be cautioned about this potential adverse effect and advised on the behavioral signs and symptoms that may indicate developing suicidality. Frequent monitoring of patients by clinicians in the early stages of treatment is essential. TCAs are particularly lethal in overdose.

The quinidine-like effect of TCAs slows cardiac conduction time and repolarization. At dosages of more than 3 mg/kg/day of imipramine, children and adolescents may develop an increased pulse and small but statistically significant ECG changes (intraventricular conduction defects, such as lengthened P-R interval, that may progress to a first-degree atrioventricular heart block and occasional widening of the QRS complex) (Wilens et al. 1996). The tendency of prepubertal children to have wider swings in blood levels may place them at higher risk for serious cardiac conduction changes. A minority of the population has a genetic defect in TCA metabolism, increasing risk for toxicity.

Anticholinergic side effects may occur in children, although less commonly than in adults. Most of these side effects are transient and/or respond to a decrease in dose. Of particular importance for children are dry mouth (which may lead to an increase in dental caries in long-term use [Herskowitz 1987]), drying of bronchial secretions (especially problematic for asthmatic children), sedation, anorexia, constipation, nausea, tachycardia, palpitations, and increased diastolic blood pressure.

Other reported side effects include abdominal pain, chest pain, headache, orthostatic hypotension (rare in young patients), syncope, mild tremors of hands and fingers, weight loss, and tics. The seizure threshold may be lowered, with worsening of preexisting EEG abnormalities and rarely a seizure. Seizures appear to be more common with clomipramine. Side effects with a probable allergic mechanism include rash, worsening of eczema, and rarely thrombocytopenia (Campbell et al. 1985).

Behavioral toxicity may be manifested by irritability, worsening of psychosis, mania, agitation, anger, aggression, forgetfulness, or confusion. CNS toxicity may be mistaken for exacerbation of the primary condition. A drug blood level is often required to differentiate the two. As depressed children, especially those who are anergic and withdrawn, improve with TCA treatment, crying and verbalizations of sadness and anger may transiently increase.

Sudden cessation of moderate or higher doses results in flu-like anticholinergic withdrawal syndrome, with nausea, cramps, vomiting, headaches, and muscle pains. Other manifestations may include social withdrawal, hyperactivity, depression, agitation, and insomnia (Ryan 1990). TCAs should therefore be tapered over a 2- to 3-week period. The short half-life of TCAs in prepubertal children often produces daily withdrawal symptoms if medication is given only once a day. These symptoms also may indicate that poor compliance is resulting in missed doses. Because of the predictability of TCA-induced electrocardiographic changes, a rhythm strip is useful in monitoring compliance.

The physician should be alert to the risk of intentional overdose or accidental poisoning, not only by the patient but by other family members, especially young children.

Cautionary note on the use of desipramine. Seven cases of sudden death have been reported in children being treated with desipramine, three of whom died immediately after physical exertion (Varley and McClellan 1997). A causal relationship between the medication and the deaths has not been established. Cardiac etiology is often suspected; however, a review of cardiovascular changes in children treated with TCAs (Wilens et al. 1996) concluded that although changes in blood pressure, heart rate, and ECG parameters are identifiable, they are probably of minor significance.

A study of the effects of desipramine on cardiac function during exercise concluded that desipramine had only minor effects on the cardiovascular response to exercise and that these effects did not appear to be age related (Waslick et al. 1999). A further study by Walsh et al. (1999) showed that desipramine reduced parasympathetic input to the heart as measured by

R-R interval variability. While this reduction in para-sympathetic tone could, theoretically, increase vulner-ability to cardiac arrhythmias, the R-R interval vari-ability did not differ with age in the 42 subjects (ages 7–66 years) who were studied. Nevertheless, because other safe and effective medications are available, the use of desipramine in children is discouraged.

Mood-Stabilizing Agents

Lithium is a natural element and alkali metal that pos-sesses antimanic properties and has been approved for use in the United States since 1970 for the treatment of mania in patients 12 years of age and older. The anti-epileptic drugs carbamazepine, oxcarbazepine, dival-proex sodium, lamotrigine, and clonazepam have been used for a variety of (non–FDA approved) psy-chiatric indications, although divalproex sodium has an FDA-approved indication for the treatment of ma-nia in adults, and lamotrigine is approved for mainte-nance treatment in adult bipolar disorder. The efficacy of these agents may be unrelated to their anticonvul-sant effects. Wide variations in bioavailability and rate of absorption of generic products have led to recom-mendations that the brand name (or at least a single generic) product be prescribed. Data on children and adolescents are far more limited than on adults, but side-effect patterns appear to be similar. All of the mood stabilizers, particularly the anticonvulsants, have complex interactions with multiple other drugs. Dosing guidelines for mood stabilizers that may be considered for use in pediatric patients are listed in Table 36–9.

Lithium

Indications and efficacy.   While the results of sev-eral open trials have supported the use of lithium in pediatric bipolar disorder (Kafantaris et al. 2003; Ko-watch et al. 2000), controlled trials are few. In a double-blind, placebo-controlled study of 25 adolescents with bipolar disorder and a substance dependence disor-der, Geller et al. (1998b) found that lithium signifi-cantly improved global functioning and decreased substance use compared with placebo. While a small sample size and lack of a follow-up phase limited this study, it is the first to examine the use of lithium in this particular population.

More recently, Kafantaris et al. (2004) performed a placebo-controlled discontinuation study on 40 ado-lescents who had responded to 4 weeks of treatment with lithium. During the 2-week discontinuation phase, 23 adolescents experienced an acute exacerba-tion of manic symptoms; the difference between the lithium and placebo groups was not statistically signif-icant. Several hypotheses were offered in an attempt to explain the poor performance of lithium, including the relatively brief stabilization period (4 weeks) before the discontinuation phase began, as well as the relatively small size of the study. It is clear that further studies are needed in order to better define the role of lithium in the treatment of adolescent mania.

Lithium may be more useful in the treatment of the depressive phase of pediatric bipolar disorder than in the treatment of unipolar depression in children at risk of developing bipolar disorder because of a strong family history. Patel et al. (2006) noted a significant decrease in CDRS-R scores at the conclusion of their 6-week open trial of lithium in the treatment of adoles-cents experiencing a depressive episode associated with bipolar I disorder. However, in a blinded con-trolled study of prepubertal children with major de-pressive disorder without a history of symptoms of mania but with a family history of either bipolar dis-order or multigenerational major depressive episode, Geller et al. (1998a) found that lithium was not statis-tically more effective than placebo in the treatment of depression in this group. Information on lithium aug-mentation of SSRIs is sparse. Lithium is not indicated for prophylaxis in bipolar disorder in children and adolescents unless there is well-documented history of recurrent episodes.

It is not yet clear whether lithium is efficacious for the treatment of behavior disorders without an appar-ent mood disorder in children of bipolar parents or for children and adolescents who have behavior disorders accompanied by mood swings. Lithium has been shown to be effective in some placebo-controlled stud-ies of children with severe impulsive aggression, while other controlled studies have rendered less encourag-ing results (Malone et al. 2000). Lithium may be useful in mentally retarded or autistic youths with severe ag-gression directed toward themselves or others or with symptoms suggestive of bipolar disorder (Campbell et al. 1985; Kerbeshian et al. 1987; Steingard and Bieder-man 1987).

Initiation and maintenance.   Lithium should not be prescribed unless the family is willing and able to comply with regular multiple daily doses and with blood monitoring of lithium levels. In addition to the usual detailed medical history and physical examina-tion, complete blood count (CBC) with differential, liver function tests, electrolytes, serum thyroxine and thyroid-stimulating hormone (TSH), blood urea nitro-gen (BUN), creatinine, and ECG should be determined

TABLE 36–9. **Clinical use of mood stabilizers in pediatric patients**

Generic name	Indications	Pediatric dosing range	Remarks
Lithium carbonate	Manic episodes of bipolar disorder Maintenance treatment for bipolar disorder	300–1,200 mg/day	Not approved for use in children <12 years of age. Start with 150–300 mg/day in children. Therapeutic level is 0.6–1.2 mEq/L. Baseline CBC, liver-associated enzymes, BUN, thyroid-function tests, urinalysis, and ECG are recommended before initiation of treatment and at regular intervals thereafter. Do not use in pregnancy. **Possesses "black box" warning.**[1]
Lamotrigine	Adjunctive therapy for partial seizures Monotherapy for adults with partial seizures already stabilized on certain other antiepilepsy medications* Maintenance treatment for bipolar disorder*	As adjunctive therapy for partial seizures: 1–5 mg/kg/day (maximum: 200 mg/day) in children 2–12 years on valproate 5–15 mg/kg/day (maximum: 400 mg/day) in children 2–12 years not on valproate 100–400 mg/day in children >12 years on valproate 300–500 mg/day in children >12 years not on valproate	Lamotrigine has complex dosing recommendations based on the use of concomitant medications; consult the package insert for the latest dosage guidelines. The lamotrigine dosage used in reports of its use in pediatric mood disorders ranges from 25 to 250 mg/day, depending on whether valproate is used concomitantly. Patients taking lamotrigine are at risk of developing potentially severe rashes. Slow titration of the medication appears to mitigate this risk. **Possesses "black box" warning.**[2]
Valproate	Complex partial and simple and complex absence seizures Acute mania* Prophylaxis of migraine headaches*	Initiate treatment at 250–500 mg/day in divided doses Assess level when total dosage of 15 mg/kg/day is reached Usual therapeutic dosage range is 15–60 mg/kg/day	CBC, serum chemistries with liver function tests, BUN, and creatinine are recommended before initiation of treatment and at regular intervals thereafter. Therapeutic level is 50–120 µg/mL. Do not use in pregnancy. Use with caution in patients <2 years of age. **Possesses "black box" warning**[3]

Note. Use with caution in combination with other medications, especially those that inhibit cytochrome P450 (CYP) 2D6 or other CYP isoenzymes. Please consult chapter text and manufacturers' product inserts for further prescribing information. BUN=blood urea nitrogen; CBC=complete blood count; ECG=electrocardiogram.
*Not an approved pediatric indication.
[1]Lithium toxicity is related to serum levels and can occur at levels close to therapeutic levels.
[2]Serious rashes, including Stevens-Johnson syndrome, have occurred with use of lamotrigine. The risk of this side effect is greater in children.
[3]Cases of hepatic failure resulting in death have occurred with treatment with valproate. Cases of life-threatening pancreatitis have been reported with valproate. The incidence of neural tube defects and other teratogenic effects may be increased in the offspring of women taking valproate during pregnancy.
Source. Adapted from product labeling and information available from Drugs@FDA (http://www.fda.gov/cder).

before starting lithium. Some clinicians recommend determining renal concentrating ability (urine specific gravity or osmolality after overnight fluid deprivation). A patient with a history suggesting increased risk of seizures warrants an EEG. Height, weight, TSH, creatinine, and morning urine specific gravity (or osmolality) should be obtained every 3–6 months.

Lithium levels, drawn 10–12 hours after the last dose, should be obtained twice weekly during initial dose adjustment and monthly thereafter. Three to four days are required to reach steady-state levels after a dose change. Therapeutic levels are the same as for adults, 0.6–1.2 mEq/L. The starting dose is 150–300 mg/day, gradually titrated upward in divided doses according to serum levels and clinical effects. Total daily therapeutic dosing is typically reached between 900 and 1,200 mg. Because lithium excretion occurs primarily through the kidney, and most children have more efficient renal function than adults, they may require higher doses for body weight than do adults (Weller et al. 1986). More steady blood levels may be obtained by using a slow-release formulation. Lithium should be taken with food to minimize gastrointestinal distress. Some difference may be present in pharmacokinetics between lithium carbonate and lithium citrate, and clinicians should not assume equal dosing when shifting between the two forms (Reischer and Pfeffer 1996). Given lithium's teratogenicity, the clinician should address this potential with sexually mature female adolescent patients and consider contraceptive options as appropriate.

Risks and side effects.   The younger the child, the more likely the occurrence of side effects (Campbell et al. 1991). Autistic children have more frequent and severe side effects from lithium than do children with conduct disorder, even at lower doses (Campbell et al. 1991). Children may experience side effects at serum levels that are lower than those in adults: most commonly, weight gain, vomiting, headache, nausea, tremor, enuresis, stomachache, weight loss, sedation, and anorexia (Campbell et al. 1991). Common early-onset side effects, which seem to be related to rapid increase in serum level, include nausea, diarrhea, muscle weakness, thirst, urinary frequency, a dazed feeling, and hand tremor. Polydipsia and polyuria secondary to vasopressin-resistant diabetes insipidus may result in enuresis, especially in institutionalized retarded patients (Campbell et al. 1985). In growing children, the consequences of hypothyroidism (which could resemble retarded depression) are potentially more severe than in adults. The calcium mobilization from bones that has been noted in adults might cause a significant

problem in growing children (Herskowitz 1987). Lithium's tendency to aggravate acne may be especially significant for adolescents. Lithium's effects on glucose are controversial, but both hyperglycemia and exercise-induced hypoglycemia are possible. Rarely, lithium may cause extrapyramidal side effects (EPS) in children (Samuel 1993).

Toxicity is closely related to serum levels, and the therapeutic margin is narrow. Symptoms of lithium toxicity include vomiting, drowsiness, hyperreflexia, sluggishness, slurred speech, ataxia, anorexia, convulsions, stupor, coma, and death. Adequate salt and fluid intake is necessary to prevent levels rising into the toxic range. The family should be instructed in the importance of preventing dehydration from heat or exercise and in the need to stop the lithium and contact the physician if the child or adolescent develops an illness with fever, vomiting, diarrhea, and/or decreased fluid intake. The erratic consumption of large amounts of salty snack foods may cause fluctuations in lithium levels (Herskowitz 1987). Clinicians should also be aware of potential drug–drug interactions, especially with nonsteroidal anti-inflammatory drugs, antipsychotic agents, SSRIs, and antibiotics (Kowatch and Bucci 1998).

Carbamazepine

The evidence suggesting a potential benefit of carbamazepine in the treatment of juvenile bipolar disorder is limited to a small case series (Woolston 1999) and a randomly assigned open study that compared the effect size of lithium, divalproex sodium, and carbamazepine in the treatment of bipolar I and II disorders in children and adolescents (Kowatch et al. 2000). No controlled studies have been reported. While preliminary data suggested this drug's efficacy in children with severe explosive aggression, a later double-blind, placebo-controlled study failed to demonstrate any superiority of carbamazepine over placebo in reducing aggression in this population (Cueva et al. 1996). Carbamazepine usage has largely been supplanted by other, more effective treatments in all of these disorders.

Divalproex Sodium

Indications and efficacy.   Three open-label trials of divalproex sodium in the treatment of children and adolescents with mania have been reported (Wagner et al. 2002). All studies found that divalproex sodium was generally well tolerated and beneficial in this population. As mentioned above, Kowatch et al. (2000) completed a randomly assigned open study that compared the effect size of lithium, divalproex sodium, and carbamazepine in the treatment of bipolar I and II disorders in children and adolescents. Similar to carbamazepine and lithium, divalproex sodium had a large effect size and was generally well tolerated.

Findling et al. (2003c) observed significant improvements in all outcome measures in their open trial of combination lithium and divalproex treatment in 90 children and adolescents with bipolar I or II disorder. The combination treatment was generally well tolerated, although 15 children were withdrawn from the study due to medication side effects. Findling et al. (2005a) then published the results comparing the efficacy of lithium or divalproex in a randomized study of children who initially received combination lithium and divalproex therapy. The study found no significant difference between the lithium and divalproex treatment groups in the time to relapse. Although divalproex sodium may be beneficial in the treatment of mania in bipolar disorder, larger controlled studies are required.

Initiation and maintenance. Hemoglobin, hematocrit, CBC, platelets, liver function, BUN, and creatinine should be measured before the patient begins taking valproate. Liver function tests and CBC may be repeated weekly for the first month and then every 4–6 months. For children younger than age 10 years, monthly liver function tests are advisable (Trimble 1990). Divalproex sodium may be initiated at 250 mg once or twice daily, depending on the weight of the child. Trough plasma levels should be drawn after reaching a dosage of 15 mg/kg/day dispensed in three divided doses. Dosages should be titrated to achieve a serum level within the therapeutic range (50–120 µg/mL). Clinicians are cautioned that the use of mg/kg loading doses for divalproex sodium may lead to supratherapeutic levels in overweight children (Good et al. 2001).

Risks and side effects. The most frequent adverse effects are nausea, vomiting, and gastrointestinal distress (which may be diminished by using enteric-coated divalproex sodium), sedation, weight gain, and tremor (Trimble 1990). Acute hepatic failure is almost always restricted to children younger than age 3 years, especially those who have mental retardation or who are following a regimen of anticonvulsant polytherapy. Other side effects are similar to those seen in adults. Of uncertain significance is the report of menstrual disturbances, polycystic ovaries, and hyperandrogenism in a series of women treated with divalproex sodium for epilepsy (Isojarvi et al. 1993). These

findings have been challenged in a recent review of the literature (Genton et al. 2001).

Oxcarbazepine

Oxcarbazepine is the 10-keto analog of carbamazepine, and is approved for use in children and adults as an anticonvulsant. The literature on its use in pediatric bipolar disorder consists of only a few case reports and one multicenter randomized controlled trial (Wagner et al. 2006b) in which oxcarbazepine was not found to be more effective than placebo. Any recommendations regarding its use in pediatric bipolarity must await further controlled trials.

Lamotrigine

Lamotrigine is an anticonvulsant approved for the treatment of certain seizure disorders and as maintenance therapy for adults with bipolar disorder. As with the other newer anticonvulsant agents, only a handful of reports describe its use in children with psychiatric disorders. Carandang et al. (2003) reported on their observations of a beneficial response in eight of nine adolescents with a mood disorder (predominantly bipolar or unipolar depression) treated with lamotrigine; three of the children received lamotrigine as monotherapy. Similar results in adolescent bipolar depression were described in an open-label trial by Chang et al. (2006).

Lamotrigine has the potential to induce serious, potentially life-threatening rashes in patients. This risk appears to be greater in pediatric patients treated for seizure disorders (0.8%) compared with adults (0.3%) (GlaxoSmithKline 2005). Prompt discontinuation of treatment at the first signs of rash is necessary, although this may not necessarily prevent a more serious rash from developing. Very slow titration of the medication seems to mitigate the potential for rash development. Until controlled trials establish lamotrigine's efficacy in the treatment of pediatric mood disorders, its use should be relegated to second- or third-line status.

Topiramate

Topiramate is indicated for the treatment of pediatric and adult seizure disorders, and as a prophylactic treatment for adult migraine.

Although a few retrospective reviews have suggested a possible role for topiramate in pediatric bipolar disorder, DelBello et al. (2005) aborted their double-blind, controlled study of topiramate monotherapy in 56 children and adolescents with bipolar I disorder after a controlled trial of topiramate in adult bipolar disorder (Powers et al. 2004) failed to demonstrate superiority. In the absence of demonstrated efficacy in the treatment of adult mania, and until open studies or controlled trials provide greater support for its use in children, there is little reason to consider topiramate for the treatment for pediatric bipolar disorder.

Antipsychotic Medications

Indications and Efficacy

Antipsychotic medications are more fully discussed elsewhere in this volume (see Chapter 26, "Psychopharmacology," by Martinez et al.). In addition to their use in the treatment of schizophrenia and other psychotic disorders, antipsychotic medications have been used in the pediatric population to treat bipolar disorders, conduct and other aggressive disorders, Tourette's disorder, and the behavioral manifestations of PDDs. The introduction of second-generation or "atypical" antipsychotic medications (aripiprazole, clozapine, olanzapine, quetiapine, risperidone, and ziprasidone) has added significantly to the child and adolescent psychiatrist's pharmaceutical armamentarium. Second-generation agents are increasingly being used over first-generation agents due to their more favorable side-effect profile and decreased risk of inducing EPS and tardive dyskinesia, despite the fact that studies examining the efficacy and safety of second-generation antipsychotics in children and adolescents, while promising, remain limited. Excellent reviews of the use of these agents in the pediatric population have recently been published (Cheng-Shannon et al. 2004; Findling et al. 2005b).

Psychotic disorders. Few studies examining the efficacy of first-generation antipsychotic medications in schizophrenic children exist (Findling et al. 2005b). Two controlled studies (Pool et al. 1976; Realmuto et al. 1984) with stringent diagnostic admission criteria demonstrated moderate effectiveness of antipsychotic medication in adolescent schizophrenic patients. Medication-induced side effects in both studies were substantial, particularly sedation (in low-potency agents) and EPS (in high-potency agents), supporting the belief that children may be at higher risk than adults for developing side effects with the typical antipsychotic agents. Spencer et al. (1992) reported preliminary results of the first double-blind, placebo-controlled trial of haloperidol in schizophrenic prepubertal children. Findings similarly support moderate improvement of symptoms in those taking haloperidol rather than placebo.

The more limited effects of typical antipsychotic medications, coupled with less favorable side-effect profiles (including tardive dyskinesia) in children, has led clinicians to consider the use of second-generation antipsychotics as first-line treatment of the pediatric population. Open trials and double-blind studies examining the efficacy of clozapine in adolescent patients with treatment-resistant childhood-onset schizophrenia have consistently demonstrated clozapine's superiority to standard treatments, specifically haloperidol (Kumra et al. 1996). Because treatment with clozapine is compounded by possible serious side effects (agranulocytosis, seizures, and significant weight gain), clozapine's use is reserved for treatment of those select pediatric patients who have failed to respond to trials of first-generation or other second-generation antipsychotics.

Information regarding the use of risperidone or olanzapine in the treatment of schizophrenia in the pediatric population is limited. One randomized controlled study (Sikich et al. 2004) compared risperidone, olanzapine, and haloperidol with placebo in 50 patients ages 8–19 years with a variety of psychotic disorders, including schizophrenia-spectrum disorders and mood disorders with psychotic features. Both second-generation antipsychotics were found to be as effective as haloperidol in controlling psychotic symptoms. However, side effects such as weight gain and EPS were prominent. Although a few open-label studies have suggested an improvement in positive and negative symptoms of schizophrenia with risperidone, retrospective and open-label studies of olanzapine have yielded mixed results. Further controlled studies of these medications in pediatric schizophrenia are needed.

A few open studies have found quetiapine to be useful in the treatment of children with a variety of psychotic disorders, including schizophrenia-spectrum and psychotic mood disorders. Appreciable weight gain was noted in subjects. Continued significant benefit from quetiapine at a dose of 300–800 mg/day was reported for up to 64 weeks in an open-label extension study by McConville et al. (2003). The literature on the use of aripiprazole and ziprasidone in pediatric psychotic disorders is limited to case reports only; the use of these agents in other pediatric psychiatric conditions has been more extensively studied.

Mood disorders. The beneficial use of clozapine in the treatment of pediatric bipolar disorder has only been described in single case reports or small case series (Kant et al. 2004). The literature describing the favorable use of risperidone or olanzapine in pediatric bipolar disorder is similarly limited to a few case reports and open-label studies (Biederman et al. 2005). In a randomized controlled study by DelBello et al. (2002) of quetiapine in 30 adolescents with bipolar disorder also being treated with divalproex, combination quetiapine/divalproex treatment demonstrated statistically superior reductions in Young Mania Rating Scale scores, compared with the placebo/divalproex group. And a randomized, double-blind study by DelBello et al. (2006) found quetiapine to be as effective as divalproex in treating acute manic symptoms. Pathak et al. (2005) reported benefit in 7 of 10 adolescents with major depressive disorder unresponsive to at least 8 weeks of treatment with an SSRI when quetiapine was added to their regimen. Barnett (2004) described 4 cases of children and adolescents with bipolar disorder who responded to ziprasidone after exhibiting a disappointing response to other mood stabilizers or antipsychotics. There are only a handful of reports on the use of aripiprazole in pediatric bipolar disorder.

Although several of the above studies suggest a possible role for second-generation antipsychotics in the treatment of pediatric mood disorders, primarily as adjunctive therapy, further rigorous open trials or randomized controlled trials need to be performed before the use of second-generation antipsychotic medications can be endorsed for these conditions.

Pervasive developmental disorders. Of the second-generation agents, risperidone has been the most extensively studied in this patient population. In 2002, the RUPP Autism Network (Scahill et al. 2002) published the findings of their randomized controlled trial of risperidone in 101 children and adolescents with autism. At the conclusion of the 8-week study, children in the treatment group (who received doses of risperidone between 0.5 and 3.5 mg/day) demonstrated significant reductions in the Irritability subscore of the Aberrant Behavior Checklist compared with placebo. The overall response rate was also significantly greater for the risperidone group than for the placebo group. Shea et al. (2004) conducted a similar 8-week randomized controlled trial of risperidone in 79 children with autism that reported similar results.

The RUPP Autism Network then set out to examine the longer-term efficacy of risperidone in children with autism in a two-part extension of their initial 8-week randomized controlled study (McCracken et al. 2005). During the open-label treatment phase of the study, more than 80% of the children continued to be rated as "much" or "very much" improved on the CGI–Improvement scale. During the controlled discontinuation phase, the relapse rate for the placebo

substitution group was significantly greater than for the treatment continuation group. Troost et al. (2005) replicated the findings of the above study in their smaller but similarly designed protocol. Risperidone was generally well tolerated in all of these studies, although weight gain was significant.

While the above studies demonstrate the efficacy of risperidone in controlling aggression, self-injurious behavior, and tantrums, risperidone appears to have limited benefit in treating the primary symptoms of autism. Analyzing the data from the secondary outcome measures used in the two RUPP Autism Network studies cited above, McDougle et al. (2005) found that risperidone did not improve the social or communication impairments of autism, although significant improvements in repetitive and stereotyped behaviors were observed.

Masi et al. (2001b) reported the benefits of low-dose risperidone (0.5 mg/qd) in a 16-week open trial studying preschool children with PDDs. Risperidone effectively targeted disruptive behaviors, as well as affective dysregulation, and was well tolerated. The benefits of long-term treatment with risperidone in the preschool-age group were described in a 3-year naturalistic study of 53 children with autistic-spectrum disorders, also by Masi et al. (2003).

A small randomized controlled trial suggests that olanzapine may be a safe and effective treatment of core symptoms in children and adolescents with autism spectrum disorders (Hollander et al. 2006). However, an open-label study of 25 children with autistic-spectrum disorders by Kemner et al. (2002) reported that while treatment with olanzapine improved several measures on the Aberrant Behavior Checklist, only 3 children were considered responders based on the CGI–Improvement scale. Similarly mixed results exist for quetiapine. Open-label trials (Corson et al. 2004) have suggested limited or no therapeutic benefit from quetiapine and reported serious side effects in the treatment group. However, while Hardan et al. (2005) reported that 6 of the 10 children in their retrospective study appeared to improve with quetiapine therapy, the average dose of quetiapine was over 200 mg/day higher than that used in the patients studied by Corson et al. (2004), and 6 of the 10 children were receiving other psychoactive medications in addition to quetiapine.

Reports of the use of ziprasidone and aripiprazole in PDD are even more limited. Only half of the 12 children and young adults with a PDD treated with ziprasidone in an open-label trial (McDougle et al. 2002) were deemed responders, based on ratings of "very much" or "much" improved on the CGI scale. Many of the study's subjects received concomitant psychoactive medication. One open study (Stigler et al. 2004) reported improvement in maladaptive behaviors in all 5 children with a PDD treated with aripiprazole. Both aripiprazole and ziprasidone appeared to be well tolerated.

Of all the second-generation antipsychotics, risperidone has the strongest evidence for its beneficial use in the treatment of the disruptive behaviors associated with PDDs, with efficacy being demonstrated in both controlled and open trials. The evidence for the other second-generation agents is mixed, with olanzapine and aripiprazole demonstrating some promise while the reports of benefit from quetiapine and ziprasidone are less encouraging. Further controlled study of these medications in the treatment of PDDs is clearly needed.

Tourette's disorder. Two 8-week randomized controlled trials in pediatric and adult patients with Tourette's disorder showed risperidone to be significantly superior to placebo in reducing symptom severity (Dion et al. 2002; Scahill et al. 2003). The mean daily dose of risperidone was comparable in both studies (2.5 mg/day), and risperidone was generally well tolerated. An average weight increase of 2.5 kg was reported in the treatment group of one study (Scahill et al. 2003), with no increase in weight in the placebo group. Gaffney et al. (2002) found risperidone and clonidine to be equally efficacious in reducing tic symptoms in a randomized 8-week trial of 21 children and adolescents.

Olanzapine has shown benefit in treating tics in a small open trial and an 8-week single-blind pilot study (Stephens et al. 2004). A potential role for quetiapine has been suggested by case reports and a small open-label trial (Mukaddes and Abali 2003). A pilot study comparing ziprasidone and placebo in the treatment of children and adolescents with Tourette's disorder reported significant clinical improvement and was well tolerated by the study subjects (Sallee et al. 2000). Controlled studies are needed in order to more clearly establish safety and efficacy.

Conduct disorder and aggression. In 2003, the Treatment Recommendations for the Use of Antipsychotics for Aggressive Youth (TRAAY) were developed in collaboration with the Center for the Advancement of Children's Mental Health at Columbia University, the New York State Office of Mental Health, and experts across the country (Pappadopulos et al. 2003; Schur et al. 2003). The group developed recommenda-

tions for psychosocial and pharmacological interventions in the treatment of aggressive children and adolescents. In brief, the group found that antipsychotic agents in general, and the "atypical" or second-generation antipsychotics in particular, were effective in the treatment of aggression in selected pediatric populations, but added that further studies were required.

Risperidone is the most studied second-generation antipsychotic for the treatment of pediatric aggression. A double-blind study of the use of risperidone (up to 3 mg/day) in the treatment of conduct disorder reported significant improvement in aggressive symptoms in a population of 10 youths when compared with placebo (Findling et al. 2000).

Risperidone was significantly superior to placebo in controlling disruptive behaviors in a double-blind, controlled study of 110 children with a disruptive behavior disorder and subaverage IQ by Snyder et al. (2002). The benefit from risperidone was not affected by comorbid ADHD, concomitant stimulant use, disruptive behavior disorder diagnosis, or IQ. Although somnolence was a commonly reported side effect in both the treatment and placebo groups, the beneficial effects of risperidone in controlling disruptive behaviors appeared to be independent of its sedating effects. A similarly designed companion study of 118 children by Aman et al. (2002) produced comparable results. In both studies, the mean dose of risperidone used was modest (0.98 mg/day and 1.16 mg/day, respectively).

Turgay et al. (2002) demonstrated the longer-term benefits of risperidone in this patient population in a 48-week open-label extension trial of the initial study by Snyder et al. (2002). The mean dose of risperidone in this study was 1.38 mg/day and was generally well tolerated. Weight gain was significant, and 26% of participants experienced EPS, but no cases of tardive dyskinesia were reported. A similarly designed follow-up study by Findling et al. (2004), using participants from the previously reported randomized controlled trial by Aman et al. (2002), produced comparable results. In the Findling study, the mean dose of risperidone used was 1.51 mg/day.

Literature on the use of aripiprazole (Findling et al. 2003a), clozapine (Soderstrom et al. 2002), olanzapine (Handen and Hardan 2006; Soderstrom et al. 2002), and quetiapine (Findling et al. 2007) in the treatment of aggression in pediatric patients is limited to case reports, small case series, or small open trials. Intramuscular ziprasidone was successfully used to treat acute agitation in a case report of 3 boys by Hazaray et al. (2004). The authors were quick to point out, however, that these findings must be considered in light of

Measham's (1995) report that intramuscular injections can often reduce disruptive and aggressive behavior even if placebo is administered. Further study of these medications in pediatric aggression is needed.

Initiation and Maintenance

Medication should not be used as the sole treatment in the aforementioned complex disorders. Before medication is initiated, a complete physical examination and baseline laboratory workup, including CBC with differential, serum chemistries including fasting glucose and liver-associated enzymes, TSH, lipid studies, and urinalysis, should be done. A baseline EEG is recommended in children being treated with clozapine, and a weekly white blood cell (WBC) count with differential is mandatory for at least the first 6 months of clozapine therapy. Antipsychotic medication use has been linked to the development of type II diabetes mellitus that may or may not be related to weight gain. Patients treated with atypical agents should specifically be monitored for changes in weight, as well as changes in fasting glucose levels. Both first- and second-generation antipsychotic agents have been shown to increase QT intervals on ECG, potentially leading to dysrhythmias and sudden death. Clinicians should consider ECG monitoring, when appropriate.

Doses must be titrated individually, with careful attention to positive and negative effects. Age, weight, and severity of symptoms do not provide clear guidelines. The initial dose should be very low, with gradual increments no more than once or twice a week. Although divided doses are often used during titration, in most cases, once a therapeutic dosage has been reached, a single daily dose (usually at bedtime) can be used. Children metabolize these drugs more rapidly than do adults but also require lower plasma levels for efficacy (Teicher and Glod 1990). Antipsychotic medications can interact with a wide variety of other drugs (Teicher and Glod 1990). Dosing guidelines for the second-generation antipsychotics can be found in Table 36–10.

Schizophrenia. Older adolescents with schizophrenia may require doses of medication in the adult range. Young adolescents fall in between, and doses must be empirically determined because there are few data. It may require several weeks for full efficacy to be achieved. While data are small, they are suggestive of the benefit and safety of the use of atypical antipsychotics as first-line agents in this population. Due to potential lethal side effects, clozapine should only be used in cases refractory to treatment with other first- or second-generation agents and should be started at very low dosages—12.5 mg/day or 25 mg/day—and titrated slowly to minimize side effects to an expected dosage range of 250–500 mg/day. Risperidone should be initiated at low doses (0.25–0.5 mg) and titrated slowly, to prevent development of EPS, to an expected dosage range of 2.0–4.0 mg/day. Olanzapine may be started at 5.0 mg/day and titrated to an expected dosage range of 10–15 mg/day.

Pervasive developmental disorders. It is important to give a trial of sufficient length to determine if the drug is efficacious, barring serious side effects requiring immediate discontinuation. At 3- to 6-month intervals, consideration may be given to discontinuation of the drug to observe for withdrawal dyskinesias and to determine if continued treatment is still necessary. Developmentally disturbed children treated with risperidone may benefit from dosages as low as 0.5–1.0 mg/day, with most responding to doses between 0.5 and 2 mg/day. Therapeutic daily dosages for olanzapine may range from 5 to 20 mg.

Tourette's disorder. Careful monitoring of patients with Tourette's disorder for several months before starting medication is possible, given that Tourette's is a chronic condition and not usually an emergency. This monitoring permits the clinician to establish a baseline of symptoms and to assess the need for psychological and educational interventions. Risperidone dosages in the range of 0.5–2.5 mg/day appear to be useful. Sallee et al. (2000) initiated ziprasidone at 5 mg/day, titrating as high as 40 mg/day to achieve clinical effect in the Tourette's disorder children they studied. Effective dosages of quetiapine in the two published reports ranged from 50 to 150 mg/day (Mukaddes and Abali 2003; Párraga et al. 2001). For olanzapine, dosages of 10–15 mg/day may be helpful (Stephens et al. 2004).

Risks and Side Effects

An excellent review of second-generation antipsychotic side effects in children can be found in Correll et al. (2006).

Extrapyramidal side effects. Acute EPS, including dystonic reactions, parkinsonian tremor, rigidity and drooling, and akathisia, occur as in adults and may be induced by either first- or second-generation agents. Laryngeal dystonia is potentially fatal. Acute dystonia may be treated with oral or intramuscular diphenhydramine, 25 mg or 50 mg, or benztropine mesylate, 0.5–2.0 mg. Adolescent boys seem to be more vulner-

TABLE 36–10. Clinical use of second-generation antipsychotics in pediatric patients

Generic name	How supplied	Indications	Target adult dosing	Pediatric dosing	Remarks
Aripiprazole	2-, 5-, 10-, 15-, 20-, 30-mg tablets 1 mg/mL oral solution	Schizophrenia Acute bipolar mania Maintenance treatment for bipolar disorder	10–15 mg/day 30 mg/day 15–30 mg/day	10–15 mg/day[a]	Start with a dose of 5–10 mg/day in pediatric patients. Maximum dosage is 30 mg/day.
Clozapine	12.5-, 25-, 50-, 100-, 200-mg tablets	Treatment-resistant schizophrenia	300–600 mg/day	250–500 mg/day[b]	Use only in cases where patients do not adequately respond to first- or second-generation agents. Start treatment with 12.5 mg/day; maximum dosage in adults is 900 mg/day. Patients taking clozapine are at risk of developing agranulocytosis, myocarditis, other cardiac side effects, or seizures. Frequent blood monitoring required.
Olanzapine	2.5-, 5.0-, 7.5-, 10-, 15-, 20-mg tablets[c] 5-, 10-, 15-, 20-mg orally disintegrating tablets 10 mg intramuscular	Schizophrenia Acute bipolar mania Maintenance treatment for bipolar disorder	10 mg/day 10–15 mg/day (range 5–20 mg/day) 5–20 mg/day	5–15 mg/day	Start with a dosage of 2.5 mg/day in children, 5 mg/day in adolescents, and 5–10 mg/day in adults. Dosage changes should be made weekly, due to the medication's long half-life. Maximum adult dosage is 20 mg/day.
Quetiapine	25-, 100-, 200-, 300-mg tablets	Schizophrenia Acute bipolar mania	300–400 mg/day 400–800 mg/day	300–800 mg/day[d]	Dosed bid or tid. Start with 25–50 mg/day in divided doses; increase by 25–50 mg every 1–2 days as tolerated. Maximum dosage in adults is 800 mg/day. Ophthalmological examination for cataracts is recommended before starting treatment and at 6-month intervals thereafter.

TABLE 36–10. Clinical use of second-generation antipsychotics in pediatric patients *(continued)*

Generic name	How supplied	Indications	Target adult dosing	Pediatric dosing	Remarks
Risperidone	0.25-, 0.5-, 1-, 2-, 3-, 4-mg tablets[c] 0.5, 1.0, 2.0 mg orally disintegrating tablets 1 mg/mL oral solution[c] 25-mg, 37.5-mg, 50-mg intramuscular depot	Schizophrenia Acute bipolar mania	4–8 mg/day 1–6 mg/day	2–6 mg/day	May be dosed qd or bid. Maximum adult dosage is 16 mg/day. Start with 0.25 mg in children, 0.5 mg in adolescents.
Ziprasidone		Schizophrenia Acute bipolar mania	40–200 mg/ day 80–160 mg/ day	20–120 mg/ day	Dosed bid. Usual adult starting doses are 20 mg bid in schizophrenia, and 40 mg bid in acute mania, increased every 1–2 days as tolerated. Baseline electrocardiogram, with repeat after dose stabilization, is recommended due to potential for QTc prolongation.

Note. bid=twice-daily dosing; qd=once-daily dosing; tid=three-times-per-day dosing. All second-generation antipsychotics carry a "black box" warning regarding increased mortality in elderly patients with dementia-related psychosis. None of the above medications have a U.S. Food and Drug Administration (FDA)–approved pediatric indication. Pediatric dosing guidelines are derived from available literature and are recommendations only. Dosing of these medications in pediatric patients should be titrated based on tolerability and symptom response. These medications are often used in pediatric patients for conditions other than those for which they are indicated in adults, such as for disruptive behavior disorders, pervasive developmental disorders, and Tourette's disorder. Published reports of the use of second-generation antipsychotics in conditions other than schizophrenia and acute mania are limited, especially in the pediatric age group. Reported dosage ranges vary widely when used for these other conditions and may differ from the dosage ranges used for schizophrenia or acute mania. Please consult chapter text and manufacturers' product inserts for further prescribing information.

[a]Dosages in most pediatric studies ranged from 1 to 15 mg/day.
[b]Dosages in most pediatric studies in schizophrenia ranged from 75 to 500 mg/day.
[c]Tentative FDA approval received for generic preparation as of 15 April 2006.
[d]Limited information on pediatric dosing of quetiapine is available. Individual case studies report dosages of 100–600 mg/day, with Tourette's disorder being treated by dosages of 50–150 mg/day. Larger case studies report dosages ranging from 300 to 800 mg/day, predominantly for schizophrenia or acute mania.
Source. Adapted from product labeling and information available from Drugs@FDA (http://www.fda.gov/cder).

able to acute dystonic reactions than are adult patients, so the physician may be more inclined to use prophylactic antiparkinsonian medication. In children, however, reduction of antipsychotic dose is preferable to the use of antiparkinsonian agents (Campbell et al. 1985).

For treatment or prevention of parkinsonian symptoms, adolescents may be given the anticholinergic drug benztropine mesylate, 1–2 mg/day, in divided doses. Chronic parkinsonian symptoms are often drastically underrecognized by clinicians (Richardson et al. 1991). The neuromuscular consequences may impair the performance of age-appropriate activities, and the subjective effects may lead to noncompliance with medication. Akathisia may be especially difficult to identify in young patients or those with limited verbal abilities.

Tardive and withdrawal dyskinesias.   Tardive or withdrawal dyskinesias, some transient but others irreversible, mandate caution regarding the casual use of these drugs. Tardive dyskinesia has been documented in children and adolescents after as brief a period of treatment as 5 months with a first-generation agent (Herskowitz 1987) and may appear even during periods of constant medication dose. Cases of tardive dyskinesia have also been reported in youths treated with second-generation antipsychotics (Kumra et al. 1998), indicating that patients treated with these newer medications may not be immune to this serious adverse reaction. In children with autism or Tourette's disorder, it may be especially difficult to distinguish medication-induced movements from those characteristic of the disorder. Before patients begin taking an antipsychotic medication, they should be examined carefully for abnormal movements by using a scale such as the Abnormal Involuntary Movement Scale (AIMS 1988) and should be periodically reexamined. Parents and patients (if they are able) should receive regular explanations of the risk of movement disorders.

Cardiovascular side effects.   Antipsychotic medications have been associated with prolongation of the QTc interval, torsades de pointes, and sudden death (Glassman and Bigger 2001). Certain antipsychotics may be at greater risk for causing these problems. Thioridazine possesses a "black box" warning due to its significantly greater risk for causing QTc prolongation and sudden death. Haloperidol has also been associated with torsades de pointes.

Ziprasidone has been shown to have a clear effect on cardiac repolarization, resulting in QTc prolongation that is greater than with most antipsychotic agents, but less than with thioridazine. While no evidence of serious cardiac events occurred during the premarketing testing of ziprasidone, its association with sudden death remains unclear at this time (Glassman and Bigger 2001). Blair et al. (2005) conducted a prospective open-label trial of ziprasidone use in 20 children and adolescents at relatively low dosages (≤40 mg/day). The mean QTc prolongation was 28 ms, which, the authors noted, was greater than the initially observed increases in QTc that caused the FDA to require a highlighted caution about this effect in ziprasidone's product labeling. Eight of the 20 children in the study experienced a QTc of ≥440 ms, and three experienced a QTc of ≥450 ms. Incidentally, Blair et al. also remarked on the poor correlation between manual and automated computation of the QTc interval and advised clinicians to be wary of taking a machine-calculated QTc at face value. Based on these findings, the prudent use of ECG monitoring at baseline and during dosage titration in medications that are of higher risk seems indicated.

The use of clozapine has been associated with the development of other cardiotoxicities, such as cardiomyopathy, myocarditis, and pericarditis, which have also occurred in the pediatric age group (Wehmeier et al. 2004). Clinicians entertaining the use of clozapine in pediatric patients should be mindful of the potential development of these cardiac side effects and should monitor patients accordingly.

Metabolic side effects.   Weight gain may be problematic with the use of antipsychotics, especially second-generation medications (Martin et al. 2004). The weight gain associated with risperidone, while significant, appears less than that associated with olanzapine (Vieweg et al. 2005). Distinguishing growth-related weight gain from weight gain associated with antipsychotic use can be problematic in children and adolescents, and no specific criteria have been widely adopted (Correll 2005). Measurements of height and weight and calculations of body mass index (BMI) are recommended before initiation of treatment with antipsychotic agents and at regular intervals thereafter.

Reports of children and adolescents developing hyperglycemia or diabetes mellitus after treatment with second-generation agents have been published, although polypharmacy or family histories of diabetes were present in many instances. Until further studies elucidate a clear relationship (or not) between second-generation agents and the development of hyperglycemia or diabetes mellitus in children, prudence would suggest especially cautious use of these agents in children who are already overweight or who have a strong family history of diabetes. Baseline measurement of fasting blood sugar, with occasional measurements thereafter, is recommended for all patients treated with these medications.

Other side effects. Hyperprolactinemia is a potential effect of treatment with antipsychotic agents, due to their effects on tuberoinfundibular pathways within the CNS, although this potential is theoretically lower with the second-generation agents, due to their serotonergic effects that result in decreased stimulation of prolactin secretion (Stahl 2000). Hyperprolactinemia has been associated with galactorrhea, menstrual irregularities, sexual dysfunction, and osteoporosis. Pappagallo and Silva (2004) have described several cases of elevated prolactin levels in their review of pediatric patients treated with atypical antipsychotic agents. Saito et al. (2004) prospectively studied 40 children and adolescents treated with risperidone, olanzapine, or quetiapine and found that prolactin levels after a mean of 11 weeks were significantly higher in children taking risperidone than olanzapine or quetiapine. Findling et al. (2003b) pooled the results of five clinical trials of risperidone in pediatric patients and found that while risperidone elevated prolactin levels in the early weeks of treatment, the prolactin level for girls returned to within normal limits by the 12th week of treatment, and the mean level for boys declined to just above the upper limit of normal by the 24th week of treatment. For both boys and girls, the mean prolactin level had returned to a normal range by the 48th week of treatment, although mean values were still above baseline. Findling et al. (2003b) also noted that only 13 of 592 children developed symptoms possibly attributable to hyperprolactinemia and that 9 of these children showed resolution of these symptoms by the end of the study.

With first-generation agents, another concern is behavioral toxicity, manifested as worsening of preexisting symptoms or development of new symptoms such as hyperactivity or hypoactivity, irritability, apathy, withdrawal, stereotypies, tics, or hallucinations (Campbell et al. 1985). Sedation, which is common with atypical antipsychotics, may also be experienced with low-potency first-generation antipsychotic drugs such as chlorpromazine and thioridazine and can interfere with the patient's ability to benefit from school. Children may be at greater risk of antipsychotic-induced seizures than adults because of their immature nervous systems and the high prevalence of abnormal EEGs in seriously disturbed children.

Anticholinergic side effects such as hypotension, dry mouth, constipation, nasal congestion, blurred vision, and urinary retention are most commonly experienced with low-potency first-generation antipsychotics and appear to be unusual in children. Potentially fatal neuroleptic malignant syndrome has been reported in children and adolescents (Chungh et al. 2005), with a presentation similar to that seen in adults.

Anxiolytics, Sedatives, and Hypnotics

There are few data on the safety and efficacy of anxiolytics and sedative-hypnotics in children and adolescents, although this population appears to respond similarly to adults (Spencer et al. 1995). In most cases, psychosocial interventions should precede and accompany pharmacotherapy.

Benzodiazepines

Indications and efficacy. Little research has been done on the use of benzodiazepines for pediatric psychiatric conditions. Benzodiazepines may be useful in the short-term treatment of children with severe anticipatory anxiety (Pfefferbaum et al. 1987). Although an open trial of alprazolam for children with avoidant and overanxious disorders was promising, a double-blind study did not find superiority of this drug over placebo in the context of an intensive treatment program (Simeon et al. 1992). Efficacy may have been limited by low doses and the short duration of treatment.

Preliminary evidence suggests that clonazepam may be useful in the treatment of panic disorder and neuroleptic-induced akathisia in adolescents (Biederman 1987; Kutcher et al. 1989). In a double-blind, placebo-controlled study, Graae et al. (1994) reported the clinical effectiveness of clonazepam in the treatment of anxiety disorders (predominantly separation anxiety disorder) in children. However, statistical superiority over placebo was not found, and most children evidenced side effects, notably sedation and disinhibition.

Initiation and maintenance. Infants and children absorb diazepam faster and metabolize it more quickly than do adults (Simeon and Ferguson 1985). Usual daily dose ranges for children and adolescents are as follows: lorazepam, 0.25–6.00 mg; diazepam, 1–20 mg; and alprazolam, 0.25–4.00 mg. Clonazepam has been used at 0.5–3.0 mg/day. Dosage schedule depends on age (more frequent in children) and the specific drug (Coffey 1990). When the medication is being discontinued, the dose needs to be tapered gradually to avoid withdrawal seizures or rebound anxiety.

Risks and side effects.   In addition to the risks of substance abuse and physical or psychological dependence, side effects include sedation, cognitive dulling, ataxia, confusion, emotional lability, and worsening of psychosis. Paradoxical or disinhibition reactions may occur, manifested by acute excitation, irritability, increased anxiety, hallucinations, increased aggression and hostility, rage reactions, insomnia, euphoria, and/or incoordination.

Buspirone

Buspirone is a nonbenzodiazepine anxiolytic that is reported to be less sedating and have less risk of abuse or dependence than do the benzodiazepines. It also has been reported possibly to have weak antidepressant efficacy.

Indications and efficacy.   Most reports on buspirone treatment of anxiety disorders in children are anecdotal. Other suggested uses include reducing aggression and anxiety in patients with mental retardation (Ratey et al. 1991) or PDDs (Buitelaar et al. 1998), and as a treatment for ADHD (Niederhofer 2003). Randomized controlled clinical studies are needed to assess the safety and efficacy of buspirone for pediatric psychiatric conditions.

Initiation and maintenance.   Tentative guidelines for children and adolescents suggest a starting dosage of 2.5–5.0 mg/day, increasing to three times a day over 2–3 days (Kutcher et al. 1992). The dosage may be increased gradually to a maximum of 20 mg/day in children and 60 mg/day in adolescents, in three divided doses. The therapeutic effects may be delayed for 1–2 weeks after reaching the proper dosage, with maximal effects not seen for an additional 2 weeks (Coffey 1990).

Risks and side effects.   Reported adverse effects include insomnia, dizziness, anxiety, nausea, headache, restlessness, agitation, depression, and confusion (Coffey 1990). Possible psychotic symptoms were reported in two children treated with buspirone (Soni and Weintraub 1992), indicating that clinicians should closely monitor children who are prescribed this medication.

Beta-Blocking Agents

Indications and Efficacy

A comprehensive review of the literature by Connor (1993) commented on the lack of methodologically controlled studies of β-blockers in the treatment of aggression in the pediatric population. Little has been added to the literature since then. Propranolol has been found to be effective in daily doses of 50–960 mg, with a median of 160 mg, in patients with otherwise uncontrollable rage reactions and impulsive aggression or self-injurious behavior, especially those with evidence of organicity (Williams et al. 1982). A study by Connor et al. (1997) examined the use of nadolol in the treatment of overt aggression in 12 developmentally delayed youths ages 13–24 years. Seven of the 12 participants received nadolol exclusively. In this open prospective pilot study, 10 of the 12 patients showed improvement in observer-rated measures of aggression and severity of illness. Anecdotal reports suggest that propranolol may be effective in the treatment of agitated, hyperaroused children and adolescents with PTSD (Famularo et al. 1988) and children and adolescents with "hyperventilation attacks" (Joorabchi 1977). In an open trial, a single dose of 40 mg propranolol appeared to be helpful in reducing test anxiety and improving performance in high school students (Faigel 1991). Pindolol and nadolol, with fewer side effects and longer half-lives, have been suggested as alternatives. Randomized controlled studies are needed.

Initiation and Maintenance

Initial workup should include a recent history and physical examination, with particular attention to medical contraindications: asthma, diabetes, bradycardia, heart block, cardiac failure, or hypothyroidism. Fasting blood sugar and glucose tolerance tests may be indicated if there is risk of diabetes. An ECG may be considered.

In children and adolescents, the initial dose of propranolol is 10 mg three times a day, increasing by 10–20 mg every 3–4 days, and pulse and blood pressure should be monitored (minimum pulse 50, blood pressure 80/50). The standard daily dose range is 10–120 mg for children and 20–300 mg for adolescents, divided into three doses (2–8 mg/kg/day) (Coffey 1990). The short elimination half-life in children (2–3 hours) may necessitate four doses daily. Dose is titrated to clinical effect or side effects. Maximum improvement at a given dose may not be seen for up to 8 weeks. β-Blockers should be tapered gradually, rather than abruptly discontinued, in order to avoid rebound hypertension and tachycardia. Because β-blockers may alter the blood levels of other medications, caution must be observed when β-blockers (especially propranolol, which is highly protein bound) are used in combination with other agents.

Risks and Side Effects

Side effects of β-blockers are generally the same as in adults. Tiredness, mild hypotension, and bradycardia are the most common. Decreased sexual interest and performance, dysphoria, insomnia, nightmares, or hypoglycemia (in patients with diabetes) may occur.

Naltrexone and Acamprosate

Abnormalities of endogenous opioids have been suggested to occur in persons who have autism and in mentally retarded persons who engage in self-injurious behavior. Published reports are mixed regarding the benefits of naltrexone, a potent opiate antagonist, in these conditions. Several double-blind and placebo-controlled studies have shown naltrexone to be effective in the treatment of hyperactivity in autistic children (Kolmen et al. 1995; Willemsen-Swinkels et al. 1996). Although earlier reports suggested that naltrexone treatment increased social interaction and decreased self-injury in autistic patients, these later controlled studies failed to demonstrate statistical difference from response to placebo in regard to these behaviors. A double-blind, placebo-controlled crossover study by Feldman et al. (1999) failed to demonstrate improvement in communication skills when comparing naltrexone to placebo in autistic children. However, the study was limited by a short period of assessment per drug (2 weeks). In their randomized, placebo-controlled crossover study of 25 patients with Rett syndrome who received naltrexone, Percy et al. (1994) showed a worsening of motor function and a more rapid progression of the disorder in 40% of those individuals taking naltrexone compared with none of the individuals taking placebo.

Case reports and a small open-label study (Deas et al. 2005) suggest that naltrexone may be of benefit in alcohol dependence in adolescents. All of the patients were treated with naltrexone 50 mg/day. These reports, while anecdotal, suggest that naltrexone may have a place in the treatment of alcohol dependence in adolescents, as it does in adults, although further study is needed.

In doses of 0.5–2.0 mg/kg/day, naltrexone appears to be safe, with only mild side effects noted. No changes in any laboratory measures, ECG, or vital signs have been demonstrated in children or adolescents.

Acamprosate is a glutamate receptor modulator recently approved in the United States for the treatment of alcohol dependence in adult patients who are abstinent at the time of initiation of treatment. A small double-blind, placebo-controlled study of adolescents with alcohol dependence by Niederhofer and Staffen (2003) reported that, at the end of the 3-month study, 7 of the 13 adolescents treated with acamprosate remained abstinent, compared with 2 of the 13 adolescents treated with placebo. Larger controlled trials of the use of acamprosate in alcohol-dependent adolescents are needed.

Desmopressin

Desmopressin (DDAVP) is an analog of antidiuretic hormone administered as a nasal spray or oral tablet to treat nocturnal enuresis. DDAVP acts by increasing water absorption in the kidneys, thereby reducing the volume of urine. Onset of action is rapid, and side effects are mild (nasal mucosal dryness or irritation, headache, epistaxis, and nausea) in patients with normal electrolyte regulation. In their review of the literature, Thompson and Rey (1995) concluded that DDAVP is superior to placebo in the treatment of nocturnal enuresis. They further noted that behavioral methods are more effective and that the relapse rate after cessation of DDAVP is high. Most of the studies cited at that time were of brief duration, usually 2 weeks. A year-long open study by Hjalmas et al. (1998) supports the safe and effective longer-term use of DDAVP.

The usual dosage is 20–40 μg intranasally at bedtime or 0.2–0.4 mg orally. Randomized, double-blind studies have demonstrated that oral DDAVP is equally efficacious to the intranasal preparation and may be better tolerated. (Janknegt et al. 1997; Skoog et al. 1997). Relapse is likely upon discontinuation of treatment. Water intoxication is rare, but children should be encouraged to limit fluid intake in the evenings when taking DDAVP.

Electroconvulsive Therapy

Electroconvulsive therapy (ECT) is currently reserved for the treatment of adolescents who have not responded to more conservative interventions (such as several trials of medication) or whose symptoms (such as severe and persistent suicidal intent) require an urgent treatment response. Experience in the use of ECT in adolescents is limited and is extremely rare in prepubertal children. The current AACAP practice parameter on the use of ECT in adolescents (Ghaziuddin et al. 2004) offers a thorough review of the literature and guidelines for the use of this treatment modality in adolescents.

Psychotherapy

Introduction

An increasing focus on evidence-based medicine has resulted in more attention being paid to the research and practice of psychotherapy. While psychotherapy for children has been shown to be effective when performed in a research setting (Kazdin 2000; Weisz 2000), the results are often less favorable when psychotherapy provided in the clinical or office setting is studied (B. Weiss et al. 2000; Weisz and Jensen 2001). Compared with children seen in research environments, children seen in "real world" clinical practice are often more symptomatic, have other comorbid conditions, have more psychosocially stressed families, and receive more eclectic forms of psychotherapy (Borkovec and Miranda 1996; Kazdin 2000; Weisz 2000).

Several methodological challenges also arise in research examining the efficacy of psychotherapy for children and adolescents. Donenberg (1999) outlined some of these challenges, which include accounting for the many influences in children's lives that affect treatment and functioning, as well as determining what (or who) should be the focus of change (e.g., parent, child, style of parenting). Moreover, how should outcomes in psychotherapy be measured, and who (e.g., parent, child, teacher) should do the measuring? Finally, how does the ongoing development of the child influence the effectiveness of therapy? The importance of an examination of the different issues related to psychotherapy research is that it will inform our understanding of how the biological, psychological, and social changes brought about by psychotherapy provide relief for suffering children and their families.

Psychotherapies are classified according to theoretical model, target of intervention, duration, or goals of treatment. There are presently more than 550 therapeutic techniques used in child and adolescent psychotherapy (Kazdin 2000). More data are emerging regarding the use and efficacy of specific forms of psychotherapy for particular disorders, especially depressive and anxiety disorders. The following sections describe, in very general terms, some of the more common forms of psychotherapy used in children. These therapies are also listed in Table 36–11. More thorough explanations of the various techniques of psychotherapy as they are applied to children may be found in therapy-specific reference materials and treatment manuals.

TABLE 36–11. Varieties of psychotherapy

Theoretical foundations
  Cognitive-behavioral (CBT)
  Behavioral or social learning
  Developmental
  Interpersonal (IPT)
  Family systems
  Psychoanalytic
Target of intervention
  Individual
  Parent
  Family
  Group
Duration
  Short (4–6 sessions)
  Intermediate (up to 6 months)
  Long (6 months to years)
Goals of therapy
  Crisis intervention
  Support
  Symptom removal
  Relief of developmental arrests

Note. CBT = cognitive-behavioral therapy; IPT = interpersonal therapy.

Individual Psychotherapy

All individual therapies have certain common themes (Strupp 1973):

- Relationship with a therapist who is identified as a helping person and who has some degree of control and influence over the patient
- Instillation of hope and improved morale
- Use of attention, encouragement, and suggestion
- Goals of helping the patient to achieve greater control, competence, mastery, and/or autonomy; to improve coping skills; and to abandon or modify unrealistic expectations of himself or herself, others, and the environment

In the treatment of children, it is essential to consider the patients' environment and family dynamics. In most cases, work with parents and school, and often pediatricians, welfare agencies, courts, or recreation leaders, must accompany individual therapy. The cooperation of parents, and often teachers, is required to maintain the child in treatment and to remove any secondary gain resulting from the symptoms. The therapist must be aware of a patient's level of physical, cognitive, and emotional development in order to understand the symptoms, set appropriate goals, and tailor effective interventions.

Communication With Children and Adolescents

Children are less able to use abstract language than are adults. They use play to express feelings, to narrate past events, to work through trauma, and to regress. It is less threatening and anxiety provoking if the therapist works in the displacement, uses the metaphor of the play, and bases questions and comments on characters in the play rather than on the child (even if the connection is clear to the therapist). Effective communications are tailored to the child's stage of language, cognitive, and affective development. The therapist must be aware that the vocabulary of some bright and precocious children exceeds their emotional understanding of events and concepts.

Dramatic play with dolls or puppets, drawing, painting, or modeling with clay, as well as questions about dreams, wishes, or favorite stories or television shows, can provide access to children's fantasies, emotions, and concerns. Adolescents may prefer creative writing or more complex expressive art techniques.

The Resistant Child or Adolescent

It is not surprising that many children or adolescents do not cooperate in therapy, because most are brought to treatment by adults. These young patients often do not wish to change themselves or their behaviors and view their parents' and teachers' complaints as unreasonable or unfair. In addition, a child or adolescent may refuse to participate in or may attempt to sabotage therapy for a variety of dynamic reasons (Gardner 1979). Effective interventions are tailored to the cause of the resistance.

A child who is feeling anxious or having difficulty separating from a parent may be helped by initially permitting the parent to remain in the therapy room. When a child or adolescent does not talk, whether from anxiety or opposition, the therapist often addresses this reluctance, either directly or through play. Long silences are not generally helpful and tend to increase anxiety or battles for control. Attractive play materials help to make therapy less threatening and to encourage participation while the therapist builds an alliance. However, the therapist must guard against

the danger of sessions becoming mere play or recreation instead of therapy. A variety of techniques incorporate therapeutic activities with storytelling, drama, and game boards (Gardner 1979). Using behavioral contingencies in therapy also may improve motivation and cooperation.

Types of Individual Psychotherapy

Psychodynamic psychotherapies. In *psychoanalysis*, a relatively infrequently used treatment modality for children and adolescents, neurotic symptoms are viewed as arising from internalized intrapsychic conflict, nonorganic developmental arrest, or regression. The goals are to remove those symptoms that have become independent of their original context, through structural changes in defensive organization and personality. The analyst functions as a transference object. The principal technique for producing change is interpretation of unconscious content, resulting in greater conscious awareness and adaptive control of emotions and behavior. The expense, frequency of sessions, length of treatment, and often lack of immediate symptom relief have contributed to the decreased use of psychoanalysis.

Psychodynamically oriented psychotherapy is grounded in psychoanalytic theory but is more flexible and emphasizes the real relationship with the therapist and the provision of a corrective emotional experience rather than the transference. Frequency is typically once or twice a week, most commonly over a period of 1–2 years, although shorter, time-limited dynamic psychotherapies are also available (Dulcan 1984). Interaction between the parents and the therapist is more active. Goals of therapy include symptom resolution, change in behavior, and return to normal developmental process. Change occurs via transference interpretation and maturation of defenses, catharsis, development of insight, ego strengthening, improved reality testing, and sublimation (Adams 1982). The therapist forms an alliance with the child or adolescent, reassures, promotes controlled regression, identifies feelings, clarifies thoughts and events, makes interpretations, judiciously educates and advises, and acts as an advocate for the patient (Adams 1982).

Dynamically oriented individual therapy alone is much more likely to be effective for children and adolescents who are in emotional distress or who are struggling to deal with a stressor than for those children with behavior problems. Children and adolescents with attention-deficit, oppositional, or conduct disorders rarely acknowledge their problem behaviors and are usually better treated in family or group therapy, by parent training in behavior management, or in a structured milieu. Youngsters with ADHD have little insight into their behavior and its effect on others, and they may be genuinely unable to report their problems or to reflect on them. However, insight-oriented therapy may be useful for some of these youngsters to address comorbid anxiety or depression or symptoms resulting from psychological trauma. Psychoanalytic therapy is usually considered contraindicated in psychotic or very disturbed children (Sours 1978).

Supportive therapy. This type of therapy has less ambitious goals than dynamically oriented psychotherapies and is usually focused on a particular crisis or stressor. The therapist provides support to the patient until a stressor resolves, a developmental crisis has passed, or the patient or environment changes sufficiently so that other adults can take on the supportive role. There is a real relationship with the therapist, who facilitates catharsis and provides understanding and judicious advice.

Time-limited therapy. All of the various models of time-limited therapy have in common a planned, relatively brief duration; a predominant focus on the presenting problem; a high degree of structure and attention to specific, limited goals; and active roles for both therapist and patient. Length of treatment varies among models from several sessions to 6 months. The short duration is used to increase patient motivation, participation, and reliance on resources within the patient's world rather than on the therapist (Kisch 1997). Theoretical foundations include psychodynamic, crisis, family systems, cognitive, behavioral or social learning and guidance, or educational theories (Dulcan 1984; Dulcan and Piercy 1985).

The limited outcome data available indicate that time-limited treatment is at least as effective for some patients as longer-term therapy. These methods have been recommended for both multiproblem families in crisis who are unlikely to persist in longer-term treatment and well-functioning children and families who have circumscribed problems of relatively recent onset.

Although time-limited treatment is designed to be brief, children or families may return to a therapist should other problems or symptoms develop for an additional "round" of treatment. Such intermittent interaction can remain problem focused and reduce dependency on the therapist (Kisch 1997).

Interpersonal psychotherapy. A model of interpersonal psychotherapy has been modified for depressed adolescents (IPT-A) (Mufson et al. 2004a). This 12-week treatment focuses on improving interpersonal relationships in the lives of depressed adolescents through role clarification and enhanced communication. This modality has been elaborated in a treatment manual and has demonstrated efficacy in several controlled studies (Mufson et al. 2004b).

Cognitive-behavioral therapy. The CBT techniques developed for the treatment of depression in adults have been adapted for use in children and adolescents. CBT has been shown in numerous controlled trials to be efficacious in the treatment of anxiety and depressive disorders in children and adolescents (Compton et al. 2004). Other randomized studies have shown CBT to be effective in treating pediatric PTSD (Cohen et al. 2005; Smith et al. 2007). Caution is needed to ensure that homework assignments that are an integral part of this therapy are not perceived as aversive when added to homework assigned in school. Prepubertal children's more concrete cognitive processes may make this rather intellectual model impractical, although creative adaptations and the incorporation of behavioral techniques can render this approach accessible (Emery et al. 1983). Studies have also shown that cognitive self-control training may be effective in reducing aggressive behavior in adolescents (Kazdin 2000; Weisz et al. 2004).

Parent Counseling

Parent counseling or guidance is primarily a psychoeducational intervention, conducted in a mental health setting. It may be conducted with a single parent or couple, or in groups. In counseling sessions, parents learn about normal child and adolescent development. Efforts are made to help parents better understand their child and his or her problems and to modify practices that may be contributing to the current difficulties (whatever their original cause). The therapist's understanding of the parents' point of view and of the hardships of living with a disturbed child is crucial to the therapist's successful work with the child. For some parents who have serious difficulties of their own, parent counseling may merge into or pave the way for individual treatment of the adult or couple.

Virtually all parents of children with psychiatric or learning problems need and deserve education in the nature of their children's disorders, support of their own emotional needs, and help in selecting treatments and managing difficult behaviors. Parents spend far more time with their children than the therapist and can powerfully assist or impede treatment. Parents of children with chronic problems must become skilled advocates to ensure that their children receive the treatment and schooling they need. Carefully selected reading material and other resources may be extremely useful to parents.

Behavior Therapy

In behavior therapy, symptoms are viewed as resulting from bad habits, faulty learning, or inappropriate environmental responses to behavior rather than as stemming from unconscious or intrapsychic motivation. Attention is focused on observable behaviors, psychophysiological responses, and self-report statements. Behavioral approaches are characterized by detailed assessment of problematic responses and the environmental conditions that elicit and maintain them, the development of strategies to produce change in the environment and therefore in the patient's behavior, and repeated assessment to evaluate the success of the intervention.

In an operant approach, positive and negative environmental factors that increase and decrease the frequency of behaviors are identified and then modified in an attempt to decrease problem behaviors and increase adaptive ones. The token economy uses points, stars, or tokens that can be earned for desirable behaviors (and lost for problem behaviors) and exchanged for backup reinforcers. These reinforcers may be money, food, toys, privileges, or time with an adult in a pleasant activity. Token economies can be successfully used by parents, teachers, and therapists (with groups or individuals) and by staff on inpatient units.

Indications and Efficacy

Behavior therapy is by far the most thoroughly evaluated psychological treatment for children. Maximally effective programs require home and school cooperation, focus on specific target behaviors, and ensure that contingencies follow behavior quickly and consistently.

Behavior therapy is the most effective treatment for simple phobias, for enuresis and encopresis, and for the noncompliant behaviors seen in oppositional defiant disorder and conduct disorder. For youngsters with ADHD, behavior modification can improve both academic achievement and behavior, if specifically targeted. Both punishment (time-out and response cost) and reward components are required. Behavior modification is more effective than medication in improving peer interactions, but skills may need to be taught first. Many youngsters require programs that are consistent, intensive, and prolonged (months to years). A wide variety of other childhood problems, such as motor and vocal tics, trichotillomania, and sleep problems, are treated by behavior modification, either alone or in combination with pharmacotherapy.

The greatest weaknesses of behavior therapy are lack of maintenance of improvement over time and failure of changes to generalize to situations other than the ones in which training occurred. Generalization and maintenance can be maximized by conducting training in the settings in which behavior change is desired, at multiple times and places, facilitating transfer to naturally occurring reinforcers and gradually fading reinforcement on an intermittent schedule.

Parent Management Training

Effective training packages, based on social learning theory, have been developed for parents of noncompliant, oppositional, and aggressive children (Barkley 1997; Forehand and Long 2002; McMahon and Forehand 2003) and delinquent adolescents (Kazdin 2005; Patterson and Forgatch 2005). Such behaviors in children have been found to lead to inappropriately harsh or ineffective parental responses. Through training, parents are taught to give clear instructions, to positively reinforce good behavior, and to use punishment effectively. One frequently used negative contingency is the time-out, so called because it puts the child in a quiet, boring area where there is a time-out from accidental or naturally occurring positive reinforcement. The most powerful parent training programs use a combination of written materials, verbal instruction, and videotapes in social learning principles and contingency management, modeling by the therapist, and behavioral rehearsal of skills to be used. Families with low socioeconomic status, parental psychopathology (such as depression), marital conflict, and lack of a social support network require maximally potent interventions, with attention to parental problems as necessary. Other families may be able to succeed with written materials only or with manuals supplemented by group lectures. Parent management training (PMT) has been shown to be effective in improving child behavior in meta-analyses conducted by Serketich and Dumas (1996) and Montgomery et al. (2006).

Behavioral intervention can be done in the context of family therapy, in which the family learns how to negotiate and how to solve problems together. A key technique is parent–child contingency contracting, which entails a written social contract between parent and child to change behaviors in both parties, with specified contingencies (Blechman 1981).

Classroom Behavior Modification

Techniques for behavior modification in schools include token economies, class rules, and attention to positive behavior, as well as response cost programs in which reinforcers are withdrawn in response to undesirable behavior. Reinforcers such as positive recognition or stars on a chart may be dispensed by teachers or more tangible rewards or privileges by parents through the use of daily report cards. Even special education teachers rarely have sophisticated skills in behavior modification, and therapists may need to work closely with teachers and other school staff to develop appropriate programs. Effective programs for use in the classroom environment include the Academic and Behavioral Competencies (ABC) program (Pelham et al. 2005) and the Positive Behavior Support program (Sugai and Horner 2002).

Behavioral Treatment of Specific Symptoms

Behavioral treatments are useful for treating enuresis, encopresis, and certain anxiety disorders in children. An evaluation for other psychiatric disorders or trauma as well as a medical history and physical examination should precede behavioral treatment.

Enuresis.   In younger children, especially those who wet only at night, enuresis is largely a consequence of delayed maturation. While waiting for the child to outgrow it, the most useful strategy is to minimize secondary symptoms by discouraging the parents from punishing or ridiculing the child. Older children can be taught to change their own beds, thus reducing expectable negative reactions from parents. A simple monitoring and reward procedure that includes a chart with stars to be exchanged for rewards may be effective for some children who are motivated to stop wetting the bed.

Two additional programs found to be effective in treating nocturnal enuresis are the urine alarm device and dry-bed training (DBT). The urine alarm is a conditioning treatment that results in dryness in 65%–75% of children (Butler and Gasson 2005; Mikkelson 2001). The success rate can be increased and relapses minimized by the addition of various behavioral interventions (Houts 1995). DBT (Azrin et al. 1974) is an equally effective, but somewhat more cumbersome, behavioral program that includes positive practice, contingent response, and the urine alarm in combination.

Combining the urine alarm with a pharmacological treatment is particularly effective in children who are frequent bed-wetters and has been shown to be more effective than the urine alarm alone in one study (Bradbury and Meadow 1995). Butler et al. (2001) have developed a structured withdrawal program to assist in relapse prevention by systematically withdrawing medication (either desmopressin or imipramine) while using a chart to allow children to track dry nights. The program encourages children to focus on internal, rather than external, factors as contributing to their ability to remain dry without medication. Almost 75% of children remained dry in the last 2 weeks of the 10-week program (when no medication was administered), with over 70% of those remaining dry at 6 months' posttreatment.

Children who are secondarily enuretic (having previously been dry) and those who have accompanying psychiatric problems are more difficult to treat. Other interventions may be necessary before they are motivated to participate in or be responsive to behavioral techniques.

Encopresis.   The treatment of encopresis is somewhat more complex, because encopresis frequently results from chronic constipation and stool withholding, which create physiological consequences requiring medical treatment. In addition, children with encopresis more commonly have associated psychiatric disorders than do those with enuresis.

Behavioral treatment of encopresis must be integrated into a plan that also includes educational and psychological approaches (Levine 1982). Because encopresis often results in stool retention and impaction, an initial bowel cleanout is sometimes required. This regimen is followed by a bowel "retraining" program using oral mineral oil, a high-roughage diet, ample fluid intake, and a mild suppository. The behavioral program focuses on the development of a regular toileting routine with scheduled positive toilet practicing. Behaviors that progressively approximate the appropriate passing of feces in the toilet are rewarded. Routine pants checks followed by contingent positive or negative response are often included. Administration of enemas by parents is contraindicated, as that alone does not improve bowel function and is toxic to the parent–child relationship.

Anxiety disorders.   Desensitization, in vivo or in fantasy, is the treatment of choice for simple phobias, often supplemented by modeling. The principles and techniques are essentially the same as those used with adults, with modification for developmental level. In vivo desensitization, often combined with contingency management and parent guidance, may be effective in the treatment of school avoidance (school phobia) resulting from separation anxiety disorder.

Behavioral approaches using exposure and response prevention (E/RP) appear to be effective in the treatment of OCD in children and adolescents. March et al. (1994) have developed a protocoled, time-limited E/RP treatment that has demonstrated therapeutic effect in an open trial with children and adolescents with OCD. In their study of 22 children with OCD randomized to either 12 weeks of behavioral therapy or treatment with clomipramine, De Haan et al. (1998) found that behavioral therapy brought about significantly greater therapeutic improvement than clomipramine as measured by the Children's Yale–Brown Obsessive Compulsive Scale. However, no significant difference in the two treatments was found on the other primary outcome measure, the Leyton Obsessional Inventory—Child Version.

Behavioral Medicine Techniques

Behavioral methods can be used to treat somatic symptoms. These interventions should be carried out in collaboration with the primary physician and any necessary medical specialists. Children are just as sensitive as adults are to implications that their symptoms are not "real," so care must be taken to explain the interaction of psychological processes and physical symptoms and to develop a working alliance.

A variety of techniques have been used for children, in much the same way as for adults, but with adaptations for the children's level of cognitive or emotional development. Especially important is an understanding of any misconceptions youngsters may have about the disease state and its treatment. These notions vary according to a patient's stage of cognitive development and his or her unique experience.

Hypnotherapy. Children are more hypnotizable than are adults (Williams 1979). Although hypnosis is occasionally used to remove a behavioral symptom or habit, for children the most common uses of hypnosis are to treat physical symptoms with a psychological component or to help a child manage pain or nausea associated with a physical disorder or its treatment. Successful use of hypnosis to reduce pain and anxiety has not been reported in children younger than 6 years of age (Varni et al. 1986). An excellent source of information on the use of hypnotherapy in children and adolescents is the text by Olness and Kohen (1996).

Relaxation training. Four types of relaxation procedures are applicable to children and adolescents: progressive muscle relaxation, meditative breathing, autogenics (i.e., silently repeating commands or statements), and imagery-based techniques (Masek et al. 1984). The choice is determined by the characteristics of the child or adolescent and of the disorder being treated. For example, asthmatic children or adolescents may have difficulty using breathing techniques. Imagery may fit particularly well with most children's interest in fantasy. Relaxation training has been used in the treatment of pediatric migraine, juvenile rheumatoid arthritis, and hemophilia. These techniques, also called cognitive-behavioral self-regulation of pain perception, can result not only in decreased subjective experience of pain and reduced need for analgesics but also in improved mood, self-esteem, and physical and social functioning (Varni et al. 1986). Similar techniques also have been used in the treatment of children and adolescents with asthma or cystic fibrosis. Autogenic relaxation training may also be of benefit in reducing mild internalizing and externalizing symptoms in children (Goldbeck and Schmid 2003).

Pain behavior management. The strategy of pain behavior management is to use operant techniques in the treatment of chronic pain. For example, the antecedents and consequences of headaches are determined by observation and by keeping a pain diary (if the child is old enough), and then attempts are made to modify those situations and events that seem to precipitate or positively reinforce pain as the therapist works with the patient, parents, teachers, pediatrician, and significant others. Emphasis is placed on stress management techniques (Masek et al. 1984) and on normal functioning despite pain. With reduced pain and pain-related behaviors, patients experience an increased sense of control and mastery and an increase in age-appropriate positive activities (Varni et al. 1986). These techniques have been adapted to the treatment of respiratory symptoms in children and adolescents with asthma or cystic fibrosis.

Stress inoculation. Stress inoculation is a multicomponent cognitive-behavioral approach that combines education, modeling procedures, systematic desensitization, hypnosis, contingency management, and training and practice in coping skills such as imagery and breathing exercises. It is useful in preventing stress and anxiety in children before medical and dental procedures and in chronically ill children for reducing anxiety, pain, or other discomfort related to repeated procedures such as spinal taps, bone marrow aspirations, and chemotherapy injections. Before a therapist implements such a program, the medical procedure is analyzed in detail, including the rationale, details of the procedure and its sensations and side effects, and portions likely to be perceived as uncomfortable or frightening. Also important are the characteristics and previous direct or vicarious experiences of the patient (Melamed et al. 1984; Varni et al. 1986).

Family Treatment

Attempts to treat children and adolescents without considering the persons with whom they live and the patients' relationships with other significant persons are doomed to failure. Any change in one family member, whether resulting from a psychiatric disorder, psychiatric treatment, a normal developmental process, or an outside event, is likely to produce change in other family members and in their relationships. Family constellations vary widely, ranging from the traditional nuclear family to the single-parent family, a blended or step-family, an adoptive or foster family, or a group home. The term *parents* in this chapter applies to adults filling the parenting role, whatever their actual relationship to the patient.

Evaluation of Families

Data should be gathered on each person living with the patient, as well as on others who may be important or have been so in the past (e.g., noncustodial parents, grandparents, siblings who are no longer living at home). It is often useful to have at least one session that includes all significant family members. For families with young children, techniques such as the use of family drawings or puppet play or the assignment of family tasks to be carried out in the session are often useful. A variety of schemas exist by which to assess a family's structure and dynamic functioning.

The family's developmental stage offers a clue to predictable transitional crises as children are born, become adolescents, and are launched from the nuclear family (Carter and McGoldrick 1980). Important tasks for all families are listed in Table 36–12.

TABLE 36–12. **Family tasks**

- Forming a "marital coalition" to meet the needs of the adults for intimacy, sexuality, and emotional support

- Establishing a parental coalition capable of flexible relationships with the children and presenting a consistent disciplinary front

- Nurturing, enculturating, and emancipating children

- Coping with crisis

Source. Adapted from Fleck 1976.

Several different models of family assessment and evaluation exist. Whatever model is used, a family assessment should be able to identify the stage of the family life cycle and the challenges encountered therein, indicate problematic areas of family interaction that require intervention, and reveal areas of the child's development that have been at risk because of influences by the family (such as communication or poor role modeling). Other goals of a family assessment should be to define areas of parental problem or psychopathology, identify other vulnerable family members, and determine how the family may be either contributing or compensating for a child's disorder (Davidson et al. 2001).

Tasks of the initial session of a family assessment include establishing an alliance with family members; gathering data by direct questioning, by observing, and by assessing the impact of trial interventions; and proposing a provisional plan for treatment.

Family Therapy

In the most general sense, family therapy is psychological treatment conducted with an identified patient and at least one biological or functional (by marriage, adoption, and so forth) family member. Related techniques include therapy with an individual patient that takes a family systems perspective, or therapy sessions with family members other than the identified patient, based on noncompliance with treatment, severity of illness, or other factors. Some family therapists insist that all family members attend sessions, but this requirement is unnecessarily rigid. Family therapy addresses primarily the interaction *among* family members rather than the processes *within* an individual.

Most clinicians would agree that there are some situations in which family therapy is preferred over other treatments, others in which it should be combined with other treatments, and still others in which it is not possible or is relatively contraindicated. Research on this topic is limited, so accumulated clinical judgment and experience must prevail.

Family therapy may be particularly useful when there are dysfunctional interactions or impaired communication within the family, especially when these appear to be related to the presenting problem. It also may be useful when symptoms seem to have been precipitated by difficulty with a developmental stage for an individual or the family or by a change in the family such as divorce or remarriage. If more than one family member is symptomatic, family therapy may be both more efficient and more effective than multiple individual treatments. Family therapy should be considered when one family member improves with treatment but another, not in treatment, worsens. In any case, the family must have, or be induced to have, sufficient motivation to participate. When the identified patient is relatively unmotivated to participate or to change, family therapy is likely to be more effective than individual therapy. Attention to family systems issues also may be useful when progress is blocked in individual therapy or in behavior therapy.

Family therapy is contraindicated as a sole treatment method in cases of clearly organic physical or mental illness or if the family equilibrium is precarious and one or more family members are at serious risk of decompensation. In these situations, family therapy may be useful in combination with other treatments, such as medication or hospitalization. It is counterproductive to include in family therapy sessions a patient who is acutely psychotic, violent, or delusional regarding the family. Family sessions may not be helpful when a parent has severe, intractable, or minimally relevant psychopathology or when the child strongly prefers individual treatment. Children should not be included in sessions in which parents persist (despite redirection) in criticizing the children or in sharing inappropriate information, when the most critical need is marital therapy, or when parents primarily need specific, concrete help with practical affairs.

A variety of family therapies are considered when treating children and adolescents (Table 36–13).

Types of Family Therapy

Structural therapy. Structural therapy has been the model most used and studied when a child or adolescent is the identified patient. Developed by Salvador Minuchin and his colleagues at the Philadelphia Child Guidance Clinic, it has been used extensively with families of children and adolescents with eating disorders and psychophysiological disorders such as asthma. Focus is on the present, in which the identified patient's symptoms are presumed to serve a function for the family. The process of assessment includes mapping patterns of communication and the structure of the family, including the location and permeability of boundaries between family members and around the family and its subsystems. Other important variables are the character and flexibility of alignments of family members, including alliances (joining together of two or more members in a common interest or task) and coalitions (joint actions directed against one or more family members). Data are gathered on the distribution of power within the family and on the family's sources of stress and support in the environment.

TABLE 36–13. Models of family therapy
• Structural
• Multigenerational
• Strategic
• Behavioral
• Psychoeducational
• Multiple-family group

The therapist uses assigned tasks and his or her interactions with family members to provoke change in the family structure and thereby its functioning. When the symptom is no longer needed, it disappears. Relabeling (i.e., redefining a behavior or symptom to have a different, less negative meaning) opens alternative pathways for family interactions.

Multigenerational family therapy. Pioneered by Murray Bowen and grounded in his family systems theory, multigenerational family therapy emphasizes how current patterns in families are repetitions of the past. Change results from insights gained in the exploration of parents' families of origin and the relationships over several generations of the nuclear family to the extended family. Grandparents are often involved indirectly or even included in sessions.

Strategic family therapy. Strategic family therapy, developed by Jay Haley and by Mara Selvini-Palazzoli and her colleagues, produces change through a complex and indirect plan of action that is not fully shared with the family. In practice, paradoxical instructions are devised to upset the family equilibrium and permit change, especially in families resistant to more straightforward techniques. This potentially powerful model should be used only by experienced therapists.

Behavioral family therapy. Models of behavioral family therapy include Patterson's (1975), based on social learning theory, and Alexander's (1992) functional family therapy, both of which are used in the treatment of children and adolescents with conduct disorder. This model has been extended to a multisystemic approach that uses energetic outreach into the home, neighborhood, and school and adds peer group and school-based interventions to family treatment of adolescent delinquents (Henggeler and Borduin 1990; Henggeler et al. 1998).

Psychoeducational family therapy. A psychoeducational approach to family therapy has been most extensively developed in the treatment of families of adult schizophrenic patients (C.M. Anderson et al. 1980), but it has been extended to a number of childhood disorders, such as eating disorders, ADHD, and depression. Detailed didactic presentations about the disorder, in the setting of a multiple family group, are designed to improve the family's coping skills through increased understanding of the illness and its treatment, to teach home behavior management techniques, and to enhance family support networks. Ongoing treatment of individual families includes family systems interventions when educational and behavioral techniques are blocked by dysfunctional family structures or processes. The identified patient is included in family sessions when his or her clinical status permits.

Multiple-family therapy.   The multifamily approach combines features of group and family therapy. Sessions include three to five families with similar problems who may be isolated from other supports and who can benefit from the interaction with other families.

Group Therapy

Indications

Group therapy is particularly appropriate for children, who are often more willing to reveal their thoughts and feelings to peers than to adults. Also, the therapist can observe behavior with peers rather than depending on the reports of others. Establishing rewarding social relationships, a crucial developmental task for children of all ages, is especially difficult for youths with a psychiatric disorder. Group therapy offers opportunities for the clinician to model and facilitate practice of important skills and to provide youngsters with companionship and mutual support. Interventions by peers may be far more acute and powerful in their effect than those by an adult therapist. An additional benefit is the larger number of patients who can benefit from limited therapist time. A meta-analysis of 56 outcome studies published between 1974 and 1997 supports the efficacy of group psychotherapy in children and adolescents (Hoag and Burlingame 1997).

Target symptoms include absent or conflictual peer relationships, aggression, withdrawal, timidity, difficulty with separation, and deficient social interactive or problem-solving skills. These problems often are not apparent or accessible to intervention in individual therapy sessions. Group therapy can be a powerful modality in the treatment of adolescents with eating disorders or substance abuse.

On the negative side, forming an outpatient group is often tedious and time-consuming. Diverse schedules and lack of transportation make gathering a sufficient number of patients difficult. More space and preparation are required than for individual or family therapy.

Group psychotherapy is contraindicated for those who are acutely psychotic, paranoid, or actively suicidal. Adolescents with sociopathic traits or behaviors should not be included in groups with teenagers who might be victimized or intimidated. Severely aggressive or hyperactive children probably should not be included in outpatient groups because of the difficulty in controlling their behavior, the contagion of problem behaviors, and the intimidation of less assertive children. Groups should *not* be used as a repository for unmotivated, nonverbal, difficult patients.

Although group therapy may be used as the sole treatment modality, it is often used in combination with another intervention. Groups also may serve an evaluation function, particularly for preschool- and school-age children (Scheidlinger 1984).

Technical Considerations

Theoretical models.   All of the theoretical models used in individual therapy may be used with groups. Therapy may be exclusively verbal, or it may include expressive arts techniques, psychodrama, arts and crafts, and sports activities; behavioral techniques such as modeling or overt practice; or cognitive-behavioral strategies for depression (Lewinsohn et al. 1990) and anxiety disorders (Silverman et al. 1999). The skilled group therapist has an understanding of systems theory and group process, whatever the model of intervention. Contingency management (i.e., rewards and consequences) may be an essential adjunct for groups that include children with behavior disorders.

Group size.   Groups range from 4 to 10 patients, with the number varying according to the number of leaders, the age and type of pathology of the group members, and the number of suitable candidates available.

Group composition.   The composition of the group depends on its purpose. Patients in support groups are chosen because they share a single stressor—for example, sexual abuse, parental divorce, or chronic physical illness. Other groups are specifically targeted to a single disorder. Groups that focus on social skills work best with a mixture of patients.

Groups that are conducted with patients in special schools, inpatient units, or day hospitals typically include all children or adolescents enrolled in the program, although the patients may be divided by age or level of functioning. Special topic groups, such as treatment of substance abuse, or predischarge groups also may be offered in these settings.

It is useful for the group therapist to interview prospective group members individually, to assess suitability for the group, to orient patients to the goals and methods of the group, to learn more about the children or adolescents, and to begin to develop a therapeutic alliance between the patients and the leader. It also is helpful to interview the parent(s) for similar reasons. The younger the child, the more important is parental cooperation.

Group members should be in the same or adjacent developmental stage. Children change so dramatically as they develop that an age span broader than 2–3 years is unlikely to result in a therapeutic group process. In forming groups for preadolescents and early adolescents, developmental stage is often more important than chronological age, because girls are approximately 2 years ahead of boys in physical and social development, and there is great variability among youngsters of the same sex. The dynamic issues differ at various developmental stages.

Opinions on the mixing of boys and girls differ. Although some issues are easier to handle in single-sex groups, children and adolescents need to learn to get along with the opposite sex in school and in the neighborhood and often with siblings. Therefore, mixing boys and girls, although initially more difficult, may be productive.

Frequency, duration, and goals. For convenience, outpatient groups typically meet once a week. Frequency of group meetings on inpatient units varies from one to seven times per week. Groups may have a defined, limited duration from several months to an academic year or may be open-ended. Short-term groups focus on "current and explicit behavior, adaptation, coping, competency, strengths and growth… [with] emphasis on the dynamics of the 'here-and-now' corrective emotional experience, [and] on the patients' active participation in the change effort" (Scheidlinger 1984, p. 581). Long-term groups are more likely to aim for the promotion of insight, the resolution of unconscious conflicts, and the removal of developmental arrests. Although there are exceptions, short-term groups generally have a defined membership, with no new members added once the group begins. Long-term groups more often have changing membership, with patients entering and leaving as their clinical status dictates.

Group leadership. Of all modalities of therapy, the need for co-therapists is most clear in group treatment. Groups are complex, with many events occurring simultaneously, and a second observer is valuable. This arrangement also allows continuity of treatment when one leader needs to be absent. In groups of younger children, an extra pair of hands is needed. Co-leaders who differ in age, gender, race, or ethnicity expand the opportunity for different types of patient–therapist relationships.

Group rules. The nature of the group and the patients determines the optimal degree of structure. A CBT group composed of depressed or anxious adolescents will need far fewer rules than a group whose goal is to teach social skills to school-age boys with conduct problems. The leaders are responsible for maintaining control of behavior within the group. At times, this control may even require strategies such as the time-out.

The leader(s) must make explicit the rules of confidentiality for the group, as the group setting expands the risk of breach of confidentiality to include the patients' peers. This breach is of most concern to adolescents and preadolescents.

Family contact. Involving parents is especially important for preschool- and school-age children to discover important events in the children's lives and to assess progress. Adolescents are more willing and able to report and are also more sensitive to confidentiality issues. All parents should be kept apprised of the goals of the group, both in general and specifically for their child. Parent education in development and behavior management can be provided efficiently by grouping parents together. Parents also may appreciate the opportunity to meet with others whose children have similar problems.

Developmental Issues

Preschool-age groups. Young children are less able to verbalize and thus require more structure and planned activities. A group can provide a powerful context for the teaching of social skills and language, especially for children who are autistic or severely delayed.

School-age groups. Because school-age children have great difficulty bringing in outside material for discussion or engaging in introspection, verbal portions of the group are best focused on events that occur in the group itself. Games and craft activities can provide a useful framework, but the leaders must ensure that recreation does not become the only function of the group. Behavior modification and cognitive problem-solving techniques are especially useful for children this age.

Many child patients will not spontaneously attempt to relate to other children. Others have been rejected or scapegoated by peers. If the group is successful, the children will use the skills they have learned to form relationships with peers at school and in their neighborhoods.

Children with ADHD are often referred to group therapy because of their difficulty with peer relations and their lack of insight into their difficulties. Those children who are being treated with stimulant medication should receive a dose before the group meets to help them benefit from the therapy and not disrupt it for others.

Adolescent groups. Scheidlinger (1985) identified four major categories of group work with adolescents:

1. *Group psychotherapy:* Offers treatment of a balanced selection of patients, using the group as the primary modality, with goals of relief of psychological distress, modification of pathological modes of functioning, and amelioration of personality dysfunction
2. *Therapeutic groups for patients in mental health, medical, or residential settings:* Is used as ancillary treatment or as an aid in rehabilitation
3. *Human development and training groups:* Is offered to youths who are not psychiatric patients and focus on prevention and enrichment
4. *Self-help and mutual-help groups:* May or may not have professional leaders and consist of peers working together to satisfy a shared need or overcome a common handicap; extensively used in the treatment of substance abuse

Although activities may be useful, many adolescent groups can be conducted in an exclusively verbal format. If both boys and girls are included in the same group, the leader must be alert to sexual undercurrents and acting-out while facilitating the discussion of sexual concerns and practicing of heterosexual social skills (Scheidlinger 1985). To avoid scapegoating, it is important that the proportion of boys to girls not be too unequal.

Inpatient and Residential Treatment

Indications

Because children should be treated in the setting that is least restrictive and disruptive to their lives, inpatient or residential treatment is indicated only in emergencies or for youngsters who have not responded to efforts at outpatient treatment because of severity of the disorder, lack of motivation, resistance, or disorganization of patients and/or family. Programs vary widely in their criteria for admission.

Placement in a residential treatment center may be indicated for children and adolescents with chronic behavior problems such as aggression, running away, truancy, substance abuse, school phobia, or self-destructive acts that the family, foster home, and/or community cannot manage or tolerate. Some parents harbor negative attitudes toward their children or adolescents or have severe psychopathology of their own. Children for whom it is not advisable to return home—because of factors in the youngsters, their families, or both—may be referred to a residential treatment center following a hospital stay.

Short-term hospitalization is typically an acute event, stemming from immediate physical danger to self or others, acute psychosis, a crisis in the environment that reduces the ability of the caregiving adults to cope with the child or adolescent, or the need for more intensive, systematic, and detailed evaluation and observation of the patient and family than is possible on an outpatient basis or in a day program. Hospital lengths of stay have decreased significantly, often allowing only clinical stabilization of the patient before his or her discharge from the hospital. Briefer hospitalizations of severely ill child psychiatric patients require well-coordinated transfer to less restrictive levels of care in the clinical continuum (residential, day, and intensive outpatient treatments).

Longer-term hospitalization may be indicated for those patients who do not improve sufficiently in a brief period and who continue to require a secure setting and intensive treatment.

Efficacy

Systematic outcome evaluation is extremely difficult because of the complexity of the cases and the need for crisis intervention. Controlled studies that would be considered methodologically adequate comparing 24-hour treatment with no treatment or other types of treatment may not even be ethical or feasible. In general, more severely ill patients with fewer individual and family resources have a poorer outcome.

Differences in Settings

Residential treatment centers, compared with hospital units, tend to be longer term, more open to and integrated with the community, and not organized by the medical model. Usually, residential centers have a lower staff-to-patient ratio and less highly trained personnel. These centers are more likely to be based on a family group model and divided into sections or cottages.

Facilities may be under the auspices of a state, county, or city; part of a medical school; or in a private, a nonprofit, or an investor-owned hospital. Inpatient units may be located in a general hospital, pediatric hospital, or psychiatric hospital. Most settings separate children and adolescents, but others mix age groups. A relatively recent development is the psychosomatic or pediatric medical-psychiatric unit for children and adolescents with coexisting physical and psychiatric problems.

Some units are locked and can accommodate involuntary patients, as well as runaways, and highly impulsive, psychotic, or actively suicidal youths who require more security. Other units are open and admit only voluntary patients. Intensity of staffing varies widely. Units that are part of an academic medical center are the most intensively staffed because of the presence of a variety of trainees. Programs operated by state or county governments often have fewer professional staff because of budget restraints and problems in recruiting.

Inpatient units for children can be classified according to the usual length of stay on such units. The lengths of stay on brief-stay or crisis intervention units average 1–2 weeks. These units emphasize rapid evaluation, triage, stabilization, and development of a treatment plan that will be implemented on an outpatient basis or in another facility. Stays on intermediate units last several weeks to months, and more definitive treatment can be conducted. Children may stay on long-term units from several months to longer than 1 year. On these units, care for the most severely impaired youth is provided. Increasing financial pressures have resulted in reduced overall lengths of stay in all types of units.

Treatment Planning

Ideally, hospitalization forms part of a comprehensive continuum of care for children. With ever-shorter lengths of stay, rapid and efficient planning and execution of evaluation and treatment strategies are essential. The goal is not to eliminate all psychopathology but to address the "focal problem" that precipitated hospitalization and then to discharge the patient to home, residential treatment, or foster placement, where he or she can receive outpatient or day treatment (Harper 1989).

Components of Treatment

The relative emphasis placed on each treatment modality differs according to the philosophy of treatment, the nature of the patient population, the usual length of stay, and the availability of highly specialized staff. All of the following should be present in some form.

Milieu therapy. Milieu therapy includes the total environment of a structured schedule for meals, sleep, and so forth and a program of activities. The patient can be observed over an extended period of time in school, free play with peers, meals, sleep, and self-care. In the most effective milieus, all activities and interactions with staff are consistent with the treatment plan. Goals of the milieu include promoting a feeling of security through clarity of rules and regularity of schedule, and increasing self-esteem and competence through learning of skills. Most settings include a token economy or levels program, which also may be used for specific treatment or for management of behavior (e.g., encouraging a patient with anorexia nervosa to eat).

Pharmacotherapy. Hospitalization offers an ideal opportunity for systematic trials of medication in children or adolescents who have not responded to conventional treatment, who are diagnostically puzzling, who have medical problems complicating pharmacotherapy, or whose parents are noncompliant, disorganized, or unreliable reporters of efficacy or side effects. The inpatient environment allows for trials of psychotropic medication where the response to treatment can be constantly observed, and side effects promptly managed. As-needed (i.e., prn) medications administered to control aggression or other behavior problems should be used only for brief periods until more effective, ongoing treatments are begun.

Individual psychotherapy. As newer treatment methods evolve and hospital stays become ever shorter, individual psychotherapy is less often a primary treatment modality than in the past. However, regularly scheduled individual sessions with a therapist with whom the child or adolescent can develop a special relationship continue to be essential in developing a more complete understanding of the patient's intrapsychic, familial, and social dynamics and in assisting him or her to develop more adaptive methods of coping with strong emotions. The therapist may be able to help the patient to deal with past traumas and losses, to better understand his or her current difficulties, and to make use of the other treatments offered. The confidentiality that is usual in outpatient therapy is not present in a hospital or residential setting, given that all staff participate as a treatment team.

Group therapy.   In addition to general or special topic groups (e.g., 12-Step models, survivors of abuse), group therapy may include community meetings in which privileges and rules are decided, social skills are practiced, and patients learn to observe their own and others' behavior and to recognize the impact of their behavior on others.

Family treatment.   Work with families is an essential part of hospital treatment, including intensive evaluation of family functioning and deciding where the child should reside. Interventions may include family therapy, parent counseling in behavior management, and education about the nature of their child's disorder. Parents may require referral for marital therapy, individual medical or psychiatric assessment and treatment, or help with housing or income.

Education.   Virtually all children who require psychiatric hospitalization have had problems in school. The small classes and highly trained teachers of a hospital unit can provide a detailed evaluation of a youngster's academic strengths and weaknesses, incorporating data from intelligence and achievement tests and special tests for learning disabilities into direct observation of classroom behavior and learning. Educational strategies can be developed and tested. One of the most important parts of discharge planning is arranging for an appropriate educational placement and working with the new teacher to continue progress made in the hospital. The hospitalization often allows child or adolescent patients their first opportunity to experience academic success.

Many residential treatment centers have their own schools on their own grounds. As youngsters improve, they are gradually integrated into special education or mainstream programs in local public or private schools.

Additional services.   Medical evaluation and treatment must be provided. Neurological evaluation and treatment should be available through consultation as necessary.

Disposition planning and aftercare.   Disposition planning and follow-up may be the most important parts of the treatment if gains made are to be maintained and continued. A complete disposition plan includes consideration of the child's living arrangements, school placement, and continuation of individual therapy, family therapy, and/or pharmacotherapy.

Partial Hospitalization

Indications

Partial hospitalization (day treatment) may be best for the child who requires more intensive intervention than can be provided in outpatient visits but who is able to live at home. Partial hospitalization is less disruptive to the patient and family than inpatient treatment or residential placement and can offer an opportunity for more intensive work with parents, who may attend the program on a regular basis. Partial hospitalization may be used as a transition for a child who has been hospitalized or to avert a hospitalization. It may be implemented in combination with placement in a foster or group home.

Programs

Day treatment programs involve a full day, 5 days a week, and include a school or therapeutic nursery school program. The treatment plan and therapeutic focus can be integrated into the entire day. Other programs, such as intensive outpatient or "partial day" programs, may meet in the late afternoon and evening hours after patients attend community schools. It is desirable to offer all of the treatment modalities described above for an inpatient unit.

Innovative, intensive summer treatment programs have been developed for children with ADHD and associated behavior and learning problems (Pelham and Hoza 1987; Pelham et al. 2000). These programs provide positive social and recreational experiences for children who otherwise would not be able to participate in camp, while teaching parents behavior modification techniques, supplementing classroom work, and rigorously assessing medication efficacy and side effects.

Adjunctive Treatments

At times, an intervention that is not a psychiatric treatment may be recommended as part of a treatment plan. These programs may be crucial for the child's well-being and/or the treatment of the psychiatric disorder, or they may be facilitative, speeding progress or improving level of function.

Parent Support Groups

Parents of children with psychiatric disorders, together with mental health professionals and teachers, have established groups that provide education and support for parents, as well as advocacy for services and fund-raising for research. National organizations with local chapters include Parents Anonymous, for abusive or potentially abusive parents; the Association for Retarded Citizens; the Autism Society of America; Children and Adults with Attention Deficit Disorders (CHADD); and the Learning Disabilities Association of America. Recently, the National Alliance for the Mentally Ill (NAMI) established a Child and Adolescent Network (NAMI-CAN) as its concerns broadened to include children and adolescents. Local groups focused on a particular disorder or on more generic issues can provide a powerful adjunct to direct clinical services.

Special Education

Modified school programs are indicated for those children who cannot perform satisfactorily in regular classrooms or who need special structure or teaching techniques to reach their academic potential. These programs range in intensity from tutoring or resource classrooms several hours a week, to special classrooms in mainstream schools, to public or private schools that serve only children with special educational needs. Resources differ from community to community, but most communities have programs for mentally retarded youth, for those with learning disabilities (specific developmental disorders), and for those whose emotional and/or behavioral problems require a special setting for learning or for the control of their behavior. Classes are small, with a high teacher-to-student ratio and teachers who are specially trained.

Before being placed in a special class, youngsters must have an individually administered battery of psychological tests, including an intelligence test, achievement tests, and an evaluation for learning disabilities. The federal Individuals with Disabilities Education Act (IDEA) requires that all children who need them receive special services and that services be provided in the least restrictive environment (i.e., as much in the mainstream with other children and adolescents as possible). An Individualized Education Program (IEP) is developed for each eligible child and must describe the nature of the educational or developmental disability, the short-term and annual goals of treatment, and the specific educational or therapeutic interventions to be used.

Boarding schools may be useful when there is a problem between parent and child that is unresponsive to treatment. Some of these schools have special programs for children with learning disabilities or psychiatric disorders.

Recreation

Learning a sport or skill that he or she can do well is an important adjunct in the treatment of a child who lacks positive relationships with peers or adults because of social isolation or withdrawal or who is ignored or actively rejected. A relationship with an adult such as a Big Brother or a YMCA counselor, and an opportunity to interact with a normal peer group under supervision, may provide support and build self-esteem until the child is sufficiently improved to establish relationships independently. Some families have employed a high school or college student one or more afternoons a week to teach social and play skills, develop a relationship, provide structured time, and assist with homework. This approach also gives parents a respite and an opportunity to spend time with their other children.

Day or overnight summer camps may present opportunities for psychological growth in multiple domains. Some youngsters can attend regular camp, whereas others need a special program for children and adolescents with psychiatric or medical problems.

Foster Care

Placement in a foster home may be needed when parents are unwilling or unable to care for a child. Indications are clearest in cases of physical neglect or physical or sexual abuse. Other families may be unable to provide the appropriate emotional or physical environment. Court intervention is required for placement. Although foster placement can be a suitable and effective intervention, children in foster care may have a variety of unmet physical, developmental, and mental health needs, often making foster care less than optimal and clearly unsatisfactory as a long- term solution (Rosenfeld et al. 1997). Unfortunately, child welfare agencies in many communities are overwhelmed, and children and adolescents may require advocacy either for removal from home to a foster placement or for termination of foster placement and return to parents, group home placement, or release for adoption. A recent study by McMillen et al. (2005) showed that older youths in foster homes have a much higher rate of psychiatric illness, compared with age-matched peers.

Children with severe behavioral or physical problems, or older adolescents who are difficult to place or maintain in foster or adoptive homes, may be admitted to group homes. These homes vary in staffing and intensity of their programs. Some approach residential treatment, whereas others simply provide a supervised residence.

Dietary Treatments

Since the mid-1970s, advocates of dietary treatment of behavioral problems have been remarkably persistent, despite the lack of scientific evidence. A variety of food additives and food allergens have been proposed as contributory or even causal in childhood behavior disorders, especially hyperactivity and autism. Reviews of methodologically adequate studies (Rojas and Chan 2005) have consistently failed to demonstrate behavioral or cognitive improvement on the Kaiser-Permanente Diet (Feingold 1975). There are no data to support dietary treatments for autism.

Parents and primary care practitioners find dietary treatment appealing because it is more "natural" than medication. However, special diets demand extra work and often additional expense from a family already disrupted by a child's behavior problems. Given the minimal evidence of efficacy and the extreme difficulty inducing children to comply with restricted diets, such diets should not be recommended. Families who insist on trying a diet should be permitted to do so, provided the diet is nutritionally sound, because initial attempts to dissuade them may disrupt the therapeutic alliance.

A thorough meta-analysis by Wolraich et al. (1995) debunks the notion that dietary sugar contributes to hyperactivity. Caffeine, in the form of coffee or cola, has been popularly recommended by nonprofessionals for the treatment of hyperactivity, despite significant side effects and no demonstration of efficacy.

Megavitamin therapy, the prescription of vitamins in quantities greatly in excess of the recommended daily allowance (RDA) guidelines, has been suggested as a treatment for schizophrenia, autism, hyperactivity, and learning disabilities. Extreme claims have been made from uncontrolled studies. Not only is scientific evidence of effectiveness lacking, but toxic effects also are possible (Harley 1980). Parents, particularly those of autistic children, may pursue this treatment out of desperation.

Integration of Multiple Modalities

Sophisticated simultaneous or sequential use of different techniques offers substantial promise of improved treatment outcome. There is a clear need for more power and wider coverage of symptoms than any single treatment alone provides. The following are some examples.

Collaborative Therapy

In general, treatment by a single therapist is most efficient and effective. Indications for collaborative treatment (two or more therapists working as a team) in the outpatient setting include a child who is unusually concerned about confidentiality; the need for several different types of skills (e.g., individual psychotherapy, family therapy, and pharmacotherapy), which a single therapist does not have; or clear indications for different qualities in a patient's and parent's therapists (e.g., a boy who would benefit from a male role model but whose mother has great difficulty relating to men).

In collaborative treatment, in order to maintain free and open communication and to discuss and agree on treatment plans, it is essential for the therapists to avoid aligning into competitive teams. Conflicts over relative power and authority of the therapists can sabotage treatment. It is fundamentally important that the child and adolescent psychiatrist not allow himself or herself to be relegated solely to the role of pharmacotherapist.

Combined Treatments

It is increasingly clear that child psychiatric patients do not benefit from a "purist" approach to treatment that makes use of a single modality. A clinician must be able to weave together flexibly a treatment that draws from psychodynamic, behavioral, family systems, and pharmacotherapeutic approaches in order to address a child's symptoms at his or her specific developmental level (Lewis 1997).

Combined Psychotherapies

Integrating techniques from different theoretical schools (such as play, cognitive-behavioral, and psychodynamic) may be more helpful and appropriate in the treatment of children and adolescents than relying on one particular theory or approach (Silverman 1997). Models have been developed that bring together techniques to address specific clinical issues. For example, a highly structured model has been developed from a theoretical framework of ego psychoanalytic object relations theory for children with oppositional or conduct disorders who have some social bonds and a capacity for guilt. Interventions include individual supportive-expressive play psychotherapy, parent training, and play group psychotherapy, according to the child's presenting problems (Kernberg and Chazan 1991).

An ingenious model of child psychotherapy developed by Strayhorn (1988) makes explicit the identification of "psychological skills" or competencies expected for the child's age that are lacking. In this model, specific interventions are designed to address the missing skills, including verbal and play therapy, education of child and parent, and behavioral techniques such as modeling and contingency management.

Medication Plus Psychotherapeutic Intervention

Traditionally, the use of medications and psychotherapy was perceived as an either/or phenomenon, in which proponents of each modality saw their own as more valuable and the other as unnecessary or even harmful. Increasingly, we are aware of the potential synergistic effect from combining medication with psychotherapeutic interventions, because these treatments may address different aspects of a single disorder (O'Brien and Perlmutter 1997). For example, the combination of CBT and pharmacotherapy has been shown to be particularly effective in treating pediatric depression and OCD (March et al. 2004, 2006).

Attention-deficit/hyperactivity disorder. The implementation of a multimodal treatment for ADHD has traditionally been clinically encouraged. Such treatment combines medication management (most often stimulants), behavioral interventions, parent management training, appropriate school placement and school-based interventions, as well as child-focused treatments (psychotherapy, cognitive-behavioral treatment, and social skills training). More recent reports have questioned the benefit of multimodal treatment over medication alone. The initial report of the Multimodal Treatment Study of Children with ADHD (MTA Cooperative Group 1999) described significantly greater improvements in the treatment groups receiving medication or combined medication and behavioral treatment than in the groups receiving only behavioral treatment or community care. Interestingly, the combination of medication and behavioral interventions was not significantly more beneficial than medication alone for the core ADHD symptoms. A follow-up study at the 24-month point affirmed the findings of the initial study, although effect sizes were smaller (MTA Cooperative Group 2004). Behavioral treatments appear to hold added benefit for children suffering from ADHD with comorbid anxiety (Jensen et al. 2001).

Autistic disorder. Children with autism require a comprehensive therapeutic plan that may include psychoeducation of the parents and family, special education placement, speech and language therapies, behavioral management approaches, social skills training, and pharmacotherapy. An individualized treatment should take into account the particular deficits of the child, as well as individual and family strengths.

Depression. Current recommendations for treatment of depression include individual or group psychotherapy (CBT, interpersonal psychotherapy, or a psychodynamically oriented psychotherapy), in addition to parental and family therapies. Pharmacotherapy may also have a role, although treatment with medication only is discouraged. Treatments should be individualized, based on presumed etiology, severity of illness, and individual/family strengths.

Anxiety disorders. Suggested approaches for treatment of older children and adolescents with anxiety disorders include the combined use of behavioral, cognitive-behavioral, psychodynamic, and supportive psychotherapies; family therapy; and pharmacotherapy tailored to the child's clinical needs (Bernstein et al. 1996).

Obsessive-compulsive disorder. The combination of CBT and pharmacotherapy appears optimal in the treatment of OCD. The POTS (March et al. 2004) demonstrated that CBT combined with sertraline was more effective than either alone in treating OCD symptoms.

Schizophrenia and psychotic disorders. While pharmacotherapy is an essential component in the treatment of pediatric psychotic disorders, psychosocial interventions should always be included as part of a comprehensive treatment plan. Supportive psychotherapy and social skills training, tailored to age and developmental level, may help children and adolescents to better understand their illness and improve social interactions with friends and family. Family education and therapy will help all family members comprehend the illness of a child or sibling and its impact on the family unit and its individual members. Liaison with the school or other caregivers should also be considered.

Conclusion

The treatment of psychiatric disorders in children and adolescents is both an art and a science. Research on assessment and diagnosis, biological correlates of disorders, and outcome of traditional and newly developed techniques will continue to improve the specificity and outcome of treatment. However, a need always will exist for clinical skills in tailoring and applying psychosomatic techniques to individual patients and their families.

Key Points

- As in adults, treatment of pediatric psychiatric patients requires expertise in psychiatric evaluation and case formulation, effective use of complex treatment strategies, and a respect for the principles of informed consent and confidentiality.

- An understanding of human development is key to the successful treatment of pediatric psychiatric patients, to include an appreciation of the differences between youngsters and adults as well as the developmental differences between children of all ages.

- Ideally, treatments identified specifically for children and adolescents should reflect evidence-based practices. However, many have been developed by applying known effective adult treatments to the pediatric population.

- Pediatric psychopharmacology research remains limited despite escalations in the use of psychiatric medications in children. Caution should be exercised to prescribe medications in a safe and monitored fashion.

- Decisions regarding the use of psychoactive medications in children, as in adults, are best supported through double-blind, placebo-controlled efficacy trials and through the collection of longitudinal data regarding medication safety. Clinicians should avoid the routine use of medication in youngsters that is based solely on case report or uncontrolled drug trials.

- Parents should be carefully informed of the presence or absence of scientific evidence supporting the use of a specific medication in a child, as well as that medication's possible side effects and adverse effects.

- Psychotherapy remains a mainstay in the effective practice of child and adolescent psychiatry and may be used solely or in combination with other treatments, depending on a patient's treatment needs.

- Further studies are required to demonstrate which types of psychotherapy are most effective for which child psychiatric diagnoses. Such efficacy studies remain methodologically challenging.

- Although each psychotherapy is based on its own theoretical constructs and purported therapeutic principles, all psychotherapies tend to rely on several similar precepts: the importance of the relationship with the therapist, an emphasis on hopefulness, the use of therapist attention and suggestion, and the expectation of change in one or more realms—psychological makeup, cognition, behavior, sense of self, or emotional experience.

Suggested Readings

General

Barkley RA: Attention-Deficit Hyperactivity Disorder: A Handbook for Diagnosis and Treatment, 3rd Edition. New York, Guilford, 2006

Connor DF, Meltzer B: Pediatric Psychopharmacology: Fast Facts. New York, WW Norton, 2006

Dulcan MK, Wiener JM (eds): Essentials of Child and Adolescent Psychiatry. Arlington, VA, American Psychiatric Publishing, 2006

Dulcan MK, Martini, DR, Lake MB: Concise Guide to Child and Adolescent Psychiatry, 3rd Edition. Arlington, VA, American Psychiatric Publishing, 2003

Mash EJ, Barkley RA (eds): Treatment of Childhood Disorders, 3rd Edition. New York, Guilford, 2006

Rating Scales

Collett B, Ohan J, Myers K: Ten-year review of rating scales, V: scales assessing attention-deficit/hyperactivity disorder. J Am Acad Child Adolesc Psychiatry 42:1015–1037, 2003

Collett B, Ohan J, Myers K: Ten-year review of rating scales, VI: scales assessing externalizing behaviors. J Am Acad Child Adolesc Psychiatry 42:1143–1170, 2003

Myers K, Winters N: Ten-year review of rating scales, I: overview of scale functioning, psychometric properties, and selection. J Am Acad Child Adolesc Psychiatry 41:114–122, 2002

Myers K, Winters N: Ten-year review of rating scales, II: scales for internalizing disorders. J Am Acad Child Adolesc Psychiatry 41:634–659, 2002

Ohan J, Myers K, Collett B: Ten-year review of rating scales, IV: scales assessing trauma and its effects. J Am Acad Child Adolesc Psychiatry 41:1401–1422, 2002

Rush AJ, First MB, Blacker D (eds): Handbook of Psychiatric Measures, 2nd Edition. Arlington, VA, American Psychiatric Publishing, 2008

Winters N, Myers K, Proud L: Ten-year review of rating scales, III: scales assessing suicidality, cognitive style, and self-esteem. J Am Acad Child Adolesc Psychiatry 41:1150–1181, 2002

Winters N, Collett B, Myers K: Ten-year review of rating scales, VII: scales assessing functional impairment. J Am Acad Child Adolesc Psychiatry 44:309–338, 2005

References

Abnormal Involuntary Movement Scale (AIMS). Psychopharmacol Bull 24:781–783, 1988

Achenbach TM: Manual for the Teacher's Report Form and 1991 Profile. Burlington, University of Vermont, Department of Psychiatry, 1991

Adams PL: A Primer of Child Psychotherapy, 2nd Edition. Boston, MA, Little, Brown, 1982

Akhondzadeh S, Tavakolian R, Davari-Ashitani R, et al: Selegiline in the treatment of attention deficit hyperactivity disorder in children: a double blind and randomized trial. Prog Neuropsychopharmacol Biol Psychiatry 27:841–845, 2003

Alexander JF: An integrative model for treating the adolescent who is delinquent/acting out, in Empowering Families, Helping Adolescents: Family-Centered Treatment of Adolescents With Alcohol, Drug Abuse, and Mental Health Problems. Edited by Snyder W, Oooms T. Rockville, MD, U.S. Department of Health and Human Services, 1992, pp 101–110

Aman MG, De Smedt G, Derivan A, et al: Double-blind, placebo-controlled study of risperidone for the treatment of disruptive behaviors in children with subaverage intelligence. Am J Psychiatry 159:1337–1346, 2002

Aman MG, Buican B, Arnold LE: Methylphenidate treatment in children with borderline IQ and mental retardation: analysis of three aggregated studies. J Child Adolesc Psychopharmacol 13:29–40, 2003

Aman MG, Arnold LE, Ramadan Y, et al (Research Units on Pediatric Psychopharmacology Autism Network): Randomized, controlled, crossover trial of methylphenidate in pervasive developmental disorders with hyperactivity. Arch Gen Psychiatry 62:1266–1274, 2005

Ambrosini PJ: A review of pharmacotherapy of major depression in children and adolescents. Psychiatr Serv 51:627–633, 2000

American Academy of Child and Adolescent Psychiatry: Practice parameter for the use of stimulant medications in the treatment of children, adolescents, and adults. J Am Acad Child Adolesc Psychiatry 41 (2 suppl):26S–49S, 2002

Anderson CM, Hogarty GE, Reiss DJ: Family treatment of adult schizophrenic patients: a psycho-educational approach. Schizophr Bull 6:490–505, 1980

Anderson GM, Cook EH: Pharmacogenetics: promise and potential in child and adolescent psychiatry. Child Adolesc Psychiatr Clin N Am 9:23–42, 2000

Arnold LE, Aman MG, Cook AM, et al: Atomoxetine for hyperactivity in autism spectrum disorders: placebo-controlled crossover pilot trial. J Am Acad Child Adolesc Psychiatry 45:1196–1205, 2006

Azrin NH, Sneed TJ, Foxx RM: Dry-bed training: rapid elimination of childhood enuresis. Behav Res Ther 12:147–156, 1974

Barkley RA: Defiant Children: A Clinician's Manual for Assessment and Parent Training, 2nd Edition. New York, Guilford, 1997

Barnett MS: Ziprasidone monotherapy in pediatric bipolar disorder. J Child Adolesc Psychopharmacol 14:471–477, 2004

Barrickman LL, Perry PJ, Allen AJ, et al: Bupropion versus methylphenidate in the treatment of attention-deficit hyperactivity disorder. J Am Acad Child Adolesc Psychiatry 34:649–657, 1995

Bastiaens L: Knowledge, expectations and attitudes of hospitalized children and adolescents in psychopharmacological treatment. J Child Adolesc Psychopharmacol 3:157–171, 1992

Bastiaens L: Compliance with pharmacotherapy in adolescents: effects of patients' and parents' knowledge and attitudes toward treatment. J Child Adolesc Psychopharmacol 5:39–48, 1995

Bernstein GA, Borchardt CM, Perwien AR: Anxiety disorders in children and adolescents: a review of the past 10 years. J Am Acad Child Adolesc Psychiatry 35:1110–1119, 1996

Bernstein GA, Borchardt CM, Perwien AR, et al: Imipramine plus cognitive-behavioral therapy in the treatment of school refusal. J Am Acad Child Adolesc Psychiatry 39:276–283, 2000

Biederman J: Clonazepam in the treatment of prepubertal children with panic-like symptoms. J Clin Psychiatry 48 (suppl):38–41, 1987

Biederman J, Quinn D, Weiss M, et al: Efficacy and safety of Ritalin LA, a new, once daily, extended-release dosage form of methylphenidate, in children with attention deficit hyperactivity disorder. Paediatr Drugs 5:833–841, 2003

Biederman J, Mick E, Hammerness P, et al: Open-label, 8-week trial of olanzapine and risperidone for the treatment of bipolar disorder in preschool-age children. Biol Psychiatry 58:589–594, 2005

Biederman J, Boellner SW, Childress A, et al: Lisdexamfetamine dimesylate and mixed amphetamine salts extended-release in children with ADHD: a double-blind, placebo-controlled, crossover analog classroom study. Biol Psychiatry 62:970–976, 2007a

Biederman J, Krishnan S, Zhang Y, et al: Efficacy and tolerability of lisdexamfetamine dimesylate (NRP-104) in children with attention-deficit/hyperactivity disorder: a phase III, multicenter, randomized, double-blind, forced-dose, parallel-group study. Clin Ther 29:450–463, 2007b

Birmaher B, Greenhill LL, Cooper TB, et al: Sustained release methylphenidate: pharmacokinetic studies in ADHD males. J Am Acad Child Adolesc Psychiatry 28:768–772, 1989

Birmaher B, Axelson DA, Monk K, et al: Fluoxetine for the treatment of childhood anxiety disorders. J Am Acad Child Adolesc Psychiatry 42:415–423, 2003

Black B, Uhde TW: Treatment of elective mutism with fluoxetine: a double-blind, placebo-controlled study. J Am Acad Child Adolesc Psychiatry 33:1000–1006, 1994

Blair J, Scahill L, State M, et al: Electrocardiographic changes in children and adolescents treated with ziprasidone: a prospective study. J Am Acad Child Adolesc Psychiatry 44:73–79, 2005

Blechman EA: Toward comprehensive behavioral family intervention: an algorithm for matching families and interventions. Behav Modif 5:221–236, 1981

Borkovec TD, Miranda J: Between-group psychotherapy outcome research and basic science. Psychotherapy and Rehabilitation Research 5:14–20, 1996

Bradbury MG, Meadow SR: Combined treatment with enuresis alarm and desmopressin for nocturnal enuresis. Acta Paediatr 84:1014–1018, 1995

Brent DA, Birmaher B: British warnings on SSRIs questioned. J Am Acad Child Adolesc Psychiatry 43:379–380, 2004

Broderick-Cantwell JJ: Accidental clonidine patch overdose in attention-deficit/hyperactivity disorder patients. J Am Acad Child Adolesc Psychiatry 38:95–98, 1999

Brown RT, Sexson SB: Effects of methylphenidate on cardiovascular responses in attention deficit hyperactivity disordered adolescents. Journal of Adolescent Health Care 10:179–183, 1989

Buitelaar JK, van der Gaag RJ, van der Hoeven J: Buspirone in the management of anxiety and irritability in children with pervasive developmental disorders: results of an open-label study. J Clin Psychiatry 59:56–59, 1998

Butler RJ, Gasson SL: Enuresis alarm treatment. Scand J Urol Nephrol 39:349–357, 2005

Butler RJ, Holland P, Robinson J: Examination of the structured withdrawal program to prevent relapse of nocturnal enuresis. J Urol 166:2463–2466, 2001

Caballero J, Nahata MC: Atomoxetine hydrochloride for the treatment of attention-deficit/hyperactivity disorder. Clin Ther 25:3065–3083, 2003

Campbell M, Green WH, Deutsch SI: Child and Adolescent Psychopharmacology. Beverly Hills, CA, Sage, 1985

Campbell M, Silva RR, Kafantaris V, et al: Predictors of side effects associated with lithium administration in children. Psychopharmacol Bull 27:373–380, 1991

Carandang CG, Maxwell DJ, Robbins DR, et al: Lamotrigine in adolescent mood disorders. J Am Acad Child Adolesc Psychiatry 42:750, 2003

Carlson GA, Dunn D, Kelsey D, et al: A pilot study for augmenting atomoxetine with methylphenidate: safety of concomitant therapy in children with attention-deficit/hyperactivity disorder. Child Adolesc Psychiatry Ment Health 1(1):10, 2007. Available at: http://www.capmh.com/content/1/1/10. Accessed October 9, 2007.

Carter E, McGoldrick M (eds): The Family Life Cycle: A Framework for Family Therapy. New York, Gardner, 1980

Chang K, Saxena K, Howe M: An open-label study of lamotrigine adjunct or monotherapy for the treatment of adolescents with bipolar depression. J Am Acad Child Adolesc Psychiatry 45:298–304, 2006

Charach A, Ickowicz A, Schachar R: Stimulant treatment over five years: adherence, effectiveness, and adverse effects. J Am Acad Child Adolesc Psychiatry 43:559–567, 2004

Cheng-Shannon J, McGough J, Pataki C, et al: Second-generation antipsychotic medication in children and adolescents. J Child Adolesc Psychopharmacol 14:372–394, 2004

Cherland E, Fitzpatrick R: Psychotic side effects of psychostimulants: a 5-year review. Can J Psychiatry 44:811–813, 1999

Chungh DS, Kim BN, Cho SC: Neuroleptic malignant syndrome due to three atypical antipsychotics in a child. J Psychopharmacol 19:422–425, 2005

Clein PD, Riddle MA: Pharmacokinetics in children and adolescents. Child Adolesc Psychiatr Clin N Am 4:59–75, 1995

Coffey BJ: Anxiolytics for children and adolescents: traditional and new drugs. J Child Adolesc Psychopharmacol 1:57–83, 1990

Coffey BJ: Ethical issues in child and adolescent psychopharmacology. Child Adolesc Psychiatr Clin N Am 4:793–807, 1995

Coffey BJ, Shader RI, Greenblatt DJ: Pharmacokinetics of benzodiazepines and psychostimulants in children. J Clin Psychopharmacol 3:217–225, 1983

Cohen JA, Mannarino AP, Knudsen K: Treating sexually abused children: 1 year follow-up of a randomized controlled trial. Child Abuse Negl 29:135–145, 2005

Compton SN, March JS, Brent D, et al: Cognitive-behavioral psychotherapy for anxiety and depressive disorders in children and adolescents: an evidence-based medicine review. J Am Acad Child Adolesc Psychiatry 43:930–959, 2004

Conners CK, Casat CD, Gualtieri CT, et al: Bupropion hydrochloride in attention deficit disorder with hyperactivity. J Am Acad Child Adolesc Psychiatry 35:1314–1321, 1996

Conners C, Sitarenios G, Parker JD, et al: The revised Conners' Parents Rating Scale (CPRS-R): factor structure, reliability, and criterion validity. J Abnorm Child Psychol 26:257–268, 1998a

Conners C, Sitarenios G, Parker JD, et al: Revision and restandardization of the Conners' Teacher Rating Scale (CTRS-R): factor structure, reliability, and criterion validity. J Abnorm Child Psychol 26:279–291, 1998b

Connor DF: Beta blockers for aggression: a review of the pediatric experience. J Child Adolesc Psychopharmacol 3:99–114, 1993

Connor DF: Preschool attention deficit hyperactivity disorder: a review of prevalence, diagnosis, neurobiology, and stimulant treatment. J Dev Behav Pediatr 23 (1 suppl):S1–S9, 2002

Connor DF, Ozbayrak KR, Benjamin S, et al: A pilot study of nadolol for overt aggression in developmentally delayed individuals. J Am Acad Child Adolesc Psychiatry 36:826–834, 1997

Connor DF, Fletcher KE, Swanson JM: A meta-analysis of clonidine for symptoms of attention-deficit hyperactivity disorder. J Am Acad Child Adolesc Psychiatry 38:1551–1559, 1999

Connor DF, Barkley RA, Davis HT: A pilot study of methylphenidate, clonidine, or the combination in ADHD comorbid with aggressive oppositional defiant or conduct disorder. Clin Pediatr (Phila) 39:15–25, 2000

Cook EH, Wagner KD, March JS, et al: Long-term sertraline treatment of children and adolescents with obsessive-compulsive disorder. J Am Acad Child Adolesc Psychiatry 40:1175–1181, 2001

Correll CU: Metabolic side effects of second-generation antipsychotics in children and adolescents: a different story? J Clin Psychiatry 66:1331–1332, 2005

Correll CU, Penzner JB, Parikh UH, et al: Recognizing and monitoring adverse events of second-generation antipsychotics in children and adolescents. Child Adolesc Psychiatric Clin N Am 15:177–206, 2006

Corson AH, Barkenbus JE, Posey DJ, et al: A retrospective analysis of quetiapine in the treatment of pervasive developmental disorders. J Clin Psychiatry 65:1531–1536, 2004

Cozza KL, Armstrong SC, Oesterheld JR: Concise Guide to Drug Interaction Principles for Medical Practice: Cytochrome P450s, UGTs, P-Glycoproteins. Washington, DC, American Psychiatric Publishing, 2003

Cueva JE, Overall JE, Small AM, et al: Carbamazepine in aggressive children with conduct disorder: a double-blind and placebo-controlled study. J Am Acad Child Adolesc Psychiatry 35:480–490, 1996

Davidson B, Quinn WH, Josephson AM: Assessment of the family: systemic and developmental perspectives. Child Adolesc Psychiatr Clin N Am 10:415–429, 2001

De Haan E, Hoogduin KA, Buitelaar JK, et al: Behavior therapy versus clomipramine for the treatment of obsessive-compulsive disorder in children and adolescents. J Am Acad Child Adolesc Psychiatry 37:1022–1029, 1998

DelBello MP, Schwiers ML, Rosenberg HL, et al: A double-blind, randomized, placebo-controlled study of quetiapine as adjunctive treatment for adolescent mania. J Am Acad Child Adolesc Psychiatry 41:1216–1223, 2002

DelBello MP, Findling RL, Kushner S, et al: A pilot controlled trial of topiramate for mania in children and adolescents with bipolar disorder. J Am Acad Child Adolesc Psychiatry 44:539–547, 2005

DelBello MP, Kowatch RA, Adler CM, et al: A double-blind randomized pilot study comparing quetiapine and divalproex for adolescent mania. J Am Acad Child Adolesc Psychiatry 45:305–313, 2006

Deas D, May K, Randall C, et al: Naltrexone treatment of adolescent alcoholics: an open-label pilot study. J Child Adolesc Psychopharmacol 15:723–728, 2005

Dion Y, Annable L, Sandor P, et al: Risperidone in the treatment of Tourette syndrome: a double-blind, placebo-controlled trial. J Clin Psychopharmacol 22:31–39, 2002

Donenberg GR: Reconsidering "Between-Group Psychotherapy Outcome Research and Basic Science": applications to child and adolescent psychotherapy outcome research. J Clin Psychol 5:181–190, 1999

Duff G (2003a): Safety of Seroxat (paroxetine) in children and adolescents under 18 years—contraindication in the treatment of depressive illness. June 10, 2003. Available at: http://www.mhra.gov.uk/home/groups/pl-p/documents/drugsafetymessage/con019507.pdf. Accessed April 30, 2006.

Duff G (2003b): Safety of venlafaxine in children and adolescents under 18 years in the treatment of depressive illness. September 19, 2003. Available at: http://www.mhra.gov.uk/home/groups/pl-p/documents/drugsafetymessage/con019503.pdf. Accessed April 30, 2006.

Duff G (2003c): Selective serotonin reuptake inhibitors—use in children and adolescents with major depressive disorder. December 10, 2003. Available at: http://www.mhra.gov.uk/home/groups/pl-p/documents/drugsafetymessage/con019492.pdf. Accessed April 30, 2006.

Dulcan MK: Brief psychotherapy with children and their families: the state of the art. Journal of the American Academy of Child Psychiatry 23:544–551, 1984

Dulcan MK (ed): Helping Parents, Youth, and Teachers Understand Medications for Behavioral and Emotional Problems: A Resource Book of Medication Information Handouts, 3rd Edition. Washington, DC, American Psychiatric Publishing, 2006

Dulcan MK, Piercy PA: A model for teaching and evaluating brief psychotherapy with children and their families. Professional Psychology: Research and Practice 16:689–700, 1985

Dulcan MK, Martini DR, Lake M: Concise Guide to Child and Adolescent Psychiatry, 3rd Edition. Washington, DC, American Psychiatric Publishing, 2003

Dummit ES, Klein RG, Tancer NK, et al: Fluoxetine treatment of children with selective mutism. J Am Acad Child Adolesc Psychiatry 35:615–621, 1996

Elia J, Borcherding BG, Rapoport JL, et al: Methylphenidate and dextroamphetamine treatments of hyperactivity: are there true nonresponders? Psychiatry Res 36:141–155, 1991

Emery G, Bedrosian R, Garber J: Cognitive therapy with depressed children and adolescents, in Affective Disorders in Childhood and Adolescence: An Update. Edited by Cantwell DP, Carlson GA. New York, Spectrum, 1983, pp 445–471

Emslie GJ, Heiligenstein JH, Wagner KD, et al: Fluoxetine for acute treatment of depression in children and adolescents: a placebo-controlled, randomized clinical trial. J Am Acad Child Adolesc Psychiatry 41:1205–1215, 2002

Emslie GJ, Heiligenstein JH, Hoog SL, et al: Fluoxetine treatment for prevention of relapse of depression in children and adolescents: a double-blind, placebo-controlled study. J Am Acad Child Adolesc Psychiatry 43:1397–1405, 2004

Emslie GJ, Wagner KD, Kutcher S, et al: Paroxetine treatment in children and adolescents with major depressive disorder: a randomized, multicenter, double-blind, placebo-controlled trial. J Am Acad Child Adolesc Psychiatry 45:709–719, 2006

Emslie GJ, Findling RL, Yeung PP, et al: Venlafaxine ER for the treatment of pediatric subjects with depression: results of two placebo-controlled trials. J Am Acad Child Adolesc Psychiatry 46:479–488, 2007

Faigel HC: The effect of beta blockade on stress-induced cognitive dysfunction in adolescents. Clin Pediatr (Phila) 30:441–445, 1991

Famularo R, Kinscherff R, Fenton T: Propranolol treatment for childhood posttraumatic stress disorder, acute type. Am J Dis Child 142:1244–1247, 1988

Feigin A, Kurlan R, McDermott MP, et al: A controlled trial of deprenyl in children with Tourette's syndrome and attention deficit hyperactivity disorder. Neurology 46:965–968, 1996

Feingold BE. Why Your Child Is Hyperactive. New York, Random House, 1975

Feldman HM, Kolmen BK, Gonzaga AM: Naltrexone and communication skills in young children with autism. J Am Acad Child Adolesc Psychiatry 38:587–593, 1999

Findling RL, McNamara NK, Branicky LA, et al: A double-blind pilot study of risperidone in the treatment of conduct disorder. J Am Acad Child Adolesc Psychiatry 39:509–516, 2000

Findling RL, Blumer JL, Kauffman R, et al: Aripiprazole in pediatric conduct disorder: a pilot study. Eur Neuropsychopharmacol 13 (suppl 4):S335, 2003a

Findling RL, Kusumakar V, Daneman D, et al: Prolactin levels during long-term risperidone treatment in children and adolescents. J Clin Psychiatry 64:1362–1369, 2003b

Findling RL, McNamara NK, Gracious BL, et al: Combination lithium and divalproex sodium in pediatric bipolarity. J Am Acad Child Adolesc Psychiatry 42:895–901, 2003c

Findling RL, Aman MG, Eerdekens M, et al: Long-term, open-label study of risperidone in children with severe disruptive behaviors and below-average IQ. Am J Psychiatry 161:677–684, 2004

Findling RL, McNamara NK, Youngstron EA, et al: Double-blind 18-month trial of lithium versus divalproex maintenance treatment in pediatric bipolar disorder. J Am Acad Child Adolesc Psychiatry 44:409–417, 2005a

Findling RL, Steiner H, Weller EB: Use of antipsychotics in children and adolescents. J Clin Psychiatry 66 (suppl 7): 29–40, 2005b

Findling RL, Reed MD, O'Riordan MA, et al: A 26-week open-label study of quetiapine in children with conduct disorder. J Child Adolesc Psychopharmacol 17:1–9, 2007

Fleck S: A general systems approach to severe family pathology. Am J Psychiatry 133:669–673, 1976

Forehand R, Long N: Parenting the Strong-Willed Child: The Clinically Proven Five-Week Program for Parents of Two- to Six-Year-Olds, Revised and Updated Edition. New York, Contemporary Books, 2002

Gadow KD: Effects of stimulant drugs on academic performance in hyperactive and learning disabled children. J Learn Disabil 16:290–299, 1983

Gadow KD: Pediatric psychopharmacology: a review of recent research. J Child Psychol Psychiatry 33:153–195, 1992

Gaffney GR, Perry PJ, Lund BC, et al: Risperidone versus clonidine in the treatment of children and adolescents with Tourette's syndrome. J Am Acad Child Adolesc Psychiatry 41:330–336, 2002

Gardner RA: Helping children cooperate in therapy, in Basic Handbook of Child Psychiatry, Vol 3: Therapeutic Interventions. Edited by Harrison SI. New York, Basic Books, 1979, pp 414–433

Garland EJ, Baerg EA: Amotivational syndrome associated with selective serotonin reuptake inhibitors in children and adolescents. J Child Adolesc Psychopharmacol 11:181–186, 2001

Geller B, Cooper TB, Zimerman B, et al: Lithium for prepubertal depressed children with family history predictors of future bipolarity: a double-blind, placebo-controlled study. J Affect Disord 51:165–175, 1998a

Geller B, Coper TB, Sun K, et al: Double-blind and placebo-controlled study of lithium for adolescent bipolar disorders with secondary substance dependency. J Am Acad Child Adolesc Psychiatry 37:171–178, 1998b

Geller B, Reising D, Leonard HL, et al: Critical review of tricyclic antidepressant use in children and adolescents. J Am Acad Child Adolesc Psychiatry 38:513–516, 1999

Geller DA, Biederman J, Steward SE, et al: Which SSRI? A meta-analysis of pharmacotherapy trials in pediatric obsessive-compulsive disorder. Am J Psychiatry 160:1919–1928, 2003

Genton P, Bauer J, Duncan S, et al: On the association between valproate and polycystic ovary syndrome. Epilepsia 42:305–310, 2001

Gepertz S, Nevéus T: Imipramine for therapy resistant enuresis: a retrospective evaluation. J Urol 171:2607–2610, 2004

Ghaziuddin N, Kutcher SP, Knapp P, et al: Practice parameter for use of electroconvulsive therapy with adolescents. Work Group on Quality Issues, AACAP. J Am Acad Child Adolesc Psychiatry 43:1521–1539, 2004

Gibbons RD, Hur K, Bhaumik DK, et al: The relationship between antidepressant medication use and rate of suicide. Arch Gen Psychiatry 62:165–172, 2005

Gittelman R, Klein DF, Feingold I: Children with reading disorders, II: effects of methylphenidate in combination with reading remediation. J Child Psychol Psychiatry 24:193–212, 1983

Glassman AH, Bigger JT: Antipsychotic drugs: prolonged QTc interval, torsade de pointes, and sudden death. Am J Psychiatry 158:1774–1782, 2001

GlaxoSmithKline: U.S. product labeling for Lamictal (lamotrigine). August 2005. Available at: http://us.gsk.com/products/assets/us_lamictal.pdf. Accessed June 3, 2006.

Goldbeck L, Schmid K: Effectiveness of autogenic relaxation training on children and adolescents with behavioral and emotional problems. J Am Acad Child Adolesc Psychiatry 42:1046–1054, 2003

Good CR, Feaster CS, Krecko VF: Tolerability of oral loading of divalproex sodium in child psychiatry inpatients. J Child Adolesc Psychopharmacol 11:53–57, 2001

Gordon CT, State RC, Nelson JE, et al: A double-blind comparison of clomipramine, desipramine, and placebo in the treatment of autistic disorder. Arch Gen Psychiatry 50:441–447, 1993

Graae F, Milner J, Rizzotto L, et al: Clonazepam in childhood anxiety disorders. J Am Acad Child Adolesc Psychiatry 333:372–376, 1994

Greenhill LL: Attention-deficit hyperactivity disorder. Child Adolesc Psychiatr Clin N Am 4:123–168, 1995

Greenhill LL, Findling RL, Swanson JM: A double-blind, placebo-controlled study of modified-release methylphenidate in children with attention-deficit/hyperactivity disorder. Pediatrics [serial online] 109:e39, 2002. Available at: http://www.pediatrics.org/cgi/content/full/109/3/e39. Accessed January 16, 2006.

Greenhill LL, Kollins S, Abikoff H, et al: Efficacy and safety of immediate-release methylphenidate treatment for preschoolers with ADHD. J Am Acad Child Adolesc Psychiatry 45:1284–1293, 2006a

Greenhill LL, Muniz R, Ball RR, et al: Efficacy and safety of dexmethylphenidate extended-release capsules in children with attention-deficit hyperactivity disorder. J Am Acad Child Adolesc Psychiatry 45:817–823, 2006b

Haapasalo-Pesu KM, Vuola T, Lahelma L, et al: Mirtazapine in the treatment of adolescents with major depression: an open-label, multicenter pilot study. J Child Adolesc Psychopharmacol 14:175–184, 2004

Hagerman RJ, Murphy MA, Wittenberg MD: A controlled trial of stimulant medication in children with the fragile X syndrome. Am J Med Genet 30:377–392, 1988

Handen BL, Hardan AY: Open label, prospective trial of olanzapine in adolescents with subaverage intelligence and disruptive behavior disorders. J Am Acad Child Adolesc Psychiatry 45:928–935, 2006

Handen BL, Feldman HM, Jurier A, et al: Efficacy of methylphenidate among preschool children with developmental disabilities and ADHD. J Am Acad Child Adolesc Psychiatry 38:944–951, 1999

Hardan AY, Jou RJ, Handen BL: Retrospective study of quetiapine in children and adolescents with pervasive developmental disorder. J Autism Dev Disord 35:387–391, 2005

Harley JP: Dietary treatment of behavioral disorders. Advances in Behavioral Pediatrics 1:129–151, 1980

Harper G: Focal inpatient treatment planning. J Am Acad Child Adolesc Psychiatry 28:31–37, 1989

Hazaray E, Ehret J, Posey DJ, et al: Intramuscular ziprasidone for acute agitation in adolescents. J Child Adolesc Psychopharmacol 14:464–470, 2004

Hazell PL, Stuart JE: A randomized controlled trial of clonidine added to psychostimulant medication for hyperactive and aggressive children. J Am Acad Child Adolesc Psychiatry 42:886–894, 2003

Health Canada (2005a): Health Canada suspends the market authorization of Adderall XR, a drug prescribed for attention deficit hyperactivity disorder (ADHD) in children. February 9, 2005. Available at: http://www.hc-sc.gc.ca/ahc-asc/media/advisories-avis/2005/2005_01_e.html. Accessed June 3, 2006.

Health Canada (2005b): Health Canada allows Adderall XR back on the Canadian Market. August 24, 2005. Available at: http://www.hc-sc.gc.ca/ahc-asc/media/nr-cp/2005/2005_92_e.html. Accessed June 3, 2006.

Henggeler SW, Borduin CM: Family Therapy and Beyond: A Multisystemic Approach to Treating the Behavior Problems of Children and Adolescents. Belmont, CA, Brooks/Cole, 1990

Henggeler SW, Schoenwald SK, Borduin CM, et al: Multisystemic Treatment of Antisocial Behavior in Children and Adolescents. New York, Guilford, 1998

Herskowitz J: Developmental neurotoxicology, in Psychiatric Pharmacosciences of Children and Adolescents. Edited by Popper C. Washington, DC, American Psychiatric Press, 1987, pp 81–123

Hjalmas KI, Hanson E, Hellstrom AL, et al: Long-term treatment with desmopressin in children with primary monosymptomatic nocturnal enuresis: an open multicentre study. Swedish Enuresis Trial Group (SWEET). Br J Urol 82:704–709, 1998

Hjalmas K, Arnold T, Bower W, et al: Nocturnal enuresis: an international evidence based management strategy. J Urol 171:2545–2561, 2004

Hoag MJ, Burlingame GM: Evaluating the effectiveness of child and adolescent group treatment: a meta-analytic review. J Clin Child Psychol 26:234–246, 1997

Hollander E, Wasserman S, Swanson EN, et al: A double-blind placebo-controlled pilot study of olanzapine in childhood/adolescent pervasive developmental disorder. J Child Adolesc Psychopharmacol 16:541–548, 2006

Horrigan JP, Barnhill LJ: Guanfacine and secondary mania in children. J Affect Disord 54:309–314, 1999

Houts AC: Behavioural treatment for enuresis. Scand J Urol Nephrol 173 (suppl):83–86, 1995

Hughes CW, Emslie GJ, Crimson ML, et al: Texas Children's Medication Algorithm Project: update from Texas consensus conference panel on medication treatment of childhood major depressive disorder. J Am Acad Child Adolesc Psychiatry 46:667–686, 2007

Hunt RD, Capper S, O'Connell P: Clonidine in child and adolescent psychiatry. J Child Adolesc Psychopharmacol 1:87–102, 1990

Hunt RD, Lau S, Ryu J: Alternative therapies for ADHD, in Ritalin: Theory and Patient Management. Edited by Greenhill LL, Osman BB. New York, Mary Ann Liebert, 1991, pp 75–95

Isojarvi JI, Laatikainen TJ, Pakarinen AJ, et al: Polycystic ovaries and hyperandrogenism in women taking valproate for epilepsy. N Engl J Med 329:1383–1388, 1993

Janknegt RA, Zweers HMM, Delaere KPJ, et al: Oral desmopressin as a new treatment modality for primary nocturnal enuresis in adolescents and adults: a double-blind, randomized, multicenter study. J Urol 157:513–517, 1997

Jensen PS: Current concepts and controversies in the diagnosis and treatment of attention deficit hyperactivity disorder. Curr Psychiatry Rep 2:102–109, 2000

Jensen PS, Hinshaw SP, Kraemer HC, et al: ADHD comorbidity findings from the MTA study: comparing comorbid subgroups. J Am Acad Child Adolesc Psychiatry 40:147–158, 2001

Jensen PS, Arnold LE, Swanson JM, et al: 3-year follow-up of the NIMH MTA study. J Am Acad Child Adolesc Psychiatry 46:989–1002, 2007

Joorabchi B: Expressions of the hyperventilation syndrome in childhood. Clin Pediatr (Phila) 16:1110–1115, 1977

Kafantaris V, Coletti DJ, Dicker R, et al: Lithium treatment of acute mania in adolescents: a large open trial. J Am Acad Child Adolesc Psychiatry 42:1038–1045, 2003

Kafantaris V, Coletti DJ, Dicker R, et al: Lithium treatment of acute mania in adolescents: a placebo-controlled discontinuation study. J Am Acad Child Adolesc Psychiatry 43:984–993, 2004

Kant R, Chalansani R, Chengappa KNR, et al: The off-label use of clozapine in adolescents with bipolar disorder, intermittent explosive disorder, or posttraumatic stress disorder. J Child Adolesc Psychopharmacol 14:57–63, 2004

Kazdin AD: Developing a research agenda for child and adolescent psychotherapy. Arch Gen Psychiatry 57:829–835, 2000

Kazdin AD: Parent Management Training: Treatment for Oppositional, Aggressive, and Antisocial Behavior in Children and Adolescents. New York, Oxford University Press, 2005

Keller MB, Ryan ND, Strober M, et al: Efficacy of paroxetine in the treatment of adolescent major depression: a randomized, controlled trial. J Am Acad Child Adolesc Psychiatry 40:762–772, 2001

Kemner C, Willemsen-Swinkels SH, de Jonge M, et al: Open-label study of olanzapine in children with pervasive developmental disorder. J Clin Psychopharmacol 22:455–460, 2002

Kerbeshian J, Burd L, Fisher W: Lithium carbonate in the treatment of two patients with infantile autism and atypical bipolar symptomatology. J Clin Psychopharmacol 7:401–405, 1987

Kernberg PF, Chazan SE: Children With Conduct Disorders: A Psychotherapy Manual. New York, Basic Books, 1991

Kisch EH: Brief psychotherapy with children, adolescents, and their families. Child Adolesc Psychiatr Clin N Am 6:137–150, 1997

Klein RG, Koplewicz HS, Kanner A: Imipramine treatment of children with separation anxiety disorder. J Am Acad Child Adolesc Psychiatry 31:21–28, 1992

Kolmen BK, Feldman HM, Handen BL, et al: Naltrexone in young autistic children: a double-blind, placebo-controlled crossover study. J Am Acad Child Adolesc Psychiatry 34:223–231, 1995

Kowatch RA, Bucci JP: Mood stabilizers and anticonvulsants. Pediatr Clin North Am 45:1173–1186, 1998

Kowatch RA, Suppes T, Carmody TJ, et al: Effect size of lithium, divalproex sodium, and carbamazepine in children and adolescents with bipolar disorder. J Am Acad Child Adolesc Psychiatry 39:713–720, 2000

Kratochvil CJ, Heiligenstein JH, Dittman R, et al: Atomoxetine and methylphenidate treatment in children with ADHD: a prospective, randomized, open-label trial. J Am Acad Child Adolesc Psychiatry 41:776–784, 2002

Kratochvil CJ, Wilens TE, Greenhill LL, et al: Effects of long-term atomoxetine treatment for young children with attention-deficit/hyperactivity disorder. J Am Acad Child Adolesc Psychiatry 45:919–927, 2006

Kumra S, Frazier JA, Jacobsen LK, et al: Child-onset schizophrenia: a double-blind clozapine-haloperidol comparison. Arch Gen Psychiatry 53:1090–1097, 1996

Kumra S, Jacobsen L, Lenane M, et al: Case series: Spectrum of neuroleptic-induced movement disorders and extrapyramidal side effects in childhood-onset schizophrenia. J Am Acad Child Adolesc Psychiatry 37:221–227, 1998

Kutcher SP, Williamson P, MacKenzie S, et al: Successful clonazepam treatment of neuroleptic-induced akathisia in older adolescents and young adults: a double-blind, placebo-controlled study. J Clin Psychopharmacol 9:403–406, 1989

Kutcher SP, Reiter S, Gardner DM, et al: The pharmacotherapy of anxiety disorders in children and adolescents. Psychiatr Clin North Am 15:41–67, 1992

Leckman JF, Ort S, Caruso KA, et al: Rebound phenomena in Tourette's syndrome after abrupt withdrawal of clonidine: behavioral, cardiovascular, and neurochemical effects. Arch Gen Psychiatry 43:1168–1176, 1986

Leckman JF, Hardin MT, Riddle MA, et al: Clonidine treatment of Gilles de la Tourette's syndrome. Arch Gen Psychiatry 48:324–328, 1991

Levine MD: Encopresis: its potentiation, evaluation and alleviation. Pediatr Clin North Am 29:315–330, 1982

Lewinsohn PM, Clarke GN, Hops H, et al: Cognitive-behavioral treatment for depressed adolescents. Behav Ther 21:385–401, 1990

Lewis O: Psychological factors affecting pharmacological compliance. Child Adolesc Psychiatr Clin N Am 4:15–22, 1995

Lewis O: Integrated psychodynamic psychotherapy with children. Child Adolesc Psychiatr Clin N Am 6:53–68, 1997

Lipinski F, Mallya G, Zimmerman P, et al: Fluoxetine-induced akathisia: clinical and theoretical implications. J Clin Psychiatry 50:339–342, 1989

Malone RP, Delaney MA, Luebbert JF, et al: A double-blind placebo-controlled study of lithium in hospitalized aggressive children and adolescents with conduct disorder. Arch Gen Psychiatry 57:649–654, 2000

Mandoki MW, Tapia MR, Tapia MA, et al: Venlafaxine in the treatment of children and adolescents with major depression. Psychopharmacol Bull 33:149–154, 1997

March JS, Mulle K, Herbel B: Behavioral psychotherapy for children and adolescents with obsessive-compulsive disorder: an open trial of a new protocol-driven treatment package. J Am Acad Child Adolesc Psychiatry 33:333–341, 1994

March JS, Foa E, Gammon P, et al: Cognitive-behavior therapy, sertraline, and their combination for children and adolescents with obsessive-compulsive disorder. The Pediatric OCD Treatment Study (POTS) randomized controlled trial. JAMA 292:1969–1976, 2004

March JS, Silva S, Vitiello B: The Treatment for Adolescents with Depression Study: methods and message at 12 weeks. J Am Acad Child Adolesc Psychiatry 45:1393–1403, 2006

Martin A, Scahill L, Anderson G, et al: Weight and leptin changes among risperidone-treated youths with autism: 6-month prospective data. Am J Psychiatry 161:1125–1127, 2004

Masek BJ, Spirito A, Fentress DW: Behavioral treatment of symptoms of childhood illness. Clin Psychol Rev 4:561–570, 1984

Masi G, Toni C, Mucci M, et al: Paroxetine in child and adolescent outpatients with panic disorder. J Child Adolesc Psychopharmacol 11:151–157, 2001a

Masi G, Cosenza A, Mucci M: Open trial of risperidone in 24 young children with pervasive developmental disorders. J Am Acad Child Adolesc Psychiatry 40:1206–1214, 2001b

Masi G, Cosenza A, Mucci M, et al: A 3-year naturalistic study of 53 preschool children with pervasive developmental disorders treated with risperidone. J Clin Psychiatry 64:1039–1047, 2003

McConville B, Carrero L, Sweitzer D, et al: Long-term safety, tolerability, and clinical efficacy of quetiapine in adolescents: an open-label extension trial. J Child Adolesc Psychopharmacol 13:75–82, 2003

McCracken JT, Biederman J, Greenhill LL, et al: Analog classroom assessment of a once-daily mixed amphetamine formulation, SLI381 (Adderall XR), in children with ADHD. J Am Acad Child Adolesc Psychiatry 42:673–683, 2003

McCracken JT, Aman MG, McDougle CJ, et al (Research Units on Pediatric Psychopharmacology Autism Network): Risperidone treatment of autistic disorder: longer-term benefits and blinded discontinuation after 6 months. Am J Psychiatry 162:1361–1369, 2005

McDaniel KD: Pharmacological treatment of psychiatric and neurodevelopmental disorders in children and adolescents, I. Clin Pediatr (Phila) 25:65–71, 1986

McDougle CJ, Kem DL, Posey DJ: Case series: use of ziprasidone for maladaptive symptoms in youths with autism. J Am Acad Child Adolesc Psychiatry 41:921–927, 2002

McDougle CJ, Scahill L, Aman M, et al: Risperidone for the core symptom domains of autism: results from the study by the Autism Network of the Research Units on Pediatric Psychopharmacology. Am J Psychiatry 162:1142–1148, 2005

McGough JJ, Biederman J, Wigal SB, et al: Long-term tolerability and effectiveness of once-daily mixed amphetamine salts (Adderall XR) in children with ADHD. J Am Acad Child Adolesc Psychiatry 44:530–538, 2005

McGough JJ, Wigal SB, Abikoff H, et al: A randomized, double-blind, placebo-controlled, laboratory classroom assessment of methylphenidate transdermal system in children with ADHD. J Atten Disord 9:476–485, 2006

McMahon R, Forehand R: Helping the Noncompliant Child: Family-Based Treatment for Oppositional Behavior, 2nd Edition. New York, Guilford, 2003

McMillen JC, Zima BT, Scott LD, et al: Prevalence of psychiatric disorders among older youths in the foster care system. J Am Acad Child Adolesc Psychiatry 44:88–95, 2005

Measham TJ: The acute management of aggressive behavior in hospitalized children and adolescents. Can J Psychiatry 40:330–336, 1995

Melamed BG, Klingman A, Siegel LJ: Individualizing cognitive behavioral strategies in the reduction of medical and dental stress, in Cognitive Behavior Therapy With Children. Edited by Meyers AW, Craighead WE. New York, Plenum, 1984, pp 289–313

Mikkelson EJ: Enuresis and encopresis: ten years of progress. J Am Acad Child Adolesc Psychiatry 40:1146–1158, 2001

Mohammadi MR, Ghanizadeh A, Alaghband-rad J, et al: Selegiline in comparison with methylphenidate in attention deficit hyperactivity disorder children and adolescents in a double-blind, randomized clinical trial. J Child Adolesc Psychopharmacol 14:418–425, 2004

Montgomery P, Bjornstad G, Dennis J: Media-based behavioural treatments for behavioural problems in children. Cochrane Database Syst Rev (1):CD002206, 2006

MTA Cooperative Group: A 14-month randomized clinical trial of treatment strategies for attention-deficit/hyperactivity disorder. Arch Gen Psychiatry 56:1073–1086, 1999

MTA Cooperative Group: National Institute of Mental Health Multimodal Treatment Study of ADHD Follow-up: 24-month outcomes of treatment strategies for attention-deficit/hyperactivity disorder. Pediatrics 113:754–761, 2004

Mufson L, Dorta KP, Moreau D, et al: Interpersonal Psychotherapy for Depressed Adolescents, 2nd Edition. New York, Guilford, 2004a

Mufson L, Dorta KP, Wickramaratne P, et al: A randomized effectiveness trial of interpersonal psychotherapy for depressed adolescents. Arch Gen Psychiatry 61:577–584, 2004b

Mukaddes NM, Abali O: Quetiapine treatment of children and adolescents with Tourette's disorder. J Child Adolesc Psychopharmacol 13:295–299, 2003

Newcorn JH, Spencer TJ, Biederman J, et al: Atomoxetine treatment in children and adolescents with attention-deficit hyperactivity disorder and comorbid oppositional defiant disorder. J Am Acad Child Adolesc Psychiatry 44:240–248, 2005

Newman TB: A black box warning for antidepressants in children? N Engl J Med 351:1595–1598, 2004

Niederhofer H: An open trial of buspirone in the treatment of attention-deficit disorder. Hum Psychopharmacol Clin Exp 18:489–492, 2003

Niederhofer H, Staffen W: Acamprosate and its efficacy in treating alcohol dependent adolescents. Eur Child Adolesc Psychiatry 12:144–148, 2003

Nilsson M, Joliat MJ, Miner CM, et al: Safety of subchronic treatment with Fluoxetine for major depressive disorder in children and adolescents. J Child Adolesc Psychopharmacol 14:412–417, 2004

O'Brien JD, Perlmutter I: The effect of medication on the process of psychotherapy. Child Adolesc Psychiatr Clin North Am 6:185–196, 1997

Olfson M, Marcus SC, Weissman MM, et al: National trends in the use of psychotropic medication by children. J Am Acad Child Adolesc Psychiatry 41:514–521, 2002

Olness K, Kohen DP: Hypnosis and Hypnotherapy With Children, 3rd Edition. New York, Guilford, 1996

Pappadopulos E, MacIntyre JC, Crimson ML, et al: Treatment recommendations for the use of antipsychotics for aggressive youth (TRAAY), Part II. J Am Acad Child Adolesc Psychiatry 42:145–161, 2003

Pappagallo M, Silva R: The effect of atypical antipsychotic agents on prolactin levels in children and adolescents. J Child Adolesc Psychopharmacol 14:359–371, 2004

Párraga HC, Párraga MI, Woodward RL, et al: Quetiapine treatment of children with Tourette's syndrome: report of two cases. J Child Adolesc Psychopharmacol 11:187–191, 2001

Patel NC, DelBello MP, Bryan HS, et al: Open-label lithium for the treatment of adolescents with bipolar depression. J Am Acad Child Adolesc Psychiatry 45:289–297, 2006

Pathak S, Johns ES, Kowatch RA: Adjunctive quetiapine for treatment-resistant adolescent major depressive disorder: a case series. J Child Adolesc Psychopharmacol 15:696–702, 2005

Patterson GR: Families: Applications of Social Learning to Family Life. Champaign, IL, Research Press, 1975

Patterson GR, Forgatch M: Parents and Adolescents Living Together: The Basics, 2nd Edition. Champaign, IL, Research Press, 2005

Pearson DA, Santos CW, Roache JD, et al: Treatment effects of methylphenidate on behavioral adjustment in children with mental retardation and ADHD. J Am Acad Child Adolesc Psychiatry 42:209–216, 2003

Pelham WE Jr, Hoza J: Behavioral assessment of psychostimulant effects on ADD children in a summer day treatment program, in Advances in Behavioral Assessment of Children and Families, Vol 3. Edited by Prinz R. Greenwich, CT, JAI Press, 1987, pp 3–33

Pelham WE, Gnagy EM, Greiner AR, et al: Behavioral versus behavioral and pharmacological treatment in ADHD children attending a summer treatment program. J Abnorm Child Psychol 28:507–526, 2000

Pelham WE, Massetti GM, Wilson T, et al: Implementation of a comprehensive schoolwide behavioral intervention: the ABC Program. J Atten Disord 9:248–260, 2005

Percy AK, Glaze DG, Schultz RJ, et al: Rett syndrome: controlled study of an oral opiate antagonist, naltrexone. Ann Neurol 35:464–470, 1994

Pfefferbaum B, Overall JE, Boron HA, et al: Alprazolam in the treatment of anticipatory and acute situational anxiety in children with cancer. J Am Acad Child Adolesc Psychiatry 26:532–535, 1987

PhysiciansMedGuide: The Use of Medication in Treating Childhood and Adolescent Depression: Information for Physicians. Available at: http://www.physiciansmedguide.org/physiciansmedguide.htm#c12. Accessed April 30, 2006.

Pliszka SR: A double-blind, placebo-controlled study of Adderall and methylphenidate in the treatment of attention-deficit/hyperactivity disorder. J Am Acad Child Adolesc Psychiatry 39:619–626, 2000

Pliszka SR, Crismon ML, Hughes CW, et al: The Texas Children's Medication Algorithm Project: revision of the algorithm for pharmacotherapy of attention-deficit/hyperactivity disorder. J Am Acad Child Adolesc Psychiatry 45:642–657, 2006

Pool D, Bloom W, Mielke DH, et al: A controlled evaluation of Loxitane in seventy-five adolescent schizophrenic patients. Curr Ther Res Clin Exp 19:99–104, 1976

Poulton A: Growth on stimulant medication; clarifying the confusion: a review. Arch Dis Child 90:801–806, 2005

Powers PS, Sachs BS, Kushner SF, et al: Topiramate in adults with acute bipolar I mania: pooled results. Presented at the 157th annual meeting of the American Psychiatric Association, New York, NY, May 1–6, 2004

Rapoport JL: Antidepressants in childhood attention deficit disorder and obsessive-compulsive disorder. Psychosomatics 27 (suppl):30–36, 1986

Ratey J, Sovner R, Parks A, et al: Buspirone treatment of aggression and anxiety in mentally retarded patients: a multiple-baseline, placebo lead-in study. J Clin Psychiatry 52:159–162, 1991

Realmuto GM, Erickson WD, Yellin AM, et al: Clinical comparison of thiothixene and thioridazine in schizophrenic adolescents. Am J Psychiatry 141:440–442, 1984

Reischer H, Pfeffer CR: Lithium pharmacokinetics. J Am Acad Child Adolesc Psychiatry 35:130–131, 1996

Richardson MA, Haugland G, Craig TJ: Neuroleptic use, parkinsonian symptoms, tardive dyskinesia, and associated factors in child and adolescent psychiatric patients. Am J Psychiatry 148:1322–1328, 1991

Riddle MA: Paroxetine and the FDA. J Am Acad Child Adolesc Psychiatry 43:128–130, 2004

Rojas NL, Chan E: Old and new controversies in the alternative treatment of attention-deficit hyperactivity disorder. Ment Retard Dev Disabil Res Rev 11:116–130, 2005

Rosenfeld AA, Pilowsky DJ, Fine P, et al: Foster care: an update. J Am Acad Child Adolesc Psychiatry 36:448–457, 1997

Ryan ND: Heterocyclic antidepressants in children and adolescents. J Child Adolesc Psychopharmacol 1:21–31, 1990

Ryan ND: The pharmacological treatment of child and adolescent depression. Psychiatr Clin North Am 15:29–40, 1992

Rynn MA, Siqueland L, Rickels K: Placebo-controlled trial of sertraline in the treatment of children with generalized anxiety disorder. Am J Psychiatry 158:2008–2014, 2001

Safer DJ: Changing patterns of psychotropic medications prescribed by child psychiatrists in the 1990s. J Child Adolesc Psychopharmacol 7:267–274, 1997

Saito E, Correll CU, Gallelli K, et al: A prospective study of hyperprolactinemia in children and adolescents treated with atypical antipsychotic agents. J Child Adolesc Psychopharmacol 14:350–358, 2004

Sallee F, Stiller R, Perel J, et al: Targeting imipramine dose in children with depression. Clin Pharmacol Ther 40:8–13, 1986

Sallee FR, Kurlan R, Goetz CG, et al: Ziprasidone treatment of children and adolescents with Tourette syndrome: a pilot study. J Am Acad Child Adolesc Psychiatry 39:292–299, 2000

Samuel RZ: EPS with lithium (letter). J Am Acad Child Adolesc Psychiatry 32:1078, 1993

Sanchez LE, Campbell M, Small AM: A pilot study of clomipramine in young autistic children. J Am Acad Child Adolesc Psychiatry 35:537–544, 1996

Saul RC: Nortriptyline in attention deficit disorder. Clin Neuropharmacol 8:382–384, 1985

Scahill L, Chappell PB, Kim YS, et al: A placebo-controlled study of guanfacine in the treatment of children with tic disorders and attention deficit hyperactivity disorder. Am J Psychiatry 158:1067–1074, 2001

Scahill L, McCracken JT, McGough J, et al (Research Units on Pediatric Psychopharmacology Autism Network): Risperidone in children with autism and serious behavioral problems. N Engl J Med 347:314–321, 2002

Scahill L, Leckman JF, Schultz RT, et al: A placebo-controlled trial of risperidone in Tourette syndrome. Neurology 60:1130–1135, 2003

Scahill L, Aman MG, McDougle CJ, et al: A prospective open trial of guanfacine in children with pervasive developmental disorders. J Child Adolesc Psychopharmacol 16:589–598, 2006

Scharko AM: Selective serotonin reuptake inhibitor-induced sexual dysfunction in adolescents: a review. J Am Acad Child Adolesc Psychiatry 43:1071–1079, 2004

Scheidlinger S: Short-term group psychotherapy for children: an overview. Int J Group Psychother 34:573–585, 1984

Scheidlinger S: Group treatment of adolescents: an overview. Am J Orthopsychiatry 55:102–111, 1985

Schur SB, Sikich L, Findling RL, et al: Treatment Recommendations for the Use of Antipsychotics for Aggressive Youth (TRAAY), part I: a review. J Am Acad Child Adolesc Psychopharmacol 42:132–144, 2003

Seedat S, Stein DJ, Ziervogel C, et al: Comparison of response to a selective serotonin reuptake inhibitor in children, adolescents, and adults with posttraumatic stress disorder. J Child Adolesc Psychopharmacol 12:37–46, 2002

Serketich WJ, Dumas JE: The effectiveness of behavioral parent training to modify antisocial behavior in children: a meta-analysis. Behavioral Therapy 27:171–186, 1996

Shea S, Turgay A, Carroll A, et al: Risperidone in the treatment of disruptive behavioral symptoms in children with autistic and other pervasive developmental disorders. Pediatrics 114:634–641, 2004

Shire U.S. Inc: U.S. product labeling for Daytrana (methylphenidate transdermal system). Available at: http://www.daytrana.com/pdf/pdf1.pdf. Accessed June 25, 2006.

Sikich L, Hamer RM, Bashford RA, et al: A pilot study of risperidone, olanzapine, and haloperidol in psychotic youth: a double-blind, randomized, 8-week trial. Neuropsychopharmacology 29:133–145, 2004

Silver LB: Alternative (nonstimulant) medications in the treatment of attention-deficit/hyperactivity disorder in children. Pediatr Clin North Am 46:965–975, 1999

Silverman WK: Using what works to help children manage stress and anxiety: an appeal for pragmatism. Session: Psychotherapy in Practice 3:103–108, 1997

Silverman WK, Kurtines WM, Ginsburg GS, et al: Treating anxiety disorders in children with group cognitive-behavioral therapy: a randomized clinical trial. J Consult Clin Psychol 67:995–1003, 1999

Simeon JG, Ferguson HB: Recent developments in the use of antidepressant and anxiolytic medications. Psychiatr Clin North Am 8:893–907, 1985

Simeon JG, Ferguson HB, Knott V, et al: Clinical, cognitive, and neurophysiological effects of alprazolam in children and adolescents with overanxious and avoidant disorders. J Am Acad Child Adolesc Psychiatry 31:29–33, 1992

Singer HS, Brown J: The treatment of attention-deficit hyperactivity disorder in Tourette's syndrome: a double-blind placebo-controlled study with clonidine and desipramine. Pediatrics 95:74–81, 1995

Skoog SJ, Stokes A, Turner K: Oral desmopressin: a randomized double-blind placebo controlled study of effectiveness in children with primary nocturnal enuresis. J Urol 158:1035–1040, 1997

Smith P, Yule W, Perrin S, et al: Cognitive-behavioral therapy for PTSD in children and adolescents: a preliminary randomized controlled trial. J Am Acad Child Adolesc Psychiatry 46:1051–1061, 2007

Snyder R, Turgay A, Aman M, et al: Effects of risperidone on conduct and disruptive behavior disorders in children with subaverage IQs. J Am Acad Child Adolesc Psychiatry 41:1026–1036, 2002

Soderstrom H, Rastam M, Gillberg C: A clinical case series of six extremely aggressive youths treated with olanzapine. Eur Child Adolesc Psychiatry 11:138–141, 2002

Sokolski KN, Chicz-Demet A, Demet EM: Selective serotonin reuptake inhibitor-related extrapyramidal symptoms in autistic children: a case series. J Child Adolesc Psychopharmacol 14:143–147, 2004

Soni P, Weintraub AL: Case study: buspirone-associated mental status changes. J Am Acad Child Adolesc Psychiatry 31:1098–1099, 1992

Sours JA: The application of child analytic principles to forms of child psychotherapy, in Child Analysis and Therapy. Edited by Glenn J. New York, Jason Aronson, 1978, pp 615–646

Spencer EK, Kafantaris V, Padron-Gayol MV, et al: Haloperidol in schizophrenic children: early findings from a study in progress. Psychopharmacol Bull 28:183–186, 1992

Spencer T, Biederman J, Steingard R, et al: Bupropion exacerbates tics in children with attention-deficit hyperactivity disorder and Tourette's syndrome. J Am Acad Child Adolesc Psychiatry 32:211–214, 1993

Spencer T, Wilens T, Biederman J: Psychotropic medication for children and adolescents. Child Adolesc Psychiatr Clin N Am 4:97–121, 1995

Spencer T, Biederman J, Wilens T, et al: Pharmacotherapy of attention-deficit hyperactivity disorder across the life cycle. J Am Acad Child Adoles Psychiatry 35:409–432, 1996

Spencer T, Biederman J, Coffey B, et al: A double-blind comparison of desipramine and placebo in children and adolescents with chronic tic disorder and comorbid attention-deficit/hyperactivity disorder. Arch Gen Psychiatry 59:649–656, 2002

Spencer T, Newcorn JH, Kratochvil CJ, et al: Effects of Atomoxetine on growth after 2-year treatment among pediatric patients with attention-deficit/hyperactivity disorder. Pediatrics [serial online] 116:e74–e80, 2005. Available at: http://www.pediatrics.org/cgi/doi/10.1542/peds.2004-0624. Accessed March 17, 2006.

Stahl SM: Essential Pharmacology: Neuroscientific Basis and Practical Applications, 2nd Edition. New York, Cambridge University Press, 2000, pp 246–255

Standaert DG, Young AB: Treatment of central nervous system degenerative disorders (Chapter 20), in Goodman and Gilman's The Pharmacological Basis of Therapeutics, 11th Edition. Edited by Brunton LL. New York, McGraw-Hill, 2006. Available at: http://www.accessmedicine.com. Accessed May 2, 2006.

Steingard R, Biederman J: Lithium responsive manic-like symptoms in two individuals with autism and mental retardation. Journal of the American Academy of Child Psychiatry 26:932–935, 1987

Steingard R, Biederman J, Spencer TJ, et al: Comparison of clonidine response in the treatment of attention-deficit hyperactivity disorder with and without comorbid tic disorders. J Am Acad Child Adolesc Psychiatry 32:350–353, 1993

Stephens RJ, Bassel C, Sandor P: Olanzapine in the treatment of aggression and tics in children with Tourette's syndrome—a pilot study. J Child Adolesc Psychopharmacol 14:255–266, 2004

Stigler KA, Posey DJ, McDougle CJ: Aripiprazole for maladaptive behavior in pervasive developmental disorders. J Child Adolesc Psychopharmacol 14:455–463, 2004

Strayhorn JM Jr: The Competent Child: An Approach to Psychotherapy and Preventive Mental Health. New York, Guilford, 1988

Strupp HH: Psychotherapy: Clinical, Research, and Theoretical Issues. New York, Jason Aronson, 1973

Sugai G, Horner RH: Introduction to the special series on positive behavior support in schools. J Emotional Behavioral Disorders 10:130–136, 2002

Swanson JM, Gupta S, Williams L, et al: Efficacy of a new pattern of delivery of methylphenidate for the treatment of ADHD: effects on activity level in the classroom and on the playground. J Am Acad Child Adolesc Psychiatry 41:1306–1314, 2002

Swanson JM, Greenhill LL, Lopez FA, et al: Modafinil film-coated tablets in children and adolescents with attention-deficit/hyperactivity disorder: results of a randomized, double-blind, placebo-controlled, fixed-dose study followed by abrupt discontinuation. J Clin Psychiatry 67:137–147, 2006

Swanson JM, Elliott GR, Greenhill LL, et al: Effects of stimulant medication on growth rates across 3 years in the MTA follow-up. J Am Acad Child Adolesc Psychiatry 46:1015–1027, 2007

Teicher MH, Glod CA: Neuroleptic drugs: indications and guidelines for their rational use in children and adolescents. J Child Adolesc Psychopharmacol 1:33–56, 1990

Thompson S, Rey JM: Functional enuresis: is desmopressin the answer? J Am Acad Child Adolesc Psychiatry 34:266–271, 1995

Tourette's Syndrome Study Group: Treatment of ADHD in children with tics: a randomized controlled trial. Neurology 58:527–536, 2002

Trimble MR: Anticonvulsants in children and adolescents. J Child Adolesc Psychopharmacol 1:33–56, 1990

Troost PW, Lahuis BE, Steenhuis MP, et al: Long-term effects of risperidone in children with autism spectrum disorders: a placebo-discontinuation study. J Am Acad Child Adolesc Psychiatry 44:1137–1144, 2005

Turgay A, Binder C, Snyder R, et al: Long-term safety and efficacy of risperidone for the treatment of disruptive behavior disorders in children with subaverage IQs. Pediatrics [serial online] 110:e34, 2002. Available at: http://www.pediatrics/org/cgi/content/full/110/3/e34. Accessed April 2, 2006.

U.S. Food and Drug Administration (2003a): FDA statement regarding the antidepressant Paxil for pediatric population. June 19, 2003. Available at: http://www.fda.gov/bbs/topics/ANSWERS/2003/ANS01230.html. Accessed March 19, 2006.

U.S. Food and Drug Administration (2003b): FDA issues public health advisory entitled: Reports of suicidality in pediatric patients being treated with antidepressant medications for major depressive disorder (MDD). October 27, 2003. Available at: http://www.fda.gov/bbs/topics/ANSWERS/2003/ANS12356.html. Accessed March 19, 2006.

U.S. Food and Drug Administration (2004a): FDA updates its review of antidepressant drugs in children. August 20, 2004. Available at: http://www.fda.gov/bbs/topics/ANSWERS/2004/ANS01306.html. Accessed March 19, 2006.

U.S. Food and Drug Administration (2004b): Center for Drug Evaluation and Research. Transcript of the joint meeting of the CDER psychopharmacological drugs advisory committee and the FDA pediatric advisory committee. September 14, 2004. Available at: http://www.fda.gov/ohrms/dockets/ac/04/transcripts/2004–4065T2.pdf. Accessed April 30, 2006.

U.S. Food and Drug Administration (2004c): FDA statement on recommendations of the psychopharmacological drugs and pediatric advisory committees. September 16, 2004. Available at: http://www.fda.gov/bbs/topics/news/2004/NEW01116.html. Accessed January 8, 2006.

Van Putten T, Marder SR: Behavioral toxicity of antipsychotic drugs. J Clin Psychiatry 48 (suppl):13–19, 1987

Varley C, McClellan J: Case study: two additional sudden deaths with tricyclic antidepressants. J Am Acad Child Adolesc Psychiatry 36:390–394, 1997

Varni JW, Jay SM, Masek BJ, et al: Cognitive-behavioral assessment and management of pediatric pain, in Handbook of Psychological Treatment Approaches. Edited by Holvman AD, Turk ED. New York, Pergamon, 1986, pp 168–192

Vieweg WVR, Sood AB, Pandurangi A, et al: Newer antipsychotic drugs and obesity in children and adolescents. How should we assess drug-associated weight gain? Acta Psychiatr Scand 111:177–184, 2005

Vitiello B, Severe JB, Greenhill LL, et al: Methylphenidate dosage for children with ADHD over time under controlled conditions: lessons from the MTA. J Am Acad Child Adolesc Psychiatry 40:188–196, 2001

Wagner KD, Weller EB, Carlson GA, et al: An open-label trial of divalproex in children and adolescents with bipolar disorder. J Am Acad Child Adolesc Psychiatry 41:1224–1230, 2002

Wagner KD, Ambrosini P, Rynn M, et al: Efficacy of sertraline in the treatment of children and adolescents with major depressive disorder—two randomized controlled trials. JAMA 290:1033–1041, 2003

Wagner KD, Robb AS, Findling RL, et al: A randomized, placebo-controlled trial of citalopram for the treatment of major depression in children and adolescents. Am J Psychiatry 161:1079–1083, 2004a

Wagner KD, Berard R, Stein MB, et al: A multicenter, randomized, double-blind, placebo-controlled trial of paroxetine in children and adolescents with social anxiety disorder. Arch Gen Psychiatry 61:1153–1162, 2004b

Wagner KD, Jonas J, Findling RL, et al: A double-blind, randomized, placebo-controlled trial of escitalopram in the treatment of pediatric depression. J Am Acad Child Adolesc Psychiatry 45:280–288, 2006a

Wagner KD, Kowatch RA, Emslie, GJ, et al: A double-blind, randomized, placebo-controlled trial of oxcarbazepine in the treatment of bipolar disorder in children and adolescents. Am J Psychiatry 163:1179–1186, 2006b

Walkup JT, Labellarte M: Complications of SSRI treatment. J Child Adolesc Psychopharmacol 11:1–4, 2001

Walkup JT, Labellarte MJ, Riddle MA, et al: Fluvoxamine for the treatment of anxiety disorders in children and adolescents. N Engl J Med 344:1279–1285, 2001

Walsh BT, Greenhill LL, Elsa-Grace V, et al: Effects of desipramine on autonomic input to the heart. J Am Acad Child Adolesc Psychiatry 38:1186–1193, 1999

Waslick BD, Walsh BT, Greenhill LL, et al: Cardiovascular effects of desipramine in children and adults during exercise testing. J Am Acad Child Adolesc Psychiatry 38:179–186, 1999

Wehmeier PM, Schüler-Springorum M, Heiser P, et al: Chart review for potential features of myocarditis, pericarditis, and cardiomyopathy in children and adolescents treated with clozapine. J Child Adolesc Psychopharmacol 14:267–271, 2004

Weiss B, Catron T, Harris V: A 2-year follow-up of the effectiveness of traditional child psychotherapy. J Consult Clin Psychol 68:1094–1101, 2000

Weiss M, Tannock R, Kratochvil C, et al: A randomized, placebo-controlled study of once-daily atomoxetine in the school setting in children with ADHD. J Am Acad Child Adolesc Psychiatry 44:647–655, 2005

Weisz JR: Agenda for child and adolescent psychotherapy research. On the need to put science into practice. Arch Gen Psychiatry 57:837–838, 2000

Weisz JR, Jensen AL: Child and adolescent psychotherapy in research and practice contexts: review of the evidence and suggestions for improving the field. Eur Child Adolesc Psychiatry 10 (suppl 1):I/12–I/18, 2001

Weisz JR, Hawley KM, Doss AJ: Empirically tested psychotherapies for youth internalizing and externalizing problems and disorders. Child Adolesc Psychiatric Clin N Am 13:729–815, 2004

Weller EB, Weller RA, Fristad MA: Lithium dosage guide for prepubertal children: a preliminary report. Journal of the American Academy of Child Psychiatry 25:92–95, 1986

Whalen EH, Henker B: Social impact of stimulant treatment for hyperactive children. Journal of Learning Disabilities 24:231–241, 1991

Whittington CJ, Kendall T, Fonagy P, et al: Selective serotonin reuptake inhibitors in childhood depression: systematic review of published versus unpublished data. Lancet 363:1341–1345, 2004

Wigal S, Swanson JM, Feifel D, et al: A double-blind, placebo-controlled trial of dexmethylphenidate hydrochloride and d,l-threo-methylphenidate hydrochloride in children with attention-deficit/hyperactivity disorder. J Am Acad Child Adolesc Psychiatry 43:1406–1414, 2004

Wigal S, McGough J, McCracken JT, et al: A laboratory school comparison of mixed amphetamine salts extended release (Adderall XR) and atomoxetine (Strattera) in school-aged children with attention deficit/hyperactivity disorder. J Atten Disord 9:275–289, 2005

Wilens TE, Spencer TJ, Swanson JM, et al: Combining methylphenidate and clonidine: a clinically sound medication option. J Am Acad Child Adolesc Psychiatry 38:614–622, 1999

Wilens TE, Biederman J, Baldessarini RJ, et al: Cardiovascular effects of therapeutic doses of tricyclic antidepressants in children and adolescents. J Am Acad Child Adolesc Psychiatry 35:1491–1501, 1996

Wilens TE, Biederman J, Kwon A, et al: A systematic chart review of the nature of psychiatric adverse events in children and adolescents treated with selective serotonin reuptake inhibitors. J Child Adolesc Psychopharmacol 13:143–152, 2003

Wilens T, McBurnett K, Stein M, et al: ADHD treatment with once-daily OROS methylphenidate: final results from a long-term open-label study. J Am Acad Child Adolesc Psychiatry 44:1015–1023, 2005

Willemsen-Swinkels SH, Buitelaar JK, van Engeland H: The effects of chronic naltrexone treatment in young autistic children: a double-blind placebo-controlled crossover study. Biol Psychiatry 39:1023–1031, 1996

Williams DT: Hypnosis as a psychotherapeutic adjunct, in Basic Handbook of Child Psychiatry, Vol 3: Therapeutic Interventions. Edited by Harrison SI. New York, Basic Books, 1979, pp 108–116

Williams DT, Mehl R, Yudofsky S, et al: The effect of propranolol on uncontrolled rage outbursts in children and adolescents with organic brain dysfunction. Journal of the American Academy of Child Psychiatry 21:129–135, 1982

Winsberg BG, Perel JM, Hurwic MJ, et al: Imipramine protein binding and pharmacokinetics in children, in The Phenothiazines and Structurally Related Drugs. Edited by Forrest IS, Carr CJ, Usdin E. New York, Raven, 1974, pp 425–431

Wolraich ML, Wilson DB, White JW: The effect of sugar on behavior or cognition in children: a meta-analysis. JAMA 274:1617–1621, 1995

Wolraich ML, Feurer I, Hannah JN, et al: Obtaining systematic teacher reports of disruptive behavior disorders utilizing DSM-IV. J Abnorm Child Psychol 26:141–152, 1998

Wolraich ML, Lambert W, Doffing MA, et al: Psychometric properties of the Vanderbilt ADHD diagnostic parent rating scale in a referred population. J Pediatr Psychol 28:559–568, 2003

Woolston JL: Case study: carbamazepine treatment of juvenile-onset bipolar disorder. J Am Acad Child Adolesc Psychiatry 38:335–338, 1999

Zahn TP, Rapoport JL, Thompson CL: Autonomic and behavioral effects of dextroamphetamine and placebo in normal and hyperactive prepubertal boys. J Abnorm Child Psychol 8:145–160, 1980

Zito JM, Safer DJ, dosReis S, et al: Trends in the prescribing of psychotropic medications to preschoolers. JAMA 283:1025–1030, 2000

37

TREATMENT OF SENIORS

Dan G. Blazer, M.D., Ph.D.

Psychiatrists who work with older adults encounter diagnostic and therapeutic problems that are more complex than those encountered in young adult and middle-aged patients. Most older patients with psychiatric disorders do not fit easily into the diagnostic categories of DSM-IV-TR (American Psychiatric Association 2000) because they experience multiple symptoms that affect both physical and psychiatric functioning. This is especially true when treating the oldest members of this population (Blazer 2000). Once the problem is formulated by the clinician, usual treatment approaches must be modified both to manage the functional disability that results from the psychiatric problem and to reverse the underlying disorder.

Multiple system involvement and functional impairment are not unique to geriatric psychiatry. Geriatricians must manage equally complex disease presentations that involve a range of dysfunctions, from the molecular to the psychosocial. For example, the onset of type 2 diabetes mellitus in an older adult disrupts not only glucose metabolism but also lifelong patterns of food intake and exercise. Educational and psychotherapeutic interventions, as well as diet and medication prescription, are necessary to treat the patient successfully. Type 2 diabetes cannot be cured, so the goal for the clinician is to maintain overall function of the older adult in the presence of the chronic illness.

In an era in which specific psychiatric disorders are emphasized, psychiatrists working with older adults can benefit from the syndromal approach to impairment, a paradigm shift developed by geriatricians to structure diagnostic and therapeutic strategies for older patients. Geriatricians deemphasize specific *diagnoses* and concentrate instead on *geriatric syndromes*, including incontinence, dizziness, falling, failure to thrive, and constipation (Hazzard 1994). In this chapter, I follow this syndromal approach by identifying seven psychiatric syndromes that are most prevalent among older individuals—acute confusion, memory loss, insomnia, anxiety, suspiciousness and agitation, depression, and hypochondriasis—and describing them within the context of managing the resultant impairment (Table 37–1). Because the psychiatric disorders that contribute to these syndromes are described elsewhere in this text, emphasis will be placed on the aspects of the syndromes that are unique to late life and on the management of the older adult with these syndromes.

TABLE 37–1. **Geriatric psychiatric syndromes**

Acute confusion
Memory loss
Insomnia
Anxiety
Suspiciousness and agitation
Depression
Hypochondriasis

Acute Confusion

Acute confusion, or delirium, is a transient organic brain syndrome characterized by acute onset and global impairment of cognitive function. The older person with acute confusion exhibits a decreased ability to maintain attention to environmental stimuli and has difficulty shifting attention from one set of stimuli to another (Table 37–2). Thinking is disorganized, speech becomes rambling, and a decreased level of consciousness is exhibited. Emotional disturbances often, but not always, accompany acute confusion and may be the presenting problem in late life. These emotional disturbances include anxiety, fear, irritability, and anger. Some older persons, in contrast, are apathetic and withdrawn during an episode of delirium and thus are much more difficult to diagnose. Acute confusion, by definition, is brief, usually lasting a few hours but possibly lasting weeks, such as in the case of confusion secondary to medications.

Frequency and Origins

The frequency of delirium among the older population is difficult to estimate because many episodes are undetected due to their brevity. Most estimates of incidence range from 15% to 25% on medical and surgical wards (Martin et al. 2000). The incidence is higher on intensive care units and among persons recovering from cardiovascular surgery. When delirium is diagnosed in a hospitalized older patient, the hospitalization is usually prolonged, and both in-hospital and posthospital mortality rates are increased. Mortality at 2-year follow-up approaches 50%.

Acute confusion in late life is the common outcome of a cascade of biological, cognitive, and environmental contributors (Table 37–3). Biological brain function declines with age, although functional capacity varies greatly within age groups. Degenerative changes, such as those characteristic of Alzheimer's disease, render the older person more susceptible to physiological changes secondary to aging and disease. These physiological changes include drug intoxication, electrolyte disturbance, infection, dehydration, hypoalbuminemia, and hypoxia. Visual and hearing impairment may also contribute to delirium. For example, an older adult with early primary degenerative dementia and loss of eyesight may experience congestive heart failure. The vulnerable nervous system cannot adapt to the decreased delivery of oxygen and glucose during failure because of a decreased reserve capacity, and acute confusion emerges. Common external biological

TABLE 37–2. Characteristics of acute confusion
Acute onset
Decreased ability to maintain attention
Difficulty shifting attention
Disorganized thinking and speech
Memory disturbance
Altered levels of consciousness
Sleep–wake cycle disturbance
Anxiety, fear, irritability, and anger
May appear apathetic and withdrawn
Fluctuating course usually brief in duration

stressors that precipitate acute confusion in older adults at risk are listed in Table 37–3.

Cognitive contributors to delirium include a predisposition to hallucinations and delusions, such as that in an aging patient with a history of schizophrenia. Environmental contributors include the unfamiliar surroundings of a hospital or long-term-care facility and social isolation. Therefore, the hospital, where the convergence of these contributors is likely, is a high-risk environment for delirium. Additional factors that may contribute to delirium in the hospital include physical restraint and bladder catheter (S. Inouye 2000).

Treatment

General therapy for the confused older individual, to be administered in parallel with specific therapy for the underlying cause of the acute confusion, begins with medical support (Table 37–4). Vital signs and level of consciousness should be closely monitored (S.K. Inouye et al. 1999). All medications that are not critical should be discontinued. Vasopressor agents may be needed to increase blood pressure, and excessive fever should be treated with ice baths and alcohol sponges. When the syndrome of acute confusion is recognized and the precipitant of the confusion is established through history, physical examination, and laboratory studies, the clinician can begin therapy. Laboratory tests should be ordered as indicated, including thyroid function tests, measurement of drug levels, toxicology screen, measurement of ammonia or cortisol levels, electrocardiogram (ECG), and neuroimaging (S. Inouye 2006). Acute confusion may present as a psychiatric emergency that threatens permanent brain damage. Severe hypoglycemia, hypoxia, and hyperthermia are examples of critical conditions

TABLE 37–3. Common external biological stressors that precipitate acute confusion in the at-risk older adult

Intoxication

Drugs (anticholinergic agents, sedative-hypnotics, anxiolytics, hypertensive agents, alcohol)

Withdrawal symptoms

Medications (sedative, hypnotic, anxiolytic)

Alcohol

Metabolic disorders

Hypoxia

Hypoglycemia

Failure of vital organs, such as liver and kidney

Nutritional disorders

Vitamin deficiency (thiamine, vitamin B_{12}, folate)

Fluid and electrolyte imbalance

Dehydration

Alkalosis or acidosis

Hypernatremia or hyponatremia

Endocrine disorders

Hyperthyroidism or hypothyroidism

Addison's disease or Cushing's syndrome

Pituitary hypofunction

Cardiovascular disorders

Congestive heart failure

Cardiac arrhythmia

Myocardial infarction

Infections

Pneumonia

Influenza

AIDS

Physical injury

Hyperthermia or hypothermia

TABLE 37–4. Treatment of acute confusion

Monitor levels of consciousness with brief bedside tests (serial 7s and digit span)

Check vital signs

Discontinue all nonessential medications

Establish an adequate airway (if necessary)

Administer 100 mL of 50% dextrose plus 100 mg of thiamine intravenously

Leave lights on in the room

Avoid unnecessary stimuli (e.g., keep the room quiet and simply furnished)

Use antipsychotic medications (haloperidol 0.5–1.0 mg po, bid 0.5–1.0 mg IM prn)

tion. Order and simplicity in the environment are critical to the management of the confused older patient, who should be maintained in a quiet, simply furnished, and well-lit room. Lights should be left on at night. Care can best be facilitated by constant attention from familiar persons such as family members, who should frequently orient the patient to time, place, and person. Physicians, nurses, and other hospital personnel should explain all procedures. Restraints should be kept to a minimum. Behavioral agitation generally can be managed by judicious use of antipsychotic medications, such as risperidone, in low doses (administered either intramuscularly or orally).

Memory Loss

The syndrome of memory loss (the dementia syndrome) is one of the more frequent and disabling syndromes experienced by older adults (Table 37–5). Late-life memory loss is usually accompanied by a more or less sustained decline in cognitive function from a previously obtained intellectual level, usually with an insidious onset. Other cognitive capacities that decline with memory include language (e.g., aphasia), spatial or temporal orientation, judgment, executive function, and abstract thought. State of consciousness is usually not altered until very late in the memory loss syndrome, which is in contrast with acute confusion.

Frequency and Origins

Disabling memory loss may begin in midlife, but it is much more frequent in persons older than 75 years than in those between 65 and 74 years of age. Preva-

that may present as acute confusion. Therefore, the initial treatment should include the establishment of an adequate airway to ensure that the patient is breathing and the administration of 100 mL 50% dextrose plus thiamine 100 mg intravenously if hypoglycemia and Wernicke's encephalopathy cannot be ruled out.

The clinician also must pay special attention to reducing the demands that excess and conflicting environmental stimuli make on the patient's cerebral func-

TABLE 37–5. Clinical characteristics of memory loss
Memory impairment (difficulty recalling previously learned information and difficulty learning new information)
Language disturbance (seen in late phases—cannot complete a sentence)
Difficulty carrying out motor activities (despite intact motor function)
Failure to recognize objects (despite intact sensory function)
Difficulty with calculations (inability to perform serial 7s)
Focal neurological signs (in vascular dementia)
Disturbances in executive function (e.g., planning a trip to three different places)
Fluctuating course (especially in vascular dementia)
Hallucinations and delusions (prominent visual hallucinations frequent in Lewy body dementia)

TABLE 37–6. Differential diagnosis of memory loss
Dementia of the Alzheimer's type
Vascular dementia
Dementia due to HIV disease
Dementia due to head trauma
Dementia due to Parkinson's disease
Dementia due to Huntington's disease
Dementia due to Pick's disease
Lewy body dementia

lence estimates from community samples of memory impairment are generally 5%–15%, with most investigators estimating memory impairment in at least 10% of persons older than 65 years in the community and in 30%–50% of institutional residents (Evans et al. 1989; Small et al. 1997). Alzheimer's disease (AD), the most common disorder contributing to the dementia syndrome, has been estimated to be prevalent in 6%–8% of community-dwelling persons older than 65 years, with more than 30% of persons 85 years or older having AD. Prevalence estimates of AD include both mild and severe cases, so significant memory impairment may be found in only a proportion of persons identified as having the condition in community samples. Until age 75 years, the life expectancy of persons with AD or vascular dementia is reduced by one-half. After 75 years of age, life expectancy is less affected by memory loss.

Other causes of memory loss include vascular dementia, Lewy body dementia, dementia associated with Parkinson's disease, and alcohol-related dementias (Table 37–6). Although the clinical presentation of memory loss does not always provide clear evidence for the etiology, there are some distinguishing characteristics, such as the increase in visual hallucinations in Lewy body dementia and sudden declines in memory with vascular dementia. Even those persons who have AD may experience significant decline over an interval, only to enter a plateau in functioning for a subsequent interval that may last for many months. Some

dementing disorders, however, do not lead to inevitable decline in function. For example, alcohol-induced amnestic disorder can be arrested if the person stops drinking and returns to a nutritional diet.

More than 50% of persons with chronic memory loss will, at autopsy, exhibit the changes of AD only. AD is characterized by neurofibrillary tangles, deposition of β-amyloid, and brain atrophy. The next most common contributor to the syndrome is vascular dementia, characterized by multiple small infarcts of the brain. Clinically and pathophysiologically, it is difficult to disaggregate the dementias. Vascular dementia frequently is comorbid with AD. In contrast to AD, however, vascular dementia is more common in males than in females. Many patients with Parkinson's disease develop brain changes late in the course of the disease similar to those changes found in AD. Clinically, except for their parkinsonian symptoms, these patients cannot be distinguished from patients with AD. In addition, many patients with AD exhibit changes in the substantia nigra at autopsy. Approximately 5% of older persons experience memory loss as a result of alcohol-induced amnestic disorder. A variant of AD is Lewy body dementia, characterized by synaptophysin-containing cytoplasmic inclusions outside the substantia nigra. In addition to memory impairment, fluctuating cognitive function is characteristic of this disorder.

The primary risk factors for AD are age and family history, with the prevalence of AD, as mentioned previously, being an exponential function of age. Other risk factors for AD include Down syndrome, head trauma, and possibly lack of education. (Use of statins and/or nonsteroidal anti-inflammatory drugs [NSAIDs] may be protective [Breitner and Zandi 2001].) Genetic risk factors have received much attention in recent years, especially the relationship between the disease and the ε4 allele of the apolipoprotein E (APOE) gene (Roses 1994). Persons who carry at least one copy of the APOE ε4 allele are at increased risk for AD. A proposed pathophysiological pathway for the ε4 allele's role in the disease is that the ε4 allele increases the deposition of β-amyloid, which in turn damages oligodendrocytes, the cells that produce myelin. Much less common forms of AD have been linked to chromosomes 14 and 1 (presenilin 1 and 2 genes). Most cases of AD, however, cannot be attributed to one etiological agent. Male sex, hypertension, and possibly black race are risk factors for vascular dementia. Alcohol use regularly over many years is the primary cause of alcohol-induced amnestic disorder.

Diagnostic Workup

The diagnostic workup of the older adult with memory loss begins with a history, the most important component of the evaluation (Table 37–7). A history should be obtained from both family members and the patient. The nature and severity of memory loss should be assessed in conjunction with a chronological account of the onset of the older adult's problems and specific behavioral changes. Patient and family should be asked about common problems resulting from memory loss, such as becoming lost in a familiar place, having difficulties with driving, becoming repetitious, and losing objects. Medical history should include inquiries about relevant systemic diseases, trauma, surgery, psychiatric problems, diet, and alcohol and drug use. (A thorough documentation of prescription and over-the-counter drugs is essential.) Family history should include questions about relatives who have memory loss, Down syndrome, alcohol problems, and psychiatric disorders. The physical examination should include not only a thorough neurological examination but also a general physical workup to determine the health of the patient.

The nature and degree of the cognitive dysfunction should be assessed by both a thorough mental status examination and objective cognitive testing. Standardized mental status examinations, such as the Mini-Mental State Examination (Folstein et al. 1975) are available and are useful quantitative means of documenting memory loss at the initial evaluation.

The in-office or hospital-based initial assessment of memory and cognitive functioning is followed by a more in-depth evaluation of cognition with tests of specific functions such as executive functioning (Trail Making Test), language (Boston Naming Test), memory (Wechsler Memory Scale), and spatial ability (tests of constructional praxis). Performance on short screening and on more in-depth neuropsychological testing provides a baseline from which decline in function

TABLE 37–7. Diagnostic workup of memory loss

Detailed history from the patient and a family member

A mental status exam, such as the Mini-Mental State Examination

A physical, including a thorough neurological exam

Report of all medications and frequency of use

More complex neuropsychological exams

Routine laboratory exam: complete blood count, electrolytes, liver function tests, thyroid function tests, vitamin B_{12}, and folate

Magnetic resonance imaging or computed tomography scan

Routine genetic testing is not recommended

and/or response to therapeutic intervention can be determined.

Routine laboratory examination is essential, with special focus on findings that could contribute to memory loss, such as hypothyroidism, anemia, and (in rarer cases) vitamin deficiencies, such as deficiency of vitamin B_{12}. Magnetic resonance imaging (MRI) or computed tomography scans are now routine in the initial evaluation of memory loss. The positive yield of clinically significant findings from these scans (except for cerebral atrophy or microinfarcts in vascular dementia) is minimal. Much interesting research is emerging to explore the association of memory loss and functional imaging (e.g., positron emission tomography), but these functional scans are not as yet appropriate for routine clinical care. Although screening for reversible causes is essential, the yield from many of these tests is sparse. Reports suggesting that a large percentage of patients who initially see clinicians because of memory loss experience a return to previous function with treatment are misleading. Genotyping a patient with AD or a patient's family members cannot be justified at this time, despite the emerging evidence of a hereditary predisposition with certain genotypes such as APOE 4/4 (Roses 1997).

Treatment

Most pharmacological therapies are based on the cholinergic hypotheses of memory and include primarily cholinesterase inhibitors (Table 37–8). Tacrine, donepezil, rivastigmine, and galantamine are available to physicians in office-based practice. (Tacrine is rarely used due to side effects, specifically liver dysfunction.)

These drugs have proven moderately effective in reducing decline in memory up to 6 months after administration, but their long-term ability to retard memory loss is questioned. Studies are now emerging to suggest that cognitive function among subjects using these agents is indistinguishable from that among control subjects after 1–2 years. Memantine, an N-methyl-D-aspartate (NMDA) receptor antagonist, has been approved for the treatment of moderate to severe AD (based on the theory that glutamatergic overstimulation may cause excitotoxic neuronal changes). Other strategies used frequently with less objective evidence of efficacy include the use of NSAIDs in low doses, estrogen replacement therapy, and antioxidants such as vitamin E. Patients in late life who have memory loss may be referred to specialized centers (memory disorder clinics) where they can be evaluated and, if they meet criteria, enrolled in a clinical trial where they may receive a number of experimental agents, including estrogens.

Psychotropic medications are used extensively in patients with memory loss, primarily because of secondary symptoms such as verbal or physical aggression, anxiety, depression, psychoses, and severe agitation or regressive behavior (see "Suspiciousness and Agitation" section later in chapter) (Katz et al. 1999). Other secondary behaviors, however, such as wandering, inappropriate verbalization, repetitive activities (touching), obstinacy in following suggestions or commands, hoarding of materials, stealing, and inappropriate voiding, are not as amenable to medication. Therefore, the first step for the clinician treating the patient with memory loss is to assess what symptoms might be responsive to a medication.

After determining that the emerging behavioral problem cannot be handled through nonpharmacological means and is ongoing, medication can be prescribed with caution. The specifics of medication use can be found in other portions of this textbook. Agitation and anxiety can be treated with antianxiety agents (e.g., short-acting benzodiazepines), neuroleptics (e.g., risperidone and olanzapine), anticonvulsants (e.g., carbamazepine), β-blockers, lithium, buspirone, and occasionally low doses of antidepressant agents (e.g., trazodone) at night. Clonazepam may be of benefit in agitated patients with vascular dementia; however, the episodic mood swings and acute confusion that often accompany such dementia are not as responsive to medications.

The antipsychotics are the most effective psychotropic agents for controlling severe agitation, aggressive behavior, and psychoses. Most neuroleptics are

TABLE 37–8. Medications for the primary treatment of memory loss

Cholinesterase inhibitors

　Donepezil (begin with 5 mg and attempt dosage of 10 mg/day)

　Rivastigmine (begin with 1.5 mg bid and increase to at least 3 mg bid)

　Galantamine (begin with 4–8 mg/day and increase to 16–24 mg/day)

N-methyl-D-aspartate (NMDA) receptor agonist

　Memantine (begin with 5 mg/day and increase to 20 mg/day)

effective but produce side effects, and therefore the selection of a drug is usually determined by the side-effect profile least adverse for a given patient. The atypical antipsychotic agents, such as olanzapine and risperidone, are the preferred drugs at present primarily because of the lower immediate side-effect profile. The most troublesome side effects that result from using antipsychotic agents are postural hypotension (and the risk of falling) and tardive dyskinesia, both of which are less frequent among users of the atypical antipsychotics. These agents and their side effects are discussed in more detail later in this chapter (see section "Suspiciousness and Agitation").

Because depression (even the syndrome of major depression) is frequent among patients with chronic memory loss, the use of an antidepressant agent is often indicated (Reifler et al. 1989). In general, the antidepressant agent will not lead to an improvement in memory. Postural hypotension and anticholinergic side effects are the major concern when using the antidepressant medications. For this reason, selective serotonin reuptake inhibitors (SSRIs) with the fewest potential side effects are preferred (e.g., sertraline, escitalopram).

Whatever medication is prescribed to the older adult with memory loss, it should be tapered slowly on a periodic basis to determine whether the medication continues to be required. If the drug is not required, then an unnecessary and potentially dangerous drug can be eliminated from the medication regimen. Careful documentation of the target symptoms for the medication and monitoring of the effectiveness of the medication in reversing these symptoms assist the physicians and nursing staff in identifying drugs that can be discontinued.

Behavioral management of the patient with memory loss not only is useful to the patient but also provides the patient's family with a sense of accomplishment in the presence of an illness that tends to leave a family feeling helpless and bewildered. The family and the physician should develop behaviors that promote both patient and family security. Familiar routines and consistent repetition of instructions usually enhance security. The family, as much as possible, should provide moments of fun with the patient, even when these brief moments of relief are quickly forgotten by the patient. Families can substitute for the patient's lost abilities by performing tasks for the patient such as putting out clothes in the morning. Families should not hesitate to "do for" these patients, because patients with memory loss are truly more dependent than other elderly persons. Families must also compensate for the loss of impulse control that accompanies memory loss. One means is distraction; the patient who is about to remove his or her clothes or masturbate in public can be distracted by being engaged in conversation or by being asked to walk with a family member. Patients with memory loss can usually assist in household tasks, even when the disorder is moderately severe. Although the older adult with memory loss cannot prepare a meal alone, he or she can work with the spouse or other family members in routine tasks.

Management of memory loss must include a review of the patient's environment for safety. Typical safety problems include behaviors such as becoming lost or wandering into busy traffic, using medicines erratically or accidentally, falling (secondary to poor lighting or slippery surfaces), having accidents while driving, and leaving things unattended (e.g., leaving appliances turned on). Home visits by geriatric nurse specialists are most hopeful in reviewing the household for potential problems.

Perhaps the most important long-term component for managing the older adult with memory loss is support of the family. Families are the primary caregivers of elderly persons with memory loss until the memory loss becomes severe enough to lead to institutionalization. With proper support, the older person can remain at home for a longer period of time, and the family can function more effectively in the midst of the devastation of the severe memory loss. Education of the family about the expected progression of memory loss, and the many behaviors that accompany such loss but that may not be intuitively recognized as resulting from the illness, is key to family support. Excellent educational materials are available and support groups are located throughout the world to assist the family of the patient with memory loss. In addition, families must be monitored for caregiver stress. If the clinician is not sensitive to the potential for stress in caregivers, then family members may exceed their limits and experience burnout, which could lead to neglect and/or abuse of the older adult. Respite for the caregiver, education, and therapy are essential in keeping the care system operative.

Insomnia

Insomnia is more frequent in the elderly population than in any other age group; 28% report difficulty falling asleep, and 46% report symptoms of difficulty both falling asleep and staying asleep and use of more sedative-hypnotic medications (Foley et al. 1995). Both the lack of sleep and the subsequent medication use frequently lead to deterioration in daytime alertness and functioning. The most common causes of sleep disturbances are listed in Table 37–9.

Sleep changes characteristic in late life include decreased total sleep time, frequent arousals, increased percentages of Stage 1 and Stage 2 sleep, decreased percentages of Stage 3 and Stage 4 sleep, decreased rapid eye movement (REM) latency, decreased absolute amounts of REM sleep, and a tendency to exhibit a redistribution of sleep across the 24-hour day (e.g., napping during the day). Many of these sleep changes are similar to those that occur in depression and dementing disorders, although not as severe. Older persons are also more likely to phase-advance in the sleep cycle, with a phase tendency toward "morningness."

TABLE 37–9. Sleep disturbances leading to insomnia in the elderly

Primary insomnia

Sleep-disordered breathing (i.e., sleep apnea)

Nocturnal myoclonus or periodic leg movements

Sleep–wake schedule disorder

Secondary causes of insomnia

    Sleep problems secondary to medication use

    Anxiety disorders

    Mood disorders

    Dementing disorders

    Comorbid physical illness (e.g., congestive heart failure, chronic obstructive pulmonary disease, nocturia)

Frequency

Approximately 5% of all elderly persons who initially report no sleep problems report new symptoms each year (Ancoli-Israel 2000). The proportion of older persons living in long-term care facilities who have sleep problems and take sedative-hypnotic agents is much higher than in the community. Sleep apnea is more prevalent in elderly men than women, with the apnea index (i.e., the number of apneic episodes per hour of sleep) being 5 or greater in 25%–35% of elderly persons in the community. The prevalence of periodic leg movement disorder (experienced most commonly as leg kicks and cold feet along with insomnia) probably ranges from 25% to 50% among healthy elderly persons in the community and generally requires polysomnography to confirm the diagnosis. Restless legs syndrome is equally frequent but does not require polysomnography. There is no adequate study of the prevalence of sleep–wake schedule disorder, but the experience of this disorder is frequently reported by elderly persons, especially in long-term care facilities.

Diagnostic Workup

The diagnostic workup of an older person with insomnia begins with a recognition of the severity of the sleep disturbance (Table 37–10). Screening questions during the interview should include an assessment of the patient's satisfaction with his or her sleep, daytime napping, fatigue during usual daily activities, and complaint by a bed partner or other observer of unusual behavior during sleep (e.g., snoring, pauses in breathing, periodic myoclonic movements). A careful medical and psychiatric history is necessary to identify or rule out serious diseases that contribute to the sleep problem.

A medication history is essential in determining the etiology of insomnia. Prescribed medications, especially sedative-hypnotics and anxiolytics, as well as alcohol, have significant effects on sleep and also may impair cardiopulmonary function. Symptoms of the major psychiatric disorders affecting older persons, such as dementia, depression, or severe anxiety, may also lead to insomnia. If a sleep–wake cycle dysfunction is suspected, patients may be asked to keep a log of napping, going to sleep, and awakening. Physical and neurological examinations are necessary, especially when sleep apnea is suspected. Heavy snoring requires a thorough examination of the nose and throat, usually by an otolaryngologist.

Although primary care physicians can usually recognize most sleep disorders and manage them effec-

TABLE 37–10. Diagnostic workup of insomnia in later life

Screening (satisfaction with sleep, daytime napping, sleep–wake cycle problems, fatigue, and complaints [e.g., snoring] from a bed partner)

Medical history

Psychiatric history

Medication use

Polysomnography

Previous treatments of insomnia

tively, specialized evaluation of sleep disorders is sometimes required. Referral to a psychiatrist or neurologist with special interest in sleep disorders is indicated. Upon referral, most patients, after a thorough history and physical examination and withdrawal from medication, are evaluated by polysomnography. Polysomnographic techniques have been improved in recent years; patients can now be fitted with a portable recording instrument and returned home to sleep for 2 evenings. Polysomnography, followed by a multiple sleep latency test, can be used to quantify daytime sleepiness as well as to document sleep apnea.

Treatment

The cornerstones of effective treatment of insomnia in late life are management of the underlying causes of the sleep disturbance and improved sleep hygiene. For example, a significant portion of older adults experiencing chronic insomnia also experience psychiatric disorders, especially depression and alcohol problems. Both of these conditions are responsive to therapy. Physical problems such as hypothyroidism or arthritis may not be reversed, but the symptoms can be relieved with medications or other therapeutic interventions. Nocturnal myoclonus or restless legs syndrome may respond to medication such as dopamine agonists (e.g., pergolide), anticonvulsants (e.g., carbamazepine), benzodiazepines (e.g., clonazepam), and opiates in severe and otherwise treatment-resistant cases. Sleep apnea syndrome that does not respond to conservative management (e.g., the use of positive-pressure breathing) may require surgery to improve flow in the nasopharyngeal region.

Institution of good sleep hygiene is the next step in managing insomnia among elderly patients (Table 37–11). First, the patient should be encouraged to initiate sleep at the same time every night, preferably at a later rather than an earlier time (to prevent early-morning wakefulness). The bedroom should be used primarily for sleeping and not for napping. Therefore, if the elderly patient has difficulty sleeping at night, the bed should be made up in the morning and the patient should be encouraged not to nap in the bed and to spend as little time as possible in the bedroom during the day. Exercising can facilitate sleep, but exercise should not be initiated after later afternoon. Alcohol and caffeine should be avoided in the evenings, and the evening meal should be moderate and at least 2–3 hours before bedtime. Fluid intake should also be limited during the 2–3 hours before bedtime (to prevent nocturia).

Bedrooms should generally be maintained at a temperature between 65°F and 72°F. To maintain a cool bedroom, many elderly persons who cannot afford air conditioning are forced to leave their windows open at night, possibly exposing them to noises that are likely to disturb sleep. One means for decreasing the potential of noise to disrupt the night's sleep is to institute white noise (e.g., a waterfall or rain sounds) using specially built devices or to run a fan during the night. If the elderly person still cannot sleep at night, he or she is encouraged to get up, go to another room, and engage in some nonstimulating activity (e.g., reading, listening to music). When the elderly person again becomes drowsy, he or she should return to the bedroom and attempt to initiate sleep once again. If the individual experiences a difficult night of sleep, he or she should make extra efforts the next day to avoid napping.

Methods of relaxation training can be used successfully in enabling the insomniac elderly patient to initiate sleep. Progressive relaxation involves the alternate tensing and relaxing of muscle groups coupled with visualizing a relaxing scene. Elderly patients can be trained in such relaxation techniques by means of training tapes (instructing in progressive relaxation) or directly by a health care professional. However, an elderly patient should not habitually use training tapes to initiate sleep but rather be encouraged to shift to autoregulation of sleep.

A number of medications can be used to facilitate sleep in the elderly population, although these medications should be used with care (Table 37–12). If the elderly patient is taking medications that adversely affect sleep (e.g., long-term use of a sedative-hypnotic agent), the pharmacological approach to treatment is to discontinue that medication (usually over about 10 days for a sedative-hypnotic). If the sleep problem is secondary to a medical problem, then optimal man-

TABLE 37–11. Sleep hygiene in the elderly

Initiate sleep at the same time each night.

Use the bed for nighttime sleeping, not for daytime napping.

Exercise, but not in late afternoon.

Avoid alcohol and caffeine during the evenings.

Eat a moderate evening meal at least 2–3 hours before bedtime.

Keep bedroom temperature between 65° and 72°F.

Use "white noise" to overcome disruptive nighttime sounds.

If unable to sleep, get out of bed and engage in some nonstimulating activity, such as reading or listening to music.

TABLE 37–12. Medications and recommended doses for treating late-life insomnia

Trazodone (25–50 mg)

Zolpidem (Ambien) (5 mg)

Temazepam (Restoril) (15 mg)

Zaleplon (Sonata) (10 mg)

Eszopiclone (Lunesta) (1–2 mg)

agement of the medical problem with medications can assist the patient with sleep. For example, adequate treatment of arthritis with analgesics can improve sleep.

The antidepressant agents not only are useful in managing the older adult with insomnia secondary to depression but also can be used as sedative agents, especially if prescribed in low doses. For example, 25–50 mg of trazodone may be preferable to using a long-term benzodiazepine if chronic use of a sedative is indicated. Trazodone, however, has not been proven efficacious in clinical trials, and withdrawal may lead to rebound insomnia (in addition, the drug reduces time spent in REM sleep). In general, short- to medium-acting benzodiazepines are preferred over those that are more extended in length of action. Therefore, shorter-acting agents such as zolpidem (5 mg) and temazepam (15 mg) are preferred as a sedative-hypnotic. A new benzodiazepine receptor agonist, zaleplon (10 mg), has the shortest half-life among these agents and does not appear to cause rebound insomnia or adversely affect psychomotor function (Ancoli-Israel 2000).

Eszopiclone (1–2 mg), although approved for long-term use to improve sleep, should be used with the same caution as other agents. Each of the newer agents has been proven to be safe and effective in older adults (Ancoli-Israel and Ayalon 2006).

Anxiety

Anxiety is a frequent symptom among older persons secondary to physical illness such as hyperthyroidism, comorbid with other psychiatric disorders such as depression, or as the primary symptom of a disorder such as generalized anxiety disorder (Blazer 1997). Many of the anxiety disorders, however, are relatively less frequent in late life. Although phobia disorders can affect persons at all stages of the life cycle, the more severe phobias, such as agoraphobia and social phobia, begin early in life and are more common in children and young adults than in older persons. Generalized anxiety disorder is a frequent diagnosis regardless of age, yet generalized anxiety is often comorbid with other psychiatric disorders such as major depression. Panic disorder is relatively frequent and severe among younger persons but much less so among older persons (although data documenting a lower prevalence among older persons are sparse). Posttraumatic stress disorder can occur at any age but is found more frequently in younger persons than older persons. Obsessive-compulsive traits are common throughout the life cycle, although the severe manifestations of this disorder are less likely to be observed in older persons. Therefore, the management of anxiety symptoms in older persons usually consists of managing the symptoms in older persons of generalized anxiety that are the primary problem or comorbid with other disorders.

Frequency and Origins

Community surveys of individuals with anxiety symptoms estimate that approximately 5% of older persons meet DSM-III (American Psychiatric Association 1980) criteria for the diagnosis of generalized anxiety disorder (Blazer et al. 1991). (There have been no large community studies of generalized anxiety using DSM-IV [American Psychiatric Association 1994] criteria, but a comparison of criteria suggests that the prevalence of generalized anxiety would be somewhat lower using the new criteria.) Approximately 20% of older persons report some cognitive or somatic symptoms of anxiety in community surveys, with somatic symptoms being more prevalent than cognitive symptoms. In a survey in North Carolina, DSM-III simple phobia was found in 10% of persons 65 years or older compared with 13% of persons in middle age (Blazer et al. 1985). Yet these phobias are generally not disabling, for the older adult usually finds convenient ways to avoid the phobic situation. Agoraphobia was found in 5% of the 65-or-older group, compared with 7% of the middle-age group (Blazer et al. 1991). Anxiety and depression are frequently comorbid, reaching nearly 50% in some studies (Beekman et al. 2000).

Anxiety results from a number of medical (Table 37–13) and psychiatric conditions. Hyperthyroidism with an atypical presentation may be mistaken for a psychogenic anxiety disorder. Cardiac arrhythmias may produce palpitations and shortness of breath in older persons in a syndrome resembling generalized anxiety, with episodic exacerbations and remissions depending on the status of the heart. Pulmonary emboli, if not severe, may present as shortness of breath and subjective anxiety.

Many medications lead to symptoms of anxiety. Caffeine is a frequent cause of anxiety, and older persons are often not aware of the multiple sources of caffeine in their diet or medications. Over-the-counter sympathomimetic medications (e.g., ephedrine) may lead to palpitations and subsequent subjective symptoms of anxiety. Anticholinergic agents, when they impair memory, lead to anxiety that is secondary to the memory loss and confusion. Older persons also may experience significant anxiety on withdrawal from certain substances and medications, especially alcohol and anxiolytic agents. Postural hypotension may lead to dizziness and shortness of breath, which may be interpreted by the older person as episodic anxiety. Hypoglycemia 4–5 hours after a large meal is another contributor to anxiety.

TABLE 37–13. **Medical causes of anxiety in the elderly**

Hyperthyroidism

Cardiac arrhythmia

Pulmonary emboli

Hypoglycemia

Medications

    Caffeine

    Over-the-counter sympathomimetic drugs

    Anticholinergic agents

    Withdrawal from anxiolytic agents

Many psychiatric disorders are manifested, in part, by symptoms of anxiety. Moderate to severe acute confusion is usually associated with anxiety and agitation, especially when the older person is in an unfamiliar place. Anxiety is a common accompaniment of major depression; older patients who experience major depression also meet the criteria for generalized anxiety disorder in more than 50% of the cases. Hypochondriasis is associated with anxiety, especially when dependency needs are not met by family and health care professionals. Dementing disorders, especially in the early and middle stages, are associated with anxiety and agitation. Later in the dementing disorder, the agitation is episodic and the cognitive, subjective anxiety is less well documented. Late-life schizophrenia with acute paranoid ideation is usually accompanied by agitation and anxiety, especially in the evenings when the older person is home alone. In addition, some older persons experience acute panic attacks and meet the criteria for panic disorder, and some exhibit symptoms of generalized anxiety without apparent biological or psychosocial causation.

The clinician must not overlook the possibility that the anxiety symptoms may be secondary to appropriate fear. Many older persons must expose themselves daily to situations that threaten their security. Older adults living in inner cities often fear being attacked as they walk the streets. Those with memory loss who live alone may fear that they will get lost driving to the doctor's office. Individuals who have lost the acuteness of their reflexes fear driving on busy, crowded highways.

Treatment

The use of nonpharmacological therapies such as relaxation training, cognitive restructuring, and activity structuring for the treatment of anxiety in older adults has not been studied extensively. Nevertheless, the danger of medication, as well as the successful application of cognitive-behavior therapies to other psychiatric disorders in late life (especially depression), suggests that nonpharmacological therapies may be applicable to anxiety disorders. Older persons who do not have cognitive dysfunction may be good candidates for relaxation training and biofeedback. No evidence has been forthcoming to suggest that older persons are less capable of taking advantage of these therapies than are middle-aged persons. Cognitive restructuring, based on the cognitive therapy described originally for depression, has not been adapted for anxiety in older adults to date. However, there is little evidence that nonstructured psychotherapy is of benefit in treating generalized anxiety or panic episodes in late life.

The cornerstone of pharmacological therapy for the anxiety disorders is the benzodiazepines (Table 37–14). These drugs repeatedly have been demonstrated to be effective for the control of anxiety when compared with a placebo and are relatively free of side effects. They are generally well tolerated by persons of all ages but present unique problems when prescribed to older persons. For example, the half-life of the benzodiazepines may be increased dramatically in late life, with diazepam (2.5–5.0 mg) having a half-life nearing 4 days in persons in their 80s. Older persons are also more susceptible to potential side effects of benzodiazepines such as fatigue, drowsiness, motor dysfunction, and memory impairment. Clinicians must be especially careful when prescribing benzodiazepines to older individuals who drive. Therefore, the shorter-acting benzodiazepines, such as alprazolam (0.25 mg), oxazepam (15 mg), and lorazepam (0.5 mg), given two to three times a day, have been preferred agents in late life. Nevertheless, short-acting drugs in some older patients may lead to brief withdrawal episodes during the day and a rebound of anxiety.

TABLE 37–14. Medications and typical starting doses for treating anxiety in the elderly

Alprazolam (begin with 0.25 mg twice a day)

Oxazepam (begin with 15 mg twice a day)

Lorazepam (begin with 0.5 mg twice a day)

Buspirone (begin with 5 mg twice a day and increase to a total of 20–30 mg/day)

Selective serotonin reuptake inhibitors (see Table 37–20 for dosages)

Propranolol (begin with 10 mg twice a day)

Other agents are generally less effective in controlling late-life anxiety. Buspirone (10 mg three times a day) is relatively safe, with few side effects, and does not appear to lead to abuse or dependency. Nevertheless, it takes 3–4 weeks for the therapeutic effect to become manifest. Older adults who perceive that they have benefited from benzodiazepines generally do not accept buspirone as an alternative. The antidepressant agents are useful in treating anxiety mixed with depression. Nevertheless, in many older persons with a mixed anxiety–depression syndrome, the depressive symptoms improve while the antidepressant is being used, yet the anxiety symptoms persist. Therefore, a combination of a benzodiazepine and an antidepressant is sometimes used. Gabapentin, 100 mg two or three times a day, has been used by some to control symptoms of anxiety in the elderly, but its efficacy has yet to be demonstrated. Some have suggested that β-blockers such as propranolol (10 mg twice daily) are valuable in treating anxiety disorders. These drugs must be monitored carefully, given their propensity to slow the heart rate. Buspirone and the β-blockers may be more effective in controlling agitation and behavioral problems in patients with dementia than in controlling generalized anxiety.

Suspiciousness and Agitation

A frequent symptom in older adults, especially older adults experiencing cognitive impairment, is suspiciousness, which may range from increased cautiousness and distrust of family and friends to overt paranoid delusions. Among suspicious or paranoid older persons, a unique group has been described, especially in the European literature, for many years. *Late-life paraphrenia* (or, as more recently labeled, *very-late-onset schizophrenia*) has been distinguished from both chronic schizophrenia and dementia and is characterized by marked paranoid delusions in older adults who nevertheless maintain function in the community for months or even years (Almeida et al. 1995). Persons experiencing paraphrenia are predominately women and often live alone. However, marked suspiciousness and overt psychosis in conjunction with cognitive impairment are a more common manifestation of the syndrome. There is sparse empirical justification for disaggregating late-life paraphrenia from other psychotic disorders.

The predominant delusions encountered in older persons are persecutory delusions and somatic delusions. Persecutory delusions often revolve around a single theme or a series of connected themes, such as family and neighbors conspiring against the older person or a delusion of sexual abuse. Somatic delusions often involve the gastrointestinal tract and frequently reflect the older person's fear that he or she is experiencing cancer. Regardless of the etiology of suspiciousness and paranoid delusions, when older persons believe they are threatened from the social environment, often because they do not understand what is happening in that environment, agitation becomes paramount. Agitation in the suspicious older person is an acute symptom that may require emergency management, as described later in this discussion.

Frequency and Origins

Suspiciousness and paranoid behavior were found in 17% of persons in one community survey (Christenson and Blazer 1984; Lowenthal 1964), and a sense of persecution was reported in 4% in another survey (Christenson and Blazer 1984). Thus, the perception by older persons that they live in a hostile social environment is common and represents a much larger proportion of older individuals than those who would be diagnosed with schizophrenia or suspiciousness secondary to cognitive impairment. Some of these suspicions may be justified if the older person lives in an unsafe community or has been the victim of fraud. Among persons in the community, fewer than 1% have schizophrenia or a paranoid disorder.

Many different disorders may lead to suspiciousness, delusions, and agitation (Table 37–15). Chronic schizophrenic disorder, which has its onset earlier in life and persists into late life, is perhaps the most easily identified cause of late-life suspiciousness (Jeste et al. 2004). As schizophrenia tends to be characterized by a decline in social function over the life cycle and a shorter life expectancy (although the prognosis of schizophrenia varies greatly from person to person), chronic schizophrenia that persists into late life and yet leaves the older person relatively free of other symptoms is uncommon. Nevertheless, persons may experience severe symptoms of schizophrenia in early life or midlife and then enter a period of remission from which they do not relapse with further schizophrenic behavior until late life. Schizophrenia-like illness also may have its first onset in late life. These patients are less likely to experience negative symptoms and neuropsychological impairment and often respond to lower doses of antipsychotic medication. Usually, depression and organic mental disorders do not contribute to these late-onset schizophrenia-like states. In contrast, organic mental disorders and late-onset depression are frequently associated with some psychotic symptoms.

TABLE 37–15. Causes of suspiciousness, delusions, and agitation in the elderly

Schizophrenia disorder
Late-onset delusional disorder
Organic delusional syndrome
Delirium

Late-onset delusional disorder, with mild to moderate symptoms, is a more frequent cause of suspiciousness in late life. Delusions, often of being persecuted by family and friends, usually center on a single theme or a connection of themes. For example, an older woman may become convinced that her daughter was instrumental in the death of her husband (or that the daughter neglected her father during a chronic illness). That woman, in turn, may not listen to reason regarding the daughter's behavior and may never forgive the daughter for the perceived abuse or neglect. These delusions may lead to a withdrawal of affection, financial support, and social contact with the daughter.

Another common cause of suspiciousness in late life is organic delusional syndrome (or dementia with psychosis). These delusions, in contrast to late-onset delusional disorder, wax and wane over time in severity and in content. In some cases, the older adult functions well and does not appear to be disturbed by the delusional thoughts, though the thoughts are frequently expressed. Imagined infidelity by a marriage partner is a common example. If the delusion does not create subjective stress and/or problems in management, regular evaluation of the patient and family without the use of medications is the preferred intervention. Persecutory delusions are most common and often emerge when the older person's environment is changed. Organic delusional syndrome frequently derives from medications or from localized brain damage (e.g., in alcohol abuse and Huntington's chorea). Suspiciousness, however, usually results from the dementing disorders. For some persons with AD, paranoid thoughts may dominate other symptoms of the dementing illness, especially in the early stages. Perhaps the most common encounter psychiatrists have with suspicious older persons is with patients with dementia who have become a management problem because of suspiciousness and agitation. Suspiciousness and agitation are also frequent symptoms of delirium, as described earlier.

Despite the range of disorders that may lead to suspiciousness in older persons, some investigators have suggested common psychobiological contributors to the syndrome in late life. A family history of suspiciousness and delusional thought is uncommon among suspicious older persons, and therefore hereditary contributions are probably less important than at earlier stages of the life cycle. Degeneration of subcortical tissues with aging may disrupt neurotransmission and higher brain functions, which in turn contributes to a deficiency in maintaining attention and filtering information, symptoms that have been asso-

ciated with psychotic thinking. That women are more likely to experience more severe syndromes of suspiciousness than men in late life (in contrast to the equal sex distribution of psychoses earlier in life) has led some investigators to suggest that menopause and the resultant decrease in estrogen binding to dopamine receptors may place women at risk who were previously protected from developing suspicious thinking. Sensory deprivation also has been identified as a potential risk factor for suspiciousness, regardless of the underlying disorder. Social isolation also may contribute to suspiciousness.

Diagnostic Workup

The key to the diagnostic workup of the suspicious older person is the psychiatric evaluation. Delusional thinking and agitation usually render the patient's history inaccurate, and therefore family members should be interviewed to review the patient's behavior, especially any change in behavior. Previous psychotic or delusional episodes should be documented, as well as previous treatment. Clinicians evaluating the suspicious older person should remember that older adults are occasionally abused by family members and that the seemingly delusional description of family behavior by the older individual may contain some truth.

Treatment

The management of suspiciousness in older adults requires 1) ensuring a safe environment; 2) initiating a therapeutic alliance; 3) considering and, if appropriate, instituting pharmacological therapy (Table 37–16); and 4) managing acute behavioral crises. The clinician must first decide whether hospitalization is necessary. In general, paranoid older persons do not adapt well to the hospital. Change from familiar surroundings and interaction with strange persons tend to exacerbate the suspiciousness. Nevertheless, older patients often are so disabled in their behavior secondary to schizophrenic or delusional disorder that hospitalization is necessary.

Once the older patient is hospitalized, the clinician must initiate a therapeutic alliance. With the older patient, this alliance is best accomplished by taking a medical approach to the patient and expressing concern about all of the patient's physical and emotional concerns. Most suspicious older patients are quite accepting of medical care and are trusting of physicians. It is rarely necessary for clinicians to confront patients regarding suspicions or delusional thinking; therefore, older patients' responses to questions can be support-

TABLE 37–16. Medications for the management of suspiciousness and agitation in the elderly

Atypical antipsychotic agents

    Risperidone (Risperdal) 1–3 mg/day

    Olanzapine (Zyprexa) 5–15 mg/day

    Quetiapine (Seroquel) 50–100 mg/day

Older antipsychotic agents

    Haloperidol (Haldol) 0.5–2.0 mg/day

TABLE 37–17. Suggestions for preventing aggressive and violent behavior in the older adult

Psychologically disarm the patient by helping him or her to express his or her fears.

Distract the attention of the older patient.

Provide directions to the patient in simple terms.

Communicate clearly and concisely.

Communicate expectations.

Avoid arguing and defending.

Avoid threatening body language or gestures.

Remain at a safe distance from the patient until help is available.

ive, and clinicians do not need to agree with statements made by the patients that are known to be untrue.

The cornerstone of managing the moderately to severely suspicious older patient is medication, especially antipsychotic agents (see Table 37–16). Medications most frequently used to treat older persons are risperidone (1–3 mg/day), olanzapine (5–15 mg/day), quetiapine (50–100 mg/day), and haloperidol (0.5–2.0 mg orally three times a day). Dosage of these agents is relatively small initially, and one-half of the dose should be given during the evening. In a large controlled study, lower doses of risperidone (1 mg/day) significantly improved symptoms of psychosis and aggressive behavior with fewer side effects compared with 2 mg/day (Katz et al. 1999). Doses can be increased if necessary. Recent reports suggest that older adults taking both the typical and atypical antipsychotic agents for the treatment of dementia-related behavioral disorders may be at some increased risk for mortality, leading to a black-box warning from the U.S. Food and Drug Administration. Physicians who prescribe antipsychotic medications for the treatment of suspiciousness in an older adult should carefully monitor the success of these agents and should discuss the potential benefits and potential risks with the patient and family. If the drug is deemed not successful—for example, if the target symptoms do not change with the medication—then it should be discontinued, given the significant side effects that may result. Tardive dyskinesia is five to six times more prevalent in elderly than in younger patients (Jeste 2000).

Finally, the physician must be prepared to deal with severe agitation and violent behavior (Table 37–17). Medications alone will not control these behaviors. Physicians must work with the nursing staff to prevent such behavior in patients at risk while they are in the hospital and must instruct families on methods of prevention when these patients are at home.

Periods of severe agitation are usually brief and, if managed properly, are soon forgotten by the older patient. Then the physician once more can work toward establishing a sustained therapeutic relationship with the patient.

Depression

Depression is one of the more frequent and the second most disabling geriatric psychiatry syndrome (after memory loss) experienced by older adults (Blazer 2002, 2003). Late-life depression that is not comorbid with physical illness and/or a dementing disorder is characterized by symptoms similar to those experienced at earlier stages of the life cycle, with some significant differences (Table 37–18). Depressed mood is usually apparent in the older adult but may not be a spontaneous complaint. Older persons are more likely to experience weight loss (as opposed to weight gain or no change in weight) during a major depressive episode and are less likely to report feelings of worthlessness or guilt. Although older persons experience more difficulty with cognitive performance tests during a depressive episode, they are no more likely than persons in midlife to report cognitive problems subjectively. Complaints of cognitive dysfunction are common in more severe depressive episodes regardless of the person's age. Persistent anhedonia associated with a lack of response to pleasurable stimuli is a common and central symptom of late-life depression. Older persons are also more likely than younger persons to exhibit psychotic symptoms during a depressive episode. Recent studies have suggested that executive function is impaired in older adults with depression and that this impairment may be associated with a higher likelihood of relapse and recurrence of symptoms (Alexopoulos et al. 2000).

TABLE 37–18. Characteristics of seniors with depression

Do not complain of depression spontaneously

Lose but rarely gain weight

Complain of insomnia but rarely of sleeping too much

Complain of problems with concentration and memory loss

Test positive for impairment on psychological testing

Suffer from anhedonia

May exhibit psychotic symptoms more frequently than middle-aged adults

Frequency and Origins

In community surveys, older adults are less likely to be diagnosed as having major depression than are persons in young adulthood or middle age. Depressive symptoms, however, are about equally prevalent across the life cycle. Standardized interviews reveal that 1%–3% of persons in the community are diagnosed as having dysthymia (Blazer et al. 1987). Major depression is much more prevalent among older persons in the hospital and in long-term care facilities, ranging from 10% to 20% (Koenig et al. 1988).

Late-life depression fits well in the biopsychosocial model of psychiatric disorders (Blazer and Hybels 2005). Although a hereditary predisposition to depression is less likely among persons in late life who are experiencing a first onset of depression, a number of biological factors are associated with late-life depression. Poor regulation of the hypothalamic-pituitary-adrenal axis, as well as disruption of the sleep cycle and other circadian rhythms, is more likely to be present among older persons than among younger persons. These problems also have been associated with major depression. In recent years, considerable attention has been directed to the association of depression with lesions in subcortical structures and their frontal projections in the brain (Alexopoulos et al. 1997; Krishnan et al. 1997). Most older persons are satisfied with their lives and are not psychologically predisposed to depression. Nevertheless, some experience a demoralization and a despair resulting not only from incapacities due to aging but also from a sense of not having fulfilled their life expectations. Older persons must adapt to many adverse life experiences, especially losses of relatives and friends, yet they are often more likely to respond to these losses without difficulty than

are persons who are younger. Older persons, for example, expect that they will lose family and friends through death, and those family and friends whom they do lose often have suffered chronic illnesses for some time, thus allowing older persons to grieve the loss, in part, before the actual loss.

Major depression is relatively infrequent among older persons, yet it can be a challenging disorder to manage. Older persons also may experience bipolar disorder, with a first-onset manic episode after age 65 years. Psychotic depressions are more common in late life than at other stages of the life cycle (Meyers 1992). Other common causes of late-life depression include organic mood disorder, such as a depressed mood secondary to antihypertensive medications, and the depression associated with the common dementing disorders, such as primary degenerative dementia and vascular dementia. Medical illness, such as hypothyroidism, frequently leads to an organic mood disorder. An adjustment disorder with depressed mood secondary to physical disability and/or chronic illness is among the most frequent causes of depressed mood among older individuals.

Diagnostic Workup

As with the diagnosis of other geriatric psychiatry syndromes, the patient's history and a collateral history from a family member are the keys to making the diagnosis of depression in late life. Although older persons may exhibit some tendency to "mask" their depressive symptoms, a careful interview almost invariably reveals significant depression if it is present. The history should be complemented by a thorough mental status examination with attention to disturbances of motor behavior and perception, presence or absence of hallucinations, disturbances of thinking, and thorough cognitive testing. Psychological testing may be implemented to distinguish depression from dementia but should not be performed in the midst of a severe depressive episode. The laboratory workup of the depressed older adult is presented in Table 37–19. Some tests, such as the blood count and measurement of vitamin B_{12} and folate levels, are useful in screening for medical illnesses that may present with depressive symptoms. The thyroid panel is essential in the diagnosis of the depressed older patient, given that subclinical hypothyroid disorders are frequently uncovered in the workup.

Although the abnormalities in sleep associated with depression frequently parallel those associated with normal aging, experienced polysomnographers can distinguish them. MRI is optional despite the as-

TABLE 37–19.   Laboratory workup of the depressed older adult

Routine

    Complete blood count (CBC)

    Urinalysis

    Triiodothyronine (T_3), thyroxine (T_4), free thyroxine index, thyroid-stimulating hormone (TSH)

    Venereal Disease Research Laboratory test (VDRL)

    Vitamin B_{12} and folate assays

    Chemistry screen (sodium, chlorine, potassium, blood urea nitrogen, calcium, glucose creatine)

    Electrocardiogram

Elective

    Polysomnography

    Magnetic resonance imaging or computed tomography scan

    Thyroid-releasing hormone stimulation test (TRHS)

    Screening for HIV

TABLE 37–20.   Antidepressant therapy for seniors with typical starting doses

Selective serotonin reuptake inhibitors

    Fluoxetine (Prozac) (10 mg/day)

    Sertraline (Zoloft) (50 mg/day in divided doses)

    Paroxetine (Paxil) (10 mg/day)

    Citalopram (Celexa) (10 mg/day)

    Escitalopram (Lexapro) (10 mg/day)

    Trazodone (Desyrel) (50 mg at night)

Serotonin and norepinephrine reuptake inhibitors

    Venlafaxine (Effexor) (37.5 mg/day)

    Duloxetine (Cymbalta) (20 mg once or twice a day)

Tricyclic antidepressants

    Nortriptyline (50–75 mg at night)

    Desipramine (50–75 mg at night)

sociation of subcortical white matter hyperintensities with late-life depression. The physician ordering laboratory tests for a depressed older patient also must consider the potential adverse health consequences for an older adult experiencing a severe or chronic mood disorder. For example, major depression is associated with decreased bone mineral density, placing older women with depression at greater risk for osteoporosis (Michelson et al. 1996).

Treatment

Clinical management involves pharmacotherapy, electroconvulsive therapy (ECT), psychotherapy, and work with the family. The pharmacological treatment of choice at present is one of the new-generation antidepressant medications (Table 37–20). Despite the advent of these newer agents, some geriatric psychiatrists still prefer to first administer one of the secondary amines, such as nortriptyline or desipramine, in healthy older adults. Each has relatively low anticholinergic effects and is known to be an effective antidepressant. Postural hypotension is the most troublesome side effect that older adults usually encounter

when treated with the tricyclic antidepressants. The lower cost of the tricyclic antidepressants compared with the cost of newer agents is one factor in prescribing them. The SSRIs fluoxetine, sertraline, paroxetine, citalopram, and escitalopram can be used at somewhat lower dosages than are prescribed at earlier stages of the life cycle (e.g., 10 mg/day for paroxetine). The most common adverse effects that limit the use of SSRIs are agitation and persistent weight loss. Paroxetine has been shown to significantly (but not dramatically) improve the symptoms of minor depression and dysthymia at dosages between 10 and 40 mg/day (Williams et al. 2000). The use of antidepressant medications, primarily the SSRIs, has increased dramatically in recent years, with more than 10% of elderly persons 75 years and older taking antidepressants at any given time (Blazer 2000). If treatment with an SSRI is not successful, then the second-choice medications are usually the serotonin–norepinephrine reuptake inhibitors (SNRIs), such as venlafaxine (beginning at around 37.5 mg/day) or duloxetine (beginning with 20 mg/day) (Alexopoulos et al. 2001).

The older person who does not respond to antidepressant medications or who experiences significant side effects from the medications may be a candidate for ECT. Depressed older persons who are candidates for ECT should be experiencing a severe depressive episode and are especially likely to respond if they are experiencing psychotic symptoms. With proper medical support, ECT is a safe and effective treatment for older adults. Despite a higher level of physical illness and cognitive impairment, even the oldest patient with severe major depression may tolerate ECT as well as younger patients do and may demonstrate similar or better acute response. Unilateral nondominant ECT is preferred. If the treatment is successful, then maintenance ECT at progressively extended intervals is a method of preventing relapse.

Several studies have demonstrated the effectiveness of cognitive and behavioral therapies (including interpersonal psychotherapy) in outpatient treatment of older persons who have major depression without melancholia (Lynch and Aspnes 2004). Cognitive therapy also may be an adjunct for severe melancholic depressions that are treated concomitantly with medications. In a large controlled trial of patients older than 59 years with major depression, maintenance therapy with interpersonal therapy and paroxetine was significant in preventing or delaying recurrence (Reynolds et al. 2006). For long-term maintenance, medications were more effective than psychotherapy. Cognitive-behavioral therapy is well tolerated by older people because of its limited duration and educational orientation, as well as the active interchange between the therapist and the patient.

Any effective therapy for depression in older persons must include work with the family. Families are often the most important allies of the clinician working with depressed older patients. Families should be informed as to the danger signs, such as potential for suicide, in a severely depressed older family member. In addition, the family can provide structure for reengaging a withdrawn and depressed older person into social activities.

Hypochondriasis

Hypochondriasis among older persons is one of the more common and frustrating of the somatoform disorders encountered by health care professionals. An essential feature of hypochondriasis in older persons is their belief that they have one of several serious illnesses (Table 37–21). This belief derives from an exaggerated interpretation of physical signs and sensations. The medical workup often will reveal some physical abnormality but does not support a medical diagnosis that can account for the severity and breadth of symptoms experienced. However, hypochondriacal symptoms do not reach the level of somatic delusions. The distinction between a psychotic disorder mani-

TABLE 37–21. Characteristics of hypochondriasis in the elderly

Belief of suffering from one or more serious illnesses

Exaggerated interpretation of physical signs

Chronic course

Symptoms frequently focused in the abdominal and genitourinary areas

Concerns not relieved by reassurance from the physician

Exaggerated side effects from medications

fested by somatic delusions and hypochondriasis is usually easy to make because the delusion either is unrelated to any physical sensation or in no way relates to the symptoms reported. To meet criteria for a diagnosis of hypochondriasis, older persons must experience the disorder for at least 6 months; when most physicians encounter hypochondriacal older patients, their symptoms have lasted far longer than 6 months. Hypochondriacal symptoms in older persons usually are described as being in the gastrointestinal or genitourinary area. Exaggerated concerns regarding constipation, difficulty with eating because of gastric problems, abdominal pain, and genitourinary pain are among the most frequent. As with individuals who have hypochondriasis at other stages of life, older persons with this disorder do not experience relief when assured by a physician that the medical problem is not severe.

Frequency and Origins

In community surveys, exaggerated concern about health is found among 10% of older persons (Blazer and Houpt 1979). In contrast, another 10% usually perceive their health as being significantly better than it actually is. Most older persons assessed their health accurately, with no trend for older individuals inaccurately perceiving their health as being worse than it actually is. There are no community surveys that accurately estimate the prevalence of hypochondriasis. That hypochondriacal older persons are frequently encountered by primary care physicians should not lead to the assumption that hypochondriasis is a common problem among this population. Hypochondriacal older persons overuse health care services, and therefore one or two hypochondriacal older patients in a primary care physician's practice may occupy an appreciable amount of time, leading the physician to believe that hypochondriasis is a common condition.

The etiology of hypochondriasis is, by definition, not biological. This does not mean, however, that hypochondriacal older persons do not experience physical illness or that the symptoms reported by some older individuals are not, to some degree, the expression of actual physical problems. Exaggeration of symptoms (as opposed to the invention of symptoms) is the manifestation of hypochondriasis.

Contributing Factors

Several mechanisms may contribute to hypochondriasis in older persons. First, the symptoms may be used to shift anxiety from specific psychological conflicts to more concrete problems with body functioning. An older person may fear the loss of his or her mind, the loss of a spouse, the loss of personal capabilities, or the loss of a social role. Fear of these losses is then replaced by a preoccupation with physical health in hypochondriasis. Some older persons may use hypochondriacal symptoms as a means of punishing themselves for unacceptable hostile feelings or behaviors in the past for which they now feel guilty. If an older person has engaged in some type of indiscretion, such as a sexual indiscretion, genitourinary pains or concerns may predominate as hypochondriacal symptoms later in life. Unfortunately, interpreting the connection between past guilt and present concern usually does not alleviate the problem of hypochondriasis.

Social factors are probably the major reason that aging persons are at risk for developing hypochondriasis. Older persons often have difficulty meeting personal and/or social expectations. Family members may wish the older family member to participate in activities that are beyond his or her capability, such as taking a long walk, lifting luggage, or preparing a meal. Failure to meet these family expectations, or perhaps anger at the family for insisting that these expectations be met, can lead the older person to focus on his or her physical problems to the exclusion of facing the issue directly. Older persons also use hypochondriasis as a means of adapting to the real problem of isolation. Preoccupation with physical problems and help-seeking for those physical problems in some cases become the center of the older person's life. Frequent visits to the physician require assistance with transportation from family or friends and provide social contact with persons in the health care professional's office. The older patient also learns that physical complaints facilitate communicating with others because they provide the individual with a topic of conversation. Isolated older persons may feel they have little else to contribute to conversa-

tions and therefore focus on their physical problems.

The clinician working with a hypochondriacal older patient must be vigilant for the presence of more severe psychopathology. Depression is frequently accompanied by exaggerated physical concerns, regardless of age. If an older person exhibits both significant depressive symptoms and symptoms of hypochondriasis, then the clinician must be alert to the possibility of suicide. Suicide has been demonstrated to be more common in persons exhibiting both depression and exaggerated physical concerns compared with those with depressive symptoms alone. Hypochondriasis also may mask emerging difficulties with memory. Older persons may avoid direct challenges to their cognitive status by focusing on their physical concerns.

Diagnostic Workup

The diagnostic workup of the hypochondriacal older patient consists of a thorough history and a routine physical examination. Routine laboratory studies should be performed, but once the clinician is assured that the patient does not have a severe or undetected physical problem that contributes to the symptoms, then he or she should limit further laboratory studies. The differential diagnosis includes major depression and dysthymia, anxiety disorders (both generalized anxiety and panic), schizophrenic disorder (if the exaggerated physical concern expressed by the patient borders on delusional thinking), and dementing disorders. The diagnosis of hypochondriasis does not exclude the diagnosis of other psychiatric disorders. Many older persons with hypochondriasis meet criteria for a somatoform disorder and, for example, a dementing disorder.

Treatment

Working with the hypochondriacal older patient requires both tact and patience. The development of a management strategy should be based on management goals (Table 37–22). Older patients with hypochondriasis are best managed by a primary care physician as opposed to a psychiatrist. After the initial evaluation, the hypochondriacal older patient should be seen for relatively brief but regularly scheduled visits, in general lasting no more than 10–20 minutes each. Emphasis during the follow-up visits initially should be on a brief review of interval historical information coupled with a brief physical examination (including checking pulse and blood pressure). The remainder of the visit should be relatively unstructured and should focus on events in the patient's life. The clinician should refrain from interpretations connecting the physical problems with specific life events, instead encouraging the patient to discuss concerns about family, friends, perceived isolation, and so forth. The clinician may prescribe medications but must recognize that older patients with hypochondriasis are at increased risk for becoming dependent on psychotropic medications. Placebos are generally not appropriate, because discovery that a placebo has been prescribed undoubtedly will destroy the relationship between patient and doctor.

Medications that can be used for treating the hypochondriacal older patient include those that have relatively few side effects and those that have been demonstrated to be at least minimally effective in alleviating the symptoms expressed by the patient. For example, L-tryptophan can be prescribed for problems with sleeping (2 grams of this drug at night would be an appropriate dose). Another mildly sedating drug is trazodone, given at a dose of 25–50 mg (taken at night). Neither of these drugs will lead to habituation.

TABLE 37–22. Goals for managing hypochondriasis in the older adult

Control excessive use of health care services.

Decrease concern and anxiety in the patient.

Provide assurance of professional commitment to managing the patient's condition.

Decrease family stress and facilitate capability of family to provide social support.

Decrease the anxiety, anger, and frustration of the health care professional treating the patient.

Prescribe medications with caution.

The concept of "treatment" for hypochondriasis is actually misleading. Whatever treatment plan is instituted, it is, in fact, a *management* plan with the goals of 1) controlling and decreasing the use of health care services, 2) decreasing the concern and anxiety expressed by the hypochondriacal older person about the availability and commitment of health care professionals, 3) decreasing strain on the family, 4) increasing the capabilities of the family to provide a supportive environment to the hypochondriacal older person, 5) decreasing conflicts within the family, and 6) decreasing anxiety expressed by the health care professional. Given these goals, it is essential that the hypochondriacal older person be treated within the context of the family when family members are available. Hypochondriacal symptoms often disappear during the process of aging. As older persons resolve conflicts with family, and as they accept their one and only life for what it is, anxiety decreases and appropriate social interactions increase.

Conclusion

The seven geriatric symptoms discussed in this chapter account for most of the psychopathology that both psychiatrists and geriatricians encounter while working with older adults. The syndromal approach permits the clinician to focus on the functional impairment that results from psychopathology and on the day-to-day management of the older person in both the hospital and the outpatient clinic. A syndromal approach also provides a more realistic conceptualization of late-life psychopathology, which often is comorbid across psychiatric diagnoses and comorbid with physical illnesses.

Key Points

- Acute confusion is much more common in hospitalized older adults than usually recognized. Careful screening is necessary to identify these patients.
- Working with the family of the patient with memory loss is key to easing the suffering of the patient and preventing institutionalization prior to when absolutely necessary.
- Good sleep hygiene is more important than pharmacological management of insomnia in older adults.
- Generalized anxiety is usually comorbid with other conditions, such as depression or physical illness. Diagnosing comorbid conditions is the first step to managing anxiety in older adults.
- Suspiciousness and agitation are the most disruptive symptoms of dementing disorders.
- Uncomplicated depression in late life is as responsive to treatment as in midlife. Depression comorbid with physical illness or memory loss is much more difficult to treat.
- Implementing a structured approach to each patient contact with a hypochondriacal patient can reduce the overuse of health care services significantly.

Suggested Readings

Alexopoulos GS, Katz IR, Reynolds CF 3rd, et al: The Expert Consensus Guideline Series. Pharmacotherapy of depressive disorders in older patients. Postgrad Med (Special Issue: Pharmacotherapy):1–86, 2001

Blazer DG: Generalized anxiety disorder. Harv Rev Psychiatry 5:18–27, 1997

Blazer DG: Psychiatry and the oldest old. Am J Psychiatry 157:1915–1924, 2000

Blazer DG: Depression in late life: review and commentary. J Gerontol A Biol Sci Med Sci 58:249–265, 2003

Blazer DG, Hybels CF: Origins of depression in later life. Psychol Med 35:1241–1252, 2005

Blazer DG, Steffens D, Busse E (eds): The American Psychiatric Publishing Textbook of Geriatric Psychiatry, 3rd Edition. Washington, DC, American Psychiatric Publishing, 2004

Inouye S: Delirium in older persons. N Engl J Med 354:1157–1165, 2006

Jeste D, Wetherell J, Dolder C: Schizophrenia and paranoid disorders, in The American Psychiatric Publishing Textbook of Geriatric Psychiatry, 3rd Edition. Edited by Blazer DG, Steffens D, Busse E. Washington, DC, American Psychiatric Publishing, 2004, pp 269–281

Roses A: Genetic testing for Alzheimer disease: practical and ethical issues. Arch Neurol 54:1226–1229, 1997

References

Alexopoulos GS, Meyers BS, Young RC, et al: "Vascular depression" hypothesis. Arch Gen Psychiatry 54:915–922, 1997

Alexopoulos GS, Meyers BS, Young RC, et al: Executive dysfunction increases the risk for relapse and recurrence of geriatric depression. Arch Gen Psychiatry 57:285–290, 2000

Alexopoulos GS, Katz IR, Reynolds CF 3rd, et al: The Expert Consensus Guideline Series. Pharmacotherapy of depressive disorders in older patients. Postgrad Med (Special Issue: Pharmacotherapy):1–86, 2001

Almeida O, Howard R, Levy R: Psychotic states arising in late life (late paraphrenia): psychopathology and nosology. Br J Psychiatry 166:205–214, 1995

American Psychiatric Association: Diagnostic and Statistical Manual of Mental Disorders, 3rd Edition. Washington, DC, American Psychiatric Association, 1980

American Psychiatric Association: Diagnostic and Statistical Manual of Mental Disorders, 4th Edition. Washington, DC, American Psychiatric Association, 1994

American Psychiatric Association: Diagnostic and Statistical Manual of Mental Disorders, 4th Edition, Text Revision. Washington, DC, American Psychiatric Association, 2000

Ancoli-Israel S: Insomnia in the elderly: a review for the primary care practitioner. Sleep 23 (suppl 1):S23–S30, 2000

Ancoli-Israel S, Ayalon L: Diagnosis and treatment of sleep disorders in older adults. Am J Geriatr Psychiatry 14:95–103, 2006

Beekman A, de Beurs E, van Balkom A: Anxiety and depression in later life: co-occurrence and communality of risk factors. Am J Psychiatry 157:89–95, 2000

Blazer DG: Generalized anxiety disorder. Harv Rev Psychiatry 5:18–27, 1997

Blazer DG: Psychiatry and the oldest old. Am J Psychiatry 157:1915–1924, 2000

Blazer DG: Depression in Late Life, 3rd Edition. New York, Springer, 2002

Blazer DG: Depression in late life: review and commentary. J Gerontol A Biol Sci Med Sci 58:249–265, 2003

Blazer DG, Houpt J: Perception of poor health in the healthy older adult. J Am Geriatr Soc 27:330–334, 1979

Blazer DG, George L, Landerman R, et al: Psychiatric disorders: a rural/urban comparison. Arch Gen Psychiatry 42:651–656, 1985

Blazer DG, Hughes D, George L: The epidemiology of depression in an elderly community population. Gerontologist 27:281–287, 1987

Blazer DG, Hughes D, George L: Generalized anxiety disorder, in Psychiatric Disorders in America. Edited by Robins L, Regier D. New York, Free Press, 1991, pp 180–203

Blazer DG, Hybels CF: Origins of depression in later life. Psychol Med 35:1241–1252, 2005

Breitner J, Zandi P: Do nonsteroidal anti-inflammatory drugs reduce the risk of Alzheimer's disease? N Engl J Med 345:1567–1568, 2001

Christenson R, Blazer D: Epidemiology of persecutory ideation in an elderly population in the community. Am J Psychiatry 141:1088–1091, 1984

Evans D, Funkenstein H, Albert M: Prevalence of Alzheimer's disease in a community population of older persons: higher than previously reported. JAMA 262:2551–2556, 1989

Foley D, Monjan A, Brown S, et al: Sleep complaints among elderly persons: an epidemiological study of three communities. Sleep 18:425–432, 1995

Folstein M, Folstein S, McHugh P: Mini-Mental State: a practical method for grading the cognitive state of patients for the clinician. J Psychiatr Res 12:189–198, 1975

Hazzard W: Introduction: the practice of geriatric medicine, in Principles of Geriatric Medicine and Gerontology, 3rd Edition. Edited by Hazzard W, Bierman E, Blass J, et al. New York, McGraw-Hill, 1994, pp xxiii–xxiv

Inouye S: Prevention of delirium in hospitalized older patients: risk factors and targeted interventions. Ann Intern Med 32:257–263, 2000

Inouye S: Delirium in older persons. N Engl J Med 354:1157–1165, 2006

Inouye SK, Bogardus ST Jr, Charpentier PA, et al: A multicomponent intervention to prevent delirium in hospitalized older patients [see comments]. N Engl J Med 340:669–676, 1999

Jeste D: Tardive dyskinesia in older patients. J Clin Psychiatry 61 (suppl 4):27–32, 2000

Jeste D, Wetherell J, Dolder C: Schizophrenia and paranoid disorders, in The American Psychiatric Publishing Textbook of Geriatric Psychiatry, 3rd Edition. Edited by Blazer D, Steffens D, Busse E. Washington, DC, American Psychiatric Publishing, 2004, pp 269–281

Katz I, Jeste D, Mintzer J, et al: Comparison of risperidone and placebo for psychoses and behavioral disturbances with dementia: a randomized double-blind trial. Risperidone Study Group. J Clin Psychiatry 60:107–115, 1999

Koenig H, Meador K, Cohen H, et al: Depression in elderly hospitalized patients with medical illness. Arch Intern Med 148:1929–1936, 1988

Krishnan K, Hays J, Blazer D: MRI-defined vascular depression. Am J Psychiatry 154:497–501, 1997

Lowenthal M: Lives in Distress. New York, Basic Books, 1964

Lynch T, Aspnes A: Individual and group psychotherapy, in The American Psychiatric Publishing Textbook of Geriatric Psychiatry, 3rd Edition. Edited by Blazer D, Steffens D, Busse E. Washington, DC, American Psychiatric Publishing, 2004, pp 443–458

Martin N, Stones M, Young J: Development of delirium: a prospective cohort study in a community hospital. Int Psychogeriatr 12:117–127, 2000

Meyers B: Geriatric delusional depression. Clin Geriatr Med 8:299–308, 1992

Michelson D, Stratakis C, Hill L: Bone mineral density in women with depression. N Engl J Med 335:1176–1181, 1996

Reifler B, Teri L, Raskind M, et al: Double-blind trial of imipramine in Alzheimer's disease patients with and without depression. Am J Psychiatry 146:45–49, 1989

Reynolds C, Dew M, Pollock B, et al: Maintenance treatment of major depression in old age. N Engl J Med 354:1130–1138, 2006

Roses A: Apolipoprotein E affects the rate of Alzheimer disease expression: beta-amyloid burden is a secondary consequence dependent on APOE genotype and duration of disease. J Neuropathol Exp Neurol 53:429–437, 1994

Roses A: Genetic testing for Alzheimer disease: practical and ethical issues. Arch Neurol 54:1226–1229, 1997

Small G, Rabins P, Barry P: Diagnosis and treatment of Alzheimer's disease and related disorders: consensus statement of the American Association of Geriatric Psychiatry, the Alzheimer's Association, and the American Geriatric Society. JAMA 278:1865–1870, 1997

Williams J, Barrett J, Oxman T, et al: Treatment of dysthymia and minor depression in primary care: a randomized controlled trial in older adults. JAMA 284:1519–1526, 2000

TREATMENT OF LESBIAN, GAY, BISEXUAL, AND TRANSGENDER PATIENTS

Jack Drescher, M.D.

Benjamin H. McCommon, M.D.

Billy E. Jones, M.D., M.S.

This chapter focuses on some issues raised in the psychiatric treatment of lesbian, gay, bisexual, and transgender (LGBT) patients. Before the 1970s, the psychiatric focus on LGBT patients often aimed to 1) "cure"—that is, change an individual's homosexual orientation to a heterosexual one—or 2) assist those with gender atypical behavior to conform to gender stereotypes. This emphasis began to change in 1973, when the American Psychiatric Association removed homosexuality from the seventh printing of DSM-II (American Psychiatric Association 1968).

Cultural normalization of homosexuality (and, to a lesser degree, transgenderism) began to emerge in the aftermath of the American Psychiatric Association decision. For example, at the time of this writing, the issue of marriage equality has been settled affirmatively in Belgium, Canada, the Netherlands, Spain, and the state of Massachusetts in the United States. In addition, there has been a tremendous expansion in academic gay and lesbian studies in the past three decades. In the fields of medicine and psychiatry, there is a growing literature of anecdotal accounts and small sample research studies. Yet much more needs to be done.

Why is it important for psychiatrists to know the sexual orientation or gender identity of the patients they treat? First, sexuality plays an important role in human development, psychology, and relationships. Sexual drives, sexual coping mechanisms, sexual object choices, and social grouping all unfold in relationship to an individual's sexual identity. Yet, as most psychiatrists have discovered, formal training in human sexuality is minimal—usually consigned to a few lectures in medical school and residency training.

In the biopsychosocial model of psychiatry, the *meanings* of an individual's sexual orientation or gender identity will be shaped by cultural factors and need to be understood as such. To understand the lives and mental health issues of LGBT patients is to embark upon a cross-cultural exploration (Drescher 2007). This chapter will address some of the general and specific issues that inevitably are encountered when a patient grows up as a member of a sexual minority. In fact, growing up LGBT constitutes a different cultural experience—and perhaps many different cultural experiences—relative to growing up as a member of the heterosexual majority. It is the scope of this chapter to introduce clinicians to some of the cultural aspects of LGBT individuals' lives and some of their mental health concerns, and to provide resources and references for further study.

Definitions

The psychiatric treatment of LGBT patients requires clinicians to be familiar with both scientific and cultural beliefs about sexuality and gender. The following colloquial and professional terms will assist mental health practitioners in their clinical practice with LGBT patients as well, and most of these terms are discussed further in this chapter (Table 38–1).

Historical Perspectives

Modern psychiatry's interest in homosexuality began in nineteenth-century Europe, as scientists, lawyers, philosophers, and physicians sought to replace traditional religious explanations of human behavior with scientific and medical understanding. Postreligious debates centered on the question of whether homosexuality is a normal variant of human sexuality or a mental disorder. American psychiatrists would not conclusively decide this debate until 1973 (see below).

In 1864, Karl Heinrich Ulrichs published a political treatise that argued against German laws criminalizing male homosexuality (sodomy laws). He maintained that homosexuality was a normal condition for some people and that these individuals constituted a "third sex." By the turn of the twentieth century, Magnus Hirschfeld (1914), an openly homosexual German psychiatrist, was the leading proponent of the third-sex theory.

In 1869, journalist Karl Maria Kertbeny, also publishing arguments against sodomy laws, coined the terms "homosexual" and "homosexuality." Neurologist Richard von Krafft-Ebing adopted Kertbeny's terminology, but he considered homosexuality to be a "degenerative" neurological disorder in his 1886 *Psychopathia Sexualis* (Krafft-Ebing 1886/1965). Krafft-Ebing believed that homosexuality's origins were biological, and he thought of it as a congenital disease.

In contrast to Hirschfeld's theory of normal varia-

tion and Krafft-Ebing's theory of pathology, Sigmund Freud put forward a different view. In "Three Essays on the Theory of Sexuality," Freud (1905/1953) took issue with Krafft-Ebing's *degeneracy theory*. He noted that homosexuality was found in people with no other mental problems and in people who were "distinguished by especially high intellectual development and ethical culture." Yet Freud also disagreed with Hirschfeld's third-sex theory and was "opposed to any attempt at separating off homosexuals from the rest of mankind as a group of special character." Instead, Freud claimed, homosexuality—as part of an innate bisexuality in human beings—was a normal phase in heterosexual development and that expressions of adult homosexuality could be attributed to an "arrested" psychosexual development.

Psychoanalytic practitioners of the mid-twentieth-century later rejected Freud's views and instead based their clinical approaches on theories put forward by Sandor Rado in 1940. Rado maintained that there was no such thing as innate bisexuality or normal homosexuality and that heterosexuality was the biological norm. He conceptualized homosexuality as a phobic avoidance of heterosexuality caused by inadequate early parenting. Rado's psychoanalytic theories had a significant impact on psychiatric thought in the mid–twentieth century and were the basis for including a diagnosis of "homosexuality" in the first and second editions of the *Diagnostic and Statistical Manual of Mental Disorders* (DSM).

In 1973, however, the American Psychiatric Association removed homosexuality from DSM-II (Drescher and Merlino 2007). The initial impetus for this change came after gay activists disrupted American Psychiatric Association meetings to protest the DSM's inclusion of the diagnosis. Those protests eventually led the American Psychiatric Association to study the issue of whether homosexuality should remain in its diagnostic manual. The scientific subcommittee addressing this issue reviewed the psychoanalytic literature on the subject. However, they also reviewed the scientific literature of sexology, which, unlike psychoanalysis of the time, supported a normal-variant view of homosexuality. Notable among sexology studies were Alfred Kinsey's reports on human sexuality in the male and female, respectively (Kinsey et al. 1948, 1953). The Kinsey reports claimed that homosexuality was more common than was generally believed. In addition, Ford and Beach's (1951) cross-cultural and ethological study confirmed Kinsey's view that homosexuality was not a rare phenomenon. Then, in 1957, Evelyn Hooker published a study that showed, again contrary

TABLE 38–1. Definitions of commonly used terms

Term	Definition
Antigay violence	Physical violence directed at people because they are gay. Colloquially referred to as *gay bashing*, the latter term is often used metaphorically to describe antigay verbal abuse as well.
Antihomosexual attitudes	Attitudes such as heterosexism, homophobia, and moral condemnations of homosexuality.
Bisexual	A broad term, applicable to men and women, used to describe 1) sexual behavior, 2) sexual identity, or 3) sexual orientation.
Closeted	A colloquial term that describes individuals who are hiding their homosexuality from others in their life. Being in the closet involves a range of psychological and behavioral activities intended to keep an individual's homosexuality a secret.
Coming out	Admitting one's homosexuality to oneself or revealing it to others. Also referred to as "coming out of the closet."
Down low (DL)	A colloquial African American term describing men who have sex with men (MSM). Men "on the down low" may engage in homosexual or bisexual behavior without adopting a gay or bisexual identity.
Gay	A sexual identity adopted by men (and some women) who openly accept, to some degree, their own homosexual orientation. Colloquially, *gay* is often used as a synonym for *homosexual*.
Gender	The psychological and social aspects of one's sex.
Gender dysphoria	Discomfort with one's biological sex.
Gender identity	An individual's psychological sense of being either a man or a woman; often erroneously confused with sexual orientation.
Gender identity disorder (GID)	Term referring to one of two DSM-IV-TR diagnoses: *GID in childhood* or *GID in adolescence or adulthood* (formerly *transsexualism*). Both diagnoses are characterized by persistent gender dysphoria, which in the case of adults may lead them to seek out sex reassignment surgery.
Heterosexism	A belief system that naturalizes and idealizes heterosexuality and either dismisses or ignores a gay subjectivity.
Heterosexual	Term describing either sexual behaviors between individuals of different sexes or their sexual orientation. When used as a noun, it may describe a sexual identity (as in "I am a heterosexual").
Homophobia	External homophobia describes the irrational fear and hatred that heterosexual individuals may have toward gay people. Internal or internalized homophobia is the self-hatred gay people have toward themselves.
Homosexual	A term first adopted by 19th-century medicine that when used as an adjective denotes either same-sex sexual behaviors or a same-sex sexual orientation. Referring to someone as "a homosexual" is considered offensive to many gay people.
Homosexuality	A broad term encompassing same-sex behaviors, orientation, attractions, and identities.
Lesbian	A sexual identity adopted by women who openly accept, to some degree, their same-sex attractions.
Men who have sex with men (MSM)	A term used in epidemiology and public health to describe men who have not necessarily accepted a gay identity but whose behavior includes sex with other men. These men may be less likely to practice safer sex (sex with a condom) and places them and their sexual partners at greater risk for exposure to HIV and other sexually transmitted infections.

TABLE 38–1.   Definitions of commonly used terms *(continued)*

Term	Definition
Moral condemnations of homosexuality	Beliefs that regard homosexual acts as intrinsically harmful to the individual, to the individual's spirit, and to the social fabric. Such beliefs are usually religious in nature, although some are secular.
Outing	Colloquially, an unwanted revelation by a third party of a closeted individual's homosexuality to others; often intended to inflict harm on the person being "outed."
Queer	Historically, a denigrating term. In recent years, *queer* has been used either as an inclusive term for all lesbian, gay, bisexual, and transgender (LGBT) individuals or as an alternative identity in itself (as in *LGBTQ*).
Sex	The biological attributes of being male or female; often used as a synonym for *gender*.
Sexual behavior	An individual's sexual activities (homosexual, heterosexual, bisexual), irrespective of sexual orientation or sexual identity.
Sexual identity	An individual's subjective experience of his or her own sexual orientation. Whereas sexual orientation is usually innate, sexual identity develops over time and in a cultural context. For example, calling oneself *gay* or *lesbian* is a subjective affirmation of one's homosexual orientation.
Sexual orientation	An individual's innate attraction to members of the same sex (*homosexual*), the opposite sex (*heterosexual*), or both sexes (*bisexual*). Recognition of one's homosexual orientation does not necessarily or automatically lead to acceptance of a gay or lesbian sexual identity.
Transgender	Colloquial term that includes transsexuals, transvestites, or any individual with a nonconventional or atypical gender presentation.
Transphobia	Hatred or lack of acceptance of transsexual or transgender individuals.
Transsexual	An individual who has undergone sex reassignment surgery, either male to female (MTF) or female to male (FTM).

to psychiatric beliefs of the time, that nonpatient homosexual men showed no more psychopathology than heterosexual control subjects.

Also emerging in the field of sexology was a growing body of research on *intersexual* (hermaphroditic) children born with ambiguous genitalia and also of adults who would later come to be known as *transsexuals*. John Money (Money and Ehrhardt 1996; Money et al. 1957) would eventually tease out the historically conflated concepts of a *gender identity* (an individual's psychological sense of being either a man or a woman) from a sexual orientation. Later, psychoanalyst Robert Stoller (1964, 1968) would introduce this concept into the psychodynamic and psychiatric literature.

In reviewing the sexology literature, the American Psychiatric Association concluded that there was greater scientific evidence supporting a normal-variant view of homosexuality than there was supporting a pathologizing one. In 1973, homosexuality was removed from the seventh printing of DSM-II. In its place appeared a new diagnosis, "sexual orientation distur-

bance" (SOD), which regarded homosexuality as an illness if an individual with same-sex attractions found them distressing and wanted to change them. This new diagnosis also allowed for the rare possibility that a person unhappy with his or her heterosexual orientation might seek psychiatric treatment to become gay. To reflect the realities of clinical practice, the 1980 revision, DSM-III (American Psychiatric Association 1980), substituted SOD with "ego-dystonic homosexuality" (EDH). However, because EDH was increasingly inconsistent with the evidence-based approach the new diagnostic system was intended to usher in, it, too, in turn was removed from the 1987 revision, DSM-III-R (American Psychiatric Association 1987).

Since 1973, the American Psychiatric Association has issued numerous position statements supporting civil rights for lesbians and gay men and opposing discrimination on the basis of sexual orientation. In its most recent statement on the matter, the American Psychiatric Association (2005) endorsed marriage equality for same-sex couples.

Development

It would be difficult, if not impossible, to delineate a developmental line for all LGBT or heterosexual patients. First, knowledge of how one acquires either a sexual orientation or a gender identity remains a subject of theoretical speculation. No definitive research yet explains the origins of homosexuality, heterosexuality, bisexuality, conventional gender identity, or gender identity disorder (GID). Second, it is unlikely that there is a developmental line that can be applied to *all* LGBT patients—even within each of the subgroups. Some individuals become aware of their sexual identity in childhood, others in adolescence, still others as young adults, and some in midlife or later. Third, since sexual *identities* are socially constructed to make meaning of one's feelings of sexual attraction or one's sense of gender, a variety of experiences lead individuals to call themselves "gay," "lesbian," "bisexual," or "transgender." In other words, there are a myriad of psychological frames of mind, interpersonal experiences, and cultural beliefs from which the diversity of modern LGBT identities are constructed.

Although it is impossible to delineate a single maturational line leading to LGBT identities, there are developmental *themes* that recur in the retrospective accounts of LGBT adults. For example, many of them look back at their lives and say they "knew" that they were lesbian, gay, bisexual, or transgender since childhood. In one retrospective study, a significant number of adult gay men and women recalled engaging in gender-atypical behavior (Bell et al. 1981). In Richard Green's (1987) "Sissy Boy Syndrome" project, a prospective study of 66 boys with gender identity disorder in childhood (GIDC), 75% of the subjects grew up identifying as gay men (not transsexuals). However, not all LGBT adults report atypical gender behavior in childhood, and the majority of gay men did not have GIDC. Consequently, it is no easy task to predict what conditions will lead a child to grow up and adopt an LGBT identity. In this section we focus on developmental themes in LGBT patients. For a more thorough review of transgender developmental issues, the reader is referred to Chapter 17 in this volume, "Gender Identity Disorders and Paraphilias," by Becker and Johnson.

Childhood

A common theme in the lives of those who, in adulthood or adolescence, come to define themselves as lesbian, gay, or bisexual (LGB) is an early memory of a same-sex attraction—a feeling they believed set them apart from others. These "children who grow up to be gay" can remember same-sex attractions or interest in members of the same sex as early as 4 years of age. Because all children are taught that they are only supposed to be attracted to the other sex, children who grow up to be gay must come to terms with heterosexual models of relatedness. The other-sex interests of future heterosexual children are naturalized and taken for granted as normal, although acting on those feelings may be discouraged until they reach a certain age or until they marry. In contrast, a child who grows up to be gay usually lacks any explanations for his or her same-sex feelings other than disparaging or stigmatizing meanings. Although what they felt as children may not have necessarily been an attraction of a sexual nature, many LGB individuals retrospectively connect their adult sexual feelings to their childhood curiosity about or a desire for intimacy with members of their own sex.

The early emerging feeling of same-sex attractions in children who grow up to be gay may generate a developmental dilemma. Early feelings that later develop into adult same-sex attraction may cause some children to question the authenticity of their assigned gender. For example, there is a common although erroneous cultural belief that a boy grows up to be gay because of gender confusion. An alternative explanation is that awareness of his spontaneous feelings for other boys may lead a young boy to question the veracity of his assigned gender. This could make it difficult for him to believe he has a masculine identity, because he possesses a trait (attraction to boys) that he has been told belongs to the other gender.

Some gay and bisexual men report a sense of childhood "otherness" that they associate with their inability to engage in "rough-and-tumble" play with other boys. It is unclear whether a feeling of otherness can lead to an inhibition of rough-and-tumble play, or vice versa, or even whether dislike of rough-and-tumble play is in any way related to feelings of same-sex attraction. It has been proposed that some boys who grow up to be gay or bisexual found rough-and-tumble play too sexually stimulating and evocative of shameful sexual feelings—leading them to avoid it altogether.

Adolescence

When children who grow up gay become teenagers, the difficulties they encounter may be compounded by the ordinary developmental challenges of adolescence. The invisibility of gay adolescents in the developmental literature stems, in part, from an assumption that adolescents are too young to have a fixed gay identity (Drescher 2002). This is not true of many LGB adults who recall strong same-sex attractions from an early age and who come out early in life. Many teenagers can and do identify themselves as gay, and by many popular and scholarly accounts (D'Augelli 1996; Savin-Williams 2005), they are coming out and doing so a much younger ages than in past generations. Puberty can sometimes provoke the first public "coming out" of these feelings, for example, when an anxious and confused adolescent tells her parents about being attracted to other girls. At other times, the parent learns about these feelings inadvertently, raising anxieties and leading to increased scrutiny of the adolescent or even coercive attempts to change her sexual orientation.

Adolescence, in general, is characterized by an increase in sexual feelings. In many cultures, there are socially sanctioned, sublimated outlets for adolescents that serve the purpose of modeling or role-playing the part of future heterosexual adults. For example, teenage dating and supervised coeducational activities such as high school dances are useful in developing the interpersonal skills required for later life and relationships. In these interactions, an adolescent's confidence may be reinforced through his or her ability to conform to conventional gender roles. This process of heterosexual socialization pervades daily life. However, while the rituals of conventional adolescence teach lessons about future adult heterosexual roles, those same rituals can generate confusion, shame, and anxiety in adolescents who grow up to be LGB. They can sometimes become anxious, superficial, or detached at a time when their heterosexual peers are learning the social skills needed for adulthood.

For example, the assumption that all youth are heterosexual leads to the separation of boys and girls during public disrobing. A gay male adolescent can be sexually overstimulated by this environment, much as a heterosexual boy would be if he were required to change in the girls' locker room. For some gay adolescents, these repeated experiences foster connections between sexual and anxious feelings.

Finally, gay teenagers may be at high risk for suicide. In one study, Remafedi et al. (1998) found that gay male adolescents were three times as likely to have suicidal intentions as their heterosexual peers.

The Closet

Those who hide their sexual identities are often referred to as "closeted" or are said to be "in the closet." LGB adolescents often develop techniques for hiding

that persist into young adulthood, middle age, and sometimes even into senescence. They hide out of fear of being subjected to antihomosexual attitudes—teasing, ridicule, or even violence.

Revealing one's LGB identity to others is referred to as "coming out" or "coming out of the closet." For example, a closeted woman can isolate her homosexual feelings and activities from herself, her acquaintances, and her family. From an intrapsychic perspective, she may be closeted to herself. Nevertheless, it can be painful to hide significant aspects of the self or to vigilantly separate aspects of the self from each other. For this reason, despite the stigma of homosexuality, many individuals find that coming out reduces their anxiety.

Sexual Identity

The developmental histories of LGB individuals frequently include periods of difficulty in acknowledging their homosexuality, either to themselves or to others. Children who grow up to be gay rarely receive family support in dealing with antihomosexual prejudices. On the contrary, beginning in childhood—and distinguishing them from racial and ethnic minorities—gay people are often subjected to the antihomosexual attitudes of their own families and communities. Antihomosexual attitudes include homophobia, heterosexism, moral condemnations of homosexuality, and antigay violence.

Closeted individuals frequently cannot acknowledge to themselves their homoerotic feelings, attractions, and fantasies. Their homosexuality is so unacceptable that it must be kept out of conscious awareness and cannot be integrated into their public persona. Consequently, these feelings must be dissociated from the self and hidden from others.

If and when same-sex feelings and attractions break into consciousness, the individual becomes *homosexually self-aware*. Such individuals can acknowledge some aspect of their homosexuality *to themselves*. However, acceptance of those feelings is not a predetermined outcome. For example, a religious homosexually self-aware woman may choose a celibate life to avoid what, for her, would be the problematic integration of her religious and sexual identities.

Individuals who are consciously prepared either to act on their homoerotic feelings or to acknowledge a homosexual identity to others usually define themselves as *lesbian, gay,* or *bisexual.* To identify as LGB, in contrast to being homosexually self-aware, is to claim a normative identity. In other words, defining oneself as LGB usually requires some measure of self-acceptance. A gay person may choose to come out to family or intimate acquaintances. Others may come out to people they have met in the gay community while keeping their gay identity separate from the rest of their lives.

Finally, a *non-gay-identified* individual may have experienced homosexual self-awareness and may have even once identified as LGB. However, such individuals find it difficult, if not impossible, to naturalize their same-sex feelings and attractions. Such persons, while recognizing that they have homosexual feelings, reject them; and despite the low odds of success, may even seek to change their sexual orientation (Erzen 2006).

Prevalence and Epidemiology

LGB people are a minority within the general population but may be disproportionately represented in some psychiatric populations. The aforementioned Kinsey studies found rates of homosexual orientation of up to 10% in men but much lower rates in women. These studies were hampered by nonrandom selection of participants and lack of population-based samples. More recent surveys (Laumann et al. 1994) have included random participant selection from large population-based samples and show lower prevalence rates. Prevalence rates have varied depending on whether homosexuality is defined as an identity or as a behavior. One analysis of two large samples in the United States showed that 2.5% of men self-identified as gay or bisexual and 1.1% of women self-identified as lesbian or bisexual. However, 4.2% of men and 2.7% of women had at least one same-sex partner over the previous 5 years. Also, examination of 1990 U.S. census data suggested that these rates may be two to three times higher in the 20 largest U.S. cities (Black et al. 2000).

Recent studies suggest that LGB people may have higher rates of certain psychiatric disorders. This should not be presumed to mean that homosexuality causes psychiatric pathology but rather that sexual orientation, like age, race, gender, and socioeconomic status, may be a risk indicator of illness (Cochran 2001). Earlier studies that did not use random selection from large population-based samples showed higher rates of depressive disorders, suicidality, anxiety disorders, substance use disorders, and eating disorders in some homosexual populations (Sandfort et al. 2006).

More recent studies using random selection from large population-based samples have produced varied results, again possibly related to whether one defines homosexuality as an identity or a behavior. A study in

the United States that examined psychiatric morbidity and self-identified sexual orientation found gay and bisexual men to have higher rates in the previous year of major depression (31% vs. 10% in heterosexual men) and panic disorder (18% vs. 4%). Lesbian or bisexual women had higher rates in the previous year of generalized anxiety disorder (15% vs. 4% in heterosexual women) (Cochran et al. 2003). Another study in the United States using same-sex sexual behavior as a marker for sexual orientation found higher rates of suicidal thoughts and drug abuse and dependence in homosexual men and higher rates of suicidal thoughts, major depression, anxiety disorders, and drug abuse in homosexual women (Gilman et al. 2001). A Dutch study that examined same-sex sexual behavior found higher rates in homosexual men in the past year for mood disorders (17% vs. 5% in heterosexual men) and anxiety disorders (20% vs. 8%) and higher rates in homosexual women in the past year for substance use disorders (14% vs. 3% in heterosexual women) and in lifetime mood disorders (49% vs. 24%) (Sandfort et al. 2001). A study in New Zealand found higher rates of major depression, generalized anxiety disorder, and substance use disorders in gay and lesbian youth ages 14–21 years (Fergusson et al. 1999).

In addition to showing higher rates of some psychiatric disorders, these studies have provided additional evidence pointing to the potential importance of sexual orientation in psychiatric care. In one study, LGB populations were more likely to see a mental health provider in the previous year (19% of gay or bisexual men vs. 8% of heterosexual men and 33% of lesbian or bisexual women vs. 11% of heterosexual women) (Cochran et al. 2003). This study and another (Sandfort et al. 2001) also showed rates of psychiatric comorbidity in homosexual populations two to four times higher than in heterosexual populations, highlighting the especial importance of thorough psychiatric evaluation for LGB patients.

Further research is needed to identify causes for mental health disparities in LGB populations. Most often, social stigma and antihomosexual bias have been proposed as causative factors. LGB people, especially LGB youth, have been reported to experience higher rates of discrimination and victimization, and this has been associated with psychological distress (Cochran 2001). Other proposed factors contributing to minority stress have included poor self-esteem (from internalization of social attitudes) and perceived inability to lead an open life, leading to loss of protective factors for mental health such as being in a steady relationship (Sandfort et al. 2006).

Diagnostic Considerations

Recent guidelines for assessing psychiatric competency in training emphasize the importance of sensitivity to a patient's sexual orientation (American Psychiatric Association 2006; Scheiber et al. 2003). As all diagnostic evaluations rely on the clinical interview, the interviewer should maintain an empathic, nonjudgmental stance; otherwise, important clinical information necessary for proper diagnosis may be missed. Therapeutic tact is paramount, and consultation is recommended if and when possible biases or limited knowledge of LGBT issues interferes with a thorough evaluation.

It is important to establish a trusting relationship with LGBT patients when discussing sexual orientation or gender identity. In fact, they may require greater assurances of confidentiality than other patients. For example, diagnostic evaluation usually requires obtaining collateral information; sources could include a same-sex partner, family members unaware of the patient's sexual identity, or LGBT-identified friends. When safety issues require contacting an LGBT patient's family or friends, the collection of necessary information does not necessarily require disclosing a patient's sexual identity. In emergency settings, however, a discharge back to family or other caregivers may require evaluating their sensitivity and responses to knowing the patient's sexual identity.

Sexual orientation may play an important role in understanding some presenting problems, such as suicidal feelings associated with coming out, substance abuse patterns of LGBT subgroup populations, or psychiatric comorbidity associated with general medical conditions such as HIV. For all patients, a complete evaluation should include a sexual history, including information about sexual orientation, intimate relationships, and sexual practices. In considering HIV risk factors, it is important that bisexual and lesbian-identified women not be excluded; they may be at risk for HIV from male sexual partners or other behaviors such as shared needles. Psychiatric diagnosis performed in the setting of a trusting working relationship can help facilitate a patient's willingness to receive appropriate medical care, including HIV testing.

A diagnostic interview of LGBT patients should include an assessment of support networks other than family and friends, including work, religious organizations, and community groups. The LGBT patient may be estranged from biological family and relying on a network of friends. She may not feel comfortable being out at work. Her religion may be welcoming, tolerant, or intolerant. She may be involved in volunteer activities with a LGBT organization or receiving services from one. A psychosocial assessment includes a history of relationships with partners, including children from current or past relationships (and for some LGBT patients, this includes past opposite-sex marriages). Legal issues for LGBT patients may include partner abuse or antigay violence (gay bashing).

DSM-IV-TR (American Psychiatric Association 2000a) stresses the importance of cultural factors for most disorders and includes an outline for cultural formulation. It is anticipated that DSM-V will emphasize sexual orientation among cultural factors pertinent to diagnosis (Alarcon et al. 2002). In particular, sexual orientation should be considered in Axis IV, which includes problems related to the social environment. Sexual orientation may be relevant here generally and also in specific Axis IV domains, including primary support group, education, housing, access to health care, and occupational, economic, and legal issues.

DSM-IV-TR contains few specific mentions of sexual orientation. Homosexual sexual orientation is an exclusionary criterion for a *transvestic fetishism* diagnosis. In an effort to focus on profound distress about gender rather than simple nonconformity to stereotypes about sexual orientation, DSM-IV-TR emphasizes that *GIDC* is not to be diagnosed merely for "tomboyish" behavior in girls or "sissyish" behavior in boys; as discussed earlier in this chapter, in one study, 75% of children with this diagnosis became homosexual or bisexual as adults (without a GID diagnosis). The diagnosis *sexual disorder not otherwise specified (NOS)* includes a category of "persistent and marked distress about sexual orientation." Because distress about sexual orientation usually does not represent a psychiatric disorder, DSM-IV-TR includes two other categories for problems related to sexual orientation. These diagnoses can be used when a patient is uncertain about sexual orientation or in the process of coming out. *Identity problem* "can be used when the focus of clinical attention is uncertainty about multiple issues relating to identity such as... sexual orientation and behavior" (American Psychiatric Association 2000a, p. 741). *Phase of life problem* "can be used when the focus of clinical attention is a problem associated with a particular developmental phase or some other life circumstance that is not due to a mental disorder" (American Psychiatric Association 2000a, p. 742).

Many social and behavioral factors are relevant to the diagnosis of psychiatric disorders in LGBT populations (Dean et al. 2000). Cultural factors include an emphasis on appearance leading to eating disorders in some gay men. There is also the problem, in communities lacking broader LGBT social infrastructures, of socialization at bars and clubs, which can contribute to increased substance use disorders, including alcohol, tobacco, and "club" drugs such as amyl nitrate, ketamine, and Ecstasy (3,4-methylenedioxymethamphetamine [MDMA]). Disclosure of sexual orientation can lead to conflicts with families of origin, lack of social supports, and physical and economic dislocation, all contributing to adjustment disorders, depressive disorders and suicidality, and anxiety disorders. As discussed above, nondisclosure of sexual orientation can lead to delayed psychiatric treatment and an incomplete psychiatric history.

Treatment Issues

General principles of psychotherapy can be applied to work with LGBT patients. However, psychotherapeutic work with LGBT patients sometimes draws attention to aspects of the therapy process that may be overlooked in doing psychotherapy with non-LGBT patients. This section discusses some of specific factors to consider when treating LGBT patients.

Respect

All patients, not just LGBT ones, can benefit from a therapeutic environment based on respectful principles. The subjects of homosexuality and transgenderism often evoke uncomfortable feelings; when these emerge in treatment, they need to be tolerated, legitimized, and treated as valuable for further exploration by the therapist. LGBT patients usually come into treatment with some history of being made to feel shame about their sexual identities. To compensate for that history, it is a prerequisite in doing psychotherapy with LGBT patients that therapists themselves be able to accept their patients' sexual orientation or gender identity without inadvertently shaming the patient.

One means of expressing respect is to be wary of psychotherapeutic interventions intended to elucidate the presumed causes of a patient's sexual orientation or gender identity, just as therapists do not usually try to determine the "causes" of a patient's heterosexuality. Also, there is little empirical evidence supporting the hypothesis that psychotherapies of any kind will reveal the "causes" of a patient's sexual orientation or gender identity—or effect changes in them. Instead, a patient's own search for "etiological explanations" may be used to bind anxieties and may limit more helpful psychotherapeutic exploration of ongoing problems in living.

Finally, many LGBT individuals internalize antihomosexual attitudes of the dominant culture. In times of stress, and regardless of where they are in their own coming-out process, LGBT individuals may become critical or condemnatory of their own homosexuality. This may lead them to regard their sexual orientation, rather than particular life circumstances, as being the cause of their distress.

Clinical Example 1

A 30-year-old gay man comes into therapy complaining of difficulty maintaining relationships. Yet in the first few sessions, his major concerns center around his mother, whom he refers to as "domineering," and how she "made me gay." The therapist explains to the patient that the causes of homosexuality are unknown; even if his mother was domineering, it is unlikely that she had anything to do with his being gay. In shifting the therapeutic focus from discussions of etiology, the patient—under the erroneous impression that psychotherapy will reveal "why he is gay"—becomes disoriented. Then the therapist interprets the patient's wish to know why he is gay as motivated by the feeling that there is something wrong with him, and it seems to the therapist that the patient is not entirely comfortable being gay. The patient agrees. Exploration of the patient's lack of self-acceptance eventually leads to more meaningful and useful explorations of the patient's ongoing interpersonal difficulties and how they make it difficult for him to maintain relationships.

Talking Sex

Another important area of specialized knowledge is a familiarity with the sexual practices of LGBT patients. A therapist would do well not to assume anything about the sexual practices of a particular LGBT patient or of any patient, for that matter. Even with heterosexual patients, talking about sexual practices that differ from those of the therapist can generate shame in a patient and countertransferential anxiety in the therapist. When LGBT patients reveal their sexual selves, they may evoke a range of countertransference responses. For example, it is one thing for a therapist to accept a patient's homosexuality in the abstract. It is another thing altogether for a therapist to feel sufficiently comfortable and nonjudgmental to listen and to take a sexual history in a way that respects the patient's dignity and avoids shaming the patient.

When conducting psychotherapy, the therapist should be aware of his or her own judgments, including the therapist's beliefs about what constitutes "normal" human sexual behavior. The therapist should also be aware of the extent to which the theory he or she has learned has embedded within it judgments about "normal" and "abnormal" sexuality.

Clinical Example 2

A 35-year-old lesbian woman entered treatment seeking relief from anxiety symptoms. Her complaints were consistent with a DSM diagnosis of generalized anxiety disorder, and she quickly experienced a reduction in symptoms after being treated with a combination of prn benzodiazepines and supportive dynamically oriented psychotherapy. As treatment proceeded, the therapeutic focus shifted to the interpersonal stressors that exacerbated her anxiety. These stressors included difficulties accepting the authority of her male employer and anxieties related to expressions of intimacy with her long-term partner.

The patient's developmental history included severe physical abuse at the hands of her mother from age 5 years and through adolescence. The patient's father was reported to have done nothing to stop the violence and made excuses to the patient that she experienced as rationalizations for his wife's behavior. At age 16 years, the patient ran away from home and never recontacted her parents. In the process of recounting this history, the patient experienced intense affective states of fear, rage, and anxiety, as well as flashbacks. This led to a modification of her diagnosis to posttraumatic stress disorder, which responded to the addition of antidepressants to her treatment.

As for her present circumstances, the patient described her lesbian relationship as "loving" and her partner's "kindness" as allowing them to stay together despite the patient's long-term difficulties with intimacy. On one occasion, she described an evening of "love-making" in which she described herself as "so happy, it was as though I had this out-of-body experience where I felt like I gravitated out of myself and I was watching me in a really happy movie."

The patient's dissociative experience during intimacy is not unusual for one who has been severely traumatized. However, the patient's intense emotions generated equally complex responses in the therapist, who found himself uncharacteristically reluctant to inquire too deeply about the sexual details of what the patient was doing when she dissociated. The therapist, a gay man, found himself unwilling to directly ask what the patient was actually doing when she felt herself "leave" her body.

Part of the therapist's reluctance came from his sense of the patient's vulnerability to intrusions. However, the therapist privately noted some internal discomfort that inhibited him from asking for descriptions of physical intimacy in his patient's lesbian relationship. He contrasted his unusual tentativeness in this case with the ease he felt in asking about intimate sexual details in the gay men he treated, even those who had been as traumatized as this lesbian patient. He decided to take the issue up in peer supervision, asking his colleagues, "How do therapists, in general, learn to comfortably talk about the intimate sexual activities of their patients if those sexual practices are dissimilar to their own?"

HIV and Risk-Taking Behavior

More than a million people in the United States are thought to be HIV-positive, and more than 20% of these may not be aware of being infected. These numbers suggest that psychiatrists can play an important role in both assessing risk factors for HIV exposure and providing education about risk reduction and HIV testing.

Although there have been increasing rates of HIV exposure worldwide due to unprotected heterosexual sex, in the United States, unprotected sex between men remains an important risk for HIV transmission (Forstein et al. 2006). Adequate assessment of HIV risk factors includes 1) obtaining a risk history (especially high-risk behavior such as penile–vaginal intercourse without a condom or penile–anal intercourse without a condom), 2) considering the need for HIV antibody testing, 3) encouraging risk reduction, and 4) encouraging appropriate medical treatment (American Psychiatric Association 2000b).

Issues that may arise when HIV test counseling gay men include 1) fear of learning one has HIV, 2) fear of having exposed one's partners to HIV, 3) fear of having one's sexual "indiscretions" exposed, 4) fear of abandonment if found to be HIV-positive, and 5) concerns about informing sexual partners. Some studies have found higher rates of suicidal ideation in the immediate posttest period, so an assessment of suicide risk factors is important (Ostrow 1996).

Some male patients who do not self-identify as gay may nonetheless have sex with men (MSM) and may also need education and encouragement about safer sex. Psychosocial factors associated with unsafe sex in gay men include self-esteem, social supports, mood, optimism, fatalism, age, education, and alcohol or drug use (Dean et al. 2000; Halkitis et al. 2005; Wainberg et al. 2006). Internalized antihomosexual attitudes may play a role in the failure of gay men to be protective of their health (Gay and Lesbian Medical Association and LGBT Health Experts 2001).

Men who have unprotected sex with men and who frequently change partners may be at especially increased risk of HIV exposure. Also, the presence of other sexually transmitted infections (STIs) may increase the risk of HIV transmission, so inquiring about STIs should be part of HIV risk assessment. Appropriate treatment referrals should be made if STIs are present. Because minority populations—in particular, Latino and African American populations—are overrepresented among individuals who are HIV-positive, it is especially important to ensure that adequate risk assessment and counseling are performed for minority patients (Gay and Lesbian Medical Association and LGBT Health Experts 2001).

Small studies have found low rates of woman-to-woman transmission of HIV, but more research is needed (Gay and Lesbian Medical Association and LGBT Health Experts 2001). In assessment of HIV risk factors, it is important to assess not just risky sexual behaviors but also injection drug use or other drug use that may make risky sexual behavior more likely (Forstein et al. 2006).

Psychiatrists can play a role in monitoring and encouraging treatment adherence to complicated medication regimens. In addition, comorbidity of HIV and psychiatric disorders may play an important role in treatment nonadherence. In general, individuals who are HIV-positive and have a depressive disorder are at risk for poor outcomes such as worsened disease or death (Forstein et al. 2006).

Clinical Example 3

An asymptomatic HIV-positive gay man, feeling depressed and anxious, presented for a psychiatric consultation. The patient was also using crystal methamphetamine (CMA) and engaging in risky sexual behaviors, including unprotected anal intercourse (UAI), colloquially referred to as "barebacking" (Halkitis et al. 2005). As the psychiatrist took a sexual history, the patient blandly described his unsafe sexual activities, making no direct connection between those behaviors and his depressive and anxious symptoms. The psychiatrist, feeling uncomfortable as the patient's history unfolded, said nothing about her inner responses and just listened and asked neutral questions.

Toward the end of the session, the patient reported a feeling of dread that had kept him awake the night before. He did not know its source. The therapist responded that she had experienced feelings of dread earlier in the session. While listening to the patient's account of his self-damaging activities, the therapist felt frightened and out of control. She said this directly to the patient, wondering if her feelings made sense to him.

The patient responded that he, too, felt out of control. He also felt shame and guilt that he might be infecting others. Since childhood, however, he had developed a bland facade as a way to live with his alcoholic parents' physical and verbal abuse. He had experienced being diagnosed HIV-positive as traumatic; by pretending he had *no feelings* about his positive serostatus, the patient was trying to dissociate himself from thinking about anything that might remind him of HIV.

The psychiatrist listened to the patient and made no rush to judgment, allowing the patient to talk about his feelings to her. Her remarks at the end of the session induced anxiety in the patient but nevertheless succeeded in drawing his attention to his feeling that he lacked agency in controlling his own behavior. This exchange allowed him to both hear and

make efforts to follow her treatment plan: a harm reduction approach to CMA abuse (Wainberg et al. 2006), as well as getting into a substance abuse treatment program; frank conversations about the use of condoms and the incentives and risks of barebacking (Halkitis et al. 2005); and finally, treatment of his underlying depressive disorder with combined psychotherapy and pharmacotherapy.

Distinguishing Sexual Orientation From Sexual Identity

Sexual orientation is defined as the sum of an individual's sexual attractions and fantasies over a demarcated period of time. If the accumulated experiences of sexual attractions are toward the same sex, the orientation is *homosexual;* if the attractions are primarily toward a different anatomical sex, then the orientation is defined as *heterosexual.* If one has significant periods of attraction to or fantasies about members of both sexes, one's orientation is defined as *bisexual.*

A *sexual identity* (see above) is a more subjective concept and includes one's feelings and attitudes toward one's gender and sexual attractions. A sexual identity can change when an individual *changes perspective about his or her sexual feelings.* For example, when a gay person decides she is "ex-gay," her sexual attractions may not have changed, nor may they ever change; what can change, however, is her attitudes about her own homosexuality from subjective acceptance to rejection (Erzen 2006).

Double-Minority Status

In a white male–dominated society, being black, Hispanic, Asian, or native American *and* LGBT makes one a "double minority." For many ethnic and racial minority LGBT patients, this is a significant clinical issue. These individuals present as having difficulties associated with living in a society that generally condemns homosexuality and condones racial and ethnic prejudice. Being a member of a "double minority" often entails interpersonal and familial issues, as well as intrapsychic conflicts that affect the successful development of an affirmative identity and self-esteem. These issues include not feeling accepted by either the ethnic or racial minority group or gay culture ("No group wants all of me"); having difficulty choosing a primary group identification ("Am I ethnic minority first or gay first?"); and dealing with overt and covert racism, homophobia, and sexism (within both the minority communities and the gay community). A therapist can help a double-minority patient uncover, identify, and resolve some of these conflicts.

Treatment Issues Specific to Lesbian Patients

Lesbian patients may experience discrimination and stress both as women and as gay individuals. Compared with gay men, lesbians are often subject to greater social invisibility and fewer role models. Differences in prevalence of certain psychiatric disorders have been found in lesbian women, although these findings have been inconsistent and the studies reporting them may have had methodological problems. Recent studies using population-based samples and reports of self-identified sexual orientation (rather than sexual practices) found that in comparison with heterosexual women, lesbian women reported higher daily alcohol intake (Case et al. 2004), higher rates of depression and antidepressant medication usage (Case et al. 2004; Diamant and Wold 2003), greater emotional stress as teenagers, higher rates of eating disorders, greater frequency of suicidal ideation in the past 12 months, a more frequent history of suicide attempts (Koh and Ross 2006), and more days of poor mental health within the past month (Diamant and Wold 2003).

Lesbian women may first become aware of same-sex attraction and have sex at a later age than gay men. They may heterosexually marry only to become aware of their homoerotic feelings well into the marriage. Some studies have shown decreased rates of masturbation and sex for lesbians and a relative importance of nongenital physical contact, with sexual satisfaction determined not just by frequency of sex but also by emotional factors. Lesbians in coupled relationships may show more cohesion and relatedness than gay or straight couples, according to some older studies. Rates of monogamy may be higher than in gay couples (Klinger 1996). Oral–genital and manual–genital sexual contact may be more common than vaginal sex with the use of a dildo. Some lesbian couples may face issues of sexual satisfaction that arise when both partners are relatively passive in initiating sex, and treatment may be helpful in exploring what might be making some patients reluctant to express their desire for sex (Herbert 1996).

Lesbian couples or single women considering children may be making decisions about whether to adopt or to become pregnant, and if they use donor insemination, whether to use known or anonymous donors (Mamo 2004). Family stresses in lesbian couples may include adoption issues, such as whether a female partner can legally adopt the biological child of her partner.

Treatment Issues Specific to Gay Male Patients

There are some gay men who present in treatment with "effeminate" mannerisms, gestures, or voices. Boyhood effeminacy (not to be confused with DSM's *gender identity disorder in childhood*) can sometimes be part of the normal developmental history of gay men entering treatment, even those who may appear conventionally masculine as adults. However, the social impact of marked effeminacy can be enormous; in many cultures, there is no child more despised than the "sissy." Thus it is not uncommon for gay men in treatment to report that, as children, teachers, peers, and even family members tormented them. Not only are these shaming experiences traumatic, they may also, in some cases, make it difficult for these individuals to fully trust authority figures—including mental health professionals (Sherman 2005). A psychiatrist's awareness and sensitivity to the trauma of and stigma engendered by reactions to effeminacy can be helpful in treating this subgroup of gay men.

Another treatment issue may pertain to middle-aged or older gay men living in urban gay communities who experienced multiple losses in the first decade of the AIDS epidemic. Prior to the development of today's life-prolonging antiviral drugs, mortality from HIV infection was quite high. There are older gay men who lost scores of friends and acquaintances. For some, these decimated support networks were never reconstituted. Such individuals may present in treatment with social isolation, unresolved bereavement, and even posttraumatic stress disorder.

Gay men considering having children face many of the same decisions and legal obstacles experienced by lesbian women. Adoption issues are similar for gay men, but gay men wishing to have a biological child may do so through surrogacy.

Treatment Issues Specific to Bisexual Patients

Bisexual individuals represent a small percentage of the LGB population. In treatment, bisexual patients may report alienation from both the gay and lesbian and heterosexual communities. Within the former, some have been told that they are "not really bisexual" but rather unwilling to commit to a gay or lesbian identity. Although it is true that some gay and lesbian individuals first identify as "bisexual" before coming out, some people are bisexual in both behavior and desire. At times, individuals may be "serially bisexual," that is, attracted to individuals of one sex at a time—for example, first homosexual, then heterosexual, then homosexual again (Money 1988). Some bisexual individuals enter treatment because of difficulties they may be having in accepting the conventions of marriage or monogamous relationships; some bisexual individuals may feel that having to choose a partner of one sex unfairly denies them access to partners of the other sex.

Treatment Issues Specific to Transgender Patients

As stated above, sexual orientation and gender identity are independent variables in most individuals. Consequently, knowledge of a person's gender identity indicates nothing about that person's sexual orientation. An ostensibly heterosexual individual, born with a man's body and attracted to women, may become a woman and remain attracted to women after transitioning. Another treatment issue of no small consequence to transgender patients is how to address them. For example, a preoperative trans man, even in the early stages of transitioning from a woman to a man, will probably prefer to be called by a man's name and being referred to using masculine pronouns. It is possible for such individuals to meet strong resistance to this request from family, friends, government officials, employers, and even treating psychiatrists. Transgender individuals may also require psychotherapeutic help in the process of transitioning from one gender to the other (Leli and Drescher 2004).

Clinical Example 4

A 17-year-old youth with depressive symptoms was brought to a psychiatrist for consultation. Although born a girl, at 14 years of age the patient felt more like a boy and was also attracted to girls. The adolescent began insisting on being addressed by parents, friends, and teachers as "Joe." Friends and some teachers complied; the parents refused to accept this change in gender, as did the high school administration. The patient did not wish to come out as a transgender individual in applying to college, preferring to be identified in the applications as a boy. However, the school would not agree to send letters of recommendation using either a masculine name or masculine pronouns. Nor would the parents support the patient's desire to be called by a boy's name.

The patient was diagnosed with major depression, single episode, and gender identity disorder in adolescence. The family conflict about the patient's gender identity was seen as a significant stressor in the development of depressive symptoms. In addition to treatment with antidepressants, individual and family therapy were recommended. The adoles-

cent reluctantly agreed but feared that the therapists would work to satisfy the parents' wish for psychological coercion away from a male gender identity. In family therapy, the parents began threatening to place the adolescent in a boarding school in the hopes of achieving some behavioral control. The family was at loggerheads on this issue when the adolescent ran away from home. Although the adolescent did eventually return home, the incident changed the attitude of the parents, who (at least for a while) began referring to their child as "Joe."

Countertransference and Self-Disclosure

Traditions of psychotherapeutic neutrality assert that therapists should not bring personal issues into the treatment setting. In recent years, critics have questioned concepts of neutrality and argue that a therapist's subjectivity inevitably shapes the patient narratives that emerge in treatment. From this perspective, a sexual identity, in part, can sometimes be seen as a narrative about the meaning of one's sexual feelings. This is true of both the patient and the therapist, each of whom will have a sexual identity based on life experiences.

However, the revelation of a therapist's subjectivity to a patient is still a controversial subject in some quarters. For those who argue against self-revelation, an openly gay therapist could only exist as a countertransferential enactment. Yet today many LGBT therapists are working openly in their professional communities. Their presence raises the question of whether therapists should tell patients about their own sexual identities.

It would be an error to assume that a therapist, by virtue of being LGBT, will automatically have greater insight into the issues that bring LGBT patients into treatment. Simply being gay or transgender is not a substitute for being trained to do psychotherapy. One does not need to be LGBT to treat LGBT patients any more than one needs a heterosexual identity to treat heterosexual patients. Nevertheless, in many cities, LGBT patients have the option of finding well-trained therapists, heterosexual or LGBT, who are comfortable with and knowledgeable about gay people's lives. A therapist who knows little about the lives of LGBT patients will sometimes find some who are willing to share that information. Other patients may feel that their time should not be used to educate a naive therapist.

There may be times when directly revealing the therapist's sexual identity can be helpful to a patient, although heterosexuals may be unaccustomed to the need for such declarations. Heterosexual therapists may assume that the patient cannot determine their true sexual identities. However, a sexual identity, gay or heterosexual, is more than just an orientation, and therapists always provide indirect clues about their own identities, even when they will not provide direct confirmation. Because LGBT people learn early in life that revealing one's sexual identity may be fraught with dangers, some develop an acute sensitivity—or "gay-dar"—regarding the sexual identities of others.

Gay therapists who live closeted professional lives have a particular need to hide. They also experience their own homosexuality as something secretive and shameful. Isay (1991) believes that gay and lesbian analysts should always come out to their patients lest they countertransferentially perpetuate patients' feelings of secrecy and shame. However, this is not the only meaning of coming out, nor does coming out prevent other enactments in the transference and countertransference of secrecy and shame. Any therapist, regardless of his or her own sexual identity, should evaluate a patient's need for the therapist to come out on an individual basis and should be prepared to do so when necessary.

Key Points

- Homosexuality was removed from the American Psychiatric Association's *Diagnostic and Statistical Manual of Mental Disorders* in 1973.
- The causes of heterosexuality, homosexuality, bisexuality, and transgenderism are unknown.
- *Sexual orientation* (the sex to which one is attracted) is a variable independent from *gender identity* (whether one feels like a man or a woman).
- Growing up LGBT is a different cultural experience from growing up as a member of the heterosexual majority.
- Expectations of heterosexual normativity are stressful for LGBT individuals and often lead them to hide their sexual identities.
- The prevalence of homosexuality in the United States has been estimated at 1%–4%, with rates in large cities two to three times higher.
- Some studies have found higher rates of certain psychiatric disorders, including depressive, anxiety, and substance-related disorders, among LGB individuals.
- LGB individuals may be more likely to have psychiatric comorbidity and to use psychiatric services.
- Sensitivity to sexual orientation is essential to clinical interviewing and thorough psychiatric diagnosis.
- DSM-IV-TR allows the diagnosis of *identity problem* or *phase of life problem* to be used for concerns about sexual orientation or coming out.
- *Sexual identity* reflects one's relationship (accepting or rejecting) to one's sexual orientation.
- Because LGBT patients usually have a history of being shamed, therapists should approach these patients with tact and respect.
- Some LGBT patients are members of "double minorities." Working with these patients requires careful clinical attention to cultural issues.

Suggested Readings

Bayer R: Homosexuality and American Psychiatry: The Politics of Diagnosis. Princeton, NJ, Princeton University Press, 1987

Byne W, Parsons B: Human sexual orientation: the biologic theories reappraised. Arch Gen Psychiatry 50:228–239, 1993

Cabaj RP, Stein TS (eds): Textbook of Homosexuality and Mental Health. Washington, DC, American Psychiatric Press, 1996

Coates S: Is it time to jettison the concept of developmental lines? Commentary on de Marneffe's paper, "Bodies and Words." Gender and Psychoanalysis 2(1):35–53, 1997

D'Augelli AR, Patterson CJ: Lesbian, Gay, and Bisexual Identities Over the Lifespan: Psychological Perspectives. New York, Oxford University Press, 1995

DeCecco JP, Parker DA (eds): Sex, Cells, and Same-Sex Desire: The Biology of Sexual Preference. New York, Haworth Press, 1995

de Marneffe D: Bodies and words: a study of young children's genital and gender knowledge. Gender and Psychoanalysis 2(1):3–33, 1997

Drescher J: Psychoanalytic Therapy and the Gay Man. Hillsdale, NJ, Analytic Press, 1998

Isay RA: Being Homosexual: Gay Men and Their Development. New York, Farrar, Straus & Giroux, 1989

Isay RA: Becoming Gay: The Journey to Self-Acceptance. New York, Pantheon, 1996

Jones B, Hill M (eds): Mental Health Issues in Lesbian, Gay, Bisexual, and Transgender Communities. Washington, DC, American Psychiatric Publishing, 2002

Magee M, Miller D: Lesbian Lives: Psychoanalytic Narratives Old and New. Hillsdale, NJ, Analytic Press, 1997

McWhirter DP, Sanders SA, Reinisch JM (eds): Homosexuality/Heterosexuality: Concepts of Sexual Orientation. New York, Oxford University Press, 1990

Mustanski BS, Chivers ML, Bailey JM: A critical review of recent biological research on human sexual orientation. Annu Rev Sex Res 13:89–140, 2002

Weinberg MS, Williams CJ, Pryor DW: Dual Attraction: Understanding Bisexuality. New York, Oxford University Press, 1994

Online Resources

American Psychiatric Association Facts on Gay, Lesbian and Bisexual Issues: http://www.healthyminds.org/glbissues.cfm

Association of Gay and Lesbian Psychiatrists: http://www.aglp.org

Gay and Lesbian Medical Association: http://www.glma.org

Journal of Gay and Lesbian Psychotherapy: http://www.haworthpressinc.com/store/product.asp?sku=J236

Journal of Homosexuality: http://www.haworthpress.com/store/product.asp?sku=J082

Lesbian and Gay Child and Adolescent Psychiatric Association: http://www.lagcapa.org

Society for the Psychological Study of Lesbian, Gay, and Bisexual Issues (Division 44 of the American Psychological Association): http://www.apa.org/about/division/div44.html

References

Alarcon RD, Bell CC, Kirmayer LJ, et al: Beyond the funhouse mirrors: research agenda on culture and psychiatric diagnosis, in A Research Agenda for DSM-V. Edited by Kupfer DJ, First MB, Regier DA. Washington, DC, American Psychiatric Association, 2002

American Psychiatric Association: Diagnostic and Statistical Manual of Mental Disorders, 2nd Edition. Washington, DC, American Psychiatric Association, 1968

American Psychiatric Association: Position Statement: Homosexuality and Civil Rights, December 1973. Available at: http://www.psych.org/edu/other_res/lib_archives/archives/197310.pdf. Accessed September 2007.

American Psychiatric Association: Homosexuality and Sexual Orientation Disturbance: Proposed Change in DSM-II, 6th Printing, page 44; Approved by the Board of Trustees, December 1973. Available at: http://www.psych.org/edu/other_res/lib_archives/archives/197308.pdf. Accessed September 2007.

American Psychiatric Association: Diagnostic and Statistical Manual of Mental Disorders, 3rd Edition. Washington, DC, American Psychiatric Association, 1980

American Psychiatric Association: Diagnostic and Statistical Manual of Mental Disorders, 3rd Edition, Revised. Washington, DC, American Psychiatric Association, 1987

American Psychiatric Association: Diagnostic and Statistical Manual of Mental Disorders, 4th Edition. Washington, DC, American Psychiatric Association, 1994

American Psychiatric Association: Diagnostic and Statistical Manual of Mental Disorders, 4th Edition, Text Revision. Washington, DC, American Psychiatric Association, 2000a

American Psychiatric Association: Practice Guideline for the Treatment of Patients With HIV/AIDS. Washington, DC, American Psychiatric Association, 2000b

American Psychiatric Association: Practice Guideline for the Psychiatric Evaluation of Adults, 2nd Edition. Washington, DC, American Psychiatric Association, 2006

American Psychiatric Association: Position Statement: Support of Legal Recognition of Same-Sex Civil Marriage, July 2005. Available at: http://www.psych.org/edu/other_res/lib_archives/archives/197310.pdf. Accessed September 2007.

Bell AP, Weinberg MS, Hammersmith FK: Sexual Preference: Its Development in Men and Women. Bloomington, Indiana University Press, 1981

Black D, Gates G, Sanders S, et al: Demographics of the gay and lesbian populations in the United States: evidence from available systematic data sources. Demography 37:139–154, 2000

Case P, Austin SB, Hunter DJ, et al: Sexual orientation, health risk factors, and physical functioning in the Nurses' Health Study II. J Womens Health (Larchmt) 13:1033–1047, 2004

Cochran S: Emerging issues in research on lesbians' and gay men's mental health: does sexual orientation really matter? Am Psychol 56:932–947, 2001

Cochran S, Sullivan J, Mays V: Prevalence of mental disorders, psychological distress, and mental health services use among lesbian, gay, and bisexual adults in the United States. J Consult Clin Psychol 71:53–61, 2003

D'Augelli AR: Lesbian, gay and bisexual development during adolescence and young adulthood, in Textbook of Homosexuality and Mental Health. Edited by Cabaj RP, Stein TS. Washington, DC, American Psychiatric Press, 1996, pp 267–288

Dean L, Meyer IH, Robinson K, et al: Lesbian, gay, bisexual, and transgender health: findings and concerns. Journal of the Gay and Lesbian Medical Association 4:101–151, 2000

Diamant AL, Wold C: Sexual orientation and variation in physical and mental health status among women. J Womens Health (Larchmt) 12:41–49, 2003

Drescher J: Invisible gay adolescents: the developmental narratives of gay men. Adolesc Psychiatry 26:73–94, 2002

Drescher J: From bisexuality to intersexuality: rethinking gender categories. Contemporary Psychoanalysis 43:204–228, 2007

Drescher J, Merlino JP (eds): American Psychiatry and Homosexuality: An Oral History. Binghamton, NY, Harrington Park Press, 2007

Erzen T: Straight to Jesus: Sexual and Christian Conversions in the Ex-Gay Movement. Berkeley and Los Angeles, CA: University of California Press, 2006

Fergusson D, Horwood L, Beautrais A: Is sexual orientation related to mental health problems and suicidality in young people? Arch Gen Psychiatry 56:876–880, 1999

Ford CS, Beach FA: Patterns of Sexual Behavior. New York, Harper & Row, 1951

Forstein M, Cournos F, Douaihy A, et al: Guideline Watch: Practice Guideline for the Treatment of Patients With HIV/AIDS. Arlington, VA, American Psychiatric Association, 2006

Freud S: Three essays on the theory of sexuality (1905), in Standard Edition of the Complete Psychological Works of Sigmund Freud, Vol 7. Translated and edited by Strachey J. London, England, Hogarth Press, 1953, pp 123–246

Gay and Lesbian Medical Association and LGBT Health Experts: Healthy People 2010 Companion Document for Lesbian, Gay, Bisexual, and Transgender (LGBT) Health. San Francisco, CA, Gay and Lesbian Medical Association, 2001

Gilman S, Cochran S, Mays V, et al: Risk of psychiatric disorders among individuals reporting same-sex sexual partners in the National Comorbidity Survey. Am J Public Health 91:933–939, 2001

Green R: The "Sissy Boy Syndrome" and the Development of Homosexuality. New Haven, CT, Yale University Press, 1987

Halkitis PN, Wilton L, Drescher J (eds): Barebacking: Psychosocial and Public Health Approaches. Binghamton, NY, Harrington Park Press, 2005

Herbert SE: Lesbian sexuality, in Textbook of Homosexuality and Mental Health. Edited by Cabaj RP, Stein TS. Washington, DC, American Psychiatric Press, 1996, pp 723–742

Hirschfeld M: The Homosexuality of Men and Women (1914), translated by Lombardi-Nash M. Buffalo, NY, Prometheus Books, 2000

Hooker EA: The adjustment of the male overt homosexual. Journal of Projective Techniques 21:18–31, 1957

Isay RA: The homosexual analyst: clinical considerations. Psychoanalytic Study of the Child 46:199–216, 1991

Kinsey AC, Pomeroy WB, Martin CE: Sexual Behavior in the Human Male. Philadelphia, PA, WB Saunders, 1948

Kinsey AC, Pomeroy WB, Martin CE, et al: Sexual Behavior in the Human Female. Philadelphia, PA, WB Saunders, 1953

Klinger RL: Lesbian couples, in Textbook of Homosexuality and Mental Health. Edited by Cabaj RP, Stein TS. Washington, DC, American Psychiatric Press, 1996, pp 339–352

Koh AS, Ross LK: Mental health issues: a comparison of lesbian, bisexual and heterosexual women. J Homosex 51:33–57, 2006

Krafft-Ebing R: Psychopathia Sexualis (1886), translated by Wedeck H. New York, Putnam, 1965

Laumann EO, Gagnon JH, Michael RT, et al: The Social Organization of Sexuality: Sexual Practices in the United States. Chicago, IL, University of Chicago Press, 1994

Leli U, Drescher J (eds): Transgender Subjectivities: A Clinician's Guide. Binghamton, NY, Harrington Park Press, 2004

Mamo L: The lesbian "great American sperm hunt": a sociological analysis of selecting donors and constructing relatedness, in Uncoupling Convention: Psychoanalytic Approaches to Same-Sex Couples and Families. Edited by D'Ercole A, Drescher J. Hillsdale, NJ, Analytic Press, 2004, pp 115–140

Money J: Gay, Straight, and In-Between: The Sexology of Erotic Orientation. New York, Oxford University Press, 1988

Money J, Ehrhardt A: Man and Woman, Boy and Girl. Northvale, NJ, Jason Aronson, 1996

Money J, Hampson JG, Hampson JL: Imprinting and the establishment of gender roles. Arch Neurol Psychiatry 77:333–336, 1957

Ostrow DG: Mental health issues across the HIV-1 spectrum for gay and bisexual men, in Textbook of Homosexuality and Mental Health. Edited by Cabaj RP, Stein TS. Washington, DC, American Psychiatric Press, 1996, pp 859–880

Rado S: A critical examination of the concept of bisexuality. Psychosomatic Medicine 2:459–467, 1940 (reprinted in: Marmor J [ed]: Sexual Inversion: The Multiple Roots of Homosexuality. New York, Basic Books, 1965, pp 175–189)

Remafedi G, French S, Story M, et al: The relationship between suicide risk and sexual orientation: results of a population-based study. Am J Public Health 88:57–60, 1998

Sandfort T, de Graaf R, Bijl R, et al: Same-sex sexual behavior and psychiatric disorders: findings from the Netherlands Mental Health Survey and Incidence Study (NEMESIS). Arch Gen Psychiatry 58:85–91, 2001

Sandfort T, Bakker F, Schellevis F, et al: Sexual orientation and mental and physical health status: findings from a Dutch population survey. Am J Public Health 96:1119–1125, 2006

Savin-Williams RC: The New Gay Teenager. Cambridge, MA, Harvard University Press, 2005

Scheiber SC, Kramer TA, Adamowski S: The implications of core competencies for psychiatric education and practice in the US. Can J Psychiatry 48:215–221, 2003

Sherman E: Notes From the Margins: The Gay Analyst's Subjectivity in the Treatment Setting. Hillsdale, NJ, Analytic Press, 2005

Stoller R: The hermaphroditic identity of hermaphrodites. J Nerv Ment Dis 139:453–457, 1964

Stoller R: Sex and Gender. New York, Science House, 1968

Ulrichs K: The Riddle of "Man-Manly" Love (1864). Translated by Lombardi-Nash M. Buffalo, NY, Prometheus Books, 1994

Wainberg ML, Kolodny AJ, Drescher J: Crystal Meth and Men Who Have Sex With Men: What Mental Health Care Professionals Need to Know. Binghamton, NY, Harrington Park Press, 2006

39

TREATMENT OF WOMEN

Vivien K. Burt, M.D., Ph.D.
Kira Stein, M.D.

Although overall men and women are at equal risk for developing a psychiatric disorder over their lifetime, there are gender-specific differences in the prevalence and clinical course of a number of specific mental disorders. These differences stem from a variety of factors, including biological and experiential differences between the sexes. Probably due in part to genetically primed alterations in the risk of depression in response to changing hormones during the menstrual cycle, pregnancy, and the postpartum, the heritability of major depression appears to be higher in women than in men (Kendler et al. 2006). These female-specific hormonal and physiological differences not only predispose women to certain psychiatric illnesses but also often inform treatment decisions.

Table 39–1 lists reproductive-related times that may influence the onset, course, and treatment of psychiatric disorders in women. Each of these times or transitional events presents hormonal challenges that have potential consequences in women's moods, behavior, and thought processing. For some vulnerable women, these reproductive transitions are times of great psychosocial stress that further increase the risk for depression and anxiety disorders. In some cases, endogenous hormones (e.g., thyroid hormone, estrogen and progesterone) and exogenous hormones (e.g., found in contraceptives, postmenopausal hormone treatment, fertility medications) influence the psychiatric states of women (Freeman et al. 2004; Oinonen and Mazmanian 2002). Furthermore, since more than 50% of pregnancies in the United States are unplanned, the psychiatric evaluation of reproductive-age women should always include questions about sexual activity, use and form of birth control, history of unprotected intercourse, recent missed periods, and regularity of menstrual cycles. For women who plan to become pregnant in their 30s or early 40s, recent data suggesting that current and past depression may be associated with earlier decline in ovarian function further increase the importance of treating depression robustly and to full remission (Harlow et al. 2003).

A variety of factors—including gender-specific differences in drug absorption, bioavailability, metabolism, and elimination—influence how women respond to psychotropic medications. While these differences are complicated and not fully understood, their net effect is that women tend to have greater bioavailability and slower clearance of drugs compared with men, such that optimal doses for men may be too high for women. Furthermore, women tend to be on more medications than men and are more prone to side effects associated with drug–drug interactions (Seeman 2004).

Medical, social, and developmental history have an impact on the mental health needs of women. Women with chronic medical illnesses (e.g., diabetes, epilepsy, thyroid disorders, fibromyalgia) are at in-

TABLE 39–1. Reproductive-related times and events of psychiatric consequence in women

- Phase of menstrual cycle
- Use of hormonal contraception
- Pregnancy
- Postpartum
- Breast-feeding or weaning
- Induced abortion
- Miscarriage
- Infertility treatment
- Hysterectomy
- Perimenopause

TABLE 39–2. Psychosocial issues of psychiatric consequence in women

- History of childhood physical or sexual abuse
- Lack of healthy and ego-supportive significant other, particularly in childhood
- Domestic abuse
- History of rape
- Nonsupportive or abusive partner
- Economic deprivation
- Multiple children with little support, economic or emotional
- Multiple responsibilities for multiple generations (children and parents)
- Chronic illness (e.g., diabetes, fibromyalgia, thyroid dysfunction)
- Divorce, widowhood

creased risk for mood and anxiety disorders. Sexual preference, relationship styles, current state of relationships, and emotional, physical, or sexual abuse may inform clinicians about which treatment option is most likely to be efficacious. Often, women with histories of major mental illnesses pair with men with similar disorders. Thus, depressed mothers who partner with antisocial fathers are putting their offspring at risk for psychopathology that goes well beyond the burden of having a mother with depression (Marmorstein et al. 2004). The risk of child behavior problems has been shown to increase with the extent of psychological and social difficulties experienced by mothers (mental health, substance use, domestic violence) (Whitaker et al. 2006). Psychiatric disorders independently and in association with psychosocial stressors therefore affect not just the well-being of mothers but also the emotional health of their children and the stability of their families (Table 39–2). Because women tend to display strong affiliative styles in their social relationships (Cyranowski et al. 2000), dysfunctional relationships as well as psychiatric illness impact women of all ages, regardless of whether they have children.

Premenstrual Dysphoric Disorder

In DSM-IV-TR (American Psychiatric Association 2000), premenstrual dysphoric disorder (PMDD) is listed as a *mood disorder not otherwise specified*. This condition comprises recurrent physical and emotional symptoms occurring in the late luteal phase of the menstrual cycle and remitting within the first day or two following the onset of menstruation. In addition to physical symptoms (bloating, breast tenderness, cramping, and headaches), emotional symptoms include depression, irritability, anxiety, and insomnia. PMDD, when accurately diagnosed, is characterized by prominent and disabling affective and physical symptoms. Table 39–3 lists the DSM-IV-TR criteria for PMDD.

While documenting prospective daily symptom ratings over a 2-month interval is the most accurate way to establish the diagnosis, PMDD is frequently diagnosed provisionally, and treatment commences while prospective daily ratings are in progress. PMDD should be differentiated from the more common premenstrual syndrome (PMS), consisting of premenstrual bloating, breast tenderness, and mild psychological discomfort. Although such relatively mild premenstrual symptoms are experienced by up to 70% of reproductive-age women during at least some of their cycles, only 5%–9% of women meet full criteria for PMDD. Because irritability, anger, dysphoria, and mood lability are common to a variety of psychiatric disorders, other psychiatric conditions should be ruled out, as treatment approaches for PMDD may exacerbate or precipitate other psychiatric illnesses (e.g., bipolar disorder).

Evaluation for PMDD includes documentation of the course and nature of presenting symptoms, possible precipitants, and prior treatment approaches and responses. Although by definition PMDD occurs during the luteal phase of the menstrual cycle, no consistent hormonal differences have been established in

TABLE 39–3. **DSM-IV-TR research criteria for premenstrual dysphoric disorder**

A. In most menstrual cycles during the past year, five (or more) of the following symptoms were present for most of the time during the last week of the luteal phase, began to remit within a few days after the onset of the follicular phase, and were absent in the week postmenses, with at least one of the symptoms being either (1), (2), (3), or (4):

  (1) markedly depressed mood, feelings of hopelessness, or self-deprecating thoughts

  (2) marked anxiety, tension, feelings of being "keyed up" or "on edge"

  (3) marked affective lability (e.g., feeling suddenly sad or tearful or increased sensitivity to rejection)

  (4) persistent and marked anger or irritability or increased interpersonal conflicts

  (5) decreased interest in usual activities (e.g., work, school, friends, hobbies)

  (6) subjective sense of difficulty in concentrating

  (7) lethargy, easy fatigability, or marked lack of energy

  (8) marked change in appetite, overeating, or specific food cravings

  (9) hypersomnia or insomnia

  (10) a subjective sense of being overwhelmed or out of control

  (11) other physical symptoms, such as breast tenderness or swelling, headaches, joint or muscle pain, a sensation of "bloating," weight gain

  Note: In menstruating females, the luteal phase corresponds to the period between ovulation and the onset of menses, and the follicular phase begins with menses. In nonmenstruating females (e.g., those who have had a hysterectomy), the timing of luteal and follicular phases may require measurement of circulating reproductive hormones.

B. The disturbance markedly interferes with work or school or with usual social activities and relationships with others (e.g., avoidance of social activities, decreased productivity and efficiency at work or school).

C. The disturbance is not merely an exacerbation of the symptoms of another disorder, such as major depressive disorder, panic disorder, dysthymic disorder, or a personality disorder (although it may be superimposed on any of these disorders).

D. Criteria A, B, and C must be confirmed by prospective daily ratings during at least two consecutive symptomatic cycles. (The diagnosis may be made provisionally prior to this confirmation.)

women with premenstrual emotional and physical symptoms. Physical conditions that may cause symptoms in association with the premenstrual phase of the menstrual cycle (e.g., endometriosis, fibrocystic breast disease, migraine headaches) should be ruled out. Because premenstrual symptoms tend to be familial, assessment should include a family history of premenstrual symptoms and effective treatments. Over-the-counter and prescription medications should be noted, and possible psychiatric side effects of these substances should be considered. The use of caffeine, salt, alcohol, and nicotine should be ascertained, because these may cause symptoms that mimic those of PMDD (e.g., bloating, lethargy, irritability, breast tenderness). A good psychosocial history is important as well, because an association of PMDD with stressful life events and also with past sexual abuse has been noted.

Mild premenstrual symptoms may be responsive to nonpharmacological interventions, such as sleep hygiene education, exercise, relaxation therapy and cognitive-behavioral therapy. Dietary modifications, including reduction of salty foods, caffeine, red meat, and alcohol, along with increased consumption of fruits, legumes, whole grains, and water and consumption of smaller and more frequent meals high in carbohydrates have been reported to improve tension and depression. Documentation of daily prospective ratings often alerts the patient to high-risk times during which it is best to avoid difficult decisions. Such nonpharmacological interventions are also useful to address symptoms while awaiting the results of prospective symptom ratings.

A recent case–control study derived from the prospective Nurses' Health Study II cohort suggested that a high intake of calcium and vitamin D may reduce the risk of moderate to severe premenstrual symptoms

(Bertone-Johnson et al. 2005). These data add to those from a previous large trial, which found that 600 mg of daily calcium twice a day reduced premenstrual symptoms, including depression (Thys-Jacobs et al. 1998). Although more substantive data are needed to confirm this initial finding, the other beneficial effects of adequate calcium (not exceeding 1,500 mg daily) and vitamin D intake in women (e.g., possibly reducing the risk of osteoporosis) certainly justify encouraging women to include these in their daily diets.

The depression of premenstrual dysphoric disorder is frequently as severe as that of major depression, and although these symptoms occur solely during the luteal phase, the condition recurs monthly over years, often resulting in severe suffering and dysfunction. Fortunately, about 70% of women with moderate to severe PMDD respond robustly to definitive psychopharmacological care with selective serotonin reuptake inhibitor (SSRI) medications (Yonkers et al. 2006). The SSRIs fluoxetine, sertraline, paroxetine, and citalopram have been found to effectively treat PMDD. SSRIs are often given throughout the month, although administration only during the 2 premenstrual weeks (i.e., the luteal phase) has also met with success (e.g., Steiner et al. 2006). Preliminary results suggest that treatment with an SSRI when symptoms begin until the onset of menses may also be effective, but larger studies are needed to confirm these data (Yonkers et al. 2006). Continuous (i.e., throughout the month) pharmacological treatment is best for women who have comorbid depressive or anxiety disorders or for women who tend to be incompletely compliant to intermittent therapy. Intermittent treatment with SSRIs is best for patients with symptoms that are clearly localized to the premenstrual days and who may have side effects (e.g., sexual side effects) that dissipate on days when SSRIs are not used. Premenstrual anxiety and irritability may be treated with anxiolytics such as buspirone and alprazolam.

Hormonal Contraception and Effects on Mood

Hormonal contraceptive agents include oral contraceptives (birth control pills), transdermal patches, and long-acting agents (implants and injections). Oral contraceptives are more than 99% effective when properly used, ensure regular menses, and reduce the risks for endometrial and ovarian cancer, ovarian cysts, ectopic pregnancy, and iron deficiency anemia.

Monophasic combination birth control pills con-
tain fixed doses of estrogen and progestin throughout the cycle, whereas biphasic or triphasic agents contain doses of hormones that vary according to different times in the cycle. Although progestin-only pills are somewhat less effective than combination agents and may cause menstrual irregularities, they are nevertheless indicated for breast-feeding women or women for whom estrogen is contraindicated (e.g., those with hypertension or breast cancer).

Oral contraceptive agents may be categorized according to their levels of estrogenic, progestational, and androgenic activities. Estrogenic side effects include nausea, breast tenderness, headaches, elevated blood pressure, and uterine fibroid enlargement. Side effects of progestational agents include weight gain, diminished libido, headaches, and irregular bleeding. Androgen-associated side effects include hirsutism, acne, and weight gain.

A recent addition to the oral contraceptive regimen is the extended-cycle agent, which was developed to reduce the number of menstrual periods. Such an agent (e.g., Seasonale, a combination of ethinyl estradiol and the progestin levonorgestrel) is taken daily for 84 days, followed by administration of an inert tablet for 7 days. Women on this contraceptive protocol will experience withdrawal bleeding approximately once every third month. Another reliable form of birth control involves the weekly application of a transdermal patch containing a combination of estrogen and a progestin (e.g., Ortho Evra) for 3 weeks followed by a patch-free week to allow for withdrawal bleeding.

The long-acting progestational contraceptive agents Norplant (levonorgestrel implants) and Depo-Provera (medroxyprogesterone acetate injections) have gained increasing acceptance because of their ease of use and long-lasting effectiveness. Norplant, a subdermal implant, provides up to 5 years of contraception, and Depo-Provera, an injectable agent, is administered every 3 months. Like the oral progestational agents, the potential side effects of these long-lasting progestational contraceptives include irregular bleeding and weight gain.

Many women on oral contraceptives tend to experience less mood instability than untreated women (Oinonen and Mazmanian 2002). However, oral contraceptives may precipitate recurrent symptoms in women with histories of depression, dysmenorrhea, premenstrual mood symptoms, or pregnancy-related mood symptoms. Other women at risk for oral contraceptive–associated mood instability include postpartum women and those with a family history of oral contraceptive–associated negative mood (Oinonen and Mazmanian 2002). The triphasic oral contraceptive agents are more likely to be associated with depressive symptoms, especially for women with histories of premenstrual depression (Oinonen and Mazmanian 2002).

Unrelated to depression, diminished libido has been reported in relation to the use of oral contraceptives. Also, highly progestational contraceptives (e.g., containing 1.5 mg norethindrone acetate) may cause fatigue and lethargy. Norplant and Depo-Provera have been anecdotally associated with depression, but these findings have not been supported by results of controlled studies.

For women with mood changes who have recently begun to use hormonal contraception, switching agents or using an alternative contraceptive method should be considered.

Psychological Aspects of Infertility, Induced Abortion, and Pregnancy Loss

Infertility

Up to 15% of all couples are unable to conceive after 1 year of unprotected intercourse. Infertility is probably caused by male factors in about 40%–60% of cases. In addition to the usual known female causes of infertility (ovulatory dysfunction, uterine or tubal disease, cervical problems, infectious disease, immunological factors), anorexia nervosa and stress-induced amenorrhea, which frequently result in hypothalamic hypopituitary syndrome, are associated with infertility. Furthermore, current depression or a history of depression has been found to be associated with a decline in ovarian function and therefore may also contribute to female causes of infertility (Harlow et al. 2003).

Many infertile couples experience lowered self-esteem and depression. Both members of the couple may have diminished libido. Often, they feel isolated from friends whose activities revolve around their children. The cost of the workup and treatment of infertility is great, in terms of both time and money, and frequently reduces the feasibility of vacations or social expenses that are particularly important to couples exposed to severe stress and uncertainty.

The evaluation of both members of the couple includes screening for sexually transmitted diseases and normal endocrine functioning. The infertility workup includes assessment of ovulation, quantity and quality of sperm, visualization of the woman's anatomy, and

determination of patency of ductile systems in the woman and/or the man. Tests are often repeated at different intervals over a single menstrual cycle and at subsequent menstrual cycles. The assessment invariably requires substantial reorganization of the day-to-day lives of both partners, with office visits dictated by responses to treatment, dates of ovulation, and physicians' schedules.

Treatment of Infertility

In some cases, surgery may correct mechanical blockage in the female reproductive tract. Endometriosis may be treated with gonadotropin-releasing hormone (GnRH) agonists such as leuprolide (Lupron). Ovulatory dysfunction may be reversed by oral clomiphene citrate and daily injections of human menopausal gonadotropins (follicle-stimulating hormone [FSH] and luteinizing hormone [LH]) or Metrodin (FSH). Frequently, such hormonal treatments cause fatigue, nausea, headache, diarrhea, and weight gain. The rate of multiple gestation is 5% with clomiphene citrate and rises to 20% with human menopausal gonadotropins. Pharmacological induction of ovulation is more likely to succeed if it is combined with intrauterine insemination. The success rate of these two combined procedures approximates 33%. Serial ultrasounds are used to monitor follicular development and confirm ovulation.

If these treatments do not enable the couple to achieve pregnancy, they may opt for assisted reproductive technology, such as gamete intrafallopian transfer (GIFT) or zygote intrafallopian transfer (ZIFT). In the former method, oocytes and sperm are combined in vitro and immediately deposited in the woman's fallopian tubes; in the latter method, eggs are fertilized in vitro and the resultant zygotes are placed in the fallopian tubes. In the case of in vitro fertilization (IVF), fertilized embryos are placed directly into the uterus. Serial ultrasounds monitor ovulation and posttransfer embryological development and screen for ovarian hyperstimulation, a potentially dangerous side effect. Success rates for assisted reproductive technology cycles using fresh nondonor eggs or embryos are approximately 34% live births per retrieval or transfer. The rate of multiple gestation is 25%, and there is a 6% chance of severe ovarian hyperstimulation syndrome. For unclear reasons, the use of assisted reproductive technology seems to double the risk of having an infant with a birth defect or low birth weight for gestational age (Mitchell 2002). Nevertheless, because 94% of couples who do conceive via reproductive assistance will have a normal-weight baby and 91% will have a baby with no major birth defect, many infertile couples engage in the latest technological treatments to enable them to become biological parents.

In cases of infertility due to an untreatable male factor, some couples choose donor sperm insemination. Egg donation is an option for women who do not respond to ovarian stimulation. Medications are administered to both the donor and the infertile woman in order to synchronize their cycles. The donor eggs are then fertilized with sperm through the procedures of IVF or GIFT and transferred to the infertile woman, who then carries the pregnancy. In the case of a woman who is able to ovulate but cannot carry the pregnancy, a fertilized egg may be inseminated in a surrogate mother who then will carry the pregnancy.

Psychological Implications of Infertility Treatment

The difficult and demanding aspects of infertility often have a negative impact on intimacy and spontaneity, and the daily monitoring of reproductive-related bodily functions can be overwhelming. Men may become so anxious that they have difficulty performing sexually at scheduled times. Uncertain and modest success rates and the high costs of the procedures add to the stress of treatment. A woman who postponed pregnancy for career concerns may experience significant guilt and self-blame. Complicating this situation, the medications used (clomiphene citrate, human menopausal gonadotropins, GnRH agonists) may produce negative mood changes, anxiety, and insomnia in addition to a number of physical side effects. Although infertility is not associated with the development of major depressive disorder, it does produce negative mood changes and may exacerbate any preexisting psychiatric disorders. Thus, psychiatric evaluation and treatment may be indicated (Table 39–4). Data suggesting that current or past depression may be associated with ovarian dysfunction (Harlow et al. 2003) add to the growing list of reasons that justify addressing depression promptly and effectively with remission as an important goal of treatment. For mild to moderate psychiatric symptoms, psychotherapy may be sufficient. Group psychological interventions can also be helpful and have been reported to increase pregnancy rates in infertile women. For major mood or anxiety disorders, treatment should involve psychotherapy and/or psychotropic medication. A psychiatrist also can play a role in exploring alternative parenting options, including adoption. The psychiatrist should encourage both members of the couple to participate in therapy, either jointly or individually. A referral to RESOLVE, the National Infertility Association's self-help organization

TABLE 39–4. Role of the psychiatric clinician in the treatment of the infertile couple

- Psychiatric evaluation
- Clarification of issues relevant to treatment decisions
- Facilitation of consensus between partners about treatment
- Help for patients in coping with stresses of infertility treatments
- Provision of support through treatment holidays or after unsuccessful course of treatment
- Referral of patients to support groups
- Psychopharmacological treatment

that sponsors groups and workshops for infertile couples, can help the couple feel less isolated and overwhelmed.

Induced Abortion

Since the Supreme Court decision of *Roe v. Wade* in 1973, first-trimester abortions have been a woman's legal right. In the United States, most women who elect to terminate a pregnancy by means of abortion are younger than 25 years, single, and childless. About 20% of women have had a legal abortion.

Most abortions are performed by dilation and evacuation of uterine contents by means of vacuum aspiration or curettage and are associated with a mortality rate of approximately 0.4 per 100,000 procedures. This rate is 25 times lower than the rate associated with carrying a pregnancy to term. Recently, a number of medical methods for inducing abortion have been introduced. In September 2000, a regimen of mifepristone followed 2 days later by the prostaglandin E analogue misoprostol was approved by the U.S. Food and Drug Administration (FDA) for termination of pregnancies of less than 49 days' duration. The off-label use of methotrexate in conjunction with misoprostol has also been used to induce abortion.

Reasons for termination of pregnancy include poor partner support, inability to provide financial support for a child, inability or lack of desire to bear responsibility for a child, and termination for the health of the mother. A woman may be reluctant to carry the pregnancy to term if a fetal congenital anomaly has been diagnosed or if the pregnancy resulted from rape or incest.

For most women, mood improves after an abortion and for years thereafter. Some women, however, may experience depression or other negative psychological outcomes. The strongest predictor of depression after elective abortion is a history of depression before the pregnancy. The risk for postabortion depression is also increased by ambivalence about having an abortion, in abortions after the first trimester, and in abortions due to fetal demise or severe deformity. Preabortion counseling offers a woman and her partner a chance to obtain information about the abortion procedure and possible adverse sequelae following the abortion and to learn effective contraceptive methods to prevent future unwanted pregnancies. For women whose pregnancy is the result of a rape, counseling is an important part of the recovery from the trauma of the assault.

For a woman undergoing an abortion because of congenital deformity or impending fetal demise, mourning for the loss of a wished-for baby and self-blame about having produced a deformed fetus are not uncommon. The woman may experience anxiety and ambivalence about becoming pregnant in the future and will benefit from sensitive education and support. Whenever possible, the woman's partner should be included in therapy, particularly because he also may be grieving.

When a chronically mentally ill woman seeks an abortion, a careful psychiatric evaluation should be undertaken to assess her ability to understand her condition and the various options that are available to address the pregnancy. She should be evaluated for the presence of delusions and paranoia that may affect her condition and influence her ability to decide between proceeding with either the pregnancy or an abortion. Should termination of the pregnancy be considered, the patient's psychiatric condition should first be stabilized.

Pregnancy Loss

Although clinically documented miscarriage (intrauterine death during the first 20 weeks of gestation) occurs in 12%–24% of identified pregnancies, up to 50% of pregnancies are not sustained, as many pregnancy losses occur in women who are unaware that they are pregnant. Miscarriage may be a serious traumatic event, and affected couples often feel isolated. In the 6 months following a pregnancy loss, women frequently experience anxiety and depression. Childless women, younger women, and women with prior histories of depression are at particular risk for major depression after miscarriage (Neugebauer 2003).

Understandably, pregnancy loss is most traumatic in cases of stillbirth. Although common practice for stillbirth deliveries has been to encourage parents to hold their deceased infant, in some cases this practice may be detrimental to the emotional well-being of the bereaved couple. Normal bereavement should be distinguished from psychopathology, and psychiatric follow-up should be encouraged for couples who have histories of depression or who have experienced late-trimester fetal loss. Women suffering a miscarriage who have significant histories of depression should be monitored during the next pregnancy to reduce the risk for subsequent depression.

Psychiatric Disorders in Pregnancy

Pregnancy is not necessarily a time of emotional stability, particularly if the expectant mother has a prior history of psychiatric conditions or has changed or discontinued a medication regimen that had kept her stable and functional (Cohen et al. 2006a; Flynn et al. 2006; Viguera et al. 2000). Most pregnant women with current major depressive symptoms are either untreated or undertreated (Flynn et al. 2006). The best time for women with psychiatric histories to decide among possible treatment options during pregnancy is prior to actually becoming pregnant. In this way, a treatment algorithm can be formulated that maximizes safety and well-being for both patient and fetus. If clinically feasible, discontinuation of psychiatric medications should be considered. However, clinical experience has shown that in some cases this is not feasible, because past history has shown that dose reduction or discontinuation of medication results in serious relapse, or because the patient is not fully stabilized even when provided with a comprehensive treatment regimen including psychotherapy and psychotropic medication.

Nonpharmacological interventions may not be sufficient during pregnancy, because unmedicated women with serious mood, anxiety, or psychotic disorders are often unable to care for themselves properly or to adhere to prenatal regimens. Psychiatric decompensation during pregnancy increases the risk of difficulties not only for mother but also for obstetrical complications and adverse fetal outcomes (e.g., preeclampsia, placental abnormalities, low birth weight, preterm labor, and fetal distress) (Chung et al. 2001; Evans et al. 2001; Federenko and Wadwha 2004; Jablensky et al. 2005; Kurki et al. 2000). Furthermore, antenatal psychiatric instability increases the risk for postpartum illness, when maternal responsibilities are new and particularly overwhelming for psychiatrically ill patients. Patients should be advised that the use of caffeine, nicotine, and alcohol is detrimental to the fetus and for their own well-being and strategies should be devised to ensure the opportunity for adequate sleep and healthful nutrition. Psychotherapy, group support, and family and marital counseling may be helpful, as pregnancy is a stressful time and may be particularly challenging for psychiatrically ill women, who often are so overwhelmed that they tend to decompensate during times of transition. When indicated, psychotropic medications during pregnancy are administered in order to prevent a relapse.

Before a psychotropic agent is administered to a pregnant patient, risks and benefits to both the mother and the fetus should be evaluated and shared with the patient, her partner (whenever possible), and her obstetrician. The patient and her partner should be informed that both the FDA and the American Medical Association agree that although the FDA does not endorse the safety of any psychiatric medication in pregnancy, physicians may prescribe medications according to data-based knowledge and their own best clinical judgment. Pregnancy counseling should emphasize that the goal is to weigh any risk associated with maternal treatment with medications against the known risks associated with untreated disease for mother and baby, during both pregnancy and the postpartum. Discussions should be documented, and the clinician should assess and note the patient's understanding and capacity to consent to the treatment plan.

Table 39–5 presents general guiding principles for the treatment of psychiatric illness during pregnancy.

Treatment of Depression During Pregnancy

Rates of depression have been found to be greater at 32 weeks' gestation than at 8 weeks' postpartum (Evans et al. 2001). Depression may be overlooked during pregnancy, because many of the neurovegetative symptoms of depression coincide with normative somatic complaints of pregnancy. The functional impairment that frequently occurs in association with depression is of particular concern during pregnancy, because it tends to affect the health and well-being of both the expectant mother and her fetus. Furthermore, depression during pregnancy significantly increases the risk for postpartum depression (Miller 2002). For mild to moderate depression, nonpharmacological modalities such as individual or conjoint psychotherapy and stress-reduction counseling are good first options for treatment (Spinelli and Endicott 2003). However, for severe and treatment-resistant depression, particularly

TABLE 39–5. Treatment of psychiatric illness in pregnancy

- The overall mental health of an expectant mother is an important determinant of the health of the fetus and neonate.
- Psychiatric illness that compromises maternal function increases the risk for poor obstetrical outcome.
- Depression during pregnancy substantially increases the risk for postpartum depression.
- Risk of maternal treatment with psychotropic medication should be weighed against known risks of untreated psychiatric disease for mother and baby.
- Risk–benefit decisions during pregnancy should be made on a case-by-case basis by an informed patient in combination with her partner and doctors.
- For mild to moderate psychiatric illness, try nonpharmacological interventions first:
  - Psychotherapy
  - Conjoint counseling
  - Stress-reduction strategies
  - Mobilization of psychosocial supports
  - Bright-light therapy (for depression)
- For severe, disabling psychiatric illness, the risk of psychotropic medication to both mother and infant is generally less than the risk of symptomatic illness.
- When treating psychiatrically ill pregnant women, whether on psychotropic agents or not, general maternal medical health indices, such as appetite, weight, and sleep patterns, should be carefully monitored to optimize maternal health and obstetrical outcome.

if symptoms jeopardize a patient's emotional stability and the viability of the pregnancy (e.g., if the woman is suicidal, psychotic, or not gaining weight or is reluctantly contemplating an abortion), psychopharmacological approaches to treatment are reasonable.

The use of antidepressants during pregnancy is not without some risk. As noted, antidepressant medications should be withheld if possible. Bright light therapy has been suggested as a noninvasive treatment option for antenatal depression (Oren et al. 2002). In addition to promoting fetal neurodevelopment and reducing the risk of preterm labor, omega-3 polyunsaturated fatty acids have also been suggested as a treatment for depression during pregnancy (Chiu et al.

2003). However, if a woman is experiencing severe, debilitating depression or if she has a history of chronic depression with severe relapses following medication discontinuation, antidepressants should be considered (Cohen et al. 2006a). When antidepressants are used during pregnancy, dosages should be kept at the minimum necessary to promote ongoing mood stability and normal functioning. The major issues of concern when evaluating outcomes with any medications in pregnancy, and in this case with antidepressants, are risks of congenital malformation, pregnancy loss, perinatal toxicity, length of gestation, and neurobehavioral sequelae.

In the past 5 years, there has been an upsurge in publications (both peer reviewed and non–peer reviewed) and pharmaceutical data analyses about the use of antidepressants during pregnancy. As a result, the FDA has released a number of widely reported public health advisories that have understandably prompted many women and their physicians to reconsider the use of antidepressants in pregnancy. For women with mild to moderate depression, the decision to discontinue antidepressants while being carefully followed psychiatrically has been prudent and well considered. However, many women with severe major depression or anxiety disorders are symptomatic and dysfunctional during or just prior to pregnancy. They may experience ongoing suicidal ideation (frequently passive, but deeply troubling), and some choose to abort their fetuses because they cannot remain off the medications that keep them free of disabling symptoms. In other cases, women with serious depressive histories have become so alarmed by the literature suggesting that antidepressants are harmful agents in pregnancy that they have discontinued their antidepressants, experienced recurrences, and required restabilization with antidepressants in order to regain their health during the remainder of their pregnancies (Cohen et al. 2006a). In the following discussion, which emphasizes data from peer-reviewed studies, we review what is currently known about the use of antidepressants in pregnancy. Because SSRIs are the antidepressants most widely used to treat depression, and because of the large amount of conflicting, controversial, and sometimes alarming data recently published on the subject of SSRI use during pregnancy, the discussion below emphasizes the prenatal use of these agents.

Selective Serotonin Reuptake Inhibitors

Teratogenicity. Although numerous peer-reviewed studies on the use of SSRIs in pregnancy have found no significantly increased risk of birth defects (Chambers et al. 1996; Cohen et al. 2000; Costei et al. 2002; Ericson et al. 1999; D. J. Goldstein 1995; Heikkinen et al. 2002; Hendrick et al. 2003a; Hostetter et al. 2000; Kulin et al. 1998; Laine et al. 2003; Nulman et al. 1997; Oberlander et al. 2004; Pastuszak et al. 1993; Simon et al. 2002; Sivojelezova et al. 2003), several recent studies have suggested possible teratogenicity with first-trimester exposure to SSRIs (Bérard et al. 2007; Kallen et al. 2007; Wogelius et al. 2006). Two recent large case–control studies involving almost 20,000 case infants with major birth defects and almost 10,000 control infants have revealed statistically significant increases in some rare defects involving the gastrointestinal tract, neural tube, and skull among babies born to women who recall taking SSRI antidepressants (Alwan et al. 2007; Louik et al. 2007). While these studies have significant strengths, two of the main methodological difficulties are the low numbers of exposed subjects and the low background absolute risk for uncommon defects. Thus, whereas both studies found that individual SSRIs may confer increased risks for certain specific defects, with the exception of an increased risk for cardiac defects with paroxetine, the two studies contradicted one another in regard to increased risks for specific other defects with individual SSRIs. Although the risk for certain rare congenital malformations may be increased by a factor of 2 or 3, the absolute risk for such defects is very low—probably no more than 1 in 2,500 births.

Although first-trimester exposure to paroxetine probably incurs a substantial risk of cardiac abnormality, it nevertheless appears that the risk for right-ventricle defects is not likely to exceed 1 in 100, and the risk for all congenital heart defects probably does not exceed 2 in 100. To place these data in perspective, it should be noted that any pregnancy carries about a 3% risk of having a birth defect, regardless of exposure, and that maternal stress and depression during pregnancy has also been associated with adverse reproductive outcomes (Alwan et al. 2007). Thus, as noted in an editorial accompanying the latest case–control studies, although it is impossible to delineate definitively either "no risk" or "risk" with most SSRIs (or most other medications) in pregnancy, "any increased risks of malformations in association with the use of SSRIs are likely to be small in terms of absolute risk" (Greene 2007, p. 2733).

Poor neonatal adaptability. Third-trimester exposure to SSRIs is associated with an increased risk of perinatal symptoms sometimes requiring admission to special care nurseries (including jitteriness, poor muscle tone, weak or absent cry, respiratory distress, hypoglycemia, low Apgar score, and seizures) (Chambers et al. 1996; Costei et al. 2002; Kallen 2004; Laine et al. 2003; Oberlander et al. 2002). If these symptoms occur, they are usually mild and disappear by 2 weeks of age. Seizures are rare in term infants (1 in 313 published cases) (Costei et al. 2002; Moses-Kolko et al. 2005). In April 2004, the U.S. Department of Health and Human Services Center for the Evaluation of Risks to Human Reproduction published an expert panel report on the reproductive and developmental safety of fluoxetine (Center for the Evaluation of Risks to Human Reproduction 2004). The panel affirmed that in utero use of fluoxetine may be associated with poor neonatal adaptation, but also noted the importance of evaluating possible risks of fluoxetine exposure in the context of risks associated with untreated psychiatric illness, particularly major depression. This advice presumably applies to the use of other psychiatric medications in pregnancy, especially if those medications are used to stabilize a pregnant woman whose mental condition might compromise her own safety or that of her fetus.

A recent small prospective study of children who had been exposed prenatally to SSRIs and had exhibited transient neonatal adaptability difficulties (including decreased affect expressivity) found that by 4–5 years of age, there was no difference in internalizing behaviors (e.g., anxiety/depression, withdrawal, somatic complaints) in comparison with control children (Misri et al. 2006).

Persistent pulmonary hypertension of the newborn.

A recent case–control study reported an association between use of SSRIs after the 20th week of pregnancy and a condition in which a newborn's circulation system does not fully adapt to breathing outside the womb (Chambers et al. 2006). This condition, persistent pulmonary hypertension of the newborn (PPHN), occurs at a background rate of 1–2 infants per 1,000 births and is potentially lethal, although no SSRI-exposed infants in this study died of the condition. Although case–control studies do not establish causality, the value of this study is that it raises the issue of a possible association and suggests the need for a prospective cohort study to examine the validity of this finding. However, if these data prove to be correct, exposure to SSRIs after 20 weeks of gestation may increase the rate of PPHN to 1 per 100 births. Women exposed to an SSRI late in pregnancy should be informed of this reported association, and this issue should be incorporated as part of a risk–benefit discussion of treatment of depression during pregnancy.

Shorter gestation.

Data have been mixed regarding the effect of SSRI exposure on the gestation period. Several reports have found that prenatal exposure to SSRIs is associated with an increased risk for shorter gestation (possibly preterm birth), small-for-gestational-age babies, and admission to special care nurseries (Chambers et al. 1996; Costei et al. 2002; Ericson et al. 1999; Kallen 2004; Malm et al. 2005; Oberlander et al. 2006; Simon et al. 2002; Zeskind and Stephens 2004). Some of these reports have associated these findings with third-trimester exposure to SSRIs; in other cases, antenatal SSRI use was not tracked with respect to a particular time of exposure during pregnancy. It has been suggested that the increased risk of small-for-gestational age babies may in part be explained by smaller maternal weight gain with third-trimester exposure to SSRIs (Chambers et al. 1996). It has been suggested that monitoring maternal weight gain in SSRI-treated expectant mothers may reduce the likelihood of delivering a small-for-gestational-age infant (Bodnar et al. 2006). A recently completed prospective controlled study found that SSRI use during pregnancy was associated with lower gestational age at birth, increased rate of prematurity, and admission to special care nurseries. In this study, birth weights and Apgar scores were not adversely affected by antidepressant use (Suri et al. 2007).

Neurobehavioral sequelae.

The developmental outcomes of children exposed to antidepressants in utero have been evaluated in five studies. Two prospective studies by Nulman et al. (1997, 2002) found no differences in temperament, mood, distractibility, behavior, or global IQ in children exposed to fluoxetine or tricyclic antidepressants (TCAs) compared with nonexposed control children. With regard to neurobehavioral sequelae, a prospective study that compared control children with children prenatally exposed to fluoxetine or TCAs found no differences in IQ, temperament, mood, behavior, or attention in children up to age 7 years (Nulman et al. 1997). Interestingly, the same group did report that maternal depression was associated with lower cognitive and language achievements in exposed children (Nulman et al. 2002). In a review of pediatric records of 384 infants exposed to TCAs and SSRIs antenatally compared with nonexposed control infants, there were no reported differences in developmental outcomes (Simon et al. 2002). In a study of 31 children (ages 6–40 months) of depressed mothers who took SSRIs during pregnancy, scores of psychomotor development were lower than those reported for 13 nonexposed children (Casper et al. 2003). A major drawback of this study was the young age of the children, because developmental scores in subjects younger than 5 years of age are not reliable. Finally, a recent longitudinal study found that 4- to 5-year-old children who had been exposed in utero to SSRIs (and in some cases to both SSRIs and clonazepam) and had displayed symptoms of neonatal adaptation difficulties did not show evidence of internalizing behaviors (impaired emotional reactivity, anxiety, depression, withdrawal, somatic complaints) (Misri et al. 2006).

Summary regarding use of SSRIs during pregnancy.

As noted in an important editorial on the use of antidepressant medication during pregnancy (Rubinow 2006), the treatment of depression during pregnancy presents the clinician and patient with difficult decisions. In his summary, David Rubinow points to a number of important issues to consider when faced with decisions about treatment of women at risk for depression during pregnancy. Depression during pregnancy is a very real and troubling problem, and largely because of the difficulties associated with performing methodologically and conceptually sound studies, the data regarding antidepressant use (some troubling, some reassuring) are limited and conflicting. Nevertheless, pregnancy does not protect against depression, and relapse rates are high in untreated women with recurrent illness. Maternal depression clearly is a risk factor for affective and other difficulties in offspring. As previously noted, paroxetine may increase the risk for certain cardiac defects. Although there may be a small increased risk for other rare congenital defects with SSRIs, the absolute risk is very small. Transient difficulties with neonatal adaptation must not be assumed to mean long-term difficulties, especially in the context of worsening maternal depression. Nevertheless, SSRIs may be associated with an uncommon but serious medical consequence (i.e., PPHN).

A recent FDA Public Health Advisory indicated that whereas babies exposed to SSRIs late in pregnancy may experience irritability, difficulty feeding, and (in rare cases) difficulty breathing, the advisory also clearly stated that the potential risk of relapsed depression after stopping antidepressants during pregnancy makes decisions about how to treat depression during pregnancy challenging for health care professionals and patients (U.S. Food and Drug Administration Center for Drug Evaluation and Research 2006). Although manufacturers have been directed to include the potential risk for PPHN in package inserts, the FDA has also cautioned women who are pregnant or thinking about becoming pregnant not to discon-

tinue their antidepressants without first consulting their physicians.

Tricyclic Antidepressants

Available data show no TCA-associated congenital anomalies, although transient perinatal toxicity or withdrawal symptoms have been reported when these agents are used near the time of birth (Altshuler et al. 1996). Symptoms include jitteriness, irritability, lethargy, decreased muscle tone, and anticholinergic effects such as constipation, tachycardia, and urinary retention (McElhatton et al. 1996). It may be that TCAs (like SSRIs) are associated with a shorter duration of gestation (Suri et al. 2007). If the decision is made to treat with a TCA, nortriptyline or desipramine is preferable, because there is less likelihood of anticholinergic and hypotensive side effects. Antidepressant dosages may need to be adjusted over the course of pregnancy, as blood levels may fall, particularly after the patient enters the third trimester.

Other Antidepressants

Three studies of in utero exposure to venlafaxine ($n = 150$), nefazodone ($n = 91$), or trazodone ($n = 58$) in pregnancy have failed to find an increased risk of birth defects or perinatal complications (Einarson et al. 2001, 2003; Yaris et al. 2004). In light of the data regarding the increased risk of neonatal difficulties in infants exposed in utero to SSRIs, the FDA has extended its advisory for perinatal complications to include third-trimester use of serotonin and norepinephrine reuptake inhibitors (SNRIs) such as venlafaxine in addition to SSRIs.

One study (136 cases) investigating the use of bupropion in pregnancy suggests that this agent is not associated with an increased risk of major malformations (Chan et al. 2005). Another study from the manufacturer (GlaxoSmithKline) investigated outcomes of 1,213 women who had taken bupropion in the first trimester of pregnancy and also found no increased risk for malformations (Cole et al. 2007). In the smaller study, the rate of spontaneous abortions was higher in both the group taking the drug for depression and the group taking it for smoking cessation, even when the use of nicotine was accounted for (Chan et al. 2005). More data using larger sample sizes are needed to further explore this possible association.

The published data for mirtazapine suggest that this agent does not increase the risk for gross organ malformation (Djulus et al. 2006; Saks 2001; Yaris et al. 2004). In the largest of these studies ($n = 104$ in utero mirtazapine exposures), which was prospective and compared disease-matched pregnant women diagnosed with depression taking other antidepressants and pregnant women exposed to nonteratogens, there were no statistically significant differences in the rates of spontaneous abortion, therapeutic abortion, or still births or in mean gestational weights at birth. The rate of preterm birth was higher in the mirtazapine group than in the group that was not exposed to antidepressants, but not higher than the group exposed to other antidepressants (Djulus et al. 2006). This suggests an association either with antidepressant exposure or with depression.

If at all possible, the use of monoamine oxidase inhibitors (MAOIs) during pregnancy is discouraged, as the hypertensive risk with these agents would likely be increased should tocolytic medications such as terbutaline be used to treat early labor. Furthermore, MAOIs have been associated in animal studies with an increased rate of congenital anomalies.

There are no published studies of in utero use of duloxetine.

Table 39–6 presents major summary points about the antenatal use of antidepressants, including SSRIs.

Treatment of Bipolar Disorder During Pregnancy

Although some women with bipolar disorder (particularly those with histories of treatment-responsive illness) may stabilize during pregnancy, for many bipolar women, pregnancy does not protect against mood instability when mood stabilizers are discontinued (Grof et al. 2000; Viguera et al. 2000). It may be that the course of bipolar illness both with and without mood stabilization predicts the course of the illness in the context of pregnancy. Women who are not treated with mood stabilizers during pregnancy are at substantially increased risk for postpartum decompensation. Furthermore, rapid rather than gradual antepartum discontinuation of lithium appears to increase the risk for postpartum relapse (Viguera et al. 2000).

With first-trimester use of lithium, the incidence of Ebstein's anomaly, a serious defect in the formation of the tricuspid valve of the heart, is raised from the estimated rate of 1 per 20,000 in the general population to a rate of approximately 1 per 1,000. The use of lithium during pregnancy also has been linked with other cardiac malformations, including coarctation of the aorta and mitral atresia. Additional potential adverse consequences to the neonate from lithium use in pregnancy include hypotonia, poor suck reflex, hypoglycemia, cyanosis, neonatal goiter, and diabetes insipidus.

Use of valproate and carbamazepine in the first trimester is associated with an increased risk of neural tube defects, including spina bifida (up to 5% for valproate and 1% for carbamazepine), and with developmental delay, craniofacial defects, and fingernail hypoplasia. These medications produce antifolate effects that contribute significantly to their embryotoxicity. They can also produce a deficiency in vitamin K–dependent clotting factors, thereby increasing the risk of bleeding disorders in the fetus and neonate. Vitamin K supplementation and folate should therefore be administered to women taking these agents during pregnancy. Hypoglycemia and hepatic dysfunction have also been reported in exposed neonates.

A recent evaluation of data from the North American Antiepileptic Drug Pregnancy Registry for lamotrigine monotherapy during the first trimester found a positive association between lamotrigine and oral clefts, with a prevalence rate of 8.9 per 1,000 in exposed infants (vs. a prevalence rate of 0.37 per 1,000 in the general population) of the Brigham and Women's Hospital Surveillance Program (Holmes et al. 2006). Data from several other large registries are currently being reanalyzed to provide further information regarding the possible association of oral clefts in infants exposed to lamotrigine therapy. Few human data exist on gabapentin or topiramate use during pregnancy. Table 39–7 summarizes the risks of commonly used mood stabilizers in pregnancy.

Antipsychotics are often used to treat bipolar disorder. Because decompensated bipolar disorder poses great risks to the mother and the fetus during pregnancy and the postpartum, antipsychotics are sometimes considered for use during pregnancy, particularly in cases of brittle bipolar disorder requiring prompt and sustained stabilization. Although low-potency phenothiazines have been reported to increase the risk of nonspecific congenital anomalies, high-potency antipsychotics have not been associated with major malformations. A prospective cohort study compared infants who had been exposed to atypical antipsychotics in utero with a comparison group of nonexposed infants (McKenna et al. 2005). This study of olanzapine ($n=60$), risperidone ($n=49$), quetiapine ($n=36$), and clozapine ($n=6$) found no increased risk for major malformations. Additional reviews—including a study of 23 women, several additional case reports, and data from more than 100 exposures recorded by the manufacturer for olanzapine (Gentile 2004; D.J. Goldstein et al. 2000; Mendhekar et al. 2002), as well as single case reports for risperidone and quetiapine (Ratnayake and Libretto 2002; Tenyi et al.

TABLE 39–6. Use of antidepressants in pregnancy: summary points

Antidepressant	Teratogenicity	Other adverse effects	Comments
SSRIs	Paroxetine may increase risk of congenital anomalies, particularly ventricular–septal defects. Greatest amount of data exist for fluoxetine ($n=1{,}700+$). As a group, SSRIs other than paroxetine do not appear to increase risk for major congenital malformations.	Increased risk of poor neonatal adaptability Possible increased risk of persistent pulmonary hypertension of the newborn Increased risk for shorter gestational period, preterm birth (<37 weeks' gestation) Increased risk of small-for-gestational-age birth	Paroxetine should be avoided if possible. Use of these agents is justified if history suggests that antenatal treatment is essential to keep a seriously depressed pregnant woman euthymic and functional. Targeted early-second-trimester ultrasound should be considered for exposed fetuses. Maintain awareness of possible neonatal side effects—observe exposed infants for several days beyond usual 1–2 days' postpartum. Monitor maternal appetite, weight, and other indices of maternal health.
TCAs	TCAs do not appear to increase risk for major congenital malformations.	Increased risk of poor neonatal adaptability Increased risk for shorter gestational period (<37 weeks' gestation)	Use of these agents is justified if history suggests that antenatal treatment is essential to keep a seriously depressed pregnant woman euthymic and functional. Maintain awareness of possible neonatal side effects—observe exposed infants for several days beyond usual 1–2 days' postpartum. Monitor maternal appetite, weight, and other indices of maternal health.
Other antidepressants: fluvoxamine, venlafaxine, bupropion, trazodone, nefazodone, mirtazapine, nefazodone, duloxetine	Fewer published cases; more data are needed Venlafaxine ($n=150$) does not appear to increase risk for major congenital malformations (but more data are needed). Mirtazapine ($n=154$) does not appear to increase risk for major congenital malformations (but more data are needed).	More data are needed Some suggestion that antidepressants may increase risk for shorter gestational period, preterm birth (<37 weeks' gestation)	Use of these agents is justified only if history suggests that antenatal treatment is essential to keep a seriously depressed pregnant woman euthymic and functional. Maintain awareness of possible neonatal side effects—observe exposed infants for several days beyond usual 1–2 days' postpartum. Monitor maternal appetite, weight, and other indices of maternal health.

TABLE 39–6. Use of antidepressants in pregnancy: summary points *(continued)*

Antidepressant	Teratogenicity	Other adverse effects	Comments
MAOIs	Animal data suggest teratogenicity.	MAOIs are associated with blood pressure changes that are potentially detrimental to fetus and that may compromise use of agents to prevent preterm labor and treat other obstetrical complications	MAOI antidepressants are best avoided during pregnancy.

TABLE 39–7. Commonly used mood stabilizers in pregnancy: summary points

Medication	Teratogenicity	Potential perinatal effects
Lithium	Cardiac risk—especially Ebstein's anomaly No long-term neurobehavioral sequelae	Hypotonia, poor feeding, cyanosis, neonatal goiter, diabetes insipidus
Valproate	Neural tube anomalies Craniofacial abnormalities Developmental delay Coagulopathy	Hypoglycemia Hepatic dysfunction Coagulopathy
Carbamazepine	Neural tube anomalies Craniofacial abnormalities Developmental delay Cardiovascular/coronary abnormalities Coagulopathy	Hypoglycemia Hepatic dysfunction Coagulopathy
Lamotrigine	Possible oral cleft	None known
Atypical antipsychotics	See Table 39–10	See Table 39–10

2002)—have likewise revealed no teratogenic or other adverse outcomes with these agents. Although such data are encouraging, the numbers of exposures are still too small to state definitely that atypical antipsychotics are safe in pregnancy. Furthermore, a study comparing placental passage of olanzapine, risperidone, quetiapine, and haloperidol demonstrated that whereas all four antipsychotic agents passed across the placenta into fetal circulation, quetiapine demonstrated the lowest placental passage (24.1%), while olanzapine demonstrated the highest placental passage (72.1%). This same study also suggested tendencies (not reaching statistical significance) of low birth weight and neonatal intensive care admissions among olanzapine-exposed newborns (Newport et al. 2007).

Of particular concern during pregnancy is the risk of atypical antipsychotic–induced hyperglycemia, which independently is associated with a risk of gestational diabetes. For infants exposed to traditional antipsychotic agents in utero near the time of delivery,

a transient syndrome of motor restlessness, tremor, hypertonia, hyperreflexia, irritability, dyskinesia, and poor feeding has been noted.

Table 39–8 outlines some basic principles of bipolar management during pregnancy. In cases where long periods of interepisode euthymia have been demonstrated, an attempt may be made in advance of conception to avoid mood stabilizers during the first trimester. Careful tapering may be attempted over a period of 2–4 weeks to reduce the likelihood of relapse. However, for women who have historically been unable to remain stable without pharmacotherapy, medication is generally best continued throughout pregnancy. Lithium is preferable to carbamazepine and valproate because of its lower risk of teratogenicity. It should be administered in multiple daily doses to avoid peak blood levels, and levels should be monitored closely. Measurement of nuchal translucency should be performed, as this may identify cardiovascular malformations as early as the twelfth week of

TABLE 39–8. **Treatment of the bipolar pregnant patient**

- For women with mild to moderate bipolar disorder, attempt to withhold mood stabilizers during first trimester. (Caution: Careful psychiatric supervision is needed to monitor for early relapse.)

- For women with moderate to severe bipolar disorder, continue mood stabilizers and other psychiatric medications as needed to maintain euthymia throughout pregnancy.

- Because all mood stabilizers carry some teratogenic risk and peripartum toxicity, choice of treatment should be made after a careful case-by-case analysis of the safest regimen to maintain maternal mood stability and fetal safety.

- Lithium, despite its risk of cardiovascular teratogenicity, is probably a reasonable choice for the pregnant bipolar patient. Prenatal testing (nuchal lucency, level II ultrasound at week 18–20) and other guidelines of careful management (see Table 39–9) should be followed.

TABLE 39–9. **Guidelines for management of lithium in the bipolar pregnant patient**

- Maintain maternal target lithium concentrations at minimum clinically effective levels.

- Monitor maternal serum levels of lithium carefully, particularly toward the end of pregnancy.

- If possible, avoid situations that tend to increase lithium levels:
  - Use of agents that cause increased lithium: nonsteroidal anti-inflammatory drugs (NSAIDs), diuretics, angiotensin-converting enzyme (ACE) inhibitors, calcium channel blockers
  - Sodium-restricted diet (e.g., to manage preeclampsia, edema)

- Maintain heightened awareness of possible maternal lithium toxicity in cases of:
  - Acute loss of fluids at delivery
  - Hyperemesis gravidarum
  - Preeclampsia

- Maintain high threshold of concern for fetal kidney abnormalities:
  - Oligohydramnios may result from lithium-associated fetal nephrotoxicity
  - Polyhydramnios may result from fetal diabetes insipidus

- Consider discontinuation of lithium 24–48 hours prior to scheduled cesarean section, at induction, or at onset of spontaneous labor.

- Maintain fluids throughout labor and delivery.

- Restart lithium at preconception dose as soon as mother has been stabilized postdelivery.

Source. Adapted from Newport et al. 2005.

gestation. At week 18, a structural ultrasound should be obtained to assess for cardiovascular and other anatomical anomalies. Because lithium equilibrates freely across the placenta and maternal levels higher than 0.64 mEq/L have been associated with neonatal toxicity (lower Apgar scores, longer hospital stays, higher rates of central nervous system and neuromuscular complications), serum lithium should be monitored carefully throughout pregnancy, especially toward term. Maternal lithium concentrations should be kept as low as possible while still maintaining psychiatric stability. It has been suggested that lithium should be withheld during the 1–2 days prior to a planned delivery (e.g., cesarean section) or at the start of labor (Newport et al. 2005). During labor, intravenous fluids should be administered to prevent lithium toxicity in the mother. Because bipolar women are at high risk for serious illness during the postpartum, preconception doses of lithium should be reinstated once the mother is medically stabilized following delivery. The guidelines for managing lithium in the bipolar pregnant woman are presented in Table 39–9.

If carbamazepine or valproate must be continued during pregnancy, an amniotic α-fetoprotein analysis at week 16 and an ultrasound at week 18–22 should be obtained to assess for neural tube defects. For women who experience exacerbation or escalation of symptoms, electroconvulsive therapy (ECT) may provide another option.

Treatment of Schizophrenia During Pregnancy

Although some women with schizophrenia remain stable during pregnancy, others are so disorganized and psychotic that they are at increased risk for fetal abuse or neonaticide and tend to have poor prenatal care. They may be so paranoid that they are unable to cooperate during necessary medical or obstetrical procedures, may fail to recognize labor, and are at greater risk of adverse pregnancy outcomes (abruptio placentae, prematurity, low birth weight, low Apgar scores, cardiovascular deformities) (Jablensky et al. 2005). Patients should be screened for substance abuse, psychosocial stressors, housing and financial resources, and other factors that negatively affect parenting ability. Women with schizophrenia are more likely to have low dietary folate intake and to be obese; for this reason, they are at increased risk of having a child with a neural tube defect. Particular attention should be directed toward maximizing psychosocial support to ensure proper nourishment, compliance with prenatal instructions (including daily intake of vitamins and folate), keeping obstetrical appointments, preparation for the responsibilities of motherhood, appropriate housing, and access to social services.

As with all psychotropic medications, antipsychotic medications should be used in pregnancy only when necessary (e.g., for patients with psychotic symptoms that pose a risk to the patient or fetus). Although use of antipsychotic agents on an as-needed basis may reduce the overall dose exposure of the fetus, daily dosing throughout pregnancy is often necessary for severely ill patients.

The limited data on antipsychotic medications in pregnancy have previously been detailed. Agents to treat extrapyramidal side effects should be avoided during pregnancy, because they are associated with major and minor congenital anomalies. The anticholinergic agents trihexyphenidyl and benztropine have been associated with minor congenital malformations and anticholinergic symptoms in the newborn, including functional bowel obstruction and urinary retention. Most studies suggest that diphenhydramine does not increase the risk of congenital malformations. Animal studies have reported cardiovascular malformations following in utero exposure to amantadine. Switching to a lower-potency antipsychotic medication probably reduces the likelihood of extrapyramidal symptoms.

Table 39–10 summarizes the risks associated with the use of antipsychotics in pregnancy.

Treatment of Anxiety Disorders During Pregnancy

The course of panic disorder in pregnancy is variable. Although in some cases, symptoms dissipate during pregnancy, often symptoms persist or worsen. Obsessive-compulsive disorder (OCD) has been reported to worsen during pregnancy. Although there is a dearth of data about the prevalence of generalized anxiety disorder during pregnancy, clinical experience suggests that women with this condition continue to be symptomatic during pregnancy and are particularly anxious

TABLE 39–10. Use of antipsychotics in pregnancy: summary points

Medication	Teratogenicity	Potential perinatal effects
Low-potency antipsychotic agents: Phenothiazines	Nonspecific congenital anomalies	Behavioral irritability, restlessness Impaired feeding Jaundice
High-potency antipsychotic agents	No known major congenital anomalies	Behavioral irritability, restlessness Impaired feeding
Atypical antipsychotics	Limited data reveal no major anomalies—more data needed (olanzapine, risperidone, quetiapine, clozapine)	Behavioral irritability, restlessness, tremor Hyperreflexia Impaired feeding

about the health of their fetuses. Since generalized anxiety disorder and major depressive disorder are often comorbid, it is not unusual for pregnant women with one disorder to have the other as well. Furthermore, discontinuation of anxiolytic antidepressants and other medications at the onset of pregnancy often results in relapse of symptoms. There is accumulating evidence that stress and anxiety in pregnancy increase the risk for cognitive, behavioral, and emotional alterations in babies and children (Van den Bergh et al. 2005). There appears to be a direct link between antenatal anxiety and stress and fetal behavior as observed by fetal ultrasound from 25–26 weeks' gestation onward. Severe anxiety during pregnancy may be associated with self-neglect, poor eating habits, disordered sleep, and poor maternal weight gain. Importantly, women with anxiety disorders who relapse during pregnancy are at particular risk for postpartum exacerbation. Thus, women with anxiety disorders should be provided with treatment options that relieve anxiety with the goal of maximizing their psychiatric and physical prenatal health and enabling them to manage the responsibilities of motherhood without being overwhelmed once they have had their babies.

Nonpharmacological interventions for anxiety disorders include cognitive-behavioral therapy, elimination of caffeine and nicotine, reduction of psychosocial stressors, and couples therapy. Cognitive-behavioral therapy is helpful to provide the behavioral tools to cope with worrisome ruminations, troubling obsessions, and anticipatory fears and to reduce the doses needed to dissipate symptoms or even eliminate the need for medications during pregnancy. TCAs and SSRIs are reasonable treatment options for severe intractable symptoms that do not respond to those measures. For OCD, SSRI doses generally are higher than for treatment of depression, and since women with OCD frequently are troubled by intrusive ego-dystonic thoughts having to do with harm to their fetuses, it may not be possible to adhere to low doses, even into the third trimester. For severely anxious pregnant women, particularly as an SSRI begins to take effect, occasional small doses of benzodiazepines may be necessary. Intermittent use of low doses of benzodiazepines during pregnancy, particularly after the first trimester, does not appear to increase the risk of adverse neonatal sequelae. Nevertheless, the use of benzodiazepines in pregnancy is controversial, with some researchers noting a risk of oral clefts, particularly with diazepam and alprazolam. Other studies, however, have not found this association. Nevertheless, an attempt should be made to avoid benzodiazepines during gestational weeks 5–9, because this is when formation of the fetal palate occurs. Of the benzodiazepines, lorazepam is a reasonable choice, because it has no active metabolites and seems to pass into the placenta at a lower rate than do other benzodiazepines. For patients who require longer action, clonazepam is an alternative agent to effectively treat anxiety or panic. Transient perinatal syndromes, including hypotonia, failure to feed, temperature dysregulation, apnea, and low Apgar scores, have been noted with last-trimester use of benzodiazepines. Near term, the use of benzodiazepines should generally be kept at a minimum. Whenever possible, benzodiazepine dosage changes should be gradual, to avoid precipitating in utero withdrawal.

Use of Electroconvulsive Therapy During Pregnancy

ECT is feasible for pregnant patients with severe mood disorders because it appears safe and effective and exposes the developing fetus to a minimum of psychoactive medication (Miller 1994). Special considerations in the administration of ECT to pregnant women include the need for a pelvic examination and uterine tocodynamometry to exclude uterine contractions and elevation of the right hip to ensure adequate placental perfusion. The muscle relaxant succinylcholine and the anticholinergic agent glycopyrrolate appear relatively safe to use in pregnancy (Miller 1994). Following the procedure, external fetal monitoring should continue for several hours.

Substance Abuse During Pregnancy

In addition to premature labor, abruptio placentae, stillbirth, and other obstetrical complications, teratogenic effects are associated with alcohol and its metabolite acetaldehyde. Fetal alcohol syndrome, a lifelong disabling condition that results from in utero exposure to alcohol, is found in up to 1.5 per 1,000 live births in the United States. Isolated abnormalities not reaching the full syndrome are described as fetal alcohol effects and are believed to occur three times as often as the full syndrome. Infants exposed in utero to alcohol are at risk for fetal mental retardation, microcephaly, abnormal facial features, conduct disorder, and attention-deficit/hyperactivity disorder in childhood. No safe quantity of prenatal alcohol consumption has been established.

The adverse effects of cocaine on the fetus are due at least in part to its acute toxic effects on the expectant mother. Thus, cocaine use during pregnancy is associated with preterm labor, abruptio placentae, and other obstetrical complications secondary to cocaine's vasoconstrictive effects. Although the teratogenicity of cocaine is the subject of some controversy, in utero exposure to cocaine may increase the risk for genitourinary tract malformations. A major cause of congenital anomalies in exposed fetuses is related more to lifestyle and other high-risk maternal activities than to cocaine use itself. Exposed neonates may experience a withdrawal syndrome lasting several months.

Heroin use during pregnancy is frequently associated with obstetrical complications and a perinatal withdrawal syndrome characterized by irritability, poor feeding, respiratory difficulties, and tremulousness. In utero exposure to opiates also has been linked with a greater risk of sudden infant death syndrome (SIDS). Women who are maintained on methadone and who receive prenatal care have better obstetrical outcomes than women with untreated opiate use. Although more rigorously controlled studies are needed, recent data suggest that buprenorphine treatment for pregnant opioid-addicted women may be preferable to methadone treatment, because buprenorphine is less likely to cause neonatal abstinence syndrome

(Fischer et al. 2004; Johnson et al. 2003).

Although tobacco is not an illegal drug, its prenatal use has been linked with intrauterine growth retardation, low birth weight, spontaneous abortion, and preterm delivery. Smoking 10 or more cigarettes daily has been associated with increased chromosomal instability in fetal cells isolated during amniocentesis (de la Chica et al. 2005). Similarly, caffeine may increase the risk of early spontaneous abortions (Cnattingius et al. 2000).

Postpartum Psychiatric Disorders

The 6 months following delivery is a time of increased risk for emotional instability for many women (Miller 2002). Postpartum psychiatric illness has been associated with ongoing risks for recurrent illness in the future and has serious negative effects on the infant and family. Conditions of disordered mood occurring following childbirth include postpartum blues, postpartum depression, and postpartum psychosis. The postpartum is also a time of recurrent and new-onset anxiety disorders. Postpartum panic disorder with or without agoraphobia appears to be the most frequently reported anxiety condition. Postpartum OCD also has been described. Although no specific etiology has been found to explain the onset of psychiatric illness during the postpartum period, the causes probably reside in a combination of biological/endocrinological and psychosocial factors. Because the data on postpartum anxiety disorders are sparse, the following discussions on postpartum conditions focus on postpartum mood disorders. Table 39–11 summarizes the three mood disorders that occur in the postpartum, their presentation, and treatment considerations.

Postpartum Blues

Up to 85% of mothers experience postpartum blues, a transient waxing and waning condition beginning in the first 2–4 days after giving birth, peaking between postpartum days 5–7, and dissipating by the end of the second postpartum week. Symptoms include tearfulness, mood lability, irritability, and anxiety. Although postpartum blues resolve spontaneously, because new mothers are generally discharged within 24–48 hours, all prospective and new parents should be made aware of its existence. In this way, partners, other family members, and health care providers will be prepared to provide needed support and reassurance.

Postpartum Depression

Major depression during the postpartum occurs at a rate of 12%–13%, which equals that in the general female population. However, the rate of troubling depression not meeting full criteria for major depression appears to be much higher. Although many studies of depression after delivery have included women whose symptoms began within 3–12 months after delivery, the "postpartum onset" specifier in DSM-IV-TR may be applied only for depression with onset in the first 4 weeks after childbirth. Postpartum depression, as well as depression occurring in mothers beyond the postpartum period, affects not only the woman but also her family. Depressed mothers are more likely than nondepressed mothers to engage in negative parenting behaviors, and their children are at risk for behavioral and cognitive deficits from infancy to early childhood. Nursing infants of depressed mothers gain less weight than infants of nondepressed mothers, possibly because depressed mothers do not eat properly, have more difficulty breast-feeding, and may be less sensitive to infants' hunger cries. Prompt and effective treatment of postpartum depression not only provides relief for new mothers but also reduces the likelihood of childhood behavioral problems and patterns of insecure attachment.

A history of major depression increases the risk for postpartum major depression to 24%, and depression during pregnancy further increases the likelihood of postpartum depression. Women who have had previous postpartum depression are at 50%–60% risk of another episode. Other risk factors for postpartum depression include stressful life events and lack of support from a partner or spouse or others. Thyroid function should always be evaluated in postpartum women with depression or anxiety, because the postpartum is a time of increased risk for thyroid dysfunction.

Postpartum depression is best treated comprehensively with individual and group psychotherapy, psychopharmacology, and psychoeducation. Interpersonal and cognitive-behavioral therapies are helpful in treating postpartum depression. Recent randomized, double-blind studies that compared outcomes in postpartum depressed women treated with TCAs or sertraline showed no differences in response, remission, time to response and remission, and improvement in psychosocial functioning with either of these treatments (Wisner et al. 2006). Decisions regarding medications should include consideration of whether the patient is breast-feeding (see section "Breast-Feeding and Psychotropic Medications" below). For new mothers with past histories of postpartum depression,

TABLE 39–11. **Postpartum mood disorders**

Disorder	Incidence	Presentation	Treatment
Postpartum blues	Very common—up to 85%	Mood lability, emotional hypersensitivity, no dysfunction 80% resolves by week 2, 20% evolves to become postpartum depression	Support, reassurance, clinical monitoring (particularly for women with past histories of mood disorders or postpartum disorders). If severe, disabling, or beyond 12 days, consider another diagnosis.
Postpartum depression	Approximately 12%–13% major depression; minor depressive symptoms more common	Major depression with obsessive, anxious symptoms Mother unable to sleep even when child care is provided for new baby	Individual psychotherapy (cognitive-behavioral or interpersonal), conjoint therapy to address interpersonal difficulties, group therapy for peer support, psychosocial assistance (child care, home care assistance), antidepressant, sometimes anxiolytic. For psychotic or suicidal depression, hospitalize, consider antipsychotic, ECT. Nursing mothers: educate regarding medications and breast-feeding; assess maternal and infant well-being.
Postpartum psychosis	Up to 1/1,000	Early onset, usually by day 2–3; often presents as mixed/rapid cycling with psychotic features Mother unable to sleep Caution: risk of infanticide	Hospitalize patient, educate and reassure family, emphasize medications and supportive care. Medications: mood stabilizer, antipsychotic, benzodiazepine, possibly antidepressants (caution in case of manic induction), consider ECT if refractory. In most cases, postpartum psychotic mothers should not breast-feed.

studies of the effectiveness of prophylaxis with antidepressant medications, begun within 24–48 hours after delivery, have produced mixed results. All women with a history of postpartum depression should be carefully monitored for signs of relapse throughout pregnancy and the postpartum.

Because the available data suggesting that estrogen may improve postpartum depression are limited, and because estrogen increases the risk of endometrial hyperplasia and thromboembolism and diminishes the production of breast milk in nursing mothers, estrogen should not be considered as a primary treatment of postpartum depression.

Lay advocacy groups (e.g., Postpartum Support International) offer assistance in the form of group therapy and mutual support. Interpersonal difficulties between the patient and her partner are best addressed with conjoint therapy. Assistance with household duties and child care provides the patient with opportunities to reduce sleep deprivation. Educating the patient and her family that postpartum disorders are both common and treatable is reassuring and provides a setting for family members to devise practical strategies to reduce stress in the home and assist with day-to-day household duties.

The issue of whether or not to breast-feed should be discussed thoroughly, because nursing may alter the treatment modality or may influence the choice of medication should pharmacotherapy be indicated. For patients whose depression is complicated by psychosis or suicidal thoughts, ECT is often the treatment of choice to hasten rapid improvement. Such cases generally require hospitalization until stabilization is achieved.

Postpartum Psychosis

The most serious postpartum illness, postpartum psychosis, occurs in 1–2 of every 1,000 births. Postpartum psychosis is thought to be a manifestation of bipolar disorder. The condition is characterized by mood lability, agitation, confusion, thought disorganization, hallucinations, and disturbed sleep. Women who have had an episode of postpartum psychosis are at risk for subsequent bipolar disorder, suggesting that postpartum psychosis may be a subcategory of bipolar disorder. A history of bipolar disorder is associated with approximately a 20%–35% risk of developing postpartum psychosis. Having both bipolar disorder and a prior postpartum psychotic episode increases the risk of subsequent postpartum psychosis to 50%. A family history of bipolar disorder also appears to heighten the risk for postpartum psychosis.

Because postpartum psychosis carries with it the risk of suicide, infant neglect, and infanticide, patients should be hospitalized. The initial evaluation includes a medical assessment to rule out organic etiologies such as postpartum thyroiditis, Sheehan's syndrome, pregnancy-related autoimmune disorders, HIV-related infection, and intoxication/withdrawal states. Acute pharmacological treatment includes use of a mood stabilizer, an antipsychotic agent, and a benzodiazepine as needed for agitation. Antidepressants should be administered with great caution, because they may provoke mania. Maintenance treatment for the patient whose postpartum psychosis was preceded by chronic recurrent affective illness generally involves long-term treatment with a mood stabilizer. For patients without a psychiatric history other than a single episode of postpartum psychosis, medications are often tapered and discontinued by 1 year of treatment, although these women should be followed, because they have approximately a 60% risk of recurrent affective illness. It is prudent for patients with a history of postpartum psychosis who subsequently become pregnant to be placed on a prophylactic mood stabilizer either during the third trimester or at delivery.

Breast-Feeding and Psychotropic Medications

Approximately one-half of new mothers breast-feed. Breast-feeding enhances mother–infant bonding and is an excellent source of nutrition for infants. For women who require pharmacological treatment for postpartum psychiatric disorders, the decision of whether to

TABLE 39–12. Breast-feeding: issues to consider for postpartum women with psychiatric disorders

- Breast-feeding provides the ideal form of nutrition for babies.
- Breast-feeding fosters bonding between mother and infant.
- Breast-feeding invariably results in sleep deprivation.
- For many new mothers with psychiatric illness, the best way to ensure their emotional stability is to avoid sleep deprivation. Consideration should therefore be given to ways in which to maximize sleep (e.g., formula feeding, supplementation of breast-feeding with formula).
- All psychiatric medications are excreted into breast milk.
- Amount of exposure via breast milk is invariably less than through maternal–fetal circulation (in pregnancy).
- Premature infants generally have immature P450 enzymes and therefore may be at greater risk for side effects or toxicity when exposed to medications via breast milk.
- Effect of neonatal medication exposure via breast milk on infant development is not known.
- Monitor appetite and weight in breast-feeding women on psychiatric medications to ensure maternal well-being and to optimize nutritional quality of breast milk.

forgo breast-feeding or to proceed with medications can be difficult. Table 39–12 lists issues for consideration when advising postpartum women with psychiatric illness about whether or not to breast-feed.

Data regarding the safety of psychotropic medications by breast-feeding mothers have increased substantially in the past decade. Nevertheless, no medication should be taken by a breast-feeding woman without careful assessment of risks and benefits. If it is concluded that the use of psychotropic medication is acceptable during nursing, the treating physician should review the available information with both mother and father.

Guidelines for using psychotropic medication in breast-feeding mothers include apprising the infant's pediatrician of the need to monitor the infant carefully for potential adverse effects. The infant's baseline behavior and sleep and feeding patterns should be assessed before the nursing mother uses the medication.

Infant hepatic drug clearance rises from about one-third of the mother's weight-adjusted clearance at birth to 100% at the age of 6 months. Thus, exposure to drugs through breast milk may be riskier in a neonate than in an older infant. In particular, premature infants should not be exposed to psychotropic medications through breast milk until they have reached full maturity. Medication exposure should be minimized by prescribing the lowest dosage of medication that achieves remission of psychiatric symptoms. Short-acting rather than long-acting medications are preferable, and supplementation of breast milk with formula reduces the infant's exposure to the drug. Because the clinical significance of any exposure to the baby of even small (and nondetectable) doses of psychotropic agents is unknown, the baby's clinical status should be continually monitored. Summary points for the major psychotropic drug classes are provided in Table 39–13.

Most medications, including TCAs, benzodiazepines, and antipsychotic agents, have been classified by the American Academy of Pediatrics as "drugs whose effect on nursing infants is unknown but may be of concern" (American Academy of Pediatrics Committee on Drugs 2001). Data on the use of SSRIs and TCAs have been increasingly reassuring (Burt et al. 2001; Wisner et al. 2006). Because infants nursed by mothers taking SSRIs, particularly paroxetine and sertraline, typically receive low serum levels of medication exposure, routine monitoring of serum concentrations is not necessary (Burt et al. 2001). MAOIs are best avoided, because they may cause hypertension in the infant. Women who breast-feed while taking antidepressants may experience appetite disturbances that may result in altered food intake and weight changes; this may be symptomatic of depression or, in some cases, a medication side effect and may compromise the nutritional composition of breast milk. Therefore, appetite and weight should be monitored in all depressed nursing women, including those on antidepressants (Bodnar et al. 2006).

Lithium is contraindicated by the American Academy of Pediatrics Committee on Drugs (2001) because adverse effects, including cyanosis, poor muscle tone, and electrocardiogram changes, have been noted in infants exposed to lithium through nursing. Although valproate and carbamazepine are considered by the committee to be compatible with breast-feeding, there have been rare reports of hepatic dysfunction and one possible case of transient seizure-like activity in infants exposed to carbamazepine via breast milk. While valproate accumulates in breast milk to a lesser extent

than does carbamazepine, it should be used with caution in breast-feeding mothers, because it has been associated with infant hepatotoxicity.

TABLE 39–13. Psychotropic medications in breast-feeding: summary points	
Medication	**Comment**
Antidepressants	• In general, no adverse effects of TCAs, SSRIs on breast-fed infants. • Infant serum levels typically below laboratory sensitivity. • Data for venlafaxine, duloxetine, nefazodone, mirtazapine, and bupropion are limited. • As extra precaution, monitor infant for possible side effects or toxicity.
Anxiolytics	• Benzodiazepines may accumulate in neonate due to immature hepatic (cytochrome P450) enzymes. • Occasional low doses of short-acting benzodiazepines acceptable. • Sparse data for zolpidem, zaleplon.
Antipsychotics	• Limited data. • In general, postpartum women who require antipsychotic medication should not breast-feed, as they require sleep and often are too ill to nurse.
Mood stabilizers	• Limited data. • Bipolar women require sleep to avoid postpartum relapse; breast-feeding is therefore not recommended.

Perimenopause and Menopause

Menopause refers to the cessation of ovulation and menstrual cycling and usually occurs between the ages of 44 and 55 years (average age, 51.4 years). *Perimenopause* (climacteric) describes the years before menopause when ovarian function begins to decline.

Hormonal Changes

As ovarian production of estrogen declines, the pituitary hormones LH and FSH rise. An elevated serum FSH level (approximately 13 MU/mL), especially if obtained shortly after the onset of menses (when FSH levels should be at their nadir), suggests that a woman is perimenopausal. Elevated FSH levels (i.e., 40 mU/mL or above) obtained later in the cycle can be misleading, because this hormone may rise into the menopausal range in premenopausal women, particularly at midcycle. Although very high levels of FSH indicate postmenopausal status and mildly elevated levels suggest that pregnancy might be difficult (although not impossible), there is considerable overlap of FSH ranges between perimenopause and postmenopause. Levels of estradiol, the biologically active form of estrogen, remain under 25 pg/mL following menopause.

The initial signal for menopause has long been thought to be the declining secretion of ovarian estrogen and inhibin, which causes elevation of the pituitary hormones LH and FSH. However, newer data have raised the possibility that menopause may actually be an ovarian response to age-related hypothalamic-pituitary insensitivity to estrogen (Weiss et al. 2004). The preliminary finding that a history of major depression may be associated with an earlier decline in ovarian function (Harlow et al. 2003), therefore, may reflect an ovarian response to brain changes occurring as a result of repetitive or current depression. If true, the implication that depression-associated ovarian decline may cause decreased fertility and a cascade of other events, including vasomotor symptoms, cardiovascular disease, sexual dysfunction, a decline in cognitive function, and reduced bone density, would be yet another persuasive reason to treat depression in women promptly and effectively. Other factors associated with an earlier transition to menopause include smoking cigarettes; having lower education attainment; being separated, widowed, or divorced; being unemployed; having a history of heart disease; and being on a weight-reduction diet.

Eighty percent of perimenopausal women experience hot flushes and cold sweats, which are a direct result of ovarian reduction in estrogen production. Hot flushes may be confused with a panic attack, particularly because they occur unexpectedly and may be associated with some anxiety. Night sweats may cause sleep deprivation, which subsequently may lead to decreased concentration, fatigue, and irritability. Other signs of declining ovarian estrogen production include atrophy of the urogenital tract lining, sometimes leading to infection; urinary frequency and urgency; and occasional stress incontinence. Women may experience painful intercourse and reduced libido. Particularly serious long-term consequences of low estrogen levels are osteoporosis and cardiovascular disease.

Perimenopausal Depression

Recent epidemiological data have found an increase in depressive symptoms as women passed from premenopause to postmenopause (Bromberger et al. 2003). The results of two recent independent prospective studies following a total of almost 700 endocrinologically confirmed premenopausal women for 8 years found that as they became perimenopausal, they were more likely to experience first-onset depression (Cohen et al. 2006b; Freeman et al. 2006). Furthermore, the faster the rise in FSH (i.e., the shorter the perimenopausal transition), the less likely were subjects to experience depression (Freeman et al. 2004). Although there is some indication that perimenopausal depression cannot be fully explained by vasomotor discomfort, the extent to which hot flushes and adverse life events contribute to negative mood during the menopausal transition remains unclear (Cohen et al. 2006b; Freeman et al. 2006).

Risk Factors

Risk factors for depressive symptoms at menopause include being divorced, widowed, or separated; having significant caregiving responsibilities; being socially disadvantaged; experiencing a chronic illness; having been depressed in the past; having sleep problems; and experiencing prominent vasomotor symptoms. Children leaving the home and parental death do not appear to increase the risk for perimenopausal depression. Table 39–14 summarizes the risk factors for perimenopausal depression.

Treatment

Some studies have found that estrogen produces mood-elevating effects in perimenopausal (Cohen et al. 2003; Schmidt et al. 2000; Soares et al. 2001) and surgically menopausal (Sherwin 1988) women, but not in postmenopausal women (Cohen et al. 2003; Morrison et al. 2004). More data are needed to establish the efficacy of estrogen as monotherapy of depression; at this time, estrogen alone is not accepted as effective for clinical depression. Data on the efficacy of estrogen as an augmenter of standard antidepressants in perimenopausal depressed women are conflicting (Amsterdam et al. 1999; Morgan et al. 2005; Schneider et al. 1997).

TABLE 39–14. Risk factors for perimenopausal depression

1. Slower rise in follicle-stimulating hormone (longer transition from pre- to postmenopause)
2. History of depression, including postpartum depression, severe premenstrual symptoms
3. Vasomotor symptoms
4. Sleep difficulties
5. Chronic health problems
6. Loss of significant others (death of partner or child, divorce)
7. Caretaking responsibilities
8. Financial problems
9. Unemployment
10. Lower level of education

For perimenopausal women with major depression, standard antidepressant treatment, often including psychotherapy, is therefore considered as first-line treatment. If vasomotor symptoms also are present, estrogen therapy is effective in reducing sleep disturbance due to middle-of-the-night awakening secondary to the physical symptoms of endogenous estrogen decline. For perimenopausal women with severe hot flushes or night sweats who report subclinical depression and lethargy, hormone therapy (HT) may relieve the psychological symptoms as the vasomotor symptoms become less distressing. As women experience relief from vasomotor symptoms (usually within 2 weeks of beginning hormone replacement), depressive symptoms also should improve. If, after resolution of vasomotor symptoms, depression persists or worsens, standard psychiatric treatment should be initiated. Psychosocial factors that may contribute to depressed mood also should be addressed, including caring for aging parents, new-onset health problems in the patient or her spouse, financial difficulties, and changes in sexuality of the patient or her partner.

Hormone Therapy

HT incurs both benefits and risks. In addition to providing relief of vasomotor symptoms, estrogen therapy helps protect against osteoporotic bony changes and urogenital atrophy. Although estrogen increases the risk of endometrial cancer, the addition of a progestin in women with an intact uterus negates this risk. The Women's Health Initiative (WHI), a large prospective, randomized, placebo-controlled study that evaluated the risks and benefits of hormone treatment on risks of coronary events, stroke, pulmonary embolism, breast cancer, bone health, and cognition in 27,000 postmenopausal women, found that overall, women taking estrogen and progesterone had more heart attacks, strokes, blood clots, and breast cancers and fewer hip fractures and colorectal cancers than placebo-treated subjects (Rossouw et al. 2002). In a recently published subanalysis of the Women's Health Initiative data, it was revealed that women who initiated HT closer to menopause tended to have a reduced risk for coronary heart disease compared with those who began HT more distant from the time of their last menstrual period (Rossouw et al. 2007). Data from surgically menopausal women who were treated with estrogen alone indicated that estrogen was associated with an increased risk for blood clots and fewer hip fractures. Unlike the estrogen plus progesterone–treated subjects, the estrogen-alone group had no increase in heart attacks and a possible decrease in breast cancers (Anderson et al. 2004). A subgroup of women older than 65 years was also followed for development of dementia. In both the estrogen–progesterone and the estrogen-alone groups, hormone treatment was associated with a higher incidence of dementia and no improvement in global cognition scores compared with placebo treatment (Espeland et al. 2004; Shumaker et al. 2003). Overall, the Women's Health Initiative data suggest that hormone treatment (either estrogen plus progesterone or estrogen alone) is associated with increases in strokes and blood clots.

For most women, HT involves the administration of both estrogen and progestin. The purpose of the progestin is to counteract the endometrial proliferation that occurs with estrogen and increases the risk of endometrial cancer. Women who have had a hysterectomy do not require progestin supplementation. The progestin is taken either on a daily basis with the estrogen (continuous regimen) or at a higher dose during only 12–14 days of each month (cyclic regimen). The cyclic regimen produces vaginal bleeding following withdrawal of the progestin. No monthly bleeding occurs with the continuous regimen, but irregular spotting may occur that requires endometrial biopsy to rule out hyperplasia or malignancy. Estrogen and progesterone supplementation is available in various preparations. When an estrogen and a progestin are prescribed, doses should be as low as possible to meet treatment goals.

In summary, the short-term use of estrogen for treatment of vasomotor symptoms and urogenital atrophy is acceptable. In perimenopausal and postmenopausal women who are at high risk for osteoporosis, estrogen replacement may be appropriate. However, HT as a primary long-term treatment to prevent heart disease and cognitive decline in postmenopausal women is not justified. Although preliminary data are promising, more and better studies are needed before short-term estrogen therapy can be considered a primary mode of treatment for depression in perimenopausal women.

Women Victims of Violence

Sexual Assault

Sexual assault affects women of all ages and all cultural, ethnic, and economic backgrounds. About 20%–25% of all adult women, 15% of college women, and 12% of adolescent girls report having experienced sexual abuse and/or assault during their lifetimes, and these rates are higher for African American women. Each year, more than 1.5 million women in the United States are physically and/or sexually abused by an intimate partner, and women are 10 times more likely than men to be killed by an intimate sexual partner. Despite the serious negative impact of sexual assault on physical and psychological well-being, only 10% of women who are assaulted seek professional help. In addition to physical symptoms such as tremulousness and cold sweats, initial psychological reactions to sexual assault include shock, numbness, withdrawal, and denial. Prolonged symptoms may include startle reactions, disturbed sleep, extreme fatigue, and somatic complaints. Although symptoms tend to dissipate over time, they often return intermittently over the course of ensuing months and even years. Long-term negative sequelae may include sexual dysfunction and aversion, impaired ability to establish healthy interpersonal relationships, and feelings of helplessness, shame, vulnerability, and depression. Posttraumatic stress disorder is particularly common and intense when there is a history of abuse.

Ideally, initial psychiatric assessment should include an evaluation of current symptoms, preexisting psychiatric diagnoses or emotional difficulties, and the availability of a healthy support network. If a detailed evaluation cannot be obtained in the initial aftermath of an assault, it should be completed at a later visit. If needed, provisions should be made for short-term safety. Preexisting psychiatric illnesses, if any, should be treated to reduce the risk for recurrence. Although further psychotherapeutic follow-up is often declined, it is important to offer the sexual assault vic-

tim an open opportunity for psychiatric follow-up and assistance at a later time. The mental health clinician should provide an empathic "holding environment" in which the patient may safely recount her experience and the ways in which it has altered her sense of self and impairs her ability to function. If needed, medication may be useful to treat depression, posttraumatic stress disorder, or anxiety. Patients should be educated that although disturbing symptoms tend to dissipate over time, they may recur at times of future stress. In such cases, a return to psychotherapy may be helpful. Female-specific issues associated with the evaluation and treatment of women who have been sexually assaulted are described in Table 39–15.

Domestic Violence

Up to 4 million women are assaulted by their partners each year. The rate of assaults to women by present or former partners is higher than by all other assailants combined. About 7% of pregnant women are victims of domestic violence, and pregnant women who are abused tend to be struck on the abdomen, in contrast to nonpregnant women, who tend to be struck in the face. In addition to the possibility of serious physical harm or death, female victims of domestic violence are at risk for serious psychological sequelae such as depression, anxiety, eating disorders, and alcoholism. Furthermore, children of battered mothers are also at risk for physical injury and are more likely to abuse substances, have school problems, exhibit violent and aggressive behaviors toward others or themselves, and experience impaired sleep, enuresis, and chronic somatic disorders.

Women are often reluctant to spontaneously disclose that they have been battered. As part of routine psychiatric evaluation, all women should be screened for domestic violence by asking them if they ever feel unsafe or have ever been hit or injured in their homes. Clinicians should be able to provide patients with a list of local hospital and community resources for battered women (available by calling the National Domestic Violence Hotline, 1-800-799-SAFE [7233]). Legal reporting requirements in the event that a patient is found to have been the victim of domestic abuse vary from state to state.

Typically, during a domestic assault, women fear for their lives. After the assault, experiences include shock, denial, isolation, confusion, psychological numbness, and fear. Long-term sequelae include disturbed sleep and appetite, startle responses, somatic complaints, fatigue, anxiety, and depression. A recent prospective birth cohort study of more than 1,000 chil-

TABLE 39–15. Special considerations in the evaluation and treatment of women who have been sexually assaulted

Component of examination	Issues to address

Review of symptoms	Acute symptoms
	  Somatic symptoms: tremulousness, diaphoresis, shortness of breath, palpitations
	  Psychological symptoms: shock, numbness, withdrawal, isolativeness, denial
	
	Prolonged or delayed symptoms
	  Startle reactions, disturbed sleep, fatigue, somatic complaints
	  Sexual dysfunction, impaired interpersonal relationships, depression, posttraumatic stress disorder

Assessment of preassault level of functioning	Interpersonal relationships Financial stability School and work history Ability to cope in times of acute stress
Evaluation of available supports	Assess for short-term safety Assess for long-term support system
Evaluation of preassault illness	Preexisting psychiatric illness Past treatment
Treatment	Facilitate and ensure provisions for short-term safety Treat preexisting, ongoing psychiatric illnesses Provide a safe place to review the assault and associated events Normalize negative effect on sense of self while acknowledging its negative impact Establish appropriate cognitive and behavioral mechanisms to restore function and therefore self-esteem Consider treatment with psychotropic medications to alleviate depression, posttraumatic stress disorder, anxiety disorder Explain that symptom recurrence may occur in the future Offer opportunity for psychiatric follow-up in the future

dren who were followed from age 3 through age 26 years revealed that although psychiatric disorders increased the risk for involvement in abusive relationships for both women and men, partner abuse precipitated psychiatric disorders in women but not in men (Ehrensaft et al. 2006). Treating clinicians should be aware that the existence of legal, financial, and shared parental responsibilities often makes it very difficult for women to leave the setting of their abuse. Treatment should be empathic and supportive. Pharmacotherapy may be needed to treat comorbid psychiatric conditions such as depression and anxiety and to facilitate movement out of the circle of danger. The initial therapeutic modality should be individual, because conjoint therapy tends to precipitate defensive behaviors. After the woman is in a safe setting, if there is the wish for possible resumption of an ongoing relationship between the woman and her partner, conjoint therapy should be instituted.

Gender Issues in the Treatment of Psychiatric Disorders

Table 39–16 summarizes important gender-specific differences in psychiatric disorders.

Schizophrenia

Although the incidence of schizophrenia has long been thought to be equal between the sexes, a recent meta-analysis has found that the incidence ratio for men relative to women is between 1.31 and 1.42 (Aleman et al. 2003). One reason may be that the rate of schizophrenia in men has increased in recent years, possibly associated with the precipitation of schizophrenia by illicit drug use in genetically susceptible males. Additionally, because oral contraceptives con-

TABLE 39–16. Gender differences in psychiatric disorders

Disorder	Ratios (female:male)	History, presentation, and course in women	Treatment issues in women
Schizophrenia	Previously thought to be equal, but recent data suggest that rates may be increasing in men	Compared with schizophrenic men, women have a better premorbid history, are diagnosed later, and are more likely to have a schizophrenic family history; have less substance abuse and are less likely to commit suicide; have more affective symptoms, more positive symptoms, and fewer negative symptoms; and have better language proficiency and better social functioning. 15% of women with schizophrenia have a midlife onset of disease.	Compared with schizophrenic men, women have a better treatment response but are at increased risk of antipsychotic-induced hyperprolactinemia. Schizophrenic women require birth control counseling and behavioral therapy to avoid unwanted sexual advances.
Unipolar major depression, dysthymia	1.7:1.0	Women experience an increased risk of exacerbation at times of reproductive transition (i.e., premenstruum, postpartum, perimenopause).	Treatment of depression to remission is advisable in women of childbearing age to safeguard against relapse in pregnancy and postpartum depression. Careful risk–benefit analysis for both mother and fetus is important in cases of pregnancy for women with past or current depression. Early data suggest that estrogen may be helpful for perimenopausal depression.
Bipolar disorder	Overall, approximately equal	Compared with bipolar men, women have more mixed states, more bipolar II disorder, and more comorbid PTSD. Risk of premenstrual worsening.	Compared with bipolar men, women are at increased risk of lithium-induced hypothyroidism. Bipolar women have a possibly increased risk of PCOS (due to valproate effect, independent hypothalamic-pituitary-gonadal effect, or both) and a high risk of postpartum destabilization.
Anxiety disorders	Panic disorder: 2.5:1.0 Social phobia: 4:1 Generalized anxiety disorder: 1.8:1.0 OCD: 1:1 PTSD: 2:1	Markedly increased risk for generalized anxiety in women older than 45 years. Women experience an increased risk for exacerbation at times of reproductive transition (i.e., premenstruum, postpartum, perimenopause, pregnancy [OCD]). Women with PTSD are at increased risk for PMDD.	Consider full differential as this informs treatment. Women are at increased risk for thyroid disorders, which may produce symptoms similar to those of an anxiety disorder. Assess for premenstrual anxious symptoms—differentiate PMS/PMDD from true anxiety disorder with premenstrual exacerbation. Assess for perimenopausal physical changes (e.g., vasomotor) that may mimic anxiety symptoms.

TABLE 39–16. **Gender differences in psychiatric disorders** *(continued)*

Disorder	Ratios (female:male)	History, presentation, and course in women	Treatment issues in women
Substance use disorders	Alcohol dependence: 0.4:1.0 Alcohol abuse without dependence: 0.5:1.0 Drug dependence: 0.6:1.0 Drug abuse without dependence: 0.6:1.0	Women are more likely to develop alcohol-induced medical complications and more likely to become intoxicated.	Pregnancy may offer a window for treatment due to the additional motivation of fetal health.
Eating disorders	Anorexia nervosa: 10:1 Bulimia: 11:1	Anorexia is often associated with hypothalamic amenorrhea and secondary infertility.	Pregnancy may offer a window for treatment due to the additional motivation of fetal health.
Sleep disorders	1.5:1.0	Women experience increased risk for exacerbation at times of reproductive transition (i.e., premenstruum, postpartum, perimenopause).	Differentiate sleep disorder from normative changes in sleep during pregnancy and postpartum or from sleep disruption due to menopausal vasomotor symptoms.

Note. OCD = obsessive-compulsive disorder; PCOS = polycystic ovary syndrome; PMS = premenstrual syndrome; PMDD = premenstrual dysphoric disorder; PTSD = posttraumatic stress disorder.

tain estrogen, which has dopamine-blocking effects in animal studies, the use of these agents may have had a protective effect in women. The onset of schizophrenia tends to occur approximately 5 years later in women than in men (ages 20–29 years in women versus ages 15–24 years in men). Furthermore, approximately 15% of women with schizophrenia have a midlife onset of disease, developing new-onset symptoms of schizophrenia in their mid-to-late 40s. Schizophrenia is diagnosed later in women than it is in men, possibly because women tend to have a more benign premorbid history and display more affective and positive symptoms and may therefore be thought to be experiencing a major depressive episode or bipolar disorder (Seeman 2004).

More relatives of women with schizophrenia than those of schizophrenic men are likely to develop the disorder. Neuroanatomical studies suggest that structural brain abnormalities are more likely to be found in men than in women. Thus, the heritability of schizophrenia may be greater for women, whereas environment may play a relatively greater role for men. Furthermore, the tendency of schizophrenic women to

have better language function than male counterparts may be explained by the fact that sexual brain dimorphisms in areas of the brain that subserve language are more likely to be relatively preserved in schizophrenic women than schizophrenic men (J.M. Goldstein et al. 2002).

Among sex-specific differences in the treatment of schizophrenia, some, but not all, studies suggest that women are more responsive to treatment and require lower doses of medication than men (Seeman 2004). The theory that estrogen, which in animals has antidopaminergic effects, may protect against schizophrenia is supported by observations that schizophrenia worsens during low-estrogen phases of the menstrual cycle (Bergmann et al. 2002) and in the perimenopausal years (Seeman 1986).

Hyperprolactinemia induced by certain antipsychotic agents (e.g., risperidone, haloperidol) frequently causes menstrual irregularities and amenorrhea. Amenorrhea tends to occur with prolactin levels greater than 60 ng/mL (normal prolactin levels=5–25 ng/mL). If prolactin levels exceed 100 ng/mL, an endocrine consultation should be requested to assess the possibility of a pituitary adenoma. Antipsychotic-induced hyperprolactinemia causes hypoestrogenemia, which in turn is associated with infertility and reduced bone mineral density (Seeman 2004). For antipsychotic-induced hyperprolactinemia, consideration should be given to reducing the dose of medication or switching to one of the newer antipsychotic agents, such as olanzapine, ziprasidone, aripiprazole, or quetiapine, which tend not to increase prolactin secretion. If the administered dose is necessary to control psychotic symptoms, the dopamine agonist bromocriptine (2.5–7.5 mg twice daily) or cabergoline (0.5 mg/week) may be given. A third approach is the use of an oral contraceptive, which has the triple effects of restoring menstrual cycle regularity, providing contraception, and protecting against the long-term hypoestrogenic effects of osteoporosis and heart disease. While oral contraceptives tend to reverse antipsychotic-induced hyperprolactinemia, this may not always be completely effective, thus necessitating continued prolactin evaluation.

Women with schizophrenia are at risk for pregnancy because of ineffective use of contraception and high rates of sexual assault. Schizophrenic women who become pregnant are at increased risk for stillbirth, preterm delivery, low-birth-weight neonates, and sudden infant death. In part, this may be due to poor compliance with prenatal follow-up assessments. Furthermore, maternal schizophrenia is associated with poor parenting outcomes (Abel et al. 2005). Schizophrenic women should therefore be counseled about birth control and provided with behavioral approaches to avoid unwanted sexual advances. Because schizophrenic mothers tend to do better as parents if they are healthy enough to engage in supportive marital and social relationships, obstetrical and psychiatric practitioners should carefully evaluate the nature of available interpersonal resources well in advance of childbirth (Abel et al. 2005).

Depression

Depression is more prevalent in women than men by a factor of 1.7 to 2.0. Dysthymia is twice as prevalent in women as in men. Although environmental stressors increase the risk for depression in both women and men, women tend to become depressed in response to close interpersonal difficulties, whereas men tend to become depressed in response to occupational stress (Kendler et al. 2001). Furthermore, it appears that the heritability of major depression is higher in women than in men (Kendler et al. 2006). It may be that genes that alter the risk for depression in women do so in re-

sponse to hormonal changes associated with the menstrual cycle, pregnancy, or the postpartum (Kendler et al. 2006). Seasonal affective disorder is also more frequent in women than in men. Women with one or more reproductive-related depressive conditions (e.g., oral contraceptive–induced depression, postpartum depression, PMDD, perimenopausal depression) are at increased risk for other reproductive-related depressive episodes.

Women of childbearing age who are planning to become pregnant and are likely to need continued psychotropic treatment during pregnancy and the postpartum period are best placed on a medication whose safety is such that it will not be necessary to alter medications should pregnancy occur. For those women whose depressive condition occurs throughout the month but with premenstrual exacerbation, charting of symptoms is often a useful way to document those days when an increase in antidepressant dose or addition of another agent may protect against recurrence of symptoms. Because women with histories of depression are at substantial risk for postpartum-onset depression, consideration should be given to prophylactic initiation of an antidepressant immediately upon delivery.

Bipolar Disorder

Bipolar disorder is equally prevalent in men and women. Some (Grant et al. 2005) but not all (Baldassano et al. 2005) studies report that bipolar women experience more depressive episodes and fewer manic episodes compared with bipolar men. Although mixed states may be more common in women (Grant et al. 2005), the conventionally held view that rapid cycling is approximately twice as common in women as it is in men has been questioned (Baldassano et al. 2005). Additionally, compared with men, women with bipolar disorder are more likely to have higher rates of bipolar II illness, comorbid thyroid disease, and concomitant posttraumatic stress disorder (Baldassano et al. 2005). Although more men than women with bipolar disorder abuse alcohol and substances, when comparing women and men with bipolar disorder to women and men in the general population, bipolar women were at greater risk of comorbid alcohol and substance use (Frye et al. 2003).

For some bipolar women, premenstrual relapse or exacerbation of symptoms occurs. If symptoms change over the course of the menstrual cycle, serum lithium levels should be checked during symptomatic days, and adjustments in lithium dosage may be made accordingly.

Because women who take lithium are at risk of developing lithium-induced hypothyroidism, thyroid function should be monitored at least every 6 months, and perhaps more frequently in women older than 40 years, who are at particularly increased risk for age-related thyroid dysregulation. Carbamazepine induces hormone clearance and metabolism, thereby diminishing oral contraceptive efficacy. In addition, women who take carbamazepine and who receive HT following menopause or complete hysterectomy may require higher doses of estrogen to treat menopause-related vasomotor symptoms effectively. Because lamotrigine metabolism is induced in the presence of estrogen, bipolar women on either oral contraceptives or HT may require increased doses of lamotrigine to maintain mood stability.

A number of studies have found that valproate may be associated with an increased risk for polycystic ovary syndrome (PCOS) (Betts et al. 2003; Isojarvi et al. 1993; McIntyre et al. 2003). It appears that unrelated to medication use, bipolar women are more likely than either unipolar depressed or healthy women to have retrospectively reported early-onset menstrual dysfunction (Joffe et al. 2006). Thus, it is not clear if conditions such as PCOS in bipolar women may reflect a valproate effect or an independent hypothalamic-pituitary-gonadal axis abnormality. An increased risk for osteoporosis with carbamazepine or valproate use has also been reported (Pack and Morrell 2004). Because bipolar disorder tends to be disabling when incompletely treated, the most effective agent(s) for controlling symptoms should be administered, although bipolar women should be monitored for symptoms of PCOS (e.g., menstrual irregularities, hirsutism, insulin resistance), particularly if they are taking valproate. For bone health, they should take calcium and vitamin D, get adequate (but not excessive) sunlight exposure, and do regular weight-bearing exercises.

As noted previously, bipolar disorder increases the risk for postpartum recurrence (including bipolar depression, mania, and psychosis). For this reason, it is essential to ensure that all bipolar women of childbearing age are managed carefully using the safest possible medications in pregnancy while still maximizing clinical stability.

Anxiety Disorders

Women are more likely than men to experience anxiety disorders, often with comorbid depression. As a result, they are twice as likely as men to use anxiolytic medication. For example, women are twice as likely as

men to suffer from posttraumatic stress disorder and two to three times as likely to experience panic disorder with agoraphobia. Panic disorder with agoraphobia is more common in alcoholic women than alcoholic men. Although OCD prevalence rates are roughly equal between the sexes, the onset of the illness tends to be earlier in women than men (age 25 years in women vs. age 20 years in men), and women tend to experience more obsessions related to food and weight than do men. The evaluation for anxiety should rule out medical conditions that mimic anxiety symptoms (e.g., cardiovascular disease, thyroid disorders, lupus, iron deficiency anemia). Caffeine and nicotine, which tend to exacerbate anxiety, should be restricted. Medications such as nonsteroidal decongestants, steroids, herbal supplements, and appetite suppressants may precipitate anxiety attacks. In some perimenopausal women, vasomotor symptoms (e.g., heat sensations, sweating, shortness of breath) may be mistaken for panic attacks. Although lifetime exposure to traumatic events is approximately equal between men and women, women are more likely than men to experience rape and sexual assault, whereas men experience more incidents of physical assault. While the etiology is unclear, it does appear that women with histories of trauma are at increased risk for PMDD.

Substance Abuse

Although the prevalence rate of alcoholism in men is more than twice that in women, the rate of alcoholism in women is 6% and rising (Greenfield et al. 2003). Because women have more body fat and less body water than do men, they reach higher blood alcohol levels and therefore become more intoxicated than men when they drink equal amounts of alcohol per unit of body weight. Complications from alcohol abuse, such as peptic ulcer, liver disease, anemia, and cerebral atrophy, develop more quickly in women, and women are more likely to die from alcoholism than are men (Greenfield et al. 2003). Risk factors for alcoholism in women include a history of sexual abuse, substance abuse, adult antisocial personality disorder, and depression.

Although hallucinogen and opiate abuse predominate in men, prevalence rates for cocaine and amphetamine abuse are equal between women and men. Women often use stimulants for weight control. Substance-abusing women are more likely to experience comorbid psychiatric disorders. Because many women drink to self-medicate premenstrual tension, it is important to assess for premenstrual symptoms in alcohol and drug use. Risk factors for drug abuse in women include a family history of substance abuse, antisocial personality disorder, depression, and being in a relationship with a drug-abusing or -dependent partner.

Treatment of substance abuse includes referral to self-help groups such as Alcoholics Anonymous, Cocaine Anonymous, and the all-women support group Women for Sobriety. Family and marital conflicts should be evaluated and addressed carefully, because the likelihood of a woman remaining sober is often dependent on the sobriety of significant others.

Eating Disorders

Anorexia nervosa and bulimia occur in approximately 4% of the population, with more than 90% of cases involving women. These disorders usually begin in adolescence. The symptoms of anorexia nervosa include body weight of less than 85% of expected for age and height, intense fear of gaining weight, distorted body image, and (in postmenarchal females) amenorrhea. Anorexia nervosa occurs in 0.3%–1.0% of women and is subtyped as either restricting or binge-eating/purge type. Approximately 50% of cases fall into each category (Yager and Andersen 2005).

Bulimia nervosa involves repeated uncontrollable episodes of binge eating in association with excessive concern about body image. To compensate for the food intake, patients fast; engage in excessive exercise; use laxatives, diuretics, or enemas; or self-induce vomiting. To meet DSM-IV-TR diagnostic criteria for bulimia nervosa, the binge eating and compensatory behaviors must occur at least twice a week for at least 3 months. The disorder is categorized as either purging type (i.e., involving the use of self-induced vomiting, laxatives, diuretics, or enemas) or nonpurging type. Anorexia and bulimia nervosa are frequently complicated by mood, anxiety, personality, and substance use disorders.

The evaluation of women with eating disorders should include assessments of body image; eating habits; actual and desired weight; menstrual patterns; exercise; self-induced vomiting; presence of other psychiatric disturbance; use of laxatives, diuretics, enemas, emetics, and diet pills; and abuse of alcohol and illicit substances. Medical complications that may result from anorexia and bulimia nervosa include electrocardiographic abnormalities, hypotension, atrial and ventricular arrhythmias, esophageal perforation, rectal prolapse, metabolic alkalosis, hypokalemia, amenorrhea, osteoporosis, erosion of dental enamel, parotid and submandibular gland hypertrophy, and anemia. Therefore, the evaluation should include a physical and dental examination. Laboratory tests

should be obtained, including albumin, total protein, and glucose levels (to help assess nutritional status); amylase levels (to assess the extent of self-induced vomiting); electrolytes; blood urea nitrogen; and creatinine. An electrocardiogram should be obtained, because cardiac conduction abnormalities may result from electrolyte imbalance, malnutrition, and ipecac-induced cardiomyopathy.

The treatment of eating disorders requires an interdisciplinary team of mental health professionals, primary care physicians, nutritionists, and dentists. The initial treatment goal is to stabilize serious medical problems such as malnutrition and electrolyte imbalances. Nasogastric tube feeding may be necessary for life-threatening conditions. When the patient is medically stable, treatment should focus on establishing healthful eating patterns and examining the psychosocial factors contributing to the disorder. Psychosocial interventions include family counseling, individual/couples psychotherapy, education, and group support. Cognitive-behavioral therapy and interpersonal therapy have been effective for eating disorders, particularly bulimia nervosa. Serotonergic antidepressant medications at high doses (e.g., 60–80 mg of fluoxetine) have been helpful for bulimia nervosa. SSRIs do not appear to hasten weight gain in severely underweight anorexic patients, and a recent study failed to demonstrate benefit from fluoxetine in the maintenance treatment of the disorder (Walsh et al. 2006). Nevertheless, once weight has been restored, a comprehensive approach involving cognitive-behavioral therapy and an SSRI is frequently employed, particularly because SSRIs may be useful in treating associated mood and anxiety disorders. It has been hypothesized that some anorexic patients have psychotic symptoms that include delusions and hallucinations having to do with body weight and food attributes (Powers et al. 2005). Although antipsychotic medications are frequently used to treat patients with anorexia nervosa, data for efficacy using these agents have come mainly from small open-label studies (Powers et al. 2005; Yager and Andersen 2005). Intensive treatment in an inpatient setting or day program is usually required for patients with anorexia nervosa. These settings allow patients' eating to be supervised and supported. Hospitalization will be necessary for patients who are refusing food or who experience severe medical complications.

Sleep Disorders

Women have a somewhat higher rate of insomnia than men, partly because sleep-related difficulties occur more frequently during women's reproductive phases. Sleep disruptions can result from premenstrual cramping, physical discomfort in the third trimester of pregnancy, and perimenopausal night sweats. Other common causes of insomnia include depression and anxiety disorders, medication side effects (e.g., bronchodilators, blood pressure medications, decongestants), alcohol, caffeine, nicotine, illicit drugs, and medical conditions (e.g., sleep apnea).

In the initial evaluation, the underlying cause of the insomnia should be determined. If the primary cause is a psychiatric or medical problem, this should be treated. The evaluation should also review the patient's daily use of caffeine, nicotine, and alcohol and the occurrence of daytime napping (Millman 1999). If sleep problems are associated with premenstrual discomfort, anti-inflammatory agents or low-dose oral contraceptives may help. For perimenopausal women experiencing sleep disruption as a result of night sweats, hormone replacement is effective. When sleep-promoting interventions have not succeeded, hypnotic medications may be appropriate and include benzodiazepines, zolpidem, and zaleplon. These medications should be administered for short-term use to avoid risks of addiction and rebound insomnia. Sedating antidepressants (e.g., trazodone, doxepin) are another option for treating insomnia.

Female-Specific Cancers

Both breast cancer and gynecological cancers tend to be particularly stressful for women because they affect the organs of reproduction, sexuality, and femininity. Treatment strategies include surgery, radiation therapy, and chemotherapy. Sexual problems may emerge after treatment because of the direct physical effects of these modalities, fears of recurring cancer, or a decreased sense of femininity. Although over time, women with breast cancer experience less emotional, sexual, and social impairment, quality of life may be negatively impacted long after treatment for the disease has been completed. Partners' attitudes are particularly important, because women with these types of cancer need support and encouragement.

A psychiatric consultation may be requested for women undergoing treatment for breast or gynecological cancer. For women in whom organic etiologies for mood disorders have been excluded, psychotherapy is a useful modality, particularly supportive or cognitive approaches to improve a sense of control. Standard antidepressant medications may be useful to increase appetite and sleep, because tamoxifen may reduce serum TCAs. For antidepressant-treated cancer patients who do not appear to be responding as well as expected, serum levels of parent and metabolite compounds should be assessed and compared with pre-tamoxifen-treatment levels. If antidepressant medication is necessary for a tamoxifen-treated cancer patient, consideration should be given to increasing the dosage of the antidepressant to achieve clinical efficacy.

Induced menopause secondary to radical hysterectomy or vasomotor symptoms due to tamoxifen may cause additional discomfort and may cause further sleep disruptions, with vasomotor symptoms, depression, irritability, and anxiety. In addition to effectively treating depression and anxiety, SSRIs and venlafaxine may reduce tamoxifen-induced hot flashes. Paroxetine has been noted to reduce the level of an active metabolite of tamoxifen that is found in some, but not all, women (Stearns et al. 2003), and it has been suggested that the use of SSRIs for tamoxifen-treated breast cancer patients may therefore reduce the antiestrogenic efficacy of tamoxifen. However, it appears that other active metabolites of tamoxifen that are not reduced in the presence of paroxetine may be effective antiestrogenic agents. Women with breast cancer who are taking tamoxifen should therefore discuss with their physicians the use of concomitant paroxetine or other SSRIs.

Many women with breast or gynecological cancer experience anxiety in response to the stress of difficult or uncomfortable treatment regimens and in response to the severe toll of the illness. Guided imagery and progressive relaxation techniques, in conjunction with the use of low doses of anxiolytic medication, may be helpful in the acute phase of treatment. For sleep difficulties, reviewing the basic techniques of sleep hygiene are helpful; if insomnia persists, short-acting benzodiazepines or low-dose trazodone also may be useful. Women with cancer who have a history of alcohol or substance abuse or dependence are at risk for a recurrence. Encouraging these women to participate in lay advocacy groups (e.g., Alcoholics Anonymous, Narcotics Anonymous) and providing them with the opportunity to discuss their fear, anger, and sadness in individual therapy are particularly important. Women with breast or gynecological cancer may experience a change in the quality of their sexual or marital relationships. For women whose surgery was extensive, their sense of sexuality and femininity may be called into question. Frequently, the partner also experiences a sense of loss and fear and may have difficulty viewing surgical or radiation scars. Conjoint education and counseling are often helpful.

Group support, in the form of advocacy groups such as Reach to Recovery or groups sponsored by the American Cancer Society, is helpful because it offers group members the opportunity to share common concerns, practical advice, and appreciation of the implications of having a diagnosis of cancer. Whether group therapy actually extends survival for breast cancer patients is unclear, although it does improve mood and reduce the perception of pain.

Summary

When assessing and treating women with psychiatric disorders, it is important that clinicians recognize gender-specific issues related to diagnosis, course, and treatment. These gender-specific differences are undoubtedly due to a combination of biological, genetic, and psychosocial factors. Thus, psychopharmacological and psychotherapeutic treatment modalities should address the special and changing needs of women over the course of their lives.

Key Points

- Although women and men are at equal lifetime risk of developing a psychiatric disorder, there are gender-specific differences in prevalence, clinical course, and treatment of specific psychiatric illnesses.

- Women are at particular risk for mood disorders at times of reproductive transition.

- When diagnosed properly, premenstrual dysphoric disorder responds robustly to treatment with selective serotonin reuptake inhibitors.

- The overall mental health of an expectant mother is an important determinant of the health and well-being of both mother and fetus.

- Decisions regarding the use of psychiatric medications in pregnancy are best made after assessing whether it is riskier to both mother and fetus for the mother to have symptomatic psychiatric illness or to be treated with a medication to effectively treat that illness.

- Although the antenatal use of many commonly used antidepressants have been associated with an increased risk of adverse effects in pregnancy, when balancing risks and benefits, these agents are sometimes judged to be necessary for the health and well-being of women and their fetuses.

- Up to 60% of bipolar women become unstable if their mood stabilizer is discontinued when they become pregnant.

- Bipolar women are at substantially increased risk for postpartum mood disorders, including postpartum depression and postpartum psychosis.

- Women are at increased risk for major depression as they move into and through perimenopause. That risk is particularly great if there is a past history of major depression.

- Treatment of women with psychiatric disorders requires a careful and comprehensive assessment of physiological, genetic, reproductive, medical, and psychosocial risks for current illness as well as relapse and recurrence potential. In light of this assessment, the mental health clinician can choose among varying treatment options to maximize the best possible outcome for the patients, their babies and children, and their families.

Suggested Readings

Cohen LS, Altshuler LL, Harlow, et al: Relapse of major depression during pregnancy in women who maintain or discontinue antidepressant treatment. JAMA 295:499–507, 2006

Cohen LS, Soares CN, Vitonis AF, et al: Risk for new onset of depression during the menopausal transition. Arch Gen Psychiatry 63:385–390, 2006

Cyranowski JM, Frank E, Young E, et al: Adolescent onset of the gender difference in lifetime rates of major depression. Arch Gen Psychiatry 57:21–27, 2000

Freeman EW, Sammel MD, Lin H, et al: Associations of hormones and menopausal status with depressed mood in women with no history of depression. Arch Gen Psychiatry 63:375–382, 2006

Harlow BL, Wise LA, Otto MW, et al: Depression and its influence on reproductive endocrine and menstrual cycle markers associated with perimenopause. The Harvard Study of Moods and Cycles. Arch Gen Psychiatry 60:29–36, 2003

Rubinow DR: Antidepressant treatment during pregnancy: between Scylla and Charybdis (editorial). Am J Psychiatry 163:954–956, 2006

Online Resources

Massachusetts General Hospital Center for Women's Mental Health (http://www.womensmental health.org): Web site of the Massachusetts General Hospital Reproductive Psychiatry Resource and Information Center. Provides information about psychiatric conditions in women, including premenstrual dysphoric disorder, postpartum disorders, and perimenopausal mood changes.

Motherisk (http://www.motherisk.org): Canadian organization that provides information on safety and risks of drugs in pregnancy and lactation, alcohol and other substance use in pregnancy.

National Domestic Violence Hotline (http://www.ndvh.org): Provides information about domestic violence and referrals to local shelters for victims of domestic violence.

National Eating Disorders Association (http://www.edap. org): Nonprofit organization dedicated to prevention and treatment of eating disorders. Provides referrals to patients with eating disorders and those concerned with body image and weight issues.

North American Menopause Society (http://www.menopause.org): Nonprofit organization promoting women's health during midlife and beyond, with special focus on menopausal health.

Postpartum Support International (http://www.postpartum. net): International network of individuals and organizations whose purpose is to increase awareness among public and professionals about pregnancy and postpartum related psychiatric disorders. Provides referrals for group and individual therapy, and for psychiatrists to women with postpartum disorders.

RESOLVE: The National Infertility Association (http:// www.resolve.org): National self-help organization for infertile couples. Sponsors support groups throughout the country.

References

Abel KM, Webb RT, Aalmon MP, et al: Prevalence and predictors of parenting outcomes in a cohort of mothers with schizophrenia admitted for joint mother and baby psychiatric care in England. J Clin Psychiatry 66:781–789, 2005

Aleman A, Kahn RS, Salten JP: Sex differences in the risk of schizophrenia. Evidence from meta-analysis. Arch Gen Psychiatry 60:565–571, 2003

Altshuler LL, Cohen L, Szuba MP, et al: Pharmacological management of psychiatric illness in pregnancy: dilemmas and guidelines. Am J Psychiatry 153:592–606, 1996

Alwan S, Reefhuis J, Rasmussen SA, et al: Use of selective serotonin reuptake inhibitors in pregnancy and the risk of birth defects. N Engl J Med 356:2684–2692, 2007

American Academy of Pediatrics Committee on Drugs: The transfer of drugs and other chemicals into human milk. Pediatrics 108:776–789, 2001

American Psychiatric Association: Diagnostic and Statistical Manual of Mental Disorders, 4th Edition, Text Revision. Washington, DC, American Psychiatric Association, 2000

Amsterdam J, Garcia-Espana F, Fawcett J, et al: Fluoxetine efficacy in menopausal women with and without estrogen replacement. J Affect Disord 55:11–17, 1999

Anderson GL, Limacher M, Assaf AR, et al: Effects of conjugated equine estrogen in postmenopausal women with hysterectomy: the Women's Health Initiative randomized controlled trial. JAMA 291:1701–1712, 2004

Baldassano CF, Marrangell LB, Ghaemi GG, et al: Gender differences in bipolar disorder: retrospective data from the first 500 STEP-BD participants. Bipolar Disord 7:465–470, 2005

Bérard A, Ramos E, Rey E, et al: First trimester exposure to paroxetine and risk of cardiac malformations in infants: the importance of dosage. Birth Defects Res B Dev Reprod Toxicol 80:18–27, 2007

Bergmann N, Parzer P, Nagl J, et al: Acute psychiatric admission and menstrual cycle phase in women with schizophrenia. Arch Womens Ment Health 5:119–126, 2002

Bertone-Johnson E, Hankinson SE, Brendich A, et al: Calcium and vitamin D intake and risk of incident premenstrual syndrome. Arch Intern Med 165:1246–1252, 2005

Betts T, Yarrow H, Dutton N et al: A study of anticonvulsant medication on ovarian function in a group of women with epilepsy who have only ever taken one anticonvulsant compared with a group of women with epilepsy. Seizure 12:323–329, 2003

Bodnar LM, Sunder KR, Wisner KL: Treatment with selective serotonin reuptake inhibitors during pregnancy: deceleration of weight gain because of depression or drug? Am J Psychiatry 163:986–991, 2006

Bromberger JT, Assman SF, Avis NE, et al: Persistent mood symptoms in a multiethnic community cohort of pre- and perimenopausal women. Am J Epidemiol 158:347–356, 2003

Burt VK, Suri R, Altshuler LL, et al: The use of psychotropic medications during breast-feeding. Am J Psychiatry 158:1001–1009, 2001

Casper RC, Fleischer BE, Lee-Ancajas JC, et al: Follow-up of children of depressed mothers exposed or not exposed to antidepressant drugs during pregnancy. J Pediatr 142:402–408, 2003

Center for the Evaluation of Risks to Human Reproduction: NTO-CERHR Expert Panel Report on the Reproductive and Developmental Toxicity of Fluoxetine (NTP-CERHR-Fluoxetine-04). Research Triangle Park, NC, U.S. Department of Health and Human Services, National Toxicology Program, Center for the Evaluation of Risks to Human Reproduction, April 2004

Chambers CD, Johnson KA, Dick LM, et al: Birth outcomes in pregnancy women taking fluoxetine. N Engl J Med 335:1010–1015, 1996

Chambers CD, Hernandez-Diaz S, Van Martner LJ, et al: Selective serotonin-reuptake inhibitors and risk of persistent pulmonary hypertension of the newborn. N Engl J Med 354:579–587, 2006

Chan BC, Koren G, Fayez I, et al: Pregnancy outcome of women exposed to bupropion during pregnancy: a prospective comparative study. Am J Obstet Gynecol 192:932–936, 2005

Chiu CC, Huang SY, Shen WW, et al: Omega-3 fatty acids for depression in pregnancy (letter). Am J Psychiatry 160:385, 2003

Chung TK, Lau TK, Yip AS, et al: Antepartum depressive symptomatology is associated with adverse obstetric and neonatal outcomes. Psychosom Med 63:830–834, 2001

Cnattingius S, Signorello LB, Anneren G, et al: Caffeine intake and the risk of first-trimester spontaneous abortion. N Engl J Med 343:1839–1845, 2000

Cohen LS, Heller VL, Bailey JW, et al: Birth outcomes following prenatal exposure to fluoxetine. Biol Psychiatry 48:996–1000, 2000

Cohen LS, Soares CN, Poiras JR, et al: Short-term use of estradiol for depression in perimenopausal and postmenopausal women: a preliminary report. Am J Psychiatry 160:1519–1522, 2003

Cohen LS, Altshuler LL, Harlow BL, et al: Relapse of major depression during pregnancy in women who maintain or discontinue antidepressant treatment. JAMA 295:499–507, 2006a

Cohen LS, Soares CN, Vitonis AF, et al: Risk for new onset of depression during the menopausal transition. Arch Gen Psychiatry 63:385–390, 2006b

Cole JA, Modell JG, Haight BR, et al: Bupropion in pregnancy and the prevalence of congenital malformations. Pharmacoepidemiol Drug Saf 16:474–484, 2007

Costei AM, Kozer E, Ho T, et al: Perinatal outcome following third trimester exposures to paroxetine. Arch Pediatr Adolesc Med 156:1129–1132, 2002

Cyranowski JM, Frank E, Young E, et al: Adolescent onset of the gender difference in lifetime rates of major depression. A theoretical model. Arch Gen Psychiatry 57:21–27, 2000

de la Chica RA, Ribas I, Giraldo J, et al: Chromosomal instability in amniocytes from fetuses of mothers who smoke. JAMA 293:1212–1222, 2005

Djulus J, Koren G, Einarson TR, et al: Exposure to mirtazapine during pregnancy: a prospective, comparative study of birth outcomes. J Clin Psychiatry 67:1280–1284, 2006

Ehrensaft MK, Moffitt TE, Caspi A: Is domestic violence followed by an increased risk of psychiatric disorders among women but not among men? A longitudinal cohort study. Am J Psychiatry 163:885–892, 2006

Einarson A, Fatoye B, Sarkar M, et al: Pregnancy outcome following gestational exposure to venlafaxine: a multicenter prospective controlled study. Am J Psychiatry 158:1728–1730, 2001

Einarson A, Bonari L, Voyer-Lavigne S, et al: A multicentre prospective controlled study to determine the safety of trazodone and nefazodone use during pregnancy. Can J Psychiatry 48:106–110, 2003

Ericson A, Kullen B, Wilholm BE: Delivery outcome after the use of antidepressants in early pregnancy. Eur J Clin Pharmacol 55:503–508, 1999

Espeland MA, Rapp SA, Shumaker SA, et al: Conjugated equine estrogens and global cognitive function in postmenopausal women: Women's Health Initiative Memory Study. JAMA 291:2959–2968, 2004

Evans J, Heron J, Francomb H, et al: Cohort study of depressed mood during pregnancy and after childbirth. BMJ 323:257–260, 2001

Federenko IS, Wadwha PD: Women's mental health during pregnancy influences fetal and infant developmental and health outcomes. FDA Public Health Advisory. CNS Spectr 9:198–206, 2004

Fischer G, Johnson RE, Eder H, et al: Treatment of opioid-dependent pregnant women with buprenorphine. Addiction 95:239–244, 2004

Flynn HA, Blow FC, Marcus SM: Rates and predictors of depression treatment among pregnant women in hospital-affiliated obstetrics practices. Gen Hosp Psychiatry 28:289–295, 2006

Freeman EW, Sammel MD, Liu L, et al: Hormones and menopausal status as predictors of depression in women in transition to menopause. Arch Gen Psychiatry 61:62–70, 2004

Freeman EW, Sammel MD, Lin H, et al: Associations of hormones and menopausal status with depressed mood in women with no history of depression. Arch Gen Psychiatry 63:375–382, 2006

Frye MA, Altshuler LL, McElroy SL, et al: Gender differences in prevalence, risk, and clinical correlates of alcoholism comorbidity in bipolar disorder. Am J Psychiatry 160:883–889, 2003

Gentile S: Clinical utilization of atypical antipsychotics in pregnancy and lactation. Ann Pharmacother 38:1265–1271, 2004

Goldstein DJ: Effects of third trimester fluoxetine exposure on the newborn. J Clin Psychopharmacol 15:417–420, 1995

Goldstein DJ, Corbin LA, Fung MC: Olanzapine-exposed pregnancies and lactation, early experience. J Clin Psychopharmacol 20:399–403, 2000

Goldstein JM, Seidman LJ, O'Brien LM, et al: Impact of normal sexual dimorphisms on sex differences in structural brain abnormalities in schizophrenia assessed by magnetic resonance imaging. Arch Gen Psychiatry 59:154–164, 2002

Grant BF, Stinson FS, Hasin DS, et al: Prevalence, correlated, and comorbidity of bipolar I disorder and Axis I and II disorders: results from the national epidemiologic survey on alcohol and related conditions. J Clin Psychiatry 66:1205–1215, 2005

Greene MF: Teratogenicity of SSRIs—serious concern or much ado about little? N Engl J Med 356:2732–2733, 2007

Greenfield SF, Manwani SG, Nargiso JE: Epidemiology of substance use disorders in women. Obstet Gynecol Clin North Am 30:413–446, 2003

Grof P, Robbins W, Alda M, et al: Protective effect of pregnancy in women with lithium-responsive bipolar disorder. J Affect Disord 61:31–39, 2000

Harlow BL, Wise LA, Otto MW, et al: Depression and its influence on reproductive endocrine and menstrual cycle markers associated with perimenopause. The Harvard Study of Moods and Cycles. Arch Gen Psychiatry 60:29–36, 2003

Heikkinen T, Ekblad U, Kero P, et al: Citalopram in pregnancy and lactation. Clin Pharmacol Ther 72:184–191, 2002

Hendrick V, Smith LM, Hwang S, et al: Weight gain in breastfed infants of mothers taking antidepressant medications. J Clin Psychiatry 64:410–412, 2003a

Hendrick V, Smith LM, Suri R, et al: Birth outcomes after prenatal exposure to antidepressant medication. Am J Obstet Gynecol 188:812–815, 2003b

Holmes LB, Wyszynski DF, Baldwin EJ, et al: Increased risk for non-syndromic cleft palate among infants exposed to lamotrigine during pregnancy (abstract). Birth Defects Res A Clin Mol Teratol 76:318, 2006

Hostetter A, Ritchie JC, Stowe ZN: Amniotic fluid and umbilical cord blood concentrations of antidepressants in three women. Biol Psychiatry 48:1032–1034, 2000

Isojarvi JI, Laatikainen TJ, Pakarinen AJ, et al: Polycystic ovaries and hyperandrogenism in women taking valproate for epilepsy. N Engl J Med 329:1383–1388, 1993

Jablensky AV, Morgan V, Zubrick SR, et al: Pregnancy, delivery, and neonatal complications in a population cohort of women with schizophrenia and major affective disorders. Am J Psychiatry 162:79–91, 2005

Joffe H, Kim DR, Foris JM, et al: Menstrual dysfunction prior to onset of psychiatric illness is reported more commonly by women with bipolar disorder than by women with unipolar depression and healthy controls. J Clin Psychiatry 67:297–304, 2006

Johnson RE, Jones HE, Fischer G: Use of buprenorphine in pregnancy: patient management and effects on the neonate. Drug Alcohol Depend 70 (2 suppl):S87–S101, 2003

Kallen B: Neonate characteristics after maternal use of antidepressants in late pregnancy. Arch Pediatr Adolesc Med 158:312–316, 2004

Kallen BA, Otterblad Olausson P: Maternal use of selective serotonin reuptake inhibitors in early pregnancy and infant congenital malformations. Birth Defects Res A Clin Mol Teratol 79:301–308, 2007

Kendler KS, Thornton LM, Prescott CA: Gender differences in the rates of exposure to stressful life events and sensitivity to their depressogenic effects. Am J Psychiatry 158:587–593, 2001

Kendler KS, Gatz, M, Gardner CO, et al: A Swedish National Twin Study of lifetime major depression. Am J Psychiatry 163:109–114, 2006

Kulin NA, Pastuszak A, Sage SR, et al: Pregnancy outcome following maternal use of the new selective serotonin reuptake inhibitors: a prospective controlled millimeter study. JAMA 279:609–610, 1998

Kurki T, Hiilesmaa V, Raitasalo R, et al: Depression and anxiety in early pregnancy and risk for preeclampsia. Obstet Gynecol 95:487–490, 2000

Laine K, Heikkinen T, Ekblad U, et al: Effects of exposure to selective serotonin reuptake inhibitors during pregnancy on serotonergic symptoms in newborns and cord blood monoamine and prolactin concentrations. Arch Gen Psychiatry 60:720–726, 2003

Louik C, Lin AE, Werler MM, et al: First-trimester use of selective serotonin-reuptake inhibitors and the risk of birth defects. N Engl J Med 356:2675–2683, 2007

Malm H, Klaukka T, Neuvonen PJ: Risks associated with selective serotonin reuptake inhibitors in pregnancy. Obstet Gynecol 106:1289–1296, 2005

Marmorstein NR, Malone SM, Iacono WG: Psychiatric disorders among offspring of depressed mothers: associations with paternal psychopathology. Am J Psychiatry 161:1588–1594, 2004

McElhatton PR, Garbis HM, Elephant E, et al: The outcome of pregnancy in 689 women exposed to therapeutic doses of antidepressants. A collaborative study of the European network of teratology information services (ENTIS). Reprod Toxicol 10:286–294, 1996

McKenna K, Koren G, Tetelbaum M, et al: Pregnancy outcome of women using atypical antipsychotic drugs: a prospective comparative study. J Clin Psychiatry 66:444–449, 2005

McIntyre RS, Mancini DA, McCann S, et al: Valproate, bipolar disorder and polycystic ovarian syndrome. Bipolar Disord 5:28–35, 2003

Mendhekar DN, War L, Sharma JB, et al: Olanzapine and pregnancy. Pharmacopsychiatry 35:122–123, 2002

Miller LJ: Use of electroconvulsive therapy during pregnancy. Hosp Community Psychiatry 45:444–450, 1994

Miller LJ: Postpartum depression. JAMA 287:762–765, 2002

Millman RP: Coping with insomnia: effective drug and non-drug therapies. Women's Health in Primary Care 1:737–745, 1999

Misri S, Reebye P, Kendrick K: Internalizing behaviors in 4-year-old children exposed in utero to psychotropic medications. Am J Psychiatry 163:1026–1032, 2006

Mitchell AA: Infertility treatment—more risks and challenges. N Engl J Med 346:731–737, 2002

Morgan ML, Cook IA, Rapkin AJ, et al: Estrogen augmentation of antidepressants in perimenopausal depression: a pilot study. J Clin Psychiatry 66:774–780, 2005

Morrison MF, Kallan MJ, Have TT, et al: Lack of efficacy of estradiol for depression in postmenopausal women: a randomized, controlled trial. Biol Psychiatry 55:406–412, 2004

Moses-Kolko EL, Bogen D, Perel J: Neonatal signs after late in utero exposure to serotonin reuptake inhibitors. JAMA 293:2372–2383, 2005

Neugebauer R: Depressive symptoms at two months after miscarriage: interpreting study findings from an epidemiological versus clinical perspective. Depress Anxiety 17:152–162, 2003

Newport DJ, Viguera AL, Beach AJ, et al: Lithium placental passage and obstetrical outcome: implications for clinical management during late pregnancy. Am J Psychiatry 162:2162–2170, 2005

Newport DJ, Calamaras MR, DeVane CL, et al: Atypical antipsychotic administration during late pregnancy: placental passage and obstetrical outcomes. Am J Psychiatry 164:1214–1220, 2007

Nulman I, Rovet J, Stewart DE, et al: Neurodevelopment of children exposed in utero to antidepressant drugs. N Engl J Med 336:258–262, 1997

Nulman I, Rovet J, Stewart DE, et al: Child development following exposure to tricyclic antidepressants or fluoxetine throughout fetal life: a prospective, controlled study. Am J Psychiatry 159:1889–1895, 2002

Oberlander TF, Eckstein Grunau R, Fitzgerald C, et al: Prolonged prenatal psychotropic medication exposure alters neonatal acute pain response. Pediatr Res 4:443–453, 2002

Oberlander TF, Misri S, Fitzgerald CE, et al: Pharmacological factors associated with transient neonatal symptoms following prenatal psychotropic medication exposure. J Clin Psychiatry 65:230–237, 2004

Oberlander TF, Warburton W, Misri S, et al: Neonatal outcomes after prenatal exposure to selective serotonin reuptake inhibitor antidepressants and maternal depression using population-based linked health data. Arch Gen Psychiatr 63:898–906, 2006

Oinonen KA, Mazmanian D: To what extent do oral contraceptives influence mood and affect? J Affect Disord 70:229–240, 2002

Oren DA, Wisner KL, Spinelli M, et al: An open trial of morning light therapy for treatment of antepartum depression. Am J Psychiatry 159:666–669, 2002

Pack AM, Morrell MJ: Epilepsy and bone health in adults. Epilepsy Behav 5 (suppl 2):S24–S29, 2004

Pastuszak A, Schick-Boschetto B, Zuber C, et al: Pregnancy outcomes following first-trimester exposure to fluoxetine (Prozac). JAMA 269:2246–2248, 1993

Powers PS, Simpson H, McCormick T: Anorexia nervosa and psychosis. Primary Psychiatry 12:39–45, 2005

Ratnayake T, Libretto SE: No complications with risperidone treatment before and throughout pregnancy and during the nursing period. J Clin Psychiatry 63:76–77, 2002

Rossouw JE, Anderson GL, Prentice RL, et al: Risks and benefits of estrogen plus progestin in healthy postmenopausal women: principal results from the Women's Health Initiative randomized controlled trial. JAMA 288:321–333, 2002

Rossouw JE, Prentice RL, Manson JE, et al: Postmenopausal hormone therapy and risk of cardiovascular disease by age and years since menopause. JAMA 297:1465–1477, 2007

Rubinow DR: Antidepressant treatment during pregnancy: between Scylla and Charybdis. Am J Psychiatry 163:954–956, 2006

Saks BR: Mirtazapine: treatment of depression, anxiety, and hyperemesis gravidarum in the pregnant patient: a report of 7 cases. Arch Womens Ment Health 3:165–170, 2001

Schmidt PJ, Nieman L, Danaceau MA, et al: Estrogen replacement in perimenopause-related depression: a preliminary report. Am J Obstet Gynecol 183:414–420, 2000

Schneider LS, Small GW, Hamilton SH, et al: Estrogen replacement and response to fluoxetine in a multicenter geriatric depression trial. Am J Geriatr Psychiatry 5:97–106, 1997

Seeman MV: Current outcome in schizophrenic women vs men. Acta Psychiatr Scand 73:609–617, 1986

Seeman MV: Gender differences in the prescribing of antipsychotic drugs. Am J Psychiatry 161:1324–1333, 2004

Sherwin BB: Affective changes with estrogen and androgen replacement therapy in surgically menopausal women. J Affect Disord 14:177–187, 1988

Shumaker SA, Legault C, Rapp SR, et al: Estrogen plus progestin and the incidence of dementia and mild cognitive impairment in postmenopausal women: the Women's Health Initiative Memory Study: a randomized controlled trial. JAMA 289:2651–2662, 2003

Simon GE, Cunningham ML, Davis RL: Outcomes of prenatal antidepressant exposure. Am J Psychiatry 159:2055–2061, 2002

Sivojelezova A, Schuhaiber S, Sarkissian L, et al: Citalopram in pregnancy and lactation. Clin Pharmacol Ther 72:184–191, 2003

Soares CN, Almeda OP, Jaffe H, et al: Efficacy of estradiol for the treatment of depressive disorders in perimenopausal women: a double-blind, randomized, placebo-controlled trial. Arch Gen Psychiatry 58:529–534, 2001

Spinelli MG, Endicott J: Controlled trial of interpersonal psychotherapy versus parenting education program for depressed women. Am J Psychiatry 160:555–562, 2003

Stearns V, Johnson MD, Rae JM, et al: Active tamoxifen metabolite plasma concentrations after coadministration of tamoxifen and the selective serotonin reuptake inhibitor paroxetine. J Natl Cancer Inst 95:1758–1764, 2003

Steiner M, Pearlstein T, Cohen LS, et al: Expert guidelines for the treatment of severe PMS, PMDD, and comorbidities: the role of SSRIs. J Womens Health 15:37–69, 2006

Suri R, Altshuler L, Hellemann G, et al: Effects of antenatal depression and antidepressant treatment on gestational age at birth and risk of preterm birth. Am J Psychiatry 164:1206–1213, 2007

Tenyi T, Trixler M, Keresztes Z: Quetiapine and pregnancy (letter). Am J Psychiatry 159:674, 2002

Thys-Jacobs S, Starkey P, Bernstein D, et al: Calcium carbonate and the premenstrual syndrome: effects on premenstrual and menstrual symptoms. Am J Obstet Gynecol 179:444–452, 1998

U.S. Food and Drug Administration Center for Drug Evaluation and Research: FDA Public Health Advisory. Treatment Challenges of Depression in Pregnancy and the Possibility of Persistent Pulmonary Hypertension in Newborns: List of Drug Names. July 19, 2006. Available at: http://www.fda.gov/cder/drug/advisory/SSRI_PPHN200607.htm. Accessed September 17, 2007.

Van den Bergh BRH, Mulder EJH, Mennes M, et al: Antenatal maternal anxiety and stress and the neurobehavioral development of the fetus and child: links and possible mechanisms. A review. Neurosci Biobehav Rev 29:237–258, 2005

Viguera AC, Nonacs R, Cohen LS, et al: Risk of recurrence of bipolar disorder in pregnant and nonpregnant women after discontinuing lithium maintenance. Am J Psychiatry 157:179–184, 2000

Walsh BT, Kaplan AS, Attia E, et al: Fluoxetine after weight restoration in anorexia nervosa: a randomized controlled trial. JAMA 295:2605–2612, 2006

Weiss G, Skurnick JH, Goldsmith LT, et al: Menopause and hypothalamic-pituitary sensitivity to estrogen. JAMA 292:2991–2996, 2004; erratum in JAMA 293:163, 2004

Whitaker RC, Orzol SM, Kahn RS: Maternal mental health, substance use, and domestic violence in the year after delivery and subsequent behavior problems in children at age 3 years. Arch Gen Psychiatry 63:351–360, 2006

Wisner KL, Hanusa BH, Perel JM, et al: Postpartum depression: a randomized trial of sertraline versus nortriptyline. J Clin Psychopharmacol 26:353–360, 2006

Wogelius P, Norgaard M, Gislum M, et al: Maternal use of selective serotonin reuptake inhibitors and risk of congenital malformations. Epidemiology 17:701–704, 2006

Yager J, Andersen AE: Anorexia nervosa. N Engl J Med 353:1481–1488, 2005

Yaris F, Kadioglu M, Kesim M, et al: Newer antidepressants in pregnancy: prospective outcome of a case series. Reprod Toxicol 19:235–238, 2004

Yonkers KA, Holthausen GA, Poschman KP, et al: Symptom-onset treatment for women with premenstrual dysphoric disorder. J Clin Psychopharmacol 26:198–202, 2006

Zeskind PS, Stephens LE: Maternal selective serotonin reuptake inhibitor use during pregnancy and newborn neurobehavior. Pediatrics 113:368–375, 2004

IMPORTANT CLINICAL ISSUES

40

CULTURAL ISSUES

Albert C. Gaw, M.D.

Culture is important for psychiatric diagnosis and treatment because it provides the *context* in which patients interpret their experiences and imbue them with meanings. Culture constructs the psychiatric experience of the individual, provides the template for an individual's idiosyncratic interpretation of mental phenomena, and shapes their unique expression in each individual's setting. Thus, culture defines for the patient the intrinsic meaning of the illness experience, helping him or her to make sense out of what is usually a chaotic situation. Because each individual could be considered an epitome of his or her cultural product and achievement, and because culture varies from place to place, the presentation of mental symptoms may vary among individuals and across cultural groups.

But what is *culture?* How does the study of culture inform psychiatry? Like an anthropologist who has to assume some kind of theoretical framework before embarking on the exploration of a new territory, the psychiatric clinician needs to possess some kind of *conceptual tool* in order to understand the cultural antecedents of the patient's experience. This chapter attempts to provide such a tool.

The scope of cultural psychiatry is broad. It could include behavioral phenomena in any social system with its own set of norms, developed over time by people living and working together, that are transmitted over generations. Examples of such phenomena include indigenous healing practices, influence of cul-

ture on early development and personality formation, ritualistic behavior in normal and pathological states, immigration and acculturation, religion, gender and ethnic issues, language, and ethnic variation in psychotropic drug responses. Because the thrust of this chapter is clinical and is focused on Western-oriented psychiatric practice, I devote my discussion to key cultural issues that may be most relevant to the practicing clinician in a one-to-one encounter. Thus, I begin by defining what *culture* is, delineating its essential components and features as a generic tool to understand cultural phenomena. A solid grounding on these concepts, I believe, will help equip the clinician to understand *what* to look for in the clinical encounter.

Next, I focus my discussion on five contemporary clinical areas in which cultural issues are intimately involved in the doctor–patient interaction. These areas include the clinician's approach to assessment of the patient's presenting problems as well as how the patient responds to prescribed therapeutic interventions. Culture influences those areas in the therapeutic transaction that involve ideas and habits of thinking, feeling, and behavioral patterns—functioning of the brain and mind—that are subsumed by what the anthropologist Goodenough (1961) termed the *subjective culture* or the *ideational order* of the mind. These five clinical areas are as follows:

- Cultural factors in DSM-IV-TR (American Psychiatric Association 2000)

- Cultural formulation of psychiatric problems
- Culture-bound syndromes
- Cultural factors in nonadherence to psychotropic medications
- Culture and psychotherapy

Finally, I conclude by providing a list of key points for the chapter. The DSM-IV-TR Glossary of Culture-Bound Syndromes and a Glossary of Cultural Psychiatry Terms are appended at the end of the chapter.

Concepts, Components, and Essential Features of Culture

Culture is that intervening variable between the human "organism" and its physical "environment" (Kroeber and Kluckholn 1952). As such, culture is "manmade," although genetic factors may also contribute to cultural phenomena. The concept of culture has evolved over the past century, each author adding a shade of clarification and refinement. The British anthropologist Sir Edward Burnett Tylor (1874) penned what is generally accepted as the first clear and comprehensive definition of culture. He defined *culture* as "that complex whole which includes knowledge, beliefs, arts, law, morals, custom and any other capabilities and habits acquired by man as a member of society" (p. 1). Culture is *learned* and includes the totality of human achievements.

The National Institute of Mental Health Culture and Diagnostic Group has adopted a more clinically oriented definition of culture: "Meanings, values, and behavioral norms that are learned and transmitted in the dominant society and within its social groups. Culture powerfully influences cognitions, feelings, and the 'self' concept, as well as the diagnostic process and treatment decisions" (Mezzich et al. 1993, p. 7).

Thus, the concepts of culture introduced here extend Engel's (1980) biopsychosocial framework on health and disease. It adds a *contextual* dimension, thus providing a holistic approach to patient care. *Culture* is that variable that makes us human. Within each individual's cultural *context*, biopsychosocial factors exert their influences to produce illness or effect a "cure" or recovery from illness. Thus, cultural concepts provide a paradigm of looking at mental illnesses not just as mind–body interaction but, as Kleinman (1988) pointed out, as mind–body interaction in *context*.

Components of Culture

The utility of culture can be further understood by examining its components.

Percepts

A *percept* is "an impression in the mind of something perceived by the senses, viewed as the basic component in the formation of concepts" (Morris 1970, p. 972). Our organs for sight, smell, touch, hearing, and taste continually receive sensory impressions that are conveyed to the higher centers of the brain. These impressions are subjected to cognitive interpretation based on the individual experiences that eventually give meanings to these impressions.

Concepts

Concepts are general ideas or understandings, especially ones derived from specific occurrences (Morris 1970). They are usually encoded in words. Many times, important concepts are embodied in and carry the force of laws, as in mandatory attendance in school or the right to vote in democratic societies.

Propositions

Having percepts and concepts is not enough. The mind must be able to manipulate these symbols to make sense of the relationships of things around us. The ways in which percepts and concepts are related to one another are called *propositions*. Thus, propositions allow us to use logical reasoning and inferences. The operation tells us what is happening in the world around us.

Beliefs

Beliefs are propositions considered to be *true*. Christians believe in an Almighty God incarnated in Jesus Christ. Muslims believe Mohammed to be the prophet of God. Jews believe the Torah to be inspired words from God. When beliefs are not based on reality, cannot be dislodged by objective facts, are tenaciously held, and exert a pervasive influence on the individual's perception of the world, such false beliefs are called delusions.

Values

When concepts and propositions are organized into a hierarchy of preference, the result is *value*. "Do no harm" has commanded a higher order of value than blind experimentation in the ethics of patient care. Members of the medical and psychiatric professions are expected to adhere to this standard.

Recipes or Operational Procedures

Recipes are ways in which people organize their efforts to accomplish certain tasks. As such, recipes could be explicit, as in a written memorandum, or implicit, as etiquette. We are taught to do a mental status examination, conduct a psychiatric interview, formulate a treatment plan, and prescribe medications or conduct psychotherapy. These are all operational procedures. They are part of the system of values and procedures that define who is a psychiatrist.

Ethnicity

Closely related to culture but applied in a narrower sense is *ethnicity*. Schermerhorn (1970), a sociologist, defined *ethnicity* as "a *collectivity* within a larger society having a real or putative common ancestry, memories of a shared historical past, and a cultural focus on one or more symbolic elements defined as the epitome of their peoplehood" (p. 12; italics added).

Thus, for example, Jewish people observe Passover, Americans have Thanksgiving, and the Chinese celebrate Chinese New Year. These rituals or operating procedures help to define the identity of each ethnic group and serve as reminders of one's common ancestry and bond.

Ethnicity is a powerful factor that binds people together. It also serves to differentiate a person or a group of individuals as a member(s) of an "in- or out-group." This feeling of affiliation within an "in-group" can have a significant influence in facilitating how one learns to "trust" and identify with another person during the initial clinical encounter.

Race, on the other hand, is a more biologically oriented term. It refers to a number of broad divisions of the human species into groups based on a common geographic origin, certain shared physical characteristics, and a characteristic distribution of gene frequencies (Kalow 1997).

Essential Features of Culture

The essential features of culture are summarized in Table 40–1. An elaboration of each feature follows.

1. *Culture is learned.* Unlike biological endowment, culture is learned. It includes people's assumptions about life that are widely shared and guide specific behaviors.
2. *Culture refers to systems of meanings.* Culture refers to systems of meanings—to what Geertz (1973) called the "webs of significance" that govern the conduct and understanding of people's lives; sys-

TABLE 40–1. Essential features of culture

Culture is learned.

Culture refers to systems of meanings.

Culture acts as a shaping template.

Culture is taught and reproduced.

Culture exists in a constant state of change.

Culture includes both objective and subjective patterns of human behavior.

tems of meanings are the negotiated agreements, such as the relationship between a word, behavior, or other symbol and its corresponding significance or meanings.

3. *Culture acts as a shaping template.* As a body of learned behaviors common to a given society, culture impels actions, with predictable form and content, for shaping consciousness and behavior within a human society from generation to generation.
4. *Culture is taught and reproduced.* Culture is transmitted across generations through family and human institutions.
5. *Culture exists in a constant state of change.* Culture is relativistic and is in a state of constant dynamic change. Different societies agree on different relationships and meanings at different points in time and space.
6. *Culture includes patterns of subjective and objective orders of human behaviors.* In addition to the more specific system of meanings referenced by Geertz (in item 2), Goodenough described two broad *orders of reality* in culture: the *implicit,* or *ideational,* and the *explicit,* or *phenomenal.* Both of these orders are products of human achievement. Thus, culture includes patterns of the subjective symbols or ideas of the mind as well as the objective expression of these symbols or thoughts as embodied in relics, behavior, and other products of human institution.

In summary, an understanding of culture can serve as a conceptual tool to inform psychiatry in at least the following areas:

1. It enhances diagnosis and treatment.
2. It fosters clinicians' sensitivity toward patients.
3. It increases psychiatric knowledge, particularly the symbolic system of healing.
4. It provides the context for differentiating "normal" from "abnormal" behavior.
5. It enhances general understanding of human being.

Cultural Statement for the Introduction to DSM-IV-TR

In the introductory section of DSM-IV-TR, clinicians are reminded that diagnostic assessment can be especially challenging when a clinician of one ethnic background "uses the DSM-IV classification to evaluate another person from a different ethnic or cultural group. A clinician who is unfamiliar with the nuances of an individual's cultural frame of reference may incorrectly judge as psychopathology those normal variations in behavior, belief, or experience that are particular to the individual's culture" (American Psychiatric Association 2000, p. xxxiv). For example, hallucinatory episodes induced by using peyote during a Native American religious ritual may be misdiagnosed as manifestations of a psychotic disorder. Likewise, seeing or hearing a deceased relative during the grieving process, usually a normal experience, may also be misdiagnosed. Thus, it is important to take the cultural *context* into consideration when making a diagnostic assessment.

One of the important contributions of DSM-IV-TR is the inclusion of "Specific Culture, Age, and Gender Features" among the types of information in the text. In so doing, DSM-IV-TR requires clinicians to consider cultural factors when making a diagnostic assessment. The following cultural features in the DSM-IV-TR categories are selected to highlight cultural considerations in the presentation of symptoms across ethnic groups.

Specific Cultural Considerations in DSM-IV-TR Diagnostic Categories

Disorders Usually First Diagnosed in Infancy, Childhood, or Adolescence

Mental Retardation and Learning Disorders

Because individualized testing is always required to make a diagnosis of mental retardation or a learning disorder, care should be taken that intelligence testing procedures have been validated across cultural groups.

Examiners who are familiar with aspects of the individual's ethnic or cultural background should be employed to perform the testing.

Language Disorder and Phonological Disorder (Formerly Developmental Articulation Disorders)

Care must be exercised when making judgments about the expressive language disorders of individuals growing up in a non-English-speaking or bilingual environment. The examiner should be familiar with the patient's cultural and linguistic contexts in the assessment of the development of communication abilities.

Selective Mutism

Care should be exercised not to misdiagnose immigrant children with selective mutism when they are unfamiliar with or uncomfortable with the official language of their host country and refuse to speak to strangers in their new environment.

Delirium, Dementia, and Amnestic and Other Cognitive Disorders

In the mental status examination, certain individuals may be unfamiliar with the information the test items use. Certain test items such as general fund of knowledge (e.g., names of presidents, geographic location), abstraction (e.g., proverbs), memory (e.g., date of birth, because some cultures do not celebrate birthday), and orientation (e.g., sense of placement, because location may be conceptualized differently) are useless if the information being used is unfamiliar to the individual.

Substance-Related Disorders

Substance Intoxication

The acceptance of mood-altering drugs, attitudes toward drug use, exposure, and pattern of substance use vary across cultural groups. Some cultural groups incorporate substance use as part of their rituals.

Alcohol-Related Disorders

Marked differences exist across different cultures in the quantity, frequency, and pattern of alcohol consumption. In most Asian cultures, the overall prevalence of alcohol-related disorders may be relatively low, and the male-to-female ratio may be high. Genetic differences may influence the prevalence of alcoholism. About 50% of Japanese, Chinese, and Korean people may be deficient in aldehyde dehydrogenase, the enzyme that metabolizes aldehyde, the intermediate product of alcohol, leading to high accumulation of blood aldehyde and causing symptoms of flushed face, palpitations, and dysphoria. In the United States, Caucasians and African Americans have nearly identical rates of alcohol abuse and dependence. Latino males have somewhat higher rates. Prevalence for Latino females is lower than among females from other ethnic groups.

Opioid-Related Disorders

In the late 1800s and early 1900s, opioid dependence was seen more often among white, middle-class individuals, suggesting that differences in use reflected the availability of opioid drugs and other social factors. Since the 1920s, in the United States, there has been an overrepresentation of opioid dependence among members of minority groups living in economically deprived areas.

Schizophrenia and Other Psychotic Disorders

The content, course, and outcome of the symptoms of schizophrenia may vary across cultural groups. Catatonic behavior appears to be more prevalent in non-Western cultures compared with that reported in the United States. In developing countries, an acute course and a better outcome have been noted in individuals with schizophrenia.

Mood Disorders

Depression, in some cultures, may be experienced largely in somatic terms rather than sadness or guilt. Depressive experiences may be expressed as complaints of weakness, tiredness, "imbalance" (in Chinese and Asian cultures), "nerves" and headaches (in Latino and Mediterranean cultures), or being "heartbroken" (among Hopi Native American culture). In some cultures, irritability as a symptom of depression may provoke greater concern than sadness or withdrawal. Culturally distinctive experiences (e.g., fear of being hexed or bewitched, feeling of "heat in the head" or crawling sensation of worms or ants, or being visited by deceased individuals) must be distinguished from acute hallucinations or delusions. Bipolar disorders tend to be underdiagnosed in some ethnic groups in the United States.

Anxiety Disorders

Panic Disorder With or Without History of Agoraphobia

In certain cultures, panic attacks may be precipitated by intense fear of magic or witchcraft. Some culture-bound syndromes such as *koro* may include features of panic attack associated with fear of genital shrinkage into the body.

Social Phobia

In Japan and Korea, instead of a marked persistent fear of social or performance situations in which embarrassment may occur (Criterion A in DSM-IV-TR), some individuals may develop a persistent and excessive fear of giving offense to others in social situations. In Japan, fears in social phobia in a culture-bound syndrome called *taijin kyofusho* may be in the form of extreme anxiety that blushing, eye-to-eye contact, or one's body odor will be offensive to others.

Posttraumatic Stress Disorder

Recent immigrants from areas with considerable social unrest and war may have higher rates of posttraumatic stress disorder (PTSD). In addition, these immigrants may be reluctant to divulge experiences of torture and trauma for fear of political repercussions or the risk of losing immigrant status.

Younger children may express their traumatic experiences differently from the adults. Distressing dreams of the event may change into generalized nightmares of rescuing others or of threats to self or others. Reliving of the trauma may occur through repetitive play. There may be diminished interest in daily activities, constriction of affect, a sense of foreshortened future, a belief in an ability to foresee future untoward events (omen formation), or complaints of various physical symptoms such as stomachaches and headaches. Clinicians may have to rely on reports from parents, teachers, and other observers in the evaluation of these symptoms.

Somatoform Disorders

Pain Disorder

There is considerable variation among ethnic and cultural groups in their reaction to painful stimuli and in the way they express their reactions to pain. In one classic study, Italian patients, compared with Irish patients, presented with significantly more pain symptoms, had symptoms in significantly more bodily locations, and noted significantly more types of bodily dysfunction (Zola 1966).

Body Dysmorphic Disorder

Cultural factors may influence or amplify preoccupations about an imagined physical defect. *Koro,* a culture-bound syndrome reported primarily in Southeast Asia and characterized by the preoccupation of genital retraction into the abdomen and thoughts of dying, may be related to body dysmorphic disorder but differs from it by its usually brief duration, different associated symptoms of panic and fear of death, positive responses to reassurance, and occasional occurrence in epidemic proportions.

Dissociative Disorders

Dissociative Fugue

Culture-bound syndromes with presumed dissociative features, such as *pibloktoq* (running syndrome) among the Arctic native people, *grisi siknis* among the Miskito of Honduras and Nicaragua, *frenzy* witchcraft among the Navajo, and some form of *amok* in Western Pacific cultures, have been reported. These syndromes may meet criteria for dissociative fugue and are characterized by a sudden onset of a high level of activity, a trancelike state, potentially dangerous behavior in the form of running or fleeing (homicide in *amok*), ensuing exhaustion, sleep, and amnesia for the episode.

Dissociative Disorder Not Otherwise Specified

Possession identity disorder, which involves a replacement of the customary sense of personal identity with a new identity attributed to the influence of a spirit, deity, another person, animal, or even an inanimate object, has been reported in many cultures. Possession trance with stereotypic "involuntary" movements or amnesia may be associated with *amok* (Indonesia), *bebainan* (Indonesia), *latah* (Malaysia), *pibloktoq* (Arctic), *ataque de nervios* (Latin America), and possession (India). Dissociative trance disorder should not be confused with normative-induced trance states in religious or cultural practice.

Sexual and Gender Identity Disorders

Care should be exercised in judging sexual dysfunction. An individual's ethnic, cultural, social, and religious background may influence sexual desire, expectations, and attitude about performance. In some cultures, a higher premium is placed on fertility, and sexual desire on the part of women is given less relevance.

Eating Disorders: Anorexia Nervosa

In industrialized societies, the abundance of food and the cultural idea that attractiveness is linked to thinness for females have been suggested as reasons for the higher prevalence of anorexia nervosa. Immigrants who have assimilated the thin-body idea may likewise be affected. Cultural expression of the motivation for food restriction may vary; instead of a disturbed perception of the body, individuals may complain of epigastric discomfort or distaste for food.

Sleep Disorders: Nightmare Disorder

Interpretation of the significance of nightmares varies across cultures. Some cultures consider nightmares to be signs of spiritual or supernatural phenomena, whereas others may relate it to mental or physical disturbance. A diagnosis of nightmare disorder should not be made unless there is persistent distress or impairment that warrants independent clinical attention.

Impulse-Control Disorders Not Elsewhere Classified: Pathological Gambling

Different cultures have different types of gambling activities (e.g., cockfights, paigo, horse racing, stock market). Clinicians should tailor their treatment to fit the attitude toward gambling in the patient's cultural background and the particular activity gambled on.

Adjustment Disorders

The threshold for maladaptiveness varies because various cultures have different ways of experiencing and coping with stressors and interpreting the meanings of stressors. Clinicians should consider an individual's cultural setting before making a diagnosis of adjustment disorder.

Personality Disorders

Criteria for deviancy vary across cultures. In immigrants, the factors of acculturation and the individual's customary expression of habits, customs, and political or religious values from the culture of origin should be taken into consideration when determining deviancy.

Paranoid Personality Disorder

Care should be made in diagnosing individuals as "paranoid," particularly for minorities, immigrants, political and economic refugees, and individuals from different ethnic backgrounds. These individuals may display a guarded attitude or defensive behavior due to unfamiliarity with the culture of the host society or in response to perceived neglect or indifference. Clinicians may be perceived as "agents" of the host society, thus confounding the issue of mutual trust. These factors should be distinguished from true paranoid personality disorder.

Schizoid Personality Disorder

Inhibited or defensive behavior, as found in some immigrants or migrants, should not be labeled as schizoid. The phenomenon of *emotional freezing* as an adjustment reaction to a new environment has been described in individuals moving from rural to metropolitan areas. This is characterized by solitary activities, constricted affect, and other deficits in communication and should be distinguished from schizoid personality disorder.

Dependent Personality Disorder

Some cultures emphasize passivity, politeness, and deferential treatment. The cultural norm of the individual should be taken into consideration in determining whether dependent behavior is excessive.

Cultural Formulation

DSM-IV-TR's cultural formulation is a set of guidelines that clinicians use as a process of cultural analysis that relates to every clinical encounter. It is a tool to assist the clinician in systematically evaluating and reporting the impact of cultural context in the individual's illness experience and in formulating a treatment plan that will be more congruent with the individual's cultural background. Judgment on deviancy can be inferred by the degree to which an individual behavior deviates from the norm of his or her sociocultural milieu. By being sensitive and attentive to feelings arising from the clinician's own cultural background, the clinician can use his or her understanding of cultural phenomena during the clinical encounter to cope with countertransference issues. Table 40–2 presents the DSM-IV-TR outline for cultural formulation.

Elaboration of the Cultural Formulation

Cultural Identity of the Individual

Clinicians should not make assumptions or prejudge an individual's identity based solely on the physical appearance of a person on the first clinical encounter. During the interview it is important to query how the patient defines him- or herself: "Considering your ethnic background, help me understand how you would define yourself." At the end of the interview, it is also helpful to ask, "After all that you've said, what is the one thing about you and your illness that you want me to know?" The revelations to such questions may further open important leads relevant to the presenting complaints that led the individual to seek psychiatric help in the first place.

Cultural Explanation of the Illness

To make sense out of a usually fearful chaotic experience during the course of a psychiatric illness, each afflicted individual usually has his or her own notion of the cause, nature, and remedies for the presenting problem(s). These ideas are usually concealed from the examiner due to shame (fear of being "laughed upon") or fear of being ignored. Yet such notions of illness may powerfully influence how one conceptualizes illness and seeks remedies. If an illness is deemed to be caused by the "evil spirit," a local healer, a priest or pastor, or a shaman will most likely be consulted and remedies such as shamanistic healing, other native or indigenous practices, prayers, or religious healing rituals may be sought and applied. If it is conceptualized as a "physical" illness, such as a fear of cancer, the patient will most likely seek Western-oriented medical practitioners.

Cultural Factors Related to the Psychosocial Environment of the Patient

Culture influences the construction of the social matrix of each individual. For example, Caucasians, who tend to value personal autonomy and independence, may construct their social relations and networks differently from Asians, who tend to value interdependence. A strong sense of social cohesiveness, family-orientedness, and regionalism is found among Filipinos (Sanchez and Gaw 2007, p. 811). Such sentiments have evolved out of the necessity of Filipinos living together in the various islands of the Philippine archipelago.

The degree of stress or distress caused by the disruption of such relations or networks may vary across

TABLE 40–2. DSM-IV-TR outline for cultural formulation

The following outline for cultural formulation is meant to supplement the multiaxial diagnostic assessment and to address difficulties that may be encountered in applying DSM-IV criteria in a multicultural environment. The cultural formulation provides a systematic review of the individual's cultural background, the role of the cultural context in the expression and evaluation of symptoms and dysfunction, and the effect that cultural differences may have on the relationship between the individual and the clinician.

As indicated in the introduction to the manual (see DSM-IV-TR, page xxxiii), it is important that the clinician take into account the individual's ethnic and cultural context in the evaluation of each of the DSM-IV axes. In addition, the cultural formulation suggested below provides an opportunity to describe systematically the individual's cultural and social reference group and ways in which the cultural context is relevant to clinical care. The clinician may provide a narrative summary for each of the following categories:

Cultural identity of the individual.   Note the individual's ethnic or cultural reference groups. For immigrants and ethnic minorities, note separately the degree of involvement with both the culture of origin and the host culture (where applicable). Also note language abilities, use, and preference (including multilingualism).

Cultural explanations of the individual's illness.   The following may be identified: the predominant idioms of distress through which symptoms or the need for social support are [is] communicated (e.g., "nerves," possessing spirits, somatic complaints, inexplicable misfortune), the meaning and perceived severity of the individual's symptoms in relation to norms of the cultural reference group, any local illness category used by the individual's family and community to identify the condition (see "Glossary of Culture-Bound Syndromes" below), the perceived causes or explanatory models that the individual and the reference group use to explain the illness, and current preferences for and past experiences with professional and popular sources of care.

Cultural factors related to psychosocial environment and levels of functioning.   Note culturally relevant interpretations of social stressors, available social supports, and levels of functioning and disability. This would include stresses in the local social environment and the role of religion and kin networks in providing emotional, instrumental, and informational support.

Cultural elements of the relationship between the individual and the clinician.   Indicate differences in culture and social status between the individual and the clinician and problems that these differences may cause in diagnosis and treatment (e.g., difficulty in communicating in the individual's first language, in eliciting symptoms or understanding their cultural significance, in negotiating an appropriate relationship or level of intimacy, in determining whether a behavior is normative or pathological).

Overall cultural assessment for diagnosis and care.   The formulation concludes with a discussion of how cultural considerations specifically influence comprehensive diagnosis and care.

Source.   Reprinted from American Psychiatric Association: *Diagnostic and Statistical Manual of Mental Disorders*, 4th Edition, Text Revision. Washington, DC, American Psychiatric Association, 2000, pp. 897–898. Copyright 2000. Used with permission.

individuals in different cultures with different value orientations.

Cultural Element of the Relationship Between Patient and Clinician

Cultural factors mediated through the transference/ countertransference axis can influence the expressive transaction (rapport) and instrumental transaction (technical information) between the patient and clinician. Unconscious, inherent biases may intrude upon the patient–doctor relationship and hinder interaction. Many minority patients may be extremely sensitive to the *power differential* between themselves and the clinician. How one relates to all patients, particularly during the first encounter, critically affects the perception of the patients toward the clinician. It is important to show respect, sensitivity, acceptance, openness, and interest through words and actions during the clinical interview.

Overall Cultural Assessment for Diagnosis and Care

Formulating cultural factors and issues that are related to the patient's chief complaints should be as rigorous as in the exercise of a psychodynamic formulation. A comprehensive picture of all possible antecedents of the patient's illness should emerge at the conclusion of a diagnostic interview. Possible cultural factors should be clearly noted and discussed with the patient in the formulation of the genesis of the patient's problems and in the formulation of a treatment plan (Lim 2006). The patient could be empowered by the clinician asking for his or her feedback about the diagnosis and care plan.

Culture-Bound Syndromes

In various parts of the world, there are unique patterns of aberrant behavior and troubling experiences whose clinical descriptions do not readily fit into the Western conventional diagnostic categories of DSM-IV-TR or ICD-10 (World Health Organization 1992). Yet these patterns of behavior are considered by the indigenous population as "illnesses." The form, content, and frequency of such categories uniquely reflect the culture and the social condition in which they occur. They assume salient expressions for communicating distress (idioms of expression) and may even have localized folk diagnostic names that frame coherent meanings. In certain situations, the frequency of presentation has assumed epidemic proportions, as in the occurrence of at least four *koro* epidemics in Southeast Asia in recent decades. These categories are labeled as *culture-bound syndromes,* a term coined by Yap (1969) in Hong Kong and now adopted for official use in DSM-IV-TR.

DSM-IV-TR is inconclusive about the classification of many of the so-called culture-bound syndromes. However, it does include a "Glossary of Culture-Bound Syndromes" in its Appendix I (see Appendix A at the end of this chapter) to encourage further research and refinement of diagnosis. Below I introduce some of the better-known culture-bound syndromes and suggest a provisional way of classifying them in DSM-IV-TR.

Amok

Amok is a Malaysian term for a homicidal frenzy preceded by a state of brooding and ending with somnolence and amnesia. Afflicted individuals are usually young or middle-aged males living away from home. Precipitating factors may be a recent loss, an insult, or incidences causing such a person to "lose face."

Ataque de Nervios

Ataque de nervios is characterized by sudden onset of uncontrollable shouting, trembling, heart palpitations, a sensation of heat in the chest rising to the head, fainting, and seizure-like activities in response to acute stressful experiences, such as grief during funerals, threats, the scene of an accident, or a family conflict. Often a person may temporarily lose consciousness.

Amnesia of the episode may occur upon regaining consciousness. Considered a culturally sanctioned response to acute stresses among Puerto Ricans and Latinos, *ataque* usually afflicts socially disadvantaged women older than 45 years with less than a high school education. It is unclear how *ataque* should be classified in DSM-IV-TR.

Brain Fag

Brain fag is characterized by complaints of the brain being "fatigued," with unpleasant head symptoms of burning, a crawling sensation, and a feeling of "vacancy"; visual symptoms of blurry vision, eye pain, and excessive tearing; an inability to grasp the meaning of printed symbols or spoken words; poor memory retention; and fatigue and sleepiness in spite of adequate rest. The term originated in West Africa, and the condition affects primarily male students under the stress of schooling. Brain fag has been compared with *neurasthenia* in Chinese, *hwa-byung* in Koreans, and *susto* in Latinos. Cases of brain fag have been reported to respond to antidepressants, antianxiety medications, and relaxation therapy. Many scholars consider brain fag to be a culturally mediated anxiety, depressive, or somatoform syndrome.

Hwa-Byung

Hwa-byung means "fiery illness" in Korean. Because "fire" is an Asian metaphysical expression of anger, *hwa-byung* is literally translated as an "illness of anger." Afflicted individuals complain of a feeling of oppression or pressure in the chest, a "mass" in the epigastrium or stomach, a hot sensation traveling up the chest or in the body, indigestion, dyspnea, fatigue, sighing, and headache. Emotional symptoms include fearfulness, panic, dysphoria, sad mood, nihilistic thoughts, loss of interest, suicidal ideas, and guilt. The illness affects women more than men.

Kim (1993) attributes *hwa-byung* to suppression of chronic anger and indignation in Korea, where there is a long history of foreign colonization and subjugation and a culture in which open expression of feeling is not encouraged.

Koro

Koro is characterized by the sudden onset of acute anxiety and panic associated with the fear of genital retraction into the abdomen and the idea of dying as a result. The condition generally affects lower-educated males, but female cases of concern of labial or breast retractions have also been reported (Bernstein and Gaw 1990). Epidemics of *koro* have been reported in Singapore, Thailand, Hainan Island of China, and India. During such epidemics, patients may be brought into the emergency department with family members, relatives, or the patient himself holding the patient's penis or using wooden clamps or strings to prevent the penis from "retracting" into the abdomen. The condition is self-limiting and could be relieved by persuasion, explanation, and education.

The term *koro* is believed to derive from a Malaysian word meaning "tortoise." The symbolic association of *koro* with the phenomenon of the retraction of the head of the turtle into its body is readily apparent. Similar conditions are described as *suk-yeong* in Cantonese Chinese, *suo-yang* among Mandarin Chinese, *jinjinia bemar* in Assam, and *rok-joo* in Thailand.

Latah

Latah is characterized by hypersensitivity to sudden fright or startle, often with echopraxia, echolalia, command obedience, and dissociative or trancelike behavior. Afflicted individuals typically respond to a sudden stimulus with an exaggerated startle, sometimes dropping or throwing objects held in the hand and often uttering obscene words. Such individuals are often the objects of amusement. Most cases of *latah* are in women of low socioeconomic status.

Latah is well described among the Malays. Outside Malay, similar conditions include *amurakh, irkunii, ikota, olan, myriachit, menkeiti, bahtschhi, imu, mali-mali, silok,* and *jumping.* Simons and Hughes (1985) consider *latah* to be a culture-specific elaboration of the potential of the startle reflex.

Pibloktoq

Pibloktoq, also called *arctic hysteria,* is characterized by abrupt episodes of extreme excitement often followed by "seizures" and transient "coma." It is reported among the Arctic and Subarctic Eskimos and affects women more than men. Afflicted individuals may show prodromes of tiredness, depressive silences, vagueness of expression, and confusion for several days. During attacks, individuals may exhibit superhuman strength and aberrant motor and verbal behaviors such as tearing off clothing and becoming partially or completely nude, fleeing, rolling in snow, jumping into water, picking up or throwing things, performing mimetic acts, and engaging in choreiform movements, glossolalia, and coprophagia. Following attacks, individuals may weep, show body tremor, become feverish with bloodshot eyes, and have a high pulse rate. The exhausted individual may sleep for hours. Rational behavior is resumed after waking.

Consistent with Eskimo culture, afflicted individuals, particularly women, are thought to express their sense of acute helplessness and traumatized ego with panic or anxiety in a regressive fashion.

Possession Disorder

Possession disorder is characterized by the experience of one's identity being taken over by another entity that may involve a person, god, demon, spirit, animal, or even an inanimate object. Afflicted individuals may have a single or episodic disturbance of consciousness, identity, or memory associated with loss of control over their actions, loss of awareness of their surroundings, change in the tone of their voice, and loss of perceived sensitivity to pain (Gaw et al. 1998). Women are more often affected than men. Afflicted individuals usually are of lower socioeconomic and educational background.

Possession disorder is found worldwide and in all cultures. Possession states are considered normal when the phenomenon occurs in the context of a broadly accepted collective cultural or religious practice.

Shenjing Shuairuo

Shenjing shuairuo is characterized by feelings of physical and mental exhaustion, difficulty in concentration, memory loss, fatigue, dizziness, insomnia, loss of appetite, sexual dysfunction, irritability, and headaches. The term in Mandarin Chinese literally means "weakness of the nervous system." It is a prominent syndrome among Chinese. It is also known also as *neurasthenia* in the West. Although neurasthenia currently is not an official category in DSM-IV-TR, it is officially included in the *Chinese Classification of Mental Disorders, Second Edition* (Chinese Society of Psychiatry 1989), and in ICD-10.

Taijin Kyofusho

Taijin kyofusho is characterized by an extreme concern that one's body, body parts, or bodily functions may offend, embarrass, or displease others. Symptoms include fear of embarrassment; blushing; causing discomfort by one's gaze, facial expression, or body odor; or offending others by speaking one's thoughts aloud. Considered a culture-specific social phobia among Japanese, the condition primarily affects young people, particularly in interpersonal situations.

Proposed Classification of Culture-Bound Syndromes in DSM-IV-TR

To arrive at a diagnosis of a culture-bound syndrome in DSM-IV-TR, the following criteria have been proposed:

1. The disorder must be a discrete, well-defined syndrome.
2. It must be recognized as a specific illness in the culture with which it is primarily associated.
3. The disorder must be expected, recognized, and to some degree sanctioned as a response to certain precipitants in the particular culture.
4. A higher incidence or prevalence of the disorder must exist in societies in which the disorder is culturally recognized, compared with other societies.

It is important before arriving at a diagnosis of a culture-bound syndrome that presenting complaints mimicking diagnostic categories in Axes I, II, and III are ruled out. A true culture-bound syndrome diagnosis should be reserved for a clinical entity that fulfills the criteria just proposed. Figure 40–1 presents a proposed decision tree for arriving at such a diagnosis.

Cultural Factors in Nonadherence to Psychotropic Medications[1]

Nonadherence is defined as "the extent to which the patient's behavior (in terms of taking medications, following diets, or executing other life-style changes) *does not* coincide with medical or health advice" (Haynes et al. 1979, p. 1, italics added). It is a widespread and serious challenge in the United States and elsewhere in the world. Sackett and Haynes (1976) estimated that at least 50% of patients do not adhere to physicians' prescribed medication regimens. In various cultural settings, psychotropic medication nonadherence is also a serious and prevalent problem among psychiatric patients. A follow-up study of 406 patients 2 years after discharge from a psychiatric hospital in South Africa revealed nonadherence rates for oral phenothiazines

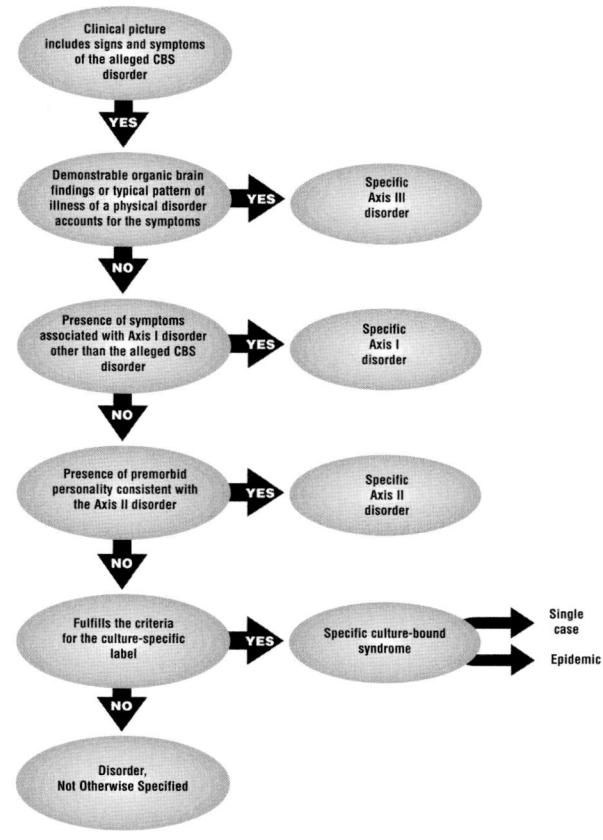

FIGURE 40–1. Proposed decision tree for culture-bound syndromes (CBSs) in DSM-IV.

Source. Reprinted from Gaw AC: *Concise Guide to Cross-Cultural Psychiatry.* Washington, DC, American Psychiatric Publishing, 2001, p. 92. Copyright 2001, American Psychiatric Publishing. Used with permission.

were about two-thirds for black patients, one-half for mixed racial ("colored") patients, and one-quarter for white patients (Gillis et al. 1987).

Nonadherence to medication regimens should be addressed just like any other pressing clinical challenge. The challenge is for the physician and other health professionals to understand the various potential reasons behind a patient's refusal of medications and to systematically examine the challenge from the perspective of the patient. The differential diagnosis of factors contributing to nonadherence and the formulation of appropriate intervention strategies should be as rigorous as the exercise in arriving at a clinical diagnosis.

---

[1] I wish to acknowledge John A. Nichols, Psy.D., for his contributions to this section.

Sociocultural Factors Affecting Psychopharmacotherapy and Nonadherence

Physicians prescribing medications and drug researchers interested in the efficacy of medication effects have long noted the importance of "nonpharmacological" factors such as placebo effect in patients' responses to medications (Lin et al. 1993). These supposedly "nonbiological" effects, thought to be mediated through a symbolic mechanism, are estimated to range from 30% to 70% among the therapeutic responses with any treatment method. In spite of this, Lin et al. (1993) noted that, paradoxically, in the midst of the current fervor of pharmacological research, less is known about and directed toward the sociocultural and symbolic factors that affect drug responses than about biological mechanisms mediated through kinetics, genetics, and dynamics. What meager information we have is unsystematic and mostly anecdotal. In spite of this, it is important to begin addressing these "nonpharmacological variables" in drug responses. Some of the factors, such as health beliefs and nonadherence, were mentioned earlier in the chapter and are further elaborated here. Table 40–3 lists some of the key sociocultural factors that influence noncompliance with psychotropic medications.

Physician Biases in Diagnosis and Prescribing

Physicians' biases in prescribing are reflected in reports of racial differences in psychiatric diagnosis and psychotropic drug responses for many diagnostic categories. For example, although the U.S. Epidemiologic Catchment Area study (Robins et al. 1991) revealed no significant differences in the prevalence of affective disorders between African Americans and Caucasians, African Americans are more likely to receive a diagnosis of schizophrenia rather than affective disorder in clinical practice (Adebimpe 1994). A number of anxiety disorders, including obsessive-compulsive disorder, panic disorder, phobic disorder, and PTSD, are often underrecognized or underdiagnosed in African Americans compared with Caucasians (Lawson 1996a, 1996b). The reasons for misdiagnosis remain unclear. However, the consequences of such misdiagnosis for African American patients are serious and can include delay in the implementation of appropriate medications such as lithium therapy for bipolar disorder, the prescribing of antipsychotic medications when not indicated, the use of higher dosages of antipsychotic medications and more frequent use of as-needed medications, and the greater likelihood of receiving a depot medication.

TABLE 40–3. Key sociocultural factors contributing to nonadherence to psychotropic medications

Physician biases in diagnosis and prescribing

Health beliefs

Concomitant use of herbal and Western medicine

Diet

Religious beliefs

Placebo effect

Cost and availability of medications

Similarly, Hispanics with a confirmed diagnosis of bipolar disorder were far more likely to receive an initial diagnosis of schizophrenia (Mukherjee et al. 1983). Heterogeneity among the Hispanic subgroups and the presence of culture-bound syndromes may also confound the diagnostic picture (Mendoza et al. 1991). Some studies suggest that the dosage requirements for tricyclic agents among Hispanic women may be different from those of their Caucasian counterparts. A retrospective chart review of Hispanic female clinic patients showed a comparable treatment outcome when given only half the dosage of tricyclic antidepressant (Marcos and Cancro 1982). Thus, if the customary dosage of tricyclic antidepressants used for Caucasians were prescribed for this population, the possibility of more complaints of side effects may occur. Indeed, more Hispanic patients in this cohort were found to complain of side effects (78% vs. 33% for Caucasian patients) and to prematurely discontinue their medication.

Among Asian patients, failure to factor in body size and potential variance due to poor metabolization of certain enzymes may lead to more reports of side effects when patients are given the usual recommended *Physicians' Desk Reference* dosages.

Thus, among ethnic patients in the United States, some studies suggest that drug dosages, patterns of drug usage, and drug nonadherence may differ from mainstream middle-class Caucasian patients. Clinicians who are increasingly involved in the care of ethnic patients need to be cognizant of such variations to drug reactions.

Health Beliefs and Alternative Healing Traditions and Practices

In many non-Western cultures, long traditions of indigenous systems of healing coexist with modern Western scientific medical healing systems. Examples of indigenous healing systems include the Traditional

Chinese Medical System and Asian Indian Ayurvedic Medicine. These traditional medical practices may influence patients' choices and reactions to modern treatment modalities, including drugs. For example, Chinese medical concepts such as *chi* and "energy flows" often shape the conceptions and responses of Chinese patients in the use of Western medicine (Gaw 1993). Indeed, discordance between professional and lay conceptions of causal attributions may determine the patient's satisfaction with treatment, medication adherence, and clinical outcome (Lin et al. 1993).

The study by Sing Lee (1993) in Hong Kong is instructive and illustrates that patients' reactions to the side effects of medications may vary according to their health beliefs. In a biocultural study of the report of side effects among 70 Hong Kong Chinese patients receiving chronic lithium therapy, Sing Lee found that there was "an imperfect correspondence between biomedically prescribed and culturally endorsed psychotropic side effects" (p. 301). Contrary to the usual reports of Western patients, Hong Kong patients did not usually regard the side effects of polydipsia and polyuria as bothersome symptoms or translate them into metaphors used to express undesirable side effects. Although complaints of tiredness, drowsiness, and poor memory were common, their frequency was significantly lower than in control subjects. Chinese patients had no conceptual equivalent for the complaint of "loss of creativity." Complaints of "missing of highs," loss of assertiveness, and fear of weight gain were rarely encountered.

Health beliefs are often reflected in varying ethnic expectations of Western and herbal drug actions. With the trend toward greater popularity of "alternative" or nontraditional healing methods, many individuals may simply reject the notion of introducing any "non-organic" chemical substance into the body. Many ethnic patients regard Western medications as providing quicker action and therefore being most appropriate for treating acute illness (Lin et al. 1993). In contrast, some patients regard herbal drugs as having less tendency to induce side effects, and thus they delay or avoid taking necessary Western medications. Concerns about the addictive and toxic effects of drugs among Hispanics and African Americans in the United States may lead them to avoid taking needed medications for a longer period and may lead to premature termination of medications and psychiatric care. On the other hand, in many Asian countries where concoctions of multiple herbal drugs, as in traditional medical practice, are usually prescribed, polypharmacy may come to be an accepted norm of medical practice.

Concomitant Use of Herbal and Western Medications

With the increasing popularity of alternative healing methods in Western countries, the use of herbal drugs has also increased (Eisenberg et al. 1993). More patients are now resorting to concomitant use of herbal drugs and Western medicines. In the United States, this is especially true in some minority communities. Some herbal drugs have been shown to possess active pharmacological properties that may interact with current psychotropic medications (Lin et al. 1993). Some Chinese herbal drugs were found to induce cytochrome P450 hepatic enzymatic actions (Allen et al. 1977). Other herbs have inhibitory effects.

Diet

That different cultural groups have varying food preferences is a widely accepted fact. In recent years, more studies have documented the effect of diet on liver microsomal enzymes and the drugs metabolized by these enzymes. Cross-cultural differences of diet on metabolizing enzymes have been ably documented in a study comparing differences in biotransformation of drugs between Asian Indians living in India and those who have immigrated to Great Britain. Biotransformation of both antipyrine and clomipramine was shown to take longer among Asian Indians maintained on their traditional vegetarian diet as compared with those who had switched to a British diet (Allen et al. 1977; Fraser et al. 1979).

Religious Beliefs

Certain religious groups discourage members from taking medications. Patients with such strong religious beliefs who present with psychiatric symptoms such as uncontrollable bipolar mood swings may feel extremely conflicted and guilty when asked to take mood regulators. The chance that such patients will avoid or discontinue medications is high, and special efforts are needed to address their religious concerns and beliefs.

Placebo Effects

Placebo effects are presumably mediated through symbolic mechanisms and are estimated to account for 30%–70% of the therapeutic responses to any treatment (Lin et al. 1993). When responses of a matched group of patients with endogenous depression to the tricyclic antidepressants trazodone and imipramine versus placebo were compared between whites and blacks in the United States and Colombia, no significant differences were found between trazodone and placebo in any of the three groups. Response to imipramine was significantly better than that to placebo in all three groups, and the Colombian patients improved more regardless of treatment, including the placebo treatment (Escobar and Tuason 1980). Thus, ethnic variation even in placebo effects should be kept in mind when assessing drug response.

Cost and Availability of Medications

The escalating costs and limitations on availability of psychotropic medications have been found to be factors in nonadherence (Pi and Gray 1998). When patients are on limited fixed incomes and are faced with a choice between food and medications, the need for medications often loses out. In an effort to control escalating costs of psychotropic medications, agencies and managed care companies have often resorted to the use of a drug formulary as a means of controlling cost. When it is determined which drugs will be included or excluded in the drug formulary, the factor of ethnic variation in response to psychotropic drugs is often ignored. As a result, drugs that have been found useful for certain ethnic groups may be made unavailable or may be discouraged from being prescribed.

Quantity and Quality of Social Support

The quality and quantity of social support have been linked to treatment outcome and drug responses. Depending on the quality of family involvement, patients whose family members have high expressed emotion (characterized by frequent criticism, hostility, and emotional overinvolvement) were found to be more likely to relapse on standard neuroleptic dosages (Anderson et al. 1986; Falloon et al. 1984). Although limited, some data revealed that various ethnic groups vary on their expressed emotion ratings. Some studies showed Caucasian American families more likely to have higher expressed emotion scores compared with their British counterparts. Hispanic families tended to score lower than Caucasian Americans and Caucasian Britons (Jenkins and Karno 1992; Keefe et al. 1978). Whether these findings translate into true causative factors for certain mental illness remains to be seen. Clinically, it is not difficult to appreciate the fact that when family members subject mentally ill patients to frequent negative criticisms, the patients would experience more stress and may be more at risk of relapse despite adequate neuroleptic dosages. Indeed, Lieberman and Strauss (1984) have shown that when bipolar patients were subjected to intense interpersonal conflicts, they experienced more relapses despite receiving adequate lithium dosages.

On the contrary, the findings from two multinational follow-up studies on the outcome of schizophrenia by the World Health Organization revealed a more favorable outcome in non-Western patients and indicated that they have more social support as compared to their Western counterparts (Jablensky et al. 1992). These findings lent credence to the postulate that social support influences the course of mental illness and the degree of adherence to psychotropic medications.

Strategies for Enhancing Medication Adherence

Considering the just-mentioned factors affecting nonadherence, a clinical protocol, "Clinician's Inquiry Into the Meanings of Taking Psychotropic Medications" (Table 40–4), may be helpful in enhancing adherence. This format can be integrated into the interview when exploring the patient's potential reaction to medications or when the problem of nonadherence emerges. Once the reason for nonadherence is identified, therapeutic strategies can be accordingly directed to it.

Culture and Psychotherapy

Defining Psychotherapy

Jerome Frank defined *psychotherapy* as "a planned, emotionally charged, confiding interaction between a trained, socially sanctioned healer and a sufferer" (Frank 1982, p. 10). Given that psychotherapists seek to interpret and transform the meanings of patients' communications, Frank (1987) concluded that psychotherapy resembles rhetoric and hermeneutics:

> All psychotherapeutic endeavors, whatever their form, transpire entirely in the realm of meanings. All psychotherapies depend on the fact that human thinking, feeling, and behavior are guided by the person's assumptions about reality, that is, meanings that he or she attributes to events and experiences, rather than their objective properties (p. 10).

Because the meanings of the events and experiences of an individual are rooted in the cultural milieu, culture provides the *context* against which an individual's event or experience is interpreted and imbued with meaning—that is, the "internal reality" to which the individual responds (Frank 1982). The job of the therapist is to "decipher" this meaning system and reframe it in a manner that will make sense for the patient. Cultural metaphors, language, and explanations that are con-

TABLE 40–4. Clinician's inquiry into the meanings of taking psychotropic medication

1. Do you have any feelings about taking medication(s)? What does it mean for you to take medication(s)?

2. What would your family, friends, (or your significant others) think of you if you take medication(s)?

3. What, if any, are your concerns about the effects and/or side effects of your medication(s)?

4. Do you have any religious beliefs regarding the taking of medications?

5. What are the benefits of taking medications?

6. What are the benefits of not taking medications?

7. Would the color, size, or form of medications mean anything to you?

8. Do you have any concerns about losing control if you take medication? (If yes, please elaborate.)

9. Does the possibility of change, even if it is positive change, make you worried or uncomfortable? (If yes, please elaborate.)

10. Would taking medication change the way you view yourself? (If yes, please elaborate.)

11. Would taking medication affect your self-esteem? (If yes, please elaborate.)

12. Can you tell me more about your specific worries or dilemmas you have when thinking about medication?

Source. Reprinted from Gaw AC: *Concise Guide to Cross-Cultural Psychiatry.* Washington, DC, American Psychiatric Publishing, 2001, p. 158. Copyright 2001, American Psychiatric Publishing. Used with permission.

gruous with the patient's background become important venues to transmit these messages. The skillful therapist pays attention to these communication devices to convey meanings and hopefully assists the patient to take appropriate actions toward recovery.

The meaning of an illness varies according the cultural background of the individual. For example, a white, athletic, middle-class male who regards his body as a "perfect machine" may develop depression as a result of a heart attack if his self-esteem is so tied up with his body image that he perceives his newly injured body to be a "broken machine." He may sense the threat to his self-esteem and body integrity with all the ramifications of such a threat to himself, his family, and his job. As a result, he may feel "vulnerable" and psychologically impotent and have lower self-esteem.

These thoughts could spiral downward to the point that he may feel life is worthless and meaningless and thus becomes depressed.

For an Asian immigrant holding traditional family values, the impact of a heart attack may assume a different meaning, as the following case illustrates:

An elderly Chinese woman developed severe depression after having a heart attack and was admitted to a local hospital in Boston. The patient refused to talk, eat, or drink. She was slowly slipping into metabolic difficulties. A psychiatric consultation was initiated to consider the possibility of electroconvulsive therapy. In the course of psychiatric interview, the patient revealed that she had developed chest pain after she returned from a visit to New York City during which she had been ignored by her son and daughter-in-law, both of whom had to work during the day. She was left alone in the apartment and felt very lonely and rejected. When she returned home, she suffered a heart attack and was literally "broken hearted." She sank into a state of severe depression.

The meaning of the heart attack for this Chinese woman was the rejection she felt from an unfilial son. She became "broken hearted." Discovery of this meaning led to an intervention in which the wishes of the patient and the dynamic meaning of the illness were communicated to the son and his family. A family meeting was arranged in which reconciliation was made. The patient began to take sips of tea and ate the food brought in by her son. With active family intervention, she eventually pulled out of depression without the use of medications or electroconvulsive therapy.

Providing Psychotherapy Across Cultural Groups

When providing psychotherapy to persons of different cultural backgrounds, it is important to appropriately apply cultural knowledge to the particular therapeutic process in the context of the patient's/client's culture. Sue and Zane (1987) studied two basic elements in the therapeutic process in which cultural knowledge can provide positive influence: credibility and giving. *Credibility* refers to the client's perception of the therapist as an effective and trustworthy helper. The therapist's credibility is imparted through two elements:

1. *The position or role assigned by others.* Diplomas, certificates of specialty board examination, plaques of recognition, and certificates of affiliation or membership in professional organizations all convey certain impressions regarding the competency of the therapist and supposedly confer status. These cultural symbols, when used appropriately, enhance the therapist's credibility and are called *ascribed status.*

2. *The skills the therapist applies to the therapeutic process.* The ability to make a correct diagnosis, prescribe drugs that ameliorate symptoms, make appropriate interpretations of hidden meanings of dysfunctional behavior, and use language to motivate the patient to change maladaptive patterns of thinking, feeling, and behaving are therapeutic skills consolidated through years of experience and are called *achieved credibility.*

Knowledge of culture can strengthen the therapist's credibility in at least three ways:

1. Conceptualizing the client's problem in a manner that is congruent with the client's belief systems
2. Providing culturally appropriate means for problem resolution
3. Defining goals that are compatible between therapist and client (Sue and Zane 1987)

Giving is the client's perception that something is received from the therapist during the clinical encounter. The act of giving could be something as concrete as prescribing drugs or giving drug samples, or it can involve verbal interventions such as interpretation of puzzling symptoms, assurances, clarification of life goals, advice about coping strategies, or recommendations about diet or exercise. These symbolic "gifts" must be culturally appropriate to achieve their maximum therapeutic impact.

The above case example of the Chinese woman with depression and the therapeutic intervention strategies guided by knowledge of Asian cultural values illustrates the usefulness and power of applying appropriate cultural knowledge in the treatment process.

Implications for Psychotherapists and Counselors

The following points are useful to keep in mind when conducting psychotherapy across cultures:

1. *Psychotherapy is culture-bound.* Both patients and therapists are the epitome of their unique cultural heritage. It behooves both patients and therapists to understand how their respective cultural heritages affect the therapeutic encounter.
2. *Transference and countertransference phenomena may be accentuated in the cross-cultural encounter.* Conducting therapy across cultural groups is both a rewarding and demanding experience. Variation in cultural percepts and concepts, propositions, values, beliefs, and operating procedures may accentuate transference and countertransference feelings.

3. *Therapists must be cognizant of the micro- as well as macro-sociocultural issues that may influence the structure and processes of the therapeutic relationship.* The demands of third-party payers and institutional requirements may intrude on the therapeutic relationship and undermine trust and confidentiality.
4. *There is a need for comparative research on psychotherapy across cultures.* Both the structure and processes of symbolic healing in psychotherapy need to be examined across cultures.

In conclusion, placed in a cultural context, both the structure and processes of psychotherapy could be examined with an emphasis on elucidation of the power of symbolic healing. Psychotherapists practicing in increasingly diverse cultures should be cognizant of the cultural variables that affect their interactions with patients, and vice versa. Understanding of cultural factors can be maximized to enhance the therapeutic process and outcomes.

Conclusion

This chapter has addressed cultural issues that enable psychiatrists and mental health clinicians to gain perspectives on the context of their patients' psychiatric experiences and the meanings of their illnesses. Sociocultural knowledge aids the diagnostic process and the formulation of treatment plans that are congruent with the patient's background.

DSM-IV-TR has begun to include more cultural information. It has provided an outline of cultural formulation that can serve as a template in eliciting and organizing cultural data in the diagnostic workup as well as a glossary of culture-bound syndromes for further research consideration, and it requires the clinician to consider "Specific Culture, Age, and Gender Features" when making a diagnostic assessment.

This chapter adds breadth and depth to the efforts advanced by DSM-IV-TR's Cultural Task Force. It explicates the concepts of culture, elaborates DSM's cultural formulation, and discusses technical aspects of the psychiatric interview in eliciting cultural data. It also provides a more in-depth discussion of the better-known culture-bound syndromes and proposes a scheme to integrate and incorporate the culture-bound syndromes into the DSM-IV-TR diagnostic categories. Furthermore, the chapter addresses key cultural clinical issues faced by psychiatrists in the clinical encounter: cultural factors in nonadherence to psychotropic medications and cultural issues in psychotherapy.

Key Points

- Culture aids psychiatric diagnosis and treatment by providing a *context* to understand a patient's distress and its symbolic meanings.

- Culture is a set of standards for behavior that a group or individual uses to orient him- or herself and that guides a person's behavior in all social circumstances, including illness behavior.

- Components of culture include percepts, concepts, propositions, beliefs, values, and operational procedures (recipes).

- Essential features of culture include the following:
  - It is learned.
  - It refers to systems of meanings.
  - It acts as a shaping template.
  - It is taught and reproduced.
  - It exists in a constant state of change.
  - It includes patterns of both subjective and objective elements of human behavior.

- DSM-IV-TR's cultural formulation is a tool to elicit pertinent cultural data in the clinical encounter.

- Culture-bound syndromes are recurrent, locality-specific patterns of aberrant behavior and troubling experiences that are indigenously considered to be "illnesses," or at least afflictions. They are generally limited to specific societies or culture areas.

- Most culture-bound syndromes could be included in the "disorders not otherwise specified" in each of the relevant DSM-IV-TR diagnostic categories.

- Sociocultural factors that may influence drug prescribing and the taking of drugs include (but are not limited to) physician biases, patient beliefs and expectations, placebo effects, cost and availability of medications, family support, and patient adherence or nonadherence to medications.

- Sociocultural factors in psychotropic drug nonadherence are less well studied than biological factors, but they exert powerful influences on drug nonadherence.

- The phenomenon of psychotropic drug nonadherence could be understood. The contributing factors of nonadherence should be as rigorously addressed as other challenging clinical problems.

- Psychotherapy conducted across diverse cultures can be exciting, but it also is more demanding, because it requires knowledge and sensitivity to local cultural norms.

Suggested Readings

American Psychiatric Association: Diagnostic and Statistical Manual of Mental Illness, 4th Edition, Text Revision. Washington, DC, American Psychiatric Association, 2000

Gaw AC (ed): Culture, Ethnicity, and Mental Illness. Washington, DC, American Psychiatric Press, 1993

Gaw AC: Concise Guide to Cross-Cultural Psychiatry. Washington, DC, American Psychiatric Press, 2001

Kleinman A: Rethinking Psychiatry. New York, Free Press, 1988

Lim RF (ed): Clinical Manual of Cultural Psychiatry. Arlington, VA, American Psychiatric Publishing, 2006

Lin KM, Poland RE, Nakasaki G (eds): Psychopharmacology and Psychobiology of Ethnicity. Washington, DC, American Psychiatric Press, 1993

References

Adebimpe VR: Race, racism, and epidemiologic surveys. Hosp Community Psychiatry 45:27–31, 1994

Allen JJ, Rack PH, Vaddadi KS: Differences in the effects of clomipramine on English and Asian volunteers: preliminary report on a pilot study. Postgrad Med J 53 (suppl):79–86, 1977

American Psychiatric Association: Diagnostic and Statistical Manual of Mental Disorders, 4th Edition, Text Revision. Washington, DC, American Psychiatric Association, 2000

Anderson CM, Reiss DJ, Hogarty GE (eds): Schizophrenia and the Family: A Practitioner's Guide to Psychoeducation and Management. New York, Guilford, 1986

Bernstein RL, Gaw AC: Koro: proposed classification for the DSM-IV. Am J Psychiatry 147:1670–1674, 1990

Chinese Society of Psychiatry: Chinese Classification of Mental Disorders, 2nd Edition (in Chinese). Hunan, China, Hunan Medical University, 1989

Eisenberg DM, Kessler RC, Foster C, et al: Unconventional medicine in the United States: prevalence, costs, and patterns of use. N Engl J Med 328:246–252, 1993

Engel GL: The clinical application of the biopsychosocial model. Am J Psychiatry 137:535–544, 1980

Escobar JI, Tuason VB: Antidepressant agents: a cross-cultural study. Psychopharmacol Bull 16:49–52, 1980

Falloon IRH, Boyd JL, McGill CW (eds): Family Care of Schizophrenia: A Problem-Solving Approach to the Treatment of Mental Illness. New York, Guilford, 1984

Frank JD: Therapeutic components shared by all psychotherapies, in Psychotherapy Research and Behavior Change (Master Lecture Series, Vol 1). Edited by Harvey JH, Parks MM. Washington, DC, American Psychological Association, 1982, pp 9–37

Frank JD: Psychotherapy, rhetoric, hermeneutics: implications for practice and research. Psychotherapy 24:293–302, 1987

Fraser HS, Mucklow JC, Bulpitt CJ, et al: Environmental factors affecting antipyrine metabolism in London factory and office workers. Br J Clin Pharmacol 7:237–243, 1979

Gaw AC (ed): Culture, Ethnicity and Mental Illness. Washington, DC, American Psychiatric Press, 1993

Gaw AC, Ding Q-Z, Levine RE, et al: The clinical characteristics of possession disorder among 20 Chinese patients in the Hebei province of China. Psychiatr Serv 49:360–365, 1998

Geertz C: The Interpretation of Cultures. New York, Basic Books, 1973

Gillis LS, Trollip D, Jakoet A, et al: Noncompliance with psychotropic medications. S Afr Med J 72:602–606, 1987

Goodenough WH: Comments on cultural revolution. Daedalus 90:521–528, 1961

Haynes RB, Taylor DW, Sackett DL (eds): Compliance in Health Care. Baltimore, MD, Johns Hopkins University Press, 1979

Jablensky A, Sartorius N, Ernberg G, et al: Schizophrenia: manifestations, incidence and course in different cultures: a World Health Organization ten-country study. Psychol Med Monogr Suppl 20:1–97, 1992

Jenkins JH, Karno M: The meaning of expressed emotion: theoretical issues raised by cross-cultural research. Am J Psychiatry 149:9–12, 1992

Kalow W: Pharmacogenetics in biological perspective. Pharmacol Rev 49:369–379, 1997

Keefe SE, Padilla AM, Carlos ML: Emotional support systems in two cultures: a comparison of Mexican Americans and Anglo Americans. Los Angeles, CA, University of California Spanish Speaking Mental Health Center, 1978

Kim LIC: Psychiatric care of Korean Americans, in Culture, Ethnicity and Mental Illness. Edited by Gaw AC. Washington, DC, American Psychiatric Press, 1993, pp 347–375

Kleinman A: Rethinking Psychiatry. New York, Free Press, 1988

Kroeber AL, Kluckholn C: Culture: a critical review of concepts and definitions, in Papers of the Peabody Museum of American Archeology and Ethnology, Harvard University. Cambridge, MA, Harvard University Museum, 1952

Lawson WB: The art and science of the psychopharmacotherapy of African Americans. Mt Sinai J Med 63:301–305, 1996a

Lawson WB: Clinical issues in the pharmacotherapy of African Americans. Psychopharmacol Bull 32:275–281, 1996b

Lee S: Side effects of chronic lithium therapy in Hong Kong Chinese: an ethnopsychiatric perspective. Cult Med Psychiatry 17:301–320, 1993

Lieberman PB, Strauss JS: The recurrence of mania: environmental factors and medical treatment. Am J Psychiatry 141:77–80, 1984

Lim RF (ed): Clinical Manual of Cultural Psychiatry. Arlington, VA, American Psychiatric Publishing, 2006

Lin KM, Poland RE, Nakasaki G (eds): Psychopharmacology and Psychobiology of Ethnicity. Washington, DC, American Psychiatric Press, 1993

Marcos LR, Cancro R: Pharmacotherapy of Hispanic depressed patients: clinical observations. Am J Psychiatry 36:505–513, 1982

Mendoza R, Smith MW, Poland RE, et al: Ethnic psychopharmacology: the Hispanic and Native American perspective. Psychopharmacol Bull 27:449–461, 1991

Mezzich JE, Kleinman A, Fabrega L, et al. (eds): Revised Cultural Proposals for DSM-IV (technical report). Pittsburgh, PA, National Institute of Mental Health Culture and Diagnostic Group, 1993

Morris W (ed): The American Heritage Dictionary of the English Language. New York, American Heritage Publishing Company, 1970

Mukherjee S, Shukla S, Woodline J: Misdiagnosis of schizophrenia in bipolar patients: a multi-ethnic comparison. Am J Psychiatry 140:1571–1574, 1983

Pi EH, Gray GE: A cross-cultural perspective on psychopharmacology. Essential Psychopharmacology 2:233–262, 1998

Pike K: Language in Relation to a Unified Theory of the Structure of Human Behavior, 2nd Revised Edition. Paris, France, Mouton & Co., 1967, pp 37–72

Robins LN, Locke B, Regier DA: An overview of psychiatric disorders in America, in Psychiatric Disorders in America: The Epidemiologic Catchment Area Study. Edited by Robins LN, Regier DA. New York, Free Press, 1991, pp 328–366

Sackett DL, Haynes RB (eds): Compliance With Therapeutic Regimens. Baltimore, MD, Johns Hopkins University Press, 1976

Sanchez F, Gaw AC: Mental Health Care of Filipino Americans. Psychiatr Serv 58:810–815, 2007

Schermerhorn RA: Comparative Ethnic Relations: A Framework for Theory and Research, Chicago, IL, University of Chicago Press, 1970

Simons RC, Hughes CC (eds): The Culture-Bound Syndromes. Dordrecht, Netherlands, Reidel, 1985

Sue S, Zane N: The role of culture and cultural techniques in psychotherapy. Am Psychol 42:37–45, 1987

Tylor E: Primitive Culture, Vol 1. Boston, MA, Estes & Lauriat, 1874

World Health Organization: International Statistical Classification of Diseases and Related Health Problems, 10th Revision. Geneva, Switzerland, World Health Organization, 1992

Yap PM: The culture-bound reactive syndromes, in Mental Health Research in Asia and the Pacific. Edited by Caudill W, Lin TY. Honolulu, HI, East-West Center Press, 1969, pp 33–53

Zola IK: Culture and symptoms: an analysis of patients' presenting complaints. Am Sociol Rev 31:615–630, 1966

Glossary of Culture-Bound Syndromes

The term *culture-bound syndrome* denotes recurrent, locality-specific patterns of aberrant behavior and troubling experience that may or may not be linked to a particular DSM-IV diagnostic category. Many of these patterns are indigenously considered to be "illnesses," or at least afflictions, and most have local names. Although presentations conforming to the major DSM-IV categories can be found throughout the world, the particular symptoms, course, and social response are very often influenced by local cultural factors. In contrast, culture-bound syndromes are generally limited to specific societies or culture areas and are localized, folk, diagnostic categories that frame coherent meanings for certain repetitive, patterned, and troubling sets of experiences and observations.

There is seldom a one-to-one equivalence of any culture-bound syndrome with a DSM diagnostic entity. Aberrant behavior that might be sorted by a diagnostician using DSM-IV into several categories may be included in a single folk category, and presentations that might be considered by a diagnostician using DSM-IV as belonging to a single category may be sorted into several by an indigenous clinician. Moreover, some conditions and disorders have been conceptualized as culture-bound syndromes specific to industrialized culture (e.g., anorexia nervosa, dissocia-tive identity disorder), given their apparent rarity or absence in other cultures. It should also be noted that all industrialized societies include distinctive subcultures and widely diverse immigrant groups who may present with culture-bound syndromes.

This glossary lists some of the best-studied culture-bound syndromes and idioms of distress that may be encountered in clinical practice in North America and includes relevant DSM-IV categories when data suggest that they should be considered in a diagnostic formulation.

amok

A dissociative episode characterized by a period of brooding followed by an outburst of violent, aggressive, or homicidal behavior directed at people and objects. The episode tends to be precipitated by a perceived slight or insult and seems to be prevalent only among males. The episode is often accompanied by persecutory ideas, automatism, amnesia, exhaustion, and a return to premorbid state following the episode. Some instances of *amok* may occur during a brief psychotic episode or constitute the onset or an exacerbation of a chronic psychotic process. The original reports that used this term were from Malaysia. A similar behavior pattern is found in Laos, Philippines, Polynesia (*cafard* or *cathard*), Papua New Guinea, and Puerto Rico (*mal de pelea*), and among the Navajo (*iich'aa*).

ataque de nervios

An idiom of distress principally reported among Latinos from the Caribbean but recognized among many Latin American and Latin Mediterranean groups. Commonly reported symptoms include uncontrollable shouting, attacks of crying, trembling, heat in the chest rising into the head, and verbal or physical aggression. Dissociative experiences, seizurelike or fainting episodes, and suicidal gestures are prominent in some attacks but absent in others. A general feature of an *ataque de nervios* is a sense of being out of control. *Ataques de nervios* frequently occur as a direct result of a stressful event relating to the family (e.g., news of the death of a close relative, a separation or divorce from a spouse, conflicts with a spouse or children, or witnessing an accident involving a family member). People may experience amnesia for what occurred during the *ataque de nervios,* but they otherwise return rapidly to their usual level of functioning. Although descriptions of some *ataques de nervios* most closely fit with the DSM-IV description of panic attacks, the association of most *ataques* with a precipitating event and the frequent absence of the hallmark symptoms of acute fear or apprehension distinguish them from panic disorder. *Ataques* span the range from normal expressions of distress not associated with having a mental disorder to symptom presentations associated with the diagnoses of anxiety, mood, dissociative, or somatoform disorders.

bilis and colera (also referred to as muina)

The underlying cause of these syndromes is thought to be strongly experienced anger or rage. Anger is viewed among many Latino groups as a particularly powerful emotion that can have direct effects on the body and can exacerbate existing symptoms. The major effect of anger is to disturb core body balances (which are understood as a balance between hot and cold valences in the body and between the material and spiritual aspects of the body). Symptoms can include acute nervous tension, headache, trembling, screaming, stomach disturbances, and, in more severe cases, loss of consciousness. Chronic fatigue may result from the acute episode.

boufée delirante

A syndrome observed in West Africa and Haiti. This French term refers to a sudden outburst of agitated and aggressive behavior, marked confusion, and psychomotor excitement. It may sometimes be accompanied by visual and auditory hallucinations or paranoid ideation. These episodes may resemble an episode of brief psychotic disorder.

brain fag

A term initially used in West Africa to refer to a condition experienced by high school or university students in response to the challenges of schooling. Symptoms include difficulties in concentrating, remembering, and thinking. Students often state that their brains are "fatigued." Additional somatic symptoms are usually centered around the head and neck and include pain, pressure or tightness, blurring of vision, heat, or burning. "Brain tiredness" or fatigue from "too much thinking" is an idiom of distress in many cultures, and resulting syndromes can resemble certain anxiety, depressive, and somatoform disorders.

dhat

A folk diagnostic term used in India to refer to severe anxiety and hypochondriacal concerns associated with the discharge of semen, whitish discoloration of the urine, and feelings of weakness and exhaustion. Similar to *jiryan* (India), *sukra prameha* (Sri Lanka), and *shen-k'uei* (China).

falling-out or blacking out

These episodes occur primarily in southern United States and Caribbean groups. They are characterized by a sudden collapse, which sometimes occurs without warning but sometimes is preceded by feelings of dizziness or "swimming" in the head. The individual's eyes are usually open, but the person claims an inability to see. The person usually hears and understands what is occurring around him or her but feels powerless to move. This may correspond to a diagnosis of conversion disorder or a dissociative disorder.

ghost sickness

A preoccupation with death and the deceased (sometimes associated with witchcraft) frequently observed among members of many American Indian tribes. Various symptoms can be attributed to ghost sickness, including bad dreams, weakness, feelings of danger, loss of appetite, fainting, dizziness, fear, anxiety, hallucinations, loss of consciousness, confusion, feelings of futility, and a sense of suffocation.

hwa-byung (also known as wool-hwa-byung)

A Korean folk syndrome literally translated into English as "anger syndrome" and attributed to the suppression of anger. The symptoms include insomnia, fatigue, panic, fear of impending death, dysphoric affect, indigestion, anorexia, dyspnea, palpitations, generalized aches and pains, and a feeling of a mass in the epigastrium.

koro

A term, probably of Malaysian origin, that refers to an episode of sudden and intense anxiety that the penis (or, in females, the vulva and nipples) will recede into the body and possibly cause death. The syndrome is reported in south and east Asia, where it is known by a variety of local terms, such as *shuk yang, shook yong,* and *suo yang* (Chinese); *jinjinia bemar* (Assam); or *rok-joo* (Thailand). It is occasionally found in the West. *Koro* at times occurs in localized epidemic form in east Asian areas. This diagnosis is included in the *Chinese Classification of Mental Disorders,* Second Edition (CCMD-2; Chinese Society of Psychiatry 1989).

latah

Hypersensitivity to sudden fright, often with echopraxia, echolalia, command obedience, and dissociative or trancelike behavior. The term *latah* is of Malaysian or Indonesian origin, but the syndrome has been found in many parts of the world. Other terms for this condition are *amurakh, irkunii, ikota, olan, myriachit,* and *menkeiti* (Siberian groups); *bah tschi, bah-tsi,* and *baah-ji* (Thailand); *imu* (Ainu, Sakhalin, Japan); and *mali-mali* and *silok* (Philippines). In Malaysia, *latah* is more frequent in middle-aged women.

locura

A term used by Latinos in the United States and Latin America to refer to a severe form of chronic psychosis. The condition is attributed to an inherited vulnerability, to the effect of multiple life difficulties, or to a combination of both factors. Symptoms exhibited by persons with locura include incoherence, agitation, auditory and visual hallucinations, inability to follow rules of social interaction, unpredictability, and possible violence.

mal de ojo

A concept widely found in Mediterranean cultures and elsewhere in the world. *Mal de ojo* is a Spanish phrase translated into English as "evil eye." Children are especially at risk. Symptoms include fitful sleep, crying without apparent cause, diarrhea, vomiting, and fever in a child or infant. Sometimes adults (especially females) have the condition.

nervios

A common idiom of distress among Latinos in the United States and Latin America. A number of other ethnic groups have related, though often somewhat distinctive, ideas of "nerves" (such as *nevra* among Greeks in North America). *Nervios* refers both to a general state of vulnerability to stressful life experiences and to a syndrome brought on by difficult life circumstances. The term *nervios* includes a wide range of symptoms of emotional distress, somatic dis-

turbance, and inability to function. Common symptoms include headaches and "brain aches," irritability, stomach disturbances, sleep difficulties, nervousness, easy tearfulness, inability to concentrate, trembling, tingling sensations, and *mareos* (dizziness with occasional vertigo-like exacerbations). *Nervios* tends to be an ongoing problem, although variable in the degree of disability manifested. *Nervios* is a very broad syndrome that spans the range from cases free of a mental disorder to presentations resembling adjustment, anxiety, depressive, dissociative, somatoform, or psychotic disorders. Differential diagnosis will depend on the constellation of symptoms experienced, the kind of social events that are associated with the onset and progress of *nervios,* and the level of disability experienced.

pibloktoq

An abrupt dissociative episode accompanied by extreme excitement of up to 30 minutes' duration and frequently followed by convulsive seizures and coma lasting up to 12 hours. This is observed primarily in arctic and subarctic Eskimo communities, although regional variations in name exist. The individual may be withdrawn or mildly irritable for a period of hours or days before the attack and will typically report complete amnesia for the attack. During the attack, the individual may tear off his or her clothing, break furniture, shout obscenities, eat feces, flee from protective shelters, or perform other irrational or dangerous acts.

qi-gong psychotic reaction

A term describing an acute, time-limited episode characterized by dissociative, paranoid, or other psychotic or nonpsychotic symptoms that may occur after participation in the Chinese folk health-enhancing practice of *qi-gong* ("exercise of vital energy"). Especially vulnerable are individuals who become overly involved in the practice. This diagnosis is included in the CCMD-2.

rootwork

A set of cultural interpretations that ascribe illness to hexing, witchcraft, sorcery, or the evil influence of another person. Symptoms may include generalized anxiety and gastrointestinal complaints (e.g., nausea, vomiting, diarrhea), weakness, dizziness, the fear of being poisoned, and sometimes fear of being killed ("voodoo death"). "Roots," "spells," or "hexes" can be "put" or placed on other persons, causing a variety of emotional and psychological problems. The "hexed" person may even fear death until the "root" has been "taken off" (eliminated), usually through the work of a "root doctor" (a healer in this tradition), who can also be called on to bewitch an enemy. "Rootwork" is found in the southern United States among both African American and European American populations and in Caribbean societies. It is also known as *mal puesto* or *brujeria* in Latino societies.

sangue dormido ("sleeping blood")

A syndrome found among Portuguese Cape Verde Islanders (and immigrants from there to the United States) that includes pain, numbness, tremor, paralysis, convulsions, stroke, blindness, heart attack, infection, and miscarriage.

shenjing shuairuo ("neurasthenia")

In China, a condition characterized by physical and mental fatigue, dizziness, headaches, other pains, concentration difficulties, sleep disturbance, and memory loss. Other symptoms include gastrointestinal problems, sexual dysfunction, irritability, excitability, and various signs suggesting disturbance of the autonomic nervous system. In many cases, the symptoms would meet the criteria for a DSM-IV mood or anxiety disorder. This diagnosis is included in the CCMD-2.

shen-k'uei (Taiwan); shenkui (China)

A Chinese folk label describing marked anxiety or panic symptoms with accompanying somatic complaints for which no physical cause can be demonstrated. Symptoms include dizziness, backache, fatigability, general weakness, insomnia, frequent dreams, and complaints of sexual dysfunction (such as premature ejaculation and impotence). Symptoms are attributed to excessive semen loss from frequent intercourse, masturbation, nocturnal emission, or passing of "white turbid urine" believed to contain semen. Excessive semen loss is feared because of the belief that it represents the loss of one's vital essence and can thereby be life threatening.

shin-byung

A Korean folk label for a syndrome in which initial phases are characterized by anxiety and somatic complaints (general weakness, dizziness, fear, anorexia, insomnia, gastrointestinal problems), with subsequent dissociation and possession by ancestral spirits.

spell

A trance state in which individuals "communicate" with deceased relatives or with spirits. At times this state is associated with brief periods of personality change. This culture-specific syndrome is seen among African Americans and European Americans from the southern United States. Spells are not considered to be medical events in the folk tradition but may be misconstrued as psychotic episodes in clinical settings.

susto ("fright" or "soul loss")

A folk illness prevalent among some Latinos in the United States and among people in Mexico, Central America, and South America. *Susto* is also referred to as *espanto, pasmo, tripa ida, perdida del alma,* or *chibih. Susto* is an illness attributed to a frightening event that causes the soul to leave the body and results in unhappiness and sickness. Individuals with *susto* also experience significant strains in key social roles. Symptoms may appear any time from days to years after the fright is experienced. It is believed that in extreme cases, *susto* may result in death. Typical symptoms include appetite disturbances, inadequate or excessive sleep, troubled sleep or dreams, feeling of sadness, lack of motivation to do anything, and feelings of low self-worth or dirtiness. Somatic symptoms accompanying *susto* include muscle aches and pains, headache, stomachache, and diarrhea. Ritual healings are focused on calling the soul back to the body and cleansing the person to restore bodily and spiritual balance. Different experiences of *susto* may be related to major depressive disorder, posttraumatic stress disorder, and somatoform disorders. Similar etiological beliefs and symptom configurations are found in many parts of the world.

taijin kyofusho

A culturally distinctive phobia in Japan, in some ways resembling DSM-IV social phobia. This syndrome refers to an individual's intense fear that his or her body, its parts or its functions, displease, embarrass, or are offensive to other people in appearance, odor, facial expressions, or movements. This syndrome is included in the official Japanese diagnostic system for mental disorders.

zar

A general term applied in Ethiopia, Somalia, Egypt, Sudan, Iran, and other North African and Middle Eastern societies to the experience of spirits possessing an individual. Persons possessed by a spirit may experience dissociative episodes that may include shouting, laughing, hitting the head against a wall, singing, or weeping. Individuals may show apathy and withdrawal, refusing to eat or carry out daily tasks, or may develop a long-term relationship with the possessing spirit. Such behavior is not considered pathological locally.

Glossary of Cultural Psychiatry Terms

alloplastic

An approach in psychotherapy with the goal of effecting changes in the external environment. See also *autoplastic*

autoplastic

An approach in psychotherapy with the goal of changing oneself to accommodate the external circumstances. See also *alloplastic*

credibility

A term introduced by psychologists Stanley Sue and Nolan Zane (1987) that refers to the patient's/client's perception of the therapist as an effective and trustworthy helper. Credibility is one of the two elements (the other element is *giving*) in the therapeutic process, in which appropriate application of cultural knowledge is thought to result in effective intercultural psychotherapy.

cross-cultural psychopharmacology

The special area of pharmacology that deals with the variation in psychotropic drug responses in different populations and the contribution of pharmacological factors to such variation.

culture

Meanings, values, and behavioral norms that are learned and transmitted in the dominant society and within its social groups. Culture powerfully influences cognitions, feelings, and the "self" concept as well as the diagnostic process and treatment decisions (DSM-IV-TR). Culture is a set of standards for behavior that a group of people attribute to those around them and that they use to orient their behavior.

culture-bound syndrome

Recurrent, locality-specific patterns of aberrant behavior and troubling experiences, indigenously considered to be "illness" or at least affliction, generally limited to specific societies or culture areas. These are localized, folk diagnostic categories that frame coherent meanings for certain repetitive, patterned, and troubling sets of experiences and observations. These

include named categories in folk nosological systems as well as "idioms of distress," or culturally salient expressions for communicating symptoms (DSM-IV-TR).

demoralization hypothesis

A concept introduced by psychiatrist Jerome Frank (1982) to explain how psychotherapy works. It posits that patients, whatever their symptoms, share a type of distress that responds to components common to all schools of psychotherapy. Demoralization suggests a state of mind characterized by one or more of the following: subjective incompetence, loss of self-esteem, alienation, hopelessness (feeling that no one can help), or helplessness (feeling that other people could help but will not). Demoralization is thought to manifest itself through subjective symptoms (anxiety, depression, loneliness) or behavioral disturbance (interpersonal conflicts). Frank suggested that improvement resulting from psychotherapy lies in its ability to restore the patient's morale, with the consequent diminution or disappearance of symptoms.

emic

A term derived from phon*emic* and one of the two (see also *etic*) contrasting levels of data or methods of analysis introduced by Kenneth L. Pike (1967) that explains the ideology or behavior of members of a culture according to indigenous definitions. Emic models are culture specific.

emotional freezing

An adjustment reaction to a new environment sometimes observed among individuals moving from rural to metropolitan areas. It is characterized by solitary activities, constricted affect, and other deficits in communication, features that may mimic characteristics of a schizoid personality disorder.

ethnicity

A collectivity of people within a larger society defined on the basis of common origins, shared symbols, and standards for behavior.

etic

A term derived from phon*etic* and one of two (see also *emic*) contrasting levels of data or methods of analysis based on criteria from outside a particular culture. Etic models are held to be universal.

expressive transaction

The human interaction and rapport between the two persons in psychotherapy. Expressive transaction rests heavily on the personality attributes of the two individuals. See also *instrumental transaction*

extensive metabolizers

Individuals with a normal amount of metabolizing enzymes. See also *poor metabolizers*

giving

A term introduced by Sue and Zane (1987) referring to a patient's/client's perception that something is received from the therapeutic encounter. See also *credibility*

haan

A Korean term that refers to an individual and collective subconscious emotional complex among the Korean people involving suppressed feelings of anger, rage, despair, frustration, holding of grudges, indignation, and revenge. The syndrome is believed to result from victimization of a Korean person both as an individual and collectively as people and is thought to be an important factor in the development of *hwa-byung* ("anger disease"). See also *hwa-byung* in Appendix A, "Glossary of Culture-Bound Syndromes in DSM-IV."

inducers

Substrates that increase the synthesis of cytochrome P450 enzymes and have the effect of increasing the rate of biotransformation and reducing the serum level of the parent compound.

inhibitors

Substrates that decrease the synthesis of P450 enzymes and that usually result from competition between two or more drugs for the active site of the same enzyme. The resulting effects are an increased serum level of the less metabolized parent compound, prolonged pharmacological effect, and increased incidences of drug-induced toxicities.

instrumental transaction

The special knowledge, skills, and procedures imparted by the therapist in the process of healing between the two persons in psychotherapy. See also *expressive transaction*

operating culture

Standards a person used at a particular time with significant others.

operating procedure (also called *recipe*)

Ways in which people organize their effort to accomplish certain purposes.

pharmacodynamics

The biochemical and physiological effects of drugs at their loci of actions in the body.

pharmacogenetics

The special area of biochemical genetics that deals with variation in drug response and the contribution of genetics to such variation.

pharmacokinetics

The general bodily responses to the presence of a foreign substance (xenobiotics) such as a drug in the human body. It is the study of the biochemical and physiological processes involved in the absorption, distribution, metabolism, and excretion of a drug, the summation of which determines the drug's final plasma concentration.

polymorphism

The condition in genetics when two or more alternative genotypes are present in a population, each at a frequency greater than that which could be maintained by recurrent mutation alone. It is reflected in a bimodal or trimodal distribution of the activity of a drug-metabolizing enzyme. Polymorphism may result in deficient or impaired enzymatic activities.

poor metabolizers

Individuals with deficient metabolizing enzymes. See also *extensive metabolizers*

psychotherapy

A planned, emotionally charged, confiding interaction between a trained, socially sanctioned healer and a sufferer.

race

A number of broad divisions of the human species into groups based on a common geographic origin, certain shared physical characteristics, and a characteristic distribution of gene frequencies.

subculture

Narrower sets of standards that govern how one acts within a smaller range of behavior with a particular set of actors.

windigo

An Algonkian Indian's idiom of distress often associated with the idea of the mystery and great concerns over a lost person. It is often cited in the literature as referring to the idea of cannibal compulsion among Algonkian Indians.

41

PSYCHIATRY AND THE LAW

Robert I. Simon, M.D.
Daniel W. Shuman, J.D.

The legal principles applied to the practice of psychiatry do not differ from those applied to medicine in general. Nevertheless, the diagnosis, treatment, and management of patients with psychiatric disorders present unique concerns that may pit the psychiatrist's duty to the patient against the psychiatrist's duty to the community. For instance, the competence of psychiatric patients to make health care decisions is often an issue in psychiatric care, as well as the risks that patients pose to others and how best to reduce those risks. Issues such as informed consent, the duty of confidentiality, the right to treatment, the right to refuse treatment, substitute decision making, and advance directives are commonly confronted by clinicians when treating psychiatric patients.

The mental threshold for criminal prosecution may demand a psychiatric assessment of the defendant. To ensure fairness and accountability, we demand that regardless of whether defendants wish to accept a plea bargain and waive trial or proceed to trial, they must meet minimal standards for competence. The legal standard is functional and does not confuse diagnosis with legal competence. Defendants with psychiatric impairments may not meet the competency standard. Once the issue is raised, however, they may require pretrial evaluations of their mental capacity to understand the charges brought against them and their ability to assist counsel in their own defense. Mental state or capacity is also central in deciding criminal responsibility and sentencing. The impact of a psychiatric disorder may be to reduce or avoid criminal responsibility for an act or to shape the length or the terms of confinement following conviction.

In the civil realm, psychiatrists, like all other professionals who render a service, are subject to damage claims by disgruntled clients. Specific areas of psychiatric practice are more vulnerable to psychiatric malpractice suits. Table 41–1 describes the malpractice claims experience of the American Psychiatric Association (APA)–sponsored Professional Liability Insurance Program prior to 1996 (Benefacts 1996). Somatic therapies, patient suicides, assessment and management of violent patients, techniques to recover memories of sexual abuse, sexual misconduct, boundary violations, premature discharge of potentially violent patients, and managed care settings are all areas of heightened risk for liability claims against the psychiatric practitioner.

The chance of a psychiatrist being sued in the 1980s was 1 in 25 per year (Benefacts 1996). Through 1995, however, the odds increased to about 1 in 12 psychiatrists per year. In some states, psychiatrists are sued at the rate of 1 in 6 per year. The APA Professional Liability Insurance Program identifies several factors to account for the increase in malpractice suits:

1. Psychiatrists are treating "sicker" patients in managed care settings.
2. The media scrutinizes so-called recovered memories and ritual satanic abuse cases.
3. Tort reform legislation has failed.
4. Psychiatrists are specializing in new practice areas such as geriatric psychopharmacology, adolescent addiction medicine, multiple personality disorder, pain management, and adult children of alcoholic persons.
5. Psychiatrists are providing more primary care, such as in the management of patients with diabetes, hypertension, and a wide variety of acute general medical illnesses.

With the advent of managed care, psychiatrists treat a large volume of patients for brief visits, creating greater liability exposure. When the psychiatrist spends less time with a patient, a working alliance may not develop. Among primary care physicians, it was reported that those with no malpractice claims used more statements of orientation, laughed and used more humor, and engaged patients more in a give-and-take dialogue than did colleagues who had been sued (Levinson et al. 1997). Primary care physicians with no claims also spent more time in routine visits than did those who had been sued (mean: 18.3 vs. 15.0 minutes). The length of the visit was an independent factor in predicting claims status.

Patient suicides are an unavoidable occupational hazard of psychiatric practice. They account for numerous malpractice suits filed against psychiatrists and the highest percentages of settlements and verdicts covered by professional liability insurers (Figure 41–1). Nonetheless, it remains difficult for a claimant to persuade a jury that, more likely than not, a psychiatric error occurred and that it caused the patient's suicide. Although the potential for malpractice suits remains high for psychiatrists who treat suicidal and violent patients, the plaintiff's success rate in malpractice actions is only 2 or 3 out of every 10 litigated claims.

Psychiatrist–Patient Relationships and the Law

General Contours of the Relationship

Informed Consent

The decision to initiate a treatment or diagnostic procedure belongs to the patient, who has the right to deter-

TABLE 41–1. Recent allegations of malpractice (approximate frequency of claims)

Allegation	Frequency, %
Incorrect treatment	33
Attempted/completed suicide	20
Incorrect diagnosis	11
Improper supervision	7
Medication error/drug reaction	7
Improper commitment	5
Breach of confidentiality	4
Unnecessary hospitalization	4
Undue familiarity	3
Libel/slander	2
Other (e.g., abandonment, electroconvulsive therapy, third-party injury)	4

Source.   Data from Benefacts 1996.

mine what will be done to his or her body (Schloendorff v. Society of New York Hospital 1914). Concomitantly, a physician occupies a fiduciary role to assist in the patient's decision. The law seeks to make that decision meaningful by requiring a physician to inform the patient about the available choices, known as an *informed consent.* Included among factors to be disclosed are the potential benefits, risks, alternatives, and consequences of the diagnostic or treatment procedure. The failure to satisfy this requirement of informed consent is a breach of the duty that the physician owes a patient and is actionable as a tort (Appelbaum et al. 1987).

The courts typically require that a decision be knowing, intelligent, and voluntary to satisfy the requirements of informed consent (Long v. Jaszczak 2004). We use "competency" instead of "intelligence" and "information" instead of "knowing," believing them to be more practical psychiatric considerations for clinical psychiatrists. We do not, however, intend to change the substantive requirements:

- Competency (intelligence)
- Information (knowing)
- Voluntariness

Usually, clinicians provide the first level of screening in identifying patient competency and in deciding whether to accept a patient's treatment decision. The patient or a bona fide representative must be given an adequate description of the treatment. If the patient who refuses treatment appears to lack health care deci-

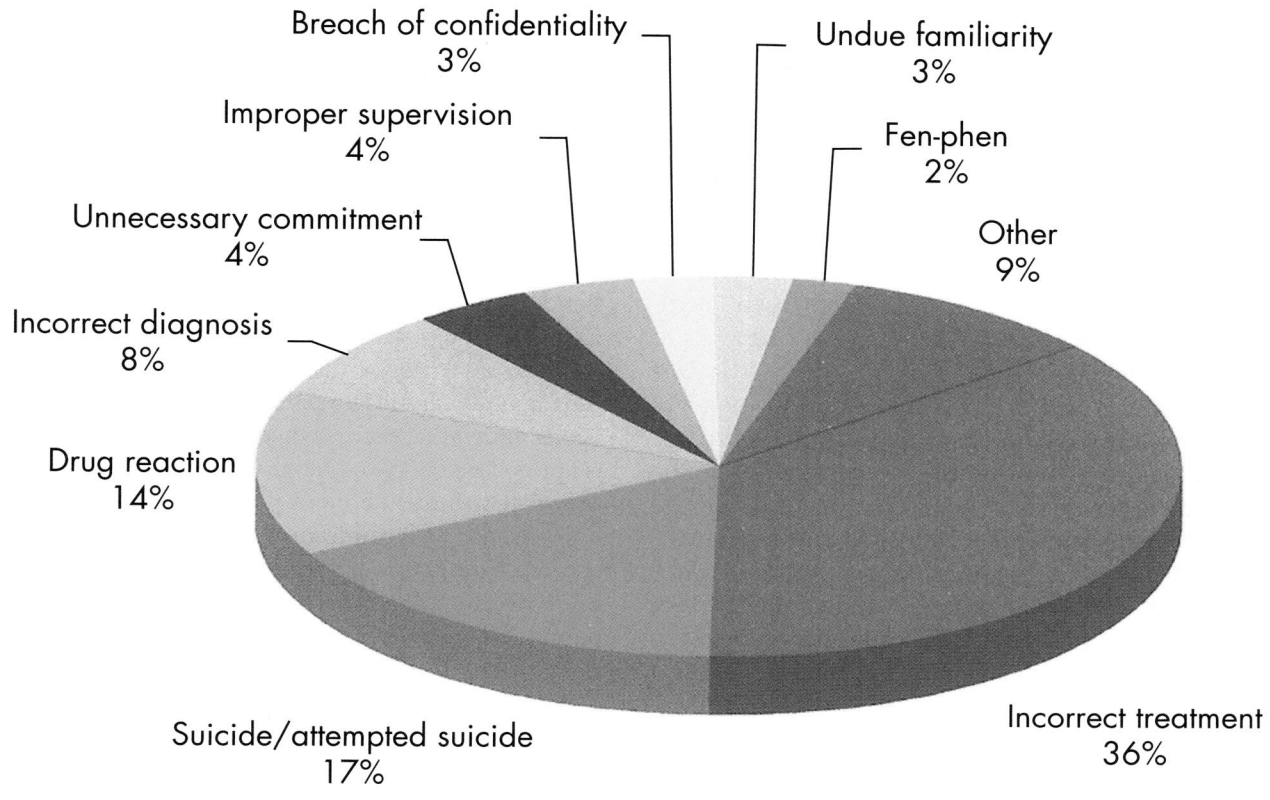

Breach of confidentiality
3%

Undue familiarity
3%

Improper supervision
4%

Fen-phen
2%

Unnecessary commitment
4%

Other
9%

Incorrect diagnosis
8%

Drug reaction
14%

Suicide/attempted suicide
17%

Incorrect treatment
36%

FIGURE 41–1.   Psychiatric claims by cause of loss: United States, 1998–2006.

The "cause of loss" represents the main allegation made in the claim or lawsuit. In almost all lawsuits, multiple allegations of negligence are asserted. These data are collected based on the chief allegation or complaint. Thus, the category of "incorrect treatment" may be alleged in a lawsuit based on a patient suicide but the main or chief allegation/complaint is stated as "incorrect treatment." Suicide and attempted suicide is the most frequently identifiable cause of loss. The "drug reaction" category used here encompasses all types of drug/medication misadventures, including errors in prescribing, adverse reactions to medications, mismanagement of a patient's medication regime, or other unanticipated outcomes related to medication use. "Other" includes Vicarious Liability "PC", Libel/Slander, Other/Not specific, Third Party (e.g., parents), Administrative, Lack of Informed Consent, Abandonment, Tarasoff, Forensic, Premises Liability, Boundary Violation.
Source.   The Psychiatrists' Program, managed by Professional Risk Management Services (PRMS; www.prms.com).

sion-making capacity, it does not mean that the patient cannot be treated. An appropriate substitute decision maker can provide (or withhold) consent. To be able to provide informed consent, the patient or substitute decision maker should be told about the risks, benefits, and prognosis both with and without treatment, as well as alternative treatments and their risks and benefits. In addition, the competent patient must voluntarily consent to or refuse the proposed treatment or procedure.

The legal doctrine of informed consent is consistent with the provision of good clinical care. The informed consent doctrine allows patients to become partners in making treatment determinations that accord with their own needs and values. In the past, physicians operated under the "do no harm" principle. Today, psychiatrists are increasingly required to practice within

the model of informed consent and patient autonomy. Most psychiatrists find increased patient autonomy desirable in fostering development of the therapeutic alliance that is so essential to treatment. Furthermore, patient autonomy is the goal of most psychiatric treatments (Beahrs and Gutheil 2001).

Competency (intelligence).   It is clinically useful to distinguish the terms *incompetence* and *incapacity*. *Incompetence* refers to a court adjudication, whereas *incapacity* indicates a functional inability as determined by a clinician (Mishkin 1989). Legally, only competent persons may give informed consent. An adult patient is presumed competent unless adjudicated incompetent or temporarily incapacitated because of a medical emergency. Incapacity does not prevent treatment; it merely requires the clinician to obtain substitute consent or an exception to the requirement of informed consent. Absent an emergency, treating an incompetent patient without substituted consent is not permitted.

Legal competence is typically thought to refer to cognitive capacity. The conception derives largely from the laws governing transactions. Important clinical concepts such as affective incompetence are not usually recognized by the law as dispositive. For example, a severely depressed but cognitively intact patient may be regarded as competent to refuse antidepressant medication. Manic patients tend to emphasize the risks of medications while downplaying their benefits. Schizophrenic patients tend to be fearful that medication will cause them serious harm. These patients may be unable to make a balanced assessment that considers both the risks and the benefits of a proposed drug. One study, in which three instruments were used to assess competency for treatment decisions, found that the schizophrenia and depression groups demonstrated poorer understanding of treatment disclosures, poorer reasoning in decision-making regarding treatment, and a greater likelihood of failing to appreciate their illness or the potential treatment benefits (Grisso and Appelbaum 1995a). Denial of illness often interferes with insight and the ability to appreciate the significance of information provided to the patient. In *In the Guardianship of John Roe* (1992), the Massachusetts Supreme Judicial Court recognized that denial of illness can render a patient incompetent to make treatment decisions.

Competency is not a scientifically determinable state and is situation specific. The issue of competency arises in a number of civil, criminal, and family law contexts. Although there are no hard-and-fast definitions, the patient's ability to do the following is legally germane to determining competency:

- Understand the particular treatment choice being proposed
- Make a treatment choice
- Communicate that choice verbally or nonverbally

A review of case law and scholarly literature reveals four standards for determining incompetency in decision making (Appelbaum et al. 1987). In order of increasing levels of mental capacity required, these standards are as follows:

1. Communication of choice
2. Understanding of relevant information provided
3. Appreciation of available options and consequences
4. Rational decision making

Patients with severely mental disorders frequently deny their illness. Although they may communicate a choice and understand the information provided, these patients may lack the insight or ability to appreciate the information provided (Grisso and Appelbaum 1995b). Rational decision making is impaired as well. For example, patients with schizophrenia tend to fear some idiosyncratic harm from the treatment while ignoring the actual risk of medication side effects.

Most psychiatrists prefer a rational decision-making standard in determining incompetency. Most courts prefer the first two standards mentioned earlier but often combine competency standards. A truly informed consent that considers the patient's autonomy, personal needs, and values occurs when rational decision making is applied by the patient to the risks and benefits of appropriate treatment options provided by the clinician.

Grisso and Appelbaum (1995a) found that the choice of standards determining competence affected the type and proportion of patients classified as impaired. When compound standards were used, the proportion of patients identified as impaired increased. These authors advised that clinicians be aware of the applicable standards in their jurisdictions.

A valid consent can be either *expressed* (oral or in writing) or *implied* from the patient's actions. The competency issue is particularly sensitive when dealing with minors or mentally disabled persons who lack the requisite cognitive capacity for health care decision making. In both cases, it is generally recognized in the law that an authorized representative or guardian may consent for the patient.

Information (knowing).   The standard for exercising a legally sufficient disclosure varies from state to state. Traditionally, the duty to disclose was measured by a professional standard: either what a reasonable physician would disclose under the circumstances or what the customary disclosure practices of physicians are in a particular community. In the landmark case *Canterbury v. Spence* (1972), a patient-oriented standard was applied. This standard focused on the "material" information that a *reasonable* person in the patient's position would want to know to make an informed decision. An increasing number of courts have applied this standard, and some have expanded "material risks" to include information regarding the consequences of not consenting to the treatment or procedure (Truman v. Thomas 1980). Even in patient-oriented jurisdictions, there is no duty to disclose every possible risk. A material risk is defined as one in which a physician knows or should know what would be considered significant by a reasonable person in the patient's position.

Voluntariness. For consent to be considered legally voluntary, it must be given freely by the patient and without coercion, fraud, or duress. In evaluating whether consent is truly voluntary, the courts typically examine all the relevant circumstances, including the psychiatrist's manner, the environmental conditions, and the patient's mental state.

Malcolm (1992) noted subtle differences in the concepts of persuasion and coercion. *Persuasion* is defined as the physician's aim "to utilize the patient's reasoning ability to arrive at a desired result" (p. 241). *Coercion* occurs "when the doctor aims to manipulate the patient by introducing extraneous elements which have the effect of undermining the patient's ability to reason" (p. 241).

Exceptions and liability. There are two basic exceptions to the requirement of obtaining informed consent. When immediate treatment is necessary to save a life or prevent serious harm, and it is not possible to obtain either the patient's consent or that of someone authorized to provide consent for the patient, the law typically presumes that the consent would have been granted. Two considerations are relevant when applying this exception. First, the emergency must be serious and "imminent"; second, the patient's condition, and not the surrounding circumstances (e.g., adverse environmental conditions), determines the existence of an emergency.

The second exception, *therapeutic privilege,* excepts informed consent if a psychiatrist determines that a complete disclosure of possible risks and alternatives might have a deleterious impact on the patient's health and welfare. Jurisdictions vary in their application of this exception. Absent specific case law or statutes outlining the factors relevant to such a decision, a doctor must substantiate a patient's inability psychologically to withstand being informed of the proposed treatment. Some courts have held that therapeutic privilege may be invoked only if informing the patient will worsen his or her condition or will so frighten the patient that rational decision making will be precluded (Canterbury v. Spence 1972; Natanson v. Kline 1960). Therapeutic privilege cannot be used as a means of circumventing the legal requirement for obtaining informed consent from the patient before initiating treatment.

Waivers. A physician need not disclose risks of treatment when the patient has competently, knowingly, and voluntarily waived his or her right to be informed (e.g., when the patient does not want to be informed of drug risks). This is not an exception to the requirement of informed consent but rather a patient choice to decide with limited information.

Absent a waiver or an exception, treatment without an adequate informed consent opens the door to a damage claim for an intentional tort if the treatment is initiated without consent or a negligence tort if treatment is initiated without an adequate consent.

Confidentiality and Privilege

Confidentiality refers to the right of a patient, and the correlative duty of a professional, of nondisclosure of relational communications to outside parties without implied or expressed authorization. The duty of confidentiality limits the actions of the professional but does not limit the power of a judge to compel disclosure of relevant relational confidences. *Privilege,* or more accurately *relational privilege,* is a limitation on the power of the judge to compel disclosure of relational confidences. A psychiatrist–, psychotherapist–, or physician–patient privilege may be recognized by case law (Jaffee v. Redmond 1996) but is more typically a statute or rule of evidence that permits the holder of the privilege (e.g., the patient) to prevent the person to whom confidential information was given (e.g., the psychiatrist) from being compelled by a judge to disclose it in a judicial proceeding.

Confidentiality. Although the law relating to confidentiality of health information has been state law, the Health Insurance Portability and Accountability Act of 1996 (HIPAA) adds a layer of federal law to protect patient health care information. If state and federal laws conflict, the more protective rule prevails. HIPAA limits disclosure of patient health information without patient authorization except as necessary for treatment, payment, and health care operations; however, the limitation is not absolute. For example, HIPAA permits disclosure in a judicial or administrative (e.g., workers' compensation or Social Security) proceeding when there is 1) the patient's written consent, 2) a subpoena, or 3) a court order signed by a judge. A separate consent is required to permit the disclosure of psychotherapy notes.

Clinical–legal foundation. Relational privileges require courts to compromise their search for truth by not availing themselves of relevant evidence. Thus courts have typically been reluctant to recognize a privilege and quick to find an exception applicable (Shuman and Weiner 1987). Indeed, the common law did not recognize physician–patient or psychotherapist–patient privilege. When courts have done so, it has been because they have been convinced of its necessity to further a relationship of great utility to society. For example, in 1996 the U.S. Supreme Court ruled that confidential communications between psychotherapist and patient are privileged and, unless an exception applies, may not be compelled in federal trials (Jaffee v. Redmond 1996). In the majority of cases where a privilege is recognized by statute or rule of evidence, there is typically an acknowledgment of similar reasoning.

Breaching of confidentiality. Once the doctor–patient relationship has been created, the professional assumes a duty to safeguard a patient's disclosures. This duty is not absolute, and there are circumstances in which breaching confidentiality is both ethical and legal.

Patients also waive confidentiality in a variety of situations, especially in managed care settings. Medical records may be sent to potential employers or to insurance companies when benefits are requested. A limited waiver of confidentiality ordinarily exists when a patient participates in group therapy. Whether one group member can be compelled in court to disclose information shared by another group member during group therapy is still unsettled legally (Slovenko 1998). Many state confidentiality statutes provide statutory exceptions to confidentiality between the psychiatrist and the patient in one or more situations (Brakel et al. 1985) (Table 41–2).

If a patient gives the psychiatrist good reason to believe that a warning should be issued to an endangered third party, the duty of confidentiality of the communication that gave rise to the warning may be limited. Psychiatrists who have issued warnings have been compelled to testify in criminal cases (Leong et al. 1992), although the obligation to breach confidentiality may not resolve the privilege issue at trial.

Privilege.   The patient, not the psychiatrist, is the holder of the physician–, psychiatrist–, or psychotherapist–patient privilege and is entitled to determine whether to assert it. Relational privileges govern disclosures in the judicial setting (e.g., deposition, trial); the duty of confidentiality governs disclosures in extrajudicial settings (e.g., cocktail parties, memoirs, visits by the police). Privilege statutes or case law recognition represents recognition by the state of the importance of protecting information provided by a patient to a psychotherapist. This recognition moves away from the essential purpose of the American system of justice (e.g., "truth finding") by insulating certain information from disclosure in court. This protection is justified on the basis that the special need for privacy in the psychotherapist–patient relationship outweighs the unbridled quest for an accurate outcome in court.

Privilege statutes usually are drafted with reference to one of the following four relationships, depending on the type of practitioner:

TABLE 41–2.	Common limitations of testimonial privilege
Valid patient consent	
Civil commitment proceedings	
Criminal proceedings	
Child custody disputes	
Court-ordered report	
Patient-litigant exception	
Child abuse proceedings	

Source.   Reprinted with permission from Simon RI: *A Concise Guide to Psychiatry and the Law for Clinicians,* 3rd Edition. Washington, DC, American Psychiatric Publishing, 2001, p. 54.

1. Physician–patient (general)
2. Psychiatrist–patient
3. Psychologist–patient
4. Psychotherapist–patient

Privilege statutes also specify exceptions to testimonial privilege. Although exceptions vary, the most common are summarized in Table 41–2.

The last exception, known as the *patient-litigant exception,* commonly occurs in the insanity defense, will contests, workers' compensation cases, child custody disputes, personal injury actions, and medical malpractice actions.

Liability.   An unauthorized or unwarranted breach of the duty of confidentiality can cause a patient emotional harm and result in a claim based on at least four theories:

1. Malpractice (breach of professional duty of confidentiality)
2. Breach of statutory duty of confidentiality
3. Invasion of privacy
4. Breach of (implied) contract

Right to Refuse Treatment

Buttressed by constitutionally derived rights to privacy and freedom from cruel and unusual punishment, the common law tort of battery, and the doctrine of informed consent, mentally disabled persons have been afforded protections typically available for patients of nonpsychiatric physicians—the right to refuse treatment. This right often collides with clinical judgment (i.e., to treat and protect). As a result of this conflict, the courts vary considerably regarding the parameters of this right and the procedures to be followed if it is to be overridden.

Two landmark cases illustrate this point. In *Rennie v. Klein* (1978), the Third Circuit Court of Appeals recognized a right to refuse treatment in the state of New Jersey. The court concluded, however, that this right could be overridden and antipsychotic drugs administered "whenever, in the exercise of professional judgment, such an action is deemed necessary to prevent the patient from endangering himself or others." In the second case, *Rogers v. Commissioner of Department of Mental Health* (1983), the Massachusetts high court decided that in the absence of an emergency (e.g., serious threat of extreme violence or personal injury), any person who has not been adjudicated incompetent has a right to refuse antipsychotic medication. Incompetent persons have a similar right, but it must be exercised through a "substituted judgment treatment plan" that has been reviewed and approved by the court.

These two decisions are often viewed as legal bookends to the issue of the right to refuse treatment. The cases suggest parameters for other courts attempting to define such a right. The *Rennie* case became the model for subsequent legal decisions that adopted a treatment-driven rationale for the right to refuse treatment. *Rogers* became the basis for rights-driven approaches taken by some courts in litigating the right to refuse treatment.

Numerous state and federal decisions have tackled aspects of this issue. Generally speaking, there is recognition of an involuntarily hospitalized patient's right to refuse medication absent an emergency or an adjudication of incompetence made in conjunction with the order of commitment. Case law criteria for emergencies range from a risk of "imminent" harm to self or others to a deterioration in the patient's mental condition if treatment is halted. Until either more states enact legislation or the U.S. Supreme Court squarely rules on this issue, jurisdictions will continue to vary regarding the substance of the right to refuse treatment and the procedures by which such a right can be implemented.

Another context in which this issue of right to refuse treatment arises is when the government wishes to medicate a nonconsenting pretrial detainee found incompetent to stand trial. In *Sell v. United States* (2003), the U.S. Supreme Court set forth the findings that the trial court is required to reach before the government may administer antipsychotic drugs to render a nonconsenting defendant competent to stand trial. The court acknowledged that its decisions in *Riggins v. Nevada* (1992) and *Washington v. Harper* (1990)

had recognized a constitutionally protected liberty interest in avoiding unwanted antipsychotic drugs that might be overridden in limited circumstances. It concluded that these decisions permit the trial court to authorize the involuntary administration of drugs to restore the defendant's competence only when four requirements are met:

1. There are important state interests served by bringing the defendant to trial through the involuntary administration of these drugs that would not be served by long-term commitment.
2. Involuntary medication is likely to restore the defendant's competence but not interfere with the ability to assist counsel.
3. There is no less intrusive treatment likely to serve the government's interests.
4. Administration of these drugs would serve the defendant's best medical interests.

Competency

The ability to effectively exercise rights recognized by the law demands a minimal mental capacity or competence. One articulation of the meaning of *competency* is "having sufficient capacity, ability…[or] possessing the requisite physical, mental, natural, or legal qualifications" (Black 1990, p. 285). This conceptualization is deliberately vague because *competency* is a broad concept encompassing many different legal issues and contexts. As a result, its requirements can vary widely depending on the circumstances in which it is being measured (e.g., making health care decisions, executing a will, or confessing to a crime).

Competency refers to a *minimal* mental, cognitive, or behavioral ability, trait, or capability required to perform a particular act (e.g., waive counsel) or to assume a particular role (e.g., practice dentistry). A determination of incompetency is ultimately a judicial determination. The term *incapacity*, which is often interchanged with *incompetency*, refers to an individual's functional inability to understand or to form an intention with regard to some act as determined by health care providers (Mishkin 1989).

The legal designation of "incompetent" is applied to an individual who fails one of the mental tests of capacity and is therefore considered *by law* to be not mentally capable of performing a particular act or assuming a particular role. The adjudication of incompetence by a court is now, more commonly, subject or issue specific. For example, the fact that a psychiatric patient is adjudicated incompetent to drive does not automatically render that patient incompetent to do other things, such as consent to treatment, testify as a witness, marry, or enter into a contract.

Generally, the law only gives effect to decisions by a competent individual and seeks to protect incompetent individuals from the harmful effects of their acts. Adults (age 18 years or older; U.S. Department of Health and Human Services 1981) are presumed to be competent (Meek v. City of Loveland 1929). This presumption, however, may be rebutted by evidence of incapacity (Scaria v. St. Paul Fire and Marine Ins. Co. 1975). For the psychiatric patient, perception, short- and long-term memory, judgment, language comprehension, verbal fluency, and reality orientation are mental functions that a court will scrutinize when the issues of "capacity" and "competency" have been raised.

As a matter of law, incompetency may not be presumed from either treatment for mental illness (Wilson v. Lehman 1964) or institutionalization (Rennie v. Klein 1978). Mental disability or illness does not necessarily render a person incompetent in any or in all areas of functioning. Instead, scrutiny is given to determine whether specific functional incapacities exist that render a person incapable of making a particular kind of decision or performing a particular type of task.

Respect for individual autonomy (Schloendorff v. Society of New York Hospital 1914) demands that individuals be allowed to make decisions of which they are capable, even if they are seriously mentally ill, developmentally arrested, or organically impaired. A judicial determination of incompetence must precede an abridgement of that decision-making authority. Physical and mental illness is but one factor to be weighed in determining competency.

Guardianship

Guardianship is a method of substitute decision making for individuals who have been judicially determined to be unable to act for themselves (Brakel et al. 1985). Historically, the state or sovereign possessed the power and authority to safeguard the estate of incompetent persons (Regan 1972). This traditional role still reflects the purpose of guardianship today. In some states, there are separate provisions for the appointment of a "guardian of one's person" (e.g., health care decision making) and for a "guardian of one's estate" (e.g., authority to make contracts to sell one's property; Sale et al. 1982). The latter type of guardian is frequently referred to as a *conservator,* although this designation is not uniformly used throughout the United States. A further distinction, also found in some jurisdictions, is between *general (plenary)* and *specific* guardianship (Sale et al. 1982). As the name implies, the specific guardian is restricted to exercising decisions

about a particular subject area. For instance, he or she may be authorized to make decisions about major or emergency medical procedures, with the disabled person retaining the freedom to make decisions about all other medical matters. General guardians, in contrast, have total control over the disabled individual's person, estate, or both (Sale et al. 1982).

Guardianship arrangements are increasingly used with patients who have dementia, particularly AIDS-related dementia and Alzheimer's disease (Overman and Stoudemire 1988). Under the Anglo-American system of law, an individual is presumed to be competent unless adjudicated incompetent. Incompetence is a legal determination made by a court of law on the basis of evidence provided by health care providers and others that the individual's functional mental capacity is significantly impaired. The Uniform Guardianship and Protective Proceedings Act (UGPPA) or the Uniform Probate Code (UPC) is used as a basis for laws governing competency in many states (Mishkin 1989). Drafted by legal scholars and practicing attorneys, the uniform acts serve as models for the purpose of achieving consistency among the state laws by enactment of model laws (UGPPA § 5–101). *General incompetency* is defined by the UGPPA as meaning "impaired by reason of mental illness, mental deficiency, physical illness or disability, advanced age, chronic use of drugs, chronic intoxication, or other cause (except minority) to the extent of lacking sufficient understanding or capacity to make or communicate reasonable decisions."

Some patients with psychiatric disorders may meet the preceding definition. Generally, the appointment of a guardian is limited to situations in which the individual's decision-making capacity is so impaired that he or she is unable to care for personal safety or provide such necessities as food, shelter, clothing, and medical care, with the likely result of physical injury or illness (In re Boyer 1981). The standard of proof required for a judicial determination of incompetency is *clear and convincing evidence.* Although the law does not assign percentages to proof, if it did, clear and convincing evidence would likely be in the range of 75% certainty (Simon 1992a).

States vary on the extent of their reliance on psychiatric assessments. Nonmedical personnel such as social workers, psychologists, family members, friends, colleagues, and even the individual who is the subject of the proceeding may testify.

Health Care Decision Making

Because psychiatric patients frequently have impaired mental capacity, the difficulty associated with obtaining a valid informed consent to proposed diagnostic procedures and treatments can be both challenging and frustrating. The need to obtain competent informed consent is not negated simply because it "appears" that the patient is in need of medical intervention or would likely benefit from it. Instead, clinicians must assure themselves that the patient or an appropriate substitute decision maker has given a competent consent before proceeding with treatment. An increasing number of states require a judicial determination of incompetence and the court's substituted consent prior to the administration of antipsychotic medications to a patient who is deemed by a health care provider to lack the functional mental capacity to consent (Simon 1992a).

Only a *competent* person is legally able to give informed consent. Competent patients must not be treated against their objections. Health care providers work with patients who sometimes are of questionable competence because of mental illness, narcotic abuse, or alcoholism. When psychiatrists treat patients with neuropsychiatric deficits, the responsibility to obtain a valid informed consent can be clinically daunting because of the vacillating and unpredictable mental states associated with many central nervous system disorders.

Psychiatric patients who have been determined to lack the requisite functional mental capacity to make a treatment decision (Frasier v. Department of Health and Human Resources 1986) should have an authorized representative or guardian appointed to make health care decisions on their behalf (Aponte v. United States 1984). A number of consent options may be available for such patients, depending on the jurisdiction.

Right to Die

Legal decisions addressing the issue of a patient's "right to die" can be divided into two categories: decisions dealing with individuals who were incompetent at the time removal of life support systems was sought (In re Conroy 1985; In re Quinlin 1976) and decisions dealing with competent patients.

Incompetent patients. The U.S. Supreme Court ruled, in *Cruzan v. Director, Missouri Department of Health* (1990), that the state of Missouri may refuse to remove a food and water tube surgically implanted in the stomach of Nancy Cruzan without clear and convincing evidence of her wishes. Ms. Cruzan was in a persistent vegetative state for 7 years. Without clear and convincing evidence of a patient's decision to have life-sustaining measures withheld in a particular circumstance, the state has the right to maintain that individual's life, even to the exclusion of the family's wishes.

The importance of the *Cruzan* decision for physicians treating severely or terminally impaired patients is that physicians must seek clear and competent instructions regarding foreseeable treatment decisions. For example, a psychiatrist treating a patient with progressive degenerative diseases should attempt to ascertain the patient's wishes regarding the use of life-sustaining measures *while that patient can still competently articulate those wishes.* This information is best provided in the form of a living will, durable power-of-attorney agreement, or health care proxy. Although physicians may fear civil or criminal liability for stopping life-sustaining treatment, liability may also arise from overtreating critically or terminally ill patients (Weir and Gostin 1990). Legal liability may occur for providing unwanted treatment to an autonomous patient or treatment that is against the best interests of a nonautonomous patient.

Competent patients. A growing body of cases has emerged involving *competent* patients—with excruciating pain and terminal diseases—who seek the termination of further medical treatment. Beginning with the fundamental tenet that "no right is held more sacred...than the right of every individual to the possession and control of his own person" (Schloendorff v. Society of New York Hospital 1914; Union Pacific Realty Co. v. Botsford 1891), courts have taken this principle of autonomy seen in informed consent cases and applied it to right-to-die cases.

The right to decline life-sustaining medical intervention, even for a competent person, is not absolute. As noted in *In re Conroy* (1985), four countervailing state interests generally exist that may limit the exercise of that right: 1) preservation of life, 2) prevention of suicide, 3) safeguarding of the integrity of the medical profession, and 4) protection of innocent third parties. Balancing autonomy and these countervailing state interests, the trend has been to support a competent patient's right to have artificial life-support systems discontinued (Bartling v. Superior Court 1984; Bouvia v. Superior Court 1986; In re M.B. 2006; In re Farrell 1987; In re Jobes 1987; In re Peter 1987; Tune v. Walter Reed Army Medical Hospital 1985).

As a result of the *Cruzan* decision, courts now focus on the reliability of the evidence proffered in establishing the patient's competence, specifically the clarity and certainty with which a decision to withhold medical treatment is made. When a fully informed, competent terminally ill patient has chosen to forgo any further medical intervention, courts are less likely to overrule the patient's decision.

Advance Directives

The use of advance directives such as a living will, health care proxy, or durable medical power of attorney is recommended to avoid ethical and legal complications associated with requests to withhold life-sustaining treatment measures (Simon 1992a; Solnick 1985). The Patient Self-Determination Act, which took effect on December 1, 1991, requires hospitals, nursing homes, hospices, managed care organizations (MCOs), and home health care agencies to advise patients or family members of their right to accept or refuse medical care and to execute an advance directive (LaPuma et al. 1991). These advance directives provide a method for individuals, while competent, to choose proxy health care decision makers in the event of future incompetency. A living will can be contained as a subsection of a durable power of attorney agreement. In the ordinary power of attorney created for the management of business and financial matters, the power of attorney generally becomes null and void if the person creating it becomes incompetent.

The right to formulate an advance directive is determined by state law. All 50 states and the District of Columbia permit individuals to create a *durable* power of attorney (i.e., one that endures even if the competence of the creator does not) (Cruzan v. Director, Missouri Department of Health 1990). Several states and the District of Columbia have durable power of attorney statutes that expressly authorize the appointment of proxies for making health care decisions (Cruzan v. Director, Missouri Department of Health 1990).

Generally, a durable power of attorney has been construed to empower an agent to make health care decisions. Such a document is much broader and more flexible than a living will, which covers only the period of a diagnosed terminal illness, specifying only that no "extraordinary treatments" be used that would prolong the act of dying (Mishkin 1985). To rectify the sometimes uncertain status of the durable power of attorney as applied to health care decisions, a number of states have passed or are considering passing health care proxy laws. The health care proxy is a legal instrument akin to the durable power of attorney but specifically created for health care decision making. Despite the growing use of advance directives, there is increasing evidence that physician values rather than patient values are more decisive in end-of-life decisions (Orentlicher 1992).

In a durable power of attorney or health care proxy, general or specific directions are set forth about how future decisions should be made in the event a person becomes unable to make these decisions. The determination of a patient's competence is not specified in most durable power of attorney and health care proxy statutes. Because this is a medical or psychiatric question, the examination by two physicians to determine the patient's ability to understand the nature and consequences of the proposed treatment or procedure, ability to make a choice, and ability to communicate that choice is usually minimally sufficient. This information, like all significant medical observations, should be clearly documented in the patient's file.

Several states have enacted laws that authorize a person to designate in writing a health care surrogate to make health care decisions reflecting that person's values, which comes into effect when the person authorizing the surrogate is determined to be incapacitated. Some states authorize separate surrogates for mental health care decisions. Unless time limited on its face, the authorization continues until revoked. If the person who executed the designation attempts to revoke it when a psychiatric disorder exists and it is not clear whether he or she is incapacitated, it may be appropriate to obtain a judicial determination of the capacity to revoke.

Substituted Judgment

Psychiatrists often find that the time required to obtain an adjudication of incompetence is unduly burdensome and that the process frequently interferes with the provision of quality treatment. Moreover, families are often reluctant to face the formal court proceedings necessary to declare their family member incompetent, particularly when sensitive family matters are disclosed. A common solution to both of these problems is to seek the legally authorized proxy consent of a spouse or relative serving as guardian when the refusing patient is believed to be incompetent. Proxy consent, however, is becoming less available as a consent option (Simon 1992a). Many states exclude surrogate authorizations for the treatment of mental disorders.

There are clear advantages associated with having the family serve as decision makers (Perr 1984). First, use of responsible family members as surrogate decision makers maintains the integrity of the family unit and relies on the sources who are most likely to know the patient's wishes. Second, it is more efficient and less costly than an attempt to prove incompetency. There are some disadvantages, however. Proxy decision making requires synthesizing the diverse values, beliefs, practices, and prior statements of the patient for a given specific circumstance (Emanuel and Emanuel 1992). As one judge characterized the problem, any proxy decision making in the absence of specific directions is "at best only an optimistic approximation" (In re Jobes 1987). Ambivalent feelings, conflicts within the family and with the patient, and conflicting economic interests may make certain family members suspect as guardians (Gutheil and Appelbaum 1980). Also, relatives may not be available or may not want to get involved. Moreover, next of kin may possess dubious competence or even less competence than the patient.

The President's Commission for the Study of Ethical Problems in Medicine and Biomedical and Behavioral Research (1982) recommended that the relatives of incompetent patients be selected as proxy decision makers for the following reasons:

1. The family is generally most concerned about the good of the patient.
2. The family is usually most knowledgeable about the patient's goals, preferences, and values.
3. The family deserves recognition as an important social unit to be treated, within limits, as a single decision maker in matters that intimately affect its members.

Several states permit proxy decision making by statute, mainly through informed consent statutes (Solnick 1985). Some state statutes specify that another person may authorize consent on behalf of the incompetent patient, whereas others mention specific relatives.

Unless proxy consent by a relative is provided by statute or by case law authority in the state where the psychiatrist practices, it is not recommended that the good-faith consent by next of kin be relied on in treating a psychiatric patient believed to lack health care decision-making capacity (Klein et al. 1983). The legally appropriate procedure to follow is to seek judicial recognition of the family member as the substitute decision maker.

A debate continues about the theory of substitute decision making. Should the substitute decision maker (i.e., guardian, designated surrogate) act in the patient's best interest (the "objective test"), or should he or she rely on what the patient would have decided if competent (the "subjective" or "substituted judgment" approach)? The increasingly used subjective test is difficult to implement for patients who have never been competent, who have made improvident or less than competent decisions in the past, or who have never openly stated choices to be implemented by others. Also, the values of substitute decision makers can be easily substituted for the patient regardless of which test is used (Roth 1985). Both the best interests and the substituted judgment standards lead to predictable biases by those who implement them. Use of the best interests standard leads to treatment of pa-

tients and sustaining life. Application of the substituted judgment standard favors treatment refusal and the upholding of civil liberties (E.D. Robertson 1989).

The substituted judgment standard has found considerable judicial favor. It is based on the incompetent person's "right to privacy" translated into the medical context as the right to refuse treatment. The right to privacy is the constitutional expression of the autonomy Americans claim as free persons living in a free society. On this point, courts find authority and inspiration from John Stuart Mill:

> The only purpose for which power can be rightfully exercised over any member of a civilized community against his will, is to prevent harm to others. His own good, either physical or moral, is not a sufficient warrant. He cannot rightfully be compelled to do or forebear because it will be better for him to do so, because it will make him happier, because in the opinion of others, to do so would be wise, or even right. (Mill 1859/1951)

Physician-Assisted Suicide

With increasing legal recognition of physician-assisted suicide, psychiatrists are likely to be called on to become gatekeepers. Such a role is a radical departure from the physician's code of ethics, in which doctors are prohibited from participating in any intervention that hastens death. Previously, the U.S. Supreme Court ruled in *Cruzan* that terminally ill persons could refuse life-sustaining medical treatment. Courts and legislatures will determine whether hastening death is an unwarranted extension of the right to refuse treatment. Every proposal for physician-assisted suicide requires a psychiatric screening or consultation to determine the terminally ill person's competence to commit suicide. The presence of psychiatric disorders associated with suicide, particularly depression, will have to be ruled out as the driving factor behind the request. Much controversy rages over the ethics of this gatekeeping function (American Medical Association 1994).

The most recent chapter in this debate is *Gonzales v. Oregon* (2006), in which the U.S. Supreme Court held that the federal Controlled Substances Act did not authorize the U.S. Attorney General to prohibit physicians in Oregon from prescribing regulated drugs for use in physician-assisted suicide, as authorized by the Oregon Death With Dignity Act. Although much of the opinion turns on a technical reading of the federal law and the authority granted under it, the opinion is also grounded in the states' authority to regulate the practice of medicine to the point of permitting physicians to assist in the administration of lethal doses of drugs.

High-Risk Relationships

Psychiatric Malpractice

Medical malpractice is a tort (i.e., a civil wrong not grounded in criminal or contract law). Most medical malpractice claims are based in negligence rather than intentional torts (e.g., battery, false imprisonment), if for no other reason than to avoid the exclusionary language in most professional liability policies for intentional acts. *Negligence,* the fundamental concept underlying most malpractice claims, is the failure to act reasonably under the circumstances. In the case of medical malpractice, negligence involves either doing something that a physician should not have done with a patient under the circumstances or failing to do something that a physician should have done with a patient under the circumstances. However, acting unreasonably is not alone sufficient to support a negligence claim.

For a psychiatrist to be found *liable* to a patient for malpractice, the four fundamental elements of a negligence claim must be established by a preponderance of the evidence (i.e., more likely than not). Each of these four elements must be met for the claim to prevail. A psychiatrist may have rendered substandard care, but if the jury finds it caused no legally recognized harm or that any harm was caused by another actor or condition, the claim fails.

In most states, whether the psychiatrist's duty to his or her patient has been breached turns on whether the fact finder decides that the defendant acted with the degree of skill and care of the average physician in that specialty under the circumstances (Stepakoff v. Kantar 1985). The use of a somatic therapy, including electroconvulsive therapy (ECT), is evaluated no differently from the use of any other medical treatment or procedure with respect to potential liability. The same standard of the degree of skill and care of the average physician practicing that specialty governs the assessment of whether a psychiatrist's use of or failure to use a somatic intervention is negligent.

It is generally acknowledged within the psychiatric profession that there is no *absolute standard* protocol for the administration of psychotropic medication or ECT. Nevertheless, the existence of professional treatment guidelines and procedures that are generally accepted or used by a significant number of psychiatrists should alert clinicians to consider such guidelines as practice reference sources. For example, the APA has published comprehensive findings and guidelines such as the task force reports concerning ECT (American Psychiatric Association 2001a), tardive dyskinesia (American

Psychiatric Association 1992), and the treatment of psychiatric disorders (American Psychiatric Association 2004). Official guidelines are relevant evidence in setting the standard but neither bind the fact finder at trial nor preempt sound professional judgment in attending to the specific clinical needs of patients.

Guidelines and procedures publications of private nongovernmental organizations cannot bind the courts and thus do not establish the standard of care by which a psychiatrist's actions must be measured in malpractice litigation. Along with expert testimony, they are sources of relevant information for the fact finder to consider in setting the standard of care (Shuman 2001). Therefore, a reasonable psychiatrist should be familiar and should have considered APA and other similar guidelines (Stone v. Proctor 1963).

There is less professional autonomy and flexibility associated with the use of ECT. Usually, the reasonable care standard applied to psychiatric treatment is construed in a fairly broad manner. Some psychiatric treatments such as ECT, however, are more rigidly regulated than others. For instance, the Joint Commission on Accreditation of Healthcare Organizations (JCAHO) considers ECT a *special treatment* procedure to be regulated by written policies. Whenever ECT is used, the procedure must be adequately justified and documented in the patient's medical chart (Joint Commission on Accreditation of Healthcare Organizations 2006a). The ECT policies of treatment facilities as well as judicial decisions and statutory regulation of ECT can also serve as establishing the basis for liability, if violated.

The standard for judging the use and administration of medication, on the other hand, appears to be consistent with the more flexible and general reasonable care requirement. Another reference source is the *Physicians' Desk Reference* (PDR), which may be used to establish or dispute the reasonableness of a psychiatrist's pharmacotherapy procedures. The PDR is a commercially distributed and privately published reference of medication products used in the United States. The U.S. Food and Drug Administration (FDA) requires that drug manufacturers have their official package inserts reported in the PDR (Simon 1992a). Accordingly, psychiatrists consult publications such as the PDR as needed to keep abreast of current and accurate medication information. Although numerous courts have cited the PDR as a credible source of medication-related information in the medical profession, the PDR does not by itself establish the standard of care (Gowan v. United States 1985; Witherell v. Weimer 1986). Instead, it is simply relevant evidence to establish the standard of care in a particular situation (Callan v. Norland 1983; Doerr v. Hurley Medical Center 1984). Courts generally follow the reasoning in *Ramon v. Farr* (1989), holding that drug inserts alone do not set the standard of care. They are only one element to be considered, along with previous clinical experience, the scientific literature, approvals in other countries, expert testimony, and other pertinent factors. The presence of a substantial scientific literature that justifies the clinician's treatment is more persuasive than FDA approval. The PDR or any other reference cannot serve as a substitute for the psychiatrist's sound clinical judgment.

Courts recognize the importance of professional judgment and give psychiatrists, like other medical specialists, latitude in explaining special diagnostic or treatment considerations that guide their decision making. For instance, the clinical data regarding pharmacological treatment of rapid-cycling bipolar disorder indicate that a variety of potentially useful drug therapies exist, some of which are considered experimental or on the cutting edge (Simon 1997). Various drugs and hormones are useful as mood stabilizers, such as carbamazepine, clozapine, thyroid and estrogen replacement, calcium channel blockers, antihypertensives, neuroleptics, atypical antipsychotics, and other anticonvulsants (lamotrigine, valproate, gabapentin).

The courts do not demand professional orthodoxy. Evidence that a treatment procedure is accepted by at least a respectable minority of professionals in the field can establish that a particular treatment is a reasonable professional practice (Simon 1993). The standard of care associated with the use of a somatic therapy to treat a psychiatric patient, *at a minimum*, is summarized in Table 41–3.

Theories of liability. The potential for negligence by a psychiatrist is greatest in clinical situations involving the use of psychotropic medication. Unlike talk therapies, in which the causation of harm is more diffuse (i.e., whether a different talk therapy likely would have produced a different result), medication errors tend to be more stark and their consequences easier to trace. Although no reliable compilation of malpractice claims data has been published, anecdotal information suggests that medication-related lawsuits constitute a significant share of claims filed against psychiatrists. As noted earlier, claims data from the APA Professional Liability Insurance Program showed that medication error and drug reaction constituted 7% of malpractice allegations. Allegations of drug mismanagement are a

TABLE 41–3. Required minimum standard of care for a somatic treatment of a psychiatric patient

Pretreatment

Complete clinical history (medical, psychiatric)

Complete physical examination as clinically indicated (performed by another physician or, if necessary, by the psychiatrist)

Administration of necessary laboratory tests and review of past test results

Disclosure of sufficient information to the patient to obtain informed consent, including information about the risks and benefits both of treatment and of no treatment

Thorough documentation of all treatment decisions, informed consent information, pertinent patient responses, and other relevant treatment data

Posttreatment

Careful monitoring of the patient's response to treatment, including adequate follow-up evaluations and appropriate laboratory testing

Prompt adjustments in treatment, as clinically indicated

Arrangement for additional informed consent when treatment is altered appreciably or new treatment initiated

significant contributor to "incorrect treatment," the most common malpractice category.

A review of the relevant case law indicates that various mistakes, omissions, and poor medication treatment practices commonly result in malpractice actions brought against psychiatrists. The following discussion, although not intended to be exhaustive, provides a framework for identifying problem areas associated with medication treatment.

Failure to adequately evaluate. Sound clinical practice requires that before any form of treatment is initiated, the patient should be adequately evaluated. The nature and extent of an evaluation are largely dictated by the type of treatment being contemplated and the medical and psychiatric condition of the patient. A physical examination should be conducted or obtained, if clinically indicated. A recently performed physical examination may suffice, or patients may be referred elsewhere if the psychiatrist does not perform physical examinations. The duty to ensure that proper informed consent is obtained can be fulfilled at this time.

Failure to monitor. Probably the most common act of negligence associated with pharmacotherapy is the failure to monitor the patient while he or she is taking medication, including carefully following the patient for adverse side effects. Once psychotropic medication is prescribed, it is the psychiatrist's duty to monitor the patient. Consultation or referral may be necessary according to the clinical needs of the patient. Monitoring may require the use of laboratory testing. Serum drug levels are obtainable for a number of psychotropic medications. The primary indications for these laboratory tests include assessment of therapeutic and toxic levels of medication and patient compliance with treatment. The use of carbamazepine, valproate, and clozapine requires periodic monitoring of the hematopoietic system and the liver. Failure to supervise patients to ensure that they are taking medications properly can delay or prevent the detection of harmful side effects or the necessity to change to more effective treatment. If a patient is harmed, a malpractice action might result (Chaires v. St. John's Episcopal Hospital 1984; Clifford v. United States 1985; Kilgore v. County of Santa Clara 1982; Muldrow v. Re-Direct, Inc. 2005).

Split treatment. Split-treatment situations require that the psychiatrist stay fully informed of the patient's clinical status as well as of the nature and quality of treatment the patient is receiving from the nonmedical therapist (Sederer et al. 1998). In a collaborative relationship, responsibility for the patient's care is shared according to the qualifications and limitations of each clinician. The responsibilities of each discipline do not diminish those of the other disciplines. Patients should be informed of the separate responsibilities of each discipline. Periodic evaluation by the psychiatrist and the nonmedical therapist of the patient's clinical condition and needs is necessary to determine whether the collaboration should continue. On termination of the collaborative relationship, the patient should be informed by the clinicians either separately or jointly. In split treatments, if negligence is claimed on the part of the nonmedical therapist, it is likely that the collaborating psychiatrist will be sued, and vice versa (Woodward et al. 1993).

In managed care or similar treatment settings, the mere prescribing of medication without an informed, working doctor–patient relationship does not meet generally accepted standards of good clinical care. Fragmented care, in which the psychiatrist functions only as a prescriber of medication while remaining uninformed about the patient's overall clinical status, constitutes substandard treatment. Such a practice may diminish the efficacy of the drug treatment itself or even lead to the patient's failure to take the prescribed medication.

Psychiatrists who prescribe medications in split-treatment arrangements should be able to hospitalize patients if necessary. If the psychiatrist does not have admitting privileges, prearrangements should exist with other psychiatrists who can hospitalize patients if emergencies arise.

In managed care settings, psychiatrists may be required to prescribe medications from a restrictive or closed formulary. Psychiatrists, in their professional discretion, should determine which medications will be prescribed according to the special clinical needs of the patient. Split treatment is increasingly used by managed care companies and is a potential malpractice minefield (Meyer and Simon 1999).

Negligent prescription practices. The selection of a medication, determination of initial dosage and form of administration, and other related procedures are all decisions left to the professional discretion of the treating psychiatrist. In managed care settings, psychiatrists should vigorously resist attempts to limit their choice of drugs. The prescribing of specific medications should be determined by the psychiatrist and the clinical needs of the patient. An appeal should be filed if a drug that is not formulary approved is denied. The law recognizes that the physician is in the best position to "know the patient" and to determine what course of treatment is best under the circumstances. The standard by which a psychiatrist's prescription practices will be evaluated is reasonableness. In administering psychotropic medication, psychiatrists need only conform their procedures and decision making to those that are *ordinarily* practiced by other psychiatrists under similar circumstances.

A review of cases involving allegations of negligent prescription procedures reveals several common practices representing potential deviations from generally accepted treatment practice (Table 41–4).

TABLE 41–4. Common negligent prescription practices
Exceeding recommended dosages without clinical indications
Prescribing multiple drugs inappropriately
Prescribing medication for unapproved uses without a documented rationale
Prescribing unapproved medications
Failing to disclose medication risks

As stated earlier, any physician who prescribes medication has a duty to first obtain the informed consent of the patient (Table 41–5). Obtaining competent informed consent may be complicated by the fact that some psychiatric patients have compromised mental capacity for health care decision making. Patients lacking such decision-making capacity require consent for treatment by substitute decision makers (Table 41–6).

Each time a medication is changed and a new drug is introduced, informed consent should be obtained. Failure to inform a patient properly of the risks and benefits of a prescribed medication is a ground for a malpractice action if the patient is injured as a result (Karasik v. Bird 1984; Moran v. Botsford General Hospital 1984; Wright v. State 1986).

Other medication-related issues that have resulted in legal action include 1) failure to treat side effects after they have been recognized or should have been recognized, 2) failure to monitor a patient's compliance with prescription limits, 3) failure to prescribe medication or appropriate levels of medication according to the treatment needs of the patient, 4) failure to refer a patient for consultation or treatment by a specialist when indicated, and 5) negligent withdrawal from medication and unclear or illegible prescriptions.

Tardive dyskinesia. The development of neuroleptic medications in the mid-1950s dramatically improved the treatment and management of patients with schizophrenia. Shortly after the introduction of neuroleptic medications as therapeutic agents, however, researchers and clinicians observed unusual muscle movements in some patients, referred to as *tardive dyskinesia.*

The risk of developing tardive dyskinesia is approximately 4%–7% per year of neuroleptic use (Lohr et al. 1986). These projections are even higher for elderly patients (Kane et al. 1982; Klawans and Barr 1982). Because the atypical antipsychotic drugs are used more frequently, the risk of developing tardive dyskinesia may be lower.

Despite the possibility of a large number of tardive dyskinesia–related lawsuits, relatively few psychiatrists have been subject of a malpractice claim arising out of tardive dyskinesia. One possible reason may be that patients who develop tardive dyskinesia may not have the physical and psychological stamina required to pursue litigation.

Allegations of negligence after a patient develops tardive dyskinesia are based on the same legal requirements as any other malpractice action. The bases for negligence include but are not limited to the following:

- Failure to evaluate and monitor a patient properly.
- Failure to obtain informed consent.

TABLE 41–5. **Informed consent: reasonable information to be disclosed**

Although there exists no consistently accepted set of information to be disclosed for any given medical or psychiatric situation, five areas of information are generally provided:

1. Diagnosis: Description of the condition or problem
2. Treatment: Nature and purpose of proposed treatment
3. Consequences: Risks and benefits of the proposed treatment
4. Alternatives: Viable alternatives to the proposed treatment, including risks and benefits
5. Prognosis: Projected outcome with and without treatment

Source. Reprinted with permission from Simon RI: *Clinical Psychiatry and the Law,* 2nd Edition. Washington, DC, American Psychiatric Press, 1992, p. 128.

TABLE 41–6. **Common consent options for patients lacking the mental capacity for health care decisions**

Proxy consent of next of kin, as permitted by state law[a]

Adjudication of incompetence and appointment of a guardian

Substituted consent of the court

Advance directives (living will, durable power of attorney, health care proxy)

[a]May be excluded for treatment of mental disorders.

Source. Adapted with permission from Simon RI: *Clinical Psychiatry and the Law,* 2nd Edition. Washington, DC, American Psychiatric Press, 1992, p. 109.

- Negligent diagnosis of a patient's condition. For instance, in *Hyde v. University of Michigan Board of Regents* (1986), a patient was awarded $1 million from a medical center because it misdiagnosed her condition as Huntington's chorea instead of tardive dyskinesia; the verdict was later reversed on the basis of a subsequent case that expanded the state's sovereign immunity coverage (Ross v. Consumer Power Company 1985).
- Wrongful prescription of neuroleptic medication. For example, in *Dovido v. Vasquez* (1986), a net award of $700,000 went to a 42-year-old plaintiff who developed tardive dyskinesia as a result of the defendant psychiatrist's negligent prescription of extremely high doses of fluphenazine.

- Failure to monitor medication side effects. For example, in *Clites v. State* (1982), the plaintiff was a mentally retarded man who had been institutionalized since age 11 years and treated with major tranquilizers from age 18 to age 23 years. Tardive dyskinesia was diagnosed at age 23 years. The family subsequently sued, claiming the defendants negligently prescribed medication, did not inform the patient of the possibility of developing tardive dyskinesia, and failed to monitor and subsequently treat the patient's resulting side effects. The jury returned a verdict for the plaintiff and awarded damages in the amount of $760,165. This award was affirmed on appeal. The court ruled that the defendants were negligent because they deviated from the standards of the industry. Specifically, the court cited various omissions in ordinary psychiatric practice that, they concluded, reasonable psychiatrists would have provided. Among the deviations they noted were failure to conduct regular physical examinations and laboratory tests, failure to intervene at the first sign of tardive dyskinesia, inappropriate use of multiple medications at the same time, use of drugs for convenience rather than therapy, and failure to obtain informed consent.

Patients receiving neuroleptic medication need to be frequently monitored. No stock answer can be given to the question of how frequently the psychiatrist should see a patient. Generally, psychiatrists should schedule return visits with a frequency that accords with the patient's clinical need. The longer the time between visits, however, the greater the risk of missing adverse drug reactions and untoward developments in the patient's condition.

The defenses and preventive measures applicable to tardive dyskinesia–related malpractice claims are consistent with those used in cases alleging negligent drug treatment. Sound clinical practice accompanied by the patient's competent informed consent, appropriately documented in the medical chart, serves as an effective foil to allegations of negligence should tardive dyskinesia develop (Chandler v. Simpson 2000).

Electroconvulsive therapy.   With the current shortened length of stay in hospitals, use of ECT appears to be increasing. Legal actions alleging negligence associated with ECT are infrequent. Litigation involving ECT-related injuries represent a variety of circumstances in which negligence has occurred. These cases can be categorized into three groups: pretreatment, treatment, and posttreatment.

Pretreatment. Although pre-ECT evaluations vary somewhat, the following procedures recommended by the APA Task Force on Electroconvulsive Therapy (American Psychiatric Association 2001a) generally should be performed:

1. Psychiatric history and examination to evaluate the indications for ECT
2. Medical examination to determine risk factors
3. Anesthesia evaluation
4. Informed consent (written)
5. Evaluation by a physician privileged to administer ECT

Although these recommendations by the APA Task Force on ECT do not define in absolute terms the standard of care for ECT, they may be proffered as evidence of the standard of care in malpractice suits involving ECT. Official treatment guidelines, however, should not be a substitute for the psychiatrist's sound clinical judgment.

Treatment. Psychiatrists are not liable for a mere mistake in judgment, nor is a psychiatrist held to a standard of 100% accuracy or perfect performance (Smith 1986; see also Holton v. Pfingst 1976). A bad result does not automatically establish a claim for malpractice (Howe v. Citizens Memorial Hospital 1968). Lawsuits involving ECT-related injuries in which the negligence is related to the actual treatment process include the following errors:

- Failure to use a muscle relaxant to reduce the chance of a bone fracture
- Negligent administration of the procedure
- Failure to conduct an adequate evaluation of the patient before continuing treatment

Posttreatment. It is common for patients treated with ECT to experience side effects such as temporary confusion, disorientation, and memory loss immediately after its administration. Because of these temporary debilitating effects, sound clinical practice requires that psychiatrists provide reasonable posttreatment care and safeguards. The failure to attend properly to a patient for a period of time after administering ECT may result in malpractice liability. The following are examples of posttreatment circumstances that may constitute a basis for a lawsuit:

- Failure to evaluate complaints of pain or discomfort following treatment

- Failure to evaluate a patient's condition before resuming ECT treatments
- Failure to monitor a patient properly to prevent falls
- Failure to supervise properly a patient who was injured as a result of ECT

ECT-related civil damage claims are infrequent today and do not represent a significant malpractice risk for psychiatrists. Nevertheless, Perlin (1989) has cautioned that "recent developments in right-to-refuse treatment law and statutory regulation of intrusive therapy are likely to insure that any future ECT litigation will still be considered carefully" (pp. 47–48).

National Practitioner Data Bank

On September 1, 1990, the National Practitioner Data Bank established by the Health Care Quality Improvement Act of 1986 went into effect. The data bank tracks disciplinary actions, malpractice judgments, and settlements against physicians, dentists, and other health care professionals (Johnson 1991).

Hospitals, health maintenance organizations, MCOs, professional societies, state medical boards, and other health care organizations are required to report any disciplinary action taken against providers lasting more than 30 days. Disciplinary actions include limitation, suspension, or revocation of privileges or professional society membership. MCOs are not required to report physicians to the data bank if they do not follow treatment protocols. However, when a physician is deselected by an MCO for a quality-of-care issue, the MCO must report it ("The National Practitioner Data Bank and MCOs" 1999). Medical malpractice payments account for approximately three-quarters of reports made to the data bank. Under the Health Care Quality Improvement Act, immunity from liability is granted for health care entities and providers making peer review reports in good faith (Walzer 1990).

Hospitals are required to request information from the data bank concerning all physicians applying for staff privileges. Every 2 years, a query of the data bank is required concerning each physician or other practitioner on the hospital staff. Hospitals that do not comply face loss of immunity for professional peer review activities.

The public does not have access to the data bank. Plaintiffs' attorneys can have access to the data bank only if they can prove that the hospital failed to query the data bank about the physician in question. The information obtained can be used only to sue the hospital for negligent credentialing. Physicians can request information from the data bank about their own file. A study found that hospital reporting of actions taken regarding clinical privileges from 1991 to 1995 declined, raising concerns about underreporting (Baldwin et al. 1999).

The Suicidal Patient

The most common malpractice claim arising from psychiatric care is the failure to provide reasonable protection to patients from harming themselves. There are categories of negligent failings that are frequently asserted: diagnostic failures (i.e., assess the potential for suicide), treatment failures (i.e., use reasonable treatment interventions and precautions), and implementation failures (i.e., carry out treatment properly and not negligently).

These categorical failings, each of which applies to inpatient and outpatient settings, are simply different ways in which the practitioner's duty of care may have been breached by unreasonable conduct. Claims for conduct resulting in the death of a patient are governed by the same tort principles that apply when a living patient brings a malpractice claim. However, because tort claims at common law did not survive the death of a patient, most states have legislation permitting the survival of such actions by the former patient's estate under the banner of wrongful death. Although they apply traditional tort principles, most wrongful-death actions brought for patient suicides turn on the legal concepts of *foreseeability, reasonableness,* and *causation.* As a general rule, a psychiatrist who exercises reasonable care in compliance with accepted medical practice will not be held liable for any resulting injury. Thus, if the fact finder concludes that a patient's suicide was not reasonably foreseeable, that the precautions taken by the psychiatrist were reasonable, or even if they were not that the suicide was caused by an unforeseeable intervening factor, the claim will fail.

Foreseeable suicide. The evaluation of suicide risk is one of the most complex, difficult, and challenging clinical tasks in psychiatry (Simon 2004). Suicide is a rare event. A systematic assessment of a patient's suicide risk forms the basis of a sound clinical management plan. Using reasonable care in assessing suicide risk can preempt the problem of predicting the actual occurrence of suicide, for which professional standards do not exist. Standard approaches to the assessments of suicide risk are described in the psychiatric literature (Simon and Hales 2006). Time attenuates suicide risk assessments, requiring that assessment be a process, not an event.

As an accepted standard of care, an evaluation of suicide risk should be done with all patients, regardless of whether they present with overt suicidal complaints. A review of case law shows that reasonable care requires that a patient who is either suspected of being or confirmed to be suicidal must be the subject of certain affirmative precautions. A failure either to reasonably assess a patient's suicide risk or to implement an appropriate precautionary plan after the suicide potential becomes foreseeable is likely to render a practitioner liable if the patient is harmed because of a suicide attempt. The law permits the fact finder to conclude that suicide is preventable if it is foreseeable. Foreseeability, however, should not be confused with preventability. In hindsight, many suicides seem preventable that were clearly not foreseeable.

When suicide risk assessments are competently performed and recorded, the psychiatrist demonstrates careful and thorough management of the suicidal patient. Moreover, evidence of a reasonable suicide risk assessment also demonstrates that the psychiatrist adhered to the prevailing standard of care. Although psychiatrists cannot ensure favorable outcomes with suicidal patients, they can ensure that the process of suicide risk assessment was competently performed (Simon 2002).

Inpatients. Intervention in an inpatient setting usually requires the following:

- Screening evaluations
- Development of an appropriate treatment plan
- Implementation of that plan
- Ongoing case review by clinical staff

Careful documentation of assessments and management interventions with changes responsive to the patient's clinical situation are evidence of clinically and legally sufficient psychiatric care. Assessing suicide risk and protective factors is only half of the equation. Documenting the benefits of a psychiatric intervention (e.g., ward change, pass, discharge) against the risk of suicide permits an evenhanded approach to the clinical management of the patient.

Psychiatrists are more likely to be sued successfully when a psychiatric inpatient commits suicide. The law permits the fact finder to conclude that the opportunities to foresee (i.e., anticipate) and control (i.e., treat and manage) suicidal patients are greater in the hospital (Hofflander v. St. Catherine's Hospital 2003).

Outpatients. Psychiatrists are expected to reasonably assess the severity and imminence of a foresee-able suicidal act. The result of the assessment dictates the treatment and safety management options. Psychiatrists are not strictly liable whenever an outpatient commits suicide (Speer v. United States 1981). Instead, the reasonableness of the psychiatrist's efforts is determinative.

Suicide prevention pacts. Suicide prevention contracts created between the clinician and the patient attempt to develop an expressed understanding that the patient will call for help rather than act out suicidal thoughts or impulses. These contracts have no legal authority; although they may be helpful in solidifying the therapeutic alliance, they may falsely reassure the psychiatrist. Suicide prevention agreements between psychiatrists and patients must not be used in place of adequate suicide assessment (Simon 1999).

Legal defenses. A psychiatrist's Answer to a malpractice claim arising out of a patient suicide may consist of a denial of allegations in the plaintiff's Complaint, from which the fact finder might reject the allegation that the psychiatrist breached a duty that proximately caused the patient's suicide. In addition, the defendant's Answer to the Complaint might include affirmative defenses that have the legal effect of defeating the claim even if the defendant's negligence proximately caused the patient's suicide.

One approach to denying a crucial allegation of the plaintiff's case is to prove that the care and supervision provided were reasonable. One example of that denial of negligence is the best-judgment defense asserting that the patient was properly assessed and treated for suicide risk but committed suicide anyway (J.D. Robertson 1991). In some cases the treatment may appear to contribute to the risk. This has proved to be controversial in the use of the "open door" policy in which patients are allowed freedom of movement for therapeutic purposes. In these cases, the individual facts and reasonableness of the staff's application of the "open door" policy appear to be paramount. Nevertheless, courts have difficulty with abstract treatment notions such as personal growth when faced with a dead patient.

The plaintiff must persuade the fact finder that the psychiatrist's negligence more likely than not caused the patient's suicide. Thus proof that the suicide was caused by an unforeseeable intervening cause negates a critical element of the claim. For example, a fact finder may find a psychiatrist not liable for the suicidal act of a borderline patient who experienced a traumatic loss of a romantic relationship between therapy sessions and then impulsively attempted suicide without trying to contact the psychiatrist.

Affirmative defenses, like the statute of limitations, bar untimely claims regardless of their merits. Governmental or sovereign immunity, where it exists, bars claims regardless of the strength of the plaintiff's claim.

The Violent Patient

As a general rule, absent a special relationship, one person has no duty to control the conduct of a second person to prevent that person from harming a third person (Restatement [Second] of Torts 1965). Applying this rule to psychiatric care, psychiatrists traditionally have had only a limited duty owed to third persons to control their patients. Included in this limited class of duty to third persons for the acts of their patients is negligent discharge of a dangerous patient who harms a third person or the failure to warn a patient about the risks of driving while taking certain medications, resulting in injury to others (Felthous 1990). After *Tarasoff* (Tarasoff v. Regents of the University of California 1976), the therapist's legal duty and potential liability significantly expanded in the outpatient setting in many, but not all, states (Thapar v. Zezulka 1999). In *Tarasoff*, the California Supreme Court reasoned that a duty to protect third parties was imposed when a special relationship existed between the individual whose conduct created the danger and the defendant. Finding this special relationship requirement met in this setting, the court concluded that "the single relationship of a doctor to his patient is sufficient to support the duty to exercise reasonable care to protect others [from the violent acts of patients]." Critical to recognizing a duty in this situation was the court's assumption about mental health professionals and the foreseeability of violence.

Psychiatrists do not have the ability to predict violence with any accuracy. Violent behaviors are the result of the complex interplay among social, clinical, and personality factors that vary significantly across situations and time (Widiger and Trull 1994). Nonetheless, clinical methods for assessing the risk of violence exist that reflect the current standard of care (Baxter and Beck 1998; Monahan and Steadman 1994; Simon 1992a; Tardiff 2002).

Assessment of risk of violence is essentially a clinical judgment. Because the validity of violence risk assessments is only modestly greater than chance, the MacArthur Violence Risk Assessment Study was established. The purpose of the study was to improve clinical risk assessment validity, enhance effective clinical risk management, and provide data on mental disorders and violence for informing mental health law

and policy (Monahan et al. 2001). In this study, violence risk assessments were found to have a validity that was modestly better than chance. Until more studies are available, sound clinical practice requires that thorough violence risk assessments be routinely performed with potentially violent patients on the basis of current knowledge of violence risk factors. Although violence risk assessments need to be made at such critical points as the initiation of ward status changes, passes, and discharge, violence risk assessment is more of a continuing process rather than a solitary event. All such assessments should be duly recorded.

The index of suspicion for potential violence should be high in patients with a past history of violence who are currently making serious threats of harm toward specific individuals. The potential for violence is further heightened if the patient is acutely psychotic, substance abusing, angry, or fearful of being harmed or is experiencing delusions of being controlled or influenced (Link and Stueve 1994).

Following *Tarasoff*, courts in other jurisdictions have interpreted the case variously. Some states have adopted the *Tarasoff* holding, whereas others have limited or extended its scope and reach. In most states, psychotherapists have a duty, established by case law or statute, to act affirmatively to protect an endangered third party from a patient's violent or dangerous acts. A few courts have declined to find a *Tarasoff* duty in a specific case, whereas some courts have simply rejected the *Tarasoff* duty (Evans v. United States 1995; Green v. Ross 1997). In *Thapar v. Zezulka* (1999), the Texas Supreme Court ruled that the state statute on confidentiality *permits* but does not *require* disclosures by therapists of threats of harm to endangered third parties by their patients.

When courts have found a duty to protect, they have required an "imminent" threat of serious harm to a foreseeable victim. The term *imminent*, however, is a problematic construct for assessing violence (Simon 2006). Just as the decisions have sought to narrow the time frame within which the violence that triggers the duty might arise, so they have sought to limit the persons who are at risk. Only a small minority of courts have held that a duty to protect exists for the population at large; most require an identifiable victim to be at risk. In some jurisdictions, courts have held that the need to safeguard the public well-being overrides all other considerations, including confidentiality. Despite the fact that the *Tarasoff* duty is still not law in some jurisdictions and is subject to different interpretations by individual courts, the duty to protect is, in effect, a national standard of practice.

Several states have enacted statutes that immunize the psychiatrist from legal liability arising from a patient's violent acts toward others when the psychiatrist facing this predicament takes certain action such as warning the endangered third party and/or notifying the authorities (Appelbaum et al. 1989). The duty-to-protect language stated in some statutes allows for a greater variety of clinical interventions.

Evolving trends.   An important evolving trend is the application of the *Tarasoff* duty to sexual abuse cases by an alleged pedophile. A psychiatrist was denied dismissal of a claim against him by a child patient who was abused by his psychiatric resident/patient for not reporting to the medical school that his student/patient was a pedophile (Garamella v. New York Medical College 1998). The resident/patient molested the child at a hospital crisis center. The court reasoned that the defendant psychiatrist's control over the psychiatric resident was far greater than in the typical psychiatrist–patient relationship, leaving for trial whether the plaintiff "was within a foreseeable class of victims to whom Dr. Ingram [the residency supervisor] might owe a duty of care arising from DeMasi's [the resident] disclosure. The issue of foreseeability is a disputed one, properly reserved for the trier of fact" (pp. 174–175).

A *Tarasoff* duty was also found where a spouse had knowledge of her husband's sexually abusive behavior against children in the neighborhood (J.S. v. R.T. 1998; Touchette v. Ganal 1996). In another case, the court found that a *Tarasoff* duty could exist but declined to find the parents of a babysitter liable for his dangerous sexual behavior (People v. Rose 1998). The court determined that no evidence existed that the parents knew of their son's proclivity to commit a sexual assault.

Release of potentially violent patients.   Under managed care, discharging violent or potentially violent inpatients presents unique challenges for treating psychiatrists (Simon 1998). The treatment of psychiatric inpatients has changed dramatically in the managed care era (Lazarus and Sharfstein 1994). Most psychiatric units, particularly in general hospitals, have become short-stay, acute-care psychiatric facilities. Generally, only suicidal, homicidal, or gravely disabled patients with major psychiatric disorders pass strict precertification review for hospitalization (Tischler 1990). Close scrutiny by utilization reviewers permits only short hospitalization for these patients (Wickizer et al. 1996). The purpose of hospitalization is crisis intervention and management to stabilize patients and to ensure

their safety, and the treatment of patients is provided by a variety of mental health professionals. Nonetheless, the psychiatrist often must bear the ultimate burden of liability for treatments gone awry ("Why Are Liability Premiums Rising?" 1996). Limited opportunity usually exists during the hospital stay to develop a therapeutic alliance with patients. The ability to communicate with patients—the psychiatrist's stock-in-trade—is often severely curtailed. All of these factors contribute to a greatly increased risk of malpractice suits against psychiatrists that allege premature or negligent discharge of patients due to cost-containment policies.

There is more control over the patient in the hospital than is available in an outpatient setting. Courts closely evaluate decisions made by psychiatrists treating inpatients that adversely affect the patients or a third party. Liability imposed on psychiatric facilities that had custody of patients who injured others outside the institution after escape or release is clearly distinguishable from the factual situation of *Tarasoff*. Duty-to-warn cases generally involve patients in outpatient treatment. Liability arises from the inaction of the therapist who fails to take affirmative measures to warn or protect endangered third parties. In negligent-release cases, liability may arise from the allegation that the institution's affirmative act in releasing the patient caused injury to the third party. Moreover, allegations may be made that a psychiatrist or hospital personnel failed, prior to the patient's discharge, to warn individuals known to be at risk of harm from that patient. Lawsuits stemming from the release of foreseeably dangerous patients who subsequently injure or kill others are roughly five to six times more common than outpatient duty-to-warn lawsuits (Simon 1992b).

The psychiatrist's liability is determined by reference to professional standards. Consultation with other psychiatrists may provide additional protection when the discharge of a potentially violent patient appears problematic. Consulting with an attorney may help clarify legal obligations, but clinicians ultimately must exercise their professional judgment.

The patient's willingness to cooperate with the psychiatrist is critical to maintaining follow-up treatment. The psychiatrist's obligation focuses on structuring the follow-up visits in such a manner as to encourage compliance. A study of Department of Veterans Affairs (VA) inpatient referrals to a VA mental health outpatient clinic showed that of the 24% of inpatients who were referred, approximately one-half failed to keep their first appointments (Zeldow and Taub 1981). Nevertheless, limitations do exist on the extent of the psychiatrist's ability to ensure follow-up care. Most patients retain the right to refuse treatment. These limitations must be acknowledged by both the psychiatric and legal communities (Simon 1992a). The American Medical Association Council on Scientific Affairs has developed evidence-based discharge criteria for safe discharge from the hospital (American Medical Association 1996).

In either the outpatient or inpatient situation, psychiatrists are in compliance with the responsibility to warn and protect others from potentially violent patients if they reasonably assess the patients' *risk* for violence and make clinically appropriate interventions based on their findings. Professional standards do exist for assessment of the risk factors for violence (Simon 2001), but no standard of care exists for the prediction of violent behavior. The clinician should assess the risk of violence frequently, updating the risk assessment at significant clinical junctures (e.g., room and ward changes, passes, discharge). A risk–benefit assessment should be conducted and recorded before a pass or discharge is issued. Assessing the risk of violence is a "here and now" determination performed at the time of discharge. After the patient is discharged, the potential for violence against self or others depends on the nature and course of the mental illness, adequacy of future treatment, adherence to treatment recommendations, and exposure to unforeseeable stressful life events.

Involuntary Hospitalization

Involuntary hospitalization of persons with mental disorders is limited to statutorily defined criteria in all states. Based on the state's decision to exercise its constitutional authority, all states have authorized civil commitment of individuals who are mentally ill and dangerous to self or others, and some states also permit commitment of individuals who are mentally ill and unable to provide for their basic needs. Generally, each state spells out which criteria are required and what each means. Terms such as *mentally ill* are often loosely described, thus placing the responsibility for appropriate diagnosis on the clinical judgment of the petitioner.

Some states have enacted legislation that permits involuntary hospitalization of three other distinct groups in addition to individuals with mental illness: developmentally disabled persons, substance-addicted persons, and mentally disabled minors. Special commitment provisions may exist governing requirements for the admission and discharge of mentally disabled minors as well as numerous due-process rights afforded these individuals (Parham v. J.R. 1979).

Involuntary hospitalization of psychiatric patients usually arises when violent behavior threatens to erupt toward self or others and when patients become unable to care for themselves. These patients frequently manifest mental disorders and conditions that meet the substantive criteria for involuntary hospitalization.

Courts, not clinicians, have the authority to commit patients. The psychiatrist initiates the process that brings the patient before the court, usually after a brief period of hospitalization for evaluation or after an evaluation of a prospective patient at the request of the court. The psychiatrist must be guided by the treatment needs of the patient in seeking involuntary hospitalization, within the constraints of commitment standards.

Commitment statutes do not require involuntary hospitalization but are permissive (Appelbaum et al. 1989). The statutes enable mental health professionals and others to seek involuntary hospitalization for persons who meet certain substantive criteria. The duty to seek involuntary hospitalization is a standard-of-care issue. Patients who are mentally ill and pose a serious threat to themselves or others may require involuntary hospitalization as a primary psychiatric intervention.

Liability. Because psychiatrists are often granted conditional immunity for their good-faith participation in involuntary hospitalization proceedings, it is not surprising that most malpractice claims involving involuntary hospitalization allege an absence of good faith in the psychiatrists' behavior. Often these lawsuits are brought under the theory of false imprisonment. Other areas of liability that may arise from wrongful commitment include assault and battery, malicious prosecution, abuse of authority, and intentional infliction of emotional distress (Simon 1992a).

The use of reasonable professional judgment is perhaps the best evidence that the psychiatrist's actions were taken in good faith (Mishkin 1989). Performing a careful examination of the patient, abiding by the requirements of the law, and ensuring that sound reasoning motivates the certification of the patient are good clinical practice and only secondarily good risk management. Evidence of willful, blatant, or gross failure to adhere to statutorily defined commitment procedures may expose a psychiatrist to a lawsuit.

Rights of involuntarily hospitalized patients. Most states recognize the right of inpatients to refuse treatment. Even though the patient is involuntarily hospitalized, the order for hospitalization, without a more specific finding, does not negate a presumption of competence. In most states, patients involuntarily hospitalized who refuse medication are entitled to a separate court hearing for an adjudication of incompetence and the provision of substituted consent by the court. In a civil rights action by a state prisoner challenging involuntary treatment with antipsychotic drugs without a prior judicial hearing (Washington v. Harper 1990), the U.S. Supreme Court ruled involuntary treatment of a prisoner was constitutionally permissible when the prisoner was found to be a serious danger to himself or others as the result of a mental illness and the treatment was in the prisoner's medical interest. The Court found that, in lieu of a judicial hearing, administrative procedures that included review by an administrative panel satisfied procedural due process requirements.

Hospitalized patients possess other rights. Patients possess rights of visitation, although these rights can be temporarily suspended for proper cause relating to a patient's care and treatment. Free communications of hospitalized patients through mail, telephone, or visitors are considered a right, unless protection of the patients or others requires supervision of communications. The right to privacy includes allowing patients to have secure locker space, private toilet and shower facilities, and a minimum square footage of floor space. Protection of confidentiality is also included. Economic rights include the right to have and spend money and to handle one's own financial affairs responsibly. In most jurisdictions, involuntarily hospitalized patients do not lose their civil rights, such as the right to manage their own money. Hospitalized patients must be paid for their work unless it is truly therapeutic labor (i.e., intended to benefit the patient, not the hospital). "Patients' rights" are not absolute and often must be tempered by the clinical judgment of the mental health professional. Inevitably, disputes over perceived or real violations of patients' rights arise. In some jurisdictions, a civil rights officer or ombudsman is mandated by statute to mediate these disputes.

Seclusion and Restraint

The psychiatric legal issues surrounding seclusion and restraint are complex. Seclusion and restraint have both indications and contraindications as clinical management tools (American Psychiatric Association 1985; see Tables 41–7 and 41–8). The legal regulation of seclusion and restraint has become increasingly more stringent over the past decade.

Legal challenges to the use of seclusion and restraints have been made on behalf of the institutionalized mentally ill and the mentally retarded. Fre-

---

TABLE 41–7. Indications for seclusion and restraint

1. Prevent harm to the patient or others.

2. Prevent disruption to treatment program or physical surroundings.

3. Assist in treatment as part of ongoing behavior therapy.

4. Decrease sensory overstimulation (seclusion only).

5. Respond to patient's reasonable voluntary request.[a]

[a]First seclusion; then, if necessary, restraints.

Source. Adapted with permission from Simon RI: *Concise Guide to Psychiatry and Law for Clinicians,* 3rd Edition. Washington, DC, American Psychiatric Publishing, 2001, p. 114.

TABLE 41–8. Contraindications to seclusion and restraint

1. Unstable medical and psychiatric conditions[a]

2. Delirious patients or patients with dementia who are unable to tolerate decreased stimulation[a]

3. High-risk suicidal patients[a]

4. Patients with severe drug reactions or overdoses or patients requiring close monitoring of drug dosages[a]

5. For punishment of the patient or for convenience of staff

[a]Unless close supervision and direct observation are provided.

Source. Adapted with permission from Simon RI: *Concise Guide to Psychiatry and Law for Clinicians,* 3rd Edition. Washington, DC, American Psychiatric Publishing, 2001, p. 117.

---

quently, these lawsuits do not stand alone but are part of a challenge to a wide range of alleged abuses within a hospital.

Generally, the courts have held that seclusion and restraints are an intrusion on a patient's constitutionally protected interests and may be implemented only when a patient presents a risk of harm to self or others and no less restrictive alternative is available. Some courts have also required the following:

1. Restraint and seclusion may be implemented only by a written order from an appropriate medical official.

2. Orders must be confined to specific, time-limited periods.

3. A patient's condition must be regularly reviewed and documented.
4. Any extension of an original order must be reviewed and reauthorized.

In addition to these substantive limitations, some courts and state statutes articulate procedural due-process requirements that must precede implementation of a seclusion or restraint order. Typical due-process considerations include some form of notice, a hearing, and the involvement of an impartial decision maker. The process that is due is context dependent; thus, what may be called for in a 3 A.M. emergency will differ from what may be called for at 3 P.M.

The acceptability of seclusion or restraint for the purposes of training was recognized in the landmark case *Youngberg v. Romeo* (1982). *Youngberg* involved a challenge to the "treatment" practices at the Pennhurst State School and Hospital in Pennsylvania. The U.S. Supreme Court held that patients could not be restrained except to ensure their safety or, in certain undefined circumstances, "to provide needed training." Although it recognized that the defendant had a liberty interest in safety and freedom from bodily restraint, the Court added that these interests were not absolute and were in conflict with the need to provide training. The Court also held that decisions made by appropriate professionals regarding restraining the patient would presumptively be considered correct. The Court recognized that professionals, rather than the courts, are best able to determine the needs of patients, including when restraint is appropriate.

Most states have enacted statutes regulating the use of restraints, normally specifying the circumstances in which restraints can be used. Most often, those circumstances occur only when a risk of harm to self or danger to others is "imminent." Statutory regulation of the use of seclusion is far less common. Most states with laws regarding seclusion and restraint require some type of documentation of their use.

The federal government's Center for Medicare Services, JCAHO (Joint Commission on Accreditation of Healthcare Organizations 2006b), and most states have developed requirements designed to minimize and avoid the use of seclusion and restraint (Simon and Hales 2006). Where they apply, federal requirements establish a floor but may be superseded by more restrictive state laws. The requirements define *seclusion* and *restraint* as follows: *Seclusion* is the involuntary confinement of a person alone in a room where the person is physically prevented from leaving or the separation of the patient from others in a safe, con-

tained, controlled environment. *Restraint* is the direct application of physical force to an individual, with or without the individual's permission, to restrict his or her freedom of movement. Physical force may involve human touch, mechanical devices, or a combination thereof. Under the federal rules, the use of these interventions is regarded as presenting an inherent risk to the patient's physical safety and well-being and therefore may be used only when there is "imminent risk" that the patient may inflict harm to self or others. As do many states, federal law includes the use of drugs in the definition of restraint (Simon and Hales 2006). Federal law permits the use of seclusion and restraint only as a last resort to protect the patient's safety and dignity and never for the convenience of the staff.

Specifically, federal requirements permit qualified staff members to initiate seclusion or restraint for the safety and protection of the patient and staff only if they obtain an order from the licensed independent practitioner as soon as possible within 1 hour of initiation. Stringent requirements for face-to-face evaluation of the patient within 1 hour of initiation and for assessment, frequency of reassessment, monitoring, time-limited orders, notification of family members, discontinuation at the earliest possible opportunity, and debriefing with patient and staff members have been carefully defined by the Center for Medicare Services and JCAHO.

The treatment of psychiatric inpatients has changed in the managed care era. Most psychiatric units, particularly those in general hospitals, have become short-stay, acute-care psychiatric facilities. Generally, only suicidal, homicidal, and gravely disabled patients with major psychiatric disorders pass strict precertification review for hospitalization. Approximately half of these patients have comorbid substance-related disorders. The purpose of hospitalization is crisis intervention and management to stabilize patients and to ensure their safety as soon as possible (Simon and Hales 2006).

The clinical staff can become temporarily overwhelmed by the rapid admission of very sick patients. The psychiatric unit may need to briefly restrict or curtail new admissions. Patients should not be placed in seclusion or restraint for the convenience of the staff or because of insufficient staffing. The indications and safety precautions for seclusion and restraint should be thoroughly documented. Seclusion and restraint should be used only when all other treatment and safety measures have failed.

The indications and contraindications for seclusion and restraint are discussed elsewhere (American Psychiatric Association 1985). Seclusion and restraint may be necessary for the patient assessed at high risk for suicide in order to prevent self-harm. If the patient can be engaged by the staff shortly after admission, a nascent therapeutic alliance may develop. Appropriate medications given at therapeutic levels often stabilize the high-risk patient. If the suicidal patient is placed in seclusion and restraint, direct observation is required, according to regulatory and hospital policies. Seclusion rooms should have windows or audiovisual surveillance capability (Lieberman et al. 2004). Open-door seclusion is preferable when clinically appropriate.

Sexual Misconduct

Therapist–patient sex is usually preceded by progressive boundary violations in treatment (Simon 1989). As a consequence, patients are often psychologically damaged by the precursor boundary violations as well as the eventual sexual misconduct of the therapist (Simon 1991). An excellent account of the gradual erosion of treatment boundaries leading to near loss of control with a client is given by Rutter (1989).

General boundary guidelines exist for conducting psychiatric treatment (Simon 1992c). Awareness of these guidelines and of their transgression may help alert the therapist to progressive boundary violations (Simon 1994). Sexual misconduct does not occur in isolation but usually involves a variety of negligent acts of omission and commission.

Three types of legal responses to sexual misconduct have been enacted: reporting, civil liability, and criminal prosecution. *Reporting statutes* require a therapist who learns of any past or current therapist–patient sex to disclose this information. Some states have enacted *civil statutes* that make it explicit that sexual misconduct is a violation of the standard of care and authorize a damage claim (Bisbing et al. 1995). *Criminal statutes* addressing sexual misconduct have also been enacted. They may be appropriate given the therapist's behavior and may be the only remedy for exploitative therapists who do not have malpractice insurance, therapists who are unlicensed, or therapists who do not belong to professional organizations.

Civil liability. Psychiatrists who sexually exploit their patients are subject to civil and criminal sanctions as well as ethical and professional licensure disciplinary proceedings. *The Principles of Medical Ethics With Annotations Especially Applicable to Psychiatry* (American Psychiatric Association 2001b) states that sex with a current or former patient is unethical (Section 2, Annotation 1). However, a malpractice claim is probably the most common legal response.

In a medical malpractice claim for sexual misconduct, in order to prevail the plaintiff has the burden of proving, by a preponderance of the evidence (i.e., "more likely than not"), among other things, that the exploitation took place. This burden can be met by corroborating evidence such as letters, pictures, hotel receipts, and identification of incriminating body markings of the exploited, as well as the testimony of other abused (former) patients. The plaintiff is also required to demonstrate that the misconduct caused harm such as a worsened psychiatric condition, suicide attempts, or the necessity for hospitalization. Expert psychiatric testimony is usually required to establish the type and extent of psychological damages as well as to establish whether a breach of the standard of care occurred.

A few states have enacted civil statutes proscribing sexual misconduct (Simon 1992a). Several states make therapist sexual misconduct a crime (Bisbing et al. 1995). Some states prosecute sexual exploitation suits under their sexual assault statutes. A number of states have enacted statutes that provide civil and criminal remedies to patients who were sexually abused by their therapists (Appelbaum 1990; Strasburger et al. 1991). For instance, Minnesota enacted legislation that states the following:

> A cause of action against a psychotherapist for sexual exploitation exists for a patient or former patient for injury caused by sexual contact with the psychotherapist if the sexual contact occurred: 1) during the period the patient was receiving psychotherapy...or 2) after the period the patient received psychotherapy...if a) the former patient was emotionally dependent on the psychotherapist; or b) the sexual contact occurred by means of therapeutic deception. (Minn. Stat. Ann. § 148A.02 2005)

A person who engages in sexual penetration with another person is guilty of criminal sexual conduct in the third degree if any of the following circumstances exists:

> (h) the actor is a psychotherapist and the complainant is a patient of the psychotherapist and the sexual penetration occurred: (i) during the psychotherapy session; or (ii) outside the psychotherapy session if an ongoing psychotherapist-patient relationship exists. Consent by the complainant is not a defense. (Minn. Stat. Ann. § 609.344 2005)

It is not a recognized defense to these common-law or statutory remedies that the patient was aware that sex was not a part of treatment, that the sex occurred outside the treatment setting, that treatment ended before the sexual relationship began, or that the patient consented to the sexual contact. Patients cannot consent to malpractice. In sexual misconduct cases, the issue is never patient consent but always breach of fiduciary trust by the therapist and the harm it caused.

There is no "respected minority" in the profession that claims sexual relations with patients is therapeutic. This position had a few adherents at one time but is no longer publicly advocated by credible mental health professionals.

Criminal sanctions. Sexual exploitation of a patient may be classified as rape or sexual assault (Hoge et al. 1995). Many of the new wave of statutes criminalizing therapist–patient sexual misconduct assume, as a matter of law, that a current patient is incapable of giving consent to sexual relations with his or her therapist and treat all sexual relations between therapist and patient as a criminal act committed by the therapist (Minn. Stat. Ann. § 609.344 2005). In states without such a provision, sex with a current patient may be criminally actionable under sexual assault statutes if the state can prove that the patient was coerced into engaging in the sexual act. Typically, this type of evidence is limited to the use of some form of substance (e.g., medication) either to induce compliance or to reduce resistance. Anesthesia, ECT, hypnosis, drugs, force, and threat of harm have been used to coerce patients into sexual submission (Schoener et al. 1989). To date, claims of psychological coercion through the manipulation of transference phenomena have not been successful in establishing the coercion necessary for a criminal case. In cases involving a minor patient, the issue of consent or coercion is irrelevant because minors and adult incompetent persons are considered unable to provide valid consent. Therefore, sex with a child or an incompetent person is automatically considered a criminal act.

Professional disciplinary action. For the purposes of adjudicating allegations of professional misconduct, licensing boards are typically granted certain regulatory and disciplinary authority by state statutes. As a result, state licensing organizations, unlike professional associations, may discipline an offending professional by suspending or revoking his or her license to practice. There is no cost to a patient to seek redress through this means, nor are licensure boards constrained by statutes of limitations. A review of published reports of sexual misconduct cases adjudicated before licensing boards revealed that in the vast majority of cases, the evidence was reasonably sufficient to substantiate a claim of exploitation, leading to revocation of the professional's license or suspension

from practice for varying lengths of time, including permanent suspension.

Patients can bring ethical charges against psychiatrists before the district branches of the APA at any time. Ethical violators who are members may be reprimanded, suspended, or expelled from the APA. All national organizations of mental health professionals have ethically proscribed sexual relations between therapist and patient.

Psychiatry in the Courtroom
The Psychiatrist as a Witness
Forensic Psychiatry

Definition and scope. *Forensic psychiatry* is defined as "a subspecialty of psychiatry in which scientific and clinical expertise is applied to legal issues in legal contexts embracing civil, criminal, correctional or legislative matters" (American Academy of Psychiatry and the Law 1989/1991, p. x). The subspecialty of forensic psychiatry is burgeoning. The past decade has witnessed enormous growth in interest in this specialty as demonstrated by the proliferation of journals devoted exclusively to forensic psychiatry, the development of forensic psychiatry fellowships, and the establishment of board certification. The American Board of Medical Specialties has recognized forensic psychiatry as a subspecialty of psychiatry. The American Board of Psychiatry and Neurology has conducted examinations for certification in the subspecialty of forensic psychiatry since 1994. In the United States, the majority of forensic psychiatric services are performed by general psychiatrists who are not board certified in forensic psychiatry (Simon 2004).

Just a few of the major areas in which forensic psychiatrists evaluate cases and provide testimony include malpractice litigation, will contests, personal injury litigation, competency determinations (both civil and criminal), criminal responsibility, and presentencing hearings. Many other areas of law and psychiatry also require the professional services of the forensic psychiatrist. In the course of practice, the forensic psychiatrist often evaluates unusual, challenging cases not ordinarily found in the general outpatient or inpatient practice of psychiatry. A list of suggested readings in forensic psychiatry is provided before the references at the end of this chapter.

Forensic psychiatric evaluation. The forensic psychiatric evaluation of the injured claimant differs in several significant ways from the traditional psychiatric evaluation. As noted previously, the differences between the roles of treating psychiatrist and forensic evaluator must be firmly maintained in the litigation context. Problems in both treatment and testimony invariably arise for the clinician when these roles are confused.

Equities usually exist on both sides of cases that reach the courts. The opposing party's conflicting evidence as well as the opinions of opposing experts should be carefully considered.

Team approach. The forensic psychiatrist who is evaluating the claimant may require the input of a neurologist, psychologist, neuropsychologist, and internist or general practitioner. Depending on the complexities of the case, representatives of a number of other disciplines may need to be consulted. The forensic evaluator should review the findings of other examinations performed at the request of opposing counsel. The burgeoning number of ever-more-complicated brain studies currently available makes consultation with a qualified neurologist or neuroradiologist virtually a necessity in cases involving claims of brain injury.

Absence of doctor–patient relationship. The psychiatrist should inform the claimant at the time of examination that no doctor–patient relationship will be formed—that is, the psychiatrist will not *treat* the claimant. The psychiatrist should explain that he or she has been retained by (name the specific party) to perform an independent psychiatric examination. The sole purpose of the examination is to provide information to the party retaining the psychiatrist and potentially to the court.

Absence of confidentiality. The claimant must be informed that, unlike the traditional doctor–patient relationship, confidentiality surrounding the forensic evaluation may not exist. Once the retaining attorney decides to disclose the findings of the evaluation in litigation or in some instances if a claim or defense is relying on a mental state, the information will be made available to court and counsel. A Protective Order issued by the court may require that the forensic psychiatrist maintain the confidentiality of specified records and documents.

Standard diagnostic schema. The diagnostic evaluation of claimants should be made according to the multiaxial classification system contained in DSM-IV-TR (American Psychiatric Association 2000). All five axes

should be employed, where applicable. Axis I permits the clinician to consider the major clinical psychiatric syndromes, either singly or multiply. It is not unusual for the claimant to have concurrent Axis I diagnoses that may have preexisted or may be exacerbated.

Axis II forces the clinician to consider personality disorders that can be overlooked or ignored in the forensic evaluation of a claimant. The occurrence of significant head injuries is high in the violent criminal population, where there is an increased incidence of antisocial personality disorder. Borderline personality disorder presents a challenge to the forensic examiner, especially distinguishing between the claimant's narrative truth and the historical truth. It is difficult to diagnose or rule out personality disorders because forensic psychiatric examinations are usually time limited. Psychological testing can be of assistance.

On Axis III, the relationship of medical disorders and their treatments to the claimant's clinical presentation on Axis I must be carefully evaluated. The claimant may have a number of injuries requiring extensive pharmacotherapy that may further complicate the clinical picture. Moreover, a host of medical disorders may present with or have associated symptoms of cerebral dysfunction. Prior head injuries or preexisting central nervous system disorders may exist. For example, a young adult who has a history of learning disabilities or attention-deficit disorder may become seriously impaired after sustaining a traumatic brain injury (TBI).

Axis IV permits the evaluation of multiple psychosocial stressors, usually occurring within the year preceding the current evaluation, that may have contributed to the development of a new mental disorder, recurrence of a prior mental disorder, or exacerbation of a preexisting psychiatric disorder. It is the rare claimant who has a single psychosocial stressor affecting his or her life. Injury often occurs in the context of other preexisting psychosocial stressors such as interpersonal difficulties, financial problems, occupational distress, or other personal losses.

Finally, functional impairment should be assessed on Axis V according to the Global Assessment of Functioning Scale in combination with other standard methods of evaluation of psychiatric impairment discussed later.

DSM-IV-TR contains a cautionary statement about its use in litigation. Lawyers and courts refer to DSM-IV-TR extensively. Psychiatrists perform an important service to the judicial system by appropriately applying DSM-IV-TR in litigation. Lawyers and courts have a tendency to apply clinical guidelines and diagnostic criteria in a cookbook manner and to become more, rather than less, confused by its application. Therefore, before preparing a written report or testifying to a DSM diagnosis, the forensic expert must consider whether the use of diagnosis is helpful to the fact finder given the relevant legal criteria (Greenberg et al. 2004).

Collateral sources of information. In the treatment situation, the psychiatrist relies almost exclusively on the subjective reporting of the patient. The patient is presumed to be candid. In litigation, however, the claimant naturally favors his or her own legal case. The possibility of malingering should always be kept in mind (Table 41–9). Malingering is not limited to the fabrication of symptoms. More often, malingering is manifested by the *exaggeration* or even *minimization* of symptoms. Thus, the psychiatrist should consider a broad array of information.

During the course of legal discovery by both parties to a lawsuit, a great deal of information usually is developed. The forensic examiner should request that the retaining lawyer provide all relevant information. Going to court with incomplete information will likely be exposed by opposing counsel, undercutting the psychiatrist's testimony and possibly damaging the claimant's case. The forensic psychiatrist should review all data carefully before coming to a conclusion. The collateral sources of information listed in Table 41–10, although not exhaustive, indicate major areas of inquiry.

Traumatic brain injury. When evaluating the mental status of the TBI claimant, the psychiatrist conducts a thorough mental status examination. The mental status assessment is an integral part of the psychiatric examination that cannot be delegated to others. If possible, the examination should be conducted in divided sessions over the course of a few days because of likely fluctuations in the mental status of the TBI claimant. Neuropsychological assessment can be a valuable adjunct to the neuropsychiatric assessment of the TBI claimant (Becker and Kay 1986). Nevertheless, the neuropsychological findings should compliment but not replace competent mental status examination. The mental status examination as described by Strub and Black (1985) provides a scored, comprehensive, reliable format for the evaluation of mental status.

The role of neuropsychological testing must be critically evaluated in each case. Neuropsychological tests are not totally objective. Thus, the clinicians' motivation is critical. Low test scores may be caused by factors other than brain damage (Table 41–11). Clinicians, not tests, make diagnoses. A neuropsychological test score by itself cannot be used to point to a specific

TABLE 41–9. Increased index of suspicion for malingering

Litigation context (financial compensation, evasion of criminal prosecution)

Marked discrepancy between clinical findings and subjective complaints

Lack of cooperation with evaluation and treatment

Antisocial personality traits or disorder

Overdramatization of complaints

History of recurrent accidents or injuries

Evidence of self-induced injuries

Vaguely defined symptoms

Poor work history

Inability to work but retention of capacity for pleasurable activities

Source. Reprinted with permission from Simon RI: "Legal and Ethical Issues in Traumatic Brain Injury," in *Textbook of Traumatic Brain Injury.* Edited by Silver JM, McAllister TW, Yudofsky SC. Washington, DC, American Psychiatric Publishing, 2005, p. 598.

TABLE 41–10. Collateral sources of information

Other physicians and health care providers (reports, direct discussions)

Hospital records

Family

Other third parties

Military records

School records

Police records

Witness information

Work records

Work products (letters, work projects)

Legal discovery (depositions, legal documents)

Prior medical and psychiatric records

Prior psychological and neuropsychological evaluations

Source. Reprinted with permission from Simon RI: "Legal and Ethical Issues in Traumatic Brain Injury," in *Textbook of Traumatic Brain Injury.* Edited by Silver JM., McAllister TW, Yudofsky SC. Washington, DC, American Psychiatric Publishing, 2005, p. 598.

cause of the litigant's injury. Moreover, in litigation, causation is ultimately a question for the fact finder.

Base rate neuropsychological deficits are typically demonstrated in the normal population. If impairments are noted without evaluation of the claimant's prior history and level of neuropsychological functioning, overinterpretation of the test data is likely. The critical review of education and work records to determine the prior level of intellectual functioning is important in establishing baseline performance. Neuropsychological impairments observed among a normal population increase with the age of the population. Lower IQ scores and slower responses are also associated with normal aging.

Comorbidity and drug effects also should be considered when evaluating the results of neuropsychological test assessments. Questionable results will be obtained in the neuropsychological testing if the impact of concurrent psychiatric disorders and medications on the neuropsychological data is not considered.

Brain injury mimics. A number of psychiatric disorders may produce symptoms indistinguishable from those of TBI. Some of the more common look-alike conditions include conversion, factitious, somatization, and depressive disorders presenting with symptoms of neurological and cerebral dysfunction. Conversion disorder symptoms classically imitate those of neurological disease. Dissociative symptoms may present with amnesia or atypical memory loss. Depressive pseudodementia is a recognized clinical disorder in elderly patients. Posttraumatic stress disorder (PTSD) manifesting symptoms of difficulty in concentration and psychogenic amnesia can also mimic brain injury. Similarly, anxiety disorders may be associated with memory complaints secondary to the inability to concentrate. TBI can also cause anxiety and depression.

To complicate matters, litigants may be receiving psychoactive substances. Antipsychotics, antidepressants, lithium, and particularly benzodiazepines can produce side effects that suggest neurological and brain disorders. Psychoactive substances can cause serious memory difficulties, either directly by effects on brain chemistry or indirectly through sedation. Various combinations of medications can interact to produce a host of side effects that involve the central nervous system. Psychoactive drug abuse is also distressingly common in these cases, especially when the litigant complains of persistent pain. Narcotic and nonnarcotic pain medications are commonly abused.

Disability determinations. In addition to the psychiatric diagnosis, an assessment of functional impair-

TABLE 41–11. Major factors influencing neuropsychological test findings
Original endowment
Environment (e.g., education, occupation, life experiences)
Motivation (effort)
Physical health
Psychological distress
Psychiatric disorders (e.g., depression, dissociative disorders)
Medications (e.g., anticonvulsants, psychotropics)
Qualifications and experience of neuropsychologist
Errors in scoring
Errors in interpretation

Source. Reprinted with permission from Simon RI: "Legal and Ethical Issues in Traumatic Brain Injury," in *Textbook of Traumatic Brain Injury.* Edited by Silver JM, McAllister TW, Yudofsky SC. Washington, DC, American Psychiatric Publishing, 2005, p. 599.

ment and disability must be made. In litigation, it is the degree of functional impairment, not the psychiatric diagnosis per se, that is determinative. There is a difference between *impairment* and *disability.* An impaired individual may not necessarily be disabled. Psychiatric impairment is considered disabling only when a psychiatric disorder limits a person's capacity to meet the demands of living. A traumatic blow to the eye of a company president that causes mild, uncorrectable visual impairment may significantly impair occupational functioning. The same injury to a major league baseball player may be totally disabling and career ending.

Similarly, a patient may have moderate impairment but only mild disability in social or occupational functioning, owing to the development of compensatory coping mechanisms. Clinicians, however, see patients who have mild impairment but who are seriously disabled. This situation is common in litigation. For claimants presenting such a picture, the psychiatrist should pay particular attention to the possible presence of concurrent personality disorders, psychosocial stressors, comorbidity, substance abuse, medication effects, and litigation issues on the clinical presentation of the claimant.

Standard impairment assessment methods can be used in combination with the DSM-IV-TR Axis V Global Assessment of Functioning. The credible psychiatric assessment of functional impairment avoids strictly subjective conclusory pronouncements about the examinee's impairment and the need for future treatment. Instead, whenever possible, the examinee's functional impairment and future treatment needs should be evaluated according to the American Medical Association's (2001) *Guide to the Evaluation of Permanent Impairment.* The guide closely follows the Social Security Administration's guidelines for the assessment of disability. Assessment of permanent impairment should not be made until maximal medical or psychiatric improvement has been achieved.

Child custody. Psychiatrists are often involved in child custody cases throughout the separation and divorce processes (Billick and Kerry 1994). Psychiatrists may be asked to give opinions regarding the following:

- Custody decisions (request by parents before litigation)
- Child custody litigation
- Assistance for a guardian *ad litem* (attorney appointed by the court to represent a child)
- Child care agency (usually court ordered after allegations of abuse have been made)
- Divorce mediation procedures
- Visitation
- Psychiatric treatment of parent, child, or both

The prevailing standard in child custody decisions is the "best interests of the child." Psychiatrists who become involved in child custody decisions should have specialized training in child psychiatry. Adequately trained general psychiatrists may also be able to perform child custody evaluations. The general psychiatrist, however, must recognize limitations in training and experience in performing child psychiatric evaluations (Simon and Wettstein 1997). Consultation with or referral to a child psychiatrist may be necessary. The APA provides guidelines for child custody evaluations (American Psychiatric Association 1982).

When performing child custody evaluations, if possible, the psychiatrist should see both parties to the litigation before offering a comparative opinion. The ethical guidelines of the American Academy of Psychiatry and the Law (1989/1991, Section IV) state the following:

> In custody cases, honesty and striving for objectivity require that all parties be interviewed, if possible, before an opinion is rendered. When this is not possible, or if for any reason not done, this fact should be clearly indicated in the forensic psychiatrist's report and testimony. Where one parent has not been seen, even after deliberate effort, it may be inappropriate

to comment on that parent's fitness as a parent. Any comments on that parent's fitness should be qualified and the data for the opinion be clearly indicated.

Child custody disputes often result in "hardball" litigation. If one parent accuses the other of child sexual abuse, a "war" between the parties often develops. Many psychiatrists refuse to perform child custody evaluations because they fear being excoriated by aggressive attorneys. Forensic training is helpful for psychiatrists to function effectively in this stressful setting.

Child custody evaluation presents special challenges and rewards. Psychiatrists must be willing to commit the time necessary to do extensive interviewing as well as manage the emotional strain of child custody cases. Evaluators should be careful to identify and correct personal biases and not allow themselves to be influenced by importuning attorneys. Recommendations made by the psychiatrist can have a profound influence on the rest of the child's life. The psychiatrist maintains a position of advocate for the child's needs. Professional and personal gratifications are achieved when the psychiatrist's evaluation provides the potential for healthy child development and a sound foundation for adult life.

After a divorce is final, absent an order for joint custody, one parent usually is granted primary custody of any minor children. The primary custodial parent typically holds the nonemergency health care decision-making power. Psychiatrists may be asked to perform an examination or evaluation of a minor child at the request of the noncustodial parent or co-custodial parent lacking health care decision-making power. Psychiatrists who perform such examinations expose themselves to legal action (Simon 1992a). Before performing an evaluation or examination on a minor child, the psychiatrist should obtain the consent of the primary custodial parent and, when appropriate, ask for copies of the divorce decree.

Posttraumatic Stress Disorder

In criminal cases, one disorder has been relied upon by both the prosecution and the defense. Defendants who committed a crime while experiencing a dissociative behavioral reenactment of a prior traumatic event have successfully relied on PTSD to support an insanity defense (Sparr 1990). The diagnosis of PTSD has also been relied on by experts for the state to bolster the credibility of the victim, by showing how other victims similarly respond or to reason backward from PTSD symptoms to establish the occurrence of a traumatic stressor (e.g., rape). Victims of criminal acts who develop PTSD or other psychiatric disorders may institute claims under criminal injuries compensation acts. PTSD has bolstered the supporters of "victims' rights," whose advocacy poses a threat to the constitutional rights of defendants (Stone 1993). Guidelines for the assessment of PTSD in litigation have been proposed (Simon 2003).

Psychiatry and Criminal Law: Criminal Proceedings

Individuals charged with committing crimes may display significant psychiatric and neurological impairment that played a causal role in the commission of the crimes or was precipitated by the charges against them. The causal connection between brain damage and violence, however, remains frustratingly obscure. Violent behavior spans a wide spectrum from a normal response to a threatening situation to violence emanating directly from an organic brain disorder. Moreover, violent behavior is often the result of the interaction between an individual and a specific situation. Brain damage and mental illness may or may not play a significant role in this equation.

Criminal Intent (*Mens Rea*)

Under the common law, criminal culpability for most serious crimes requires 1) the mental state or level of intent to commit the act (known as the *mens rea*, or guilty mind), 2) the act itself or conduct associated with committing the crime (known as *actus reus*, or guilty act), and 3) a concurrence in time between the guilty act and the guilty mental state (Bethea v. United States 1977). To convict a person of a particular crime, the state must prove beyond a reasonable doubt that the defendant committed the criminal act with the requisite intent. All three elements are necessary to satisfy the threshold requirements for the imposition of criminal sanctions.

The defendant's intent determines not only the culpability for an offense but also the gravity of the offense. For instance, a person who deliberately plans to commit a crime is subject to more serious prosecution and punishment than one who does so impulsively. The difficulty, of course, is in assessing intent retrospectively (Simon and Shuman 2002).

Traditionally, legislative definitions of offenses required proof of general intent for some crimes and proof of specific intent to meet the *mens rea* requirement for others. *Specific intent* refers to the *mens rea* in crimes in which a *further intention* exists beyond the presence of a general criminal intent. For instance, the intent necessary for first-degree murder typically includes a "specific intent to kill" (Rogers and Shuman 2005). Unlike general intent, specific criminal intent may not be presumed from the unlawful criminal act alone. Because of the difficulties inherent in these categories, modern statutory codes have created more precise criteria for defining mental states that distinguish intentional, knowing, reckless, and negligent behavior (Rogers and Shuman 2005).

Mental handicaps or impairments present a host of problems across the criminal justice system. From assessing appropriateness of diversion to the specialized mental health courts or the mental health system, the risks posed by release on bail, or competence to stand trial to face criminal charges (Dusky v. United States 1960); to addressing *mens rea* or an affirmative defense of insanity and the disposition of an insanity aquittee (M'Naughten's Case 1843; United States v. Brawner 1972); to sentencing of convicted offenders and determination of eligibility for a sentence of death (Penry v. Lynaugh 1989; Tennard v. Dretke 2004), as well as competence to be executed (Ford v. Wainwright 1986), the impact of mental impairment pervades the criminal justice system. The first and most common context in which mental impairment arises is competence to stand trial. We do not require every defendant to be assessed and found competent before a trial begins; competence is presumed. However, when as the result of the defendant's conduct a question arises, the defense counsel, prosecutor, or judge may raise the issue, thus requiring the court to decide whether the defendant understands the charges brought against him or her and is capable of rationally assisting counsel with the defense.

Competency to Stand Trial

The legal standard for assessing pretrial competency was established by the U.S. Supreme Court in *Dusky v. United States* (1960). To be competent to make decisions during the pretrial process, at trial, and during an appeal, the court succinctly and without embellishment required that the defendant have "sufficient present ability to consult with his lawyer with a reasonable degree of rational understanding" and "has a rational as well as factual understanding of the proceedings against him" (Dusky v. United States 1960). Subsequent decisions have clarified that the level of understanding required need not be sophisticated.

Although the *Dusky* test does not require the absence of understanding resulting from the presence of a mental disease or defect, that is typically the case. However, a defendant may be found incompetent to stand trial even if he or she does not have a mental disease or defect as defined by the latest version of the DSM, as in the case of a physical illness that affects cognition.

Although most impairments implicated in competency examinations are functional rather than organic (Reich and Wells 1985), various forms of neuropsychiatric impairments typically raise questions about a defendant's competency to stand trial. In *Wilson v. United States* (1968), the defendant had no memory of the time of an alleged robbery because he had permanent retrograde amnesia. This impairment was caused by injuries he sustained in an automobile accident that occurred as he was being pursued by the police after the offense. Of the various criteria that the court established in determining the defendant's competency to stand trial, the following are directly relevant to the issue of neuropsychiatric impairment (Wilson v. United States 1968):

1. The extent to which the amnesia affected the defendant's ability to consult with and assist his lawyer
2. The extent to which the amnesia affected the defendant's ability to testify in his own behalf

Any disorder, whether functional or organic, that significantly impairs a defendant's cognitive and communicative abilities is likely to have an impact on competency. Nevertheless, it is the actual *functional* mental capability to meet the minimal standard of trial competency, and not the severity of the deficits, that determines whether an individual is cognitively capable to be tried. For example, Slovenko (1995) questioned whether psychiatric diagnosis is relevant to competency to stand trial. The presence or absence of a mental illness is irrelevant if the defendant is capable of meeting competency requirements. It is legal criteria, not medical or psychiatric diagnosis, that govern competency. Diagnosis is relevant only to the question of restoring the defendant's competency to stand trial with treatment.

Checklists and structured interviews have been developed to assess specific psychological factors applicable to the competency standards established in *Dusky*. The Interdisciplinary Fitness Interview, designed for use by lawyers and mental health professionals (Schreiber et al. 1987), provides for a detailed examination of psychopathology and legal knowledge using explicit scales for rating each response to the competency evaluation. *Evaluating Competencies: Forensic Assessments and Instruments,* by Thomas Grisso (1986), is a standard reference in the field.

A defendant's impairment in one particular function, however, does not automatically render him or her incompetent. For example, the fact that the defendant is manifesting certain deficits because of damage to the parietal lobe does not necessarily mean that he

or she lacks the requisite cognitive ability to aid in his or her own defense at trial (Tranel 1992). The ultimate determination of incompetency is for the court to decide (United States v. David 1975). Moreover, the impairment must be considered in the context of the particular case or proceeding. Mental impairment that may render an individual incompetent to stand trial in a complicated tax fraud case might not for a misdemeanor trial.

Psychiatrists and psychologists who testify as expert witnesses regarding the effect of psychiatric problems on a defendant's competency to stand trial are most effective if their findings are framed according to the degree to which the defendant is cognitively capable of meeting the standards enunciated in *Dusky*.

Insanity Defense

One of the most controversial issues in American criminal jurisprudence is the insanity defense. Defendants with functional or organic mental disabilities who are found competent to stand trial may seek acquittal claiming that they were not criminally responsible for their actions because of insanity at the time the offense was committed. The retrospective assessment of the offender's mental state at the time of the crime in insanity defense cases is one of the most challenging evaluations that the forensic psychiatrist performs (Simon and Shuman 2002).

Criminals may commit crimes for many reasons, but the law presumes that they do so of their own free will and that is therefore just to impose punishment. Some offenders, however, are so mentally disturbed in their thinking and behavior that they are thought to be incapable of making a choice that could have been deterred by the criminal law and for which retribution is justified. Historically, albeit controversially, the common law has long recognized some form of limitation on the punishment of a "crazy" or insane person (Blackstone 1769; Coke 1680). Larger in legend than in life, the insanity defense is rarely used and even more rarely successful. Approximately 1% of criminal defendants plead not guilty by reason of insanity; of these, only 10%–25% are successful. The chance of exculpation is greatest when the criminal defendant was found to be psychotic at the time of the crime by the pretrial assessment (Brakel et al. 1985).

A universally accepted definition of legal insanity does not exist. Over the years, tests of insanity have been subject to much controversy, modification, and refinement (Brakel et al. 1985). Thus, there is variability in the insanity defense standard in the United States, depending on which state's or jurisdiction's law applies.

Following the acquittal by reason of insanity of John Hinckley Jr. on charges of attempting to assassinate President Reagan and murder others, an outraged public demanded changes in the insanity defense. Federal and state legislation to accomplish that result ensued. Between 1978 and 1985, approximately 75% of all states made some sort of substantive change in their insanity defense (Perlin 1989). Nevertheless, a number of states continued to adhere to the American Law Institute (ALI) insanity defense standard or some version of it. The ALI test provides that a person is not responsible for criminal conduct if at the time of such conduct, as a result of mental disease or defect, he or she lacks substantial capacity either to appreciate the criminality (wrongfulness) of his or her conduct or to conform that conduct to the requirements of law. As used in this article, the terms *mental disease* or *defect* do not include an abnormality manifested only by repeated criminal or otherwise antisocial conduct (Model Penal Code § 4.01 [1962]).

This standard contains both a cognitive and a volitional prong. The *cognitive prong* derives from the 1843 M'Naughten rule exculpating the defendant who does not know the nature and quality of the alleged act or does not know the act was wrong. The *volitional prong* is a vestige of the irresistible impulse test, which states that the defendant who is overcome by an irresistible impulse that leads to an alleged act is not responsible for that act.

By contrast, defendants tried in a federal court and most state courts are governed by a cognitive, pre-ALI standard. The federal standard is contained in the Comprehensive Crime Control Act (CCCA) of 1984 (P.L. 98–473 1984), which provides that it is an affirmative defense to all federal crimes that, at the time of the offense, "the defendant, as a result of a severe mental disease or defect, was unable to appreciate the nature and quality or the wrongfulness of his acts. Mental disease or defect does not otherwise constitute a defense." This codification eliminates the volitional or irresistible impulse portion of the insanity defense—that is, it does not allow an insanity defense based on a defendant's inability to conform his or her conduct to the requirements of the law. The defense is limited to defendants who are unable to appreciate the wrongfulness of their acts (i.e., the *cognitive portion* of the defense). The rule applicable in the federal courts requires the defendant to prove insanity by clear and convincing evidence. The standard of persuasion varies among the states. In a minority of states, the prosecution has the burden of proving beyond a reasonable doubt that the defendant was sane. In most states, the

defendant must bear the burden of proving by a preponderance of the evidence that she or he was insane (Melton et al. 1997). A few states have abolished the affirmative defense of insanity, leaving defendants who claim that their mental state at the time of the crime should render them not responsible to attempt to negate *mens rea* with a more formidable burden.

Depending on the definitions contained the criminal code or case law, the lack of capacity due to mental defects other than mental illness may be sufficient. For instance, mental retardation may represent an adequate basis for the insanity defense under certain circumstances. However, the impulse disorders—intermittent explosive disorder, kleptomania, pathological gambling, and pyromania—have not fared well under an insanity defense both because some of these disorders are specifically excluded in some states and because in jurisdictions with only a cognitive test, these disorders do not satisfy the cognitive impairment requirement. Absent class-wide exclusions of these disorders and with a volitional prong applicable, case by case scrutiny is appropriate. Pathological gambling has had little success as a basis for an insanity defense (Rosenthal and Lorenz 1992). McGarry (1983) pointed out that the lack of volitional control over the isolated act of gambling does not assume a lack of control concerning criminal acts committed in the service of the impulse to gamble. Compulsive gambling, however, has been raised as a mitigating factor at sentencing (Rosenthal and Lorenz 1992).

Depending on the severity of the functional or organic mental disorder and its effect on an offender's cognitive and affective processes, a defense of insanity might be warranted. At the least, the presence of a psychiatric disorder should be investigated as a *mitigating* factor that may have caused the offender to have diminished capacity.

Diminished Capacity

Because the insanity defense is an affirmative defense, it is only presented in a case after the prosecution has presented sufficient evidence to persuade a reasonable juror that the state has met its burden of proof on *mens rea* and *actus reus*. There are, however, degrees of mental impairment that are relevant to *mens rea* but do not negate it. In recognition of this, the concept of *diminished capacity* was developed (Melton et al. 1997).

Diminished capacity, where it is recognized, permits the accused to introduce medical and psychological evidence relating directly to the *mens rea* for the crime charged without having to assert a defense of insanity (Melton et al. 1997). Typically, when this is available, it applies to specific intent crimes. When a defendant's *mens rea* for the crime charged is nullified by psychiatric evidence, the defendant is acquitted only of that charge but is likely held responsible for an offense requiring a lesser *mens rea*, such as manslaughter (Melton et al. 1997). Patients with psychiatric disorders who commit criminal acts may be eligible for a diminished capacity defense.

Guilty But Mentally Ill

In a number of states, an alternative verdict of *guilty but mentally ill* has been established. Under these statutes, if the defendant pleads not guilty by reason of insanity, this alternative verdict is available to the jury. Under an insanity plea, the verdict may be

- Not guilty
- Not guilty by reason of insanity
- Guilty but mentally ill
- Guilty

Guilty but mentally ill is an alternative verdict that is not different in its legal effect from finding the defendant guilty. The court must still impose a sentence on the convicted person, and the length of sentence and terms of confinement are not altered. Although the verdict directs that the convicted person receive necessary treatment, treatment should also be available to any prisoner with a mental disorder. The frequent unavailability of appropriate psychiatric treatment for prisoners adds to the spuriousness of this verdict.

Exculpatory and Mitigating Disorders

Psychotic disorders of differing etiology form the most common basis for an insanity defense. In addition to the major psychiatric and organic brain disorders, other conditions may provide a foundation for an insanity or diminished capacity defense.

Automatisms. For conviction of a crime, there must be not only a criminal state of mind (*mens rea*) but also the commission of a prohibited act (*actus reus*). The physical movement necessary to satisfy the *actus reus* requirement must be conscious and volitional. In addition to statutory and common law in many jurisdictions, Section 2.01(2) of the Model Penal Code (1962) specifically excludes from the *actus reus* the following: "(a) a reflex or convulsion; (b) a bodily movement during unconsciousness or sleep; (c) conduct during hypnosis or resulting from hypnotic suggestion; [and] (d) a bodily movement that otherwise is not the product of the effort or determination of the actor."

Automatism is a defense claiming that the commission of a crime was an involuntary act. The classic, although rare, example is the person who commits an offense while "sleepwalking." Courts have held that such an individual does not have conscious control of his or her physical actions and therefore acts involuntarily (Fain v. Commonwealth 1879; H.M. Advocate v. Fraser 1878). A conscious reflexive action carried out under stressful circumstances may qualify for an automatism defense. Situations relevant to psychiatry in which the defense might be used arise when a crime is committed during a state of altered consciousness caused by a concussion after a head injury, involuntary ingestion of drugs or alcohol, hypoxia, metabolic disorders such as hypoglycemia, or epileptic seizures (Low et al. 1982).

There are limitations to the automatism defense. Voluntary actions by the defendant (e.g., alcohol, drugs) leading to an altered state of consciousness have not qualified for this defense. Additionally, if the defendant was aware of the condition prior to the offense and failed to take reasonable steps to prevent the criminal occurrence, the defense is not available. For example, if a defendant with a known history of uncontrolled epileptic seizures loses control of a car during a seizure and kills someone, that defendant will not be permitted to assert the defense of automatism.

Intoxication. Ordinarily, intoxication is not a defense to a criminal charge. Because intoxication, unlike mental illness, mental retardation, and most neuropsychiatric conditions, is usually the product of a person's own actions, the law is cautious about viewing it as a defense or mitigating factor. Most states view voluntary alcoholism as relevant to the issue of whether the defendant possessed the *mens rea* necessary for a specific intent crime. The mere fact that the defendant was voluntarily intoxicated will not justify a finding of automatism or insanity. A distinct difference arises when, because of chronic, heavy use of alcohol, the defendant has an alcohol-induced psychotic disorder, withdrawal delirium, amnestic disorder, or dementia. If competent psychiatric evidence is presented that an alcohol-related neuropsychiatric disorder caused significant cognitive or volitional impairment, a defense of insanity or diminished capacity may be considered.

Temporal lobe seizures. Another "mental state" defense occasionally raised by defendants charged with assault-related crimes is that the assaultive behavior was involuntarily precipitated by abnormal electrical brain patterns. This condition is frequently diagnosed as temporal lobe epilepsy (Devinsky and Bear 1984). Episodic dyscontrol syndrome (Elliott

1978, 1982) has also been advanced as a neuropsychiatric condition causing involuntary aggression. Studies have hypothesized that there are "centers of aggression" in the temporal lobe or limbic system—primarily the amygdala. This hypothesis states that sustained aggressive behavior by these persons may be the product of an uncontrollable, randomly occurring, abnormal brain dysrhythmia, hence the claim that these individuals should not be held accountable for their resulting aggressive actions. Despite its simplicity and occasional success in the courts, few empirically significant studies exist to support this theory at the present time (Blumer 1984).

Metabolic disorders. Defenses based on metabolic disorders have also been tried. In 1979, the so-called Twinkie defense was used as part of a successful diminished capacity defense of Dan White in the murders of San Francisco Mayor George Moscone and Supervisor Harvey Milk. This defense was based on the theory that the ingestion of large amounts of sugar contributed to a state of temporary insanity (People v. White 1981). The forensic psychiatric report stated that the defendant had been "filling himself up with Twinkies and Coca-Cola" (Blinder 1981–1982). A jury found White guilty only of voluntary manslaughter. In 1981, California repealed the defense of diminished capacity (Slovenko 1995).

Hypoglycemic states also may be associated with significant psychiatric impairment (Droba and Whybrow 1989). When substantial glucose depletion occurs, a wide variety of responses may occur, including episodic and repetitive dyscontrol, temporary amnesia, depression, and hostility with spontaneous recovery (i.e., quick recovery after the consumption of appropriate nutrients). The degree of mental abnormality associated with hypoglycemic states varies from mild to severe according to the blood glucose level. It is the degree of disturbance, not the mere presence of an etiological metabolic component, that is determinative in a mental state defense. This principle also applies to mental dysfunctions produced by disorders originating in the hepatic, renal, adrenal, and neuroendocrine systems (e.g., premenstrual syndrome; Parry and Berga 1991).

Psychiatry and Civil Law: Personal Injury Litigation

Assessment of Sexual Harassment

Psychiatrists perform evaluations of litigants and provide testimony in court in a number of areas of civil lit-
igation. As an example, civil suits alleging sexual harassment are burgeoning. Psychiatrists are being called on to testify in these cases, which present emerging, complex psychological and social issues (Gold 2004).

The statutory basis for sexual harassment claims is found in Title VII of the Civil Rights Act of 1964. Section 703(a)(1) of Title VII, 42 U.S.C. § 2000e-2(a) reads as follows: "It shall be an unlawful employment practice for an employer…to fail or refuse to hire or to discharge any individual, or otherwise to discriminate against any individual with respect to his compensation, terms, conditions, or privileges of employment, because of such individual's race, color, religion, sex, or national origin." In 1980, the Equal Employment Opportunity Commission (EEOC) issued guidelines that declared sexual harassment to be a violation of Section 703 of Title VII. The guidelines propounded criteria for determining unwelcome conduct of a sexual nature that constituted sexual harassment, defined the circumstances under which an employer may be held liable, and suggested affirmative steps that an employer should take to prevent sexual harassment (Guidelines on Discrimination Because of Sex, 29 C.F.R. §1604.11).

In defining sexual harassment, Title VII does not proscribe all conduct of a sexual nature in the workplace. Only unwelcome sexual conduct that is a term or condition of employment constitutes a violation. The EEOC's guidelines define two kinds of sexual harassment: "quid pro quo" and "hostile environment." Sexual conduct constitutes sexual harassment when "submission to such conduct is made either explicitly or implicitly a term or condition of an individual's employment" (Guidelines on Discrimination Because of Sex, 29 C.F.R. §1604.11 [a][1]). *Quid pro quo* harassment takes place when "submission or rejection of such conduct by an individual is used as the basis for employment decisions affecting the individual" (Guidelines on Discrimination Because of Sex, 29 C.F.R. §1604.11 [a][2]). The EEOC guidelines also recognize that unwelcome sexual conduct that "unreasonably interfere[s] with an individual's job performance" or creates an "intimidating, hostile, or offensive working environment" can constitute sex discrimination, even if it causes no tangible or economic job consequences (Guidelines on Discrimination Because of Sex, 29 C.F.R. §1604.11 [a][3]).

The U.S. Supreme Court, in *Harris v. Forklift Systems, Inc.* (1993), ruled unanimously that a woman who claims she was sexually harassed on the job need not prove she was psychologically injured to win monetary damages. The court defined unlawful harassment as creating a work environment that a reasonable person would find "hostile or abusive." The broadly written ruling will likely make it easier for employees to bring suits for sexual harassment.

Psychiatrists who become involved in sexual harassment litigation usually are asked to determine the veracity of harassment complaints, the psychological consequences of harassment, and the treatment needs and prognosis for women or men who have been sexually harassed. Binder (1992) presented examples of cases in which psychiatric testimony was provided to help decision making in assessing damages secondary to the psychological effects of sexual harassment. Guidelines have been proposed for conducting a credible forensic psychiatric evaluation in sexual harassment litigation (Simon 1996).

Expert Testimony

Civil litigation in psychic injury and head trauma cases may require the evaluation and testimony of psychiatrists, often working in conjunction with neurologists, other physicians, psychologists, neuropsychologists, and allied mental health professionals. Psychiatrists become involved in litigation as witnesses in one of two ways: as treaters (fact witnesses) or as forensic experts.

The treating clinician.   The treating psychiatrist and the forensic psychiatric expert have different roles in litigation. Treatment and expert roles do not mix (Greenberg and Shuman 1997; Strasburger et al. 1997). The treating psychiatrist must rely heavily on the subjective reporting of the patient. In the treatment context, psychiatrists are interested primarily in the patient's perception of his or her difficulties, not necessarily the objective reality. As a consequence, treating psychiatrists usually do not speak to third parties or check pertinent records to gain additional information about a patient or to corroborate the patient's statements. The law, however, is interested in truth as scrutinized by the crucible of the adversary system. Uncorroborated patient reports relied on by a treating psychiatrist are vulnerable to attack as unreliable.

Credibility issues also abound. The treating psychiatrist is, and must be, an ally of the patient. This bias *in favor of* the patient is a proper treatment stance that fosters the therapeutic alliance. The psychiatrist looks for mental disorders to treat. A treatment rather than a litigation agenda is the appropriate stance for the treating psychiatrist.

In court, credibility is critical. Opposing counsel may attempt to portray the treating psychiatrist as an advocate for the patient-litigant, which may or may not be true. Also, court testimony by the treating psychiatrist may compel the disclosure of information that is not *legally* privileged but nonetheless is viewed as intimate and confidential by the patient. This disclosure by a trusted therapist is bound to cause psychological damage to the therapeutic relationship (Strasburger 1987). In addition, psychiatrists must be careful to inform patients about the consequences of releasing treatment information, especially in legal matters. Section 4, Annotation 2, of *The Principles of Medical Ethics With Annotations Especially Applicable to Psychiatry* (American Psychiatric Association 2001b) states, "The continuing duty of the psychiatrist to protect the patient includes fully apprising him/her of the connotations of waiving the privilege of privacy. This may become an issue when the patient is being investigated by a government agency, is applying for a position, or is involved in legal action."

Finally, when the treating psychiatrist testifies concerning the need for further treatment, a conflict of interest is readily apparent. In making such treatment prognostications, the psychiatrist stands to benefit economically from the recommendation of further treatment. Although this may not be the intention of the psychiatrist, opposing counsel will be sure to point out that the psychiatrist has a financial interest in the case.

The American Academy of Psychiatry and the Law (1989/1991), in its ethics statement, advises that "a treating psychiatrist should generally avoid agreeing to be an expert witness or to perform an evaluation of his patient for legal purposes because a forensic evaluation usually requires that other people be interviewed and testimony may adversely affect the therapeutic relationship" (p. xii). The treating psychiatrist should attempt to remain solely in a treatment role. If it becomes necessary to testify on behalf of the patient, the treating psychiatrist should testify only as a fact witness rather than as an expert witness. As a fact witness, the psychiatrist will be asked to describe the number and length of visits, the diagnosis, the treatment, and the prognosis. The treatment relationship does not provide an adequate basis for going beyond these issues. Psychiatrists must remain ever mindful of the many double-agent roles that can develop when mixing psychiatry and litigation (Simon 1987, 1992a).

The forensic expert.   The forensic expert is usually free from the encumbrances of the treating psychiatrist in litigation. No doctor–patient relationship, with its treatment biases toward the patient, is created during forensic evaluation. The forensic expert typically reviews various records and looks to multiple sources of information to verify the factual assumptions that underlie any opinions drawn (Shuman and Greenberg 2003). Furthermore, the forensic expert considers the possibility of exaggeration or malingering because of a clear appreciation of the litigation context and the absence of treatment bias. Finally, the forensic psychiatrist does not face a conflict of interest for recommending treatment from which he or she would personally (i.e., financially) benefit. However, this same absence of a traditional doctor–patient relationship may subject the expert to being labeled as a "hired gun."

Conclusion

The legal issues surrounding the treatment and management of psychiatric patients are challenging and complex. The forensically informed psychiatrist is in a stronger position to provide good clinical care to the patient within the regulation of psychiatry by the courts and through governmental legislation. Moreover, psychiatrists will be increasingly required to testify in court concerning psychiatric patients. Familiarity and comfort with the role of a fact or expert witness will facilitate competent psychiatric testimony.

Key Points

- While the risk of being sued is inherent in the practice of psychiatry, spending time and talking with patients reduces the chances of being sued when things go bad.

- Except in an emergency, a psychiatrist must obtain informed consent—intelligent, knowing, and voluntary—from a competent patient before providing treatment. If the patient is not competent, an alternative method of consent (e.g., advance directive, guardianship) must be used.

- Patient confidences are sacrosanct and may be disclosed only when authorized in writing by the patient, ordered by the court, or excepted by law (e.g., elder or child abuse).

- Although psychiatrists may be competent in many roles, they should avoid conflicting roles such as forensic expert and therapist for the same patient-litigant.

- The psychiatrist who remains informed about the legal regulation of psychiatry can more effectively manage complex clinical-legal issues that inevitably arise with patients.

Suggested Readings

American Psychiatric Association: The Principles of Medical Ethics With Annotations Especially Applicable to Psychiatry. Washington, DC, American Psychiatric Association, 2001

Appelbaum PS, Gutheil TG: Clinical Handbook of Psychiatry and the Law, 3rd Edition. Baltimore, MD, Williams & Wilkins, 2000

Lifson LE, Simon RI (eds): The Mental Health Professional and the Law: A Comprehensive Handbook. Cambridge, MA, Harvard University Press, 1998

Melton GB, Petrila J, Poythress NG, et al: Psychological Evaluation for the Courts, 2nd Edition. New York, Guilford, 1997

Monahan J, Steadman HJ, Silver E, et al: Rethinking Risk Assessment. New York, Oxford, 2001

Morris R, Sales BD, Shuman DW: Doing Legal Research: A Guide for Social Scientists and Mental Health Professionals. Thousand Oaks, CA, Sage, 1996

Rogers R, Shuman DW: Fundamentals of Forensic Practice: Mental Health and Criminal Law. New York, Springer, 2005

Sales BD, Shuman DW: Experts in Court: Accommodating Law, Science and Expert Knowledge. Washington, DC, American Psychological Association, 2005

Schoener GR, Milgrom JH, Gonsiorek JC, et al: Psychotherapists' Sexual Involvement With Clients. Minneapolis, MN, Walk-In Counseling Center, 1989

Shuman DW: Psychiatric and Psychological Evidence, 3rd Edition. Rochester, NY, Thomson West, 2005

Simon RI: Assessing and Managing Suicide Risk: Guidelines for Clinically Based Risk Management. Washington, DC, American Psychiatric Publishing, 2004

Simon RI, Gold LH (eds): American Psychiatric Publishing Textbook of Forensic Psychiatry. Washington, DC, American Psychiatric Publishing, 2004

Simon RI, Hales RE (eds): American Psychiatric Publishing Textbook of Suicide Assessment and Management. Washington, DC, American Psychiatric Publishing, 2006

Simon RI, Shuman DW: Predicting the Past: The Retrospective Psychiatric Assessment of Mental States in Litigation. Washington, DC, American Psychiatric Publishing, 2002

Slovenko R: Psychotherapy and Confidentiality: Testimonial Privileged Communication, Breach of Confidentiality, and Reporting Duties. Springfield, IL, Charles C Thomas, 1998

Slovenko R: Psychiatry in Law, Law In Psychiatry. New York, Brunner-Routledge, 2002

References

American Academy of Psychiatry and the Law: Ethical Guidelines for the Practice of Forensic Psychiatry. Adopted May 1987. Revised October 1989, 1991

American Medical Association: Physician-Assisted Suicide. Code of Medical Ethics Reports, Vol 5, No 2. Chicago, IL, American Medical Association, July 1994, pp 269–275

American Medical Association: Report of the Council on Scientific Affairs: Evidence-Based Principles of Discharge and Discharge Criteria (CSA Report 4-A-96). Chicago, IL, American Medical Association, 1996

American Medical Association: Guide to the Evaluation of Permanent Impairment, 5th Edition. Chicago, IL, American Medical Association, 2001

American Psychiatric Association: Child Custody Consultation. Washington, DC, American Psychiatric Association, 1982

American Psychiatric Association: The Psychiatric Uses of Seclusion and Restraint (APA Task Force Report No 22). Washington, DC, American Psychiatric Association, 1985

American Psychiatric Association: Tardive Dyskinesia: A Task Force Report of the American Psychiatric Association. Washington, DC, American Psychiatric Association, 1992

American Psychiatric Association: Diagnostic and Statistical Manual of Mental Disorders, 4th Edition, Text Revision. Washington, DC, American Psychiatric Association, 2000

American Psychiatric Association: The Practice of Electroconvulsive Therapy: Recommendations for Treatment, Training, and Privileging. A Task Force Report of the American Psychiatric Association, 2nd Edition. Edited by Weiner RD. Washington, DC, American Psychiatric Association, 2001a

American Psychiatric Association: The Principles of Medical Ethics With Annotations Especially Applicable to Psychiatry. Washington, DC, American Psychiatric Association, 2001b

American Psychiatric Association: Practice Guidelines for the Treatment of Psychiatric Disorders. Washington, DC, American Psychiatric Association, 2004

Appelbaum PS: Statutes regulating patient–therapist sex. Hosp Community Psychiatry 41:15–16, 1990

Appelbaum PS, Lidz CW, Meisel A: Informed Consent: Legal Theory and Clinical Practice. New York, Oxford University Press, 1987, pp 84–87

Appelbaum PS, Zonana H, Bonnie R, et al: Statutory approaches to limiting psychiatrists' liability for their patients' violent acts. Am J Psychiatry 146:821–828, 1989

Baldwin LM, Hart LG, Oshel RG, et al: Hospital peer review and the National Practitioner Data Bank. JAMA 282:349–355, 1999

Baxter P, Beck JC: The violent patient: minimize your risk, in Practicing Psychiatry Without Fear: Guidelines of Liability Prevention. Edited by Lifson LE, Simon RI. Cambridge, MA, Harvard University Press, 1998

Beahrs JO, Gutheil TG: Informed consent in psychotherapy. Am J Psychiatry 158:4–10, 2001

Becker B, Kay GG: Neuropsychological consultation in psychiatric practice. Psychiatr Clin North Am 9:255–265, 1986

Benefacts. A Message from the APA-sponsored Professional Liability Insurance Program. Psychiatric News, April 19, 1996, pp 1, 26

Billick SB, Kerry CD: Role of the psychiatric evaluator in child custody disputes, in Principles and Practice of Forensic Psychiatry. Edited by Rosner R. New York, Chapman and Hall, 1994, pp 271–281

Binder RL: Sexual harassment: issues for forensic psychiatrists. Bull Am Acad Psychiatry Law 20:109–118, 1992

Bisbing SB, Jorgenson LM, Sutherland PK: Sexual Abuse by Professionals: A Legal Guide. Charlottesville, VA, Michie, 1995

Black HC: Black's Law Dictionary, 6th Edition. St Paul, MN, West Publishing, 1990

Blackstone W: Commentaries, Vol 4, 1769, pp 24–25

Blinder M: My examination of Dan White. Am J Forensic Psychiatry 2:12–22, 1981–1982

Blumer D: Psychiatric Aspects of Epilepsy. Washington, DC, American Psychiatric Press, 1984

Brakel SJ, Parry J, Weiner BA: The Mentally Disabled and the Law, 3rd Edition. Chicago, IL, American Bar Foundation, 1985

Coke E: Third Institute 6, 6th Edition, 1680

Devinsky O, Bear D: Varieties of aggressive behavior in temporal lobe epilepsy. Am J Psychiatry 141:651–656, 1984

Droba M, Whybrow PC: Endocrine and metabolic disorders, in Comprehensive Textbook of Psychiatry/V, Vol 2, 5th Edition. Edited by Kaplan HI, Sadock BJ. Baltimore, MD, Williams & Wilkins, 1989, pp 1209–1221

Elliott FA: Neurological aspects of antisocial behavior, in The Psychopath: A Comprehensive Study of Antisocial Disorders and Behaviors. Edited by Reid WH. New York, Brunner/Mazel, 1978, pp 146–189

Elliott FA: Neurological findings in adult minimal brain dysfunction and the dyscontrol syndrome. J Nerv Ment Dis 170:680–687, 1982

Emanuel EJ, Emanuel LL: Proxy decision making for incompetent patients: an ethical and empirical analysis. JAMA 267:2067–2071, 1992

Felthous AR: The duty to warn or protect to prevent automobile accidents, in American Psychiatric Press Review of Clinical Psychiatry and the Law, Vol 1. Edited by Simon RI. Washington, DC, American Psychiatric Press, 1990, pp 221–238

Gold LH: Sexual Harassment: Psychiatric Assessment in Employment Litigation. Washington, DC, American Psychiatric Publishing, 2004

Greenberg SA, Shuman DW: Irreconcilable conflict between therapeutic and forensic roles. Journal of Professional Psychology: Research and Practice 28:50–56, 1997

Greenberg SA, Shuman DW, Meyer RG: Unmasking forensic diagnosis. Int J Law Psychiatry 27:1–15, 2004

Grisso T: Evaluating Competencies: Forensic Assessments and Instruments. New York, Plenum, 1986

Grisso T, Appelbaum PS: Comparison of standards for assessing patients' capacities to make treatment decisions. Am J Psychiatry 152:1033–1037, 1995a

Grisso T, Appelbaum PS: The MacArthur treatment competence study, III: abilities of patients to consent to psychiatric and medical treatments. Law Hum Behav 19:149–174, 1995b

Gutheil TG, Appelbaum PS: Substituted judgement and the physician's ethical dilemma: with special reference to the problem of the psychiatric patient. J Clin Psychiatry 41:303–305, 1980

Gutheil TG, Simon RI: Risk management principles in recovered memory cases: the importance of the clinical foundation. Psychiatr Serv 48:1403–1407, 1997

Hoge SK, Jorgenson L, Goldstein N, et al: APA resource document: legal sanctions for mental health professional–patient sexual misconduct. Bull Am Acad Psychiatry Law 23:433–448, 1995

Johnson ID: Reports to the National Practitioner Data Bank. JAMA 265:407–411, 1991

Joint Commission on Accreditation of Healthcare Organizations: Comprehensive Accreditation Manual for Behavioral Healthcare Hospital Accreditation Standards PC 13.50. Oak Brook Terrace, IL, Joint Commission on Accreditation of Healthcare Organizations, 2006a

Joint Commission on Accreditation of Healthcare Organizations: Comprehensive Accreditation Manual for Behavioral Healthcare Restraint and Seclusion Standards for Behavioral Health. Oak Brook Terrace, IL, Joint Commission Accreditation of Healthcare Organizations, 2006b

Kane JM, Weinhold P, Kinon B, et al: Prevalence of abnormal involuntary movements ("spontaneous dyskinesia") in the normal elderly. Psychopharmacology (Berl) 77:105–108, 1982

Klawans HL, Barr A: Prevalence of spontaneous lingual-facial-buccal dyskinesia in the elderly. Neurology 32:558–559, 1982

Klein J, Onek J, Macbeth J: Seminar on Law in the Practice of Psychiatry. Washington, DC, Onek, Klein and Farr, 1983

LaPuma J, Orentlicher D, Moss RJ: Advance directives on admission: clinical implications and analysis of the Patient Self-Determination Act of 1990. JAMA 266:402–405, 1991

Lazarus JA, Sharfstein SS: Changes in the economics and ethics of health and mental health care, in American Psychiatric Press Review of Psychiatry, Vol 13. Edited by Oldham JM, Riba MB. Washington, DC, American Psychiatric Press, 1994, pp 389–413

Leong GB, Eth S, Silva JA: The psychotherapist as witness for the prosecution: the criminalization of *Tarasoff*. Am J Psychiatry 149:1011–1015, 1992

Levinson W, Roter DL, Mullooly JP, et al: Physician–patient communication: the relationship with malpractice claims among primary care physicians and surgeons. JAMA 227:553–559, 1997

Lieberman DZ, Resnik HL, Holder-Perkins V: Environmental risk factors in hospital suicide. Suicide Life Threat Behav 34:448–453, 2004

Link BG, Stueve A: Psychotic symptoms and the violent/illegal behavior of mental patients compared to community controls, in Violence and Mental Disorder: Developments in Risk Assessment. Edited by Monahan J, Steadman H. Chicago, IL, University of Chicago Press, 1994, pp 137–159

Lohr JB, Wisniewski A, Jeste DV: Neurological aspects of tardive dyskinesia, in Handbook of Schizophrenia, Vol 1: Neurology of Schizophrenia. Edited by Nasrallah H, Weinberger DR. Amsterdam, The Netherlands, Elsevier, 1986, pp 97–119

Low P, Jeffries J, Bonnie R: Criminal Law: Cases and Materials. Mineola, NY, The Foundation Press, 1982, pp 152–154

Monahan J, Steadman HJ, Silver E, et al: Rethinking Risk Assessment: The MacArthur Study of Mental Disorder and Violence. New York, Oxford University Press, 2001

Malcolm JG: Informed consent in the practice of psychiatry, in American Psychiatric Press Review of Clinical Psychiatry and the Law, Vol 3. Edited by Simon RI. Washington, DC, American Psychiatric Press, 1992, pp 223–281

McGarry AL: Pathological gambling: a new insanity defense. Bull Am Acad Psychiatry Law 11:301–308, 1983

Melton GB, Petrila J, Poythress NG, et al: Psychological Evaluations for the Courts: A Handbook for Mental Health Professionals and Lawyers, 2nd Edition. New York, Guilford, 1997

Meyer DJ, Simon RI: Split treatment: clarity between psychiatrists and psychotherapists. Psychiatr Ann 29:241–245, 327–332, 1999

Mill JS: On liberty (1859), in The World in Literature. Atlanta, GA, Scott, Foresman and Company, 1951, pp 316–333

Mishkin B: Decisions in Hospice. Arlington, VA, The National Hospice Organization, 1985

Mishkin B: Determining the capacity for making health care decisions, in Issues in Geriatric Psychiatry (Advances in Psychosomatic Medicine, Vol 19). Edited by Billig N, Rabins PV. Basel, Switzerland, S Karger, 1989, pp 151–166

Monahan J, Steadman H (eds): Violence and Mental Disorder: Developments in Risk Assessment. Chicago, IL, University of Chicago Press, 1994

The National Practitioner Data Bank and MCOs, in Psychiatric Practice and Managed Care, Vol 5, No 5. Washington, DC, American Psychiatric Association, 1999, pp 1, 9–10

Orentlicher D: The illusion of patient choice in end-of-life decisions. JAMA 267:2101–2104, 1992

Overman W Jr, Stoudemire A: Guidelines for legal and financial counseling of Alzheimer's disease patients and their families. Am J Psychiatry 145:1495–1500, 1988

Parry BL, Berga SL: Neuroendocrine correlates of behavior during the menstrual cycle, in Psychiatry, Vol 3. Edited by Cavenar JO. Philadelphia, PA, JB Lippincott, 1991, pp 1–22

Perlin ML: Mental Disability Law: Civil and Criminal, Vol 3. Charlottesville, VA, Michie, 1989

Perr IN: The clinical considerations of medication refusal. Legal Aspects of Psychiatric Practice 1:5–8, 1984

President's Commission for the Study of Ethical Problems in Medicine and Biomedical and Behavioral Research: Making Health Care Decisions, Vol 1: A Report on the Ethical and Legal Implications of Informed Consent in the Patient–Practitioner Relationship. Washington, DC, U.S. Government Printing Office, October 1982

Regan M: Protective services for the elderly: commitment, guardianship, and alternatives. William Mary Law Rev 13:569–573, 1972

Reich J, Wells J: Psychiatric diagnosis and competency to stand trial. Compr Psychiatry 26:421–432, 1985

Robertson ED: Is "substituted judgment" a valid legal concept? Issues Law Med 5:197–214, 1989

Robertson JD: The trial of a suicide case, in American Psychiatric Press Review of Clinical Psychiatry and the Law, Vol 2. Edited by Simon RI. Washington, DC, American Psychiatric Press, 1991, pp 423–441

Rogers R, Shuman DW: Fundamentals of Forensic Practice: Mental Health and Criminal Law. New York, Springer, 2005

Rosenthal RJ, Lorenz VC: The pathological gambler as criminal offender: comments on the evaluation and treatment. Psychiatr Clin North Am 15:647–660, 1992

Roth LH: Informed consent and its applicability for psychiatry, in Psychiatry, Vol 3. Edited by Cavenar JO. Philadelphia, PA, JB Lippincott, 1985, pp 1–17

Rutter P: Sex in the Forbidden Zone: When Therapists, Doctors, Clergy, Teachers and Other Men in Power Betray Women's Trust. Los Angeles, CA, JP Tarcher, 1989

Sale B, Powell DM, Van Duizend R: Disabled Persons and the Law: State Legislative Issues. New York, Plenum, 1982, p 461

Schoener GR, Milgrom JH, Gonsiorek JC, et al: Psychotherapists' Sexual Involvement With Clients. Minneapolis, MN, Walk-In Counseling Center, 1989

Schreiber J, Roesch R, Golding S: An evaluation of procedures for assessing competency to stand trial. Bull Am Acad Psychiatry Law 155:187–203, 1987

Sederer LI, Ellison J, Keyes C: Guidelines for prescribing psychiatrists in consultative, collaborative, and supervisory relationships. Psychiatr Serv 49:1197–1202, 1998

Shuman DW: Expertise in law, medicine, and health care. J Health Polit Policy Law 26:267–290, 2001

Shuman DW, Greenberg SA: Expert witnesses, the adversary system, and the voice of reason: reconciling impartiality and advocacy. Professional Psychology: Research and Practice. 34:219–224, 2003

Shuman DW, Weiner MF: The psychotherapist-patient privilege: a critical examination. Springfield, IL, Charles C Thomas, 1987

Simon RI: The psychiatrist as a fiduciary: avoiding the double agent role. Psychiatr Ann 17:622–626, 1987

Simon RI: Sexual exploitation of patients: how it begins before it happens. Psychiatr Ann 19:104–112, 1989

Simon RI: Psychological injury caused by boundary violation precursors to therapist–patient sex. Psychiatr Ann 21:614–619, 1991

Simon RI: Clinical Psychiatry and the Law, 2nd Edition. Washington, DC, American Psychiatric Press, 1992a

Simon RI: Clinical risk management of suicidal patients: assessing the unpredictable, in American Psychiatric Press Review of Clinical Psychiatry and the Law, Vol 3. Edited by Simon RI. Washington, DC, American Psychiatric Press, 1992b, pp 3–63

Simon RI: Treatment boundary violations: clinical, ethical, and legal considerations. Bull Am Acad Psychiatry Law 20:269–288, 1992c

Simon RI: Innovative Psychiatric Therapies and Legal Uncertainty: A Survival Guide for Clinicians. Psychiatr Ann 23:473–479, 1993

Simon RI: Treatment boundaries in psychiatric practice, in Forensic Psychiatry: A Comprehensive Textbook. Edited by Rosner R. New York, Van Nostrand Reinhold, 1994

Simon RI: The credible forensic psychiatric evaluation in sexual harassment litigation. Psychiatr Ann 26:139–148, 1996

Simon RI: Clinical risk management of the rapid cycling bipolar patient. Harv Rev Psychiatry 4:245–254, 1997

Simon RI: Psychiatrists' duties in discharging sicker and potentially violent patients in the managed care era. Psychiatr Serv 49:62–67, 1998

Simon RI: The suicide prevention contract: clinical, legal and risk management issues. J Am Acad Psychiatry Law 27:445–450, 1999

Simon RI: Concise Guide to Psychiatry and the Law for Clinicians, 3rd Edition. Washington, DC, American Psychiatric Publishing, 2001

Simon RI: Suicide risk assessment: what is the standard of care? J Am Acad Psychiatry Law 30:340–344, 2002

Simon RI (ed): Posttraumatic Stress Disorder in Litigation: Guidelines for Forensic Assessment, 2nd Edition. Washington, DC, American Psychiatric Publishing, 2003

Simon RI: Assessing and Managing Suicide Risk: Guidelines for Clinically Based Risk Management. Washington, DC, American Psychiatric Publishing, 2004

Simon RJ: The myth of "imminent" violence in psychiatry and the law. University of Cincinnati Law Review 75:631–644, 2006

Simon RI, Hales RE (eds): American Psychiatric Publishing Textbook of Suicide Assessment and Management. Washington, DC, American Psychiatric Publishing, 2006

Simon RI, Shuman DW (eds): Retrospective Assessment of Mental States in Litigation: Predicting the Past. Washington, DC, American Psychiatric Publishing, 2002

Simon RI, Wettstein RM: Toward the development of guidelines for the conduct of forensic psychiatric examinations. J Am Acad Psychiatry Law 25:17–30, 1997

Slovenko R: Assessing competency to stand trial. Psychiatr Ann 26:392–393, 397, 1995

Slovenko R: Psychotherapy and Confidentiality: Testimonial Privileged Communication, Breach of Confidentiality, and Reporting Duties. Springfield, IL, Charles C Thomas, 1998

Smith JT: Medical Malpractice: Psychiatric Care. Colorado Springs, CO, Shepard's/McGraw-Hill, 1986

Solnick PB: Proxy consent for incompetent nonterminally ill adult patients. J Leg Med 6:1–49, 1985

Sparr LF: Legal aspects of posttraumatic stress disorder: uses and abuses, in Posttraumatic Stress Disorder: Etiology, Phenomenology, and Treatment. Edited by Wolf ME, Mosnaim AD. Washington, DC, American Psychiatric Press, 1990, pp 22–34

Stone AA: Posttraumatic stress disorder and the law: critical review of the new frontier. Bull Am Acad Psychiatry Law 21:23–36, 1993

Strasburger LH: "Crudely, without any finesse": the defendant hears his psychiatric evaluation. Bull Am Acad Psychiatry Law 15:229–233, 1987

Strasburger LH, Jorgenson L, Randles R: Criminalization of psychotherapist–patient sex. Am J Psychiatry 148:859–863, 1991

Strasburger LH, Gutheil TG, Brodsky A: On wearing two hats: role conflict in serving as both psychotherapist and expert witness. Am J Psychiatry 154:448–456, 1997

Strub RL, Black FW: The Mental Status Examination in Neurology, 2nd Edition. Philadelphia, PA, FA Davis, 1985

Tardiff K: The past as prologue: assessment of future violence in individuals with a history of past violence, in Retrospective Assessment of Mental States in Litigation: Predicting the Past. Edited by Simon RI, Shuman DW. Washington, DC, American Psychiatric Publishing, 2002

Tischler GL: Utilization management of mental health services by private third parties. Am J Psychiatry 147:967–973, 1990

Tranel D: Functional neuroanatomy: neuropsychological correlates of cortical and subcortical damage, in The American Psychiatric Press Textbook of Neuropsychiatry, 2nd Edition. Edited by Yudofsky SC, Hales RE. Washington, DC, American Psychiatric Press, 1992, pp 70–75

U.S. Department of Health and Human Services: The Legal Status of Adolescents 1980. Washington, DC, U.S. Department of Health and Human Services, 1981

Walzer RS: Impaired physicians: an overview and update of legal issues. J Leg Med 11:131–198, 1990

Weir RF, Gostin L: Decisions to abate life-sustaining treatment for nonautonomous patients: ethical standards and legal liability for physicians after Cruzan. JAMA 264:1846–1853, 1990

Why Are Liability Premiums Rising? Psychiatric News, June 21, 1996, pp 1, 24–25

Wickizer TM, Lessler D, Travis KM: Controlling inpatient psychiatric utilization through managed care. Am J Psychiatry 153:339–345, 1996

Widiger TA, Trull TJ: Personality disorders and violence, in Violence and Mental Disorder: Developments in Risk Assessment. Edited by Monahan J, Steadman H. Chicago, IL, University of Chicago Press, 1994, pp 203–226

Woodward B, Duckworth K, Gutheil TG: The pharmacotherapist-psychotherapist collaboration, in Annual Review of Psychiatry, Vol 12. Edited by Oldham J. Washington, DC, American Psychiatric Press, 1993

Zeldow PB, Taub HA: Evaluating psychiatric discharge and aftercare in a VA medical center. Hosp Community Psychiatry 32:57–58, 1981

Legal Citations

Aponte v. United States, 582 F.Supp 65 (D PR 1984)

Bartling v. Superior Court, 163 Cal.App.3d 186, 209 Cal.Rptr. 220 (1984)

Bethea v. United States, 365 A.2d 64 (D.C. App. 1976), cert. denied, 433 U.S. 911 (1977)

Bouvia v. Superior Court, 179 Cal.App. 3d 1127, 225 Cal.Rptr. 297 (1986)

Callan v. Norland, 114 Ill.App.3d 196, 448 N.E.2d 651 (1983)

Canterbury v. Spence, 464 F.2d 772 (D.C. Cir. 1972), cert denied, Spence v. Canterbury, 409 U.S. 1064 (1972)

Chaires v. St. John's Episcopal Hospital, No. 808/75 N.Y. Cty.Sup.Ct (N.Y. Feb 21, 1984)

Chandler v. Simpson, 100 Wn. App. 1034 (2000)

Civil Rights Act of 1964, 42 U.S.C. §§ 2000a–2000h

Clifford v. United States, No 82-5002 USDC (SD 1985)

Clites v. State, 322 N.W.2d 917 (Iowa App. 1982)

Cruzan v. Director, Missouri Department of Health, 497 U.S. 261 (1990)

Doerr v. Hurley Medical Center, No 82–674–39 NM Mich Aug (1984)

Dovido v. Vasquez, No 84–674 CA(L)(H) 15th Jud. Dist. Cir. Ct., Palm Beach Cty. (FL Apr 4, 1986)

Dusky v. United States, 362 U.S. 402 (1960)

Evans v. United States, 883 F.Supp. 124 (SD Miss 1995)

Fain v. Commonwealth, 78 Ky. 183 (1879)

Ford v. Wainwright, 477 US 399 (1986)

Frasier v. Department of Health and Human Resources, 500 So.2d 858, 864 (La. Ct. App. 1986)

Garamella v. New York Medical College, 23 F.Supp. 2d 167 (D Conn 1998)

Gonzales v. Oregon, 126 S.Ct. 904 (2006)

Gowan v. United States, 601 F.Supp. 1297 (D. Or. 1985)

Green v. Ross, 691 So.2d 542 (Fla. 2d DCA 1997)

Guidelines on Discrimination Because of Sex, 29 C.F.R. §1604.11

Harris v. Forklift Systems, 510 U.S. 17 (1993)

Health Care Quality Improvement Act of 1986, 42 U.S.C. §11101 (Supp v. 1987)

H.M. Advocate v. Fraser, 4 Couper 70 (1878)

Hofflander v. St. Catherine's Hospital, 664 N.W.2d 545 (WI 2003)

Holton v. Pfingst, 534 S.W.2d 786, 789 (Ky. App. 1976)

Howe v. Citizens Memorial Hospital, 426 S.W.2d 882 (Tex. Civ. App. Corpus Christi 1968), rev'd, 436 S.W.2d 115 (Tex. 1968)

Hyde v. University of Michigan Board of Regents, 426 Mich. 223, 393 N.W.2d 847 (1986), revised in accord with Ross v. Consumer Power Company, 420 Mich. 567, 363 N.W.2d 641 (1986)

In the Guardianship of John Roe, 411 Mass. 666 (1992)

In re Boyer, 636 P.2d 1085, 1089 (Utah 1981)

In re Conroy, 98 N.J. 321, 486 A.2d 1209, 1222–23 (1985)

In re Farrell, 108 N.J. 335, 529 A.2d 404 (1987)

In re M.B., 2006 WL 721511, Court of Appeals N.Y., Mar 23, 2006

In re Jobes, 108 N.J. 394, 529 A.2d 434 (1987)

In re Peter, 108 N.J. 365, 529 A.2d 419 (1987)

In re Quinlin, 70 N.J. 10, 355 A.2d 647, cert denied, 429 U.S. 922 (1976)

Jaffee v. Redmond, 518 U.S. 1 (1996)

J.S. v. R.T., 714 A.2d 924 (N.J. 1998)

Karasik v. Bird, 98 A.D.2d 359, 470 N.Y.S.2d 605 (1984)

Kilgore v. County of Santa Clara, No. 397–525 (Santa Clara Cty. Super. Ct. Cal. 1982)

Long v. Jaszczak, 688 N.W.2d 173 (N.D. 2004)

Meek v. City of Loveland, 85 Colo. 346, 276 P. 30 (1929)

Minn. Stat. Ann. § 148A.02 (West 2005)

Minn. Stat. Ann. § 609.344 (West 2005)

M'Naughten's case. 10 Cl. & Fin. 200, 8 Eng. Rep 718 (HL 1843)

Model Penal Code (1962)

Moran v. Botsford General Hospital, No. 1 81–225–533, Wayne Cty. Cir. Ct. (MI Oct. 1, 1984)

Muldrow v. Re-Direct, Inc., 397 F.Supp.2d 1 (D.D.C. 2005)

Natanson v. Kline, 186 Kan. 393, 350 P.2d. 1093 (1960)

P.L. 98–473, 1984

Parham v. J.R., 442 U.S. 584 (1979)

Penry v. Lynaugh, 492 U.S. 302 (1989)

People v. Rose, 573 N.W.2d 765 (Neb 1998)

People v. White, 117 Cal.App.3d 270, 172 Cal. Rptr. 612 (1981)

Ramon v. Farr, 770 P.2d 131 (Utah 1989)

Rennie v. Klein, 462 F.Supp. 1131 (D. N.J. 1978), remanded, 476 F.Supp. 1294 (D. N.J. 1979), aff'd in part, modified in part and remanded, 653 F.2d 836 (3d. Cir. 1980), vacated and remanded, 458 U.S. 1119 (1982), 720 F.2d 266 (3rd Cir. 1983)

Restatement [Second] of Torts 315(a) (1965)

Riggins v. Nevada, 504 U.S. 127 (1992)

Rogers v. Commissioner of Department of Mental Health, 390 Mass. 489, 458 N.E.2d 308 (Mass. 1983)

Ross v. Consumer Power Company, 363 N.W. 2d 641 (Mich 1985)

Scaria v. St. Paul Fire and Marine Ins. Co., 68 Wis.2d 1, 227 N.W.2d 647 (1975)

Schloendorff v. Society of New York Hospital, 211 N.Y. 125, 105 N.E. 92 (1914), overruled, Bing v. Thunig, 2 N.Y.2d 656, 143 N.E.2d 3, 163 N.Y.S.2d 3 (1957)

Sell v. United States, 539 U.S. 166 (2003)

Speer v. United States, 512 F.Supp. 670 (N.D. Tex. 1981), aff'd, Speer v. United States, 675 F.2d 100 (5th Cir. 1982)

Stepakoff v. Kantar, 473 N.E.2d 1131 (Mass. 1985)

Stone v. Proctor, 259 N.C. 633, 131 S.E.2d 297 (1963)

Tarasoff v. Regents of the University of California, 17 Cal.3d 425, 551 P.2d 334; 131 Cal. Rptr. 14 (1976)

Tennard v. Dretke, 542 U.S. 274 (2004)

Thapar v. Zezulka, 944 S.W.2d 635 (Tex. 1999)

Touchette v. Ganal, 922 P.2d 347 (Haw. 1996)

Truman v. Thomas, 27 Cal.3d 285, 611 P.2d 902, 165 Cal. Rptr. 308 (1980)

Tune v. Walter Reed Army Medical Hospital, 602 F.Supp. 1452 (D.D.C. 1985)

Uniform Guardianship and Protective Proceedings Act (1997)

Union Pacific Realty Co. v. Botsford, 141 U.S. 250, 251 (1891)

United States v. Brawner, 471 F.2d 969 (D.C. Cir. 1972), superseded by statute, see Shannon v. United States, 512 U.S. 573 (1994)

United States v. David, 511 F.2d 355 (D.C. Cir. 1975)

Washington v. Harper, 494 U.S. 210 (1990)

Wilson v. Lehman, 379 S.W.2d 478, 479 (Ky. 1964)

Wilson v. United States, 391 F.2d 460, 463 (D.C. Cir. 1968)

Witherell v. Weimer, 148 Ill. App.3d 32, 499 N.E.2d 46 (1986), rev'd on other grounds, 118 Ill. 2d 515 N.E.2d 68 (1987)

Wright v. State, No. 83-5035 Orleans Parish Civ. Dist. Ct. (LA April 1986)

Youngberg v. Romeo, 457 U.S. 307 (1982); on remand, Romeo v. Youngberg, 687 F.2d 33 (3rd Cir. 1982)

Glossary of Legal Terms

Action
See civil action.

Adjudication
The formal pronouncement of a judgment or decree in a cause of action.

Assault
Any willful attempt or threat to inflict injury.

Battery
An intentional and wrongful physical contact with an individual without consent that causes some injury or offensive touching.

Beyond a reasonable doubt
The level of proof required to convict a person in a criminal trial. This is the highest level of proof required (90%–95% range of certainty).

Breach of contract
A violation of or failure to perform any or all of the terms of an agreement.

Brief
A written statement prepared by legal counsel arguing a case.

Burden of proof
The legal obligation to prove affirmatively a disputed fact (or facts) related to an issue that is raised by the parties in a case.

Capacity
The status or attributes necessary for a person so that his or her acts may be legally and responsibly acknowledged and recognized.

Case law
The aggregate of reported cases as forming a body of law on a particular subject.

Cause in fact
The requirement of fact that without the defendant's wrongful conduct, the harm to the plaintiff would not have occurred.

Cause of action
The grounds of an action—that is, those facts that, if alleged and proved in a suit, would enable the plaintiff to attain a judgment.

Civil action
A lawsuit brought by a private individual or group to recover money or property, to enforce or protect a civil right, or to prevent or redress a civil wrong.

Civil law
As contrasted with criminal law, a system for enforcement of private rights arising from sources such as torts and contracts.

Clear and convincing
A proof that results in reasonable certainty of the truth of an ultimate fact in controversy (75% range of certainty); for example, the minimum level of evidence necessary to involuntarily hospitalize a patient.

Common law
A system of law based on customs, traditional usage, and prior case law rather than codified written laws (statutes).

Compensatory damages
Damages awarded to a person as compensation, indemnity, or restitution for harm sustained.

Competency
The mental capacity to understand the nature of an act.

Consent decree
An agreement by a defendant to cease activities asserted as illegal by the government.

Consortium
The right of a husband or wife to the care, affection, company, and cooperation of the other spouse in every aspect of the marital relationship.

Contract
A legally enforceable agreement between two or more parties to do or not do a particular thing upon sufficient consideration.

Criminal law
The branch of the law that defines crimes and provides for their punishment. Unlike civil law, penalties include imprisonment.

Damages
A sum of money awarded to a person injured by the unlawful act or negligence of another.

Defendant
A person or legal entity against whom a claim or charge is brought.

Due process (of law)
The constitutional guarantee protecting individuals from arbitrary and unreasonable actions by the government that would deprive them of their basic rights to life, liberty, or property.

Duress
Compulsion or constraint, as by force or threat, exercised to make a person do or say something against his or her will.

Duty
The legal obligation that one person owes another. Whenever one person has a right, another person has a corresponding duty to preserve or not interfere with that right.

False imprisonment
The unlawful restraint or detention of one person by another.

Fiduciary
A person who acts for another in a capacity that involves a confidence or trust.

Forensic psychiatry
A subspecialty of psychiatry in which scientific and clinical expertise is applied to legal issues in legal contexts embracing civil, criminal, correctional, or legislative matters.

Fraud
Any act of trickery, deceit, or misrepresentation designed to deprive someone of property or to do harm.

Guardianship
A legal arrangement wherein one individual (the guardian) possesses the legal right and duty to care for another individual (the ward) and his or her property.

Hold harmless
An agreement to protect a party from damages.

Immunity
The freedom from duty or penalty.

Incompetence
A lack of ability or fitness for some legal qualification necessary for the performance of an act (e.g., being a minor, lacking mental competence).

Informed consent
A competent person's voluntary agreement to allow something to happen that is based upon full disclosure of facts needed to make a knowing decision.

Intentional tort
A tort in which the actor is expressly or implicitly judged to have possessed an intent or purpose to cause injury.

Judgment
The final determination or adjudication by a court of the claims of parties in an action.

Jurisdiction
The legal right by which courts or judicial officers exercise their authority.

Malpractice
Any professional misconduct or unreasonable lack of skill in professional or fiduciary duties.

***Miranda* warning**
Refers to the *Miranda v. Arizona* decision that requires a four-part warning to be given prior to any custodial interrogation.

Negligence
The failure to exercise the standard of care that would be expected of a normally reasonable and prudent person in a particular set of circumstances.

Nominal damages
Generally, damages of a small monetary amount indicating a violation of a legal right without any important loss or damage to the plaintiff.

Parens patriae

The authority of the state to exercise sovereignty and guardianship of a person with legal disability so as to act on his or her behalf in protecting health, comfort, and welfare interests.

Plaintiff

The complaining party in an action; the person who brings a cause of action.

Police power

The power of government to make and enforce all laws and regulations necessary for the welfare of the state and its citizens.

Power of attorney

A document giving someone authority to act on behalf of the grantor.

Preponderance of evidence

Superiority in the weight of evidence presented by one side over that of the other (51% range of certainty); the level of certainty required in order to prevail in civil trials.

Privileged communication

Those statements made by certain persons within a protected relationship (e.g., doctor–patient) that the law protects from forced disclosure.

Proximate cause

The direct, immediate cause to which an injury or loss can be attributed and without which the injury or loss would not have occurred.

Proxy

A person empowered by another to represent, act, or vote for him or her.

Punitive damages

Damages awarded over and above those to which the plaintiff is entitled, generally given to punish or make an example of the defendant.

Respondeat superior

The doctrine whereby the master (i.e., employer) is strictly liable in certain cases for the wrongful acts of his or her servants (i.e., employees).

Right

A power, privilege, demand, or claim possessed by a particular person by virtue of law. Every legal right that one person possesses imposes corresponding legal duties on other persons.

Sovereign immunity

The immunity of a government from being sued in court except with its consent.

Standard of care (negligence law)

In the law of negligence, that degree of care that a reasonably prudent person should exercise under the same or similar circumstances.

Stare decisis

The duty too adhere to precedents and not to unsettle principles of law that are established.

Statute

An act of the legislature declaring, commanding, or prohibiting something.

Subpoena

A writ commanding a person to appear in court.

Subpoena ad testificandum

A writ commanding a person to appear in court to give testimony.

Subpoena duces tecum

A writ commanding a person to appear in court with particular documents or other evidence.

Tort

Any private or civil wrong by act or omission, not including breach of contract.

United States Code (U.S.C.)

The compilation of laws derived from federal legislation.

Vicarious liability

See *respondeat superior*.

42

ETHICAL ASPECTS OF PSYCHIATRY

Laura Weiss Roberts, M.D., M.A.
Jinger G. Hoop, M.D., M.F.A.
Laura B. Dunn, M.D.

> Ethics is an endeavor. It refers to ways of understanding what is good and right in human experience. It is about discernment, knowledge, and self-reflection, and it is sustained through seeking, clarifying, and translating. It is the concrete expression of moral ideals in everyday life. Ethics is about meaning, and it is about action.
>
> Roberts 2002a, p. 525

The importance of ethics to psychiatry is rooted in the powerful and intimate role that psychiatrists play in the lives of their patients. Patients living with mental illnesses that may be profoundly impairing, deeply stigmatizing, and potentially life-threatening place great trust in their caregivers not only to do what is right as healers but also to value and respect them as human beings. Psychiatrists often carry their patients' most closely held thoughts, hopes, and fears. Across the spectrum of severity, people with mental illness, and their families, have to muster courage and take risks to seek help, typically battling various forms of stigma as well as systemic societal barriers to care (Link and Phelan 2006). Moreover, ill individuals have often struggled alone for years, are frequently misdiagnosed before coming to psychiatric attention, and may need substantial efforts in terms of time and attention in order for a clinician to earn their confidence. Becoming worthy of that trust also requires, at its foundation, that psychiatrists develop and work to maintain a deep capacity for self-reflection and a sensitivity to the ethical nuances of their work (Roberts and Dyer 2004; Roberts et al. 1996).

The high value of ethics to psychiatry also stems from the unique place of psychiatry within the house of medicine and all of society. As physicians who are well-trained observers of human behavior, psychiatrists are given special credence to make decisions about complex situations that require an understanding of ethics, medicine, and psychology and of psychosocial aspects of daily life. Psychiatrists are thus often called upon to help clarify and resolve ethical dilemmas that arise in the care of medical patients, to join ethics committees, and to reflect publicly on ethical questions confronted by society. For all these reasons, cultivating an understanding of ethics is vital to providing competent and compassionate psychiatric care and to fulfilling psychiatrists' complex and varied duties and roles.

Furthermore, ethical behavior is a core feature of what it means to be a medical professional. While *professionalism* has been defined in multiple ways (Table 42–1), a key element of many definitions is a willing acceptance of an ethical obligation to place the patient's and society's interests above one's own (Roberts and Dyer 2004). Ethics education therefore is strongly linked to the development of professionalism in trainees; for psychiatrists, special privileges and obligations accompanying their roles make ethics education a crucial component of training in psychiatry and lifelong learning. The knowledge, skills, and professional attitudes relevant to ethical behavior, analysis, and problem-solving are critical components of psychiatric training (Roberts et al. 2004). Model curricula for the teaching of ethics to psychiatric residents regarding both clinical and research-related ethics have been developed, and ongoing work is needed to refine and test such models (Chen 2003; Rosenstein et al. 2001).

TABLE 42–1. Definitions of professionalism

- Being a professional is an ethical matter, entailing devotion to a way of life, in the service of others and of some higher good (Kass 1983).

- A profession is a socially sanctioned activity whose primary object is the well-being of others above the professional's personal gain (Racy 1990).

- A profession has three features: training that is intellectual and involves knowledge, as distinguished from skill; work that is pursued primarily for others and not for oneself; and success that is measured by more than the amount of financial return (Brandeis 1993).

- Professionalism is not a matter of *trying* but of *being* (LaCombe 1993).

- A profession is a set of values, attitudes, and behaviors that results in serving the interests of patients and society before one's own (Reynolds 1994).

- Professionalism means aspiring to altruism, accountability, excellence, duty, service, honor, integrity, and respect for others (Stobo and Blank 1994).

Source. Adapted from Roberts LW, Dyer AR: "Ethics: Principles and Professionalism," in *Concise Guide to Ethics in Mental Health Care.* Washington, DC, American Psychiatric Publishing, 2004, pp. 15–16.

Essential Ethical Skills of Psychiatrists

The clinical skills and personal abilities of well-trained psychiatrists translate readily into a natural facility with ethical problem solving that goes beyond a simple adherence to written guidelines, laws, and codes. Clinical training and, frequently, natural aptitude typically enable psychiatrists to attend to subtleties and nuances, to look beyond the surface for hidden motivations, and to form the habits of self-reflection and self-scrutiny. These abilities readily translate into a sensitivity to moral issues and an ability to solve ethical dilemmas in a systematic and thoughtful way.

Psychiatrists whose work embodies the highest ethical standards tend to rely on a set of six core "ethics skills" that are learned during or before medical training and are continually practiced and refined during their professional careers (Table 42–2) (Roberts and Dyer 2004; Roberts et al. 1996). Acquiring these skills in support of professional conduct in psychiatry is itself a developmental process, with certain predictable issues and milestones that occur in relation to the nature of our work and roles we are entrusted with in society (Fann et al. 2003; Hoop 2004; Roberts et al. 1996).

TABLE 42–2. Essential ethics skills in clinical practice

The ability to identify the ethical features of a patient's care

The ability to see how the clinician's own life experience, attitudes, and knowledge may influence the care of the patient

The ability to identify one's areas of clinical expertise (i.e., scope of clinical competence) and to work within these boundaries

The ability to anticipate ethically risky or problematic situations

The ability to gather information and to seek consultation and additional expertise in order to clarify and, ideally, to resolve ethical conflicts

The ability to build ethical safeguards into the patient care situation

Source. Reprinted from Roberts LW, Dyer AR: "Clinical Decision-Making and Ethics Skills," in *Concise Guide to Ethics in Mental Health Care.* Washington, DC, American Psychiatric Publishing, 2004, p. 20. Copyright 2004, American Psychiatric Publishing. Used with permission.

The first of these core skills is the ability to *identify ethical issues* as they arise. For some this will be an intuitive insight (e.g., the internal sense that "something isn't right"), and for others it will be derived more logically (e.g., the foreknowledge that involuntary treatment or the care of "VIP" patients poses specific ethical problems). The ability to recognize ethical issues requires some familiarity with key ethics concepts and the emerging interdisciplinary field of bioethics. As a corollary, this ability presupposes the psychiatrist's capacity to observe and translate complex phenomena into patterns, using the common language of the profession (e.g., conflicts between autonomy, beneficence, and justice when a person with mental illness threatens the life of a specific individual and is thus held for an evaluation against his preferences) (Tables 42–3 and 42–4).

The second skill is the ability to *understand how the psychiatrist's personal values, beliefs, and sense of self may affect his or her care of patients.* Just as psychiatrists must be able to recognize and deal with countertransference in the therapeutic setting, they must also be able to understand how their own personalities and experiences may influence their ethical judgment. For instance, a psychiatrist who places a high value on her ability to "do good" as a healer should recognize that this may subtly influence her judgment when evaluating the decisional capacity of patients who refuse medically necessary treatments. A psychiatrist with a strong commitment to personal self-care and athleticism may have difficulty accepting patients who do not share this commitment and engage voluntarily in high-risk behaviors that themselves have ethical consequences. This skill, of appreciating this aspect of the doctor–patient relationship, is important in safeguarding the ethical decision making of the professional in serving the needs and best interests of the patient.

Another key ethics skill is an *awareness of the limits of one's own medical knowledge and expertise and a willingness to practice within those limits.* Providing competent care within the scope of one's expertise fulfills both the positive ethical duty of doing good and the negative obligation to "do no harm." In some real-world situations, however, psychiatrists may at times feel compelled to perform services outside their area of competence. Such circumstances are often encountered in geographically isolated communities, where treatment providers may be faced with the dilemma of providing care for which they lack adequate training, treating people with whom they have other relationships (e.g., local businesspeople), or being unable to treat all of the patients who need help (Roberts and Dyer 2004). In such settings, clinicians may feel ethically justified in

choosing to do their best in the clinical situation while simultaneously trying to resolve the underlying problem (American Psychiatric Association 2001b). For example, a rural psychiatrist may expand her zone of competence by obtaining consultation by telephone.

The fourth skill is the ability to *recognize high-risk situations in which ethical problems are likely to arise,* often in circumstances in which the psychiatrists must step out of the usual treatment relationship to protect the patient or others from harm. These situations include initiating involuntary treatment and hospitalization, reporting child or elder abuse, and informing a third party of a patient's intention to inflict harm.

The fifth skill is the *willingness to seek information and consultation* when faced with an ethically or clinically difficult situation, and the ability to *make use of the guidance offered by these sources.* Just as psychiatrists should tackle clinically difficult cases by reviewing the psychiatric literature and consulting with more experienced colleagues, they should clarify and solve ethically difficult situations by referring to ethics codes and guidelines and consulting with colleagues and ethics committees.

The final essential skill for psychiatrists is the ability to *build appropriate ethical safeguards into their work.* For example, psychiatrists who treat children and adolescents are wise to routinely inform new patients and their parents—at the onset of treatment—about the limits of confidentiality and the physician's legal mandate to report child abuse (Belitz 2004). Similarly, clinical researchers can prevent some ethical conflicts from arising in the course of their research by designing protocols that incorporate safeguards, such as careful training for research staff, participant education sessions in conjunction with the informed consent process, operating procedures that protect personal information gathered from study volunteers (e.g., data encryption), and a priori "exit" criteria for disenrolling participants (Roberts 1999).

Conceptual and Empirical Foundations of Psychiatric Ethics

Principles of Moral Behavior

Because the ability to identify ethical issues when they arise is an essential skill for clinical practice, it is important for psychiatrists to be fluent in the language of ethics discourse (Table 42–5). Contemporary ethics

TABLE 42–3. Ethical tensions in common clinical situations

Clinical situation	Relevant ethical principles	Conflicts and tensions
A patient refuses a medically indicated treatment	Autonomy and beneficence	The patient's right to make his or her own decisions is in tension with the physician's duty to do good by providing medically indicated treatment
A patient tells his psychiatrist that he plans to harm another person	Confidentiality and beneficence	The physician's duty to guard his patient's privacy must be balanced against the obligation to protect the threatened third party
A close friend asks a psychiatrist to write a prescription for a sleep medicine	Nonmaleficence	The desire to oblige a friend may conflict with the psychiatrist's duty to avoid harm by prescribing without conducting a medical evaluation and establishing a treatment relationship
The parent of an adolescent patient asks the psychiatrist for information about the patient's sexual activity and drug or alcohol use	Confidentiality and beneficence	The psychiatrist's duty to guard his patient's privacy may be in tension with the psychiatrist's desire to do good by educating the parent about the child's high-risk behaviors
A patient asks a psychiatrist to document a less-stigmatizing diagnosis when filling out insurance forms	Veracity and nonmaleficence	The psychiatrist's obligation to document the truth may be in tension with the desire to avoid the harm that may occur if the insurance company learns of the diagnosis
A rural psychiatrist's patient needs a treatment the psychiatrist is not competent to provide; no other practitioner is available	Nonmaleficence	The psychiatrist's duty to avoid harming the patient by practicing outside his scope of competencies is in conflict with the obligation to avoid harming the patient by leaving him without any treatment provider
A medical student performs a lumbar puncture for the first time on a patient	Nonmaleficence and beneficence	The medical student's obligation to avoid harming the patient by performing a procedure without sufficient expertise must be balanced against the student's need to "learn by doing" in order to help future patients
A psychiatrist treating a physician believes the patient is too impaired to practice medicine safely; the patient/physician refuses to close his practice because he has no other source of income	Confidentiality, nonmaleficence, and beneficence	The psychiatrist's duty to guard his patient's privacy and to avoid harming him is in tension with the obligation to protect the impaired physician's patients by reporting the impairment to the proper authorities
A pharmaceutical company offers a psychiatrist a large fee for referring patients to a research trial	Fidelity	Financial self-interest threatens the psychiatrist's duty to remain faithful to the goals of treatment and to the role as a healer
A psychiatrist transfers care of a "difficult" patient to another provider	Fidelity, nonmaleficence, and beneficence	The psychiatrist's obligations to remain faithful to the goals of treatment and to avoid the harm of patient abandonment must be balanced against the duty to do good by transferring care to a more competent or appropriate provider when clinically necessary

TABLE 42–4. Key ethical challenges in special clinical circumstances

Clinical circumstance	Key ethical challenges
Academic psychiatry	Conflicts between clinical and supervisory roles of faculty and between clinical and student roles of trainees Financial conflicts of interest related to managed care contracts and relationships with industry Duty to provide competent care despite trainee status of resident physicians and medical students
Addiction psychiatry	Confidentiality, due to adverse legal and social consequences of addictive behaviors Justice, because of the lack of equitable treatment for persons with addictive disorders compared with other conditions
Child and adolescent psychiatry	Confidentiality and truth telling for patient and guardians Informed consent for treatment, which may require the consent of guardians
Forensic psychiatry	Conflicts between roles as forensic expert and physician
Geriatric psychiatry	Informed consent for treatment when decisional capacity may be impaired End-of-life issues, including assisted suicide and treatment withdrawal
Military psychiatry	Conflicts between roles as physician and member of the military
Psychotherapy and psychoanalysis	Confidentiality, due to the intensely private nature of patient disclosures Maintenance of therapeutic boundaries
Public psychiatry	Duty to provide competent care despite limited resources Justice, in terms of the need to distribute social resources fairly
Rural psychiatry	Confidentiality in a setting where "everyone knows everyone" Conflicts among multiple roles of physician and patients within community Duty to provide competent care in the absence of specialists Nonabandonment of patients in a setting in which there may be a lack of qualified clinicians to provide backup coverage
Treatment of "difficult" patients	Duty to provide competent care to patients with clinically challenging psychopathology Nonabandonment despite countertransference feelings or physician burnout

Source. Adapted from Roberts and Dyer 2004.

discussions often center on a set of moral principles that physicians are considered duty bound to uphold. The key principles of moral behavior with special importance to the field of medical ethics include nonmaleficence, beneficence, autonomy, respect for persons, justice, fidelity, and the linked concepts of privacy and confidentiality (Beauchamp and Childress 2001).

Nonmaleficence is a modern term for the old, perhaps ancient, rule of *primum non nocere* (first, do no harm). In medical ethics, *harm* is defined broadly, including killing, causing physical or emotional suffering, or depriving others of beneficial things.

Beneficence refers to the belief that individuals should try to do good, to try to seek benefit for others.

Beneficence encompasses the notion of *utility,* the duty to act in a way that provides the greatest positive consequences and the least negative consequences.

Autonomy, which means "self-rule," suggests a moral principle based on the importance of respecting others' right to personal self-governance. To be autonomous, an individual must be free from coercive influences and capable of making independent decisions and actions. To respect a patient's autonomy requires one to behave in a way that allows for and enhances the ability of the patient to make voluntary decisions on his or her own behalf (Roberts 2002b).

Respect for persons is a broad concept that encompasses respect for autonomy plus a deep regard for the

TABLE 42–5. Glossary of ethics terms

Altruism   The virtue of acting for the good of another rather than for oneself, at times entailing self-sacrifice.

Autonomy   Literally, "self-rule." In medical ethics, autonomy is the ability to make deliberated or reasoned decisions for oneself and to act on the basis of such decisions.

Beneficence   An action done to benefit others. The principle of beneficence in medicine signifies an obligation to benefit patients and to seek their good.

Coercion   The use of some form of pressure to persuade or compel an individual to agree to a belief or action.

Compassion   Literally, "suffering with" another person, with kindness and an active regard for his or her welfare. Compassion is more closely related to empathy than to sympathy, as sympathy connotes the more distanced experience of "feeling sorry for" the individual.

Confidentiality   The obligation of physicians not to disclose information obtained from patients or observed about them without their permission. In clinical care, it entails taking precautions to protect the personal information of patients. Confidentiality is a privilege linked to the legal right of privacy and may at times be overridden by exceptions stipulated in law.

Conflict of interest   In medicine, a situation in which a physician has competing roles, relationships, or interests that could potentially interfere with the ability to care for patients. Such situations may naturally occur in clinical care and research, and they are not inherently unethical but must be recognized and managed appropriately to safeguard the well-being of vulnerable individuals (e.g., patients, research participants) and to prevent exploitative practices.

Empathy   The act of entering into someone else's frame of reference in terms of thoughts, feelings, and experiences, to gain an authentic understanding of the other person's experiences imaginatively as one's own.

Euthanasia   A form of physician-assisted death in which the physician deliberately and with compassionate intent acts to end the life of a person with an incurable and progressive disease that will cause imminent death.

Fidelity   The virtue of promise keeping, truthfulness, and honor. In clinical care, it refers to the faithfulness with which a clinician commits to the duty of helping patients and acting in a manner that is in keeping with the ideals of the profession.

Fiduciary   An entity in a position of trust with a duty to act on behalf of another, for the other's good. Physicians are fiduciaries with respect to their patients.

Honesty   A virtue in which one conveys the truth fully, without misrepresentation through deceit, bias, or omission.

Human dignity   The belief that every person, intrinsically, is valued and worthy of respect. In medical ethics, every patient is believed to have innate and inalienable worth as a human being that requires he or she be treated with respect and compassion and full interpersonal regard as expressed in attitudes, behaviors, and nondiscriminatory practices.

Informed consent   In the clinical setting, a legal and ethical obligation for clinicians to inform patients about their illness and alternatives for care and to assist them in making reasoned, authentic decisions about treatment. In the research setting, a similar obligation for a researcher to inform participants about the research protocol and help them make reasoned, authentic decisions about research participation.

Integrity   A virtue literally defined as wholeness or coherence. It connotes professional soundness and reliability of intention and action.

Justice   The ethical principle of fairness. Distributive justice refers to the fair and equitable distribution of resources and burden throughout society.

Medical decision making   The intentional process associated with making a choice in clinical care. It pertains to a patient's capacity to make decisions related to his or her health or health care and to the clinician's process of deliberation, consultation, and data gathering that results in the development of a diagnosis and of therapeutic alternatives for a patient.

TABLE 42–5. **Glossary of ethics terms** (continued)

Medical negligence   The legal concept of a breach of duty of medical care. It rests on the existence of a duty of care, failure to fulfill that duty, and the existence of harm.

Nonmaleficence   The duty to avoid doing harm.

Personhood   Having full moral status as a human being.

Quality of life   The expression of a value judgment regarding the experience of life as a whole or some aspect of it by an individual.

Respect   The virtue of fully regarding and according intrinsic value to someone or something. In clinical care, it is reflected in treating another individual with genuine consideration and attentiveness to that person's life history, values, and goals.

Self-understanding   The awareness of one's own values and motivations. Self-understanding based on insight and careful self-scrutiny is a key ethical skill of special importance to mental health care ethics.

Therapeutic boundaries   The set of concepts, rules, and duties that structures the clinician–patient relationship to ensure psychological safety, to optimize therapeutic benefit, and to prevent potentially exploitative practices.

Trustworthiness   A virtue that pertains to a disposition that inspires confident belief in and reliance upon the physician's character and ability to act beneficently and honestly.

Voluntary   The attribute in which a belief or act derives from one's own free will and is not coerced or unduly influenced by others.

Vulnerability   The capacity to be wounded or hurt physically, emotionally, spiritually, or socially and being without the means to defend or advocate for oneself fully.

Source.   Adapted from Roberts LW, Dyer AR: "Appendix A," in *Concise Guide to Ethics in Mental Health Care.* Washington, DC, American Psychiatric Publishing, 2004, p. 319.

worth and dignity of all human beings. The protection of potentially vulnerable groups of people represents a key aspect of respect for persons and is embodied in specific ethical guidelines.

Justice is a moral principle that relates to treating people fairly and, in modern society, without prejudice. Distributive justice refers to equitable distribution of benefits and burdens among members of society. "Parity" legislation that seeks to ensure the provision of insurance for mental illness and related conditions that is equal or equivalent to insurance for physical illness illustrates a real-life effort at distributive justice in the United States.

Veracity refers to honesty or truth telling. Upholding the moral ideal of veracity involves both a "positive" ethical duty (i.e., being truthful in one's statements), as well as a "negative" ethical duty (i.e., not telling lies *and* avoiding misimpression or misrepresentation, such as misleading others by withholding the truth or some aspects of it).

Fidelity is the ideal of faithfulness. In medicine, physicians who demonstrate fidelity are steadfast in their role of healer. They do not abandon or exploit patients, and they do not place self-interest or the interest of third parties above patients' needs.

Privacy generally refers to the right to be free from the intrusions of others upon one's physical body, one's mind, or one's personal information. In medicine, *confidentiality* is the privilege of having one's privacy protected by a physician. Keeping the confidences of patients has been a professional duty of physicians from at least the time of Hippocrates. The privilege of confidentiality is suspended under certain circumstances, such as danger to third parties. On the other hand, it is important to protect patient confidentiality to whatever extent it is possible, even when there are legal requirements to share information. To give just one example, one should never turn over a patient's entire medical record to, say, a police officer who is investigating the circumstances of a sexual assault—providing only the salient elements of the medical record is sufficient and appropriate according to both ethical and legal directives and prevents inadvertent disclosure of irrelevant (but perhaps very sensitive) personal material.

Philosophical Foundations

Several theories of moral behavior form the philosophical foundation of contemporary medical ethics.

Each theory delineates an aspect of ethics that is relevant to particular situations or conditions in biomedical ethics. Although the theories described below are often discussed separately, in practice the value of understanding them arises from the ability to draw upon them as a toolkit; that is, different tools or considerations derived from different theories may need to be combined to approach complex ethical dilemmas faced in psychiatric practice, in the development of professional guidelines, and in policy-making related to mental health.

Kantianism is a philosophical theory based on the work of Immanuel Kant (1724–1804). Kantianism suggests that the morality of an action may be independent of its consequences and that some actions, such as telling the truth, are morally obligatory in almost all circumstances. To be ethical, a person must follow these moral obligations unconditionally. Kantian theory is at the core of how contemporary bioethicists think about ethical behavior in patient care (i.e., serving the needs and interests of each individual patient above other goals in a clinical situation). For instance, most Western physicians believe that it is always important to tell patients the truth, even though the truth in some circumstances may be difficult to speak or painful to hear. Kantian ideals may be challenging to live out in some real-world medical situations, however, where there are scarce resources (e.g., allocation of organs for transplantation or of highly expensive medications). Oftentimes, these situations involve conflicting moral obligations, such as balancing the needs of others or of the community against the preferences of an individual (e.g., insisting upon involuntary treatment in the care of a mentally ill person voicing a homicidal threat toward a specific person).

Utilitarianism refers to an ethical theory supported by the writings of Jeremy Bentham (1748–1832) and John Stewart Mill (1806–1873). Utilitarian philosophy posits that the most ethical actions and rules are those that bring about the greatest good for the most people—that is, those actions that have the greatest utility. Utilitarian philosophy emphasizes the importance of the consequences of one's actions and highlights beneficence and justice as guiding ethical principles. While Kantianism is particularly relevant to the ethical treatment of individuals, utilitarianism is vital to ethical reasoning about larger systems. The principles of utility and justice are the ethical foundation of public health policies, for example. However, a rigidly utilitarian viewpoint could justify practices that most people would consider immoral—for example, coercing a small, randomly selected group of people to enroll in a risky medical research trial in order to derive significant benefits for the rest of the population.

Principle-based ethics, as described by contemporary theorists James Childress and Thomas Beauchamp, suggests that ethical dilemmas should be resolved through the specification and balancing of the principles of nonmaleficence, beneficence, respect for autonomy, and justice (Beauchamp and Childress 2001). By contrast, *casuistry* describes a "bottom up" approach to ethical decision making in which ethicists focus first on the details of a particular case rather than overarching rules and principles. Casuistry also highlights the importance of ethical reasoning by analogy with similar cases from the past (Jonsen and Toulmin 1988).

Other philosophical approaches to biomedical ethics include *virtue ethics,* which defines as ethical the actions of virtuous people; *relationship* or *care ethics,* which emphasizes commitments and relationships to others as the basis of ethical life; and *communitarian ethics,* which defines morality based on social values and traditions (Roberts and Dyer 2004).

Practical Ethical Problem Solving

Many clinicians use an eclectic approach to ethical problem solving that intuitively makes use of both principle-based ethics and casuistry through a combination of inductive and deductive reasoning. Such an approach does not typically yield one "right" answer but, rather, an array of possible and ethically justifiable approaches that may be acceptable in the current situation.

In the clinical setting, a widely used approach to ethical problem solving is the "four-topics method" described by Jonsen et al. (1998). This method entails gathering and evaluating information about 1) clinical indications, 2) patient preferences, 3) patient quality of life, and 4) contextual or external influences on the ethical decision-making process (Figure 42–1). This model has the advantage of being pragmatic, offering an implicit prioritization of issues that arise in complex real-world situations, and having been successfully utilized to analyze ethical issues in a variety of clinical settings and decision contexts. The approach has been widely disseminated, and many ethics committees in hospitals use the model in their evaluations and decisions regarding ethical dilemmas. In the psychiatric context, less attention has been paid to developing ethical decision-making models specifically addressing the unique characteristics of psychiatric patients, settings, and decisions (Roberts et al. 1996). With practice, however, the four-topics method can be

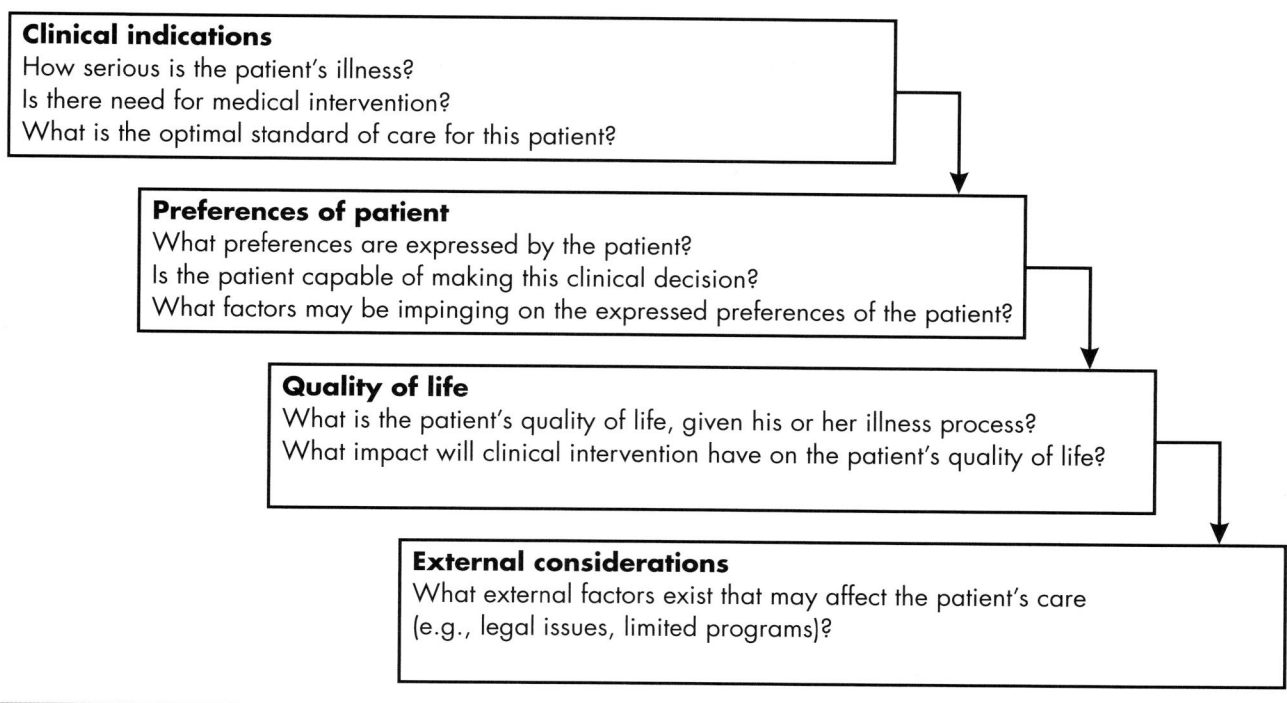

FIGURE 42–1.   A model for ethical decision making.

Source.   Reprinted from Roberts LW, Dyer AR: *Concise Guide to Ethics in Mental Health Care.* Washington, DC, American Psychiatric Publishing, 2004, p. 307. Used with permission.

used to help psychiatrists and other mental health professionals think through both straightforward and complex ethical cases. Strategies for systematically evaluating ethical issues in clinical supervision of multidisciplinary colleagues and clinicians-in-training may also be helpful in academic and community-based patient care settings (Roberts et al. 2003b).

Many ethical dilemmas in clinical care involve a conflict between the first two topics of the four-topics model: clinical indications and patient preferences (see Table 42–3). These dilemmas include situations in which an elderly cancer patient refuses life-prolonging chemotherapy, a psychotic adolescent is brought to a hospital for treatment against his will, or a young mother refuses a lifesaving blood transfusion on religious grounds. In each situation, the preferences of a patient are at odds with what is medically beneficial, creating a conflict for the physicians between their duties of beneficence and respect for patient autonomy. To work through such dilemmas, it is first necessary to fully and thoughtfully explore the patient's preferences as well as the clinical indications. Why does the patient refuse treatment? Does the patient have the cognitive and emotional capacity to make this decision at this time? What is the full range of options that are

medically beneficial? How urgent is the clinical situation, and is time available for discussion, collaboration, and perhaps compromise? If the patient does not have decision-making capacity, the dilemma is at least temporarily resolved by identifying an appropriate alternative decision maker. If the patient does have the ability to provide informed consent—involving capacity for decision making and capacity for voluntarism—then, under most foreseeable circumstances, his or her preferences must be followed. However, by engaging the patient in a meaningful dialogue in which the physician describes the full range of treatment options and demonstrates sensitivity to the reasons for the patient's refusal, it may often be possible to discover a solution that the patient can willingly accept and the physician can justify as medically beneficial.

Empirical Foundations of Clinical and Research Ethics

Empirical data as well as conceptual theory have become increasingly important in understanding ethical aspects of clinical practice and clinical research. Perhaps the most influential early empirical ethics work was Henry Beecher's 1966 article in the *New England*

Journal of Medicine in which he provided descriptions of 22 published biomedical research projects with significant ethical violations, including studies in which individuals were injected with cancer cells or deliberately infected with hepatitis. Interestingly, none of these studies involved psychiatric research or mentally ill individuals, though some of the projects included developmentally disabled individuals (e.g., the Willowbrook study).

Empirical studies can provide valuable support for more rigorous ethical decision making broadly throughout the field of biomedicine. Scientific evidence can establish the utility of medical interventions, can facilitate respect for persons by surveying the perspectives and values of patients and research volunteers, and can describe how the benefits and burdens of a health care policy are distributed among members of society (Roberts 2000). Such studies provide much-needed data to inform, support, test, and refine ethical guidelines and public policies. Further, ethics studies can help us to fulfill our ethical obligations of respect for persons and justice by offering empirical evidence on the perspectives, experiences, and attributes of the individuals who will enact or live with the consequences of the guidelines and policy approaches that are envisioned. For these reasons, and because people with mental illness often remain "unheard," are societally disadvantaged, and face heightened challenges in advocating for themselves, psychiatric ethics research has a distinct and important ethical justification.

In terms of the four-topics method for clinical ethical decision making, empirical evidence relevant to understanding a patient's clinical situation has long been gathered. These data concern disease prognosis, the relative efficacy of treatment options, and the treatments' risks and benefits. More recently, investigators have begun to compile data that may be helpful in understanding patient preferences, quality-of-life issues, and contextual features. For example, a handful of empirical studies have examined how psychiatric patients who have undergone involuntary treatment reflect on the experience afterward. Schwartz et al.'s (1988) survey of 24 psychiatric patients who had been involuntarily medicated found that at the time of hospital discharge, 70% believed the involuntary treatment had been appropriate. More recently, a survey of 433 involuntarily hospitalized patients (Gardner et al. 1999) demonstrated that 52% of those who believed they did not need hospitalization 2 days after admission decided by 4–8 weeks after discharge that hospitalization had been appropriate, though they felt the experience was coercive. Another study, though small,

demonstrated that patients felt it was of great importance to experience a sense of relatedness and caring human contact during an involuntary hospitalization (Olofsson and Norberg 2001).

Empirical studies have also been helpful in identifying and working through some of the complex ethical issues that arise in psychiatric research. For example, in the MacArthur Treatment Competence Study, Appelbaum and Grisso (1995) assessed the decision-making abilities of people with major depression, schizophrenia, or ischemic heart disease and a control group of nonpatient volunteers. The results of this landmark project revealed areas of decision-making capacity that were more difficult for acutely ill psychiatric patients than for the medically ill patients or members of the control group. This study demonstrated that decisional capacity was most impaired among the psychotic psychiatric patients but, very importantly, also showed that clinical treatment significantly improved the deficits in the decisional capacity of the acutely ill psychiatric patients. Roberts and colleagues' semistructured interviews with schizophrenia patients regarding their opinions about medical research demonstrated that persons with severe and persistent mental illness may have a nuanced understanding of the goals, risks, and benefits of research participation (Roberts et al. 2000, 2002b). Other work has shown that the public's view of psychiatric research may be fueled by stigma: a large online survey of U.S. adults found that mentally ill research participants were viewed as less capable of making independent research participation decisions compared to medically ill individuals (Muroff et al. 2006).

Finally, empirical findings have also been helpful as a guide to monitor the ethical attitudes and behaviors of psychiatrists and trainees and to suggest educational interventions. One survey project (Roberts et al. 1996) of 181 psychiatry residents training in 10 U.S. programs found that 92% believed that their prior ethics training had helped them respond appropriately to clinical ethical dilemmas and 76% had encountered an ethical problem for which they felt unprepared. This study and others, including surveys of 121 psychiatry chief residents and training directors (Coverdale et al. 1992), demonstrated enthusiasm among medical trainees for additional ethics training in medical school and/or residency. Roberts et al.'s (2005) ethics education study of 336 medical students and residents at the University of New Mexico demonstrated that trainees perceived a need for more education about ethical and professional dilemmas that occur during medical training and the practice of medicine. Compared with male participants, women expressed a greater desire for increased ethics education. In addition, psychiatry residents reported a greater need than residents in other specialties for more education about specific ethical problems that occur during training, including dealing with conflicts between residents and attending physicians and performing work outside the trainees' area of competence (Roberts et al. 2005).

Codes of Ethical Conduct
Ethical Codes for Clinicians

Practical guidelines for the ethical conduct of physicians have been codified in various forms since the Hippocratic Oath was documented about 2,500 years ago. Hippocratic writings describe the importance of beneficence, confidentiality, and nonmaleficence and proscribe exploitation of patients, euthanasia, and abortion. In 1803, the English physician Tomas Perceval published the *Code of Institutes and Precepts*, and this document formed the basis of the American Medical Association's (AMA) first code of medical ethics (American Medical Association 2005a). More recently, the AMA also drafted a Declaration of Professional Responsibility, stating professional duties of physicians to patients, society, and future generations of physicians (see "Online Resources" at end of chapter).

The American Psychiatric Association (APA) code of medical ethics was first published in 1973 in the form of annotations to the AMA's *Principles of Medical Ethics*. The APA ethical guidelines are described as "not laws but standards of conduct, which define the essentials of honorable behavior for the physicians" (American Psychiatric Association 2001a). All psychiatrists should be familiar with *The Principles of Medical Ethics With Annotations Especially Applicable to Psychiatry* (selections from this brief document are shown in Table 42–6, and the complete guideline is available online at http://www.psych.org/psych_pract/ethics/ethics.cfm). This document is currently in revision, and there are several related resource and policy documents of value to psychiatrists available through the APA as well as the American Psychological Association (1992). Complaints of unethical behavior by a member of the APA are investigated by local ethics committees, who conduct reviews of documents and testimony, offer education-oriented supportive interventions, and, when necessary, may render sanctions as serious as expulsion from membership of the APA. State legislatures have also imposed legal sanctions against some forms of physician ethical misconduct, such as sexual relations

with patients (Milne 2002). In addition to the ethics codes for psychiatry and medicine, other health professionals have their own written statements describing the ethical rules by which their members must abide. These organizations include the American Psychological Association, the National Association of Social Workers, and the American Nursing Association.

A cardinal feature of a profession is its ethical obligation to monitor the ethical conduct of its members. Nevertheless, it is important to recognize that professional codes of ethics exist for a number of reasons, not only the promotion or assurance of high ethical standards (Fulford and Bloch 2003). First and foremost, they serve to enhance the public trust. They are resources for professionalism education in the early and ongoing training of psychiatrists (Schreiber et al. 2003). In addition, they may have a secondary impact by influencing the economic goals of the members of a profession. Dyer (1988) examined the issue of restrictions on physician advertising as an example of the dual aims of professional codes. Until its 1980 revision, the AMA code explicitly prohibited advertising, with the statement, "A physician…should not solicit patients" (American Medical Association Judicial Council 1957). This restriction can be seen as upholding an ethical standard by not allowing members to falsely claim exceptional abilities. However, the U.S. Federal Trade Commission and the courts viewed the prohibition as an unfair restriction on trade, one that potentially results in fewer choices for patients and higher fees for physicians (Dyer 1988).

Codes of Research Ethics

Codes of ethics formulated in the past century to govern research involving human volunteers form the basis for modern-day ethical practices in the design, conduct, and oversight of biomedical research. The most famous code of ethics related to medical research is the Nuremberg Code. Developed after World War II in response to experimentation on humans conducted under the Nazis (Annas and Grodin 1992), the Nuremberg Code was a 10-point statement intended to protect human subjects in research. Its famous first sentence is, "The voluntary consent of the human subject is absolutely essential" (Annas and Grodin 1992). Necessary elements of informed consent were also emphasized as part of this first point, including requirements for legal capacity to give consent, the absence of coercion, and comprehension of the "nature, duration, and purpose" of the research, the procedures involved, the reasonably foreseeable risks, and the possible effects on the participant's health. Table 42–7 describes the major

TABLE 42–6. **Selections from The Principles of Medical Ethics With Annotations Especially Applicable to Psychiatry**

Section 1: "A physician shall be dedicated to providing competent medical service with compassion and respect for human dignity."

Section 1.2: "A psychiatrist should not be a party to any type of policy that excludes, segregates, or demeans the dignity of any patient because of ethnic origin, race, sex, creed, age, socioeconomic status, or sexual orientation."

Section 1.4: "A psychiatrist should not be a participant in a legally authorized execution."

Section 2: "A physician shall uphold the standards of professionalism, be honest in all professional interactions and strive to report physicians deficient in character or competence, or engaging in fraud or deception to appropriate entities."

Section 2.1: "Sexual activity with a current or former patient is unethical."

Section 2.3: "A psychiatrist who regularly practices outside his/her area of professional competence should be considered unethical."

Section 2.4: "Special consideration should be given to those psychiatrists who, because of mental illness, jeopardize the welfare of their patients and their own reputations and practices. It is ethical, even encouraged, for another psychiatrist to intercede in such situations."

Section 4.2: "A psychiatrist may release confidential information only with the authorization of the patient or under proper legal compulsion."

Section 4.14: "Sexual involvement between a faculty member or supervisor and a trainee or student, in those situations in which an abuse of power can occur, often takes advantages of inequalities in the working relationship and may be unethical because (a) any treatment of a patient being supervised may be deleteriously affected; (b) it may damage the trust relationship between teacher and student; and (c) teachers are important professional role models for their trainees and affect their trainees' future professional behavior."

Section 7.3: "On occasion, psychiatrists are asked for an opinion about an individual who is in the light of public attention, or who has disclosed information about himself/herself through public media. In such circumstances, a psychiatrist may share with the public his/her expertise about psychiatric issues in general. However, it is unethical for a psychiatrist to offer a professional opinion unless he/she has conducted an examination and been granted proper authorization for such a statement."

Source.   American Psychiatric Association: *The Principles of Medical Ethics With Annotations Especially Applicable to Psychiatry,* 2006 Edition. Washington, DC, American Psychiatric Association, 2006 (available at: http://www.psych.org/psych_pract/ethics/ppaethics.cfm).

principles articulated in the Nuremberg Code in 1947 and other major ethics codes promulgated in the past century regarding biomedical experimentation.

In 1964, the World Medical Association issued the Declaration of Helsinki (which has undergone several revisions and clarifications since then; see the World Medical Association Web site at http://www.wma.net/e/policy/b3.htm). The Declaration of Helsinki substantially expanded upon several areas that were either not discussed or only briefly mentioned in the Nuremberg Code, including issues of undue influence and coercion in recruitment, potential vulnerability in research subjects, and surrogate consent (which was not mentioned by the Nuremberg Code). It has also

been a source of disagreement because of its stance (including a recent clarification in 2004) on the ethics of placebo-controlled trials in the situation where standard treatments already exist.

The Belmont Report, issued in 1979 by the National Commission for the Protection of Human Subjects of Biomedical and Behavioral Research (1979), is another important document in the history of research ethics. It set out three core principles of research with human subjects—respect for persons, beneficence, and justice—and discussed the potential for tensions and conflicts among the principles, described particular applications flowing from these principles (e.g., informed consent), and highlighted gaps where ethical issues remained.

TABLE 42–7. **Major codes of research ethics**

Code	Major principles articulated
Nuremberg Code (Katz 1972)	Voluntary participation, legal capacity for informed consent, elements of informed consent Results must be useful to society and unobtainable by other means Human research must be justified based on animal research and other knowledge informing the basis of the planned study Must avoid unnecessary physical and mental suffering Must not occur if there is reason to believe that death or disabling injury will occur Degree of risk should be justified by the importance of the research question Even remote possibilities of injury should be protected against Qualified people must conduct the experiment Voluntary withdrawal by participant at any time Termination of study by researcher if continuation is likely to result in injury, disability, or death
Declaration of Helsinki (World Medical Association 1964)	Physician duty to protect life, health, privacy, and dignity of the human subject Scientific basis and validity of methods of medical research Respect for environment and animals Independent protocol review and monitoring Qualified and supervised persons must conduct the research Assessment of risks and burdens must precede the research; risks must be managed; termination of study if positive and conclusive evidence of benefit Favorable risk–benefit ratio Voluntary informed consent Protection of privacy, confidentiality Elements of informed consent Safeguards for informed consent process Provision for informed consent from legally authorized representative in the case of minors or individuals who are legally incompetent because of physical or mental incapacity Other provisions for proxy consent: requirement of scientific necessity of enrolling the decisionally incapable population, assent from incompetent individual Ethical obligations of authors and publishers: accuracy, publication of negative findings, sources of funding and possible conflict of interests declared Provisions for combining of research with clinical care New method should be tested against best currently available methods; access at end of study to best methods identified by study (placebo-controlled trial acceptable in specific circumstances: "Where for compelling and scientifically sound methodological reasons its use is necessary to determine the efficacy or safety of a prophylactic, diagnostic or therapeutic method"; or for minor condition with no additional risk of serious harm to those receiving placebo Inform patients which aspects of clinical care are research Ability, based on physician judgment, to use unproven or new methods in some situations; ideally should be focus of research
Belmont Report (National Commission for Protection of Human Subjects of Biomedical and Behavioral Research 1979)	Respect for persons: Treat individuals as autonomous agents; protect those with diminished autonomy Beneficence: Do no harm; maximize possible benefits/minimize possible harms Justice: Addresses principles of fairness in recruitment and in distribution of fruits of knowledge gained

Key Ethical Issues in Clinical Psychiatry

Ethical decision making can be extremely challenging in the field of psychiatry because of the complexities of the doctor–patient relationship in this medical specialty, the need for careful attention to ethical safeguards when working with people with disorders and treatments that affect mental processes, and the legally authorized power of psychiatrists to use involuntary treatment and hospitalization. For instance, maintaining treatment boundaries is important for all who work therapeutically with others, but it is especially so in the intimacy of the psychotherapeutic setting. Similarly, the concept of doctor–patient confidentiality is an important safeguard in all of medicine, but it is particularly relevant to patients with illnesses that are socially stigmatized and for whom treatment may involve revealing deeply private, often "shaming," information about themselves. As another example, the process of informed consent for treatment may require more careful efforts in psychiatry because of the possibilities that patients with severe and persistent mental illness may suffer episodic, fluctuating, and/or progressive impairments of decisional capacity (Carpenter et al. 2000; Kovnick et al. 2003; Moser et al. 2002; Palmer et al. 2005). Finally, all physicians have an obligation to use their power ethically, but only psychiatrists must routinely and appropriately use the legal power to impose involuntary treatment and hospitalization. These and other key ethical issues in psychiatry are discussed in more detail in the following sections.

Maintenance of Therapeutic Boundaries

The intimate nature of the psychotherapeutic relationship requires psychiatrists to establish and adhere to appropriate professional boundaries, which have been defined as the "edge or limit of appropriate behavior by the psychiatrist in the clinical setting" (Gabbard 1999, p. 142). Therapeutic boundaries are important in any type of clinical work, but they have been most thoroughly defined in the context of psychoanalysis and psychodynamic therapy (Gabbard 1999; Gabbard and Lester 1995). These boundaries include temporal and spatial limits: therapeutic encounters typically occur at the physician's office during business hours, except in crisis situations. Limits are also observed in the nature of the relationship, which involves the psychiatrist being paid for services and acting as a *fiduciary*, a

professional who is worthy of the patient's trust. Nontherapeutic encounters, including business arrangements, social relationships, and sexual activity, are forbidden. Within the therapeutic relationship, limits are also observed. The patient is encouraged to share intimate feelings, thoughts, and memories, while the physician generally avoids self-disclosure and adopts a posture of neutrality. Physical contact other than handshakes is avoided.

Boundary violations are actions by a psychiatrist that are outside normal professional limits and that have the potential to harm a patient. The most widely studied boundary violation is sexual contact. Although sexual and romantic entanglements between psychiatrists and patients were not uncommon in the early days of psychiatry (Gabbard and Lester 1995), the damage such relationships may cause has become increasingly clear over the past several decades (R.S. Epstein 1994). Sexual contact between patients and physicians has been prohibited by the APA since 1973 (American Psychiatric Association 2001a), and it is illegal in many states (Milne 2002). A review of qualitative and quantitative studies of therapists who had sexual relations with their patients suggests that risk factors for such behavior include inadequate training, isolation from colleagues, and narcissistic pathology (R.S. Epstein 1994). Gabbard classified these errant therapists into four groups based on the underlying psychodynamics: 1) psychotic individuals whose sexual transgression stems from a delusion; 2) therapists with predatory psychopathology and paraphilias who prey on patients because they are easy to exploit; 3) "lovesick" therapists whose own psychological vulnerabilities cause them to become infatuated with a particular patient; and 4) therapists who give in to a patient's demands for sex as a form of masochistic surrender (Gabbard 1999; Gabbard and Lester 1995).

Sexual contact with *former* patients is also understood as inherently exploitative, as there has been growing recognition that transference feelings do not disappear when treatment ends (American Psychiatric Association 2001a). In addition, sexual or romantic involvement with key third parties to a treatment, such as the parent or spouse of a patient, threatens the therapeutic relationship and presents a conflict of interest that should be avoided (American Psychiatric Association 2001b).

Nonsexual boundary violations have been less well studied than sexual violations. These transgressions include seeing patients outside normal office hours and in nonclinical locations, engaging in social or business relationships with patients, accepting gifts from them, and having nonsexual physical contact (Gabbard 1999; R.S. Epstein 1994). Any of these violations carry the potential to exploit the patient or to harm the treatment relationship and should therefore be avoided. The term *boundary crossing* has been used to describe a subtle nonsexual transgression that is helpful to the patient because it advances the treatment (Gutheil and Gabbard 1993, 1998). As an example of a boundary crossing, Gabbard describes a guarded, paranoid patient who offers her psychiatrist a cookie. By accepting this token gift graciously, the psychiatrist helps the patient feel more relaxed in the treatment setting and more willing to discuss her symptoms. Boundary crossings such as this are common and not unethical, but differentiating such crossings from actual boundary violations may be difficult in the course of treatment (Gabbard 1999). The "exploitation index" (R.S. Epstein and Simon 1990) is a useful tool for educating clinicians—in particular, those involved in analytically oriented psychotherapy—about potential boundary violations in their own practices (Table 42–8).

TABLE 42–8. Warning signs of problems maintaining therapeutic boundaries

- Doing any of the following for your family members or social acquaintances: prescribing medication, making diagnoses, offering psychodynamic explanations for their behavior

- Accepting gifts or bequests from patients

- Engaging in a personal relationship with patients after treatment is terminated

- Making exceptions for a patient, such as providing special scheduling or reducing fees, because you find the patient attractive, appealing, or impressive

- Touching patients (other than shaking hands or performing appropriate medical procedures)

- Using information learned from patients, such as business tips or political information, for your own financial or career gain

- Asking patients to do personal favors for you (e.g., bring lunch, mail a letter)

- Arranging business deals with patients

- Accepting for treatment persons with whom you have had social involvement

- Disclosing sensational aspects of a patient's life to others (even when protecting the patient's identity)

- Accepting a medium of exchange other than money for professional services (e.g., work on your office or home, trading of professional services)

- Making exceptions in the conduct of treatment because you feel sorry for a patient or because you believe that the patient is in such distress or so disturbed that there is no other choice

- Recommending treatment procedures or referrals that you do not believe to be necessarily in the patient's best interests but that may instead be to your own direct or indirect financial benefit

- Making exceptions for a patient because you are afraid that the patient will otherwise become extremely angry or self-destructive

- Failing to deal with the following patient behavior(s): Paying the fee late, missing appointments on short notice and refusing to pay for the time (as agreed), seeking to extend the length of sessions

- Telling patients personal things about yourself

- Trying to influence patients to support political causes or positions in which you have a personal interest

- Seeking social contact with patients outside of clinically scheduled visits

- Joining in an activity with a patient that may serve to deceive a third party (e.g., misleading an insurance company)

Source. Adapted from Epstein RS, Simon RI: "The Exploitation Index: An Early Warning Indicator of Boundary Violations in Psychotherapy." *Bulletin of the Menninger Clinic* 54:450–465, 1990.

Patient Nonabandonment

According to accepted ethical standards in medicine, except in emergencies, physicians are "free to choose whom to serve" (American Psychiatric Association 2001a). Once an ongoing doctor–patient relationship has been established, however, the physician may not ethically abandon the patient. As a practical matter, this means that psychiatrists must arrange for clinical coverage when on vacation and must give adequate notice to patients when closing their practices (American Psychiatric Association 2001b). It is not considered patient abandonment to transfer a patient's care to another physician if the treating psychiatrist is not able to provide necessary care and if the situation is not an emergency. This may occur because the treating doctor is not trained in the therapeutic modality that the patient needs or because, despite diligent work, it has not been possible to form a therapeutic alliance. Nevertheless, psychiatrists must be aware that a covert, even unconscious, form of patient abandonment may occur when countertransference issues or burnout cause a psychiatrist to subtly encourage a difficult patient to leave treatment. Self-reflective clinicians who recognize this pattern benefit their patients by seeking consultation or supervision (Roberts and Dyer 2004).

Informed Consent

Informed consent is the process by which individuals make free, knowledgeable decisions about whether to accept a proposed psychiatric treatment or whether to participate in a medical research study. Informed consent is thus a cornerstone of ethical practice in both treatment and research settings. While informed consent is a legal requirement in both contexts, its philosophical roots as a medicolegal doctrine are deeply embedded in our societal and cultural respect for individual persons, in affirming individuals' freedom of self-determination. An adequate process of informed consent thus reflects and promotes the ethical principle of autonomy.

Yet autonomy without the incorporation of other key ethical principles would embody neither the spirit nor the intent of informed consent, which is to enhance meaningful decision making. The principle of beneficence is therefore also crucial in this context and entails a thorough appraisal, on the part of the clinician or investigator, of the degree to which the informed consent process has adequately met the patient's needs. These needs are not just informational. Providing individuals with meaningful, interactive opportunities to learn about their diagnosis, prognosis, and treatment options better enables them to discuss choices and arrive at a treatment plan that is most consistent with their own authentic understanding, preferences, and values (Roberts 2002b).

Viewing informed consent as more than a medicolegal requirement also helps frame it as part of an overall therapeutic relationship and as a further opportunity for respectful dialogue and interaction. Informed consent thus represents not only an ethical obligation but also an opportunity to enhance the provider–patient relationship and patient care. When performed in a way that is attuned to the full intent of informed consent, the process consists of repeated opportunities, over time, to gather relevant clinical information and to discuss and clarify patients' (and often families') values, preferences, informational needs, decisional abilities, and decision-making processes.

Ideally, informed consent represents "shared" or "participatory" decision making (R.M. Epstein et al. 2004). As distinct from paternalistic models of decision making formerly dominant in medicine (Faden and Beauchamp 1980), shared decision making represents a formal recognition of the professional's respect for the individual; awareness and incorporation of personal, familial, and sociocultural dimensions of the patient–provider relationship; and compassion for the often difficult decision-making processes that patients encounter. Patients' fuller participation in decision making about treatment has been associated with higher levels of treatment adherence, more engagement in their own care, and better physician–provider communication (R.M. Epstein et al. 2004).

Standards for Consent

Informed consent has been conceptualized as consisting of three distinct yet related features: information, decisional capacity, and voluntarism (Figure 42–2) (Faden et al. 1986). Each of these is discussed in turn below. Recently, the focus on these primarily cognitive aspects of informed consent has been increasingly criticized as an overly narrow focus (particularly in the research context), neglecting the importance of emotional aspects of motivation and decision making (Glannon 2006; Roberts et al. 2000, 2002b). Thus, the construct of informed consent, while foundational to the ethical practice of psychiatry and psychiatric research, will and should remain an important topic of both conceptual and empirical work (Appelbaum 2006; Dunn et al. 2006).

Although there is no clear index for deciding how stringent the standard for consent should be, a general rule of thumb is to use a "sliding scale" approach

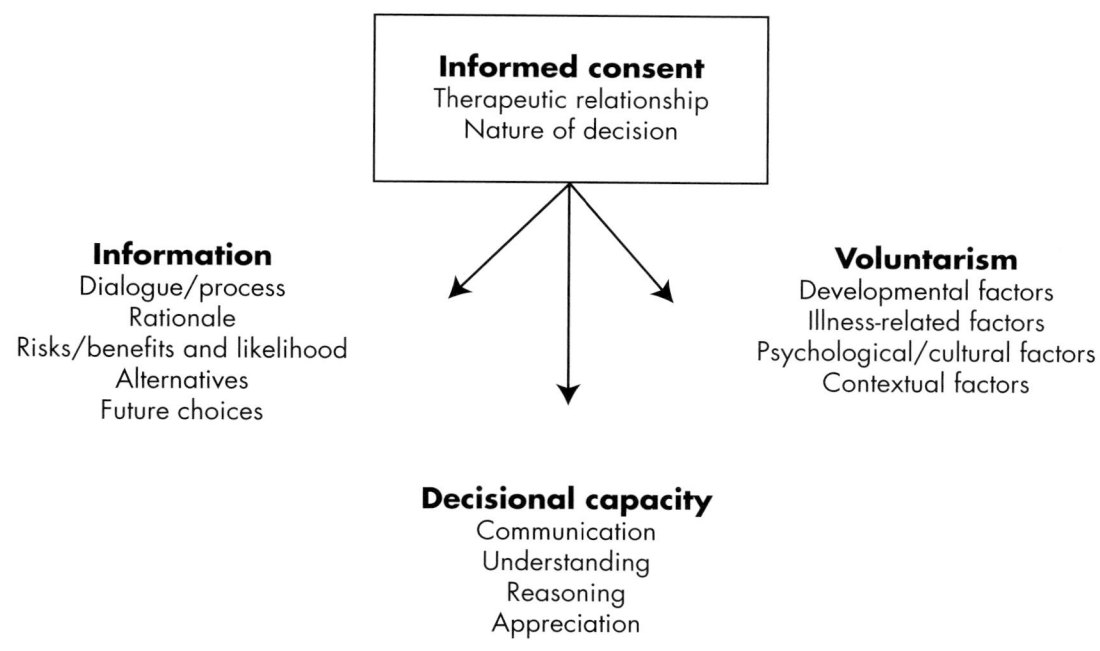

FIGURE 42–2.   Elements of informed consent.

Source.   Reprinted from Roberts LW, Dyer AR: *Concise Guide to Ethics in Mental Health Care.* Washington, DC, American Psychiatric Publishing, 2004, p. 52. Used with permission.

(Drane 1984), titrating the expectation for consent to the potential risk of the decision. Figure 42–3 depicts this concept: decisions involving higher risks or greater risk–benefit ratios generally require a more stringent standard for decisional capacity, whereas more routine, lower-risk decisions generally require a less rigorous standard for decisional capacity. This "sliding scale" concept and the three critical elements comprising informed consent—information provision, decisional capacity, and voluntarism capacity—pertain both to the informed consent process for a treatment-related decision and to research-related decisions.

Information.   *Information provision,* or information sharing, the first element, refers to a dialogue in which the patient or potential research participant is given all relevant information about treatment options, proposed tests, or the research protocol. Although the legal standard for how much information should be provided differs among jurisdictions, many states use the "professional standard," referring to the information (amount and content) that would be disclosed by most physicians. Another standard used in other states is the "reasonable person standard"—indicating the need to disclose what a reasonable person would want to know. Such information must include the purpose, the procedures involved, any foreseeable risks, and

potential benefits. The issues that need to be covered include immediate issues, but "potential benefits" may include eligibility for other forms of treatment in the future, and "foreseeable risks" may encompass ineligibility for future treatment as well. In many instances, particularly for some research protocols, the possibility of no benefit is a key piece of information that must be provided. In clinical trials of early experimental therapies, in fact, there may be no expectation of benefit and some clear expectation of risk or harm to the volunteer, such as in "toxicity" studies. In the research context, it is crucial that participants understand which procedures are experimental and which are standard and what the usual standard of care is. A thorough consent process requires that alternatives be described as part of information sharing, including the option of nonintervention (i.e., no treatment or preexisting treatment). This point is worth emphasizing, as empirical studies in which clinicians in training are observed obtaining informed consent and retrospective interviews with former study subjects suggest that "alternatives" are one information category more often forgotten than other content areas (Advisory Committee on Human Radiation Experiments 1996; Roberts et al. 1999, 2003a).

Increasingly, the *process* of the information-sharing component of informed consent is emphasized in both

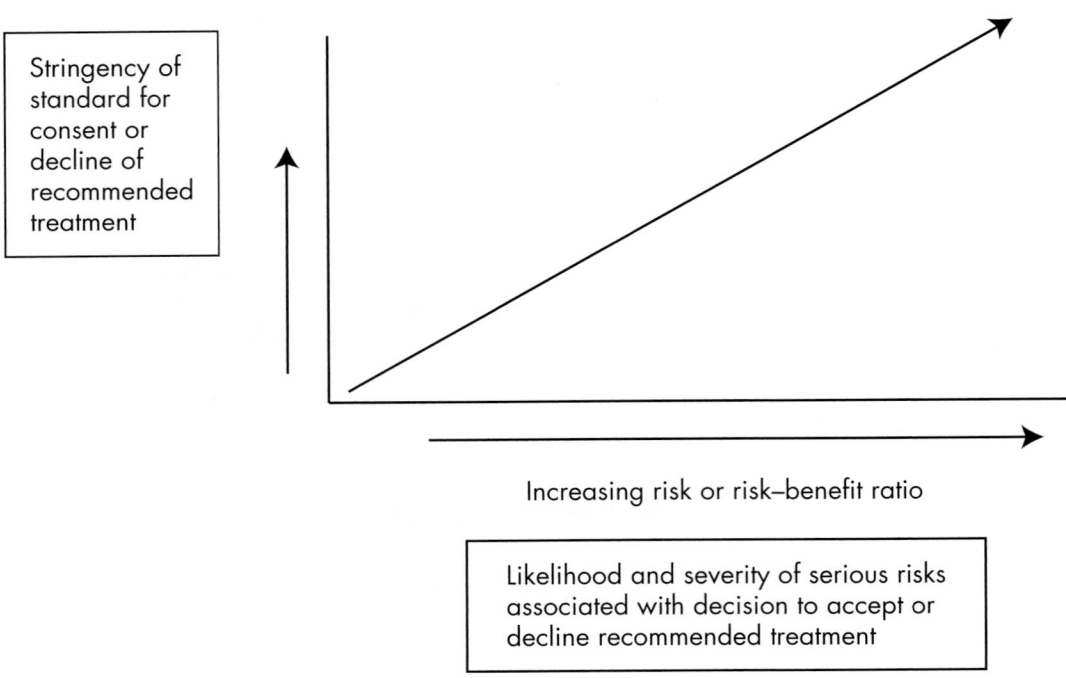

FIGURE 42–3. The "sliding scale" of consent standards.

Source. Reprinted from Roberts LW, Dyer AR: *Concise Guide to Ethics in Mental Health Care.* Washington, DC, American Psychiatric Publishing, 2004, p. 61. Used with permission.

clinical and research settings. As described above, this has benefits for the patient/participant, the provider/investigator, and the overall relationship they have. The process provides the opportunity for patients to ask questions; to involve family, friends, or other important third parties in their decision-making process; and to become active participants in making what may be a very complex decision. It is important for mental health care providers to realize, however, that different individuals have varying levels of desire to be involved in decision making for their own condition. In addition, the inherent power differential in the doctor–patient relationship may make many patients uneasy about asking questions during the informed consent process or stating that they do not understand health-related information. Rather than substituting the provider's own preferences for that of an indecisive or hesitant patient, the provider is ethically obligated to try to provide information in an easily understood form, to try to ensure that the patient has grasped the information provided, and to help the patient clarify his or her own parameters for the decisions.

Decisional capacity. Decisional capacity can be described as a "sociocultural construct" (Dunn et al. 2007) consisting of intrapersonal elements, aspects re-

lated to the quality of the consent process (deriving from the information-sharing component described above as well as from the professionalism of the physician), and the complexity of the information and the decision at hand. For example, figuring out whether or not to undergo electroconvulsive therapy for severe psychotic depression is a difficult decision. The disease process itself, as well as other individual factors (such as age and cognitive functioning), may substantially impair patients' abilities to make a fully informed, meaningful choice about this treatment; on the other hand, empirical evidence suggests that many people with severe depression may commonly have adequate abilities to make such a decision (Lapid et al. 2003). Thus, a judgment of capacity cannot reside in the diagnosis alone nor in the severity of the illness; a targeted assessment, which can be aided by capacity assessment tools designed to help guide such evaluations, is the most valid way to determine a patient's capacity to make a specific decision at a specific time. At times, particularly when a clinical situation is rapidly fluctuating or progressing, the best course of action (while also ensuring that the patient is safe) is to try to delay a decision to permit greater clarity, because the clinical circumstances may change (e.g., a manic patient becomes more stable; a delirious patient's delirium resolves). There is thus often a need to reassess capacity, which is best viewed not as a static trait but, rather, as a state that may fluctuate over time depending on various individual, clinical, and contextual factors.

The phrase "decision-making capacity" differs from the term *competency* in that competency to perform a specific function or for a particular life domain is a legal determination made through a judicial or other legal process. It should be noted, however, that some legal jurisdictions have different standards for establishing "competency" (Appelbaum and Grisso 1995). Decisional capacity refers to a determination made by a clinical professional with knowledge of and experience in assessing the key abilities necessary for making a specific medical decision.

Decisional capacity has been defined by experts as consisting of four standards (Appelbaum and Grisso 1995). The first ability, communication of a preference, is the least stringent standard, requiring that a person be able to express or state a decision. This standard was originally conceived as a basic physical ability to communicate—a capability that is sometimes lost when a patient is experiencing catatonia or in patients who are comatose, poststroke, or post–spinal injury. Some have come to view this standard differently and as relating to the ability to communicate a stable choice, and there are certainly circumstances where even this standard is not met—for example, a patient with delirium whose attention waxes and wanes, affecting her ability to focus on a discussion of her treatment options; or a patient who is ambivalent or erratic by virtue of his illness process.

The second standard, understanding or comprehension of the information necessary for the specific decision at hand, is primarily a cognitive ability and has been shown to be correlated with cognitive functioning in people with a variety of psychiatric illnesses (Carpenter et al. 2000; Kovnick et al. 2003; Moser et al. 2002; Palmer et al. 2005). Cognitive disorders such as dementia clearly affect the ability to understand relevant information (Kim et al. 2001). It is important to note additionally that sociocultural factors, such as literacy, numeracy, and educational background, clearly influence the ability to understand health decision information. It is thus critical that psychiatrists strive to communicate health information in ways that can be more readily understood by patients (Roberts and Dyer 2004).

The third ability or standard is "appreciation." This generally is considered to refer to the patient's awareness of the implications and significance of the information provided or the choice being made for his or her own life circumstances. Appreciation is a concept tightly linked with the psychiatric notion of insight, a patient's knowledge that his or her symptoms are abnormal or the product of illness. Insight is often eroded in diverse mental illnesses, personality disorders, and disabling conditions. Lack of insight may create a situation in which an individual has an understanding of factual information but cannot apply it to his or her own situation, in which case appreciation would be lacking. An example is the patient who can demonstrate an understanding that an untreated infection could lead to death but who believes that this information does not apply to him—for example, because he has supernatural powers that will protect him.

The capacity for appreciation is seen as the most personal, the most influenced by individual values and experiences, and thus often the most difficult to assess in clinical contexts; the basis for an apparent lack of appreciation might be religious beliefs or idiosyncratic personal beliefs, in which cases it has been more difficult to derive consensus about what constitutes lack of appreciation. It has also been more difficult to operationalize in the form of standardized questions as it is a less factually based standard. Nonetheless, it is important to try to assess the degree to which a patient integrates the information about the decision with his or her own values and personal beliefs.

The fourth standard is the ability to reason—to weigh information, comparing options and considering their consequences. An assessment of reasoning abilities should include evaluating whether the patient understands the consequences of alternative treatment choices and also of no treatment. A patient does not need to be able to calculate probabilities but should be able to weigh options. The patient also need not come to the "rational" choice as a result of the reasoning process. A patient who refuses treatment but whose understanding, appreciation, reasoning, and indication of a choice are adequate has the right to refuse treatment. Involuntary treatment is predicated, in part, on the absence of intact decision-making capacity, and thus careful assessment of these component abilities is key in evaluating the appropriateness of seeking involuntary treatment for a given patient.

Voluntarism. The third key part of informed consent is voluntarism. Being able to make an authentic, free decision—a decision that is most concordant with an individual's own values, history, and circumstances—is a fundamental aspect of autonomy. Four spheres, or domains of influence, have been proposed as a framework for thinking about those issues that may affect an individual's ability, in a given set of circumstances, to make a voluntary decision (Roberts 2002b). These domains include developmental factors; illness-related factors; cultural, religious, and psychological factors; and external pressures or features (Figure 42–4). For example, an adolescent who is asked to volunteer as a healthy control for a research study on a disease afflicting his sibling may be influenced by numerous factors that could impair his voluntarism—including his youth and relative immaturity; feelings of guilt, anger, concern, competitiveness, and/or love toward the sibling; religious and cultural beliefs regarding the meaning of disease and the importance of helping family members and society; and overt or covert pressure from family members, treating physicians, or research personnel.

The existence of such influences does not mean that voluntary decisions are not possible; rather, awareness of possible influences on decision making can help clinicians tune in to and explore issues they may not have previously considered as affecting their patients' choices. The clinician's attention to upholding voluntarism also represents acts of beneficence and justice. As with other ethical principles, voluntarism is rooted in a sociocultural consensus of the rights of individuals to self-determination and "involves philosophical ideals of freedom, independence, personhood, and separateness" (Roberts 2002b). Yet there are also unresolved issues related to how voluntarism applies in various contexts (including both treatment and research), and voluntarism remains an understudied ethical principle and topic compared to decision-making capacity.

Alternative Decision Making and Advance Directives

In cases where an individual is deemed, via a clinical assessment or legal decision, to lack the ability to make a particular decision or set of decisions related to his or her care, a surrogate, proxy, or alternative decision maker is asked to step in and make choices for that person. Alternative decision making has received some empirical attention in the ethics literature, with the perhaps surprising finding that alternative decision makers' choices do not closely align with what the patient him- or herself would have decided (Sachs et al. 1994). Alternative decision makers are, in fact, asked to do what is a very challenging task: make a treatment or research decision on behalf of another person, often in the absence of any information about that person's wishes in such a situation.

Advance directives are documents that describe an individual's wishes regarding future care in the event that the person loses decisional capacity. Advance directives are typically used to help in end-of-life decision making. The existence of an advance directive does not necessarily increase the accuracy of an alternative decision maker's choices, as one study showed (Ditto et al. 2001).

Psychiatric advance directives may be useful for persons with mental illnesses that cause fluctuating or progressive impairment. For example, a patient with a history of severe bipolar disorder or recurrent psychotic depression may create an advance directive requesting hospitalization and involuntary medication treatment if he or she becomes incapable of decision making during a future relapse. Psychiatric advance directives represent a means for patients with chronic and severe illnesses to maintain control over their treatment despite periods of incapacity. However, advance directives are used only when patients lack decisional capacity, and patients can change their advance directives at any time.

In the context of psychiatric treatment and research, there has been relatively little work examining alternative decision making and advance directives, although there appears to be increasing interest in developing guidelines and policies for these mechanisms in both contexts (Srebnik et al. 2004, 2005). In the final analysis, policies regarding alternative decision making and advance directives must adhere to and advance the same fundamental ethical principles that are requirements for individually based decision making.

Ethical Use of Power

The relationship between physician and patient is inherently one of inequity. Relative to the population at large, the psychiatrist holds a position of power because of his or her education and socioeconomic standing, by the role as healer and keeper of confidences, and by the special powers granted by the state—the ability to involuntarily hospitalize patients and to stand as a gatekeeper to health care services such as prescribed medication. Conversely, individuals who seek psychiatric care are relatively disempowered compared with the general population. Psychiatric disorders may impair one's abilities to reason, feel, and behave in an effective manner. Most individuals enter psychiatric treatment at a time of great personal vulnerability, and some psychotherapeutic treatments may encourage further regression as a step toward eventual healing. Such a highly unequal power relationship can leave the weaker party less able to advocate for his or her interests and needs and thus more potentially vulnerable to exploitation.

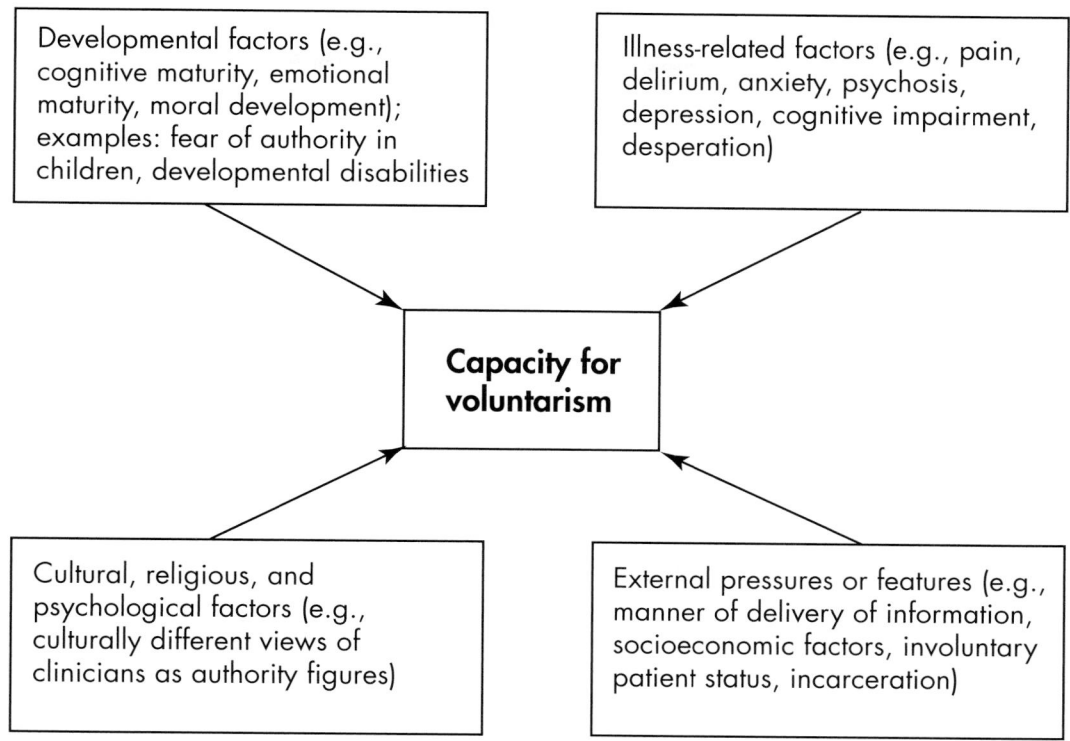

FIGURE 42–4. Conceptual model of voluntarism: four domains of potential influences.

Source. Adapted from Roberts LW: "Informed Consent and the Capacity for Voluntarism." *American Journal of Psychiatry* 159:705–712, 2002b. Used with permission.

The most egregious ethical violations in the history of psychiatry have been blatant abuses of power. Some have involved individual sociopathic practitioners who exploit their patients for financial gain, sexual gratification, or sadistic pleasure (Gabbard and Lester 1995). Others have involved entire communities of psychiatrists who have allowed their skills and legal powers to be misused to harm patients. In Nazi Germany, psychiatrists killed thousands of patients in mental hospitals in the name of eugenic goals (Gottesman and Bertelsen 1996). Also in the past century, psychiatrists in the Soviet Union diagnosed political dissidents as suffering from dubious "mental disorders" and subjected them to unnecessary treatments, including long-term involuntary hospitalization (Bloch and Reddaway 1984). Similar accusations have more recently been made against psychiatrists in other countries (e.g., Kahn 2006).

Involuntary Treatment

Far more subtle but nonetheless important ethical issues surround the use of power in high-risk situations by well-meaning and thoughtful clinicians. An example of such a high-risk situation is psychiatrists' legally authorized use of involuntary treatment (e.g., inpatient hospitalization, outpatient commitment, or involuntary medication treatment), which is sometimes necessary in the care of patients whose mental illness makes them a danger to themselves or others. Involuntary treatment is a clear example of conflicting ethical principles: the obligation to respect patient autonomy and the obligation of beneficence. Choosing not to override a patient's treatment refusal is an expression of respect for patient autonomy, but blind adherence to a patient's wishes about treatment may not be ethically justifiable—and in fact, it may cause harm. The suicidal patient who refuses hospitalization, the patient who expresses homicidal ideas, and the patient whose mental illness seriously jeopardizes his or her health (e.g., the psychotically depressed patient who refuses to eat due to a somatic delusion) are all examples of patients for whom involuntary treatment may be necessary and justifiable.

Legal statutes and mechanisms for providing treatment on an involuntary basis vary from state to state (Roberts and Dyer 2004). The ethical use of involuntary treatment in such situations has been a matter of much discussion among psychiatrists, legal scholars, the public, and policy makers (Bartlett 2003; Levenson 1986–1987; Rosenman 1998). Indeed, a major transformation in the United States mental health care system occurred in the latter half of the twentieth century, when many involuntary long-term patients in state psychiatric hospitals were released and transferred to community settings (Burnham 2006). Although some civil rights advocates and psychiatrists have argued that *any* involuntary treatment is an unethical violation of individual rights (Szasz 1976), a middle ground has emerged, supported by most psychiatrists, as well as by major patient advocacy organizations (e.g., the National Alliance for the Mentally Ill), using the guideposts of clear and specific indications for involuntary treatment (as opposed to merely the presence of a serious mental disorder); careful assessment, documentation, and review of the justification for involuntary treatment; and ongoing monitoring and reevaluation of treatment progress and the involuntary status (Roberts and Dyer 2004).

In the outpatient setting, involuntary treatment poses special challenges. Deinstitutionalization and a fragmented mental health care system have led to a crisis of lack of access to quality continuous care. As a result, individuals with mental illnesses living in the community appear to frequently fall through cracks in the system (U.S. Department of Health and Human Services 1999); some of these individuals' safety may be in jeopardy for reasons of lack of access or nonadherence to treatment.

In recognition of the needs of many seriously psychiatrically ill individuals for outpatient treatment, and spurred by the tragic death of a young woman in New York City, a new mandatory outpatient treatment program was signed into law in New York State in 1999 (New York State Office of Mental Health 2005). Known as "Kendra's Law," this legislation provided mechanisms for identifying and providing care to individuals with a treatment history of nonadherence, who were unlikely to voluntarily engage in treatment and whose current behavior indicated that without assisted outpatient treatment, they were at risk of clinical deterioration likely to result in harm to themselves or others. This has been viewed as a proactive but compassionate approach to involuntary community-based care. Through the end of 2004, approximately 3,800 individuals had received services under this law. A recent report from the New York State Office of Mental Health documents that most of the recipients (71%) had a diagnosis of schizophrenia, and over half also had a co-occurring alcohol and/or substance use disorder (New York State Office of Mental Health 2005).

The use of assisted outpatient treatment under the law was associated with improvements in a number of life domains for the participants. Many of those receiving court-ordered services expressed anger (54%) or embarrassment (53%) about being in mandatory treatment, although 62% also said that being in mandatory treatment had been a good thing for them (New York State Office of Mental Health 2005). These mixed views serve as a reminder of the frequently conflicting feelings that patients have about receiving care against their stated wishes.

Overall, the ethical use of involuntary therapies, regardless of setting, must be approached with care and with careful regard for the balancing of duties that should characterize assessments of the need for involuntary treatment. Clinicians hold great power in their relationships with patients, and lines can be crossed in sometimes subtle ways. The ethical use of power in therapeutic relationships is a topic of central importance for psychiatrists at all levels. Table 42–9 summarizes key strategies for providing ethical care in involuntary treatment.

TABLE 42–9.   Working therapeutically in the setting of involuntary treatment

- Understand treatment refusal as a possible expression of distress
- Ascertain the reasons for refusal
- Allow the patient to discuss his or her preferences and fears
- Explain the reason for the intervention in simple language
- Offer options for the disposition of treatment
- Appropriately enlist the assistance of family and friends
- Request support from nursing and support staff
- Assess decisional capacity and if necessary have recourse to the courts
- Attend to side effects—both long-term and short-term, serious and bothersome
- Employ emergency treatment options where available
- Work to preserve the therapeutic alliance
- Utilize treatment guardians where appropriate

Source.   Adapted from Roberts LW, Dyer AR: "Ethical Use of Power in High-Risk Situations," in *Concise Guide to Ethics in Mental Health Care.* Washington, DC, American Psychiatric Publishing, 2004, p. 93. Used with permission.

Confidentiality

Respect for the privacy of patients' personal information has been an established ethical duty of physicians for millennia. Hippocrates stated the ethical duty of confidentiality as follows: "What I may see or hear in the course of treatment…in regard to the life of men… I will keep to myself, holding such things to be shameful to be spoken about" (Hippocratic Writings, *The Oath*). Patients entrust their physicians with the most intimate details of their lives, often telling their doctors things they have never told—or would never tell— anyone else. Effective treatment, and in particular effective psychotherapy, would not be possible if patients did not feel free to disclose intensely personal information under the assumption of confidentiality.

From the standpoint of U.S. law, doctor–patient confidentiality is a legal privilege granted to patients. The privilege requires physicians to keep patient information private, unless the doctor is legally compelled to make a disclosure or the patient waives the privilege. Although this may sound straightforward, in practice there are many gray areas in which a physician's legal and ethical duties may conflict. In remote rural settings, where clinicians and their patients are also neighbors, lifelong friends, and even relatives by blood or by marriage, confidentiality poses extraordinary challenges (Roberts et al. 1999). This is true in other small communities in which individuals have multiple and overlapping roles (Roberts 2004). In another example, a psychiatrist may protest a specific legal mandate to provide otherwise protected patient information, believing that the disclosure would be unethical. Such disagreements have led to numerous court cases, and the legal protection of confidentiality between patients and psychotherapists has thus evolved over the past 50 years, culminating in a 1996 U.S. Supreme Court decision recognizing the legal privilege between patient and psychotherapist (Jaffee v. Redmond 1996). With the Health Insurance Portability and Accountability Act (HIPAA) of 1996, specific protections for personal health information, including a higher level of protection for psychotherapy notes, were also enacted (U.S. Department of Health and Human Services 1996).

What remains unclear, however, is whether, to what degree, and how special privacy protections for mental health treatment will continue to be guarded in an emerging era of electronic health records, digitized medical information, and a push toward national health identifiers (Flynn et al. 2003; Griener 2005). Ensuring privacy of genetic and genomic data stored electronically is another evolving issue that promises to raise new challenges related to confidentiality in psychiatric care (Sax and Schmidt 2005).Thus, the ethical obligation of confidentiality will continue to be a topic of concern and should be a matter of heightened attention on the part of psychiatrists as health information technology evolves. Guarding one's passwords has now become critical to guarding patient confidentiality.

There is a broad recognition of several limits on confidentiality. When patients consent to specific limited disclosures of their information (e.g., for third-party payment or for a court proceeding), disclosure may occur. In these instances, the amount of information to be revealed should be the minimum amount necessary for the specific situation (i.e., a rigorously upheld "need to know" approach). Patients should be informed of limits to confidentiality when entering treatment (although there is disagreement about how best to enact this duty). Patients should not be asked to sign a blanket waiver of general consent to disclosure, as many patients would not want all of their personal mental health information being disclosed to a third-party payer, for example (Mosher and Swire 2002).

There are other instances when a nonconsenting patient may have the privilege of confidentiality suspended, based on the physician's overriding duties to others. These situations typically involve breaching patient confidentiality in order to protect third parties in cases of child or elder abuse or threatened violence. The notion that psychiatrists have a "duty to protect" members of the public from the violent intentions of their patients was demonstrated by the legal case *Tarasoff v. Regents of the University of California, 1974 and 1976* (see Chapter 41, "Psychiatry and the Law," by Simon and Shuman). From an ethical standpoint, the *Tarasoff* ruling gives more weight to the importance of beneficence (preventing harm to a third party) than to fidelity and confidentiality (protecting the confidences of one's own patient).

In general, however, patients should reasonably be able to expect that the information they tell their psychiatrist or other mental health professional will be kept confidential and that disclosure will not occur without their consent. Unfortunately, several studies have shown that many patients are not informed about specific safeguards for their confidentiality and that many do not seek treatment out of fears about lack of confidentiality (Roberts and Dyer 2004). A useful list of *dos* and *don't*s for safeguarding patient confidentiality related to specific issues has been compiled by Roberts et al. (2002a) and is shown in Table 42–10.

TABLE 42–10. Eight dos and don'ts for protecting confidentiality

Confidentiality Issue	Do	Don't
Patient information	Do provide accurate information to your patients about the "realities" of confidentiality in your clinical care situation.	Don't assure your patients that whatever they tell you is confidential.
Medical records	Do explain that the *purpose* of the medical record is to be read so that optimal care may be given.	Don't assure your patients that the medical record—whether printed or electronic—is confidential.
Stigmatizing conditions	Do strategize explicitly with your patients about potential confidentiality problems.	Don't avoid discussing the difficult issues that surround stigmatizing disorders.
Practices such as tailoring the charts and gaming the system	Do consider how to reconcile accuracy and privacy in all forms of documentation.	Don't use these protective practices without considering the consequences.
Significant others	Do remember to inquire about the patient's important relationships.	Don't talk to significant others without permission from the patient.
Law and professional standards	Do actively work to change laws and policies regarding confidentiality you think are unethical.	Don't break the law or violate professional standards in the process of respecting confidentiality.
Lifelong learning	Do continue to learn about professional aspects of medicine and share your knowledge with colleagues.	Don't neglect your commitment to lifelong learning—including ethics.
Consultation	Do seek consultation and direction from other sources: books, articles, continuing medical education, Web sites, ethics consultants, and ethics committees.	Don't feel that you are on your own when confronting difficult confidentiality questions.

Source. Adapted from Robert LW, Geppert C, Bailey R: "Ethics in Psychiatric Practice: Essential Ethics Skills, Informed Consent, the Therapeutic Relationship, and Confidentiality." *Journal of Psychiatric Practice* 8:290–305, 2002. Copyright 2002, Lippincott Williams & Wilkins. Used with permission.

Management of Dual Roles and Conflicts of Interest

By virtue of their skills and training, psychiatrists are naturally invited to participate in a variety of roles in the medical community and in society. Psychiatrists are educators of medical students and residents, administrators of academic programs and health care systems, clinical researchers and basic scientists, and consultants to industry. Because the ethical duties required by one role may not align precisely with the duties of another role, psychiatrists in multiple roles may face ethical binds. The conflicts of interest that arise are not necessarily unethical, but they must be managed in a way that allows the psychiatrist to fulfill professionalism expectations and maintain a fiduciary rela-

tionship with patients. There are many strategies for helping to ensure that role conflicts do not distort the judgments of professionals, such as disclosure and documentation, focused supervision and oversight committees, retrospective review, and other safeguards (Roberts and Dyer 2004).

Financial Conflicts of Interest Pertaining to Patient Care

Among the most obviously unacceptable conflicts of interest are those in which physicians have a clear-cut financial arrangement that could adversely influence how they treat patients. For example, fee-splitting arrangements in which a psychiatrist is paid to refer patients to a consultant are unethical because the payment may compromise the psychiatrist's judgment about the clinical merits of the referral. In a similar fashion, accepting lavish bonuses from hospitals for referring patients suggests that the physician's professional judgment may be co-opted. Physicians who work in managed care organizations may also face a financial conflict of interest, particularly with plans that provide incentives if physicians order less expensive treatments and tests. Guidelines for ethical practice in organized settings established by the APA in 1997 require that managed care psychiatrists disclose such incentives to patients (American Psychiatric Association 2001a).

Relations With Industry

The possibility of conflicts of interest arising from accepting gifts or other forms of support from industry is the subject of much controversy in all of medicine. A meta-analysis of 29 studies on physician–pharmaceutical company interactions demonstrated that physicians' attitudes toward a medication and/or their prescribing practices are influenced by having personal contact with pharmaceutical sales representatives, attending sales presentations, attending continuing medical education (CME) conferences sponsored by pharmaceutical companies, and using industry funding for travel and housing expenses to attend professional meetings (Wazana 2000).

Currently, various organizations within medicine differ in their approaches and guidelines for dealing with relationships with industry (American Medical Association 2005b). At minimum, psychiatrists should be aware of the issues that may be of unique concern to patients (e.g., patients may note that the name of the medication being prescribed matches that on the pen being used to prescribe it) and should attend to these concerns. Each psychiatrist should also learn and work within the guidelines specified by his or her own organizations and work environments. Academic departments of psychiatry and psychiatric residency training programs increasingly play an important role in educating physicians about the ethical issues involved in relationships with the pharmaceutical industry (Christensen and Tueth 1998).

Dual Agency

Another type of conflict of interest arises for psychiatrists who have additional professional duties that may not be fully congruent with the role of physician. Such conflicts are sometimes referred to as "dual agency" situations. An extreme example is the forensic psychiatrist who may be asked to evaluate a death-row inmate to determine whether he or she is sane

enough to be executed (Guntheil 1999). Ethical binds occur with many other types of dual roles. Research psychiatrists who provide clinical care for their study volunteers may struggle to maintain the integrity of the doctor–patient relationship in the face of the demands of the research protocol (Lo 2005). Similarly, medical trainees, supervisors, and administrative psychiatrists may find that their roles as students, teachers, and managers challenge their ability to put the needs of patients first (Hoop 2004; Roberts and Dyer 2004). In public health settings, for example, psychiatrists may find it challenging to balance fidelity to individual patients with the legitimate need to be good stewards of social resources and to distribute them fairly (Sabin 1994). Managing these multiple roles requires physicians to recognize the potential for ethical binds, institute safeguards when possible, and fully inform patients (Roberts and Dyer 2004).

Social Stigmatization of Mental Illness

Stigma sits at the intersection of several ethical issues in psychiatry. Stigma diminishes the profession's ability to fulfill the principle of justice by reducing access to care, at both the individual (care seeking) and the systemic (care providing, financing) level. It also may impede patient autonomy by interfering with people's abilities to enact their personal wishes for care and recovery. Finally, stigma may affect medical students' decisions to enter (or not) the field of psychiatry, and it may influence an individual practitioner's ability to "do good" throughout his or her career because of barriers and challenges experienced by patients who are stigmatized. In a related way, providers of all specialties need to be particularly attuned to their own feelings toward psychiatric illnesses and patients. Most psychiatrists have at some point or another felt the sting of stigma simply by working in the field. It has also been shown that psychiatric diagnoses place patients at risk of receiving inadequate medical treatment: for instance, a large study found a significantly lower likelihood of receiving a coronary revascularization procedure after acute myocardial infarction among patients with a psychiatric diagnosis compared to those without such a diagnosis (Druss et al. 2000).

In light of the fact that the indirect and direct costs of mental illness exceed 100 billion dollars each year (Rice and Miller 1996; Rice et al. 1992), the importance of stigma is not to be underestimated. Stigma relating to mental illness has been conceptualized and measured in many different ways (Link et al. 2004); its presence, however, is not in dispute. Insurance parity for covering mental health remains elusive, despite the massive strides made by the field in demonstrating treatment effectiveness and cost-effectiveness of providing care. The evidence base relating to stigma and mental illness has been steadily increasing over the past several decades and has had a significant impact upon the field (Link et al. 2004). Important findings have come from studies documenting the role of stigma as a barrier to accessing care, such as that seen among some cultural and ethnic minority groups (Ojeda and McGuire 2006; Schraufnagel et al. 2006; U.S. Department of Health and Human Services 2001); research demonstrating the impact of stigma upon the self-esteem of people with psychiatric illnesses (Link et al. 2001); work exploring the perceptions and effects of stigma on family members (Ostman and Kjellin 2002; Phelan et al. 1998); and findings showing the ongoing complicating effects of stigma upon mental health treatment of those affected, such as individuals dually diagnosed with substance abuse and mental illness (Link et al. 1997).

AMA and APA ethics codes state that a physician "shall recognize a responsibility to participating in activities contributing to an improved community" (American Psychiatric Association 2001a). Many psychiatrists feel ethically compelled to speak out against social injustice that harms psychiatric patients, such as mental health insurance nonparity, stigmatization and discrimination, and public policies that neglect the needs of the mentally ill.

Ethical Interactions With Colleagues and Trainees

As members of a profession, psychiatrists are expected to behave ethically toward their colleagues individually and collectively. The AMA *Principles of Medical Ethics* explicitly states that physicians should "deal honestly" with colleagues, "respect the rights" of colleagues, and "strive to expose those physicians deficient in character or competence, or who engage in fraud or deception" (American Psychiatric Association 2006) (see Table 42–6). While the first two statements in the ethics code encourage collegial behavior, the third suggests the importance of self-governance in the medical professions and the need to report colleague misconduct and impairment.

Reporting of Colleague Misconduct and Impairment

When colleagues bring legitimate cases of physician misconduct to light, they are fulfilling the ideals of be-

neficence and nonmaleficence by protecting the physician's current and future patients. Nevertheless, a number of psychological barriers to reporting colleague impairment have been identified, including overidentification with the impaired physician, collusion with the colleague's denial and minimization, and a tendency to overvalue confidentiality and to protect the colleague's reputation and career at the expense of safety (Roberts and Miller 2004). The early roots of this code of silence were suggested by Roberts et al.'s (2000) study of more than 1,000 medical students at nine medical schools. When asked to consider hypothetical scenarios involving medical students with severe illnesses such as uncontrolled diabetes, suicidal depression, and substance dependence, approximately one-third said they would protect the student's privacy rather than actively intervening or reporting the problem.

To help psychiatrists overcome their reluctance to report a colleague's improper behavior, Overstreet (2001) suggested a useful four-step procedure for working through the issue. First, the psychiatrist should become informed about the reporting requirements of his or her state. In some localities, physicians have a legal mandate to report colleague misconduct, and they may suffer penalties if they fail to do so. Second, the psychiatrist should seek to more fully understand the situation, including how his or her own feelings may complicate the ability both to observe the colleague's behavior objectively and to report it. Third, all options that fulfill the duty to "strive to expose" the misconduct should be identified. Just as there is a range of physician misbehaviors, there can be a range of appropriate responses. These may include speaking privately with the colleague about one's concerns, informing the colleague's supervisor or administrative chief, filing an ethics complaint with the district APA branch, and/or notifying the state licensing board. Finally, the physician should choose the most appropriate option or options as a first step, knowing that others are available should the situation persist (Overstreet 2001).

It is important to note that a reporting physician is not expected to make a definitive judgment about whether or not a colleague is practicing competently. Worrisome professional behavior should instead be investigated by appropriate professional bodies such as the APA and state licensing boards (American Psychiatric Association 2006). Furthermore, as a practical matter, an impaired physician may in fact be greatly helped by the impetus to accept treatment. To that end, many states have enacted laws regarding physician impairment based on model legislation proposed by the AMA Council on Mental Health. These statutes are designed to encourage appropriate treatment and rehabilitation rather than approaches that may be seen as merely punitive (Roberts and Dyer 2004).

Ethical Issues of Concern to Medical Faculty and Trainees

The ethical obligations of psychiatric faculty toward trainees involve many of the same requirements as relations with colleagues, plus the added obligations of a "fiduciary-like" relationship with trainees (Mohamed et al. 2005). The connection between an attending physician and a resident or medical student has some similarities with the doctor–patient relationship, though the two are of course not identical. In both, there is a power differential, the possibility of transference feelings, and in some cases the potential for the weaker party to be exploited. The propriety of sexual relationships between supervising physicians and trainees therefore has become increasingly controversial, due to the potentially negative impact on the trainee, the patients whose care is being supervised, and the training program as a whole (American Psychiatric Association 2006).

Medical school and residency training also give rise to specific ethical issues because of the need for trainees to provide care that is beyond their current level of expertise. The third-year medical student who performs a lumbar puncture for the first time, the new intern responsible for evaluating the suicide risk of a patient in an emergency room, the inexperienced resident with a severely regressed therapy patient—all must provide medical care outside their current zone of competence in order to learn skills that will benefit future patients. The process requires treating patients as a means to an end—a violation of the principle of respect for persons—and yet the thorough training of psychiatrists is clearly beneficent from a public health standpoint. Handling this ethical dilemma requires the informed consent of patients as willing participants in the educational setting, as well as safeguards to ensure that trainees practice only marginally beyond their current capabilities and with adequate supervision (Fry 1991; Hoop 2004; Roberts and Dyer 2004; Vinicky et al. 1991).

Ethical Concerns in Psychiatric Research

The suffering of persons with mental illnesses, the distress of their families, and the economic impact of psychiatric diseases on society justify heroic research efforts (Roberts and Roberts 1999). Many currently available treatments, while providing some benefits, do not "cure" the disorder in question; moreover, while providing some relief, they may be accompanied by difficult-to-tolerate or long-term side effects. Additionally, there is a great need, in psychiatry as in medicine more generally, for data about the effectiveness of various treatments in broader, more representative samples and in more real-world contexts and settings (Tunis et al. 2003).

During the past two decades, increasing attention has been paid to the ethics of psychiatric research (Carpenter et al. 1997, 2003; Charney 1999; Frank et al. 2003; Miller 2000; National Bioethics Advisory Commission 1998; Roberts 2002a; Roberts et al. 2001; Rosenstein and Miller 2003). In general, concerns have centered on issues of scientific design (e.g., the use of medication washout periods, the use of placebo controls), research safeguards (institutional review practices, study monitoring, and debriefing), and informed consent (Dunn and Roberts 2005). In addition, the nature of psychiatric illnesses—which may cause some individuals to have impaired decision-making abilities, to have decreased insight into the need for and potential benefits of treatment, and to be subject to involuntarily imposed treatments—raises ethical concerns about the recruitment and enrollment of those with serious psychiatric disorders into clinical research protocols.

Because psychiatric illnesses are highly stigmatized, research involving individuals with psychiatric illnesses also tends to receive intense public scrutiny (Kong and Whitaker 1998; National Bioethics Advisory Commission 1998). In some cases, heightened concerns and attention are justified. On the other hand, blanket restrictions or protections targeting psychiatric research or people with psychiatric diagnoses considering research enrollment have repeatedly been shown to be unjustified. There are several reasons that such diagnostic-driven restrictions are problematic. First, a substantial amount of research has now been amassed demonstrating that problems with informed consent are frequently due to a combination of factors (e.g., overly complex and lengthy consent forms, inadequate efforts to ensure that information provided during the consent process is actually understood) and not just impaired decision-making capacity (Dunn and Jeste 2001; Flory and Emanuel 2004). Indeed, in certain circumstances, such as acute medical illness (Raymont et al. 2004), or in desperate or catastrophic circumstances (Dermatis and Lesko 1990; Roberts 2002b), previously decisionally capable individuals may actually be "vulnerable" and unable to give informed consent.

Furthermore, when persons with mental illness lack an adequate understanding of informed consent, educational interventions have been shown to enhance comprehension, generally up to the level of non–mentally ill comparison subjects (Carpenter et al. 2000; Moser et al. 2006). A corollary of this finding is a concern held by numerous psychiatric research ethics investigators—namely, that the danger in seeking perfect or near-perfect comprehension of consent from people with mental illnesses who are considering research participation holds these populations to an unreasonable standard, one that is not asked of people with medical illnesses or of healthy people who enroll in research trials.

Concerns about the potential vulnerability of psychiatrically ill research subjects, as well as about the risks of further stigmatizing the mentally ill by developing policies and practices in the absence of empirical research on these issues, have fueled numerous research groups' endeavors to examine specific ethically relevant issues in psychiatric research (Dunn and Roberts 2005; Dunn et al. 2006). These studies, taken as a whole, have affirmed that patients with serious neuropsychiatric disorders are generally able to provide adequate informed consent for research, that enhancements to consent procedures result in improved understanding of research consent, and that participants' motivations for enrolling in psychiatric research are very similar to those of people with medical illnesses.

Attention to the detailed application of ethical principles to psychiatric research is vital not just for the protection of patient-volunteers; it is also critical to upholding and enhancing public trust in research, which has come under increased strain in recent years. As psychiatric research expands and takes on more potentially ethically fraught areas of inquiry, such as the genetic bases of disease risk and treatment response, there will be a growing need for the field to develop ethically sensitive and nuanced approaches to research (Appelbaum 2004; Biesecker and Peay 2003; Dinwiddie et al. 2004; Wilson and Stanley 2006). Unfortunately, specific guidance on how to deal with these issues and other issues in psychiatric research is lacking in federal laws and regulatory guidelines. Two novel frameworks for evaluating the ethics of clinical research protocols have been recently articulated. Emanuel et al. (2000) described seven required aspects of ethical clinical research (Table 42–11), including value, scientific validity, fair subject selection, favorable risk–benefit ratio, independent review, informed consent, and respect for enrolled subjects. The basis of each of these requirements can be discerned in research ethics codes. For example, the first requirement, value, reflects the second point of the Nuremberg Code (Emanuel et al. 2000).

Roberts has also enumerated a framework useful for investigators to identify ethical dimensions and potential pitfalls in research protocols (Roberts 1999), emphasizing the need for investigators to view consideration of these ethical aspects as a critical proactive endeavor. The Roberts RePEAT method (*Research Protocol Ethics Assessment Tool*) suggests that research protocols be analyzed on 24 topics in the following categories: scientific merit and design issues; expertise, commitment, and integrity issues; risks and benefits; confidentiality; participant selection and recruitment; informed consent and decisional capacity; and incentives and other issues (Table 42–12).

Future Directions

For the past several decades, major topics of ethical reflection in psychiatry have included boundary issues in psychotherapy, informed consent, and involuntary treatment. More recently, several new avenues for ethical inquiry have opened. First, technological advances, as in medicine as a whole, continue to create new and unforeseen ethical challenges. For example, scientific research in genetics and molecular and cellular neuroscience hold the potential to produce new technologies for diagnosing predispositions to mental illness. Both the risks and the benefits of such diagnostic testing could be substantial, and empirical and conceptual ethics research is needed to guide its proper use. Another example is presented by emerging invasive treatments (including surgical interventions) for psychiatric disorders such as severe depression. Issues pertaining to patient selection, informed consent for both research and treatment options, and maintenance of an ongoing therapeutic relationship with such patients are just beginning to be described.

A second trend in psychiatry with important ethical implications is the field's increasing reliance on the pharmaceutical industry to subsidize psychiatric education and clinical research. Psychiatrists, academic departments of psychiatry, and editors of peer-reviewed journals must successfully manage this potential conflict of interest or risk damaging the public trust.

Finally, psychiatrists as a group, and psychiatric practice settings and patterns, have changed considerably since the first APA ethics code was published in 1973. U.S. psychiatrists are now more culturally and ethnically diverse, with more women and fewer psychotherapists. Many psychiatrists practice in managed care settings, in psychiatric group practices, or within governmental agencies. It seems reasonable to expect

TABLE 42–11. **Requirements for ethical clinical research**

Value	Research must have the potential to lead to improved knowledge or health; it must answer a nontrivial question.
Scientific validity	Methods must be scientifically rigorous.
Fair subject selection	Communities and people should not be exploited for research purposes; inclusion criteria and study sites should be determined with these principles in mind; burdens and benefits of research participation should be equitably distributed.
Favorable risk–benefit ratio	Risks of research should be minimized; potential benefits (to individuals and knowledge gained for society) should be enhanced; potential benefits should exceed risks.
Independent review	People not associated with the research must evaluate it and have the authority to monitor it and, if necessary, terminate it.
Informed consent	Consent to research must be voluntary and must follow a complete discussion of the research.
Respect for enrolled subjects	There must be respect for the privacy of enrolled participants and ongoing monitoring of participants.

Source. Adapted from Emanuel EJ, Wendler D, Grady C: "What Makes Clinical Research Ethical?" *Journal of the American Medical Association* 283:2701–2711, 2000.

TABLE 42–12. **Questions to consider regarding the ethical acceptability of psychiatric research protocols**

1. **Scientific issues**

   - Is the study scientifically valuable?
   - Will the hypotheses be tested adequately?
   - Can the design yield meaningful data?
   - Does the protocol employ accepted scientific methods?

2. **Research team and institutional issues**

   - Does the investigative team have enough expertise and institutional and other support to successfully complete the experiment?
   - Are the researchers aware of research ethics issues and potential problems related to the protocol?
   - Are they in good standing within the scientific and professional communities?
   - What conflicting roles and conflicts of interest exist in relation to this protocol? How will they be dealt with?
   - Are the documentation features of the protocol adequate to monitor procedures and the professional accountability of the research team?

3. **Design issues related to risk and benefit**

   - Does the design minimize experimental risks to participants? Do alternative designs pose less risk?
   - Does the protocol pose excessive risk to individual participants, the community, and/or larger society?
   - If participants are likely to have emerging symptoms as a result of protocol involvement, have appropriate mechanisms for following symptom progression been developed? Are there clear criteria for disenrollment, and have alternative mechanisms for treatment been provided?
   - What benefits exist for participants? Is the likelihood of benefit accurately described?
   - Is it expected that any benefits derived from the protocol will be applicable to the specific population being studied?

(continued)

TABLE 42–12.   Questions to consider regarding the ethical acceptability of psychiatric research protocols *(continued)*

4. **Confidentiality**
    - Is participant information carefully safeguarded during the collection, storage, and analysis stages of the study?
    - Is the participant aware of potential disclosure obligations of the researchers?
    - Are research records kept separate from clinical records? If not, is there a sound justification for this practice?
    - Are there important "overlapping relationships" between investigative staff and participants? How will these be dealt with in terms of confidentiality protections?

5. **Selection, exclusion, and recruitment issues**
    - Does the process of selection, exclusion, and recruitment ensure that members of vulnerable populations are included in a manner consistent with federal guidelines and only if essential to the study's scientific hypotheses?
    - Are understudied populations inappropriately excluded from participation (i.e., are selection and recruitment practices potentially biased)?
    - Is the recruitment process itself noncoercive?

6. **Informed consent and decisional capacity issues**
    - Is the consent form concise, readable, accurate, and understandable?
    - Does the informed consent disclosure process include all relevant information, such as
        - the study's purpose and the nature of the illness or the phenomenon being studied
        - who is responsible for the scientific and ethical conduct of the study
        - why the individual may be eligible for participation
        - the proposed intervention and its associated risks and benefits and their relative likelihood
        - alternatives to participation
        - key study design features (e.g., placebo use, randomization, medication-free intervals, frequency of visits, confidentiality, plans for use of data)
    - Is there reasonable assurance of adequate decisional capacity of participants with respect to the ability to understand, analyze, and appreciate the meaning of the research decision?
    - If a participant has (or is at risk for) diminished decisional capacity at any time during protocol participation, are efforts to identify and follow the participant's capacity in place? Have specific interventions intended to enhance or restore the diminished capacity been built into the protocol?
    - Does the protocol include an appropriate mechanism for advance decision making by the participant or for identifying an alternative decision maker for the participant? Is it clear when the advance directive or alternative decision maker should be put into effect?
    - Is there reasonable assurance that individuals will not experience coercive pressure to participate in the project or continue in the project?

7. **Incentive issues**
    - Are incentives for participation sufficient and timed so that they compensate research participants without being coercive?
    - If health care is an incentive, how will the patient's health care needs be met if disenrollment becomes necessary?

8. **Institutional and peer/professional review issues**
    - Is the institutional context sufficient to allow the research to be conducted successfully?
    - Has the protocol undergone appropriate scientific and ethical review?
    - Should the protocol undergo any additional review steps (e.g., by community leaders)?
    - Does the protocol have features (e.g., very high-risk, very vulnerable participants) that merit ongoing external monitoring?

(continued)

TABLE 42–12. Questions to consider regarding the ethical acceptability of psychiatric research protocols *(continued)*

9. **Data presentation issues**

   - Will the presentation of the data describe the ethical safeguards employed in the protocol?
   - Will the presentation of the data meet current ethical standards (e.g., authorship, accurate disclosure of conflicting roles and conflicts of interest)?
   - Will participants' identities be adequately protected in data presentation?

Source. Reprinted from Roberts LW, Geppert CMA, Brody JL: "A Framework for Considering the Ethical Aspects of Psychiatric Research Protocols." *Comparative Psychiatry* 42:5 351–363, 2001. Copyright 2001, Elsevier. Used with permission.

that such sweeping changes would be reflected in the field's ethical and professional standards in the future. Although based on enduring principles of human morality, the application of bioethics principles is a dynamic enterprise, evolving with changes in the scientific, social, and cultural landscape.

Conclusion

In summary, ethics is intrinsic to the practice of psychiatry. In the professional life of a psychiatrist, ethics informs myriad day-to-day choices—not only the decisions surrounding clearly problematic situations such as involuntary treatment, mandatory reporting, or high-risk research but also the routine decisions of clinical practice, from the care we take when making a diagnosis or delivering an interpretation to the breadth of treatment options we envision for patients and explore with them. Through each of these actions, and through our ongoing attempts to become more discerning, more self-aware, and more respectful of others, we embody ethics for our patients, our profession, and ourselves.

Key Points

- Ethical decision making is a skill that can be taught and learned.

- Key moral principles that provide a foundation for contemporary discussions of medical ethics are autonomy, respect for persons, beneficence, nonmaleficence, justice, veracity, fidelity, and privacy.

- Psychiatrists have an ethical duty to provide competent care, treat patients with respect and dignity, and uphold ethical and professional obligations of confidentiality and truth telling.

- Sexual contact with patients and former patients is unethical.

- Physicians have an ethical duty to report the improper behavior of colleagues.

- Informed consent represents not only a legal and ethical requirement but also an opportunity to enhance physician–patient communication, assess patient preferences and values, and optimize treatment planning through a process of shared decision making.

- Individuals with psychiatric diagnoses are heterogeneous in terms of their decision-making abilities for treatment and research and should not be presumed to lack decisional capacity.

- Information about decisions should be provided in a manner that is appropriate to the individual patient.

- A "sliding scale" approach should be used for assessing decision-making capacity: a higher level of capacity may be needed for higher-risk or risk–benefit ratio decisions.

- The ethical use of involuntary treatment and hospitalization balances the duties of trying to do good, avoiding harm, and respecting autonomy.

Suggested Readings

American Psychiatric Association: Ethics Primer of the American Psychiatric Association. Washington, DC, American Psychiatric Association, 2001a

American Psychiatric Association: Opinions of the Ethics Committee on The Principles of Medical Ethics. Washington, DC, American Psychiatric Association, 2001b

American Psychiatric Association: The Principles of Medical Ethics With Annotations Applicable to Psychiatry. Washington, DC, American Psychiatric Association, 2006

Appelbaum PS, Grisso T: Assessing patients' capacities to consent to treatment. N Engl J Med 319:1635–1638, 1988

Beauchamp TL, Childress JF: Principles of Biomedical Ethics, 5th Edition. New York, Oxford University Press, 2001

Emanuel EJ, Wendler D, Grady C: What makes clinical research ethical? JAMA 283:2701–2711, 2000

Grisso T, Appelbaum PS, Hill-Fotouhi C: The MacCAT-T: a clinical tool to assess patients' capacities to make treatment decisions. Psychiatr Serv 48:1415–1419, 1997

Jonsen AR, Siegler M, Winslade WJ: Clinical Ethics, 4th Edition. New York, McGraw-Hill, 1998

Roberts LW, Dyer AR (eds): Concise Guide to Ethics in Mental Health Care. Washington, DC, American Psychiatric Publishing, 2004

Roberts LW, Mines J, Voss C, et al: Assessing medical students' competence in obtaining informed consent. Am J Surg 178:351–355, 1999

Roberts LW, Warner TD, Carter D, et al: Caring for medical students as patients: access to services and care-seeking practices of 1,027 students at nine medical schools. Collaborative Research Group on Medical Student Healthcare. Acad Med 75:272–277, 2000

Roberts LW, Geppert CM, Bailey R: Ethics in psychiatric practice: essential ethics skills, informed consent, the therapeutic relationship, and confidentiality. J Psychiatr Pract 8:290–305, 2002

Rubenstein L, Pross C, Davidoff F, et al: Coercive US interrogation policies: a challenge to medical ethics. JAMA 294:1544–1549, 2005

Schouten R: Impaired physicians: is there a duty to report to state licensing boards? Harvard Rev Psychiatry 8:26–39, 2000

Online Resources

AMA Declaration of Professional Responsibility: http://www.ama-assn.org/ama/upload/mm/369/decofprofessional.pdf

AMA Principles of Medical Ethics: http://www.ama-assn.org/ama/pub/category/2512.html

AMA Virtual Mentor: Ethics Education Resources: http://virtualmentor.ama-assn.org

APA Principles of Medical Ethics With Annotations Especially Applicable to Psychiatry: http://www.psych.org/psych_pract/ethics/ethics.cfm

Declaration of Helsinki, World Medical Association: http://www.wma.net/e/policy/b3.htm

The Belmont Report: http://www.hhs.gov/ohrp/humansubjects/guidance/belmont.htm

References

Advisory Committee on Human Radiation Experiments: The Human Radiation Experiments. New York, Oxford University Press, 1996

American Medical Association: AMA (Professionalism) E-History. August 1, 2005a. Available at: http://www.ama-assn.org/ama/pub/category/8291.html. Accessed June 22, 2006.

American Medical Association: AMA Ethical Opinions and Guidelines: Gifts to Physicians from Industry. January 26, 2005b. Available at: http://www.ama-assn.org/ama/pub/category/4001.html. Accessed June 12, 2006.

American Medical Association Judicial Council: Principles of Medical Ethics. Chicago, IL, American Medical Association, 1957

American Psychiatric Association: Ethics Primer of the American Psychiatric Association. Washington, DC, American Psychiatric Association, 2001a

American Psychiatric Association: Opinions of the Ethics Committee on The Principles of Medical Ethics. Washington, DC, American Psychiatric Association, 2001b

American Psychiatric Association: The Principles of Medical Ethics With Annotations Applicable to Psychiatry. Washington, DC, American Psychiatric Association, 2006

American Psychological Association: Ethical Principles of Psychologists and Codes of Conduct. 1992. Available at: http://www.apa.org/ethics/code2002.html. Accessed December 19, 2006.

Annas GJ, Grodin MA: The Nazi Doctors and the Nuremberg Code. New York, Oxford University Press, 1992

Appelbaum PS: Ethical issues in psychiatric genetics. J Psychiatr Pract 10:343–351, 2004

Appelbaum PS: Decisional capacity of patients with schizophrenia to consent to research: taking stock. Schizophr Bull 32:22–25, 2006

Appelbaum PS, Grisso T: The MacArthur Competence Study I, II, III. Law Hum Behav 19:105–174, 1995

Bartlett P: The test of compulsion in mental health law: capacity, therapeutic benefit and dangerousness as possible criteria. Med Law Rev 11:326–352, 2003

Beauchamp TL, Childress JF: Principles of Biomedical Ethics, 5th Edition. New York, Oxford University Press, 2001

Beecher H: Ethics and clinical research. N Engl J Med 274:1354–1360, 1966

Belitz J: Caring for children, in Concise Guide to Ethics in Mental Health Care. Edited by Roberts LW, Dyer AR. Washington, DC, American Psychiatric Publishing, 2004, pp 119–135

Biesecker BB, Peay HL: Ethical issues in psychiatric genetics research: points to consider. Psychopharmacology (Berl) 171:27–35, 2003

Bloch S, Reddaway P: Soviet Psychiatric Abuse. Boulder, CO, Westview Press, 1984

Brandeis LD: Business: A Profession. Boston, MA, Hole, Cushman & Flint, 1993

Burnham JC: A clinical alternative to the public health approach to mental illness: a forgotten social experiment. Perspect Biol Med 49:220–237, 2006

Carpenter WT, Schooler NR, Kane JM: The rationale and ethics of medication-free research in schizophrenia. Arch Gen Psychiatry 54:401–407, 1997

Carpenter WT, Gold JM, Lahti AC, et al: Decisional capacity for informed consent in schizophrenia research. Arch Gen Psychiatry 57:533–538, 2000

Carpenter WT, Appelbaum PS, Levine RJ: The Declaration of Helsinki and clinical trials: a focus on placebo-controlled trials in schizophrenia. Am J Psychiatry 160:356–362, 2003

Charney DS: The National Bioethics Advisory Commission Report: the response of the psychiatric research community is critical to restoring public trust. Arch Gen Psychiatry 56:699–700, 1999

Chen DT: Curricular approaches to research ethics training for psychiatric investigators. Psychopharmacology (Berl) 171:112–119, 2003

Christensen RC, Tueth MJ: Pharmaceutical companies and academic departments of psychiatry: a call for ethics education. Acad Psychiatry 22:135–137, 1998

Coverdale JH, Bayer T, Isbell P, et al: Are we teaching psychiatrists to be ethical? Acad Psychiatry 16:199–205, 1992

Dermatis H, Lesko LM: Psychological distress in parents consenting to child's bone marrow transplantation. Bone Marrow Transplant 6:411–417, 1990

Dinwiddie SH, Hoop J, Gershon ES: Ethical issues in the use of genetic information. Int Rev Psychiatry 16:320–328, 2004

Ditto PH, Danks JH, Smucker WD, et al: Advance directives as acts of communication: a randomized controlled trial. Arch Intern Med 161:421–430, 2001

Drane JF: Competency to give an informed consent. A model for making clinical assessments. JAMA 252:925–927, 1984

Druss BG, Bradford DW, Rosenheck RA, et al: Mental disorders and use of cardiovascular procedures after myocardial infarction. JAMA 283:506–511, 2000

Dunn LB, Jeste DV: Enhancing informed consent for research and treatment. Neuropsychopharmacology 24:595–607, 2001

Dunn LB, Roberts LW: Emerging findings in ethics of schizophrenia research. Curr Opin Psychiatry 18:111–119, 2005

Dunn LB, Candilis PJ, Roberts LW: Emerging empirical evidence on the ethics of schizophrenia research. Schizophr Bull 32:47–68, 2006

Dunn LB, Palmer BW, Karlawish JHT: Frontal dysfunction and capacity to consent to treatment or research: conceptual considerations and empirical evidence, in The Human Frontal Lobes: Functions and Disorders, 2nd Edition. Edited by Miller B, Cummings JL. New York, Guilford, 2007, pp 335–344

Dyer AR: Ethics and Psychiatry: Toward Professional Definition. Washington, DC, American Psychiatric Press, 1988, pp 20–27

Emanuel EJ, Wendler D, Grady C: What makes clinical research ethical? JAMA 283:2701–2711, 2000

Epstein RM, Alper BS, Quill TE: Communicating evidence for participatory decision making. JAMA 291:2359–2366, 2004

Epstein RS: Psychological characteristics of therapists who commit serious boundary violations, in Keeping Boundaries: Maintaining Safety and Integrity in the Psychotherapeutic Process. Washington, DC, American Psychiatric Press, 1994, pp 239–254

Epstein RS, Simon RI: The Exploitation Index: an early warning indicator of boundary violations in psychotherapy. Bull Menninger Clin 54:450–465, 1990

Faden RR, Beauchamp TL: Decision-making and informed consent: a study of the impact of disclosed information. Soc Indic Res 7:313–336, 1980

Faden RR, Beauchamp TL, King N: A History and Theory of Informed Consent. New York, Oxford University Press, 1986

Fann JR, Hunt DD, Schaad D: A sociological calendar of transitional stages during psychiatry residency training. Acad Psychiatry 27:31–38, 2003

Flory J, Emanuel E: Interventions to improve research participants' understanding in informed consent for research: a systematic review. JAMA 292:1593–1601, 2004

Flynn HA, Marcus SM, Kerber K, et al: Patients' concerns about and perceptions of electronic psychiatric records. Psychiatr Serv 54:1539–1541, 2003

Frank E, Novick DM, Kupfer DJ: Beyond the question of placebo controls: ethical issues in psychopharmacological drug studies. Psychopharmacology (Berl) 171:19–26, 2003

Fry S: Is health-care delivery by partially trained professionals ever morally justified? J Clin Ethics 2:42–44, 1991

Fulford KWM, Bloch S: Psychiatric ethics: codes, concepts, and clinical practice skills, in New Oxford Textbook of Psychiatry. Edited by Gelder M, Lopez-Ibor JJ, Andreasen N. Cambridge, UK, Oxford University Press, 2003, pp 27–32

Gabbard GO: Boundary violations, in Psychiatric Ethics, 3rd Edition. Edited by Bloch S, Chodoff P, Green SA. New York, Oxford University Press, 1999, pp 141–160

Gabbard GO, Lester EP: The early history of boundary violations in psychoanalysis, in Boundaries and Boundary Violations in Psychoanalysis. New York, Basic Books, 1995, pp 68–86

Gardner W, Lidz CW, Hoge SK, et al: Patients' revisions of their beliefs about the need for hospitalization. Am J Psychiatry 156:1385–1391, 1999

Glannon W: Phase I oncology trials: why the therapeutic misconception will not go away. J Med Ethics 32:252–255, 2006

Gottesman II, Bertelsen A: Legacy of German psychiatric genetics: hindsight is always 20/20. Am J Med Genet 67:317–322, 1996

Griener G: Electronic health records as a threat to privacy. Health Law Rev 14:14–17, 2005

Guntheil TG: Ethics and forensic psychiatry, in Psychiatric Ethics, 3rd Edition. Edited by Bloch S, Chodoff P, Green SA. New York, Oxford University Press, 1999, pp 345–362

Gutheil TH, Gabbard GO: The concept of boundaries in clinical practice: theoretical and risk-management dimensions. Am J Psychiatry 150:188–196, 1993

Gutheil TH, Gabbard GO: Misuses and misunderstandings of boundary theory in clinical and regulatory settings. Am J Psychiatry 155:409–414, 1998

Hoop JG: Hidden ethical dilemmas in psychiatric residency training: the psychiatry resident as dual agent. Acad Psychiatry 28:183–189, 2004

Jaffee v Redmond, 518 U.S. 1, 116 S. Ct.1923, 135 L. Ed. 2d 337, 1996

Jonsen AR, Toulmin S: The Abuse of Casuistry: A History of Moral Reasoning. Berkeley, CA, University of California Press, 1988

Jonsen AR, Siegler M, Winslade WJ: Clinical Ethics, 4th Edition. New York, McGraw-Hill, 1998

Kahn J: Sane Chinese put in asylum, doctors find. New York Times, March 17, 2006

Kass LR: Professing ethically: on the place of ethics in defining medicine. JAMA 249:1305–1310, 1983

Katz J: Experimentation With Human Beings. New York, Russel Sage Foundation, 1972

Kim SY, Caine ED, Currier GW, et al: Assessing the competence of persons with Alzheimer's disease in providing informed consent for participation in research. Am J Psychiatry 158:712–717, 2001

Kong D, Whitaker R: Doing harm: research on the mentally ill. Boston Globe, November 15–18, 1998

Kovnick JA, Appelbaum PS, Hoge SK, et al: Competence to consent to research among long-stay inpatients with chronic schizophrenia. Psychiatr Serv 54:1247–1252, 2003

LaCombe MA: On professionalism. Am J Med 94:329, 1993

Lapid MI, Rummans TA, Poole KL, et al: Decisional capacity of severely depressed patients requiring electroconvulsive therapy. J ECT 19:67–72, 2003

Levenson JL: Psychiatric commitment and involuntary hospitalization: an ethical perspective. Psychiatr Q 58:106–112, 1986–1987

Link BG, Phelan JC: Stigma and its public health implications. Lancet 367:528–529, 2006

Link BG, Struening EL, Rahav M, et al: On stigma and its consequences: evidence from a longitudinal study of men with dual diagnoses of mental illness and substance abuse. J Health Soc Behav 38:177–190, 1997

Link BG, Struening EL, Neese-Todd S, et al: Stigma as a barrier to recovery: The consequences of stigma for the self-esteem of people with mental illnesses. Psychiatr Serv 52:1621–1626, 2001

Link BG, Yang LH, Phelan JC, et al: Measuring mental illness stigma. Schizophr Bull 30:511–541, 2004

Lo B: Resolving Ethical Dilemmas: A Guide for Clinicians. Philadelphia, PA, JB Lippincott, 2005

Miller FG: Placebo-controlled trials in psychiatric research: an ethical perspective. Biol Psychiatry 47:707–716, 2000

Milne D: Psychologists' disciplinary failure leads to new law in Ohio. Psychiatr News 37:18, 2002

Mohamed M, Punwani M, Clay M, et al: Protecting the residency training environment: a resident's perspective on the ethical boundaries in the faculty-resident relationship. Acad Psychiatry 29:368–373, 2005

Moser DJ, Schultz SK, Arndt S, et al: Capacity to provide informed consent for participation in schizophrenia and HIV research. Am J Psychiatry 159:1201–1207, 2002

Moser DJ, Reese RL, Hey CT, et al: Using a brief intervention to improve decisional capacity in schizophrenia research. Schizophr Bull 32:116–120, 2006

Mosher PW, Swire PP: The ethical and legal implications of Jaffee v Redmond and the HIPAA medical privacy rule for psychotherapy and general psychiatry. Psychiatr Clin North Am 25:575–584, 2002

Muroff JR, Hoerauf SL, Kim SY: Is psychiatric research stigmatized? An experimental survey of the public. Schizophr Bull 32:129–136, 2006

National Bioethics Advisory Commission: Research Involving Persons With Mental Disorders That May Affect Decisionmaking Capacity. Rockville, MD, National Bioethics Advisory Commission, 1998

National Commission for the Protection of Human Subjects of Biomedical and Behavioral Research: The Belmont Report: ethical principles and guidelines for the protection of human subjects of research, 1979. Available at: http://www.hhs.gov/ohrp/humansubjects/guidance/belmont.htm. Accessed June 12, 2006.

New York State Office of Mental Health: Kendra's Law: final report on the status of assisted outpatient treatment. New York, Office of Mental Health, 2005

Ojeda VD, McGuire TG: Gender and racial/ethnic differences in use of outpatient mental health and substance use services by depressed adults. Psychiatr Q 77:211–222, 2006

Olofsson B, Norberg A: Experiences of coercion in psychiatric care as narrated by patients, nurses and physicians. J Adv Nurs 33:89–97, 2001

Ostman M, Kjellin L: Stigma by association: psychological factors in relatives of people with mental illness. Br J Psychiatry 181:494–498, 2002

Overstreet MM: Duty to report colleagues who engage in fraud or deception, in Ethics Primer of the American Psychiatric Association. Washington, DC, American Psychiatric Association, 2001, pp 51–56

Palmer BW, Dunn LB, Appelbaum PS, et al: Assessment of capacity to consent to research among older persons with schizophrenia, Alzheimer disease, or diabetes mellitus: comparison of a 3-item questionnaire with a comprehensive standardized capacity instrument. Arch Gen Psychiatry 62:726–733, 2005

Phelan JC, Bromet EJ, Link BG: Psychiatric illness and family stigma. Schizophr Bull 24:115–126, 1998

Racy J: Professionalism: sane and insane. J Clin Psychiatry 51:138–140, 1990

Raymont V, Bingley W, Buchanan A, et al: Prevalence of mental incapacity in medical inpatients and associated risk factors: cross-sectional study. Lancet 364:1421–1427, 2004

Reynolds PP: Reaffirming professionalism through the education community. Ann Intern Med 120:609–614, 1994

Rice DP, Miller LS: The economic burden of schizophrenia: conceptual and methodological issues, and cost estimates, in Handbook of Mental Health Economics and Health Policy, Vol 1: Schizophrenia. Edited by Moscarelli M, Rupp A, Sartorious N. New York, John Wiley & Sons, 1996, pp 321–324

Rice DP, Kelman S, Miller LS: The economic burden of mental illness. Hosp Community Psychiatry 43:1227–1232, 1992

Roberts LW: Ethical dimensions of psychiatric research: a constructive, criterion-based approach to protocol preparation. The Research Protocol Ethics Assessment Tool (REPEAT). Biol Psychiatry 46:1106–1119, 1999

Roberts LW: Evidence-based ethics and informed consent in mental illness research. Arch Gen Psychiatry 57:540–542, 2000

Roberts LW: Ethics and mental illness research. Psychiatr Clin North Am 25:525–545, 2002a

Roberts LW: Informed consent and the capacity for voluntarism. Am J Psychiatry 159:705–712, 2002b

Roberts LW: Caring for people in small communities, in Concise Guide to Ethics in Mental Health Care. Edited by Roberts LW, Dyer AR. Washington, DC, American Psychiatric Publishing, 2004, pp 167–184

Roberts LW, Dyer AR (eds): Concise Guide to Ethics in Mental Health Care. Washington, DC, American Psychiatric Publishing, 2004

Roberts LW, Miller MN: Ethical issues in clinician health, in Concise Guide to Ethics in Mental Health Care. Edited by Roberts LW, Dyer AR. Washington, DC, American Psychiatric Publishing, 2004, pp 233–242

Roberts LW, Roberts B: Psychiatric research ethics: an overview of evolving guidelines and current ethical dilemmas in the study of mental illness. Biol Psychiatry 46:1025–1038, 1999

Roberts LW, Hardee JT, Franchini G, et al: Medical students as patients: a pilot study of their health care needs, practices, and concerns. Acad Med 71:1225–1232, 1996

Roberts LW, Battaglia J, Smithpeter M, et al: An office on Main Street. Health care dilemmas in small communities. Hastings Cent Rep 29:28–37, 1999

Roberts LW, Warner TD, Brody JL: Perspectives of patients with schizophrenia and psychiatrists regarding ethically important aspects of research participation. Am J Psychiatry 157:67–74, 2000

Roberts LW, Geppert CM, Brody JL: A framework for considering the ethical aspects of psychiatric research protocols. Compr Psychiatry 42:351–363, 2001

Roberts LW, Geppert CM, Bailey R: Ethics in psychiatric practice: essential ethics skills, informed consent, the therapeutic relationship, and confidentiality. J Psychiatr Pract 8:290–305, 2002a

Roberts LW, Warner TD, Brody JL, et al: Patient and psychiatrist ratings of hypothetical schizophrenia research protocols: assessment of harm potential and factors influencing participation decisions. Am J Psychiatry 159:573–584, 2002b

Roberts LW, Geppert C, McCarty T, et al: Evaluating medical students' skills in obtaining informed consent for HIV testing. J Gen Intern Med 18:112–119, 2003a

Roberts LW, McCarty T, Roberts BB, et al: Clinical ethics training in psychiatric supervision. Focus 1:435–444, 2003b

Roberts LW, Green Hammond KA, Geppert CM, et al: The positive role of professionalism and ethics training in medical education: a comparison of medical student and resident perspectives. Acad Psychiatry 28:170–182, 2004

Roberts LW, Warner TD, Green Hammond KA, et al: Becoming a good doctor: perceived need for ethics training focused on practical and professional development topics. Acad Psychiatry 29:301–309, 2005

Rosenman S: Psychiatrists and compulsion: a map of ethics. Aust N Z J Psychiatry. 32:785–793, 1998

Rosenstein DL, Miller FG: Ethical considerations in psychopharmacological research involving decisionally impaired subjects. Psychopharmacology (Berl) 171:92–97, 2003

Rosenstein DL, Miller FG, Rubinow DR: A curriculum for teaching psychiatric research bioethics. Biol Psychiatry 50:802–808, 2001

Sabin JE: A credo for ethical managed care in mental health practice. Hosp Community Psychiatry 45:859–860, 1994

Sachs GA, Stocking CB, Stern R, et al: Ethical aspects of dementia research: informed consent and proxy consent. Clin Res 42:403–412, 1994

Sax U, Schmidt S: Integration of genomic data in Electronic Health Records—opportunities and dilemmas. Methods Inf Med 44:546–550, 2005

Schraufnagel TJ, Wagner AW, Miranda J, et al: Treating minority patients with depression and anxiety: what does the evidence tell us? Gen Hosp Psychiatry 28:27–36, 2006

Schreiber SC, Kramer TAM, Adamowski SE: Core Competencies for Psychiatric Practice: What Clinicians Need to Know (A Report of the American Board of Psychiatry and Neurology). Washington, DC, American Psychiatric Publishing, 2003

Schwartz HI, Vingiano W, Perez CB: Autonomy and the right to refuse treatment: patients' attitudes after involuntary medication. Hosp Community Psychiatry 39:1049–1054, 1988

Srebnik D, Appelbaum PS, Russo J: Assessing competence to complete psychiatric advance directives with the competence assessment tool for psychiatric advance directives. Compr Psychiatry 45:239–245, 2004

Srebnik DS, Rutherford LT, Peto T, et al: The content and clinical utility of psychiatric advance directives. Psychiatr Serv 56:592–598, 2005

Stobo JD, Blank LL: American Board of Internal Medicine's Project Professionalism: staying ahead of the wave. Am J Med 97:1–3, 1994

Szasz TS: Involuntary psychiatry. University of Cincinnati Law Review 45:347–365, 1976

Tunis SR, Stryer DB, Clancy CM: Practical clinical trials: increasing the value of clinical research for decision making in clinical and health policy. JAMA 290:1624–1632, 2003

U.S. Department of Health and Human Services: Health Insurance Portability and Accountability Act of 1996. Available at: http://aspe.hhs.gov/admnsimp/pl104191.htm. Accessed November 21, 2006.

U.S. Department of Health and Human Services: Mental Health: A Report of the Surgeon General—Executive Summary. Rockville, MD, U.S. Department of Health and Human Services, Substance Abuse and Mental Health Services Administration, Center for Mental Health Services, National Institutes of Health, National Institute of Mental Health, 1999

U.S. Department of Health and Human Services: Mental Health: Culture, Race, and Ethnicity—A Supplement to Mental Health: A Report of the Surgeon General. Rockville, MD, Department of Health and Human Services, Substance Abuse and Mental Health Service Administration, Center for Mental Health Services, 2001

Vinicky J, Connors R, Leader R, et al: Patients as "subjects" or "objects" in residency education? J Clin Ethics 2:35–41, 1991

Wazana A: Physicians and the pharmaceutical industry: is a gift ever just a gift? JAMA 283:373–380, 2000

Wilson ST, Stanley B: Ethical concerns in schizophrenia research: looking back and moving forward. Schizophr Bull 32:30–36, Jan 2006

World Medical Association: Declaration of Helsinki: ethical principles for medical research involving human subjects. Ferney-Volatire, France, World Medical Association, 1964. Available at: http://www.wma.net/e/policy/b3.htm. Accessed June 12, 2006.

43

SUICIDE

Robert I. Simon, M.D.

There are two kinds of clinical psychiatrists: those who have had patient suicides, and those who will have patient suicides. Every patient suicide is also a tragedy for the clinician and for the suicide survivors. Patient suicide is an occupational hazard of psychiatric practice, accompanied by increased malpractice liability exposure (see Figure 41–1 in Chapter 41, "Psychiatry and the Law," by Simon and Shuman). The only way to avoid patient suicide attempts or patient suicides is to not treat patients.

Suicide Statistics

The suicide rate in the United States for the year 2004 was 11.1 per 100,000. The suicide rate for males was 17.7 per 100,000 and for females 4.6 per 100,000 (American Association of Suicidology 2006). Suicide ranks eleventh as a cause of death. It is the eighth leading cause of death in the United States for all men (National Center for Injury Prevention and Control 2006). Women attempt suicide about three times as often as men (Table 43–1). In 2004, there were 3.7 male suicides for each female suicide and 3 female attempts for each male attempt (American Association of Suicidology 2006). Suicide completions occur on an average of one person every 16.6 minutes. For young persons, on average, one person commits suicide every 2 hours and 11 minutes.

It is estimated that 811,000 suicide attempts occur annually in the United States (25 attempts for every

TABLE 43–1. Suicide statistics, United States (2004)

Suicide rates	
Males	17.7 per 100,000
Females	4.6 per 100,000
Total	11.1 per 100,000
Gender ratios	
Suicide completions	3.7 male suicides for each female suicide
Suicide attempts	3 female attempts for each male attempt

Source. American Association of Suicidology 2006.

suicide). In 2002, 132,353 persons were hospitalized after suicide attempts; 116,659 were treated in emergency departments and released (American Association of Suicidology 2006). Based on more than 754,570 suicides between 1980 and 2004, it is estimated that the number of suicide survivors in the United States is 4.5 million (1 of every 64 Americans in 2002; American Association of Suicidology 2006).

The most common methods of suicide in 2004 were firearms (51.6%), suffocation/hanging (22.6%), and poisoning (17.9%; American Association of Suicidology 2006). Firearms accounted for 16,750 suicides in 2004. Guns in the home substantially increase the risk of suicide in psychiatric patients, as does the recent purchase of a firearm, especially a handgun purchase for women (Brent 2001; Wintemute et al. 1999).

Statistical data reveal that suicide is a rare event (see Table 43–1). For example, as noted earlier, the national suicide rate in the general population for the year 2004 was 11.1 per 100,000. The suicide rate for individuals with bipolar disorders is estimated at 193 per 100,000 (absolute risk), or 18 times higher (relative risk) compared with the suicide rate for the general population (Baldessarini 2003). Reframing these data, of every 100,000 patients with bipolar disorder, 99,807 will *not* commit suicide. Statistical data are static factors that can be useful in supplementing assessment of suicide risk.

Suicide Risk Assessment

Suicide risk assessment is a core competency that psychiatrists are expected to acquire during their residency training (Scheiber et al. 2003). The purpose of suicide risk assessment is to identify modifiable, treatable risk and protective factors that inform the patient's treatment and safety management needs.

A standard of care does not exist for the prediction of suicide (Pokorny 1983, 1993). Attempting to predict who will commit suicide creates false-positive and false-negative predictions (R.I. Simon 2004). The standard of care for suicide risk assessment is an elusive concept (R.I. Simon and Shuman 2006). An examination of what constitutes the standard of care for suicide risk assessment reveals differences of opinion among competent clinicians, academics, and researchers who testify as experts in suicide cases. Clinicians are expected to perform reasonable suicide risk assessments (R.I. Simon 2002). The bedeviling question is—what is reasonable?

A number of suicide risk assessment methods have been proposed (Beck et al. 1998; Clark and Fawcett 1999; Jacobs et al. 1999; Linehan 1993; Mays 2004; Rudd et al. 2001; Shea 2004; R.I. Simon 2004). No suicide risk assessment method has been empirically tested for reliability and validity (Busch et al. 1993). Clinicians can create their own systematic suicide risk assessment methodology reflecting their training, clinical experience, and knowledge of the evidence-based psychiatric literature. A systematic suicide risk assessment, whichever method is used, should more than meet the standard of care.

Systematic suicide risk assessment encourages the clinician to gather sufficient information to perform a competent assessment. Risk and protective factors are assessed dimensionally as low, moderate, or high according to the clinical presentation of the patient. An overall assessment of the level of suicide risk is determined. The assessment of suicide risk and protective factors creates an individualized mosaic of the patient's overall suicide risk. The clinician assesses the acute high-risk suicide factors, especially the response to treatment, over the patient's clinical course. Protective factors are also monitored. *Acute* is defined as the magnitude and intensity of the symptom, for example, early-morning waking versus debilitating global insomnia. A high-risk factor is supported by an evidence-based strong association with suicide.

The suicide risk assessment method in Table 43–2 is only one way of *conceptualizing* risk assessment. It is *not* intended to be used as a suicide risk assessment form or protocol. Obviously, suicidal patients may present with only a few risk factors or with risk factors not identified on a form or protocol. No form or protocol can encompass all possible risk factors. Using stand-alone risk assessment forms may lead to robotic assessments that fail to capture the highly individual risk and protective factors presented by every patient at risk for suicide. Invariably, crucial risk factors are omitted.

Standardized suicide risk prediction scales do not identify which patient will attempt or commit suicide (Busch et al. 1993). Single scores on suicide risk assessment scales and inventories should not be the sole basis for clinical decision making. Structured or semistructured suicide scales may complement but are not a substitute for systematic suicide risk assessment (American Psychiatric Association 2003). Malone et al. (1995b), however, found that semistructured screening instruments improved routine clinical assessments in the documentation and detection of lifetime suicidal behaviors. Oquendo et al. (2003) discussed the advantages and limitations of research instruments in assessing suicide risk. The standard of care does not require that specific psychological tests or checklists be used as part of systematic suicide risk assessment (Bongar et al. 1992).

The standard of care requires psychiatrists and other mental health professionals to reasonably assess patients at risk for suicide. It is foreseeable that failing to perform a reasonable suicide risk assessment can harm the patient. Suicide risk assessment is an integral part of the psychiatric examination. Systematic suicide risk assessment that evaluates both risk and protective factors should exceed any reasonable definition of "adequate" (G.E. Simon et al. 2006). Systematic suicide assessment is an inductive process, reasoning from specific patient data to arrive at a clinical judgment that informs treatment and safety management.

TABLE 43–2. **Systematic suicide risk assessment: conceptual model**

Assessment factors[a]	Risk	Protective
Individual		
Unique clinical features		
Clinical		
Current attempt (lethality)		
Panic attacks[b]		
Psychic anxiety[b]		
Loss of pleasure and interest[b]		
Alcohol abuse[b]		
Depressive turmoil (mixed states)[b]		
Diminished concentration[b]		
Global insomnia[b]		
Suicide plan		
Suicidal ideation (command hallucinations)[c]		
Suicide intent[c]		
Hopelessness[c]		
Prior attempts (lethality)[c]		
Therapeutic alliance		
Psychiatric diagnoses (Axis I and Axis II)		
Symptom severity		
Comorbidity		
Recent discharge from psychiatric hospital		
Drug abuse		
Impulsivity		
Agitation		
Physical illness		
Family history of mental illness (suicide)		
Mental competency		
Interpersonal relations		
Work or school		
Family		
Spouse or partner		
Children		

TABLE 43–2. **Systematic suicide risk assessment: conceptual model** (continued)

Assessment factors[a]	Risk	Protective
Situational		
Living circumstances		
Employment or school status		
Financial status		
Availability of guns		
Managed care setting		
Statistical		
Age		
Gender		
Marital status		
Race		
Overall risk ratings[d]		

[a]Rate risk and protective factors present as low (L), moderate (M), high (H), nonfactor (0), or range (e.g., L–M, M–H).
[b]Risk factors statistically significant within 1 year of assessment.
[c]Associated with suicide 2–10 years following assessment.
[d]Judge overall suicide risk as low, moderate, high, or a range of risk.

A certain analogy exists between suicide risk assessment and weather forecasting (Monahan and Steadman 1996; R.I. Simon 1992). Suicide risk assessments are "here and now" determinations made for the purpose of treatment and management; they are not predictions. Moreover, there are no suicide risk factors for "imminent" suicide. *Imminence* is another word for a short-term prediction that is not supported by evidence-based research (R.I. Simon 2006). Like weather forecasts, suicide risk assessments require frequent updating. The analogy, however, is imperfect. Weather forecasters can predict the weather with reasonable accuracy, but they cannot change it. Psychiatrists cannot predict who will commit suicide, but they can reduce or even eliminate the threat of suicide through treatment and safety management.

Professional organizations have developed practice guidelines for the assessment and management of individuals at risk for suicide. The American Academy of Child and Adolescent Psychiatry (2001b) has published practice parameters for children and adolescents with suicidal behaviors. The American Psychiatric Association (2003) has also developed practice guidelines for the treatment and management of patients at suicide risk.

Suicide Risk and Protective Factors

Risk Factors

Suicide is the result of multifaceted determinants, including diagnostic (psychiatric and medical), psychodynamic, genetic, familial, occupational, environmental, social, cultural, and contextual factors. No pathognomic risk factors exist. A single risk factor does not have the statistical power upon which to base a suicide risk assessment. General risk assessment factors have been identified through retrospective community-based psychological autopsies and studies of completed suicides (Fawcett et al. 1993). To be useful, general risk factors must be adapted to the clinical presentation of the individual patient. Evidence-based research finds that high-risk factors associated with attempted suicide in adults include depression, prior suicide attempts, hopelessness, suicidal ideation, alcohol abuse, cocaine abuse, and recent loss of an important relationship (Murphy et al. 1992).

Short-term suicide risk factors derived from a 10-year prospective study of patients with affective disorders were statistically significant within 1 year of assessment (Fawcett et al. 1990). The short-term risk factors were panic attacks, psychic anxiety, loss of pleasure and interest, moderate alcohol abuse, depressive turmoil, diminished concentration, and global insomnia. Short-term risk factors were predominantly severe, anxiety driven, and treatable by a variety of drugs (Fawcett 2001). Acute suicide risk factors are usually treatable or modifiable. For example, treating anxiety or severe insomnia in a depressed patient can rapidly lower suicide risk. Modifying just a few acute risk factors can significantly reduce a patient's risk for suicide (Table 43–3).

TABLE 43–3. Examples of modifiable and treatable suicide risk factors

Depression	Impulsivity
Anxiety	Agitation
Panic attacks	Physical illness
Psychosis	Difficult situations
Sleep disorders	(e.g., family, work)
Substance abuse	Lethal means
Command hallucinations	(e.g., guns, drugs)

Source. Reprinted from Simon RI: *Assessing and Managing Suicide Risk: Guidelines for Clinically Based Risk Management.* Arlington, VA, American Psychiatric Publishing, 2004, p. 26.

Long-term suicide risk factors in patients with major affective disorders were associated with suicides completed 2–10 years after assessment (Fawcett et al. 1990). Long-term risk factors include suicidal ideation, suicidal intent, severe hopelessness, and prior suicide attempts.

Clarity of diagnosis is essential in suicide risk assessment. All mental disorders except mental retardation are associated with an increased risk of suicide. Harris and Barraclough (1997) abstracted 249 reports from the medical literature on the mortality of mental disorders. They compared the observed number of suicides with the expected rate. A standardized mortality ratio (SMR) was calculated for each disorder. The SMR determines the relative risk of suicide for a particular disorder compared with the expected rate in the general population. It is calculated by dividing the observed mortality by the expected mortality (Table 43–4).

Patients with Axis I psychiatric disorders such as schizophrenia, anxiety disorders, major affective disorders, and substance abuse disorders (especially alcohol) often present with acute (state) suicide risk factors. Sareen et al. (2005) demonstrated that a pre-existing anxiety disorder is an independent risk factor for the onset of suicidal ideation and attempts. Patients with Axis II disorders often display chronic (trait) suicide risk factors. Exacerbation of a personality disorder or comorbidity with an Axis I disorder (including substance abuse) can transform a chronic suicide risk factor into an acute factor. Suicide risk increases with the total number of risk factors, providing a quasi-quantitative dimension to suicide risk assessment (Murphy et al. 1992).

Personality disorder, recent negative life events, and Axis I comorbidity were found in a large sample of suicides (Heikkinen et al. 1997). Recent stressful life events, including workplace problems, family strife, unemployment, and financial trouble, were highly represented among patients with personality disorder. Personality disorders associated with depressive symptoms and substance abuse disorders are highly represented among patients who complete suicide (Isometsa et al. 1996).

Patients with personality disorders have a sevenfold increased risk of suicide compared with the general population (Harris and Barraclough 1997). Cluster B personality disorders, especially borderline and antisocial personality disorders, place patients at increased risk for suicide (Duberstein and Conwell 1997). In borderline patients, impulsivity was associated with a high number of suicide attempts, after controlling for substance abuse and a lifetime diagnosis of depressive

TABLE 43–4. Suicide risk associated with various mental and physical disorders

Disorder	Standardized mortality ratio[a]
Eating disorders	23.14
Major depression	20.35
Sedative abuse	20.34
Mixed drug abuse	19.23
Bipolar disorder	15.05
Opioid abuse	14.00
Dysthymia	12.12
Obsessive-compulsive disorder	11.54
Panic disorder	10.00
Schizophrenia	8.45
Personality disorders	7.08
AIDS	6.58
Alcohol abuse	5.86
Epilepsy	5.11
Child and adolescent psychiatric	4.73
Cannabis abuse	3.85
Spinal cord injury	3.82
Neuroses	3.72
Brain injury	3.50
Huntington's chorea	2.90
Multiple sclerosis	2.36
Malignant neoplasms	1.80
Mental retardation	0.88

[a]Standardized mortality ratio is calculated by dividing observed mortality by expected mortality.
Source. Adapted from Harris and Barraclough 1997.

disorder (Brodsky et al. 1997). Impulsivity can be assessed clinically by asking patients about violent rages, assaultive behaviors, arrests, destruction of property, spending sprees, speeding tickets, sexual indiscretions, and other indicia of poor impulse control.

The lifetime suicide rate for schizophrenia is between 9% and 13%. The lifetime rate for suicide attempts is between 20% and 40%. The estimated number of suicides annually in the United States among schizophrenic patients is 3,600, or 12% of total suicides. Suicide is the leading cause of death among persons with schizophrenia who are younger than 35 years (Meltzer 2001). Suicide tends to occur in the early stages of a schizophrenic illness and during acute exacerbations (Meltzer 2001). Suicide remains a risk throughout the individual's life cycle. Palmer et al. (2005), in a reexamination of the psychiatric literature, estimated that 4.9% of schizophrenic patients will complete suicide, usually near the onset of illness. Recent studies have found an increased rate of suicide among patients with psychotic disorders (Radomsky et al. 1999; Warman et al. 2004). No differences exist in rates of suicide between depressed patients with and without melancholic features (Kessing 2003).

Prior suicide attempts by any method had the highest SMR of 38.36. Suicide risk was highest in the 2 years after the first attempt (Harris and Barraclough 1997). Between 7% and 12% of patients who make suicide attempts complete suicide within 10 years. Thus, a suicide attempt is a significant risk factor for suicide. Most suicides, however, occur in patients with no prior history of attempts (Malone et al. 1995a).

Suicidal ideation is an important risk factor. Suicidal *ideation* should be differentiated from suicide *intent*. *Suicidal ideation* can be passive, fleeting, intermittent, active, and intense, with or without the intent to die. *Suicide intent* is the subjective expectation and desire to die by a self-destructive act. *Lethality* refers to the danger to life posed by a suicide method or act. An individual who takes 10 aspirins in the mistaken belief that he or she will die forms the intent to complete suicide even though the method is not lethal. A person who accidentally dies by hanging, as in autoerotic asphyxia, does not intend to die.

In the National Comorbidity Survey, the transition from suicide ideation to suicide plan was 34% and from plan to attempt was 72% (Kessler et al. 1999). The transition from suicide ideation to an unplanned attempt was 26%. Approximately 90% of unplanned and 60% of planned first attempts occurred within 1 year of the onset of suicide ideation. Mann et al. (1999) found that the severity of suicidal ideation is an indicator of risk for attempting suicide. Beck et al. (1990) discovered that when patients were asked about suicidal ideation at its worst point, patients with higher scores were 14 times more likely to complete suicide than patients with lower scores.

Approximately 25% of patients who are at risk for suicide do not admit having suicidal ideation to clinicians but do tell their families (Robins 1981). When patients withhold permission to speak with families, the psychiatrist can listen to families without violating confidentiality. Hall et al. (1999) found that 69 of 100 patients had only fleeting or no suicidal thoughts before they made a suicide attempt. No patient reported a specific plan before making an impulsive suicide attempt. A prior suicide attempt had not occurred in 67% of the patients. Patients who are determined to commit suicide regard the psychiatrist and other mental health professionals as the enemy (Resnick 2002). Thus, a patient's denial of suicidal ideation requires additional assessment for the presence of other suicide risk factors.

A family history of mental illness, especially of suicide, is a significant suicide risk factor. The offspring of patients with mood disorders who attempt suicide are at a markedly increased risk for suicide (Brent et al. 2002). Genetic and familial transmission of suicide risk is independent of the transmission of psychiatric illnesses (Brent et al. 1996). The Copenhagen Adoption Study showed that adoptees who completed suicide had a sixfold increased rate of suicide among their biological relatives compared with matched adoptees who did not commit suicide (Schulsinger et al. 1979). Trémeau et al. (2005) found that a family history of suicide was associated with an increased risk for suicide attempt, with lethality of method, with repeated attempts, and with the number of attempts. Mann et al. (1999) proposed a stress–diathesis model of suicide behavior. For suicide to occur, a trigger (stress)—usually a psychiatric disorder and a preexisting vulnerability to suicidal behaviors (diathesis)—must be present. The neurobiology and genetics of suicide are reviewed by Mann et al. (2001).

Protective Factors

A competent suicide risk assessment evaluates both risk and protective factors (R.I. Simon 2004). The self-report Reasons for Living Inventory measures beliefs that may act as preventive factors against suicide (Linehan et al. 1983). The preventive factors include survival and coping skills, responsibility to family, child-related concerns, fear of suicide, fear of social disapproval, and moral/religious values. Other protective factors may include availability and community access to effective clinical care for mental, physical, and substance abuse disorders; adherence with recommended treatments; family and community support; life-affirming cultural values that discourage suicide; skills in problem solving and nonviolent con-

flict resolution; children at home; and pregnancy (Goldsmith et al. 2001). The inventory can be used to monitor patients at chronic high suicide risk and to assess the effectiveness of treatment. Dervic et al. (2004) found that religious affiliation was associated with less suicide behavior in depressed patients. Severely depressed patients, however, may feel angry and abandoned by God or that "God will understand," increasing their risk of suicide.

The presence of a therapeutic alliance can be an important protective factor against suicide (R.I. Simon 1998). The therapeutic alliance is influenced by a number of factors, especially the nature and severity of the patient's mental disorder. It can change from session to session. It cannot be assumed, therefore, that a therapeutic alliance will remain a protective factor between sessions. Clinicians are shocked and bewildered when a patient with whom they believed they had a sustaining therapeutic alliance attempts or completes suicide between sessions. The absence of a therapeutic alliance with a patient at risk for suicide is a significant risk factor (R.I. Simon 2004).

Protective factors, like risk factors, vary with the clinical presentation of the individual patient at suicide risk. An ebb and flow exists between risk and protective factors. Protective factors are easier for patients to talk about and thus tend to be overvalued by the patient and the clinician. Protective factors can be overcome, however, by the acuteness and severity of the patient's illness. Identification and marshalling of protective factors are important aspects of patient discharge planning.

Patients display distinctive suicide risk and protective factors. Suicide patterns can be identified by obtaining a detailed history of the patient's past suicide crises or attempts. Understanding a patient's psychodynamic responses to past and current life stressors is also important. Identifying a patient's recurrent prodromal symptomatology provides the clinician with insight in treating and managing the patient's current clinical condition.

A suicide attempt, especially if recent, may be a rehearsal for completed suicide. Although a patient may repeat the method of prior attempts, there is no assurance that a subsequent attempt will use the same methods. Isometsa and Lonnqvist (1998) found that 82% of suicide attempters used at least two different methods in subsequent suicide attempts and completions. Sixty-two percent of males and 38% of females died in their first attempt. The risk of suicide is highest during the first year after a suicide attempt.

Populations at Suicide Risk

Children and Adolescents

Practice parameters are available for the assessment and treatment of children and adolescents with suicidal behavior (American Academy of Child and Adolescent Psychiatry 2001a). Risk factors for adolescents' suicide include prior attempts, affective disorder, substance abuse, living alone, male gender, age 16 years or older, and a history of physical and/or sexual abuse. Adverse childhood experiences such as emotional, physical, and sexual abuse are associated with an increased risk of attempted suicide throughout the life span (Dube et al. 2001). More suicidal women than suicidal men experienced childhood abuse (Kaplan et al. 1995). Brent (2001) described a framework for the assessment of suicide risk in the adolescent that can be used to determine immediate disposition, intensity of treatment, and level of care.

The Elderly

In adults older than 65 years, risk factors for late-life suicide include depression, physical illnesses, functional impairment, personality traits of neuroticism, social isolation, and loss of important relationships (Conwell and Duberstein 2001). The suicide rate for men 85 years and older rises substantially. Forty-one percent of older adults had seen their primary care physician within 28 days of committing suicide (Isometsa et al. 1995). Thus, primary care is an important point of suicide prevention for elders at high risk (Loebel 2005).

Sexual Minorities

No studies have examined the rates of completed suicide among gay, lesbian, and bisexual individuals. Recent studies have consistently found that gay, lesbian, and bisexual youths have a greater risk of suicide attempts than matched heterosexual comparison groups (American Psychiatric Association 2003). In HIV-positive men, suicide rates are only moderately elevated and comparable with other medically ill populations since the advent of antiretroviral treatments (American Psychiatric Association 2000; Marzuk et al. 1997).

Suicide risk may be increased in individuals who experience high stress concerning the experiences of homophobia, harassment, and disclosure of sexual orientation to family and friends and other difficulties associated with gender nonconformity (American Psychiatric Association 2003).

Jail and Prison Inmates

Between 8% and 19% of prison inmates have psychiatric disorders (Metzner and Hayes 2006). Another 15%–20% require some form of psychiatric intervention while incarcerated. Substance abuse and use disorders are highly prevalent among prisoners.

The suicide rate in jails (rural and city jails and police lockups) is high in comparison with that among prison inmates. In 1986 the suicide rate for jail inmates was 107 per 100,000, or approximately nine times greater than in the general population. In 1999, the suicide rate for prison inmates was 14 per 100,000, compared with 55 per 100,000 among jail inmates. The profile of a jail suicide victim is a young, white, single, first-time nonviolent offender who is intoxicated, has a substance abuse history, is in isolated jail housing, hangs him- or herself with bed clothing, and dies within 24 hours of arrest (Metzner and Hayes 2006). Thus, the focus of suicide prevention must begin with the inmate jail population.

Treatment

Treatment of the patient at risk for suicide requires a full commitment of time and effort by the clinician. A realistic self-appraisal should help the clinician decide whether such a commitment can be made. The treatment of patients at risk for suicide can be emotionally taxing and professionally threatening. Some clinicians decline to treat suicidal patients, if at all possible. Countertransference reactions often occur during the treatment of suicidal patients; these reactions need to be identified and constructively managed so as not to interfere with treatment. Anger, despair, frustration, hopelessness, hate, and a threat to one's competence are some of the feelings evoked in clinicians (Gabbard and Allison 2006). Acting as a savior and attempting to re-parent the patient are countertransference traps. Clinicians must be able to effectively manage the inevitable anxieties and vicissitudes that arise in the treatment of suicidal patients.

Psychotherapies

Psychotherapies have an essential role in the treatment and management of patients at risk for suicide. Evidence-based research has identified psychotherapeutic treatments that reduce the risk of suicide attempts or completions in psychiatric patients. In a randomized controlled trial, cognitive therapy was found effective in preventing suicide attempts for adults who had recently attempted suicide (Brown et al. 2005).

Linehan et al. (2006) demonstrated, in a 2-year randomized controlled trial, that dialectical behavior therapy (DBT) was uniquely effective in reducing suicide attempts. In comparison with therapy by experts for suicidal behaviors and borderline personality disorder, DBT was associated with better outcomes during a 2-year treatment and follow-up period.

Guthrie et al. (2001, 2003) randomly assigned 119 patients who were seen in the emergency department after deliberate self-poisoning to either psychodynamic interpersonal therapy or treatment as usual (outpatient follow-up by a general practitioner). The patients who received therapy experienced a significantly greater reduction in suicidal ideation at a 6-month follow-up as compared with the control subjects. Also, they were less likely to report repeat self-harm attempts.

Treatment of borderline personality disorder using a randomized, controlled trial of psychodynamically based partial hospitalization demonstrated dramatic reductions in suicide behavior (Bateman and Fonagy 2000, 2004). Ninety-five percent of the sample of 39 borderline patients attempted suicide in the 6 months before the beginning of the study. Only 5.3% made attempts in the 6 months after treatment.

There is, however, limited evidence-based research for treatments that effectively prevent recurrent suicide attempts (Hawton et al. 2005). Nonetheless, psychosocial interventions are critically important in the treatment and management of suicidal patients.

Somatic Therapies

Lithium significantly decreases suicide risk in patients with bipolar disorder (Baldessarini et al. 2001). The risk of suicide attempts in bipolar patients taking lithium is more than eight times lower than among patients not taking the medication. Even with lithium, however, the completed suicide rate among bipolar patients is still 10 times higher than the suicide rate in the general population (Baldessarini 2003). The potential for lethal overdose should guide the quantity of lithium prescribed for a patient at risk for suicide. In some responders, antidepressant medication can have a significant therapeutic benefit within several weeks. Most responders require 8–12 weeks for maximum benefit following the initiation of antidepressant treatment (Gelenberg and Chesen 2000). Patients should be informed that an antidepressant requires time to become effective, and educating patients about the "ups and downs" in depressive symptoms that commonly occur in the course of improvement helps combat hopelessness. According to some researchers, other than prior suicide attempts, hopelessness is the best indication of suicide risk (Beck et al. 1985; Malone et al. 1995b). During this "down time," the patient must be carefully monitored.

Clozapine reduces the suicide attempt and completion rates in schizophrenia and schizoaffective disorder (Meltzer 2001; Meltzer et al. 2003). The U.S. Food and Drug Administration (FDA) has approved clozapine for the treatment of recurrent suicidal behaviors in patients with schizophrenia or schizoaffective disorder.

Suicidal ideation, intent, and plan in selected patients with mood and psychotic disorders are indications for electroconvulsive therapy (ECT), especially when alternative treatments are not appropriate or have not been effective (American Psychiatric Association 2001). ECT should be the treatment of choice when rapid results are needed for the patient at high risk for suicide for whom a delay would be life-threatening. A rapid clinical response with reduction or resolution of suicidal behaviors often occurs with ECT, presumably by treating the underlying psychiatric disorder (Prudic and Sackheim 1999). A study by Kellner et al. (2005) showed that suicidal intent in depressed patients was rapidly relieved by ECT. The authors recommended that ECT be given earlier consideration rather than thought of as a last option.

There is little evidence that ECT imparts long-term beneficial effects on suicidal behaviors or completed suicide (Sharma 1999). Administration of inpatient ECT may be followed by outpatient maintenance ECT. The effectiveness ascribed to ECT can be difficult to distinguish from the coadministration of pharmacotherapy. As with any treatment, there is a certain percentage of patient nonresponders.

Baldessarini et al. (2001) asserted that the extensive use of antidepressant and antimanic treatments has not reduced the long-term rates of suicide or premature mortality from other causes of illness. For example, the suicide rate in the United States between 1901 (11.8 per 100,000) and 2000 (10.6 per 100,000) dropped by only 1.2 per 100,000 despite the availability of antidepressants and other treatments since the 1950s (Silverman 2003). Because 90%–95% of individuals who completed suicide were mentally ill before their deaths, psychiatric interventions have not substantially reduced the suicide rate over 99 years (Barraclough et al. 1974).

In contrast, Isacsson (2000) examined the overall suicide rates in Sweden from 1978 to 1996, determining that suicide rates decreased with increased antidepressant use. In a 22-year prospective study of patients hospitalized with mood disorders, long-term medication (antidepressants, lithium, and neuroleptics alone or in combination) significantly lowered the suicide rates, despite the fact that more severely ill patients were treated (Angst et al. 2002). G.E. Simon et al. (2006) reviewed the computerized health plan records of 65,103 patients with 82,285 episodes of antidepressant treatment between January 1, 1992, and June 30, 2003. They found that risk of suicide was not "significantly" higher in the months following initiation of antidepressant medications than in later months. The patients' risk of suicide was highest in the month prior to starting medication, declining steadily after they started antidepressant treatment.

The antidepressant treatment of depressed patients at risk for suicide is often inadequate. Thus, the ability to measure the antisuicidal efficacy of antidepressants in naturalistic studies is undermined (Oquendo et al. 2003). Whether psychopharmacological agents reduce the long-term risk of suicide remains inconclusive. It is a clinical reality, however, that improvements in the quality of life and the prevention of patient suicide attempts or completions result from treatment with antipsychotic, antimanic, and antidepressant drugs and ECT.

In 2004, the FDA began requiring black-box warnings of increased suicide risk for children and adolescents with major depressive disorders and other psychiatric disorders during the first few months of treatment with selective serotonin reuptake inhibitors (SSRIs). In 2005, the FDA issued similar warnings for adults treated with antidepressants. Hammad et al. (2006) reviewed all placebo-controlled trials submitted to the FDA, consisting of 4,582 patients in 24 trials. The trial periods ranged from 4 to 16 weeks. They found that the use of antidepressant medications is associated with a "modestly" increased risk of suicide.

The FDA has told manufacturers of antidepressants to issue stronger warnings on their labels regarding the monitoring of both pediatric and adult patients for the emergence of suicidal ideation and the worsening of depression. Precursors to worsening depression and suicidal ideation include symptoms of activation syndrome such as anxiety, agitation, panic attacks, insomnia, irritability, hostility, impulsivity, akathisia, hypomania, and mania. Psychiatrists should document the rationale, including risk–benefit assessments, for prescribing an antidepressant drug to a child or adolescent. At a minimum, FDA monitoring requirements should be followed. Hopelessness and suicide may be averted by informing all patients and the parents of children and adolescents that activation symptoms can be a drug reaction, a worsening of the psychiatric dis-

order, or some combination of both. Close follow-up by the clinician is indicated according to the clinical needs of the patient. The practitioner's clinical experience, the consensus experience of colleagues, and case reports in the psychiatric literature are important guides to prescribing drugs for children and adolescents. For further discussion of antidepressant use in children and adolescents, see Ash (2006) and Kim et al. (2006).

A study by Gibbons et al. (2007) demonstrated an association between decreased SSRI prescriptions for children and adolescents and increased suicide cases in this population in the United States and Finland. SSRIs continue to be considered the first-line treatment for depression with associated suicidal behaviors. While psychiatrists wait for further studies to definitively settle the question, the risks and benefits of SSRIs should be thoroughly explained (with documentation) to patients and their families, according to the current state of scientific knowledge.

The psychiatrist's clinical focus must necessarily be on treating the patient's current condition. Treatment of the patient's current episode of psychiatric illness is frequently successful in decreasing or eliminating the associated acute risk of suicide. Factors unrelated to the efficacy of psychiatric treatment also affect suicide mortality rates in the long run. For example, Ostamo and Lonnqvist (2001), in a 5-year follow-up study of patients treated in hospitals after suicide attempts, found an increase in mortality from suicide, homicide, and other causes. The nature of the patient, the efficacy of treatments, and the adherence and access to or availability of mental health resources are central to determining treatment outcomes.

Collaborative or Split Treatment

Assessment and management of patients at risk for suicide are especially challenging in collaborative or split-treatment arrangements. The hospital length of stay is brief for most psychiatric patients. Patients referred to partial hospitalization are discharged rapidly to outpatient split treatment.

The medication management of patients at risk for suicide who are in split treatment requires close monitoring. Psychiatrists owe a duty of care to their patients for the duration of their drug prescriptions. The patient may be given a 90-day prescription that can be mailed to a pharmacy. Such "mail-away" bulk prescriptions lower the cost of medication. In addition, the patient's copayment is reduced from once a month to once every 90 days. However, the prescription of large quantities of medications for patients at risk for suicide can be lethal. For example, a patient is prescribed 1,000 mg/day of an anticonvulsant mood stabilizer; 1,500 mg/day of lithium; 15 mg/day of an atypical antipsychotic; and 900 mg/day of sleep medication. A 90-day prescription or a 30-day prescription renewable three times gives the patient 90,000 mg of anticonvulsant mood stabilizer, 135,000 mg of lithium; 1,350 mg of an atypical antipsychotic, and 81,000 mg of sleep medication. Even a 30-day supply of these medications would be lethal. The potential lethality of the medications prescribed for the patient should be conveyed to the psychotherapist (Silk 2001).

Patients at risk for suicide commonly have more than one psychiatric diagnosis and often are taking several medications. If the patient is scheduled for a 15-minute medication check once every 30, 60, or 90 days, the risk for suicide may increase over this period. The psychiatrist must rely on the psychotherapist's assessment and management of suicide risk during the 90-day period. The "we are in this together" part of split treatment is negated unless frequent communication between psychiatrist and therapist is maintained according to the clinical needs of the patient. Close monitoring of patients at risk for suicide who are taking potentially lethal amounts of medication should be standard psychiatric practice (R.I. Simon 2004).

Safety Management

In the safety management of suicidal patients, the tension between providing safety and allowing freedom of movement creates uncertainty (R.I. Simon 2006). Clinicians also experience dissonance between the need to provide adequate supervision for patients at suicidal risk and the denial of insurance coverage by third-party payers for these services. As noted earlier, the only certainty is that effective treatment and safety management of the suicidal patient require the clinician's full commitment of time and effort.

Systematic suicide risk assessment informs the safety management of patients at risk for suicide. Patients who are determined to commit suicide will find a way (Fawcett et al. 2003). Fawcett et al. (2003), in a review of 76 inpatient suicides, found that 42 of these patients were on 15-minute checks. Nine percent of patients were on one-to-one observation or with a staff member at the time of suicide. Deception and lack of patient cooperation complicate safety assessments.

Gun safety management may be necessary. The psychiatrist usually asks a responsible family member to remove and secure guns and ammunition outside the home. Guns may also be kept by the suicidal patient in his or her car or office or at another location. The psychiatrist must receive a timely call-back from the responsible person confirming that the guns and ammunition have been removed and separately secured according to plan. A call-back is essential. The complex subject of gun safety management is discussed in detail elsewhere (R.I. Simon 2007).

Outpatients

The ability to exercise control over outpatients at suicide risk, including those attending partial hospitalization programs, is limited. In outpatient settings, patient safety is usually managed by clinical intervention such as increasing the frequency of visits, strengthening the therapeutic alliance, providing or adjusting medications, and involving family or other concerned persons in the treatment, if the patient permits. Voluntary or, if necessary, involuntary hospitalization remains an option for suicidal patients at high suicide risk who can no longer be safely treated as outpatients. In the managed care era, most suicidal patients at moderate suicide risk and even some patients at high risk are treated in outpatient settings.

Whether to hospitalize a patient can be a trying decision for the clinician. The decision is considerably more complicated when the need for hospitalization is clear but the patient refuses. The action that the clinician takes at this point is critical for the patient's treatment and for risk management.

The clinician, after systematic suicide risk assessment, may determine that the suicidal patient requires hospitalization. The risks and benefits of continuing outpatient treatment are weighed against the risks and benefits of hospitalization, and these are shared with the patient. If the patient agrees, arrangements for immediate hospitalization are made. The patient must go *directly* to the hospital, accompanied by a responsible person. The patient should not stop to do errands, get clothing, or make last-minute arrangements. A detour can provide the patient with the opportunity to attempt or to complete suicide. If the patient is driven to the hospital, an additional passenger may be needed to prevent the patient from jumping out of the car. In some cases, clinicians have accompanied the patient to the hospital. The clinician, however, has no legal duty to assume physical custody of the patient (Farwell v. Un 1990).

Involuntary Hospitalization

If the patient rejects the clinician's recommendation for hospitalization, the matter is immediately addressed as a treatment issue. Because the need for hospitalization is acute, a prolonged inquiry into the patient's reasons for rejecting the recommendation for hospitalization is not feasible. Furthermore, the therapeutic alliance may be strained. Consultation and referral are options for the clinician to consider, if time and the patient's condition permit. It is this situation that tries the professional and personal mettle of the clinician.

The failure to involuntarily hospitalize a patient judged to be at high risk for suicide who subsequently attempts or completes suicide may result in a malpractice suit against the clinician. The uncompensated time required, the inconvenience, the disruption of the clinician's schedule, the possibility of a court appearance, and the fear of a lawsuit by the patient may dissuade the clinician from initiating involuntary hospitalization. State commitment statutes grant clinicians immunity from liability when they use reasonable judgment, follow statutory commitment procedures, and act in good faith.

Documenting suicide risk assessment and the rationale for involuntary hospitalization represents good clinical care and provides sound risk management. When involuntary hospitalization is sought on reasonable clinical grounds, it must be left to the courts to resolve uncertainty about commitment. The clinician's proper focus is the patient's treatment and safety.

Inpatients

There must be a rational nexus between patient autonomy in the hospital setting and the patient's diagnosis, treatment, and safety needs. With patients at risk for suicide, standard safety precautions must be observed where indicated, such as removal of shoelaces, belts, sharps, glass products, and even pillowcases that can be used for suffocation and other potentially lethal instruments. A thorough search for contraband is standard procedure on admission. Psychiatric units are usually fitted, at a minimum, with non-weight-bearing fixtures and shower curtain rods, very short cords for electrical beds (properly insulated), cordless telephones or telephones with safety cords, jump-proof windows, barricade-proof doors, and closed-circuit video cameras. The most common and available method of committing suicide by inpatients is strangulation, usually accomplished by a belt, articles of clothing, shoelaces, or a bed sheet hooked up to the patient's bed, door, or bathroom fixtures. Safe installation of plumbing pipes for toilets and use of solid ceilings are necessary to diminish the risk of hanging. The most dangerous place on the psychiatric unit is the patient's room, especially the bathroom. Seclusion rooms should have windows or audiovisual surveillance capability (Lieberman et al. 2004).

Determining safety precautions is complicated by court directives that require highly disturbed patients to be treated by the least restrictive means (R.I. Simon 2000). In *Johnson v. United States* (1976), the Court noted that an "open-door" policy creates a higher potential for danger. The Court went on to say:

> Modern psychiatry has recognized the importance of making every effort to return a patient to an active and productive life. Thus, the patient is encouraged to develop his self-confidence by adjusting to the demands of everyday existence. Particularly because the prediction of danger is difficult, undue reliance on hospitalization might lead to prolonged incarceration of potentially useful members of society.

The tension between promoting individual freedom and preventing self-injury introduces an inherent uncertainty in the safety management of suicidal patients (Amchin et al. 1990). In malpractice suits, the individual facts of the case and the reasonableness of the staff's application of the open-door policy are determinative.

Suicide Prevention Contracts

The suicide prevention contract has achieved wide acceptance, although no studies demonstrate that it is effective in preventing suicide (Stanford et al. 1994). The suicide prevention contract can increase patients' risk of suicide when used in place of adequate suicide risk assessments. Suicide risk assessment is a *process*, whereas contracts tend to be *events*. The suicide prevention contract goes by a variety of names, such as the "no-harm contract," the "no-suicide contract," or the "contract for safety." It is frequently used by mental health professionals in outpatient and inpatient settings and in hospital emergency departments. In managed care settings, a criterion for admission to an inpatient unit may be based on a patient's refusal to sign a suicide prevention contract. If the patient is willing to sign a no-harm contract, third-party payers may not authorize admission. Suicide prevention contracts are frequently used in nursing assessments (Egan 1997).

A suicide prevention contract is a clinical, not a legal, contract. It is a mutual understanding reached between the clinician and the patient regarding collaboration to prevent suicide. The trustworthiness of the arrangement is contingent upon many variables. The contract establishes that the patient is at risk of suicide but does not establish that suicide risk has been assessed.

With the advent of the managed care era, mental health professionals have come to rely on suicide prevention contracts to manage patient risk for suicide (R.I. Simon 1999). In both outpatient and inpatient settings, patients are treated only briefly. The average length of stay for patients in acute care psychiatric units and hospitals is often less than 5 days. Only severely mentally ill patients who are at high risk for suicide are admitted. The admission requirements usually exceed substantive criteria for involuntary hospitalization. Suicide prevention contracts provide only an illusion of safety for newly admitted high-risk patients.

The therapeutic alliance often fails to develop in managed care settings because of limitations on treatment sessions and an increased reliance on medications. Empathic interaction, pivotal to the development of a therapeutic alliance, is difficult to maintain in inpatient or outpatient settings where a large volume of mentally ill patients are rapidly treated, stabilized, and discharged. Yet these settings are precisely where such contracts are heavily utilized.

Suicide prevention measures work best when a therapeutic alliance exists between the psychiatrist and patient. The therapeutic alliance is a dynamic, changeable interaction between the clinician and the patient that is influenced by the course of the patient's illness as well as situational and other factors. The therapeutic alliance that supports a patient's safety during one session may dissipate before a next scheduled session due to an acute exacerbation of the illness. The status of the therapeutic alliance should be assessed regularly and documented. The presence or absence of a therapeutic alliance can be a key preventive or suicide risk factor.

Health care decision-making capacity, the foundation for the patient's ability to cooperate with a suicide prevention contract or plan, often varies with the patient's clinical course. Mental capacity should be assessed as necessary and documented. The existence and terms of agreement (including time limit) of the suicide prevention contract or plan also require documentation. If suicide prevention contracts are used, mental health personnel should be trained in their appropriate use (Chiles and Strosahl 2005).

Suicide Aftermath

Suicide aftermath presents the clinician with conflicting tensions between maintaining patient confidentiality, providing support to the suicide survivors, and implementing risk management principles that limit liability exposure. After a patient's death, the duty to maintain confidentiality of the patient's record continues unless a court decision or statute provides otherwise. Careful documentation and maintenance of confidentiality of the patient's records provide a sound defense in malpractice litigation, in administrative hearings, and in ethics proceedings.

Gutheil recommends family outreach by the clinician as crucial for devastated family members following a patient's suicide (T.G. Gutheil, personal communication, October 1989). This recommendation, which is based primarily on humanitarian concerns for survivors, has important risk management implications. Gutheil pointed out that "bad feelings" combined with a bad outcome often lead to litigation. The persons who lived with the patient before the suicide not only experience intense emotional pain currently but also shared it with the patient before death. Some lawsuits are filed because of the clinician's refusal to express, in some way, feelings of condolence, sympathy, and regret for the patient's death.

In Massachusetts, an "apology statute" exists that renders various benevolent human expressions such as condolences, regrets, and apologies "inadmissible as evidence of an admission of liability in a civil action" (Mass. Gen. Laws 1986). Slovenko (2002) noted that Texas and California enacted legislation similar to that in Massachusetts. The highest courts of Georgia and Vermont provided apology protection by judicial opinions in 1992. Regehr and Gutheil (2002) stated that "the current empirical evidence is insufficiently solid to support the proposition that apology by oppressors, perpetrators, and a defendant is a panacea leading to healing of trauma under all circumstances" (pp. 429–430).

A fine line exists between a psychiatrist's apology and the perception by others that fault is being admitted. Admissions of wrongdoing may void insurance coverage (Slovenko 2002). Moreover, another party may be found ultimately at fault in litigation, not the psychiatrist. A skillful lawyer may take feelings of genuine sympathy and turn them against the psychiatrist as an admission of fault. To say "I am sorry" is certainly the appropriate human response, but in a litigation context, it may backfire. The psychiatrist must be guided by good judgment, not by guilt-driven feelings or masochistic impulses.

Attorneys advise psychiatrists variously about suicide aftercare. Following a bad outcome, some attorneys recommend that the case be sealed and no communication be established with the family. Other attorneys encourage judicious communication, consultation, or even treatment of family members. The treatment of family members by the psychiatrist who also treated the patient before his or her suicide is ill advised and likely doomed from the start by insurmountable transference and countertransference reactions. The family should be referred elsewhere for treatment. In meeting with family members, the psychiatrist should focus on addressing the feelings of family members rather than the specifics of the patient's care.

Suicide aftercare is similar to any other grief-related therapy or consultation. The value of such consultation in healing grief is important enough for clinicians to consider providing humanitarian support to the survivors of patient suicide. The clinician may justifiably worry that contact with survivors of suicide will increase the risk of a lawsuit. Outreach to survivors of patient suicides should not be undertaken primarily for risk management purposes. No easy answers exist for managing the complex and often conflicting tensions between suicide aftercare and risk management.

Psychiatrist reactions to a patient's suicide often include shame, guilt, anger, avoidance behaviors, intrusive thoughts, questioning of one's competency, and litigation fears (Gitlin 1999; Hendin et al. 2000). The American Association of Suicidology's Clinician Task Force makes available a number of resources to clinicians who have had patients complete suicide (see http://www.suicidology.org).

Risk Management

Risk management is a reality of psychiatric practice, especially in the assessment and management of patients at risk for suicide. Many risk management guidelines are derived from malpractice cases, often recommending *ideal* or *best* liability prevention practices. The actual standard of care required of a psychiatrist is the skill and care "ordinarily provided" or reasonable, prudent care. These standards can be confused by expert witnesses who testify in malpractice cases (R.I. Simon 2005). Moreover, suicide cases are fact specific, challenging, multifaceted, and nuanced, making it difficult to provide precise assessment and management guidelines. Although most risk management guidelines commonly set forth best practices, clinical risk management is embedded in the provision of sound clinical care and the use of common sense.

Clinically based risk management is patient cen-

TABLE 43–5. Basic elements of clinically based risk management

Patient centered

Supports treatment and the therapeutic alliance

Working knowledge of legal regulation of psychiatry

Clinical management of psychiatric–legal issues

Wellness, not legal agenda

"First do no harm" ethic

Consultation, "never worry alone"

Source. Adapted from Simon RI: *Assessing and Managing Suicide Risk: Guidelines for Clinically Based Risk Management.* Arlington, VA, American Psychiatric Publishing, 2004, p. 19.

tered. It supports the treatment process and the therapeutic alliance (Table 43–5). At a minimum, it follows the fundamental ethical principle in medicine of "first do no harm." A working knowledge of the legal regulation of psychiatry enables the psychiatrist to manage clinical-legal issues more effectively. Clinically based risk management provides the psychiatrist with a significant measure of practice comfort that permits continued maintenance of the treatment role with patients at risk for suicide.

Performing systematic suicide risk assessments that inform treatment and management interventions is good clinical care and, secondarily, sound clinically based risk management. Documentation of the risk assessments supports good patient care and substantiates clinical judgment (American Psychiatric Association 2003). The argument can be made in court by plaintiff's counsel that a suicide risk assessment that was not documented was not performed. Documentation of suicide risk assessments can be done efficiently (Table 43–6). Important clinical assessments require documentation. It is worth repeating that good care of patients at suicidal risk requires the clinician's full commitment to the patient's evaluation, treatment, and management. The clinical imperative holds true as well in collaborative treatment relationships with other mental health professionals.

Risk management practices that are not clinically tempered and patient centered can interfere with the patient's treatment and undermine the therapeutic alliance. They are undertaken to avoid malpractice liability or to provide a legal defense against a malpractice claim. For example, an undue reliance on suicide prevention contracts may be the result of the clinician's attempt to reduce the anxiety associated with

TABLE 43–6. Sample suicide risk assessment note: contents

Suicide risk factors assessed and weighed (low, moderate, high)

Protective factors assessed and weighed (low, moderate, high)

Overall assessment rating (low, moderate, high, or range)

Treatment and management intervention informed by the assessment

Effectiveness of interventions evaluated

Source. Reprinted from Simon RI: "Suicide Risk: Assessing the Unpredictable," in *The American Psychiatric Publishing Textbook of Suicide Assessment and Management.* Edited by Simon RI, Hales RE. Arlington, VA, American Psychiatric Publishing, 2006, p. 25.

treating suicidal patients (Miller et al. 1998). Some mental health professionals erroneously believe that the suicide prevention contract provides a legal defense or legally binds the patient to refrain from self-harm. A suicide prevention contract does not provide a legal defense if the patient attempts or completes suicide and the clinician is sued. The contrary is true. Suicide prevention contracts may falsely reassure the clinician, preempting adequate suicide risk assessment and increasing the patient's risk for suicide (R.I. Simon 2004).

Defensive psychiatry can be divided into preemptive and avoidant practices (R.I. Simon 1985). Deviant preemptive defensive practices utilize procedures and treatments designed to prevent or limit liability—for example, unnecessarily hospitalizing a patient at moderate risk for suicide who could effectively and safely be treated as an outpatient with careful monitoring. Errant avoidant defensive practices forgo clinically indicated procedures or treatments for fear of being sued, even though the patient will likely benefit from these interventions. An example of avoidant defensiveness is failing to prescribe an SSRI to an adolescent patient with recurrent depression, despite the fact that the drug was effective in resolving an earlier depression. The fear of legal liability should not be allowed to paralyze clinical judgment.

Consulting with a colleague is good clinical practice when the clinician is confronted with complex diagnostic, treatment, and management issues. As a clinically based risk management technique, consultation also supports and guides good clinical care by providing "a biopsy" of the standard of care. The clinician's uncertainty, even anxiety, must be contained within reasonable limits to effectively treat the suicidal patient. The clinician should "never worry alone" (T.G. Gutheil, personal communication, December 2002). In some instances, consulting with a risk manager or an attorney may be necessary when managing difficult clinical-legal dilemmas. Clinically based risk management helps the psychiatrist avoid defensive practices that are harmful to both the patient at risk for suicide and the clinician. The focus must be trained on providing good care, but at the same time, the clinician should carry good malpractice insurance.

Conclusion

Suicide risk assessment is a core competency. Systematic suicide risk assessment identifies risk and protective factors that inform the patient's treatment and management. Suicide risk factors must be aggressively treated and protective factors rapidly mobilized. The treatment and management of the suicidal patient require the clinician's full commitment of time and effort.

Patient suicides are an occupational hazard of clinical practice. The psychiatrist should carry comprehensive malpractice insurance from an established professional liability insurer.

Key Points

- Systematic suicide risk assessment informs treatment and management for patients at risk for suicide. It is secondarily a risk management technique.

- Treatable and modifiable acute suicide risk factors should be identified early and treated aggressively.

- Systematic suicide assessment identifies and weights the clinical importance of both risk and preventive factors.

- Suicide risk assessment is a process, not an event. Psychiatric inpatients should have suicide risk assessments conducted at admission and discharge and at other important clinical junctures during treatment.

- Suicide prevention contracts must not take the place of conducting systematic suicide risk assessments.

- Contemporaneous documentation of suicide risk assessments is good clinical care and standard practice.

- Systematic suicide risk assessment performed at the time of discharge informs the patient's postdischarge plan.

- During the treatment of patients at significant risk for suicide, it may be necessary to contact family members or others to facilitate hospitalization, to mobilize support, and to acquire information of clinical importance to the clinician. Whenever possible, this should be done with the patient's permission.

- Suicide risk assessment is the responsibility of the psychiatrist. It should not be delegated to others.

- The treatment and management of the patient at risk for suicide require the clinician's full commitment of time and effort, despite denial of services and cost containment policies of third-party payers.

Suggested Readings

American Academy of Child and Adolescent Psychiatry: Summary of the practice parameters for the assessment and treatment of children and adolescents with suicidal behaviors. J Am Acad Child Adolesc Psychiatry 40:495–499, 2001

American Psychiatric Association: Practice guidelines for the assessment and treatment of patients with suicidal behaviors. Am J Psychiatry 160 (suppl):1–60, 2003

Berman AL, Jobes DA, Silverman M: Adolescent Suicide: Assessment and Intervention, 2nd Edition. Washington, DC, American Psychological Association, 2006

Chiles JA, Strosahl KD: Clinical Manual for Assessment and Treatment of Suicidal Patients. Arlington, VA, American Psychiatric Publishing, 2006

Goldsmith SK, Pellman TC, Kleinman AM, et al. (eds): Reducing Suicide: A National Imperative. Washington, DC, National Academies Press, 2001

Rudd MD, Joiner T, Rajab MH: Treating Suicidal Behavior: An Effective, Time-Limited Approach. New York, Guilford, 2001

Shea SC: The delicate art of eliciting suicidal ideation. Psychiatr Ann 34:385–400, 2004

Simon RI: Assessing and Managing Suicide Risk: Guidelines for Clinically Based Risk Management. Washington, DC, American Psychiatric Publishing, 2004

Simon RI, Hales RE (eds): Textbook of Suicide Assessment and Management. Washington, DC, American Psychiatric Publishing, 2006

References

Amchin J, Wettstein RM, Roth LH: Suicide, ethics, and the law, in Suicide Over the Life Cycle. Edited by Blumenthal SJ, Kupfer DJ. Washington, DC, American Psychiatric Press, 1990, pp 637–663

American Academy of Child and Adolescent Psychiatry: Practice parameter for the assessment and treatment of children and adolescents with suicidal behavior. J Am Acad Child Adolesc Psychiatry 40 (7 suppl):24S–51S, 2001a

American Academy of Child and Adolescent Psychiatry: Summary of the practice parameters for the assessment and treatment of children and adolescents with suicidal behaviors. J Am Acad Child Adolesc Psychiatry 40:495–499, 2001b

American Association of Suicidology: Suicide Statistics Archive 1996–2002. Available at: http://www.suicideinfo.ca/csp/90/aspx. Accessed February 5, 2006.

American Psychiatric Association: Practice Guideline for the Treatment of Patients with HIV/AIDS. Washington, DC, American Psychiatric Association, 2000

American Psychiatric Association: The Practice of Electroconvulsive Therapy: Recommendations for Treatment, Training, and Privileging. A Task Force Report of the American Psychiatric Association, 2nd Edition. Edited by Weiner RD. Washington, DC, American Psychiatric Association, 2001

American Psychiatric Association: Practice guidelines for the assessment and treatment of patients with suicidal behaviors. Am J Psychiatry 160 (suppl):1–60, 2003

Angst F, Stassen HH, Clayton PJ, et al: Mortality of patients with mood disorders: follow-up over 34–38 years. J Affect Disord 68:167–181, 2002

Ash P: Children and adolescents, in The American Psychiatric Publishing Textbook of Suicide Assessment and Management. Edited by Simon RI, Hales RE. Washington, DC, American Psychiatric Publishing, 2006, pp 35–56

Baldessarini RJ: Lithium effects on depression and suicide. J Clin Psychiatry (visuals), January 2003

Baldessarini RJ, Tondo L, Henner J: Treating the suicidal patient with bipolar disorder: reducing suicide risk with lithium. Ann NY Acad Sci 932:24–38, 2001

Barraclough B, Bunch J, Nelson B, et al: A hundred cases of suicide: clinical aspects. Br J Psychiatry 125:355–373, 1974

Bateman AW, Fonagy P: Psychotherapy for Borderline Personality Disorder: Mentalization-Based Treatment. Oxford, England, Oxford University Press, 2000

Bateman AW, Fonagy P: Mentalization-based treatment of BPD. J Personal Disord 18:36–51, 2004

Beck AT, Steer RA, Kovacs M, et al: Hopelessness and eventual suicide: a 10-year prospective study of patients hospitalized with suicidal ideation. Am J Psychiatry 142:559–562, 1985

Beck AT, Brown G, Berchick RJ, et al: Relationship between hopelessness and ultimate suicide: a replication with psychiatric outpatients. Am J Psychiatry 147:190–195, 1990

Beck AT, Steer RA, Ranieri WF: Scale for suicidal ideation: psychometric properties of a self-report version. J Clin Psychol 44:499–505, 1998

Bongar B, Maris RW, Bertram AL, et al: Outpatient standards of care and the suicidal patient. Suicide Life Threat Behav 22:453–478, 1992

Brent DA: Assessment and treatment of the youthful suicidal patient. Ann NY Acad Sci 932:106–131, 2001

Brent DA, Bridge J, Johnson BA, et al: Suicidal behavior runs in families. Arch Gen Psychiatry 53:1145–1152, 1996

Brent DA, Oquendo M, Birmaher B, et al: Familial pathways to early onset suicide attempt. Arch Gen Psychiatry 59:801–807, 2002

Brodsky BS, Malone KM, Ellis SP, et al: Characteristics of borderline personality disorder associated with suicidal behavior. Am J Psychiatry 154:1715–1719, 1997

Brown GK, Ten Have T, Henriques GR, et al: Cognitive therapy for the prevention of suicide attempts. JAMA 294:536–570, 2005

Busch KA, Clark DC, Fawcett J, et al: Clinical features of inpatient suicide. Psychiatr Ann 23:256–262, 1993

Chiles JA, Strosahl KD: Clinical Manual for Assessment and Treatment of Suicidal Patients. Washington, DC, American Psychiatric Publishing, 2005

Clark DC, Fawcett J: An empirically based model of suicide risk assessment of patients with affective disorders, in Suicide and Clinical Practice. Edited by Jacobs DJ. Washington, DC, American Psychiatric Association, 1999, pp 55–73

Conwell Y, Duberstein PR: Suicide in elders. Ann NY Acad Sci 932:132–150, 2001

Dervic K, Oquendo MA, Grunebaum MF, et al: Religious affiliation and suicide attempt. Am J Psychiatry 161:2303–2308, 2004

Dube SR, Anda RF, Felitti VJ, et al: Childhood abuse, household dysfunction and the risk of attempted suicide throughout the lifespan: findings from the Adverse Childhood Experiences Study. JAMA 286:3089–3096, 2001

Duberstein P, Conwell Y: Personality disorders and completed suicide: a methodological and conceptual review. Clinical Psychology: Science and Practice 4:359–376, 1997

Egan MP: Contracting for safety: a concept analysis. Crisis 18:23, 1997

Farwell v. Un, 902 F.2d 282 (4th Cir. 1990)

Fawcett J: Treating impulsivity and anxiety in the suicidal patient. Ann NY Acad Sci 932:94–105, 2001

Fawcett J, Scheftner WA, Fogg L, et al: Time-related predictors of suicide in major affective disorder. Am J Psychiatry 147:1189–1194, 1990

Fawcett J, Clark DC, Busch KA: Assessing and treating the patient at suicide risk. Psychiatr Ann 23:244–255, 1993

Fawcett J, Busch KA, Jacobs DG: Clinical correlates of inpatient suicide. J Clin Psychiatry 64:14–19, 2003

Gabbard GO, Allison SE: Psychodynamic treatment, in The American Psychiatric Publishing Textbook of Suicide Assessment and Management. Edited by Simon RI, Hales RE. Washington, DC, American Psychiatric Publishing, 2006, pp 221–234

Gelenberg AJ, Chesen CL: How fast are antidepressants? J Clin Psychiatry 61:712–721, 2000

Gibbons RD, Brown CH, Hur K, et al: Early evidence on the effects of regulators' suicidality warnings on SSRI prescriptions and suicide in children and adolescents. Am J Psychiatry 164:1356–1363, 2007

Gitlin MJ: A psychiatrist's reaction to a patient's suicide (clinical case conference). Am J Psychiatry 156:1630–1634, 1999

Goldsmith SK, Pellman TC, Kleinman AM, et al (eds): Reducing Suicide: A National Imperative. Washington, DC, National Academies Press, 2001

Guthrie E, Kapur N, Mackway-Jones K, et al: Randomized controlled trial of brief psychological intervention after deliberate self-poisoning. BMJ 323:135–138, 2001

Guthrie E, Kapur N, Mackway-Jones K, et al: Predictors of outcome following brief psychodynamic-interpersonal therapy deliberate self-poisoning. Aust N Z J Psychiatry 37:532–536, 2003

Hall RC, Platt DE, Hall RC: Suicide risk assessment: a review of risk factors for suicide in 100 patients who made severe suicide attempts: evaluation of suicide risk in a time of managed care. Psychosomatics 40:18–27, 1999

Hammad TA, Laughren T, Raloosin J: Suicidality in pediatric patients treated with antidepressant drugs. Arch Gen Psychiatry 63:332–339, 2006

Harris CE, Barraclough B: Suicide as an outcome for mental disorders. Br J Psychiatry 170:205–228, 1997

Hawton K, Townsend E, Arensman E, et al: Psychosocial and pharmacological treatments for deliberate self-harm. Cochrane Database Syst Rev (2):CD001764, 2005

Heikkinen ME, Henriksson MM, Erkki T, et al: Recent life events and suicide in personality disorders. J Nerv Ment Dis 185:373–381, 1997

Hendin H, Lipschitz A, Maltsberger JT, et al: Therapists' reactions to patients' suicides. Am J Psychiatry 157:2022–2027, 2000

Isacsson G: Suicide prevention: a medical breakthrough? Acta Psychiatr Scand 102:113–117, 2000

Isometsa ET, Lonnqvist JK: Suicide attempts preceding completed suicide. Br J Psychiatry 173:531–535, 1998

Isometsa ET, Heikkinen ME, Martunen MJ, et al: The last appointment before suicide: is suicide intent communicated? Am J Psychiatry 152:919–922, 1995

Isometsa ET, Henriksson ME, Heikkinen ME, et al: Suicide among subjects with personality disorders. Am J Psychiatry 153:667–673, 1996

Jacobs DG, Brewer M, Klein-Benheim M: Suicide assessment: an overview and recommended protocol, in Guide to Suicide Assessment and Intervention. Edited by Jacobs DJ. San Francisco, CA, Jossey-Bass, 1999, pp 3–39

Johnson v. United States, 409 F.Supp. 1283 (M.D. Fla. 1976); revised, 576 F.2d 606 (5th Cir. 1978); cert denied, 451 U.S. 1019 (1981)

Kaplan M, Asnis GM, Lipschitz DS, et al: Suicidal behavior and abuse in psychiatric outpatients. Compr Psychiatry 36:229–235, 1995

Kellner CH, Fink M, Knapp R, et al: Relief of expressed suicidal intent by ECT: a consortium of research in ECT study. Am J Psychiatry 162:977–982, 2005

Kessing LV: Subtypes of depressive episodes according to ICD-10: prediction of risk of relapse and suicide. Psychopathology 36:285–291, 2003

Kessler RC, Borges G, Walters EE: Prevalence of and risk factors for lifetime suicide attempts in the National Comorbidity Survey. Arch Gen Psychiatry 55:617–626, 1999

Kim HF, Marangell LB, Yudofsky SC: Pharmacological treatment and electroconvulsive therapy, in The American Psychiatric Publishing Textbook of Suicide and Management. Edited by Simon RI, Hales RE. Washington, DC, American Psychiatric Publishing, 2006, pp 199–220

Lieberman DZ, Resnik HLP, Holder-Perkins V: Environmental risk factors in hospital suicide. Suicide Life Threat Behav 34:448–453, 2004

Linehan MM: Cognitive Behavioral Treatment of Borderline Personality Disorder. New York, Guilford, 1993

Linehan MM, Goodstein JL, Nielsen SL, et al: Reasons for staying alive when you are thinking of killing yourself: the Reasons for Living Inventory. J Consult Clin Psychol 51:276–286, 1983

Linehan MM, Comtois KA, Murray AM, et al: Two-year randomized controlled trial and follow-up of dialectical behavior therapy vs therapy by experts for suicidal behaviors and borderline personality disorder. Arch Gen Psychiatry 63:757–766, 2006

Loebel JP: Completed suicide in late life. Psychiatr Serv 56:260–262, 2005

Malone KM, Haas GL, Sweeney JA, et al: Major depression and the risk of attempted suicide. J Affect Disord 34:173–185–1995a

Malone KM, Szanto K, Corbitt EM, et al: Clinical assessment versus research methods in the assessment of suicidal behavior. Am J Psychiatry 152:1601–1607, 1995b

Mann JJ, Waternaux C, Haas GL, et al: Toward a clinical model of suicidal behavior in psychiatric patients. Am J Psychiatry 156:181–189, 1999

Mann JJ, Brent DA, Arango V: The neurobiology and genetics of suicide and suicide attempts: a focus on the serotonergic system. Neuropsychopharmacology 24:467–477, 2001

Marzuk PM, Tardiff K, Leon AC, et al: HIV seroprevalence among suicide victims in New York City, 1991–1993. Am J Psychiatry 154:1720–1725, 1997

Mass. Gen. Laws, Ch. 233, Sec 23D (1986)

Mays D: Structured assessment methods may improve suicide prevention. Psychiatr Ann 34:367–372, 2004

Meltzer HY: Treatment of suicidality in schizophrenia. Ann NY Acad Sci 932:44–58, 2001

Meltzer HY, Alphs L, Green AI, et al: Clozapine treatment for suicidality in schizophrenia. Arch Gen Psychiatry 60:82–91, 2003

Metzner JL, Hayes LM: Suicide prevention in jails and prisons, in The American Psychiatric Publishing Textbook of Suicide Assessment and Management. Edited by Simon RI, Hales RE. Washington, DC, American Psychiatric Publishing, 2006, pp 139–156

Miller MC, Jacobs, DG, Gutheil TG: Talisman or taboo: the controversy of the suicide prevention contract. Harv Rev Psychiatry 6:78–87, 1998

Monahan J, Steadman HJ: Violent storms and violent people: how meteorology can inform risk communication in mental health law. Am J Psychol 51:931–938, 1996

Murphy GE, Wetzel RD, Robins E, et al: Multiple risk factors predict suicide in alcoholism. Arch Gen Psychiatry 49:459–462, 1992

National Center for Injury Prevention and Control: Suicide fact sheet. Available at: http://www.cdc.gov/ncipc/factsheets/suifacts.htm. Accessed February 5, 2006.

Oquendo MA, Halberstam, Mann JJ: Risk factors for suicidal behavior: the utility and limitation of research instruments, in Standardized Evaluation in Clinical Practice. Edited by First MB (Review of Psychiatry Series, Vol 22; Oldham JM and Riba MB, series eds). Washington, DC, American Psychiatric Publishing, 2003, pp 103–130

Ostamo A, Lonnqvist J: Excess mortality of suicide attempters. Soc Psychiatry Psychiatr Epidemiol 36:29–35, 2001

Palmer BA, Pankratz S, Bostwick JM: The lifetime risk of suicide in schizophrenia. Arch Gen Psychiatry 62:247–253, 2005

Pokorny AD: Predictions of suicide in psychiatric patients: report of a prospective study. Arch Gen Psychiatry 40:249–257, 1983

Pokorny AD: Suicide prediction revisited. Suicide Life Threat Behav 23:1–10, 1993

Prudic J, Sackheim H: Electroconvulsive therapy and suicide risk. J Clin Psychiatry 60 (suppl):104–110, 1999

Radomsky ED, Haas GL, Mann JJ, et al: Suicidal behavior in patients with schizophrenia and other psychotic disorders. Am J Psychiatry 156:1590–1595, 1999

Regehr C, Gutheil TG: Apology, justice and trauma recovery. J Am Acad Psychiatry Law 30:425–429, 2002

Resnick PJ: Recognizing that the suicidal patient views you as an adversary. Current Psychiatry 1:8, 2002

Robins E: The Final Months: Study of the Lives of 134 Persons Who Committed Suicide. New York, Oxford University Press, 1981

Rudd MD, Joiner T, Rajab MH: Treating Suicidal Behavior: An Effective, Time-Limited Approach. New York, Guilford, 2001

Sareen J, Cox BJ, Afifi TO, et al: Anxiety disorders and risk for suicidal ideation and suicide attempts: a population-based longitudinal study of adults. Arch Gen Psychiatry 62:1249–1257, 2005

Scheiber SC, Kramer TSM, Adamowski SE: Core Competence for Psychiatric Practice: What Clinicians Need to Know. Washington, DC, American Psychiatric Publishing, 2003

Schulsinger F, Kety SS, Rosenthal D, et al: A family study of suicide, in Origins, Prevention and Treatment of Affective Disorders. Edited by Schou M, Stromgen F. London, England, Academic Press, 1979, pp 277–287

Sharma V: Retrospective controlled study of inpatient ECT: does it prevent suicide? J Affect Disord 56:183–187, 1999

Shea SC: The delicate art of eliciting suicidal ideation. Psychiatr Ann 34:385–400, 2004

Silk K: Split (collaborative) treatment for patients with personality disorders. Psychiatr Ann 31:615–622, 2001

Silverman MM: Understanding suicide in the 21st century. Preventing Suicide: The National Journal 2(2), March/April 2003

Simon GE, Savarino J, Opersklaski B, et al: Suicide risk during antidepressant treatment. Am J Psychiatry 163:41–47, 2006

Simon RI: Coping strategies for the "unduly" defensive psychiatrist. Int J Med Law 4:551–561, 1985

Simon RI: Clinical Psychiatry and the Law, 2nd Edition. Washington, DC, American Psychiatric Press, 1992

Simon RI: The suicidal patient, in The Mental Health Practitioner and the Law: A Comprehensive Handbook. Edited by Lifson LE, Simon RI. Cambridge, MA, Harvard University Press, 1998, pp 329–343

Simon RI: The suicide prevention contract: clinical, legal and risk management issues. J Am Acad Psychiatry Law 27:445–450, 1999

Simon RI: Taking the "sue" out of suicide: a forensic psychiatrist's perspective. Psychiatr Ann 30:399–4071, 2000

Simon RI: Suicide risk assessment: what is the standard of care? J Am Acad Psychiatry Law 30:340–344, 2002

Simon RI: Assessing and Managing Suicide Risk: Guidelines for Clinically Based Risk Management. Washington, DC, American Psychiatric Publishing, 2004

Simon RI: Best practices or reasonable care? J Am Acad Psychiatry Law 33:8–11, 2005

Simon RI: Patient safety versus freedom of movement: coping with uncertainty, in The American Psychiatric Publishing Textbook of Suicide Assessment and Management. Edited by Simon RI, Hales RE. Washington, DC, American Psychiatric Publishing, 2006, pp 423–439

Simon RI: Gun safety management with patients at risk for suicide. Suicide Life Threat Behav 37:518–526, 2007

Simon RI, Shuman DW: The standard of care in suicide risk assessment: an elusive concept. CNS Spectr 11:442–445, 2006

Stanford EJ, Goetz RR, Bloom JD: The no harm contract in the emergency assessment of suicidal risk. J Clin Psychiatry 55:344–348, 1994

Slovenko R: Psychiatry in Law/Law in Psychiatry. New York, Brunner-Routledge, 2002

Trémeau F, Staner L, Duval F, et al: Suicide attempts and family history of suicide in three psychiatric populations. Suicide Life Threat Behav 35:702–713, 2005

Warman DM, Forman E, Henriques GR, et al: Suicidality and psychosis: beyond depression and hopelessness. Suicide Life Threat Behav 34:77–86, 2004

Wintemute GJ, Parham CA, Beaumont JJ, et al: Mortality among recent purchasers of handguns. N Engl J Med 341:1583–1589, 1999

44

ASSESSMENT OF DANGEROUSNESS

Charles L. Scott, M.D.
Cameron D. Quanbeck, M.D.
Phillip J. Resnick, M.D.

The term *dangerousness* is not a psychiatric diagnosis; the concept of dangerousness is a legal judgment based on social policy. In other words, dangerousness is a broader concept than either violence or dangerous behavior; it indicates an individual's propensity to commit dangerous acts (Mulvey and Lidz 1984). Unfortunately, no psychological test or interview can predict future violence with high accuracy. Relatively infrequent events (e.g., homicide) are more difficult to predict than more common events (e.g., domestic violence) because they have a low base rate of occurrence. The accuracy of a clinician's assessment of future violence is related to many factors, including the circumstances of the evaluation and the length of time over which violence is predicted.

In a classic review of clinicians' accuracy at predicting violent behavior toward others, Monahan (1981) concluded that psychiatrists and psychologists were accurate in no more than one out of three predictions of violent behavior among institutionalized patients followed over many years who both had committed violence in the past and were diagnosed as mentally ill (Monahan and Steadman 1994). However, more recent studies indicate that clinicians' accuracy in assessing future violence improves when the prediction is limited to briefer periods of time. For example, Lidz et al. (1993) found that the accuracy of clinicians' predictions of violence by male patients (but not female patients) examined in an acute psychiatric emergency room significantly exceeded chance based on patient self-reports of violent incidents, corroborating information from someone who knew the patient well, and a review of official records.

When conducting a violence risk assessment, the clinician should consider dividing the concept of dangerousness into the five components outlined in Table 44–1.

TABLE 44–1. **Components of dangerousness**

- Magnitude of harm
- Likelihood harm will take place
- Imminence of harm
- Frequency of aggressive behavior
- Situational factors associated with violence

In humans, two primary subtypes of aggression have been described: 1) reactive aggression characterized by an emotionally laden, uncontrolled outburst of aggressive behavior that is impulsive in nature, and 2) planned or predatory aggression that is controlled, purposeful, and premeditated, with little associated emotion (Weinshenker and Siegel 2002). In reactive (impulsive) aggression, the violence is often externally provoked, with subsequent feelings of remorse and confusion. In contrast, premeditated aggressive acts are not usually considered to have a large emotional component but are more "cold blooded" in nature. The aggression is goal oriented and requires a degree of forethought or planning (Stanford et al. 2003). Predatory violence is more dangerous because there is usually an absence of observable antecedent behaviors that foreshadow the aggression (Meloy 1987). The predator usually has no remorse and is comfortable using violence to retaliate against others, to gain a sense of control, or to obtain a desired goal.

Risk Factors Associated With Violence

Demographic Factors and Violence Risk

The clinical assessment of dangerousness requires a review of several risk factors that have been associated with an increased likelihood of future violence. Table 44–2 highlights demographic risk factors associated with violence.

Males in the general population perpetrate violent acts approximately 10 times more often than females (Tardiff and Sweillam 1980). However, among people with mental disorders, men and women do not significantly differ in their base rates of violent behavior. In fact, rates are remarkably similar and in some cases slightly higher for women (Lidz et al. 1993; Newhill et al. 1995).

The MacArthur Violence Risk Assessment Study monitored male and female psychiatric inpatients (ages 18–40 years) released into the community for acts of violence toward others (MacArthur Foundation 2001). During the 1-year follow-up, men were "somewhat more likely" than women to be violent, but the difference was not large. Women were more likely than men to target their aggression toward family members in the home environment. Violent acts by men were more likely to result in an arrest or a need for medical treatment (MacArthur Foundation 2001). Re-

TABLE 44–2. Demographic factors associated with violence

- Younger age (Swanson et al. 1990)
- Male gender (in non–mentally ill individuals)
- Lower socioeconomic status (Borum et al. 1996)
- Concentrated poverty in neighborhood (E. Silver et al. 1999)
- Lower intelligence and mild mental retardation (Borum et al. 1996; Quinsey and Maguire 1986)
- Less education (Borum et al. 1996; Link et al. 1992)

search examining the relationship of gender and violence committed by psychiatric inpatients also concluded that both men and women have similar rates of aggression in this setting. In their study of 155 male and 67 female psychiatric inpatients, Krakowski and Czobor (2004) found that a similar percentage of women and men had an incident of physical assault in the hospital. However, women had a higher frequency of physical assaults during the first 10 days of the study period, and men were more likely to perpetrate assaults that resulted in an injury.

Past Violence History

A past history of violence is the single best predictor of future violent behavior (Klassen and O'Connor 1988). The evaluator should determine the answers to the questions described in Table 44–3 when conducting an assessment of past violence.

Criminal and court records are particularly useful in evaluating the person's past history of violence and illegal behavior. For example, the age at first arrest for a serious offense is highly correlated with persistence of criminal offending (Borum et al. 1996). Each prior episode of violence increases the risk of a future violent act (Borum et al. 1996). Given four previous arrests, for example, the probability of a fifth is 80% (Wolfgang et al. 1987).

Additional sources of information relevant in assessing a person's potential for violence include a military and work history. For those individuals who have served in the military, the clinician should review any history of fights, absences without leave (AWOL), and disciplinary measures (Article XV in the Uniform Code of Military Justice), as well as the type of discharge. An evaluation of the work history should review frequency of job changes and reasons for each termination. Frequent terminations increase the risk for violence. Persons who are laid off from work are six

TABLE 44–3. Evaluation of past history of violence

- What is the most aggressive act you have ever committed?

- What are triggers for your anger and violence?

- Have your targets of aggression been people, property, or both?

- Who are the victims of your aggression?

- What weapons have you used when violent?

- Were you under the influence of alcohol or another substance when you were aggressive?

- Were you experiencing any type of mental health symptom when violent?

- If you were on psychiatric medications, were you taking them when you became violent?

- What have been the legal consequences of your violence in the past?

- What have been the social consequences of your violence in the past?

- How do you feel about the violent acts you have committed?

- What factors have helped you control your aggression?

times more likely to be violent than their employed peers (Catalano et al. 1993).

A person who has used weapons against others in the past may pose a serious risk of future violence. The main difference between assault and homicide is the lethality of the weapon used. Loaded guns have the highest lethality of any weapon. An assault with a gun is five times more likely to result in a fatality than an attack with a knife (Zimring 1991). According to the U.S. Department of Justice, an estimated 40% of U.S households contain a gun and 20% of all gun-owning households keep the gun loaded and unlocked (Cook and Ludwig 1997). Subjects should be asked whether they own or have ever owned a weapon. The recent movement of a weapon, such as transferring a gun from a closet to a nightstand, is particularly ominous in a paranoid person. The greater the psychotic fear, the more likely the paranoid person is to kill someone he or she misperceives as a persecutor.

Substance Use and Violence Risk

Drugs and alcohol are strongly associated with violent behavior (MacArthur Foundation 2001). The majority of persons involved in violent crimes are under the influence of alcohol at the time of their aggression (Murdoch et al. 1990). At least half of all violent events, including murders, were preceded by alcohol consumption by the perpetrator of a crime, the victim, or both (Roth 1994). Stimulants such as cocaine, crack, amphetamines, and phencyclidine (PCP) are of special concern. These drugs typically result in feelings of disinhibition, grandiosity, and paranoia. Among psychiatric patients, a coexisting diagnosis of substance abuse is strongly predictive of violence (MacArthur Foundation 2001). In a study comparing discharged psychiatric patients and nonpatients in the community, substance abuse tripled the rate of violence in nonpatients and increased the rates of violence in discharged patients by up to five times (Steadman et al. 1998).

Mental Disorders and Violence Risk

Studies examining whether individuals with mental illness are more violent than individuals without mental illness have yielded mixed results (Steadman et al. 1998; Torrey 1994). In a study of civilly committed psychiatric patients released into the community, most mentally ill individuals were not violent (Monahan 1997). Although a weak relationship between mental illness and violence was noted, violent conduct was greater only during periods in which the person was experiencing acute psychiatric symptoms. Individuals with a diagnosis of schizophrenia had lower rates of violence compared with individuals with a diagnosis of depression or of bipolar disorder. In addition, Monahan et al. (2001) noted that substance abuse was a much greater risk factor for violence than mental illness.

Psychosis and Violence Risk

Specific psychiatric symptoms and diagnoses should be carefully reviewed when conducting a violence risk assessment. The presence of psychosis is of particular concern when evaluating a person's risk of future violence. In paranoid psychotic patients, violence is often well planned and in line with their false beliefs. The violence is usually directed at a specific person who is perceived as a persecutor. Relatives or friends are often the targets of the paranoid individual. In addition, paranoid persons in the community are more likely to be dangerous because they have greater access to weapons (Krakowski et al. 1986).

Do specific delusions increase the risk that a person will behave violently? Research examining the contribution of delusions to violent behavior does not provide a clear answer to this question. Earlier studies suggested that persecutory delusions were associated with an increased risk of aggression (Wessely et al. 1993). Delusions noted to increase the risk of violence were those characterized by threat/control-override symptoms. These delusions involve the following beliefs: that the mind is dominated by forces beyond the person's control; that thoughts are being put into the person's head; that people are wishing the person harm; and that the person is being followed (Link and Stueve 1995). Similarly, Swanson et al. (1996), using data from the Epidemiologic Catchment Area surveys, found that people who reported threat/control-override symptoms were about twice as likely to engage in assaultive behavior as those with other psychotic symptoms.

By contrast, results from the MacArthur Study of Mental Disorder and Violence (MacArthur Foundation 2001; Monahan et al. 2001) showed that the presence of delusions did not predict higher rates of violence among recently discharged psychiatric patients. In particular, a relationship between the presence of threat/control-override delusions and violent behavior was not found. In a study comparing male criminal offenders with schizophrenia found not guilty by reason of insanity with matched controls of nonoffending persons with schizophrenia, Stompe et al. (2004) also found that threat/control-override symptoms showed no significant association with the severity of violent behavior, nor did the prevalence of threat/control-override symptoms differ between the two groups. However, nondelusional suspiciousness, such as misperceiving others' behavior as indicating hostile intent, was associated with subsequent violence (Monahan et al. 2001). Factors that have demonstrated an association between delusions and violence are summarized in Table 44–4.

A careful inquiry about hallucinations is required to determine whether their presence increases the person's risk to commit a violent act. In general, the presence of hallucinations is not related to dangerous acts, but certain types of hallucinations may increase the risk of violence (Zisook et al. 1995). Patients with schizophrenia are more likely to be violent if their hallucinations generate negative emotions (anger, anxiety, sadness) and if the patients have not developed successful strategies to cope with their voices (Cheung et al. 1997a).

In a review of seven controlled studies examining the relationship between command hallucinations and violence, no study demonstrated a positive relationship between command hallucinations and violence, and one found an inverse relationship (Rudnick 1999).

TABLE 44–4. Factors associated with delusionally driven violence

Associated negative emotional states (Appelbaum et al. 1999):
- Unhappiness
- Fear
- Anxiety
- Anger

Prior history of acting on delusional beliefs (Monahan et al. 2001)

A positive relationship between violence in the presence of command hallucinations was found when the voice was familiar to the person and when the act commanded was less serious. In contrast, McNiel et al. (2000) reported that in a study of 103 civil psychiatric inpatients, 33% reported having had command hallucinations to harm others during the prior year and 22% of the patients reported that they complied with such commands. The authors concluded that patients in their study who experienced command hallucinations to harm others were more than twice as likely to be violent.

Junginger (1990) reported that command hallucinations were more likely to be followed in the presence of a delusion whose content was related to the hallucination. In the MacArthur Violence Risk Assessment Study (MacArthur Foundation 2001), there was no relationship between the presence of general hallucinations or nonviolent command hallucinations and violence. However, there was a relationship between command hallucinations to commit violence and actual violence (MacArthur Foundation 2001; Monahan et al. 2001). In addition to evaluating positive symptoms of psychosis, clinicians should also assess their patients' insight into their illness and into the potential legal complications of their illness. Buckley et al. (2004) found that violent patients with schizophrenia had more prominent lack of insight regarding their illness and the legal complications of their behavior compared with a nonviolent comparison group.

Delusions and hallucinations are prominent diagnostic symptoms of schizophrenia. Although the majority of individuals with schizophrenia do not behave violently (Walsh et al. 2002), there is emerging evidence that a diagnosis of schizophrenia is associated with an increase in criminal offending. In a retrospective review of 2,861 Australian patients with schizophrenia followed over a 25-year period, Wallace et al. (2004) found that patients with schizophrenia accumulated a greater total number of criminal convictions and were significantly more likely to have been convicted of a criminal offense (including violent offenses) relative to matched comparison subjects. These authors noted that the criminal behaviors committed by schizophrenic patients could not be entirely accounted for by comorbid substance use, active symptoms, or characteristics of systems of care (Wallace et al. 2004). In data from the CATIE (Clinical Antipsychotic Trials of Intervention Effectiveness) project, researchers clinically assessed and interviewed 1,410 schizophrenia patients about violent behavior. Definitions of violence were those used in the MacArthur Community Violence Interview and are outlined in Table 44–5. The 6-month prevalence of any violence was 19.1%, with 3.6% of individuals reporting serious violence. Positive symptoms, including persecutory ideation, increased the risk of both minor and serious violence. By contrast, negative symptoms, such as social withdrawal, actually lowered the risk of serious violence (Swanson et al. 2006).

Mood Disorders and Violence Risk

Depression may result in violent behavior, particularly in depressed individuals who strike out against others in despair. After committing a violent act, the depressed person may attempt suicide. Depression is the most common diagnosis in murder–suicides (Marzuk et al. 1992). One pattern of murder–suicide involves depressed or psychotic parents (particularly mothers of very young children) who kill their children prior to attempting to take their own lives (Resnick 1969). Murder–suicide in couples is associated with feelings of jealousy and possessiveness (Rosenbaum 1990). In murder–suicides, the homicide is often an extension of the suicidal act. The individual can no longer endure life without what is perceived to be a vital element (i.e., spouse, family, or a job). The perpetrator cannot bear the thought of other persons carrying on without him, so he forces others to join him in death.

Patients with mania show a high percentage of assaultive or threatening behavior, but serious violence itself is rare (Krakowski et al. 1986). Additionally, patients with mania show considerably less criminality of all kinds than patients with schizophrenia. Patients with mania most commonly exhibit violent behavior when they are restrained or have limits set on their behavior (Tardiff and Sweillam 1980). However, active manic symptoms appear to play a substantial role in criminal behavior. In a study of 66 inmates with bipolar disorder, 74% were manic and 59% were psychotic at the time of their arrest (Quanbeck et al. 2004).

TABLE 44–5. MacArthur Community Violence Interview: definitions of violence

Serious violence
- Any assault using a lethal weapon
- Any assault resulting in injury
- Any threat with a lethal weapon in hand
- Any sexual assault

Other aggressive acts (minor violence)
- Battery that did not result in injury

Source. MacArthur Foundation 2001.

Cognitive Impairment and Violence Risk

Brain injury or illness can also result in aggressive behavior. After a brain injury, formerly normal individuals may become verbally and physically aggressive (National Institutes of Health 1998). Characteristic features of aggression resulting from a brain injury are outlined in Table 44–6.

Personality Factors and Violence Risk

Violence is also associated with certain personality traits and disorders. While borderline personality disorder (Tardiff and Sweillam 1980) and sadistic personality traits (Meloy 1992) are associated with increased violence, the personality disorder most commonly associated with violence is antisocial personality disorder (MacArthur Foundation 2001). The violence by individuals with antisocial personality disorder is often motivated by revenge or occurs during a period of heavy drinking. Violence among these persons is frequently cold and calculated and lacks emotionality (Williamson et al. 1987). Low IQ and antisocial personality disorder are a particularly ominous combination for increasing the risk of future violence (Heilbrun 1990). It is important to assess for the presence of antisocial personality disorders in individuals with a major mental illness. Compared with schizophrenic patients without antisocial personality disorder, offenders with both schizophrenia and antisocial personality disorder are less likely to have violence that is prompted by psychotic symptoms. Their violence is more likely to be associated with alcohol use, involve an altercation with the victim prior to violence, and be perpetrated against a victim who is not a family member (Joyal et al. 2004).

Adults may have personality traits that increase their risk for violent behavior but may still not meet the criteria for a personality disorder. Personality traits

TABLE 44–6. Characteristics of aggression associated with brain injuries

- Reactive behavior triggered by trivial stimuli
- Lack of planning or reflection
- Nonpurposeful action with no clear aims or goals
- Explosive outbursts without a gradual buildup
- Episodic pattern with long periods of relative calm
- Feelings of concern and remorse following episode

TABLE 44–7. Components of threat evaluation

- Obtain detailed information regarding how threat is to be carried out.
- Evaluate what other steps (if any) the person has taken to solve the situation prior to initiating threat.
- Review whether prior threats have been acted on.
- Determine what steps have been taken to enact current threat.
- Inquire as to the person's expected personal consequences if threat is enacted.
- Review any grudge lists, which may include unidentified potential victims.
- Investigate person's violent fantasies.
- Assess suicide risk, particularly history of violent suicide attempts.

associated with violence include impulsivity (Borum et al. 1996), low frustration tolerance, inability to tolerate criticism, repetitive antisocial behavior, reckless driving, a sense of entitlement, and superficiality. The violence associated with these personality traits usually has a paroxysmal, episodic quality. When interviewed, these people often have poor insight into their behavior and frequently blame others for their difficulties (Reid and Balis 1987).

In addition to DSM-IV-TR (American Psychiatric Association 2000) personality disorders or traits, the clinician should also be familiar with the psychological construct known as psychopathy. The term *psychopath* was described by Cleckley (1976) as an individual who is superficially charming, lacks empathy, lacks close relationships, is impulsive, and is concerned primarily with self-gratification. Hare and colleagues developed the Psychopathy Checklist—Revised (PCL-R; Hare 1991) as a validated measure of psychopathy in adults. The concept of psychopathy is important, because the presence of psychopathy is a strong predictor of criminal behavior generally and violence among adults (Salekin et al. 1996).

Assessment of Current Dangerousness

When conducting an assessment of current dangerousness, pay close attention to the individual's affect. Individuals who are angry and lack empathy for others are at increased risk for violent behavior (Menzies et al. 1985). In the MacArthur Study of Mental Disorder and Violence, subjects with high anger scores, as measured by the Novaco Anger Scale, were twice as likely as subjects with low anger scores to have engaged in violent behavior (Monahan et al. 2001).

All threats should be taken seriously and details fully elucidated. Table 44–7 outlines important elements to consider when evaluating a particular threat.

As noted in Table 44–7, the clinician should assess the suicide risk in any patient making a homicidal threat. Violent suicide attempts increase the likelihood of future violence toward others (Convit et al. 1988). One study found that 91% of outpatients who had attempted homicide also had attempted suicide and that 86% of patients with homicidal ideation also reported suicidal ideation (Asnis et al. 1997).

When organizing strategies to decrease those risk factors that may contribute to future violence, the clinician should distinguish static from dynamic risk factors. By definition, static factors are not subject to change by intervention. Static factors include such items as demographic information and past history of violence. Dynamic factors are subject to change with intervention and include such factors as access to weapons, psychotic symptoms, active substance use, and living setting. The clinician may find it helpful to organize a chart that outlines known risk factors, management and treatment strategies to address dynamic risk factors, and the current status of each risk factor. This approach will assist in the development of a violence prevention plan that addresses the unique combination of risk factors for each particular patient. As shown in Table 44–8, an organized risk management chart allows the practitioner to identify the factors that continue to increase the person's risk of future violence so that treatment interventions can be more effectively monitored.

TABLE 44–8. Sample violence risk management chart

Risk factor	Intervention	Status
Paranoia	Antipsychotic medication	Treated for 7 days; symptoms decreased but are still present.
Gun at home	Removal of gun	Brother removed all guns from home, and gun is now under lock and key.
Cocaine abuse	Substance use treatment Random urine drug screens	Refusing substance groups. Positive urine for cocaine.
Marital conflict	Marital therapy	Two marital sessions completed; jealousy of wife persists.
Antipsychotic medication nonadherence history	Antipsychotic intramuscular depot injection	Client agreed to depot medication.

Psychiatric Inpatients and Risk of Violence

Assaultive behavior committed by psychiatric inpatients is a significant problem in terms of staff injury and the use of seclusion and restraint. Each year, nearly one in four public psychiatric nurses suffers a disabling injury from a patient assault, making it one of the most dangerous occupations for work-related injuries (Love and Hunter 1996). Patients who perpetrate violence are adversely affected as well. Seclusion and restraint are often used to manage aggressive behaviors (Kaltiala-Heino et al. 2003) despite the possibility that their use presents psychological and physical risks to patients. Because release from civil and forensic psychiatric facilities is often based on risk of future dangerousness, inpatient violence can result in a prolonged involuntary confinement. Despite the magnitude of this problem, current understanding of the causes and optimal treatments for aggression remains limited. To appropriately assess and minimize the risk of violence, the clinician should be familiar with common characteristics of assaultive inpatients, categories of aggression, and motivations that underlie violent inpatient behavior.

Common Characteristics of Assaultive Inpatients

Past research has consistently shown that a small percentage of patients are responsible for the majority of assaults in institutional settings (Cheung et al. 1997b; Convit et al. 1990). In addition, these patients inflict serious injuries at a rate 10 times higher than that of patients who assault less frequently. Identifying characteristics of this high-risk group provides clinicians an opportunity to focus efforts on reducing overall levels of institutional aggression. In contrast to gender ratios of violence in the general population, mentally ill male psychiatric patients are not more violent than their female counterparts. Therefore, gender is not considered a distinguishing risk factor for violence in the psychiatric inpatient setting (Krakowski and Czobor 2004). Factors in the literature that have been associated with psychiatric inpatient aggression are summarized in Table 44–9.

TABLE 44–9. Common characteristics of assaultive psychiatric inpatients

- Younger age (Flannery 2002; Rabinowitz and Mark 1999)
- Prior history of aggression (Klassen and O'Connor 1988; Soliman and Reza 2001)
- Previous violent suicide attempt (Flannery 2002)
- Victim of childhood physical abuse and/or other deviant upbringing (Hoptman et al. 1999)
- Schizophrenia (Tardiff and Sweillam 1982)
- Personality disorder (Tardiff and Sweillam 1982)
- Impulse-control disorder (Tardiff and Sweillam 1982)
- Mental retardation (Tardiff and Sweillam 1982)
- Neurological impairment (Tardiff and Sweillam 1982)
- Abnormal electroencephalogram (Convit et al. 1988)

Categories and Motivations for Violent Inpatient Aggression

As described earlier in this chapter, aggression has been categorized as primarily reactive or predatory in nature. A study in a New York psychiatric state hospital examined inpatient assaults to determine whether these aggression subtypes were applicable to this population (Nolan et al. 2003). Assaults occurring in a common area of the inpatient unit were videotaped so that motivations and triggers for the aggression could be examined. After the assault, the assailant and victim were interviewed separately in an attempt to identify the underlying reason for the aggressive act. Three primary categories of assaultive behavior were described: 1) disordered impulse control; 2) psychopathic (planned/predatory) behavior; and 3) underlying psychotic symptomatology. Psychotic assaults were generally committed by an individual acting under the influence of delusions, hallucinations, and/or disordered thinking.

In a more recent study of inpatient assaults, researchers reviewed more than 1,000 aggressive acts committed by chronically assaultive inpatients at a large California state psychiatric hospital (Quanbeck et al. 2007). The three categories of violent behavior (impulsive, predatory/planned, and psychotic) were also observed in this study. More than 40% of all assaults were impulsive in nature. Specific triggers, such as a staff member directing the patient to go to his or her room or refusing the patient something he or she wanted, were common precipitants to the impulsive act. Organized or planned assaults were the second most common reason inpatients were aggressive and accounted for over 25% of all assaults. These aggressive acts were frequently motivated by the patient's desire to seek revenge or retaliate against another patient or staff member. Psychotic assaults were the least common type (15%) of all assaults. Psychotic aggression was usually committed by patients acting under the paranoid belief that the victim intended to harm them (e.g., by poisoning), was stealing from them, or was talking about/laughing at them (Quanbeck et al. 2007). Characteristics that distinguish impulsive, organized, and psychotic assaults are detailed in Table 44–10.

Structured Risk Assessments of Violence

Standardized risk assessment instruments for the prediction of violence are increasingly being used by clinicians in conjunction with their clinical violence risk assessments. The goals of these prediction schemes are to assist clinicians in gathering appropriate data and to anchor clinicians' assessments to established research. One of the most validated risk assessment instruments is the Psychopathy Checklist. The PCL-R (Hare 1991) is a clinical construct rating scale designed to measure psychopathic attributes in individuals. Individuals who score higher on this measurement of psychopathy have been shown to have higher rates of violent recidivism. The PCL-R uses a semistructured interview, case history information, and specific scoring criteria to rate each of 20 items on a 3-point scale (0, 1, 2) according to the extent to which it applies to a given individual. Total scores (ranging from 0 to 40) reflect an estimate of the degree to which the individual matches the prototypical psychopath. In North America, the cutoff score for psychopathy is 30 or greater. A screening version of the PCL-R, known as the PCL-SV, has also been developed. The PCL-SV has been shown to have good predictive validity for institutional violence (Hill et al. 1996) and community violence (Monahan et al. 2001). Concerns about using the PCL-R as the sole assessment of dangerousness include its inability to capture protective, mediating, and moderating factors against future violent behavior (Rogers 2000) and a potential to overpredict violent behavior (Freedman 2001).

The Violence Risk Appraisal Guide (VRAG; Webster et al. 1994) is another actuarial risk assessment instrument that consists of 12 items, one of which is psychopathy as defined by the PCL-R. The VRAG instrument was derived from information about 618 patients at a maximum-security hospital providing assessment and treatment services for persons received from the courts, correctional services, and other provincial psychiatric hospitals in Canada (Webster et al. 1994). A third risk assessment instrument is the Historical Clinical Risk–20 (HCR-20; Webster et al. 1997), which combines the assessment of historical risk factors and clinical judgment regarding risk management. The HCR-20 is a broadband violence risk assessment instrument with 20 items divided into historical, clinical, and risk management items. One of the items is the presence or absence of psychopathy as determined by the PCL-R. An assessment tool commonly used in correctional settings is the Level of Service Inventory—Revised (LSI-R; Andrews and Bonta 1995). The LSI-R is a combined risk and needs assessment tool developed in Canada whose measurements have been validated in North America. The LSI-R consists of 54 items and is composed of 10 subscales. The LSI-R score indicates the likelihood of recidivism and suggests interventions based on the score.

TABLE 44–10. **Characteristics of impulsive, organized, and psychotic assaults**

Assault type	Impulsive	Organized	Psychotic
Triggering event	Stressor immediately precedes assault	Delay between triggering event and assault	Psychotic misperception of reality, resulting in sudden and unexpected assault
Behaviors preceding assault	Agitated, pacing, clenched jaw, yelling, verbally threatening	Calm, minimal signs of emotional escalation, controlled behavior, "surprise attack" on victim	Isolated, pacing, mumbling, disorganized speech, hallucinating, fearful, anxious
Motivation for assault	Impulsive reaction with no long-term motive or secondary gain	Clear motive or self-serving goal (e.g., extortion of goods, retaliation, dominance of others)	Psychotic motivation stemming from fear, paranoia, or misperceived need to act in self-defense
Insight regarding assaultive behavior	Remorseful and may recognize reaction was in excess of stressor	Limited insight or superficial expression of remorse and minimization of harm to others	Limited insight due to psychotic symptoms

A recently developed tool for the purpose of assessing the violence risk of individuals discharged from civil psychiatric facilities is known as the Iterative Classification Tree (ICT; Monahan et al. 2001). This approach utilizes a sequence of questions related to risk factors for potential violence. Contingent on the answer to a question, one or another second question is posed, until the individual is classified into a category of high or low risk of future violence. In a sample of 939 male and female civil psychiatric patients followed after hospital discharge, the ICT classified 72.6% of the sample as either low risk or high risk. This tool shows promise in the assessment of future violence for periods up to 20 weeks. However, the extent to which the accuracy of the ICT generalizes to other types of clinical settings, such as forensic hospitals, is currently unknown.

Actuarial models have inherent limitations when used exclusively. Specific criticisms of actuarial instruments include the following: They provide only approximations of risk; their use is not generalizable beyond the studied populations on which they are based; they are rigid and lacking sensitivity to change; and they fail to inform violence prevention and risk management (Douglas et al. 2003). Although actuarial models attempt to standardize the practice of dangerousness assessment, they are not designed to be the sole standard for violence assessment. Actuarial tools are useful in assisting clinicians in reaching reasonable conclusions based on research findings (Borum et al. 1996), but the evaluator must also consider the imminence and severity of violence that may not be reflected in an actuarial instrument alone (Glancy and Chaimowitz 2005). Furthermore, in his review comparing actuarial and clinical methods of risk prediction, Litwack noted that many of the actuarial assessments also incorporate factors requiring clinical judgment (Litwack 2001).

Pharmacological Management of Chronic Aggression

The treatment focus of emergent aggression is rapid sedation and calming of the agitated patient. In contrast, the primary objective of the pharmacological treatment of chronic aggression is the prevention of future assaultive acts without adversely affecting other areas of functioning. As of September 2007, no medication had been approved by the U.S. Food and Drug Administration (FDA) for the treatment of chronic aggression. Utilizing medication for this purpose is considered "off-label" prescribing. Therefore, physicians who prescribe medications to help manage chronic assaultive behavior should consider utilizing the systematic approach outlined in Table 44–11.

A wide variety of pharmacological agents have been prescribed in an attempt to decrease violent and aggressive behaviors, and their treatment efficacy in this population is summarized below. Suggested off-label uses for a variety of medications are summarized in Table 44–12.

TABLE 44–11. Systematic approach to the pharmacological treatment of chronic aggression

- Choose medication with empirical evidence of antiaggressive effects.
- Document informed consent regarding potential risks and benefits.
- Utilize an objective measure to record aggressive acts and monitor treatment outcome.
- Change medications one at a time when possible.
- Use adequate dosage for appropriate time period.
- Have modest expectations for treatment improvement.

TABLE 44–12. Off-label pharmacotherapy interventions for aggression

Medication class	Target symptoms
Selective serotonin reuptake inhibitors	Irritability, impulsivity, negative affect–triggered aggression
Anticonvulsants	Paroxysmal rage attacks, impulse-control disorders, aggression triggered by poor information processing or head injury
Lithium	Aggression triggered by negative affect or head injury, impulsivity, violence associated with mental retardation
Antipsychotics	Hostility associated with psychosis, potential use in aggression associated with borderline personality disorder
β-Adrenergic blockers	Aggression associated with schizophrenia, akathisia, or head injury

Selective Serotonin Reuptake Inhibitors

Selective serotonin reuptake inhibitors (SSRIs) have shown some benefit in reducing impulsivity and aggression in a variety of patient populations. In a study of 51 "normal" individuals (defined as not meeting criteria for an Axis I disorder), 25 "normals" treated with paroxetine over a 4-week period were less hostile, less irritable, and more socially cooperative compared with 26 "normals" treated with placebo (Knutson et al. 1998). Paroxetine has also been shown to decrease the number of aggressive and impulsive responses in a sample of adult males with antisocial personality characteristics playing a computer game (Cherek et al. 2002). Other SSRIs have been shown to decrease measures of aggression in persistently assaultive inpatients with schizophrenia (Vartiainen et al. 1995), a sample of personality disorder patients (Coccaro and Kavoussi 1997), and patients with dementia and brain injury (Kim et al. 2001). The antiaggressive properties of the SSRIs may be mediated by their ability to stabilize mood, reduce negative affects (Knutson et al. 1998), and improve impulse control (Hollander and Rosen 2000).

Anticonvulsants

Anticonvulsant medications have demonstrated efficacy in decreasing aggressive behavior in individuals with a wide variety of psychiatric symptoms and diagnoses. In a study of prisoners exhibiting impulsive aggression, phenytoin reduced the frequency and intensity of violence among the impulsive group but had no effect on violence committed by prisoners whose aggression was premeditated. Carbamazepine has shown some efficacy in reducing the severity of "rage attacks" in a sample of patients with a variety of diagnoses including antisocial and borderline personality disorders, substance use disorders, attention-deficit disorder, intermittent explosive disorder (Mattes 1984), and aggressive behavior subsequent to traumatic brain injury (Azouvi et al. 1999). Oxcarbazepine had a significant benefit in the treatment of outpatients with clinically significant impulsive aggression (Mattes 2005).

In a review of 17 uncontrolled studies that used valproic acid to treat impulsive aggression, 77% of individuals treated with valproic acid had a 50% reduction in violent acts (Lindenmayer and Kotsaftis 2000). In another study, researchers compared the behavioral effects of three anticonvulsants (phenytoin, carbamazepine, and valproate) in impulsive-aggressive men. In this double-blind, placebo-controlled study, a significant reduction in impulsive aggression was demonstrated for all three anticonvulsants compared with placebo (Stanford et al. 2005).

Impulsive-aggressive behaviors account for a substantial portion of the morbidity and mortality associated with borderline personality disorder (Goodman and New 2000). Several well-designed placebo-controlled studies indicate that anticonvulsants may play a role in treating assaultive behavior by decreasing irritability, anger, and aggression (Frankenburg and Zanarini 2002; Hollander et al. 2001; Nickel et al. 2004, 2005; Tritt et al. 2005). Anticonvulsants are sometimes used as an adjunctive treatment for patients with schizophrenia. Valproic acid is the only mood stabilizer considered to be a first-line augmenting agent for patients with schizophrenia who are persistently aggressive (Volavka 2002).

Lithium

In a classic study examining the efficacy of lithium in decreasing violence, inmates convicted of a violent offense and engaging in impulsively aggressive acts while in prison were randomly assigned to placebo or Eskalith CR (a slow-release form of lithium) (Sheard et al. 1976). The lithium-treated inmates had a significant decrease in the number of major violent infractions. Lithium has also demonstrated efficacy in open and controlled trials in reducing aggressive behavior in those with mental retardation and brain injury (Volavka 2002). In the above studies, lithium levels were maintained in a range lower than typically used to treat mania (0.5–1.0 mEq/L). Because this relatively low lithium level is not commonly associated with sedation and impaired cognition, the decrease in aggressive behaviors may be due to specific antiaggressive properties of lithium rather than decreased violence due to sedation.

Antipsychotics

Clozapine has demonstrated efficacy superior to that of atypical antipsychotics (risperidone and olanzapine) and haloperidol in reducing hostility (Citrome et al. 2001) and reducing the number and severity of aggressive incidents (Volavka et al. 2004) in treatment-resistant patients diagnosed with chronic schizophrenia or schizoaffective disorder. In these studies, the antiaggressive effect of clozapine was independent from measures of sedation and positive psychotic symptoms. Risperidone (Aleman and Kahn 2001) and quetiapine (Volavka 2002) are superior to typical antipsychotics (haloperidol) in reducing hostility in patients with schizophrenia. In one study, atypical antipsychotics (clozapine, risperidone, olanzapine) significantly reduced the risk of violent behavior in persons with schizophrenia in community-based treatment, whereas treatment with conventional neuroleptics did not have the same beneficial effect (Swanson et al. 2004). This positive effect was primarily attributable to

fewer adverse side effects and increased medication adherence. The propensity of typical neuroleptics (particularly at high doses) to cause akathisia has been linked to irritability and increased violence (Volavka 2002) and therefore may have the effect of increasing rather than decreasing assaultive behaviors.

Atypical antipsychotics may also have a role in the treatment of aggression in borderline personality disorder. Risperidone significantly reduced self-rated aggression in an open trial of patients with borderline personality disorder and a history of aggression (Rocca et al. 2002). A randomized controlled trial of female patients with borderline personality disorder treated with olanzapine over a 6-month period found a significant improvement on many core symptoms including aggression and hostility (Zanarini and Frankenburg 2001). In both of these studies, the mean dose was lower than would be used in the treatment of schizophrenia (e.g., risperidone 3 mg, olanzapine 5 mg). In a chart review study, the effects of clozapine were examined in a diagnostically heterogeneous group of persistently violent patients (including patients whose primary diagnosis was a personality disorder). Clozapine treatment resulted in marked decreases in violent episodes and the use of seclusion and restraint. These data suggest a possible role for clozapine in treatment-refractory, persistently violent patients irrespective of DSM diagnosis (Kraus and Sheitman 2005).

Beta-Adrenergic Blockers

β-Adrenergic blockers are medications designed to treat high blood pressure by reducing the sympathetic tone in the circulation. There is evidence that the adjunctive use of propranolol (J.M. Silver et al. 1999) and nadolol (Ratey et al. 1992) decreases aggressive behavior in schizophrenia. This finding suggests that β-adrenergic blockers may mediate antiaggressive effects by treating the motor symptoms of akathisia (Lipinski et al. 1988). Propranolol has demonstrated efficacy in reducing organically driven aggression (e.g., head injury) but at variable and often high dosages (from 30 to 1,600 mg/day). In addition, the effect may require an extended trial lasting up to 2 months (Greendyke and Kanter 1986; Greendyke et al. 1986; Yudofsky et al. 1981). When used as an antihypertensive, propranolol can cause fatigue, lethargy, and drowsiness, and these side effects were not measured in the above studies. Subsequently, it is unclear if nonspecific sedation mediates the antiaggressive effects of β-blockers. Further, the use of propranolol requires careful monitoring of blood pressure and heart rate during titration and is contraindicated in certain medical conditions (e.g., asthma, heart failure, bradycardia). Pindolol, a β-adrenergic blocker with partial agonist effect, has fewer cardiovascular side effects. Studies indicate that pindolol reduced assaultiveness and hostility in patients with dementia without causing lethargy (Greendyke and Kanter 1986) and significantly reduced the number and severity of aggressive incidents in patients with schizophrenia who had been repetitively assaultive (Caspi et al. 2001).

Benzodiazepines

Past animal research examining the effect of benzodiazepines on aggressive behavior found a bidirectional dose–response effect—lower doses increase aggression, while higher doses decrease aggression (Volavka 2002). In humans, early research indicated that benzodiazepines may hold promise in managing aggressive behavior. Chlordiazepoxide and diazepam appeared to exert a general calming effect on state hospital inpatients with a variety of psychiatric diagnoses. A subsequent small randomized controlled trial investigating the use of clonazepam as an augmenting agent in schizophrenia found no benefit. Surprisingly, several patients became aggressive who had no history of aggression in the past (Karson et al. 1982). A number of case reports have appeared in the literature where patients treated with benzodiazepines developed paradoxical "rage reactions" (French 1989; Gutierrez et al. 2000; Mathew et al. 2000). In a randomized clinical trial examining the effects of benzodiazepines on aggressive behavior, researchers compared the willingness of men treated with benzodiazepines or placebo to shock an imaginary opponent in a reaction-time test (Weisman et al. 1998). Surprisingly, subjects treated with benzodiazepines delivered more severe shocks than did subjects on placebo, particularly diazepam-treated subjects. The effect of benzodiazepines on aggression is complex and difficult to predict. Because there is no substantial evidence that the long-term use of benzodiazepines reduces the risk of violence, their use should probably be reserved for the management of acute aggression and agitation.

Psychotherapeutic Approaches to Treating Chronic Aggression

Determining the psychotherapeutic approach most appropriate for a chronically aggressive mental health patient should be based on careful assessment of the type of aggressive behavior exhibited, psychiatric diagnosis, and intellectual ability. Patients with chronic schizophrenia with a suboptimal response to medication and those with organic brain disease (mental retardation, dementia, autism, brain injury) are most effectively treated by behavioral approaches. For personality disorder patients whose aggression is secondary to difficulties in regulating emotional states, cognitive-behavioral techniques may be more effective than other types of psychotherapy (Alpert and Spillmann 1997).

Behavioral Interventions

In chronic institutionalized psychiatric patients, social learning programs have been effective in decreasing aggression, the need for seclusion and restraint, and time to discharge (Goodness and Renfro 2002). These programs are based on social learning theory, which holds that social behaviors are learned and acquired over time through two mechanisms: 1) experiencing success or failure as the result of one's own actions, and 2) observing the positive and negative consequences of others' behaviors (Bandura 1977).

The goal of behavioral intervention is to restructure the consequences of a patient's actions so that the link between aggressive behavior and its reinforcers is weakened while the link between alternate prosocial behaviors is reinforced. The token economy is one type of behavioral management approach used to foster the development of prosocial behavior. In this system, a patient's socially appropriate behavior is positively reinforced by earning tokens or points that can be exchanged for rewards (e.g., privileges, games, TV time, snacks). A token can be earned by attending groups, taking medications, and refraining from or reducing aggressive behavior for a specified period of time. Maladaptive aggressive behavior results in a loss of tokens or privileges, or "time-outs" in which a patient is temporarily placed into a calmer environment. This type of program requires a careful assessment of behaviors targeted for change, clearly defined objectives for the patient, and consistent positive reinforcement by staff.

Social skills training is often used in conjunction with a behavioral program to accelerate progress by teaching patients new behaviors to replace dysfunctional interactions. Patients learn assertiveness and self-control skills in individual or group settings. Important elements of social skills training are summarized in Table 44–13.

TABLE 44–13. Essential components of social skills training

- Focused education on the specific behavior desired
- Modeling of how to perform expected behavior
- Rehearsal and role-playing of expected behavior
- Positive reinforcement of desired behaviors and corrective actions for inappropriate behaviors
- Practicing of skills in real-life situations

Cognitive-Behavioral Approaches

Treatments of aggression involving cognitive-behavioral techniques have been predominantly based on anger management techniques (Alpert and Spillmann 1997). Novaco's cognitive-behavioral model of anger proposes that anger and aggression are mediated by an individual's perception of threat from others. The treatment assists the person in formulating strategies to managing conflict in a nonaggressive manner (Novaco 1997). This technique has shown efficacy in violent forensic patients (Holbrook 1997; Serin and Kuriychuk 1994) and in those with mild borderline intellectual functioning (Lindsay et al. 2003). A potentially beneficial cognitive-behavioral approach to aggression in those with borderline personality disorder has recently been identified. Male forensic patients with borderline personality disorder who participated in a dialectical behavior therapy program modified to target violence and anger had significant reductions in the seriousness of violence-related incidents and in self-report measures of hostility and anger (Evershed et al. 2003). Key components of successful anger management treatment are described in Table 44–14.

TABLE 44–14. Key components of anger management skills training

- Imagining angry scenarios, then using relaxation techniques
- Identifying and challenging cognitive distortions
- Identifying personal warning signs of anger
- Recognizing potentially provocative situations
- Implementing nonaggressive responses to provocative situations
- Building a repertoire of behavioral skills for managing conflict

Prosecution of Inpatient Assaults

Overview

As a last resort, psychiatric facilities can consider filing criminal charges against patients for inpatient assaults. Criminal prosecution of violent inpatients is a recent phenomenon, with the first case report appearing in the literature in 1978 (Appelbaum and Appelbaum 1991). In the past, prosecution was rarely considered as a viable option because of the prevailing belief that hospitalized psychiatric patients are not responsible for their actions and any violence is the result of staff negligence or incompetence (Norko et al. 1991).

Rationale for Prosecuting Inpatient Assaults

The "criminalization" of inpatient assaults has been a controversial issue because it poses an ethical dilemma. Clinicians are expected to act in a patient's best interests; prosecution removes a patient from a therapeutic milieu and places him or her in the punitive atmosphere of a jail or prison. Nonetheless, this approach may be ethically justifiable in certain circumstances. The Supreme Court has determined that patients are entitled to safe conditions, which obligates hospitals to protect the physical safety of patients (Appelbaum and Appelbaum 1991). Under *Tarasoff* reasoning, mental health professionals who believe a third party is endangered must take steps to protect the intended victim. An involuntarily confined patient who is endangered by another patient does not have the freedom to escape the situation; removing the dangerous patient from the hospital may be an appropriate clinical intervention.

Psychiatric institutions also have an interest in providing for the safety of hospital personnel. In U.S. public-sector psychiatric hospitals, the risk of injury to staff from assault is higher than the risk of injury from all causes combined in other occupations (Dinwiddie and Briska 2004). Assaulted staff may have higher rates of substance misuse, posttraumatic stress disorder, and other anxiety disorders (Coyne 2002). Ignoring assaults can lead to poor staff morale and performance, which interfere with the therapeutic aims of the hospital (Norko et al. 1991).

Prosecution should be reserved for repetitively violent patients who may be unmotivated for change and when the usual treatment approaches are not effective. These patients engage in repeated acts of planned aggression to achieve short-term goals (Dinwiddie and Briska 2004). Such patients may have learned that assaults on staff or patients brings few punishments or sanctions (Coyne 2002), and consequently their antisocial behaviors are reinforced (Miller and Maier 1987). A strong argument exists that patients, despite living in a hospital environment, are autonomous individuals who are expected to be responsible for their behavior and function within societal rules. Prosecution can serve as a form of limit setting and motivate a change in behavior. Failing to address these behaviors may ultimately harm these patients when they reenter society with the belief that acts of violence do not result in serious consequences (Dinwiddie and Briska 2004).

Development and Implementation of a Policy for Prosecution of Assaults

Psychiatric facilities should develop a clear, consistent policy regarding prosecuting patients for assault. The policy should be uniform and objective and allow patients an opportunity to change their behavior before resorting to the filing of criminal charges. The approach should not make some patients feel as if they have been singled out (Norko et al. 1991).

Elements outlined in Table 44–15 can be helpful in developing a policy to deal with repetitively assaultive inpatients or patients with an egregious calculated violent act. Assaultive behavior that a patient's illness prevents him or her from controlling (e.g., a profound disruption in reality testing [psychosis] or severe mood dysregulation) should not be prosecuted (Dinwiddie and Briska 2004; Miller and Maier 1987). Other interventions, short of prosecution, have also demonstrated efficacy. For example, patients could be taken to a judge who admonishes them about their behavior and warns them that any future violence will result in criminal charges. The creation of a "probationary status" for violent inpatients has been successful in prompting patients to change their behavior (Hoge and Gutheil 1987).

Summary

The assessment of potential violence is an important area when evaluating psychiatric patients in both an

TABLE 44–15. Policy considerations for prosecuting inpatient assaults

- Provide written documentation to patient of his or her rights and responsibilities, which include respect for others and lawful behavior (Norko et al. 1991).
- Conduct a thorough assessment of assailant's state of mind during and motivation for the assault by reviewing the following:
  - Was the patient acting under the influence of delusions or hallucinations?
  - Was the assault provoked?
  - Did the assailant appear to lose control of his or her behavior?
  - Was the violence planned?
  - Was the assailant attempting to use violence for a specific goal or purpose?
- Carefully document each assault in the medical record.
- Obtain forensic consultation to review whether prosecution is appropriate.
- Weigh the following factors when considering prosecution:
  - Nature/severity of violence
  - Adequacy of prior treatment attempts and results
  - Clinical impact on patient and likelihood of response to further intervention
  - Probable legal outcome (chances of conviction)
  - Possible effects on or risks to staff and other patients

outpatient and inpatient setting. Despite improvements in this field, the prediction of violence remains an inexact science. Predicting violence has been compared to forecasting the weather. Like a good weather forecaster, the clinician does not state with certainty that an event will occur. Instead, he or she estimates the likelihood that a future event will occur. Like weather forecasting, predictions of future violence will not always be correct. However, gathering a detailed past history and using appropriate risk assessment instruments help make the risk assessment as accurate as possible.

Key Points

- The best predictor of future violent behavior is a past history of violent behavior.
- Mental disorders, particularly paranoia and suspiciousness, increase the risk of violence.
- Substance use represents a major risk factor for future violent behavior.
- Actuarial risk assessment instruments can assist the evaluator in more accurately predicting future violence.
- Inpatient violence includes impulsive, planned, and psychotic assaults.
- Treatment interventions should match type of assaultive behavior.

Suggested Readings

Lidz CW, Mulvey EP, Gardner W: The accuracy of predictions of violence to others. JAMA 269:1007–1011, 1993

Litwack TR: Actuarial versus clinical assessment of dangerousness. Psychol Public Policy Law 7:409–443, 2001

Monahan J, Steadman HJ: Violence and mental disorder: developments in risk assessment. Chicago, IL, University of Chicago Press, 1994

Monahan J, Steadman HJ, Silver E, et al: Rethinking Risk Assessment: The MacArthur Study of Mental Disorder and Violence. New York, Oxford University Press, 2001

Swanson JW, Holzer CE III, Ganju VK, et al: Violence and psychiatric disorder in the community: evidence from the Epidemiologic Catchment Area surveys. Hosp Community Psychiatry 41:761–770, 1990

Swanson JW, Swartz MS, Van Dorn RA, et al: A national study of violent behavior in persons with schizophrenia. Arch Gen Psychiatry 63:490–499, 2006

References

Aleman A, Kahn RS: Effects of the atypical antipsychotic risperidone on hostility and aggression in schizophrenia: a meta-analysis of controlled trials. Eur Neuropsychopharmacol 11:289–293, 2001

Alpert JE, Spillmann MK: Psychotherapeutic approaches to aggressive and violent patients. Psychiatr Clin North Am 20:453–472, 1997

American Psychiatric Association: Diagnostic and Statistical Manual of Mental Disorders, 4th Edition, Text Revision. Washington, DC, American Psychiatric Association, 2000

Andrews D, Bonta J: LSI-R: The Level of Service Inventory: Revised Users Manual. Toronto, ON, Canada, Multi-Health Systems, 1995

Appelbaum KL, Appelbaum PS: A model hospital policy on prosecuting patients for presumptively criminal acts. Hosp Community Psychiatry 42:1233–1237, 1991

Appelbaum PS, Robbins PC, Roth LH: Dimensional approach to delusions: comparison across types and diagnosis. Am J Psychiatry 156:1938–1943, 1999

Asnis GM, Kaplan ML, Hundorfean G, et al: Violence and homicidal behaviors in psychiatric disorders. Psychiatr Clin North Am 20:405–425, 1997

Azouvi P, Jokic C, Attal N, et al: Carbamazepine in agitation and aggressive behavior following severe closed-head injury: results of an open trial. Brain Inj 13:797–804, 1999

Bandura A: Social Learning Theory. Englewood Cliffs, NJ, Prentice Hall, 1977

Borum R, Swartz M, Swanson J: Assessing and managing violence risk in clinical practice. Journal of Practical Psychiatry and Behavioral Health 4:204–215, 1996

Buckley PF, Hrouda DR, Friedman L, et al: Insight and its relationship to violent behavior in patients with schizophrenia. Am J Psychiatry 161:1712–1714, 2004

Caspi N, Modai I, Barak P, et al: Pindolol augmentation in aggressive schizophrenic patients: a double-blind crossover study. Int Clin Psychopharmacol 16:111–115, 2001

Catalano R, Dooley D, Navaco RW, et al: Using ECA survey data to examine the effect of job layoffs on violent behavior. Hosp Community Psychiatry 44:874–879, 1993

Cherek DR, Lane SD, Pietras CJ, et al: Effects of chronic paroxetine administration on measures of aggressive and impulsive responses of adult males with a history of conduct disorder. Psychopharmacology (Berl) 159:266–274, 2002

Cheung P, Schweitzer I, Crowley K, et al: Violence in schizophrenia: role of hallucinations and delusions. Schizophr Res 26:181–190, 1997a

Cheung P, Schweitzer I, Tuckwell V, et al: A prospective study of assaults on staff by psychiatric inpatients. Med Sci Law 37:46–52, 1997b

Citrome L, Volavka J, Czobor P, et al: Effects of clozapine, olanzapine, risperidone, and haloperidol on hostility in patients with schizophrenia. Psychiatr Serv 52:1510–1514, 2001

Cleckley HM: The Mask of Sanity. St. Louis, MO, Mosby, 1976

Coccaro EF, Kavoussi RJ: Fluoxetine and impulsive aggressive behavior in personality-disordered subjects. Arch Gen Psychiatry 54:1081–1088, 1997

Convit A, Jaeger J, Lin SP, et al: Predicting assaultiveness in psychiatric inpatients: a pilot study. Hosp Community Psychiatry 39:429–434, 1988

Convit A, Isay D, Otis D, et al: Characteristics of repeatedly assaultive psychiatric inpatients. Hosp Community Psychiatry 41:1112–1115, 1990

Cook PJ, Ludwig J: Guns in America: National Survey on Private Ownership and Use of Firearms. May 1997. Available at: www.ncjrs.org/txtfiles/165476.txt. Accessed June 2005.

Coyne A: Should patients who assault staff be prosecuted? J Psychiatr Ment Health Nurs 9:139–145, 2002

Dinwiddie SH, Briska W: Prosecution of violent psychiatric inpatients: theoretical and practical issues. Int J Law Psychiatry 27:17–29, 2004

Douglas KS, Ogloff JR, Hart SD: Evaluation of a model of violence risk assessment among forensic psychiatric patients. Psychiatr Serv 54:1372–1379, 2003

Evershed S, Tennant A, Boomer D, et al: Practice-based outcomes of dialectical behavior therapy (DBT) targeting anger and violence, with male forensic patients: a pragmatic and non-contemporaneous comparison. Crim Behav Ment Health 13:198–213, 2003

Flannery RB Jr: Repetitively assaultive psychiatric patients: review of published findings, 1978–2001. Psychiatr Q 73:229–237, 2002

Frankenburg FR, Zanarini MC: Divalproex sodium treatment of women with borderline personality disorder and bipolar II disorder: a double-blind placebo-controlled pilot study. J Clin Psychiatry 63:442–446, 2002

Freedman D: False prediction of future dangerousness: error rates and psychopathy checklist—revised. J Am Acad Psychiatry Law 29:89–95, 2001

French AP: Dangerously aggressive behavior as a side effect of alprazolam. Am J Psychiatry 146:276, 1989

Glancy GD, Chaimowitz G: The clinical use of risk assessment. Can J Psychiatry 50:12–17, 2005

Goodman M, New A: Impulsive aggression in borderline personality disorder. Curr Psychiatry Rep 2:56–61, 2000

Goodness KR, Renfro NS: Changing a culture: a brief program analysis of a social learning program on a maximum-security forensic unit. Behav Sci Law 20:495–506, 2002

Greendyke RM, Kanter DR: Therapeutic effects of pindolol on behavioral disturbances associated with organic brain disease: a double-blind study. J Clin Psychiatry 47:423–426, 1986

Greendyke RM, Kanter DR, Schuster DB, et al: Propranolol treatment of assaultive patients with organic brain disease: a double-blind crossover, placebo-controlled study. J Nerv Ment Dis 174:290–294, 1986

Gutierrez MA, Roper JM, Hahn P: Paradoxical reactions to benzodiazepines. Am J Nurs 101:34–39, 2000

Hare RD: The Hare Psychopathy Checklist—Revised. Toronto, ON, Canada, Multi-Health Systems, 1991

Heilbrun AB Jr: The measurement of criminal dangerousness as a personality construct: further validation of a research index. J Pers Assess 54:141–148, 1990

Hill CD, Rogers R, Bickford ME: Predicting aggressive and socially disruptive behavior in a maximum security forensic psychiatric hospital. J Forensic Sci 41:56–59, 1996

Hoge SK, Gutheil TG: The prosecution of psychiatric patients for assaults on staff: a preliminary empirical study. Hosp Community Psychiatry 38:44–49, 1987

Holbrook MI: Anger management training in prison inmates. Psychol Rep 81:623–626, 1997

Hollander E, Rosen J: Impulsivity. J Psychopharmacol 14:S39–S44, 2000

Hollander E, Allen A, Lopez RP, et al: A preliminary double-blind, placebo-controlled trial of divalproex sodium in borderline personality disorder. J Clin Psychiatry 62:199–203, 2001

Hoptman MJ, Yates KF, Patalinjug MB, et al: Clinical prediction of assaultive behavior among male psychiatric patients at a maximum-security forensic facility. Psychiatr Serv 50:1461–1466, 1999

Joyal CC, Putkonen A, Paavola P, et al: Characteristics and circumstances of homicidal acts committed by offenders with schizophrenia. Psychol Med 34:433–442, 2004

Junginger J: Predicting compliance with command hallucinations. Am J Psychiatry 147:245–247, 1990

Kaltiala-Heino R, Tuohimaki C, Korkeila J, et al: Reasons for using seclusion and restraint in psychiatric inpatient care. Int J Law Psychiatry 26:139–149, 2003

Karson CN, Weinberger DR, Bigelow L, et al: Clonazepam treatment of chronic schizophrenia: negative results in a double-blind, placebo-controlled trial. Am J Psychiatry 139:1627–1628, 1982

Kim KY, Moles JK, Hawley JM: Selective serotonin reuptake inhibitors for aggressive behavior in patients with dementia after head injury. Pharmacotherapy 21:498–501, 2001

Klassen D, O'Connor WA: A prospective study of predictors of violence in adult male mental health admission. Law Hum Behav 12:143–158, 1988

Knutson B, Wolkowitz OM, Cole SW, et al: Selective alteration of personality and social behavior by serotonergic intervention. Am J Psychiatry 155:373–379, 1998

Krakowski M, Czobor P: Gender differences in violent behaviors: relationship to clinical symptoms and psychosocial factors. Am J Psychiatry 161:459–465, 2004

Krakowski M, Volavka J, Brizer D: Psychopathology and violence: a review of literature. Compr Psychiatry 27:131–148, 1986

Kraus JE, Sheitman BB: Clozapine reduces violent behavior in heterogeneous diagnostic groups. J Neuropsychiatry Clin Neurosci 17:36–44, 2005

Lidz CW, Mulvey EP, Gardner W: The accuracy of predictions of violence to others. JAMA 269:1007–1011, 1993

Lindenmayer, JP, Kotsaftis A: Use of sodium valproate in violent and aggressive behaviors: a critical review. J Clin Psychiatry 61:123–128, 2000

Lindsay WR, Allan R, MacLeod F, et al: Long-term treatment and management of violent tendencies of men with intellectual disabilities convicted of assault. Ment Retard 41:47–56, 2003

Link BG, Stueve A: Evidence bearing on mental illness as a possible cause of violent behavior. Epidemiol Rev 17:172–181, 1995

Link BG, Andrews H, Cullen FT: The violent and illegal behavior of mental patients reconsidered. Am Sociol Rev 57:275–292, 1992

Lipinski JF Jr, Keck PE Jr, McElroy SL: Beta-adrenergic antagonists in psychosis: is improvement due to treatment of neuroleptic-induced akathisia? J Clin Psychopharmacol 8:409–416, 1988

Litwack TR: Actuarial versus clinical assessment of dangerousness. Psychol Public Policy Law 7:409–443, 2001

Love CC, Hunter ME: Violence in public sector psychiatric hospitals. Benchmarking nursing staff injury rates. J Psychosoc Nurs Ment Health Serv 34:30–34, 1996

MacArthur Foundation: The MacArthur Violence Risk Assessment Study Executive Summary. 2001. Available at: http://macarthur.virginia.edu/risk.html. Accessed August 11, 2002.

Marzuk PM, Tardiff K, Hirsch CS: The epidemiology of murder-suicide. JAMA 267:3179–3183, 1992

Mathew VM, Dursun SM, Reveley MA: Increased aggressive, violent, and impulsive behavior in patients during chronic–prolonged benzodiazepine use. Can J Psychiatry 45:89–90, 2000

Mattes JA: Carbamazepine for uncontrolled rage outbursts. Lancet 2(8415):1164–1165, 1984

Mattes JA: Oxcarbazepine in patients with impulsive aggression: a double-blind, placebo-controlled trial. J Clin Psychopharmacol 25:575–579, 2005

McNiel DE, Eisner JP, Binder RL: The relationship between command hallucinations and violence. Psychiatr Serv 51:1288–1292, 2000

Meloy JR: The prediction of violence in outpatient psychotherapy. Am J Psychother 41:38–45, 1987

Meloy JR: Violent Attachments. Northvale, NJ, Jason Aronson, 1992

Menzies RJ, Webster CD, Sepejak DS: The dimensions of dangerousness: evaluating the accuracy of psychometric predictions of violence among forensic patients. Law Hum Behav 9:49–70, 1985

Miller RD, Maier GJ: Factors affecting the decision to prosecute mental patients for criminal behavior. Hosp Community Psychiatry 38:50–55, 1987

Monahan J: Predicting violent behavior: an assessment of clinical techniques. Beverly Hills, CA, Sage Publications, 1981

Monahan J: Actuarial support for the clinical assessment of violence risk. Int Rev Psychiatry 9:167–170, 1997

Monahan J, Steadman HJ: Violence and mental disorder: developments in risk assessment. Chicago, IL, University of Chicago Press, 1994

Monahan J, Steadman HJ, Silver E, et al: Rethinking Risk Assessment: The MacArthur Study of Mental Disorder and Violence. New York, Oxford University Press, 2001

Mulvey EP, Lidz CW: Clinical considerations in the prediction of dangerousness in mental patients. Clin Psychol Rev 4:379–401, 1984

Murdoch D, Pihl RO, Ross D: Alcohol and crimes of violence: present issues. Int J Addict 25:1065–1081, 1990

National Institutes of Health: Rehabilitation of Persons with Traumatic Brain Injury, National Institutes of Health Consensus Development Conference Statement. October 26–28, 1998. Available at: http://consensus.nih.gov/1998/1998TraumaticBrainInjury109html.htm. Accessed May 31, 2006.

Newhill CE, Mulvey EP, Lidz CW: Characteristics of violence in the community by female patients seen in a psychiatric emergency service. Psychiatr Serv 46:785–789, 1995

Nickel MK, Nickel C, Mitterlehner FO, et al: Topiramate treatment of aggression in female borderline personality disorder patients: a double-blind, placebo-controlled study. J Clin Psychiatry 65:1515–1519, 2004

Nickel MK, Nickel C, Kaplan P, et al: Treatment of aggression with topiramate in male borderline patients: a double-blind, placebo-controlled study. Biol Psychiatry 57:495–499, 2005

Nolan KA, Czobor P, Roy BB, et al: Characteristics of assaultive behavior among psychiatric inpatients. Psychiatr Serv 54:1012–1016, 2003

Norko MA, Zonana HV, Phillips RT: Prosecuting assaultive psychiatric inpatients. Hosp Community Psychiatry 42:193–194, 1991

Novaco R: Remediating anger and aggression with violent offenders. Legal and Criminological Psychology 2:77–88, 1997

Quanbeck CD, Stone DC, Scott CL, et al: Clinical and legal correlates of inmates with bipolar disorder at time of criminal arrest. J Clin Psychiatry 65:198–203, 2004

Quanbeck CD, McDermott BE, Lam J, et al: Categorization of aggressive acts committed by chronically assaultive state hospital patients. Psychiatr Serv 58:521–528, 2007

Quinsey VL, Maguire A: Maximum security psychiatric patients: actuarial and clinical prediction of dangerousness. J Interpers Violence 1:143–171, 1986

Rabinowitz J, Mark M: Risk factors for violence among longstay psychiatric patients: national study. Acta Psychiatr Scand 99:341–347, 1999

Ratey JJ, Sorgi P, O'Driscoll GA, et al: Nadolol to treat aggression and psychiatric symptomatology in chronic psychiatric inpatients: a double-blind, placebo-controlled study. J Clin Psychiatry 53:41–46, 1992

Reid WH, Balis GU: Evaluation of the violent patient, in Psychiatry Update: The American Psychiatric Association Annual Review, Vol 6. Edited by Hales RE, Frances AJ. Washington, DC, American Psychiatric Press, 1987, pp 491–509

Resnick PJ: Child murder by parents: a psychiatric review of filicide. Am J Psychiatry 126:325–334, 1969

Rocca P, Marchiaro L, Cocuzza E, et al: Treatment of borderline personality disorder with risperidone. J Clin Psychiatry 63:241–244, 2002

Rogers R: The uncritical acceptance of risk assessment in forensic practice. Law Hum Behav 24:595–605, 2000

Rosenbaum M: The role of depression in couples involved in murder–suicide and homicide. Am J Psychiatry 147:1036–1039, 1990

Roth JA: Psychoactive substances and violence (publication NCJ 145534). U.S. Department of Justice, National Institute of Justice, 1994. Available at: http://www.ncjrs.gov/txtfiles/psycho.txt. Accessed June 1, 2006.

Rudnick A: Relation between command hallucinations and dangerous behavior. J Am Acad Psychiatry Law 27:253–257, 1999

Salekin RT, Rogers R, Sewell KW: A review of meta-analysis of the Psychopathy Checklist and Psychopathy Checklist—Revised: predictive validity of dangerousness. Clinical Psychology: Science and Practice 3:203–213, 1996

Serin RC, Kuriychuk M: Social and cognitive processing deficits in violent offenders: implications for treatment. Int J Law Psychiatry 17:431–441, 1994

Sheard MH, Marini JL, Bridges CI, et al: The effect of lithium on impulsive aggressive behavior in man. Am J Psychiatry 133:1409–1413, 1976

Silver E, Mulvey EP, Monahan J: Assessing violence risk among discharged psychiatric patients: toward an ecological approach. Law Hum Behav 2:237–255, 1999

Silver JM, Yudofsky SC, Slater JA, et al: Propranolol treatment of chronically hospitalized aggressive patients. J Neuropsychiatry Clin Neurosci 11:328–335, 1999

Soliman AE, Reza H: Risk factors and correlates of violence among acutely ill adult psychiatric inpatients. Psychiatr Serv 52:75–80, 2001

Stanford MS, Houston R, Villemarette-Pittman N, et al: Premeditated aggression: clinical assessment and cognitive psychophysiology. Pers Individ Diff 34:773–781, 2003

Stanford MS, Helfritz LE, Conklin SM, et al: A comparison of anticonvulsants in the treatment of impulsive aggression. Exp Clin Psychopharmacol 13:72–77, 2005

Steadman HJ, Mulvey EP, Monahan J, et al: Violence by people discharged from acute psychiatric inpatient facilities and by others in the same neighborhoods. Arch Gen Psychiatry 55:393–401, 1998

Stompe T, Ortwein-Swoboda G, Schanda H, et al: Schizophrenia, delusional symptoms, and violence: the threat/control-override concept reexamined. Schizophr Bull 30:31–44, 2004

Swanson JW, Holzer CE 3rd, Ganju VK, et al: Violence and psychiatric disorder in the community: evidence from the Epidemiologic Catchment Area surveys. Hosp Community Psychiatry 41:761–770, 1990

Swanson JW, Borum R, Swartz M: Psychotic symptoms and disorders and risk of violent behavior in the community. Crim Behav Ment Health 6:317–338, 1996

Swanson JW, Swartz MS, Elbogen EB: Effectiveness of atypical antipsychotic medications in reducing violent behavior among persons with schizophrenia in community-based treatment. Schizophr Bull 30:3–20, 2004

Swanson JW, Swartz MS, Van Dorn RA, et al: A national study of violent behavior in persons with schizophrenia. Arch Gen Psychiatry 63:490–499, 2006

Tardiff K, Sweillam A: Assault, suicide, and mental illness. Arch Gen Psychiatry 37:164–169, 1980

Tardiff K, Sweillam A: Assaultive behavior among chronic inpatients. Am J Psychiatry 139:212–215, 1982

Torrey EF: Violent behavior by individuals with serious mental illness. Hosp Community Psychiatry 45:653–662, 1994

Tritt K, Nickel C, Lahmann C, et al: Lamotrigine treatment of aggression in female borderline patients: a randomized, double-blind, placebo-controlled study. J Psychopharmacol 19:287–291, 2005

Vartiainen H, Tiihonen J, Putkonen A, et al: Citalopram, a selective serotonin reuptake inhibitor, in the treatment of aggression in schizophrenia. Acta Psychiatr Scand 91:348–351, 1995

Volavka J: Neurobiology of Violence. Washington, DC, American Psychiatric Publishing, 2002

Volavka J, Czobor P, Nolan K, et al: Overt aggression and psychotic symptoms in patients with schizophrenia treated with clozapine, olanzapine, risperidone, or haloperidol. J Clin Psychopharmacol 24:225–228, 2004

Wallace C, Mullen PE, Burgess P: Criminal offending in schizophrenia over a 25-year period marked by deinstitutionalization and increasing prevalence of comorbid substance use disorders. Am J Psychiatry 161:716–727, 2004

Walsh E, Buchanan A, Fahy T: Violence and schizophrenia: examining the evidence. Br J Psychiatry 180:490–495, 2002

Webster CD, Harris GT, Rice ME: The Violence Prediction Scheme: Assessing Dangerousness in High-Risk Men. Toronto, ON, Centre of Criminology, University of Toronto, 1994

Webster CD, Douglas KS, Eaves D, et al: HCR-20: Assessing the Risk for Violence (Version 2). Vancouver, BC, Mental Health, Law, and Policy Institute, Simon Fraser University, 1997

Weinshenker N, Siegel A: Bimodal classification of aggression: affective defense and predatory attack. Aggression and Violent Behavior 7:237–250, 2002

Weisman AM, Berman ME, Taylor SP: Effects of clorazepate, diazepam, and oxazepam on a laboratory measurement of aggression in men. Int Clin Psychopharmacol 13:183–188, 1998

Wessely S, Buchanan A, Reed A, et al: Acting on delusions, I: prevalence. Br J Psychiatry 163:69–76, 1993

Williamson S, Hare R, Wong S: Violence: criminal psychopaths and their victims. Canadian Journal of Behavioral Sciences 19:454–462, 1987

Wolfgang ME, Thornberry TP, Figlio RM: From Boy to Man, From Delinquency to Crime. Chicago, IL, University of Chicago Press, 1987

Yudofsky S, Williams D, Gorman J: Propranolol in the treatment of rage and violent behavior in patients with chronic brain syndromes. Am J Psychiatry 138:218–220, 1981

Zanarini MC, Frankenburg FR: Olanzapine treatment of female borderline personality disorder patients: a double-blind, placebo-controlled pilot study. J Clin Psychiatry 62:849–854, 2001

Zimring FE: Firearms, violence, and public policy. Sci Am 265:48–54, 1991

Zisook S, Byrd D, Kuck J, et al: Command hallucinations in outpatients with schizophrenia. J Clin Psychiatry 56:462–465, 1995

Appendix

DSM-IV-TR CLASSIFICATION

DSM-IV-TR Classification

NOS = Not Otherwise Specified.

An *x* appearing in a diagnostic code indicates that a specific code number is required.

An ellipsis (. . .) is used in the names of certain disorders to indicate that the name of a specific mental disorder or general medical condition should be inserted when recording the name (e.g., 293.0 Delirium Due to Hypothyroidism).

Numbers in parentheses are page numbers.

If criteria are currently met, one of the following severity specifiers may be noted after the diagnosis:

> Mild
> Moderate
> Severe

If criteria are no longer met, one of the following specifiers may be noted:

> In Partial Remission
> In Full Remission
> Prior History

Disorders Usually First Diagnosed in Infancy, Childhood, or Adolescence

MENTAL RETARDATION

Note: These are coded on Axis II.

317	Mild Mental Retardation
318.0	Moderate Mental Retardation
318.1	Severe Mental Retardation
318.2	Profound Mental Retardation
319	Mental Retardation, Severity Unspecified

LEARNING DISORDERS

315.00	Reading Disorder
315.1	Mathematics Disorder
315.2	Disorder of Written Expression
315.9	Learning Disorder NOS

MOTOR SKILLS DISORDER

315.4	Developmental Coordination Disorder

COMMUNICATION DISORDERS

315.31	Expressive Language Disorder
315.32	Mixed Receptive–Expressive Language Disorder
315.39	Phonological Disorder
307.0	Stuttering
307.9	Communication Disorder NOS

PERVASIVE DEVELOPMENTAL DISORDERS

299.00	Autistic Disorder
299.80	Rett's Disorder
299.10	Childhood Disintegrative Disorder
299.80	Asperger's Disorder
299.80	Pervasive Developmental Disorder NOS

ATTENTION-DEFICIT AND DISRUPTIVE BEHAVIOR DISORDERS

314.xx	Attention-Deficit/Hyperactivity Disorder
.01	Combined Type
.00	Predominantly Inattentive Type
.01	Predominantly Hyperactive-Impulsive Type
314.9	Attention-Deficit/Hyperactivity Disorder NOS
312.xx	Conduct Disorder
.81	Childhood-Onset Type
.82	Adolescent-Onset Type
.89	Unspecified Onset
313.81	Oppositional Defiant Disorder
312.9	Disruptive Behavior Disorder NOS

FEEDING AND EATING DISORDERS OF INFANCY OR EARLY CHILDHOOD

307.52	Pica
307.53	Rumination Disorder
307.59	Feeding Disorder of Infancy or Early Childhood

TIC DISORDERS

307.23	Tourette's Disorder
307.22	Chronic Motor or Vocal Tic Disorder
307.21	Transient Tic Disorder
	Specify if: Single Episode/Recurrent
307.20	Tic Disorder NOS

ELIMINATION DISORDERS

—.—	Encopresis
787.6	With Constipation and Overflow Incontinence
307.7	Without Constipation and Overflow Incontinence
307.6	Enuresis (Not Due to a General Medical Condition)
	Specify type: Nocturnal Only/Diurnal Only/Nocturnal and Diurnal

OTHER DISORDERS OF INFANCY, CHILDHOOD, OR ADOLESCENCE

309.21	Separation Anxiety Disorder
	Specify if: Early Onset
313.23	Selective Mutism
313.89	Reactive Attachment Disorder of Infancy or Early Childhood
	Specify type: Inhibited Type/Disinhibited Type
307.3	Stereotypic Movement Disorder
	Specify if: With Self-Injurious Behavior
313.9	Disorder of Infancy, Childhood, or Adolescence NOS

Delirium, Dementia, and Amnestic and Other Cognitive Disorders

DELIRIUM

293.0	Delirium Due to . . . [Indicate the General Medical Condition]
—.—	Substance Intoxication Delirium (refer to Substance-Related Disorders for substance-specific codes)
—.—	Substance Withdrawal Delirium (refer to Substance-Related Disorders for substance-specific codes)

———.— Delirium Due to Multiple Etiologies
(code each of the specific etiologies)
780.09 Delirium NOS

DEMENTIA

294.xx Dementia of the Alzheimer's Type, With
Early Onset (also code 331.0 Alzheimer's disease
on Axis III)
.10 Without Behavioral Disturbance
.11 With Behavioral Disturbance

294.xx Dementia of the Alzheimer's Type, With Late
Onset (also code 331.0 Alzheimer's disease on
Axis III)
.10 Without Behavioral Disturbance
.11 With Behavioral Disturbance
290.xx Vascular Dementia
.40 Uncomplicated
.41 With Delirium
.42 With Delusions
.43 With Depressed Mood
Specify if: With Behavioral Disturbance

*Code presence or absence of a behavioral disturbance in the
fifth digit for Dementia Due to a General Medical Condition:*

0 = Without Behavioral Disturbance
1 = With Behavioral Disturbance

294.1x Dementia Due to HIV Disease
(also code 042 HIV on Axis III)
294.1x Dementia Due to Head Trauma
(also code 854.00 head injury on Axis III)
294.1x Dementia Due to Parkinson's Disease
(also code 331.82 Dementia with Lewy bodies on
Axis III)
294.1x Dementia Due to Huntington's Disease
(also code 333.4 Huntington's disease on Axis III)
294.1x Dementia Due to Pick's Disease
(also code 331.11 Pick's disease on Axis III)
294.1x Dementia Due to Creutzfeldt-Jakob Disease
(also code 046.1 Creutzfeldt-Jakob disease on
Axis III)
294.1x Dementia Due to . . . [Indicate the General Medical Condition not listed above] (also code the
general medical condition on Axis III)
———.— Substance-Induced Persisting Dementia
(refer to Substance-Related Disorders for substance-
specific codes)
———.— Dementia Due to Multiple Etiologies
(code each of the specific etiologies)
294.8 Dementia NOS

AMNESTIC DISORDERS

294.0 Amnestic Disorder Due to . . . [Indicate the
General Medical Condition]
Specify if: Transient/Chronic
———.— Substance-Induced Persisting Amnestic
Disorder (refer to Substance-Related Disorders
for substance-specific codes)
294.8 Amnestic Disorder NOS

OTHER COGNITIVE DISORDERS

294.9 Cognitive Disorder NOS

Mental Disorders Due to a General Medical Condition Not Elsewhere Classified

293.89 Catatonic Disorder Due to . . . [Indicate the
General Medical Condition]
310.1 Personality Change Due to . . . [Indicate the
General Medical Condition]
Specify type: Labile Type/Disinhibited Type/
Aggressive Type/Apathetic Type/Paranoid Type/
Other Type/Combined Type/Unspecified Type
293.9 Mental Disorder NOS Due to . . . [Indicate the
General Medical Condition]

Substance-Related Disorders

*The following specifiers apply to Substance Dependence as
noted:*

[a]With Physiological Dependence/Without
Physiological Dependence
[b]Early Full Remission/Early Partial Remission/
Sustained Full Remission/Sustained Partial
Remission
[c]In a Controlled Environment
[d]On Agonist Therapy

*The following specifiers apply to Substance-Induced
Disorders as noted:*

[I]With Onset During Intoxication/[W]With Onset
During Withdrawal

ALCOHOL-RELATED DISORDERS

Alcohol Use Disorders

303.90 Alcohol Dependence[a,b,c]
305.00 Alcohol Abuse

Alcohol-Induced Disorders

303.00	Alcohol Intoxication
291.81	Alcohol Withdrawal
	Specify if: With Perceptual Disturbances
291.0	Alcohol Intoxication Delirium
291.0	Alcohol Withdrawal Delirium
291.2	Alcohol-Induced Persisting Dementia
291.1	Alcohol-Induced Persisting Amnestic Disorder
291.x	Alcohol-Induced Psychotic Disorder
.5	With Delusions[I,W]
.3	With Hallucinations[I,W]
291.89	Alcohol-Induced Mood Disorder[I,W]
291.89	Alcohol-Induced Anxiety Disorder[I,W]
291.89	Alcohol-Induced Sexual Dysfunction[I]
291.82	Alcohol-Induced Sleep Disorder[I,W]
291.9	Alcohol-Related Disorder NOS

AMPHETAMINE (OR AMPHETAMINE-LIKE)–RELATED DISORDERS

Amphetamine Use Disorders

304.40	Amphetamine Dependence[a,b,c]
305.70	Amphetamine Abuse

Amphetamine-Induced Disorders

292.89	Amphetamine Intoxication
	Specify if: With Perceptual Disturbances
292.0	Amphetamine Withdrawal
292.81	Amphetamine Intoxication Delirium
292.xx	Amphetamine-Induced Psychotic Disorder
.11	With Delusions[I]
.12	With Hallucinations[I]
292.84	Amphetamine-Induced Mood Disorder[I,W]
292.89	Amphetamine-Induced Anxiety Disorder[I]
292.89	Amphetamine-Induced Sexual Dysfunction[I]
292.85	Amphetamine-Induced Sleep Disorder[I,W]
292.9	Amphetamine-Related Disorder NOS

CAFFEINE-RELATED DISORDERS

Caffeine-Induced Disorders

305.90	Caffeine Intoxication
292.89	Caffeine-Induced Anxiety Disorder[I]
292.85	Caffeine-Induced Sleep Disorder[I]
292.9	Caffeine-Related Disorder NOS

CANNABIS-RELATED DISORDERS

Cannabis Use Disorders

304.30	Cannabis Dependence[a,b,c]
305.20	Cannabis Abuse

Cannabis-Induced Disorders

292.89	Cannabis Intoxication
	Specify if: With Perceptual Disturbances
292.81	Cannabis Intoxication Delirium
292.xx	Cannabis-Induced Psychotic Disorder
.11	With Delusions[I]
.12	With Hallucinations[I]
292.89	Cannabis-Induced Anxiety Disorder[I]
292.9	Cannabis-Related Disorder NOS

COCAINE-RELATED DISORDERS

Cocaine Use Disorders

304.20	Cocaine Dependence[a,b,c]
305.60	Cocaine Abuse

Cocaine-Induced Disorders

292.89	Cocaine Intoxication
	Specify if: With Perceptual Disturbances
292.0	Cocaine Withdrawal
292.81	Cocaine Intoxication Delirium
292.xx	Cocaine-Induced Psychotic Disorder
.11	With Delusions[I]
.12	With Hallucinations[I]
292.84	Cocaine-Induced Mood Disorder[I,W]
292.89	Cocaine-Induced Anxiety Disorder[I,W]
292.89	Cocaine-Induced Sexual Dysfunction[I]
292.85	Cocaine-Induced Sleep Disorder[I,W]
292.9	Cocaine-Related Disorder NOS

HALLUCINOGEN-RELATED DISORDERS

Hallucinogen Use Disorders

304.50	Hallucinogen Dependence[b,c]
305.30	Hallucinogen Abuse

Hallucinogen-Induced Disorders

292.89	Hallucinogen Intoxication
292.89	Hallucinogen Persisting Perception Disorder (Flashbacks)
292.81	Hallucinogen Intoxication Delirium
292.xx	Hallucinogen-Induced Psychotic Disorder
.11	With Delusions[I]
.12	With Hallucinations[I]
292.84	Hallucinogen-Induced Mood Disorder[I]
292.89	Hallucinogen-Induced Anxiety Disorder[I]
292.9	Hallucinogen-Related Disorder NOS

INHALANT-RELATED DISORDERS

Inhalant Use Disorders

304.60	Inhalant Dependence[b,c]
305.90	Inhalant Abuse

Inhalant-Induced Disorders

292.89   Inhalant Intoxication
292.81   Inhalant Intoxication Delirium
292.82   Inhalant-Induced Persisting Dementia
292.xx   Inhalant-Induced Psychotic Disorder
    .11   With Delusions[I]
    .12   With Hallucinations[I]
292.84   Inhalant-Induced Mood Disorder[I]
292.89   Inhalant-Induced Anxiety Disorder[I]
292.9   Inhalant-Related Disorder NOS

NICOTINE-RELATED DISORDERS

Nicotine Use Disorder

305.1   Nicotine Dependence[a,b]

Nicotine-Induced Disorders

292.0   Nicotine Withdrawal
292.9   Nicotine-Related Disorder NOS

OPIOID-RELATED DISORDERS

Opioid Use Disorders

304.00   Opioid Dependence[a,b,c,d]
305.50   Opioid Abuse

Opioid-Induced Disorders

292.89   Opioid Intoxication
    Specify if: With Perceptual Disturbances
292.0   Opioid Withdrawal
292.81   Opioid Intoxication Delirium
292.xx   Opioid-Induced Psychotic Disorder
    .11   With Delusions[I]
    .12   With Hallucinations[I]
292.84   Opioid-Induced Mood Disorder[I]
292.89   Opioid-Induced Sexual Dysfunction[I]
292.85   Opioid-Induced Sleep Disorder[I,W]
292.9   Opioid-Related Disorder NOS

PHENCYCLIDINE (OR PHENCYCLIDINE-LIKE)–RELATED DISORDERS

Phencyclidine Use Disorders

304.60   Phencyclidine Dependence[b,c]
305.90   Phencyclidine Abuse

Phencyclidine-Induced Disorders

292.89   Phencyclidine Intoxication
    Specify if: With Perceptual Disturbances
292.81   Phencyclidine Intoxication Delirium
292.xx   Phencyclidine-Induced Psychotic Disorder
    .11   With Delusions[I]
    .12   With Hallucinations[I]
292.84   Phencyclidine-Induced Mood Disorder[I]
292.89   Phencyclidine-Induced Anxiety Disorder[I]
292.9   Phencyclidine-Related Disorder NOS

SEDATIVE-, HYPNOTIC-, OR ANXIOLYTIC-RELATED DISORDERS

Sedative, Hypnotic, or Anxiolytic Use Disorders

304.10   Sedative, Hypnotic, or Anxiolytic Dependence[a,b,c]
305.40   Sedative, Hypnotic, or Anxiolytic Abuse

Sedative-, Hypnotic-, or Anxiolytic-Induced Disorders

292.89   Sedative, Hypnotic, or Anxiolytic Intoxication
292.0   Sedative, Hypnotic, or Anxiolytic Withdrawal
    Specify if: With Perceptual Disturbances
292.81   Sedative, Hypnotic, or Anxiolytic Intoxication Delirium
292.81   Sedative, Hypnotic, or Anxiolytic Withdrawal Delirium
292.82   Sedative-, Hypnotic-, or Anxiolytic-Induced Persisting Dementia
292.83   Sedative-, Hypnotic-, or Anxiolytic-Induced Persisting Amnestic Disorder
292.xx   Sedative-, Hypnotic-, or Anxiolytic-Induced Psychotic Disorder
    .11   With Delusions[I,W]
    .12   With Hallucinations[I,W]
292.84   Sedative-, Hypnotic-, or Anxiolytic-Induced Mood Disorder[I,W]
292.89   Sedative-, Hypnotic-, or Anxiolytic-Induced Anxiety Disorder[W]
292.89   Sedative-, Hypnotic-, or Anxiolytic-Induced Sexual Dysfunction[I]
292.85   Sedative-, Hypnotic-, or Anxiolytic-Induced Sleep Disorder[I,W]
292.9   Sedative-, Hypnotic-, or Anxiolytic-Related Disorder NOS

POLYSUBSTANCE-RELATED DISORDER

304.80   Polysubstance Dependence[a,b,c,d]

OTHER (OR UNKNOWN) SUBSTANCE–RELATED DISORDERS

Other (or Unknown) Substance Use Disorders

304.90   Other (or Unknown) Substance Dependence[a,b,c,d]
305.90   Other (or Unknown) Substance Abuse

Other (or Unknown) Substance–Induced Disorders

292.89   Other (or Unknown) Substance Intoxication
    Specify if: With Perceptual Disturbances
292.0   Other (or Unknown) Substance Withdrawal
    Specify if: With Perceptual Disturbances
292.81   Other (or Unknown) Substance–Induced Delirium

292.82 Other (or Unknown) Substance–Induced Persisting Dementia

292.83 Other (or Unknown) Substance–Induced Persisting Amnestic Disorder

292.xx Other (or Unknown) Substance–Induced Psychotic Disorder

.11 With Delusions[I,W]

.12 With Hallucinations[I,W]

292.84 Other (or Unknown) Substance–Induced Mood Disorder[I,W]

292.89 Other (or Unknown) Substance–Induced Anxiety Disorder[I,W]

292.89 Other (or Unknown) Substance–Induced Sexual Dysfunction[I]

292.85 Other (or Unknown) Substance–Induced Sleep Disorder[I,W]

292.9 Other (or Unknown) Substance–Related Disorder NOS

Schizophrenia and Other Psychotic Disorders

295.xx Schizophrenia

The following Classification of Longitudinal Course applies to all subtypes of Schizophrenia:

Episodic With Interepisode Residual Symptoms (*specify if:* With Prominent Negative Symptoms)/Episodic With No Interepisode Residual Symptoms

Continuous (*specify if:* With Prominent Negative Symptoms)

Single Episode In Partial Remission (*specify if:* With Prominent Negative Symptoms)/ Single Episode In Full Remission

Other or Unspecified Pattern

.30 Paranoid Type

.10 Disorganized Type

.20 Catatonic Type

.90 Undifferentiated Type

.60 Residual Type

295.40 Schizophreniform Disorder

Specify if: Without Good Prognostic Features/ With Good Prognostic Features

295.70 Schizoaffective Disorder

Specify type: Bipolar Type/Depressive Type

297.1 Delusional Disorder

Specify type: Erotomanic Type/Grandiose Type/ Jealous Type/Persecutory Type/Somatic Type/ Mixed Type/Unspecified Type

298.8 Brief Psychotic Disorder

Specify if: With Marked Stressor(s)/Without Marked Stressor(s)/With Postpartum Onset

297.3 Shared Psychotic Disorder

293.xx Psychotic Disorder Due to . . . *[Indicate the General Medical Condition]*

.81 With Delusions

.82 With Hallucinations

—.— Substance-Induced Psychotic Disorder (*refer to Substance-Related Disorders for substance-specific codes*)

Specify if: With Onset During Intoxication/With Onset During Withdrawal

298.9 Psychotic Disorder NOS

Mood Disorders

Code current state of Major Depressive Disorder or Bipolar I Disorder in fifth digit:

1 = Mild

2 = Moderate

3 = Severe Without Psychotic Features

4 = Severe With Psychotic Features

Specify: Mood-Congruent Psychotic Features/ Mood-Incongruent Psychotic Features

5 = In Partial Remission

6 = In Full Remission

0 = Unspecified

The following specifiers apply (for current or most recent episode) to Mood Disorders as noted:

[a]Severity/Psychotic/Remission Specifiers/ [b]Chronic/[c]With Catatonic Features/[d]With Melancholic Features/[e]With Atypical Features/[f]With Postpartum Onset

The following specifiers apply to Mood Disorders as noted:

[g]With or Without Full Interepisode Recovery/ [h]With Seasonal Pattern/[i]With Rapid Cycling

DEPRESSIVE DISORDERS

296.xx Major Depressive Disorder

.2x Single Episode[a,b,c,d,e,f]

.3x Recurrent[a,b,c,d,e,f,g,h]

300.4 Dysthymic Disorder

Specify if: Early Onset/Late Onset

Specify: With Atypical Features

311 Depressive Disorder NOS

BIPOLAR DISORDERS

296.xx   Bipolar I Disorder
- .0x   Single Manic Episode[a,c,f]
  Specify if: Mixed
- .40   Most Recent Episode Hypomanic[g,h,i]
- .4x   Most Recent Episode Manic[a,c,f,g,h,i]
- .6x   Most Recent Episode Mixed[a,c,f,g,h,i]
- .5x   Most Recent Episode Depressed[a,b,c,d,e,f,g,h,i]
- .7   Most Recent Episode Unspecified[g,h,i]

296.89   Bipolar II Disorder[a,b,c,d,e,f,g,h,i]
Specify (current or most recent episode):
Hypomanic/Depressed

301.13   Cyclothymic Disorder

296.80   Bipolar Disorder NOS

293.83   Mood Disorder Due to ... *[Indicate the General Medical Condition]*
Specify type: With Depressive Features/With Major Depressive–Like Episode/With Manic Features/With Mixed Features

—.—   Substance-Induced Mood Disorder
(refer to Substance-Related Disorders for substance-specific codes)
Specify type: With Depressive Features/With Manic Features/With Mixed Features
Specify if: With Onset During Intoxication/With Onset During Withdrawal

296.90   Mood Disorder NOS

Anxiety Disorders

300.01   Panic Disorder Without Agoraphobia

300.21   Panic Disorder With Agoraphobia

300.22   Agoraphobia Without History of Panic Disorder

300.29   Specific Phobia
Specify type: Animal Type/Natural Environment Type/Blood-Injection-Injury Type/Situational Type/Other Type

300.23   Social Phobia
Specify if: Generalized

300.3   Obsessive-Compulsive Disorder
Specify if: With Poor Insight

309.81   Posttraumatic Stress Disorder
Specify if: Acute/Chronic
Specify if: With Delayed Onset

308.3   Acute Stress Disorder

300.02   Generalized Anxiety Disorder

293.84   Anxiety Disorder Due to ... *[Indicate the General Medical Condition]*
Specify if: With Generalized Anxiety/With Panic Attacks/With Obsessive-Compulsive Symptoms

—.—   Substance-Induced Anxiety Disorder
(refer to Substance-Related Disorders for substance-specific codes)
Specify if: With Generalized Anxiety/With Panic Attacks/With Obsessive-Compulsive Symptoms/With Phobic Symptoms
Specify if: With Onset During Intoxication/With Onset During Withdrawal

300.00   Anxiety Disorder NOS

Somatoform Disorders

300.81   Somatization Disorder

300.82   Undifferentiated Somatoform Disorder

300.11   Conversion Disorder
Specify type: With Motor Symptom or Deficit/With Sensory Symptom or Deficit/With Seizures or Convulsions/With Mixed Presentation

307.xx   Pain Disorder
- .80   Associated With Psychological Factors
- .89   Associated With Both Psychological Factors and a General Medical Condition
  Specify if: Acute/Chronic

300.7   Hypochondriasis
Specify if: With Poor Insight

300.7   Body Dysmorphic Disorder

300.82   Somatoform Disorder NOS

Factitious Disorders

300.xx   Factitious Disorder
- .16   With Predominantly Psychological Signs and Symptoms
- .19   With Predominantly Physical Signs and Symptoms
- .19   With Combined Psychological and Physical Signs and Symptoms

300.19   Factitious Disorder NOS

Dissociative Disorders

300.12   Dissociative Amnesia

300.13   Dissociative Fugue

300.14   Dissociative Identity Disorder

300.6   Depersonalization Disorder

300.15   Dissociative Disorder NOS

Sexual and Gender Identity Disorders

SEXUAL DYSFUNCTIONS

The following specifiers apply to all primary Sexual Dysfunctions:

Lifelong Type/Acquired Type
Generalized Type/Situational Type
Due to Psychological Factors/
  Due to Combined Factors

Sexual Desire Disorders

302.71   Hypoactive Sexual Desire Disorder
302.79   Sexual Aversion Disorder

Sexual Arousal Disorders

302.72   Female Sexual Arousal Disorder
302.72   Male Erectile Disorder

Orgasmic Disorders

302.73   Female Orgasmic Disorder
302.74   Male Orgasmic Disorder
302.75   Premature Ejaculation

Sexual Pain Disorders

302.76   Dyspareunia (Not Due to a General Medical Condition)
306.51   Vaginismus (Not Due to a General Medical Condition)

Sexual Dysfunction Due to a General Medical Condition

625.8   Female Hypoactive Sexual Desire Disorder Due to . . . *[Indicate the General Medical Condition]*
608.89   Male Hypoactive Sexual Desire Disorder Due to . . . *[Indicate the General Medical Condition]*
607.84   Male Erectile Disorder Due to . . . *[Indicate the General Medical Condition]*
625.0   Female Dyspareunia Due to . . . *[Indicate the General Medical Condition]*
608.89   Male Dyspareunia Due to . . . *[Indicate the General Medical Condition]*
625.8   Other Female Sexual Dysfunction Due to . . . *[Indicate the General Medical Condition]*
608.89   Other Male Sexual Dysfunction Due to . . . *[Indicate the General Medical Condition]*
——.—   Substance-Induced Sexual Dysfunction *(refer to Substance-Related Disorders for substance-specific codes)*
    Specify if: With Impaired Desire/With Impaired Arousal/With Impaired Orgasm/With Sexual Pain
    Specify if: With Onset During Intoxication
302.70   Sexual Dysfunction NOS

PARAPHILIAS

302.4   Exhibitionism
302.81   Fetishism
302.89   Frotteurism
302.2   Pedophilia
    Specify if: Sexually Attracted to Males/Sexually Attracted to Females/Sexually Attracted to Both
    Specify if: Limited to Incest
    Specify type: Exclusive Type/Nonexclusive Type
302.83   Sexual Masochism
302.84   Sexual Sadism
302.3   Transvestic Fetishism
    Specify if: With Gender Dysphoria
302.82   Voyeurism
302.9   Paraphilia NOS

GENDER IDENTITY DISORDERS

302.xx   Gender Identity Disorder
   .6   in Children
   .85   in Adolescents or Adults
    Specify if: Sexually Attracted to Males/Sexually Attracted to Females/Sexually Attracted to Both/Sexually Attracted to Neither
302.6   Gender Identity Disorder NOS
302.9   Sexual Disorder NOS

Eating Disorders

307.1   Anorexia Nervosa
    Specify type: Restricting Type; Binge-Eating/Purging Type
307.51   Bulimia Nervosa
    Specify type: Purging Type/Nonpurging Type
307.50   Eating Disorder NOS

Sleep Disorders

PRIMARY SLEEP DISORDERS

Dyssomnias

307.42   Primary Insomnia
307.44   Primary Hypersomnia
    Specify if: Recurrent
347.00   Narcolepsy
780.57   Breathing-Related Sleep Disorder
327.xx   Circadian Rhythm Sleep Disorder
   .31   Delayed Sleep Phase Type
   .35   Jet Lag Type
   .36   Shift Work Type
   .30   Unspecified Type
307.47   Dyssomnia NOS

Parasomnias

307.47	Nightmare Disorder
307.46	Sleep Terror Disorder
307.46	Sleepwalking Disorder
307.47	Parasomnia NOS

SLEEP DISORDERS RELATED TO ANOTHER MENTAL DISORDER

327.02	Insomnia Related to . . . *[Indicate the Axis I or Axis II Disorder]*
327.15	Hypersomnia Related to . . . *[Indicate the Axis I or Axis II Disorder]*

OTHER SLEEP DISORDERS

327.xx	Sleep Disorder Due to . . . *[Indicate the General Medical Condition]*
.01	Insomnia Type
.14	Hypersomnia Type
.44	Parasomnia Type
.8	Mixed Type
—.—	Substance-Induced Sleep Disorder *(refer to Substance-Related Disorders for substance-specific codes)*

Specify type: Insomnia Type/Hypersomnia Type/Parasomnia Type/Mixed Type

Specify if: With Onset During Intoxication/With Onset During Withdrawal

Impulse-Control Disorders Not Elsewhere Classified

312.34	Intermittent Explosive Disorder
312.32	Kleptomania
312.33	Pyromania
312.31	Pathological Gambling
312.39	Trichotillomania
312.30	Impulse-Control Disorder NOS

Adjustment Disorders

309.xx	Adjustment Disorder
.0	With Depressed Mood
.24	With Anxiety
.28	With Mixed Anxiety and Depressed Mood
.3	With Disturbance of Conduct
.4	With Mixed Disturbance of Emotions and Conduct
.9	Unspecified

Specify if: Acute/Chronic

Personality Disorders

Note: *These are coded on Axis II.*

301.0	Paranoid Personality Disorder
301.20	Schizoid Personality Disorder
301.22	Schizotypal Personality Disorder
301.7	Antisocial Personality Disorder
301.83	Borderline Personality Disorder
301.50	Histrionic Personality Disorder
301.81	Narcissistic Personality Disorder
301.82	Avoidant Personality Disorder
301.6	Dependent Personality Disorder
301.4	Obsessive-Compulsive Personality Disorder
301.9	Personality Disorder NOS

Other Conditions That May Be a Focus of Clinical Attention

PSYCHOLOGICAL FACTORS AFFECTING MEDICAL CONDITION

316	. . . *[Specified Psychological Factor] Affecting . . . [Indicate the General Medical Condition]*

Choose name based on nature of factors:

Mental Disorder Affecting Medical Condition

Psychological Symptoms Affecting Medical Condition

Personality Traits or Coping Style Affecting Medical Condition

Maladaptive Health Behaviors Affecting Medical Condition

Stress-Related Physiological Response Affecting Medical Condition

Other or Unspecified Psychological Factors Affecting Medical Condition

MEDICATION-INDUCED MOVEMENT DISORDERS

332.1	Neuroleptic-Induced Parkinsonism
333.92	Neuroleptic Malignant Syndrome
333.7	Neuroleptic-Induced Acute Dystonia
333.99	Neuroleptic-Induced Acute Akathisia
333.82	Neuroleptic-Induced Tardive Dyskinesia
333.1	Medication-Induced Postural Tremor
333.90	Medication-Induced Movement Disorder NOS

OTHER MEDICATION-INDUCED DISORDER

995.2	Adverse Effects of Medication NOS

RELATIONAL PROBLEMS

V61.9	Relational Problem Related to a Mental Disorder or General Medical Condition
V61.20	Parent-Child Relational Problem
V61.10	Partner Relational Problem
V61.8	Sibling Relational Problem
V62.81	Relational Problem NOS

PROBLEMS RELATED TO ABUSE OR NEGLECT

V61.21	Physical Abuse of Child *(code 995.54 if focus of attention is on victim)*
V61.21	Sexual Abuse of Child *(code 995.53 if focus of attention is on victim)*
V61.21	Neglect of Child *(code 995.52 if focus of attention is on victim)*
—.—	Physical Abuse of Adult
V61.12	(if by partner)
V62.83	(if by person other than partner) *(code 995.81 if focus of attention is on victim)*
—.—	Sexual Abuse of Adult
V61.12	(if by partner)
V62.83	(if by person other than partner) *(code 995.83 if focus of attention is on victim)*

ADDITIONAL CONDITIONS THAT MAY BE A FOCUS OF CLINICAL ATTENTION

V15.81	Noncompliance With Treatment
V65.2	Malingering
V71.01	Adult Antisocial Behavior
V71.02	Child or Adolescent Antisocial Behavior
V62.89	Borderline Intellectual Functioning *Note:* This is coded on Axis II.
780.93	Age-Related Cognitive Decline
V62.82	Bereavement
V62.3	Academic Problem
V62.2	Occupational Problem
313.82	Identity Problem
V62.89	Religious or Spiritual Problem
V62.4	Acculturation Problem
V62.89	Phase of Life Problem

Additional Codes

300.9	Unspecified Mental Disorder (nonpsychotic)
V71.09	No Diagnosis or Condition on Axis I
799.9	Diagnosis or Condition Deferred on Axis I
V71.09	No Diagnosis on Axis II
799.9	Diagnosis Deferred on Axis II

Multiaxial System

Axis I	Clinical Disorders Other Conditions That May Be a Focus of Clinical Attention
Axis II	Personality Disorders Mental Retardation
Axis III	General Medical Conditions
Axis IV	Psychosocial and Environmental Problems
Axis V	Global Assessment of Functioning

INDEX

*Page numbers printed in **boldface** type refer to tables or figures.*

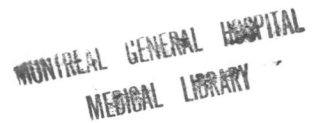